W9-BLC-803

Medical-surgical nursing

CONCEPTS AND CLINICAL PRACTICE

Edited by

WILMA J. PHIPPS, R.N., B.S., A.M., Ph.D.
Professor and Chairperson of Medical-Surgical
Nursing, Frances Payne Bolton School of Nursing,
Case Western Reserve University;
Director of Medical-Surgical Nursing,
University Hospitals of Cleveland,
Cleveland, Ohio

BARBARA C. LONG, R.N., M.S.N.
Associate Professor of Nursing,
Frances Payne Bolton School of Nursing,
Case Western Reserve University,
Cleveland, Ohio

NANCY FUGATE WOODS, R.N., M.N., Ph.D.
Associate Professor, School of Nursing,
University of Washington, Seattle, Washington;
formerly of Duke University School of Nursing,
Durham, North Carolina

Medical-surgical nursing

CONCEPTS AND CLINICAL PRACTICE

with **731** illustrations

THE C. V. MOSBY COMPANY

ST. LOUIS • TORONTO • LONDON 1979

■ **To our students, families, and friends**
for all their support while this book was in progress

Printed in the United States of America

The C. V. Mosby Company
11830 Westline Industrial Drive, St. Louis, Missouri 63141

Library of Congress Cataloging in Publication Data

Phipps, Wilma J 1925-
Medical-surgical nursing.

Bibliography: p.
Includes index.
1. Nursing. 2. Surgical nursing. I. Long, Barbara C., 1926- joint author. II. Woods, Nancy Fugate, joint author. III. Title. [DNLM: 1. Nursing care. WY150 P573m]
RT41.P56 610.73 78-27863
ISBN 0-8016-3932-8

C/VH/VH 9 8 7 6 5 4 02/A/218

Contributors

Jane E. Anderson, R.N., M.S., Doctoral Student, University of Michigan School of Nursing, Ann Arbor, Michigan; formerly Assistant Professor of Nursing, Duke University, Durham, North Carolina

Shirley Potts Bourbous, R.N., M.S.N., Nurse Practitioner, Veterans Administration Hospital; formerly Assistant Professor of Nursing, Duke University, Durham, North Carolina

Linda Anne Broseman, R.N., M.S.N., Assistant Professor of Medical-Surgical Nursing, Frances Payne Bolton School of Nursing, Case Western Reserve University; Associate in Nursing, University Hospitals of Cleveland, Cleveland, Ohio

Frances R. Brown, R.N., M.S.N., Assistant Clinical Professor of Nursing, Frances Payne Bolton School of Nursing, Case Western Reserve University; Nurse Clinician, Cardiovascular Nursing, University Hospitals of Cleveland, Cleveland, Ohio

Dorothy J. Brundage, R.N., M.S.N., Assistant Professor of Nursing, Duke University, Durham, North Carolina

Patricia Buergin, R.N., B.S.N., Senior Clinical Nurse, University Hospitals of Cleveland, Cleveland, Ohio

Mary E. Bushong, R.N., M.S.N., Assistant Professor of Operating and Recovery Room Nursing, Frances Payne Bolton School of Nursing, Case Western Reserve University; Assistant Director, Recovery Room Nursing, University Hospitals of Cleveland, Cleveland, Ohio

Virginia Cassmeyer, R.N., M.S.N., Assistant Professor of Medical-Surgical Nursing, Frances Payne Bolton School of Nursing, Case Western Reserve University; Associate in Nursing, University Hospitals of Cleveland, Cleveland, Ohio

Ella Cinkota, R.N., Ed.M., Consultant Nurse, Bureau of Maternal and Child Health, New York State Department of Health, Albany, New York

Linda Craig, R.N., M.S.N., Assistant Professor of Nursing, Hartwick College, Oneonta, New York

Barbara J. Daly, R.N., M.S.N., Assistant Clinical Professor of Medical-Surgical Nursing, Frances Payne Bolton School of Nursing, Case Western Reserve University; Assistant Director of Medical-Surgical Nursing, University Hospitals of Cleveland, Cleveland, Ohio

Gretchen Kramer Dery, R.N., M.S.N., Assistant Professor of Nursing, Duke University, Durham, North Carolina

Nancy Durham, R.N., M.S.N., Formerly Assistant Professor of Medical-Surgical Nursing, Frances Payne Bolton School of Nursing, Case Western Reserve University, Cleveland, Ohio

Janet Larson Gelein, R.N., M.S., Assistant Professor of Nursing, University of Rochester, Rochester, New York

Jean Goeppinger, R.N., Ph.D., Director of Primary Nursing Care in Society, University of Virginia School of Nursing, Charlottesville, Virginia

Sister Paula Gonzales, Ph.D., Professor of Biology, College of Mount Saint Joseph, Cincinnati, Ohio

C. Joan Gowin, R.N., M.A., Associate Professor of Nursing, Frances Payne Bolton School of Nursing, Case Western Reserve University; Director of Operating and Recovery Room Nursing, University Hospitals of Cleveland, Cleveland, Ohio

Judith L. Greig, R.N., M.S.N., Assistant Professor of Medical-Surgical Nursing, Frances Payne Bolton School of Nursing, Case Western Reserve University; Nurse Clinician, Operating Room Nursing, University Hospitals of Cleveland, Cleveland, Ohio

Donna Hewitt, R.N., M.N., Assistant Professor of Nursing, Duke University, Durham, North Carolina

Rosemarie Hogan, R.N., M.S.N., Assistant Professor of Medical-Surgical Nursing, Frances Payne Bolton School of Nursing, Case Western Reserve University; Associate in Nursing, University Hospitals of Cleveland, Cleveland, Ohio

Patricia Humphrey, R.N., M.P.H., Assistant Professor of Nursing, Duke University, Durham, North Carolina

Virginia Burke Karb, R.N., M.S.N., Assistant Professor of Medical-Surgical Nursing, University of North Carolina, Greensboro, North Carolina

Jane Steinman Kaufman, R.N., M.S., Assistant Professor of Nursing, Duke University, Durham, North Carolina

Marjorie Kinney, R.N., M.S.N., Assistant Professor of Nursing, Wright State University, Dayton, Ohio

Mary K. Kirkpatrick, R.N., M.N., Assistant Professor of Nursing, East Carolina University, Greenville, North Carolina

Donna J. Kuklo, R.N., M.S.N., Assistant Clinical Professor of Medical-Surgical Nursing, Frances Payne Bolton School of Nursing, Case Western Reserve University; Senior Infection Surveillance Nurse, University Hospitals of Cleveland, Cleveland, Ohio

Mariann Lavacca, R.N., M.A., Assistant Professor of Nursing, Duke University, Durham, North Carolina

Juanita Long, R.N., M.S.N., Assistant Professor of Nursing, Duke University, Durham, North Carolina

Lynn Chenoweth McWilliams, Formerly Assistant Professor of Medical-Surgical Nursing, Frances Payne Bolton School of Nursing, Case Western Reserve University, Cleveland, Ohio

Paula Lambrecht Miller, R.N., M.S., Assistant Clinical Professor of Medical-Surgical Nursing, Frances Payne Bolton School of Nursing, Case Western Reserve University; Assistant Director of Medical-Surgical Nursing, University Hospitals of Cleveland, Cleveland, Ohio

Carol J. Mitten, R.N., M.S.N., Assistant Clinical Professor of Medical-Surgical Nursing, Frances Payne Bolton School of Nursing, Case Western Reserve University; Assistant Director of Medical-Surgical Nursing, University Hospitals of Cleveland, Cleveland, Ohio

Brenda Martin Morgan, R.N., M.S., Assistant Professor of Nursing, Duke University, Durham, North Carolina

Janice Neville, D.Sc., Professor and Chairman of Nutrition, Case Western Reserve University, Cleveland, Ohio

Joan Nivinski, R.N., M.S.N., Assistant Clinical Professor of Pediatric Nursing, Frances Payne Bolton School of Nursing, Case Western Reserve University; Nurse Clinician, Pediatric Nursing, University Hospitals of Cleveland, Cleveland, Ohio

Alice Norman, R.N., M.S.N., Assistant Clinical Professor of Medical-Surgical Nursing, Frances Payne Bolton School of Nursing, Case Western Reserve University; Nurse Clinician, Pulmonary Nursing, University Hospitals of Cleveland, Cleveland, Ohio

Catherine O'Malley, R.N., Supervisor of Specialty Units, Cleveland Metropolitan General Hospital, Cleveland, Ohio

Antoinette T. Ragucci, R.N., Ph.D., Associate Professor of Medical-Surgical Nursing, Frances Payne Bolton School of Nursing, Case Western Reserve University; Associate in Nursing, University Hospitals of Cleveland, Cleveland, Ohio

Sally Schafer, R.N., M.S.N., Assistant Professor of Nursing, Duke University, Durham, North Carolina

Katherine Schenk, R.N., Ed.D., Associate Professor of Nursing, Duke University, Durham, North Carolina

Barbara Soltis, R.N., M.S.N., Assistant Professor of Medical-Surgical Nursing, Frances Payne Bolton School of Nursing, Case Western Reserve University; Associate in Nursing, University Hospitals of Cleveland, Cleveland, Ohio

E. Ronald Wright, Ph.D., Associate Professor of Microbiology and Administrative Officer, Instructional Development Programs, Case Western Reserve University, Cleveland, Ohio

May Wykle, R.N., M.S.N., Associate Professor of Psychiatric Nursing, Frances Payne Bolton School of Nursing, Case Western Reserve University; Associate in Nursing, University Hospitals of Cleveland, Cleveland, Ohio

Rosemary Craycroft Yeganef, R.N., B.S.N., Formerly Staff Nurse, University Hospitals of Cleveland, Cleveland, Ohio

Karen K. Yoder, R.N., M.N., Doctoral Student, University of Michigan School of Nursing, Ann Arbor, Michigan; formerly Assistant Professor of Nursing, Duke University, Durham, North Carolina

Deanna Melton Xistris, R.N., M.S.N., Clinical Instructor in Medical-Surgical Nursing, Frances Payne Bolton School of Nursing, Case Western Reserve University; Nurse Clinician, Oncology Nursing, University Hospitals of Cleveland, Cleveland, Ohio

Marie J. Zimmer, R.N., M.S.N., F.A.A.N., Director of Nursing Service, University of Wisconsin Hospitals, Madison, Wisconsin

Preface

The social environments in which nursing is practiced have undergone considerable change in recent years, and as a result the knowledge base necessary to practice nursing has grown considerably. Today there are many facets to the nursing role, and nurses practice in more diverse environments than ever before. Central to all of these environments is an encounter between the nurse and the patient or client. In order to enhance the effectiveness of this encounter, the nurse needs information drawn from a wide variety of sources. The purpose of this book is to present information that we believe is relevant to the practice of medical-surgical nursing today.

This book is divided into three major parts. In Part One, "Perspectives for Nursing Practice," there are two units. Unit I examines social, cultural, and environmental perspectives that can be applied to nursing practice, whether it be in the community or in the hospital. In this unit, concepts of health and illness; the systems approach; family, culture, and society; health care delivery systems; ecology and health; and an epidemiologic approach to health care are presented. These concepts can broaden the base from which nursing is practiced and are relevant to nursing students and practicing nurses alike.

Unit II looks at those concepts and processes in wide use today. First, the components of the nursing process are presented, with emphasis on the steps of assessment, including data collection and analysis. Key concepts in nurse-client interactions are presented next, followed by an introduction to the problem-oriented system for organizing data. The last chapter in Unit II looks at the issues involved in quality assurance programs and the monitoring of client outcomes. This introduction to client or patient outcomes should prepare the reader to understand the reason for, and the importance of, the outcome criteria presented in the chapters in Part Three of this book.

Throughout the book we have referred to the persons who are recipients of the services of nurses as clients or patients. In our minds the term *client* is most generally accepted as a referrant to persons in nonhospital settings, while *patient* is more commonly used to denote those who are in hospitals or other health care institutions. We recognize that some nurses are more comfortable with one term than the other, and for this reason we have used both terms in this text.

In Part Two, "Stress and Adaptation," concepts necessary to understanding these processes are presented in Unit III, "Adaptation," with a stress and adaptation framework presented first. Next, mechanisms necessary to understanding the integration of the body, biologic defense mechanisms, and mechanisms for maintaining a dynamic equilibrium are discussed. This is followed by chapters on adaptive and maladaptive behavior, adaptation throughout the life cycle, and death and dying.

Common stressors and their management are discussed in Unit IV. These include fluid and electrolyte imbalance, infection, pain, trauma in the form of surgical intervention, and trauma due to accidents, injuries, and disasters. Other stressors included in this unit are neoplasia, sensory overload and deprivation, altered levels of consciousness, alterations in body image, and prolonged illness. Like the chapters in Part One, these chapters present concepts essential to the practice of nursing in a wide variety of settings.

Part Three of this text, "Clinical Management of Persons with Medical-Surgical Problems," presents material traditionally found in medical-surgical books. The content is divided into seven units to reflect common problems encountered as pathophysiologic changes occur relative to certain essential body processes. Failure of integrative mechanisms resulting in regulatory problems are presented first, followed by sensorimotor problems, gas transport problems, problems of nutrition, problems of elimination, problems related to sexuality and reproduction, problems related to impaired protective mechanisms, and care of the critically ill. The units were organized in the above manner to allow the content to be presented in a relevant and useful manner. In each of these units a nursing process format is used, with an assessment chapter of the systems involved being presented first, followed by a management chapter, which discusses care of persons with that impairment. Thus the management chapters present most of the interventions that might otherwise be repeated over and over again in relation to certain pathologic processes. For example, Chapter 45, "Management of the Person with Impaired Oxygen–Carbon Dioxide Exchange," discusses general care whether the cause be cardiac, pulmonary, or peripheral vascular in origin. Following the management chapters are problem chapters that present the basic pathophysiologic changes causing specific disease processes.

Throughout this text the emphasis is on assisting the patient or client to improve his or her health by providing appropriate physical care, emotional and social support, and information necessary for self-care. We believe that the patient's or client's significant others, be they family or friends, provide essential support to that person, and therefore we make reference to involving them as appropriate in the care of the individual patient or client.

Readers who are familiar with *Medical-Surgical Nursing* by Shafer et al. will recognize that some of the material presented in this book is drawn from that classic text. For example, the chapter "Ecology and Health," which was originally conceived for that book, is also presented in this text.

It is our hope that the content presented in this book will assist nursing students and practicing nurses to provide person-centered care appropriate to each patient's or client's health status.

We wish to thank the many persons who contributed chapters to this book. We are grateful to each of them.

We also wish to thank the illustrators whose drawings are presented within: William Holmes, Ellen Sands, and James T. Suchy of Cleveland, Robert DeVoe, Jr., of Durham, and Jack P. Tandy of St. Louis.

The typing of the manuscript was done by Debbie Ryall and Pam McNitsky of Durham, and by Janet Mitchell and Sondra Patrizi of Cleveland, who deserve special thanks for their help with every aspect of the preparation of this manuscript. We are also grateful to Mrs. Geraldine Mink who assisted with the library work in Cleveland.

Wilma J. Phipps
Barbara C. Long
Nancy Fugate Woods

Contents

PART ONE

Perspectives for nursing practice

UNIT I

Social, cultural, and environmental perspectives

Health and illness, when considered from a clinical perspective, frequently bring to mind definitions rooted in biology. Because they are biologic organisms, people's physical bodies, organs, cells, and even subcellular components are intimately involved with their health statuses; however, the experience of health and illness is inexorably linked to the social, cultural, and physical environments in which they live. This unit explores definitions of *health, illness,* and *disease* from lay as well as professional perspectives. One approach to foster a holistic view of humanity, the *systems perspective,* is considered. The *influence of society and culture on behavior* in times of health and illness is examined. This is followed by exploration of *systems of health care delivery* with an emphasis on models for the delivery of nursing care. After examining the influence of the environment on humans and that of humans on the environment (ecology), the unit concludes with a description of an *epidemiologic perspective* for health care, stressing the need for a multicausal approach to understanding health and illness.

1

Concepts of health and illness

GRETCHEN KRAMER DERY

Nicole Peters is 3 months old. She was born with an umbilical hernia. Mr. and Mrs. Peters have been informed by their pediatrician that this is not uncommon. The physician recommends observation as the best approach, since many hernias of this type will resolve without intervention.

Stephen Walters is 7 years old. He was born with no right leg. He walks with crutches and is able to play with the children in his neighborhood. He is not able to be involved in some of the children's more strenuous and highly competitive activities. He attends the neighborhood school and is making satisfactory progress in his studies.

Craig Wellons is a 35-year-old successful insurance salesperson. He is married and has two children. He and his family are financially comfortable and view their life situation as very positive. Unknown to him, atherosclerotic plaques are insidiously forming in his coronary arteries.

Each of the persons described above could be defined as ill or healthy, depending on the perspective of the definer. The purpose of this chapter is to explore concepts of health and illness from the perspective of the patient or client as well as that of the health professional. This chapter begins with a comparison of definitions of health, illness, and disease from lay and medical perspectives. This is followed by an exploration of concepts of health including high-level wellness and a consideration of behavior in health and illness.

■ LAY AND PROFESSIONAL PERSPECTIVES

Lay persons and health professionals alike have notions of health, illness, and disease that guide their behavior. In some instances, the lay and professional definitions vary significantly, which leads to difficulty in communication between the professional who desires to deliver acceptable health care and the lay person who desires to receive health care.

□ Health

The medical profession has concentrated on defining the nature of aberrant functioning rather than health. Consequently, "normal" has come to imply the opposite of "abnormal." At one pole is health, which is normal and denoted by the absence of pathologic signs and symptoms. At the opposite pole is disease, which is abnormal and denoted by the presence of pathologic signs and symptoms. Thus some health professionals define health as a negative concept, the absence of disease, the uninteresting opposite of disease.[51]

Lay definitions of health reflect both positive and negative aspects. Three orientations to health include:

1. The feeling state orientation, described as "feeling good"
2. The symptom orientation, characterized by lack of general or specific symptoms of disease
3. The performance orientation, defined as activities that a person who is healthy should be able to perform[5]

Thus the lay view of health is multidimensional.

□ Disease and illness

The professional orientation defines disease as objective, observable, and quantifiable. Disease involves change in the structure or function of the body or mind of the human organism. A knowledge of anatomy and physiology is essential for studying disease. Objective changes in structure and function are called *signs* of disease. Although the medical profession also looks at subjective information concerning disease, this type of data is often considered as a secondary source for diagnosis. Subjective information about disease is called *symptoms* and includes reports such as perception of pain, anxiety, and nausea. Such perceptions are difficult to quantify and tend to be influenced by a variety of factors, which are not necessarily directly related to the disease process. Thus subjective reports are considered by some professionals to provide less reliable diagnostic information than objective signs. The signs and symptoms of certain diseases tend to recur among geographic, cultural, social, and socioeconomic populations. The frequent recurrence of combinations of signs and symptoms is labeled a clinical *syndrome*. There are, in addition to signs and symptoms, other characteristics of disease, including incidence, onset, course, prognosis, duration, and communicability.[52] *Incidence*, or frequency with which the disease occurs (or more accurately, is diagnosed), results in such labels as "common childhood diseases" and the "common cold" versus such entities as "rare blood dyscrasias." The *onset*, or beginning appearance of signs and symptoms, can be insidious, obvious, gradual, or rapid. The *course*, or path, may be smooth, rough, predictable, or unpredictable. The *prognosis*, or ultimate outcome, can be hopeful or guarded or can range from poor to excellent. The *duration*, or length, can be short, long, or permanent. *Acute* and *chronic* are words frequently used to describe duration but have such a diversity of interpretation that there is little universal agreement on their precise meaning. "Acute" is generally used to describe both diseases with rapid onset and those with severe consequences. "Chronic" is generally applied to diseases of a long-term nature. *Communicability* refers to the contagious or transmissible quality of a disease. Contrasting examples of communicability are gastric ulcer and venereal disease, the former being noncommunicable and the latter considered highly communicable. The terms *disease* and *illness* are commonly used interchangeably by the medical profession.

The lay person experiencing a disease regards it from a completely different framework than does the professional treating the disease. Whereas the medical diagnostician considers disease in terms of medical knowledge and objectively evaluates the meaning of signs and symptoms, the lay person generally tends to perceive disease from a subjective, personalized, and *phenomenologic* framework. That is, illness is perceived by the lay person in terms of its meaning to that particular individual.

In a study of lay perceptions of illness, research has tried to determine at what point health problems are considered illness by lay persons. The findings suggested that for middle-class Americans being ill meant *having an ailment of recent origin that interfered with one's usual activities*. Interference with usual activities seemed to be the most important criterion lay persons applied to the definition of illness.[1] In another study it was noted that lay persons often perceived disease as *an object or thing that invaded the body*. These individuals regularly referred to a wide spectrum of diseases as objects, that is, invading and foreign "its." They impersonalized both the symptoms and organs involved through the use of depersonalized language.[9]

Disease can occur in an individual without the person's awareness of illness and without others perceiving illness. On the other hand, a person can feel very ill even though no pathologic processes can be identified.[11]

■ CONCEPTS OF HEALTH

Although much of the medical and nursing literature describes disease and illness, increased attention is being devoted to health. Two contemporary concepts of health are Maslow's hierarchy of needs and Dunn's notion of high-level wellness.

□ Maslow's hierarchy of needs

Maslow[26] describes a hierarchy of needs in which the physiologic needs are considered as most basic, followed by safety, love, esteem, and self-actualization needs. A need that is not satisfied constitutes a motivating factor for an individual.

Needs are generally more unconscious than conscious. Basic needs are not seen as being exclusive determinants of behavior(s), since almost all behaviors have social, cultural, and biologic motivations. Any particular behavioral incident is more likely to be influenced by all the needs in varying degrees than by a single need.

It is necessary to recognize that for most people the needs in the hierarchy exist simultaneously and in differing degrees and that new needs emerge not suddenly but very gradually. At varying times an individual will have different amounts of various needs being met. Lower level needs do not need to be met *completely* before higher level needs can emerge. Maslow suggests that the degree of need satisfaction is positively related to mental health and that, theoretically, total need gratification and ideal health are synonymous.

Physiologic needs

Physiologic needs include hunger, thirst, sleep, and rest. Totally deprived human beings would generally find the physiologic needs to be their major motivating force. All other needs would be pushed into the background or cease to exist for those persons. However, once physiologic needs are satisfied, the higher level needs begin to emerge, and when they are satisfied, new and still higher level needs are manifested.

Safety needs

Safety needs are the second level of needs. For the majority of citizens of developed countries these are not the prime motivators of human behavior. Societies usually succeed in protecting their members from extremes in temperature and from such forms of aggression as assault, murder, and tyranny. In the lower socioeconomic groups of these same societies it is possible that safety needs may not be met and that these safety needs may become the prime motivators of behavior within these segments of the society. In general, however, safety needs are seen as prime motivators only in times of national, natural, or personal crises, for example, war, natural disasters, and illness. When safety needs are satisfied, the need for love and belonging emerges.

Love and belonging needs

Love is associated not only with sexual behavior but also with a desire for affectionate relationships with people in general. Deprivation of love and belonging needs is believed to cause the basic maladjustment seen in the more severe psychopathologies, while less severe thwarting of these needs is seen among those who are lonely.

Esteem needs

Esteem needs consist of two subsets. The first includes a desire for strength, achievement, adequacy, mastery, competence, and independence. The second subset is geared toward reputation or prestige entities received from others, as in status dominance, recognition, attention, importance, and appreciation. Thwarting of these needs produces negative feelings such as inferiority, weakness, and helplessness. Satisfaction of self-esteem needs leads to positive feelings of being useful and necessary in the world.

Self-actualization need

Self-actualization is the highest need and describes persons continually moving toward achieving their potential. Few persons achieve self-actualization, a need more commonly met during the mature years.

While there is generally a progression in the hierarchy of needs, it is not a rigid scheme of classification. A person who has had basic needs satisfied for a consistent period throughout life demonstrates ability to withstand the thwarting of needs. However, a person's aspiration level may be permanently lowered by consistent deprivation; for example, chronically unemployed persons may be totally satisfied as long as they have enough food, and they may cease to strive for more than that. When a need has been long satisfied and then is deprived, its importance may be underevaluated. For example, many people who have met their physiologic and higher needs throughout life may find the fact that they presently have only one meal a day *not* a potent motivator. Such a situation can frequently be observed among our aged population today.

□ Dunn's high-level wellness

Dunn describes high-level wellness in relation to the individual, family, community, environment, and society.

Individual high-level wellness is described as integrated functioning oriented toward maximizing individual potential while maintaining balance and purposeful direction in the environment. It includes three components: an upward and forward direction toward higher functional potential; an open-ended future containing challenges to achieve higher potential; and an integrated being, that is, body-mind-spirit participating in the functioning process.[16]

Nature of people

Dunn's view of wellness is based on a philosophy of the nature of people that includes the following five aspects. First, each individual functions as a *total personality.* Next, each person possesses enormous *dynamic energy.* Third, each person has and must maintain *peace with inner and outer worlds.* Fourth, each person has a *relationship* between *energy use* and *self-integration*, when self-integration is defined as the interweaving of all the known aspects of life. Finally, each individual possesses an *inner* and an *outer world.* The inner world can be described as each and every body cell composing an organized whole. The outer world refers simply to the individual's environment with all its components. A person must find his or her being and belonging in both worlds. Questions to be explored are: "What and why am I?" and "Where am I going?"

Dunn maintains that humans have the capacity to recognize certain *processes* that help provide them with the answers to the above questions. These processes are being, belonging, becoming, and befitting. In *being*, one can recognize oneself after the neonatal period as something separate and distinct from the remainder of the world. Additionally, if one is a separate part, there must be a whole to which one *belongs.* People grow and develop in all spheres of their being; that is, they are *becoming.* As people grow and become, they individually and selectively make choices; that is, they *befit* themselves for the future.

Cellular commonwealth

From a physiologic standpoint, a person is composed of a cellular commonwealth organized into systems. The optimal functioning of the cellular commonwealth is an essential component of wellness. Each of the body's cells is seen as a unique totality, is made of energy, has an inner and outer world, and is an open system. Protoplasm, the main constituent of cells, has six qualities, which then become qualities of each cell. These qualities or functions are:

1. Irritability: the ability to attract or repel
2. Mobility: the ability to move about, sacrificed by some cells in the name of organization and cooperation

3. Metabolism: the ability to perform chemically
4. Growth and reproduction: the abilities to expand and replicate
5. Adaptability: the ability to be interdependent and to maintain an organized whole

Systems have several functions to perform if the cellular needs are to be met, including keeping ports of entry and exit open, transforming energy and waste, growing, reproducing, and problem solving (including the storage, integration, and use of information).

The overall function served by the commonwealth of cells is maintenance of unity.

Mind

The *mind,* called the emergent mind because of its developing state, is characterized by its potential for problem solving in daily living. The mind's total functioning is not yet fully understood. Problem solving, its chief function, involves eight components: communication, storage, values, imagination, concept of self, integration of self, maturity in wholeness, and purpose.

High-level wellness cannot exist without *communication* and freedom to pick and choose solutions. One of society's greatest crimes against a biologic person is constriction of channels of communication so that the individual cannot problem solve.

Three types of *storage mechanisms* exist for people: memory stored in the nervous system, memory stored in muscles as tension patterns, and chemical memory of cells. Dunn believes that pain and fear can be locked into body tissues and can constitute an ongoing source of increasing tension. Trapped physical pain can raise tension and prevent tissue healing; trapped emotional pain can prolong grieving. For the storage mechanism to function, access to data must be maintained. Blocked accesses must be cleared. Long-standing barriers may require psychotherapy or other therapeutic measures. New blocks caused by recent physical or emotional pain can be diminished or dispersed through discussion and sharing.

Values are essential problem-solving components because they provide a means for selection of options and decision making. The ultimate goal of people can be seen as seeking enhancement of the value attributes or experiences.

Imagination refers to mental synthesis of new ideas from elements experienced separately and appears to be a uniquely human phenomenon. Imagination helps people see alternatives; for example, when problems arise the mind perceives similarity to situations previously encountered, and possible solutions are postulated with freedom of choice. Creative imagination is one part of the problem-solving process whereby people can explore their futures and maximize their potential to reach high-level wellness.

The "self" in the problem-solving process provides the reason for choosing. Although the *self-concept,* or how we see ourselves, tends to be rigid, every "self" is continually changing. If one does not periodically bring the "self" and the self-concept into focus, the "self" idea of oneself may become less and less reality oriented. Self-fulfillment and satisfaction come from what one is, not what one was. Health requires that one is capable of facing the facts about one's self.

Integration of self is the sixth component of problem solving. Integration of body-mind-spirit is more feasible when body and mind are in balance. Rest, sleep, relaxation, and leisure are necessary for body-mind-spirit balance. Mental health, physical health, spiritual health, and social health are possible only when there is balance between the interacting and integrated energy fields of the body-mind-spirit and the environment.

Maturity in wholeness is related to how the body-mind-spirit grows. It is not an end point but varies at different points in the life cycle. The principal expressions of maturity in wholeness lie in the development of conceptual thought, formation of knowledge, self-integration, group integration, and development of purpose. Maturity in wholeness involves understanding of and harmony between the individual and others.

The final component of the problem-solving mechanism is *purpose.* It is in the pursuit of purpose that humans boldly attempt to solve complex problems.

Family, community, and social high-level wellness

To this point high-level wellness has been discussed in relation to the individual. The concept is easily applied to groups. The family is an essential group in our society that fulfills several functions: reproduction, rearing of children, and provision of an emotional setting for the stabilization of the adult personality. Family wellness is reflected in the degree to which the family unit succeeds in providing security for all members; love characterized by caring, responsibility, knowledge of other family members, and shared values; a future with the opportunity to develop to full potential; and integration so that problem solving can be done in unity.

Community wellness does not involve only good sanitation, water supply, living space, lack of crime, or sound businesses but might include concern for beauty and wildlife, an environment conducive to interchange between generations, and decentralization of industry to decrease long commuting hours. *High-level environmental wellness* includes more than absence of air, water, and noise pollution; it assumes people's cooperation with nature.

Social wellness involves a forward direction in *progress*, an open-ended expanding future, and the integration of the society into a total personality. Dunn maintains that societies would benefit from learning to fight *for* things and not against them and that problems must be dealt with on a world basis, for there is no possible unilateral human survival.

The concept of high-level wellness can be applied by health professionals, especially nurses, as they begin to focus attention on the wellness of people rather than focusing exclusively on sickness. To shift the emphasis in this fashion, wellness needs to be viewed not as a simple category or static entity but as a dynamic process ranging along a continuum.

An acceptance of the holistic approach outlined in this chapter will not allow the nurse-client relationship to be superficial. It will not be sufficient to know only the name and health care need of the person to be served. A functional relationship will be replaced by one of care and concern for the total person, incorporating full consideration of both inner and outer worlds.[22]

■ BEHAVIOR IN HEALTH AND ILLNESS

Health and illness are usually considered from their clinical perspectives, but it is the social system perspective that has provided practitioners with a wealth of insight into the behavioral aspects of health and illness. Social scientists have examined health and illness in terms of the statuses and roles involved. *Status* refers to the position that could be occupied by members of a society, and *roles* are behaviors of persons who fill a particular status. The individuals of a particular social system share certain common expectations about how people of a specific status should behave in the performance of their roles. These expectations, called *role expectations*, are different for each status. All of these expectations together form the normative framework of a social system. The *norms* outline the expected behaviors for a status. These norms may impose a behavior as obligatory, may prohibit a behavior, or may allow the individual a choice about certain optional behaviors.[30] A summary of the social science descriptions of human behavior in health and illness roles follows.

□ Health behavior

Health behavior is defined as any activity undertaken by persons who believe they are well for the purpose of preventing or detecting disease.

Categories of health behavior

Health behaviors can be classified into three general categories: behaviors geared toward the individual's health, health behavior related to the source and utilization of health care, and individual health behavior in relation to the larger community and health care system as a whole. Each of the three categories describes behaviors geared toward prevention and detection of illness.[25]

The first category, *behaviors geared toward the individual's health,* is admittedly very broad and in need of further research. Preventive behaviors include eating a well-balanced diet, obtaining proper rest, and participating in a daily exercise program. Some detection behaviors in this category could include monthly self-examination of the breasts by women, taking one's temperature, weighing oneself regularly, and a host of other activities.

The second category, *health behavior related to the source and utilization of health care,* has received a great deal of study.[21] Preventive behaviors in this category include such activities as receiving immunizations, seeking information about health problems such as warning signals of cancer, or fluoride treatment for teeth. Examples of health behaviors directed toward detecting illness in this category include seeking routine screening of vision and hearing, Pap smears, physical examinations, chest x-ray studies, and prenatal and postpartum care.

The third category, *individual health behavior in relation to the larger community and health care system as a whole,* has received comparatively little attention. These behaviors might include individual involvement in health legislation, service as a volunteer in health programs, financial support of health organizations, and voting on health proposals.

Changed health attitudes and resultant changed behaviors could become a major preventive resource. Prevention of chronic disease now depends more on changing life styles than on modifying the physical world. Health is determined more by what people do to themselves than by what an external infectious agent does to them.

Health belief model

One widely used model for describing health behavior is the health belief model (Fig. 1-1) designed to explain the widespread failure of people to accept low-cost or free health screening and detection measures for asymptomatic disease.

Health behavior, viewed from the perspective of this model, is influenced by several variables. All variables are interpreted from the phenomenologic viewpoint. The major components of the model are individual perceptions about the threat of the disease; modifying factors, including demographic variables and cues to action; and the likelihood of action.

Individual perceptions. The perceived threat of disease results from two factors: perceived susceptibility and perceived seriousness. *Perceived susceptibility* is the

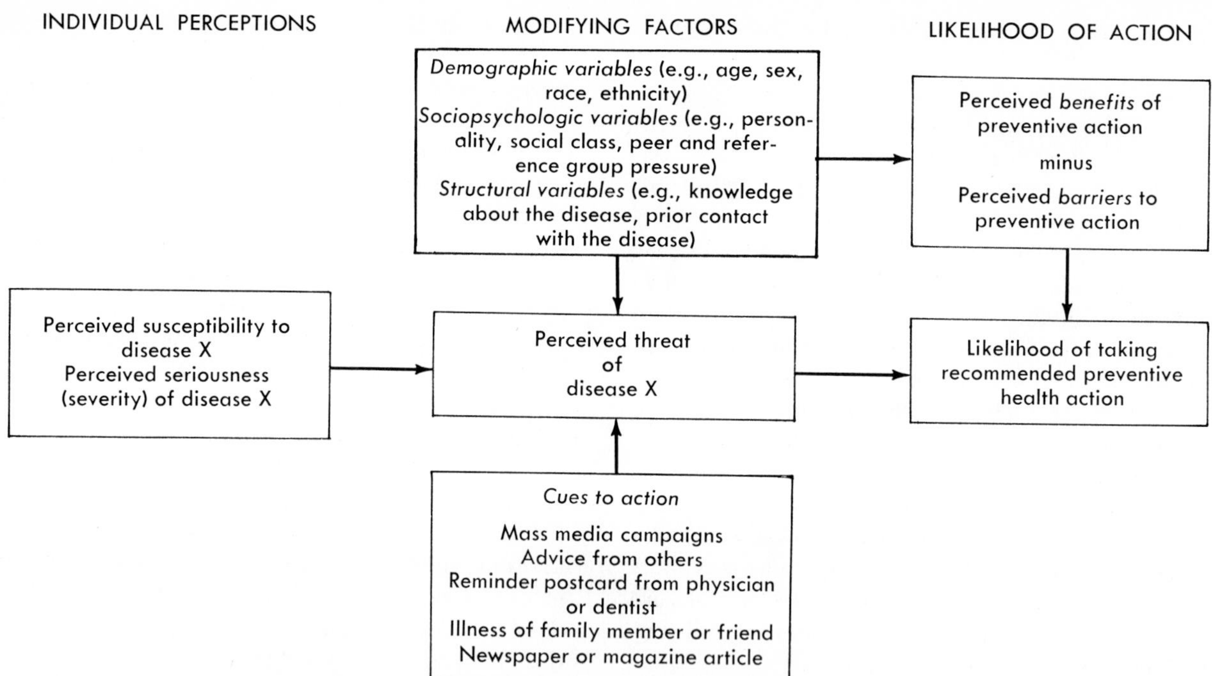

Fig. 1-1. Health belief model. (From Becker, M. H., Drachman, R. H., and Kirschit, J.: Am. J. Public Health **64**:205-216, 1974.)

extent to which individuals feel threatened with contraction of a disease. Since this is a phenomenologic or subjective assessment, the individual's perception of risk may be similar to or vary widely from the perception of a health professional. Perceived susceptibility could conceivably range from being very afraid one will contract a certain condition to complete denial of any risk and feelings of invulnerability. Persons who smoke two packages of cigarettes each day may see themselves as highly susceptible to lung cancer or they may deny the risk of contracting the disease.

Perceived *seriousness*, the second factor comprising the perceived threat, can be viewed from two perspectives: inherent seriousness and impact on one's life style. A disease such as a brain tumor may be seen as inherently serious inasmuch as the disease process could lead to extensive physical disability or death. The impact of this disease on the person's life style may also be judged as quite serious inasmuch as it can necessitate drastic adjustments in employment, function, and ability to care for oneself. Perceived seriousness is calculated on the basis of knowledge about a particular condition and constitutes a force leading to action. The actual performance of a particular recommended action is further influenced by two factors: the individual's conviction that performing the health behavior will prevent or modify the disease, and the person's perception of the unpleasantness or cost of performing the health behavior as compared with taking no action. These two factors can be combined in several ways, providing a large range of resultant behaviors.

Modifying factors and likelihood of action. Even though the *perceived threat of the disease* and the *perceived value of the action* are both high, it is possible that the individual involved may elect to engage in no health behavior at all. Cues seem to be necessary to initiate health behavior. These cues are most likely to be external and may take a wide variety of forms, such as a discussion with a friend, a television or newspaper message, or a postcard reminder from the dentist.

People are thought to vary in their susceptibility to cues.[37] In a situation where the perceived value of action and the perceived threat are high, a weak cue may be effective in eliciting health behavior. In another situation where the perceived value of the action and the perceived threat are low, a strong cue would be needed to be effective. The role of cues has been very difficult to determine because of their transient nature.

Other modifying factors include demographic, sociopsychologic, and structural variables. Thus such variables as sex, age, race, ethnic origin, education, occupation, income, and amount of knowledge are considered influential in health behavior. In general, services for prevention and detection in the United States are used most by the young or middle-aged, by those with higher income and greater formal education, and by whites.[38]

Assessment of health belief model

The health belief model is not without problems and limitations. Health services comprise only one of many possible arenas for health behaviors, and there is a vast array of health providers other than those trained as professionals. The health belief model is based on perceived threat of disease, very much in the manner of the medical-clinical model. It does not attempt to provide a mechanism to study causal factors in achieving higher levels of health where perceived threat of a disease entity is not an important variable.

The model is supposedly applied in situations where the behavior is purely voluntary and the individuals are symptom free, yet much of health behavior is a result of social pressure, legal compulsion, and job requirements.[38] It is conceivable that only a small proportion of the population presently takes voluntary health action to detect or prevent disease in the absence of symptoms. But careful study of these people could lead to an understanding of health behavior that would allow health teaching to increase the number of people who would take preventive action. Looking at how people utilize preventive or detection health services does not explain *why* they use such services. Little is known about the stability of health beliefs over time or about the acquisition of health beliefs. There may be different patterns of behavior for beliefs established early in life versus those established later in life. The usefulness of the model may lie less in predicting who will undertake health actions and more in determining the extent to which health beliefs can be modified in a planned way to meet the needs of the people described by the model.

Other research has suggested that health behaviors, no matter how well described and analyzed, might in fact *not* be predictably related to the impetus to seek preventive or diagnostic services.[14] Several other factors may also be of significant importance for health behavior. These could include life style, working conditions, and housing.

□ At-risk role

Research describes four states in which individuals can find themselves while fluctuating between various states of health and illness: being healthy, at risk, convalescent, or ill. The term *healthy*, as applied by this study, is reserved for those persons who pursue no dangerous habits such as smoking, who do not engage in certain activities that involve directly some health hazard, and who are not in an age range in which there is a high risk from some designated health threat. Those persons who participate in activities that elevate their risk to a significant degree but who are neither convalescent nor ill are termed *at risk*. Convalescents are those who need treatment or rehabilitation prior to regaining their full working capacity. *Ill* persons are defined as persons under medical treatment or as individuals who must perform certain activities in addition to receiving medical treatment. Thus those individuals who according to the study are not healthy, convalescent, or ill constitute a group whose health status warrants their behaving in a way that will reduce their risk of illness, that is, assuming the at-risk role.[3]

Phases of the at-risk role

The above study describes four phases of the at-risk role. The first phase involves acquiring information related to a threat through mass media or through participating in screening procedures and applying that data to one's specific situation. The second phase involves validating the credibility of and attitudes toward both the threat and the recommended preventive action in the social milieu, that is, the lay system. The third phase involves pursuing medical validation of the threat and its applicability to the individual. The fourth phase is acceptance of the high-risk status and is accompanied by compliance with behaviors recommended in relation to the threat.[3]

Appraisal of the at-risk role

The tendency of healthy persons to accept the at-risk role is limited by several factors. First, the at-risk role possesses no rights, only responsibilities. The person at risk is expected to maintain the usual healthy-role responsibilities, to change or modify present behavior, and to do this with no right to social recognition for any achievements. Besides these disadvantages, the at-risk role is not time limited. Its appropriate behaviors could be required over a long period. Results of behaviors are not immediately evident, although they may have a positive outcome that is likely to be manifested in the remote future. Further, the at-risk role is *noninstitutionalized*, and the assumption of it depends solely on the individual. That is, the person at risk must take action to reduce the risk status without the benefits of social reinforcement.

Many times the social environment will negatively reinforce the behaviors necessary for the at-risk role by tempting individuals to deviate from those necessary behaviors. Positive reinforcement, if there is any, could come in the form of additional information concerning the health threat.

Two final disadvantages of the at-risk role exist. First, the at-risk role is based on a statistical probability (as opposed to cause and effect) between certain behaviors and the health threat and often relates to diseases for which no cure exists. The role allows for no transfer of responsibility for cure to the medical profession, since the individual could be blamed for his or her own illness.

The research recommends that three criteria be met before the at-risk role can be implemented and produce viable results in achieving increased levels of wellness in our society. The first involves recognition and acceptance of the at-risk role. The second involves institutionalization of the at-risk role. All medical practitioners, since they are considered to be the legitimizing institution, would need to confirm the at-risk status and reinforce it periodically. The third criterion is the development of norms related to the at-risk role; that is, society would need to begin to regulate the demands and expectations related to this role. This would provide a basis for the social network of the person at risk to exert pressure on him to conform to those expectations.

Nursing could become involved in implementing the recognition and acceptance of the at-risk role by focusing on the value system of nursing. The validity of the nursing profession could become a significant part of the legitimizing force. Nurse practitioners, community health nurses, and others are presently discovering and validating the existence of the at-risk role in individuals and providing reinforcement to persons who have assumed the at-risk role. The concept of the at-risk role is presently utilized by many nurses teaching in clinics for birth control, hypertension, and obesity. It could easily become an integral part of every nurse's function to assess clients for their at-risk status and to follow through by reinforcing appropriate behaviors.

□ Illness behavior

Behavior during illness can be considered as a process with distinguishable phases or stages.

Stages of illness

The illness process can be viewed as a five-stage model that facilitates consideration of social, cultural, and psychologic implications of the illness experience. The five stages are symptom experience, assumption of the sick role, medical care contact, dependent patient role, and recovery or rehabilitation. The decisions, behaviors, and outcomes associated with each phase are summarized in Fig. 1-2.[46]

Symptom experience begins as the person makes a *decision* that something is wrong. This decision has three components: physical, cognitive, and emotional. The *physical* aspects include the presence of signs or symptoms, such as nausea, vomiting, or a rash. The *cognitive* aspects include the personal meaning that the signs and symptoms have for the individual. The *emotional* responses to the physical experience and cognitive interpretation constitute the third aspect.

A community survey based on this model demon-

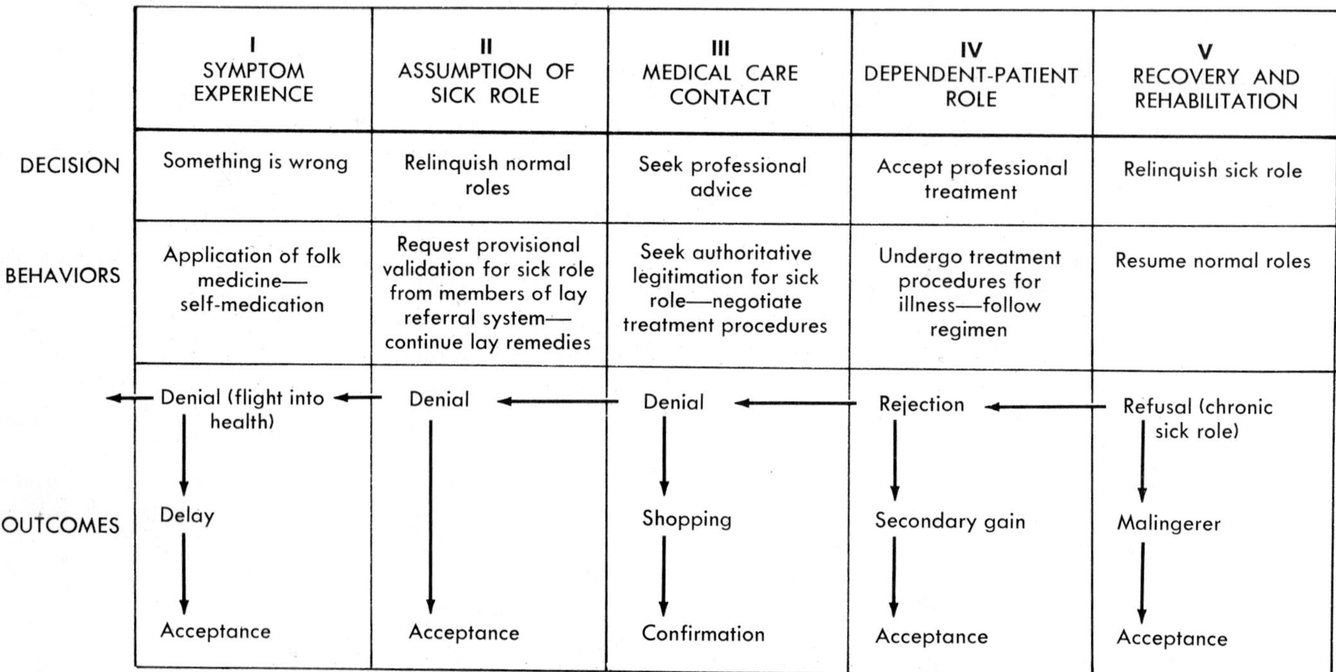

	I SYMPTOM EXPERIENCE	II ASSUMPTION OF SICK ROLE	III MEDICAL CARE CONTACT	IV DEPENDENT-PATIENT ROLE	V RECOVERY AND REHABILITATION
DECISION	Something is wrong	Relinquish normal roles	Seek professional advice	Accept professional treatment	Relinquish sick role
BEHAVIORS	Application of folk medicine—self-medication	Request provisional validation for sick role from members of lay referral system—continue lay remedies	Seek authoritative legitimation for sick role—negotiate treatment procedures	Undergo treatment procedures for illness—follow regimen	Resume normal roles
OUTCOMES	← Denial (flight into health) ←	Denial ←	Denial ←	Rejection ←	Refusal (chronic sick role)
	↓ Delay	↓	↓ Shopping	↓ Secondary gain	↓ Malingerer
	↓ Acceptance	Acceptance	↓ Confirmation	↓ Acceptance	↓ Acceptance

Fig. 1-2. Stages of illness experience. (From Coe, R.: Sociology of medicine, New York, © 1970, McGraw-Hill Book Co. Used with permission of McGraw-Hill Book Co.)

strates that pain was the most significant symptom experienced during the first phase, followed by fever and chills and shortness of breath. The initial signs and symptoms were extremely difficult to ignore, were usually severe, were continuous, and could not be alleviated by lay interventions. Most of the individuals, when faced with frightening and serious symptoms, thought immediately of seeking professional health care. This observation supports the premise that the severity of the symptoms determines the rapidity with which the ill individual seeks care from professionals.

Aspects of symptom experience that have meaning to health care professionals include the results of symptom denial, delay in seeking treatment, and possibly the use of illness for social or psychologic purposes as in hypochondriasis. It becomes a problem to establish a suitable balance between denial of symptoms and overreaction to symptoms (hypochondriasis) at this stage. While chronic illness is insidious in its onset and not immediately productive of serious or incapacitating effects, it is nevertheless a major concern, and it is important that persons thus afflicted be encouraged to seek early health care.

The second stage of illness, the *assumption of the sick role,* involves a decision that one is ill and needs competent care. The ill individual now consults with selected respected lay persons. This serves two purposes. Validation is provided (or not provided) by the friend or relative consulted that the person really is sick. If validation is given, there is a *provisional excuse* for nonperformance of usual role obligations. It is provisional because American society requires that a health professional legitimize one's entrance into the sick role.

The ill person seeks *advice* as well as validation. It was found that the majority of people in the survey did discuss their illnesses, usually with one other person, most often their spouse. This discussion occurred prior to seeking medical help, and almost all discussion took place as soon as the signs and symptoms were noticed.

The majority of the persons consulted by the sick individual also interpreted the signs and symptoms as illness, and most of them recommended seeking professional assistance. Sick persons tended to follow the options suggested by the lay consultant, whether the advice was to seek medical assistance, begin self-treatment, or await further developments. On the whole the discussion process provided a necessary and usually positive impetus toward seeking adequate care.

The *medical care contact stage* involves the decision to seek medical care, that is, to obtain a diagnosis, prognosis, and treatment plan from a medical source. It is here that the person receives authoritative permission to assume the sick role. If such validation is not forthcoming, the sick individual either returns to normal role and status obligations or continues seeking professional opinions until an acceptable diagnosis is found. During this stage most of the individuals in the survey did in fact receive diagnoses, prognoses, and plans of care that they were able to accept.

The fourth stage, the *dependent patient role stage,* includes the ill individual's decision to delegate control to the physician and to cooperate with the prescribed therapy. Now the sick person becomes a patient and tends to look on this role with ambivalence because of the dependency component of the role. While the role in itself is almost always deemed undesirable, it is often looked on as the only means to the desired end, that is, a cure. Patients expressed difficulty with the assumption of this role. While they were willing to follow the physician's recommendations, they displayed concern and expressed a desire to be kept informed.

It remains unclear how much of the dependency and regression imposed on the person during this phase is essential to the patient and how much fulfills the needs of the patient's significant others and health professionals. Issues that await further research include:

1. Why much of the decision making tends to be delegated to the medical profession
2. What benefits could derive from leaving more decision making and autonomy with the patient
3. How helpful it would be to offer the well-informed patient the choice of feasible, promising treatments rather than leave the selection entirely to the professional

The fifth and final stage, *recovery and rehabilitation,* involves the decision to relinquish the sick role. During this phase the individual resumes normal roles and tasks and rejoins the world of the well. In acute limited illness, there are generally no major problems encountered in resuming normal roles. In chronic illness, however, this can be more demanding and the return to normal roles more difficult.

During this phase the majority of persons were being cared for at home and reported satisfaction with their care. It was concluded that most patients are either satisfied with their care or reluctant to complain. Patients who do not successfully accomplish the tasks of this final stage are identified as malingerers.

The major and recurrent concerns of persons during the entire illness experience were variations of questions about chances of full recovery, residual effects of the illness, ability to carry on usual activities, and method of payment for services.

Types of illness behavior

Illness behavior can be of various types. The individual can take action for symptom relief, take no action, vacillate, or take counteraction.[52]

Illness behavior involves symptom perception, evaluation, and response. The individual reacts or does not react to such cues or symptoms as pain, discomfort, or malfunction. Not only is the form of illness extremely variable, but the individual's definition and recognition of and response to the illness are highly complex, interrelated, and diverse. Persons who decide to *take action* can seek help from either health care professionals or non-health-oriented professionals, such as a minister or some identifiably significant person in the community whom people consult for guidance in various sorts of problems. When one decides to *take no action*, there are several possible reasons. Perhaps the appearance of symptoms is just not that important to the individual. In this instance the person recognizes the symptom but does not feel that it is significant enough to warrant action. On the other hand, it could be that fear, lack of resources (or knowledge about the resources), or dislike of entering the health care system leads the individual to delay initiation of help-seeking behavior. Should the symptom subside, the person will usually consider the procrastination effective and adequate. Should the symptom continue and intensify, most people will then take action. Inability to decide either way can cause one to *vacillate*. The situation reflects conflict. The desire to take action is present, but some type of cost to the individual remains a significant deterrent. *Taking counteraction* is a form of denial. It consists of attempting to demonstrate that no illness exists. This behavior opposes definition and assessment of the symptoms and resists action to alleviate or correct them. This type of response to illness can be labeled *deviant illness behavior*. The term does not apply, however, to the behaviors demonstrated by persons who, perhaps due to lack of knowledge of the situation, do not realize that the symptoms could be illness related.[52]

The type of illness behavior demonstrated by the individual is probably determined by a number of variables, such as:

1. Visibility and importance of the symptoms
2. Perceived seriousness of the situation
3. Degree of description caused by the symptoms
4. Tolerance threshold of the individual experiencing the symptoms
5. Interpretation of the symptoms
6. Availability and accessibility of treatment resources.[28]

Utility of studying illness behavior

Since almost all health care is delivered on the initiative of individuals who choose to seek professional help, the study of illness behavior is very important. If we are to understand how persons select themselves for professional health care, then we must learn more about how they define themselves as ill and decide to take action. Attention needs to be focused on the nonusers of health care. If too much attention is devoted to examining the characteristics of those who do seek professional care while relatively little attention is turned to those who do not seek care, an unbalanced, or biased, understanding of illness behavior could result. Once the motivating factors influencing both use or nonuse of professional health care are understood, improved educational programs geared toward increasing options for those experiencing illness can be developed. The study of illness behavior can also increase the accuracy of history taking. Response tendencies that are a part of a person's illness behavior pattern, such as denial, adversely influence the diagnostic process. Illness behavior patterns could influence the patient's response to varying treatment modalities; an awareness of these response patterns could improve compliance with therapy regimens.

□ Sick role

Being sick may result in the person's inability to perform normally expected roles and tasks. Our society has institutionalized a set of expectations and sanctions regarding the behavior of persons unable to perform their usual roles because of illness: the sick role.

Components of the sick role

On assuming the sick role the person is exempted from normal social roles and responsibilities as necessitated by the kind and severity of the illness. Being exempted from normal social roles requires that the illness be legitimized, usually by a physician. The sick person is not considered responsible for an aquired illness; that is, the individual cannot be expected to get well by personal volition. "He can't help it." Being ill is seen as undesirable; the sick person is expected to want to get well and to seek technically competent help.[32]

Three factors produce variations in the sick role: the unique background and experience of the individual, the specific disease process and its severity, and the interactional context in which the person seeks to assume the role. It has been suggested that the demands placed on the individual by roles other than the sick role may cause the greatest variation in assumption of the sick role.[27]

The necessity for legitimizing the illness and seeking competent help confers on the therapeutic agency a method for social control. These agencies are allowed to regulate and define the individual illness process as well as facilitate recovery from the illness state.[32] *Negative control* is exerted through isolating the sick person, both from other sick persons and from the healthy. This accomplishes two goals: the sick cannot reinforce the illness behavior of others, and there does not develop a subculture of sick people; and it decreases the visibility of the sick role and thus decreases the likelihood that healthy people will choose to imitate it.

Society exerts *positive control* by having sick persons place themselves under the control of therapeutic agencies. This places the ill persons in a situation of dependency on health professionals, not on others who are ill.

Assessment of the sick role paradigm

Questions have been raised about the applicability of the sick role paradigm to all types of illnesses.[27] It could be argued that the sick role paradigm is less applicable to the person with a mental illness than to the person with a physical illness, since the mentally ill are seen as more responsible for their illness, mental illness is less acceptable than physical illness as a legitimized illness, and those who are mentally ill often maintain the ability to perform their normal social roles.

Similar concerns have been raised regarding the applicability of the sick role paradigm to the chronically ill. Health professionals do not encourage the chronically ill to define their states as undesirable but to accept and learn to live with their limitations. The chronically ill often are able to perform some of their social roles and thus are not exempted from total responsibility to society. The maintenance care required by the chronically ill person requires that the individual assume a great deal of responsibility for his or her own condition rather than having the health professional assume such responsibility. The utility of the sick role paradigm has also been questioned for those who are aging, abusing drugs or alcohol, suicidal, or pregnant.

The legitimated sick role requires the seeking of technically competent help, yet most persons do not consult a health professional when ill. Often their illnesses are legitimized by family members or friends. Some individuals simply exempt themselves from their usual roles by going to bed. Individuals with some acute illnesses, such as venereal disease, may desire to get well, seek technically competent help, but continue to perform their usual roles.

Several aspects of the sick role require further research. These include:

1. Whether different groups of people have different expectations of the sick role
2. Which specific role and task exemptions are permissible with which types of illnesses
3. How significant others influence sick role expectations
4. Whether different illnesses elicit different types of sick role behavior
5. Whether people accept responsibility for contracting certain illnesses[39]

□ Deviance, health, and illness

Deviance implies the violation of the norms of a group or society.[48] Persons who are ill might be considered deviant if they are no longer able to meet the expectations associated with their roles.

Deviant behaviors violate norms, nondeviant behaviors do not. Variant behaviors depart from specified norms but are still within a permissible or acceptable range.[48] In this context primary deviance occurs when a person defined as normal commits a deviant act; for example, a non-drug-user experiments once with drugs. Secondary deviance occurs when a person defined as deviant commits a deviant act; for example, a "drug abuser" habitually uses drugs.

Labeling a person as deviant alters the expectations that the person will behave normally and may perpetuate the deviance. Labeling the chronically ill or physically handicapped as deviant results in stereotypic expectations that they will not be able to perform adequately in certain situations. Employers and others may consequently deny the chronically ill or handicapped the opportunity to demonstrate their abilities.

Illness can be differentiated from other forms of deviance, for example, crime and sin. The criminal and the sinner commit their acts volitionally, whereas ill persons lack voluntary control over their health state. The social response to sin and crime is punishment in hopes of eliciting conformity. The social response to the sick person is to use some form of therapy to change the factors that prevent that person from conforming. In all situations there are role changes inasmuch as the sinner, criminal, and ill person are pronounced incapable of accepting full responsibility for their behavior: others must intervene to control their behavior.

Several investigators have criticized the *deviance model* of illness,[18,34,48] yet others believe that the deviance model has utility for the health field.[2] The deviance model allows labeling of populations as deviant rather than labeling individuals. The labeling of populations, such as smokers, as deviant would then allow health professionals the right and give them the responsibility to change unhealthy situations. This change would be accomplished by social sanctions and pressures and education to change the deviants into conformists. However effective it might be, this approach does little to foster individual autonomy and responsibility for health.[3]

Medicine as an institution is increasingly assuming more responsibility for controlling deviant behaviors.[32,48] Some behaviors that in previous eras would have been defined as sin or crime and controlled by religious or legal institutions are now being defined as illness and being controlled through medical institutions.

Simultaneously, legal and religious institutions are increasingly adopting medical approaches to control deviance. Churches utilize the mental health model of deviance to provide pastoral counseling similar to psychotherapy. The legal profession often chooses confinement to mental institutions rather than imprisonment, and prisons now frequently define rehabilitation rather than punishment as their goal.

Szasz,[47] a psychiatrist and well-known crusader for the rights of individuals, warns against this medicalization of social deviance. In his view medicine, sociology, psychiatry, and psychology should have nothing to say about whether a person ought to be free to use drugs, commit suicide, engage in homosexual acts, or have delusions. The potential ability to injure or destroy oneself is a basic freedom and there are no grounds for regarding self-injury as a crime to be controlled by police power. Szasz warns of the "therapeutic state," a society in which government, advised by health professionals, increasingly makes individuals' decisions for them. Self-determination is replaced by a powerful medicopsychiatric complex, a subtle and yet real threat to individual liberty. The medicopsychiatric complex has grown in the last decades to a government monopoly that has a strong voice in public policy and legislative decisions. It is armored with vast federal funds to provide therapy when people get out of line.

Maslow asks for studies of the *positive effects* of deviance, a much neglected area of study. Culture can never be advanced without persons who are not afraid to be different. He asks why these persons are usually seen as pathologic and if deviance can be healthy.[26]

The labeling of behavior as deviant can be confined to those areas that impinge on the rights of others. Certain behaviors that have been labeled deviant are presently being reconsidered. Homosexuality can be used to illustrate this. At one time homosexuality was defined as a psychiatric illness. Now it has been removed from this illness status and is considered one of the variations of normal. Nursing could be a force in preventing the labeling of behaviors as deviant when in fact they are only variant, thus increasing individual freedom and the number of acceptable options available to people.

■ SUMMARY

Several models of health, disease, and illness have been presented. As health professionals, nurses need to be familiar with such models and the research based on them to enhance the conceptual bases of their practice. If the goal of nursing is to help people move toward improvement of their health status, then the practitioner needs to ascertain the patient's or client's philosophy of health and illness and also the professional's own view of health and illness. The client's concept of health and illness will be an influential modifier of behavior and will be a prime determinant of goals relative to health. How nurses define health and illness will influence the goals they try to set with clients. The nursing interventions selected by individual nurses, and indeed by the nursing profession as a whole, will be determined largely by theoretical beliefs about health and illness. The effective functioning of nurses may be based on their ability to bring their own and their clients' beliefs, theories, and attitudes to the conscious level. At this level the nurse and client can examine, refine, add, or modify knowledge and attitudes of the health and illness process.

REFERENCES AND SELECTED READINGS

1. *Apple, D.: How laymen define illness, J. Health Soc. Behav. **1**:219-225, 1960.
2. Baric, L.: Conformity and deviance in health and illness, Int. J. Health Educ. **12**:2-12, 1969.
3. *Baric, L.: Recognition of the at-risk role: a means to influence behavior, Int. J. Health Educ. **12**:24-34, 1969.
4. Barker, R. G., Wright, B. A., and Gonick, M. R.: Adjustment to physical handicap and illness: a survey of the social psychology of physique and disability, New York, 1946, Social Science Research Council.
5. Bauman, B.: Diversities in conceptions of health and physical fitness, J. Health Soc. Behav. **2**:39-46, 1961.
6. *Becker, M. H., Drachman, R. H., and Kirschit, J.: A new approach to explaining sick-role behavior in low income populations, Am. J. Public Health **64**:205-216, 1974.
7. Blakiston's Gould Medical Dictionary (Osol, A., editor), ed, 3, New York, 1972, McGraw-Hill Book Co.
8. Brown, J., and Raulinson, M.: Relinquishing the sick role following open heart surgery, J. Health Soc. Behav. **16**:12-27, 1975.
9. *Cassel, E. J.: Disease as an "it": concepts of disease revealed by patients' presentation of symptoms, Soc. Sci. Med. **10**:143-146, 1976.
10. Chalfant, P., and Kurtz, P.: Alcholics and the sick-role: assessments by social workers, J. Health Soc. Behav. **12**:66-72, 1971.
11. Coe, R.: Sociology of medicine, New York, 1970, McGraw-Hill Book Co.
12. Cole, S., and Lejune, R.: Illness and the legitimation of failure, Am. Sociol. Rev. **37**:347-356, 1972.
13. Dolfman, M.: Toward an operational definition of health, J. Sch. Health **43**:206-209, 1974.
14. Dowie, J.: The portfolio approach to health behavior, Soc. Sci. Med. **9**:619-631, 1975.
15. *Dubos, R.: Man overadapting, Psychol. Today **4**:50-53, 1971.
16. *Dunn, H.: High-level wellness, Arlington, Va., 1961, R. W. Beatty, Ltd.
17. *Fabrega, H.: Toward a model of illness behavior, Med. Care **11**:470-484, 1973.
18. Gerson, E.: The social character of illness: deviance or politics? Soc. Sci. Med. **10**:219-224, 1976.
19. Hern, W. M.: The illness parameters of pregnancy, Soc. Sci. Med. **9**:365-372, 1975.

*References preceded by an asterisk are particularly well suited for student reading.

20. *Jago, J.: Hal—old word—new task, Soc. Sci. Med. **9**:1-6, 1975.
21. *Kasl, S. V., and Cobb, S.: Health behavior, illness behavior, and sickrole behavior, Arch. Environ. Health **12**:246-266, Feb. 1966.
22. Kaufman, M.: High-level wellness, a pertinent concept for the health professions, Ment. Hygiene **47**:57-60, 1962.
23. Kurtz, R., and Giacopassi, D. J.: Medical and social work students' perceptions of deviant conditions and sick role incumbency, Soc. Sci. Med. **9**:249-255, 1975.
24. *Lederer, H.: How the sick view their world. In Skipper, J., and Leonard, R.: Social interaction and patient care, Philadelphia, 1965, J. B. Lippincott Co.
25. Lewis, W. R.: Health behavior and quality assurance, Nurs. Clin. North Am. **9**:359-366, 1974.
26. *Maslow, A. H.: Motivation and personality, New York, 1954, Harper & Row, Publishers.
27. *McKinlay, J.: The sick-role: illness and pregnancy, Soc. Sci. Med. **6**:561-572, 1972.
28. Mechanic, D.: Medical sociology: a selective view, New York, 1968, The Free Press.
29. *Mechanic, D.: The concept of illness behavior, J. Chron. Dis. **15**:189-194, 1962.
30. Mechanic, D.: Illness behavior and medical diagnosis, J. Health Soc. Behav. **1**:86-94, 1960.
31. Mercer, J. R.: Who is normal? Two perspectives on mild mental retardation. In Jaco, E. G.: Patients, physicians and illness, New York, 1972, The Free Press.
32. *Parsons, T.: Definitions of health and illness in the light of American values and social structure. In Jaco, E. G.: Patients, physicians and illness, New York, 1958, The Free Press.
33. Patrick, D. L., Bush, J. W., and Chen, M.: Toward an operational definition of health, J. Health Soc. Behav. **14**:6-23, 1973.
34. Pflanz, M., and Rhode, J.: Illness: deviant behavior or conformity, Soc. Sci. Med. **4**:645-653, 1970.
35. The Random House Dictionary of the English Language (Stein, J., editor), New York, 1967, Random House, Inc.
36. Roget's college thesarusus (Morehead, A., editor), New York, 1962, The New American Library Inc.
37. Rosenstock, I.: Historical origins of the health belief model, Health Educ. Monogr. **2**:328-335, 1974.
38. *Rosenstock, I.: The health belief model and preventive health behavior, Health Educ. Monogr. **2**:354-386, 1974.
39. *Segall, A.: The sick-role concept: understanding illness behavior, J. Health Soc. Behav. **17**:163-170, 1976.
40. *Segall, A.: Sociocultural variation in sick-role behavioral expectations, Soc. Sci. Med. **10**:47-51, 1976.
41. *Shuval, J., and Antonovsky, A.: Illness: a mechanism for coping with failure, Soc. Sci. Med. **7**:259-265, 1973.
42. Sorochan, W. D.: Health concepts as a basis for orthobiosis, J. Sch. Health **38**:673-682, 1968.
43. Steadman's medical dictionary, ed. 23, Baltimore, 1976, The Williams & Wilkins Co.
44. Suchman, E. A.: Accidents and social deviance, J. Health Soc. Behav. **11**:4-15, 1970.
45. Suchman, E. A.: Health attitudes and behavior, Arch. Environ. Health **20**:105-110, 1970.
46. *Suchman, E. A.: Stages of illness and medical care. J. Health Soc. Behav. **6**:114-128, 1965.
47. *Szasz, T.: Our despotic laws destroy the right to self-control, Psychol. Today **8**:19-127, 1974.
48. *Twaddle, A. C.: Illness and deviance, Soc. Sci. Med. **7**:751-762, 1973.
49. White, K. L.: Life, death and medicine, San Francisco, 1973, W. H. Freeman and Co. Publishers.
50. Williams, J. S.: Disease as deviance, Soc. Sci. Med. **5**:219-226, 1971.
51. Wilson, R.: The sociology of health: an introduction, New York, 1970, Random House, Inc.
52. *Wu, R.: Behavior and illness, Englewood Cliffs, N. J., 1973, Prentice-Hall, Inc.

2

Introduction to the systems approach

JANET LARSON GELEIN

Biomedicine is a term applied to medicine in Western nations; it encompasses knowledge, practice, organizations, and social roles.[15] The biomedical model that guides beliefs and actions today in health care has been predominantly influenced by the science of molecular biology. The influence of molecular biology on medicine and the study of disease has resulted in the assumption that disease may be fully accounted for by deviations of measurable biologic variables from the norm. The assumption seems to be that many of the values of key physiologic and chemical variables in humans conform to narrow ranges that are common to the entire species. Deviations from health are viewed in physicalistic terms: the sciences of chemistry and physics are used to explain the phenomena accompanying disease.[15] The limitations of this approach are that it separates the body and the mind and that it neglects the social, psychologic, and behavioral dimensions of illness.

When an individual experiences an alteration in health, that individual's past experiences will determine reactions to the illness and the actions taken in an attempt to regain health. Likewise, society and the culture in which the individual lives will affect perception of and give meaning to the altered states of functioning. "The level of function, the efficiency, and the flexibility of a biologic system are affected by the kind of environment in which the individual lives."[14] Thus, cultural, social, and psychologic variables as well as biologic phenomena need to be considered in conjunction with alterations in health. The tendency to ignore these variables and to separate the psyche from the soma may be attributable to the lack of models that integrate the various sciences into a unified, holistic perspective of humanity and health.

■ GENERAL SYSTEMS THEORY

General systems theory provides a perspective for the consideration of humanity and nature in the context of wholes. It is a model for organizing and examining holistic relationships, an alternative to the reductionistic, physicalistic models that have promoted illness care by specialization around organ systems. (In reality there is little, if any, health care practiced today.) The purposes of this chapter are to describe general systems theory and identify fundamental qualities of open systems, to consider the development of a systems approach for nursing, and to explore the application of systems concepts to the developing science of nursing.

Von Bertalanffy, a theoretical biologist, is generally credited with the development of the science of systems. The systems sciences consider a number of different interacting characteristics of nature and examine these characteristics as whole under diverse conditions. The systems sciences grew out of diversity and ever-increasing specialization. Scientists from many disciplines, independent of one another, were studying similar problems and exploring similar concepts. However, a common language that would enable investigators from multiple disciplines to communicate with each other was lacking. The development of general systems theory enabled scientists to derive principles that apply to any system, irrespective of the particular properties or elements of the system involved. These principles are valid for systems in general, whatever the nature of their component elements or the relationship of forces between them.

□ Living systems: basic concepts

A system may broadly be defined as a set of units with relationships among them.[31] These *components*, or units, interact with each other and possess a *boundary*, which is capable of filtering both the kind and rate of flow of inputs that enter the system and outputs that leave the system.[4]

The *state* of a system refers to the value that is given to a set of system variables at a given instant in time. The state of a system changes continuously over time.[25]

One way to evaluate the state of a system is by classifying the system as closed or open. A *closed system* is one that does not exchange matter or energy with its environment. Conventional physics and physical chemistry are limited to the examination of processes in closed systems. The laws of thermodynamics apply only to closed systems. In fact, the second law of thermodynamics states that in a closed system entropy will increase to a maximum and eventually the process will come to a stop at a state of equilibrium.[31] *Entropy,* the energy cost that cannot be recovered from any reaction, accumulates in closed systems. Because matter, energy, or information cannot enter or leave a closed system, the system becomes increasingly disorganized as the amount of stored energy is utilized. In closed systems, entropy is always increasing. As a result order is continuously destroyed.[31]

Living systems are open systems. An *open system* exchanges matter, energy, and information with its environment, has inputs into its boundaries and outputs into the environment, and constantly builds up and breaks down its material components.[31] Although living systems have some characteristics similar to those of closed systems, or systems in equilibrium, we cannot consider living systems as in equilibrium, or closed systems. Even though cells have a certain composition and react to disturbances in ways similar to chemical reactions, there is a fundamental difference between chemical equilibria and metabolizing, living organisms. The organism is *not* a static system for it is not closed to the environment and does not always contain identical components. Rather, it is an open system in a quasi-steady state.

The *steady state* of open systems is maintained by means of a continuous exchange of component matter and energy. Matter is continually entering from the environment and leaving the system to the environment. The openness of a system, then, refers to the ability of the system to exchange matter, energy, or information with its environment.

The steady state of an open system may be defined as a relative state of balance: a dynamic equilibrium. Von Bertalanffy believes that a steady state exists when the composition of the system is relatively constant despite continuous exchange of matter.[31]

Open systems have the capability to import matter as the potential carrier of free energy, or "negative entropy."[31] Negative entropy, or *negentropy,* is the capability of open systems to take in inputs of matter or energy that are higher in complexity of organization than their outputs. Negentropy makes it possible for an open system to restore energy and prevent breakdowns. Living systems adapt through maintaining a steady negentropic state.

Along with the ability to adapt, open systems exhibit a dynamic process called *equifinality.* Whereby closed systems eventually reach thermodynamic equilibrium, open systems may attain a steady state that has a value equifinal or independent of initial conditions. In other words, independent states or goals in open systems may be reached from different initial conditions in different ways at the same time. One example of this concept may be seen in the development of a human being, which may occur from the fertilization of one whole ova or from the fertilization of a divided ovum as with identical twins. Both processes may eventually result in the birth of a normal human infant. Likewise, two infants of different heights and weights may arrive at the same final state, a certain species-specific adult size, despite possible intervening variables disturbing or inhibiting growth in childhood.[31]

☐ Hierarchy of systems

The systems view allows us to understand that humanity is one species with values and intrinsic worth in a hierarchy of nature. Life begins with complex macromolecules, such as genes and viruses, which may be organized and integrated with chemical substances to form cells. Cells may be organized into tissues and organs, which may be further integrated into organisms that are capable of organization into groups, organizations, communities, and societies. This hierarchy of complexity can extend to multinational systems.[25a]

When using systems theory it is imperative to identify the level of reference one is using. To avoid confusion the following terms are used in this chapter to identify the level of reference for systems analysis. *System* refers to the identified level on which we are focusing. *Suprasystem* refers to the level above the focal system, and *subsystem* refers to the level below the identified system. All systems tend to function by maintaining steady states, keeping an orderly balance among subsystems within the system, their environments, and suprasystems. There are inputs across the boundary of a system to the subsystems; internal processes that utilize energy, matter, or information; and outputs from the system to suprasystems. Humanity is considered as one system in a hierarchical structure of nature that occurs in multiple levels, each level reflecting its own variant of general systems characteristics.

☐ Fundamental qualities of open systems

When defining an open system consideration should be given to three fundamental qualities: structure, process, and function. *Structure* refers to the arrangement of all defined components of a system at a given moment in time. Miller[25] defines the structure of a system as three dimensional, remaining relatively fixed or changing depending on the characteristics of the process of the system at that particular time.

The model of a simple feedback control scheme in Fig. 2-1 illustrates the basic structure of an open system. The *environment* external to an open system consists of

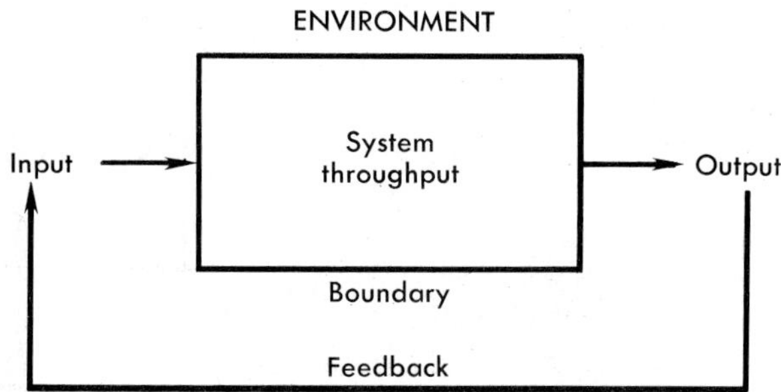

Fig. 2-1. Simple control scheme involves input, throughput, and output. Feedback provides a self-regulating mechanism for the organism.

all those elements that affect the system and are likewise affected by the system. The *boundary* of a system is permeable and delineates intrasystemic processes from extrasystemic elements. All boundaries of open systems are dynamic in that they function by continually exchanging information, energy, or matter with their environments.[31] The boundary of a system may be viewed as a filter through which inputs and outputs must pass and it functions in a manner that differentiates processes within the system from those outside the boundaries of the system. The boundary controls both the rate and flow of inputs and ouputs. The processes within the boundaries of the system (subsystem processes) are mutually attracted or balanced in a way that permits the system to function as a whole. The exchange of energy or the intensity of interaction is greater between elements within the boundary of a system than between those elements outside of the boundary.

Process refers to the transformation of energy, information, or matter in a system over time and incorporates the function of a system. *Function* relates to the interaction between component parts.

The exchange of matter, energy, or information between the environment and the identified system occurs through the processes of input, throughput (systems processing), output, and feedback. *Input* to a system occurs when matter, energy, or information is obtained by the system. Once the system absorbs this input, it processes or transforms the information or energy in a way that is useful to its function in a process called *throughput* and then expels or discharges matter, information, and energy in the process of output. *Output* is energy, matter, or information disposed of by the system as a consequence of its function.

Feedback refers to the process of self-regulation in open systems and involves the system's ability to control input and output. Negative feedback reduces deviation from the kinetic state, and positive feedback amplifies deviation from the steady state. If the system's negative feedback is disrupted, its steady state vanishes, and ultimately its boundary disappears and the system terminates. Feedback mechanisms in open systems allow them to maintain steady states and to adapt.[25]

Adaptation to the environment may be accomplished by means of certain boundary maintenance functions. The boundary can contain undesirable elements in the environment; obtain needed matter, energy, or information (inputs); retain these are necessary; and dispose of unwanted or unnecessary matter (outputs).[6]

It is also suggested that integration and decision making are processes critical to the survival of a system. Integration of the components of a system is essential for the system to function effectively and to persist. The integration of components requires patterns of interaction between the components. Decision making refers to the process by which resources for adaptation and integration are allocated.

■ DEVELOPMENT OF A SYSTEMS APPROACH FOR NURSING

□ Historical perspective

If we closely examine publications of early nursing leaders we find that some of them seemed to view disease as it more recently was described from a systems perspective. Von Bertalanffy describes disease as a life process that regulates toward normalcy after a disturbance, this regulation toward normalcy being attributable to the equifinality of biologic systems.[31] In 1859 Florence Nightingale expressed similar beliefs about disease. She asserted that all disease was a reparative process and was not necessarily accompanied by suffering. Nightingale conceived of disease as an effort of nature to repair destructive processes.[26] When disease is viewed as a life process moving toward normalcy, roles of health professionals can be viewed as supplementary to this process.

Von Bertalanffy considers the role of medicine to be an expression of dynamic systems and thus, to the extent possible, maintaining and reestablishing the steady state.[31] Again comparing Von Bertalanffy's ideas about the role of medicine with Florence Nightingale's, we find some similarities. Nightingale considered medicine as doing nothing more than assisting nature—only nature was believed to cure. She suggested that nursing's goal was to assist the patient to attain the optimum condition for nature to act.[26] In 1885, Clara Weeks Shaw, another nursing leader, expressed a view similar to that of Nightingale's. She spoke of the role of the nurse as keeping the patient in the state most conducive for natural reparative tendencies.[28] Even though the concepts of systems theory were not refined by Von Bertalanffy until 1968, there are similarities between his statements about disease and medicine and Nightin-

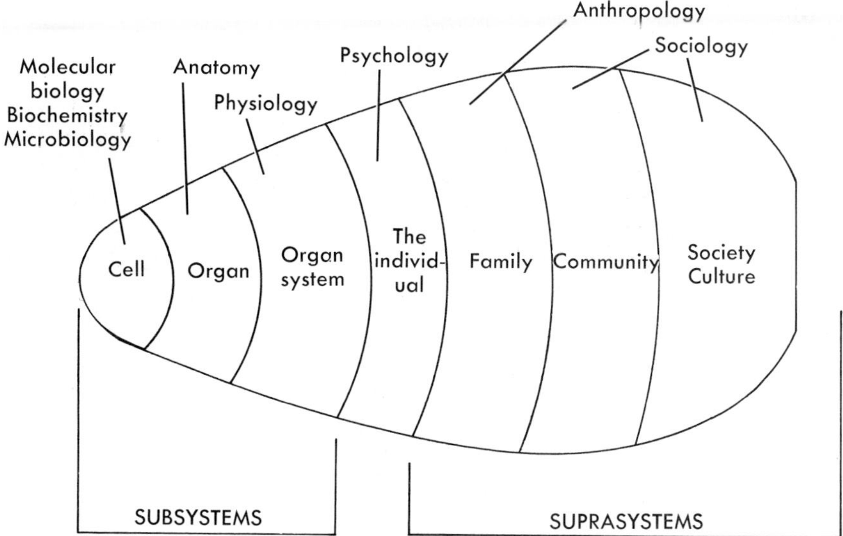

Fig. 2-2. Sciences influencing nursing practice. Molecular biology, biochemistry, microbiology, anatomy, and physiology support our understanding of human subsystems. Knowledge of psychology, anthropology, and sociology contribute to our understanding of humankind as a holistic entity in context of suprasystems.

gale's and Shaw's earlier descriptions of disease and the role of nursing.

Rogers[27] would probably be identified as the first nurse to introduce a theoretical basis for nursing that recognized the person as a system whose characteristics are identifiably those of the whole. She proposed a conceptual model for nursing that envisioned the individual as an open system: more than and different than the sum of the parts, continually exchanging matter and energy with the environment.

Since Rogers' writings, several texts have been published in nursing that consider a systems perspective for nursing practice.[3,8,18] The reader is encouraged to consult these or other texts for alternative viewpoints on the application of systems theory to nursing practice. The remainder of this chapter *considers one conception* for the application of systems theory to nursing practice. First nursing will be defined and then a systems model for nursing explicated.

☐ Systems definition of nursing

From a systems perspective nursing may be defined as a process that supports, maintains, or helps restore, insofar as possible, the desired steady state of an identified system. As defined earlier, when an identified system is in a steady state, it is in a relative state of balance or in a dynamic state of equilibrium. This relative state of balance, or steady state, does not negate the presence of disease; rather, it assumes a state of wellness. Wellness, on the other hand, assumes integration of social, cultural, psychologic, and biologic functioning in a manner that is oriented to maximize the potential capabilities of the identified system.[13] The goal of nursing is to promote the maximum health potential of a system and is directed toward supporting, maintaining, or restoring, insofar as possible, a dynamic state of equilibrium: the steady state of an identified system.

Maximum health potential and the steady state of an identified system are dependent on system variables. For example, if the identified system is an individual, the nurse would assess and define the structure, process, and function of this system. Are there subsystem or suprasystem variables that influence the systems' ability to achieve maximum health? If so, what can the nurse and the client design that will support, maintain, or restore a desired steady state? These questions, basic to the process of nursing, are central to a systems perspective for nursing. The following sections of this chapter explicate the application of systems concepts.

☐ Applied science of nursing today

Nursing as a developing science draws on many disciplines for knowledge to assist with the assessment of systems and the dynamics associated with health. Fig. 2-2 illustrates the bodies of knowledge useful to nursing and the potential focal systems to which they pertain. Since the biomedical model dominates health care in most Western nations, medicine and nursing are still influenced by the biologic sciences such as anatomy, physiology, biochemistry, microbiology, and molecular biology. One can see from Fig. 2-2 that the microscopic orientation of the biologic sciences restricts our notions of humanity and health to the subsystem levels of reference. However, if the individual were identified as the focal system (as in Fig. 2-2), organ systems, organs, and cells would be seen as subsystems and the family, community, society, and culture as relevant suprasystems. This approach enables us to examine health from a perspective that includes the relevant suprasystems and illustrates that knowledge of the social sciences is essential for nursing practice. This concept can be explored further through some self-assessment.

Subsystem focus

Nurses are familiar with the structure, function, and processes of many organ systems and with the organs, cellular functions, and alterations that frequently occur with disease. For example, systems theory concepts can be readily applied to the cardiovascular system.

STRUCTURE
Heart, blood vessels, lymphatic vessels and nodes, red bone marrow

FUNCTION
Transportation, protection, regulation

PROCESS
Homeostatic mechanisms related to structures of organ system

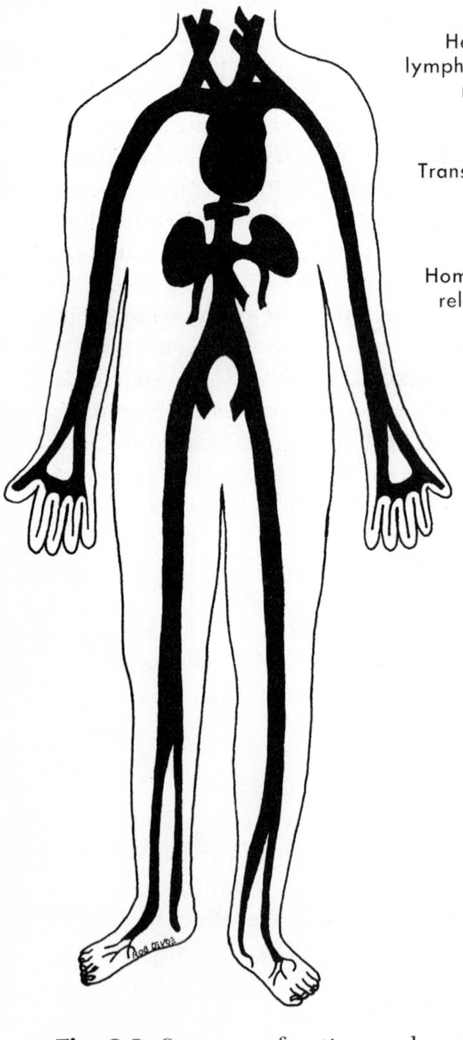

Fig. 2-3. Structure, function, and process of cardiovascular system.

The cardiovascular system meets the criteria for a system, since it is a complex of elements in purposeful interaction. The structure of this organ system is composed of the heart, blood vessels, lymphatic vessels and nodes, and the red bone marrow by virtue of its hematopoietic function (Fig. 2-3). The functions of the cardiovascular system are to transport various substances to and from the body cells, to protect the body against invading microorganisms, and to regulate body heat. System processes are accomplished through homeostatic mechanisms related to structures in the organ system: the heart, blood vessels, and blood cells. Starling's law of the heart would be one example of such a process: energy set free at each contraction of the heart is a simple function of the length of the fibers composing its muscular walls.

Individual as a system

The individual as a focal system requires a variety of different inputs from subsystems and suprasystems to maintain a state of health. For example, one conception of humankind and health identifies a hierarchy of needs that the individual as a system is motivated to fulfill. Maslow conceives of full health as individuals actualizing and fulfilling their natural potentialities (see Chapter 1). As shown in Fig. 2-4, the natural potentials of individuals are fulfilled through the satisfaction of five basic needs: physiologic, safety, love and belongingness, self-esteem, and self-actualization needs.[24] The individual's environment—the suprasystems of family, community, society, and culture—provide a variety of inputs to satisfy the development of these needs. For example, food, fluids, and oxygen nourish cells and promote physiologic functions. A safe environment provides protection, order, and predictability in the world, nurturing survival of the organism. These two needs, physiologic and safety needs, are considered as lower level needs or prerequisites of all living animal systems. Lower level needs require a form of energy that is similar to what Berrien refers to as "maintenance input" in social systems. Maintenance input energizes the system and makes it ready to function.[4] All living systems require some type of maintenance input to survive. However, what distinguishes the human from all other living systems is the motivation to fulfill upper level needs.

The motivation to pursue a range of upper level needs—love and belongingness, self-esteem, and self-actualization—is unique to human beings. Gratification of these needs results in increased happiness, serenity, and richness of inner life. The lack of input to gratify these needs is the most commonly identified core of low level of health in our society.[24] The form of energy processed from the suprasystem to promote upper level needs may be similar to the input that Berrien has described in social systems as "signal input."[4] *Signal input* is energy-information processed by social systems to produce an output to the suprasystem. This form of energy that promotes upper level needs, along with the interchange of energy between humans and the environment, advances humanity. Upper level need fulfillment cultivates apperception: self-perceptive consciousness and creativity.

Suprasystem focus: the family

One of the suprasystems of the individual identified in Fig. 2-2 is the family. Like the human subsystems and the individual as a focal system, the family may also be analyzed from a systems perspective. Let us consider one perspective of the family as the focal system and apply some of the concepts of systems theory to this suprasystem of humanity.

Function. The family as a social system performs several essential functions: socialization, selection, recreation, protection, and reproduction.[19] As was discussed earlier, the function of a system relates to the interaction between component parts and cannot always be readily distinguished from system processes. One way to describe the function of the family is to consider the family as an open, adaptive, organizationally complex, information-processing system.[20] Families as organizationally complex systems involve networks of interdependent, causal relations governed by feedback control mechanisms. Like other systems, the family changes as it responds to input from the environment. As an open system the family interchanges matter, energy, and information with the environment and adapts through these frequent processes.

The information processing of family systems involves the relationship between sets, or ensembles, of structured variety. The process of feedback informs parts of the family how to function toward purposive, goal-seeking activity. What distinguishes family systems from other biologic or mechanical systems is the feedback process, which involves primarily psychic, complex communication processes of information exchange.[7]

Structure. The structure of family systems has been conceptualized in a variety of ways.[2,19,23] To explicate the application of systems concepts, only one systems perspective for the analysis of families will be discussed. Kantor and Lehr[20] describe the family system as one that is composed of three subsystems: the personal subsystem, the family-unit subsystem, and the interpersonal subsystem. These three subsystems interact with each other as well as with systems outside their boundaries.

The *personal subsystem* refers to an individual family member and incorporates self-interests, desires, meanings, and needs of individual, similar to those discussed earlier. In addition to the characteristics of an individual, or the personal subsystem, members of a family are also part of the family unit subsystem. *Family-unit subsystem* refers to selected architectural boundaries and social space perimeters that the family uses to establish family territory. Besides the same name and address, families have neighborhoods and associated community elements such as schools, libraries, town centers, and churches. One component of structure related to the family unit is the social space, or the structural enclosure where the family process takes place. The social space perimeter of "territory" of families is evidenced in the behaviors they signal to others around them. Even though there are no physical walls to block entrance, one is usually aware of the extent to which the family wants

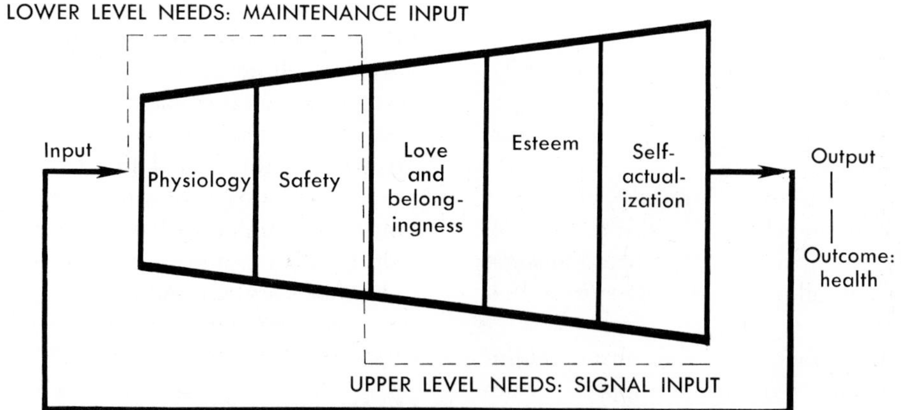

Fig. 2-4. Individual as system: hierarchy of needs. Lower level needs require maintenance input into system, whereas upper level needs require and produce signal input.

others to impinge on their family boundaries. High fences, doorbells, and privately listed telephone numbers all function to limit access to the social space of family subsystems.

Even when others have been admitted to a family unit's space there is no guarantee that they will be allowed to enter the family's *interpersonal* subsystem. The family's interpersonal subsystem involves the interrelationships between individual family members in the realization of three goals: *affect* (intimacy and nurturance), *power* (freedom to decide and acquire money or skills), and *meaning* (philosophical framework for guiding reality).

Process. According to Kantor and Lehr, family members regulate access to power, affect, and meaning through time, space, and energy. Families regulate space through defining safety zones to protect privacy, property, and relationships among family members. Time in families is structured as clock or calendar time, and an understanding of temporal relationships in families is facilitated through examining the family's basic rhythmic patterns. Energy in families is both static and kinetic: kinetic when members expend supplies of energy and static when energy is stored and available for use. The assessment of energy in families provides insight into the balance between supply and demand and the amount of energy available to facilitate the target goals of affect, power, and meaning. The family that has energy to process information and matter to maintain goals so that no one subsystem is consistently denied actualization enables individual family members and the family unit to grow and develop in a healthy way.[20]

■ ALTERATIONS IN BASIC HUMAN NEEDS: STRESS, INSTABILITY, AND DISEASE

Let us return to the individual as the focal system and examine the distinction mentioned earlier between maintenance and signal input, since this often provides insight into the decay and deterioration of social systems. It is postulated that for varied periods of time open systems may be impervious to signal inputs and appear relatively isolated and closed. Human systems, like social systems, begin to deteriorate if they do not interact purposefully with their environments.

To reach full health potential a human system must interact with the environment to satisfy a hierarchy of needs. If individuals are impaired or obstructed in some way from achieving their full potential, their systems become stressed.

Stress is experienced when there is a substantial imbalance between what the environment supports or demands and what the system needs. If matter, energy, or information is lacking or there is an underload of input, the system may experience stress. Likewise, if there is an excess or overload of input, the system must act to correct this excess of matter, energy, or information. Since individual systems have a range of stability within which they function and process inputs of energy, there is a wide range of adaptive potentials. However, there are limits to a system's ability to function and process stress.

One outcome for a system that is stressed is *instability*. A system that is unstable responds by changing its own state or that of its environment so as to increase its efficiency with respect to its function.[1] Instabilities in an open system do not lead to random behavior; rather, they tend to drive the system to a new dynamic regimen that corresponds to a new state of complexity. When a system is in such a transition it acquires new possibilities for action.[17] If the system were closed it would monotonously increase entropy, and the development of maximum disorder would reach a state of equilibrium or rest: death. Open systems, through the exchange of energy with the environment, move through instabilities, fluctuations, transitions, and mutations to new regimens of metabolizing activity for life. Instability promotes order through fluctuation, which mutates toward new dynamic regimens.

The traditional view of disease is that of a deranged condition in an affected organ or organ system, usually precipitated by an agent external to the system. From a systems perspective disease is a life process related to the structure and functions of humanity, due to the equifinality of open systems. Disease is manifest when basic human needs are impeded either through self-selected actions or environmental demands and constraints that obstruct basic need satisfaction. When individuals' basic needs are such that they fail to make rapid enough a perfect adaptive response to the new environments in which they elect to live and function, disease ensues. Dubos cautions that disease cannot be kept at bay through environmental and medical control, since humans cannot control all cosmic forces and because of the human propensity to move on to the unknown.[12] Humans will never live in an environment that is static. Instability is an inevitable outcome as humanity changes and evolves. Disease is one outcome of instability for individuals as they adapt to stress, a transitional state, a time when the system promotes order through fluctuation. In this framework, nursing assists the individual to help restore, insofar as possible, the steady state of the individual's system and provides support during transitions from one dynamic regimen to another dynamic regimen.

■ SUMMARY

This chapter has considered systems theory as one theory for guiding nursing practice. As the science of nursing evolves, various theories will be defined to explain nursing phenomena. Systems theory as a theory of theories could provide the framework for classifying and defining knowledge as it develops in nursing and assist in relating this knowledge to other disciplines, thus expediting nursing's endeavors to promote the health of the individual as a holistic system.

Education, research, and nursing practice often tend to focus on the subsystem level. The recognition and exploration of psychologic, social, and cultural variables in promoting health will assist nursing exploration of suprasystem variables and encourage options other than the reductionistic, physicalistic, subsystem approach to health care that exists today. Systems theory constructs could guide the understanding of systems and the integration of physical and psychologic principles, since it provides a perspective for considering humanity and nature in the context of wholes.

Basic concepts for living systems were defined, including steady state, negentropy, equifinality, and the distinctions between open and closed systems. The fundamental qualities of an open system—structure, process, and function—were examined, along with boundary and the processes of input, throughput, output, and feedback. System, subsystem, and suprasystem were defined.

A systems perspective for nursing was explicated. Nursing was described as a process that supports, maintains, or helps restore, insofar as possible, the steady state of an identified system. The applied science of nursing was considered as it relates to humanity's subsystems, to an individual system, and to a suprasystem with the family as a focal system. Systems concepts were applied to the subsystem, system, and suprasystems of human beings.

REFERENCES AND SELECTED READINGS

1. Ackoff, R., and Emory, F.: On purposeful systems, Chicago, 1972, Aldine Publishing Co.
2. Anderson, R., and Carter, I.: Human behavior in the social environment, Chicago, 1974, Aldine Publishing Co.
3. *Auger, J.: Behavioral systems and nursing, Englewood Cliffs, N.J., 1976, Prentice-Hall, Inc.
4. *Berrien, K.: General and social systems, New Brunswick, N.J., 1968, Rutgers University Press.
5. Boulding, K.: General systems theory, Management Sciences **2**:197-208, 1956.
6. Bredemeier, H. C. cited in Smoyak, S. A.: Toward Understanding nursing situations: a transactional paradigm, Nurs. Res. **18**:405-411, 1969.
7. Buckley, W.: Sociology and modern systems theory, Englewood Cliffs, N. J., 1967, Prentice-Hall, Inc.
8. Byrne, M. L., and Thompson, L.: Key concepts for the study and practice of nursing, ed. 2, St. Louis, 1978, The C. V. Mosby Co.
9. *Cassel, J.: Psychiatric epidemiology. In Caplan, G.: An American handbook of psychiatry, New York, 1973, Basic Books, Inc., Publishers.
10. Dickoff, J., James, P., and Wiedenbach, E.: Theory in a practice discipline, Nurs. Res. **17**:415-435, 1968.
11. Dubos, R.: Man adapting, New Haven, 1965, Yale University Press.
12. Dubos, R.: Mirage of health, New York, 1959, Doubleday and Co., Inc.
13. Dunn, H.: High-level wellness, Arlington, Va., 1961, R. W. Beatty, Ltd.
14. Fabrega, H.: Toward a theory of human disease. J. Nerv. Ment. Dis. **162**:299-312, 1976.
15. Fabrega, H.: The need for an ethnomedical science, Science **189**:969-975, 1975.
16. Guyton, A.: Textbook of medical physiology, Philadelphia, 1975, W. B. Saunders Co.
17. Jantsch, E.: Design for evolution: self-organization and planning in the life of human systems, New York, 1975, George Braziller, Inc.
18. *Hall, J., and Weaver, B.: A systems approach to community health, Philadelphia, 1977, J. B. Lippincott Co.
19. Horton, T. E.: Conceptual basis for nursing intervention with human systems. In Hall, J., and Weaver, B.: A systems approach to community health, Philadelphia, 1977, J. B. Lippincott Co.
20. Kantor, D., and Lehr, W.: Inside the family, San Francisco, 1975, Jossey-Bass, Inc., Publishers.
21. Kuhn, T.: The structure of scientific revolutions, Chicago, 1962, The University of Chicago Press.
22. *Laszlo, E.: The systems view of the world: the natural philosophy of the new developments in the sciences, New York, 1972, George Braziller, Inc.
23. Lewis, J., et al.: No single thread: psychological health in family systems, New York, 1976, Brunner/Mazel, Inc.
24. Maslow, A. H.: Motivation and personality, New York, 1954, Harper & Row, Publishers.
25. *Miller, J. G.: Living systems: basic concepts. In Gray, W., et al.: General systems theory and psychiatry, Boston, 1969, Little, Brown and Co.

25a. Miller, J. G.: Living systems, New York, 1978, McGraw-Hill Book Co.

26. Nightingale, F.: Notes on nursing: what it is and what it is not, London, 1859 and 1914, Harrison.
27. Rogers, M.: The theoretical basis of nursing, Philadelphia, 1970, F. A. Davis Co.
28. Shaw, C. W.: A textbook of nursing, ed. 3, New York, 1885 and 1902, D. Appleton and Co.
29. Svalastoga, K.: The social system, (translated), Copenhagen, 1974, Akademisk Forlag.
30. *Vickers, G.: Is adaptability enough? Behav. Sci. **4**:219-234, 1959.
31. *Von Bertalanffy, L.: General systems theory: foundations, development, and applications, New York, 1968, George Braziller, Inc.

*References preceded by an asterisk are particularly well suited for student reading.

3

Social and cultural dimensions of health and illness

ANTOINETTE T. RAGUCCI
JEAN GOEPPINGER

Health maintenance, illness, and death are universals of the human condition. Preventive, diagnostic, and curing behaviors have characterized all human groups' responses in coping and adapting to threats to the biologic integrity of the body. The diversity of human responses to events associated with illness, disease,* and death and the adaptive arrangements that must be made by individuals and groups need to be taken into account in nursing interventions. Health and illness behaviors may be viewed as social and cultural categories as well as physiologic and psychologic.

The purpose of this chapter is to examine the interconnections between acute and chronic disease entities that affect a person's biologic integrity and some social and cultural variables that need to be considered in planning nursing interventions on behalf of patients and clients. Some concepts and findings derived from the specialty areas of medical anthropology and medical sociology will be explicated. These include the physical anthropology, or biocultural dimensions, of disease and the social and cultural determinants of health-seeking behavior. To facilitate identification of universal features of human responses to illness as well as responses unique to a group or subculture, a cross-cultural comparative approach is used.

The specialty areas cited above are engaged in the development of a body of knowledge that will advance theoretical as well as applied interests in health and illness care. Medical anthropologists, for the most part, have directed their attention to cultural phenomena associated with illness events and health-seeking behaviors. On the other hand, the medical sociologists' prime focus has been on society and social class variables.[29] Both areas of study use an essentially comparative approach to facilitate the identification of differences and similarities in group responses to health and illness events.

A comparative approach is developing within nursing. One nurse-anthropologist advocates a transcultural nursing approach, which offers a frame of reference that "can offer insight, new relationships, new foci and new dimensions of caring about one's own culture in relation to another."[50] Transcultural health care is defined as an evolving body of knowledge and practices regarding health-illness caring patterns from a comparative perspective of two or more cultures to determine major care features and the health services of cultures.[50]

Psychologic, cultural, and social phenomena are analytically distinct categories. A review of the nursing literature reveals that these dimensions of nursing care are usually subsumed under the headings *psychosocial* or *sociocultural* needs or components. In addition some medical-surgical nursing literature appears to treat sociocultural or psychosocial considerations of patient care almost as an afterthought. Nursing interventions directed toward ameliorating discomfort and the problems associated with social and cultural variables are usually phrased in general terms of "shoulds" and "oughts." Failure of nurses to distinguish analytically between the physiologic, psychologic, social, and cultural determinants of health-seeking behavior and their interconnections has resulted in many instances of less attention being paid to the social and cultural components of nursing care.

Fig. 3-1 presents a model delineating the various dimensions of health-seeking behaviors. It can be noted that the extrapersonal factors (social and cultural) affect and in turn are influenced by intrapersonal factors (biologic and psychologic) and environmental factors (ecologic and demographic). The model is intended to convey the analytical distinctiveness of the variables that determine human behaviors.

*Following Fabrega[25,26] a distinction is made between the terms "disease" and "illness." *Disease* refers to pathology as defined by Western biomedical science. *Illness* is conceptualized as the perception of pathology in the context of a particular culture, that is, the layman or folk definition.

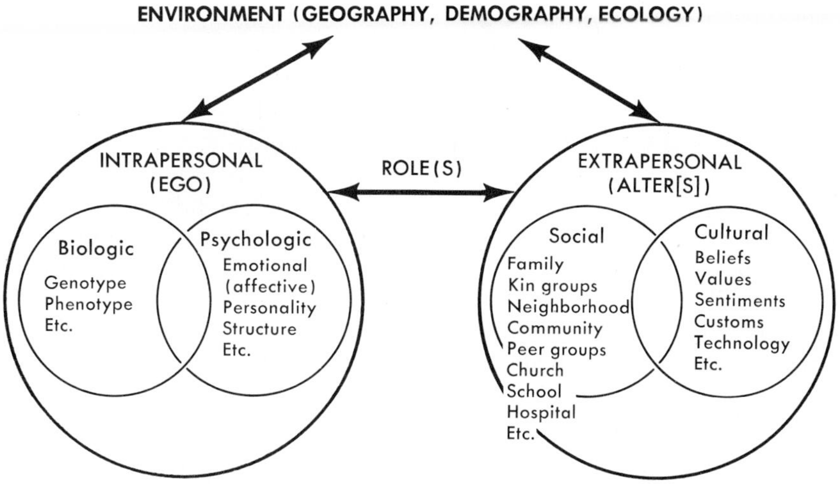

Fig. 3-1. Dimensions of health-seeking behaviors.

■ SOCIAL PHENOMENA

Social phenomena are conceptualized as those human actions and interactions that involve two or more persons. Subsumed under the category *social* are the constructs of social structure, social system, and social organization. These constructs are variously defined by sociologists, anthropologists, and other behavioral theorists. In general *social structure* refers to ongoing, recurring, or patterned relationships. The concept is applied to small groups (such as the nuclear family) as well as to large organizations or aggregates (such as the community and society).[38] A social structure consists of arrangements of positions or statuses variously created and maintained or a network of relationships among persons.

A *social system* is made up of the interactions of a number of individuals whose relationships to each other are defined and mediated by a system of culturally structured and shared expectations. Thus the analytical unit of the social system is the role (or role sets) that serves to link or relate the individual (ego) to one or more others or alter(s).[74] Role is differentiated from status, which may be interpreted as a unit of society. Status defines a person's place or position within a social group or society.[53]

Social roles may be further defined as goal-directed configurations of acts patterned in accordance with cultural value orientations[100] and conforming to the position (status) a person holds in a social group or situation. The behavioral expectations within a role differ across cultures. The underlying assumption of the above definition of social roles is that roles never exist within a vacuum but are considered from the perspective of a social group or context. Roles form social systems that are reciprocally geared by the acts of role partners, such as nurse-patient (dyadic) or nurse-patient-physician (triadic).

Social organization can be defined as the actions of any individual resulting from personal choices and decisions and the actions of others.[28] Social organization is conceptualized as consisting of the working arrangements of a society or processes involved with ordering actions and relationships toward given social goals. Social organization refers to those actions that are directed toward the integration of a society.[28] It is through social organization that the work of a society or cultural group is accomplished. Some categories of social organization are political parties and economic, legal, and health care institutions (hospitals) (Fig. 3-1). The analysis of the hospital as a social system would be concerned with delineating relationships between individuals and groups of individuals according to their social roles, which are culturally defined.

■ CULTURAL PHENOMENA

Cultural phenomena include those objects or events that are patterned and arranged into a cultural system whose different parts are interrelated to form values, beliefs, and symbolic systems (Fig. 3-1). The concept of culture is variously defined as the ways of life or designs for living common at any one time to all humankind, the ways of living peculiar to a group or societies between whom there is a greater or lesser degree of interaction, the patterns of behavior peculiar to a group, or special ways of behaving characteristic of a segment of a large and complex society. The classical definition of culture is that of Sir Edward Tylor, who defined culture as "that complex whole which includes knowledge, belief, art, morals, law, custom and any other capabilities and habits acquired by man as a member of society."[109] The notions of holism, continuity, and diversity are implicit in the concept of culture. Kluckhohn and Kelly define culture as a "historically derived system of explicit and implicit designs for living which tend to be shared by all or specifically designated members of a group."[48] Culture is learned behavior transmitted with modifications from generation to generation. Some categories of culture are technology, beliefs, values, and symbols associated with religion, medicine, nursing, politics, and so on.

The concept of *subculture* refers to specific social units or groupings within a society. For example, in America the following may be viewed as subcultures: socioeconomic strata (lower, middle, upper), regional populations (the South, New England), community types (rural or urban), occupational groupings, religious groups, and political groups. When considered within the context of American society, a subcultural group may also be defined as one that retains its identity and to a varying degree the customs and language or dialects of the country or region of origin. The term *ethnic* refers to a common and distinctive culture and people whose origins are from the same or related racial, linguistic, and cultural groups.

The construct of *health culture* has been developed to refer to "all of the phenomena associated with the maintenance of well-being and problems of sickness with which people cope in traditional ways, in their own social networks."[113] Distinction is also made between popular, lay, or folk health cultures and the orthodox, or "scientific," health culture. Freidson has suggested the use of Redfield's concepts of the "great" and "little" traditions to differentiate modern medical knowledge from that possessed by the layman.[31] In an era characterized by technologic innovation and complexity and increasing professional specialization, the medical or cultural lag between lay and professional knowledge can be expected to increase rather than decrease. According to Freidson, professional knowledge, then, is the "great tradition" of the contemporary era, and the "little tradition" of medicine refers to the layman's perceptions and interpretations of modern medical knowledge and practices as well as to traditional or indigenous healing practices.

The social and cultural dimensions of health-seeking behavior (Fig. 3-1) and their linkage to biologic and environmental variables are discussed next. The psychologic correlates of health-seeking behavior are discussed in Chapter 16.

■ BIOCULTURAL DIMENSION OF HEALTH AND ILLNESS

The analysis of direct relationships between culture and specific disease entities provides a fertile field for anthropologic, epidemiologic, and health research. A new field, *biocultural ecology*, has as a major focus the study of human adaptation and homeostasis. The effort is to transcend the fragmentation inherent in the separation of culture, human biology, and ecology or environment.[5]

The study of human populations using this three-way interaction system focuses on specific, localized individuals and populations for whom the environment is taken to represent all relevant variables, external and internal, to the people under study (Fig. 3-1).

□ Ecologic influences on genetics

Subcultural and ethnic peoples within America, linguistic groups in Africa, and tribal people of North and South America and New Guinea provide a number of population groups that are sufficiently distinct to provide the demographic isolates or units required for purposes of study of certain disease entities. For example, the study of the distribution of the sickle cell trait in Africa illustrates the changed ecologic conditions that have led to selective pressures and subsequent evolutionary and genetic changes.[58] Sickle cell polymorphism provides the classic example of cultural and ecologic effects on the genetic and demographic structure of human populations. The introduction of the technologic innovations, iron working, and slash-and-burn agriculture changed the tropical rain forest, resulting in stagnant pools of water that served as breeding grounds for mosquitoes carrying the malarial parasite. This ecologic change led to the balanced polymorphism and relatively high frequencies of the allele (alternate gene forms in one chromosome) for hemoglobin S. In the contemporary era, the introduction of another cultural object, DDT, for control of malaria has altered selective processes and resulted in demographic changes whose effects on morbidity, mortality, and perhaps fertility have not yet been fully studied[5] (see Chapter 5 for further discussion).

The study of many genetic conditions requires consideration of changing social and cultural variables, especially those relating to nutrition or drugs. A well-known case is glucose-6-phosphate dehydrogenase (G6PD) deficiency. The highest frequency of this sex-linked condition occurs in malarial belts, reaching slightly over 70% in a population of Kurdish Jews on the northern Iraqui border. It is generally assumed that G6PD-deficient individuals possess resistance to malaria in these regions.[5] Over 80 different G6PD variants have been found, many of which are associated with nonspherocytic hemolytic anemia on ingestion of natural foods (fava beans) or administration of certain antimalarial and antibiotic medications.

Attention to seemingly esoteric cultural practices associated with ritual cannibalism in the Fore tribe in New Guinea provided data instrumental in gaining knowledge about the causative factors that may be operating in some so-called slow-virus diseases. Kuru, a neurologic disease, was originally believed to be of genetic origin. Instead, cannibalism was found to be responsible for the epidemic spread of the disease through the tribes and neighboring groups with whom tribal members intermarried. The incidence of kuru was found to be higher for women and for children of both sexes. Kuru was rare in the men who did not participate in the rituals carried out as marks of respect for the dead. Clinical disease followed 4 to 20 years after eating poorly cooked tissues containing the viral agent.[34,59] Observations in the field combined with epidemiologic and genealogic observations over time and the transmission of kuru to chimpanzees by the oral route did not support the original postulate of genetic origin of the disorder.[34] The Fore tribe provided the natural setting for gaining insight into the probable causes of some neurologic disorders prevalent in Western countries today.

□ Biocultural dimensions of disease

It has been stated that the word *adaptation* connotes fitness to a particular environment or the possession of traits or attributes that make it possible for individuals to function effectively and to reproduce in this environment.[20] Adaptation, however, may be bought at a high price, and certain peculiarities that are assets in some geographic areas may be handicaps in others. The sickle cell hemoglobin deficit is an example of such a change. Cancer, heart disease, disorders of the cerebral system, and diabetes have all been referred to as diseases of civilization. Many types of *neoplastic disease* have been traced to environmental factors. The incidence of cancer has been shown to vary according to culture and social class.[20] Lung cancer is a common cause of death in the United States, England, Wales, and several other Western countries where cigarette smoking is common. Stomach cancers account for 50% of cancer among men in Iceland and Japan but only 10% in the United States. Liver cancer comprises one half of all causes of death among the Bantus in Africa and less than 4% in Europe. Breast cancer is eight times more common in Israel than among the women of Japan.[20] Regional variations have been found for skin and lip cancer in the United States and Russia. There are more cases in the South than in the North for both countries.

The etiologic factors in *diabetes* are still poorly understood. Some epidemiologic and genetic evidence suggests that viruses may be involved in causing at least one type of diabetes.[60] Both genetic and environmental factors are believed to play an important role in the high incidence of diabetes in some cultural groups. The high incidence of obesity among some populations is also correlated with the prevalence of diabetes. Changes in the specific components of a cultural groups' diet and activity patterns have been identified as leading to an increased expression of diabetes.[70,90] The data accumulating about geographic and cultural differentials in the incidence of diabetes and pathologic complications raise questions relative to the nature of humankind's adaptation to culture change.[77] The increased incidence of diabetes reported for rural migrants to urban centers in Israel,[12] South Africa,[81] and Canada[89] has led some to label diabetes a disease of civilization.[46]

The relationship between increasing urbanization and diabetes morbidity reinforces Neel's hypothesis of diabetes as a "thrifty" genotype.[70] The theory holds that in prehistoric times the prediabetic individual was better equipped to adapt to the environment. The gene or genes responsible for diabetes mellitus permitted gaining extra weight during times of relative plenty and therefore enhanced survival during times of famine. Once these factors no longer existed the diabetic gene once considered functional for survival became a liability.

Studies of the differences in population frequencies of *lactase deficiencies* suggest a genetic as well as an acquired basis.[8] Adults of cultures as diverse as the Thai, Japanese, Andean Indians, and Chinese have inadequate levels of lactase. In the United States the rate for lactase deficiency among adults of predominantly European ancestry is between 10% and 20%. This contrasts with 70% lactase deficiency among adults of African descent.[39] The geographic distribution of the trait supports the hypothesis that primary adult hypolactasia arose after the cultural innovation of the domestication of milk-producing animals and large-scale milk production.[61] McCracken believes that all human populations were originally lactase deficient[14] and that with the development of milk-producing cultures and uninterrupted consumption of milk during the transition years from infancy to childhood, those individuals who could metabolize milk enjoyed a reproductive advantage over those who could not.

Given the high nutritional value placed on milk and milk products in the United States and the inclusion of these nutrients in special diets, a reassessment of milk consumption is indicated. Individuals with the enzyme deficiency suffer discomforts such as flatulence, bloating, and diarrhea after ingesting milk; thus, contrary to the popular slogan, some people do outgrow their need for milk, especially those of African and Asian origin.

□ Social and economic influences on disease

The interaction between social class, culture, and illness has been identified in several studies. For example, some social and economic correlates of diabetes mellitus have been identified. Economic deprivation is associated with an increased incidence of diabetes.[17] Diabetes per se may intensify economic deprivation because of the increased cost of carrying out prescribed medical and dietary regimens. In addition there is increased probability of work limitations because of sickness, absenteeism, or disability rising out of diabetic complications.[67,69]

Sexual and racial differentials in the incidence of diabetes have been found. A period of steady increase in diabetic rates for whites was noted in the 1930s. The rates leveled off in 1940 and have varied little since then. On the other hand, the rates for nonwhites were lower than the rates for whites during most of the century. The pattern began to change in the 1960s. Now the rate for nonwhites is higher, 23 per 100,000 versus 17 to 18 per 100,000 for whites.[82] Other demographic contrasts relative to the diabetic death rate (age adjusted) are those found to exist in different regions and states within the United States. Alaska has the lowest incidence of deaths, Delaware the highest. Death rates were higher in the eastern and central states and lower in the Mountain and Pacific states.[82]

The influence of socioeconomic conditions on developmental adaptation has been studied. Poor socioeconomic conditions associated with nutritional limitations represent an environmental stress that is known to influence body size. Using anthropometric* and demographic measures,† researchers studied highland and lowland migrants living in new settlements (barriados) in a city slum in Peru. They found that parents of small body size (particularly the mother) had significantly greater offspring survivals than parents of large body size. It was hypothesized that women with low growth potential are better adapted to a poor environment than those who grow fast and become tall.[32]

In the American urban setting, the diversity of ethnic and social class groups provides the basis for comparative studies of within-group and between-group similarities and differences. Premigration patterns as well as postmigration histories are available. A study of ethnic differences in the prevalence of anencephaly (cranial neural deficit) and spina bifida (vertebral neural deficit) in Boston revealed the highest rates for children born to mothers who had emigrated from Ireland and lower rates for children of Jewish and Italian origins. There was a marked association with father's occupation, and the rates were twice as high for children born to mothers in ward accommodations than to mothers in private accommodations. The findings suggest cultural determinants as well as the fact that those in the lower socioeconomic group may have had increased exposure to an as yet unidentified environmental factor.[68]

This section provides some data that nurses may find useful for the identification of those groups or populations at risk. Nursing interventions may then be directed toward educational and care activities that will ameliorate or prevent the occurrence of these health care problems.

■ SOCIAL CONTEXT OF HEALTH AND ILLNESS BEHAVIOR

The articulation of lay and professional knowledge and roles has been studied from the point of view of status differentials in reciprocal, or dyadic, role relationships of patient and physician (see Chapter 9). This section discusses some functions of family, kin, and community social units in health care systems and social class and cultural variables associated with the "sick role" and the place of the sick in society (see Chapter 1 for definition and discussion of the sick role).

□ Social class and health and illness

According to social scientists, the utilization of complex medical services calls for a medically sophisticated population with a degree of knowledge and understanding that is lacking in groups with low levels of education.[92,105] The greater the social and cultural distance between participants in a social system the less likely that they will perceive each other in terms of ideal role types. Therapeutic relations should function at optimum where the professional and the patient are of the same status and hold common values.[105]

A number of sociologic studies have identified some social and psychologic characteristics of the poor that may influence health-seeking behaviors. People in the lower socioeconomic strata are perceived as being less likely than those in the middle class to engage in preventive health behavior and to defer gratification in the interest of long-term goals. The poor tend to have a fatalistic nonachievement orientation with a focus on adjustment or resignation rather than control over natural events or forces. The kin or peer group is preferred to professionals for consultation for solution of common human problems.[49,65,92] For example, a study of the concepts of health and illness in a Nova Scotian community revealed that when compared with the more affluent members of the society, the lower socioeconomic groups were less informed about illness and health care, were more skeptical of modern medical care, expected a good deal of illness in their lifetime, and had greater difficulty internalizing the sick role.[18]

Studies by nurses of class values as determinants of health-seeking behavior both support and refute the findings relative to class differences in values and

---

***anthropometric** science and technique of human measurements, specifically anatomic and physiologic factors.

†**demographic** (from demography) study of vital and social statistics and their application.

health-seeking actions. Based on the findings of a study of maternal activity patterns, it was concluded that a clearer explication of the values of people in the lower class category is needed.[65] In particular, the variations that exist within this class in the ranking or preference for values, the informal social organization, and patterns of communication require further study.[65] The use of preventive health services by low-income women studied by Triplett revealed "ample evidence that there is no magic formula, no convenient stereotype, no generalizations to be made that can relieve the nurse of her responsibility for a careful assessment of each patient."[107] It has also been found that low-income mothers of high-risk infants had values concerning health similar to those of nurses.[7] Nurses, however, perceived the values held by clients as dissimilar, and it was suggested that this misperception by nurses may be a barrier to communication.[7]

□ Cultural dimension of the sick role

A cross-cultural comparative study of three communities (each with a rural and urban component) in England, Yugoslavia, and the United States tested empirically the notion of cultural relativity in the definition of illness and the assumption of the sick role.[10] It was found that a substantial amount of perceived illness is handled outside the framework of the sick role. A large number of people were validated by the medical profession as ill without the individuals' assuming the privileges of the sick role. The study showed that in the English and American communities fewer than one third sought professional advice or reported limitation of usual activities. On the other hand, the proportion reporting limitation of usual work activities in the Yugoslavian community was 59%. In Yugoslavia over half of those who reported limitation of activities failed to seek medical treatment. In a summary of the international cooperative effort to study the cultural dimensions of the sick role, it was concluded that to define people as being ill solely in terms of social adjustment is to disregard a number of people who, using a different set of nonclinical criteria, also define themselves as ill and in some cases as seriously ill.[10]

Gassow and Tracy's study of "impression management" by patients with leprosy describes patients' attempts to alter and control the negative social and emotional responses of others to this stigmatized disease. Impression management refers to efforts people make to create a desired image about themselves and to control the conduct of others by controlling what they say and hear. Patients have developed theories that redefine the disease so that it may be removed from its position as the "idealized maximal horrible illness." Patients function in the role of educators in the attempt to change the public image of the leper. The development of these "educational specialists" has led to a new concept that is descriptive of their function: the career patient status.[35]

The destigmatizing ideology and the concept of a career patient status may be applied to other disease entities. Social organizations such as the "ostomy clubs" (see p. 1253), the Lost Chord Club for laryngectomees (see p. 1103), and Alcoholics Anonymous are among those groups that use career patients who employ their own theories and concepts to facilitate their adaptation as well as to bring about changes in society's attitudes.

□ Illness referral systems

A concept or construct that may be useful for analysis of people's health and action systems within a community context is that of illness referral systems. An *illness referral system* is conceptualized as a subsystem of the medical system and includes all health factors and their actual or expected behavior in illness situations.[111] Summarizing the definitions of a number of investigators and theorists, Weaver has defined a *medical system* as being comprised of the "whole complex of a people's beliefs, attitudes, practices and roles associated with concepts of health and disease and with patterns of diagnosis and treatment."[111] The patterns and modes of treatment have meaning only when the totality of social, structural, and group actions are taken into account.

This construct of an illness referral system is similar to Freidson's conceptualization that a *lay referral system* consists of a "variable lay culture and a network of personal influence along which the patient travels on his way to the physician."[30,111] Two variants of the lay referral system are identified: an extended and a truncated or modified form.[30] The former is found most often among certain indigenous and low socioeconomic cultural groups. The modified version is one in which individuals participate directly with the professional health care giver.

Four distinct phases of the illness referral system as it functioned in a Spanish community have been identified. These phases were used differently by traditional and acculturated Spanish-Americans. The typical traditional Spanish-American family or patient would progress through the following phases: the *self-addressed* phase, or self-perception of a change in health status; the *kinship phase,* in which consultants are members of the patient's own social group; the *community phase,* in which friends, neighbors, and influential community members are sought for help and diagnostic and curing advice; and a *folk specialist* phase, in which culturally recognized practitioners are consulted.[30,111]

This account of the referral system used by Spanish-Americans residing in a southern Rocky Mountain community bears similarity to the system used by residents of immigrant origin, that is, first generation of an Italian-

American community in an eastern city.[78] The "home medical specialists" in the Spanish-American subcultural group, who treated minor ailments within the home or neighborhood, functioned in ways that were similar to the "therapeutic women" and "lay medical specialists" in the Italian-American community.[78] The therapeutic women gave traditional or folk prescriptions for the reported emotional or physical ailments of the elderly Italian immigrant women. Most of the therapeutic women were immigrants themselves. On the other hand, the lay medical specialists were women of the second generation, or American-born offspring of Italian parents. These women had assumed the functional role of intermediary between the immigrant who lacked language and literary skills in English and the American medical and health care systems. The lay medical specialists were among the first to be consulted by the elderly for help in making a decision about seeking professional medical assistance. In addition they interpreted prescribed medical and dietary regimens and often were depended on to administer treatments such as eyedrops or insulin injections. Their ability to make preliminary or differential diagnoses was enhanced by the intermediary role relationships in which they functioned.

Thus far health and illness actions have been discussed from the perspective of the social context in which these actions take place. Reciprocal role relationships of patient and health care giver, the consequences of environmental and cultural influences on certain disease entities, and the use of alternate health care referral systems have been discussed. Knowledge of family variations in social structural roles and functions provide another dimension for assessing the social and cultural correlates of health-seeking behavior.

□ Family in health and illness

The family is a basic unit of society. It is probably the single most important social context in which health and illness occur, health-protective activities are performed, illness is identified and resolved, and professional health care is implemented. During the last two decades the family has been studied as an independent, dependent, and intervening variable in the illness and treatment of physically and emotionally ill family members and as a basic unit of health services utilization.[55] The development of interest in familial health and self-care has been more recent.[47,62,66]

A focus on the family, irrespective of whether the family unit or an individual family member is considered the client or patient, is mandatory for nurses. The site where the nurse practices (hospital, health center, private practice, or home), the thrust of health care offered at the site (primary, secondary, or tertiary), and the nurse's own expertise determine how the nurse incorporates the family into health care. The purpose of this section is to contribute to effective family-oriented nursing by (1) defining the family and sketching a useful frame of reference for the nurse working with families and their members, (2) presenting family-oriented nursing interventions, and (3) discussing family competence and its consequences for behavior in health and illness.

Family

The American family may be defined by three criteria: kinship, function, and location. The family is generally characterized by (1) any one occurrence or combination of sexual or marital, parental, and sibling relationships; (2) intensive and inclusive relationships; and (3) cohabitation. Each criterion can be specified more precisely.

In the first criterion of relationships the three dyads with biologic or genealogic correlates (sexual or marital, parental, and sibling) imply the existence of three positions or locations for the individual within the family structure: husband-father, wife-mother, and child-sibling. Two conventional forms of family structure are the nuclear, or conjugal, family and the stem family. The *nuclear family* consists of a man, his wife, and their unmarried or nonadult children. It is based on marital, parental, and sibling dyads and is restricted to a depth of two generations. The *stem family* grouping encompasses three generations: grandparents, parents, and children. Other forms of family structure such as the single-parent family and the affiliated family exist, as do counterculture forms such as communes and group marriages and the urban kin networks of impoverished blacks.* Each of these family forms also includes individuals occupying sexual or marital, parental, and sibling positions.

The second criterion defining the family, *intensive and inclusive relationships*, is often contrasted with diffuse and segmented, temporary and expedient relationships. Intensive and inclusive family relationships are notable for their persistence over a substantial period and for their concern with basic domestic tasks, for example, the pooling of income, the socialization of the children, the taking of rest or leisure, and the preparation and serving of meals. The criterion also suggests closeness, warmth, and affection as opposed to social distance and compelling moral obligation. The intimate emotional quality of family life results from its chronologic depth and from continuous interaction to ensure that tasks are allocated and completed.

The final criterion, *cohabitation*, may be defined as

*References 22, 72, 96, 104, 107.

common or at least proximate residence. Family members usually have one address, sleep under one roof, and eat at the same table.

Frame of reference for family-oriented nursing practice

Since 1960 a number of family theories and conceptual frameworks have been developed.[9,11,43,71] The *developmental* and *interactional* approaches to family analysis, in particular, have been extensively developed.[2,21,41,84]

These two approaches are salient to family-oriented nursing. They suggest that nurses be attentive to such basic concepts as stages of family development; family tasks or functions; individual members' positions and roles within the family; the norms constraining the making, taking, and playing of family roles; kin networks; and certain basic interaction processes such as conflict, decision making, and problem solving. Each of these concepts and their relevance to nursing is discussed in turn.

The *stages of family development* are the sequential phases in the family life cycle. The time periods encompass the natural history of most nuclear families, beginning with the simple husband-wife pair, becoming more complex as children are born, stabilizing briefly, becoming less complex after the launching of adult children into jobs and marriage, and eventually dissolving with the deaths of the original conjugal pair. Seven stages are identified in the family life cycle: the beginning family, the childbearing family, the family with preschool children, the family with school-aged children, the family with teenagers and young adults, the postparental family, and the aging family.[1]

Family behavior is expected to change predictably as families move from one developmental stage to the next, and a book of research efforts testing the utility of this concept has been published.[1] The research indicates that some family behaviors can be predicted by knowing the developmental stage of the family. Other family behaviors are relatively constant, while still others are situational or circumstantial. Prediction is possible because certain family tasks or functions are specific to each stage of the family life cycle. The findings support the proposition that the achievement of a developmental task at one period affects family life at a later period.

Family tasks or functions are the activities carried out by the family: the allocation of economic and material resources; the reproduction, recruitment, and release of family members; education and socialization; physical maintenance and protection; and the exchange of affection. The accomplishment of these tasks is imperative for the social life of communities and for the growth of individual family members. At each stage of family development the tasks that have primacy and those that are secondary can be highlighted. Thus, for the aging family in contemporary America the tasks of ensuring economic survival on a fixed income, of reallocating household responsibilities, and of maintaining or rediscovering intimacy are crucial.

To accomplish these tasks the family develops an organization. The key elements of the family organization are *positions, roles,* and *norms.* The husband-father, wife-mother, child-sibling positions are common to the nuclear family. Each position is composed of roles, or prescriptions for interpersonal behavior. The husband-father position in the nuclear family often consists of breadwinner, sex partner, companion, teacher, and disciplinarian roles. The role content of a position changes over the family life cycle, as occurs, for instance, with the retirement of the husband-father from active employment. Roles are distinguished from one another by norms (social expectation for behavior). For example, the normative power structure in the modern family is thought to be egalitarian; an authoritarian role is no longer expected of many husband-fathers. Nurses may properly investigate a family's organization to ascertain if positions are filled and roles developed and played in ways that enhance the functioning of individual family members, the family unit, and the community. Intervention may be required to support or modify a family's organization to better accomplish its tasks.

Interaction processes are another fundamental construct. Interaction between the family and the surrounding society is critical. The family must negotiate for income and services; in turn it must supply society with productive, responsible members. The nurse may be required to mediate between a family and society when its own activities are inadequate or inappropriate to healthful living.

The family's interaction with noncohabitating kin is also significant. Kin relationships among families range from integrated to isolated. Notwithstanding the current spate of research efforts to prove that the American family is isolated from its kin, relatives do keep in touch, celebrate rituals and ceremonies associated with death and weddings, and exchange gifts and services.[28,57,104,107] Nurses may need to intervene to mobilize kin in situations of family crisis, as kin are frequently an essential source of support.[16]

Intrafamilial interaction processes are equally important. Family conflict is as basic an interaction process as family cohesion. The management of family conflict, not the avoidance or resolution of strife and disharmony, has been proposed as essential to healthy family life.[85,101,103] The nurse might be essential to successful conflict management during transitions from one family development stage to another, the transition to parenthood for example.

Family problem solving, those behaviors selected and implemented by families to accomplish desired tasks, is the final concept to be considered. Family problem-solving efforts are perhaps less rational than those of other small work groups or committees and are less problem than solution oriented. The elements in the problem situation are often not open to manipulation and change.[1,42,106,112] It is believed that families seldom explicitly define a situation as a problem, seek satisfying solutions, and take action. Rather, they handle the most resistant, unsettling features of the situation in the ways past experience has suggested may be effective. The daily routines and the constant pressure of problematic situations force the family to solve but not to analyze their problems. In addition, many family problems arise either from economic and political events that the family alone is powerless to control or from interpersonal relationships that would require personality changes if solutions were to endure. Families facing the unexpected protracted illness of the breadwinner may, for instance, require nursing assistance to reach workable solutions for problems ranging from the care of the ill individual and role reversal to income maintenance.[15] Families may also benefit from nursing intervention related to problems of everyday life.[97]

The concepts presented above provide one frame of reference for family-oriented nursing practice. They suggest broad areas of assessment and intervention that are necessary if the family is to be incorporated into nursing care. The need to develop a clinically salient holistic measure of effective family functioning or competence and to examine its relationship to individual, family, and community well-being is obvious, and several recent studies indicate that attempts in this direction have begun.[6,98]

Competent family in health and illness

One expert has approached the competent family from the perspective of the family's effective functioning as a social unit, "a unit created to allow people to live together and rear children who are themselves physically well and have qualities accepted as desirable by the community concerned."[66] Another expert conceptualized family competence as including seven dimensions: the commitment of family members to family group objectives, communication, pride in the family, self-confidence, judgment, creativity-resourcefulness, and participation.[6] Still another approach was taken by two experienced clinicians whose concept of family functioning included the components of communication, togetherness, closeness, decision making, and child orientation.[76]

All three approaches imply that the family, whether it is a healthy family or a family in trouble, must be treated as a social unit; that effective family functioning or competence may be equated roughly with family health; and that the nature, that is, the health or competence, of the family unit has an impact on individual and societal well-being.

The family may play a part in defining and legitimizing members' rights to assume the sick role and in deciding not only whether a family member will receive care but if it should be provided at home. The process of becoming a patient includes a series of decisions involving family, friends, and health care providers.[4] In general the role the family may play in the process varies over time and is contingent on the disease condition, its severity and chronicity, the family members involved, and the degree of familial concern. The mother, for example, may exhibit a great deal of reluctance to accept the sick role. It has been observed that mothers are more likely to seek medical care and advice for their children than for themselves and that they are more willing to define their children rather than themselves as sick.[63] It is easy to speculate that the mother, the pivotal member of many families, experiences considerable difficulty in fulfilling her obligations when she is ill and thus tends to postpone labeling herself as sick.

The decision as to whether a family member's illness should be treated at home or with the assistance of professional health care providers also tends to be negotiated within the family setting. In one study approximately half of the respondents of low-income urban households consulted a household member about what they should do in the case of a particular symptom.[83] Another study found that the decision to seek professional care for an ill family member generally rested with the wife-mother; half of the respondents would find it fairly difficult to care for a sick member at home for any protracted period of time and would be willing to relinquish the care of the sick to the hospital.[55,56] The ultimate success of the family's involvement in home diagnosis, treatment, and referral to professional sources of care may revolve around restoration of its ability to do the task and preparation to do so. The self-help movement and the parallel disenchantment with the cure-rate and iatrogenic effects of "scientific" medicine as reported in the literature may stimulate the family to care for itself more effectively.[44,52]

In summary, the family as a unit of society functions within cultural systems that convey values, beliefs, and customary ways of accomplishing tasks and roles (Fig. 3-1). Some concepts by which the family is linked to the wider society and culture are discussed next. The focus is on the cultural dimensions of health and illness.

■ CULTURAL DIMENSIONS OF HEALTH BELIEFS AND PRACTICES

□ Effects of cultural health beliefs and practices

Every culture provides a set of significant questions and potential answers and procedures for arriving at answers to cope with illness events. Effective communication directed toward therapeutic nursing intervention requires that the nurse know something about how the patient and family members perceive and define the illness, its cause, and therapy in general. Assessment of the level of patients' knowledge and understanding of what ails them will permit nurses to identify the medical or cultural lag or discrepancy between lay and professional knowledge. Nursing care actions may then be directed toward closing the knowledge gap.

The articulation for comparative purposes of folk or lay and modern medicine, that is, the "little tradition" and the "great tradition" (p. 26), has not received much attention by medical-surgical nurses. The reason for this may be a lack of knowledge or the general disregard of many health professionals for folk or layman's expressed beliefs and practices. Folk healing actions and beliefs are variously perceived by some health professionals as esoteric, quaint, irrelevant, or scientifically unproved. Yet cultural and individual beliefs about the cause of disease do determine, to a greater or lesser degree, what actions people will take to ameliorate or prevent illness and whether they will comply with prescribed regimens.

People living in traditional or nontechnologically developed societies have had a long history of medicinal contributions, particularly in pharmacology. It has been estimated that more than 220 medicines have been contributed to the official *U.S. Pharmacopoeia* by indigenous Indian healers of North and South America.[110] Rational therapy employing indigenous botanical drugs was extensive among these Indian groups, and medicinal preparations, such as insulin and penicillin, were anticipated. An effective remedy for scurvy was in use in the New World at a time when the then great tradition of European medicine believed it to be caused by bad air. Among the well-known medicinal preparations contributed by South American Indians are cinchona, coca, curare, and ipecac. The American variety of foxglove was used for its cardiac stimulant qualities hundreds of years before digitalis was discovered in England.[110]

Belief systems do interfere with therapy. For example, in a multidisciplinary study of Quechua Indians living at high altitudes in the Andes, the people gave unexpected resistance to giving blood samples and having blood pressures taken.[3] It was determined that the people believed that blood removal was detrimental because once removed it would not be replaced, and the blood pressure cuff was perceived as extracting blood.

On the other hand, one would expect some resistance to giving blood samples from laymen whose beliefs about the generation of blood differ from those of conventional modern medicine. One study of southern black migrants in Tucson revealed that people held notions about blood, such as that new blood is constantly being formed, used blood is eliminated through sweat in men and menses in women, and blood loss is weakening.[99] It is reasonable to assume that in any hospital or clinic setting the perception of individuals relative to the common procedure of drawing blood samples will vary according to idiosyncratic or cultural variables.

□ Assessment of health beliefs

Lay concepts and categories can be arrived at by noting the answers and responses to eight dimensions expressed as questions about illness episodes[13]:

1. What kind of illness is it (i.e., its name)?
2. How has it been treated (or how will it be treated, or how should it be treated)?
3. What caused the illness?
4. How serious is it?
5. Does the sickness pose a threat to others?
6. Will the condition endure (i.e., acute or chronic)?
7. Was the illness inherited?
8. Is the condition appropriate to the afflicted individual?

These questions originally used for a Malayan population by Colson[13] may be adapted for patients in the American health and medical setting.

The illness referral system, which defines the social process by which people seek therapy, has been discussed. Cultural responses to the above questions will supply the cognitive categories, the theories about illness causation, prevention, treatment, and prognosis. Cultural categories and criteria for defining illness may be studied by the use of an approach called ethnomedicine. Ethnomedicine is a domain of *ethnoscience*, an approach that seeks to discover and describe the concepts and behavioral system of a given culture in accordance with concepts derived from that culture. *Ethnomedicine* is an attempt to elicit the layman's own definitions of the illness situation without the imposition of a priori categories by health professionals. Clients may not use the same sets of criteria or expectations as members of the health professions for the same illness event. For example, a study of emergency department admissions revealed that laymen and professionals differed in their definition of what constituted a medical emergency.[23]

Beliefs concerning cause of illness

Beliefs about causation of illness reveal variations across cultural groups. Americans in general attribute illness to physiologic and psychologic causes. People as diverse as the Gadsup of New Guinea[51] and the Azande of Africa[24] stress the social and cultural causes of a number of illnesses. Some ethnic groups, particularly those in the lower socioeconomic class and of rural origin, attribute illness to fate, destiny, or God's will.

Cultural themes pertaining to curing and healing, particularly in regard to nutrition or foods, have been identified. A study of Puerto Rican families in New York revealed that the hot-cold notions associated with the Hippocratic humoral theories continued to find expression.[40] Health, according to the humoral theoretical orientation, was defined as a state of balance among four bodily humors, namely, blood, phlegm, black bile, and bile. An imbalance in these humors results in illness, which causes the body to become excessively dry, cold, hot, wet, or a combination of these qualities. Foods and medicinal herbs are classified as having hot or cold qualities and are prescribed to return the body to its proper balance.

Vestiges of theories directed toward correcting body imbalance form the basis for treatment within a number of ethnic and cultural groups. The New England Yankee, for example, uses apple cider and honey to maintain proper acid-base balance.[45] In a Guatemalan community two concepts, *fresco* (fresh or cool) and *alimento* (highly nutritive substance), were used to accommodate and reinterpret modern health and nutritional beliefs.[14] Fresh or cool substances (carrot juice, tea, chicken, rice) rather than cold were considered the best treatment for "hot" illnesses. Many of the health professionals working with the Guatemalans were not aware of the distinctions people made between highly nutritive substances (alimento) and other foods. The wet-dry polarity forms the basis of the therapeutic beliefs about foods of several eastern and western European groups.[78,87] A balance in the wet and dry foods is believed to be important in maintaining a healthy state. Meals or prescribed diets lacking soups, dark green leafy vegetables, and fresh fruits are perceived as "too dry" and detrimental in maintaining the body in its proper state.

The identification by nurses of cultural themes associated with caring and curing behaviors is facilitated within settings such as the hospital, where these behaviors would be more likely to be manifested. Acknowledgement and respectful recognition by nurses of the functional nature of folk or laymen's beliefs aid in decreasing the social and cultural distance between patient and professional. Beliefs and practices that reinforce or interfere with the physician's prescriptions require identification. Nurses may then be able to develop therapeutic plans of care working within the patient's belief system. For example, it was found that Puerto Rican patients receiving diuretics discontinued use of orange juice, a needed source of potassium, when they had a cold because of its "cold" quality.[40] In such cases nurses can suggest alternate potassium-rich foods that do not fall into the "cold" category.

□ Behaviors associated with pain

The pain experience is a universal component of the human condition, and the phenomena associated with pain have been encountered by all nurses. Health professionals tend to be aware of the psychologic, social, and cultural components of patient pain responses (see Chapter 22 for further discussion of pain). Differences in responses to pain in relation to the variables of ethnicity, religious affiliation, and race have been the subject of several studies.[64,114,115] Zborowski's study was one of the earliest to focus on differentials in cultural responses to pain. The findings of this study are still applied without question by some nurses. However, the study has been criticized for its failure to distinguish between pain as a basically physiologic phenomenon and the "pain experience," which has affective and emotional components.[114] Social class and generation variables were not adequately controlled in the study, and subsequent studies revealed that immigrant and other groups (e.g., religious and racial) will follow the patterns of the majority group in the society if the subjects are made aware of the ethnic or religious differences.[114] A comprehensive review of research of cultural factors and pain responses concluded that there is a paucity of adequately controlled experimental studies of the pain experience; any attempt to delineate cultural factors in human responses should be made in the wider context of cultural attitudes toward sickness and health; and religious attitudes, insofar as they "influence perception of the physical self," may be an important variable for study.[114]

□ Pollution behaviors

Beliefs and cultural health practices categorized under the construct *pollution behaviors* are another universal component of human behavior, yet it is a relatively little researched topic in nursing and health literature. The word *pollution* conveys notions of uncleanness, dirty, untouchable, defilement, taboo, contamination, and disease, especially communicable disease. All cultures have elaborated definitions and rules relative to behaviors to ensure a clean or pure state and means by which the unclean or impure may be restored. Most pollution rules spell out proscriptions and prohibitions in relation to food and contact with certain objects or persons. Pollution theories and practices probably have been most fully elaborated for the occupational caste and outcaste systems of India. Food taboos and prohibitions about contact, however, find expression throughout the world.[95] Most nurses are familiar with kosher dietary rules and the food proscriptions of other religious groups, such as the Seventh Day Adventists.

Study of pollution within a cultural context has led to the delineation of some concepts that may be useful for nurses in understanding some of the underlying dynamics of the subtle yet pervasive behaviors associated with pollution.[19] Pollution as a concept has affective and cultural components. All pollution behaviors are perceived as the reaction to any event that is likely to confuse or contradict "cherished classifications" or the usual order of things. Implicit in the pollution concept is the notion of "things out of place" (deviant). Ambiguity and cultural dissonance are other qualities associated with the concept. Cultures have evolved pollution rules (ways of behaving) as an attempt to impose order on existence. Pollution beliefs reinforce the cultural norms and social structure and reduce dissonance.[19]

Rules and rituals that regulate behaviors for the avoidance of pollution vary cross-culturally. In some cultures rules about menstrual blood or the menstruating woman have been elaborated. In other cultures the bodies of the dead, certain body excretions, and a wide variety of foods may be avoided or treated in such a way that contact is minimized.

Pollution and pollution behaviors are relevant constructs for nursing. Illness or disease may be viewed as a deviance (deviance from a healthy state), and with illness there is a disruption of the social order (see the discussion of the sick role in Chapter 1.) Some disease entities or physiologic states more than others may be viewed as "dirty" or "things out of place." Leprosy is the classical disease in which affective and cultural behaviors are manifested. Other conditions are colostomy and ureterostomy (see Chapter 57). Pathologic conditions in which there are increased secretions and incontinence may be viewed as "things out of place." Some persons with diabetes consider diabetes a "dirty" disease because of the need for contact with urine and urine-testing equipment. The fear of defilement or pollution with body secretions and excretions appears to be deeply imbedded. Nurses need to be aware of the culturally specific ways in which these beliefs and behaviors are expressed. Nursing care plans may then be developed to assist patients and their families in developing techniques to minimize the distressing features of self-care functions.

Most theoretical formulations and empirical research about people's modes of coping with the "unclean" or pollution have been carried out by anthropologists among peoples of non-Western, technologically less developed societies. There has been little research about pollution beliefs and behaviors and their consequences on health care within large urban medical and community centers in America, and thus there is a need for future research in this area. Nurses have a unique opportunity as they work with clients to systematically collect data about these beliefs and behaviors and share them with other health care providers.

■ SUMMARY

The social and cultural correlates of health-seeking behavior have been discussed. Social class differences, family organization and practices, and cultural beliefs and values do affect health caring behaviors and actions directed at the prevention, treatment, and amelioration of symptoms of disease. Beliefs about the causation of illness vary according to cultural groups (ethnic or subcultural) and social class. The consideration of similarities and differences within and between groups aids in the identification of health beliefs and actions that are either universal for all people, specific or unique for a group or social class, or idiosyncratic, that is, applicable only to an individual. This comparative frame of reference, which focuses on group variations as well as similarities, will help to decrease the tendency toward stereotyping the behavior of clients. In addition the cultural or "medical" lag between lay (folk) and professional knowledge and action may be determined. Nursing interventions that acknowledge the discrepancy between these two levels of knowledge may then be planned and instituted.

REFERENCES AND SELECTED READINGS

1. Aldous, J.: The developmental approach to family analysis, 2 vols, Minneapolis, 1975, The University of Minnesota Press (mimeographed).
2. Aldous, J., editor: Family problem solving, Hinsdale, Ill., 1971, The Dryden Press.
3. Baker, P. T., and Little, M.: Man in the Andes, Strodsburg, Penn., 1976, Dowden, Hutchinson & Ross, Inc.
4. Becker, M., editor: The health beliefs model and personal health behavior, Thorofare, N.J., 1974, Charles B. Slack Co.
5. Bennett, K. A., Osborne, R. H., and Miller, R. J.: Biocultural ecology: annual review of anthropology, Palo Alto, Calif., 1975, Annual Reviews Inc.
6. Boardman, V.: School absences, illness and family competence, Ph.D. dissertation, Chapel Hill, N.C., 1972, University of North Carolina.
7. *Brinton, D. M.: Value differences between nurses and low-income families, Nurs. Res. **21**:46-52, 1972.
8. Brock, D. J. H.: Inborn errors of metabolism. In Brock, D. J. H., and Mayo, O.: The biochemical genetics of man, New York, 1972, Academic Press, Inc.
9. Broderick, C. B.: Beyond the five conceptual frameworks: a decade of development in family theory, J. Marriage Fam. **33**:139-159, 1971.
10. *Butler, J. R.: Illness and the sick role: an evaluation in three communities, Br. J. Sociol. **21**:241-261, 1970.
11. Christenson, H. T., editor: Handbook of marriage and the family. Chicago, 1964, Rand McNally & Co.
12. Cohen, A. M.: Prevalence of diabetes among different ethnic Jewish groups in Israel, Metabolism **10**:50, 1961.

*References preceded by an asterisk are particularly well suited for student reading.

13. Colson, A. C.: The prevention of illness in a Malay village: an analysis of concepts and behavior, Overseas Research Center Developing Nations, Monograph series 2, no. 1, Winston-Salem, N.C., 1971, Wake Forest University.
14. Cosminski, S.: Alimento and fresco: nutritional concepts and implications for health care, Hum. Org. **36**:203-207, 1977.
15. Craven, R. F., and Sharp, B. H.: The effects of illness on family functions, Nurs. Forum **11**:187-193, 1972.
16. *Croog, S. H., Lipson, A., and Levine, S.: Help patterns in severe illness: the roles of kin network, non-family resources and institutions, J. Marriage Fam. **34**:32-41, 1972.
17. Davidson, J. K.: Diabetes in socioeconomically deprived neighborhoods. In Diabetes mellitus: diagnosis and treatment, New York, 1971, American Diabetes Association, pp. 207-210.
18. Davidson, K. R.: Conceptions of illness and health practices in a Nova Scotia community, Can. J. Publ. Health **61**:232-242, 1970.
19. Douglas, M.: Pollution. In UNESCO: a dictionary of the behavioral sciences, New York, 1969, The Free Press, Inc.
20. Dubos, R.: Man, medicine, and environment, New York, 1968, Mentor Books, The New American Library Inc.
21. Duvall, E. M.: Family development, ed. 4., Philadelphia, 1971, J. B. Lippincott Co.
22. Ellis, A.: Group marriage: a possible alternative? In Otto, H.: The family in search of a future, New York, 1970, Appleton-Century-Crofts.
23. *Evaneshko, V., and Bauwens, E.: Cognitive analysis and decision-making. In Leininger, M.: Medical emergencies in health care dimensions, Philadelphia, 1976, F. A. Davis Co.
24. Evans-Pritchard, E. E.: Witchcraft, oracles and magic among the Azande, Oxford, England, 1936, Oxford Clarendon Press.
25. *Fabrega, H.: The need for an ethnomedical science, Science **189**:969-975, 1976.
26. Fabrega, H.: On the specificity of folk illness, Southwestern J. Anthropol. **26**:304-314, 1970.
27. Firth, R., Hubert, J., and Forge, A.: Families and their relatives, Atlantic Highlands, N.J., 1970, Humanities Press, Inc.
28. Firth, R.: Essays on social organization and values, Atlantic Highlands, N.J., 1969, Humanities Press, Inc.
29. Foster, G.: Medical anthropology: some contrasts with medical sociology, Med. Anthropol. Newsl. **6**:1-6, 1974.
30. Friedson, E.: Patients' view of medical practice, New York, 1961, Russell Sage Foundation.
31. Freidson, E.: Client control and medical practice, Am. J. Sociol. **65**:374-382, 1960.
32. Frisancho, A. R., et al.: Adaptive significance of small body size under poor socio-economic conditions in southern Peru, Am. J. Phys. Anthropol. **39**:255-261, 1973.
33. Frisancho, A. R., et al.: Influence of developmental adaptation on lung function at high altitudes, Human Biol. **45**:583-594, 1973.
34. Gajdusek, D. C.: Unconventional viruses and the origin and disappearance of Kuru, Science **197**:943-960, 1977.
35. *Gassow, Z., and Tracy, G. S.: Status, ideology and adaptation to stigmatized illness: a study of leprosy, Hum. Org. **27**:316-325, 1968.
36. Goffman, E.: Stigma, Englewood Cliffs, N. J., 1963, Prentice-Hall, Inc.
37. Goffman, E.: The presentation of self in everyday life, New York, 1959, Doubleday & Co., Inc., Anchor Books.
38. Gould J., and Kolb, W. L.: A dictionary of the social sciences, UNESCO, New York, 1969, The Free Press, Inc.
39. Harris, M.: One man's food is another man's whitewash, Nat. Hist. **81**:12-13, 1972.
40. Harwood, A.: Hot-cold theory of disease, J.A.M.A. **216**:1153-1158, 1971.
41. Heiss, F.: Family roles and interaction: an anthology, ed. 2., Chicago, 1976, Rand McNally & Co.
42. Hill, R.: Decision-making and the family life cycle. In Sheras, E., and Schreib, G.: Structure and the family, Englewood Cliffs, N.J., 1965, Prentice-Hall, Inc.
43. Hill, R., and Hansen, D.: The identification and conceptual frameworks utilized in family study, Marriage and Family Living **22**:299-311, 1960.
44. Illich, I.: Medical nemesis: the expropriation of health, New York, 1976, Pantheon Books, Inc.
45. Jarvis, D. C.: Folk medicine, Greenwich, Conn., 1958, Fawcett World Library: Crest Books.
46. Judkins, R., and Lieberman, L.: Specialist reports: biomedicine and nutrition, Med. Anthropol. Newsl. **6**:14-17, 1974.
47. Kaplan, F. H., and Cassel, J. C., editors: Family and health: an epidemiological approach, Chapel Hill, N.C., 1975, University of North Carolina Press.
48. Kluckhohn, C., and Kelly, W.: The concept of culture. In Linton, R.: The science of man in the world crisis, New York, 1945, Columbia University Press.
49. Kluckhohn, F., and Strodtbeck, F.: Variations in value orientations, Evanston, Ill., 1961, Row Peterson & Co.
50. Leininger, M.: Transcultural health care: issues and conditions, Philadelphia, 1976, F. A. Davis Co.
51. *Leininger, M.: The culture concept and its relevance to nursing, J. Nurs. Educ. **6**:27-37, 1967.
52. Levin, L. S., Katz, A. H., and Holst, E.: Self care: lay initiatives in health, New York, 1976, Neale Watson Academic Publications, Inc., PRODIST.
53. Linton, R.: The cultural background of personality, New York, 1945, Appleton-Century-Crofts.
54. Linton, R.: The study of man, New York, 1936, Appleton-Century-Crofts.
55. Litman, T. J.: Health care and the family: a three-generation analysis. In Sussman, I. B.: Sourcebook in marriage and the family, ed. 4., Boston, 1974, Houghton Mifflin Co.
56. *Litman, T. J.: The family as a basic unit in health and medical care: a social-behavioral overview, Soc. Sci. Med. **8**:495-519, 1974.
57. Litwak, E.: Extended kin relationships in an individual democratic society. In Sheras, E., and Shreib, G.: Social structure and the family, Englewood Cliffs, N.J., 1965, Prentice-Hall, Inc.
58. Livingstone, F. B.: Anthropological implications of sickle cell gene distribution in West Africa, Am. Anthropol. **60**:533-562, 1958.
59. Matthews, J. D., et al.: Kuru and cannibalism, Lancet **2**:449-452, 1968.
60. Maugh, T. H.: Diabetes: model systems indicate virus a cause, Science **188**:436-438, 1975.
61. McCracken, R. D.: Lactase deficiency: an example of dietary evolution, Curr. Anthropol. **12**:479-517, 1971.
62. McEwen, P.: The social approach to family health, Soc. Sci. Med. **8**:487-493, 1974.
63. Mechanic, D.: Influence of mothers on their children's health attitudes and behavior, Pediatrics **33**:4-15, 1964.
64. Meehan, J. P., Stoll, A. M., and Hardy, J. P.: Cutaneous pain threshold in native Alaskan, Indian and Eskimo, J. Appl. Physiol. **6**:397-400, 1954.
65. Milio, N.: Values, social class and community, Nurs. Res. **16**:26-31, 1967.
66. Miller, F. J. W.: The epidemiological approach to the family as a unit in health statistics and the measurement of community health, Soc. Sci. Med. **8**:479-482, 1974.
67. Mills, J. W., Saunders, K., and Martin, F. I. R.: Socioeconomic

problems of insulin dependent diabetes, Med. J. Aust. **2**:1040-1044, 1973.

68. Naggan, L., and MacMalton, B.: Ethnic differences in the prevalence of anencephaly and spina bifida in Boston, Massachusetts, N. Engl. J. Med. **277**:1119-1123, 1967.
69. Nasr, A. N. M., et al.: Absentee experience in a group of employed diabetics, J. Occup. Med. **8**:621-625, 1966.
70. Neel, J. V.: Diabetes mellitus: a "thrifty" genotype rendered detrimental by progress, Am. J. Hum. Genet. **14**:353-362, 1962.
71. Nye, F. I., and Besordo, F. M.: Emerging conceptual frameworks in family analysis, New York, 1966, Macmillan, Inc.
72. Otto, H. A.: Communes: the alternative life style, Sat. Rev. April 23, 1971, pp. 16-21.
73. Parsons, T.: Definitions of health and illness in the light of American values and social structure. In Jaco, G. E.: Patients, physicians and illness, New York, 1957, The Free Press, Inc.
74. Parsons, T., and Shils, E.: Toward a general theory of action, New York, 1962, Harper & Row, Publishers, Torchbooks.
75. Pell, S., and D'Alonzo, C. A.: Sickness and injury experience of employed diabetics, Diabetes **9**:303-310, 1960.
76. Pless, I. B., and Satterwhite, V.: A measured family function and its application, Soc. Sci. Med. **7**:613-621, 1973.
77. Prosnitz, L. R., and Mandell, G. L.: Diabetes mellitus among Navajo and Hopi Indians: the lack of vascular complication, Am. J. Med. Sci. **253**:700-705, 1967.
78. Ragucci, A. T.: Generational continuity and change in the concepts of health, curing practices and ritual expressions of the women of an Italian American enclave, Ph. D. dissertation, Boston, 1971, Boston University.
79. Redfield, R.: Peasant society and culture, Chicago, 1960, The University of Chicago Press.
80. Reid, J. M., et al.: Nutrient intake of Pima Indian women: relationship to diabetes mellitus and gallbladder disease, Amr. J. Clin. Nutr. **24**:1282-1289, 1971.
81. Remoin, D. L.: Ethnic variability in glucose tolerance and insulin secretion, Arch. Int. Med. **124**:695-700, 1969.
82. Report of National Commission on Diabetes, vol. 3., U.S. Department of Health, Education and Welfare, No. (NIH) 76-1019, 1975.
83. Richardson, W.: Measuring the urban poor's use of physicians' services in response to illness episodes, Med. Care **18**:132, 1970.
84. Rodgers, R. H.: Family interaction and transaction: the developmental approach, Englewood Cliffs, N. J., 1973, Prentice-Hall, Inc.
85. Safilias-Rothschild, C.: The study of family power structure: a review, 1960-1969, J. Marriage Fam. **32**:539-552, 1975.
86. Salsedo, A. J.: Book reviews, Med. Anthropol. Newsl. **8**:22-23, 1977.
87. Sanders, I.: Balkan Village, Lexington, Ky., 1949, University of Kentucky Press.
88. Sarbin, T. R., and Allen, V. L.: Role theory. In Lindsey, G., and Aronson, E.: Handbook of social psychology, ed. 2, Reading, Mass., 1968, Addison-Wesley Publishing Co., Inc.
89. Schaefer, O.: The changing health picture in the Canadian North, Can. J. Ophthalmol. **8**:196-204, 1973.
90. Schaefer, O.: When the Eskimo comes to town, Nutrition Today **6**:8-16, 1971.
91. Scott, E.: Family and social network, ed. 2, New York, 1971, The Free Press, Inc.
92. Shostak, A. B., and Gomberg, W.: Blue-collar world: studies of the American workers, Englewood Cliffs, N. J., 1964, Prentice-Hall, Inc.
93. Shostak, A. B.: Blue collar life, New York, 1969, Random House, Inc.
94. *Sigerist, H.: The special position of the sick. In Roemer, M. I.: Henry E. Sigerist on the sociology of medicine, New York, 1960, M. D. Publications.
95. Simoons, F. J.: Eat not this flesh, Madison, 1967, University of Wisconsin Press.
96. Skolnick, A. S., and Skolnick, H.: Family in transition: rethinking marriage, sexuality, child rearing and family organization, Boston, 1971, Little, Brown and Co.
97. Smiley, O.: The family centered approach: a challenge to public health nurses, Can. J. Publ. Health **63**:424-426, 1972.
98. *Smilkstein, G.: The family in trouble—how to tell, J. Fam. Pract. **2**:19-24, 1975.
99. Snow, L. F.: Folk medical beliefs and their implications for care of patients, Ann. Int. Med. **81**:82-96, 1974.
100. *Spiegel, J.: Transaction: the interplay between individual, family and society, New York, 1971, Science House Inc.
101. Sprey, J.: Family power structure: a critical comment, J. Marriage Fam. **34**:235-238, 1972.
102. Sprey, J.: On the management of conflict in families, J. Marriage Fam. **33**:722-731, 1971.
103. Sprey, J.: The family as a system in conflict, J. Marriage Fam. **31**:699-706, 1969.
104. *Stack, C.: All our kin: strategies for survival in a black community, New York, 1974, Harper & Row, Publishers.
105. Suchman, E. A.: Social factors in medical deprivation, Am. J. Publ. Health **55**:1725-1733, 1965.
106. Sussman, M. B.: Relationships of adult children with their parents in the United States. In Sheras, E., and Shreib, G.: Social structure and the family, Englewood Cliffs, N.J., 1965, Prentice-Hall, Inc.
107. Tallman, I.: The family as a small problem solving group, J. Marriage Fam. **32**:94-104, 1970.
108. Triplett, J.: Characteristics and perceptions of low-income women and use of preventive health services, Nurs. Res. **19**:140-146, 1970.
109. Tylor, E.: Primitive culture, vol. 2, English edition, New York, 1974, New York Publ.
110. Vogel, V. L.: American Indian medicine, Norman, Okla., 1970, University of Oklahoma Press.
111. Weaver, T.: Use of hypothetical situations in a study of Spanish American illness referral system, Hum. Org. **29**:140-154, 1970.
112. Weick, K.: Group processes, family processes and problem solving. In Aldous, J.: Family problem solving, Hinsdale, Ill., 1971, The Dryden Press.
113. Weidman, H. H., and Egland, J.: A behavioral science perspective in the comparative approach to the delivery of health care, Soc. Sci. Med.**7**:845-860, 1973.
114. *Wolff, B. B., and Langley, S.: Cultural factors and the response to pain: a review, Am. Anthropol. **70**:494-501, 1968.
115. Zborowski, M.: Cultural components in response to pain, J. Soc. Issues **8**:16-30, 1952.

4

Systems of health care delivery

KATHERINE SCHENK

■ HEALTH CARE IN THE UNITED STATES

The system through which health care is obtained by those who need it in the United States is mixed and fragmented. It has been said by some that there is no "health care system," by others that there are many "systems," which are only poorly articulated with each other. The latter is probably more nearly correct. Centers of excellent medical (illness) care are scattered throughout the country, yet many areas of the country are unserved or underserved by health care personnel and facilities. These centers of excellence are the finest in the world; they are usually in the close environs of universities that have schools of medicine, nursing, and other health sciences. These are also the centers of research in the health sciences. Paradoxically, it is not unusual for many of the underserved to live close to these centers in the urban ghettos.

Persons with the means and know-how or those who meet certain specific qualifications (such as chronic renal failure) can obtain the finest medical and health care ever known. Other citizens of the United States are more poorly served than those in many other modern countries today where there is a broad base of at least minimal service for all.

The great diversity of care in the United States is not hard to understand in view of the pluralistic nature of the society—the many national and cultural origins of the citizens, each with varying expectations about health, how it is attained and retained, and the part played by self, family, and others in maintaining health.

In contrast one might look at Denmark. It is a comparatively small nation, with a population of about 5 million, compared with 235 million in the United States. It encompasses only about 1/200 of the U.S. land mass. In addition it has a much more homogeneous population in terms of a common cultural heritage. Many more customs and values are commonly understood and accepted as Danish than is true in the United States. A broadly accepted national approach to dealing with social problems such as housing and unemployment extends to health care. There is a centrally designated institution, the National Board of Health, through which most decisions regarding the national heath system are coordinated. This involves all care for citizens, from maintenance and preventive services through surgery and acute care. It involves health personnel from the highly skilled specialists through all preventive and supportive levels to the least skilled. It is concerned with determining what facilities and personnel are needed and with providing the educational facilities for the personnel. Although there are some additional care givers such as medical and surgical specialists outside of this system, and although change and conflict and rising medical care costs are no more foreign to this system than to others in our changing world, there is nevertheless a sense of order and wholeness to Denmark's health care system.

In contrast the supersystem designated the United States of America has a large aggregate of illness care systems, only a few of which articulate with each other. There is, as yet, no specific commitment to either health or illness care on an overall basis, although we appear to be moving toward such commitment. One factor responsible for the fact that the United States is the only major industrialized country today that does not have an identifiable system for delivering health care to every citizen is our traditional emphasis on local decision making, on states' rights and communities' rights to determine their own needs and how they should be met. Although health care is not mentioned in the Constitution, a good case can be made that the well-known and accepted right of each citizen to life, liberty, and the pursuit of happiness cannot be achieved without provision for adequate health care.

Still another factor in the health care dilemma in the United States is the private enterprise concept of operation and the fact that, except for those conditions that affect the health of large segments of the population and thus come under the aegis of public health (such as safe drinking water or protection from communicable disease), the delivery of health care has tended to be a service performed as a charity or for private profit.

Most illness care is provided by physicians in private practice operating on a fee-for-service basis. Many communities within the supersystem have hospitals for care of the ill. A few of these receive some tax support, and many were built with large amounts of federal funding. However, the majority are operated through payment from those they care for (this payment being managed by means of "health" insurance) plus community fund drives and charitable bequests of various kinds. It is these hospitals that presently employ the largest number of registered nurses in the United States. Associated with these hospitals are the largest number of private, practicing physicians.

There are other illness-care systems. The Veterans Administration hospitals and nursing homes are completely tax supported for the use of veterans. Some labor unions, such as the United Mine Workers, have provided similar services for their members, supported by dues or company contributions to their welfare funds.

Care of the elderly and chronically ill in the United States has gradually assumed a place of major importance as our society has moved to a higher and higher median age. Institutional care for the aged was not greatly needed when the country was younger. Most of the few elderly who did survive to old age lived with their own families. A few unfortunate persons were relegated to "old folks' homes" or poor farms, supported by taxes, where some minimal health care was provided. The major focus of health and illness care was on infants and children and their mothers. A Children's Bureau was established within the federal government. Health care providers for many reasons preferred to devote their knowledge and skills to caring for the young, and the needs of the aging were often ignored.

More people are now living beyond retirement into the seventh, eighth, and ninth decades of life. While less than 5% become institutionalized, the needs of both those living in the community and those needing some type of institutional care are not being met in the same manner that the needs of children were met in the past. The majority of professional health care providers —physicians, nurses, and others—are not interested in caring for the elderly. There is now some evidence that this attitude is changing as some physicians and many nurses turn to the specialty of gerontology.

For the aging who remain in their own homes or elsewhere in the community, it is evident that additional facilities for their care and well-being, including health care, must be provided. A comparative newcomer on the scene, the day care center for the chronically ill and the elderly, shows evidence of becoming an important part of the health care scene. In addition there are a large number of nursing homes for care of the chronically ill, especially the elderly. It is unfortunate that many of these day care centers and nursing homes are developing as private profit-making enterprises along lines similar to that of private practice medicine and that they often are not closely associated with other health-illness care facilities.

Another very old model of illness care, but one that has an important element of health promoting care, is the Visiting Nurse Association or Public Health Nursing Agency, together referred to as community nursing. Although the original idea was to provide care for illness in the home, health promotion has always been an important focus of these organizations. They may be supported by voluntary gifts, by taxes, or both. Recently the term Home Health Agency has been used to indicate expanded services available to clients in their homes.

All states and many communities have departments of public health, which are supported by tax funds and employ physicians, nurses, and other health care workers. Their primary purpose is to protect the health of the total community; thus they are preventative in focus. Goals and activities of many health departments have been changing and expanding in recent years in response to the changing conditions of our society. In former years communicable disease control was the primary focus; now other environmental threats such as pollution are of greater significance.

Lately a model of health care has emerged that is truly focused on health promotion and illness prevention, at least to the point where the financial advantage to both provider and client is *wellness*. This is the *health maintanence organization (HMO)*. Early models included the Health Insurance Plan of New York, the Ross-Loos plan, and the Kaiser-Permanente Foundation. Employees of Kaiser-Permanente in California were provided with preventive and health maintenance facilities and ambulatory care clinics as fringe benefits of their employment. This model has been adopted by other industries and also by some private medical practices, many of which include nurses. In these systems clients pay a set fee for regular preventive and screening services as well as for illness care. The HMO fares best financially when clients are kept well and out of hospitals. An additional feature, accountability to the public, has been built into the HMOs that have been financed in their beginning stages by the federal government. Peer review of the quality of care provided is a requirement and a condition of funding.

Despite all of the above resources many of the very poor as well as people with nontraditional life styles have often felt they did not or could not obtain health care or preventive services from any of the establishment facilities and organizations. In recent years many nurses as well as physicians have worked in so-called *free* or *nontraditional agencies* such as storefronts and other community-based clinics. Many of these were originally funded through federal grants available in the late 1960s and early 1970s and have now fallen on hard times in regard to funding. Ideas and lessons learned from such experimental approaches to health care will not be lost, however, and may be built into future health care planning.

In our society individuals and families are responsible for their own health and when concerned about health, or frank illness, are expected to seek the health care provider or agency of their choice. This plan presupposes either the ability to pay the chosen health care provider or possession of insurance to cover the payment. Today many persons do have health insurance, and for many it is provided as a fringe benefit of employment. Again, nearly all insurance is directed at coverage for illness. Those who are unemployed or medically indigent are nominally covered for illness care through Medicaid, a plan associated with the welfare systems of each of the 50 states and supplemented by federal funds. But as with other welfare plans such as Medicare, which is the system for illness care for the elderly and others receiving Social Security benefits, there are many gaps and inadequacies, and many persons do not meet the qualifications set by individual states.

In view of such wide differences of philosophy, expectations, and objectives, plus much entrenched existing self-interest in maintaining present systems, national planning for health care delivery has been very difficult. The picture is changing as more and more segments of our society recognize their own needs and interests and demand health care as a right, not a privilege. John Bryant has suggested a principle of justice for health care as follows:

> Whatever health care is available should be equally available to all. Departures from that equality of distribution are permissable only if those worse off are made better off. . . . There should be a floor, or minimum of health services for all. Resources above the floor should be distributed according to need.[5]

Traditionally nursing has supported this philosophy. Primary prevention of illness and maintenance of high-level wellness has long been a goal of organized nursing. More recently it has been reiterated by nursing interest groups such as those concerned with maternity and infant nursing, pediatric nursing, gerontologic nursing, and psychiatric and mental health nursing. Still further commitment was made by the establishment of the Commission on Human Rights as a permanent component of the American Nurses' Association at the 1976 biennial convention. Nurses have reaffirmed their position that the fulfillment of their national purpose depends on quality health care for every citizen.[22]

The problem of financing such care is now one of the major issues that must be faced. The United States presently spends a greater percent of its gross national product (GNP) for illness care than any other country, yet many feel that resources are being wasted and misused. Although there has been increasing financial support for health care, this support has been provided through the existing health care systems. Legislation that provided funding for Medicare and Medicaid continued the use of presently existing models. One outcome of this has been the greatly increased costs. As the most conspicuously rising factor in the cost of living within the past decade, health care (illness care) is a target for considerable criticism. Writers outside the health care establishment, for example, Ivan Illich,[14] as well as many within believe that only willingness of individual citizens to assume responsibility for their own health including adopting healthy life styles and taking preventive measures can contain health care costs. Nursing has been moving in the direction of promoting and facilitating clients' self-health care. This philosophy has been extensively developed by Orem[27] and other members of the Nursing Development Conference Group.

On the national level the federal government has for many years supported the education and training of health care providers; programs of research and education for certain special illnesses, such as heart disease, cancer, and stroke; and considerable basic medical research. More recently systems of delivery of care have been financed on a demonstration basis, such as the HMOs and programs such as those to prepare nurse practitioners and physician assistants.

In contrast it is useful to look at a model such as that suggested by Leininger for providing health care to a specific population, for example, to all the people within a given country or state or community (Fig. 4-1). This model would begin by examining the needs for service and care of the specified population across a broad spectrum: physiologic, psychologic, sociocultural, politico-economic. It would then identify those factors relevant for that population and would classify the levels of care appropriate for identified needs. It would next obtain or develop through education and training the providers and the facilities to meet these needs.

Our traditional approach has been exactly the opposite. Especially in medicine, the supersystem has supported the preparation of increasing numbers of specialists in an increasing array of subspecialty areas and then identified the need for their services. This is not a good economic model for the consumer, although it may be for the provider, and there is increasing evidence that it cannot continue unchecked. Recent legislative

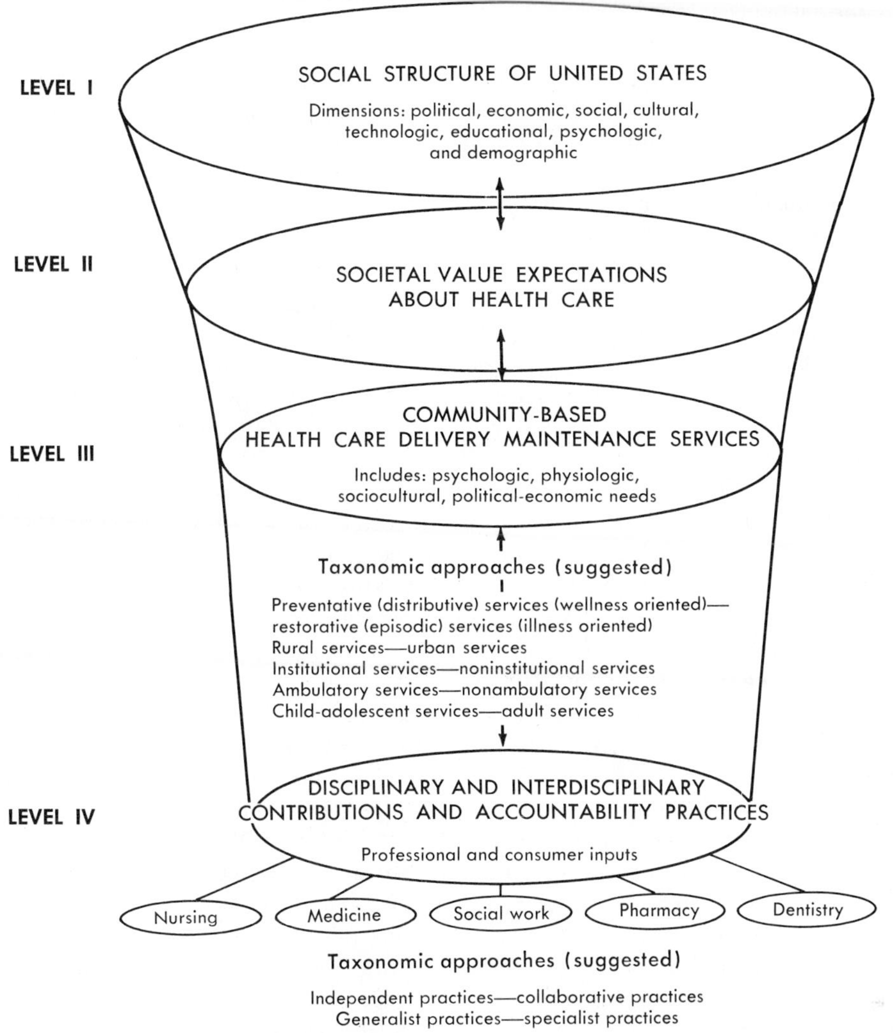

Fig. 4-1. Structural framework for health care maintenance services. Conceptual model developed by Professor Madeleine Leininger, University of Utah, 1973. (From Leininger, M.: Transcultural nursing: theories and practices, New York, 1977, John Wiley & Sons, Inc.)

moves have indicated a change in direction. In the 1974 Health Planning and Resources Development Act (PL 93-641) signed into law in January 1975 the Congress, influenced by constituent dissatisfaction with health care, mandated regional planning in the context of the Leininger model. This law lists several national health priorities, including providing for people in underserved areas and the sharing and coordinating of existing facilities. State and local health service planning agencies have been set up under the provisions of this law, and consumers as well as health care providers must be represented on the planning committees. In addition the Department of Health, Education and Welfare in its *Forward Plan for Health* for the years 1977 to 1981[29] stated five major target areas for the 5-year period. These include planning, cost containment, and better distribution of services to all of the people of the nation. Although health care planning is in the early stages and there is recognition that it will not be easily accomplished; it is a change in direction and a move to bring some measure of order and articulation into decision making relating to health care delivery.

NURSING WITHIN THE HEALTH CARE SYSTEM

Historically in the United States nursing has been provided in a variety of models. Within institutional settings it has been in acute and chronic care hospitals, in long-term care facilities, and in community nursing agencies. The heyday of private duty nursing was in the early part of this century when it was the major employment opportunity for nurses. In this model of practice nurses were private entrepreneurs. Even though they often depended on the favor and recommendations of specific physicians, they provided service for a fee and were paid directly by the clients they served. From before the turn of the century this service was frequently provided in the homes of the affluent; but as the care of the ill moved into hospitals, so did private duty nursing, still generally for the financially advantaged. It was total patient care and was more art than science. Even when employed by the hospital, the registered nurse of pre–World War II usually did everything prescribed for and needed by the patients, since there were few other health care providers. By far the greatest amount of care to those in hospitals was provided by nursing students. Private duty nursing suffered a mortal blow in the Great Depression of the 1930s.

With the shortage of registered nurses during the war years of the 1940s, this total patient care gave way to the functional method of practicing in which each nurse or nursing student in the interest of efficiency of time did a particular task, for example, administering medications to every patient on a unit. This was the beginning of the wide support for and the increasing preparation of licensed practical (vocational) nurses. Although continued long after the war and even into the present, the functional model of nursing care is generally considered both by health care providers and by patients to be unsatisfactory and fragmented. It was succeeded by team nursing, in which a group of health care providers with a variety of preparations (registered nurse, licensed practical [vocational] nurse, and the nursing assistant or aide) cared for a designated group of patients, using the skills of each to best advantage. In concept this was the ideal way to care for patients with a variety of needs. In practice it often did not work as well as conceptualized. One of the main problems seemed to be finding time for the needed team planning and conferences essential for good team nursing. The guidance and coordination of the team by the professional nurse, an essential component of the plan, was often sketchy or completely lacking. There were and still are places where team nursing is felt to be a rewarding and satisfactory way of delivering nursing care, both within acute and chronic hospital settings and in community settings, when the basic concepts and plans can be implemented.

The most recent development in the care of clients in organizational settings (which includes the community health agency) is called *primary nursing.* (This term must be distinguished from primary care giver, which will be discussed later.) In this model one professional nurse is totally responsible for planning and evaluating the care given to a relatively small number of clients. To those who were active in nursing before World War II this does not appear to be a new method but a coming full circle. The model has been well demonstrated at the Loeb Center for Nursing and Rehabilitation where for many years nurses have been providing care through the primary nursing model.[3] Many other agencies are also moving to primary nursing as it is shown to be more satisfactory to the health care provider and to the clients.[19,20]

Thus there have been many attempts to find the ideal way of providing nursing care to groups of clients designated as ill or in need of care. It is likely that all of these will continue to be used in one way or another, even coexisting within the same organization, in accordance with the philosophies of individual health care providers.

With the development of scientific and theoretically based nursing within recent years, several distinctive models of professional practice that fit clients' health care needs as currently identified have been developed and tested. Such terms as *extended* and *expanded* roles have been used. The question has been raised: Are these terms accurate, or are client needs expanding and is nursing moving to provide for these needs?[27] The much used terms *nurse clinician* and *nurse practitioner* have also been critically questioned by nursing leaders. If professional nurses are prepared and licensed to practice nursing, are they not in fact nurse practitioners? And if nurses must practice in a clinical setting in order to be practicing at all, must they not be nurse clinicians?

Although the above is undeniably true, the new terms are in vogue and are understood by many to have some specific meaning, even though there may be disagreement about the exact meaning. According to the American Nurses' Association (ANA) definitions of clinician and practitioner, both are skilled in obtaining a health history from clients and in assessing client needs. *Clinicians* manage the care of a case load of clients, usually in a hospital setting such as a coronary care unit, an acute respiratory care unit, or an orthopedic unit. They plan care on the basis of immediate and long-term needs; this care may sometimes be carried out by others. They supervise care given by others and help them perform certain functions and skills in a conceptual frame very closely akin to that of good team nursing. Clinicians also communicate with other disciplines relative to the needs of clients and their families.

Practitioners, in the current definition of the term, usually practice in a broader area than do clinicians, such as an ambulatory care setting or in the community. Thus they may be expected to be aware of even more factors in the larger social systems that impinge on client needs and care. They are expected to be skillful in taking a health history, to be able to do physical assessment, and to recognize abnormal signs and symptoms. They are closely associated with a physician, whether within an institutional setting or in the community. Nurse practitioners usually become members of health care groups such as HMOs, but they may work alone in remote areas with backup of centrally located physicians. The pediatric nurse practitioner is one outstanding example of this model.[31]

According to a recent survey by the American Nurses' Association[2] the majority of pediatric nurse practitioners responding were graduates of baccalaureate nursing programs and had received educational preparation to function as practitioners in short-term continuing education programs. A large number work with high-risk populations such as children in Head Start programs, day care centers, and neighborhood clinics. Such facilities are often supported by tax funds to provide services to clients who may not normally have access to private physicians.

Other models include practitioners working with adults who have chronic diseases and with aging clients. Many health care systems are presently using nurse practitioners to provide *primary care*. This is the term used to describe the first contact of a client needing care with the health care system. It is also used to describe the care needed by most of the people most of the time. It may be preventive, including identification of health problems at an early stage, or care of minor, noncritical, and chronic illnesses. Most primary care is for those who are ambulatory (not occupying beds in hospitals or other inpatient settings), and most, but not all, ambulatory care is primary care. Several studies have shown that primary care provided by nurses is at least as good as the care provided by physicians and is highly valued by clients.[32] The same positive results have been found when nurse practitioners work with clients who have chronic and long-term health problems.[33]

With additional education leading to a master's degree the nurse may become a *clinical specialist* in a specific area. In contrast to the titles mentioned above, this title is widely accepted, with considerable agreement regarding functions and qualifications. Some examples are the cardiovascular, renal, and orthopedic nurse specialists, most of whom are employed by hospitals and other health care agencies (Fig. 4-2). Such nurses are well prepared to practice with a great

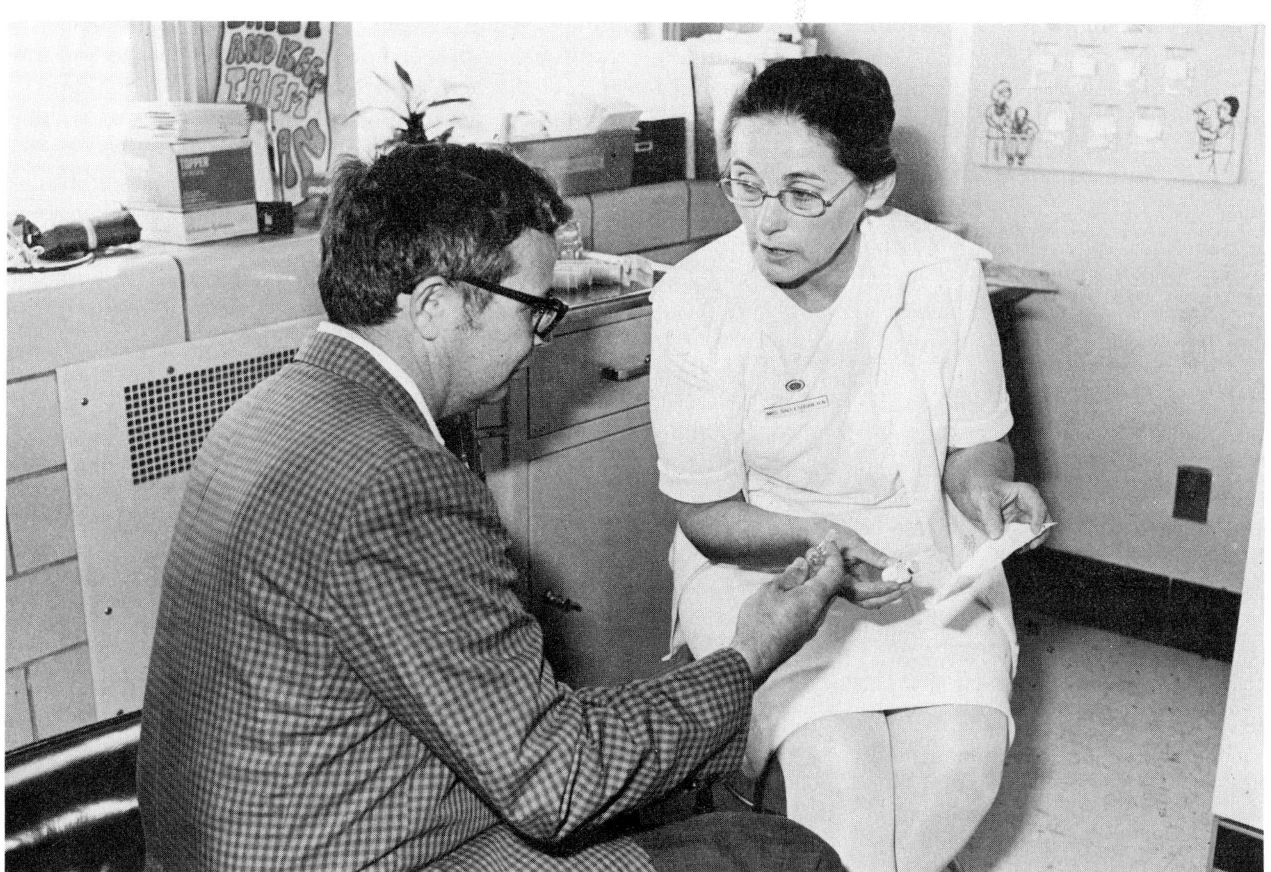

Fig. 4-2. Clinical specialist confers with client about chemotherapy regimen. Clinical specialist possesses ability to manage caseload of clients with needs for clinical expertise in areas such as oncology.

deal of autonomy, and some have set up an independent practice and accept clients, who may contact them on their own initiative or may be referred by physicians.[16,17]

The issues of responsibility and accountability for one's own professional actions are vital in this type of practice. To some extent it is governed by individual state laws related to medical and nursing practice, although most state laws allow the nurse to practice *nursing* independently. A more telling restriction has been the payment of fees for service. Most third-party payers (Blue Cross/Blue Shield, Medicare, Medicaid, and other insurers) will not reimburse nurses for independent nursing services. There is legislation pending to change reimbursement for nursing services. Scores of such clinical specialists currently are practicing independently. Mainly because of the fee-for-service problem, it is presently more common to find the nurse clinical specialist in a group practice with other nurses, physicians, or other professionals. Others are employed in agencies such as a mental health center or a community nursing service.

Within the United States nursing has in the past identified populations at risk and set up systems of health care delivery to serve these populations. The educational focus and the broad humanistic approach of caring for individuals and families, with emphasis on primary prevention of illness and disease, led to the establishment of agencies such as the Frontier Nursing Service and the Henry Street Settlement in New York City, which was that city's first community nursing service. These were systems developed by nurses in response to identified needs of clients. Much of the focus in those early days was on children and on the neonatal period. Nurses in these systems expanded their activities to meet the needs of the clients; nurses in the Frontier Nursing Service delivered babies in areas only accessible by horseback. While the needs of mothers, infants, and children remain important, nurses now also identify additional groups of vulnerable persons, notably those with long-term and chronic illness and the aged. Care for such identified populations at risk has become a major concern of specific groups of nurses.

The struggle to bring order out of the confusion among the health care delivery systems and to make access to health care more realistic to all within the supersystem has been greatly enhanced by the recent developments in nursing. We might illustrate the activities of the several different nursing models identified above by describing a conference held recently at a community hospital in a medium-sized city in a midwestern state. This hospital is the referral point for clients from the city and the surrounding countryside, which includes several small communities. The conference is held on a regular basis to plan for the continuity of care of clients to be admitted to a rehabilitation unit, either from their homes or from the hospital, or who were returning home from that unit. Among those present were the nurse clinician from a specific hospital unit, the staff physician, the dietitian, the social worker, the occupational therapist, and the physical therapist. Also present was a staff nurse from the community health agency of the city. They discussed Mr. W., who had suffered a stroke 2 weeks previous and had been admitted by way of the emergency room to the hospital.

The nurse clinician from the neurology unit discussed the progress Mr. W. had made and his present status. On that unit the staff practiced primary nursing, and Mr. W. was one of a small number of patients to whom this nurse gave total care. She reported not only on his physical state, which was improving, but on his emotional state and his motivation, both of which were good at that time. She recommended his admission to the special rehabilitation unit for care before returning home.

The staff nurse from the community agency had cared for Mr. W. and his wife in the past. She was familiar with the home situation and offered pertinent data related to the prospect for his continued progress at home. Because of special skills she had acquired in a continuing education course, she had the title of Nurse Practitioner; she had a case load of families in the community for whom she was the primary care provider, the health professional whom they contact first when they need care. She was the person called by Mrs. W. when her husband suffered his stroke, and it was she who referred him to the emergency room of the local hospital.

The nurse who coordinated the rehabilitation unit had a master's degree in rehabilitation nursing. He was a clinical specialist and was expected to be responsible for planning the program for Mr. W. in the rehabilitation unit, arranging for the special services such as physical and occupational therapy and medical care. He also was responsible for communicating with the community nurse practitioner about Mr. W.'s plans to return home.

Although the more familiar modes of nursing practice by which care is given to those who are ill, injured, and infirm in acute and chronic care settings will continue to exist, it is expected that the proportion of nurses presently employed within hospitals in contrast to outside of hospitals will change. Client awareness and demand is likely to cause a shift from receiving care in places and settings more convenient for *providers* to those settings that better meet needs of *consumers*. At the same time, cost effectiveness of care in inpatient settings is being compared with cost of care received in clients' own homes and communities.[12] Skilled nurses will increasingly provide care in these settings, meeting health care needs as they have done through the past hundred years or more. Increasingly nurses are preparing themselves to practice in these settings.

Health and the prevention of illness are inexorably joined to the culture and the life style of an individual. In our present society there are very few diseases or problems, especially in adulthood, for which a totally external cause can be identified and eliminated. Yet people continue to live and to think of health and illness as if this were not true. To some extent the providers of health care have supported this idea, and many have gained great advantage and power in the society from their image as great healers, as possessors of almost magical knowledge and ability.

A majority of nurses have been caught up in this myth for generations. The reasons are many: none of us can escape our own culture, nor are we usually even aware of the culture as more than the way things are ordained to be. The changes that have occurred in nursing's image of itself are enormous and only beginning to be felt in the supersystem.

Few are gifted with sight into the future, but it is impossible to believe that the significant beginnings that have been made will not continue and expand, or that the numbers of well-prepared and assertive young people in professional nursing today will be held back by the existing power structure in health care systems from offering and practicing the skills they have in helping to improve the health of our society.

Thus in an era when citizens and clients, the consumers of health care, are becoming better informed, more critical of existing care, and more active as decision makers in the kind and quality of care they need and want, nurses are being prepared through a variety of models to contribute to that care. The concept that nursing has a unique service to offer the health care consumer has been held by nurses throughout history. Through research and through demonstration, the reality of that concept is presently in evidence and is continuing to be affirmed.

REFERENCES AND SELECTED READINGS

1. American Academy of Nursing: Long-term care in perspective: past, present, and future directions for nursing, American Academy of Nursing Papers Presented at Annual Meeting, Sept. 22-23, 1975.

1a. American Nurses' Association: A national policy for health care: principles and positions, Publ. No. G-130, Kansas City, Mo., 1977, The Association.

2. American Nurses' Association: Pediatric nurse practitioners: their practice today, Kansas City, Mo., 1975, The Association.

3. Bower-Ferres, S.: Loeb Center and its philosophy of nursing, Am. J. Nurs. **75:**810-815, 1975.

4. Brown, E. L.: Nursing reconsidered: a study of change, part 1, Philadelphia, 1970, J. B. Lippincott Co., pp. 45-54.

5. Bryant, J. H.: Some interrelations between the evolving health care system and nursing practice and education. Paper presented at Duke University School of Nursing Conference on Distributive Nursing and Mental Health, Durham, N.C., Sept. 20, 1973.

6. Cambridge Research Institute: Trends affecting the U.S. health care system, U.S. Department of Health, Education and Welfare, No. (HRA) 76-14503, vol. 1, 1975.

7. Chopoorian, T., and Craig, M. M.: Nursing and health care delivery, Am. J. Nurs. **76:**1988-1989, 1976.

8. Craven, R. F.: Primary health care: six nurses talk about what they do in a variety of settings, Am. J. Nurs. **76:**1958-1968, 1976.

9. Donabedian, A.: Issues in national health insurance, Am. J. Public Health **66:**342-350, 1976.

10. Donabedian, A.: Models of organizing the delivery of personal health services and criteria for evaluating them, Milbank Mem. Fund Q. **50:**103-154, 1972.

11. Edwards, J., Curtis, J., Ortman, K., et al.: The Cambridge-Council concept or two nurse practitioners make good, Am. J. Nurs. **72:**460-465, 1972.

12. Hapgood, D.: What people like you and me are doing to get better health care, *The Washington Monthly*, Oct. 1976, pp. 21-31.

13. Hellman, C.: The making of a clinical specialist, Nurs. Outlook **22:**165-167, 1974.

14. Ilich, I.: Medical nemesis: the expropriation of health, New York, 1976, Pantheon Books, Inc.

15. Isaacs, G.: The family nurse and primary health care in rural areas. In Nolan, R. L., and Schwartz, J. L.: Rural and Appalachian health, Springfield, Ill., 1973, Charles C Thomas, Publisher.

15a. Kennedy, E. M.: Congress and the national health policy, Rosenhaus lecture, Am. J. Public Health **68:**241-244, 1978.

16. Kinlein, M. L.: Independent nursing practice with clients, Philadelphia, 1977, J. B. Lippincott Co.

17. Lane, H.: Promoting an independent nursing practice, Am. J. Nurs. **75:**1319-1321, 1975.

18. Lehman, E. W.: Coordinating health care: explorations in interorganizational relations, Beverly Hills, Calif., 1975, Sage Publications, Inc.

19. Manthey, M., Ciske, K., Robertson, P., et al.: Primary nursing, Nurs. Forum **9:**65-83, 1970.

20. Marram, G. D., Schlegel, M. W., and Bevis, E. O.: Primary nursing: a model for individualized care, St. Louis, 1974, The C. V. Mosby, Co.

20a. Mauksch, I. G.: On national health insurance, Am. J. Nurs. **78:**1323-1327, 1978.

21. Mauksch, I. G., and Young, P. R.: Nurse-physician interaction in a family medical care center, Nurs. Outlook **22:**113-119, 1974.

22. Members named to Commission on Human Rights: Editorial, Am. Nurse **8:**11, 1976.

23. Miller, C. A.: Societal change and public health: a rediscovery, Am. J. Public Health **66:**54-60, 1976.

24. Navarro, V.: A critique of the present and proposed strategies for redistributing resources in the health sector and a discussion of alternatives, Med. Care **12:**721-742, 1974.

25. Nursing Development Conference Group: Concept formalization in nursing: process and product, Boston, 1973, Little, Brown and Co.

26. Olendski, M. C.: Cautionary tales, Wakefield, Mass., 1973, Contemporary Publishing.

27. Orem, D. E.: Nursing: concepts of practice, New York, 1971, McGraw-Hill Book Co.

28. Ozimek, D., and Yura, H.: Who is the nurse practitioner? New York, 1975, National League for Nursing.

29. Public Health Service: Forward plan for health: FY 1977-81, U.S. Department of Health, Education and Welfare, No. (OS) 76-50024, 1975.

30. Saward, E. W., and Greenlick, M. R.: Health policy and the H.M.O. In Leininger, M.: Barriers and facilitators in quality health care: health care dimensions, Philadelphia, 1975, F. A. Davis Co.
31. Silver, H. K., Ford, L. C., and Stearly, S. G.: A program to increase the health care for children: the pediatric nurse practitioner program, Pediatrics **39:**756-760, 1967.
32. Spitzer, W. O., Sackett, D. L., Sibley, J. C., et al.: The Burlington randomized trial of the nurse practitioner, N. Engl. J. Med. **290:**251-256, 1974.
33. Stoeckle, J. D., Noonan, B., Farrisey, R. M., and Sweatt, A.: Medical nursing clinic for the chronically ill, Am. J. Nurs. **63:**87-89, 1963.
34. Walters, W. J.: State level comprehensive health planning: a retrospect, Am. J. Public Health **66:**139-144, 1976.
35. White, K. L.: Health care arrangements in the United States: AD 1972, Milbank Mem. Fund Q. **50:**17-40, 1972.

5

Ecology and health

SISTER PAULA GONZALES

HOMEOSTASIS IN THE BIOSPHERE: THE BALANCE OF NATURE

Through modern communications technology, millions of persons around the globe have witnessed the earth from a spectacular perspective—from space. Through this occurrence we have been given the opportunity to go far beyond an intellectual understanding of ecologists' description of our finite planet; we have experienced it. Recent events such as the oil embargo and natural gas shortage are making us increasingly aware that we are dependent on the earth's vulnerable supplies of air, water, soil, and energy, which can only be preserved through care, conservation, work, and love we give to our earth and environment.

The need is urgent and it challenges each of us to change from the "frontiersman" mentality that has characterized the growth and progress of industrialized nations to an "astronaut" outlook through which it may be possible to assure the continuation of life on our finite planet.

Composition of biosphere

Environ systems

The biosphere is the thin "layer" of air, water, and soil on the planet Earth within which all living things exist. Fig. 5-1 establishes the components of the biosphere and suggests their interrelationships. John McHale, the eminent futurist, calls the material components of ecosystems *environ systems* to distinguish them from the human systems, which we will survey later. In each of the biosphere compartments there are both living and nonliving portions, which interact in energy-dependent interrelationships to form a complex, interconnected web. Urbanization and industrialization place a severe strain on many of the natural cycles in the biosphere, as illustrated by contrasting a typical forest area with a city (Fig. 5-2). Note that in the forest large amounts of oxygen are being produced as a result of photosynthesis. This maintains the normal ratios of the atmospheric gases. In the urban area oxygen is consumed in much greater quantities than it is produced. Also, carbon dioxide and other materials are present in concentrations that often can be harmful. This example dramatically points up an important ecologic principle: the cyclic nature of almost all events in the biosphere.

A look at the water cycle (Fig. 5-3) illustrates not only this cycling activity but also the integral interrelatedness of the major biosphere compartments: *hydrosphere, atmosphere,* and *lithosphere.* Not only are water molecules being constantly cycled through the soil, air, and water, but many other substances are being transported with the water, thus constantly influencing the chemical composition of all three compartments. Water serves as one of the chief instruments both in the building of soil through weathering of rock and in its breakdown through erosion. We shall see later how even a slight imbalance in one of the compartments affects not only that compartment but the others also.

Physical processes such as those involved in the water cycle can cause significant and often dramatic changes in the three biosphere compartments; consider the effects of such events as volcanic eruption, earthquake, and tornado. However, when weather conditions are relatively normal the chief factors affecting the homeostatic, or steady-state, condition of any ecosystem are the activities of the living organisms that inhabit the area. All ecosystems (e.g., oceans, deserts, grasslands, forests) have a characteristic structure and organization: (1) a typical combination of abiotic factors, such as soil or water composition, temperature, altitude, and humidity, and (2) specific populations of living organisms, the variety and number being dependent to a large extent on the combination of abiotic factors characteristic of a given region.

Biotic factors and energy flow

The biotic components of any ecosystem in the biosphere (plants, humans and other animals, and microbial organisms) exist in what is fundamentally an energy-

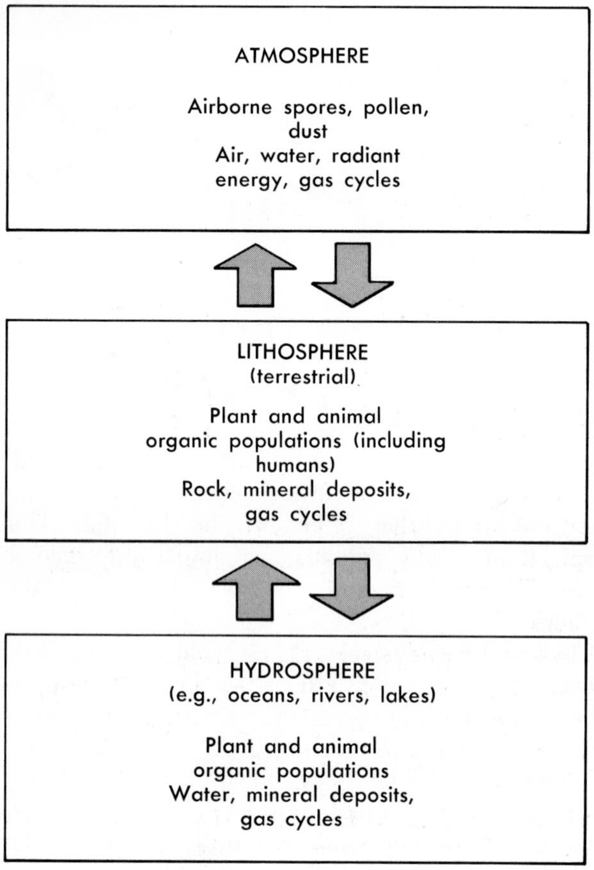

ATMOSPHERE

Airborne spores, pollen, dust
Air, water, radiant energy, gas cycles

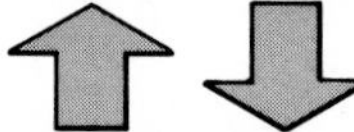

LITHOSPHERE
(terrestrial)

Plant and animal organic populations (including humans)
Rock, mineral deposits, gas cycles

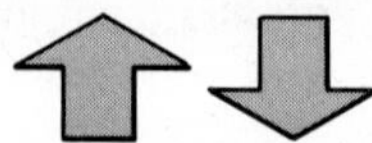

HYDROSPHERE
(e.g., oceans, rivers, lakes)

Plant and animal organic populations
Water, mineral deposits, gas cycles

Fig. 5-1. Material components of biosphere. (Modified from McHale, J.: World facts and trends, ed. 2, New York, 1972, Macmillan, Inc.)

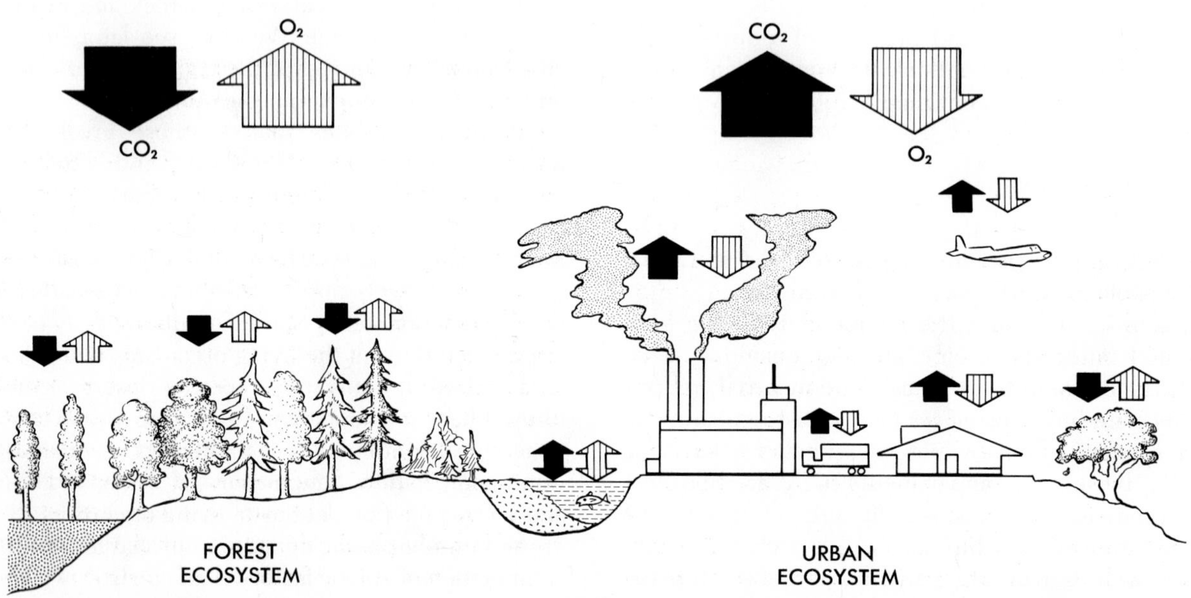

Fig. 5-2. Carbon oxygen cycle. Summary of events in forest ecosystem and in urban ecosystem. Atmosphere and bodies of water serve as reservoirs of carbon dioxide and oxygen. Carbon dioxide is produced by animal respiration, burning fuels, and dissolving carbonates and is used by plants in photosynthesis. It is consumed in process of plant photosynthesis and combustion of fuels.

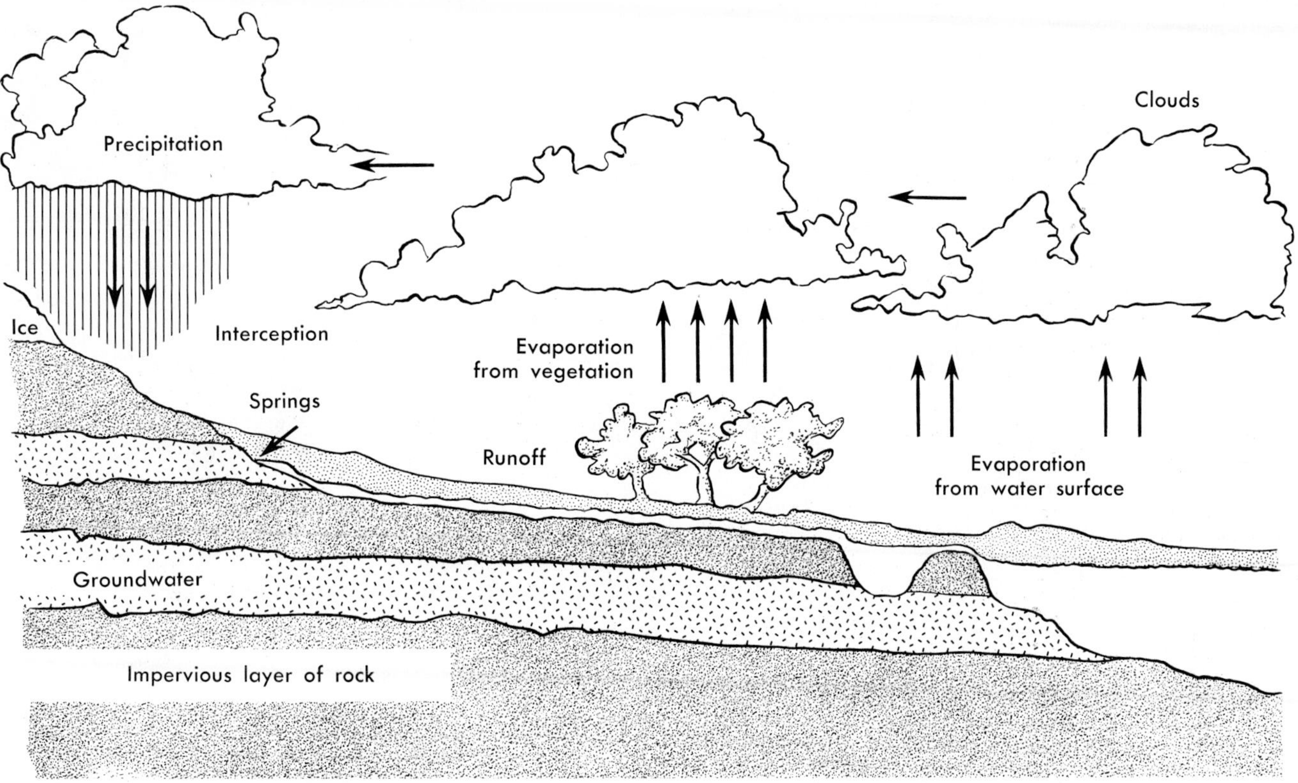

Fig. 5-3. Water cycle activity and its interrelatedness to major biosphere compartments. (Redrawn from Humphrey, C. C., and Evans, R. G.: What's ecology? Northbrook, Ill., 1971, Hubbard Press.)

dependent interrelationship. Radiant energy in the form of sunlight is the ultimate source of energy for all ecosystems. When sunlight enters the biosphere, it is used in the process of photosynthesis through which carbon dioxide and water are converted into energy-rich carbon compounds such as carbohydrates, proteins, and lipids. Green plants are the organisms that perform this function in each ecosystem; thus they are called *producers* and are said to be *autotrophic* (self-feeding). They form the first link in the many and diversified food chains that characterize ecosystems. Almost all other organisms are said to be *heterotrophic* (other feeding), since their nutritional needs are met by feeding on other organisms. There are two groups of heterotrophs: the *consumers* and the *decomposers*.

In the consumer group, those that derive their nutrition directly from plants are called *herbivores* (primary consumers); those that obtain nourishment by consuming herbivores are called *carnivores* (secondary consumers); and in some food chains there may be one or two other levels of carnivores. In Fig. 5-4 these organism-energy interrelationships are illustrated clearly through use of what ecologists call a *pyramid*, in which the number of organisms or the amounts of available energy at each of the trophic levels is represented by blocks of decreasing width. It should be evident that the reason there are only a few types of food chains with second- and third-level carnivores and that the number of these is very low is because of the enormous loss of available energy that occurs from one trophic level to the next.

Decomposers are the other heterotrophs and include chiefly bacteria and fungi. These organisms do not ingest food as do the consumers; rather, they produce and release enzymes into dead plant and animal material and then absorb some or all of the digested products. Aside from assuring their own survival, these organisms contribute an invaluable service to an ecosystem by releasing to the environment (soil or water) various minerals found in protoplasm, thereby making them available for reuse by producers. Thus in all ecosystems two processes are always proceeding simultaneously: the noncyclic flow of energy with much of it lost as heat and the cycling of nutrient elements such as carbon dioxide, water, and minerals. Fig. 5-5 shows the realization not only of the complexity of the interrelationships in the "web of nature" but also of the fact that the slightest

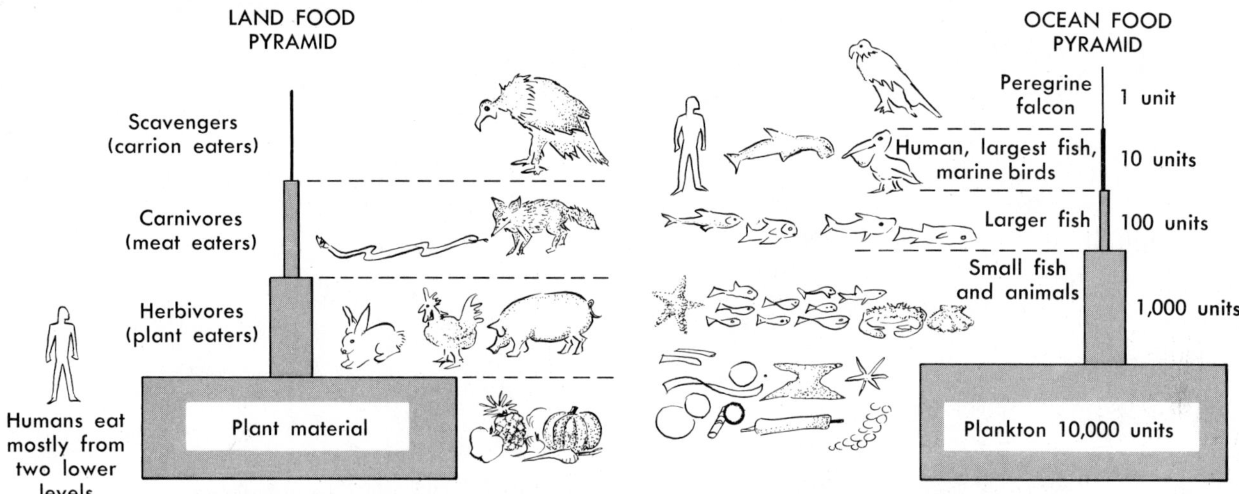
LAND FOOD PYRAMID
Scavengers (carrion eaters)
Carnivores (meat eaters)
Herbivores (plant eaters)
Humans eat mostly from two lower levels
Plant material
OCEAN FOOD PYRAMID
Peregrine falcon
1 unit
Human, largest fish, marine birds
10 units
Larger fish
100 units
Small fish and animals
1,000 units
Plankton 10,000 units

Fig. 5-4. Ecologic pyramids. *Left,* relative amounts of matter available at each tropic level for conversion into energy. *Right,* 90% reduction in available energy in ascending steps of food pyramid. (Redrawn from Humphrey, C. C., and Evans, R. G.: What's ecology? Northbrook, Ill., 1971, Hubbard Press.)

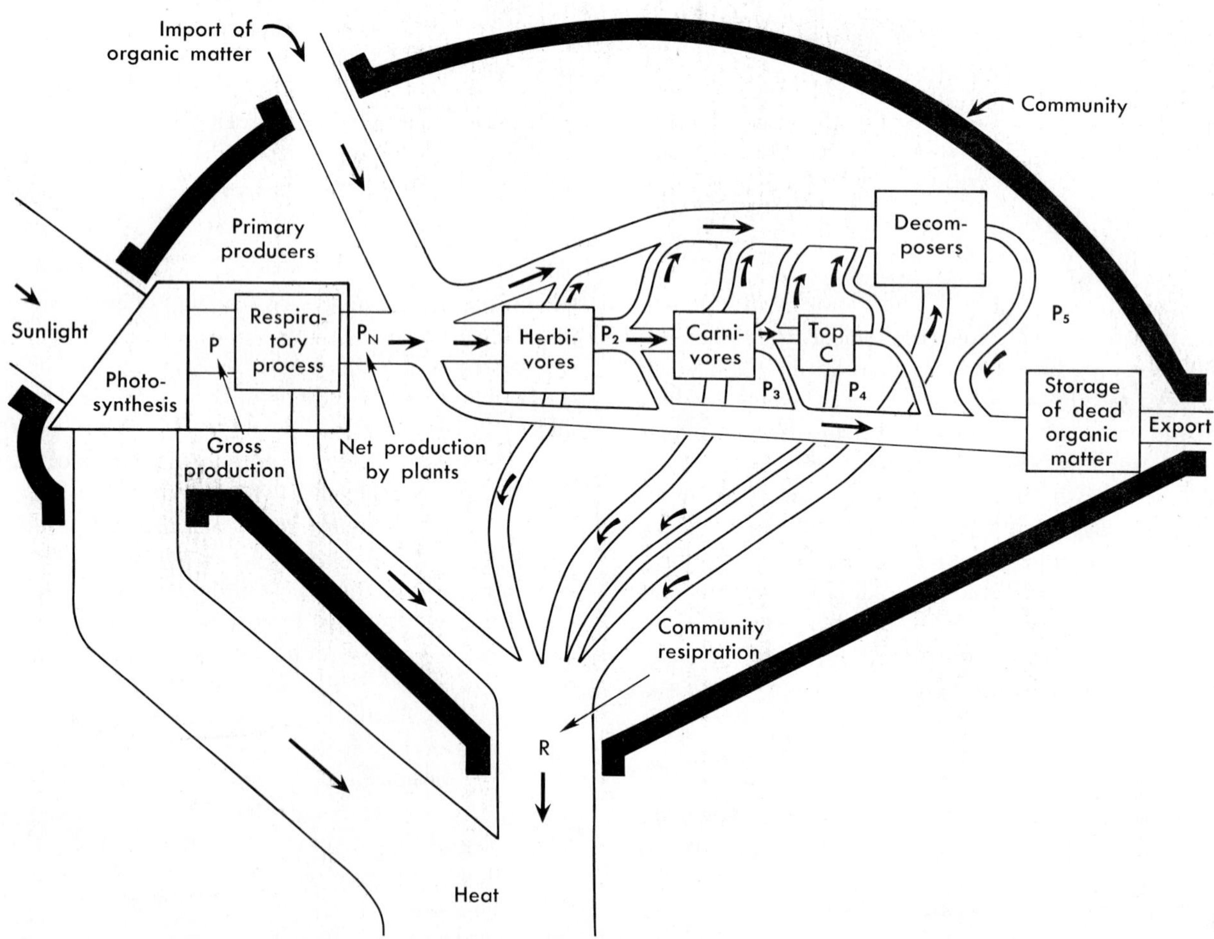

Fig. 5-5. Energy flow in ecosystem. (Modified from Odum, E. P.: Fundamentals of ecology, ed. 2, Philadelphia, 1959, W. B. Saunders Co.)

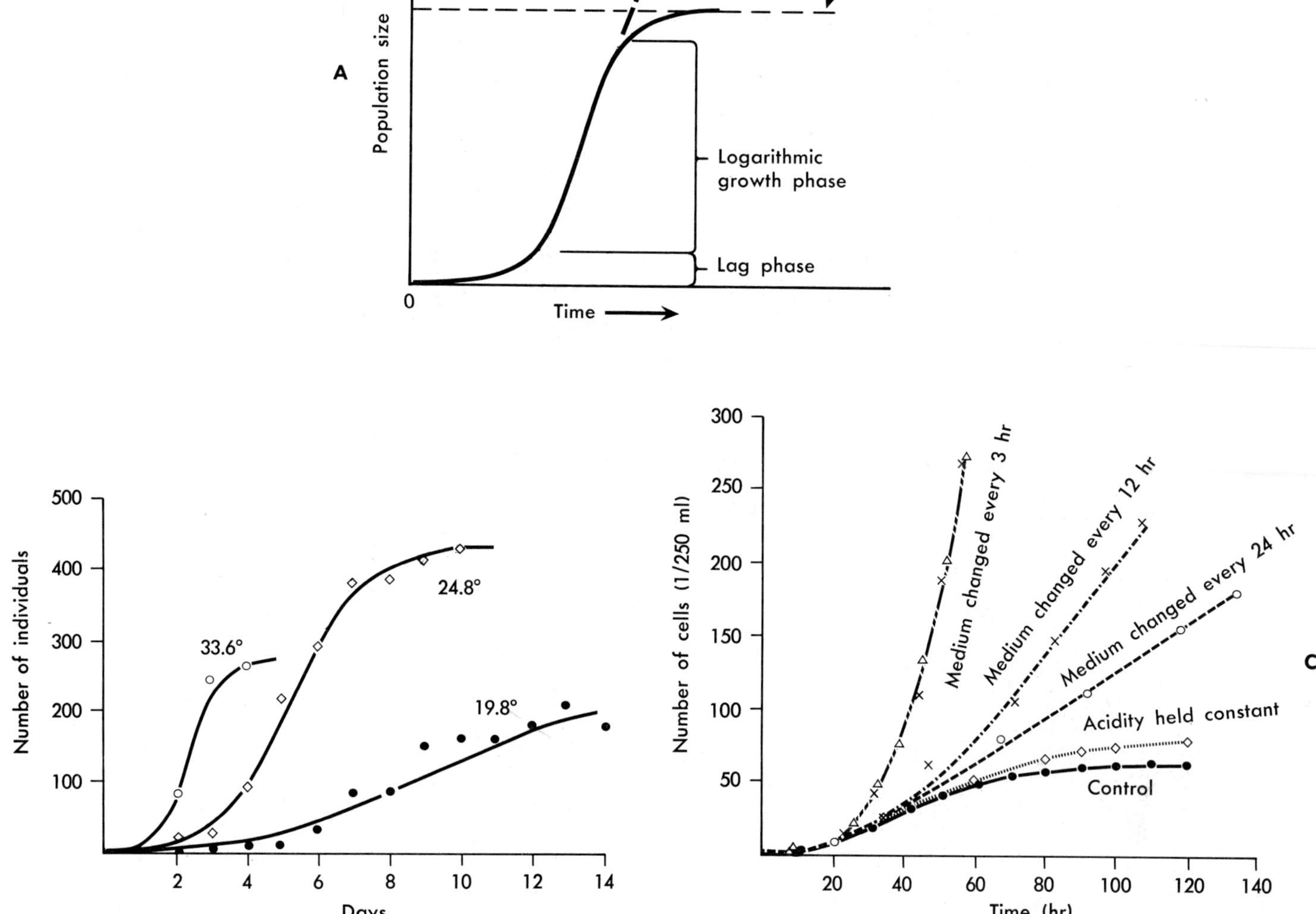

Fig. 5-6. Growth curves under varying conditions. **A,** Generalized growth curve. **B,** Growth at various temperatures. **C,** Influence of nutrients available. (**B** after Terao and Tanaka [1928]; modified from Kormondy, E. J.: Concepts of ecology, Englewood Cliffs, N.J., 1969, Prentice-Hall, Inc.)

change at any point will necessarily produce some effect in the entire system.

Figs. 5-4 and 5-5 also suggest that a wide variety of factors can influence the number of organisms that can survive simultaneously at each trophic level. Any decrease in availability of energy to the producers (through the influence of clouds, smog, changes in temperature, and so forth) will automatically influence the number of herbivores and in turn the carnivore population. Other great influences on the populations at each level are factors such as predation; parasitism; and competition for nutrients, mates, and space. Fig. 5-6 shows the effects of some of these factors on population growth. Fig. 5-6, *A*, shows a generalized growth curve. Fig. 5-6, *B*, shows typical S curves and illustrates the difference in rate of growth as well as the final number within populations as influenced by an abiotic factor, temperature. The enormous influence of nutrient availability is shown in Fig. 5-6, *C;* if these curves were shown for a longer time, one would expect the "equilibrium" (stationery phase)

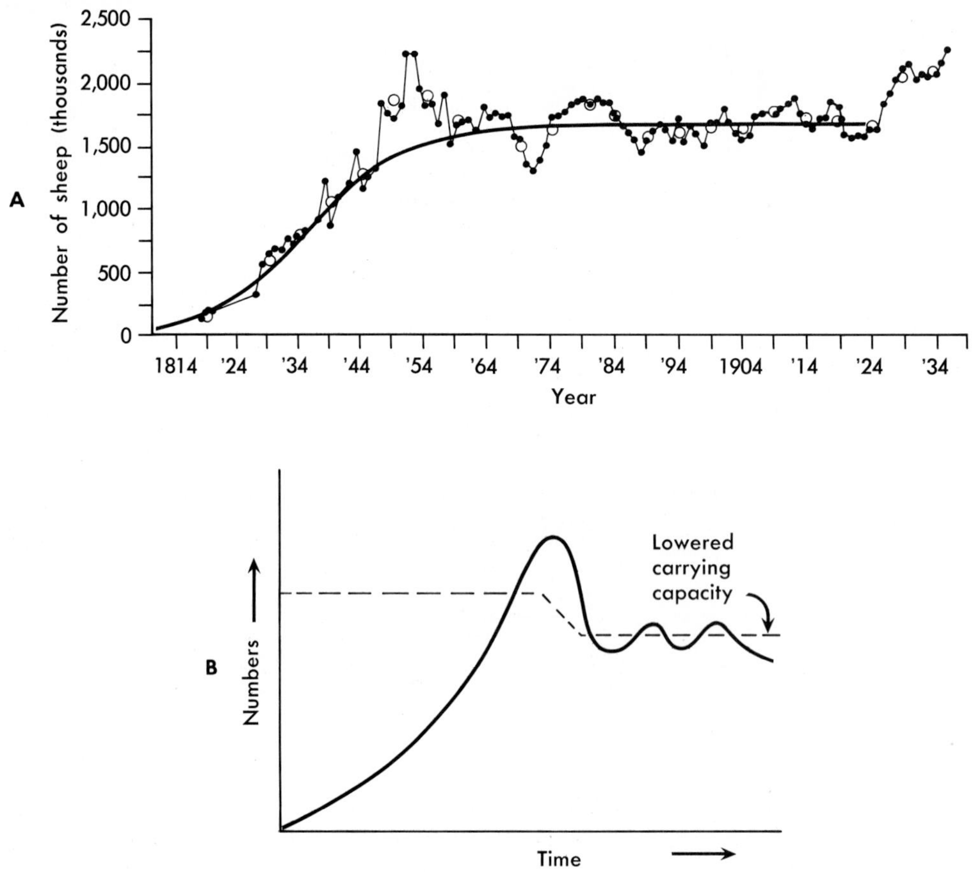

Fig. 5-7. Population curves as related to carrying capacity of system. **A,** Seasonal fluctuations in population showing relatively stable carrying capacity. **B,** Drop in population due to diminished carrying capacity. (**A** after Davidson [1938]; modified from Kormondy, E. J.: Concepts of ecology, Englewood Cliffs, N.J., 1969, Prentice-Hall, Inc.)

population of the typical S curve to become established (as in Fig. 5-6, *B*) due to lack of space and accumulation of toxic metabolic wastes.

The combination of factors that exists during the equilibrium portion of the curve is called the *carrying capacity* of the particular system. In animals with longer life cycles this equilibrium actually represents a series of seasonal fluctuations, as seen in Fig. 5-7, *A*. If the carrying capacity deteriorates permanently, the equilibrium level population will decrease, as shown in Fig. 5-7, *B;* the implications of this figure for the subsequent brief study of pollution effects should be obvious. There are many other aspects of population dynamics that would better enable us to understand the interrelationships among living organisms, but they are beyond the scope of this brief survey. You may wish to consult some of the readings suggested at the end of this chapter to gain more information.

□ Human systems

Humanity, as we have just seen, is an integral part of the particular ecosystem in which it exists. However, it is vital to human survival that more and more of us recognize that we alone are in a position both to realize our role in the biosphere and to plan and control our influence on it. Fig. 5-8 shows a simple scheme that might be used as we proceed to look at the interrelationships between humanity and nature. Each component of this "human ecology" cycle suggests the many ways in which people, especially in industrialized nations, will have to change their life styles in order to restore homeostasis in the biosphere.

Fig. 5-9 graphically depicts some of the various aspects of human complexity and the interrelationships involved; these are aptly described as *internal and external human metabolism.* Humanity's basic biophysical functions are similar to those of many other organisms in

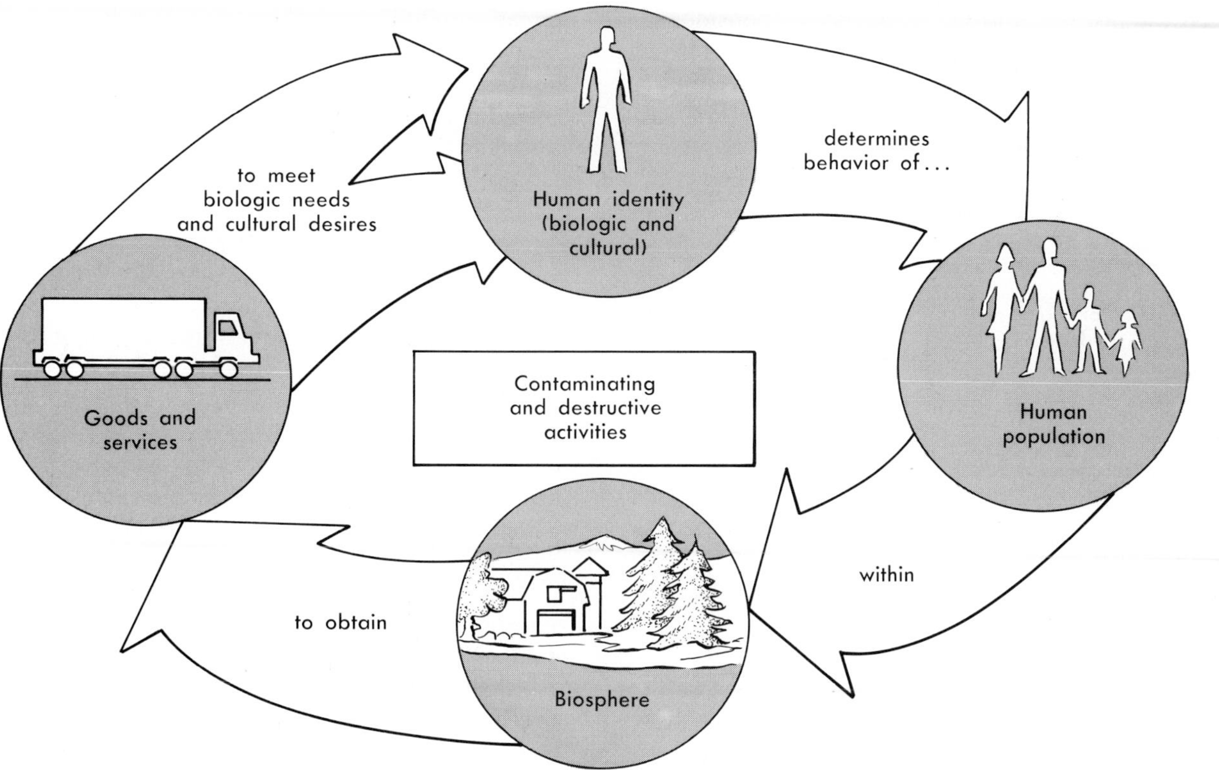

Fig. 5-8. Human ecology cycle. Simple scheme showing interrelationships between humans and nature. (From Humphrey, C. C., and Evans, R. G.: What's ecology? Northbrook, Ill., 1971, Hubbard Press.)

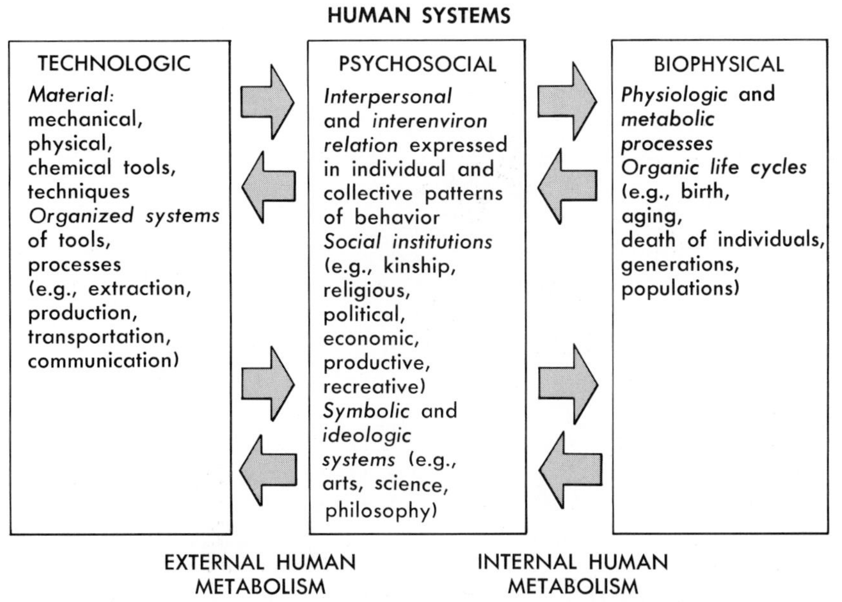

Fig. 5-9. Unique interactions of human populations in biosphere. (Modified from McHale, J.: World facts and trends, ed. 2, New York, 1972, Macmillan, Inc.)

the ecosystems we inhabit. Ecologically considered, people are heterotrophs who can consume food from any and all levels of the food pyramid and can survive only within very narrow ranges of temperature, pressure, and other factors of the abiotic environment. But people are human and find personal meaning largely in the psychosocial sphere, more by a sense of belonging to the larger human society and to a particular cultural heritage than by understanding that we are organisms of a particular species within an ecologic population. Even when we attempt objectivity, we perceive the environment from a uniquely human perspective; our uniqueness is evident in the use of language to interpret and communicate the reality of what we experience.

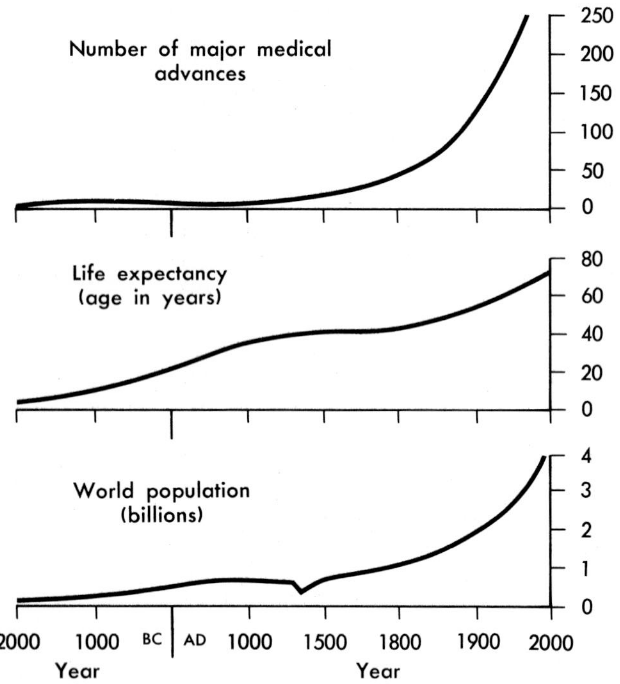

Fig. 5-10. Medical advances and effect on life expectancies and population. (Modified from McHale, J.: The future of the future, New York, 1969, George Braziller, Inc.)

Through technology humans have learned to transcend their physical limitations by controlling their environment so well that for brief periods they can live in considerable comfort even in outer space. Since the nineteenth century, medical advances have significantly lowered mortality in infants and in those with infectious diseases (Fig. 5-10). The result has been an unprecedented rise in the rate of human population growth during a very brief period.

Fig. 5-11 shows that it took hundreds of thousands of years for the human population to reach the current level of 3.8 billion; yet United Nations projections, even at a "medium" rate, suggest that the gobal population will exceed 6 billion by the year 2000—a doubling in less than 30 years!

This is more clearly seen in Fig. 5-12 and can alert us to an important implication: the projected growth will not be evenly distributed. Rather, the populations of the underdeveloped regions, with their much higher birth rates, will increase much more rapidly than those of the industrialized areas, where the birth rate has become more stabilized. As the underdeveloped nations make agricultural, industrial, and medical advances, the total world population will probably grow for generations at a

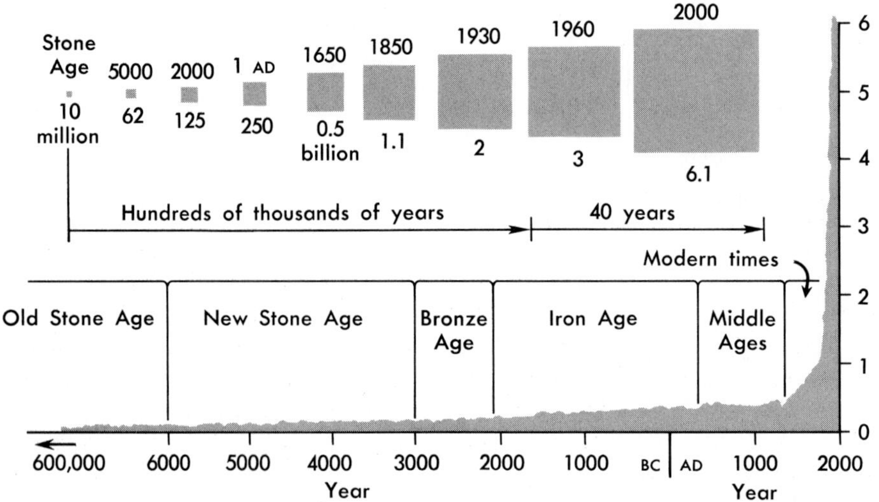

Fig. 5-11. Growth of human numbers. (Modified from Desmond, A.: Pop. Bull. **18:**5, 1962.)

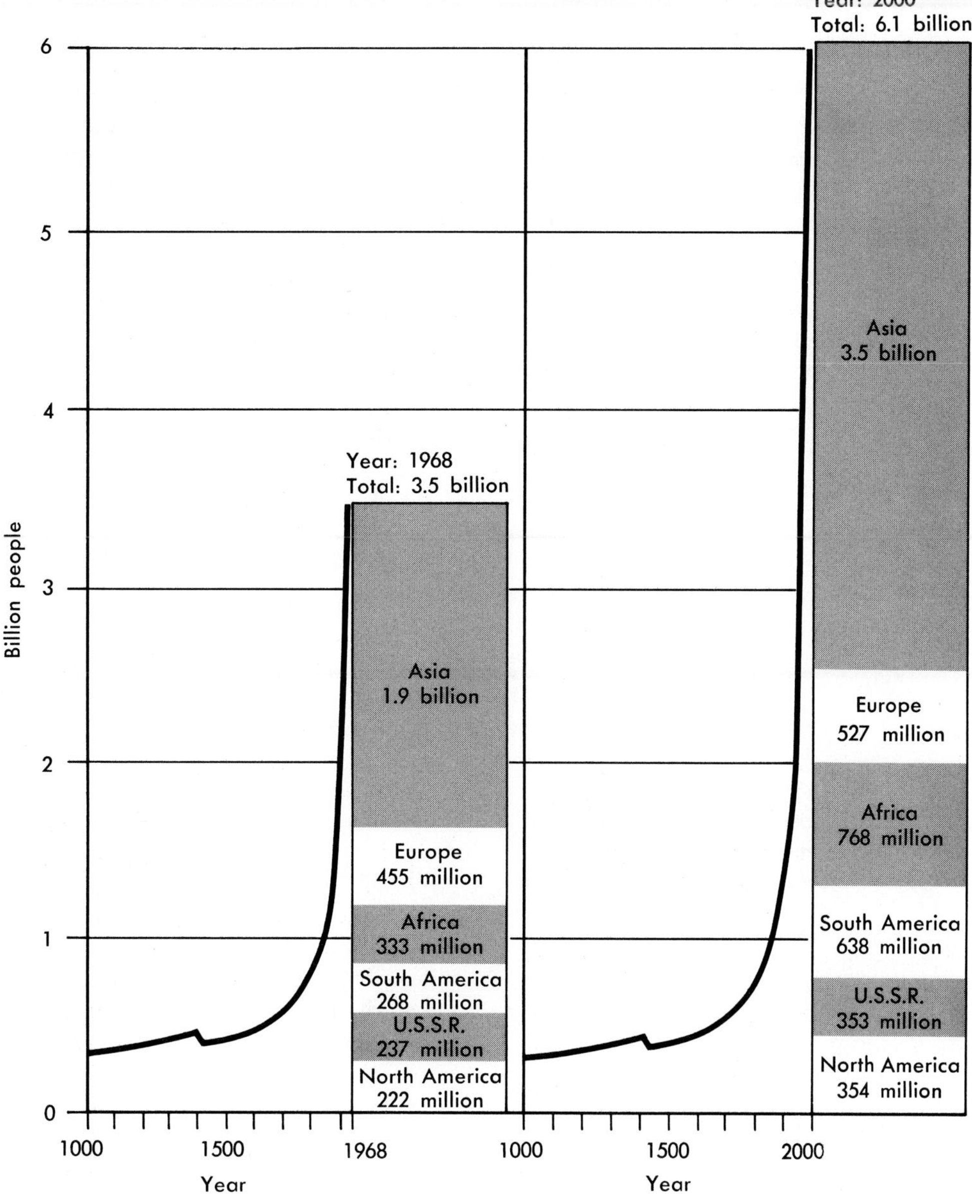

Fig. 5-12. Growth of human population from 1000 AD to 2000 AD showing population distribution. (Modified from McHale, J.: World facts and trends, ed. 2, New York, 1972, Macmillan, Inc.)

rate even greater than the present one before the lowered birth rates indicative of increased development occur.

A brief review of Fig. 5-7, *B*, should clearly point out the importance of understanding that the increasing deterioration of the earth's carrying capacity by pollution, mining, deforestation, urbanization, and so forth, along with the current rate of population increase, cannot be tolerated if human life as we have known it is to continue. Our immediate prospects can be reasonably optimistic, but it will call for greater personal and social discipline. Technology and proper management of resources can eliminate many of the current insults to the environment, but this will require a commitment to the restoration and maintenance of environmental quality that can only result if major changes in personal values are accepted. These assume major adjustments in consumption patterns, income, and life styles, especially for us in the United States, for though we make up only 5.3% of the world's population, we consume 40% to 80% of its various resources. In the context of the ecologic crisis in which the global populations of the next few dec-

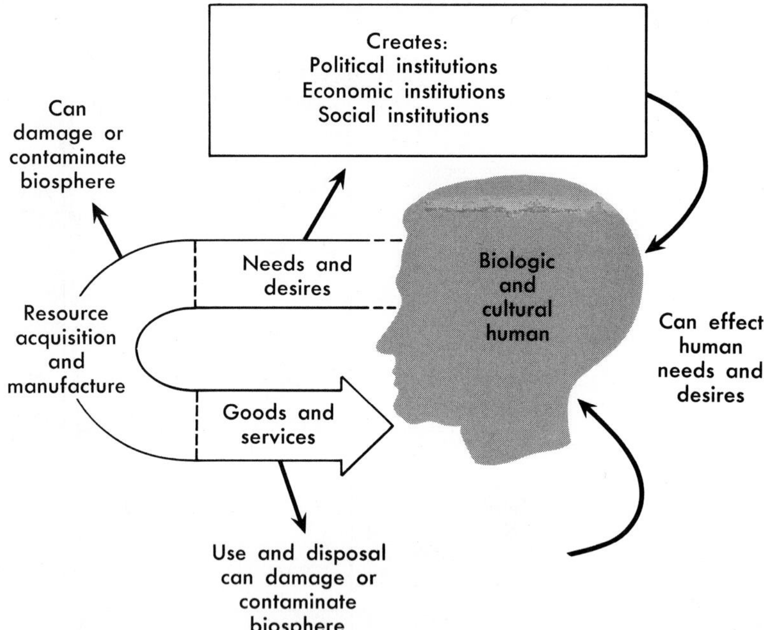

Fig. 5-13. Unique position of humans in biosphere. (From Humphrey, C. C., and Evans, R. G.: What's ecology? Northbrook, Ill., 1971, Hubbard Press.)

ades will live, Fig. 5-13 summarizes simply the unique position of humanity in the biosphere; it is humankind —political, economic, and social—who will determine whether our planet will regain homeostasis.

IMBALANCE: AFFLUENCE AND POLLUTION

An ecosystem can be studied in much the same way as an organism. In the preceding section we have looked briefly at the "anatomy and physiology" of that collectivity of ecosystems called the biosphere and we have found it to be an amazingly complex steady-state system. Homeostasis can be maintained only if energy supplies are adequate and if the cyclic feedback processes that regulate the system are all operating properly. Some of the major strains and imbalances on various compartments of the biosphere result from urbanization, industry, agricultural methods, and affluence. In Fig. 5-14 twentieth century humanity in industrial societies is affected far more by technologic and psychosocial factors than by those that unite us to the more fundamental cycles of the particular ecosystems in which we live. Affluence has been defined as "that state of societies or of individuals in which materials and facilities are available in excess of those necessary for the maintenance of physical and psychological health."[58] Increasingly we are beginning to see that the unbridled production and consumption associated with affluence are not only damaging the physical compartments of the biosphere but are endangering humanity's interrelationships in the psychosocial sphere through serious imbalances in the distribution of global resources.

Damaged atmosphere

The air we breathe is part of the tropospheric layer of the atmosphere, which extends outward about 6 to 10 miles. It functions as a great reservoir within which move all the great wind systems, carrying water, gas, and particulate materials that are constantly circulated from one part of the globe to another. Air in its natural state is very pure; it is essentially a mixture of approximately 79% nitrogen and 20% oxygen with small amounts of carbon dioxide and argon and traces of other gases including water vapor. However, since the time of the discovery of fire humans began to contaminate the air with smoke, the volume of which continually increased as people moved into cooler latitudes where combustion of fuel was necessary to provide heat. Urbanization and the industrial revolution have resulted in the addition of many foreign substances to the atmosphere. Industrial growth, internal combustion, jet engines, and incineration of refuse have only served to multiply these effluents through the ever-increasing combustion processes required to serve our desire for warmth, power, and material goods. The enormous magnitude of the problem, if current trends continue, is dramatically illustrated in a recent projection (Fig. 5-15). In spite of governmental efforts to prevent and control pollution through such measures as the Clean Air Act of

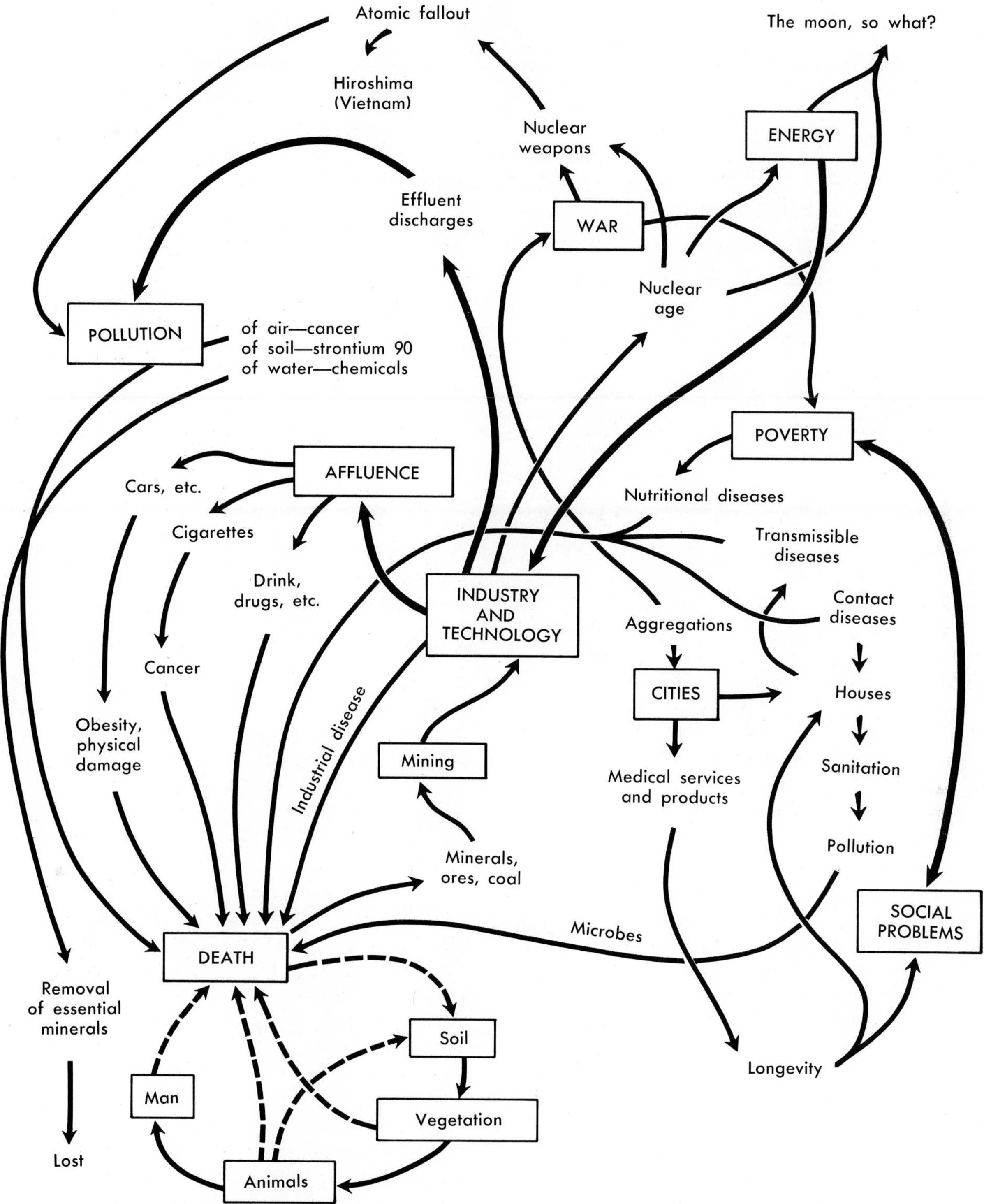

Fig. 5-14. Effects of technologic and psychosocial facts on twentieth-century humans. (Modified from Arthur, D. R.: Man and his environment, London, 1969, The English Universities Press.)

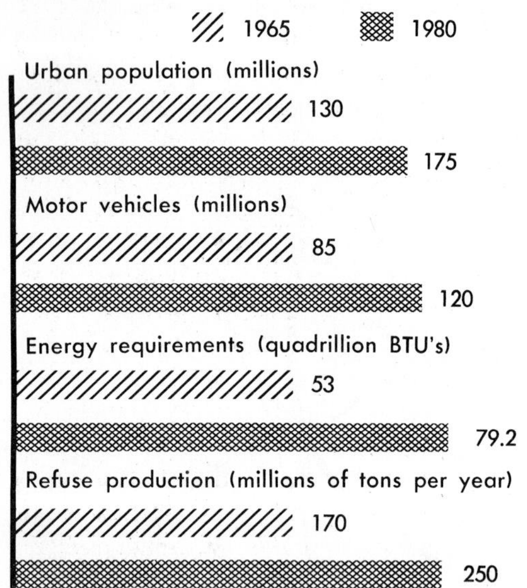

Fig. 5-15. Current trends affecting air pollution in United States. (Modified from Middleton, J.: Pop. Bull. **24:**117, 1968.)

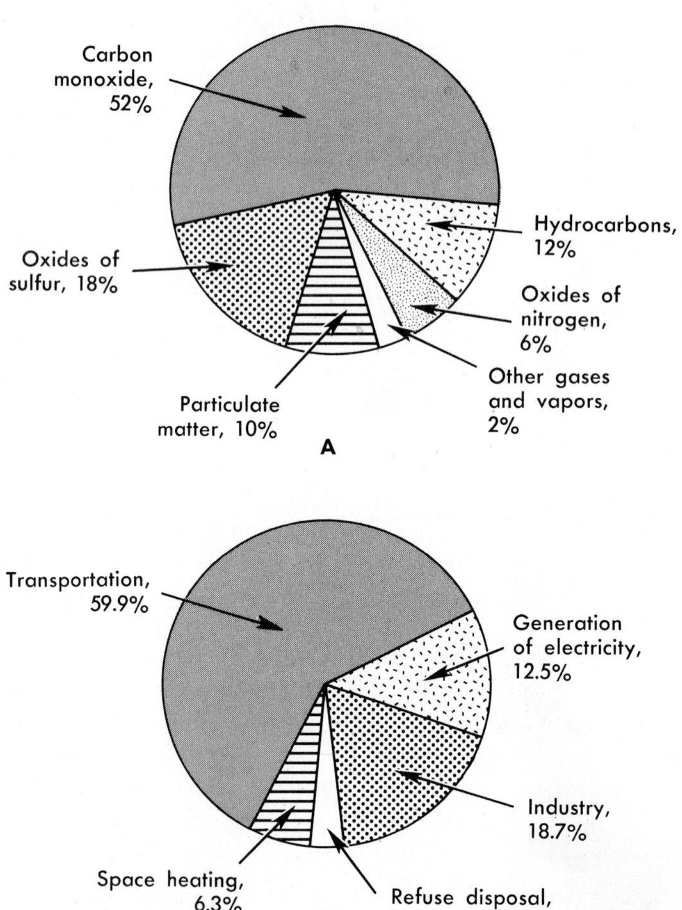

Fig. 5-16. Air pollution in United States. **A,** Types of pollutants. **B,** Source of pollutants. (Modified from Marx, W.: Man and his environment: waste, New York, 1971, Harper & Row, Publishers.)

1963 with its several amendments, it is unlikely that the degree of improvement in air quality that is urgently needed will be achieved unless there is a considerable change in the life style of many individuals.

The types and quantities of pollutants and the sources of these materials in the air are shown in Fig. 5-16. It is interesting to note that the total tonnage of pollutants in the air exceeds our annual steel production. Soot, hydocarbons, oxides of nitrogen and sulfur, carbon dioxide, and carbon monoxide all result from fossil-fuel combustion; the latter two are relatively stable, but the other substances are unstable and can react with one another, making air both toxic and corrosive. For example, hydrocarbons and oxides of nitrogen are relatively harmless, but when combined in sunlight they can generate large volumes of ozone. Other substances that can accumulate to potentially toxic levels are sulfuric acid mists, lead aerosols from gasoline and paints, asbestos fibers, pesticide sprays, and radioactive emissions. The effects of these toxic agents are often intensified by atmospheric turbidity, both sulfur-based smog such as that found over New York and London and the photochemical smog typical of areas such as Los Angeles, which results largely from the action of sunlight on auto emissions such as hydrocarbons and oxides of nitrogen.

We can see, then, that most of the pollutants originate in metropolitan areas. In the past we have relied on wind movement to disperse and dilute the contaminants, a rather efficient process where air temperatures decrease rapidly with altitude. Commonly, however, temperatures may decrease only slightly with height or be even warmer above than near the surface, a condition known as *inversion*. This situation is frequent at night, especially over large urban areas, and because it is often coupled with very weak winds, it may last several days and become very dangerous to health. It has not yet been fully established to what extent pollutants interfere with global and local climates, but careful study of the effects of increasing accumulations of carbon dioxide and particulates is important lest these result in major global temperature changes or marked rises in sea level. With regard to effects on human health, the establishment of specific causes and effects is difficult because poor air quality is primarily a characteristic of urban areas, where there are so many other factors that contribute to physiologic stress. However, there seems to be little doubt that air pollution increases both the incidence and seriousness of many respiratory disorders, and more and more evidence suggests a high incidence of carcinogenic factors in the total environmental complex of airborne chemicals to which we are exposed.

The recovery and maintenance of clean air will be increasingly expensive, as pollution can be effectively controlled only by decreasing pollutant levels at their source; most of this economic burden will be borne by the consumer of goods and services. Because dispersion of air depends on wind movements, control measures must be undertaken at least on a regional basis and should eventually become international in scope. How vital these efforts will become should be evident if we consider not only the direct effects of air pollution on a global scale but also the influences of the many foreign chemicals, particulates, and radioactive products as precipitation washes them into the lithosphere and hydrosphere.

□ Degraded waters

Everyone has discussed water pollution at one time or another, each person having a personal concept of what it is. The term may have meanings ranging all the way from occasional litter in a body of water to bacteriologic content so high as to make the water seriously dangerous to living organisms, including people. Even natural waters are never pure, and they range in quality from tasty, safe water to poisonous drinking water and from fresh rainwater to ocean water. Because of the enormous quantity of water in the hydrosphere, the ability of bodies of water to rid themselves of wastes through natural processes such as dilution, water movement, and bacterial decomposition has been too heavily relied on in many areas. Fig. 5-17 will make us aware that much of the domestic and industrial sewage and the agricultural runoff that constitute water pollution are received primarily by the surface waters; these make up only about 0.02% of the total water in the world! Most of the organic wastes from cities are highly concentrated and enter rivers and lakes through pipes so large that they produce concentrations of materials that can completely exhaust the dissolved oxygen content of the waterway. Once a body of water's capacity to meet the biologic oxygen demand (BOD) is exceeded, most of the living organisms die and are decomposed by anaerobic bacteria, producing a septic condition often accompanied by very foul odors. Undecomposed wastes can settle to the bottom and build up sludge bands. Natural reaeration occurs downriver, but the number of outfall discharges along major waterways, particularly in our highly industrial regions, often makes impossible the recovery of conditions suitable for maintaining most living organisms. Some of our rivers and lakes have enormous populations of the very few species of organisms that can survive in polluted conditions instead of the rich diversity of living things characteristic of freshwater ecosystems; some have virtually no living organisms at all.

Domestic and industrial sewage can be treated to lower its biologic oxygen demand level and still release large quantities of waste products such as the plant nutri-

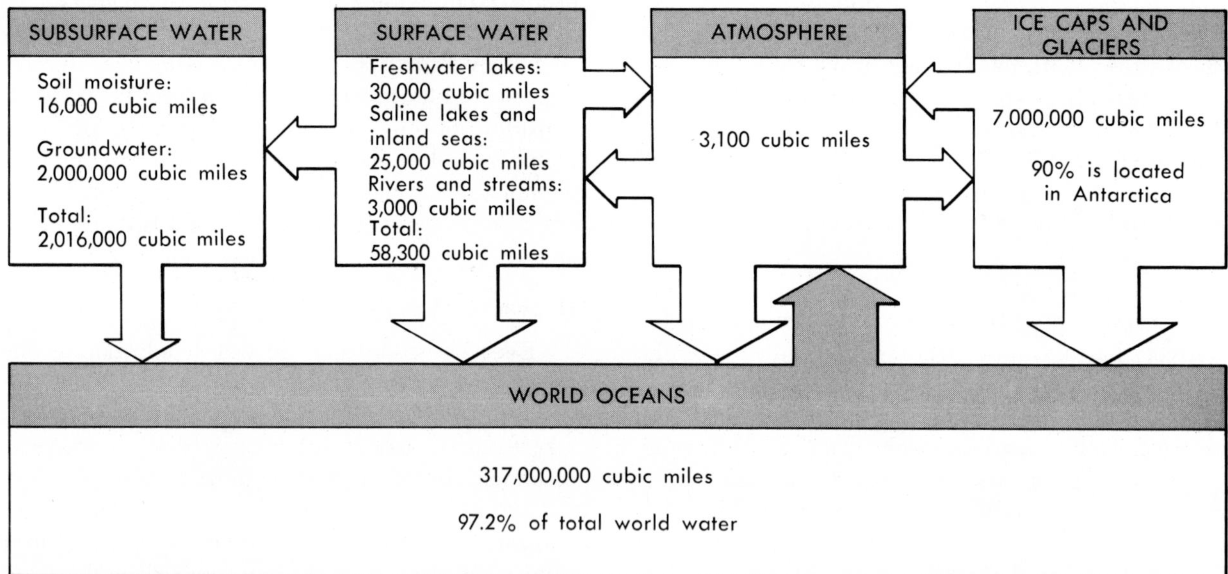

Fig. 5-17. Distribution of global water. (Modified from McHale, J.: The ecological context, New York, 1970, George Braziller, Inc.)

ents from artificial fertilizers and detergents. An idea of the scope of the problem can be gained from Fig. 5-18. Lakes are particularly prone to excessive enrichment, or eutrophication, because reaeration cannot occur as rapidly as it does in rivers and streams. A body of water may be overwhelmed not only by organic wastes but also by enormous loads of inorganic and nonbiodegradable materials. Many human activities, such as strip mining and bulldozing for highways and subdivisions, greatly increase sediment loads to a point where they cannot be diluted. The increased water turbidity can interfere with algal photosynthesis with resultant effects all the way up the food chains. It can also produce amounts of silt that are very injurious to gill-breathing organisms and eventually form sediments capable of completely burying such forms as clams and oysters. In addition such sediments can carry tremendous loads of toxic wastes such as DDT, PCB, and other pesticides; herbicides; acid drainage from mines; heavy metal residues; and a host of organic compounds from industrial processes. Many of these materials, even if present only in trace quantities, can become severely toxic by being taken up in the food web and concentrated through the process of biologic magnification. As Fig. 5-19 shows, concentrations have been recorded that are sufficient to affect reproduction in some waterfowl.

Reports have shown that radioactive materials in

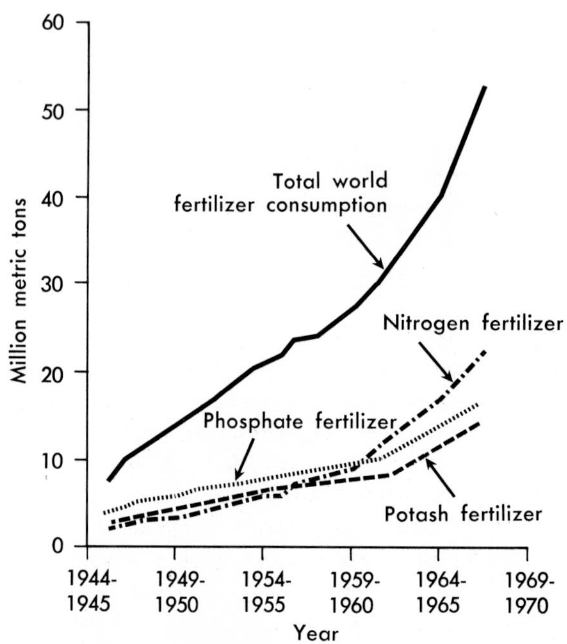

Fig. 5-18. Increase in fertilizer consumption. (From Brown, L. R.: Human food production as a process of the biosphere, Sci. Am. **223:**161, 1970. Copyright © by Scientific American, Inc. All rights reserved.)

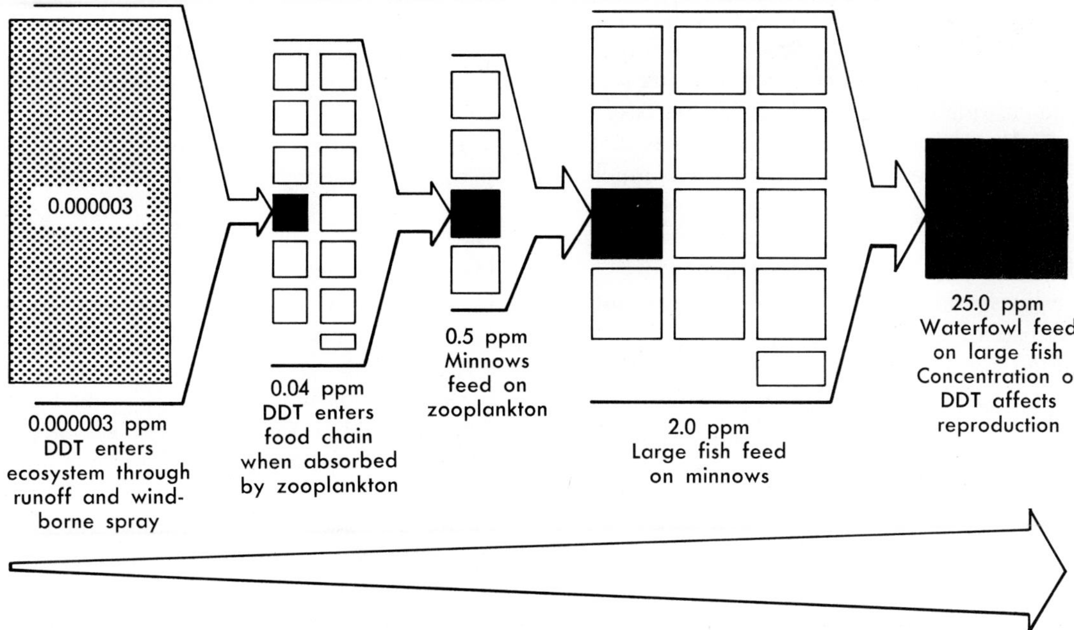

Fig. 5-19. Biologic magnification of DDT. Concentration of DDT and effect on reproduction through food chain. Adapted from Time, The Weekly Newsmagazine, July 11, 1969. Copyright Time Inc.)

water also tend to be concentrated by aquatic organisms, although the pattern of concentration does not seem to show the magnification of pesticide residues. However, even relatively low levels of accumulation in fish and other organisms consumed by humans may become a more serious threat as increasing numbers of nuclear power plants become operative to ease the energy crisis. More nuclear plants probably result also in increased thermal pollution. Both conventional and nuclear power plants and many industries remove millions of gallons of water from lakes and rivers to cool electric generating processes and then return the water to its original source several degrees warmer. Aquatic ecosystems are often severely disrupted by these temperature changes.

Dangers to the marine environment come not only from dumping radioactive wastes from land-based nuclear reactors far out at sea but also from the increasing number of nuclear-powered ships. According to the Committee on Effects of Atomic Radiation on Oceanography and Fisheries, 300 nuclear-powered ships had come into service by 1975.

Although the oceans are enormous, pollution conditions similar to those in fresh water are becoming increasingly present at ocean outflow sites, causing considerable damage to coastal ecosystems and even to marine life at enormous depths through dispersion of nonbiodegradable chemicals. Recent oil spills of millions of gallons have dramatized the global nature of the effects of such pollution of the oceans. Sizable oil slicks have been found at every latitude. International agreement on safety codes for offshore drilling and tanker specifications are urgently needed, for despite their vastness even the oceans can become ecologic disaster areas if people are as careless with them as we have been with surface waters. Perhaps the most serious effects of these oil spills are yet to be seen: the potential accumulation in human food of long-term poisons, such as the carcinogens that can be derived from crude oil.

□ Land degradation

The surface of the lithosphere is being influenced constantly by the action of wind and water; thus many of the pollutants just discussed are transferred to the land and then percolate into the groundwater through the soil. Groundwater and soil also can be contaminated by acid or radioactive wastes from surface mining of metals and uranium, pesticide residues, synthetic chemicals, heavy-metal salts, and other soluble materials. Data showing the adverse effects on human health of chemicals used as pesticides, herbicides, and fertilizers have been accumulating for two decades.

Historically, humankind has used the surface of the land in its natural condition as rangeland or forest; with an increasing world population, more and more of these regions have been converted into croplands. Table 5-1 shows some international projections for land use that make the finiteness of land surface on the planet readily apparent. In addition the exploitation of the soil to produce large crops at a minimum cost is producing a drop in the nutritional quality of crops in many parts of the United States. For example, evidence indicates that in Kansas the protein concentration of corn fell as much as 22% between 1910 and 1950 although the period was marked by substantial increases in corn yields—a corn with a much higher carbohydrate-to-protein ratio.

Intensive livestock-raising techniques have resulted in increased use of antibiotics to protect animals in closely confined conditions and antibiotics and various hormones to encourage rapid growth. Consumption of feeds containing these materials is resulting in emergence of antibiotic-resistant strains of bacteria and the accumulation of antibiotic and hormone residues in foods. Although it is unlikely that concentrations of hormones from food will reach a level where the metabolic changes associated with the hormone become apparent, other effects may provide threats to health. It is difficult to assess the effects on health that may develop from the increasing use of synthetic chemicals by both industry and agribusiness, as "disease" effects may be subtle or may not show up until a future generation.

Table 5-1. Present and potential uses of land surface of planet (percent of total area)*

Use	Present	Potential
Croplands	11	24
Rangelands	20	28
Managed forests	10	15
Reserves (80% forest)	26	0
Not usable	33	33
Total	100	100

*From Matthews, W. H., et al., editors: Man's impact on terrestrial and oceanic ecosystems, Cambridge, Mass., 1971, The M.I.T. Press.

Increasingly the loads of wastes resulting from the production characteristic of affluent societies produce solid-waste disposal problems that are critical, especially in densely populated areas. The rate at which the problem is growing is evident from Fig. 5-20, a projection resulting from a 1969 Atomic Energy Commission study. Solid wastes fall into five major categories: urban, which includes domestic, commercial, and muncipal; industrial; agricultural; mineral; and those from federal establishments. The mountains of urban wastes—garbage, paper, furniture, abandoned cars, ashes, dead animals, street sweepings, materials resulting from construction and demolition, and the many nonbiodegradable "disposable" products—not only utilize enormous amounts of land surface but also tend to be esthetically offensive because of the appearance and odor, and they enhance the multiplication of disease-producing organisms and create fire and explosion hazards. Improvements in management are beginning to be evident in a few cities

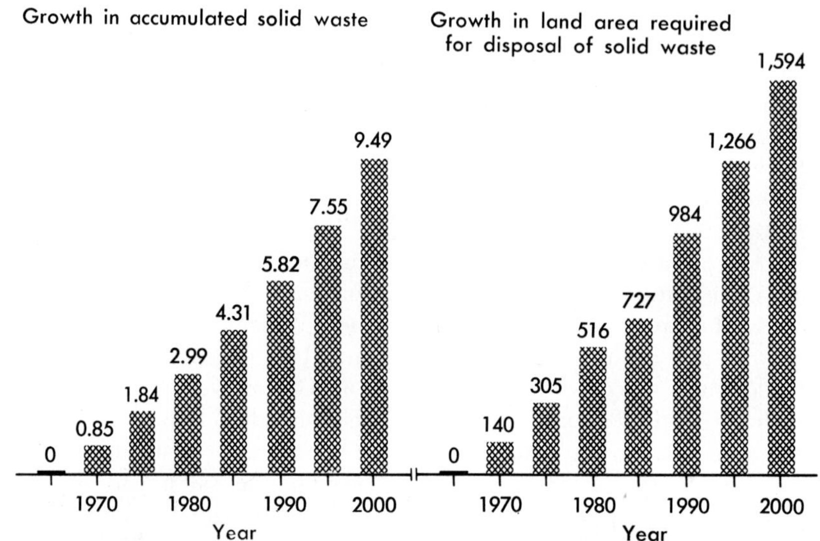

Fig. 5-20. Projected scope of solid waste disposal problem in United States. Accumulated solid waste shown in billion tons. Land area shown in square miles at 15-ft deep density of 32 lb/cu ft. (Modified from Closing the cycle from use to reuse: the fusion torch, Washington, D.C., 1969, U.S. Atomic Energy Commission.)

through use of sanitary landfills, composting, metal reclamation, and other recycling efforts, but open dumping remains by far the most widely used means of urban waste disposal. Industrial concerns are struggling to cope with up to 115 million tons of waste yearly, such as waste plastics, scrap metals, paper wastes, and large inventories of offgrade products, sludges, and slags. Most of these materials cannot be processed and reintroduced into use.

Wastes from agriculture and forestry include animal manures and residues from such activities as crop harvesting, pruning, fertilizing, and spraying. Domestic animals produce close to 2 billion tons of animal wastes annually, as much as 50% of which is generated in concentrated growing and feeding operations close to urban areas.

Mountains of mineral wastes such as submarginal-grade ores, coal waste piles, tailing slag, and wastes from chemical processing are produced by about 80 mineral industries, with the copper, iron, steel, phosphate rock, bituminous coal, lead, zinc, and anthracite industries generating the most wastes. Dredging and strip mining also produce large-scale pollution and destruction of the land; by 1980 it is estimated that more than 5 million acres will have been defaced by strip-mining operations alone. Research in solid-waste disposal will increase as an urgent need, and it is to be hoped that a unified, comprehensive approach to solid-waste management will be sought if the enormous cost of effective management is to be reduced. Some idea of the projected cost of

Table 5-2. Composition of municipal refuse*

Type of refuse	Percent of total
Rubbish	64.0
Paper	42.0
Dry leaves	5.0
Grass	4.0
Street refuse	3.0
Wood and bark	2.4
Brush	1.5
Green cuttings	1.5
Household dirt	1.0
Oils and paint	0.8
Plastics	0.7
Rags	0.6
Rubber	0.6
Leather goods	0.3
Linoleum	0.1
Miscellaneous	0.5
Food Wastes	12.0
Garbage	10.0
Fats	2.0
Noncombustibles	24.0
Ashes	10.0
Metals	8.0
Glass and ceramics	6.0

*After Gough, W. C.: Why fusion? U.S. Atomic Energy Commission, 1970.

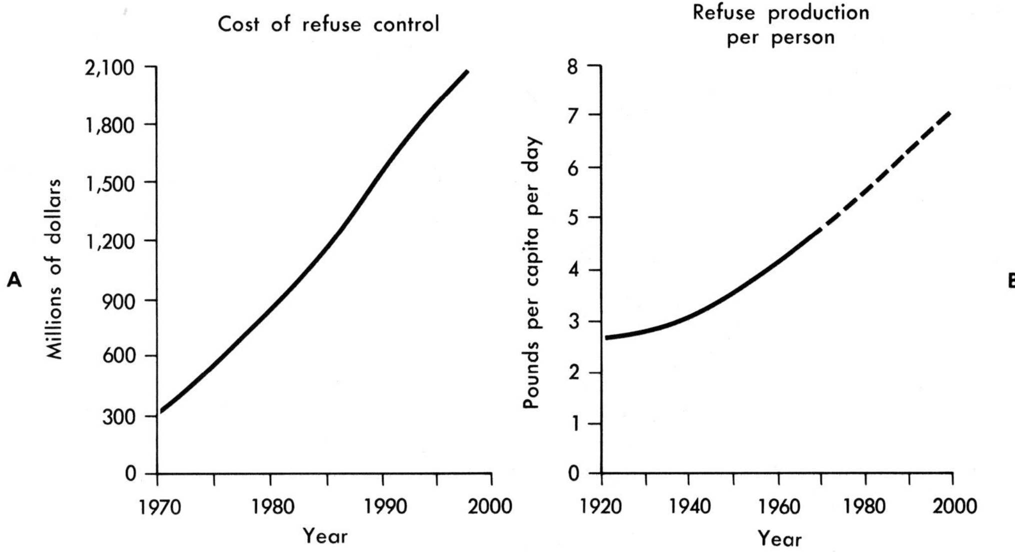

Fig. 5-21. Solid waste management and cost in United States. (**A** modified from Waste management and control, pub. no. 1400, Washington, D.C., 1966, National Academy of Sciences; **B** modified from Gough, W. C.: Why fusion? Washington D.C., 1970, U.S. Atomic Energy Commission.)

solid-waste control can be gained from a recent study by the National Academy of Sciences (Fig. 5-21, *A*). The projected figure probably includes support of the new technologies that will be required to ensure that recycling techniques are made effective enough to reduce significantly the pollution of all compartments of the biosphere. Fig. 5-21, *B*, indicates, however, that recent trends have shown nearly a doubling of refuse production per person; so much of the economic burden projected is due to the increasing "throwaway" mentality of an affluent society. Table 5-2 reveals that most of this accumulation of trash could be avoided if each person made a careful evaluation of the wastefulness of his or her lifestyle and began to utilize increasing amounts of recycling in everyday habits.

It is becoming more and more apparent that the environmental crisis confronting us today has a cultural basis. Industrial humankind's affluence, technology, urbanization, increasing individual wealth, and exploitive attitude toward nature are wrecking the environment. If we are concerned about our own physical, mental, and social health as well as the welfare of generations yet unborn, our attitudes toward nature must change enough to result in new individual behavior and new institutions; both of these must be enlightened by the global perspective that social justice demands.

People must come to a recognition of the interdependence of all creatures and a respect not only for life in all its forms but also for the nonliving components of the biosphere (Fig. 5-22). We must learn to live as part of the community of life—as the steward of the planet, not its master.

■ PERSPECTIVES FOR HUMAN HEALTH

□ Metabolic hemeostasis and health

Health is often thought of as freedom from disease, weakness, or malfunction. Viewed positively, however, it is quite appropriate to equate it with homeostasis, or steady-state functioning. In many ways the human body can be likened to an ecosystem, with the metabolic systems accomplishing the producer-decomposer roles, the musculoskeletal complex and (on a less consistent basis) the reproductive system being the consumers of much of the energy produced by the metabolic systems, and the entire interacting "ecosystem" under exquisite neuroendocrine control. Such an analogy is shown schematically in Fig. 5-23.

Just as in an ecosystem, an imbalance or malfunction

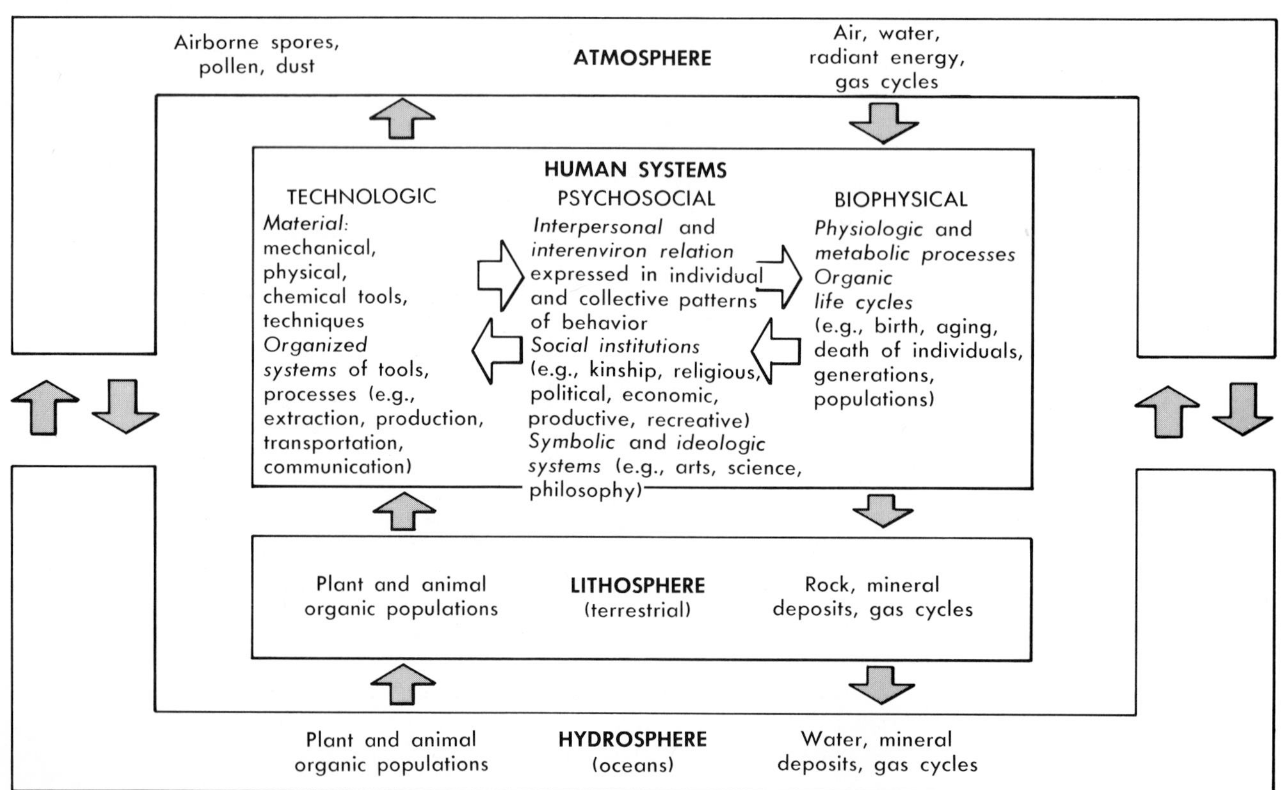

Fig. 5-22. Integral interrelatedness of environ systems and human systems in biosphere. (Modified from McHale, J.: World facts and trends, ed. 2, New York, 1972, Macmillan, Inc.)

in part of this steady-state complex is reflected throughout the organism; this we know as disease or illness. Historically, people have suffered primarily from the infectious diseases caused by invading microorganisms, and to a large extent this is still true in many of the Third World regions. In the developed nations, however, especially since the discovery of antibiotics (Fig. 5-24), infectious disease has been all but eradicated. Yet simultaneously the incidence of chronic metabolic and degenerative disease continues to rise in the more affluent areas of the world (Table 5-3). Data such as these reflect a complex interaction of factors characteristic of affluent, highly industrialized urban regions. Many persons in such regions show high cholesterol levels and obesity coupled with decreased activity. Heavy cigarette smoking seems to be more prevalent in sophisticated, urban cultures, and the deleterious effects of smoking are significantly aggravated by intake of polluted air characteristic of these densely populated regions. Noise tends to produce psychologic trauma of varying seriousness by limiting efficiency, interfering with sleep, and generally adding to the many other stressful conditions from which industrial peoples suffer. Thus it is difficult to implicate

Table 5-3. International mortality statistics: comparison of death rates from arteriosclerotic and degenerative heart diseases per 100,000 population in developed and underdeveloped countries, 1966*

Developed countries		Underdeveloped countries	
Scotland	366.5	Venezuela	47.8
Denmark	327.7	Mauritius	46.5
Eire	326.1	Costa Rica	45.8
United States	320.0	Singapore	35.9
England and Wales	317.0	Mexico	16.9
Australia	290.0	Philippines	14.5
Canada	240.1		
Switzerland	218.6		
Netherlands	184.5		
France	81.4		

*From Smith, G., and Smyth, J. C., editors: The biology of affluence, Edinburgh, 1972, Oliver & Boyd, Ltd.

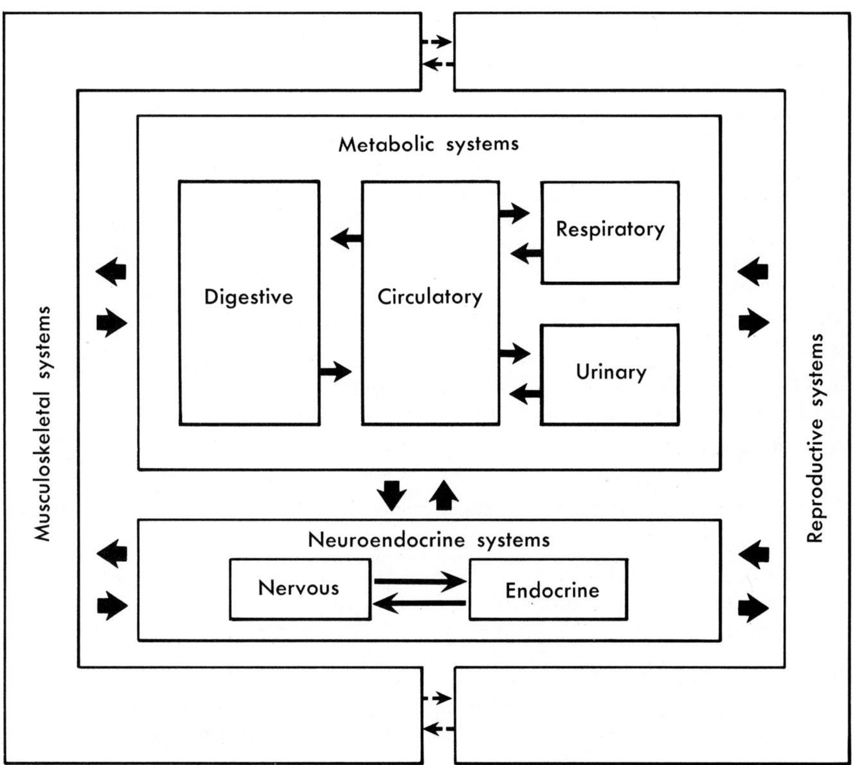

Fig. 5-23. Human body viewed as "ecosystem."

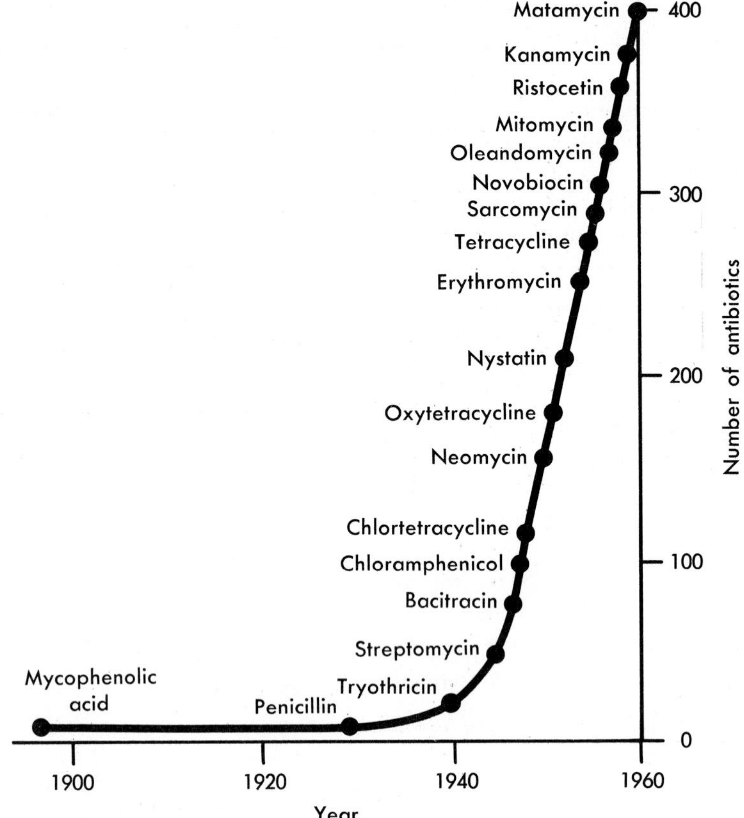

Fig. 5-24. Years in which antibiotics were developed and number in use. (Modified from McHale, J.: The future of the future, New York, 1969, George Braziller, Inc.)

individual environmental factors directly as causative of specific disease conditions.

The task of studying the environment as it relates to human health is enormous because it requires simultaneous handling of a multitude of variables that can be understood only as a whole system rather than as separate parts. This is a staggering realization to researchers, since historically medical research investigations have been those of individual scientists testing effects of one variable at a time on test animals and sometimes on humans. Only through the use of integrated team efforts, aided by systems analysis and projection possible through computer use, is there any hope that humanity will arrive at an understanding of the many cause-effect relationships between humans and their environment.

Institutional response has begun to be evident in the new departments of community medicine and environmental health being formed in some medical schools and schools of public health. Such programs evidence the growing realization that today's health personnel should not simply restore clients to health but should be instrumental in helping to educate them concerning the many environmental factors that can influence their health directly or indirectly.

The global nature of the problem is beginning to be addressed by such meetings as the 1974 International Symposium on Recent Advances in the Assessment of the Health Effects of Environmental Pollution. This meeting, which was organized by the World Health Organization, the Commission of the European Communities, and the U.S. Environmental Protection Agency, gathered 800 representatives from 40 countries and 12 international organizations to assess techniques and need for measurement and monitoring of environmental effects and the scope of the scientific data base required for global decision making to protect human health. The 2,400-page proceedings of this meeting illustrate clearly that recognition of the "many-sided and complex character of environmental problems and the need to develop a common methodological approach to tackle them" has barely begun.[64] But this beginning is a milestone, perhaps most of all because of the recognitions that "one of the major problems confronting us is how to improve our knowledge of the long-term and

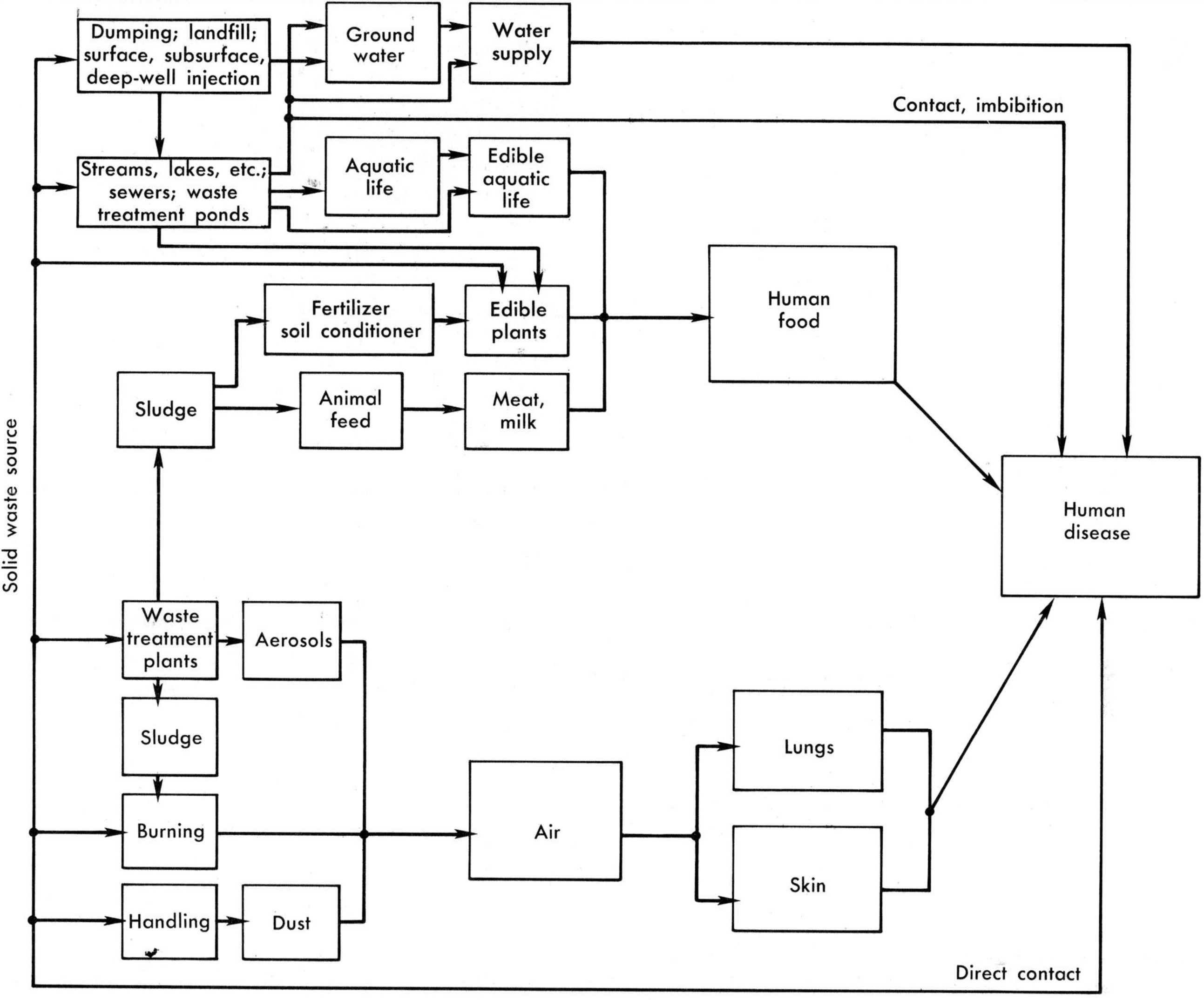

Fig. 5-25. Relationship between chemical waste and disease. Schema showing how any source of waste can contaminate air, food, or water. (Modified from Marx, W.: Man and his environment: waste, New York, 1971, Harper & Row, Publishers.)

hereditary effects of pollution" and that vital as objective analysis of scientific phenomena are, "the results of scientific observations must not become the all-important factors in legislative and political decisions."[56]

Pollution and physiologic imbalance

Because of the complexity of the interacting body-environment systems that must be studied, there is very little solid evidence to date of cause-effect relationships between specific pollutants and particular disease processes. To clarify the effects of chronic, low-level exposure to pollutants, fundamental research must include (1) basic studies on the physiologic effects of pollutants on various body tissues and organs, (2) animal experimentation on the effects of these substances on susceptibility to infectious diseases, (3) industrial and urban-rural morbidity studies in relation to known exposures, and (4) controlled epidemiologic studies. To date the only concerted research efforts that fulfill these criteria have been made in two areas: the relationship of smoking to health and the somatic and genetic effects of radioactivity. We shall study these in greater detail later in an effort to comprehend how difficult it will be to marshal sufficient interest and financial backing to make the necessary investigations for the enormous number of compounds that would have to be tested. But first let us survey briefly a few of the pollutant-disease relationships that have come under suspicion, usually through a dramatic incident such as a localized air-pollution episode or an industrial or research accident that exposed victims to unexpected quantities of a hazardous material.

The entry site for disease-producing pollutants is always one of the body surfaces exposed to the environment: the digestive and respiratory tracts and the skin. A general indication of how easily any of the wastes that we surveyed earlier can enter the body is seen in Fig. 5-25. Note that because of the integral interrelationships among the biosphere compartments any waste from any source can eventually influence the food and water ingested and the air taken in by the respiratory tract and be potentially disease producing.

Two groups of substances that enter the mouth are *intentional* and *incidental* food additives. In our affluent society we have come to expect enormous variety in our diet, regardless of seasonal availability and location of production. To make this possible, processors add a large variety of materials to color, flavor, sweeten, ripen, add firmness, thicken, soften, moisten, dry, emulsify, enrich, hasten chemical reactions, or retard oxidation and rancidity in foods. In many cases such intentional additives have enhanced nutritional health. For example, addition of potassium iodide to table salt has all but eliminated simple goiter, and the enrichment of bread with B vitamins has greatly cut down the incidence of pellagra in the United States.

In many other cases, however, laboratory tests, usually performed on animals, have strongly suggested that particular additives of both incidental and intentional types may be dangerous to human health. In 1958 the Food, Drug and Cosmetics Act was amended by the so-called Delaney Clause: No additive shall be deemed safe if it is found, after tests which are appropriate for the evaluation of safety of food additives, to induce cancer in man or animal.

Among the incidental additives that find their way into food are pesticides and herbicides, chemicals introduced into animal feed, substances that might diffuse from packaging materials, heavy metals, and radioactive materials from fallout and other sources. Just before Thanksgiving in 1959 all cranberries and cranberry products were removed from the market because it was feared that they might contain residual aminotriazole, an herbicide that had been found to induce cancerous growth in the thyroid glands of rats. The death rate from pesticides is estimated at 150 persons yearly, 50% to 75% being children who have accidentally eaten lethal doses. A more subtle effect is illustrated by the finding that the 18- to 23-year old daughters of mothers who were treated with diethylstibestrol (DES) to prevent threatened abortion have a significantly higher uterine cancer rate. In 1974 the Food and Drug Administration (FDA) approved use of DES in poultry raising. Soon 85% of the cattle feed used in the United States had this synthetic estrogen as a feed supplement to enhance growth. In 1973 residues of DES were found in beef; almost as soon as the FDA banned its use, attempts to have the ban lifted began in the courts.

In March 1977 spirited controversy arose in the United States concerning the potential threat to health from incidental addition to potentially carcinogenic chemicals from plastic soft-drink bottles and intentional use of saccharin, the only remaining FDA-approved artificial sweetener since the 7-year-old cyclamate ban. The possibility of an FDA ban on production and use of both of these products raised a great outcry. The bottle manufacturers claimed that under the physical conditions in which the bottles would normally be used there is no danger of toxic contamination of the bottle contents. Within 1 week after the ban on saccharin was announced, vehement public outrage spurred the introduction of several bills in the Congress either to repeal the Delaney amendment outright or to write detailed standards for the FDA to follow so that results of tests announced from individual laboratories might be assessed in a more reasonable manner. The fact that to be subjected to a quantity of saccharin such as that which produced bladder cancer in rats in the recent Canadian study would require the consumption of 800 cans of diet soda daily suggested that more specific guidelines are necessary for the FDA than the Delaney amendment provided.

Consumer stockpiling of saccharin-sweetened products rapidly emptied supermarket shelves following the announcement of the ban, and public reaction indicated the real possibility of bootleg production of diet soda and black-market distribution of other saccharin-sweetened products. The economic implications of this type of ban on various industries that would result in this one case along if the proposed July 1, 1977, ban went into effect was well illustrated by the threatened shutdown of plastic-bottle manufacturing plants, soft-drink bottling plants, and saccharin production and distribution firms. Diet-soft-drink sales of $1.5 billion yearly represent 15% (the fastest growing segment) of the total United States soft-drink market. This example points up the enormous complexity of the problems underlying the entire question of "internal pollution," which is only beginning to emerge as an issue in national and international seminars and symposia. It is difficult to assess the effects of increasing industrial and agribusiness use of synthetic chemicals on our food supply, for the harm to health may be subtle or may show up only in generations to come.

The dilemmas raised by the use of pesticides and

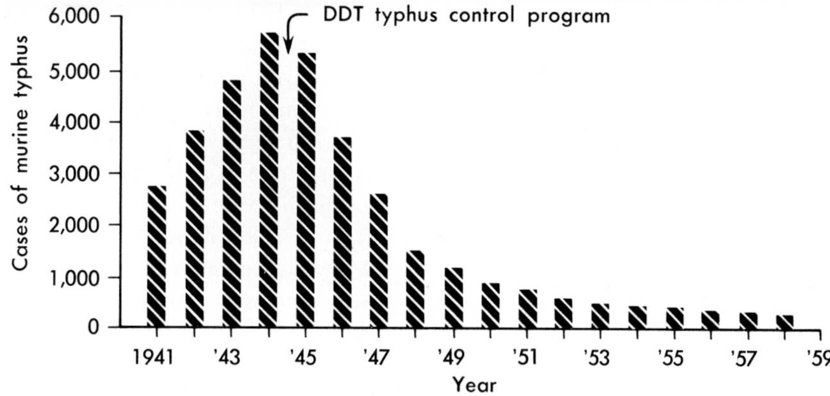

Fig. 5-26. Impact of control programs. Effect of DDT on incidence of typhus. (Redrawn from Bernarde, M. A.: Our precarious habitat, New York, 1970, W. W. Norton & Co., Inc.)

their possible incidental addition of potentially harmful chemicals to the food supply are of the same nature. Danger of acute exposure has often been thought to be limited to very few persons: spray pilots, insecticide producers, and greenhouse personnel. Recently, however, the migrant workers who pick the crops have been agitating for improved working conditions, including more protection from insecticides and herbicides. In addition to direct effects, the potential dangers of low-level exposure over long periods must be considered. All of the hazards must be weighed against the benefits to health (Fig. 5-26) and the enormous rise in global food productivity that have been made possible. Such increases in food production are essential if we are to achieve the projected increases in total food supply needed just to maintain present diet levels: a 50% increase by 1985 and a 75% increase by the year 2000. This is just one more example of the complexity of every problem that involves some trade-off between adverse effects to environment and health and the increased productivity necessitated by rising population numbers.

Exposure to lead and mercury poisoning has attracted much attention. Incidences of lead poisoning from paints ingested by children begin to rise in spring and peak in July and August. It is thought that this seasonal pattern arises because increased temperature and ultraviolet light are thought to act on old paint chips and result in increased intestinal absorption of lead. Evidence of severe damage to the nervous system has been seen among many employees of an industrial complex in Japan where industrial wastes loaded with mercury were discharged into the water and underwent magnification through the food chain. No amount of financial settlement by the industry involved can ever reverse the misery of the weakened, grotesquely deformed victims of Minamata disease. It has been suggested that several other metals, such as cadmium, vanadium, and beryllium, might be implicated in disease, and although the extent and effects of exposure to these and many other suspected materials may not be known for some time, there is certainly reason for caution.

Chemicals added by those wishing to market nearly spoiled goods are called "malicious" additives; these may be dangerous particularly because of the concentrations in which they are often used.

People can survive for weeks without food and for

Table 5-4. Deaths during acute episodes of air pollution*

Date	Place	Sulfur dioxide value—peak (ppm)	Mortality
Feb. 1880	London	—	1,000
Dec. 1930	Meuse Valley	9.6-38.4†	63
Oct. 1948	Donora	2.0	17‡
Dec. 1952	London	1.47	4,000
Jan. 1956	London	—	1,000
Dec. 1957	London	—	700-800
Dec. 1962	London	Same as 1952	700
Nov. 1953	New York	0.86	200
Jan.-Feb. 1963	New York	0.40-1.50	200-400
Nov. 1966	New York	0.69-0.97-1.02	168

*From Battigelli. M. C.: Sulfur dioxide and acute effects of air pollution. Paper presented at the Air Quality Criteria Symposium, New York, June 4-5, 1968.

†Assumed retrospectively.

‡These deaths are usually counted in the literature as 20. Actually, only 19 occurred during the week, and two deaths were the usual expected per week.

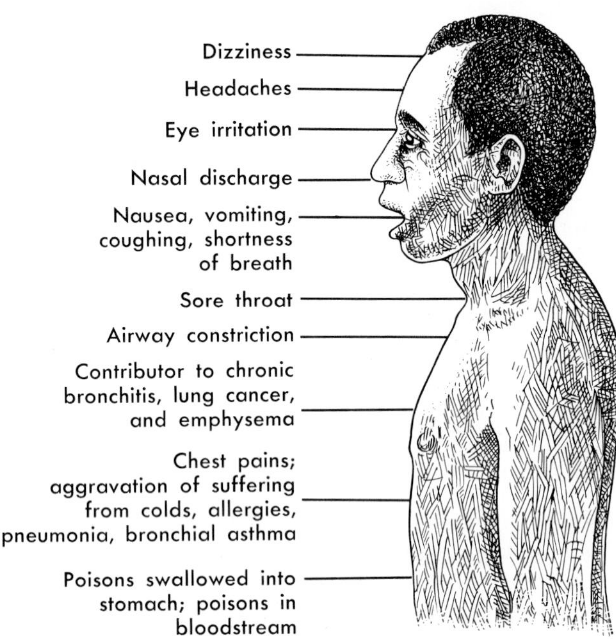

Fig. 5-27. Some possible effects of air pollution on human body. (From Living in the environment: concepts, problems, and alternatives by Miller, G. T., Jr. Copyright © 1975 by Wadsworth Publishing Co., Inc., Belmont, Calif. Reprinted by permission of the publisher.)

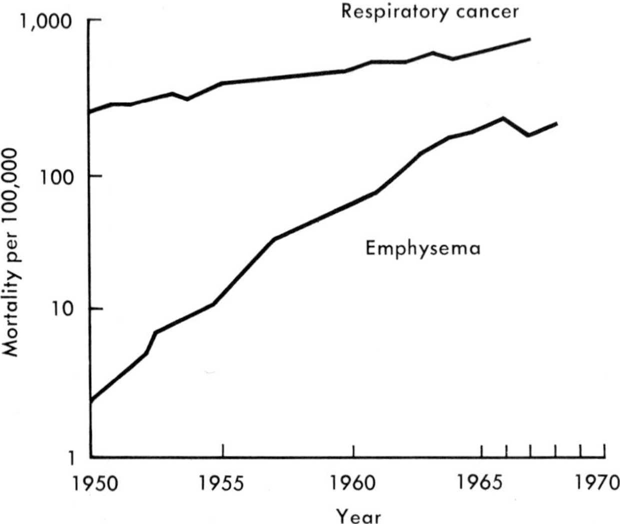

Fig. 5-28. Trends in respiratory cancer and emphysema in California. (After K. E. F. Watt; from Biology and society by Ehrlich, P. R., et al. Copyright 1976, McGraw-Hill Book Company, New York. Used with permission of the publisher.)

about 5 days without water, but we cannot survive even 5 minutes without air. Perhaps this is why the adverse effects of air pollution on health and comfort (Fig. 5-27) and on property first generated more public concern and research activity than any other type of pollution. A major piece of evidence of the health implications of air pollution came in 1930 when the Meuse Valley in Belgium was blanketed by a heavy smog and 63 persons died as a result of the dense layer of fog and smog that hung low and bottled up comtaminants for nearly 4 days. Similar weather conditions occurred in 1948 in Donora, Pennsylvania, where almost half of the city's 14,000 residents were seized by fits of coughing and vomiting; 19 persons died, 17 more than the average number of deaths a week in this small town. Several other acute episodes of this type (Table 5-4) have made public health officials very aware that although it is usually impossible to implicate a particular component of polluted air as causative, there is no doubt that air pollution can kill and disable people and that the effects could easily become a great deal more widespread. To date there have been no acute air-pollution episodes resulting from the ozone-rich Los Angeles type of smog that have resulted in recorded fatalities. However, the irritating effects on mucous membranes, the reduced visibility and increased ozone concentrations, and the observed trends in respiratory cancer and emphysema (Fig. 5-28) that are constant experiences of inhabitants of these regions, along with the damage to plants and to residential and industrial properties, make a strong economic case for air-pollution abatement before a deadly disaster occurs.

It is not simply a case of mustering the scientific and medical personnel needed to analyze the potential health effects of each component of polluted air; even if this nearly impossible task could be accomplished, it would not provide a solution. The constituents of polluted air are very complex and are constantly varying in concentration. They have the potential for additive, synergistic action among themselves, and in addition their effects may be related to many other factors such as climate and age, occupation, and state of health of those exposed and whether they are habitual smokers. That synergistic action is significant in the prevalance of chronic bronchitis is clear from Fig. 5-29. It is important to realize that acute exposures such as those indicated in Table 5-4 may be a much less serious health threat than continuous exposure to low-level but cumulative contaminants that may produce or aggravate chronic disease conditions. These possibly hasten the degenerative conditions that are characteristic of aging in various organs and tissues.

In the *Proceedings of the U.S. Technical Conference on Air Pollution* published in 1952 each and every paper on health aspects indicated that although there seemed

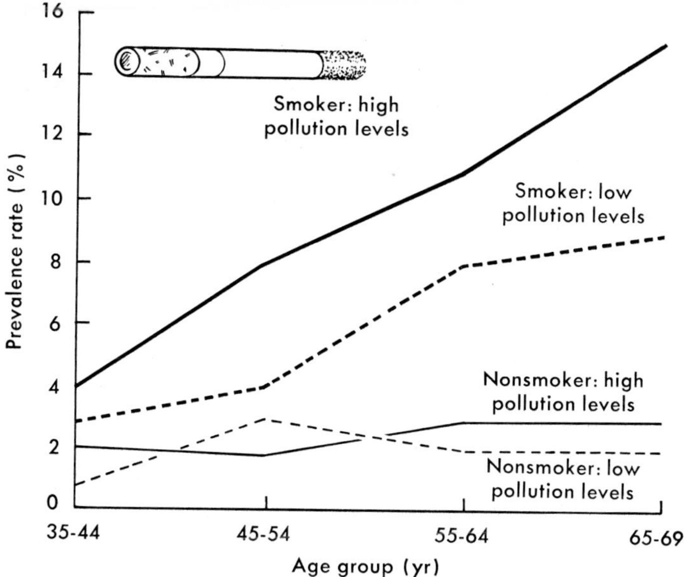

Fig. 5-29. Air pollution and smoking may increase bronchitis separately or they may interact synergistically so that their net effect is greater than sum of their separate effects. (After Lambert and Reid, 1970; from Living in the environment: concepts, problems, and alternatives by Miller, G. T., Jr. Copyright © 1975 by Wadsworth Publishing Co., Inc., Belmont, Calif. Reprinted by permission of the publisher.)

to be a relationship between polluted air and incidence of bronchitis and lung cancer, there had been no clear causal relation demonstrated between any specific air pollutant and chronic disease. By 1961, in a symposium at the University of California School of Medicine, the following was recognized:

> Most of the major medical problems today are not episodic, at least etiologically. Cancer, heart disease and of course the host of degenerative diseases of old age have their roots far back in the life history of the patient. In order to understand these diseases we are learning, slowly, to think of medicine not in terms of organs and diseases, but in terms of interactions in time. We are approaching an ecologic conception of medicine, a conception which emphasizes environment and interaction, to understand the process of life as processes. . . .*

By 1973 air pollution was assumed to be damaging to health in spite of the lack of hard scientific data that would implicate specific pollutants, with a few exceptions such as those determined as causative factors in lung cancer in smokers. The extent of the effects observed is evident in the report of the Council on Environmental Quality, which projected damage, avoidance, transaction, and abatement costs for environmental pollutants. That damage to health is one of the most significant components of estimated damage costs is illustrated in Table 5-5. The costs, which cannot be projected in dollars, suggest the magnitude and complexity of the problem as indicated in the report:

> Many types of environmental damage will create both tangible and intangible costs. By damaging health, air pollution affects tangible resources by causing lost production and by consuming equipment, supplies, and the time of highly skilled manpower required to restore good health. The illness, as well as the threatened loss of in-

*From Farber, M., and Wilson, R. H. L., editors. The air we breathe, Springfield, Ill., 1961. Charles C Thomas, Publisher.

Table 5-5. Estimated national air pollution damage costs with no pollution control, 1968 and 1977 (in billions of dollars)*

Damage class	1968†	1977‡
Health	6.1	9.3
Residential property	5.2	8.0
Materials and vegetation	4.9	7.6
Total	16.2	24.9

*From The economics of clean air, Senate Document No. 92-67. Washington, D.C., 1972, U.S. Government Printing Office.
†In 1968 dollars.
‡In 1970 dollars.

Table 5-6. Common noise levels*

Examples	Decibels (dbA)	Relative sound intensity	Effect with prolonged exposure
Jet takeoff (close range)	150	1,000,000,000,000,000	Eardrum ruptures
Aircraft carrier deck	140	100,000,000,000,000	
Armored personnel carrier	130	10,000,000,000,000	
Thunderclap, jet takeoff (200 feet)	120	1,000,000,000,000	Human pain threshold
Steel mill, live rock music, riveting, auto horn (3 feet)	110	100,000,000,000	
Jet at 1,000 feet, subway, outboard motor, power mower, motorcycle (25 feet), farm tractor, printing plant, jackhammer, blender	100	10,000,000,000	Serious hearing damage (8 hours)
Busy urban street, diesel truck	90	1,000,000,000	Hearing damage (8 hours)
Garbage disposal, clothes washer, average factory, freight train (50 feet), noisy office, dishwasher	80	100,000,000	
Freeway traffic (50 feet), vacuum cleaner	70	10,000,000	Annoying
Conversation in restaurant, typical suburb	60	1,000,000	Intrusive
Quiet suburb (daytime), conversation in living room	50	100,000	Quiet
Library	40	10,000	
Quiet rural area (nighttime)	30	1,000	
Whisper, rustling leaves	20	100	Very quiet
Breathing	10	10	
	0	1	Threshold of audibility

*From Living in the environment: concepts, problems, and alternatives by Miller, G. T., Jr. Copyright © 1975 by Wadsworth Publishing Co., Inc., Belmont, Calif. Reprinted by permission of the publisher.

> come security, may also arouse anxiety and fear in the individual and his family and friends. These are some of the psychic costs of air pollution—costs that are rarely included in damage estimates.
>
> Although probably comprising a significant portion of total damage costs, psychic costs, unfortunately, cannot be accurately quantified. Further, they change over time. Opinion surveys indicate that the degree of concern about such problems as air and water pollution has increased substantially in less than a decade . . . . In the past, people were less aware of the extent and dangers of environmental degradation and had less interest in the amenities offered by a clean environment. Even as we improve our environment, the psychic costs may be higher than before because of this heightened concern.*

In reference to this "psychic cost," perhaps one of the most ignored types of pollution is noise. As can be seen from Table 5-6, urban living imposes a burden on the human ear that often exceeds mere annoyance and causes serious impairment of hearing. A realization of the extent of this potential damage should force us to examine with great care the projected increased use of supersonic jet aircraft, a consideration that at present has enormous implications for international relations. The importance of pointing out to young people the extent of the permanent damage that their highly amplified music may be causing is obvious, as is the duty of industry to safeguard the hearing of all who work in noisy surroundings (see Chapter 38).

Even a partial cataloging of substances suggested to be associated with various diseases is not possible in this brief chapter, for we would have to consider many types of materials, both chemicals and particulates; nitrogen and sulfur-containing chemicals; particulates such as soot, asphalt, rubber, and asbestos; gases such as hydrogen sulfide, chlorine, and fluorine; heavy metals such as cadmium, vanadium, and lead; and many others.

*From Council on Environmental Quality: Fourth annual report on environmental quality, Washington, D.C., 1973, U.S. Government Printing Office.

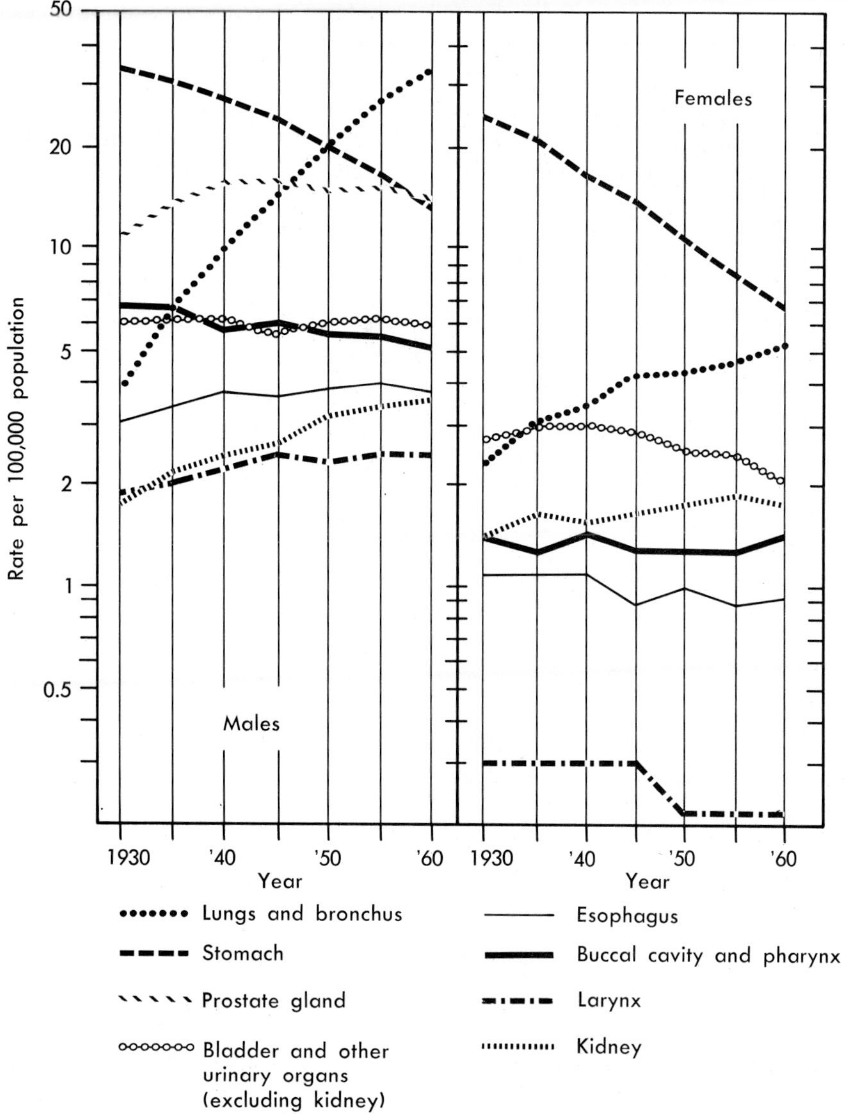

Fig. 5-30. Trends in age-adjusted mortality for selected cancer sites by sex in United States, 1930 to 1960. (Data from U.S. Department of Health, Education and Welfare, Public Health Service: Smoking and health, Washington, D.C., 1964, U.S. Government Printing Office.)

It is interesting and somewhat alarming to note that what is perhaps the most definitive report of cause-effect relationships between pollutants and specific diseases, the Surgeon General's report *Smoking and Health,* has not produced any lasting reduction in smoking in the United States. This indication of attitude is particularly significant if we consider that it has been estimated in a report to the Muskie Subcommittee on Air and Water Pollution in 1968 that persons breathing the air of the average large city probably receive at least as much carcinogens as if they smoked one pack of cigarettes a day. In heavily polluted areas the risk of simply breathing may produce an accumulation of known carcinogens equal to that of inhaling two packs of cigarettes daily. The gravity of the situation for the urban smoker should be obvious.

Reports, even in the late 1950s, indicated that epidemiologic studies revealed a worldwide increase in the prevalence of lung cancer, with a greater incidence in males and urban residents and especially in those with a history of prolonged or excessive cigarette smoking. Thus urban air alone was associated with an increased risk of developing lung cancer. This rise in lung cancer was described to the Muskie Subcommittee as "a dramatic increase . . . now approaching epidemic proportions." The dramatic nature of the increase is evident in Fig. 5-30, which clearly illustrates the summary of the report: "Cigarette smoking is causally related to lung cancer in men; the magnitude of the effect of cigarette smoking far outweighs all other factors. The data for women, though less extensive, point in the same direction."[63] Among the other findings summarized were the establishment that "cigarette smoking is the most important of the causes of chronic bronchitis in the United States and increases the risk of dying from chronic

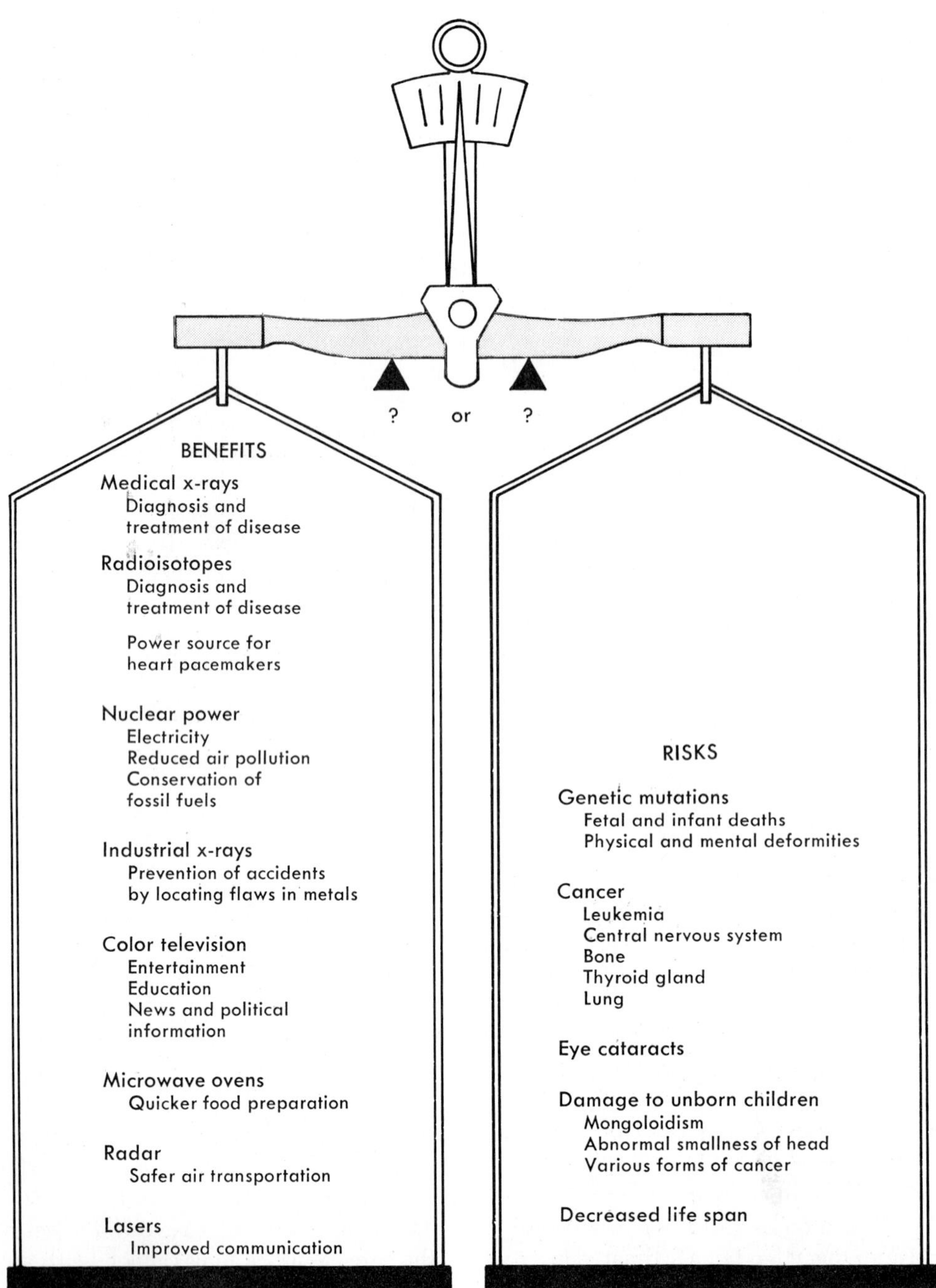

Fig. 5-31. Benefits versus risks of exposure to man-made sources of radiation. (From Living in the environment: concepts, problems, and alternatives by Miller, G. T., Jr. Copyright © 1975 by Wadsworth Publishing Co., Inc., Belmont, Calif. Reprinted by permission of the publisher.)

bronchitis." A correlation was definitely found between pulmonary emphysema and cigarette smoking, but the facts did not definitely implicate smoking as causal. That cigarette smoking is a "significant factor in the causation of laryngeal cancer in the male" and associated with cancer of the esophagus and urinary bladder also can be seen in Fig. 5-30. No relationship was established between cigarette smoking and stomach cancer.

Among the other conditions though to be aggravated are ulcers, the association being greater for gastric than for duodenal ulcer, and pulmonary emphysema. For all of these conditions, as well as for cirrhosis of the liver, increased mortality of smokers has been shown in the seven prospective studies that were carried out on 1,123,000 men. These studies have shown clearly that cigarette smoking, besides causing lung cancer and chronic bronchitis, at least predisposes to or aggravates a large number of the degenerative conditions that are the major causes of death in industrialized, economically affluent regions.

One of the most potent of all the carcinogens now known is benzopyrene. It has been shown to be one of the two most potent of the seven carcinogens listed. Since 1933 it was known to be the coal tar constituent that evoked skin cancer when applied to the skin of mice. The particular significance of this single finding is that benzopyrene is one of the gaseous hydrocarbons found in automobile emissions and thus reaches high concentrations in urban air. The concentration in cities such as New York, Chicago, and Los Angeles has been reported to be as much as 50 million times that of Grand Canyon National Park.

A recent report by the genetic study section of the National Institutes of Health suggests that the danger of birth defects from airborne chemicals may dwarf even the well-documented dangers of radiation. Since the effects of air contaminants may be much less acute than those of radiation, the danger may be even greater because the increased mutation rates might spread over many generations and include ill-defined abnormalities such as subtly increasing aging and susceptibility to diseases such as leukemia and cancer. It is significant to note in this regard that benzopyrene has been shown to produce many malformations in mice. Although knowledge of chemical mutagenesis and teratogenesis in humans is much less certain than that of radiation, a number of chemicals have been discovered that are known to induce genetic or teratogenic effects in some organisms.

It is outside the scope of this brief chapter to consider in any detail the well-documented genetic and somatic hazards of long-term exposure to low-level ionizing radiation. Somatic effects involve mostly the induction of cancer. Whether there is a threshold below which exposure to radioactivity has no somatic effects has been a major uncertainty. If the relationship between exposure and cancer induction can be extrapolated back to the very light exposure to which the general population could be subjected under current radiation standards, an impressive number of deaths would be attributable to radiation if the maximum permissible levels were reached for everyone. It is not likely that we will reach such levels from reaction operation, but the problem of disposing of the enormous increases of radioactive wastes for thousands of years presents hazards of a social and political nature.

In Fig. 5-31 the question marks suggest (as they do in so many other environmental risk-benefit considerations) that the current state of our knowledge is still very limited as we strive to determine whether we may have to sacrifice some of these benefits in favor of improved health for ourselves and those who will come after us.

The fundamental causes of environmental problems, as we have seen, are in the psychosocial and technologic spheres. In the final analysis it is political, economic, and social humankind who will determine whether to pay the price required to restore the biosphere to homeostasis. The choice is in our hands. The implications of the problem that postindustrial humanity faces are indicated in Fig. 5-32. This relationship has been experienced by many Americans in recent years in the increased cost of

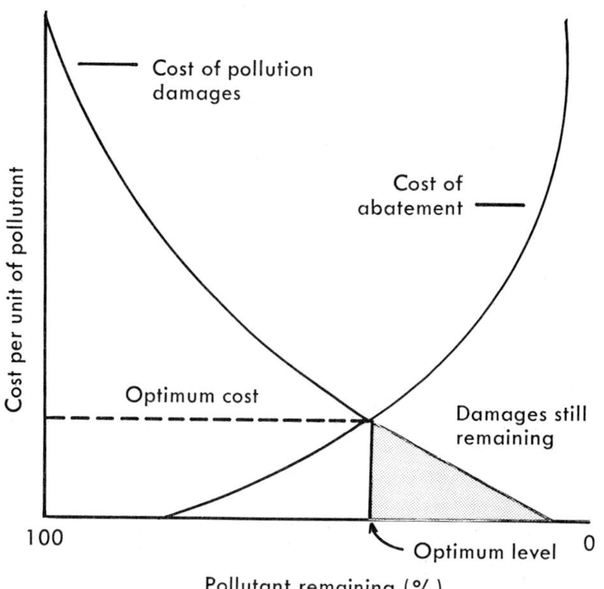

Fig. 5-32. Balancing pollution damages and pollution costs. Shaded area shows that some damages remain, but removing these residual damages would raise pollution abatement costs to prohibitive levels. (From Living in the environment: concepts, problems, and alternatives by Miller, G. T., Jr. Copyright © 1975 by Wadsworth Publishing Co., Inc., Belmont, Calif. Reprinted by permission of the publisher.)

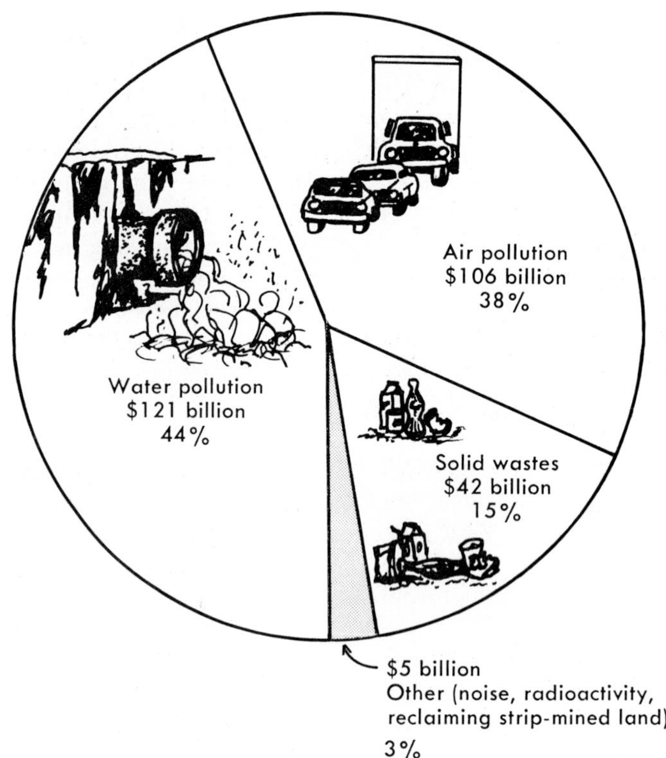

Fig. 5-33. Estimated amount of private and federal spending needed for environmental protection between 1972 and 1982. (Data from Council on Environmental Quality, 1973. From Living in the environment: concepts, problems, and alternatives by Miller, G. T., Jr. Copyright © 1975 by Wadsworth Publishing Co., Inc., Belmont, Calif. Reprinted by permission of the publisher.)

automobiles because of all the pollution-control devices introduced to comply with the Clean Air Act. The shaded area reminds us that our affluent life style will probably always have some degree of adverse effect on human living. In Fig. 5-33 we can get some idea of the actual magnitude of that cost, and even this enormous expenditure will result in meeting standards for air, water, and soil quality that are far from ideal according to many biologists. The choice of "how clean" is sure to be one of the most controversial questions of the next decade.

REFERENCES AND SELECTED READINGS

1. American Chemical Society: Cleaning our environment: the chemical basis for action, Washington, D.C., 1969, The Society.
2. *Arther, D. K.: Man and his environment, New York, 1969, American Elsevier Publishing Co., Inc.
3. *Barbour, I. G., editor: Western man and environmental ethics, Reading, Mass., 1973, Addison-Wesley Publishing Co., Inc.
4. Beranek, L.: Noise, Sci. Am. **215**:66-76, 1966.
5. *Bernarde, M. A.: Our precarious habitat, New York, 1979, W. W. Norton & Co., Inc.

*References preceded by an asterisk are particularly well suited for student reading.

6. *Blau, S. D., and Rodenbeck, J. von B.: The house we live in, New York, 1971, Macmillan, Inc.
7. *Bookchin, M.: Our synthetic environment, New York, 1974, Harper & Row, Publishers, Colophon Books.
8. Boughey, A. S.: Ecology of populations, New York, 1968, Macmillan, Inc.
9. Cailliet, G., et al.: Everyman's guide to ecological living, New York, 1971, Macmillan, Inc.
10. Carson, R: Silent spring, Boston, 1962, Houghton Mifflin Co.
11. Chute, R. M.: Environmental insight, New York, 1971, Harper & Row, Publishers.
12. *Clark, J.: Thermal pollution, Sci. Am. **220**:18-27, 1969.
13. Colinvaux, P. A.: Introduction to ecology, New York, 1973, John Wiley & Sons, Inc.
14. *Commoner, B.: The closing circle: nature, man and technology, New York, 1971, Alfred A. Knopf, Inc.
15. Commoner, B.: Science and survival, New York, 1966, The Viking Press, Inc.
16. Council on Environmental Quality: Fourth annual report on environmental quality. Washington D.C., 1973, U.S. Government Printing Office.
17. *Curtis, R., and Hogan, E.: Perils of the peaceful atom, New York, 1970, Doubleday & Co., Inc.
18. Dansereau, P.: Challenge for survival: land, air, and water for man in megalopolis, New York, 1970, Columbia University Press.
19. Dasmann, R. F.: Man and the biosphere: a challenge for UN-

ESCO in a new international program, Washington D.C., 1970, The Conservation Foundation.
20. DeBell, G., editor: The environmental handbook, New York, 1970, Ballantine Books, Inc.
21. *Deevey, E. S.: The human population, Sci. Am. **203**:194-204, 1960.
22. Detwyler, T. R.: Man's impact on environment, McGraw-Hill series in geography, New York, 1971, McGraw-Hill Book Co.
23. Dubos, R.: So human an animal, New York, 1968, Charles Scribner's Sons.
24. Dubos, R.: The mirage of health, New York, 1961, Doubleday & Co. Inc.
25. Ehrlich, P. R., and Ehrlich, A. H.: Population, resources, and environment: issues in human ecology, San Francisco, 1970, W. H. Freeman and Co., Publishers.
26. *Ehrlich, P. R., Holm, R. W., and Brown, I. R.: Biology and society, New York, 1976, McGraw-Hill Book Co.
27. Fabun, D.: The dynamics of change, Englewood Cliffs, N. J., 1970, Prentice-Hall, Inc.
28. Frakes, G. E., and Salberg, S. B.: Pollution papers, New York, 1971, Appleton-Century-Crofts.
29. Galbraith, J. K.: The affluent society, Boston, 1958, Houghton Mifflin Co.
30. *Handler, P., editor: Biology and the future of man, London, 1970, Oxford University Press, Inc.
31. Hanks, T. G.: Solid waste–disease relationships, Washington D.C., 1967, U.S. Department of Health, Education and Welfare.
32. Helfrich, H. W., Jr., editor: The environmental crisis, New Haven, Conn., 1970, Yale University Press.
33. *Holt, S. J.: The food resources of the world, Sci. Am. **221**:180-194, 1969.
34. *Hulett, H. R.: Optimum world population, Bioscience **20**:160-161, 1970.
35. Humphrey, C. C., and Evans, R. G.: What's ecology, Northbrook, Ill., 1971, Hubbard Press.
36. *Hutchinson, G. E.: The biosphere, Sci. Am. **223**:44-58, 1970
37. *Johnson, H. D.: No deposit—no return, Reading, Mass., 1970, Addison-Wesley Publishing Co., Inc.
38. Kahn, H., et al.: The year 2000, New York, 1967, Macmillan, Inc.
39. Kormondy, E. J.: Concepts of ecology, Englewood Cliffs, N. J., 1969, Prentice-Hall, Inc.
40. *Lucas, J.: Our polluted food, New York, 1974, John Wiley & Sons, Inc.
41. Marquis R. W., editor: Environmental improvement (air, water, and soil), Washington D.C., 1966, U.S. Department of Agriculture.
42. Marx, W.: Man and his environment: waste, New York, 1971, Harper & Row, Publishers.
43. Matthews, W. H., et al., editors: Man's impact on terrestrial and oceanic ecosystems, Cambridge, Mass, 1971, The M.I.T. Press.
44. McCabe, L. C.: Air pollution, Proceedings of the U.S. Technical Conference on Air Pollution, New York, 1952, McGraw-Hill Book Co.
45. *McDermott, W.: Air pollution and public health, Sci. Am. **205**:49-57, 1961
46. *McHale, J.: World facts and trends, ed. 2, New York, 1972, Macmillan, Inc.
47. McHarg, I.: Design with nature, New York, 1969, Natural History Press.
48. Miller, G. T.: Living in the environment: concepts, problems, alternatives, Belmont, Calif., 1975, Wadsworth Publishing Co. Inc.
49. Mumford, L.: The myth of the machine, New York, 1967, Harcourt Brace Jovanovich, Inc.
50. Murphy, E. F.: Man and his environment: law, New York, 1971, Harper & Row, Publishers.
51. National Association of Science–National Research Council: Rapid population growth, Baltimore, 1971, The Johns Hopkins University Press.
52. National Association of Science–National Research Council: Resources and man: a study and recommendation, San Francisco, 1969, W. H. Freeman and Co. Publishers.
53. Novick, S.: The careless atom, Boston, 1969, Houghton Mifflin Co.
54. *Odum, E. P.: Fundamentals of ecology, ed. 2, Philadelphia, 1959, W. B. Saunders Co.
55. Packard, V.: The waste makers, New York, 1964, Pocket Books.
56. Proceedings of the Symposium on Recent Advances in the Assessment of the Health Effects of Environmental Pollution, vol IV, Paris, 1974, Commission of the European Communities, U.S. Environmental Protection Agency, World Health Organization, pp. 2465-2466.
57. Shepard, P., and McKinley, D., editors: The subversive science, Boston, 1968, Houghton Mifflin Co.
58. Smith, G., and Smyth, J. C., editors: The biology of affluence, Edinburgh, 1972, Oliver & Boyd, Ltd.
59. Teilhard de Chardin, P: The future of man, New York, 1964, Harper & Row, Publishers.
60. Toynbee, A.: Surviving the future, New York, 1971, Oxford University Press, Inc.
61. *Tullar, R. M.: The human species, New York, 1977, McGraw-Hill Book Co.
62. *Turk, A., et al.: Ecology, pollution, environment, Philadelphia, 1972, W. B. Saunders Co.
63. U.S. Department of Health, Education and Welfare, Public Health Service: Smoking and health, Washington D.C., 1964, U.S. Government Printing Office.
64. *U.S. Department of Health, Education and Welfare, Environmental Health Service/Public Health Service: Environmental health problems, Washington D.C., 1970, U.S. Government Printing Office.
65. *U.S. Department of Interior: Man . . . an endangered species? Conservation yearbook no. 4, Washington D.C., 1968, U.S. Government Printing Office.
66. U.S. Public Health Service: Today and tomorrow in air pollution, Publ. no. 1555, Washington D.C., 1966, U.S. Government Printing Office.
67. Waldbott, G. L.: Health effects of environmental pollutants, ed. 2, St. Louis, 1978, The C. V. Mosby Co.
68. Williams, J. S., and et al.: Environmental pollution and mental health, Washington D.C., 1973, Information Resources Press.
69. *Woodwell, G. N., Toxic substances and ecological cycles, Sci. Am. **216**: 24-31, 1967
70. World Health Organization: Health Hazards of the human environment, Geneva, 1972, The Organization.
71. World Health Organization: Global environmental health monitoring, Geneva, 1970, The Organization.
72. World Health Organization: WHO Stat. Rep. **22**:448-476, 1969.

6

An epidemiologic approach to health care

BRENDA MARTIN MORGAN

Epidemiology is the study of the occurrence, distribution, and determinants of health conditions in human populations. This general definition adequately describes the two principal ways that most epidemiologists and others who use the concepts of epidemiology view this field. Epidemiology describes both the methods needed to investigate health conditions for groups of people and a body of theory and knowledge necessary to understand the information derived using those methods.

■ EVOLUTION OF EPIDEMIOLOGY

Epidemiologists investigate, define, and describe the occurrence of specific health and illness states. When carrying out these functions, epidemiologists often depend on other professionals to aid them in the definition of the existence of particular conditions. They seek out microbiologists to confirm the presence of microorganisms, physicians for diagnosis of illness, pharmacologists and biochemists to determine levels of drugs or chemicals within the body or in the environment, nurses for evaluation of health status and health care delivery, psychologists for definitions of behavior, and sociologists to describe family, group, or community characteristics. In addition epidemiologists identify such facts as age, sex, race, and circumstances of residence for those people who experience a common condition. In many studies differences in these variables are noted between those people who experience the condition and those who do not. A full description of the occurrence of any specific health or illness state is the first step in understanding the factors that contribute to its occurrence and may eventually lead to prevention or promotion of its future occurrence.

Although describing the occurrence of health and illness conditions and the multiple and perhaps unique circumstances surrounding these occurrences is important, the task is not completed until *meaning* is assigned to the descriptive information. For example, to say that one group of people experiences 50% fewer fatal automobile accidents than another without also including the knowledge that the driving habits of the group with less fatalities includes use of seatbelts more often than the other group and that this greatly affected the fatality rate of this group would make the initial descriptive statement inaccurate and nearly useless. It is necessary to collect the significant data surrounding a particular event, to identify what specific elements of the situation are associated with the occurrence of the event, and then to discuss whether there is a causal relationship between these factors. The epidemiologic approach to study defines what event has happened to whom and under what circumstances, why the event happened, what the likelihood is of it happening again, and how and what intervention may encourage or discourage this event or a similar one in the future.

With the advance of scientific and medical knowledge the scope of epidemiologic study has moved from "epidemics" of infectious disease to "epidemics" of noninfectious disease and other health conditions. The existence of disease in humans has been noted, recorded, and hypothesized about for a long time by many people from many points of view. Just exactly when the systematic use of scientific inquiry into disease causes and cures became epidemiology is not agreed on, but the subject that was under study is known: the widespread existence of infectious diseases that plagued people wherever they lived.

Several hundred years ago a few people began to suggest that some diseases could be passed from one person to another or that persons coming into contact with certain geographic areas or "bad water" would become ill. Later, even before bacteria or viruses had been discovered, laws were written to keep diseased persons from traveling to areas where disease had not spread. At the same time some writers began to describe the circumstances around the disease epidemics, putting forth the conclusions that the occurrences were not just random, but that there were patterns to disease development. It was observed that not everyone became ill, that some who became ill did not die, and that those who had had a particular disease at one time were likely not to get the disease again (the beginning of the idea of immunity). Progress in the understanding of disease during the eighteenth and nineteenth centuries was impressive, although the concept of contagion was not universally accepted until bacteria were isolated and identified using the microscope.

THEORIES OF SINGLE AND MULTIPLE CAUSALITY

With the study of infectious diseases the evolution of disease causality began. At first, manipulation of the environment became an important part of disease control. It became apparent that careful handling of food and waste water, keeping drinking water free of waste contamination, and isolating contaminants and ill people resulted in less disease occurrence. Later, the development of the ability to immunize against disease increased greatly the possibilities of controlling diseases. The great force behind the movements of environmental control and development of immunizations was the image of the *dangerous agent:* if the agent were controlled, the problem would be solved. The overwhelming success of this theory in improving the health of large populations has firmly implanted the idea of *single causality,* or the germ theory of disease: for any disease there is a cause; if one finds that cause, the disease can be controlled.

After many years of observing infectious diseases, two conclusions began to emerge: (1) that germs are immensely resourceful, for no sooner was one controlled than another appeared, and (2) the germ, though a necessary condition for infectious disease, was not sufficient to cause that disease. Investigators recognized that although specific microorganisms caused disease, other factors needed to be present. These were virulent organisms, a susceptible host, and a means by which the organisms could be transmitted to the host. Fig. 6-1 illustrates the widely held theory of transmission of infectious disease. If any point of the cycle was interrupted, control of the disease was possible. When people began to recognize that several factors had to be present before some diseases were manifested, the theory of *multiple causality* began to evolve.

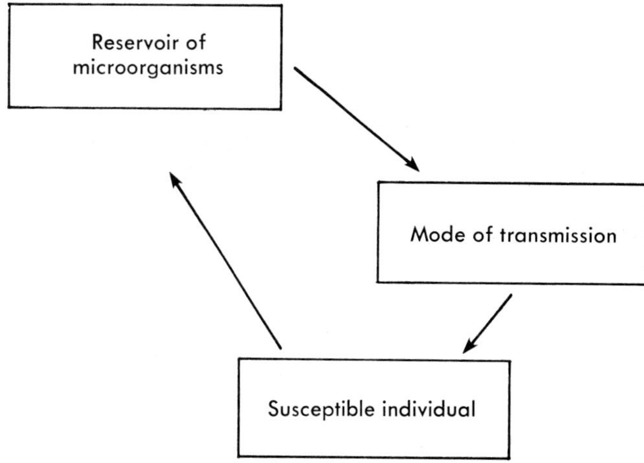

Fig. 6-1. Basic components of infectious disease model. Reservoir of organisms, mode of transmission, and susceptible individual were once thought to be sufficient for causation of disease.

The infectious disease model generally describes a direct cause-effect relationship between a single agent (microbe) and an outcome (disease). Studies of noninfectious diseases have concluded that this model is not helpful. The search for a single cause for heart disease or cancer or highway deaths has brought frustration, although the general population has found it hard to accept that a "cause" cannot be found for these and other current plagues of humans.

From the theory of single causality, scientific inquiry has moved to a theory of multiple causality: multiple agents working and interacting together to bring about most noninfectious diseases. To control these diseases many causes have to be identified and the way the causes work together defined. This situation results in a seemingly endless number of possibilities that must be carefully evaluated. In the future we may need to redefine some disease conditions taking into account findings of multiple causality.

Although there is much evidence to support the model of multiple causality, it has not entirely replaced the single-causality theory. It is important to recognize that for infectious disease control to have occurred, it was important that everyone believe in a single cause for disease. It still has applicability to the control of infectious diseases today. However, for health workers to look for "the reason" why people do not take their medication, why hypertension occurs, or why children are abused illustrates the failure to recognize that many social, psychologic, biologic, and environmental factors may contribute to their occurrence.

CURRENT EPIDEMIOLOGIC INQUIRY

With study of infectious disease the methods and knowledge of association and causality were developed and refined. Epidemiologic focus had been on the identification of physical, chemical, and microbial factors thought to be directly pathogenic to humans. Once these factors were seen to give only a partial explanation of the occurrence of some health problems, social, cultural, and psychologic factors were included as potential contributors to disease. Epidemiologic study now encompasses the physical, chemical, microbial, psychologic, and sociocultural environments of health and disease.

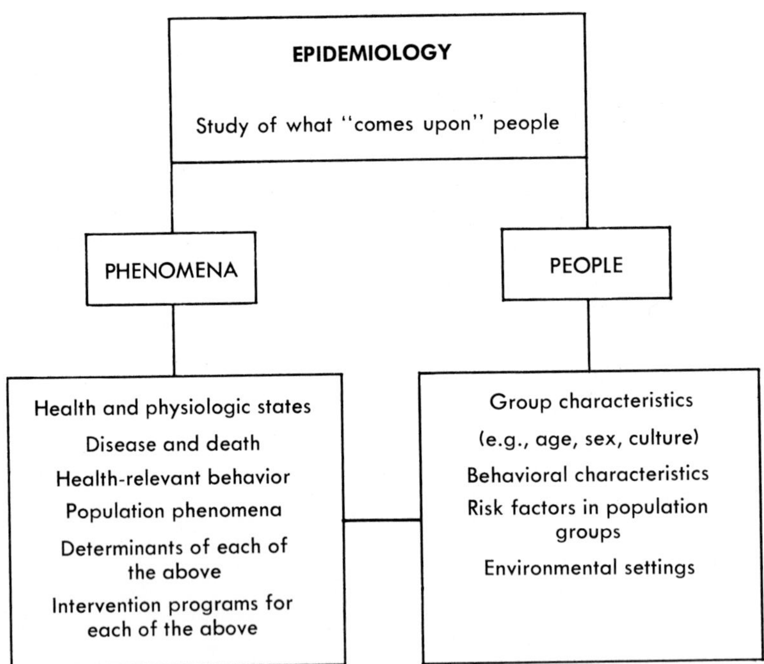

Fig. 6-2. Scope of epidemiology. (From Abdel R. Omran, editor, Community medicine in developing countries, p. 5. Copyright © 1974 by Springer Publishing Company, Inc., New York. Used by permission.)

Just as the study of disease determinants has expanded, so has the scope of disease entities that epidemiologic study considers. An accelerated pace of studying noninfectious diseases and general health conditions has occurred within the past three or four decades. At first, study involved diseases such as cancer, coronary heart disease, diabetes, and mental illness. Recently epidemiologists have studied such concerns as automobile accidents, overpopulation, street violence, compliance behavior, child growth and development, and the maintenance of health. It is not simple to define either what health is or what contributes to keeping people in a healthy state. As people have greater opportunities to live longer, the development of such measures becomes essential.

One of the major achievements of epidemiologic inquiry has been identifying factors in the human environment that influence health. The desirability of identifying cause-effect relationships is obvious. Once the relationships between cause and effect are defined, means to intervene can be developed. Epidemiologic concepts that can be used by health care providers in their practice and the application of these concepts to the practice of nursing are discussed later in this chapter.

□ Epidemiologic method

Epidemiologic knowledge and methods always involve groups of people, not individuals. At the same time epidemiologists always relate or seek to identify an experience *common* among these people. Fig. 6-2 is a simple illustration of the scope of epidemiology.

The epidemiologist looks for the commonalities of human experiences, the patterns by which certain health and illness conditions occur. The basic assumption continues to be that which was put forth a long time ago: health and illness do not occur randomly but occur as a result of identifiable forces acting in identificable circumstances to identifiable people. Although a great many of these factors are not yet identified, the search continues, and over time the identifiable patterns are emerging.

The search for patterns of health conditions usually starts with *identifying what conditions affect which groups of people.* It is important to note the relative importance of the conditions to the people, the frequency with which the conditions occur, whether this frequency is subject to sudden fluctuation or is fairly stable, and whether the conditions are widespread or localized to one group. The occurrence of sunburn in groups of sunbathers is important to the individuals concerned, but it is not an important event to the larger community. On the other hand, the occurrence of even one case of poliomyelitis in a community has relevance to the larger community because of concern that it might spread, especially if immunization levels are low.

Additional health patterns are determined by identifying the *characteristics of the people* within the groups who are most affected by the condition. The scope of these characteristics begins with the demographic data such as age, sex, and race of the affected persons and usually goes on to include a growing list of other characteristics such as personality type, family configuration or type, type of employment, social interaction, and cultural beliefs. Just as important in determining the sought-after patterns are identifying the same characteristics of the people within the groups who are *not* affected by the condition. Epidemiologic inquiry seeks to know why some people are affected and others are not when all are exposed to the same or similar set of circumstances.

After a period of study, hypotheses are usually generated concerning the relationship between certain characteristics of a group of people and the occurrence of a particular condition. Tests of these hypotheses determine their accuracy and general applicability to other groups of people. In addition potential interventions that might alter one or more of the factors identified as contributing to the condition are tested and evaluated. New knowledge of association and causation is thus gained for use by many practitioners.

☐ Epidemiologic terms

Whether one decides to use epidemiologic methods to study specific problems or only uses the findings of such studies, it is necessary to understand some of the terms most commonly involved. These terms have such widespread applicability that they are sometimes used to describe situations far removed from health:

population at risk a term applied to those persons having a common characteristic to whom an event could have happened, whether it did or not.

risk factor if the presence of a particular factor increases the likelihood of some event happening, then for that event the factor is a risk factor, and people with that factor are at high risk for the event.

relative risk the risk of an event occurring in the presence of a certain factor compared with its occurrence in the absence of that factor.

The following example illustrates several of the terms and concepts used in epidemiologic inquiry. A group of 40 people ate lunch, 20 of whom (group I) ate food contaminated with salmonella and 20 of whom (group II) ate uncontaminated food. Because of their common characteristic (risk factor) of eating the contaminated food, group I became a population at risk for developing a gastrointestinal disturbance. Of that group, five persons actually became ill. Of group II, one person also became ill after eating. To determine the relative risk of becoming ill following a lunch of contaminated food, it is helpful first to put the information in a 2 × 2 contingency table,

Ate contaminated food	Became ill: Yes	Became ill: No	Total
Yes (group 1)	5 (a)	15 (b)	20 (a + b)
No (group 2)	1 (c)	19 (d)	20 (c + d)
Total	6 (a + c)	34 (b + d)	40 (a + b + c + d)

Fig. 6-3. Data presentation in 2 × 2 table. Considering epidemiologic data in 2 × 2 table allows one to study association between two variables. Relative risk can be computed by comparing ratios between a/a + b and c/c + d.

as in Fig. 6-3. Such a table allows the association between two variables to be studied.

Once the table is constructed, relative risk can be computed following the formula:

$$\frac{a}{a+b} \div \frac{c}{c+d} \text{ or } \frac{5}{20} \div \frac{1}{20} = \frac{100}{20} = 5$$

In this situation the relative risk was 5, meaning those who ate contaminated food were at a risk of becoming ill five times greater than those who ate uncontaminated food.

Other commonly used concepts are:

rate a fraction made by dividing all the events that happened by all the population to whom the event could have happened and then connecting to a base denominator, such as 100, 1,000, or 100,000. Incidence and prevalence are commonly used rates.

incidence a measurement of only the *new* cases of a disease or other event during a given time period. Incidence rates have new cases as the numerator and the population at risk as the denominator. In the above example the incidence rate for illness after eating contaminated food was 25 per 100 (5/20).

prevalence a measurement of *all* (new and old) cases of disease or other events present at a given time. Prevalence rates are computed like incidence rates. In our example there were no old cases; therefore the prevalence rate was the same as the incidence rate.

association the relationship of events in some way that makes them appear together more often than they would by chance alone.

Our example showed that eating contaminated food was associated with becoming ill. (This could also be shown by means of statistical tests of association.) If we had not known that the food was contaminated but only that it came from restaurant A, we might have concluded that eating food from restaurant A was associated with becoming ill. Depending on our knowledge at the time, both associations were correct.

□ Epidemiologic designs

Epidemiologic method includes three general designs that are useful when studying groups of people. These are *cohort,* or *prospective,* studies; *case history,* or *retrospective,* studies; and *cross-sectional* studies. The particular problem to be studied, the circumstances surrounding the occurrence of the problem, and the resources available to the investigator all contribute to the decision as to which design to use. The final use to which the results of epidemiologic studies are put is largely determined by the design used.

Prospective studies

The cohort, or prospective, study is used to determine the relationship between a particular condition and a characteristic of the population, usually a relationship that the investigator has reason to suspect exists. The cohort study begins with a group of people who *do not have the condition* (lung cancer, for instance), *but some of whom have the characteristic* thought to be related to the development of the condition (cigarette smoking). For a period of time the cohort (the original group of people) is followed to determine how many develop cancer of the lung. The general form of this study design is illustrated in Fig. 6-4 using the example of lung cancer. A population free of lung cancer, composed of both smokers and nonsmokers, is followed for a period of time (probably years). At the end of that time all people who have developed lung cancer are identified, both smokers and nonsmokers. The data can be put in a 2 × 2 table such as Fig. 6-3. Incidence rates of lung cancer in smokers and nonsmokers, the relative risk of developing lung cancer for smokers versus nonsmokers, and the association between smoking and lung cancer can be computed.

The advantages of a prospective, or cohort, design are several. First, it is possible to determine which came first, the condition or the characteristic. Next, it reduces several types of bias (influences that may alter the outcome of the study). The disadvantages, however, include the large amount of time necessary to follow clients for the development of some conditions; the loss of participants from the beginning to the end of the study due to death, moving, or loss of interest in participating; and the need to be fairly certain of characteristics that might be related to specific conditions before the study begins. All of these factors and many others must be weighed by the investigator before selecting this design.

Retrospective studies

The case history (case-control), or retrospective, study also investigates the relationship between a condition and a characteristic but is the opposite of the cohort design. In case history studies people who have the condition are identified, and then it is determined whether

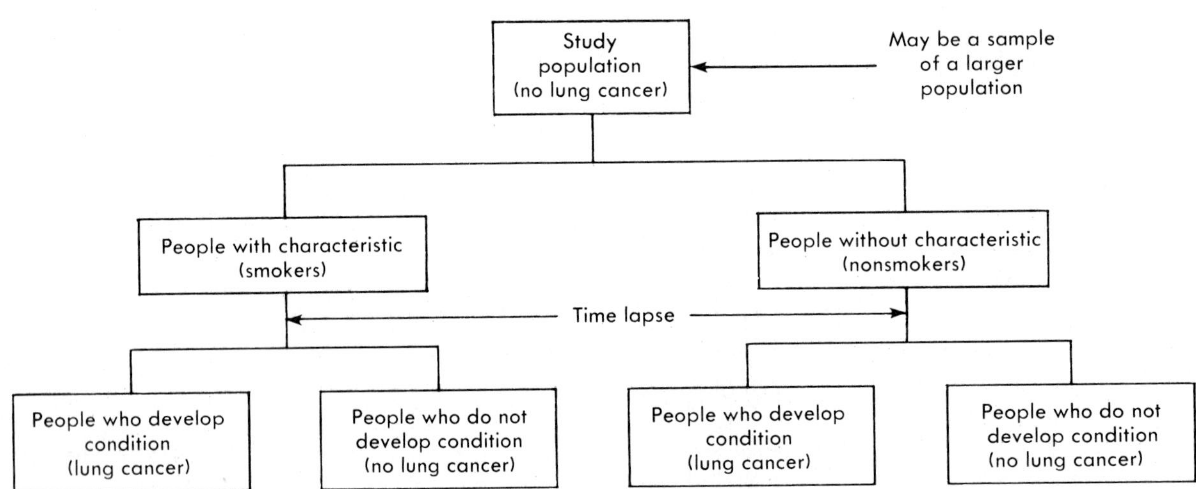

Fig. 6-4. Cohort, or prospective study design. This study design involves following population free of disease under study. Characteristic (e.g., smoking) of population is determined. After period of time elapses, investigator determines proportion of people who developed condition (e.g., lung cancer). Comparisons are made between those with characteristic and those without characteristic to determine whether characteristic is associated with condition.

they have or have had a particular characteristic. Further, people without the condition, known as controls, are also identified and a determination made as to whether they have the characteristic. Fig. 6-5 illustrates the general design of the retrospective study using the example of child abuse. A group of parents who abuse their children and a similar group of parents who do *not* abuse their children are identified. An assessment is made to determine whether the parents were themselves abused as children. The incidence rate of abuse as children for the cases and for the controls can be calculated. A large difference between the two groups might lead the investigator to hypothesize for further testing an association between the characteristic and the condition.

This design has the advantages of being less costly than the cohort design in time, money, and subjects; study participants are not usually lost during the study; and it can be used to study conditions that occur rarely or occur throughout a large geographic area. The disadvantages include (1) difficulty in identifying the true impact of the characteristic if the control group is not similar to the cases, (2) difficulty in defining the *risk* of developing the condition when the characteristic is present, and (3) the lack of general applicability of the study results to other populations. Very often a case history study develops hypotheses of association or causation that are tested later in a cohort study.

Cross-sectional studies

The third epidemiologic design is the cross-sectional study. This design includes many of the advantages of the two previously discussed designs, but it has some disadvantages as well. Generally speaking, the investigator using the cross-sectional approach selects a small sample from a larger population and determines the presence of both the condition and the characteristic *at the same time*. Fig. 6-6 illustrates this design using elevated blood pressure as the condition and being overweight as the characteristic. As was the situation in the

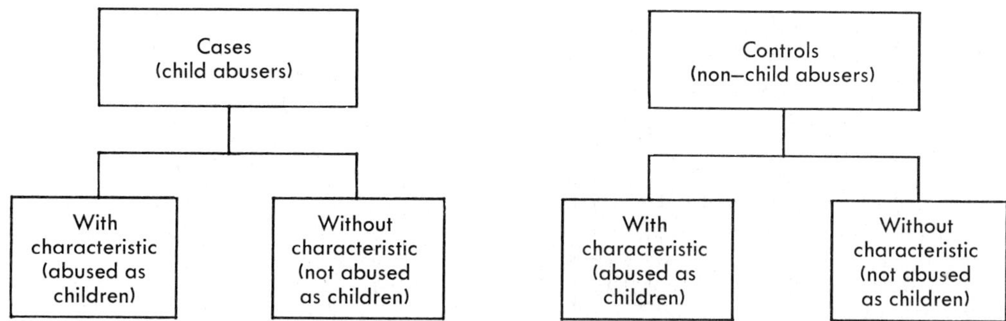

Fig. 6-5. Case control, or retrospective study design. This study design involves comparing those who have condition with those who do not to determine association between characteristic (having been abused as children) and condition (child abuse).

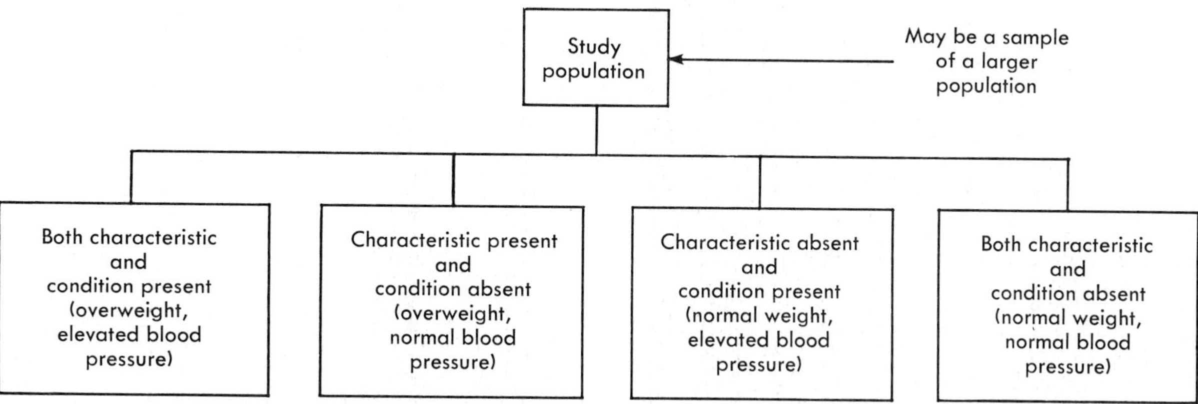

Fig. 6-6. Cross-sectional study design. This design involves gathering information about characteristic (being overweight) and condition (high blood pressure) simultaneously.

cohort study, the prevalence of both elevated blood pressure and overweight in the study population can be determined. It may also be possible to define the relative risk of developing elevated blood pressure when overweight (if the data were to show such a risk) as well as association between the two. One of the major problems of this type of design, however, is that it is not always possible to determine whether the condition or the characteristic occurred first.

Cross-sectional studies, like retrospective studies, are less costly than cohort studies, since they are usually short term. This advantage may be diminished, however, by the two major difficulties of this design: the survival of the persons with the condition and the timing of the measurement for the presence of the characteristic. Using the example from Fig. 6-6, if elevated blood pressure (the condition) were to cause death in some subjects in a short time, the study population would have too few people in it with that condition at any point in time, thus making it possible to incorrectly describe the relationship between being overweight to elevated blood pressure. If, on the other hand, people recover from elevated blood pressure, an underestimate of the occurrence of the condition would occur, and again the relationship between the condition and the characteristic might be incorrect. Similar difficulties arise with the characteristic. If being overweight for at least 3 years is necessary before elevated blood pressure occurs, a cross-sectional study would probably inaccurately describe the extent of the relationship of being overweight to elevated blood pressure.

■ APPLICATION TO NURSING PRACTICE

The application of epidemiologic concepts and methods by nurses can give them a strong theoretical base for their practice and consistent ways to handle the data for which they are responsible. The use of the concepts may be formal or informal, in simple or complex situations. However they are used, the results should provide direction to nursing practice and greater benefits for the clients nurses serve.

Often nurses find themselves struggling to solve a patient care problem that seems to defy solution. Applying a basic epidemiologic concept, that a *full description of the occurrence of a specific event* is the first step toward understanding that event, should lead to greater success in overcoming these problems. For example:

> Nurses who worked in an intensive care unit noticed that almost every day some of the patients developed tachycardia. When the concept of full description was applied, the problem (and potential solution) became clearer. It became apparent to the nursing staff through planned observations that the episodes of tachycardia occurred almost always during or immediately following staff rounds. It was also observed that the tachycardia occurred in patients who during rounds were those who appeared not to be oriented or who were unable to speak due to intubation. Further, there was usually some physical contact made to arouse these patients. With additional observations it was determined that those patients who were not purposely aroused or were involved in some discussion with the health care team did not experience tachycardia. An alternative approach to planning patient care was devised based on these observations.

Another epidemiologic concept useful in nursing is that there are *identifiable patterns to the occurrence of events*. Looking for these patterns can be beneficial both to individual practice and to cumulative nursing knowledge. The observation that certain events occur more often to some clients than to other clients leads to the use of another concept, *identifying clients at particular risk* and applying specific interventions to them. Public health nurses have always identified clients at risk and concentrated their efforts with these clients. An example would be giving priority to working with mothers of low-birth-weight babies to prevent this occurring in future births. In hospital settings the nurse has many opportunities to identify populations at risk. A nurse who recognizes that patients who undergo a particular diagnostic test require a predictable amount of care (a previously identified pattern) will arrange activities so as to be able to provide the care.

□ Use of multiple causality

Consistent *use of the theory of multiple causality* directs the nurse to view many aspects of the client's condition. During client assessment, nurses must gather information about and be alert to a large variety of factors that may have an impact on the client's situation. Concentrating on biologic variables (such as temperature, blood pressure, or breath sounds) to the exclusion of sociologic and psychologic variables denies the client an opportunity to have a nursing diagnosis made with full knowledge of all the multiple factors that, working together, result in the condition. A negative response to the question, "Are you taking your medicine?" may be a result of having no money to buy it, no transportation to a drugstore, no knowledge of the prescription or understanding of why it is important, no faith in medicines, severe side effects, or a combination of these and other factors. Looking for a single reason for most situations is serious and dangerous, as it can lead to an erroneous conclusion because all the contributing factors are not known. Nursing practice must use a multiple-causality approach.

Following assessment, the theory of multiple causality continues to guide nursing *intervention*. Identifying many potential ways to achieve a particular treatment goal promotes creativity in the nurse and responsiveness in the client. Interventions can be tailored to the particular and individual needs of each client only if there are many available from which to choose. When nurses are heard to say, "When there is an elevated temperature, we always . . . ; sometimes it works and sometimes it doesn't," this probably reflects the use of one intervention to reach a treatment goal each time that goal appears. This kind of nursing practice disregards the need for thinking, devising and modifying nursing action depending on the particular causal or related factors. Improvement in health care is dependent on designing and implementing intervention related to the multiple causes of health conditions.

It is equally imperative that nursing consider many aspects of *outcomes of care* during evaluation. Evaluating in one sphere, just as assessing or intervening in one sphere, does not contribute to good nursing practice. For example, many people are concerned that evaluation of health care in terms of life without considering the quality of that life is evaluation in one sphere only. Finding out whether a client follows a diet without determining whether the health condition changed because of the diet does not consider the multiple facets of evaluation. To be thorough, consistent, and accurate, nursing evaluation must examine (1) the accuracy of the original assessment data, (2) the applicability of the treatment goal, (3) the effectiveness of the interventions toward achievement of the treatment goal, (4) and the side effects of the interventions or of goal achievement.

□ Populations at risk

Nursing practice based on identification of target populations and tailoring care for these target populations (e.g., adolescent maternity clinics, surgical recovery rooms) has existed for decades. As health care potential continues to expand with the concurrent problem of increased cost, even greater use of the concept of populations at risk must be implemented. It is and will continue to be impossible to make available to all people unlimited amounts of technologic advances, most of which will not ever be needed by most people. Rather, it is possible to identify potential health care needs of particular populations and provide those services to them. On a large or small scale, nurses can be involved in identifying high-risk populations and planning care to address these populations. The overall effect should be more efficient use of all resources (knowledge, personnel, time, space) with greater possibilities of improved health.

□ Care of groups

Another epidmiologic concept long in practice by some practitioners, but usually not nurses, is providing care to *groups of people* rather than to individuals. Professional nursing care on a one-to-one basis is very expensive in terms of cost, space needed, time, and energy requirements of the nurse. It is necessary to provide this kind of care for particular people at very specific times; overall, however, few people may require that kind of intensive professional care. Many people do not need individual nursing care and may even benefit more from care as a member of a larger group. Professional nurses who target their care to groups of clients who have similar needs will find themselves having a greater and perhaps more lasting effect on the health of people.

□ Systematic inquiry

Perhaps the greatest impact epidemiology can have on the practice of nursing is the value to be placed on *systematic tabulation of observations.* Nurses continuously make professional assessments in multiple spheres, but they generally do not describe that information in a manner that allows for comparisons of findings between practitioners. Identification of such patterns as client and nurse behavior, successful and unsuccessful patient outcomes, and client care needs could greatly improve both nursing and health care delivery in general. Carefully describing all the parameters of specific situations, developing concise questions and problem statements, supporting intuitive beliefs with more objective data, and promoting the acquisition of new knowledge from the findings of others can all lead to the development of improved nursing care. The basic methods of how to achieve better documentation are available; it is now up to nurses to use and profit from them.

REFERENCES AND SELECTED READINGS

1. Fisher, F.: An introduction to epidemiology, ed. 1, New York, 1975, Appleton-Century-Crofts.
2. *Friedman, G. D.: Primer of epidemiology, New York, 1974, McGraw-Hill Book Co.
3. *Lilienfeld, A. M.: Foundations of epidemiology, New York, 1976, Oxford University Press, Inc.
4. *MacMahon, B., and Pugh, T.: Epidemiology, Boston, 1970, Little, Brown and Co.
5. Morris, J. N.: Uses of epidemiology, New York, 1975, Churchill Livingstone.
6. Omran, A. R.: Community medicine in developing countries, New York, 1970, Springer Publishing Co., Inc.
7. *Susser, M.: Causal thinking in the health sciences: concepts and strategies in epidemiclogy, New York, 1973, Oxford University Press, Inc.
8. White, K. L., and Henderson, M. editors: Epidemiology as a fundamental science: its uses in health services planning, administration, and evaluation, New York, 1976, Oxford University Press, Inc.

*References preceded by an asterisk are particularly well suited for student reading.

UNIT II

Concepts and processes

As nursing practice becomes increasingly sophisticated, nurses are seeking more specialized knowledge as a basis for decision making. Despite increasing specialization, there remains a group of concepts and processes that are common to nursing practice regardless of the clinical practice area.

The focus of this unit is on concepts and processes common to the practice of nursing in a variety of clinical areas. A systematic approach to nursing care, commonly termed *nursing process,* is addressed as this serves as the basic framework for the latter part of the book. The overall process in terms of assessment, intervention, and evaluation is addressed first, followed by a more in-depth discussion of *assessment* with special emphasis on data collection and analysis. Since much of nursing assessment and intervention involves interaction between nurse and client or patient, *nurse-patient relationships* are considered. The last two chapters deal with the use of a *problem-oriented system* for both planning and recording health information and the monitoring of patient/client outcomes by means of *quality assurance programs.*

7

Nursing process

JANE E. ANDERSON
KAREN K. YODER

Nursing process is a rational, scientifically based framework for nursing. It provides organization and direction to various elements of nursing practice and an accurate means of predicting outcomes, prescribing action alternatives, and evaluating results. Nursing process is a way of thinking about nursing care. It provides a more rational basis for nursing practice than intuition. Furthermore, nursing process provides a method for establishing standards of nursing care. These standards constitute a means for judging the quality of nursing services given to patients and clients. Thus the quality of nursing care is monitored on the basis of objective data and scientific criteria.[2] In addition nursing process provides a framework for identifying recurring nursing problems, relationships between data, and various nursing care approaches. This information in turn initiates research that further contributes to the theoretical basis of nursing.

The most commonly designated steps or phases of the nursing process are assessment, planning, intervention, and evaluation. Some experts eliminate planning as a step because they believe planning is essential to all phases of the nursing process. Thus *assessment, intervention*, and *evaluation* appear in all formulations of nursing process as noted in Fig. 7-1.

Nursing process has several characteristics. The following attributes should be integral parts of nursing process as a whole and each of its phases:

1. Systematic: characterized by the use of an orderly procedure
2. Purposeful: guided by a definite aim
3. Interactional: involves reciprocal actions between nurse and client
4. Specific: formulated precisely
5. Theoretically based: determined according to an assumed set of facts or principles
6. Based on priorities: established according to preferential rating
7. Validated: well grounded; conclusions reached by the nurse are verified with the client
8. Dynamic: characterized by continuous change
9. Mutually derived: formed by both nurse and client
10. Generalized: rendered applicable to a wide class of clients

Another feature of nursing process is that there are no constraints as to who or what entities are defined as participants in the process or in what setting the process occurs. The client may be defined as an individual, family, group, community, organization, or society. The process may be applied to populations defined on the basis of characteristics such as physical, social, or economic. The process occurs in multiple settings such as homes, schools, clinics, or hospitals.

■ ASSESSMENT

The first phase of the nursing process is assessment, which involves systematic data collection and data analysis. This phase is usually initiated when there is a discrepancy between what is and what should be in relation to optimum health for the client. Either the nurse or the client identifies the discrepancy and provides the impetus for change. The felt need for change, then, provides the initial input to establish a data base derived from a variety of sources.[1]

□ Collection of data

To provide a comprehensive data base, the information gathered must reflect the perceptions of both the client and the nurse regarding the individual, the subsystem, and the suprasystem. When the client is the family, for example, data is collected about the family (client), each member of the family (subsystems), and the community of the family (suprasystem). The family's self-report of their perceptions is *subjective data*. The data obtained by the nurse is *objective data*. Specific examples of subjective and objective data for each aspect of a client system are listed in Table 7-1.

Primary and *secondary* sources provide data about the client's present and past status. The client provides

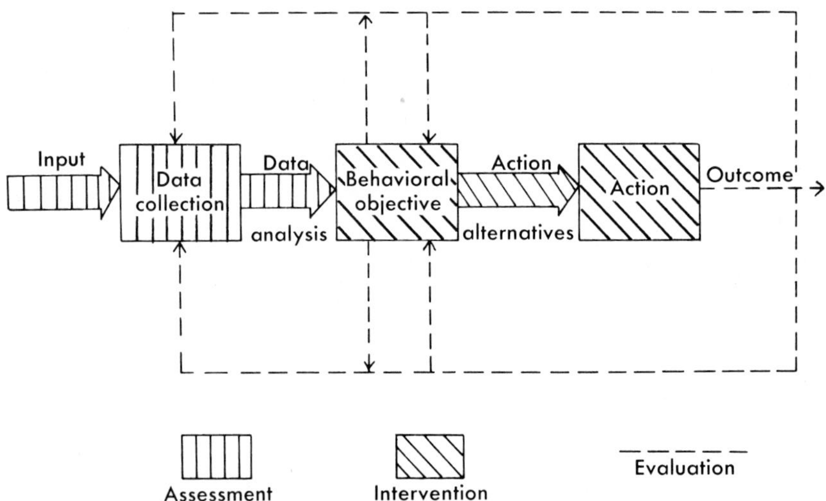

Fig. 7-1. Model of nursing process.

Table 7-1. Examples of subjective and objective data collected for each aspect of a client system

Client	Subjective data	Objective data
Individual	Results of interview, such as symptoms, feelings about wellness-illness, attitudes toward hospitalization	Results of inspection, palpation, percussion, auscultation
Family	Values, norms, status	Communication patterns, roles
Community	Culture, folkways, customs	Population characteristics, geographic factors, facilities

primary data, and sources related to the client contribute secondary data. The following sources of data are defined as either primary or secondary depending on the client system being considered: significant others, written records about the client, nursing personnel and other members of the health team, and relevant humanistic and scientific literature.

Data is collected through interview, observation, examination, and literature review. Although data may be collected from the client in an informal manner, there is evidence that a systematic approach results in a more complete data base. Since no one method or tool is sufficient to gather all the necessary information, the vehicle for data collection is determined by considering the nature of the situation and the time available to collect the data. Examples of comprehensive data collection forms can be found in Chapters 8 and 10. References providing information on other published forms can be found in the list of references following Chapter 8.

An important feature of the assessment is that it is mutually derived by the nurse and the individual. If nurses do not verify their perceptions with the client system, they are practicing in an automatic, nontherapeutic manner.[8] Nursing assessment conducted in consultation with the individual is more likely to yield effective nursing interventions than if the client is not given opportunity to participate in the assessment.[4]

□ Analysis of data

Data analysis involves *sorting* and *organizing* the collected data into a logical framework. This procedure makes the accumulated data more meaningful and easier to manage, suggests missing data, prevents omission of relevant data, and saves time and energy for both the nurse and the client.

Analysis of the data focuses on actual and potential interferences with the client's health status. *Actual interferences* indicate difficulties present at the time the assessment is made, while *potential interferences* allude to difficulties that the individual is at unusually high risk of developing or experiencing.[5]

The framework utilized for organizing the data is determined by the amount and type of data collected, the client, and the nurse's knowledge and philosophy about nursing. The data may be analyzed according to several approaches. Nursing diagnoses may be made or assets and limitations may be identified (see Chapter 8 for additional discussion). A list of health problems may be generated (see Chapter 10 for additional discussion).

Conclusions from data analysis indicate how well the client is dealing with the situation. The conclusions indicate that the individual is successfully handling the situation or is utilizing preventive measures, needs help but is getting it, or is unable to handle the situation or prevent it with personal resources. If the client is successfully handling the situation alone or by means of other resources, the nurse concludes that nursing intervention is not currently needed. If the individual cannot handle or prevent the situation, the nurse intervenes by determining what help is needed and who can provide it.[6]

□ Establishment of priorities

After the data have been analyzed, priorities are determined. The establishment of priorities allows the nurse to make rational choices at any given time when several problems or needs compete for attention.[6] Priorities usually reflect differentiation between life-threatening problems and problems of lesser importance or those that are long term in nature.[3]

One hierarchy that can be used in setting priorities for the client follows.[3] Consideration is first given to the problems that threaten the *life*, *dignity*, and *integrity* of the individual. Examples of such problems for the various client systems are:

Individual: Lack of patent airway
Family: Difficulty affecting whole unit that contributes to conflict and breakdown
Community: Epidemic

Secondary consideration is given to the problems that threaten to destructively change the client. Examples of such problems are:

Individual: Metabolic imbalance, abnormal cell growth, or retreat from social contacts
Family: Breakdown of communication
Community: Drug abuse

Finally, consideration is given to the problems that affect the normal growth and development of the client. Examples of such problems are:

Individual: Nutritional deprivation
Family: Lack of defined rules
Community: Lack of resources

The above hierarchy indicates how priority is given to situations where *illness* is prevalent. Establishment of another priority is necessary in *wellness* situations where the emphasis is on preventive health care. One suggestion is that the priority be reversed in wellness situations. Primary consideration in wellness situations, therefore, pertains to interferences with the normal growth and development of the individual. Secondary consideration in wellness situations is given to interferences in the client's status that have the potential to destructively change the person. Then, at the point where the interferences actually do change the individual's status, the priority indicated in the hierarchy is initiated. While collecting and analyzing the data, the individual may make a request or the nurse may recognize the need for an action. The nurse, therefore, may be tempted to intervene during the assessment phase. However, if the nurse waits to intervene until the data is analyzed and specific interventions are planned, more complete and accurate conclusions can usually be drawn. The components of the assessment phase are illustrated with vertical lines in Fig. 7-1.

■ INTERVENTION

The second phase of the nursing process is intervention, which includes the following components: formulation of behavioral objectives, generation and selection of alternative courses of action, and implementation of an action alternative(s).

Clients have the capacity to participate in varying degrees in the intervention phase. As in the assessment phase, it is important that the client system, subsystem, and suprasystem work toward the same objectives and that their efforts are not in conflict. Mutual derivation of objectives and action alternatives enhances the effectiveness of nursing interventions.

□ Formulation of objectives

The first component of the intervention phase involves the formulation of behavioral objectives. These objectives provide guidelines for determining the aim of intervention, or what is to be accomplished as a result of intervention. When stated behaviorally, objectives indicate desired client outcomes that can be observed, demonstrated, heard, or felt. The desired outcomes, therefore, provide standards for evaluating client progress.

Behavioral objectives contain the following elements: client, action verb, and criterion or condition under which performance occurs. The designated client (individual, family, group, or community) indicates who is to perform the desired behavior. A specific measurable action verb then states what the client needs to do to indicate achievement of the objective. By stating the criterion or condition in relation to a time period or accuracy of performance, the standards for judging the outcome behavior are defined. An example might be that "Mrs. Jones states the procedure for instilling her eyedrops with 100% accuracy." Objectives provide the scope and focus for delineation of alternatives for action.

□ Formulation of action alternatives

The action alternatives are hypothesized solutions that indicate how to achieve the desired outcome. The complexity of the situation and the desired outcome usually influence the number and quality of alternatives. The alternatives proposed for a singular or isolated event, for example, may be decreased in number and quality. If the situation is complex, however, the quantity and quality of the alternatives are likely to be increased.[3]

The determination of action alternatives is based on concepts and principles in the literature, the nurse's clinical experience, observation of what others are doing, and the nurse's creative inclinations. Alternatives are proposed through brainstorming: one idea stimulates the formation of another idea.[1]

After the action alternatives are proposed, it is necessary to select among the alternatives. The selection is facilitated by considering the consequences of each action. Since consequences are conclusions that result from reason, a sound theoretical base is essential to identify all the consequences of the action.

The consequences of proposed alternatives are ranked in relation to probability and desirability. Probability provides an estimate of the likelihood that the consequences of a proposed alternative will occur. This ranking is derived from the subjective experience of self and others and from objective recorded information. The desirability of the consequences of an alternative is also considered. An alternative is considered desirable if the preferred intent is likely to be accomplished, no harmful side effect is apt to occur, and the means for accomplishing the goal is efficient and appropriate.[3] Consideration of the side effect or risk is especially crucial. When considering risk, the negative aspect of the safety issue often becomes the critical criterion for decision making. Safety then tends to assume unrealistic proportions and overrides consideration of other more positive consequences. As a result, the potential outcome for the individual may be compromised at a low level of attainment. In ranking the consequences of alternatives according to risk, factors in addition to safety must be considered to maximize the client's potential. Thus when the consequences of action alternatives are considered, the alternatives selected for implementation usually reflect high probability and desirability.

□ Implementation of action

The last component of the intervention phase is to implement the selected alternative. During implementation there are potential ramifications and outcomes for all levels of the system (client system, subsystem, and suprasystem). When a family is the client system, for example, actions designed to alleviate family stressors will also have an effect on the individual (subsystem) and the community (suprasystem).

When the action is occurring, several health care providers may be interacting with the individual. The actions taken by these providers of health care may potentially be in conflict and may hinder the individual's progression toward optimal health. The action, therefore, should be sufficiently detailed to provide consistency in the implementation. The components of the intervention phase, formulation of behavioral objectives and action, are illustrated by the diagonal lines in Fig. 7-1.

■ EVALUATION

The last phase of the nursing process is evaluation, which involves appraisal of the actual outcome that results from the action. The actual outcome is compared with the behavioral objective (desired outcome) through the evaluation feedback loop. This comparison yields the following possible results:

1. Objective (desired outcome) successfully accomplished
2. Objective partially accomplished: some of the variables in the objective not accomplished
3. Objective not successfully accomplished and corrective action in the process necessary
4. Objective accomplished and data collected regarding other outcomes

If the actual outcome is consistent with the desired outcome, the actual outcome becomes part of the data collection. However, if there is a discrepancy between actual and desired outcomes, revision of the process is essential. In accordance with the progression of the feedback loop (as indicated by dotted lines in Fig. 7-1), revision may be appropriate at various points. Solutions for the revision, therefore, may include the following procedures:

1. Redesigning the behavioral objective
2. Selecting and implementing another action alternative
3. Collecting and analyzing more data to evolve new nursing diagnoses (or problems), behavioral objectives, action alternatives, and actions.

For the evaluation process to be successful, the participants must be able and willing to receive the feedback. Therefore from the beginning, plans for evaluation involve the client system, subsystem, and suprasystem. Mechanisms are established to make the evaluation reliable and replicable. For example, a high degree of agreement on evaluation tools is established before they are used by the nursing staff.

This last phase of the nursing process, therefore, is not an end in itself. Evaluation provides a means to facilitate processing and reprocessing by means of corrective mechanisms. The cyclical quality of evaluation contributes to the dynamic nature of nursing process and is shown by the dotted lines in Fig. 7-1.

■ RELATIONSHIP OF NURSING PROCESS TO OTHER APPROACHES TO THINKING

Since nursing process is a way of thinking, the elements of the process are inherent in other guidelines

Table 7-2. Comparison of guidelines for thinking with phases of nursing process

Guidelines for thinking	Phases of nursing process		
	Assessment	Intervention	Evaluation
General systems perspective	Input	Throughput	Output, feedback
Scientific method	Identify and define problem, collect data	Formulate a hypothesis; evaluate the hypothesis; test the hypothesis	Form conclusions
ANA Standards of Practice	Collect data systematically and continuously about health status of client; communicate and record data	Implement nursing actions that provide client participation in health promotion, maintenance, and restoration	Reassess, reorder priorities, set new goal, and revise plan based on progress or lack of progress
Problem-oriented record	Collect a data base, derive a problem list.	Establish an initial plan.	Write progress notes, including: Subjective: what client says Objective: information observed by another or measured by instruments Assessment: interpretation, evaluation Plan: decisions for immediate or future action

for thinking: general systems perspective, scientific method, American Nurses' Association Standards of Practice, and problem-oriented record. The common elements of assessment, intervention, and evaluation are evident when comparing the other guidelines to thinking, as noted in Table 7-2.

SUMMARY

The nursing process provides a rational, scientifically based framework for nursing practice. Each level of the system (client, subsystem, and suprasystem) is considered throughout the process. Input from the nurse or client regarding the need for change initiates the assessment phase. During the assessment phase data are collected and analyzed. During the intervention phase behavioral objectives are formulated to designate the desired outcome and alternative actions are proposed to indicate how the desired outcome may be achieved. After reviewing the proposed alternatives the selected actions are implemented. During the evaluation phase the actual outcome is compared with the behavioral objectives (desired outcome). If the actual outcome is consistent with the desired outcome, the actual outcome becomes part of the data collection. However, if there is a discrepancy between actual and desired outcomes, the process begins anew at assessment or intervention. The nursing process, therefore, is a means for providing dynamic, scientifically based client care.

Each phase is considered as a separate step; however, in reality the phases occur concurrently. To the beginning nurse practitioner, each phase of the nursing process may seem time consuming. With practice, however, the time involved in utilizing the various phases is minimized.

REFERENCES AND SELECTED READINGS

1. *Bailey, J. T., and Claus, K. E.: Decision making in nursing: tools for change, St. Louis, 1975, The C. V. Mosby Co.
2. *Becknell, E., and Smith, D.: System of nursing practice, Philadelphia, 1975, F. A. Davis Co.
3. *Bower, F. L.: The process of planning nursing care: a model for practice, ed. 2, St. Louis, 1977, The C. V. Mosby Co.
4. *Dumas, R., and Leonard, R. C.: The effect of nursing on the incidence of postoperative vomiting, Nurs. Res. **12:**12-15, 1963.
5. *Mayers, M.: A systematic approach to the nursing care plan, ed. 2, New York, 1972, Appleton-Century-Crofts.
6. *Mitchell, P.: Concepts basic to nursing, ed. 2, New York, 1977, McGraw-Hill Book Co.
7. *Mundinger, M., and Jauron, G.: Developing a nursing diagnosis, Nurs. Outlook **23:**94-98, 1975.
8. *Orlando, I. J.: The dynamic nurse-patient relationship, New York, 1961, G. P. Putnam's Sons.

*References preceded by an asterisk are particularly well suited for student reading.

8

Assessment process: data collection and analysis

JANE STEINMAN KAUFMAN

Assessment is the crucial foundation on which the future steps of the nursing process depend. Assessment includes two phases: the collection of data from multiple sources and analysis of the data into nursing care problems or diagnoses. Data are collected systematically, subjectively and objectively, through interview and physical examination. A complete data base assures that the nurse will be aware of the patient's problems and will be able to plan care based on the data. When the data base is incomplete the nurse may assume incorrectly that the client's problems are adequately identified and can be appropriately addressed. In other words, the nursing plan is only as complete and accurate as the data on which it is based.

The process of assessment is a complex one that most beginning practitioners find extremely time consuming. Identifying and analyzing a patient's nursing care problems requires a knowledge base on which to make judgments, the ability to compare data with established norms and standards, and the ability to think analytically.

■ DATA COLLECTION

Data collection is initiated with the first patient contact. During all succeeding contacts the nurse continually collects information relevant to the nursing care of a client. Observations range in complexity from the gross observation that a patient is bleeding to more intricate mental noting of nonverbal cues emitted by a client.

In our everyday lives data collection and observation occur constantly, often in a random pattern: one often observes something by chance. In nursing one collects data systematically in order to improve accuracy, to avoid missing cues, and to ensure a complete data base.

There are three basic components of systematic data collection. First, it is *purposeful.* The nurse has particular reasons for collecting the data. Second, data collection is *planned systematically* with criteria or methodology outlined in advance. For example, if the nurse is assessing the normal growth and development of a 6-month-old child, criteria used to evaluate children of this age need to be available. The data to be collected are also ordered, or organized. Third, systematic data collection requires *accurate observations* in order to draw valid conclusions.

To assess systematically decisions are made concerning (1) the areas of daily living about which information will be sought, (2) the methods of collecting information that are most appropriate to the situation, (3) the priorities for collecting data and for instituting therapy, and (4) the means to be used for organizing and analyzing the data.[42]

□ Fact versus inference

When gathering data, facts or descriptive data are collected before meaning is attached to the information. Facts are objective and noncontroversial. Conversely, inference allows one to attach meaning to the information or behavior that is more useful than the information itself. Various inferences can be made from one item of data.[14] The nurse asks, "What could this behavior mean?" Consider a patient who is teary eyed, has a downcast head, and is curled up in bed. Inferences could include: (1) the patient is depressed, (2) the patient is homesick, (3) the patient is in pain.

Inferences must be validated before the nurse acts on them. There are four main approaches to validation. The best way to validate is to *refer to an authoritative source.* For example, one might compare findings with an expert nurse clinician or a reference book to determine if the observations are concordant. The nurse may think a newborn baby has a skin infection; however, an obstetrics textbook may reveal that this is a normal characteristic of a newborn called *milia.*

Second, the nurse can determine if all other cues are *consistent.* For example, the patient may be picking at food, not sleeping well at night, and constantly looking downcast. It may be inferred that the client is depressed. However, other cues need to be checked to see if they are consistent with the picture of depression. For example, it should be determined whether the patient has recently experienced some type of loss or has a major physical problem. From the other cues it may be determined whether depression is the correct diagnosis or inference.

Third, the nurse can *clarify inferences* with the client. The nurse asks specific, pointed questions when validating inferences. For example, the nurse may see an elderly man sitting in his room with his food tray out of reach. The nurse may walk into the room and say, "You can't eat?" If the patient says, "No," the nurse may then offer to cut up the patient's food and move the tray closer. However, this man's real problem may be that he cannot eat because of nausea. In this case the nurse made the wrong inference because precise, pointed questions were not used.

Fourth, the nurse can *seek consensus* from the appropriate reference group. For example, the nurse may validate the inferences with other nurses in team conference or with the physical therapist or physicians. However, each of *these* individuals also may have made incorrect inferences. Therefore it is advisable to use other methods of validating an inference prior to seeking consensus.

□ Factors affecting data collection

As a nurse observes and collects data about a client, there are a variety of factors, both environmental and personal, that may influence the data collected. Awareness of these factors enhances objectivity in data collection.

One of the most important factors influencing data collection is *selective perception*. Due to our unique perceptual fields, we all see selected aspects of a situation. We may see more detail in familiar than unfamiliar situations. We also tend to see only what we know. It is much easier to see the superficial aspects of a situation than the more covert aspects.

One also tends to remember items that conform to one's own picture of a situation. One may *stereotype* or distort what is seen due to preconceived ideas or past experiences with a situation. Error or bias may occur because of the invention of items or omission of items. Bias often occurs with random observations; stereotyping often distorts our view. Unfortunately, nurses may stereotype or "label" individuals. For example, a nurse who equates confusion and senility with old age may label an elderly man who is up walking at night as "confused." In actuality the man may be merely seeking the bathroom or stretching his legs.

Finally, *anxiety* may affect data collection inasmuch as it may narrow one's perceptual field. The hospital and certain areas in the community may contain unfamiliar and frightening situations. These environments may cause nurses to feel anxious and subsequently to omit or invent observations.

The nurse's *biologic*, *psychologic*, and *sociocultural systems* influence data collection and observation skills. Biologic examples include hunger, illness, or fatigue. The nurse who is tired may overlook significant observations.

The nurse's *mood*, beliefs, needs, or motivation may influence the data collected. For example, the nurse may assist the patient with activities of daily living that the patient is capable of doing independently. One inference might be that the patient likes to be dependent. It may be, however, that the nurse has a particular need to be liked or to be seen as helpful.

Numerous *sociocultural factors* such as language, role, mores, or socioeconomic class may influence observations. A common sociocultural factor that widely influences new practitioners is *role*. Often the beginning nurse is unsure of the parameters of the nurse role and what can and cannot be done within it. The nurse may be uncomfortable with data collection methods, such as the history, that require asking the patient questions about such things as financial situation, which may be viewed as invasion of privacy. Examining the rash on a patient's buttocks may be seen as too intrusive.

The factors discussed above may be present in the patient as well as the nurse, since a person's biologic and psychologic state does affect the way in which data collection is approached.

The client's level of understanding, ability to remember, fear, or embarrassment may be psychologic factors that influence the data that can be collected. The individual may be extremely afraid to offer information during the nurse's history or examination because of fear of hospitals. Clients may be embarrassed to offer particular information if they think it will reflect poorly on their characters. For example, a middle-aged woman from a middle-class family who fears she may have contracted tuberculosis may be reluctant to discuss her symptoms with the nurse. She may be embarrassed because of the stigma that was placed on having tuberculosis when she was a young child.

The client's family and culture also influence the data collected, and the nurse and patient may be from very different cultural backgrounds. They may differ in terms of their language, customs, and beliefs. For example, nurses may not realize the importance to the Italian family of having numerous family members in attendance when a patient is admitted to the hospital. The family may be very important to the patient, who may not divulge necessary information without the family members being present.

□ Data collection roles

The extent of interaction between the nurse and clients affects the accuracy of data collected. Generally nurses are *participant observers*. That is, the nurse participates in the daily life of clients while simultaneously collecting data. The role of participant observer has advantages and disadvantages. The *advantages* are that the nurse can validate clients' feelings with them and that people are more likely to be themselves when the observer is participating in their care. The nurse is therefore more likely to observe behavior that is characteristic of the patient's usual way of behaving.

Participant observation also has *limitations*. It is more difficult to be objective when interacting with a person. The nurse may draw inferences without validating them. Being emotionally involved in the situation may also bias observations, since the nurse's feelings may affect the client's feelings and responses.

It is important to record data as soon as possible after obtaining it. Otherwise important information may be forgotten and thus omitted. Whenever possible the data should be recorded as close to the source as possible. There is a trend to place the portions of the client's records on which nurses record closer to the patient's bedside. Thus it is not unusual for flow sheets and even nurse's notes or progress sheets to be placed outside the client's room or at a minicharting area geographically removed from the nursing station on the division. When this is done the nurse is encouraged to record the data as soon as possible rather than waiting to do it all at the end of the shift.

Nurses can also assume the *nonparticipant observer role*. This role entails observing only, not participating. For example, nurses practicing in nursery schools or elementary schools may observe a particular age group in an unobtrusive way in order to determine stages of growth and development. In this situation the individuals being observed may or may not know that they are being observed.

There are also advantages and limitations to the nonparticipant observer role. One advantage is greater objectivity in data collection. A greater number of cues may be absorbed and more accurate data can be collected without the need to attach meaning to it. Additionally the observations can be recorded immediately. This should improve the accuracy and validity of the data, since the nurse is performing only one role and thus can concentrate all energies on that role.

A limitation of the nonparticipant observer role is that the nurse is unable to clarify and validate with the individuals being observed. Therefore the nurse cannot investigate the subjective feelings of those observed. The nurse's mere presence in the environment may also influence the behavior of those being observed. For example, the children in the nursery school may behave quite differently when a stranger is present. Therefore data collected may not represent their usual behavior. Finally, because nurses are accustomed to being participants many find the nonparticipant observer role difficult to tolerate.

□ Data resources

Nurses have begun to expand their data collection methods. They are becoming more sophisticated not only in using themselves but also in using a variety of assessment instruments. The nurse has numerous resources available for the assessment process.

Self

One use of self is in the use of the five senses as a means of data collection. *Sight* is probably the sense that most nurses learn to use first. Using sight to make observations is called *inspection*. Sight is also involved in the use of equipment such as the otoscope and the ophthalmoscope. *Hearing* is employed in listening to patients when they express feelings and when they talk with other persons, such as family members. Environmental noises that nurses hear may be disturbing to patients,

Table 8-1. Types of data obtained with assessment instruments

Instrument	Data obtained
Sphygmomanometer (blood pressure cuff)	Status of respiratory, cardiovascular, and renal systems; psychologic state
Thermometer	Body temperature
Tape measure	Girth of body parts such as abdomen, leg
Light source	Constriction of pupils in response to light; status of oral cavity (e.g., inflamed or obstructed)
Reflex hammer	Presence of and degree of reactivity of reflexes
Otoscope	Status of eardrum and ear canal
Ophthalmoscope	Status of retina (e.g., variations in veins and arteries)
Chemically treated papers or reagent tablets	Presence of chemical substances in blood, urine, stool, and other body fluids (e.g., Clinitest indicates level of glucose in urine)

and they are often pleased to learn that others are aware of these noises and might be able to do something about them. Another use of hearing is in *auscultation* of sounds through the stethoscope. *Touch* is frequently used to collect data, as in *palpation* in which an area is felt to determine whether body parts are of normal size, contour and texture. *Percussion* may be used to distinguish the relative density of tissues. Although the sense of *taste* is seldom used, the sense of *smell* can be used to detect fetid wounds or the fruity breath of a person with ketoacidosis.

Various *mechanical instruments* are used by the nurse to expand the scope of data collection and to permit greater accuracy of observations. These instruments and the types of data they are used to obtain are listed in Table 8-1.

Client's family

Another important data source is the client's family. The client is considered a member of the family system, recognizing that what affects one part affects all parts. It is often essential to collect information from family members regarding their response to the client's illness. Family members are vital when working with clients who are unable to communicate effectively, such as children or adults who are unable to communicate either because of age or physical impairment.

The nurse may also find that the client and family members do not have the same perceptions, since a question asked of both elicits different information. The family's perception of how the client's life style may have changed because of an alteration in health may be quite different from that of the client. In addition family members are often helpful in giving the nurse insight about the client's past behavior and current level of coping with the health alteration.

Other resources

The patient's past and present *medical records* often contain data that are helpful in assessment. The nurse uses data from the medical history and other health care workers' notes rather than subjecting the patient to repeated questioning on the same topic.

The physician can provide data about the patient's health alteration and assist the nurse with some trouble shooting for predicting other potential or existing problems. The beginning nursing student is often somewhat hesitant to contact the physician and collect information.

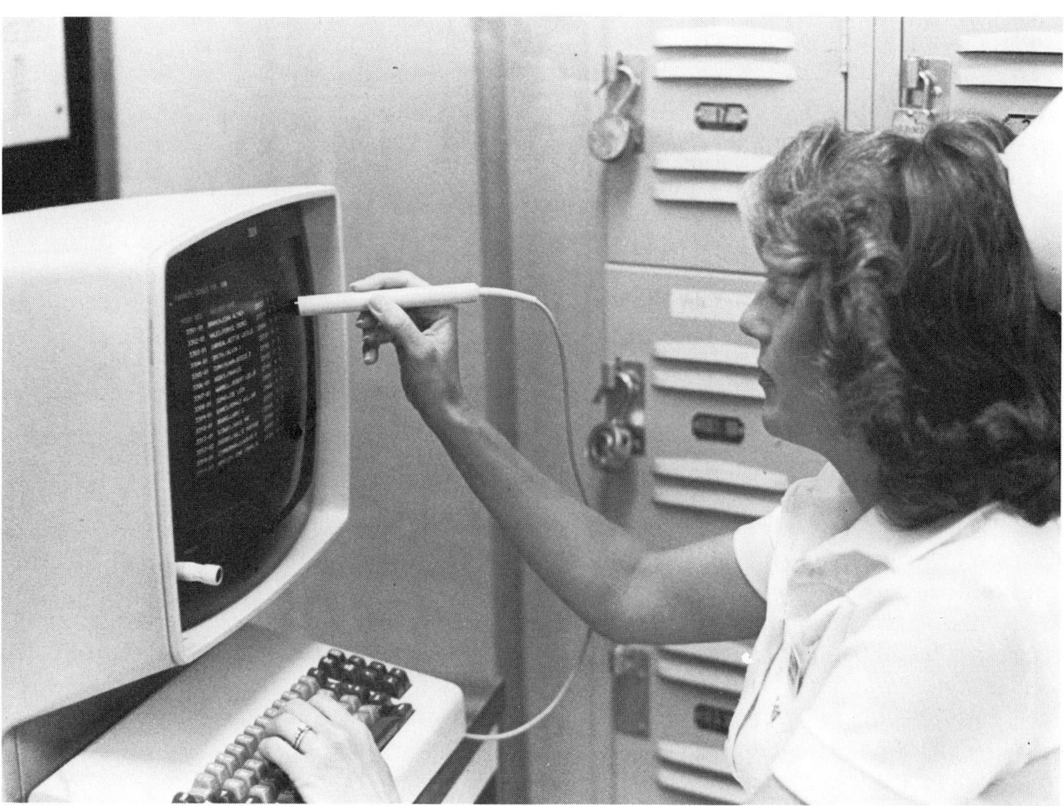

Fig. 8-1. Nurses have access to vast data resource by means of computer.

Often this occurs because of preconceived ideas about physicians and perhaps the aloof reception the student expects to receive from them. However, most nursing students find that physicians will respond positively to requests made of them.

Other health care workers have a wealth of useful information. Nurses who have worked with the client in the past or are currently working with the client are most likely to have relevant information that can add to or clarify the nurse's assessment. In addition the physical therapist, social worker, respiratory therapist, dietitian, chaplain, and many other health care workers can provide information about the patient from the perspective of their own disciplines.

Some hospitals record patient histories in a computer as the patient responds to a series of questions. The patient's answers are stored in the computer, and the nurse or other health care providers can retrieve the data from the computer anytime they need particular information. It is predicted that computers will be used more and more in the future for storage of vital client information, and for this reason nurses can expect to be more involved in using them.

The literature (books, journals, monographs) is a vital source of information. Data can be obtained here to explain or validate information collected from the patient.

□ Subjective data collection: assessment interview or history

Data collected are both subjective and objective. Subjective data are reported by the client but are not directly observable. Objective data are those items of information that can be gathered by a second party, in this case the nurse. Subjective data are obtained through the *nursing history,* while objective data are obtained by *physical examination* of the client.

In order for a nursing history to be complete and comprehensive it must be well organized and used systematically. The history contains a series of questions designed to obtain information needed to plan nursing care. Questions are asked about the client's present functional abilities and how this compares with previous ability to function. In addition questions may be asked about how the functions have been impaired [29,39,41] and what *adaptive processes* the client is using to cope with alterations in health. The client should also be asked about self-*perception* of present health status and what effect this has on personal life style.

In summary, the purpose of the nursing history is to obtain data as a basis for determining potential or existing nursing care requirements or client problems, which in turn will guide nursing actions. The nursing history also provides data that enable nurses to personalize care based on the individual's values, life style, and patterns of living. Thus nurses acquire a unique data base that focuses on the total person and that person's health maintenance.

For example, a nurse may ask questions about the patient's syncope and its frequency, precipitating factors, and time of occurrence. Because the nurse realizes the safety factors necessitated with fainting, the questions determine what changes in the patient's environment need to be made. On the other hand the physician may also inquire about the syncope but for a different purpose. A diagnosis may be sought about a mitral valve problem with syncope recognized as a symptom.

The type and level of information collected by the nurse depends on numerous factors. The nurse's educational preparation and years of experience will affect the kind of information sought. Other factors influencing the content of the history are the nurse's and employing agency's philosophy about nursing and the nurse's level of practice. If nurses view their practice as fairly autonomous, their data base will emphasize information related to the independent aspects of practice. The clients who are the recipients of health care also dictate the content of the history. For example, an elderly person would be asked different questions than a 5-year-old. Each history should contain questions appropriate to the client's bio-psycho-sociocultural systems and life experience.

Interviewing

Interviewing is a method used to collect information for the history. It is purposeful communication that focuses on specific content. The assessment interview usually occurs early in the nurse-client relationship; therefore the nurse needs to begin to establish a trust relationship with the client and set mutually agreed on goals from the beginning. The process of establishing a relationship with a client is vital to the nursing process (see Chapter 9 for explanation of the process).

Functions of an interview may be to:

1. Assess the client's bio-psycho-sociocultural status and needs
2. Understand the (client's) perceptions of self and others
3. Gain information about teaching needs
4. Assist the client to identify needs, conflicts, or problems
5. Review with the client usual coping mechanisms
6. Identify the alternatives open to the client in managing the present situation

Assessment interviewing or history taking encompasses each of these functions. However, the primary purpose involves gathering information to determine the individual's bio-psycho-sociocultural status and to identify the patient's unique perception of the present situation and coping mechanisms. Because the subjective data (history) is often obtained in situations where the client is actively seeking help in coping with a problem, he or she may be anxious to have these problems solved. Also, there may be other factors that are affecting coping. For example, a woman may come to a clinic seeking additional treatment to control the pain of rheumatoid arthritis when in reality her major problem is inability to observe rest periods as ordered because her invalid mother requires increasing hours of physical care. It is the latter concern that the client may dwell on during the history while expressing frustration with her mother. If the nurse were to concentrate on this concern exclusively in an attempt to help the client solve the problem, the nurse would be engaging in another type of interviewing, therapeutic interviewing. Although the nurse's assessment interview may have components of support and therapy, the *primary emphasis* of assessment interviewing is to collect data about the patient's current health status. Therapeutic counseling may be offered after the assessment is completed and goals are established for the nurse and client to work together. During the history the nurse needs to acknowledge the patient's concerns and indicate a willingness to discuss them later. In the above example the nurse could acknowledge the individual's concern about her mother and later discuss ways the patient might receive help in caring for her mother. In other words, the nurse needs to keep in mind the primary purpose of the assessment interview while at the same time noting the patient's plea for help.

Guidelines for interviewing. In preparing for the interview the nurse may wish to review mentally the purposes of the interview and the approach to be taken, thus internalizing the *role of interviewer*. The client needs to have a simple explanation of the purpose of the interview and how the nurse will use the information obtained.

The following principles may be used as guidelines for the interview.

1. *Content to be explored is clearly delineated and systematically outlined in advance.* The nurse decides whether the data can be collected best through direct or indirect means. For example, the client may be asked directly, "Does your stomach burn after ingesting spicy foods?" This is an example of a *closed* question requiring little elaboration other than yes or no. Content in the history that is noncontroversial or not open to interpretation can be sought by this method. Questions about the client's social system such as number of children, address, and church affiliation or items pertaining to certain symptoms such as fainting, headache, or nausea can be appropriately asked in a very direct, or closed, manner.

On the other hand, if the nurse wants the client to express feelings or describe a particular behavior, the information is best sought through an indirect, or *open* method, since it may uncover the client's true feelings and perceptions, which may not be ascertained by the direct method. If the client is asked directly, "Do you resent your wife's lack of attention?" he may respond in the negative. However, if the client is asked, "Tell me about your relationship with your wife," it is hoped he will express some of the negative feelings as he tells the story. A series of indirect statements may be needed in order to elicit feelings.

2. *Interviewing is facilitated by establishing rapport with the client.* Rapport implies that there are mutual feelings of comfort, confidence, and harmony. A variety of modes can be used to foster rapport. First, the nurse can extend common courtesy to the client. An introduction of self, greeting the client by name, and extending one's hand can initially place both the nurse and client at ease. The nurse can offer a few general comments to help the client be recognized as an individual. Comments on the client's pictures or flowers, or even comments about the weather can be phrased to relax both individuals.

3. *The purpose of the interview and examination is clarified with the client.* If the client understands how the obtained data is relevant to care, he or she is more apt to cooperate. The client may not have previously experienced a nurse asking numerous questions. Therefore the client needs to be informed that the questions are asked in order to provide the best nursing care. It might also be noted that the questions will determine not only health-related difficulties the client is experiencing but also ways to keep the client as healthy as possible. The nurse informs the client that if any aspect of the question is not understood, it will be clarified by the nurse at any point during the history. The nurse may inquire as to the client's thoughts about notes being taken during the interview. Notes are helpful to the nurse, as specific facts can be recorded immediately and are less biased than on later recall. Most clients will not object to the nurse taking notes as reminders of the content. Taking notes in view of the client helps keep the atmosphere open.

4. *"The climate the nurse creates influences the substance of the interviews."*[6] Climate refers to the immediate conditions, both physical and psychologic, that surround an individual. One component of a climate conducive to effective interviewing is appropriate timeing. The initial history is usually taken soon after admission or contact with a health facility. However, the acuteness of the client's state will affect the timing and type of interview obtained. For example, a nurse would not obtain a lengthy initial history from someone with a ruptured appendix when immediate care is essential.

The length of time needed to complete the history

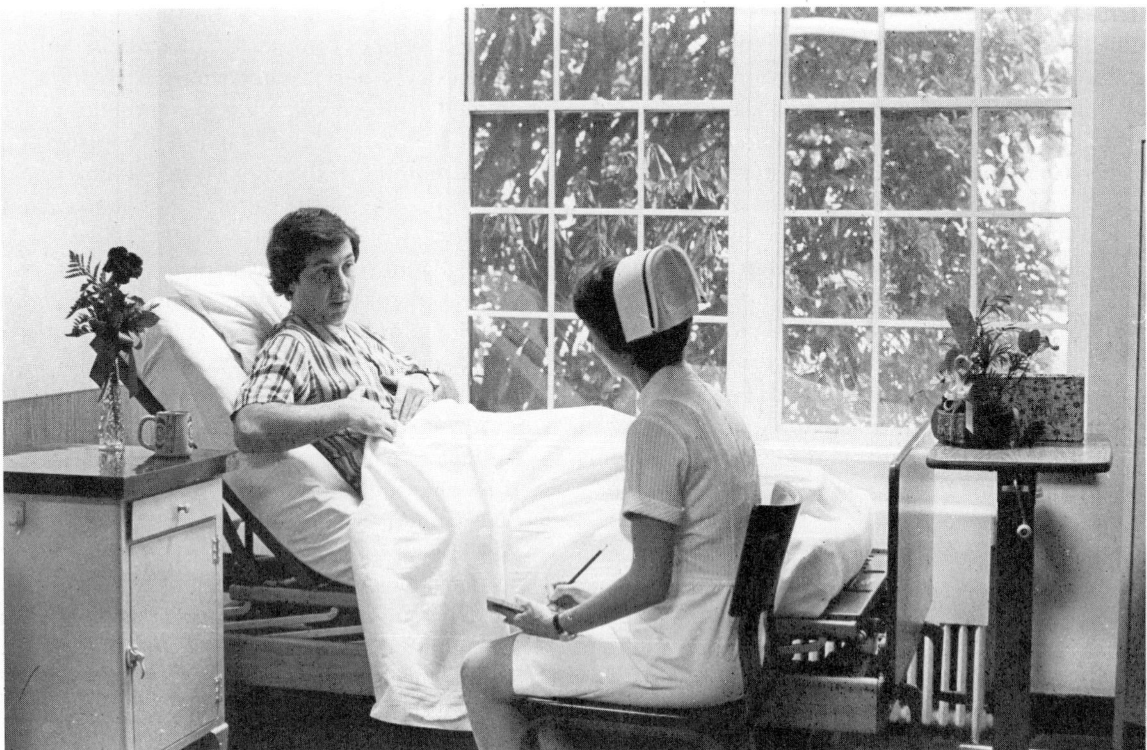

Fig. 8-2. Sitting in chair facing client enhances comfort of both during history taking.

and examination should be communicated to the client. The length of time needed to complete the data collection will depend on a variety of factors such as the nurse's skill, amount and complexity of assessment, the content covered, and the client's willingness to converse and participate. In any case the nurse allows sufficient uninterrupted time that is as anxiety free as possible for the client. For example, the busy preoperative morning would not be an effective time for an assessment interview.

A comfortable climate is facilitated by creating environmental privacy. Closing the client's door or pulling the curtains between beds will help the interviewer and client feel more at ease. Environmental noise should be kept at a minimum. The nurse may also ask that the client's family leave for certain segments of the history and examination. Frequently, beginning nurses who feel somewhat unsure of their roles will hesitate to ask the family to step out of the room while they proceed. However, families are excellent data resources and can often validate or refute baseline information collected by the nurse *after* the interview has concluded.

Physical comfort of both nurse and client contributes to a positive climate. The nurse can assist the client to the bathroom, have water available, or adjust the bed pillows. The nurse will find that sitting in a chair facing the client will facilitate comfort of both nurse and client (Fig. 8-2). As the chair is placed for the interview, the nurse is aware of the personal space surrounding individuals. Various cultures proscribe different meanings to space surrounding the body. An individual from the Middle East may feel quite comfortable speaking with a stranger at a distance of 6 to 18 inches, whereas an American would consider that improperly close.[22] The nurse observes these distances as the interview proceeds. This is not to say that touch should not be utilized. To the contrary, a touch of the hand can be quite effective in an interview to relay warmth and concern for a client.

5. *The interview is initiated with those topics that are the least threatening to the patient and easiest to discuss.* Questioning that moves from the least personal to the most personal items helps to gain the patient's confidence and cooperation. For example, the nurse might be more effective if the beginning question refers to the patient's occupation rather than bowel habits.

6. *Questions should be brief and limited to a single idea.* Only one question should be asked at a time. If questions are too lengthy the patient may become confused and stop listening. The client may be unsure of the

relevant data on which to concentrate. Also, if more than one question is asked the patient will be unsure of which is to be answered.

7. *Leading questions should be avoided.* A leading question may place the client in an uncomfortable position and squelch spontaneity. For example, a question such as, "Do you still smoke?" places the client in a double bind in which either a yes or no answer fails to convey that the client never did smoke.

8. *Language used should be understood by the client.* Patients may be too embarrassed to admit they do not understand the words used by the nurse and may give inaccurate information. Medical terminology is a type of jargon that can be quite confusing to the layman. The client may not comprehend that up ad lib means he can be up walking at his liberty. After beginning the interview the nurse will be able to determine major language patterns of the client, noting if the language needs to be simple and concrete or if more complex ideas can be utilized.

Not only does the nurse need to communicate clearly to the patient, but the language used by the patient needs to be clarified and clearly understood by the nurse. Often words used by clients are quite descriptive or are a play on words, yet may be unfamiliar terms to the nurse. For example, I have heard the following terms used by clients: "cascading" for vomiting, "avalanche" for ambulance, "falling out" for fainting, "fireballs in the universe" for fibroids of the uterus. (See Robert Whalen's article "Medical Malaprops"[59] for an interesting and humorous history and play on words as told by the client and interpreted by the physician.)

9. *Allow an appropriate amount of time for the client to answer.* Experience and judgment are required to determine when the client is leading into discussing perceptions and feelings relevant to the care versus "rambling." The difference between the two is subtle. The nurse allows the client to tell the story in the client's own words; repeated themes or obvious omissions of data can give the nurse clues as to what is important information versus rambling. The nurse who is learning to obtain histories would be wise to allow too great versus too little rambling until more experience is gained in recognizing themes of communication.

10. *Keep the interview purposeful and focused on the topic of discussion until necessary data have been obtained.* If the interview moves abruptly from one topic to another, both parties may become lost in the maze of conversation. The neophyte interviewer who is insecure in the role may focus too little, and the interview may tend to become social chit-chat. If this occurs the nurse may refocus (e.g., "Before we discuss your job, I'd like to find out more about your dizziness.").

11. *Maintain momentum and move to the next interview section once the data have been obtained.* Perhaps the client has expressed all he or she possibly can about feelings about a job loss. The nurse may lose the patient's interest and cooperation if the point is belabored.

12. *Specific answers should be obtained.* Words such as "good," "sometimes," and "regular" have many different interpretations; therefore clarification is sought. Do regular dental checkups mean once or twice a year or every 3 years?

13. *Transitional comments are made when moving from one section of the interview to the next.*[5,p.46] This helps the history flow smoothly rather than jumping from one part to another. The patient will also realize that it is time to move to a new topic. For example, the nurse may say, "I have all the information I need about your daily activity. Could we move on to discuss your employment?"

14. *At the end of the history the nurse states that the information needed to plan care has been obtained.*[5,p.56] A courteous manner will help the client feel a sense of cooperation in volunteering the needed information. The nurse might say, "Thank you for giving the information I need to plan your care more effectively."

15. *Before leaving the patient the nurse should summarize the major ideas offered by the patient and inform him when contact will be made.* The nurse may state, "It sounds like you have most trouble with shortness of breath and decreased physical activity. I will talk with the other nurses about helping you with this. Also, I will be back at 7:00 AM tomorrow and will help you with your care then." This will help the client validate any misconceptions gained by the nurse. Also the patient will know when to expect the nurse again.

Special guidelines for interviewing children. For the most part the guidelines previously listed are also applicable for children. However, depending on the child's developmental level and presence of a parent, some special guidelines are warranted.

1. *Try to have the parent present for the interview.* The parent is essential when working with newborns and schoolagers. The limited vocabulary of a toddler can make history taking futile. However, with older children separate and combined interviews may be necessary. The adolescent may be extremely hesitant to express true feelings about a topic with the parent present.

2. *Rapport needs to be established not only with the child but also with the parent.* Often the parent's anxiety and concern is greater than the child's. Therefore establishing a warm, trusting relationship is paramount to obtaining the information needed in the history. It is often said in pediatrics that there are two patients, the child and the parent. As the nurse proceeds with the interview this phrase needs to be remembered. A quiet,

confident tone of voice may allay both the parent's and the child's anxiety.

Implementing the interview

When the nurse is actually faced with obtaining a patient's history or data base, the variety of forms available in texts and articles may be overwhelming. The educational preparation of the nurse, the setting, the psychophysical condition, and the developmental level of the client influence the type of information collected.

Two basic types of history forms for the data base are found in the literature: the structured and the semistructured. The *structured* format may consist of a *questionnaire* that the patient fills out on entry into the health care system. This format will save the nurse time but allows for little free expression by the patient. However, this format may yield more complete data than an unstructured interview administered by the nurse. The structured format may also be initiated by the nurse and may consist of a list of specific questions related to various bio-phycho-sociocultural systems where the nurse directly records answers, or client's responses may be typed into a teletypewriter to allow for computerizing the information. In a study comparing the use of a self-completed questionnaire with unstructured interviews conducted by nurses, the nurses made significantly more errors of omission than the patient.[3]

A structured interview may also list *specific topics* about each patient's system. The nurse then decides how to phrase the particular question. This method allows for more individuality in the interview yet assures that certain topics will be covered (see references 35 and 39 for examples).

The other main type of interview method is the *semistructured* interview. Here the nurse will investigate *broad* categories of data. The questions to be asked may be open or closed and are developed by the nurse in the process of interviewing. The nurse may record a few brief notes but usually writes up the data *after* the interview. The main difficulty with this approach is that it is time consuming. It does allow for free expression of the client's feelings but may not be conducive to obtaining specific, precise data necessary for valid inferences. Research has elicited that the structured interview yielded significantly more data than the unstructured and took half the time.[37]

The box below describes data to be collected under one system (gastrointestinal-nutritional habits) and may serve to clarify the differences between the methods of structured (questionnaire and topics) and semistructured data collection.

Structured—questionnaire

1. How many meals do you eat each day?
2. What do you typically eat for breakfast? Lunch? Dinner? Snacks?
3. What foods do you like?
4. What foods do you dislike?
5. How many glasses of fluid do you drink each day?

Structured—topics

1. Number of meals and snacks.
2. Amount of basic four food groups daily.
3. Amount of daily fluid intake.
4. Likes.
5. Dislikes.

Semistructured

Nutritional habits, food-fluid intake.

Systems framework for assessment

As stated in the previous section, the data base, or history, may be collected in a structured or semistructured manner. The important point is to make sure the data are collected in a comprehensive and organized fashion. The approach used in this chapter seeks to obtain objective and subjective data by means of a nurse-initiatied, semistructured, bio-psycho-sociocultural systems format. For our purposes the individual is seen as a system with subsystems or suprasystems (Fig. 8-3, *top row*). However, components other than the individual may be identified as the system, thus shifting the definitions of corresponding sub- and suprasystems (Fig. 8-3, *middle row*). For example, if the organ system is identified as the system of interest, the individual and higher systems on the continuum become the suprasystems.

Fig. 8-3 *bottom row,* illustrates the subsystems of the individual's bio-psycho-sociocultural systems and where each falls along the continuum. The biologic systems are largely related to organ systems, organs, and cells. The psychologic systems (cognitive and emotional) are related to the individual. The social systems relate to the individual, family, community, and society. Subsystems can be noted in each bio-psycho-sociocultural system. For example, "respiratory" is listed under organ system and biologic systems, whereas "work" is part of community and social system. The placement of these subsystems is somewhat arbitrary, since several items involve numerous levels of the individual. For example, sexual development is listed under the individual system and the psychosystem. However, there are certainly biologic and social components of sexual development.

When the nurse utilizes the systems approach, the concept of the individual as an open system needs to be uppermost in the mind. As the nurse collects data within the bio-, psycho-, or social systems, it is assumed that these areas are not isolated but affect and are affected by other named subsystems or suprasystems. The reader

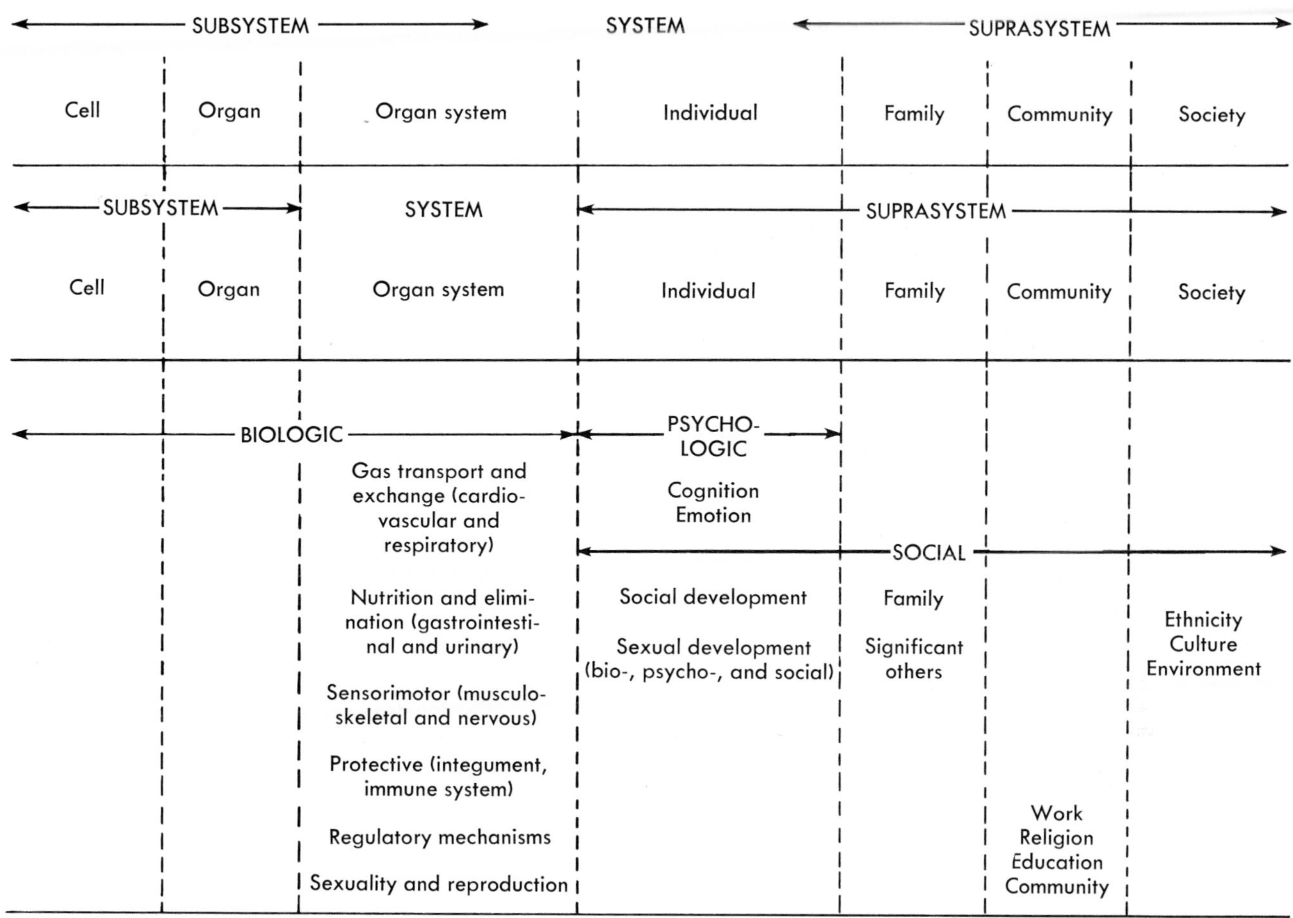

Fig. 8-3. Systems framework for assessment. *Top row,* focal system as individual. *Middle,* focal system as organ system. *Bottom,* individual with corresponding bio-psycho-social subsystems. (Adapted from Byrne, M. L., and Thompson, L. F.: Key concepts for the study and practice of nursing, ed. 2, St. Louis, 1978, The C. V. Mosby Co.)

will note that the vertical lines between the systems in Fig. 8-3 are dotted and not solid, denoting a constant exchange between systems. As the nurse explores one system, decisions need to be made about which other supra- or subsystems also need to be explored. For example, the nurse gathering data about the gastrointestinal system of a patient not only inquires about and examines the biologic system of anatomical organs from the mouth to the stomach to the rectum but also collects data about food intake, a phenomenon largely influenced by the social system, that is, social development, religion, work-economics, and culture.

Using the systems approach, specific topics for a structured interview have been listed for each subsystem of biologic, psychologic, and social systems. Although the format may look overwhelming at first glance, it can be modified to fit the setting, particular client, and experience of the nurse. Since what affects one system affects all systems, data for each of the subsystems need to be collected to prevent missing important information.

A health history is outlined in the box on pp. 103-105. Key data to be collected for each client are marked with an asterisk; these data are especially appropriate for clients being admitted to an inpatient facility. Data not marked are collected if the key data reveal a dysfunction in a subsystem. For example, a patient may state that he or she has chronic bronchitis, experiences shortness of breath after walking 100 feet, and coughs up 2 tablespoons of mucus each morning. The nurse would then inquire about data not asterisked for the respiratory system, such as orthopnea, fever (infection), frequency of sore throat and colds, and factors affecting breathing. Also during the examination the color of nails, and skin and sputum characteristics are noted. Additional data not listed here may need to be collected if a dysfunction is found.

Practice improves the nurse's ability to determine which subsystems require greater investigation with particular clients. Certain health needs may require depth in particular areas of assessment. For example, an elderly individual on bed rest would warrant particular inquiry about the integumentary system to check for dryness, areas of redness, and lesions. In contrast, a young child entering a clinic for a well-child examination would most likely not require as great an inquiry into the same system. The integument of the child might be noted for cleanliness and lesions and little else.

Beginning the interview

As with other aspects of the assessment process, the setting and condition of the client will influence how the interview is begun. The nurse should utilize a specific tool rather than rely on intuition.

The nurse can begin with an open-ended, fairly nondirective statement such as "What brings you to the health care setting?" This is also known as the *chief complaint*. The complaints reflect the patient's subjective perception of the situation. The chief complaint should be noted in a brief statement that includes limited symptoms and their duration.

Within this context the patient should be encouraged to elaborate on the specific symptom, duration, and chronologic history of the problem or a history of present illness. Specific data to investigate about the symptom would include:

1. Location in the body and extension to other body parts
2. Character, both quality and quantity (what is it like and how severe is it?)
3. Time chronology (when did it begin and what course has it followed?)
4. Circumstances of occurrence
5. Aggravating or alleviating factors (what makes it better or worse?)
6. Associated complaints
7. Previous clinicians consulted and effects of prescribed therapies
8. Disability rendered by the chief complaint

Many of the above items are asked by the physician. The nurse may also wish to inquire about the details of the patient's main concern, as the version told to the nurse is often quite different from that told to the physician. For example, the patient's chief complaint may be "increasing shortness of breath over the past 6 weeks." The nurse may determine from the patient's elaboration on the shortness of breath a concern about inability to socialize with friends. The nurse may capitalize on this issue and center interventions around increasing the patient's social network. On the other hand, the physician would delve into determining the cause of the breathing difficulty.

If the nurse obtains the history several days after the admission, it should be remembered that what brought the patient to the hospital and the current chief complaint may be different. To illustrate, the patient may have entered the hospital with a complaint of "a red, swollen, painful left lower leg," which was diagnosed as thrombophlebitis. The nurse needs to collect data about this problem but also note that the patient may think of the current main problem as the "bad food."

After inquiry is made into the chief complaint, data about the individual's *social system* are obtained. As noted in the health history, the categories of data are not extremely personal. Information about family, work, and so forth, gives one a picture of the patient's suprasystems and allows the patient to be seen in another role, as a person. Often this section of the history facilitates the development of rapport with the patient. Another term for this part of the history is the *patient profile*.

Next the nurse can inquire about data listed under the *psychologic systems*. Direct, open-ended questions are asked about some of the categories; for example, "What feelings do you have about this hospitalization?" However, much of the data about the cognitive and emotional systems, such as mood and attention span, will surface indirectly through the course of questioning in the other systems or during the physical appraisal. Often much of the data in this section are not gained by direct questioning.

The final subjective data to be collected relate to the *biologic systems*. This section is also called the *review of systems*. As one develops skill in the assessment process, parts of the biologic systems history may be done during the physical appraisal. For example, the patient's pharynx may appear erythematous on examination. At that point the nurse may inquire about soreness and difficulty in swallowing. With practice the nurse can determine what data is effectively asked before and during the physical appraisal.

It is important to note that with increased knowledge and practice the nurse will improve the ability to recognize patients' significant behavior cues. The questioning will also become more precise in areas related to those behavioral cues.

Subjective data collection (history) does not occur only in the initial encounter with the patient but is ongoing. Initially questions are asked to gather information to plan care. In ongoing assessment questions are asked in those areas where deficits were initially identified, such as a problem with diet. Often as nursing care is given the patient may develop new complaints. Sub-

HEALTH HISTORY: A SUBJECTIVE DATA BASE

I. Chief complaint of client
  A. Location
  B. Character
  C. Chronology
  D. Situational determinants
  E. Aggravating or alleviating factors
  F. Previous attempts at therapy and their effectiveness
  G. Disability resulting from this complaint
II. Social systems
  A. Social development
    *1. Age
    *2. Sex
    *3. Developmental tasks
    *4. Psychosocial personality development (Erickson's Eight Stages of Man)
    *5. Diversional, recreational interests (what to do to pass time while ill)
    *6. Roles in family, community, work and perceived performance of them
    *7. Degree of independence-dependence
    *8. Child's favorite play activity
    *9. Socially oriented habits (include alcohol, drugs), frequency of use, and response to use
  B. Family or significant others
    *1. Others in living group
    *2. Significant others outside living group
    *3. Visiting preferences and who is able to visit
    *4. Marital status
    *5. Alterations for family's life style because of ill member
    *6. Interaction patterns (observe this also)
    *7. Presence of disease in other family members
  C. Work
    *1. Occupation
    *2. Source of income
    *3. Insurance (hospitalization)
    *4. Changes in work pattern because of illness
    *5. Feelings about work and being away from productivity and routine
  D. Religion
    *1. Religious affiliation
    *2. Desire for chaplain visit
    *3. Practices or beliefs that might affect reaction to health care (proscriptions against immunization or blood transfusion, dietary laws, beliefs, about disease causation, death)
  E. Education
    *1. Formal education
    *2. Satisfaction and progress with school
  F. Community
    *1. Type of housing
    *2. Contacts or previous referrals to social agencies
    *3. Availability and pattern of utilization of health care facilities (physician, dentist), frequency and reason for visits
    *4. Immunizations (type, date)
  G. Ethnic-cultural system
    *1. Factors that my influence reaction to hospitalization, therapy, illness
    *2. Food preferences
    *3. Response to stress (e.g., pain)
  H. Environment
    *1. Effect of present environment on health status and developmental level (e.g., lighting, noise, activity, color—variation, consistency excessive or absent)
    *2. Arrangement of environmental in relation to functional abilities or disabilities
    *3. Safety factors
      a. Mobility (arrangement of objects in physical environment)
      b. Use of prosthetic or supportive devices (e.g., crutches, wheelchair)
    *4. Infection control
      a. Ready sources of infection
      b. Barriers to infection (isolation technique, handwashing facility)
III. Psychologic systems
  A. Cognition
    *1. Level of consciousness (response to sensory stimuli)
    *2. Orientation to time, place, person
    *3. Mental skills
      a. Ability to read and write
      b. Vocabulary
      c. Ability to comprehend and follow directions
      d. Attention and memory span
    *4. Intellectual development relative to chronologic age (e.g., Piaget's formulation)
    *5. Understanding of and reaction to health concern and goals of medical-nursing therapy
    *6. Desired information about present tests and treatment
    *7. Previous experience with and reaction to illness and hospitalization
    *8. Name child or adolescent prefers

*Key data to collect for all clients. Data not marked are collected if dysfunction is found in system.

Continued.

HEALTH HISTORY: A SUBJECTIVE DATA BASE—CONT'D

B. Emotion
  *1. Quality of mood, expression, intensity of reaction
  *2. Activity level (active, sluggish, hyperactive)
  *3. Effect of illness on life style and expectation of future effects
  *4. Feelings about hospitalization
  *5. Coping patterns in stressful situations (describe stressful situations); availability, need for, and effectiveness of internal-external support systems
  *6. Special concerns or fears
  *7. Patterns of relating to others (e.g., verbal, congenial)
  *8. Self-concept (body image prior to and in relation to current health problem)
  *9. Comfort, rest and sleep patterns (hours, time, nap periods, feeling of being rested) before and since illness
  *10. Aids used to sleep
  *11. Presence of pain or discomfort (location, duration, degree, character, precipitating factors, change in pattern)
  *12. Use of aids to relieve pain

IV. Biologic systems
  A. Gas transport and exchange
    1. Cardiovascular
      *a. Past or present disease of cardiovascular system
      *b. Syncope
      *c. Dizziness
      *d. Fatigue, activity tolerance
      *e. Chest pain
        (1) Type
        (2) Pattern
        (3) Precipitating factors
        (4) Relief measures
      *f. Subjective feeling of warmth or coldness of body parts
      *g. Medications taken to affect CV system
      *h. Edematous body parts
    2. Respiratory
      *a. Past or present diseases of respiratory system
      *b. Cough
        (1) Frequency
        (2) Duration
      *c. Sputum
        (1) Color
        (2) Odor
        (3) Amount
      *d. Shortness of breath
        (1) Precipitating factors
        (2) Frequency
        (3) Effect on activity
      *e. Allergies
      *f. Smoking
        (1) Amount
        (2) Duration
        (3) Attempts and success at stopping
      *g. Medications taken to affect respiratory system
      h. Orthopnea
      i. Hemoptysis
      j. Fever
      k. Frequency of colds and sore throat
      l. Activity tolerance
      m. Factors affecting breathing
        (1) Emotion
        (2) Pollution
        (3) Position
  B. Nutrition and elimination
    1. Gastrointestinal
      *a. Past or present disease of GI system
      *b. Dietary habits
        (1) Amount of basic four food groups
        (2) Amount of fluid intake daily
        (3) Likes
        (4) Dislikes
        (5) Number of meals and snacks
        (6) Time of meals
        (7) Assistance needed with eating
        (8) Alcohol intake
      *c. Appetite, thirst, stability of weight
      *d. Factors related to ingestion
        (1) Nonoral intake
        (2) Chewing
        (3) Swallowing
        (4) Oral hygiene habits
      *e. Factors related to digestion
        (1) Ease
        (2) Nausea
        (3) Vomiting
        (4) Belching
        (5) Pain in abdomen
      *f. Bowel elimination pattern
        (1) Time and frequency of bowel movements
        (2) Degree of child's independence in toileting
        (3) Words used by child regarding elimination
        (4) Character of stools
        (5) Ease (constipation, diarrhea)
        (6) Hemorrhoids
        (7) Passage of flatus, blood
      *g. Abdominal pain and characteristic

HEALTH HISTORY: A SUBJECTIVE DATA BASE—CONT'D

- *h. Medicines taken to alter digestion and metabolism of foods
- 2. Urinary
  - *a. Past or present diseases of urinary system
  - *b. Fluid intake
  - *c. Urination pattern
    - (1) Amount
    - (2) Color
    - (3) Odor
    - (4) Frequency, night or day urgency
    - (5) Dysuria
  - *d. Vaginal or urethral discharge
  - *e. Degree of independence in toileting
  - *f. Edema
- C. Sensorimotor
  - 1. Musculoskeletal
    - *a. Past or present diseases of musculoskeletal system
    - *b. Abnormal innervation to muscles (paralysis, weakness, spasticity)
    - *c. Activity endurance
    - *d. Method of ambulation
      - (1) Assistance needed with dressing, hygiene
      - (2) Safety measures needed
    - *e. Range of motion limitation
    - *f. Muscle weakness
    - *g. Medicines taken to affect musculo-skeletal subsystem
  - 2. Nervous
    - *a. Past or present diseases of nervous system
    - *b. Visual status
      - (1) Acuity
      - (2) Deficits and corrective devices
    - *c. Auditory status
      - (1) Deficits and corrective devices
      - (2) Unusual sensations (ringing, buzzing, vertigo, pain)
    - *d. Olfactory status
    - *e. Gustatory status
    - *f. Tactile status (ability to discriminate sharp-dull, light-firm, heat-cold sensations)
    - *g. Mobility (coordination, balance)
    - *h. Medicines taken to affect nervous system
- D. Protective mechanisms
  - 1. Integument
    - *a. Past or present diseases of integumentary system
    - *b. Factors predisposing to skin break-down
    - *c. Personal hygiene
      - (1) Bathing (kind, type, frequency)
      - (2) Frequency, time of shaving
      - (3) After bath skin care
    - *d. Medicines taken to affect integumentary system
  - 2. Immune mechanism
    - *a. Past or present allergy
    - *b. Past or present sensitivities to drugs or other agents (pollens, insect bites)
    - *c. Past or present high susceptibility to infection
- E. Endocrine mechanisms
  - *1. Abnormal function of endocrine gland(s) and effect; past or present diseases
  - *2. Growth patterns
  - *3. Medicines taken to affect endocrine system
- F. Sexuality and reproduction
  - *1. Past or present alterations of reproduction system
  - *2. Reproductive data
    - a. Number of pregnancies
    - b. Live births
    - c. Living children
    - d. Family planning (methods used)
    - e. Menstrual pattern
    - f. Menopause (age of onset and associated factors)
  - *3. Breast self-examination routine
  - *4. Frequency of Pap smears
  - *5. Sexual libido and performance
  - *6. Level of sexual development
  - *7. Attitudes toward own sexuality
  - *8. Medicines taken to affect reproductive system

sequently, relevant areas within the subsystem and suprasystem related to the complaint are investigated to increase the data pool. For example, the patient may complain of constipation. Rather than immediately administering a laxative the nurse evaluates factors with the suprasystem of the gastrointestinal system, such as level of exercise and comfort in using a bedpan in a two-bed room. Subsystem factors such as dietary intake, bowel movement frequency, and fluid intake are also assessed.

□ Objective data collection: physical appraisal

A controversy exists concerning the level and scope of physical assessment skills appropriate to nursing practice. Many nursing programs now include these skills as a basic part of the curriculum.

The physical appraisal skills are an important adjunct to the assessment process. Even though a thorough history generally yields more data, the physical appraisal (or objective data collection) contributes to the nurse's inferences about the patient's strengths and limitations. These skills also offer measures to evaluate nursing interventions.

Techniques

The four techniques utilized in physical appraisal are inspection, palpation, percussion, and auscultation.

The skill of *inspection,* or visual examination, was alluded to earlier. This examination technique considers the general appearance and specific characteristics of the patient's body. Notations may be made about color, shape, position, size, and symmetry (to name a few). Inspection begins on first meeting the patient and may be integrated with other techniques. Of the four techniques inspection may be the most difficult to use, but it yields the most relevant, important data.

Palpation capitalizes on the sense of touch for the purpose of determining the characteristics of tissues or organs. Characteristics such as movement, pain, edema, consistency, temperature, form, vibration, and texture

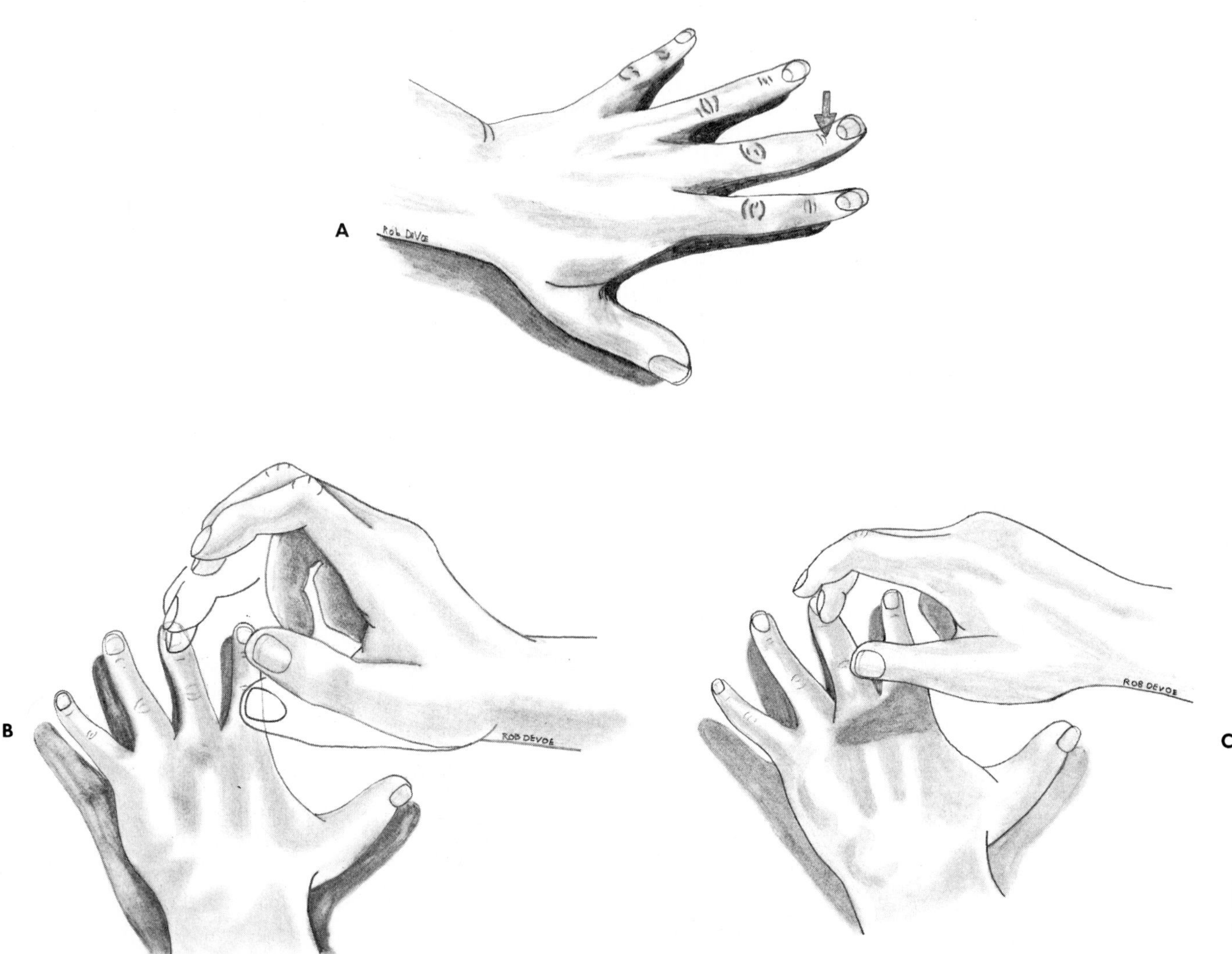

Fig. 8-4. Percussion. **A,** Middle or index finger is placed on body surface with palm and other fingers held away from skin. **B,** Tip of middle finger of opposite hand strikes base of distal portion of finger next to body surface. **C,** Wrist is flexed with forearm in stationary position.

can be assessed. Different parts of the hands are used for different aspects of the appraisal. The fingertips are the most sensitive part of the hand and are the best for fine, tactile discriminations such as texture of skin and size of lymph nodes. The dorsum of the finger has thin skin and is most sensitive to temperature. The palmar aspects of the hands are the most sensitive to vibration. Palpation is also used to check for symmetry of a body part. Pressure is applied with the warmed hands in a deliberate, gentle manner, first using light then deep palpation.

The skill of *percussion* involves tapping a body surface to produce sounds that determine the position or density of an underlying structure. The usual method is direct percussion. The middle or index finger of the nondominant hand is placed against the body surface with the palm and the other fingers of the same hand off the skin. The tip of the middle finger of the opposite hand strikes the base of the distal phalanx of the finger on the patient's skin. The stroke delivered is sharp, with the wrist flexing and the forearm stationary; the striking finger is immediately removed (Fig. 8-4). The sound is then evaluated to determine the type of substance or location of structure percussed. For example, dense solid tissue such as muscle has a flat sound. Air-filled cavities such as the lungs have a resonant sound. The more dense a tissue, the shorter and softer the sound.

The sense of hearing is used in *auscultation* to delineate the sounds of organs such as heart, lungs, and intestines. Characteristics of sounds, such as frequency, intensity, quality, and duration, are evaluated. The stethoscope is used in auscultation, with the diaphragm evaluating high-pitched sounds and the bell low-pitched sounds. Auscultation is performed in a quiet, warm environment with the listener concentrating on one sound at a time.

Guidelines for physical appraisal

The guidelines for assessment interviewing are appropriate here also. It is important that the client understand the purposes for the appraisal and that physical privacy is maintained.

As mentioned earlier, the parent should be present when children are examined. Maintain eye level contact with the child. Children are informed of each procedure

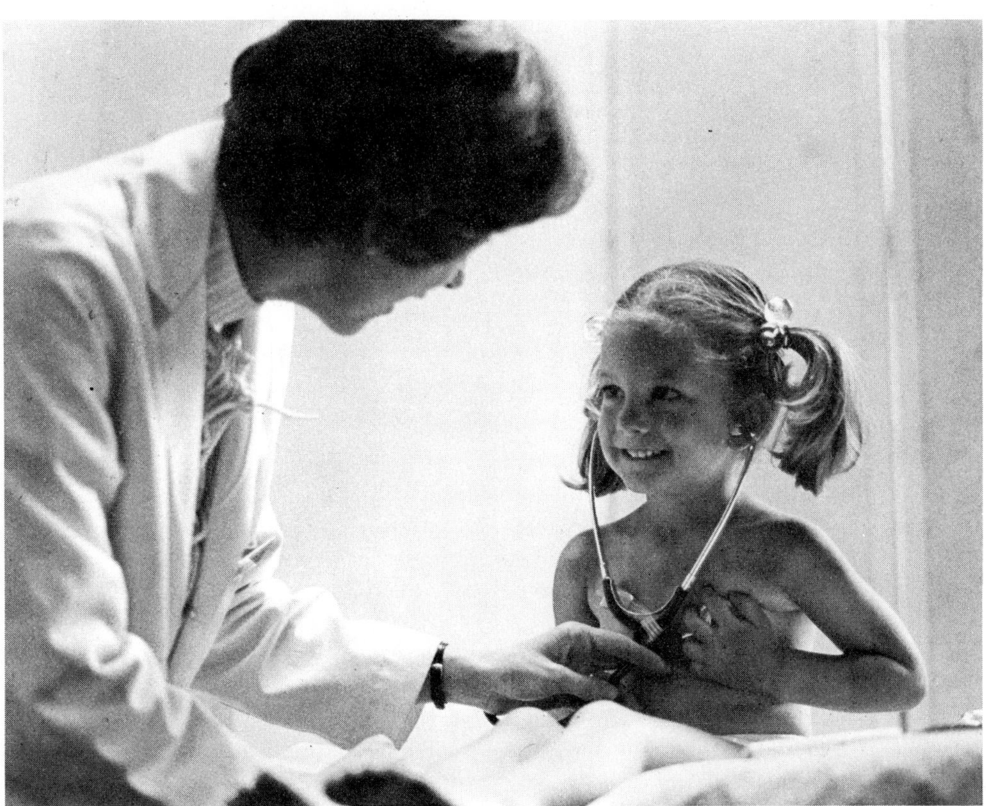

Fig. 8-5. Physical examination of child is enhanced by eye contact, explanation of procedures, and opportunity to handle equipment. Parent's presence is encouraged.

in the examination and are allowed to handle the examination equipment, when appropriate, to decrease fear (Fig. 8-5). When procedures are announced, the examiner follows through with them.

The clinician makes commands for the child's performance in positive statements. This informs the child of what *can* versus what *cannot* be done. For example. "Sit on the table" yields a more positive result than "Don't stand on the table!"

Commands are stated in *specific* terms rather than general ones. When the child is asked to perform, be patient and allow time.

The child's participation in the appraisal is encouraged. The bulk of conversation with school-aged and older children is directed toward the child rather than the parent.

Carrying out the physical appraisal

The key to completing a worthwhile appraisal is to be systematic and thorough. For adults, collecting data in a head-to-toe fashion is best utilized during the initial assessment (see box, pp. 109-111).

The physical appraisal or examination according to biologic systems is best utilized when specific concerns or problems of the patient evolve. For example, the patient may complain of a productive cough. The nurse would then key into data specific to the respiratory system (see Chapter 44) versus completing a head-to-toe examination.

Before beginning the appraisal a general overview of the patient can yield many clues about significant data to be collected later. Proceeding from head to neck to thorax to abdomen to extremities provides a systematic framework for data collection.

With infants the nurse may start with the feet and move to the head, since they object less strongly to a peripheral-to-central examination. The infant and toddler sits on the mother's lap during the appraisal, as they usually react strongly to being separated from mother. This age group may resent intrusion of body parts by an unfamiliar person. Therefore the systematic approach may be quite jumbled. Their mouths may not open when you ask but can be examined at an unsuspecting moment or when the child cries. Nurses must be adaptable!

■ DATA ANALYSIS

The second aspect of nursing assessment is data analysis. This component of the nursing process is perhaps the most important yet was relatively overlooked until the mid-1970s. Few books are written on data analysis. Also there has been considerable disagreement in the nursing field as to the labeling of this component. For example, when the nurse analyzes the data, is it called identifying needs, problems, strengths, and liabilities or is it diagnosis? Regardless of the terminology, this aspect of the nursing process is finally receiving more attention both in the literature and in active investigation by nurses.

Data analysis requires high-level thinking, such as inductive and deductive reasoning, synthesis, and comparison of data with norms and standards to determine their significance. Each data analysis method *must* be substantiated by a sound theoretical rationale. To utilize the above-mentioned thinking processes, nurses need a sound knowledge base. Data analysis is closely linked with inference making, described earlier. Data analysis is farther reaching than inference making but permits greater specificity. Whereas the inference might be "patient fearful," the data analysis might be "patient fearful of death, especially of dying alone." The latter was attained by considering a wider range of clinical behaviors and required synthesis. The nurse may also utilize the four methods of validation here as described for validating inferences.

□ Strengths and liabilities

One method used by nurses is to group the collected raw data into strengths and liabilities according to each system listed on the tool. For example, the history and examination of the integumentary system may reveal strengths and liabilities as follows:

Strengths

1. No past history of problem
2. Clean, intact body skin with pleasant odor
3. Normal hair distribution
4. Bathes self every day (sponge bath)
5. Warm, dry, pink skin

Liabilities

1. Thin, 76-year-old woman requiring bedrest
2. Hair oily with 1/4-inch white scaly patches on scalp
3. Dry, flaky skin on extremities

After completing the process with each system, the nurse has a view of the patient's overall status. Plans can be made to correct the liabilities.

□ Needs and problems

Before beginning to establish patient goals, the nurse critiques the raw data or strengths and liabilities and delineates patient *needs* or *problems*, a second major method of data analysis. The nurse must ask: What kind of needs or problems does the data reflect?

At times needs and problems are used interchangeably. However, a need is a requirement that an individual often defines in relationship to society's norms. Orlando defines need situationally "as a requirement of

SYSTEMATIC PHYSICAL APPRAISAL: A HEAD-TO-TOE APPROACH

I. General survey (60-second impression regarding immediate status of patient on entering room)
  A. Apparent state of health
  B. Signs of distress
  C. Skin color
  D. Stature and body build
  E. Posture, motor activity, and gait
  F. Dress, grooming, and personal hygiene
  G. Odors of body and breath
  H. Manner, mood, and relationship to persons and things around client
  I. Speech
  J. State of awareness, consciousness
  K. Presence of supportive or monitoring devices and their function
  L. Facial expression

II. Vital signs
  A. Blood pressure
  B. Temperature
  C. Radial pulse
    1. Quality
      a. Equal on both sides
      b. Thready, bounding, weak, strong
    2. Rhythm
      a. Regular
      b. Irregular-irregular
      c. Irregular-regular
    3. Rate
  D. Respiration
    1. Rate
    2. Rhythm
    3. Depth
    4. Ease
  E. Height, weight, head circumference

III. Head
  A. Hair, scalp, skull
    1. Texture, cleanliness, quantity, distribution, pattern of loss or gain of hair
    2. Scalp condition (scaly, lumpy, other lesions)
    3. Skull contour, head circumference
    4. Condition of fontanels (infants)
  B. Face
    1. Facial expression
    2. Symmetry, involuntary movements, edema, lesions, masses
  C. Eyes
    1. Position and alignment of eyes
    2. Position of eyelids in relation to eyeballs
    3. Eyelid (closed completely [ptosis], edema, lesions)
    4. Eyelashes (presence, direction of growth)
    5. Eyes
      a. Conjunctiva, sclera, color
      b. Lens
      c. Iris
      d. Pupil (size pre- and poststimulation, shape, equality, reaction to light and accommodation)
    6. Visual fields by confrontation method
    7. Corrective or prosthetic devices
    8. Test range of extraocular movement through six cardinal fields of gaze
  D. Ears
    1. Auricle color, lumps, lesions
    2. Patency of canal and color (use otoscope)
    3. Weber and Rinne tests
  E. Nares
    1. Inhales through nose or mouth
    2. Flaring, patency, position of septum
    3. Palpate for sinus tenderness
  F. Mouth
    1. Lips (color, moisture, lumps, ulcers, cracking)
    2. Mucous membranes (ulcers, nodules, color, moistness)
    3. State of teeth and gums
    4. Tongue
      a. Coated
      b. Lesions (including floor of mouth; palpate if found)
      c. Edema
      d. Symmetry of movement
    5. Tonsils, uvula
      a. Color, exudate
      b. Edema
      c. Symmetry

IV. Neck
  A. Lymph nodes
  B. Jugular vein (distention)
  C. Carotid pulse (palpate)
  D. Trachea (inspect and palpate for deviation)

V. Thorax
  A. Inspection: lungs
    1. Shape of chest, deformity of thorax, spine contour, symmetry of chest expansion
    2. Use of accessory muscles and retraction of intercostal muscles
    3. Presence of cough
    4. Sputum
      a. Color
      b. Odor
      c. Amount
    5. Local lag or impairment of respiratory movement
    6. Position of comfort
  B. Inspection and palpation: heart
    1. Point of maximal intensity (PMI) (location, amplitude)
    2. Pulsations over chest wall

Continued.

SYSTEMIC PHYSICAL APPRAISAL: A HEAD-TO-TOE APPROACH—CONT'D

C. Inspection: breasts, nipples
  1. Female clients
    a. Size, contour
    b. Puckering, dimpling, flattening
    c. Discharge, nipple crusting
    d. Inspect as patient sits, raises arm over head, presses hands against hips
  2. Male clients
    a. Nodules, swelling, ulceration
D. Palpation: lungs
  1. Distance of chest wall excursion
  2. Tenderness around pain or lesions
  3. Fremitus
E. Palpation: breast (periphery, tail, areola), nipple
  1. Note consistency, induration, tenderness
  2. Nodules (size, location, shape, mobility, tenderness, consistency)
  3. Elasticity of nipple
F. Percussion: lungs
  1. Symmetry of chest wall sound
  2. Abnormal areas (identify, localize, describe)
  3. Diaphragmatic excursion
G. Auscultation: Lungs (NOTE: Examination of respiratory system is done anteriorly and posteriorly.)
  1. Presence and loudness of breath sounds throughout lung fields (symmetry)
  2. Breath sounds (quality, intensity)
    a. Vesicular
    b. Bronchial
    c. Bronchovesicular
  3. Adventitious sounds
    a. Rales
    b. Rhonchi, including wheezes
H. Auscultation: heart
  1. First and second heart sounds at aortic, pulmonic, mitral, tricuspid areas
  2. Heart rate, rhythm
  3. Apical, radial pulses
  4. Extra sounds or murmurs

VI. Abdomen (NOTE: Order of examination: inspection, auscultation, percussion, palpation)
  A. Inspection
    1. Abdominal contour
    2. Scars, striae
    3. Umbilicus, contour, signs of inflammation
    4. Pulsations
    5. Hernia
  B. Auscultation
    1. Bowel sounds (frequency, character)
  C. Percussion
    1. Abdominal distention
    2. Distended bladder (in suspected individuals)
  D. Palpation
    1. Tenderness (including rebound tenderness)
    2. Abdominal masses and organs in four quadrants
    3. Distended bladder (in suspected individuals)
    4. Sacral edema

VII. Perineal area
  A. Inspection
    1. Vaginal or urethral discharge (amount, color, odor)
    2. Indication of bladder or bowel incontinence
    3. Presence and size of hemorrhoids
    4. Infant/toddler: configuration of genitalia
    5. Male clients: penis skin, foreskin, scrotum, hernias
    6. Female clients: labia, clitoris, vaginal orifice, perineum

VIII. Extremities
  A. Inspection: arms
    1. Size, symmetry
    2. Color and blanching of nail beds
    3. Bilateral hand grasp
    4. Movement of limbs on command, symmetry of movement
    5. Degree of strength to raise and lower arms against resistance
    6. Degree of range of motion
  B. Palpation: arms
    1. Brachial, ulnar pulses (if arterial insufficiency suspected)
    2. Edema
  C. Inspection: legs
    1. Size, symmetry
    2. Hair distribution of legs, feet, toes
    3. Color of skin of lower legs and ankles
    4. Color, temperature of feet
    5. Color of toenails and blanching
    6. Degree of range and motion
    7. Degree of strength to raise and lower legs and flex and extend feet and legs against resistance
    8. Flexor plantar reflex (Babinski)
    9. Homan's sign
  D. Palpation: legs
    1. Tenderness of thigh and calf muscles
    2. Varicosities
    3. Presence of edema (pretibial, medial malleolus, dorsum of foot)

SYSTEMIC PHYSICAL APPRAISAL: A HEAD-TO-TOE APPROACH—CONT'D

4. Femoral, popliteal, posterior tibial, dorsalis pedis pulses (normal, diminished, absent)

IX. Skin
  A. Inspection
    1. Hair distribution
    2. Vascularity (bleeding, bruising, varicosities)
    3. Mobility, turgor, thickness, texture
    4. Color
    5. Edema
    6. Odor, excretions, cleanliness
    7. Moisture, dryness
    8. Lesions (color [note nevi], drainage, distribution)
  B. Palpation
    1. Temperature

X. Concomitant observations
  A. Degree of orientation by the appropriateness and clarity of patient's responses
    1. Speech perception and formation
    2. Auditory deficits
    3. Level of consciousness (persons, place, time)
  B. Cognitive-emotional systems
    1. Restlessness
    2. Hostility
    3. Apprehension
  C. Condition of neuromuscular system
    1. Level of consciousness (persons, place, time)
    2. Muscle mass
    3. Abnormal innervation to muscles (paralysis, weakness, spasticity)
    4. Ability to discriminate sharp-dull, light-firm, heat-cold sensations
    5. Mobility (gait, balance, coordination, method of ambulation)
    6. Activity endurance
    7. Presence-absence of primitive reflexes (infants)
    8. Visual acuity using Snellen chart
  D. Laboratory tests relevant to each body system

the patient which, if supplied, relieves or diminishes his immediate distress or improves his immediate sense of adequacy or well-being."[46] Examples might be a need for oxygen, which may be deficient and could relieve distress. There may be a need for a positive self-image, which could improve one's sense of adequacy.

Maslow's hierarchy of needs is very applicable in the clinical setting (see Chapter 1). The nurse may identify liabilities from the data, such as inadequate hydration and loneliness. By using Maslow's hierarchy the problem of inadequate hydration reflects a block in the need for the physiologic need of fluid. Plans are then made to provide fluids for the patient. The difficulty of loneliness reflects inadequate meeting of the need for belongingness-love.

Maslow's hierarchy not only helps the nurse identify needs but also places priority, or order of importance, on needs. For example, the nurse should meet the patient's need for fluid before concentrating on the need for love. Likewise, if a patient is bleeding the nurse should attend to that physiologic need before talking to the patient about retirement. In establishing priority of needs the patient should be actively included, when appropriate.

Another aspect of the second method of data analysis is identifying patients' *problems*. Problems reflect a difficult situation with which the person usually requires outside help for effective coping. Problems may be actual or potential negative alterations in a person's biopsycho-sociocultural health or steady state. Problems may reflect an unmet need or a conflict between two needs. In the previous example inadequate hydration is the problem and adequate fluid intake is the need. When an individual or family does not realize that a need exists or is meeting the need ineffectively, a problem exists as identified by objective data. A young mother may not realize that her 18-month-old child needs nutritional intake in addition to milk. Therefore the need for food is reflected in the problem of inadequate nutritional intake, namely, vitamins and iron.

Problems may be overt or covert. Overt problems are readily identifiable, such as immobility or inadequate urinary output. Covert problems are more difficult to identify, require greater synthesis of a variety of data, may be masked by other problems, or lack objectivity. A patient's crying may have a variety of meanings. The nurse may need to collect a variety of data to determine that this patient is not crying because of postoperative pain but because of a sense of loss because today is the first anniversary of her mother's death.

Problems may be identified through inductive or deductive reasoning. With induction the nurse critiques the data collected in each system. Then a generalization is made (similar to inference making) that has support from a theoretical base. For example, a postoperative patient may be seen with weak, thready, increasing pulse of 98 beats per minute; cool, pale, dry skin; decreasing blood pressure to 98/40; respiratory rate of 36 per minute; and apprehension. The nurse may delineate the problem as hemorrhagic shock based on knowledge of its manifestations.

With the deductive method the nurse moves from generalizations to specifics. For example, the patient may be immobile because of a fracture. The nurse then delineates problems indicative of immobility that should be validated such as stasis of pulmonary secretions, constipation, skin breakdown. Then the nurse proceeds to establish goals based on the defined problems.

□ Nursing diagnosis

The final method of data analysis to be discussed here is nursing diagnosis. Nursing diagnosis is a fairly apt synonym for patient problems that are based on needs, a judgment or conlcusion about the individual's or other's perception of an actual or potential alteration in the client's health status, and the identified cause of the alteration. The alteration may occur in the bio-psycho-sociocultural systems. For example, a diagnosis may be "pain secondary to abdominal surgery for laparotomy." One should keep in mind also that the conclusion reached may not be a problem. The conclusion reached may be that the patient is in normal health and growth-development status, as one may find on a well-child visit.

A difference exists between a medical and nursing diagnosis. Both medical and nursing diagnoses imply a shortcut method of describing a cluster of signs and symptoms. Signs are objective manifestations of disease, such as vomiting, purulent sputum, or agitated motor activity. Symptoms are subjective manifestations of disease, such as pain or nausea. The medical diagnosis of bacterial pneumonia implies a grouping of signs and symptoms, as does the nursing diagnosis of impaired mobility.

Medical diagnoses generally focus on defining the cause of the impairment or pathologic condition, whereas the nursing diagnosis considers the effect of the impairment on the individual's daily functioning in bio-psycho-sociocultural systems. Gordon aptly defines nursing diagnoses as those "made by professional nurses, which describe actual or potential health problems which nurses, by virtue of their education and experience are capable and licensed to treat."[21]

A nursing diagnosis may be indicative of a medical diagnosis. For example, respiratory distress may be indicative of the medical diagnosis of status asthmaticus.

In acute settings both diagnoses may be the same, but the treatment usually evolves differently because the knowledge needed and the approach used to treat are different. Treatment implies implementing modes of nursing or medical therapy. A nurse may clearly identify pulmonary edema or ventricular fibrillation as the patient's problem. However, by Gordon's definition, these conclusions should not be viewed as nursing diagnoses, since the nurse is not licensed to treat them. However, the nurse may implement therapy and collaborate with the physician. In these situations it is difficult to draw a clear-cut line between what a physician and a nurse should do. Collaboration is mandatory!

The diagnosis or problem is stated precisely and concisely. The diagnosis of "impairment of skin integrity" could be supplemented by more descriptive terms. For example, the impairment of skin integrity may be related to superficial laceration, compound fracture, excess pressure due to immobility, or dry skin leading to cracking. Each of these contributing factors requires a different intervention. Therefore, listing the contributing factors allows for greater precision as the nurse plans care.

The diagnosis is stated in terms of the patient's state rather than the nurse's. For example, "Needs to be turned in bed" describes a nursing activity rather than the patient's problem of "impaired mobility, unable to turn in bed."

Little and Carnevali[31] list some helpful guidelines that describe what a nursing diagnosis is *not:*

1. Not the medical diagnosis (e.g., cirrhosis)
2. Not the diagnostic test (e.g., barium enema)
3. Not the medical treatment (e.g., colostomy)
4. Not the equipment (e.g., catheter)
5. Not the nurse's problem with the client (e.g., uncooperative)

The integration of data analysis with the problem-oriented system is discussed in Chapter 10.

■ SUMMARY

This chapter has considered how to systematically assess patient's bio-psycho-sociocultural systems in an effective manner. Both data collection and analysis have been discussed. It is the nurse's responsibility to develop the skills mentioned here in order to provide a data base and problem list that can support individualized nursing care.

REFERENCES AND SELECTED READINGS

1. Alexander, M. M. and Brown, M. S.: Physical examination: history taking, part 2, Nursing '73 **3**:35-39, 1973.
2. Aspinall, M. J.: Nursing diagnosis: the weak link, Nurs. Outlook **24**:433-437, 1976.
3. Aspinall, M. J.: Development of a patient completed admission questionnaire and its comparison with the nursing interview, Nurs. Res. **24**:377-381, 1975.

*References preceded by an asterisk are particularly well suited for student reading.

4. Bates, B., and Lynaugh, J.: Teaching physical assessment, Nurs. Outlook **23**:297-302, 1975.
5. Becknell, E. P., and Smith, D. M.: System of nursing practice, Philadelphia, 1975, F. A. Davis Co.
6. Bermosk, L. S., and Mordan, M. J.: Interviewing in nursing, New York, 1964, Macmillan, Inc., p. 46.
7. Bircher, A. U.: On the development and classification of diagnosis, Nurs. Forum **14**:10-29, 1975.
8. Bower, F. L.: The process of planning nursing care: a model for practice, ed. 2, St. Louis, 1977, the C. V. Mosby Co.
9. Byrne, M. L., and Thompson, L. F.: Key concepts for the study and practice of nursing, ed. 2, St. Louis, 1978, The C. V. Mosby Co.
10. Carrieri, V. K., and Sitzman, J.: Components of the nursing process, Nurs. Clin. North Am. **6**:115-124, 1971.
11. Chambers, W.: Nursing diagnosis, Am. J. Nurs. **62**:102-104, 1962.
12. Chinn, P. L., and Leitch, C. J.: Handbook for nursing assessment of the child. Salt Lake City, 1973, University of Utah Press.
13. Crane, J.: Physical appraisal: an aspect of the nursing assessment. In Sana, J. M., and Judge, R. D.: Physical appraisal methods in nursing practice, Boston, 1975, Little, Brown and Co.
14. Culver, C. M., and Dunham, F.: The inference process, unpublished paper prepared in conjunction with USPHS grant no. 81-1362, 1964, pp. 1-34.
15. Dugas, B. W.: Introduction to patient care, ed. 3, Philadelphia, 1977, W. B. Saunders Co.
16. *Durand, M., and Prince, R.: Nursing diagnosis, process and decision, Nurs. Forum **5**:50-64, 1966.
17. Fuller, D., and Rosenaur, J. A.: A patient assessment guide, Nurs. Outlook **22**:460-462, 1974.
18. Garant, C.: A basis for care, Am. J. Nurs. **72**:699-701, 1972.
19. Gebbie, K., and Lavin, M. A., editors: Classification of nursing diagnoses, St. Louis, 1975, The C. V. Mosby Co.
20. Gebbie, K., and Lavin, M. A.: Classifying nursing diagnosis, Am. J. Nurs. **74**:250-253, 1974.
21. Gordon, M.: Nursing diagnosis and the diagnostic process, Am. J. Nurs. **76**:1298-1300, 1976.
22. Hall, E. T.: The hidden dimension, New York 1966, Doubleday & Co., Inc., p. 110.
23. Hamdi, M. E., and Hutelmyer, C. M.: A study of the effectiveness of an assessment tool in the identification of nursing care problems, Nurs. Res. **19**:354-358, 1970.
24. Hazzard, M. E.: An overview of systems theory, Nurs. Clin. North Am. **6**:385-393, 1971.
25. Helfer, R. E., Black, M. A., and Helfer, M. E.: Pediatric interviewing skills taught by nonphysicians, Am. J. Dis. Child **129**:1053-1057, 1975.
26. Hermone, R. H.: How to get results from an interview, Hosp. Topics **49**:88-89, 1971.
27. Johnson, I.: The art of history taking, J. Neurosurg. Nurs. **2**:5-17, 1970.
28. Johnson, M. M., and Davis, M. L.: Problem solving in nursing practice, ed. 2, Dubuque, Ia., 1975, William C. Brown Co., Publishers.
29. Langer, S. R.: The nursing process and the interview, Occup. Health Nurs. **21**:19-23, 1973.
30. Lewis, L.: Planning patient care, ed. 2, Dubuque, Ia., 1976, William C. Brown Co., Publishers.
31. Little, D., and Carnevali, D.: Nursing care planning, ed. 2, Philadelphia, 1976, J. B. Lippincott Co., pp. 157-159.
32. MacFarlane, J.: Pediatric assessment and intervention: some simple how-to's for ambulatory settings, Nursing '74 **4**:66-68, 1974.
33. Mahoney, E., Verdisco, L., and Shortridge, L.: How to collect and record a health history, Philadelphia, 1976, J. B. Lippincott Co.
33a. *Malasanos, L., Barkauskas, V., Moss, M., and Allen, K. S.: Health assessment, St. Louis, 1977, The C. V. Mosby Co.
34. Mansell, E., and Stokes, S.: Patient assessment: taking a patient's history, Am. J. Nurs. **74**:293-324, 1974.
35. Manthey, M. E.: A guide for interviewing, Am. J. Nurs. **67**:2088-2090, 1967.
36. Marriner, A.: The nursing process: a scientific approach to nursing care, St. Louis, 1975, The C. V. Mosby Co.
37. Marshall, J. C., and Feeney, S.: Structured versus intuitive intake interview, Nurs. Res. **21**:269-272, 1972.
38. Maslow, A.: Motivation and personality, New York, 1969, Harper & Row, Publishers.
39. McCain, R. F.: Nursing by assessment—not intuition, Am. J. Nurs. **65**:82-84, 1965.
40. McCloskey, J. C.: The nursing care plan: past, present and uncertain future; a review of the literature, Nurs. Forum **14**:364-382, 1975.
41. McPhetridge, L. M.: Nursing history: one means to personalize care, Am. J. Nurs. **68**:68-75, 1968.
42. Mitchell, P. H.: Concepts basic to nursing, New York, 1977, McGraw-Hill Book Co., p. 76.
43. Mumford, E.: A brief program: the nurse as observer, Nurs. Outlook **15**:56-60, 1967.
44. Mundinger, M. O., and Jouron, G. D.: Developing a nursing diagnosis, Nurs. Outlook **23**:94-98, 1975.
45. Murray, M.: Fundamentals of nursing, Englewood Cliffs, N. J., 1976, Prentice-Hall, Inc.
46. Orlando, I. J.: The dynamic nurse-patient relationship, New York, 1961, G. P. Putman's Sons, p. 5.
47. Pearsall, M.: Participant observation as role and method in behavioral research, Nurs. Res. **14**:37-42, 1965.
48. Peplau, H. E.: Talking with patients, Am. J. Nurs. **60**:964-966, 1960.
49. Prange, A. J., Jr., and Martin, H. W.: Aids to understanding patients, Am. J. Nurs. **62**:98-100, 1962.
50. Rothberg, J. S.: Why nursing diagnosis? Am. J. Nurs. **67**:1040-1042, 1967.
51. Roy, Sister C.: A diagnostic classification system for nursing, Nurs. Outlook **23**:90-94, 1975.
52. Roy, Sister C.: Introduction to nursing: an adaptation model, Englewood Cliffs, N. J., 1976, Prentice-Hall, Inc.
53. Roy, Sister C.: The impact of nursing diagnosis, A.O.R.N. J. **21**:1023-30, 1975.
54. Ryan, B. J.: Nursing care plans: a systems approach to developing criteria for planning and evaluation, J. Nurs. Admin. **3**:50-58, 1973.
55. Seedor, M. M.: The physical assessment: a programmed unit of study for nurses, New York, 1974, Teachers College Press.
56. Sobol, E. G., and Robischon, P.: Family nursing: a study guide, St. Louis, 1975, The C. V. Mosby Co.
57. Wagner, B. M.: Care plans: right, reasonable, and reachable, Am. J. Nurs. **69**:986-990, 1969.
58. Wesseling, E.: Automating the nursing history and care plan, J. Nurs. Admin. **2**:34-38, 1972.
59. Whalen, R.: Medical malaprops, J.A.M.A. **177**:158-160, 1961.

9

Nurse-client interactions

LINDA CRAIG

■ COMMUNICATION THEORY

The ability to analyze the dynamics of nurse-client interactions is a skill basic to all areas of nursing. This chapter focuses on the dyadic (two-person) interpersonal communication process within these interactions and discusses the elements the nurse needs to understand, namely, the self, the client, and the interactions between self and client. The development, over time, of the nurse-client relationship is also studied.

The concept of communication is difficult to define because of its breadth. Researchers from many fields have viewed communication from various perspectives and have developed different definitions and models. While many of these definitions are complementary, others conflict, especially with regard to the inclusiveness of the concept, the intentions of the communicators, and the success of the messages sent. Some researchers define communication to include all behavior, and others limit the meaning to the *purposive* behavior of persons in *conscious* interaction. There is a disagreement whether intent to send a message is a requirement and whether success of the message is essential to the definition.[11] Success of the message requires that the message sent be the one the sender intended and that the receiver perceive the message correctly.

If dyadic interpersonal communication is defined as *the exchange, with acknowledgment, of messages between two persons*, then the scope is limited to acknowledged behavior, the intent to communicate does not have to be conscious, and the accuracy of the message perception is irrelevant so long as the message is acknowledged. Fig. 9-1 shows the dyadic interpersonal communication model.

For dyadic interpersonal communication there must be a *receiver*, a *sender*, *encoded* and *decoded messages*, *channels*, *feedback*, and *context*. There is no real separation between the sender and the receiver roles in dyadic interpersonal communications, as two people are communicating as a system. A person is simultaneously receiver and sender because the communication is *dynamic*, involving active response from the receiver, which in turn influences the sender's message. This concept is essential to the understanding of the *circular* model of communication, as depicted in Fig. 9-1, as opposed to the earlier *linear* model. In the circular model, communication occurs *simultaneously between* person A and person B, whereas in the linear model, communication goes *from* person A *to* person B.

The *message* or *feedback* may be verbal or nonverbal, conscious or unconscious, intentional or unintentional. Usually more than one message is sent at a given time. One message may confirm or contradict other messages. A single message (meaning) may be sent over more than one channel. Messages are *encoded* and *decoded* by the sender-receiver. Encoding refers to how one symbolizes ideas in order to send them via a channel. This includes the selection of verbal and nonverbal symbols to convey the messages. Decoding refers to the process of interpreting incoming verbal and nonverbal messages. *Feedback* includes what has been referred to as acknowledgment of the message. Each message or instance of feedback affects the sender-receiver and alters subsequent messages or feedback. Feedback or acknowledgement of a message is crucial to establishing that communication has occurred. Lack of acknowledgement of another person's message is, in a way, a rejection of that person.

Human communication is multichanneled. All the sensory (and perhaps extrasensory) modalities are used in communicating. Facility in the use of all the channels enables people to be more flexible in their communication. Good judgment in the choice of channels increases the effectiveness of communication and requires knowledge of the total communication system.

Dyadic interpersonal communication always occurs within a *context* or setting. This refers to the environment around the interaction, including the physical setting, atmosphere, and the presence or absence of other people. The nurse and the client communicate within the context of other systems, for example, the client's

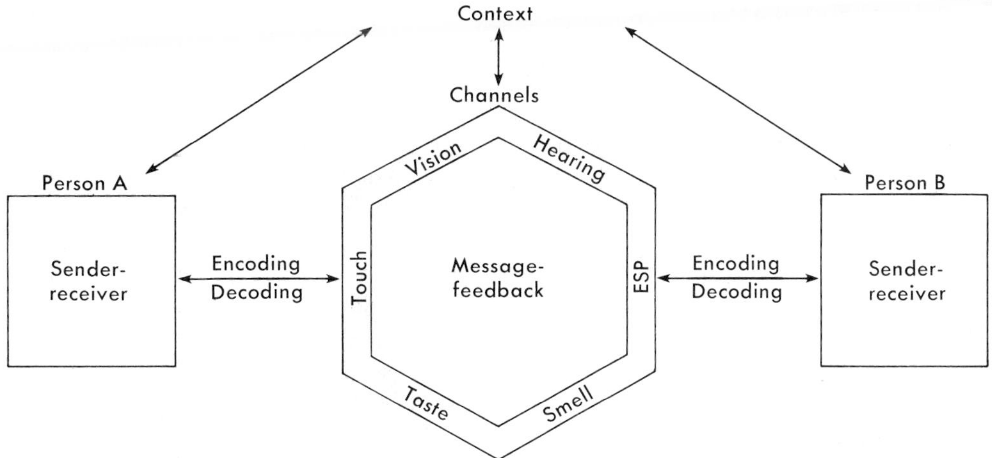

Fig. 9-1. Model of dyadic interpersonal communication.

family system, the hospital unit administration, the community health care system, the political system, and the ecosystem.

□ Nonverbal communication

Nonverbal communication is the most basic form of communication. It is the most primitive form of communication as well as the first form of communication learned by the child. Some have estimated that two-thirds of all information transferred between people is exchanged on the nonverbal level.[5] Nonverbal communication is continuous when two persons are interacting. It is the major channel for the communication of feelings, as language often falls short of words to express nuances of feelings. Nonverbal communication is much less subject to conscious control than verbal communication. It tends to reflect more accurately the sender's true thoughts and feelings. Nonverbal communication includes gestures, mannerisms, physical appearance, dress, facial expression, eye contact, body sounds, intonation of voice, demeanor, bearing, posture, gait, touch, and silence.

Communication is obviously enhanced when verbal and nonverbal messages are consistent. When verbal and nonverbal messages contradict each other, however, the receiver is confronted with a *verbal-nonverbal split* and must decide which of the two messages was probably intended. One can respond verbally or nonverbally to either the verbal or nonverbal message, or to both the verbal and nonverbal messages, perhaps pointing out the inconsistency. One can also choose *not* to respond to verbal or nonverbal messages. The choice of response will be influenced by the receiver's needs and goals as well as by the receiver's perception of the sender's needs and goals.

Nonverbal communication has a greater chance of being misinterpreted. Interpretation of nonverbal messages varies with the receiver's culture, age, needs, awareness, past experiences with nonverbal communication, and so on. Past experiences within the family group are especially influential in determining how a person uses and interprets nonverbal messages. The interpretation the receiver assigns to the sender's nonverbal message determines the manner of response to the message.

Touch is a special kind of nonverbal message and one quite necessary to the health professions. Touch is the chief way a person can attempt to communicate love, safety, and security to a little child who does not yet understand words. The infant understands touch directly. However, the adult understands touch more through past associations, connotations, and experiences, especially those related to closeness, sexuality, and comforting than through the gesture alone. The well-intended use of touch has the potential of decreasing or increasing anxiety. For example, touch may be associated with procedures, pain, and the use of restraint in the health profession as well as with gestures of kindness. Touch, as with other forms of nonverbal communication, has less chance of being misunderstood when it is accompanied by verbal messages that are congruent with the kind of touch.

Communication by use of symbols is yet another form of nonverbal communication. This is culturally learned. The significance and interpretation of symbols is dependent upon the conventions of the culture that uses the symbols, so the meanings must be learned. The serving of food and drink to guests can be symbolic, and the wearing of black by mourners is symbolic. There is often no intrinsic significance to the association of meanings that constitute an accepted symbol. Thus there can be and are cultures that wear white for mourning. The atmosphere of a place or situation communicates to the beholder and often imperceptibly influences the thinking and behavior elicited. This is also a form of symbolic communication.

□ Verbal communication

Verbal messages allow for the communication of more sophisticated concepts. Despite our highly developed language of word symbols, it is often difficult to convey intended messages through words. This may be because of inconsistencies in the use of language, provincial forms of speech, inadequacy of vocabulary for thorough and precise descriptions, multiple meanings of words, and so on.[5]

The effectiveness of verbal communication is closely tied to one's knowledge of and facility with the language. Effectiveness is also dependent on factors already cited —context, judgment in choice of symbols (in this case, words), and knowledge of the receiver's attitudes, values, cultural beliefs, and customs. It has long been recognized that the personality of the sender influences effectiveness in communicating. The same words said by two different people may convey two different meanings.

□ Obstacles to effective communication

One common problem in communication is the sending of contradictory messages, such as the verbal-nonverbal split. If a nurse reflects to a client that he seems to be angry, and the client scowls and uses a very angry-sounding tone of voice to protest, then the message of anger is nonverbally affirmed while verbally denied. Although there is the option to believe the verbal message, the nurse will probably tend to believe the nonverbal message. We learn as we grow that nonverbal messages are usually accurate reflectors of feelings. The child is particularly confused by verbal and nonverbal splits—confused about how to interpret them and how to respond to them.

The sender may seek to disguise the meaning of a message because of fears of rejection by the receiver or perhaps because the sender finds the message unacceptable or uncomfortable. This might result in the sender actually saying the opposite of what he means. This coping mechanism is called reaction formation. (See Chapter 16.)

Numerous problems exist in the area of encoding and decoding messages. We typically have peculiarities (idiosyncrasies) in these areas that are specific to us as individuals. *The more aware we are of our own peculiarities and the more sensitive we are to the peculiarities of others in the area of encoding and decoding, the better chance we have of successful communication.* For example, some people decode touch from nonintimate friends as being forward or taking liberties, whereas others might interpret that same touch as an indication of warmth and acceptance and perhaps comfort on the part of the sender.

Difficulty in receiving the message constitutes another obstacle to effective communication. This may stem from a number of related problems including distaste for the channel over which the particular message came, unwillingness to accept the content of the message, inability to perceive the message because of a physical handicap such as blindness or deafness, decreased receptivity to *any* messages because of fatigue, illness or preoccupation with other thoughts, and emotional reaction to a message, which interferes with reception of the cognitive content. For example, when strong affect (feeling) such as fear exists in a person, he may shut off any incoming stimuli that he feels might further increase his fear. His need to feel secure causes him to *selectively inattend* to incoming stimuli.[44] Thus he may not decode the messages, or if he does, he does not acknowledge them.

Hidden agendas create another problem area of communication. These agendas are suspected when persons communicating are not straightforward and direct in their purposes or goals for interacting. Their stated or *manifest* reasons for communicating are not their primary reasons. Their messages may be confusing and misunderstood by the receiver because they are not being interpreted with knowledge of the total context. Consider the employee who is unexpectedly praised by her employer and given a small merit raise. A bit bewildered, the employee nevertheless concludes that she must have been doing an outstanding job. A day later the employer asks the employee to do a personal favor that could seriously jeopardize the reputation of the employee. The employee may now interpret the praise and salary increase differently. Obstacles to effective communication may occur as a result or consequence of sending contradictory messages or disguised messages, experiencing encoding and decoding problems or difficulty in receiving messages, or because of hidden agendas.

■ NURSE-CLIENT RELATIONSHIP

As a *relationship*, the nurse-client relationship is more than just an *interaction*. An interaction refers to any contact between two people by which these individuals mutually influence each other. An interaction can be superficial, automatic, helpful, voluntary, or inconsistent. A relationship, however, implies a *series of experiences* between two people, and this experience is *mutually significant*.[46] Moreover, relationships develop over time.

Not all interactions between nurses and clients develop into relationships. Some of these contacts are one-time interactions. This does not imply that they are not therapeutic, as one interaction may be all that is needed by the individual. Often nurse-client interactions are interrupted by unexpected discharge or transfer of the individual, change of nurse assignment, nurse vacations, and other circumstances that force premature terminations of relationships or abort the establishment of relationships.

A nurse-client relationship has specific purposes to identify the client's needs, to help the client promote his or her health, and to assist the client in preventing or coping with illness and suffering. The latter may include helping the client achieve a peaceful death. A nurse-client relationship differs from the social relationship in that it is designed to meet the needs of the client, not the nurse. The social relationship usually allows for focus on the needs of both persons. While nurse-client relationships may allow for the meeting of nurse needs, they are not designed to focus on the needs of the nurse per se. The nature of the nurse's obligation differs from that of a friend. Nurses are obligated to use their knowledge and skills to assess the client's health care needs and to provide quality nursing care. The very establishment and maintenance of the nurse-client relationship may be the nurse's responsibility alone, since illness may preclude the individual's initiating interaction with the nurse.

The *structure* of the nurse-client relationship varies according to the client's needs, nurse and client goals, and the context of the relationship. Structuring an interaction involves making interactions predictable and purposeful; subsequent interactions can be tested, trust can begin to grow, and a relationship becomes established.

The *nature* of the nurse-client relationship varies with the context. The extended role of the nurse has increased the range of contexts within which nursing is practiced. Nursing is no longer practiced primarily within highly structured and controlled environments such as hospitals, where roles are usually well defined for both nurse and client. Nurses may be faced with defining their own employment roles for themselves, their employers, and their clients. Nurses who choose to open new roads for nursing need to be quite skillful at defining their roles in very open, undefined areas of practice. Nurses need to interpret their roles effectively to all people. Clients may be uncomfortable with nurse roles in new contexts, such as the nurse functioning as a primary care practitioner in areas where other health professionals are not readily accessible.

The *context* of the nurse-client relationship differs greatly in inpatient as opposed to outpatient settings. The individual is in a potentially better position to control his affairs and make his own decisions as an outpatient. Nurses in outpatient settings function increasingly as consultants and teachers, even though they may give direct physical and psychosocial care. The nurse who enters a client's home is a guest in that home, a status quite different than the status of the nurse who treats clients in a clinic or cares for the patient in a hospital. In the hospital, individuals often feel that they have little or no control and assume very dependent roles. This dependency can foster regression and interfere with physical and psychosocial recovery. Nurses strive to give clients maximum input into planning their care and controlling their immediate environment, for example, their room or area of a room. The issue of control over the environment is thus a significant factor in determining the nature of the nurse-client relationship in different contexts.

The nurse-client relationship involves acceptance of the client's needs, values, rights, and dignity. It is *dynamic* in that it is everchanging, requiring continuous assessment and evaluation. The nurse-client relationship utilizes both *affective* and *cognitive* levels of interaction, as the nurse teaches and provides physical and psychosocial care. The relationship is *time-limited* and geared to the time needed to accomplish mutually defined goals. It is *honest* and *responsible*, requiring both nurse and individual to examine their behavior and be accountable to one another.

The nurse-client relationship is a series of *mutually significant* experiences with a specific purpose. It is *structured* to accomplish its purpose in varying contexts.

□ Phases in nurse-client relationships

A nurse-client relationship develops over time and proceeds through predictable phases or stages. These phases are not discrete, but may overlap one another. They are sometimes omitted, and regression to an earlier phase may occur, especially at stressful points.

The basic phases of the nurse-client relationship—*establishment, development,* and *termination*—correspond roughly to the beginning, middle, and end of the nurse-client relationship.[37] Each phase will be explained in greater detail.

Establishment phase

As the establishment phase begins, the nurse and the client are strangers. Both nurse and client may be anxious. If anxiety is high, communication may be difficult. Client and nurse may have different ideas of what the client's problem is. There may be a great tendency on the part of the nurse to do something before adequate data collection is accomplished. The nurse may also be overcome with "rescue fantasies."

During the establishment phase the nurse establishes initial structure, making clear the purpose, timing, and context of the relationship. To establish predictability, it is necessary to define certain unknowns. The client needs to know who the nurse is, what the nurse's roles entail, the purpose of the interaction, how long the nurse will stay, if and how often the nurse will return, and where they will meet. Basically the nurse states "who," "what," "when," "where," and "why," so that realistic mutual expectations can be established. The nurse can give the client a good indication of the probable duration of the relationship. In this way termination is begun from the onset, establishing a valuable foundation for the last phase. This initial structure need not be *announced* to the client, but may be *discussed* with the client, seeking his input and suggestions. Thus a climate of mutual respect and flexibility can be created.

The structure of the relationship will, of course, be open to revision when there is agreement by nurse and client that revision is needed. The degree of responsibility the nurse expects from the client in helping to establish and maintain the structure will vary according to the client's abilities and the context of the nurse-client relationship.

During the establishment phase the nurse and client together define the client's problem and set goals to work toward, with some time estimate in mind. Some authors refer to this as *contracting* with the client. Such contracts are often verbal, but on occasion may be written. The purposes of contracting (or setting goals) with the client are to clarify or reinforce roles and purposes and to facilitate coordinated efforts toward common goals. Otherwise, nurse and client may work at odds, inefficiently, and with limited success toward different goals.

The nurse collects much data about the client during the establishment phase. It is the responsibility of the nurse to respect the client's dignity and rights and to assure that this information will be treated confidentially. It is also the nurse's responsibility to protect the client's privacy while collecting data. This involves being mindful of others in the environment and being sensitive to the client's feelings and need for privacy. The following illustrates an episode from the establishment phase of a nurse-client relationship.

EPISODE 1. ESTABLISHMENT PHASE

Mr. Winston, a 58-year-old married man, was admitted to a medical inpatient unit with the complaints of dyspnea, cough, rusty-colored sputum, and pain on inspiration. He is a manager of a local supermarket and had been working until a week ago. At this time he consulted his general practitioner, who told him he must be evaluated in the hospital for possible lung cancer. Mr. Winston is very apprehensive. Under pressure from his wife, he has just given up cigarettes. He is often found pacing in his room and wringing his hands.

Ms. Ames, R.N., met Mr. Winston yesterday when she admitted him to the unit. She and the physician collected appropriate admission data. Ms. Ames will be directly responsible for Mr. Winston's care during his hospitalization. She decides to set aside 15 minutes today to initiate the nurse-client relationship with Mr. Winston. The following interaction takes place.

Dialogue	Analysis
Ms. A.: *(stops at Mr. Winston's door and knocks)* Mr. Winston, I'll have some time to spend with you in about a half hour. I'd like to come in and talk with you for a few minutes then. Will you be in your room?	Ms. A. warns Mr. W. of her presence. She respects his privacy. She explains her plan to speak with him so he can cooperate if he chooses, allowing him some control of his environment. She makes herself predictable, setting up a structure to which she will adhere. This is useful groundwork for the establishment of trust. Yet Ms. A. does not explain the purpose of the interaction. Lack of this element of structure increases anxiety.
Mr. W.: *(pacing the room, frowning, sweating, and wringing his hands)* Where else do you suppose I'd be? *(gruffly and only glancing up)* Do you have a thousand more questions to ask? I told you everything yesterday.	Mr. W. lashes out verbally at Ms. A. He sounds irritated. He implies he has no choice over where he will be. He seems to have been angered yesterday by all the data collection. He does not seem to want to engage in conversation with the nurse. Perhaps he sees no need to.
Ms. A.: *(feels defensive, attacked, angry)* No, Mr. Winston. I don't have any specific questions, but I wanted to talk with you about how we can work together toward your recovery while you're in the hospital.	Ms. A. does not feel that the attack is justified, so she wonders where the feelings originate. Perhaps if she had clarified her purpose from the start, Mr. W.'s response might have been different. Perhaps not. The nurse accepts Mr. W.'s anger without judgment or retaliation. She explains her purpose. If Mr. W. sees this purpose as fulfilling a need he

Dialogue	Analysis
	has, then motivation for the relationship is established.
Mr. W.: *(no response)*	Mr. W. does not acknowledge Ms. A.'s messages. This leaves her feeling rejected.
Ms. A.: *(feels rejected)* I'll be back in a half hour to talk with you.	Ms. A. establishes a basis for predictability. She might have added, "We'll see how you feel then," giving him the chance to change his mind.
Mr. W.: *(no response)*	Mr. W. may still be angry—unwilling to accept Ms. A.'s help. He may be testing to see if she cares enough to come despite his lack of enthusiasm.
(One half hour later)	
Ms. A.: *(knocks)* Mr. Winston?	It is very important that the nurse returns when she said she would. Ms. A. has been predictable. Again she respects his privacy by knocking.
Mr. W.: Yeah. *(head down, sitting on bed)*	
Ms. A.: May I come in to talk with you?	By asking his permission to talk, Ms. A. gives Mr. W. some sense of control over his immediate environment. Ms. A. remembers that she and the client are still strangers, even though Mr. W. has given her considerable data the day before.
Mr. W.: Umm . . .	Mr. W. is noncommittal.
Ms. A.: *(sits in chair near door)* You seem upset today. I guess yesterday was long and tiring for you and you went for chest x-rays this morning, right?	Ms. A. sits at a distance from Mr. W., respecting his body space, allowing him time to get to know her. Ms. A. should have let Mr. W. know of her time limit of 15 minutes today. Ms. A. tries to explore other sources of Mr. W.'s angry feelings. She tries to show understanding of his experiences.
Mr. W.: Yeah.	
Ms. A.: How did that go?	Ms. A. again attempts to explore other possible sources for Mr. W.'s feelings.
Mr. W.: Okay. Tomorrow they're gonna operate. *(with emphasis and looking fearful)*	Mr. W. reveals a source of fear.
Ms. A.: *(surprised)* Operate?	
Mr. W.: He said they're gonna take me to the operating room and do a bronchoscopy. What's that anyway? What does that mean—that I have cancer? *(looks worried)*	Mr. W. reveals his misunderstanding of the bronchoscopy. This seems to be his immediate problem.
Ms. A.: A bronchoscopy is a test, Mr. Winston. They are still doing tests to see what you do have. They do this particular test in the operating room. They are prepared there to give you anesthesia and deal with any unforeseen complications. Also, the doctor needs a dark room so he can better see the tissues lighted by the bronchoscope. Did your doctor explain the procedure of the test?	Ms. A. clarifies, explains, collects data about what he knows, and teaches Mr. W. about the procedure.
Mr. W.: Yes, he did. I can't tell you what he said, though.	Mr. W.'s response may indicate that the doctor did not explain well or that the client, being very anxious, used *selective inattention* and did not "hear" the explanation. This factor must always be considered in teaching the client.
Ms. A.: I will go with you for the procedure tomorrow if you like, Mr. Winston.	This is a supportive act designed to reduce Mr. W.'s anxiety.
Mr. W.: *(surprised)* You will?	
Ms. A.: Yes. Would you like that?	
Mr. W.: *(looking quite relieved)* Yes.	Mr. W.'s attitude toward Ms. A. has changed. This could be because his most pressing need was met. It could be because the nurse has accepted his anger and given of herself without requiring anything of him. Also the client could feel that Ms. A. really cares and can meet some of his needs.
Ms. A.: Mr. Winston, I will be responsible for your nursing care during the day shift—7:00 to 3:30—while you are in the hospital. I know this will be a difficult time for you while they are	Ms. A., taking advantage of her leverage, decides to introduce the nurse-client relationship idea. She defines the nature of the relationship. She says that she is responsible for his care while he is in the hos-

Dialogue	Analysis
doing many diagnostic tests to find your problem.	pital. This is not correct, as her responsibility for him is contingent on his being on this division. She inadvertently promises more than she can deliver.
Mr. W.: Umm . . .	
Ms. A.: You must be very worried about the possibility of having cancer and what can be done.	Ms. A. suggests that Mr. W. has needs and opens up the topic of his feelings about the prospects of cancer.
Mr. W.: Yes . . . it's awful to think about. God! What would I *do?* I had a buddy who died of cancer of the colon. His wife is a wreck now—torn up with grief.	When Mr. W. indicates readiness to explore this right now, Ms. A. has a conflict. Her hidden agenda was to suggest topics they could discuss at another time so as to establish a need for the nurse-client relationship and have Mr. W. agree to the relationship today.
Ms. A.: *(first silent, listening; then, wanting to get back to her task to defining the nurse-client relationship, she shakes her head sadly)* Yes, it is sad and scary to think about. Yet, we don't know for sure whether you have cancer.	Ms. A. tries to respond to his feelings but ends up cutting him off by saying that it isn't time to worry yet. Mr. W. may well have been confused as to her intent. She needs to get her hidden agenda on the table and tell him that she wants to discuss this with him—that today she has limited time but wants to set up times to get together regularly to discuss his problems, feelings, and so on. Then Mr. W. would understand why he was being cut off. Ms. A. could also have helped Mr. W. to see that having cancer does not necessarily mean you will die, as was the case with his friend.
Mr. W.: *(hesitantly)* No . . .	
Ms. A.: Mr. Winston, I'd like to set aside some time each day for us to talk about how things are going and what we can do together to make your stay here as comfortable as possible and . . . just to talk about how you are feeling and what your concerns are.	Now Ms. A. gets her hidden agenda out into the open by telling Mr. W. what she wants. She defines the purpose of the relationship.
Mr. W.: Um hm . . .	
Ms. A.: I have some other patients, too, so it would be a good idea if we could agree on a regular time.	Ms. A. asks for Mr. W.'s input as to time.
Mr. W.: Well, yes, but I never know when they'll come take me for tests.	
Ms. A.: That's true. Perhaps we should leave it flexible but agree to save a half hour each day for talking together.	Ms. A. allows her client to participate in the defining of the structure of the relationship. Again, this allows Mr. W. more control and may increase his motivation to adhere to the structure.
Mr. W.: That's okay.	
Ms. A.: Do you think we can talk here in your room without disturbing your roommate?	Ms. A. was trying indirectly to ask Mr. W. where he'd prefer to meet, thinking of his need for privacy and confidentiality. This intent did not come through. It sounded more like concern for his roommate. The nurse should have been more direct. She could ask, "Will you be comfortable talking here with your roommate nearby, or would you prefer the privacy of the office down the hall?"
Mr. W.: Oh, yes. He doesn't hear well.	
Ms. A.: Okay.	

Development phase

The next phase of the nurse-client relationship is the *development* phase. After initial structure has been defined by the client and nurse, both will test to determine the reliability of the other. Both may wonder: "Will he do what he said he would?" and "Does he refrain from doing what he said he wouldn't do?" Through the process of structuring, testing, and consistent behavior, the nurse and client develop mutual trust. The nurse begins to discover whether the client is committed to working on the defined problems and whether the client's part of the contract will be fulfilled. Trust takes time to develop and is established to varying degrees in nurse-client relationships. Without some degree of trust, it is extremely difficult to establish a working relationship. Testing need not be interpreted as an affront to the nurse, but as a chance for the nurse to establish credibility with this particular client.

During the development phase the client will begin to depend upon the nurse to some degree. The nurse's response to this dependence is crucial to the relationship. The nurse must assess the degree of dependency necessary to help the individual meet the goals of the nurse-client relationship. Allowing too much dependency may frighten the client or lead to a conclusion that the nurse is not confident of the person's ability to be independent. Not allowing dependency may interfere with the development of trust and may lead the individual to conclude that the nurse does not want to help.

During the development phase, nurse and client get to know one another better. While they began to set goals in the establishment phase, they now formulate plans around their goals, putting the plans into action and evaluating the results. As the nurse becomes more involved with the client, it is often easy to get caught up in the individual's problems. The nurse may begin to experience the individual's feelings of hopelessness and helplessness. This might be termed the "vacuum-sweeper syndrome," assimilating all the feelings expressed by the client with loss of professional objectivity.

When this occurs, it is necessary that objectivity be reestablished. This is accomplished by the nurse examining his or her own feelings and trying to understand their origins, by examining his or her own needs and how these needs are influencing behavior, and revalidating the abilities and limitations of the client.

Development can be a rewarding phase, as the client trusts enough to dare to try new approaches to problem solving. Yet both nurse and client cannot expect all progress and no regression. There will be setbacks in the growth process. Nurse and client should discuss this as they plan, so that they are prepared for problems in implementation. Nurses can help clients learn the problem-solving process so that clients can better solve problems after termination of the relationship. The following illustrates an episode from the development phase.

EPISODE 2. DEVELOPMENT PHASE

After 5 days of hospitalization, Mr. Winston has been diagnosed as having bronchogenic carcinoma. Ms. Ames has just learned this, and she is quite upset, having learned to like Mr. Winston very much in 5 days. She has supported him through several unpleasant diagnostic procedures, and he has come to rely on her.

Dialogue	Analysis
Mr. W.: *(smoking a cigarette)*	
Ms. A.: Hello, Mr. Winston. *(looks very disapproving)* I see you are smoking.	The nurse's opinion is communicated to Mr. W. nonverbally. She decides not to remind him that smoking is hazardous to his health, as she knows that he must be very upset just now. Thus she sets a priority of present needs.
Mr. W.: Hell, what difference does it make? The damage is done. *(laughs)*	Mr. W. indicates hopelessness and resignation. He may laugh instead of cry—a reaction-formation.
Ms. A.: The damage?	Ms. A. prompts him to continue. Mr. W. here shows a typical verbal-nonverbal split. The feeling tone he communicates nonverbally does not coincide with the content of his verbal message. While the nonverbal is usually the truer message, as it is less subject to conscious control, it appears to be a defense here—an attempt to avoid facing his real feelings. Ms. A. infers this because she knows how worried Mr. W. has been about the possibility of cancer.
Mr. W.: The doctor just told me the tests proved I had a cancer . . . tumor. . . . I just couldn't believe it at first. *(laughs)* I kept asking him over . . . to repeat himself.	Mr. W. expresses his initial disbelief and shock, a characteristic initial defensive reaction to a crisis. This is a prime example of one of the obstacles to communication—difficulty receiving the message. The laugh seems to be defensive again, defending against his sadness and grief.

Dialogue	Analysis
Ms. A.: I'm *very* sorry to to hear you do have lung cancer, Mr. Winston.	Ms. A. expresses her own feelings about the diagnosis. Perhaps the nurse model will help Mr. W. express his feelings.
Mr. W.: *(silence, smoking, inhaling deeply)*	Mr. W. cannot respond to Ms. A.'s feelings verbally but shows nonverbal signs of increasing anxiety. His sad feelings may be surfacing. Ms. A. allows him time to deal with sad feelings and anxiety they engender.
Ms. A.: *(pause)* What else did the doctor say?	Ms. A. tries to get him to to focus on the facts to ascertain his understanding of his condition.
Mr. W.: He thinks he can get it all out if he operates. . . . He doesn't think it's spread.	
Ms. A.: That's hopeful.	Ms. A. comments on the hopeful, partly to reassure herself. She went into this interaction upset by just hearing the news herself, and she is beginning to "catch" Mr. W.'s fear.
Mr. W.: *(staring straight ahead, blank facial expression)* Umm . . .	Mr. W. is not reassured or cheered by the hope. He shows little feeling at all.
Ms. A.: Are you feeling kind of numb from hearing all of this?	Ms. A. interprets this as a defensive withdrawal of feelings to protect the self. She allows him to feel numb—or not to feel.
Mr. W.: Yes. *(pause)* I have to decide soon about surgery.	Ms. A. stays silent during the pause to communicate acceptance of his feelings and give him time to organize his thoughts. Mr. W. now brings up a pressing problem that is also on his mind and perhaps one reason why he hesitates to express his feelings. He may be afraid that his feelings will interfere with his ability to make a very important decision in a rational way.
Ms. A.: What are your thoughts about it now?	Ms. A. encourages him to think about his decision, as it is imminent.
Mr. W.: It's not without risk. I've got heart damage from a heart attack.	
Ms. A.: Yes.	
Mr. W.: But there's not a lot of choice. Untreated, he said I'd have less than a year . . . *(begins to cry)* . . . my poor wife . . .	Mr. W. reveals his concerns and fear of death. With this he begins to express his feelings, yet indicates that it is his wife that he's worried about. Perhaps he feels he should not grieve over his own potential loss, just his wife's. Perhaps he is grieving over the possible separation from his wife.
Ms. A.: *(feeling very sad and hopeless, reaches over and puts her hand on client's hand, pats it briefly)*	Ms. A. uses touch to communicate caring.
Mr. W.: I don't want to die yet. I wanted to work till I was 62, retire, and enjoy life. *(crying)*	Mr. W. uses the past tense "wanted" as if his wishes were no longer possible.
Ms. A.: *(weakly)* It is still possible, perhaps.	Ms. A. picks up on this but is not convinced. She is beginning to experience the "vacuum-sweeper syndrome." She is losing her objectivity and perspective.
Mr. W.: I feel like I have a death sentence, that I'm rotting inside. Who knows what they'll find when they cut in. Oh, it would be awful to rot away slowly.	Mr. W. continues to express how badly he sees things. He needs the nurse to accept that he sees such a black picture, but does not need her to be convinced by him that it *is* necessarily that black.
Ms. A.: *(also feeling hopeless, stays silent; feels like crying; feels afraid for Mr. W.; feels helpless; wants to comfort him; cannot find words; anxiety level very high)* When will your wife be in?	Ms. A. is becoming more distressed; her anxiety level is increasing. She has difficulty coping with her feelings of despair, hopelessness, and helplessness, so she changes the subject.
Mr. W.: *(first silence, then muttering)* Oh God, I don't know—about an hour I guess. What am I gonna tell her?	
Ms. A.: Mr. Winston, I will be back shortly so we can talk about this some more—so much has happened today. *(leaves)*	Ms. A. finally removes herself from the situation, recognizing she cannot meet Mr. W.'s needs until she meets her own. She tries not to do this in a rejecting way, indicating her intent to return and continue the conversation. Considering her needs at the time, she ended the conversation as best she could. She was able to return later, after she had her feelings better under control, and help the client and his wife with their feelings.

Termination phase

Termination, the last phase of the nurse-client relationship, occurs logically when the nurse and client agree that they have accomplished the goals of the relationship. *Termination with resolution* occurs when the client becomes more independent. Both the actual and felt need for the nurse are less. Resolution is a freeing process, freeing the client to manage again without a nurse.[37] In termination with resolution, both the client and the nurse feel that the time has come to end the relationship, even though it may be difficult to give up the relationship. The degree of mutual involvement experienced influences the depth of pain and anxiety felt at separation.

The nurse and client conjointly evaluate the total relationship and the learning that has occurred. Nurses can assist clients to transfer this learning to other aspects of their lives as applicable, helping them to integrate their experiences into their general life experiences. If clients see their learning as isolated events out of the context of general life experiences, they will have difficulty utilizing the learning that has occurred. Nurses and clients benefit from sharing their feelings at termination. Although this may be difficult and uncomfortable, it provides valuable feedback to both nurse and client.

Sometimes, even if feelings are strong, defenses may shelter individuals from their feelings. This may be the case when a client cannot understand why he does not feel sad when he expected he would. Another manifestation of defense is minimizing the importance of the relationship. It may be easier to give up a relationship if its meaning is denied.

Feelings at termination are generally mixed. There may be relief that the relationship is over; joy in the new, more independent position; sadness or anger at giving up the comfortable security of the predictable relationship; pride in accomplishment of goals; or fear and arousal of old insecurities. The latter may produce temporary regressions prior to termination.

Unfortunately, *termination* often occurs *without resolution.* This occurs when the nurse or client leaves the relationship before resolution, for example, the nurse is transferred, the client is discharged, the client or nurse voluntarily withdraws because of dissatisfaction with the relationship, death, and so on. These situations arouse all the feelings of termination and, in addition, frustration. If circumstances of termination are beyond nurse or client control, it is hard to know where to direct the feelings of frustration or anger. Feelings are often displaced; for example, the nurse may become unjustifiably angry with the family of the client if the client dies. Rejection and anger on the part of the person who is "left," guilt on the part of the person "leaving," and perhaps relief on both parts may also occur.

If possible, the nurse and client summarize and evaluate the relationship, recognizing and dealing with their feelings as time permits. In general, the nurse terminates the relationship by accomplishing all the tasks of the phase that are appropriate. The following illustrates an episode from the termination phase.

EPISODE 3. TERMINATION PHASE

Ms. A. returned yesterday afternoon and had a long talk with Mr. W. and his wife. They discussed the diagnosis, prognosis, surgery, and their feelings. Mr. W. seemed to be deciding that he should have the surgery. The doctor was to speak with him this morning.

Dialogue	Analysis
Ms. A.: Good morning, Mr. Winston.	
Mr. W.: Good morning, Ms. Ames. *(smiling)* Well, I've decided to have the surgery.	Mr. W. seems proud of his decision. He announces it to Ms. A. immediately.
Ms. A.: You have! *(smiling)* You look as if you feel good about your decision.	Ms. A. acknowledges his message that he is pleased with the decision; that is, she acknowledges his verbal and his nonverbal messages.
Mr. W.: Yes. Can't say I'm not scared, but if there's a possibility of a cure, I guess I should risk it.	Mr. W. admits that not all the scared feelings are gone and that he still has needs.
Ms. A.: I'm glad to hear you are feeling optimistic!	Ms. A. puts a value on his optimism by praising it. This could cause problems. Mr. W. may feel that optimism is more acceptable than fear and hopelessness and therefore may be reluctant to express these latter feelings again. He may feel badly about having been so dejected yesterday.
Mr. W.: Yes, I feel better today. I was pretty down yesterday.	This may indicate that Mr. W. does feel bad about being so dejected yesterday.
Ms. A.: So was I. I feel better today too. *(smiles and pats his shoulder; sits down on chair; thinks about client's transfer)* Tell me, did your doctor say when you might have surgery?	Ms. A. alludes to her own "down" feelings yesterday, which is helpful in that Mr. W. may have received that impression from her nonverbal messages yesterday anyway. However, Ms. A. must be careful not to leave Mr. W. feeling guilty for having upset her. Ms. A. uses nonverbal communica-

Dialogue	Analysis
	tion to convey her warm feelings. Feelings are more often communicated nonverbally. Ms. A. begins to prepare Mr. W. for termination of their relationship.
Mr. W.: Well, he said that if I felt sure, he could schedule me for this week. I told him to go ahead. I guess the sooner I get the operation, the better it will be.	
Ms. A.: *(feeling very sad to see him leave the unit)* I wish I could go with you, Mr. Winston.	
Mr. W.: Why, what do you mean?	Mr. W. does not seem aware that his surgery will signal the end of the relationship with Ms. A.
Ms. A.: That I would have liked to have gone with you to surgery and stayed with you in the Recovery Room.	Ms. A. is able to express feelings of sadness at Mr. W.'s leaving.
Mr. W.: *(shocked)* You won't be there?	Mr. W. is shocked. He has not expected the termination.
Ms. A.: No. You will be going to a surgical unit for your operation.	Ms. A. assumes he knows the hospital policy of first assigning nurses to divisions and then assigning nurses to clients. Assumptions should be validated with the client.
Mr. W.: I know, but I thought you were my nurse for my whole hospitalization. Wasn't that what you said in the beginning?	Mr. W. reveals the source of his confusion. This also indicates the importance he attached to the initial structure, which is why it is so crucial to structure carefully.
Ms. A.: *(recalling her initial structure)* Yes, I think I did, Mr. Winston. What I meant was during your stay on this unit . . . . I'm sorry that I didn't make that clear. *(feeling very guilty, afraid client will lose trust)*	Ms. A. admits her mistake and clarifies the structure. Ms. A.'s feelings of guilt over her mistake are increased by her natural feelings of guilt at termination, especially termination without resolution.
Mr. W.: *(mumbling)* Oh, it's okay. *(louder)* It's just that you've been through a lot with me already, and I'd like to have you there when I go under.	Mr. W. sounds angry. He says he still needs her. His problems are not yet resolved. He indicates his trust in her based on the development of their relationship. His tone communicates an appeal to Ms. A. to come with him anyway.
Ms. A.: *(feeling very guilty, like she is abandoning Mr. W., and wondering how he will do without her)* Perhaps I could go up and speak to the nurse who will be responsible for your care on the surgical unit. She may want to come down and talk with you before your transfer.	Ms. A.'s guilt leads her to wonder if Mr. W. can manage without her, though cognitively she knows that he can and that another nurse will assist. Both her guilt and fears and positive concern for Mr. W. motivate her to offer to identify her substitute, which does facilitate continuity of care.
Mr. W.: I guess so. That would be nice. *(doctor arrives and tells Mr. W. that a bed is ready for him on the surgical unit and that he will be taken there directly; the situation forces abrupt termination, as is often the case in the hospital; Mr. W.'s surgery is is scheduled for 2 days later)*	Ms. A. does not deal with his angry feelings at all. She might have said, "I can see you are upset with me, Mr. W., which is understandable. You expected I would stay with you until you were ready to go home. I'm sorry I misled you." She could then allow him time to respond with his feelings. Feelings are more likely to be left undiscussed and unresolved when the relationship is terminated abruptly. There is not time for resolution of feelings.
Ms. A.: Well, I guess we will not have much time to say our goodbyes.	
Mr. W.: No. Things happen in a hurry around here.	
Ms. A.: Mr. Winston, I've enjoyed getting to know you, and I think you are a fine person.	Ms. A. begins to summarize the relationship briefly and to share her feelings—tasks of termination.
Mr. W.: Why, thank you, Ms. Ames. You've helped me through a lot and have always been willing to listen when I got upset, and I've been a lot of that lately. It was nice knowing you were my nurse. You explained things to me—let me know what was going on. That helped.	Mr. W. is quite able to take part in this process, despite his disappointment and lack of preparation for the termination. He gives Ms. A. quite specific feedback about what he liked about the relationship.
Ms. A.: I'm glad it helped. You've been through a lot in a short time. You've coped very well. The surgery won't be easy, but I know you'll cope with that too.	Ms. A. attempts to help him put the relationship in a time perspective—what he's already come through and what has ahead of him. This is a variation of integration—another task of termination. It is not appropriate *at this time* to focus on integrating this

Dialogue	Analysis
	experience into Mr. W.'s total life experience. Yet this will be crucial after surgery, before hospital discharge.
Ms. W.: Yes.	
Ms. A.: I'll try to get up to visit you when I can during my shift. But I will be a visitor then. You will have another nurse. *(feels guilty that she cannot go with Mr. W.)*	Ms. A. explains that the nurse-client relationship is terminated, even though she will see the client again. She redefines the nature of the relationship. She might anticipate having to be more specific about what she can and cannot do in the new relationship when she visits Mr. W. later. He may test the new structure. For example, he might say, "My nurse is busy now, Ms. Ames. Would you speak to my doctor about getting me a laxative?" Ms. A. will need to think ahead about how she will define the limits of her new role and establish mutual expectations. Again, she will need to be consistent and predictable. As she has already established trust, this process may be shortened. However, it will *not* be eliminated, as the *relationship* is new.
Mr. W.: *(smiles)* I hope she's like you. *(feels very sad to leave Ms. A.)*	
Ms. A.: Thank you, Mr. W. I hope things work out well for you.	Mr. W.'s new nurse should anticipate that Mr. W. will need to discuss his feelings about terminating with Ms. A. before he is ready to reengage in a new nurse-client relationship. This is one of the side effects of termination without resolution—it interferes, even if briefly, with establishment of subsequent relationships.

THE NURSE IN THE NURSE-CLIENT RELATIONSHIP

As should be clear from the discussion of the nurse-client relationship, *one of the nurse's most valuable tools is the self. The self is the part of the health care system over which the nurse has the most control.* The concept of therapeutic use of self is not new to nursing. It refers to the nurse's ability to help the client by the way the nurse interacts and relates as opposed to using such tools as medications and treatments. The nurse consciously makes use of knowledge, communication skills, and a unique personality to bring about a desired client outcome. This outcome is therapeutic when it helps individuals cope with their problems and alleviates their suffering.

To use the self therapeutically the nurse needs a knowledge and awareness of self, the ability to reflect upon and analyze nurse and client behavior, and the ability to alter one's behavior when evaluation indicates the need to do so. The second and third tasks are obviously facilitated by the accomplishment of the first task.

Increasing one's self-awareness is not always easy or pleasant, since not every insight will please the self. Sometimes a person cannot even admit to certain of his own characteristics. Sullivan's "good-me," "bad-me," and "not-me" conception of the self serves to elucidate this. The "good-me" is the self a person likes and prefers to identify with, the ideal self. The "bad me" is the part of the self the person has learned to dislike, the part of which he is ashamed. The "not me" is the part of the self the person considers to be so bad that he cannot admit to it.[44]

One of the purposes of increasing self-awareness is to decrease the percentage of the "not me" so that the person sees more of the total self, thus making it possible to change this part of the self. In order to bring more "not me" into awareness, the person needs an adequate percentage of "good me." Bringing into awareness areas of the self which were so unacceptable that they were blocked out of awareness (not me) increases anxiety. Increasing the percentage of "good me" enables the person to cope with the anxiety generated by recognizing the "not me" and may require the help of another person who can serve as a listener-counselor.

The process of increasing self-awareness takes time and patience; it involves focusing on needs, knowledge and skills, self-concept, roles, beliefs and values, and feelings. Each of these will be discussed in more detail.

□ Needs

As stated earlier, the nurse-client relationship allows for the meeting of nurse needs but is not designed to *focus* on the nurse's needs, since the primary reason for the nurse-client relationship is to focus on the client's needs. If the nurse happens to meet some needs as a result of helping the client meet his needs, there is no problem. Problems do arise when the nurse's needs begin to interfere with helping the client meet his needs, especially when this happens outside of the nurse's awareness. A nurse who needs to be needed (loved) may inadvertently encourage inappropriate dependency in the client, whose need is for increased independence (self-esteem and self-actualization). The nurse who needs to be praised may be effectively manipulated by the thankful but demanding client. To reduce such problems to a minimum, it is necessary that nurses gain awareness of their own needs and satisfy them as much as possible outside the nurse-client relationship.

□ Knowledge and skills

The knowledge required to practice nursing is vast and ever increasing. Nurses cannot gain in their professional schools all of the knowledge they will need in practice. To keep abreast they must have the desire and ability to continue to learn independently as long as they practice.

Nurses need to assess honestly their level of knowledge and ability. If nurses have learned to value their clients and to practice nursing with integrity, they will make sure that their knowledge and skills are sufficient to the needs of their clients. Of course, practitioners can actively seek to increase their knowledge and skills by engaging the assistance and consultation of colleagues to assure the quality of their care.

□ Self-concept: personal and professional

"What kind of person am I?" The self-concept is an important variable in determining the nurse's behavior. For example, nurses with very negative self-concepts will not be able to utilize effectively their knowledge and skills because they lack self-confidence. They may spend considerable energy trying to present a desirable picture of themselves to others. Nurses with positive self-images may find it easier to be closer to others and to share more of themselves.

Both the client and the nurse have their own personal self-concepts, which are largely products of their past experiences. The self-concept is formed early in life and is based on reflected appraisals of significant others as well as the person's own estimate of himself.[44] A self-concept is not static, but fluctuates with daily experiences. In the healthy person, however, it is relatively stable, with smaller fluctuations than those of the more vulnerable or less healthy person. A stable self-concept that is realistic and generally positive is perhaps the nurse's most valuable resource. It sustains the nurse through problems, disappointments, and failures and allows the nurse to use more energy for learning and self-growth.

Closely related to the personal self-concept is the professional self-concept—the evaluation of one's performance in the professional role. What is my professional ideal, and how do I measure up to that ideal? Nurses' ideas about the role of the nurse undergo much growth and development during their basic educational preparation. As nurses begin to bring their ideal closer to reality, they might begin to discover that they do not like all of their clients, that some of their clients do not want their help, or that they are unable to help some of their clients. Often nurses then begin to identify and define their strengths, their limitations, and their potential for growth.

Striking a good balance between reality and the ideal is crucial for the nurse, especially during the first year of employment, a period termed "reality shock."[27] Many nurses withdraw from active nursing practice because they cannot sustain a very idealistic professional self-concept in the reality of initial employment. They lack the supervision and support systems necessary to sustain their positive professional self-concept as it is undergoing a stressful test. However, most nurses do survive and continue in nursing.

□ Roles

The roles nurses assume in their work depend upon the context of the health care system, the clients' abilities and concept of their client role, and the nurses' abilities and concept of the nurse role. Nurses' personalities influence the types of roles they assume most comfortably or successfully. The reticent nurse who desires to please others and who prefers to avoid conflict rather than problem solve probably will not function well as a team leader, whereas the more assertive nurse may function well as a team leader. It is important to remember that new behavior patterns can be learned.

Just as the nurse has certain expectations of self in the nurse role (such as to be kind, patient, understanding, sensitive, and fair), the nurse has certain expectations of the client in the client role (such as to be appreciative, able to define his problem, to help in his care, and to want to get well). It is very helpful for nurses to examine just what they expect from their clients, how the clients meet these expectations, how this affects abilities to function in the nurse role, and their feelings in this regard.

□ Beliefs and values

One's expectations of self and others are influenced strongly by one's beliefs and values. Culture has a decided impact on one's beliefs and values. Common values in the United States include the value of work, individuality, social welfare, status, material wealth, and youth. Since values often conflict, priorities must be established. A nurse who values life as well as individual freedom must struggle with conflicting values when working with a suicidal client.

The nurse's social class also influences values and beliefs. Health workers typically come from the middle class and are often accused of imposing their middle-class values on clients. A community nurse committed to zero population growth might urge a postpartum client to consider tubal ligation, although the woman may desire a third child.

Nurses can become aware of their own beliefs and values and be alert to the ways in which these influence clinical inferences and behavior. It is necessary to evaluate one's own value system as well as to gain an appreciation of and respect for the values of others.

□ Feelings

All of the variables mentioned (needs, knowledge and skills, self-concept, roles, and beliefs and values) influence the nurse's feelings. Nurses can examine their feelings in general (e.g., happy, excited, disappointed, depressed, angry) as well as their feelings about particular clients (e.g., like them or feel uneasy about them). Awareness and acceptance of feelings can facilitate a nurse's understanding of how feelings may color perceptions. Acknowledging these feelings should increase the nurse's objectivity.

The nurse's increased self-awareness results in an increased capacity to understand the client. Since the nurse's perception is influenced by past experience, knowledge, needs, and expectations, it follows that *the more the nurse knows about these aspects of the self, the greater can be the reliability of the nurse's inferences about the client.* In systems terms, the more variables that can be defined in the communication network (the nurse, message, channel, and context), the easier it will be to identify what aspects of the systems' process are caused by the undefined variable (the client). If an interpersonal problem arises in the nurse-client relationship, the nurse will be better able to differentiate between the parts played by the client and the nurse.

One's knowledge of self is not akin to knowledge of a fixed variable. An individual is dynamic and changing and, hopefully, ever growing. Therefore knowledge of the self is not static. Personality patterns, typical defense mechanisms, areas of perceptual blindness, and areas of vulnerability in self-concept can be anticipated, and their effects on the nurse-client relationship can be recognized more quickly with increased self-awareness.

■ THE CLIENT IN THE NURSE-CLIENT RELATIONSHIP

Like nurses, clients have needs, knowledge and skills, self-concepts, roles, beliefs and values, and feelings. These client variables influence clients' behavior and nurses' behavior.

□ Needs

One of the first steps in the nursing process is assessment of client needs. Clients cannot always verbalize what their needs are, but they may indicate their needs by their behavior. The nurse collects data and makes inferences, which can then be validated with the client. The client who is unusually irritable, complaining, unhappy, and sarcastic could be expressing fear of his diagnosis, prognosis, treatment, decreased mobility, or any number of things. The client may be unaware of his fear, being preoccupied with the symptoms as opposed to his actual problem. The nurse might attempt to clarify the problem source by saying, "Mr. Jones, you seem out of sorts this morning. Are you worried about the outcome of your tests?" This gives the client a chance to reflect on his feelings and validate (or refute) the nurse's inference. In general, the nurse's goal is to define the individual's needs and help him meet them, not necessarily to increase the client's insight into how his needs influences his behavior, although this may be a therapeutic side effect. (When working with clients with special problems in communicating, the nurse's goal may be to increase the client's insight into his behavior.)

□ Knowledge and skills

Clients differ in their knowledge levels—knowledge of the health care system, of daily hygiene, of illnesses, of treatments, of diets, and of medications. The client's present level of knowledge is assessed before teaching begins. Increased knowledge about illness can serve to increase *or decrease* the client's ability to cope with his illness. Lack of knowledge of an illness usually will increase a client's anxiety because of fear of the unknown. This varies with the client. Therefore the nurse assesses carefully what to teach the client and when to teach him. Learning goals for the client need to be clear and related directly to the promotion of the client's health. For example, the nurse preparing to do preoperative teaching will need to assess the client's readiness for learning. This will include (1) assessing the client's anxiety, (2) determining his present level of knowledge, (3) deciding upon any further knowledge the client needs, (4) determining the best time to teach him, (5) choosing the best method, (6) teaching him, and (7) evaluating the teaching process, the client's level of learning, and any observable effect of the learning on the client. The same process applies to the client's learning of skills, such as the person who is newly diagnosed as being diabetic learning to give his own insulin.

The nurse is cognizant of the client's coping abilities in the present as well as his *potential*. The client's abilities and limitations may well differ from his pre-illness status and recovery status. In some instances illness accentuates limitations. In others, crisis may increase the client's capabilities.

□ Self-concept

The client's self-concept will influence his ability to request and accept help from another person. If the client has a poor self-concept, he may feel unworthy of attention and decline to make requests. Thus he may deny his own needs or attempt to meet them on his own. This may consume unnecessarily the energy needed for recovery. The client whose self-concept is threatened by an illness (and its implications for changes in the person's life style) may be demanding of help, may stubbornly refuse help, or may accept help reluctantly. Clients often fear the dependency of forced immobility, especially if their former independence contributed strongly to their positive self-concepts. Clients may also fear change of body image because of surgery or loss of bodily function. These clients need help accepting their altered bodies while still maintaining self-esteem. Other strengths can be identified and developed to help compensate for the loss, thus broadening the basis of self-esteem.

□ Roles

The client may have a preconceived notion of the "client role." For instance, a client may expect to present a problem to the nurse and expect the nurse to take care of it. The idea of mutual problem solving and the enlisting of the nurse as a resource person may be foreign to the client, so he may resist interacting with the nurse in this manner. Clarification of this issue will avert many problems if the nurse can learn about the client's perceptions of his roles by clarifying mutual expectations during the establishment phase of the nurse-client relationship.

□ Beliefs and values

The client's beliefs and values influence his reactions to illness and treatment. A client could have the religious belief that God is using illness as a means of bringing him into contact with a hospital roommate whose needs are greater than his. Thus the client may view himself as an instrument of God and illness as a means to God's ends. There is nothing to be gained by the nurse's countering the client's beliefs, especially if the client's beliefs do not interfere with meeting the client's other needs (or with meeting the roommate's needs). Even when the client's beliefs interfere with meeting health needs, such as might be the case when a Christian Scientist refuses emergency treatment, the client has the right to refuse individual treatment. Other values that influence the client's response to illness include independence, youth, productivity, family life, and socioeconomic status. The nurse can be instrumental in helping the client define how illness will affect his individual life style and values and how to make the best adjustment, considering the realities of the situation.

□ Feelings

The client's feelings are influenced by all of the previously mentioned factors. The client has feelings about illness, prognosis, treatment, the health care facility, the health team members, his family, and so on. The client's feelings about the nurse may stem from past experiences with nurses or attitudes about the health professions. These feelings will color perception of the nurse-client relationship and attitudes about cooperation. The client may displace feelings about his general situation onto the nurse because the nurse is a convenient target. The client may scream at the nurse when he learns that his exploratory laparotomy uncovered cancerous tissue.

Even when feelings seem irrational, the nurse tries to accept them and seeks to help the client express and resolve them. The nurse's judgment and sense of timing are crucial. The nurse would not encourage a previously anxious client to explore his feelings immediately before taking him to the operating room. The nurse would instead seek to alleviate his anxiety by reassuring him, staying with him, using touch, structuring, and listening. However, the nurse recognizes this as a stopgap measure and would try to discuss the client's feelings with him after the operation and initial recovery. In this way the client is given an opportunity to review his feelings in a less threatening situation and to understand their origin. This is valuable preparation for future crises that may arouse similar feelings.

■ CONCLUSION

Nurses very often engage in short-term nurse-client relationships, especially in inpatient medical and surgical divisions. While short-term relationships have their frustrations, they can be highly rewarding for client and nurse. Hospitalization can be a very stressful experience for clients. To have a nurse interested enough to become therapeutically involved can be a major impact on the client's physical and psychologic status. Nurses can remember that they are their own best tools, especially when some might be inclined to say, "There is nothing I can do." Nursing involves, most crucially, the ability to comfort, to lend strength, and to help clients cope with problems, including terminal illness and death. Realizing one's potential in therapeutic use of self requires time, experience, and flexibility, and the ability to assume for the moment the other person's perspective, without completely losing one's own. Sharing another person's fears, sorrows, joys, and hopes has a humbling effect that most health workers find therapeutic for themselves.

REFERENCES AND SELECTED READINGS

1. Bird, B.: Talking with patients, ed. 2, Philadelphia, 1973, J. B. Lippincott Co.
2. Birdwhistell, R. L.: Kinesics and context: essays on body motion communication, New York, 1970, Ballantine Books, Inc.
3. Birdwhistell, R. L.: Communication, Int. Encycl. Soc. Sci. **3**:24-29, 1968.
4. *Bothamley, V. A.: Communication and the ventilated patient, Nurs. Times **71**:628-630, 1975.
5. *Brill, N.: Working with people: the helping process, Philadel-1973, J. B. Lippincott Co.
6. Buber, M. (Smith, R. G., translator): I and thou, ed. 2, New York, 1958, Charles Scribner's Sons.
7. *Carlson, C. E., coordinator: Behavioral concepts and nursing intervention, ed. 2, Philadelphia, 1978, J. B. Lippincott Co.
8. *Carson, R. C.: Interaction concepts of personality, Chicago, 1969, Aldine Publishing Co.
9. *Carter, F. M.: Psychosocial nursing, ed. 2, New York, 1976, Macmillan Publishing Co., Inc.
10. Chapman, J. E., and Chapman, H. H.: Behavior and health care: a humanistic helping process, St. Louis, 1975, The C. V. Mosby Co.
11. Dance, F. E. X.: The "concept" of communication, J. Commun. **20**:201-210, 1970.
12. Darnell, D. K., and Brockriede, W.: Persons communicating, Englewood Cliffs, N.J., 1976, Prentice-Hall, Inc.
13. *Dorroh, T. L.: Between patient and health worker, New York, 1974, McGraw-Hill Book Co.
14. *Eisenberg, A. M.: Living communication, Englewood Cliffs, N.J., 1975, Prentice-Hall, Inc.
15. Finkelman, A.: Commitment and responsibility in the therapeutic relationship, J. Psychiatr. Nurs. **13**:10-14, 1975.
16. Fisher, S.: Body consciousness: you are what you feel, Englewood Cliffs, N.J., 1973, Prentice-Hall, Inc.
17. Florer, R. M.: Nurse-patient relationships in general nursing, Nurs. Mirror **136**: 41-43, 1973.
18. *Francis, G., and Munjas, B.: Manual of socialpsychologic assessment, New York, 1976, Appleton-Century-Crofts.
19. *Garrett, A.: Interviewing: its principles and methods, ed. 2, New York, 1972, Family Service Association of America.
20. Goffman, E.: Strategic interaction, Philadelphia, 1969, University of Pennsylvania Press.
21. Goffman, E.: Interaction ritual: essays on face-to-face behavior, New York, 1967, Doubleday & Co., Inc.
22. Goffman, E.: The presentation of self in everyday life, New York, 1959, Doubleday & Co., Inc.
23. Gowan, N. G., and Morris, M.: Nurses' responses to expressed patient needs, Nurs. Res. **13**:68-71, 1964.
24. Hall, E. T.: The silent language, New York, 1973, Doubleday & Co., Inc., Anchor Books.
25. Hollister, W. G., and Edgerton, J. W.: Teaching relationship: building skills, Am. J. Publ. Health **64**:41-46, 1974.
26. Johnson, F. C., and Klare, G. R.: General models of communication research: a survey of the developments of a decade, J. Commun. **11**:13-26, 1961.
27. Kramer, M.: Reality shock: why nurses leave nursing, St. Louis, 1974, The C. V. Mosby Co.
28. Laing, R. D., Phillipson, H., and Lee, A. R.: Interpersonal perception: a theory and a method of research, New York, 1966, Harper & Row, Publishers.
29. Maslow, A.: Motivation and personality, New York, 1969, Harper & Row, Publishers.
30. Mehrabian, A.: Significance of posture and position in the communication of attitude and status relationships, Psychol. Bull. **71**:359-372, 1969.
31. Mercer, L. S., and O'Connor, P.: Fundamental skills in the nurse-patient relationship: a programmed text, ed. 2, Philadelphia, 1974, W. B. Saunders Co.
32. Minter, R. L.: A denotative and connotative study in communication, J. Commun. **18**:26-36, 1968.
33. Mitchell, P. H.: Concepts basic to nursing, New York, 1977, McGraw-Hill Book Co.
34. *O'Brien, M. J.: Communications and relationships in nursing, ed. 2, St. Louis, 1978, The C. V. Mosby Co.
35. *Pasquali, E.: East meets West: a transcultural aspect of the nurse-patient relationship, J. Psychiatr. Nurs. **12**:20-22, 1974.
36. Pearce, W. B., and Sharp, S. M.: Self-disclosing communication, J. Commun. **23**:409-425, 1973.
37. Peplau, H. E.: Interpersonal relations in nursing, New York, 1952, G. P. Putnam's Sons.
38. Rawlinson, M. E.: Projection in relation to interpersonal perception, Nurs. Res. **14**:114-118, 1965.
39. Ruesch, J., and Bateson, G.: Communication: the social matrix of psychiatry, New York, 1968, W. W. Norton & Co., Inc.
40. Scheflen, A. E.: How behavior means, New York, 1974, Doubleday & Co., Inc., Anchor Books.
41. Shannon, C. E., and Weaver, W.: The mathematical theory of communication, Urbana, Ill., 1949, University of Illinois Press.
42. *Skipper, J. K., and Leonard, R. C., editors: Social interaction and patient care, Philadelphia, 1965, J. B. Lippincott Co.
43. Spiegel, J. P.: Messages of the body, New York, 1974, The Free Press.
44. Sullivan, H. S.: The interpersonal theory of psychiatry, New York, 1953, W. W. Norton & Co., Inc.
45. Ticho, E. A.: Donald Winnicott, Martin Buber and the theory of personal relationship, Psychiatry **37**:240-253, 1974.
46. *Travelbee, J.: Interpersonal aspects of nursing, ed. 2, Philadelphia, 1971, F. A. Davis Co.
47. Ujhely, G. B.: Current technological advances and the nurse-patient relationship, J. N.Y. State Nurs. Assoc. **5**:25-28, 1974.
48. Wallston, K. A., and Wallston, B. S.: Nurses' decisions to listen to patients, Nurs. Res. **24**:16-22, 1975.

*References preceded by an asterisk are particularly well suited for student reading.

49. Wiener, N.: Cybernetics, New York, 1948, John Wiley & Sons, Inc.
50. Zefron, L. J.: The history of the laying-on of hands in nursing, Nurs. Forum **14**:350-363, 1975.

AUDIOVISUAL RESOURCE

*Concept Media: Nurse-patient interaction series, slide cassettes, Costa Mesa, Calif., Concept Media.

10

The problem-oriented system

GRETCHEN KRAMER DERY

Professional nursing practice uses a problem-solving process, commonly referred to intraprofessionally as the "nursing process." This problem-solving process originated in the scientific method that has been used successfully by many professions for decades.

The purpose of this chapter is to explore a specific method of recording client health and illness data within the context of the problem-solving method. Problem-oriented record keeping is not merely a mechanism for preserving specific data, although this is indeed part of the system. The problem-oriented system stipulates a defined and structured manner of procuring and communicating information and will ultimately influence and mold the system of health care provided.

Within the traditional hospital setting, nurses, physicians, social workers, physical therapists, and others have labored to provide illness care for those in need. There has been a tendency for the care provided to be fragmented, divided, and delivered within the context of departments or professions within the bureaucratic setting. Even with the best intentions, there is a lack of communication between health and illness care personnel. Nurses identify and work with nursing problems, the physician defines medical problems, and other groups define problems from other perspectives. There has recently been a trend to attempt to define health and illness care problems from the client's perspective, since in fact the problems *are* the client's. The problem-oriented system allows different professions to identify, from their particular frame of reference, problems relating to the client's past, present, and future situation. It additionally allows the client and professionals involved in the client's care to plan and problem solve together. Because of increasing complexity and specialization, health and illness professionals must develop some understanding of each other's skills and abilities, learn to value the contributions of differing professions, and develop an effective method of communication.

The nursing process consists of three steps: assessing, intervening and evaluation (see Chapter 7). The problem-oriented system is easily incorporated into the nursing process and complements the traditional problem-solving approach to client care.[29] Its use can facilitate understanding and application of the nursing process by adding specific form to parts of the process.[26] As specific components of the problem-oriented record are presented and discussed, articulation with the nursing process will be highlighted.

Each profession tends to develop its own language, which facilitates intraprofessional communication, but this can be a formidable barrier to interprofessional communication. Unless this communication barrier is minimized, it may be impossible for the client or other professionals to understand what is being said.

Traditional charting reflects a separatist philosophy. It is "source oriented"; that is, information is recorded according to where it originated. Nurses write on "nurses' notes" or "progress notes"; physicians write on physicians' "order sheets" and "progress notes"; radiologists report on "x-ray sheets"; the laboratory personnel report in the "lab report" section. This system illustrates the communication barriers between and among disciplines.[39]

Nursing has used both written and verbal mechanisms for communication, but has relied more heavily upon verbal means.[7] Verbal communication has some drawbacks as a primary mode of communication: it can be time consuming because of frequent repetition; it is not highly organized; it cannot easily be retrieved; it is more subject to misinterpretation; and it has no value in the courtroom situation.[1]

Is there a need for written records? In the hospital setting the increasing complexity of care, the increasing amount of data collected about each patient, and the increasing number of personnel caring for patients necessitates written means of communication. Written records serve to communicate information, document the patient's status, allow for the measurement of change, record interventions that might account for changes in the client's status, describe what is done in a manner that makes the logic apparent to others, serve as a means for storing information, and allow for auditing.[38]

To a great extent, nursing notes have been an exercise in futility. Nurses have in the past been socialized not to analyze the data collected but merely to act as a vehicle for data transmission, especially in the written record. Most notations were preceded by qualifiers, giving the observation, but not risking an inference. A typical situation might involve a patient grimacing, groaning, moaning, and holding her operative site. The nurse's note would read: "Ms. Thompson is holding her operative site and moaning and groaning." To say that the patient was in pain was considered paramount to making a medical diagnosis and was not encouraged.

Thus charting became a routinized task and suffered from many shortcomings. Notes were disorganized, disconnected, long, random, dissociated, and written in terms of specific events that occurred rather than an overall scheme or plan. Additionally, they were repetitious and unused by other professional colleagues. Attempts were made to minimize the repetition by charting only significant data and omitting all other data, thus practically no charting was done. Perhaps the most significant difficulty was, and still is, the fact that nurses' notes reflected written response *only* to delegated medical interventions rather than nursing interventions. Such things as administering prescribed medications and carrying out prescribed treatments were and are well documented, but *nursing* functions were not.

The nursing care plan, a close ally to the nursing note, suffers from another set of difficulties, and there has been a growing disenchantment with its use.[26] Common criticisms of the nursing care plan include the following complaints: they are limited in physical size, they are unused, they do not individualize care, and they are too difficult to write and maintain. There are two features of nursing care plans that are problematic. The nursing care plan is often separate from the remainder of the patient's record (i.e., in a Kardex) and is relatively inaccessible or unused rather than visible and available to other health and illness professionals. Data can only be useful if it can be used. The second feature is that nursing care plans are written in pencil, updated by erasures, and destroyed when the patient is discharged from the institution. The nursing care plan never becomes a permanent part of the patient's record, and one cannot retrospectively use the data for a subsequent admission or for evaluation of outcomes of nursing care. Thus nursing care plans are disposable and transient—certainly not the material from which accountability is made. However, saying that nursing care plans may not be the best tool to accomplish client-care planning does in no way negate the value of the nursing process per se.[26]

If the nursing care plan and traditional mechanisms for charting have been ineffective methods for communication, what are the alternatives? One alternative, based specifically upon the writings of Weed, advocates the use of the "problem-oriented" record.[36] The problem-oriented record is a method of record keeping, which requires several ongoing processes to be operant. The components of the problem-oriented record include a data base, problem list, initial plans, progress notes, flow sheets, and periodic summaries (including a discharge summary for institutions that do not provide for ongoing health and illness care for clients). All professionals contributing to health or illness care for clients can successfully utilize this method, and its use is not restricted to hospitals or institutions. The method has been used by health and illness care professionals in a variety of settings including federally operated hospitals, community hospitals,[18] physicians' practices, and public health agencies.[17] The method encourages a multidisciplinary approach, which has led to use by nurses, social workers, dieticians, physical therapists, pharmacists, and physicians.[28]

In the discussion of the problem-oriented record, each of the component parts will be defined and discussed, and the relationship between the problem-oriented record and the nursing process will be detailed. Because of the nature of the illness problems presented within this text, the example used to illustrate these component parts will be one exemplifying the stressors commonly found in a medical-surgical hospital setting.

■ DATA BASE

The data base is the information gathered about a client and is one part of the assessment component of the nursing process. The data base is acquired *before* the identification of client problems begins. It consists of all information necessary to begin to determine the client's health or illness status. A data base provides a nurse with information that will serve as a beginning point for planning nursing interventions. Those concerned with the delivery of specified care to a selected population need to identify the components of the data base before the method is instituted.[32] Weed suggests that the initial data base be as complete as possible and only be constrained by three factors: expense, discomfort, and possible hazard.[36] Gathering a data base generally can include three basic processes: interviewing, physical examination, and laboratory tests.

One frequently asked question is "who collects the data base?" The answer may vary from situation to situation, but in the hospital setting it seems imperative that a minumum of four people be involved. These four people would include employees from the *admitting office* (to help with insurance and other very real necessities involved in the process of hospitalization in this country), the *physician* (who must be involved to a greater or lesser extent to ascertain that the information needed to make a medical diagnosis is available), and a *nurse* (to ascertain that the information needed to make a nursing diagnosis is available). For a hospitalized patient this is the minimum involvement. In addition, the *patient* (or other substitute) should be *actively* involved in the gathering of the data base.[39] In many situations in the community the private practitioner (nurse or physician) and the client will be the primary persons involved.

Perhaps the most important issue is not necessarily who collects the data base. In some hospitals nurse-practitioners collect the majority of the data base, and in some the task is more equally shared. The crucial issue is *what* information *is* gathered, and whether it is sufficient for the professions involved to formulate a problem list.

Different groups or institutions have a variety of forms or mechanisms that assist in the data-collection process. In some instances a one-to-one interview is done, in some instances a computer "interviews" a client, and in some instances the patient simply responds to a paper and pencil tool. In the majority of cases several of the above options are combined.

A hospital-defined data base usually contains three major categories of information: the patient's *history* (including a review of systems), a *physical examination*, and *laboratory findings*. The patient history has several components: (1) reason for contact, (2) patient profile, (3) family illness history, (4) present patient illness history, (5) past patient illness history, and (6) patient's current health practices. The patient's significant others such as spouse, family, or friends can help supply the history component of the data base.

The *reason for contact*, the first part of the defined data base, is generally simply stated in the patient's own words. Throughout the following discussion, an example of the component parts of a problem-oriented record for a patient entering a small community hospital will be used for illustration.

Date: July 1, 1978

I. PATIENT HISTORY

A. Reason for contact

"I have been having stomach pains and upsets."

The second section of the patient history, the *patient profile*, might include data related to name, age, sex, race, occupation, place of residence, admitting physician, number of children and their state of health, marital history, significant others, financial matters, living conditions, education, dietary habits, interests, future plans, fears, handicaps, and response to illness.

B. Patient profile

Ms. Melissa Smith is a 45-year-old caucasian female. She presently does not work outside the home, but was an elementary school teacher. She has not been actively involved in teaching for twelve years. She lives in the immediate suburban area. Dr. Mary Jane Long is her admitting physician. Ms. Smith has two female children, ages 21 and 22. Both children are in college out of state.

Ms. Smith has been recently widowed (6 months ago). She has no present financial difficulties and owns her own four bedroom home. Her late husband's insurance provides her with a continued adequate income to maintain her present life style, and she possesses comprehensive health insurance. Money had been secured for the children's edution prior to her husband's death. She feels she has "no financial concerns at the present." Ms. Smith is a college graduate. She is a "protestant," but "religion does not serve a significant function in my life."

She spends an "average day" in the following manner: She wakes up early, but arises around 10:00 a.m. She does not eat breakfast or lunch, but watches TV or reads. She takes a walk in the afternoon or goes to the movies occasionally. She fixes supper, generally convenience foods, retires about 1:00 AM, but has trouble "falling asleep and never feels rested." She used to be interested in growing plants, needlework, and painting landscapes. She states she "has not felt like doing anything" since her husband's death. She "has no future plans, finds it enough of a challenge to get through one day at a time." She voices no fears at the present time, but is "concerned about her stomach upsets." She has not been hospitalized since her last childbirth experience and does not know what the "rules and regulations" are for this hospital.

Ms. Smith has no visible handicaps.

A *family illness history* could include data about ages and illness or cause of death in parents, siblings, and children. Some information about diseases such as diabetes, heart disease, hypertension, stroke, renal disease, cancer, arthritis, tuberculosis, drug or alcohol abuse, epilepsy, and mental disorders is usually collected. This gives information that could be related to genetic transmission or exposure or problems that have increased "familial occurrence."

C. Family illness history

Parents

Mother: Age 68—living—arthritis

Father: Age 70—deceased—coronary heart disease

Siblings

Brother: Age 45—living and well

Children

Daughter: Age 23—living and well
Daughter: Age 21—living and well

The *current illness status* generally includes information related to each current illness problem perceived by the client. Data is gathered around such parameters as onset, progression, signs and symptoms, any attempts by the patient to treat the problem, and the client's understanding of the problem.

D. Current illness status

Ms. Smith states that she has had an "upset stomach" for the past 3 months. It began gradually, but now she feels nauseated, especially upon arising. She vomits occasionally, that is, four or five times a week. This almost always occurs in the morning. She has noticed a recent change in her bowel habits alternating between diarrhea and constipation. This has occurred in the last 2 weeks. Also during the last 2 weeks she has been having "burning" pain in her stomach. She has been taking aspirin for her stomach pain, 0.64 g, three or four times daily. She feels that she is "not well" and states that "it may be due to the fact that I have not been taking care of myself lately."

The patient's *past illness history* generally includes any significant illness episodes, a description of all illnesses requiring hospitalization, any major surgical procedures, previous developmental problems, and information related to foreign travel, which may be implicated in the etiology of certain diseases such as malaria that are not commonly found in this country.

E. Past illness history

Ms. Smith has had the following childhood diseases: mumps, rubella, and chicken pox. No noted sequelae. She has been hospitalized twice for childbirth, both uncomplicated. She has had no major surgical procedures, and has not traveled out of the country in the past 5 years. Ms. Smith is in her middle-adult period and appears to have had an unremarkable growth and development until the present period.

The *current health practices* section describes health maintenance or preventative health behaviors undertaken by the patient either to increase the level of wellness or prevent illness episodes.

F. Current health practices

Ms. Smith has had her personal and family primary health care needs met by Dr. Long for the past 10 years. She has a physical examination, including pap smear, every year. She performs a monthly self-breast examination. She sees the dentist routinely every 6 months.

The next section of most hospital-based patient histories is the *review of systems.* The review of systems is the patient's verbal or written response to an orderly systematic group of questions primarily related to the body's biosystems. The specific details of a review of systems may vary, but the overall characteristics are generally similar from setting to setting. The reader will note that although the general topics included in the review of systems in Chapter 8 are similar to these, the specific bits of data vary.

II. SYSTEM REVIEW

Please check (√) "yes" or "no." If "yes," give further data in "Comments" section.

A. General	**Yes**	**No**	**Comments**
1. Weight loss or gain	√		Past 3 to 6 months (20 lb.)
2. Fever or chills		√	
3. Weakness		√	
4. Malaise	√		Past 3 months
B. Integument—skin			
1. Color changes		√	
2. Pigmentation		√	
3. Temperature changes		√	
4. Dryness		√	
5. Bruising		√	
6. Pruritus		√	
7. Scaling		√	
8. Abnormal perspiration		√	
Integument—hair			
1. Color		√	
2. Texture		√	
3. Distribution		√	
4. Abnormal growth or loss		√	

Integument—nails	Yes	No	Comments
1. Color changes		√	
2. Brittleness		√	
3. Ridging		√	
4. Pitting		√	
5. Curvature		√	

C. Head

	Yes	No	Comments
1. Headache		√	
2. Migraine		√	
3. Trauma		√	
4. Syncope		√	
5. Seizures		√	

D. Eyes

	Yes	No	Comments
1. Pain		√	
2. Discharge		√	
3. Visual loss		√	
4. Color blindness		√	
5. Trauma		√	
6. Diplopia		√	
7. Glasses or contacts (date of refraction)		√	

E. Ears

	Yes	No	Comments
1. Pain		√	
2. Discharge		√	
3. Hearing changes		√	
4. Vertigo		√	
5. Tinnitus		√	

F. Nose

	Yes	No	Comments
1. Pain		√	
2. Epistaxis		√	
3. Discharge		√	
4. Obstruction		√	

G. Throat

	Yes	No	Comments
1. Pain		√	
2. Soreness		√	
3. Voice changes		√	
4. Hoarseness		√	

H. Mouth

	Yes	No	Comments
1. Sore throat		√	
2. Sore tongue		√	
3. Bleeding gums		√	
4. Dentures		√	

I. Neck

	Yes	No	Comments
1. Swelling		√	
2. Pain		√	
3. Limitation of motion		√	
4. Enlargement of lymph nodes		√	

J. Breasts

	Yes	No	Comments
1. Lumps		√	
2. Pain or tenderness		√	
3. Nipple discharge		√	

Breasts—cont'd	Yes	No	Comments
4. Gynecomastia		√	
5. Nipple change		√	
6. Normal development and lactation history	√		Breastfed both children for 12-month period
7. Dimples		√	

K. Respiratory system

	Yes	No	Comments
1. Cough		√	
2. Sputum		√	
3. Dyspnea		√	
4. Shortness of breath		√	
5. Orthopnea		√	
6. Wheezing		√	
7. Pain		√	
8. Hemoptysis		√	

L. Cardiovascular system

	Yes	No	Comments
1. Claudication		√	
2. Palpitations		√	
3. Edema		√	
4. Chest pain/discomfort		√	
5. Tachycardia		√	
6. Irregularities of rhythm		√	

M. Gastrointestinal system

	Yes	No	Comments
1. Change in appetite	√		Decreased appetite since husband's death—past 6 months
2. Dysphagia		√	
3. Heartburn		√	
4. Nausea and vomiting	√		Especially in early morning and with increased frequency
5. Hematemesis		√	
6. Melena		√	
7. Jaundice		√	
8. Food intolerance		√	
9. Abdominal pain	√		Burning in epigastrium
10. Changes in bowel habits	√		Alternating diarrhea and constipation

N. Genitourinary system

	Yes	No	Comments
1. Frequency		√	
2. Nocturia		√	
3. Dysuria		√	
4. Incontinence		√	
5. Polyuria		√	
6. Hematuria		√	
7. Pyuria		√	
8. Urinary retention		√	
9. Passage of stones		√	

O. Genitourinary system—menstruation

Last menstrual period: 5/20/77 Gravida/para/abortion: 2:2:0
Age at onset of menses: 12
Last Pap smear: ____ Positive ____ Negative _√_

	Yes	No	Comments
1. Abnormal menses		√	
2. Vaginal discharge		√	
3. Dyspareunia		√	
4. Pelvic pain		√	
5. Itching		√	
6. Burning		√	
7. Menorrhagia		√	
8. Metrorrhagia		√	
9. Contraception	√		Has diaphragm
10. Menopause		√	

P. Musculoskeletal system

	Yes	No	Comments
1. Backache		√	
2. Joint pain		√	
3. Stiffness		√	
4. Joint swelling		√	
5. Muscle weakness		√	

Q. Neurologic system

Cranial nerves

	Yes	No	Comments
1. Changes in smell (I)		√	
2. Changes in vision (II, III, IV, VI)		√	
3. Orofacial parathesias or chewing difficulties (V)		√	
4. Facial weakness or taste disturbances (VII)		√	
5. Disturbances in hearing or equilibrium (VIII)		√	
6. Disturbances in speech, swallowing, and taste (IX, X, XII)		√	
7. Limitation in neck motion (XI)		√	

Sensory nerves

	Yes	No	Comments
8. Paresthesia		√	
9. Hyperesthesia		√	
10. Hypesthesia		√	
11. Anesthesia		√	

Motor nerves	**Yes**	**No**	**Comments**
12. Paralysis		√	
13. Atrophy		√	
14. Involuntary movements		√	
15. Incoordination		√	
16. Gait disturbances		√	
17. Convulsions		√	

R. Mental status

	Yes	No	Comments
1. Memory change		√	
2. Sleep disturbance	√		As in history
3. Crying spells	√		Cries easily—almost everyday
4. Anxiety		√	
5. Depression	√		Feels "down" almost all the time
6. Hallucinations		√	
7. Social withdrawal	√		"Doesn't fit in well" without husband
8. Difficulties with sex life	√		No interest in sex since husband's death

---

The physical examination comprises the second major part of the data base. It can be performed in a manner similar to the review of systems, that is, either a head-to-toe or body-systems fashion. The extent and depth of the physical examination will also vary from setting to setting, based upon the types of services offered.

II. PHYSICAL EXAMINATION

A. General

1. Height: 5′8″
2. Weight: 115 lb. Normal weight: 135 lb.
3. Temperature: 37 C (98.6 F)
4. Pulse: 84
5. Blood Pressure: 100/80
6. Respiration: 14

Check all examined areas normal or abnormal. If abnormal, please explain under "comments."

B. Integument	**Normal**	**Abnormal**	**Comments**
1. Turgor	√		
2. Lesions	√		
3. Hair	√		
4. Nails	√		

	Normal	Abnormal	Comments
C. Head			
1. Skull	√		
2. Scalp	√		
D. Eyes			
1. Vision (Snellen test)	√		
2. Extraocular movements	√		
3. Eyelids	√		
4. Conjunctivae	√		
5. Cornea	√		
6. Sclera	√		
7. Lens	√		
8. Pupils	√		
9. Fundi	√		
E. Ears			
1. Auditory acuity	√		
2. External ear	√		
3. Canals, drums	√		
F. Nose			
1. External	√		
2. Mucosa	√		
3. Septum	√		
4. Turbinates	√		
G. Mouth and throat			
1. Lips	√		
2. Breath	√		
3. Teeth, gums	√		
4. Tongue	√		
5. Mucosa	√		
6. Tonsils	√		
7. Pharynx	√		
8. Speech	√		
9. Salivary glands	√		
H. Neck			
1. Range of motion	√		
2. Appearance	√		
3. Trachea	√		
4. Thyroid	√		
5. Masses	√		
I. Breasts			
1. Masses	√		
2. Nipples	√		
J. Nodes			
1. Cervical	√		
2. Axillary	√		
3. Inguinal	√		
K. Chest			
1. Configuration of thorax	√		
2. Respiratory movements	√		

	Normal	Abnormal	Comments
3. Percussion	√		
4. Inspiratory breath sounds	√		
5. Expiratory breath sounds	√		
L. Vascular			
1. Carotid pulse	√		
2. Radial pulse	√		
3. Femoral pulse	√		
4. Posterior tibial pulse	√		
5. Dorsal pedal pulse	√		
6. Popliteal pulse	√		
7. Neck veins	√		
8. Peripheral veins	√		
Ieart			
1. Impulse	√		
2. Palpation	√		
3. Rhythm	√		
4. Auscultation	√		
N. Abdomen			
1. Abdominal wall	√		
2. Distension	√		
3. Tenderness		√	Abdominal tenderness noted over epigastrium
4. Liver	√		
5. Spleen	√		
6. Kidneys	√		
7. Other masses	√		
8. Bowel sounds	√		
O. Rectal			
1. Anus and sphincter	√		
2. Rectum	√		
3. Prostate	N/A	N/A	
P. Genitalia			
Male			
1. Penis	N/A	N/A	
2. Scrotum	N/A	N/A	
3. Testes	N/A	N/A	
4. Epididymis	N/A	N/A	
5. Inguinal canal	N/A	N/A	
Female			
6. External genitalia	√		
7. Urethra	√		
8. Vagina	√		
9. Cervix	√		
10. Uterus	√		
11. Adnexa	√		
Q. Extremities			
1. Muscles	√		
2. Joints	√		

Extremities—cont'd	Normal	Abnormal	Comments
3. Edema	√		
4. Ambulation	√		
5. Coordination	√		
6. Amputation; deformities	√		
R. Spine			
1. Configuration	√		
2. Mobility	√		
3. Tenderness	√		
S. Neurologic system			
1. Cranial nerves	√		
2. Gait	√		
3. Biceps reflex	√		
4. Triceps reflex	√		
5. Patellar reflex	√		
6. Achilles reflex	√		
7. Plantar response	√		
8. Peripheral nerves	√		
9. Sensory	√		
T. Mental status			
1. Orientation	√		
2. Memory	√		
3. Mood		√	Has been very "depressed" since husband's death, which coincided with youngest daughter's departure for college
4. Consciousness	√		

The last section of most data bases for hospitalized patients is *routine admission laboratory work*. In most settings this will minimally include a urinalysis and a complete blood count.

III. LABORATORY REPORTS

Ms. Smith's CBC and urinalysis were within normal limits.

MASTER PROBLEM LIST

The next section of a problem-oriented record is the *master problem list*. The problems are derived from the data base, and the more adequate the data base, the more comprehensive the problem list.

The formulation of problems is similar to the assessment phase of the nursing process. The problems are not just a numbering of information contained in the data base, but a conclusion or decision resulting after careful investigation, examination, and analysis of the data.[4]

Problems can be defined as anything that causes concern to the client or those professions providing care.[38] They can include any situation or condition in which a person requires help to maintain or regain a state of health or achieve a peaceful death.[4]

Problems can include physical abnormalities, symptoms, physical findings, laboratory abnormalities, psychologic disequilibrium, socioeconomic difficulties, demographic variables. past illnesses, potential problems, or incomplete data.[2]

Every problem identified may not be treated, but it can be identified and examined in relation to its effect upon the patient's situation. Since the focus of the patient and the providers of illness care can differ, what constitutes a problem may differ, depending upon the perspective involved. But all problems that belong on the problem list *are* the patient's problems, and it is generally important when several professions are involved with providing care for an individual that their perspective be shared *interprofessionally* and *with the patient*. This helps to avoid having those involved working in isolation and at differing purposes. Thus all involved are responsible for identifying and adding problems to the problem list.

Several general categories of problems can be defined. *Active problems* are those problems that require attention or treatment at the present time. *Inactive or resolved problems* are those that have caused previous significant difficulties and may recur or lead to other problems.[36] Minor problems of short duration can be identified as *temporary problems*. Later, if they prove to be of significant magnitude, they can be added to the permanent problem list. *Potential problems* are those that have an increased likelihood of occurring because of the characteristics and number of factors present in the situation.

Problems should be worded at the level of sophistication that the data supports. Problems are not defined as a probable or possible medical diagnosis. Until the medical diagnosis is confirmed, the problem is stated in terms reflecting the health team's level of certainty. Once the diagnosis is confirmed, it is entered as a problem. For an active or current problem, the date of onset should be recorded, and the date of resolution should be recorded for resolved or inactive problems.

One format for recording problems is to title, number, and list permanent active and inactive problems at the front of the chart on a master problem list. However, some persons feel numbering problems quickly becomes cumbersome in multiproblem patients, and they prefer to list problems by title alone.

The problem list must be dynamic if it is to serve its purpose of structuring communication between professionals. It is updated by any professional member of the patient care team as new information is obtained, new problems are identified, and as active problems become inactive.[32]

MASTER PROBLEM LIST

Active problems	Date of onset	Date of resolution	Inactive or resolved problems
Gastrointestinal symptoms	3/1/78		
Nausea and vomiting	3/1/78		
Decreased appetite	3/1/78		
Burning pain in stomach	1/1/78		
Change in bowel habits	1/1/78		
Weight loss	3/1/78		
Sleep difficulties and lethargy	3/1/78		
Lack of future orientation	3/1/78		
Social withdrawal	3/1/78		
Poor dietary habits	3/1/78		

PLAN

The third major section of the problem-oriented record is the initial plan. The initial plan is formulated through the description and assessment of each problem and a proposed action to be taken in relation to the problem. These actions are usually described as diagnostic, therapeutic, or educational. An additional category of actions is seeking further information. This part of the problem-oriented process incorporates aspects from the assessment and intervention phases of the nursing process.

The initial plan is written on the progress note. The "SOAP" format is used in formulating the initial and all subsequent plans. The "S" represents subjective data and is a description of the problem from the patient's view. The "O" represents objective data and includes information gathered from inspection, percussion, auscultation, and laboratory and other tests. The "A" represents assessment and is the analysis of the subjective and objective components. The "P" represents the plan and can include diagnostic plans, therapeutic plans, and patient education plans.

From this point forward all subsequent data is recorded in the body of the record under the specific related problem. Thus all further assessment and interventions will be related to the appropriate problem in the progress note or will be the stimulus for the definition of a new problem.

Laboratory work, medications, diet, activity modification, and procedures all are related to the specific problems. Unchanged unremarkable events are not recorded in the problem-oriented system.

The initial statement of plans establishes the need for further data and the type of treatment to be given. Nursing and medical and other plans need to be complementary, and plans of the involved professions should be integrated and written as notes under the specific problems.[39] The patient profile and the complete problem list need to be reviewed before any discipline makes plans for a single problem. Plans made without understanding of overall problems and the patient's life style are likely to be ineffective, even though they might seem appropriate when related to a single isolated problem.[36]

INITIAL PLAN

Date: July 1, 1978 (admission day)

Problem 1: GI symptoms

S: Early morning nausea and vomiting; lack of appetite, burning pain in stomach; weight loss; bowel function changes
O: Tenderness in epigastric area on palpation; thin
A: Gastrointestinal distress
P: Regular diet with no spicy foods; record types and amounts of foods eaten; weigh daily in early morning before breakfast; note frequency, color, and consistency of stools; Maalox, 1 oz., q 2 to 3 hr. p.r.n. for burning; stool for guaiac; upper and lower GI series

Problem 2: Sleep difficulties and lethargy

S: Unable to sleep well at night, feels tired all day
O: Looks and acts lethargic
A: Inadequate sleep
P: Talk further with patient about her usual sleep patterns and routines; try to keep active during daytime; observe but do not awaken at night; schedule interventions for time when patient is awake

Problem 3: Lack of future plans or goals

S: "It seems as if I am no use to anyone any more—no one needs me."

O: None

A: Situational crisis—husband's death and daughter's leaving home; still grieving loss of husband and children

P: Let patient verbalize her feelings about her present situation and changes it has made in her life style; assess her readiness or ability and motivation to explore new directions for her life.

Problem 4: Social withdrawal

S: "My husband's gone, my daughters don't need me. I don't fit in with my friends anymore. I tried to go out when my friends invited me—but they are couples and I am alone."

O: Tearful, sad

A: Separation from "significant others"; self-isolation

P: Allow one consistent nurse to care for Ms. Smith to allow for establishment of solid relationship; in light of problems 2 and 3, might consider the nurse-clinician for this

Problem 5: Poor dietary habits

S: Eats only one meal per day, usually convenience foods

O: None

A: May be secondary to problem 1, lack of appetite, or may be result of other factors

P: Schedule interview with dietitian sometime this week for purpose of gathering more data

Temporary problem: Unfamiliar with hospital routine

S: "I don't know the rules and regulations."

O: Appears to be anxious lest she do something "against the rules"

A: None

P: Thorough orientation today regarding visiting hours, mealtimes, physical layout, access to other areas of hospital, and her upcoming activities

M. J. Long, M.D.
J. Belein, R.N., Primary Nurse

PROGRESS NOTES

After the initial plan for each problem is formulated and recorded, the next section for the problem-oriented record is what has been traditionally called "progress notes." In the problem-oriented record there are three types of progress notes: the *narrative note*, the *flow sheet*, and the *discharge summary*.

Each *narrative note* should relate directly to a problem and should be titled (or numbered) accordingly. Progress notes can be used to record the patient's progress, resolution of old problems, and development of new problems.[27] Progress notes follow the same SOAP format as the initial plan.[27] Nurses, social workers, physical therapists, physicians, and all other professions providing care for the client record their data in relation to a specific problem and in sequence with all other data related to that problem. Thus the helping professions assume an integrated role in the solution of patient problems, and each profession avoids establishing the kind of identity that permits or encourages the possibility of dealing with problems out of context.

Narrative notes do not need to be made on each problem daily, only when indicated. Two problems can be combined in a progress note, as long as it is clearly noted that this is being done. If this happens frequently, it may indicate that the two problems are actually subparts of another problem. And it is not always necessary to use each step of the SOAP formula with each note.

Progress notes contain the ongoing elements of evaluation—the final phase of the nursing process. As plans for particular problems are executed, the ongoing results should be visible in the data collected in the progress notes.

PROGRESS NOTES

2nd hospital day
Monday: 2 PM

Problem: Unfamiliar with hospital routine

S: "I feel more comfortable here now—I know visiting hours, mealtimes, physicians visiting times, and the plans for the next two days."

O: Nervous movement of hands; anxious look of face

A: Appears more comfortable with hospitalization routine; still somewhat apprehensive

P: Continue to be alert for need to inform patient of varying aspects of her care

J. Gelein, R.N., Primary Nurse

2nd hospital day
Monday: 8 PM

Problem: Sleep difficulties and lethargy

S: Unable to sleep last night, even after two sleeping pills.

O: Patient awake all night, even after repeated dose of Seconal; had not napped during day

A: May be due to first night in strange place; seems to have unusual tolerance to sedatives

P: Talk again with patient about current medications being taken; observe again this evening for response

N. Yates, R.N.

2nd hospital day
Monday: 8 PM

New problem: Anxious, irritable, hallucinating

S: "I am very nervous. I hear my daughters. I need a drink."

O: Patient's face and body tense; answers questions in tense manner; hearing voices of persons not present; blood pressure 114/110, pulse 128, respirations 26; nauseated and vomiting

A: Possible drug withdrawal

P:
1. Notify Dr. Long immediately; request p.r.n. sedation orders
2. Observe for changes (↑) in V.S.
3. Establish a relaxed atmosphere—prevent excessive fear and anxiety
   a. Medicate patient per physician's orders
   b. Remain with patient
   c. Assure patient that "voices" are only her mind playing tricks on her
   d. Keep the room well lighted and avoid shadows
   e. Keep out loud noises and unnecessary traffic
   f. Calm patient by lowering voice, speaking slowly, and moving deliberately
   g. Remain firm with patient and assure her she can be responsible for her behavior
   h. Encourage patient to drink 8 oz. fluid (juices) to maintain blood sugar and electrolytes
   i. Offer small high-protein snacks q 4 h after nausea and vomiting abate
   j. Encourage ambulation with assistance q 1 to 2 h to bathroom; change position in bed frequently
   k. Use touch as in backrubs for comfort
   l. Frequent mouth care
   m. Seizure precautions

P. Craig, R.N.

Date: Monday
Time: 11 PM

Problem: Anxious; irritable; hallucinating; increase in blood pressure, pulse, and respirations; and nausea and vomiting

S: Hallucinating, feels very nervous, admits to drinking 5 to 10 drinks per day since husband died

O: Agitated; increased blood pressure, pulse, and respirations; vomiting

A: Acute alcohol withdrawal

P:
1. Valium 25 mg IM stat and q 4 h p.r.n.
2. Phenergan 25 mg intramuscularly for nausea and vomiting stat and q 4 h p.r.n.
3. Laboratory work: chemistry 12, stat.

M. J. Long, M.D.

Flow sheets, the second form of the progress note, are used to record significant data in a tabular or graphic manner. Flow sheets are predesigned and variable. They help to facilitate interpretation of rapidly changing interrelated variables. Flow sheets also serve as a place to record everyday activities, such as mouth care, bathing, and ambulation, that need documentation but require no other comment (p. 142).

Flow sheets are a permanent part of the patient's record. All entries on the sheet are signed and dated. They have several advantages. Specifically, they prevent overlooking important items of information. Once designed, they cause a series of actions to be completed automatically, rather than requiring a person to plan each action. They may be the only record for certain rapidly changing variables. They save a tremendous amount of time trying to unravel and assemble disorganized data. Flow sheets can be used as an evaluative tool for certain interventions by outlining results, and they allow for some consistency of data gathered from patient to patient by allowing analysis of data for more than one patient. They can also provide structure for new persons giving care to the patient.

Common examples of flow sheets are vital sign sheets, intake and output records, medication sheets, diabetic records, and treatment records. In some situations (i.e., ICU, CCU) a great variety of data is kept on a very large flow sheet that shows several interrelated variables for 15-minute time spans (see Chapter 70). Thus such parameters as drugs, intravenous fluids, laboratory work, vital signs, and urinary output can be easily visualized almost on a minute-to-minute basis, and changes in one variable can be related to changes in others.

The third and final section of the progress note is the *discharge planning summary*. Discharge summary notes from the hospital are merely final narrative notes that relate the overall assessment of progress while hospitalized and plans for the patient's continued follow-up or referral. The SOAP format provides a systematic method for reviewing what was identified (subjective and objective), what interventions were planned (assessment), and what must still be done (plan). The discharge summary should be problem oriented and should include only that information from the data base necessary for ongoing management of a problem.[36] Discharge summaries can help facilitate continuity of care from the hospital to other agencies or professionals who will continue to provide care for the patient or client (p. 143).

FLOW SHEET

Name: Ms. Smith
Date: Tuesday/month/year Wednesday/month/year Thursday/month/year

Parameter observed	Hour				
	9 PM	**11 PM**	**1 AM**	**3 AM**	**4 PM**
Vital signs					
Blood pressure	140/100	130/100	128/98	130/100	110/80
Pulse	126	120	118	122	80
Respirations	26	24	24	22	16
Fluid intake					
PO	Refused	120 cc OJ	Refused	150 cc	OJ 240 cc
IV	—	—	—	—	—
Protein snacks	Nauseated	Nauseated		One cheese cracker	Peanut butter crackers
Fluid output					
Urine	—	100 cc	—	200 cc	400 cc
Emesis	50 cc	—	—	100 cc	—
Other	—	—	—	—	—
Patient's behavior state	Hearing voices Moving nervously about in bed	Somewhat calmer; still having auditory hallucinations	Unchanged	Increased restlessness; visual hallucinations	Some tremulousness; embarrassed
Activity	Position changed	Up with assistance to bathroom	Turned	Turned	Up walking and in chair
Sedation	Valium	—	Valium	—	—
Antiemetics	Phenergan	—	Phenergan	—	—
Mouth care	Done	Done	Done	Done	Self-care
	P. Craig, R.N.	P. Craig, R.N.	J. Fugate, R.N.	N. Yates, R.N.	J. Belein, R.N.

CONCLUSION

Are there advantages to using the problem-oriented process? Are there disadvantages? What threats to professionals are implicit in this process? And what, if any, are the long-term implications for clients and professionals?

There are several suggested advantages to using the problem-oriented record. It is well established that this type of record keeping provides a means for permanent documentation of the thinking process of those involved in health and illness care. It can be and has been used as an evaluative tool for the peer review process and as a means for auditing for quality control; thus it logically should lead to provision of improved quality of care.

Quality of care, however, is a very nebulous phenomenon and lacks adequate definition. A distinctly causal relationship between using the problem-oriented record and subsequent improvement in patient care is at best difficult to prove.

The problem-oriented record allows for several modifications that facilitate the teaching-learning process. Since the problem-oriented record reflects problem-solving behavior, one can use it to evaluate students' knowledge and understanding. It allows for self-teaching in that a learner can review in depth one patient's record or several records cross sectionally. Because of its inherent logic and flow, it facilitates learning by making explicit the decision-making process used in giving patient care.

The problem-oriented record allows for another person to grasp easily the important aspects of a patient situation and to see quickly the plans in progress for each

DISCHARGE PLANNING SUMMARY

Date: Time
Friday: 10th hospital day

Problem: Acute/chronic alcoholism (GI symptoms, sleep difficulties, and poor dietary habits)

S: "I feel much better now. I know I have to work through several problems, but at least I am beginning to realize that drinking has not helped me solve anything."

O: Patient suffered withdrawal symptoms 28 hours after admission for GI distress; tolerated withdrawal with no untoward affects; blood chemistries and vital signs now within normal limits; stools guaiac negative and back to her normal routine; eating three meals per day with snacks; weight gain of 8 lb.; occasional burning in stomach controlled with Maalox; minimal nausea; no vomiting; taking no medication except Maalox p.r.n.; able to sleep most of the night with relaxation techniques

A: Has made considerable progress; recognizes and admits her dependence on alcohol; feel future prognosis is guarded, but she is an excellent candidate for rehabilitation; needs to increase her self-esteem

P:
1. Return appointment with Dr. Long in 2 weeks
2. Refer to Dr. Ann Spencer, psychiatrist, for follow-up
3. Continue emphasis on diet; have dietitian who has been following Ms. Smith review diet before she completes discharge; she is going to keep a diet history to help keep her nutrition needs foremost in her mind; she has an adequate knowledge base about good nutrition and seems to be motivated

Problem: Social withdrawal

S: Perhaps I have been overly sensitive about not having a partner. My friends have shown their concern throughout my hospital stay. If I still feel strange in some social situations, perhaps I need to make some new friends who won't always think of me as John's wife. I know my daughters can't stay home with me."

O: Patient able be verbalize concerns and feelings

A: Still actively grieving loss of husband, daughters (to college), and life style; will need continued support to complete the grief process, since losses involve so much of previous valued ways.

P:
1. Suggest possibility of going to "widow's group" as additional social support
2. Work with Dr. Spencer on this problem

Problem: Lack of future orientation

S: "I know I felt I had no future. I still do not know if I can find an important reason for being other than my husband and children, but I was a whole person before I had them and perhaps I can be again. I realize I either have to take control of my life or just let things happen."

O: Patient had previous marketable skills, is intelligent, and able to recognize the possibility of functioning in different manner than before—but still have a satisfying situation.

A: Alcohol noneffective coping mechanism for "empty-nest" syndrome and grieving process; new awareness on Ms. Smith's part that she is not the only person who has ever experienced these problems or sought a similar solution; support needed to assume active life style built around some aspect other than nuclear family

P:
1. Dr. Spencer to help with further development of self-concept separate from deceased husband and living children
2. After return appointment with Dr. Long, Ms. Smith is going to "tutor" students with long-term goal of returning fulltime to the teaching profession

Mary Jane Long, M.D.
Janet Belein, R.N., Primary Nurse

person. Thus when a person must substitute temporarily or permanently for a specified care giver, the transition is eased. Such occurrences result from many instances in the daily lives of professionals, such as illness, vacations, moving, and so on.

Another presumed benefit resulting from this process is increased collaboration among professionals. This in turn remains significant primarily in terms of improved patient care. In a situation involving several different health and illness care professions, each practitioner can advantageously utilize the problem-oriented method to document his or her particular contribution to the patient's progress and plan of care, or it is possible for it to be used as traditional charting has been—only to document the client's response to medical intervention.

One major shortcoming of the problem-oriented process and record is focus on problems. It appears that there is little room for careful assessment of the strengths of the client or patient in relation to the problem-solving process. The management of a problem from the client's perspective will depend heavily on what strengths and assets this person brings to the situation, and building upon those assets may be a crucial function of health and illness care professionals. Additionally, attempts to help clients attain a higher level of wellness does not appropriately appear to fall into a "problem" category.

The one inherent threat for professionals in the use of the problem-oriented record is that it exposes the practitioner to criticism. Information collected is explicit and easily retrieved. Lack of judgment or ignorance is readily apparent. Inadequacies become obvious, and practitioners have to admit when they lack knowledge or understanding. While exposure is an inherent threat in this system, it also can be viewed as having a positive aspect in its tremendous potential for growth.

One possible threat to clients that is inherent in the use of this system is the permanent keeping of easily retrievable, confidential information related to a person. This method of record keeping has the potential of being and in some instances has been computerized. Information could be collected and stored from birth to death in a well-organized fashion. In one manner this could provide for the possibility of continuity of care throughout a lifetime. On the other hand, the potential for possible invasion of privacy and use of data for reasons other than those specifically requested by the client presents possible abuses.

Other implications for the use of the problem-oriented record revolve around the areas of research, licensure, and third-party payment. The need for research in education and practice is obvious. Adequate record keeping is a prerequisite to all forms of research, including nursing. A format that outlines problems and assigns names to them can easily serve as a source of statistical data in reviewing care from records. Additionally, problems can be categorized and used to study the complementary care given by various health and illness care personnel. A review of multiple records might reveal common client problems, effective versus ineffective approaches used in meeting them, and the complementary roles of the varying professionals contributing to the care. Predictive outcomes of approaches to clients' problems can then be made in various situations.

The problem-oriented record has implications for licensure. The potential for peer review and audit may contain the essence of a more valid approach for determining licensure or certification. The possibility of evaluation based upon documented performance, with or without other "tests," may allow for more definite and well-defined evaluation criteria.

Another possible implication for the problem-oriented record involves third-party payment systems. The thorough documentation of the skilled contributions made by the participating health care personnel may allow for more equitable distribution of health-insurance remunerations. Nursing especially has not been visible in this area and has generally been unable to seek remuneration for services rendered. This may be a crucial issue with the close advent of some type of national health insurance.

In conclusion, Weed has stated that form leads to economy of time in almost all human endeavors.[36] While this cannot be denied, it must also be remembered that form is restrictive and any form is derived from the basis of a set of assumptions. In this particular case the assumptions are influenced by a person's background of knowledge, past experiences, and definition of health and illness care. If one can recognize the assumptions underlying this process of thinking and method of record keeping, then one can intelligently accept or reject the problem-oriented record as a mechanism for improving health and illness care.

REFERENCES AND SELECTED READINGS

1. *Atwood, J., Mitchell, P. H., and Yarnall, S. R.: The problem-oriented record: a system for communication, Nurs. Clin. North Am. **9**:229-234, 1974.
2. Bauman, K.: The problem-oriented medical record: a self-instructional manual for nurses, Chapel Hill, N.C., 1975, U.N.C.
3. Beckman, L. J.: Alcoholism problems and women: an overview. In Greenblatt, M., and Schuckit, M.: Alcoholism problems in women and children, New York, 1976, Grune & Stratton, Inc.
4. Becknell, E. P., and Smith, D. M.: System of nursing practice: a clinical assessment tool, Philadelphia, 1975, F. A. Davis Co.
5. *Berni, R., and Nicholson, C.: The POR as a tool in rehabilitation and patient teaching, Nurs. Clin. North Am. **9**:265-270, 1974.
6. *Bloom, J.: Problem oriented charting, Am. J. Nurs. **71**:2144-2148, 1971.
7. Bronkowski, M. S.: Adopting the POMR to community child health care, Nurs. Outlook **20**:515-518, 1972.
8. Calobrisi, A.: Treatment programs for alcoholic women. In Greenblatt, M., and Schuckit, M.: Alcoholism problems in women and children, New York, 1976, Grune & Stratton, Inc.
9. Carroll, J. F.: "Mental illness" and "disease": outmoded concepts in alcohol and drug rehabilitation, Community Ment. Health J. **11**:418-429, 1975.
10. Chavigny, C.: Self-esteem for the alcoholic: an epidemiologic approach, Nurs. Outlook **24**:636-639, 1976.
11. Degowin, E. L., and Degowin, R. L.: Bedside diagnostic examination, New York, 1969, Macmillan Publishing Co., Inc.
12. Ditzler, J.: Rehabilitation for alcoholics, Am. J. Nurs. **76**:1772-1775, 1976.
13. Field, F. W.: Communication between nurse and physician, Nurs. Outlook **20**:722-725, 1972.
14. *Gane, D.: Sparky: a success story, Am. J. Nurs. **73**:1176-1177, 1973.
15. Gerken, B., Molitor, A. M., and Reardon, J.: Problem oriented records in psychiatry, Nurs. Clin. North Am. **9**:289-300, 1974.
16. Heinemann, E., and Estes, N.: Assessing alcoholic patients, Am. J. Nurs. **76**:785-789, 1976.
17. *Kelly, M. E., and McNutt, H.: Implementation of problem-oriented charting in a public health agency, Nurs. Clin. North Am. **9**:281-287, 1974.
18. *Kinney, S., Smith, C., and Barnes, R. H.: The problem-oriented record: a community hospital approach, Nurs. Clin. North Am. **9**:247-254, 1974.
19. Larkin, P. D., and Backer, B. A.: Problem oriented nursing assessment, New York, 1977, McGraw-Hill Book Co.
20. Leonard, P., Cowan, D. B., and Mattingly, P. H.: The POR as a means of collaboration between pediatric nurse practitioner and other health team members, Nurs. Clin. North Am. **9**:271-279, 1974.
21. Lewis, L.: Recognizing the alcoholic, Nurs. 77 **7**:59, 1977.
22. Lewis, L.: The hidden alcoholic: a nursing dilemma, Nurs. 75 **5**:20-30, 1975.

*References preceded by an asterisk are particularly well suited for student reading.

23. Luke, B.: The nutritional implications of alcohol abuse, R.N. **39**:32-34, 1976.
23a. *Marshall, J. C., and Feeney, S.: Structural versus intuitive intake interview, Nurs. Res. **21**:269-272, 1972.
24. Mahoney, E. A., Verdisco, L., and Shortridge, L.: How to record a health history, Philadelphia, 1976, J. B. Lippincott Co.
25. Malloy, J. L.: Taking exception to problem oriented nursing care, Am. J. Nurs. **76**:582-583, 1976.
26. *McCloskey, J. C.: The problem-oriented record vs. the nursing care plan: a proposal, Nurs. Outlook **23**:492-495, 1975.
27. *Mitchell, P. H.: A systematic nursing progress record: the problem oriented approach, Nurs. Forum **12**:187-210, 1973.
28. National League for Nursing: The problem oriented system: a multidisciplinary approach, New York, 1974, Department of Hospital and Related Institutional Nursing Services (NLN #20-1546).
29. *Niland, M. B., and Bentz, P. M.: A problem-oriented approach to planning nursing care, Nurs. Clin. North Am. **9**:235-245, 1974.
30. Nursing Grand Rounds: The alcoholic surgical patient, Nurs. 77 **7**:56-61, 1977.
31. *Payne, S., McBarron, R. A., and O'Connor, E. J.: Implementation of a problem-oriented system in a CCU, Nurs. Clin. North Am. **9**:255-263, 1974.
32. Schell, P. L., and Campbell, A. T.: POMR—not just another way to chart, Nurs. Outlook **20**:510-514, 1972.
32a. *Stevens, B. J.: Why won't nurses write nursing care plans? J. Nurs. Admin. **2**:6-7, 91-92, Nov.-Dec. 1972.
33. Strong, M. L.: Evaluation of problem-oriented nursing notes, J. Nurs. Admin. **2**:50-58, May-June 1972.
34. Thoma, D., and Pittman, K.: Threats of the WEED system, N. Engl. J. Med. **284**:925, 1971.
34a. *Walker, H. K., Hurst, J. W., and Woody, M. F.: Applying the problem-oriented system, New York, 1973, Medcom Books, Inc.
35. Walter, J. B., Pardee, G. P., and Molbo, D. M.: Dynamics of problem-oriented approached: patient care and documentation, Philadelphia, 1976, J. B. Lippincott Co.
36. *Weed, L. L.: Medical records, medical education, and patient care, Cleveland, 1971, Case Western Reserve University Press.
37. *Woody, M., and Mallison, M.: The problem-oriented system for patient-centered care, Am. J. Nurs. **73**:1168-1175, 1973.
38. Woolley, F., Warnick, M., Kane, R., and Dyer, E.: Problem-oriented nursing, New York, 1974, Springer Publishing Co., Inc.
39. *Yarnall, S., and Atwood, J.: Problem oriented practice for nurses and physicians: general concepts, Nurs. Clin. North Am. **9**:215-228, 1974.
40. Zelechowski, G. P.: Helping your patient sleep: planning instead of pills, Nurs. 77 **7**:62-65, 1977.

11

Quality assurance programs: monitoring patient/client outcomes

MARIE J. ZIMMER
WILMA J. PHIPPS

Nurses, the persons who are the recipients of the human service that nurses deliver, the fiscal intermediaries who pay for these services, the health professionals from other disciplines who deliver care to the same patient populations, and the community that determines the allocation of resources to health care delivery are results-oriented people. They wish to know (1) what kinds of health and wellness problems nurses help patients or clients to solve; (2) what patient care processes nurses use in nurse-patient encounters; (3) what changes in patient health and wellness and family status result from these encounters; (4) what it costs to achieve these results; and (5) if these are the best patient care processes and benefits considering the current status of the science and art of nursing and other health or health-related sciences?

■ EXPECTATIONS OF NURSES

Each registered nurse is expected to give an accounting of the results of his or her professional services to patients or clients. Since there is a health care resources *cost* attached to each nurse-patient encounter or series of encounters, people want to know if use of these resources was necessary and if the results were of the best available quality.

Until now few registered nurses have applied organized and formalized procedures to the evaluation of a patient's progress toward desired health and wellness outcomes at the time periods at which change would best be observable. There have been only a few studies of populations of patients to determine the patient health and wellness outcomes, the nursing interactions that helped achieve the outcomes, or the interventions that did not appear to influence the outcomes. Few nurses have calculated the cost of nursing interventions in relation to benefits to patients and their significant others. Now and in the future, these evaluations are an expectation of all health care professionals.

■ ACCOUNTABILITY

In the past the orientation of health science professionals was to *personal accountability*. Presently health care professionals are experiencing a change to *public accountability*. Society, which gives health science professionals the authority to deliver a human service, is asking them to account for an array of outcomes or benefits of their services, and society has a right to do so. The Professional Standards Review Organization (PSRO) legislation (Medicare legislation) that is contained in PL 92-603, Social Security Amendments of 1972, established a nationwide network of organizations for review of patient care financed by the federal government.[8] The stated purpose of PSRO review is to determine if services were medically necessary, if the quality of the services meets professionally recognized standards, if the services could be provided effectively on an outpatient basis, or if the services could be provided more economically in a different type of inpatient facility. In other words, the emphasis is on having all patients or clients receive care in the setting most appropriate to their individual needs. In some areas of the country, third-party payors such as Blue Cross and other private insurance companies are establishing standards for review of the care for which they make payment.

■ QUALITY ASSURANCE

Quality assurance is a process that involves evaluating the degree of excellence of the results of care delivered. In health care delivery the purpose of evaluation is to appraise an ongoing program to find out the extent to which predetermined standards are met. The findings are used to make a decision about changes that are to be implemented by the persons carrying out the program. The aims for evaluation may differ, depending on what information about the quality is sought. *Quality* is a distinguishing characteristic or attribute. People may inquire about whether the patient health and wellness benefits; the processes used in diagnosis, treatment, prognosis, or care; the place; the accessibility; the costs; and other attributes of health care delivery conform to predetermined standards. For each attribute a range of dimensions (usually 0% to 100%) can be measured. Before setting standards, the questions the evaluation is to answer have to be determined along with the kinds of information that will be needed to fully answer the questions.

Although the aim of evaluation studies may differ, quality assurance is always a two-part process. One part *compares actual results of practice with standards.* The other uses the negative findings from the comparison (deficiencies) to *generate recommendations for improvement* to be implemented in the program of care.

Nurses who are engaged in delivery of health care cannot escape inclusion of quality assurance review in their practice responsibilities. Proficiency in evaluation must become part of nurses' repertoire of skills, and there must be evaluation study and restudy results that show that this skill is an ongoing part of practice. Nurses who are expert in the care of specific patient populations possess the knowledge necessary to determine desired health and wellness outcomes for specific patient populations. They know what direct care processes to employ in encounters with patients and significant others in order to assist them to move toward health and wellness. They also know what observable changes in patients' problems should occur at certain time periods in episodes of care. Most nurses are not expert in the methodology that is needed to conduct evaluation studies and must rely on nurse experts to help them define desired outcomes.

In quality assurance review, nurses may conduct nursing studies or they may participate in health review with other health professionals who are active in care of the same patient population. Understanding of the following terms is desirable. Among the terms that are used are utilization review, audit, concurrent review, and retrospective review.

In *utilization review,* each patient's diagnosis or problem is assessed at the time of admission to determine whether the type of facility to which the patient is being admitted is judged to be the most appropriate one economically. Also, the length of the patient's stay is monitored so that it does not exceed the number of days that can be justified for persons with the same type of illness. This process is referred to as concurrent review, since the assessment occurs while care is in progress.

In *audit,* standards that focus on quality are prepared either by peers (audit committee) who are involved together in delivering care to the patient population that is to be studied, or by regional or national groups such as the American Nurses' Association. The standards may cover many parameters of care such as criteria for admission, diagnosis, treatment, prognosis, complications, preparation for discharge, and desired patient outcomes. Information that is documented in the records of a sample of persons who have received care in an agency such as a hospital are compared with the stated standards to determine the degree to which the standards were met. This is referred to as *restrospective review (retrospective chart audit* or *closed review),* which means that the reviewers examine care that was previously given based on documentation in patients' records. Thus it is obvious that accurate detailed documentation is crucial to retrospective audit, since care that is not documented cannot be assumed to have been given. The steps involved in retrospective chart audit are discussed in detail following the next paragraph.

Analysis of standards that are used in audits is needed in order to draw conclusions about the results of particular audits. Until recently the majority of standards were process oriented rather than *outcome oriented;* that is, they dealt with activities (nursing interventions) rather than with patient outcomes. Process standards can be used to measure patient health and wellness outcomes if there is research that establishes the connection between a process (intervention) or group of processes (interventions) and a particular outcome. These process standards are used in *concurrent audit,* which is also referred to as a *process audit, peer review,* or *open audit,* since it is carried out while the patient is still in the hospital. Details of concurrent audit are presented on p. 149.

□ Retrospective chart audit

One audit format that is widely used is that developed by the Joint Commission on the Accreditation of Hospitals (JCAH). In the JCAH format, outcome criteria are defined for a group of patients in terms of their status at discharge on three parameters: *health, activity,* and *knowledge.* In addition, complications commonly occurring during the hospitalization of the selected patient population and the critical management of these complications are reviewed as part of the audit process. In order to establish a retrospective audit system the following steps are necessary:

1. Select a patient population for audit.
2. Determine patient outcomes in terms of health status, activity, and knowledge at discharge.
3. Audit charts for desired outcomes or transmit audit criteria to data retriever.
4. Review feedback on how well stated outcomes

were met and where deficiencies were identified.
5. Analyze deficiencies and make plans for improving deficiencies.
6. Inform nursing staff on patient care units of the results of the audit and the plans for improving the deficiencies such as classes about outcome criteria, necessary documentation, and practices that need to be improved.
7. Carry out the plans outlined to improve deficiencies.
8. Review audit criteria in preparation for reaudit and revise as necessary.
9. Establish date for reaudit.
10. Repeat steps *2* to *4* to determine if there is improvement in the deficiencies identified in the first audit.

Audit committees are appointed or volunteers nominate themselves for the committees. An audit committee is best composed of nurses who possess expertise about the nursing interventions appropriate to a specific patient population. In medical-surgical nursing the patient populations are usually centered around diagnostic categories. For example, the patient populations to be audited might be insulin-dependent diabetics or persons with myocardial infarction, cerebral vascular accidents, chronic obstructive pulmonary disease, total hip arthroplasty, and so on. Thus in many inpatient areas several audit committees may be working simultaneously, with each committee working on a specific audit topic. A committee may be of any size desired by an agency, but committees of more than five persons may find it difficult to arrange a time when all members can be present. Where possible, fulltime faculty members from schools of nursing assigned with students to the hospital or community health agency may provide valuable input as members of audit committees.

The first task of the audit committee is to determine the patient outcomes at time of discharge in terms of *health, activity, knowledge*, and *complications*. Next the committee decides what percentage of the patient population should be expected to achieve the stated outcomes. In the JCAH system the standard for attainment of outcomes is either 100% or 0%. The 100% standard is used for desired outcomes such as the ability of the person to carry out self-care after discharge, while the 0% standard is used for undesired outcomes such as complications. Thus while it would be desired that 100% of insulin-dependent diabetics be able to give their own insulin safely, it would also be desired that 0% of these persons would develop a urinary tract infection while hospitalized. By setting the standards at either 100% or 0% it is easy for the person(s) retrieving the data from the charts to report back to the committee the *number* and *percentage* of the audit population meeting the stated outcomes.

Because it would be obvious that some patients would have associated conditions that would prevent them from attaining the desired outcomes, the audit committee lists *exceptions* that will be considered as legitimate reasons for the outcome not being achieved. These often include such conditions as *physical, mental,* or *intellectual impairment* present on admission. For example, if the desired outcome is that the person be able to resume ADL (activities of daily living) on discharge, a physical impairment that would be identified during data retrieval would be the person being discharged with an indwelling catheter. In this instance the person would be listed as an exception to the 100% standard. At the same time, the data retriever would list documentation that states that alternate plans were made. This would include such notations as "patient and wife instructed in the management of the Foley catheter and leg bag; referral made to VNA."

The JCAH format also provides space for the audit committee to list *special instructions* for the data retriever if the data is to be retrieved from the charts by other than the audit committee members themselves. Many larger hospitals hire persons whose sole job is to retrieve data from charts. They sometimes have the title of medical data analysts (MDAs). Some persons employed in these positions are nurses, while others are specially prepared lay persons. The special instructions tell the retriever where in the patient record the data being sought can best be found. For example, with the current emphasis on discharge summaries by nurses, the discharge summary should speak to each of the desired outcomes and thus would be the prime source for retrieval of the desired data. The nursing discharge summary may be charted either in the nurse's notes, when nursing personnel chart on a separate part of the patient record, or it may appear in the progress notes when all disciplines including nursing chart on the same progress record.

Under the *complications and critical management and reporting* section of the JCAH form, the committee lists complications most likely to occur with that specific patient population and the nursing actions to be taken when each complication occurs. Some examples of these may be found in Table 11-1. The elements of critical management and reporting are also audited in terms of the number and percentage of the population with the complications receiving the stated critical management and reporting. Thus it is possible for the audit committee to analyze the deficiencies in management and reporting and to make plans for improvement of them.

Table 11-1. Examples of complications and critical management and reporting for persons with insulin-dependent diabetes

Complications	Critical management and reporting
Insulin reaction	Charts signs and symptoms Gives sugar-base beverage Notifies physician
Ketoacidosis	Charts signs and symptoms Checks urine for sugar and acetone and documents same Notifies physician
Nosocomial infection	Documents observations Notifies physician

□ Analysis of deficiencies

Once the data is retrieved, the audit committee meets to analyze the findings in order to make plans for improvement of deficiencies. As part of the data retrieval process, the chart numbers of patients exhibiting variations from the desired criteria are listed. This makes it possible for the committee to pull those patient records and have them present at the time of analysis. The committee then determines whether a deficiency does, in fact, exist and whether the deficiency is in *documentation* or in *practice*. A determination is also made as to the type of deficiency; that is, whether it is a deficiency related to *knowledge* or one related to *performance*.

Once a determination is made of the above, plans are made to provide feedback from the audit to nursing personnel on units from which the patient population was drawn. Along with the feedback, plans for improving the identified deficiencies are discussed with the staff. When retrospective chart audit is first begun, it is not uncommon for many of the deficiencies to be attributed to poor documentation. This is especially so if the outcome criteria have not been made available to the nursing staff prior to the first audit. The advantage in not making the outcome criteria available before the first audit is that this audit then serves as baseline data on the quality of care being provided. Subsequent reaudit after the outcome criteria have been shared with the nursing staff provides a comparison in the changes in level of care over time.

After the audit criteria are shared with the staff, most nurses become acutely aware of the need to improve the documentation of patient outcomes, since it can no longer be assumed that patient outcomes that are not documented were, in fact, achieved. The same is true for other aspects of the audit such as documentation of complications and the nursing actions taken when they occur.

NURSING ACTIONS	Yes	No	Not applicable
1. Initial assessment form is completed.			
2. Admission note is on patient's chart.			
3. Patient problems are identified and problem lists started.			
4. Nursing interventions are congruent with identified problems and stated desired patient outcomes.			
5. Documentation indicates that physicians orders are being executed properly			

PATIENT INTERVIEW

1. Is the patient aware of some of the problems identified for inclusion on the problem list?
2. Can the patient state some of the interventions being used for each problem and give the reason for them?
3. Does the patient know the desired outcomes to be achieved by the time of discharge?
4. Does the patient perceive that his or her needs are being met?

Although all the nuances of retrospective chart audit cannot be discussed in this chapter, the above discussion outlines the salient points necessary to understand what is involved in retrospective audit.

□ Concurrent audit (peer review)

As the name implies, the patient's nursing care is audited while the person is still receiving care. As mentioned previously, this type of audit is also referred to as a process audit or an open audit. Before carrying out a concurrent audit, criteria must be established for the parameters to be audited (see boxed material above). In carrying out the audit, the patient's chart and nursing care plan are reviewed and the patient is interviewed to determine how well the patient believes that the established criteria are being met. In some settings the nurse responsible for the patient may be asked to present the nursing care plan and discuss the interventions being provided (or those being anticipated) with the persons conducting the peer review.

The JCAH now advocates that both retrospective and concurrent audits be used. A recent study by Trussell and Stand[10] compares the results of audits of the two types and it is evident that more comparative studies are necessary. At the same time, McClure[6] raises some interesting questions about carrying peer review beyond a concurrent audit to examining the practice of individual practitioners so that those who are not competent are not allowed to practice.

■ SUMMARY

The issues and procedures outlined in this chapter are applicable to nurses no matter where they practice. All professionals have to be responsible for assuring that all patients or clients receive the highest quality of care possible. The reader will note that specific outcome criteria are presented in chapters throughout this book. It is hoped that the outcome criteria presented in these chapters will assist the reader to be more aware of desired patient outcomes as nursing interventions are planned and delivered.

REFERENCES AND SELECTED READINGS

1. Anderson, M. I.: Development of outcome criteria for the patient with chronic heart failure, Nurs. Clin. North Am. **9**:349-358, 1974.
2. Berg, H. V.: Nursing audit and outcome criteria, Nurs. Clin. North Am. **9**:331-335, 1974.

2a. Bloch, D.: Evaluation of nursing care in terms of process and outcome, Nurs. Res. **24**:256-263, 1975.

2b. Davidson, S.: PSRO: utilization and audit in patient care, St. Louis, 1976, The C. V. Mosby Co.

2c. Diddie, P.: Quality assurance: a general hospital meets the challenge, J. Nurs. Admin. **6**:6-16, July-August 1976.

2d. Froebe, D., and Bain, J.: Quality assurance programs and controls in nursing, St. Louis, 1976, The C. V. Mosby Co.

3. Helger, E. E.: Developing nursing outcome criteria, Nurs. Clin. North Am. **9**:323-330, 1974.
4. Hover, J., and Zimmer, M. J.: Nursing quality assurance: the Wisconsin system, Nurs. Outlook **26**:242-249, 1978.
5. Lewis, W. R.: Health behavior and quality assurance, Nurs. Clin. North Am. **9**:359-366, 1974.

5a. Lindeman, C.: Measuring quality of nursing care, J. Nurs. Admin. **6**:7-9, June 1976, and **6**:16-19, Sept. 1976.

6. *McClure, M. L.: The long road to accountability, Nurs. Outlook **26**:47-50, 1978.
7. *McClure, M. L.: Quality assurance and nursing education: a nursing service director's view, Nurs. Outlook **24**:267-269, 1976.

7a. Phaneuf, M.: The nursing audit: self-regulation in nursing practice, ed. 2, New York, 1976, Appleton-Century-Crofts.

8. P.S.R.O.: the law (PL-92-603, Title XI), Laws of the 92nd Congress, Second Session, October 1972.

8a. Selveggi, L., Ericksen, L., Keon, P., and MacKinnon, H.: Implementing a quality assurance program in nursing, J. Nurs. Admin. **6**:37-43, Sept. 1976.

9. Taylor, J.: Measuring the outcomes of nursing care, Nurs. Clin. North Am. **9**:337-348, 1974.
10. Trussell, P. M., and Strand, N.: A comparison of concurrent and retrospective audits on the same patients, J. Nurs. Admin. **8**:33-38, 1978.

10a. Watson, A., and Mayers, M.: Evaluating the quality of patient care through retrospective chart audit, J. Nurs. Admin. **6**:17-21, March-April 1976.

11. *Zimmer, M. J.: Guidelines for development of outcome criteria, Nurs. Clin. North Am. **9**:317-321, 1974.

*References preceded by an asterisk are particularly well suited for student reading.

PART TWO

Stress and adaptation

UNIT III

Adaptation

Individuals with medical-surgical problems are exposed to multiple stressful events in the course of their illnesses and therapy. Exposure to these stressors may enhance their growth or be detrimental to their health. It is important for nurses to identify those variables that foster positive outcomes as well as those that may intensify the individual's response to a stressor.

This unit begins with a framework for reviewing the relationships between *stressful* life events, the person's perception of and responses to these stressors, and their means of coping with stressful episodes. Levels of *adaptation* and factors that may mediate the effects of stressors are also discussed. Biologic mechanisms that facilitate adaptation are explored next, including the integrative mechanisms of the autonomic nervous system and endocrine organs; biologic defense mechanisms, including *immunologic responses;* and mechanisms for maintaining *dynamic equilibrium* such as the mechanisms regulating fluid and electrolyte balance. *Adaptive behavior* with an emphasis on cognitive and noncognitive coping mechanisms, and *maladaptive behavior* or inadequate coping are addressed. *Adaptation throughout the life cycle* follows with emphasis on age-specific adaptations required of the individual. The unit concludes with a discussion of *coping with death,* emphasizing the ways in which nurses can be supportive and facilitate adaptation to this event.

12

Stress, coping, and adaptation

JANET LARSON GELEIN
SHIRLEY POTTS BOURBOUS

Stress is a state that is not only ever present in humans, but is also necessary for their survival. Indeed, Selye[31] says that complete freedom from stress exists only in death. Stress becomes intensified by changes or threats with which individuals must cope. The intensity of stress is believed to be a determinant of health outcomes, with development of certain diseases being attributed to intensely stressful episodes.

Individuals are constantly subjected to a variety of agents capable of inducing stress. These agents are commonly referred to as stressors. A *stressor* may be defined as input of matter, energy, or information that, through lack or excess of some characteristic, forces a system's variables beyond the range of stability.[25] Stressors may be physical, biologic, psychologic, or social in nature, or a combination of these, as for example, psychosocial. Examples of physical or biologic stressors include trauma (such as surgery), heat, cold, noise, overcrowding, fluid or electrolyte imbalance, or cancer. Some of these stressors are discussed in detail in later chapters. Psychosocial stressors may include paternal deprivation, divorce, retirement, or death of a friend or family member.

The relationship between psychosocial stressors and the occurrence of disease has been investigated and several methods for documenting and scaling life style have been developed.[17] There appears to be a significant relationship between the magnitude of life changes and the time and onset of disease. It is postulated that psychosocial stressors evoke adaptive responses, and if these responses are faulty in kind or duration, they lower bodily resistance and enhance the probability of disease occurrence.

Although a relationship between exposure to stressors and development of illness has been demonstrated to exist, the exposure to stressors does not always result in a negative outcome. We live in an environment that constantly provides inputs that are capable of inducing stress, yet it is only when stressors force system variables beyond their range of stability that one experiences stress. Exposure to stressors may enhance growth or be detrimental to health. Because individuals with medical-surgical problems are exposed to multiple stressors in the course of their therapy and because their illnesses are often induced or exacerbated by stressful events, it is important for nurses to identify those variables that foster positive outcomes as well as those that may intensify the individual's response to a stressor. The purposes of this chapter are to present a model for viewing the relationships between stressors, the person's perception of such events, coping processes, mediating factors, and adaptation; and to illustrate the utility of this model in caring for the person with a medical-surgical problem.

A model illustrating adaptation to stressors is shown in Fig. 12-1. It can be seen that the relationship between exposure to stressors and subsequent adaptation is not a direct one. *Adaptation* is the end result of adjustments made in response to internal or external environmental changes. It depends on the individual's perception of the stressor(s), the coping processes, and the biologic adaptive responses used to deal with the stressor. Both perception and coping processes are modified by factors internal and external to the individual. The suprasystem may provide resources that support the individual during stressful episodes, or it may make additional demands, possibly increasing stress or instability. These supports or demands are termed *external mediating factors*. Likewise, factors unique to the individual, *internal mediating factors*, may either nurture the system during stressful episodes or force system variables toward increasing instability. Each component of the model will now be explored in detail.

■ PERCEPTION

Humans are vulnerable to stress because they react not only to the actual existence of danger, but also to

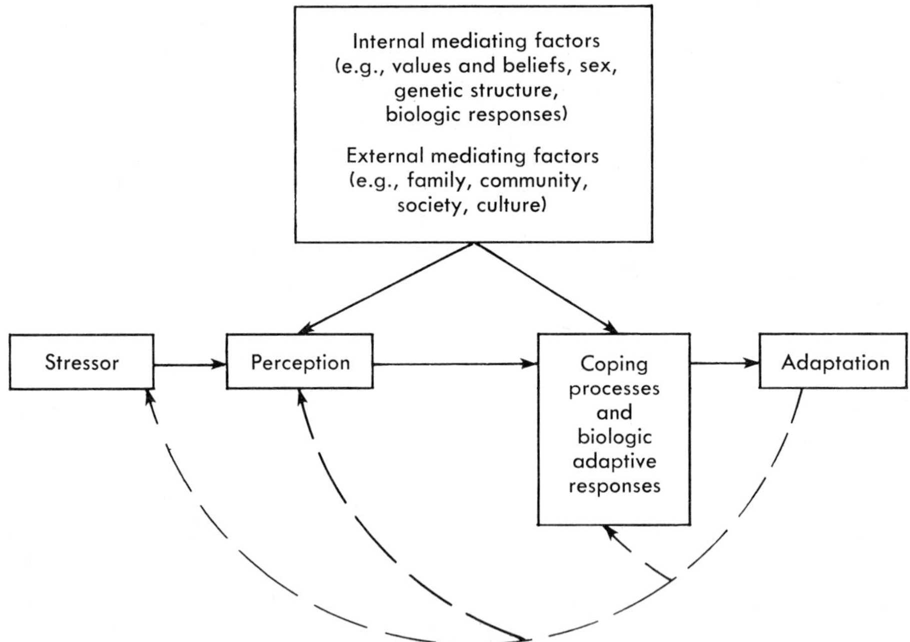

Fig. 12-1. Adaptation to stressors is influenced by perception, coping processes, and biologic adaptive responses. The individual's perception of the stressor and his coping responses are influenced by internal and external mediating factors. The outcome (adaptation) may influence further encounters with stressors, may alter the individual's perception of a stressor, or may influence the coping processes and biologic adaptive responses used in the future.

threats and symbols of danger experienced in their past. Perception, an essential concept in the consideration of stress, involves distinguishing potentially harmful input from input that may be beneficial or irrelevant. It consists of selecting and organizing input, appraising the meaning attached to the input, and then acting upon these meanings. The outcome of perception, purposeful decisions and actions, assumes consciousness of the environment and self along with some memory of previous situations. Piaget[27] viewed perception as a framework into which incoming data could be fit—the integrated knowledge and experience that underlie a person's repertoire of responses. It is a framework that is continually changing, the better to absorb incoming data.

Upon careful examination, one soon realizes that perception may not be an absolute factor in adapting to stress. In some specific cases where an individual is, at that point in time, unable to perceive stressors impinging upon his physiologic functioning, the stressors will continue, and the system will adapt. One need only look at a neurologically impaired individual developing stress ulcers to fully appreciate the body's ability to react regardless of its ability to perceive.

To acquire insight into stress experienced by an individual, nurses seek to understand that person's perception of a stressor. When certain stressors make demands on a person, stress will occur only if the person anticipates that he will not be able to cope, believes that he will not be able to cope with them adequately, or believes he will not be able to cope with them without endangering other goals. Consequently, to adequately assess adaptation to stress, the nurse cannot rely on only an objective analysis of the demands and supports of an individual, but must assess that person's perception of these demands and supports.

There are numerous factors within the mediating process affecting perception that will enhance the nurse's understanding of perception. An individual's attitudes and beliefs are prime factors in perception, since much of the meaning attached to our perceptions is influenced by them.

■ INTERNAL MEDIATING FACTORS

□ Values and beliefs

Values may be defined as conditions of being that a person seeks to actualize. Beliefs are expressed choices.[6] We may have beliefs about values or value beliefs, but values are unspoken, directly intuited, and expressed in the choices the person makes.

When an individual is stressed, the available courses of action are those that the individual believes are true. The individual may be in error, but nevertheless the parameters open are the ones believed relevant. Nurses may use Ackoff's[2] conception of beliefs when assessing an individual system in stress through seeking answers to the following questions:

1. What actions does the individual perceive are available to reduce stress?
2. What are the potential outcomes available from these courses of action?
3. What are the possible states of a choice environment (an ideal situation)?
4. What is the probability of the choice environment being true?
5. How does the individual perceive the efficiency of each course of action for each outcome in each possible state of the choice environment?
6. What is the relative value of specified outcomes?

A close analysis of the answers given to these questions provides insight into what the individual believes about a stressor and the options he believes may alter stress.

□ Sex and role expectations

One example of the way values influence perception relates to the way traditional sex roles are viewed in our society. American society socializes children to become men and women that meet society's ideal norm. As a result, they may be exposed to different types of stressors and learn to cope with stress in varying ways. They also may receive different types of support from the suprasystem when stressed. Sex roles are influential in health and illness.

Female behaviors such as dependency, sexual timidity, self-sacrifice, and maternality are identified as behaviors that devalue women and contribute to a double standard for mental health. Patient "careers" of women coping with stress are quite different than their counterparts: lengthy hospital stays with recurring and frequent commitments characterize the female "career."[13] Sex and role expectations then may not only influence the type of stressors that one is exposed to, but also the process of coping with stress, and the supports offered for deviations from expected role behaviors also seem to be influenced by gender.

Genetic structure

The inheritance of basic biologic material influences the individual's processes and functions. Factors such as physical characteristics, autonomic reactivity, and energy level are believed to be determined by genetic constitution. Consequently, genetic structure may influence the type of input an individual receives and reacts to in his environment, and the amount of maintenance energy available to function as a system. For example, a boy who is "handsome," energetic, and personable will probably have his needs and desires more readily met by the suprasystem than a boy who lacks these characteristics. Children with genetic abnormalities are subject to a variety of inputs that may be quite different in nature and number than infants without these abnormalities. Depending on the resources available to them from the suprasystem and the structure and function of the genetic malformation, individuals with abnormalities achieve various levels of wellness.

□ Education and intelligence

American society places high value on education. Much of the knowledge and many of the skills required for adulthood are provided through socialization in educational systems. Educational resources in the suprasystem may provide the person with a repertoire of problem-solving abilities that could assist the processing of stressful life events. If an individual is aware of options open to decrease the number of stressors in any situation, the outcome may be quite different than that for a person unaware of those options.

Intelligence also exerts an influence on development throughout the life cycle (see Chapter 18). How we view ourselves and others, the degree of mastery and competence achieved, and the opportunities available all bear a relationship to intelligence and intellectual development. Like education, intelligence may promote problem-solving skills for manipulating the environment and learning new behaviors in response to stress.

Closely intertwined with education is social and economic status. Education is one variable that influences occupation, income, and consequently, social and economic status. When confronted by a stressor that may threaten health, an individual must have knowledge about availability of health resources, how to enter the health care delivery system, and the financial resources to pay for the resources. Many health resources that are available to assist individuals under stress are not available to those unable to pay for them.

□ Coping style and ego strength

Coping processes may be regarded as problem-solving efforts of an individual that are used to decide on the actions that are most relevant to his or her welfare. Over time, individuals develop functions that facilitate coping with stress. These functions tend to be stable over time and are referred to as "coping styles." A style of coping is distinguished from coping processes in that the process of coping is related to an outcome. A style of coping is a descriptive term related to the variety of actions or decisions an individual has made in the past that may or may not have promoted a steady state. Ego strength, on the other hand, refers to certain personality traits that are traditionally assumed by an individual when confronting a stressor. It involves the ability to use inherent resources along with environmental supports to reduce threat and facilitate optimal forms of coping.[23]

Biologic resources

Biologic resources constitute a final set of internal mediating factors. These include an intact central nervous system (CNS), a functioning autonomic nervous system, pituitary-adrenal sufficiency, and adequate biologic defense mechanisms (see Chapter 14). While these resources, with the exception of the CNS, do not directly impinge on the individual's ability to problem solve, they do influence the organism's ability to respond to biologic stress that frequently accompanies stressful life events. (These are discussed in detail in Chapters 13 to 15.)

The assessment of individual traits that allow us to estimate and predict stress and the outcomes related to health is difficult. It is necessary, however, if nurses are to help people experiencing stress and advance the practice of nursing with those confronting stressors. Along with ego strength, coping style, and the other internal mediating factors identified above, there is a need to examine the suprasystems of humans and identify factors that may externally mediate the perception of stressors and stress.

EXTERNAL MEDIATING FACTORS

The suprasystem, like selected aspects of the individual, functions to mediate stress. Society, culture, community, family, and the structural setting all influence the type of input an individual receives and the actions and decisions taken to mediate a stressor. Each may support the person when confronting a stressor or place additional demands on the person in stress.

Social support systems

Social support systems may be defined as continuing social groups or aggregates that provide individuals with opportunities for feedback and validation of themselves, which may offset demands within the larger community.[9] Support systems may be structured, as with professional systems of care, or they may be unstructured, as with nonprofessional caregivers. Both imply enduring patterns of continuous or intermittent relationships that promote psychologic and physical integrity of the individual over time. Natural or nonprofessional caregivers include family, co-workers, friends, or neighbors. They also may include such individuals as store clerks, bartenders, hairdressers, or more organized support networks such as Parents Without Partners, Alcoholics Anonymous, or Weight Watchers. They all have a common element of providing for the reassurance of worth.

Caplan describes support systems as functioning in two ways. First, they collect and store information about the suprasystem and offer guidance and direction to the individual that he may fail to comprehend without such help; second, social support resources function as a refuge or sanctuary for the individual to rejuvenate energy during times of stress.[9] One example of support systems as sources of energy relates to those individuals in transitions.

Individuals in transitional states, referred to as "marginal people," are believed to receive input that is either insufficient or too demanding. Such people as those recently divorced, widowed, or retired are at risk of developing physical and emotional illness unless support is provided to facilitate cognitive guidance and mobilize psychologic resources. A variety of organized support systems have been developed to assist individuals in transition with stressors. Some of the more notable include programs like the Harvard Widow-to-Widow Program,[32] the Chicago Looking Glass,[21] the Portland (Oregon) "Natural Neighbors"[16] program, the Palo Alto (California) "Peer Counseling"[20] program, and the Harvard Laboratory of Community Psychiatry project with the Episcopal Church.[10] Often these organized groups provide to the person in transition a combination of cognitive material, support, and an assured place in a temporary community. Support systems developed to nurture people experiencing a transition provide some of the same qualities a family gives to an individual in stress: they seem to buffer the stress that an individual experiences.

More research is needed to prove the relationship between social support and illness. Several studies have indicated that individuals with adequate support systems have a lower incidence of mental and physical illness as compared to those without such support. This lowered incidence of illness with support seems to be even more pronounced under conditions of acute and chronic stress associated with social or physical changes.[12] Apparently such social support from the suprasystem functions somewhat similar to antibodies in the subsystem of humans. Like tissues with specific antibodies for pathologic antigens, individuals with adequate social support from the suprasystem appear to have more resistance against stressors.

COPING

Coping is a process by which an individual deals with stressors in his own unique manner. Through coping, individuals decide on actions that are relevant to their welfare. Coping processes may be described as problem-solving efforts to decide on the actions or decisions that are most relevant to the individual's welfare when the individual is stressed.[15] These processes are influenced by a myriad of decisions and actions previously employed by the organism to deal with stress.

There are two types of coping measures: cognitive and noncognitive.[7] *Cognitive measures* include learning and problem solving, in which the primary focus is dealing with the cause of the stressor with a secondary emphasis on the uncomfortable emotional response the organism experiences. Although an individual may not always be able to cope cognitively, teaching the individual cognitive coping measures is a common method of intervention in nursing.

Noncognitive coping measures are automatic and focus on relief of discomfort rather than the cause of the stressor. Such measures are also known as defense mechanisms or security operations. Aggression, withdrawal, and somatization are examples of noncognitive ways of coping. Several problems are associated with the use of noncognitive responses. First, the response that worked on one occasion may fail to prevent stress in the future when the individual encounters the same or similar sets of stressors. Because no cognitive activity took place, the individual learned nothing about himself and his method of coping. Second, noncognitive coping responses result in behavior that may seriously alter the person's interactions with others who are essential to meeting his needs. The classic "demanding patient" usually drives away the very people he is trying so desperately to contact. Finally, the individual may generalize too freely from one situation to another, automatically employing noncognitive coping measures and thus bypassing any potential self-growth through cognitive learning. (These coping mechanisms are discussed in greater detail in Chapters 16 and 17.)

Coping processes are influenced by perception, individual or internal mediating factors, and elements external to the system. To promote an understanding of the process of coping, an analogy between coping processes and the optic nerve in the eye may help to emphasize the central, key function that coping processes serve to mediate between internal and external system elements.

The eye is a receptor that initiates impulses that are conducted over specialized nerve tissues in the body to stimulate the sensation of vision. A variety of structures and processes internal and external to the eye enable it to make the necessary responses for vision to occur. For the conscious experience of vision one must first perceive an image external to the eye and then transmit and process this image through internal structures. The optic nerve, a key central structure in vision, mediates between impulses that leave the retina and those that enter the visual cortex in the calcarine area of the occipital lobe of the brain. For optimal vision to initiate a behavioral response the eye functions as a whole, integrating structures and processes within the visual and motor centers of the brain. However, for vision to occur there must be stimuli external to the eye: without a visual field to process the eye would not have a function.

If one of the structures of the eye is damaged, the function may be altered and the individual could be threatened with the loss of vision. Visual loss, depending upon the nature of the threatening agent, may be temporarily alleviated or completely corrected through supportive devices. For example, support may be external in the form of eyeglasses or internal with a medication such as pilocarpine with glaucoma. In both forms of therapy, adaptation of the eye and visual acuity are dependent upon the structures within the individual and factors external to the eye.

An individual confronting a stressor is also dependent upon internal and external structures for the mediation of stress. Identification of stressors and mediating factors enables the nurse to reduce or eliminate stressors and to strengthen internal and external supports. By direct intervention to enhance the individual's problem solving or indirect intervention by interaction with the social structural setting (family, community, society, or culture), the nurse may support, maintain, or help restore, as far as possible, the steady state of the individual.

■ BIOLOGIC ADAPTIVE RESPONSES

Although stressors in the social milieu or threats to the person's integrity elicit coping processes such as problem solving, they also induce biologic responses. For purposes of this discussion, biologic responses will be discussed separately from coping. However, it should be noted that the two are inexorably intertwined. There are two systems primarily responsible for the physiologic or biologic response to stress—the endocrine system and the autonomic nervous system. These are discussed in detail in Chapter 13.

A localized tissue assault will produce a *local adaptation* such as the inflammatory response seen as the result of a small incision.[30] Blood vessels in the area of the incision dilate, producing increased blood flow to the area. Vascular cell walls become more permeable, resulting in fluid and white blood cells shifting into the interstitial spaces. Connective tissue proliferates in the area to isolate it and prevent the spread of microorganisms. Chemical substances are secreted to neutralize poisons, kill bacteria, and absorb debris. Granulation tissue then begins to grow because of the interruption of tissue integrity.

Close assessment of a surgical incision allows the nurse to note visible changes indicating that adaptation has occurred. The area becomes warm, red, and edematous. Pain occurs because of trauma to nerves as well as pressure on nerve endings resulting from edema.

Movement may be decreased as a result of pain. Pus then may accumulate, resulting in an abscess.

There would be major problems if the local adaptation syndrome continued at a massive rate and in multiple sites. The extensive vessel dilatation and movement of vascular fluid to the interstitial tissue would produce circulatory collapse. When the individual must cope with such widespread stressors, the *general adaptation syndrome*, as described by Selye, becomes essential.[31] The nonproductive inflammatory process is halted as ACTH and the mineralocorticoids (aldosterone and desoxycorticosterone [DOCA]) cause sodium and water to be retained and potassium to be excreted to reestablish the relationship between blood volume and vascular capacity. Glucocorticoids (cortisone and cortisol) are released to act on the vascular cell membrane to decrease permeability and maintain vascular tone.

In addition to the endocrine system, the autonomic nervous system assists in adaptation. Any unusual, extreme, or threatening situation that calls for immediate resolution of stressors or a reallocation of energies so that adaptation can occur, stimulates the autonomic nervous system. The resultant responses are called nonspecific because of the fact that they occur regardless of the type of stressor—pain, intense emotion, forced exercise, hemorrhage, or surgery. These responses prepare the organism for emergency action, be it fight or flight. Physical sensory modalities (tactile, visual, auditory, and so on) pick up the stressor stimulus, which travels up the nerve pathways to the reticular activating system (RAS), producing arousal. The RAS sends the stimulus up to the cortex, at which level it is identified as a threat to the system. The adrenal gland is stimulated by the sympathetic branch of the autonomic nervous system. Epinephrine is released, resulting in increased cardiovascular output. Blood flow to areas of the body and organs not essential for immediate survival is decreased. Digestion and excretion is decreased. Sodium and water are retained to increase blood volume. Muscle tone and respiratory rate and depth is increased. The pupils dilate and metabolism (such as glycogenolysis) is increased for immediate energy needs. Dissipation of body heat is increased and sweating occurs.

■ ADAPTATION

Realistic coping and unrealistic coping represent two sides of the same coin. The outcomes of this process are influenced by internal and external structures and function along with the processes that interrelate the two. *Adaptation* represents the end result of the coping process. It can be said to refer to the state of the organism at any point in time. The organism has no choice of whether it will adapt. An organism can only control, to some extent, *how* it will adapt. When usual coping responses fail, the organism may achieve adaptation in four different ways: by learning a new behavior, altering the environment, withdrawing from the environment, or altering its desired state.[32a]

Birth is adaptation to a specific set of circumstances that, if allowed to occur, propels the organism into an everchanging world of adaptation. Death is also an adaptation of the organism to a specific set of circumstances, whether a carcinoma or self-induced poisoning. Thus in this discussion adaptation refers to the current state of the organism.

Redman describes *four adaptive levels* nurses can use when assessing the adequacy of the individual's adaptive response. These are based on a level of adaptation that is potentially achievable. The first or lowest level is *economy*. The responses here are aimed at self-preservation and conservation of energy. *Compensation* is the second level. Adaptations occur internally, such as by means of defense mechanisms. The next level is *mobility*, in which adaptive responses are externally focused. The individual manipulates the environment to meet its needs or goals, The last and highest level is *growth*. Here the responses are aimed at self-actualization. Evaluation of an individual's adaptive responses is made with an awareness of the individual's potential. One could argue that using such adjectives as "maladaptive" is inappropriate, since at any point in time an individual has adapted. Death resulting from a surgical assault constitutes adaptation, although it may be viewed as a less than optimal adaptation (Chapter 19).

■ NURSING APPLICATION

The model illustrated in Fig. 12-1 can be used to guide nursing assessments of individuals exposed to stressors and to plan nursing management. The example of a woman experiencing therapy for breast cancer will be used to illustrate the utility of the model.

In this instance the woman is exposed to the *stressor* of a radical mastectomy. Her *perception* of the situation may vary, depending on her value system, beliefs about her self-worth, and the value she assigns to the breast that will be surgically removed. No absolute value can be assigned to the stressor, since the woman's perception is highly individual. For example, if she has had previous experience with surgery, does not believe that her femininity is totally dependent upon her body, and believes that the surgery will cure her condition, then she may be more inclined to perceive the surgery as less threatening than a woman who is convinced that her value as a person depends heavily on her body.

The woman in this example may *cope* by consenting to the surgery. Her ability to cope with the situation may be facilitated by suprasystem variables: sustained emotional support from her spouse, continued teaching of new abilities by nurses, and sharing experiences with women who have had similar surgery.

Postoperatively the woman may demonstrate several indicators of *biologic adaptive responses* to the surgery. Her pulse and blood pressure increase slightly. Because of vasoconstriction, her skin is pale, cool, and clammy. After anesthesia is dissipated, her oxygen consumption increases, producing a concomitant increase in the rate and depth of respirations. Her nailbeds are pale and her mouth is dry. Her skeletal muscles are kept rigid in an attempt to splint her wound. Her body temperature has increased slightly. Peristalsis may be decreased or absent for as long as 12 to 48 hours postoperatively. Gas pains and abdominal distension may be present, as well as the inability to defecate. Inability to void or difficulty in voiding is likely to occur. After the effects of anesthesia disappear and the intellectual processes become operational, the woman may demonstrate *coping processes* integrated with the biologic responses. She may actively seek to alter her environment, keeping out visitors to enhance her physical comfort. She may learn new behaviors that allow her to accommodate the changes in her body: wearing a prosthesis and exercising to compensate for the loss of muscular tissue as a result of the surgery. Finally, she may withdraw from social activities for a period of time in order to become physically stronger or to avoid situations she would consider especially stressful.

The *level of adaptation* exhibited by the woman in the above example would predictably change over time. Initially the adaptive level was one designed to conserve energy. Later, there may be evidence of compensation if she denies the importance of the surgery. Still later there may be mobility and growth as the woman resumes her preoperative activities within prescribed limits, and as her relationship with her spouse becomes characterized by increased communication.

Finally, the outcome of dealing with the stressor of a mastectomy (adaptation) constitutes feedback. Adaptation to this stressor may alter the woman's ability to cope with future stressors by altering internal mediating factors, external mediating factors, and coping processes that are used in the future. A positive outcome may change the way in which she perceives the stressor of hospitalization, may increase the social support available to her, and may improve her health status.

CONCLUSIONS

To assist individuals to deal with life's inevitable stressors, nurses should be familiar with a variety of stressors with which individuals must cope. Several methods of documenting and scaling life events have been developed to investigate the relationship between certain life events and disease. Efforts are currently being made to document the events surrounding hospitalization that are perceived as stressful.[33] These methods can be valuable tools to nurses during their initial assessment of patients. As part of assessment, nurses attempt to ascertain relevant stressors impinging on individuals as well as their perceptions of these stressors. Biologic, psychologic, and social resources require exploration in order to determine the individual's potential for coping.

Cognitive, self-actualizing coping processes are worth striving to attain. Assisting individuals to identify realistically their coping resources will facilitate attaining this objective. Nurses need to recognize and utilize other resources when available, particularly the significant others who are supportive to the person. Perhaps the biggest contribution nurses can make is helping the individuals to augment their coping resources by allowing individuals to try out new responses while providing nonjudgmental support. Finally, nurses may manipulate the environment to foster a positive response. This may vary from adjustment of light and temperature to encouraging a social environment conducive to mutual support among patients.

There is some evidence that nursing intervention to structure the individual's perception of a stressor may decrease the stress attendant with the procedure. Teaching programs have not only decreased tension levels experienced by patients but have also decreased the length of their hospital stays.[22,28] Nursing intervention can be evaluated either subjectively or objectively. Eliciting the individual's perception of the outcome of a stressful episode will provide essential input into the nurse's evaluation. The nurse's own feelings, based on professional experience, should not be discounted. In addition, objective biologic indices can be utilized in evaluating nursing interventions. Foster[18] suggests using the sodium-to-potassium ratio in urine to evaluate the effectiveness of measures to decrease stress. Other autonomic nervous system indices may be incorporated into evaluation. Finally, assessing the effectiveness of nursing intervention in producing changes in the individual's coping behavior is another approach to evaluation.

REFERENCES AND SELECTED READINGS

1. Aakster, C. W.: Psycho-social stress and health disturbances, Soc. Sci. Med. 8:77-90, 1974.
2. Ackoff, R., and Emory, F.: On purposeful systems, New York, 1972, Aldine Publishing Co.
3. Bertalanffy, L.:. General systems theory: a critical review, In Buckley, W.: Modern systems research for the behavioral scientist, Chicago, 1968, Aldine Publishing Co.
4. Bertalanffy, L.: General systems theory: foundations development and applications, New York, 1968, George Braziller, Inc.
5. Buckley, W.: Sociology and modern systems theory, Englewood Cliffs, N. J., 1967, Prentice-Hall, Inc.

6. Bugenthal, J.: Values and existential unity. In Buhler, C.: The course of human life, New York, 1968, Springer Publishing Co., Inc.
7. Burd, S.: A psychological approach to adaptation. In Murphy, J.: Theoretical issues in professional nursing, New York, 1971, Appleton-Century-Crofts.
8. *Caplan, G.: Support systems and community mental health: lectures on concept development, New York, 1974, Behavioral Publications.
9. *Caplan, G.: Support systems and mutual help: multidisciplinary explorations, New York, 1976, Grune & Stratton, Inc.
10. Caplan, R., Caplan, G., et al.: Helping the helpers to help, New York, 1972, The Seabury Press, Inc.
11. Casey, R. L., Masuda, M., and Holmes, T.: Quantitative study of recall of life events, J. Psychosom. Res. **11**:239-247, 1967.
12. *Cassel, J.: Psychiatric epidemiology. In Caplan, G.: American handbook of psychiatry, vol. 2, ed. 2, New York, 1974, Basic Books, Inc., Publishers.
13. Chesler, P.: Women and madness, New York, 1972, Doubleday & Co., Inc.
14. *Coe, W.: Challenges of personal adjustment, San Francisco, 1972, Holt, Rinehart & Winston, Rinehart Press.
15. Coehlo, G., Hamburg, D., and Adams, J.: Coping and adaptation, New York, 1974, Basic Books, Inc., Publishers.
16. Collins, A.: Natural delivery systems: accessible sources of power for mental health. Paper presented at 45th annual meeting of the American Ortho-Psychiatric Association, Detroit, Mich., April 5-8, 1972.
17. *Dohrenwend, B., and Dohrenwend, B.: Stressful life events: their nature and effects, New York, 1974, John Wiley & Sons, Inc.
18. *Foster, S. B.: An adrenal measure for evaluating nursing effectiveness, Nurs. Res. **23**:118-124, 1974.

*References preceded by an asterisk are particularly well suited for student reading.

19. Guyton, A.: Textbook of medical physiology, ed. 5, Philadelphia, 1975, W. B. Saunders Co.
20. *Hamburg, B. A., and Varenhorst, B. B.: Peer counseling in the secondary schools: a community mental health project for youth, Am. J. Orthopsychiatry **42**:566-581, 1972.
21. *Hansell, N.: Explorations of service methods of a volunteer counseling group. Discussions with staff of Looking Glass in Chicago, 1971, Northwestern University Medical School, Department of Psychiatry.
22. *Johnson, J.: Effects of structuring patients' expectations on their reactions to threatening events, Nurs. Res. **21**:499-504, 1972.
23. Lazarus, R.: Psychological stress and the coping process, New York, 1966, McGraw-Hill Book Co.
24. Lipowski, Z. J.: Psychosocial aspects of disease, Ann. Intern. Med. **71**:1197-1206, 1969.
25. Miller, J.: Living systems: basic concepts. In Gray, W., et al.: General systems theory and psychiatry, Boston, 1969, Little, Brown & Co.
26. Murphy, J.: Theoretical issues in professional nursing, New York, 1971, Appleton-Century-Crofts.
27. Piaget, J.: Mechanisms of perception, New York, 1969, Basic Books, Inc., Publishers.
28. *Putt, A.: One experiment in nursing adults with peptic ulcers, Nurs. Res. **19**:484-494, 1970.
29. *Rahe, R. H., Mahan, J. L., Jr., and Arthur, R. J.: Predictions of near-future health change from subjects' preceding life changes, J. Psychosom. Res. **14**:401-406, 1970.
30. *Redman, B.: Why develop a conceptual framework? J. Nurs. Educ. **13**:2-10, 1974.
31. Selye, H.: The stress of life, New York, 1956, McGraw-Hill Book Co.
32. Silverman, P.: The widow-to-widow program: an experiment in preventive intervention, Ment. Hyg. **53**:333-337, 1969.
32a. Vickers, G.: Is adaptability enough? Behav. Sci. **4**:219-234, 1959.
33. *Volicer, B. J.: Patients' perception of stressful events associated with hospitalization, Nurs. Res. **23**:235-238, 1974.
34. Wolf, S., and Goodell, H.: Stress and disease, Springfield, Ill., 1968, Charles C Thomas, Publisher.

13

Integrative mechanisms

VIRGINIA CASSMEYER

To remain healthy and functioning the human cell must have a stable internal environment with an adequate supply of oxygen, nutrients, water, and electrolytes and a constant temperature. The maintenance of a stable internal environment requires the integrated functioning of all body systems. There are many stressors that are constantly changing the internal environment. Survival of humankind is dependent on the integrative mechanisms. The integrative mechanisms constantly monitor the internal environment and activate appropriate body responses to maintain a stable internal environment. The nervous and endocrine systems are responsible for the integrative mechanisms in the body. These two systems can function dependently, independently, and interdependently. These two systems have other complex functions, which will be discussed in chapters in Units V and VI.

This chapter focuses on the parts of the systems involved in the integration of body functions necessary to maintain a stable internal environment. The first section focuses on a description of the components of the integrative mechanisms; the second section describes how the integrative mechanisms maintain energy, water, electrolytes, oxygen, and temperature balance on a minute-to-minute basis; and the third section describes the integrative mechanisms' responses to major stressors.

PHYSIOLOGIC CONCEPTS

The hypothalamus is the master controller of the integrative mechanisms. It is a relatively small area of the brain that receives input directly or indirectly from almost all parts of the brain.[8] The body has multiple receptors, which monitor the blood levels of oxygen and carbon dioxide, the blood levels of sodium and water, the pressure within the vascular bed, the level of glucose, and body temperature. Increases or decreases in any of these are transmitted to the hypothalamus either directly or indirectly. The perception of threat or danger by the cerebral cortex is also transmitted to the hypothalamus. Once stimulated the hypothalmus can activate the endocrine system (through the pituitary gland) and the autonomic nervous system. The somatic neural efferent systems may also be involved. The two mechanisms that play a major role in the body's response to stress are the sympathetic–adrenal medullary mechanism and the pituitary-adrenocortical mechanism.

□ Sympathetic–adrenal medullary mechanism

The sympathetic–adrenal medullary mechanism is stimulated when impulses are conducted from the hypothalamus to the thoracolumbar segment of the autonomic nervous system. Impulses are transmitted from these ganglia to various effectors necessary to maintain vital functions. When stimulated the sympathetic (adrenergic) fibers release the chemical mediator *norepinephrine* and the adrenal medulla secretes *norepinephrine* and *epinephrine*. The effects of sympathetic–adrenal medullary stimulation are summarized in Table 13-1. Overall, complete stimulation of this system suppresses functions nonessential to life and augments functions essential for life.

Epinephrine and norepinephrine differ somewhat in their effects. Norepinephrine is a more potent vasoconstrictor and subsequently increases peripheral resistance to a greater extent, while epinephrine has a greater effect on cardiac activity and on metabolism.

□ Pituitary-adrenocortical mechanism

The second mechanism activated by the hypothalamus is the pituitary-adrenocortical mechanism. The relationship between the hypothalamus, pituitary gland, and other endocrine glands is described in Chapter 30. The hypothalamus releases *corticotropin-releasing* factor (CRF) (p. 538). CRF causes the anterior pituitary gland to release adrenocorticotrophic hormone (ACTH), which in turn causes an outpouring of adrenocorticosteroid hormones.

The release of adrenocorticosteroid hormones has four major effects on the internal environment. First, it

Table 13-1. Effects of sympathetic–adrenal medullary stimulation on body organs

Effect	Organ
Heart	Increased rate and stroke volume
Blood vessels	Dilation of cardiac arteries; vasoconstriction of peripheral arterial and venous systems
Brain	Increased alertness
Skin	Increased sweat production
Gastrointestinal tract	Inhibition of production of GI secretions; decreased motility
Pancreas	Inhibition of enzyme and hormone secretion
Liver	Increased glycogenolysis
Spleen	Contraction
Lungs	Increased rate and depth of respiration; dilation of bronchioles
Eyes	Dilation of pupils and relaxation of ciliary bodies

provides additional nutrients for metabolism. The majority of nutrients are provided by the process of gluconeogenesis. In this process extrahepatic tissue proteins are broken down into amino acids, taken to the liver, and synthesized into glucose. Glucocorticoids also provide nutrients by mobilizing fatty acids and stimulating fatty acid oxidation. Second, glucocorticoids help to maintain fluid and electrolyte balance by conservation of sodium and water. Third, glucocorticoids indirectly help to maintain blood pressure because they are required for the vasoactive effects of norepinephrine. And fourth, glucocorticoids increase the ability of skeletal muscles to maintain contractions and delay the onset of fatigue.

□ Additional hormones

Although the major protection of the body's environment during stress is due to the stimulation of the sympathetic–adrenal medullary mechanism and the pituitary-adrenocortical mechanism, additional hormones are frequently released when the internal environment is changed. These additional hormones are *aldosterone*, *antidiuretic hormone* (ADH), *growth hormone*, and *thyroxine*.

Aldosterone is a hormone produced by the adrenal cortex. Aldosterone secretion may be stimulated by increased ACTH secretion, but most of its production is due to the stimulation of the reninangiotensin system. Stimulation of the sympathetic–adrenal medullary mechanism leads to vasoconstriction of renal arterioles. This vasoconstriction causes the release of *renin* from the *juxtaglomerular apparatus*. Renin acts on the plasma protein *angiotensinogen* to convert it to *angiotensin*. Angiotensin stimulates the adrenal cortex to release aldosterone.

Aldosterone aids in the body's response to stress by the conservation of sodium and water. This increases the amount of fluid available for the transportation of needed products to vital organs.

ADH, growth hormone, and thyroxine secretion are controlled by the hypothalamus (see Chapter 30). The antidiuretic hormone aids in water retention, and thyroxine and growth hormone aid in meeting energy needs during stress.

The relationship between the hypothalamus, sympathetic–adrenal medullary system, and various endocrine glands involved in the body's response to stress is depicted in Fig. 13-1.

■ NUTRIENTS, WATER, OXYGEN, AND TEMPERATURE BALANCE

Even in states of health the body has a very limited ability to withstand inadequate replacement of nutrients, water, and oxygen from the environment or variations in the temperature of the body. In everyday life the integrative mechanisms are frequently called into action to maintain internal balance when deviations occur. The following section describes what happens when nutrients, water, oxygen, and temperature needs for not being adequately met.

□ Food and water

A well-nourished young adult can exist without food for several weeks if necessary. The baby and young child must have daily replacement of nutrients because their needs are great and their reserves minimal. Elderly persons need a constant supply of nutrients because they may have impaired circulation, which makes the distribution of nutrients to cells inefficient. In addition vital organs such as the heart and kidneys may be functioning near maximum capacity and be less able to withstand inadequate cellular nutrition. If adequate food is not available the body burns its own tissues to supply its energy needs. It cannot do this for any length of time without imbalances occurring.

A complete absence of water can be tolerated by an adult for several days. A baby or child can tolerate the absence of water for no more than 1 day because of the proportionately smaller fluid reserve and the need for proportionately more fluids than an adult needs. To maintain essential body functions, the adult uses at least 1,700 ml of water a day, an infant about 300 ml, and a child about 500 ml. Water produced from the burning of tissues (oxidation) and water pulled from the interstitial spaces can be used to maintain the body's needs for a short time. The kidneys too can conserve some water. However, since only 150 ml a day is produced by oxida-

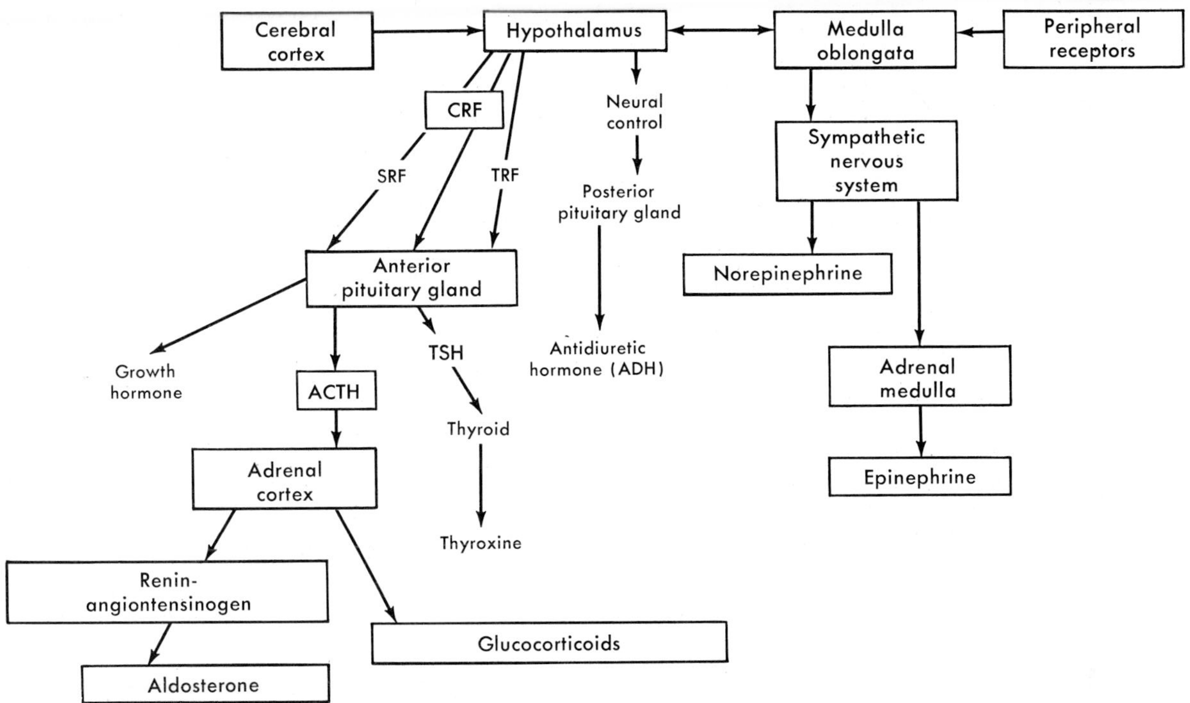

Fig. 13-1. Relationship between hypothalamus, sympathetic–adrenal medullary system, and various endocrine glands involved in body's response to stress. Principal hormonal and nervous components are boxed.

tion (proportionately less in infants and children despite their higher metabolic rate), the available supply is rapidly depleted and the patient can become seriously ill.

Lack of adequate food and water is a stressor. The perception of lack of water and food by the body leads to the stimulation of the hypothalamus and a resultant stimulation of the sympathetic–adrenal medullary mechanism and the pituitary-adrenocortical mechanism. To supply its energy needs the body first burns its glycogen stores, fats are then oxidized, and finally body proteins are mobilized and burned for energy. The burning of body fats produces ketones, and as proteins are burned nitrogen and potassium are liberated. If at the same time a lack of fluid is present, the stimulation of the sympathetic–adrenal medullary mechanism and the pituitary-adrenocortical mechanism leads to the conservation of sodium and water and the end products of metabolism will not be adequately excreted.

The release of norepinephrine, epinephrine, and glucocorticoids provides needed energy and water for a short time; however, symptoms of fluid and electrolyte imbalance will occur. The ketones produced will lead to metabolic acidosis (p. 327), the blood urea nitrogen level will rise (p. 310), and symptoms of hyperkalemia (p. 310) and hypernatremia (p. 308) can result.

Although it is possible to live for short periods without food and fluid, the results can lead to an internal imbalance and can be very serious for the person who is ill. In stress, energy requirements increase, which quickly compounds the problems. Therefore, seeing that food and fluid intake is maintained is of primary importance in the care of any patient.

□ Oxygen

Although the body must always have a supply of oxygen, it normally can make some adjustments to decreased amounts of available oxygen. For example, people who live at high elevations where less oxygen is available to the body gradually develop an increased number of red blood cells. This compensatory mechanism provides for greater oxygen transport in the blood, and although each blood cell may carry less oxygen than normal, the increased number of carriers may provide for adequate oxygenation of tissues.

Since travel has become so rapid and widespread, it is important to teach the public the implications of this adjustment, which normally is slow. Because extreme or unusual exercise or stressful situations always require extra oxygen supplies, care should be taken to avoid these situations for several days after arriving in a place where the altitude is higher than that to which a person is accustomed. In high altitudes the atmospheric pressure is low, and at low atmospheric pressures less oxygen diffuses across the alveoli into the blood, while carbon dioxide diffuses more rapidly than usual from the blood, causing respiratory alkalosis. If precautions are not taken before the body has had an opportunity to compensate by increasing the number of red blood cells, the tissues may not receive enough oxygen. Persons whose work takes them to places where the altitude is high are likely to have serious difficulty if they contract respiratory illness. They also need to avoid strenuous physical activity for several days after arrival.

Because of the dangers accompanying atmospheric pressure changes, most airplanes now have pressurized cabins as well as additional oxygen supplies. It is unwise for anyone who would be susceptible to the development of problems due to a low concentration of oxygen to travel in an airplane without these protections. Elderly persons and those persons who have circulatory or respiratory diseases often tolerate atmospheric pressure changes poorly. They should be advised to consult their physician before planning a trip that entails going to mountainous regions.

A precipitous change from an area of high pressure to one of low pressure can cause rupture of the alveoli because of the expansion of the gases in them. This type of pressure change also causes a decrease in the solubility of the nitrogen in the blood, causing the nitrogen to form bubbles that obstruct blood flow. The latter condition is commonly known as "the bends" (*decompression sickness* or *caisson disease*) and may be a problem for pilots, divers, and others such as "sand hogs" who work underwater for long periods of time. Unless pressurized cabins or tanks are used, descent from airplanes or ascent from diving should be gradual enough to allow time for accommodation to pressure changes. Informing the public about this reaction is very important because many people today engage in flying and diving for recreation.

The preceding discussion shows that if given time the body can make some adjustments to decreased amounts of available oxygen. But in everyday life situations leading to an inadequate supply of oxygen or a buildup of carbon dioxide can occur quickly. In addition in stress situations there is a need for a rapid exchange of oxygen and carbon dioxide. In both of these instances the respiratory center in the medulla oblongata is directly or indirectly stimulated to fire more rapidly. The multiple influences on the respiratory center are described in Chapter 15. Increased firing by the respiratory center leads to increased rate and depth of respiration. Respiration may become gasping, allowing more air to be inspired. The bronchioles in the lungs dilate to enhance the gaseous exchange unless disease prevents dilation. The heart rate increases, allowing for more rapid transportation of oxygen to the vital organs.

Although the body has mechanisms to help assure an adequate supply of oxygen, the person suffering from an oxygen deficit should be protected from any additional stress. The body may be functioning at maximal capacity, and stress will increase oxygen needs further.

If the body is unable to accommodate to an inadequate oxygen supply in the external environment or if, even though oxygen is available, the blood is unable to carry adequate amounts of it because of a low hemoglobin level (anemia), oxygen may be administered. Usually adequate amounts can be provided by face mask, nasal catheter, or cannula. Occasionally oxygen must be administered under positive pressure, and hyperbaric oxygen chambers also may be used.

□ Temperature

For normal body function the body temperature must be maintained around 37 C (98.6 F). Various parts of the body have different temperatures. The extremities are generally cooler than the rest of the body. The magnitude of the temperature difference between body parts varies with the environmental temperature. The rectal temperature is representative of the temperature at the core of the body and varies least with the environmental temperature.

There is a clear circadian rhythm in body temperature. The normal human core temperature undergoes a regular diurnal fluctuation, being lowest during sleep and highest during the waking state. In women the temperature pattern follows the menstrual cycle, with a rather sharp rise in temperature occurring at the time of ovulation (see Chapter 60).

The body produces heat as a result of a variety of basic chemical reactions that include metabolic processes and the ingestion and metabolism of food. The major source of heat, however, is from the contraction of skeletal muscles. Epinephrine and norepinephrine produce a rapid but transient increase in heat production; *thyroxine* causes a slowly developing but prolonged increase in heat production. Body heat is lost by various processes such as radiation, conduction, and vaporization from perspiration, respiration, urination, and defecation.

The maintenance of normal body temperature is dependent on maintaining a balance between heat production and heat loss. The primary integrating area for temperature regulation is located in the hypothalamus. There are two neural pathways to the hypothalamus: the skin receptors and the thermoreceptive properties of the

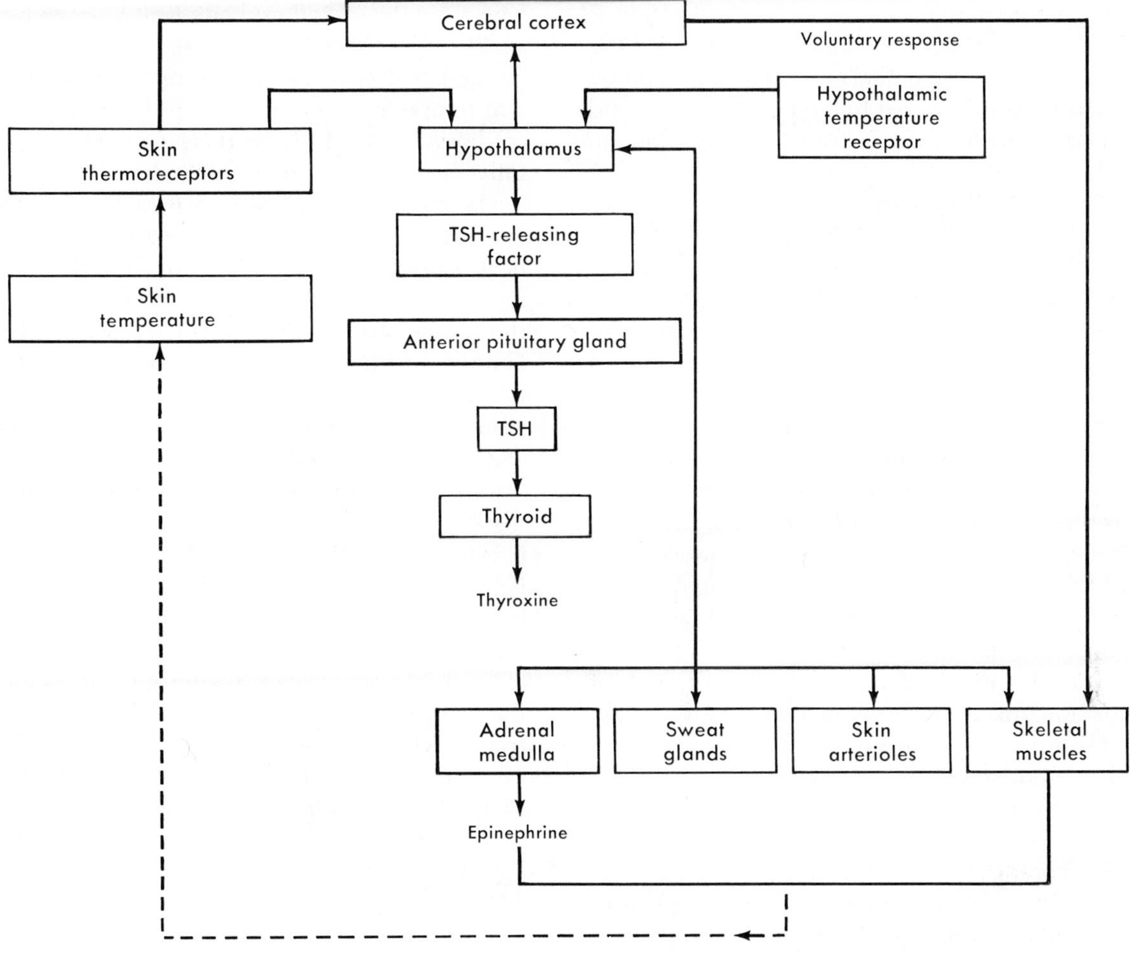

Fig. 13-2. Summary of temperature-regulating mechanisms in body. (Adapted from Vander, A. J. et al.: Human physiology: the mechanisms of body functions, New York, 1975, McGraw-Hill Book Co.)

hypothalamus itself. The stimulation of the hypothalamus results in efferent output from the hypothalamus to bring about appropriate responses. Fig. 13-2 summarizes the temperature-regulating mechanisms in the body. As can be seen from the figure, in addition to the control exerted by the hypothalamus, humans exert voluntary control by increasing skeletal muscle activity when cold and decreasing skeletal muscle activity when hot.

When the environment is hot, body temperature rises. Skin receptors and the hypothalamic thermoreceptors are stimulated by the increased temperature. This information is transmitted to the hypothalamus by afferent fibers. The efferent output from the hypothalamus leads to dilation of blood vessels in the skin so that heat can be released. Sweat is produced, and as the moisture evaporates the air enveloping the skin is cooled so body heat can radiate to the environment. Respirations increase, with a resultant release of heat and moisture. When the body temperature is decreased to normal this information is sensed by the skin receptors and the hypothalamic thermoreceptors. This information is transmitted by afferent fibers to the hypothalamus and measures leading to heat loss are stopped.

When the internal environment is cold, body temperature begins to drop. Skin receptors and the hypothalamic thermoreceptors are stimulated. This information is transmitted to the hypothalamus by afferent fibers. The efferent output from the hypothalamus leads to constrictions of blood vessels so that heat is retained. If too much heat is still being lost, shivering occurs. Shivering increases heat production. In some cases epinephrine, norepinephrine, and thyroxine may be secreted, causing elevation in basal metabolic rate and increasing heat production. When the body temperature is increased to normal this information is sensed by the skin receptors and the hypothalamic thermoreceptors. This information is transmitted to the hypothalamus and measures leading to heat conservation and production are stopped.

The ability to regulate body temperature varies with age. Infants have no difficulty with the production of heat but do have difficulty regulating heat loss. This difficulty is due to their scanty layer of insulating fat, smaller size, and greater surface–to–body weight ratio as compared with adults. The elderly are capable of maintaining constancy of their internal temperature under conditions of favorable environmental temperature, but their response to extreme environmental temperatures is less efficient than in younger adults. The reasons for this are believed to be a slowing of the circulation and structural and functional changes that occur in the skin as the result of aging. Even the normal person may be unable to compensate for extremely high or extremely low environmental temperatures. If compensatory mechanisms are ineffective, heat syncope, heat exhaustion, sunstroke, or freezing may occur (see Chapter 24). Heat syncope results from the extensive peripheral vasodilation combined with orthostatic hypotension to produce cerebral ischemia. Drugs that cause vasodilation, such as those used to lower blood pressure, may predispose an individual to heat syncope. In addition sedative and tranquilizing drugs suppress or interfere with temperature regulation.

Temperature regulation is affected by diseases that cause pathologic changes in blood flow, including congestive heart failure (p. 1031), Raynaud's disease (p. 1003), Buerger's disease (p. 1031), other arteriosclerotic diseases, dysfunction of the autonomic nervous system caused by drugs, surgery, or injury, and diseases of the hypothalamus or medulla.

Fever

Fever is a state of hyperthermia. It may result from faulty regulation of body temperature because of age, circulatory disturbances, or dysfunction of the autonomic nervous system, hypothalamus, or medulla from injury, disease, or drugs. Fever also can occur even though regulatory mechanisms are normal. It is a cardinal sign of many diseases. The cause of fever in these situations is thought to be due to a "resetting" of the hypothalamus thermostat. The patient regulates body temperature in response to heat and cold but at a higher level. The "resetting" of the hypothalamic thermostat is thought to be due to effects on it by endogenous pyrogens released by injured body cells.

Measures may need to be taken with some patients to help the body regulate its temperature. Persons who have a tendency to lose body heat need to be protected against the cold, such as by the use of light, warm clothing and bed coverings. Persons who may have ineffective temperature regulatory mechanisms because of age or disease need to have their body temperatures carefully checked at frequent intervals.

In giving nursing care to patients it is important to avoid measures that counteract the natural defenses for heat control. For example, providing too much warmth for a patient who has a fever yet feels chilly may cause the temperature to rise higher. However, if the patient is not protected enough to prevent shivering, the temperature also will be increased. If shivering occurs as a result of the "resetting" of the hypothalamic thermostat, adding warmth will not stop the shivering. Sudden warming of a person whose body temperature has been markedly lowered may actually cause it to drop farther because unless the environment is very warm, the heat is lost through the dilated vessels. The temperature control mechanism is especially ineffective when there is a wide swing in environmental temperature or when a fever-producing disease is present. The temperature of the external environment needs to be carefully controlled when giving care to any patient with the above problems, and treatment to reduce fever needs to be instituted promptly (see Chapter 21).

■ GENERALIZED RESPONSE TO MAJOR STRESSORS

The body responses essential for life and controlled by the integrative mechanisms will be activated in the presence of any major stressor. Examples of major stressors include trauma, surgery, disease, and anger, frustration, or fear. Inadequate supplies of water, nutrients, and oxygen also serve as major stressors. Any of these situations if perceived as a stressor will lead to the activation of the sympathetic–adrenal medullary mechanism and the pituitary-adrenocorticoid mechanisms. Aldosterone, ADH, growth hormone, and thyroxine may also be released.

The intensity of the response to the stressor is related to the extent and severity of the stressor. The response activated by the integrative mechanisms is a generalized nonspecific response to the stressor. This means that the same response occurs regardless of the initiating event. The body's response in most instances does not eradicate the stressor but only allows the body to contain or resist the stressor until it is alleviated naturally or by outside interventions.

First described in 1936, this defense mechanism was referred to as the stress syndrome or the *general adaptation syndrome (GAS)*.[9] Three stages were identified in the general adaptation syndrome. The first stage is called the *alarm reaction*. During this stage the nervous and hormonal mechanisms are activated and the body's response to this activation is initiated. Stage two is the *stage of resistance*. During this stage the body has reached its full ability to fight or resist the stressor, and the stressor is controlled by the body's response. Stage three is the *stage of exhaustion*. If the stressor continues, the body's ability to fight or contain it is exhausted. The stressor overrides all the efforts of the neural and hormonal mechanisms to contain or resist it. Death may ensue.

In addition to adapting to general systemic stressors, the body is able to adapt to localized stressors. This is called the *local adaptation syndrome (LAS)*. Inflammatory response is an example of the local adaptation syndrome.

□ Signs and symptoms

The signs and symptoms seen in the presence of major stressors are due both to the stressor and to the neural and hormonal activation of body responses. The person appears pale, skin is cool and moist, pupils are dilated, pulse is full and rapid, systolic blood pressure is elevated, and respirations are deep and their rate is increased. The person may be keenly alert and have tense muscles. The person may have abdominal distention, be nauseated, may vomit, and may have diarrhea. These signs and symptoms are mainly due to the activation of the sympathetic–adrenal medullary mechanism.

Other signs and symptoms are due to the activation of the pituitary-adrenocortical mechanism and to the release of the hormones aldosterone, ADH, growth hormone, and thyroxine. One sign is decreased urine output. The urine will be very concentrated. Blood glucose levels, fatty acids, and proteins may be elevated. Muscle wasting will occur in long-term stress situations. Overall, the person is ready for "flight or fight." In times of minor stress or danger the body's response may be minimal or so short-lived as not to produce any symptoms.

□ Interventions

Any hospitalized patient may show signs and symptoms associated with the body's response to stress because of the stress of illness or the fears associated with the illness. Without an understanding of the body's mechanisms for handling stressors, nursing actions may impede rather than complement or supplement the protective mechanisms. It should be remembered that the purpose of the initial response to stressors is to help the person escape the stress-producing situation or mobilize all defenses to resist it. Nursing measures designed to support the protective mechanisms are necessary. Rest is promoted, since activity can impede maintenance of body functions essential to life. The patient is kept comfortably warm but never overly warm, because overheating causes vasodilation, counteracting arteriolar constriction , which assures an adequate blood supply to the vital organs.

Measures to prevent additional physical or emotional stress are necessary, because although the patient may be able to cope with one stress-producing situation, his or her body may not be able to adapt to further stressors. Special care needs to be taken to prevent further trauma, superimposed infection, anxiety, or fear. Extraordinary thoughtfulness is necessary, since the patient is likely to be very alert. Anxiety-producing conversations with the patient or in the vicinity of the patient are to be avoided. Noise, bright lights, and disturbances should be kept to a minimum. Pain should be alleviated.

Even minor stress reactions cause annoying discomforts such as backache, generalized muscle tension, and headache. These discomforts can act as additional stressors, and comfort measures such as back rubs, position changes, and support to relax the muscles are indicated. During severe stress oral food and fluids may need to be withheld until nausea subsides and gastrointestinal tract activity returns to normal.

While caring for a patient who is facing a stressful event or is experiencing a major stressor, the nurse is alert to symptoms and signs of stress. The sudden appearance or the worsening of these signs and symptoms may be the first indication that the patient's condition is deteriorating. Transitory signs and symptoms of stress such as a temporary rise in systolic blood pressure and pulse rate and periodic deep breathing may be a signal that there is an increase in emotional stress or that the patient is overexerting physically.

□ Conditions in which the stress response is detrimental or ineffective

The body's response to stress may be detrimental to some persons or ineffective in others. The response may be detrimental in persons with heart disease, generalized arteriosclerosis, or aneurysms because they may be unable to tolerate the increased stress on the cardiac muscles or blood vessel walls. The person with diabetes mellitus may have difficulty with control of disease because epinephrine and the gluccocorticoids cause an increase in blood sugar.

The frequent occurrence of moderate to severe responses to stress can lead to permanent damage to the body. For example, constant exposure to emotional stress is thought to cause gastric ulcers, coronary heart disease, or hypertension in some people. It also appears to play a part in the responsiveness of some people to allergenic substances.

The body's response to stress may be ineffective in patients with inadequate adrenocorticoid hormones and in patients with disease of the liver. In both situations the necessary energy supplies may not be available and the homeostatic regulation of body fluid and electrolyte balance is inadequate. It is also known that persons do not tolerate stress equally well at all times of the day. The adrenocorticosteroid output is decreased during the night hours and increased in the early mornings. The nurse can be instrumental in scheduling stress-producing situations such as diagnostic tests early in the day when steroid levels are higher.

The original stressor may be so damaging to the body that it is impossible for the defense mechanisms to be effective. Examples of extreme stress situations are arterial bleeding, pressure on the hypothalamus, overwhelming infections, and blockage of a major branch of the coronary artery. In these situations the primary condition must be controlled promptly or death will occur. Persons with diseases in which the response to stress is detrimental or ineffective may need help to plan their lives so as to avoid unnecessary stress.

REFERENCES AND SELECTED READINGS

1. *Axelrod, J.: Neurotransmitters, Sci. Am. **230**:58-71, 1974.
2. Beck, W. S.: Human design: molecular, cellular, and systematic physiology, Chicago, 1971, Harcourt Brace Jovanovich, Inc.
3. Carlson, L. D., and Hsieh, A. C. L.: Control of energy exchange, New York, 1970, Macmillan, Inc.
4. Devney, A. M., and Kingsbury, B. A.: Hyperthermia: fact and fantasy, Am. J. Nurs. **72**:1424-1425, 1972.
5. *Frohman, I. P.: The adrenocorticosteroids, Am. J. Nurs. **64**:120-123, 1964.
6. Goodman, L. S., and Gilman, A.: The pharmacological basis of therapeutics, ed. 5, New York, 1975, Macmillan, Inc.
7. Guillenin, R., and Burgus, R.: The hormones of the hypothalamus. In Organic chemistry of life, San Francisco, 1973, W. H. Freeman and Co. Publishers.
8. Mountcastle, V. B.: Medical physiology, ed. 14, St. Louis, 1979, The C. V. Mosby Co.
9. Selye, H.: The stress of life, New York, 1956, McGraw-Hill Book Co.
10. *Selye, H.: The stress syndrome, Am. J. Nurs. **65**:97-99, 1965.
11. Some psychological effects of medical and surgical advances, Front. Hosp. Psychiatry **3**:1, 1966.
12. Sotaniemi, E.: Environmental temperature and the incidence of myocardial infarction, Am. Heart J. **82**:723-724, 1971.
13. Sotaniemi, E., Palva, I. P., and Hakkarainen, H.: Effect of environmental temperature on hospital admissions for cerebrovascular accidents, Ann. Clin. Res. **4**:233-235, 1972.
14. Tepperman, J.: Metabolic and endocrine physiology, ed. 3, Chicago, 1973, Yearbook Medical Publishers, Inc.
15. Thorn, G. W., et al.: Harrison's principles of internal medicine, ed. 8, New York, 1977, McGraw-Hill Book Co.
16. Vander, A. J., et al.: Human physiology: the mechanisms of body function, ed. 2, New York, 1975, McGraw-Hill Book Co.
17. Williams, S. R.: Nutrition and diet therapy: a learning guide for students, ed. 3, St. Louis, 1977, The C. V. Mosby Co.

*References preceded by an asterisk are particularly well suited for student reading.

14

Biologic defense mechanisms

E. RONALD WRIGHT

CONCEPT OF BIOLOGIC DEFENSE

The human body exists within a milieu of antagonistic environmental forces that are constantly attacking and threatening the integrity of the individual. In response to these onslaughts, the body exhibits a wide array of adaptations (structures, mechanisms, and responses) designed to provide a defense against these encroachments. These mechanisms serve to protect the body from both external and internal deleterious agents. This chapter deals with those anatomic and biologic mechanisms that provide protection against environmental factors that physically threaten the client's body. The implications and applications of the functions of these systems are also discussed.

Knowledge of the basic structures and mechanisms that provide this protection helps in the understanding of (1) resistance to infectious disease, (2) diagnosis of disease and physiologic state, (3) rejection of tissue transplants, (4) prevention of the development of malignancies, (5) adaptations in the aging process, (6) immunization against infectious disease, (7) expression of diseases of autoimmunity or immundeficiency, (8) development of allergic reaction, and (9) significance of the localized or systemic inflammatory response. Much of preventive and restorative nursing practice is built on the maintenance or restoration of the cells, systems, and mechanisms that provide defenses against harmful factors in the external environment.

Self versus nonself

Each human being can be regarded as a genetically and immunologically unique collection of cells and molecules that comprise a biologic unit of *self*. It is the function of the biologic defense mechanisms of the body to protect the integrity of self from encroachment by *nonself* (or foreign) materials. These mechanisms (Fig. 14-1) serve to protect self from both external and internal destructive agents by:

1. *Exclusion* of harmful agents from the body
2. *Recognition* of harmful agents within the body
3. *Response* designed to rid the body of the harmful agents that do gain access

The sources of these harmful nonself materials are generally external. These external agents include nonliving materials of the environment such as potentially harmful inorganic chemicals and compounds produced by other living organisms. The most serious external threats to biologic integrity, however, come from the living organisms that constantly surround the body. Some of these organisms pose no real threat because the mechanical, biochemical, and metabolic processes of the human body will not support them or offer them shelter. There are a myriad of living forms, on the other hand, for which the human body is an ideal haven for growth and survival. Most of these organisms if allowed to penetrate the body would wreak havoc on the normal functionings of the body. The living forms that come to mind in this regard are the organisms classified as pathogenic (disease causing). While it is true that the progress of these organisms in the body can be altered by external agents such as antibiotics, the eradication of the offending organism from the body must be accomplished by the host's own adaptive mechanisms.

In addition to protection against external agents, the defense mechanisms also protect against the accumulation of damaged or dysfunctional self-material. If it were not for these processes that carry out the systematic, specific removal of damaged or worn out cellular material, the body would become clogged with debris. Still another general function of these systems is that of recognition of the alteration of self to a potentially dangerous state. When this defense function falters, the tragedy of malignancy (cancer) results.

Scope of defense mechanisms

The array of defense mechanisms that have been adapted to protect the normal human body is formidable and complex. For the sake of orderly presentation they

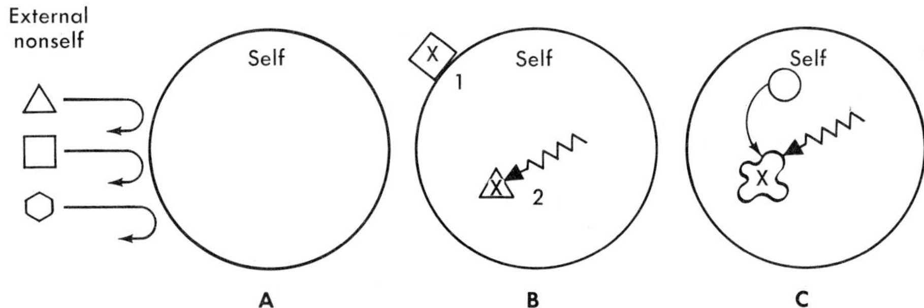

Fig. 14.1. Mechanisms of biologic defense in human body. **A,** Exclusion of external nonself. **B,** Destruction of external nonself by *(1)* nonspecific external mechanisms and *(2)* nonspecific or specific internal mechanisms. **C,** Destruction of altered self. *X* indicates nonspecific mechanisms; ⟿ indicates specific mechanisms.

Table 14-1. Biologic defense mechanisms

Nonspecific mechanisms	Specific mechanisms
External	
A. Mechanical exclusion	A. Immunoglobulin A
1. Physical structures	1. In mucosal secretions
a. Skin	2. In mucosal cells
b. Mucous membranes	
c. Specialized structures	
2. Physical actions	
B. Biochemical factors	
1. Body secretions	
2. pH	
3. Lysozyme	
C. Microbial antagonism	
Internal	
D. Reticuloendothelial system	B. Antigen-processing by macrophage
E. Blood	C. Primary immune response
1. Cellular components	1. Humoral immune response
2. Fluid components	a. Synthesis of circulating antibodies by B cells
a. Opsonins	b. Interaction of antibodies with antigen
b. Complement	2. Cell-mediated immune response
c. Properdin	a. Sensitization of T cells
d. C-reactive protein	b. Lymphokines
3. Phagocytosis	3. Combined immune response
F. Inflammatory response sponse	D. Secondary immune response
G. Interferon	

may be divided mechanistically into *nonspecific* and *specific* mechanisms (Table 14-1). The specific and nonspecific mechanisms can be further divided on the basis of where the lines of defense are formed, that is, *external* for the mechanisms of mechanical exclusion, biochemical destruction, and microbial competition and *internal* for the physiologic reactions. The nonspecific mechanisms are nonselectively directed against *any* foreign substance. The specific mechanisms are specifically elicited by *unique* substances to which the body has *acquired* the ability to respond.

□ Concept of immunity

The objective of the biologic defense mechanisms is to provide the host with protection. The ultimate protection would be total resistance to encroachment or damage by an organism or agent; this is usually termed *absolute immunity.* Absence of such protective barriers is called *susceptibility.* Although these terms are generally applied to immunity from infectious organisms, they can be used to describe the relative susceptibility to encroachment by any external agent. *Nonspecific immunity* (or *innate immunity*) is provided when the external and internal nonspecific defense mechanisms serve as the barrier excluding or destroying the invading agent. *Specific immunity* protects against a single unique agent through the development of specific antibodies or responsive cells in the body. It is *acquired* from prior contact with that agent (antigen) or through the introduction of specifically protective antibodies or cells into the body.

The acquisition of specific immunity may result from *natural* encounter or by *artificial* introduction. Immunity acquired naturally means under natural conditions such as recovery from a disease. Immunity acquired artificially means that the antigen or protective antibodies were purposely introduced into the body (for example, by vaccination). The immunity may be an *active* or *passive* immunity. When an individual is producing the an-

Table 14-2. Types of acquired specific immunity

Type of immunity	Acquisition of immunity	Protection	Examples
Active: antibodies synthesized by body in response to antigenic stimulation	*Natural:* natural contact with antigen through clinical or subclinical case	*Development:* develops slowly; protective levels reached in a few weeks *Duration:* longterm; often lifetime *Spectrum:* specific to antigen contacted	Recovery from childhood diseases (e.g., chickenpox, measles, mumps)
	Artificial: immunization with antigen	*Development:* develops slowly; protective levels reached in a few weeks *Duration:* several years; extended protection with "booster" doses *Spectrum:* specific to antigen immunized against	Immunization with live or killed vaccines; toxoid immunization
Passive: antibodies produced in one individual are transferred to another	*Natural:* transplacental and colostrum transfer from mother to child	*Development:* immediate *Duration:* temporary; several months *Spectrum:* to all antigens that mother has immunity	Maternal immunoglobulins in neonate
	Artificial: injection of serum from immune human or animal	*Development:* immediate *Duration:* temporary; several weeks *Spectrum:* to all antigens that source has immunity	Injection of pooled human gammaglobulin; injection of animal hyperimmune sera

tibodies within his or her own body, the immunity is termed active. When an individual receives the protective antibodies from some other source, the immunity is termed passive. Thus when antibodies are transferred from the mother across the placenta, the child is said to have a natural passive immunity; or when a vaccine is given, so that antibodies are produced within the body, the immunized individual is characterized as having an artificial active immunity. Table 14-2 summarizes the different types of specific acquired immunities.

Specific or nonspecific immunity to harmful agents is a relative state. The effect of different dosages of an infectious organism or the toxic products of such organisms in experimental studies clearly demonstrate that administration of sufficiently large numbers of an organism or high dosages of a toxin can overwhelm even the most highly immunized animal. Further, when the normal mechanisms of defense are breached, even in the highly resistant host, disease can result. Thus acquired immunity to infection is not always an absolute condition but depends on a large number of complex variables. These include not only the defense mechanisms of the host but also the dose, route of contact, and virulence of the harmful agent.

■ EXTERNAL NONSPECIFIC DEFENSE MECHANISMS

□ Anatomic structures and mechanical actions

Skin and mucous membranes

The first line of defense against penetration by foreign materials, including pathogenic microorganisms, is the skin. When the skin is intact it serves as an extremely efficient physical barrier to harmful agents and environmental forces such as heat, cold, and trauma. This protection is afforded by the keratinized surface cells, which provide a tough, dense, waterproof covering. Beneath this outermost layer is a dense layer of highly vascularized connective tissue (see Fig. 65-1).

Even though some of the fatty acids derived from sebaceous gland secretions have antimicrobial activity, the environment provided by the skin does allow the growth of microorganisms on its upper layers and within hair follicles and sweat glands. For the most part these resident microorganisms are nonpathogenic; however, when these organisms gain entrance to the tissues of a host exhibiting reduced resistance, they may cause significant problems. Because even thorough scrubbing with soap and water removes only the surface organisms, the skin can never be considered sterile.

Any time the physical integrity of the skin is broken, such as in surgery, indwelling venous catheterization, or physical irritation or trauma, there is significant risk of microorganisms gaining entrance to the body. The skin must be kept relatively dry, since the continued presence of moisture tends to cause maceration of the skin. Further, when essential oils are lost from the skin surface they should be supplemented by lotions to maintain the resilience and unbroken texture of the surface cells. Adequate care of the skin of the hospitalized patient is not just a luxury but a necessity for the provision of an extremely important aspect of biologic defense.

Mucous membranes protect the eye and line all body tracts that have external openings. When intact the mucous membranes, like the skin, are basically impervious to foreign materials and microorganisms. The surfaces are covered by a viscous secretion that tends to trap and inactivate microorganisms. The mucous membrane of the respiratory tract is further protected by the surface activity of the ciliated epithelial cells, which sweep foreign material out of the tract. The mucous membranes are highly vascularized so that the internal defense mechanisms are readily available to attack any microorganisms that do gain access to the surface of these cells.

Also found in the mucosal secretions and in high concentration within the secretory mucosal cells of the respiratory and intestinal tracts are a specific class of immunoglobulins (antibodies) known as immunoglobulin A (IgA). These specific antibodies are secreted from the mucosal cells and have antibacterial, antiviral, and antitoxic properties. These antibodies serve to prevent microbial adherence and colonization of these tracts by pathogens.

Specialized structures and mechanical functions

Other structures and functions of the human body that are generally taken for granted actually serve extremely important roles in defense. The filtration action of the nasal hairs serves to trap particles and microorganisms. The flushing action of saliva and urine prevents the buildup of organisms. The eyes are protected from the entrance of dirt particles and organisms by the lids and lashes. Foreign material that does gain entrance to the eye tends to be washed out by tears. The constant movement of foods through the stomach and intestines prevents the buildup of organisms or toxic waste products. Even the action of vomiting and the watery stools of diarrhea are active mechanisms of removal of harmful products from the gastrointestinal tract. Dysfunction or blockage of any of these processes means that special measures must be taken to protect against the establishment of pathogenic organisms and the buildup of toxic materials.

□ Biochemical factors

Many areas of the body are protected not only by mechanical barriers but also by the presence of specific antimicrobial chemicals that provide added protection.

Skin

The acetic acid and salt concentration of perspiration is toxic to many pathogenic microorganisms. Some of the fatty acids released to the skin surface by the sebaceous glands also serve to inhibit the growth of some microorganisms.

Gastrointestinal tract

In the stomach the acidity (approximate pH 2) of the gastric juice kills many organisms and detoxifies certain potentially toxic substances. For this reason, when gastric acidity is low special precautions must be taken to avoid introduction of organisms through the nose and mouth. Low gastric acidity is characteristically encountered in neonates; therefore special care should be taken in feeding and handling babies to prevent exposure to pathogens by the oral route. The upper intestine is generally freed of organisms by the action of bile and other proteolytic enzymes.

Vagina

Vaginal secretions allow certain harmless acid-producing bacteria to colonize the vagina and create an acidic environment. This reduces the chance of the colonization of the vagina by pathogens. When either the amount or acidity of the vaginal secretions is reduced, there is a much greater chance that a vaginal infection will develop. Since vaginal secretions are not present prior to puberty and are greatly reduced after menopause, both young girls and older women are more prone to vaginitis. The use of birth control pills causes a shift in the composition and pH of the vaginal secretions, which increases the possibility of colonization of the vagina, especially by the causative agent of gonorrhea, *Neisseria gonorrhoeae.*

Lysozmye

The most ubiquitous antimicrobial factor in the body is the enzyme lysozyme. It is capable of lysing (splitting) the bacterial cell wall of many gram-positive organisms, causing their destruction. The enzyme is present in mucus, tears, saliva, and skin secretions and is also found

Table 14-3. Distribution of normal microbic flora

Region of body	Sterile areas	Nonsterile areas	Microorganisms
Skin	None	All skin	*Staphylococcus, Bacillus, Corynebacterium, Mycobacterium, Streptococcus,* transient environmental organisms
Respiratory tract	Larynx, trachea, bronchi, bronchioles, alveoli, sinuses	Nose, throat, mouth	*Staphylococcus, Candida, Streptococcus, Neisseria, Pneumococcus,* oral organisms
Gastrointestinal tract	Esophagus, stomach, upper small intestine	Esophagus and stomach (transiently), large intestine	Gram-negative rods, *Streptococcus, Bacteroides, Proteus, Clostridium, Lactobacillus*
Genitourinary tract	Cervix, uterus, fallopian tubes, ovaries, prostate gland, epididymis, testes, bladder, kidney	External genitalia, anterior urethra, vagina	Skin organisms, *Lactobacillus, Bacteroides*
Body fluids and cavities	Blood, pleural fluid, synovial fluid, spinal fluid lymph, etc.	None	

in many of the internal fluids and cells of the body. Within the body it tends to work in combination with complement and other blood factors to destroy bacteria directly.

❑ Microbial antagonism

The skin and mucosal surfaces offer varying nutritional and environmental conditions for the growth and multiplication of certain microbial cells. Although the surfaces of the body are constantly exposed to temporary contamination by organisms from the environment, most of these organisms, known as *transient flora,* do not find conditions suitable for the colonization of the body; however, there are many microorganisms that do colonize the skin and mucosal surfaces. These organisms comprise what is known as the *normal microbic flora.* Although this normal flora varies from site to site within the body and may vary in response to environmental, hygienic, and physiologic changes, it is capable of reestablishment and reflects a fairly predictable pattern. Table 14-3 provides an overview of the body areas normally colonized and shows which organisms most often make up the normal flora of the various areas.

The maintenance of this balanced microbic flora serves to make it difficult for pathogenic organisms to establish themselves on the body surfaces. Since the normal flora have a selective advantage in their environmental niche, they compete for nutrients and space. Some release antimicrobial substances to retard the growth of transient organisms seeking to occupy the same site. These microbial interferences are known as *microbial antagonism.*

Most of the normal microbic flora are basically nonpathogenic; however, some overtly pathogenic organisms such as *Staphylococcus aureus* and *Streptococcus pyogenes* can be part of the normal flora. The individual who harbors such organisms without demonstrating any symptoms of disease is known as a *carrier.* This carrier state is of significance because the carrier may be unknowingly shedding organisms into the environment and infecting others.

The protective effects of the normal microbic flora become most apparent when something upsets the microbic balance within the body. The use of broad-spectrum antibiotics sometimes creates such an effect. The imbalance may allow a segment of the normal flora to gain ascendency, causing adverse reactions. An example of this phenomenon is seen when certain oral antibiotics induce marked shifts in the normal intestinal flora, allowing organisms that are generally suppressed by the growth of competitors to thrive to an unusual degree. This imbalance may induce uncomfortable gastrointestinal tract problems or even allow gastroenteritis to develop.

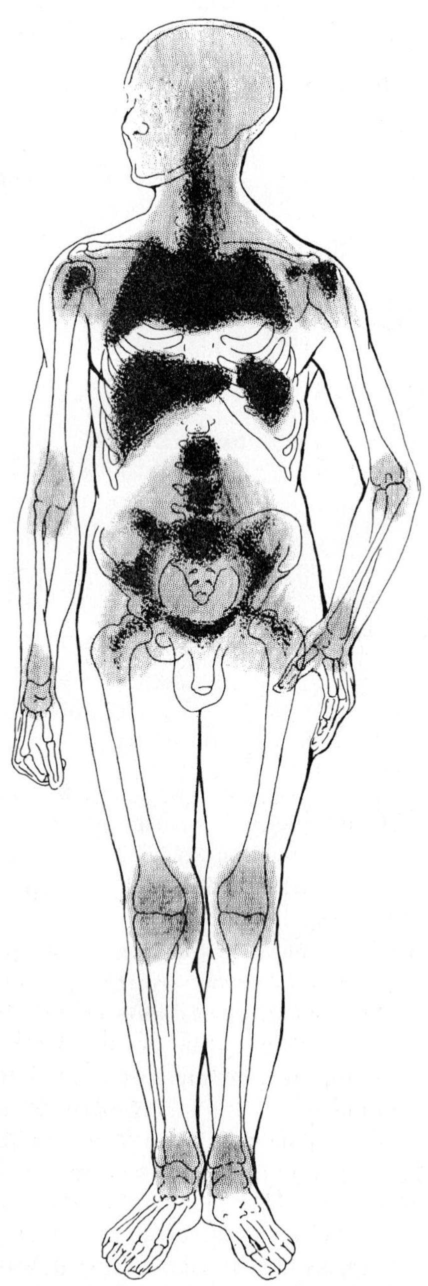

Fig. 14-2. Reticuloendothelial system. Note anatomic distribution of maximal activity in system, as indicated by black areas over body. To produce such an image certain radioactive colloidal particles are given to subject, and radiation detection techniques delineate tissue uptake. Note definition of liver, spleen, and active bone marrow in axial skeleton and proximal parts of long bones. (From Smith, A. L.: Microbiology and pathology, ed. 11, St. Louis, 1976, The C. V. Mosby Co.)

Table 14-4. Distribution and names of macrophages in various tissue sites

Tissue	Name
Peripheral blood	Monocyte
Loose connective tissue	Histiocyte
Liver	Kupffer cells
Spleen and reticuloendothelial system	Wandering or fixed macrophage
Lung	Alveolar macrophage or dust cell
Granulomatous tissue	Epithelioid and giant cells
Peritoneal cavity, pleural cavity, and bone	Macrophages

■ INTERNAL NONSPECIFIC DEFENSE MECHANISMS

Once a foreign agent (living or nonliving) penetrates the external resistance barriers, it is met by an even more complex array of defense mechanisms, which provides for the recognition, capture, and disposal of the foreign material. The key to this process is the specific recognition and vigorous action taken against the foreign material while at the same time protecting the host tissues from extensive damage. The physiologic reactions that serve to contain and inactivate the foreign agent are carried out through interactions of cells and molecules of the blood, reticuloendothelial system, vascular system, and body tissues.

□ Reticuloendothelial system

The reticuloendothelial system (RES) is a widespread system of phagocytic cells (devouring cells) scattered throughout various body tissues (Fig. 14-2). The role of these cells is to ingest and digest foreign particulate matter and damaged host tissues. Some of the phagocytic cells are *fixed* in a variety of tissues, such as lymphoid tissue, liver, spleen, bone marrow, lungs, and blood vessels. Within the different tissues these anchored cells have been given unique names (Table 14-4). It is the function of the fixed cells to capture and destroy foreign materials found in the fluids of their environment.

Other cells comprising the reticuloendothelial network are not stationary and are given the name *wandering macrophages*. Depending on where they are found, they may be known as monocytes (in the bloodstream) or histiocytes (in loose connective tissues). The wandering macrophages carry out the important role of final cleanup of à damaged site in preparation for repair. The cells have the capacity to engulf and destroy virtually any type of foreign material or debris within the body. The macrophages also play an important role in the specific response mechanisms.

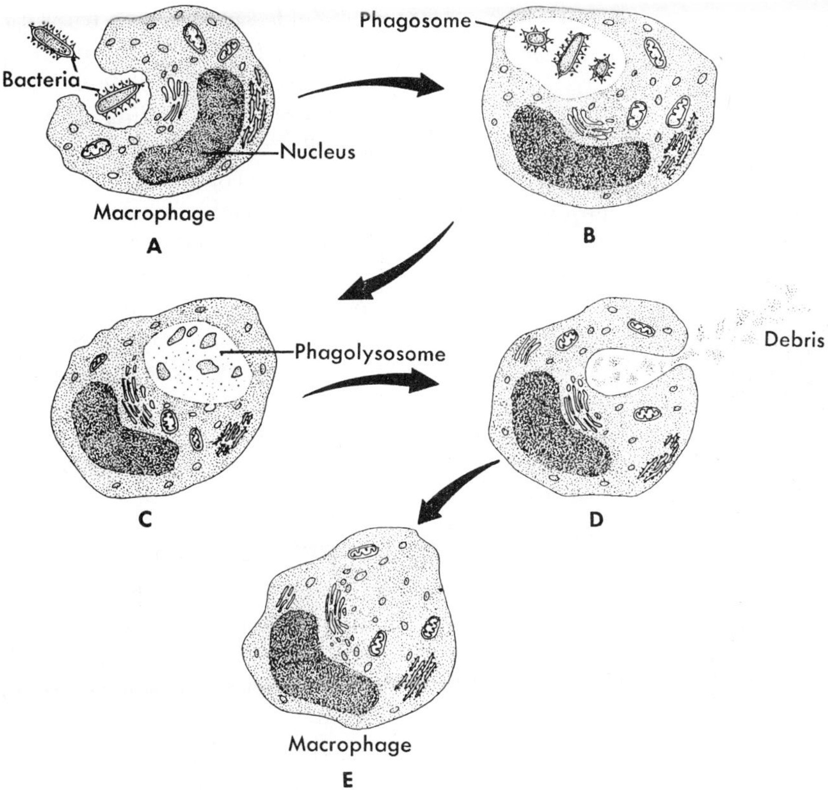

Fig. 14-3. Phagocytosis sketched in macrophage. **A,** Opsonized bacteria engulfed by phagocyte (macrophage). **B,** Phagosome formed. **C,** Phagosome becomes phagolysosome; bacteria digested. (To this point process of phagocytosis is comparable in either macrophage or neutrophil, not shown.) **D,** Debris is egested. (Neutrophil would succumb here.) **E,** Macrophage returns to resting state. (From Smith, A. L.: Microbiology and pathology, ed. 11, St. Louis, 1976, The C. V. Mosby Co.)

□ Blood

Blood is one of the primary sources of elements designed to provide protection against injurious agents. The blood transports these active factors to the site of an injury or intrusion and through specific vascular changes concentrates these materials at the site. Both the fluid and cellular constituents of blood contain these factors.

Cellular components

The cellular components of blood that are of importance in this nonspecific response include granulocytes, lymphocytes, monocytes, and thrombocytes (platelets). The granulocytes, also referred to as polymorphonuclear leukocytes (PMNs), and the monocytes are of the most importance because of their phagocytic activity.

One of the key methods of nonspecific defense is the ingestion of microorganisms and other particulate matter by the phagocytic white blood cells. The phagocytes carry out the process of *phagocytosis* in several discrete steps (Fig. 14-3). Most infecting microbes are quickly and efficiently destroyed by phagocytosis; however, some pathogens exhibit methods of escape from this destruction. Some bacteria such as strains of the streptococci and staphylococci and *Bacillus anthracis* (anthrax) actually produce factors that will kill the phagocyte. Other organisms resist ingestion or digestion. Some organisms may survive within the phagocytes or reticuloendothelial cells and multiply there. This may lead to the transport of the organism to other sites in the body or serve as a chronic focus of continued infection.

The granulocytes can be divided on the basis of their structure and function into neutrophils, eosinophils, and basophils. The "granules" found within these cells represent discrete packets of degradative enzymes used to digest the ingested materials. The neutrophils are the most numerous in circulation and are the most efficient and responsive phagocytic cells involved in the inflammatory process. Where there is adequate blood supply to a region, the phagocytes are constantly available to move from the blood vessels to the site of injury or infection. The neutrophils and monocytes are actually attracted to the scene by chemicals released during infection or injury. This cellular response to chemical attractants is known as *chemotaxis*, and the substances released are called *chemotactic substances*.

Fluid factors

The fluid portion of uncoagulated blood is called *plasma*. Some of the components of plasma provide important constituents for the internal defense mechanisms. Plasma transports the *circulating antibodies* produced in specific response to antigenic stimulation. These antibodies when bound to their specific antigens enhance the ability of white blood cells to engulf the clumped and sticky antigens. The antibodies of the blood that create this coating effect are known as *opsonins*. Another plasma constituent, *fibrin*, may create a meshwork around the injured area causing the sealing off of the area. Microorganisms may also become trapped within this meshwork where they are more easily captured by the phagocytic cells.

One of the most important constituents of plasma is a complex series of 11 proteins known by the singular name of *complement*. The primary role of complement is to provide specific lysis (rupturing) of cell membranes. The initiation of the "complement cascade" is most often triggered by the binding of the first complement protein to complement-binding antibodies that have already bound to their antigens. Thus complement serves to accentuate or complete the action of an antibody. The antibody by itself cannot produce cell lysis, but with the recruitment of complement to join in the reaction the cell may be ruptured. However, other substances of a nonimmune nature can also activate complement. Complement is considered a nonspecific component of the plasma because it is not increased by immunization. In addition to its cytolytic effects, complement is involved in leukocyte chemotaxis, release of histamines, enhancement of phagocytosis by PMNs, viral neutralization, and bactericidal activity.

The classical activities ascribed to complement depend on the sequential interaction of nine protein subunits (C1 to C9), the first component of which consists of three subfractions termed C1q, C1r, and C1s (thereby accounting for the 11 separate proteins mentioned above). When the first component, C1 is bound by an

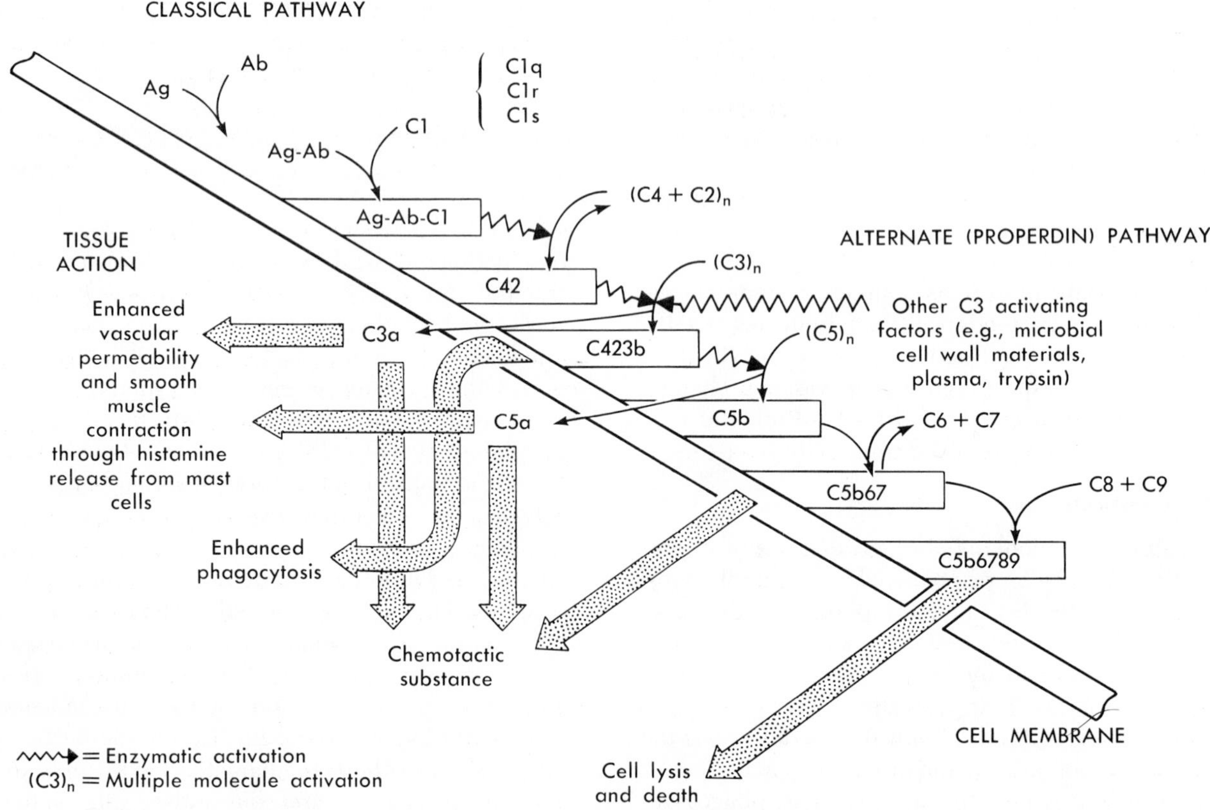

Fig. 14-4. Classical and alternate complement cascade. Sequence of complement activation generates multiple biologically active intermediate molecules, which are active in inflammatory response.

antigen-antibody complex on the surface of a cell, it acquires the enzymatic ability to activate several molecules of the next components in the sequence, C4 and C2, to form an active C42 complex (Fig. 14-4). (Unfortunately the numbering system of the complement components reflects their order of discovery and not their sequential additive pattern.) Each of the activated C42 complexes is then able to act on the next component, and so on, producing both a cascade effect and greatly amplifying the reaction. As each component is added there is created new enzymatic activity to initiate the next step. The final component, C89, has the ability to create a lesion in the cell membrane, and if enough lesions are created on the membrane, cell death results.

The intermediate stages in the complement sequence also give rise to complexes and fragments with other significant biologic activities. Fig. 14-4 depicts the generation of some of these activities. These include:

1. *Histamine release.* Histamines cause an extreme increase in vascular permeability and contraction of smooth muscle. A fragment (C3a) split off during the activation of C3 and another fragment (C5a) created by the activation of C5 are released into the surrounding tissues where they cause the release of histamine from mast cells. The histamines in turn exert their physiologic effects on the smooth-muscle tissues and vascular system. Because these histamine-mediated reactions are the same as those created during anaphylactic shock (p. 196), these fragments are called *anaphylatoxins.*
2. *Enhanced phagocytosis.* One of the intermediate activators in the cascade, C423b, makes the labeled antigen tend to stick to the surface of cells so that it is more easily phagocytosed.
3. *Chemotactic substance formation.* Several of the fragments and intermediate factors serve as chemotactic substances to attract phagocytes to the site of the reaction.

All of these activities are central to the inflammatory response.

The plasma fraction contains several proteins that inhibit the action of the activated components of complement in the fluid phase, that is, off of the membrane surface. Such inhibitors serve to localize the effects of the membrane surface and thereby to protect the "innocent bystander" membranes.

In addition to the activated C42 complement complex, a number of other enzymes exhibit *C3 convertase* activity. These include trypsin, plasmin, and thrombin as well as bacterial endotoxins and a factor derived from cobra venom. Each leads to alterations of C3, which are similar to if not identical with those produced by the complement cascade–derived C3 convertase. These activations are mediated through a plasma component known as *properdin* and are referred to as the *alternative* or *properdin pathway.*

C-reactive protein is a beta globulin found in the serum of individuals suffering from any type of severe inflammatory process. Both infectious and noninfectious inflammations will elicit the formation of this protein in the plasma. The protein will form a precipitate with a constituent of the cell wall of *Streptococcus pneumoniae* known as the C polysaccharide; hence its name. The amount of C-reactive protein found in the serum is roughly proportional to the severity of the inflammation; therefore a test for this protein is useful in diagnosis and management of hard to differentiate diseases that have a hidden inflammatory aspect such as bacterial endocarditis, cryptic abscesses, rheumatic fever, and certain types of cancer.

□ Interferon

Interferon is a low-molecular-weight protein produced by certain virally infected cells. The protein is released into the extracellular environment, and when taken up by uninfected cells it can protect those cells from viral multiplication. This antiviral action is exerted before the antibody levels can reach protective levels. The interferons are synthesized by the cells of many different animal species, but they are species specific; that is, bovine interferon will not protect human cells. In general the product of a viral infection is the same regardless of the viral agent that initiated its formation. Therefore interferons can be described as being host specific but viral nonspecific.

Interferons are produced by cells infected with infectious viral particles, infectious inactivated viruses, or even laboratory-synthesized double-stranded polynucleotides. Virtually all tissue cells are capable of producing interferons when properly stimulated. The stimulation seems to be tied to the recognition of the "foreign" nucleic acid, which signals the infected cells to synthesize and liberate interferon for a few hours (up to about 24 hours). The interferon acts on the uninfected cells, causing them to synthesize another protein that remains within the protected cell. This protein inhibits the synthesis of the viral particle without blocking normal cell synthetic functions (Fig. 14-5). The interferon itself has no direct effect on the viral particles, nor does it interfere with the entry of the viral particle into the interferon-protected cell. This interferon-mediated protection lasts for only about 24 hours.

While viruses seem to be the most potent inducers of interferon production, other microorganisms also stimulate its synthesis. Included in this group are the causative agents of malaria, rickettsial diseases, brucellosis, and tularemia.

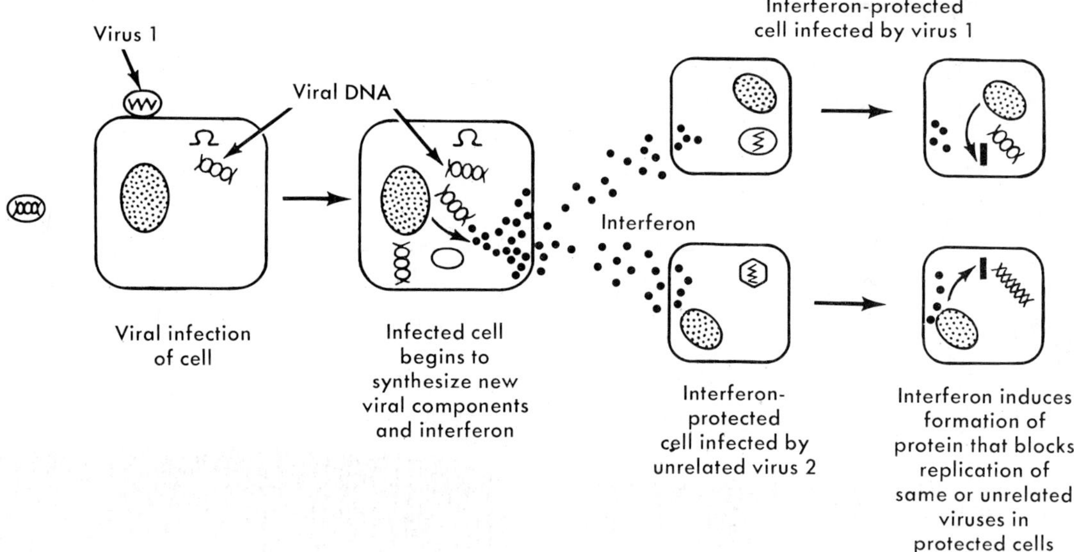

Fig. 14-5. Mechanism of interferon action.

Interferon does not inhibit all viruses equally; some are more readily inhibited than are others. Among the viruses that seem to be especially sensitive are the arboviruses, influenza, and smallpox viruses.

That interferon plays a significant role in the recovery from viral infections seems inescapable; however, it has never been shown conclusively that interferon is a necessary part of defense against viral infection. Since naturally occurring deficiencies have never been demonstrated and since there is no mechanism for selective inhibition in experimental animals, it is not possible to evaluate specifically the role of interferon as a defense mechanism.

Because of its general protective effect against a wide range of viruses and its low toxicity and antigenicity, interferon has great potential as a prophylactic and therapeutic agent. At the present time, however, its limitations make it of little clinical significance. These limitations include (1) its species specificity, which means that it would have to be produced in tissue cultures of human cell lines, which is both difficult and expensive; (2) the difficulty in purification, which makes the recovery of large enough quantities impractical; (3) the lack of any effect on viral synthesis already in progress; (4) the inability to deliver protective doses to susceptible host cells; and (5) its short duration of activity. If some means can be found to stimulate interferon production within the host to maintain effectively protective levels, the control of a number of viral infections might be obtained.

□ Inflammatory response

When injury occurs in the body, all of the nonspecific and to some degree the specific defense mechanisms are directed toward localizing the effects of the injury, protecting against microbial invasion at the site, and preparing the site for repair. This process is called *inflammation*. When an inflammation occurs at a particular site in the body, the addition of the suffix *-itis* is added to the site designation to indicate the pathologic state; for example, an inflammatory response on the pericardium is termed pericarditis; of the bladder, cystitis.

The *inflammatory response* can be initiated by any type of injury: heat, cold, irradiation, chemicals, trauma, infection, immunologic injury, or neoplasia. Whatever the stimulus, the response of the body is the same, but the extent of the involvement of the various facets of the nonspecific response system depends on the extent and severity of the injury.

Three major physiologic responses occur during the inflammatory process: vascular response, fluid exudation, and cellular exudation (Table 14-5). The *vascular response* consists of a transitory vasoconstriction (stress response) followed immediately by vasodilation. This occurs as a result of chemical substances such as histamine or kinins released at the site of injury or invasion. The amount of blood flow to the area is thus increased *(hyperemia)*, causing redness and heat. Blood flow slows as the capillaries dilate. There is increased permeability of the capillary walls facilitating fluid and cellular exudation. *Fluid exudation* from the capillaries into the inter-

Table 14-5. Summary of the steps of the inflammatory response

Steps	Mediators	Outcome
1. Injury	Physical, chemical, biologic, immunologic stimulus	Cell and tissue injury
2. Vascular response		
a. Vascular dilation	Histamine, plasmin, serotonin, kinins, prostaglandins released or activated by injury	Dilation of vessels causing stasis of blood and margination of leukocytes
b. Fibrin clot formation	Activation of clotting mechanism	Containment of irritants
3. Fluid exudation	Histamine, kinins, prostaglandins cause opening of venule–endothelial cell junction	Fluid exudation into tissues
4. Cellular exudation		
a. Leukocyte exudation	Chemotactic substances released by complement activation, clot formation, and injured cells	Passage of leukocytes from blood to site of injury and accumulation there
b. Attack and engulfment of foreign materials	Neutrophils and macrophages	Removal and digestion of bacteria, foreign particles, and damaged tissues
5. Healing	Fibroblasts produce collagen fibers and tissue regeneration	Resolution of inflammation and formation of scar tissue

stitial spaces begins immediately and is most active during the first 24 hours after injury or invasion. Initially the fluid exudate is primarily serous fluid, but as the capillary wall becomes more permeable, protein (albumin) is lost into the interstitial spaces. This increases the colloid osmotic pressure in the interstitial spaces, which encourages more fluid exudation. The swelling of the tissue from the fluid in the interstitial spaces is called *edema* (p. 303). *Cellular exudation* refers to the migration of white blood cells (leukocytes) through the capillary walls into the affected tissue. An increased number of white blood cells are attracted to the vessels in the affected area as a result of chemotactic substances being released from the tissues by cell injury and complement activation. The white blood cells adhere to the capillary wall and then pass ameboid fashion through the widened endothelial junctions of the capillary wall. Neutrophils (polymorphonuclear leukocytes), which comprise about 60% of the circulating white blood cells, are the first leukocytes to respond, usually within the first few hours. The neutrophils ingest the bacteria and dead tissue cells *(phagocytosis);* then they die, releasing proteolytic enzymes that liquefy the dead neutrophils, dead bacteria, and other dead cells (pus). Monocytes and lymphocytes appear later. The macrophages continue the phagocytosis, and the lymphocytes play a role in the antigen-antibody response at the site.

The five cardinal symptoms of inflammation were identified many centuries ago. These are redness *(rubor)* and heat *(calor)* due to the hyperemia, swelling *(tumor)* due to the fluid exudate, pain *(dolor)* due to the pressure of the fluid exudate and to chemical (bradykinin) irritation of the nerve endings, and loss of function of the affected part due to the swelling and pain.

The inflammatory response serves to prepare the tissue for healing and to contain the spread of bacterial invasion. To prevent the spread of bacteria, fibroblasts are attracted to the area and secrete fibrin, a threadlike substance that encircles the affected area to wall if off from healthy tissue. If there is interference with this walling-off process, bacteria can spread into the surrounding tissue. This explains why an abscess should not be incised and drained until it has "come to a head" or until the walling-off process is completed.

Bacteria may fail to be contained locally and spread to other parts of the body by means of the lymph system or bloodstream. If picked up by the lymph stream, the bacteria will be carried to the nearest lymph node. These nodes are located along the course of all lymph channels, and here too bacteria can be ingested and destroyed. If the bacteria are virulent enough to resist the action in the lymph nodes, leukocytes are brought in by the bloodstream to attack and engulf the bacteria in the node. The node then becomes swollen and tender because of the accumulation of phagocytes, bacteria, and destroyed lymphoid tissue. This is known as *lymphadenitis*. Swollen lymph nodes can be palpated primarily in the neck, axilla, and groin (p. 340).

Moderate to severe inflammatory responses can produce generalized systemic effects. Products from the breakdown of bacteria and white blood cells can affect the temperature-regulating center in the hypothalamus and produce fever. A severe infection without an accompanying fever may suggest a poor prognosis. Loss of appetite (anorexia) and fatigue may be due to conservation of body energy needed to resist the infection. The body increases the production of white blood cells to help fight the infection and *leukocytosis* (serum white blood cell levels greater than 10,000/cu mm) may occur. With infection there is also an increased blood sedimentation rate; that is, when an anticoagulant is added to the blood in the laboratory, the red blood cells settle to the bottom of a test tube more rapidly than normal. This increase in the sedimentation rate is believed to be caused by an increase in fibrinogen (a blood protein essential to the healing process). The sedimentation rate is elevated during the acute inflammatory stage of infection. Its elevation is an indication that the body's defense mechanism for the repair of damaged tissue is operating. Because the sedimentation rate gradually returns to normal as tissues heal, it also is used to determine when physical activity can be safely resumed following an acute infection.

Inflammations can be classified as acute or chronic. *Acute* inflammations are characterized by a sudden onset and an increase in the fluid exudative response. *Chronic* inflammations have a slower more insidious onset and are characterized by increased cellular exudation.

Knowledge of the physiologic changes that occur during the inflammatory process helps the nurse to understand the changes that occur in a wide variety of diseases. For example, whenever cells die as a result of injury or disease *(necrosis)* such as during a myocardial infarction (p. 992), the inflammatory process will occur. Fat deposits (atheromas) on blood vessel walls cause injury to the lining of the vessel wall and initiate an inflammatory response. Irritation of the peritoneum by trauma or bacterial invasion can cause inflammation of the peritoneum *(peritonitis)*.

No healing will occur until inflammation has subsided and pus and dead tissue have been removed. Pus is a local accumulation of dead phagocytes, dead bacteria, and dead tissue. The bacteria most commonly causing this reaction are the staphylococci, streptococci, *Neisseria*, and *Pseudomonas aeruginosa (pyocyanea)*. A collection of pus that is localized by a zone of inflamed tissue is called an *abscess* (Fig. 14-6). An inflammation that involves cellular or connective tissue is called *cellulitis*, whereas an inflammation in which pus collects in a preexisting cavity such as the pleura or gallbladder is called *empyema*. When infection forms an abscess within the body, develops a suppurating channel, and ruptures onto the surface or into a body cavity, it is called a *sinus*. If the infection forms a tubelike passage from an

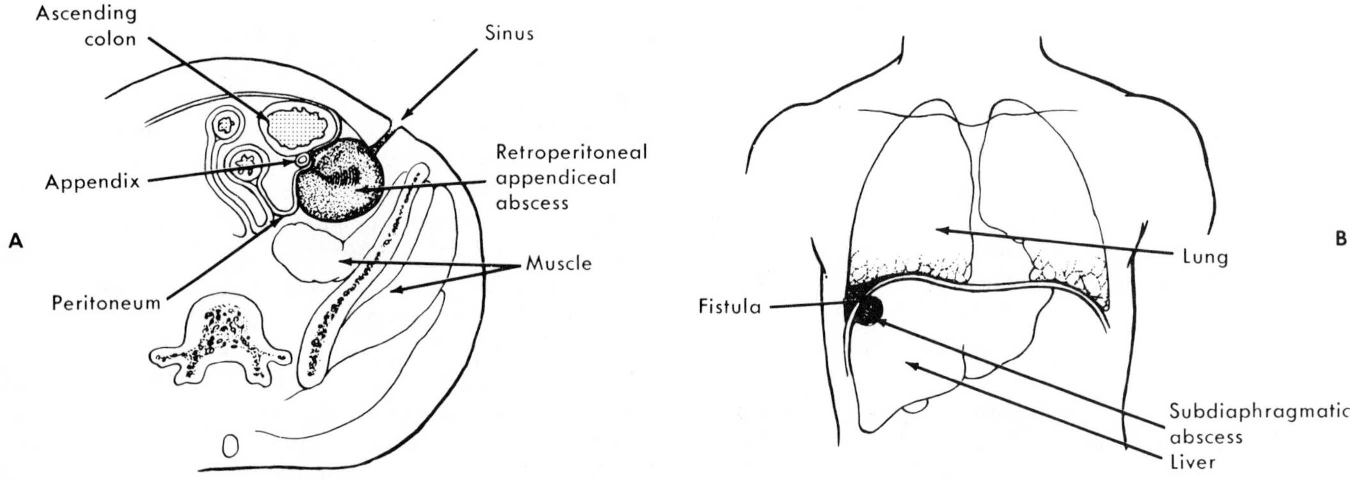

Fig. 14-6. A, Cross section of torso showing appendiceal abscess with sinus that has developed through abdominal wall. **B,** Subdiaphragmatic abscess that has developed fistula opening into pleural cavity.

epithelium-lined organ or normal body cavity to the surface or to another organ or cavity, it is called a *fistula* (Fig. 14-7).

After the infected area is clean, new cells are produced to fill in the space left by the injury. They may be the normal structural cells or they may be fibrotic tissue cells known as *scar tissue*. If they are fibrotic cells, they will not function as formerly but only serve to fill in the injured area. Some body cells readily regenerate; for instance, after the bowel has healed it is almost impossible to find the injured area. The respiratory tract also regenerates its tissues readily. Liver tissue has the capacity to regenerate its tissue, but over a longer period of time. Some nerve cells are always replaced with fibrous tissue. If a large amount of tissue is destroyed, structural cells may not be replaced, regardless of the type of tissue. (See Chapter 23 for discussion of wound healing.)

Some people, especially those with brown or black skin, are prone to excessive scar formation. Such tissue formation, known as a *keloid*, is hard and shiny in appearance and may enlarge to a surprising degree. It may cause disfigurement or undergo malignant degeneration and for this reason is usually excised surgically. Serous membranes sometimes become adherent during inflammatory and healing processes, and as the inflammation subsides, fibrous tissue forms, holding the membranes together. This fibrous tissue is called an *adhesion*. Adhesions may occur in the pleura, the pericardium, about the pelvic organs, and in many other parts of the body. They often occur in and about the intestinal tract, where they may cause an obstruction.

Instead of healing there may be necrosis, or death of the tissue. Bacteria, both pathogens and nonpathogens, often invade the necrotic tissue and cause decomposition, which is called *gangrene*. The body defenses are useless in preventing or curing gangrene because no blood can get to the area. Gangrenous tissue must be completely removed before healing can occur.

■ SPECIFIC DEFENSE MECHANISMS

□ Concept of an adaptive specific immune system

Specific defense mechanisms within the body provide specific protection against a particular microorganism or molecular entity. This mechanism of protection leads to what is termed *immunity*. Depending on the relative levels of protection, the body may be able to defend itself totally or only partially from damage by the agent. The *immune system*, which is composed of many of the same organs, cells, and molecular entities that are operative in providing nonspecific defense, works in concert with the nonspecific mechanisms to focus and amplify the general mechanisms of defense against specifically recognized foreign materials.

The fundamental nature of the specific immune response is characterized by *diversity*, *specificity*, *recognition*, *memory*, and *action*. Among the most intriguing aspects of immune response is its *diversity of ability to respond* while at the same time responding with *specificity of action*. Almost any conceivable organic molecular array on the surface of a molecule has been shown to be able to induce a series of cellular events culminating in the production of *antibodies*. These antibodies combine with the inducing *antigen* by virtue of combining sites on the antibody molecule, which exhibit an extremely narrow specificity. The remainder of the antibody molecule is chemically and structurally quite similar to all other antibody molecules with distinctly different combining site specificities. *Recognition* and *mem-*

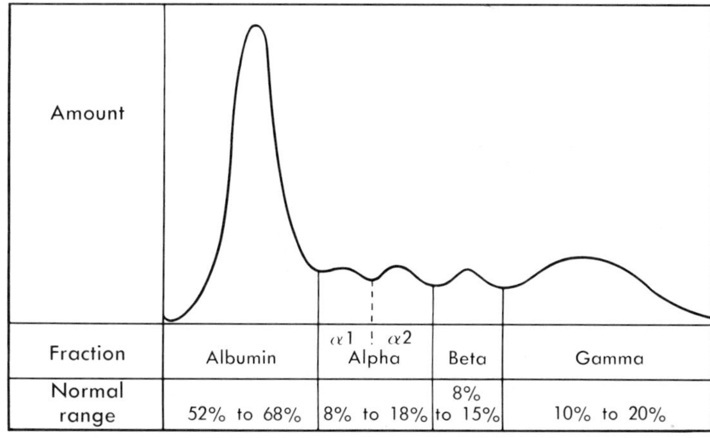

Fig. 14-7. Electrophoretic separation of major serum proteins. Majority of antibody activity lies within gamma globulin fraction. Gamma globulin fraction will rise with active synthesis of antibodies in response to antigenic stimulation.

ory are two other aspects of this system that make it unique. The normal organism recognizes its own antigenic makeup and will not produce antibodies against its own antigens. This is known as *recognition of self.* At the same time this intricate system of self-recognition must be able to recognize extremely subtle changes in its own cells when incipient tumors that differ only slightly in antigenic constitution are forming. Further, once the immune system has responded to an antigen, subsequent encounters with that antigen will produce an even more vigorous and rapid response. This response includes a wide variety of mechanisms designed to take *action* against the offending agent. Many of these actions are among the most potent biochemical and cellular reactions that the body can produce, yet they are focused so discretely that the foreign agent is rapidly destroyed with a minimum of damage to the host.

☐ Antigens and antibodies

Antigens

An antigen is defined as a substance that when introduced into an animal elicits the formation of antibodies or specifically sensitized cells. The antigen must be recognized as "nonself" or "foreign" material within the body. While most antigens are naturally occurring proteins of at least 10,000 molecular weight, other substances such as polysaccharides, nucleoproteins, lipoproteins, and glycoproteins may also serve as antigens. The bulk of the antigen consists of subsurface molecular structures that do not elicit an immune response but do serve as carrier for the multiple *antigenic determinants* on the surface. Most antigens have multiple antigenic determinants and are termed multivalent antigens; however, some molecules may be monovalent.

Certain molecules because of their small size cannot by themselves induce the synthesis of antibodies; however, when coupled with a high-molecular-weight carrier, they can serve as antigenic determinants. These molecules are *incomplete antigens,* or *haptens.* These molecules take on special significance in the consideration of hypersensitivities (allergies to low-molecular-weight compounds such as certain drugs and antibiotics) (p. 198).

Antibodies

The body's response to the introduction of an antigenic substance is the production of a specific, soluble *antibody* or a sensitized (antigen reactive) lymphocyte population. The type of antigen introduced will determine the immune response: antibody synthesis, antigen-reactive lymphocyte, or a combination of both.

The circulating antibodies represent modified (that is, antigen specific) globulin proteins found in blood serum. The serum contains several distinct protein frac-

Table 14-6. Properties of immunoglobulin classes

Property	Immunoglobulin class				
	IgG	IgM	IgA	IgE	IgD
Physicochemical					
Percent of Ig	82	7	10	0.002	1
Configuration	Monomer	Pentamer	Monomer, dimer	Monomer	Monomer
Half-life in serum (days)	23	5	6	2	3
Functional antigen-binding sites	2	5	2	2	?
Biologic					
Principal site found	Internal body fluids	Serum	Serum and exocrine secretions	Tissue bound	?
Fixes complement	Yes	Yes	No	No	No
Crosses placenta	Yes	No	No	No	No
Principal functions	Agglutination, detoxification, virus neutralization; enhances phagocytosis	Agglutination, cytolysis; enhances phagocytosis	Protection of mucosal surfaces	Mediates immediate-type hypersensitivity	?

tions, which are separable on the basis of their net electrical charge, molecular size, and molecular conformation into several fractions: albumin, alpha globulins, beta globulins, and gamma globulins (Fig. 14-7). The antibody activity of the serum is characteristically associated with the gamma globulin fraction. Those gamma globulins with the ability to bind antigens are called *immunoglobulins*. The immunoglobulins can be further subdivided into different *classes* on the basis of structure and function of the molecules. The generic symbol for immunoglobulins is Ig, and each of the classes is designated by a letter of the alphabet: IgA, IgD, IgE, IgG, and IgM (Table 14-6).

The basic pattern of structure for all immunoglobulins is based on a four-peptide-chain monomeric unit (Fig. 14-8). Two of the chains are of higher molecular weight and are termed *heavy* (H) *chains;* two are of lower molecular weight and are called *light* (L) *chains*. Each L chain is linked by disulfide (—ss—) bonds to an H chain, and in turn the H chains are linked to each other by a disulfide bond. When immunoglobulin monomers are visualized by electron microscopy, they are seen to have a Y-shaped structure. At the ends of the two arms of the Y are the sites where antigen is bound. Both the H and L chains participate in the formation of these *antigen-binding* sites. Thus most monomers of immunoglobulin have two antigen-binding sites and are termed *bivalent*. The two arms of the Y are designated the *Fab* (for fragment, antigen-binding) *regions*. The base of the Y is called the *Fc region* (for fragment, crystallizable). In the region of the disulfide bond joining the H chains the molecule seems to be flexible, and this region is known as the *hinge region*.

The predominant class of immunoglobulins in normal adult serum is IgG. It makes up about 75% to 85% of the immunoglobulin fraction. Because of its structure and biologic activity, it is also found in the extravascular fluids of the body (Table 14-6). IgG is capable of crossing the placenta to provide the newborn with temporary natural passive immunity to those diseases against which the mother has circulating antibodies. It functions in the processes of toxin neutralization and virus and bacterial inactivation and in the formation of antigen-antibody-complement immune complexes associated with certain types of hypersensitivity (p. 197). IgG is the immunoglobulin class primarily responsible for the rise in serum antibodies during a secondary (anamnestic, booster) response (p. 188).

IgM structurally is composed of five monomeric units attached to each other at the Fc region. Thus the star-shaped molecule with the antigen-binding sites pointed outward that results from this macromolecular arrangement is termed a pentamer. Sometimes this immunoglobulin class, which constitutes about 7% of the immunoglobulin in serum, is called the *macroglobulins* because of its molecular size. As a result of its size it is confined primarily to the intravascular fluids. IgM, like IgG, is capable of binding the C1 component of comple-

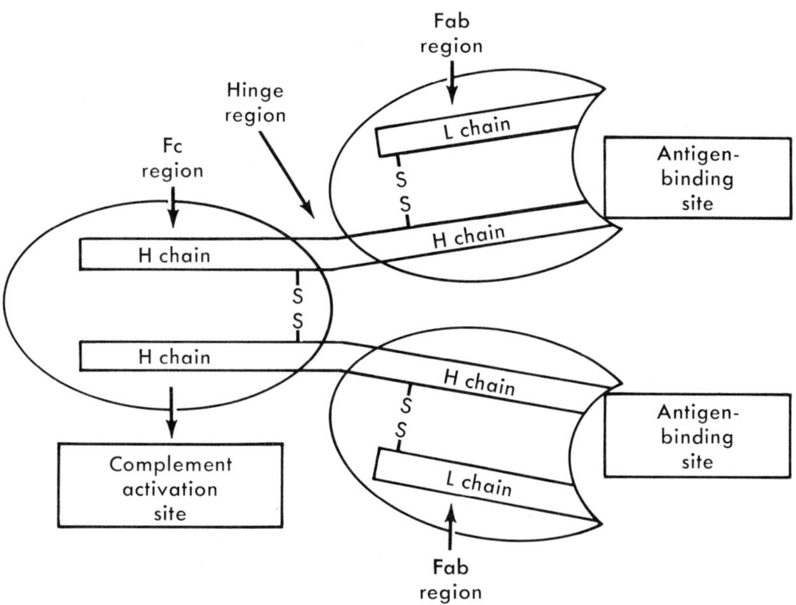

Fig. 14-8. Basic structure of IgG immunoglobulin monomer. All immunoglobulin classes are composed of variations of this basic structure with combination to form dimers (IgA) or pentamers (IgM).

ment and initiating the complement cascade. In each antigenic stimulation IgM antibodies are the first to appear, but they do not reach the levels of IgG, nor do they exhibit an anamnestic response on subsequent antigen contact. They are primarily involved in providing protection against viral and bacterial invaders in the blood. Because of their ability to bind complement, they too are responsible for certain immune complex hypersensitivities and autoimmune diseases such as rheumatoid arthritis.

IgA constitutes about 10% of the total immunoglobulin in serum. It can be found in a variety of polymeric forms (primarily monomer in serum and dimer in exocrine secretions). IgA is also termed the *secretory immunoglobulin* because it is found in the exocrine secretions of the body (milk, mucin, saliva, tears). Within these secretions IgA provides specific protection of the mucosal surfaces of the respiratory, digestive, and genital tracts from pathogenic invasion.

IgD makes up about only 1% of the immunoglobulin fraction of serum. Its biologic functions are unknown. It may be an early receptor or precursor necessary for the later development of IgM and IgG.

IgE is present in the serum in extremely small amounts (0.002%). This is the result of the predilection this immunoglobulin class has for attachment to the surface of mast cells and basophils. Once bound by the Fc region of the monomer to the surface of these cells, which are rich in the potent physiologically active substances histamine, kinins, and serotonin, IgE serves to mediate the severe and occasionally fatal anaphylactic type of hypersensitivities. These include anaphylactic shock, allergic asthma, and hay fever (p. 196). The protective role of these immunoglobulins is not clear, but they may be effective in providing protection against certain parasitic worms.

Antigen-antibody interactions

When an immunoglobulin comes in contact with its specific antigen, there is a physical interaction between the two causing a reversible binding of the antibody to the antigen. The affinity that the antibody has for the antigen and the avidity, or tightness, of the binding depend on the location and spatial arrangement of the antigenic determinants on the surface of the antigen and how well the antigen-combining site on the antibody molecule "fits" the antigenic determinant. Since the antigen is usually multivalent and the antibody is generally at least bivalent, the antigen molecules may be crossbound and clumped (agglutinated, precipitated) by antibody molecules (Fig. 14-9).

Within the body the binding of antibody to the antigen can have direct beneficial effects such as detoxification of toxins, inactivation of viruses, or, coupled with complement, the direct lysis of cells. However, in most cases the antigen-antibody combination initiates and facilitates the nonspecific defense mechanisms (phagocytosis, complement, inflammatory response, and so forth).

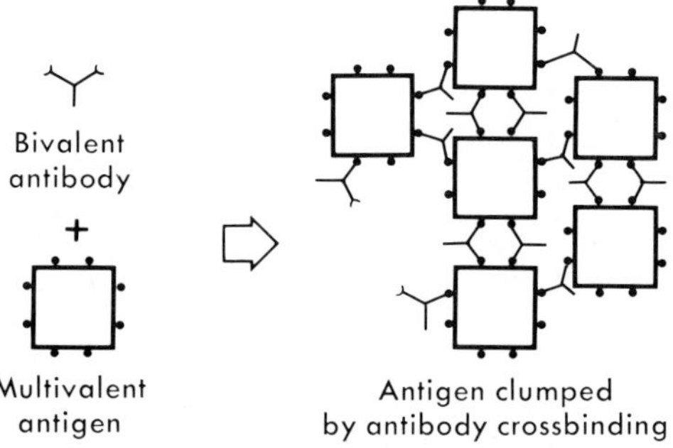

Fig. 14-9. Clumping of multivalent antigen by its specific antibody.

□ Immune response system

Cells involved

The cells involved in the specific immune response are all derived from the original undifferentiated stem cells of the bone marrow. The stem cell has the possibility of developing into any of the blood cells of the body depending on various signals and influences. The primary cells of the immune response system develop from the lymphocytic cell population (Fig. 14-10). One population of lymphocytic cells undergoes differentiation under the influence of the thymus gland and becomes known as *thymus-dependent lymphocytes*, or *T cells*. These cells become responsible for mediating the *cell-mediated immune responses* (CMI). Another population of lymphocytes matures in the lymphoid tissues and is referred to as *thymus-independent lymphocytes*, or *B cells*. The designation B cell comes from the fact that in the chicken, where this process was first detected, there is a single site where this differentiation occurs, the *bursa of Fabricius*. No such singular lymphoid organ is found in humans, but it is believed that the gut-associated lymphoid tissues such as the tonsils, the Peyer's patches of the intestine, and the appendix serve as the equivalent sites in humans. The B cells are responsible for the production of the immunoglobulins and the provision of the *humoral immune response*.

The role of the lymphocytes (B or T cells) is to recognize the presence of an antigen and to initiate specific mechanisms of disposal. Just as important, the lymphocyte must recognize a component of host tissue as *self* and protect that tissue from immunologic response reactions.

The *macrophage* appears to act nonspecifically, but

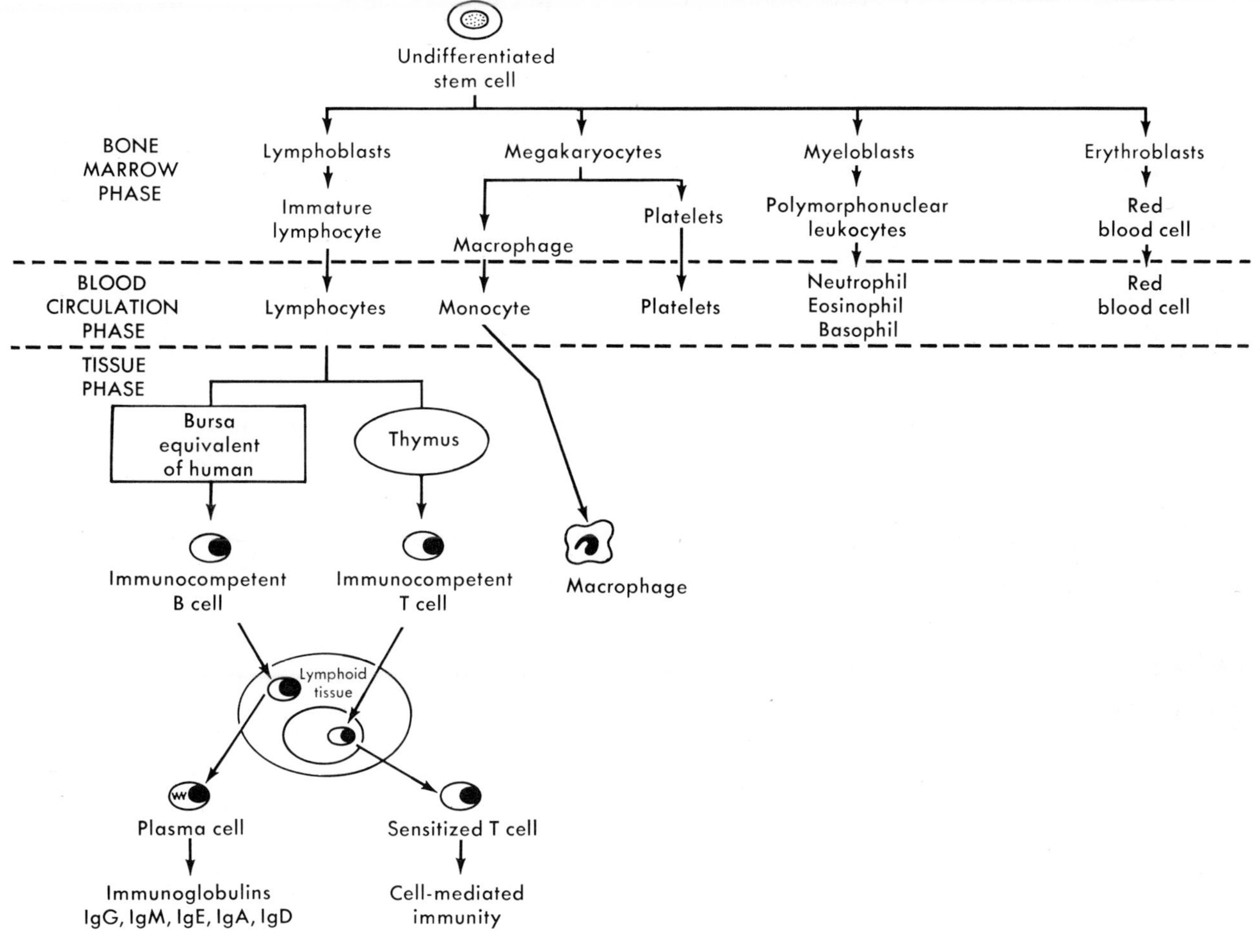

Fig. 14-10. Development of B and T cell lymphocytes.

its role in the immune response is critical. First, the macrophage seems to be responsible for initially capturing, processing, and presenting the antigen to the lymphocytes. Capture of the antigen occurs by phagocytosis as described earlier in this chapter. The processing of the antigen is a poorly understood mechanism, but there is evidence that the macrophage digests and concentrates the antigen and then couples the antigen to an RNA. This processed signal is transferred to the surface of the macrophage for presentation to lymphocytes. Antigen presented to lymphocytes in this manner triggers the series of events within the lymphocytes that leads to full immunologic response. Antigen that escapes this macrophage processing will stimulate only a weak immune response or no response at all.

At the other end of the immune response the macrophage is activated to its maximum of phagocytic efficiency by the release of stimulatory, soluble substances, known as *lymphokines*, by activated lymphocytes (Table 14-7). In this way the macrophage is stimulated at the site of an immune reaction. Other of the soluble lymphokines serve to attract the macrophages to the site by chemotaxis.

Table 14-7. Lymphokines liberated by activated T cell lymphocytes

Lymphokine	Function
Lymphocyte-derived chemotactic factors	Chemotactic for macrophages
Lymphocytotoxins	Nonspecific lysis of cells
Macrophage inhibition-activation factors	Maintains macrophage at site and activates it
Interferon	Inhibits replication of viruses
Lymphocyte-activating factors	Activates nonsensitized lymphocytes

Organs and tissues involved

The organs and tissues of the specific immune response system include the central organs (bone marrow, thymus, and gut-associated lymphoid tissues) and the peripheral organs (lymph nodes, spleen, and lymphatic vessels). Within the central organs the immune response cells are synthesized and matured, while within the peripheral organs the mature cells are concentrated.

The *thymus* serves as the control organ of the immune system. It is the site of differentiation of the T cell lymphocytic populations and through certain soluble thymic hormones serves to regulate the overall immune system. The activity of the thymus reaches it peak in childhood, and the organ begins to shrink in size after puberty. If the thymus is removed (thymectomy) very early in the life of an animal, a severe state of immunodeficiency is induced and T cell–mediated immunity never develops. The thymectomized animal develops a wasting disease characterized by stunted growth, diarrhea, and death from massive infection by intestinal or respiratory tract normal flora. The B cell function is also reduced, pointing to a cooperative effect between the two basic systems. The loss of the thymus from the adult animal creates less severe reactions. This is probably due to the establishment of an already functional, long-lived population of T cells.

The *lymph nodes* and *spleen* serve as the primary sites of localization of the immune response cells. The lymph node serves to filter the lymph drained from a region of tissue. The structure of the lymph node (Fig. 14-11) consists of an inner medullary and paracortical region comprised primarily of T cells and an outer cortex composed of clusters, or germinal centers, of B cells known as follicles. The spleen is structured on somewhat the same pattern with diffusely packed T cell areas and germinal centers of tightly packed B cells. In certain types of antigenic stimulation, either the T cell areas or the B cell areas will show tissue proliferation, while the other area remains quiescent. By the same principle, if a person is suffering a basic primary immunodeficiency of one system, the corresponding area of lymph nodes and spleen may degenerate.

During the course of the immune response reaction, within the lymph nodes there is significant proliferation of specific cells and migration of phagocytic cells to the site, which may lead to lymph node enlargement. Enlargement of the lymph nodes in a region may be the result of (1) infections, (2) immune diseases, (3) intrinsic neoplasms of the lymph node itself, or (4) metastatic spread of malignant cells to the node. The presence of an enlarged spleen or enlarged lymph nodes is virtually always an important clinical finding.

□ Immune response

Primary immune response: antigenic challenge

When an antigen is introduced into the body, it can trigger a wide or narrow spectrum of the response mechanisms. The specific pattern of response is dependent on (1) the amount of antigen introduced, (2) the site of introduction, and (3) the type of antigen introduced.

Small amounts of a noninvasive, large, particular antigen introduced at a single body site are quickly and efficiently handled at a local site with little or no systemic involvement beyond the local lymph node. Since the inflammatory response and local lymph node can localize the spread of the antigen, the immune response may go completely unnoticed by the host organism. Larger, particulate antigens are readily cleared, but small, soluble antigens are more difficult to clear from the circulation.

Large amounts of an antigen may allow the antigen to escape from the local site by simply overwhelming the

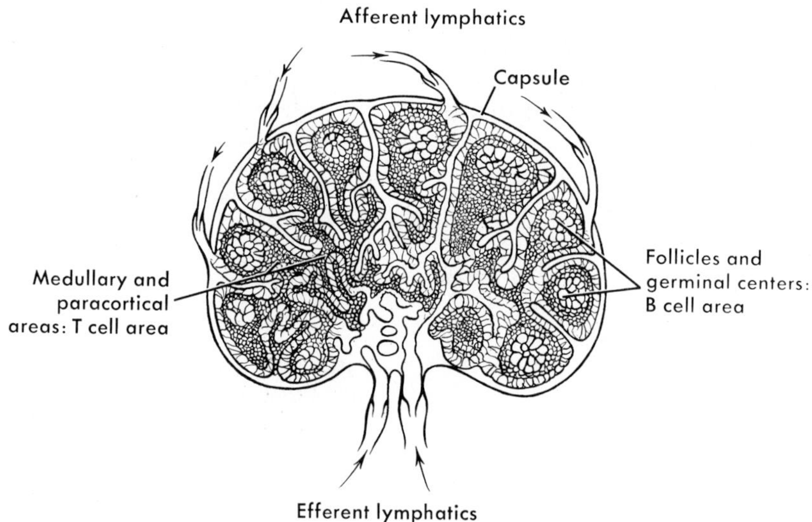

Fig. 14-11. B and T cell areas of lymph node.

local defense mechanisms. Even though the lymph nodes and reticuloendothelial organs can clear 80% to 90% of an antigen on a single pass, if the amount of the antigen is extremely large some antigen may escape the local site. An excessively large, sustained antigen dose can exhaust not only the local site but the entire reticuloendothelial system as well. This greatly reduces the body's ability to respond to even minor invasive challenges and renders the host vulnerable to secondary infections.

Highly invasive antigens (e.g., bacteria such as *Staphylococcus aureus* or *Streptococcus pyogenes*) or those introduced directly into the bloodstream by blood transfusion, intravenous catheterization, or injection can immediately establish a systemic type of immune response. This is why extreme care must be exercised in the use of any type of medical procedure that would allow the introduction of organisms into the general circulation. The localization action of the immune response is critical to efficient functioning of the response.

Primary humoral response

When the antigen is introduced for the first time, one of three basic mechanisms of response will be elicited: (1) a response mediated primarily by B cells, the humoral response; (2) a response in which the T cells are primarily involved, the cell-mediated response; or (3) a combined type of response.

If the antigen is of the type that triggers a humoral response, the first time the body is exposed to the antigen the B cell system responds with the synthesis of circulating immunoglobulins (Fig. 14-12). The encroaching antigen is phagocytosed by a lymph node macrophage or tissue-active macrophage. The macrophage processes the antigen and presents the antigenic stimulus to a B cell, which has been preprogrammed to respond to the introduced antigen. These antigen-specific B cells bear receptors on their surface, which allows them to recognize their antigenic stimulant. Only a few lymphocytes within a lymph node have the ability to respond to the antigen. The stimulated B cell then begins a process of

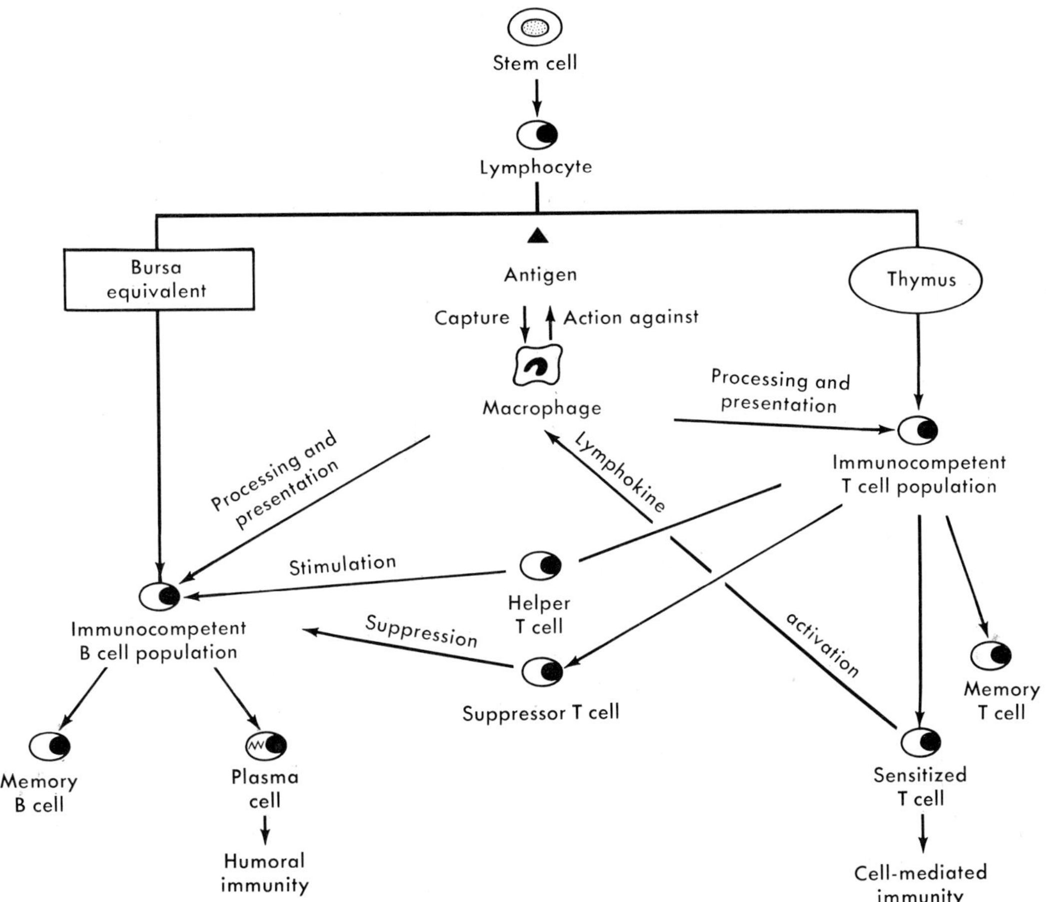

Fig. 14-12. Combined response of B and T cell systems.

proliferation (increase in number) and differentiation (change in structure and function). The progeny of the stimulated cell increase in number within the lymph node, forming *clones* of specifically adapted lymphocytes. With each generation of new cells within the clone, the lymphocytes become more differentiated toward a cell population ideally suited for the synthesis and release of immunoglobulin. These cells are known as *plasma* cells. With the development of this cell population in the lymph node (several days after the introduction of the antigen), antibodies can be detected in the lymph node. However, it is not until about 1 to 2 weeks after the antigenic challenge that detectable levels of specific antibodies appear in the serum. The plasma cell population of the lymph node and the levels of antibody in the blood continue to increase for another 2 to 3 weeks, and then both begin to retreat. Some of the lymphocytes of the activated clone become "memory cells," which are much more responsive, both in time of reaction and efficiency of antibody synthesis, to subsequent contact with the antigen.

The humoral response serves to protect the body from such agents as microbial toxins, bacteria within the extravascular spaces in the blood and on mucosal surfaces, and viruses that must pass through the circulatory system to reach their site of infection (such as poliomyelitis virus).

Primary cell-mediated response

Certain antigens trigger a response mediated by T cell proliferation and reaction. A T cell that has received its antigenic stimulus is referred to as a *sensitized T cell lymphocyte* (Fig. 14-12).

The initial steps of the cell-mediated response, those involving the antigen processing by the macrophage, seem to be the same as in the humoral response. Following the presentation of the antigenic stimulus to lymph node T cells, there is proliferation in the T cell domain. There is no release of circulatory antibodies; rather, sensitized lymphocytes are released into the circulation. These cells migrate to the site of the entrance of the antigen into the body where the invading agent or residual antigen is found. These activated lymphocytes along with macrophages infiltrate the regions of the tissue and begin a direct attack on the antigen or tissue cells labeled with the antigen. The T cells participating in this direct attack are known as *killer T cells*.

To amplify the site reaction further, the sensitized lymphocytes activate the nonspecific phagocytotic cells (macrophages, PMNs, and noncommitted lymphocytes) in the region of the antigen. This is accomplished through the release of the soluble lymphokines (Table 14-7), which marshall this additional cellular involvement to attack the antigenic materials.

The cell-mediated response is especially effective in protection against diseases that grow and do their damage intracellularly where the circulating immunoglobulins cannot reach them. Diseases of this type include viral and rickettsial diseases and those produced by certain chronic types of infective agents, fungal pathogens and the tubercle bacillus being the most outstanding examples. One other important function of this system is the provision of *cancer cell surveillance* (p. 201).

Combined-type primary immune response

Most antigens do not cause a purely humoral or purely cell-mediated response; rather, both types of response are evoked. Likewise, our protection against most harmful antigens is the result of both of these specific response systems being brought to bear on the antigen involved. In the *combined type of response* there is an initial perturbation within the T cell areas of the lymph node. This becomes obvious within about 2 days after the introduction of the antigen. About 3 to 5 days later the B cell areas begin to proliferate.

To mount a maximal immune response, the cooperative action of the three central cell types is necessary. The macrophage serves to capture, process, and present the antigen to immunocompetent cells of both T and B cell ancestry. The T cells aid in the direct cell-mediated response, but there also seems to be a population of T cells that serves to interact with the B cell population to control the development of an effective immune response. A *helper T cell* population cooperates with the B cells by some as yet undefined mechanism to enhance the activation and proliferation of the immunoglobulin synthesizing cells. The existence of the helper T cell explains the observation noted earlier in this chapter that the removal of the thymus from the neonate not only comprises the cell-mediated immune response but also significantly reduces the host's ability to mount a humoral immune response.

Secondary immune response

As was emphasized at the outset of this section, one of the touchstone characteristics of the specific response system is the ability of the system to remember prior contact with an antigen and to provide a more complete protective reaction on subsequent contact. The first contact between the immune response system and an antigen leads to what is termed the *primary* response, the events of which have been laid out in the preceding paragraphs. When antibody synthesis is measured in a primary response, there is a significant lag time to the appearance of antibodies in the circulation (Fig. 14-13). Immunoglobulins of the IgM class are the first to appear, but they maintain protective levels for only a short period. Specific IgG antibodies follow and reach protec-

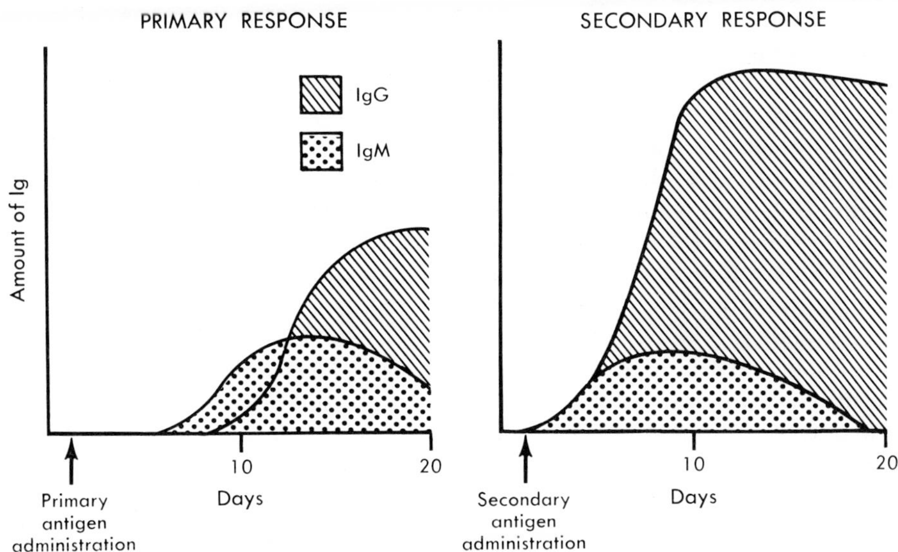

Fig. 14-13. Primary and secondary humoral responses.

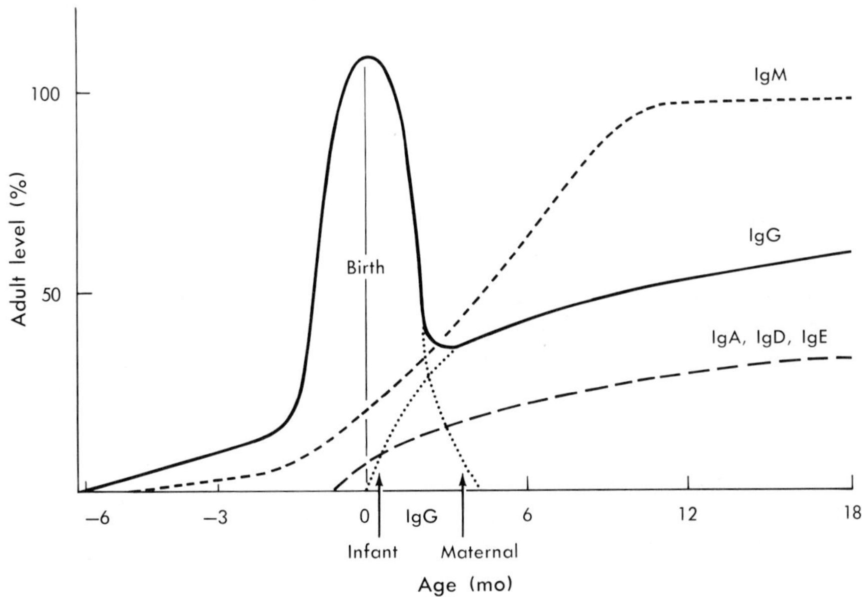

Fig. 14-14. Immunoglobulin levels in fetus and neonate.

tive levels within 12 to 14 days, but they too fall off fairly quickly with only this initial exposure. When the "primed" immune response system encounters the antigen again, a *secondary response* ensues, which is more rapid, of greater intensity, and longer lasting than the primary response. This secondary response is also termed an *anamnestic response*. This "remembered" response is a characteristic of both the B and T cell systems. The prior contact with the antigen is stored in special memory cells of both cell lines. This phenomenon provides the basis for active immunization and "booster" doses to maintain the protective levels of immunity. In an immunized individual the memory cells elicit the rapid response in time for the immune system to overwhelm the pathogen or toxin before it can produce its damage.

Developmental aspects of the immune response

Lymphoid cells first appear in the fetus as stem cells in the fetal liver at about the end of the first trimester.

The lymphoid tissues of the thymus also develop fairly early in the fetus. At birth, however, the lymph nodes and spleen are still underdeveloped, but T and B cell responsiveness is fully functional. The fetus is capable of some immune response if challenged by an in utero (within the uterus) infection such as in the case of congenital syphilis or rubella. Unless the fetus has been exposed to a congenital infection, at birth the neonate-synthesized immunoglobulin levels are low (Fig. 14-14). The child does have high levels of transplacentally acquired maternal IgG antibodies. These maternal antibodies have a half-life of about 30 days in the child, and this coupled with the increase in blood volume in the growing infant leads to a drop in the IgG levels of the blood over the first 3 months. Thereafter the rate of the child's own synthesis of IgG provides for a steady increase in the immunoglobulin concentration within the serum. IgM levels reach adult concentrations by about the age of 9 months.

Numerous studies in both animals and humans have shown that during the aging process there is a progressive loss of immunologic vigor. The prime immunologic age probably is achieved during the late teen years when virtually the full complement of immunities have been developed and the responsiveness of the system peaks. The middle years are characterized by a plateau and slowly falling curve until the later years of life when a sharp decline becomes evident. This decline is seen in both the cell-mediated and humoral response systems. This loss in immunologic sensitivity is associated with an increasingly less effective and more misdirected immune response. There is an increasing frequency of autoimmune disease, susceptibility to pathogenic and opportunistic microorganisms, and incidence of cancer.

Development of immune tolerance

Immune tolerance is defined as the state of immunologic nonresponsiveness. By some mechanisms the body becomes tolerant to self while maintaining responsiveness to foreign materials. Evidence establishes the fact that self-tolerance is acquired during embryonic development; however, the exact mechanisms by which it develops remain an issue. During fetal development the immune system is presented with antigens from the developing tissues; these become identified as self-antigens, so that when exposed to these antigens postnatally the individual is tolerant of them. One proposed mechanism by which this state could be induced is known as the *clonal selection theory*. This theory states that when potentially responsive clones of B or T cells come into contact with an antigen prenatally, the responsive cell line is killed, thus eliminating the responsiveness to that antigen from the body. This produces a state of *natural tolerance*. This theory is supported by experimental data that show that by exposing experimental animals to foreign antigens in utero a tolerance to that antigen is developed; however, some antigens introduced in this manner are found to be more *tolerogenic* (capable of inducing tolerance) than are others. Further, the clonal selection theory does not explain how it is possible to break tolerance in adults as indicated in certain experimental studies or as in the case of certain of the autoimmune diseases. In some cases at least, tolerance is not due to the total elimination of specifically reactive cells but to the blocking of expression of temporary inactivation of the responsive cells. The action of suppressor T cells or the failure of mobilization by helper T cells may play a significant role in maintaining the state of self-tolerance.

■ APPLICATIONS AND IMPLICATIONS OF IMMUNE RESPONSE

□ Immunization

Long before the mechanisms of immune response were worked out, it was recognized that recovery from certain diseases conferred protection against subsequent exposure to that disease. Dating from the days of Jenner's vaccination with cowpox exudate to protect against smallpox (1798), through the success of Pasteur with anthrax and rabies (1880s), up to the present, the specific protective mechanisms of the immune system have been used to protect against serious infectious diseases.

Passive immunization

Temporary protection, usually measured in days or at most weeks, is afforded by the acquisition of preformed anitbody from another host. As the acquired antibodies are used up through binding with antigen or by being catabolized, the protection is lost.

Transplacental passive immunization occurs through the transfer of IgG antibodies from the maternal circulation across the placenta to the fetal blood. There is also some acquisition of immunoglobulins through the colostrum of the mother's milk.

Artificial passive immunization may be necessary if the individual to be immunized has suffered exposure to a serious infectious agent to which he or she has no immunity or if the individual's own immune system is impaired or deficient. The sources of these preformed antibodies are pooled human adult gamma globulin or heterologous (from another species) globulin fractions. Pooled human gamma globulin has been used to modify the effects of measles, particularly in premature infants, in children with primary immunodeficiencies, and in patients undergoing immunosuppressive therapies. Persons who have contact with persons with hepatitis and smallpox may also be protected by this method. It should be noted, however, that isolated gamma globulin preparations tend to form small protein aggregates, and these, if injected intravenously, could lead to severe anaphylactic reactions (p. 195). For this reason the material *is always administered intramuscularly.*

The most commonly used heterologous antibody fractions are antitetanus and antidiphtheria antisera derived from horse globulins. Since these are foreign proteins, they can lead to the development of serum sickness (p. 197). Serum sickness is more likely to occur in subjects already primed by previous contact with horse globulin; thus multiple use of hetereologous sera is to be avoided.

Active immunization

The objective of active immunization is to provide effective long-term immunity by establishing within the individual's own body the capacity to produce effective levels of immune response and to establish a population of sensitive cells that can respond to subsequent antigenic contact.

Immunizing agents ideally should be noninjurious to the individual being immunized. To accomplish this the pathogenic effects must be modified while at the same time maintaining the antigenicity of the agent. Bacteria exotoxins such as those produced by the diphtheria and tetanus bacteria can be successfully detoxified by formaldehyde treatment without destroying the major antigenic determinants on the protein molecule. Such detoxified antigenic materials are called *toxoids.* The use of *killed vaccines* of viruses and bacteria can also provide a safe antigen for immunization. Killed vaccines include those for pertussis (whooping cough), typhoid and cholera, and the Salk poliomyelitis vaccine. The protection conferred by these vaccines is generally inferior to that produced by live vaccines. A number of the most successful vaccines consist of living organisms that have been modified so that they are nonvirulent. The *attenuated live vaccines* provide excellent protection, but there is some risk in their use due to the possibility of reversion to the virulent form of the organism. Live vaccines of importance are those for measles, mumps and tuberculosis (BCG) and the Sabin poliomyelitis vaccine.

The provision of protective levels of residual immunity depends on the inducement of (1) the right type of response (i.e., cell mediated or humoral), (2) in sufficient amounts, (3) at the right place (i.e., where the immune response can contact the antigen), and (4) against the right antigenic determinants (i.e., the antibodies formed produce an inactivating effect). Simply the induction of an immune response is not sufficient to provide protection. For example, the early killed virus measles vaccines elicited a splendid production of circulating antibodies against the measles virus, but protection against measles is most effectively mediated by cellular immune responses. The humoral protection did not prevent infection.

Another problem of immunization for which provision must be made is the *interference* that one antigen may have with another if the two are given simultaneously. The live virus vaccines occasionally interfere with each other; when measles and smallpox vaccines are administered at the same time, they each interfere with the development of immunity by the other. This is probably the result of interferon production. Some live virus vaccines contain more than one strain of the virus and these can cross-inhibit. In the case of the Sabin oral polio vaccine three separate dosages are required because there are three strains within the same vaccine. With the initial dosage, immunity to only one strain may develop if that strain interferes with the other two.

Complications of immunization

Although immunization is the most successful approach to the control of many infectious diseases, there are small but still real risks involved. The development of postvaccination encephalitis or other neural autoimmune complications is a serious risk with such vaccines as those for smallpox or rabies. Children with immunodeficiencies may be overwhelmed by vaccination with live vaccine. With viral vaccines, which are produced in monkey kidney of human cell culture, there is a slight risk of the introduction of oncogenic (cancer causing) viruses. A fetus may be significantly at risk if the mother receives a live virus vaccine during pregnancy. Such vaccines as smallpox and live influenza should never be administered to a pregnant woman. It is still unclear whether the rubella virus vaccine harms the fetus or not, so it too should be avoided. Besides these rather serious risks, general discomfort is to be expected from some forms of immunization. The typhoid vaccine, for instance, is composed of large numbers of killed salmonella bacteria; since the endotoxic cell wall materials of these cells is a pyrogenic (fever producing) substance, fever and malaise are not uncommon sequelae. The influenza vaccines often produce febrile reactions in children.

□ Immunologic disorders

As expected in such an interrelated, complex system as is operative in the mechanisms providing biologic defense, there are innumerable points at which the system may malfunction. The immunologic disorders that have been characterized reflect nonresponsiveness, blocked responsiveness, limited responsiveness, misdirected responsiveness, and overresponsiveness. The underlying causes of the disorders may be attributed to developmental defect, infection, malignancy, trauma, metabolic state, or pharmacologic intervention. The severity of the

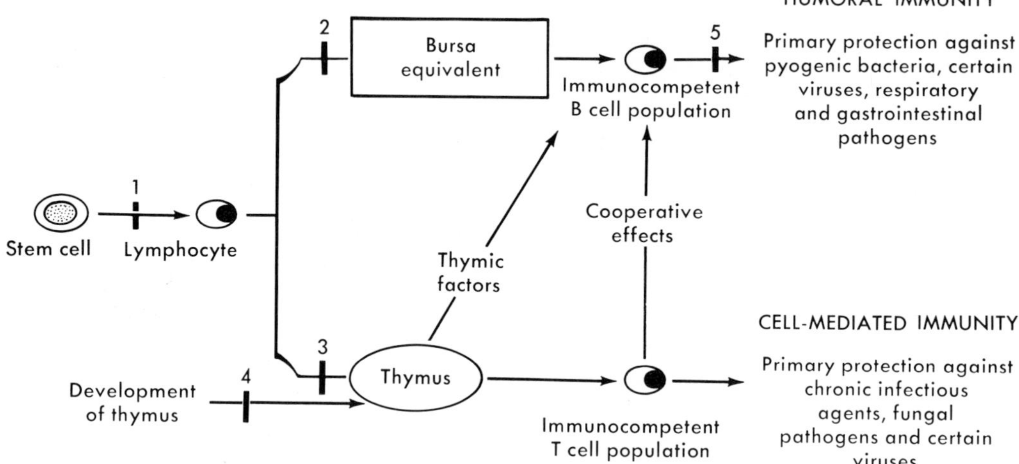

Fig. 14-15. Causes of immunodeficiencies. Abnormalities at *1* result in combined humoral and cell-mediated immunodeficiency. Blockage at *2* produces agammaglobulinemia. Blockage at *3* or *4* results in drastic reduction in T cell–mediated function and, because of cooperative effects on B cell system, some reduction in humoral response. Abnormalities in synthesis of specific immunoglobulin classes are reflected by blockage at *5*. While some blockages result in complete deficiency, others show up as reduction in response.

disorders ranges from creation of a minor nuisance (such as mild hay fever) to a life-threatening situation (such as anaphylactic shock). The disorders may be classified into the following general categories:

1. Immunodeficiencies: deficiencies in the proper expression of the immune response system, parts of the system, or individual cell types within the system
2. Gammopathies: abnormal production of immunoglobulins.
3. Hypersensitivities: exaggerated or inappropriate response to specific antigens.
4. Autoimmunities: the immunologic attack on self-antigens.

Each of these categories is briefly discussed.

Immunodeficiencies

Since the cells and tissues of the immune response system develop in sequential fashion, if a defect in that development appears, the severity of the resulting deficiency reflects the stage of development at which the abnormality arose (Fig. 14-15). Deficiencies exist in phagocytosis, immunoglobulin synthesis, cellular immune functions, or a combination of deficiencies. The deficiencies resulting from the improper development of the immunoresponsive cells and tissues are termed *primary immunodeficiencies*. The nonspecific depression of immune responsiveness as a secondary result of some interference with the immune system produces a *secondary immunodeficiency*.

Primary immunodeficiencies. Chronic granulomatous disease in children is an example of a *defect in phagocytosis*. The disease is characterized by the development of abscesses and granulomas containing plasma cells and macrophages. In patients exhibiting this defect the polymorphonuclear leukocytes will ingest organisms and particles, but because they lack a specific digestive enzyme, killing and digestion do not occur. The defect is a sex-linked recessive genetic characteristic appearing only in males; however, the female carriers of the trait have somewhat reduced leukocytic activity.

In the severe *B cell deficiency* known as infantile sex-linked agammaglobulinemia, the production of immunoglobulin is grossly depressed and the follicular areas of the lymph nodes lack plasma cells. This disease too is found only in boys and is manifested in childhood by multiple infections with pyogenic bacteria. Pneumonia, otitis media, sinusitis, and septicemias are quite common and recurrent in these children. The cell-mediated immune response is intact and provides adequate protection against antigens eliciting a T cell response.

DiGeorge's syndrome produces a classical *T cell deficiency*. The basis of the disease is the absence of the thymus in the neonate. Stem cells cannot differentiate to become T lymphocytes; therefore the T cell areas of the lymph nodes are underdeveloped. Circulating antibodies are present but at a somewhat reduced level. Sometimes this defect is reversible by the transplant of a fetal thymus into the immunodeficient neonate.

The most severe type of immunodeficiency is a *combined type* in which there is a lack of responsiveness from both immune systems. Lymphopenic agammaglobulinemia, also known as Swiss-type immunodeficiency syndrome, characterizes this type of defect. Neither T nor B cells develop, and the infant is immunologically incompetent. On any exposure to the environment, even nonpathogenic organisms can initiate a fatal infection. The basis of this deficiency is a stem cell defect that creates an inability to develop lymphocytes.

These severe types are encountered almost exclusively in children. The reason for this highlights how vitally dependent a host is on the immune response system: survival past the first few years of life is almost impossible in children exhibiting any of these three syndromes.

Other types of partial immunodeficiencies are much more frequently encountered. Depending on the severity of the deficiency, a spectrum of inability to mount a normal immune response is exhibited.

Secondary immunodeficiencies. Any factor that can interfere with the normal growth or expression of the immune response system can lead to a *secondary immunodeficiency.* In the nursing care of the adult, these types of immunodeficiencies, though not as dramatic, are of greater significance than the primary deficiencies. Cell-mediated responses are impaired by malnutrition. This probably accounts for the greater incidence of chronic diseases such as tuberculosis in the malnourished. Patients with Hodgkin's disease also frequently develop profound impairments in cellular immunity. These patients frequently develop severe infections of fungal or viral etiology. Viral infections themselves can produce a suppression in the ability of the body to respond immunologically. This probably is the result of direct cytotoxic damage to lymphoid cells by viruses such as the measles virus. Many of the medical therapies and chemotherapeutic agents are significantly immunosuppressive. Irradiation, certain antibiotics, cancer chemotherapy, and corticosteroids all can reduce or alter the immune response.

Gammopathies

Gammopathies, better termed *hypergammaglobulinemias,* are elevated levels of gamma globulin in serum resulting from the overproduction of whole gamma globulin or nonassociated heavy chains (H chains) or nonassociated light chains (L chains). The normal synthesis of an immunoglobulin is the result of the proliferation and plasma cell differentiation of a single clone of B cells in response to an antigenic signal. In gammopathies a single clone or multiple clones of plasma cells begin to overproduce immunoglobulin product. If the gammopathy involves a single B cell clone, it is termed a *monoclonal gammopathy,* and the electrophoretic pattern will be characterized by a single sharp peak in the gamma globulin region (Fig. 14-16). *Polyclonal gammopathies* are more common, and they involve the overproduction of virtually all classes of immunoglobulins in response to inappropriate antigenic stimulation.

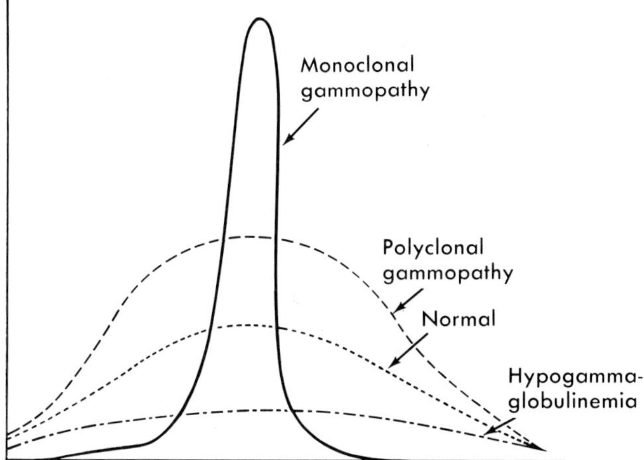

Fig. 14-16. Electrophoretic peaks of gamma globulin fractions in monoclonal gammopathies, polyclonal gammopathies, and hypogammaglobulinemia. Obtained by electrophoresis of gamma globulin fraction of serum.

Monoclonal gammopathies, which are most often seen in older patients, often lead to the development of *multiple myeloma.* Multiple myeloma is a widespread osteolytic (skeletal destroying) neoplasm of the bone marrow. The disease leads to weight loss, hypercalcemia, proteinuria, recurrent bacterial infection, and renal involvement. Another form of monoclonal gammopathy, involving the overproduction of IgM, is known as *macroglobulinemia.* This disease can produce increased blood viscosity (due to the size of the IgM molecule), which can lead to serious circulatory impairments, neurologic disorders, weakness, and fatigue. The monoclonal gammopathies are also called plasma cell dyscrasias.

The development of high levels of dysfunctional gamma globulins depresses the synthesis of normal immunoglobulins. This renders the hypergammaglobulinemic individual susceptible to infection. Bacterial pneumonias and pyogenic bacterial septicemias are extremely frequent, often producing fatal results.

Hypersensitivity reactions

The immune response system, which has been immunologically primed or sensitized, is designed to provide an immediate, effective, protective reaction to subsequent encounter with the sensitizing antigen. This of course is a positive factor in the provision of immunity; however, under a given set of conditions or due to an idiotypic reactivity to a particular antigen, the response of the immune system may produce detrimental effects. This inappropriate response is usually manifest as a tissue-damaging overreaction to the antigen; thus it is termed *hypersensitivity*, or allergy. The antigenic stimulants invoking the reactions are referred to as *allergens*. Hypersensitivities, then, are classic expressions of the immune system, but they take place in inappropriate sites, in excessive amounts, or with inappropriate involvement of nonspecific tissues. Whether an allergic response occurs and to what degree is dependent on a combination of interrelated factors:

1. *Responsiveness of the host to the allergen.* If the host's sensitivity is extremely high, there is far greater chance a tissue-damaging reaction will occur.
2. *Amount of the allergen.* Generally speaking, the greater the amount of allergen contacted the more severe the reaction.
3. *Nature of the allergen.* Most are complex, high-molecular-weight, multivalent proteins, but some may be low-molecular-weight nonprotein materials, which exert a haptenic effect when coupled with a normal tissue protein carrier.
4. *Route of entrance of the allergen.* The greatest proportion of allergens enter through the respiratory tract; however, others may enter by epidermal or mucosal contact, injection, or through the digestive tract.
5. *Timing of exposure to the allergen.* If the host's contacts with the allergen are widely separated (such as years apart), the immunologic mediators (antibodies or sensitized cells) may be so dilute that there will be less response.
6. *Site of the allergen-immune mediator reaction.* If certain antigen-antibody reactions occur in the tissues, there is no untoward effect, whereas the same reaction occurring within the bloodstream can lead to intravascular inflammation.

Hypersensitivities can be broadly divided into two categories based on the components of the immune system involved in mediating the hypersensitivity reaction: humoral response (B cell mediated) or cellular response (T cell mediated) (Table 14-8). This basic division corresponds with the older clinical symptom division of *immediate* and *delayed*, which was developed prior to the elucidation of the mechanisms. The terms immediate or

Table 14-8. Summary of hypersensitivity reactions

	Hypersensitivity type			
	Immediate			Delayed
Property	**I Anaphylactic**	**II Cytotoxic**	**III Immune complex**	**IV Cell mediated**
Immune system mediators	IgE (IgG) bound to mast cells	IgG or IgM (+ complement)	IgG or IgM + complement	T cells, macrophages
Allergens	Exogenous antigens	Foreign cells or alteration of cell surface antigens	Soluble antigens	Infectious agent, contact allergens, foreign tissues, cancer cells
Response to intradermal skin test	Wheal and flare within 30 min, edema	Not done	Erythema and edema within 3 to 8 hr	Erythema and induration within 24 to 48 hr
Pathophysiologic effects	Release of histamines, kinins, SRS-A from mast cells, which affect smooth muscle shock organs	Direct cytotoxic destruction of cells	Acute inflammatory reaction; primary PMNs	Tissue destruction, primarily lymphocytes and macrophages
Examples	Systemic anaphylaxis, atopic allergies, hayfever, insect sting reactions	Hemolytic disease of the newborn (Rh), transfusion reactions	Serum sickness, Arthus reaction, glomerulonephritis	Tuberculin reaction, skin graft rejection, poison ivy

delayed were assigned to describe the timing of the appearance of clinical symptoms and the speed of skin test reactions when a host was challenged with various allergens. This terminology is still used today, but it has taken on new significance in relation to the understanding of the basic mechanisms at work.

It is possible to subcategorize the different manifestations of the humorally mediated hypersensitivities. The most widely used scheme of classification is presented in Table 14-8. As can be seen from this table, the type I, II, and III reactions are mediated by the humoral system, while type IV reactions are those of the cell-mediated system. Since types I, II, and III hypersensitivities are the result of interactions involving circulating antibodies, these reactions can be transferred from a sensitized host to a nonsensitized host by serum transfer. Type IV sensitivities can be transferred by lymphocyte exchange only.

Type I anaphylactic, IgE-dependent hypersensitivity. The most serious and life-threatening hypersensitivity diseases are associated with the reactions mediated by the IgE class of immunoglobulins. These antibodies, also called *reaginic antibodies*, have a predilection for attachment to the surface of mast cells and basophils. The mast cells are found in virtually all tissues of the body and often in close proximity to blood vessels, while the basophils are found circulating as one of the leukocytes within the blood. Mast cells are particularly abundant in the skin, nasal region, and lungs. Both mast cells and basophils harbor within their cells numerous, membrane-bound vacuoles containing potent, pharmacologically active substances (histamine, bradykinin, serotonin, and other vasoactive amines). When IgE immunoglobulins bind to the surface of these cells by the Fc portion of the immunoglobulin molecule, the antigen-binding site of the molecule is left exposed to bind the allergen at the surface of the cell (Fig. 14-17). When the allergen is bound to the IgE, the cell is induced to undergo *degranulation*, which releases the internal agents into the environment of the mast cell or basophil. These mediators then cause increased vascular permeability and smooth-muscle contraction.

Of the agents released, histamine seems to be the most important. The direct injection of histamine can mimic many of the symptoms of the type I hypersensitivity, and in the hypersensitive individual a reaction may be assuaged by antihistamines. Other physiologically similar substances are released as well. Thus in type I reactions the detrimental symptoms are not at the site of the antigen-antibody reaction but at the site of the *shock organs* where the pharmacologically active *anaphylactic mediators* exert their action. If those mediators remain confined to a local area, the tissue reactions remain localized and are referred to as *local anaphylaxis*. The local hypersensitivity that most people demonstrate to a mosquito bite is the classic example of this type of reaction; the intradermal injection of the mosquito anticoagulants produces a wheal-flare type of reaction within a matter of minutes. If, on the other hand, the mediators become released systemically the response is known as *systemic anaphylaxis*, which can produce *anaphylactic shock*. As is illustrated by the mosquito bite, the mediators are quickly broken down in the body and their effects are reversible.

For type I reactions to occur, the hypersensitive individual must initially come into contact with the allergen that triggers the synthesis of the specific antiallergenic IgE antibodies. This primary contact is known as a *sensitizing dose*. With the synthesis of the IgE antibodies and their attachment to mast cells and basophils, the individual is rendered hypersensitive. On subsequent contact with the allergen (termed the *shocking* or *challenging dose*), the individual exhibits the symptoms of type I sensitivity. The severity of those symptoms depends on a number of factors: the amount and route of entrance of the sensitizing dose, the amount and distribution of the IgE antibodies, and the amount and route of entrance of the shocking dose.

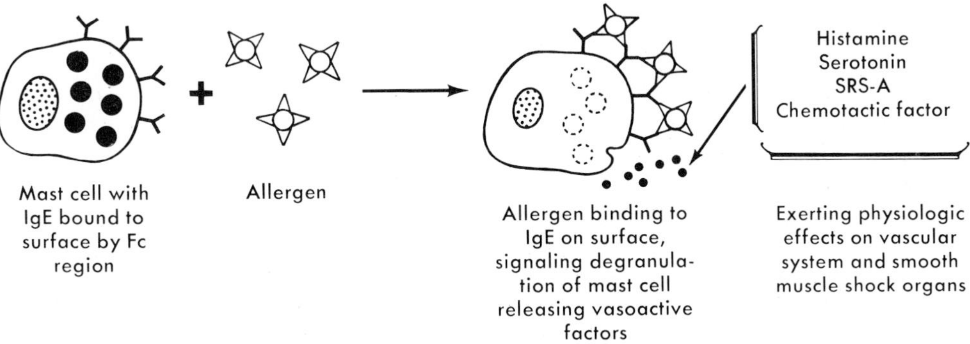

Fig. 14-17. Mediators of type I hypersensitivity.

Anaphylactic shock. The most severe form of type I hypersensitivity in humans is systemic anaphylaxis. The initial symptoms of anaphylactic shock are edema and itching about the site of the infection, apprehension, and sneezing. These mild reactions are rapidly followed, sometimes in a matter of seconds or minutes, by edema of the face, hands, and other parts of the body, wheezing respirations, cyanosis and dyspnea, dilation of the pupils, rapid weak pulse, and falling blood pressure. Death may follow in a few minutes. The respiratory and circulatory symptoms are caused by constriction of smooth muscle by histamine and other substances released from the mast cells in large amounts.

Parenteral injections of penicillin are the most frequent cause of anaphylactic shock. Animal serum used in the preparation of antitoxins and extracts of allergenic substances used for testing or desensitization of an allergic patient also frequently cause it. Sudden death resulting from a bee sting is due to anaphylactic shock. Contrast media containing iodide, such as those used for intravenous pyelograms and angiograms, may produce this serious allergic response. Persons also have been known to develop anaphylactic reactions to acetylsalicylic acid (aspirin) as it is absorbed in the the bloodstream. Therefore this drug is not as innocuous as many people believe.

Since people with a history of allergies are more likely to develop anaphylactic reactions to drugs than are those without such a history, all patients should be questioned about allergies and sensitivity to drugs before drugs are initiated. If there is any positive history, the physician should be consulted before a new drug is started, and if it is given the patient should be watched closely for allergic response. In hospitals it is now common practice to have the fact that the patient is sensitive to certain substances posted conspicuously on the outside of the chart where it cannot be overlooked by anyone responsible for the care of the pateint. In addition many hospitals use a special color identification bracelet for the patient who is sensitive to certain substances. This alerts personnel throughout the hospital to the patient's hypersensitivity.

People who are known to be allergic or who have received a specific type of animal serum and who must rereceive antiserum should be given another type if it is available in order to lessen the possibility of an allergic response. When it is necessary to use animal serum, the individual should first be tested for sensitivity to the substance. An intradermal skin test, preceded by a scratch or eye test, is recommended. In persons who have a positive reaction to any of these tests, desensitization may be undertaken.

Any time animal sera, allergenic extracts, or contrast media containing iodide are given, a syringe containing 1:1,000 epinephrine hydrochloride (Adrenalin) should be at hand. An antihistamine such as tripelennamine (Pyribenzamine) or diphenhydramine (Benadryl), aminophylline, and isoproterenol (Isuprel) also should be available, and the patient should be kept under surveillance for at least 20 minutes. Any reaction that occurs within a few minutes forewarns of an impending emergency. At the first sign of untoward symptoms (redness and itching about the injection site, itching of the eyes, nasal symptoms, tightness in the chest) epinephrine, 1:1,000 (0.01 ml/kg), is administered subcutaneously or intramuscularly. In case of a more severe reaction an antihistamine is given parenterally, a tourniquet is applied above the injection site and epinephrine is injected into the site. Additional epinephrine may be given at intervals until the reaction subsides or tachycardia develops. Aminophylline may have to be given to relax the bronchial spasm and a vasopressor to raise the blood pressure. ACTH or corticosteroids may also be administered. Sometimes to counteract shock the patient's lower limbs are elevated, oxygen may be given by positive pressure mask, and an infusion is started. If there is tracheal edema, an endotracheal tube may be inserted or a tracheostomy may be done.

A less severe form of type I hypersensitivity is exhibited in *atopic allergies*, which have hereditary influences. Ten percent to 30% of the population suffer overt clinical symptoms of hypersensitivities involving localized anaphylactic reactions. The allergens vary and include spores, pollens, animal danders, foods, cosmetics, animal stings, and drugs. The diseases also vary widely in their severity, and the symptoms reflect the site of interaction between the allergen and the sensitized tissues.

Hay fever (allergic rhinitis) is the most common clinically evident type I hypersensitivity and is primarily due to the histamine release by mast cells within the upper respiratory tract and conjunctiva. A more severe atopy is *allergic asthma*. In this case the sensitized mast cells are found in the bronchial lumina, and their degranulation results in bronchospasm, excessive viscid mucus secretion, and loss of lung compliance. Since antihistamines are only marginally successful in alleviating the symptoms of asthma, the mast cell mediator known as *slow-reacting substance of anaphylaxis* (SRS-A) is probably the most active agent in the creation of the bronchial blockage through smooth-muscle constriction of the bronchioles. Some types of *urticaria* (hives) may occur following exposure to certain types of allergens. The symptoms of urticaria are the classic wheals (hard, raised swelling) and erythematous (reddened) flare covering large areas of the skin. These lesions are often pruritic (severely itching), and there may be local edema. The allergens implicated in urticarial reactions are varied, but among the more common are foods, cosmetics, and pharmaceuticals.

Type II cytotoxic hypersensitivities. The underlying mechanism of these hypersensitivities involves the direct binding of IgG or IgM immunoglobulins to an antigen on the surface of a cell. This antibody labeling then triggers the destruction of the cell by phagocytic attack, nonspecific lymphocytic attack, or lysis of the cell through the operation of the full complement cascade.

Transfusion reactions. The type II hypersensitivity is classically illustrated by the reactions that occur in mismatched blood transfusion reactions. Within the serum, individuals possess naturally occurring antibodies to the red blood cell surface antigens of the ABO blood groups that are not present on their own erythrocytes. Thus a person with type A blood will possess anti-B antibodies within the serum. These antibodies, called *isohemagglutinins*, are usually of the IgM class. They are thought to arise through a natural immunization to the glycopeptide antigens on the red blood cell surface through contact with similar glycopeptide found on the surface of the cell walls of bacteria that make up the natural flora of the gut. Antibodies formed in this way are capable of cross-reacting with the A or B antigens on the surface of the "foreign" ABO types. Since these antibodies are naturally present in the serum, on transfusion mismatched blood will be immediately coated by the isohemagglutinins, causing agglutination of the introduced cells and the rapid lysis of the cells by complement. The products released by the lysed cells are then dumped into the bloodstream.

After having received about 50 ml of incompatible blood, the patient usually complains of fullness in the head, severe pain in the back, and a sensation of constriction in the chest. Nausea and vomiting may occur, and the patient's pulse usually becomes rapid and blood pressure drops. If the transfusion is discontinued at this point, these symptoms will disappear, but a few hours later the urine becomes red (port-wine urine) and the urinary output is diminished. The urine contains red blood cells and albumin. This reaction is thought to be caused by the release of a toxic substance from the hemolyzed blood that causes a temporary vascular spasm in the kidneys, resulting in renal damage and blockage of the renal tubules by the hemoglobin precipitated out in the acid urine (hemoglobinuria). If the patient receives more than 100 ml of incompatible blood, irreversible shock with complete renal failure may occur, and death may follow. This renal failure is similar to the renal damage that sometimes results from ingestion of poisons and highly toxic drugs (p. 1321).

At the first sign of a reaction the blood transfusion should be discontinued and the physician notified. Epinephrine hydrochloride, 1:1,000, is given at once, and the urine is rapidly alkalized by an intravenous injection of sterile 1/6M sodium lactate solution. This procedure reduces the precipitation of hemoglobin in the kidneys.

As blood cells disintegrate (lyse), large amounts of potassium are released into the bloodstream, and if the renal function is impaired, hyperkalemia (excessive amount of potassium in the blood) will develop (p. 1310). If this condition occurs, the patient may be treated with an artificial kidney machine (p. 1335).

Type III immune complex hypersensitivities. The pathogenesis of the type III hypersensitivities lies in the union of soluble antigen and immunoglobulins of the IgM and IgG classes. The complexes formed in these interactions are not properly cleared by the reticuloendothelial system because of the small size of the complexes, which tend to defy phagocytosis. They are deposited in the body tissues. The complexes can then bind complement with all the attendant reactions of an internal, often intravascular, inflammatory response. The chemotactic factors released with the involvement of complement lead to an influx of phagocytes, which tend to intensify the inflammation. The clinical symptoms observed are the result of the amounts and relative proportions of the antigens and antibodies and the distribution of the complexes within the body.

The repeated subcutaneous injection of a highly antigenic soluble antigen can lead to the formation of such *immune complexes*, which trigger a localized inflammatory response known as the *Arthus reaction*. The region exhibiting the Arthus reaction shows the following sequential tissue changes: reduction of blood flow, development of microthrombi in the venules, increased permeability of the venule to the point that red blood cells escape into the surrounding tissues, development of edema, massive infiltration of the site by PMNs, and tissue destruction. Arthus reactions are not of great clinical importance, since strongly antigenic substances are not usually administered in repeated subcutaneous injections. However, a disseminated type of intravascular inflammation, known as allergic vasculitis, sometimes occurs in patients undergoing therapy with certain drugs (for example, sulfonamides, iodides, thioureas, and penicillin).

A type III hypersensitivity of clinical significance can develop 6 to 12 days after the administration of a large amount (more than 10 ml) of foreign serum. The condition, known as *serum sickness*, is characterized by fever, polyarthritis, urticaria, and enlargement of the spleen and lymph nodes. A severe, acute glomerulonephritis may also occur. The critical factor in this hypersensitivity reaction is a large amount of a persisting soluble antigen, the foreign serum proteins. The antigen initiates an immune response, and the resultant antibodies begin to appear in the blood about 1 week later where they interact with the antigen still present in the bloodstream. The complexes are deposited within the blood vessel walls, particularly the vessels of the renal glomeruli. Complement is bound, and an intravascular inflammation occurs.

Type IV cell-mediated (delayed type) hypersensitivities. The cell-mediated immune mechanisms, as has been noted previously, function in host defense against chronic bacterial and fungal infections, in rejection of foreign tissue cells, and in surveillance for cancer cells; however, it can also produce adverse effects in the form of delayed-type hypersensitivity. Three major areas of clinical concern are (1) hypersensitivity reactions in response to infections by certain bacteria, fungi, or viruses; (2) contact dermatitis reactions; and (3) tissue transplant rejections.

The body's reaction to the tubercle bacillus *(Mycobacterium tuberculosis)* is a classical example of a type IV hypersensitivity. The organism itself is not directly toxic to human cells or tissues. As a result the tubercle bacillus may invade the tissues of a nonsensitized host and establish residence in the host tissues, causing virtually no damage. However, in the course of time, as the organism sheds antigenic material, the cell-mediated immune response system is triggered. The sensitized lymphocytes and the activated macrophages attack not only the organism but also the tissues surrounding the organism. This process is aimed at destroying the foreign organism, but in the course of the attack tissue destruction may result. The lesions associated with tuberculosis, such as caseation necrosis cavitation, and general toxemia are a result of the hypersensitivity.

Following the initial sensitization with the infectious organism, subsequent contact with the tuberculosis organism or even an extract of a purified protein from the organism will elicit a hypersensitivity reaction. This is the basis of the Mantoux tuberculin skin test (p. 1117). The skin rashes of smallpox and measles and the lesions of herpes simplex virus and tuberculoid leprosy have all been attributed to an infectious type IV hypersensitivity.

Allergic contact dermatitis is one of the most commonly encountered types of human allergic disease. Usually both the route of sensitization and the display of symptoms are produced by direct dermal contact with the allergen. Many simple chemicals can serve as contact allergens. Among those most often implicated are industrial chemicals, topical ointments, soaps, dinitrochlorobenzene (DNCB), nickel, mercury, topical antibiotics, cosmetics, and the catechols of poison ivy, poison oak, and poison sumac.

Many of the contact allergens are of a size (less than 10,000 molecular weight) and structure that do not allow them to serve as a complete antigen (p. 182). It is most probable that the compound attaches to proteins of the skin and functions as a hapten to stimulate the proliferation of a T cell population sensitized to the compound. Following sensitization, subsequent contact with the contact allergen leads to the formation of an erythematous, vesiculated (blistered) lesion. The inflamed area itches, burns, or stings. Scratching the lesion may further spread the allergen or infect the site. There is often a serous exudate.

Tissue graft rejections, which are also an expression of type IV hypersensitivities, are discussed next.

Graft rejection. The rejection of foreign cells and tissues by the body is a beneficial function of the immune system primarily mediated by a type IV hypersensitivity. If it were not for this mechanism, the human body would be a haven for the inappropriate establishment of growth of any animal cell that penetrated the external defense mechanisms. However, this process is regarded as a disservice when it operates to prevent the positive aspects of the exchange of tissues between hosts.

The transfer of healthy tissues and organs from one individual to replace damaged or diseased tissues of another has been surgically possible for many years. The early attempts at tissue graft failed because of the rejection process. With the growing knowledge of the immune response, the mechanisms of this rejection process became more apparent, and it is now possible to make judgments and predictions concerning the likelihood of success of such an endeavor. Recently with this newly acquired knowledge it has become possible to control the course of the graft transfer process to favor the acceptance of the transplanted tissues. Today certain tissues can be transferred with a high expectation for success if the "rules" for prevention of rejection are followed.

The following terminology has been derived to describe transplants between individuals and species. It is based on the genetically derived discrepancies and similarities between the donor and the recipient.

autograft transfer of tissue from one site on an individual to another site; since this simply means the rearrangement of self, immunologically there is little concern.

isograft transfer of tissue between syngeneic (identical genetic makeup) individuals, such as identical twins; again since there is no genetic discrepancy in antigens, the immunologic factors favor success.

allograft transfer of tissues between allogeneic (members of the same species but exhibiting different genetic makeup) individuals; since the tissues of the donor are foreign to the recipient, they are antigenic and subject to rejection.

xenograft transfer of tissues between xenogeneic (different species) individuals; since the genetic differences are enormous, there is virtually no chance of avoiding immunorejection.

The allograft tissue transfer offers the most promise for organ and tissue replacement and is the one currently receiving the most experimental attention. Blood transfusion is the most common allografting procedure used today, and notwithstanding the problems associated with transfusion (p. 1542), it is carried out daily with success. Solid-tissue grafts such as skin and organs, however, introduce considerably greater problems.

The antigenic determinants of the tissues that lead to graft rejection are primarily found on the surface of the cells within the transplanted tissues. These antigens are known as *histocompatibility antigens* and are controlled by independently segregating genes within the chromosomal structure of the animal. They are also called *HL-A antigens* (human leukocyte antigens). Some of the histocompatability antigens are more antigenic than are others; thus some antigens are referred to as major and others as minor. The major transplantation antigens are those of the ABO and Rh blood groups and the HL-A antigens.

In preparation for an allograft the closest match of donor-recipient transplantation antigens is sought. This is done by *tissue typing* for the major antigenic determinants (ABO, Rh, and HL-A). If there are no significant discrepancies in these antigens, the recipient's serum is mixed with the lymphocytes from the donor, or the lymphocytes from the donor and recipient are cultured together to detect minor (but significant) cross-reactions. This is known as a *mixed lymphocyte reaction* (MLR).

The process of graft rejection is as complicated and exquisite as the immune response system that brings it about. It has been best characterized in the case of skin allograft rejections. In this case, when the nonmatched skin is transferred to the new host, it settles down and becomes vascularized within 2 to 3 days; however, within 6 to 10 days sensitized lymphocytes appear in the regional lymph nodes and the lymph nodes begin to enlarge. The initial signs of rejection appear in about 10 to 14 days with the appearance first of sensitized lymphocytes and then macrophages at the site. Within 12 to 14 days the vascular bed begins to deteriorate and the graft becomes necrotic and is sloughed off. *This is known as first-set rejection.* If another skin graft is taken from the *same* donor and is transplanted to a different site on the same recipient, the graft rejection is much more rapid. This accelerated reaction, known as *second-set rejection*, is so rapid that the graft may never even be vascularized before it is sloughed. In second-set rejection circulating antibodies as well as the sensitized lymphocytes play a role. The antibodies create a direct cytotoxic attack on the graft. This is analagous to a type II immediate hypersensitivity reaction.

Some allografts circumvent immunorejection because of their site in the body. Corneal grafts survive without the need for immunosuppression because the site is avascular. Cartilage grafts enjoy the same privilege. Grafts into these types of sites are referred to as *privileged-site grafts.* By some as yet unknown mechanism, the fetus developing within the uterus enjoys this privileged-site status.

Graft rejection can be minimized by the use of chemical or physical agents that nonspecifically or specifically interfere with the development of an immune response reaction against the allograft. Clinically, three types of immunosuppressive agents are effective in providing the transitional protection needed to promote the graft establishment.

Antimetabolites and alkylating agents, such as *azathioprine* (Imuran) and *cyclophosphamide* (Cytexan) act nonspecifically against rapidly dividing cells within the body, and for this reason they are also used for cancer chemotherapy. They interfere with DNA synthesis. Azathioprine, which is the most commonly used and least toxic, has both immunosuppressive and antiinflammatory actions. Both agents nonspecifically interfere with both the B cell and T cell systems.

Glucocorticosteroids, especially *prednisone,* are significantly antiinflammatory and impair lymphocyte (B and T cell) activation and function. Prednisone exerts a wide spectrum of activity against all immune response and inflammatory response mechanisms. Though it suppresses the cell-mediated system to a greater degree than the humoral system, the continued high dosage needed to maintain cell-mediated suppression creates significant risks in reducing the responsiveness of the humoral system. Other side effects (fluid retention, hypertension, behavior alterations, peptic ulcers, and osteoporosis) also obviate its use for prolonged periods at high dosage. Often lower dosages of prednisone and azathioprine are used together because they seem to act synergistically.

A more specific immunosuppression of the T cell system is achieved with the use of *antilymphocytic serum* (ALS). This antiserum is prepared by immunizing horses with human fetal thymocytes obtained from aborted fetuses. The antibody-containing globulin fraction is extracted and used to block the action of the sensitized cells in circulation while leaving the lymph node B cell system only slightly suppressed. This leaves the host with protection against the humorally protected infectious agents while providing protection against the most active rejection system. Since ALS contains foreign proteins itself and since it must be administered in fairly high repeated dosages, an Arthus reaction (p. 197) frequently occurs.

Autoimmune diseases

When the mechanisms for recognition of self versus nonself are subverted or altered, immune attack on self

Table 14-9. Some diseases with autoimmune aspects

Disease	Autoantigen	Comments
Pernicious anemia	Intrinsic factors of parietal cells	Specific autoantibodies detectable
Autoimmune hemolytic anemia	Antigens on the surface of RBC	RBC surface antigens may be altered by drugs, etc.
Systemic lupus erythematosus	Nucleoproteins, DNA, many other antigens	Multiple autoimmune responses
Guillain-Barré syndrome	Myelin	
Glomerulonephritis	Cross-reactive streptococcal antigens	May also result from direct attack of glomerular basement membrane
Rheumatic fever	Cross-reactive streptococcal antigens	
Rheumatoid arthritis	Immunoglobulin G	Rheumatoid factor is an IgM that reacts with IgG
Ulcerative colitis	Colon cells	
Myasthenia gravis	Skeletal and heart muscle	Thymectomy improves
Male infertility	Sperm cell	Agglutinins formed against sperm cells
Multiple sclerosis	Brain cells	Not proved to be autoimmune
Sympathetic uveitis	Uveal tissues	Release of sequestered uveal antigen
Autoimmune thyroiditis	Thyroid hormones and tissues	Autoantibodies and sensitized lymphocytes

may result. The chance that the control mechanisms will be lost increases with the age of the individual. The symptoms of such a self-attack are referred to as *autoimmune disease* or *autohypersensitivity*. For the most part these self-reactions are not immunologically initiated; the etiologic (causative) agent lies outside the immune system, but the immune response serves as the pathogenic mechanism. Many diseases for which no etiologic agent could be identified have been classified as autoimmune, only to be removed from that category when some cryptic, latent, or slow-growing agent was identified within the cells or tissue under attack. Some of the diseases listed as autoimmune-associated diseases in Table 14-9 will probably be removed from that list as the initiating factor or microorganism is identified.

The meaning of the demonstration of *autoantibodies* and *autosensitive T cell clones* is not always clear. These self-reactive immunoglobulins are often associated with certain pathologic states in the body but many times can also be isolated from the serum of "normal" individuals as well. Autoantibodies have been demonstrated against nuclear material in systemic lupus erythematosus, against gamma globulins in rheumatoid arthritis, against gastric parietal cells in pernicious anemia, and against platelets in autoimmune thrombocytopenia. Sensitized lymphocytes have been demonstrated in the Guillain-Barré syndrome and autoimmune thyroiditis.

Some of the theoretical mechanisms by which the immunologic tolerance might be broken include:

1. *Release of sequestered antigens*. If an antigen does not come into contact with the immune system during fetal development when the tolerance to self normally develops (either because of anatomic site or later development), it is not registered as a self-antigen, and clones of immunoresponsive cells to that antigen remain reactive. As a result of trauma or infection these antigens may be exposed to the immune system. If this occurs they will elicit an immune response. Examples of this include thyroiditis, aspermia (male infertility), and uveitis.
2. *Activation of suppressed clones*. If one of the functions of the suppressor T cell is to suppress the activation of certain clones of potentially self-reactive T or B cells, it is possible through some loss of suppressor function that these "forbidden" clones are allowed to proliferate. There is no currently identified experimental disease model to support this hypothesis, but it is theoretically feasible.
3. *Synthesis of cross-reactive antibodies*. Antibodies synthesized in response to certain foreign antigens may have cross-reactivity with some similar antigenic components within human tissues. Contact with antigens called *heterophile antigens* may trigger the production of autoantibodies. This seems to be a mechanism of rheumatic heart disease, where the antibodies produced against certain streptococcal antigens during scarlet fever, streptococcal sore throat, or other streptococcal infections cross-react with myocardial tissue, producing a myocardial inflammation.

4. *Alteration of self-antigens.* Normal body proteins may be altered by chemicals, infectious organisms, or therapeutic drugs to present new antigenically active groups to the immune system. The autoimmune hemolytic anemia associated with alpha-methyldopa (Aldomet) treatment of hypertension probably results from the alteration of the Rh antigens of the red blood cell rendering it antigenic. Certain antibiotics such as the penicillins and cephalosporins can have the same effect.

□ Cancer immunology

One of the primary functions of the cell-mediated immune response system seems to be the recognition and destruction of cancer cells within the body. By the same mechanisms that are operative in allograft rejection, it is postulated that the immune system continually protects against the establishment of tumor growths. The recognition of these cells as nonself is based on the appearance of "new" surface antigens that allow identification. There is a growing body of evidence to support the view that this is a vital function of the immune system. Patients in whom the cellular immune system is impaired (immunosuppressed) or defective (immunodeficient) for significant periods are at especially high risk of certain neoplastic diseases. To these data are coupled the observation that cancers are most prone to appear early in life before the immune system is fully functional or in later life as the system becomes less effective.

Cancers may become established in the body by escaping the surveillance mechanisms or by growing so rapidly that they outdistance the immune system's ability to respond. Experimentally if a few thousand tumor cells are transferred from one animal to a noncancerous animal, the latter is capable of responding and destroying the tumor; however, if the tumor cell load is increased to several billion cells, the tumor may become established. The humoral immune system may actually serve to protect the developing cancer by producing noncytotoxic antibodies *(enhancing antibodies)* that coat the tumor cell surfaces and mask the surface from recognition by sensitized lymphocytes. As a tumor grows it is capable of both specific and nonspecific suppression of the immune system. This further reduces the effectiveness of a response. For example, as the tumor burden increases, the ability to respond to dinitrochlorobenzene (DNCB) type IV hypersensitivity decreases.

Some of the new surface antigens (known as *tumor specific transplantation antigens* (TSTA) appearing on the cancerous cell are shed into the circulation and can be immunologically detected there. Some of these antigens such as carcinoembryonic antigen (CEA) and alpha-fetoprotein (α-FP) are present during fetal development but are not expressed in the adult. The reappearance lends support to the theory that cancer represents a dedifferentiation to a more primitive cell. These antigens, termed oncofetal antigens (OFA), are of some significance in early detection, diagnostic confirmation, and determination of malignant disease progress.

Some very early progress has been made in stimulating, both specifically and nonspecifically, the body's immunologic response to cancers in the hope of preventing further growth of the tumors. With further knowledge of both the cancer process and the immune response mechanisms, the possibility of utilizing immunotherapy, immunoprophylaxis, and immunodiagnosis as specific tools against malignancies seems quite realistic.

REFERENCES AND SELECTED READINGS

1. Abdou, N. I., Lisak, R. P., Zweiman, B., et al.: The thymus in myasthenia gravis: evidence for altered cell populations, N. Engl. J. Med. **291**:1271, 1975.
2. Acherson, G. F.: Immunodeficiency disorders, Practioner **214**: 494, 1975.
3. *Alexander, J. W., and Good, R. A.: Fundamentals of clinical immunology, Philadelphia, 1977, W. B. Saunders Co.
4. American Academy of Pediatrics: Report of the Committee on Infectious Disease, ed. 17, Evanston, Ill., 1974, The Academy.
5. Amos, H. E.: Allergic drug reactions, London, 1976, Edward Arnold, Ltd.
6. *Barr, S. E.: Allergy to hymenoptera stings, J.A.M.A. **228**:718, 1974.
7. Barrett, J. T.: Textbook of immunology: an introduction to immunochemistry and immunobiology, ed. 3, St. Louis, 1978, The C. V. Mosby Co.
8. Benacerraf, B.: Immunogenetics and immunodeficiency, Baltimore, 1975, University Park Press.
9. Bernstein, I. D.: Immunologic defenses against cancer, J. Pediatr. **83**:906, 1973.
10. Booth, B., et al.: Modern concepts in clinical allergy, New York, 1973, Medcom Books, Inc.
11. *Boyd, R. F., and Hoerl, B. G.: Basic medical microbiology, Boston, 1977, Little, Brown and Co.
12. Brown, S. M., Stimmel, B., Taub, R. N., et al.: Immunologic dysfunction in heroin addicts, Arch. Intern. Med. **134**:1001, 1974.
13. Buckley, C. E., III, and Roseman, J. M.: Immunity and survival, J. Am. Geriatr. Soc. **24**:241, 1976.
14. *Bunting, F. W.: Immunity against infectious disease, Nurs. Times **67**:634, 1971.
15. *Burke, D. C.: The status of interferon, Sci. Am. **236**:42, 1977.
16. *Burnet, F. M.: Immunology, San Francisco, 1976, W. H. Freeman and Co.
17. Burnet, F. M.: Auto-immunity and autoimmune disease, Philadelphia, 1972, F. A. Davis Co.
18. *Child, J., Collins, D., and Collins, J.: Blood transfusions, Am. J. Nurs. **72**:1602, 1972.
19. *Cleland, V., Cox, F., Berggren, H., et al.: Prevention of bacteriuria in female patients with indwelling catheters, Nurs. Res. **20**:318, 1971.

*References preceded by an asterisk are particularly well suited for student reading.

20. Cochrane, C. G., and Koffler, D.: Immune complex disease in experimental animals and man, Adv. Immunol. **16**:186, 1973.
21. *Craven, R. F.: Anaphylactic shock, Am. J. Nurs. **72**:718, 1972.
22. *Cunningham, B. A.: The structure and function of histocompatibility antigens, Sci. Am. **237**:96, 1977.
23. Danilevicius, Z.: HL-A system and rheumatic disease, J.A.M.A. **231**:283, 1975.
24. *Dharan, M.: Immunoglobulin abnormalities, Am. J. Nurs. **76**:1626, 1976.
25. *Donley, D. L.: Nursing the patient who is immunosuppressed, Am. J. Nurs. **76**:1619, 1976.
26. Edelman, G. M.: Antibody structure and molecular immunology, Science **180**:290, 1973.
27. Eisen, H. N.: Immunology, New York, 1974, Harper & Row, Publishers.
28. Evans, H. E., Akpata, S. O., Baki, A., et al.: Flora in newborn infants: annual variation in prevalence of *Staphylococcus aureus, Escherichia coli*, and streptococci, Arch. Environ. Health **26**:275, 1973.
29. Fahey, J. L., Brossman, S., Ossorio, R. C., et al.: Immunotherapy and human tumor immunology, Ann. Intern. Med. **84**:454, 1976.
30. Faktor, M. A., et al.: Hypersensitivity to tetanus toxoid, J. Allergy Clin. Immunol. **52**:1, 1973.
31. *Faulk, W. P., Demaeyer, E. M., and Davies, A. J.: Some effects of malnutrition on immune response in man, Am. J. Clin. Nutr. **27**:638, 1974.
32. *Francis, B. J.: Current concepts in immunization, Am. J. Nurs. **73**:646, 1973.
33. Gatti, R. A., and Good, R. A.: Occurrences of malignancy in immunodeficiency diseases, Cancer **28**: 89, 1971.
34. Gell, P. G. H., et al.: Clinical aspects of immunology, ed. 3, Oxford, 1975, Blackwell Scientific Publications.
35. Gordon, B. L.: Essentials of immunology, ed. 2, Philadelphia, 1974, F. A. Davis Co.
36. *Hardy, C. S.: Infection control: what can one nurse do?, Nursing '73 **3**:18, 1973.
37. Heath, R. G., and Krupp, I. M.: Schizophrenia as an immunologic disorder, Arch. Gen. Psychiatr. **16**:1, 1967.
38. Idsoe, O., Guthe, T., Wilcox, R. R., et al.: Nature and extent of penicillin side reactions with particular reference to fatalaties from anaphylactic shock, Bull. W.H.O. **38**:159, 1968.
39. Kaplan, M. M., and Webster, R. G.: The epidemiology of influenza, Sci. Am. **237**:88, 1977.
40. *Kelly, J. F., and Patterson, R.: Anaphylaxis, course, mechanisms, and treatment, J.A.M.A. **227**:1431, 1974.
41. Makinodan, T.: Immunobiology of aging, J. Am. Geriatr. **24**:249, 1976.
42. *Marples, M. J.: Life on the human skin, Sci. Am. **220**:108, 1969.
43. Marx, J. L.: Tumor immunology: the host's response to cancer, Science **184**:552, 1974.
44. *Maugh, T. H.: Leukemia: much is known but the picture is still confused, Science **185**:48, 1974.
45. *McAllen, M. K.: Hayfever, Nurs. Mirror **138**:63, 1974.
46. Medawar, P. B.: The new immunology, Hosp. Prac. **9**:48, 1974.
47. Metz, D. H.: The mechanism of action of interferon, Cell **6**:429, 1975.
48. *Mims, C. A.: The pathogenesis of infectious disease, New York, 1977, Academic Press, Inc.
49. *Moody, L.: Asthma: physiology and patient care, Am. J. Nurs. **73**:1212, 1973.
50. *Morse, L. J., and Schonbeck, L.: Hand-lotions: a potential nosocomial hazard, N. Engl. J. Med. **287**:376, 1968.
51. Murillo, G. J.: Synthesis of secretary IgA by human colostral cells, South. Med. J. **64**:1333, 1971.
52. *Nysather, J. O., Katz, A. E., and Lenth, J. L.: The immune system: its development and function, Am. J. Nurs. **76**:1614, 1976.
52a. *Oettgen, H. F.: Immunotherapy of cancer, N. Engl. J. Med. **297**:484, 1977.
53. *Old, L. J.: Cancer immunology, Sci. Am. **236**:62, 1977.
54. Park, A. K., et al.: Immunosuppressive effect of surgery, Lancet **1**:53, 1971.
55. Pierce, J. C., Madge, G. E., Lee, H. M., et al.: Lymphoma, a complication of renal allotransplantation in man, J.A.M.A. **219**:1593, 1972.
56. Remington, J. S.: The compromised host, Hosp. Pract. **7**:59, 1972.
57. Richards, F. F., Konigsberg, W. H., Rosenstein, R. W., et al.: On the specificity of antibodies, Science **187**:130, 1975.
58. Roberts-Thomson, I. C., Whittingham, S., Youngchaiynd, U., et al.: Aging, immune response and mortality, Lancet **2**:368, 1974.
59. *Roitt, I. M.: Essential immunology, ed. 2, Oxford, 1975, Blackwell Scientific Publications.
60. Rose, N. R., and Friedman, H.: Manual of clinical immunology, Washington, 1976, American Society for Microbiology.
60a. *Rosenberg, L. E., and Kidd, K. K.: HLA and disease susceptibility, N. Engl. J. Med. **297**:1060, 1977.
61. Sell, S.: Immunology, immunopathology, and immunity, ed. 2, New York, 1975, Harper & Row, Publishers.
62. *Shaffer, J. H., and Sweet, L. C.: Allergic reactions to drugs, Am. J. Nurs. **65**:100, 1965.
63. Smith, A. L.: Microbiology and pathology, ed. 11, St. Louis, 1976, The C. V. Mosby Co.
64. Solomon, G. F., and Amkraut, A. A.: Emotions, stress and immunity, Front. Rad. Ther. Onc. **7**:84, 1974.
65. Stossel, T. P.: Phagocytosis, N. Engl. J. Med. **290**:833, 1974.
66. Tarnawski, A., and Balko, B.: Antibiotics and immune processes, Lancet **1**:674, 1973.
67. Thaler, M. S., et al.: Medical immunology, Philadelphia, 1977, J. B. Lippincott Co.
68. Weiss, H. J.: Aspirin: a dangerous drug? J.A.M.A. **229**:1221, 1974.
69. Yunis, E. J., Fernandes, G., and Greenberg, L. J.: Tumor immunology, autoimmunity and aging, J. Am. Geriatr. **24**:253, 1976.
70. Zweifach, B. W., et al.: The inflammatory process, ed. 2, New York, 1974, Academic Press, Inc.

15

Mechanisms for maintaining dynamic equilibrium

VIRGINIA CASSMEYER

Humans live in two environments, an external one that is changing constantly and a much more stable internal environment. The human machinery, steered by the integrative mechanisms (see Chapter 13), is constantly adapting to changes on the cellular level to maintain a stable environment. Cellular growth and functioning can occur only when the internal environment has an adequate supply of oxygen, nutrients, and electrolytes. The amount and characteristics of body fluid bathing the cells must be kept relatively stable to provide the cells with the requirements necessary for survival and growth. The process of maintaining this relatively constant environment is the process of *dynamic equilibrium*. Functioning body systems that can provide oxygen and remove carbon dioxide, provide nutrients, maintain fluid and electrolyte balance, excrete waste, and transport needed products to cells and waste products to elimination sites are necessary to maintain dynamic equilibrium.

The nurse must know how body systems function to maintain dynamic equilibrium in order to help persons maintain health and to give supportive nursing care when disease or injury upsets the body's ability to maintain its checks and balances.

■ MAINTAINING ADEQUATE OXYGEN–CARBON DIOXIDE EXCHANGE

□ Cellular need for oxygen

Maintenance of adequate oxygen–carbon dioxide exchange is dependent on the process of respiration. Of all body functions involved in maintaining cellular growth and functioning, the maintenance of normal respiration probably has the greatest immediate significance. All body functions require energy. The most important energy component in cellular work is adenosine triphosphate (ATP).

ATP is formed from the metabolism of carbohydrates (CHO), fats, and proteins. Carbohydrates, fats, and proteins are catabolized completely to carbon dioxide, water, and ATP only if there is an adequate supply of oxygen. For example, in the absence of oxygen 1 molecule of glucose yields only 2 molecules of ATP, whereas in the presence of oxygen 1 molecule of glucose can proceed through the Krebs cycle to yield 38 molecules of ATP.

The metabolism of neutral fat to produce ATP also requires oxygen. Neutral fat is first broken down into glycerol and fatty acids. The glycerol enters the glycolytic pathway and the fatty acid is then broken down to acetyl coenzyme A (acetyl CoA) and carrier $—H_2$ molecule.[75] The acetyl CoA enters the Krebs cycle and in the presence of oxygen releases ATP. The carrier $—H_2$ molecule in the presence of oxygen transfers hydrogen to the electron transport chain and ATP is synthesized.

Proteins not necessary for growth and repair of body tissues are broken down into intermediary metabolites that enter the Krebs cycle and synthesize ATP. As is true with carbohydrate and fat metabolism, oxygen is necessary for this synthesis to occur. The reader is advised to consult physiology and biochemistry texts for more detailed information.

□ Mechanisms for providing oxygen

The oxygen necessary to maintain adequate levels of ATP for energy and thus for cellular function must be obtained from the environment and transported to the cells. This is accomplished through the process of *respiration*. Respiration is defined as the gas exchange (O_2 and CO_2) between an organism and its environment. There are three components of respiration: *ventilation*, *perfusion*, and *diffusion*.

Ventilation

Ventilation is a mechanical process by which air is moved in and out of the lungs. There are two phases to ventilation: inspiration and expiration.

Inspiration occurs because of rhythmic impulses arising from the inspiratory center in the medulla that stimulate the phrenic and intercostal nerves. Stimulation of the phrenic nerves causes the diaphragm to contract and move downward. Stimulation of the intercostal nerves causes the external intercostal muscles to contract, moving the ribs upward and out. The net result is an enlarged thoracic cavity and a decrease in the intraalveolar (intrapulmonary) pressure to less than atmospheric pressure (760 mm Hg), and air moves into the lungs.

As the lung tissue is stretched, the *Hering-Breuer* stretch receptors are stimulated. Impulses from the stretch receptors are transmitted by way of the vagus nerve to the inspiratory center in the medulla. The center sends inhibitory impulses to the inspiratory center to inhibit further lung expansion. The elastic recoil of the alveoli and chest wall returns the chest to its normal resting positon and *expiration* occurs.

Control of breathing

In addition to the neural controls described above, breathing is influenced by the levels of CO_2 and pH in the cerebral spinal fluid. The normal stimulus for respiration is CO_2. However, when CO_2 is retained in the alveoli and the level of CO_2 rises, the respiratory center can become depressed by too high levels of CO_2, resulting in a condition known as *CO_2 narcosis*. In this situation the *peripheral chemoreceptors* in the carotid and aortic bodies, which are sensitive to decreases in arterial oxygen tension, stimulate the respiratory center to maintain breathing. Since respiration in this situation is being maintained by a decrease in the Po_2, it is important that high doses of oxygen not be administered to these patients or the mechanism that is keeping them breathing will be removed. In patients with the potential for developing CO_2 narcosis, only low-flow oxygen (1 to 3 liters/minute) is administered (p. 1135). If the oxygen needs cannot be met with low-flow oxygen, mechanical ventilation is necessary (p. 935). A summary of the neural and chemical influences on the respiratory center is presented in Fig. 15-1.

Perfusion

Perfusion is the movement of blood to and from the alveolar capillary bed. The pulmonary circulation is derived from the main pulmonary artery, which receives

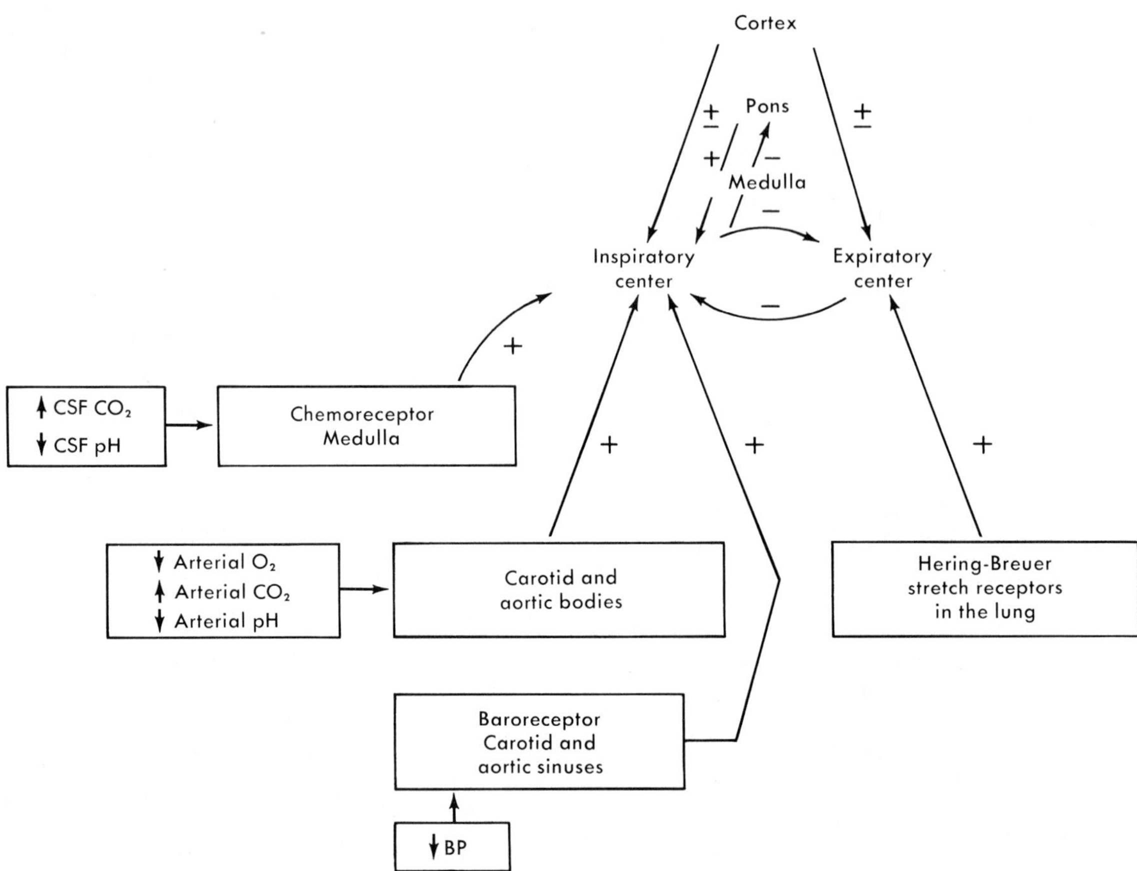

Fig. 15-1. Nervous and chemical influences on medullary center. +, stimulates; −, inhibits.

venous blood from the *right* ventricle. The pulmonary artery branches following the bronchial tree to form the capillary plexus surrounding the alveoli. The capillary plexus reunites to form the pulmonary vein, which returns blood to the *left* side of the heart.

The pulmonary vascular bed is a low-pressure system as compared with the systemic circulation. The pulmonary capillaries are surrounded only by gas, and they collapse or distend if the pressure within or outside of them changes. The pulmonary capillary vascular bed is responsive to changes in alveolar oxygen levels, blood pH, and sympathetic outflow. The perfusion of all the alveoli is not uniform, and at any one time not all alveoli are being perfused. The important determinant of oxygen–carbon dioxide exchange is the ratio of ventilation to perfusion. This ratio is usually designated by symbols: ventilation by $\dot{V}$ (gas volume per unit of time) and perfusion by $\dot{Q}$ (volume flow of blood per unit of time). The normal $\dot{V}/\dot{Q}$ is about 1. This is derived from the fact that $\dot{V}$ is normally 500 ml/minute (tidal volume) and $\dot{Q}$ is normally about 600 ml/minute. Certain disease processes cause changes in ventilation, perfusion, or both (see Chapter 50 for discussion).

Diffusion

Diffusion is the process by which oxygen and carbon dioxide are exchanged across the alveolar-capillary membrane. Oxygen and carbon dioxide diffusion is passive, since the two gases diffuse with a pressure gradient (from greater pressure to less pressure). Fig. 15-2 shows the Po_2 and Pco_2 levels in the alveolus and the capillary. Diffusion is a rapid process, and oxygen enters the red blood cell in less than 1 second.[79] Carbon dioxide diffuses about 20 times faster than oxygen. The diffusion of oxygen into blood is limited only by the amount of perfusion. After oxygen diffuses into the blood it reacts with hemoglobin to form oxyhemoglobin. It is in this manner that the majority of oxygen is carried to the tissue.

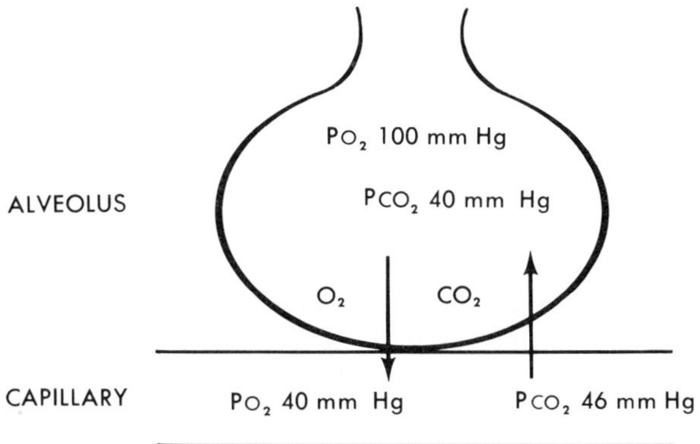

Fig. 15-2. Oxygen and carbon dioxide levels in alveolus and pulmonary capillaries.

Oxygen deficit or carbon dioxide excess or both can be caused by a variety of conditions that interfere with ventilation, perfusion, or diffusion (see box below). In addition anemia can lead to oxygen deficit, since the amount of hemoglobin present is inadequate to carry the amount of oxygen necessary for cellular metabolism.

Early signs of inadequate oxygenation include restlessness, dyspnea, tachycardia, and confusion. Although cyanosis is a classic sign of hypoxia, it is unreliable because it does not occur until there are 5 g or more of reduced hemoglobin in the blood. Also severe hypoxia may be present even when arterial oxygen level is satisfactory, as occurs in polycythemia. In the presence of hypoxia the nurse carries out measures to enhance optimum oxygenation such as positioning to facilitate breathing and assisting the patient to clear and maintain the airway and to perform appropriate breathing exercises. When these measures are not effective, nasotracheal suctioning (p. 960) and ventilatory support (p. 955) may be necessary.

Adequate respiration is necessary not only to maintain adequate oxygen levels but also to maintain acid-base balance. The respiratory system helps eliminate acids by the excretion of carbon dioxide. In conditions leading to hyperventilation the level of carbon dioxide and thus the hydrogen ion level decreases, causing respiratory alkalosis. In some diseases carbon dioxide is trapped in the alveoli, and the serum level of carbon dioxide and hydrogen ions increases, causing respiratory acidosis.

CAUSES OF OXYGEN DEFICIT OR CARBON DIOXIDE EXCESS FROM INTERFERENCE WITH VENTILATION, PERFUSION OR DIFFUSION

Ventilation

Inhibition of thorax or lung (bronchioles, alveoli) expansion
Decrease in elastic recoil

Perfusion

Circulatory collapse, shock
Blockage of pulmonary capillaries (emboli)
Compression of pulmonary capillary bed (increase in alveolar pressure)
Vasoconstriction from alveolar hypoxia
Decrease in blood pH
Destruction of capillary bed

Diffusion

Decrease in alveolar surface area; thickening of alveolar membrane
Increase in fluid/secretions in interstitial space or alveoli

The respiratory system also serves as a compensatory mechanism for metabolic acid-base imbalances. In metabolic acidosis the respiratory system can excrete increased amounts of hydrogen ions in the form of carbon dioxide. Respirations will be deep and rapid (Kussmaul breathing). In metabolic alkalosis the respiratory system can conserve increased amounts of hydrogen in the form of carbon dioxide. Respirations will then be slow and shallow.

■ MAINTAINING ADEQUATE NUTRIENT LEVELS

□ Basal metabolic needs

Adequate energy production requires adequate nutrients such as carbohydrates, fats, and proteins in addition to its oxygen requirements. Enzymes (biologic catalysts) are also essential ingredients for producing energy. Enzymes are special proteins built under genetic control, and some of them function only when specific minerals and vitamins (coenzymes) are available. Thus for adequate energy production all nutrients must be available.

The healthy man of average size who lives in a moderate climate needs 1,500 calories a day to maintain the basic functions essential to life, that is, those functions that continue even while a person is at rest. Basic caloric needs vary with age, sex, body size, climate, and body temperature. Additional physical activities require additional calories. Normally an adequate diet with selections of food from the various food groups will supply the energy needs and provide nutrients for cell growth.

The body always meets its energy needs before nutrients are used for any other purpose. Extra caloric intake is necessary in any situation in which extra energy is being used either because of increased physical activity or illness. Energy production is so important that if adequate nutrients are unavailable from outside sources or if the body is unable to utilize the nutrients, the body will burn its own tissue. The normal body usually has stores of excess nutrients in the form of fats and glycogen, and these can meet energy needs for a short time, but eventually tissue breakdown *(catabolism)* due to burning of body protein will occur. Some diseases lead to specific abnormalities. For example, in diabetes mellitus (a condition in which carbohydrates are not metabolized effectively) excess fats are burned for energy. Because the body is unable to dispose of the increased acid end products of fat metabolism, acidosis may develop (p. 327). The same situation occurs with starvation. In other diseases (renal failure and cirrhosis) the body may be unable to handle the nitrogen waste products, and protein must be restricted. Only minimal amounts of proteins are then available for cell growth and repair. If enough calories are not ingested in the form of carbohydrates or fats, however, the protein ingested will be used for energy and nitrogen waste products will accumulate.

□ Effects of stress on nutrient needs

Under all conditions of stress some of the body's proteins will be burned. When there is extensive tissue damage, this metabolic process seems to be accelerated and usually continues for 7 to 10 days despite adequate intake of food. The acceleration is probably due to the action of the adrenocortical hormones. The burning of proteins can cause serious chemical imbalances because of the loss of large amounts of nitrogen and potassium. For the kidneys to be able to handle the increased amounts of urea (end products of protein catabolism) an increased fluid intake is necessary. The adrenocortical hormones tend to cause sodium and water retention; therefore in stress situations when intravenous fluids are often required there is an increased risk of circulatory overload. The status of the patient must be monitored closely so that signs of fluid overload can be detected early.

When calories cannot be taken by the alimentary route, calories are provided parenterally. It is not possible to meet even the basic energy requirements of a person by the administration of glucose alone. For example, 1,000 ml of 5% dextrose in water contains 50 g of glucose, or the equivalent of 200 calories. To provide even basic caloric needs for the average man 7,500 ml of fluid would be needed. This amount of fluid would severely compromise the circulatory system. For this reason total parenteral nutrition (hyperalimentation), which can supply approximately 1,000 calories/liter of fluid, is being more widely used when persons must be maintained on parenteral nutrition for a prolonged period (p. 321).

Amino acids that can be given parenterally are not complete proteins; therefore they cannot be used to synthesize proteins. For this reason it is important to resume feeding orally as soon as possible.

The metabolic process by which proteins are synthesized is called *anabolism.* All body cells are basically proteins, and anabolism makes possible the development of new cells for tissue growth and repair. Anabolism cannot take place until energy requirements are met.

A nutritious diet should be given as soon as the patient is able to tolerate it. The diet needs to be relatively high in calories (2,000 to 3,000 calories per day) despite limited physical activity because extra energy is being expended by the increased metabolism secondary to stress (early) and tissue repair (later). The diet should also be high in protein. Persons who are ill at home or are returning home after an illness are instructed to continue this high-caloric diet until they regain their normal weight. Caloric and protein intake should then be reduced to normal. When it is expected that someone will be unable to eat for several days, as after certain surgical procedures, special emphasis is placed on maximizing nutritional status preoperatively (see Chapter 23).

■ MAINTAINING FLUID AND ELECTROLYTE BALANCE

In order to survive, body cells must be bathed in a normal fluid and electrolyte concentration. In health, fluid and electrolyte balance is maintained without difficulty by multiple body systems. As mentioned (p. 206), any stressor can cause some fluid and electrolyte imbalance. Normal fluid and electrolyte *balance* are discussed next; fluid and electrolyte *imbalance* are discussed in Chapter 20.

□ Body fluid and electrolyte compartments, distribution, and functions

Fluid and electrolytes are found in the body either within the cell *(intracellular)* or outside the cell *(extracellular)*. The extracellular fluid is contained in two compartments: the *interstitial* fluid (fluid between the cells) and the *intravascular* fluid (fluid in the blood vessels). A third type of fluid, *transcellular*, denotes fluid separated by a layer of epithelial cells from other extracellular fluid.[45] Transcellular fluid includes digestive juices, water and solutes in the renal tubules and bladder, intraocular fluid, and cerebral spinal fluid. Some authorities consider this to be a part of the extracellular compartment, and others consider it to be a separate compartment. Transcellular fluid makes up 1% to 3% of body weight.

Body water is the largest single constituent of the body, representing 45% to 75% of body weight. The volume and distribution of body water varies with age and sex (Fig. 15-3). In the newborn infant almost three fourths of the body weight is water, with the greatest percentage found in the extracellular compartment. The volume and distribution change over time, and by adulthood in the young male only 60% of body weight is water and two thirds of this is in the intracellular compartment. In the average young female only approximately 50% of body weight is water. This difference between males and females is due to increased amount of fat in the female. Fat is essentially water free.

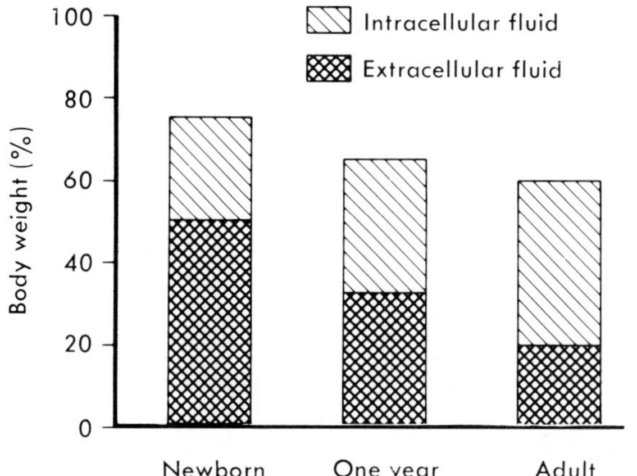

Fig. 15-3. In newborn more than half of total body fluid is extracellular. As child grows, proportions gradually approximate adult levels.

Body water has multiple functions. The extracellular water maintains blood volume and serves as the body's transport system to and from cells. Intracellular fluid provides the internal aqueous medium for cellular chemical function. Adequate body water balance is necessary for the maintenance of normal body temperature and for the elimination of waste products.

All body fluids contain electrolytes. Electrolytes are chemical compounds in solution that have the ability to conduct an electrical current. In solution electrolytes break into charged particles called *ions*. Positively charged ions are called *cations*, and negatively charged ions are called *anions*. Electrolytes are distributed in different concentrations in the intracellular, intravascular, and interstitial compartments (Table 15-1). Transcellular fluids have very distinct patterns of electrolyte concentration. For example, gastric secretions have a high hydrogen ion concentration, pancreatic secretions have a high bicarbonate concentration, and renal tubular and bladder fluid vary on a daily basis. Gastric, pancreatic, and intestinal juices and bile all contain high concentrations of sodium. In all fluid compartments, although the concentration of electrolytes will vary, electrical neutrality will be maintained; that is, the solution will contain equal quantities of anions and cations.

Each electrolyte has specific functions. The general functions of all electrolytes are to (1) promote neuromuscular irritability, (2) maintain body fluid volume and osmolality, (3) distribute body water between fluid compartments, and (4) regulate acid-base balance.

□ Normal exchange of fluid and electrolytes

In health body fluids (water and electrolytes) are constantly being lost and must be replaced in order to maintain normal processes. The fluid that is lost is not "pure water" but always contains some electrolytes; thus both water and electrolytes must be replaced daily. By knowing the concentration of fluid and electrolytes in the various compartments, the nurse can anticipate which fluid and electrolyte imbalance will most probably occur if abnormal losses occur from any particular site.

Loss and gain

In a state of health body fluids are lost daily from the kidneys, lungs, gastrointestinal tract, and skin, with neg-

Table 15-1. Normal electrolyte content of body fluids*

Electrolytes (anions and cations)	Extracellular: Intravascular (mEq/liter)	Extracellular: Interstitial (mEq/liter)	Intracellular (mEq/liter)
Sodium (Na^+)	142	146	15
Potassium (K^+)	5	5	150
Calcium (Ca^{++})	5	3	2
Magnesium (Mg^{++})	2	1	27
Chloride (Cl^-)	102	114	1
Bicarbonate (HCO_3^-)	27	30	10
Protein ($Prot^-$)	16	1	63
Phosphate ($HPO_4^=$)	2	2	100
Sulfate ($SO_4^=$)	1	1	20
Organic acids	5	8	0

*Note that the electrolyte level of the intravascular and interstitial fluids (extracellular) is approximately the same and that sodium and chloride contents are markedly higher in these fluids, whereas potassium, phosphate, and protein contents are markedly higher in intracellular fluid.

Table 15-2. Normal fluid intake and loss in an adult eating 2,500 calories/day (approximate figures)

Intake: Route	Intake: Amount of gain (ml)	Output: Route	Output: Amount of loss (ml)
Water in food	1,000	Skin	500
Water from oxidation	300	Lungs	350
Water as liquid	1,200	Feces	150
		Kidney	1,500
TOTAL	2,500	TOTAL	2,500

ligible amounts being lost in saliva and tears. Two processes demand continual expenditure of water: control of body heat and excretion of metabolic waste products. The volume of fluid used in these processes depends on such things as external temperature, humidity, metabolic rate, and physical activities. In normal fluid balance the output of fluid equals the intake of water. In addition a balanced diet (see Chapter 51) provides excess amounts of electrolytes; the excess is excreted, and electrolyte balance is maintained.

Table 15-2 summarizes the normal routes of gains and losses in an adult eating approximately 2,500 calories per day. It should be noted that approximately two fifths of the normal fluid intake are obtained from water in food, or "preformed water." Solid foods such as meat and vegetables are 60% to 90% water. The fact that a large quantity of water is obtained from food has important implications if a person's food intake decreases substantially.

Approximately two fifths of the fluid lost daily is lost through the insensible route (skin, lungs, and gastrointestinal tract). Insensible loss through the skin refers to invisible perspiration. When visible perspiration occurs, such as that following heavy physical activities or with shock, the loss of water through the skin is greater than the normal 500 ml. Fecal loss increases in the presence of diarrhea or watery stools. Persons with certain pulmonary problems lose more than the normal amount of fluid (350 ml) during respiration. Increased loss of fluids through these insensible routes also results in the loss of electrolytes.

□ Internal regulation of body water and electrolytes

Fluid and electrolyte balance is dependent on an adequate intake and output. This means that the intake must equal the output. The control of intake and output is regulated by various internal mechanisms. In this section the regulation of body water and major electrolytes is discussed. The reader is referred to physiology texts for a more in-depth review.

Sodium and water

Thirst. The major control of actual fluid intake is thirst. The thirst center in the brain is stimulated by extracellular and intracellular fluid loss, decreased cardiac output, dryness of the mouth, and angiotensin (p. 209). How these factors cause the thirst center to be stimulated is not fully understood. It is felt that when the cells in the thirst center become dehydrated (shrink), this causes stimulation of the neurons, which creates the sensation of thirst. Most of the time thirst is not thought of as a control because social and cultural habits greatly influence the quantity of liquid humans drink. Persons who are dependent on others to supply their intake of fluid or persons who have a sudden increase in fluid loss

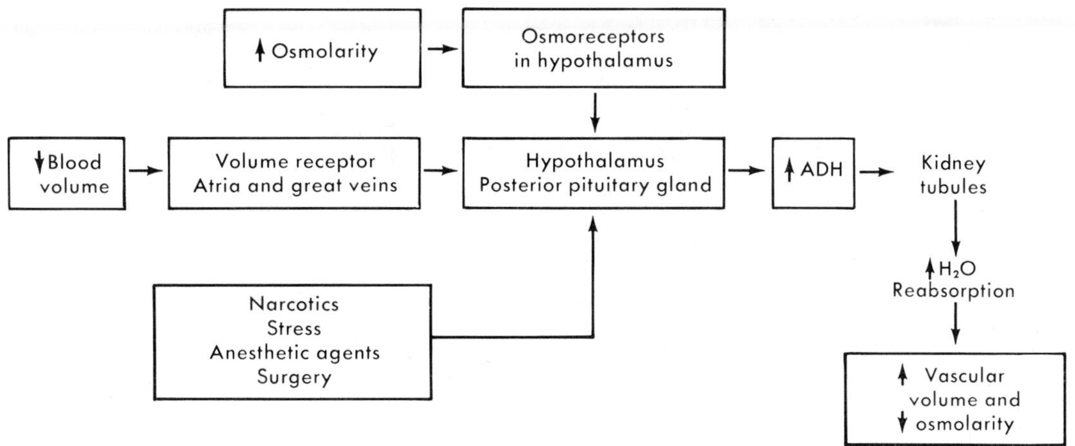

Fig. 15-4. Factors and mechanisms involved in ADH production and effect of ADH.

(bleeding, increased sweating) will complain of being thirsty. Also there is some evidence that humans have a salt appetite; that is, when persons are deprived of or have a deficit in salt, they will have a craving for salt.

Kidney. The major organ controlling output is the kidney, which is under the influence of several control mechanisms. The kidney is responsible for regulating the volume and osmolarity of body fluids. The osmolarity of body fluids is predominantly dependent on sodium and its associate anions. The maintenance of water and sodium balance is dependent on glomerular filtration rate (GFR), antidiuretic hormone (ADH), and the aldosterone-renin-angiotensin system.

Glomerular filtration. Glomerular filtration is an involved topic, and the reader is urged to consult references 45, 75, and 76 for more information. Three factors determine glomerular filtration: glomerular capillary blood pressure, Bowman's capsule hydrostatic pressure, and plasma protein concentration. Many factors and pathophysiologic states can affect these three factors and thus change glomerular filtration. Diseases such as shock and hypertension change glomerular capillary blood pressure. Changes in Bowman's capsule pressure can be caused by urinary obstruction. Protein deficiency can occur with increased loss, decreased intake, or decreased production.

Antidiuretic hormone. ADH is a hormone produced by the hypothalamus and released from the posterior pituitary gland. The neurons in the hypothalamus receive input from volume receptors in the left atrium and great veins and from osmoreceptors in the hypothalamus. Volume receptors are stimulated by changes in atrial blood volume. Impulses from the volume receptors are transmitted by afferent nerve fibers to the hypothalamus. Increased volume increases the firing of the volume receptors, stimulates the hypothalamus, and inhibits ADH production. Conversely, decreased blood pressure decreases the firing of the volume receptors and increases ADH production.

Osmoreceptors are stimulated by changes in cell size. If pure water is added to the body fluids, this changes the size of the cells in the osmoreceptors and leads to the inhibition of ADH production. A loss of pure water causes the cells to shrink and stimulates the secretion of ADH. ADH secretion is also stimulated by angiotensin, narcotics, stress, and anesthetic agents. Fig. 15-4 depicts the factors and mechanisms involved in ADH production and the results of ADH production.

ADH causes the renal tubules to conserve water. The conservation of water increases blood volume and blood pressure and decreases osmolarity. Since ADH can be secreted in response to factors other than a deficit of water (narcotics, anesthetic agents, stress) fluid overload can occur. Patients who are at high risk of inappropriate ADH secretion need to be monitored closely by the nurse. This would include postoperative patients (see Chapter 23).

Aldosterone-renin-angiotensin system. Aldosterone is a hormone produced by the adrenal cortex. It affects the kidney's reabsorption of sodium and thus water. In the complete absence of aldosterone a person may excrete 25 g of sodium per day, whereas if large quantities of aldosterone are present no sodium will be excreted.

The major stimulus for aldosterone production is a reflex initiated by the kidney. Cells in the kidney monitor sodium levels and blood volume. When the serum sodium level or the blood volume decreases, the juxtaglomerular cells in the kidney secrete a protein, *renin.*

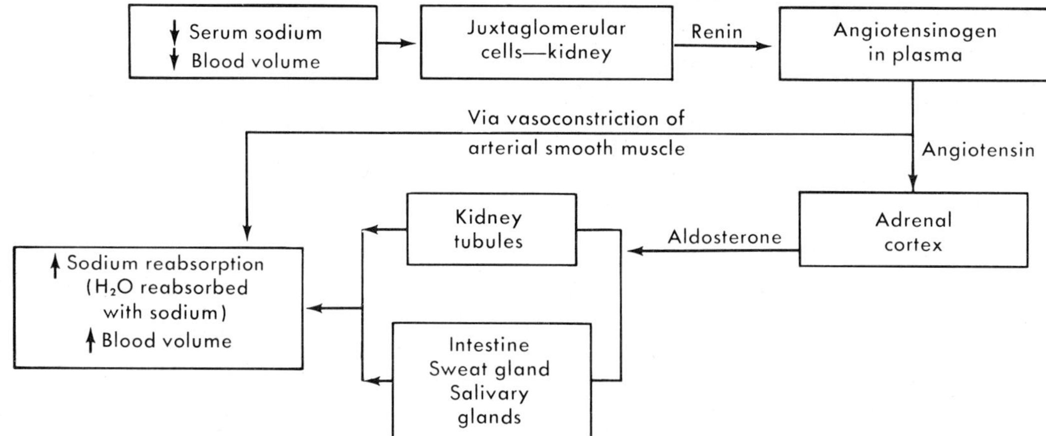

Fig. 15-5. Factors and mechanisms involved in aldosterone production and effects of aldosterone production.

Renin acts as an enzyme that splits off a small polypeptide, *angiotensin,* from the plasma protein *angiotensinogen.* Angiotensinogen is produced by the liver and is circulating in the blood at all times. It is only activated by renin. Angiotensin stimulates the adrenal cortex to secrete aldosterone. Aldosterone causes the retention of sodium by the kidneys, intestines, and sweat and salivary glands. In addition angiotensin causes vasoconstriction of arterial smooth muscles, thus decreasing the glomerular filtration rate. Aldosterone is also secreted in response to ACTH (p. 161). Another important fact is that aldosterone is catabolized by the liver, and with liver failure inappropriate amounts of aldosterone may lead to sodium and water retention because of ineffective catabolism. Fig. 15-5 depicts the factors and mechanisms involved in aldosterone production and the effects of aldosterone production.

Third factor. Glomerular filtration, ADH, and the aldosterone-renin-angiotensin system do not explain the kidney's complete control of sodium and water reabsorption and excretion. It is hypothesized that a "third factor" is involved in the control of sodium and water balance.[75,76] The term *third factor* is used because there is little known about this mechanism. At present there seems to be three other factors that assist in the control of sodium and water: (1) a natriuretic hormone, (2) intrarenal physical factors, and (3) redistribution of blood flow. Research is ongoing in this area.

Potassium

Potassium (K^+) is the major intracellular cation and regulates intracellular osmolarity. Potassium is very important in conduction of nerve impulses and promotion of proper skeletal and cardiac muscle activity. Because of potassium's role in the excitability of nerves and muscles, it is important that the extracellular concentration of potassium be maintained within the normal range.

The major excretion site of excess potassium is the kidney. The majority of excess potassium (80% to 90%) is excreted in the urine, and the remainder is excreted by the gastrointestinal tract. Potassium is completely filtered by the kidney, but most of the potassium filtered is reabsorbed in the proximal tubules and the loop of Henle. Glomerular filtration of potassium plays only a minimal role in normal potassium excretion. The control of renal excretion of potassium resides in the distal tubular cells' ability to secrete potassium into tubular fluid. As extracellular potassium levels rise more potassium moves into all cells including the distal tubular cells. This higher concentration in the cells facilitates potassium secretion into tubular fluid because of the gradient difference between the distal tubular cell and the fluid in the tubular lumen. Conversely, if potassium intake is low or if there is increased loss of potassium through the gastrointestinal tract the potassium level in the distal tubular cell is decreased. This causes a decrease in the gradient, and less potassium is secreted.

Even though glomerular filtration plays only a minimal role in the amount of potassium excreted in the urine, it is an important point to remember. Certain situations interfere with the reabsorption of the filtered potassium in the proximal tubules, and this can lead to an increased loss of potassium. Osmotic diuretics and disease states that produce osmotic diuresis are examples of situations in which there is interference with the reabsorption of potassium in the proximal tubules.

Aldosterone can increase the amount of potassium secreted by the distal tubules. The aldosterone-secreting cells of the adrenal cortex are sensitive to the extracellular concentration of potassium. If the extracellular concentration of potassium increases, aldosterone is produced and stimulates the distal tubular cells to secrete more potassium. The renin-angiotensin system is not involved in this stimulation of aldosterone.

It is apparent that a conflict arises when potassium levels and sodium levels are high, since these changes stimulate aldosterone production to move in different ways. What happens in such a situation is unknown. This is not the only conflict that can arise between different electrolytes. Hydrogen ion concentration affects potassium levels. The existence of a low hydrogen ion concentration increases potassium excretion and leads to potassium depletion. The presence of a high hydrogen ion concentration decreases potassium excretion and can cause potassium excess (hyperkalemia).

Calcium and phosphorus

Calcium (Ca^{++}) plays a major role in the promotion of neuromuscular irritability and muscular contractions. Calcium and phosphorous are found in the body primarily in the bones and teeth (99%) and dissolved in the blood (1%). The amount of dissolved calcium and phosphorous are in an inverse relationship. As one increases the other decreases. The inverse relationship must be maintained because if both are elevated at the same time they form an insoluble precipitate. The dissolved portion of calcium is carried in the blood in two forms: bound to protein and ionized. The serum levels usually reported measure both the ionized portion and the bound portion. Only the ionized fraction is involved in promotion of neuromuscular irritability.

The ionized portion must be maintained within fine limits because a decrease in ionized calcium has profound effects on the body, such as *tetany* (p. 312). The level of calcium is dependent on three hormones: parathormone, vitamin D, and calcitonin. *Parathormone* is a hormone produced by the parathyroid gland, and decreased calcium and possibly increased phosphorous levels stimulate the production of it. Parathormone causes increased movement of calcium from the bone, increased absorption of calcium from the gastrointestinal tract, and increased reabsorption of calcium in the renal tubules, all of which lead to an increase in calcium levels. Parathormone also increases the excretion of phosphorous by the kidneys.

Vitamin D is a hormone that is formed by the action of sunlight on a provitamin in the skin or is obtained from dietary sources. Vitamin D is hydroxylated by reactions in the liver and kidney to its active form. Vitamin D is essential for the absorption of calcium from the gastrointestinal tract. Parathormone cannot increase the absorption of calcium from the gastrointestinal tract unless activated vitamin D is present. Vitamin D also significantly increases the effectiveness of parathormone in bone resorption. In addition vitamin D and parathormone are interlinked in another way. The major control point for the blood concentration of active vitamin D is the hydroxylation step in the kidney, which is stimulated by parathormone. Therefore a low calcium level stimulates the secretion of parathormone, which then activates vitamin D; both then increase the absorption of calcium from the gastrointestinal tract and the resorption of calcium from the bone.

Calcitonin, a hormone produced by the thyroid gland, decreases calcium levels by preventing bone resorption of calcium. It opposes the effects of parathormone and vitamin D. High calcium levels stimulate the thyroid gland to release calcitonin, which inhibits the release of calcium from the bone and thus lowers serum calcium levels.

Acid-base status

Hydrogen ions are vital to life and health. The concentration of hydrogen in the body is far lower than that of other ions (0.00004 mEq/liter). Hydrogen ion concentration is expressed as pH. Normal arterial body pH is 7.35 to 7.45. A reading less than 7.35 is present in acidosis and a reading greater than 7.45 is present in alkalosis. Limits of pH compatible with life are 7.0 to 7.8.

Hydrogen circulates throughout the body fluids in two forms: the volatile hydrogen of carbonic acid and the nonvolatile form of hydrogen in organic acids such as sulfuric, pyruvic, phosphoric, and lactic acids. In a day's time many acids are produced as the end products of metabolism. In the normal person the lungs excrete 13,000 to 30,000 mEq/day of hydrogen in carbonic acid (H_2CO_3), and the kidneys excrete approximately 50 mEq/day of nonvolatile acids.

Buffer systems. The body cells are very sensitive to changes in hydrogen ion concentration (pH), and the pH is kept relatively constant by the *buffer systems* in the body. A buffer is a substance that can act as a chemical sponge, either soaking up or releasing hydrogen ions so that the pH remains stable. The main buffer systems of the extracellular fluid are hemoglobin, protein, and the carbonic acid–bicarbonate buffer system. The carbonic acid–bicarbonate buffer system is the system that is monitored clinically. If this buffer system is stable the other buffer systems are stable.

The ability to maintain a stable pH relies essentially on maintenance of the normal ratio of 20 parts bicarbonate to 1 part carbonic acid. The normal serum bicarbonate is 24 to 28 mEq/liter. The carbonic acid level is determined by taking the P_{CO_2} (normally 40 mm Hg) and multiplying it by the constant 0.03. This constant is the dissolvability factor of a gas. This computation gives an approximate figure of 1.2. From these figures it can be seen that the normal bicarbonate–carbonic acid ratio is 20:1 (Fig. 15-6).

This ratio of 20:1 is maintained by the lungs and the kidneys. The carbonic acid concentration is controlled by the lungs' excretion of the gas carbon dioxide. The depth and rate of respiration changes in response to changes in carbon dioxide (p. 204). The bicarbonate concentration is controlled by the kidneys, which selectively retain or excrete bicarbonate in response to the body's needs.

Compensation. The kidneys and lungs serve a compensatory function in relation to maintaining acid-base balance. Many disease conditions can affect the excretion and retention of carbon dioxide and bicarbonate (see Chapter 20). In a disease state that leads to an acid-base imbalance the normal ratio of 20:1 will be lost. In compensation the system not involved (kidneys or lungs) will conserve or excrete the products it controls to bring the ratio back to normal. Fig. 15-7 illustrates what happens in metabolic acidosis and how compensation of acid-base imbalance can occur.

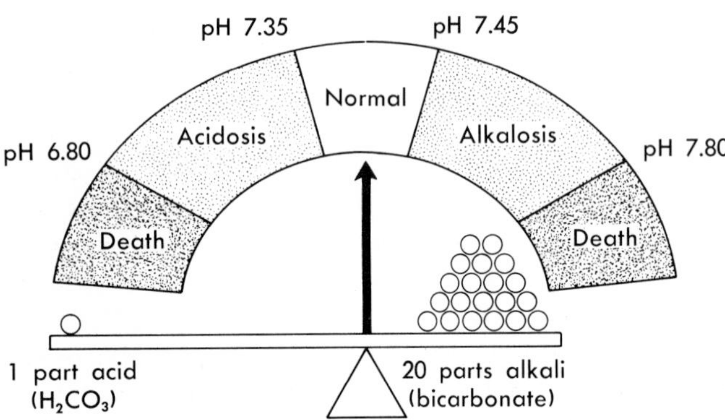

Fig. 15-6. Note that relationship of 1 part carbonic acid to 20 parts bicarbonate will maintain hydrogen ion concentration (pH) within normal limits. Increase in H_2CO_3 or decrease in HCO_3 will cause acidosis; similarly, decrease in H_2CO_3 or increase in HCO_3 will cause alkalosis. (Redrawn from Fluid and electrolytes, Abbott Laboratories, North Chicago, Ill., 1970.)

□ Movement of fluids between compartments

The preceding discussion has referred to the fact that water and solutes are in various compartments. The water and solutes in these compartments are not static but are constantly moving between compartments. The movement of water and solutes is how needed materials are carried to the cells and waste products are removed from the cells.

Fluid and solute transport between the extracellular and intracellular compartments

Fluids and electrolytes flow between the extracellular and intracellular compartments by diffusion, osmosis, and active transport. Some electrolytes and other solutes flow between the two compartments with a concentration gradient by the process of diffusion. Other solutes, to move into the cell, must flow against a concentration gradient by active transport. *Active transport* is not well understood but implies that solutes are moving against a concentration gradient or an electrical potential gradient. The mechanism involves the expenditure of energy. It has been shown that with the expenditure of 1 high-energy phosphate bond from adenosine triphosphate (ATP) (p. 203), 3

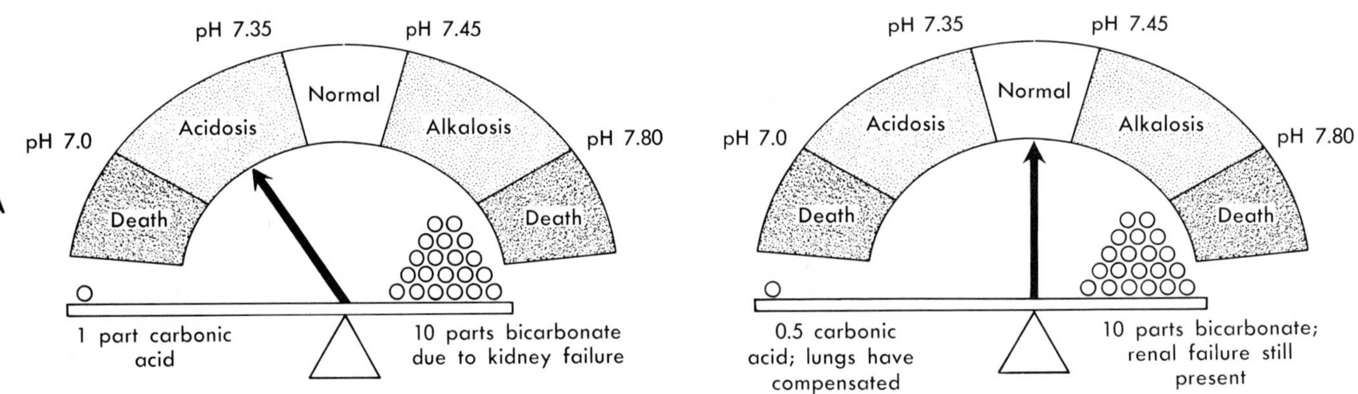

Fig. 15-7. A, Example of metabolic acidosis. Bicarbonate decreased because of renal failure. Carbonic acid normal ratio 10:1; acidosis present. **B,** Example of compensation. Note bicarbonate is still decreased, but now carbonic acid is also decreased. Ratio return to 20:1; pH normal.

sodium ions move out of the cell and 2 potassium ions move into the cell. Active transport uses a large percentage of the energy formed each day because sodium is constantly diffusing into the cell and potassium is constantly diffusing out of the cell. Active transport is required to keep the concentration of the two electrolytes in the appropriate amounts within the cell.

Water, like solutes, moves between the extracellular compartment and the intracellular compartment. The movement of water is controlled by the osmolarity of the two compartments. Osmolarity relates to the number of dissolved particles in the solution (p. 299). Sodium is the main regulator of extracellular osmalarity, and potassium is the main regulator of intracellular osmolarity.

Water moves from an area of high concentration of water (low concentration of solutes) to an area of low concentration of water (high concentration of solutes) This process is called *osmosis*. The movement of water will continue until the osmolarity between the two compartments is approximately equal. Therefore if the water content increases in the extracellular compartment or the solute concentration decreases in the extracellular compartment, water moves into the cells to equalize the osmolarity. Likewise if the water content decreases in the extracellular compartment or the solute concentration increases in the extracellular compartment, water moves from the cells to equalize osmolarity. Solutes are moving back and forth between the two compartments, but the cell membrane is more permeable to water than it is to solutes.

The mechanisms that control water and sodium levels control osmolarity and thus the movement of fluid between the extracellular compartment and the interstitial compartment. Various disease states can change the osmolarity and cause cellular edema or cellular dehydration. These processes are discussed in Chapter 20.

Fluid transport between the vascular and interstitial spaces

The control of fluid movement between the vascular and interstitial spaces is governed by Starling's law of capillaries. Two different types of pressures influence the flow of fluid between the vascular space and the interstitial space. These are hydrostatic pressure and colloid osmotic pressure (oncotic pressure). *Hydrostatic pressure* is that pressure caused by the blood pressing against the walls of the blood vessels. Hydrostatic pressure also exists in the tissue but is very minimal; thus hydrostatic pressure effectively *pushes* fluid out of the vascular bed into the interstitial space.

Colloid osmotic pressure is the pressure needed to overcome the pull of the proteins in the blood. The proteins do not pass freely through the walls of the capillaries because of their size. There are a few proteins in the interstitial space but a much larger concentration is in the vascular space. The colloid osmotic pressure within the vascular space serves as a force to *pull* or *absorb* fluid from the interstitial space.

The difference between the hydrostatic pressure and the colloid osmotic pressure determines the movement of fluid between the vascular and interstitial spaces. The hydrostatic pressure at the arteriole end of the capillary (approximately 32 mm Hg) is greater than the hydrostatic pressure at the venule end of the capillary (approximately 12 mm Hg). The colloid osmotic pressure stays approximately the same throughout the vascular bed and equals about 22 mm Hg.

The difference between the hydrostatic pressure and

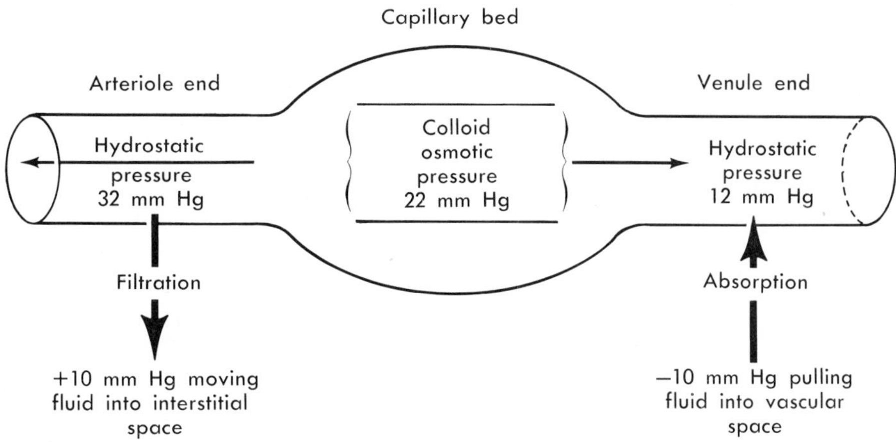

Fig. 15-8. Pressure difference across capillary providing for movement of fluid, nutrients, and waste between interstitial and vascular space.

colloid osmotic pressure at the arteriole end of the capillary is +10 mm Hg (32 mm Hg − 22 mm Hg = 10 mm Hg) and favors the movements of fluid out of the vascular compartment. The difference between the hydrostatic pressure and colloid osmotic pressure at the venule end of the capillary is − 10 mm Hg (12 mm Hg − 22 mm Hg = −10 mm Hg) and favors the movement of fluid into the vascular compartment (Fig. 15-8).

Overall, this system allows fluids high in nutrients and oxygen to diffuse out of the vascular bed at the arteriole end and fluids containing waste products to move back into the vascular bed at the venule end of the capillaries. The lymphatic system picks up the small amount of excess fluids that remain in the tissues and returns them to the vascular space.

Multiple factors affect the hydrostatic pressure. At the arteriole end of the capillary the hydrostatic pressure is dependent on the volume of blood, viscosity of the blood, force of the heart, and resistence of the blood vessels. Hydrostatic pressure at the venous end is dependent on the venous pressure. The venous pressure in turn is dependent on the condition of the veins, respiration, and skeletal muscle contractions. The colloid osmotic pressure is dependent on the protein level, which is dependent on the dietary intake, the liver's ability to produce proteins, and the fact that excess proteins are not lost from the body. Various disease states can interfere with any of these multiple factors and result in edema. Edema is discussed in detail in Chapter 20.

■ MAINTAINING ADEQUATE CIRCULATION

The delivery of oxygen, nutrients, and electrolytes to cells and the delivery of waste products to elimination sites is dependent on an adequate circulatory system. Adequate circulation requires a functioning pump (the heart) to propel approximately 5 liters of fluid (blood) continuously through channels (vascular beds). The circulatory system is a closed-circuit system. Blood is continuously perfused through the body, traveling from the heart through arteries and arterioles and back to the heart through venules and veins. Between the arteries and veins lie approximately 60,000 miles of capillaries.[75,76] Every tissue is permeated by capillaries. It is in the capillaries that oxygen, nutrients, and electrolytes diffuse from the blood into cells and waste products diffuse from the cells into the blood. It is evident that not all capillaries can be perfused at the same time. The distribution of blood through the capillaries is controlled by the arterioles. The arterioles are normally slightly constricted, but they have the ability under nervous and hormonal control to constrict and shunt blood around capillary beds.

The survival of cells is dependent on a circulatory system that has an adequate pump, an adequate vascular volume, and a vascular bed that constricts and dilates as necessary. Severe malfunction of any of these components can lead to a state of shock.

■ INTERFERENCE WITH MAINTENANCE OF CIRCULATION

□ Shock

Shock is a pathologic syndrome characterized by inadequate perfusion and oxygenation and inadequate cellular metabolism. Shock results from a wide variety of conditions that interfere with one of the components of the circulatory system. Conditions such as severe cardiac and pulmonary disease, burns, dehydration, hemorrhage, anaphylaxis, and spinal injury all interfere with at least one component of the circulatory system. Severe infection and sepsis can also cause shock.

Classification and susceptible clients

Shock has been classified in a variety of ways. Classification helps in identifying the most likely cause so that preventive care can be instituted. The most commonly used classification is according to the altered component. Using this classification the types of shock are: hypovolemic, cardiogenic, neurogenic, vasogenic, and septic.

Hypovolemic shock. In hypovolemic shock the vascular volume is decreased so drastically that there is inadequate volume to perfuse cells. Hypovolemic shock occurs when vascular volume has decreased 15% to 25%. Common causes of vascular deficit are hemorrhage resulting from rupture or injury of a blood vessel such as in gastrointestinal bleeding; after surgery; erosion of a vessel by drainage tubes, tumors or infections; or some interference with clotting. Vascular deficit also occurs from fluid loss due to burns, losses from the gastrointestinal tract seen with severe vomiting or diarrhea, and losses from fistulas.

Cardiogenic shock. Cardiogenic shock results in hypoperfusion, cellular anoxia, and inadequate metabolism because of failure of the heart to pump an adequate amount of blood to the tissues. Cardiogenic shock most frequently results from failure of the heart following myocardial infarction. Approximately 15% of all patients suffering from myocardial infarction develop cardiogenic shock. Cardiogenic shock can also occur secondary to left ventricular failure, cardiac tamponade, or pulmonary emboli.

Neurogenic shock. Neurogenic shock is a rare phenomenon as compared with other types of shock. Neurogenic shock results from the sudden vasodilation of the vascular bed because of interference with sympathetic nervous control of the arterioles. The vasodilation increases vascular capacity, and a relative hypovolemia occurs. Neurogenic shock can occur as a result of damage to the sympathetic nervous system from spinal cord injury and rarely from brain damage, blockage of sympathetic activity by spinal anesthesia and other ganglionic blocking agents, or psychic trauma resulting in fainting. Barbiturate and other drug intoxications cause the same type of response.

Vasogenic shock. Vasogenic shock results from massive vasodilation of the vascular bed because of direct interference with the vessels. In this instance a foreign protein such as histamine or some other agent is acting directly on the arterioles, causing vasodilation. Anaphylactic reactions to drugs or blood transfusion are the common causes of vasogenic shock.

Septic shock. Septic shock following infection with gram-negative organisms is becoming increasingly common (see Chapter 21). The mechanism by which septic shock causes cellular hypoxia and inadequate metabolism is not fully understood. In most instances of septic shock normal cardiac output is present, and apparently some impairment of the cell membrane prevents cells from utilizing glucose, oxygen, and electrolytes. In addition, although cardiac output may be normal there may be abnormal shunting of blood around capillary beds through arteriovenous fistulas. A relative hypovolemia may also occur because of the leakage of fluids and plasma into the infected or inflamed area. Septic shock most frequently occurs in the elderly or immunosuppressed person who develops a gram-negative infection. Common organisms causing septic shock are *Escherichia coli, Klebsiella, Aerobacter, Pseudomonas, Proteus,* or coliform species.[44] Shock can also occur secondary to a gram-positive infection with *Staphylococcus aureus* or streptococcus organisms. Yeast and fungus can also cause septic shock.

In general, although shock occurs in a wide variety of conditions, the very young and the elderly are more likely to develop septic and hypovolemic shock following surgery or trauma than the young healthy adult. The person with a chronic disease such as diabetes mellitus or cardiovascular disease also is at increased risk of developing shock. Persons with diseases of the immune system receiving glucocorticoid replacement therapy, receiving glucocorticoids or other drugs for their immunosuppressive effect, or who have recently had glucocorticoids discontinued are at increased risk of developing septic shock because of an actual or potential depressed immune response. In addition persons receiving glucocorticoids are at higher risk for developing shock following any injury or surgery because they may have decreased compensatory mechanisms.

Cellular response in shock

Although the pathologic mechanisms vary in different types of shock, the common elements are cellular anoxia, altered metabolism, and cell death. Schumer and Sperling[59] summarized the cause of cell death as follows.

First there is decreased oxygen to the cells, which then causes a disarrangement of metabolic pathways resulting in decreased adenosine triphosphate (ATP) production and increased acid production. The decreased production of ATP causes malfunction of the sodium and potassium pump with sodium entering the cell and potassium leaving the cell. The influx of sodium and water into the cell causes cellular edema and further interferes with cellular function. The increased acid end products cause intracellular acidemia, which causes lysosomal membranes to rupture and lytic enzymes to be released. The lytic enzymes degrade protein, carbohydrate, and fat, and death of the cell occurs. With cellular death multiple substances are released into the bloodstream that can destroy other cells directly or increase the degree of cellular hypoxia.

Body response in shock

Shock is often insidious and slow in developing. Regardless of the cause of shock, the blood pressure will decrease temporarily, which will stimulate the integrative mechanisms (see Chapter 13). Stimulation of the integrative mechanisms may result in the blood pressure being brought back to normal for varying lengths of time. This increase in blood pressure is due to a variety of effects of the integrative mechanisms: the heart rate increases, vasoconstriction and shunting of blood from periphery to the major arteries is increased, sodium and water are conserved by the kidney, and fluid moves from the interstitial space back to the vascular space. There is also movement of extra red blood cells from the liver and spleen into the vascular space.

Signs and symptoms of shock

When compensatory mechanisms are working, the classic symptom of decreased blood pressure may be seen only as shock progresses. Early indications of shock are behavioral changes (restlessness, apprehension, and feeling of fright) and increased pulse rate, decreased urinary sodium and increased urinary osmolarity, and respiratory alkalosis.

Shock stimulates the medullary respiratory center, causing hyperventilation and an increased excretion of carbon dioxide. The skin usually is cool and clammy in hypovolemic and cardiogenic shock but warm and flushed in neurogenic, vasogenic, and septic shock. The temperature will vary with the type of shock.

As the shock state progresses the compensatory mechanisms will not be able to sustain the blood pressure. Urinary volume will be reduced secondary to continued vasoconstriction and the presence of aldosterone and ADH. Persistent shock will cause permanent renal damage.

Metabolic acidosis occurs as the shock state continues. It is the result of the original hypoperfusion, compensatory vasoconstriction, and in later stages stagnation and pooling of blood in the microcirculation. Permanent organ damage can occur, and signs and symptoms of failure of various organs are seen. Stagnation and clotting of the blood in the microcirculation occurs as shock progresses. Clotting factors can become depleted, and disseminated intravascular coagulation can occur (p. 1070).

The progression of shock will vary with the underlying disease, the health status of the patient, and the type of shock. The compensatory mechanisms activated by the integrative mechanisms are not equally effective in maintaining essential body functions in all types of shock. The best compensation occurs in hypovolemic shock. It must be remembered that although the compensatory mechanisms can be beneficial in early shock, if allowed to persist they can increase the degree of tissue anoxia and lead to cellular death in the same manner as the original insult does.

Organ damage in shock

Organ damage in shock occurs from the original insult and because of the hypoperfusion associated with the shunting of blood and pooling of blood and vasoconstriction. As a result organ hypoxia and cell death occur. Most prone to damage in shock are the kidneys, lungs, and liver.

Kidney damage. The presence of shock leads to vasoconstriction and the stimulation of glucocorticoids, ADH, and aldosterone. Perfusion of the kidneys is decreased and sodium and water are conserved. The decreased excretion of sodium and water also prevents the kidneys from excreting excess amounts of electrolytes and waste products. The continual shunting of blood from the kidneys can lead to acute tubular necrosis. Signs of renal failure may occur even though no actual renal damage is present.

Lung damage. Damage to the lungs begins very early in shock and results in a variety of problems. These include acute respiratory distress syndrome, atelectasis, and pulmonary edema. The pulmonary vascular system may become plugged with white blood cells, red blood cells, and platelets. Very early in shock, anoxia causes damage to the epithelial cells of the alveoli and capillaries and fluid leaks out of the capillaries into the alveoli. The leakage of fluid and decreased blood flow can cause a decrease in surfactant. Surfactant is a lipoprotein secreted by the alveoli epithelium cells (type II cells). It is important in normal pulmonary function because it decreases the work of expanding the lung and helps to maintain stability of the alveoli. When there is a decrease in surfactant the alveoli may collapse. Pulmonary edema resulting from overhydration and a decrease in ventricular function can also be present. The decreased frequency of deep breathing and sighing can result in atelectasis. The pulmonary damage increases tissue hypoxia, since the amount of oxygen that can be diffused across the alveolar-capillary membrane is decreased.

Liver damage. The tissue hypoxia occurring during shock leads to liver damage. Normally the reticuloendothelial system (RES) of the liver rapidly and effectively picks up toxic elements from the blood. In shock this does not occur. The loss of the RES in the liver increases susceptibility to all types of infections. The loss of the RES may result in a septic component being added to the original shock. Loss of liver function also prevents lactic acid conversion, which further compounds the metabolic acidosis.

Intestinal damage. In shock the gastrointestinal tract seems to be exceptionally susceptible to vasoconstriction, which leads to ischemic damage and loss of the bowel integrity. The loss of intestinal integrity allows the bacteria normally present in the gastrointestinal tract to be released into the general circulation. The seeding of the circulatory system by bacteria from the gastrointestinal tract is believed to play a role in the shock state moving to an irreversible stage. Another consequence of shock is gastrointestinal tract bleeding, which may be due to a destruction of the gastric mucosal barrier secondary to ischemia, increased acid production, or decreased clotting factors.

Cardiac damage. In shock the myocardium is depressed and the coronary vascular bed seems to lose its autoregulatory ability and becomes entirely pressure dependent.[72] This loss easily leads to ischemic changes, arrhythmias, and cardiac failure. The myocardial depression decreases cardiac output farther and may be responsible for shock entering into the irreversible stage. When organ damage occurs, a wide variety of other signs and symptoms such as those seen in renal failure, respiratory insufficiency, gastrointestinal bleeding, and myocardial damage are seen.

Assessment

The management of shock will depend on the results of the continuous monitoring of the status of the patient. To pick up subtle changes, a flow sheet on which data from all parameters can be recorded should be used. The box on p. 217 lists parameters to be monitored. The assessment of multiple parameters is necessary to obtain an adequate evaluation of the adequacy of tissue perfusion. Not all parameters will necessarily be measured on any one person. The following section discusses some of the special monitoring techniques that may be used.

PARAMETERS FOR ASSESSING STATUS OF THE PATIENT IN SHOCK

Hemodynamic monitoring
Blood pressure
Pulse
Central venous pressure (CVP)
Pulmonary wedge pressure (PWP)
Cardiac output (CO)
Electrocardiogram

Respiratory monitoring
Respiratory rate, depth
Breath sounds
Blood gases
  pH
  PO_2
  PCO_2
  Percent saturation

Fluid and electrolyte monitoring
Serum electrolytes
Blood lactate and pyruvate levels
Intake
Output
  Urinary
  Gastrointestinal tract
  Sweating
  Dressings
Weight
Creatinine serum level
Blood urea nitrogen level (BUN)
Serum and urinary osmolarity
Urinary specific gravity

Neurologic monitoring
Alertness
Orientation

Hematologic monitoring
Erythrocytes
Hematocrit and hemoglobin levels
Leukocytes
Platelets
Prothrombin and partial thromboplastin time
Clotting time

Others
Bowel sounds
Skin temperature

Hemodynamic monitoring. The *blood pressure* may be monitored by auscultation; however, auscultation may give inaccurate results because of the vasoconstriction or the poor stroke volume that occurs with shock. The vibration produced by the blood may be too minimal to produce audible sounds. Other methods may be necessary to monitor the blood pressure. Intraarterial monitoring is used often. An intraarterial line is inserted into the radial, brachial, or femoral artery and attached to a transducer and monitor. If transducers are not available, there is another simple way of measuring intraarterial pressure, as described in other literature.[11,72]

Central venous pressure (CVP) may be monitored in all types of shock but is most helpful in hypovolemic shock. The CVP assists in assessing the adequacy of the vascular volume, the function of the right ventricle, and venous return. There are several pointers that must be remembered to gain the most information from CVP monitoring. The technique and important points in obtaining an accurate CVP reading are discussed on p. 923. Normally the function of the right and left ventricles is similar, but in shock the left ventricle may be deficient, and this deficiency will not be picked up by monitoring the CVP.

Accurate information about left ventricular function is obtained by measuring the *pulmonary artery pressure* (PAP) and the *pulmonary wedge pressure* (PWP). To obtain the PAP a Swan-Ganz catheter is inserted into the pulmonary artery by way of the superior vena cava. The Swan-Ganz catheter has an inflatable balloon. Normally the catheter floats in the pulmonary artery, but it can be advanced with the balloon inflated into the wedged position to give the PWP. The catheter is attached to a transducer and recorder, which gives constant pressure readings. The exact location of the catheter is determined by the pressure readings. The normal PWP is approximately 12 mm Hg. If left ventricular failure is suspected, PWP monitoring is necessary because the PWP can be dangerously elevated even though the CVP is low or normal. This is discussed further in Chapter 50.

Cardiac output measurements can assist in the assessment of the status of the patient and in evaluating the effectiveness of therapy. Cardiac output can be measured in several ways. A common way is the thermodilution technique. In this method a Swan-Ganz catheter with a thermistor electrode on the tip is placed in the pulmonary artery and a known amount of cold solution is injected through the lumen of the same catheter into the right atrium. The thermistor, which is positioned in the pulmonary artery, picks up the temperature of the solution when it reaches that area. The better the cardiac function the less the temperature change will be.[4]

Respiratory monitoring. The importance of an

adequately functioning respiratory system has been discussed. The person in shock is suceptible to a wide variety of pulmonary problems, and pulmonary status must be continually assessed. This is accomplished by evaluating breath sounds (p. 933), measuring blood gas levels (p. 935), determining lung compliance and airway resistance (p. 936), and measuring pulmonary shunting.

The passage of blood from the pulmonary artery to the pulmonary vein without being oxygenated is called pulmonary shunting. A certain amount of shunting occurs normally, but an increased amount of shunting can occur in shock because of lung damage. The amount of shunting is determined by measuring the PO_2, PCO_2, and hemoglobin.

Fluid and electrolyte monitoring. Some of the parameters discussed under hemodynamic monitoring assess fluid status. In addition to the previously described monitoring elements, the serum and urine osmolarity are measured frequently. The presence of injuries, wounds, trauma, or internal bleeding can result in significant amounts of undetected fluid loss. The patient in shock cannot tolerate even minute changes in fluid balance. All potential sites of fluid loss must be monitored, dressings should be weighed, and the number of times bed linens or gowns need to be changed should be recorded. This will help approximate fluid loss by perspiration. The output from the gastrointestinal tract (nasogastric drainage, diarrhea, and vomitus) must also be measured. Since some fluid losses can only be approximated, accurate body weights are necessary.

The status of the kidney plays a major role in the ability to maintain fluid and electrolyte balance during shock. The status of the kidneys can also be used as an indicator of perfusion to other organs. Because of the vasoconstriction and shunting of blood that occurs during shock, renal damage can be easily precipitated. The patient should have an indwelling catheter, and output must be measured continuously on an hourly basis. Other tests valuable in determining renal status are blood urea nitrogen (BUN), creatinine, serum and urinary osmolarity, and the specific gravity of urine.

Neurologic monitoring. The neurologic status can be affected by a number of factors. Neurologic changes occur because of the original injury, shock state, respiratory malfunction, acidosis, or compensatory mechanisms. Changes in neurologic status may be the earliest signs of shock and should be assessed on a continual basis to judge the adequacy of cerebral blood flow.

Hematologic monitoring. Hematologic changes can occur because of blood loss, hemodilution and concentration, and disseminated intravascular coagulation (DIC) (p. 1070). The red blood cell count and hematocrit and hemoglobin levels are used as guides to fluid status and need for blood replacement. The other factors listed in the box on p. 217 will assist in detecting the onset of DIC or other possible causes of continuous blood loss.

Other monitoring. Skin temperature will vary depending on the type and stage of shock, the amount of physiologic compensation, and the treatment. Changes in skin temperature may help to assess the limited or improved state of tissue perfusion. With continual sympathetic stimuli, vasoconstriction, and the shunting of blood, the normal peristaltic movement of the gastrointestinal tract is decreased. Assessment of bowel sounds help determine adequacy of blood flow to the gastrointestinal tract.

Intervention

The management for every patient in shock is unique and depends on the patient's status as determined by the data gathered from continuous assessment. There is no one type of management, but there are general principles of management, which are discussed. The patient's care is guided by four major outcomes:

1. The patient's tissue perfusion, cellular oxygenation, and cellular metabolism will return to normal.
2. The patient will have decreased metabolic needs.
3. The patient and significant others will be free of avoidable anxiety.
4. The patient will be free of avoidable injuries.

The particular criteria used by the health team to measure the effectiveness of therapy will depend on the individual patient.

Outcome: *Tissue perfusion, cellular oxygenation, and cellular metabolism will return to normal*

Fluid replacement. Almost all patients in shock, no matter what type, will require some fluid replacement because of the pooling of vascular fluid in the microcirculation. The type of fluid replaced depends on the type and amount lost. Blood, plasma, albumin, hydroxyethyl starch, dextran, 5% dextrose, and electrolyte solutions are used.

Most persons can tolerate blood losses of 500 ml to 1,000 ml without difficulty. Blood is replaced if the loss exceeds this amount. In addition the etiology of the blood loss must be identified and corrected. Measures to control hemorrhage are discussed on p. 221.

Plasma, dextran, hydroxyethyl starch, or albumin are used if the initiating event is a disorder such as pancreatitis, peritonitis, or severe burns where there is an excessive loss of plasma. These solutions are preferred over glucose solutions because the molecules are larger and will remain in the vascular bed. These solutions also are used to expand the vascular volume while waiting for blood to be typed and cross matched. They are not without risk. Viral hepatitis can be transmitted by plasma; normal human-weight dextran causes red blood cell aggregation; and high- and low-molecular-weight dextran and hydoxyethyl starch can interfere with the clotting mechanisms. Albumin is the safest plasma expander but is ten times as expensive as the commercially made plasma expanders.[73]

The type of solution used will depend on the patient's serum and electrolyte levels. Bicarbonate solutions are used to correct metabolic acidosis, and dextrose is given to provide some of the needed calories. Saline solutions may have to be limited if cardiac disorders are present.

Most patients will receive a combination of fluids, blood, and plasma expanders. The amount of fluids given will depend on the CVP and the PWP. Patients require sufficient fluids to make up for vasodilation, pooling, and extravasation of fluids out of the vascular bed. With adequate fluid replacement a gradual but not extreme rise in CVP and PWP will occur. Care must be taken to prevent hypervolemia and pulmonary edema.

Vasopressors and vasodilators. The role of vasopressors in the treatment of shock is controversial. Some physicians believe vasopressors cause additional problems and organ damage because, at least in some shock states, the patient is already in a state of severe vasoconstriction.

Vasopressors increase vasoconstriction and increase blood flow to vital organs by shunting blood past other tissues. The failure to perfuse these other tissues interferes with cellular metabolism. In addition vasopressors can lead to cardiac arrhythmia because of their cardiac stimulant affects.

On the other hand, cerebral circulation is not adequate if the arterial blood pressure is below 60 mm Hg. If fluid replacement does not succeed in increasing the blood pressure, vasopressor agents will be used. The five vasopressors commonly used are epinephrine, norepinephrine (Levophed), dopamine, isoproterenol hydrochloride (Isuprel), and metaraminol bitartrate (Aramine). All five vary in their vasoconstrictor effects. Norepinephrine, epinephrine, and metaraminol at high doses and dopamine at very high doses cause vasoconstriction of the arterial and venous vasculature. Dopamine at low to moderate doses exerts a dopaminergic action, which causes vasodilation of the renal, mesenteric, cerebral, and coronary vessels. Isoproterenol does not cause vasoconstriction.

Vasopressors are usually given intravenously, and the rate of infusion is titrated to keep the mean blood pressure at 80 mm Hg. The blood pressure may need to be monitored as frequently as every 5 minutes because the action of some of these drugs varies with the dosage and because the goal is to give the least amount necessary. The amount needed to maintain the blood pressure must be carefully documented. The rate of administration should be mechanically controlled by an intravenous infusion pump to prevent too rapid infusion. Also the nurse must keep in mind that tissue sloughing can result from the extravasation of some vasopressors, especially norepinephrine.

If vasoconstriction is thought to be a major cause of inadequate tissue perfusion, oxygenation, and metabolism, vasodilators will be given. The hypothesis is that vasodilators, by decreasing vasoconstriction, will increase tissue perfusion. To prevent hypotension from vasodilation, provision is made for rapid fluid replacement as the vasodilator drug is given. Common vasodilators are phenoxybenzamine hydrochloride (Dibenzyline), phentolamine mesylate (Regitine), chlorpromazine hydrochloride (Thorazine), and sodium nitroprusside (Nipride).

Cardiac support. Other measures to augment tissue perfusion and oxygenation may be used. If ventricular arrhythmias occur, antiarrhythmic therapy is given. Cardiac glycosides (digitalis) may be given to strengthen cardiac contractility. If severe left ventricular dysfunction is present an intraaortic counterpulsation balloon may be used. The catheter with balloon is inserted into the femoral artery and threaded into the aorta to the approximate level of the thoracic aorta. The balloon inflates at the beginning of diastole and deflates just prior to systole. The inflation at the beginning of diastole pushes blood into the coronary arteries and into the periphery. The deflation just prior to systole decreases the resistance in the aorta so that the ventricle does not have as much resistance to overcome.

Respiratory support. To ensure adequate oxygenation, oxygen administered by mask, catheter, or with a respirator may be needed. Po_2 should be maintained at a minimum of 60 mm Hg. Respiratory support may also be necessary to prevent or treat acid-base imbalance.

Oxygen in high levels can cause alveolar damage; therefore only the amount of oxygen necessary to maintain a Po_2 of 60 is given. If a high fraction of forced inspiratory oxygen (FIO_2) is necessary to maintain a Po_2 of 60, added ventilatory support such as positive end-expiratory pressure (PEEP) may be necessary (p. 1137).

In addition the nurse must remember that oxygen is very drying, and adequate humidity must always be provided. In addition to supplemental oxygen, good respiratory care consisting of helping the patient to cough and deep breathe is necessary. If the patient is unable to cough effectively, nasotracheal suctioning is necessary.

Renal support. One of the primary organs affected by the vasoconstrictive effects of the compensatory mechanisms and administration of vasopressor drugs is the kidneys. Adequate renal function is necessary to prevent major fluid, electrolyte, and acid-base imbalance. If fluid replacement and establishment of adequate blood pressure do not increase urine output to an adequate level, diuretics may be given. Urine output should be at least 25 to 30 ml/hour. Commonly used diuretics are mannitol (Osmitrol) and furosemide (Lasix).

Reticuloendothelial support. In septic shock and in almost all other types of shock, broad-spectrum antibiotics are used. A combination of antibiotics to cover both gram-positive and gram-negative organisms is given. In sepsis, cultures of urine, sputum, blood, and secretions from any other orifice that is a possible site for sepsis are obtained prior to instituting antibiotic therapy.

Additional measures. Other measures that assist in promoting adequate tissue perfusion, oxygenation, and metabolism are positioning of the patient and use of steroids. In the past the Trendelenburg position (head-low position) often was used to increase the flow of blood to the brain. However, this position has been found to inhibit cardiac output and respirations because the visceral organs push up against the diaphragm. Many physicians now prefer that the lower extremities be elevated at a 45-degree angle from the hip, with the knees straight and the head level with or slightly higher than the chest. This position promotes increased venous return from the legs without interfering with the cardiac output. The nurse should assess each situation to determine the position of maximum physiologic effect and comfort. In some settings in which the nurse is functioning there may be policies concerning positioning of the patient in shock; nevertheless the nurse should assess the patient's response to such positioning and take appropriate action as necessary.

Glucocorticoids are used in some patients with shock. Their use is still controversial. Several beneficial effects of the glucocorticoids have been hypothesized. Glucocorticoids stabilize mitochondrial lysosomal membranes. They seem to strengthen cardiac contractility, and they have a mild alpha-adrenergic blocking effect, thus causing some vasodilation and improvement in tissue perfusion. Glucocorticoids also increase lactic acid conversion to glycogen and increase ATP production.[72]

Outcome: *Metabolic needs are decreased*

To achieve this outcome, all the necessary interventions must be carried out, yet rest periods must be provided. Only the essential physical care needs should be met. Unnecessary activities should be eliminated and sedatives may be given to increase rest and comfort. Pain and discomfort increase restlessness and thus metabolism. Morphine sulfate may be used to decrease pain. It should be given intravenously, since in shock it may be absorbed too slowly or may accumulate in the tissues.

The patient is kept warm, not hot or cold. Decreased temperature causes chilling and shivering and thus increases metabolic needs. Increased temperature leads to vasodilation, which can cause hypoperfusion because of movement of blood to the body surface. Sweating accompanies increased temperature and also increases metabolic needs.

Outcome: *The patient or significant others are free of avoidable anxiety*

Measures to decrease or eliminate anxiety must be incorporated into the care of the patient. Questions from the patient or significant others should be answered and all interventions should be explained. Talking around the patient should be eliminated. Time to sit down and talk with the patient and family should be planned for so that they have an opportunity to verbalize their fears. The nurse must remember that anxiety can stimulate the body's compensatory mechanisms and increase metabolic needs. The environment of an intensive care unit (ICU) increases anxiety (p. 1556), and the nurse plays a major role in controlling the environment and in eliminating anxiety insofar as possible.

Outcome: *The patient is free of avoidable injuries*

The patient in shock has the potential of developing multiple injuries. Three common avoidable injuries are those due to immobility, those due to infection from invasive procedures, and those due to the accidental dislodgement of tubes and lines.

These patients have decreased resistance to infection. In addition the presence of multiple tubes (intravenous, intraarterial, nasogastric, and endotracheal) increases the risk of infection. Sterile handling of all tubes is of primary importance. Tracheal suctioning, if necessary, must be done with sterile technique (p. 960). Intraarterial and intravenous tubing should be changed on a regular basis. A routine for appropriate care of intravenous and intraarterial insertion sites should be planned and instituted on a continuous basis.

The patient in shock may be confused and often is restless and anxious. These behavioral changes make the patient very vulnerable to accidents. The patient can easily fall if side rails are not used. A more frequent injury results from dislodgement of the various lines and tubes by the patient. The tubes and lines are irritating, and the patient may not be able to understand the purpose of them and may accidently or intentionally remove them.

Soft restraints or mittens may be necessary. They should only be used if the patient's cooperation cannot be obtained. Usually if restraints or mittens are used they can be removed while the staff is with the patient. They should be removed at least every 4 to 8 hours so that the extremities can be moved and inspected.

Outcome criteria for the patient in shock

A. Tissue perfusion, cellular oxygenation, and cellular metabolism will return to normal
   1. Mean BP will be >80 mm Hg
   2. Pulse will not be >10 of baseline
   3. Cardiac arrhythmias will be controlled
   4. Cardiac output will be normal
   5. CVP will be >6 cm of H_2O and <15 cm of H_2O
   6. PWP will be >10 mm Hg and <20 mm Hg
   7. Urinary osmolarity will be > serum osmolarity
   8. Urinary output will be ≥ 25 ml/hr
   9. Serum electrolytes will be within normal limits
   10. BUN and creatinine levels will not increase and will decrease toward normal
   11. Serum lactic acid will return to normal
   12. Temperature will be normal
   13. Skin will be warm and dry without cyanosis or mottling
   14. Blood gas results will be:
       Po_2 60 to 100 mm Hg
       Pco_2 38 to 42 mm Hg
       CO_2 content (plasma) 25 to 32 mEq/liter
       HCO_3^- 23 to 25 mEq/liter
       pH 7.38 to 7.42
       O_2 saturation 97%
   15. Mental status will return to preshock state
   16. Respiratory rate will be 16 to 22/min, regular deep
   17. Breath sounds will be clear in all lobes
   18. Physiologic shunting will be <15%
   19. Red blood cell count and hematocrit and hemoglobin levels will be normal or at least at the preshock levels
   20. Coagulation factors and platelets will be within normal range
   21. White blood cell count will be normal or returning to normal
B. The patient will have decreased metabolic needs
   1. Will have periods of REM sleep
   2. Will be free of discomfort
   3. Will be warm, not hot or cold
C. The patient or significant others are free of avoidable anxiety.
   1. Will receive explanations of all interventions
   2. Will be informed of the client's status
   3. Will not exhibit behavior showing anxiety (e.g., restlessness, inappropriate movements)
   4. Will be able to verbalize fears and feelings
D. The patient will be free of avoidable injuries
   1. Will not develop a nosocomial infection from venous or arterial lines; from the presence of an indwelling catheter, endotracheal or tracheostomy tubes, or ventilator; or from suctioning.
   2. Will not develop deleterious effects of immobility (e.g., foot drop, contractures, atelectasis)
   3. Will not injure self (e.g., by pulling out tubes, developing skin abrasions)

□ Hemorrhage

A second major insult to the circulatory system is hemorrhage. Hemorrhage if not controlled can lead to shock, discussed above. This section deals with measures to control blood loss.

Hemorrhage is the loss of a large amount of blood from the bloodstream due to rupture or injury of a blood vessel; slipping of a ligature from a blood vessel postoperatively; erosion of a vessel by a drainage tube, tumor, or infection; or some interference with the clotting mechanism of the blood such as occurs in hemophilia. A person may lose small amounts of blood over a long period or may lose a large amount of blood in a short period. The bleeding may be arterial (bright red and spurting), venous (continuous flow of dark red blood), or capillary (oozing). The blood may be expelled from any body orifice, from an incision, or from the site of an injury, or it may collect under the subcutaneous tissues as a tumor mass *(hematoma)* or in a body cavity such as the peritoneal cavity.

Assessment

Symptoms of massive hemorrhage, both internal and external, are apprehension, restlessness, thirst, pallor, a cold, moist skin, drop in blood pressure, increased pulse rate, subnormal temperature, and rapid respirations. As hemorrhage continues, the lips and conjunctivae become pale and the patient may complain of spots before the eyes, ringing in the ears, and extreme weakness. If the hemorrhage is not controlled, shock and finally death will occur.

Intervention

The treatment of hemorrhage is directed toward stopping the bleeding if possible and replacing blood loss. When bleeding occurs the vessel walls constrict, narrowing the lumen of the vessels, and a clot forms over the end of the bleeding vessel. Clotting usually occurs much earlier in the child and very young person than in older persons because the blood vessels of children and young persons are more elastic. In arterial bleeding the clotting phenomenon is not possible until there has been enough blood loss to decrease the pressure of the blood circulating through the bleeding vessel. However, pressure against the artery proximal to the bleeding point decreases the flow of blood through it and permits clotting to take place. Elevation of the part also may decrease arterial bleeding. *Direct pressure* at the site of the bleeding also decreases the blood flow and encourages clotting. This method is frequently used in superficial wounds, and a gelatin sponge (Gelfoam) also may be applied to help form a clot. The principle of direct pressure may also be used to control hemorrhage from esophageal varices. An esophageal balloon is inserted and then inflated until it compresses the bleeding vessels. In a similar way bleeding from the prostate gland such as may occur following prostatectomy is controlled by direct pressure. A Foley catheter is inserted and the balloon inflated to compress bleeding vessels.

Cold applications are often used to control bleeding into tissues or into body cavities, since the cold causes the small vessels to constrict. In uterine hemorrhage an ice bag may be applied to the abdomen over the uterus. In gastric hemorrhage cold can be applied by irrigating the stomach with iced solution through a gastric tube. (See p. 1209 for additional information.)

Very *hot applications* cause reflex vasoconstriction and control bleeding temporarily. This method is often used during surgery in which there is considerable vascular oozing. To control the bleeding permanently, large vessels usually have to be ligated, and smaller ones may be electrically cauterized. A ruptured organ such as the spleen may have to be removed to control bleeding. Removal of the spleen also may be necessary to control bleeding due to a blood dyscrasia such as idiopathic thrombocytopenic purpura.

When the bleeding is caused by a prothrombin deficiency, such as occurs in liver diseases in which hepatic ducts are obstructed or in biliary duct obstruction, *vitamin* K_1 is given parenterally. Vitamin K_1 is helpful in controlling hemorrhage following overdoses of bishydroxycoumarin (Dicumarol). Protamine sulfate is given after overdoses of heparin.

If possible the blood loss should be measured so that the physician can prescribe replacement more accurately. Dressings saturated with blood can be weighed, and bloody vomitus, which may be bright red or coffee-ground color, and drainage from gastric tubes should be measured. Whenever possible tarry stools and bright blood discharged from the rectum should be measured. If this is not feasible the amount should be estimated. The physician often will want to see evidence of bleeding, such as bloody stools or urine, vaginal clots, and bloody vomitus.

Blood replacement usually is started before complete hemostasis has been accomplished, since the restoration of blood volume is imperative in preventing the occurrence of irreversible shock. Blood plasma or a plasma expander may be given until whole blood is available. The physician's determination of the amount of blood to be given depends on the amount of blood loss, the central venous pressure, and the condition of the patient. When large amounts of blood must be given rapidly, the blood should be warmed to body temperature, since cold blood can act as a hypothermic agent. A decrease in the body temperature may cause cardiac slowing, with decreased cardiac output or the development of ventricular fibrillation. The speed at which blood is given depends on the patient's condition. If the blood pressure is very low, the blood may be given very rapidly and may even be pumped in under pressure by the physician.

The patient is usually very apprehensive because of the hemorrhage and because of the emergency measures that follow it. Every attempt should be made to keep the patient quiet, reassured, and comfortable. He or she should never, under any circumstances, be left alone while a hemorrhage is occurring. Morphine sulfate is often ordered as a sedative. Evidences of bleeding should be removed from the bedside, and stained linen and clothing should be replaced. Noise and excitement should be kept to a minimum, and all treatments and procedures, such as frequent blood pressure readings, transfusions, the use of unusual positions, and, if necessary, restriction of food and fluids, should be explained to the patient and family. The patient with a massive hemorrhage usually is given nothing to eat or drink until the hemorrhage is controlled, since surgery may be necessary. Food and fluid also are often withheld when the bleeding is from the gastrointestinal tract.

REFERENCES AND SELECTED READINGS

1. *Abbey, J. C.: Nursing observations of fluid imbalances, Nurs. Clin. North Am. **3**:77-86, 1968.
2. Andersson, B.: Thirst and brain control of water balance, Am. Sci. **59**:408-415, 1971.
3. Ando, S., Guze, L. B., and Gold, E. M.: ACTH release in vivo and in vitro: extrapituitary mediation during *Escherichia coli* bacteremia, Endocrinol. **74**:894-901, 1964.
4. *Andreoli, K. G., Hunn, V. K., Zipes, D. P., and Wallace, A. G.: Comprehensive cardiac care: a text for nurses, physicians, and other health practitioners, ed. 3, St. Louis, 1975, The C. V. Mosby Co.
5. Ashbough, D. G., and Petty, T. L.: Positive and expiratory pressure: physiology, indication and contraindications, J. Thorac. Cardiovasc. Surg. **65**:165-170, 1973.
6. Beck, W. S.: Human design: molecular, cellular, and systematic physiology, New York, 1971, Harcourt Brace Jovanovich, Inc.
7. Beland, I. L., and Passos, J. Y.: Clinical nursing: pathophysiological and psychosocial approaches, ed. 3, New York, 1975, Macmillan, Inc.
8. Bergersen, B. S., and Goth, A.: Pharmacology in nursing, ed. 13, St. Louis, 1976, The C. V. Mosby Co.

*References preceded by an asterisk are particularly well suited for student reading.

9. Berne, R. M., and Levy, M. N.: Cardiovascular physiology, ed. 3, St. Louis, 1977, The C. V. Mosby Co.
10. *Betson, C.: Blood gases, Am. J. Nurs. **68:**1010-1012, 1968.
11. Brand, L.: A practical approach to infection surveillance in the intensive care unit. Heart Lung **5:**788-790, 1976.
12. *Brand, L., and Wilson, R. F.: Shock. In Meltzer, L. E., et al.: Concepts and practices of intensive care for nurse specialists, Bowie, Md., 1976, The Charles Press.
13. Brooks, S. M.: Basic facts of body water and ions, ed. 3, New York, 1977, Springer Publishing Co., Inc.
14. Brown, W. J.: A classification of microorganisms frequently causing sepsis, Heart Lung **5:**397-405, 1976.
15. Brown, W. J.: The increasing incidence of sepsis and antibiotic resistance, Heart Lung **5:**593-597, 1976.
16. Burgess, R. E.: Fluids and electrolytes, Am. J. Nurs. **65:**90-95 1965.
17. Cohn, H. D.: Hemostasis and blood coagulation, Am. J. Nurs. **65:**116-119, 1965.
18. *Cohn, J. N.: Monitoring techniques in shock, Am. J. Cardiol. **26:**565-569, 1970.
19. Comroe, J. H.: Physiology of respiration, Chicago, 1965, Year Book Medical Publishers, Inc.
20. Cushing, R.: Pulmonary infection, Heart Lung **5:**611-613, 1976.
21. Davis, B. D., et al.: Microbiology, ed. 2, New York, 1973, Harper and Row, Publishers.
22. Dicken, M. L.: Fluid and electrolyte balance: a programmed text, ed. 2, Philadelphia, 1970, F. A. Davis Co.
23. *Duff, J. H.: Cardiovascular changes in sepsis, Heart Lung **5:**773-776, 1976.
24. Dutcher, I. E., and Hardenburg, H. C., Jr.: Water and electrolyte imbalances, In Meltzer, L. E., et al.: Concepts and practices of intensive care for nurse specialists, Bowie, Md., 1976, The Charles Press.
25. Fisher, E. J.: Antimicrobial therapy: some guidelines, Heart Lung **5:**437-448, 1976.
26. Fisher, E. J.: Surveillance and management of hospital-acquired infections, Heart Lung **5:**784-787, 1976.
27. Fluid and electrolytes, North Chicago, Ill., 1968, Abbott Laboratories.
28. Golderger, E.: A primer of water, electrolyte and acid-base syndromes, ed. 5, Philadelphia, 1975, Lea & Febiger.
29. Goldmann, D. A., and Maki, D. G.: Infection control in total parenteral nutrition, J.A.M.A. **223:**1360-1364,
30. Goldmann, D. A., Maki, D. G., Rhame, F. S., et al.: Guidelines for infection control in intravenous therapy, Ann. Int. Med. **79:**848-850, 1973.
31. Goodman, L. S., and Gilman, A.: The pharmacological basis of therapeutics, ed. 5, New York, 1975, Macmillan, Inc.
32. Guyton, A. C.: Textbook of medical physiology, ed. 5, Philadelphia, 1975, W. B. Saunders Co.
33. Holliday, R. L.: Intra-abdominal sepsis, Heart Lung **5:**781-783, 1976.
34. *Hoshal, V. L., Jr.: Intravenous catheters and infection, Surg. Clin. North Am. **52:**1407-1417, 1972.
35. Jacobson, E. D.: A physiologic approach to shock, N. Engl. J. Med. **278:**834-839, 1968.
36. *Jahre, J. N.: Medical approach to the hypotensive patient and the patient in shock, Heart Lung **4:**577-587, 1975.
37. Kee, J. L.: Fluids and electrolytes with clinical applications: a programmed approach, New York, 1976, John Wiley & Sons, Inc.
38. King, O. M.: Care of the cardiac surgical patient, St. Louis, 1975, The C. V. Mosby Co.
39. Lauter, C. B.: Opportunistic infections, Heart Lung **5:**601-606, 1976.
40. Ledgerwood, A.: Hepatobiliary complications of sepsis, Heart Lung **5:**621-623, 1976.
41. Lillehei, R. C., and Dietzman, D. H.: Circulatory collapse and shock. In Schwartz, S. I., et al.: Principles of surgery, New York, 1974, McGraw-Hill Book Co.
42. Linton, A. L.: Diagnosis and treatment of infections of the urinary tract, Heart Lung **5:**607-610, 1976.
43. Mason, J. W., Kleeberg, U., Dolan, P., et al.: Plasma kallikrein and Hageman factor in gram negative bacteremia, Ann. Int. Med. **73:**545-551, 1970.
44. Meltzer, L. E., et al.: Concepts and practices of intensive care for nurse specialists, Bowie, Md., 1976, The Charles Press.
45. Mountcastle, V. B.: Medical physiology, ed. 13, St. Louis, 1974, The C. V. Mosby Co.
46. *Murray, J., and Smallwood, J.: CVP monitoring, Nurs. '77 **7:**42-47, 1977.
47. Petersforf, R. G.: Septic shock. In Thorn G. W., et al.: Harrison's principles of internal medicine, New York, 1977, McGraw-Hill Book Co.
48. Petersdorf, R. G., and Dale, D. C.: Infections in compromised host. In Thorn, G. W., et al.: Harrison's principles of internal medicine, New York, 1977, McGraw-Hill Book Co.
49. *Phipps, W. J., et al.: Respiratory insufficiency and failure. In Meltzer, L. E., et al.: Concepts and practices of intensive care for nurse specialists, Bowie, Md., 1976, The Charles Press.
50. Pitts, R. F.: Physiology of the kidney and body fluids, ed. 3, Chicago, 1974, Year Book Medical Publishers, Inc.
51. Potassium imbalance: programmed instruction, Am. J. Nurs. **67:**343-366, 1967.
52. Rodman, M. J., and Smith, D. W.: Clinical pharmacology in nursing, Philadelphia, 1974, J. B. Lippincott Co.
53. Roellig, S.: Management of patients with contagious illness, Heart Lung **5:**596-600, 1976.
54. *Rosenberg, I. K.: Renal hemodynamic effects of sepsis, Heart Lung **5:**777-780, 1976.
55. Sargis, N. M.: Cardiogenic shock, N.Y. State J. Nurs. Assoc. **3:**22-28, 1972.
56. Schuler, J. J., Erve, P. R., and Schumer, W.: Glucocorticoid effect on hepatic carbohydrate metabolism in the endotoxin-shocked monkey, Ann. Surg. **183:**345-354, 1976.
57. *Schumer, W.: Metabolism during shock and sepsis, Heart Lung **5:**416-421, 1976.
58. Schumer, W., and Sperling, R.: Steroids in the treatment of clinical septic shock, Ann. Surg. **184:**333-341, 1976.
59. *Schumer, W.: Shock and its effect on the cell, J.A.M.A. **205:**75-79, 1968.
60. Schumer, W., Erve, P. R., Kapica, S. K., et al.: Endotoxin effect on respiration of rat liver mitochondria, J. Surg. Res. **10:**609-612, 1970.
61. Schumer, W., and Nyhus, L. M.: Corticosteroid effect on biochemical parameters of human oligemic shock, Arch. Surg. **100:**405-408, 1970.
62. Schwartz, S. I., and others: Principles of surgery, ed. 2, New York, 1974, McGraw-Hill Book Co.
63. Shoemaker, W. C.: Cardiorespiratory patterns in complicated and uncomplicated septic shock, Ann. Surg. **174:**119-125, 1971.
64. Shubin, H., and Weill, M. H.: Touchstones in critical care medicine: an introduction, Crit. Care Med. **2:**281-282, 1974.
65. Sibbald, W. J.: Bacteremia and endotoxemia: a discussion of their roles in the pathophysiology of gram-negative sepsis, Heart Lung **5:**765-771, 1976.
66. Silva, J.: Anaerobic infections, Heart Lung **5:**406-410, 1976.
67. *Snively, W., and Roberts, K. T.: The clinical picture as an aid to understanding body fluid disturbances, Nurs. Forum **12:**132-159, 1973.

68. Sodeman, W. A., Jr., and Sodeman, W. A.: Pathologic physiology: mechanisms of disease, ed. 5, Philadelphia, 1974, W. B. Saunders Co.
69. Strout, V., et al.: Fluid and electrolytes: a practical approach, Philadelphia, 1974, F. A. Davis Co.
70. *Taylor, C. M.: When to anticipate septic shock, Nurs. '75 **5**:34-38, 1975.
71. Tepperman, J.: Metabolic and endocrine physiology, ed. 3, Chicago, 1973, Year Book Medical Publishers, Inc.
72. Thal, A. P., et al.: Shock: a physiologic basis for treatment, Chicago, 1971, Year Book Medical Publishers, Inc.
73. Thompson, L.: Management of shock: rational use of plasma substitutes, Vols. 1 and 2, Therapeutic topics, University Hospitals of Cleveland, 1975.
74. Thorn, G. W., et al.: Harrison's principles of internal medicine, ed. 8, New York, 1977, McGraw-Hill Book Co.
75. Vander, A. J., et al.: Human physiology: the mechanisms of body function, ed. 2, New York, 1975, McGraw-Hill Book Co.
76. Vander, A. J.: Renal physiology, New York, 1975, McGraw-Hill Book Co.
77. Voda, A. M.: Body water dynamics: a clinical application, Am. J. Nurs. **70**:2594-2601, 1970.
78. Wade, J. F.: Respiratory nursing care: physiology and technique, ed. 2, St. Louis, 1977, The C. V. Mosby Co.
79. West, J. B.: Respiratory physiology: the essentials, Baltimore, 1974, The Williams & Wilkins Co.
80. Widmann, F. K.: Goodale's clinical interpretation of laboratory tests, ed. 7, Philadelphia, 1973, F. A. Davis Co.
81. Williams, S. R.: Nutrition and diet therapy, ed. 3, St. Louis, 1977, The C. V. Mosby Co.
82. Wilmore, D. W.: Alimentation in injured and septic patients, Heart Lung **5**:791-792, 1976.
83. Wilson, J. A.: Infection control in intravenous therapy, Heart Lung **5**:430-436, 1976.
84. Wilson, R. F.: Endocrine changes in sepsis, Heart Lung **5**:411-415, 1976.
85. *Wilson, R. F.: The diagnosis and management of severe sepsis and septic shock, Heart Lung **5**:422-429, 1976.
86. *Wilson, R. F.: The diagnosis and treatment of acute respiratory failure in sepsis, Heart Lung **5**:614-620, 1976.

AUDIOVISUAL RESOURCE

Trainex: Fluids and electrolytes: clinical application. Film strips, Trainex Corp., Garden Grove, Calif., PC261-PC264, 1970.

16

Adaptive behavior

MAY WYKLE

■ PERSONALITY AND BEHAVIOR

Personality refers to all that a person is, feels, and does, either consciously or unconsciously, as manifested in interactions with the environment. Behavior is an expression of personality and is defined as all the activity of which a human being is capable. It is a person's never-ending attempt at adjustment to the enviornment and is determined by unmet needs. Thus according to the humanists, all behavior is motivated, purposeful, and meaningful.

Behavior is the manner in which an organism responds to a need stimulus. Once the stimulus is gratified, the organism changes its behavior. Unmet needs create frustration, which leads to increased anxiety. This anxiety is then released as behavior.

If the behavior is such that the anxiety is resolved in an acceptable manner to the person and those around him it is termed *adaptive*. Persons who display adaptive behavior are those who make better use of their coping mechanisms and do not need to resort to symptoms in order to relieve anxiety. Those with *maladaptive* behavior are at the other end of the spectrum (Fig. 16-1) and resort to the use of psychiatric symptoms to deal with increased stress.

Humans are social beings, and one of their basic needs is to feel secure and accepted by others in a social group. An individual's entire life from birth to death consists of a series of adjustments to meet biologic and emotional needs in socially acceptable ways. Because human behavior is characterized by a powerful tendency to repeat itself, especially if the behavior is rewarded, it is essential that health care professionals possess a thorough knowledge of human behavior and factors that influence it. Not only must care givers understand client behavior, but they also need to have reasonable insight into their own behavior. Responses to people are influenced by many factors, particularly early life experiences with significant others. Parents, teachers, neighbors, heroes, and peers all have had a part in shaping a person's behavior and have had some effect on why people behave as they do. Often personal problems and feelings of health care providers produce conflict in the work setting. Sometimes it is necessary for an outsider (client, friend, co-worker) to point this out, yet the more a person knows about himself, the more capable he becomes in establishing working relationships with co-workers and clients. An awareness of what shapes their own behavior, how they manage stress, and how their behavior affects others will facilitate care givers' effectiveness in implementing nursing interventions.

□ Illness and behavior

It is essential that nurses not underestimate the psychosocial aspects of health care. Emotional stress may accentuate physical symptoms in patients. Because of this effect alone, nurses need to have a working knowledge of the dynamics of behavioral responses to illness.

Illness stimulates certain kinds of behavior based on the person's previous adjustment patterns, degree of physical impairment, abruptness of illness onset, prognosis, and meaning of the part of the body affected. All illness is a threat to self and evokes some anxiety, but an acute illness can create a crisis situation for the patient. A necessary part of total care therefore is to support the person's adaptive behaviors and prevent further decompensation.

The anxiety resulting from the stress of illness is manifested as an energy that must be discharged in order to restore equilibrium of the individual. This energy is discharged through behavioral reactions (Fig. 16-1). The type of behavioral reaction that occurs is influenced by psychosociocultural factors such as basic personality development, past experiences, values, and economic status.

When anxiety is markedly increased, the ego attempts to manage the disequilibrium through coping behaviors that will either reduce the anxiety or make the tension tolerable to the individual. The organism can handle the stress by fight, flight, or immobility. The in-

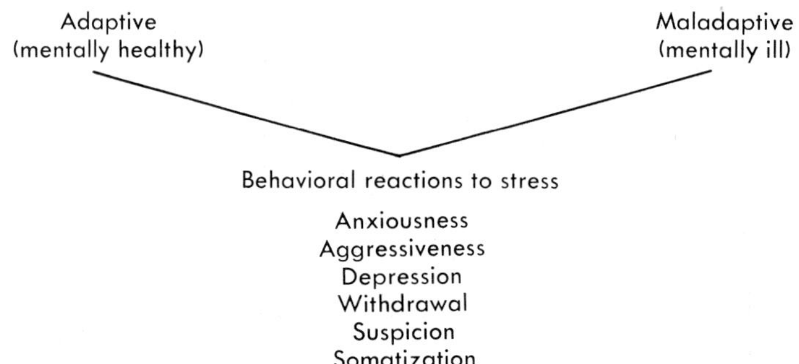

Fig. 16-1. Behavioral responses of persons experiencing anxiety from stress such as illness range from behavior that is adaptive to that which is maladaptive.

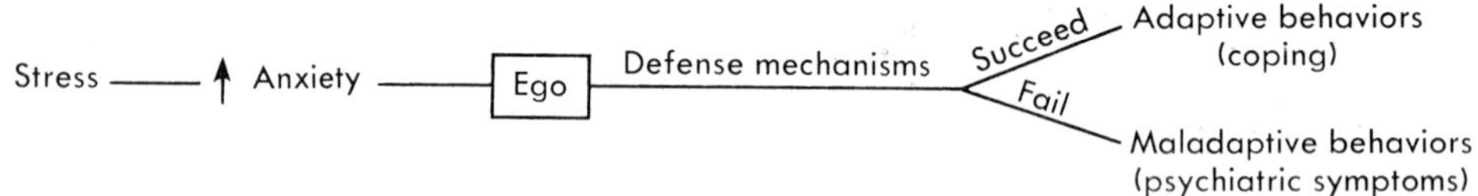

Fig. 16-2. When increased anxiety occurs from stress such as illness, the ego attempts to decrease anxiety by means of defense mechanisms. If these mechanisms fail, the ego resorts to psychiatric symptoms (maladaptive behaviors) as a means of coping.

crease in anxiety calls for the use of defense mechanisms (p. 227). Failure of these mechanisms to solve conflict may lead the ego to utilize psychiatric symptoms, which are considered to be maladaptive (Fig. 16-2).

The capacity to tolerate stress varies among individuals. Whether behavior is adaptive or maladaptive will depend on the amount of stress, the strength of the ego, and its ability to use coping mechanisms. Since behaviors reflect how well stress is being managed, an assessment of behavioral reactions is essential for planning nursing care. Nursing intervention is geared toward support of the person's coping mechanisms, which prevents further escalation of anxiety.

□ Defense mechanisms

Defense mechanisms are unconscious processes used by individuals in adjustment to life stresses. They evolve during personality development and serve to protect the personality, to satisfy emotional needs, to maintain harmony between conflicting tendencies, and to reduce tension of anxiety by modifying reality to make it more acceptable. Defense mechanisms are compromise solutions.

There are two levels of defense mechanisms: those that are considered more primitive and those that are of a higher level (see box, p. 227). Defense mechanisms are used by mentally healthy people as well as by those who are neurotic or psychotic. In the mentally healthy the mechanisms are used less frequently and those mechanisms of a more primitive kind are avoided. Defense mechanisms become pathologic when they are overused.

A defense mechanism is effective when it succeeds in easing intrapsychic tension. When lower level defense mechanisms fail, a more pathologic process evolves and the person exhibits psychiatric symptoms. All defense mechanisms are unconscious with the exception of suppression. Two defense mechanisms, denial and repression, are discussed in more depth as they are more frequently manifested by the hospitalized patient.

Denial

One of the defense mechanisms used frequently in dealing with the stress of illness is denial. This mechanism occurs during the early stages of crisis after the initial stressful impact. Denial of the illness helps the person deal with increased tension and protects the ego (self). The pattern used by the person is similar to the child who closes his eyes and believes no one can see him: "It's not there because I don't see it."

During denial intolerable thoughts are disowned. The ego gets rid of unwelcome facts (such as an illness) while still retaining its faculty for reality testing. The patient manifests denial by disowning any body changes. For example, the patient with coronary disease may say that he did not have a heart attack and will blame his dis-

DEFENSE MECHANISMS

Higher level: less primitive mechanisms

repression ideas painful to consciousness are forced into the unconscious.

suppression thoughts or desires are consciously inhibited.

sublimation energy of repressed tendencies is transformed and directed to social acceptable goals.

identification person assumes the personal qualities or elements of the personality of another.

compensation person makes up, covers up, or disguises real or fancied inadequacies in another area.

displacement an emotion is transferred or displaced from its original object to a more acceptable substitute that is less threatening.

rationalization plausible explanations are given to account for a belief or behavior motivated from unconscious sources.

Lower level: more primitive mechanisms

denial person refuses to admit the reality of the situation.

regression person reverts to a lower level of development.

conversion painful emotional experience is repressed and later is expressed in the form of a physical symptom.

projection that which is emotionally unacceptable within the self is rejected and attributed to others.

introjection person absorbs the emotional attitudes, wishes, ideals, or personality of others into oneself; the aspirations and self restraints of others are incorporated into the personality.

reaction formation person adapts attitudes and behaviors that are opposite to those he cannot accept.

comfort on indigestion. The patient may even deny the severity of the pain and act as though no pain were present.

Denial works well for the person who has been independent and has a self-image of a strong, self-made individual or who views sickness as a sign of weakness. Denial can be complete or partial and includes a "splitting" of thoughts, feelings, and actions; for example, the patient may own the thoughts but deny the feelings.

Intervention for denial is vital if improvement in the patient's physiologic condition depends on his gaining some awareness of the seriousness of the illness or at least enough insight so that he can participate in nursing care. At one time it was believed necessary to confront the patient's denial; however, *direct* attack usually makes the patient more defensive. A patient will give up the need to deny once he feels supported by others and the anxiety is lessened. Denial, although a more primitive mechanism, can be very useful to the person in the face of sudden crisis. The patient should be given reasons for his needed cooperation, but the nurse does not dwell on the patient's dependency or fearfulness. The patient need not agree that the treatment procedures are necessary for him, but neither can his participation cause any harm.

Limits are set firmly but kindly when denial behavior interferes with treatment. The person experiencing denial needs control over those routines not vital to his care and needs reassurance that it is all right to ask for help because the nurse is there for assistance. Nursing care is given in a manner that emphasizes the patient's worthwhileness as a human being although in a dependent state. When the patient gets enough support and reassurance, he will be able to give up some of the denial and face reality.

Regression

Regression is a defense mechanism seen often in persons who are ill, since it facilitates acceptance of the patient role. Regression makes a dependency relationship possible by reversion of the individual to an earlier level of development. Illness necessitates that the person place himself in the hands of competent others. The person often becomes self-centered and concerned only with his own needs and interests. These interests are focused on what is happening to him and his acceptance or rejection by care givers. Often regression is a help to patients in that it promotes conservation of energy.

■ BEHAVIORAL RESPONSES TO STRESS

□ Anxiety

The state of anxiousness is the behavioral manifestation of anxiety. Although the ego attempts to deal with anxiety through defense mechanisms, a certain amount of anxiety manifests itself through anxious behavior. This behavior is usually seen following the initial impact of an acute illness. The level of anxiety engendered and its manifestations will depend on the individual's maturity, understanding of the illness, level of self-esteem, and coping mechanisms.

There are four levels of anxiety according to Peplau.[11] The *mildly* anxious person is more alert, exhibits quick eye movements, and has increased hearing ability. The field of awareness is enlarged, and the person sees, hears, and grasps more of the environment. As anxiety increases to the second stage, *moderate* anxiety, the person sees, hears, and grasps less detail of his surroundings. He may focus on a few details of the illness and ignore the rest. He is able to recall only with clues from the nurse. In the third stage, *severe* anxiety, the nurse may notice disturbances in the person's thought patterns. Thoughts, feelings, and actions may not be congruent; for example, a patient may know he is supposed to stay in bed but may still get out of bed and go to the bathroom or walk in the hall. The fourth stage of anxiety is one of pure *panic*. Perceptions of what is actually happening to the person are blown out of proportion, and the patient may be described literally as "climbing the walls." Persons can vacillate between several stages of anxiety.

Since anxiety is felt empathetically and communicated interpersonally, it is imperative that the nurse take steps to reduce a patient's anxiety to a lower stage. If anxiety is not lowered, other patients and staff are caught up in the tension. Recognition of the effects that the patient's anxiety is having on the nurse, followed by problem-solving steps to reduce anxiety in self, will in turn help to reduce some of the patient's anxiety.

Assessment of anxiety level

In assessing a patient, the nurse observes appearance, behavior, and conversation for signs of anxiety (see boxed material). The conclusion that the patient is demonstrating anxious behavior can be made when several of the signs of anxiety are present. With mild anxiety the signs are fewer and less prominent, and it is important to validate the conclusion with the patient. Signs of anxiety will be more overt in persons experiencing severe anxiety or who are in a state of panic.

Interventions to prevent and release anxiety

The type of intervention used by the nurse will depend on the level of the patient's anxiety and include the following.

Explanations. Structure decreases anxiety. Explanations are one method of providing structure, which is helpful for the person experiencing mild or moderate anxiety. The newly admitted patient is usually anxious; therefore orienting him (and his family) to the hospital environment and routines tends to minimize anxiety. Each new experience should be explained to the patient and, if possible, related to familiar experiences. It is helpful to inform the patient how to call the nurse, when he will see his physician, the hours the religious adviser is available, and how he may contact his family. In addition the family should be told how to obtain information concerning the patient, when they may visit, and any immediate plans for the patient.

If a patient is to have a treatment or test, he must be given some idea of what will be done, the preparation involved, and the reasons why the procedure is necessary. To remove the water pitcher and inform a patient that he cannot have any more water until after his x-ray examination can generate many anxious thoughts: "What x-ray examination?" "I wonder when it is?" "What will it be like?" "It must be something special if I can't have any water." Lack of knowledge as a cause of anxiety reflects the nurse's lack of consideration for the patient's rights as an individual.

Explanations should be given in the patient's own terms at appropriate times and repeated as necessary. If the patient is very anxious, repeated explanation may be necessary, since extreme anxiety reduces intellectual function. It is useless to give detailed explanations to patients who are severely anxious or sedated or to those who have high temperatures or severe pain. Repetition

SIGNS OF ANXIETY

Appearance
↑Muscle tension (rigidity)
Skin blanches, pales
↑Perspiration, clammy skin
Fatigue
↑Small motor activity (e.g., restlessness, tremor)

Behavior
↓Attention span
↓Ability to follow directions
↑Acting out
↑Somatizing
↑Immobility

Conversation
↑Number of questions
Constant seeking of reassurance
Frequent shifting of topics of conversation
Describes fears with sense of helplessness
Avoids focusing on feelings
Focuses on equipment or procedures

Physiologic signs mediated through autonomic nervous system
↑Heart rate
↑Rate or depth of respirations
Rapid extreme shifts in body temperature, blood pressure, menstrual flow
Diarrhea
Urinary urgency
Dryness of mouth
↓Appetite
↑Perspiration
Dilation of pupils

Signs of anxiety are dependent on the degree of anxiety. Mild anxiety heightens the use of capacities, whereas severe and panic states severely paralyze or overwork capacities.

is often required for older persons and children because they may have a short memory span.

Time spent in giving explanations to relatives is not wasted. Not only does it relieve their anxieties, which may be transmitted to the patient, but it also saves having to untangle misinformation. Often the family is helpful in interpreting necessary instructions to the patient in such a manner that the patient understands and accepts them.

Exploration of feelings. In most instances a large part of the nurse's work is to encourage the patient to express anxieties, to help the patient see the universality of fear in his situation, to help him seek outlets for his fears and tensions, and to allay them whenever possible. Nurses should provide opportunities for the patient to talk, but they should not probe. There is a difference between prying into a patient's thoughts and beliefs and eliciting information that will aid in the understanding of his behavior and in planning for his care. Without seeming unduly curious, one can usually find some topic of personal interest to the patient that will provide an opening. A picture on the bedside table may create such an opening. Then nurses who listen with sincere interest and without making judgments about the patient may begin to gain insight into the patient as a person. And more important, the patient may begin to speak about his fears.

As soon as the patient begins to talk about his feelings, the nurse should proceed with conversation, taking cues from what the patient offers. The nurse who feels inadequate or anxious may cut off the conversation. For instance, if a patient says, "You know, I don't think I'll ever get to see my little boy again," a common response is "Oh, don't say that, certainly you will; you're going to be all right." The patient may very well not be all right. Would it not be better to respond, "What makes you feel this way?" Such a response helps the patient explore the subject and leaves opportunity for the patient to examine this fear himself. It also gives the nurse a chance to find out what the patient fears. The nurse who is willing to listen to patients, to be guided by their reactions, and to work with them rather than to make decisions for them will give them needed emotional support. Solving patients' problems for them, even if it were possible, is not the aim of nursing. Indeed it would tend to make patients less healthy psychologically.

The art of meaningful communication involves more than just listening: it includes moving the conversation so that the patient's attempts to communicate are assisted. Observing the patient for facial changes and general body movements provides opportunities for the nurse to discover from the individual the full meaning of the situation. For example, consider the patient who sucks in air while talking. His mouth becomes drier and drier; his tongue seems to stick in his mouth. He is not at ease and shows anxiety even though his words may be quite innocuous. A simple statement such as, "Your mouth seems very dry; would a glass of water help?" allows the nurse to clarify observations made. Such an approach gives the patient a chance to tell what he is experiencing, and he may gain understanding by talking about it.

The nurse is prepared only to help the patient look at those problems that he himself is able to bring into awareness. Underlying problems should be handled by people trained in psychotherapy. A nurse needs to be able to recognize normal anxiety reactions and to report exaggerated reactions that may indicate the need for psychiatric referral. Stuttering and blocking of words may indicate increasing tension.

Intervention for severe anxiety

When any patient's anxiety increases to a high level, the nurse may need to sit with the patient. The nurse's very presence is often reassuring. If possible the patient is helped to recognize the anxiety by the nurse asking, "Are you uncomfortable?" or "What are you feeling?" In severe anxiety and panic, being there is most important, and touch may be used as a means of reassurance. Some severely anxious persons, however, view touching as an intrusion of their personal boundary, and the nurse needs to keep this in mind. When the patient is able to talk, the nurse helps the patient to describe what he thinks is happening, what has happened to him, and what he expects will happen.

□ Crisis model

Overwhelming anxiety may be indicative of a crisis situation that demands specific intervention. Nurses may be confronted with clients in crisis in a variety of settings: emergency rooms, intensive care units, cardiac or surgery units, community health centers, and clinics. Awareness of what occurs during a crisis helps the nurse understand the behavior occurring when a person experiences a crisis.

When the *ego* is met with overwhelming anxiety created by biologic, physiologic, or social threats to the *self*, a crisis ensues. The ego is not able to cope successfully with the sudden disequilibrium. Several authors[1,5,13] have described what occurs during crisis and what is involved in assisting the client so that he can utilize the situation as a growth experience.

A crisis occurs when a person is unable to utilize customary methods of coping when faced for a time with what seems to be an unsurmountable obstacle to an important life goal.[5] A period of disorganization ensues, a period of upset during which many abortive attempts at solutions are made.

Phases of crisis

Shontz describes several phases or stages that occur during crisis.[16] These stages are similar to the stages of death and dying as described by Kubler-Ross.

1. *Initial impact.* During this phase the client experiences shock and depersonalization as reality is clearly perceived. Functioning is organized and automatic with individual centering and docility.
2. *Realization.* In the second phase there is a collapse of the existing self-structure. Reality seems overwhelming, and the person experiences high anxiety, panic, and helplessness. There is inability to plan, reason, or understand the situation.
3. *Defensive retreat.* The third phase is one of regression in which there is an attempt to establish previous identity, to return to better times. There is an avoidance of reality, and denial and wishful thinking may ensue to relieve the anxiety. When challenged the ego reacts with anger and may experience rage and disorientation. Thinking is situation-bound, and there is a resistance to change.
4. *Acknowledgement.* This is the "yes" stage: "It has happened to me." The individual experiences depression and self-depreciation. Reality imposes itself again and looms large in relating the event to one's life. Without intervention the client may become more disorganized, depressed, and suicidal.
5. *Adaptation.* This is the stage when change occurs if help is adequate. New identity appears along with hope and a renewed sense of personal worth. There is a subsequent decrease in anxiety and an increase in satisfaction due to the stabilization and reorganization. Functional improvement is noted without actual change in disability status.

The above model is a useful approach for explaining what a patient experiences during an illness crisis, even though reactions to crisis are individual. Patients are not equally vulnerable to all categories of stress, but there is thought to be some commonality in the reactions. Knowledge about the commonalities can facilitate plans for nursing intervention.

Crisis intervention

The essential element of crisis intervention is the intensive nature of support required to help the ego maintain its integrity and its ability to use coping mechanisms. Crisis, according to Caplan,[5] is self-limiting. Early intervention can prevent maladaptive behavior, and the person can emerge a stronger person. Acute illness or catastropic illness often precipitates a crisis reaction. The outcome of a crisis is governed by the kind of interaction that takes place between the individual and key figures in the environment during the time of crisis.

Often because of changes in society, previous guidelines for behavior in stressful situations render the individual helpless. In crisis the individual is helped to find ways to facilitate efforts to enlarge on the experience. A state of disequilibrium produces a felt need to reduce anxiety. The following balancing factors have been identified as being necessary to resolve the problem and to avert crisis: (1) a realistic perception of the event, (2) adequate situational support (staff and family), and (3) adequate coping mechanisms.[1] When one or more of these balancing factors are absent, the result is an increase in anxiety, with immobilization and an inability to avert the crisis (Fig. 16-3).

In crisis, help should be immediate. Staying with the person, talking through the situation, and encouraging catharsis facilitate recognition of feelings, expression of feelings, and subsequent relief of guilt. Strengthening of coping mechanisms is crucial in preventing the formation of symptoms. Growth in the client is facilitated by using problem-solving skills and a hierarchy of needs framework to help the client set priorities. Nurses are in strategic positions to observe clients in crises and add to a theory of behavioral reactions to illness and to the prevention of maladaptive behavior.

■ MANAGEMENT OF NORMAL BEHAVIORAL RESPONSES TO STRESS

Many persons are able with the added support from health professionals to maintain behavior within the adaptive range when subjected to the stress of illness. In order for support to be provided, for the ego to achieve balance, the client's coping mechanisms and dependency needs are assessed. By reinforcing existing coping mechanisms that are appropriate to the reduction of anxiety and by supporting problem-solving skills, the nurse can draw on the inherent strengths of the person.

Giving persons an opportunity to express their feelings enables them to identify consciously their fears or concerns about illness that may be influencing their behavior. Care givers can assist persons to maintain control of their behavior through the use of problem-solving and behavior modification techniques.

Gains are accrued by the nurse as well as the patient when the nurse intervenes in deliberative interventions planned to help a person cope with the stress of illness (Fig. 16-4).

□ Problem solving

The problem-solving approach is a useful nursing intervention for behavioral reactions to illness and during

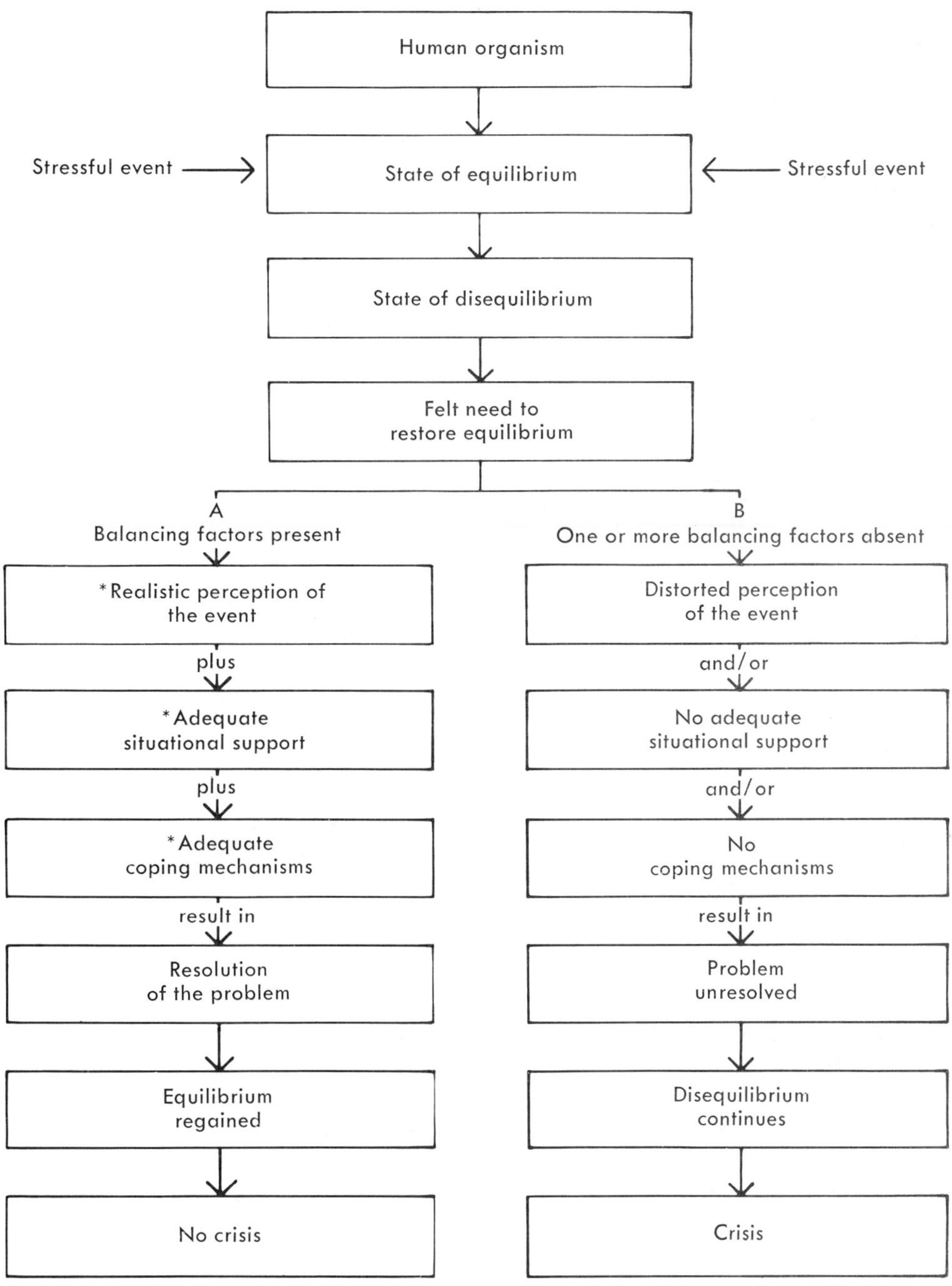

Fig. 16-3. Paradigm: effect of balancing factors in stressful event. (From Aguilera, D. C., and Messick, J. M.: Crisis intervention: theory and methodology, ed. 3, St. Louis, 1978, The C. V. Mosby Co.)

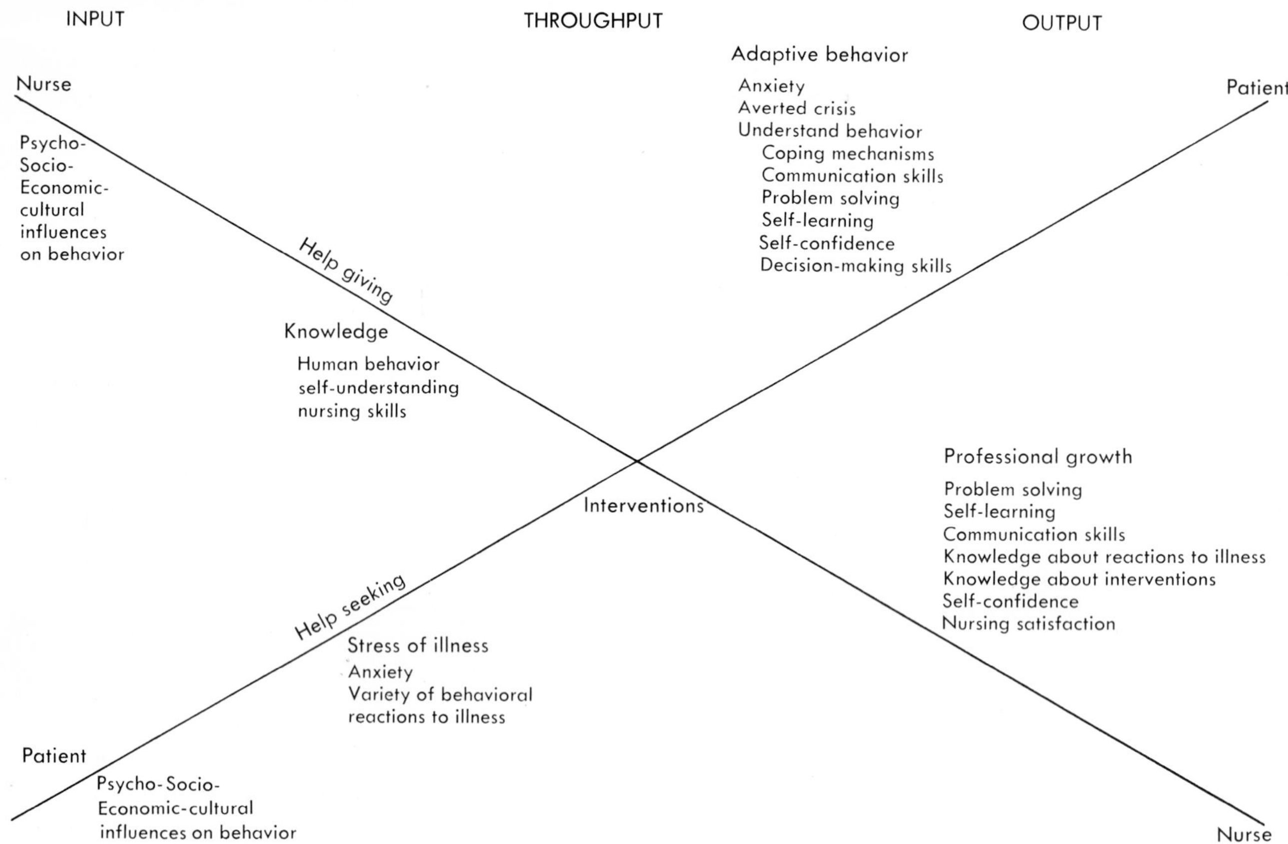

Fig. 16-4. Nursing care is a two-way learning process. Professionals who understand themselves use skills and knowledge to teach patients to become aware of self, assets, deficits, and needs. Both nurses and patients grow from the experience.

crisis. A crucial aid in problem solving is the establishment of a nurse-client relationship (for further information see Chapter 9). The nurse's approach is one of openness and warmth; being nonjudgmental and exhibiting a sense of caring are crucial.

The first step of problem solving includes the nurse's and client's assessment of the stage of the client's reaction to the stress of illness. The nurse promotes reality orientation and provides the client with an opportunity to air feelings and talk through concerns using a problem-solving framework. Clients vary in their ability to identify the problem and in their desire to discuss personal feelings, although it is widely accepted that talking does help. If the client is pushed indiscriminately to talk about problems, the relationship will become superficial and mechanical. Identification and description of problems is followed by analysis, which consists of looking at possible causes. Formulation of alternatives and consequences precedes action aimed at solving the problem. Problem solving reduces ambiguity and feelings of loss of control; the way back to health is a learning process.

When using the problem-solving approach with patients, nurses need to consider the patient's family and others in the support system. Assessment of the family network often provides the client with avenues of support he may have neglected. In addition attention given to families, who often have similar behavioral reactions as the client, will prevent potential conflicts between client and family.

□ Behavior modification

Behavior modification principles may be useful in planning nursing interventions related to emotional aspects of illness. The focus of this approach is to change the behavior of the patient. Thoughts, feelings, and actions normally are syntonic; therefore a change in one affects the other two. Behavior modification provides an approach to growth in patients.

Essentially behavior modification consists of deciding which behaviors exhibited by a particular client are desirable and which are undesirable; actions are then taken to increase the frequency of the desirable behaviors and to decrease the frequency of the undesirable behaviors. Basically people behave in ways that will fulfill their needs; the task is to help select those behaviors that are most helpful and most socially acceptable. For example, the patient who becomes demanding and puts on the call light every 5 minutes would benefit from the use of the principle of saturation. In this situation, if the call light is consistently answered each time it is put on or the patient is seen before he puts on the light, the patient's needs are anticipated and the demanding behavior will cease. The patient's need for attention through turning on the light becomes saturated. The behavior must be tolerated and handled in a nonhostile manner. Interacting with the patient before he puts the light on becomes a reward for positive behavior. The focus of intervention is on building up desirable behavior and not on why the patient is hostile. Saturation works well with over-dependency. Once dependency needs are saturated, the patient will be able to give up overdependent behavior.

Behavior modification focuses on reinforcing behaviors that are curative for patients. The nurse can plan with the patient and agree on which behaviors should be strengthened. Weight reduction through behavior modification using positive and negative reinforcement is beginning to gain popularity as a successful, nonharmful way to lose weight. (For more information see reference 18 at the end of this chapter.)

NURSING INTERVENTION FOR SPECIFIC BEHAVIORAL REACTIONS TO ILLNESS

The five behaviors presented in this section are all adaptive behaviors that are normal reactions to illness, both acute and chronic (Fig. 16-1). Anxious behavior is discussed on p. 228. Intervention is aimed at preventing further disintegration and crisis.

□ Aggressive behavior

Whenever there is a threat to self-concept, such as occurs with illness, the individual may respond by aggression, a way that make him feel less helpless and more powerful. Aggression is another way of handling anxiety. The person is often angry at the loss of health status and questions what is happening to him. He becomes irritable and uncooperative and may project his anger onto the staff and become demanding. It is important that staff accept the patient's hostility without retaliation and that the patient not be made to feel guilty for his actions. Limits should be set and the patient's demands anticipated. Expression of anger in socially acceptable ways prevents anger from being turned inward, causing depression. The patient should be given reasonable control of his environment and the opportunity to participate in planning and implementing his own care.

□ Depressed behavior

Depression is a normal response to illness, once the illness has been accepted. In making an assessment of the person who is depressed, the nurse needs to be aware of the clinical signs of depression. The patient is quiet and may show some confusion. He is apt to lack interest in the surroundings or activities around him. He may voice concern about the illness or the amount of care his illness requires and may express wishes or concerns about dying. The patient's behavior may be extremely dependent and his activity and conversation are slowed. Complaints of weakness and fatigue are common.

Intervention requires that the nurse approach the patient in a serious mood, conveying through actions and communication an understanding of what he must feel. The nurse helps the patient express feelings and conveys acceptance of his right to feel sad. When the patient shows signs of readiness, he is helped to focus on interested areas outside of the illness. The patient may need to talk about activities that he was involved in prior to hospitalization. This is particularly true for persons who have chronic illness. It is important to *listen* to the person who is depressed complain about his problems so that he may turn his anger outward.

Dependency, a common behavior of the depressed patient, is a reaction that may follow the stage of accepting an illness. The patient readily places himself in the hands of others. While dependency is a form of regression, it is also a part of learning to trust. The patient does not want to do much for himself and accepts total care, although he may not demand it. Supportive care is indicated in the early stages with gradual advancement from doing *for* the patient to doing *with* the patient, and then his doing for himself. Thus the patient returns gradually to helping himself.

Overdependency exists when the patient shows physical readiness to progress but prefers to remain dependent. Nurses need to assess the difference through deliberate observation and then set limits kindly on those nursing interventions that continue to promote the dependency. Appropriate interventions at this time include the use of saturation along with helping the patient develop cognitive awareness of his physical ability to do more for himself. The nurse also makes it clear that the patient will not be abandoned and that support in the form of the presence of a member of the nursing staff will be available as he does more for himself.

□ Withdrawn behavior

Withdrawn patients usually do not pose as many problems and are apt to be labeled "good" patients. They demand little from others and thus may be overlooked. Withdrawn patients regress more easily to earlier levels of behavior at which they can accept the patient role. Withdrawn patients need gentle encouragement to talk, to express feelings, and to relate to the staff. Spending time sitting with these patients, often in silence, does much to increase their sense of self-worth.

□ Suspicious behavior

Suspicious patients have difficulty with trust. They may have had previous experiences in which they learned to distrust care givers. They may be suspicious of staff, the routines, the medicine, and the procedures. They need to talk about these concerns but should not be forced to do so. It is imperative that staff keep promises made to these patients and avoid an overzealous approach. Explanations of procedures and establishment of expected routines are helpful. Whispering and talking about the patients within their field of hearing is avoided as the communication may be misinterpreted.

□ Somatic behavior

A familiar reaction to illness is one that can be labeled as a flight into illness. The patient somatizes his concerns; that is, he has learned to express anxiety through complaints about a variety of physical symptoms. He may be preoccupied with bodily functions and feelings of pain. Vague complaints of backache, headache, or fatigue may be expressed in order to legitimize the attention he needs. Support and acceptance by allowing the patient to talk about his symptoms with some limit setting will decrease his anxiety.

Staff often become angry at patients expressing somatic behavior because of their vague symptomatic complaints and because they feel "caught" if they "play down" such symptoms, since there is always the possibility that the complaints are truly connected with the illness. Guilt on the part of staff prevails for some time if a complaining patient who was ignored is diagnosed as having a physical illness. It is wise for the staff to accept all symptoms and report them. Time spent with the patient, listening to him and using the saturation technique (p. 233) will help lessen this behavior.

REFERENCES AND SELECTED READINGS

1. *Aguilera, D. C., and Messick, J. M.: Crisis intervention: theory and methodology, ed. 3, St. Louis, 1978, The C. V. Mosby Co.
2. Bailey, D. S., and Dreyer, S. O.: Therapeutic approaches to the care of the mentally ill, 1977, Philadelphia, F. A. Davis Co.
3. Bellak, L., and Small, L.: Emergency psychotherapy and brief psychotherapy, New York, 1955, Grune & Stratton, Inc.
4. Caplan, G.: Principles of preventative psychiatry, New York, 1964, Basic Books Inc., Publishers.
5. Caplan, G.: An approach to community mental health, New York, 1961, Grune & Stratton, Inc.
6. *Carlson, C. E., editor: Behavioral concepts and nursing interventions, Philadelphia, 1978, W. B. Saunders Co.
7. Erickson, E. H.: Childhood and society, New York, 1963, W. W. Norton & Co., Inc.
8. Frank, A.: Psychoanalysis and psychotherapy, New York, 1956, W. W. Norton & Co., Inc.
9. Janis, I.: Psychological stress: psychoanalytical behavioral studies of surgical patients, New York, 1958, John Wiley & Sons, Inc.
10. Maslow, A. H.: Toward a psychology of being, New York, 1968, D. Van Nostrand Co.
11. *Peplau, H.: A working definition of anxiety. In Burd, S., and Marshall, M., editors: Some clinical approaches to psychiatric nursing, New York, 1963, Macmillan, Inc.
12. Programmed Instruction: helping depressed patient in general nursing practice, Am. J. Nurs. 77:1-32 (Suppl.), 1977.
13. Rappaport, L.: The state of crisis: some theoretical considerations, Chicago, 1972, University of Chicago Press.
14. *Robinson, L.: Liason nursing: psychological approach to total care, Philadelphia, 1974, F. A. Davis Co.
15. Schwartz, L. H., and Schwartz, J. L.: The psychodynamics of patient care, Englewood Cliffs, N.J., 1972, Prentice-Hall, Inc.
16. *Shontz, F.: The psychological aspects of physical illness and disability, New York, 1975, Macmillan, Inc.
17. Simmons, J. A.: The nurse-client relationship in mental health nursing, Philadelphia, 1976, W. B. Saunders Co.
18. *Snyder, J. C., and Wilson, M. F.: Elements of psychological assessment, Am. J. Nurs. 77:235-239, 1977.
19. Strain, S.: Psychological care of the medically ill, New York, 1975, Appleton-Century-Crofts.
20. *Stuart, R. B., and Davis, B.: Slim chance in a fat world: behavioral control of obesity, Champaign, Ill., 1972, Research Press.

*References preceded by an asterisk are particularly well suited for student reading.

17

Maladaptive behavior

MAY WYKLE

The individual with a well-integrated personality has learned to live in relative harmony with the environment. Poor adjustment leads to difficulty in interpersonal relationships. Maladjustments vary in degree from occasional withdrawal to overt psychosis. Many individuals with such emotional problems have nevertheless made marginal adjustments within a particular environment. The additional stress accompanying illness may threaten their security enough to disrupt their personalities, causing personality disorganization and disintegration. This disintegration has been referred to over the years as a "nervous breakdown" by most people and is classified *medically* as mental illness.

It is important to remember that the well-integrated person may have intense emotional responses to illness. The main difference is that these reactions are usually reversible, while the maladaptive individual has an underlying problem that has been "instigated" by stress. Removal of the stress may stop the specific difficulty, but it will seldom if ever change the basic maladaptive behavior pattern.

Since the signing of the Community Mental Health Centers Act in 1963 the number of patients in public mental hospitals declined from 558,922 to 215,566 in 1974. The National Institute of Mental Health has helped fund some 600 community centers, increasing services available to 41% of the nation's population. Nevertheless over 50% of hospital beds in the United States are occupied by patients whose primary diagnosis is mental illness. Another 25% are taken by patients with psychophysiologic diseases such as peptic ulcers, colitis, and asthma; some experts include essential hypertension, arthritis, and other somatic complaints in this classification.

Drug substance abuse and alcoholism are often seen in persons with maladaptive behaviors. These conditions frequently cause physical illness severe enough to require hospitalization.

It is sometimes difficult to differentiate maladaptive behavior from physical illness because of the intimate relationship between the mind and the body. Illness of one always affects the other. Physical illness is usually organic, while mental illness is termed functional. These terms are used when trying to determine the cause of behavior. For example, there may be similarity in the behavior of the patient with an adrenal tumor and the individual with schizophrenia, as can be seen in the following case history.

An 18-year-old high school student had been in a general hospital for diagnosis and treatment of "blackout spells." No organic basis for these spells was found. She was transferred to a private psychiatric hospital with a diagnosis of schizophrenic reaction, catatonic type. She appeared somewhat shy, especially with her peer group. Occasionally she was difficult to rouse in the morning, and she took frequent naps. One morning the nurses decided to try some TLC while attempting to wake her. She was brought a glass of chocolate milk and fed with a spoon, being assured that people cared about her and wanted to help her face the day. Her response was much more rapid than usual, and the nurses felt they had hit on a solution to her problem. The psychiatrist was impressed with their reports but questioned whether the response to the milk was psychologic or physiologic and ordered blood to be drawn for blood sugar level testing the next time she was "catatonic." This was done. The sugar level was 37 mg/100 ml serum (normal 75 to 105 mg/100 ml serum). The patient was transferred to a general hospital for further diagnostic workup. It was determined that she had a left adrenal tumor. This was surgically removed, and she took up life as a relatively normal, healthy young woman.

This case history demonstrates that careful observation, laboratory studies, and even surgery may be necessary to determine the cause of a disease.

Naturally, maladaptive individuals are subject to injury and physical illness, and when they are sick they may need treatment in a general hospital. Many general and community hospitals have set aside a few rooms with special safety provisions to meet the particular needs of clients who are emotionally disturbed.

Basic courses in personality development provide an understanding of normal behavior of patients, but specialized help may be necessary when caring for persons with maladaptive behavior. If the hospital has a psychiatric division it may be possible for the psychiatric nurses to consult with the medical and surgical nurses regarding the care of patients who are mentally ill. Many hospitals do not have such experts available, however, and nurses must depend largely on their own integrated knowledge and resources. When a nurse is assigned to care for patients with severe emotional problems, textbooks, journal articles, audiovisual resources, and other materials on psychiatric nursing provide excellent information. This chapter contains only a brief discussion of a few important principles or criteria to follow in caring for clients with maladaptive behavior.

■ BEHAVIOR

The behavior of the maladjusted individual does not differ in kind from that of the defined normal person; it differs only in degree.[49] Many clients with maladaptive behavior appear quite normal on casual observation and conversation, and it is only on more prolonged contact that abnormalities of personality may be evident. Consequently the nurse needs to take time to assess the patient. On the other hand the patient's interactions with others and his self-control may have deteriorated to a point where he is conspicuous. This type of behavior is often manifested during an acute psychotic episode.

The nurse who for the first time encounters a patient in an acute psychotic episode may be unprepared for the behavior demonstrated. Nurses have been accustomed in their daily living and in their dealings with patients to meeting persons who are able to face challenges to their security with a normal amount of assurance, thus keeping themselves in harmonious association with others. In the hospital the client is often expected to repress fears, irritations, and aggressive impulses to a socially acceptable degree and to be a "good" patient. Because the normal patient has a reasonably well-integrated personality and anticipates a short stay in the hospital, he usually is able to live up to these expectations. The client who has a severe emotional disturbance may be unable to control emotional responses and may react freely and impulsively. He may be out of contact with reality at times, expressing bizarre ideas *(delusions)*, and he may have false sensory perceptions *(hallucinations)*. Hallucinations are usually auditory or visual, but they may be tactile, olfactory, or gustatory. The individual may also feel pain for no apparent physical reason. Regardless of the unreality of these sensations, they are real to the patient. Hearing voices is very common, and patients often answer the voices or respond to the directions given by them. Tactile sensations usually are of crawling objects, and patients may try to flick them away or to run from them.

It is quite common for an emotionally disturbed person to be *severely depressed.* This depression is much deeper than that experienced in varying degrees by normal people. It is described as a feeling of utter hopelessness or as a living death. The individual feels exhausted and is dejected in posture, facial expression, gait, and verbal reactions. He loses interest in his physical surroundings and personal appearance. His appetite is poor, and constipation may develop. Although the individual may be quiet and lie for hours with eyes closed, the severely depressed patient seldom enters a deep-sleep state. At times a depressed patient may become quite tense and restless, showing signs of agitation such as pacing the floor and wringing his hands. He may be tearful and express feelings of inadequacy, unworthiness, and guilt. A depressed patient may mention and often contemplate suicide. Any severely depressed person who suddenly seems much better should be watched carefully, since this improvement often means only that he has decided on a means of escape that may be suicide

Research has shown that the individual contemplating suicide almost always shows warning symptoms in a desperate plea for help. He may talk about death or dying; get his affairs in order; ask to see business associates, family members, or friends; and if hospitalized often make a point of saying good-bye to the nurse who is going off duty or preparing him for sleep.

For the last several years suicide has been among the 10 leading causes of death in the United States. In 1971 there were more than 23,000 reported suicides in this country. Suicide accounted for one of 17 deaths per 100,000 population in the United States in 1973.[9] Interesting studies have shown that by the mid-1980s the fastest growing rate of suicide will be among teenagers and the elderly. The actual number of suicides is probably much higher than figures indicate, since many experts consider many automobile accidents and other accidental deaths as possible suicides (drownings and carbon monoxide poisoning, for example).

The emotionally disturbed patient may be *hyperactive* (manic) or aggressive in his behavior. He may flit from one activity or one subject of conversation to another, and it may be impossible to hold his attention for more than an instant. Profanity and vulgarity are common, and the patient may be critical of the hospital and the personnel as well as sarcastic, caustic, and domineering. The *manic* has the exaggerated behavior of the noisy, demanding patient and may become irritated easily and express his irritation in assaultive behavior. *Hyperactivity* may become so pronounced as to cause exhaustion.

Suspicion (paranoid reactions) may be exhibited by some maladjusted patients. They may appear suspicious, critical, and watchful of every move others make, and they may question activities and refuse medications, treatment, and even food. At the same time they may feel persecuted and neglected if left out of an activity.

Some people with maladaptive behavior show *obsessive-compulsive behavior*. They are compelled to follow certain rituals or behavior patterns that are far beyond normal but that in some way serve to relieve inner tensions. For example, it is normal for many persons to count fence posts as they walk down the road. However, a compulsion neurosis is evident when a person cannot ever walk down a road without counting and touching each post. Ritualistic compulsions in such matters as bathing, washing hands, and dressing in certain sequence are common and, even when carried to great extremes, may sometimes be successfully concealed from the outside world.

The maladjusted individual may become overconcerned and preoccupied with body functions. This type of behavior is known as *hypochondriasis*.

Hysteria is an abnormal behavior pattern that has been recognized for centuries. Despite the lack of physical cause, the person may not be able to do such things as void or move a particular limb. He may have areas of numbness, lack of one of the special senses, or a variety of other physical complaints. He may have apparent convulsive seizures, although unlike the patient with a true convulsive disorder he is not likely to injure himself during an attack.

Anxiety states are common among emotionally disturbed patients. The individual may have an abnormal fear of impending disaster, and this fear may be expressed in bodily signs such as flushing, tachycardia, and excessive perspiration. Although there may be no rational basis for his fear, it is very real to the patient and cannot be dissipated by rational explanation. A word or two picked out of a statement made by his physician may serve as a basis for worries and fears. If anxiety becomes too great, *panic*—complete disorganization of behavior in the face of overwhelming terror—may result. The client then loses complete control of himself and is unable to perceive, communicate, or control motor actions. The environment is often misinterpreted, and the client may try to escape from what he imagines is acute danger around him. This behavior may lead to physical injury such as may be sustained from disconnecting intravenous tubes, removing drainage tubes, or falling out of bed. The client may not be intent on suicide but may destroy himself as he attempts to flee from imagined danger unless special precautions for his safety are taken. The individual in a panic may attack hospital personnel in the belief that they are endangering his life. He acts quickly and impulsively and therefore should be carefully observed and assessed.

■ INTERVENTION FOR PATIENTS WITH MALADAPTIVE BEHAVIORS

□ General principles for nursing care

The care needed by a patient with maladaptive behaviors on a medical or surgical unit is no different from that needed by any other patient. He needs acceptance as a person, provision for physical needs, and provision for safety. Bizarre, socially unacceptable behavior can often be handled by a clear statement of recognition of the behavior and its importance to the patient. This will not necessarily change the behavior, but it will often help prevent further disintegration. It is important that the patient not lose self-esteem; therefore he should be protected from the curious eyes of staff and other patients. Many drugs are available that can help the disturbed client be more comfortable, and when he is more comfortable he can be more cooperative. The nurse who approaches the disturbed patient with an objective, nonprejudiced attitude communicates acceptance and concern. A positive, assertive, expectant manner will shore up the patient's self-respect and help him to be less fearful in a foreign environment.

Emotional care

The client with maladaptive behavior benefits from calmness, consistency, and uniformity in his environment. Procedures should be explained calmly and sometimes repeatedly, even though the individual may not appear attentive or concerned. Even the smallest details of necessary medical or surgical treatment should be explained before they are undertaken. The equipment used for procedures should be reduced to a minimum, but basic principles such as aseptic technique used in changing dressings should not differ from those used in safe nursing anywhere. The client must also be prepared for routine nursing measures; for example, when lights are to be turned out, a meal is to be presented, or a visit to the bathroom is to be made, the patient should be told what is going to occur.

Anything that increases the individual's anxiety may be harmful to him. The use of technical language and discussion of disease and technical procedures should be avoided. Subjects that appear to increase the patient's anxiety are assessed carefully, and mention of them should be made in the nurse's records. Religion is commonly associated with anxiety or feeling of guilt. Also sexual maladjustment is common in persons who are maladaptive. Discussion of close members of the family may produce anxiety. Often the final failure in interpersonal relationships occurs in the family environment, among those whose acceptance is most valued by the patient. It is safest to let the patient volunteer the information he wishes. If he shares personal information, the nurse must let him know that his confidences will be kept and that his disclosures, regardless of their nature, will not be judged.

The nurse should assess change in behavior indicating that anxiety is increasing and panic may develop.[42] These may include failure to hear people speaking, muscular tension, perspiring for no observable reason, failure to make connections between details in conversation or conduct, headaches, nausea, trembling, and weakness.[38] At this time intervention should be taken to help the patient release tension. The patient should be constantly assessed, and if possible he should be removed from the situation that induces the increased anxiety. Activities such as walking, talking, counting, describing something, or playing a simple game reduce anxiety. It also helps to increase the patient's awareness of his surroundings.[38] If panic does occur the patient can often be handled best by two people calmly approaching him, firmly but slowly addressing him, and leading him away from the situation. Large groups should not suddenly approach a greatly disturbed or active patient unless emergency measures are needed to protect him and others. The patient then should be placed in an environment as free from stimuli as possible, and a practitioner should constantly assess him until he becomes calmer. When he is left alone again he should be assured of immediate response if he should need help.

It is useless to argue with the maladaptive individual or to attempt to simply talk him out of his delusions by reasoning with him. He has lost the ability to understand the psychotic nature of his ideas or to see the fallacies in them. No attempt should be made to explain his behavior to him. Many patients become confused and disoriented and may be terrified by their delusions or hallucinations. The nurse can best support the patient by confirming what is real to the individual. For example, the most bizarre concept usually has some element of reality in it. Listening and reflection of the real portion of the patient's experience will help him with his reality testing. It is useless to ask a confused person such questions as time and place. It is better to tell him in a general, conversant manner, "It is 3:00 PM, Mr. Smith. I'll be leaving at 3:30, and I wanted to see if you would like to sit up for a while before I go."

Nonspecific reassurance should be avoided. Simply telling the client that he is not going to die or that he is worthy of his family may do more harm than good, since it may destroy a picture of himself that it is necessary for him to have at the moment. However, specific reassurance that produces a calm, quiet, accepting environment is always of value. The patient should feel that he will not be censured or rejected because of his behavior. He should be given security by assurance of consistency in routine, of the conduct of others toward him. He may gain reassurance from consistency in the way in which he is encouraged to express negative feelings. He may show such feelings by disliking the nurse, for example. He may dislike the nurse without fear of retaliation that would be present if he disliked his spouse or any other close member of the family. Thus hostility toward personnel may be a healthy sign and should be accepted as such by the nurse. Effort should be made to have the patient feel that his behavior is understood even though it may not be approved. The right of the patient to want to behave as he does is acknowledged. For example, the patient may have the right to want to hurl his water pitcher, but he should know that the staff will continue to prevent him from harming himself or others.

Drug therapy

Adequate control of behavior can usually be maintained by the use of antipsychotic drugs (Table 17-1). These drugs are in the phenothiazine group and have side effects that may be uncomfortable to the patient such as dry mouth, blurred vision, and photophobia. It is especially important to observe the patient for extrapyramidal reactions such as tremors, shuffling gait, masklike face, drooling, and restlessness. Severe reactions may cause extreme muscle spasm, particularly of the upper body and frequently limited to one side. This reaction can be quickly alleviated by the use of antiparkinsonian drugs such as benztropine mesylate (Cogentin), biperiden (Akineton), or trihexyphenidyl hydrochloride (Artane) administered intramuscularly or intravenously. In psychiatric facilities patients receiving phenothiazines often are given anticholinergic drugs prophylactically. The appearance of side effects may necessitate changing the dosage or even the drug. Intolerance to one drug does not necessarily indicate intolerance to other tranquilizers. Tranquilizers derived from compounds other than phenothiazines and used for mild to moderate anxiety states include chlordiazepoxide hydrochloride (Librium), diazepam (Valium), and meprobamate (Equanil, Miltown).

Antidepressant drugs, often referred to as psychic energizers, produce feelings of well-being in depressed persons. Amitriptyline (Elavil), imipramine hydrochloride (Tofranil), and phenelzine sulfate (Nardil) are some of the common ones prescribed. Antidepressant drugs may produce any of the more severe as well as the less severe side effects that are observed in patients taking tranquilizers. Since all of these drugs can produce serious side effects, the nurse is cautioned to be aware of average doses and individual tolerance to the drugs. The nurse should also teach patients the purpose, dosage, and side effects of medications prescribed.

Medications are often refused by the maladaptive patient, who may be exceedingly clever at concealing drugs

Table 17-1. Drugs commonly used with persons exhibiting maladaptive behavior

Type of agent	Generic name	Trade name	Average daily dosage (mg)
Antipsychotic agents (phenothiazines)	Chlorpromazine hydrochloride	Thorazine	30 to 1,200
	Thioridazine hydrochloride	Mellaril	30 to 800
	Fluphenazine dihydrochloride	Prolixin	1 to 20
	Trifluoperazine hydrochloride	Stelazine	2 to 20
	Prochlorperazine	Compazine	15 to 150
Antianxiety agents	Chlordiazepoxide hydrochloride	Librium	15 to 300
	Diazepam	Valium	4 to 10
	Meprobamate	Equanil, Miltown	200 to 1,200
Antidepressant agents	Amitriptyline	Elavil	75 to 150
	Imipramine hydrochloride	Tofranil	100 to 300
	Phenelzine sulfate	Nardil	15 to 75

not swallowed. When staff have reason to believe the patient is not taking his medication, pills may be crushed and dissolved unless their bitter taste precludes this measure. Serious problems in giving medications orally must be reported to the physician so that he or she may order another method of administration.

Safety needs

The confused or psychotic patient may be unable to comprehend medical orders such as bed rest or intravenous feedings. Repeated clear explanation of treatments and, most important, frequent short contracts with the patient will do much to gain cooperation. If the patient is unable to comply with medical orders, it may be necessary to restrain him. For instance, if a catheter is in place and the patient repeatedly pulls it out, there is a danger of injury to the bladder and urethra. In this instance soft restraints may be enough of a reminder to prevent the patient from removing the catheter.

Severe restriction of motion such as by leather restraints should be avoided unless there is real danger to the patient or others. Restraining patients often causes increased anxiety, and increased anxiety decreases the patient's ability to deal rationally with his environment. A family member, friend, or staff member who can stay with the patient provides the best way to help the agitated patient adjust to the hospital.

Physical needs

When a patient in a general hospital becomes maladaptive, there is a tendency to become overconcerned with his behavior and to neglect his physical needs. It must be remembered that the patient needs good general nursing care, including mouth care and attention to hygiene. Even if the patient is physically able to carry out these tasks for himself, he is likely to need help, since he may be too preoccupied with thoughts or with other activities to care for himself completely or safely. Patients have been known to lean against a hot radiator and sustain a severe burn or to step into a tubful of very hot water without flinching. Dressings must be changed and medications administered. Often patients will not even ask for a bedpan or urinal or for medication for pain, and the nurse must be responsible for providing for these needs.

For some time before hospitalization the depressed patient may have eaten improperly. He may refuse to eat or he may hide his food to give the impression that he has eaten. The hyperactive patient may be too frightened or preoccupied to eat, yet he may require more than the usual amount of food. An assessable record of *food* and *fluid intake* should be kept on all patients with maladaptive behavior. A record of *urinary* and *bowel elimination* is also necessary. The patient who is depressed often suffers from constipation, and the hyperactive patient may delay going to the bathroom because of his many preoccupations.

Sleep is necessary for the mentally ill patient but is sometimes hard to achieve. Adequate sleep and good general physical health make it easier for him to face his problems and attempt to solve them. Patients with acute mental illness may require large doses of sedatives or tranquilizers to control daytime behavior, although these drugs may actually interfere with sleep, particularly dream (REM, or rapid eye movement) sleep. Exercise outdoors, a quiet environment, a back rub or warm bath, and warm drinks are often surprisingly helpful.

Observations and recordings

The nurse's records are very important to the care of the maladaptive patient. The nurse is around the patient more than any other professional person and may be the only one who observes and assesses him during evening and night hours. Recorded observations can be of great help to the psychiatrist in management of the patient. These notes should be remarkable for their quality rather than their length, but it is best to err on the side of length than of brevity. They should contain actual expressions of the patient, using quotation marks and taking care that the words recorded are exactly those of the patient. Notes should be recorded immediately after significant conversation or behavior has been observed and assessed so that details will be fresh in mind. Although the specialty of psychiatry has a complete vocabulary of its own, it is wiser to clearly record actual statements and situations rather than label the patient's symptoms as delusions or hallucinations. Factual statements such as "States over and over, 'I see men at the window, they are wearing red, they have come to kill me.' " can provide a clearer understanding of the patient's mental state. The nurse's notes should also contain detailed accounts of what the patient does, such as "Sat at the window grimacing and smiling for 2½ hours this evening; keeps saying as he smiles, 'I'll be dead tomorrow.' "

□ Special needs of the depressed patient

The deeply depressed patient may require almost complete physical care to sustain him, and he may be almost totally unresponsive to any attempts to communicate with him. Nevertheless the patient needs human contact both physically and interpersonally even though he may seem oblivious to it. Observant nurses usually will be able to determine to some extent what type of activity or conversation seems to help a particular patient, and they must try to provide it. Overcheerfulness, overt solicitude, abruptness, or a dictatorial manner on the part of personnel is particularly upsetting to depressed patients. A deeply disturbed patient may be depressing to the nurse or other personnel caring for him. If so, personnel should plan their contacts with the patient so that they can provide continuity of care, prevent evident avoidance of the patient, and still retain reasonable emotional personal comfort.

If there is just one person who consistently shows he or she cares for the patient, this fact may be enough to prevent him from coming to the point where he considers *suicide* as the only means of escape from his untenable situation. Even though he is unable to ask for help openly, the depressed patient wants someone to be concerned about his welfare. He wishes to be protected from himself and his possible impulsive behavior. In contemplating suicide he does not necessarily really want to die but to express the urgency of escape from an unbearable situation.

It is not true that persons who talk about suicide rarely attempt it. At least a third of those committing suicide talk about it or give some indirect indication of their intent. Mention of suicide intent by the patient should be taken calmly by the nurse but should be reported to the physician at once and recorded in the patient's record. The patient should immediately be given increased attention, with sympathetic and serious concern. By showing more concern for the patient, the nurse indicates to him that he really matters. It is exceedingly important that the nurse not answer the patient in a way that appears to dare him to carry out his threat. A comment such as, "I know you don't mean that" leaves the patient with the possible choice of carrying out his threat to prove the seriousness of his statement.

Prevention of suicide or other injury requires alert observations and assessment on the part of the nurse. Pocketknives and objects such as nail files, razor blades, belts, drugs, and any pieces of equipment that might be used either impulsively or with premeditation are removed. If the patient is known to be suffering from maladaptive behavior, such belongings should obviously be removed on admission, as is done in mental wards and hospitals. If windows can be raised enough so that the patient could crawl through them, they must be equipped with stop devices to prevent complete opening, and occasionally protection over the glass is necessary. Doors should be fitted with locks that cannot be turned from the inside. Electrical fixtures must be out of reach of the patient who might attempt to electrocute himself by tampering with the socket or who might injure himself with glass from bulbs.

The physician is responsible for ordering constant observation if it is necessary because of the danger of suicide or injury to others. The newspapers bear testimony to many instances of patients leaping from windows or otherwise destroying themselves in the few brief moments when the nurse's back was turned. A decrease in the patient's tension should not cause a relaxation of observation, since decision on a plan of action may be its cause.

The nurse must find a way to observe and assess the suicidal patient carefully and sympathetically without making him feel that he is under constant scrutiny. The patient may resent constant observation, believing that he is being spied on or that he is in danger from the observer. The least conspicuous way to observe a patient is by observing him in a group, but such an arrangement may not be feasible on the medical and surgical unit because of the patient's other illness. The nurse may appear to be busy with a patient in an adjoining room while watching the maladaptive patient. Sometimes locating the observer outside the patient's room may cause the least annoyance. Efforts should be made to convey to the patient that he is being given special attention because the nurse cares about him and feels he needs this attention. When nurses consistently make a genuine and serious effort to find the best way to help a patient, their interest and concern may be crucial in keeping him alive.

Individuals who have made unsuccessful suicide attempts are often admitted to general hospitals for emergency care by means by community rescue services, mobile intensive care units, or private ambulance services. The immediate care depends on the attempts made and the physical emergency care provided at the scene. Patients are frequently treated for drug overdose and other poisoning, severed arteries, and gunshot wounds. They must now face not only the original problem that precipitated the suicide attempt but the consequences of the act. Special care needs to be taken to avoid a repeated attempt, and psychotherapy usually is instituted. Family members, too, often need help in understanding and accepting the patient's problems. Sometimes they need the help of the physician, mental health consultant, social worker, or member of the clergy in planning for the role they will take in the future in helping the patient.

☐ Special needs of the aggressive individual

A patient with aggressive behavior is often overactive and fares best in a nonchallenging and nonstimulating environment. Noise should be kept at a minimum and distraction and irritations of all kinds should be avoided.

The aggressive patient needs to be allowed to express his feelings in a calm, accepting atmosphere. Although he may be most annoying, he must not be allowed to feel that he is a nuisance or is unliked. He should not be prevented from verbalizing his annoyances, and no attempt should be made to talk him out of his attack or to defend the person or situation being verbally attacked. The patient should never be compared with other patients or with himself on previous occasions, as the comparison may make him feel rejected. Answers to questions should be simple and direct. The nurse should avoid encouraging stimulating conversation, while still conferring a feeling of warmth and interest. This encouragement may lead to provocation of aggression when the conversation is ended and the patient assumes rejection.

The aggressive patient may not respond favorably to direct requests. He usually is happier associating with quiet patients, since his aggressiveness often calls forth aggression in others. Attempts should be made to channel the aggressive patient's energy into constructive activity, but he must be observed carefully to detect signs of approaching exhaustion and to prevent upsetting situations from arising because of the possibility of injury to the patient or others. Establishing a relaxed atmosphere in a darkened, quiet room may be helpful for the overactive, aggressive patient, and a sedative may also be given.

☐ Special needs of the patient who focuses on physical symptoms

The patient with a psychoneurosis concerning physical symptoms requires infinite patience and understanding. He also needs firm and thoughtful management. Usually he has told his physical symptoms endless times to numerous people and has worn out his welcome with all. The nurse should listen attentively for a reasonable time and should then try to direct the patient's conversation away from discussion about himself. The nurse should not be trapped into implying that there is nothing wrong with the patient, and it is well to avoid discussion of any medical subject. Activity therapy that can be undertaken at the bedside often helps divert conversation away from the patient and also may result in creativity that earns recognition for him.

The nurse should watch for any attempts the patient may make to aggravate his physical ailment or to produce symptoms. So great may be his need to maintain an acceptable outlet for his problems through illness that he may go to surprising lengths to delay a cure. Patients have been known to hold their thermometers against light bulbs, add water to urine collection bottles, tamper with their wounds to cause infection, and even subject themselves to needless surgery. The nurse has the responsibility to report to the physician if there is reason to believe that a patient is attempting to falsify his clinical picture. An example of such behavior is seen in the following case history.

A 39-year-old unmarried woman who resided with her mother was admitted to the medical service for severe diarrhea and blood loss through her ileostomy. Initially the staff was concerned about fluid loss and dehydration although there was no clinical evidence such as weight loss, poor skin turgor, or changes in laboratory findings. The patient kept her own intake and output record. In one 24-hour period she recorded 450 ml intake and 4,700 ml output, including 28 loose stools, none of which was observed by a staff member. The ileostomy site was reddened and bleeding. The patient in the next bed reported seeing her using a rat-tail comb to irritate the site.

In an attempt to provide more healthy attention-getting activities a very active occupational therapy program was initiated. The patient was quite talented artistically and received many honest compliments on her work. She accepted an invitation to work as a volunteer in the children's ward. Since the intake-output record served no purpose, it was discontinued. No questions were asked about loose stools. She was weighed routinely and without comment about her weight. The patient was most responsive to this regimen and after discharge returned to the hospital weekly for occupational and group therapy. She also entered therapy with a psychologist. The improvement was maintained for 3 months, at which time her mother had a serious fall. The patient was admitted to a surgical floor with an acute exacerbation of symptoms. (The patient had had 27 prior surgical procedures in over 40 hospital admissions.)

To assure reasonable success of this type of approach, each staff member must be well informed about what is being done and why. This prevents the patient from "using" one staff member against another to defeat the program and thus himself.

■ DISORDERS NOT RELATED TO MALADJUSTED PERSONALITY

Organic psychoses are due to disease processes that have produced physical changes. Among the common causes of organic psychoses are neurologic syphilis, arteriosclerosis, and epilepsy with deterioration. Brain tumors, brain trauma, Huntington's chorea, and encephalitis are other examples of organic origins of mental illness.

Toxic reactions or *toxic delirium* may occur when high temperature is present or when toxins have accumulated in the body from disease (for example, uremia). When such factors are the cause, the toxic reaction is *endogenous*. When psychosis results from a reaction to drugs such as bromides, anesthetics, and alcohol, the reaction is *exogenous*.

Toxic reactions are the most common of the psychoses seen in general hospitals. They usually come on suddenly and may disappear as quickly, particularly if the cause can be found and eliminated. Patients with toxic reactions almost always suffer from confusion, hallucinations, and delusions that usually cause fear and sometimes panic.

■ SPECIFIC DISORDERS RELATED TO MALADJUSTED PERSONALITY

□ Functional psychoses

Functional psychoses have no demonstrable organic cause, although it is suspected that eventually one may be found. The emotional disorders commonly classified as functional psychoses include involutional psychotic reaction (involutional melancholia), manic-depressive reaction, schizophrenia (dementia praecox), and paranoia. Functional psychoses are rarely classified as distinct entities, since most patients have a mixture of reactions. Both schizophrenia and paranoia are serious mental illnesses for which the patient often needs long-term care in a special psychiatric facility. Patients with involuntional melancholia and manic-depressive reactions have a fairly good prognosis for recovery from an attack, but attacks tend to recur. If it is known that a patient has suffered from a functional psychosis, the nurse should be alert for early signs of recurring emotional illness, since mental health is taxed by physical illness.

□ Psychoneuroses

Patients with psychoneuroses are seen most often in general hospitals. This is because their behavior, although exasperating to the physician and to all who must help them solve their health problems, is seldom such that care in a mental hospital is necessary. The patient suffering from a psychoneurosis conforms to social standards and is able to appreciate the rights of others in a general sense. He is oriented as to time and place. However, in compromising his desires with social demands he has failed to make a satisfactory emotional adjustment and has escaped from the untenable demands of living by developing psychoneurotic behavior. This behavior may take the form of hypochondriasis, anxiety states, hysteria, or obsessive compulsive behavior. Although the patient may have a physical disease that may or may not be related to his basic emotional disturbance, the emotional problem is predominant and is the one that is really important to the patient. He is less upset by his symptoms than would be expected, and even when extensive diagnostic procedures and surgery are performed, he usually is surprisingly philosophic about the whole experience.

The nurse or anyone else caring for psychoneurotic patients should not assume that these patients are willfully sick. Unfortunately they are too often considered problems by members of the staff who lack the insight to recognize their need to be ill. The patient does feel real pain and discomfort even though no physical cause may be found. Psychoneurotic patients are large consumers of medical care and all related services. It is probable that the economic cost to society of this group of patients is greater than the cost for all the psychoses combined.

□ Alcoholism

Alcoholism is very common and may compound the problems of a person experiencing other health disorders. Excessive alcohol intake may lead to coma or near death from acute alcohol poisoning, or if it occurs over a period of time may lead to numerous other health disorders. Alcoholism is recognized today as a treatable entity. Significant changes in the identification and treatment[22] of alcoholism point toward advances that are having an important impact on this major health problem.

Epidemiology

Alcoholism in the United States is on the increase. Conservative estimates are that 90 million people use alcohol and about 9 million people are afflicted with alcoholism. Alcoholism is defined as "a continuing problem (with alcohol) that affects the person's life, such as his family, his work and/or his social activities." Also, an alcoholic "cannot predict with 100% accuracy what his behavior will be after his first drink."[31] The second definition has to do with the individual's control of the amount he drinks. The nonalcoholic can say he will have one or two drinks and stick to his plan, whereas the alcoholic may not be able to do so. In defining alcoholism one can extrapolate from the quantity-frequency-variability information on alcohol intake, on the presence or absence of physical addiction, or the presence of alcohol-related life problems.[21]

Industries lose at least $10 billion yearly because of alcoholism. This figure includes the cost of time lost, misjudgments, spoiled materials, broken machines, and other factors. Many companies have special programs for the treatment and rehabilitation of employees with alcoholism. Referrals are made by supervisors and managers on the basis of decreased productivity, thus eliminating the need for them to make a diagnosis.

Recent court rulings have declared that the alcoholic is sick and entitled to medical treatment, not imprisonment. Unfortunately there are not enough facilities to treat the alcoholic; treatment is long, expensive, and often unsuccessful.

Etiology

There is no one cause of alcoholism, but alcoholics have been classified empirically into three groups: those whose alcoholism is a symptom of mental disease, those for whom alcohol is a physiologic poison, and those who develop from social drinkers. Persons in the latter group may appear well adjusted until some trouble arises to cause excessive drinking, or they may drift slowly and unknowingly into alcoholism. The alcoholic is likely to be basically insecure and to face realities with difficulty. Alcohol may become a means of escaping the demands of life. The person who is becoming an alcoholic tends to be untruthful about his drinking and to defend himself by rationalizations and pretenses. Alcoholism, like mental illness, is in no way related to social or economic class. It is equally common among the rich and the poor, the intelligent and the mentally limited, the successful and the unsuccessful.

Effects of alcohol

Alcohol contains calories but no vitamins, proteins, or minerals. It is absorbed rapidly from the stomach wall into the bloodstream. However, there is a limited rate at which body cells can use alcohol as food. Any taken in excess of the limit remains in the bloodstream, where it acts as a depressant and an anesthetic, which in turn slows down cellular metabolism. The anesthetic action of alcohol can have serious consequences. The margin of safety for the person anesthetized by alcohol is very small. Unless stimulants are given, alcohol is removed from the stomach, and attention is paid to respiratory function, death may occur.

Assessment

Habitual drunkenness is the main symptom of the disease of alcoholism. Usually alcoholism develops slowly, over a period of 10 to 20 years, until the person reaches a point where he "drinks to live and lives to drink." At this point he tends to be irritable and unreasonable. He may lack judgment and develop physical as well as mental ailments.

The true alcoholic is more interested in alcohol than in food. The person who drinks a great deal may get as much as a third of his daily intake of calories from alcohol, and the alcoholic may get more calories from alcohol than from any other source. When he obtains the alcohol he wishes, he may be too intoxicated to eat or he may have no appetite for normal food. Alcohol is also the most common cause of acute gastritis that results in severe vomiting, which contributes to poor nutrition. Malnutrition may therefore contribute greatly to the alcoholic's physical and mental decline. The alcoholic may be in a general state of poor health with vitamin deficiency, anemia, liver changes, and debility. His resistance to infectious disease is low, and contact with infection is likely during severe bouts of drinking. Consequently he is often admitted to the hospital with infectious disease such as pneumonia or tuberculosis.

Many alcoholics have neurologic symptoms (polyneuropathy) that may include severe pain in the legs and arms and burning of the soles of the feet. Foot drop and wrist drop may develop, and walking and use of the hands may be seriously limited or made impossible. Many alcoholics develop pellagra with its characteristic skin changes of redness, dryness, scaling, and edema. Both pellagra and polyneuropathy are due to vitamin deficiency and are treated with massive doses of vitamin B complex. Weakening of the heart muscle and resultant heart enlargement ("beer heart") is believed to be caused largely by vitamin deficiency. Symptoms of acute heart failure may bring the patient to the hospital. Cirrhosis of the liver occurs often in persons who are alcoholic, and it is believed that the cause is primarily malnutrition—a lack of protein and perhaps other food constituents that are not contained in alcohol.

Chronic alcoholics often exhibit personality changes and general deterioration of thinking processes. They may be emotionally unstable, suspicious, quick to take offense, and unpredictable in social and related situations. Serious impairment of memory may occur. Severe tremor, visual hallucinations, and loss of memory may develop even if nutrition has been adequate.

Any hospitalized patient who is not known to be an alcoholic but who does not respond normally to preoperative medication, to anesthetics, or to sedatives should be observed carefully for signs of alcoholism. The alcoholic patient usually requires large doses of sedatives and anesthetic agents for effect, and he is likely to be overly excited and active as he reacts from anesthesia. The most apparent signs of chronic alcoholism that may be noted by the nurse are a tremor that is worse in the morning and morning nausea. The patient feels "jittery," and were alcohol available he would probably have a drink or two to "steady his nerves" before eating.

Intervention

Alcohol may be prescribed for alcoholic patients during their hospitalization, particularly during an acute illness when reaction to deprivation is severe. However, close observation is necessary because even the patient receiving alcohol as prescribed may be extremely resourceful in obtaining an additional supply. If a patient appears to be obtaining unauthorized alcohol, the physician should be notified, since additional alcohol may interfere with the medical regimen. Any alcoholic patient admitted to the general hospital for an acute medical or surgical condition should be observed closely for signs of impending delirium tremens. Early treatment may prevent the development of an acute psychosis.

Regardless of the circumstances surrounding his hospitalization, the alcoholic patient often feels hopeless, guilty, and apprehensive. If his physical ailment is related directly to alcoholism, he is usually quite ill before he consents to be hospitalized. Often he wishes to talk to someone, but the person must be someone who seems to accept him as he is and to understand his problem. The nurses caring for him need to be patient and willing to listen. They should not appear critical of the patient or offer specific advice but must try to make him feel that he is ill and that help is available. The patient is more likely to be able to accept help if he feels that he still has his self-respect.

It is only when the patient truly desires and seeks help with his alcohol problem that treatment is useful. The nurse frequently is the person present at the time the patient is most ready for help—when he has "reached the bottom" and is suffering from the embarrassment and discomfort of a physical misfortune brought on by drinking. It may be at this time that he is a little more ready to face reality than he has been for some time in his recent past. Nurses' attitudes toward the patient and their knowledge of facilities for treatment of alcoholism may be crucial to the life of the patient and for his family.

The objective of all treatment is to induce the patient to stop drinking alcohol. When the alcoholic does stop drinking, he can *never take one single drink* on any occasion without serious danger of relapsing. He is never considered cured, and abstinence is his only course. Sedatives and tranquilizers may be administered until he recovers from the nervous agitation and insomnia caused by the withdrawal of alcohol. Vitamins and a diet high in calories, proteins, and carbohydrates may be prescribed to improve nutrition and to help overcome weakness and fatigue. Psychotherapy may be helpful to the patient in overcoming the desire to drink.

Because alcoholism is a major health concern, nurses need to be aware of community efforts and resources for its treatment. Most facilities do not require a physician's referral; the patient simply presents himself. If the nurse encounters an alcoholic person in the community who is seeking help, he should be directed to sources of help. If the patient is hospitalized, the nurse would work through the physician in charge and often through the social worker. Alcoholics Anonymous (AA) is a group of self-acknowledged alcoholics whose aim is to stay sober and to help other alcoholics gain sobriety. There are AA groups in most communities, and usually regular meetings are held. These groups are open to anyone who has a problem with alcohol, and there are no charges involved. Local groups are listed in the telephone directory for each community. A phone call at any hour of the day or night will bring an AA member to see any alcoholic desiring help. Some communities have subgroups of AA that also hold regular meetings. They include Al-Anon for relatives and friends of alcoholics and Al-Ateen for children of alcoholics. Many communities have alcoholic clinics where medical and psychiatric help are available, and many industries now have medical and rehabilitation programs for alcoholics. Information on alcoholism and programs for alcoholics and others are available for interested individuals and groups.*

Delirium tremens, an acute alcoholic psychosis, can occur when the confirmed alcoholic is denied a regular supply of alcohol, or it may develop when the patient is taking alcohol regularly. It may follow injury, infectious disease, anesthesia, or surgery and may develop in the patient who has not revealed his alcoholic status to his doctor. Delirium tremens is a serious mental illness and

*National Council on Alcoholism, 2 Park Ave., New York, N.Y. 10016; North American Association of Alcoholism Programs, 1130 17th St. S.W., Washington, D.C. 20036; Alcoholics Anonymous World Service, Inc., Box 459, Grand Central Station, New York, N.Y. 10017; Al-Anon Family Group Headquarters, Box 182, Madison Square Station, New York, N.Y. 10010.

may cause the death of the patient. Signs of acute alcoholic psychosis include severe uncontrollable shaking and hallucinations. The patient often says that he sees insects on the wall and that rats or mice are on his bed and sometimes that they are biting him. He becomes extremely restless and apprehensive and perspires freely; sometimes true panic occurs. The treatment consists of tranquilizing drugs such as chlordiazepoxide; sedatives such as paraldehyde given rectally, intramuscularly, or orally; and a high-caloric and high-vitamin diet that may have to be given by nasogastric tube. The patient must be protected from physical injury and observed carefully for signs of cardiac failure. ACTH and cortisone may be given. Recovery usually takes from 1 to 2 weeks.

□ Drug abuse and narcotic addiction

In recent years drug abuse has risen sharply. There are no reliable statistics on drug abusers, and experts disagree as to what actually constitutes drug abuse. Some would include repeated use of any drug, while others limit it to those drugs that used repeatedly lead to habituation or addiction. The Alcohol, Drug Abuse and Mental Health Administration estimates that there are 25 million narcotic addicts and drug abusers in the United States.[53]

Drug traffic has particularly increased among adolescents and young adults, and drugs are readily available on most elementary and secondary school and college campuses. The use of marijuana is widespread. There is much controversy as to whether it is addicting; many experts say that it is not. There have been many reports of actual psychotic episodes following the use of drugs such as LSD (lysergic acid diethylamide) or other hallucinogenic drugs such as peyote or mescaline. It must be remembered that the person using drugs may have an underlying personality problem that is aggravated by the drug, not necessarily caused by it. Drugs commonly taken in an attempt to "get high" include barbiturates, sedatives, amphetamines, synthetic analgesics, and cough syrups.

While there is no general agreement on a definition for drug addiction, the World Health Organization has suggested the following:

> Drug addiction is a state of periodic or chronic intoxication produced by the repeated consumption of a drug (natural or synthetic). Its characteristics include an overpowering desire or need (compulsion) to continue taking the drug or to obtain it by any means; a tendency to increase the dose; a psychological and gradually a physical dependence on the effects of the drug; and a detrimental effect on the individual and on society.*

*From Expert Committee on Addiction-Producing Drugs: Seventh report, Technical report series no. 116, Geneva, 1957, World Health Organization.

Heroin, an opium derivative that quickly produces addiction, is the drug used most often by American addicts today. There is uncertainty as to the extent of the narcotic problem because many narcotic users are not known. In New York City alone it is believed that there are over 100,000 heroin addicts. Federal agents estimate that heroin addiction in persons below age 25 years rose by 40% from 1968 to 1969 in the United States.[26] There are many reported cases of children aged 14 years and under who admit to heroin addiction. There has been a shift toward younger addicts and an increase in the percentage of whites using heroin. In 1975, 51% of addicts in the United States were white, compared with 44% in 1959. The average age has dropped from 35 years in 1950 to 23 in 1975.

The use of drugs is not limited to any socioeconomic group. The problem has long existed in the ghetto, and today it has spread to the affluent suburbs and homes of middle-class Americans. Increased social pressures, stresses of puberty and the search for self, frustration, and even boredom can lead adolescents to try drugs as they seek something to ease the pain of growing up.

One of the obstacles to early detection and treatment of addiction is the reluctance of parents to admit that their son or daughter is a drug user. Even members of the health professions "overlook" the often obvious symptoms of drug addiction or, having confronted the user, fail to report their findings to the parents or authorities. The incidence of drug addiction is high also among health care professionals, probably because drugs are more available to them than to other groups of people. Occasionally a patient who must be given narcotics to control pain over a long period of time becomes an addict. It is rare, however, that addiction develops in those given narcotics for real pain, and the nurse should not let fear of the development of addiction keep her from administering prescribed narcotics to patients hospitalized and in severe pain.

Assessment

Early indications of drug use vary with the individual but frequently include (1) abrupt changes in behavior, mood swings; (2) loss of interest in school, sports, dates, other activities; (3) frequent talking and reading about drugs; and (4) loss of appetite, increased thirst, and constipation. When the drug is actually present in the body, the user may seem drowsy or inebriated and be unconcerned about painful stimuli; the pupils of the eyes may be constricted to pinpoints.

After the individual has developed a tolerance, he may appear quite normal, converse easily, and be able to work. Constipation and appetite loss persist, and he may look undernourished. If the person has been "mainlining'" (injecting the drug directly into the vein), needle marks, scars, or small scabs can be seen on the hands and forearms or the instep. Addicts often wear long sleeves to hide such marks. However, many other veins are used as points of entry to conceal addiction, including such inconspicuous areas as the dorsal vein of the penis or the conjunctival artery of the eyelid.

When the addict goes without the drug for a period longer than he can tolerate, he displays *withdrawal symptoms*. These include (1) restlessness, twitching, excessive yawning, sweating, and running eyes and nose; (2) severe abdominal cramps, diarrhea, and vomiting; and (3) dilation of the pupils. Complete withdrawal of the drug without the substitution of another drug is called "cold turkey" and is a very uncomfortable physical and psychologic condition that may last up to 3 days.

Because of the expense involved, users often sell their belongings or steal to get the money to buy a "fix." Many addicts spend from $200 to $300 a day to maintain their habit. Each day abuse of drugs in the United States costs the economy $27.7 million. Property loss through crimes connected with drugs is estimated at $17.3 million. The disappearance of such items as transistor radios, watches, jewelry, and other similar objects from the home should arouse the suspicion of parents and friends.

Intervention

In the United States the addiction to narcotics has been considered a crime ever since the passage of the Harrison Narcotic Act in 1914. The general feeling of the Council on Mental Health of the American Medical Association is that narcotic addiction should be considered and treated as an illness. The present methods of treating narcotic addicts are not satisfactory, and the incidence of relapse is high.

One approach to the treatment of narcotic addiction is the methadone maintenance program. Methadone is a synthetic drug, and the average narcotic user's daily dose is inexpensive. The drug is given legally as a part of a rehabilitation program that includes group or individual therapy or both. The drug reduces the severity of the heroin withdrawal, and the user can often maintain employment while undergoing treatment. Methadone itself is addictive and must be tapered off or the user may continue the habit the rest of his life. Because this drug is easily available through legal channels and permits the person to work, methadone advocates feel its use is essentially the same as that of the diabetic taking insulin or that of persons on maintenance doses of other drugs such as steroids or digitalis. A newer drug, acetylmethadol, may prove to be superior to methadone.

One of the most effective means of treatment to evolve recently is the use of residential communities, usually run by ex-addicts, with or without professionals. Synanon is such a community. It was founded in California in 1958, and there are now several chapters across the country. In New York there are the Phoenix and Horizon Houses. Marathon House serves the Rhode Island–Massachusetts area. In Chicago the program is available under the name of Gateway Houses. Such services are usually listed in local telephone directories, and the organizations often have literature for distribution and will provide speakers for groups.* The treatment in such communities consists of helping the person through the withdrawal state and then attempting to help him to increase his self-understanding and to change his life pattern. Therapy is provided by the group. Rules of the community are strict, and breaking them results in severe consequences. The programs range in length from 18 to 36 months. Many addicts stay in the community after they no longer use the drug and help to rehabilitate other addicts. This provides support, and a good number of former users can "stay clean." Of those who leave the community, many return to drug use.

There are two federal narcotics hospitals, one in Lexington, Kentucky, and the other in Fort Worth, Texas. Most of the patients in these institutions are there by court order and have little motivation for giving up drugs. Treatment is conservative. More than 90% of these patients return to heroin use. There is much controversy as to the merits of the various programs. Financial problems are serious, and there is much competition for the limited available funds.

Although patients receiving treatment for drug addiction usually are housed in special units of psychiatric facilities, the nurse on a medical or surgical unit may have patients who are drug addicts. The drug addict may develop any of the medical and surgical ailments that any other person may have. Because of their poor nutritional state, many addicts have lowered resistance to disease and infection. The use of contaminated syringes and needles often causes hepatitis. In addition the drug addict, in an attempt to get drugs, may seek admission to a general hospital. He may complain of severe pain such as that from renal colic or back strain, since these are disorders for which narcotics often are given even before a specific diagnosis is made.

*Additional information on drugs and drug abuse can be obtained from the National Institute of Mental Health, Box 1080, Washington, D.C. 20013.

REFERENCES AND SELECTED READINGS

1. A pot primer for parents: Time **95:**56, Feb. 23, 1970.
2. *Ayd, F. J., Jr.: The chemical assault on mental illness: the major tranquilizers, Am. J. Nurs. **65:**70-78, 1965; The minor tranquilizers, Am. J. Nurs. **65:**78-84, June 1965.
3. *Bahra, R.: The potential for suicide, Am. J. Nurs. **75:**1782-1788, 1975.
4. Bailey, D., and Dryer, S.: Therapeutic approaches to the care of the mentally ill, Philadelphia, 1977, F. A. Davis Co.
5. Beck, A. T.: The diagnosis and management of depression, Philadelphia, 1973, University of Pennsylvania Press.
6. *Bowles, C.: Children of alcoholic parents, Am. J. Nurs. **68:**1062-1064, 1968.
7. *Brooks, B. R.: Aggression, Am. J. Nurs. **67:**2519-2522, 1967.
8. *Burd, S. F., and Marshall, M. A.: Some clinical approaches to psychiatric nursing, New York, 1963, Macmillan, Inc.
9. Carter, F. M.: Psychosocial nursing, New York, 1971, Macmillan, Inc.
10. Christoffers, C. A.: An existential encounter, Perspect. Psychiatr. Care **5:**174-181, 1967.
11. *Clarke, A. R., editor: Conference on hostility in the nurse-patient interaction, Perspect. Psychiatr. Care **7:**150-187, 1969.
12. *Ditzler, J.: Rehabilitation for alcoholics, Am. J. Nurs. **76:**1772-1775, 1976.
13. Dixson, B. K.: Dealing with passive-aggressive behavior, Nurs. Forum **3:**277-285, 1969.
14. Dulcher, I. E., and Hakerem, H. M.: Mother-child interaction in psychosomatic illness, Nurs. Forum **7:**173-189, 1968.
15. *Eiseman, B., Lam, R. C., and Rush, B.: Surgery on the narcotic addict, Ann. Surg. **159:**748-757, 1964.
16. *Farberow, N., and Shneidman, E. S.: The cry for help, New York, 1961, McGraw-Hill Book Co.
17. *Field, W. E., Jr.: When a patient hallucinates, Am. J. Nurs. **63:**80-82, 1963.
18. *Fowler, G. R.: Understanding the patient who uses alcohol to solve his problems, Nurs. Forum **4:**6-15, 1965.
19. *Gerdes, L.: The confused or delirious patient, Am. J. Nurs. **68:**1228-1233, 1968.
20. *Haber, J., et al.: Comprehensive psychiatric nursing, New York, 1978, McGraw-Hill Book Co.
21. *Heinemann, E., and Estes, N.: Assessing alcoholic patients. Am. J. Nurs. **76:**785-789, 1976.
22. Industrial Service Department of National Council on Alcoholism: Prevalence of alcoholism among employees, New York, 1968, National Council on Alcoholism.
23. *Jourard, S. M.: Living and dying, suicide: the invitation to die, Am. J. Nurs. **70:**273-275, 1970.
24. *Kalkman, M. E.: Recognizing emotional problems, Am. J. Nurs. **68:**536-539, 1968.
25. Kaufman, R., and Levy, S. B.: Overdose treatment, J.A.M.A. **227:**411-413, 1974.
26. *Kids and heroin: the adolescent epidemic, Time **95:**16-25, March 16, 1970.
27. Klimenko, A.: Multifamily therapy in the rehabilitation of drug addicts, Perspect. Psychiatr. Nurs. **6:**220-223, 1968.

*References preceded by an asterisk are particularly well suited for student reading.

28. *Kline, N., and Davis, J. M.: Psychotropic drugs, Am. J. Nurs. **73:**54-62, 1973.
29. *Long, B.: Sleep, Am. J. Nurs. **69:**1896-1899, 1969.
30. Manfredo, L., and Krampetz, S.: Psychiatric nursing, Philadelphia, 1977, F. A. Davis Co.
31. Mann, M.: New primer on alcoholism, ed. 9, New York, 1968, Holt, Rinehart & Winston, Inc.
32. *McCown, P. P., and Wurm, E.: Orienting the disoriented, Am. J. Nurs. **65:**118-119, 1965.
33. Mereness, D. A., and Taylor, C. M.: Essentials of psychiatric nursing, ed. 10, St. Louis, 1978, The C. V. Mosby Co.
34. *Mertz, H.: How the nurse helps the patient in his experience with psychiatric care, Perspect. Psychiatr. Nurs. **6:**260-263, 1968.
35. *Mueller, J. F.: Treatment for the alcoholic: cursing or nursing, Am. J. Nurs. **74:**245-247, 1974.
36. *Muhlenkamp, A. F.: Personality characteristics of drug addicts, Perspect. Psychiatr. Nurs. **6:**213-219, 1968.
37. *Nelson, K.: The nurse in a methadone maintenance program, Am. J. Nurs. **73:**870-874, 1973.
38. *Newson, B., and Oden, G.: Nursing intervention in panic, emergency intervention by the nurse, No. 1, New York, 1962, American Nurses' Association.
39. *Nowlis, H. H.: Why students use drugs, Am. J. Nurs. **68:**1680-1685, 1968.
40. Parley, K.: Supporting the patient on LSD day, Am. J. Nurs. **64:**80-82, 1964.
41. *Parry, A. A., McNatt, J., and Sahler, S.: Alcoholism and caring for the alcoholic, Am. J. Nurs. **65:**111-116, 1965.
42. *Peplau, H.: Interpersonal techniques: the crux of psychiatric nursing, Am. J. Nurs. **62:**53-55, 1962.
43. *Price, G. M.: Alcoholism—a family, community and nursing problem, Am. J. Nurs. **67:**1022-1025, 1967.
44. Roberts, S. L.: Territoriality: space and the schizophrenic patient, Perspect. Psychiatr. Nurs. **7:**29-33, 1969.
45. Scarpitti, F. R., et al.: Public health nurses in a community care program for the mentally ill, Am. J. Nurs. **65:**89-95, 1965.
46. Shneidman, E. S.: Preventing suicide, Am. J. Nurs. **65:**111-116, 1965.
47. Tallent, N., Kennedy, G. F., Jr., and Hurley, W. T.: A program for suicidal patients, Am. J. Nurs. **66:**2014-2016, 1966.
48. *Thomas, B. J.: Clues to patients' behavior, Am. J. Nurs. **63:**100-102, 1963.
49. Topalis, M., and Aguilera, D.: Psychiatric nursing, ed. 7, St. Louis, 1978, The C. V. Mosby Co.
50. *Ujhely, G.: Nursing intervention with the acutely ill psychiatric patient, Nurs. Forum **3:**311-325, 1969.
51. Ujhely, G.: The nurse and her problem patients, New York, 1963, Springer Publishing Co., Inc.
52. *Umscheid, Sister Theophane: With suicidal patients caring for is caring about, Am. J. Nurs. **67:**1230-1232, 1967.
53. U.S. Department of Health, Education and Welfare: Meeting America's needs, Alcohol, Drug Abuse and Mental Health Administration, Washington, D.C., 1975, U.S. Government Printing Office.
54. *Vaillot, Sister Madeleine Clemence: Living and dying: hope, the restoration of being, Am. J. Nurs. **70:**268, 270-273, 1970.
55. *Wilner, D. M., and Kassebaum, G. G., editors: Narcotics, New York, 1965, McGraw-Hill Book Co.

18

Adaptation throughout the life cycle

PATRICIA HUMPHREY
DONNA HEWITT

Each client that the nurse meets in any setting is engaged in the process of growth, from the pregnant mother and her growing fetus to the toddler, the adolescent, and the aged grandmother. Growth encompasses physical, mental, and emotional spheres; therefore in planning nursing care it is just as important to provide for the patient's growth and development needs as it is to meet needs generated by the client's illness. Each contact that a nurse has with a child or a family is an opportunity for developmental assessment.

Diseases and disorders requiring medical or surgical treatment afflict persons of all ages, from newborn infants to octogenarians. The age of a patient influences his nursing needs and must always be considered in planning and providing care for him. Each person, regardless of age and whether he is sick or well, has needs related to his physical and emotional welfare. These include being fed, clothed, and housed, being safe and comfortable both physically and spiritually, and being important to others.

In the United States two age groups have received a great deal of society's attention: children and the elderly. These groups of people were easier to study because they were in institutions such as schools or rest homes. The adult population has not been quite so easy to study. It is only in recent years that we are seeing more information in the literature regarding young adults and middle-aged persons. The number of elderly people in the United States has increased steadily over the past 50 years. Approximately 21.8 million persons are 65 years of age or over.[21] By 2000 it is estimated that this number will reach or surpass 30 million. At present those persons 75 years of age or over are increasing proportionately faster than the total age group who are over 65. The increasing number of elderly persons has come about primarily through the decrease in infant mortality, the prevention and control of communicable disease during childhood, the improved treatment of adult acute and chronic disease, and improvements in medical care in general. At the same time the birth rate in the United States is declining; in 1973 it was slightly above the zero population growth level.

The growth rate of the older population has been consistently faster than that of persons under 65. Every day approximately 4,000 Americans turn 65; every day 3,000 Americans 65 years or older die. Thus every day there is a net increase of 1,000 persons in the older population.[21]

■ CYCLES OF HUMAN GROWTH

Growth may be defined as a change in body structure or size. Physical growth is a continuous process from the moment of conception until the organism reaches adulthood. Growth takes place by the development and integration of differentiated cells and tissues. *Development* denotes increases in functional capacity evolved from maturation of physical and mental capacities and learning. *Maturation* implies the replacement or rejection of a previously learned appropriate behavior in order to replace that behavior with one more appropriate to the age of the changing individual. In all children development takes place as growth takes place—regularly and in a predictable, continuous pattern. Every child moves through the same developmental stages in a characteristic human way. As mentioned, development is dependent on physical maturation. The organism must reach a certain level of physical growth before certain developmental tasks are possible. One illustration is that infants can make primitive stepping motions but cannot walk because the bones and muscles of the legs are not physically mature enough to support the body weight.

While allowing for individual variations, development is always governed by a few principles. There is a cephalocaudal (from head to toe) and proximodistal (from

Table 18-1. Cephalocaudal development during first year of life

First year	Development
First quarter	Control of eyes and head
Second quarter	Control of upper trunk and arms
Third quarter	Control of lower trunk and fine prehensile grip
Fourth quarter	Erect posture and bipedal locomotion begin

the midline of the body outward) progression of development (Table 18-1).

Development also proceeds from the general to the specific. The infant possesses the gross or large muscle movements long before fine motor skills are developed.

■ NEONATE AND INFANT

The greatest risk of death is in the period immediately following birth when the transition must be made from intrauterine symbiotic existence to extrauterine independent life.[28] Neonates must make several adaptations in order to survive. They must establish respiration and adapt their circulatory system to function independently of the placenta.

On the other hand some systems are able to function very well at birth. For example, the gastrointestinal system is able to handle complex sugars in human milk. The infant can digest carbohydrates for energy in the first 5 hours of life, and fat becomes an important source of energy by the second day. It is not until the third day that protein metabolism begins.[5] The liver is immature at birth and has limited ability to conjugate bilirubin and corticosteroid. The nervous system of the newborn, while functioning primarily at a reflex level, is fully functional in a life-sustaining sense.

Assessment of the neonate

Assessment begins at birth. Apgar scoring charts available in most delivery rooms evaluate five signs of a healthy neonate: a heart rate of 120 to 160 beats per minute, a good strong cry, well-flexed extremities, irritable reflexes, and a healthy pink color. An initial assessment is made at 60 seconds, and a second assessment, which gives some measure of the infant's adjustment to extrauterine life, is made at 5 minutes (Table 18-2).

Gross physical anomalies such as cleft lip or palate, omphalocele, or club foot may be observed on initial examination at birth.

More detailed assessment of the infant may be conducted at this time if the infant is stable, or may be de-

Table 18-2. Apgar scoring

Sign	Score		
	0	1	2
Heart rate	Absent	Slow (below 100)	Over 100
Respiratory effort	Absent	Weak cry, hypoventilation	Good; strong cry
Muscle tone	Limp	Some flexion of extremities	Active motion, extremities well flexed
Reflex irritability	No response	Grimace	Cry
Color	Blue, pale	Body pink, extremities blue	Completely pink

DISAPPEARANCE OF INFANTILE REFLEXES

Reflex	Disappearance
Sucking	Persists throughout infancy, particularly during sleep
Rooting	3 to 4 months while awake; many persist during sleep for 9 to 12 months
Palmar grasp	5 to 6 months
Plantar grasp	9 to 12 months
Moro reflex	4 to 7 months
Stepping	3 to 4 months
Placing	10 to 12 months
Incurvation of trunk	2 to 3 months

layed until a later time. Nursing care during the immediate postnatal period is directed toward provision of warmth, safety, adequate respiration, and nutrition.

Infancy is the most rapid period of physical growth during life. The average infant increases in length by 50% during the first year. Most infants double their birth weight by 6 months and triple their birth weight by 1 year. During infancy neurologic development proceeds from reflexive behavior, which is normal during the early months of infancy, to voluntary control as association pathways begin to develop (see box above).

The relatively immature gastrointestinal tract of the infant matures and the rapid emptying time begins to slow by the end of the first year. Because the rate of water turnover is great during infancy, an increased amount of fluid must be ingested each day to keep pace with the normal fluid loss. Water needs are generally met if the infant is fed properly, as most sources of food

NUTRITIONAL NEEDS OF INFANTS

Calories	100 calories/kg wt
Protein	2 to 3.5 g/kg wt
Vitamin A	2,000 to 2,500 IU/day
Thiamine	0.4 mg/day
Riboflavin	0.6 mg/day
Niacin	10 mg/day
Vitamin C	20 to 30 mg/day
Vitamin D	400 to 800 units/day

TASKS TO BE MASTERED DURING INFANCY

Stabilization of newly independent physiologic processes
Developing control of muscular and nervous system
Learning to understand and control the physical world through exploration
Beginning to acquire language
Establishing self as separate entity
Learning to trust
Developing independent emotional relationships with others

for infants are very dilute. The infant's need for calories, fluids, and all nutrients is greater proportionately than that of persons of other age groups (see box above). Due to limited reserves of fat, glycogen, and extracellular water, the infant cannot tolerate loss of fluid or omission of food or fluids for more than a few hours without experiencing acidosis and dehydration.

The infant generates large amounts of heat because of an active metabolism. However, infants lose proportionately larger amounts of fluid than older persons when dissipating heat. Thus there is a danger of rapid dehydration when the infant is febrile. In addition the infant's poor control of vascular dilation and constriction interferes with body heat retention. Thus the infant chills easily. Both fluid balance and temperature control warrant special concern by those providing infant care.

Psychosocial growth

Infants are primarily egocentric beings and are concerned only with themselves and the satisfaction of their own needs and desires. Most of their reactions are based on the "pleasure principle."

Basic to emotional development during infancy is the acquisition of a *sense of trust* (Fig. 18-1). Most often the mother, who is the primary caretaker, is the most significant person involved in the achievement of basic trust. When the mother provides nurturance, familiarity, security, and continuity of experience, the infant is able to develop a sense of trust of the world around him and the people in it. A sense of mistrust of the environment and the people in it may result if an inadequate mothering relationship is present. Erikson feels this experience is irrevocable and influences the way subsequent stages evolve.[10]

Research in learning indicates that early stimulation during infancy is important for the future learning capacity of the individual.[13] According to Piaget's theory of cognitive development, the period of infancy is termed the period of *sensorimotor development*. During the first month of life the infant acts on the ready-made sensorimotor schemata consisting primarily of reflexes and the innate capacities for performance. From 1 to 4 months infants act primarily on events that are centered around their own bodies. They begin sucking as the bottle approaches, show signs of recognition, and may respond to a familiar toy. Objects have no permanence as attested to by the fact that an infant makes no search when a toy disappears from the visual field. Between 4 and 8 months, building on the schemata of the first two periods, infants develop the ability to perceive objects as separate from themselves and become more active in causing events to happen. In the last 4 months of the first year of life the infant continues refinement of characteristics acquired during the third period. They begin to develop a more mature notion of causality and of the concept of means-end relationships.

Language development begins shortly after birth with the ability to cry. Infants develop different cries to communicate specific needs such as hunger, pain, or being wet. By 3 months of age most infants develop the beginnings of prelanguage, vocalizing by babbling and cooing. Before the age of 6 months infants respond to their names and begin to respond to simple instructions such as "Come here." At 7 months of age the infant is able to vocalize four different syllables and makes talking sounds in response to the talking of others. The 8-month-old babbles to produce consonant sounds and says "dada" or "mama." By 11 months the infant initiates definite speech sounds and uses jargon. At this age he communicates a great deal by pointing at objects. By the end of the first year the child can say a few simple words and jabbers expressively. The tasks to be mastered during infancy are shown in the box above.

Health concerns during infancy

During the first year or two of life the infant's endocrine functions are sluggish. Their fluid and electrolyte balance is easily upset, and they have little resistance to infection or stressors of any kind. Babies therefore respond quickly and critically to illness. They may be ap-

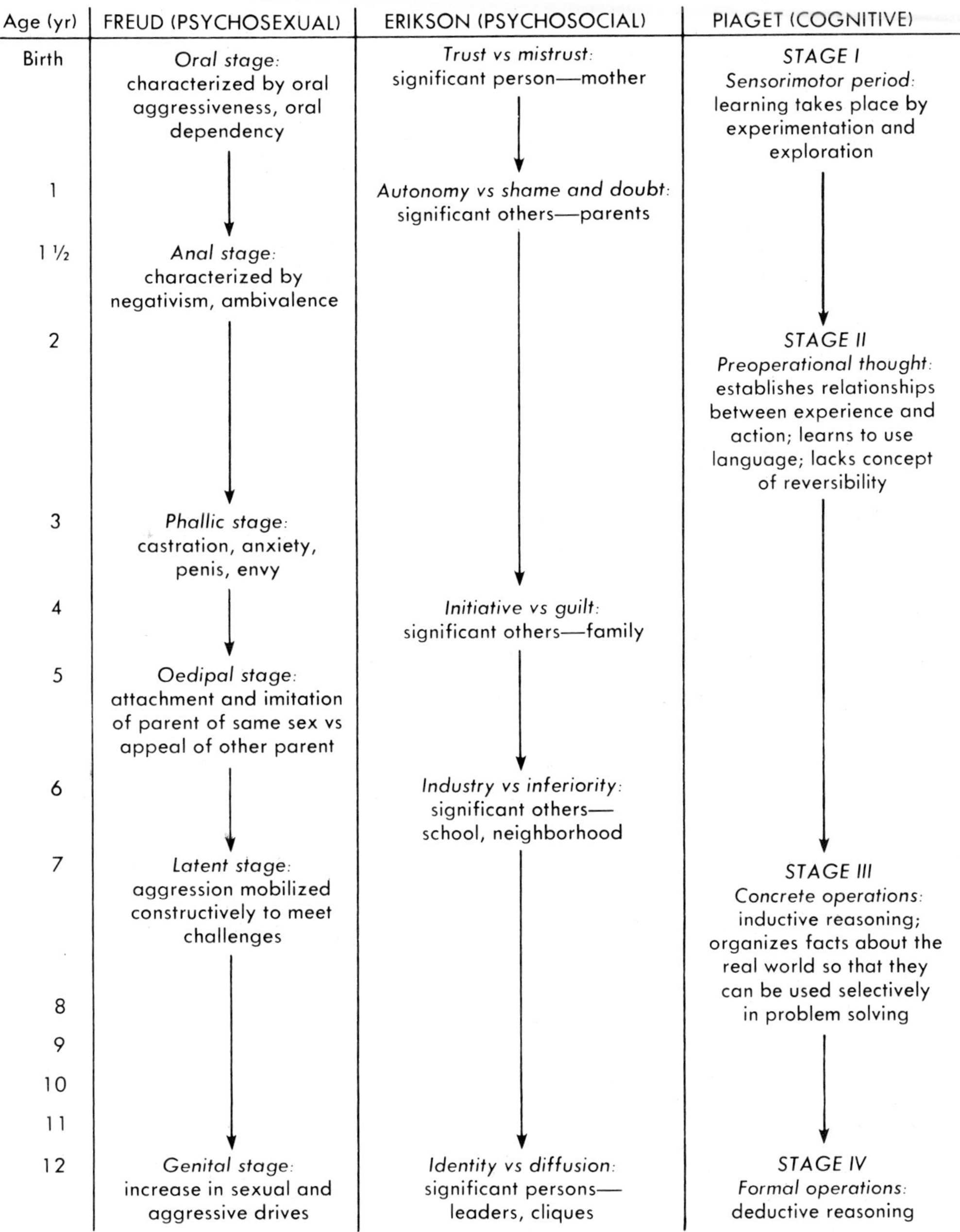

Fig. 18-1. Summary of psychosocial development in early life.

parently well one moment and an hour later seriously ill. The younger the child, the more pronounced is this response.

Hydration

Because of the immature system, loss of fluids and the accompanying loss of electrolytes present a serious hazard for the infant. During infancy and early childhood there is an increased percentage of fluid in the extracellular spaces, which makes the infant more vulnerable to fluid losses. The resulting imbalance in fluid and electrolyte composition of the interstitial and intracellular spaces presents serious threat. Fluid loss in infants and young children from diarrhea and vomiting, which may occur in association with many illnesses during infancy, is initially assumed to be isotonic for purposes of immediate therapy. Since electrolyte composition of the extracellular spaces of the infant and young child differs significantly from that of the older child and adult, replacement needs must be estimated correctly. Care must be taken not to cause overhydration.

The clinical signs of the state of hydration in the young infant may be difficult to determine. Chinn lists the following signs of dehydration for the infant and young child:

1. Dry skin, parched tongue, sunken eyeballs, sunken fontanel
2. Decreased urinary output
3. Specific gravity of urine greater than 1.030
4. Recent weight loss of over 6% of initial body weight[5]

Signs of overhydration include:

1. Increased urinary output
2. Weakness, lethargy, drowsiness
3. Vomiting
4. Edema, sudden weight gain
5. Coma and delirium (resulting from intracellular edema)
6. Convulsions[5]

Respiratory tract infections. The most common cause of illness in infancy and early childhood is upper respiratory tract infections. These infections range from the minor ones that cause minimal distress to the severe life-threatening infections.

Infants are prone to the common cold, with the incidence being up to eight per year for many infants. The invading organisms most commonly are the rhinoviruses. Proper care and intervention by the family is important in order to prevent complications.

Tonsillitis, adenoiditis, laryngitis, pharyngitis, epiglottiditis, laryngotracheobronchitis (croup), bronchiolitis, pneumonitis, and pneumonia are common during early childhood. While definitive diagnosis falls within the realm of medical practice, nursing management continues for nursing problems such as fever, fluid depletion, maintenance of an adequate airway, and comfort.

Croup, which often has an acute onset, is very frightening to parents. Infection usually involves a combination of sites including the epiglottis, larynx, trachea, and bronchi. The most characteristic sign of croup is a hoarse "barking" cough that is urgent and persistent. Because of inflammation, swelling, and narrowing of the lumen of the passage of the airway there is a trapping of air in the lungs, some degree of respiratory distress, and some oxygen hunger. High humidity levels and oxygen usually give some immediate relief. When the epiglottis is involved surgical intervention to provide an adequate airway may be required.

Acute bronchiolitis, characterized by inflammation of the bronchioles and small bronchi, is most common in infants under 6 months. It causes lower airway obstruction. This infection most commonly occurs in epidemics during the winter and spring.

Supportive measures including fluids to prevent dehydration and to liquefy mucus in the lower respiratory tract are usually successful. If significant respiratory distress is present hospitalization may be necessary to provide humidified oxygen. Careful attention should be given to infants with bronchiolitis in order to prevent complications such as pneumonia.

Fever. Fever often accompanies illness during infancy and childhood. The hypothalamus, which is the center for temperature control, is immature during early life. A temperature of 42.5 C (104 F) carries critical risk of febrile convulsions.

Treatment of the cause of the fever and symptomatic relief are the major objectives of nursing management. Nursing interventions aimed at symptomatic relief may involve the use of environmental measures to increase body heat loss, the use of drugs such as acetylsalicylic acid, or both.

Congenital malformations. Congenital malformations result from problems in early morphogenesis. Fortunately most malformations are early ones leading to unrecognized pregnancy, spontaneous abortion, or stillbirth. At present only about 2% of live neonates are recognized as having serious malformations at birth. This rises to 4% by the end of the first year and continues to rise slowly until school age. Congenital malformation ranks second after prematurity as the leading cause of death in infants.

The birth of a malformed child produces an emotional reaction in the family, which may be expressed in a variety of ways including grief, resentment, guilt, and blame. The nurse may help the parents to identify the meaning the malformation holds for them and allow the parents to grieve for the normal child they expected. When working with the parents of a malformed baby it is important to allow additional time with parents so they can be encouraged to verbalize their feelings.

Recent advances in medicine offer increased hope of assistance for many malformed infants. The parents can be made aware of what can be done for the child as soon after birth as indicated and should be directed to the appropriate resources within the community. When the malformation is genetically linked, genetic counseling is appropriate.

For a more detailed discussion of specific malformation the reader should consult one of the pediatric textbooks listed at the end of this chapter.

Problems of national concern

Sudden infant death syndrome. Sudden infant death syndrome (SIDS) is the leading cause of death between the ages of 1 and 12 months and accounts for up to

10,000 infant deaths per year in the United States.[23] Until recently physicians had no idea what caused the sudden death of these apparently healthy babies. Recent studies indicate that the victims of crib death are not completely normal, as once was thought. There is evidence that these infants have subtle physiologic defects, probably in mechanisms that control breathing.[23] Many adults and infants have periods of apnea during sleep, and the question of what constitutes a dangerously long apneic episode is as yet unanswered. It is hypothesized that infants who die of crib death may be prone to prolonged periods of apnea during sleep. Other investigators have found that the formation of certain chemicals involved in the transmission of nerve impulses that control breathing are impaired in premature infants with apnea, and this may be a contributing factor to SIDS in these infants. Most investigators believe that there is more than one cause of SIDS. At present major efforts are being directed toward applying this new information to devise tests that will predict which infants are at risk of SIDS.

Nurses are concerned primarily with preventive mental health care and family advocacy. In order to work effectively with these families the nurse must have adequate knowledge of the concepts of grief and loss and counseling skills and be willing to become involved.

Child abuse. In 1961 Kempe coined the phrase "battered child" and began a campaign that brought national attention to the problem of child abuse. While it may be due in part to better reporting and an increased awareness of the problem, child abuse appears to be on the incline in the United States. The problem of child abuse is multifactorial. Numerous studies of the late 1960s and early 1970s provide health professionals with better guidelines for identifying potential child abusers and abused children (see box).

GUIDELINES FOR IDENTIFYING POTENTIAL CHILD ABUSERS

One or both parents were often abused as children. Studies indicate over 90% of abusive parents were abused children.

Parents tend to be lonely adults, attracted to each other as they search for loving parent figures.

Extreme personal and social isolation. These parents lack group and community integration and most often lack family support.

Unstable marital relationship. Parents lack positive feedback and support.

Low self-esteem.

Parent-child role reversal. The parents want the infant to meet their unfulfilled needs for mothering.

Unrealistic expectations of infants. Parents expect children to act older.

Parents unable to reach out and ask for help.

SPECIAL TRAITS THAT MAKE A CHILD VULNERABLE TO ABUSE

Usually young child, under 3 years of age.

Something different about child (i.e., pregnancy or delivery uncomfortable, child unwanted, premature birth).

Child is extremely irritable or cries often.

Birth order. Most often it is the first or last child who is abused.

Health care personnel need to be alert to the clinical pathology of the battered child such as surface marks (e.g., abrasions, bruises, burns), musculoskeletal injuries (e.g., multiple fractures in varying stages of repair), and visceral injuries (e.g., head injury, ruptured liver or spleen).[4]

For treatment to be effective health personnel must regard the family as a unit, and rehabilitation of the family as a viable unit must be the aim of intervention. Unless the abusive cycle is broken completely one can expect the act to be repeated. Studies show that approximately one half of the small children who are abused will be brain injured or dead within 1 year if returned to unchanged environments.[30]

Health workers and others in society must exercise care not to exhibit feelings of disgust and repulsion toward abusive parents. Abusive parents are often frightened, defensive, and angry. They need help and most often want help but do not know how to face the reality of the problem. Many communities now have Parents Anonymous and other groups that both potential abusers and abusers find to be a great source of help. Information about local groups can be obtained from child welfare agencies. One such group is CALM (Child Abuse and Listening Mediation, Inc.).*

Maternal deprivation. Early in the nineteenth century astute physicians wrote about children who suffered under institutional conditions. By the late 1950s and the 1960s recognition of the problem of maternal deprivation became more apparent. Maternal deprivation exists when an infant is deprived of the opportunity of forming an initial tie with a mother figure or when an infant is deprived of the mother figure after a meaningful tie has been formed.

While many of the studies done in this area are beset with methodologic difficulties, the majority of studies

*P.O. Box 718, Santa Barbara, Calif. 93102.

point out the damaging effects to the infant in motor, intellectual, and emotional development resulting from separation from the mother figure during the early years (see Chapter 26). The extent of damage depends on the degree of emotional and sensory deprivation, the stage of development of the child, and the quality of the relationship with the mother prior to separation.

Such studies indicate the need for continuity of the relationship and emphasize the desirability of rooming-in for mothers with sick infants or young children.

Nursing the infant

Whenever possible, facilities for rooming-in should be available for mothers of hospitalized infants. When the mother is present she is encouraged to participate in the infant's care as much as possible, which makes the infant more secure and helps the mother to become more comfortable with a sick child. When possible one staff member should work consistently with the mother and the child. Such a plan helps the mother to continue her mothering responsibilities under stress and will make her more comfortable if it is necessary for her to leave the infant. When the mother is unable to be present the staff member should take over the mothering. Infants need cuddling, verbalization, and stimulation.

The nursing assessment may include questions relative to eating habits, the home routine, and methods of comforting the baby. The home routine should be followed as much as possible to facilitate the development of the infant's sense of trust. If the infant has a favorite blanket or toy, parents should be encouraged to bring it to the hospital.

The hospital staff can make certain the parents are informed relative to the care of their infant. All procedures need to be carefully explained to the parents.

■ TODDLER (1 to 3 years)

Physical growth

Probably one of the most significant occurrences during the toddler stage is that the child develops the ability to move about unassisted. Physically the musculoskeletal system expands and matures to allow the child to develop a standing posture and to walk. Previously the child could only lie or sit. The world now contains a new facet. Locomotion allows for development in a variety of ways including running and jumping and a variety of other motor skills.

Self-regulatory activities such as bowel-bladder control, eating, sleeping, and physical manipulative skills become important during the toddler period. Neurologic maturation of the bowels and bladder, occurring between 18 and 24 months, allows the toddler to develop an awareness of the sensations related to elimination. Not until neurologic maturation is complete will toilet training be successful or meaningful to the child. By $2^{1}/_{2}$ years daytime bowel and bladder control is usually possible, but nighttime control is more difficult to master.

After the first year of life the growth rate slows and stabilizes, with gains in height and weight occurring slowly. There are also proportional changes in the body contour as the child loses subcutaneous fat. The arms and legs grow longer as ossification and growth in the epiphyseal centers of the long bones occur. The trunk and head grows at a slower rate. Toward the end of the toddler period the protruding abdomen and lumbar lordosis disappears.

Psychologic development

Language development. During the toddler stage the child makes rapid strides toward becoming a social being. The ability to communicate increases as the toddler acquires language. The voice structures develop to a point that allows for the formation of words. As the brain structures mature, new behavior patterns are possible and the child begins to build a vocabulary.

Cognitive development. The child continues to operate on a sensorimotor level until about 2 years of age (Fig. 18-1). The next stage of cognitive development, the period of preconceptual thought, is a period of preparation for conceptual thought. The child begins to understand simple abstractions, but thinking remains basically concrete and literal. The child begins to associate certain objects as being representative of other objects. This is easily seen in symbolic play where dolls are given the roles of babies or mothers and where the sandbucket becomes the garbage can as the child plays at being the garbage collector.

The child has no clear conception of quantity but operates on the principle that if it looks like more, it is more. The child of 2 or 3 years is likely to think 100 ml of orange juice in a tall glass is more than 100 ml of juice in a shorter, wider container. The child has not yet mastered the concept of conservation of matter (Fig. 18-2).

The child of this age has not yet formed concepts of time and space. Time is now and space is what he sees at this moment. Children's stories begin with "once upon a time" or "long, long ago" because time and space are felt by the young child, not measured.

Emotional development. Egocentrism remains a major characteristic of early childhood. Toddlers are very much concerned with their own importance, constantly seeking attention, approval, and their own goals. They are only poorly able to take another person's point of view. At this age they exhibit a great deal of testing behavior in their quest for independence. They lack any self-control over exploratory impulses and rely on their parents to help them develop safe and socially acceptable behaviors. They require the attention and approval of

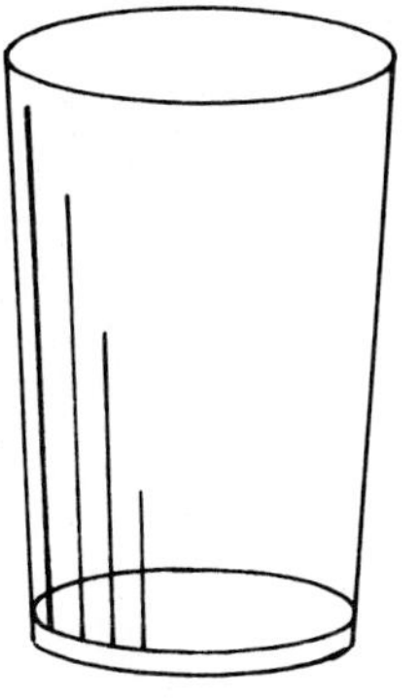

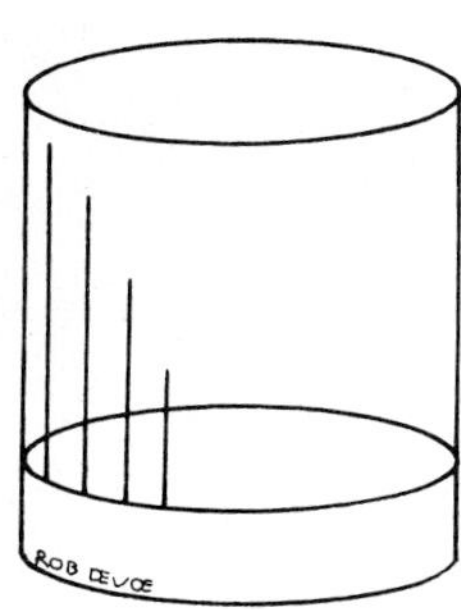

Fig. 18-2. Which is more? Child of 2 or 3 years is likely to choose taller glass on left rather than shorter glass on right, even though glasses hold same volume.

TASKS OF THE TODDLER

Learning to control socially unacceptable emotional impulses
Learning appropriate sex role distinction
Tolerating separation from the mother
Learning to differentiate self from other people and things
Reaching a stable physiologic state
Becoming enculturated

parents, as it is one of the main motivational forces in socialization and ego development.

According to Erikson, the developmental crisis of this age level is achieving autonomy versus shame and doubt. Autonomy is achieved as the toddler gains self-control over motor abilities and sphincter muscles. It can be seen as the child develops some measure of control over self and learns to make and carry out decisions, to cope with small problems, to wait patiently, and to share.[10]

Rituals in activities performed are at a peak at $2^1/_2$ to 3 years, especially those associated with feeding and bedtime. Rituals contribute to developing autonomy because the child learns to master tasks through rituals.

Negativism and dawdling are ways toddlers learn to control their own bodies. They often continue in an activity over parents' objections or say no even as they are doing what they have been asked to do.

If the child fails to develop a positive self-concept and a sense of autonomy, shame and doubt predominate. It is important that parents create an atmosphere in which expectations are reasonable and in which criticism, blame, and punishment are not excessive. The major developmental tasks of the toddler are outlined in the box above.

Nursing the toddler

With the well child the nurse's role is primarily one of assessing and evaluating to determine whether growth and development are proceeding in a normal pattern. The nurse serves as a resource person providing anticipatory guidance and teaching. Intervention can be undertaken when needed to promote and foster the child's developmental potential. Another vital role the nurse plays is serving as a sounding board for parents who have concerns about their child's behaviors or just need to ventilate their feelings.

Special needs of the hospitalized child. If hospitalization is necessary, the child of any age should be prepared for the experience by his parents. The nurse in the physician's office or clinic should be sure the parents know how to prepare him. They should tell the child truthfully about the hospital and why he must go there. He should not be frightened about the experience, but neither should he be led to expect the experience to be completely pleasant. He should be told about the high beds, bedpans, urinals, bed baths, eating in bed, the attire of nurses and physicians, and the play facilities in a matter-of-fact and reassuring way. If possible the preparation for hospitalization should be done gradually. Well-written storybooks concerning hospitalization are available in bookstores and may be helpful in introducing the topic (Fig. 18-3). In addition many children's hospitals have written their own books for patients.

Children, especially those between 2 and 5 years of age, tend to form attachments to inanimate objects such as well-loved toys or blankets. Such an object, whatever it may be, gives the child comfort and security. Even a sick child of school age may want to bring some favorite object to the hospital. He should be allowed to do so, and no one should worry if it is old or ragged. The object is the child's link with home, and he should be free to take it with him wherever he goes, even to treatment rooms and to the operating room.

It is important too for parents to allow children of any age, prior to their departure for the hospital, to help prepare for their return home again. Often the child can pack a bag with clothes that he will wear when he is discharged from the hospital, or he may help prepare the room where he will stay while he is recuperating.

During the toddler stage attachment to the mother is quite strong, and this group experiences the greatest amount of regression due to separation anxiety. The effects of hospitalization and illness can be severe. Health care providers, especially nurses, can make every effort to make hospitalization as pleasant an experience as possible and to minimize emotional trauma.

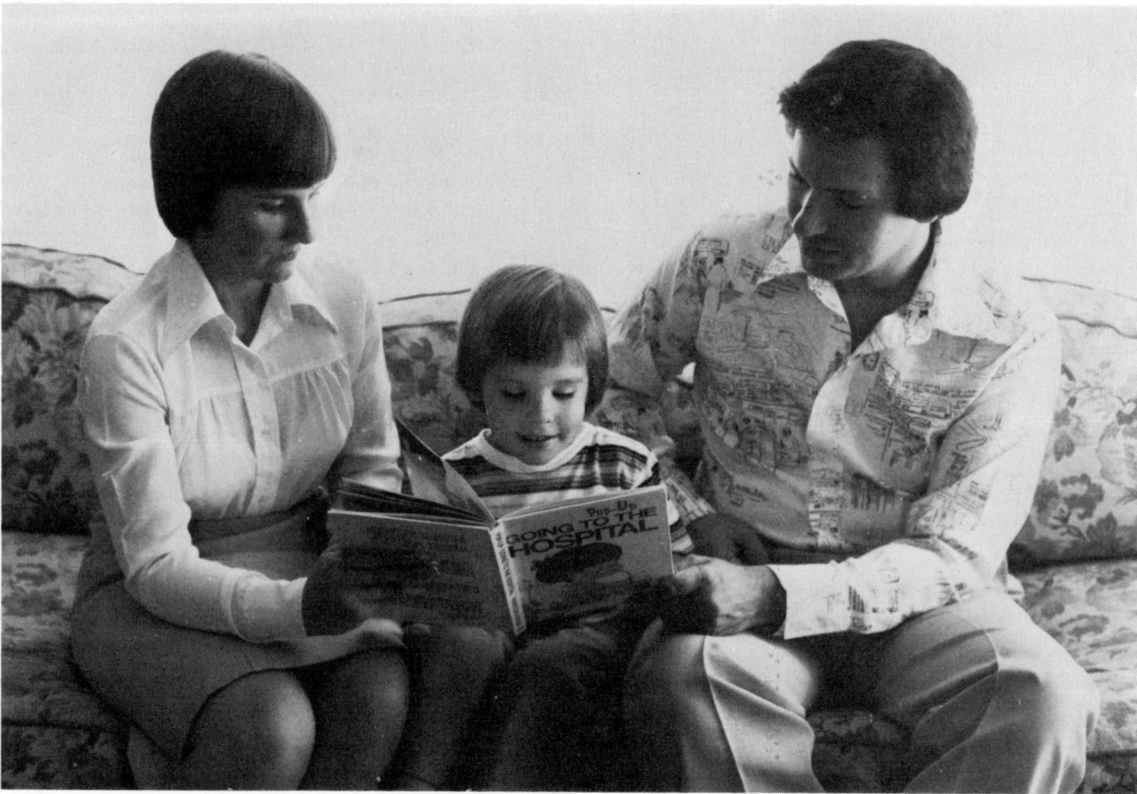

Fig. 18-3. Parents preparing child for hospitalization. Parents can make important contribution to child's hospitalization by proper preparation.

Parents need to leave their children. They should be given permission to leave the child and help in separating from him. They should not try to sneak out but should tell the child they are leaving and when they will return relative to his activities. Leaving personal articles with the child helps to assure him that parents will return. The clinging behavior generally subsides after the parents set up a pattern of reappearance and keep promises.

The initial nursing history should include assessment data relative to toilet training, and every effort should be made to continue the routine carried out at home. Potty chairs should be available for the child who is trained.

If the 2- or 3-year-old is still drinking from a bottle, do not attempt to change his habits while he is in the hospital.

If the procedure will be uncomfortable, a parent or a nurse who is well liked by the child should be present to comfort and firmly hold him as necessary. A child of any age should be told truthfully what type of sensation he may expect, and it usually is advisable to tell him when he is about to be hurt. Restraining techniques such as "mummying" (use of blanket restraints) occasionally must be used for the safety of a toddler who is overactive, but usually just talking to the child and holding him firmly is all that is needed.

Health care concerns during toddlerhood

Nutrition. As the growth rate slows, the appetite decreases and the child loses subcutaneous fat. Mothers often express concern about this behavior and feel the child is not healthy. Anticipatory guidance can prepare mothers for this change in eating habits and alleviate much of their worry. Toddlers are finicky eaters and are given to food jags. When they are hospitalized special care should be taken to see that they are served familiar foods. It is most unlikely they will eat unfamiliar foods or foods that do not resemble those served at home. They often dawdle and play with their food.

Injuries. Accidents are the leading cause of death in children from 1 to 14 years of age. Some 15 million children are brought for treatment for accident-related injuries each year. Automobile accidents account for the largest number of deaths. Many smaller children are hit by cars and trucks while playing or crossing streets. The most frequently occurring injuries are fractures and concussions.

Burns are a significant cause of mortality and morbidity in children. Unfortunately it is often the action of the child that causes the injury. As concerned citizens nurses must push for better education of the public relative to fire prevention. Care of the burned client is discussed in Chapter 67.

Poisoning. The 2-year-old is the most common victim of accidental ingestion of *poisons.* Most often the poison is a drug or household product. These products should be kept in their original containers and locked up or placed on high shelves out of reach of toddlers. Care of the person who has ingested poisons is discussed in Chapter 24.

Illnesses. Respiratory infections remain a problem during the toddler years. Otitis media (see Chapter 49) is seen most commonly in young children because their eustachian tubes are short and straight, permitting easier passage of bacteria from the nasopharynx to the middle ear. The use of antibiotics has markedly decreased the incidence of mastoiditis frequently seen in young children in previous decades.

Recognition and treatment of otitis media are extremely important to prevent hearing loss and subsequent emotional and learning difficulties. Unrecognized otitis media results in persistent fluid in the middle ear, which leads to glue-ear syndrome (sequelae of serous otitis media often leading to hearing loss).

■ PRESCHOOL YEARS (3, 4, and 5 years)

Physical growth

The refinement of motor skills occurs during the preschool years and allows the child to do progressively more difficult things and to achieve integrated motor and perceptual control. Physical activity becomes goal directed. The child makes rapid progress toward the perfection of certain skills such as improving his ability to comprehend and communicate, forming simple concepts of social and physical reality, learning how to behave toward persons and things, learning to distinguish right from wrong, and developing a value judgment system (conscience).

The gain in height is faster than the weight gain; thus the child changes from a chubby toddler to a thinner, sturdier child. The child is also losing his baby look and maturing into the kind of person he is going to be in later life.

By 5 years of age the child is beginning to lose the deciduous teeth. Vision is improving; however, the preschooler remains far-sighted. It is normal for a 5-year-old to have 20/50 or 20/40 vision on Snellen chart testing. It is very important that vision screening be done during the preschool years so that defects such as strabismus and amblyopia can be identified and corrected so that permanent damage can be prevented or minimized.

Psychosocial growth

A major developmental task of the preschool period is the *emergence* of the *child* as a *social being.* The child now spends more time in association with his peers. The 4-year-old child is imaginative and creative, often talking and playing with imaginary companions. These children are struggling with fact and fantasy and are fond of telling long and elaborate stories, which are mostly imaginary. During this period the child changes from a self-centered being to a person who can relate to others in play and is ready for group experiences such as nursery school, playgroups, and kindergarden.

Another important task of this period is the process of *identification* and gender identity. During the phallic stage children become aware of anatomic differences between the sexes (Fig. 18-1). Development of sexuality comes to the forefront during the oedipal stage. Children become interested in the appearance and function of their bodies. The child first assigns sex on the basis of the appearance of men and women.

Identification is imitation of behavior of the parent of the same sex. The child tries to imitate the role of mother or father. Identification is influenced by the attitudes about sexual, moral, social, and occupational roles and values dominant in the culture.

Erikson's developmental task of *initiative versus guilt* is dominant during the preschool period. The child who does not develop a sense of initiative, the ability to assure himself, to plan and control his own activity, is likely to feel a sense of anger or defeatism. If the guilt and anger persist the child develops a rigid superego.

Cognitive development remains in stage II, *preoperational thought.* The intuitive phase, beginning at age 4, is a period during which the child begins to think more completely and elaborates his concepts more. A concept is formed when a word comes to define an area of experience. At this age the child becomes more flexible in use of language; he uses the word "because" and makes simple associations between ideas. "Centering" is still very characteristic, with the child's attention being centered on one detail of an event to the exclusion of other parts of the event. The child of this age is unable to cope intellectually with problems of time, space, causality, measurement, numbers, quantity, or movement. He thinks everything is just as it appears.

Language development continues during the preschool years with increasing use of more complex words and sentences. By 5 years of age most children have a vocabulary of approximately 2,000 words.

Children of this age sometimes project their own feelings onto their playthings; toys are used as safety valves for aggressive feelings. Parents are sometimes distressed at this behavior and need to be told that it is normal.

In summary, the preschool age is a period of relative calm with a steady gain in height and weight, refinement of motor skills with increasing control over the body, and development of social relationships with peers. Self-care activities greatly improve as a result of improved physical skills. The human organism is transformed in 5 short years from a helpless infant to a sturdy and complicated being capable of communication, conceptualization, and complex social and motor behavior.

Nursing the preschooler

As with younger children, it is desirable to have one nurse assigned to the hospitalized child as consistently as possible. Mothers should be encouraged to participate in the child's care, as this indicates to the child that mother approves of hospital routine.

Castration and mutilation fantasies are common to this age group. The preschooler often feels that he is in the hospital as punishment for something bad that he did. It is important to reassure the child repeatedly that he is not to blame for his illness or hospitalization. The fears commonly expressed before age 5 include abandonment, loss of control over usual routines, pain, and invasion of body orifices.

Play is extremely helpful with this age group. Dolls may be used to demonstrate the external appearance postoperatively. Children of this age enjoy the opportunity to manipulate equipment and will often act out their feelings with toys. Storytelling and puppet play are also useful in teaching preschoolers to express their feelings.

The 5-year-old is just mastering self-care activities and should be encouraged to take care of self-hygiene as much as possible. This sense of accomplishment is threatened when the child must relinquish self-care activities to others.

Health concerns during the preschool years

Upper respiratory tract infections continue to be the most common cause of illness in children between 3 and 5 years of age. Toward the end of the preschool years the child's respiratory tract matures, and infections are localized to a greater degree.

Entrance into nursery school and kindergarten exposes the child to a variety of infections, particularly the common communicable diseases of chickenpox, measles, and mumps. All children should receive early immunization against measles because of its severe complications (see Chapter 14).

Accidents and burns continue to remain a major health concern during the preschool years as the child gains greater mobility and moves into new environments. The preschooler should be taught some very basic rules of safety and what to do should there be an accident on the playground.

MIDDLE CHILDHOOD

The period between 6 years and the onset of puberty is a phase of gradual growth and development. It is a steady period in both physical and emotional aspects.

Physical growth

During the first few years of school, the gross motor activities such as running and climbing of the earlier years become increasingly directed to more specialized activities and games requiring particular motor and muscular skills. The child refines skills, especially those dealing with neuromotor coordination, that is, those involving fine coordination of the hands, eyes, and cerebral cortex.

Development of the facial bones continues actively during the school years, particularly with enlargement of the sinuses. The frontal sinuses have usually made their appearance by the seventh year. The face begins to change, taking on a more adult appearance.

The first of the permanent teeth, the first-year molars, most often erupt during the sixth year. With the so-called *six-year molars* in place, the shedding of the deciduous teeth begins, following approximately the same sequence as their acquisition. They are replaced at a rate of about four teeth a year over the next 7 years. The second permanent molars are commonly erupted by the fourteenth year, and the third molars, irregular in occurrence and time of eruption, may not appear until the early twenties.

Lymphatic tissues are at the peak of their development during these years and generally exceed the amount of such tissue present in adults.

Visual development should be completed by the sixth or seventh year. The child should have fully developed peripheral vision and be able to discriminate fine differences in shades of colors. A maximum level of acuity, at least 20/30 in each eye by Snellen chart testing, is normal by 7 years of age. The child learns to coordinate eye movements, to see a single image, and to associate incoming visual stimuli with past and present mental images and functions.

The physical growth rate is slow and steady. There may be considerable variation in height and weight among children, depending on genetic and environmental influences. During the early school years the child gains an average of 3 kg (6 to 7 pounds) yearly and increases in height by about 6 cm ($2^1/_2$ inches) yearly.

Nutritional needs

The nutritional requirements of the schoolchild remains relatively greater than the adult's. Approximately 80 calories/kg wt daily are required by the young schoolchild. This gradually decreases to 70 calories/kg wt daily by age 12 years. The caloric needs for a child can be calculated as 1,000 calories for the first year and 100 calories for each additional year.[24]

Protein requirements remain high, with 50 to 80 g needed daily. A large intake of calcium (1.5 to 2 g) and vitamin D (40 units) is needed daily because the child is constantly building new bony tissue.

Psychosocial growth

Middle childhood is characterized by three great outward pushes:

1. Socially the child makes his way out of the family environment into a peer group society.
2. Physically the child moves into a world of games and activities requiring neuromuscular skills.
3. Mentally the child is thrust into school and a world of concepts, symbols, logic, and communication.

Influence of school. The school is the one agency in the United States that reaches, by compulsion of law, all the community's children. The objectives of schools are the teaching of certain subject matter, the promotion of health, the development of character, and preparation for citizenship. It may be said that school is the child's business or job and that attitudes about school are very important in later life.

Children begin increasingly to live independently and to look outside the home for goals and standards of behavior. They find new role models, such as their school teachers.

Emergence of peer groups. During the school years there is a tendency for children to form into groups or clubs. This is the child's first experience with a society of his own making. During the early school years these groups are characteristically limited to members of the same sex. Being accepted and being active with the peer group is very important for healthy development. Around the age of 9 or 10 years the chum stage emerges, when the affection shifts from the peer group to a special friend of the same sex and age.

Emotional development. The developmental crisis of the school-aged child is that of industry versus inferiority. *Industry* is achieved as the child successfully learns to problem solve, develops reasonable work habits and attitudes, and masters age-appropriate tasks. Children compare themselves with peers, and if they cannot perform as well as others, they will eventually perceive themselves in a negative manner. If this continues and age-appropriate tasks are not mastered, a sense of inferiority will develop.

Cognitive development. By 6 years of age most children are able to understand the use of abstract concepts, permitting the beginning contact with the subjects of reading, writing, and arithmetic. Academic education is also made possible by the child's progress in the emotional aspects of development.

Intellectual behavior evolves descriptively from activity without thought to thought with less emphasis on activity. Cognitive behavior evolves from doing to doing knowingly. In earlier years when told, "Don't touch the stove" or, "Wash your hands" the child performs the task because of commands to do so. By 6 years of age there is learning of the whys behind these activities.

By 7 years of age the child is in stage III (Fig. 18-1), the period of concrete operations, which is characterized by the ability to solve concrete problems. Systematic reasoning about actual or imagined situations is now possible. Classification, seriation, and multiplication are characteristic operations during this stage. *Classification* involves the placement of objects in groups depending on their attributes such as size, shape, or color. *Seriation* involves the placement of objects in an increasing series relative to characteristics such as height and weight. *Multiplication* involves simultaneous classification and seriation, or the use of two attributes together. During stage III, *reversibility*, the performance of operations or actions with the same problem or situation becomes possible. This allows the child to move into mathematics.

At this age, children recognize that other people see things differently from the way they do. A value system and social interaction are necessary; children must interact socially to grow intellectually, because without social life they will never succeed in understanding the viewpoints of others.

Language. During the school years vocabulary is increased and more complex sentences are used. Consensual or syntatic communication is used when cause-and-effect relationships are seen in an objective logical way. Observations are validated by others.

Male-female differences. In latency girls are likely to be a year or two ahead of boys in social and emotional maturity and perhaps in the capacity to use intellectual abilities. Schools in the United States have been accused of fostering this and being female oriented. Looking at school performance, one finds that girls generally are better achievers in the early years of school when language development, reading, and writing are heavily stressed. In the latter years when the concepts of mathematics and science are introduced, boys improve in performance. To what extent these differences are fostered by the sociolization process is open to question.

To summarize middle childhood:

1. It is a period of steady growth and steady emotions; the child is developing *self-control.*
2. There is an outward shift, and school and peer groups become very important; the child is developing *increased independence.*
3. It is a time for building a wholesome concept of

the self; the child is developing a sense of *self-worth.*

Health and middle childhood

Middle childhood is ordinarily characterized by health and well-being. Many of the problems encountered during the school years are preventable and subject to nursing intervention. Nurses are most likely to have contacts with the well child of this age through the schools, in pediatrician's offices, and in well-child nurse clinics. As with the younger child, assessment of the pattern of growth and development is an important factor. Vision, speech, hearing, and dental problems appear during these years and should be identified as early as possible for correction to be most effective. Screening programs for such defects should be part of all school health programs and should be included in assessment during routine physical examinations.

Nursing the school-aged child

Hospitalization apparently is not too psychologically traumatic for school children, especially if they have been adequately prepared for it. Unless the child is acutely ill or will be having an operation, the constant attendance of the mother is rarely necessary. However, parents should be urged to visit regularly or, if frequent visits are not possible, to keep in regular contact by telephone or letter.

When preparation has been adequate, hospitalization can be an educational and social experience. By middle childhood the child is capable of learning a great deal from contacts with staff and other children. Children of this age are capable of verbalizing their feelings and concerns. These children can be reasoned with, since they are capable of understanding cause-and-effect relationships.

Preoperative teaching and preparation for diagnostic procedures are important. The child of this age is interested in the scientific approach and likes to learn scientific terminology for body parts and medical procedures. Useful guidelines for teaching the school-aged child are available.[26]

If a child of school age is hospitalized or is sick at home for a long period of time (usually over 2 weeks), most boards of education provide visiting teachers. Parents need to be reminded of this service. Continuing with schoolwork not only provides diversion for the child but also assures keeping up with classmates.

The school-aged child may be interested in reading, listening to records, observing and caring for birds or fish, making such objects as model planes or jewelry, painting, or taking part in competitive activities. Playing with others usually is possible even for the bedridden child. Care should be taken that the child does not overexert or become overtired. Educational play activity and play with others are especially important for the child who has a prolonged illness because they assure continued mental and social development.

Health concerns during middle childhood

Respiratory tract disease. Minor respiratory tract diseases spread rapidly among children in the close proximity of classrooms. Many of the respiratory tract illnesses discussed with previous age groups continue to occur frequently during middle childhood. The more mature structures of the respiratory tract are not as prone to communicate infection from one area of the system to another; thus the older child has increased capacity to localize infection. The anatomy of the ear now begins to approach adultlike proportions, resulting in a decline in the incidence of otitis media. Colds occur 3 or 4 times a year.

Communicable diseases. The incidence of many of the communicable diseases has greatly decreased due to immunizations. Public health officials are concerned, however, with the breakdown in immunizations occurring in the United States in recent years. Small epidemics of childhood diseases have occurred in some areas of the United States, and the Public Health Service has launched a massive program to increase the level of immunization. Some states have passed laws barring children who are not immunized from school in order to emphasize the seriousness of the problem. The National League for Nursing (NLN) and its constituent members sponsored immunization clinics in many areas of the United States in 1977.

Streptococcal infections are a major health problem among school-aged children, with the highest incidence occurring between 6 and 12 years of age. Incidence is highest in areas where the weather is temperate and during the winter months. Transmission occurs primarily by direct contact with an infected person. Serious sequelae can result as a response to streptococcal infection; therefore prevention and control of the spread of this infection among children is very important.

Tonsillitis, pharyngitis, scarlet fever, and skin eruptions such as impetigo are the primary forms of streptococcal infections. Streptococcal infection is characterized by an abrupt onset, which may be accompanied by fever, abdominal pain and vomiting, headaches, and chills. With scarlet fever the typical skin rash appears within 12 to 48 hours after the onset of throat and constitutional symptoms.

An accurate diagnosis depends on positive throat culture results. Nurses working in settings with children may carry supplies for collecting throat cultures. Many school systems have developed plans for obtaining cultures from the entire student body when the incidence of streptococcal infections is high. Antibiotic (penicillin) therapy should be instituted within 7 days of onset to prevent deleterious sequelae. In order to effectively prevent rheumatic and renal sequelae the antibiotic must be administered for at least 10 days.

For a detailed discussion of rheumatic fever and renal sequelae the reader is referred to a pediatric text on communicable disease.

Skin and skeletal injuries. As the child becomes increasingly mobile, active, and more daring and is exposed to greater danger, injuries to the skin and skeletal system increase. Broken bones, dislocated joints, and muscle and ligamentous injuries are prevalent. The nature of the injury should be carefully assessed, and measures should be taken to prevent bleeding, promote comfort, and protect the injured area from further insult during efforts to move or reposition. The child should receive treatment from a specialist in skeletal trauma care.

■ ADOLESCENCE

Following World War II the American public became increasingly conscious of adolescents. It was during this period that the word "teenager" was coined and became popular. The adolescent, who is no longer a child but not yet adequately prepared for the adult world, is searching for emotional and social maturity on his own terms. Adolescents have acquired specific identity as a population in the United States. Adolescence varies depending on the culture. In the United States the length of this period has extended even more than formerly. Adolescence is seen in most countries in which the level of affluence permits a prolongation of dependent behavior beyond puberty.

U.S. Bureau of Census estimates for 1972 show 42 million people between the ages of 10 and 19 who can be labeled adolescents. If present trends continue, it is projected that by the year 2000 the number of adolescents in the United States will reach 54 million.[36]

It may be said that adolescence begins in biology and ends in culture. Many people have proposed various definitions for the adolescent. One nurse-author comments that a friend of hers defines an adolescent as "someone who doesn't have his act together yet."[12] In many ways this is an appropriate definition.

Adolescence refers to a specific stage or period in the life cycle. It is the outgrowth of childhood and the prelude to adulthood. It consists of the psychologic, social, and cognitive maturational processes initiated by puberty. Puberty may be defined as the biologic stage of sexual development at which one is able to bear or beget children.

Adolescence is a developmental phenomenon unique to the higher primates. Our nature as interdependent social animals, with unique adaptations of culture and society, has its basis in a specifically human pattern of biologic maturation. The delay in attainment of full growth and sexual maturity in humankind would appear to be essential to our longer and richer development, and on this basis it has been suggested that adolescence is an important evolutionary trait.

Physical growth

The most important concept to remember when dealing with adolescent is that of *individuality of growth.*

Biologic changes. Puberty refers to maturational, hormonal, and growth processes occurring within the body. Sexual maturation becomes evident in the first

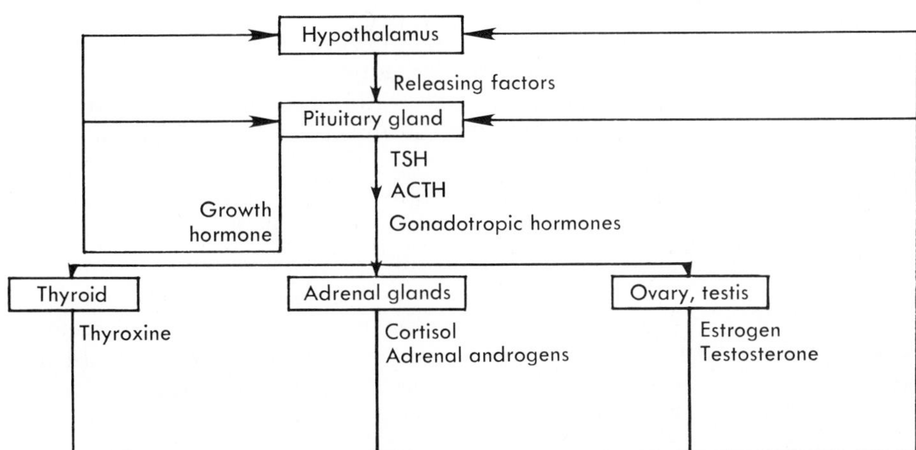

Fig. 18-4. Endocrine control at adolescence. Activating hormones from pituitary gland stimulate other endocrine glands, activating their own growth-related hormones. These hormones in turn provide for orderly and progressive physical and psychologic changes of adolescence.

PUBERTAL STAGES ACCORDING TO TANNER

Boys: genital development

Stage 1 Preadolescent: testes, scrotum, and penis are about the same size and proportion as in early childhood.

Stage 2 Scrotum and testes are enlarged. Skin of scrotum reddened and changed in texture. Little or no enlargement of penis is present at this stage.

Stage 3 Penis is slightly enlarged, which occurs at first mainly in length. Testes and scrotum are further enlarged.

Stage 4 Increased size of penis with growth in breadth and development of glands is present. Testes and scrotum larger; scrotal skin darker than in earlier stages.

Stage 5 Genital adult in size and shape.

Girls: breast development

Stage 1 Preadolescent: elevation of papilla only.

Stage 2 Breast bud stage. Elevation of breast and papilla as small mound. Enlargement of areola diameter.

Stage 3 Further enlargement and elevation of breast and areola with no separation of their contours.

Stage 4 Projection of areola and papilla to form a secondary mound above the level of the breast.

Stage 5 Mature stage: projection of papilla only, due to recession of the areola to the general contour of the breast.

Both sexes: pubic hair

Stage 1 Preadolescent: vellus over the pubes is not further developed than that over the abdominal wall (i.e., no pubic hair).

Stage 2 Sparse growth of long, slightly pigmented downy hair, straight or curled, chiefly at the base of the penis or along labia.

Stage 3 Considerably darker, coarser, and more curled. The hair spreads sparsely over the junction of the pubes.

Stage 4 Hair now adult in type, but area covered is still considerably smaller than in the adult. No spread to the medial surface of thighs.

Stage 5 Adult in quantity and type with distribution of the horizontal (or classically "feminine") pattern. Spread to medial surface of thighs but not up linea alba or elsewhere above the base of the inverse triangle.

Stage 6 Spread up linea alba.

(From Tanner, J. M.: Growth and endocrinology of the adolescent. In Gardner, L. I., editor: Endocrine and genetic diseases of childhood, Philadelphia, 1969, W. B. Saunders Co. Cited in The approach to the adolescent patient, Pediatr. Clin. North Am. 20:4, 1973.)

phase of adolescence. Puberty is initiated by the liberation of hormonal secretions in response to hypothalamic stimuli. The pituitary gland (master gland) sends out messages to certain parts of the body causing activation of TSH, ACTH, gonadotropic, and growth hormones. These in turn stimulate other endocrine glands activating their own growth-related hormones. Fig. 18-4 illustrates the hormonal pathways believed to be involved at adolescence.

The sequence of events occurring at adolescence has been well documented by the work of Tanner and others (see box). All humans seem to follow this sequence of development of breasts, genitalia, and pubic hair. The age at which these physical changes occur varies by sex. By comparing the ages of development one notes that physical changes in adolescent girls precede those of boys (Fig. 18-5). Both are considered reproductively mature, however, at almost the same age.

Changes in bodily dimensions. Virtually all parts of the skeletal and muscular structures take part in the growth spurt. The head, hands, and feet achieve adult form earliest; this is why one often thinks junior high school basketball players are all hands and feet. The arms and legs achieve adult form next. Adult trunk length is achieved last but accounts for the greatest proportion of the increase in height; adolescent boys often outgrow the coat of a suit while the pants still fit.

Ossification of bones. During adolescence a great deal of the cartilage in the body calcifies. This process is speeded up during the growth spurt and is completed more rapidly by girls. By 17 years of age an average girl's bones are mature in size and ossification. Boys do not

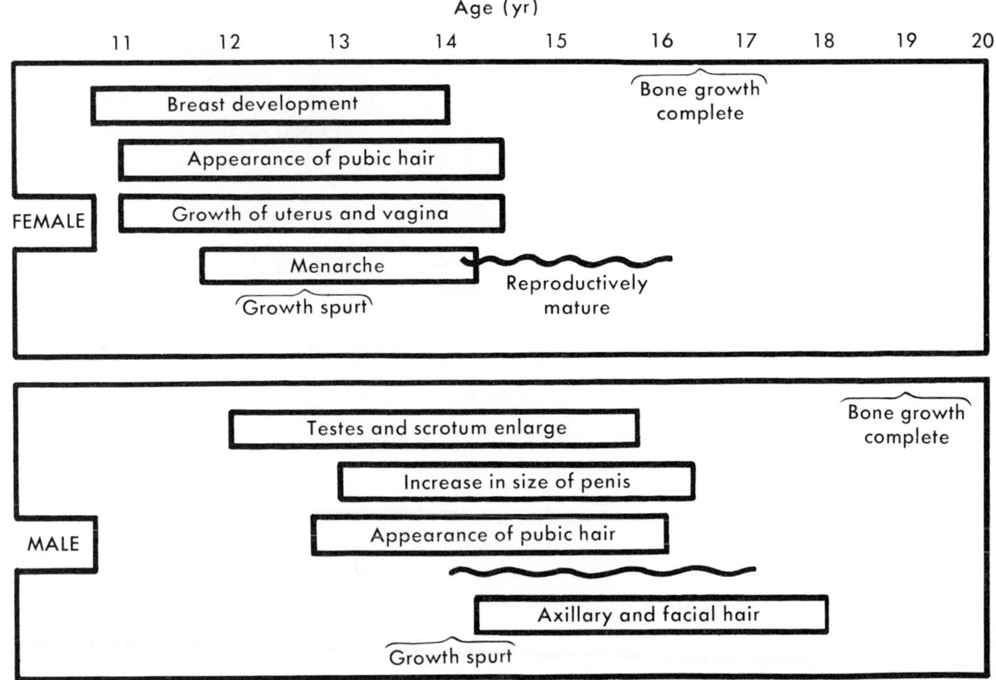

Fig. 18-5. Physical changes of adolescence by age and sex.

complete bone growth until late adolescence or early adulthood.

Differential development of muscle and fat. Increased muscular development occurs in both sexes. The overall gain, however, is greater for boys and remains so during the adult years.

During adolescence there is an overall decrease in the *rate* of development of fat. In girls this decrease in the rate is not so great as to eliminate a modest gain in fat. In boys the rate of decline is so great that it produces an actual, though temporary, loss of fat in the months preceeding and following the point of peak velocity in height.

Changes in strength and exercise tolerance. The increase in strength and exercise tolerance is greater for boys than for girls. Relative to size, boys develop larger hearts and lungs, an increase in systolic blood pressure, a greater capacity for carrying oxygen in the blood, a decreased heart rate at rest, and a greater power for neutralizing the chemical products of muscular exercise such as lactic acid, which manifests itself in fatigue. Since women have had the opportunity to participate in sports activities we have begun to question the physiologic basis for greater strength and exercise tolerance of males. Females may have equal potential for the development of increased strength and exercise tolerance, given the opportunity to participate equally in sports and exercise programs. Many of the outstanding female athletes appear to have a capacity equal to that of their male counterparts.

Basal metabolic rate. The basal metabolic rate (BMR) declines during adolescence. This decline is less in boys, probably due to greater muscular development, which requires greater oxygen consumption, and because of hormonal differences.

Types of physical growth. The four chief types of physical growth are as follows:

1. *Lymphoid:* reaches peak between 10 and 12 years. Gradually declines to steady point by 20 years.
2. *Brain and head:* reaches peak at 6 years with small gradual increase up to 20 years.
3. *General:* increases to 6 years then levels off until 12 years. Increases steadily until 20 years, then reaches steady point.
4. *Reproductive:* gradual increase until 11 to 12 years, then rises rapidly until age 20 years.

Nutritional needs. Nutritional needs are greatly accelerated during this period of rapid growth. The need for increased calories is greater than for any period of life except for during pregnancy and lactation. The increased need for protein, calcium, and iron is especially important for building of bones and muscles. There is increased need for calories, especially carbohydrates, to provide fuel for the increased energy needs (Table 18-3).

Table 18-3. Recommended daily dietary allowances

	Age (yr)	Weight (kg)	Height (cm)	Calories	Protein (g)	Calcium (mg)
Male ♂	9 to 12	32.4	139.7	2,400	50 to 60 or 15% of calorie intake	1,300
	12 to 15	44.1	154.9	3,000		
	15 to 18	60.3	172.7	3,400		
Female ♀	9 to 12	32.4	139.7	2,200	50 to 60 or 15% of calorie intake	1,300
	12 to 15	46.4	157.5	2,500		
	15 to 18	52.7	162.6	2,300		

Earlier maturation and larger size. During the last 100 years there has been a trend toward accelerated maturation in height and weight in both boys and girls. Full growth is now achieved at a much earlier age: 18 to 19 years rather than 25 years or older as was the case several decades ago. Since 1850 there has been a downward trend in the age of menarche. This downward trend occurs at the rate of about 4 months per decade.

There has been much speculation that these phenomena may create psychologic and social problems. One needs to look at other factors that influence this downward trend. When the age of menarche is compared across generations reared under nearly identical conditions, no dramatic continuing downward trend in menarcheal age is found. In the United States it appears that there has been a tapering off of this downward trend in the last 20 years; that is, it has reached a plateau.

Apparently nutrition plays an important part in determining when menarche occurs. During and following World War II when many countries experienced periods of nutritional deprivation, a number of European countries reported that the age of menarche was significantly retarded. Contrary to myth, there is no evidence to support the direct influence of climate on maturational rate; however, maturational age may be related to genetic factors that vary from one individual or group to another.

Psychosocial growth

Ego identity. The central problem in adolescence is Erikson's *ego identity*, or the development of one's identity as a person. This requires a perception of the self as *separate* from others, hence the breaking away from the family. Ego identity is a feeling of wholeness and of self-consistency. Erikson theorizes that the youth culture has developed in technologic societies as an attempt to establish identity formation. Dedication to the adolescent culture provides a means of moving into and through the identity crisis period. The circle of significant others for adolescents includes leaders and cliques, which are a very important part of their lives. In later adolescence the youth is working on a sense of intimacy, and the circle of significant others now focuses on developing a love relationship with a member of the opposite sex.

The primary risk of this stage is identity confusion, which occurs when adolescents feel self-conscious and have doubts about themselves as human beings and their roles in life. When identity confusion is great, delinquent behavior or borderline psychotic episodes may occur.

In a sense the identity crisis involves a restaging of each of the previous stages of development. The extent to which the earlier tasks were successfully resolved influences the adolescent's success in finding identity.

Accelerated outward shift. With the onset of adolescence there is an accelerated shift from dependence on the family to dependence on the peer group as a major source of security and status.

Many authorities have described the adolescent group as a marginal group with the characteristic of being uncertain in itself. As a marginal group there is much emphasis on conformity. Adolescents have highly idealized norms for physical appearance and skills for male and female roles. These roles conform largely to culturally determined stereotypes of males and females.

Intellectual and cognitive development. According to Piaget the *formal operation stage* begins at around 12 years of age. At this stage thought proceeds from combination of possibility, hypothesis, and deductive reasoning. By this age the person can deal with problems not related to real or current situations. Purely abstract and verbal problems can be solved without the presence of actual referents.

There are also quantitative gains. The adolescent is capable of accomplishing more easily, more quickly, and more efficiently intellectual tasks that as a child or preadolescent were accomplished only slowly.

Sexual maturation. It is extremely important to consider the psychologic aspects of menstruation. It involves a great deal more than simple physiologic readjustment. Menstruation is a symbol of sexual maturity and for some a symbol of preparation for the role of future wife and mother. It is very important that negative reactions to menstruation be avoided. Most girls usually become capable of ovulating once the menstrual cycle is regularly established (see Chapter 60). In some cases it is suspected that ovulation occurs prior to the first menstrual flow.

Nocturnal emission may concern the boy as much as menstruation does the girl. Boys have as great a need for information about the growth and development of their bodies as do girls. All too often this may be neglected in our society and is taught by the peer group. Boys are capable of producing mature sperm about a year after the first nocturnal emissions (see Chapter 60).

Very early or very late maturation can create problems for the adolescent. Studies show that it is usually the early maturing girl and the late maturing boy who experience the greatest difficulty.

Body image changes. Adolescence is a time of change in body image (see Chapter 28). Rapid growth in height, weight, and sexual maturation demands that the adolescent deal with a changing body image. Adolescents are very much aware of and concerned about their changing bodies. One way they integrate this change in body image is by spending a long time in front of mirrors, in personal hygiene, and in grooming and dressing.

Adolescents are very sensitive and are often upset by their clumsy movements, acne, and early signs of sexual development. They need the support of the adults around them, especially their parents. They need help in accepting the positive and negative aspects of their bodies so that they can develop a healthy body image.

Influence of family, society, and culture on adolescents. The psychosocial implications of adolescence are greatly influenced by the culture in which one lives. The culture determines whether the period of adolescence is long or short, whether the social demands represent an abrupt change or only a gradual transition from earlier stages of development. In many of the more traditional cultures where people are still taught by apprenticeship, adolescence simply represents a gradual change with an increase in responsibilities and work expectations. The culture may also influence whether these changes become a source of pride or a source of anxiety and confusion. Many cultures practice puberty rites or rites of passage to adulthood. The Bar and Bas Mitzvah ceremonies, graduation from high school, and the Debutante Ball may be viewed as rites of passage.

In the United States the difference between a child and an adult is emphasized sharply by social and legal institutions. The Twenty-sixth Amendment gives 18-year-olds the right to vote, and many states have redefined the beginning of adulthood as 18 years of age.

The change from one mode of interpersonal relationship to another creates discontinuity in the growth process. Attitudes, values, and skills learned as a child must be redefined as an adult. For example, sexual taboos must be unlearned and the way one relates to parents of the opposite sex is changed.

In Western society the major changes that occur during adolescence are (1) responsible versus nonresponsible status role, (2) dominance versus submission, and (3) contrasted sexual role.

In terms of the influence of the modern family and society on adolescence, the greater the rate of social change the larger the generational gap. In the developed countries the rate of social change in the past 25 years has been greater than at any other period in history. In the previous generation the extended family and neighborhood ties were very prevalent and important. Geographic mobility was limited. Today families are quite mobile, with one in three moving every 5 years. Nuclear families and single-parent families are more common. Families of the adolescent's peers are unlikely to know one another, much less be friends. Parents are less likely to be united in rules for the conduct of adolescents.

Health and the adolescent

It was not until the 1950s that the special health needs of adolescents gained recognition. Dr. Rosewell Gallagher of Boston called attention in his writings to the medical problems peculiar to adolescents. He advocated special support and companionship for adolescents needing health care. In response to his suggestions several health agencies opened adolescent outpatient clinics centered around diseases prevalent in this age group. These clinics met with much success.

Prior to the late 1950s adolescence had been viewed as a relatively healthy period with few true "medical" illnesses or diseases. Between 1965 and 1975 the existing health facilities were not prepared to deal with the health needs of adolescents, either in numbers or scope. Few adolescents receive adequate or appropriate health care, yet every adolescent deserves the best possible health care.

Nursing the adolescent

The role of the nurse varies and includes assessment of normal growth and development with appropriate intervention when needed, counseling and teaching in areas such as nutrition, health habits, sexuality, and family planning, and caring for the pregnant adolescent or the hospitalized adolescent.

The adolescent client must be accepted and understood as an individual and allowed as much independence as he can handle. Although some limits must be imposed due to hospitalization, whenever possible choices should be allowed. It is most important to be alert to the adolescent patient's concern about his body and to give thorough explanations about procedures. A working knowledge of the theories of cognitive development enables nurses to plan for teaching that is age appropriate.

The teenager's relative maturity must be acknowledged by nurses. The adolescent is likely to be flattered by being talked to as an adult and usually responds well. The teenager is usually interested in his health problem even though he may appear very blasé and even disinterested. Unless nurses make a deliberate effort this attitude may cause them to be negligent about exploring the true reaction of the patient to his condition and even about explaining procedures to him. Actually the teenager usually is eager for health teaching and is likely to accept it well and often enjoys discussions of a scientific nature.

Adolescent health concerns

Acne. Acne is the most common skin disease of adolescence, and almost every adolescent experiences some skin eruption. A very common, minor ailment, it is of great significance to the adolescent who has it. Acne can affect popularity, decrease self-confidence, and keep the individual from activities that might bring friends and success. Acne is thought to be associated with the increased androgen level. It is important for health care professionals to remember that no matter how insignificant the acne appears, it is a major concern to the adolescent (see Chapter 68 for a further discussion of acne).

Fatigue. Adolescents use their energy for activity and growth. Activity includes daily work and play. When energy is used rapidly for growth, as occurs during adolescence, there is less energy for activity and the adolescent shows signs of fatigue. The nurse can help the adolescent make changes in the daily schedule to allow for more rest. The adolescent should be reassured that the fatigue is normal and does not indicate that one is in poor health.

Faulty nutrition. Much has been written about the poor eating habits of the adolescent population. Studies show that many adolescents have adequate knowledge of what foods are good for them but are often too busy to eat or eat on the run and rely on the foods available. Often the most readily available foods are obtained from vending machines. There is a need for concerned citizens and health professionals to encourage vending companies to make good, healthful foods available instead of junk foods.

Both consistent overeating (obesity) and chronic loss of appetite (anorexia nervosa) may result from emotional problems during the adolescent years. These behaviors may be conditioned by the culture in which one is reared.

Obesity (overnourishment). Obesity is common among adolescents who live in societies where food availability is not severely limited by costs or scarcity. Obesity is defined as an excess of body fat. The male with 20% to 25% excess body fat and the female with 25% to 30% excess body fat are classified as obese.[1]

Obesity prevalence rates range from 11% to 30% in high school populations according to several recent studies. It is estimated that between 80% to 90% of obese children become obese adults.

Obesity is multifactorial in etiology. Factors contributing to obesity operate in varying degrees and combinations. Some factors that have been identified include:

1. Constitutional factors such as genetic and structural makeup
2. Cultural factors such as reactions to food and being fat
3. Psychologic factors such as the values of food and obesity to the person
4. Activity level of the individual

The earlier one can identify the obese state and institute treatment, the better the hope for a rational program of dietary control. Adolescent obesity is best managed with a combination of moderate diet and exercise. Rigid restrictions of food or crash diets should be discouraged because the rapid growth process at this time requires a high caloric intake and rigid dietary restrictions could interfere with growth.

Motivation, which is difficult to achieve, may be provided with group counseling and group activities with other overweight adolescents. Cooperation and understanding from the parents is essential. A family history of obesity suggests that eating habits may be firmly entrenched, and weight loss will be much more difficult.

Undernutrition may be due to a rapidly increasing basal metabolism rate. These children may not be eating enough to meet all the body's needs during this period of rapid growth. The underweight adolescent may need to slow down and get more rest. Mammer and Eddy found that approximately 20% of teenagers are underweight.[1]

Orthopedic problems. While orthopedic problems may show up during the school years, many tend to surface during adolescence.

Abnormal curvatures of spine. Kyphosis, lordosis, and scoliosis are the most commonly encountered disorders of the spine. *Kyphosis*, a a fixed flexion deformity, most often occurs in the thoracic and upper lumbar parts of the spine. Adolescent kyphosis is a self-limiting process and often goes undiagnosed, with the child being accused of having "poor posture" or "round shoulders." Should the curvature progress, moderate back pain will be felt. Treatment is usually conservative and includes spine-stretching exercises and sleeping without a pillow and with a board under the mattress. In severe cases the Milwaukee brace may be modified to treat kyphosis. In rare cases spinal fusion may be necessary.

Lordosis, a fixed extension deformity, often forms to compensate for other abnormalities. It it often present with kyphosis. Treatment is generally conservative.

Structural scoliosis is caused by changes in the vertebral bodies. *Idiopathic scoliosis*, which accounts for 80% of scoliosis, is a hereditary condition occurring five to six times more often in girls. It is most commonly seen between the ages of 8 and 15 years, and most often a right thoracic curve occurs.

Treatment must be instituted to prevent progression of mild scoliosis and to stabilize or correct the more severe curvature. Without treatment pulmonary function may be impaired and back pain may be a problem in later life. The older the age at which the curvature begins and the milder the curvature at initial diagnosis and treatment, the better the prognosis.

Conservative treatment with the Milwaukee brace and exercise is the choice of treatment. Surgical intervention is required when the deformity is progressive and does not respond to conservative measures. The aim of surgery is to correct the curvature and stabilize that area of the spine. A variety of surgical procedures including Harrington's rod or other instrumentation, spinal fusion, and immobilization in a body cast for several months may be employed.

The nursing care of these patients is similar in many cases to the care of adult patients having spinal fusions (see Chapter 42). The psychosocial implications of scoliosis are most important. The alteration in body image caused by the disease and by most modes of treatment creates anxiety and concern for most adolescents. Treatment may also impose restrictions on the activities of the adolescent, and he may feel left out. It is important to help the adolescent devise ways to remain active with his peer group. Kalafatich[18] presents an excellent case history dealing with the management of an adolescent hospitalized with scoliosis.

Slipped femoral epiphysis. In *slipped femoral epiphysis* a weakness of the epiphyseal plate allows the epiphysis to slip off the femoral neck in reaction to force. It is more common in boys than in girls and occurs between the ages of 10 and 16 years. Treatment consists of internal fixation with an epiphyseal plate. Without treatment a permanent limp and degenerative hip disease in adulthood may result.

Athletic injuries. A variety of orthopedic injuries may result from athletic injuries caused by either internal or external forces. Many of these injuries are preventable by proper conditioning and training of athletes, and many occur during unsupervised sports activities. In 1973 adolescents sustained 12,591 football-related injuries.[12] It is important to teach young people the principles of first aid to be employed in case of injuries. Another source of sport-related injuries are bicycle accidents, which numbered 17,411 in 1973.[12] Good preventive care demands that young people be taught the basics of bicycle safety and maintenance of the bicycle, as many accidents are the results of defective brakes or other mechanical failures.

Accidents. Between the ages of 15 to 24 years, accidents are the leading cause of death. In 1972 the motor vehicle accident mortality for this age group was 47.4 per 100,000 population.[36] Many adolescents injured in automobile accidents must be hospitalized for extended periods of time due to orthopedic injuries (see Chapter 42 for discussion of nursing care). If a friend or relative is killed in the accident, the nursing staff are often the ones who must help the adolescent deal with grief and guilt. It is important to allow the adolescent to express feelings about loss and death and to assist the individual to vent feelings.

Pregnancy. If pregnancy occurs before a girl completes her own physical growth, she is at increased risk both biologically and emotionally. According to recent studies pregnant adolescents have higher rates for toxemia, prolonged labor, pelvic disproportion, and cesarean section. Mortality is much higher for infants born to very young mothers.

The pregnant adolescent requires more intensive maternity care than older women. While she is still dealing with the crisis of adolescence, she is thrust into another crisis situation, that of pregnancy. The pregnant teenager has all the needs and wants of any adolescent. At a time when she is trying to deal with her recent growth and body image change, pregnancy creates yet another disturbance in the self-concept. At a time when peer association is at a peak, the pregnant teenager is often isolated from her peers by school regulations or social sanctions. As mentioned earlier, nutrition is often less than ideal among adolescents, and this is of special concern during pregnancy because the girl's own physical growth is incomplete. Her nutritional needs may suffer if nutritional intake is not sufficient to meet both her needs and those of the fetus.

Progressing through her pregnancy the adolescent will experience all the physical and emotional changes that the adult pregnant woman experiences. The teenager most often has less knowledge and understanding about these changes, and the need for prenatal teaching is especially important.

To prevent future unwanted pregnancies it is important that the pregnant adolescent have adequate information regarding contraception. Acceptable family planning services should be available to and used by the sexually active teenager. For more detailed information on contraceptive devices the reader is referred to Chapter 61.

Venereal disease. The incidence of venereal disease among the adolescent population in the last decade has been frightening. Gonorrhea has reached epidemic proportions among teenagers, and the incidence of syphilis among adolescents continues to increase.

Teenagers who suspect that they have contracted a venereal disease should be encouraged to seek medical help as soon as possible. Most cities have free VD clinics, and emergency departments in general hospitals screen for venereal disease. Adolescents need to understand that in many states they do not need parental consent to be treated and that information about their disease will be kept confidential and their parents will not be informed by those treating them. See Chapter 62 for further information about venereal disease.

Drug abuse. There is now evidence of a decrease in the use of hard drugs by older adolescents, while the use of drugs among very young adolescents may be increasing. Like many other problems among teenagers the explanations for the use of drugs are varied and include experimentation, escapism, rebellion, and pursuit of new meanings for human existence.

There is a high rate of recidivism (recurrence of the problem), and rehabilitation for drug addicts is expensive. Rehabilitative and preventive programs developed with the cooperation of young people appear to be the most promising avenue for combating drug abuse.

According to Dr. Morris E. Chafetz, former director of the National Institute on Alcohol Abuse and Alcoholism, alcohol was the most abused drug in the United States in the mid-1970s. It appears that the young are switching from drugs to alcohol, which is more readily available and has less severe legal penalties for illegal use. Alcohol problems among teenagers have resulted in development of many Alcoholics Anonymous groups for teenagers in this country.

Mental health. There appears to be an increase in mental health disorders among adolescents. Many of the complaints of clients attending adolescent clinics have an emotional cause.[36]

Probably the most dramatic indicator of emotional instability is the increasing incidence of suicide. The suicide rate for white males between the ages of 15 and 24 years was 11.4 per 100,000 in 1973 according to the National Center for Health Statistics.[36] Suicide is the third leading cause of death in older adolescents.

To combat the high morbidity and mortality, there is a need for preventive mental health programs that include early identification and surveillance of those most likely to be susceptible to stresses within the environment. Patient assessment should include questions about the adolescent's emotional state. Other clues are a family history of mental illness, alcoholism, or drug abuse. Difficulty with interpersonal relationships and a preference for solitary pursuits are also clues that the adolescent may need special help.

■ ADULT YEARS

Adulthood is one of the most stable periods in the life span. Even though various physical and psychologic changes occur during these years, there is relative stability in values, attitudes, and feelings about the self and others. The adult has developed a sense of self-utilization to achieve desired goals as contrasted with the self-consciousness of the adolescent.[33]

While dramatic changes in physical development are few, the main physiologic event of the adult years is the menopause. The psychologic changes that may occur are largely responses to changing life events.

Early and middle adulthood covers a long period of life, extending approximately from ages 20 to 65. Because circumstances and expectations are not the same in the first 25 years as they are in the second 20 years, adulthood is separated into three stages: young adulthood, middle adulthood, and late maturity.

□ Young adulthood

The young adult years, extending from approximately 20 to 45, is a complex period of life, a time in which the achievement of personal goals is the primary focus. The young adult years are referred to as the expansion years in which energies are directed toward career fulfillment, social involvement, and the initiation and maintenance of a family.[33]

Physical development

Full growth and development are completed by the mid-twenties, and most body systems are functioning at maximum levels. Of those changes that occur in adulthood, some begin early and others not until later in middle age; some are abrupt and some are gradual.

Intellectual development

Cross-sectional studies have shown that the highest overall intelligence test performance occurs at some time between the late teens and late twenties. People in their thirties, forties, and fifties tend to score somewhat lower. Longitudinal evidence has shown that general intelligence either remains the same or increases slightly during the adult years.[34] Certain factors may influence intellectual development and performance, such as education and other sociocultural factors.

Sexuality in young adulthood

Sexuality is an integral part of self-concept. Competence in the area of one's sexuality is of prime importance during the adult years. Sexuality may be defined as a "deep pervasive aspect of the total person, the sum total of one's feelings and behavior as a male or female, the expression of which goes beyond genital response."[24] Young adulthood is normally the time when the body's sexual response is powerful and there is a need to find adequate and satisfactory expression. It is known that a man reaches his peak sexual capacity at about 18 years of age. Women, however, reach their peak of sexual capacity in their early thirties.

If the expression of sexual feelings is restricted, perhaps because of illness or injury, causing a felt or imagined change in body image, sexual concerns may become paramount. Nurses frequently are asked by young adults for assistance with marital or sexual concerns. Unless the nurse is secure in his or her own sexual identity and has had adequate preparation to deal with such matters, clients should be referred to appropriate persons who can deal with these concerns.

Psychosocial development

Adulthood is often equated with maturity and is characterized by a sense of responsibility, maintenance of appropriate impulse control, ability to plan and implement realistic goals, and the capacity to enter into intimate relationships.

The nurse needs to understand that everyone does not arrive at young adulthood with the same level of maturity. Emotional maturity varies from person to person, as do intellectual ability and physical characteristics. In addition an adult who appears reasonably mature under usual circumstances may when under stress exhibit certain immature behavior. For example, a person may become more demanding or very critical or lose his temper.

In Erikson's *eight ages of man*, the first adult stage is characterized by *intimacy versus isolation* (Fig. 18-6). Intimacy is seen as sharing the self to form a commitment to an intense lasting relationship with another person, a cause, or a creative effort without fearing the loss of identity. Intimacy requires responsibility, impulse control, the ability to plan, and also the ability to trust. The inability to develop some form of intimacy draws the person into increasing feelings of isolation, alienation, and self-absorption.

The successful resolution of this phase of the life cycle is dependent on a positive self-concept. How a person feels about himself affects relationships as well as the choices made during this period. A person who feels adequate and competent in setting and achieving goals tends to experience more positive outcomes than one whose self-concept is that of inadequacy and incompetency. These negative feelings tend to foster withdrawal and the inability to mobilize resources for positive gains. When caring for the young adult it is therefore important to assess the individual's self-perception. These data not

Age	FREUD (PSYCHOSEXUAL)	ERIKSON (PSYCHOSOCIAL)	PIAGET (COGNITIVE)
Young adulthood	*Young adulthood*	*Intimacy vs isolation:* significant objects—persons, causes	*STAGE IV continued formal operations:* development beyond this stage has not been studied
Adulthood	*Adulthood*	*Generativity vs stagnation:* Significant persons—spouse, grandchildren, friends	↓
Maturity	*Maturity*	*Integrity vs disgust, despair:* significant persons—spouse, family members, friends	↓

Fig. 18-6. Summary of psychosocial development in later life.

only provide information as to motivation potential but are a basis for nursing intervention to help increase the individual's self-esteem.

Body image, an important aspect of self-concept, is a mental picture of the body's appearance as well as the attitudes, emotions, and personality of the individual. At a period of life when acceptance by others is most important, and with society's emphasis on youth, beauty, and physical fitness, any alteration in body function or structure poses a threat to a positive body image. Adaptation to these alterations depends on the nature and meaning of the threat, coping mechanisms, and available support systems.

Therefore nursing intervention to help someone deal with a threat to or change of body image involves (1) careful assessment of the individual's perception of the condition, (2) assistance in helping the individual maintain a realistic perception of the threat in relation to the person's total self-image, (3) assistance in identifying useful coping mechanisms, and (4) identification of support systems (see Chapter 28).

Developmental tasks

Other psychologic and social aspects of the young adult's development can be gleaned from the developmental tasks common to this period. The developmental tasks of early adulthood, most concretely seen in the choice of a vocation and a marriage partner, clearly involve a certain choice of life style. While fairly clear boundaries have been established between self and parents by this time, parental attitudes and value systems have been internalized in the young adult to become a salient part of his identity, thus affecting future life choices. Inherent in these choices is the quest for independence from family, social, and economic dependence.

Occupational choice. An occupation represents much more than a set of skills and functions. It is a way of life that determines much of the environment, both physical and social, in which a person lives.[22] Occupational choice plays a significant part in further shaping the personality by providing a social system, status, roles, and a life style. The choice of an occupational role often necessitates consideration of appropriate educational preparation, and thus educational goals and achievements become a very important part of this choice.

At a time in life when involvement in an occupation is of prime importance, unemployment may cause the individual to feel that he or she is not needed or wanted, thus breeding feelings of inadequacy and failure. When caring for an individual it is very important for the nurse to be as sensitive to the concerns and anxieties of those who are employed and face many pressures as to those who are faced with the problems of unemployment.

The Women's Liberation Movement has exerted a significant influence on women relative to occupational choices. As a result it is now more socially acceptable for a woman to choose a career goal as an alternative or as a supplement to the traditional housewife-mother roles. Among married young adults there is a growing tendency to delay having children until career goals are more solidified. Some married women in this age group may choose to have an abortion if they become pregnant at a time that is not convenient relative to their career or other anticipated goals or when children are not desired (see Chapter 62 for further information about family planning and abortion).

Marital choice. Another major decision of early adulthood is whether to marry or not to marry. Our society continues to strongly support marital status among young adults. However, some people are choosing not to marry, enjoying the independence and freedom of single living. While there may be many reasons for entering into the marital relationship, marriage is generally recognized as a close and loving partnership between two people where intimacy and affection exist in a free and equal relationship as opposed to only a social institution where the man is the undisputed head of the house and the wife is the childbearer.[24]

The arrival of the first child transforms the spouses into parents as they take on the roles and parenting behavior learned from parents. Parenthood is experienced as a joy as well as a crisis: a joy because a child is the product of their common bond and fulfillment of goals; a crisis because the child necessitates adjustments in daily routine and lifestyle, which is often seen as a burden. Preparation for parenthood has not been widespread in our society. It is therefore difficult for an individual to anticipate many of the stresses of being a parent and the changes required in themselves and their marital relationship. If the nurse assesses that an individual is experiencing undue stress and an inability to cope, resources for this kind of assistance can be made available.

While personality characteristics and interpersonal problems are primary sources of difficulties in adjustment to marriage and parenthood, cultural and societal variables often make these adjustments difficult. For instance, the mobility of our society results in a dispersal of family members and close relatives, with less available help from these significant others in times of need and stress.

While the institutions of marriage and family are the most socially acceptable, there is an increasing tolerance for diversity relative to optional living patterns such as communes as a temporary way of life, living together, staying single, becoming a bachelor mother or remaining a childless couple, and experimenting with bisexuality or homosexuality.[29] It is important that the nurse be in touch with his or her attitudes about varying life styles and choices and remain nonjudgmental, refraining from imposing one's own values on others.

Health needs

The cessation of physical growth and development by the time a person reaches the young adulthood period of life, together with the changes in life styles, necessitates certain alterations in physical and psychosocial needs.

Three aspects of physical needs dealt with here relate to *nutrition, exercise,* and *rest* and *sleep.*

The young adult's *nutritional needs* are not the same as those of adolescents. The cessation of physical maturation necessitates a reduction in some nutritional requirements such as calcium and protein, while an increase in some nutrients is needed. Young men should increase their consumption of foods high in vitamin C, E, B_6, and riboflavin. In young women the needs for protein, vitamins A, E, B_6, B_{12}, and riboflavin remain about the same, but the need for vitamin C increases. In relation to the need for iron in the diet, the man needs only 10 mg of iron daily and the woman 18 mg. Sometimes dietary modifications are indicated, especially for young adults at risk of heart disease. Foods high in cholesterol and saturated fats should be limited in the diet of the young adult, since they contribute to the formation of atheromatous plaques in the blood vessels resulting in cardiovascular problems.[7] Nutritional problems of young adults frequently stem directly from their life styles, such as busy schedules, limited income, and job or educational demands. The increased demands placed on the young adult (job, home, children, economics) often lead to poor nutritional choices and habits.

The nurse can help the young adult understand the importance of adequate nutrition and of adjusting schedules to allow more time for meals. An understanding of how illnesses and prolonged recovery periods can be related to inadequate nutritional intake is important. Young wives may need suggestions about planning nutritionally adequate meals that are as economical as possible.

Exercise serves several functions in the young adult. It helps to regulate appetite, release tension, aid sleep, retard aging, and keep body muscles firm and it protects the heart. It is important to note that exercise should be regular and appropriate to the individual's physical condition. Too often adults think they have worked hard all day and feel they have gained the necessary exercise. Many sport activities such as tennis, horseback riding, and swimming provide physical exercise and exertion. However, sporadic involvement in these activities is not as effective as a regularly planned physical exercise program.[24] Sporadic exertion often produces sudden demands on body systems, not allowing the body to compensate adequately and adjust to the demands. A gradual increase in the intensity of exertion allows the body to adapt to the physical demands, while regularity contributes to sustained maintenance and optimal functioning of body systems.

As the demands of jobs, social acitivities, family responsibilities, and educational pursuits increase, the young adult's need for adequate *rest and sleep* also increases, but in actuality the young adult often goes without proper rest and sleep. While an individual can adjust to a lack of sleep for a length of time, prolonged periods of lack of sleep and rest can contribute to altered mental and physical functions resulting in illness and slowed recovery periods.

Health concerns

Research has shown relationships between physical adaptation and illness and sociocultural experiences. Death rates from cancer, diabetes, tuberculosis, heart disease, and multiple sclerosis in urban populations are inversely proportional to income, implying that stresses of poverty may be determinants of such diseases. Accidents are the leading cause of death of young adults.[24] Among young men industrial accidents and drownings also rank high as major causes of accidental death.[24] Many injuries require restriction of activity, which presents the young adult with social and economic problems.[24]

Acute conditions such as upper respiratory tract infection and influenza occur more frequently in the young adult than do other acute illnesses. With young adults the primary responsibility of the nurse lies in the teaching of preventive measures. Prevention is directed at supporting the body defenses and reducing the person's susceptibility. Avoiding environmental pollutants, including cigarette smoke, as much as possible and keeping alcohol intake at an acceptable level as well as observing basic health practices (adequate rest, sleep, exercise, and nutritious diet) should be stressed.

Physiologic and psychologic changes resulting in unusual or disturbed adaptive behavior patterns occur when the young adult is unable to cope with the newly acquired tasks and responsibilities. Mate selection, marriage, childbearing, college, job demands, social expectations, and independent decision making are all stressors, carrying the threats of insecurity and possibly some degree of failure. Some of these stress reactions take the form of physical illness. Related to the stresses of achievement in the young adult years is the occurrence of gastric and duodenal ulcers. Prevention here is directed at reinforcement of appropriate diet, exercise, and rest. When stressors are perceived as overwhelming, they may result in self-destructive behavior such as drug abuse and addiction, alcoholism, excessive smoking, and suicide (ranking as one of the leading causes of death among this age group).

Sensitivity to the many pressures and responsibilities

facing the young adult is vital to good nursing care. The patient's major concern often is not about himself. He or she may be the breadwinner of a family. How is the family being supported during the illness? How are the medical bills to be paid? The patient may be a mother of small children. Who will care for them? If she is hospitalized, she is often concerned about how her family is getting along at home. The patient may have no family. Who will look in on him if he is ill at home? Who will care for him during convalescence? These are only a few of the problems frequently facing the young adult patient. Some problems of hospitalized patients may be alleviated by providing the use of a telephone or by arranging a visit with a family member, friend, or business associate. Help needed by the patient may be available through other support systems such as social services in the hospital or through family service or public health agencies. It is important also for the nurse in a physician's office or clinic to be alert for clients who need this kind of assistance.

The adult patient is often expected "to act like an adult," and this is especially true if he is a man. Social expectations have made it difficult for men to cry or reveal their emotions. Thus when ill they may become irritable, withdrawn, and depressed because they may be concealing their true feelings. The nurse needs to be able to convey sincere interest in the patient as a unique human being and acceptance of his behavior.

Providing the opportunity for the patient to express feelings and concerns is very therapeutic in helping the person deal with problems and anxieties. Appropriate intervention also entails helping patients identify coping mechanisms that have been useful to them in times of stress as well as the various support systems that can assist in meeting their needs.

□ Middle adulthood

While the transition from young adulthood to the middle years involves more of a state of mind than some dramatic bodily change, it is generally agreed that middle adulthood comprises those years between 45 and 65 years of age. As the young adulthood phase begins to taper off in the middle to late thirties, a change begins to occur in the perceptions of time left to live, productivity, self, and others. The middle years are approached with a sharpened sense of awareness as the individual begins to take stock of life. Has it been fulfilling? Am I doing what I really want to be doing? What are my goals from now on? How the individual evaluates the quality of life already lived and the potential outlook for the future may have a significant influence on further adaptation in the succeeding years.

Erikson has described adaptation to this stage in terms of the resolution of the crisis, *generativity versus stagnation* (Fig. 18-6). He sees generativity as "primarily the concern in establishing and guiding the next generation."[10] Generativity also includes productivity, creativity, and concern for others in the broadest sense. When this enrichment and fulfillment is not experienced, stagnation and personal impoverishment occur to the point of isolation and preoccupation with self.[29]

Many variables affect the degree to which one experiences productivity or stagnation. The discussion that follows focuses on some of those physiologic and psychosocial variables that influence one's adaptation to this stage of the life cycle.

Physical development

The adult usually approaches this phase of life functioning at near peak efficiency. As the middle years progress gradual physiologic changes occur. The individual becomes aware of the appearance of gray hairs, small creases or lines, and dry skin that begins to show signs of decreasing elasticity. There is a redistribution of fatty tissue regardless of a change in diet or exercise patterns. The skeletal muscles increase in bulk until about the age of 50 and do not begin to degenerate until approximately 60 years of age. Smooth muscles, on the other hand, change very little with age; therefore the vital organs can, by and large, be kept healthy until death.[19]

The sense organs undergo change in the middle years, one of the most noticeable being the eyes. The necessity to wear bifocals, trifocals, or reading glasses is brought on by a condition called presbyopia, characterized by a reduction in the elasticity of the lens of the eye resulting in decreased accommodation for near points of vision. During the middle years there is a gradual deterioration and hardening of the auditory cells and nerves resulting in some loss of auditory acuity.

Hormonal deficiencies associated with menopausal changes in women take place, on the average, between 40 and 55 years of age. As ovarian function gradually diminishes, decreased amounts of estrogen and progesterone are produced by the ovaries, while other body tissues continue to produce small amounts of estrogen for several years after ovarian function ceases. Some of the symptoms associated with menopause are "hot flashes," the cause of which is unknown; atrophic vaginitis in which the vaginal mucosa becomes thin and dry, contributing to itching, burning, and possible discharge; and osteoporosis, which is not necessarily a product of menopause but often accompanies or follows menopause as bone demineralization is accelerated in the absence of estrogens.[11]

The psychologic changes that often accompany menopause may not be precipitated by the hormonal deficiency but may be more appropriately related to the adjustments and adaptations of the middle years.[11] Mood swings may be apparent. The middle-aged woman can be laughing one minute and crying the next. Nervousness, insomnia, and fatigue are common complaints at this time. There may be mild depression, but this is usually transitory. This depression may be a reaction to the loss of generativity, at which times stages of the grief process may be observed.[11]

There are no physical changes in men comparable to the menopausal changes in women, although some emotional changes occur in men during this period of life. This is not, however, the result of hormonal deficiency, as androgen levels decline very slowly.[19] Reproductive capabilities continue into the later years, and any loss of sex drive or potency may be more a state of mind than a result of some physical change.

As activity and metabolism slow down during this period, the weight gain that often results may have detrimental effects on other body systems. The incidence of diabetes, kidney disease, and gallstones increases during this period. While adults get fewer respiratory tract infections than children do, the decreased elasticity of the lungs results in certain chronic respiratory diseases. The loss of elasticity and changes in the structure of the arteries lead to many cardiovascular problems. The middle-aged adult needs more time for recovery from both minor and serious ailments.[19]

Patient education about these potential threats to health and knowledge of how these problems may be prevented is a necessary part of nursing care of the middle-aged adult. It is important to encourage these individuals to receive physical examinations at least yearly in order that sound health might be maintained throughout the remaining years of their lives.

Intellectual development

Contrary to some popular beliefs, mental capacity if used is unimpaired in the middle years. Data suggests that there is little or no decrement in learning capability and memory function.[34] Cerebral capacity deteriorates slowly and only begins to weaken at about the age of 70 years.[19] Active utilization of mental capacity throughout the years will contribute to mental productivity in the later years. It is therefore important that the nurse provide mental stimulation as a part of nursing care and encourage the middle-aged adult to continue with involvement in activities that will facilitate mental productivity.

Sexuality in middle adulthood

The physical aspects of aging, together with the many pressures that are common to this stage of life, affect the attitudes about one's sexuality and sexual functioning.

Some adults expect that with middle age (particularly after menopause) comes the end of their physical attractiveness and thus a decline in sexual interest and the capacity for competent sexual functioning. It has been found that this is more a psychologic phenomenon than an actual physical occurrence. It seems that cultural influences have been significant in perpetuating the idea that with the aging process comes decline of sexual interest and activity. Ambivalence about oneself growing older in a youth-oriented society often breeds feelings of inadequacy relative to one's sexuality. As a result some adults may become depressed and sexually unresponsive. Others may feel a need to retrieve that sense of youthfulness by behaving and dressing in a youthful manner or by having an affair with a younger person.

The middle-aged adult who approaches these years with self-acceptance and appreciation is more apt to continue into the later years with a satisfying and fulfilling sexual life.

Some of the physical changes that accompany the menopause may affect the pleasure of sexual intercourse. For example, delay in the production of vaginal lubrication caused by the decrease in steroids may result in some discomfort during intercourse, and on occasion the irritation may cause cystitis. There may be a tendency to refrain from sexual activity because of discomfort. If such problems exist the nurse can explain their causes, suggest use of a water-soluble lubricant during intercourse, and advise the woman to consult her physician. Carefully monitored estrogen replacement therapy is recommended for some women, although controversy exists regarding its risk.

As men age, certain social and psychologic factors influence their sexual responsiveness. Masters and Johnson noted several recurrent themes in interviews about waning sexual responsiveness: monotony in the sexual relationship or a feeling of being taken for granted, concerns with economic or career pursuits, mental and physical fatigue, physical or mental illness of the individual or spouse, overindulgence in food or drink, and fear of failure.[35] They suggest that practice of sexual activity contributes to quality of the sexual relationship as well as to the continuation of sexual activity into the later years.[31]

In another study of persons aged 45 to 69 years, previous sexual experience was the most significant contributing factor to current sexual functioning, including interest in, frequency, and enjoyment of sexual relations.[9]

Because of prevailing cultural attitudes about waning sexual interest in the middle years, sexual concerns are often ignored in the care and rehabilitation of the middle-aged adult. It is very important therefore that health care providers become knowledgeable about and sensitive to the sexual needs of patients, particularly those who experience injury or illness that restricts physical activity. The nurse can help the patient deal with these anxieties by providing the opportunity to discuss these concerns. If the nurse does not feel competent to discuss such matters, someone with more proficiency in this area can be sought.

It may be helpful for nurses to avail themselves of opportunities to learn more about sexuality in health and illness in order to better assist patients with these concerns.

Psychosocial development

The psychologic and social development of an individual in the middle years is best exemplified in the various developmental tasks that are common to this stage of life.

Many of the developmental tasks associated with the middle years involve role transitions, which may involve some alteration in self-image, life style, values, and attitudes.

The ability to shed roles and take on new roles smoothly contributes to a more creative and productive life during the middle years. With the maturation of children comes the transition of parental attitudes, values, and actions that formerly were child oriented to those more appropriate to an adult relationship. In those instances where the focus of life revolved solely around the children, the outcome of their departure from home may be an experience of loss. Often referred to as the "empty nest syndrome," this sudden loss frequently leads to depression in women. What is lost is not only the grown child but all the attachments associated with the mother role, resulting in altered perceptions of the self as being needed.[25]

Not only is the role transition relative to one's offspring complex, but this may also be a time when the health status of one's parents is changing. Illnesses and perhaps impending death often necessitate assuming the role of parent to one's own parent(s). The decision making regarding the care of aging parents may necessitate changes in life style if the parents come to live in the home.

While the adult must deal with many changes and alterations during these middle years, this is the time when renewal and full development of relationships can occur. It is a time of altering the patterns of child-centered days and of nurturing the intimate relationship of husband and wife. If throughout previous years a couple has not developed mutual support, open communication, and awareness of each other's needs, the development of an enriching relationship may be difficult if not impossible to achieve.

At the same time that the individual may be enjoying the enrichment of new and renewed relationships and a new sense of freedom, there is the inevitable experience of loss of significant others. Death begins to take friends, parents, and spouse, necessitating alterations in relationships and life styles.

For some adults the middle years are a time when peak social influence, prosperity, economic success, and stability are experienced. But for many the middle years are approached with a sense of frustration and failure if goals and expectations set in earlier years have not been reached and are not realistically attainable. The realization that the time has passed for significant achievement of status and success is often a crisis-producing situation. For example, limited upward career mobility is experienced as younger individuals move up more quickly and are selected for the more choice positions and jobs.

Stock taking and reevaluation often result in ambivalence and uncertainties associated with everyday tasks, reflecting a change in values and attitudes. The adult who previously perceived daily responsibilities to be fulfilling and enjoyable may at this time begin to complain about being trapped and hemmed in, with few rewards. It may not be, however, the job or situation that has changed, but the individual.

Wives who perceived their status relative to the success of their husbands may become dissatisfied with themselves for not being involved in self-fulfilling activities. At this time many wives previously linked only to the home embark on new careers in search of self-fulfillment and satisfaction. The women's movement has contributed much to women's motivation to seek heightened self-fulfillment, satisfaction, and usefulness.

Development of creativity may have been impeded during the childrearing and career development days. Productive use of leisure may be a source of contentment for some adults with the exploration and development of new hobbies and areas of talent and skill. The adult may now have more time to invest in outside activities such as clubs, organizations, church, and politics.

The new and renewed relationships and increased involvement in outside activities is demonstrative of the external orientation to those things outside the individual characteristic of this period of life. This is compared with the internal orientation of the young adult years in which the individual is more preoccupied with achieving mastery of goals and responsibilities and gaining approval from the outside world.

When there is a lack in the cultivation of various relationships and areas of interest that contribute to the meaningfulness and satisfaction of life, stagnation and immobilization often occur. It is the mobilization of one's inner resources that generates the kind of creativity and productivity that facilitate continued growth throughout the remaining years.

Health needs

One important reason for studying growth and development is to gain a better understanding of those physical and psychosocial variables that determine the health needs of individuals as they progress through life. For as individuals change, so do their health needs.

Consideration of the needs of proper *nutrition, rest,* and *exercise* are most important during these middle years. Reduced energy requirements together with reduced physical activity dictate a lesser demand for calories. Improper nutrition, excessive to the physical demands, may result in obesity and atherosclerosis, which are risk factors for such diseases as coronary artery disease, chronic hypertension, renal failure, and diabetes. Thus the middle-aged adult needs to be aware of the fact that biophysical changes necessitate a reduction in calories, saturated fats, and cholesterol. The diet should contain the basic four food groups with an emphasis on protein, minerals, and vitamins; the caloric intake should be based on age, body build, size, and activity patterns. Diet counseling should include specific examples of polyunsaturated oils, dairy products, and meats that can be substituted for those that are high in saturated fats and cholesterol.[17] Adequate fluid intake and an appropriate diet help prevent constipation, and dietary discretion will help maintain weight control.

Changes in life style may result in mental strain and frustration and a lack of exercise, restful sleep, and relaxation. It is important that rest and sleep be balanced with physical activity in order to keep the body functioning at its optimum. Exercise helps to promote relaxation and improves muscle tone, strength, and coordination. It improves work performance, reduces chronic fatigue, and improves the efficiency of the cardiopulmonary system. An assessment of daily activities may give some indication as to the kind and amount of exercise necessary. Exercise activities that are performed incorrectly and cause overexertion can be detrimental to one's health. The regularity of exercise is of great importance; sporadic exercising is not as effective. Middle-aged individuals should take certain precautions: (1) increase exercise gradually, (2) exercise consistently, and (3) avoid overexertion. Ten minutes after exercising, the heart rate and respirations should return to their normal status. Prior to instigating any exercise program a physician should be consulted if the person is overweight, has a personal or family history of cardiovascular or respiratory tract disease, or has led a physically inactive life.

Middle-aged adults should be encouraged to have a thorough medical examination which that includes not only a careful medical history and physical assessment of body systems but also blood and urine tests, electrocardiogram, chest x-ray examination, and rectal or proctoscopic examination; women should have Pap smear tests. Routine dental, vision, and hearing examinations should also be done because periodontal disease, glaucoma, and hearing loss may be prevented or treated if detected early.[17]

Health concerns

The gradual changing physical characteristics may account for the high incidence of accidents among middle-aged adults. Fractures and dislocations are leading causes of injuries to both sexes.[24] Motor vehicle accidents, occupation-related accidents, and falls in the home are leading causes of death.[24] Respiratory conditions are frequent causes of absenteeism from work. Generally, middle-aged women have more disability days from work because of respiratory and other acute disorders, while men have more disability days from injury.[24]

The main health problems of this age group are cardiovascular disease, cancer, pulmonary disease, diabetes, obesity, alcoholism, anxiety, and depression. Mounting statistical evidence points to excessive smoking as an influence in lung cancer, cardiovascular disease, chronic obstructive pulmonary disease, and peptic ulcer.

The close interrelationship between physical and psychologic makeup of the human body is exemplified in the climacteric (change of life) phase. How a woman reacts to the menopause depends a great deal on her feelings about herself and her womanhood. If over the years procreation and motherhood have been her major sources of self-esteem, equated with youth and femininity, she may have a much more severe reaction to menopause than a woman who has other sources of self-esteem. Some women who cannot adapt to their physical changes and changing life circumstances may become severely depressed (involutional melancholia) and may need treatment, as the danger of suicide is great. Reactions to menopause may vary depending on the woman's past use of measures to control reproduction. If sterilization occurred earlier in her life, the woman may not perceive menopause as the loss of her femininity.

It is helpful to allow the client to discuss her feelings about herself and this phase of her life. It is also important to help the patient identify those strengths and inner resources on which she can focus and build up her self-esteem.

While men do not experience the same physiologic menopausal phenomena as women, they often go through a kind of psychologic "change of life." Symptoms may include fatigue, headaches, increased moodiness, impatience, worry, and psychosomatic complaints such as indigestion, heartburn, rapid or irregular heart beat, urinary problems, respiratory difficulties, and insomnia. Many of these symptoms are often related to emotional depression and anxiety that may be associated with a preoccupation with thoughts of aging, anticipation of retirement, loss of career status, and a general feeling of worthlessness.

For the middle-aged person who feels depressed, trapped, frustrated, or isolated, easily accessible escapes may be alcoholism, drugs, or excess food intake. Illness or accident proneness may also become escape mechanisms as a means of avoiding responsibility or resolving serious difficulties. Hypochondriasis is a common symptom of the self-absorbed adult and may become a means of getting attention. Suicide is a leading cause of death among the middle aged. The nurse therefore should be alert and sensitive to any communication that might be suggestive of suicidal thoughts.

Nursing the adult

When encountering the adult individual experiencing physical or emotional stress, it is important to make a careful assessment not only of the major problem at hand but also of the physical, psychologic, and situational variables relative to the individual's current developmental status. These data are important in that they provide guidance in understanding those factors that may be affecting the individual's response to stress as well as feelings and attitudes about recovery. For example, if an individual unconsciously uses injury, disability, or illness as a way to escape problems or responsibility, progress and treatment may be slowed. Again, the self-absorbed individual is likely to demonstrate regressed, immature behavior resulting in increased dependency needs. Situations such as these are often frustrating for the nurse because there is the tendency to think that adults should react to situations in a mature, logical manner, making appropriate decisions about their welfare. When adults do not react according to our expectations, there is the danger of treating them as children, thereby reinforceing dependency and regression. It is important that the nurse demonstrate acceptance of the adult's behaviors and attitudes, realizing that this may be the individual's manner of coping with stress. Usually when certain needs are met or problems are resolved or dealt with, the individual returns to more mature behavior patterns. Thus facilitating the individual's expression of fears, anxieties, and concerns is often very therapeutic relative to emotional as well as physical healing.

Adulthood is a time when productivity, achievement, and responsibilities are dominant concerns in the individual's life. When goals and expectations are thwarted by illness or disability a crisis often results. This crisis may not affect just a single individual but the family as well. When stress is intense, problem solving may be diminished. The nurse can be helpful at this time by assisting the individual or family in making some decisions by offering options and resources that will help meet their needs, while at the same time being careful to foster and maintain independence by facilitating the client's participation in care planning and decision making.

Sensitivity to the concerns and anxieties brought about by illness or disability is of utmost importance. For example, the paraplegic who is impotent as a result of a spinal cord injury is concerned about his sexuality and adequacy as a man. The woman who must have a mastectomy or hysterectomy is also concerned about her self-image and sexuality. The adult who must be hospitalized for a long period of time may worry about financial support for the family or child care. Coping, like healing, is more than a physical process. Thus genuine acceptance and enlightened concern rather than indifference or pity can be of incalculable benefit to the patient.

While it is a fact that the nurse cannot meet all of an individual's needs, it should be emphasized that nursing is concerned with the total picture of a person's needs. Therefore the nurse who is knowledgeable about all aspects of growth and development and incorporates that knowledge into nursing care planning and intervention is better able to deal with more of the individual's needs and concerns.

□ Late maturity

Although 65 years of age is usually considered the beginning of late maturity or old age, tremendous individual variation exists. Age is really a sociocultural concept and not wholly physiologic and chronologic. Chronologic age is related to but not identical with aging because individual and personal variables enter the picture. The U.S. Department of Health, Education and Welfare has defined age in terms of three classes. These classes are biologic age (a person's position in time relative to his potential life span), psychologic age (the individual's capacity for adapting to his environment), and social age (a person's role in the family, at work, and in his community as well as his interests and activities).[32] Some people may be old at 45 years of age, while others are not old at 80.

Characteristics of aging

Aging is a normal process in which certain *anatomic* and *physiologic changes* take place. The changes are associated with a decline in the effectiveness and functioning of the organism that eventually results in death. The speed with which aging occurs varies and depends on hereditary factors and the stresses of life. The genetic factor in these biologic processes determines the time of onset, the course and direction, and the time sequences of the various aging processes.

Aging is now being explored by many researchers.

Many models of aging have been hypothesized. These models are generally divided into three classes. The first concerns models centered around aging due to *loss of cellular synthesis*. The loss of cellular synthesis can be attributed to genetic damage (DNA), loss of messenger synthesis ability of the cells, or a loss of message-translating ability. A second class of models to explain aging concerns *loss of cellular function*. The loss of function can occur because of loss of function of cellular organelles, insufficiency of growth factors, or an accumulation of inhibitors. Finally, the third class of models or hypotheses centers around *loss of intercellular coordination*. Reasons hypothesized to explain this include physical alteration, decreased cell responsiveness due to loss of receptor sites or cells, or just cell loss. Total cell loss with age may average 10% to 40% in some parts of the body. This cell loss occurs to the greatest extent in the nervous and endocrine systems. Kidney, liver, heart, and muscle tissue seem affected to a lesser degree.

Biologic aging leads to different responses in the older person. Healing takes place more slowly, and the body's response to infection is less rapid and apparently less effective. Tissues gradually lose their elasticity, leading to a decreased speed of muscle response and decreased strength. Loss of tissue elasticity also causes increased rigidity of such body structures as the rib cage. This rigidity in turn may cause decreased lung expansion and predisposes the aged person to lung congestion. Bones become rarefied in the aging process and fractures occur easily. This is true particularly of the vertebral bodies and the neck of the femur, which begin to lose their density while a person is in his thirties.

Cardiovascular changes that began during middle age begin to present symptoms in the older years. The elasticity of the blood vessels lessens, and the cardiac output decreases as the cardiac muscle strength is less; thus the heart in the elderly person must work harder to provide adequate oxygenation. Arteriosclerosis and atherosclerosis, prevalent in the elderly, may result in ischemia and eventually in death of the tissue in one or more organ systems.

Peripheral resistance increases with age despite a reduction in cardiac output. Blood pressure may show a marked increase with age, both in systolic and diastolic readings. The elderly person does not tolerate radical changes in position such as lowering of the head for postural drainage or elevation of the feet above heart level. Vessels in the head may become engorged, and there is inadequate circulation to the lower extremities. With prolonged standing, blood may accumulate in the lower extremities so that not enough is provided for the brain. Dizziness and accidents may follow.

There is gradual degeneration and atrophy of the nervous system in old age, leading to lessened nerve acuity and impaired sensation. There is a generalized loss of neurons with age and a progressive decrease in the weight of the brain. The older person's gag reflex may be less acute than that of a younger person, and therefore aspiration of mucus or other foreign material such as food may occur easily. He may be unaware of burning himself or of pressure on soft tissues. Bed rest causes the elderly person's circulation to slow; consequently many elderly people become confused when they must stay in bed. This is noticeable in some even after several hours of sleep. Loss of interest in life may also make an elderly person appear dull mentally. Oftentimes these individuals will become more bright and alert when stimuli are increased by contact with others. Therefore it is often preferable to put the elderly person in a room with others rather than in a single room by himself.

The acuity of the senses begins to decline with old age. As with all the changes associated with the aging process, the amount of decline varies with the individual. One in four persons over 65 years of age has some type of hearing problem.[3] Sensitivity to sound decreases with age, and there is some selective loss of hearing of the higher pitches. Such changes are usually not reversible because they are due to neurologic decline. If the loss is due to ossification of the bones of articulation in the middle ear, some hearing may return following surgery and the use of a hearing aid (see Chapter 38 for information about hearing aids).

More light is required for the aged retina to produce the same physiologic sensation as was produced in the younger years. Adaptation to light and dark requires more time. Visual acuity, especially for close reading, is impaired as a result of changes in the structure of the eyeball and its muscles. Twice as many elderly people have visual impairments as have hearing loss.

The sense of taste appears to decline with age, which is often one explanation for the aging person's lack of appetite or loss of interest in foods that were once favorites.

The senses of touch and smell also decline as a part of the aging process. Since aromas often stimulate eating, the decline in the sense of smell contributes to the appetite decline in many aging persons. Decline in the senses of touch and smell present certain safety hazards that need to be discussed with the aging individual and his family.

The liver, heart, kidneys, and other vital organs of many elderly people may be working hard to maintain normal function with little margin available for adaptability to stress. Any additional burden may be enough to tip the balance unfavorably unless particular care is given. The physiologic controls of fluid and electrolyte balance and temperature also are less adaptable in the aged. Faintness and shock may follow relatively short periods without food and fluid because of fluid and electrolyte imbalances. Therefore the elderly person should receive medical attention for even apparently slight indispositions.

Psychosocial development

Psychologic and social development continue during maturity. Psychologic and socioeconomic concepts of aging are most important for all who work with the aged. A knowledge of the crises occurring in this stage of life is useful if one is to assist clients and their families in attainment of developmental tasks.

Developmental tasks to be achieved during maturity consist of:

1. Accepting life with serenity
2. Adjusting to new limitations of declining physical strength and declining health
3. Adjusting to retirement and changed financial status
4. Adjusting to reorganized family patterns
5. Adjusting to a new pattern of social and civic responsibilities
6. Adjusting to death of spouse and other loved ones
7. Establishing affiliation with one's age group
8. Maintaining satisfactory living arrangements
9. Accepting death with serenity and assisting others to accept death

Emotional development is reflected in Erikson's description of the mature years, *integrity versus disgust or despair.*[10] As the individual looks back and perceives life to have been rich and fulfilling, with purpose and meaning, that individual will experience a sense of satisfaction and contentment in the remaining years. If one does not evaluate his life as such the final years will be faced with despair.

Another kind of emotional and psychologic response is often seen as the elderly individual looks forward to contemplate the subsequent brevity of and end to life. Cumming described this response as *disengagement*, characterized by a "mutual withdrawal or disengagement" when the individual perceives the reality of being mortal and death.[31] This behavioral response may be initiated by the individual or by others in the social system, with the outcome being a movement away from involvement, achievement, and productivity on the part of the mature individual.[31]

Many younger people falsely assume that older people have no interest in sex and lack the ability to perform sexually. Men and women of all ages are capable of sexual arousal and orgasm. Masters and Johnson emphasized the consistency of sexual behavior for the maintenance of sexual activity in old age.[31] Studies conducted at the Duke University Center for the Study of Aging revealed sexual activity in the eighth and ninth decades. Often the aged person becomes sexually inactive due only to a lack of an acceptable partner.

The basic *psychologic needs* of the elderly are no different from those of adults. In one survey,[15] elderly persons were asked what they considered essential for their happiness. They mentioned good health, a place to live, enough money to live comfortably, recognition by others, participation with others, and opportunity for a variety of experiences. However, the elderly typically have greater difficulty obtaining their desires than do younger adults. Both their desires and the difficulties that must be overcome to obtain them should be considered in planning the nursing care of elderly people. The primary objective in caring for the elderly person is to help him make the adjustments necessary to make life worth living. Each patient has different limitations and frustrations, and each will react to them differently. In general the elderly person will react essentially as he has reacted to other stresses throughout his life.

Health needs in late maturity

Most diseases from which the aged suffer are chronic, and most patients have several chronic ailments. Some of these ailments are not particularly troublesome. Most have developed slowly and usually take time to alleviate. Heart disease, cancer, renal disease, vascular disease such as cerebrovascular accident, chronic obstructive pulmonary disease such as emphysema, and accidents are the most common problems that bring older patients to the hospital. Other common chronic ailments such as arthritis, skin disorders, and mild neuromuscular conditions are usually cared for while the client is ambulatory. The most prevalent acute illnesses of later life are acute respiratory conditions such as pneumonia and pulmonary edema.

When the elderly person becomes ill, he is particularly apprehensive and worried, probably because his security is more profoundly affected by illness than that of younger persons. He often fears helplessness and physical dependence on others. The elderly patient may face many adjustments that make it difficult and sometimes impossible for his basic emotional needs to be met. In addition to illness and the depleted physical energy almost always accompanying it, he may have no family and few friends, or his spouse may be ill also. He often has an inadequate income and housing problems. Even before his illness, he may have been depressed because of feeling unwanted and useless.

Illness may break down psychologic defenses that have been built up over a lifetime. The aged individual may be overwhelmed with fear of increased dependency needs or other problems to which he may react with extreme irritability. If his self-esteem is low due to years of suffering from economic or emotional deprivation, he may use his illness aggressively as a means of revolt. A trivial and purely incidental event may precipitate irritability. Other individuals, even those who had been quite active, may develop excessive lethargy with the onset of illness and may seem to give up all hope and desire to live.

Similarities between childhood and old age should not be assumed, because they are not valid. Even in the matter of helplessness there is no similarity. The child is in ascendance; he is developing new power daily and marking up achievements over his environment. The aged person's helplessness is infinitely more frustrating because it is increasing rather than decreasing.

Nursing the elderly patient

The goal of medical and nursing care is to keep the patient functioning at the highest possible level for his age. This includes living with chronic ailments and continuing degenerative changes. The nurse who views aging as a normal, inevitable process, one requiring adjustments in living patterns but not a withdrawal from life, is best prepared to work with the aging patient. The nurse's philosophy of aging can be one of ever-changing life that eventually will end in death, not one of approaching death.

Necessary nursing care depends on the physiologic and anatomic changes that have taken place, the disease from which the patient is suffering, and his own emotional makeup and apparent adjustment to his particular situation. In planning nursing care for elderly patients, consideration is given to each patient's physical, social, economic, and psychologic capacities and limitations. The older patient frequently talks at length about his family and the past to the nurse who is willing to listen. His conversation may give clues to interests that should be encouraged and of problems that are confronting him. These clues are evaluated and plans made to help the patient maintain as much independence as possible despite his limitations.

When giving nursing care to elderly patients, it is necessary to take special care *to build up and protect their sense of worth and their feelings of adequacy.* Remembering the names of patients and calling them by name instead of using such terms as "grandma" or "grandpa" helps. Giving clear and slow explanations to the patient may spare him the embarrassment of mistakes caused by misunderstanding. Since many elderly patients experience some loss of hearing special care must be taken to be sure the patient has heard the explanation. The best method to use to ensure that he hears and understands should be recorded on his nursing care plan. The nurse should always face an elderly patient when speaking and speak distinctly so that he can lipread inconspicuously if necessary. If hearing is better in one ear than the other, the nurse should talk into the good ear. It usually does no good to shout in an attempt to help the elderly person to hear, since with shouting the voice frequency increases and the elderly have the greatest difficulty hearing sounds in the higher frequency range. If the patient uses a hearing aid, care should be taken to assure that it is working properly. Written instructions are helpful for some elderly patients. The nurse should also be thoughtful about repeating instructions because the short-term memory span decreases with age.

Placing equipment conveniently so that assistance need not be requested also makes the elderly patient feel more adequate. Self-help devices may help him maintain some degree of independence. For example, an overbed trapeze or side rails on the bed may allow him to pull himself about in bed. Handrails along hallways and in the bathroom or a walkerette may make it possible for him to walk alone. Sturdy chairs with arms and wooden seats make it easier for many elderly patients to get into and out of chairs themselves. Electric beds also allow them to be more independent. If the patient uses a cane, glasses, hearing aid, or dentures, these devices should be readily available. Showers or bathtubs equipped with handrails and with nonskid strips may make it possible for some patients to bathe independently.

Many adjustments can be made to help the patient who is confined to a wheelchair retain some measure of independence. If the patient is able to transfer himself to the toilet, having a bathroom fixed in such a way that his maneuver is possible may be desirable. Some patients, especially if they have urinary frequency or incontinence, appreciate their wheelchair or chair being fixed as a a commode. Removal of door sills may make it possible for an elderly patient confined to a wheelchair to move about the house. Elderly patients are often unable to propel their chair manually. They may, however, be able to use a motorized wheelchair.

Elderly patients often need help with personal care such as arranging the hair, applying cosmetics, shaving, and dressing. Personal appearance is important to everyone's morale.

Many elderly patients can give most or all necessary *physical care* to themselves. Some may need encouragement to do so; others resent not being allowed to care for themselves. The nurse or the family member caring for them, however, must be patient and give them adequate time. The older patient often is exceptionally slow in the morning and, in fact, geriatricians instruct their patients to take twice the usual time to shave, to dress slowly, and to avoid hurry of any kind, particularly in the morning hours. Since the elderly patient may tire easily, the nurse should be sure that the individual is physically able to give his own care.

If the patient is in a general hospital, a slow pace is often hard to assume. For example, many diagnostic procedures must be carried out in the morning, and breakfast must usually be served with that of other patients. When possible many hospital routines can be adjusted for the elderly patient. For instance, he may prefer to bathe and shave in the afternoon or early evening. The nursing care plan for physical care of each elderly patient should include what self-care is possible, what assistance is needed, the method used, and the schedule the patient follows. Most elderly patients find comfort in familiar things and processes. It is therefore important to maintain routine as much as possible. The elderly are not unable to make changes but require more time to adjust to new routines. The patient should participate in planning the schedule, and whenever possible it should parallel the pattern of care at home.

Since *physical change* occurs in the aging process, elderly people need to use somewhat different hygienic practices than an adult uses to maintain an optimum physical condition. The *skin* of an elderly person is usually thin, delicate, and sensitive to pressure and trauma. The loss of subcutaneous fat and the hardening of the tiny arterioles near the surface cause the skin to be wrinkled, sagging, and sallow. Sweat glands atrophy and the excretory function of the skin is lessened, making the skin dry and flaky and sometimes causing it to itch. Color changes occur in the skin with aging. Seborrheic keratoses, which are lesions resembling darkened, greasy warts, are common. These lesions are nonmalignant but should be inspected frequently for signs of any irritation or change.

Because the skin is likely to be very dry, daily bathing is often contraindicated for the elderly. Usually one or two baths a week are sufficient, although the patient who is incontinent needs local sponging at frequent intervals and perhaps more frequent baths. Because regular soaps can be irritating, mild superfatted soaps are preferred. Bath oils may be used, or lanolin or body lotions can be applied after bathing.

If the patient is confined to bed, an alternating pressure mattress, flotation pad, or flotation mattress may be extremely helpful in maintaining the skin in good condition. Above all, the patient's position should be changed frequently, and bony prominences and weight-bearing areas should be massaged at least every 2 hours. Sheepskin pads placed under bony prominences are also used to relieve pressure and to prevent irritation of the skin. Every effort should be made to get the elderly out of bed as much as possible. This not only helps to redistribute pressure over the body and improve circulation but can also give patients a psychologic boost.

Because of dryness, poor circulation, and low resistance to infection, the skin of elderly persons readily becomes infected. Elderly persons often need assistance in drying their feet after bathing and in cutting and caring for their toenails. Nails are often hard and scaly; soaking the feet in warm water or applying oil to the nails for a day or two prior to cutting softens them and makes cutting easier and safer. A podiatrist should be asked to care for very hard nails and other conditions such as calluses, corns, and bunions.

As the tissues age and circulation becomes sluggish, the *hair* becomes thin, dry, and colorless. Massage of the scalp and daily brushing with a soft-bristled brush help to preserve its beauty. Frequent shampooing should be avoided. Every 2 to 4 weeks is sufficient for most elderly persons, although some people who have washed their hair more frequently throughout their lives may wish to continue to do so.

Changes occur in the *eyes* with aging. There is a decrease in the conjunctival secretions, and sometimes the lower lid droops (ectropion), causing the moistening fluid of the eye to be lost. Therefore irritation of the conjunctivae and tearing are common complaints of the aged. Smoke also may be more irritating to their eyes than to those of younger persons. Eyedrops are frequently ordered as a comfort measure.

An accumulation of secretions at the inner canthus of the eye may be present, particularly on awakening, and may be uncomfortable and unsightly. A sterile cotton sponge moistened with a physiologic solution of sodium chloride can be used to cleanse the eyes. Care must be taken not to press on the eyeballs or to irritate any exposed conjunctiva.

The lens of the eye loses its ability to accommodate effectively as aging progresses. Most people over 60 years of age need glasses, at least for reading. Care of glasses, making certain that they are not lost or broken, is important in the nursing care of the elderly. It is advisable to label glasses with the patient's name. They should also be kept clean. Smudged glasses rather than failing vision may be the cause of difficulty in seeing. The patient should have his glasses available at all times, since confusion and inability to deal with situations in an adequate fashion may result if they become misplaced. The eyes of older people also accommodate more slowly to changes in light. Bright lights or sunlight may be almost unbearable to some elderly people. Many elderly persons see very poorly in the dark. Therefore nightlights should always be used to reduce confusion in patients and to prevent those who get up during the night from having accidents.

Cataracts, failing vision, and actual blindness are common in the aged (see p. 755 for care of the patient with visual impairment).

The elderly person should be urged to give special attention to the care of his *mouth* and *teeth*. Free hydrochloric acid in the stomach may be decreased, predisposing the elderly to poor oral health as well as to impaired digestion. The gums become less elastic and less vascular. They may recede from the remaining teeth, exposing areas of a tooth not covered with enamel. These areas are sensitive to injury from brushes and coarse dentifrices. In addition, diseases of the gum that may have been progressing symptom free for years may cause loss of teeth. Many elderly persons have decayed, broken, or missing teeth. This leads them to avoid foods that are difficult to eat but that may be necessary for the health. The effect of oral health on nutrition is very real; definite improvement in appetite has followed correction of unhealthy conditions in the mouth.

By 70 years of age, the loss of teeth is common, necessitating dentures. Many individuals over 65 years of age have oral lesions of which they are unaware. Some of these lesions are potentially malignant.[2] Consequently, care of dentures and prevention of their loss are part of the general nursing care of most elderly patients. Patients may be encouraged by their dentists to keep dentures in place while they sleep as well as when they are awake, since this helps to preserve the normal contours of the face. Dentures should be cleansed following each meal. Because dental plates may be conductors of heat and since the mouths of aged patients are often not too sensitive to excessive heat, they should be urged not to consume very hot food or fluids. Care should be taken that dentures are not lost, as they are costly. Dentures can also be easily mixed up, especially if the patient removes them frequently and then forgets where he puts them. Dentures should be marked, and there is equipment now available to do this.

The feet and legs usually show the results of limitation in peripheral circulation before any other body part. Therefore it is important for the aging person to *exercise the feet and legs regularly,* to avoid constriction or stasis of the circulation to their lower extremities, and to avoid injury and infections of their feet and legs. Precautions similar to those described for the patient who has peripheral vascular disease (p. 1023) should be taken by all elderly people.

As the muscles become less active in age, slumped posture may result. The abdomen may sag, the spine becomes rounded, and the chest and shoulders droop forward. Lessened elasticity of tissue tends to make these changes fixed. Attention to preventive posture is therefore essential. Although corrective postural exercises and general exercise must be prescribed carefully by a physician, teaching good posture and encouraging deep breathing are part of the daily nursing care of all elderly patients. Any improvement in posture will enable the elderly person to use his diminishing resources to better advantage. Good body alignment adds to the comfort of the patient confined to bed as well as decreasing the need for corrective exercises later. A firm mattress is usually preferable and helps to make the use of pillows more effective. If greater stability is needed, a fracture board can be placed under the mattress. Bedcovers should be light and warm and should be tucked loosely, giving sufficient room for the patient to move about in bed. A block or board placed at the foot of the bed helps to keep covers off the toes and provides something firm against which the patient may press his feet and thereby get some exercise. A pillow placed lengthwise under the head and shoulders helps to bring the chest forward, thereby permitting good chest expansion. Pillows placed under the arms support the muscles of the shoulder girdle and provide comfort for the patient who must have the head of the bed raised for long periods of time.

Unless there is some particular contraindication, exercises for the arms and legs, exercises to keep abdominal and gluteal muscles in good tone, and exercises to strengthen the extensor muscles of the spine should be performed several times each day by every bed patient. The patient is taught to flex, abduct, adduct, and extend each leg separately and both legs simultaneously. The heel of one foot can be placed on the knee of the opposite leg and then the heel passed slowly down the leg to the ankle. This can then be repeated, alternating the legs. Arm, hand, neck, and shoulder movements can be encouraged by having the patient first raise and lower his head, neck, and shoulders from a flat supine position without a pillow and then by having the patient extend his arms in front of his chest, followed by raising them above his head. Each of these exercises should be done, if possible and if not contraindicated, in time to regular, deep respiration to encourage deep breathing while bedfast. These exercises should be taught to the patient by the nurse, and they should be supervised daily by the nurse or the family member caring for the patient. The regular performance of exercises will help to prevent the loss of muscle tone that occurs in all bed patients, regardless of age, unless activity is continued. If the elderly person is unable to do active range-of-motion exercises independently, the nurse should assist with them or do passive range of motion exercises.

The elderly person should wear the *clothing* that is comfortable for him. He often feels cold and may wear woolen clothing even when it seems very warm to others. The hospitalized patient often wishes to wear socks, woolen underwear, a bed jacket, a cap, or other items of clothing to which he is accustomed. Some provision must be made for the care of this clothing. Sometimes members of the family are glad to care for special clothing that the patient needs.

Elderly women often appreciate assistance with altering their clothes. They may be unable to afford new ones, but they are often interested in remaining stylish. Wearing a well-fitted brassiere and corset not only improves the elderly woman's appearance, but the support given to sagging tissues may make her more comfortable.

The elderly person should be encouraged to wear firm well-fitted shoes with good support to prevent damage to the arches of the feet, since the muscles are often weak. Hospitalized patients should have their shoes and should wear them when they are up. If an elderly person wears slippers, they should also fit well and be firm, since the person is less likely to slip or stumble and fall.

Fresh air is especially necessary for the elderly person because with his diminished chest expansion poorly oxygenated air may not provide him with a sufficient blood level of oxygen. The aged, however, may be susceptible to drafts not even noticed by younger persons; consequently, they may dislike open windows.

Protective adipose tissue under the skin disappears with age, and the volume of circulating blood, particularly to the small outer arteries, may be diminished, thus affecting the ability to withstand chilling without discomfort. Decreased activity also lessens circulatory function, resulting in lowering of skin temperature and susceptibility to chilling. Many elderly people suffer from mild arthritis and fibrositis, which produce vague muscle and joint pains, and these conditions are aggravated by chilling. Measures to provide fresh air but to avoid drafts and chilling are essential.

Rest is essential for the aged. However, confusion, decubitus ulcers, lung congestion, and general deterioration may result from prolonged bed rest. Circulation to the brain as well as to the body in general is markedly slowed during long periods of inactivity, and therefore rest should be alternated with activity. It is undesirable for an elderly patient to be confined to bed, and even acutely ill elderly people are often gotten up in a chair for most of the day. They may even be encouraged to walk. When the patient is being cared for by his family, the nurse should try to impress on them the great importance of keeping the patient active, since they may be oversolicitous of the patient or it may seem to require too much effort to get him in and out of bed.

Elderly people usually *sleep* lightly and intermittently with frequent waking. At home the aged person may get out of bed, read, wander about the house, and even prepare something to eat at odd hours. Actually this activity is probably good, since it prevents excessive slowing of circulation. Some wakefulness, therefore, can be expected in the elderly patient who is hospitalized. If the patient is allowed out of bed, it probably is best for him to get up as he would at home. However, a low bed, nightlights, and adequate supervision should be employed to avoid accidents, and the nurse should be sure that the patient is not constantly wakeful. Elderly patients, similar to all others, may be unable to sleep. They are rarely given sedation, however, since many become excited rather than sedated by it.

Many elderly people are undernourished, and for this reason a great deal of emphasis is placed on *nutrition* for the aged. Other than acute and chronic illness, possible causes of malnutrition in the elderly are limited financial resources, psychologic factors such as boredom and lack of companionship when eating, edentia, lifelong faulty eating patterns, fads and notions regarding certain foods, lack of energy to prepare foods, and lack of sufficient knowledge of the essentials of a well-balanced diet. Many elderly persons, particularly those living alone, subsist on a diet high in carbohydrates and low in vitamins, minerals, and protein. Often they think that because they are elderly they do not need much food. A diet composed largely of tea and toast may seem sufficient to them.

The nurse should instruct the patient and those responsible for his care in the essentials of a well-balanced diet (Chapter 51). Dietary patterns should not be changed too quickly, and it is useless to attempt to change many established food patterns. Simply prepared and easily digested foods are best, and meals should be distributed throughout the day. Usually elderly persons do not tolerate fried food. Large amounts of roughage should be avoided, but bulk is necessary. Fluid intake is important, yet many do not drink much water. Tea, coffee, and other beverages are usually preferred. Drinks prepared with dry skim milk supply essential protein and are useful in helping to meet the protein and calcium needs of older patients without supplying too many calories.

Some elderly persons are obese even though they may be undernourished. Excess weight burdens the heart, liver, kidneys, and musculoskeletal system and should be avoided. Weight reduction for the aged person, however, should be gradual and must be supervised by a physician. Sudden loss of weight is poorly tolerated by many elderly persons whose vascular system has become adjusted to the excess weight. Sudden weight reduction may lead to serious consequences, including confusion associated with lowered blood pressure, exhaustion, and vasomotor collapse.

Elderly patients may worry about their *bowel function*. They tend to forget that less food and less activity will result in reduced bowel function. Any marked change in bowel habits, however, and any unusual reactions to normal doses of laxatives should be reported, since malignancies of the large bowel and diverticulitis are fairly common among this age group.

Regularity in going to the toilet is important, since it provides stimulus to evacuate the bowel. Motor activity of the intestinal musculature may be decreased with age, and supportive structures in the intestinal walls become weakened. Sense perception is less acute, so that the signal for bowel elimination may be missed. Constipation may occur and in turn lead to impactions. The very elderly and somewhat confused patient should be reminded to go to the bathroom following meals. If the patient is constipated, it may be necessary occasionally to carefully insert a gloved finger into the rectum to be certain impaction has not occurred.

Frequency of voiding is common with aging and becomes a problem during illness. The ability of the kidneys to concentrate urine during sleeping hours usually decreases slowly with age. In addition decreased muscle tone in the bladder with resultant impairment of emptying capacity may result in residual urine in the bladder and subsequent infection. It may be necessary to catheterize the patient to check for residual urine. One of the first signs of diminishing or failing kidney function is frequency of micturition during the night. Frequency and slight burning on urination are symptions of bladder infection.

Elderly women have relaxation of perineal structures, which may also interfere with complete emptying of the bladder and predispose to bladder infection. Some elderly patients have decreased sensation and do not realize when the bladder must be emptied. Periodic dribbling of urine suggests that the bladder is not being emptied completely. The nurse should observe the very elderly patient for distention of the bladder and consult the physician about it.

Unless there is a definite contraindication to high fluid intake, the elderly patient should be urged to take sufficient fluids to dilute urine and decrease its irritating properties. Fluids may be limited in the evening if nocturia is troublesome and is interfering with sleep. If the patient is quite feeble, it is well to offer a urinal or bedpan during the night.

Involutional changes in the lining of the vagina lead to lessened resistance to invasion of organisms. Mild infections with troublesome discharge are not unusual in elderly women. This condition should be reported to the physician, who may order specific therapy for it. Frequent local bathing may be helpful in allaying itching. Application of cornstarch also relieves itching. Embarrassment may prevent the elderly patient from reporting symptoms. The nurse should be aware of the symptoms of this condition and watch for them.

Almost all elderly men have hypertrophy of the prostate gland, which makes urination difficult. The nurse must report or must urge the patient to report such complaints to his physician because specific treatment is often necessary and can be safely administered even when the patient is far advanced in years.

Incontinence of urine or feces is twice as common among women as men.[27] It is a particularly upsetting problem not only to the patient and his family but also to the nursing staff. Every effort should be made to institute and maintain the patient on a bowel and bladder training regimen. Specific details about bladder and bowel training can be found in Chapter 57.

An important part of nursing care for the elderly is helping to meet their *emotional needs*. Elderly patients are often lonely, and individual attention should be given to them. They often appreciate just talking with others. If possible the nurse should plan time to visit with them daily. Volunteers may also be used to visit the elderly. Some patients appreciate visits with a clergyman.

When visiting with elderly patients, one should remember that, although they commonly talk about events and activities in their own past, they usually are interested in the activities of young people and of the world about them. These interests often must be satisfied for them through the eyes and ears of others. If the patient is unable to see well enough to read, he may enjoy being read to by others.

Provision should be made for the patient who requires long hospitalization to maintain his family contacts. A grandfather or grandmother often wishes to see a grandchild, and a visit should be arranged, if possible. Sometimes plans can be made for the patient to make a short visit outside the hospital. This is especially important if a wife or husband is physically unable to visit the patient. Arranging for telephone conversations with family members also is desirable.

If the elderly patient likes to read, reading materials should be provided. If he is unable to see to read, talking books available through public libraries may be appreciated. It is also possible to get books and magazines with large print for persons with reduced vision. Television and radio also provide desirable diversion and stimulation.

Elderly people often are interested in doing useful tasks. There are many tasks in which even the elderly person who is ill may be able to participate. Women may enjoy mending or knitting. If they are at home they may be able to help with dishes or meal preparation. Men may be interested in repairing toys or making useful gadgets for the house. Many elderly persons enjoy painting. The older person may be quite slow in all his activities, and great care must be taken not to show impatience, which may discourage further participation.

Elderly patients are usually aware of death as an imminent possibility and sometimes see it as a welcome event. The nurse should not avoid this issue. If the nurse senses that the patient is genuinely concerned about death, he can be urged to discuss his feelings about it. He may also wish to see a clergyman, a family member, or the physician or perhaps to arrange to transact some unfinished business. The nurse must always be responsive to such requests, since they frequently are more important for the patient's peace of mind than his medical treatment. The feelings of the family of the elderly person must also be considered in dealing with the question of death. They may find it a very uncomfortable subject.

Special precautions related to diagnosis and treatment

Elderly persons usually tolerate *medications* poorly and may have bizarre reactions to them. This occurs for several reasons. Older persons experience a reduction in metabolic turnover so that a lower dosage of a drug produces the desired effect. A second factor to be considered with drug therapy in the elderly is the altered response of medication on the central nervous system. The decreased blood flow to the brain is a contributing factor to this response. Medication that produces sedation in younger adults may cause extreme confusion in the elderly. This is especially true of the barbituarates.

Many elderly persons maintain a delicate balance between normal and abnormal because of impairments of homeostatic mechanisms, especially if disability or impairment is already present. Drugs given may produce toxic effects that occur quickly and may have far-reaching manifestations. One of the most common of these manifestations is drug-induced hypotension, which can lead to ataxia, falls, and possible injuries. Another factor that affects medication therapy in the elderly is the decreased blood flow to the kidneys and liver. This leads to decreased function of both organs, and drugs are not detoxified and eliminated as quickly as in the healthy adult. Toxic concentrations of drugs may occur because of the cumulative effects. One drug that does this easily is digitalis. With an elderly person who is maintained on a medication for a prolonged length of time, frequent checks of blood levels should be made. Another factor is that the delayed effects of drugs may be observed in the elderly weeks or even months after the drug has been discontinued.

Drug treatment in the elderly has its definite place in the therapeutic regimen, but it must be handled carefully. One general principle in treatment of the elderly with medication is that the drug level should be built up gradually.

The nurse should carefully check for untoward reactions from medications and report them to the physician. If the patient is emaciated or of very advanced years, the use of full adult doses of drugs should be questioned.

Many elderly patients must administer medicines to themselves. The nurse should carefully determine their ability to do so and should report to the physician if the practice does not seem to be safe so that other plans can be made. In planning self-administration of drugs with the elderly patient, it is frequently helpful to determine the easiest time for him to remember to take medication. This time is usually tied in with some incident of daily living such as arising or taking meals. The use of a medication check sheet is helpful in reminding some patients. Plans may also include placement of the medication so that seeing it will be a reminder. Special care needs to be taken, however, to put it where it will not accidentally be taken in place of another drug or where other family members such as small children may take it. Some elderly persons have found it helpful to use something such as an egg carton with the days marked. One dose is put into each hole, and it is easy to know if the medication has been taken.

Elderly persons should understand the medications they are taking. They should be cautioned against taking extra doses of the medication because some believe that if one tablet or pill helps, two will be better.

Elderly patients who are undergoing *diagnostic tests* requiring withholding of meals or the use of enemas or cathartics should be attended unless they are in their beds because they often become quite weak and dizzy. No elderly patient should ever be left unattended on a treatment table, and he should be helped on and off the table. Since he often is quite dizzy, it is advisable for him to arise slowly and sit on the edge of the table for a few moments before standing. The dizziness is caused by the slow compensation of inelastic blood vessels. Older patients with cardiovascular disease may also be orthopneic and cannot tolerate lying flat for examinations.

Because of the rapidity with which they develop pressure ulcers, elderly patients who must lie on x-ray, treatment, or operating room tables for lengthy periods of time need pads placed under the normal curves of their backs and a pad of material such as sponge rubber placed under bony prominences. Skin over bony prominences should be rubbed occasionally to improve the circulation to the area. On return to the unit the patient's skin should always be checked for pressure areas, and if any signs of pressure are evident, these areas should be massaged frequently until the tissue appears normal in color. If possible the patient should be kept off these areas until signs of pressure disappear. If the patient is placed in lithotomy position, care must be taken to place both legs in the stirrups at the same time to prevent undue pull on unresilient muscles. The same principle applies when removing the legs from the stirrups. Care must also be taken to prevent hyperextension and hyperflexion of the joints, since many elderly patients have arthritis.

The kind of nursing care given to the elderly may be influenced by the attitudes one has toward the elderly and aging. Societal attitudes have yielded a stereotype of the elderly that says that they are slow, cannot think as well as in earlier years, are consumed by mental confusion, do not want to learn anything new, are plagued by disease, are most dependent, behave in a childlike manner, and are burdens to family and society. If these attitudes are also held by the nurse, the elderly individual may be approached with condescending tolerance, thereby reinforcing his often felt feelings of inferiority.

It is most helpful when the nurse can deal with the individual in an empathetic manner, demonstrating a willingness to listen, explain, comfort, and support independent functioning. Accepting elderly individuals as they are and where they are in terms of their developmental status as well as suspending youth-oriented attitudes and standards that may be inappropriate are essential elements in adequately meeting the elderly person's needs and fostering a better quality of life.

While many of the changes discussed above do necessitate special nursing approaches for the elderly, it should be emphasized that all of these changes do not occur with all aging persons. Indeed many older persons are very healthy and actively engaged in the world around them.

REFERENCES AND SELECTED READINGS

1. Berengerg, S. R., editor: Puberty: biologic and psychosocial components, Netherlands, 1974.
2. Bhaskar, S.: Oral lesions of the aged population, Geriatrics **23**:137-149, 1968.
3. Burnside, I.: Nursing and the aged, New York, 1976, McGraw-Hill Book Co.
4. Cameron, J. M: The battered baby, Nurs. Mirror **9**:32-37, 1972.
5. Chinn, P.: Child health maintenance: concepts in family centered care, The C. V. Mosby Co.
6. Diekelman, N. L.: The young adult: the choice is health or illness, Am. J. Nurs. **76**:1272-1277, 1976.
7. Diekelman, N. L.: The middle-years: emotional tasks of the middle adult, Am. J. Nurs. **75**:997-1001, 1975.
8. Diekelman, N. L., and Galloway, K.: The middle years: a time of change, Am. J. Nurs. **75**:994-996, 1975.
9. Dresen, S. E.: The middle years: the sexually active middle adult, Am. J. Nurs **75**:1001-1005, 1975.
10. Erikson, E. H.: Childhood and society, ed. 2., New York, 1963, W. W. Norton & Co., Inc.
11. Galloway, K.: The middle years: the change of life, Am. J. Nurs. **75**:1006-1011, 1975.
12. Giffra, M.: Demystifying adolescent behavior, Am. J. Nurs. **75**:1724-1727, 1975.
13. Goldfarb, W.: Effects of psychological deprivation in infancy and subsequent stimulation, Am. J. Psychiatr. **102**:18, 1945.
14. Gould, R.: Adult life stages: growth toward self tolerance, Psychology Today, 74-78, Feb. 1975.
15. Hargreaves, A. G.: Life in the middle years: making the most of the middle years, Am. J. Nurs. **75**:1772-1776, 1975.
16. Havinghurst, R. H., et al.: Psychology of aging, Bethesda Conference, Public Health Rep. **70**:837-856, 1955.
17. Johnson, L.: The middle years: living sensibly, Am. J. Nurs. **75**:1012-1016, 1975.
18. Kalafitch, A.: Approaches to care of adolescents, Englewood Cliffs, N.J., 1975, Appleton-Century-Crofts.
19. Kaluger, G., and Kaluger, M. F.: Human development: the span of life, St. Louis, 1974, The C. V. Mosby Co.
20. Knox, A. B.: Adult development and learning, San Francisco, 1977, Jossey-Bass, Inc., Publishers.
21. Lawton, M. P., et al.: Community planning for an aging society, Stroudsburg, Pa., 1976, Dowden, Hutchinson & Ross, Inc.
22. Lidz, T.: The person, New York, 1968, Basic Books, Inc., Publishers.
23. Marx, J.: Crib death: some promising leads but no solution yet, Nurs. Digest **4**:12-15, 1976.
24. Murray, R., and Zentner, J.: Nursing assessment and health promotion through the life span, Englewood Cliffs, N. J., 1975, Prentice-Hall, Inc.
25. Paplau, H. E.: Life in the middle years: mid-life crises, Am. J. Nurs. **75**:1761-1765, 1975.
26. Petrillo, M., and Sanger, S.: Emotional care of hospitalized children, Philadelphia, 1972, J. B. Lippincott Co.
27. Roznoy, M. S.: The young adult: taking a sexual history, Am. J. Nurs. **76**:1279-1282, 1976.
28. Scipien, G., et al.: Comprehensive pediatric nursing, New York, 1975, McGraw-Hill Book Co.
29. Sheehy, G.: Passages, New York, 1974, E. P. Dutton & Co., Inc.
30. Shydro, J.: Child abuse, Nursing '72 **2**:37-41, 1972.
31. Starr, B. D., and Goldstein, H. S.: Human behavior and development, New York, 1975, Springer Publishing Co.
32. Stosky, B. A.: The elderly patient, New York, 1968, Grune & Stratton, Inc.
33. Sze, W. C.: Human life cycle, New York, 1975, Jason Aronson, Inc.
34. Troll, L. E.: Early and middle adulthood, Monterey, Calif., 1975, Brooks/Cole Publishing Co.
35. Woods, N. F.: Human sexuality in health and illness, St. Louis, 1975, The C. V. Mosby Co.
36. U.S. Department of Health, Education and Welfare: Approaches to adolescent health care in the 1970's, No. (HSA) 75-5014, 1975.
37. U.S. Department of Health, Education and Welfare: Working with older people, Public Health Service, No. 1459, Vol. 2, Washington, D.C.; 1970, U.S. Government Printing Office.

AUDIOVISUAL RESOURCES

1. A visit with Clipper: Media Center, Children's Hospital National Medical Center, Washington, D.C. 20009.
2. Aging: 16-mm color film, CRM educational films, 1104 Camino Del Mar, Del Mar, California 92014
3. Denver developmental screening test: Series of films, Ladoca films, Denver.
4. Patient mental health, psychological growth and adjustment: Color filmstrip and audiotape, Westinghouse Learning Corp., Oaklawn, Ill. 60453
5. Perspectives on aging: Concept media.
6. Play in hospital: 16-mm color film, Campus Film Distributors Corp., 2 Overhill Road, Scarsdale, New York 10583.
7. To prepare a child: 16-mm color films, Media Center, Children's Hospital National Medical Center, Washington, D.C. 20009.

19

Death and dying

JANET LARSON GELEIN

This chapter is about death and the process of dying in America. Birth and death are two processes that are inevitable to all people. Birth is generally perceived as a joyous, exciting event in our society; death is often something dreaded, feared, and denied. For nurses who have the responsibility of assisting individuals with the event of death, an assessment of their own feelings and reactions is as important as the assessment of the individual who is facing death. Only after nurses acquire an awareness of and appreciation for their own values and beliefs can they reach out to help others. An examination of the factors in American society that affect attitudes toward dying can help nurses gain an awareness of not only their own, but also their clients' beliefs about death and dying.

■ FACTORS AFFECTING ATTITUDES ABOUT DEATH AND DYING

Recently a newspaper revealed the following account:

> Mr. S.'s son died November 8 of injuries suffered in an auto accident. He won't be buried. Instead, Mr. S. said, the body will remain in a casket with a clear plastic top in a room off the family's kitchen. Mr. S. went on to say: "There are three especially painful moments at the death of a loved one. The first is at the news of the death, the second when you see the body in the casket at the funeral home, and the third and most difficult is when you have to turn away from the grave site and know you'll never see that person again. We simply decided not to go through that last step."*

In the following pages, four characteristics of life in America that may have influenced the attitudes and behaviors of Mr. S. and his family will be explored. The four factors implied by the acronym LIFE are *L*ongevity, *I*solation, *F*amily life, and *E*nvironment for the dying. This discussion will consider how these social phenomena influence those persons and their families who are confronting death, as well as those who care for the dying.

□ Longevity

America may be described as a nation of aging citizens. Today the average life expectancy is 72 years, as compared to 1900 when it was 47 years. Low infant mortality, control of infectious diseases, and improved socioeconomic conditions have prolonged life. A decreasing birthrate has produced an increased proportion of older persons in our society.

Mortality control has facilitated technology and has modernized American society. Medical sciences have developed the technology for extending life. Intensive care units, kidney dialysis, heart-lung machines, respirators, artificial pacemakers, and transplanted organs have all prolonged lives. These technologies have created a dilemma for nursing and medicine: no longer can clinical death be clearly defined. Although technologies directed toward prolongation of life have received much emphasis in medical research, there have been few investigations of the quality of the lives our technologies have extended.

The "modernization" of our society implies career specialization and social mobility.[22] Long-term planning is demanded of modern economies; as a consequence, society values youth and invests energy and resources in the education of children to prepare for the specialized careers and leadership positions of tomorrow. The modernization of an aging American society, with an emphasis on youth, has evolved—but not without consequences.

The aged, who in many ways provide us with physical proof of our own mortality, are increasingly relegated to institutions or retirement villages that shield us from the realities of aging and approaching death. In 1939 there were 1,200 homes for the aged, with 25,000 beds; this number grew to 21,329 by 1973, with 1,277,000 beds in such institutions.[44,56]

---

*From *Durham Morning Herald,* July 25, 1975, Louisville, Ky. Printed with permission of The Associated Press.

Decreased mortality and increased segregation of the elderly reduce regular confrontations with death. "When death is confined largely to the elderly—those retired from work, finished with direct parental responsibilities—and handled within specialized bureaucracies, mortality becomes removed from the daily business of social life. . . . The 'nonpresence' of death in modern societies physically and socially removes the death of man from the life of society."[22] According to one author, the modern emphasis on youth, health, sports cars, long vacations, and longevity has led people to see death as an infringement upon their basic rights to both life and the pursuit of happiness.[18]

□ Isolation

Americans live in a culture that in many ways isolates them from direct confrontation with death. The most recent national data indicate that over half of all deaths in this country occur in institutions: either hospitals, convalescent homes, nursing homes, or other domiciliary institutions.[36]

Contemporary burial customs also isolate individuals from the dead. Mittford[42] provides insight into the burial customs and practices in America. What one may assume to be accepted custom, elaborate funeral arrangements, commercially prepared flowers, and so on, may be designed for profit of the funeral director, rather than for support of the next-of-kin. There is little resemblance between the funeral practices of today and those of even 50 to 100 years ago.

From colonial times to the nineteenth century, funeral practices were almost exclusively a family affair. Friends of the family and family members were responsible for the body after death. After washing, wrapping, and placing the body in a wooden casket, it was placed in the family parlor for all mourners to grieve over. What today is viewed as the funeral director's responsibility was yesterday largely the task of the family and close friends.

This observed change in family responsibility for care after death is only one outcome of the changes in the structure of family life over the past century. Several other features of the family in modern society have changed our relationship to the dying and beliefs and attitudes about death.

□ Family life

Families, as a unit of American society, provide an environment for their young members to learn social roles and acquire values. Some changes in family life in our society that have influenced value systems and role relationships within the family are the size of the family unit, mobility, and the decline in the influence of religion.

In societies with high mortality rates, social organization and identification is around kinship units. Extended families are necessary for survival; they function to allocate status, distribute goods, and exercise power. With the immediate threat of death always present, isolated individuals without support are prone to a precarious existence. In American society, families are often isolated from extended kin and lack their close support when confronting death.

In traditional, early American society an extended family provided multiple resources for a single family member facing death. The dying individual and his family were often supported by grandparents, aunts, uncles, and other relatives. This extended family provided a system of relationships that drew together resources in times of need. Today family members must depend on each other for assistance, manage by themselves, or cope with a crisis through the utilization of resources provided within the community. For some single persons, friends become the significant others and serve in lieu of the family.

A family's ability to utilize community resources is somewhat dependent upon its familiarity with available resources and its knowledge and skill in using them. Rapid social mobility of families has influenced these skills. With a change in residence comes the need for developing new social relationships and the ability to orient oneself quickly to the resources within a community. If the family lacks these relationships or abilities to allocate and procure supports, they may cope with death or dying in relative isolation. To some families, their religion and church may be support in such times of need.

Studies of American culture tend to reflect an emerging secular attitude toward death. Today death has become a subject for scientific investigation and rationalization. The decline of religious influence has been cited as one of the factors contributing to the fragmentation of caring for the dying and their significant others.[30] One writer suggests that the decline of religions and the emergence of secularism is related to the needs that religion satisfies in American society. If a society is confronted with frequent deaths and life is precarious, social institutions are needed to explain death. When mortality is decreased and concentrated among the elderly, as is in this society, the need to explain why we should die is decreased.[5]

Recent literature suggests a return to more spiritual and, in some instances, mystical concerns. Moody[43] has documented the religious experiences of those who have survived life-threatening events. Descriptions of those persons have included "life-after-life" or "out-of-body" experiences. These persons reported observing events surrounding their "deaths" and related feelings of moving toward a deity or toward a peaceful "out-of-body" existence. The lay literature also contains references to faith healing and therapies that transcend clinical sciences. Perhaps literature such as this indicates a trend away from the secularization of death and a movement toward a more spiritual orientation toward death.

□ Environment for dying

Increasingly people are dying in health care institutions. More than half of the deaths in America occur within an institutional setting. Removed from a familiar home dwelling, individuals facing death are often subjected to a mechanical, dehumanized environment in an institutional setting. Kübler-Ross speaks about the person dying in an institutional environment and the reactions of health care providers:

> He may cry for rest, peace, and dignity, but he will get transfusions, a heart machine, or tracheostomy if necessary. He may want one single person to stop for one single minute so that he can ask one single question—but he will get a dozen people around the clock, all busily preoccupied with his heart rate, pulse, electrocardiogram or pulmonary functions, his secretions or excretions but not with him as a human being. He may wish to fight since all this is done in the fight for his life, and if they can save his life they can consider the person afterwards. Those who consider the person first may lose precious time to save his life! At least this seems to be the rationale or justification behind all this—or is it? Is the reason for this increasingly mechanical, depersonalized approach our own defensiveness? Is this approach our own way to cope with and repress the anxieties that a terminally or critically ill patient evokes in us? Is our concentration on equipment, on blood pressure our desperate attempt to deny the impending death which is so frightening and discomforting to us that we displace all our knowledge onto machines, since they are less close to us than the suffering face of another human being which would remind us once more of our lack of omnipotence, our own limits and failure, and last but not least perhaps our own mortality?*

■ CONFRONTATION WITH DEATH: A HOLISTIC APPPROACH

The primary goal of the nurse assisting an individual who is confronting death is to *maximize the coping processes of the dying person in order to promote an appropriate death.* An appropriate death implies that the individual completes the act of dying in a manner that is meaningful to his existence. This goal protects an individual's autonomy and personal dignity and provides a climate for the person to express his needs and control his own destiny. The following discussion may assist the nurse with an assessment of factors influencing the coping processes in individuals confronting death.

□ Coping processes

Death may occur at various ages, at different rates, and with a different degree of participation from the individual involved. Coping processes are the strategies used by an individual when confronting a crises such as death. The strategy used will depend upon the individual's perception of death and the anticipated threat or harm associated with death. Unless death is perceived as an agent of harm, direct forms of coping such as avoidance or attack are not possible—one must be able to identify the threat if one is to avoid or attack it.[35]

In some circumstances death is not a threat but a release or welcome relief from a painful existence. To the person contemplating suicide, life may be more painful than the prospect of death itself. However, for the individual who appraises death and defines it as threatening, the process of coping is initiated to reduce, eliminate, or master the anticipated harm. Coping is mobilized by the realization that life, health, cherished relationships, or wealth are in danger.[35] The individual's response to death may be influenced by perception, beliefs and value systems, developmental level, sex and social role, education and intellectual resources, ego strength and coping style, and time and mode of dying along with situational supports and the social structural setting in which the individual dies. An assessment of each of these variables and their influence on the person facing death can provide the nurse with insight into the coping processes available to a person who is dying.

In caring for the individual who is confronting death, it is useful to consider three sets of variables: (1) factors related to the *configuration of death,* (2) elements within the *psychologic structure of the individual,* and (3) characteristics of the *situational and social structural setting* in which the individual is facing death. These variables may influence the coping process in the individual confronting death (Fig. 19-1).

Configuration of death

The configuration of death or the stimulus that promotes confrontation with death may be *external* or *internal* in nature. For example, an individual may confront death through an accident, homicide, or suicide (situational—external in nature) or through genetic factors or illness (biologic—organic or internal in nature). These two classifications are not mutually exclusive, and often situational and organic processes interact simultaneously to promote death. For example, an individual with a terminal illness may be experiencing such intense pain and turmoil that he commits suicide to hasten dying.

*From Kübler-Ross, E.: On death and dying, New York, 1969, Macmillan Publishing Co., Inc., p. 8. Copyright © 1969 by Elisabeth Kübler-Ross.

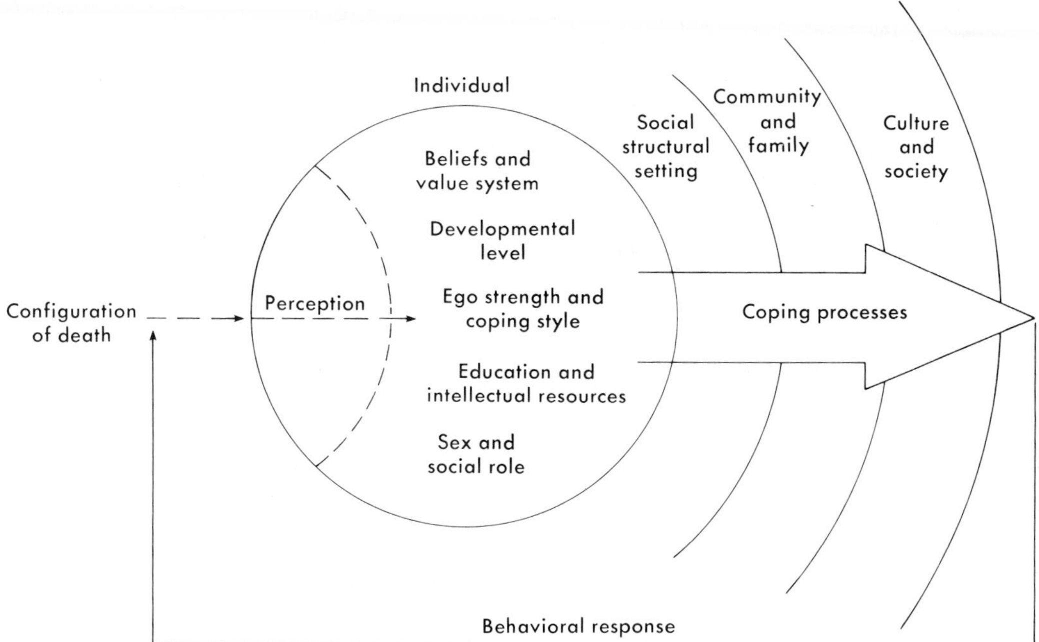

Fig. 19-1. Confrontation with death: a holistic approach.

Another factor related to the configuration of death is the *temporal aspect of dying*, which refers to the time when certain death will occur, or when uncertain death will be resolved. Glaser and Strauss, who have studied the temporal features of dying in hospitals, have identified four types of death expectations associated with dying. These death expectations refer to the "degree of certainty" or the degree to which the defining person is convinced the patient will die and the time expectations related to this certainty, which may vary from minutes to months. Four types of death expectations based on certainty and time are (1) certain death at a known time, (2) certain death at an unknown time, (3) uncertain death but a known time when certainty will be established, and (4) uncertain death and an unknown time when the question will be resolved.[19] These time variables, along with expectations of persons confronting death, may affect the interactions and coping mechanisms of the dying individual.

Psychologic structure of the individual

Aspects of the psychologic structure of an individual that may influence coping and behavior when confronting death are perception, beliefs and value systems, developmental level, ego strength and coping style, education and intellectual resources, and sex and social role. Selected aspects of these will be discussed next.

Perceptions. Perceptions vary when one examines confrontations with death. Cognitive appraisal of the configuration of death involves an interaction between the individual, his judgment about the meaning and future significance of death or dying, and the properties of the situation in which he confronts death. Coping processes are initiated first through perception, and then mediated through situational-environmental elements that result in an observable behavioral response. The nurse interacting with an individual coping with death, and concerned with maximizing this individual's resources in this confrontation, will be cognizant of those factors believed to influence perception of death.

Perception involves the process of appraisal, which requires the cognitive activities of choice, discrimination, and judgment. The statement "I will die" implies the ability to formulate concepts such as the following:

1. I am an individual with a life of my own, a personal existence.
2. I belong to a class of beings, one of whose attributes is mortality.
3. Using the intellectual process of logical deduction, I arrive at the conclusion that my personal death is a certainty.
4. There are many possible causes of my death, and these causes might operate in many different combinations. Although I might evade or escape one particular cause, I cannot evade all causes.

5. My death will occur in the future. By the future, I mean a time-to-live that has not yet elapsed.
6. But I do not know when in the future my death will occur. The event is certain; the timing is uncertain.
7. Death is a final event. My life ceases. This means that I will never again experience, think, or act, at least as a human being on this earth.
8. Accordingly death is the ultimate separation of myself from the world.*

How an individual perceives a confrontation with death will partially depend on his appraisal of this constellation of abstract concepts. One factor influencing this appraisal is the developmental level of the individual.

Developmental level. Appraisals of death seem to vary throughout the life span. The examination of perceptions and the development of death conceptions will be reveiwed considering three broad areas of growth and development: childhood, adulthood, and late maturity. Perceptions of death or deathlike attributes are considered to be the forerunners of death conceptions.

Infancy and early childhood. Conceptions of death in childhood may be roughly divided into three broad age categories: infancy and early childhood (birth to 5 years), middle and late childhood (5 to 10 years), and adolescence (10 to 20 years). Mauer has proposed that selected processes associated with being and nonbeing are evident even in the *newborn infant.* Periodic sleeping and waking cycles are considered to be the first introduction to an appreciation of being and nonbeing. This phenomenon is followed by infant experimentation involving a variety of disappearance-and-return games such as "peekaboo" and "all-gone." (Peekaboo is believed to have originated from an Old English phrase meaning "alive or dead.") Through such activities the infant begins to develop a conception of self and organismically becomes involved in states of being and nonbeing.[38]

The *infant* and *young child* are exposed to a variety of feelings toward death; however, it is generally accepted that a child of this age does not have a conception of personal mortality.[1,11,19] Nagy, in her studies on Hungarian children, made one of the most important contributions to the psychology of children and their conceptions of death. Her work considered children from 3 to 10 years of age. The first stage she described, from 3 to 5 years, is a time when the child views death as continuous with life. Death is not recognized as final; rather, the child in this stage explains death as a reversible or temporary departure. Even though the child may recognize death as a physical event, he cannot separate it from life; he considers death as gradual or temporary.[46]

*From Kastenbaum, R., and Aisenburg, R.: The psychology of death, New York, 1972, Springer Publishing Co., Inc.

DEVELOPMENTAL STAGES AND SELECTED RESPONSES OF CHILD TO DEATH[23]

Developmental stage	Selected response to death
Birth	Physiologic reaction to "death agony"
5 to 6 months	Reacts to disease symptoms and treatment procedures
2 to 4 years	Aware of changes in personal self: separateness, "me," "I," "not me"
5 to 7 years	Appreciates death as a final separation from life; reacts to prognosis; changes in social role and relationships.

Middle and late childhood. Sometime between the ages of 5 and 10 the child begins to comprehend that death is final. Death to a child at the beginning of this stage of development is often metaphorically personified as a "death man" or person. Children may describe death as the boogeyman, a skeleton, angel, or witch. Generally, death is conceived as reversible and something that can be avoided. To the child in middle childhood, death is still something separate from his own being. "Run faster than the death-man, lock the door, trick him, somehow, elude Mr. Death and you will not die."[30]

In later childhood, around age 9 or 10, children come to develop the conception of death as final, universal, and inevitable.[46] Anthony found two dominant themes in a child's conceptions of death at this age: sorrowful separation and the ultimate result of aggression.[2] Children in late childhood may be concerned about their own deaths and the death of parents or pets. Zeligs believes that children around this age fear death and keep it at a distance.[67]

A child's perception of death is influenced by his developmental capacity to conceive the meaning of death; however, he responds to selected aspects of death long before he conceptualizes "I will die" (see boxed material). Since the young child does not conceptualize death, his perceptions upon confronting death are often associated with the reactions of others, bodily instincts, and sensations. As one advances up the scale of growth and development, behavior becomes increasingly dependent upon learning rather than instinct.

Adolescence. One particularly relevant conception about death acquired during this age span is the conception of time. An adult conception of time is achieved around age 13 to 15; however, *adolescents* seem to prefer to limit their conceptions of time to the immediate future.[29,59] To the adolescent the prospect of death is a threat to future identity; in an attempt to deny this possibility, he prefers to live in the present or near future. The rationale for this orientation may be that death threatens the adolescent's possibility of becoming the self he values and seeks to become. The adolescent cannot bolster his sense of identity by looking back on a lifetime, nor is he at a stable point in his current existence. Instead, he is emerging.[30]

To the adolescent, death is something that exists in the future. Through extending the time between life today and death sometime in the distant future, the adolescent successfully creates a psychologic distance between himself and death. One study indicated that adolescents who displayed high manifest concern over death were limited in their abilities to project into the future.[10] Time appears to serve as an insulation between the adolescent's present self and eventual death. A direct confrontation with death in adolescence may promote one of several responses. The early adolescent (ages 10 to 14) with a growing need for independence is vulnerable to rejection and loneliness when confronting death. Growing away from parental and family ties and moving toward peer groups, gangs, and crowds for support, the dying adolescent may feel rejected by parents and isolated from peers. Midadolescence (ages 14 to 16) brings increased self-confidence and an achievement of self-identity: the adolescent now follows his own standards. To the competent adolescent who has just begun to feel mastery, death represents defeat.[11] Finally, approaching adulthood, the late adolescent (ages 17 to 20), alive and in love with the world, is likely to perceive death as the loss of rich and meaningful relationship that he has just attained.[11]

Adulthood. Erikson suggests that young adulthood is a time of intimacy in which the individual emerges from the search for and insistence on identity and is ready to fuse his identity with that of another.[13] It is also a period when physical and mental vigor are at the peak of development. To the adult who has expanded his ego and become less egocentric, and who may have a spouse and family, confrontation with death may intensify feelings about loss of physical and mental control, body image disturbances, and role expectations.

Another author describes a crisis of midadulthood that accompanies the realization that one is growing old and approaching the latter half of life. Paradoxically, the adult is at a midpoint in life: he simultaneously enters the prime of life and a stage of fulfillment and recognizes that death lies beyond.[26]

There is relatively little literature about the adult confronting death in comparison to the literature on children and the elderly. Perhaps the dying adult is too close to the lives of those who are involved in the research on death. Choron suggests that humans tend to suppress the part of reality emphasizing finitude rather than adjusting to death.[6] One of the early studies on adult attitudes toward death demonstrated that the adult considers death in much the same way as a child. This study revealed that the adult conceived of death as an unnatural end of life: the result of a violent act, either an accident or catastrophe.[5]

Kastenbaum and Aisenburg describe a contemporary personification of death in adults. The automaton is an image of death, an unfeeling instrument in the guise of a human. The automaton advances an automatic or soulless apparatus devoid of emotion.[30] If personifications tell us something about an individual's conception of his place in the universe and the meaning of life, there is something rather absurd about the personification of death as a nonperson. The automaton may be part of a broader image of the universe—a vast chamber whose design is indifferent to the feelings and purposes of humans.[30] Perhaps this orientation to humans accounts for some of the dehumanized, mechanical care the dying often receive from adult health care professionals in an institutional setting.

Late maturity. From a developmental perspective, the unique feature of old age is the inevitability of death, bringing with it the task of integrating one's past life and the acceptance of one's own death. To the elderly person who has formed basic values, achieved life goals, and developed a conception of self, one of the final tasks of life is the achievement of integrity. Elderly individuals with a sense of integrity are ready to defend the dignity of their own life styles against physical and economic threats. In such final consolidation, Erikson notes that death loses its sting.[13] Several studies on the attitudes of elderly people toward death indicate that only a small number of old people fear death.[17,27,45]

The meaning given to aging and approaching death is dependent to a great extent on one's interpretation of the immediate and total life situation. Elderly persons who do not develop or socially inherit adequate modes for shaping experience may experience aging as a marking of time that is devoid of purpose; losses and impairments appear without pattern from both the self and environment.[28] In one context the distinction between modes of relating potentialities is referred to as the "clinging person" and the "letting-go person." The "clinging person" is secretly frightened by the passage of time and his own mortality. These are events that he cannot personally subdue or control. The "letting-go person" allows himself to experience the passage of time and his own aging, with its bodily manifestations. His feeling life, unlike his aging limbs, need not become rigid and arthritic.[68]

The possible importance of one's ability to grasp the concept of a future and, with this, death, may play more of a role in present behavior than we now assume. A contemporary novel about the lives and deaths of several aging individuals depicts how some elderly individuals reflect anxiety toward approaching death while others recount that to remember one's death is in short, a way of life.[56] Death, a universal and inevitable experience, is a fact of human existence.

Sequential responses to death. Coping processes used by individuals confronting death have been described by authors, poets, clinicians, and investigators involved with various aspects of death and dying. Generally the processes used by individuals facing death have been analyzed from two perspectives: as *sequential* responses to death and as *tactics* unique to the life style of the person confronting death. Examples of the sequential responses to coping with death include the theories of Kübler-Ross, Engel, and Weisman.

Kübler-Ross has delineated five psychologic stages related to the process of dying. Stage one is characterized by *shock* and *denial:* "No, not me." The second stage involves *anger* and *rage:* "Why me?" During the third stage, *bargaining* occurs: "Yes, me, but. . . ." Stage four is characterized by *depression* and *preparatory grief:* "It *is* me . . . what's the use?" Stage five, *acceptance*, could be characterized by "I am ready"; it is seen as a final rest before the long journey.[11] Kübler-Ross has stimulated deep concern among many health care professionals for a humanistic approach in the care of the dying. However, clinical research on the process of dying has not supported a predictable order to the five stages described by her theory.[53] Rather, it has been observed that these stages may vary in their order, and may even recur in a cyclic fashion. In any case, her work has provided health professionals with a heightened awareness of the way people adapt to impending death, and the fact that *hope* may be the single most important factor in this process.

Weisman, who examined the psychodynamics of death, found that denial occurred in four sequential steps. First, the person accepts the public perception that death may occur. Next, a portion of the shared meaning of that public perception is repudiated. Third, the dying person replaces the repudiated meaning with a more congenial version that is acceptable to him. Finally, the individual reorients himself within the scope of the total meaning in order to accommodate his revised reality.[63] These steps in the development of denial seem to result in the constant interplay between disbelief and hope. Interactions between acceptance and denial, understanding that one is dying and magically disbelieving it, may reflect a deeper dialogue of the human mind that involves different layers of the conscious awareness: knowing, yet needing not to know.[54]

Engel provides a framework for viewing those who are *bereaved*. The sequence of events comprising normal grief reactions include: shock and disbelief, developing awareness, and restitution. The first reaction, *shock* and *disbelief*, helps the bereaved gradually become aware of the loss. It can be characterized as "numbness." As *awareness* develops, the bereaved demonstrates sadness and anger in ways modulated by culture. Finally, *restitution* involves resolving the loss and idealizing the person who was lost.[12] *Mourning* may continue for several years, and the process cannot be accelerated.

Furthermore, it is important for nurses to recognize that just as the individual's response to the threat of death varies, so does the family's response. It is also important to bear in mind that the individual's and family's responses may be at variance with one another; the family may have accepted the individual's death as inevitable whereas the individual is still denying it. This is illustrated well by the family who has accepted the inevitable death of their loved one and subsequently has their hopes resurrected by remission of a terminal illness. The individual may continue to live with a family who is mourning his loss.

These sequential responses to death that incorporate the defense mechanisms of anger, denial, shock, and depression provide useful frameworks for the assessment of coping activity. However, nurses must also consider several other factors related to the individual that are equally influential in the process of coping.

Life-style approach. An alternative perspective of coping activity and death is termed the life-style approach. Life style, a term that has been popularized in the gerontology literature, refers to a general attribute of the social system of individuals, governing the person's investment and involvement in areas of living.[66] It is believed that all people develop a primary style of living that influences their expectations and interactions with others. One's life style affects attitudes and beliefs about living and may influence choices related to the process of dying.

McCoy explores the relationship between life style and the final achievement of death. She describes the following styles of living: *accepting, defiant, sensual, humorous, tragic,* and *questing*. Each life style has positive and negative aspects. Each individual prepares for death in much the same manner as he participates in life. This does not mean that an individual cannot change his life style or process of coping, or that he has a predestined style of dying. Rather, each person, through being aware of the self, expresses a style of living that has implications for his death. Although one cannot choose to avoid death indefinitely, one may be able to make choices about how to die, and die in one's own style.[41]

Social structural setting

Humans, when confronting death, are influenced by their environment—social structural setting, family, community, society, and culture—and likewise affect their environment through behavioral responses. Structures unique to the individual and external structures affect the coping process and resultant behavior. This discussion explores the social structural setting as a factor in the individual's confrontation with death.

The social structural setting where a person dies will influence coping and behavior in the process of dying. A major factor influencing the person who is dying in an institutional environment is the *loss of control:* the power to influence awareness, the information received about one's health or illness, and the means to relieve pain, suffering, isolation, and loneliness.

Awareness. Many physicians believe in being reticent with the dying. Studies report that 69% to 90% of physicians are opposed to telling a patient the truth, while 77% to 89% of all patients with a terminal illness want to be told.[15] In a sample of 52 terminally ill patients, one author found that 82% wanted to be informed about their condition for such reasons as "to settle affairs," "to make various financial and family arrangements," because they "don't want to be denied the experience of realizing that I am dying," and because they want to "have time to come to live with the idea, and to learn to die."[15]

Two sociologists have examined information given to terminal patients and the resultant patterns of interaction between staff and patients in an institutional setting. They use the term "awareness context" to describe what each interacting person knows of the patient's defined status, as well as each person's perception of the others' awareness of his definition. The total picture of an awareness context is complex and changes over time. The following types of awareness are described: *closed awareness, suspicion awareness, mutual pretense,* and *open awareness.* Each awareness context includes tactics for interaction that guide communication and behavior based on what each person knows and with what degree of certainty.[21]

In a *closed awareness* context the patient does not recognize his impending death even though hospital personnel have this information. Initially the patient believes he will recover and continues to live as though he had a temporary illness; however, as new symptoms develop and continued treatment and medication are required, the person begins to question his diagnosis. The potential consequence of this context is a feeling of betrayal and a loss of trust in care givers when, and if, the truth is revealed.

Suspicion awareness is the situation that exists when the patient does not know but suspects in varying degrees that others believe him to be dying. Continued therapy along with deteriorating bodily changes arouse suspicions of terminality. This context becomes a fencing match with the patient on the offensive and the health team on the defensive. The staff will determine whether the patient will play a mutual pretense game or move to an open awareness context.

Mutual pretense is the context in which both staff and patient are aware that the patient is dying but choose to pretend otherwise. This context is the most predominant one seen in an institutional setting. In some ways this pretense may yield a measure of dignity or privacy for the patient, since it minimizes the interactional strain that could exist in an open awareness between staff, patient, and family. Since many staff members are uncomfortable in their interactions with dying patients and their families, this context is one that promotes safe topics of discussion—conversation about most anything but death. The consequence of this context is that it does not allow the patient to express needs or share feelings related to dying. Observations on terminally ill, institutionalized elderly persons suggest that they wish to express their thoughts about death but do not have anyone to listen to them.[31]

Open awareness exists when both staff and patient know that the patient is dying and acknowledge it in their actions. This context provides the patient an opportunity to close his life according to his own ideas of dying. However, open awareness is not a context that necessarily promotes adaptation. Certain potential consequences also exist, since once the patient is aware of his diagnosis, he is held responsible for his actions as a dying person. Glaser and Strauss observed that health professionals perceive certain standards of proper conduct for dying such as courageous, decent behavior, relative composure, and cheerfulness.[21]

Should nurses expect all people to accept death with courage and composure? How do nurses react to patients who fear death or that rage with anger when death draws near? Nurses who promote a social structural setting for an appropriate death do not assume that all individuals will accept death. A nurse who shared some lessons from a dying patient revealed: "And the question must still remain: Must there be a 'happy' ending, or isn't the struggle not to die as much a successful adjustment for some as is a peaceful death for others?"[54]

The social structural setting that provides for an appropriate death is one that enhances the individual's right to express emotions and feelings as he chooses. A closed or *suspicion awareness* context does not enhance the expression of needs; in these contexts those around the patient are in control. They have decided to withhold selected information about the individual, and through making such a decision, the individual does not have the right to control the last phase of his life. However, information about health or illness is not a sole prerequisite for the expression of needs related to dying. The individual confronting death may elect to establish a *mutual pretense* context and feel most comfortable discussing topics unrelated to illness or approaching death. The nurse does not assume that all people will be open with their feelings about dying. "Tacit communication can actually be quite successful: the patient is grateful for being spared the emotional pain of discussing his fate."[62] Nurses participating in a *mutual pretense* context, however, must be comfortable enough with their own feelings and beliefs about death to be attuned to cues that a patient desires to change the context from mutual pretense to open awareness. Often a nurse's own anxiety about dying patients prevents the establishment of an open awareness context. Hackett and Weisman have observed that some patients prefer to avoid the truth rather than risk the withdrawal of those who cannot confront death.[24]

Pain and suffering. Chapter 22 describes the assessment of pain and nursing interventions for pain. This discussion will review selected issues related to the form of suffering we call pain as it is experienced by the dying. Pain accompanies birth, growth, disease, and death, and thus is intertwined with most of human existence.[3] Pain is an individual experience; and like death, pain can only be defined introspectively, as each person defines it for himself.

Although pain is an individual experience, the social structural setting in which the individual experiences pain may influence his perception and response to pain. Saunders, an authority on the nature and management of pain in the terminally ill, advocates constant pain control to permit dying persons to take part in suitable activities and enjoy open visiting hours with their families.[51] One of the most difficult aspects of pain in the terminally ill is that it appears to be meaningless as well as endless, often bringing a sense of isolation and despair. Regular doses of analgesics seem to decrease the threat and anxiety associated with this pain, and reduce the guilt and despair of family members.[52]

When an individual is in an institution that discourages self-control of pain, pain relief is frequently in the form of a "demand schedule." The demand schedule is usually referred to as prn medication for pain, meaning "whenever the nurse judges the patient needs pain relief." A demand schedule can constitute a very demoralizing experience for both the patient and the nurse. The nurse must watch for symptoms of pain; the patient must withstand more pain before it is reduced by the nurse's action.[21] Alternatives to this demand schedule are self-administration of pain medication or a regimen that provides constant control of pain, such as that advocated by Saunders.

Suffering is a response to pain. Pain has been conceived of as a universal language: it produces an outcry that evokes help from others.[3] The nature of this help may influence the perception of pain and suffering. Sometimes the inability of helpers to relate to those who are dying and to ease pain through the therapeutic use of self results in the oversedation and tranquilization of those in need of help. Kübler-Ross, in discussing the use of psychopharmacologic agents for the dying patient and the bereaved, expressed the belief that the dosage and number of drugs prescribed might be used as an index of the comfort (or discomfort) of the prescribing physician. She equates sedation of the dying with the health professional's discomfort in caring for them.[33] Perhaps if nurses gave more of themselves, rather than sedatives and tranquilizers, the pain and suffering that accompanies some dying could be eased. As the next discussion on loneliness and isolation will explore, the art of caring may decrease suffering.

Loneliness and isolation. The beginning of this chapter explored characteristics of American society that influence attitudes and behaviors toward death and dying. The following discussion will consider how the dying individual perceives the actions of others. A dying professor shared these perceptions: "The nonverbal response, the avoidance itself, generates considerable anxiety, fear, confusion on the part of any patient in that kind of situation."[47] Another young girl dying of cancer expressed these feelings, "I don't think dying would be so tough if it could be shared with those around you. There are times when I feel people are really avoiding me and it is a sinking sensation to feel you are being isolated." It is widely accepted that for many who confront death, death itself is often less of a threat than the process of dying and the perception of loneliness and isolation.

The perception of loneliness and isolation is enhanced by many rituals that exist within an institutional setting. Hospital practices such as limiting visitors, moving the dying to single rooms, rotating assignments of personnel, closing doors, and "hushing" discussions on deaths of patients are all strategies for decreasing the anxiety associated with dying. These practices limit interaction between the dying individual, his family, and the staff. They also decrease the possibility of threatening questions to the staff. As the father of a dying child revealed, "Death always brings one suddenly face to face with life. . . . It raises all the infinite questions, each answer ending in another question."[49] Inability to feel at ease with these questions is one reason for isolation of the dying—rituals and formalities in hospitals promote a comfortable distance between the nurse and death.

Isolation of the dying creates feelings of loneliness. The basic reason for loneliness is that the human being experiences the self out of his relatedness to other persons; without other persons, he fears he will lose the experience of being a self.[39] Loneliness has been described as a response to a relational deficit and the product of emotional or social isolation.[64] If the process of dying results in the loss of a truly intimate tie, such as the lack of relationships with a child, parent, spouse, or lover, the individual may experience *emotional isolation.* The loneliness of *social isolation* is a consequence of the lack of a network of involvement with peers, fellow workers, kinfolk, neighbors, or friends.[63] Loneliness that results from social or emotional isolation has been decreased in some settings that provide care for the terminally ill. St. Christopher's Hospice in Sydenham, England, is probably best known for the care given there to dying persons.

The hospice, unlike the hospital that treats sick people, is a place where people come to die. This concept of a hospice is just beginning to develop in the United States. St. Christopher's Hospice, of which Dr. Cicely Saunders is the founder and medical director, has few rituals and institutional rules. To decrease social and emotional isolation and loneliness, visiting hours are unlimited, except for Monday—the "family day off." Children are welcomed as visitors, and there is no age limit on visitations. Family pets also frequent the hospice. Families are encouraged and helped to care for their loved ones.[25]

At St. Christopher's the staff understands and practices the concept of caring. One nurse who visited the setting reflected, "The secret of the care of patients is still caring."[25] Patients are encouraged to have as much control over their daily lives as possible. When a resident dies, the staff makes a point of giving the others in a ward the chance to talk about it. Things do not take precedence over people; the nurse takes time to care, to see the person as an individual, and hear and respond to questions of worried families. This caring part of St. Christopher's can be emulated in any setting. For the individual confronting death, the issue seems to be not *how many days*, but *what kind of days* are left.[67]

Health professionals. Several studies indicate that not all nurses respond in the most supportive manner with dying patients. One psychologist who examined the amount of time required to respond to call bells at the bedside of hospitalized patients found that nurses took longer to respond to requests for help from pateints with terminal prognoses.[28] Another study found that nurses displayed a variety of behavioral strategies to maintain "professional demeanor" in work situations with the dying.[21] Yet another study demonstrated that nursing students with the least experience in caring for dying persons were actually better able to provide human comfort during lengthy assignments to dying patients than those with more experience.[48] Nurses need to ask themselves if rather than providing humanistic care, do they become less human with continued personal contact with the institutionalized dying individual. Also, they need to discern whether their own anxieties and concerns about death are preventing them from humanely caring for those most often dependent on them for their needs—those who are dying.

Caring. If nurses are attuned to their own beliefs and feelings as well as those of the individual who is dying, they will create a social structural setting that facilitates an appropriate death. Such a setting would be one in which the nurse cares enough to help the person die in a manner that is meaningful to his existence. This element of caring was succinctly summarized by a dying student nurse, "Please believe me, if you care, you can't go wrong. Just admit that you care. That is really for what we search. We may ask for why's and wherefores, but we really don't expect answers. Don't run away . . . wait . . . all I want to know is that there is someone to hold my hand when I need it. . . . Then, it might not be so hard to die . . . in a hospital . . . with friends close by."[9]

Caring for another person is a process that involves development such as that involved as a friendship emerges: through mutual trust and through a deepening and qualitative transforming of the relationship.[40] Mayeroff describes eight major ingredients of caring: *knowing, alternating rhythms, patience, honesty, truth, humility, hope,* and *courage.*[40] These ingredients can be applied to the nurse who cares for the dying in the following ways:

1. *Knowing.* To respond to another who is in need and to care, I must first know myself. I continue to refine my philosophy of life and death and recognize my powers and limitations. I also understand the necessity of knowing the beliefs, values, and needs of those I care for, along with their limitations and strengths.
2. *Alternating rhythms.* I invest my energy in caring for another in a way that meets his needs, maintaining or modifying my behaviors to better help him.
3. *Patience.* I patiently participate with another in the process of caring, believing that he will grow in a way that is meaningful to his existence. Patience also allows for growth of myself.
4. *Honesty.* I care for the other in a way that facilitates an appropriate death: one that is defined by the individual, a death that gives meaning to his

existence. I am honest with myself in that I do not believe that another should die in a manner that I define. "In caring I am honest in trying to truly see."

5. *Trust.* Trust allows me to give the type of care that enables the other to grow in his own way and time. Besides trusting the other, it involves the courage to believe and trust in my own capacity to care.
6. *Humility.* I believe that each encounter with a dying person or his family brings a new, novel learning experience. Each encounter requires the readiness and willingness to learn and care. Humility also means accepting myself, being open to others, and recognizing that others have an integrity of their own.
7. *Hope.* Hope is an expression of belief in "now," the plentitude of the moment, alive with a sense of the possible. Hope also implies that my caring for another is a commitment: a commitment to a relationship that exists in this moment for the realization of the other through my caring.
8. *Courage.* I communicate courage when I take existential anxiety upon myself. The anxiety associated with death and the unknown belongs to existence. Courage takes the anxiety of nonbeing into itself: "The courage to be enrooted in the God who appears when God has disappeared in the anxiety of doubt."[60] "Courage gives me the trust I have in myself to care, and the trust I have in the belief that the other who is confronting death will grow."*

■ SUMMARY

In summary, this chapter has examined the process of dying in American society. It has reviewed selected characteristics of American culture that influence attitudes and beliefs about death and dying: longevity, isolation, family life, and the environment for dying. A holistic approach to the confrontation with death has been explicated. Consideration has been given to the individual's perceptions, psychologic structure, and the coping processes. Selected factors related to the social structural setting that may influence coping during the process of dying have been described, including awareness, pain and suffering, isolation, loneliness, and attitudes of health professionals. The individual confronting death relies on factors within himself and elements external to his being for adaptation. Through caring the nurse develops a relationship with the dying individual that encourages him to grow and die in a manner that is meaningful to his total existence.

Implementation of humanistic caring for the dying requires not only an awareness of those actions fostering death with dignity, but also introspection on the part of the practitioner. Examination of one's own feelings, attitudes, and values about death and dying contributes to one's abilities to care and grow. Just as the dying may suffer from isolation and grow by sharing their experiences with others, so do nurses suffer when they are unable to share their losses with colleagues. Practitioners often find it helpful, if not essential, to share their feelings about death and their dying patients with others who can listen supportively.

*Abridged and adapted from pp. 9-20 of On caring, by Milton Mayeroff, vol. 43 of World Perspectives series. Planned and edited by Ruth Nanda Anshen. Copyright © 1971 by Milton Mayeroff. By permission of Harper & Row, Publishers, Inc.

REFERENCES AND SELECTED READINGS

1. Anthony, S.: The discovery of death in childhood and after, London, 1971, Penguin Press.
2. Anthony, S.: The child's discovery of death, New York, 1940, Harcourt Brace Jovanovich, Inc.
3. Bakan, D.: Disease, pain and sacrifice: toward a psychology of suffering, Chicago, 1968, The University of Chicago Press.
4. Bowers, M., Jackson, E., Knight, J., and LeShan, L.: Counseling the dying, New York, 1964, Thomas Nelson & Sons.
5. Bromberg, W., and Schilder, P.: Attitudes to death and dying, Psychoanal. Rev. **20:**133-185, 1933.
6. Choron, J.: Modern man and mortality, New York, 1964, Macmillan Publishing Co., Inc.
7. *Craven, J., and Wald, F.: Hospice care for dying patients, Am. J. Nurs. **75:**1816-1822, 1975.
8. *Craytor, J.: Talking with the persons who have cancer, Am. J. Nurs. **69:**744-748, 1969.
9. *Death in the first person, Am. J. Nurs. **70:**336, 1970.
10. Dickenstein, L., and Blatt, S.: Death concern, futurity and anticipation, J. Consult Clin. Psychol. **30:**11-17, 1966.
11. Easson, W.: The dying child, Springfield, Ill., 1970, Charles C Thomas, Publisher.
12. *Engel, G.: Grief and grieving, Am. J. Nurs. **64:**93-98, 1964.
13. Erikson, E.: Childhood and society, ed. 2, New York, 1950, Norton and Co.
14. Family balking at "last step." *Durham Morning Herald,* July 25, 1975, Louisville, Ky.
15. Feifel, H.: The function of attitudes toward death, J. Long Island Cons. Center **5:**26-29, 1967.
16. Feifel, H., Hanson, S., et al.: Physicians consider death. Proceedings from 75th annual convention of the American psychological Association, Washington, D.C., 1967.
17. Feifel, H.: Older persons look at death, Geriatrics, **11:**127-130, 1956.
18. Fulton, R.: Attitudes of American public toward death. In Fulton, R.: Death and identity, New York, 1965, JOhn Wiley & Sons, Inc.
19. Gesell, A., and Ilg, F.: The child from five to ten, New York, 1946, Harper & Row, Publishers, Inc.
20. Glaser, B., and Strauss A.: Time for dying, Chicago, 1968, Aldine Publishing Co.
21. Glaser, B., and Strauss, A.: Awareness of dying, Chicago, 1965, Aldine Publishing Co.
22. Goldscheider, C.: The mortality revolution. In Shneidman,

*References preceded by an asterisk are particularly well suited for student reading.

E. S.: Death: current perspectives, Palo Alto, Calif. 1976, Mayfield Publishing Co., p. 187.
23. Grollman, E.: Explaining death to children, Boston, 1967, Beacon Press.
24. Hackett, T., and Weisman, A.: Reactions to the imminence of death. In Grosser, G. H., Weehsler, H., and Greenblatt, H.: The threat of impending disaster, Cambridge, Mass., 1964, The MIT Press.
25. *Ingles, T.: St. Christopher's hospice, Nurs. Outlook.**74**:759-763, 1974.
26. Jaques, E.: Death and the mid-life crisis. In Ruitenbeck, H.: The interpretation of death, New York, 1973, Jason Aronson, Inc.
27. Jeffers, F., Nichols, C., and Eisdorfer, C.: Attitudes of older persons toward death: a preliminary study, J. Gerontol. **16**:53-56, 1961.
28. Kastenbaum, R.: Theories of human aging: the search for a conceptual framework, J. Soc. Issues **21**:13-36, 1965.
29. Kastenbaum, R.: Time and death in adolescence. In Feifel, H.: The meaning of death, New York, 1959, McGraw-Hill Book Co.
30. Kastenbaum, R., and Aisenburg, R.: The psychology of death, New York, 1972, Springer Publishing Co., Inc.
31. Kastenbaum, R. and Weisman, A.: The psychological autopsy: a study of the terminal phase of life, monograph series no. 4, Comm. Ment. Health J., New York, 1968, Behavioral Publications, Inc.
32. *Kneisal, C.: Thoughtful care of the dying, Am. J. Nurs.**68**:550-553, 1968.
33. Kübler-Ross, E.: On the use of psychopharmacologic agents for the dying patient and the bereaved. In Goldberg, I., Malitz, D., and Kutscher, A.: Psychopharmacological agents for the terminally ill and bereaved. New York, 1973, Columbia University Press.
34. *Kübler-Ross, E.: On death and dying, New York, 1969, Macmillan Publishing Co., Inc., p. 8.
35. Lazarus, R.: Psychological stress and the coping process, New York, 1966, McGraw-Hill Book Co.
36. Lerner, M.: When, why and where people die. In Shneidman, E. S.: Death: current perspectives, Palo Alto, Calif., 1976, Mayfield Publishing Co.
37. Livingston, R., and Zimet, C.: Death anxiety, authoritarianism, and choice of specialty in medical students, J. Nerv. Ment. Dis. **140**:222-230, 1965.
38. Maurer, A.: Maturation of concepts of death, Br. J. Med. Psychol. **39**:35-41, 1966.
39. May, R.: Man's search for himself, New York, 1953, Norton and Co.
40. Mayeroff, M.: On caring, New York, 1971, Harper & Row, Publishers, Inc.
41. McCoy, M.: To die with style, Nashville, Tenn., 1974, Abingdon Press.
42. *Mittford, J.: The American way of death, New York, 1963, Simon & Schuster, Inc.
43. Moody, R.: Life after life, New York, 1976, Stockpole Books.
44. Moroney, R., and Kurtz, H.: The evolution of long-term care institutions. In Sherwood, S.: Long-term care, New York, 1975, Spectrum Publications, Inc.
45. Munnichs, J.: Old age and finitude, Basel, Switzerland, 1966, S. Karger.
46. Nagy, M.: The child's view of death. In Feifel, H.: The meaning of death, New York, 1959, McGraw-Hill Book Co.
47. *Notes on a dying professor, Nurs. Outlook **23**:503-506, 1972.
48. *Quint, J.: The nurse and the dying patient, New York, 1967, Macmillan Publishing Co.
49. *Quint, J.: Obstacles to helping the dying, Am. J. Nurs. **66**:1568-1571, 1966.
50. *Roose, L.: To die alone, Ment. Hyg. **53**:321-326, 1969.
51. Saunders, C.: A therapeutic community: St. Christopher's Hospice. In Schoenberg, B., Carr, A., Peretz, D., and Kutscher, A.: Psychosocial aspects of terminal care, New York, 1972, New York, 1972, New York University Press.
52. Saunders, C.: The nature and management of terminal pain. In Shotter, E.: Matters of life and death, Great Britain, 1970, Darton, Longman & Todd Ltd.
53. Schulz, R., and Aderman, D.: Clinical research on the stages of dying, Omega **5**:137-143, 1974.
54. *Sharp, D.: Lessons from a dying patient, Am. J. Nurs. **68**:1517-1520, 1968.
55. Shneidman, E. S.: Death work and stages of dying. In Shneidman, E. S.: Death: current perspectives, Palo Alto, 1976, Mayfield Publishing Co.
56. Spark, M.: Momento mori, New York, 1964, Meridian Books, World Publishing Co.
57. Statistical abstracts for the United States: 1975, Washington, D.C., 1975, U.S. Bureau of the Census.
58. Strauss, A., and Glaser, B.: Anguish: a case history of a dying trajectory, Mill Valley, Calif., 1970, The Sociology Press.
59. Sturt, M.: The psychology of time, New York, 1925, Harcourt Press.
60. Tillich, P.: The courage to be, New Haven, Conn., 1952, Yale University Press.
61. U.S. Department of Health, Education, and Welfare: Facts about older Americans 1975, no. OHD 75-20006, Office of Human Development, Administration on Aging, National Clearing House on Aging.
62. *Verwoerdt, A., and Wilson, R.: Communication with fatally ill patients: tact or explicit? Am. J. Nurs. **67**:2307-2310, 1967.
63. Weisman, A.: On dying and denying, New York, 1972, Behavioral Publications, Inc.
64. Weiss, R.: Loneliness: the experience of emotional and social isolation, Cambridge, Mass, 1973, The MIT Press.
65. *Wentzel, K.: The dying are the living, Am. J. Nurs. **76**:956-957, 1976.
66. Williams, R., and Wirths, C.: Lives through the years, New York, 1965, Atherton Press, Inc.
67. Zeligs, R.: Children's attitudes toward death, Ment. Hyg. **51**: 393-396, 1967.
68. Zinker, J., and Hollenback, C.: Notes on loss, crises and growth, J. Gen. Psychol. **73**:347-354, 1965.

UNIT IV

Common stressors and their management

Persons with medical-surgical problems encounter many stressful situations in conjunction with their illnesses and the interventions necessary to their treatment. This unit explores common stressors that occur regardless of the pathologic entity or biologic system involved. Emphasis is placed on the effects of the stressors and on nursing interventions to modify effects that are detrimental to health.

Fluid and electrolyte imbalance considers such stressors as excesses and deficiencies of water and electrolytes. In the chapter on *infectious agents* and the adaptive responses, emphasis is placed on nosocomial infections, and persons with minimal adaptive potential are identified. *Pain* is explored as a stressor, and adaptation is discussed from biologic as well as psychosocial perspectives. Nursing measures for pain relief are emphasized. The stress resulting from *trauma* is discussed from two standpoints, the needs of the person experiencing surgery, and the effects incurred from accidental injury. The overwhelming effects of large-scale disasters are also explored. The effects of having a malignant disease regardless of location are discussed in the chapter on *neoplasia.* Information relative to specific malignant diseases is dealt with in later chapters.

Sensory deprivation and overload are also common stressors and are discussed in terms of nursing assessment and management. Changes in *level of consciousness* are explored, emphasizing the protective interventions necessary for the dependent unconscious patient. Many of the diseases seen in persons with medical-surgical problems or interventions to treat these problems result in alteration in *body image,* and the adaptive responses this elicits are discussed. The experience of having a *prolonged illness,* of being chronically ill, including altered roles and adaptation to long-term impairments, is also explored.

20

Fluid and electrolyte imbalance

BARBARA SOLTIS

Almost all medical and surgical conditions threaten fluid and electrolyte equilibrium. In some instances, imbalances are minor and can be corrected by merely adjusting a pateint's food and fluid intake. In other instances, imbalances are life threatening and require prompt medical treatment to prevent death.

Although a physician prescribes medical therapy to prevent and treat imbalances, nurses have many vital functions to carry out in this area: (1) recognize situations that are likely to cause imbalances; (2) intervene to prevent imbalances from developing; (3) carry out preventive and therapeutic measures ordered by the physician, and monitor patients' responses to these measures; (4) recognize signs and symptoms of fluid, electrolyte, and acid-base disturbances; (5) monitor patients to prevent and recognize imbalances related to their specific conditions or treatments; and (6) alleviate the effects of disturbances on patients' comfort and safety.

The reader is referred to Chapter 15 for a description of normal fluid and electrolyte balance and some of the control mechanisms that maintain this balance. This chapter deals with the causes, prevention, assessment, and management of imbalances of body fluids, sodium, potassium, calcium, magnesium, and hydrogen ions. Each imbalance will be discussed separately, although in most instances a disturbance in one is accompanied by a disturbance in the balance of one or more of the others.

Normally the body receives oxygen through the lungs, and water and various organic and inorganic substances through the gastrointestinal tract. After utilizing what is needed for healthful functioning, any excesses are excreted along with the waste products of metabolism through the body's excretory organs, the skin, lungs, kidneys, and gastrointestinal tract (see Chapter 15). When these normal processes of intake, utilization, and excretion are disrupted, fluid, electrolyte, and acid-base imbalances result. These imbalances are manifest as excesses, deficits, or abnormal shifts among body compartments.

Excesses result from increased intake or decreased loss, and deficits result from decreased intake or excess loss of fluids or electrolytes. Either an excess or a deficit can result from abnormal shifts of fluids or electrolytes among the body compartments. For example, excesses occur when the intake of fluids and electrolytes exceeds the ability of the body's control and excretory mechanisms to eliminate the amounts that are not needed. Fluids, electrolytes, and metabolic wastes are retained when kidney function is impaired. An excess of carbon dioxide accumulates when there is inadequate respiratory function.

On the other hand, deficits develop when an individual is unwilling or unable for some reason to take in adequate fluids and food. Excessive amounts of fluids and electrolytes are lost through the skin due to diaphoresis or to oozing from severe wounds or burns. Fluids and electrolytes are lost from the gastrointestinal tract when profuse diarrhea or vomiting occurs and when the gastrointestinal tract is drained by intubation or purged with cathartics or enemas. In hemorrhage, body fluids and electrolytes are always lost.

Deficits may also result from the inability to utilize needed substances, such as when fluids with their electrolyte constituents are trapped in the body by edema or intestinal obstruction. They are therefore not available for normal processes.

■ TYPES OF FLUID IMBALANCES

Osmotic pressure of the extracellular fluid (ECF) varies proportionately with its sodium concentration. When there is a change in the sodium-to-water ratio, a disturbance in osmolality results; that is, the extracellular fluid becomes more dilute *(hyposmolar)* or more concentrated *(hyperosmolar)* than normal. A considerable change in the concentration of solutes other than sodium in the extracellular fluid can also effect osmolar disturbances.

Hyposmolality of the ECF causes water to move into

Table 20-1. Water and sodium imbalances

Osmolar imbalances				Isotonic volume imbalances	
Hyperosmolar		Hyposmolar		Volume excess	Volume deficit
Water deficit: water ↓ in relation to sodium and other solutes	Sodium or solute excess: sodium or other solutes ↗ in relation to water	Water excess: water ↗ relation to sodium and other solutions	Sodium deficit: sodium ↓ in relation to water	ECF volume excess (edema): water and sodium ↗ proportionately	ECF volume deficit: water and sodium ↓ proportionately

body cells by osmosis to equalize the concentration of fluid on both sides of the cell membrane. Hyperosmolality of the ECF causes water to move out of the cells to dilute the ECF and to equalize concentration in both compartments.

When there are changes in the volume of ECF but no change in osmolality, an *isotonic* volume disturbance results. There is no significant change in the sodium-to-water ratio; sodium deficits or excesses are accompanied by proportional water deficits or excesses. There is no appreciable movement of water between the intracellular fluid (ICF) and ECF compartments, and the imbalance is essentially restricted to the ECF compartment. Table 20-1 shows the types of fluid imbalances that are likely to occur.

□ Hyperosmolar imbalances: extracellular water deficit and solute excess

An extracellular water deficit occurs when the amount of extracellular water is diminished in proportion to the amount of solute contained therein. The solute excess raises the osmolality to above the normal 300 mOsm/liter.

Etiology. Imbalances may originate in either the fluid or the solute portion of the extracellular fluid. There may be (1) decreased intake of water, (2) excess loss of water without proportionate loss of solutes, (3) increased solute intake without sufficient water, and (4) excess accumulation of solutes secondary to a particular disease condition.

Any person who does not have fluids available to drink, cannot take fluids independently, or who does not respond to thirst will be likely to develop a water deficit.

In a disaster such as shipwreck, flood, or earthquake, a supply of drinkable water may not be available. Any patient who is unable to ask for fluids, to identify his own need for fluid, or to swallow easily may develop a fluid deficit. Thus a patient with a cerebral vascular accident and aphasia may not be able to communicate his desire for fluids or may have difficulty swallowing fluids that are offered to him. A confused or disoriented patient may not be aware that he is thirsty. Patients who are comatose, weak, or catatonic may also develop fluid deficits.

Although loss of body water is usually accompanied by loss of electrolytes, there are a number of conditions in which water is lost in excess of electrolytes. These include increased loss through the lungs in hyperventilation or in secretions from a tracheostomy, through the skin with a high fever, through the gastrointestinal tract when there is watery diarrhea, or in urine when the kidneys fail to concentrate solutes.

When solutes are taken in without sufficient water, hyperosmolality results, such as occurs with intake of tube feeding solutions, which are high in protein, dextrose, and electrolytes. The excess of solutes causes an *osmotic diuresis*, the body's attempt to excrete a solute load through the kidneys by excreting a large volume of urine. Formation of the urine in this process requires the use of a great deal of water and interferes with the normal water conservation mechanisms resulting in a water deficit.

Several conditions lead to endogenous (internal) addition of excess solutes—large amounts of glucose can accumulate in the blood in the disease diabetes mellitus, and glucose and ketone bodies can accumulate in the blood in diabetic ketoacidosis (p. 590). A large volume of nitrogenous waste products results from metabolism of a high-protein diet. All of these solute excesses cause large water losses during osmotic diuresis.

When an extracellular water deficit occurs, water moves out of the cells to replace water lost from the extracellular compartment, thus maintaining an adequate circulating blood volume. If the water deficit is not corrected, the cells eventually become unable to compensate for extracellular losses, and circulation begins to fail. As both intracellular and extracellular fluids decrease, cell function is impaired because food, oxygen, and waste products are diffused inadequately. Brain cells are particularly sensitive to these changes and a disruption of brain cell function develops, manifested as mental changes in the patient.

Prevention. Prevention is crucial in the nursing care

Table 20-2. Signs and symptoms of water deficit

	Moderate deficit	Severe deficit
Skin	Flushed, dry	Cold, clammy
Mouth	Dry mucous membranes	Dry, cracked tongue; sordes
Eyes	Decrease in tears	Soft, sunken eyeballs
Cardiovascular system	—	Tachycardia, low blood pressure, rapid respirations
CNS	Apprehension, restlessness	Lethargy, coma
Blood	—	Hemoconcentration, increase in hematocrit, BUN, electrolytes
Urine	High specific gravity, scant amount (except with osmotic diuresis)	Oliguria
Other	Thirst, weight loss	Thirst, weight loss, fever

of patients who are at risk of developing a water deficit. The nurse is alert to those patients who may not be receiving adequate fluid intake, monitors their intake and output, and plans a schedule for offering fluids to them. Patients who are hyperventilating for long periods of time, regardless of the reason, should have their fluid intake increased somewhat because they are losing more fluid than usual through the lungs. Those receiving high-protein tube feedings need sufficient water to prevent water deficit and osmotic diuresis.

Assessment. Thirst and weight loss are early symptoms of water deficit and become more pronounced as the deficit increases. Body temperature begins to rise as less water is available for temperature regulation. When cells are not able to continue providing water to replace extracellular fluid losses, signs of collapse of the circulatory system appear. Signs and symptoms of water deficit are shown in Table 20-2.

Intervention. Goals of treatment are to treat the underlying causes to prevent further water loss and to replace lost fluid.

The physician can use several methods, such as those based on serum sodium concentration or change in the patient's weight, to calculate the volume of water loss.[16] For instance, if a patient has lost 4 kg of body weight, his fluid deficit equals 4 liters (1 kg weighs 1 liter). Therapy will require replacement of the volume lost plus about 1.5 liters of fluid to supply current daily need. Often the replacement is administered over a period of several days, since too rapid infusion of fluid may cause sudden intercompartmental shifts of water and pulmonary edema.

When water deficit is not severe, fluids can be replaced orally if the patient is able to drink fluids. Otherwise, intravenous fluids are given.

Intravenous glucose and water are usually given first to replace the water loss and increase urinary flow. Urinary output must be adequate so that electrolytes in excess of body needs can be excreted. Solutions containing electrolytes are therefore not given until renal function is established. Normal saline or half-strength saline (0.45%) can be given with other ions—potassium, calcium, and lactate—as needed.

In addition to providing fluids and participating in the treatment of conditions underlying water loss, nurses employ measures to decrease discomfort and assure patient safety. Mouth care is especially important to relieve dryness and remove sordes (foul debris on lips and teeth) from oral mucous membranes. Safety measures such as side rails on beds are necessary for patients who have developed restlessness, confusion, lethargy, or other mental changes as a result of water deficit. Monitoring intake and output and changes in the patient's weight and vital signs will indicate whether the patient's condition is improving or deteriorating.

A state of adequate hydration will be evidenced by mental alertness, moist mucous membranes, and urine output that is approximately equal to fluid intake.

□ Hyposmolar imbalance: water excess or water intoxication

When there is an excess of water in relation to solutes in the extracellular fluid, a hyposmolar imbalance exists known as *water excess* or *water intoxication*. Although this imbalance is not common, it can develop when water intake exceeds the ability of the kidneys to excrete it. Usually there is a concomitant increase in secretion of ADH, which promotes water retention and aggravates the water excess.

Under normal conditions, a decrease in osmotic

pressure suppresses ADH production and permits free water to be excreted by the kidneys.

Etiology. One or more of the following conditions exist when water intoxication develops: (1) excess intake of electrolyte-free fluid, (2) increased secretion of ADH, or (3) decreased or inadequate output of urine.

Water excess can be caused by ingestion of large amounts of tap water by a person who is hysterical or psychotic. This behavior is called *psychogenic polydipsia.* The ingestion of frequent sips of tap water by one who is not able to tolerate food or other fluids because of illness can also lead to water excess. Some treatments that lead to excessive water intake are multiple tap water enemas and absorption of water from irrigating solutions during transurethral resection of the prostate gland.

Excess or inappropriate secretion of ADH occurs in response to stress, drugs, and anesthetics. (See Chapter 15 for more information on ADH.) It can also accompany inflammatory conditions of the lung (tuberculosis, pneumonia) and brain (encephalitis, meningitis), endocrine disturbances and tumors in the lungs (especially oat cell carcinoma), pancreas, duodenum, and other body organs.[16] Inadequate kidney function or renal failure will potentiate the development of water excess.

A low serum sodium or sodium deficit can also produce a hyposmolar imbalance. This condition is discussed under sodium deficit (p. 307). Hyposmolar water excess in the extracellular compartment quickly becomes an *intracellular water excess.* Decrease in extracellular osmotic pressure causes water to enter the cells to equalize concentration on both sides of the cell membrane.

Prevention. Water intoxication can be anticipated by identifying patients who present one or more risk factors. Daily weights and careful monitoring of intake and output will help to detect the developing problem before it becomes severe.

Assessment. Since brain cells are particularly sensitive to the increase in intracellular water, the most common symptoms are manifestations of changes in the patient's mental status.

In acute water intoxication there is swelling of the cells, which may develop rapidly and dramatically. Signs of water intoxication include changes in behavior, confusion, incoordination, convulsions, hyperventilation, sudden weight gain, and warm, moist skin. When the condition develops more slowly, there may be apathy, sleepiness, anorexia, nausea, and vomiting. A low serum sodium concentration is a usual finding. Signs of increasing intracranial pressure may develop—slow, bounding pulse and rising pulse pressure as the systolic blood pressure rises and the diastolic pressure falls. Some peripheral edema may be present, but it is not marked.

Intervention. The patient will usually recover with only careful water restriction. When severe symptoms (coma and convulsions) develop, a small amount of intravenous hypertonic saline, along with the fluid restriction, will hasten the return to normal water balance.

Providing for the safety of patients with this imbalance is a priority nursing function because of the confusion and other mental changes that exist. Any patient who is receiving a large amount of water orally, rectally, or intravenously needs to be monitored carefully for signs of water intoxication, especially if a condition of excess ADH prevails.

□ Isotonic volume deficit: extracellular fluid deficit

Conditions causing a loss of water together with a loss of electrolytes lead to *isotonic volume deficit,* also known as *extracellular fluid depletion.*

Etiology. Water and electrolytes are lost in hemorrhage and profuse sweating. About 8 liters of fluid circulate through the gastrointestinal tract per day (Table 20-3). These fluids are derived from the extracellular fluid; therefore vomiting, diarrhea, draining intestinal fistulas, and surgical openings such as ileostomy and cecostomy result in extracellular fluid loss. Severe losses can deplete the extracellular compartment rapidly.

In isotonic volume deficit the extracellular osmolality does not change because sodium, the chief contributor to extracellular osmolality, is lost along with water. Consequently, water content of the cells is not affected, and the deficit remains restricted to the extracellular compartment. Fluid movement is from extracellular compartment to outside the body, depleting blood and interstitial volume.

Prevention. Nurses are responsible for identifying and monitoring patients who are likely to develop isotonic fluid deficit. Taking postural (orthostatic) blood pressures helps to detect this deficit before more severe cardiovascular symptoms develop. Postural blood pres-

Table 20-3. Fluid composition of total internal secretions*

	Approximate ml of fluid (daily)
Saliva	1,500
Gastric juice	2,500
Intestinal juice	3,000
Pancreatic juice	700
Bile	500
TOTAL	8,200 ml/24 hr

*Adapted from Fluid and electrolytes, North Chicago, Ill., 1968, Abbott Laboratories.

Note that approximately 8 liters of fluid are used daily for digestive purposes. Normally most of this fluid is reabsorbed. Some of each of the ions found in blood plasma is present in each of the fluids listed, but the individual concentration varies with each fluid.

sures are a comparison of a patient's blood pressure measured first in a lying position and then in a sitting position. A drop in blood pressure of 10 mm Hg or more in the upright position is significant. The healthy person who is perspiring profusely needs extra salt in his diet and should drink extra fluids. Patients on low sodium diets and those with draining gastrointestinal fistulas are especially likely to experience sodium depletion. They should always be taught to increase their salt intake slightly whenever they perspire profusely. Patients who have hot packs applied to large areas of the body also lose sodium and water, although the loss may not be readily noticeable as perspiration. Attention to ingesting more salt and water than usual in situations of excessive heat, climatic or otherwise, may prevent heat exhaustion.

Assessment. The most prominent symptoms are manifest in the cardiovascular system as a result of volume depletion. Following is a listing of the symptoms of extracellular fluid depletion:

1. Skin: poor turgor
2. Mouth: dry mucous membranes
3. Cardiovascular: postural hypotension (early), low blood pressure, tachycardia, increased respiration, decreased vein filling
4. Weight: loss
5. Urine: low output, increased specific gravity

Intervention. Treatment consists of identifying and correcting the underlying cause to prevent further fluid and electrolyte loss and replacing those fluids and electrolytes that have been lost. Hemorrhage must be controlled (see Chapter 15). Vomiting may be treated with antiemetics, such as trimethobenzamide hydrochloride (Tigan) and prochlorperazine (Compazine), and diarrhea with antidiarrheal drugs (Lomotil, paregoric, Kaopectate).

Any patient who is losing body fluids through perspiration, fever, or loss of gastrointestinal fluid should be given salty fluids to drink. Meticulous mouth care will relieve the discomfort of dry mucous membranes.

As blood volume decreases, postural hypotension develops, and the patient's safety may be threatened by the resultant weakness, dizziness, or fainting on standing upright.

Isotonic volume excess: extracellular fluid excess and edema

If there is an excess of body water with a concomitant increase in sodium, the excess fluid will be retained in the *extracellular* compartments and lead to the formation of edema. *Edema* is the accumulation of fluid in the interstitial spaces. In the normal tissue there is a negative interstitial fluid pressure, and cells are held in close approximation to facilitate the exchange of gases, nutrients, and waste products between the cells and capillaries. If fluid accumulates in the interstitial space and is not removed either by direct return to the blood vessel or through the lymph system, a positive interstitial fluid pressure develops, and cells are pushed further apart. In the healthy individual, edema does not develop immediately after the initial inflow of fluid into the interstitial spaces because of the body's compensatory mechanisms, which include the existing negative interstitial fluid pressure and the lymph system, which removes excess fluids and proteins (p. 1077).

A review of normal capillary dynamics will help the nurse to understand the various factors that can cause the development of edema. Two different types of pressures influence the flow of fluid across a capillary membrane: *fluid pressure* (pressure resulting from the hydrostatic force of fluid) and the colloid osmotic pressure, or *oncotic pressure* (pressure resulting from the presence of the proteins that do not diffuse across the membrane wall). Fluid pressure within the capillary is much greater than fluid pressure within the interstitial space; Thus fluid is forced out of the capillary. Since there are a larger number of proteins in plasma than in interstitial fluid, the oncotic pressure within the capillary serves as a force to *absorb* fluid back into the capillary (Fig. 20-1). According to Starling's law of the capillaries, there is an equilibrium between the forces filtering fluid out of the capillary and the forces absorbing fluid back into the capillary. The *fluid hydrostatic pressure gradient* (the difference between the fluid pressures inside and outside the capillary) should equal the oncotic pressure gradient (Fig. 20-1). If there is a change in the oncotic pressure in or out of the capillary or in the capillary fluid pressure, there will be a rapid fluid flow across the capil-

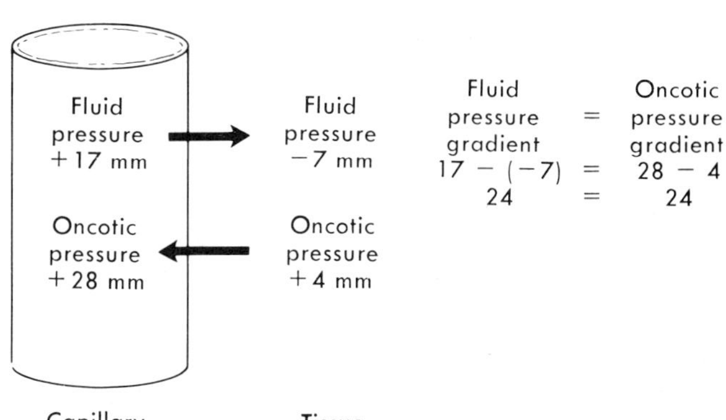

Fig. 20-1. Starling's law of capillaries. An equilibrium exists between forces filtering fluid out of capillary and forces absorbing fluid back into capillary. Note that fluid pressure within capillary is greater than fluid pressure in tissue. This differential (fluid pressure gradient) serves as a filtering force. Note also that oncotic pressure (colloid osmotic pressure) is greater within capillary. This serves as an absorbing force.

Table 20-4. Causes of edema according to underlying physiologic mechanism

Fluid pressure	Oncotic pressure
Increased capillary fluid pressure	*Decreased capillary oncotic pressure*
Increased venous pressure	Loss of serum protein
Vein obstruction	Burns, draining wounds, fistulas
Varicose veins	Hemorrhage
Thrombophlebitis	Nephrotic syndrome
Pressure on veins from casts, tight bandages, or garters	Chronic diarrhea
Increased total volume with decreased cardiac output	Decreased production of protein
Congestive heart failure	Malnutrition (kwashiorkor)
Fluid overloading	Cirrhosis of liver
Sodium and water retention: increased aldosterone due to	*Increased interstitial oncotic pressure*
Decreased renal blood flow	Increased capillary permeability to protein
Congestive heart failure	Burns
Renal failure	Inflammatory reactions
Increased production of aldosterone	Trauma
Cushing's syndrome	Infections
Aldosterone added to system	Allergic reactions (hives)
Corticosteroid therapy	Blocked lymphatics: decreased removal of tissue fluid and protein
Inability to destroy aldosterone	Malignant diseases
Cirrhosis of liver	Surgical removal of lymph nodes
	Elephantiasis

lary membrane, creating a change in the interstitial fluid pressure until an equilibrium is reached again.*

Etiology. Edema was defined earlier as an accumulation of fluid in the interstitial spaces creating a positive fluid pressure. Thus edema can be produced by any of the following: increase in capillary fluid pressure, decrease in capillary oncotic pressure, increase in interstitial oncotic pressure, and any condition that increases the amount of aldosterone circulating in the blood. Causes of edema with clinical examples are shown in Table 20-4.

The same mechanisms that create edema in the interstitial spaces can create fluid collection in *potential fluid spaces,* spaces between two membranes that normally contain only traces of fluid. The main potential fluid spaces are *intrapleural* (lung and chest wall), *pericardial* (heart and pericardial sac), *peritoneal* (intestines and abdominal wall), and joint capsules. The symptoms of fluid collection in these spaces are caused by the pressure of the collected fluid on adjoining organs or walls. Large amounts of fluid can collect in an operative site and in tissues surrounding an injury. Fluid that collects in the intrapleural space is termed *pleural effusion,* and in the pericardial space, *pericardial effusion.* Fluid high in protein and electrolytes that accumulates in the peritoneal space is termed *ascites.* An accumulation of fluid in all body tissues is a generalized edema or *anasarca.*

Overloading of the vascular system with fluid causes an increase in the hydrostatic pressure of the blood, resulting in generalized tissue edema. More important, if the increase in hydrostatic pressure is great enough, large amounts of fluid will be pushed across the alveolar-capillary membrane into the alveoli of the lungs. *Pulmonary edema* can occur unless it is rapidly treated and the process reversed.

Overloading of the vascular system may be caused by giving too much fluid within a short period of time to a person who, because of circulatory or renal disease, cannot dispose of the surplus. Infants and young children can also be overloaded easily because they normally have little extravascular fluid reserve. Elderly people tolerate increases in blood volume very poorly, since with inelastic vessels only relatively small increases in volume are needed to markedly increase the hydrostatic pressure.

---

*For example, a decrease in capillary oncotic pressure to 16 mm could produce the following (see Fig. 20-1):

$$17 - (x) = 16 - 4$$
$$17 - x = 12$$
$$x = 5 \text{ mm of interstitial fluid pressure}$$

Fluid would filter rapidly into the interstitial space until a pressure of 5 mm is reached. This would then effect a balance of 12 mm of fluid pressure gradient and 12 mm of oncotic pressure gradient.

Monitoring the central venous pressure is the best way to determine if overloading is occurring.

Overloading of the vascular system also may be caused by increasing the oncotic (pull) pressure of the intravascular fluid by giving proteins so rapidly that the body cannot dispose of those that are in excess of its need. This overloading causes fluids to be pulled into the intravascular compartment from other body fluid compartments. The blood volume increases rapidly, neutralizing the oncotic pressure but increasing the hydrostatic pressure of the vascular system and the oncotic pressure of the interstitial fluid compartment. Fluid is then pushed into the tissues. Overloading the vascular system is a risk when fluids such as plasma, plasma expanders, albumin, or blood are given to any patient regardless of age or state of health.

Prevention. The nurse is especially alert to overhydration whenever intravenous fluids are being given and should consider it in planning "forced fluid" regimens for these patients. Patients with renal or circulatory impairment can easily be overhydrated. Such patients usually must restrict fluid and sodium intake.

Any patient on a low sodium diet needs to know which foods to avoid. He should read labels on all prepared foods because many contain large amounts of sodium. He may need assistance in planning ways of adhering to a specified fluid restriction regimen. If medications are to be taken with minimal medical supervision over a period of time, the patient should know the purpose of each drug and its usual side effects. He should also record the fluid taken with medications, monitor his own weight daily at home, and notify his physician if there is a significant change.

Assessment. In general, weight gain is the best indicator of an extracellular volume excess, since several liters of fluid can be retained without visible evidence of edema. Because hydrostatic pressure in the capillaries is greatest at the lowest parts of the body, edema will collect in these areas. This is called *dependent* edema. When one is standing, or sitting with feet on the floor, edema develops in the ankles and feet; when in a supine position edema fluid collects in the sacral area of the back.

If a finger is pressed over an edematous area, the indentation made by the finger will remain briefly as the fluid is pushed to another area; this is called *pitting edema.* Fluid refills the interstitial space in the "pit" area gradually. A subjective measure is sometimes used to describe pitting edema on a scale from "one plus" (+) to "four plus" (++++), with the latter indicating severe pitting edema because it takes longer for fluid to move into the pit area. Skin over parts of the body with marked edema is usually tight, smooth, and shiny. It is cool and pale because of poor circulation. If edema is very severe, fluid will leak out of pores when the skin is pressed. This is called *weeping* edema.

Overhydration causes neck vein engorgement, so that these veins will appear distended even when the patient is in an upright position. Pulmonary edema is a medical emergency requiring rapid and knowledgeable treatment (see p. 1004). In pulmonary edema the symptoms are dramatic—the patient gasps for air, is anxious and frightened, has moist "gurgling" respirations, coughs up frothy sputum, and shows signs of cyanosis. The symptoms are related to the fact that the alveoli are filled with fluid and oxygen is unable to diffuse across the alveolar-capillary membrane.

Intervention. The treatment of edema depends on the condition that has caused it. Congestive heart failure is usually treated with digitalis, diuretics, and sodium and fluid restriction (p. 1003). Cirrhosis of the liver is also treated with diuretics and sodium and fluid restriction (p. 607), and renal failure requires severe restrictions of water and electrolytes (p. 1329).

Reducing sodium intake alone may reduce edema because the supply of body sodium is reduced, and that which remains appears to be needed to maintain isotonicity of the blood.

Malnutritional edema responds to adequate dietary intake, especially the addition of protein to the diet, unless the condition is far advanced, as occurs in starving children and adults in famine areas where kwashiorkor is a common cause of death. Edema associated with infection and burns resolves over time as the underlying cause responds to treatment.

Diuretics. Edema is often treated with diuretics that act on the kidneys. Thiazide diuretics, the most commonly used, inhibit reabsorption of sodium and chloride in the proximal renal tubules, thus promoting excretion of sodium and water, or *diuresis.* Potassium is usually lost along with sodium and water unless a potassium-sparing diuretic is used. Fluid and electrolyte imbalances are undesirable, but are rather common side effects of diuretic therapy. When diuretics are given, a large amount of fluid is lost from the vascular compartment, decreasing its hydrostatic pressure and causing fluid to be pulled back into it from the tissues.

Before excess fluid in the interstitial spaces can be excreted, it must be moved back into the vascular compartment, otherwise, diuresis causes serious vascular depletion. Table 20-5 shows some diuretics and their effects.

Excess fluid in the tissues results in poor cellular nutrition as cells are pushed further apart and away from capillaries. Normal exchange of nutrients and wastes is interrupted. Edematous tissues therefore are poorly nourished, susceptible to trauma and infection, and heal poorly.

Table 20-5. Common diuretics and their effect on fluid and electrolyte balance

Generic name	Trade name	Method of administration	Peak effect	Probable effects on fluid and electrolyte balance
Thiazides				
Chlorothiazide	Diuril	Oral	4 hours	Hyponatremia
				Hypokalemia
				↓ ECF volume
				Hyperglycemia
				Hyperuricemia
Hydrochlorothiazide	Esidrix HydroDiuril	Oral	3 to 4 hours	Hypomagnesemia
Loop diuretics (act mainly on ascending loop of Henle)				
Furosemide	Lasix	IM or IV	½ hour	Hypokalemia
				Hyperuricemia
		Oral	2 to 4 hours	↓ ECF volume
Ethacrynic acid	Edecrin	Oral	2 to 4 hours	Hyponatremia
		IV	½ hour	
Aldosterone antagonist (opposes potassium-losing action of aldosterone)				
Spironolactone	Aldactone	Oral	72 hours	Hyperkalemia Hyponatremia
Potassium-conserving action				
Triamterene	Dyrenium	Oral	4 to 8 hours	Hyperkalemia
Osmotic agent				
Mannitol	Osmitrol	IV infused over 24-hour period	—	Hyponatremia Hypochloremia ↑ ECF volume

Caution must be taken to protect edematous parts of the body from prolonged pressure, injury, and extremes of heat and cold. Skin over these parts should be kept well lubricated to prevent dryness. If edematous areas are exposed to extensive moisture from incontinence or perspiration, they should be kept dry to prevent maceration. When edema is caused by venous stasis, elevating dependent body parts and applying supportive stockings to the legs helps promote venous return. Extremities that become edematous as a result of surgery or trauma should also be elevated and supported.

■ ELECTROLYTE IMBALANCE

No single electrolyte can be out of balance without causing other electrolytes to be out of balance also. This fact should be kept in mind while reading this section.

Sodium, potassium, and calcium are all essential for the passage of nerve impulses. Whenever the concentrations of any of these cations are increased or decreased in body fluids, the increase or decrease is reflected in the nerve stimulation of muscles by nerves. The muscles may become weak and atonic because of inadequate stimulation, or they may become somewhat spastic because of excess stimulation. A decrease in calcium concentration in body fluids may cause the stimulus to be irregular, and muscle spasms result. Gastrointestinal and cardiac symptoms so often produced by electrolyte imbalances result in part from changes in neural stimulation of the muscles of these systems.

With cation imbalances, the distribution of body fluids frequently is upset. Abnormal collections of fluid may cause gastrointestinal symptoms such as nausea, vomiting, and diarrhea. Decreased amounts of fluid may cause anorexia, dyspepsia, and constipation, It is thought that edema of cerebral tissues may be responsible for headache, convulsions, and coma.

□ Sodium

The normal concentration of sodium in the blood is 138 to 145 mEq/liter. Sodium is the most prevalent cation in the extracellular fluid and controls the osmotic pressure of this compartment. It is essential for neuromuscular functioning, for many intracellular chemical reactions, and for helping to maintain acid-base bal-

Table 20-6. Comparison of serum sodium levels with total body sodium*

Condition	Serum sodium	Total body sodium
Edema (cardiac, renal, hepatic disease)	Low (hyponatremia)	High
Prolonged sweating	Low	Low
Diuretics and low sodium diets	Low	Low
Addison's disease	Low	Low
Edema (cardiac, renal, hepatic disease)	Normal	High
Excretion of dilute urine, early stages of GI sodium loss	Normal	Low
Excess oral or IV sodium intake	High (hypernatremia)	High
Water and sodium loss with water loss > sodium loss	High	Low

*Note that a low or high serum level does not necessarily correspond with the total body sodium.

ance in the body. The sodium gradient theory states that sodium must be present in order for glucose to be transported into cells.[18]

As previously mentioned, aldosterone causes reabsorption of sodium in the kidney tubules (p. 209). When sodium supply becomes low, renal loss of sodium drops to zero. Aldosterone does not greatly influence sodium *concentration*, however, because as sodium is reabsorbed, water is also reabsorbed in equal proportions.

Deficit

A low sodium level in the blood, *hyponatremia*, can result from either a sodium loss or a water excess.

Physiology. Sodium loss from the intravascular compartment causes fluid from the blood to diffuse into the interstitial spaces. As a result, the sodium in the interstitial fluid is diluted. In response to this reduction in sodium concentration in the extracellular fluid, potassium moves out of the intracellular fluid. Therefore the patient with sodium imbalance is also likely to have potassium imbalance.

The decreased osmolality of extracellular fluid that exists with sodium loss creates a condition similar to water excess; water moves into the cells by osmosis and leaves the extracellular compartment depleted. It differs from water intoxication because there is not an excess of total body water, but an intercompartmental movement of water and depletion of the extracellular compartment.

The laboratory test for plasma sodium does not always give an accurate indication of total body sodium. Some clinical conditions in which the level of serum sodium is not an accurate indicator of total body sodium can be seen in Table 20-6.

Etiology. Sodium depletion results most often from the loss of gastrointestinal secretions. This can occur through vomiting, diarrhea, gastrointestinal or biliary drainage, or fistulas. Symptoms of sodium depletion appear rapidly in patients with profuse ileostomy drainage. Diarrhea in infants is extremely dangerous. Infants normally have large sodium losses through the skin; therefore when large amounts of sodium are lost through the bowel as well, their sodium supply quickly becomes depleted. Sodium depletion can also occur in the shifting of body fluids so that the sodium and water are "trapped" in certain body areas and are not accessible for use. This can occur in massive edema, ascites, burns, or small bowel obstruction.

Anyone who is perspiring profusely because of climate, exercise, or fever is losing large amounts of both sodium and water. A form of chronic renal disease, "salt-wasting nephritis," also causes large daily losses of sodium ions. Sodium depletion caused by any of the above conditions is aggravated by a low sodium diet.

Prevention. Athletes and persons who work in very hot environments are advised to take salt tablets along with water or to ingest fluids containing sodium and to add some salty foods to their diets. If salt is not replaced with water, such as when thirst is quenched by drinking large amounts of tap water, water intoxication can occur. Diuretics such as the thiazides eventually may cause sodium depletion; therefore the patient who is receiving extensive diuretic treatment should be observed for symptoms of sodium depletion. Since many patients receiving diuretics are at home, they should be taught to report symptoms of sodium depeletion to the physician. These patients should not be on severely restricted sodium diets.

Assessment. The symptoms of sodium depletion are headache, muscle weakness, fatigue, apathy, postural hypotension, anorexia, nausea and vomiting, and abdominal cramps. In contrast to water excess, in which there is a weight gain, with sodium deficit there is a loss of weight. As the sodium loss becomes more severe, the increase in intracellular fluid and decrease in circulating blood volume produces symptoms of mental confusion, delirium, coma, and shock. If the onset of sodium depletion is rapid, shock can ensue quickly from the sudden decrease in blood volume.

Intervention. Treatment of shock, if present, is the first concern of the physician. Saline solution, usually 0.9% sodium chloride, is given intravenously at a rapid rate. Plasma expanders may also be infused.

If other electrolytes (potassium, calcium, bicarbonate) have been depleted, these also need to be replaced. Treatment that alleviates the underlying cause will prevent further sodium loss. Salt or salty foods are added to the diet for sodium depletion, which develops slowly or follows profuse perspiration (diaphoresis) or vomiting. (See Chapter 15 for a more detailed description of the treatment.)

Safety measures, such as the use of side rails on the bed, supervision of ambulation, and frequent observation, are necessary if the patient becomes weak, confused, or experiences marked hypotension.

Excess

A serum sodium level greater than 145 mEq/liter is known as *hypernatremia.* There are actually two kinds of sodium excess, edema or hypernatremia. When there is a sodium and water excess, edema exists; when there is an excess of sodium in relation to water in the extracellular compartment, hypernatremia exists. As seen in Table 20-6, hypernatremia does not necessarily indicate an excess of total body sodium.

Physiology. If sodium becomes concentrated in the extracellular fluid, osmolality rises, water leaves the cells by osmosis and enters the extracellular compartment to dilute fluids there, and the cells are water depleted. The presence of hypernatremia will suppress aldosterone secretion, and sodium will be excreted in the urine.

Etiology. Hypernatremia occurs when more water than sodium is lost from the body and sodium concentration in the blood rises. It can also result from an abnormally large oral intake of sodium, such as when a child accidentally eats many salt tablets, or when intravenous saline is infused so rapidly that the body cannot excrete the amount not needed.

Prevention. Sodium excess can be prevented in persons whose ability to excrete it is impaired. Persons with kidney failure, congestive heart failure, or increased aldosterone production need to have sodium intake restricted. Whenever intravenous electrolyte solutions are being given, the urinary output must be adequate so that portions of the electrolytes not needed by the body can be excreted. This usually means that fluid intake should not exceed urinary output.

Assessment. Hypernatremia causes dry, sticky mucous membranes, low urinary output, and firm, "rubbery" tissue turgor. If adequate fluid is not given to dilute the sodium, and if excretion of sodium is not increased, severe fluid and electrolyte imbalances will occur, and manic excitement, tachycardia, and eventual death will ensue.

Intervention. Water alone is given in the treatment of sodium excess. If cardiac and renal function are normal, liberal amount of water is administered orally or 5% dextrose in water is given intravenously. In the absence of normal cardiac and renal function, hydration must be carried out with caution to prevent fluid overloading in the patient.

Diuretics are of value in removing sodium. If sodium excess is severe, with or without excess water retention, and does not respond to other treatment, renal dialysis may be necessary.

□ Potassium

The normal concentration of potassium in the blood is 3.5 to 5.0 mEq/liter. Because most of the potassium in the body is intracellular, the serum potassium does not necessarily indicate the total body potassium content. Maintenance of serium potassium within normal range, however, is vital to normal body functions.

Potassium has a direct effect on the excitability of nerves and muscles, contributes most to the intracellular osmotic pressure, and helps maintain acid-base balance and normal kidney function. A potassium deficit is associated with excess alkalinity (alkalosis) of the body fluids, and a potassium excess accompanies an excess of acid (acidosis). These conditions are discussed later in this chapter.

Potassium is the major cation of the cells. During the formation of new tissues (anabolism) or when glucose is converted to glycogen, potassium enters the cell. With tissue breakdown (catabolism) such as occurs with trauma, dehydration, or starvation, potassium leaves the cell. The body conserves potassium less effectively than it conserves sodium, and the kidneys excrete potassium even when the body needs it. Normally about 5% of the total body potassium is excreted each day.

Deficit

A low serum potassium, below 3.5 mEq/liters, is known as *hypokalemia.*

Physiology. Movement of sodium (inward) and potassium (outward) across the cell membrane causes depolarization of the membrane and initiates an action potential creating nerve and muscle activity. When extracellular potassium is low, the resting membrane potential increases and the cell becomes less excitable. For this reason the major symptoms of hypokalemia are muscle weakness and atony.

Potassium is involved in acid-base balance because it

moves out of the cells when hydrogen ions move to the intracellular compartment in acidosis; therefore hyperkalemia accompanies acidosis. As the acidosis is treated, potassium moves back into the cells and hypokalemia may develop. In alkalosis, hypokalemia usually develops because of movement of potassium into cells and also because potassium is excreted by the kidneys while hydrogen ions are being retained.

Whenever sodium is being retained in the body through reabsorption by the kidney tubules, potassium is excreted. Thus whenever aldosterone secretion is increased such as in stress, potassium will be excreted. Potassium may also be lost in the urine when there is considerable urinary output and as a result of certain diuretics such as the thiazide derivatives, the latter being the most common cause of hypokalemia.

Etiology. The patient who has food withheld for several days, is dehydrated, or is given large amounts of parenteral fluids with no replacement of potassium develops potassium depletion. The parenteral administration of 5% dextrose in water without the addition of potassium tends to dilute the potassium in the extracellular tissues. This dilution, in addition to the lack of a balanced diet and to potassium loss caused by catabolism of body proteins, accounts for many instances of electrolyte imbalance in the postoperative patient. Patients who eat an inadequate diet, or take no food for an extended period of time, or those who are losing large amounts of

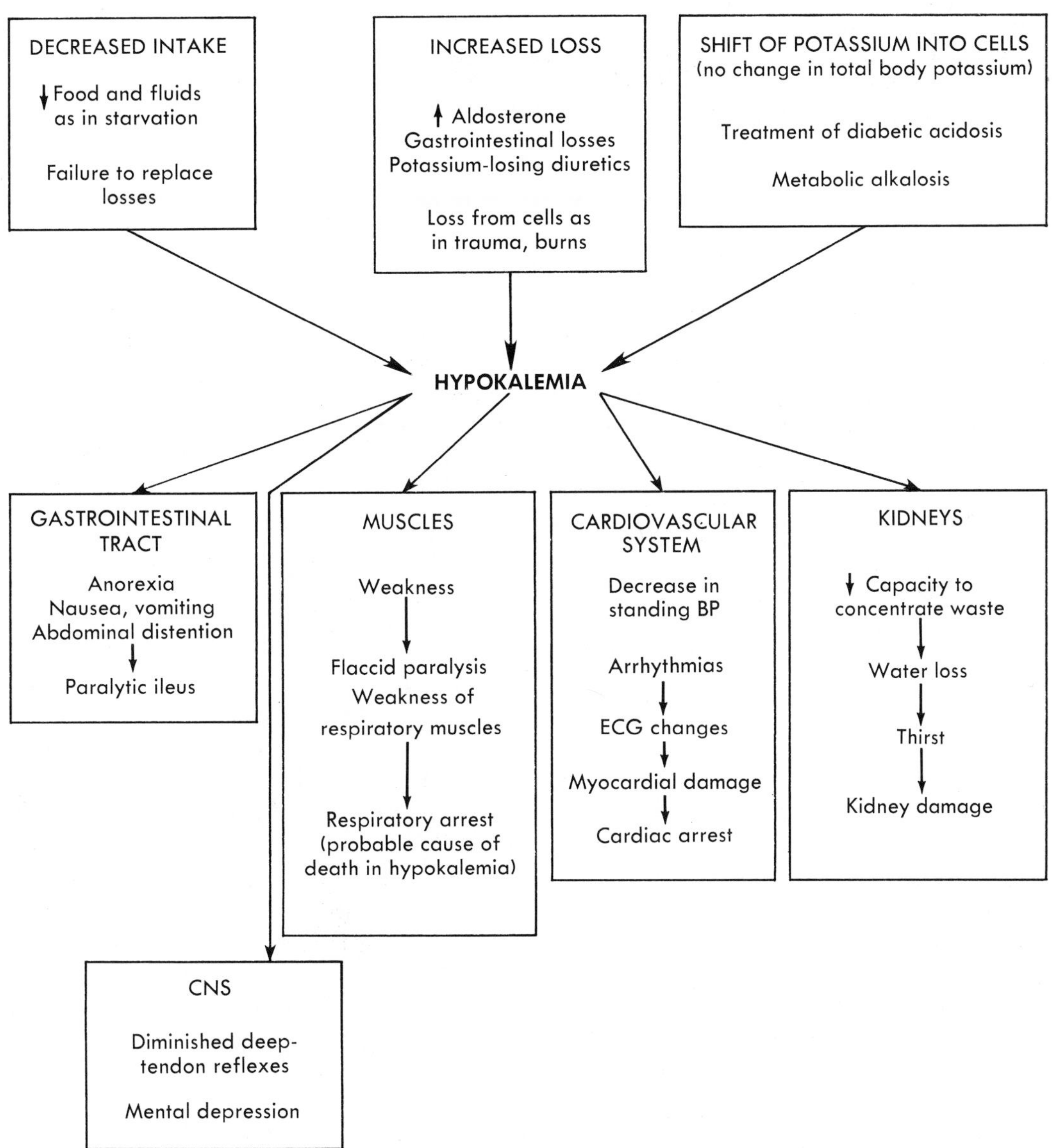

Fig. 20-2. Causes and effects of hypokalemia.

fluid from the gastrointestinal tract usually are given intravenous glucose solutions containing potassium.

The practice of giving multiple enemas is becoming much less common because it is now known that some of the enema fluid is absorbed through the bowel wall diluting the potassium in the interstitial compartment. Hypertonic enema solutions may damage cells in the bowel mucosa, causing potassium loss. Fig. 20-2 summarizes the causes and effects of hypokalemia.

Prevention. Hypokalemia can be prevented by being alert to the conditions that cause potassium depletion—vomiting, diarrhea, diuretics—and by monitoring the patient for early warning signs. If there is an order for enemas until results are clear, the nurse should not give more than three enemas to a patient without consulting the physician, since this treatment may result in water intoxication or potassium loss.

Assessment. The patient with potassium deficit will show characteristic electrocardiographic changes of flattened or inverted T waves with prolonged QT segments. (See p. 922 for discussion of a normal ECG.) The most striking symptom of hypokalemia is muscle weakness. Other symptoms are apathy, abdominal distention, and paralytic ileus.

Digitalis toxicity can occur in persons taking digitalis if they develop hypokalemia (p. 1007). If potassium deficit persists over a period of time, kidney and heart damage will result.

Intervention. With severe hypokalemia the patient may die unless potassium is administered promptly. The safest way to administer potassium is orally. Fresh fruits (especially oranges and bananas) or foods high in protein are good sources of potassium. When potassium is given intravenously, the rate of flow must be monitored closely in order to prevent hyperkalemia and atrial arrest. The usual rate of infusion should not exceed 20 mEq/liter of potassium per hour. Since potassium is irritating to the veins, it is given very diluted, usually 20 to 40 mEq/liter of intravenous solution.

Persons who are receiving potassium-losing diuretics (p. 306) should be instructed to include foods high in potassium in their diet (Table 20-7). If low serum potassium levels are shown to result from diuretic therapy, a potassium supplement may be ordered by the physician, usually in the form of potassium chloride (elixir of potassium chloride), or a potassium-sparing diuretic such as triamterene (Dyrenium) may be used. Persons taking diuretics at home should be taught to recognize symptoms of potassium depletion, such as muscle weakness, anorexia, nausea and vomiting, and to report these symptoms to the physician. Patients taking digitalis must be monitored carefully for toxicity, since hypokalemia enhances the action of digitalis preparations.

Excess

A serum potassium level greater than 5.0 mEq/liter is termed *hyperkalemia.* This condition does not occur as frequently as hypokalemia, especially if renal function is normal.

Physiology. Hyperkalemia in the extracellular fluid has the opposite effect from hypokalemia on the resting cell membrane. The membrane potential is decreased and the cell becomes more excitable. Potassium excess therefore causes nerve and muscle irritability. Severe hyperkalemia, however, soon leads to muscle weakness and flaccid paralysis.

Etiology. As previously stated, whenever there is severe tissue damage, potassium is released from the cells into the extracellular fluid. If it is not excreted quickly, hyperkalemia results.

Since shock often accompanies tissue damage, renal function is reduced, promoting hyperkalemia. There is great danger in giving extra potassium to any patient with poor renal function. If the patient is dehydrated or

Table 20-7. Good dietary sources of potassium

Beverages	Fruits	Vegetables*	Protein foods	Miscellaneous
Cocoa	Citrus fruits	Greens	Meat	Chocolate
Cola	Bananas	Tomatoes	Poultry	Nuts
Coffee	Melons	Potatoes	Fish	Molasses
Wine	Canned fruit juices (apple, grape, tomato)	Beans (lima, navy, kidney, chili)		
Milk	Dried fruits (dates, raisins, figs)	Winter squash		
Buttermilk		Carrots		

*Most raw vegetables contain potassium, but it is lost in the water during cooking.

has lost vascular fluid, glucose and water or plasma expanders usually are given until renal function returns. Untreated adrenal insufficiency also is a contraindication for giving potassium. If the patient who has potassium intoxication needs a blood transfusion, fresh blood must be used. Cells in blood that has been kept for several days tend to release potassium during storage. Administration of stored blood may increase the patient's blood potassium level still further. Fig. 20-3 shows the causes and effects of hyperkalemia.

Prevention. Hyperkalemia can be anticipated and prevented in patients who for any reason have a significant decrease in urinary output, especially if they are receiving oral or intravenous potassium preparations.

Assessment. The patient with potassium intoxication develops spasticity of muscles because of their overstimulation by nerve impulses. The patient complains of nausea, colic, diarrhea, and skeletal muscle spasms. The muscles later become weak because overstimulation produces an accumulation of lactic acid and because potassium is lost from the muscle cells.

If the condition is not controlled, overstimulation of the cardiac muscle will cause the heartbeat to become irregular and eventually stop. ECG evidence of potassium elevation includes tall, peaked, symmetric, or tented T waves with a short QT segment. As the blood potassium level increases further, the QRS complex spreads and atrial arrest occurs.[1]

Intervention. When potassium intoxication occurs, the patient is allowed nothing orally, and an infusion of 10% glucose with 50 units of insulin is often given to induce transfer of potassium from the serum to the intracellular fluid. If the patient is in a state of acidosis, correction of the acidosis will result in movement of potassium back into the cell (p. 328). Cation exchange resins such as sodium polystyrene sulfonate (Kayexalate) may also be given. If the patient is in acute renal failure, dialysis may be necessary. Calcium, given intravenously, will antagonize the effect of potassium on the heart.

The patient with potassium excess is placed on bed rest and receives complete nursing care until the potassium blood level returns to normal.

Patients who retain potassium secondary to renal failure or decrease in aldosterone will need instruction in restricting foods high in potassium (Table 20-7). If salt substitutes are being used, patients need to be aware that these usually contain potassium as a substitute for sodium.

Cation exchange resins act by exchanging other cations in the resin for potassium in the intestine; the potassium is then excreted in the stool. Maintenance of

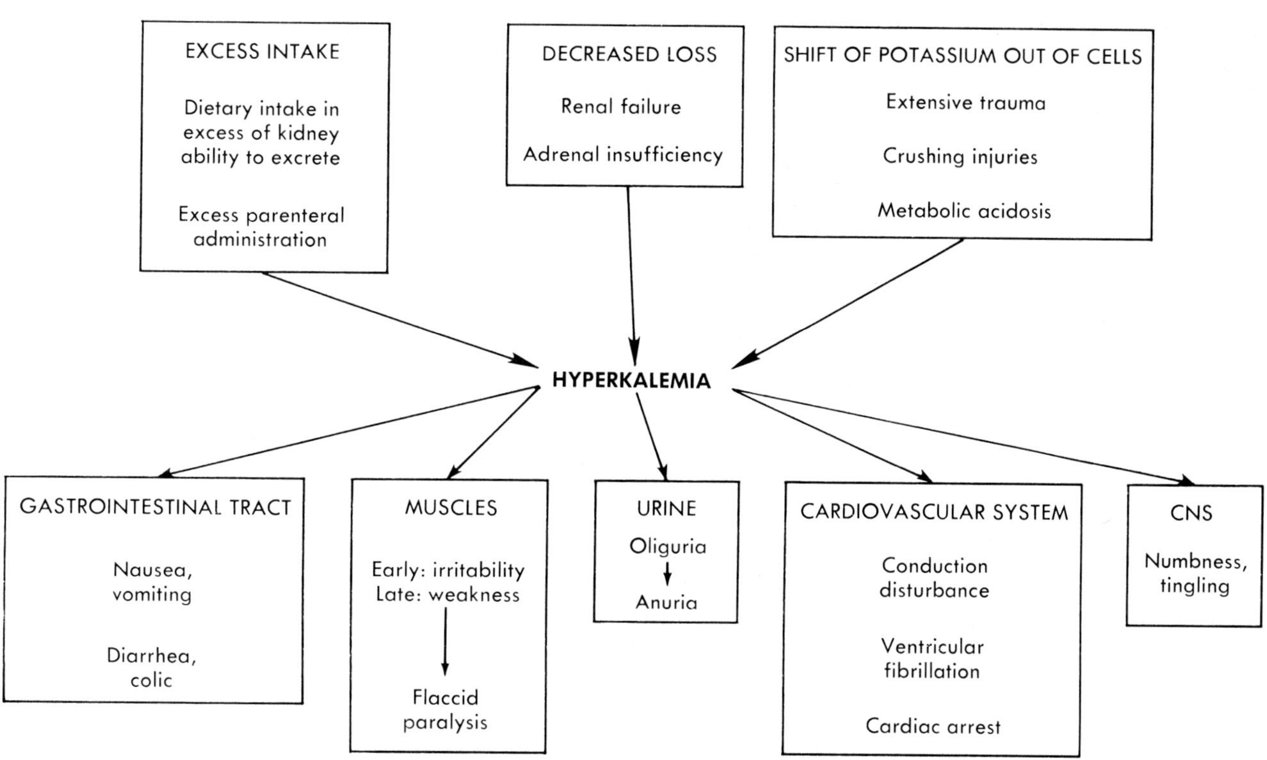

Fig. 20-3. Causes and effects of hyperkalemia.

good bowel function is necessary for this therapy to be effective.

☐ Calcium

The normal calcium level in the blood is 4.5 to 5.8 mEq/liter. Calcium in the blood is in two forms: ionized and bound to plasma proteins. Free, ionized calcium is needed for (1) blood coagulation, (2) smooth, skeletal, and cardiac muscle function, (3) nerve functions, and (4) bone and teeth formation. Only the ionized calcium is physiologically active. *Vitamin D* is necessary for absorption of calcium from the gastrointestinal tract and in mobilization of calcium from bones.

Both vitamin D and parathyroid hormone must be present for calcium absorption from the gastrointestinal tract (p. 552). Calcium is excreted principally through the gastrointestinal tract, with very small amounts being lost in the urine.

Deficit

Hypocalcemia is the decrease of serum calcium below 4.5 mEq/liter.

Physiology. It is thought that calcium ions line the pores of cell membranes. Since both calcium and sodium ions carry a positive charge, they tend to repel each other. The presence of calcium in the pores of cells (especially neurons), through which sodium must pass for depolarization to take place, has a blocking effect on this permeability to sodium. When calcium levels in the blood are low, this blocking effect is minimized, sodium moves more easily into the cell, and depolarization with resulting action potential takes place more readily[18] The result is increased excitability of the nervous system leading to muscle spasm, tingling sensations, and if severe, to convulsions and tetany. Skeletal, smooth, and cardiac muscle function are all affected by overstimulation.

Etiology. Calcium deficit results from inadequate intake, vitamin D deficiency, hypoparathyroidism, interruption of normal calcium absorption from the gastrointestinal tract, and excess loss of calcium through the kidneys.

Patients with pancreatic disease or disease of the small intestine may fail to absorb calcium normally from the gastrointestinal tract, and they may excrete large amounts of calcium in the feces. Persons with chronic pancreatitis have persistent hypocalcemia. Draining intestinal fistulas also cause excess calcium loss. These causes and effects are shown in Fig. 20-4.

Prevention. Calcium deficiency can be prevented by alertness to conditions of inadequate intake, excess calcium loss, or vitamin D deficiency. Patients who are on extremely poor diets or who have calcium-depleting conditions should be monitored for signs of hypocalcemia. Teaching persons with low calcium and vitamin D intake to include more of these nutrients in the diet is an important nursing action.

Assessment. Tetany is the most characteristic sign of severe hypocalcemia. The patient who has calcium deficiency usually complains first of numbness and tingling of the nose, ears, fingertips, or toes. If he is not given calcium at this time, painful muscular spasms, especially of the feet and hands (carpopedal spasm), muscle twitching, and convulsions may follow (tetany).

There are two tests used to elicit signs of calcium deficiency. *Trousseau's sign* is elicited by grasping the patient's wrist to constrict the circulation for a few minutes. If his hand goes into a position of palmar flexion (carpopedal spasm), he probably has a serious calcium deficit. *Chvostek's sign* is elicited by tapping the patient's face lightly over the facial nerve (just below the temple). A calcium deficit is probably present if the facial muscles twitch.

Intervention. The drug of choice in treating calcium deficiency is a 10% solution of calcium gluconate given slowly.[2] In milder cases, high calcium diet or oral calcium salts may be sufficient. When decreased parathyroid hormone or vitamin D are causative factors, these substances must be supplied. When the serum phosphorus level rises, the calcium level falls; aluminum hydroxide gel can be given to lower a high serum phosphorus concentration.

Any patient who has had thyroid surgery must be watched very closely for symptoms of calcium deficiency (tetany), since there is a possibility that parathyroid glands may have been inadvertently removed with the thyroid tissue or may be temporarily suppressed by local edema.

Since chronic hypocalcemia can result in loss of calcium from bone to replenish low serum calcium, persons with this condition must be carefully moved, turned, or ambulated to prevent fractures of the demineralized bone. Calcium preparations must be given with caution to cardiac patients, since calcium has an effect on the heart similar to digitalis.

Excess

Serum calcium above 5.8 mEq/liter is called *hypercalcemia.*

Physiology. The blocking effect of calcium on cell membrane permeability, as previously discussed, is accentuated in the presence of high serum calcium levels. Nerve and muscle activity is depressed. The activity of cardiac muscle is depressed, gastrointestinal motility decreases, and skeletal and smooth muscles become fatigued. Deep tendon reflexes are decreased or absent.[45]

When a person is immobilized for any reason, cal-

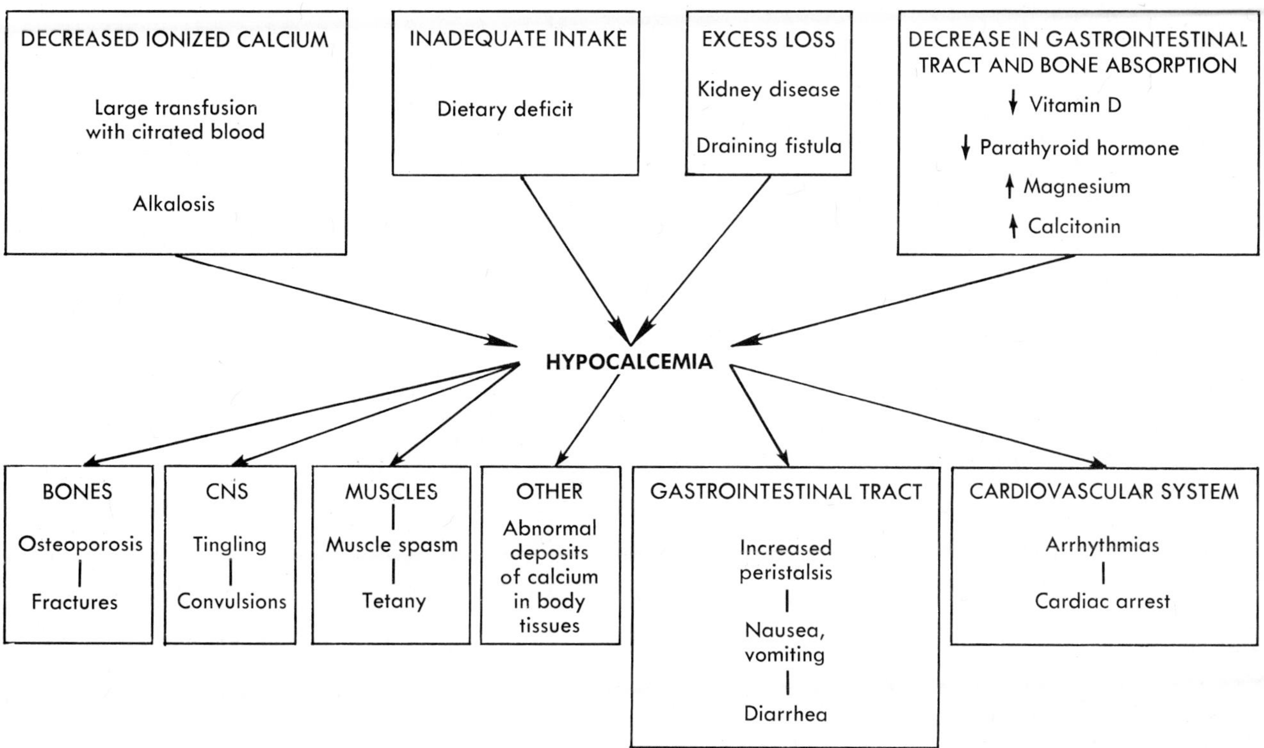

Fig. 20-4. Causes and effects of hypocalcemia.

cium leaves the bone and concentrates in the extracellular fluid. Normal retention of calcium in the bones is believed to be caused by the pressure exerted on bones by active movement or exercise. When a large amount of calcium accumulates in the extracellular fluid and passes through the kidneys, calcium can precipitate and form stones (calculi), a not infrequent complication of immobilization.

Calcium precipitates more readily in alkaline solution. This can be a problem in a urinary tract infection, which increases the alkalinity of the urine, since renal calculi are more likely to be formed. Metastatic carcinoma, multiple myeloma, hyperparathyroidism, and other diseases with extensive bone involvement also produce marked hypercalcemia.

Etiology. Hypercalcemia can result from excessive intake of calcium, especially in milk and absorbable calcium-containing antacids (milk-alkali syndrome), from excessive vitamin D intake, and from conditions that promote release of calcium from the bones into the extracellular fluid. These causes and their effects are shown in Fig. 20-5.

Prevention. Hypercalcemia can be alleviated in persons who are immobilized by helping them to exercise muscles in uninvolved parts of the body. A tilt table may be used to put a patient who is unable to stand unassisted in an upright, weight-bearing position so as to provide pressure on the bones. Patients who are immobilized in a back-lying position should be encouraged to use a trapeze bar, and all patients who are able should move about as much as possible and, with the use of side rails and other means, engage in activities that require muscle action.

Assessment. The patient with hypercalcemia commonly complains of severe thirst and has polyuria. Gastrointestinal symptoms, including anorexia, nausea, vomiting, and constipation, may also develop. Without treatment the patient may become lethargic and confused, and he may become comatose. There may be deep bone pain and roentgenographic evidence of bone cavitation.

Hypercalcemia crisis is an emergency condition that is signaled by intractable nausea and vomiting, dehydration, stupor, coma, and azotemia.[35]

Intervention. The only definitive treatment is removal of the cause. Because calcium excretion is promoted by excretion of sodium, hypercalcemia is treated with intravenous saline and a diuretic (furosemide). If this treatment fails, inorganic phosphate preparations given orally or intravenously may be effective. Mithramycin (Mithracin), a potent antitumor drug, has been used successfully to reduce serum calcium.

Because persons with marked hypercalcemia often are losing calcium from their bones or have malignant

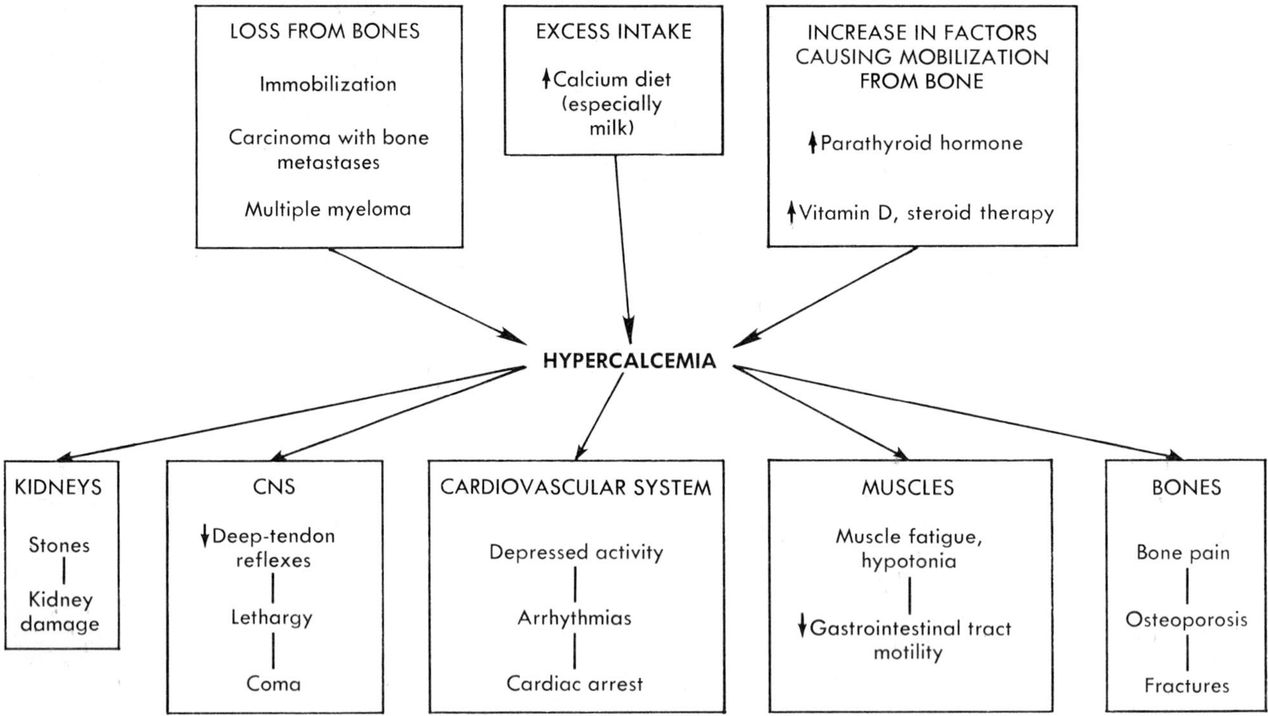

Fig. 20-5. Causes and effects of hypercalcemia.

involvement of bone, special care should be taken to prevent pathologic fractures. Even the pressure used in giving a back rub must sometimes be avoided.

Careful attention must be directed to the prevention of calcium stone formation in the kidneys. Acid-ash fruit juices, cranberry and prune juice, or ascorbic acid can be given to promote urinary acidification and discourage stone formation. Urinary tract infections must be avoided. Good perineal care and meticulous technique in inserting and caring for Foley catheters are mandatory.

Unless contraindicated, persons with hypercalcemia are encouraged to drink 3,000 to 4,000 ml of fluids per day to reduce the possiblity of renal calculi and to overcome the thirst that accompanies hypercalcemia.

□ Magnesium

The normal serum magnesium is within the range of 1.5 to 2.5 mEq/liter. About 50% of magnesium is located in bones, 5% in extracellular fluid, and the remaining 45% is in the intracellular compartment. It functions in the activation of enzymatic reactions, especially in carbohydrate metabolism. Magnesium has a sedative effect on the central nervous system similar to that of calcium. It has been used successfully to prevent convulsions in toxemia of pregnancy. High serum levels result in vasodilation with lowering of blood pressure.

Deficit

Hypomagnesemia is a serum magnesium level below 1.5 mEq/liter.

Physiology. A low serum magnesium level leads to increased neuromuscular irritability by increasing acetylcholine release, increasing the sensitivity of the myoneural junction to acetylcholine, diminishing the threshold of excitation of the motor nerve, and enhancing the force of contraction of the myofibril.[27]

In the presence of a large amount of calcium in the gastrointestinal tract, calcium is absorbed in preference to magnesium and the magnesium is excreted. Conversely, low calcium levels increase magnesium absorption. The kidneys effectively conserve magnesium when intake is low. Hypocalcemia and hypokalemia that are unresponsive to therapy may indicate hypomagnesemia.[13] Metabolically, magnesium is closely interrelated with both calcium and potassium.

Etiology. Hypomagnesemia may be caused by impaired absorption from the gastrointestinal tract, excess loss through the kidneys, or prolonged malnutrition states. Fig. 20-6 shows some of the causes and effects of magnesium deficit.

Prevention. Dietary teaching and management can help to prevent magnesium deficit, especially in persons with magnesium-depleting conditions. Fruits, green

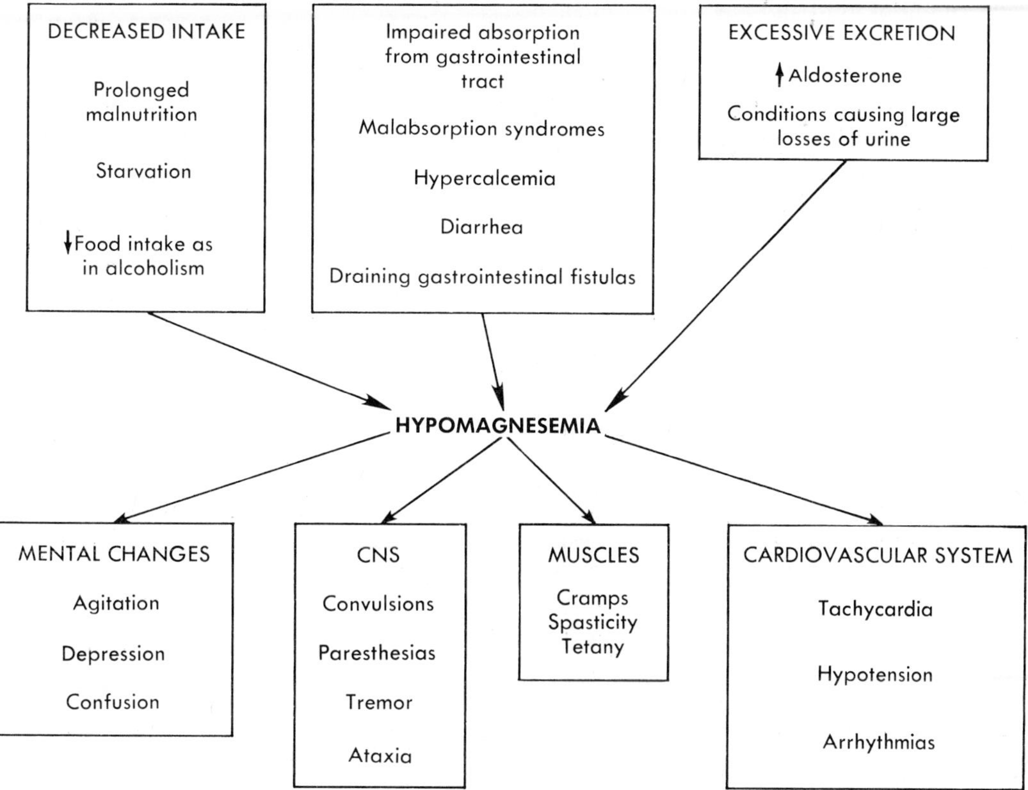

Fig. 20-6. Causes and effects of hypomagnesemia.

vegetables, whole grain cereals, milk, meats, and nuts are good dietary sources of magnesium.

Assessment. Hypomagnesemia is usually manifested by behavioral and neurologic symptoms such as confusion, hallucinations, convulsions, increased reflexes, tremors, muscle spasms, and paresthesias.

Intervention. Treatment of magnesium deficit consists of correction of the underlying cause and the administration of magnesium salts orally or parenterally. Providing for patients' safety until the magnesium deficit is corrected is the prime nursing responsibility. Careful observation and supervision of the patient who is confused or hallucinating and protective measures for patients who develop convulsions will prevent injury.

Excess

Hypermagnesemia is a serum magnesium level greater than 2.5 mEq/liter. The action of magnesium is on the myoneural junction where a high magnesium level blocks acetylcholine release, decreasing the excitability of the muscle cells. Hypermagnesemia seldom develops unless there is renal failure, although it has been identified in diabetic ketoacidosis where there is severe water loss. In persons with renal failure, frequent use of magnesium-containing antacids or cathartics can cause toxicity.

Assessment. The vasodilating effect of magnesium is accentuated in hypermagnesemia and can lead to hypotension. A very high magnesium level can cause loss of deep tendon reflexes, respiratory depression, and cardiac arrest.[13]

Intervention. Correction of the underlying cause will correct the magnesium excess. If renal failure is present, dialysis will be necessary. Intravenous calcium gluconate may be a useful temporary treatment, since calcium has an antagonistic effect on magnesium.

■ ASSESSMENT OF FLUID AND ELECTROLYTE IMBALANCE

The nurse needs to recognize the symptoms of fluid and electrolyte imbalance and make ongoing physical assessments of those patients who have a potential for fluid and electrolyte imbalances (Table 20-8). For subjective data such as headache, thirst, nausea, or dyspnea, time of onset and extent of symptoms are ascertained. Objective data can be compared to baseline assessments made at the time of the patient's entry into the health system.

Data of particular importance in assessing fluid and electrolyte imbalance are comparison of fluid intake to output and changes in the patient's weight. Acutely ill medical patients and patients undergoing major surgery

Table 20-8. Assessment of fluid and electrolyte imbalance

	Fluid excess	Fluid loss/electrolyte imbalance
Behavior	Change in behavior, confusion, apathy	Change in behavior, confusion, apathy
Head, neck	Facial edema, distended neck veins	Headache, thirst, dry mucous membranes
Upper gastro-intestinal	Anorexia, nausea, vomiting	Anorexia, nausea, vomiting
Skin	Warm, moist, taut, cool feeling where edematous	Dry, decreased turgor
Respiration	Dyspnea, orthopnea, productive cough, moist breath sounds	Changes in rate and depth of breathing
Circulation	Tire easily, loss of sensation in edematous areas, pallor*	Pulse rate changes, arrhythmias
Abdomen	Increased girth, fluid wave	Distention, abdominal cramps
Elimination	Oliguria, constipation, scrotal edema	Oliguria, diarrhea, constipation
Extremities	Dependent edema "pitting," discomfort from weight of bedclothes	Muscle weakness, tingling, tetany

*Pallor-edema decreases the intensity of skin color by decreasing the distance between the skin surface and the pigmented or vascular areas. In the dark-skinned individual, pallor is observed by absence of underlying red tones that give brown and black skin "glow." The brown skin appears more yellow-brown and the black skin appears more ashen gray.[41]

should have their fluid intake and output and daily weight closely monitored. If patients and families are given explanations, they can participate, when appropriate, in measuring and recording the intake and output. Totaling the fluid intake and output every hour, every 8 hours, or every 24 hours gives the nurse and physician additional data for determining if the patient may have a fluid imbalance.

Since symptoms of fluid and electrolyte imbalance are sometimes not very specific, a good rule is to be alert for any changes in behavior, level of consciousness, vital signs, skin turgor, muscle strength, and mucous membranes. Baseline observations made during the first encounter with a patient are essential for comparison with subsequent observations in order to be able to detect changes.

□ Intake record

The intake record should show the type and amount of all fluids the patient has received and the route by which these were administered. This includes fluids given orally, parenterally, rectally, or fluids administered by tubes. A record of solid food intake is sometimes necessary, especially with very young children. Foods that are eaten in a semisolid state but which are basically liquid, such as gelatin or ice cream, are recorded as fluids. Ice chips are recorded by dividing the amount of chips by one-half (60 ml of chips would equal 30 ml of water). Patients may receive a considerable amount of fluid intake through the frequent sucking of ice chips.

□ Urinary output

Urinary output should be recorded as to time and amount of each voiding. If renal function is a major concern, as in a severely burned patient, an indwelling catheter is used so that the amount of urinary drainage can be recorded every hour and fluid intake regulated accordingly. It has been said that nothing is more difficult to obtain in a modern hospital than an accurate record of urine output, and unfortunately this statement is often true. Conspicuous signs posted on the patient's chart and in the utility room and bathrooms will help to prevent the discarding of urine before it is measured. Flow sheets kept close to the patient's room facilitate the recording of intake and output and other patient data.

□ Wound drainage

All drainage from body orifices or artificial openings should be measured. This would include such drainage as that from an ileostomy, from a T tube following exploration of the common bile duct, or from any catheter draining a surgical area. If there is excessive drainage from a wound, it may be necessary to weigh the dressings. Fluid loss is the difference between the wet weight and the dry weight of the dressing.

□ Gastrointestinal output

Vomitus, gastrointestinal drainage, and liquid stools should be measured as accurately as possible and should be described as to color, content, and odor. Gastric secretions are watery, a pale yellowish green, and usually have a sour odor. However, if the acid-base balance has been upset, gastric secretions may have a fruity odor because of the presence of ketone bodies (acetone). Bile is somewhat thicker than gastric juice and may vary from bright yellow to dark green in color. It has a bitter taste and acrid odor. Intestinal contents vary from dark green to brown in color, are likely to be quite thick, and have a fecal odor. The amount of fluid retained during irrigation of nasogastric tubes is added to "intake" and needs to be subtracted from total drainage before it is recorded.

It is difficult to determine accurately the amount of water lost in the stools, but a description of their consistency and a record of the number of stools passed gives a good estimate. The color of stools is also recorded. Because infants are likely to lose large amounts of water in their stools, daily records usually are kept for any baby who is ill.

□ Other output

Fluid aspirated from any body cavity such as the abdomen (paracentesis) or pleural spaces (thoracentesis) must be measured. The fluid contains not only electrolytes and water but also proteins. Blood loss from any part of the body should be measured carefully.

Diaphoresis is difficult to measure without special laboratory equipment; however, it may be important to estimate the loss of fluid by this route in some patients. Careful note of "excessive" perspiration and its duration is made. If the clothing and linen become saturated, dry and wet weights may be taken. Accurate recording of body temperature helps the physician to determine how much fluid should be replaced, since fluid loss through the skin and lungs increases as the temperature rises. A patient with a high fever and who is breathing rapidly can lose as much as 2,500 ml/day through the lungs.[16]

□ Daily weight

The daily weight record is often the best way to determine the onset of dehydration or the accumulation of fluid either as generalized edema or as "hidden" fluid in body cavities. An increase of 1 kg in weight is equal to the retention of 1 liter (1,000 ml) of fluid in the edematous patient. If the weight record is to be accurate, the patient must be weighed on the same scale and at the same hour each day, and he must be wearing the same amount of clothing. Circumstances that may affect the weight should be kept as nearly identical as possible from day to day. Usually weights are taken in the early morning before the patient has eaten or defecated, but after he has voided. When extremely accurate measurements are needed, all clothing and even wound dressings are removed from the patient before he is weighed. A person maintained on intravenous fluids alone can be expected to lose approximately 0.5 kg a day (p. 206).

□ Laboratory values

Laboratory determinations of serum levels of the specific electrolytes help in making decisions concerning electrolyte excesses or deficits. When there is water excess, hemodilution will occur and the hematocrit and electrolyte levels will be decreased. With excessive fluid loss there will be hemoconcentration, and the hematocrit and electrolyte levels will be increased.

■ REPLACEMENT AND MAINTENANCE OF WATER, ELECTROLYTES, AND NUTRIENTS

Replacement of the water and electrolyte losses from the body and the necessary daily intake of these substances and other nutrients is usually accomplished by one of the following methods: (1) oral intake, (2) tube feeding (gavage), (3) intravenous infusion, (4) parenteral hyperalimentation, and (5) hypodermoclysis.

The best way to administer water, electrolytes, and nutrients is to give them orally. When fluids can be tolerated by the stomach but cannot be swallowed, a nasogastric tube may be passed, and fluids containing all the essentials of a balanced diet may be given through it. Normal saline solution or plain water also may be given by slow drip through the tube to replace fluid loss and provide for daily fluid needs.

If it is not possible for a patient to take food or fluid through the alimentary tract, the most common method of replacement is by intravenous infusion. In adults a vein in the leg or arm is commonly used, but in infants a vein in the scalp or the femoral or jugular vein may be used. An intravenous infusion may be given by introducing a needle or intracatheter into a vein and taping the needle in place or by making an incision (cutdown) and threading a polyethylene catheter (intracatheter) into the vein. The intracatheter is the method of choice for parenteral hyperalimentation in which a concentrated nutrient solution is infused into the superior vena cava.

Physiologic solutions of sodium chloride or solutions containing other electrolytes may be administered into subcutaneous tissues *(hypodermoclysis)*, although this method is performed less frequently than in the past. Infants and young children also may be given fluid intraperitoneally.

Fluids given by any route should be spaced throughout the 24-hour period. Not only does this practice help to maintain normal body fluid levels, but it also provides for better regulation of the electrolyte balance by the kidneys and prevents the end products of metabolism and toxic materials from being excreted in concentrated form. In this way the danger of renal damage, formation of calculi, and irritation of the lower urinary tract is reduced. In addition, fluid spacing prevents overloading of the circulation, which may result in dilution of body fluids, with resultant fluid and electrolyte shifts, the most serious of which causes pulmonary edema (p. 304).

Concentrated solutions of sugar or protein should always be given slowly and in small amounts at a time because they require body fluids for dilution. Hypertonic saline solutions may cause fluid to diffuse from the tissues to equalize the concentrations of salt in the vascular compartments; therefore it too should be given slowly and in small amounts. The superior vena cava is the preferred site for infusions of hypertonic solutions given by parenteral hyperalimentation because of the rapid dilution by the larger amount of blood at this site. If any of these concentrated solutions flow too rapidly into the vascular system, pulmonary edema can develop.

Giving concentrated solutions rapidly and in large amounts into the alimentary tract causes the blood volume to drop, and if large amounts of fluid are needed to dilute the substance, irreversible shock can result. The "dumping syndrome," which sometimes occurs after a gastric resection (p. 1214), is caused by this abnormal shift of fluid. Concentrated solutions sometimes are given intentionally to reduce cerebral edema (p. 673). Giving large amounts of fluid either orally or parentally is potentially dangerous even in a healthy person, and therefore fluids of any kind should never be replaced faster than they are lost.

The size of the patient should be considered when administering fluids. The small adult normally has less fluid in each body compartment, especially in the intravascular system. He therefore becomes seriously dehydrated more quickly than a larger adult and needs his fluid losses replaced more promptly. Prompt replacement is even more important in infants and young children. Because so much of their body fluid normally is extracellular, they have proportionately less reserve fluid in the cells from which to pull than has a small adult (see Table 15-1). People with small or inelastic vascular systems also become overhydrated easily. It is important to remember that the vascular system of a person who has had a large portion of his body such as a limb removed either by surgery or trauma is not the same size as previously.

□ Oral intake

Adults who have no circulatory or renal malfunction usually are given between 2,500 and 3,000 ml/day. Precautions should be taken so that the overzealous patient does not drink too much fluid in a day or that he does not take too much (3 to 4 glasses) at one time. Excessive water intake may cause water intoxication.

Many persons, when ill, find it difficult to eat or drink even though they are allowed to do so. There are many ways that the nurse can help the patient take adequate food and fluids orally and thus avoid the need for parenteral fluids. Fruit drinks, tea, coffee, ginger ale, or other soft drinks may be substituted for part of the water. Soup, bouillon, milk, eggnog, and cocoa provide both fluid and nutrients. Juicy fruits and other semisolid foods with a high fluid and nutrient content, such as custard, ice cream, or gelatin, may be more palatable than regular meals and tap water. Care must be taken, of course, that any substitutions are allowed on the diet prescribed for the patient. If a fluid record is needed, the amount of fluid given in semisolid form is estimated and recorded. A juicy orange, for example, contains about 50 ml of fluid.

The methods used in presenting food and fluids to patients may influence their consumption; often a small amount of either food or fluid offered at frequent intervals is more acceptable than is a large amount presented less often. Serving foods that the patient likes may improve his appetite. For example, carbonated beverages may be better tolerated by patients who are nauseated. Consideration should always be given to the cultural and aesthetic aspects of eating.

Vomiting and diarrhea are common symptoms of many illnesses, and most people suffer from them from time to time. Sodium and some potassium are lost in vomiting and diarrhea, while chloride is lost only in vomitus. As soon as fluids are tolerated, the patient who has vomiting or diarrhea should be served salty broth and tea or another fluid high in potassium (see Table 20-7) in order to replace the losses. This measure often keeps the patient from feeling so weak and exhausted. Dry soda crackers often are tolerated when fluids are not and can be used to replace sodium. Prompt replacement of both water and electrolytes is essential in infants, since they have limited reserves. If vomiting or diarrhea persist for even a few hours and oral foods are not tolerated, infants should have medical attention, since they may need intravenous replacement of losses.

A patient with a draining fistula from any portion of the gastrointestinal tract loses sodium, calcium, and some potassium. It is important that his diet be supplemented. Extra milk will replace all the losses, and the patient should be instructed to increase his milk intake somewhat above normal levels. For the body to use the calcium, vitamin D also must be available, but most milk is now fortified with vitamin D. Persons with a permanent fistulous opening, such as an ileostomy, need to be especially careful to supplement sodium and potassium when vomiting, diarrhea, or fever add to their already unusually large loss of electrolytes.

The nurse needs to know which foods contain large and small amounts of various essential nutrients, minerals, and vitamins (see Chapter 51). When losses must be restored, the patient needs more than is required in the usual adequate diet. It is especially important to know which foods and fluids are high or low in potassium and sodium and which foods are complete proteins. Bananas, citrus fruits, all fruit juices, many fresh vegetables, coffee, and tea are relatively high in potassium and low in sodium content. Salty broths and tomato juice provide extra sodium but have a high potassium content. Meat, milk, and eggs are all complete protein foods and contain relatively large quantities of both sodium and potassium. Current nutrition literature and the dietitian or nutritionist should be consulted as necessary.

The nurse frequently has an order to "force fluids." Since the amount required depends on the size of the patient, the amount of fluid loss, and the patient's circulatory and renal status, no standard amount can be given. The nurse must therefore make a judgment as to the desirable amount and inform members of the nursing team or family members who will care for the patient. If there is any question, the physician is consulted.

If an elderly person living at home complains of pronounced weakness without apparent cause, the nurse should ask whether he has been taking cathartics or enemas. If so, stopping this procedure, eating foods with high sodium and potassium content, and increasing the fluid intake may relieve the symptoms. Methods to combat constipation without purging should be taught.

Any patient with renal or circulatory impairment, as may occur in shock, cardiac decompensation, or constriction of blood vessels because of disease, may develop electrolyte imbalance. Sodium and water may be held in the tissues, the potassium level of the blood may rise, acidosis may develop from inadequate tissue oxygenation, or the kidneys may be unable to excrete waste products properly. The nurse should instruct patients with cardiac and renal impairment to avoid taking too much food containing sodium, potassium, or bicarbonate.

☐ Gavage (feeding by tube)

Water, a physiologic solution of sodium chloride, high protein liquids, or a regular diet that has been passed through a blender and diluted are often given by gavage to older children and adults (see Chapter 53). As previously mentioned, high-protein tube feeding can cause water deficit through osmotic diuresis. A need to increase water intake along with the tube feeding should be considered when (1) the patient complains of thirst; (2) protein content of the tube feeding is high; (3) the patient has a fever; (4) urine output is decreased or very concentrated; and (5) signs of water deficit develop.[28]

☐ Parenteral fluids

The nurse needs to know the common solutions used parenterally (Table 20-9). A solution of 5% dextrose in distilled water is often used to maintain fluid intake or to reestablish blood volume. Ascorbic acid and vitamin B (Solu-B) are frequently added. Dextrose, 5%, in saline solution may be given depending on the serum levels of sodium, and potassium chloride may be added to meet normal intake needs of potassium and to replace losses. A physiologic solution of sodium chloride is given primarily when sodium chloride has been lost in large amounts such as in loss of gastrointestinal fluids or in burns. A one-sixth molar lactate solution may be ordered

Table 20-9. Solutions for intravenous use

	Contents of solutions								
	Cations (mEq/liter)					Anions (mEq/liter)			
Type of solution	Na^+	K^+	Ca^{++}	Mg^{++}	NH_4^+	Cl^-	HCO_3^- lactate	PO_4^-	Glucose (g/liter)
5% dextrose in water									50
10% dextrose in water									100
Normal saline (0.9%)	154					154			
3% saline	513					513			
Ringer's solution	147	4	4			155			
5% dextrose in Ringer's lactate	130	4	3			109	28		50
Ringer's lactate	130	4	3			109	28		
Ammonium chloride (0.9%)					170	170			
Sodium lactate 1/6 molar	167						167		
5% dextrose in 0.2% saline	34					34			50

when sodium, but not chloride, needs replacement; ammonium chloride solution may be used to replace chlorides when added sodium is undesirable. Balanced solutions containing several electrolytes may be used. Ringer's solution and lactated Ringer's solution are examples.

Body needs for carbohydrates may be partially met by giving fructose or 10% or 20% glucose in distilled water, but these solutions are hypertonic and require additional water for excretion.

Amino acid preparations (Aminosol) are seldom given by standard intravenous methods. Whole blood is the fluid of choice to replace blood loss, but plasma, 25% salt-poor albumin, or plasma volume expanders can be given to substitute for blood protein loss and are used to reestablish normal blood volume and prevent shock. Dextran is the most generally accepted plasma volume expander. It increases the oncotic pressure of the blood, thus increasing the reabsorption of fluid from interstitial spaces and increasing plasma volume. Low molecular weight dextran decreases the viscosity of the blood, allowing greater flow of blood through the capillaries; thus it is useful in treating cardiogenic, hemorrhagic, or septic shock (Chapter 15). It may cause a prolonged bleeding time and should not be used if renal disease with severe oliguria or anuria is present or during pregnancy.[16]

Nursing responsibilities

Intravenous fluids containing electrolytes should be run slowly to allow the body to regulate their use. The patient is watched carefully for untoward signs (excess of fluids or electrolytes). Increased serum potassium (hyperkalemia) can be particularly dangerous, since it may cause cardiac arrest. When solutions containing electrolytes are given, the nurse monitors the urinary output carefully, and reports any marked decrease in the amount to the physician. Because the kidneys select the ions needed and excrete surplus ones, a normal output is essential. If the nurse is planning the sequence of intravenous fluids, hydrating fluids such as one half strength physiologic solution of sodium chloride or glucose in water solution should be given first. Renal failure and untreated adrenal insufficiency are contraindications for the use of potassium. If these conditions are known or suspected to exist, the nurse should verify orders for its administration. Many physicians do not start intravenous therapy for the day until blood chemistry results have been reported.

Usually the rate of administration of fluids is ordered by the physician and will depend on the patient's illness, the kind of fluid given, and the patient's age. An infusion is rarely run at a rate faster than 4 ml/min. If it is given continuously or if it is given when there is impaired renal function or impaired cardiac function, it is rarely run faster than 2 ml/min. The usual rate for replacement of fluid loss is 3 ml/min. This rate allows time for the fluid to diffuse into the extracellular fluid compartments and avoids overloading the circulation or raising the blood volume high enough to produce a diuretic effect. The equipment used for fluid administration may have varying numbers of drops per milliliters, and the nurse needs to check the equipment being used to determine the rate of delivery, since it is not the drops per minute but the milliliters per minute that are important.

Nurses should question the advisability of the rather common practice of speeding up the rate of flow of solutions given intravenously primarily to complete the treatment at a specified time. Every nurse should recognize the initial signs of pulmonary edema (bounding pulse, engorged peripheral veins, hoarseness, dyspnea, cough, or pulmonary rales) and should observe closely for them in those patients who are receiving concentrated solutions, those who must be given any intravenous solution rapidly, and those whose age or physical condition makes them special risks. At the first signs of increased blood volume the rate of flow of the infusion should be reduced to a "keep open" rate or barely running at 5 to 6 drops/min and the physician notified. Special care needs to be taken in giving fluids to infants, elderly patients with circulatory impairment, patients whose hearts are decompensated, those with renal impairment, those who have had plasma shifts such as burned patients, and those with extensive tissue trauma from other causes. Patients whose plasma has shifted need to be watched especially carefully because after a few days the plasma tends to shift back suddenly from the interstitial tissue to the blood, producing an increase in blood volume with resulting pulmonary edema (p. 304).

It is imperative that the nurse check the labels of fluid bottles carefully for correctness of content and record accurately the fluids given. (For details of equipment and nursing techniques needed in parenteral fluid administration refer to a textbook on fundamentals of nursing.)

Patients who are receiving fluids intravenously are observed frequently so that symptoms indicating the need to slow down, speed up, or stop the infusion may be noted. The tissue at the site of the inserted needle is checked at intervals for signs of infiltration or inflammatory reaction. If infiltration occurs, the infusion should be stopped at once and plans made to restart it. Solutions containing potassium are very irritating, and extravasation may cause tissue necrosis. When dextran or other protein solutions are being given, the patient is observed for signs of anaphylactic reaction (apprehension, dyspnea, wheezing respirations, tightness of chest, itching, hypotension) (p. 196).

□ Parenteral hyperalimentation

Parenteral hyperalimentation, also known as total parenteral nutrition (TPN), is a method of giving highly concentrated solutions intravenously to maintain the nutritional purpose of protein synthesis (Fig. 20-7). Indications for this therapy are (1) major gastrointestinal diseases, fistulas, or inflammatory diseases; (2) extensive negative nitrogen balance such as occurs with major body burns, extensive wounds, or starvation; and (3) gastrointestinal side effects from radiation therapy.

The physician initiates the infusion by inserting an intracatheter either into the brachial artery and into the subclavian vein or directly into the subclavian vein and threading it through the innominate vein into the superior vena cava. The large amount of blood in the superior vena cava helps to dilute the highly concentrated solution rapidly and thus prevent phlebitis or vein occlusion. The jugular vein is preferred in infants for ease of insertion but is too close to hair-growing areas in adults (possibility of sepsis) and is more restricting of neck movements.

Experts recommend that the patient be taken to the

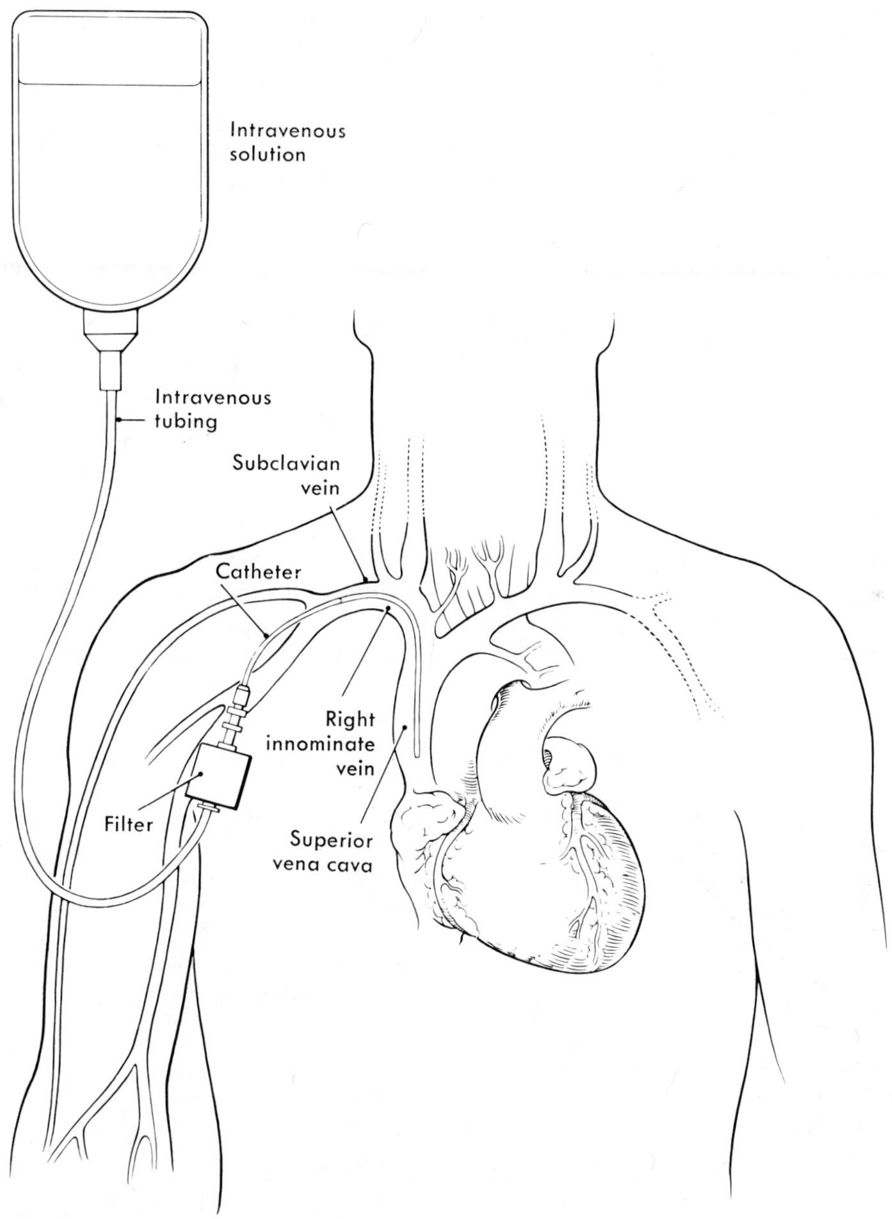

Fig. 20-7. Hyperalimentation showing catheter placed directly into subclavian vein and threaded into innominate vein and superior vena cava.

operating room for insertion of the intracatheter in order to maintain sterility. The insertion of the intracatheter is not painful, but the patient may experience a feeling of pressure. The intracatheter is sutured with one suture and covered by an air-occlusive dressing. The infusion is started with a standard intravenous fluid (5% dextrose) until a roentgenogram confirms the location of the catheter tip in the superior vena cava.

Solutions for parenteral hyperalimentation are good culture media and should be prepared under strict aseptic conditions, preferably in the pharmacy under a laminar airflow hood. The physician orders the solution contents based on the patient's nutritional needs. A sufficient amount of glucose to meet energy needs is necessary so that the amino acids are used for protein synthesis rather than for energy. The basic nutrient solution usually contains 20% to 25% glucose to which amino acids, minerals, electrolytes, and vitamins are added. The commercial preparations are relatively trouble free, but some patients do demonstrate sensitivity reactions (headache, fever, myalgia, chills, nausea and vomiting, rash, vasodilation, abdominal pain, convulsions).[7] Medication should *never* be given through the parenteral hyperalimentation line because of the need to maintain scrupulous aseptic conditions. Prepared solutions must be kept refrigerated and should be warmed to room temperature just prior to infusion.[7] Solutions should not be hung for longer than a 12-hour period.

Nursing responsibilities

Prevention of infection. Strict aseptic technique is mandatory during changing of bottles, tubings, or dressings. The nurse should be knowledgeable concerning the frequency and method of dressing changes being utilized. Some medical centers have a hyperalimentation team, and one nurse changes the dressings for all patients, usually three times weekly. The purpose of having only one nurse involved in changing the dressings is to assure consistency of technique and to reduce the chance of infection. If a dressing becomes wet, it is changed immediately to prevent transmission of bacteria by capillary action. The dressing should be air occlusive. Presence of an elevated temperature is reported immediately to the physician, and cultures are taken of the insertion site, tubing, and solutions for fungal as well as bacterial studies. Patients who experience itching under the dressing are cautioned not to scratch or disturb the dressing.

Prevention of air embolism. The possibility of air embolism is greater with use of the superior vena cava then with a peripheral vein because the decreased venous pressure as the blood approaches the heart can cause air to be sucked into the hyperalimentation tubing. All connections in the parenteral hyperalimentation set-up are taped to prevent accidental separation. Tubing changes are made quickly with the patient lying flat in bed. The patient may be asked to perform the Valsalva maneuver, forced expiration against a closed glottis, while the tube is disconnected.[7] Filters are useful for trapping air as well as bacteria.

Maintenance of fluid and electrolyte balance. The goal of parenteral hyperalimentation is a continued and uniform infusion rate of the hypertonic solution. Frequent checking (every 30 to 60 minutes) of the established drip rate and patency of the infusion are important. A decreased flow rate may be caused by a plugged filter. Changes in body position will also alter the flow rate. If the rate becomes too slow, hypoglycemia may develop. The flow rate should be maintained as ordered and never "speeded up," since overload of the hypertonic solution can cause massive dehydration of body cells. Daily weights and recording of intake and output help in monitoring fluid balance. The patient is observed for signs of fluid overload (p. 305). Sugar overload can be identified by presence of sugar in the urine. Serum electrolytes, glucose, and BUN levels are usually monitored daily initially and then at longer intervals.

Promotion of health. The patient should be encouraged to assume activities of daily living. Initially he is likely to be in a catabolic state, which increases the susceptibility to infections of the mouth and respiratory tract. If he is not allowed food or fluids orally, good mouth care is essential. Ambulation should be encouraged, if possible, as inactivity promotes catabolism and negative nitrogen balance.

Emotional support. The patient may have many fears and concerns about being fed by intravenous fluids over a long period of time. He should have an understanding of what is occurring and the reason for the frequent dressing changes. If he is not permitted food orally, he may need aid in coping with stress incurred by the smell of food or watching others eat. If he is receiving parenteral hyperalimentation over an extended period of time, he may be concerned about regaining his appetite, taste, or normal eating patterns.[12] Being fed only by tube, even though temporary, may create stress from a change in body image.

□ Hypodermoclysis

Infants and young children often are given fluids by hypodermoclysis. In adults the fluid usually is injected beneath the skin of the thigh directly into the subcutaneous tissue. In babies the thighs, scapular region, or abdomen are used. Isotonic solutions are used to prevent rapid shifts of fluid among compartments. Physiologic saline or 5% dextrose in saline are suitable for administration by this route. If the patient has a deficit of body fluid, 5% dextrose in water should not be used. This solution tends to draw sodium and, hence, water from the plasma, further depleting the circulating blood volume.

RELIEF OF SYMPTOMS

Patients with fluid and electrolyte imbalance often have extreme thirst, nausea, and vomiting. These symptoms are distressing, and the nurse should know measures that can be used to give the patient relief.

Thirst

Thirst, the first and most insistent sign of dehydration, sometimes causes the patient more misery than surgery or the symptoms of a disease. It may develop even when fluids have been withheld only for a number of hours. If fluids are being withheld intentionally, thirst often is made more bearable by explaining to the patient why the fluids are being withheld and when they will be reinstituted.

Usually thirst is relieved readily by taking fluids. When fluids cannot be taken orally, the administration of fluids parenterally usually gives relief. This is often helpful to explain to the patient. Mouth care will allay some of the discomfort from thirst. This care includes cleansing the tongue, teeth, and mucous membranes lining the oral cavity. It may be necessary to repeat the procedure every hour. Cleansing the mouth with lemon and glycerine swabs is usually helpful. If the patient can be trusted not to swallow, he may be given mouthwash, water, or ice chips to be held in the mouth and then expelled. Hard lemon candies (sour balls) often give relief even though they must be expelled. The chewing of gum helps some patients.

When fluids are not permitted, the water pitcher at the bedside is removed, and if the patient cannot be relied upon not to get up and drink at a water tap, special provisions such as constant attendance or insistence on bed rest may be necessary. Thirst sometimes compels the patient to obtain water in any way he can.

Pronounced and continued thirst, despite the administration of fluids, is not normal and should be reported. In the immediate postoperative period, this kind of thirst suggests internal hemorrhage, elevation of temperature, or some other untoward development. In the chronically ill patient it may indicate the onset of disease such as diabetes mellitus in which extra water is used by the kidneys to eliminate glucose in the urine. It also is a symptom of hypercalcemia.

Nausea and vomiting

Nausea and vomiting often are part of the body's response to insults to its integrity. They usually occur together, but occasionally, if the mechanism for vomiting is touched off by local pressure in the medulla, vomiting may be sudden and not preceded by nausea or any other warning sensation.

There are two centers in the medulla involved with vomiting: the chemoreceptor emetic trigger zone and the vomiting center.[11] The vomiting center may be stimulated directly through the vagal or sympathetic nerves. Gastrointestinal irritants, distention or injury of any of the viscera, pain, and psychic trauma cause nausea and vomiting in this manner. Increased intracranial pressure may stimulate vomiting by direct local pressure. The vomiting center also may be stimulated indirectly through the chemoreceptor emetic trigger zone. Emetic agents such as morphine sulfate, meperidine hydrochloride (Demerol), ergot derivatives, digitalis preparations, and metabolic emetic substances resulting from uremia, infection, and radiation stimulate the chemoreceptor center to produce vomiting. Labyrinthine stimulation, the primary factor in the nausea and vomiting of motion sickness, (seasickness, airsickness) is also believed to pass through the trigger center. It still is not clear by what route irritating gases such as those used in anesthesia affect the vomiting center or what specifically causes some women to vomit during the first trimester of pregnancy.

Nausea and vomiting are distressing to most people, but vomiting also can be a serious symptom. Prolonged and severe vomiting will interfere with nutrition and cause fluid and electrolyte imbalance. The act of vomiting produces a strain on the abdominal muscles, and in some postoperative patients it may cause wound separation, wound dehiscence, or bleeding. Vomiting is especially dangerous for anesthetized patients, persons in coma, and infants because they are likely to aspirate the vomitus into the lungs. Aspiration may cause asphyxia, atelectasis, or pneumonitis, especially in the elderly person whose nasopharyngeal reflexes are less acute than those of a younger person.

Treatment of nausea and vomiting depends on the cause. Medications or other substances known to cause nausea and vomiting are stopped, and fluid and electrolyte imbalances are treated. Most patients will have less vomiting if the emotional components of its cause are removed. Therefore the nurse tries to relieve the patient's anxiety. Sedation may help to quiet the patient. Nausea and gagging sometimes are relieved by taking deep breaths through the mouth. Ginger ale and other effervescent drinks seem to have a remarkable effect in controlling postoperative nausea and vomiting and often can be taken and retained long before other fluids are tolerated. Effervescent fluids also may be effective in controlling vomiting from other causes such as seasickness.

Antihistaminic drugs such as dimenhydrinate (Dramamine), meclizine hydrochloride (Bonine), and trimethobenzamide hydrochloride (Tigan) are used widely in control of motion sickness such as is encountered in air and sea travel. These medications are effective prophylactically when taken about 30 minutes before the initial motion and then continued at regular intervals. They also are ordered with varying success in the nausea and vomiting associated with illness. Tigan and prochlorperazine (Compazine) are quite effective in controlling postoperative nausea and vomiting. All these drugs are available as rectal suppositories as well as for oral administration. Any of the antihistaminic drugs may cause drowsiness and dizziness, and the possibility of these reactions should be pointed out to persons who are taking them when traveling. They are especially dangerous to use when driving.

■ ACID-BASE IMBALANCES

Control of acid-base balance in the body is accomplished by regulation of hydrogen ion in body fluids (p. 211). The pH of body fluids is normally maintained within a range of pH 7.35 to 7.45, or slightly alkaline. When pH of the blood drops below 7.35, a state of *acidosis* exists; above 7.45 a state of *alkalosis* exists. A pH below 6.8 or above 7.8 is incompatible with life (Fig. 15-6).

The major effect of acidosis is depression of the central nervous system as evidenced by disorientation followed by coma. Alkalosis is characterized by overexcitability of the nervous system, and the muscles may go into a state of tetany and convulsions. Acid-base imbalance always produces an imbalance of the body's other cations as well, therefore symptoms of these imbalances will also occur.

□ Control mechanisms

Regulation of pH is vital because even slight deviations from the normal range will cause marked changes in the rate of cellular chemical reactions. Acid-base balance is controlled by several regulatory mechanisms shown in Table 20-10. (See p. 211 for further information on regulatory mechanisms.)

Chemical buffer systems

There are three major buffer systems in cells and extracellular fluid—carbonic acid–bicarbonate, phosphate, and protein buffer systems—that act very rapidly to prevent minute-to-minute changes in pH.

Carbonic acid–bicarbonate. This system is present in extracellular fluids. Carbonic acid is formed by the combination of carbon dioxide and water $CO_2 + H_2O \rightleftarrows H_2CO_3$. When a strong base is added to the body fluids, it is buffered by carbonic acid to a bicarbonate salt and water: $H_2CO_3 + NaOH \rightarrow NaH\ CO_3 + H_2O$. When a strong acid is added to the system, a bicarbonate buffer changes it to a salt and carbonic acid: $HCl + NaH\ CO_3 \rightarrow NaCl + H_2CO_3$. The carbonic acid then dissociates into carbon dioxide and water and can be excreted by the lungs and kidneys.

Bicarbonate and carbonic acid normally exist in the extracellular fluid in a ratio of 20:1 respectively (or 134:27). This ratio is more vital to maintenance of acid-base balance than the actual amounts of the two substances. For instance, if the amount of carbonic acid increases, an increase in bicarbonate, which keeps the 20:1 ratio intact, will prevent a change from normal pH.

The carbonic acid–bicarbonate buffer system is important because concentrations of these two substances can be controlled by the respiratory and renal systems (discussed later in this chapter).

Phosphate buffer system. The phosphate buffer system is present in cells and extracellular fluids; it is especially active in the kidneys. This system is composed of sodium and other cations in combination with $H_2PO_4^-$ and HPO_4^{--}. When a strong acid is present, the following action takes place: $Na_2HPO_4 + HCl \rightarrow NaCl + NaH_2PO_4$. A hydrogen ion is excreted via the urine in the NaH_2PO_4. A strong base is buffered in the following reaction: $NaOH + NaH_2PO_4 \rightarrow Na_2HPO_4 + H_2O$. The NaH_2PO_4 is a weak base and minimizes the pH change.[19]

Protein buffer system. The protein buffer system is located in the plasma and inside cells; the protein hemoglobin in red blood cells is one of the proteins in-

Table 20-10. Mechanisms regulating acid-base balance

	Action time	Effect
Chemical buffers in cells and extracellular fluid	Instantaneous	Combine with acids or bases added to the system to prevent marked changes in pH
Respiratory system	Minutes to hours	Controls CO_2 concentration in extracellular fluid by changes in rate and depth of respiration
Kidneys	Hours to days	Regulate hydrogen ion concentration by ↑ or ↓ bicarbonate concentration in body fluids

volved. Although most protein buffers are intracellular, they assist in buffering extracellular fluid. Some of the amino acids in proteins contain free acid radicals, —COOH, which can dissociate into CO_2 + H, thus adding a hydrogen ion. Other proteins have basic radicals, —NH_3OH, which can dissociate into —NH_3^+ and OH^-; the OH^- combines with a hydrogen ion to form water, thus removing one hydrogen ion from body fluid. The protein buffer system is the most powerful buffer system in the body.[19]

Respiratory control of pH

The respiratory control center in the brain responds to increases of carbon dioxide and hydrogen ion in body fluids. Rate and depth of respiration are, in turn, controlled by the respiratory control of pH as follows: (1) when pH decreases (more acid), respiratory rate and depth are increased, and there is greater excretion of carbon dioxide through the lungs, thus less carbon dioxide is present to produce carbonic acid by the reaction: $CO_2 + H_2O \rightleftarrows H_2CO_3$, and the pH increases toward alkalinity; and (2) when pH rises above the normal range (more alkaline), the respiratory center is depressed, rate and depth of respiration decrease, carbon dioxide is retained, and more carbonic acid is formed, moving the pH toward acidity.

Because carbon dioxide is constantly being formed as a product of metabolism, the concentration of carbon dioxide in extracellular fluids must be continuously balanced between the rate of metabolism and the rate of pulmonary exretion.[19] The buffering capacity of the respiratory system is more than double that of all the chemical buffers combined.

Renal regulation of pH

Both chemical buffers and respiratory regulation have limited ability to make complete adjustments in pH, and it remains for the kidneys to make permanent adjustments in the pH of body fluids. The renal regulation of pH, is effected by control of the retention or excretion of bicarbonate and hydrogen ions. The kidneys usually excrete an acid urine because of the excess of acid metabolic products (nonvolatile acids), which must be eliminated by the renal route. Normally, almost all of the bicarbonate formed by the kidneys is retained.

Hydrogen ions, secreted by kidney tubule cells, and bicarbonate, filtered into the glomerular filtrate, combine in the kidney tubules to form carbon dioxide and water, which is excreted through exhalation (CO_2) and in urine (H_2O). There is usually an excess of hydrogen ions, however, because of the acid products of metabolism, and these hydrogen ions combine with bases and are excreted in the urine. Hydrogen ions can be exchanged for sodium and potassium ions in the kidney tubules; therefore conservation of hydrogen ions can result in imbalances of sodium and potassium.

□ Compensation

Compensation is a response that tends to reverse an abnormal trend in pH. The kidneys attempt to compensate for changes in blood CO_2 by making a corresponding change in blood bicarbonate, and the lungs attempt to

Table 20-11. Types of acid-base disturbances and compensatory mechanisms

Disturbance	Physiologic causes	Method of compensation
Respiratory acidosis	Carbonic acid excess: lungs not removing sufficient CO_2 (hypoventilation)	Bicarbonate production by kidneys is increased. Bicarbonate is retained and chloride is excreted instead by the kidneys. Secretion and excretion of hydrogen ions in urine is increased.
Respiratory alkalosis	Carbonic acid deficit: lungs removing too much CO_2 (hyperventilation)	Kidneys increase excretion of bicarbonate ions.
Metabolic acidosis	Bicarbonate deficit: retention of acid metabolites, diabetic ketoacidosis, excess acid intake (salicylate poisoning), or loss of bicarbonate	Increased rate and depth of respiration causes increased excretion of CO_2 by lungs. Formation of bicarbonate ions in the kidneys is increased.
Metabolic alkalosis	Bicarbonate excess: excess intake (sodium bicarbonate, carbonated drinks) or retention of bicarbonate Potassium depletion Loss of acid	Rate and depth of respiration is decreased. Lungs retain more CO_2. Kidneys excrete bicarbonate.

Table 20-12. Laboratory values in uncompensated and partially compensated acid-base disturbances

	pH	PCO_2	HCO_3
Respiratory acidosis			
Uncompensated	↓	↑	Normal
Partially compensated	Move toward normal, but still ↓	↑	↑
Respiratory alkalosis			
Uncompensated	↑	↓	Normal
Partially compensated	Move toward normal, but still ↑	↓	↓
Metabolic acidosis			
Uncompensated	↓	Normal	↓
Partially compensated	Move toward normal, but still ↓	↓	↓
Metabolic alkalosis			
Uncompensated	↑	Normal	↑
Partially compensated	Move toward normal, but still ↑	↑	↑

compensate for abnormal changes in blood bicarbonate by making corresponding changes in blood CO_2. Compensation is an effort to maintain the normal 1:20 ratio between bicarbonate and carbonic acid that is necessary to maintain the pH within normal range.

□ Types of acid-base disturbances

Table 20-11 shows the four types of acid-base disturbances that occur and their compensatory mechanisms.

Following are the laboratory values used in diagnosing and monitoring acid-base disturbances: pH, 7.38 to 7.42; PCO_2, 38 to 42 mm Hg; and plasma bicarbonate, 23 to 25 mEq/liter.

Bicarbonate is sometimes expressed as a CO_2 content value, which is actually the sum of all carbon dioxide dissolved in the plasma. Actual bicarbonate can be calculated from a CO_2 content value by the following formula: Bicarbonate = CO_2 content − (0.03 × PCO_2). Both pH and PCO_2 are determined from a sample of arterial blood, a blood gas analysis.

Table 20-12 shows whether laboratory values characteristic of the four types of acid-base disturbances are increased or decreased and the results of the body's compensatory efforts.

Respiratory acidosis: carbonic acid excess

Any factor that decreases the rate of pulmonary ventilation increases the concentration of dissolved carbon dioxide, carbonic acid, and hydrogen ions and results in *respiratory acidosis*. An excess of carbon dioxide can cause carbon dioxide narcosis. In this condition (as the name implies), carbon dioxide levels are so high that they no longer stimulate respirations but depress them. Associated with the decreased respiratory rate are lack of oxygen and hypoxia. During respiratory acidosis, potassium moves out of the cells, producing hyperkalemia. Ventricular fibrillation may occur if the blood potassium levels are greatly increased.

Etiology. Respiratory acidosis can result from a number of pathologic conditions: (1) damage to the respiratory center in the medulla; (2) obstruction of respiratory passages (e.g., pneumonia, chronic bronchitis); (3) loss of lung surface for ventilation (e.g., atelectasis, pneumothorax, emphysema, pulmonary fibrosis); (4) weakness of respiratory muscles (e.g., poliomyelitis, hypokalemia); and (5) severe depression of respirations (e.g., overdose of respiratory depressant drugs).

Prevention. Patients with diseases such as emphysema that limit lung excursion and therefore limit gaseous exchange should not take carbonated beverages or bicarbonate of soda. These substances tend to make the blood more alkaline than normal, and respirations are depressed in an effort to correct this imbalance. Depression of respirations is highly undesirable for these patients.

Any patient with symptoms of inadequate oxygenation or carbon dioxide retention requires medical treatment. Early recognition and treatment of the primary condition often prevents its becoming complicated by acid-base imbalance. Therefore any person with symptoms suggestive of anemia, cardiac insufficiency, chronic bronchitis, emphysema, asthma, or other obstructive diseases of the bronchioles should receive medical attention. These conditions are discussed in detail in the latter half of this book.

Assessment. Signs and symptoms of respiratory acidosis (hypercapnia) include hyperpnea, visual disturbances, and headache. Later, confusion, drowsiness, and coma can ensue. Ventricular fibrillation may be the first sign noted in some cases.

Intervention. Treatment is aimed at increasing the

alveolar ventilation rate in order to improve the exchange of carbon dioxide and oxygen. This objective is accomplished by using an intermittent positive pressure breathing (IPPB) machine to assist the patient to exhale carbon dioxide. Because the respiratory center is narcotized by the increased amounts of carbon dioxide, the lowered oxygen tension of the blood is the stimulus for respiration. If the patient then inhales large amounts of oxygen, he will remove the stimulation for respiration and breathing may cease. For this reason, oxygen is never given to patients with carbon dioxide narcosis. Low flow oxygen (1 to 3 liters/min) is given to a patient with chronic pulmonary disease who maintains a chronically high P_{CO_2}. IPPB treatments are usually given using compressed air or room air instead of oxygen in these situations (p. 1136).

If ventricular fibrillation or severe potassium excess exists, it may be necessary to administer sodium bicarbonate intravenously.

The major nursing responsibility is to recognize patients who have the potential for developing respiratory acidosis because of conditions that interefere with normal respiratory gas exchange. A patient whose airway is compromised by the presence of secretions must be encouraged to cough frequently or may need to have nasopharyngeal or tracheal suctioning.

Respiratory alkalosis: carbonic acid deficit

Etiology. Excessive pulmonary ventilation will decrease hydrogen ion concentration and thus cause *respiratory alkalosis.*[30] A common cause of respiratory alkalosis is *hyperventilation.* When the patient hyperventilates, he blows off large amounts of carbon dioxide. At the same time there are too many free cations in the blood, and they may be excreted through the kidney, leaving a deficiency.

Hyperventilation may be caused by anxiety, hysteria, or lesions affecting the respiratory center in the medulla (brain tumor, encephalitis). Some other causes of respiratory alkalosis are conditions that greatly increase metabolism (hyperthyroidism) and the overventilation of patients with mechanical respirators.

Prevention. Respiratory alkalosis can be prevented in a patient who is hyperventilating by administering a few whiffs of carbon dioxide or by having the patient breathe into a paper bag and then rebreathe his own exhaled carbon dioxide. Care should be taken in adjusting mechanical respirators so that the patient is not being breathed too deeply or rapidly.

Assessment. The patient may complain of lightheadedness and numbness or tingling of the fingers and toes. If the alkalosis becomes more severe, tetany and convulsions may be present. Serum potassium levels will be decreased because the kidneys retain hydrogen ions and excrete potassium instead.

Intervention. Treating the underlying condition usually effectively resolves the respiratory alkalosis. Respiratory alkalosis becomes especially dangerous when it leads to cardiac arrhythmias caused partly by a decreased plasma potassium. If a patient who is receiving assisted ventilation complains of dizziness or shows any signs of muscle irritability, it is likely that the depth of respiration is too great, and the respiratory rate of the machine should be decreased. If tetany is present, calcium gluconate is given intravenously (p. 313). Renal function must be maintained to promote renal compensation of the disturbance.

Metabolic acidosis: bicarbonate deficit

When excess acids are added to the body fluids, or when bicarbonate is lost, a *metabolic acidosis,* or nonrespiratory acidosis results.

Etiology. In some conditions, such as uncontrolled diabetes mellitus or starvation, glucose either cannot be utilized or is not available for oxidation. The body compensates for this by using body fat for energy, producing abnormal amounts of ketone bodies in the process. In an effort to neutralize the ketones and maintain the acid-base balance of the body, plasma bicarbonate is exhausted. The resultant acid-base imbalance is called metabolic acidosis or *ketoacidosis.* This condition can develop whenever the person does not eat an adequate diet and his body fat must be burned for energy. It is the reason why extremely low-carbohydrate or high-protein–no-carbohydrate reduction diets are criticized by nutrition experts.

Ketoacidosis develops more rapidly in infants than in adults because they have less glycogen reserves. It also can develop whenever excessive amounts of lactic acid are produced, such as in prolonged strenuous muscle exercise, or when oxidation takes place in cells without adequate oxygen, such as occurs in heart failure and shock. Loss of large amounts of alkaline intestinal secretions such as in severe diarrhea or through fistulas can also create a bicarbonate deficit.

The normal functioning kidney excretes an excess of hydrogen ions in conditions of acidosis and, in so doing, retains potassium so that hyperkalemia as well as acidosis is present. In kidney failure, metabolic acids accumulate in the blood stream. Following is a listing of the many causes of metabolic acidosis:

1. Diarrhea or draining intestinal fistulas (loss of bicarbonate)
2. Renal failure
3. Ureteroenterostomy (retention of Cl^- ions)
4. Diabetic ketoacidosis
5. Lactic acidosis secondary to strenuous exercise

6. Salicylate intoxication
7. Starvation (increased breakdown of body fat or protein-producing ketone bodies)
8. Surgical anesthesia
9. Conditions that greatly increase the body's metabolic needs (high fever, infectious disease, thyrotoxicosis)
10. Shock
11. Convulsions

Prevention. Metabolic acidosis can be prevented by careful medical management or, when possible, prevention of the conditions that lead to acidosis.

Assessment. Headache and mental dullness are early signs of acidosis. The patient in acidosis is hyperpneic and has deep respirations (Kussmaul respirations). This breathing pattern represents an attempt to blow off carbon dioxide, thus compensating for the acidosis. If the condition is untreated, disorientation, stupor, coma, and death will occur.

Hyperkalemia results from the movement of potassium out of the cells as hydrogen ions move in and from the retention of potassium by the kidneys. Aside from laboratory evidence, there may be few indications of the acidosis until the pH falls to 7.1 or lower.

Intervention. Treatment of acidosis is directed toward treating the underlying cause and restoration of electrolyte balance. If the acidosis is severe, intravenous sodium bicarbonate or sodium lactate is given. In milder cases, sodium bicarbonate may be given orally if the patient is able to retain it. Bicarbonate and lactate preparations must be administered with caution because they can induce a metabolic alkalosis and lead to tetany and convulsions.

When acidosis is caused by renal failure, renal dialysis may be necessary.

As the acidosis is corrected, potassium moves back into cells and hypokalemia develops. If a patient being treated for acidosis needs to receive potassium, it is given after the acidosis has been partially corrected and as pH is returning to normal. It is important to bear in mind that even though acidosis is accompanied by hyperkalemia, the patient may be potassium depleted. The potassium leaves the cells in exchange for the hydrogen ions, and much of it is excreted.

Maintenance of good respiratory function in a patient with metabolic acidosis will facilitate the excretion of carbon dioxide. If the kidneys are functioning well, they can help correct the acidosis by producing more bicarbonate. Since many conditions that lead to this imbalance are hyperosmolar as well, osmotic diuresis will take place and the patient will need fluid replacement along with careful monitoring of intake and output. If changes in the sensorium have resulted, safety precations are instituted.

Metabolic alkalosis: bicarbonate excess

When excessive amounts of acid substance and hydrogen ions are lost from the body, or when large amounts of bicarbonate or lactate are added orally or intravenously, the result is an imbalance in which there is an excess of base elements, *metabolic alkalosis.* This type of imbalance does not occur as often as metabolic acidosis. In alkalosis, potassium enters the cells and hypokalemia results. A potassium loss causes a metabolic alkalosis, while an alkalosis causes hypokalemia.[16] An excess of bicarbonate in distal tubular fluid causes obligatory potassium loss.

Etiology. Metabolic alkalosis can occur in the following conditions: (1) loss of hydrochloric acid from the stomach due to vomiting or gastric drainage from a nasogastric tube (loss of chloride leaves more sodium to combine with and retain bicarbonate in the kidneys); (2) loss of potassium ions through intestinal fistulas, diarrhea, or in the urine; (3) ingestion of large amounts of sodium bicarbonate or antacids to treat indigestion or ulcers; (4) infusion of excessive amounts of bicarbonate or lactate intravenously; (5) diuretic therapy; and (6) excessive mineralocorticoids.

Prevention. Persons must be cautioned against the excessive use of sodium bicarbonate to alleviate indigestion. Controlling the conditions that can cause metabolic alkalosis can prevent this imbalance from developing. If drug therapy is causing the alkalosis, these drugs should be discontinued and others substituted where possible.

Assessment. In metabolic alkalosis, breathing becomes depressed in an effort to conserve carbon dioxide for combination with hydrogen ions in the blood to raise the blood level of carbonic acid. Symptoms that can occur are mental confusion, dizziness, numbness and tingling in extremities, muscle twitching, and later, tetany and convulsions. There may be electrocardiographic changes consistent with hypokalemia.

Intervention. Treatment is aimed at correcting the cause of the metabolic alkalosis. Sodium chloride or ammonium chloride may be given orally or intravenously. If the condition is associated with loss of sodium chloride, potassium must be restored because it is lost with the sodium. It is given in the form of potassium chloride. A diuretic that acts as a carbonic anhydrase inhibitor (Diamox) may help relieve the alkalosis by increasing excretion of bicarbonate by the kidneys.

The nurse assists in maintenance of good respiratory function so that compensation can take place through this mechanism. Careful monitoring of the patient for adequate renal function and safety precautions is important in the nursing care of patients with metabolic alkalosis. Since convulsions may occur, precautions are taken for the patient's protection.

REFERENCES AND SELECTED READINGS

1. Beeson, P. B., and McDermott, W.: Textbook of medicine, ed. 14, Philadelphia, 1975, W. B. Saunders Co.
2. Bergersen, B. S.: Pharmacology in nursing, ed. 14, St. Louis, 1979, The C. V. Mosby Co.
3. *Blood gas and acid-base concepts in respiratory care; a programmed instruction, Am. J. Nurs. **76**:1-30, 1976.
4. Brobeck, J. R., editor: Best and Taylor's physiological basis of medical practice, ed. 9, Baltimore, 1973, The Williams & Wilkins Co.
5. *Brooks, S. M.: Basic facts of body water and ions, ed. 3, New York, 1973, Springer Publishing Co., Inc.
6. *Butts, P.: Magnesium sulfate in the treatment of toxemia, Am. J. Nurs. **77**:1294-1298, 1977.
7. *Colley, R., and Phillips, K.: Helping with hyperalimentation, Nursing 73 **3**:6-17, 1973.
8. Davis, L., editor: Christopher's textbook of surgery, ed. 11, Philadelphia, 1977, W. B. Saunders Co.
9. *Deitel, M.: Intravenous hyperalimentation, Can. Nurs. **69**:38-43, 1973.
10. Dickens, M. L.: Fluid and electrolyte balance; a programmed text, ed. 2, Philadelphia, 1970, F. A. Davis Co.
11. *Downs, H. S.: The control of vomiting, Am. J. Nurs. **66**:76-82, 1966.
12. *Dudrick, S. J., and Rhoads, J. E.: Total intravenous feeding, Sci. Am. **226**:73-80, 1972.
13. *Elbaum, N.: Detecting and correcting magnesium imbalance, Nursing 77 **7**:34-35, 1977.
14. *Fenton, M.: What to do about thirst, Am. J. Nurs. **69**:1014-1017, 1969.
15. Fitzsimmons, J.: Thirst, Physiol. Rev. **52**:468-548, 1972.
16. *Goldberger, E.: A primer of water, electrolytes and acid-base syndromes, ed. 5, Philadelphia, 1975, Lea & Febiger.
17. *Grant, J.: Patient care in hyperalimentation, Nurs. Clin. North Am. **8**:165-181, 1973.
18. *Grant, M., and Kubo, W.: Assessing a patient's hydration status, Am. J. Nurs. **75**:1306-1311, 1975.
19. Guyton, A.: Textbook of medical physiology, ed. 5, Philadelphia, 1976, W. B. Saunders Co.
20. *Haughey, E., and Sica, F.: Diuretics: how safe can you make them? Nursing 77 **7**:34-39, 1977.
21. *Kee, J.: Fluid imbalances in elderly patients, Nursing 73 **3**:40-43, 1973.
22. *Kee, J.: The critically ill patient and possible fluid and electrolyte imbalances, Nursing 72 **2**:6-11, 1972.
23. *Kee, J.: Fluids and electrolytes with clinical applications: a programmed approach, ed. 2, New York, 1978, John Wiley & Sons, Inc.
24. Kettel, L.: Acute respiratory acidosis, Hosp. Med. **12**:31-33, 1976.
25. Keyes, J.: Basic mechanisms in acid-base homeostasis, Heart Lung **5**:239-245, 1976.
26. Keyes, J.: Blood gas analysis and the assessment of acid-base status, Heart Lung **5**:247-255, 1976.
27. Krupp, M., and Chatton, M.: Current medical diagnosis and treatment, rev. 16, Los Altos, Calif., 1977, Lange Medical Publications.
28. *Kubo, W., et al.: Fluid and electrolyte problems of tube-fed patients, Am. J. Nurs. **76**:912-916, 1976.
29. *MacLeod, S.: The rational use of potassium supplements, Postgrad. Med. **57**:123-127, 1975.
30. *Manzi, C.: Edema, how to tell if it's a danger signal, Nursing 77 **7**:66-70, 1977.
31. *McGann, M.: Secondary hyperaldosteronism, Am. J. Nurs. **76**:634-637, 1976.
32. *Metabolic acid-base disorders: programmed instruction, part I. Am. J. Nurs. **77**:1-32, 1977.
33. *Metabolic acid-base disorders: programmed instruction, part II. Am. J. Nurs. **78**:1-20, 1978.
34. *Metheny, N.: Water and electrolyte balance in the post-operative patient, Nurs. Clin. North Am. **10**:49-57, 1975.
35. *Metheny, N., and Snively, W.: Nurses; handbook of fluid balance, ed. 2, Philadelphia, 1974, J. B. Lippincott Co.
36. Newmark, S., and Dluhy, R.: Hyperkalemia and hypokalemia, J.A.M.A. **231**:631-633, 1975.
37. *Plumer, A. L.: Principles and practice of intravenous therapy, ed. 2, Boston, 1975, Little, Brown & Co.
38. *Potassium imbalance; programmed instruction, Am. J. Nurs. **67**:343-366, 1967.
39. *Reed, G. M.: Confused about potassium? Nurs. 74 **4**:21-27, 1974.
40. Reed, G. M., and Sheppard, V.: Regulation of fluid and electrolyte balance, ed. 2, Philadelphia, 1977, W. B. Saunders Co.
41. *Roach, F. B.: Color changes in dark skin, Nurs. 72 **2**:20-22, 1972.
42. *Sharer, J.: Reviewing acid-base balance, Am. J. Nurs. **75**:980-983, 1975.
43. *Snively, V., and Roberts, K.: The clinical picture as an aid to understanding body fluid disturbances, Nurs. Forum **12**:132-159, 1973.
44. Stroot, V., Lee, C., and Schaper, C.: Fluids and electrolytes: a practical approach, Philadelphia, 1974, F. A. Davis Co.
45. *Tripp, A.: Hyper- and hypocalcemia, Am. J. Nurs. **76**:1142-1145, 1976.
46. *Wade, J. F.: Respiratory nursing care: physiology and technique, ed. 2, St. Louis, 1977, The C. V. Mosby Co.
47. Widman, F., editor: Goodale's clinical interpretation of laboratory tests, ed. 7, Philadelphia, 1973, F. A. Davis Co.

*References preceded by an asterisk are particularly well suited for student reading.

AUDIOVISUAL RESOURCES

1. Trainex: Fluids and electrolytes: clinical application, Garden Grove, California, 1970, Trainex Corp. (filmstrip and audiotape).
2. Trainex: Parenteral hyperalimentation, Garden Grove, California, 1971, Trainex Corp. (filmstrip and audiotape).

21

Infectious disease

DONNA J. KUKLO

An *infectious disease* is the result of the establishment of a host-parasite relationship within the human body that is overtly injurious to the host. The injury to the body is the result of the presence of the parasite (usually bacterium, virus, fungi, and so on) within the body or contact with the microorganism's toxic products. Many organisms that parasitize the human body do not incite any injurious body response under normal conditions of the host; these organisms are said to be *colonizing* the body (e.g., *Staphylococcus aureus* in the nasal passages). A specific parasitic organism will not always elicit the same symptoms or host responses in all infected individuals. The response is dependent upon a number of host factors and parasite factors. The development of an infectious disease is a dynamic process pitting the *resistance of the host* against the *pathogenesis of the parasite*. Chapter 14 deals with many of the factors of biologic defense exhibited by the host to prevent infection and injury, while such factors as the *invasiveness* and *toxigenicity* of the parasite favor its injurious establishment within the host. Some parasitic infectious agents are highly invasive and virtually nontoxigenic (e.g., the pneumococci); others present the other extreme—high toxigenicity but low invasiveness (e.g., *Clostridium tetani*).

With all infectious diseases a common sequence of events occurs. The infectious organism gains access to the body of the host, establishes itself within the host, creates injurious results, and exits the host. The pathogen may be introduced directly into the host; for example, through the bite of an arthropod (e.g., tick, mosquito, flea), through the injection of contaminated injectable drugs, or through the contamination of the site of an indwelling catheter. Such sources of the infecting agents are termed *vectors*. However, the most common source of the infectious agents is through contact with the organisms in the environment. The organisms contaminate the air, environmental surfaces, hands of others, inanimate objects (fomites), or food or water. Under normal states of health the human body is extremely resistant to the establishment of an infection; however, when the basic biologic defense mechanisms of the body are breached or compromised, the infectious organism has a much greater chance of creating injurious results.

Once the parasite gains access to the host organism, there is a period of time, known as the *incubation period,* before the clinical symptoms of the disease appear. During this period the organism is establishing itself, spreading to target organs or tissues, and proliferating within various body sites. This incubation period may be variable depending upon the condition of the host, but it is often quite predictable and diagnostically significant. The appearance of the symptoms will depend upon the type of injury elicited by the virulent parasite and the site of the organism within the body. The disease may be described as being *localized* (a focal point of symptoms or injury) or *generalized* (systemic involvement). The course of the disease may be *acute* or *chronic*. An acute disease often incites an immediate violent host response. The outcome of the infection (parasite over host or host over parasite) is determined within a relatively short span of time (mumps, plague, smallpox). Conversely, a chronic infection indicates a more insidious establishment of the parasite within the host, which does not cause immediate damage and tends to provoke less of a host response (tuberculosis, aspergillosis). Though the terms chronic and acute are generally useful in describing an infectious disease relationship between host and parasite, there are many examples of acute infections becoming chronic and vice versa.

An infectious disease is termed a *communicable* disease when it is highly transmissible to other persons, either through airborne droplet transmission or direct contact with the causative infectious agent.

The establishment of an infection within the human body leads to a number of specific (diagnostic symptoms) and generalized manifestations. The earliest manifestations of an infectious process are generally sensed within the host as nondescript, nonspecific reactions such as weakness, headache, lightheadedness, "stuffiness," muscle aches, pain in the joints, loss of appetite, or malaise. These sensations are broadly referred to as *prodromal symptoms*. As the infection progresses, however, other manifestations also develop. These may include fever, leukocytosis, anemia, increase in erythrocyte sedimentation rate (p. 180), appearance of C-reactive protein (p. 177), increased pulse rate, hypotension, proteinuria, and even jaundice, shock, confusion, and convulsions.

Although infectious diseases are more easily prevented and cured than any other major group of disorders, humans are not free of infectious disease and probably never will be. As specific microbial infections have been brought under control, others have emerged as problems. Some current problems in the control of infectious disease are the result of medical progress. For example, because of the availability of antibiotics, few people today die of uncomplicated pneumococcal pneumonia. It is not uncommon, however, to see patients seriously ill from diseases that are resistant to specific antibiotics or from organisms that are a part of the normal body flora of humans. New surgical procedures requiring suppression of the body's immunologic defenses against foreign proteins, or treatments such as chemotherapy or radiation that are also immunosuppressive, have a potential for producing life-threatening systemic infections.

Infections formerly seen only in children are being seen more frequently in adults because of improved sanitary conditions and the failure of the population to develop acquired immunity during early childhood. In many countries, as contact with poliomyelitis virus in childhood has decreased, poliomyelitis has become more common in young adults. The elimination of the barriers of time and distance by modern air travel has the potential for bringing a person with an infectious disease from a remote area of the world to a population center where the disease can be readily spread to a susceptible public.

COMMUNITY-ASSOCIATED INFECTIONS

In the United States there has been a marked reduction in recent years in the incidence of infectious disease, such as measles, whooping cough, and poliomyelitis, that can be prevented by immunization. Concern is being expressed, however, at the decrease in the numbers of children presently being immunized, despite the fact that these immunizations can often be obtained free of cost. The incidence of gonorrhea in the United States has shown a progressive annual increase. (See p. 1447 for further information on factors affecting the increased incidence of gonorrhea).

The dramatic control of several infectious diseases is caused by the development and use of a variety of inactivated vaccines and live attenuated antigens. The potential for eradication of common infectious diseases brings with it major responsibilities for public health agencies, physicians, and nurses. Not only must ways be found to carry out planned programs of immunization, but also to educate the public to the hazards of apathy and failure to maintain proper levels of immunization. Continued progress in control and eradication requires that there be commitment to continue to add to knowledge about immunization patterns, to evaluate effectiveness and risks of antigens used, and to monitor the levels of protection present in a population.

HOSPITAL-ASSOCIATED INFECTIONS

About 2 million of the 30 million patients admitted to the nation's hospitals each year develop hospital-associated (nosocomial) infections. In addition to the considerable morbidity and mortality caused by these infections, their diagnosis and treatment (including additional days of hospitalization) cost more than 1 billion dollars per year.[25]

Nosocomial infections are those infections that develop after the patient has been admitted to the hospital. They are most common in the very young, the very old, and persons with chronic, disabling, and potentially fatal diseases. They may occur as a secondary infection or they may be incidental to a patient's primary problem. For example, a patient with benign prostatic hypertrophy may develop a urinary tract infection and it may persist as a secondary infection until surgical intervention relieves the urinary obstruction. On the other hand, a patient with lung cancer may develop a urinary tract infection that obviously has no relationship to the primary disease.

Two factors contribute to the occurrence of nosocomial infections: a concentration of virulent forms of different organisms and presence of individuals with anatomic or physiologic defects in their immune defenses. Patients whose immune defenses are severely impaired because of irradiation, immunosuppressive therapy, or general debilitation are prone to develop infections not only from the usual organisms in the external environment (exogenous) such as staphylococci, pseudomonas, and streptococci, but also from their own internal (endogenous) organisms such as *Escherichia coli*, *Clostridium perfringens*, and *Proteus* species. In addition, organisms that are of low virulence in the environment, such as *Aspergillus* species, and viral and parasitic agents about which there is limited knowledge, such as the cytomegaloviruses and *Pneumocystis carinii*, may cause life-threatening infections. In patients undergoing chemotherapy for malignant disease, virtually any microorganism with which they come in contact is capable of producing disease because of the compromised state of their defense mechanisms. Common hospital-associated infections include (1) urinary tract infections that are usually associated with indwelling catheters; (2) pneumonia, sometimes attributed to the use of contaminated ventilatory equipment; (3) cellulitis, phlebitis, and bacteremia, all associated with the use of indwelling venous and arterial lines or contaminated intravenous fluids; and (4) postsurgical wound infections. These four categories account for 85% of nosocomial infections. Most of the causative organisms are present in the external environment of the patient and are introduced into the body through direct contact or through contaminated materials. In many instances, nosocomial infections could be prevented by strict aseptic technique when giving care to the patient and by greater restraint in the use of invasive procedures and antibiotics.

The different types of bacteria commonly responsible for nosocomial infections are listed in Table 21-1. *Staphylococcus aureus* continues to be the major problem in nosocomial infections. The reservoir for this organism is the respiratory tract and skin. Indications are that nasal carriers, especially those with respiratory infections, are potent sources of environmental and human contact contamination.[19] Careful attention to *handwashing* before and after contact with patients (particularly those with known *Staphylococcus aureus* infections) and the institution of wound isolation techniques are the two most effective measures to prevent cross-infection. The sources of spread listed in Table 21-1 bear this out.

Group A *Streptococcus* is the second gram-positive organism that has the potential for causing nosocomial infections. This organism is known for its role in causing streptococcal sore throat, scarlet fever, and streptococcal skin infections. The source of epidemic *Streptococcus* organisms in hospitals is the pharynx and nares of infected personnel and patients.

Other organisms involved in nosocomial infections include the gram-negative coliforms, *Escherichia*, *Klebsiella*, and *Enterobacter*, which live in the human intestinal tract. Although these organisms are usually susceptible to antibiotics, they have the capacity to develop antibiotic resistance. The large reservoir of coliform organisms within the general population can be a source for self-infection or for cross-infection from the hands of hospital personnel, through the ingestion of foods, or through the contamination of other materials. With such a large reservoir of organisms it is possible that new strains will be developed by colonization in patients. This is most likely to occur in patients who are receiving antibiotics and whose resident flora have been altered by antibiotics. Immune-deficient patients are particularly susceptible to colonization by these evolving strains of coliforms.

Table 21-1. Modes of transmission of some common pathogens

Pathogen	Source of spread
Gram-positive cocci	
Staphylococcus aureus	Contaminated objects, *hands* and nasal tracts of health care workers, air, self
Group A *Streptococcus* organisms	Direct contact, air, *hands*, rarely objects
Enterococcus organisms	Self, *hands* of health care workers, environmental surfaces
Gram-negative rods	
Escherichia, *Klebsiella*, *Enterobacter*	Self, *hands* of health care workers, contaminated solutions
Proteus, *Salmonella*, *Providencia*, *Serratia*, *Citrobacter*	Contaminated food and water, *hands* of health care workers, self
Pseudomonas	Contaminated environment, *hands*, self
Anaerobic bacteria	
Clostridium, *Bacteroides*	Self, contaminated environment, *hands*
Fungal organisms	
Yeasts	Self, *hands* of health care workers
Fungi	Air, contaminated environment
Viruses	
Varicella	Air, direct contact
Herpes	Self, direct contact, air
Rubella	Direct contact, air
Hepatitis B	Contaminated instruments or injectables, direct contact
Poliomyelitis	Contaminated food or water

Although *Salmonella* organisms are usually acquired outside the hospital, the organism is readily transmissible and can be the cause of nosocomial infection. It is transmitted by direct or indirect contact with an infected person or through food, dairy products, or water contaminated with the organism. Patients with sickle cell disease or malignancies are more vulnerable to infection from these organisms.

Pseudomonas aeruginosa, a gram-negative organism, is another cause of hospital-associated infection. The organism is present throughout the hospital environment, especially where there is a persistent presence of water (in sinks, irrigating solutions, nebulizers). It is more frequently found in patients with leukopenia secondary to burns, leukemia, cystic fibrosis, and various immune-deficiency syndromes. It is also known to be a significant cause of infection in patients receiving prolonged courses of antibiotics, immunosuppressive drugs, and inhalation therapy. It can be a threat to patients undergoing instrumentation (tracheostomy, urinary tract catheterization), and to recipients of renal transplants. Newborns, particularly prematures, as well as the elderly and the debilitated are the most vulnerable.[10]

■ PREVENTION

□ Control measures

On the international level, the World Health Organization (WHO), a special agency of the United Nations, has as its primary purpose to improve and standardize measures of disease prevention and control throughout the world. Its Epidemiological Intelligence Service in Geneva, Switzerland, receives immediate notification of outbreaks of infectious diseases throughout the world and is able to advise countries of impending epidemics. The *Weekly Epidemiological Record* is an official publication of the agency.

On the national level, the Center for Disease Control (CDC) of the Public Health Service, located at Atlanta, Georgia, is responsible for programs for the prevention and control of communicable and other preventable diseases in the United States. It has epidemiologic and laboratory services that provide assistance to the state health facilities upon request. The CDC enforces quarantine regulations, conducts foreign quarantine activities, administers international activities for the control of malaria, smallpox, and measles, and provides consultation to other nations in the control of preventable diseases. It also collects, tabulates, and assesses data on reportable diseases from state health departments and publishes the findings in the *Morbidity and Mortality Weekly Report.*

In the United States the control of infectious diseases at the local level is the responsibility of each state. State health officers usually delegate the activity to a division of communicable diseases. A staff of physicians, nurses, veterinarians, and sanitary engineers works closely with the state epidemiologist in detection, assessment, and control of specific reportable diseases. The American Hospital Association (AHA) and the Center for Disease Control have developed guidelines for the prevention and control of infectious diseases for use in patient care centers. In addition, the Joint Commission on the Accreditation of Hospitals (JCAH), the agency that accredits health care facilities, requires that those institutions seeking accreditation have a program of infection control centered around monitoring (1) patients with infections, (2) patient care practices, (3) antibiotic usage, (4) health of personnel, and (5) environment of the institution.

□ Other preventative measures

Immunization programs

Immunization programs have played and continue to play a primary role in the control of infectious disease throughout the world. The body can be stimulated to produce antibodies against some specific diseases without actually having the disease *(active artificial immunity).* Temporary protection sometimes can be provided by injecting antibodies produced by other persons or other animals into the bloodstream of a human being *(passive artificial immunity).*

Active immunization. Active immunity can be acquired by artificially injecting small numbers of attenuated (weakened) or dead organisms of specific types or modified toxins from the organisms into the body. This procedure is known as *inoculation.* If 90% of the population is protected against organisms that require continued passage through human beings in order to reproduce and live, the disease caused by the organism can be virtually eliminated because there are too few susceptible hosts for the organism to thrive. Smallpox has been eliminated from the United States in this way. This type of protection of a group is called *herd immunity.* It is ineffectual, however, against organisms such as tetanus bacilli that can exist independently of humans, and in this instance each person must be immunized to be protected. If the disease is one not prevalent in the environment, such as smallpox in the United States, or is not spread from person to person by direct contact, such as tetanus, the inoculation must be repeated at regular intervals to maintain protection. This inoculation is called a *booster dose,* and usually one tenth of the original inoculating dose is sufficient.

An inoculation causes a histamine response. Local symptoms of inflammation (redness, tenderness, swelling, sometimes ulcerations) appear at the site of the injection, and symptoms of widespread tissue involvement (slight febrile reactions, general malaise, muscle aching) for a day or two are common. The initial inoculation produces delayed symptoms because tissues must become sensitized to the antigen. There is an accelerated and less severe systemic reaction to subsequent inoculations because antibody production is stimulated at once. The local reaction also is less severe than that following the initial inoculation because the organisms have less opportunity to produce inflammation.

Active artificial immunization against many bacilli and viruses is now available. Every person should be encouraged to avail himself of the protection advised by health officials in the local area. Persons should be advised to keep a permanent record of the date of each immunization.

In the United States the Public Health Service recommends that all children be immunized against diphtheria, pertussis (whooping cough), tetanus, mumps, rubella, poliomyelitis, and measles. The injections are started when the baby is 2 months old, and 0.5 ml of DPT, a combination of diphtheria, pertussis, and tetanus vaccines, is given monthly for 3 months and followed by a reinforcing dose a year later. To be certain of immunity to tetanus, a booster dose of toxoid is recommended at the time of entrance into school and every 10 years thereafter. Since the immunity conferred by the toxoid has proved to be long lasting, annual booster injections are unwarranted.

Immunization against poliomyelitis may be started when the infant is 6 weeks of age or older. Salk vaccine is now rarely used, but the nurse should be familiar with the schedule by which it is given to help parents determine whether their children had a complete course. This is essential for protection. Two injections of Salk vaccine are given 1 month apart, a third injection 7 months later, and a booster dose in a year. Immunization with oral Sabin vaccine is now recommended. To provide maximum protection it should be started 2 or 3 months before the "polio season." Trivalent Oral Poliovirus Vaccine (TOPV), which contains Sabin strains types I, II, and III, is usually given. Two drops of the vaccine are taken orally either on a cube of sugar, in a small amount of distilled water, or with a spoonful of corn syrup. The first dose of trivalent vaccine is given at approximately 2 months of age; the second and third at 6- to 8-week intervals. A fourth dose should be given at approximately 18 months of age. For infants, three doses of trivalent vaccine are recommended. For the primary immunization of older children and adults, trivalent vaccine is given with an interval of 8 weeks between the first two doses, followed by a third dose 6 months to 1 year later. In the event that monovalent vaccine is used, it is given to the infant 1 to 2 months apart in the following order: type I, type III, and type II. Approximately 1 year later a single booster dose of trivalent preparation is administered.

Measles (rubeola) vaccine is not given until the child is 12 months old because antibodies from the mother make it unnecessary. One injection is given. Children who have not been immunized as infants can be given measles vaccine at any age.

Routine vaccination against smallpox is no longer recommended by the Public Health Service. Because of the low incidence of smallpox, the side effects and complications of the vaccine have become of greater concern than the danger of acquiring the disease. However, vaccination is recommended for individuals living or traveling in countries where smallpox is endemic.

Immunization to protect against other disease is given on a selective basis; that is, groups at a high risk are immunized. Because of the prevalence of influenza and its potential for causing death, the Public Health Service recommends immunization against influenza for the aged and persons with chronic cardiac, respiratory, metabolic, and renal disease. Initial protection is obtained by giving two injections of the vaccine 2 weeks apart beginning in October or November. Infants and children up to 6 years of age are given three small doses, the first and second doses 2 weeks apart and a third dose 2 months later. Yearly booster doses are needed to maintain immunity.

In 1966 the Public Health Service announced that a new vaccine against German measles (rubella) had been developed. Studies since then indicate that 95% of the susceptible individuals vaccinated develop antibodies; however, the titers are lower than those following natural infection. The duration of immunity has not been established, but it is likely to be long term. Live rubella virus vaccine is recommended for children between 1 year of age and puberty, regardless of whether there is a history of German measles. School-age children (between 5 and 9) should have priority, since they are the major source of virus dissemination in the community.

As a preventive measure, women in the childbearing years should be tested for rubella antibodies. If no antibodies are present and it is certain that the woman is not pregnant, rubella vaccine is given. The woman should agree not to become pregnant for at least 2 months after vaccination.[2]

At the present time, immunization against typhoid fever is only recommended when there is exposure to a typhoid carrier in the household, when there is an outbreak of typhoid in a community, or when traveling to countries where typhoid is endemic.[2]

Passive immunization. Antibodies produced by other persons or by other animals such as the horse, cow, and rabbit can be introduced into the bloodstream of a person to protect him against attack by a pathogen. This protection is *temporary*, usually lasting only a few weeks, and stimulates no production of antibodies by the recipient. It is called *artificial passive acquired immunity*. Artificial passive immunization is given to a person who has been exposed to a disease and has no natural or artificial active immunity. It usually is given before the disease develops, but it may be given to modify the symptoms of a disease. However, for effectiveness after the disease has developed, it must be administered early, before extensive damage to body tissue has occurred.

Passive immunization usually is reserved for situations in which the disease would be detrimental to the person. For example, it is rarely given to prevent a disease such as chickenpox or mumps in children because they are at an optimum age for the body to produce antibodies with minimal histamine response. On the other hand, an adult exposed to the same disease often would be given antibodies because adults may have a severe histamine response. Immunization is given to all age groups exposed to pathogens that cause serious diseases such as hepatitis, poliomyelitis, diphtheria, tetanus, or rabies. Antivenins, which are given to people bitten by poisonous snakes or black widow spiders, also are passive immunologic products.

Products used for passive immunization may be specific to the disease. Antitoxins and immune animal and human sera are examples. The whole blood of a patient who has recently recovered from a disease against which antibodies are produced also may be used. Antitoxins are available for diphtheria, tetanus, botulism, gas gangrene, and the venom of snakes. Immune animal serum is available against the *Haemophilus influenzae* virus and rabies; human immune serum is available for mumps, measles, pertussis, poliomyelitis, and tetanus.

Immune serum globulin (ISG), or gamma globulin, is an antibody-rich fraction of pooled plasma from normal donors. The rationale for pooling plasma is that someone among the donors will have had the diseases and will have developed antibodies against them. The globulin fraction of the plasma is believed to carry the antibodies, and because it is known not to transmit the virus of hepatitis, it is considered safe to use. Because of occasional side effects, it is now recommended that the use of immune serum globulin be limited to those disorders in which its efficacy has been definitely established. These are measles prophylaxis or modification, viral hepatitis type A (infectious hepatitis) prophylaxis or modification, and antibody deficiency diseases. Immune serum globulin is considered to be of questionable value in the following situations: (1) prevention of rubella in the first trimester of pregnancy, (2) prevention or modification of varicella in certain highrisk patients, (3) prevention or modification of viral hepatitis type B (serum hepatitis) after accidental inoculation, and (4) life-threatening bacterial infections.[2]

Special human immune serum globulins are derived from the sera of persons previously immunized or convalescing from specific diseases. Tetanus immune globulin (human) is of value in prophylaxis and treatment of tetanus. Vaccinia immune globulin (human) is used in the prophylaxis and treatment of vaccinia complication and for smallpox. Pertussis immune globulin (human) and mumps immune globulin (human) are of uncertain or unproved value in the prevention and treatment of pertussis and mumps, respectively.

Nursing responsibilities in immunization. Probably the greatest responsibility of the nurse in immunization programs is to teach the public the advantages of immunization and encourage widespread participation in programs recommended by the local public health officer.

In teaching it is advisable to provide the public with the following information: against what disease protection is being given, why immunization is desirable, and when booster doses should be obtained. The relative safety of the immunization and the advantages of immunization early in life should be stressed.

The nurse is responsible for assessing patients prior to immunization because there are some contraindications to receiving certain immunizing substances. Those that are prepared in chicken or duck embryos may cause an allergic reaction in persons who are allergic to eggs. Many people are allergic to horse serum, and substances containing horse serum, such as tetanus antitoxin, should never be given unless a small amount of the substance has been injected intradermally (a sensitivity test) and after 20 minutes produces no "hive" reaction about the injection site. Active immunologic products should not be given while a person has a cold or other infection because the histaminic reaction from the immunization will be greater than usual.

Children with histories of allergy often are *not* given routine immunization against diseases for which there is herd immunity because the danger of severe allergic response to the immunization is greater than the danger of contracting the disease. These children should be immunized against diseases such as tetanus, however, and immunization is achieved by giving the vaccine or toxoid in small doses over a period of several weeks or months. The package inserts accompanying the immunologic product should always be read carefully to determine the indications, precautions, and side effects.

Before the person leaves the clinic, he or his family should be instructed as to the expected effects and told to contact his physician or to report to a hospital emergency room if any other symptoms develop. He should be cautioned not to scratch any lesion produced by an inoculation. If a severe local reaction with redness, swelling, and tenderness occurs, the physician may order the application of hot, wet dressings. If the lesion is open, these dressings should be sterile.

When antitoxins, antisera, or antivenins are given, the patient should be kept under observation for 20 to 30 minutes. Symptoms of severe allergic response usually will appear within that period of time.

Persons employed in health care facilities should maintain their immune status against smallpox, poliomyelitis, diphtheria, and tetanus. Persons with negative tuberculin tests should be retested every 6 months, and those with positive tuberculin tests should have a yearly chest x-ray. Persons working in dialysis units and blood processing areas (laboratories, blood banks) need to guard against infection with hepatitis B virus.

Environmental measures

Preventive measures involving the environment have been accomplished through sanitation techniques related to purification of the water supply and the proper disposal of sewage and other potentially infectious material. These measures have been legislated into building codes, city planning, state laws, and federal regulations. In hospitals, cleanliness in areas where the population is at high risk such as nurseries, operating room, and intensive care units, is vital because of the potential hazard of nosocomial infections. Ample facilities for handwashing are important throughout hospitals, since *handwashing is the single most effective procedure used in preventing nosocomial infection.*[27] Routine sampling of room air or objects within patient rooms is not advocated. However, spot-culturing of nebulizers and monitoring sterilizing equipment is felt to be important in prevention and control.

Avoidance of prophylactic antibiotics

Although prophylactic antibiotics are still widely prescribed, there are more questions being raised about this practice. Because the use of prophylactic antibiotics often results in the development of secondary infections (either from the patient's own natural flora or from exogenous organisms), some experts question their use. Another factor is that in many of the infections that do develop in persons taking prophylactic antibiotics the organisms develop resistance to the antibiotic being administered.

Isolation

Various forms of isolation are used to control infectious disease. These range from enforcement of rules restricting infected food handlers from employment in eating establishments to temporary suspension of patient contact and required treatment of the hospital employee who is a carrier of an epidemic strain of an infectious disease. An example of this would be the prohibition of a member of the nursing staff who is a nasal carrier of *Staphylococcus aureus* from the newborn nursery.

Identification of susceptible hosts

Highly transmissible disease (communicable) sometimes can be controlled by limiting the contacts of infected persons with others and by identifying potentially susceptible hosts (persons likely to become infected) so that they can be protected. When there is a known epidemic of airborne disease (such as influenza, scarlet fever, or measles), health officials may close meeting places such as schools and theaters in an attempt to minimize the spread of the disease by persons who are in the incubation stage of the infectious disease.

■ ASSESSMENT

The spectrum of disease caused by infectious agents is so broad that a systematic approach to the problem is necessary. In assessing the need for intervention the nurse must be alert to clues that will assist in the prevention and control of infectious diseases and in providing comfort to the patient. By taking a careful nursing history the nurse will note systemic manifestations of infection such as fever, chills, diaphoresis, malaise, pain, suppuration, and swelling. Other pertinent data include order and progression of symptoms, response to prior therapies (reaction to intravenous therapy), antibiotics, blood transfusions, recent dental work, genitourinary examinations (such as cystoscopy), systemic and topical medications, contacts with persons having a similar illness, history of recent travel, exposure to animals, place of residence, and vocational and recreational activities.

A history of preexisting systemic or local disease may be helpful in predicting the pattern of an infection. For instance, persons who have chronic pulmonary disease are particularly susceptible to pneumonias caused by *Haemophilus influenzae* and other gram-negative organisms. Persons who are chronic alcohol abusers are prone to develop pneumococcal or *Klebsiella* pneumonia following vomiting and aspiration.

Infections in the elderly present additional problems. After about age 65 the response of the body to infection decreases because of changes in the immune response system (p. 190). Older persons, then, may exhibit symptoms quite different from the usual signs of infection, and as a result, a serious infection may go undetected. The most common hidden infections of the elderly, are influenza, pneumonia, urinary tract infections, tuberculosis, subacute bacterial endocarditis, vaginitis, suppurative arthritis, herpes zoster, and fungal infections. The nurse needs to know the baseline vital signs of the elderly patient and be alert to variations in these throughout the day. Attention also should be given to changes in the alertness, responsiveness, and general behavior of the patient.

■ PLANNING NURSING INTERVENTION FOR THE PATIENT WITH AN INFECTIOUS DISEASE

□ Isolation

Because most hospitalized patients have altered metabolic states, they are particularly susceptible to infection from both their own normal microbic flora (endogenous source) and the organisms of others (exogenous source). When a patient contracts an infection, the nurse must protect other patients from pathogens, present in or on his own body, that may spread through direct contact, through indirect contact (contaminated objects), or through the air. The way to do so is by isolation. In planning care, the nurse determines the characteristics of the pathogen or pathogens involved to decide whether the patient needs to be isolated and, if so, what type of isolation to use.[7] The determining factors are the virulence of the pathogen and its mode of transmission. The major types of isolation are strict, respiratory, wound and skin, enteric, and protective.

Strict isolation is recommended only for highly transmissible diseases that are spread by direct contact and airborne routes of transmission. Some examples of disease requiring strict isolation are burn wounds infected with *Staphylococcus aureus* or group A *Streptococcus* organisms, diphtheria, disseminated herpes zoster, staphylococcal pneumonia, *Staphylococcus aureus* or group A *Streptoccus* skin infections, smallpox, and rabies. Strict isolation requires that the patient be in a private room with the door kept closed; gowns, masks, and gloves are worn by all persons entering the room; hands are washed on entering and leaving the room; and all articles in the room must be placed in impervious plastic or paper bags and double-bagged for disinfection or sterilization.

Respiratory isolation is recommended to prevent transmission of organisms by droplets or droplet nuclei that are coughed, sneezed, or breathed into the environment. Some of the diseases for which respiratory isolation is recommended are measles, meningococcal meningitis, meningococcemia, mumps, whooping cough, and German measles. (See Chapter 50 for discussion of care of the patient with pulmonary tuberculosis.)

The precautions to be practiced in respiratory isolation include placing the patient in a private room with the door closed. Masks are worn only by persons susceptible to the disease, and gowns and gloves are not necessary. Tissues and dressings are placed in a paper or plastic bag, sealed, and then placed in an impervious plastic or paper bag before removal from the room.

Wound and skin precautions are used to prevent cross-infection where infective material is present in wounds, on body surfaces, or on heavily contaminated articles.

It is recommended for infected burn wounds except those infected with *Staphylococcus aureus* or group A *Streptococcus* organisms, which require strict isolation (p. 1516). Other infections requiring wound and skin precautions are gas gangrene (*Clostridium perfringens*). localized herpes zoster, bubonic plague, and puerperal sepsis with group A *Streptococcus* organisms isolated from the vaginal discharge. In addition, any wound or skin infection that is not covered by a dressing, or where there is copious drainage that seeps through the dressing, requires these precautions. Wound and skin precautions are also used in catheterized patients who have demonstrated colonies of *Pseudomonas* that are multidrug resistant, or when an epidemic strain of this organism is present. The urinary catheter is regarded as the "infected wound," and gloves should be worn during all perineal care and urinary catheter manipulation.[25] The emphasis is on proper handwashing before and after patient contact, and gloves are recommended for persons having direct contact with the infected area, as when changing dressings. A private room is desirable but not required. Dressings should be closed securely in an impervious plastic bag, double-bagged, and incinerated. Contaminated linen should also be double-bagged, and mattresses and pillows should be covered with impervious plastic.

Enteric precautions are recommended for patients with cholera, viral hepatitis (A and B), salmonellosis (including typhoid fever), shingellosis, staphylococcal enterocolitis, and diarrhea associated with an acute illness of suspected infectious etiology. The purpose of enteric precautions is to prevent transmission of disease through direct or indirect contact with infected feces or heavily contaminated articles. Pathogens are spread from infected hands to the mouth, where they are ingested. In this type of isolation the emphasis is placed on proper handwashing, gown technique, and excreta precautions. Gloves are recommended by some experts because of the fear that proper handwashing will not be practiced consistently.

Protective isolation (reverse isolation) is used to prevent contact between potentially pathogenic organisms and uninfected persons who have seriously impaired resistance. Patients with agranulocytosis, extensive burns, or with leukemia or lymphoma receiving radiation, steroid, or antimetabolite therapy are much more susceptible to infections than other patients, and they may need to be protected from other people and the environment. The patient should be placed in a single room with the door kept closed and provision for air flow from the room into the hall. Air should not be recirculated from other hospital areas unless it has been filtered through a high-efficiency filter. Meticulous handwashing and use of gowns, gloves, and masks are essential during each patient contact. Only procedures that are essential should be done in order to avert possible exposure to pathogenic organisms. A procedure like a catheterization is avoided, since it could result in a fatal infection in these patients. Patients whose immune response has been severely compromised must even be protected from their own body flora. The degree to which sterility of certain items such as bed linen needs to be assured depends upon the level of protection required. The Public Health Service has published a manual establishing guidelines for isolation techniques in hospitals.[22] This manual is a valuable source of information for all nurses.

□ Prevention of complications

Many of the communicable diseases commonly prevalent today are caused by viruses. Special care should be taken to protect patients with viral diseases from exposure to bacteria because tissue damaged by viral infection have increased susceptibility to bacterial invasion. Since bacterial complications frequently accompany viral diseases, and because bacteria are prevalent in hospitals, physicians may prefer to treat patients with viral diseases at home. Ear infections, meningitis, and encephalitis of bacterial origin are common complications of measles, and staphylococcal pneumonia is a common sequela of viral influenza.

Toxin-producing bacterial diseases such as streptococcal sore throat, scarlet fever, rheumatic fever, and diphtheria frequently cause serious secondary disease of the heart or kidneys. Patients with these diseases usually are given antibiotics and are kept relatively quiet until the blood sedimentation rate returns to normal.

□ Home care

Unless the pathogen is highly contagious, persons with communicable diseases frequently are cared for at home. The public health nurse often is asked to teach some family member how to care for the patient and how to protect other family members; other nurses may be consulted by friends and neighbors about protection. The same principles apply in the home as in the hospital. A smock or coverall may be used to protect the clothes, and a mask can be improvised from any closely woven, absorbable white material, or disposable ones can be purchased at a pharmacy. All liquid wastes can be flushed down the toilet. Garbage and other wastes from the room should be burned. If local laws prohibit burning of rubbish, the wastes should be wrapped in several layers of newspaper, placed in a plastic bag, and tied securely before discarding in a rubbish container. Dishes should be boiled for 10 minutes before washing. If the laundry must be isolated, it can be boiled for 10 minutes and then washed. When the patient has recovered, the room should be thoroughly aired. Depending on the type of illness, the walls, floor, and furniture may need to be washed well with a detergent or disinfectant and warm water. If materials that cannot be washed, such as books and toys, have been contaminated, leaving them in the sun and air for 24 to 48 hours usually provides sufficient protection.

□ Care of the patient with a fever

Most persons with an infectious disease develop a fever *(pyrexia)* as a generalized response of the body to the infectious agent. The factors that influence maintenance of normal body temperature are discussed on p. 164.

Assessment. The initial symptoms that occur as body temperature begins to rise result from the autonomic response of the body to the higher temperature setting. The response is similar to that which occurs when the body is exposed to cold. The person feels cold because of vasoconstriction, and he experiences shivering, which he cannot control. The shivering is not resolved by adding of blankets because the blood temperature has not yet reached the higher setting established by the hypothalamus. Piloerections (goose bumps) also occur as a mechanism to trap heat close to the skin. When the body temperature equals the higher setting, shivering ceases and the patient does not feel either hot or cold. Metabolic activity is increased by the higher temperature and causes thirst and an increased pulse and respiratory rate. Weakness, loss of appetite, and general aches or muscle soreness result from the increased energy expenditure. Headache and photophobia may also occur. The skin is dry and may feel warm to touch.

When the temperature-regulating setting resets back to the normal temperature, heat is lost from the body by radiation as the vessels dilate and provide a larger surface area close to the outer skin layers. Sweating also occurs to provide for heat loss by evaporation. The skin feels warm and moist. Thirst continues because of the fluid loss.

With prolonged fever, the tongue becomes coated because of dehydration from fluid loss, and the mouth may have an unpleasant taste. Dehydration also decreases gastrointestinal activity so that the person has anorexia despite the increased metabolic activity. Constipation may also occur. The person is extremely fatigued and loses weight because of the increased metabolic activity and decreased nutrient intake from the anorexia.

Sudden rises (spikes) in temperature are not unusual in infants and young children who have acute infections because their temperature control mechanism is so labile. They do not, however, tolerate fever well. Infants and young children are easily dehydrated because their body surface is proportionately greater than that of an adult. Consequently, they rapidly develop fluid and electrolyte imbalance.

Intervention

Reduction of fever. Correction of the underlying cause, when possible, will return body temperature to normal. When an infectious agent is the cause, antibiotics are given and continued until after the temperature has returned to normal levels. Antibiotics must be given at regular intervals to maintain constant blood levels in order to maximize their effectiveness. Since fever is an essential part of the defense mechanism, specific actions to decrease the temperature are not taken unless the temperature exceeds 39.5 C (103 F) in an older child or adult, or 39 C (102 F) in an infant or young child, or if the fever is prolonged. Acetylsalicylic acid (aspirin) reduces an elevated body temperature. The antipyretic effects are caused by either protection of the heat-regulating center against pyrogens or interference with the peripheral release or production of endogenous pyrogenic factors.

Body temperature can also be lowered by inducing heat loss by evaporation. Alcohol sponge baths, which consist of sponging alternate parts of the body with a solution of half alcohol and half *lukewarm* water, are often helpful. Cold water is not used, as the cold stimulates vasoconstriction that leads to heat retention by the body. The goal of the sponge bath is to encourage vasodilatation and loss of heat as the alcohol evaporates from the skin surface. The patient's temperature is monitored and the sponge bath is discontinued if a sudden reduction occurs. A lukewarm tub bath may also decrease an elevated temperature because of the vasodilatation.

Hypothermia may be used for patients with high, prolonged fevers from serious generalized infections, especially in patients who tolerate high fever poorly, such as infants, debilitated persons, and persons who have cardiac or renal disease. Hypothermia decreases the body's metabolic needs. The lowered body temperature also inhibits multiplication of the infecting organism, making it easier for the body's defenses and the prescribed treatment to control the infection producing the fever. (See p. 384 for management of a patient being treated with hypothermia.)

Food and fluids. Persons with high or prolonged fever experience considerable fluid loss (dehydration) from the increased respirations and diaphoresis, and from an increased need for fluid because of the accelerated metabolic processes. Sodium and potassium deficits also occur. A negative nitrogen balance results as more protein is being utilized than is being replaced, thus increasing nitrogenous wastes. (See p. 362 for further information on negative nitrogen balance.) Sufficient fluids are needed to promote normal renal function and eliminate the increased wastes. The adult patient is therefore strongly urged to take 2,500 to 3,000 ml of fluid a day. Since the patient is anorexic and usually will not eat much solid food, fluids that have high caloric, high protein, high sodium, potassium, and vitamin C content need to be substituted for some of the water intake. Fruit juices, milk shakes, milk puddings, jello, ice cream, and soups are usually well tolerated. Mouth care given prior to eating will remove the unpleasant taste that occurs with fever and will promote an increased food and fluid intake. The patient's fluid intake is closely monitored to assess the adequacy of the fluid replacement. If the patient becomes severely dehydrated, intravenous fluids may be indicated.

Elimination. Fluid output is also monitored to assess adequacy of nitrogenous waste and toxin removal. Dark-colored urine is tested for specific gravity, and the fluid intake is increased if the specific gravity is high (over 1.025).

Bowel elimination is assessed daily and compared to the patient's usual bowel pattern. Not only is gastrointestinal activity decreased, but also the colon will be attempting to conserve fluid through increased reabsorption of water, and the stool will be hard. Measures to prevent constipation and fecal impaction are carried out (see p. 1244).

Comfort. Activities must be planned to provide frequent rest periods because of the fatigue that is usually present. In some instances when fever is high, the nurse may elect to bathe the patient who is capable of bathing himself in order to conserve his energy. Tub baths, if permitted, are relaxing, but the patient usually needs assistance and close monitoring, since he may become dizzy or faint. Baths also help remove waste products that are excreted during diaphoresis and reduce fever by heat evaporation.

If headache and photophobia are present, the patient may be more comfortable if the lights are dimmed and other environmental stimuli decreased. Back rubs may ease some of the muscle soreness that occurs, although some persons prefer to be left alone. The person with a high fever sleeps more than usual; this helps to conserve energy. Bed rest is indicated for persons with temperatures greater than 38 C (100.4 F).

Safety. With very high fevers, convulsions and disorientation may occur. In these situations the patient needs to be protected from falling out of bed or injuring himself. Side rails should be raised and the patient closely monitored.

Prolonged effects. After a high or prolonged fever, most adults feel weak, perspire on physical exertion, and become tired easily. The person usually stays in bed until his temperature has been normal for 24 hours. For several days (or even weeks after a prolonged fever) the patient of any age should have extra rest and eat foods high in protein and calories. Children and young adults usually recover much more rapidly than elderly persons, even when the infection has been severe.

□ Outcome criteria

An outcome criteria for any person who is hospitalized is that the person be protected from acquiring a nosocomial infection during hospitalization.

The person with an infection or infectious disease or significant others can:

1. Describe the method of spread of the infection.
2. List common signs and symptoms so as to recognize the spread of the infection among significant others.
3. List measures to prevent spread of the infection to others.

4. Explain the need for attention to personal hygiene, such as handwashing.
5. Explain antibiotic therapy to be followed:
   a. Need to take the medication at specified intervals.
   b. Need to complete the course of antibiotic therapy as prescribed.
   c. Signs and symptoms of adverse effects or toxicity.
6. Plan menus that are high in protein and calories.
7. List signs and symptoms of possible sequelae.
8. Explain need for medical follow-up care until discharged by the physician.

■ INTERVENTION FOR LOCALIZED INFECTIONS

Most persons with localized infections are not hospitalized, and the nursing care therefore consists of teaching the person or a family member how to care for the infected or inflamed part. Some of the most common localized infections include infections of the hand, ulcers of the legs (p. 1024), furuncles and carbuncles (p. 1527), and lymphangitis and lymphadenitis.

□ Infections of the hand

Infections of the hand occur frequently because the hands are functionally involved in most activities and thus are likely to be injured or exposed to infection. These injuries and infections usually are painful, and rest is essential to healing. Therefore although the patient rarely is hospitalized, he may be partially incapacitated.

An infection involving the soft tissues around and underneath the nail is called a *paronychia* (Fig. 21-1, *A*). It usually results from the infection of a hangnail. The involved finger is very painful, and the patient complains of a continuous throbbing sensation. The pain is relieved immediately by lifting the soft tissues away from the nail with a scalpel and draining the pus. The patient then may be given an antibiotic and instructed to soak his finger in warm, sterile saline solution for 15 to 20 minutes several times a day and to refrain from using his hand.

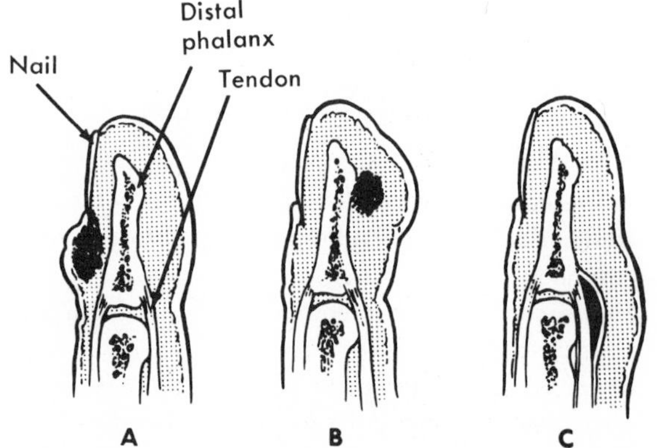

Fig. 21-1. Common infections of the finger. **A,** Paronychia. **B,** Felon. **C,** Tendon sheath infection.

An infection that involves the soft tissue of the fingertip is called a *felon* (Fig. 21-1, *B*). It often is caused when staphylococci are introduced into the finger by a pinprick and sometimes can be prevented by making pinpricks bleed. In the early stages the infection responds to warm soaks, and sometimes an antibiotic is given. If it is allowed to progress untreated, the swelling may cause obstruction of the arterial blood supply to the soft tissues of the finger, and necrosis of the tissue and underlying bone may occur. The infected area will then have to be surgically incised and drained and the necrotic tissue excised. A pricked finger should be watched carefully, and if swelling or pain develops, medical treatment should be obtained.

Infection of the tendon sheath (Fig. 21-1, *C*), particularly on the palmar surface, often follows puncture wounds of the fingers or hand. Streptococci are most often the infecting organisms. The hand becomes red and swollen along the tendon, and movement is very painful. This kind of infection usually responds to early treatment with antibiotics and hot soaks, but surgical incision and drainage may be necessary. Untreated infections of the tendon sheath lead to destruction of the tendon with resulting finger and hand deformities. If the tendon has been damaged, a tendon graft to correct deformities may be necessary after healing has occurred.

□ Lymphangitis and lymphadenitis

Lymphangitis is an inflammation of the lymphatic vessels. It is usually of streptococcal origin and is a sequela of infections of the feet, legs, hands, or arms. The first symptom to appear is a red, tender streak under the skin of the leg or forearm, indicating the spread of the infection to the lymphatic vessels. The lymph nodes above the infection (in the knee, groin, elbow, or axilla) become swollen and tender as the infectious organisms invade them. This condition is known as lymphadenitis. If the infection continues uncontrolled and bacteria reach the bloodstream, septicemia with fever, chills, malaise, and increase in the pulse rate may develop. Infections of the lymph channels are treated by drainage of the original infection, antibiotics, hot wet dressings, and elevation of the affected extremity.

□ Use of heat or cold

The application of either heat or cold are two methods of treatment for inflammatory conditions. The decision to use heat or cold depends on the desired goals, that is, enhancement or restriction of the inflammatory process.

Application of heat

Heat applied locally increases vasodilation in an inflamed area and thus augments the natural defense mechanism. The inflammatory process serves a function when an open wound or an infection is present, since it promotes removal of foreign material by the cellular defense mechanisms. (For more information on the inflammatory response, see p. 178.)

Dry heat in the form of heat lamps or diathermy may be ordered, or moist heat in the form of warm compresses or soaks may be used. Some physicians prefer massive warm, moist compresses because they insulate the part, preventing loss of body heat from the physiologically dilated vessels. Warm compresses, however, may cause reflex vasoconstriction and decrease, instead of increase, the blood supply to the affected part. Applications of heat are used rarely and with great caution for infants, because their tender skin is easily burned. If warm compresses are used for long intervals on an extensive area such as an extremity of an infant or small child, the body temperature is checked at least every 2 hours because a large percentage of the body area is exposed to extra heat and deprived of dissipation of heat. If the temperature rises, the warm compresses are discontinued and the physician notified.

Warm, moist compresses. One method for applying warm, moist compresses at home is to duplicate the method used in hospitals. This necessitates boiling forceps (or tweezers) in a pan with water for 10 minutes and using the boiled warm water for the dressing. (For details of this procedure consult a fundamentals text.) A second method is to warm a bottle of sterile water in a water bath, pour some of the warm sterile water over a sterile dressing that has been applied over the infected part, and then cover with a dry dressing. A piece of aluminum foil may be placed over the dressing and covered by a hot water bottle to help maintain the desired heat.

Warm soaks. The use of sterile or unsterile solutions for soaking a foot or hand depends on whether the skin over the infected part is intact. Clean but unsterile basins and solutions can be used for intact skin. If the infected part is open and draining, sterile basins and solutions are used. If the soak is done at home, the water is boiled for 10 minutes in the soaking pan and then allowed to cool until it is lukewarm (37.5 C or 100 F)—*not* hot. Hot water will cause vasoconstriction, which would decrease circulation to the part. If a saline soak is desired, 10 ml (2 teaspoons) of salt is added to each liter (quart) of water.

Application of cold

Vasoconstriction occurs when cold is applied to an area, decreasing the blood supply. Cold is applied when the effects of the inflammatory response serve no purpose; that is, when further tissue damage or increased pain can occur because of the increased fluid in an enclosed space. Examples of these situations are acute bursitis and the initial period after trauma such as a sprained ankle. In some instances it is desirable to slow down the inflammatory process to prevent complications. Thus if appendicitis is suspected, cold is applied to the lower abdomen to try to prevent rupture of the appendix with subsequent peritonitis and to aid in decreasing pain.

Unsterile cold compresses can be used since the skin is intact. Compresses can be placed in ice water, wrung out, applied immediately, and changed frequently. The patient can often do this himself. Cold can also be applied by means of an ice bag. One method for applying cold over curved body areas is to fill a plastic glove with crushed ice and fasten the cuff by several folds and a rubber band to prevent escape of water. Plastic sandwich bags filled with crushed ice can be used in the home for application to small areas. A cloth covering is placed between the ice bag and the patient's skin for comfort. Cold applications are applied for periods of 20 to 30 minutes for maximum effect.

REFERENCES AND SELECTED READINGS

1. Alter, H. J.: Health-care workers positive for hepatitis B surface antigen, N. Engl. J. Med. **292**:454-457, 1975.
2. American Academy of Pediatrics: Report of the Committee on the Control of Infectious Diseases, ed. 17, Evanston, Ill., 1974, The Academy.
3. *American Public Health Association: Control of communicable disease in man, ed. 12, New York, 1975, The Association.
4. Armstrong, D., et al.: Infectious diseases: diagnosis and treatment, New York, 1975, Medcom Press.
5. Baranowski, K., Greene, H. L. II, and Lamont, J. T.: Viral hepatitis—how to reduce its threat to the patient and others (including you), Nurs. 76 **6**:31-38, 1976.

5a. Barrett-Connor, E., Simon, H. J., Brandt, S. L., Dechairo, D. C.: Epidemiology for the infection control nurse, St. Louis, 1978, The C. V. Mosby Co.

6. *Beletz, E. E., and Covo, G. A.: The case of the hidden infection in the elderly, Nurs. 76 **6**:15-16, 1976.
7. *Castle, M.: Isolation-precise procedures for better protection, Nurs. 75 **5**:50-57, 1975.
8. Cody, L. D., et al.: Infection control in the cancer hospital, APIC Newsletter **4**:1-4, 1976.
9. Dale, D. C., and Petersdorf, R. G.: Corticosteroids and infectious diseases, Med. Clin. North Am. **53**:1277, 1973.
10. Farmer, J. J. III: Pseudomonas in the hospital, Hosp. Pract. **11**:63-70, 1976.
11. Feingold, D. S.: Hospital-acquired infections, N. Engl. J. Med. **283**:384, 1970.
12. Gardner, P., Oxman, M. N., and Breton, S.: Hospital management of patients and personnel exposed to communicable diseases, Pediatrics **56**:700-709, 1975.

*References preceded by an asterisk are particularly well suited for student reading.

13. Gardner, P., et al.: Manual of acute bacterial infections, New York, 1975, Little, Brown and Co.
14. Jawetz, E., et al.: Review of medical microbiology, ed. 11, Los Altos, Calif. 1974, Lange Medical Publications.
15. *Kunin, C.: Detection, prevention and management of urinary tract infections, ed. 2, Philadelphia, 1974, Lea and Febiger.
16. *Lauter, C. B.: Opportunistic infections, Heart Lung, **5**:601-606, 1976.
17. Lightfoot, R. W., Jr., and Gotschlich, E. C.: Gonococcal disease, Am. J. Med. **56**:347-356, 1974.
18. Matsen, J.: Pathogens: their sources and control. Part II: Hospitals, J.A.H.A., **49**:63-65, 1975.
19. Matsen, J.: Pathogens: their sources and control. Part I: Hospitals, J.A.H.A., **48**:71-76, 1974.
20. McInnis, M. E.: Essentials of communicable diseases, ed. 2, St. Louis, 1975, The C.V. Mosby Co.
21. Orkin, M.: Treatment of today's scabies and pediculosis, J.A.M.A. **236**:1136-1139, 1976.
22. *Public Health Service, Center for Disease Control: Isolation techniques for use in hospitals, ed. 2, U.S. Department of Health, Education and Welfare, No. (CDC) 76-8314, 1975.
23. Roellig, S.: Management of patients with contagious illnesses, Heart Lung **5**:596-600, 1976.
24. Sanford, J. P.: The hospital reservoir. Paper presented before the American College of Surgeons: Symposium on the control of surgical infections, Fort Lauderdale, Fl., March 6, 1970.
25. *Schabert, D., et al.: Epidemics of nosocomial urinary tract infection caused by multi-resistant gram-negative bacilli, J. Infect. Dis. **133**:363-366, 1976.
26. Spencer, D. J., et al.: Utilization of cost-benefit analysis in planning prevention programs, Acta Med. Scand. **576**:123, 1974.
27. *Steere, A. C., et al.: Handwashing practices for the prevention of nosocomial infections, Ann. Int. Med. **83**:683-690, 1975.
28. Thorn, G. W., et al.: Harrison's principles of internal medicine, ed. 8, New York, 1975, McGraw-Hill Book Co.
29. Wood, R. E.: Pseudomonas: the compromised hospital, Hosp. Pract. **11**:91-94, 1976.
30. U.S. Immunization Survey, Center for Disease Control and the Bureau of Census, Atlanta, 1973.
31. Youmans, G. P., et al.: The biologic and clinical basis of infectious diseases, Philadelphia, 1975, W. B. Saunders Co.

22

Pain

VIRGINIA BURKE KARB

■ INTRODUCTION

Pain is a two-edged sword. On the one hand it warns us to move away from heat, cold, and sharp objects before injury occurs and makes us aware of the presence of disease and tissue damage; thus it usually influences us to seek medical attention. On the other hand fear of pain may cause us to delay medical treatment, and if its cause cannot be located and relieved, its presence serves no useful purpose and it becomes harmful. Continuous, severe pain eventually causes physical and mental exhaustion and prevents the individual from functioning productively. Pain accompanies almost all illnesses, and perhaps no sensation is more dreaded by patients undergoing medical treatment or surgery.

Pain has never been satisfactorily defined or understood. It is an unpleasant feeling, entirely subjective, that only the person experiencing it can describe. It can be evoked by a multiplicity of stimuli (chemical, thermal, electrical, mechanical), but the reaction to it cannot be measured objectively. Pain is a learned experience that is influenced by the entire life situation of each person. What is perceived as pain and the reaction to that pain differ among people and sometimes differ in the same person from one time to another.

Care of patients suffering pain demands skill in both the science and the art of nursing. The nurse's responsibility is to make the patient as comfortable as possible physically and emotionally and to observe and report findings so that they may help the physician make a correct diagnosis and prescribe appropriate treatment.

□ Definition of pain

Sternbach describes pain as an abstract concept that refers to sensation, stimulus and response.[81] Another author points out that there is an emotion of pain in addition to the sensation of pain.[93] It is probably not necessary to have an elaborate definition of pain in order to provide nursing care to a patient in pain. McCaffery states that "pain is whatever the experiencing person says it is and exists whenever he says it does."[60] The nurse therefore will see pain frequently and must learn to assist each individual to deal as effectively as possible with it.

□ Significance and frequency of pain

Pain serves a major function by alerting us to possible harm or damage. It may or may not influence us to seek medical attention. Pain may have other meanings for an individual: the possible loss of mobility or activity, the recurrence of a particular disease, the reminder that the individual may be aging. Pain may precipitate feelings of fear, anger, uneasiness, challenge, or punishment. Other individuals may see pain as an opportunity for creative expression, self-searching, self-testing, or for fostering an appreciation of what less fortunate patients have gone through.

In general, however, most persons view pain as a negative experience. Below is a list of the top 20 words used to describe pain as listed by 148 patients:

Treacherous	Hidden	Variety of words meaning satanic
Mean	Obnoxious	Nasty
Hateful	Faceless	Sharp
Detestable	Degrading	Cunning
Sneaky	Cruel	Nervous
Intense	Inconsiderate	Persistent[18]
Dark	Invading	

Factors that influence the meaning of pain to an individual are many and varied. Some of these include age,[5] sex, cultural background,[10,23] psychosocial factors,[41,42] environmental factors, expected response, and other assorted problems and diagnoses. The setting in which pain occurs may be important. For example, the pain incurred by an athlete injured during a sports event may be severe if it also means he must leave the game and perhaps forfeit play during the remainder of the season. A soldier injured in wartime activities may associate injury and concomitant pain as relatively minor if the injury also means relief from the pressure of battle and possible return home.[4]

Pain is experienced by most individuals at various times throughout life. It may be the result of or associated with trauma, exposure to excessive heat or cold, excessive strain or use of body parts (as in the person who exercises vigorously), normal bodily functions such as labor and delivery, surgical intervention, and so on. Most individuals try to avoid pain but at the same time expect that it will occur with various activities associated with living.

Pain threshold

Pain threshold refers to the intensity of the noxious stimulus necessary for the person to perceive pain.[42] The threshold is approximately the same for all individuals.[7] The tolerance for pain, on the other hand, refers to "the duration of time or the intensity at which a subject accepts a stimulus above the pain threshold before making a verbal or overt pain response."[81]

The tolerance for pain may be raised by alcohol, drugs, hypnosis, warmth, rubbing, or distracting activities. Strong beliefs and faith seem to increase tolerance for pain, and it is sometimes difficult to judge how much pain a patient with deep religious faith is actually experiencing. Fatigue, anger, boredom, and apprehension may decrease one's ability to tolerate pain. Pain tolerance also is lowered by persistent pain such as that sometimes experienced by patients with far-advanced carcinoma. A weak, debilitated patient usually tolerates pain less well than a healthy person, although increasing debility will eventually cause mental dulling with a resultant decrease in pain perception.

Perception of pain

The perception of pain, or the actual feeling of pain, takes place in the cerebral cortex. It is known that a functioning frontal lobe of the brain is required to experience the full suffering and worry that result from pain. The reaction to the same stimuli differs widely among people and in the same person from one time to another because the final perception of pain depends more on the interpretation in the cerebral cortex than on the characteristics of the original stimuli. What the cerebral cortex interprets as pain will depend on childhood training, previous experience, cultural values, religious beliefs, physical and mental health, knowledge and understanding, attention and distraction, fatigue, anxiety, tension, fear, state of consciousness, and the frequency and intensity of pain impulses.

Atrophy of nerve endings, degenerative changes in the pain-bearing pathways, and decreased alertness may reduce the perception of pain in the elderly, and more stimulation may be required to evoke a response. Elderly persons therefore may fail to perceive tissue damage that normally would cause pain and thus alert a younger person.

The perception of a pain stimulus may be altered at many points by both normal and abnormal conditions. A pleasant environment, an enjoyable book, stimulating conversation, or other distracting activity of a pleasing nature may serve to lessen the sensation of pain. Tissue damage or inflammatory conditions at the site where the stimuli originate may increase or decrease the impulse. For example, slapping a person who has a sunburn may set off a far greater impulse than if the person were not sunburned. On the other hand, if the local nerve endings have been damaged by a severe burn the patient may not respond at all to what would ordinarily be painful stimuli. Abnormal conditions within the spinal cord such as inflammatory diseases, tumors, or injuries may prevent transmission or nerve impulses. This may occur at either the spinal or the thalamic relay stations. The impulse may also be altered at either of these two relay stations by other activity going on simultaneously within the spinal cord. This probably accounts for the fact that sometimes bruises and cuts sustained during absorbing activities go unnoticed until the activity is over. Perception in the cortex may be influenced by abnormal conditions such as inflammatory processes, degenerative changes, and depression of brain function, which may alter the original signal pattern. Anesthesia and analgesia also cause depression of sensory perceptions.

Reaction to pain

Meaning and perception of pain are accompanied by reaction to pain. Reaction to pain is influenced also by such factors as past experience, conditioning, cultural values, and physical and mental health. Consequently people will respond differently to the same stimuli. Some may accept the pain and be patient and resigned; others may become depressed and withdrawn. Some may be fearful, apprehensive, and anxious, while others are tolerant and optimistic. Some weep, moan, scream, beg for relief or help, threaten to destroy themselves, thrash about in bed, or move about aimlessly while they are in severe pain. Others lie quietly in bed and may only close their eyes, grit their teeth, bite their lips, clench their hands, or perspire profusely when experiencing pain.

Some people, by training and example, are taught to endure severe pain without reacting outwardly. American Indian men have rites in which they show their strength by the amount of pain they can endure. Such individuals probably would tolerate pain from disease or injury better than those from a culture in which free expression of feelings is encouraged. Persons from cultures in which health teaching and disease prevention are emphasized tend to accept pain as a warning to seek help and expect the cause of pain will be found and cured.

Parents' attitudes toward pain may determine their children's lifelong reaction to pain. In the American culture parents usually begin to teach their children what is expected of them in regard to courage and self-control at about the age of 2 or 3 years. They try not to appear too concerned about minor injuries and usually encourage their children not to cry when they are hurt. Children try very hard to be brave, especially in the presence of other children.

The setting in which injury occurs may influence the external response to pain. A boy may feel, for example, the pain suffered from injury during a hockey game, though perhaps severe because of its meaning to the boy, should nevertheless be borne quietly, whereas pain resulting from an automobile accident may be expressed freely.

Influence of fear

Morbid fear of a disease may intensify pain caused by it or it may lead the individual to deny pain in his eagerness to believe that nothing is wrong. Anticipation of pain based on past experience often intensifies pain. For example, the child who enters the hospital for the last of several operations may react more vigorously to postoperative pain than he did on his first encounter with the sensation.

One's personality also influences reaction to pain. A person who reacts hysterically to trying situations may find even a small amount of pain intolerable. People may sometimes use moderate pain as an escape from unacceptable life situations, or they may try to use it to control situations around them. This latter reaction is often demonstrated both in the hospital and at home.

There is more reaction to pain during the night and early morning hours when the person's physiologic processes are at low ebb and there is little distracting activity. The patient's thoughts may easily turn to concern for himself and his loved ones, and his worrying may increase his reaction to pain.

Age affects the reaction to pain. The young fear it because it may represent an unfamiliar experience, and they frequently respond to it by crying. The older person may know what to expect and accept it, or he may be withdrawn and quiet while experiencing it because of emotional exhaustion.

Theories of pain transmission

People have been studying pain and attempting to develop theories of pain transmission for centuries. Three major theories are mentioned briefly: the specificity theory, the pattern theory, and the gate control theory. None of these provides all the answers to explain pain transmission, but many recent experiments in pain therapy have been based on the gate control theory.

The *specificity theory* holds that there are certain specific nerve receptors that respond to noxious stimuli and that these noxious stimuli are always interpreted as pain. In addition this theory states that pain impulses are carried by pain fibers—fast, myelinated A-delta fibers and more slowly conducting unmyelinated C fibers—to the lateral spinothalamic tract in the spinal cord to a pain center in the thalamus. Impulses are then sent to the cerebral cortex by way of the corticothalamic tract where the actual perception of pain takes place (Fig. 22-1). Opponents of this theory point out that specific pain receptors have not been identified, nor does the body always interpret certain stimuli as noxious.[67]

The *pattern theory* suggests that pain is produced by intense stimulation of nonspecific fiber receptors. In other words, any stimulus could be perceived as painful if the stimulation were intense enough. This model does not explain, for example, the functioning of the spinal

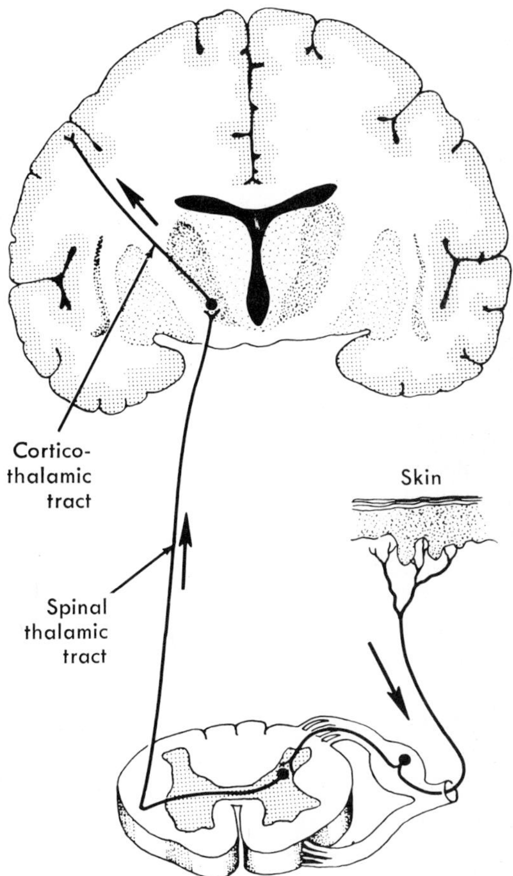

Fig. 22-1. Pathways of pain transmission according to specificity theory.

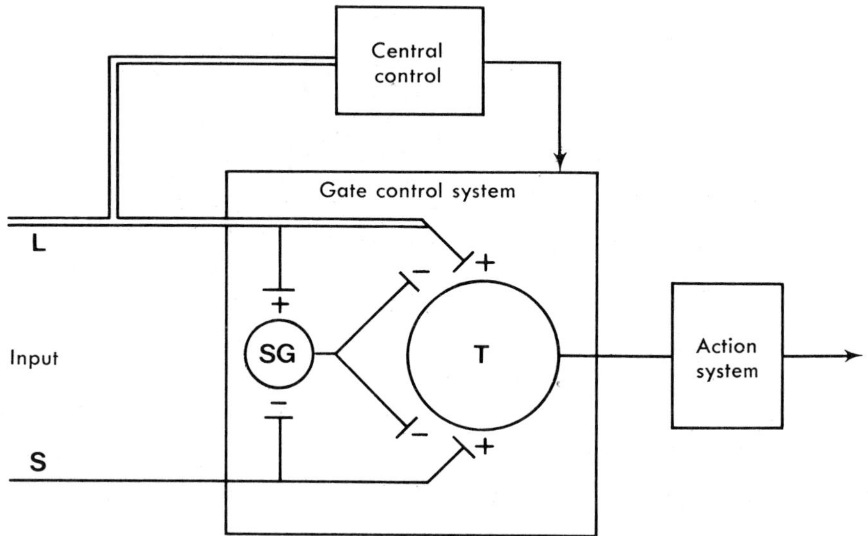

Fig. 22-2. Schema of gate control theory of pain mechanisms. L, large-diameter fibers; S, small-diameter fibers. Fibers project to SG, substantia gelatinosa, and T, first central transmission cells. Inhibitory effect exerted by SG on afferent fiber terminals is increased by activity in L fibers and decreased by activity in S fibers. Central control processes project to gate control system. They include fibers from brainstem, which have predominantly inhibitory effect, as well as fibers from cortex. T cells project to entry cells of action system. +, Excitation; −, inhibition. (From Weisenberg, M.: Pain: clinical and experimental perspectives, St. Louis, 1975, The C. V. Mosby Co.; after Melzack and Wall.)

cord in pain transmission and thus does not explain the pain relief provided by many neurosurgical therapies.

In 1965 Melzack and Wall proposed the *gate control theory*. This theory proposes that pain and its perception depend on the interaction of three systems: the substantia gelatinosa in the dorsal horn of the spinal cord, which modulates impulses entering the spinal cord; a central control system in the cortex and thalamus, which influences the impulses reaching the brain; and the neural system associated with perception of pain. The theory proposes that pain impulses are conducted over small-diameter fibers to the spinal cord, travel across an "opened gate" in the substantia gelatinosa to the anterolateral spinothalamic tract, and then ascend the tract to the thalamus and cortex where pain perception and interpretation occur. The "gate" in the substantia gelatinosa can be "closed" (Fig. 22-2) so that the contact is not made, thus interrupting the pain impulse. This gate can be closed by conflicting impulses from the skin conducted over large-diameter fibers, by impulses from the reticular formation in the brainstem, or by impulses from the entire cortex or thalamus (central control system).[80] Thus impulses from the skin, brainstem, thalamus, or cortex can effectively block the transmission of pain impulses or can intensify the impulse. In this manner thoughts (cognition), attitudes, past experiences, and so forth, can modify or intensify the pain experience.

Not all scientists accept the gate control theory, and in fact new theories are still being proposed. It would seem, though, that most new theories take as their starting point the gate control theory, and it is still the most widely accepted theory.*

□ Referred pain

Referred pain is that pain felt in areas other than those stimulated. It may occur when stimulation is not perceived in the primary area. For example, the person experiencing a heart attack may complain only of pain radiating down the left arm when in fact the tissue damage is occurring in the heart.

Referred pain seems to occur most often with damage or injury to visceral organs, and the pain is referred to cutaneous surfaces (Fig. 22-3). The exact physiologic mechanism that occurs during referred pain is not clearly understood but may relate in part to the lack of sensory nerve endings near visceral organs. The cutaneous pattern of various referred pains is fairly constant and frequently seen in practice. The nurse should be able to recognize the possibility of visceral organ disease

*References 21, 47, 65, 72, 78.

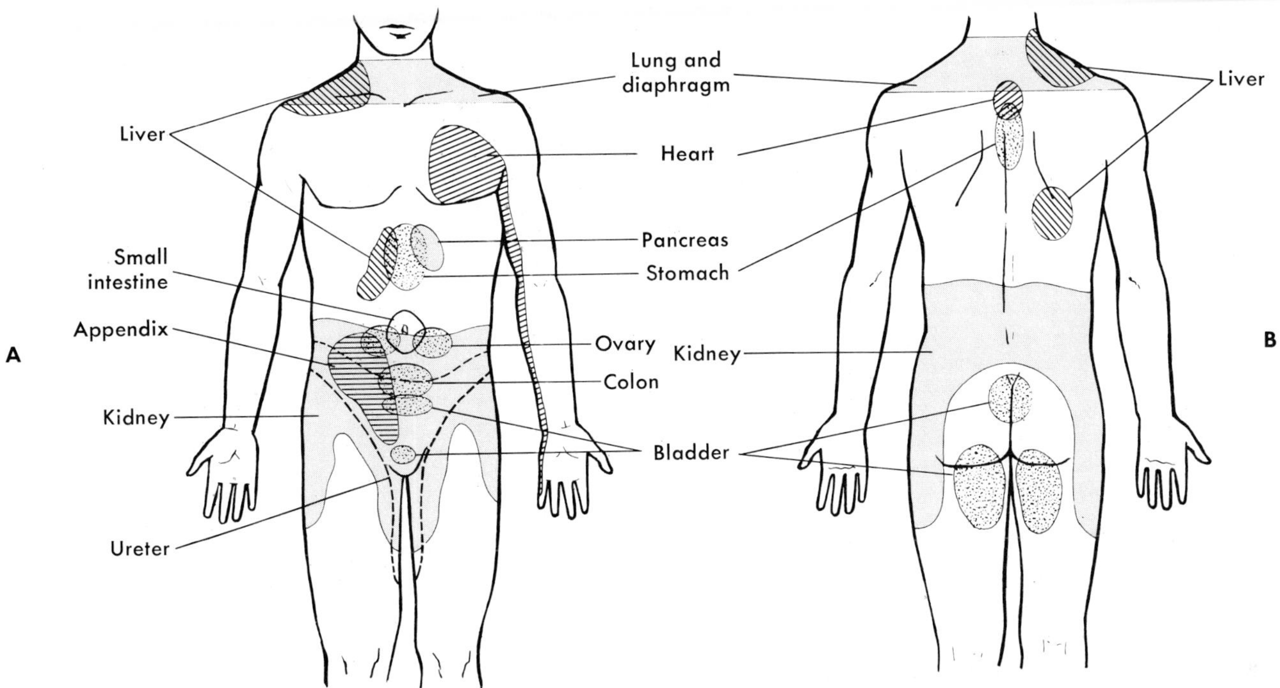

Fig. 22-3. Referred pain.

in patients with appropriate cutaneous complaints of pain.

□ Other types of pain

Some types of pain are not completely explained by present theories of pain transmission and present specific management problems. *Phantom limb* pain refers to pain or discomfort perceived by the individual to be occurring in an extremity that has been amputated. It is known that phantom limb pain:

1. Has no single cause.
2. Endures long after healing of the injured tissues.
3. Is more likely to develop in patients who suffered pain in the limb before amputation.
4. May be associated with trigger zones that when stimulated will result in the perception of this pain; the trigger zones may spread to healthy areas on the same or opposite sides of the body.
5. Is influenced by emotional factors and the sympathetic nervous system, but neither cause it.[65]

Phantom limb pain may be very difficult to treat, probably because it is not clearly understood.

Another unusual type of pain is *causalgia*, "severe, burning pain characteristically associated with rapid, violent deformation of nerves by high velocity missiles such as bullets."[65] This type of pain may gradually disappear, but a significant number of patients may still be complaining of pain a year after injury. An unusual feature of this type of pain is that it may be triggered by normally nonnoxious stimuli such as the noise created when planes fly overhead.[65]

Neuralgia refers to pain or discomfort that occurs as a result of infection or disease that damages peripheral nerves. Causalgia may be thought of as a type of neuralgia, but the converse is not true.

Headache is another type of pain that may vary significantly from one individual to another. The causes of certain headaches are fairly well understood: tension, increasing intracranial pressure as a result of a mass lesion, infection, and so on. The migraine headache is less clearly understood, as is the cluster headache characterized by severe localized pain that is intense, of short duration, and difficult to treat (see Chapter 35).

■ ASSESSMENT OF THE CLIENT WITH PAIN

□ Subjective data

Assessment of the client undergoing a pain experience begins with a careful history. Information to elicit includes characteristics and description of the pain. The client may use his own words to describe the pain, and the nurse should take care to validate with the client his exact meaning if it is unclear to the nurse. The characteristics may include the site, severity, and location of pain. If asked what he thinks may be causing the pain, the client may shed some light on possible topics for further elaboration.

The patient may also be able to say what he thinks might relieve the pain and what was effective or ineffective for pain relief at home. Careful questioning may also elicit the client's expectations of the health care team in relation to the pain. Does he hope for pain elimination or palliation? Is he opposed to surgical intervention or does he expect surgical manipulation? What does the pain mean to the patient? Has it interfered with his life style, and if so, how? At home or at work? If the client can be helped with his pain, what activity(ies) would he like to resume?

Appropriate sociocultural data to include are the client's age, religion, usual reaction to pain, position in the family (i.e., breadwinner, homemaker), and the responsibilities associated with that position. The client may be able to describe his usual coping mechanisms and the expectations he and his family may have about an appropriate response to pain.

If the patient has been taking medications for pain, what was the medication, in what dose and with what frequency was it taken, and did it provide relief?

It is always necessary to decide with each client his tolerance for an elaborate assessment. In the critically ill patient a few key questions about pain rather than the long list above may be all that is appropriate, particularly if the nurse must quickly do a total assessment.

The nurse who has an opportunity to work with the client on an ongoing basis can easily assess the client's pain and his response to it over time and during various circumstances. The ongoing assessment should still include subjective data about the location, duration, and intensity of pain. The nurse and client may also determine that there are associated factors with the pain experience: time of day, week, or month; certain body positions or actions; certain environmental situations; and so on. In every case the nurse needs to convey trust and interest in the client in order that he may feel free to discuss his pain with the nurse.

□ Objective data

The nurse needs to make careful objective observations of all clients. The objective data may help clarify the subjective client response, or it may be the only way the nurse becomes aware of the client's pain.

Physiologic signs of pain may include increased heart rate, increased frequency or depth of respiration or both, diaphoresis, increased systolic and diastolic blood pressure, pallor, dilated pupils, increased muscle tension, and piloerection (goose bumps). The client may complain of nausea or of feeling weak or sick.

If the pain is chronic or less severe, the physiologic manifestations may be less prominent and less severe. Instead the nurse may notice changes in facial expression such as frowning or gritting of teeth. The client may clench his fists and withdraw inwardly from his surroundings. The physiologic response then begins to meld with the psychologic reaction to pain: the client may complain bitterly, cry, moan, toss about in bed, assume a fetal position, clutch at the affected body part, or sit stiff and withdrawn. The friendly client may begin to appear hostile and angry. The client may or may not call the nurse for assistance with pain relief.

Observing the behavior of the young child who cannot yet talk is the only way to determine whether he has pain and where it is located. The child who tugs at his ear, doubles his body over and clasps his abdomen, or refuses to move a certain area of his body or permit it to be touched may have pain in the area. Irritability and continuous crying that is unrelieved by the usual comfort measures may mean that the child is in pain. Parents may be asked about activities they have observed that appear to cause discomfort. When signs of pain are apparent, a close examination of the child's body should be made to rule out an injury or other obvious cause of distress.

The nurse must be able to assess the patient's pain and his emotional response to it without being judgmental about his reaction to pain. The manner in which the patient perceives and reacts to pain has been influenced by his whole life, and he cannot voluntarily modify this response very much. Regardless of the cause of pain or the patient's behavior, his immediate need is for relief from pain. Knowing how the patient feels about pain helps the nurse initiate measures to make him more comfortable.

The need to assess the person with pain is ongoing, yet the nurse must begin to plan an approach to the person and the pain. The nurse is able to function independently with many interventions, but careful planning with other members of the health care team should ensure that all have the same patient outcomes or goals in mind.

■ INTERVENTIONS DIRECTED TOWARD PAIN RELIEF OR ALTERATION

The first step in developing and implementing the plan of care is to obtain the patient's trust. Ideally the nurse would have begun the initial assessment of the person with this need for trust in mind. In order to convey trust and interest, the nurse needs to remember that the pain is whatever the experiencing person says it is and that it exists whenever he says it does.[60] Thus the nurse may not always know when to anticipate that the patient will manifest pain. Patience, conveying an interest, being willing to help, and avoiding prejudging the patient are helpful. Prejudging implies tending to look for behavior associated with acute pain. Interventions can be directed at modifying the pain stimulus, altering the mode of transmission, or modifying the response to pain.

□ Modification of stimulus: changing the cognitive or sensory input

Explaining the problem

As the nurse assesses the individual it may become clear that his response to the pain is really a manifestation of lack of knowledge about what is happening to him. The nurse explains, in simple terms if necessary, what is causing the pain, if it is to be expected, and how long it may last. This explanation should continue with each new experience, for example, before each new diagnostic test. Understanding that pain is to be expected may relieve the patient's anxiety or help him alter his expectations and approach. A simple example might be the pain associated with a lumbar puncture.

Decision making

Allowing the individual to regain some control over his day may allow him to exert better control over pain. If possible and within limits, the patient should be allowed to make decisions about the frequency of certain tasks such as exercises and turning and the order of such daily events as the bath, getting out of bed, and so on. If the patient has delineated the least painful way of doing a certain activity, such as turning, this method is recorded on the plan of care and everyone working with the client is expected to follow this method.

Consistency and careful planning

Allowing the same health care team members to care for the patient regularly should result in a more consistent approach and plan of care. Between the small group of health care team members and the patient, a plan of care can be developed in which the patient's decisions are honored, the day-to-day activities are put in order, and a daily routine can be devised that will reduce anxiety and frustration about constant changes. This plan should include, if appropriate, such items as specified hours for drug administration before uncomfortable procedures, specified blocks of time for rest or napping, and coordination between various departments such as physical therapy and occupational therapy. For some patients fatigue is a great problem, so regular visits to off-unit departments should be interspersed with rest periods throughout the day; for other patients the most beneficial plan includes ensuring that they go directly from one department to the next each day so that time is not wasted getting in and out of bed or performing other painful maneuvers.

Distraction

Many individuals can be distracted from constant preoccupation with discomfort. Distraction interferes with the pain stimulus, thereby modifying the awareness of the pain. Mild or moderate pain can be modified by focusing on activity in the environment. A very quiet environment providing little or no sensory input can actually intensify the pain experience because the individual has nothing to focus on but the painful stimulus.

Severe pain requires more active participation by the individual in an effort to block out the painful stimulus. This can be enhanced by involving two or more sensory modalities such as vision, hearing, touch, or movement.[60] The distracters must be powerful enough to involve the individual's total interest without resulting in fatigue. Pain of long duration requires a variety of meaningful distracters.

Careful assessment may indicate ways in which the patient can be distracted, for example, playing games such as chess or checkers, watching television, or getting away from a particular setting. Simply talking with someone may be a sufficient distraction for some persons, and allowing time for this in a patient's daily routine may be very helpful. This same intervention can easily be used during some diagnostic procedures. With careful goal-directed questions and comments the nurse may be able to take the patient's mind off the test. Discomfort will probably still occur, but preoccupation with the pain may be lessened.

Another form of distraction that may help involves the use of rhythmic breathing. To clarify, the nurse may assist the patient to concentrate on respirations, breathing more slowly and more deeply with each respiration. The patient might practice inhaling through his nose and exhaling through his mouth. Pain reduction is enhanced by keeping the eyes open and focusing on one object.[60] This in combination with efforts to relax and breathe may help the person focus on something other than pain.

Exercise

In selected situations exercises may be prescribed to assist in the alleviation of discomfort. The individual may need frequent encouragement to do what may actually be painful or which may not seem to be working as well or as quickly as anticipated. The client should occasionally be supervised while doing the exercises to make sure he is not having unnecessary difficulty or perhaps doing them incorrectly.

Working, dressing, and eating may be strenuous exercises for someone who has been unable to do these and other activities of daily living. Reasonable expectations should be determined for the rate and frequency of exercising. Actually doing the exercises may serve as a form of distraction for the client. He may also accept the responsibility for remembering to do them, which will increase his independence and control.

Rest, relaxation, and sleep

If the client has not been able to sleep because of pain or if his daily activities are so strenuous or hectic so as not to allow rest periods, his response to the pain may reflect exhaustion or fatigue. The nurse may be able to assist in several ways. Determine the client's usual rest and sleep patterns, decide if they are adequate now, and analyze why the client is not getting sufficient rest. In consultation with the client decide what might help to change the situation and develop a plan. This plan might include decreasing the number of interruptions during the night to check vital signs and for other activities, ensuring that the environment is quiet after a certain hour, providing a warm, noncaffeinated drink before sleep, providing rest periods during the day, and administering a sleeping medication or analgesic at a regular time each night.

The nurse may need to assist the client to relax. The approach will be different with each individual but may include the following. Direct the client to assume a comfortable position (the nurse may have to assist). Make certain that this position is one the client can remain in for 2 to 3 hours. Also make certain the sheets are not constricting, the client is warm enough, and so on. Instruct the client to concentrate on each extremity, one at a time, to focus on how light and relaxed each extremity is, and to begin to breathe slowly but fully, allowing no other thoughts to enter the mind. With practice the client may be able to use the above to enable him to fall asleep.

The Lamaze method of childbirth and other forms of relaxation combined with exercise are examples of ways the patient may be assisted to relax. Just as success with Lamaze depends partly on how well the woman has practiced the exercises and relaxation, so will the same be true of the person in pain. The patient should not be led to expect success on the first couple of tries; the nurse and the patient may have to work together for a period of time before the best method for relaxation is achieved.

Waking-imagined analgesia

Waking-imagined analgesia[58,60] is defined as "imagining a pleasant situation when a noxious stimulus is applied." This intervention is similar to distraction except that with this approach the client concentrates on trying to relive the sensations that occurred during a previous pleasant experience rather than only on enumerating the events that took place. McCaffery points out that only a small percentage of the population in pain can actually use this method of analgesia; more can derive benefit from distraction alone.

Reducing social isolation

Social isolation may occur for the patient in pain for a variety of reasons: the serious nature of a patient's disease may necessitate placing him in a private room for an extended period; isolation to prevent spread of infection may have confined the patient to a single room; hospitalization far away from home may mean few family members and friends can visit; extended periods of hospitalization may result in friends losing interest in visiting; or the patient may complain so much about his problems that no one cares to visit to hear this monologue repeated.

Each of the above causes of isolation may have a different solution. In any event, careful assessment by the nurse may indicate that social isolation is a problem for the patient. Before determining the plan for decreasing this problem the patient should be consulted about his desire and need to alter his present situation.

In the hospital careful selection of roommates may provide mutual support for any two or more patients. The need for actual isolation cannot be ignored, but perhaps more frequent visits by the health care team members would help. The nurse might assist a patient to write or telephone often to family and friends so they will keep in close touch. In many cases the hospital staff almost becomes the family for the patient; each day a staff member fails to stop in to talk may contribute to feelings of loneliness for the patient.

If the patient is hospitalized or at home it may be possible to contact friends and arrange a time for them to visit regularly or even occasionally. It may be that certain friends are reluctant to come because they feel unsure of their role; the nurse may be able to reassure them or clarify expectations with them before their visits.

A careful but frank discussion with the client about his behavior around guests and family may be necessary. The nurse may be able to help the client develop new methods for coping with constant pain, and this coupled with genuine interest and support of the nurse may help the patient reduce his social isolation.

Counterirritants and cutaneous stimulation

For some individuals a change in the type of stimulation at the site of pain may result in pain relief. For example, lightly rubbing the affected area may cause significant pain reduction. The gate control theory would support changing the amount and type of sensory receptor stimulation, and the nurse with the help of the patient may be able to find a satisfactory and relatively simple stimulus modification to ease the patient's discomfort.

Associated with sensory input modification at the site of discomfort are other forms of cutaneous stimulation. Depending on the individual, various forms of touch may be helpful to diminish pain or distract the client, such as a back rub, application of heat or cold to various body parts, or simply holding the client's hand. A gentle, cool sponge bath or whirlpool massage of a body part may be helpful.

Reducing painful stimuli

With skill and adequate help the nurse usually can move the patient without causing excessive pain. Proper technique when handling the patient with generalized pain or a painful limb or other body part is important. Support to painful parts of the body is essential. Supporting the trunk and limbs in good body alignment will prevent increasing the pain by unnatural pulling on muscles, joints, and ligaments. A "turning sheet" is often useful in preventing uneven lifting or pull on patients with severe neck, back, or general trunk pain. Painful joints may be moved with less discomfort if they are placed on a pillow or otherwise supported rather than being lifted directly. If there is tenderness or pain in the shaft of the bone, in muscles, or in large skin areas, the limb should be supported at the joints when the patient moves to prevent additional pain.

Binders, surgical belts, and girdles give support to the abdomen. Body casts, corsets, and braces are used to immobilize the vertebral column and thus decrease pain. A firm bed gives support and thereby lessens pain both when the patient is at rest and when he is moving. Traction, splints, casts, and braces are used to immobilize a painful part of the body such as an ankle. Special beds (e.g., Stryker frame, Foster bed, CircOlectric bed, and Bradford frame) allow movement with minimal handling of the body and thereby help lessen pain. If the nurse in caring for a patient in pain feels that any of these mechanical devices would be of benefit, the problem can be discussed with the physician.

Reducing noise and visual stimulation

The client may be suffering from sensory overload. If nurses could stand still for 5 minutes in the client's environment and watch and listen, they might understand that some clients are simply bombarded with noise and visual stimulation. If these are problems it may be possible to change the environment. Changes include moving the individual away from a busy nurses' station, or in the home, away from a busy family room. Try to ensure that the lights are turned out or at least significantly dimmed at night. In the home or in the hospital, those around the client may need to be reminded to talk and move more quietly at night.

Television and radio can serve as wonderful distracters, but most individuals tire of them after 14 to 18 consecutive hours. It may be possible to determine a schedule based on the likes and dislikes of family members or roommates that would include periods of silence during the day. Radio and television volume should be at a level comfortable for listening.

Overtalkativeness and overoptimism are often annoying to the person in pain. This is particularly true when the patient knows or suspects that his prognosis is poor. Florence Nightingale gave the following advice on this subject:

> But the long chronic case, who knows too well himself, and who has been told by his physician that he will never enter active life again, who feels that every month he has to give up something he could do the month before—oh! spare such sufferers your chattering hopes. You do not know how you worry and weary them. Such real sufferers cannot bear to talk of themselves, still less to hope for what they cannot at all expect.[73]

Plans should be made so that a minimum number of persons enter the room of the patient in severe pain. The patient cannot possibly learn to know and trust all the individuals who enter his hospital room each day. Unless some effort is made to control traffic in and out of his room, the patient may be unable to relax and rest. The same principle applies to care of the patient in his own home where the problem of too many visitors is frequently a real one. The nurse, of all members of the health care team, is in the best position to give attention to this real need of the patient. Some patients in pain welcome interruptions and distractions, whereas others prefer privacy and seclusion. The nurse should see that the patient's wishes are respected.

□ Alteration of pain transmission

Medication to alter pain

The nurse needs to know the precise effect on the body of medications used to treat pain. The time curve of beginning effect, the height of effectiveness, and the time of declining effect must be understood. In addition the effects of the medication may vary according to the time of day it is administered and the physiologic status of the individual. A brief summary of several categories of drugs is presented here; for a more definitive discussion refer to a pharmacology text.

Medication to relieve the cause of pain. Pain may be treated by drugs that help to relieve the cause of pain. For example, the belladonna group of drugs (atropine) or synthetic substitutes such as propantheline bromide (Pro-Banthine), which cause relaxation of smooth muscle, may diminish the pain caused by spasm of the smooth muscles. If pain is due to impairment of circulation, drugs that dilate the blood vessels such as papavarine hydrochloride, nitroglycerin, and tolazoline hydrochloride (Priscoline) may do more good than analgesic drugs. A final example includes antibiotics used to reduce an infection that may be causing pain. Specific drugs are chosen based on the nature of the infection, the sensitivity of the organism to the antibiotic, and the general condition of the patient.

Salicylates. One of the most widely used analgesic drugs is acetylsalicylic acid (aspirin). This is the safest of the coal-tar products; it usually relieves headache, muscle ache, and arthritic pain. The specific action of aspirin on pain is not known, but it does not cause clouding of the sensorium. Aspirin is highly effective when given with codeine, the combined effect being much superior to the use of either drug alone. The nurse needs to be constantly aware that some persons are allergic to aspirin. Death can occur when aspirin is given to such individuals. Common side effects of acetylsalicylic acid are irritation of the gastric mucosa, ulceration of the gastric mucosa, and reactivation of peptic ulcers. Salicylism can occur in persons who take large doses of aspirin over long periods of time. Nausea, vomiting, ringing in the ears, deafness, and severe headache are common manifestations. A decreased prothrombin level with hemorrhagic manifestations can also occur. Hemorrhage is uncommon when the dose is less than 1 g/day.[6]

Aspirin products are available in a variety of combinations and forms such as timed-relief aspirin, enteric-coated aspirin, and aspirin with phenacetin or caffeine. Individuals vary widely in their response to these, but there has been little conclusive data to indicate that any form or combination is best.[36] Aspirin is also a widely used antipyretic.

Acetaminophen (Tylenol, Datril), a salicylatelike analgesic, achieved wide popularity because it causes less alteration of the prothrombin level and fewer side effects. It can, however, cause severe liver damage and should not be used indiscriminately. This drug also has antipyretic action but does not have as much antiinflammatory action as aspirin. It is frequently prescribed for persons for whom aspirin is contraindicated.

Other coal-tar analgesics such as phenacetin and acetanilid may produce toxic effects after prolonged use. They should be used only under the direction of a physician despite the fact that they can be purchased without medical prescription.

Salicylatelike antiinflammatory agents. *Phenylbutazone* (Butazolidin) is prescribed to relieve symptoms of an acute episode of gout. It has some antiinflammatory properties but is poorly tolerated by many individuals and has numerous side effects including hematologic changes, gastric irritation, and fluid and electrolyte disturbances.

Indomethacin (Indocin) also is an effective antiinflammatory drug with antipyretic action. It has many side effects but may be helpful in decreasing pain in individuals with rheumatoid arthritis, osteoarthrosis, and ankylosing spondylosis.

Propoxyphene hydrochloride (Darvon) is another widely used analgesic. It is said to be as potent as codeine, but some trials have indicated that it has little more than a placebo effect. Propoxyphene is considered nonaddictive, but dependence may occur after repeated use of high dosages. Side effects include dizziness, headache, gastrointestinal disturbances, and rashes. The effectiveness of the drug may be enhanced by use of combination preparations containing propoxyphene.

Counterirritants. Ointments, emollients, and liniments such as ethyl aminobenzoate and methyl salicylate (oil of wintergreen) are counterirritants that may be applied locally to alleviate pain. Oil of clove, used for toothaches, is another example.

Medications to control pain

Other types of pain medications are effective through modification of the response of the person experiencing the pain rather than altering the transmission of the pain stimuli. These medications are discussed in order to serve as a useful reference source for the reader.

Narcotics. The opiates are drugs most widely recognized and used for the control of pain. Morphine and codeine are usually ordered. Synthetic narcotic drugs such as meperidine hydrochloride (Demerol) and methadone hydrochloride are also widely used. When given in therapeutic doses, narcotics act by depressing brain cells involved in pain perception without seriously impairing other sensory perceptions. They also affect to some extent the patient's feeling about pain and thus affect both physical pain and the reaction to it. In addition the synthetic narcotic drugs have some antispasmodic action and thereby encourage relaxation.

The effects of narcotics vary with the physiologic state of the patient. The very young and the very old are quite sensitive to the effects of narcotics and require smaller doses to obtain relief from pain. A person of any age may be more depressed physically and emotionally by narcotics during the early morning hours (1 to 6 AM) than at any other time of the day and therefore should be watched carefully for untoward effects.

Narcotics cause lowering of the blood pressure and general depression of vital functions. This reaction can be an advantage in treating a condition such as hemorrhage in which some lowering of blood pressure may be desirable. It may be a disadvantage in treating the debilitated patient, who may go into shock from an excessive dosage of a drug. The narcotic drugs are less likely to cause shock if the patient is up and moving about and taking food and fluids, since these activities tend to maintain the blood pressure at a safe level.

So much emphasis has been placed on the danger of drug addiction (and to be sure, the danger is very real) that nurses sometimes withhold narcotic drugs and allow patients to suffer more than is advisable. The patient in severe pain will not become addicted to narcotic drugs if they are given at frequent intervals for several days. Provided there are no physical contraindications, narcotics prescribed by the physician should be given to the patient with intractable pain as often as every 3 or 4 hours regardless of the possibility of addiction. However, before giving any patient an analgesic drug, the nurse should always determine whether the patient's pain is that for which the drug was ordered. If it is a "new" pain, analgesics may mask symptoms of undiagnosed disease.

A commonly used synthetic, nonnarcotic analgesic is pentazocine (Talwin). It is often prescribed in place of morphine or meperidine for the relief of moderate to severe pain. It is given orally or parenterally. The most commonly occurring reactions are vertigo, nausea, and euphoria. Since sedation and dizziness have been noted in some instances, clients receiving pentazocine should be warned not to operate machinery, drive cars, or unnecessarily expose themselves to hazards. Pentazocine is contraindicated in persons with increased intracranial pressure, head injury, or pathologic brain conditions in which clouding of the sensorium is particularly undesirable.

Sedatives. Sometimes the patient needs a sedative drug instead of additional analgesics. This type of drug may permit him to become drowsy and relaxed enough for the analgesic to be effective. Phenobarbital, for example, often enables the patient to be comfortable with a lower narcotic dose than might otherwise be necessary. The patient with a severe emotional reaction to illness will often get relief when analgesic drugs are interspersed with sedative drugs. This arrangement has been found useful when the narcotic or other analgesic drug does not seem to quite "hold" the patient for the desired interval. Small doses of phenobarbital appear to relieve most of the discomfort expressed by infants and small children when they have pain. The effect of sedative drugs, similar to narcotics, may be increased by the slowing down of physiologic response. In the presence of fever they sometimes produce excitement rather than relaxation. This effect may occur in older patients as well. Because barbiturates may make the patient less aware of his surroundings, side rails and constant nursing supervision may be necessary to protect him from injuries such as from falls.

Ataractic drugs. Ataractic drugs, or so-called tranquilizers, which affect the mood of the patient, have been found helpful in the treatment of pain, particularly when given in combination with narcotics. This combination of drugs tends to separate the perception of pain from the reaction to pain. The sensation of pain appears less acute and therefore the reaction to it becomes less severe. When fear and apprehension appear to be the most striking features of the patient's reaction, tranquilizers alone may be sufficient to help him relax. Diazepam (Valium), prochlorperazine (Compazine), and chlordiazepoxide hydrochloride (Librium) are examples of commonly used tranquilizers. If these drugs cause lethargy and failure of normal response, this should be reported to the physician at once. The physiologic state of the person may cause a variance in response to these drugs similar to that seen with narcotics.

Placebos. Placebos are sometimes used for their psychogenic effect in relieving pain, but they should never be given without a physician's order. Although the most usual response to a placebo is positive, some persons have negative reactions and may report intensified pain or other symptoms. Therefore when a placebo is being used, the nurse should observe the patient carefully and share with the physician any information that will help determine the best treatment for the patient. Favorable response to a placebo should not lead the nurse to ignore complaints of pain, for the individual who responds to placebos is in great need of the nurse's interest and support. Furthermore the patient may have a new physical pain that needs to be evaluated. (For more information on placebos see Jourard, S. M.: The transparent self, ed. 2, New York, 1971, D. Van Nostrand Co.)

Transcutaneous electrical stimulators

A transcutaneous electrical stimulator is a battery-powered stimulator worn externally by the client. Two or more electrodes attached to the battery box are applied on, around, or near the site of pain, and the client then manually regulates the power source to vary the amplitude and frequency of electrical stimulation passing between the electrodes. The goal of the device is to modify the sensory input by blocking or changing the painful stimulation with stimulation perceived as less painful or nonpainful. Success with this device may come only after repeated trials with various electrode placements or battery-box manipulations. The nurse may be very valuable in encouraging the patient and assisting him to make these small manipulations.

Because the transcutaneous electrical stimulator is noninvasive in its application, it may be particularly useful for the person who cannot tolerate more extensive procedures. The only absolute contraindication to its use is the presence of a demand-type cardiac pacemaker.[43]

Dorsal column stimulators

The dorsal column stimulator is similar to the transcutaneous electrical stimulator except that an electrode is surgically implanted over the dorsal column of the spinal column through laminectomy and the transmitter is worn externally (Fig. 22-4). The low-voltage pulses produced by the stimulator are thought to block transmission of pain by stimulating large sensory fibers.[74] The success of this therapy and the transcutaneous stimulator

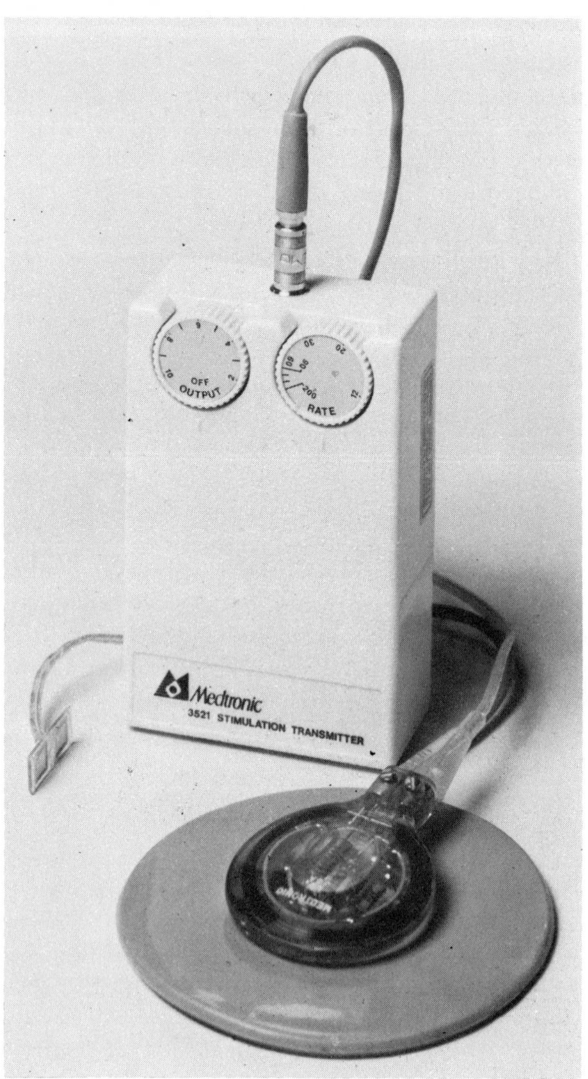

Fig. 22-4. Dorsal column stimulator. (Courtesy Medtronic, Inc., Minneapolis.)

is thought to be explained by the gate control theory of pain transmission.

In many institutions where dorsal column stimulators are implanted, candidates for this surgery are chosen only after they demonstrate success with the use of the transcutaneous stimulator. The nurse needs to be alert to postoperative complications associated with spinal cord surgery, especially infection and cerebrospinal fluid leak.

The PISCES system is a newer, less intrusive approach to spinal cord stimulation. The leads are inserted percutaneously into the epidural space with the patient under local anesthesia (Fig. 22-5).

Neurosurgical procedures

Constant, relentless pain that cannot be controlled by analgesics (intractable pain) may be reduced or abolished by one of various neurosurgical procedures.

Rhizotomy. Rhizotomy involves the surgical interruption of posterior nerve roots (i.e., the sensory roots) just before they enter the spinal canal. There are a number of disadvantages to rhizotomy: (1) because it involves major surgery (laminectomy), not all patients are appropriate candidates, (2) it is less effective for areas below the head and neck, and (3) the person loses all sensory input from the affected area after surgery. Nursing management involves the usual postlaminectomy care. Teaching the patient what to expect is important so that he can adjust his expectations accordingly. The patient must understand that the loss of sensory transmission from the area of the rhizotomy interferes with the ability to perceive heat and cold. Care must be taken when the affected area is exposed to extremes in temperature (e.g., heat used for cooking and baking).

Cordotomy. Cordotomy involves the surgical interruption of pain-conducting pathways in the spinal cord.

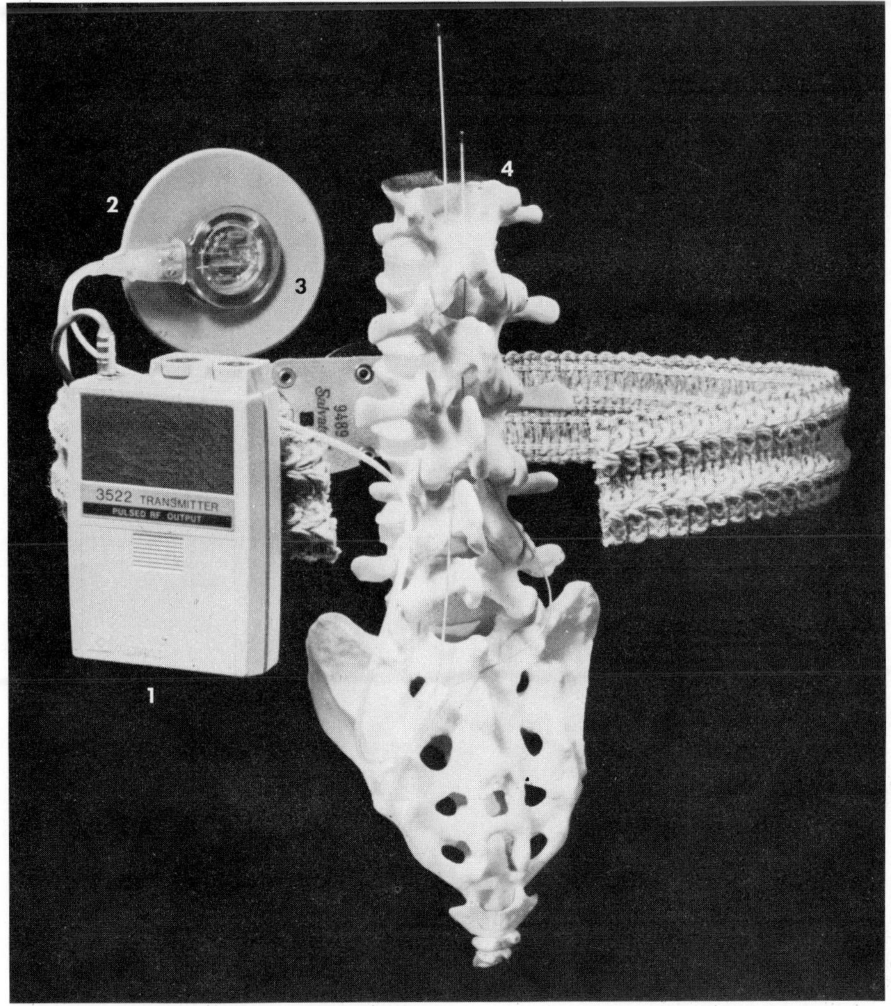

Fig. 22-5. PISCES spinal cord stimulator. *1,* Stimulation transmitter. *2,* Receiver-extension. *3,* Antenna. *4,* Leads. (Courtesy Medtronic, Inc., Minneapolis.)

This interruption involves cutting the spinothalamic portion of the anterolateral tract (Fig. 22-1). Laminectomy is usually required unless the surgeon is skilled in performing this procedure percutaneously. In this latter method needle electrodes are inserted, without the need for an incision, into the appropriate quadrant of the spinal cord, and the pathway is interrupted by electrical coagulation by means of the electrodes.

Cordotomy results in the loss of pain and temperature sensation below the level that is severed, but other sensations and motor function remain intact. It is especially effective for intractable pain of the trunk and legs. The procedure may be unilateral or bilateral. Postoperatively, even with the percutaneous approach and when done on only one side, the patient may have trouble with paralysis below the level of the lesion and with urinary retention; men may become impotent. For some, these problems are only temporary. Again special nursing management involves teaching and, especially if complications occur, emotional support.[26]

Interruption of nerve pathways in the brain. Numerous attempts have been made to alter the transmission of pain and the response to pain by surgical or stereotactic interruption of pathways in the brain. Lesions have been placed in the thalamus, the cingulum, the mesencephalon, the medulla, and the frontal lobe. The success rate has varied considerably depending on the skill of the surgeon, the type of pain, and the patient's general physical and emotional condition.

These surgeries may have complications, particularly changes in the personality of the patient. Although the assistance of a psychiatrist is helpful in managing all pa-

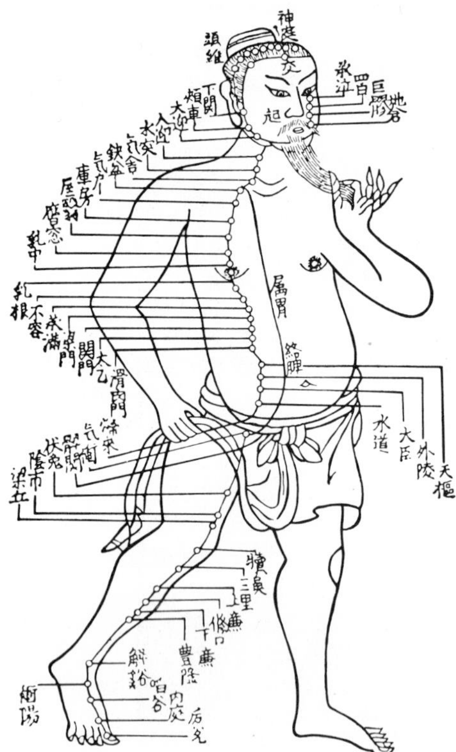

Fig. 22-6. Typical acupuncture chart showing sites for insertion of needles along several body meridians. After two or more needles are inserted, electrical current is usually passed through needles for about 20 minutes. Resulting analgesia can permit major surgery. (From Weisenberg, M.: Pain: clinical and experimental perspectives, St. Louis, 1975, The C. V. Mosby Co.; courtesy *Abbottempo*, vol. X, no. 1.)

tients with chronic pain, it is highly recommended for any surgery that may change the patient's personality.

Intrathecal phenol. Another medical intervention used at some institutions is the injection of phenol in combination with glycerin into the subarachnoid space by means of lumbar puncture. The phenol combination is heavier than the cerebrospinal fluid and will descend to lower nerve roots to block pain transmission.[52] The effect is analogous to a chemical posterior rhizotomy, and effects may last several weeks to months.[9] Side effects are common and include bladder and bowel dysfunction and various degrees of lower extremity weakness. The value of this intervention is that no major surgery is required, but its use is limited to pain in the trunk, abdomen, and lower extremities. Nursing management includes that given a patient undergoing lumbar puncture.

Acupuncture

Acupuncture is an ancient form of disease treatment that can be used for pain relief. Only recently, however, has the method been used in Western countries. Small needles are skillfully inserted and manipulated at specific body points, depending on the type and location of pain, producing often immediate and continued relief of pain. The gate control theory provides the best explanation for the success of acupuncture: the local stimulation of large-diameter fibers by the needles "closes the gate" to pain. It is not known to what extent the psyche and the power of suggestion contribute to effectiveness of this therapy. Nursing management includes careful client assessment and teaching.[13,58]

□ Modification of the response to pain

Decreasing the anxiety of the client and family

The patient in pain is often afraid. Fear may be allayed in part by the nurse's calm, quiet manner and particularly by a demonstration of competence. Confidence in the persons who care for him is a tremendous help to the patient. It is a great comfort to the patient to know, for example, that the nurse will not hurry while giving nursing care, thus increasing his pain, or be so "busy" that pain medication is not given at the prescribed intervals.

Sometimes preparation for pain helps to increase acceptance of it and in turn produces relaxation, which will decrease pain. An example is the benefit derived from special preparation for childbirth. Fear and irritability can sometimes be allayed by explaining to the patient why he has pain. This knowledge may let him relax somewhat and thereby lessen his discomfort. If he can be told honestly that the pain will probably be of short duration, this should be done. Postoperative pain is often aggravated by movement. Therefore when certain activities such as turning and coughing are necessary to prevent complications, the nurse explains this to the patient. The nurse may be able to comfort a child who is frightened by his pain by holding him, rocking him, or talking to him. Older patients also may be comforted by having someone sit quietly with them, and some patients benefit from the personal contact of holding another's hand.

It is understandable that the family will be upset when the patient is in pain. Not only may he appear uncomfortable, but he may not respond in his usual manner to those about him or relate appropriately emotionally and socially with people because his psychic energy is absorbed by the pain. Prompt attention to the patient's needs helps reduce the family's concern, and the patient's behavior should be interpreted as necessary to family and friends with simple, clear explanations. Regardless of explanations, persons who are emotionally close to the patient may need extra time to accept his behavior, and they may need repeated explanations.

Reassurance of family members is an essential part of nursing care because it may prevent them from communicating their concern to the patient. Expressions of concern by others may make the patient increasingly tense, which in turn lowers his pain tolerance. Helping the family understand the patient's behavior often reduces their demands for the patient to relate to them as usual and may help the patient feel less guilty when he cannot respond to them in his usual way.

Teaching

Teaching as a nursing role has been mentioned frequently in relation to helping the client who has pain. Just as each client's plan of care should be individualized, so should the teaching within that plan of care. Careful assessment of the client's willingness and interest to learn, coupled with his mental and physical ability to tolerate teaching, should be made before teaching is initiated. Teaching varies with each client but may include the cause of the pain, even at the physiologic level if the patient wishes to know, why or how various attempts at pain relief could or should work, and alternate ways to do daily activities that might be less painful or consume less energy. Various nursing measures, even if not primarily for pain relief, are explained.

In preparation for surgery or diagnostic procedures the client should be told honestly what to expect in terms of duration and intensity of pain *usually* experienced and what measures will be available to assist with this discomfort. If the patient must actually perform certain maneuvers or treatments, it is helpful to have him practice these before the procedure, for example, to cough and deep breathe preoperatively. If at all possible the family should be included in these teaching sessions, not only so they can support and assist the client but also so they will understand what the client will be expected to do.

Providing spiritual assistance

Even if no estimate can be made as to the duration of pain, the patient should be given encouragement that the problem will not become too great for him to accept with the assistance that is available. Many patients who have prolonged pain with no hope of relief can and do derive benefit from their religious faith. This may help them to consider pain in a more positive way and thus make it more bearable for them. The nurse can arrange for the appropriate religious advisor to be available to the patient who so desires.

In addition the nurse may become involved in doing such things as sharing in a prayer with the patient, reading from the Bible or other meaningful book, ensuring that meaningful religious medals or statues are within reach or sight, and so on.

Psychiatric assistance

In some situations the medical team will ask a psychiatrist to evaluate the client and perhaps begin ongoing psychiatric care. The individual suffering from chronic or intractable pain may appear sad, hostile, anxious, and so on. These persons often have spent years undergoing various diagnostic and surgical procedures and have seen many different physicians without significant pain relief.[8,65]

For many individuals psychiatric care is still not as acceptable as other kinds of medical care. The nurse should be supportive to the patient and help him understand why this type of therapy may be helpful. The nurse's role also includes the careful recording and reporting of objective data about the patient's behavior and his interactions with family and others.

Behavior modification

Whether used as part of the psychiatrist's plan of care or not, the nursing plan of care may outline a program designed to increase more acceptable or pleasing behavior or performance in the client and reduce unpleasant or undesired behavior. The basis for this therapy is the idea that "a behavior will tend to occur more frequently if it is consistently followed by a reward such as praise."[60] Forms of this behavior therapy are used unconsciously all the time: a child "throwing a tantrum" may be ignored, but as he becomes more appropriate in his behavior his mother may point this out and reward the child with her time and attention.

Behavior modification can be used frequently with the person in pain. For example, the nurse may praise and congratulate a client each time he remembers to perform postoperative exercises. If the client is being encouraged to try a new pain relief measure such as relaxation, it is hoped the ultimate reward will come in the form of pain relief. During the practice and learning phase, however, positive reinforcement and verbal praise and encouragement by the nurse when the client does try relaxation should stimulate the client to practice the new method regularly.

Biofeedback and autogenic training

Some persons are able to alter their body functions through mental concentration.[79] In biofeedback training the individual is repeatedly attached to a machine that monitors brain wave activity (electroencephalograph). The individual then concentrates and tries to slow his brain wave activity to rates at which pain and distress are unlikely to bother him (i.e., complete relaxation). Normal waking brain activity is in the beta range, 14 to 22 pulses per second. The goal of biofeedback is to reduce this activity to 8 to 13 pulses per second (alpha) or even slower, 4 to 7 pulses per second (theta). The biofeedback machine is regulated so that when alpha or theta ranges are reached a signal will sound to indicate success. The goal is to become adept at reaching the alpha or theta range at will and thus suppressing pain. It may take many months of regular practice to achieve the desired level of control. The nurse can be very helpful in encouraging and praising the individual's efforts.[79,80]

In autogenic training the same type of self-regulation is used to alter various autonomic nervous system functions such as pulse, blood pressure, and muscle tension. Practiced use of transcendental meditation and other methods of concentration and self-control may achieve the same degree of autoregulation without the use of sophisticated physiologic monitoring equipment. As can be seen, many of the pain relief therapies combine distraction, relaxation, self-control, and forms of behavior modification.

Hypnosis

Hypnosis had been used for decades in the treatment of various conditions, particularly when these conditions are aggravated by tension and stress. This therapy helps the individual to alter his perception of pain through the acceptance of positive suggestions made to the subconscious. Individuals vary in their suggestibility and readiness to try this approach. The skill of the hypnotist is also important. The nurse's most helpful role may be to support the client in his desire to make hypnotism work.

Nutrition

Appetite is affected by pain. When one is in continuous pain nothing, including meals, seems quite right. Care should be taken that foods the patient likes are prepared in a way that he likes. His appetite may be improved by small, attractive servings and by a sincere interest in his reactions to food. Foods that the patient does not like or that he believes disagree with him should not be offered. Very gratifying improvement in appetite has followed the control of intractable pain by surgical procedures that interrupt sensory pathways that transmit the painful sensation.

Suicide prevention

When caring for the patient who is experiencing severe, continuous, or intractable pain, the nurse must keep in mind the possibility of suicide. Pain is wearing and demoralizing, especially when it is difficult to control with medications and when the individual knows or suspects that no permanent relief will be forthcoming. The patient may dread the danger of a growing dependence on drugs, he may fear that drugs will no longer help, and he may be depressed by thoughts of being a burden and an expense to his family. He may appear to tolerate pain quite well but at the same time may be planning his own destruction. Plans for protection should be individualized for each patient and will depend on such factors as whether he is confined to bed. (For further discussion on patients who commit suicide, see p. 240.)

PAIN CLINICS

In recent years the knowledge that pain has both a physical and an emotional component, combined with increased understanding of client's needs and the treatments available, has resulted in the establishment of pain clinics. Most pain clinics or rehabilitation centers use a team approach. Physicians including internists, dolorologists (specialists in pain), surgeons and psychiatrists, nurses, physical and occupational therapists, social workers, psychologists, vocational rehabilitation counselors, and others may be available to help the client. Treatment may be on an inpatient or outpatient basis, with family members encouraged to participate in various aspects of the program.

At the Pain Rehabilitation Center in LaCrosse, Wisconsin, there are four major goals of therapy for the client: withdrawal from drugs, increased physical activity, improved emotional well-being, and a reduction in pain by 50% to 100%.[79] Each client is assessed individually, and a unique plan of care based on the needs and goals of that client is established. The plan involves most if not all of the following: progressive exercise, massage, application of heat and cold, acupuncture, external electrical stimulation, counseling, and autogenic biofeedback training.

Each pain clinic is organized slightly differently, placing greater emphasis on various aspects of pain relief and manifestation. Many of the clinics with inpatient services employ various forms of behavior modification.

The responsibility of the nurse may vary according to the team members available but often includes assisting in assessment of the patient, documenting observations, creating and maintaining a therapeutic milieu, providing emotional support to the patient and his family, and teaching the patient, family, and other nursing team members about the interventions planned for the patient. Nurses who work in pain clinics need to be skilled in nurse-client interactions, be knowledgeable about the mechanisms of pain and the effectiveness of various treatment modalities, and possess patience and understanding in order to help clients reach their goals.

OUTCOME CRITERIA FOR THE PERSON WITH PAIN

1. The client states that he is more comfortable.
2. The client or significant others can:
   a. Describe general measures for relief of pain:
      (1) State rationale for therapy.

(2) Demonstrate exercises.
(3) Describe method and frequency of specific measures.

b. Explain prescribed medications:
(1) State actions, dosage, frequency, and side effects.
(2) Describe when to seek medical assistance if pain is not relieved as expected.

c. Demonstrate correct use of transcutaneous electrical stimulator, if prescribed:
(1) State method and location for applying electrode.
(2) Describe how to adjust the frequency and amplitude controls.
(3) Demonstrate how to clean electrodes, how to change electrodes or batteries.
(4) Explain safety measures (e.g., checking for loose wire connections, not bathing while apparatus is in use).

3. The client demonstrates increased tolerance for pain as manifested by return to full- or part-time employment, decreased analgesic consumption, and independence in activities of daily living.

REFERENCES AND SELECTED READINGS

1. *Acupuncture, Am. J. Nurs. **74**:503, 1974.
2. Alfonso, D.: Assessment of pain during labor. In Anderson, E. H., Bergerson, B. S., Duffey, M., and Rose, M. H., editors: Current concepts in clinical nursing, vol. 4, St. Louis, 1973, The C. V. Mosby Co.
3. Armstrong, M. E.: Acupuncture, Am. J. Nurs. **72**:1582-1588, 1972.
4. Beecher, H. K.: Relationship of significance of wound to pain experienced, J.A.M.A. **161**:1609-1613, 1956.
5. Bellville, J. W., Forrest, W. H., Jr., Miller, E., et al.: Influence of age on pain relief from analgesics, J.A.M.A. **217**:1835-1841, 1971.
6. Bergersen, B. S., and Goth, A.: Pharmacology in nursing, ed. 14, St. Louis, 1979, The C. V. Mosby Co.
7. *Billars, K. S.: You have pain? I think this will help, Am. J. Nurs. **70**:2143-2145, 1970.
8. Black, R. G.: The chronic pain syndrome, Surg. Clin. North Am. **55**:999-1011, 1975.
9. Black, R. G., and Bonica, J. J.: Analgesic blocks, Postgrad. Med. **53**:105-110, 1973.
10. Blaylock, J.: The psychological and cultural influences on the reaction to pain: a review of the literature, Nurs. Forum **7**:262-274, 1968.
11. Bonica, J. J., editor: International symposium on pain. Advances in Neurology, vol. 4, New York, 1974, Raven Press.
12. Bonica, J. J.: Fundamental considerations of chronic pain therapy, Postgrad. Med. **53**:81-85, 1973.
13. Botton, J. E.: Neurosurgical procedures for the management of intractable pain, Clin. Orthop. **73**:101-108, 1970.
14. Brugger, M. C., and Clifford, K. M.: Dorsal column stimulator implant, A.O.R.N. J. **17**:67-76, 1973.
15. *Cady, J. W.: Dear Pain . . . , Am. J. Nurs. **76**:960-961, 1976.
16. *Cashatt, B.: Pain: a patient's view, Am. J. Nurs. **72**:281, 1972.
17. *Chambers, W. G., and Price, G. G.: Influence of nurse upon effects of analgesics administered, Nurs. Res. **16**:228-233, 1967.
18. *Copp, L. A.: The spectrum of suffering, Am. J. Nurs. **74**:491-495, 1974.
19. Crowley, D. M.: Pain and its alleviation, Los Angeles, 1962, Los Angeles School of Nursing, UCLA.
20. Crowley, D. M.: Chronic pain: social aspects. Clinical Sessions, ANA (1974), New York, 1974, Appleton-Century-Crofts, pp. 255-266.
21. Crue, B. L., editor: Pain: research and treatment, New York, 1975, Academic Press, Inc.
22. Davitz, L. J., and Pendleton, S. H.: Nurses' inferences of suffering, Nurs. Res. **18**:100-107, 1969.
23. Davitz, L. J., Sameshima, Y., and Davitz, J.: Suffering as viewed in six different cultures, Am. J. Nurs. **76**:1296-1297, 1976.
24. Derrick, W. S.: The management of chronic pain, CA **23**:269-274, 1973.
25. *Diers, D., Schmidt, R. L., McBride, M. A., et al.: The effect of nursing interaction on patients in pain, Nurs. Res. **21**:419-428, 1972.
26. *Drakontides, A. B.: Drugs to treat pain, Am. J. Nurs. **74**:508-513, 1974.
27. Dunbar, N.: Percutaneous stimulation in the treatment of acute and chronic pain, J. Neurosurg. Nurs. **8**:105-112, 1976.
28. Finneson, B. E.: Diagnosis and management of pain syndromes, Philadelphia, 1969, W. B. Saunders Co.
29. Fordyce, W. E.: Behavioral methods for chronic pain and illness, St. Louis, 1976, The C. V. Mosby Co.
30. Fordyce, W. E.: Operant conditioning in the treatment of chronic pain, Arch. Phys. Med. Rehab. **54**:399-408, 1973.
31. Freese, A. S.: Pain: the new help for your pain, New York, 1974, G. P. Putnam's Sons.
32. *Gaumer, W. R.: Electrical stimulation in chronic pain, Am. J. Nurs. **74**:504-505, 1974.
33. Glynn, C. J.: The diurnal variation in perception of pain, Proc. R. Soc. Med. **69**:369-372, 1976.
34. *Goloskov, J., and LeRoy, P.: Use of the dorsal column stimulator, Am. J. Nurs. **74**:506-507, 1974.
35. Gowell, E. C.: Transactional analysis strategies for dealing with pain, J. Psychiatr. Nurs. **12**:25-30, 1974.
35a. *Gramse, C. A.: Dorsal column stimulation, Am. J. Nurs. **78**:1022-1025, 1978.
36. Halpern, L. M.: Analgesics and other drugs for relief of pain, Postgrad. Med. **53**:91-100, 1973.
37. Hannington-Kief, J. G.: Pain relief, Philadelphia, 1974, J. B. Lippincott Co.
38. *Healy, K. M.: Does preoperative instruction make a difference? Am. J. Nurs. **68**:62-67, 1968.
39. Housepian, E. M.: Current problems in the surgical management of pain, A.O.R.N. J. **3**:70-75, 1965.
40. *Isler, C.: New approach to intractable pain . . . , RN **38**:17-21, 1975.
40a. *Jacox, A.: Pain: a sourcebook for nurses and other professionals, Boston, 1978, Little, Brown and Co.
41. Jacox, A., and Stewart, M.: Relation of psychosocial factors and type of pain, ANA Ninth Nurs. Res. Conf. March 1973, pp. 13-31.
42. Jacox, A., and Stewart, M.: Psychosocial contingencies of the pain experience, Iowa City, Ia., 1973, University of Iowa Press.
43. Johnson, I.: Transcutaneous electrical stimulation, J. Neurosurg. Nurs. **7**:87-90, 1975.
44. Johnson, I.: Radiofrequency percutaneous facet rhizotomy, J. Neorosurg. Nurs. **6**:82-96, 1974.

*References preceded by an asterisk are particularly well suited for student reading.

45. Johnson, J. E., and Rice, V. H.: Sensory and distress components of pain: implications for the study of clinical pain, Nurs. Res. **23**:203-209, 1974.
46. *Johnson, M.: Pain: how do you know it's there and what do you do? Nurs. '76 **6**:48-50, 1976.
47. Kerr, F. W.: Pain: a central inhibitory balance theory, Mayo Clin. Proc. **50**:685-690, 1975.
48. Knighton, R. S., and Dumke, P. R.: Pain, Henry Ford Hospital International Symposium, Boston, 1966, Little, Brown and Co.
49. Loeser, J. D.: Neurosurgical relief of chronic pain, Postgrad. Med. **53**:115-119, 1973.
50. Lipton, S.: The relief of intractable pain by cordotomy, Nurs. Times **69**:755-757, 1973.
51. Long, D. M.: Recent advances in the management of pain, Minn. Med. **57**:705-709, 1974.
52. Maher, R. M.: Cancer pain in relation to nursing care, Nurs. Times **71**:344-350, 1975.
53. *Mastrovito, R. C.: Psychogenic pain, Am. J. Nurs. **74**:514-519, 1974.
54. *McBride, M. A. B.: The additive to the analgesic, Am. J. Nurs. **69**:974-976, 1969.
55. McBride, M. A. B.: Nursing approach, pain, and relief: an exploratory experiment, Nurs. Res. **16**:337-341, 1967.
56. McBride, M. A. B.: "Pain" and effective nursing practice, Clinical Sessions ANA (1966), New York, 1966, Appleton-Century-Crofts, pp. 75-82.
57. McCaffery, M.: Brief episodes of pain in children. In Anderson, E. H., and others, editors: Current concepts in clinical nursing, vol. 4, St. Louis, 1969, The C. V. Mosby Co.
58. *McCaffery, M.: Intelligent approach to intractable pain, Nurs. '73 **3**:26-32, 1973.
59. *McCaffery, M.: Patients in pain, Nurs. '73 **3**:41-50, 1973.
60. *McCaffery, M.: Nursing management of the patient with pain, Philadelphia, 1972, J. B. Lippincott Co.
61. *McCaffery, M., and Moss, F.: Nursing intervention for bodily pain, Am. J. Nurs. **67**:1224-1227, 1967.
62. *McLachlan, E.: Recognizing pain, Am. J. Nurs. **74**:496-497, 1974.
63. Mehta, M.: Intractable pain, Philadelphia, 1973, W. B. Saunders Co.
64. Melzack, R.: Self-regulation of pain: the use of alpha-feedback and hypnotic training for the control of chronic pain, Exp. Neurol. **46**:452-469, 1975.
65. *Melzack, R.: The puzzle of pain, New York, 1973, Basic Books, Inc., Publishers.
66. Melzack, R., and Chapman, C. R.: Psychologic aspects of pain, Postgrad. Med. **53**:69-75, 1973.
67. Melzack, R., and Wall, P. D.: Pain mechanisms: a new theory, Science **150**:971-979, 1965.
68. *Minckley, B. B.: A study of noise and its relationship to patient discomfort in the recovery room, Nurs. Res. **17**:247-250, 1968.
69. Moertel, C. G., Ahmann, D. L., Taylor, W. F., et al.: A comparative evaluation of marketed analgesic drugs, N. Engl. J. Med. **286**:813-815, 1972.
70. Morrison, F.: Dorsal column stimulator: nursing aspects, J. Neurosurg. Nurs. **7**:18-21, 1975.
71. Moss, F. T., and Meyer, B.: The effects of nursing interaction upon pain relief in patients, Nurs. Res. **15**:303-306, 1966.
72. Nakahama, H.: Pain mechanisms in the central nervous system, Int. Anesthesiol. Clin. **13**:109-148, 1975.
73. Nightingale, F.: Notes on nursing: what it is, and what it is not, London, 1859, Harrison; Philadelphia, 1957, J. B. Lippincott Co.
74. Noel, M.: Dorsal column stimulation, J. Neurosurg. Nurs. **7**:32-36, 1975.
75. *Pain: basic concepts and assessment. Programmed instruction, Am. J. Nurs. **66**:1085-1108, 1966.
76. *Pain: rationale for intervention. Programmed instruction, Am. J. Nurs. **66**:1345-1368, 1966.
77. Rigby, B.: Transcendental meditation, Nurs. Times **71**:1240, 1975.
78. Rosenburgh, S. P.: Pain: theories and treatment by cutaneous afferent stimulation, J. Neurosurg. Nurs. **8**:80-84, 1976.
79. Shealy, C. N.: The pain game, Millbrae, Calif., 1976, Celestial Arts.
80. *Siegele, D. S.: The gate control theory, Am. J. Nurs. **74**:498-502, 1974.
81. Sternbach, R. A.: Pain: a psychophysiological analysis, New York, 1968, Academic Press, Inc.
82. *Stewart, E.: To lessen pain: relaxation and rhythmic breathing, Am. J. Nurs. **76**:958-959, 1976.
83. Strauss, A., Eagerhaugh, Y. F., and Glaser, B.: Pain: an organizational-work-interactional perspective . . . , Nurs. Outlook **22**:560-566, 1974.
84. Swerdlow, M., editor: Relief of intractable pain, New York, 1974, American Elsevier Publishing Co., Inc.
85. Szasz, T. S.: Pain and pleasure: a study of bodily feelings, New York, 1957, Basic Books, Inc., Publishers.
86. Therrian, B., and Salmon, J. H.: Percutaneous cordotomy for relief of intractable pain, Am. J. Nurs. **68**:2594-2597, 1968.
87. *Ujhely, G. B.: Nursing implications of the studies by Dr. Krieger and Dr. Jacox and Ms. Stewart, ANA Ninth Nurs. Res. Conf., March 1973, pp. 73-77.
88. *Walike, B. C., and Meyer, B.: Relation between placebo reactivity and selected personality factors, Nurs. Res. **15**:119-123, 1966.
89. Wang, R. I. H.: Control of pain, Am. J. Med. Sci. **112**:590-609, 1963.
90. Way, E. L., editor: New concepts in pain and its clinical management, Philadelphia, 1967, F. A. Davis Co.
91. Weisenberg, M.: Pain: clinical and experimental perspectives, St. Louis, 1975, The C. V. Mosby Co.
92. *Wiley, L., editor: Intractable pain: how nursing care can help (nursing grand rounds), Nurs. '74 **4**:54-59, 1974.
93. Wilson, W. P., Blazer, D. G., and Nashold, B. S.: Observations on pain and suffering, Psychosomatics **17**:73-76, 1976.
94. Zborowski, M.: People in pain, San Francisco, 1969, Jossey-Bass, Inc., Publishers.

AUDIOVISUAL RESOURCE

Movie: Pain and its alleviation, Educational Film Sales, University Extension, Berkeley, Calif., 1962, University of California.

23

Trauma: surgical intervention

BARBARA C. LONG
C. JOAN GOWIN
MARY E. BUSHONG

Persons experiencing surgery share some common experiences during the preoperative, intraoperative, and postoperative phases. This chapter deals with these commonalities and with the nurse's role in assisting patients to regain their optimal level of functioning after surgery. Patient needs and interventions specific to the types of surgery performed are described elsewhere.

■ SURGERY AS A STRESSOR

Although some operations are considered minor procedures by hospital personnel, surgery is always a major experience for the patient and family. Trauma is a stressor and produces both psychologic stress reactions (anxiety) and physiologic stress reactions (neuroendocrine responses). Surgery is a potential or actual threat to a person's integrity and can interfere with need gratification during any of the phases of surgery.

□ Anxiety related to surgery

Anxiety is a normal adaptive response to the stress of surgery. Anxiety occurs in the preoperative phase as the patient anticipates the surgery and in the postoperative phase as the patient anticipates or deals with problems such as pain and discomfort, changes in body image or function, increased dependency, loss of control, family concerns, or potential changes in life style.

The functions of the nurse in assisting the patient to cope with the stress of surgery are to assess the patient's anxiety level and adequacy of his coping responses, to prepare him physically and psychologically for surgery, to support him during the intraoperative phase, and to assist him in meeting his psychologic and physical needs during the postoperative phase.

□ Neuroendocrine responses to surgery

The neuroendocrine responses to stress are described in considerable detail in Chapter 13. It is important to remember that these responses play a major role in the reaction of a patient to the stress of trauma occurring as an accidental injury or as planned surgery.

Sympathetic nervous system

Stimulation of the sympathetic nervous system serves to protect the body from further damage. Vasoconstriction of peripheral blood vessels enables the body to compensate for blood loss and redirect blood flow to critical areas such as heart and brain. Increased cardiac output also helps to maintain blood flow. Severe trauma or excessive blood loss, however, will overwhelm the compensatory mechanisms and blood pressure will fall. Certain types of anesthetics or high spinal anesthesia may also interfere with the compensatory vasoconstriction, producing hypotension. The patient's blood pressure is therefore monitored closely during the intraoperative and early postoperative phases.

One aspect of the sympathetic response that may produce undesirable effects is the decrease in gastrointestinal activity. Psychologic stress in the preoperative period may lead to anorexia and constipation. Following the trauma of surgery the patient may experience anorexia, gas pains, and constipation from diminished peristalsis in the gastrointestinal tract. Peristalsis may cease completely after abdominal surgery following manipulation of abdominal organs.

Hormonal response

Adrenal cortical activity is increased, producing greater amounts of aldosterone and glucocorticoids. Aldosterone enhances sodium reabsorption by the kidney. This serves to retain fluid to compensate for fluid lost through blood loss, diaphoresis, and respirations. When sodium is reabsorbed by the kidneys, potassium is excreted; thus after surgery there is loss of potassium. The potassium is excreted regardless of the body's need for the potassium.

The increase in the amount of glucocorticoid from

the adrenal cortex is thought to mobilize cellular stores of fats and amino acids for energy and protein synthesis.[44] Healing tissues require protein. Glucose is released for energy with resultant hyperglycemia and glycosuria. Patients who have diabetes must be carefully monitored during the early postoperative phase for signs of ketosis.

In addition to the increase in adrenocortical hormones, there is an increase in antidiuretic hormone (ADH) by the neurohypophysis (anterior pituitary gland) during the first 24 to 48 hours after surgery. Water is reabsorbed by the kidney, and renal output is decreased. Following surgery the increased production of aldosterone and ADH is evidenced by a decreased amount of urine output as compared with fluid intake. Spontaneous diuresis occurs as the amount of ADH is decreased, usually in about 24 to 48 hours.

Metabolic responses to surgery

It can be said that following surgery the patient is in a relative state of starvation; metabolism is increased, while nutrient intake is decreased.

Carbohydrate metabolism. As a result of the increased production of glucocorticoid hormones, there is an increase in the carbohydrate metabolism following the stress of surgery. With major surgery there are periods when the patient is not permitted to eat and is given dextrose by intravenous fluids. This is not adequate to meet the body's energy needs (p. 206). Anorexia may also occur as part of the stress response, thus adding to the problem of inadequate carbohydrate intake even if food is permitted by mouth.

Fat metabolism. Glucocorticoids also have a ketogenic effect; that is, they increase the rate of mobilization of fat from the cells to make fat available as an energy source. With the decreased intake of carbohydrates and fats after surgery, body fats are metabolized for energy and the patient loses weight.

Protein metabolism. Body proteins consist of combinations of the essential amino acids, of which nitrogen is an essential component. When tissues break down during catabolism following surgery, some of the nitrogen is lost. As new tissue is formed essential amino acids are needed. If none of these amino acids are taken in, as by ingestion, the body will continue to break down some existing tissue proteins to obtain the amino acids that it needs for healing. The "leftover" amino acids not used at that time are broken down to the nitrogen end products such as urea and are excreted. A *negative nitrogen balance* results; nitrogen loss exceeds nitrogen intake. If there is little or no protein intake following surgery, nitrogen balance will be further compromised; the patient will continue to lose weight and healing will be delayed. Nitrogen is also needed for production of white blood cells and fibroblasts needed to resist infection and to repair tissue.

■ FACTORS AFFECTING PATIENT RESPONSES TO SURGERY

No two persons respond to surgery in exactly the same way. A number of variables influence physiologic and psychologic responses throughout the entire surgical experience. These include age, nutritional status, effectiveness of neuroendocrine responses, presence of disease or limiting conditions, surgical procedure performed, complications, and psychologic factors.

□ Age

Surgery can be performed on persons of any age, from the newborn to the very elderly. Persons at the extremes of age are less able to tolerate stress such as tissue trauma (surgery) or infection.

Children

The very young infant has decreased resistance to stress because of immature development (see Chapter 18). Endocrine functions are sluggish, and reserves of fat, glycogen, and extracellular water are limited. Fluid and electrolyte balance are easily upset and must therefore be monitored very carefully during the postoperative period. Resistance to infection is also limited, and measures to prevent respiratory and wound infections must be instituted.

The young child tolerates surgery well, and the postoperative course is usually rapid if no complications occur and if the child was essentially well before surgery. The tendency of the child to be active helps to prevent postoperative respiratory and circulatory complications. Young children, however, are sensitive to chilling and rough handling because of body size and immature development.

Elderly

The ability of the elderly patient to tolerate surgery depends on the extent of physiologic changes that have occurred with the aging process, the duration of the surgical procedure, and the presence of one or more chronic diseases.

Elderly persons vary greatly in the extent to which physiologic changes occur. The changes that affect responses to surgery are cardiovascular, renal, pulmonary, and musculoskeletal (Table 23-1). The greater the number of changes present, the greater the potential for the patient to develop a postoperative complication. The cardiovascular changes affect mechanisms that help the body compensate for the sympathetic nervous system response to stress. Since heart rate changes in the elderly occur more slowly than in younger persons, pulse rates

Table 23-1. Physiologic changes related to aging process that can affect surgery

Physiologic changes	Result	Potential postoperative complications
Cardiovascular		
↓ Elasticity of blood vessels ↓ Cardiac output ↓ Peripheral circulation	↓ Circulation	Shock (hypotension), wound infection, thrombophlebitis
Renal		
↓ Blood flow in kidney	↓ Kidney function	Prolonged response to anesthetic, fluid and electrolyte imbalance (especially overhydration)
Respiratory		
↓ Lung expansion	↓ Ability to cough and deep breathe	Atelectasis, pneumonia
Musculoskeletal		
↓ Muscle strength Limitation of motion	↓ Activity	Atelectasis, pneumonia, thrombophlebitis, constipation or fecal impaction

may not be a good index in assessment of shock, and a longer period of time may be necessary to wait for pulse stabilization after activity.[83] Careful monitoring of the elderly person receiving fluids parenterally is important in order to prevent overhydration (either water intoxication or pulmonary edema).

Since elderly persons tolerate stress less effectively, the duration of the surgical experience can affect the response. Surgery of short duration is more easily tolerated. Presence of chronic diseases such as pulmonary, cardiac, or central nervous system disease limits the elderly person by prolonging recovery or increasing the risk of mortality.[26]

□ Nutrition

Malnourished persons (nutrition defecits or excess) are poorer surgical risks than the well nourished and are more likely to develop postoperative complications.

Nutritional deficiency

Persons most likely to have nutritional deficiencies are the aged and the chronically ill, particularly those with gastrointestinal tract conditions or malignancies. The person who is emaciated or cachectic or who has lost considerable weight below his acceptable level usually has a prolonged postoperative recovery.

The undernourished person already has diminished reserves of carbohydrates and fats. Body proteins will be utilized to provide the necessary energy requirement to maintain metabolic functioning of cells. Nitrogen imbalances (p. 362) will be greater than normal, and less protein will be available for healing. Collagen, the connective tissue that is the substance of scar tissue, is a protein. Wound healing therefore becomes considerably delayed, and wound separation and infection may occur.

If the surgery is not an emergency and can be delayed for several weeks, the undernourished patient is placed on a high-protein, high-carbohydrate diet preoperatively. In the postoperative period he may be placed on total parenteral nutrition (hyperalimentation) (p. 321) until he is able to tolerate a high-protein, high-carbohydrate diet by mouth. High protein intake will not result in increased body protein unless there is sufficient carbohydrate to provide the necessary energy. Activity or exercise also is required for protein synthesis (p. 1170).

Nutrition-depleted patients usually have a deficiency of vitamins. Vitamins B_1, C, and K are necessary for wound healing and clot formation, and supplemental vitamins will be prescribed.

Nutritional excess

The obese patient presents several risk factors for surgery. He has enlarged organs such as heart, kidneys, liver. During surgery fluctuations of vital signs are more common in the obese person, resulting from the excessive demands on the cardiovascular system.[96] The surgeon incising through layers of fatty tissue has to exert more traction on the tissues to expose the surgical site; this increases trauma to the tissues. Incisional hernias may occur at a later date.

During the immediate postoperative period these patients often require more assistance with turning, coughing, and deep breathing. Excess fat deposits often limit movement of the diaphragm, thereby decreasing ventilation. It is also more difficult for obese persons to move about with ease, and they may require additional assistance. Both decreased activity and decreased diaphragm expansion are contributing factors to development of postoperative pulmonary complications. Decreased activity also predisposes to thrombophlebitis.

The obese person is more likely to develop wound separation and infection. Good circulation is important for the healing process to bring to the wound the white blood cells, fibrocytes, and nutrients necessary for healing. Since fatty tissue has a decreased number of blood vessels, wound healing may be impaired.

□ Neuroendocrine response ineffectiveness

The neuroendocrine response assists the person to cope with the stress of surgery. If this response is ineffective, postoperative complications such as shock and delayed wound healing may occur. In addition anesthesia may be tolerated poorly, and fluid and electrolyte imbalances are more likely to occur. Persons with diseases of the adrenal gland or the sympathetic nervous system or those who are under a great deal of stress prior to surgery may do less well postoperatively. Infants and the elderly also have diminished neuroendocrine response (p. 362).

□ Chronic diseases or disabilities

The existence of one or more chronic diseases does not necessarily increase surgical risk. The nature and extent of the disease(s) and the degree to which it is under control are the important variables.

Pulmonary disease, such as chronic obstructive pulmonary disease (COPD), may affect the person's response to the anesthetic and ability to cope with respiratory problems after surgery (see Chapter 50). In preparation for surgery the pulmonary status of persons with COPD will be carefully evaluated and measures will be instituted to improve ventilation. In persons with a history of recent respiratory infection surgery will be delayed until they are in optimum condition. Most surgeons prefer that persons who are heavy smokers decrease their smoking for a period of time prior to surgery, since smoke irritates the tracheobronchial tree, resulting in increased secretions that impinge on the airway and decrease ventilation.

Persons with chronic pulmonary problems must be very carefully monitored during surgery and in the early postoperative period to prevent atelectasis, respiratory insufficiency, and respiratory acidosis.

Cardiovascular disease can affect the individual's response to surgery. A heart that pumps effectively and blood vessels that constrict effectively are necessary for the prevention of shock and of fluid imbalances. Body responses to hemorrhage and inflammation depend on an adequate supply of red and white blood cells. Surgery is usually postponed if possible when the cardiovascular status of the patient is not at the optimal level of functioning. Measures are instituted to improve the cardiovascular status and reduce the risk of surgery. Careful monitoring for potential problems is carried out by both physician and nurse during the intraoperative and postoperative phases.

Renal insufficiency can increase the risk of surgery due to difficulty in the removal of increased amounts of electrolytes, especially potassium, and waste products from catabolism. Persons with renal disease are prone to develop fluid overload from parenteral fluids if urine production is not adequate.

Endocrine diseases that are influenced by hormonal changes occurring with the stress response can affect the patient's response to surgery. The patient with diabetes mellitus should be well controlled prior to surgery and monitored closely during and after surgery. Glucocorticoid activity and potassium changes following surgery can influence insulin utilization (see Chapter 32). If the wound is in an area where the patient may have impaired circulation, such as legs and feet, healing may be delayed. In persons who have increased levels of adrenocortical hormones such as occurs in pituitary or adrenal cortical disease or who are receiving exogenous hormones, healing may be delayed because of an antiinflammatory response. In contrast the patient with Addison's disease (hypofunction of the adrenal cortex) or patients receiving hormonal replacement will require additional replacement therapy because of the stress of surgery.

Disabilities that can influence response to surgery include those that affect or limit activity. Inability to ambulate, to exercise, or to move about freely in bed increases the risk of atelectasis, pneumonia, or thrombophlebitis postoperatively.

□ Surgical procedure

The site of the surgical procedure, the type and extent of surgery performed, and the reason for doing the surgery can all influence the patient's response.

Site

Surgery that is performed on body areas that are visible to others may leave scars that are perceived by the patient or significant others to be disfiguring. Surgery of vital organs such as the heart, lungs, and kidneys may be threatening to the patient in terms of survival. Surgery of the mouth or throat may create temporary breathing problems that can be perceived as a threat. Surgery of the extremities may create permanent changes or be perceived as creating changes in life style, especially in activities of daily living (eating, bathing, dressing, walking). Surgery on body areas that have special meaning to the person such as breasts, genitalia, or reproductive organs will have differing effects and responses.

Type and extent of surgery

Removal of organs can be perceived as a threat (especially if there is considerable meaning attached to the organ by the patient) or can create changes in life style. Surgery that creates artificial openings such as a colostomy are highly stressful to the patient and produce differing responses. The more extensive the surgery, the greater the physiologic responses that will occur. Psychologic responses are not directly related to the extent of the surgery, since they are influenced by the patient's past experiences, perceptions of what the surgery means to his self-image, and possible changes in life style.

Reasons for surgery

There are a number of reasons why surgery is done (see box below). Anxiety may be decreased if the patient perceives the surgery as a positive experience such as curing disease, relieving discomfort, or creating a more attractive physical appearance. On the other hand anxiety is usually increased when the underlying pathology is or is believed to be a malignancy or life threatening (such as open heart surgery).

□ Postoperative complications

Occurrence of complications in the postoperative period will delay recovery. Wounds that separate or become infected may take considerable time to heal, especially if other complicating factors such as inadequate nutrition are also present. Shock, cardiac aberrations, fluid and electrolyte imbalances, atelectasis or pneumonia, or thrombophlebitis can all prolong the postoperative course. These complications are discussed in more detail later in this chapter and in later chapters of this book.

REASONS FOR SURGERY

Diagnostic: to determine cause of symptoms (e.g., biopsy, exploratory laparotomy)
Curative: to remove diseased part (e.g., appendectomy)
Restorative: to strengthen weakened area (e.g., herniorrhaphy); to rejoin disconnected or injured area (e.g., hip pinning); to correct deformities (e.g., mitral valve replacement)
Palliative: to relieve symptoms without curing disease (e.g., sympathectomy, total hip arthroplasty)
Cosmetic: to improve appearance (e.g., plastic surgery)

□ Previous experience with surgery

The patient who has had previous experience with surgery may respond either positively or negatively to the present surgery. A previous negative experience can be transferred to the present experience and increase anxiety. On the other hand a previous negative experience is sometimes viewed by the patient as an entirely separate event that happened under different circumstances and thus may not influence the present experience.

□ Anxiety and coping responses

One of the major factors that creates variations in responses to surgery is the extent of anxiety that the patient experiences and the effectiveness of coping responses utilized by the patient to deal with the anxiety (see Chapter 16). Some degree of anxiety prior to surgery is normal. The degree of anxiety may range from minimal to severe and may not be directly related to the severity of the surgery. Existing and perceived factors in the environment and within the patient all influence the extent of the anxiety and the patient's responses to it.

■ PREOPERATIVE PHASE

The preoperative phase actually begins when the client first visits a physician or primary nurse for examination. The client may already have some symptoms that caused him to seek medical advice, or the need for surgery may have been identified during a routine physical examination. There may be a period of time prior to surgery during which tests are carried out to determine the necessity for surgery. Surgery that follows trauma or sudden onset of acute symptoms, such as acute appendicitis, may take place shortly following the initial medical contact. In this situation there is less time for psychologic and physiologic preparation for surgery. Preoperative management by both physician and nurse is directed toward making the surgical experience safe and comfortable for the patient (Table 23-2).

The preoperative phase extends until the patient is transferred to the operating room for surgery.

□ Psychologic preparation for surgery

Common fears related to surgery

The person facing surgery has numerous decisions to make that involve threat and are therefore anxiety provoking. The first decision may be whether to seek medical advice (fear of the unknown). Decisions may have to made concerning having specific tests made (fear of dis-

Table 23-2. Preoperative management

Physician	Nurse
Collect data	
Aid in medical diagnosis	Identify psychologic readiness for surgery
Determine need, type, and extent of surgery	Identify knowledge of events that will occur
Identify potential complications requiring medical intervention	Identify potential complications requiring nursing intervention
Obtain baseline data for future comparison	Obtain baseline data for future comparison
Psychologic preparation	
Explain need, type, and extent of surgery to patient and significant others	Verify patient's understanding and clarify as indicated
	Give explanations about tests
	Give opportunities to express feelings and concerns
	Support significant others
Physical preparation	
Prescribe and/or carry out tests	Assist patient and physician in carrying out tests
Prescribe diet, drugs	Assist patient to meet basic needs in preparation for surgery
Prescribe actions to ensure safety and comfort during surgery	Assist patient in carrying out physician's orders

comfort, fear of unknown). The decision to have surgery may be the most difficult. Having major surgery involves putting one's life under the control of others and subjecting oneself to the intrusion of the body and possible pain. It may also involve permanent changes in life style.

Some of the fears underlying preoperative anxiety are elusive, and the person may not be able to identify the cause. Others are more specific (see box above). Fear of the unknown is the most common. If the diagnosis is uncertain, fear of malignancy is frequent regardless of the probability of this being so. Fears concerning anesthesia are usually related to dying, "going to sleep and never waking up." Fears concerning pain, disfigurement, or permanent disability may be realistic or may be influenced by myths, lack of information, or lurid stories recited by friends. The patient may also have other con-

FEARS RELATED TO SURGERY

General	Specific
Fear of unknown	Diagnosis of malignancy
Loss of control	Anesthesia
Loss of love from significant others	Dying
Threat to sexuality	Pain
	Disfigurement
	Permanent limitations

ASSESSMENT OF PREOPERATIVE ANXIETY

Subjective data

1. Understanding of proposed surgery
   - Site
   - Type of surgery to be done
   - Information from surgeon regarding extent of hospitalization, postoperative limitations
   - Preoperative routines
   - Postoperative routines
   - Tests
2. Previous surgical experiences
   - Type, nature, time interval
3. Any specific concerns or feelings about present surgery
4. Religion
   - Meaning for patient
5. Significant others
   - Geographic distance
   - Perception as source of support
6. Changes in sleep patterns

Objective data

1. Speech patterns
   - Repetition of themes
   - Change of topic
   - Avoidance of topics related to feelings
2. Degree of interaction with others
3. Physical
   - Pulse and respiratory rates
   - Hand movements and perspiration
   - Activity level
   - Voiding frequency

cerns related to hospitalization such as job security, income, and care of family.

Assessment of psychologic readiness for surgery

If the person facing possible surgery has contact during the prehospitalization period with a professional nurse, data should be collected at that time to identify potential or actual sources of preoperative anxiety and to begin interventions to assist the person in coping with the threat of surgery. Communication of the data to the nurse in the hospital can provide for continuity of care. If preadmission data is not available the hospital admission or primary care nurse assesses the person's psychologic readiness for surgery.

Subjective data. Much of the data concerning knowledge and perceptions of the coming event will be obtained directly from the patient (see box, p. 366). It is necessary to know the level of the patient's understanding of the surgical event before any teaching can take place. Since the patient is responding on the basis of his perceptions, it is important to find out from him exactly how he perceives the surgery. He may not be able to identify specific concerns, and further exploration may be indicated. If the nurse has identified cues on which conclusions are drawn, these conclusions should be validated with the patient.

Knowledge of the meaning of religion for the patient can help the nurse identify a possible source of support. The effect of family members or significant others on the patient's level of anxiety needs to be determined. Some significant others increase the patient's anxiety by transmission of their own anxiety by hovering over the patient, displaying anxious behaviors, or by offering false reassurances. Others are calm, and it is observed that the patient's anxiety is reduced when they are present.

Changes in sleep patterns also provide clues about increased anxiety. Major causes of insomnia are worry, fear, and concerns about the future.

Objective data. Signs of anxiety in the presurgical patient are no different than in other persons. Signs vary from person to person and can be observed in a number of ways. The highly anxious person may talk rapidly, ask many questions without waiting for answers, repeat the same questions, or change topics frequently during the interaction. He may deny that he has any worries or fears, but his actions belie this. Some persons will not talk about the forthcoming surgery, responding only in monosyllables, while others cry and display anger; both behaviors are overt signs of anxiety. Physical signs include an increased pulse and respiratory rate, moist palms, constant hand movements, and restlessness.

Analysis of data. The degree of anxiety experienced by the patient needs to be assessed. Most surgeons will cancel surgery for a patient who is extremely anxious. Persons with anxiety levels so high that they cannot talk about and begin to cope with their anxiety before surgery frequently experience difficulty in the postoperative period. They are more apt to be angry, resentful, confused, or depressed. They are also more vulnerable to psychotic reactions than are persons with lower levels of anxiety.[95]

Lack of any emotional response to surgery may indicate denial; this precludes dealing with and coping with the anxiety before surgery. A moderate amount of anxiety enables the individual to identify and begin to cope with his feelings. These persons usually experience a smoother postoperative course.

Intervention

Outcome: *Patient identifies concerns related to surgery; he is relaxed; signs of anxiety are decreased*

Having opportunities to talk with a supportive knowledgeable person will help the patient begin to identify the reasons for his anxiety and to marshal his coping responses. It is helpful for the nurse to plan for a quiet unhurried time to sit down with the patient and give him an opportunity to ask questions and talk about his concerns. Touch is often a helpful form of communication, sending the message, "I care," and some patients will talk more readily while receiving a back rub. Knowing that a nurse is interested and cares about him as an individual helps to reduce anxiety. If the patient knows also that anxiety is a normal reaction to the threat of surgery, it may help to remove the often self-imposed expectation, "I shouldn't be nervous." Emphasis should be on accentuating the positive and helping the patient identify his own strengths and coping responses.

Loss of control is one of the fears associated with surgery. Allowing the patient to participate in decision making concerning his own care when feasible helps the patient partially meet his need for control. Identifying and carrying out measures to help the patient meet his physical needs in the preoperative phase may help to give him a feeling of security about having his postoperative needs met and thus allay some anxiety. Protection of the patient's privacy and modesty may also help.

Outcome: *Patient can explain events that will occur*

Fear of the unknown can be partly relieved by knowledge about what to expect. Too much detail or information can have an opposite effect and serve to increase anxiety. The amount of information to give preoperatively depends on the background, interest, and stress level of the patient. A good rule to follow is to ask the patient what he would like to know about the forthcoming surgery and to base responses on the types of questions asked. Persons under considerable stress such as those in considerable pain cannot cope with much added stimuli, and simple explanations would be indicated. A highly anxious person has a narrow perceptual field and may not perceive events occurring around him or information being given. It is also important to remember that giving someone information does not necessarily mean that he has perceived it or understood it.

The information helpful to most patients preoperatively relates to preoperative tests and activities, events related to the surgery to be performed, and expectations about what will happen postoperatively. Most persons are less anxious and participate more effectively if they know the reasons for the tests and preoperative activities. If discomfort is a probability, foreknowledge of the pain and that medication will be given to relieve it helps to decrease the stress response when the discomfort does occur, and the person is better prepared to cope with the discomfort.

Preoperative visits by the operating room nurse are helpful in many instances, especially in those situations when a great deal of anxiety may be expected such as in open heart surgery (Fig. 23-1). The visit promotes the feeling that "Someone in surgery knows me as an individual and will look after me." If it is known that the patient will be in intensive care for a period of time after surgery, a visit by a nurse from the intensive care unit may also help to allay anxiety. Most patients find it helpful to know when they will be taken to surgery, the length of time they will be in surgery, where they will awaken (recovery room), when they will return to their room, and where their family can wait to receive information.

Preparation of the child for surgery depends on his age and developmental level. Some 3-year-olds can be prepared ahead of time for surgery. Up to the age of 7 years, information should be given not more than a week in advance, and after age 7, as soon as the need for surgery is established or about 2 weeks before admission.[59]

The child should be told in language appropriate to his age and his development level what to expect before and after the operation and what the operative procedure will be (Fig. 23-2). The child, like the adult, should

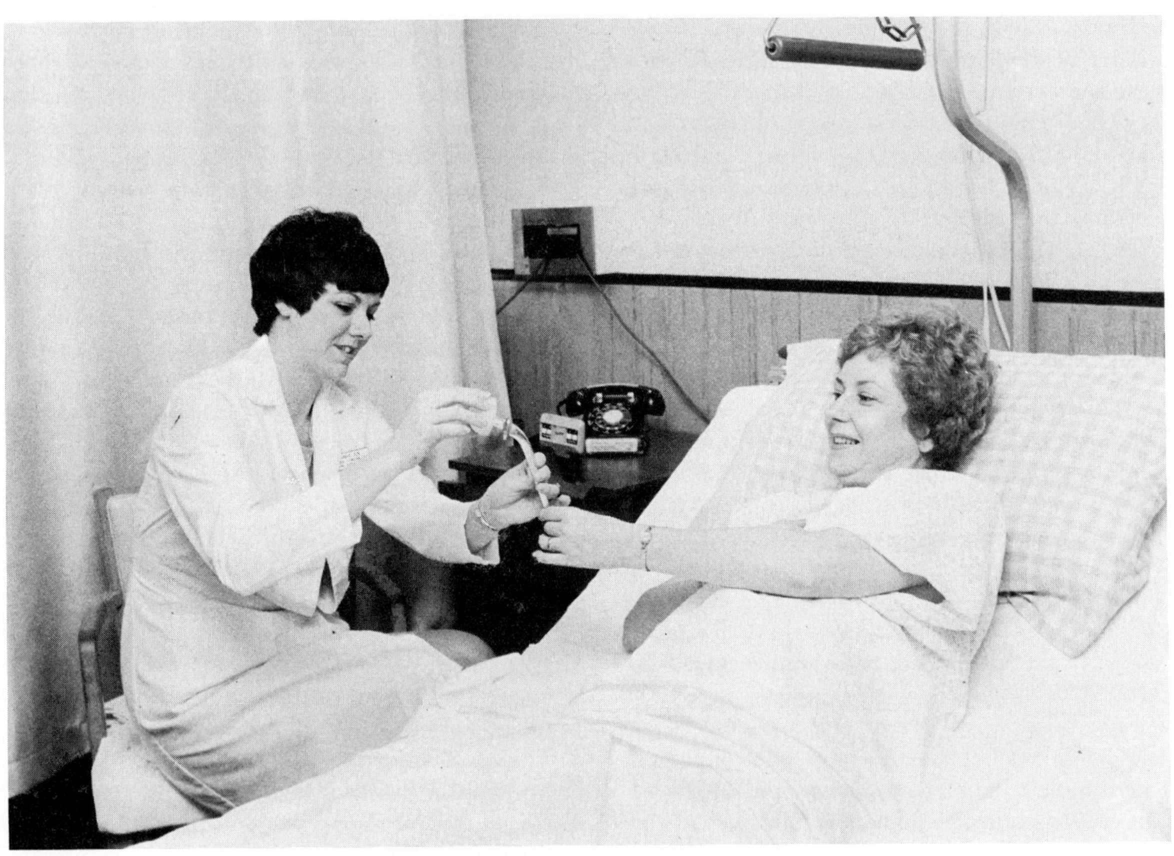

Fig. 23-1. Operating room nurse makes preoperative visit to prepare patient for joint replacement surgery.

have individualized instruction. Sometimes the preparation should be gradual, and storybooks about hospitalization and anesthesia are available and are useful for parents to use. Unless the child is old enough to have developed a perspective as to time, a small amount of factual information given shortly before the operation is best. Knowing too far ahead may only confuse the child, since his concept of time is immediate and he does not grasp the significance of a a waiting period. Parental participation in preoperative care should be encouraged. The child should never be told untruths. Honesty and simplicity concerning tests, preparations, surgery, stitches, and pain encourage the child to trust those who will be caring for him. He should know that the experience may not be entirely pleasant, but the positive aspects of the situation should be stressed. Placing a child in a room with other children usually helps him adjust to hospitalization more easily, and telling him (if it is true) that his mother will be at his bedside when he awakens helps a great deal to comfort him and allay fear. When possible the child should be allowed to bring his favorite toy, blanket, or other comfort object with him to the hospital. He should also be allowed to take this object to the operating and recovery rooms.

Outcome: *Significant others have opportunities for emotional support*

Persons who have close ties with the patient are also frequently anxious. This anxiety can be transmitted to the patient, increasing his anxiety level. The same principles described in exploring concerns and giving information to the patient hold true for significant others. If the patient needs assistance in meeting physical needs, receptive family members can be shown how they can effectively participate if they so desire. This can serve to reduce some of their own anxiety.

□ Physiologic preparation for surgery

Assessment

The nurse collects data in the preoperative phase for two reasons: to obtain baseline data for comparison during the intraoperative and postoperative phases and to identify potential postoperative problems that may require preventive nursing interventions prior to surgery.

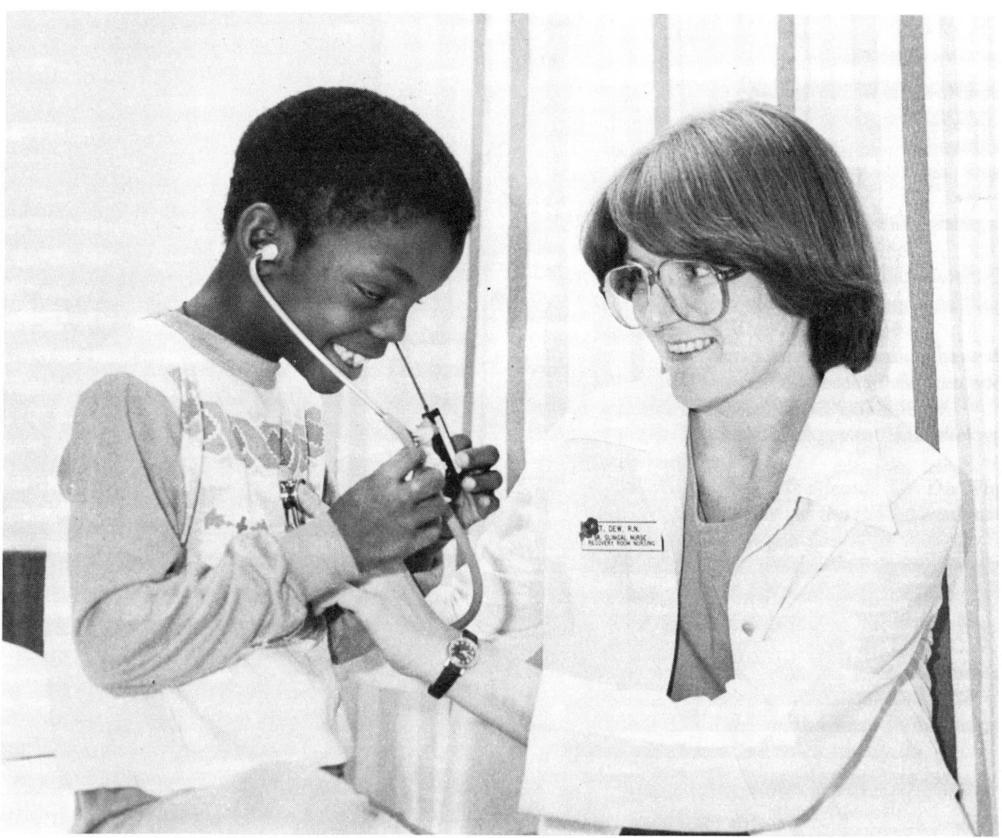

Fig. 23-2. Preoperative teaching familiarizes child with what he can expect during surgical experience.

Data of special significance during the intraoperative phase such as blood pressure readings should be recorded so that they are available for comparison.

Baseline data. The nursing history and physical assessment obtained when a patient is admitted to the hospital should contain pertinent data that can serve as baseline data for surgery. Data include height and weight, vital signs, sensory abilities, respiratory and circulatory status, elimination habits, activity status, and rest and sleep habits. Recording of these data is important so that they are available for comparison as changes occur in the patient and for planning nursing care.

Data for identification of postoperative problems. Some operative and postoperative complications can be prevented or ameliorated if persons who are at high risk of developing these complications are identified early and measures are taken to try to prevent the complications.

Respiratory. Decreased ventilation resulting in atelectasis or pneumonia is a common postoperative problem. It is important to obtain data about ventilatory status before surgery. Presence and character of breath sounds for each lobe of the lung will identify baseline status. The presence of factors indicating potential risk for developing postoperative pulmonary complications should be identified (Table 23-3). The patient's ability to use diaphragmatic breathing and to expand the chest when taking a deep breath is assessed.

The physician usually orders a chest radiograph to be sure that there is no lung disease. If interference with pulmonary function is suspected, additional tests will be ordered such as vital capacity, pulmonary function tests, and blood gas studies (Table 23-4). If signs of upper respiratory infection are present (rhinitis, pharyngitis, sore throat, fever, cough), surgery will be postponed until the symptoms abate.

Cardiovascular. Medical assessment of the cardiovascular status identifies signs of heart disease that need correction before surgery is carried out. An electrocardiogram (ECG) is ordered routinely on adults for signs of cardiac arrhythmia or heart damage. Blood studies (Table 23-4) may indicate presence of blood dyscrasias, liver disease, or electrolyte imbalances as well as serving as baseline data. Blood volume studies or central venous pressure measurements may be ordered when there is known or suspected heart disease or if the patient is elderly and fluid overload is a potential problem.

If surgery is to be performed on major blood vessels or on the extremities, presence and strength of peripheral pulses are recorded. Comparison of pre- and postoperative findings helps determine adequacy of circulation. If the patient has a low hematocrit or blood hemoglobin level or if major surgery that may involve considerable blood loss is planned, blood is drawn for typing and cross-matching so that blood will be available for transfusion as necessary.

Table 23-3. Risk factors in development of postoperative pulmonary complications

Risk factors	Effect
Increased respiratory secretions	
Smoking Intubation Inhalant anesthetics Chronic lung disease Upper respiratory infection	Irritation of lining of tracheobronchial passages Decreased ciliary action to remove secretions Secretions will block bronchial passages or alveoli
Dry sticky secretions	
Chronic lung disease Dehydration	Difficult to cough up secretions Secretions will block bronchial passages
Decreased thorax expansion	
Pain (chest, upper abdomen) Obesity Age Tight binders or casts Skeletal abnormalities (e.g., scoliosis)	Lung does not expand fully, resulting in hypoventilation of alveoli
Decreased diaphragm mobility	
Abdominal distention Surgery of chest or upper abdomen Muscle relaxants Neurologic defecit	Decreased lung expansion, leading to hypoventilation
Depression of respiratory center	
Sedatives Narcotics Acid-base imbalance	Depressed respirations result in hypoventilation
Aspiration of gastric contents	
Vomiting	Causes aspiration pneumonia

Nutrition. Since undernourished or obese persons have a greater potential for developing postoperative complications, it is important to identify these patients before surgery. Weight is compared with height and bone structure. Diet histories should be taken for high-risk patients to determine likes and usual food habits. (For further information on dietary assessment, see Chapter 51.) Presence of excessive nausea and vomiting preoperatively will dehydrate the patient and cause electrolyte imbalance. Signs of dehydration (decreased skin turgor, dry mucous membranes, soft eyeballs, high hematocrit level) should be noted.

Table 23-4. Preoperative tests to establish baselines and detect presence of diseases that can affect patient responses in intraoperative or postoperative phases

System	Test	Disease or condition
Respiratory	Chest x-ray	Tuberculosis or other pulmonary disease
	Vital capacity	Tuberculosis, chronic obstructive lung disease, bronchitis, asthma
	Pulmonary function	
	Blood gas studies	
Circulatory	Electrocardiogram	Cardiac arrhythmias, myocardial damage
	Blood studies:	
	WBC and differential	Chronic infection
	RBC, hemoglobin, hematocrit	Anemia
	Electrolytes	Electrolyte imbalances
	Platelet count, bleeding and clotting times, prothrombin	Liver disease, blood dyscrasias
	Typing and cross-matching	Compatibility for transfusion
	Blood volume	Heart disease
Renal	Urine studies	
	Bacteria	Urinary tract infection
	Albumin, specific gravity	Kidney disease
	Blood studies	
	Creatinine, BUN, NPN, electrolytes	Kidney disease
Metabolic	Blood sugar, urine sugar,	Diabetes mellitus
	acetone	Starvation

Elimination. Good renal function is necessary to maintain fluid and electrolyte balance postoperatively. Urinalysis will be ordered routinely on all patients. Presence of albumin or a low specific gravity may indicate the possibility of kidney disease, and further evaluation will be necessary. Sugar may indicate diabetes mellitus; thus blood sugar level is also obtained. Acetone may indicate diabetes mellitus or starvation. Signs of urinary tract infection include bacteriuria, fever, urgency, frequency, and burning on voiding. Urinary tract infection is treated with antibiotics before surgery if possible. Men with a history of prostatic enlargement may have difficulty voiding postoperatively.

A history of chronic constipation should be noted for vigorous follow-up in the postoperative period when decreased activity may further complicate the problem. Methods that the patient has found effective in the past to control constipation are noted. The presence of diarrhea is reported as this may lead to dehydration and electrolyte imbalances (p. 306).

Activity. Any limitations that affect the patient's ability to ambulate in the postoperative period are noted.

Comfort, rest, and sleep. The patient's perception of expected discomfort related to the surgery is explored as well as his expectations concerning relief of pain. Existing discomforts or limitations in achieving rest or sleep are assessed. Insomnia may be related to anxiety concerning the forthcoming surgery.

Table 23-5. Medications that can adversely affect anesthesia or surgery

Medication	Effect
Antibiotics	Potentiate muscle relaxants
Anticoagulants	Increase bleeding and hemorrhage
Antihypertensives	Affect anesthesia and compensatory ability (hypotension may occur)
Aspirin	↓ platelet aggregation
	Potentiates effect of anticoagulants
Diuretics (thiazides)	Possible potassium imbalance
Steroids	↓ Neuroendocrine response
	Antiinflammatory effect, may delay wound healing
Tranquilizers	Potentiate effect of narcotics and barbiturates
	Hypotension

Medications. The patient may be taking certain medications that can interfere with anesthesia or contribute to postoperative complications (Table 23-5). Some medications may need to be discontinued for a time prior to surgery.

Intervention

Prevention

Correction of existing deficiencies. Postoperative complications can be minimized if existing medical conditions are treated or under good control prior to surgery. Measures to treat wound infections are carried out prior to secondary closure or skin grafting. Dehydration from vomiting and diarrhea is treated with parenteral fluids to reestablish fluid and electrolyte balance.

Patients with chronic diseases should be at their optimal health level prior to surgery. The undernourished patient is placed on a high-protein, high-carbohydrate diet rich in vitamins B_1, C, and K. Supplementary vitamins may be ordered. The obese patient is placed on a weight-reducing diet. Both the undernourished and obese patient should understand the rationale for the diets, and they may need considerable support and encouragement to maintain the diets.

Patients with chronic obstructive pulmonary disease (COPD) are frequently placed on vigorous respiratory therapy to ensure maximum ventilation and to decrease postoperative respiratory complications. This therapy usually includes postural drainage, aerosol inhalations, and intermittent positive pressure breathing (IPPB) therapy. Smoking should be discouraged for all patients preoperatively and especially for patients with COPD. Diabetes mellitus should be under good control.

Teaching needs. Teaching is an important function of the nurse in the preoperative phase. If the person is to move toward self-care and independence, he needs to know early the what, why, and how of activities that will help him regain his optimal level of functioning after surgery. Preparation for discharge begins at the time of admission. Any assessment that identifies teaching needs should be followed with a teaching plan that starts in the preoperative period and is modified and continued in the postoperative period. Waiting until the patient has sufficiently recovered from the insult of surgery before teaching is started means considerable loss of time, and learning may be less effective. In addition the patient may be discharged before teaching is completed.

One purpose of teaching is the giving of information related to the forthcoming surgical experience (p. 367). Its goal is to decrease anxiety in the preoperative and intraoperative phases. A second purpose of teaching is to decrease postoperative discomforts or complications. A number of studies[29,30,48,55] have demonstrated that preoperative teaching has positive effects in the postoperative phase.

Principles of teaching and learning should be used. It is important to find out first what the patient already knows. Previous experiences, level of understanding, level of anxiety, and presence of distractors such as pain are assessed. Explanations are kept simple, but the rationale for what is being taught and how it will affect the patient later on is given. Planning ahead may be necessary so that a quiet area conducive to teaching is available. The patient is asked to repeat in his own words what he has learned, or he may be asked to demonstrate how to do an acitivity such as coughing, or arm exercises.

Teaching content should include what the patient can expect to occur and what will be expected of him after he wakens from anesthesia. He should know whether he will return to his own room or be in a recovery room or an intensive care unit. Special equipment such as monitors, tubes, and suction equipment that will be used postoperatively should be explained to the patient.

Outcome: *The patient will explain and carry out exercises to prevent postoperative complications*

All patients potentially at risk of developing postoperative pulmonary complications (Table 23-3) should be taught deep-breathing and coughing exercises prior to surgery. Waiting to do so until the patient is awakening from anesthesia decreases the possibility that these exercises will be carried out effectively; anesthesia and pain decrease ability to retain information. The patient should practice deep breathing using diaphragmatic breathing (p. 952) and should be shown how the incision can be splinted with a pillow, towel, or hands to decrease pain when coughing. If it is known that the patient will be using intermittent positive pressure breathing (IPPB) in the postoperative phase, it will be more effective if he has a chance to learn how to use the machine before surgery.

Pain is usually a source of concern for the patient. Many patients do not know that medication for pain can be given when necessary, and it is helpful for them to know that they can ask for medication if none has been offered and they are experiencing discomfort. The patient can be taught how to decrease pain by changing position frequently in bed. It is helpful for him to learn how to use the side rails to turn in bed. The nurse can help him role play, first how to sit up on the side of the bed and then how to stand without placing undue strain on the site where the incision will be located. Knowing beforehand what he will be expected to do can help the patient feel in control of the situation.

Muscle activity and ambulation help to prevent many postoperative complications. The patient should know that he may be sitting up on the side of the bed and possibly standing and walking the evening after surgery (except in conditions such as orthopedic surgery). Teaching

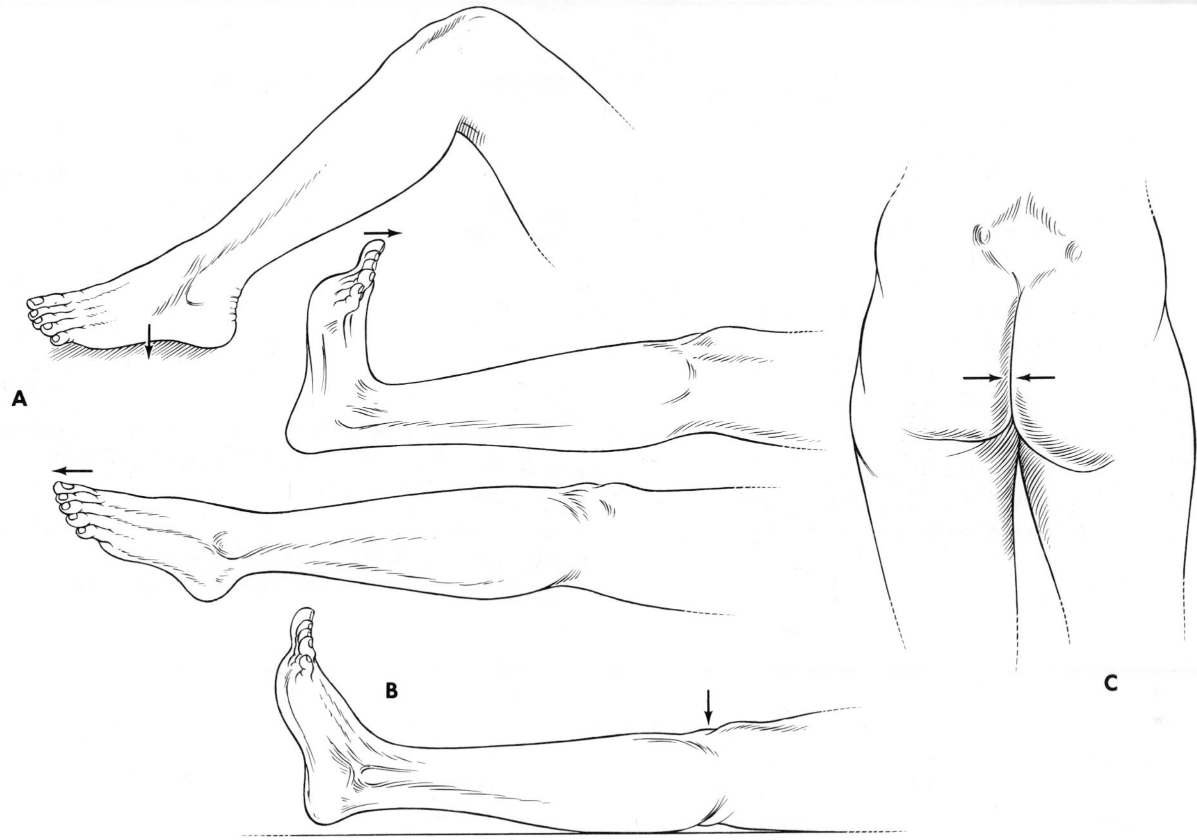

Fig. 23-3. Exercises to strengthen muscles for ambulation and to prevent thrombus formation. **A,** Knees and ankle are flexed and extended. **B,** Knee is pressed against bed and heel is lifted off bed (quadriceps setting). **C,** Buttocks are pinched together and relaxed (gluteal setting).

should include bed exercises to strengthen leg muscles for walking and to prevent venous thrombus formation (Fig. 23-3). Flexing the ankle and leg utilizes the muscles as pumps to prevent venous stasis. Quadriceps and gluteal setting exercises strengthen the muscles used for walking.

If the patient is scheduled to remain in the hospital for only a few hours postoperatively, instructions for postoperative care are best given before admission to the hospital. At this time the patient has not received medication and a family member may be present. If not done before admission, instructions should be given before premedication for surgery. The instructions should be reviewed with the patient and family postoperatively.

Preoperative management

Operative permit: informed consent. The patient will be asked to sign a statement indicating that he consents to have the operative procedure performed. This consent implies that the patient has been provided with the knowledge necessary to understand the nature of the procedure to be carried out as well as the known and possible consequences of the procedure. The individual should be informed of the options available to him and the risks associated with each. The patient has thus given his "informed consent" for the procedure to be carried out when he signs the permit. The signed consent protects the hospital and the surgeon against claims that unauthorized surgery has been performed and that the patient was unaware of the potential risks of complication involved. The permit also protects the patient from undergoing unauthorized surgery.

Sometimes the patient wishes to talk to a close family member before signing an operative permit. If so, the nurse should assist him in contacting the relative. If serious, extensive, or disfiguring surgery must be anticipated, the patient may wish to leave the hospital for a short time to confer with relatives or attend to business affairs before he signs the operative permit. The nurse should realize that signing the operative permit is a very serious step for the patient and one that is taken much more easily when the nurse conveys warmth, friendliness, and sympathy for him at this time of decision.

Permission should be obtained for each operation performed and is usually obtained for major diagnostic procedures that involve entering a body cavity such as thoracentesis, cystoscopy, and bronchoscopy. For the consent to be valid, the person giving it must be mentally competent. If a client is determined to be incapable of understanding or is intoxicated, a relative or guardian must sign for him. When mental incompetence has been determined on the basis of a judicial determination, permission must be obtained from the legal guardian appointed by the court. The legal guardian may be an individual, an institution, or an agency. If the legal guardian is not available, a court of competent jurisdiction may authorize the operative procedure.

The written permission must be witnessed by an authorized person, and who this person can be may vary from one institution to another. If a patient is unable to sign his legal signature, he may write any sort of notation that legally represents "his mark." In this event two witnesses are required. In an emergency situation the surgeon may operate without written permission of the patient or his family, although, time permitting, every effort should be made to contact a family member or guardian. Consent in the form of a telegram or telephone call is permissible in this situation. It is customary to require the signature of a parent or legal guardian for a minor child. An "emancipated minor," that is, one who is married or earning his own livelihood and retaining the earnings, can sign his own permit. The signature of the husband or wife of a married minor is also acceptable. Parenthood alone does not emancipate a minor. Consent for a procedure on the child of an unwed minor parent must be obtained from the adult who is next of kin to the unwed parent. A special informed consent form for a therapeutic abortive procedure or an operative procedure that has the express purpose of terminating reproductive capacity may be required. This form usually requires the signature of the patient and his or her spouse.

The nurse is usually responsible for seeing that the operative permit is signed and attached to the patient's chart when he goes to the operating room. The signature should be obtained without pressure and before the patient receives sedation. The patient may refuse to undergo an operation, and it is his privilege to do so.

The nurse should note whether a permit has been signed at least a day before an elective operation is scheduled. If it has not been signed or if the patient is reluctant to sign it, the nurse should notify the surgeon at once. The ultimate responsibility for obtaining the necessary permission for an operation rests with the surgeon.

Preoperative medical orders. When the patient is ready for surgery, the surgeon writes orders pertaining to gastrointestinal tract preparation, skin preparation, and medications. All preoperative medical orders are automatically cancelled when the patient leaves the unit for surgery. Following the surgical procedure the physician will write new orders. All medical orders should be written clearly and completely to prevent errors.

Outcome: *Complications related to gastrointestinal tract (aspiration, bowel obstruction, bowel trauma) are avoided*

DIET: ADULT. On the day prior to surgery there is usually no change in the patient's dietary intake. One exception is bowel surgery, in which case patients may be placed preoperatively on a low-residue diet. If general anesthesia is planned, food and fluids are usually not permitted for 4 to 8 hours prior to surgery. Presence of food or fluids in the stomach increases the possibility of aspiration of gastric contents should the patient vomit while under anesthesia. This can lead to aspiration pneumonia. If it should be discovered that the patient has consumed food or fluids when he was ordered "nothing by mouth," the surgeon should be notified as this may necessitate rescheduling of the surgical procedure. If a local or spinal anesthetic is planned, a light meal may be permitted.

Patients who are dehydrated will usually have parenteral fluids initiated prior to surgery. If it is anticipated that the patient may have decreased peristalsis after surgery (due to anesthesia or manipulation of the abdominal viscera), a nasogastric tube may be inserted prior to surgery.

DIET: CHILD. Differences in size of fluid compartments and in metabolic rates of infants and children as compared with adults necessitate different regimens. Long periods without foods or fluids preoperatively can cause hypoglycemia and dehydration. Infants usually receive formula up to 4 hours prior to anesthesia. Small children are given clear fluids up to 4 hours preanesthesia. Milk passes rapidly through the stomach in young children and is sometimes permitted in preference to clear fluids as it helps to prevent hypoglycemia.[93] No child under 8 years of age should be without supplemental glucose for more than 6 hours preoperatively. If glucose cannot be given orally, parenteral fluids are started.

BOWEL PREPARATION. Cleansing the bowel preoperatively by means of enemas is not a routine procedure. The surgeon makes the decision based on the surgical site and type of surgery to be performed. Preoperative enemas are frequently ordered prior to gastrointestinal tract surgery or surgery on the pelvic, perineal, or perianal areas. The purpose of the preoperative enema is to prevent injury to the colon and to provide better visualization of the surgical area. Enemas are seldom ordered for children. Enemas should be given if a patient has had radiographic studies involving barium immediately prior to surgery. Barium remaining in the intestinal tract may predispose to fecal impactions postoperatively. Enemas given preoperatively should be effective.

If enemas are to be given until the returns are clear, it is important to remember that fluid excess and potassium deficits can occur with repeated enemas. It is common practice to check with the physician if returns are not clear after the third enema. One method is to give up to three enemas the evening prior to surgery, then if returns are still not clear to repeate the enemas the following morning. Repeated enemas are very tiring to the patient and may irritate rectal and bowel mucosa. If antibiotic enemas are ordered for the purpose of decreasing intestinal bacteria prior to intestinal surgery, synthesis of vitamin K by the intestinal bacteria may be inhibited. Supplementary vitamin K may be given to prevent increased bleeding after surgery.

When a preoperative enema is not ordered it is important to determine that the patient has had a bowel movement in the last day or two. If he has not had a bowel movement, a mild laxative is often given. This prevents fecal impaction after surgery.

Outcome: *Wound infection due to presence of pathogenic organisms on the skin prior to surgery does not occur*

The skin is the body's first line of defense against invading microorganisms. Any break in the continuity of the skin presents the potential for an infection. The purpose of preoperative skin preparation is to free the operative site of as many microorganisms as possible. The normal flora of even very clean skin contains several types of microorganisms including staphylococcus and streptococcus.

The skin can never be completely rid of microorganisms, but the numbers can be considerably reduced by thorough cleansing, especially with hexachlorophene preparations. In many instances showering well with a hexachlorophene soap will suffice. In certain types of surgery such as orthopedic surgery where infections can lead to permanent dysfunction, a special cleansing routine with hexachlorophene preparations is often indicated. Hexachlorophene is freely soluble in organic solvents such as alcohol or soap but is insoluble in water. To retain the antiseptic properties of the hexachlorophene solutions on the skin, therefore, no soap, alcohol, or alcohol-based solutions should be used in conjunction with the hexachlorophene solutions.

The presence of hair close to the surgical incision can contribute to wound infection because of the microorganisms that cling to the hair. There is considerable difference of opinion concerning shaving of hair prior to surgery. When hair is shaved there is increased possibility of the skin being abraded or cut by the razor. This destroys the continuity of the skin and provides a site for growth of microorganisms. When the incision is made at the time of surgery, the microorganisms are introduced into the wound. Some surgeons advocate that hair be shaved only when there is excess hair that can interfere with the surgical procedure. Ideally, if hair is shaved, it should be done as close to the time of making the incision as possible. Shaving of hair should be carried out with extreme care with a sharp blade to prevent scratching or nicking the skin. Most hospitals use disposable skin preparation sets that are discarded after use. Shaving of the infant or young child is usually not done.

Shaving of hair on certain areas of the body may have a special meaning for some persons. These areas include face, head, and pubic area. If the entire head is to be shaved, this is frequently carried out after the patient has been anesthetized. The eyebrows are not shaved. Pubic hair is shaved only when necessary; the regrowth of this hair is uncomfortable to many patients.

Before carrying out any preoperative shaving, an explanation is given to the patient. The privacy of the patient is protected as much as possible. Every effort should be made to minimize discomfort and embarrassment of the patient by carrying out the skin preparation in a considerate, competent, and professional manner.

Most hospitals have specified procedures delineating the size of the area to be shaved. The surgeon usually specifies which of the areas is to be shaved. An area larger than the anticipated incision is shaved to permit flexibility in location and size of incision.

Outcome: *Patient sleeps the night before surgery*

Anxiety often causes sleeplessness and restlessness. If the patient is extremely restless a tranquilizer may be given for 1 to 2 days before surgery. Ambulation is encouraged prior to surgery in order to give the patient a feeling of well-being, to stimulate circulation and ventilation, and to maintain muscle tone. Fatigue is to be avoided, and patients with chronic illnesses may need planned periods of rest.

A sedative is usually ordered on the night before surgery to ensure a good night's rest. If additional sedation or medication for pain is given during the night, it must be given at least 4 hours before the preoperative medication.

Measures to decrease anxiety, as described earlier, are important nursing interventions. If a barbiturate or other sedative is given to an elderly patient, he should be assessed frequently during the night for signs of confusion, and measures should be instituted to protect the patient from injury.

Care of the patient on the operative day

Special needs

Outcome: *Patient states he feels comfortable*

The patient should be permitted to sleep on the morning of surgery for as long as possible and to rest undisturbed until shortly before administration of the preanesthetic medication. Many patients therefore prefer to take their bath or shower the evening before surgery rather than in the morning. If the patient has bathed the night before, he is given an opportunity to wash his hands and face and to perform mouth care. He should be reminded not to swallow water if he is not permitted fluids by mouth. A hospital gown is worn to surgery.

Comfort also implies readiness for surgery and that the patient is able to marshal effective coping mechanisms. The patient should have an opportunity to have last-minute questions answered. Explanations for last-minute routines are given if not done previously. If the surgery is to be delayed even for a short time, both the patient and his family should be informed.

It is advisable that the patient is not unduly stimulated by visitors before surgery. The patient's choice of whom he wants to see should be taken into consideration whether it be family members or a close friend. The nurse should arrange a short time of privacy for the patient and his visitors. A parent is usually encouraged to remain with a child. The patient may also desire a visit from a chaplain on the morning of surgery.

Outcome: *Patient is protected preoperatively from potential operative hazards*

A number of interventions are carried out prior to the patient's transfer to the operating room that help to promote patient safety during the intraoperative phase.

1. *Final assessment is made.* Vital signs are taken for identification of significant changes. It is normal for the pulse rate and systolic blood pressure to be increased from baseline levels due to the immediacy of the stressful situation; however, marked changes should be reported to the surgeon. Other data to be reported are temperature elevation (possible infection), signs of upper respiratory tract infection, or expressions of new or a different type of pain.
2. *Identification band is checked.* The band should be legible and secured firmly to the patient. The identification band is checked in the operative suite to ensure that surgery is performed on the right patient.
3. *Hairpins are removed; hair is protected.* Hairpins may become dislodged and injure the scalp. Hair may become tangled or interfere with equipment used for anesthetic. If the hair is long or bulky, braiding is useful. Wigs are removed as they may become lost. A disposable cap is worn by the patient during surgery to protect the hair should the patient vomit.
4. *Nail polish is removed.* The nail beds are used to observe for signs of hypoxia.
5. *Denture are removed.* Muscles of the jaw relax under anesthesia, and dentures may fall away from the gums and drop back into the pharynx causing respiratory obstruction.
6. *Hearing aid is left in place.* It is important that the operating room staff be able to communicate with the patient in the crucial minutes before surgery. The operating room nurse should be informed that the hearing aid is in place. If the patient does not speak English, an attempt should be made to locate an interpreter who can accompany the patient to the operating room and remain with him until anesthesia is induced. Many larger hospitals have foreign language registries of employees who can be called on for such assistance.
7. *Antiembolic stockings or bandages are applied to legs of high-risk patients.* The surgeon may order antiembolic stockings or bandages for patients who are elderly, who have marked varicosities, or who are to have surgical procedures that involve the pelvic area, surgery that will be time consuming, or surgery that will prevent ambulation for a time postoperatively. The stockings or bandages compress superficial veins and increase blood flow through deep veins by pressure, preventing venous stasis. This in turn helps to prevent thromboembolisms and shock.
8. *Patient's bladder is emptied.* The patient is asked to void immediately prior to leaving for the operating room. An empty bladder permits better visualization of abdominal organs and decreases the chances of inadvertent injury to the bladder. A patient who has voided shortly before being asked to do so may not be able to void again because of the fluid restrictions. If the bladder must be kept in a collapsed state throughout the surgery or if the patient has a condition that will interfere with urination postoperatively, an indwelling catheter is inserted and attached by tubing to a closed drainage system. This is frequently carried out in the operating room to ensure asepsis.
9. *Safety measures are instituted after preanesthetic medication.* After the preanesthetic medications

are administered, the patient should stay in bed as he may become drowsy, light-headed, or unsteady on his feet. He should be reminded not to smoke and be told to call the nurse if he needs anything.

Outcome: *Loss or damage of valuable objects is prevented*

Objects or prostheses taken to the operating room with the patient may become lost or damaged. Prostheses such as dentures, false limbs or false eyes, or wigs should be removed, labeled, and placed in safekeeping. Patients who desire to take religious medals to the operating room can be advised that in many instances paper emblems may be obtained from their priest. All jewelry and money should be sent home with the family if possible or removed from the bedside and locked up. The patient is permitted to wear a wedding ring, but it should be taped or tied securely to the hand.

Preanesthetic medications. The term premedication is used to signify medications that are given immediately prior to the patient's transfer to surgery and for the purpose of allaying anxiety and permitting a smoother induction of anesthesia. Some medications also serve to minimize some of the effects of anesthetic agents. The preanesthetic medications most commonly used are barbiturates, narcotics, and anticholinergic drugs. Tranquilizers may also be ordered by the physician.

The combination and dosages of the premedication vary based on factors identified by the anesthesiologist. Age is an important factor. The infant is usually given only atropine. Adults frequently receive a combination of drugs, the dosage depending on body size. Dosages are frequently decreased for the elderly.[24]

Pentobarbital and secobarbital are the barbiturates prescribed most frequently. Dosages vary from 50 to 200 mg. These drugs have a sedative-hypnotic effect with minimal depression of respiration or circulation. Other frequently used hypnotics include flurazepam hydrochloride (Dalmane), 50 mg, or chloral hydrate, 0.5 to 1.0 g.

The most commonly used narcotics are morphine sulfate, 5 to 15 mg ($^1/_{12}$ to $^1/_4$ grain) or meperidine (Demerol), 50 to 100 mg. Narcotics are useful for sedative-hypnotic effects as well as for diminishing metabolic levels, thereby decreasing the amount of anesthetic needed. If the patient is having pain prior to surgery, narcotics help reduce discomfort. Narcotics are not given preoperatively to reduce postoperative pain as the desired effect will have worn off before the patient awakens from anesthesia. Narcotics have a number of disadvantages that give rise to some disagreement as to their use as preanesthetic medications. Narcotics depress respiration, circulation, and gastric motility and may produce nausea and vomiting.

Anticholinergic drugs such as atropine or scopolamine reduce secretions and block vagal transmission, which prevents bradycardia and hypotension associated with certain anesthetic agents. With the more effective techniques of administering anesthetics and the faster acting agents used today, induction is more rapid and secretions are less of a problem.[24] Scopolamine in small doses (0.3 to 0.4 mg) is superior to atropine because it promotes amnesia and a state of indifference.

Tranquilizers such as phenothiazine derivatives are sometimes used for preanesthetic medication but are more limited in their effect. They are given mostly to allay apprehension and for their antiemetic effects. Some tranquilizers such as promethazine hydrochloride (Phenergan) potentiate the action of narcotics.

Preanesthetic medications are usually administered intramuscularly 60 to 90 minutes before the induction of anesthesia so that the maximal effect takes place. Any delay in giving the medication should be reported to the anesthesiologist. All preoperative routines should be completed before the preanesthetic medication is given. Noise and confusion are avoided in order to achieve maximum effect. It must be reemphasized that psychologic preparation of the patient for surgery is the most effective approach to help allay anxiety. Studies have shown that the administration of preanesthetic medication without any attempt at psychologic preparation may render the patient drowsy but does not reduce his anxiety.

The patient's family. The patient's family or close friends who plan to be with him the day of surgery should be made aware of the schedule and plans for the day. The nurse should share with the patient and his family the time the patient is scheduled for surgery, the time the patient will leave his room, where the family should wait while the patient is in the operating and postanesthesia recovery rooms, how they will receive information about the patient after surgery is completed, the length of time the patient is expected to be in the recovery room, policies related to recovery room visitation, and plans for the patient if transfer to an intensive care unit is anticipated postoperatively. If the family does not plan to stay in the hospital during the operative period, they should be made aware of the importance of leaving a phone number where they can be reached.

The patient and his family should be prepared for the use of any special equipment or devices that may be used in the care of the patient postoperatively (e.g., oxygen, drainage tubes from catheters, intravenous fluids, monitors). If they are prepared for these nursing care activities, the anxiety levels of both the patient and his family in the immediate postoperative period will be lessened.

Recording. Before the patient is transported to the

operating room all pertinent data should be recorded accurately and completely. It is helpful to have a form that contains space for baseline data and specific data that will be useful during the intraoperative phase (see box below). Having a form with the important data highly visible and accessible facilitates continuity of care and easy retrieval of data for later use. When such a form is not available it is important that all the data listed be put in a summary note in the nurse's notes. A checklist identifying completion of last-minute routines helps to avoid neglecting an important action.

The patient's chart must contain all the necessary information for use by the anesthesiologist and surgeon. The signed operative permit must be attached to the chart. Results of all laboratory tests, x-ray studies, and electrocardiograms should be available and any abnormal findings on late returns reported to the surgeon. It is essential that the nurse record the latest vital signs, the time premedication was given, the time that the patient voided, removal of prostheses, and the emotional response of the patient before surgery.

Transportation to the operating room. The surgical patient is usually transported to the operating room on a mobile stretcher unit or in some instances in his bed. The stretcher should be well maintained and in good working condition at all times. It is washed and made up with fresh linen between each patient use. To protect the patient from falling each stretcher should have restraint straps for over the body and side rails. Stretchers used for transporting children have head and foot rails in addition to side rails. For the tiny infant the Isolette incubator may be used. Foot extensions must be available for use with the patient who is over 6 feet tall and extends beyond the end of the stretcher.

Personnel transporting the surgical patient identify themselves to the clinical unit nursing staff and request assistance. The unit nurse assigned to prepare the patient for surgery checks the patient record, accompanies the transportation attendant to the patient's bedside, and signs the patient identification form. Before the patient is transported from his room the patient identification form is attached to the stretcher or bed. The patient is made comfortable with a pillow under his head and a blanket as a cover. Woolen or synthetic blankets should never be sent to the operating room because they are a source of static electricity. All patients should be protected from drafts, and if the patient holding area in the operating room is kept cool, additional blankets may be needed.

DATA TO BE SENT WITH PATIENT TO SURGERY

The following data are useful for the operating room and recovery room nurses as baseline data for comparison during surgery and identification of potential problems:

Name	Hearing
Age	Vision
Height and weight	Respiratory status
Consciousness level	Drainage systems
Anxiety level	Allergies
Language and speech	Special problems

■ INTRAOPERATIVE PHASE

□ Anesthesia

Usage

Anesthetics must be given by an experienced person who has been trained in the administration of anesthetic agents. Although surgical nurses do not administer anesthetic agents, they may be called on to assist the physician on the clinical unit or in a specialized area of the hospital such as the emergency room. Therefore nurses should understand anesthetic agents and their purposes and effects. The nurse should also be able to answer questions the patient may have regarding the anesthetic to be administered during surgery. It is essential for the nurse to have an understanding of drug interactions and the preanesthetic preparation of the patient and the effects of anesthetic agents given during the operative phase in order to provide effective nursing care in the postoperative period.

Anesthesia implies amnesia (loss of memory), analgesia (insensibility to pain), hypnosis (artificially produced sleep), and relaxation (rendering a part of the body less firm or rigid). Anesthetic agents that produce unconsciousness and are given by inhalation or intravenous injection are referred to as general anesthetics. Regional anesthesia produces a loss of sensation in a specific area of the body while the patient remains conscious. Regional anesthetic agents applied to the body surface (topical) and those injected around nerves interfere with the initiation and transmission of nerve impulses; thus the patient experiences no pain.

Choice

The choice of anesthetic is based on many factors: the physical condition and age of the patient; the presence of coexisting diseases; the type, site, and duration of the operation; and the personal preferences of the anesthetist. The anesthesiologist evaluates each patient carefully and selects the anesthetic agents best suited for that individual and the individual's condition. Within limits of feasibility, an important factor to consider when selecting the anesthetic to be administered is the preference of the patient; that is, many patients may have a preference for spinal, local, or general anesthesia.

An apprehensive patient may not respond well to a regional anesthetic. In some instances patients having anesthetics intravenously may respond with depression of respirations. Spinal and regional anesthetics are not practical for children as they have difficulty in holding still. It should be noted that anesthesiology is a complex and delicate discipline, and a strong knowledge of drug interaction and basic pharmacology is paramount.

Anesthesia and the patient

Patients have many anxieties related to anesthesia. They may fear going to sleep and not waking up or they may simply have a fear of the unknown. They frequently express a dislike of ether because of a previous experience and the pungent odor of the agent. They may be apprehensive regarding the effectiveness of the anesthetic and fearful of experiencing pain during the surgical procedure. Patients frequently have concern about nausea and vomiting that may occur postoperatively as a result of anesthesia. Other fears associated with anesthesia may relate to talking and revealing personal information, anticipation of a mask being placed over the face, or receiving an anesthetic that will not induce unconsciousness, that is, spinal anesthesia.

Most anxieties can be dispelled if the patient and his family are well informed about the anesthetic selected for use and the care taken by the physician and nurse in assessing the patient's physical condition. The patient should be encouraged to discuss any questions or concerns about the anesthetic with either the anesthesiologist or the surgeon.

The nurse should make the patient and family aware that the patient is under close surveillance while under anesthesia and in the immediate postoperative period. The nurse can reassure the patient that he will not be left alone until he has fully recovered from the effects of anesthesia. Very few patients talk while under anesthesia, and what is said is usually unintelligible so that talking need not be of great concern to the patient. Persistent anxiety on the part of the patient regarding his anesthetic should be discussed with the surgeon and the anesthesiologist.

General anesthesia

General anesthesia is produced by inhalation of gases or vapors of highly volatile liquids or by injection into the bloodstream of anesthetic drugs in solution. Certain drugs that produce general anesthesia such as thiopental sodium (Pentothal sodium) are used to put the patient to sleep and are almost always supplemented with other agents to produce surgical anesthesia. Other general anesthetic agents such as ether do produce surgical anesthesia but are very irritating to the respiratory tract.

Such irritation prolongs the introductory stages of anesthesia. Frequently a combination of inhalation anesthetic agents such as nitrous oxide and oxygen may be used with curare and a narcotic. The choice of agents will depend on the anesthesiologist's judgment and the individual patient's needs.

General anesthesia affects all the physiologic systems of the body to some degree. It affects chiefly the central nervous, respiratory, and circulatory systems. The anesthesiologist judges the depth of anesthesia by the changes produced in these systems. These changes are observed by monitoring heart rate with the precordial stethoscope, by ECG, blood pressure, and respiratory rate, and by blood gas determinations. Stages of anesthesia are best seen with diethyl ether. *Stage I* extends from the beginning of the administration of an anesthetic to the beginning of the loss of consciousness. *Stage II*, often called the stage of excitement or delirium, extends from the loss of consciousness to the loss of eyelid reflexes. If the patient is very apprehensive or was not given premedication correctly or on time, this stage, usually of short duration, may last longer. The patient may become excited and struggle, shout, talk, laugh, or cry. *Stage III*, the stage of surgical anesthesia, extends from the loss of the lid reflex to cessation of respiratory effort. The patient is unconscious, his muscles are relaxed, and most of his reflexes have been abolished. *Stage IV* is the stage of overdose or the stage of danger. It is complicated by respiratory and circulatory failure. Death will follow unless the anesthetic is immediately discontinued, possibly counteracting anesthetics are administered, and artificial respiration is performed. The nurse may find that some patients recovering from the effects of general inhalation anesthesia pass through stage II before becoming fully conscious and noisy and restless.

Inhalation anesthesia. Inhalation anesthesia is produced by having the patient inhale the vapors of certain liquids or gases. Oxygen is always given with these anesthetic agents. The gas mixture may be administered by mask or it may be delivered into the lungs through an endotracheal tube inserted into the trachea. The use of endotracheal intubation assures an airway can be used to aerate the lungs when the chest wall is open. The endotracheal tube has a balloon that is inflated after insertion. The balloon fills the tracheal space, lessening the chance of aspiration of gastric contents. Regardless of the skill of the anesthesiologist, an endotracheal tube cannot help causing some irritation to the trachea and subsequent edema. Because the child's trachea is smaller, edema may more easily obstruct the lumen. Therefore signs of sudden respiratory difficulty are more likely to occur postoperatively in the child than in the adult. The child's respiratory pattern must be observed carefully when an endotracheal tube has been used. Signs of respiratory embarrassment such as cyanosis or difficulty in inspiring must be reported to the surgeon at once.

Ether. Ether is a volatile, flammable liquid. It has a very pungent odor that is disagreeable to many patients. It is irritating to the mucous membranes of the pulmonary tract and the first and second stages of anesthesia are prolonged. For this reason a rapid-acting, nonirritating drug such as thiopental sodium may be used to produce sleep before ether is administered. Ether is a relatively inexpensive drug. Although it provides excellent muscle relaxation and has a greater margin of safety than some of the other anesthetic agents, it is flammable and is seldom used in the United States today.

Recovery from anesthesia with ether may be prolonged, especially if a large amount of the drug was used. The patient will require constant supervision until completely awake. Because of ether's irritating qualities, large amounts of mucus may be present, in which case the patient must be suctioned frequently. Since vomiting often occurs after the administration of ether, the patient should be placed on his side to prevent aspiration of any vomitus. If the foot of the bed is elevated, gravity will aid the flow of mucus and vomitus from the throat and mouth. Before anesthesia is started, an isotonic eye ointment in a petroleum base is frequently instilled into the eyes to prevent irritation. If an irritation does occur it should be immediately checked and, if serious, an ophthalmologist consulted. Redness or blistering of the skin, which sometimes occurs around the site of the mask, is caused by the combination of ether, moisture, and pressure. This condition can be unsightly and uncomfortable for the patient. Petroleum jelly or other ointments may be applied as ordered to relieve discomfort.

Nitrous oxide. Nitrous oxide is a nonirritating, odorless, colorless, nonflammable gas. Nitrous oxide should be given with no less than 30% oxygen. The patient becomes anesthetized quickly and recovers rapidly. This gas may be used for dental surgery and as a supplemental agent when ether is to be administered.

Nitrous oxide is also used extensively with halothane and enflurane to supplement their actions. In low concentrations nitrous oxide may provide adequate anesthesia even for intraabdominal procedures in patients who are in profound shock, debilitated, or who are critically ill and cannot tolerate other anesthetic agents. If an excessive amount of this gas is administered there is the possibility of hypoxia. Patients having open-chest surgery should have arterial oxygen determinations when inhaling high percentages of nitrous oxide.

Cyclopropane. Cyclopropane is a highly flammable and pleasant-smelling gas that quickly produces unconsciousness and produces adequate relaxation for most abdominal surgery. Because it is associated with cardiac irritability and causes arrhythmias, it should be used with caution in patients with cardiac diseases. Postoperatively the patient's pulse rate and cardiac rhythm should be checked frequently for any irregularities that might occur as a result of receiving cyclopropane gas. Emergence excitement is common. Nausea, vomiting, and headache may also occur in the postoperative period. During the administration of this gas, extreme care must be taken to prevent the production of any electric charge that might cause it to be ignited. Due to its flammability, operating room procedures should be consistent with those for other hazardous environments.

Halothane. Halothane (Fluothane) is a highly potent, nonflammable, colorless liquid with a sweet smell somewhat resembling chloroform. It is easily inhaled and usually administered through special vaporizers with nitrous oxide and oxygen. Halothane is nonirritating; thus irritation to the larynx is reduced and laryngospasm is infrequent. Induction of anesthesia is usually much faster than with ether, and the rate of emergence is more rapid.[42] An important clinical feature of halothane is the low incidence of postoperative nausea and vomiting. Emergence from anesthesia may be accompanied by shivering, probably of neurologic origin rather than the lowered body temperature commonly found.[28] Halothane can depress the circulation when high concentrations are given. It is also a respiratory depressant. Disadvantages are that it is expensive, tends to depress respiration and circulation, and may cause hepatic failure.[42] There is some evidence that in certain very rare individuals exposure to halothane may lead to sensitization so that subsequent halothane anesthesia may be followed by severe, and indeed fatal, jaundice. Some authorities recommend omitting halothane from the anesthesia sequence if multiple administrations for the same patient are anticipated.[106]

Methoxyflurane. Methoxyflurane (Penthrane) is a clear, colorless liquid with a characteristic fruity odor. It is a nonflammable agent under normal conditions of clinical anesthesia. It is a halogenated ether, and induction is prolonged. This may be overcome by injecting a quick-acting drug such as thiopental sodium before administration of methoxyflurane. Emergence from anesthesia is slow, and the need for analgesic drugs in the immediate postanesthesia period may be lessened. Methoxyflurane is associated with renal toxicity in a dose-related manner. Nausea and vomiting may occur postoperatively but to a lesser degree than after cyclopropane or ether.

Enflurane. Enflurane (Ethrane) is a clear, colorless, nonflammable liquid that has a mild, sweet odor. It is fluorinated ether used for inhalation anesthesia. Induction and recovery from anesthesia with enflurane are rapid. It does not appear to stimulate excess salivation or tracheobronchial secretions, and pharyngeal and laryngeal reflexes are readily deadened. Enflurane reduces ventilation and decreases blood pressure as the depth of anesthesia increases. It provokes a sigh response reminiscent of that seen with diethyl ether. Heart rate remains relatively constant.

Muscle relaxation is adequate for intraabdominal operations at normal levels of anesthesia, and if greater relaxation is necessary minimal doses of muscle relaxants may be used. All commonly used muscle relaxants are compatible with enflurane. Enflurane may be used for induction and maintenance of general anesthesia. It is contraindicated when the patient is subject to seizure disorders or has a known sensitivity to enflurane or other halogenated anesthetics.

Intravenous anesthesia

Thiopental sodium. Thiopental sodium (Pentothal sodium) is the drug used most frequently for induction of anesthesia. It produces unconsciousness quickly. Recovery is rapid if the total dose is small. Thiopental may also be given to relieve severe, prolonged convulsive states. Laryngeal reflexes are not depressed at light levels of narcosis, and laryngospasm may occur with stimulation of the larynx. Signs of laryngospasm are apprehension, stridor (a harsh whistling sound), retraction of the soft tissue about the neck, and cyanosis. If these signs appear in the postanesthesia period the nurse should notify the physician immediately. If large doses of thiopental have been used the patient may sleep for a long time and should be observed for signs of respiratory depression. Some individuals appear to awaken quickly only to return to the anesthetized state when undisturbed.[28] The blood pressure may drop suddenly and should be check frequently. Thiopental is detoxified in the liver and excreted by the kidneys. Therefore in patients with liver or kidney disease this drug should be used with caution.

Thiopental is used primarily to produce sleep before an inhalation anesthetic is administered. The major advantage of this agent is the smooth induction afforded the patient. This anesthetic agent may be used for brief surgical procedures such as closed reduction of a fracture or a dislocation or incision and drainage of an abscess.

Droperidol and fentanyl. Droperidol and fentanyl (Innovar) are the combination of a potent tranquilizer (droperidol) and a powerful narcotic analgesic (fentanyl). Surgical anesthesia is produced quickly, and recovery is smooth and rapid. In most patients orientation returns quickly without restlessness or emergence delirium. Incorporating droperidol and fentanyl into the anesthetic regimen will usually result in a lower incidence of postoperative nausea and vomiting. Because of its apparent lack of toxicity to the liver, kidneys, and heart, it can be given intermittently throughout a surgical procedure. Due to the tranquilizing component, droperidol, the patient requires less analgesia in the postanesthesia recovery room. Patients should be observed for hypoventilation during the immediate recovery period and may need to be urged to breathe. Postoperative narcotic orders should be reduced to one third or one fourth the usual amount. Droperidol and fentanyl may be used as premedication, as an adjunct to general anesthesia, alone, or with regional anesthesia.

Ketamine. Ketamine is a nonbarbiturate, parenteral anesthetic agent. The anesthetic state characterized by ketamine is termed *dissociative anesthesia.* It is a substance permitting surgical operations on patients who may appear to be awake, since movemment may occur and the eyes remain open. However, the individuals are anesthetized so far as recollection or awareness is concerned. Ketamine is chemically related to the hallucinogens, and unpleasant dreams during awakening and extending into the postoperative period may constitute a drawback.[3] To overcome these effects a small dose of a barbiturate is given, or more important the patient is left undisturbed during the emergence phase.[100]

Ketamine produces profound analgesia but does little to block visceral pain, which eliminates its usefulness for intraabdominal or intrathoracic procedures unless supplemented by an inhalation agent.[28] It is useful in diagnostic procedures such as neuroradiology and for superficial procedures of short duration. Ketamine has been most valuable in the anesthetic management of children and young adults.[28] Contraindications for the use of ketamine include patients with upper respiratory tract infections, prior cerebrovascular accident, hypertension, and psychiatric disorders.

Muscle relaxants. Certain drugs such as *d*-tubocurarine chloride (curare), succinylcholine chloride (Anectine), pancuronium bromide (Pavulon), and gallamine triethiodide (Flaxedil) are neuromuscular blocking agents used to provide muscle relaxation. They are employed for facilitating endotracheal intubation and may also be given as adjuncts to provide sufficient relaxation of abdominal muscles.[42]

These agents cause respiratory depression or paralysis; thus the patient must be observed closely for signs of respiratory distress during and after administration of the drug. Patients developing respiratory problems will require intubation and mechanical ventilatory assistance. All patients who are paralyzed with muscle relaxants require skilled airway management with the capability of endotracheal intubation until the patient is able to maintain his own respirations.

The drug *d*-tubocurarine is injected intravenously in the form of solutions. About one third of the amount administered is excreted unchanged in the urine, whereas the rest is metabolically altered. It is probably still the most important competitive neuromuscular blocking agent.[42]

Succinylcholine chloride is a valuable agent for producing short periods of muscular relaxation. The short duration of action of succinylcholine may be attributed to its rapid metabolic degradation. Facilities for artificial respiration are essential, since this appears to be the only effective antidotal measure to apnea.[42]

Pancuronium bromide is approximately five times as potent as *d*-tubocurarine chloride. It has little effect on the circulatory system. The most frequently reported observation is a slight rise in pulse rate. A major portion of administered pancuronium bromide is excreted unchanged in the urine.

Gallamine triethiodide is a synthetic drug that has an atropinelike effect on the cardiac branch of the vagus nerve and can produce considerable tachycardia. It is excreted unchanged in the urine and is not the agent of choice in the presence of poor renal function.

Regional anesthesia. Regional anesthesia is produced by the injection or application of a local anesthetic agent along the course of a nerve, thus abolishing the conduction of all impulses to and from the area supplied by that nerve. The patient experiences no pain in the operative area and remains awake during the entire procedure because the anesthetic affects a particular region only; it does not affect cortical functions.

Regional anesthesia is used for treatments, diagnostic measures, examinations, and surgery. The nurse usually assembles the equipment necessary for the administration of the drugs used to produce anesthesia, assists the physician during the procedure, and observes the patient for reactions to the anesthetic or to the procedure.

The drugs used to produce regional anesthesia are usually called local anesthetics. Examples are procaine (Novocain), cocaine, tetracaine (Pontocaine), dibucaine (Nupercaine), and lidocaine (Xylocaine). When these drugs are absorbed into the bloodstream they cause stimulation of the central nervous system and depression of the heart. Therefore care is taken that they are given in a localized area and in the smallest dose necessary to produce anesthesia. A barbiturate is usually given before the drugs are administered to reduce and stabilize patient anxiety. Epinephrine may be added to the solution of local anesthetic drugs to produce vasoconstriction in the area of the injection. Vasoconstriction tends to reduce the rate of absorption, to extend the length of anesthesia, and to reduce hemorrhage. Epinephrine should not be added to solutions when nerve block of the digits is contemplated.

The nurse must observe the patient for signs of excitability (laughing, crying, excessive talking), twitching, pulse or blood pressure changes, pallor of the skin, and respiratory difficulties. At the first sign of these toxic reactions an intravenous injection of a short-acting barbiturate such as thiopental sodium should be ready for the physician to administer. Oxygen may also be necessary, and it is important that a patent airway be maintained. If the reaction is due to an idiosyncrasy to the drug, circulatory failure may occur, and emergency measures such as artificial respiration must be started. Patients should be questioned regarding any previous sensitivity to these drugs, and skin tests are usually advocated before their administration.

Regional anesthesia of the limbs can be achieved by injecting an anesthetizing agent such as lidocaine into a vein in the limb to be anesthetized. A tourniquet is applied to the limb to prevent the distribution of the anesthetizing agent throughout the body.[27,47]

Topical anesthesia. Topical anesthesia is accomplished by applying or spraying a local anesthetic drug such as cocaine or lidocaine directly on the part to be anesthetized. It is used for surgical procedures on the nose and throat and to eliminate pharyngeal and tracheal reflexes during bronchoscopy and similar procedures. Topical anesthesia may be used in genitourinary procedures (urethral meatotomy, cystoscopy) and to provide anesthesia of the lower urethra.

Infiltration anesthesia. Infiltration anesthesia is accomplished by the injection of the anesthetic drug directly into the area to be incised or manipulated. This method is used for minor procedures (incision and drainage, thoracentesis). Nerve block is regional anesthesia in which the drug is injected into or around the nerve a short distance from the site of the operation. This method may be employed for patients have tonsillectomies, dental procedures, or plastic surgery.

In a pudendal block a long 20- or 22-gauge spinal needle attached to a Luer syringe is passed just below and beyond the ischial spine. Solution is then injected to anesthetize the internal pudendal nerve. The needle is partially withdrawn and then inserted laterally toward the ischial tuberosity, where more solution is injected, followed by infiltration of the labia in the same manner, which is repeated on the opposite side. Perineal muscles relax in a few minutes and the skin of the perineum is anesthetized.

Extradural anesthesia. In an epidural block the drug is injected into the epidural space and affects a band around the body, depending on the area of the vertebral columns and the dose of the drug. When a caudal block is performed, the drug is injected into the caudal canal lying below the cord and affects the nerve trunks that supply the perineal area

Spinal anesthesia. Spinal anesthesia is accomplished by the injection of a local anesthetic drug in solution into the subarachnoid space, which contains spinal fluid (Fig. 23-4). The anesthetic drug acts on the nerves as they emerge from the spinal cord. Depending on the type of

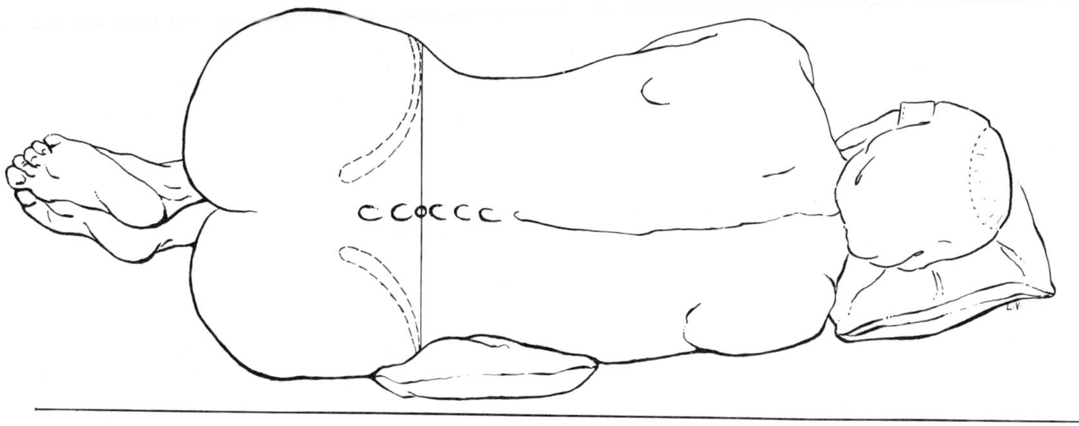

Fig. 23-4. Patient in lateral position for spinal anesthesia.

anesthesia desired, the injection is made through the second, third, or fourth interspace of the lumbar vertebrae. Anesthesia is quickly produced and provides good relaxation of muscles.

Spinal anesthesia is used for surgery of the lower limbs, perineum, and lower abdomen and sometimes for surgery in the upper abdomen such as removal of the gallbladder. It is not used for operations on the upper part of the body because it causes paralysis of the diaphragm and the intercostal muscles used in respiration. A "saddle block" is a low spinal block commonly used in vaginal deliveries. With this block, analgesia rarely extends above the tenth dermatome. The patient may be unable to move her legs for 2 to 8 hours following induction of the anesthetic. With spinal anesthesia the patient may be conscious of pulling sensations throughout the operation, but he experiences no pain. Occasionally a feeling of faintness and nausea occurs because of these sensations. One of the limitations of spinal anesthesia is that the patient may be awake during the operation, although the preoperative medication may make him quite unaware of his surroundings. A screen restricts his vision in the operating room, and a towel may be placed over his eyes. The conversation and activities of the members of the operating room staff should be carried on with the patient's consciousness in mind. It is a nursing responsibility to remind other members of the surgical team that the patient is awake and that some topics of conversation may be upsetting to him. In some hospitals a sign "Patient is Awake" is posted both in the operating room and outside the door.

Because of the sympathetic blockade, hypotension may occur with these anesthetic techniques. Vasopressor drugs such as epinephrine hydrochloride may be given if a drop in blood pressure occurs. This may also be seen with epidural anesthesia.

Following spinal anesthesia the patient should be quiet in bed in a supine position. Since sensation may not return to the anesthetized area for an hour or two, the nurse must see that the patient sustains no injuries such as burns from hot-water bottles during this time. The nurse must always be alert for signs of respiratory or circulatory depression. Although the patient is conscious, his blood pressure, pulse, and respirations should be checked frequently. Hypotension may occur as a result of relaxation of the vascular bed.

Headache following spinal anesthesia will be reduced if the patient does not sit up or assume the erect position for 8 hours. Spinal headache is thought to be due to leakage of spinal fluid from the puncture in the dura or to sterile chemical meningitis. It usually occurs 24 hours after the puncture and is more common in women than in men. It may last several days, and occasionally it persists for weeks or months. The nurse should not suggest the possibility of this complication to the patient. If it does occur the patient complains of a throbbing, pulsating headache that is aggravated by a change to the upright position or by merely coughing or sneezing; an ice bag may bring relief. To lessen discomfort analgesics and sedatives should be given as ordered. Hydration of the patient is of great importance, since it will aid in the replacement of spinal fluid. Increased oral intake should be encouraged. If the patient is receiving nothing orally, intravenous fluids will be ordered.

When the effects of the anesthetic wear off, the patient occasionally complains of a backache. His pain may be the result of the position in which he was placed on the operating table or of the insertion of the needle at the time of the puncture. The complaint is treated symptomatically, and heat applied locally often brings relief.

Fire, explosion, and electrical safety

Certain anesthetizing agents such as ether and cyclopropane are flammable and explosive. Therefore extreme caution must be taken at all times to eliminate electric charges that could ignite or explode these agents. Fire and explosion hazards have decreased in recent years as new nonflammable anesthetic agents have been developed, and flammable agents are used with much less frequency. All personnel entering the operating room must strictly adhere to the dress code regulations. Conductive shoes or boots are worn in this area.

Today the greatest hazard to the life of the surgical patient is the electrical one. The present concerns revolve around the grounding systems in operating and recovery rooms and the increasing use of electrical monitoring equipment.

Induced hypothermia

Local hypothermia. Induced local hypothermia refers to the lowering of the temperature of only a part of the body such as a limb. It is used largely to produce surgical anesthesia prior to amputation of a limb affected by arteriosclerotic gangrene. Elderly, debilitated patients and patients who have diabetes are most likely to be treated with this anesthesia. Advantages of this method are that physical shock to the patient is minimal, no inhalation anesthesia is required, and the lowered temperature reduces cell metabolism.

The extremity is packed in ice and anesthesia is usually obtained in 1$^1/_2$ to 3 hours. The duration of anesthesia produced by this method is approximately 60 minutes. The patient may be experiencing pain from the diseased limb and the weight of the ice makes him more uncomfortable; thus there is a need to administer a barbiturate or narcotic before initiating the procedure.

Another method for producing hypothermia in an extremity is through the use of a blanketlike device consisting of coils that contain circulating water. Thus the temperature of the water can be lowered to produce hypothermia and raised when the limb is to be rewarmed.

General hypothermia. General hypothermia for the patient in surgery is rarely used today. It refers to the reduction of body temperature below normal to reduce oxygen and metabolic requirements. Hypothermia is now being used widely for a variety of illnesses when extremely high temperatures occur. For example, patients with neurologic disease causing a high temperature may be kept in a state of relatively mild hypothermia (30.6 to 35 C or 87 to 95 F) for as long as 5 days.

If hypothermia is to be used as an adjunct to anesthesia during surgery, the patient usually is given meperidine hydrochloride and atropine sulfate 45 minutes to 1 hour before the procedure is to begin. Provision is made for monitoring temperature readings from different parts of the body, preferably the esophagus and rectum, by placing electric thermometers in these areas. In addition the heart is monitored with an electrocardiograph to detect cardiac arrhythmias produced by lowered temperature and the brain is monitored with an electroencephalograph to detect cerebral anoxia. The care of the patient at this time is under the supervision of the operating room team. The temperature is lowered by one of the following methods.

External hypothermia may be produced by applying crushed ice around the patient, by totally immersing the patient in ice water, or by exposing him to the cooling effects of special blankets. The most widely accepted method of hypothermia today is the use of cooling blankets. The patient is placed on and may be covered by body-sized vinyl pads containing many coils. The pads are connected to a reservoir filled with alcohol and water. A pump fills the coils and circulates the solution through the coils in the pad. A recording thermometer monitors the patient's temperature, and an electric unit heats or cools the solution to a preset temperature (Fig. 23-5).

Extracorporeal cooling, a method of bloodstream cooling, consists of removing the blood from a major vessel, circulating it through coils immersed in a refrigerant, and returning it to the body through another vessel. Bloodstream cooling is the fastest method for producing hypothermia and is used primarily for patients who are undergoing surgery. The patient is given heparin to prevent the blood from clotting during the procedure.

Nursing intervention during prolonged hypothermia. If he is conscious, the patient who is to undergo hypothermia for an elevated temperature needs reassurance that the procedure will not be too uncomfortable. Because the treatment is relatively new and is often erroneously conceived by the laity, the patient may have fears and apprehension that should be reported to the physician so that he or she can answer specific questions that may be causing worry. When hypothermia is to be continued for several days, any of the external methods for producing hypothermia may be used. Before the procedure is started the patient is given a complete bath and a thin coating of oil or cream may be applied to the skin; a cleansing enema may also be ordered. While the temperature is being lowered to the desired level and for as long as the procedure is continued the patient is observed closely. Any irregularities of pulse, temperature, or blood pressure must be reported at once. It is expected that all of these vital signs will lower gradually. If they rise, drop too suddenly, or fluctuate, the physician should be notified. The temperature is monitored by a rectal thermometer probe to determine whether a desired temperature (usually between 30 and 32 C or 86 and 89.6 F) is maintained throughout the treatment.

Shivering is a complication of hypothermia that should be avoided because peripheral vasoconstriction

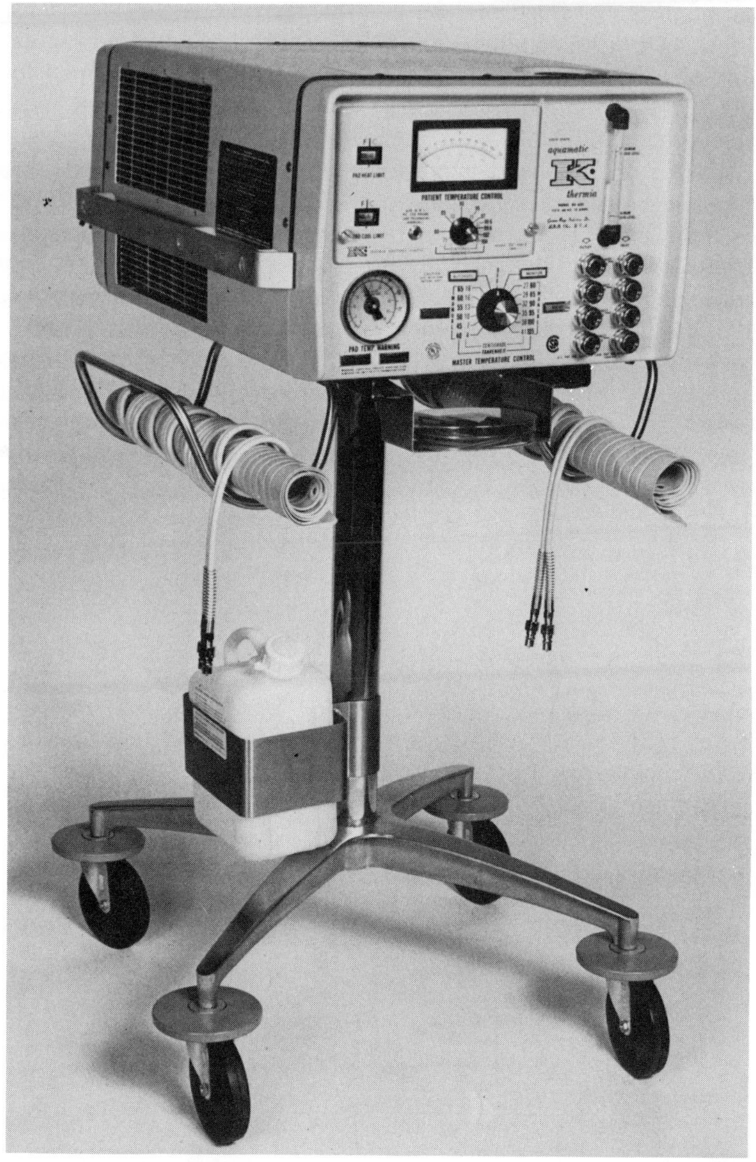

Fig. 23-5. Hypothermia can be produced by means of cooling blanket. Cold alcohol and water are circulated through coils by pressure pump.

is accompanied by an increase in body temperature, circulation rate, and oxygen consumption. Usually shivering occurs when the temperature is lowered to 30 C (86 F). To prevent shivering, chlorpromazine hydrochloride (Thorazine) usually is administered before the treatment is started and is repeated as often as every 2 hours if shivering continues. Since urinary output is decreased when the body temperature is reduced to 32 C (89 F), a retention catheter (Foley type) is inserted before hypothermia is started so that output can be measured carefully and recorded. Because the gag and other reflexes may be depressed, food and fluids are not given orally. Fluids containing glucose and electrolytes are given intravenously and usually through a polyethylene catheter that has been sutured into a vein. Depending on the method being used to produce hypothermia, the patient may be fed by means of a nasogastric tube. The patient's skin must be observed for signs of pressure, edema, and discoloration. He should be turned at least every 2 hours, and footboards and pillows should be used to prevent strain on joints and to maintain proper body alignment. Often the patient is placed on a CircOlectric bed to make possible a complete change in position. Good oral hygiene is necessary, and dried secretions should be removed from the nares. If corneal reflexes are diminished and eye secretions reduced, the eyes may need to be cleansed and covered to protect them (p. 679).

The cooling agent or blankets are removed at the termination of hypothermia and regular blankets are applied. The patient is usually allowed to warm at his own rate. The temperature must be observed carefully as it approaches normal, and blankets must then be removed. The thermometer probe is removed when the temperature becomes stable.

□ Positioning the patient for surgery

The responsibility for positioning the patient on the operating room table is one shared by the nurse, surgeon, and anesthesiologist. The nurse must be aware of the position required for each surgical procedure and understand the many physiologic changes that occur as the anesthetized patient is placed in a particular operative position.

No matter what position is to be assumed, good positioning is important to (1) adequately expose the operative area; (2) make the patient accessible for induction of anesthesia and administration of intravenous solutions or drugs; (3) minimize interference with circulation due to pressure on a body part; (4) provide protection from injury to nerves due to improper positioning of arms, hands, legs, or feet; (5) provide for the maintenance of respiratory function by avoiding pressure on the chest to allow for adequate ventilation of the lungs and by holding the jaw forward to keep it from dropping on the

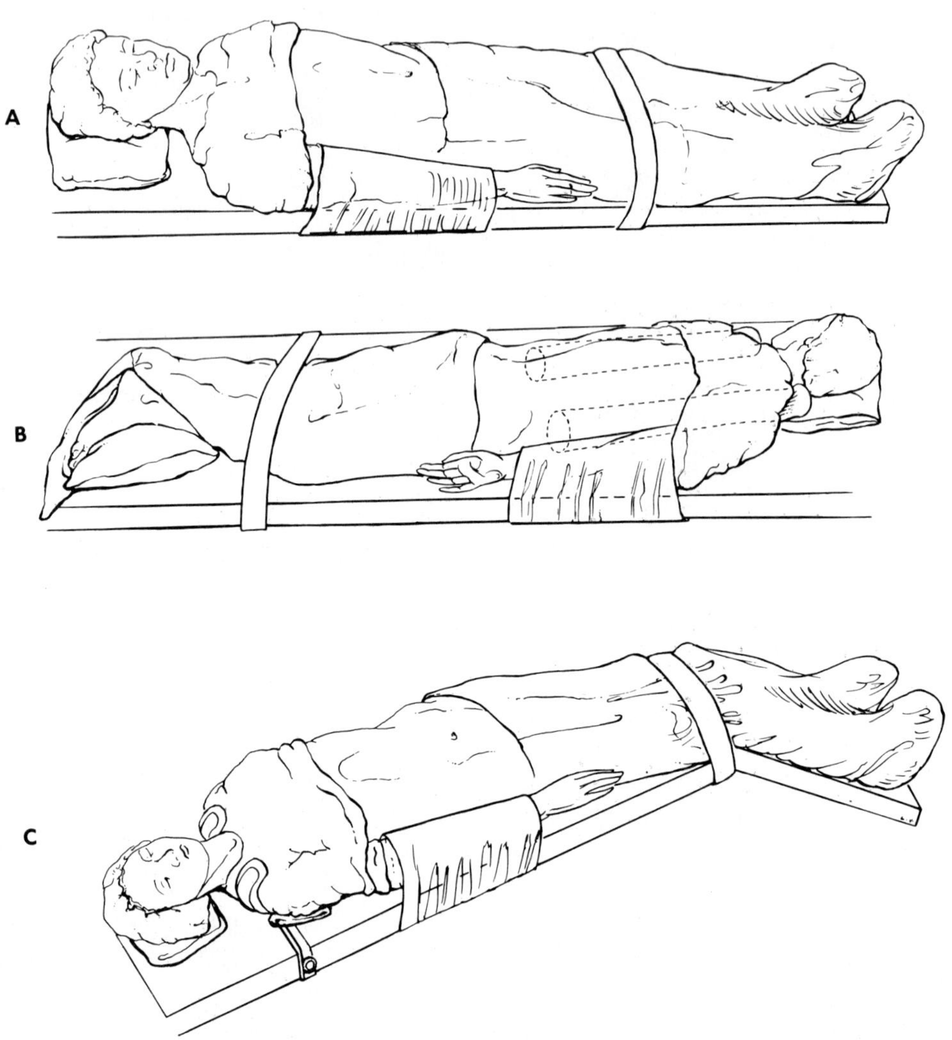

Fig. 23-6. Three commonly used operative positions. **A,** Supine. **B,** Prone. **C,** Trendelenburg.

chest; and (6) provide for the patient's individuality and his privacy by proper draping. A brief discussion of the commonly used operative positions and some of the precautions that are necessary follow.

Supine

In the supine position the patient lies flat on his back with arms at his side, palms down with fingers extended and free to rest on the table, and legs straight with feet slightly separated (Fig. 23-6, *A*). This is the most commonly used position in the operating room and is used for hernia repair, exploratory laparotomy, cholecystectomy, gastric and bowel resection, and mastectomy. Attention must be given to proper support of the patient's neck and jaw to assure the maintenance of a patent airway.

Prone

In the prone position the patient lies on his abdomen with his face turned to one side and his arms at his side with palms pronated and fingers extended (Fig. 23-6, *B*). The arms should be well protected and carefully positioned to prevent ulnar or radial nerve damage. Elbows may be slightly flexed to prevent overextension of the shoulders. The patient's feet should be elevated off the table with a small pillow or blanket roll to prevent plantar flexion and pressure on the toes. Body rolls should be placed under each side of the patient to raise the chest and permit the diaphragm to move freely and the lungs to expand. When the patient is in the prone position the restraint strap is placed below the knee. It is important that the patient's head and neck be positioned properly to assure a patent airway. This position is used for surgery on the back, spine, and rectal area. The patient is anesthetized in the supine position and then placed in the prone position. This position should be assumed gradually and usually four persons are required to turn the patient safely. Details of the turning process can be found in specialized texts and articles.[66,78a]

When the surgery is completed the patient will be returned to the supine position. This should be done gradually and slowly to allow the patient's cardiovascular system to adjust to the change in position. Rapid turning of the patient can cause a precipitous drop in the blood pressure.[66]

Trendelenburg

In the Trendelenburg position the patient's head and body are lowered into a head-down position. The knees are flexed by "breaking" the table, and the patient is held in position by padded shoulder braces (Fig. 23-6, *C*). This position is used for operations on the lower abdomen and the pelvis to obtain good exposure by a displacement of the intestines into the upper abdomen. The upward position of the viscera decreases the movement of the diaphragm and interferes with respiratory excursion. For this reason this position is not maintained any longer than necessary. The operating room table should be returned to a normal position very slowly so that the patient's cardiovascular system has time to adjust to the shift in position. When the patient is in the Trendelenburg position, blood pools in his upper torso and the blood pressure rises. As the patient is lowered to a normal position, the venous supply is shunted to the legs and a sudden drop in blood pressure may occur.

Reverse Trendelenburg

As the name implies, in this position the head is elevated and the feet are lowered. This position may be used to obtain better visualization of the biliary tract in surgery. The patient must be properly supported by a footboard, body restraints, and a lift sheet around the arms. Since blood will tend to pool in the lower extremities, caution should be used in slowly returning the patient to a normal position. A sudden influx of the pooled blood from the feet can cause an overloading of the cardiovascular system. Obviously this would be of most concern in elderly patients or in those with preexisting cardiovascular problems.

Lithotomy

In the lithotomy position the patient lies on his back with his buttocks to the break in the operating table. After the patient is anesthetized the thighs and legs are flexed at right angles and then simultaneously placed in stirrups (Fig. 23-7 A). This prevents injury, which can occur to the muscle if each leg is flexed and placed in the stirrup separately. The hands and arms may be placed over the patient's chest and secured by his gown or positioned on armboards at his side. They should not extend beyond the break in the table as they may be injured when the table is manipulated. The lower section of the table is then lowered. This position is used in perineal, rectal, and vaginal surgery.

In this position the patient has blood from his legs shunted into his torso and upper extremities. If the patient must remain in the lithotomy position any period of time, Ace bandages are often wrapped around each leg prior to surgery to lessen pooling and thrombus formation. Because of increased pressure on the sacral area, these patients may also develop pressure areas with redness and maceration of the skin.

When the surgery is completed the patient's legs must be gradually returned to a normal position. As in the Trendelenburg position, rapid lowering of the legs may cause a sudden drop in blood pressure as part of the total blood volume is shunted back into the legs.

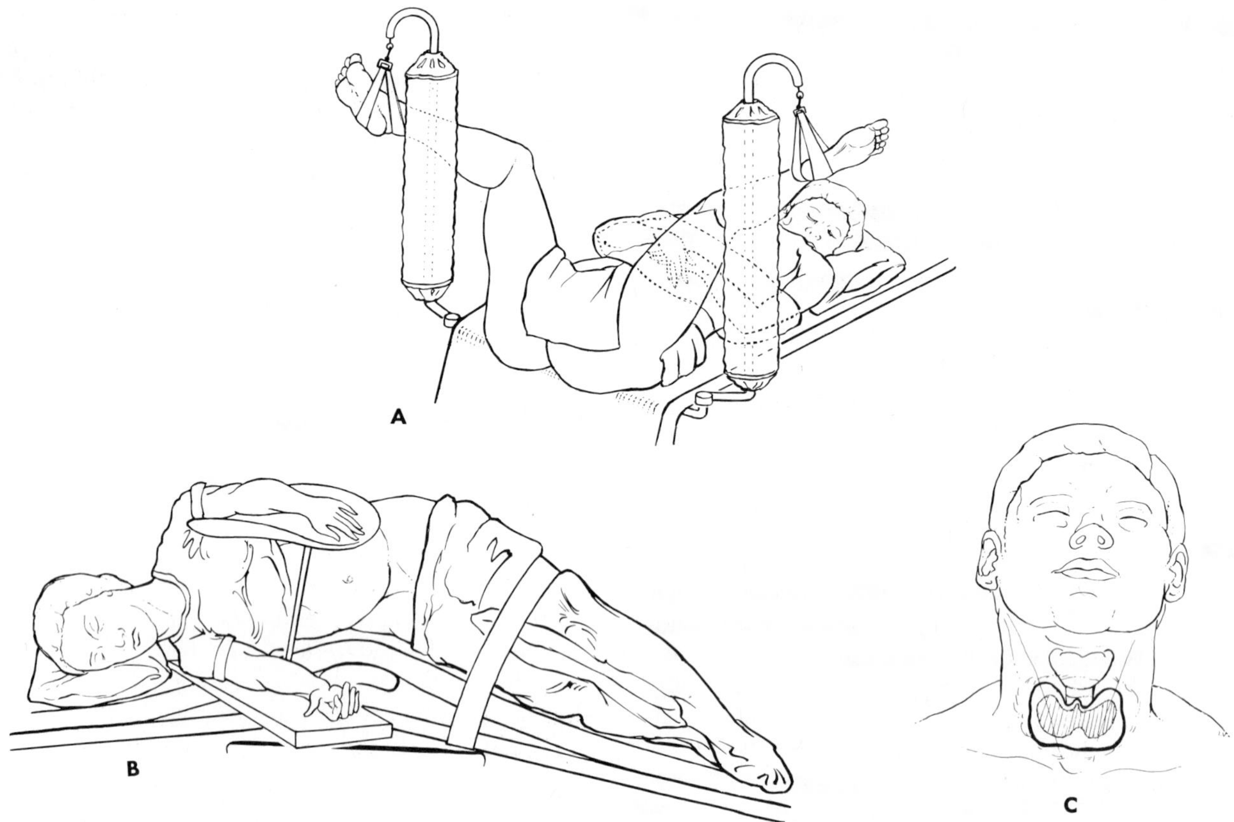

Fig. 23-7. Three operative positions for specialized surgery. **A,** Lithotomy. **B,** Lateral. **C,** Thyroid gland exposure.

Lateral positions

Various versions of the lateral position are used for surgery on the kidney and the chest. The kidney position (Fig. 23-7, *B*) is used for nephrectomy and pyelolithotomy. As can be seen, this position puts pressure on the lower arm and leg and blood pools in these areas. The position of the chest allows the upper lung to move more freely than the lower lung. This can interfere with pulmonary ventilation as the two lungs function differently. (See the current literature for further discussion of these problems.[66])

Other positions

Special positions may be necessary to place the operative site in the best possible position. One example of this would be the thyroid exposure (Fig. 23-7 *C*). In this position the patient lies on his back with his head hyperextended and a small sandbag, pillow, or thyroid rest under his neck and shoulders to provide exposure of the thyroid gland.

Special operating tables and attachments are frequently used for genitourinary, rectal, bone, endoscopy, and brain surgery. The operating room nurse, anesthesiologist, and surgeon must be well informed in the use of such tables and attachments and be aware of the desired position for each surgical procedure.

In the past few years more attention than ever has been paid to the proper positioning of the patient to minimize the physiologic changes that occur in the sedated and anesthetized patient. The nurse who is aware that these changes can occur will be more alert to situations in the operating room that can adversely affect the recovery of the patient.

■ POSTANESTHETIC PHASE

The immediate postanesthetic period is a critical one for the patient. He must be observed diligently and must receive intensive physical and psychologic support until the major effects of the anesthetic have worn off and his overall condition stabilizes. The nurse is largely responsible for the care of the patient at this time and must be prepared to meet his specific needs as they arise.

It is the practice in most hospitals that any patient who has received general, dissociative, or regional anesthesia is taken to a postanesthesia recovery room after surgery where he can be given continuous attention for a period of time. In some instances the patient who has had local anesthesia but who requires close observation in the immediate postoperative period may also be cared for in the recovery room. In such an area, specially prepared nursing personnel and all the equipment that may be necessary for the care of the patient in the postanesthetic phase are readily available. Ideally the recovery room is located on the same floor as the operating rooms or in the immediate vicinity. If there is no recovery room the nurse must prepare the patient's clinical unit with as much equipment as may be needed, considering the individual patient who will be returning to the unit.

□ Assessment

The patient should be accompanied to the recovery room or to his clinical unit by the anesthesiologist and another member of the operating room professional staff. While the anesthesiologist remains at the bedside, the nurse begins assessment of the patient by obtaining his vital signs (blood pressure, pulse rate, respiratory rate). Measuring the vital signs also includes evaluation of the pulse volume and regularity, airway patency, symmetry of chest expansion, depth of respirations, and color of the skin. The patient's level of consciousness and ability to follow commands are also ascertained at this time.

Once it has been determined that the patient's circulatory and ventilatory functions have remained adequate after the transfer from the operating room, the nurse receives a report on the patient's condition from members of the operating room team before assuming responsibility for his care (see box above). Information pertaining to the patient's preoperative status may already have been obtained if a preoperative patient visit was made by recovery room nursing personnel.

Following the report the nurse completes the overall assessment of the patient. The temperature is taken. The surgical site is inspected for dressings and for the presence of drainage or frank bleeding. Tubes and catheters including intravenous infusion lines are evaluated for patency. Drainage tubes are connected to proper collection containers and the character of all drainage is noted. The patient who has received regional anesthesia is evaluated as to his ability to move the extremity(ies) and recognize touch in the areas anesthetized. Finally assessments specific to the surgical procedure performed are carried out, and the physician's order sheet is checked for other instructions and orders for treatments and medications that need to be initiated.

It is essential that there is complete and accurate recording of the immediate postanesthetic course so that those who continue management of the patient have a thorough picture to refer to as necessary. The recording should start with a summary of the patient's status when he is admitted from the operating room, that is, the baseline assessment. Thereafter changes in the patient's status as determined by frequent reassessments need to be noted. All medications, fluids, and treatments the patient receives during this time must be recorded so that there will be no duplication that might prove harmful to the patient.

DATA TO BE OBTAINED WHEN PATIENT IS ADMITTED TO THE RECOVERY ROOM

- Surgical procedure performed
  - What, why
- Agents administered
  - Anesthetic
  - Narcotic
  - Muscle relaxant
  - Muscle relaxant reversal agent
- Complications during surgery
  - Type
  - Treatment instituted
- Fluids
  - Estimated blood loss (EBL)
  - Blood and fluid administered
- Pertinent preoperative problems
  - Physical
  - Psychologic

□ Intervention

Much of the ongoing nursing care provided in the immediate postanesthetic period is dependent on the particular surgical procedure performed and is discussed elsewhere in this text (see specific disease entities and surgical procedures). Some outcomes, however, are the same for all postanesthetic patients: pulmonary ventilation and circulation are maintained, comfort is promoted, and injury is prevented.

Outcome: *Pulmonary ventilation is maintained*

The goal of respiratory care for the postoperative patient is to maintain pulmonary ventilation that is adequate to prevent hypoxemia (a deficiency of oxygen in the blood) and hypercapnia (an excess of carbon dioxide in the blood). In the immediate postanesthetic period two of the most common causes of inadequate pulmonary exchange are airway obstruction and hypoventilation.

Airway obstruction most frequently occurs as a result of the tongue, which is relaxed from anesthesia, falling back against the pharynx or as a result of secretions or other fluids collecting in the pharynx, trachea, or bronchial tree. While caring for the postanesthetic patient it is essential for the nurse to recognize that all noisy breathing (for example, snoring, gurgling, wheezing, crowing) is indicative of some type of airway obstruction. It is equally important, however, for the nurse to realize that obstruction can occur without being accompanied by noise.

The most desirable position to ensure maintenance of a patent airway depends on the size and condition of the patient, the anesthesia used, the surgery performed, and the amount of experienced nursing care that is available. Ideally the patient should be in a position in which he can breathe normally with full use of all portions of his lungs and so that vomitus, blood, and mucus can drain out and will not be aspirated. Until protective reflexes have returned, the best position for the majority of patients is a *side-lying* or *semiprone* position with the head tilted back and the jaw supported forward. It is important to remember that aspiration can occur unless the *whole body* is turned. Turning the patient's head when his chest and shoulders remain in the back-lying position is useless. Although the side-lying position somewhat diminishes chest expansion, it has the advantages of helping to keep the tongue forward and promoting the drainage of secretions and other fluids outside the mouth. The disadvantage related to chest expansion can be minimized by turning the patient frequently and by raising the flexed upper arm and placing it on a pillow. The supine position with head hyperextended permits fullest expansion of the lungs, but as noted it is dangerous because of its potential for aspiration or obstruction from secretions. Unless absolutely necessary this position should not be used before the patient's pharyngeal reflexes have returned and he is able to manage his own secretions. When the supine position must be used, all supplies for suctioning as well as personnel to perform the procedure must be available at the bedside at all times.

An oropharyngeal or nasopharyngeal airway is often left in place following the administration of a general anesthetic to keep the passage open and the tongue forward until pharyngeal reflexes have returned. These artificial airways are made of rubber, plastic, or metal. They should be removed as soon as the patient begins to awaken and has regained his cough and swallowing reflexes. After this time their presence can be irritating and can stimulate vomiting or laryngospasm. If an artificial airway is ineffective or if one is not in place, the majority of obstructions due to the tongue falling back can be alleviated by holding the patient's jaw up and forward or by positioning him on his side as described previously. When absolutely necessary to clear the airway, the nurse can open the patient's mouth by pushing at the angle of the jaw with the thumbs and have someone insert a padded tongue depressor between the back teeth. The tongue can then be brought forward by grasping it with a piece of gauze. An endotracheal tube may need to be inserted by the physician if there is considerable difficulty maintaining a patent airway.

Excessive secretions from the nasopharynx or tracheobronchial mucosa can also lead to partial or complete airway obstruction. Unless the patient can manage these secretions by coughing them up and expectorating them, they must be removed by suctioning. Pharyngeal suctioning is often all that must be done (Fig. 23-8). If intratracheal suctioning is necessary sterile technique should be used and the patient should be hyperventilated with 100% oxygen before and after each introduction of the catheter into the trachea. Rarely, but occasionally, a bronchoscopy may be needed to remove secretions, especially if they are very inspissated. When thick secretions are a problem or potential problem, the humidity of the air breathed should be increased to keep secretions as thin as possible and to prevent dry air from further irritating the already irritated respiratory passages.

Postoperative hypoventilation results from numerous causes. Respirations can be directly depressed by drugs, which may have been administered preoperatively, intraoperatively, or postoperatively. These drugs include inhalation and intravenous anesthetic agents, narcotics, tranquilizers, and sedatives. The residual effects of muscle relaxants and of high spinal or epidural anesthesia in which paralysis of the lower rib cage muscles results can limit the patient's power to breathe. Incisional pain, obesity, chronic lung disease, gastric dilation, and constrictive surgical dressings also can interfere with lung expansion and thus with respiratory exchange.

Oxygen is usually given postoperatively because after anesthesia almost all patients have decreased pulmonary expansion and areas of atelectasis, both of which result in hypoxemia. Oxygen is administered by nasal cannula or catheter, disposable face mask or shield, or endotracheal or tracheostomy tube if one is in place. How long postoperative oxygen therapy should be continued depends on the individual patient. As a general rule all patients should receive oxygen at least until they are conscious and able to take deep breaths on command. Prolonged oxygen therapy should be guided by arterial blood gas determinations. Patients with thoracic or upper abdominal incisions or with preexisting pulmonary disease may be given oxygen for several hours, perhaps until the next day. Special care must be taken when administering oxygen to patients with chronic obstructive pulmonary disease so that hypoxemia, which is their stimulus to

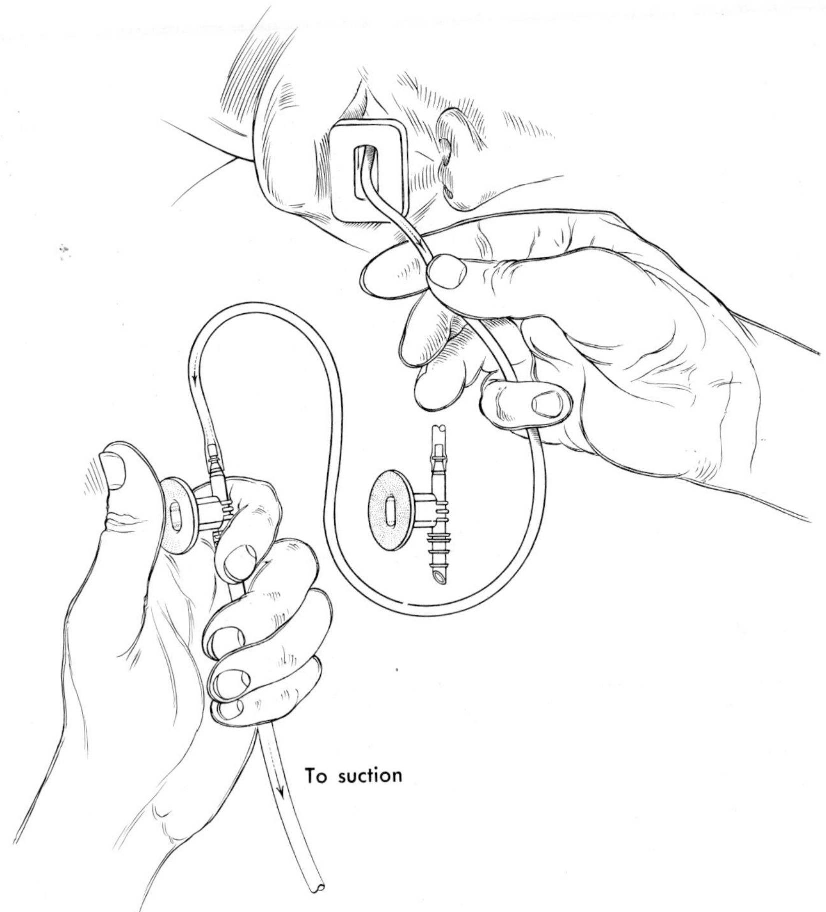

Fig. 23-8. Inserting catheter into airway of unconscious patient. Vacuum regulation hole is left open until catheter is inserted and in place. Hole is then occluded with thumb, and secretions are aspirated.

breathe, is not entirely removed (p. 1135). Any patient experiencing shivering, which increases oxygen consumption, should receive oxygen therapy until the shivering has ceased.

To help maintain normal levels of arterial blood gases and to counteract hypoventilation, all patients need to be encouraged to breathe deeply at frequent intervals. Ideally the patient will take three or four deep inhalations every 10 to 15 minutes. If the patient is unconscious or if he will not breathe deeply when stimulated, the nurse can hyperventilate his lungs passively using a breathing bag and mask.

When hypoventilation exists to the extent that hypercapnia is present, the patient must have respiratory assistance. Drug therapies that might be indicated include narcotic antagonists such as nalorphine or naloxone to counteract the respiratory depressant effects of the opiate, reversal agents such as neostigmine or edrophonium to counteract the effects of nondepolarizing muscle relaxants, and narcotics themselves if pain is causing the patient to splint his respirations. With obese patients elevation of the head of the bed is often helpful in relieving pressure on the diaphragm. Nasogastric tubes may be inserted to relieve gastric distention. Constrictive dressings must be loosened. When these measures are ineffective in improving ventilation and in instances of excessive respiratory depression from depolarizing muscle relaxant drugs or from high spinal anesthesia, the patient may need to be intubated and receive mechanical ventilator assistance.

Outcome: *Circulation is maintained*

Hypotension and *cardiac arrhythmias* are the most commonly encountered cardiovascular complications of the immediate postanesthetic period. Early recognition and management of these complications before they become serious enough to diminish cardiac output is dependent on frequent assessment of the patient's vital signs. The blood pressure, pulse, and respirations are usually taken every 15 minutes until stable, then every half hour for 2 hours, and then every 4 hours until ordered otherwise. In many hospitals the monitoring of vital signs every 15 minutes extends for as long as the patient is in the recovery room and for at least 1 hour after he leaves the recovery room. The rate, volume, and rhythm of the pulse are carefully observed and the character and rate of respiration noted.

Hypotension

Moving the patient from the operating room table to his bed, jarring during transport, reactions to drugs and anesthesia, loss of blood and other body fluids, cardiac arrhythmias, cardiac failure, inadequate ventilation, pain, and residual sympathectomy from conductive anesthesia are among the many factors that will cause circulatory changes that may result in lowering the blood pressure. A mild decrease in the patient's blood pressure from his normal preoperative range is not uncommon during the early postoperative period. It is usually well tolerated in healthy patients and does not require treatment.

Shock, however, must be prevented because the brain, heart, kidneys, and other vital organs do not tolerate long periods of hypoxemia. A weak, thready pulse with a significant drop in blood pressure may indicate hemorrhage or circulatory failure. The surgeon, anesthesiologist, or both should be notified at once if any of these signs occur, especially if the patient's skin becomes cold, moist, pale, or cyanotic or he suddenly becomes restless or apprehensive. Oxygen therapy should be started to increase the oxygen saturation of the circulating blood. Unless contraindicated, the patient's legs are elevated to facilitate venous return. Blood, plasma, or other intravenous fluids usually are ordered to increase the blood volume when the hypotension is due to hypovolemia. Vasopressor agents may be used when vasodilation is apparent. Digitalis preparations or other inotropic agents may be administered if the decrease in blood pressure is due to cardiac failure.

Cardiac arrhythmias

When a cardiac arrhythmia is detected it is important for the nurse to ascertain if the patient has a history of such a disturbance. Arrhythmias unchanged from those that existed preoperatively usually do not require treatment. When there is no history of a cardiac irregularity but one has developed postoperatively, the nurse immediately assesses the patient to determine if he is ventilating adequately. Oxygen should be started while the physician is being notified. A patient who is exchanging gases poorly should receive ventilatory assistance with a bag and mask.

Hypoxemia and hypercapnia are common causes of postoperative cardiac arrhythmias, especially premature beats and sinus tachycardia. These arrhythmias often can be suppressed by adequate ventilation. Frequent premature beats of ventricular origin, which are not decreased by oxygen therapy, are usually treated with drugs such as intravenous lidocaine (Xylocaine) or procainamide (Pronestyl). The sinus bradycardia that may follow the administration of neostigmine (Prostigmine) or edrophonium (Tensilon) is counteracted by the administration of atropine. Other common causes of postoperative cardiac arrhythmias include pain, hypovolemia, gastric distention, and acidosis. In the event that a life-threatening arrhythmia such as ventricular fibrillation or cardiac asystole occurs, resuscitation efforts must be started immediately.

Outcome: *Injury is prevented*

Following anesthesia side rails on the stretcher or bed are generally raised and are left so until the patient is fully awake. Although the patient is constantly watched, it is possible for him to turn suddenly and throw himself from the bed. Physical restraints are seldom used. If the patient is restless the nurse should remain with him and guide his movements so he does not hurt himself. Restraints can be frightening to the semiconscious individual and may stimulate him to struggle violently to get away from them.

The patient is turned frequently and placed in good body alignment to prevent nerve damage from pressure and muscle and joint strain due to lying in one position for a long time. The nurse must be constantly aware that unconscious patients and those recovering from spinal or epidural anesthesia have loss of sensation and are unable to indicate discomfort. Heating pads, heat lamps, or cast driers must be used with great care while the patient is unconscious or semiconscious so that burns do not occur. When infusions are being given the patient's arm should be secured on an armboard if the needle is in an area where it could be easily dislodged.

Outcome: *Comfort is promoted*

The immediate postanesthetic period is often a frightening time for the patient. Psychologic support is imperative for his physical as well as his emotional well-being. While awakening from anesthesia the patient needs frequent orientation as to where he is and reassurance that he is not alone. He also needs to know that his operation is over and that he is recovering from anesthesia satisfactorily. Procedures carried out should be carefully explained to him even when it appears that he is not alert. Patients who receive this type of support frequently recover from anesthesia faster, with fewer complications, and with less incisional pain. The patient who has had regional anesthesia needs the same information and needs to be reassured that the sensation and movement in his extremities will return.

Incisional pain is a common complaint after surgery, and from the patient's point of view it is probably the most significant postoperative complication. In the immediate postanesthetic period narcotic analgesics should be given for pain when warranted but should be done so with the realization that pronounced depression of the respiratory, circulatory, or central nervous systems may follow. Because the patient generally has not completely recovered from the effects of anesthetic agents, the first postoperative dose of a narcotic is usually reduced to about *one half* the dose he will be receiving after he has fully recovered from anesthesia. Pain medication for restlessness should be given only after it has been determined that the restlessness is not a result of hypoxia.

□ Discharge from recovery room

Multiple criteria are used to determine when a patient has sufficiently recovered from anesthesia to be transferred from the recovery room (see below). Complications that must be under control include excessive wound drainage, vomiting, fever, pain, or inadequate urinary output as well as complications specific to the type of surgery performed. Acutely ill patients who cannot adequately fulfill these criteria are usually transferred to an intensive care unit.

Before discharging a patient the recovery room nurse needs to determine that there is adequate nursing staff available on the clinical unit to receive and care for him. All pertinent information concerning the patient's status must be communicated to the nurse who will be continuing to provide his postoperative nursing care.

Outcome criteria for patient discharged from recovery room

1. Vital signs are stable and indicate adequate respiratory and circulatory function.
2. Patient is awake or easily aroused and can call for assistance if needed.
3. Postsurgical complications have been thoroughly evaluated and are under control.
4. The patient who has had regional anesthesia has motor as well as partial sensory return to all anesthetized areas.

POSTOPERATIVE PHASE

□ Preparation for return of patient to clinical unit

Equipment

Before the patient returns to the clinical unit from the postanesthesia recovery room, the patient's room is prepared to facilitate meeting the patient's needs in the immediate postoperative period. The bed is made so that the patient can be moved easily from stretcher to bed. The bed should have added protection in areas where drainage may be expected to occur and sufficient covers to ensure patient warmth.

The patient's room is cleared of any unnecessary equipment and a clear passageway provided for approach to the bed by the stretcher. Equipment that will be needed is placed in readiness. This equipment will depend on the type of surgery and might include such items as an intravenous pole, emesis basin, tissues, sphygmomanometer, and stethoscope. The recovery room nurse should alert the unit staff of any specialized equipment such as for suction or oxygen that may be needed.

Family

The nurse on the clinical unit should show the greatest consideration to the patient's family during the time that he is in the operating and recovery rooms. The family is kept informed of the patient's progress, particularly when the patient's return to the unit has been delayed. Information that can be shared with the patient's family helps to lessen their anxiety.

Most surgeons discuss the results of the operation with the family immediately after the surgery and also visit the patient, telling him briefly what was found and reassuring him about his condition. The family is frequently highly anxious concerning the patient's condition and may not perceive or understand all that the surgeon tells them. The patient frequently experiences periods of amnesia during the hours when he first regains consciousness and may not remember what he has been told. The nurse needs to know what information was given to the patient and family so as to be able to answer their questions. The family also needs to know what to expect when the patient returns to his bed on the unit.

□ Return of patient to clinical unit

Initial patient assessment and interventions

The recovery room nurse generally calls the unit when the patient is ready to be transferred and reports on the patient's condition. When the patient arrives the unit nurse accompanies him to his room to facilitate a smooth transfer, to make an initial assessment of the patient's status (see box, p. 394), and to carry out immediate nursing interventions.

Subjective data. The patient is asked for symptoms of discomfort after he has been transferred to the bed and positioned in supportive body alignment. This gives the nurse a quick indication of his level of alertness as well as symptoms of discomfort. An indirect question

PATIENT ASSESSMENT ON RETURN FROM RECOVERY ROOM

Respiratory status
- Patency of airway
- Respirations: depth, rate, character
- Breath sounds: presence, character

Circulatory status
- Pulse, blood pressure, temperature
- Skin color, temperature
- Capillary filling

Neurologic status
- Level of consciousness

Dressing
- Presence of drainage
- Presence of tubes to be connected to drainage systems

Comfort
- Presence of pain, nausea, vomiting
- Patient position: position of comfort, position to facilitate ventilation

Safety
- Necessity for side rails
- Call light in reach

Equipment
- Monitors connected and functioning
- Intravenous fluids: rate, amount in bag, patency of tubing
- Drainage systems (e.g., nasogastric, chest, urinary): type, patency of tubing, connection of appropriate container, character and amount of drainage

such as, "How do you feel?" will elicit data concerning nausea or pain without focusing on a specific area where there may be no discomfort. There is frequently an increase in pain perception at this time because of the movement from stretcher to bed. It is important to seek specific data concerning location, onset, and change in pain intensity and not to assume that the pain is incisional in nature.

Nausea occurs less frequently postoperatively with the use of newer anesthetics. There is greater possibility of nausea when the stomach has been manipulated extensively during the surgical procedure or if considerable amounts of narcotics have been administered. The emesis basin should be easily available but not in sight if vomiting is a possibility.

Objective data

Respiratory status. The patient's respiratory status is assessed immediately on his return to the unit. A patent airway is of primary importance during the early postoperative period until the patient is fully alert. Respirations are assessed for rate, depth, and sounds. Slow respirations may occur as a result of drugs given intraoperatively or postoperatively. Shallow rapid respirations may be due to pain, constrictive chest or abdominal dressings, obesity, or gastric dilation. If a nasal catheter is in place, oxygen should be started.

If respirations are very noisy they may be heard without the aid of a stethoscope. Noisy respirations may be due to airway obstruction from the tongue falling back against the pharynx (Fig. 23-9) or from secretions. The patient with noisy respirations should be assisted to cough and then positioned on his side if possible. Suctioning may be indicated if coughing does not clear the airway.

If the respirations are not noisy the lungs are auscultated to establish a baseline for future comparison and to identify adventitious sounds (see Chapter 44 for assessment of breath sounds). Absent breath sounds indicate hypoventilation of that lobe (Table 23-6). Coarse rales indicate secretions in air passages. Presence of adventitious sounds indicates the need for energetic ventilatory exercises. Deep-breathing and coughing measures are instituted immediately for all patients who have had general anesthesia.

Circulatory status

PULSE. The pulse is assessed for rate and quality. An increased rate usually occurs during the transfer to the bed, but the rate should return to the patient's usual range. A rapid, weak, thready pulse may indicate increased bleeding. If this is a change from the recovery room status, other signs of shock and evidence of bleeding are assessed and reported to the physician. Tachycardia may also indicate anxiety, hypoxemia, dehydration, overhydration, or acidosis. Bradycardia is usually caused by medications.

The presence and strength of peripheral pulses distal to plaster casts or the operative site on an extremity are used to measure adequacy of circulation. If the dressing is too tight it should be loosened, if this is permissible, or reported at once to the physician.

TEMPERATURE. A slight rise in body temperature to about 38 C (100 F) is commonly observed during the first 24 hours after surgery as a result of the stress reaction to the trauma of surgery. A subnormal temperature may be related to the cool air-conditioning found in most operating room and recovery room suites. A light blanket will usually provide sufficient warmth.

BLOOD PRESSURE. Although the blood pressure has usually reached a stable level before the patient is discharged from the recovery room, changes may occur due to the transfer to the clinical unit. An increase in systolic pressure may be related to anxiety concerning the transfer or to pain. Hypotensive changes may be due to shock, although other signs of shock usually appear before changes in blood pressure occur. The patient's blood pressure is taken immediately on return to his

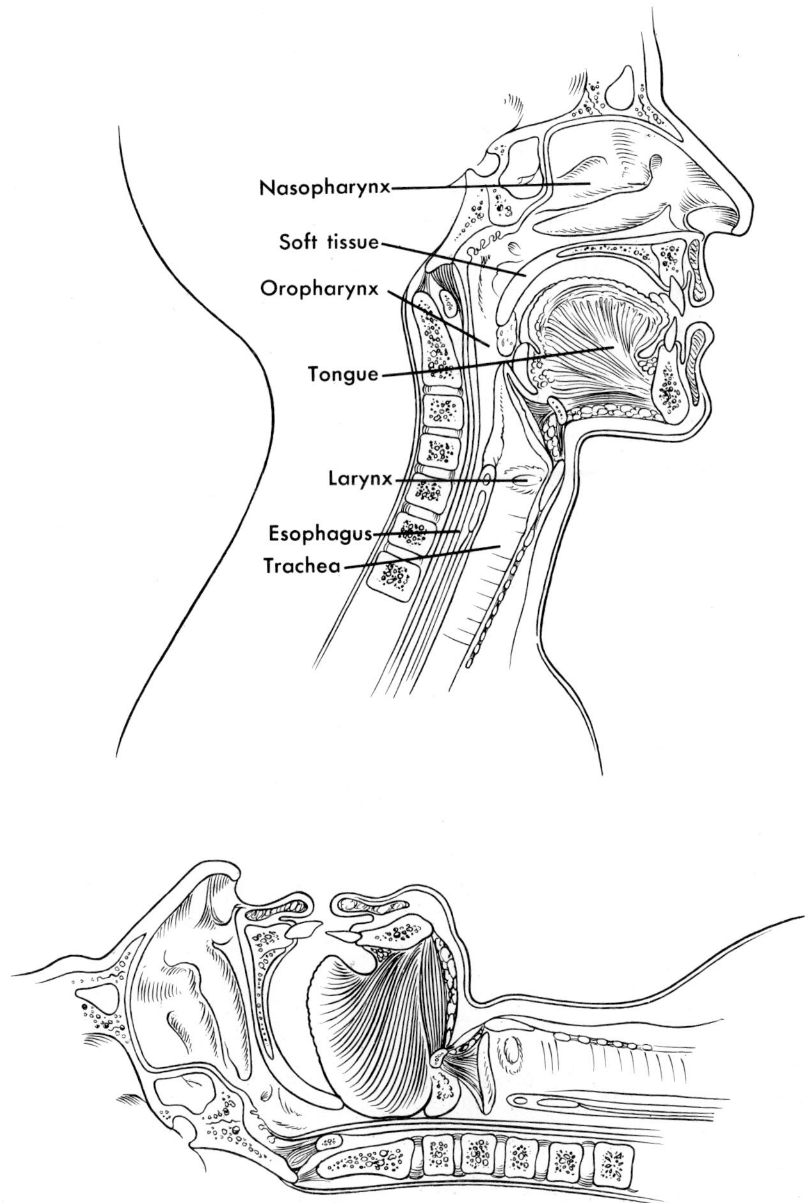

Fig. 23-9. Obstruction of airway by tongue in unconscious patient. Note how back of tongue can obstruct oropharynx in unconscious patient in supine position.

Table 23-6. Some causes of vital sign changes in early postoperative phase

Vital sign	Increase	Decrease
Temperature	Stress reaction (low-grade fever)	Cold operating room and recovery room
Pulse rate	Jarring during transfer Shock, hemorrhage Hypoventilation Acute gastric dilation Pain Anxiety Cardiac arrythmias	Digitalis overdose Cardiac arrythmias
Respiratory rate	Hypoventilation: poor positioning, tight chest or upper abdominal dressing, obesity, gastric dilation Anxiety	Drugs: anesthetics, narcotics, sedatives
Blood pressure	Anxiety (↑ systolic) Pain	Jarring during transfer Severe pain Cardiac arrhythmias Shock: fluid loss, hemorrhage, acute gastric dilation

room and comparisons are made with readings made in the recovery room.

SKIN COLOR AND TEMPERATURE. Pallor indicates decreased circulation to the skin. This is difficult to observe in dark-skinned individuals and is usually indicated by a dullness or decrease in the red tones. Vasoconstriction may result from the coolness of the recovery room suite, from a decrease in the amount of circulating blood due to blood loss, or from the neuroendocrine response to stress. Blueness of the lips, mucous membranes, or nail beds may be caused by cold or inadequate oxygenation of the blood. The nailbeds are checked for capillary return. If circulation is adequate, pinkness should return to the nail after it is "flicked" by the nurse's finger.

Skin usually feels cool to the touch after surgery due to the exposure to a cool environment. Coolness may also be due to vasoconstriction from blood loss or stress reaction. Warm moist skin may be secondary to vasodilation from excessive warmth applied after surgery or to overhydration from excess fluid replacement. The intravenous solution may be running at an excessively rapid rate, and this should be checked if overhydration is a possibility.

Level of consciousness. This can be ascertained by asking the patient to respond to simple questions or commands. Variations in consciousness level from alertness to drowsiness will be observed. If the patient is not easily aroused, these data are compared with his consciousness status at the time of discharge from the recovery room. A decrease in consciousness level may indicate shock (from jarring motions during the transfer) and should be reported to the surgeon at once along with any other pertinent data.

Dressing. The entire dressing is inspected with the covers pulled back or the patient turned as necessary. A dressing applied to the side such as for kidney surgery may appear dry on the top visible area if the patient is supine but may have excess drainage on the lower portion due to gravity. An excess amount of drainage is reported immediately. Certain types of surgery of the urinary tract normally produce large amounts of drainage; if this is a probability, Montgomery straps will have been applied after surgery so that the dressing can be changed frequently. If small amounts of unexpected drainage occur, especially bright red drainage, the area can be outlined with a pen so that the rate of increase can be easily determined. Any drainage tubes from the dressing that require connection to a drainage system are attached immediately.

For psychologic reasons and to prevent trauma the wound is covered in the operating room with a dry sterile dressing. Medicated sprays forming a transparent film on the skin may be used as a dressing over clean incisions. The film lasts 3 to 4 days; it may be removed with acetone or will flake and peel off eventually. This type of dressing is particularly useful in covering wounds in children. Occasionally surgeons leave an operative wound uncovered, believing that healing progresses best when the wound is exposed to the air.

Some surgeons and pediatricians believe that seda-

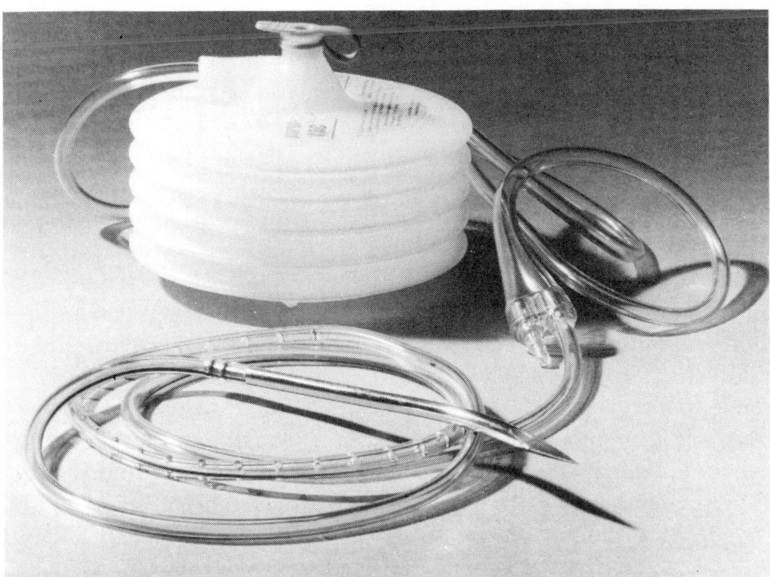

Fig. 23-10. Porto-Vac portable wound suction unit consists of bellows with top port, drain plug, and side port; x-ray opaque wound tube with needle attached; and connector tube. Needle with wound tube attached is placed in wound and brought out through healthy tissue near wound. After wound tube is cut from needle it is assembled to connector tube. To establish vacuum, connector tube is attached to side port of bellows, drain plug on top of bellows is opened, bellows are depressed against solid surface, and drain plug is reinserted. Drainage is removed by opening drain plug, inverting bellows, and pouring fluid out. (Courtesy Howmedica, Inc., Medical Division, Rutherford, N.J.)

tives and analgesic drugs in small, carefully measured doses should be given to children postoperatively to prevent pain and restlessness. The nurse should assess the need for restraints with a small child who may be tampering with the wound or dressing. The age of the child, his ability to reason, presence and anxiety level of family members, type of surgery, actions of medications given, and safety of the child are factors utilized by the nurse in assessing the need for any type of restraint.

Body position. The patient is placed in a position of comfort and one that facilitates good ventilation. Except after spinal anesthesia or in certain types of eye surgery or neurosurgery when the bed must remain flat, most patients prefer the head of the bed slightly elevated. The patient who is not very alert needs to be placed in a position of good alignment. There should not be any strain placed on the area surrounding the incision. Pillows should *not* exert pressure on the popliteal area (behind the knee) as this leads to venous obstruction. A sidelying position is used for the unconscious patient to prevent airway obstruction.

Assessment of environmental factors

Equipment. All equipment at the bedside is checked for functioning. Monitors are connected to the patient and visual patterns should be in working order. Fluids may be ordered to be given to the patient intravenously or instilled in body cavities for irrigation such as in the bladder. The contents of the fluid containers, the patency of the tubing, and the rate of fluid administration are checked. Intravenous fluids are usually given at rates ranging from minimal (to keep the line open, K/O) to 3 ml/min. If the rate is greater than 3 ml/min, and if the physician's order sheet is not available in the patient's room, the rate should be slowed, the order checked immediately, and the rate adjusted appropriately. Rate of administration varies with the amount of fluid lost, size and age of the patient, and the underlying illness (see Chapter 20). The patient and family should be instructed early concerning permissibility of fluids taken orally.

Drainage from tubes can be accomplished by either gravity or suction. Urinary bags are filled by direct gravity (see p. 1257 for care of the patient with urinary drainage). Intermittent or continuous suction may be used for nasogastric drainage. Constant suction under low negative pressure can be accomplished by a Porto-Vac (Fig. 23-10) or by electric suction. These pumps are used for drainage of incisional areas when large amounts of drainage are anticipated (urologic surgery) or when smaller amounts may delay healing (mastectomy, arthroplasty, radical neck dissection, amputation). Chest tubes drain by means of a water-seal drainage system by gravity or with added suction. The nurse should be familiar with this type of drainage system before making any connections. All tubing is connected to the drainage receptacle and checked for patency. The amount of fluid in each receptacle is marked on the receptacle and recorded as a baseline for future comparison.

Safety. Side rails of the bed should be kept raised until the patient is fully awake and responding, or if he is heavily medicated, to prevent falls. There should be easy access to the bed and patient. The patient is instructed early regarding permissibility of ambulation and the need to call for assistance for initial attempts. The call cord should be easily accessible to the patient.

Family members. If the family members are present in the room when the patient returns they may be asked to step outside until the patient has been transferred and assessed. Before leaving the patient the nurse invites the family to return, explains equipment, and describes the patient's state of awareness and comfort. Family members who understand what is occurring can offer support to the patient. Explanations should be simple but concrete and accurate.

Data from patient's chart

Once the initial patient assessments and interventions are completed, the nurse collects the following data from the patient's chart.

Surgeon's orders

1. *Activity.* Range can be from strict bed rest to up as desired. The order should state clearly the extent of activity allowed.
2. *Fluids, food.* Orders for fluids or food to be given intravenously should include type, amount, and rate. Orders for fluid or food to be taken orally should include type and time these can be started.
3. *Medications.* An order for a pain medication to be given as needed should be included if pain is a possibility. Other medications that need to be reinstituted or started immediately are noted.
4. *Other orders.* These depend on the type of surgery and anesthesia. The nurse should understand the rationale for each order.

Surgical notes

1. *Postoperative diagnosis.* The patient or his family may need interpretation of what the surgeon has told them.
2. *Type of surgery.* For interpretation to patient or family; for direction of specific nursing care.
3. *Anesthetic.*
   a. Inhalants: need for active deep-breathing measures.
   b. Muscle relaxants: assessment for respiratory distress.
   c. Spinal: supine position postoperatively; headaches may occur.
4. *Estimated blood loss and fluid replacement.* Potential for fluid and electrolyte imbalance or delayed transfusion reactions.
5. *Drains.* Drainage on the dressing can be expected if a soft Penrose drain is in place. Soiled dressings that are removed during a dressing change should not exert a pull on the drain.

Recovery room summary

1. *Vital signs before discharge.* For comparison with present data.
2. *Patient progress.* Identification of problems that may persist.
3. *Medications given.* Identify time span before next dosage permissible for prn drugs and response by the patient and if other medications have been started.
4. *Urinary output.* Identify whether patient has voided and how much. Urine suppression may occur with shock; urine retention may occur from the effects of anesthesia or surgery and may create pressure on abdominal organs or the incision.

Planning patient care

The collected data are recorded in the nursing admission note and utilized to identify the specific needs of the patient in the postoperative period. The preoperative condition of the patient, type of surgery performed, and strengths and resources of the patient are determining factors influencing the occurrence of postoperative discomforts or complications. In planning the patient's care, therefore, the nurse needs to utilize previously collected data, present data, knowledge of factors related to specific types of surgery (as illustrated in succeeding chapters of this text), and specific postoperative needs and possible postoperative complications. Identified problems and specific plans for care are written in the appropriate place on the chart or nursing care plan.

□ Needs of postoperative patient

All of the individual's basic needs can be affected by the trauma of surgery. Nursing care is directed toward achievement of specific outcomes so that each need is met and the patient has been helped to move toward his optimal level of functioning.

Safety needs

Outcome: *Patient does not fall*

Contributing factors. Next to errors in medication, falls by patients constitute the major reason for incident reports in hospitals. Patients with an increased potential for falls are those who have had extensive surgery or who have had surgery of the extremities. Elderly persons may become confused, especially on the first postoperative night, and may try to get out of bed. Each postoperative patient is assessed to determine his potential for falling.

Assessment. Areas of assessment include level of consciousness, medications given, circulatory adaptability, and physical environment.

Level of consciousness. The more alert the patient, the less the possibility of a fall (p. 418). Decreased alertness may be due to cerebral hypoxia from blood loss, fluid overload, acid-base imbalances, respiratory insufficiency, shock, hypoglycemia, or chronic brain syndrome.

Medications. Many analgesics, sedatives, or tranquilizers produce a feeling of well-being, and the patient may believe that he is stronger than he actually is and attempt to get out of bed by himself when he is still weak. Narcotics may also produce dizziness, and the patient may fall while walking or sitting up in a chair.

Circulatory adaptability. The circulatory system is under considerable stress during surgery, and wide fluctuations in vital signs during surgery are common. Orthostatic hypotension (a temporary drop in blood pressure when assuming an upright position) can occur when the patient has been lying flat and inactive for a time. The patient complains of dizziness; pallor and tachycardia can be observed. He may fall if he attempts to ambulate.

Muscle strength. If the patient has been in bed for a time, some muscle strength and tone may be lost. The quadriceps muscles of the legs should be tested for general strength before the patient gets out of bed for the first time. The patient lies flat and flexes his knee. The nurse supports the flexed leg off the bed and places one hand against the sole of the foot. The patient is then requested to extend his leg by pushing against the nurse's hand. Weak quadriceps muscles indicate decreased ability to stand and walk.

Physical environment. The room must be examined for possible physical causes for falls such as equipment or footstools in the path of ambulation to the patient's chair, door, or bathroom or water spilled on the floor.

Intervention

Patient weakness. If the patient is not alert or is very weak, side rails are raised at all times. Patients who attempt to climb over the side rails may need constant attention by a family member. The call cord can be pinned to the gown of a confused patient so that excessive movements can be checked readily. Restraints should be used judiciously and only when really necessary. A Hi-Lo bed may be left in low position to decrease the distance to the floor. An ambulatory patient who has difficulty moving because of an incision can get out of bed more easily and safely if the bed is at chair level. Patients who are receiving parenteral narcotics for pain should not ambulate alone.

Patients sitting up to "dangle" or to get up for the first time after surgery should assume a sitting position gradually, with assistance as necessary, and not be permitted to stand until the pulse has essentially stabilized to the baseline level and the patient no longer feels faint. The pulse is taken *before* the patient sits up as well as after he is sitting on the side of the bed.

Leg exercises should be carried out by the bedfast patient to prevent loss of muscle tone and to strengthen weakened muscles (Fig 23-3). Patients with weak leg muscles will need greater support during standing and walking in order to prevent a fall.

Physical environment. The equipment and furniture in the room is arranged to promote large open spaces for safe ambulation. Electrical cords should be against the walls or under the bed if possible. Footstools are used only if needed and kept under the bed when not in use. Portable poles for holding intravenous fluids should have large easily movable wheels. During early ambulation or if the patient is weak, he should not hold onto the pole when ambulating. The floor should be free of debris and water.

Outcome: *Incision heals normally; no purulent discharge*

Pathophysiology of wound healing

Result of wound healing. Wounds may heal by *regeneration* of the tissue or by *scar formation.* The type of cells that constitute the tissue determine the end result. There are three types of cells: labile cells, stable cells, and permanent cells. *Labile* cells multiply throughout life, constantly replacing similar cells being destroyed. Regrowth is through regeneration of marginal cells. Examples of labile cells are those of the skin and mucous membranes and the blood cells. *Stable* cells, occurring in bone or functional cells of glandular organs, do not usually multiply vigorously but will do so if injured. Both labile and stable cells necessitate an underlying structure; they will not grow across an empty space. Thus if the framework is intact there will be regeneration of normal structure. If the framework is destroyed, scarring will occur.

Permanent cells are the main constituents of muscle and nerve tissues. These cells rarely undergo mitotic division and are unable to regenerate. Muscle cells in striated, smooth, and cardiac muscles therefore do not regenerate. Satisfactory performance may result by hypertrophy of the preserved marginal cells. Nerve cells of the central nervous system do not regenerate. In the peripheral nervous system there is no regeneration if the cell body is destroyed. If the axon is injured there is degeneration of the injured part to the closest node of Ranvier; then regeneration will occur. Destruction of permanent cells results in scarring. A typical surgical incision cuts into muscle tissue. Although the epithelial cells regenerate over the scar tissue, the epithelial layer is so thin that the scar tissue is visible.

Types of wound healing. Tissues may heal by one of three ways: primary, secondary, or tertiary intention. Most surgical wounds heal by *primary* intention; the incision is a clean straight line and all layers of the wound (muscle, subcutaneous tissue, and epithelial tissue) are well approximated by suturing. These wounds, if they remain free of infection and do not separate, heal quickly with a minimum of scarring. Wounds such as ulcers have edges that cannot be approximated; healing occurs by a filling in of the wound by granulation tissue over a larger area. This is healing by *secondary intention.* Because these wounds are more open they have a greater possibility for infection. More granulation tissue is formed than in healing by primary intention; therefore more scarring occurs. Healing by *tertiary intention* occurs when there is a delay between injury and suturing; greater granulation tissue will be formed than with primary intention but less than with secondary intention.

Process of wound healing. Regardless of the type of wound healing, the process is the same. The difference is in the length of time for each phase of healing and the extent of granulation tissue formed.

When there is injury to tissue, two major responses occur: the stress response (see Chapter 13) and the inflammatory response (see Chapter 14). The inflammatory response serves to prepare the tissue so that wound healing can take place (Fig. 23-11). During the cellular exudation, leukocytes (white blood cells) invade the injured area to ingest bacteria and debris (phagocytosis). Fibroblasts also migrate from the blood vessels and deposit fibrin, a threadlike substance that stretches through the clot that has sealed the wound. Adjacent blood vessels begin to develop buds that stretch across the wound using the fibrin for support. When the capillary buds reach across the wound they cannulize, establishing blood flow across the wound. A thin layer of epithelial cells migrate across the wound and help to seal the wound. This is *phase I;* the wound strength is low, although sutured wounds will hold together if sutured correctly. With major surgery the patient looks and feels ill during phase I.

Phase II lasts approximately from day 3 to day 14 in surgical wounds. The leukocytes start disappearing and the fibroblasts start filling in spaces in the network with *collagen,* a white protein fiber. All layers of epithelial cells are completely regenerated in about 1 week. The

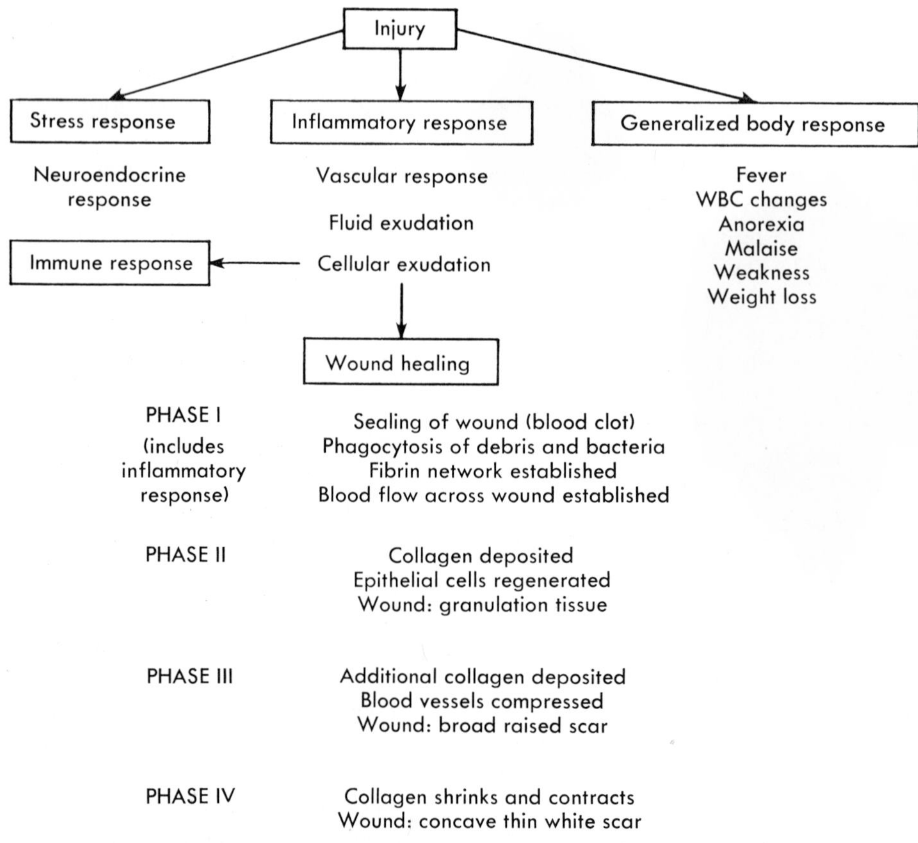

Fig. 23-11. Response of body to injury.

new tissue is a highly vascular connective tissue, reddish in color from the numerous blood vessels, and is called *granulation* tissue. If scraped this tissue will bleed readily. The patient begins to look and feel better.

The collagen that is deposited will provide good support for the wound in 6 to 7 days so that stitches can be removed, and there will be normal tissue strength by 2 weeks. Although wound union is weak until after the sixth postoperative day, the sutures permit the patient to deep breathe, cough, and move around or ambulate without danger of wound separation. It is important for the patient to know this, otherwise he may be reluctant to carry out these activities. Skin sutures (black silk thread, fine wire, or metal skin clips) are removed from abdominal wounds on about the seventh postoperative day, from neck and face wounds on about the third to the fifth postoperative day, and from wounds of the extremities on the eighth to tenth postoperative day. Retention sutures made of heavy wire and placed deep into muscle tissue usually are not removed until the fourteenth to the twenty-first postoperative day. Most patients become apprehensive when they know the sutures are to be removed. It is helpful to tell them that they will have little if any pain during the procedure; the deeper retention sutures do cause discomfort. Unless there is some seepage of fluid after the sutures are removed, a dressing is not necessary and the area may be washed.

During phase III collagen continues to be deposited. This compresses the new blood vessels and blood flow decreases. The wound at this time looks like a broad pinkish raised scar. During this phase, which lasts from about the second to the sixth week after surgery, the patient should avoid heavy use of the affected muscles.

The final phase, phase IV, lasts for several months after surgery. The patient may complain of itching around the wound. Although collagen continues to be deposited during this time, there is shrinkage and contraction of the wound. If the wound is near a joint, contractures may occur. Because of the shrinkage the wound becomes a concave thin white line. Scar tissue is acellular, avascular collagen tissue. It will not tan with sunlight nor sweat or produce hair.

Factors influencing healing. Some of the factors that affect patient responses to surgery (p. 362) are directly related to wound healing. Research to date has not discovered anything that will hasten wound healing. There are, however, a number of factors that can prolong the healing process.

Age. Wounds in children normally heal more rapidly than in adults. Children have increased metabolism and good circulation. Wounds in the elderly often heal more slowly due to decreased fibroblastic activity and impaired circulation.

Nutrition. Vitamin C is necessary for collagen formation. It is also necessary to maintain the integrity of the capillary walls. Protein is the major constituent of collagen. Persons with inadequate vitamin C or protein intake will have delayed healing.

Circulation. Adequate circulation to the injured tissue is important to provide the white blood cells, fibroblasts, and nutrients needed for healing and to remove the debris after phagocytosis. Subcutaneous tissue is poorly supplied with blood vessels; therefore wounds of obese patients may heal more slowly. Patients with peripheral vascular disease will have impaired circulation to the legs causing delayed healing of leg ulcers.

Endocrine function. Steroids have an antiinflammatory effect and delay healing by depressing the inflammatory reaction that precedes wound healing. Cortisone also interferes with collagen formation. Patients with diabetes mellitus have decreased movement of leukocytes to the site and may have impaired circulation, which will delay healing.

Presence of foreign bodies. Most foreign bodies are not sterile and create an excessive inflammatory reaction and infection when present in a wound. Foreign bodies are usually removed unless removing them will cause more damage than their being left in the tissue.

Infection. A contaminated wound usually becomes infected. There is a greater inflammatory response as the white blood cells fight the invading microorganisms. A wound that is infected will not heal until the infection is cleared up. The greater the number of bacteria or amount of necrotic tissue present, the longer healing will be delayed.

Dead space. If fluid collects in a closed area where tissue has been removed, a space will occur where tissue healing does not take place. Cells above this dead space may break down due to the absence of underlying support. This occurs in surgery such as mastectomy, radical neck dissection, or arthroplasty. Hemovac suction is often used to remove the fluid so that healing will not be delayed.

Radiation. Direct radiation of the wound after surgery may slow down the development of blood vessels through the wound. Heavy radiation may cause necrosis of the wound.

Wound separation. When dehiscence (separation of previously joined edges) occurs, the wound is resutured if infection is not present. The separated area must restart the healing process, and healing occurs by tertiary intention.

Complications of wound healing

Hemorrhage

PHYSIOLOGIC FACTORS. External or internal hemorrhage may occur. Although hemorrhage from the wound is most likely to occur within the first 48 hours postoperatively, it may occur as late as the sixth or seventh postoperative day in apparently normal wounds and after a much longer time if the wound is infected. Hemorrhage occurring soon after operation may be due to the slipping of a ligature or the mechanical dislodging of a clot, caused for example by vomiting after a tonsillectomy. During surgery small vessels may go unnoticed because of decreased blood pressure or use of a tourniquet. These vessels will not be properly obliterated and hemorrhage may occur with the reestablishment of blood flow. Hemorrhage after a few days may be due to sloughing of a clot or of tissue, to infection, or to erosion of a blood vessel by a drainage tube.

ASSESSMENT. Dressings should be checked at frequent intervals during the first 48 hours and at least once every 8 hours thereafter. Subjectively the patient may complain of a wet sensation on the skin or dressing or of feeling restless or weak. Any postoperative patient who complains of an uneasy, restless feeling, such as "Something is wrong, but I don't know what," should be checked for signs of hemorrhage.

Objective data would include signs of shock (tachycardia, weak thready pulse, cold clammy skin, fall in blood pressure or central venous pressure, or decreased urinary output). Bright red blood may be present on the dressing or coming from a drainage tube.

INTERVENTION. The physician is notified of any signs of increased bleeding or shock. A small amount of bleeding on the dressing is outlined with a pen and rechecked at 10- to 15-minute intervals for signs of change. If there is bleeding from a tube into a container (chest or urinary), the amount of drainage is marked with the time and the amount so that the rapidity of bleeding can be determined at frequent intervals. If the bleeding is profuse, measures to control bleeding are instituted if possible; for example, a pressure dressing is applied over the existing dressing and measures to treat shock are started immediately (p. 218). Constant monitoring of vital signs is important. A calm environment is necessary so that increased anxiety does not add further stress to the patient's system.

If the bleeding is from an open cavity such as the nose, the cavity may be packed or an exposed bleeder cauterized by the surgeon. The patient who is bleeding internally or in profuse amounts externally is usually returned immediately to surgery where the incision is opened and the bleeding vessel is ligated. Intravenous fluids will be started and the patient's blood typed and cross-matched for transfusion before surgery. If a preanesthetic medication is ordered, the time when the last narcotic was given should be checked. Under pressure of the emergency there is danger of the patient receiving an overdose of narcotics. It should also be remembered that during shock peripheral circulation is decreased, resulting in poor absorption of medication from the tissue. Respiratory depression can occur when the shock is corrected and narcotics in the tissue from previous injections are rapidly absorbed.

Infection

PHYSIOLOGIC FACTORS. Surgical wound infections are caused by introduction of organisms into the open wound. Streptococcus, staphylococcus, and *Pseudomonas* organisms are the most frequent causes of infection. Modern surgical suites are designed to minimize the entry of organisms during the surgical procedure. Dry dressings are usually not disturbed until the sutures are to be removed, to prevent contamination during phase I of healing. Wet dressings have a greater potential for causing infections, as the bacteria can travel by capillary action through the wet dressing to the wound. Whether a wound becomes infected depends on factors intrinsic to the patient, factors that can delay healing, and the aseptic technique utilized by health personnel (physician, nurse). Whenever there is an open or draining wound, aseptic technique must be scrupulously followed. Infection control teams in hospitals are responsible for monitoring the incidence of wound infections (see Chapter 21).

ASSESSMENT. The patient may complain of persistent pain in the incisional area and a feeling of general malaise. Pain is due to stimulation of the nerve endings from the increased inflammation and to pressure from edema. The malaise is a systemic reaction to infection.

Objective signs include fever after the third postoperative day, increased white blood cell count (leukocytosis), incisional swelling, and erythema. There may be purulent drainage on the dressing. Wound culture and sensitivity studies should be obtained from the infected wound to determine the causative organism.

INTERVENTION. Prevention of wound infection is an important nursing measure. All open wound dressing changes are carried out under sterile conditions. Sterile gloves or instruments are used when cleaning an open wound and applying the sterile dressings. Soiled wet dressings should be changed immediately to prevent tissue breakdown from maceration and infection. Sterile moist dressings are covered with a dry sterile cover. The nutritional needs of the patient are assessed and interventions carried out when a deficiency is present that may delay healing.

If a wound infection does occur, the physician may open the wound to facilitate drainage if spontaneous drainage has not already taken place. Wound discomfort usually disappears after the wound has drained. A small drain may be placed in the wound to facilitate drainage, and irrigations may be ordered to wash away debris of infection. Purulent drainage is cleansed from the skin; pus contains proteolytic enzymes that can cause skin breakdown. The pus is sent to the laboratory for culture and sensitivity studies before antibiotics are given to control the infection. To maintain adequate blood levels the antibiotics must be given at the scheduled times.

Wound dehiscence and evisceration

PHYSIOLOGIC FACTORS. Wound disruption (dehiscence) is a partial to complete separation of the wound edges. Wound evisceration is protrusion of abdominal viscera through the incision and onto the abdominal wall (Fig. 23-12).

Wound separation that occurs during phase I (first 3 days) is usually related to technical factors such as the suturing. During phase II (3 to 14 days) it is usually associated with postoperative complications such as distention, vomiting, excessive coughing, dehydration, or infection. Many of these complications can be prevented by careful assessment and continued monitoring and by the institution of vigorous preventive measures (ventilatory exercises, ambulation, adequate fluid intake, aseptic technique) on the part of the nurse. Wound separation during phase III (after 2 weeks) is usually associated with metabolic factors such as cachexia, hypoproteinemia or avitaminosis, increased age, decreased resistance to infection, malignancy, multiple trauma, or hypothermia. These factors can also cause wound separation at an earlier time.

ASSESSMENT. Subjectively the patient may complain of a "giving" sensation at the incision or a feeling of wetness. If evisceration has occurred and if a loop of bowel has obstructed, the patient will complain of severe localized pain at the incision. On inspection the dressing will be found to be saturated with clear, pink drainage.

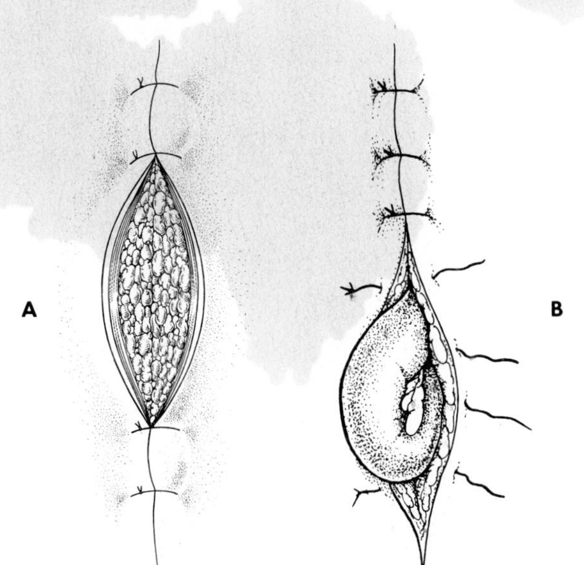

Fig. 23-12. A, Wound dehiscence. Wound edges are partially separated. **B,** Wound evisceration. Viscera protrude through incision.

The wound edges may be partially or entirely separated, and loops of intestine may be lying on the abdominal wall. Signs of shock may be present.

INTERVENTION. If the patient experiences either a wound dehiscence or wound evisceration, he is put to bed in a low Fowler's position and told to remain quiet, not to cough, and not eat or drink anything until the surgeon arrives. Protruding viscera should be covered, preferably with a warm, sterile saline dressing. Interventions for shock are initiated if signs of shock are present. The surgeon will cover the wound after inspection.

The treatment for wound dehiscence and wound evisceration is immediate closure of the wound under local or general anesthesia. If the patient is in shock the preanesthetic medication may be omitted. Convalescence is usually prolonged, although the wound usually heals surprisingly well following secondary closure.

Oxygen needs

Outcome: *Pulmonary complications do not occur; breath sounds are clear*

Physiologic factors. Many of the respiratory complications that occur in the postoperative patient can be prevented by nursing management. The most common respiratory complications are atelectasis and hypostatic pneumonia. In atelectasis a bronchiole becomes blocked by secretions and the distal alveoli collapse as the existing air is absorbed. This produces hypoventilation. A major bronchus (indicating the main stem bronchus) or many small bronchioles may be involved. The latter situation is frequently undetected due to few symptoms. The extent of the atelectasis will be determined by the site of the blockage; if the main stem bronchus to one lung is blocked, that lung will be atelectatic. If a bronchus going to a lobe is blocked, that lobe will be atelectatic. Stasis of the secretions leads to pneumonia. Both atelectasis and pneumonia decrease oxygenation, prolong recovery, and add to the patient's discomfort.

Assessment. Early in the postoperative period the patient is assessed to determine his risk for developing a pulmonary complication (Table 23-3). Pertinent data from the preoperative period are reviewed. New data in the postoperative period include anesthetic used and type of surgery performed, medications given pre- and postoperatively that will influence secretions, state of hydration, and presence of pain, vomiting, or nasogastric tube.

Inspection of the patient will determine the amount of activity being carried out (movement in bed, ambulation) and position in bed. Respirations are monitored closely. Hypoventilation is indicated by rapid shallow respirations and absent or diminished breath sounds in the lower lobes. Depth of respirations is an important criterion because the alveoli are poorly ventilated when respirations are shallow. Chest expansion is observed during inspiration; if the chest is held fairly rigid, there will be decreased ventilation.

Auscultation of the lungs allows the nurse to detect both hypoventilation of specific lobes (breath sounds will be diminished) and the presence of secretions (rales will be heard). The lungs should be free of rales, but diminished breath sounds may be present during the first 24 hours after surgery.[50]

Presence of a productive cough during the first few days postoperatively is a positive sign that the patient is able to clear the bronchial secretions that might otherwise block the bronchioles. The productiveness of the cough usually decreases as secretions diminish.

An unexplained rise in temperature is often the first sign of atelectasis. Pulse and respiratory rates increase. If a large bronchus is blocked the patient may exhibit dyspnea and cyanosis and signs of shock. Diagnosis is confirmed by chest radiography. Pneumonia also produces fever, dyspnea, chest pain, and a cough productive of mucopurulent sputum.

Intervention. Prevention of respiratory complications is an area where nursing care provides a key to a smooth postoperative recovery. The use of "routines," however, is not the answer. It is common to find postoperative routines that read "Turn, cough, and deep breath every 2 hours"; the order is never changed. In reality some patients need deep-breathing exercises more often than every 2 hours, others less. Most patients after general anesthesia will need to ventilate their lungs well at least every 2 to 3 hours the first postoperative day, then every 4 hours while awake for several days if not active. The decision for the type and frequency of preventive respiratory measures should be based on each patient's risk factors and his hour-by-hour and day-by-day response. Measures that work effectively in increasing ventilation in one patient may be less effective in another.

A plan should be developed for each patient that best meets his oxygen needs. For example, an elderly patient with a history of lung disease, who smokes and has just had high abdominal surgery with an inhalant anesthetic, may need to carry out coughing and deep-breathing exercises as often as every 15 to 30 minutes during the first few hours postoperatively. A young patient with no history of smoking or lung disease, who had preoperative medication and an inhalant anesthetic and who is up ambulating frequently after surgery, may need breathing exercises only every 2 to 3 hours the first day and none thereafter. Reassessment is important, and the plan of care should be updated as the risk factors change.

Ventilation measures. The types of ventilation measures most commonly used in the postoperative period are coughing and deep-breathing exercises, blow-bottles, rebreathing tubes, or intermittent positive pressure breathing (IPPB) (for details on the use of these measures see Chapter 45). The nurse may institute any of the first three measures and should be familiar with the advantages and disadvantages of each. It is important to remember that many patients are drowsy or have periods of amnesia during the early postoperative period, so that frequently the instructions must be repeated. Persons who have had good instruction in the preoperative phase are usually better able to carry out the measures postoperatively.

All of the ventilation measures used by the surgical patient are followed by deep coughing to remove any secretions that have been loosened. Deep breathing in itself often stimulates coughing. Coughing may be contraindicated in a few instances such as following brain, spinal, or eye surgery because of the increased intracranial or intraocular pressure that can result. Patients with incisions can be told that it may be painful to cough but that assistance will be given. Narcotics given before ventilation exercises may facilitate cooperation of the patient; on the other hand narcotics decrease the cough reflex and depress respirations. Some patients are afraid that the incision will split open while they are coughing and should be told that the incision can be splinted during coughing. Splinting of the incision can be accomplished by means of a drawsheet or towel, small pillow, or placement of the hands firmly on either side of the incision and with exertion of slight pressure (see Fig. 45-16). Such splinting prevents excessive muscular strain around the incision.

The most effective position for ventilation exercises is high Fowler's, as this decreases the pressure of the abdominal contents on the diaphragm and permits better thorax expansion. If the patient must remain flat in bed, restraining bedclothes and pillows are removed from around the chest.

A shallow cough is ineffective in mobilizing secretions and serves only to tire the patient; he should be encouraged to cough deeply and productively. If the first attempt is not successful the patient should rest, then try again. Auscultation of the lungs before and after ventilatory measures provides data for evaluation of the effectiveness. If the patient has noisy breathing but is unable to cough up secretions, he may need respiratory tract suctioning.

Positioning and turning. If the patient lies in one position with continuous pressure from his weight against the chest wall, proper ventilation and drainage of secretions on that side of the chest are not possible and atelectasis can develop (Fig. 23-13). Turning and changing of position frequently (at least every 2 to 3 hours) provide for better ventilation of the lungs. The patient should be

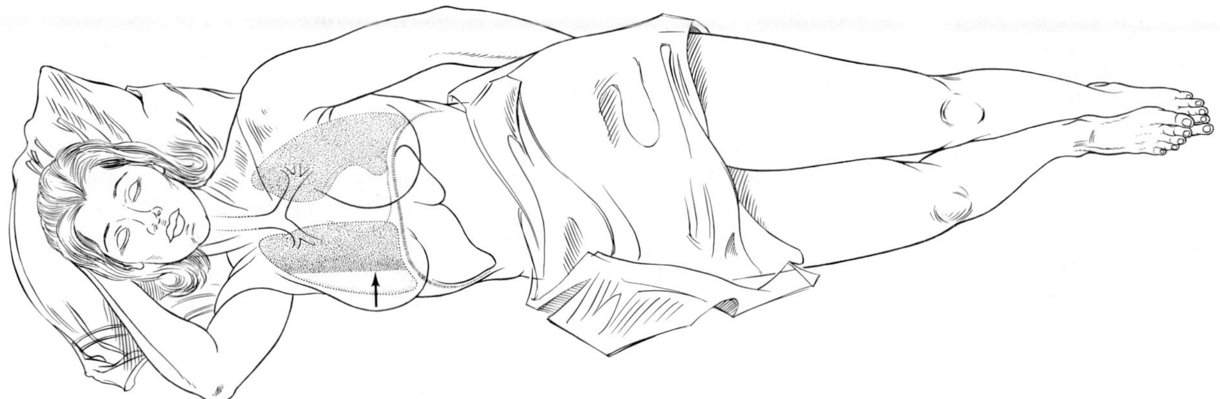

Fig. 23-13. Gravity will facilitate drainage of secretions from upper lung. In lower lung next to bed, secretions will pool in alveoli due to gravity and decreased chest expansion. Frequent turning will facilitate drainage from both lungs.

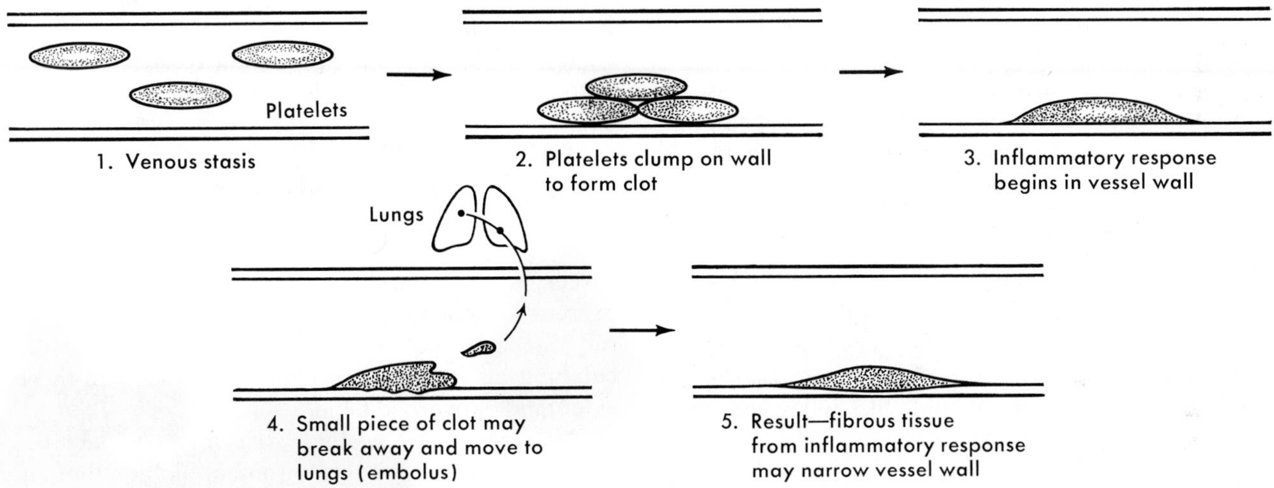

Fig. 23-14. Diagram illustrating formation of thrombus on wall of vein following venous stasis resulting in narrowing of blood vessel.

encouraged to help turn himself. Most patients assume a supine position and are not eager to change position because of the increased pain during movement. They may find side rails useful for turning during the early postoperative period. Assistance can be given by supporting a limb or helping the patient to turn in one smooth movement. Alternating the height of the bed is useful: high Fowler's position facilitates diaphragm movement; low Fowler's or a flat position facilitates drainage and expectoration of respiratory secretions.

Activity. Stimulation of the respiratory center occurs with activity because of the increased need for oxygen at the cellular level. The more active the patient, the more he will increase the depth of his respirations and ventilate the alveoli. Activity is encouraged within the prescribed limits and depending on the patient's tolerance to activity.

Outcome: *Peripheral circulation remains adequate; no calf pain or vascular changes occur*

Physiologic factors. Oxygen is needed by tissue cells for metabolism. It cannot reach the cells if blood flow to the part is curtailed. The formation of clots in the veins of the pelvis and the lower extremities, impairing circulation, is a fairly common and potentially serious postoperative complication.

Blood clots develop because of a roughness in the vessel wall such as occurs with trauma or from venous stasis (slowing of blood flow). Platelets adhere to the vessel wall, and the resulting inflammatory response stimulates blood coagulation and fibrin development, resulting in a blood clot on the vessel wall (thrombophlebitis) (Fig. 23-14). Postoperatively the clot often forms in a vein of the foot, calf, thigh, or pelvis. The clot grows, usually in the direction of the slow-moving blood. It can occur in either a deep or superficial vein. In about one of every 10 instances[44] the clot or a portion of it breaks away and flows through the heart into the pulmonary circulation until it occludes a pulmonary vessel (pulmonary embolism) (p. 1130).

Venous stasis occurs postoperatively for a number of reasons. Respiratory and circulatory depression occur from anesthesia and other drugs and from shock. Patients who have had prolonged anesthesia, considerable blood loss during surgery, or shock following surgery have a greater possibility of clot formation.[80]

Other predisposing conditions interfering with circulation are obesity, increased age, cardiovascular diseases (especially varicose veins), and malnutrition. Increased pressure on veins creating venous stasis can occur from tight dressings, casts or traction, intestinal distention, prolonged sitting, or pressure on the popliteal area from pillows. A major contribution to venous stasis is inactivity of the legs. Every time the leg is moved the muscle compresses the vein pushing the blood toward the heart (venous pump); valves prevent the blood from moving backward. Exercise therefore promotes return of venous blood to the heart and prevention of venous stasis. There is a high incidence of thrombophlebitis following cardiovascular and pelvic surgery.

Assessment. A venous blood clot may develop without any local symptoms (phlebothrombosis), and the first indication of difficulty may be a pulmonary embolism. Homan's sign, pain on dorsiflexion of the foot, indicates a phlebothrombosis, but this may not always be present. Pain and local tenderness in the leg are signs of thrombophlebitis.

If a superficial vein is involved, thrombophlebitis can be noted as a reddened line along the vessel route, which feels firm on gentle palpation. If it forms in the femoral or iliac veins, the entire limb becomes swollen, pale, and cold. There is usually exquisite tenderness along the course of the vein. The swelling and coldness are caused by lymphatic obstruction and arterial spasm. The body temperature often rises. If the thrombophlebitis is confined to the saphenous vein, the accompanying edema is not so marked, but pain and tenderness are just as severe, and heat and redness can be noted along the inflamed vein.

Signs of a pulmonary embolism depend on the size of the blood vessel that has been occluded. Any complaints of sudden sharp thoracic or upper abdominal pain or dyspnea or any signs of shock are reported immediately to the physician.

Intervention

Prevention. Many circulatory postoperative complications can be prevented by nursing management. Patient education of the causes of thrombophlebitis will help ensure greater participation in preventive measures. Elastic stockings or bandages should be worn both in and out of bed by high-risk patients. These stockings compress superficial veins, increase blood flow through deep veins by pressure, and prevent venous pooling. The stockings are removed at least once daily to permit washing and inspection of the legs.

Patients should not sit in one position for a long time and should elevate their feet on a stool to facilitate venous return by gravity. No pressure should be permitted on the popliteal area such as by pillows. When supporting legs on pillows, pressure should be equally distributed along the entire leg. Because of the danger of dislodging a clot, the muscle portion of a patient's leg should not be massaged postoperatively. If a patient is noted to be rubbing his leg, he should be questioned about his discomfort.

Bed exercises (Fig. 23-3) and early ambulation are known to minimize the effects of venous stasis caused by bed rest, and they usually are contraindicated only in the presence of thromboembolic diseases or after vascular surgery such as anastomosis of a blood vessel. Specific exercises for the upper extremities are not usually necessary, since the patient uses his arms in eating, bathing, combing his hair, and reaching for articles on the bedside stand or overbed table.

Management of postoperative thrombophlebitis. At the first sign of a possible thrombophlebitis the patient should return to bed and remain there until seen by a physician. Rest, heat, and elastic bandages are usually prescribed. The patient may also be given anticoagulant therapy.

Nutritional needs

Outcome: *Fluid balance is maintained*

Physiologic factors. Fluid is lost during surgery through blood loss and increased insensible fluid loss through the lungs and skin. During the surgical procedure the blood loss is estimated and fluids are replaced intravenously. Gastrointestinal tract function may be slowed. Fluids are started orally as soon as the patient can tolerate them and if active peristalsis is present. Surgery of the gastrointestinal tract or on closely related organs within the abdomen usually decreases peristalsis, and paralytic ileus (intestinal obstruction due to cessation of peristalsis) may occur.

For at least the first 24 to 48 hours after surgery,

fluids are retained by the body due to the stimulation of antidiuretic hormone (ADH) as part of the stress response to trauma and the effect of anesthesia. Overhydration can occur with vigorous fluid replacement, especially in the infant or small elderly person. Both water intoxication and pulmonary edema can occur depending on the type and amount of fluids given (for further information on fluid overload see p. 303).

Assessment. All patients who have had major surgery and those receiving fluids intravenously after surgery need careful monitoring of fluid balance. Fluid intake will exceed fluid output during the first 24 to 48 hours. After this initial period fluid intake should essentially equal fluid output for the patient taking solid foods. The patient receiving fluids intravenously is monitored for signs of pulmonary edema (dyspnea, cough) or water intoxication (change in behavior, confusion, warm moist skin). Weight is monitored in those patients receiving fluid intravenously over a period of several days postoperatively. Sudden weight gain indicates fluid retention. Small elderly persons may need central venous pressure monitoring of fluid volume. The presence of bowel sounds, passing of flatus, or belching indicates the return of peristalsis.

Intervention. As soon as the patient has recovered fully from anesthesia, he is offered sips of water if this is permitted. Some persons cannot tolerate iced fluids well but can tolerate sucking on ice chips. Ice chips must be recorded as intake (2 parts of ice equal 1 part water). Intravenous fluids are monitored carefully so that fluids are given evenly over the entire 24-hour period (for further information on intravenous fluids see p. 319).

Outcome: *Electrolyte balance is monitored*

Physiologic factors. Sodium and potassium depletion can occur in the postoperative patient with the loss of blood or body fluids during surgery or the loss of gastrointestinal secretions by vomiting and through nasogastric tubes. Potassium is also lost during catabolism (tissue breakdown). Loss of gastric secretions can result in chloride loss producing a base-bicarbonate excess (metabolic alkalosis).

Assessment and intervention. The patient is monitored for signs of sodium and potassium deficit (p. 308). Potassium is usually added to intravenous fluids of postoperative patients. High-protein foods and fresh fruits, high in potassium, are encouraged when foods are permitted by mouth.

Outcome: *Patient's normal weight is maintained; protein and vitamin C intake is enhanced*

Physiologic factors. The best way to supply essential foods is orally. Solid food can promote the flow of saliva during mastication, aiding digestion and encouraging the stomach to empty. This process in turn stimulates peristalsis of the lower gastrointestinal tract. Ingestion of solid food also helps to prevent the occurrence of nonepidemic parotitis, an inflammation of the salivary glands that occurs occasionally in debilitated patients who have poor oral hygiene and who also may be dehydrated.

Two food substances of special importance in wound healing are protein and vitamin C. During catabolism in the early postoperative period, a negative nitrogen balance occurs; more nitrogen is lost than is taken in (p. 362). Protein intake is necessary to restore nitrogen balance and to provide the necessary amino acids for anabolism. Vitamin C is necessary for tissue healing (p. 401).

Assessment. Daily weight measurement for patients not eating a full meal at least three times a day will give an indication of the degree of tissue loss. Rapid weight gain indicates fluid retention; rapid loss indicates dehydration. A gradual loss of about $^1/_3$ to $^1/_2$ pound per day indicates tissue loss.[64] There is usually an increase in blood urea nitrogen (BUN) levels during catabolism, but unless the patient has renal insufficiency he excretes the excess urea in the urine. Meal trays of surgical patients should be inspected to identify those patients who are not eating foods high in protein and vitamin C.

Intervention. Patients receiving standard intravenous fluids containing dextrose do not have sufficient caloric intake. This is essentially a "starvation diet." As soon as fluids can be tolerated foods are started. Most patients quickly resume their usual diet. Elderly persons or persons who have had stomach surgery may tolerate a soft diet and six small feedings more easily than a standard diet. Urging solid food when the patient has no appetite may induce vomiting and may lessen the desire to eat. The anorexic patient is encouraged to select foods he prefers and which are high in protein. Carbohydrate is also needed to provide energy expended in early ambulation. After even a few days of enforced starvation the patient may be somewhat indifferent to food, and it may take 2 to 3 days on a well-balanced diet to overcome this. The patient who was malnourished before surgery and who has extensive gastrointestinal surgery is a candidate for hyperalimentation.

The usual home diet of elderly persons living alone is frequently low in protein and vitamins. Patient education concerning the increased need for these food substances in the weeks following surgery may be indicated.

Elimination needs

Outcome: *Urinary output resumes normal pattern; urinary tract infection does not develop*

Physiologic factors. If the patient is well hydrated, urinary function usually returns within 6 to 8 hours after surgery. Although 2,000 to 3,000 ml of intravenous solution usually are given on the operative day, the first voiding may not be more than 200 ml and the total urinary output for the operative day may be less than 1,500 ml. The small amount of urinary output is due to the loss of body fluid during surgery, increased insensible fluid loss, vomiting, and increased secretion of antidiuretic hormone (ADH). As body functions stabilize, fluid and electrolyte balance returns to normal in about 48 hours.

Urinary retention, or the inability to void, may also occur in the early postoperative period. The difficulty may be due to the recumbent position, nervous tension, the effects of anesthetics that interfere with bladder sensation and the ability to void, the use of narcotics that reduce the sensation of bladder distention, the pain caused by movement onto the bedpan, or pain at the site of operation if it is near the bladder or urethra. Inability to void is a common occurrence following surgery of the rectum or colon and following gynecologic procedures, since the innervation of the bladder musculature may be temporarily disturbed, and local edema may increase the difficulty.

Urinary tract infections may occur in patients who must be on prolonged bed rest following surgery, who have a history of urinary tract infections, who have had pelvic surgery, or who have indwelling catheters.

Assessment. Urine output is closely monitored after surgery until normal urinary function is reestablished. During the oliguric phase the specific gravity is high as the usual amount of solutes are excreted in less water. The bladder is palpated for distention when output is low to identify urinary retention. The distended bladder rises out of the pelvis just above the symphysis pubis. This may be difficult to palpate when the patient is obese. Occasionally the overdistended bladder expels just enough urine to relieve the pressure within it temporarily. This is known as retention with overflow. The patient voids frequently in small amounts. This differs from frequency seen in urinary tract infections; in the latter the bladder is not distended, the patient complains of burning on urination, and may have fever.

Intervention. Suppression of urine after the initial oliguric phase postoperatively requires medical intervention (p. 1254). If the patient is well hydrated and has no cardiovascular or renal problems, the inability to void past the first 6 to 8 hours is usually due to urinary retention. This requires nursing intervention. Voiding may be facilitated by measures such as offering fluids, placing the patient on the bedpan frequently or getting him up to the bathroom or commode if possible, running water in the bathroom, pouring water over the perineum, and assuring the patient of time and privacy. Many men can void if they are allowed to stand at the side of the bed. If these measures are not effective the physician may order catheterization. Because of the emotional trauma to the young child, the possibility of reproductive tract infections in men, and the danger of urinary infection in all patients, catheterization may be delayed longer than the usual 8 hours postoperatively in the hope that the patient will void normally. Bethanechol chloride (Urecholine) may be ordered by the physician for acute postoperative retention. It may be given orally or subcutaneously but not by intramuscular injection as this may induce circulatory collapse.

If the patient must be catheterized repeatedly after surgery, an indwelling catheter may be inserted and fluids forced. Good perineal care of a patient with an indwelling catheter will help to prevent ascending infection. Bacteria can move up the outside of the catheter by means of capillary action. Patients who exhibit signs of urinary tract infection should have a urine specimen sent to the laboratory for culture and sensitivity. Fluids are encouraged up to 3,000 ml, unless contraindicated, to prevent urinary stasis.

Outcome: *Bowel patterns are reestablished*

Physiologic factors. Decreased peristalsis from the neuroendocrine response to the stress of surgery and from the effect of anesthesia and narcotics or from hypokalemia may lead to constipation in the early postoperative period. Inactivity and decreased intake of foods that provide roughage are contributing factors. Peristalsis will be decreased in all patients with abdominal or pelvic surgery for at least 24 hours and will be delayed for several days if the patient had surgery of the gastrointestinal tract. For some surgical patients, having a bowel movement may be painful and the patient may be reluctant to pass stool.

A patient receiving therapy intravenously may have bowel movements if peristalsis is present. Stool is composed of 75% water plus waste products, both of which are present in the hydrated patient. Because of the lack of ingested roughage, stools will occur less frequently and may be hard. The longer stool remains in the colon, the more water is reabsorbed and the harder the stool becomes.

Assessment. Return of peristalsis of the lower gastrointestinal tract is indicated by presence of bowel sounds, gas pains, and passing of flatus. Absence of bowel sounds does not indicate absence of peristalsis as the sounds may be occurring only occasionally and may be missed. On the contrary, the presence of bowel sounds does not indicate active peristalsis but may only be gas moving in segments of bowel.

Stool is examined for amount and consistency; small, hard stool indicates constipation. A small amount of diarrhea may be indicative of a fecal impaction. If present in the rectum, a fecal impaction can be identified by digital examination; this is contraindicated following surgery of the rectum.

Assessment should also be made of the frequency

with which narcotics are given, extent of activity, amount of fluid intake, and previous bowel problems to determine the patient's potential for developing constipation.

Intervention. Signs indicating the return of intestinal peristalsis are recorded after abdominal surgery. No attempt is made to hasten bowel evaucation for the first 2 to 3 days after peristalsis fully returns, but preventive measures should be instituted. Fluids are encouraged to 2,000 to 3,000 ml per day unles contraindicated. Maximum activity is encouraged within the prescribed limits. Bathroom privileges are provided as early as possible.

If there are no results after 3 to 4 days, a mild laxative may help reestablish function. Fruit juices, especially prune juice, may be effective. If these are not effective, a hypertonic (Fleet) enema or small soapsuds enema will usually stimulate defecation. If a fecal impaction is suspected, a mineral oil enema may preceed a soapsuds enema to soften the stool. A bowel movement may be intentionally delayed following burns of the buttocks or extensive rectal surgery by the administration of paregoric orally.

Comfort needs

Outcome: *General discomforts are minimized*

Vomiting

Physiologic factors. Nausea and vomiting in the postoperative patient may be related to a number of factors: effect of certain anesthetics on the stomach, decreased peristalsis producing a collection of fluid and gas in the stomach, drinking fluids before peristalsis returns, psychologic factors in patients who anticipate postoperative vomiting, drug idiosyncracies, pain, or disturbances in electrolyte balance.

Persistent postoperative vomiting is usually a symptom of pyloric obstruction, intestinal obstruction, or peritonitis. Vomiting tires the patient, puts a strain on the incision, and causes excessive loss of fluids and electrolytes. Choking while vomiting may lead to aspiration pneumonia.

Intervention. Postoperative vomiting is one of the most distressing problems that a patient encounters. To prevent possible aspiration the patient who is vomiting should lie on his side. He should be advised not to take food or fluid for several hours and to lie quietly in bed. The emesis basin and soiled linen are cleaned and changed. Frequent oral care is provided. When vomiting has subsided, and unless contraindicated, sucking on ice chips, taking sips of ginger ale or hot tea, or eating small amounts of dry solid food may relieve nausea. Antiemetics such as trimethobenzamide hydrochloride (Tigan) or prochlorperazine dimaleate (Compazine) may be administered by injection. Since vomiting can be a sign of drug idiosyncrasy, presence of other side effects should be observed and the pattern of vomiting in relation to administration of drugs noted. Accurate recording of intake and output of fluids and electrolyte balance is important.

Hiccoughs

Physiologic factors. Hiccoughs interfere with eating and sleeping and are among the most exhausting postoperative complications. The exact cause of postoperative hiccoughs is not known, but it is known that dilation of the stomach, irritation of the diaphragm, peritonitis, and uremia cause either reflex or central nervous system stimulation of the phrenic nerve. Fortunately hiccoughs are not a common postoperative complaint. They usually disappear within a few hours.

Intervention. Hiccoughs may be relieved by such a simple measure as having the patient breathe his own carbon dioxide at 5-minute intervals by inhaling and exhaling into a paper bag held tightly over his nose and mouth. Carbon dioxide inhalations, using 5% carbon dioxide and 95% oxygen, may also be ordered for 5 minutes every hour. If dizziness occurs they should be discontinued, since an overdose of carbon dioxide may cause convulsions and coma. Aspiration of the stomach will stop hiccoughs caused by gastric dilation. Chlorpromazine hydrochloride is used to treat mild cases of hiccoughs. If the hiccoughs are persistent and do not respond to these treatments, local infiltration of the phrenic nerve with 1% procaine may be necessary, or in extreme cases surgical crushing of the phrenic nerve may be done.

Abdominal distention and gas pains

Physiologic factors. Postoperative distention is a result of an accumulation of nonabsorbable gas in the intestines caused by a reaction to the handling of the bowel during surgery, by swallowing of air during recovery from anesthesia and as the patient attempts to overcome nausea, and by passing of gases from the bloodstream to the atonic portion of the bowel. Distention will persist until the tone of the bowel returns to normal and peristalsis resumes. It is experienced to some degree by most patients after abdominal and renal surgery.

"Gas pains" are caused by contractions of the unaffected portions of the bowel in an attempt to move the accumulated gas through the intestinal tract.

Assessment. Patients with abdominal distention complain of diffuse abdominal pain. High distention may cause dyspnea by pressure on the diaphragm and lead to atelectasis. Abdominal girth is increased due to the collection of gas; this can be measured with a tape measure to determine progress. Percussion produces a drumlike (tympanic) sound as compared with a dull sound occurring with ascites or obesity. Acute gastric dilation may produce signs of shock (restlessness; rapid, weak, thready pulse; hypotension) and overflow vomiting. Gas pains in the intestinal tract usually occur as peristalsis is beginning to return and can be extremely painful. Bowel sounds are usually audible on auscultation.

Intervention. Ambulation is one of the most effective means for stimulation of peristalsis and expulsion of flatus. Dilation of the stomach can be relieved by aspiration of fluid or gas with a nasogastric tube.

Gas in the lower bowel may be removed by a lubricated rectal tube inserted into the rectum. This tube should be inserted just past the rectal sphincter and should be removed after approximately 20 minutes. If necessary it may be used every 4 hours. Heat applied to the abdomen in the form of a hot-water bottle or heating pad may be used in conjunction with the use of a rectal tube. A hypertonic enema is often effective in relieving gas pains postoperatively. If this fails, small carminative enemas of milk and molasses or of glycerin, magnesium sulfate, and water sometimes are ordered to stimulate the expulsion of flatus.

If the distention progresses and the flatus is not expelled after 48 hours, a paralytic ileus is suspected. The patient is given nothing by mouth. Nasogastric suctioning is started and continued until peristalsis returns.

Outcome: *Postoperative pain is minimized*

Physiologic factors. Pain is a common occurrence after nearly all types of surgical procedures in which there has been cutting, pulling, or manipulations of tissues and organs. It may be caused by stimulation of nerve endings by chemical substances released at the time of surgery or to tissue ischemia caused by interference of blood supply to the part such as by pressure, muscle spasm, or edema. Trauma to the nerve fibers in the skin produces sharp localized pain. Extensive dissection and prolonged retraction of muscle and fascia produce deep long-lasting pain. Pain originating in a visceral organ may be referred to a distant portion of the body surface or deeply in a different area. It is usually characterized as a deep, aching pain. A hollow visceral organ such as the ureter or bile duct can develop muscle spasms characterized as cramping pain.

Following surgery other factors can add to the pain sensation. These include pressure from tissue edema, infections, distention, muscle spasms surrounding the incisional area, and tight dressings or casts. Postoperative pain usually lasts 24 to 48 hours but may continue longer depending on the extent of the surgery, the pain threshold of the patient, and his response to pain (p. 344). The presence of pain can prolong convalescence, since it may interfere with return to activity.

Assessment. When the patient complains of pain in the postoperative period, one must not assume that the pain is incisional by nature. It is important to try to ascertain the possible cause of the pain. Subjective data include origin, area involved, nature of the pain, and possible cause from the patient's viewpoint. Objective data include observation of facial expressions, body position, activity, muscle rigidity, and pulse rate.

Pain with fever may be due to wound infection. Pain with vomiting and abdominal distention is a result of gas collecting in the intestinal tract. Pain with fullness about the symphysis pubis is due to a full bladder. Pain with coldness, parathesia, or numbness of a part is a result of decreased circulation from a tight bandage or cast or venous stasis. If the patient is experiencing severe pain the assessment should be made gently and quickly but thoroughly.

Intervention. It is not often possible to prevent the occurrence of postoperative pain, but it can be alleviated so that the patient is relatively comfortable. Patients who have had adequate preoperative instructions and who have confidence in the surgeon, in the nurse, and in the outcome of the surgery usually have less postoperative pain than the apprehensive patient because they have less tension. Measures to reduce anxiety and apprehension will also help reduce any pain that is present.

If the cause of pain is determined to be other than incisional, measures are taken to relieve the cause. Emptying a full bladder can relieve what was thought to be pain from a lower abdominal incision. Elevation of a part may relieve venous stasis. Loosening of a tight bandage if permissible will relieve ischemic pain.

Incisional pain can be relieved by nursing measures and by analgesics. Spasms and pain from surrounding muscles being continually contracted contributes to incisional pain. Many patients find a position that is tolerable and then hesitate to move for fear of increased pain. Muscles used to hold this position and guard the incision become strained. If the patient understands what is occurring and is helped and encouraged to move frequently, pain will be decreased. Patients with surgery of the trunk should avoid twisting the body; they may be more comfortable if the trunk is moved as one unit. Side rails are helpful for the patient to hold onto when turning over. A limb that has been operated on should be supported. If hands are used for supporting a limb, the broad palms rather than fingers, which dig into painful tissue, are more comfortable for the patient. Pillows serve as useful "splints" during movement of a limb. Autogenic techniques for control of pain such as the "relaxation response" technique (p. 350) may be helpful for some patients.

Medications. In addition to making the patient as comfortable as possible, it is usually necessary during the first 12 to 48 hours after major surgery to administer a narcotic. The goal is to keep the patient fairly comfortable without overmedicating him. Analgesics have greater effect if they are administered before pain becomes severe. If severe pain is expected, medication should be offered to the patient within the prescribed limits before he has to ask for it.

Addiction to narcotics is *not* a probability if given during the first few postoperative days for severe pain. Although certain narcotics such as morphine depress the respiratory center, the patient in pain may be breathing shallowly or splinting the chest and not moving about in bed adequately. Relief of pain may encourage the patient to move and breathe more deeply, thus preventing postoperative complications. During early ambulation patients receiving meperidine hydrochloride (Demerol) may develop orthostatic hypotension.

After the first 48 to 72 hours, pain usually decreases in severity and may be controlled with a less potent analgesic. Because of the variability in perception and reaction to pain, each patient must be assessed individually. It is the custom in some hospitals for physicians to write prn orders for different analgesics, thus permitting the nurse to select the one that best meets the immediate needs. If this is the practice, careful patient assessment and monitoring to prevent overlapping of drugs given is important. Some communities do not permit this practice, considering it to be prescription of drugs and therefore not under the legal jurisdiction of nursing.

Activity needs

Outcome: *Maximum activity is carried out within established limits*

Physiologic factors. Early ambulation has been a significant factor is hastening postoperative recovery and preventing postoperative complications. Numerous benefits accrue from the exercise of getting in and out of bed and walking during the early postoperative period (Fig. 23-15). Increases in rate and depth of breathing improve ventilation, helping to prevent atelectasis and hypostatic pneumonia. Oxygen intake increases and with the increased circulation more oxygen reaches the brain, increasing mental alertness. Cardiac output increases; more blood flows through the capillaries, providing the wound with substances needed for healing; and venous return is enhanced, decreasing venous stasis. Kidney function is increased due to the increased circulation. Activity also promotes micturition.

Metabolism increases as muscles are stimulated, preventing loss of muscle tone. Nitrogen loss is decreased, thus helping to restore nitrogen balance. Activity stimulates peristalsis in the gastrointestinal tract, promoting passage of fluids and gas and thus helping to prevent abdominal distention, gas pains, and constipation. Pain is decreased over time as the chemical stimuli are removed through increased circulation and strained muscles around the incision, neck, back, and legs relax. Morale is also affected as the patient sees function returning. Ambulation is usually contraindicated when there is a severe infection or thrombophlebitis.

Exercises in bed facilitate strengthening of muscle tone (Fig. 23-3). Moving around in bed, if carried out actively by the patient with minimal help, will offer some of the same benefits but to a much less extent. Moving to different positions also helps prevent tissue ischemia from pressure.

Assessment. A postoperative patient who is to get out of bed needs to be alert enough to follow directions. Asking the patient simple questions or to follow simple commands will help to determine his level of alertness.

Assessment of the patient's cardiovascular status includes obtaining baseline pulse and respiratory rate and rhythm. A change in position from supine to sitting or standing may produce orthostatic hypotension. Pulse and respiratory rates will increase as the result of sympathetic stimulation. The patient's face may become pale and he may complain of dizziness. He should not attempt ambulation until the pulse and respirations stabilize at close to their baseline level.

Assessment of motor status includes muscle strength (p. 399) and sitting ability. Sitting ability will give an indication of the patient's ability to maintain his balance while ambulating. This is assessed by asking the patient to maintain an erect position while he is gently pushed sideways while sitting on the side of the bed.

It is also important to know of any limitations to ambulation that the patient had preoperatively. The patient with arthritis or arteriosclerosis may take longer to move and to adjust to standing and walking. The patient who used a walker preoperatively will need assistance for a longer time before progressing to using the walker again.

Intervention. Muscle strengthening exercises should be carried out by patients who are not permitted to or cannot ambulate for a period of time. Exercises of the lower extremities will also prevent venous stasis. The patient is taught to bend his knees, to lower them, and to push the backs of the knees hard against the bed. The nurse's hand can be slipped under the popliteal area while the patient pushes hard against it. The same thing can be accomplished by having the patient alternately contract and relax his calf and thigh muscles. This should be done at least 10 times, and a brief period of rest should follow each contraction and relaxation. The cycle is contract, relax, and rest. Bed exercises should be carried out several times a day. If the patient is unable to do active exercises, passive range-of-motion exercises should be carried out.

When the patient is permitted to be out of bed, he is assisted to sit up on the side of the bed and dangle his legs over the side to become accustomed to an upright position. Orthostatic hypotension may occur at this time.

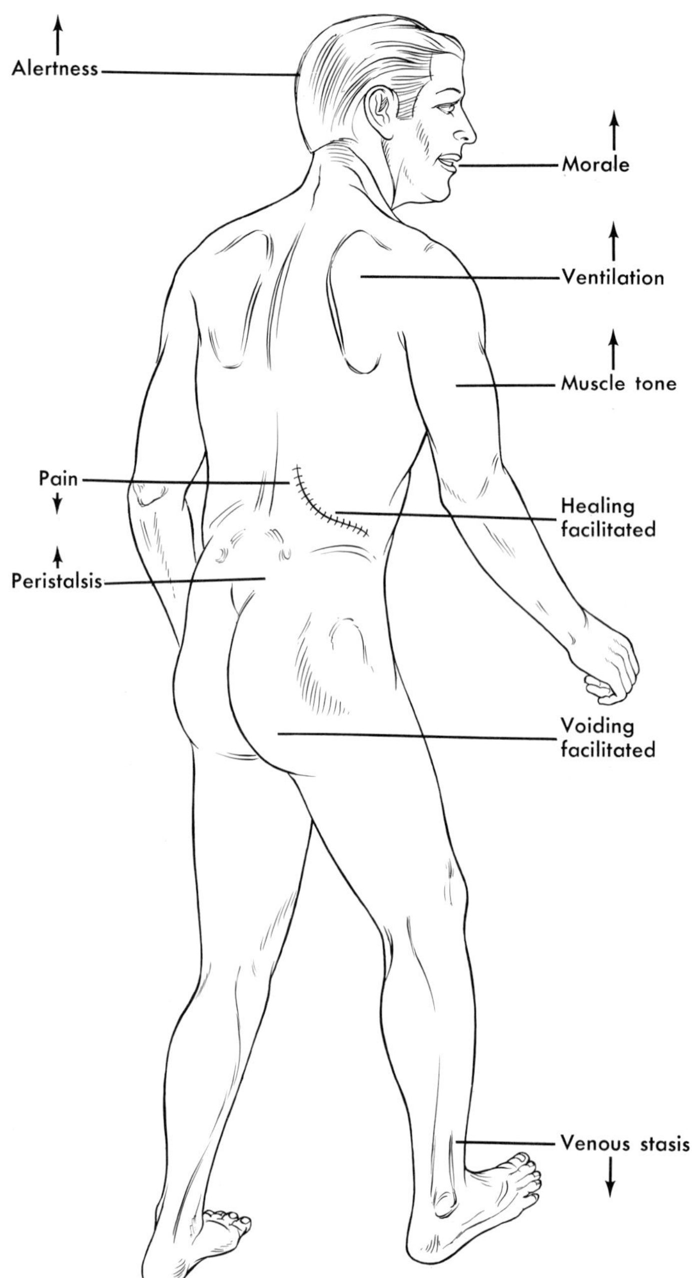

Fig. 23-15. Benefits from early postoperative ambulation.

After the pulse has stabilized and the patient is ready to move, he is assisted to stand and walk a few steps. Each time he gets up he is encouraged to increase the distance walked. There should be ample space available for walking. A very weak patient may need two helpers, one to assist the patient and the other to manage the intravenous fluid pole or other equipment. The patient is assisted and supervised in getting out of bed and walking until he is able to do this without difficulty or danger of injury. Small goals can be set each day to give the patient something to work for and a sense of achievement.

Children usually recover quickly from the effects of surgery and often sit up and walk around in their cribs without urging. Older children occasionally are fearful of injuring the operative site and must be encouraged to leave the bed and move about freely.

Treatments need not interfere with helping the patient out of bed. If the patient is receiving an infusion, the bottle of infusion fluid can be hung on a movable pole that can be wheeled by the nurse as the patient walks. Permission is usually given by the physician to clamp off nasogastric tubes for a short period of time. Urethral catheters should remain attached to the closed drainage system. Plastic drainage bags make ambulation for these patients possible.

The word ambulate means to move from place to place, to walk. Sitting in a chair is not considered ambulation. After ambulating, the patient may sit in a chair if permitted but should be advised to stand and walk at intervals and to elevate his legs while sitting to prevent venous pooling in the extremities. Sitting in a chair for long periods is to be avoided.

Outcome: *Patient returns to optimal functioning in activities of daily living*

Encouraging the patient to carry out activities of daily living (washing, combing hair, dressing) promotes activity and helps move the patient from a dependent to an independent level. Pain and tiredness are useful criteria in determining when to step in and take over for the patient. Priorities must be set between the need for activity and the need for rest. Family education is important; if the family members do not understand the basis for encouraging the patient to do for himself, the family member may become upset or step in and do for the patient. This may prolong hospitalization and the recovery period.

Psychologic needs

Outcome: *Concerns related to surgery are identified and examined*

Psychologic factors. Some of the concerns that were present in the preoperative period may continue into the postoperative period. These concerns fall into essentially three different categories.

Concerns specific to the surgery performed. Sometimes a patient doubts the information that has been given to him. He may still worry that he has cancer but nobody is telling him the truth. If he does have cancer he may think that it was more extensive than he is being told. He may wonder if he really needed the surgery in the first place.

Concerns over loss of a body part. Surgery frequently means removal of tissue. If an organ such as the uterus or part of the colon is removed or if part of a limb, breast, or face is removed, the patient is faced with a change in self-image (Chapter 28). He may experience grief over the lost part (p. 292). For complete recovery the patient needs to identify his feelings and cope with the changes that he perceives.

Concerns about the future. The patient may have concerns about changes in sexuality, economic status, prognosis, or permanent effects. Sexuality may be threatened by the enforced absence from home or a specific surgery such as a colostomy. These concerns may center around the effect of the surgery on the spouse or parent relationship or on the effect of surgery on sexual performance itself. Economic worries center on loss of income during hospitalization, cost of the surgery, and so forth. Fears also exist relating to prognosis. Is the surgery really going to correct the original problem? Am I going to die? Will the problem recur? Will there be more pain? What permanent effects will occur? How will my life change?

Assessment. Anxieties will be expressed in many different ways. It must be remembered that expressions such as anger, resentfulness, crying, excessive joking, inappropriate laughter, or withdrawal may all be signs of anxiety and are often seen in the postoperative period. Some of these feelings may be projected against the surgeon, nurse, housekeeping aide, food, and so forth.

Intervention. Sitting down and talking with a surgical patient about his concerns is as important a nursing action in many instances as any of the physical activities. Time must be planned for this. If a specific concern is expected, such as sexual functioning after a perineal prostatectomy, the topic may have to be introduced by the nurse who has established rapport with the patient in order to let the patient know that it is permissible to talk about this topic.

Some patients will talk freely about the cancer or the heart operation but never really face their feelings about the surgery. No patient is forced to do so, but the alert nurse will watch for cues that the patient is beginning to move from a cognitive thinking level to a feeling level and may need some support while he is identifying and learning to cope with these feelings.

□ Discharge planning

Discharge planning is an important part of nursing care postoperatively. Plans for the patient's discharge may have been discussed and begun preoperatively, but most of the teaching, arrangements, and preparations are done after surgery. The patient, his family, and the members of the health team responsible for the care of the patient during his hospitalization should participate in the long-range planning. Outcome criteria for the patient at discharge are given on p. 414.

As a result of early resumption of ambulation and a nutritious diet, most patients regain their strength rapidly, and the average hospital stay following surgery is 7 to 10 days. During this time the patient and his family should be prepared for any care that must be given at home, and any necessary arrangements for convalescent care should be completed several days prior to discharge. The patient is helped to become as self-sufficient as possible before being discharged so that he does not have to depend any more than necessary on the assistance of relatives and friends.

After surgery the nurse consults with the physician regarding the anticipated discharge plans for the patient. The nurse assesses the patient's ability to participate in the care to be given at home, the interest and the desire of the family to help, and the home situation and its facilities. Whenever possible both the patient and a member of his family should be taught all treatments and exercises that must be done at home. Sometimes arrangements should be made for a member of the family to come to the hospital to observe and perhaps practice procedures, to talk to the dietitian, to consult with the physician, to discuss problems with the social worker, and to plan with the nurse about home care. The patient and his family should have ample opportunity to ask questions.

The nurse should try to anticipate any problems that might arise and help the patient and his family plan for them. For example, if a colostomy irrigation must be given and there are no bathroom facilities, extra equipment will be necessary so that it can be done in the room available. If the patient is reluctant or unable to give himself an injection, some member of the family must be taught how to give injections or arrangements must be made for a public health nurse to give them. If the patient does not understand English an interpreter may be needed to explain diets, medications, or treatments. If dressings are needed the patient should be given a 48-hour supply to take home unless a family member has already obtained them from the hospital. The patient and his family must know where in the community they can get dressings and other needed materials. If treatment of almost any kind is to be done at home, it is advisable for the nurse to discuss with the surgeon and with the patient the advisability of having a public health nurse visit the patient in his home soon after he leaves the hospital. A written referral should be made, and the report returned by the public health nurse helps the nurse in the hospital to learn how effective her teaching of the patient has been.

If the patient lives alone or has no relatives or friends to care for him, he may need to go to another hospital for further treatment or for terminal care, or he may need nursing home care. Since these institutions usually have long waiting lists and since it takes time to arrange for such transfers, referrals should be made as early as possible. Thus as soon as the need for a specific type of care is established, the physician should discuss it with the patient and family. If the health team includes a social worker, he will explore community resources, present alternate plans (if there are any) for consideration, and help with the referral. Both the patient and the family may need a great deal of support to help them accept the plan that seems best.

On discharge the patient is given an appointment for a follow-up examination in the surgeon's office or in the outpatient department of the hospital. This appointment is usually for 1 to 2 weeks after discharge. The nurse should make sure that the patient understands the importance of returning for the medical examination and that he can make arrangements to come in at this time.

With modern surgical techniques the wound is usually well healed by the time of discharge from the hospital. Therefore the convalescent period usually is relatively short, and most patients may return to their usual activities and occupation within 2 to 4 weeks postoperatively. During this time the patient should rest when he becomes tired and should increase his activity gradually. When the patient visits the physician after discharge, the healing of the wound and the patient's general physical condition are checked. Depending on the outcome of this examination and the type of work the patient does, the surgeon will decide when it will be desirable for the patient to resume his usual activities.

■ OUTCOME CRITERIA FOR THE PATIENT WHO HAS HAD SURGERY

1. No injury has occurred during hospitalization.
2. The incision heals normally without infection.
3. No avoidable complications (atelectasis, pneumonia, thrombophlebitis) have occurred.
4. Elimination patterns are reestablished.
5. The patient carries out activities of daily living at his optimal level of functioning; he may still tire easily.
6. The patient has had an opportunity to explore his concerns.
7. The patient or significant others can explain and carry out any treatments to be carried out at home or medication program resulting from the surgery.
8. The patient or significant others can explain any dietary changes required by the surgery after discharge.
9. The patient or significant others can explain activity limits incurred by the surgery and any exercise programs to be followed at home.
10. The patient or significant others can explain health maintenance or therapeutic follow-up programs; they know where and when the patient is to see the surgeon.
11. The patient or significant others can explain how to obtain any needed professional or community resources.

REFERENCES AND SELECTED READINGS

1. Abram. H. C.: Psychological aspects of surgery, Boston, 1967, Little, Brown and Co.
2. American College of Surgeons: Manual of preoperative and post-operative care, ed. 2, Philadelphia, 1971, W. B. Saunders Co.
3. Anderson, H. C.: Newton's geriatric nursing, ed. 5, St. Louis, 1971, The C. V. Mosby Co.
4. Auld, M., Craven, R., and West, J.: Wound healing, Nurs. 72 2:36-40, 1972.
5. Bakutis, A.,: Anesthetic reactions, Nurs. '72 **2**:16-19, 1972.
6. Ballinger, W. F., Treybal, J. C., and Vose, A. B.: Alexander's care of the patient in surgery, ed. 5, St. Louis, 1972, The C. V. Mosby Co.
7. *Barnett, L. A.: Preparing your patient for the operating room, A.O.R.N. J **18**:534-539, 1973.
8. Bastasaraswathi, K. and El-Etr, A. A.: Preoperative evaluation of drug history, A.O.R.N. J. **23**:616;620, 1976.
9. Beal, J. M., et al.: Intensive and recovery room care, New York, 1969, Macmillin, Inc.
10. Belleville, J., et al.: Influence of age on pain relief from analgesics, J.A.M.A. **217**:1835-1841, 1971.
11. Bergersen, B. A., and Goth, A.: Pharmacology in nursing, ed. 14, St. Louis, 1979, The C. V. Mosby Co.
12. *Berry, E. C., and Kohn, M. F.: Introduction to operating room technique, ed. 4, New York, 1972, McGraw-Hill Book Co.
13. *Betschman, L. L.: Handbook of recovery room nursing, Philadelphia, 1967, F. A. Davis Co.
14. *Blackwell, A., and Blackwell, W.: Relieving gas pain, Am. J. Nurs. **75**:1474-1475, 1975.
15. *Brinling, T.: Tearing down a wall, Am. J. Nurs. **71**:1406-1409, 1971.
16. *Brownsberger, C.: Emotional stress connected with surgery, Nurs. Forum **4**:46-55, 1965.
17. Bushnell, S. S.: Respiratory intensive care nursing, Boston, 1973, Little Brown and Co.
18. *Castillo, P.: Care of the patient under local anesthia, A.O.R.N. J. **18**:283-285, 1973.
19. *Castle, M.: Wound care, Nurs. '75 **5**:40-44, 1975.
20. Clark, R. B.: The case for spinal anesthesia, Am. J. Nurs. **67**:294-297, 1967.
21. Codd, J., and Grohar, M.: Postoperative pulmonary complications, Nurs. Clin. North Am. **10**:5-15, 1975.
22. *Collart, M. E., and Brenneman, J. K.: Preventing postoperative atelectasis, Am. J. Nurs. **71**:1982-1987, 1971.
23. Creighton, H.: Law every nurse should know, ed. 3, Philadelphia, 1975, W. B. Saunders Co.
24. Cullen, S., and Larson, C. P.: Essentials of anesthetic practice, Chicago, 1974, Year Book Medical Publishers, Inc.
25. *Damsteegt, D.: Pastoral roles in presurgical visits, Am. J. Nurs. **75**:1336-1337, 1975.
26. Denny, J., and Denson, J.: Risk of surgery in patients over 90, Geriatrics **27**:115-118, 1972.
27. Dickler, D. J., Friedman, P. L., and Susman, I. C.: Intravenous regional anesthesia with chloroprocaine, Anesthesiology **26**:244-245, 1965.
28. Dripps, R. D., Eckenhoff, J. E., and Bandam, L. D.: Introduction to anesthesia ed. 5, Philadelphia, 1977, W. B. Saunders Co.
29. Dumas, R. G., and Leonard, R. C.: The effect of nursing on the incidence of postoperative vomiting, Nurs. Res. **12**:12-15, 1963.

*References preceded by an asterisk are particularly well suited for student reading.

30. Egbert, L. D., Battit, G. E., Welch, C. E., et al.: Reduction of postoperative pain by encouragement and instruction of patients: a study of doctor-patient rapport, N. Engl. J. Med. **270**:825-827, 1964.
31. Eisele, J. H.: Recognizing and treating respiratory problems in the surgical patient, A.O.R.N. J. **17**:80-87, 1973.
32. Fay, M. R.: Nursing process in the recovery room. A.O.R.N. J. **24**:1069-1075, 1976.
33. Felton, G., Huss, K., Payne, E. A., et al.: Preoperative nursing intervention with the patient for surgery: outcomes of three alternative approaches, Int. J. Nurs. Stud. **13**:83-96, 1976.
34. *Field, L. W.: Identifying the psychological aspects of the surgical patient, A.O.R.N. J. **17**:86-90, 1973.
35. Fitzmaurice, J. B., and Sashara, A. A.: Current concepts of pulmonary embolism: implications for nursing practice, Heart Lung **3**:209-218, 1974.
36. Fochtman, D., and Raffensperger, J. G.: Principles of nursing care for the pediatric surgery patient, ed. 2, Boston, 1976, Little, Brown, and Co.
37. Fortin, F., and Kirovac, S.: A randomized controlled trial of preoperative patient education, Int. J. Nurs. Stud. **13**:11-24, 1976.
38. *Garrett, J.: Oliguria in postoperative patients, Nurs. Clin. North Am. **10**:59-67, 1975.
39. Ginsberg, R., et al.: A manual of operating room technology, Philadelphia, 1966, J. B. Lippincott Co.
40. Goodman L. S., and Gillman, A.: The pharmacological basis of therapeutics ed. 5, New York, 1975, Macmillan, Inc.
41. *Gordon, M.: Assessing activity tolerance, Am. J. Nurs. **76**:72-76, 1976.
42. Goth, A.: Medical pharmacology: principles and concepts, ed. 9, St. Louis, 1978, The C. V. Mosby Co.
43. *Gruendemann, B.: The impact of surgery on body image, Nurs. Clin. North Am. **10**:635-643, 1975.
44. Guyton, A.: Textbook of medical physiology, ed. 5, Philadelphia, 1977, W. B. Saunders Co.
45. *Halsell, M.: Moist heat for relief of postoperative pain, Am. J. Nurs. **67**:767-770, 1967.
46. Hanamey, R.: Teaching patients breathing and coughing techniques, Nurs. Outlook **13**:58-59, 1965.
47. *Harris, W. H., Slater, E. M., and Bell, H. M.: Regional anesthesia by the intravenous route, J.A.M.A. **194**:1273-1276, 1965.
48. *Healy, K. M.: Does preoperative instruction make a difference? Am. J. Nurs. **68**:62-67, 1968.
49. Johnson, J. F., Dabbs, J. M., Jr., and Leventhal, H.: Psychosocial factors in the welfare of surgical patients, Nurs. Res. **19**:18-29, 1970.
50. *Johnston, M.: Outcome criteria to evaluate postoperative respiratory status, Am. J. Nurs. **75**:1474-1475, 1975.
51. *Knudsen, K.: Play therapy: preparing the young child for surgery, Nurs. Clin. North Am. **10**:679-686, 1975.
52. Laird, M.: Techniques for teaching pre- and postoperative patients, Am. J. Nurs. **75**:1338-1340, 1975.
53. LeMaitre, G., and Finnigan, J. A.: The patient in surgery, ed. 3, Philadelphia, 1975, W. B. Saunders Co.
54. *Libman, R. H.: Relieving airway obstruction in the recovery room, Am. J. Nurs. **75**:603-625, 1975.
55. Lindeman, C. A., and Van Aerman, B. H.: Nursing intervention with the presurgical patient: the effects of structured and unstructured preoperative teaching, Nurs. Res. **20**:319-332, 1971.
56. *Lipman, M.: Informed consent and the nurse's role, RN **35**:50, 1972.
57. Lisboa, J. M.: Role of the special care unit nurse in a preoperative teaching program, Nurs. Clin. North Am. **7**:389-395, 1972.

58. Litsky, B.: Infection control and hospital design. Sup. Nurse 3:23, 1972.
59. *Luciana, K.: The who, when, where, what and how of preparing children for surgery, Nurs. '74 **4**:64-65. 1974.
60. Mason, J., Gau, F., and Bryne, M.: General surgery. In Steinberg, F. U., editor: Cowdry's the care of the geriatric patient, ed. 5, St. Louis, 1976, The C. V. Mosby Co.
61. *McConnell, E. A.: Meeting with special needs of diabetics facing surgery, Nurs. '76 **6**:30-37, June 1976.
62. *McConnell, E. A.: After surgery, Nurs. '77 **7**:32-39, 1977.
63. McCredie, J. A., editor: Basic surgery, New York, 1977, Macmillan, Inc.
64. *Metheny, N.: Water and electrolyte balance in the postoperative patient, Nurs. Clin. North Am. **10**:49-57, 1975.
65. Mezzanotee, E. J.: Group instruction in preparation for surgery, Am. J. Nurs. **70**:89-91, 1970.
66. *Minckley, B. A.: Physiologic hazards of position changes in the anesthesized patient, Am. J. Nurs. **69**:2606-2611, 1969.
67. *Mitchell, J. A., and Cragin, C. L.: Informed consent: a doctor's dilemma, A.O.R.N. J. **18**:810-826, 1973.
68. Mitchell, M. A.: An RR experience: as nurse and patient say it, RN **38**:46-47, 1975.
69. *Moore, C., and Marion, R.: Working with children and their families to help them through a long-anticipated surgical experience. In Bergersen, B., Anderson, E. H., Duffey, M., and Lohr, M., editors: Current concepts in clinical nursing, vol. 2, St. Louis, 1969, The C. V. Mosby Co.
70. Morgan, D.: Prepared patients make faster surgical recovery, Can. Hosp. **50**:45-49, 1973.
71. Murphy, J. W., Riu, R., and Ponka, J. L.: Local anesthesia for gastric surgery in aged patients, J. Am. Geriatr. Soc. **16**:673-679, 1968.
72. *Nielson, M. A.: Intra-arterial monitoring of blood pressure, Am. J. Nurs. **74**:48-53, 1974.
73. *Nursing care of the patient in the O.R., Somerville, N.J., 1972, Ethicon Co.
74. Olson, E. V., et al.: The hazards of immobility, Am. J. Nurs. **67**:779-797, 1967.
75. *Parsons, M. C., and Stephens, G.: Postoperative complications: assessment and intervention, Am. J. Nurs. **74**:240-244, 1974.
76. *Patrick H.: Electrical hazards in the operating room. A.O.R.N. J. **18**:1127-1130, 1973.
77. Peacock, E. E., and Van Winkle, W.: Wound repair, ed. 2, Philadelphia, 1976, W. B. Saunders Co.
78. Powell, M.: An environment for wound healing, Am. J. Nurs. **72**:1862-1865, 1972.
78a. *Rhodes, M., Gruendemann, B. J., and Ballinger, W. F.: Alexander's care of the patient in surgery, ed. 6, St. Louis, 1978, The C. V. Mosby Co.
79. *Ross, R.: Wound healing, Sci. Am. **220**:40-50, 1969.
80. Sabiston, D. C., editor: Davis-Christopher's textbook of surgery, ed. 11, Philadelphia, 1977, W. B. Saunders Co.
81. Saylor, D.: Understanding presurgical anxiety, A.O.R.N. J. **22**:624-636, 1975.
82. Schmitt, F. E., and Woolridge, P. J.: Psychological preparation of surgical patients, Nurs. Res. **22**:108-116, 1973.
83. *Schwab, Sister M.: Caring for the aged, Am. J. Nurs. **73**:2049-2053, 1973.
84. Schwarz, S., et al.: Principles of surgery, Ed. 2, New York, 1974, McGraw-Hill Book Co.
85. Scully, H. F., and Martin, S. J.: Anesthetic management for geriatric patients, Am. J. Nurs. **65**:110-112, 1965.
86. Shaw, W. M.: Positional control of immediate postanesthetic vomiting, Anesthesiology **26**:359, 1965.
87. *Smith, R. B., Petruscak, J., and Solosko, D.: In a recovery room, Am. J. Nurs. **73**:70-73, 1973.
88. Smith, R. M.: Anesthesia for infants and children, ed. 3, St. Louis, 1968, The C. V. Mosby Co.
89. Starving children before operation, Br. Med. J. **3**:213-216, 1974.
90. *Strauss, R. J., et al.: Operative risks of obese patients: nursing care, A.O.R.N. J. **25**:1053-1057, 1977.
91. *Symposium on perspectives in operating room nursing, Nurs. Clin. North Am. **10**:613-686, 1975.
92. *Symposium on postoperative nursing care, Nurs. Clin. North Am. **10**:1-67, 1975.
93. Thomas, D.: Hypoglycemia in children before operation: its incidence and prevention, Br. J. Anesthesiol. **46**:66-68, 1974.
94. Tinker, J., and Wehner, R.: Postoperative recovery and the neuromuscular juntion, Am. J. Nurs. **74**:74-75, 1974.
95. Travelbee, J.: Interpersonal aspects of nursing, ed. 2, Philadelphia, 1971, F. A. Davis Co.
96. Vain, E.: Obesity in surgery, A.O.R.N. J. **16**:85-88, 1972.
97. Walter, C. W.: Safe electric environment in the hospital, Bull. Am. Coll. Surg. **54**:4, 1969.
98. Weiler, Sister C. M.: Postoperative patients evaluate preoperative instruction, Am. J. Nurs, **68**:1464-1467, 1968.
99. *William, J., et al.: The psychological control of preoperative anxiety, Psychophysiology **12**:50-54, 1975.
100. Williams, S. R.: Nutrition and diet therapy, ed. 3, St. Louis, 1977, The C. V. Mosby Co.
101. Willig, S. H.: The nurse's guide to the law, New York, 1970, McGraw-Hill Book Co.
102. *Winslow, E., and Fuhs, M.: Preoperative assessment for postoperative evaluation, Am. J. Nurs. **73**:1372-1374, 1973.
103. *Wolfer, J. A., and Davis, C. E.: Assessment of surgical patients: preoperative emotional condition and postoperative welfare, Nurs. Res. **19**:402-414, 1970.
104. Wolfer, J. A., and Visintainer, M.: Pediatric surgical patients and parents' stress responses and adjustments, Nurs. Res. **24**:244-245, 1975.
105. Wound care, Postgrad. Med. **55**:171-177, 1974.
106. Wylie, W. D., and Churchill-Davidson, H. C.: A practice of anesthesia, ed. 3, Chicago, 1972, Year Book Medical Publishers, Inc.
107. *Zepernick, R. G.: New trends in anesthesia, Nurs. Forum **4**:41-45, 1965.

24

Trauma: emergencies and disasters

BARBARA C. LONG

There are many different situations in which a nurse is called on to provide emergency care to persons experiencing a health crisis. A number of books are available that deal with this topic alone (see references). The purpose of this chapter is to identify major points in the delivery of emergency care, assessment and interventions of common emergencies, and principles of management in disasters.

■ TRAUMA AS A STRESSOR

The physiologic and psychologic responses of the person experiencing accidental trauma are the same as those resulting from surgery, since both involve body trauma (see Chapter 23). The "fight-flight" response of the neuroendocrine system enables the body to fight off or flee from the situation causing the trauma. Thus the effectiveness of the body to cope with the stressor(s) determines the person's response to the emergency situation. When there is massive trauma such as that occurring in a severe motor vehicle accident, the stressors are multiple and the effectiveness of coping responses is decreased (see Chapter 71).

■ EPIDEMIOLOGIC DATA

Accidents in the United States claim over 100,000 lives each year. Of these deaths 45% are due to motor vehicle accidents.[67] There has been a significant trend in recent years to decreased mortality from motor vehicle accidents, thought by some to be due to the 55-mph speed limits on highways. Accidents remain one of the leading causes of death (9% of all deaths), exceeded only by heart disease, cancer, and strokes in adults.[5] Accidents are the leading cause of death in children.

In terms of morbidity, approximately *60 million* persons are injured in the United States every year, or about 30 of every 100 persons. Approximately 13% are injured at work, 37% at home, and 50% in motor vehicle accidents.[67] Millions of dollars are spent annually on medical expenses, property damage, and administrative costs related to accidents. Money lost from potential earnings or disability adds to this figure.

Accidents that result in injury or death involve human suffering that cannot be measured in dollars and includes pain, long-term rehabilitation, disabilities (temporary or permanent), loss and grief, and family disruption. Accidents are for the most part preventable and require attention of health care professionals not only as to their causes and the environment in which they occur but also to the victim's physical, social, and psychologic state and his readiness to avoid accidents.

■ DELIVERY OF EMERGENCY CARE

Health crises that demand immediate interventions can occur anywhere—in the home, other parts of the community, or in the hospital itself. The nurse may be the sole giver of care until medical care is available, or the nurse may be working with other paramedical personnel.

□ Community

In recent years there has been increased awareness by communities of inadequacies in the delivery of emergency care. In the past, persons who usually responded to emergency calls were either police or drivers from funeral homes who also doubled as private ambulance drivers. The preparation for care of the injured varied from nothing to elementary first-aid training. Victims who might have survived if more advanced care had been available have died on the way to a hospital.

Many communities are now preparing and utilizing emergency medical technicians (EMTs) or paramedics to respond to emergency calls. EMTs have had preparation beyond basic first-aid training but do not carry out intrusive procedures. Paramedics have had more training than EMTs and can carry out such skills as starting intravenous fluids, giving medications, and defibrillation. The preparedness of personnel responding to emergency calls and the responsibilities that are legally permissible vary among states and communities within each state.

The National Safety Act of 1966 requires each county to appoint an emergency medical care committee. The effectiveness of these committees varies greatly, influenced to a large extent by citizen interest and political activity.[73] Every community needs an organized emergency care system with support and input from community health organizations and community political elements. Once an organization is established there should be continued evaluation of the effectiveness of the emergency care provided. Nurses should become actively involved in all phases of activities that can influence the level of emergency care in their own communities.

The American Heart Association has been instrumental in developing a program to educate large numbers of persons who are certified to administer cardiopulmonary resuscitation (CPR). This increases the possibility of a trained person being available to initiate resuscitation early in a larger number of emergency situations.

□ Hospitals

Hospitals that receive financial support from government sources are required to provide emergency departments open to the public. In many emergency departments more than half of the persons seeking medical attention are not actually in need of emergency care. These are persons who do not have a private physician or are unable to obtain the services of their physician at the hour or day when they feel they need medical attention. Persons requiring immediate care are treated first. If there are a large number of patients, those with nonacute symptoms often have to wait a considerable time. Newer approaches to delivery of both emergency and nonacute health care are being explored.

Many emergency departments have direct radio communication with rescue personnel in the community. Treatment can be initiated at the site of injury under medical direction and hospital personnel can be better prepared to receive the injured. This helps to eliminate some of the delays in initiation of care.

The role of the nurse in the emergency department has changed considerably in recent years due to the increased utilization of emergency departments by persons seeking medical attention and the increased sophistication of therapeutic management. Emergency department (ED) nurses are developing skills in assessment and *triage* (sorting patients to determine priority of need for medical attention); in management of persons with high levels of anxiety; and in carrying out specialized technical skills such as initiating parenteral fluids, defibrillation, resuscitation, intubation, or operating monitoring devices, and interpreting selected laboratory findings and electrocardiograms and acting on these findings.

■ LEGAL ASPECTS OF EMERGENCY CARE

Nurses who intervene to assist victims in an emergency situation should be aware of the legal ramifications that can ensue as a result of their actions. Many states have enacted "Good Samaritan" laws in an effort to protect health personnel who aid accident victims. These laws vary in coverage among states as to the classes of people who are protected from liability, types of situations, geographic limits, and extent of immunity.[28] The classification of persons covered varies in specificity from any person who stops at the scene of an accident to only those registered nurses licensed in that state. Thus in the latter situation giving nursing care in an emergency situation could be construed in that state to practicing nursing without a license. One state (Vermont) allows criminal penalties for failure to stop and give assistance, although the victim cannot sue if the nurse fails to stop.

Good Samaritan laws serve to identify in statutory language those persons or situations that provide some degree of immunity from liability, many of which already exist by common law. Persons are judged as not liable unless they act willfully with gross negligence.[28] Negligence is the key word. Negligence, according to common law, involves four concepts: duty, breach of duty, damage, and proximal cause.[28] In an emergency a nurse is not dutybound to stop and render aid (except in Vermont) unless the nurse was the cause of the accident. The moral issue of whether to stop and render aid is the nurse's decision. If the nurse does render aid, then duty is implied and failure to continue rendering aid until the victim is released to another competent person can result in breach of duty (abandonment). Some Good Samaritan laws permit releasing the care of the victim to a qualified ambulance attendant (EMT). Damage must occur if negligence is to be proved, and the actions of the nurse must be the proximal cause of the damage.

"Reasonable care" provided by the nurse at the scene of an accident is usually judged as that care given by another similar nurse *under the prevailing situation*. Thus the care provided on a back road on a dark rainy night would not be judged the same as that given in an emergency room. In an emergency situation a nurse can perform medical acts to save life. It may be necessary later, however, to prove that a true emergency did exist. Good Samaritan laws will not protect the nurse in this situation.[23] Malpractice and liability claims can be filed even if Good Samaritan laws exist.

■ PREVENTION OF ACCIDENTS

Accident prevention is a major public health goal, and both the Public Health Service and the American

Public Health Association (APHA) are active in promoting accident prevention. Community groups can be helpful in investigating accident statistics in their local area and in disseminating information to encourage accident prevention. Nurses have an important role in accident prevention, both through their roles as professionals and as residents of a community. The influence of nurses can be extended in many areas because nurses are represented in schools, industry, community nursing programs, and hospitals.

There are a number of resources for information concerning accident prevention. The *Statistical Abstracts* published by the U.S. Bureau of the Census is a helpful reference. Local health departments can provide local data, health education materials, and other resource materials. Engineers can be a valuable resource for consultation on safety hazards in the home, hospital, or community.

□ Home

Accidents in and about the home cause almost one third of all accidental deaths each year. Falls account for about half the number, and fires, burns, and poisonings account for most of the remainder. Many aged persons who fall do so when walking from room to room. Some fall because of heavily waxed floors, loose rugs, poor lighting, scattered toys, and other conditions that could have been corrected. People fall from roofs, windows, high ladders,and steps and are fatally burned or otherwise injured while using solvents and cleansing agents without proper knowledge of their hazards.

The number of electric appliances used in the home has increased the danger of electric shock and fire from overloaded circuits. Many persons die in fires caused by burning cigarette ashes dropped on furniture or rugs or discarded in waste containers and by cigarettes that are dropped as the smoker falls asleep. Attention needs to be given to teaching homeowners with older heating systems to have the equipment checked periodically for gas leaks and other unsafe features. All persons in a household should be aware of what to do in the event of fire, and fire evacuation drills are encouraged.

Homes with young children should be made as accident-proof as possible. Prevention of poisoning is discussed on p. 427. Safety rules should be taught to children at an early age. Children sustain injuries during their play and exploring activities. The possibility of child abuse must be considered, however, when children, especially those under the age of 3 years, are seen with injuries such as bruises, fractures, or burns. When child abuse is suspected, health care professionals have a responsibility to protect the child from further injury by reporting their suspicions. At the same time it is important that help be sought for the parent or parents involved. In several communities, groups have been organized for parents who are child abusers. Since it has been found that most parents who abuse their children were abused as children themselves, this form of group therapy is often helpful in assisting parents to ventilate deep-seated feelings. Information about local groups can be obtained from child welfare agencies. One group working in this area is CALM (Child Abuse and Listening Mediation, Inc.), located in California.* Another group, Parents Anonymous, has local chapters in many cities.

The community health nurse has an opportunity to assess safety hazards during home visits and to teach not only the client but also members of the family about general accident prevention as well as specific measures for the safety of the ill person.

□ Community

Community action can best be effected by group action, but it often takes persistent individuals to interest and stimulate group action. Parent-teacher associations, recreational associations, and religious and social groups are usually interested in accident control. Support by governmental groups is important. Efforts should be made to use existing agencies and groups and to work with them in order that the sincere efforts of small groups of enthusiastic citizens will not be dissipated. Phases of accident prevention that should be of community interest include (1) teaching of accident prevention in the public schools, (2) better control and inspection of homes for the aged and prisons, (3) rigid enforcement of driving regulations, (4) improvement of street lighting and traffic signals at busy intersections, (5) periodic inspection of all automobiles, and (6) promotion of laws pertaining to fire-proofing of buildings and laws protecting the public from flammable clothing, potentially harmful toys, and similar items.

□ Hospital

Assessing the need for safety in the general environment and for the safety of specific patients and taking measures to prevent injury are important functions of the nurse. The nurse can participate in policy making and safety monitoring through membership on hospital safety committees.

Falls

The major cause of hospital-incurred injury is falling. Hospitalized persons are in unfamiliar surroundings with strange furniture and equipment, may be weak for many reasons, or may become confused, all of which may contribute to falls. Elderly persons are at high risk for falls.

---

*P.O. Box 718, Santa Barbara, Calif. 93102.

All patients should be assessed for the potential of falling, and preventive measures should be instituted.

The following safety measures help to prevent falls. Handrails in hospital corridors and in bathrooms give weak persons something to hold onto for support. Chairs with arms are safer than armless chairs. Stools in showers and adjacent to tubs provide safety for patients who become tired or who develop hypotension from vasodilation. There should be call systems in the bathrooms and lounges as well as at the patient's bedside. Hi-Lo beds should be used whenever possible, and the bed should be in low position when the patient is ambulatory.

Elderly persons often become confused at night, a time when sensory input is decreased. Sedation may increase the confusion. A night light in the room can be useful for sensory input. The bed should be in low position; in the event that the patient attempts to climb out of bed, the bed will be at the same height as his bed at home. The use of the side rails is a nursing decision. Side rails should be kept raised for all infants and unconscious patients. A confused patient may attempt to climb over the side rail and thus have farther to fall; a jacket restraint may be more useful.

Patients who are weak may need frequent reminders to seek assistance before ambulating. Some patients do not want to "bother the nurse" and attempt to walk to the bathroom unaided, especially at night. All patients should use supportive slippers; paper slippers can be a hazard.

Fire

All hospital and nursing homes must have established fire-prevention routines and all personnel must be familiar with these routines. Participation in fire drills should be taken seriously and evaluation should follow each drill.

Fires usually occur due to smoking or to faulty electrical equipment. Since smoking is also hazardous to one's health, many hospitals are restricting smoking in patient's rooms and in many public areas. If smoking is permitted in the patient's room, ashtrays should be available and the patient and visitors instructed about not emptying them. Patients who are careless smokers or who may drop a cigarette or ash are to be monitored while smoking. Faulty electrical equipment is not used. Any questions about smoke should be investigated and reported immediately.

If a fire should occur, the nurse in charge who is most familiar with the patients' conditions should be in charge of any evacuation. Until evacuation is necessary, the doors and windows of all patient rooms are closed. If evacuation is deemed advisable, patients closest to the fire are evacuated to the opposite end of the floor (horizontal evacuation), then downward by the stairway (vertical evacuation) if necessary. Death usually occurs from inhaling the superheated air. Doors that are excessively hot should not be opened. The rescuer should keep as low as possible and, if necessary, use wet cloths around the nose and mouth if the air is hot.

Infection

Prevention of infection is another preventive safety measure. Good aseptic technique, including frequent handwashing, is especially important to help prevent hospital-acquired (nosocomial) infection (see Chapter 21).

■ ASSESSMENT

When an emergency occurs or on arriving at the emergency scene, it is important to assess the situation, the patient, and the environment before initiating action. Some conclusions can be drawn from the immediate environment. If there is multiple trauma, all victims should be assessed before any but lifesaving interventions are initiated. Overt clues such as an automobile accident, report of falling, or ingestion of poison can give direction to probable types of injuries. A complete head-to-toe assessment is carried out, if possible, before moving the victim so that additional injuries or conditions requiring intervention can be identified.

PRIORITY ASSESSMENT

Level of consciousness
Response to voice and touch

Respiratory status*
Presence of respirations
Respiration rate, depth, and character
Use of accessory muscles for breathing
Presence of foreign body, vomitus, loose dentures in mouth
Cyanosis

Circulatory status*
Presence of carotid pulse
Pulse rate, strength, rhythm
Skin color, temperature, moisture
Presence of hemorrhage

Pupils
Equal or unequal
Dilated or constricted
Response to light

Medic alert tag
Presence if victim unconscious

*Respiratory and circulatory status are assessed simultaneously.

□ Data collection

A person who is not breathing, who has no palpable pulse, or who is hemorrhaging needs immediate assistance. Obtaining data to identify these circumstances is the first priority in assessment (see box, p. 420). This is sometimes referred to as the ABCs of emergency assessment (*a*irway, *b*reathing, *c*irculation). Assessing the general level of consciousness can be done as the approach is made to the victim. The carotid pulse can be checked at the same time as breathing is checked. If pulse and breathing are absent, cardiopulmonary resuscitation is initiated.

Hemorrhage is treated with direct pressure to the wound, and if shock is present the legs are assessed, then elevated if there are no signs of fracture. The victim is protected from chilling. Before the victim is moved or turned, it is important to assess for possible fracture of the neck and spine (see box).

Before starting the head-to-toe assessment, observe the victim's general position, any obvious deformities or asymmetry, or any purposeful movements. Ask him to indicate any pain or discomfort and assess these areas first. During the overall assessment continue to monitor for changes in level of consciousness and respiratory status. Ask the victim or any relatives or friends present to describe the preceding events; the presence of any medical conditions such as heart or lung disease, epilepsy, or diabetes; or any special medications taken by the victim that may have a bearing on the present situation.

If there is more than one person on the scene, the nurse or paramedic should remain with the victim while others are given directions to assess the environment for additional signs of danger and to call for any needed transportation.

HEAD-TO-TOE ASSESSMENT

Head and neck

- Assess pupils
- Examine ears, nose, mouth for bleeding, other drainage, foreign body
- Palpate* cervical spine for pain (do not move head)
- Examine head for bleeding, lacerations, contusions, depression of skull
- Palpate jaw for fracture (pain, deformity)
- Ask about stiffness of neck (if no history of trauma, assess movement)
- Examine neck for distended neck veins, presence of tracheal stoma, tracheal deviation

Chest and spine

- Palpate clavicles for fracture (pain, deformity)
- Examine chest for external injury
- Observe chest movements for symmetry of expansion and character of respirations
- Palpate ribs for fracture (pain)
- Palpate spine for point tenderness (do not move victim)

Abdomen and pelvis

- Palpate pelvis for pain in groin when pressure applied over pelvis
- Ask about abdominal pain
- Examine abdomen for external injury, rigidity, distention

Extremities

- Examine for signs of external injury
- Ask about pain in extremities
- If no obvious injury, ask victim to move each limb
- Test for sensation in each limb
- Assess presence and strength of peripheral pulses

*All palpations should be carried out gently.

□ Data analysis

Patient data

Level of consciousness. Determine whether the person responds immediately to voice and touch, responds only to painful stimuli, or does not respond. Unconsciousness may be due to many causes (see box, p. 422).

When shock or respiratory insufficiency occurs, there is decreased oxygenation of the brain, either because there is insufficient amount of blood to carry the oxygen or because there is decreased oxygen taken in. This can lead to loss of consciousness, and the pupils will be equal and may be dilated.

When unconsciousness occurs because of the effect of drugs or chemicals, the pupils are equal and may be constricted or dilated depending on the effect of the specific drug. Information from relatives may elicit data concerning history of diabetes, liver or kidney disease, and medication taken by the victim. Environmental data such an empty pill container can be useful in the identification of unconsciousness from drug overdose.

If there has been trauma to the brain, it is important to ascertain level of consciousness at different times. Temporary loss of consciousness followed by alertness and equal pupils usually indicates a concussion. If there is no skull fracture present, the patient is simply observed for 24 hours. Alertness after injury followed by increasing loss of consciousness usually indicates an intracranial hematoma. The pupils are usually *unequal.* Medical attention is urgent if an intracranial hematoma is suspected. The pupils may also be unequal if the patient has had a cerebral vascular accident (stroke).

An unconscious person should be placed in a position that facilitates patency of the airway (side-lying position

POSSIBLE CAUSES OF UNCONSCIOUSNESS

Hypoxia (decreased oxygen to brain)
1. Respiratory insufficiency
   - Airway obstruction from foreign body, secretions
   - Pneumothorax
   - Spinal cord injury
2. Shock
   - Cardiogenic: cardiac arrest
   - Hypovolemic: hemorrhage

Metabolic (chemical brain depressants)
1. Extrinsic
   a. Drugs: alcohol, narcotics, barbiturates, antihistamines, tranquilizers
   b. Poisons: carbon monoxide, carbon tetrachloride, hydrocarbons, methane gas
2. Intrinsic
   a. Ketones: diabetic ketoacidosis, starvation
   b. Glucose: hypo-, hyperglycemia
   c. Ammonia: liver failure
   d. Urea: kidney failure
   e. Hormonal hypofunction: hypothyroidism, Addison disease
   f. Electrolyte imbalance: sodium, potassium, calcium, hydrogen ions

Brain pathology
1. Trauma: concussion, brainstem contusion, intracranial hematoma
2. Seizures: epilepsy, tumors, idiopathology
3. Cerebral vascular accident: cerebral hemorrhage, thrombosis
4. Tumors: benign, malignant
5. Infections: meningitis, encephalitis

is preferred unless contraindicated), and the respiratory status should be constantly monitored (see Chapter 27).

Respirations. Noisy breathing characterized by wheezing or stridor is caused by air flowing through a narrowed passage. Edema of the air passages or partial obstruction by the tongue or a foreign body may be the cause. Bronchospasm secondary to an allergic response or to asthma also can cause wheezing and stridor. If obstruction is severe or if the victim is in need of oxygen because of circulatory collapse, breathing will be labored and gasping, neck muscles will be prominent, and accessory muscles of breathing will be utilized. During shock, respirations will be rapid and are usually shallow. Kussmaul respiration, or air hunger, is seen with metabolic acidosis, as occurs with diabetic ketoacidosis. If sputum is present and is frothy and blood tinged, fracture of the ribs with lung injury is suspected. This also occurs with pulmonary edema and pulmonary embolus.

Shock. Victims who sustain major trauma or a major stressor to the system such as a myocardial infarction usually develop shock (p. 214). Signs of shock include restlessness, pale cold moist skin, rapid thready pulse, and rapid shallow respirations. Nausea and vomiting may occur. With anaphylactic shock the victim may complain of itching or burning of the skin, a tightness in the chest, and difficulty in breathing. Wheals may develop on the skin, and the face and tongue may develop edema (see Chapter 14).

Sensation and movement. Pain following trauma usually indicates severe tissue contusion or possible fracture. The painful area should be examined gently and carefully. Pain may occur with tissue anoxia, such as with obstruction of blood vessels or frostbite. Loss of sensation in a painful limb may be due to obstruction of a main artery. Loss of sensation below a suspected fracture indicates possible nerve damage. Loss of sensation in a limb in the absence of pain and with loss of movement occurs with injury to the spinal cord or following a cerebral hemorrhage. Injury to the abdominal viscera may produce abdominal pain and rigidity of abdominal muscles.

Behavioral manifestations. Trauma is a stressful event, and victims and significant others respond in many different ways when accidental trauma occurs. No one really knows how he or she will respond until the situation occurs. The exhibited behavior is not always proportional to the degree of injury (p. 423). The behavior of bystanders may interfere with the assessment being carried out, and if so these persons may be given small tasks to do such as setting out flares or searching for drug bottles.

Other data

Analysis of the data should include the type of injury or medical emergency that has probably occurred, the urgency of the need for medical attention, the availability of resources for carrying out necessary interventions, the availability of transportation, and the time factor before medical attention can be obtained. For example, the type of interventions that will be carried out for someone with a fractured tibia when splints are available and an ambulance is standing by for transportation to a nearby hospital are quite different than if the same injury occurs during a wilderness hiking expedition.

■ INTERVENTION

□ General intervention

Outcome: *Lifesaving measures are instituted immediately in an attempt to restore breathing and circulation; further injury does not occur*

Some general principles of management when accidental injuries or sudden illnesses occur serve as guidelines when giving first aid:

1. Remain calm and think before acting.
2. Identify oneself as a nurse to victim and bystanders.
3. Do a rapid assessment for *priority* data (cessation of breathing or heartbeat, hemorrhage, poisoning).
4. Carry out lifesaving measures as indicated by the priority assessment.
5. Do a head-to-toe assessment before initiating general first-aid measures.
6. Keep the victim lying down or in the position in which he is found (unless orthopnea present), protected from dampness or cold.
7. If victim is conscious, explain what is occurring. Assure him that help will be given.
8. Avoid unnecessary handling or moving of the victim; move him only if danger is present.
9. Do not give fluids if there is possibility of abdominal injury or if anesthesia will be necessary within a short time.
10. Do not transport victim until all first-aid measures have been carried out and appropriate transportation is available.

Lifesaving measures (described on succeeding pages) are carried out first when the initial assessment indicates that breathing or circulatory difficulties are present or that poisoning has occurred. After breathing has been reestablished and excessive bleeding controlled, other interventions are carried out when the head-to-toe assessment is completed.

Victims are kept in a supine or sitting position, depending on symptoms, until all necessary interventions are carried out. Wounds are covered and fractures splinted before the victim is transported. Since shock is a possibility when major injuries occur, the victim should be protected from chilling. On a cold day he will need protection underneath him and enough covering to keep him warm but not hot. The goal is to prevent vasodilation while promoting conservation of body warmth. Oral fluids are only given to a conscious person showing signs of shock if there will be a considerable delay before medical care can be obtained and if abdominal injury is not present.

Psychologic needs of victims and significant others

Accidental trauma can be a threat to life and there is a potential threat of pain and disability. The victim may be concerned about economic problems such as the cost of medical care and loss of time from work. Accidental trauma is therefore anxiety producing. In addition many persons have been found to have already been experiencing some other temporary anxiety and were under stress immediately prior to the time of the accident.[8]

The very nature of the experiences following the emergency contribute additional anxieties. The victim is transported, perhaps by strangers, in an ambulance to a hospital emergency department. Significant others are relegated to long periods in a waiting room with little information provided. The victim sees or hears other persons who are upset. He may be alone. He may wait for long periods for medical attention while other higher priority victims are receiving care and for results of tests or treatment. Small incidents become blown out of proportion and a casual remark may be misinterpreted. Five minutes can seem like an hour.

Health personnel who work with accident victims from the primary point of input into the health care system until the emergency is over are prepared to meet the physical life-threatening needs. Because these needs assume priority, it is not difficult to overlook the psychologic needs of the victim and significant others. A calm, interested approach that conveys concern to the victim as a person is helpful for him. Giving information frequently during all phases of emergency care to both victim and significant others will help them understand what is occurring and that help is being provided, thus decreasing some of the anxiety.

Varying levels of tolerance to stress are found in different individuals. The highly anxious person may need someone to stay with him. At the scene of an accident a calm bystander can be helpful. Some hospitals provide selected volunteers for that purpose. All health personnel need to evaluate frequently their own effectiveness in assessing anxiety and in conveying understanding and emotional support to the victim and significant others during an emergency.

□ Cardiopulmonary problems

Outcome: *Pupils react to light; respirations and pulse are present; hemorrhage is controlled*

For life to be maintained, oxygen must be taken in by the lungs and pumped to the tissues; carbon dioxide must be returned from the tissues to the lung and exhaled. Thus any obstruction that interferes with the diffusion of these gases, failure of the heart as a pump, or inadequate blood to carry the oxygen to the tissues is a threat to life and demands immediate emergency intervention. Airway patency, breathing facilitation, and circulation maintenance are the ABCs of emergency care and take first priority in assessment and intervention.

Airway obstruction and breathing difficulties

Asphyxia occurs if the airway is obstructed suddenly by foreign bodies or the tongue, by edema of the tissues (as with burns or inflammation of airway passages), or by laryngospasm occurring with croup. Interference with respiration can also occur if an open chest wound or flail chest is present. In an open wound air rushes into the pleural cavity between the lung and chest wall creating positive pressure rather than the normal negative pressure, and the lung cannot expand to take in air. A flail chest is a closed chest injury in which ribs are broken creating an unstable chest wall. Paradoxical breathing will occur and lead to hypoxia.

Presence of fluid in the alveoli can interfere with diffusion of gases to and from the circulation in the lung. This can occur with drowning, secretions from infection (pneumonia), or pulmonary edema (p. 1009). Hypoxia can also occur if there is depression of the respiratory center in the brain such as with drug overdose.

Assessment. Pupils that constrict when exposed to light indicate adequate oxygenation of the brain. This will not occur with some drugs or in some elderly persons. Brain damage has occurred if the pupils remain widely dilated and do not respond to light.[66]

Signs of hypoxia are related to the efforts made by the victim to take in air. As the anoxic condition persists, signs of decreased oxygenation to tissue occur. The person with asphyxia will be struggling to get air. Neck muscles will be prominent, but little or no air may be moving in or out of the nose and mouth. Intercostal rib retractions will occur as the intercostal muscles pull against resistance. Infants may show sternal retraction. If the passageway is not totally blocked, respirations will be noisy and a wheezing sound will be heard as the air moves through the narrowed passageway. As less oxygen is taken in, skin color will become first pale then eventually cyanotic (grayish blue). This can be observed first in mucous membranes, lips, and nailbeds.

If an open chest wound is present, a sucking noise may be heard with inspiration. The chest should be inspected for signs of bleeding or a wound. Paradoxical breathing is denoted by the fact that the chest cage at the site of fractures moves in the direction opposite from normal during inspiration and expiration (p. 1132). Noisy respirations, rales, or rhonchi may be heard with auscultation if fluid is present in the alveoli. Excess fluid may be coughed up; secretions will be mucoid with infection, watery and frothy or blood tinged with pulmonary edema. Dyspnea will be present.

Depression of the respiratory center will be evidenced by bradycardia and slow shallow respirations. In respiratory arrest, breathing ceases completely.

Intervention

Open airway. A conscious victim may need assistance to facilitate removal of a foreign body obstructing the airway. Four forceful blows to the back between the shoulder blades may dislodge the object. If this is not effective, the Heimlich maneuver may be attempted (Fig. 24-1). The rescuer stands behind the victim encircling his arm around the victim's waist. The rescuer then places a fist between the umbilicus and the xiphoid process with the thumb against the abdomen. The fist is grasped with the other hand and pressed into the abdomen with quick upward thrusts.[40] Unless it is known positively that there is a foreign body obstructing the trachea, time should not be wasted examining for one. The first step in assisting a person who is not breathing or is having extreme difficulty breathing is to position him to assure a maximum airway. If the person is unconscious, his neck may be observed to be in a position of flexion with the back of the tongue obstructing the airway (Fig. 23-9). If there is no trauma suggesting a neck fracture, the neck is extended by placing one hand on

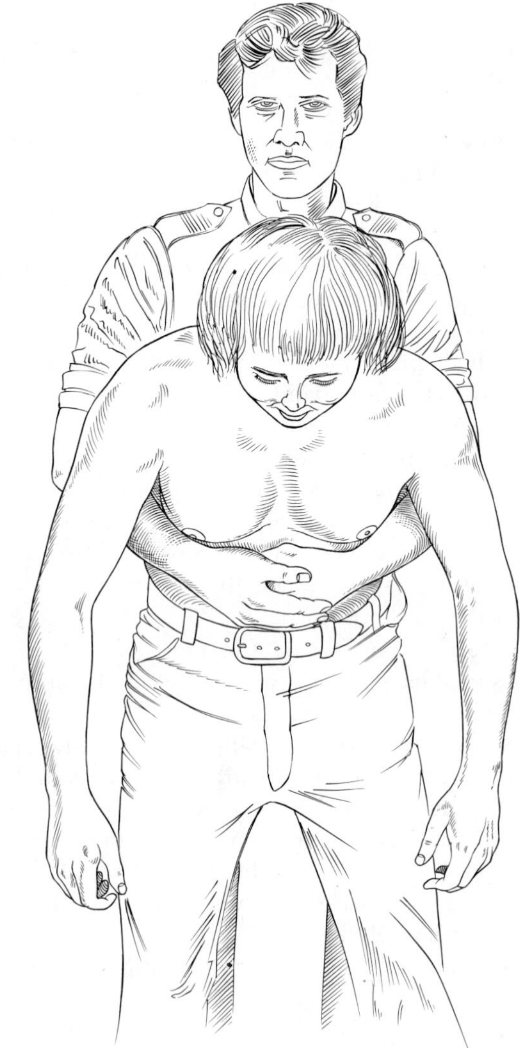

Fig. 24-1. Heimlich maneuver. Rescuer places fist between umbilicus and xyphoid process with thumb pressed against abdomen.

the forehead and the other hand under the neck and tilting the head back. If a neck fracture is suspected, the jaw can be pulled forward while the neck remains in a stable position. Either of these maneuvers will pull the back of the tongue away from the pharynx. Sometimes this maneuver alone may be enough to open the airway.

If extension of the head and neck does not initiate breathing, artificial ventilation must be initiated immediately (p. 964). Failure of the chest to rise with ventilation indicates that the airway is obstructed by a foreign body. The victim is rolled onto his side and given four sharp blows between the shoulder blades. If this fails to dislodge the object, the victim is turned on his back and given a series of eight abdominal thrusts. The rescuer kneels at the victim's hips (not straddling) and places the heel of one hand between the xiphoid process and the umbilicus. With the second hand on top of the first hand, he or she presses into the abdomen with quick upward thrusts.[66]

The mouth is then quickly checked for the presence of a foreign body that may have been forced up by the abdominal thrusts. The foreign body may be removed by sweeping a hooked finger across the back of the throat. Artificial ventilation is then attempted (3 to 5 breaths). These maneuvers are repeated if chest expansion does not resume.

Cardiopulmonary resuscitation. With the absence of both breathing and heartbeat, cardiopulmonary resuscitation is initiated (p. 963). All nurses, no matter where they work, should be certified by the American Heart Association in all phases of cardiopulmonary resuscitation (CPR). All nurses and physicians who work in emergency departments should be trained and certified in basic and advanced life support. Advanced life support includes endotracheal intubation, cardiac monitoring, defibrillation, and initiating and maintaining intravenous infusions.[66]

Oxygen. Supplemental oxygen is given after breathing resumes to treat the resultant hypoxemia. Oxygen is also given for other types of hypoxemia following trauma or stress such as with smoke inhalation, carbon monoxide poisoning, chest injuries, near drowning, or myocardial infarction.

Special cardiopulmonary problems

Myocardial infarction. The person suspected of experiencing a myocardial infarction needs immediate attention. The greatest risk of mortality occurs within the first 2 hours after onset.[66] Some communities have established mobile coronary units that respond immediately in these situations with advanced life-support systems. In the absence of such a unit the victim needs immediate safe transport to a medical center. If the heart ceases to beat, cardiopulmonary resuscitation is instituted immediately. If the patient is breathing, he may be more comfortable in a well-supported sitting position. Oxygen is useful if available. A calm atmosphere is of utmost importance, and the patient should never be left alone. Fear will add an additional stress to the already overburdened heart (see Chapter 46).

Drowning. The person who is drowning holds his breath until the carbon dioxide level rises to the point of stimulating the respiratory center causing him to breathe. Water is then aspirated into the lungs, irritating the lining of the airway and causing pulmonary edema and collapse of some alveoli. Fresh water is rapidly absorbed into the circulation, causing dilution of the blood constituents and hemolysis of red blood cells. Ventricular fibrillation will occur. Salt water, because of its hypertonicity, pulls fluid into the lungs, producing extensive pulmonary edema and hypovolemia.[54] Some persons develop severe laryngospasm and asphyxia without water entering the lungs.

If the victim of drowning has ceased breathing, artificial ventilation is initiated as soon as possible, even before he has been completely removed from the water. If the carotid pulse is absent, cardiac resuscitation is started as soon as possible. Time should not be wasted trying to remove water from the lungs. The person removed from salt water should be placed in a head-lowered position if possible. If distention of the abdomen from swallowed water is present and is interfering with adequate ventilation, the victim can be rolled onto his stomach and lifted with pressure over the stomach to force the water out.[66]

Persons who have experienced near drowning need close observation for several hours, even if they indicate that they feel all right. Pulmonary edema can develop a few hours later.

Electric shock. Electricity can cause injury in a number of ways. Depression of the respiratory center results in temporary or prolonged paralysis of respiration. Ventricular fibrillation occurs when the electric current hits the heart at the end of the refractory period. This can occur with a low current. Powerful muscle contraction from the effect of the electric current can cause bone or muscle injury that may persist for many months. Since the body acts as a conductor, electricity has an entrance point, travels through the body, and exits at a distant point. Burns with resultant necrosis of tissue occur at both entrance and exit points.

The extent of injury from electricity depends on the point in the heartbeat cycle that is stimulated by the electricity, the intensity of the current, and skin resistance. Moisture decreases skin resistance; therefore greater damage occurs when skin is moist with water or perspiration.

The victim must be removed from the source of electricity with the rescuer being careful to avoid contact with the electric charge. The rescuer must never have direct contact with the body of the victim because the charge may be transmitted. He should use a long, dry stick and stand on a dry board to roll the victim away from the electric charge. Asbestos or heavy dry gloves are needed if the victim must be moved away from an electric wire. Cardiopulmonary resuscitation is started immediately (if breathing and pulse are absent) and continued even when there is no evidence of response. Defibrillation is indicated for ventricular fibrillation.

Hemorrhage

As stated earlier, maintenance of an adequate blood flow to carry oxygen to the tissues is vital to support life. External bleeding is readily visible and if profuse needs immediate attention. It can occur with lacerations, crushing injuries, amputations, fractures, and nosebleeds. Internal bleeding is more difficult to identify and can occur with chest or abdominal trauma such as a ruptured spleen, trauma to large muscle masses of the extremity (thigh), or with certain medical conditions such as esophageal varices or bleeding ulcers. The thigh can hold 2 to 4 liters of blood after a fractured femur.[54]

When a blood vessel is severed, there is an immediate contraction of the vessel wall reducing the size of the opening and decreasing blood loss. Platelets begin to adhere to the roughened edges until a platelet plug is formed. A clot begins to form within 1 to 2 minutes. By 3 to 6 minutes that clot has filled the end of the blood vessel blocking blood flow.[39] Direct pressure over a bleeding vessel for 5 to 6 minutes will help stop the blood flow to permit clot formation. If a major artery is severed, ligation (tying off) of the artery may be necessary for continued cessation of bleeding. Pressure (digital pressure or tourniquet) applied to an artery proximal to the wound may also slow or stop the blood flow. This also slows or stops blood perfusion to the tissue between the pressure point and the wound producing tissue damage. Direct pressure over the bleeding vessel is therefore the action of choice unless bleeding cannot be controlled in this manner. Large arteries have musculature that can produce considerable vasospasms. Amputation of a leg, for example, may produce minimal bleeding. Veins and capillaries have thinner walls, and bleeding of these vessels can usually be controlled by direct pressure.

Assessment. External bleeding, if excessive will saturate the clothing and be readily visible. If the person is wearing bulky outer garments, bleeding may be concealed. The examiner should run the hands quickly over the entire body under the outer clothing, being sure to check underneath the victim. Saturated clothing may need to be cut away to examine the area of bleeding. Three types of bleeding can be observed: spurting of bright red blood indicates arterial bleeding, continuous flow of darker blood indicates venous bleeding, and oozing indicates capillary bleeding. The scalp is very vascular, and what appears to be considerable bleeding may occur from a small scalp laceration.

Internal bleeding may be difficult to identify. Bleeding into the thorax (hemothorax) may inhibit respirations and chest pain may be present. Abdominal bleeding may be evidenced by rigidity of abdominal muscles and abdominal pain. Hemoptysis or hematemesis indicates internal bleeding.

Shock occurs with severe internal or external bleeding. The victim is assessed for weak rapid pulse, slow shallow respiration, cold clammy skin, anxiety, restlessness, and thirst. The pupils are equal, may be dilated, and respond slowly to light.

Intervention. Direct pressure is applied to the site of external bleeding. If a sterile dressing is not available, a clean handkerchief, sanitary pad, or clean cloth may be used. The dressing is held in place by a tight bandage for continued pressure. The bare hand can be used to apply direct pressure until an adequate dressing is available. If

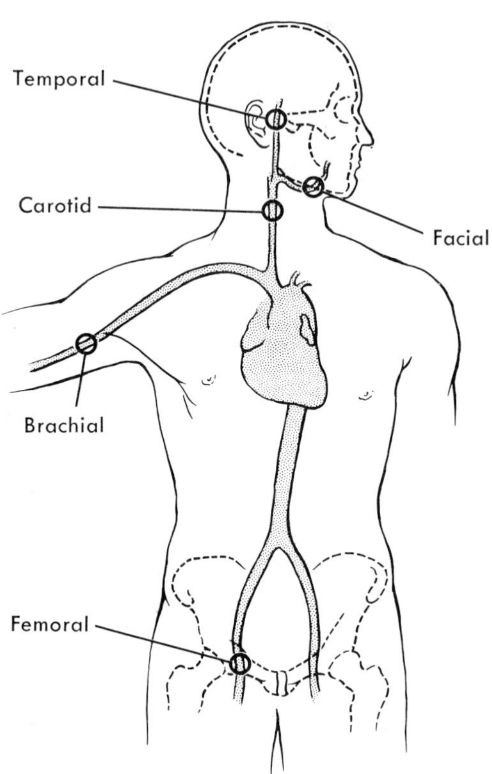

Fig. 24-2. Pressure points—locations at which large blood vessels may be compressed against bones to help control hemorrhage.

severe arterial bleeding cannot be controlled by direct pressure, or if direct pressure cannot be applied, pressure-point control over a bony prominence proximal to the point of hemorrhage can be attempted (Fig. 24-2).

Tourniquets are rarely necessary as they may cause further damage and can result in loss of an arm or leg.[2] If a tourniquet must be used, it should be applied with the following precautions. A triangular bandage should be folded at least 3 to 4 inches wide, six to eight layers thick, and wrapped twice around the extremity.[2] A stick or similar object is tied on by the ends of the bandage and twisted to tighten the tourniquet just enough to stop the bleeding but no tighter. A blood pressure cuff makes a useful tourniquet. Once the tourniquet is applied, it should be released only by a physician. The tourniquet is never covered, and a notation is made and attached to the patient giving the location and time of application. At the scene of an accident a large TK is written on the victim's forehead with lipstick to identify the presence of a tourniquet.

□ Poisoning

Poisoning, either accidental or deliberate, remains a major cause of accidental deaths. On the average there are 5,000 deaths from poisoning in the United States each year.[67]

Poisoning among children usually results from accidental ingestion. Children are naturally curious, and as they begin to crawl and walk they explore their widening horizons. Bottles or containers containing brightly colored pills or liquids are examined, and if the container can be opened the substance is put into the mouth and swallowed. Older children mimic the pill taking of adults either in their play activities or as a relief for symptoms for which they have received medication in the past. They may also take pills as an attention-getting device.

Poisoning in adults commonly occurs from not checking medication labels (overdose or wrong medication), from lack of knowledge (such as taking alcohol and sedatives together), by taking an excess amount in an attempt to obtain a desired effect, or as a suicide attempt.

Prevention of poisoning

There has been a decrease in the number of fatalities from poisoning in children under the age of 5 years.[56] This has been due to safety packaging of medications and to better education of the public about preventive measures. The Food and Drug Administration established regulations in 1970 that require that hazardous medicines be enclosed in containers with child-proof safety closure caps. The cap must be squeezed in or pushed down before it can be released. Originally the Safety Packaging Law applied to aspirin and drugs containing aspirin. Later it was extended to include narcotics and barbiturates; as of the spring of 1974, all prescription drugs are included with the exception of nitroglycerin and isosorbide dinitrate (Isordil).

Barbiturates are often recorded as the cause of accidental death by poisoning, In a 17-month period ending in December 1972 there were 1,711 barbiturate suicides and 3,475 overdoses and injury cases reported in 32 states. Because of the high potential of the abuse of certain barbiturates, the U.S. Justice Department's Drug Enforcement Agency (DEA) (formerly the Bureau of Narcotics and Dangerous Drugs) established stricter control methods for five of the barbiturates. As of December 1973 prescriptions for amobarbital (Amytal), pentobarbital (Nembutal), secobarbital (Seconal), sodium amobarbital (Amytal sodium), and Tuinal may not be refilled. In addition these drugs must be stored in a locked narcotic cabinet.

Another activity of the Drug Enforcement Administration was project DAWN (Drug Abuse Warning Network), which was set up to gather data on drug abuse. This project surveyed approximately 750 emergency rooms from July to October of 1973 in an attempt to learn the most common substances cited as the reasons for drug abuse visits to emergency departments. The survey showed that the six most commonly abused substances were diazepam (Valium), alcohol (in combination), aspirin, heroin, chlordiazepoxide (Librium), and secobarbital. These reports reinforce the need for nurses to take an active role in discouraging the public from the injudicious use of drugs. It is also important that the public be reminded to store all drugs and other dangerous substances out of reach of children.

Education of the public is directed toward increasing their awareness of safety hazards in the home. Medicine cabinets, kitchen cupboards, and laundry closets are the places from which children most often take poisons. Sleeping pills and tranquilizer tablets left on bedside tables and in handbags also are a potential source of poisoning. Cleaning compounds should be kept away from food storage areas and out of reach of children. Nonpotable liquids should be kept in their original containers, tightly capped, and *never* placed in a soft-drink bottle, drinking glass, or cup.

Aspirin remains the substance most often ingested in quantity by children. There has been a decrease in the ingestion of insecticides and bleaches but an increase in the ingestion of soaps, detergents, plants, perfumes, vitamins, and cold medicines by children.[56] Lead poisoning remains a problem in preschool children in low economic areas who live in pre–World War II housing, a time when lead based paints were commonly used.[24]

In recent years education about drug abuse has been aimed at school-aged children. A comparison of four studies of an existing drug education program indicated that drug education at the secondary school level may fail to decrease the illegal use of drugs. Drug abuse education should be aimed at the younger child, who appears more easily influenced by drug education than older students. During the 1960s there was a rapid increase in the number of persons using hallucinogenic drugs, but this leveled off by the mid 1970s. A considerable number of young persons become addicted and may experience overdoses.

Assessment of poisoning

A *rapid* assessment is made to determine whether poisoning or overdosage has occurred so that immediate action can be taken to prevent or diminish the effect of the poison or drug. It is important to identify (1) cues that poisoning is a possibility and (2) the type and quantity of the poisonous agent.

Poisoning is suspected when there is a sudden onset of symptoms, especially in a very young child. These symptoms may include nausea and vomiting, abdominal pain, convulsions, change of consciousness, and decreased respirations or pulse rate. If poisoning is suspected, the lips and mouth are examined for signs of burns, excessive salivation, or difficulty in swallowing. The breath is noted for an odor such as from petroleum products or cleaning compounds.

If the victim is conscious he should be questioned for information concerning what and how much was taken. The victim may not be conscious, as coma occurs with many drug overdosages. Not much time should be spent looking for needle marks as drugs may be injected by addicts in unusual places such as the penis or feet.[35] Identification of the poison or drug can be facilitated by asking others to look for clues while you are examining the victim. Empty containers, spilled fluids, open medication bottles, or syringes may provide needed information. *All* potential agents should be gathered in their original containers and taken to the hospital with the victim. The physician may need to know the ingredients of the agent for those situations when an antidote is indicated. Assessment data should also include the expected time before medical help can be obtained.

Intervention

Outcome: *Absorption of poison is minimized*

General intervention. Immediate action is necessary if poisoning is suspected; in some instances delay of a few minutes may make a difference between life and death. If the victim is *unconscious,* he must be transported *without delay* to the nearest medical facility. This is one instance where waiting for an ambulance for transportation is not advisable if another means of transportation such as a car is available. Keep the victim warm.

If the victim is *conscious,* ascertain his age and identify the type, method, and estimated amount of poison or drug taken. Have someone call a physician immediately if possible. If a private physician is not available, a poison control center can give rapid and accurate information. Most large cities have poison control centers, which maintain an extensive file on the most common substances and drugs. The telephone number is usually easily obtained from a list of emergency numbers in the front of the telephone directory.

Management consists of stopping absorption of the poisonous substance or drug. Poisonous substances can be inhaled, absorbed from the skin or mucous membranes, ingested, or injected. The type of intervention depends on the method by which the poison entered the system.

Specific intervention

Inhaled poison. Persons who have inhaled a toxic gas first need to be removed from the site to fresh air and given oxygen if available. As in any emergency, cardiopulmonary status should be assessed and resuscitation started if indicated. The victim is transported immediately to a medical center.

Carbon monoxide is one of the more common of the toxic gases. It is odorless and occurs as a result of incomplete combustion such as during fires or from automobile exhaust. It cannot be filtered by the use of a cloth face mask. Toxicity occurs because of the higher affinity of hemoglobin for carbon monoxide than for oxygen. The victim becomes profoundly hypoxic and loses consciousness. Carboxyhemoglobin has a deep red color and is seen in the mucous membranes of all victims and by a red coloring of white or light-colored skin.

Contact poison. Poisonous substances absorbed through the skin or mucous membranes should be rinsed off immediately with copious amounts of water without taking time to remove garments. Following this the garments containing the substance are removed and the skin is rinsed again.

Ingested poison. The most common form of poisoning is by ingestion of a poisonous substance or an excessive amount of a drug. Absorption of the agent can be prevented by inducing vomiting or by gavage to eliminate the agent and by giving a substance that will make the poisonous agent inert or move it rapidly through the gastrointestinal system so that it can be excreted.

VOMITING. The best way to eliminate an ingested poison is by vomiting. This is *contraindicated* in certain situations (see box, p. 429). Corrosive substances such as strong acids or bases can cause as much damage to the esophagus during regurgitation as they did during swallowing. Substances containing petroleum products, such as cleaning compounds or paints, can cause aspiration pneumonitis following vomiting. The victim must be

ACTIONS IN SELECTED SITUATIONS WITH A CONSCIOUS VICTIM WHO HAS INGESTED POISON

Corrosive substances
- Household cleaners: do *not* induce vomiting; give milk
- Paint (liquid); do *not* induce vomiting; give milk
- Ammonia: do *not* induce vomiting; give *citrus juice*

Noncorrosive substances
- Insecticides: induce vomiting; give milk
- Medicines: induce vomiting; give milk
- Cosmetics: induce vomiting; give milk
- Plants: induce vomiting; give milk

METHODS OF INDUCING VOMITING

1. Give 1 or 2 glasses of warm water followed by tickling the back of the throat.
2. Give 1 tbsp (15 ml) syrup of Ipecac followed by 1 glass of water. (Dose can be repeated once only if vomiting does not occur within 15 to 20 min.)
3. Give 1 tbsp salt *or* 1 to 2 tsp mustard in 1 glass of *warm* water. (Mix dry mustard with water just before drinking.)
4. Physician's order: Apomorphine hydrochloride 0.03 mg/lb subcutaneously. (Contraindicated if respiratory depression present.)

conscious for vomiting to be induced; victims who are convulsing or unconscious may aspirate or choke on vomitus. Vomiting can be induced in a number of ways (see box above). There should be no delay in transporting the victim to the nearest medical center.

GAVAGE. In the hospital, gastric lavage by means of a large-bore tube may be instituted if the victim is unconscious. A cuffed endotracheal tube is inserted before gavage in the unconscious person to prevent aspiration of gastric contents.

ACTIVATED CHARCOAL. In recent years there has been a rekindling of interest in the use of activated charcoal, which is usually given after the victim has vomited. Activated charcoal will adsorb a drug and prevent it from being absorbed into the body by way of the gastrointestinal tract. It varies in its adsorptive action but has a high affinity for analgesics (especially aspirin), barbiturates and other hypnotics, and amphetamines.[19] Activated charcoal should be administered within 30 minutes of poisoning to achieve maximum effect but can be given later with good results.

Activated charcoal, which is not the same as a blackened piece of toast, can be purchased at a drugstore. The major drawback is the color of the solution. Children will drink it, however, if it is presented with a positive approach.[19]

ANTIDOTES. If it is known exactly what poisonous substance or drug has been ingested, a specific antidote may be given in some cases by the physician. (Common poisons and antidotes are discussed in pharmacology and toxicology texts). The use of a "universal antidote" has not proved to be effective.

CATHARTIC. Once a substance has passed through the stomach, some absorption can be prevented if a saline cathartic is given to move the substance more quickly through the gastrointestinal tract. In the home, 1 tbsp of Epsom salts (magnesium sulfate) in one to two glasses of water can be given. Cathartics are especially useful after the ingestion of sleeping medications, narcotics, tranquilizers, and food poisoning (unless diarrhea is already present).

Injected poison. Poisonous substances can be injected through the skin, such as by insect bites or drug overdose by needle injection. Drugs most commonly injected are heroin, barbiturates, and amphetamines. Stimulants such as the amphetamines produce hyperactivity and "uncooperative" behavior. Overdosage may produce tachycardia, chills, and collapse. Depressants such as heroin or barbiturates produce respiratory depression resulting in coma and death. Overdosage often occurs because the victim is unaware of the potency of the drug purchased illegally.

INSECT BITES. The most common insect bites that can produce severe reactions are those of wasps and bees. Death can occur either because of the multiplicity of bites (especially in young children) or from anaphylactic shock if the victim is allergic to the protein in the venom. The reaction may be slow in developing or sudden and acute. Persons who know that they are allergic to insect stings should avoid areas where bees and wasps are found and should have epinephrine (Adrenalin) available for immediate use parenterally if anaphylaxis occurs. The wearing of a Medic-Alert tag facilitates emergency care if the victim is unconscious.

When a person is stung by a bee, the stinger with the venom bag is left in the skin. The stinger should be removed immediately because venom continues to be pumped into the skin from the bag. Removal of the stinger by grasping and pulling is to be avoided as this pushes more venom into the skin. The stinger is removed by a scraping motion.[73] Ice can be applied to prevent absorption of the venom (heat should be avoided). A paste of sodium bicarbonate and water or a weak solution of ammonia may help by counteracting the formic acid present in the venom.

Tick bites can cause tick fever by transmission of a

toxin, a virus as in Colorado tick fever, or rickettsiae as in Rocky Mountain spotted fever. Sudden removal of a tick will result in its mouthpiece remaining. Applying gasoline or turpentine to the head of a tick or applying the hot end of a previously lighted match to the body will cause the tick to drop off within 10 minutes. Ice can be applied to reduce absorption of toxin.

Supportive care. Good nursing care of the acutely poisoned patient may make the difference between a favorable and a fatal outcome. The patient is kept warm and observed extremely closely for changes in physical signs such as rapid thready pulse, respiratory distress, cyanosis, diaphoresis and other signs of collapse, vasogenic shock, or impending death. Changes are reported to the physician immediately. Vital signs are usually monitored at least every 15 minutes for several hours. Nausea, vomiting, and abdominal pain are recorded, and all vomitus is observed for signs of blood and saved for study. Stools and urine are checked for abnormal constituents such as blood. Intravenous fluids are usually prescribed.

If the patient has marked depression of respiration, oxygen may be given, and sometimes a mechanical ventilator is necessary. A suction machine should be on hand at all times as suctioning of the bronchial tree may be necessary. Unconscious patients are turned frequently to provide drainage from each bronchus.

If the poisoning was a suicide attempt, adequate safety precautions should be instituted. A psychiatric consultation is often recommended. Persons addicted to heroin or morphine derivatives who have overdosed should be observed for signs of withdrawal. Symptoms usually appear within 12 to 18 hours and include yawning, sweating, shaking, vomiting, diarrhea, lacrimation, runny nose, abdominal pain, backache, and other flu-type symptoms.

Food poisoning

A number of toxicants occur in plants and animals ingested as food. Some toxicants are introduced by mistake as pesticides during plant growth, as food additives, or as part of food packaging. Commercially packaged foods are monitored closely, and products are withdrawn from the market if contamination is suspected.

Plant poisoning. Poisoning from plants is usually not a problem, as people have learned to identify poisonous foods. Mushroom poisoning still occurs, however, when people eat uncultivated mushrooms thinking that they are of a safe variety. Two types of mushroom poisoning can occur. One type contains the alkaloid muscarine, which has a parasympathetic effect. Symptoms develop immediately after eating and are characterized by sweating, lacrimation, salivation, dyspnea, vomiting, and muscle tremors. Respiratory and circulatory depression may occur. The second type of mushroom poisoning has an atropinelike effect. Symptoms occur 6 to 24 hours after ingestion and are characterized by nausea and vomiting, bloody diarrhea, dehydration, and muscle weakness. Circulatory system collapse and central nervous system involvement may occur.

First-aid treatment of mushroom poisoning is the same as for drug poisoning: induce vomiting, give fluids, then give activated charcoal. Thirty milligrams (1 ounce) of magnesium sulfate (Epsom salts) may be given in water by mouth to hasten evacuation. Medical care should be obtained.

Bacterial food poisoning. Food poisoning occurs more frequently than is reported because the majority of persons recover quickly without treatment.[38] The incidence of food poisoning from commercially prepared foods has become relatively uncommon in the United States, but food poisoning due to home-cooked foods or improper handling of foods still occurs.

Bacteria such as *Staphylococcus aureus* or *Clostridium botulinum* can produce a toxin that acts as a poison causing acute gastrointestinal tract upset. The toxin of S. *aureus* does not spread through the body, and the symptoms are therefore limited. The toxin of *C.* botulinum does spread and can be fatal (Table 24-1). *Salmonella* organisms introduced in food multiply in the intestines causing acute gastrointestinal tract upset and infection. Food poisoning is not caused by food that has spoiled or decomposed unless the food happens to contain disease-causing bacteria. The majority of food poisonings are due to S. *aureus*.

Prevention. Acute food poisoning can be prevented. Rigid controls of slaughterhouse practices have decreased the incidence of food poisoning. Pasteurization of milk destroys salmonellae. Rigorous enforcement of sanitary practices by food handlers can decrease food poisoning by *Staphylococcus* and *Salmonella* organisms. Food handlers should not be allowed to work if they have even minor infections on their hands or do not adhere to the requirements for handwashing after using the toilet. Toilets should not be adjacent to kitchens.

Health teaching should include the proper handling and cooling of foods. Home canning has become increasingly popular, but many people are unaware of the need to process low-acid foods (foods other than tomatoes or fruits) under pressure to prevent botulism. The U.S. Department of Agriculture, state agricultural departments, the home economics departments of schools, or newspapers may have booklets available on home canning methods. Any can that is bulging should be discarded. If there is a question, the food can be *boiled* for 15 minutes before eating, since this will destroy the toxin.

Table 24-1. Bacterial food poisoning

Symptoms	Causative agent	Source	Comments
Nausea and vomiting, diarrhea, abdominal pain, lowered temperature	*Staphylococcus aureus:* enterotoxin	Fish and meats (especially ham), dehydrated milk, unrefrigerated mayonnaise and cream-filled foods; skin and respiratory tract of food handlers	Mortality low Toxin heat stable Incubation 1 to 6 hours Symptoms last 24 to 48 hours Treatment: bedrest, fluids
Nausea and vomiting, diarrhea, abdominal pain, chills and fever, weakness	*Salmonella:* multiply in gut and produce toxin	Inadequately cooked eggs, poultry, meat (especially pork)	Mortality low Organism killed by heat Incubation 10 to 24 hours Symptoms: last 2 to 3 days Treatment: bedrest, fluids (no antibiotics; they produce resistant strains)
Nausea and vomiting; double vision; flaccid paralysis of of face, eyes, mouth, throat; dryness of skin, mouth, throat	*Clostridium botulinum:* exotoxin; spores germinate under anerobic conditions and produce toxin	Improperly canned vegetables, meat (low-acid foods); spiced, smoked, vacuum-packed, or canned alkaline foods eaten without cooking	Mortality high Toxin heat labile Incubation 12 to 72 hours Death due to respiratory failure or cardiac arrest

Additional measures to prevent food poisoning include avoiding slow cooling of meat dishes; avoiding cooking of extremely large chunks of meat (especially pork) unless a meat thermometer is used that measures the heat of the core of the meat; or allowing meats, fish, mayonnaise, or cream-filled foods to remain unrefrigerated for periods of time. Foods that are rewarmed should be boiled, as merely warming will rapidly increase bacterial growth.

Intervention. If abdominal pain and diarrhea accompany the nausea and vomiting, with or without fever, the causative organisms are either *Staphylococcus* or *Salmonella.* If the symptoms are very mild, no interventions are indicated. If fluid loss is severe, fluid balance should be restored and bed rest may be indicated. Fluids such as tea or broth may be well tolerated. If severe dehydration occurs, intravenous fluids may be necessary.

There is no emergency first-aid treatment suitable for *C. botulinum* poisoning. The victim should be taken to a hospital for medical care. Data should be obtained concerning the source of the poisoning, and any other persons who might have eaten the contaminated food should be contacted immediately. Medical treatment consists of supportive therapy and the administration of botulinum antitoxin. Antitoxin cannot undo damage that has already occurred but can prevent further damage. Approximately 65% of these patients die within 3 to 16 days after onset of symptoms. Fortunately this type of poisoning is now quite rare.

☐ Environmental injuries: heat, cold, radiation

Exposure to extremes of temperature affects both the general reaction of the body to the stress and the local reaction of the skin. General reactions occur more readily when the individual has not conditioned himself to the extremes in temperature. Incidences of overexposure to heat, for example, occur more often in the early part of a hot spell before the individual is acclimated.

General reactions to heat and cold

Three general reactions can occur with heat: heat cramps, heat exhaustion, and heat stroke (sunstroke). Cold produces a general cooling of the body.

Heat cramps. Heat cramps are sudden muscle pains caused by loss of sodium chloride in perspiration during strenuous exercise in hot weather. The best treatment is prevention by taking extra salt when severe exertion is anticipated. The immediate treatment consists of salty fluids and foods by mouth, extra water, and rest for a few hours.

Heat exhaustion. Heat exhaustion is vasomotor collapse due to inability of the body to supply the peripheral vessels adequately with sufficient fluids to produce the perspiration needed for cooling and yet meet vital tissue requirements. The condition usually follows an extended period of vigorous exercise in hot weather, particularly when an individual has not had a period of acclimatization. The symptoms are faintness, weakness, headache, and sometimes nausea and vomiting. The skin is pale and moist. Temperature is normal or subnormal. Heat exhaustion can often be prevented by taking extra salt and extra fluid during hot weather and by tempering physical activity during very hot weather. Emergency care consists of treating for shock and transporting the victim to a medical center. Fluids should be given, preferably containing salt, although the condition is not primarily caused by lack of salt.[2]

Heat stroke (sunstroke). Heat stroke is a serious condition in which excessive body heat is retained, and it requires immediate emergency treatment. It is due to a failure of the perspiration-regulating mechanism in the hypothalamus. The person undergoing vigorous exercise in intense heat may perspire profusely for some time and then become dehydrated and fail to produce sufficient perspiration to maintain normal body temperature. The skin is dry, hot, and flushed in contrast to the pale moist skin of the person suffering from heat exhaustion. The victim becomes confused, dizzy, and faint and may quickly lose consciousness.

Without treatment most heat stroke victims will die, but with prompt and vigorous treatment almost all will recover. Treatment consists of actions to reduce the body temperature immediately while transporting the victim to a medical center. The victim should be placed in a cool place, such as an air-conditioned room, while awaiting transportation. Cold moist applications applied to the body and a fan to increase evaporation are helpful. These measures are continued during transportation.

If the elevated temperature is allowed to persist, serious permanent damage is done to the brain and the entire nervous system. A temperature of 40.5 C (105 F) or higher means that treatment is essential. Treatment should be continued until the temperature has been lowered to at least 39 C (102 F), and the temperature must then be checked carefully for several hours for sudden rise. The patient should respond when the temperature lowers. Failure to do so may indicate that brain damage has occurred. Persons do not recover from heat stroke as quickly as from heat exhaustion. Often there is faulty heat regulation for days and a lowered tolerance to heat for years and sometimes for the rest of the individual's life. The person who has had a heat stroke should be advised to plan his living so that repeated long exposures to heat are avoided.

General cooling of the body. The extent of the cooling effect that occurs with exposure to extreme cold depends on the temperature and exposure time, the thermal conductivity of the environment, and the amount of air current present. Moisture is a good conductor; air is not. Wet clothing therefore contributes to increased cooling of the body. Several light layers of clothing to provide air insulation will keep a person warmer than one heavy layer. Air movement contributes to heat loss. Lower environmental temperatures can be tolerated better in the absence of wind (wind-chill factor).

When the body is exposed to cold, shivering occurs to produce heat by increased metabolism. As the cold increases, shivering ceases and heat loss exceeds heat production. The individual becomes listless, apathetic, and sleepy. He may become indifferent to his surroundings and not seek adequate protection. Pulse and respirations become slower as metabolism decreases. Freezing of the extremities, unconsciousness, and finally death will result if help is not received.

The victim needs to be kept warm while being transferred to a medical facility. Wet clothing is removed immediately and warmed blankets applied. If a tub bath is given, the temperature should be approximately 41 C to 43 C (105 F to 110 F). Warmer temperatures can cause skin damage due to the decreased circulation to the skin.[39] Rubbing of the skin is to be avoided as this can also cause skin damage. Hot liquids may be given if the victim is conscious.

The person suffering hypothermia should be monitored closely during rewarming. Hypovolemic shock can occur due to vasodilation. If intravenous fluids are given, overloading of the circulation is a potential complication. Vital signs are monitored for sudden changes. Cardiac monitoring may also be indicated during the rewarming period for signs of ventricular fibrillation and cardiac arrest.

Local reactions to heat and cold

Burns. Burns may be caused by direct heat, chemicals, electricity, or radiation (sun or nuclear rays). Heat burns are treated by immersion in cool water or application of clean, cool wet packs. Clothing should not be removed nor ointments applied. Shock may occur with severe burns due to fluid shifts. (For more detailed information on burns, see Chapter 67.)

Frostbite. Cellular injury occurs with exposure to extreme cold. Cell water freezes and the resulting ice crystals damage the cell. The degree of injury depends on the depth of freezing. Frostbite occurs most frequently in exposed areas such as the nose, cheeks, ears, and fingers and can be prevented by adequate covering with loose-fitting dry clothing. Toes are also susceptible due to dampness and to tight pressure from shoes or boots. Persons with circulatory problems are more prone to develop frostbite.

Frostbite can be classified as incipient, superficial, or deep.[2] *Incipient frostbite* often goes unnoticed and is evidence by paleness or loss of color of the skin. Removing the victim to a warm room, cupping the injured part with the hands, or placing fingers in the armpit for warmth may be all that is needed. Tingling occurs with warming.

Superficial frostbite may develop if incipient frostbite is not noticed. Freezing extends into the superficial tissue below the skin. The frozen part is soft, and white skin does not redden with pressure. Dark skin has a dull ashen shade. Blisters may form and pain and edema may develop and last for several weeks. The frozen part may be warmed by covering. Heat is not applied as this may damage the injured tissue, but the frozen part may be immersed gently in warm water (43 C [110 F]). Contrary to popular belief, the frozen part should never be rubbed with snow as this increases the trauma to the injured tissue.

Deep frostbite is evidenced by hardness of the frozen tissue because deep subcutaneous tissue is injured. The victim should be taken to a medical center as soon as possible. The care is then similar to that for vascular disease of the extremities (p. 1020). Efforts are made to decrease the oxygen needs of the tissues while healing takes place, to improve blood supply by the use of drugs, and to prevent infection of open lesions. Necrotic tissue may have to be debrided for healing to occur.

Radiation exposure and injury

Accidental injury through radiation is an ever present potential as a result of nuclear energy and the use of nuclear materials in industry. Considerable precautions are employed in areas where nuclear materials are used. The likelihood of accidental injury is greater while these materials are being transported from one area to another.[2]

Radiation injury is caused by exposure to gamma rays and neutrons from radioactive material. Persons can become contaminated by the rays as a result of a nuclear explosion or directly through the air from unshielded radioactive material or inhaled or swallowed on particles of contaminated dust or smoke. The amount of radiation that a person receives depends on the strength of the radiation source, the distance of the victim from the source, the duration of the exposure, the area of the body exposed to the radiation source, and the amount and type of shielding that is present.[2]

Prevention of radiation injuries. Special precautionary measures should be used whenever radioactive materials are being utilized. All persons having contact with these materials should become knowledgeable concerning preventive measures. Exposure to radiation is carefully monitored; for example, personnel who work with radioactive materials or x-rays (gamma rays) wear special monitoring badges.

Rescue workers who must remove a victim from an area of radioactivity need to protect themselves from radiation exposure. Since radioactive particles can be carried on dust, all skin areas must be covered and a filtering mask worn by rescue workers following an explosion involving nuclear materials. The greater the time of exposure, the greater the potential for injury; therefore the victim must be removed immediately to a less hazardous environment. Some of the basic principles of emergency care may have to be violated when there is danger of other explosions or when fires occur. The rescue worker should remove all contaminated clothing at the edge of the contaminated area and any exposed skin areas are washed throughly. A shower should be taken as soon as possible as an additional preventive measure.[2]

Intervention for radiation injury. Radiation rays can cause a local inflammatory reaction of the skin similar to a burn. The involved area may be washed gently with soap and water and a dry sterile dressing applied. No antiseptic or disinfectant solutions should be used and no debridement should be attempted.[32]

Radiation sickness will not become apparent until several days after exposure. There may be nausea and vomiting shortly after exposure, but this ceases spontaneously. Because radiation affects the body's immune response, later symptoms may include severe inflammation and sometimes sloughing and hemorrhage of the mucous membranes of the mouth and throat, bloody diarrhea, purpura (hemorrhagic spots under the skin), and alopecia (loss of hair). A severe leukopenia quickly follows exposure to large amounts of radiation.

There is no specific treatment for radiation sickness. The patient needs the same care as one who receives radiation treatment (p. 470). This care includes rest, protection from superimposed infection, good mouth care, fluid and electrolyte replacement, and a high-caloric bland diet.

□ Musculoskeletal injuries

Soft-tissue injuries

Injury to soft tissue may result in either open or closed wounds. Types of open wounds include abrasions, avulsions, incisions or lacerations, and puncture wounds. In a closed wound the skin is not broken, but there is injury to underlying tissue. A contusion (bruise) is a closed wound.

Open wounds usually become infected. This develops 1 to 2 days after injury, but in grossly contaminated wounds signs of infection can be observed in 8 to 12 hours.[73] Signs of infection include erythema, edema, and pain, and a purulent exudate is present. The patient may develop fever and lymphadenopathy.

General management of open wounds consists of control of bleeding, thorough cleansing with soap and water to prevent infection, irrigation of deep wounds to remove foreign material, and suturing, if possible, to approximate skin edges and hasten healing.

Types of wounds

Abrasions. An abrasion is a scraping of the skin surface commonly referred to as a "floor burn." It involves only a partial thickness of the skin. Abrasions are commonly experienced by active children and athletes and in motorcycle accidents. When a large area of skin has been denuded, an abrasion can be painful. Good cleaning of the wound with soap and water is important to remove all pieces of imbedded foreign matter, which can delay healing and cause scarring. An antiseptic ointment can be applied. If the wound can be kept clean, no covering is necessary. Covering with a sterile dressing may be indicated for children.

Avulsions. A flap of skin and subcutaneous tissue that has been torn loose is called an avulsion. Large flaps can be torn loose from any part of the body especially the head and extremities. Avulsions must be cleaned thoroughly and irrigated well to remove any foreign material before they are sutured.

Lacerations. A jagged cut through skin and other tissue is termed a laceration. A sharp knife will produce a straight cut, or *incision.* Lacerations or incisions vary in depth and may involve muscles and tendons.

The laceration or incision is cleaned well and sutured through each layer. Any gap left through nonapproximation of the wound may delay healing. Incisions usually heal more quickly with less scar formation than lacerations because the edges can be better approximated. Suturing should be carried out within the first few hours after injury to obtain maximum healing with less complications or scarring. If the wound is grossly contaminated, the decision may be made to delay suturing for a few days to permit thorough cleansing. Healing then occurs by tertiary intention (p. 400). Suturing may not be necessary for superficial lacerations. The edges of the wound can be approximated by the use of one or more butterfly adhesive strips (Fig. 24-3).

Puncture wounds. A puncture wound is caused by a sharp, pointed, narrow object such as a nail, pin, bullet, splinter of wood, or animal bite. As the tissues are penetrated by the object, pathogenic organisms may be introduced. Since the skin quickly seals over, the wound rarely bleeds enough to wash out organisms. Bacteria such as *Clostridium tetani,* which thrive without air, may infect these wounds. Because anaerobic bacterial infections are extremely serious, a physician should be consulted if the punture was made by a dirty object.

Puncture wounds received from objects such as contaminated needles used for any parenteral treatment also should be reported to the physician as viral hepatitis may be contracted from this type of injury. Immune serum globulin may be given as prophylaxis.

Puncture wounds are treated by soaks. A small amount of bleeding is encouraged in small puncture wounds to assist in washing out microorganisms. The wound should be observed for signs of infection. Prophylaxis against tetanus is instituted (p. 437).

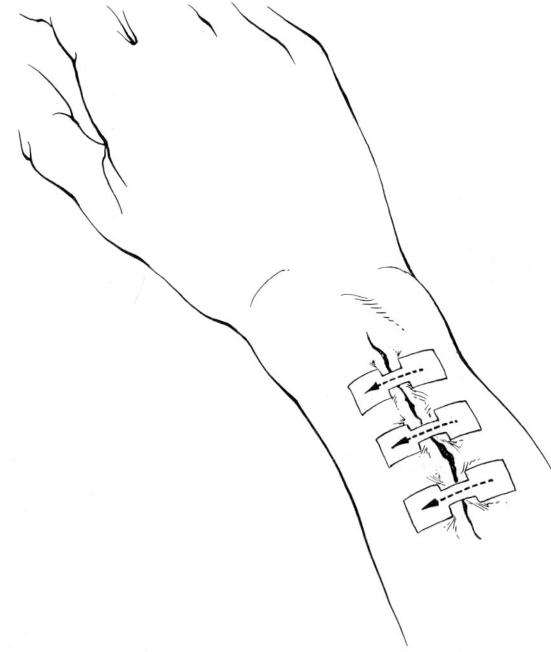

Fig. 24-3. Use of butterfly adhesive strips to approximate skin edges in laceration of forearm. Note irregular wound edges and placement of adhesive. Arrows indicate direction of pull used to partially close wound.

Stab wounds are a form of puncture wound. An object such as a knife, stick, or piece of glass can become impaled in the body. The impaled object should *not* be removed except by a physician in a medical facility, usually in the operating room. If there is severe bleeding, pressure points may be used to control loss of blood. The object should be stabilized before transportation to prevent accidental dislodgement and further trauma.

Contusions. Blunt objects may injure underlying tissue without breaking the skin. Edema may develop from trauma to the injured cells; this is usually "brawny" edema because it does not "pit." Blood vessels usually rupture, and the blood seeps into the tissue creating a hematoma. The skin acquires a black-and-blue appearance from the extravasated blood. Pain is usually present. Rest of the injured part is advised, and analgesics may be helpful if pain is severe. Application of ice during the first 24 to 48 hours encourages vasoconstriction, decreasing blood seepage and edema.

Special wounds

Chest wounds. Open wounds of the chest create a problem if there is intrusion into the pleural cavity. Air is drawn into the pleural space because of the existing negative pressure but does not escape. The resultant positive pressure causes *pneumothorax* (collapse of the lung) (p. 1133). A sucking noise is heard as the air is drawn in. Respirations are impaired. Immediate action is indicated to cover the opening. A nonporous material must be used as air can pass through a standard dressing or material. Plastic wrap, which is not only nonporous but tends to cling to the skin, is excellent. Aluminum foil or the cellophane covering of a cigarette pack can also be used. If a dressing is used, it must be covered with petrolatum to create an air barrier. After the chest wound has been sealed, a pressure dressing is applied. Continual monitoring of respirations is indicated.

Abdominal wounds. Blows to the abdomen can rupture underlying organs. The spleen is often lacerated, and the intestines, liver, kidney, and bladder may also sustain injury. Symptoms include abdominal pain and rigidity, nausea and vomiting, shock, and contusions on the abdominal wall. The victim may be more comfortable in a position with his knees drawn up toward the abdomen. If there is an open wound, evisceration may occur. If the abdominal organs are exposed to the air and become dry, necrosis can result. The abdominal organs lying outside the abdominal cavity should therefore be covered by a warm, moist, preferably sterile covering. If a sterile dressing is not available, it is better to cover the organs with a clean moist cloth and risk infection than not to cover the organs, resulting in loss of tissue.

Amputations. Traumatic amputations are treated as other wounds by controlling hemorrhage and applying pressure dressings. Severe bleeding does not always occur. The amount of bleeding is dependent on the extent of trauma that occurs. The greater the amount of trauma, such as the amputation of a limb by a crushing injury, the greater will be the amount of muscle spasm in the arterial walls (vascular spasm).[39] This causes the artery to contract and bleeding is decreased. A limb or appendage that is severed cleanly by a sharp object such as a knife will bleed more profusely. If a tourniquet is necessary, it should be applied close to the site of the amputation to decrease potential injury to intervening tissue. The amputated portion should be taken with the victim to the hospital as replantation is sometimes possible. The amputated part is placed in a plastic bag and kept cool during transportation, such as in a camping cooler. It should never be frozen, cleaned, disinfected, debrided, or perfused.[46]

Bites. Approximately 1 million Americans are bitten by animals every year, mostly by dogs.[20] Most animal bites produce puncture wounds, but lacerations can occur as the individual attempts to pull away from the animal. Human bites also occur; they have a high potential for infection because of the high bacterial count in the human mouth.

The immediate local wound care of animal and human bites consists in thorough washing with soap and water and copious rinsing under running water. After all traces of soap have been removed, the wound may be flushed with 1% benzalkonium chloride (Zephiran). Antibiotic therapy is usually given for large contaminated animal bites or for human bites. Prophylaxis against tetanus is also given (p. 437). Data related to the potential for rabies is collected.

Snakebites. There are four kinds of poisonous snakes in the United States. Three of them, the copperhead, the cottonmouth moccasin, and the rattlesnake, belong to the group known as pit vipers and are distinguished by a pit resembling a second nostril between the eyes and the nostril and by a broad, flat, triangular head. Everyone should know the kinds of poisonous snakes found in the part of the country in which he lives and how to recognize them. The copperhead, named for its color, is about 3 feet long and is found in the eastern and southern states. The cottonmouth moccasin is grayish in color and blends with its surroundings. It is found in marshy country in the southeastern states. Rattlesnakes are probably found in every state in the United States and are responsible for the largest number of bites and the largest number of deaths. One antivenin is effective for all pit vipers.

The fourth poisonous snake, the coral snake, is small with coral, yellow, and black rings encircling its body. It is found in North Carolina and other southern states, particularly around the Gulf of Mexico. The snake is shy and seldom bites, but its venom is deadly and affects the nervous system. No specific antivenin is prepared for the bite of the coral snake, but cobra antivenin, kept in most zoos, is effective.

PREVENTION. Poisonous snakes in North America will almost always move away when disturbed and will not bite unless suddenly molested without warning. Snakebites can often be prevented by wearing high leather boots and thick trousers when walking through snake-infested areas. Heavy gloves should be worn and the greatest care taken when climbing because hands may be placed on ledges that cannot be seen, and reptiles often sun themselves on rocky ledges.

ASSESSMENT. Snakebites can be classified as mild, moderate, or severe.[4] Scratches made by the teeth of the snake (but no fang marks) are visible in mild cases. Moderate and severe snakebites are distinguished by two fang marks above the horseshoe-shaped array of tooth marks. Immediate severe pain and swelling distinguish the bite of a poisonous snake from that of a nonpoisonous one, even when swelling and discoloration are so sudden as to make the fang marks impossible to see.

Ecchymosis may be extensive, and bullae and petechiae may develop. Systemic symptoms such as anxiety, nausea and vomiting, vertigo, dyspnea, and dimness of vision accompany the severe bite. If the venom is injected directly into a major blood vessel, a fatal reaction may occur within 15 minutes.

INTERVENTION. The mild bite (no fang marks) is treated as an abrasion with good cleaning with soap and water. No further treatment is necessary.[4] Treatment for moderate and severe poisonous snakebites consists of the immediate application of a flat tourniquet just above the bite. This tourniquet should not be tight enough to prevent venous return in deep vessels or arterial supply to the part but should be tight enough to prevent superficial venous circulation of blood and lymph, thus stopping absorption of the poison. The tourniquet is not removed.[4] If less than 30 minutes has elapsed since the bite, a ½-inch incision is made lengthwise through the fang marks, extending only into the subcutaneous tissue about ¼ inch deep. (No incision is made if the bite marks are near a major blood vessel.) If emergency snakebite equipment is not available, suction must be applied by mouth. This procedure is safe unless there are open lesions in the rescuer's mouth, since the venom is not poisonous if swallowed. Constant suctioning is continued for 20 to 30 minutes.

Antivenom, if available, is given only for severe snakebites, since severe reactions to the antivenom can occur. Antivenom is given intravenously, not injected into the tissue around the bite as it will not neutralize the venom.

The victim of the moderate or severe snakebite should lie very quietly to lessen circulatory flow and absorption of the poison. He should be observed for signs of shock. If no nausea or vomiting are present, warm but not hot fluids can be given. Alcohol is contraindicated, since it increases circulation and thus speeds up the absorption of the poison. The injured limb should be placed in a dependent position. Cold but not ice may be applied; cold will diminish circulation, but ice may freeze the injured tissue.

The victim should be transported quickly to the hospital. There he is treated with antivenom if indicated. Tetanus prophylaxis is instituted and antibiotics are given to combat infection. Analgesics are given for pain; however, the initial severe pain may diminish to a numbness after a few hours. Fluid balance is monitored and therapy for shock instituted as indicated. Oxygen should be available for use as needed. Massive sloughing of the tissues may occur following snakebite. The skin under the large bullae that form may resemble a severe burn.[73] Frequent dressing changes may be indicated. Snakebite wounds heal slowly, and in severe cases amputation may be necessary.

Rabies. Rabies is an acute infectious viral disease that affects the nervous system, primarily the brain. The disease has been known for centuries. In the twentieth century BC the Eshnunna code of ancient Mesopotamia set forth strict regulations about the obligations of dog owners who let mad dogs bite persons, thereby causing death. Rabies is usually fatal, although there have been a few documented survivals.[14]

The rabies virus is transmitted to humans through bites of carnivorous animals. The most frequent source in the United States since the advent of required inoculation of dogs is wild animals, primarily skunks, foxes, bats, and raccoons.[20] Bats can frequently be found in urban as well as rural areas. Rabies does not usually occur following bites by members of the rodent family (rats, squirrels, chipmunks, or rabbits). There has been an increase in the incidence of rabies found in cattle. The virus can also be transmitted from the saliva of the rabid animal to a person through an existing break in the victim's skin.

Not all rabies-infected animals are mad. There are two types of rabies. In one type the animal may be restless, barking, and biting. In the other, so-called dumb rabies, the animal may be quiet and stay close to its master. In the latter type, paralysis, which begins in the throat and lower jaw, may lead the animal's owner to suspect that something harmful has been swallowed. If he tries to investigate the trouble, some of the highly infectious saliva may enter an abrasion on his hand.

Prevention. The control of rabies is a public health responsibility. The police and health departments must be notified at once if it is thought that a rabid animal is at large. In England and the Scandinavian countries the disease has been almost entirely eliminated by rigid enforcement of laws that prohibit allowing dogs to run about unleashed. Rabies could be controlled by compulsory vaccination of all dogs and cats kept as household pets, capture and confinement of stray animals, and destruction of wild animal reservoirs of infection under the supervision of wildlife experts. How long the immunity lasts following vaccination is not known for certain. Immunization in humans is thought to last about 12 months and in animals up to 39 months.

Rabies can be prevented in humans by immunization whenever the possibility of developing rabies is present. The decision for postexposure prophylaxis is made by the physician after comparing the potential for developing rabies with the potential for serious reaction to prophylaxis. Prophylaxis is initiated if the bite was from a wild animal, from an unprovoked attack by a domestic animal that cannot be observed for 10 days, or from an animal observed to develop signs of rabies. Every attempt is made to capture the animal by competent authorities, and wild animals are killed for analysis. The presence of *Negri* bodies in the brain of an animal is conclusive evidence of rabies. The effectiveness of postexposure prophylaxis decreases over time; therefore a prompt decision to start treatment for prevention of rabies is important.[20]

The United States Public Health Service Advisory

Committee on Immunization Practices has developed standards for prophylactic treatment. There are two types of prophylactic treatment for rabies: antirabies serum and rabies vaccine. In most situations both the serum and the vaccine are given to the victim. The vaccine may be given alone for nonbite exposures to escaped cats and dogs.[20]

Hyperimmune rabies *serum* is a form of passive immunity for rabies. Until recently the antirabies serum (ARS), a horse serum, has been the recommended serum. Since horse serum causes allergic reactions in at least 20% of those receiving it, hypersensitivity testing must be done before it is administered. Serum sickness occurs in 15% children and 40% of adults who receive ARS.[20] At least half of the ARS given is used to infiltrate around the wound and the remainder is given intramuscularly. There is a new hyperimmune rabies immune globulin (HRIG), but it is not yet readily available.[20] The benefit of the new serum is that it is not a horse serum so the danger of anaphylaxis is not present.

Rabies *vaccine* produces active immunity. Two vaccines are in common use at this time and one new vaccine is being tested. Nerve tissue vaccine (NTV) is used worldwide but seldom in the United States as it is associated with central nervous system reactions. The vaccine approved for use in the United States at this time is duck embryo vaccine (DEV). Injections are given subcutaneously in rotating sites in the abdomen or lateral aspects of the thighs for 21 doses over 14 to 21 days, followed by two booster doses on the tenth and twentieth days after the initial series is completed. Anaphylaxis occurs in 0.9% of persons, and systemic reaction (fever, malaise, myalgia) in 33%.[58] All patients experience local reactions (pain, erythema). Major complications are uncommon, but central nervous system reactions can occur.

The new human diploid cell vaccine (HDCV) shows promise as a possible replacement for DEV. Since the origin is from human cells, anaphylaxis is prevented. Systemic reactions occur in a smaller number of persons. The vaccine has been found to produce effective antibody titers after a four-dose schedule.[58] HDCV vaccine is given intramuscularly, and local soreness does develop as with DEV.

Corticosteroids should not be given to the person receiving any type of rabies vaccine unless the situation is life threatening.[20] Corticosteroids are antiinflammatory and interfere with the development of active immunity.

Assessment. The incubation period of the disease in humans is from 10 days to more than a year.[12] The involvement, as in animals, is in the central nervous system. The disease is ushered in with a few days of melancholia, depression, pain at the site of the animal bite, and a feeling of impending danger. Acute symptoms (difficulty in swallowing, excessive salivation, muscle spasm, often maniacal fear, difficulty in breathing, and convulsions) then appear. A terrific, painful spasm of the muscle of deglutition occurs when there is an attempt to swallow water, hence the name hydrophobia. Even the mention of water is often enough to bring on an attack. Aerophobia is also present, and convulsions can be produced by a draft of air on the skin. Death from rabies has been reduced in the United States to several cases per year.

Intervention. The nursing care of the patient with acute rabies is difficult but of short duration. Most patients die from heart failure or respiratory difficulty within 3 or 4 days of the acute onset of symptoms. The patient is restless, irritable, and fearful, with episodes of uncontrolled fear and mania alternating with periods of calm. Every effort is made to keep the patient quiet. The room is darkened, and the noises in the halls outside the room should be eliminated. Side rails are placed on the bed and are sometimes padded to help prevent injury during episodes of uncontrolled thrashing about. Sedatives, including chloral hydrate, morphine, and the barbiturates, are given. Anesthetics may be given intravenously. Fluids often are given intravenously, and it is important to bandage the arm securely on a board to prevent injury in the event of a convulsion or an attack of mania while a needle is in the vein. The head of the bed is sometimes lowered in an attempt to facilitate drainage of saliva, and often suctioning must be used. All persons caring for the patient should be aware of contamination from saliva, and a gown and rubber gloves should be worn.[3] Relatives of the patient must be prepared for the fact that the patient cannot talk. Sometimes the visits of relatives bring on severe painful muscle spasm in the throat of the patient, who is usually conscious up to the time of death even though he is unable to speak.

Tetanus. Tetanus, or lockjaw, is an infectious disease caused by the gram-positive anaerobic spore-producing bacteria *Clostridium tetani*, which are normal inhabitants of the intestinal tracts of humans and other animals and which can survive for years in soil and dirt. They enter the bloodstream of human beings through wounds and travel to the central nervous system. They produce a powerful toxin that acts at the myoneural junction causing prolonged muscular contractions. Tetanus is a highly fatal disease; almost one fourth of persons who develop tetanus die, even with rigorous treatment.

Prevention. The only sure method of prevention of tetanus is through immunization. Tetanus prophylaxis is part of the planned immunization program for children. Persons who have had previous tetanus immunizations within 10 years are given a booster dose after sustaining a contaminated or deep puncture wound. Nonimmunized persons are given a tetanus immunizations series and are also given tetanus immune globulin (human) (TIGH).

Assessment. The symptoms of tetanus appear from 3 days to several weeks after the introduction of the bacteria into the wound. The patient first notices stiffness of the jaws and then develops difficulty in opening his mouth. He complains of rigidity of the facial and sternocleidomastoid muscles. The muscles become hypertonic and cause stiffness of the neck and spasm of the facial muscles, which produces the characteristic sardonic smile *(risus sardonicus).* The abdominal and lumbar muscles also become rigid, and opisthotonos (arching of the back) occurs. Painful muscle spasms may occur on the slightest stimulation (a draft, jarring the bed, touching the bedclothes).

Intervention. Treatment is directed toward neutralizing the toxin with TIGH administered intramuscularly with part of the dose infiltrated around the wound. Tetanus antitoxin (TAT) of equine origin is used only when TIGH is not available, as hypersensitivity to the horse serum may be present with the potential for anaphylaxis. Penicillin G or tetracycline is often administered to reduce the number of vegetative forms and to control secondary infection.[3]

Other therapy includes constant care in a quiet semidark room, sedation, and muscle relaxants to reduce the severity and frequency of muscle spasms. The treatment of choice in severe disease is *d*-tubocurarine (curare) to produce paralysis of muscles and sedation with diazepam (Valium). Tracheostomy and artificial ventilation may be necessary.

Fractures

Injury to the musculoskeletal system may result in fractures or dislocations of the bones, strained muscles, or torn ligaments (see Chapter 42 for a complete discussion of these injuries). Emergency care consists in assessment of injury and interventions to prevent further trauma until medical help is available.

Assessment. Pain localized over a bone or joint should be considered a fracture until a definitive diagnosis is made. Obvious deformity can be either a dislocation (if at a joint) or a fracture. In a compound fracture the bone may be protruding through the skin. Ecchymosis (bluish discoloration) of the skin may occur with any musculoskeletal injury due to rupture of blood vessels at the time of injury. The ability to move an extremity or digit does not negate a fracture, although the victim usually refrains from movement because of pain. Shock may occur with severe fractures, either from the stress of the trauma or from blood loss such as the extravasation of blood in the thigh following injury.

The victim should not be moved when being examined for fracture of the spine (neck or back). The examiner slides his or her hand under the victim and checks for point tenderness along the length of the spine. Bruises on the head may indicate that a force has been exerted that could cause a neck fracture. Bruises on the shoulder, back, or abdomen are frequently seen with back fractures. A spinal fracture can be present in the absence of any bruises. If the spinal cord has been damaged there may be loss of movement or sensation of the extremities.

Skull fractures may vary from a small linear fracture with few symptoms to severe depression of bone fragments into the brain. Basilar skull fractures may be accompanied by bleeding or draining serous fluid from the nose or ears or both. Fractures of facial bones may interfere with respiration if the air passages become blocked.

Pain or deformity at the hip can be caused by either a fracture or dislocation. The leg will be shortened in both instances but turned outward if there is a fracture and inward with a dislocation. Fractures of the extremities may be accompanied by loss of circulation or sensation if blood vessels or nerves are pinched by the bone fragment. Circulation distal to the fracture is assessed by observing skin color and presence of pulses. A neurologic check for sensation and circulatory system checks should be repeated after splinting and during transportation.

Intervention

General management of fractures. Dressings are applied to an open wound at the site of a fracture before splinting is carried out in order to prevent infection and minimize bleeding. The fractured bone should be well supported and moved as little as possible during application of dressing and splint. Unless there is imminent danger of further accidental injury, such as by fire or explosion, the victim is not moved until the fracture is splinted.

Fractures are splinted as they are found with the exception of severely angulated fractures of the *shafts* of bones of the extremities. The severe angulation is straightened by placing one hand just below the fracture and the other farther down the extremity and applying gentle traction.[2] The purpose of straightening a severe angulation is not to reduce the fracture but to decrease the spasm of the muscles and prevent damage to blood vessels and nerves. The sooner the traction is applied, the less the discomfort to the victim as some numbness occurs immediately following the injury.[2] Traction is maintained until the extremity is splinted. Deformities of a joint (shoulder, elbow, wrist, knee) are *never* straightened because of the presence of major blood vessels and nerves at a joint.

Splints are applied to include the joint above and below the fracture. Rigid splints such as boards or cardboard are padded for comfort and to prevent pressure areas. Soft splints such as pillows can be reinforced by a rigid material such as boards or magazines for added firmness. Air splints, if available, are inflated only by the mouth, not a pump, to a point where the thumb makes a slight dent. Toes and fingers should remain free for assessment of circulation. Gentleness and support of the fractured part are imperative during handling as careless handling can add to the severity of the original injury and increase the potential for shock.

Fracture of the spine. Any questionable injury to the neck or back is treated as a fracture of the spine. Two problems can occur from a fractured spine: damage to the spinal cord and neurogenic shock. If the cervical spine is fractured, there may be interference with respiration so that respirations must be continually monitored. The victim may use diaphragmatic breathing for a short period of time but be unable to sustain this. Artificial ventilation is more difficult because the neck cannot be hyperextended as this can cause further injury to the spinal cord. The head can be extended by gentle traction and the jaw pulled forward to open the airway. Traction must be maintained until the neck can be supported in this position. The neck should never be flexed, twisted, or hyperextended. If the victim is not having difficulty with respiration, the neck can be splinted in the position in which it was found.

Transportation of a person with a potential spine fracture must be on a firm base, preferably a back board. Forward or backward bending of the spine is to be avoided to prevent further trauma to the spinal cord. The victim should be slid, not rolled, in straight alignment onto the back board. It takes several persons working together to move the victim safely. The victim remains on the back board during the initial diagnostic tests in the emergency room.

□ Rape

Rape is one of the violent crimes for which an increasing number of people, primarily women, are seeking help. Despite the increasing number of rapes being reported, it is estimated that unreported rape ranges from 200% to 300% more than reported rape.[63] There are many reasons why women do not report rape. In the past, women who were raped were often thought to have encouraged it or to have been secretly desiring rape. This belief still persists among some people.

In past years if the victim pursued the matter of rape in the courts, she was often embarrassed and humiliated; the rapist would then often be acquitted. The rise of the feminist movement has provided an impetus to make changes. These changes are occurring, more rapidly in some places than in others, but there is still much to be accomplished.[60] Legal definitions are being changed. The court procedure is still one of great trauma psychologically for the victim, and she needs to know what is actually involved before she makes the decision to press charges.

Rape crisis centers have been formed in many large cities. These centers differ in their functions but usually have one or all of three main functions (1) victim service, (2) service to professional agencies (health, law), and (3) community education. The victim service is the primary role for which the centers have been formed. Since this service is not adequate to change the system for the victim, services for education of professionals serving rape victims and education of the community to increase public awareness of the problems of rape victims are being developed. The victim service consists of volunteers, many of whom have been raped themselves, who serve as victim advocate through the medical examination and police interview. Some form of follow-up service such as counseling may be available. Some rape crisis centers have volunteer attorneys who can offer the victim legal advice or representation.

It is difficult to obtain statistics concerning the sociologic variables relating to rape because of the large number of unreported cases. There are many misconceptions concerning rape. The facts are that rape is common to all classes (there is a higher incidence of reported rape among the lower class), that rape occurs mostly *intra*racially rather than interracially, and that a majority of rapes are committed by someone the victim knows.[7] This latter reason is one major factor why many rapes go unreported. Often the victim fears for her own safety, is made to feel that she is the cause of the incident, or fears the stigma involved. The majority of rape victims are females, but males, especially young boys, may also be rape victims. The attacker is usually another male. Rape of males is a major problem in prisons in the United States. Some prison reform groups are actively addressing this problem with the major emphasis being on protecting the young and the vulnerable from attack.

Trauma of rape

Rape is a traumatic event for the victim physically, psychologically, and socially. Physical force is often employed; a weapon may be used either as a threat or to injure the victim, or the hands or fists may be used to beat the victim or threaten choking. Injury can also occur as the victim is attempting to defend herself or while struggling on the ground or floor. The vagina and perineum may be injured by force used during the sexual attack, and the rectum may also be lacerated if anal sex has been attempted. The latter is more common in rape of males.

Psychologic trauma is usually severe; the rape victim is in a state of crisis. Fear is a dominant theme as the victim perceives the event as life threatening.[45] Other feelings expressed by victims are depersonalization, shame, degradation, defilement, violation, guilt, humiliation, anger.[17,63] The victim has not only been under threat of harm but has also been subjected in many instances to multiple sexual assaults, some natural, some perverted, by one or more persons. Fellatio (oral sex) is frequently demanded by the rapist. Some rapists will urinate on the victim before leaving her.

The rape victim also experiences a sociologic crisis. If the woman is married, marital relationships may be affected. If she is single she is often in fear of repeated occurrences and may feel the need to move, especially if the attack occurred in her home or apartment. Decisions have to be made concerning whom to tell about the incident as loss of needed support by significant others may occur. Job security or relationships with co-workers may be threatened. If a child is the victim, social relationships within the family may be altered. Problems of a sociologic nature take considerable time to be resolved, but concerns related to these potential problems may occur in the initial emergency period.

Types of rape victimization

Burgess and Holmstrom[17] have identified three types of rape victimization from their research: (1) rape or sex without consent, (2) accessory to sex or inability to give consent, and (3) sex stress situation or sex with initial consent. The first type is easily identified as rape; the victim is attacked suddenly (blitz rape) or the rapist gains the victim's confidence but then takes advantage of her. Some persons are unable to give consent because of their cognitive or personality development. They are lured by the rapist by offers of material goods such as candy or by offers of pleasure or human contact. In the third group are persons who agree to a sexual relationship, but either perversion occurs or the victim or family becomes worried at a later time concerning possible consequences. All of these situations produce victims in need of help.

Prevention

All women need to know the measures they can take to help prevent rape from occurring (see box). It would also be helpful for every woman to learn methods of self-defense. Some communities are beginning to introduce both the issue of rape and self-defense into secondary school curricula. Many YWCAs teach classes in self-defense. Rape crisis centers can provide information on availability of classes in the community. Women learning physical defense skills need to learn to value themselves so they can justify the need for self-defense and have confidence in their ability to defend themselves.

RAPE PREVENTIVE MEASURES

Prevention of attack

- Set house lights to go on and off by timer
- Keep light on at all entrances
- Place safety locks on windows and doors
- Have key ready before reaching door of house or car
- Look in car before entering
- Insist on identification before letting a stranger in house; check identification with agency if suspicious
- Do not list first name on mailbox or in telephone directory
- Make arrangements with neighbor for needed assistance
- Be alert when walking in street; walk in lighted areas
- Walk down center of street if possible
- Avoid lonely or enclosed areas

If attacked

- Run toward a lighted house; yell, "Fire"
- Spit in rapist's face; act bizarre; vomit
- Rip off rapist's glasses
- Step hard on his foot (instep)
- Aim at eyes—try to gouge eyes, scrape face
- Hit throat at Adam's apple (larynx)
- Use fighting and screaming with caution; this may scare some rapists, encourage others
- Try talking to avoid rape
- If powerless, make close observations about rapist, car, location.

Health care

Persons who are raped may seek medical help directly or call the police, who will then take the victim for medical examination. Some victims fear reprisal by the rapist or are unwilling for others to know about the rape and therefore do not seek medical attention. Victims need to be encouraged to report the incident. They need considerable support during both the acute emergency and the long-term consequences, and knowledgeable nurses are able to provide appropriate support.

Many hospitals have developed protocols for care of the rape victim in the emergency department. If such a protocol does not exist, it behooves the nurses in the emergency department to work toward development of a protocol. Rape crisis centers can be helpful in this regard. The protocol includes high priority in triage, provisions for privacy without leaving the victim alone, provision of a victim advocate such as a woman from a rape crisis center if desired, continual emotional support by nonjudgmental health personnel, and routines to assure the protection and comfort of the victim. These routines delineate which personnel have priority for contacts with the victim. If no injury is present that threatens life, the nurse may be designated to have primary contact with the victim and make the decision as to when the victim is ready for medical examination or police interview. Large city police departments often have women police officers assigned to interview rape victims, since many girls and women become very upset when asked to talk with a male police officer.

Assessment

Subjective data. The person who has been raped goes through the same phases as any person facing a crisis situation (p. 230). The initial phase is one of shock and disbelief that rape has occurred and of emotional disequilibrium manifested in many different ways. After the initial acute phase there is a period of pseudo-equilibrium when the victim rationalizes the event or attempts to suppress thoughts concerning the rape. During the long-term phase there are periods of depression, phobic reactions, nightmares, and changes in life style.[17,32]

The victim will be asked many questions by the physician to identify the type of assault and potential for injury. If the victim has been threatened, she may have succumbed through fear, and this needs to be elicited. Victims often talk freely to the nurse about their feelings; their fears concerning injury, mutilation, or death at the time of assault; or present fears concerning pregnancy or venereal disease. Other feelings of degradation, feeling "dirty," shame, guilt, and so forth, may be expressed. Anger may be directed at the assailant or projected toward medical care or personnel. Pain may be local at the site of assault or generalized and diffuse. The victim may complain of a sore throat if choking was used as a threat or following oral sex. Nausea may also be reported.

Objective data. One of the myths concerning rape is that all women are hysterical after rape. Burgess and Holmstrom[17] in their research identified two different types of responses with about half of the victims falling in each category. The first type they labeled "expressed style." These women were emotionally labile as evidenced by crying, shaking, restlessness, tenseness, smiling or laughing inappropriately. The other group, labeled "controlled style," appeared calm, composed, or subdued. The full impact of the experience often hit them at a later time.

A head-to-toe assessment for signs of physical trauma is usually carried out by the physician. The clothing will be inspected and described and is often requested by the police for evidence. Clothing should not be washed or discarded. Other data needed by the police usually include samples of the assailant's hair from combing of pubic hair and fingernail deposits for samples of the assailant's tissue.

Tests. Papanicolaou smears of the vagina, mouth, or rectum and saline suspensions are done for the presence of sperm. An acid phosphatase test will demonstrate recency of intercourse. Tests will be inconclusive if the victim has bathed or douched since the rape. Tests for venereal disease are done at the initial visit to obtain baseline information for comparison at 3 to 6 weeks.

Intervention

All personnel who have contact with the rape victims need to refine their skills in providing support to the victim using a nonjudgmental approach. Knowledge of the problems and experiences of other victims as well as rapists is helpful in understanding what is being experienced by the victim (see references listed at the end of the chapter). Interdisciplinary conferences involving health care providers, volunteers from rape crisis centers, and the police help clarify issues and problems.

Emotional support. Initially the victim needs time to marshal her coping responses. Most victims have a need to talk and a need to know that someone cares what is happening to them. The nurse utilizes crisis intervention theory as the basis for deciding how best to help the victim (see Chapter 16). Many hospitals have contacts with a rape crisis center. The victim is given the choice of having a victim advocate from the center be with her during the entire procedure, and medical examination or interviews by the police are not begun until the volunteer arrives.

Preparation for the physical examination is carried out in advance. Having a pelvic examination after a sexual assault can be a traumatic experience for the victim, and some girls or women have never had a pelvic examination previously.

Comfort. *After the victim has been examined,* she will probably have a need to wash herself. Mouthwash is appreciated, especially if there has been oral sex. A change of clothing may be needed if the police want her clothing for evidence, which is not uncommon.

Sexuality. The victim has many concerns related to her sexuality. Time is needed to work through these concerns, and long-term counseling is helpful to many victims.

Concern about possible pregnancy depends on the circumstances: whether she is in the child-bearing years, whether birth control is in effect at the time of sexual attack, and at what point in the menstrual period the rape occurs. If pregnancy is a possibility, diethylstilbestrol (DES) may be given. Side effects may include nausea, vomiting, and cramplike chest pains.

Concern about venereal disease is common. An antibiotic is given following the initial examination as a preventive measure. The victim needs to know that medical follow-up is important and that she should be retested for venereal disease in about 3 weeks unless symptoms occur earlier. In addition the victim may experience vaginal discharge, itching, and burning sensation due to an acute vaginal infection (vaginitis). This infection may become chronic.[17]

Discharge. The victim should not go home to an empty house or apartment. The volunteer from the rape crisis center, the social worker, or police can all facilitate arrangements for transportation to her home or to the home of family or friends. Frequently the victim goes to the police station after medical care is completed to follow up with the police report. The victim needs to know about the availability of follow-up medical services and counseling services. In some medical centers there are psychiatrists who are especially interested is assisting rape victims with counseling as desired.

Outcome criteria for the woman who has been raped

The victim:

1. Has means for transportation and someone to accompany her to a self-designated destination.
2. Can state why, when, and where to obtain medical follow-up for venereal disease.
3. Knows resources for obtaining temporary and long-term support or counseling.

■ DISASTERS

Disasters are sudden catastrophic events that disrupt patterns of life and in which there is possible loss of life and property in addition to multiple injuries. Disasters can be either natural phenomena or caused by people (see box).

□ Effect of disasters

The effects of disasters are multiple. People are killed or injured and separated from their families. Many become homeless. In a large-scale disaster confusion and chaos occur during the early stages. Panic rarely occurs, but when it does it is because the involved persons believe that escape routes are limited and may be closing off. Effective leadership and communication can usually prevent panic from occurring.[34]

Transportation difficulties are created as streets and roads become clogged by persons trying to get away from the impact area or others trying to get in. Persons within the area are trying to flee or to find friends, family, or medical assistance. Persons outside of the disaster area are either trying to move in to help, to find relatives, or just because of curiosity. Sightseers can present a serious problem to maintenance of open roads in and out of the area.

Food and water supplies can become contaminated or nonexistent. Medical supplies can be inadequate to meet the sudden increased need. Utilities can become disrupted. Law enforcement is necessary to prevent looting and other civil disorders. Establishment of a communication system takes first priority to prevent chaos.

TYPES OF DISASTERS

Natural	Man-made
Air	*Transportation*
Tornado	Air
Hurricane	Land
Blizzard	Water
Land	*Fire*
Earthquake	Housing
Volcanic eruption	Forest
Avalanches	Explosions
Cave-ins	*Disease*
Water	Epidemics
Floods: slow rising	*Civil disorders*
and flash floods	Riots
Tidal waves	Wars (nuclear attack)

□ Roles of nurses in disasters

The actual role assumed by a given nurse at a disaster will depend on (1) the abilities of the nurse and (2) the specific situation. The nurse may not be able to reach a specific location where his or her services may be most useful, so the needs of victims may then be better served by the nurse functioning in a different capacity.

Nurses can participate in a disaster in many ways. Nurses with leadership ability and experience may be needed to serve in this capacity. Any nurse may be in a position of being the only health care provider in a given area and be responsible for giving initial first-aid treatment or supervising the activities of others. It therefore behooves nurses to continually update their first-aid skills. Because of their education and experience in assessment and intervention for psychosocial problems, professional nurses can be especially helpful in aiding victims to cope with their emotional reactions to the disaster. Nurses may be asked to serve at emergency morgues for support of families experiencing loss of loved ones.

As shelters are established, nurses are needed to staff the shelters to help meet the health needs of victims separated from their homes and families. The American Red Cross, which assumes an active role during disasters along with governmental agencies, operates shelters for victims. They provide supplies and food as well as service personnel (shelter manager, nurses, physicians, food helpers). Nurses interested in serving during disasters at home or in other parts of the country may contact the local American Red Cross office. Other services provided by the American Red Cross include emergency services on an individual family basis and aid for recovery.

When the disaster occurs in the nurse's own geographic area, the ability of the nurse to function is influenced by the impact of the disaster on self and on family. The nurse may be unable to contact or reach his or her own family and may be in a position of having to provide health care while actively concerned about the family's safety and welfare. The nurse may also be experiencing the emotional impact of the crisis situation, and this may limit the effectiveness of the care provided.

□ Prevention

Preparedness for disasters includes community planning to identify and, it is hoped, to prevent disasters that can occur and education of the public to minimize the number of casualties.

Community planning

Most states have disaster service agencies, which are outgrowths of civil defense organizations. These agencies act as coordinating agencies for the local agencies. Every community should have a disaster planning group as part of the emergency medical care committee. There should be representation by all groups who will be active participants should a disaster occur. This would include governmental groups (political, law enforcement, fire), health groups (hospitals, physicians, nurses, pharmacists, social workers), official groups (American Red Cross), and nonofficial groups (telephone company, parent-teacher organization, religious organizations). The disaster planning committee identifies the types of disasters that may occur in the local community, organizes a plan to be followed for different situations and arranges for simulated drills to test the effectiveness of the plans, and determines need for education or updating of necessary skills of participants. Nurses need to be active participants in the planning, implementation, and evaluation phases.

During a disaster the local hospitals become actively involved and need their own disaster plan to cope with the sudden influx of persons needing emergency care. Any time a large number of injured persons are in need of emergency care, hospital disaster plans are put into effect. Testing of hospital disaster plans at specified intervals by simulated drills is useful for determining if the plans are effective and what changes, if any, are needed.

Public education

Public awareness of potential community disasters is needed for effective community preparedness for disasters. Disaster planning committees need support and participation by community members. Individual persons need to know what they should do in the event of a disaster. Most radio and television stations regularly notify communities of potential disasters and give directions for preventive actions to be taken and for methods of obtaining further information should the disaster occur. Since electricity may be cut off, battery-operated radios should be available in all homes for continued communication.

All homes should have an emergency food cabinet with sufficient nonperishable foods to meet nutritional needs for several days. Supplies are rotated with current supplies to prevent these supplies from spoiling or becoming outdated.

□ Assessment

Triage

Triage during disasters differs from that at other times because of the large numbers of injured persons. The injured are sorted according to the following priority for treatment and transportation.

Urgent. These victims have a reasonable chance of survival only if they receive immediate treatment. First-aid treatment is started immediately and continued during transportation. This category includes victims with respiratory insufficiency, cardiac arrest, hemorrhage, and severe abdominal injury.

Serious. These victims can wait for transportation after they receive initial first-aid treatment. They include victims with immobilized closed fractures, soft-tissue injuries without hemorrhage, and burns on less than 40% of the body.

Minimal. Victims in this category are ambulatory, have minor tissue injuries, and may be dazed. They can be treated by nonprofessionals and held for observation if necessary.

Delayed or expectant. If the injuries are of such magnitude that there is a question of survival, transportation for these victims is given low priority during an overwhelming disaster. This rarely occurs in civilian life.[54] The number of victims in the serious or urgent category must greatly outnumber the health and transportation personnel available. Victims in this category are reclassified as the emergency situation changes. Priority is then given to those victims with the greatest chance of survival. Examples are victims with massive damage to the respiratory tract or central nervous system.

Disaster syndrome

The behavior of victims following the impact of disaster can be characterized as progressing through four phases: shock, awareness, euphoria, and anger.[34] The victims are experiencing loss; therefore the phases are similar to those experienced by others during any kind of loss (grieving).

The shock phase may last only a few minutes or up to several hours after impact. The victim is dazed and unable to comprehend what is occurring. He cannot follow even simple directions. Persons prepared to function in emergencies are less apt to spend much time in the shock phase.[34]

The awareness phase may last up to several days. The victim becomes aware that he has survived and tries to help others, minimizing his own injuries or losses. During this stage guilt feelings may arise because others died while he survived. The victim is high suggestible, can follow simple directions, but cannot carry out problem solving effectively. For example, following one major earthquake a young woman who had run outdoors on a chilly night clad only in a thin nightgown was told to put on something warm. Her solution was to wrap a warm scarf around her neck.

The euphoria phase may last for several weeks. The victim feels a sense of brotherhood with the community and participates willingly in helping others with plans for recovery.

Before resolution occurs, the victim may go through the "Why me?" or anger phase that occurs because of the experienced loss. The anger is often projected against helping persons from the outside who were not personally affected by the disaster. It is especially important for nurses who may be assisting victims during the recovery phase to understand that the anger is part of the loss experience. As the victim copes with the losses incurred by the disaster and his life returns to more normal patterns, the anger will disappear.

□ Intervention

Emergency aid stations

The number, size, and staffing of emergency aid stations depends on the type and extent of the disaster. There must be one person who is designated as the leader and who is responsible for making decisions for maximum effectiveness of the unit. Medical supplies and food for personnel must be available. One person is designated for triage. In the absence of a physician, a nurse assumes leadership of the first-aid care that is rendered. Transportation teams will bring some victims to the station and transport victims to a medical center for follow-up care. Unfortunately many victims will go directly to a medical center, bypassing a first-aid unit and thus creating a logistics problem at the medical center and decreasing the effectiveness of the care that can be given.

The types of injuries that occur will depend on the type of disaster. Soft-tissue and bone injuries are common in most natural disasters. Respiratory insufficiency may occur with airway injuries. Fear resulting from the disaster can precipitate cardiac arrests. Childbirth may also be precipitated. If the weather is inclement, additional injuries and disease may occur after the immediate crisis is over. If tear gas has been used, the victim should not be placed in a closed environmment near other victims. Health personnel will be unable to function if they are affected by the tear gas.

Victims are not transported until first-aid care has been given, as in any emergency. If hemorrhage has not been controlled or fractures splinted, the victim may arrive at the medical center in shock that could have been prevented or minimized, and surgical intervention will not take place until measures to treat shock are instituted and the patient's condition is stable. If first-aid measures are instituted before the victim is transported, he can be taken to surgery at the earliest opportunity. Records indicating all treatment given at an emergency aid center *must* accompany a victim if he is referred or transported to a medical center or any other health care facility. The information is attached to the victim if he is not responsible and should include his name, age, address, name of nearest relative, assessment made, and treatment given.

Shelters

Most shelters are set up in schools, which can house a large number of people. Toilet facilities, running water, and cooking facilities must be available. The role of the nurse in a shelter is to assess and provide for health needs of the shelter population. Persons with infectious diseases need to be isolated from other persons.

Elderly persons may become confused by the rapidly changing events and strange surroundings. Many elderly have chronic illnesses and very often their medications have been left at home. They may not be able to see well if their glasses have been lost or eat well if dentures are missing. Because elderly persons may have decreased resistance, they are more susceptible to disease following a disaster.

Any victims who have chronic illnesses must be identified. If they are receiving replacement therapy such as insulin, this must be obtained. Arrangements must be made for the care of pregnant women and infants. Formulas must be obtained and special dietary needs arranged. Immunization of shelter occupants may also be necessary. Occupants should be monitored for signs of developing health problems.

Assessment of safety factors in the environment is also a nursing responsibility. The nurse is part of the shelter team and advises the shelter manager of any potential health hazards. The care of victims in a disaster is a team effort, and the nurse is an important member of this team.

REFERENCES AND SELECTED READINGS

1. Accident facts, Chicago, 1976, National Safety Council.
2. American Academy of Orthopedic Surgeons, Committee on Injuries: Emergency care and transportation of the sick and injured, Chicago, 1971, The Academy.
3. American Academy of Pediatrics: Report of the Committee on Infectious Diseases, ed. 17, Evanston, Ill., 1974, The Academy.
4. American College of Surgeons, Committee on Trauma: Early care of the injured patient, ed. 2, Philadelphia, 1976, W. B. Saunders Co.
5. American Council of Life Insurance: Life insurance fact book, New York, 1976, The Council.
6. American Hospital Association: Principles of disaster preparedness for hospitals, rev. ed., Chicago, 1971, The Association.
7. Amir, M.: Forcible rape. In Schultz, L.: Rape Victimology, Springfield, Ill., 1975, Charles C Thomas, Publisher.
8. Anderson, R.: The behavioral aspects of safety, Am. Assoc. Indust. Nurse J. **14:**9-11, 1966.
9. Baer, E.: Civil disorder: mass emergency of the 70's, Am. J. Nurs. **72:**1072-1076, 1972
10. Baker, G. W., and Chapman, D. W., editors: Man and society in disaster, New York, 1962, Basic Books, Inc.
11. Beall, A. C., Jr., Noon, G. P., and Harris, H. H.: Surgical management of tracheal trauma, J. Trauma **7:**248-256, 1967.
12. Beeson, P. B., and McDermott, W., editors: Textbook of medicine, ed. 14, Philadelphia, 1975, W. B. Saunders Co.
13. Bergersen, B. S., and Goth, A.: Pharmacology in nursing, ed. 14, St. Louis, 1979, The C. V. Mosby Co.
14. Bhatt, D.: Human rabies, Am. J. Dis. Child **127:**862-869, 1974.
15. Bishop, G., and Hynek, R.: Rape. In The Boston Women's Health Book Collective, editors: Our bodies, ourselves: a book by and for women, ed. 2, New York, 1976. Simon & Schuster, Inc.
16. Burgess, A., and Holmstrom, L.: Crisis and counseling requests of rape victims, Nurs. Res. **23:**196-202, 1974.
17. Burgess, A., and Holmstrom, L: Rape: victims of crisis, Bowie, Md., 1974, Robert Brady Co.
18. Burgess, A., and Holmstrom, L.: The rape victim in the emergency ward, Am. J. Nurs. **73:**1741-1745, 1973.
19. Corby, D., and Decke, W.: Management of acute poisoning with activated charcoal, Pediatrics **54:**324-329, 1974.
20. Corey, L., and Hattwick, M.: Treatment of persons exposed to rabies, J.A.M.A. **232:**272-276, 1975.
21. Cosgriff, J. H., Jr.: Emergency nursing, Supervisor Nurse **5:**30-37, 1974.
22. Cosgriff, J. H., Jr., and Anderson, D.: The practice of emergency nursing, Philadelphia, 1975, J. B. Lippincott Co.
23. Creighton, H.: Law every nurse should know, Philadelphia, 1970, W. B. Saunders Co.
24. Croft, H., and Frenkel, S.: Children and lead poisoning, Am. J. Nurs. **75:**102-104, 1975.
25. *Division of Health Mobilization, Public Health Service: The role of the nurse in national disaster, U.S. Department of Health, Education and Welfare, No. 1071-1-5, 1965.
26. Dreisbach, R. H.: Handbook of poisoning, diagnosis and treatment, ed. 8, Los Altos, Calif., 1974, Lange Medical Publications.
27. Eckert, C.: Emergency room care, ed. 3, Boston, 1976, Little, Brown and Co.
28. Ede, L., and Nelson, R.: The "Good Samaritan" law and the nurse's immunity for emergency care, Occup. Health Nurs. **20:**10-15, 1972.

*References preceded by an asterisk are particularly well suited for student reading.

29. Elliman, V. B., editor: Disaster nursing, Nurs. Clin. North Am. **2:**285-358, 1967.
30. *Emergency medicine (special fifth anniversary edition): Common emergencies in daily practice, 1974.
31. Erdman, K.: Keeping the consumer informed, FDA, Ohio's Health, vol. 19-22, July-Aug. 1973.
32. Flint, T. and Cain, H. D.: Emergency treatment and management, ed. 5, Philadelphia, 1975, W. B. Saunders Co.
33. Fox, S., and Scherl, D.: Crisis intervention with victims of rape. In Schultz, L.: Rape victimology, Springfield, Ill., 1975, Charles C Thomas, Publisher.
34. Garb, S., and Eng, E.: Disaster handbook, ed. 2, New York, 1969, Springer Publishing Co., Inc.
35. Gay, G.: Immediate care in the drug scene. In Stephenson, H. E., Jr.: Immediate care of the acutely ill and injured, ed. 2, St. Louis, 1978, The C. V. Mosby Co.
36. Genigeorgis, C., and Riemann, H.: Food safety and food poisoning, World Rev. Nutr. Diet. **16:**363-397, 1973.
37. Gosselin, T., et al.: Clinical toxicology of commercial products, ed. 4, Baltimore, 1976, The Williams & Wilkins Co.
38. Gunn, A.: Food poisoning. Nurs. Times **72:**842-844, 1976
39. Guyton, A.: Textbook of medical physiology, ed. 5, Philadelphia, 1977, W. B. Saunders Co.
40. Heimlich, H. J.: Death from food-choking prevented by a new life-saving maneuver, Heart Lung **5:**755-758, 1976.
41. Heimlich, H. J.: Pop goes the café coronary, Emergency Med. **6:**154-155, 1974.
42. Hess, F., and Jones, G.: Broadening our approach to emergency nursing care, Nurs. Clin. North Am. **5:**559-607, 1970.
43. Hill, G. J. II, editor: Out-patient surgery, Philadelphia, 1973, W. B. Saunders Co.
44. Hinkhouse, A.: Craniocerebral trauma, Am. J. Nurs. **73:**1719-1722, 1973.
45. Holmstrom, L., and Burgess, A.: Assessing trauma in rape victim, Am. J. Nurs. **75:**1288-1291, 1975.
46. Jaffe, S., Earle, A. S., Fleegler, E. J., et al.: Replantation of amputated extremities: report of five cases, Ohio State Med. J. **71:**381-386, 1975.
47. Kerr, A.: Orthopedic nursing procedures, ed. 3, New York, 1972, Springer Publishing Co., Inc.
48. *Kilpatrick, H. M.: The frightened patient in the emergency room. Am. J. Nurs. **66:**1031-1032, 1966.
49. Lee, J. M.: Emotional reactions to trauma, Nurs. Clin. North Am. **5:**577-587, 1970.
50. MacDonald, J.: Rape: offenders and their victims, Springfield, Ill., 1971, Charles C Thomas, Publisher.
51. *Mahoney, R. F.: Emergency and disaster nursing, ed. 2, New York, 1969, Macmillan, Inc.
52. *Manheimer, D. I., Dewey, J., Mellinger, G. D., et al.: 50,000 child-years of accidental injuries, Public Health Rep. **81:**519-533, 1966.
53. Marcus, H.: The accident repeater: a comparative psychiatric study, Int. J. Indust. Med. Surg. **37:**768-733, 1968.
54. Miller, R. H., and Cantrell, J. R.: Textbook of basic emergency medicine, St. Louis, 1975, The C. V. Mosby Co.
55. Mofenson, H., and Greensher, J.: Keeping up with the trends in childhood poisoning, Clin. Pediatr. **14:**621, 1975.
56. Mofenson, H., and Greensher, J.: The unknown poison, Pediatrics **54:**336-342, 1974.
57. Moore, M.: Medical emergency manual: differential diagnosis and treatment, Baltimore, 1972, The Williams & Wilkins Co.
58. Plotkin, S., Wiktor, T. J., Koprowski, H., et al.: Immunization schedules for the new human diploid cell vaccine against rabies, Am. J. Epidemiol. **103:**75-80, 1976.

59. Replantation of digits, Point of View (Sommerville, N.J., Ethicon Inc.) **13**:11, 1976.
60. Report of District of Columbia Task Force on Rape. In Schultz, L.: Rape victimology, Springfield, Ill., 1975, Charles C Thomas Publisher.
61. Romano, T.: Trauma Nurse Specialist, Am. J. Nurs. **73**:1008-1011, 1973.
62. Romano, T., and Boyd, D.: Illinois trauma program, Am. J. Nurs. **73**:1004-1007, 1973.
63. Schultz, L.: Rape victimology, Springfield, Ill., 1975, Charles C Thomas, Publisher.
64. Slater, R. R.: Triage nurse in the emergency department, Hospitals **44**:50-52, 1970.
65. Sovie, M., and Fruehan, C.: Protecting the patient from electrical hazards Nurs. Clin. North Am. **7**:469-480, 1972.
66. Standards for cardiopulmonary resuscitation and emergency cardiac care, J.A.M.A. **227**:796-797, 1974. (Supplements available from local chapters of the American Heart Association; 10¢ each if 100 or more copies ordered.)
67. Statistical abstract of the United States, 1975, ed. 76, Washington, D.C., 1975, U.S. Bureau of the Census.
68. Stephenson, H. E., Jr., editor: Immediate care of the acutely ill and injured, ed. 2, St. Louis, 1978, The C. V. Mosby Co.
69. Symposium on Trauma, Surg. Clin. North Am. **57**:1-226, 1977.
70. Tennant, F. S., Jr., Weaver, S. C., and Lewis, C. E.: Outcomes of drug education: four case studies, Pediatrics **52**:246-251, 1973.
71. *Wagner, M., guest editor: Emergency nursing. Nurs. Clin. North Am. **1**:377-466, 1973.
72. Walker, L.: Why do patients use the emergency room? Hosp. Topics **53**:19-21, 1975.
73. Warner, C. G., editor: Emergency care: assessment and intervention, ed. 2, St. Louis, 1978, The C. V. Mosby Co.
74. Wintrobe, M. M., et al., editors: Harrison's principles of internal medicine, ed. 8, New York, 1977, McGraw-Hill Book Co.

25

Neoplasia

ROSEMARIE HOGAN

Cancer was recognized in ancient times by skilled observers who gave it the name "cancer" (L., *cancri*, crab) because it stretched out in many directions like the legs of a crab. The term is somewhat general and is used interchangeably with malignant tumor and malignant neoplasm. It denotes a tumor caused by cell growth. Forms of cancer are found in plants and in humans and other animals. It would be good if the image of the crab, suggested by Hippocrates for superficial cancer in the advanced stages, could be dropped because it helps maintain a legend of incurability[13]

Few diseases cause greater feelings of anxiety and apprehension than cancer. Its physiologic and psychologic impact on patients and their families results in profound changes in their life style. Cancer may spell death to some and mutilation to others. The legends surrounding malignant disease, often focusing on incurability, help foster feelings of hopelessness and dread. Yet much progress has been made in prevention, early detection, and treatment of cancer, and research continues in these areas.

Nurses too may have the same negative attitudes that exist in society. For this reason it is extremely important that all nurses examine their own feelings about cancer and try to work them through, both by increasing their knowledge of the disease and its treatment and by discussing feelings openly with members of the health team. Nurses who have worked through their feelings are more able to be of assistance to patients and their families than nurses who have not done so.

The nurse's role in helping cancer patients is broad in scope and areas of influence. The nurse must have correct knowledge of prevention, control, and treatment of cancer and be able to apply this information in a variety of settings. Teaching about cancer is not limited to the hospital or clinic setting but takes place in industry, at PTA meetings, and other public forums. In addition to teaching about prevention, the nurse has an active role in treatment and control programs in all settings in which clients are found. Clients and their families look to the nurse for assistance and guidance in all phases of illness from detection to terminal care.

To be effective as a helping person the nurse must be aware of the emotional impact that the diagnosis of cancer has on the patient and family because this emotional response affects every aspect of nursing care. Cancer nursing is a challenge to the creativity, skill, and commitment of the nurse.

■ EPIDEMIOLOGY OF CANCER

Cancer is a disease that is universal in scope. It has existed since the beginning of history and affects humans wherever they live and whatever their race, color, level of culture, and material progress.[2]

Cancer ranks second to heart disease as the cause of death in the United States, but significant progress has been made in prevention and treatment. Twenty-five years ago, one in four patients with cancer survived 5 years. Today one in three will be saved, a gain of 55,000 lives each year. Success can be attributed to (1) the diagnosis of more cancers in the early localized stage, (2) the treatment of more patients within 4 months of diagnosis, and (3) the development of new diagnostic and treatment modalities, especially chemotherapy.

Despite these advances, in 1975 an estimated 110,000 persons died of cancer who might have been cured by early detection followed by prompt treatment.[1] Although in general cancer shows no respect for economic or social status, there are some variables with regard to sex, site, age, race, and geographic location.

□ Sex and site

The average incidence of cancer is similar in both sexes. The overall incidence (excluding carcinoma in situ of the uterine cervix and nonmelanoma skin cancer) has decreased slightly during the past 25 years. Cancers of the stomach, esophagus, rectum, uterus, ovary, and bladder (female) have declined while cancers of the lung,

Table 25-1. Reference chart: leading cancer sites, 1977*†

Site	Estimated new cases 1977	Estimated deaths 1977	Warning signals: (if you have one see your doctor)	Safeguards	Comment
Breast	90,000	34,000	Lump or thickening in the breast or unusual discharge from nipple	Regular checkup, monthly breast self-exam	Leading cause of cancer death in women.
Colon and rectum	101,000	51,000	Change in bowel habits, bleeding	Regular checkup including proctoscopy, especially for those over 40	Considered a highly curable disease when digital and proctoscopic examinations are included in routine checkups.
Lung	98,000	89,000	Persistent cough or lingering respiratory ailment	Eighty percent of lung cancer would be prevented if no one smoked cigarettes	Leading cause of cancer death among men and rising mortality among women.
Oral (including pharynx)	24,000	8,000	Sore that does not heal, difficulty in swallowing	Regular checkup	Many more lives should be saved because the mouth is easily accessible to visual examination by physicians and dentists.
Skin	10,000‡	5,000	Sore that does not heal or change in wart or mole	Regular checkup, avoidance of overexposure to sun	Skin cancer is readily detected by observation and diagnosed by simple biopsy.
Uterus	47,000§	11,000	Unusual bleeding or discharge	Regular checkup including pelvic examination with pap test	Uterine cancer mortality has declined 65% during the last 40 years with wider application of the pap test. Postmenopausal women with abnormal bleeding should be checked.
Kidney and bladder	45,000	17,000	Urinary difficulty, bleeding, in which case consult physician at once	Regular checkup with urinalysis	Protective measures for workers in high-risk industries are helping to eliminate one of the important causes of these cancers.
Larynx	9,000	3,000	Hoarseness, difficulty in swallowing	Regular checkup including laryngoscopy	Readily curable if caught early.
Prostate gland	57,000	20,000	Urinary difficulty	Regular checkup including palpation	Occurs mainly in men over 60. The disease can be detected by palpation at regular checkup.
Stomach	23,000	14,000	Indigestion	Regular checkup	A 40% decline in mortality in 25 years for reasons yet unknown.
Leukemia	21,000	15,000	Leukemia is a cancer of blood-forming tissues and is characterized by the abnormal production of immature white blood cells. Acute lymphocytic leukemia strikes mainly children and is treated by drugs which have extended life from a few months to as much as 10 years. Chronic leukemia strikes usually after age 25 and progresses less rapidly.		
Lymphomas	22,000	16,000	These cancers arise in the lymph system and include Hodgkin's disease and lymphosarcoma. Some patients with lymphatic cancers can lead normal lives for many years. Five-year survival rate for Hodgkin's disease increased from 25% to 54% in 20 years.		

*From American Cancer Society: 1977 Cancer facts and figures, New York, 1976, The Society.

†All figures rounded to nearest 1,000. Incidence estimates based on rates from NCI Third National Cancer Survey, 1969 to 1971.

‡Estimated new cases of nonmelanoma skin cancer about 300,000.

§If carcinoma in situ is included, cases total over 87,000.

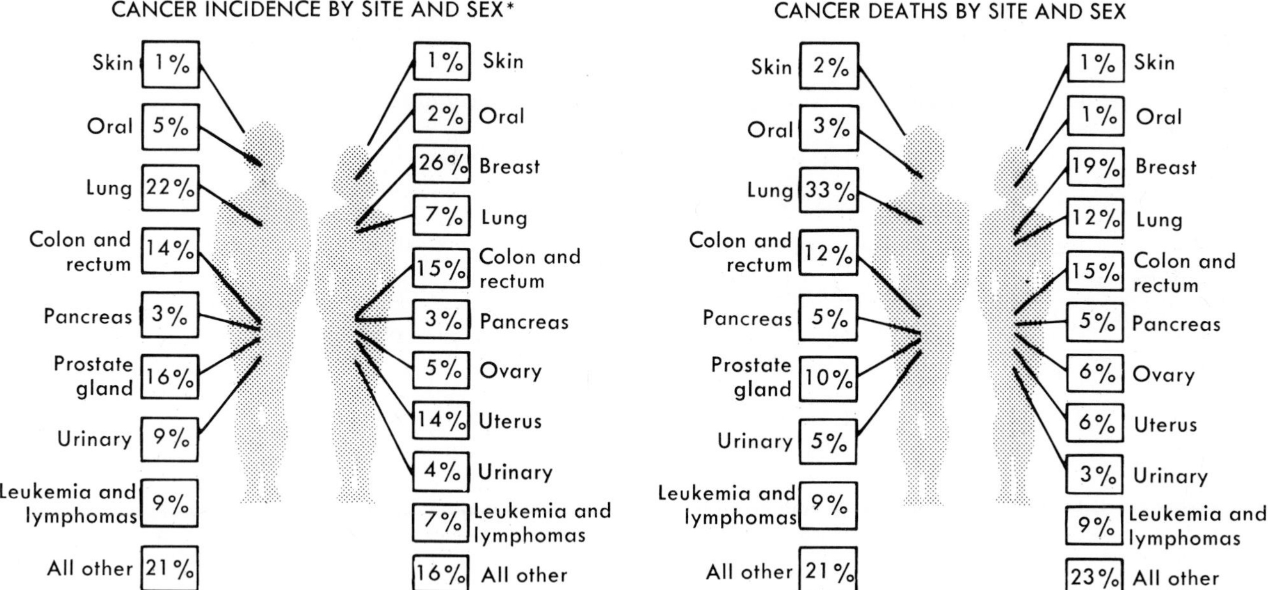

Fig. 25-1. Comparison of cancer incidence and deaths by site and sex (1978 estimates). (From American Cancer Society: 1977 Cancer facts and figures, New York, 1976, The Society.)

pancreas, colon (male), prostate gland, and bladder (male) have increased (Table 25-1).

Overall survival rates for some cancers have increased, such as those for cervical cancer, whereas rates for most other cancers have leveled off in the past 25 years. Dramatic increases in survival have occurred for cancers of the prostate gland, uterine corpus, thyroid gland, kidney, bladder, and larynx, and for melanoma of the skin, Hodgkin's disease, and chronic leukemia.

The average cancer mortality in developed countries is higher for men than for women. During the past 40 years there has been a decrease of 13% in mortality from cancer among American women due to a sharp reduction in mortality from uterine cancer. Among men a 40% mortality increase is due to a 1,400% increase in lung cancer.[1] It is revealing to note that there has been an increase in the incidence of lung cancer in women from 6 to 12 cases per 100,000 women between 1947 and 1969. This appears to be related to increased cigarette smoking by American women.

The death rate from cancer involving the female genital tract has dropped from between one third to one half the rate of 25 years ago, and there is ample evidence that the increased use of the Papanicolaou test to detect lesions of the cervix before symptoms develop has resulted in early treatment and a higher rate of cure (Fig. 25-1).

□ Age

Although more than half of the deaths due to cancer occur in persons over 65 years of age, cancer is the leading cause of death in women between 30 and 54 years of age and more school-aged children die of it than of any other disease.

In children, cancer death rates have declined from 8.4 per 100,000 population under 15 years of age in 1950 to 5.3 in 1974. The actual number of deaths, as well as the rate, has also decreased during the period.[1] Although no age group is totally exempt from cancer, the death rate shows a rapid increase with aging, and some researchers believe that if one lives long enough, he will eventually develop cancer.[2] (Table 25-2).

□ Race

There has been an increase in the incidence of cancer in black males, but in black females there has been little change. However, controlling cancer is more difficult in the black population than in the white population. Blacks are developing more cancers, and their prospects for diagnosis in a localized stage are poorer. Survival rates are poorer and death rates are higher. Most differences in the cancer rates of black and white populations are attributed to environmental and social factors rather than to inherent biologic characteristics.[1]

Table 25-2. Most frequent type of cancer by age (except for nonmelanoma skin cancer)*†

Age (yrs)	Site
0 to 10	Leukemia, cancer of the brain and kidney, lymphoma, cancer of the eye and connective tissue
10 to 20	
Males	Leukemia, Hodgkin's disease, cancer of the brain, bone, and testis
Females	Carcinoma in situ of cervix, leukemia, cancer of the brain, Hodgkin's disease, cancer of the thyroid
20 to 30	
Males	Hodgkin's disease, cancer of the testis, leukemia, melanoma of skin, cancer of the brain
Females	Cancer of the uterus, thyroid, and breast, Hodgkin's disease, melanoma of skin
30 to 40	
Males	Cancer of the lung, testis, colon and rectum, Hodgkin's disease, melanoma of skin
Females	Cancer of the uterus, breast, thyroid, ovary, and melanoma of skin
40 to 50	
Males	Cancer of the lung, colon and rectum, bladder, brain, and larynx
Females	Cancer of the breast, uterus, colon and rectum, ovary, and lung
50 to 60	
Males	Cancer of the lung, colon and rectum, prostate gland, bladder, and larynx
Females	Cancer of the breast, uterus, colon and rectum, lung, and ovary
60 to 70	
Males	Cancer of the prostate gland, lung, colon and rectum, bladder, and stomach
Females	Cancer of the breast, colon and rectum, uterus, lung, and ovary
Over 70	
Males	Cancer of the prostate gland, colon and rectum, lung, bladder, stomach
Females	Cancer of the colon and rectum, breast uterus, stomach, and pancreas

*From National Cancer Institute: Third National Cancer Survey, 1969 to 1971.
†Nonmelanoma skin cancer is omitted from this table, since there is seldom adequate reason for failure to diagnose it correctly and early.

□ Geographic factors

Differences in the geographic distribution of cancer occur. For example, primary cancer of the liver is common in Indonesia and parts of Africa and Asia but rare in other regions. Cancer of the breast is more frequent in the United States and Western Europe than it is in Japan. Genetic differences between populations may contribute to international variations but are not likely to be the only reason, since migration from one country to another results in major changes in the cancer pattern.[2]

■ FACTORS AFFECTING PROGNOSIS OF CANCER

Trends are being evaluated to determine why the incidence of certain cancers has decreased, increased, or remained the same. There is reason to believe that the cure rate and the prognosis of cancer would improve substantially with earlier recognition and more complete reporting of early signs. Success in treating many cancers awaits better and more sensitive diagnostic aids to detect lesions in their early stages. In some parts of the body such as the skin and cervix, early recognition and prompt treatment often result in cure.

The prognosis is also affected by the intrinsic characteristics of the tumor such as histologic type and grade, size, and rate of growth. Another important factor is the general condition of the patient. The presence of debilitating conditions such as infection, diabetes, or malnutrition may adversely affect the outcome[13]

Cancer is not only a threat to life, but its cost in loss of income and disruption of the lives of families cannot be estimated. Nurses must be in the forefront of the thousands of health professionals who are working to eradicate the disease.

■ PATHOPHYSIOLOGY OF TUMORS

□ Characteristics of normal cells

Normal tissue contains large numbers of mature cells of uniform size and shape, each containing a nucleus of uniform size. Within each nucleus are the chromosomes, a specific number for the species, and within each chromosome is *deoxyribonucleic acid (DNA).* DNA is a giant molecule whose chemical composition controls the characteristics of *ribonucleic acid (RNA),* which is found both in the *nucleoli* of cells and in the cytoplasm of the cell itself and which regulates cell growth and function. When ovum and sperm unite, the DNA and RNA within the chromosomes of each will govern the differentiation and future course of the trillions of cells that finally develop to form the adult organism. In the development of various organs and parts of the body, cells undergo differentiation in size, appearance, and arrangement; thus the histologist or the pathologist can look at a piece of prepared tissue through a microscope and know the portion of the body from which it came.

In the normal cell, multiplication takes place by an orderly process, mitosis. It consists of successive changes that result in a complicated rearrangement and splitting of chromosomes, ending with the formation of a new cell from each set of halved chromosomes. Normal cell multiplication occurs in response to a need and then stops.

□ Characteristics of malignant cells

A malignant cell is one in which the basic structure and activity have become deranged in a manner that is unknown and from a cause or causes that are still poorly understood. It is believed, however, that the basic process involves a disturbance in the regulatory functions of DNA. It is know that the DNA molecule is affected by radiation in certain instances, and it is speculated that it may be affected by other factors as well.

In the neoplastic cell, normal restraints on growth are defective. It is believed that malignant neoplasms occur as the result of faulty mechanisms inside the cell nucleus.[7]

DNA, the permanent genetic material in nuclear chromosomes, contains information necessary for cell replication, the chemical code for cell growth and development. To convey this information, *RNA* serves as a messenger. Any small change in *DNA* (mutation) causes a distortion of biologic information, which results in the affected cells running wild. Malignant neoplasm is the result.[7] The malignant cells lose the normal specialized function of the normal cell or may take on new characteristics and functions.

A characteristic of malignant cells that can be observed through a microscope is a loss of differentiation, or a likeness to the original cell (parent tissue) from which the tumor growth originated. This loss of differentiation is called *anaplasia*, and its extent is a determining factor in the degree of malignancy of the tumor. Other characteristics of malignant cells that can be seen through a microscope are the presence of nuclei of various sizes, many of which contain unusually large amounts of chromatin (hyperchromatic cells), and the presence of mitotic figures (cells in the process of division), which denotes rapid and disorderly division of cells (see box below for characteristics of malignant cells).

CHARACTERISTICS OF NEOPLASTIC CELLS[7,73]

1. Nuclei are larger and irregular in shape.
2. DNA is coarsely distributed and tends to appear near nuclear membrane.
3. Nucleoli are large, usually increased in number, and contain more chromatin than usual.
4. Mitosis is increased and atypical in appearance.
5. Abnormal multipolar mitoses and multinucleated cells may appear.
6. Cytoplasm is comparatively scanty and stains more deeply than normal cytoplasm, indicating greater RNA concentration.
7. Cells vary in size from normal cells.

□ Classifying and naming neoplasms

Tumors derive their names from the types of tissue involved (Table 25-3), but classification of malignant tumors is difficult, since many contain several types of cells and may have benign tissue incorporated within them as well. Benign (nonmalignant) tumors are not in themselves lethal but cause death only by their pressure on vital structures within an enclosed cavity such as the cranium. In general the names of benign tumors carry the suffix *-oma* following the name of the parent tissue, for example, neuroma or fibroma; there are some exceptions.

Cancers may be classified according to cell type origin. Two main types are those of epithelial and of mesenchymal (connective tissue) origin. The term *carcinoma* denotes a malignant tumor of epithelial cells, and the term *sarcoma* denotes a malignant tumor of connective tissue cells. When a malignant tumor contains all three types of embryonal tissue, it is called a *teratoma*.

Tumors are also classified according to cellular maturity. When there is complete loss of identity with the tissue of origin, the tumor is called *undifferentiated* (anaplastic). Some tumors are known by the names of the scientists who first described them, for example Hodgkin's disease and Wilms' tumor. Other tumors are named after the organ from which they arise, for example, hepatoma and thymoma.

□ Characteristics of malignant and benign tumors

Malignant tumors have no enclosing capsule; thus they invade adjacent or surrounding tissue, including lymph and blood vessels, through which they may spread to distant parts of the body to set up new tumors *(metastases)*. Unless completely removed or destroyed, they tend to recur after treatment, and their continued presence causes death by replacing normal cells and by other means not fully understood.

There is considerable difference in the rate of growth of malignant tumors. Occasionally one grows so slowly that it can be removed completely after a long period of time. This characteristic probably accounts for the good results obtained in a few circumstances even when treatment has been delayed. No physician, however, ever relies on this possibility to justify delay in treat-

Table 25-3. Classification of neoplasms

Parent tissue	Benign tumor	Malignant tumor
Epithelium		
Skin and mucous membrane	Papilloma	Squamous cell carcinoma
	Polyp	Basal cell carcinoma Transitional cell carcinoma
Glands	Adenoma Cystadenoma	Adenocarcinoma
Endothelium		Endothelioma
Blood vessels	Hemangioma	Hemangioendothelioma Angiosarcoma
Lymph vessels	Lymphangioma	Lymphangiosarcoma Lymphangioendothelioma
Bone marrow		Multiple myeloma Ewing's sarcoma Leukemia Lymphosarcoma
Lymphoid tissue		Reticulum cell sarcoma (difficult to classify due to cell embryology) Lymphatic leukemia
Connective tissues		
Embryonic fibrous tissue	Myxoma	Myxosarcoma
Fibrous tissue	Fibroma	Fibrosarcoma
Adipose tissue	Lipoma	Liposarcoma
Cartilage	Chondroma	Chondrosarcoma
Connective—cont'd		
Bone	Osteoma	Osteogenic sarcoma
Synovial membrane	Synovioma	Synovial sarcoma
Muscle tissue		
Smooth muscle	Leiomyoma	Leiomyosarcoma
Striated muscle	Rhabdomyoma	Rhabdomyosarcoma
Nerve tissue		
Nerve fibers and sheaths	Neuroma Neurinoma (neurilemoma) Neurofibroma	Neurogenic sarcoma Neurofibrosarcoma
Ganglion cells	Ganglioneuroma	Neuroblastoma
Glia cells	Glioma	Glioblastoma Spongioblastoma
Meninges	Meningioma	
Pigmented neoplasms		
Melanoblasts	Pigmented nevus	Malignant melanoma Melanocarcinoma
Miscellaneous		
Placenta	Hydatidiform mole	Chorionepithelioma (choriocarcinoma)
	Dermoid cyst	Embryonal carcinoma Embryonal sarcoma Teratocarcinoma

ment. Occasionally a malignant tumor grows slowly for a long time and then undergoes change, and the rate of growth increases enormously.

Benign or nonmalignant tumors are composed of adult or mature cells growing slowly and in an orderly manner within a capsule, not invading surrounding tissues, causing harm only by pressure, remaining localized and not entering the bloodstream. Benign tumors do not recur on removal. (See box on p. 453 for differences between benign and malignant tumors.)

□ Types of metastases

Cancer spreads in several different ways; the first is local spread or invasion into surrounding tissues. For this reason any excision of cancer must include a margin of surrounding tissues to ensure that all malignant cells have been removed.[13]

Cancer also spreads by lymphatic permeation and embolization. Once cells have invaded the lymph vessels, they then may detach and become emboli, which lodge in the lymph node forming a metastatic lesion.

DIFFERENCES BETWEEN BENIGN AND MALIGNANT NEOPLASMS

Benign	Malignant
Limited growth potential	May proliferate rapidly or grow slowly
Localized	Spreads (metastasizes) throughout the body
Fibrous capsule	No enclosing capsule
Rarely recurs after removal	May recur even after treatment
Usually regular in shape	Irregular shape with poorly defined border
Cells similar to cell of parent tissue (well differentiated)	Cells much different than parent cells (poorly differentiated)
Expansive growth	Infiltrative growth

Spread continues to the next group of nodes and into the other organs. The presence of cancer in the lymph nodes is certain evidence of spread, but even if there is no lymph node metastases, there still may be dissemination of malignant cells. The cell may pass through the lymph node without leaving a trace, to grow in other areas. Vascular embolism of malignant cells may occur through the veins to any part of the body but particularly to the lungs, the bone, and the liver.[2]

Finally, cancer can spread by implantation, the spread of clumps of cancer cells from the surface of the tumor by mechanical means. This type of spread is particularly prevalent in serous cavities such as the abdominal or the pleural cavity. In the peritoneal cavity cells tend to gravitate to the pelvis. Cancer cells can also be implanted by the surgeon into the operative area, causing metastatic lesions.[7, 13]

☐ Sites of metastases

The site of metastatic spread depends on the venous drainage of the organ involved, the type of cancer, and the tissue from which the cancer arises.[2] Cancer of an organ that ordinarily drains into systemic veins usually metastasizes to the lungs. Various body tissues seem to have different attraction for metastases, common sites being, in order, the liver, lungs, bone marrow, brain, and adrenal glands. Spleen, muscle, and skin are rarely involved.[13]

☐ Methods of classifying tumors and extent of spread

The degree of malignancy (stage) may be estimated by histologic criteria. Tumors may be graded by roman numerals into four grades; the higher the grade the worse the prognosis.[13] A grade 1 tumor is the most differentiated (most like the parent tissue) and therefore the least malignant, whereas grade 4 is the least differentiated (unlike parent tissues) and has a high degree of malignancy. These classifications are useful to the physician in knowing whether the tumor may be expected to respond to radiation treatment as well as in planning all other aspects of the patient's treatment. Usually malignant tissue is slightly more sensitive to irradiation than normal tissue.

Determination of the extent of the spread of cancer (staging) and the site of the original tumor is vital for planning therapy. The International Union Against Cancer has devised the TNM system of classification: *T*, tumor; *N*, regional lymph nodes; *M*, distant metastases.

Adding a number to the letters (e.g., T1, T2, N1, N2) indicates the extent of the malignancy.[13] Staging may also be classed in a I to IV manner, I indicating that the tumor is localized and IV that distant metastasis is present.

☐ Nurse's responsibility regarding pathophysiology

As individuals take more responsibility for their own health care and as their knowledge of disease processes grows, they want more explanation of and information about their illness. Physicians may give adequate explanation about cancer and its treatment, but the patient may not understand because of anxiety or misinterpretation of vocabulary. The nurse can clarify information for both patient and family, using appropriate but understandable terms and illustrations. If there is any question of the patient's or the family's understanding of the information given by the physician, the nurse clarifies with the physician what the patient and family have been told. The nurse may also interpret to the physician the patient's or family's readiness for more information.

■ PREVENTION AND HEALTH EDUCATION

☐ Carcinogenesis

The factors that contribute to the development of cancer are many and at the present time are not fully understood; however, certain health practices are known to decrease the possibility that cancer may occur. Knowledge of and communication of this information to the public is one of the health teaching responsibilities of nurses in all practice settings. Factors involved in carcinogenesis include host susceptibility, environmental carcinogens, habits and customs, and viruses.

Host susceptibility

Genetic factors. Certain conditions and predispositions of the individual seem to contribute to the development of cancer. Studies of genetic factors have focused on specific cancer sites and the disease in general. Retinoblastoma occurs with frequency in some families.

Familial polyposis of the colon, a precursor of cancer, is indisputably hereditary. There is also a high incidence of breast cancer in a vertical line of descent, such as from mother to daughter.[2] Risk of breast cancer in the first-degree relatives of a patient is five times that of the general population. Heredity in some way seems to be connected with bronchogenic cancer. It seems to interact with cigarette smoking to cause a synergistic effect.[39]

Studies have shown that the pattern of inheritance is not usually that of a single mendelian gene, and it is still not known whether the incidences of many specific cancers are due to a combination of genetic or environmental factors.[51]

Hormonal factors. Some evidence suggests that hormones may in some way be connected with the development of certain cancers. Some breast cancer, for example, is hormone dependent.[2] In addition hormonal factors are capable of restraining or enhancing tumor growth.[51]

Precancerous lesions. Certain benign lesions and tumors have a tendency toward malignant change. These cancers are preventable if minor precursor conditions are treated carefully. These precancerous conditions include leukoplakia of the oral cavity, polyps of the colon and rectum, certain pigmented moles, dysplasias of the cervical epithelium, Paget's disease of the bone, and radiodermatitis and senile keratosis.[2]

Chronic irritation. It is also known that cancer may follow chronic irritation of any part of the body. There are many ways to prevent irritation that may lead to cancer. Effort is being made in industry to protect workers from coal-tar products known to contain carcinogens. Masks and gloves are recommended in some instances, and workers are urged to wash their hands and arms thoroughly to remove all irritating substances at the end of the day's work. Industrial nurses participate in intensive educational programs to help workers understand the need for carrying out company rules that may help prevent cancer.

Prolonged exposure to wind, dirt, and sun may also lead to skin cancer. Skin cancer of the face and hands is particularly frequent among farmers and cattle ranchers who have fair complexions and who do not protect themselves from exposure.

Any kind of chronic irritation to the skin should be avoided, and moles that are in locations where they may be irritated by clothing should be removed. Shoelaces, shoetops, girdles, brassieres, and shirt collars are examples of clothing that may be a source of chronic irritation. Glasses, earrings, dental plates, and pipes that are in repeated contact with skin and mucous membrane may contribute to cancer. Chewing food thoroughly is recommended to lessen irritation in the throat and stomach. Cancer of the mouth is sometimes associated with rough jagged teeth and the constant irritation of tobacco smoke. The habit of drinking scalding hot or freezing cold liquids is also thought to be irritating to the mouth and to the esophagus. Indiscriminate use of laxatives is believed to have possible carcinogenic effects on the large bowel.

Immunologic factors. Immunologists have been increasingly aware of the role of the immune system in the natural history of malignant disease. It may be possible that failure of the normal immune mechanism may predispose to certain cancers.[45] (The role of the immune system and cancer therapy is discussed later in this chapter and in detail in Chapter 14).

Environmental factors

Many years ago it was observed that skin cancers developed more often in men who were employed as chimney sweeps in English homes in which coal was burned in fireplaces. It was then learned that when the suspected substance (methylcholanthrene) contained in the sweepings was repeatedly painted on the ears of experimental animals, cancer developed.

There are several types of chemical and physical carcinogens (cancer-producing substances). Various carcinogens may have an additive or enhancing effect on one another, and even small amounts of these substances in the environment may constitute a hazard. Carcinogens act on different organs depending on the portal of entry and the distribution in the body.[1]

Ionizing radiation. Radiographs and radium may cure cancer, but in other cases they cause it. Ionizing radiation consists of electromagnetic waves or material particles that have sufficient energy to ionize atoms or molecules (that is, remove electrons from them) and thereby alter their chemical behavior.[71] In adequate amounts it destroys the cells.

Every living thing from the beginning of time has been exposed to small amounts of radiation from the sun and from certain natural elements in the earth, such as uranium, that emit gamma rays in the process of their decay. This is called natural background radiation.[71] No problem regarding radiation existed until after 1895, when the roentgen-ray (x-ray) machine was developed and became widely used in diagnosis of disease. The development of this machine was followed by the discovery of radium and the use of both radium and radiographs for treatment of diseases such as cancer. With developments in the field of nuclear energy, it has been possible to produce radioactive isotopes of a number of the elements, although only a few of them such as gold, iodine, cobalt, and phosphorus have medical application at the present time. The problem of overexposure and possible harm to patients and to personnel caring for them has increased greatly with the increased use of radiographs in diagnosis and treatment and the more recent use of radioisotopes in diagnosis and treatment. Also radiation in the environment resulting from atomic testing has become a widely feared and much debated subject in many parts of the world.

No one really knows how much exposure to radiation is safe for persons working with patients and for patients having repeated radiograph films taken for various purposes. Relatively small amounts of exposure have produced serious damage in experimental animals, but humankind has not lived through enough generations of relatively high exposure for conclusive evidence of safe levels to be obtained. It is reasonable to assume that the less exposure one has the better. This does not mean that a patient receiving radiation treatment should not receive adequate nursing care. There are ways to protect persons from exposure, and hospitals are required to have protective procedures and guidelines for persons who care for patients receiving radiation therapy. All nurses should be familiar with the procedures used in the institution in which they are employed.

The ionizing effect of radiation on the body cells remains, so that exposure is cumulative throughout life. Exposure of the entire body enormously increases the amount of radiation received. For this reason all of the body except the part being treated is protected from exposure when relatively high doses are given for therapeutic purposes.

The National Committee on Radiation Protection has accepted *5 R (roentgens)* per year as the maximum permissible dose considered safe for well people over 18 years of age.[42] The United States National Academy of Sciences and the United Nations have estimated that the average person receives a total of 3 to 5 R from background radiation between birth and 30 years of age. They also estimate that additional exposure for medical and dental work probably doubles this amount in the Western world. The amount of exposure the patient receives from a series of radiographs taken for diagnostic purposes depends on the machine used and the technical skill involved. Usually the fluoroscopic examination entails more exposure than radiography. To prevent excessive exposure with fluoroscopy, the physician allows time for his or her own eyes to accommodate to the darkened room so that the patient can be observed with a lower intensity of the machine. The exposure of the average nurse working in a hospital and occasionally assisting a patient while a radiograph is taken is almost negligible.

Radiation effects. Systemic reactions to excessive radiation exposure are leukopenia, leukemia, and sterility or damage to the reproductive cells. Leukemia is an occupational disease among radiologists, with one study showing that its incidence is nine times higher among radiologists than among other physicians.[42] Because of the increased risk, badges are worn by persons whose daily work exposes them to radiation. The badge, which contains photographic film capable of absorbing radiation, is developed each month. A darkening or blackening of the film indicates excessive exposure. Personnel who are becoming overexposed are removed, at least temporarily, from direct contact with radiation.

Because of the possible danger to the fetus, particularly between the second and sixth weeks of life, radiographs are seldom taken of pregnant women. If they must be taken, the lower abdomen is carefully protected. Also, pregnant women usually are not employed in radiology departments or in caring for patients receiving radioactive materials internally.

Nurses who work where they are exposed to x-rays repeatedly or who care for patients receiving radioactive substances must take responsibility for learning how to protect themselves from too much exposure.

Effects of the sun. Our society at times seems sun addicted and a tanned skin is eagerly sought by many, yet sunlight is the most universal carcinogen.[15] Skin cancer occurs mostly in people who work in the open air, such as sailors and farmers, and on areas of the body most exposed to sunlight. Light-complected individuals are the most cancer susceptible.[13]

Chemical pollutants. Air pollution has been blamed for the rising cancer incidence in the twentieth century (see Chapter 5). Ten polycyclic aromatic hydrocarbons have been recognized as carcinogenic.[13]

In addition to the high incidence of epithelioma of the scrotum among the chimney sweeps mentioned earlier, tar and pitch and their derivatives as well as mineral oils containing aromatic hydrocarbons were discovered to be carcinogenic many years ago.

Skin cancers due to arsenic have been found among farmers and vineyard workers who handle arsenicals. Bladder cancer from aromatic amines is an occupational disease of workers in the rubber industry. The risk of contacting lung cancer is 15 to 30 times greater among those exposed to the chromium compounds. Other common occupational cancers are respiratory cancers from asbestos and leukemia resulting from long-term inhalation of benzol.[13]

Many nitrosamines cause a variety of cancers in different species. Nitrates are commonly used as food additives, while nicotine may be a source of amines. A new liver carcinogen, aflatoxin 13, has been isolated from a common mold that grows on peanuts, soybeans, fruit, some meats, and mild and cheddar cheese. The most recently indicated carcinogenic agents are chloromethyl methyl ether and vinyl chloride (a basic precursor of polyvinyl plastics). A rare form of vaginal cancer in young women has been linked to the ingestion by their mothers of diethylstilbestrol (DES) prescribed to prevent spontaneous abortion.[33]

Various red dyes used in the coloring of food products have been banned because they may be potentially carcinogenic. In late 1969 cyclamates, which were widely used as sugar substitutes, were banned when experimental studies revealed that in high doses they could produce cancer of the bladder in mice. Saccharin has also been identified as being carcinogenic in a study of rats, and the Federal Drug Administration (FDA) has recommended that it not be used as an artificial sweetener. In 1977 the United States Congress approved an 18-month moratorium on the proposed ban to allow for further scientific study of the effects of saccharin because of questions raised about the validity of applying the results of the study to humans.

Health practices

Smoking. There is now no question that excessive cigarette smoking is linked with the increased incidence of lung cancer. More and more reports are appearing that incriminate moderate and heavy cigarette smoking as a predisposing factor in the development of lung cancer, which now causes 14 times as many deaths each year as it did 30 years ago. In 1976 lung cancer killed approximately 83,000 persons in the United States (63,500 men and 17,600 women).[1] These figures represent an increase of 3% in men and 10% in women over the 1973 figures. Although the rate of increase of lung cancer in men has been alarming, separate and independent studies have noted a rise in the rate of lung cancer in women. The rise appears to parallel an increase in women smokers, particularly teenage girls, over the last 5 years. In 1968 the number of girl smokers between the ages of 12 and 18 was about half the number of teenage boys who smoked. By 1972 there was only a 2.4% difference. The rise in number of women smokers has captured the attention of cigarette manufacturers, who have increased their advertising efforts in this direction to the point of designing cigarettes expressly for women. An enormous amount of effort is being made by both private and public agencies concerned with the health of the public to alert everyone, smokers as well as nonsmokers, to the dangers of cigarette smoking.

It has also been demonstrated that there is a correlation between cancer mortality and the number of cigarettes smoked daily, number of years an individual has smoked, and the age at which he or she began to smoke cigarettes.[13] Smoking has also been connected with esophageal cancer and possibly bladder cancer.[13,74] If smoking is discontinued even after a habit of 30 years, there is a decrease in the evidence of lung cancer.[75]

After the release of the Surgeon General's Report on Smoking and Health in 1964, the National Interagency Council on Smoking and Health was formed. This group, composed of 27 public and private health, educational, and youth organizations, has as its major objective combating smoking as a health hazard. Several of these participating organizations have produced films and other educational materials that are available to schools, organizations, and individuals. Assistance in securing films and other materials can be obtained from the Library, National Clearinghouse for Smoking and Health, Public Health Service.* One of the main concerns of the Interagency Council is how to convince young people not to start smoking. A new film, *Breathing Easy*, was produced by the American Lung Association† especially for the preteen group. The American Cancer Society is designing smoking cessation clinics for places of employment and for schools. Antismoking education drives in schools are conducted through school courses, assemblies, and exhibits.

As of January 2, 1971, no cigarette advertising is permitted on either television or radio. On the same date the warning on cigarette packages was changed from "Caution: cigarette smoking may be hazardous to your health" to "Warning: the Surgeon General has determined that cigarette smoking is dangerous to your health." While the campaign to convince people to stop smoking has been slow and arduous, there has been change noted in smoking patterns. There is a trend toward increased use of filter cigarettes and pipes among smokers. The two thirds of the population who are nonsmokers have been active and in some instances successful in getting smokers to refrain from smoking in public places such as specified sections of airplanes and public buildings. In 1972 the Surgeon General of the United States declared that smoking in the presence of a nonsmoker might be considered an act of aggression. Experiments have shown that cigarette smokers in a crowded, ill-ventilated room or automobile can raise the level of carbon dioxide to the point that all within the area can experience trouble discriminating time intervals and visual and sound cues as well as difficulty with eye-hand coordination. Action in the form of bills, ordinances, and restrictions on smoking and the sale of tobacco in places of public assembly are being instituted at all government levels on a nationwide basis.

Nurses have a responsibility, both as well-informed citizens and as professional persons, to be aware of the most recent antismoking programs and to interpret them to the public. One of the best ways for nurses to do this would be to stop smoking themselves. Although there are no figures available on the number of nurses who

---

*5401 Westbord Ave., Bethesda, Md. 20016.

†1740 Broadway, New York, N.Y. 10019.

have stopped smoking, the American Cancer Society estimates that 50,000 physicians have done so.

Nutrition. Nutritional habits are increasingly being investigated and implicated in the cause of cancer. A high incidence of cancer of the colon occurs in populations whose diet is high in refined food and low in nonabsorbable cellulose "roughage" or fiber. Evidence indicates that there is a low incidence of colonic carcinoma among persons who eat a largely vegetarian diet with relatively little animal products.[31,63]

Many food substances contain additives, contaminants, and naturally appearing substances such as aflatoxin, which may be carcinogenic. Food additives being studied include food dyes, flavoring agents, and antimicrobial preservatives such as sodium and potassium nitrite and nitrate. Although some potential carcinogens are present in the diet, the time trends do not indicate that additives now in use are significant in the cause of cancer. The present government policy is to keep the levels of potential carcinogenic agents in food as low as feasible, recognizing that it is almost impossible to state with absolute certainty that any ingested chemical is safe.[31]

Alcohol. There is a significant association between high alcohol intake and cancer of the mouth, pharynx, larynx, and esophagus. However, alcoholism is often associated with smoking and with vitamin and dietary deficiencies, whose roles in the cause of cancer are not known.

Sexual practices. Carcinoma of the uterine cervix is less common in virgins than in married women. It is higher in those who have first coitus at an early age, who have an early first marriage, and who have had multiple sex partners. Cervical cancer is more frequent in women who have had multiple pregnancies, but this factor decreases in importance when the groups of women compared started their sex life at the same age. The development of cancer seems to be connected with coitus rather than pregnancy.

Carcinoma of the penis is virtually unknown among circumcised men. The means by which circumcision provides protection is not clear, but it is probably related to better hygiene. There is also a lower incidence of cancer of the uterine cervix in women whose sexual partner has been circumcised and in cultures in which the men, even though not circumcised, have a high standard of genital hygiene.[13]

The correlation with sexual experience and breast cancer is the reverse of that for the uterine cervix. Breast cancer patients have usually been married and become pregnant later in life. Lactation may provide some protection against breast cancer, since women who have breast-fed their infants show a lower incidence of breast malignancy. Cancer of the breast is reported to be unknown among Eskimo women and to be relatively rare among Japanese women; both cultures practice breastfeeding.

Viruses

Studies in animals have established that there is a viral role in carcinogenesis, but proof that humans are affected has not been definitely established.[2,64,73] Viruses have been isolated and identified as the cause of cancer in mice, rabbits, and frogs.

Cervical cancer may result from a virus introduced into the cervix during sexual intercourse. This virus may be a member of the herpes group, *herpesvirus hominis (HV-2).* Carriers of HV-2 in the population are generally uncircumcised males with poor personal hygiene.[73]

Herpeslike viruses have been visualized by electron microscopy in Burkitt's tumor and Hodgkin's disease cells. Investigators, however, have been unable to demonstrate human oncogenic viruses from human tumors. This may be a technical problem, since the ideal laboratory conditions for the isolation of tumor viruses have not been found.

The viruses found in animal tumors indicate that viruses may act individually or as co-carcinogens in causing malignancy in humans.[73] The question is no longer, however, whether viruses have a role in the cause of cancer but when they will be definitely implicated and whether one or many will be involved.[64]

Conclusions

Carcinogenesis is a dynamic process that is influenced by many independent and poorly defined variables. The initial molecular changes are irreversible, but they may not be expressed when cooperative conditions are absent. Changes in these conditions may alter the carcinogenic process, resulting in either acceleration, inhibition, or even reversal of the process.[33] Fig. 25-2 illustrates the relationship between various carcinogenic factors in the cause of cancer.

Nurses have a vital role to play in communicating to the public the factors involved in carcinogenesis. They can clarify misconceptions as well as do health teaching so that known carcinogenic practices may be eliminated. They can also set an example of good health practices for the general public, perhaps a more difficult role to assume. As knowledgeable and concerned citizens. nurses must be initiators and supporters of efforts to have carcinogens removed from the environment.

□ Health teaching

The American public is more widely read and informed about health problems than ever before. Health-seeking behavior and a desire to be more knowledgeable about health problems are indicated by the fre-

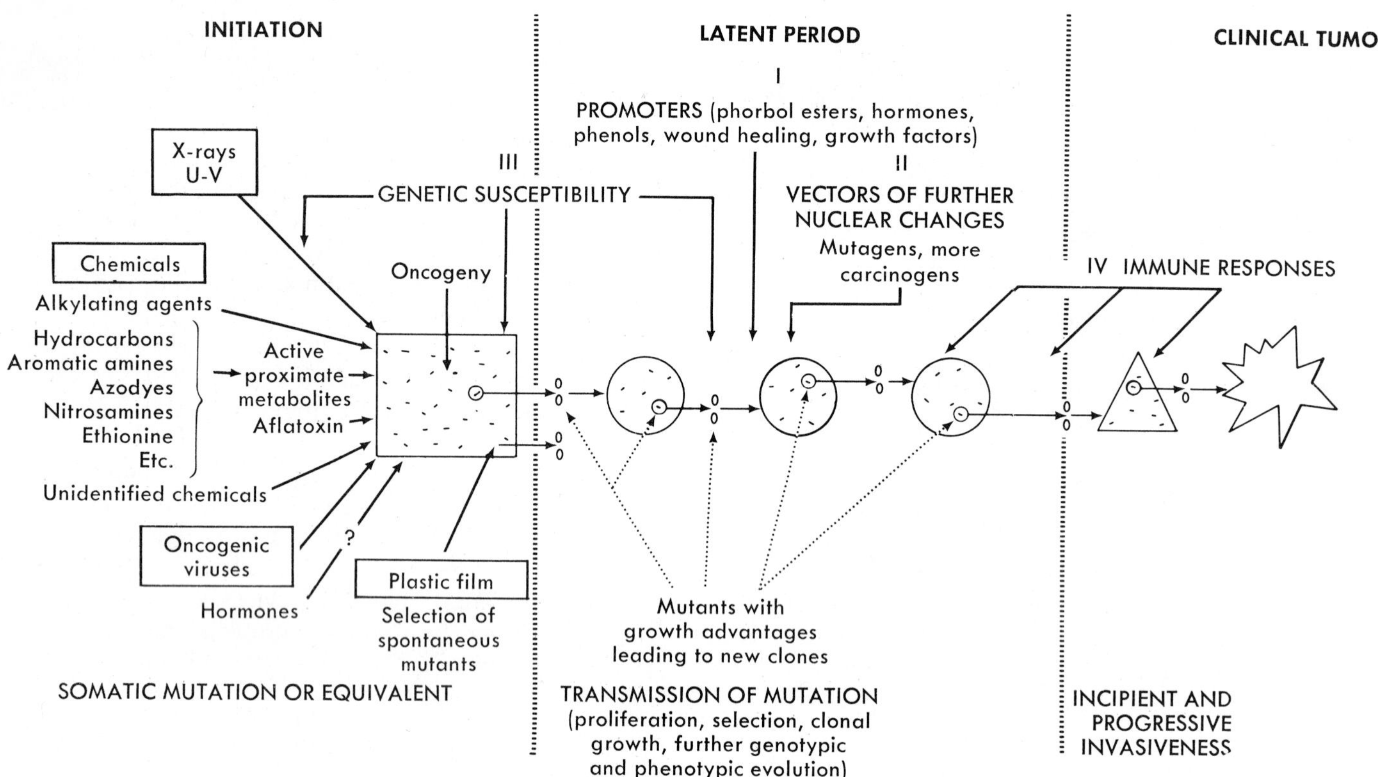

Fig. 25-2. Physical, chemical, and viral carcinogens may cause damage in cells of target organs *(dots in square)*. Changes are transmitted by cell division resulting in clones of modified cells *(small circles)*. These cells undergo further genotypic and phenotypic changes due to exposure to same or different carcinogens. Promoters of proliferation, whether chemical, hormonal, or viral, enhance carcinogenic process. Successive selection of new clones *(large circles)* leads to premalignant state. From complex interplay of host and tumor, affected by genetic, endocrine, immunologic, and other environmental factors, populations of cells characteristic of clinical tumors arise. (From Ryser, H. J.: CA **24**:358-359, 1974.)

quency of articles about topics such as cancer in the lay press. The topic of cancer is also discussed more openly than ever before. Nurses have a major responsibility in the prevention of cancer. Because of their knowledge about the disease and their opportunity for contact with the public in the inpatient and outpatient setting, nurses have the opportunity to teach about cancer and to help motivate patients to seek treatment.

Case finding is a responsibility of all nurses. The nurse must be able to (1) counsel and direct patients to the proper sources of help, (2) have information about those conditions that are known to predispose to the development of the disease, and (3) be able to educate the public about these factors. In addition the nurse must be sensitive to the needs of patients who may be afraid and embarrassed when confronted with the possibility of cancer.

Since prevention of cancer is a primary goal of health professionals, the nurse must be aware of and be able to communicate to others the importance of good health habits and the importance of avoiding conditions that predispose to cancer.

Early detection and treatment

The approach to early detection of cancer is worldwide. General criteria for cancer screening and testing programs have been drawn up by the epidemiology section of the American Public Health Association, and these criteria have been adapted by the World Health Organization. Multiphasic screening and a periodic health examination are being accepted by the public. In some cases diagnosis can be made months before the development of symptoms causes the person to seek care.[61]

Cancer detection is not inexpensive. Education of the public often includes convincing them that a periodic health examination is a sound investment. Some cities have cancer detection centers where a complete physical examination including chest radiograph, Papanicolaou smear, breast examination, proctoscopy, urinalysis, and blood count are performed for a moderate fee. Nurses should be aware of clinics in their area where persons needing such resources may be referred.

Early detection of cancer can decrease mortality. The nurse must know and be able to explain the significance of the seven warning signs of cancer, stressing that any of these signs should be reported immediately to a physician. These warning signs as listed by the American Cancer Society are:

1. Change in bowel and bladder habits
2. A sore that does not heal
3. Unusual bleeding or discharge
4. Thickening or a lump in the breast or elsewhere
5. Indigestion or difficulty in swallowing
6. Obvious change in a wart or mole
7. Nagging cough or hoarseness

It should be emphasized that any of these signs should be investigated medically (Table 25-1), but their occurrence does not necessarily mean that the person has cancer.

All persons should know the most common sites of cancer. In women these are the breast, uterus (cervix), and gastrointestinal tract (Fig. 25-1). Women should be taught to examine their breasts each month immediately after the menstrual period or, if postmenopausal, on a designated day each month. Such self-examination (Fig. 53-2) is a much better method of detecting early breast cancer than an annual physical examination.

Women of all ages should know the importance of reporting any abnormal vaginal bleeding or other discharge occurring between menstrual periods or after the menopause (see p. 1387 for details of early symptoms of cancer of the female reproductive system). All women should have a pelvic examination annually and a cervical smear taken for testing by the Papanicolaou stain. Some physicians advise that the Pap test be done every 6 months for women over the age of 30. Women should request that the test be done if it has inadvertently been overlooked by the health care provider. If the test is done early, cancer may be diagnosed before metastasis occurs (see Chapter 60).

The most common sites of cancer in men are the skin, lungs, gastrointestinal tract, and prostate gland. All men 40 years of age and over should have a physical examination every 1 to 2 years that includes search for diseases in these locations. In many cancer detection clinics, proctoscopic examinations are done on all men 35 years of age or over because of the high incidence of cancer of the lower bowel in men of this age group. (Further information about cancer of specific organs can be found in appropriate chapters in Part Three of this book.)

Two common misconceptions that lead the patient to ignore symptoms should be corrected. The first is a belief that a disease as serious as cancer must be accompanied by weight loss. Weight loss is usually a late symptom of cancer, yet the patient often remarks, "I wasn't losing weight so I thought nothing serious could be wrong." Another reason for neglect of cancer is that it may not cause pain, and again the patient believes the absence of pain means that his indisposition is minor. It must be repeatedly emphasized to the public that pain is not an early sign of cancer and that cancer often is far advanced before pain occurs.

In addition to being knowledgeable about measures for prevention and early detection of cancer, nurses must be aware of current therapeutic modalities and their rationales. Because of lack of information, misinformation, or fear of the effects of treatment, patients may put off seeking help. Clearly presented information about therapy will help to allay the patient's anxiety and confusion.

Factors that interfere with health-seeking behavior

Even though there is more widespread knowledge of cancer, a more positive attitude toward the disease is essential if individuals are to follow good health practices and seek help when warning signs of cancer are noted.

Unfortunately anxiety and fear may immobilize the individual. Despite all the public announcements that have been made in the last few decades, there are still people who think of cancer as a disgraceful disease that must be hidden from others. Cancer is talked about in whispers by some people who look on it as a punishment for past sins, a shameful disease, or a disgrace to the family. This attitude stems partly from the fact that cancer in its terminal stages may be a painful and demoralizing disease that is sometimes accompanied by body odor and other signs of physical debility that are deeply etched on the consciousness of friends and relatives. Actually there is no characteristic odor of cancer, although diseased tissue that breaks down and becomes infected with odor-producing organisms will be as unpleasant as any other infected wound. The essential point—so often missed by the public—is that this tragic situation is by and large an unusual one.

Some people fear cancer and shun persons who have the disease because they believe it is contagious. Scientific speculation on the possibility that a virus may be the cause has added to this fear. At this time there is no conclusive evidence that a virus or any other communicable agent contributes in any way to the development of cancer.

The positive aspects of cancer care should be emphasized. It is estimated that approximately one third of the persons for whom a diagnosis is made are cured by medical treatment. Another one third could perhaps be cured by medical treatment if the cancer is diagnosed early enough. Only a third have cancer occurring in locations in which the disease advances beyond permanent medical aid before sufficient signs appear to warn the patient of trouble. In spite of these facts, some persons think it is useless to report symptoms early, since they believe that if they do have cancer they cannot be cured. It can only be hoped that the recent publicity given to well-known persons who have been treated for cancer will help overcome some of these beliefs. If nothing else, the open discussion of the diagnosis and treatment in all types of media should result in a better informed public than ever before.

Cancer quackery

Fatal delay in seeking medical care may occur because of the patient's reliance on a "quick, painless cure." Despite public education and efforts of the medical profession to control extravagant claims of a few unethical practitioners, cancer quackery still exists, feeding on the ignorance and fear of the cancer patient and his family.[2,68]

Quacks rely on testimonials of people they have "cured." Books and testimonials in magazines may be so appealingly written that the reader may get the impression that the content is factual and accurate. Electronic gadgets, dietary regimens, and various drugs and enzymes have all been purported to cure cancer.

Two drugs still available mostly outside the United States are krebiozen and Laetrile, a substance derived from apricot kernels. Use of Laetrile for cancer therapy has been outlawed by the FDA, whose regulations prohibit the transportation of Laetrile across state lines. In response to active lobbying by various groups, however, 11 states in 1977 passed legislation legalizing use of Laetrile within their borders. The American Cancer Society and the American Medical Association do not recommend use of Laetrile or krebiozen, as neither drug has been scientifically demonstrated to result in objective benefit to the person or show evidence that metastatic growth has been controlled. The tragedy in the use of these drugs is the false security the treatment gives to patients. The security results in delay in seeking medical care until it is too late.[34]

Federal legislation is aimed at controlling quackery. The nurse must teach the danger of unproved methods of treatment in contacts with individuals and families.

□ Cancer research

Cancer research is multifaceted. Investigations are ongoing into the cause, prevention, and treatment of cancer. Research on the cause of cancer has explored the effect of several factors acting together to stimulate aberrant cell growth, the role of chemicals and other environmental pollutants, genetic factors, and the role of viruses in the development of cancer.

Many investigators are focusing their interest on subcellular components. There is increasing interest in changes in the chromosome and in the nucleic acids, essential cell constituents, DNA (deoxyribonucleic acid) and RNA (ribonucleic acid). In addition investigations using animals yield much useful information. For example, a strain of mice has been developed in which all the mice develop breast cancer. Evidence obtained through animal experimentation, however, does not necessarily prove that human beings react in the same way, but it raises the possibility that they may do so.

Immunologists in cancer research have become increasingly aware of the role of the immune system in both the natural history and the therapy of malignant disease. They suggest that it is possible to strengthen the body's natural responses so that the body would be able to destroy malignant cells when they first appear. The discovery that human neoplasms contain tumor-specific antigens not found in normal cells has opened up new avenues of therapy in controlling the progression and in inducing the regression of human neoplasms.

Around the world many research centers are developing better treatment modalities. Use of a combination of surgery, radiation, and chemotherapy has shown that there may be significant prolongation of life and in some instances complete cure of children with Wilms tumor, an extremely malignant embryonal tumor of the kidney. Continued study of the use of chemotherapeutic drugs has resulted in effective new combination therapies for many types of cancer.

Future research against cancer will probably be directed toward developing and screening new drugs that can act alone or with other drugs; applying new forms of radiation such as laser beams that spare normal tissue and are not carcinogenic themselves; developing new regimens for the use of bacille Calmette-Guérin (BCG) vaccine and other forms of immunotherapy, both alone and in combination; developing new combinations of known effective drugs; and combining treatment modalities such as surgery, irradiation, chemotherapy, and immunotherapy.[64]

Research in cancer nursing is in its infancy. In the past 10 years only 33 cancer research studies have been reported by nurses.[4] Nurses are working with others in clinical centers specializing in cancer, and they must report their findings. Too often effective nursing care practices have been passed on by word of mouth rather than being validated by careful investigation. There are many topics that if diligently and imaginatively studied might result in increased comfort to patients and their families. The psychologic response of patients and families, innovative approaches to care, and attitudes of care givers are just a few of the topics that might be investigated.

□ Organizations involved in cancer education, detection, and rehabilitation

Federal organizations

Federal recognition of the need to give intensive assistance to educational programs in cancer began in 1926 when Congress proclaimed April of each year as National Cancer Control Month. In 1937 the National Cancer Institute was created within the National Institutes of Health. This institute, with generous support from the federal government, conducts an extensive program of research in the field of cancer.

Cancer patients may also obtain help from both Medicare and Medicaid. The Community Services Administration provides services through state agencies such as Welfare and Aging or by direct grants. The Rehabilitation Services Administration will arrange and pay for services that help the cancer patient return to productive living.[2] With the passage of the National Cancer Act of 1971, impetus was given for the development of Cancer Clinical Research Centers. The goal was to translate research results into medical practice so that no one will be denied professional advice and care because of lack of facilities and knowledge. These centers combine research capability, demonstration of recent techniques and therapy, and community outreach programs.[69]

Nurses can be articulate speakers for the cause of cancer care and cure, since they are intimately aware of the effects of cancer in threat to life and cost in dollars, disrupted lives, and human suffering. Nurses must assertively express to their representatives in government the importance of a combined effort to eradicate cancer.

American Cancer Society

The American Cancer Society, Inc., (ACS), a large national voluntary organization, has branches in all states and in 11 major cities. It was organized in 1913 as the National Society for the Control of Cancer with the major objective of combating the fear, shame, and ignorance that were outstanding obstacles in the early treatment of the disease. This huge organization, which is supported by voluntary gifts, has expanded its functions and now has three main objectives: research, education, and services to cancer patients.

Research is a major focus, and the Society finances studies that seek the cause of cancer and the development of better methods of treatment. As part of its education efforts, ACS publishes booklets and pamphlets for the use of health care providers and it stimulates better preparation of professional persons in the care of patients with cancer by sponsoring institutes and other programs for these special groups. Information about available teaching materials may be obtained from the main office of the Society or from state or local offices.*

In addition the American Cancer Society strives constantly to educate the public. It works intensively through magazines, radio, television, women's clubs, insurance companies, state departments of health, and medical and nursing organizations in an effort to reach all the population with the educational message of how cancer may be prevented and controlled. A large amount of literature for the laity is prepared and distributed annually. Also many excellent films for use in public education may be borrowed from the Society.

The Society also performs services for patients and their families. Branches in most communities provide assistance for cancer patients who cannot afford to pay for adequate care and for those who, although they can presently afford to pay, will eventually leave their families with too great a financial burden. Depending on how much community support is given to the society, the services may include dressings, transportation to and from clinics and physicians' offices, special drugs such as expensive hormones, blood, prostheses, and the loan of equipment such as hospital beds. In some communities homemaking, visiting nurse, and rehabilitation services are also provided. Of the money collected, 60% remains with the local chapter for the community's use. The remaining 40% supports the activities of the national office. Patients and their families should know about these services before their own resources are depleted, and local citizens should be urged to support the Society.

Other voluntary organizations

In addition to the American Cancer Society, some large cities have other voluntary organizations that serve only cancer patients. For example, Cancer Care, a large voluntary organization in New York City, confines its activities solely to the tremendous needs of patients with advanced cancer and to the needs of their families. The nurse who works in a small community or a rural area may learn of the resources available to cancer patients through local or state health departments.

Lists of available films for both professional and lay use can be obtained from the American Cancer Society and from state and local health departments. Some insurance companies, such as the Metropolitan Life Insurance Company and the John Hancock Insurance Company, prepare very useful pamphlets on control of cancer

*Headquarters: 291 E. 42nd St., New York, N.Y. 10017.

and the care of persons who have the disease. These pamphlets are useful to nurses in conducting health education programs and in teaching relatives of a patient with cancer how to care for him.

Cancer patients' groups

Patient groups have been organized to help others with the same disability. Lost Chord Clubs (laryngectomy patients), Reach to Recovery (mastectomy patients) and ostomy clubs have been formed in many cities. Individuals share what they have learned about coping with the problems resulting from therapy of their conditions. They visit patients either in the hospital or at home and hold regular group meetings.

Public health agencies

Many other agencies may be needed for the rehabilitation of the cancer patient. Community health nurses have a vital role in helping patients and families adjust after the cancer patient returns from the hospital. It is by the coordinated effort of hospital and community nurses that the patient and his family can return to a satisfying and self-fulfilling life.

■ ASSESSMENT

□ Subjective data

The physician obtains a careful medical history inquiring into family history to determine those with a familial tendency for cancer, social history, marital and sex history, habits, occupation, and past medical history, since all may provide valuable clues to identify the presence of cancer.

It is especially important that the nurse obtain baseline data in relation to the cancer patient's health and health habits, since the treatment of cancer often involves complex changes in the patient's ability to meet psychologic, physiologic, and sociologic health needs. By careful collection of data the nurse can plan and carry out the complex nursing care that may be needed by the patient with cancer.

Knowledge of diagnosis

Some initial data are needed to plan care. The first important question to be answered is whether the patient knows he has cancer. Whether the patient has been told that he has cancer should be recorded on the nursing care plan and discussed with other health team members. This will ensure that the person does not receive different answers to the same questions from the health care providers. Some hospitals have partially overcome this problem by having regular meetings of all the members of the professional staff at which the information given to each patient is reviewed. If meetings of this type are not being held, nurses should take the initiative in planning such a meeting.

The nurse should also elicit from both the patient and the physician what the patient has been told. Because of anxiety and the need for denial to protect the ego, the patient may have only heard part of the information given him by the physician or he may have misinterpreted what he did hear. The nurse can identify any discrepancies in order to plan the care on the basis of the patient's perceptions of the illness.

Members of the medical profession differ in their opinions as to whether the patient with cancer should be told the diagnosis. The decision is usually made by the physician after consultation with the patient's family. The present trend is toward telling the patient he has cancer, although studies show that fewer than 50% of physicians do tell their patients.[53] One detailed study indicates that the reasons are related much more to the physician's own attitudes and emotional reactions than to concern about the patient's reactions.[53] The nurse may help by discussing with the physician the reactions of the patient and the feelings he expresses. It is the nurse's responsibility and sometimes a challenge to work effectively for the ultimate benefit of the patient within the seeming limitation it may impose.

Many spiritual advisers recommend telling the truth. Some persons, however, may not want to know the diagnosis and may ask, then answer their own questions negatively. Some do not ask for the diagnosis because they do not wish to have confirmed what they already suspect. Some insist on knowing the diagnosis and are preoccupied with every detail of their progress and treatment in a detached but completely abnormal fashion. Finally there are some who wish to know the facts and who can accept them in a realistic way when given an opportunity to discuss their feelings with others. Some physicians prepare the patient over a period of time and tell him the complete truth when they feel he is ready to accept it.

It is also important to determine how long the patient has known the diagnosis. If the patient has just been told, he may be going through the initial grief reactions. If he has known for many years, he may have made a realistic adaptation and may see cancer as a chronic disease and not as a death sentence. The nurse should ascertain from the physician whether the cancer has already metastasized and, if so, whether the patient is aware of this fact. Responses of the patient with metastatic cancer will be different from those of the patient who can be more hopeful of a cure.

Coping skills

Coping skills should be identified, for in no other disease are the person's inner resources and those of friends and families tested to a greater degree. Some persons cope by directly verbalizing fears and seeking support from others, while other persons are less direct. Some deal with problems with a problem-solving approach, while others try to avoid dealing with the problem.

The patient's and family's interpersonal, physical, and financial resources must be determined. What kind of support can be expected from the family? (See Chapter 3 for discussion of family.) The financial burden the patient anticipates because of the therapy may affect his reaction to the disease.

Psychologic response to cancer

Once the diagnosis of cancer has been made, the patient and his family may be overwhelmed and immobilized. As one patient stated, "I cried all day Saturday, Sunday, and Monday. My daughter and my husband wanted to help but they didn't know what to do or say. I know my daughter was scared that she'd get cancer, too." Not all patients can openly express their feelings. Consequently the nurse may have difficulty gathering data in order to assess and plan intervention. Some individuals are stoical, feeling it is a sign of weakness to display their psychologic devastation in public. The nurse must be alert for subtle cues that may indicate that intervention is needed.

Grief. The general psychologic responses to a diagnosis of cancer are those accompanying the grieving process (see Chapter 19). The patient and his family may go through a period of denial, during which there may be a delay in beginning therapy. Anxiety, depression, regressive behavior, and anger may all be manifested (see Chapter 16).

To many the diagnosis of cancer signifies the end of life itself, the ultimate loss. Nurses must be careful that they do not communicate any negative reactions to cancer. Beginning practitioners must look at their own attitudes toward the disease.

Guilt. Guilt is also a frequent psychologic response. The cancer patient may feel that his disease is punishment for actions of his past life. He may also feel guilty if he has delayed seeking treatment (see Chapter 16).

Sense of isolation. Perhaps one of the most prevalent reactions described by patients with cancer is a sense of isolation, of being cut off from those persons and things that are important to them. Patients with cancer may report that there is a gradual break in relationships.[16] In some cases the isolation is patient initiated,[22,38] in others it may result from actions of significant others because of their negative attitude toward the disease. Perhaps the most profound isolation is psychologic isolation, an inability to relate to and derive comfort from others, the feeling of being alone in a crowd.

Sexual disequilibrium. Nurses must be comfortable with their own sexuality and sensitive to the patients' responses, which may indicate that sexual tension is present (see Chapter 64).

Fantasies of death and dying. Some patients report that they are overwhelmed with fantasies of death and dying. Most patients are more concerned about the process of dying, fearing pain, mutilation, and deterioration in both their physiologic and psychologic status, than with death itself. Patients may be open about their fantasizing, but they are more apt to communicate this in less obvious ways. Patients may focus their attention and discussion on the suffering and pain of others. They may express concern about the future of their families and may speculate what will happen to their loved ones. The nurse must be alert to these signs that the patient needs to talk about his view of his future (see Chapter 19).

□ Objective data

Local effects

Benign tumors cause serious problems if they obstruct the lumen of tubular structures such as the ureter, trachea, or intestinal tract. Intraspinal and intracranial tumors cause problems because of the pressure they exert in a closed space. Tumors may also degenerate or by the pressure they exert cause atrophy and ulceration of overlying epithelium.

Malignant tumors may produce the same problems as benign tumors. In addition, because of their size and ability to infiltrate and destroy surrounding tissue, there is danger of obstruction, hemorrhage, ulceration, and secondary infection.

Systemic effects

Systemic effects of malignant tumors are varied and depend in part on the organ or organs involved. For example, patients with cancer of the gastrointestinal tract often develop anemia secondary to chronic blood loss and malabsorption. Tumors of the endocrine glands usually cause an increase in secretion from the glands, resulting in various syndromes such as Cushing's disease or hyperthyroidism. In addition some malignant tumors of the lung secrete trophic hormones, which can result in conditions resembling Cushing's syndrome.[13]

When there is a metastatic implant in the peritoneal or pleural cavity, this causes an increased production of serous fluid, and the patient develops either pleural effusion or ascites (peritoneal).

Degenerative changes can occur in the central nervous system of patients with advanced cancer, even in the absence of metastases to the area. The patient may show signs of cerebellar disease and peripheral neuritis. There may be severe muscle weakness or dermatomyositis, and hemorrhage may occur if blood vessels are eroded by the growing tumor.

Anemia, leukopenia, and platelet deficiency may result from replacement of bone marrow by cancer cells. Patients with advanced cancer have an increased susceptibility to infection.[2] Cachexia is usually a sign of advanced cancer. There may be gradual or rapid weight loss, signs of muscular weakness, and anorexia. Along with this may be insomnia and a feeling of hopelessness.[7]

Contrary to popular belief, pain is frequently the last symptom to appear. Cancer may cause distortion and destruction of tissue activating pain fibers. Infiltration and occlusion of arteries, veins, and lymphatics may cause obstruction of their lumens, producing pain by distention of the vessels. Partial or complete occlusion of an artery may cause pain from ischemia and gangrene. Inflammatory changes in the stomach, ovary, bladder, and bowel may also be pain producing, as is infection and necrosis of tissue[7] (see Chapter 22).

□ Diagnostic studies

The nurse needs to be able to give a simple description of various diagnostic procedures to patients and families. The tests may involve the use of complex equipment as well as the injection or ingestion of various substances. The patient's anxiety may be high, and the nurse's ability to give factual information often will help decrease his anxiety. Several of the most widely used tests are discussed below.

X-ray, isotope, and scanning procedures

X-ray and isotope studies are usually ordered. Chest radiography is absolutely necessary if the patient is a smoker. Gastrointestinal series, intravenous pyelogram, and mammography may be done depending on areas where lesions are expected to be present.[13]

Lymphangiography is a newer development in radiology. It is useful in diagnosing lymphoma and metastatic cancer. A mixture of vital blue stain and Novocain is injected in the skin of the web between the first and second toes to show lymphatic drainage of the lower extremities. If the upper extremity is to be investigated, the injection is made in the web between the index and second finger.

Five to 10 minutes following the injection of the dye, the skin of the dorsum of the foot or hand is prepared. An incision is made and the lymphatics that can be visualized are dissected. Ethyl ester iodinated poppyseed oil (Ethiodol) is injected. Normal lymphatics appear as thin beaded vessels. Lymphomatous nodes are usually enlarged and sometimes have a "foamy" or "lacy" architecture. "Moth-eaten" is the term used to describe the appearance of metastatic nodes.[13] Skin discoloration from the dye may persist for a week after the procedure.

Xeroradiography, taking of an x-ray picture on a plate of selenium-coated metal, results in a detailed picture of soft tissue. Another examination used to visualize soft tissue is *tomography,* an x-ray technique with ability to penetrate dense shadows.[2] *Thermography* is a method of constructing photographic images of surface temperature; localized skin temperature elevations that occur over inflammatory or malignant lesions are sharply delineated.

Computerized axial tomography (CAT) of the brain is a new method for diagnosing intracranial lesions by the use of an x-ray beam in conjunction with a computer. It produces a detailed study of the brain without patient discomfort (p. 650).

Radioisotope studies

Various scanning procedures that involve the introduction of a radioactive substance into the body are used to detect primary or metastatic cancer. The radioisotope either concentrates in the tumor and shows up as a "hot spot" in the scan of the organ, or the tumor does not concentrate the isotope and a "cold spot" surrounded by normal tissue that did concentrate the isotope is found.

Radioactive iodine is a commonly used isotope employed in the diagnosis of thyroid gland disease. Researchers are also experimenting with it in other diagnostic tests. Radioactive iodine-tagged albumin has proyed useful in locating tumors in the brain, and it is frequently used to determine blood volume.

In diagnostic procedures a tracer dose of the radioactive iodine either is taken by mouth or is injected intravenously as radioactive iodine-tagged albumin. The test is dependent on either the percentage of the dose picked up (blood volume) or on the rate of excretion (hyperthyroid studies). This is only one example of the advances that have occurred in the diagnostic use of radioactive isotopes. The scanning technique, which permits the mapping of organs by the detection and measurement of radioactive substances, plays an important part in the evaluation of the patient with cancer (see Figs. 30-9 and 34-20).

Ultrasound

Ultrasound probing, or *echography,* is done by an electronic instrument that detects and records echoes of sound when they are reflected at the junction of tissues with different densities. The procedure is helpful in differentiating between cystic and solid tumors.

Endoscopy

Hollow metal tubes equipped with a light are used to illuminate various body cavities and to permit visual inspection of the interior of the cavity being examined. These instruments are commonly referred to as scopes and are named for the organs they are to visualize. Thus a bronchoscope is used to examine the bronchus, a gastroscope is used to visualize the stomach, and a proctoscope to visualize the anus and sigmoid colon. A biopsy of tissue or secretions is usually obtained during these endoscopic procedures. A local anesthetic that diminishes the gag reflex is used prior to bronchoscopy or gastroscopy. Usually no anesthetic is necessary for sigmoidoscopy.

A newer technique, peritonoscopy, is being employed to examine the peritoneal cavity. It is particularly helpful in visualizing peritoneal metastasis. A local anesthetic is used with this procedure.

Cytology

In 1942 Dr. George Papanicolaou demonstrated that the diagnosis of cancer can be made from the study of cells that have sloughed or exfoliated from a tumor. These cells are found in body secretions such as cervical discharges, sputum, gastric washings, pleural fluid, and urinary washings. The secretion is spread on a slide, stained, and examined by a pathologist. The main use of the Pap smear, as it is often called, is to diagnose cancer in an asymptomatic person and to identify precancerous lesions or noninvasive cancer. If suspect cells are found, a biopsy must be performed to diagnose cancer.[1,13] The Pap smear is most widely used in routine examination of the cervical washings.

Biopsy

Biopsy is the only definitive way that cancer can be diagnosed. *Incisional biopsy* is the surgical removal of a section of the neoplasm. If the tumor is small the entire growth may be removed, a procedure called an *excisional biopsy*. When possible an *aspiration biopsy*, removing a small plug of tumor by use of a needle or syringe, is used to avoid the larger incisional or excisional biopsy.

The biopsy specimen is examined under a microscope to obtain a histologic diagnosis as to the type of cancer. In some cases it may be possible to determine the degree of malignancy.

Contrary to a belief sometimes expressed by patients, a biopsy, properly taken, adds little or no risk of causing the spread of cancer. Nurses must be careful to dispel the idea that biopsy should be avoided.

General laboratory tests

The patient's general health status must be determined in addition to determining the presence of cancer. Routine blood and urine studies are done. In addition tests that are especially valuable in cancer detection are employed. Measurement of an enzyme, acid phosphatase, which is produced almost entirely by the prostate gland, gives evidence of the extent of prostatic disease. Another enzyme, alkaline phosphatase, is elevated in individuals with bone metastases and sometimes in those with liver metastases. Blood in the stool, identified by the guaiac test, may be a sign of gastrointestinal cancer.

□ Nursing intervention during assessment phase

The emotional climate produced during the period of diagnostic examination and initial treatment is very important in determining whether the patient will continue diagnostic examination, treatment, or repeated follow-up care after discharge. The care he receives in the hospital may shape his attitudes toward his disease and may determine whether he can return home and either care for himself or be cared for by his family. An important nursing function in care of the patient with cancer is building up his faith in the physician and in the clinic or the medical center where he receives care. The patient needs to feel certain that everything possible is being done for him and that new measures will be tried if there is any promise whatsoever of their being helpful.

Many patients must undergo extensive diagnostic examination and surgery in large medical centers a long distance from their homes. Some patients have reported that, although they were confident that they were in "good medical hands," such confidence did not make up for the feeling that they were not always known as individuals. They needed desperately to feel that at least one person knew and understood them. Some patients experience near panic at the thought of their loved ones coming to visit and being unable to locate them. The nurse who works with the patient in the community, in the small hospital, or in the physician's office can help the patient by preparing him for what he may experience in the large medical center. In most instances it is best for the patient to be accompanied by a relative or a close friend. It should also be recognized that even a patient in familiar surroundings may feel very much alone when awaiting diagnostic tests or surgical treatment for known or suspected cancer.

The patient needs something to help pass the time while he is awaiting completion of diagnostic tests and treatment and between steps of treatment such as surgery or x-ray therapy.

The family also needs to keep busy while awaiting the results of diagnostic tests and the outcome of surgery or of other treatment. One woman, on learning that her husband had far advanced carcinoma, went home immediately and made his favorite cake, even though he was in the hospital and unable to enjoy it. Psychologic relief may sometimes come from keeping occupied with usual daily activities. Anxious relatives also receive satisfaction from doing things that the patient would do if he could, thus preserving parts of cherished routines. Taking the dog for his daily walk is an example. Members of the family often need direction in their activity when they have just learned that a loved one has cancer. They may need to talk over immediate and long-term plans with someone not close to the family situation. The nurse can sometimes be this listening person. At other times the family can best be served by a social caseworker, who will help them talk through and think through a course of action (see Chapter 16).

■ INTERVENTION

□ Planning care

A sound personal philosophy and an objective, positive attitude toward the disease based on knowledge will help the nurse who is caring for the patient with cancer. The nurse should be able to give support and hope to the patient and to his significant others.

Four principles should be considered by the nurse when planning nursing interventions that are patient or client centered: (1) the person has a right to be part of the treatment team, (2) the person has the right to choose the degree of privacy or communiction that he wants, (3) the nurse must respect the coping mechanisms of the patient who is trying to maintain himself through a difficult illness, and (4) the nurse must remember not to give the appearance of hurrying, thus blocking communications and "turning the patient off."

□ Meeting psychologic needs

Cancer nursing demands not only caring *for* the patient but also caring *about* the patient, who may be angry, depressed, and perhaps physically unattractive because of the effects of the disease or its treatment. Communication is vital in meeting the needs of the cancer patient and his family. Validating assumptions and assisting patients to describe, clarify, and identify reasons for feelings are important to promote communication, In addition the nurse must try to make explanations clear and uncomplicated. Getting feedback from the patient is one way to ensure that he has received the message.

Nursing intervention to help the patient cope

Since the threat to life and the potential for other losses are so great for patients with cancer, they need especially to have their existing coping mechanisms supported or to receive support if coping mechanisms are inadequate to meet their needs.

Each patient's reaction to cancer is unique, so there can be no easy formula for care. The nurse must be able to work with and accept patients' behavior and coping style. Avoidance of false reassurance and pat answers that block communication will contribute to patient comfort. Openness, honesty, and creativity of the nurse are essential. In working with the patient the inexperienced nurse may find it helpful to turn to an instructor, head nurse, or supervisor with problems that appear too great to handle alone. The nurse reinforces patients' hope but is careful to avoid giving false hope, which can be more devastating than none at all. At times patients may need to deny their illness, while at other times they may want to talk about it.

Trusting patients' resilience and their will to try and helping them live as fully as possible are all appropriate interventions. When patients complain, perhaps the best response is, "Tell me how you feel. Perhaps we can do something about it." Self-esteem is maintained by fostering patients' independence, even if this only involves taking part in decision making about the care to be given.

Persons working with these patients must have confidence in themselves and the ability to suspend their own concerns, needs, and desires in order to concentrate on patients' problems. In order to do this one must be able to tolerate a high level of anxiety and to look at problems on both a feeling (affective) and a thinking (cognitive) level.

Listening carefully and attentively to concerns of patients helps to calm fears. In addition nurses who are knowledgeable about cancer, who can answer questions and clear up misconceptions, help promote the patient's psychologic well-being.

Nursing interventions to help the family cope

The interventions that help the patient cope are also important in helping the family cope. The nurse must get to know them and their reactions. They may feel guilty, helpless, and angry just as the patient does. Letting them know that their feelings are normal may increase their comfort. Families should not be pushed into responsibilities that they cannot handle. Some want to participate in care, others are overwhelmed by the disease and are afraid to or may not want to help. Their feelings need to be respected.

Teaching the family is a major responsibility. They should be reminded not to cut the patient off from family activities and concerns. If possible the patient should be included in family decision making and planning. In their desire to help their loved one, families may unintentionally contribute to the patient's sense of isolation by shielding him from family concerns.

Interdisciplinary approach to care

The skills of many members of the health team may be required to meet the needs of the cancer patient. Clear, concise communication of ideas about care and the planned interventions is essential for coordination, continuity, and integration of care. Team conferences are helpful in promoting the sharing of expertise.[62] The social worker, occupational therapist, minister, and psychologist may all be needed to contribute to the patient's well-being. The nurse, who spends the most time with the patient, may be the first to recognize that the patient and his family could benefit from the services of other health team members.

Rehabilitation of the cancer patient to his optimal level of functioning through the efforts of many health team members results in a more satisfying life for the patient and the family. Often the community health nurse is called on to give care, teach, counsel, and support the patient and family after discharge.

□ Therapeutic regimens

Often several physicians are involved in determining the appropriate treatment for cancer. The medical team decides on the choice of treatment on the basis of the biologic characteristics of the tumor, its clinical stage (p. 453), and the condition of the patient.[13] The histologic type of tumor is particularly important in determining the treatment to be used.

Therapy may be curative (removal of all traces of the disease from the body) or palliative (directed only toward relieving symptoms). At the present time there are three major forms of treatment: surgery, radiotherapy, and chemotherapy. The newest type of treatment is immunotherapy, which holds promise for the treatment of cancer.[13,45,73] Combination therapy (surgery, radiotherapy, and chemotherapy) is often employed in curing or controlling cancer.

□ Surgical intervention

Surgery, the oldest method of treating cancer, may be either curative or palliative. The best treatment for cancer at the present time is complete surgical removal of all malignant tissues before metastasis occurs. Surgery must often be extensive and may require adjustments beyond that needed in many other conditions. The person with cancer does not have the privilege of electing surgery. This fact alone makes the person feel trapped and seriously threatened. There is not time to accustom oneself gradually to the idea of surgery and the effect it can have on one's body and on one's life style. The individual often faces the prospect of mutilating surgery with only the hope that it will cure the cancer and be lifesaving. Concern about what will happen to his family may be utmost in the patient's mind. Obviously the individual and family need empathy and understanding as they attempt to accept the recommendation for immediate surgery.

The operative procedures used to treat various types of cancer are discussed in Part III of this book under the particular systems.

□ Radiotherapy

Radiotherapy, or the use of radiation in the treatment of disease, has been used in the treatment of cancer for about 70 years. The principal radiation agents are: (1) x-ray, which consists of electromagnetic radiation produced by waves of electrical energy traveling at a very high speed; (2) radium, which is a radioactive isotope occurring freely in nature; and (3) the artificially induced radioactive isotopes produced by bombarding the isotopes of elements with highly energized particles in a

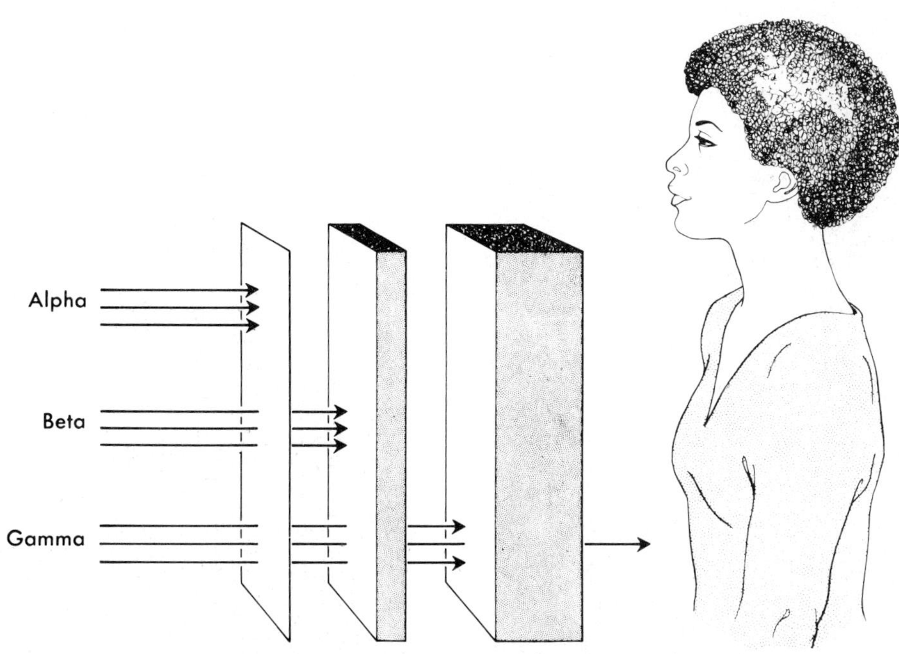

Fig. 25-3. Relative penetrating power of three types of radiation. (From Bouchard, R., and Owens, N. F.: Nursing care of the cancer patient, ed. 2, St. Louis, 1972, The C. V. Mosby Co.)

cyclotron. One of the most useful of these radiation agents is radioactive cobalt (cobalt 60, irradiated cobalt), which is now used in external radiation therapy.

Radiotherapy is effective in curing cancer in some instances; in other instances it controls the growth of cancer cells for a time. Because it may deter the growth of cancer cells, it may relieve pain even when extension of the disease is such that cure is impossible.

Principle underlying radiotherapy

Radiotherapy is based on the fact that rapidly reproducing malignant cells are more sensitive to radiation than are normal cells. Therapeutic doses of radiotherapy are calculated to destroy or delay the growth of malignant cells without destroying normal tissue. Rotation of either the target site in the patient or the radiation beam makes it possible to deliver a high total dose to the tumor while at the same time only part of the dose reaches the noncancerous tissue surrounding it.

The radiation used medically consists of alpha, beta, and gamma rays (Fig. 25-3). Alpha and beta rays cannot pass through the skin. Gamma rays, however, have been found to penetrate several inches of lead, although lead shielding offers a considerable degree of protection. X-rays, which are similar to gamma rays, require lead protection.

Radiation can be delivered to the patient *externally* by exposure to rays, such as from an x-ray machine or from cobalt 60, or *internally*, either by placing radioactive material such as radium within the tissues or body cavity (sealed internal radiation) or by administering the materials intravenously or orally so that they are distributed throughout the body (unsealed internal radiation).

Protection of health workers from radiation hazards

Radiation delivered externally (including x-rays) can do harm to persons working with the patient *only during* the time that the patient is being treated. This is true also of the radiation from some radioactive substances used for other methods of treatment (p. 454). Patients with internal radiation who emit gamma rays, however, may expose other persons to radiation for varying periods of time, and the time one can be exposed safely to the patient is important in planning care. The time interval required for the radioactive substance to be half dissipated is called its *half-life* (Table 25-4). This period varies extremely widely, but as the end of the half-life is reached, danger from exposure decreases.

There are three ways by which exposure to radiation can be controlled: *time, distance*, and *shielding*. All emanations are subject to the physical law of inverse-square. For example, if a person stands 2 meters away

Table 25-4. Characteristics and uses of some commonly used radioactive agents

Radiation source	Half-life (where applicable)	Rays emitted	Appearance or form	Method of administration
X-ray	—	Gamma	Invisible rays	X-ray machine
Radium	1,600 years	Alpha Beta Gamma	In needles, plaques, molds	Interstitial (needles) Intracavitary (plaques, molds)
Radon	4 days	Alpha Beta Gamma (low intensity)	In seeds, needles	Interstitial (seeds, needles)
Cesium (^{137}Cs)	33 years	Beta Gamma	In needles, capsules	Interstitial (needles) Intracavitary (capsules)
Cobalt (^{60}Co)	5 years	Beta Gamma	External (cobalt unit) Internal (needles, seeds, molds)	Machine (teletherapy) Interstitial (needles, seeds)
Iodine (^{131}I)	8 days	Beta Gamma (low intensity)	Clear liquid	By mouth
Phosphorus (^{32}P)	14 days	Beta	Clear liquid	By mouth, intracavitary, intravenous
Gold (^{198}Au)	3 days	Beta Gamma	Purple liquid	Intracavitary
Iridium (^{192}Ir)	74 days	Beta Gamma (low intensity)	In needles, wires, seeds	Interstitial
Yttrium (^{90}Y)	3 days	Beta	Beads, needles	Interstitial

from the source of radiation, he receives only one fourth as much exposure as when standing only 1 meter away. At 4 meters he receives only one sixteenth of the exposure. Therefore increasing the distance from the emanations decreases the exposure (Fig. 25-4). When a patient such as an infant must be held for x-ray treatment, the nurse or person who holds him must be careful to keep at arm's length or as far away as possible and to avoid having any body part in the direct path of the rays. *Lead-lined gloves and a lead apron, which act as a shield to reduce exposure, should be worn by anyone who attends patients during x-ray treatment or during examination by fluoroscopy.*

When the nurse knows the kind of substance used, the kind and amount of rays it emits, its half-life, and its exact location in the patient and considers these facts in relation to control of exposure, safe and adequate care for the patient can be planned.

Nurses wishing to know about radioactive substances can obtain information from the Division of Radiological Health of the Public Health Service or from their state health department. Several drug companies also publish phamphlets that contain helpful information. In cities with large medical facilities a radiation physicist may be consulted.

External radiotherapy

Preparation of the patient. The patient who is to have x-ray or radioactive cobalt therapy needs an adequate explanation so that he will know what to expect before, during, and after the treatment. It is helpful if the nurse can observe the patient receiving therapy, since this will enable the nurse to answer the patient's questions about the therapy more intelligently. The patient should know that he will be placed on a table in a room by himself and that the equipment, although somewhat similar to what he has probably seen during a routine x-ray examination, will be larger and more complicated. He should also know that the radiologist or the radiotherapist will be stationed outside the room, will observe him throughout the treatment, and can communicate with him by means of an intercommunication system. After he is positioned by the radiologist, the patient must remain absolutely still. This is a very trying experience for many patients, and the sympathetic understanding of the nurse will be appreciated.

The patient should also be told that there is no pain associated with radiation therapy. He may have heard that the treatment causes nausea or skin burns or irritation. If he asks about these problems, the nurse can ex-

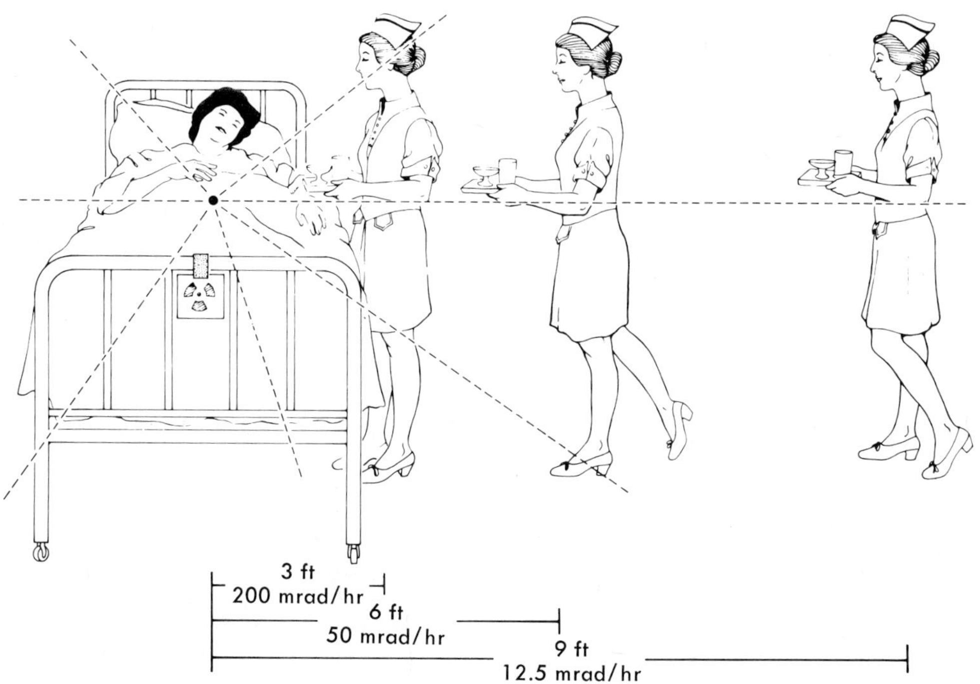

Fig. 25-4. Nurse nearest source of radioactivity (patient) is exposed to more radioactivity. (From Bouchard, R., and Owens, N. F.: Nursing care of the cancer patient, ed. 2, St. Louis, 1972, The C. V. Mosby Co.)

plain that with the carefully controlled dosages now given, they seldom occur.

The patient may be curious as to how many treatments he will receive. It is best not to give a definite answer. Radiation dosages may be difficult to estimate accurately if the growth is deep within the body. Sometimes treatment must be discontinued because of local skin reaction or other reasons; thus the patient who has been told the number of treatments planned to assure successful recovery may become depressed when treatment is discontinued. The patient also becomes concerned if he learns he is to receive more treatments than were originally planned.

Procedure. In giving treatment, rays can be directed at the tumor from several different angles so that normal tissue receives a minimum of exposure. The areas through which rays pass are known as *ports*. Different ports may be used on different days, or the position may be changed at intervals during a daily treatment so that only a certain amount is given through each of several ports. The patient may be placed on a rotating device such as a rotating chair so that although the tumor mass receives the full dose of radiation, skin areas receive less exposure.

In medical centers where hyperbaric oxygen chambers are available, patients may receive radiation therapy while receiving hyperbaric oxygen. The rationale for this combined therapy is that malignant cells, in which the oxygen tension is increased, are more susceptible to the effects of radiation. At the same time the sensitivity of normal cells to the radiation effects is not increased.[3,48,49] Several excellent texts on the use of hyperbaric oxygen can be found in the references at the end of this chapter.

Early reaction. When radiation therapy is used some degree of radiation reaction may occur. Early reactions include blanching or erythema of the skin and mucous membranes, possibly progressing to dry or moist desquamation. If the mucosa of the mouth, pharynx, bladder, or rectum is affected there may be pain, inhibition of the normal secretions, and impairment of function.[13]

When treatment is directed toward abdominal organs or any deep tissues there is almost always some skin reaction. There may be itching, tingling, burning, oozing, or sloughing of the skin. The term "burn" should never be used in referring to this reaction, since it implies incorrect dosage. Reddening may occur on or about the tenth day, and the skin may turn a dark plum color after about 3 weeks. The skin may also become dry and inelastic and may crack easily.

Gastrointestinal reactions to radiation therapy are more common when treatment includes some part of the gastrointestinal tract or when the ports lie over this system. The patient may have nausea, vomiting, anorexia, malaise, and diarrhea. This difficulty is usually not discussed with the patient before treatment is started because it is thought that the power of suggestion may contribute to symptoms. Almost all patients who receive moderate or large doses of radiation, however, have these symptoms in varying degrees.

Radiation therapy also causes depression of the hematopoietic system and in turn a low white blood cell count, predisposing the patient to infection. Sloughing of tissue and subsequent hemorrhages are complications that must be considered when radiation is used in any form. Hemorrhage is not mentioned to the patient, but if he is ambulatory he is told that he should call the physician at once should any sloughing of tissue occur.

Late reaction. Effects of radiation may be apparent months or years after therapy. Genital tissue, muscles, and kidneys may be affected resulting in painful radionecrosis.[13] Radiation causes destruction of fine vasculature, and the skin may show signs of atrophy (thinning and blanching), pigmentation, and telangiectasis. If there is severe vascular damage or if there are other complications that require further surgery, the irradiated tissues may fail to heal.[13]

Nursing intervention for patients receiving external radiation

Preventing skin breakdown. Skin preparation for external radiation therapy includes removal of any ointment and dressing and thorough cleansing of the skin. This procedure usually is followed by an alcohol rub. After this preparation nothing should be used on the skin. The area to be treated is usually outlined by the radiologist at the time of the first treatment. Occasionally a small tattoo mark is used instead of the conspicuous skin markings when treatment is given to exposed parts of the body. Marks must not be washed off until the treatment is completed because they are important guides to the radiologist (Fig. 25-5). If the patient is ambulatory he is instructed not to wash the skin in the area being treated or to remove the marks. Sponge bathing of other parts of the body must replace showers and tub baths. A vegetable fat or oil may be ordered to protect the affected skin.

Medicated solutions or ointments and even powders that may contain heavy metals such as zinc are not permitted on the skin until the series of treatments is completed because they may increase the radiation dosage. Cornstarch may be used instead of powder.

The radiologist is consulted about skin care when a local radiation reaction occurs. The area may be cleansed gently with sterile mineral oil, but crusts should not be removed. Lanolin or petroleum jelly may be used to protect the area, and healing ointments containing vitamins

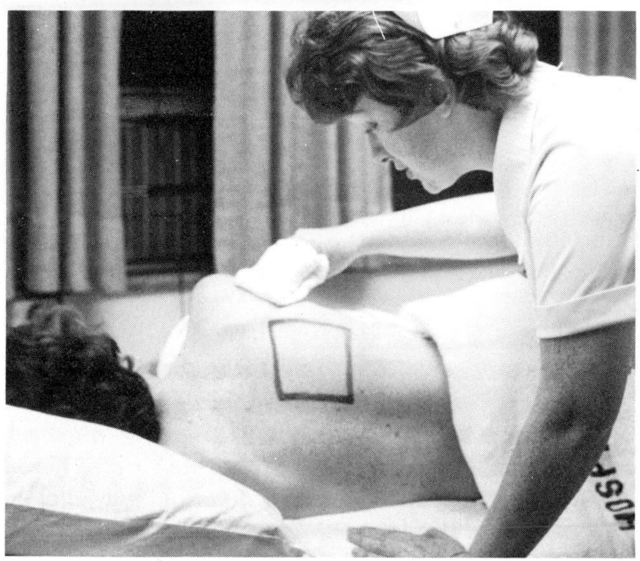

Fig. 25-5. When bath is given, care must be taken not to remove skin markings used to guide radiologist in giving x-ray treatments.

A and D and healing oils such as cod liver oil may be used if breakdown of superficial tissues occurs. Healing usually starts approximately in the fifth week of treatment and should be completed about a month later.

Ointments are best applied by spreading them on a piece of sterile gauze and fastening the gauze to the patient's clothing. If this procedure is not possible, dressings may be bandaged loosely or anchored to healthy skin outside and beyond the treatment ports. If tape must be used instead of a bandage, a nonirritating tape is used. In removing dressings the greatest care must be taken to pull toward the middle of the area and thus avoid any pull on affected skin. Dressings should be loose to permit circulation of air and to avoid pressure on the skin.

Because the skin exposed to radiation treatment may become irritated and break down easily, it should be protected from constricting clothing or friction of any kind. For example, the patient receiving treatment to the trunk should not wear a girdle, tight panty hose, or a constricting trouser or skirt belt during the period of treatment and for several weeks thereafter. During the period of treatment, excesses of heat and cold to affected skin surfaces should be avoided. Hot-water bottles and ice caps should not be used, and exposure to the sun should be avoided. Some physicians advise that no water be used on the skin for at least 2 weeks after the completion of treatment.

If the radiation dosage has been high and blanching or discoloration of the skin has resulted, the patient may be advised to avoid exposure to temperature changes for several years. The patient may have to take much cooler baths or showers than formerly, and he may have to avoid sunbathing or any other extreme of temperature. If x-ray treatment has been given to a woman's face, she must be cautioned regarding the use of cosmetics to cover discolored skin. They may contain heavy, irritating oils and should not be used until the physician believes they are safe.

When treatment must be given to any part of the head, women may ask about the danger of loss of scalp hair and men about loss of beard. Whether hair will return after falling out depends on the amount of radiation received. Attractive scarves and wigs are useful for patients with permanent baldness or until such time as the normal hair returns.

Decreasing gastrointestinal tract upset. Many patients find that resting just before meals and lying down immediately after eating help to control nausea and vomiting. Frequent small meals instead of the usual three a day may be more helpful. Some patients find that it helps to avoid food for 2 or 3 hours before and about 2 hours after each treatment. Sour beverages and effervescent liquids may also relieve nausea. Usually breakfast is the meal best tolerated. Therefore it should be substantial, and the patient should be encouraged to eat as much as possible. Problems related to radiation therapy in specific body locations are discussed in the appropriate sections of this book.

Intravenous solutions of glucose in physiologic solution of sodium chloride are used for nausea, anorexia, and dehydration. Pyridoxine (vitamin B_6), dimenhydrinate (Dramamine), chlorpromazine (Thorazine), and trimethobenzamide hydrochloride (Tigan) relieve nausea in some patients. Camphorated tincture of opium (paregoric) may be used to control diarrhea, but drugs such as bismuth subcarbonate are not given because they contain a heavy metal that will increase radiation dosage.

Preventing infection. As previously mentioned, radiation therapy depresses the hematopoietic system, thus reducing the white blood count and making the patient more vulnerable to infection. If the client is at home and receiving treatment on an ambulatory basis, he and his family are cautioned to avoid persons with upper respiratory tract or other infections. In the hospital he should never be in the same room with patients who have an infection, and a private room and even protective isolation may be required if the white blood cell count is very low. Antibiotic drugs may be ordered to be given prophylactically both during and following a course of treatment.

Promoting psychologic comfort. To many people radiotherapy and cancer are synonymous. It is natural, then, that the patient may react with panic to news that this treatment is necessary. Sometimes the patient is told that the treatment is necessary "to cure a growth that may become cancerous if not so treated." Often he does not really believe this statement. The nurse should give the patient who is about to receive radiation therapy an opportunity to talk about the therapy and to ask questions.

Internal radiotherapy

Internal radiation may be delivered by sealed or unsealed methods. In either type special precautions may be necessary. Whether the patient receiving internal radiation will be treated under radiation precautions and the nursing time with him will be restricted depends on the amount of radioactive material used, its location, and the kind of rays being emitted (Table 25-4). Special precautions may be taken if more than a tracer diagnostic dose has been given. Hospitals in which therapeutic doses of radioactive isotopes are administered are required to have a radiation safety officer. Quite often this person is a physicist. The radiation safety officer determines the precautions to be observed in each situation. Most hospitals have printed instruction sheets stating the precautions to be followed for each substance used. Personnel should be fully acquainted with all precautions and should be supervised in carrying them out. Generally the patient will be placed in a single room or in a double room with another patient who is also receiving radiation therapy. A radiation precaution sign should be placed on the door to the patient's room, and visitors should be restricted.

Sealed internal radiotherapy. Radium, a naturally occurring radioactive isotope, and cobalt and iridium that have been made radioactive artificially are used to deliver sealed internal radiotherapy to certain malignant lesions that can be expected to respond to this kind of treatment. These radioactive substances may be used in the form of molds, plaques, needles, wires, special applicators, or ribbons that are carefully placed and left in position for a specified length of time (Fig. 25-6). Emanations from the radioactive substances may also be sealed in tiny gold tubes (seeds) and left indefinitely within the tissues into which they are inserted (Fig. 25-7). The half-life of the seeds is much less than that of the substances from which their emanations come. Radium is extremely costly, and its use is being replaced with the use of radioactive cobalt and other radioactive materials.

A fairly common site for the implantation of seeds is the mouth. Plaques and molds also are used for lesions in the mouth (see Chapter 54). Sealed internal radiation also is used widely in treatment of cancer of the cervix (p. 1431).

Prevention of radiation hazard: sealed radiotherapy. Safe practice for the nurse caring for a patient receiving

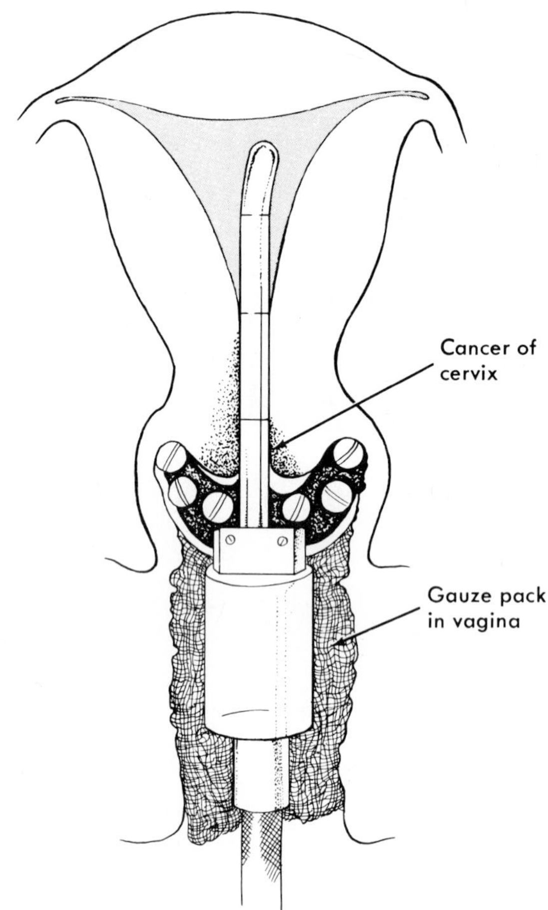

Fig. 25-6. Ernst applicator in place for treatment of cancer of cervix. Note gauze packing in vagina to help maintain applicator in position.

sealed internal radiotherapy depends on the principles of time, distance, and shielding (p. 468). Radioactive materials for sealed internal therapy usually are kept in a lead-lined container in the radiology department and are inserted into the patient in the operating room. They should never be touched with bare hands. When the nurse handles these products a pair of forceps at least 14 inches long is used and the radioactive materials are held at arm's length and above waist level. A pair of forceps should be kept in the patient's room for use in case the radioactive implant becomes dislodged.

Sealed radioactive material is often reused. On removal from a patient the radioactive material should be cleansed using the precautions just described and returned to the radiology department in a lead-lined container at once so that it may be safe from accidental handling or loss. Even if it is not to be reused, it is returned in a lead-lined container. To prevent accidental loss in cleansing, radioactive material is cleansed in a basin of

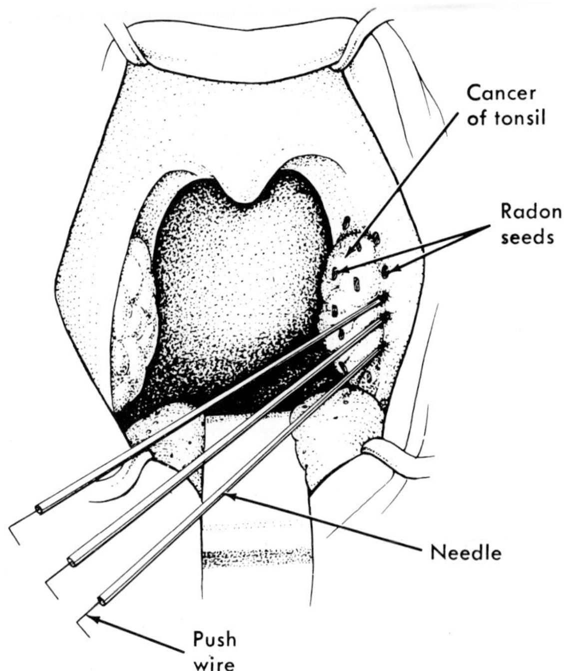

Fig. 25-7. Radium emanations may be sealed in tiny gold tubes (radon seeds) and left indefinitely within tissue into which they are inserted. Schema shows insertion into tonsil.

water instead of in an open sink. If a brush must be used, it must be grasped with forceps so that close contact with the material is avoided.

Exposure is sometimes termed external in that it can occur only by direct exposure to the encased radioactive substance. It cannot result from contact with linen, vomitus, or urine or from touching the patient. Knowing where the radioactive material is implanted helps the nurse to plan activities of care. If, for example, the substance is in the patient's mouth, there is less exposure if one stands toward the foot of the bed. If it is in the uterus or bladder, standing at the head of the bed is safer.

Unsealed internal radiotherapy. Unsealed internal radiation is delivered to the patient by mouth as an "atomic cocktail" or as a liquid instilled into a body cavity. Exposure for persons caring for the patient can result from direct contact with emanations from the substance in the patient (external exposure) or from contact with the patient's discharges that contain the radioactive substances (internal exposure). It may be inhaled, ingested, or absorbed through the skin. The exposure varies with each of the substances used, and safety for the nurse and for other persons caring for the patient depends on a thorough knowledge of the substance used and its action within the body. If only tracer doses (very small amounts) of radioactive substances are used, as for diagnostic purposes, no precautions are necessary.

The substances used most often at the present time are radioactive iodine (^{131}I), radioactive phosphorus (^{32}P), and radioactive gold (^{198}Au). None of them cures cancer, but they sometimes control the disease to some extent and lessen pain. They are used in selected cases of cancer along with other forms of treatment such as surgery and x-ray therapy.

Prevention of radiation hazards: unsealed radiotherapy. Radioactive iodine (^{131}I) is a clear liquid with a half-life of 8.1 days. Originally it was hoped that it might destroy malignant cells in the thyroid gland, but results of its use have been disappointing because malignant thyroid cells do not concentrate iodine as well as normal thyroid cells. Therefore the treatment of the original tumor in the thyroid gland or its areas of metatasis with radioactive iodine is not effective. It is often used, however, in conjunction with surgical removal of the thyroid gland.

Most of the radioactive iodine is eliminated through the kidneys, but small amounts will be present in sputum, vomitus, perspiration, and feces. Special precautions are needed only for the *urine*, which usually is collected in a lead-lined container. It is transported daily on a special cart to the radioisotope laboratory, where it is stored until it can be disposed of safely. An indwelling catheter may be inserted before the radioactive iodine is given, and urine may be released at intervals directly into the lead-lined container. It is important that all urine be collected carefully, because it is the quantitative determination of the amount of radioactive substance excreted that determines when the patient may be removed from isolation. The nurse should know the approved hospital procedure to safely dispose of any urine that may be spilled on the floor accidentally.

No linen or equipment should be removed from the room until it is monitored with a Geiger-Muller counter for contamination. If the isolation gown and linen show contamination, they are placed in a special container labeled "Radioactive" and stored in lead containers in the isotope laboratory, or they are burned. Dishes are washed thoroughly and then monitored, or paper dishes are used and then burned. In some institutions the dishes are sent to the kitchen if the monitor reading is less than 6 mR (milliroentgens) per hour. If the nurse's skin should become contaminated, it should be washed thoroughly with soap and water and then monitored. If contamination remains, washing should be continued until monitoring shows that additional cleansing is not necessary. Because washing is essential to prevent or to lessen contamination, the patient must be in a room that has running water. Nurses may be required to wear rubber gloves when handling linen to lessen the possibility of contamination.

When the patient is removed from isolation, all equipment is monitored and carefully scrubbed by attendants who have been instructed in safe methods by persons who are in charge of the administration of the radioactive substance. It is then remonitored. The room is aired until monitoring shows that radioactivity is negligible and that the room is safe for any other patient. Airing takes at least 24 hours.

Radioactive phosphorus (^{32}P) is a clear liquid with a half-life of 14 days. It is used in the treatment of polycythemia vera and leukemia. It may be given intravenously, orally, or directly into a body cavity. Sources of contamination are vomitus and seepage from wounds. There is no danger from external exposure because the beta rays emitted by this substance are absorbed by the patient's body. Vomitus and dressings are placed in a lead-lined container and taken to the radioisotope laboratory for disposal. Care of contaminated equipment and the procedures used when staff members are exposed by contamination on the skin are similar to those described for radioactive iodine contamination.

Radioactive gold (^{198}Au) is a purple liquid with a half-life of 2.7 days. It is used largely for treatment of cancer of the lung that has caused effusion into the pleural cavity and for peritoneal ascites due to generalized carcinoma. It is injected into the body cavity, and the patient is turned every 15 minutes for 2 hours so that the radioactive gold will spread evenly within the cavity. In addition to beta rays, the substance emits gamma rays, so that special isolation precautions may be necessary to prevent external exposure.

If a purple stain appears, it indicates that some of the radioactive gold is escaping from the wound or the site of injection. Wearing rubber gloves, the nurse should apply dressings over the site of injection or the wound. Linen that has been in contact with the wound or the site of injection is placed in a special container clearly marked for care in the isotope laboratory or other facilities provided by the hospital. Dressings and cleansing tissues are burned immediately or sent for disposal in special containers to the isotope laboratory.

The patient who receives radioactive gold is usually terminally ill. If he dies soon after receiving ^{198}Au, a notation that the patient was receiving radioactive gold immediately before death is made on a tag, and the tag should be conspicuously placed on the body for the protection of the coroner and the mortician. If the nurse has any questions about precautions that should be taken, the radiation safety officer is consulted.

Nursing intervention for patients receiving internal radiotherapy

Teaching the patient. It is important to explain the routine to the patient and the reason for the precautions that are to be taken. He is kept in his own room for the period of isolation so that danger of contamination to others is minimized and so that his reaction to the radioactive substance can be studied and controlled. He should know that isolation is temporary, that the restrictions will be removed on a certain day, and that members of the nursing staff will be available for anything that he needs, but that they will work quickly and will remain in the room only long enough to carry out essential activities. The patient can assist in notifying his significant others about the restriction on visitors and how long it will last. The patient should know how the radioactive substance he takes is eliminated lest he fear that he will be dangerous to other people indefinitely and become concerned about social isolation or about the possibility of harming his loved ones when he returns home.

Many patients anticipate cure from radioactive isotopes. The nurse can learn what the patient understands about the treatment and should report any misunderstandings on his part to the physician.

Decreasing patient isolation. Occasionally no direct contact with the patient is permitted. If so, the patient's room must be equipped with an intercommunication system and all supplies he may need during isolation. The room should have a window through which the patient can be observed and through which he can see other people. It should have a telephone so that he can talk to family members if he is able and wishes to do so. Food and other items the patient desires or needs usually are passed into the room through a special porthole.

A radio or television will help the patient keep in contact with outside happenings. The patient needs to see the nursing staff, however, and if treatment permits they should speak to him from the open doorway. If isolation is complete, they should come to the observation window frequently and speak to him through the intercommunication system.

Trips made in haste into the patient's room are disturbing to him psychologically because they imply that he is not acceptable to others. The nurse who plans thoughtfully might deliver a letter, a telephone message, an ice cap, fresh water, and the newspaper and make pertinent observations in much less time than the one who plans less well and must make several trips into the patient's room.

Promoting physical and psychologic comfort. There are many things the nurse can do to add to the patient's physical and emotional comfort during the period of restricted nursing contact. Before treatment is given, his immediate environment is checked. Are the bed and bedside table in the most convenient location for self-help? Can any arrangement be made so that the patient may draw his own blinds or curtains? Are extra covers readily available? Are reading materials and lighting adequate and conveniently located? Are plants and flowers receiving care and is it possible to arrange their location so that the patient may care for them himself if he feels able?

Before treatment requiring a period of precaution or isolation is started, the patient should have a complete bath, since bathing will not be permitted for a few days. The bed is made with clean linen, and all personal linen should be fresh. If the patient is very ill and requires help in turning and moving, a turning sheet may be placed under him so that the nursing staff can turn him and raise him in bed in the shortest possible time and with little close contact. Sometimes a laxative or an enema is ordered to obviate the need for an enema or attention to bowel elimination for a few days. If treatment requires lying still in a specified position, measures for comfort should be anticipated. For example, if the patient is receiving treatment to the cervix and must lie on her back, a small pillow should be provided for use against the curve of the back before fatigue and discomfort become a major problem.

Outcome criteria for patient receiving external radiotherapy

1. The patient is free from infection on discharge from the hospital.
2. The patient or significant others can:
   a. Describe measures to prevent skin breakdown.
   b. Describe the measures to decrease nausea and vomiting and increase food and fluid intake.
   c. List the components of an adequate diet.
   d. Describe measures to prevent infection.

□ Chemotherapy

Surgery and radiation, when used with early diagnosis, are still the most important treatments for cancer. Some cancers, either by their nature or by their extent at the time of diagnosis, are too widespread to be treated successfully with surgery or radiation or both. For these patients chemical control of the cancer is the primary therapeutic method.

The more pronounced the proliferative activity of cells, the greater are their sensitivity to chemotherapeutic agents. Drugs used in chemotherapy are nonspecific; that is, they are cytotoxic to both neoplastic and normal cells. Normal cells that proliferate rapidly such as those of the hematopoietic system, the intestinal mucosa, and the hair are particularly affected by the cytotoxic action of the drugs.

Chemotherapeutic drugs are administered in relation to the cancer cell's reproductive cycle; specific drugs are effective at different points of cell growth. Among the major conceptual advances in the treatment of cancer in the past decade have been those of combination chemotherapy, the realization that the stage of mitotic activity of the cancer target cell may determine the metabolic effects of chemotherapeutic agents, and that the dose scheduling of drugs is as important as the drug itself in achieving therapeutic benefit and lessening the toxic response by normal tissue.[47]

The goal in using combination chemotherapy is to produce an effect that is greater than that from the sum of each agent alone (synergism). An example of synergism in cancer chemotherapy is the combination of vincristine and prednisone in acute lymphocytic leukemia. By using the drugs singly, the observed remission rate is approximately 80%, whereas combination therapy effects 90% remission rate. Combination chemotherapy decreases the potential for the development of resistant cells. There is less likelihood of the evolution of mutations resistant to several drugs than of mutations resistant to single drugs. Only a combination of drugs may be capable of destroying all the malignant cells.

Combination chemotherapy is of greatest advantage when it is used to exploit different toxicities of the chemotherapeutic agents. Suppression of bone marrow activity is an important limiting factor in the use of these agents. By using combinations of drugs that have different toxicities to bone marrow, the dose of each drug can be given in combination at full doses.[74]

Zubrod[77] states that "chemotherapy has arrived at a stage where it is clearly responsible for producing normal life expectancy in 10 of the 100 or more types of cancer. These are generally cancers of the young and are uncommon, yet high on the list of causes of childhood deaths. In a number of more common tumors of older age groups, chemotherapy is producing an increasing percentage of complete remissions of significant duration—milestones on the road to normal life expectancy."[77] The effectiveness of chemotherapy in cancer has been best demonstrated in the treatment of the lymphomas and leukemias. The trend today is to use a dose schedule of antitumor drugs in combination and as an adjunct to other treatment modalities. Cancer chemotherapy is gradually being confined to special centers where experience and facilities are concentrated. Many such centers around the world are actively devising and testing multiple-drug schedules for all forms of advanced cancer and are applying more sophisticated techniques of biochemistry and cell kinetics directly to the problems of human cancer.

Chemotherapeutic agents

The five large classes of chemotherapeutic agents in use today are alkylating agents, antimetabolites, plant alkaloids, antibiotics, and hormones (Table 25-5). A discussion of each follows.

Table 25-5. Highlights of commercially available cancer chemotherapeutic drugs*

Drug	Usual dosage and route of administration	Toxicity: Acute	Toxicity: Delayed	Major indications
Alkylating agents				
Busulfan (Myleran)	2 to 8 mg/day for 2 to 3 weeks PO; stop for recovery; then maintenance	None	Bone marrow depression	Chronic granulocytic leukemia
Chlorambucil (Leukeran)	Start 0.1 to 0.2 mg/kg/day PO; adjust for maintenance	None	Bone marrow depression (anemia, leukopenia, and thrombocytopenia) can be severe with excessive dosage	Chronic lymphocytic leukemia, Hodgkin's disease, non-Hodgkin's lymphoma, trophoblastic neoplasms
Cyclophosphamide (Cytoxan)	40 mg/kg IV in single dose or in 2 to 8 daily doses or 2 to 4 mg/kg/day PO for 10 days; adjust for maintenance	Nausea and vomiting	Bone marrow depression, alopecia, cystitis	Hodgkin's disease and other lymphomas, multiple myeloma, lymphocytic leukemia, many solid cancers
Mechlorethamine (nitrogen mustard; HN_2, Mustargen)	0.4 mg/kg IV in single or divided doses	Nausea and vomiting; vesicant	Moderate depression of peripheral blood count	Hodgkin's disease and other lymphomas, bronchogenic carcinoma
Melphalan (1-phenylalanine mustard; Alkeran)	0.25 mg/kg/day for 4 days PO; 2 to 4 mg/day as maintenance or 0.1 to 0.15 mg/kg/day for 2 to weeks	None	Bone marrow depression	Multiple myeloma, malignant melanoma, ovarian carcinoma, testicular seminoma
Thio-TEPA (triethylenethiophosphoramide)	0.2 mg/kg IV for 5 days	None	Bone marrow depression	Hodgkin's disease, bronchogenic and breast carcinomas
Antimetabolites				
Cytarabine hydrochloride (arabinosyl cytosine; Cytosar)	2 to 3 mg/kg/day IV until response or toxicity or 1 to 3 mg/kg IV over 24 hours for up to 10 days	Nausea and vomiting	Bone marrow depression, megaloblastosis	Acute leukemia
Fluorouracil (5-FU, FU)	12.5 mg/kg/day IV for 3 to 5 days or 15 mg/kg/wk for 6 weeks	Nausea	Oral and gastrointestinal ulceration, stomatitis and diarrhea, bone marrow depression	Breast, large bowel, and ovarian cancer
Mercaptopurine (6-MP; Purinethol)	2.5 mg/kg/day PO	Occasional nausea and vomiting; usually well tolerated	Bone marrow depression, occasional hepatic damage	Acute lymphocytic and granulocytic leukemia, chronic granulocytic leukemia
Methotrexate (amethopterin; MTX)	2.5 to 5.0 mg/day PO; 0.4 mg/kg rapid IV daily 4 to 5 days (not over 25 mg) or 0.4 mg/kg rapid IV twice/wk	Occasional diarrhea, hepatic necrosis	Oral and gastrointestinal ulceration, bone marrow depression (anemia, leukopenia, thrombocytopenia), cirrhosis	Acute lymphocytic leukemia, choriocarcinoma, carcinoma of cervix and head and neck area, mycosis fungoides, solid cancers

*From Carter, S. K., and Kershner, L. M.: Cancer chemotherapy: what drugs are available? Resident and Staff Physician Jan. 1976, pp. 56-65.

Table 25-5. Highlights of commercially available cancer chemotherapeutic drugs—cont'd

Drug	Usual dosage and route of administration	Toxicity: Acute	Toxicity: Delayed	Major indications
Antimetabolites—cont'd				
Thioguanine (6-TG)	2 mg/kg/day PO	Occasional nausea and vomiting; usually well tolerated	Bone marrow depression	Acute leukemia
Plant alkaloids				
Vinblastine sulfate (Velban)	0.1 to 0.2 mg/kg/wk IV or every 2 weeks	Nausea and vomiting; local irritant	Alopecia, stomatitis, bone marrow depression, loss of reflexes	Hodgkin's disease and other lymphomas, solid cancers
Vincristine sulfate (Oncovin)	0.01 to 0.03 mg/kg/wk IV	Local irritant	Areflexia, peripheral neuritis, paralytic ileus, mild bone marrow depression	Acute lymphocytic leukemia, Hodgkin's disease and other lymphomas, solid cancers
Antibiotics				
Doxorubicin (Adriamycin)	60 to 90 mg/sq m IV, single dose or over 3 days; repeat every 3 weeks to total dose 550 mg/sq m	Nausea, red urine (not hematuria); vesicant	Bone marrow depression, cardiotoxicity, alopecia, stomatitis	Soft tissue, osteogenic and miscellaneous sarcomas, Hodgkin's disease, non-Hodgkin's lymphoma, bronchogenic and breast carcinoma, thyroid cancer
Bleomycin (Blenoxane)	10 to 15 mg/sq m/week or twice/week IV or IM to total dose 300 to 400 mg	Nausea and vomiting, fever, very toxic	Edema of hands pulmonary fibrosis, stomatitis, alopecia	Hodgkin's disease, non-Hodgkin's lymphoma, squamous cell carcinoma (head and neck), testicular carcinoma
Dactinomycin (actinomycin D; Cosmegen)	0.015 to 0.05 mg/kg/week (1 to 2.5 mg) 3 to 5 weeks IV; wait for marrow recovery (3 to 4 wks), then repeat course	Nausea and vomiting; local irritant, vesicant	Stomatitis, oral ulcers, diarrhea, alopecia, mental depression, bone marrow depression	Testicular carcinoma, Wilms' tumor, rhabdomyosarcoma, Ewing's and osteogenic sarcoma, other solid tumors
Mithramycin (Mithracin)	0.025 to 0.050 mg/kg IV every 2 days for up to 8 doses	Nausea and vomiting, hepatotoxicity	Bone marrow depression (thrombocytopenia), hypocalcemia	Testicular carcinoma, trophoblastic neoplasms
Mitomycin C (Mutamycin)	0.05 mg/kg/day IV for 5 days	Nausea and vomiting, flulike syndrome	Bone marrow depression, skin toxicity; pulmonary. renal, CNS effects	Squamous cell carcinoma of head and neck, lungs, and cervix; adenocarcinoma of the stomach, pancreas, colon, rectum; adenocarcinoma and duct cell carcinoma of breast

Continued.

Table 25-5. Highlights of commercially available cancer chemotherapeutic drugs—cont'd

Drug	Usual dosage and route of administration	Toxicity: Acute	Toxicity: Delayed	Major indications
Other synthetic agents				
Dacarbazine (DTIC-Dome; DIC)	4.5 mg/kg/day IV for 10 days; repeated every 28 days	Nausea and vomiting, flulike syndrome	Bone marrow depression (rare)	Metastatic malignant melanoma
Hydroxyurea (Hydrea)	80 mg/kg PO single dose every 3 days or 20 to 30 mg/kg/day PO	Mild nausea and vomiting	Bone marrow depression	Chronic granulocytic leukemia
Mitotane (ortho-para-DDD, o-*p*-DDD; Lysodren)	6 to 15 mg/kg/day PO	Nausea and vomiting	Dermatitis, diarrhea, mental depression	Adrenal cortical carcinoma
Procarbazine hydrochloride (methylhydrazine; ibenzmethyzin; Matulane)	Start 1 to 2 mg/kg/day PO; increase over 1 wk to 3 mg/kg; maintain for 3 weeks, then reduce to 2 mg/kg/day until toxic	Nausea and vomiting	Bone marrow depression, CNS depression	Hodgkin's disease, non-Hodgkin's lymphoma, bronchogenic carcinoma
Hormones				
Diethylstilbestrol (DES)	15 mg/day PO (1 mg in prostate gland cancer)	None	Fluid retention, hypercalcemia, feminization, uterine bleeding; during pregnancy may cause vaginal carcinoma in offspring	Breast and prostate gland carcinomas
Ethinyl estradiol	3 mg/day PO	None	Fluid retention, hypercalcemia, feminization, uterine bleeding	Breast and prostate gland carcinomas
Fluoxymesterone	10 to 20 mg/day PO	None	Fluid retention, masculinization, cholestatic jaundice	Breast carcinoma
Medroxyprogesterone acetate	100 to 200 mg/day PO; 200 to 600 mg twice weekly	None	None	Endometrial carcinoma; renal cell, breast cancer
Prednisone	10 to 100 mg/day PO	None	Hyperadrenocorticism	Acute and chronic lymphocytic leukemia, Hodgkin's disease, non-Hodgkin's lymphomas
Testolactone (Teslac)	100 mg IM three times weekly	None	Fluid rentention, masculinization	Breast carcinoma
Testosterone propionate	50 to 100 mg IM three weekly	None	Fluid retention, masculinization	Breast carcinoma

Alkylating agents (mustards). These agents act on already formed nucleic acids. Interference with the function of the nucleic acids, particularly DNA, accounts for the inhibition of proliferative activity of certain normal and neoplastic cells. The various types of nitrogen mustards in use have essentially similar action on normal and malignant cells. They differ mainly in local tissue irritation, degree of stimulation of the vomiting center, absorption from the gastrointestinal tract, and, consequently, routes of administration. At effective dosage levels all produce some degree of bone marrow depression.

Antimetabolites. The antimetabolites act by interfering with the synthesis of chromosomal nucleic acid necessary for new tumor cell production. This group includes mercaptopurine, fluorouracil, cytarabine hydrochloride (arabinosyl cytosine), and the folic acid antagonists such as methotrexate. Their toxic reactions include anorexia, oral ulceration, gastrointestinal disturbances such as diarrhea, and bone marrow depression.

Plant alkaloids. Vincristine sulfate and vinblastine sulfate are plant alkaloids that act as mitotic inhibitors. In addition to transient bone marrow depression, these drugs may cause alopecia, nausea and vomiting, severe constipation, paralytic ileus, peripheral neuritis, and psychomotor disturbances.

Antibiotics. Antibiotics become incorporated in the cancer cell's DNA, causing interference with the synthesis of RNA from DNA, the initial step of protein synthesis.[10]

Doxorubicin (Adriamycin) is the newest member of this family of drugs. It has demonstrated effectiveness against hematologic cancer, sarcomas, and cancer of the breast and lung.[10]

Dactinomycin (actinomycin D) is produced by a species of *Streptomyces*. It has been used to control metastasis of Wilms' tumor (nephroblastoma), testicular tumors, and choriocarcinoma. Side effects include bone marrow depression and gastrointestinal tract irritation. Infiltration during intravenous administration produces a severe local irritation.

Hormones. It is believed that steroid hormones may determine the time of development or trigger the growth of certain malignant tumors, provided other factors within the cell are present. They may also be necessary for the continued growth of certain tumors of the secondary sexual gland tissues. Attempts to alter the hormonal influences on the tumor consist of either removing the glands producing the hormones (ovaries, testicles, adrenal glands) or the endocrine gland controlling their secretion (pituitary gland) or negating the action of these respective hormones by giving their antagonists. Thus men with carcinoma of the prostate gland may be given a female hormone such as stilbestrol, and women who have carcinoma of the breast with metastasis may be given a male hormone such as testosterone. These persons may also be given large doses of hormones of their own sex to prevent stimulation of the pituitary gland and to prevent their own sexual glands from producing the hormone.

Adrenocorticosteroids such as hydrocortisone or prednisone are used as a specific therapy for certain leukemias, lymphomas, multiple myeloma, other blood dyscrasias, and metastatic cancer of the breast. They are also often employed terminally in many diverse cancers for their nonspecific ability to temporarily improve appetite and sense of well-being.

Methods of administration of chemotherapeutic drugs

Infusion. Most of the chemotherapeutic drugs may be given as an intravenous infusion for their general suppressive effect on an advanced malignancy. More recently they have been given in this way at the time of surgery for their suppressive effect on any malignant cells that might be released into the bloodstream or remain after surgery. They may also be given by infusion along with radiation therapy in order to hasten or increase its effect.

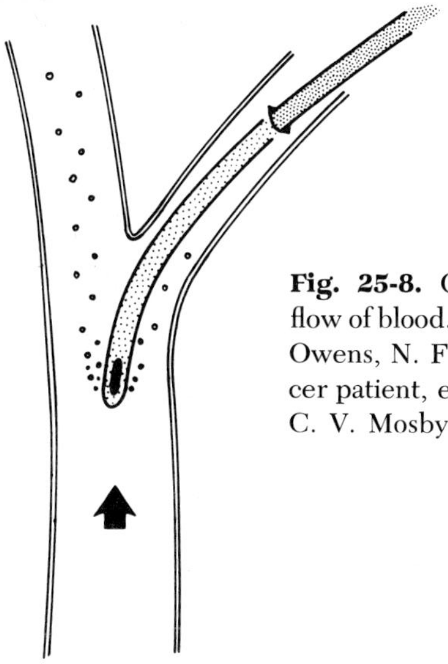

Fig. 25-8. Catheter inserted against flow of blood. (From Bouchard, R., and Owens, N. F.: Nursing care of the cancer patient, ed. 2, St. Louis, 1972, The C. V. Mosby Co.)

Perfusion. By means of several variations of a procedure known as perfusion, it is now possible to deliver an extremely large dose of one of the alkylating agents directly to a tumor. *Intraarterial perfusion* differs from the usual intravenous method only in that the drug is introduced under pressure and inserted into an artery flowing directly into the area to be treated. Thus the full strength of the drug reaches the tumor before it enters the general circulation and is distributed throughout the body.

Intraarterial perfusion is used for cancers of the head and neck, for liver metastasis, and as adjuvant chemotherapy with radiotherapy for advanced cancer of the cervix. This method provides for prolonged administration and exposure of neoplastic cells to the drug at a time when rapid mitosis is occurring (Fig. 25-8). Intraarterial infusion can be accomplished in ambulatory patients by means of a portable infusion pump slipped over the patient's head and anchored at the waist (Fig. 25-9).

Complications include hemorrhage from the artery at the site of injection, either during or after the treatment, and renal failure. If a lesion in the head is being treated, temporary baldness may occur on the affected side several weeks after treatment and may be most distressing to the patient. Some clinicians have found that applying a tourniquet around the hairline before the administration

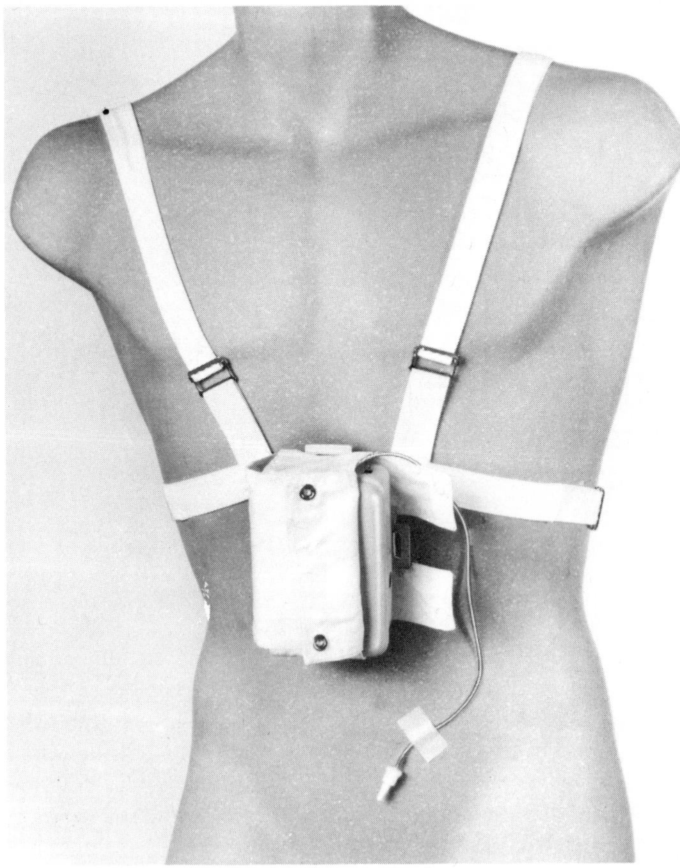

Fig. 25-9. Torso showing lightweight battery-operated infusion pump. Flow rate is variable and may be set exactly by means of plug-in meter. Power pack supplies current to operate pump for 7 days without recharging or replacement. (Courtesy Sigmamotor, Inc., Middleport, N.Y.)

of chemotherapy decreases the hair loss experienced by patients.

In the special technique known as *extracorporeal perfusion* or *isolation perfusion,* a portion of the body to be treated may be isolated in its blood supply from the rest of the body during the time of treatment. This measure makes it possible to give much larger doses more directly to the tumor than would be tolerated if they were introduced into the general circulation. For example, a tumor of the lower leg can be treated by applying a tourniquet to the upper portion of the thigh. the drug is injected directly into an artery leading to the tumor, and venous blood is removed from the area being treated through a catheter, circulated through an oxygenator to provide oxygen, and then returned under pressure to the artery. After the drug has been circulated, the blood in which the drug circulated may or may not be replaced by a fresh transfusion, depending on the condition of the patient, the amount of drug used, and its toxicity.

If the tumor to be treated is in the abdomen or lower pelvis, an abdominal operation may be required, and the entire procedure becomes much more difficult. The blood supply to the cancerous area is isolated and blocked from systemic circulation by means of pneumatic tourniquets and clamps to prevent distribution of the drug throughout the body. Catheters are inserted into the artery and vein supplying the area to be treated, and the agent is introduced through the arterial catheter as near to the tumor as possible. The venous catheter is attached to a pump oxygenator that provides for oxygenation of the blood and pumps it back into the arterial system through the arterial catheter. This procedure is essential for tissue viability (Fig. 25-10). When the treatment is complete and fresh blood has been supplied by transfusion if necessary, the vessels are unclamped, catheters and tourniquets are removed, and the surgical wound is closed.

Postoperative concerns are related to the local tissue

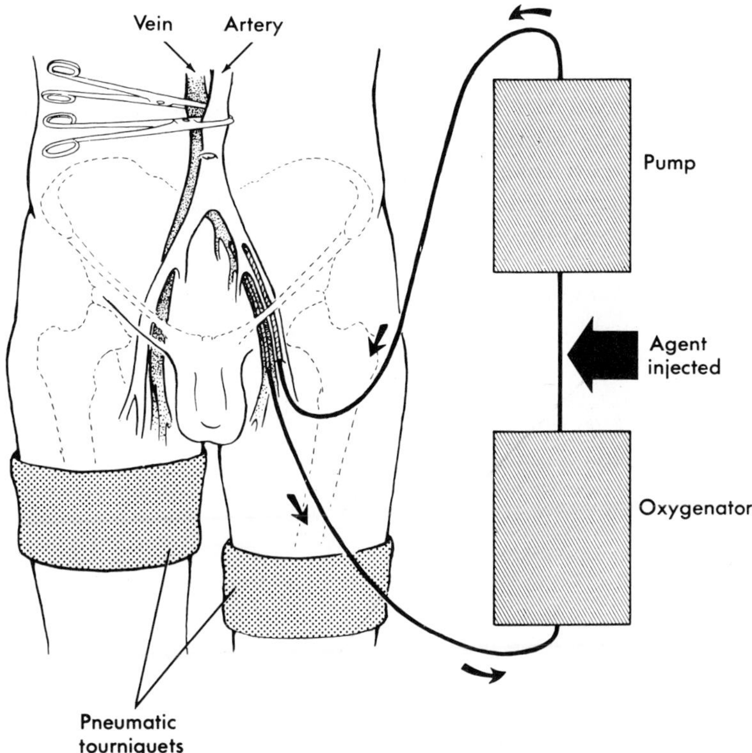

Fig. 25-10. Schema showing regional perfusion for pelvic tumor. (From Bouchard, R., and Owens, N. J.: Nursing care of the cancer patient, ed. 2, St. Louis, 1972, The C. V. Mosby Co.)

tolerance and the amount of leakage of the agent used. Local tissues can be permanently damaged, and thrombosis and phlebitis may occur at or near the site of treatment. Reactions of significance appear as tanning, erythema, or blistering of skin over tissues that have been perfused. These reaction resemble toxic reactions to radiation. The toxic effects of leakage may cause bone marrow depression, and infection such as septicemia can occur. The general signs of circulatory disturbance that sometimes occur after cardiac surgery should be watched for and reported promptly if they occur (p. 975). Renal function must be checked carefully. Following extracorporeal perfusion of an extremity, color and warmth of the extremity must be observed. Pain in the extremity is a danger signal and often indicates that there has been severe tissue damage.

The patient who undergoes perfusion procedures needs thoughtful care and encouragement. Usually his disease is advanced and the procedure is only palliative, although it is done only when there is reasonable assurance that metastasis has not spread throughout the body. Sometimes the patient develops lesions elsewhere after the perfusion seemed to control the growth satisfactorily.

Nursing intervention for patients receiving chemotherapy

The administration of chemotherapeutic drugs involves proper psychologic preparation of the patient and a frank discussion of their possible effects. Nursing intervention at this point must be supportive. There are times when the nurse may strongly disagree with such radical drug therapy, and such an attitude can be easily transmitted to the patient. Preparation of the patient for the administration of nitrogen mustard (Mustargen), for example, can greatly aid in its effectiveness or at least diminish some of its side effects.

If it appears that the toxic effects of these agents have been stressed rather than the therapeutic effects, it is only because the nurse must be concerned with creating an environment in which these agents can be safely used.

Cancer chemotherapy nursing is difficult and often discouraging; however, it is expected that chemotherapy for cancer will grow in importance and effectiveness as the result of continued research in this area.

Planning care. Before chemotherapy is initiated, careful planning of patient care is necessary. Data about the patient's food likes and dislikes, leisure activities that are satisfying, and the patient's attitude toward therapy help the nurse select appropriate interventions. The toxic effects of chemotherapy may affect the patient's ability to maintain fluid and electrolyte balance and meet nutritional needs. The bone marrow depression and subsequent leukopenia and thrombocytopenia require that the patient be protected from infection and trauma. Oral ulcerations may occur as a result of the effects on the mucous membrane, and effective methods of coping with the problems of oral hygiene need to be instituted (see Chapter 54). Caring for the patient receiving chemotherapy is a challenge to the nurse.

Maintaining fluid and electrolyte balance and nutritional needs. In order to maintain essential nutrition and fluid and electrolyte balance, several factors need to be considered, including preventing hemorrhage, decreasing nausea and vomiting, and promoting adequate nutrition. Each of these is discussed in detail.

Preventing hemorrhage. Both radiotherapy and chemotherapy may result in depression of bone marrow resulting in thrombocytopenia. Frequent blood counts may be ordered, since hemorrhage may be a fatal complication of treatment. Anemia may result from frank blood loss, from destruction of red blood cells, or from deficiencies of the precursors necessary for red blood cell production. Blood transfusions may be ordered, and if there is decreased prothrombin production vitamin K may be ordered.

To prevent hemorrhage the patient is instructed to avoid bumps, bruises, and falls. Injections may be prohibited, or if needed, small-gauge needles should be used and several minutes of pressure should be applied at the site of the injection. Soft-bristled toothbrushes should be used. The patient should be taught to avoid sneezing or blowing his nose forcefully. The patient and his family are taught to be alert for signs of bleeding in the skin, stool, urine, sputum, and nasal secretions. Women who still menstruate should report menorrhagia (excessive menstrual bleeding).

Treatment of hemorrhage for accessible sites includes application of pressure, packing, ice, and topical application of epinephrine (Adrenalin). Putting the patient at physical and emotional rest decreases blood pressure and enhances clot formation.[7,18]

Decreasing nausea and vomiting. Many chemotherapeutic drugs cause gastrointestinal tract toxicity with subsequent nausea and vomiting. This side effect of the drugs is usually not communicated to the patient *before* therapy, since the power of suggestion may produce the condition. Nitrogen mustard (Mustargen) is particularly irritating to the gastrointestinal tract. It is usually given in the evening, and supper is either omitted or is limited to fluids. Administration of an antiemetic drug and a sedative prior to the treatment may prevent nausea and vomiting. The dose is adjusted according to the patient's weight and also his previous experience, if any, with agents that depress bone marrow. Adequate fluid intake is felt by some to prevent hyperuricemia, thought to be a consequence of sudden cytolysis.[67] If hyperuricemia is considered to be a serious threat, allopurinol, a drug inhibiting uric acid formation, is given several days before chemotherapy is begun.

The nurse must be creative in identifying nursing measures to decrease the patient's discomfort. Treatment should not be given near mealtime. Placing the patient in a semi-Fowler's position rather than flat seems to be helpful.

Good mouth care after any emesis and use of sour balls and breath fresheners may all promote comfort. Emesis basins are emptied and removed immediately. The room should be free from any disagreeable sights and odors.

Nursing measures are used to decrease the patient's anxiety. Involvement in distracting activities may aid in lowering the patient's awareness of nausea. A careful record of intake and output must be kept, and the patient is observed for signs of dehydration if vomiting persists.

Promoting adequate nutrition. The effects of the illness and of chemotherapy may cause severe anorexia. Smaller quantities of foods that the patient likes and more frequent feedings may increase the patient's intake. It is important to maintain a positive nitrogen balance in the face of increased metabolic demands that cancer places on the body (see Chapter 23). The patient's diet should be high in protein foods (see Chapter 51).

Preventing infection. Large portions of functioning bone marrow may be depressed by many chemotherapeutic drugs, resulting in severe leukopenia and a depression of the body's immune defenses.[13,18] Frequent white blood cell counts may be ordered by the physician. If granulocytes are decreased radically, treatment may be stopped. The nurse should also be aware that the white blood cell level may drift down for days or weeks after treatment is stopped. In addition, since pus does not form in the absence of granulocytes, the patient may have a localized infection without abscess formation. This infection may not remain localized but develop into septicemia.[18] Fever may be the first clue that an infection is present.

Body areas with high potential for infection should be inspected daily. The skin and mucous membranes, especially the mouth, axillae, and perineal areas, are especially infection prone. Assessment of the respiratory tract is also important to identify early signs of respiratory infection. In preventing all types of infection, good medical asepsis and especially careful handwashing by the medical and nursing staff is important.

Maintaining intact skin and mucous membranes. Nursing intervention includes teaching the patient to avoid bumping and breaking the skin. Injections are usually avoided. Aseptic technique must be scrupulously maintained during intravenous infusions and dressing changes. It is important that the nurse keep fingernails short or small skin breaks may result while giving care.

Patients should be taught the proper method of wiping after a bowel movement to help prevent urinary tract or vaginal infections. Sexual counseling may be necessary. The importance of good perineal hygiene is stressed. Avoiding excessive friction and providing proper vaginal lubrication during sexual activity is emphasized.[18] Anal intercourse should be avoided, since the area is very prone to abscess formation if any breaks in the tissue occur. Enemas, rectal medications, and rectal temperatures are also contraindicated.[18]

The mouth is also very infection prone. Teeth and gums should be in good condition before therapy begins. Fastidious oral hygiene with use of a soft toothbrush is essential. Petroleum jelly or other lubricants can be used to prevent drying and cracking of the lips.

The patient's mouth is inspected daily for ulcers and white patches, which may indicate moniliasis. Nystatin (Mycostatin) mouthwash may be used, or Mycostatin tablets, usually used for intravaginal infections, may be sucked.[18] Antiseptic sprays, mouthwashes, and oral irrigations help keep the mouth clean. Irrigating devices such as a Water Pik may be recommended to maintain oral cleanliness.

Maintaining optimal respiratory function. Patients are susceptible to middle-ear infections, sinusitis, and pharyngitis. Pneumonia is especially prevalent in patients with leukemia and in elderly persons.[18] Families of patients are instructed not to visit if they have colds.

Use of patient isolation. Reverse isolation may be ordered, but it is not usually effective unless life islands or laminar air flow units are used. The life island consists of a special large plastic canopy placed around and over the patient's bed. All equipment is sterilized and the air is filtered to remove airborne bacteria. Objects are passed in and out through locks irradiated by ultraviolet light. Patient contact is through arm-length gloves built into the side of the canopy.[18]

Laminar air flow units are rooms that have a constant

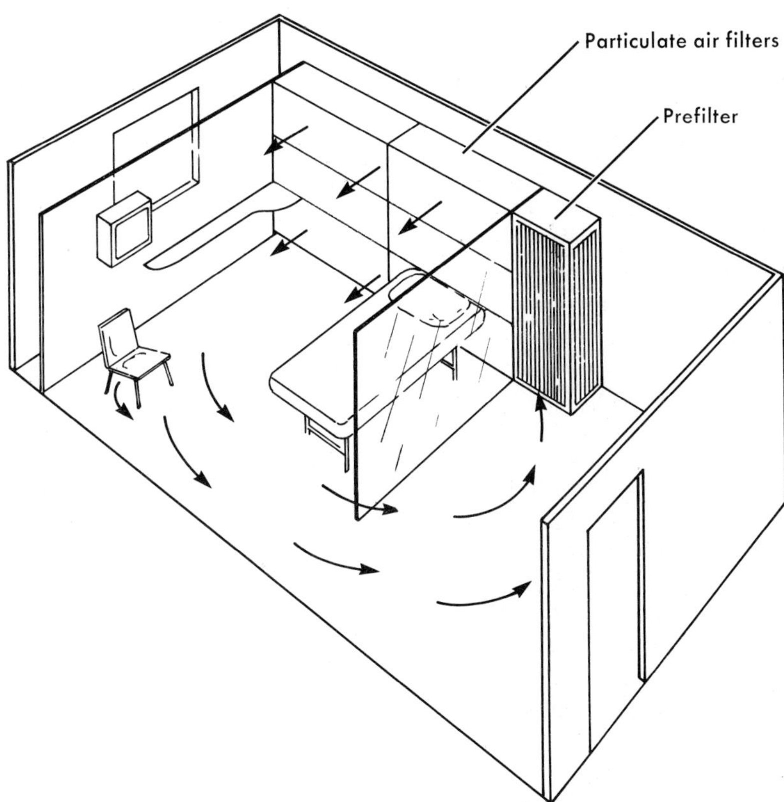

Fig. 25-11. In laminar air flow units constant flow of purified air flows across width and breadth of room. (From American Cancer Society, Proceedings of the National Conference on Cancer Nursing, 1973.)

flow of purified air flowing across the width and breadth of the room (Fig. 25-11). Anyone in the room remains downstream from the patient. If the patient must be touched a mask, cap, and gown is worn. The advantage of the laminar air flow room is that it is large and allows more freedom of movement than the life island.[18]

One danger of any type of isolation is that the patient may experience psychotic episodes because of sensory deprivation. In addition the patient may react adversely when allowed out of the unit. He may feel unsafe, vulnerable, and angry because he is removed from the protected environment.

Outcome criteria for patient receiving chemotherapy

1. The patient is free from infection on discharge from the hospital.
2. The patient or significant others can:
   a. State the name of the drug or drugs being given.
   b. State the times that each drug is to be taken.
   c. List the signs and symptoms of the side effects and complications of each drug.
   d. Describe whether the drug is to be taken before or after meals or with antacids, milk, and so forth.
   e. List the foods the patient should try to eat daily.
   f. State plans for ongoing care.

Effect of immunotherapy

The role of immunotherapy in the prevention and treatment of cancer is growing in importance. Many scientists believe cancer occurs in the body more frequently than once in a lifetime; however, in most cases clinical evidence of the disease is not apparent. It is postulated that there is a natural immunity against the development of the disease and that cancer cells are destroyed almost as fast as they develop.[65] Clinical malignancy may occur as a result of failure in the immunologic surveillance system of the body (see Chapter 14).

Studies of cancer in lower animals and in humans show that when the normal cell becomes malignant it often undergoes biochemical changes resulting in formation of new cellular antigens that cause an immune response.

This response has two major components. The first, or *cellular immune response,* produces lymphocytes capable of destroying tumor cells on contact. These lymphocytes (called T cells because they mature in the thymus gland, although they originate in the bone marrow) undergo division and are released into the bloodstream when stimulated by an antigen. In addition to destroying cancer cells on contact, T cells may release cytotoxins, which cause holes in the cell membrane, eventually resulting in lysis or death of the malignant cell.

Another important cell, which collaborates with the T cell, is the macrophage. The macrophage, which is attracted to the immune lymphocyte, is immobilized in its vicinity and then activated by the lymphocyte. It is a relatively nonspecific cell that seems to have the ability to kill selectively malignant cells with which it comes in contact.

The second component of the immune response is *antibody production* resulting from activation of lymphocytes, called B cells, which originate in and mature in the bone marrow. When stimulated by antigen, B cells proliferate and differentiate into plasma cells, which are the major source of antibody production.

The cells involved in the immune response interact and seem to exchange signals at both cellular and humoral levels.[46] Antigenic human tumors such as carcinomas of the skin, colon, lung, stomach, esophagus, breast, and thyroid and parathyroid glands have been identified. Some leukemias, sarcomas, and melanomas have been responsive to immunotherapy.

Approaches used in immunotherapy

There are three major approaches to immunotherapy. The first, *nonspecific immunotherapy,* uses substances such as BCG (bacille Calmette-Guérin) vaccine and *Corynebacterium parvum,* which appear to increase the general immune capacity of the patient. Experimentally these agents prevent tumor growth and halt the growth of small tumors. BCG vaccine has been used against acute leukemia, malignant malanoma, and soft-tissue sarcoma.

Specific immunotherapy, the second type of immunotherapy, uses substances that are antigenically related to the tumor or its products. These substances may be (1) killed tumor cells from the same patient or from another patient with an antigenically similar tumor, (2) tumor cells that have been altered in vitro, making them more immunogenic, and (3) antigen substance extracted from tumor cells.

The third type of immunotherapy is accomplished by *transfer of tumor immunity,* either by transfering lymphocytes from one tumor patient to another or more recently by transferring tumor immunity at the informational level. Two sources of informational molecules recovered from lymphoid cells are immune RNA and transfer factor. Their advantage is that, unlike intact lymphoid cells, they are nonimmunogenic and therefore do not produce a host immune response[46] (Fig. 25-12).

The ultimate goal of immunotherapy is to immunize the patient effectively against his own tumor. A perhaps more utopian goal is prophylactic immunization. When more is known about the cause of some tumors, use of attenuated virus or tumor antigen may be a real possibility.[45]

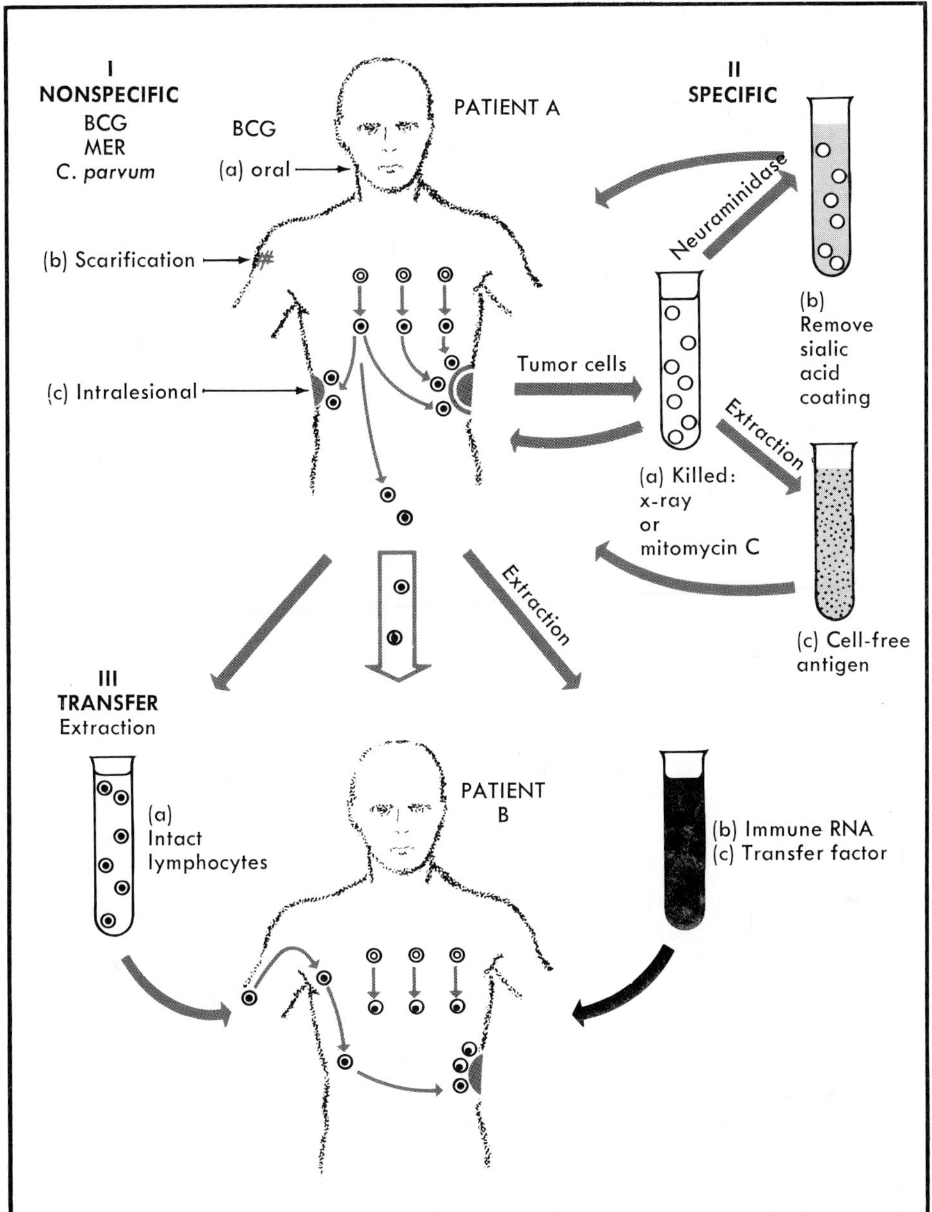

Fig. 25-12. Three major approaches to immunotherapy are active nonspecific immunization, active specific immunization, and transfer of immunity. In each case nonimmune lymphoid cells (◎) are converted to specifically or nonspecifically sensitized cells (◉), which are then capable of attacking tumor. Specific immunotherapy requires inactivating or killing tumor cells and then returning killed cells to host in multiple injections. Cells may be altered with such materials as neuraminidase, which removes surface coating of sialic acid, thus increasing immunogenicity, or cell-free antigen extracts made from tumor cells. Nonspecific and specific immunization are carried out in original tumor-bearing individual, while transfer of immunity delivers specific immune capacity to another individual with similar tumor by intact lymphoid cells or with extracts of immune RNA or transfer factor made from such cells. (From McKhann, C. F., and Yarlott, M. A.: CA **25**:196, 1975.)

At the present time the immune response can handle only a limited number of tumor cells, up to 10 million. After a growth to 100 million cells the immune response is not capable of preventing further growth. Once the cancer is large, it cannot be totally controlled by the immune system, so immunotherapy cannot be the primary mode of cancer therapy at the present time. It is used after surgery, radiotherapy, and chemotherapy have removed the bulk of the tumor.[65]

Complications of immunotherapy

Some complications of immunotherapy may occur. Intratumor injection of BCG vaccine has resulted in fever, chills, localized abscesses, and draining sinuses. Regional lymphadenitis, systemic infections, anaphylactic reactions, malaise, and influenzalike reactions may also occur. Fewer problems (mild fever, malaise) have arisen with the intradermal multiple-tine technique of administration. There has been some evidence of liver dysfunction, although the incidence is low.[50] Immunotherapy holds promise for the future prevention as well as treatment of cancers.

□ Supportive care of the patient with advanced cancer

Planning care

When all possible surgery and maximum radiation therapy have failed to control the spread of cancer, the patient and his family have many special problems. They need encouragement and help in living as normally as possible, in planning for the late stages of the patient's illness, and in adjusting to death and its implications for the family.

Before nurses can help the patient and his family, they must have developed a mature philosophy that allows acceptance of death as an eventual reality for everyone. This philosophy is not acquired overnight. The nurse needs the opportunity to discuss feelings about caring for the patient whose death is imminent, since the nurse's attitude toward death and suffering will affect the ability to plan and give care to the patient with advanced cancer. (See Chapter 19 for discussion of death and dying.)

No one can say with certainty when death will come. The patient may ask about the length of time he is expected to live, but no absolute answer can be given. Physicians may have made a statement to the patient about his life expectancy. The nursing staff should know what the patient has been told, since the patient's willingness to participate in his care and his attitude toward his illness may be influenced by his perception of his life expectency.

It is important not to "give up" on a patient or to abandon him.[23,32] Planning, doing, and achieving is the best way to prevent the hopelessness and despair that may overwhelm the patient. Every effort must be put forth to meet the patient's physiologic needs so that higher order psychologic needs may be expressed. The patient who is in pain or feels "dirty" will have difficulty making known his concerns and his fears.

Other factors to consider in planning care are the personality of the patient, his feelings about death and illness, and the reactions of those significant others whose opinion the patient values.[18] The goal of nursing care should be to relieve physical, mental, and spiritual distress.

Planning for home care

At least half of all deaths from cancer occur in the patients' homes. Planning for home care of the patient without completely disrupting the rest of the family takes the concerted efforts of many people. The patient must always be consulted, and his wishes should be respected in the early stages of the disease. In the final stages he may be too ill to be bothered or concerned with making decisions. The physician, the social worker, and the nurse must work together with the local community nursing agencies, such as the American Cancer Society, to ensure continuity of care from the hospital to the home. The principles governing suitability for home care are similar to those for any patient receiving home care, although the patient with cancer may not live as long as many others with chronic long-term illnesses. The patient must be under medical supervision, it must be possible to give the care he needs in his home, he must want to be home, his family must want him home and be able to assist with care, and the home facilities must be suitable (p. 532). Rehabilitation teams may also be sent into the home to help the patient and his family.

The concept of the hospice, a place where patients may come for short or long periods for nursing care and then return to their homes as their condition warrants is exciting. The hospice tries to maintain a homelike setting while relieving the family of the emotional and physical burden of constant care.[25]

Nursing interventions to meet the psychologic needs of patients with advanced stages of cancer

Avoiding false hope. Very occasionally there is a mistake in diagnosis or the disease is in some way arrested for a long time. If the patient assumes that one of these occurrences may take place in his case, the nurse should not try to help him face probable reality. The nurse must, however, avoid encouraging false hopes. Many patients accept their prognosis philosophically, with the hope that a cure for cancer will be found before their disease is far advanced. Some patients are better able to accept the situation if their religious faith can be strengthened. Some patients and their families find it helpful to live each day as fully as possible without looking too far ahead. Sometimes patients with cancer have few symptoms and are able to carry on quite well until shortly before death.

Encouraging social and vocational activities. Patients with advanced cancer should resume their regular work if they can possibly do so, for work makes them feel as though they are still an active part of their group and worthy of the approval of others. It was said many centuries ago that employment is man's best physician, and this concept applies particularly to persons whose existence is seriously threatened by cancer. Social activities and all experiences associated with normal family life should be continued whenever possible. There is probably no greater service the nurse can give to the patient with uncontrollable cancer than to help him to continue in any way possible. Family members often need guidance in seeing the patient's need to live as normally as possible. Sometimes the patient appears almost unduly concerned with the details of some aspect of his immediate treatment and almost oblivious to his entire problem. Such a patient senses that success with the immediate treatment is his only way to remain up and about or to carry on as well as he is at that time.

Giving realistic reassurance about pain control. The patient with advanced cancer often worries about whether he will have severe pain and whether such pain can be alleviated. He should know that medical science now has several ways of controlling pain. Hormones, radiation therapy, and a number of analgesic drugs are available and helpful in most instances. Synthetic substitutes for the opiate drugs make it possible to alternate drugs so that their benefit is not lessened by tolerance and so that toxic reactions can be avoided. The patient and family are sometimes told of operations that can be performed if pain becomes too severe to control by other means (see Chapter 22).

Decreasing fear of helplessness. The patient may be haunted by fear of brain involvement, loss of mental faculties, and the possibility that he may become completely helpless and dependent on others.[18] By these fears he expresses a basic human wish: the wish to leave the world with as much dignity as possible. The nurse should urge the patient and his family to discuss such fears with the physician. The patient may feel that the physician is too busy and that his questions are too trivial to justify the use of the physician's time. Some questions, however, are not trivial at all, and a satisfactory answer to them adds tremendously to the patient's peace of mind. Metastasis to the brain in persons who have other metastases is somewhat rare, and some patients suffer more from fear of damage to the brain than is justified. The patient should know that good general hygiene, good nutrition, being up and about for part of each day, and doing deep-breathing exercises with attention to posture all help to prevent helplessness. A positive approach to all problems certainly shortens the time of helplessness and makes the patient more content.

Nursing interventions to meet physiologic needs of patients with advanced stages of cancer

Increasing comfort. Giving good nursing care to the patient with advanced cancer is challenging. Promoting the patient's comfort should be high on the list of goals. Nursing measures that increase rest and sleep and reduce pain will help maintain the patient's physical and psychologic well-being.

Maintaining nutrition. Cachexia is a frequent problem. Anorexia may accompany therapy, and the increased protein needs of the body resulting from tumor growth may be difficult to meet. Mealtimes should be incorporated with family visiting, or patients can eat together if possible.

Maintaining elimination. Diarrhea may be a problem, but constipation is more likely. If the patient is receiving narcotics, especially opium derivatives, peristalsis is decreased. Patients receiving the plant alkaloid vincristine (Oncovin) may develop neurotoxicity, causing a high fecal impaction.[18] Increasing the intake of roughage and fluids in the diet, maintaining activity, and using stool softeners may be helpful. Enemas and laxatives may be necessary.

Maintaining personal hygiene. Careful and meticulous hygiene is essential. Careful bathing and attention to skin, hair, and clothing will all promote self-esteem in the patient. Odors from body exudates, draining wounds, and incontinence may occur. Soiled dressings and bed linen are changed immediately. Judicious use of deodorizers is helpful, but deodorizers do not take the place of good hygiene.

Preventing the effects of immobility. Pressure sores may be a severe problem. The combination of inactivity, poor nutrition, and incontinence seen in patients with advanced cancer predisposes to skin breakdown. Maintaining the patient's activity by getting him out of bed as much as possible will prevent pressure and also promote the patient's joint mobility and muscle strength.

Teaching the patient and family. The nurse is involved in teaching during most interactions with the patient and his family.[54] Careful explanations about care and sensitivity to what the patient thinks and feels about his disease contribute to the nurse's effectiveness in promoting change in the patient's behavior. When possible, self-care activities should be emphasized. Maintaining the patient's independence whenever possible should be the goal while recognizing that the time may come when dependence is necessary.

Outcome criteria for the patient with advanced cancer

The following patient outcomes occur to the extent that is physically and emotionally possible:

1. The patient makes his own decisions as long as he cares to do so.
2. Skin does not break down.
3. Pain is minimized.
4. Hope is maintained.

REFERENCES AND SELECTED READINGS

1. American Cancer Society: 1977 Cancer facts and figures, New York, 1976, The Society.
2. American Cancer Society: A cancer source book for nurses, New York, 1975, The Society.
3. Augenstein, D.: Hyperbaric oxygen radiation therapy, Nurs. Forum **12:**324-335, 1968.
4. Ayers, R., Baker, V., and Padilla, G.: Research in cancer nursing. In Proceedings of the National Conference in Cancer Nursing, American Cancer Society, New York, 1974.
5. *Boeker, E. H., editor: Symposium on radiation uses and hazards, Nurs. Clin. North Am. **2:**1-113, 1967.
6. *Boeker, E. H.: Radiation safety, Am. J. Nurs. **65:**111-116, 1965.
7. Bouchard, R. E., and Owens, N. F.: Nursing care of the cancer patient, ed. 3, St. Louis, 1976, The C. V. Mosby Co.
8. Burt, A. L.: The role of the public health nurse in the care of the cancer patient, Nurs. Clin. North Am. **2:**683-689, 1967.
9. Cancer Statistics, 1976, CA **26:**14-23, 1976.
10. Carter, S. K., and Kershner, L. M.: Cancer chemotherapy: what drugs are available, Resident and Staff Physician **22:**56-65, 1976.
11. Cline, M. J.: Cancer chemotherapy, ed. 2, Philadelphia, 1975, W. B. Saunders Co.
12. Cobb, A. B.: Medical and psychological problems in the rehabilitation of the cancer patient. In Hardy, R. E., and Cull, J. G.: Counseling and rehabilitating the cancer patient, Springfield, Ill., 1975, Charles C Thomas, Publisher.
13. Committee on Professional Education of International Union Against Cancer, editors: Clinical oncology: a manual for students and doctors, New York, 1973, Springer-Verlag Co.
14. Croll, M. N., and Brady, L. W., editors: Recent advances in nuclear medicine, New York, 1966, Appleton-Century-Crofts.
15. Daniels, F. J.: Sunlight. In Schottenfeld, D.: Cancer epidemiology and prevention, Springfield, Ill., 1975, Charles C Thomas, Publisher.
16. Davis, M. Z.: Patients in limbo, Am. J. Nurs. **66:**746-748, 1966.
17. *Donaldson, S. H., Fletcher, W. S., and Nowak, P. A.: The treatment of cancer by isolation perfusion and nursing care in isolation perfusion, Am. J. Nurs. **64:**81-88, 1964.
18. Donovan, M. I., and Pierce, S. G.: Cancer care nursing, New York, 1976, Appleton-Century-Crofts.
19. *Downs, H. S.: The control of vomiting, Am. J. Nurs. **66:**76-82, 1966.
20. Egan, R. L.: Mammography, Am. J. Nurs. **66:**108-111, 1966.
21. Fitzpatrick, G. M., and Shorkin, J. M.: Pelvic perfusion, Am. J. Nurs. **61:**79-81, 1961.
22. Francis, G. M.: Cancer: the emotional component, Am. J. Nurs. **69:**1677-1681, 1969.
23. Freihofer, P., and Felton, G.: Nursing behaviors in bereavement, Nurs. Res. **25:**332-337, 1976.
24. Cahart, B. L.: Intravenous medications: a handbook for nurses and other allied health personnel, ed. 2, St. Louis, 1977, The C. V. Mosby Co.
25. Galton, V.: Cancer nursing at St. Christopher's Hospice. In Proceedings of the National Conference on Cancer Nursing, American Cancer Soceity, 1974.
26. George, M. M.: Long-term care of the patient with cancer, Nurs. Clin. North Am. **8:**623-631, 1973.
27. *Greenwald, E. S.: Cancer chemotherapy, ed. 2, Flushing, N.Y., 1973, Medical Examination Publishing Co., Inc.
28. Greenwald, E. S.: Cancer chemotherapy, N.Y. State J. Med. **72:**2541-2556, 1972.
29. Helping cancer patients effectively, Horsham, Pa., 1977, Nursing '77 Books.
30. Hensinkveld, K.: Cues to the communication with the terminal cancer patient, Nurs. Forum **11:**105-113, 1972.
31. Higginson, J., Terracini, B., and Agthe, C. Nutrition and cancer: ingestion of foodborne carcinogens. In Schottenfeld, D.: Cancer epidemiology and prevention, Springfield, Ill., 1975, Charles C Thomas Publisher.
32. Hoffman, E.: "Don't give up on me!" Am. J. Nurs. **71:**60-62, 1971.
33. Hughes, J., and Ryser, P.: Chemical carcinogenesis, CA **24:**351-360, 1974.
34. Isler, C.: Cancer quackery, RN **37:**55-59, 1974.
35. Isler, C.: The cancer nurses: how the specialists are doing it RN **35:**28-34, 1972.
36. *Kautz, H. D., Storey, R. H., and Zimmerman, A. J.: Radioactive drugs, Am. J. Nurs. **64:**124-128, 1964.
37. *Kegeles, S. S., Kirscht, J. P., Haefner, D. P., et al.: Survey of beliefs about cancer detection and taking Papanicolaou tests, Public Health Rep. **80:**815-823,1965.
38. Klagsbrun, N. C.: Communications in the treatment of cancer, Am. J. Nurs. **71:**944-948, 1971.
39. Knudson, A. G.: Genetic differences in human tumors. In Becker, F. F.: Cancer: a comprehensive treatise, New York, 1975, Plenum Press.
40. *Koons, S. B.: The future of cancer nursing, RN **39:**23, 1976.
41. *Kyle, Sister M. Willa: The nurse's approach to the patient attempting to adjust to inoperable cancer: effective therapeutic communication in nursing, Clinical Session 8, 1964, American Nurses' Association.
42. *Lieben, J.: The effects of radiation, Nurs. Outlook **10:**336-338, 1962.
43. *Livingston, B. M.: How clinical progress is made in cancer chemotherapy research, Am. J. Nurs. **67:**2547-2554, 1967.
44. Marino, E. B., and LeBlanc, D.: Cancer chemotherapy, Nursing '75 **5:**22-32, Nov. 1975.
45. McKhann, C. F.: Immunotherapy of cancer. In Gottlieg, A. A., Plescia, P. J., and Bishop, D. H.: Fundamental aspects of neoplasia, New York, 1975, Springer-Verlag Publishing Co.
46. McKhann, C. F., and Yarlott, M. A.: Tumor immunology, CA **25:**187-197, 1975.
47. Modell, W., editor: Drugs of choice 1978-1979, St. Louis, 1978, The C. V. Mosby Co.
48. Molbo, D. M.: The nurse's role in hyperbaric therapy. In Bergersen, B. S., et al., editors: Current concepts in clinical nursing, vol. 1, St. Louis, 1967, The C. V. Mosby Co.
49. Molbo, D. M., and von Elk, J.: Hyperbaric oxygenation. In Meltzer, L. E., Abdellah, F. G., and Kitchell, J. R., editors: Concepts and practices of intensive care, Philadelphia, 1969, The Charles Press, Publishers.
50. Morton, D. L., and Golub, S. H., Sulit, H. L., Gupto, R. K.,

*References preceded by an asterisk are particularly well suited for student reading.

Elber, F. R., Holmes, E. C., and Sparks, F. C.: Response to active immunotherapy of malignant melanomas. In Gottlieb, A. A., Plescia, O. J., and Bishop, D. H.: Fundamental aspects of neoplasia, New York, 1975, Springer-Verlag Publishing Co.

51. Newell, G. R.: Prologue: the national cancer plan and its relationship to basic research. In Gottlieb, A. A., Plescia, O. J., and Bishop, D. H.: Fundamental aspects of neoplasia, New York, 1975, Springer-Verlag Publishing Co.
52. Niles, A. G., and Paulen, A. E.: A humanistic approach to nursing care, Supervisor Nurse **4**:42-44, 1973.
53. Oken, D.: What to tell cancer patients: a study of medical attitudes, J.A.M.A. **175**:1120-1128, 1961.
54. Paulen, A. E.: Patient and family teaching in the hospital. In Proceedings of the National Conference on Cancer Nursing, American Cancer Society, 1974.
55. Prosnitz, L. R.: Radiation therapy: treatment for malignant disease, RN **34**:42-47, 1971.
56. *Quimby, E. H.: Safe handling of radioactive isotopes in medical practice, New York, 1960, Macmillan, Inc.
57. *Rhoads, P. S.: Management of the patient with terminal illness, J.A.M.A. **192**:661-665, 1965.
58. Rodman, M. J., and Smith, D. W.: Clinical pharmacology in nursing, Philadelphia, 1974, J. B. Lippincott Co.
59. *Rumerfield, P. S., and Rumerfield, M. J.: What you should know about radiation hazards, Am. J. Nurs. **70**:780-786, 1970.
60. Ryser, H. J.: Special report: chemical carcinogenesis, CA **24**:351-360, 1974.
61. Sackett, D.: Periodic examination of patients at rest. In Schottenfeld, D.: Cancer epidemiology and prevention, Springfield, Ill., 1975, Charles C Thomas, Publisher.
62. Shepardson, J.: Team approach to the patient with cancer, Am. J. Nurs. **72**:488-491, 1972.
63. Shills, M. E.: Nutrition and cancer: dietary deficiency and modifications. In Schottenfeld, D.: Cancer epidemiology and prevention, Springfield, Ill., 1975, Charles C Thomas, Publisher.
64. Shinkin, M. B.: Reporting on cancer research, CA **25**:105-106, 1975.
65. Silverstein, M. J., and Morton, D. L.: Cancer immunotherapy, Am. J. Nurs. **73**:1178-1181, 1973.
66. Teitelbaum, A. C.: Intra-arterial drug therapy, Am. J. Nurs. **72**:1634-1637, 1972.
67. Ultmann, J.: Chemotherapy of lymphoma, Semin. Hematol. **3**:131-153, 1966.
68. Unproven methods of cancer management: cancer quackery, CA **25**:66-71, 1975.
69. U.S. Department of Health, Education and Welfare: The cancer centers program, Division of Cancer Research Resources and Centers, National Cancer Institute, November 1973.
70. *Vernick, J., and Lunceford, J. L.: Milieu design for adolescents with leukemia, Am. J. Nurs. **67**:559-561, 1967.
71. Warren, W.: Ionizing radiation and medicine, Sci. Am. **201**:154-176, 1959. (Entire issue devoted to radiation, including articles on what it is, its circulation in the body, and how it affects the cell, evolution, and the whole animal.)
72. *Welsh, M. S.: Comfort measures during radiation therapy, Am. J. Nurs. **67**:1880-1881, 1967.
73. Winters, W. D., and Morton, D. L.: Immunobiology. In Schottenfeld, D.: Cancer epidemology and prevention, Springfield, Ill., 1975, Charles C Thomas, Publisher.
74. Wintrobe, M. M., et al.: Harrison's textbook of medicine, ed. 8, New York, 1977, McGraw-Hill Book Co.
75. Wynder, E. L., and Mabuch, K.: Tobacco and cancer epidemiology and prevention. In Schottenfeld, D.: Cancer epidemiology and prevention, Springfield, Ill., 1975, Charles C Thomas, Publisher.
76. *Zaino, C.: Eliminating the hazards from radiation, Am. J. Nurs. **62**:60-61, 1962.
77. Zubrod, C. G.: The basis for progress in chemotherapy, Cancer **30**:1474-1479, 1972.

AUDIOVISUAL RESOURCES

1. Audiotape: Highlights of the National Conference on Cancer Nursing, Chicago, 1973, American Cancer Society, 2 cassette-audiotapes.
2. Cancer: Series 1 (kit), Concept Media, 1971, Costa Mesa, Calif.
   1. The malignant cell: physiology of disordered function.
   2. The malignant cell: etiology of disordered function.
   3. The malignant neoplasm: growth, invision metastasis.
   4. The malignant neoplasm: interactions with the host.
   5. Diagnostic procedures.
3. Cancer: Series 2: Focusing of feelings, Concept Media, 1971, Costa Mesa, Calif.
   4 filmstrips, 4 cassettes.
   1 and 2. Viewpoint: the nurse.
   3 and 4. Viewpoint: the cancer patient.

26

Sensory overload and sensory deprivation

MARIANN LAVACCA

Individuals as open systems are continuously interacting with the environment. Their boundaries, as unique systems, have been developmentally defined through their sensory apparatus. It is through their senses that individuals learn to differentiate themselves as separate entities.

Infants initially respond to the environment almost exclusively through their skin, as the first nerve endings to be myelinated are those of touch, temperature, and pain.[8] Eventually, as the sensory apparatus develops and refines, children perceive their boundaries as separate from the environment and learn to use their senses to expand their knowledge of the world. It is this very process of receiving and responding to environmental cues that an individual uses throughout the life cycle to form the basis for adaptive responses.

Since our sensations are such an integral part of our ability to perceive and interact with our environment, it follows that any alteration of this process will result in system disequilibrium. As open systems, individuals constantly receive inputs or cues from the environment. If these inputs were suddenly altered, either diminished or overloaded in some way, the normal method of receiving environmental cues would be affected, and the individual would have to adapt to this sudden change. As anyone knows who has played childhood games involving patching of the eyes, the immediate response on the part of the patched individual is to place his arms in a frontal position to obtain from the environment through touch those cues no longer available through vision. This illustrates one way in which the organism adapts to a loss of sensation from one modality by obtaining data through another modality.

Clients in health care settings may also experience system disequilibrium. The mechanized hospital environment may result in altered sensory input and may be compounded further by the physiologic alterations of illness, which add further stress to the client system.

The purpose of this chapter is to explore sensory alteration and its resultant disequilibrium for both theoretical and clinical perspectives.

Interest in the area of sensory alteration began in the 1950s. Early experiments manipulated the environment in an attempt to seek some answers to the phenomena of brainwashing and the effects of monotony on an individual's performance.[32] The findings indicated that by manipulating the amount of sensory-perceptual inputs, behavioral changes could be elicited from experimental subjects. When exposed to sensory and perceptual deprivation, subjects experienced hallucinations, difficulty in cognitive tasks, disorientation, anxiety, and somatic complaints.

Since these first studies, interest in sensory deprivation has grown considerably. Nurses have also evidenced particular interest in what happens to clients experiencing sensory deprivation and, to some extent, sensory overload. Although the nursing profession requires additional rigorous clinical research to substantiate some of the nursing interventions proposed for clients with a sensory alteration, it is useful to consider a model of sensory overload and underload for intervening with clients whose behavior often seems confusing and perplexing to the nurse. In viewing this model of sensory overload and underload from a systems perspective, it enables the nurse to use a systematic approach for processing inputs that could be possible system stressors and to intervene to assist the client in making adaptive responses.

■ SENSORY PROCESS

□ Sensory perception

Humans orient themselves to their environment through their ability to receive and organize sensory stimuli. This *reception* and *organization of stimuli* is collectively known as *sensory perception.* The process of sensory perception is dependent upon several factors: a stimulus, adequate sensory receptors, intact neural pathways, and adequate processing by the brain to interpret the stimulus input.

A stimulus is received by a sensory receptor which then synapses with a cranial, peripheral, or autonomic nerve. The nerve then either synapses with sensory nerve tracts in the spinal cord or with areas of the brain. The exact mechanism by which the brain interprets sensory input is not known, but there is evidence that the *reticular activating system (RAS)* plays an integral role in processing sensory input. The RAS is composed of a network of neurons, called the reticular formation, which forms a central core extending from the medulla of the lower brain to the thalamus in the diencephalon.[31] The RAS can be stimulated by two major sources: cortical impulses and sensory stimulation from visual, auditory, olfactory, somatic, and visceral sources.[31] It controls general central nervous system activity and selectivity of attention (arousal) to the environment. It serves a monitoring function for both inputs and outputs to the human system.

It is believed that the RAS in conjunction with the thalamus and hypothalamus collects and combines sensory input. *Perception* takes place when the sensory input is received, decoded (synthesized), and interpreted by the cortex. When interpretation occurs, a conscious awareness of sensation begins. Perception provides the individual with an awareness of reality, which then serves as a basis for determining if an adaptive or maintenance action is required. To clarify this further, consider the following example: if the cortex interprets an auditory stimulus to be loud, unpleasant, and painful, the individual becomes consciously aware of his discomfort and may adapt be covering his ears or moving to a quieter environment. If the cortex interprets an auditory stimulus to be pleasant, the client becomes consciously aware of this sensation and may utilize a maintenance action of remaining stationary in the pleasant environment.

It is important to note that without the function of the ascending reticular activating system, perception does not occur. Lindsley[23] gives the example of an individual who is under barbiturate anesthesia: the sensory pathways can conduct their messages to the primary receiving areas, but discrimination and perception do not occur. Thus it is seen that the RAS not only plays an important role in providing a mechanism for general arousal and alerting of the individual, but it must also be stimulated for perception to take place.

If sensory inputs are adequate, the RAS is stimulated and an alert aroused state is created in the individual—a state that allows perception and adaptive responses to occur. If there is inadequate stimulation of the RAS, disorientation, confusion, boredom, drowsiness, and sleep may occur (Fig. 26-1).

In viewing the sensory process from a systems perspective, the input would be the stimulus; the sensory receptors, neural pathways, and cerebral decoding necessary for processing (the RAS) would be throughput; and the resulting adaptive response or behavior of the individual would be output (Fig. 26-2).

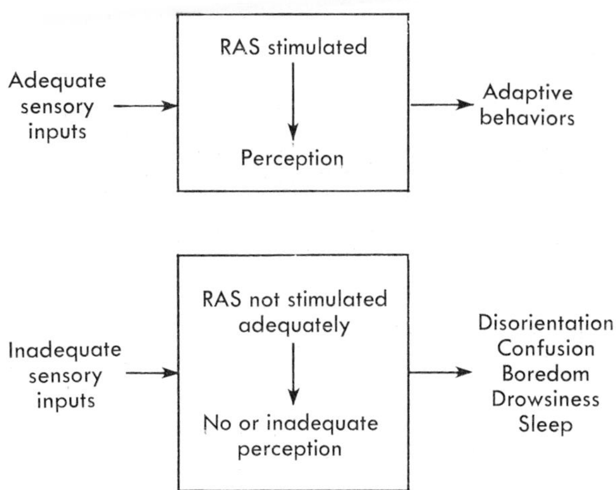

Fig. 26-1. Relationship between sensory inputs, arousal, and outcome.

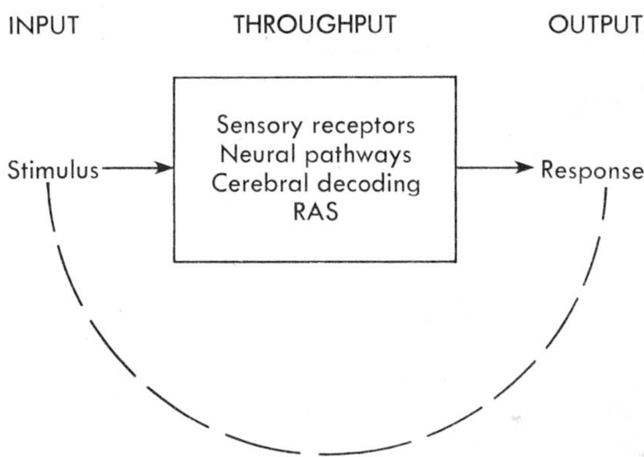

Fig. 26-2. Sensory process from a systems perspective.

□ Sensory apparatus and modalities

The sensory apparatus provides stimulus inputs into the system; the eyes, ears, nose, skin, tongue, muscles, and visceral organs all provide information relevant to system functioning. It is not hard to imagine what would happen if one of the sense organs was no longer providing cues about the environment. It is easy to see, then, the relevance of this function to everyday life situations.

Sensory *modalities* can be broadly classified as either originating internally or externally (Table 26-1). The internal souces of stimuli are *kinesthetic*, such as those arising from muscles and specialized neural tissue, or

Table 26-1. Sources of sensory inputs, modalities, and their functions

Source and function of stimulus inputs	Sense organs	Modality
Internal: provide internal environmental cues	Muscle and specialized neural tissue	Kinesthetic
	Hollow organs	Visceral
External: provide external environmental cues	Eyes	Visual
	Ear	Auditory
	Nose	Olfactory
	Skin	Tactile
Internal and external: provide internal and external environmental cues	Tongue	Gustatory

visceral, originating from hollow organs. These internal sensations provide information about our placement and position in space, that is, where parts of the body are in relation relation to one another. These internal sensations are primarily involved with the sensations of pain and with the regulatory mechanisms of the internal environment of the body.

The external sources of stimulation arise from the eyes, ears, nose, and skin, while the tongue provides both internal and external inputs of stimulation.

It is important to emphasize that sensation has both internal and external components, as both sources contribute to the overall sensory information processed by the brain. An alteration in the amount of stimulation received from either an internal or external source will affect the amount of sensory input to the brain and may necessitate an adaptive response. The importance of this will be more evident in the discussion of the clinical applications of sensory alteration.

□ Sensoristasis

Schultz[31] has defined *sensoristasis* as a drive state of cortical arousal that propels the awake individual to seek an optimal level of sensory variation. In other words, each individual has a drive or need for a constant range of varied sensory input. This varied input is required for the organism to function optimally. Schultz[31] compares sensoristasis as being similar to the homeostasis concept of Cannon[4]—a dynamic changing condition that adapts to subject and task variables, but which also has a relatively constant pattern. The RAS appears to play a monitoring function by its mediation of system inputs and outputs in maintaining the sensoristatic equilibrium. This equilibrium, however, can be disturbed under conditions of sensory restriction or overload, and the organism must then use adaptive behaviors to restore the balance. For example, if sensory stimulation is below the optimal level, the organism will adapt to seek alternative stimuli or become more sensitized to existing stimuli. If stimulation is greater than the optimal level, the organism will adapt by attempting to decrease system inputs.

Schultz[31] lists four major corollaries of his sensoristatic model:

1. The drive or need mechanism implemented in the sensoristasic concept is equivalent with arousal as mediated by the RAS.
2. An optimal range of external stimulation exists that influences cortical arousal. Only when this optimal level is maintained can the organism function adaptively with its environment. If there is alteration of stimulation, there is a disruption of learned responses and prevention of new learning.
3. An organism behaves in a way that will maintain this optimal arousal level.
4. The optimal range of sensory stimulation can alter depending upon several factors: the task to be performed, the present status of the organism, and the preceding level of stimulation. Also, there may be individual differences in need for sensory inputs and differences also over time within the same individual.

There seems to be general agreement that there is an optimal level of arousal required to maintain perceptual and adaptive functions; however, it is still unclear what the exact limits of normal sensory stimulation are. What is considered optimal seems to vary widely among individual subjects.

■ DEPRIVATION AND OVERLOAD

□ Definitions

The term sensory deprivation has been used synonymously in the literature with many different terms, ranging from social deprivation to restricted stimulation and solitude. For the purposes of this discussion, *sensory deprivation* is defined as a state of being in which the amount or intensity of sensory inputs is below the individual's range of tolerance. Tolerance is the unique range each person has for tolerating every type of sensation and enables them to function well and comfortably. The state of being in which the sensory inputs exceed the optimal range of tolerance is termed *overload.*

Deprivation refers to the general concept of decreasing sensory inputs, but in the specific case of a reduction in the pattern of meaningfulness of stimuli, the term

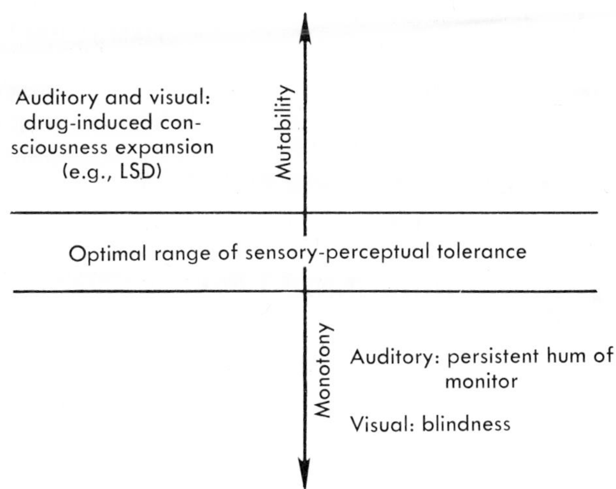

Fig. 26-3. Sensory-perceptual deprivation. Change in patterning of sensory input may create mutability or monotony.

perceptual deprivation is employed. This occurred in experimental studies when subjects wore translucent goggles or translucent halved Ping-Pong balls as eye shields to produce diffused, unpatterned light. The subject saw light, but the form and pattern did not alter. Another example is the consistent hum of a monitor in the ICU. The state of being in which the patterning of sensory input is below the individual's optimal range of tolerance is defined as *monotony;* that which is above the optimal range is termed *mutability* (Fig. 26-3). It should be emphasized that both sensory and perceptual deprivation refer to a reduction of stimulation from a previous condition and not the total absence of all stimulation, which is logistically impossible.

□ Effect of early alteration on growth and development

Deprivation or overload of system inputs will affect an individual's capacity for adaptive responses. Experimental literature indicates that there are effects on adult behavior from alteration of sensory stimulation early in life.[27,36] The normal growth and maintenance of neural structures is dependent upon adequate stimulation at an early level of development.[27,30] Experimental work with cats, monkeys, and chimpanzees demonstrated that organisms reared in restricted sensory environments show perceptual visual deficits, which may never be eliminated.[27] The primates also reacted violently to a marked increase in stimulation. From these studies it appears that the adaptive capacity of an organism is severly limited, if not totally absent, when there is early sensory deprivation.

Studies of institutionalized children reveal that early childhood deprivation results in behavioral changes and developmental problems. When children who spent their first 3 years in an institution before being placed in a foster home were compared with children raised continuously in a foster home, the children who were institutionalized experienced less intellectual and emotional capacity.[13] The institutionalized children demonstrated aimlessness, poor concentration, poor impulse control, and a decreased capacity for abstract thinking as compared with the control group. Thus it is evident that a decrease in critical inputs from a consistent source, such as a mother, adversely influenced the emotional and intellectual development of these children.

Another study compared the developmental patterns of institutionalized children with children raised in their own homes for the first year of life. Children were observed in two different institutions. The first was a foundling home where children had only minimal brief contacts with a nurse. The other institution was a nursery located in a penal institution for delinquent girls, where the children had consistent, frequent contacts with their own mothers.[33] The children raised in a foundling home began at a normal developmental level, but did not maintain it, and eventually fell behind the other children in social, perceptual, and motor development. Both of these studies indicate the critical nature of early sensory inputs from a consistent source and the importance of perceptual and social stimulation to normal human development.

Another study investigated the effects of increased sensory input on infants. It found that infants who had experienced increased handling and exposure to objects within their visual field demonstrated "visually directed reaching" and "visual attentiveness" earlier than infants who had not been exposed to such stimuli.[38,39]

It has been suggested that early levels of stimulation influence the optimal level of sensory variation in the adult. The child's level of stimulus variation will influence the arousal of the RAS for adaptive behavior as an adult. Thus adaptation levels may be determined by the amount and variety of early sensory input. This may explain individual differences in the optimal level of stimulation within which the organism can function effectively.[31]

The fact that early sensory input is critical to the normal growth and development of children has definite implications for nurses, who may be called upon to assess the amount of stimulation available to an infant in his home environment.

The same assessment process is called for when children are hospitalized. Nurses are entrusted with the care of hospitalized children whose needs include a stimulating sensory environment to enhance normal development. Contact with families, other children, play therapy and various sensory stimulators such as mobiles, toys, colors and patterns on walls, curtains, and furniture all contribute to adequate sensory inputs.

□ Adaptive and maladaptive responses

When system inputs either exceed or fall short of the optimal range for the organism, the overload or deprivation state is considered a system stressor. Any conditions that alter sensory inputs would also be considered stressors. These can be environmental, social, physical, psychologic, or developmental factors. For example, anxiety, immobilization, paralysis, body casts, isolation, and neurologic deficits alter sensory inputs and can be categorized as system stressors. The degree to which each individual tolerates system stressors differs, and this influences how a client will respond—whether in an adaptive or maladaptive manner. Roy[29] defines adaptation as a human's positive response to a changing environment. An adaptive response maintains client integrity, while a maladaptive response does not and is disruptive to the individual.

Mitchell[25] cites examples of adaptive behaviors by newly blinded individuals who can no longer perceive traffic lights through their visual apparatus. These individuals can adapt and obtain environmental cues through other sensory modalities, such as their auditory sense by listening to traffic patterns to determine if traffic has stopped, or through their sense of touch by becoming aware of the motion against their person as the crowd begins to move across the street. A maladaptive response to the same situation would occur if this individual became anxious, confused, and immobilized on the street corner and unable to utilize alternative environmental cues (Fig. 26-4).

Stressors that exceed the optimal tolerance level of the client will result in maladaptive responses, which can be cognitive, perceptual, motor, or affective disturbances.

Cognitive changes experienced by subjects range from poor concentration, altered sequencing of thoughts, or unusual ideas to bizarre or primary process thinking—defined as the instinctual thought patterns experienced in dreams. There is also alteration in ability to perform unstructured cognitive tasks.[31,43]

Perceptual changes include visual and auditory distortions, perceived movement of stable objects, warping and curvature of surfaces and lines, changes in color and form, and changes in bodily sensations such as numbness. More elaborate distortions have also been reported where clients perceive their bodies to be floating or experience olfactory sensory distortions—exemplified by cooking or burning odors.[10,11,17] There is a difference of opinion among researchers as to whether these can be considered hallucinatory experiences, since they are not psychotic episodes but more accurately episodic occurrences where the subjects are aware that their experiences are not truly reflective of reality. It has been contended that the term "perceptual distortions" is more accurate a description than hallucinations. Ellis[11] uses the term "indeterminate stimulus experience" (ISE) to describe such distortions where a perceptual disturbance occurs for which there is no known stimulus. This can occur without disorientation to time, place, or person.

The experimental literature supports the contention that sensory and perceptual alteration will produce changes in *motor* coordination. Dexterity, other measures of eye-hand coordination, balance, and body coordination have been found to be negatively affected by deprivation conditions.[37,44]

Affective disturbances noted by researchers include anxiety, fear, mood swings, irritability, depression, exaggerated emotional responses, and anger.[31] The in-

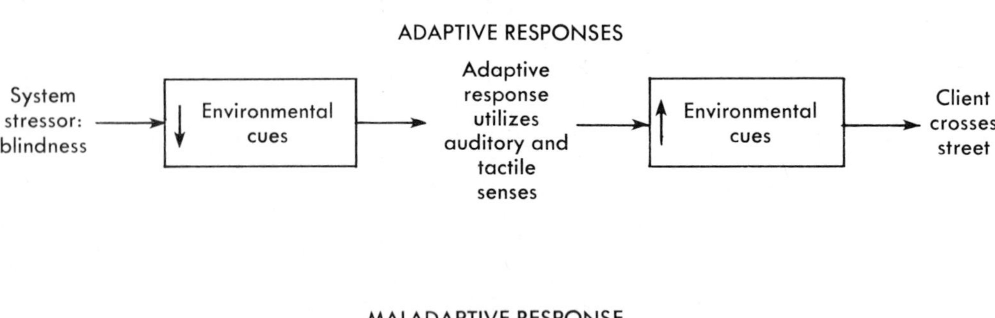

Fig. 26-4. Adaptive versus maladaptive responses to blindness.

tensity of the disturbances vary from mild discomfort to panic.

Additional responses include somatic complaints and noncompliant behavior. Noncompliant behavior would include actions clients display that are contrary to the instructions of health care providers and detrimental to the client. A study of postoperative eye surgery patients identified behaviors such as removing eye patches and getting out of bed as noncompliant.[42]

It should be emphasized that clients may not openly or easily share with staff some of these disturbances, such as perceptual distortions, because of the anxiety or embarrassment that may accompany such experiences. The nurse must be alert for maladaptive responses and investigate further, seeking additional data from the client if the situation warrants intervention.

It is also important for the nurse to be aware that clients in a hospitalized setting can display maladaptive behaviors in response to an altered sensory environment. It is not unlikely that the nurse may be in a situation where an apparently "normal" client is exhibiting psychotic-life behavior such as confusion, noncompliance, disorientation, anxiety, mood swings, or perceptual distortions. This does not mean the client has suddenly become psychotic, tonic, or senile, but he may be responding to an altered sensory environment. However, in applying research findings to the clinical situation, certain limitations must be noted. Although it is hypothesized that responses are correlated with alterations in sensory inputs, this hypothesis needs further testing. It is not a ready explanation but a framework to use in attempting to assess and understand client behavior.

Goals of nursing are to promote harmonious interaction between humans and their environment, to strengthen the integrity of the individual, and to direct and redirect patterning for maximum health potential.[28] With this aim in mind, the nurse must assess each individual client for his unique responses to stressors and if maladaptive behaviors are exhibited, the nurse must intervene to assist the client in achieving an adaptive state.

ASSESSING FOR SENSORY ALTERATIONS

In assessing for altered sensory inputs, the nurse includes both individual and environmental variables, as both contribute to the total amount of sensory input. Data can be collected either by direct questioning or by observation of the client.

☐ Individual factors

Following are individual factors to be considered:

1. *Sensory status of visual, auditory, olfactory, gustatory, and tactile modalities:* Does the client have normal visual and auditory functions? Are there any impairments, defects, or corrective devices required such as glasses or a hearing aid? Can the client discriminate between odors and various taste sensations? Can he perceive changes in temperature, feel pain, and discriminate between various forms of touch such as sharp, light? Does he have the ability to define his placement or position in space?

2. *Neurologic status:* What is the client's level of consciousness? (See Chapter 28.) Are the normal pathways and processing functions intact? Are there any neurologic deficits that would affect sensory inputs, such as spinal cord injuries, stroke conditions, or hyperirritability of neural tracts, that would cause excessive stimulation?

3. *Motor status:* Is the client capable of independent movement? Is there any alteration due to illness, such as paralysis, casts, immobilizations?

4. *Cognitive status:* Can the client perceive, process information, and respond appropriately to his environment? Can he read or write and follow simple commands?

5. *Communication status:* Is his ability to communicate within normal range? Can he understand and initiate speech? Can he respond to verbal communications? Is there any impairment of speech organs or neural pathways necessary for verbal communications?

6. *Age and development level:* What is appropriate for the client in terms of his age and developmental level?

7. *Psychologic status:* Is the client an independent, self-reliant person? What coping mechanisms does he use? Does he appear anxious, irritable, angry? Is he oriented to time, place, person?

8. *Utilization of drugs:* Has the client been exposed to central nervous system depressants, such as alcohol or narcotics, which decrease awareness of the environment? Has he utilized stimulants, such as amphetamines or consciousness expanding drugs such as LSD, which would alter perception?

9. *Presence of maladaptive behaviors:* Are there any cognitive, perceptual motor, or affective disturbances noted?

10. *Presence of specific stressors:* Are there any additional specific stressors to which the client is exposed that would further alter sensory input? This could include pain, drug toxicity, immobilization, isolation, or specific system disorders such as alterations in gas exchange or regulatory mechanisms?

☐ Environmental factors

Two variables are considered when assessing the effect of environment on sensory input: (1) the amount and intensity of environmental inputs and (2) the increase or reduction of pattern or meaningfulness of sensory inputs from the environment. It is important to assess whether these two variables are sufficient to maintain an arousal state in the individual, which permits adaptive responses to occur.

Much of the clinical literature concerns itself with two alterations that can occur in the environment of the client. The environment can be analyzed on the basis of being either a therapeutically restricted environment or a socially restricted environment.

Therapeutically restricted environment

Because of particular health care needs, clients may be placed in a therapeutic environment that is at the same time restrictive. Mitchell[25] cites the following clinical situations:

1. Clients who are kept isolated in sterile environments to protect them or others from pathogenic organisms constitute one major category of clients. Their environments are generally unchanging, and contacts with staff are minimal and often directed through gowns and masks.
2. Clients with orthopedic or neurologic injuries are often placed in traction, casts, or on Stryker or Foster frames, which obviously limits their mobility and commonly confines them to bed. They are not only restricted in movement but can also be restricted visually, as their position may not afford them a changing environment. They may be positioned, for example, on their backs, with the major visual field being the ceiling.
3. Clients placed in intensive care units or coronary care units comprise another category of individuals with a restricted environment. These clients are removed from their familiar world often under an acute crisis situation that did not allow time for client preparation or a transitional period. They are exposed to unfamiliar repetitious sounds, constant light, constant activity, immobilization, strange equipment, and are commonly further stressed by the alterations of illness, pain, sleep, and anxiety. This restricted environment may also be one that predisposes to sensory overload.

Socially restricted environment

Living circumstances that lead to social deprivation are also restrictive to clients. Several variations of this condition have been cited:[25]

1. Infants raised in nonstimulating institutions with minimal contact with care givers or infants raised by families who do not provide an adequately stimulating environment
2. Institutionalized individuals of any age whose living situation is devoid of adequate social or perceptual inputs
3. The depressed or psychotic client, the elderly, or the chronically ill individual constitute another group who may live in their own homes but are physically, socially, or emotionally unable to venture out or whose home environment is restricted or monotonous.

In summary, all factors considered, both individual and environmental variables should be assessed as possible contributory factors to sensory alteration.

■ CLIENTS PREDISPOSED TO SENSORY ALTERATION

It appears that many clinical situations contain elements of sensory deprivation or overload. It also appears that certain clients are prone to developing cognitive and behavioral impairments. There is no research to support specific predictions of exactly who will experience the effects of sensory alteration, but there is evidence to suggest the categories of clients that might be considered as possible risks.

Clients experiencing *eye surgery* are the most common situations discussed in the literature, the majority of which have had cataract surgery.[16] These clients were relatively immobilized postoperatively and wore eye patches, a combination that greatly reduced sensory input. These clients experienced anxiety, perceptual and thought disturbances, confusion, and exhibited noncompliance behavior such as getting out of bed and removing their bandages.[16,18] Nursing interventions that were reported to be most useful in these situations were reassurance, reality orientation, and providing information to the client.

Immobilized clients also experienced sensory impairments. The hallucinatory behavior of clients with bulbar poliomyelitis confined to tank-type respirators has been described as exemplifying the possible effects of sensory alteration.[22] It has been suggested that immobility with the reduction of kinesthetic input produces perceptual and motor abnormalities. Downs[10] investigated the effects of bed rest on young, healthy adults. The subjects, who were relatively immobile for a fixed period of time, experienced difficulty in concentration, disorientation in time and place, olfactory distortions, and "indeterminate stimulus experiences" (ISEs). Similar effects may also be seen in orthopedic clients immobilized for long periods of time.

The third category discussed in the literature are those clients placed in *intensive care units* (ICU). The environment of the ICU has received attention as a possible stressor. The constant light, noise, physical examinations, and constant activity to which clients were exposed were found to be conducive to physical overstimulation and emotional deprivation.[9] Clients interviewed stated that they felt restricted by the monitoring equipment and experienced a feeling of being trapped—that they could not escape. Researchers have also found that noise levels of the ICU and recovery room environment have potential for both sensory overload to the client and as a possible stressor for the staff's own work environment.[12,40] The psychotic-like symptoms exhibited by open-heart surgical clients has prompted researchers to analyze the ICU for psychologic hazards.[20] It has been suggested that critical care areas be designed to promote the client's sense of well being and to promote appropriate adaptive response. Health care providers should influence decisions regarding architectural details, such as isolating utility areas from client areas, providing adequate privacy for individual clients, and utilizing carpeting and drapes to absorb sound. Interventions can also be initiated by staff to promote client adaptation. Preparing the client for the ICU environment when appropriate (prescheduled surgery, for example), freeing the client from restrictive equipment as soon as possible or placing equipment in such a way to diminish noise levels, limiting conversation to that which is essential, and speaking in a normal tone are all appropriate interventions.

The three conditions of eye surgery, immobilization, and exposure to the ICU environment are the primary alterations considered in the clinical literature for client predisposition to sensory alteration. However, in considering the experimental literature, we can hypothesize that the research results are also applicable to other clients. This would encompass clients with a sudden alteration in one or more sensory modalities such as acute blindness, neurologically impaired clients, spinal cord injuries, stroke victims, surgical clients who may be experiencing multiple stressors, clients in drug induced states that alter perception of the environment, and clients experiencing social isolation.

NURSING INTERVENTION

There are no clear-cut differences between clinical manifestations of sensory deprivation or overload. The nurse may be in a position where an individual client's unique situation must be assessed and the nurse must utilize professional judgement in making a decision to either increase or decrease sensory inputs as an intervention measure. It may be a trial and error approach until the client responds adaptively.

In managing manifestations of sensory alteration, the logical first step in the process is to perform an assessment including both individual and environmental variables, as discussed previously in this chapter. In addition, the nurse would consider the temporal variable. Is it an *acute* manifestation or is it indicative of a *chronic* condition, such as social restrictions that can occur with institutionalization?

Consider the following clinical example: M. H. is an 84-year-old woman recovering from abdominal surgery, which was performed yesterday. She is in a private room. Although she was alert on admission, the staff has noted that since surgery she has become disoriented—she does not recognize her visitors and calls staff by her granddaughter's name. She appears confused and has been combative with staff when they approach to check her dressing. She has pulled out both her IV and Foley catheter. She is complaining of pain and is presently receiving medication for both pain and sedation. Restraints have been applied.

In assessing M. H. the following data was gathered:

1. This is her first hospital admission. She is unfamiliar with this environment and was not prepared for hospitalization because of the emergency nature of her illness. She requires glasses to visualize the environment clearly and has diminished hearing.
2. This client, whose sensory input is generally altered because of the aging process, has suddenly been placed in a strange environment where familiar orienting clues are not available. Sensory inputs have been further altered by the presence of pain, sedatives and pain medication, immobility due to restraints, and the physiologic stressors of illness. The problem has been further compounded by being placed in a private room where social contacts are minimal.
3. The sudden manifestation of the behavior, plus the supporting assessment data, are indicative of an acute reaction to sensory alteration. This can occur after exposure to a restricted environment and generally occurs more frequently with an older client, although it can occur regardless of age or diagnostic factors.
4. This condition can clear spontaneously or, in the specific situation of M. H., nursing intervention can be initiated by staff, such as increasing sensory inputs in the form of environmental stimulations—night-light, radio, increased social contacts with family members and staff, and frequent orientation to reality.

☐ Specific client problems

Perceptual disturbances

Clients experiencing hallucinations or perceptual disturbances are often frightened and anxious, even when the client has an awareness that the experience is not reality based. The nurse should not indulge or appease the client in an attempt to allay anxiety. A more useful intervention is to encourage the client to describe his experience and to allow him to ventilate his feelings. It may also be helpful to the client for the nurse to clarify possible environmental stimuli that were misinterpreted, such as an intercom message, and for the nurse to remain in the room with the client to provide reassurance.

Delusional thinking

Clients may articulate beliefs that are contrary to reality, such as the staff is persecuting or mistreating them.

This generally is an episodic occurrence that passes when the client becomes reoriented. The client should not be ridiculed, dismissed, or strongly confronted when such beliefs are expressed. Instead, it would be more helpful to allow the client to verbalize his thoughts and, when appropriate, be presented with the nurse's perception of the facts.

Confused, combative clients

When the client's behavior indicates confusion or combativeness, attempts should be made to reorient the client repeatedly to time, place, and person. Explanations should also be provided regarding identification of staff, tasks to be performed, and environmental stimuli to which the client is exposed. If the client is combative and requires restraints, the rationale for the restraints should be given and reassurance provided to the client that he is not being punished. Restraints that allow the most freedom in movement (body versus limb restraints) should be utilized and safety measures should be taken regarding careful supervision and protection of the client. *Restraints should not be utilized indiscriminately, but only when the client's condition absolutely necessitates it.*

Decreased sensory inputs

As stated throughout this chapter, the nurse has many options at his or her disposal to increase sensory inputs when conditions necessitate such interventions. In summary, the nurse can intervene with both individual and environmental variables. Visual inputs can be increased through the utilization of mobiles, pictures, greeting cards, flowers, color, or something as simple as providing the client with his glasses to enable him to see his environment clearly. Auditory inputs can be increased through the use of radio, TV, and increased verbal interaction with staff, family, or other clients. Tactile stimulation can be provided by administering back rubs or allowing the client to explore objects in his environment through his own sense of touch. Social contacts can be initiated through group activities. Group sessions with the chronically ill have been described as one way to increase social interactions.[7] Also, utilizing natural meeting places in the hospital environment for staff and patients, such as a solarium or day room, appears to increase social stimulating and client satisfaction.[5] Clarifying and providing meaning to the environment through the use of calendars, clocks, and other measures to provide reality orientation is an additional source of increasing sensory inputs.

Increased sensory inputs

If inputs are above the client's range of tolerance, the nurse can intervene to reduce the amount and intensity of stimuli by reducing noise, light, or social contacts. The pattern of stimuli may also require a change. It appears that this is most problematic in critical care areas where the client's condition often necessitates constant monitoring. Interventions that can be instituted by the nurse have been discussed previously, and the reader is referred to that section.

REFERENCES AND SELECTED READINGS

1. Bellak, L.: Overload, New York, 1975, Human Sciences Press.
2. Berrien, K. F.: General and social systems, New Brunswick, N.J., 1968, Rutgers University Press.
3. Brownfield, C. A.: Isolation: clinical and experimental approaches, New York, 1965, Random House, Inc.
4. Cannon, W.: The wisdom of the body, New York, 1932, W. W. Norton & Co., Inc.
5. *Carlson, S.: Selected sensory input and life satisfaction of immobilized geriatric female patients. In ANA clinical sessions, New York, 1968, Appleton-Century-Crofts.
6. Chodil, J., and Williams, B.: The concept of sensory deprivation, Nurs. Clin. North Am. **5**:453-459, 1970.
7. Cockburn, K.: Sensory stimulation in the nursing care of chronic schizophrenic patients. In ANA regional clinical conference, New York, 1967, Appleton-Century Crofts.
8. Cohen, S.: Contact deprivation in infants, Psychosomatics, **7**:85-88, 1966.
9. DeMeyer, J.: The environment of the intensive care unit, Nurs. Forum **6**:262-272, 1967.
10. *Downs, F.: Bed rest and sensory deprivation, Am. J. Nurs. **74**:434-438, 1974.
11. *Ellis, R.: Sensory and thought disturbances after cardiac surgery, Am. J. Nurs. **72**:2021-2025, 1972.
12. *Falk, S. A., and Woods, N. F.: Hospital noise: levels of potential health hazards, N. Engl. J. Med. **289**:274-281, 1973.
13. Goldfarb, W.: Emotional and intellectual consequences of psychological deprivation in infancy: a reevaluation: psychopathology of childhood, Proceedings of American Psychopathological Association, New York, 1955, Grune & Stratton, Inc.
14. *Haslam, P.: Noise in hospitals: its effect on the patient, Nurs. Clin. North Am. **5**:715-724, 1970.
15. *Hearth, K.: Beyond the curtain of silence, Am. J. Nurs. **74**:1060-1961, 1974.
16. Jackson, C. W.: Clinical sensory deprivation: a review of hospitalized eye-surgery patients. In Zubek, J. P.: Sensory deprivation: 15 years of research, New York, 1969, Appleton-Century-Crofts.
17. *Jackson, C. W., and Ellis, R.: Sensory deprivation as a field of study, Nurs. Res. **20**:49, 1971.
18. Jackson, C. W., and O'Neil, M.: Experiences associated with sensory deprivation reported for patients having eye surgery. In Jeffries, J. E., editor: Disturbances in sensory input in nursing practice and research, Columbus, Ohio, 1966, Ross Laboratories.
19. *Kornfeld, D.: Psychological hazards of the internal care unit, Nurs. Clin. North Am. 3:41-51, 1968.
20. *Kornfeld, D., Maxwell, T., and Momrow, D.: Psychological hazards of the intensive care unit, Nurs. Clin. North Am. 3:41-51, 1968.
21. Kornfeld, D., Zimberg, S., and Malm, J.: Psychiatric com-

*References preceded by an asterisk are particularly well suited for student reading.

plications of open-heart surgery, N. Engl. J. Med. **273**:287-292, 1965.

22. Leiderman, H., et al.: Sensory deprivation: clinical aspects, Arch. Med. **101**:389-396, 1958.
23. Lindsley, D.: Common factors in sensory deprivation, sensory distortion and sensory overload. In Solomon, P., et al.: Sensory deprivations, Cambridge, Mass., 1961, Harvard University Press.
24. Lipowski, Z. J.: Sensory overloads, information overloads and behavior, Comp. Psychiatry **16**:199-220, 1975.
25. Mitchell, P. H.: Concepts basic to nursing, New York, 1977, McGraw-Hill Book Co.
26. Perron, D.: Deprived of sound, Am. J. Nurs. **74**:1057-1059, 1974.
27. Riesen, A.: Excessive arousal effects of stimulation after early sensory deprivation. In Solomon, P., et al.: Sensory deprivation, Cambridge, Mass., 1961, Harvard University Press.
28. Rogers, M.: An introduction to the theoretical basis of nursing, Philadelphia, 1970, F. A. Davis Co.
29. Roy, C.: Introduction to nursing: an adaptation model, Englewood Cliffs, N.J., 1975, Prentice-Hall, Inc.
30. Sackett, G.: Innate mechanisms, rearing condition, and a theory of early experience effects in primates. In Jones, M.: Miami symposium on the prediction of behavior, Coral Gables, Fla., 1970, University of Miami Press.
31. Schultz, D.: Sensory restriction, New York, 1965, Academic Press, Inc.
32. Solomon, P., et al.: Sensory deprivation, Cambridge, Mass., 1958, Harvard University Press.
33. Spitz, R.: Hospitalism: an inquiry into the genesis of psychiatric conditions in early childhood, Psychoanal. Study Child **1**:53-74, 1945.
34. Suedfeld, P.: The benefits of boredom: sensory deprivation reconsidered, Am. Sci. **63**:60-69, 1975.
35. *Thompson, L. R.: Sensory deprivation: a personal experience, Am. J. Nurs. **73**:266-268, 1973.
36. Thompson, W. R., and Schaefer, T.: Early environmental stimulation. In Fiske, D. W., and Maddi, S. R., editors: Functions of varied experience, Stonewood, Ill., 1961, Dorsey Press.
37. Vernon, J., McGill, T., Gulick, W., and Candland, D.: The effect of human isolation upon some perceptual and motor skills. In Solomon, P., et al.: Sensory deprivations, Cambridge, Mass, 1961, Harvard University Press.
38. White, B. L.: Human infants: experience and psychological development, Englewood Cliffs, N.J., 1971, Prentice-Hall, Inc.
39. White, B. L.: An experimental approach to the effects of experience in early human behavior, Minn. Symp. Child Psychol. **1**:201-226, 1967.
40. *Woods, N. F., and Falk, S. A.: Noise stimuli in the acute care area, Nurs. Res. **23**:144-150, 1974.
41. Ziskind, E.: A second look at sensory deprivation, J. Nerv. Ment. Dis. **64**:223-230, 1964.
42. Ziskind, E., Jones, H., Filante, W., and Goldberg, J.: Observations on mental symptoms in eye patched patients: hypnagogic symptoms in sensory deprivation, Am. J. Psychiatry **116**:893-900, 1960.
43. Zubek, J., editor: Sensory deprivation: 15 years of research, New York, 1969, Appleton-Century-Crofts.
44. Zubek, J. P., Sansom, W., and Prysiazniuk, A.: Intellectual changes during prolonged perceptual isolation, Can. J. Psychol. **14**:233-243, 1960.

27

Altered levels of consciousness

JUANITA LONG

Caring for a client with an altered consciousness is one of the most demanding situations in nursing practice. The unconscious patient is totally dependent upon the skill and good judgment of the nurse who spends a large amount of time with the patient. There is no way to get valid subjective cues from the patient, so all care is based on objective data and the conclusions that can be drawn from that data. It is the purpose of this chapter to explore altered states of consciousness, their causes, assessment, and care.

DEFINING LEVELS OF CONSCIOUSNESS

One should distinguish between the level of consciousness (LOC) and the content of consciousness. Plum and Posner[23] refer to the two aspects of consciousness as *arousal* and *content*. Levels imply a continuum from greatest to least awareness. When the content is disturbed, the person is said to be *confused*. The problems of caring for the patient experiencing confusion will be discussed later in the chapter, apart from the problems of altered LOC.

The *conscious* person is able to respond to sensory stimuli, has subjective experiences, exercises his will, and is capable of thought and reasoning. Consciousness may also be defined as self-awareness: being able to function mentally and physically in a manner appropriate to the level of one's normal ability and to experience life to the fullest degree. Guyton[18] proposes that each instant of awareness can be defined as a thought, and the awareness itself as consciousness.

In contrast, to be *unconscious* implies that there is no response to sensory stimuli—no thinking and no feelings or emotions. The conscious person is aware of what is going on in the environment; the unconscious person is unaware of self and the environment. To differentiate between consciousness and unconsciousness is relatively easy, but between these two ends of the continuum are many levels of awareness and mental ability not so easily defined or precisely described.

While it is not known what the neural mechanisms are that make awareness possible, it is known that many different parts of the nervous system work together to determine the nature of one's awareness. Any impairment, reduction, or absence of consciousness indicates a serious dysfunction of the brain. The presence of consciousness is dependent on a normally functioning interplay between certain neurons, the brain, and the reticular activating system (RAS).[18] Impulses from the RAS keep us active and serve as an alerting system. When the effects of an insult impinge upon the RAS, the state of consciousness can be altered. As the severity of the insult or dysfunction increases, the client experiences an increasing impairment of responsiveness to events in the internal and external environment. If the dysfunction is great enough, unconsciousness or coma will result.

Consider a continuum with awareness and consciousness at one extreme and unawareness and coma at the other. Inasmuch as consciousness is a complex expression of the mind, and not just a single function, there will be a wide spectrum of levels of consciousness between the two ends of the continuum: consciousness and coma. To set these levels into neatly defined patterns is impossible. The use of such common terms as "alert," "confused," "stuporous," "drowsy," "light coma," and "deep coma" is likely to lead to misunderstanding on the part of the health team providing care, as there is overlap in behaviors from one term to another.

Since the nomenclature used to describe the various levels of consciousness is vague and ill defined, communication between health care providers is often tentative when labels are used. One therefore avoids the use of labels and clearly states the behavior observed. Clear descriptions of the things the patient can do and say will be much more likely to indicate the changing status of the patient and will afford him the best opportunity for prompt, high-quality care.

While it is better that one should not use labels, it is still incumbent on the nurse to have an understanding of them in order to have some idea of what is being said when they are encountered. *Stupor* has been described

Table 27-1. Commonly used states of awareness and associated behaviors

State	Conscious-aware		Semiconscious-semicomatose		Unconscious-comatose	
Level	**Alert**	**Confused**	**Drowsy**	**Stupor**	**Light coma**	**Deep coma**
Behaviors	Normal activity Aware; mentally functional	Poor coordination Delirium Hallucinations Restlessness Excitable May be combative Short attention span Inappropriate actions and judgments Decreased awareness Disorientation	Sleepy Very short attention span Can respond appropriately if aroused	Apathetic Slow moving Blank expression Drooping head Staring Aroused only by vigorous stimuli	Not oriented to time, place, or person Aroused only by painful stimuli Response is only to grunt, grimace, or withdraw limb from pain	No response except decerebrate or decorticate reflexes

as unresponsiveness from which the subject can be aroused only by vigorous and repeated stimuli, whereas *coma* is unarousable responsiveness.[23]

Table 27-1 places the commonly utilized terms for altered levels of consciousness into an organizational framework to help provide an understanding of how each level relates to the others. It also describes some of the behaviors often observed for each of the levels cited.

Impaired consciousness may be the result of two general types of pathological processes: first, conditions that widely and directly depress the function of the cerebral hemispheres, and second, conditions that depress or destroy the brain stem activating mechanisms that lie in or near the central core of the gray matter of the diencephalon, midbrain, and rostral pons.[23]

A single stressor, then, is not the cause of an altered LOC. Indeed, an altered LOC may be the end result of any one of a number of causes typified by the two types of processes. Following are possible causes of alterations in LOC:

1. Vascular lesions: epidural hematomas, subdural hematomas, subarachnoid hematomas, thrombosis, embolism
2. Pressure: tumors (malignant or benign) that compete for limited space within the cranium, hydrocephalus, compression fractures of the skull
3. Trauma: contusions of the brain, concussion (this is more likely to cause confusion), ruptured aneurysm
4. Toxins: barbiturates, narcotics, alcohol, anesthetics, gases, malfunctioning kidneys or liver causing excess of usually normal substances
5. Deficits: decreased oxygen as in respiratory diseases or with overexertion, decreased blood flow in arteriosclerotic conditions, fluid and electrolyte imbalance causing reduced amounts of normal substances
6. Infections: bacterial or viral infiltration of the meninges and brain tissue, cerebral edema, very high temperatures
7. Epilepsy: grand mal or petit mal seizures
8. Shock: diabetic, electrical, hematogenic, sunstroke, emotional stress
9. Nonorganic diseases: mental illness

As can be seen, causes for altered levels of consciousness are many, and nursing care will need to be individualized according to the cause and the symptoms manifested. The brain must be protected against serious damage, which would occur through loss of oxygen or glucose needed to meet cerebral metabolic needs.[23] However, the fact that the patient has a decreased ability to think and plan for himself leads to certain general guidelines for nursing care regardless of the cause of the altered LOC.

■ NURSING INTERVENTION FOR THE PERSON WITH AN ALTERED LEVEL OF CONSCIOUSNESS

Following are general guidelines for caring for the person with an altered level of consciousness.

1. *Provide for alert and knowledgeable assessment.* Technology is valuable for monitoring individual aspects of the patient's response. Machinery gives objective data, but nurses make judgments that may be lifesaving. Assessment will vary according to the client's changing level of consciousness and whether it is an initial or subsequent assessment.

2. *Prevent complications resulting from altered biopsychosocial functioning.* The nurse asks, "Will the patient be safe? What precautions should be taken? Will the patient move frequently enough? Will he eat properly? What will happen if he does not eat, move, etc.?"

3. *Support normal physiologic functioning wherever there is a need.* The nurse thinks beyond the evident, asking such questions as "What will this patient be unable to do because of his deficit in reasoning? What are the routine requests from any rational patient, and which of those requests might this patient be unable to make? Are all essential bodily functions taking place?"

4. *Support and participate in the medical therapy directed at eliminating the cause of the problem.* This will be dictated by the cause and the prescribed therapy.

ASSESSMENT OF THE PATIENT MANIFESTING DECREASING CONSCIOUSNESS

When a patient begins manifesting a decreased LOC, an initial baseline of information is gathered against which later assessments may be compared. This baseline includes a measurement of history, vital signs, and LOC.

Elicit the *history* from the patient (recognizing that his sensorium is impaired and the data may not be accurate) *and* any other person (family member, friend, another client) with such knowledge. Since changes in the sensorium emanate from so many sources, what the nurse will monitor may be varied according to clues found in the assessment.

Vital signs include blood pressure, temperature, pulse and respiration, as well as a pupil check. The anatomic proximity of brain stem areas controlling consciousness to areas controlling the pupils makes pupillary changes a valuable guide to the presence and location of pathologies causing coma[8,23] (Chapter 34). Also, the size and reaction of the pupils to light provide a reliable indication of increased intracranial pressure.

Another aspect of the assessment is to establish the *level of consciousness*, the best indicator of the function of the entire brain.[8] The ability of the nurse to note changes in the LOC and interpret them could mean the difference between life and death. The nurse is sensitive to where the patient is on the continuum between awareness and coma, and he or she knows how long the patient has been at that level, the direction in which change is taking place, and how fast the change is occurring. If the patient is unconscious, the nurse needs to know how long the condition has existed, for the length of unconsciousness and speed of change will give valuable clues to the severity of the problem.

Accuracy is best attained when a systematic approach is used by all persons involved in the continuing assessments. Although some efforts have been made to develop scales to measure LOC, there is a paucity of tools.

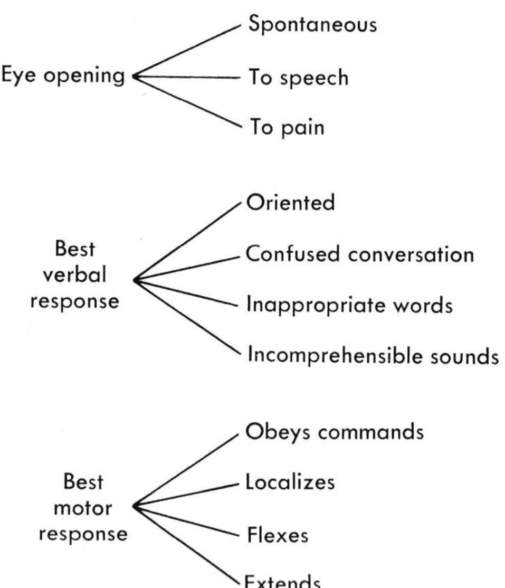

Fig. 27-1. Glasgow coma scale. (From Teasdale, G.: Nurs. Times **71**(24):914-917, 1975.)

What is vital is that all persons in a facility consistently use a single technique (Fig. 27-1). The patient's state is usually described in terms of three aspects of behavior: eye opening, verbal response, and motor response. The clues or evidence that might lead to the use of a descriptive term are recorded or reported as opposed to the descriptive term itself.

When the onset of unconsciousness is *not* immediate, as it is with fainting or extreme shock or trauma, there is usually a consistent pattern of deterioration, although each patient is unique and may depart somewhat from the usual pattern. In the early stages of a deteriorating LOC the changes are so subtle they may not be noted. The behavior may appear to be a normal mood change. For instance, there may be less interest in the surroundings or in events taking place; the client may seem bored or drowsy, inattentive or irritable, and restless. If these behaviors are noted and if there is any history that could lead one to suspect altered brain function, further exploration is necessary.

When checking the LOC, the nurse explains to the patient the content and purpose of the examination. With a small child, verbal assessment is unlikely to be valid; therefore a check of motor ability should be used. With the adult patient, however, there is a sequence of questions and examinations to be used in assessing awareness.

Procedure for assessing level of consciousness

The procedure for assessing level of consciousness is outlined in Fig. 27-2. One begins by determining the patient's orientation by means of several questions regard-

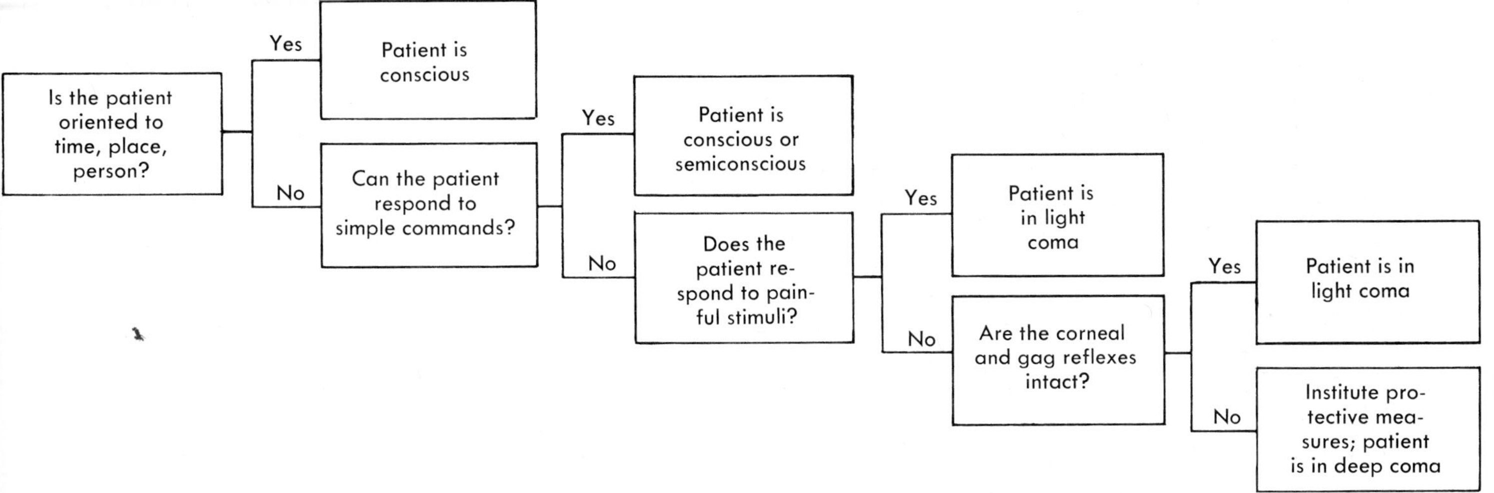

Fig. 27-2. Procedure for assessing level of consciousness.

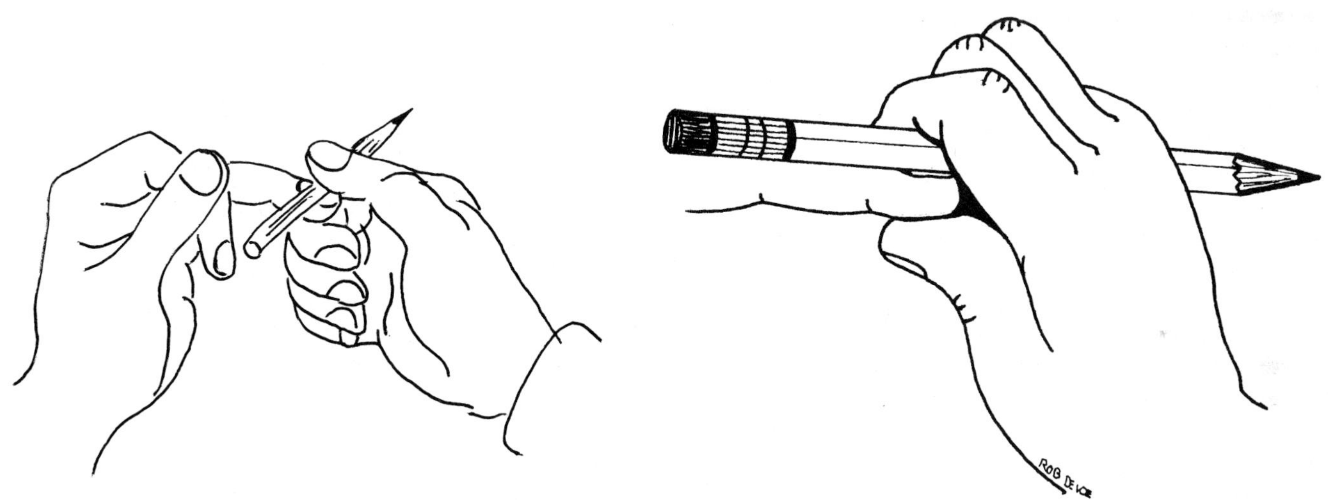

Fig. 27-3. Fingertip pressure stimulation.

ing time, place, and person. The month and year are more readily recalled than days and dates. One can be satisfied if the patient knows he is in a hospital even if he cannot recall the name of the institution. The person can be asked his name and occupation.

Next the person is requested to respond to simple commands such as blinking his eyes or touching the nose or ear with his fingers. Lack of symmetry can be noted by testing both sides of the body. This is important in localizing some lesions. The person can be asked to squeeze your hand with first his right and then his left hand, or to lift both feet simultaneously. If the person cannot perform in response to these commands, then proceed to assess the response to pain.

There are several techniques for checking response to pain that do not cause trauma to the patient. Pinching and pricking may damage tissues and are avoided when possible. Other ways to test for pain include use of supraorbital pressure, pressure on the fingertips, and on the trapezius muscle. To perform the supraorbital pain maneuver, put the thumb on the upper edge of the bony groove of the eye socket about one third the distance from the inner aspect of the orbit and press. Probably the best check and the one with the least potential for harm is shown in Fig. 27-3. One can apply pressure to the nailbed using a pencil held between the examiner's thumb and the patient's finger. One can also apply pressure to the trapezius by pinching it between the patient's neck and the shoulder. (Practice on yourself to see how much pressure is necessary.) The response showing the highest level of consciousness is for the patient to withdraw from the stimulus or try to push it away. If he responds with grimaces or by moving or thrashing around but in a nonpurposeful manner, the level of awareness is lower. Finally, with very deep coma there may be no response at all. Regardless of the response, be sure to record the type of stimulus and the response behavior.

If none of the pain stimuli lead to responses, the final check is of reflexes, since they will be the last responses to be lost. To check the corneal reflex, hold the eyelid open and gently stroke the eye with a thin wisp of cotton. A positive reflex is indicated by immediate blinking. Checking the cornea more than once or twice a day is avoided, since the cornea is quite sensitive and may easily be irritated. The gag reflex is checked by touching the posterior of the pharynx with a cotton swab or tongue depressor.

As the status changes, dependency needs become either greater or lesser, based on the direction of change. Assessments may need to be made every 15 minutes—more frequently if the level of consciousness is decreasing or less frequently if the level is maintained over time or is improving. The nurse independently institutes more frequent observations when the patient's status so indicates.

CARE OF THE COMATOSE PATIENT

The nurse who cares for an already unconscious patient is constantly aware of the *patient's total dependency* on others. Aside from involuntary motor activities such as cardiac, respiratory, and gastrointestinal actions, the patient is unresponsive. It then becomes paramount for others to provide for additional life-sustaining requirements including nourishment, elimination, and protection of tissues.

Since *hearing is probably the last sense to be lost,* the monitoring of what is said in the presence of the unconscious person is vitally important. At present there is no sure device to assess when a patient is no longer able to hear; therefore, even when the patient appears incapable of receiving messages, he may still understand what is said. Grave prognoses or flippant comments are best kept outside a patient's range of hearing. In fact, positive and hopeful comments made in the patient's presence may give the patient motivation to struggle back to consciousness. Thus the nurse speaks to the patient and explains what is being done as if the patient were fully aware.

The third factor to consider is the *therapeutic effect of touch.* The patient is spoken to before he is touched and is handled with gentleness. Because there is no pain response to remind care providers when stress is increased, the tendency is to move the unconscious patient without consideration of soft tissue. Touch is one of the first sensations experienced by the human organism, and without proper touch, normal development would not take place.[21] Touch is a medium for communication. Holding and cuddling infants seems to make them more tranquil and content. Research has shown positive results from the use of touch with disoriented and some mentally ill persons. It is highly possible that some of the same positive responses can be elicited in the unconscious patient. Using a firm hand grasp while talking to the patient about the day or the environment, smoothing the hair away from the face with the full palmar surface of the hand, or tucking the bed covers snuggly around the patient may stimulate the feeling of being cared for or encompassed.

A fourth concern relates to the environment. The *environment should be low key,* with loud noises kept to a minimum. Soft music may be beneficial, but unnecessary sounds should be eliminated. The unconscious person with improving awareness often has an overly excitable nervous system response and is unable to attend to multiple stimuli. To facilitate the patient's ability to focus on any stimulus, eliminate all but necessary noises.

Assessment of the comatose patient

The assessment of the patient who is comatose for an extended period of time is similar to the assessment of a patient with a changing level of consciousness, but is broader in scope, focusing on needs for health maintenance. Following is a guideline for assessment of the comatose patient:

1. General impressions
   a. Skin
      (1) Color and consistency of color
      (2) Temperature
   b. Olfactory cues
      (1) Odor of breath
      (2) Other odors (e.g., incontinence)
   c. Activity level
      (1) Presence of movement
      (2) Character and symmetry of movement
2. Specific aspects of assessment
   a. Pupillar response
      (1) Size and equality
      (2) Reaction to light
      (3) Consensual movement of eyes
   b. Respiratory status
      (1) Breath sounds
      (2) Excursion of chest, abdomen
      (3) Respiratory rate
   c. Muscular status
      (1) Tonus
      (2) Symmetry of paralysis
      (3) Posturing—decorticate or decerebrate

d. Elimination
   (1) Presence of incontinence
   (2) Skin irritation
   (3) Palpation of abdomen for impaction
e. Cardiovascular status
   (1) Pulse rate
   (2) Rhythm

One begins with a general inspection of the patient's body. *Skin color* and *consistency of color* is noted. A bluish area or swelling may indicate trauma in the comatose patient and be significant in determining the cause of unconsciousness. Redness may indicate beginning skin breakdown.

A significant change from normal *skin temperature* prompts the nurse to take the body temperature. A gradual increase in temperature may indicate that an infection is beginning. Infections may develop in wounds but are equally prone to develop in the urinary tract (especially in the presence of an indwelling catheter) or lungs (because of decreased movement of secretions caused by immobility and the inability to cough voluntarily). Dehydration may cause an elevated temperature. Rarely the temperature-regulating center in the hypothalamus is disturbed by pressure or trauma, and there will be significant increase or decrease in temperature.

The *olfactory sense* may provide cues. A sweet acidotic breath may indicate hyperglycemia. An objectionable odor may signify the need for better mouth care, signal bleeding gums, or indicate incontinence.

Next note the *activity level*. Watch the patient from a short distance. Is the patient motionless or moving? Are the movements purposeful or jerky and erratic? Convulsive movements may indicate increasing intracranial pressure. Movement on one side and not the other may indicate hemiplegia. Observe fingers, eyelids, and lips for tremors, as these may be a prelude to a seizure. Report any changes to the physician to allow for preventive intervention or further evaluation. General restlessness may indicate increasing cerebral pressure, discomfort from a distended bladder, a tight bandage, or poor positioning. Restlessness may also be a positive sign indicative of an increasing awareness.

Next one determines if the *pupils* are equal in size and reaction. Their size is recorded in millimeters, and the reaction to light is noted for symmetry and speed. Sluggish responses are reported. Findings are compared with the patient's "normal" or predetermined standard. Being unaware that the patient has an artificial eye or pupil that does not respond to light as readily as the other may lead to erroneous inferences. The unconscious patient will usually stare straight ahead without eye movements, but from time to time the eyes will move. When this happens the eyes should move consensually. If there is deviation of either eye from the midline (disconjugate), toward the midline (strabismus), or back and forth oscillation (nystagmus), this is significant to report.

Next one listens to *breath sounds* and observes the *rise and fall of the chest or abdomen*. The pattern and rate of breathing and character of respiration (easy or labored, fast or slow, regular or irregular, deep or shallow) are noted. Many different parts of the brain influence respirations. Trauma to the brain or reactions to drugs and toxins may cause abnormal and inadequate breathing.

Next the *muscle tone* is noted. Are the muscles tight? Flaccid? Each arm and leg is put through passive range of motion, comparing one side to the other side and upper extremities with lower extremities. Changes or asymmetry give clues about the location of the problem and are reported. When the arms are lifted and allowed to fall, the paralyzed arm will fall faster than the unaffected arm. When the patient's heels are placed on the bed and the legs flexed and released, the paralyzed leg will fall outward.

Unusual movements such as decorticate or decerebrate rigidity are observed. *Decorticate* rigidity is characterized by stiff, extended legs, with arms flexed on the chest, and is caused by damage to the pyramidal motor tract above the brain stem. Upper brain stem damage may cause the *decerebrate* position, with all limbs extended and arms hyperpronated. This indicates a grave condition.

Finally the patient is inspected for *incontinence*. Continued contact of the skin with either feces or urine exposes the patient to skin problems such as rashes or decubitus ulcers and should be avoided stringently. A consistent check will enable quick care to prevent skin breakdown or to plan intervention when there has been no elimination over a period of time. The abdomen is palpated daily to check for fecal buildup and impaction.

Palpation may also be used to check the *pulse* for rate and rhythm. A slow pulse may indicate increasing intracranial pressure or overreaction to medication. The significance of pulse in relation to electrolyte imbalance may be found in Chapter 20.

□ Management of the comatose patient

Intervention begins even as assessment and goal setting are being accomplished. There are two functions of intervention on behalf of the patient experiencing a diminished level of consciousness—maintenance and prevention. As consciousness begins to improve, intervention may include rehabilitative measures also.

Maintenance

While there is often overlap in the maintenance and prevention functions, maintenance may be thought of as that care essential to the support of life. It is often described as those activities carried out when a person is suddenly rendered unconscious, before the body has returned to a state of dynamic equilibrium. An example of maintenance would be to provide sufficient oxygen to maintain life processes. This would require the nurse to clear the air passages, loosen clothing, position the patient in such a way that breathing and circulation are facilitated, and, if necessary, turn the patient on the side to facilitate drainage from the oral cavity. See Chapter 24 for an in-depth discussion of other emergency measures. Maintenance intervention for the patient experiencing coma of long duration includes provision of adequate nutrition, promotion of regular elimination, promotion of adequate circulation, and control of body temperature.

Nutrition. When a patient is experiencing rapidly decreasing awareness, nutrition is not a primary concern; however, if the patient becomes comatose and remains so for an extended period of time, nutritional support becomes a major concern. For the first few days of unconsciousness the patient will probably be maintained on intravenous fluids, as prescribed by the physician. Close observation of the needle site for inflammation or infiltration, as well as attention to flow rate to prevent excessive fluid intake, are essential. After 2 or 3 days a nasogastric tube may be inserted into the stomach through which nourishment will be supplied in liquid form (p. 1184). Feedings are usually prescribed every 2 to 3 hours in small amounts to decrease the possibility of regurgitation and aspiration. The tube should be changed every 5 to 7 days unless it becomes clogged sooner, but the naris through which the tube is placed should be cleaned daily with warm water and lubricated with a water soluble lubricant to decrease the formation of crusts.

The presence of a tube in the nostril is irritating and may cause tissue damage, so if coma lasts for an extended period of time, there may be a need for a gastrostomy tube to provide a means for feeding. The gastrostomy tube is inserted through the abdominal wall into the stomach. A catheter with an inflatable tip (to prevent the tube from slipping out of the stomach) is then sutured in place. This tube remains clamped or plugged except during feedings, and the area around the tube is cleaned daily and covered with a dry dressing (p. 1212).

Elimination. Measures must be taken to assist in elimination and maintain the tone of the bowel muscles. Without intervention, the tendency is for the comatose patient to become constipated and possibly impacted. Routinely palpate the abdomen to determine when a fecal mass is present. This palpation may also serve to stimulate peristalsis and induce a bowel movement. If possible, determine the patient's normal elimination schedule and place him on a bedpan at that hour. If a suppository is needed, administer it about 30 minutes prior to the regular elimination schedule. Dulcolax (bisacodyl) is an effective suppository to use for bowel training. When laxatives are needed, a mild one such as milk of magnesia is often used and can be administered via the nasogastric tube.

Sometimes it becomes necessary to give a cleansing enema. Usual techniques for administering an enema are used; however, it may be necessary to hold the patient's buttocks together to prevent expulsion of the solution before the enema is ready to be expelled. The enema may also be administered through a Foley catheter placed in the rectum. The balloon is inflated before the fluid is introduced, thus preventing the expulsion of the fluid until the desired amount has been administered. The balloon is deflated (before removing the catheter) to allow expulsion of the enema. When placing the patient on the bedpan, care is taken to align the body correctly and to protect the skin. Gentle massage of the abdomen along the path of the transverse and descending colon will assist in the expulsion of the fecal mass. Stool softeners such as dioctyl sodium sulfosuccinate (Colace) administered via the nasogastric tube will also help facilitate elimination. Assuring an adequate liquid intake helps keep the fecal mass soft, and juices that have a laxative effect, such as prune juice, may be included in the diet. In the event that an impaction does occur, a retention enema is administered. If this is unsuccessful, the impaction may require manual removal; that is, using a gloved, lubricated finger to remove small pieces of the fecal material until the mass is eliminated.

The need for communication between health care providers is especially great with reference to bowel function. Only when bowel movements are carefully recorded as to time, amount, and consistency can the nurse make competent judgments about laxatives and enemas.

Circulation. Circulation can be assisted in several ways. Conscientiously turning the patient from side to side at least every 2 hours will enhance circulation, for muscle movement stimulates circulation. Careful attention to positioning so that there are no constricted areas, as would be caused by twisted clothing, tight bedclothes, or a misplaced limb, will allow for maximum circulation. Joints bent at sharp angles slow circulation and should be avoided. Passive range-of-motion exercises planned into the nursing care regimen at least every 8 hours will increase blood flow. Padding of dependent bony prominences when they are being laid upon decreases pressure and helps to maintain good circulation. Back massage with application of increasing pressures toward the level of the heart and decreasing pressure away from the heart is thought to increase circulation to the skin. A commonly overlooked area is the ear. If it is folded over, circulation to the outer area is occluded and tissue necrosis occurs quickly. Always check the lower ear after turning the patient. Frequent monitoring of infusions to prevent overloading the circulatory system will also enhance good circulation. The use of elastic stockings or wraps from toe to thigh on the lower extremities decreases the potential for stasis. These should be removed every 8 hours and the skin observed. They can be replaced after 30 minutes. When putting them on, raise the leg above the heart level to assist in having the volume of blood as near normal as possible before putting on the wrap.

Temperature. A normal body temperature is generally considered to range from 36 C (98.6 F) to 38 C (99 F). Since the comatose patient is unable to say when he is either too cold or too warm, it becomes the nurse's responsibility to monitor the body temperature at least every 4 hours and more frequently if a problem arises. If the heat center in the hypothalamus is disturbed, as it often is by trauma or by certain medical problems, the temperature may change rapidly. When the temperature is excessively elevated, it is called *hyperthermia*. An elevated temperature may also be indicative of an infection or dehydration. When a patient is experiencing hyperthermia, the nurse can assist in maintaining the temperature within a normal range by removal of bedclothes and lowering the room temperature. If necessary, remove all of the patient's clothes except enough to protect his modesty and the family's sense of propriety. Antipyretics may be given via the nasogastric or gastrostomy tube or by suppository. Ice bags covered with protective wraps to prevent tissue damage may be placed on the groin and axilla where there is a large blood supply. This helps to hasten body cooling. Sponging the body with a water and alcohol solution causes evaporation and subsequent cooling. The use of a fan to blow over the patient while being sponged further enhances cooling. Electrically controlled hypothermia blankets are now available and are often used to reduce fever when a patient suffers from hyperthermia. The patient should not be allowed to get chilled and shiver, since shivering increases body metabolism and produces heat, thus raising the temperature. Continued hyperthermia will result in brain damage and ultimately death, so the temperature is kept as near normal as possible. On the other end of the continuum, a subnormal temperature (hypothermia) may be experienced. Additional clothing and covers and increased room temperature will help. Warmed blankets may help to elevate temperature in the hypothermic patient.

Prevention

Preventive interventions include safety measures and those actions aimed at avoiding damage to the eyes, ears, nose, mouth, and hair, as well as to the musculoskeletal, gastrointestinal, integumentary, urinary, and cardiovascular systems.

Safety. Numerous activities of the nurse are geared toward providing a safe environment for the comatose patient experiencing a changing level of consciousness. Side rails are kept up at all times for the unconscious patient unless the nurse is present. When the patient is restless and likely to be thrashing about, the railing should be padded. Equipment is placed far enough from the bed that a confused patient would be unlikely to interfere in its operation. Any prosthetic device such as false teeth, an artificial eye, or contact lenses should be removed and carefully stored in a safe place until the patient is lucid enough to use them appropriately. Restraint should be avoided unless the patient is agitated enough to harm himself. When any type of restraint is used, caution should be taken that it is put on properly and is not too tight. Periodic checks should be made for tissue damage.

Musculoskeletal positioning. To protect musculoskeletal integrity, there are numerous possible interventions and aids. Perhaps the most crucial is positioning. Improper positioning can lead to contractures, foot drop, wrist drop, and other deformities (p. 840). The preferred position of the comatose patient is in the *side-lying position*.

The comatose patient is at risk of pulmonary complications. Therefore frequent changes of position are essential. Turning the patient from side-to-side at frequent intervals prevents pooling of pulmonary secretions. In some instances, tracheal suctioning may be necessitated by the patient's inability to cough. Unless neurologic complications contraindicate it, postural drainage may be initiated.

Patients who are comatose may be placed in a prone or supine position; however, care must be taken to ensure a patent airway. The reader is referred to a text on fundamentals of nursing for information about turning and positioning patients.

Exercise. Passive range-of-motion exercise is done a minimum of twice daily and ideally several times a day (p. 818). One way to accomplish this is to put the upper side through complete range-of-motion each time the patient is turned. Doing it systematically helps assure that it is not postponed and subsequently overlooked. This too will increase circulation and decrease the likelihood of thrombi.

When the physical condition is stable enough and the patient conscious, he should sit in a chair at least once and preferably twice a day. The upright posture fosters weight-bearing on the long bones, thus limiting calcium loss, and enhances pulmonary expansion, circulation, and digestive motility. Unless the patient is small enough for two people to manage, use a mechanical lift.

Position the patient so that he is seated squarely on the buttocks with the spine straight and feet flat on the floor or footrest. Support the arms and head with pillows. Use a chest harness support tied behind the chair or secure the patient's torso by wrapping a sheet around the torso and the chair.

Skin care. The integument of the comatose patient is prone to many assaults: being pulled and slid across bed linens, lying too long on bony prominences, dryness or moisture, and increased bacteria from incontinence of urine and feces. A warm water bath daily is recommended. While tub baths are not always feasible, when the patient becomes conscious and stable, he can be placed in a tub or shower if there is an adequate number of people to manage him without incurring injury. Until such time, a daily bed bath should include a brisk rub (except when the skin is fragile) with sparing use of soap and a thorough rinse. Soap residue causes dryness and skin irritation, and moisture increases the potential for skin breakdown.

To prevent dryness, place a lotion (such as Alpha-Keri oil or Jeri-Bath) in the bath water. If this is not sufficient, rub the body with a lanolin preparation or other cream. The family may suggest a lotion the patient has used routinely.

The skin of the feet is especially prone to drying, and the nails harden with decreased circulation. Rub the feet daily with a lubricant such as Vaseline. Never use alcohol unless specially indicated, for it make the skin extremely dry. Comatose patients perspire just as alert patients do. If talcum powder is used, it tends to hold this perspiration. Since moist skin is more prone to necrosis, avoid using talcum.

Linens are kept dry and crumb free. Keep them pulled taut so there will be no wrinkles underneath the patient that might cause decubitus ulcers. Protect the patient's skin from the shearing effect of sliding on the sheets by positioning the head of the bed at not more than a 10° angle so that the patient will not constantly be sliding down in bed. Additional ways to prevent decubitus ulcers include the use of lamb's wool under pressure areas. A water or air mattress to equalize pressure can be used, although if the patient is turned carefully, this is not needed. Be sure never to use a doughnut or rubber ring, as it simply causes a circle of pressure and cuts down on the blood supply to the area within that circle, making skin breakdown more likely.

Incontinence. A condom catheter connected to a urinary elimination bag may be placed on the male patient. The condom is unrolled on the penis and secured by an elasticized piece of tape around the penis. Care should be taken that the tape is not placed on the skin, but on the condom, and is wrapped around the penis snuggly enough to prevent the condom from slipping, but not so tight as to interfere with circulation. Tactile stimulation may cause a temporary engorgement of the penis. When the size of the penis diminishes, the condom may slip off unless it has been securely wrapped. The condom is removed and the penis cleansed with soap and water daily.

An indwelling catheter with closed drainage may be needed for the female patient. Consult the physician prior to using this method. While the catheter remains in, continual observation for signs of infection, chills, or fever is required. Accurately monitor intake in relation to output. Irrigation of the bladder through an indwelling catheter increases the possibility of introducing organisms; therefore irrigate as seldom as possible. When irrigation must be done, observe scrupulous sterile technique. Infections from prolonged use of an indwelling catheter cause the urine to become alkaline. This in turn causes inorganic materials such as phosphorus and calcium to settle out, and as a result, bladder stones may form. A fluid intake of at least 3,000 ml/day will keep the urine dilute enough to lessen the risk of bladder stones.

The catheter should be changed before mineral deposits plug the lumen or tip of the catheter. If no manufacturer's information is available regarding how frequently the catheter must be changed, a safe estimate is every 10 days.

Hair. Shampoos are indicated every 1 or 2 weeks, unless contraindicated by the patient's underlying problems, for the scalp of the comatose patient continues to secrete oils and perspiration; the hair becomes sour-smelling and difficult to manage when not properly cleansed. Comb hair daily, and braid or arrange long hair to prevent matting. Take care that there are no lumps of hair on the part of the head where the patient lies.

Hair care for black persons differs from that recommended for white persons. For the black person, cleansing the hair with a warm solution of one part alcohol with four parts of mineral oil is followed by an application of warm olive oil, baby oil, or Vaseline oil to the scalp and hair.[17] Excess oil may be removed with a towel. Long hair can be braided; very short hair can be left loose after combing. Afro combs make combing less uncomfortable.

Hair care is important to the patient's sense of well-being and comforting for the family because a well-groomed patient conveys that he is "cared about" as well as "cared for."

Mouth and teeth. The unconscious patient is often a mouth breather and therefore has a dry mouth. Regardless of how he breathes, the patient experiencing a decreased level of consciousness will require mouth care. When not cleansed, the mouth becomes inflamed and prone to other infections. Mucus and bacteria form plaque. Plaque, tartar, and food debris collect in gingival crevices around the teeth and cause mechanical and bacterial irritation. The tissue becomes swollen and inflamed. In time, gingival tissue will separate from the teeth and form pockets where still more debris can accumulate.[24] Teeth may be lost and bone may become involved. Elderly persons have thinner oral membranes and less flow of salivary juices to help wash the mouth, so their problem is compounded. Refer to Chapter 54 for oral care guidelines.

Nose. The nares should be cleansed daily to help keep them patent. Inspect for secretions and note the type. If crusts are forming, gently remove with a moist applicator unless the patient's condition contraindicates. A thin application of a water-soluble lubricant helps decrease accumulation of debris. This is especially important when a nasogastric tube is in place, for it causes some trauma to the tissues, and inflammation may ensue if the naris is not kept cleaned.

Ears. The folds of the ears should be cleansed and dried carefully. The area behind the ear is easily overlooked when drying, but is prone to skin irritation when soap or moisture is not removed. Check the ears for wax while bathing the patient. Over a period of time large amounts of wax may accumulate, but are easily removed with a small wire loop. When head trauma is the basis of coma, be very cautious about introducing anything into the ear until it has been ascertained that there is no damage within the ear.

Eyes. When a person becomes unconscious, one of the first interventions is to remove contact lenses (p. 759). When properly done, there is little likelihood of causing damage. The cornea receives its oxygen supply primarily through exchange of gases in the atmosphere. When eyes are closed during sleep, the metabolic rate of the cornea goes down and the oxygen supply from the blood system is adequate to maintain health. When contact lenses are worn, however, the metabolic rate of the cornea increases. If the eyes are closed for a long time with the contact lenses in place, the cornea cannot remain healthy. The damage will be directly related to the time the lenses have been in place and the extent of interference with metabolic rate of the tissue.[15] The contact lenses, having been removed, should be stored either in saline solution or distilled water, keeping the right and left lens separated and labeled.

Since the eyes are very precious and cannot be replaced, special caution should always be given to prevent any damage occurring to them. Pull the lid back and check the eyes several times a day. Make sure they do not become dried out. Cleanse them with clear water or one of the commercial lubricants. Keep the eyelids closed. If there is any problem with keeping the eyelid closed, shield the eye to prevent irritation from scratching or from dryness.

□ Support of significant others

The unconscious patient has no awareness of the severity of his situation, but the alert family does. This awareness creates great anxiety and stress. It is difficult for family members to understand what is going on, and it is very frightening to stand by feeling inadequate and unable to help. The family then becomes part of the responsibility of the nurse. From the beginning, they need special understanding and special consideration. For them it may be a crisis. They can be helped to cope by becoming involved in the patient's care.

A good way of involving the family in the care of the patient is by asking for help with positioning the patient. They are usually quite capable of doing an excellent job of monitoring and maintaining position and are often with the patient extended periods of time when the nurse cannot be. The involvement not only ensures more consistent care for the patient, but it is very beneficial to the family, giving them a sense of accomplishment and purpose. The hours of waiting are lessened for significant others when they feel they are needed and involved. For this reason, carefully explain what is to be done and the principles underlying the actions; then allow them to help you, not only with positioning but in other aspects of care as they desire. The value of their contributions is acknowledged.

Family members often will wish to stay at the bedside. If they do, share with them that their talking is providing sensory stimulation to the patient. The assumption is made that some of this talking may be filtering through to the awareness of the patient even though he is unable to respond to it.

The nurse conveys to the family a willingness to listen, to be involved, and to help them explore their thoughts. Keeping the family informed of what is being done, what is planned, and the changing condition is very crucial. Provide the family with a comfortable environment. An expression of a willingness to help is frequently all that is required.

When a patient begins to recover, the first response often is to a familiar voice or face, and this may be in the form of a verbal comment. He will need the security of knowing that his family, friends, and the staff are concerned. He will need much support and encouragement, as well as explanation. Nurses should take the time to encourage and to assist, for each little accomplishment is of great consequence to the patient.

□ Outcome criteria for the person who has been comatose

The patient will:

1. Demonstrate no further signs of brain damage attributable to lack of oxygen or glucose.
2. Exhibit minimal loss of body weight.

3. Be free of fecal impaction, urinary tract infection, decubitus ulcers, thrombi, effects of pulmonary infiltrates, corneal abrasions, hyperthermia, joint contractures, and oral and dental problems resulting from inability to provide self-care.
4. Be free of bodily injury from falls or other accidents.

CONFUSED OR DISORIENTED PATIENT

When one has a disturbed consciousness, rather than a decrease in the level of consciousness, one is said to be experiencing a confused or disoriented state. It is the *content* of consciousness that is altered. The disoriented person may experience hallucinations or have illusions or delusions. With *disorientation* the patient is awake, but perceives phenomena incorrectly. Thinking and reasoning are inappropriate, and remembering is difficult.

A *hallucination* is an impression on any of the senses in the absence of a stimulus. The patient believes he sees, hears, tastes, feels, or smells something, but the source of this occurrence is within the patient's thinking rather than in reality. Confusion and hallucinations may be caused by injury, drugs, psychologic problems, or organic problems. Organic causes may be acute infections with high fever, drug toxicity from alcohol or psychedelic drugs, withdrawal from drugs, brain tumors, senility, or exhaustion.

It is well to consider the causes of confusion in the *elderly* apart from the other confused states. It is probable that much of the confusion of the elderly may be the result not of insult, but of normal physiologic aging of tissues and organs. In the aged person the lungs do not expand as well as in the younger person, thereby decreasing the ability to cough and deep breathe. Cardiovascular changes in the myocardium of the older person prohibit the heart from responding quickly to stress with a resulting decrease in blood flow throughout the body. This decreased oxygen supply to the brain tissue may bring about a lowering in sensory perception, making contact with reality more difficult. A new environment such as a hospital or nursing home increases the likelihood of misperceptions. This is especially true in the elderly. When drugs that are eliminated through the kidney are given to the elderly, unless there are fully functioning nephrons, there may be accumulations of the drug. In increased amounts, many drugs have the capacity to cause confusion. The nurse is advised to be aware of the changed physiology in older persons and mediate the care given accordingly. It is more common that disorientation in the elderly manifests itself during the evening and night hours.

An *illusion* is a sensory experience based on fact, but misinterpreted. This may happen when one of the senses is faulty or when environmental conditions prohibit a true interpretation of what is sensed. For example, the older person who has failing vision may think there is someone in the room with him when a shadow moves.

The care of the *confused* patient begins with a thorough assessment to determine the cause and needs. There may be some metabolic imbalance or deficit in circulation or respiration, or the client may be experiencing pain. Try to determine if the patient has been eating and eliminating. The patient's reply to such inquiries may not be reliable if he is already confused, hence it is extremely important for all staff to be accurate in recording all objective data. Check on other possibilities: Is the client positioned in poor body alignment? Is there an elevated temperature? Is the client experiencing an overload or deficit that might create a confused state? When causes are found, one makes adjustments, trying to eliminate the cause.

Establish communication with the patient. A good way to get the patient's attention is through touch. Once the contact is made, use a calm, quiet, unhurried voice. To keep the patient oriented, explain in advance what you will do. Include the patient in planning and discussions. See that the room is well lighted. Keep a calendar in view. Introduce yourself each time you care for the patient. Talk slowly and distinctly and use short statements. Face the patient and stay within a conversational distance of 4 feet. When speaking to the patient, eliminate extra stimuli such as the radio and television, which would tend to clutter the sensory field and might prevent a clear communication between the nurse and patient. When it is possible, provide consistency by having the same staff members care for the patient every day. It is advisable to keep decision making at a minimum for the confused person.

Help family members or significant others to understand what is happening and what such behavior might imply. Let them know that their presence provides a familiar stabilizing force. Let them make plans for the patient's care in the hospital and at home. Support them as much as possible in whatever they decide.

Delirium is exemplified by disorientation, fear, agitation, irritability, excitement, insomnia, misperception of sensory stimuli, and often illusions. High fevers, fear, drug overdose, alcoholism, and physical or mental shock may induce the delirious state. The patient's behavior is erratic and impulsive. To care for the patient experiencing delirium, the nurse assists in the treatment of the cause as well as symptoms. Such efforts might be directed at lowering an elevated temperature or facilitating proper elimination.

Regardless of the specific treatments, the nurse provides safety for the patient and protects him from self-injury. This may include keeping the environment quiet and nonstimulating or using side rails if the patient is to be left alone. If side rails disturb the patient by their presence, as they sometimes do, a judgment must be made whether to use them and risk increased agitation or not use them and risk a fall. Occasionally it becomes necessary to restrain the patient.

One also monitors the physiologic processes, ensures the adequate intake of fluid and food, and monitors and supports elimination. Speak slowly and clearly. This facilitates communication with the person who experiences delirium. Recognizing that the patient cannot control his behavior fosters acceptance and patience.

□ Outcome critera for the person who has been confused or disoriented

The patient will:

1. Be free of bodily injury, either self-inflicted or from falls.
2. Be free of physiologic effects attributable to inability to perform self-care tasks related to nutrition, elimination, and mobility.

REFERENCES AND SELECTED READINGS

1. *Adam, N. R.: Prolonged coma: your care makes all the difference, Nurs. 77 **7**:21-27, 1977.

1a. *Alexander, M., and Brown, M.: Physical examination. Part 18. Neurological examination. Nurs. 76 **6**:50-55, April 1976.

2. *Baxter, S.: Psychological problems of intensive care-1, Nurs. Times **71**:22-23, 1975.
3. *Burton, G.: Families in crisis, Nurs. 75 **5**:36-43, Dec. 1975.
4. *Cahall, J., and Smith, D.: Considerate care of the elderly, Nurs. 75 **5**:38-39, Sept. 1975.
5. *Canning, M.: Care of the unconscious patient, Nurs. Mirror **139**:61-62, 1974.
6. Conway, B. L.: Carini and Owens' neurological and neurosurgical nursing, ed. 7, St. Louis, 1978, The C. V. Mosby Co.
7. Downie, P.: Physiotherapy and the care of the progressively ill patient-2. The unconscious and bedridden patient, Nurs. Times **69**:922-923, 1973.
8. Erickson, R.: Cranial check: a basic neurological assessment, Nurs. 74 **4**:67-72, Aug. 1974.

*References preceded by an asterisk are particularly well suited for student reading.

9. *Field, W., and Ruelke, W.: Hallucinations and how to deal with them, Am. J. Nurs. **73**:638-640, 1973.
10. Fuerst, E., Wolff, L., and Weitgel, M.: Fundamentals of nursing, Philadelphia, 1974, J. B. Lippincott Co.
11. *Gerdes, L.: The confused or delirious patient, Am. J. Nurs. **68**:1228-1233, 1968.
12. Gifford, R., and Plant, M.: Abnormal respiratory patterns in the comatose patient caused by intracranial dysfunction, J. Neurosurg. Nurs. **7**:57-61, July 1975.
13. *Gifford, R., and Plant, M.: On describing altered states of consciousness, J. Neurosurg. Nurs. **5**:18-20, 1973.
14. *Glass, S. J.: Nursing care of the neurosurgical patient: head injuries, J. Neurosurg. Nurs. **5**:49-55, Dec. 1973.
15. *Gould, H.: How to remove contact lenses from comatose patients, Am. J. Nurs. **76**:1483-1485, 1976.
16. *Grant, M., and Kubo, W.: Assessing a patient's hydration status, Am. J. Nurs. **75**:1306-1311, 1975.
17. Grier, M.: Hair care for the black patient, Am. J. Nurs. **76**:1781, 1976.
18. Guyton, A. C.: Textbook of medical physiology, ed. 5, Philadelphia, 1976, W. B. Saunders Co.
19. Hafey, L., and Keane, B.: Patients with acute insult to the central nervous system—an observation tool, Nurs. Clin. North Am. **8**:743-749, 1973.
20. Mitchell, P. H.: Concepts basic to nursing, ed. 2, New York, 1977, McGraw-Hill Book Co.
21. Montague, M. F. A.: Touching: the human significance of the skin, New York, 1971, Columbia University Press.
22. *Norsworthy, E.: Nursing rehabilitation after severe head trauma, Am. J. Nurs. **74**:1246-1250, 1974.
23. Plum, F., and Posner, J.: Diagnosis of stupor and coma, contemporary neurology series, ed. 10, Philadelphia, 1972, F. A. Davis Co.
24. Reitz, M., and Pope, W.: Mouth care, Am. J. Nurs. **73**:1728-1730, 1973.
25. Robinson, L.: Coping with psychiatric emergencies, Nurs. 73 **3**:42-44, July 1973.

25a. *Rudy, E.: Early omens of cerebral disaster, Nurs. 77 **7**:59-62, 1977.

26. Scarbrough, D.: Reality orientation: a new approach to an old problem, Nurs. 74 **4**:12-13, Nov. 1974.
27. *Schwab, M.: Caring for the aged, Am. J. Nurs **73**:2049-2053, 1973.
28. Swift, N.: Head injury: essentials of excellent care, Nurs. 74 **4**:926-933, Sept. 1974.
29. Teasdale, G.: Acute impairment of brain function-1. Assessing conscious level, Nurs. Times **71**:914-917, 1975.
30. *Wahe, S.: Only a concussion, Nurs. 76 **6**:44-45, Jan. 1976.

28

Altered body image

DOROTHY J. BRUNDAGE

Body image is the mental idea a person has of his body at any moment and is based on past as well as present perceptions. This mental picture of one's body develops over time and is derived from internal sensations, postural changes, contact with outside objects and people, emotional experiences, and fantasies.[34] According to Gorman, the body image is formed by the interaction between the perceptual pool and the experiential pool.[15] The perceptual pool consists of all present and past sensory experiences, while the experiential pool consists of all experiences, affects, and memories. The body image is conceived as being a changing, dynamic entity. Modification occurs with new percepts and new experiences.[30] It varies with age as well as state of health.

Change in the structure, function, or appearance of the body requires modification of the image of the individual's body. The idea of body image disturbances arises from observations that persons with altered structure, function, or appearance may fail to perceive the changes and to adapt to the body as it exists.[20]

Current clinical literature related to persons with altered structure, function, or appearance includes studies of patients following amputation,[13,27] heart attacks,[39] and facial disfiguration.[2,25] Such studies frequently have direct application to patient assessment and intervention by a variety of the health professions involved in rehabilitation of the physically disabled.

A major assumption underlying this chapter is that physical disability or a change in bodily structure that results in altered function or appearance or both are accompanied by an alteration in the person's body image. Interventions by the health team to help the patient manage the results of the physical change must include help in the psychosocial areas of life also affected. Much of the effort made in this latter area is focused on helping the patient recognize, accept, and live with the change in self-concept, which includes both body image and self-esteem. These conditions occur not only in the young but also in the older person. Often there are multiple handicaps, and the financial situation may border on the poverty level. The chronicity of the problem often requires drastic changes in life style.[23]

This chapter will focus on (1) physical causes of alterations in body image; (2) reactions to such alterations; (3) responses to physical disability by the patient, family, health team, and community; and (4) nursing interventions and desired patient outcomes when changed body image occurs. The content of this chapter will be limited to acquired physical alterations. Please refer to pediatric texts for information about congenital problems.

■ PHYSICAL DISABILITY AND CHANGE IN BODY IMAGE

The nature of the change causing altered body image may include (1) altered appearance; (2) altered patterns of eating, breathing, communicating, and elimination; (3) action and motion limitation; (4) deformity; (5) discomfort; (6) stigma; (7) social isolation; and (8) vocational threat.[5]

□ Altered structure: change in function and appearance

Physical changes in body structure may be temporary or permanent. If temporary, the patient generally adjusts and waits out the period of disturbance. The major problems requiring body image alteration are the result of permanent changes in structure. These alterations may be readily visible, as in an amputation of an extremity or facial disfigurement. They may, however, not be visible at all, as in impaired cardiac function after myocardial infarction.

Physical disability can cause loss of function or change in appearance or both. Complete loss of function occurs in paraplegia, hemiplegia, and chronic renal failure. Partial loss of function occurs in chronic respiratory insufficiency and chronic cardiac disease. Renal, respiratory, and cardiac problems show relatively few visible signs of their presence until the problems are far advanced. Appearance is modified in paraplegia as the muscles of the legs atrophy and contractures occur. Fa-

SELECTED CAUSES OF BODY IMAGE ALTERATIONS

Injuries from accidents or war
- Amputation
- Burns: scars and contractures
- Lacerations: scars

Sensorimotor system disease
- Paralysis: paraplegia, hemiplegia
- Blindness, deafness
- Parkinsonism, muscular dystrophy, multiple sclerosis

Change in body structure
- Cardiac, renal, respiratory disease
- Cushing's syndrome
- Rheumatoid arthritis
- Cancer: colostomy, ileostomy, laryngectomy
- Excessive overweight or underweight

cial muscles may droop and the hands may appear flaccid or spastic on the affected side of a patient with hemiplegia. Change in appearance without loss of function occurs with a traumatic injury to the external ear that leaves hearing unimpaired and with facial scarring after multiple lacerations received in an automobile accident. Enucleation of the eye and amputation of an extremity cause marked changes in both function and appearance.

While some physical changes are immediately visible, some must be disclosed during the activities required to replace the functional loss or to improve appearance. A patient with chronic renal failure who requires hemodialysis two or three times a week cannot hide this fact except from strangers. The person with an artificial eye, ear, or nose may under some circumstances (such as hospitalization) be forced to share this information.

□ Causes of body image alteration

Major causes of conditions that result in physical disability and altered body image are (1) injuries from accidents and war, (2) diseases of the sensorimotor systems, and (3) changes in body structure from toxic or metabolic disorders (see boxed material). Body image changes related to these conditions may also include the need to incorporate external or internal prosthetic devices or a donated body part.

■ REACTIONS TO BODY IMAGE CHANGES AND LOSSES

Individuals are disturbed when serious threats to or actual deficits in the structure, function, or appearance of the body occur. They must revise long-accepted assumptions about their bodies. Life patterns may need to be changed. The patient faces problems regarding work, social activities, and family. Sexual activities may require modification. The patient may believe that goodness is lost, the ability to accomplish is lost, and that valued skills and talents are impaired. They may feel they are receiving "deserved punishment." One reaction that may interfere with recovery is expectation of rejection and separation. The individual also may feel vulnerable, resigned, rebellious, defiant, rejected, dependent, avoided, resentful, timid, self-conscious, unhappy, humiliated, stigmatized, inferior, and hypersensitive. Indecision, decreased self-respect, bitterness, and cynicism also occur. The hostility of a disabled person toward the healthy may interfere with communication. The attitudes of disabled persons toward themselves are more important than the nature and extent of their disabilities.

□ Grief and mourning

Several authors note that the loss of a valued body part or function is followed by a period of reaction and adjustment that can be compared to the grief and mourning process that follows the death of a loved one[9,16,22,36,43] (see also Chapter 19). Grief is the subjective state of one who has sustained the loss of a valued object, in this instance, physical function or bodily appearance or both. Mourning is the psychologic process by which one works through to acceptance (ideally) of the loss. The subjective reactions to grief include helplessness, loneliness, hopelessness, sadness, guilt, and anger. Mourning usually leads to relinquishing that which was lost. Eventually the person looks at the past realistically and comfortably.

Rubin describes the losses associated with body image change as the loss of the *capacity for functioning* and the loss of the capacity for *control of functioning* in time and place.[33] A sense of shame accompanies such losses. This reaction reflects a private judgment of failure. The intensity of the emotional response seems to be related to the intensity of the struggle to maintain control.

Different responses occured to the same type of deformity in patients with acquired facial disfiguration.[25] A seemingly exaggerated response was found in patients with a slight defect. There was no "typical" response to bodily changes.

□ Important determinants of reactions

The physiologic status of the person, that is, amount of pain, extent of disability, and the realistic expectations of therapy, influence the outcomes of a change in body image.[29] The major categories of psychosocial determinants are (1) the person's premorbid personality and coping behavior, (2) the nature and meaning of the change, (3) the responses from significant others, and (4) the help available to the person and his family.

The physiologic status is relatively fixed for the specific disability. Therefore this section will explore the broader psychosocial factors that are amenable to intervention by health professionals.

Premorbid personality and coping behaviors

Consider the following questions:

1. What are the individual's attitudes toward his body?
2. What concept of illness is held?
3. What experience has there been with illness?
4. How has the patient faced adversity in the past? Rejection? Acceptance? Surrender?
5. What were the attitudes of the patient toward disability before the disability occurred?
6. What is the patient's age and sex?
7. What is the patient's socioeconomic, educational, religious, and cultural background?

Health problems have different meanings at different stages in the life cycle. However, the same problem may be perceived quite differently by persons of the same age. By age 4 the body image is becoming stabilized and will be affected by changes in the body. Special care must be taken to assess the child's perception of his body image because it indicates his personality organization and ego strength.[31] The level of psychosocial development, the quality of the child's relationship with the parents, and previous adjustment are important.[12] In adolescence the body image undergoes a massive upheaval. Physical changes in the body caused by accident or illness place an enormous strain on the coping abilities of the young person.[7]

Murray outlines development of body image through adulthood.[28] The physical changes and the psychologic tasks of those years are described using Erikson's model. The young adult needs independence. The nurse who wishes to "care for" rather than permit self-care may precipitate conflicts. Young veterans with injuries at a time of high physical capability find adjustment very difficult.[6] Aggressive behavior is common. Concern for sexual identity is prominent. Older patients face the changes of aging: physical and social losses and death. The ability to view one's life as having had value helps patients face physical disability.

Meaning of the change

What is the value to the individual of what was lost? What meaning does the part or function have? How intense are the feelings? A person may attribute the successes in life to specific bodily features. When there is an overvaluation and reliance upon security through bodily beauty or activity, alteration in the body image is likely to cause severe emotional disturbances. Women appear to be less disturbed by threats to the body than men.[10] Women are often concerned about cosmetic effects.[36] Men are especially concerned about masculine adequacy, job, and earning capacity.

What effect will the change have on the occupation, social group membership, and habitual ways of interacting? Work is important to a sense of achievement. Work may become "something one is" as well as "something one does."

The extent of the change is an important factor. How severe is the loss? How different will one be from one's peers in appearance, action, and motion? Is it a loathsome mutilation? A change that is recognized by all demands adjustment. The patient may feel isolated, excluded, stigmatized, helpless, ashamed, and lowered in self-esteem and security. What is most important is the patient's perception or definition of the situation. The face has social value and an important role in interpersonal relationships. Physical unattractiveness is associated with social devaluation, denied opportunities, inaccurate judgments of worth, and attacks on self-esteem.

What is the expected duration of the change, its permanency, finality, irrevocability? A loss that carries the threat of future loss obviously creates a greater impact. A mastectomy for cancer carries with it the threat of a recurrence of cancer or death.

The rapidity of onset is quite important. A sudden, unexpected change may be very devastating. A slow progression, as in rheumatoid arthritis or peripheral vascular disease, allows time for anticipatory mourning.

The source of the change, its type, and the opinions of others are important. Hirschfield describes acceptable and unacceptable disability following accidents.[18] Changes resulting from heroic sacrifice are viewed differently from changes resulting from socially unacceptable activities. The loss of a leg saving a comrade in battle is viewed quite differently from loss of a leg in a motorcycle accident during a high-speed chase from the scene of a crime. Sterility following venereal disease may be viewed as deserved punishment, while sterility caused by exposure to prescribed radiation therapy carries no stigma. The cause of the disability (active combat injury versus the sequelae of venereal disease), the type of disability (paralysis versus weakness or anxiety), and the opinion of others (sympathy versus scorn) make the difference.

Responses from significant others

What are the attitudes of others, including parents, siblings, and peers, toward physical disability? Satisfactory social adaptation to a bodily defect depends to a great extent upon family relationships and cultural attitudes toward the body structures involved. The sociocultural milieu is important. What are the specific bodily values of the subculture of the patient? What prejudices are there related to wholeness, independence, and attractiveness?

Does stigma accompany the change? A stigma is an attribute that is deeply discrediting. Goffman discusses the idea of being discredited, that is, having a disability fairly readily noted, and being discreditable, that is, having a disability that may be discovered.[14]

Myths and misconceptions abound regarding one whose body is scarred or misshapen by disease, or is distorted during movement. There is an over-abundance of largely unfounded opinion and folklore regarding physical disability. A strange belief exists that suffering and misfortune somehow make one "a better person." It is also believed that the disabled person mysteriously develops untapped assets and achieves a new depth of understanding and sensitivity.

Help available to patient and family

How a client deals with the loss may well depend on the kind of help available. The help available from the health team and specifically the nurse's role in helping clients with altered body image is discussed later in this chapter. Much of the outcome will depend on whether the patient can and does make use of the help offered.

The rehabilitation program generally has as its goal the recovery of physical function. Psychosocial diagnoses and psychosocial therapy are often secondary. Kutner and Abramson speak strongly for considering the person needing rehabilitation as a complete person with a partial disability.[21] They believe that attempts should be made to strengthen the individual's inner resources and the relationship between the individual and his immediate family. A family assessment should be made and family therapy instituted, if necessary.

■ RESPONSES TO BODY IMAGE CHANGES

What are the expected responses to physical changes that require body image alterations? Adaptive and maladaptive responses of patients are considered next. The responses of family, community, and health team follow. The last part of this section examines the effect of reactions to disability on rehabilitation.

□ Adaptive responses

Those responses in which the patient works through and accepts the loss are considered adaptive. Most commonly the period of crisis is followed by unrealistic defenses, gradual acceptance, and then reduction of the problem to manageable proportions. Responses depend on the number and intensity of the stresses in comparison to the degree of emotional support and the strength of personal attributes. Patients are helped to meet the challenge of disability if they are mature and secure from the start. An acute sense of proportion helps them recognize reality. A sense of humor helps them live with reality. The urge to fight back and pick up the pieces of an interrupted life may motivate the patient. Hunt has edited a series of essays written by persons with disabilities that provide profound insights into their perceptions of living with a disability.[19]

Gruendeman uses Engel's stages of grieving in her discussion of the problems of physical loss.[16]

Stage 1: apprehending the loss. The immediate response is shock and disbelief. This stage may last minutes, hours, or several days. The patient's reactions at first are almost invariably negative. This may or may not be unhealthy. Some denial early in the process is helpful. If prolonged, it may interfere with recovery. The patient is preoccupied with the loss. Crying helps them acknowledge the loss. Depression is common. Uncertainty and pain increase the stress. The early reactions help protect the client from overwhelming stress.

Stage 2: trying to deal with the loss. Patients are aware of sadness, anxiety, and anger both in themselves and others. Preoccupation with the loss is expected. They recognize limits to life. Perhaps limited movement, loss of independence, and restricted choices face the patient. Loss of self-esteem and withdrawal from others may occur.

The time since the loss is important in this stage. As time passes, efforts are directed toward managing the loss. At first the acceptance may be intellectual and on the surface. Usually the client moves on to work through the loss realistically.

Stage 3: resolution of the loss. Eventually the patient looks at the change, the disability, and remembers the past realistically and comfortably. Healthy adaptation includes willingness to discuss the problem, accept offers of help, and use prosthetic devices. Mutual support between the client and his family and the health team is important. Appropriate plans are made for changing jobs, homes, and financial arrangements. When one's emotional investment in the external world is great, bodily losses will be less distressing.[32] The goal is not to give up trying. There is a happy balance between acceptance and dissatisfaction that will assist making the best use of the capabilities one has.

□ Maladaptive responses

When the patient is unable to look at reality, maladaptive responses occur (Chapter 17). Grief is unresolved. The wish to maintain the preexisting body image guides response. Denial of disfigurement and a refusal to accept prosthetic devices are thought to be indications of an unhealthy response. Complete denial may be manifested by withdrawal and aloofness, joking and laughter, or superficial self-confidence.

The loss may be acknowledged, but its significance is denied. The situation is intellectualized. The client may project concern to others: "My wife is very upset about my having to change jobs." Tasks may be avoided. Overcompensation for the loss may occur. Previously learned defense mechanisms may operate: repression and introjection or projection of hostile feelings may interfere with acceptance. The resumption of a social, sexual, and emotional life may be impossible. The disabled person may reject love perceived as adulterated with pity.

Is there obvious disfigurement of the body or hidden disfigurement of the personality? The patient may try to hide the disability and forget it. He pays a high price often for such a futile endeavor. Exaggerated independency, overdependency, and pseudocooperation are responses that interfere with the necessary acceptance of help from the family and health team.

The disability may be used as a crutch. This will cause problems if the defect is corrected.[17] For example, a patient may attribute failures in life to an external facial feature, and when this feature is changed by plastic surgery, he may be forced to face his own shortcomings. A similar situation may exist following changes from illness and injury. In both cases extreme emotional upsets are possible.

Another strategy is to focus attention on a healthy part in order to deny or shut out the damaged part. Idealizing normal standards commits the disabled person to repeated feelings of inferiority. On the other hand, overidentification with the disabled may occur and limit efforts toward achievable levels of rehabilitation. The patient may use the disability as the excuse for early retirement. A return to work can thus be avoided. Another defensive response is the illusion of restoration of the part (phantom).[10] A complete rejection of reality is a psychotic response and may require intense and prolonged therapy.

The effects of the disability may spread beyond the specific structure, function, or change in appearance to other areas of life and activity and increase the patient's limitations. Perceptions of being incompetent, unlovable, insecure, and unworthy reflect low self-esteem. The person's perception of the situation, the responses received from others, and previous experience with losses determine the level of self-esteem and affect coping mechanisms.

The initial response of the family to the loss depends on many factors already discussed. The *rapidity of onset*, the *specific loss*, and *its meaning* are especially important. The patient is the center of attention, and the family is unified by dread, numbness, a sense of unreality, and the shared threat of loss. During the time the patient is denying the situation, the family may also be denying it. Fear and anger may be directed at the staff. The family may lose interest and patience. They may urge the patient to make a more rapid recovery.

The *degree and quality of support* are important. Sometimes families deal well with the immediate threat but have difficulty with the long-term kinds of help needed. The family must acknowledge the change in the patient, their way of life, and the patient's reactions. Family conflicts over the prescribed regimen occur. Families may use the patient's changed state to keep the patient dependent. Rejection by the family complicates the life of a disabled person. They may attempt to conceal the defect by avoiding and isolating the patient. They may be angry, blaming, and rejecting or indifferent. Ambivalence is not uncommon.

The family must acknowledge the change in the patient and deal with changes in the interpersonal reactions within the family. Constructive, supportive attitudes in the family increase the possibilities for successful adaptation for compensatory development without personality disorder.

How does the disability meet or thwart family desires either for the patient or the family? What role reversals are occurring and how acceptable are they? If the patient is the pivotal point in the family, panic may ensue. As the patient moves to reorganize his life, the family reexamines interactions, modifies living arrangements, encourages social activities, and tries to improve family relationships.

□ Community responses

Society values youth and beauty, good looks in facial features, physical wholeness and activeness, and social discrimination against those who are different is common. Physical disability, its thought and reality, provoke stereotyped responses in the general public. The type of deformity rather than its severity evokes the stereotypic response. Subtle and overt negative reactions occur. Repulsion, revulsion, rejection, contempt, ridicule, taunts, discrimination, patronizing aversion, tactless curiosity, staring, questioning, and devaluing pity are frequent.

Reactions to one who is physically disabled may range from overly sympathetic to unsympathetic. One takes on the attitude of others toward one's body. Negative feelings already present about one's body thus may be reinforced by society.

Visible handicaps alter social and psychologic functioning in important ways. Confronting a damaged face disrupts one's sense of inner security. The thought of disfigurement or scarring causes fear of public reaction in most people, and not without cause. Social ostracism is a real possibility. Physical disability is accompanied by a fear of being unable to perform one's regular routines, the fear of loss of control of oneself. It the disability is not visible, it may not be considered to be important by others.

Attitudes toward body structures affect responses to those with physical disabilities. The attitudes of well people affect the social adaptation of those with bodily defects. Disapproval may be present when those persons with disability appear not to be helping themselves. Generalized indifference rejects the reality of the person facing real threats. Studies show that women are more accepting than men, while adolescents are less accepting than those of college age of persons with disability.[26] No significant difference in attitude was found according to socioeconomic status.

Goffman describes two sets of sympathetic others: those who share stigma and the "wise" who are normal but are acquainted intimately with the secret life of the stigmatized.[14] The latter includes family members and professional persons involved in the patient's care.

□ Health team responses

Members of the health team are not immune to negative attitudes toward the disabled. They may subscribe to certain stereotypes, especially with regard to sexual functioning in persons with disabilities. Condescension, resentment, insensitiveness, and aloofness can be found in those "dedicated to help." The health team may expect a passive, compliant, dependent patient. They may feel protective or they may react with superiority. Examples of negative attitudes are reflected in the use of such labels as "unmotivated" as justification for closing a case. The use of stereotype labels—"CPs," "CVAs," "quads"—reflects obvious disregard for the individuality of the patient. The reactions of health professionals may include embarrassment, undefined anxiety, relief if the patient is cheerful, abandonment by disregarding stress signals, and maintenance of a superficial atmosphere to being thoughtful, understanding, and helpful. Anger at being unable to help is a recurring phenomenon.

Health professionals can contribute to a patient's lowered self-esteem when they express openly or covertly negative reactions to the change in structure, function, or appearance. A patient's loss of control threatens the health professional's control. Sarcasm covered with saccharine sweetness and teasing may be signs of displaced anger. People reject what they cannot cope with, and they may withdraw from the situation. Health professionals should honestly explore their feelings toward the patient with bodily changes.

Little investigation of health team attitudes has been done. This is unfortunate, for as McDaniel says, the health team probably is more important in shaping the patient's response than any other group.[26] Persons who work with the disabled should try to be as sensitive and perceptive as possible about their own responses to disability and the disabled and about the patient's emotional reactions to his problems.

□ Reactions to physical disability and rehabilitation

Rehabilitation attempts to enable the disabled person to live within the limits of his disability but to the full extent of his capacity. How do reactions to physical disability affect the rehabilitation of the physically disabled?

Rehabilitation will be impeded if the person with the disability feels inferior, self-conscious, frustrated, preoccupied with the deformity, hypersensitive, anxious, hostile, or paranoid. One measure of the capacity to adapt is the person's willingness to participate in a program of restoration or rehabilitation.[36]

Disability may be perceived by some as deserved punishment or by others as a source of pride: the person is specially selected by God to suffer. Dependency in disability may be hard to accept or be welcomed, temporary or permanent. The exemptions and privileges of illness may be tempting, and some patients find it to their advantage to be disabled.[10] Such a person gains the satisfaction of security and other psychosocial needs without stigma or shame attached to the role change.

■ NURSING MANAGEMENT FOR PERSONS WITH ALTERED BODY IMAGE

Persons with changes in structure, function, and appearance face problems related to (1) physical limitations and failures; (2) discomfort from appliances, abnormal sensations, and fatigue; (3) visual or auditory changes in appearance; (4) vocational and economic limitations; and (5) social interaction limitations.

□ Assessment

Bernstein has delineated six axes for adjustment to disability[2]: (1) active coping—passive surrender; (2) leading and comanaging treatment—resisting treatment; (3) loving exchange—rage; (4) denial—overawareness; (5) adaptive defenses—maladaptive defenses; and (6) mental (activity) mode—physical (activity) mode. Along each axis are important variables. Complex interwoven patterns form within a matrix of factors including money, education, family support, religious help, and rehabilitation services. Bernstein has found this framework helpful in looking at the catastrophe of burn disfigurement.

The patient's perception of the situation and his usual pattern of adapting must be considered in planning nursing intervention. How does the patient deal with stress? What threats are seen as dangerous? What are the patient's goals? Consider the patient's personality, values, needs, and readiness for learning.

Does the patient cry? If not, consider the following possibilities. The patient cannot cry or does not want to cry or perhaps the loss will not be missed. Usually, however, there is ambivalence with feelings of guilt and shame.

Recognize the energy used to handle the enforced

awareness of the disability. Be aware of how far the patient has come and the distance yet to go.

Appraise the response of family members and significant others. Identify the patient's support systems—those people and resources that may assist during the period of adaptation. Consider the importance of the patient's peers.

Transitional points of entry and termination are critical points of emotional adjustment—they reflect periods of change. The move from rehabilitation center to home for a patient with paraplegia or the first hemodialysis treatment at home for a patient with chronic renal failure are examples of such points.

□ Intervention

Nursing care is important during the *acute, convalescent,* and *rehabilitative* phases following disability.[5] During the acute phase the nursing focus is on activities such as life-saving techniques, assisting with diagnosis, and preoperative and postoperative care. Most frequently the patient is hospitalized. The goal is to save life, halt illness, and to prevent helplessness and deformity.

During the convalescent phase nursing activities include assisting the patient to adjust to change, maintaining physical abilities through occupational therapy and physical therapy, and home planning with the family, community health nurse, and social worker. The patient may still be hospitalized but may be at home. The goal is to prepare for the rehabilitative phase.

The rehabilitative phase includes coordination of specialized services (as needed) of the physiatrist (specialist in rehabilitation medicine), speech therapist, prosthetist, psychologist, vocational counselor, and social worker. The patient may be an outpatient or an inpatient in a rehabilitation center. The goal is to complete the maximum rehabilitation of the patient, including sexual functioning.

Physical function should not be considered to the exclusion of the affective implications of the disability. During the acute phase, the nurse should not expect clear reasoning. A quiet, reassuring manner that focuses on reality and short, truthful answers are appropriate in this early phase. Help the patient verbalize his feelings, avoid despair, and plan realistically for the future. Do not reinforce negative behavior. Try to identify the causes of the patient's behavior. Bring reality to the patient in manageable steps. Nonjudgmental, reassuring approaches used with persistence help maintain the rapport needed for the patient to work through to the reality of the situation. Meet the patient's needs, but avoid perpetuating dependency.

□ General aspects of nursing care

The person with a disability needs understanding. Assume that the patient is coping with an overwhelming experience, support the self-esteem necessary to reorganize the body image, and permit crying in such a manner that the patient still has a sense of self-respect and worthiness. Give the patient time, and help him confront the problem in manageable steps. Acknowledge appropriate feelings, recognize assets and strengths, and provide support to the extent needed, that is, the degree mutually agreed upon.

Let the patient ventilate, helping him clarify misconceptions. Promote a sense of trust, respect, security, and comfort. It is essential for the patient to come to terms with the change. Reassurance that "you'll be as good as new" delays adjustment and raises false hopes. Do not encourage the patient to blame others; rather, assist the patient to accept help with everyday tasks. Counteract the effects of deprivation and immobilization by helping the patient understand what is occurring and maintaining the remaining body integrity. The focus of care is on what is left—not what is lost.

Be accepting within appropriate limits. Assure the patient that grief is normal. The patient must also accept the fact that permanently unattainable goals exist. Privacy and a safe environment are necessary for the patient to achieve control of a lost or altered body function. Avoid overprotection and unnecessary restrictions. Explore realistic alternatives rather than being overly optimistic or pessimistic. Help the patient find the facts, as speculating can be worse than the truth. Help the patient develop compensatory personality traits.

Predict the occurrence of body image problems, prevent them where possible, and be ready to intervene to help solve them when necessary. Anticipatory guidance and preventive intervention help to promote the capacity of individuals to cope with life crises. Prepare patients before surgery or before receiving drugs that alter body image. Consider various influencing factors. Recognize the need for grief and mourning. Help the patient strengthen both coping mechanisms and problem-solving skills.

□ Health team

All the health team members must work through their feelings regarding loss, disability, and disfigurement, and examine their behaviors used in coping with such threats. If this conscious self-examination is omitted, feelings and behaviors may interfere with the patient's rehabilitation and may result in the professional's leaving this field of service. Staff responses to persons with disability should be honest, patient, consistent, realistic, and firm, but not hostile. Often they must accept the patient despite his hostility and rejection toward them. Every effort must be made to avoid reinforcing the person's low self-esteem. Special preparation is needed for open, honest discussion of the patient's problems with sexuality.[42] Consistent support promotes the trust vital to learning to cope with altered structure, function, and appearance.

□ Evaluation

Positive attitudes of the patient toward rehabilitation, the staff, and program of help are desirable. Acceptance and use of prosthetic devices are expected. Desired patient outcomes include self-assurance, confident behavior, self-reliance, stable motivation, self-acceptance, and adequate social interactions. It is generally accepted that a person is happier if involved in productive activities.

Siller suggests that one outcome measure of the acceptance of the loss is the degree that the reconstituted self is oriented toward self-approval and is responsive to reality.[38]

Some dependency may be legitimate, and some physical help may be needed. Retirement from gainful employment may be required, or reduced household responsibilities and a sharp curtailment of social activities may be unavoidable.

Litman's study of family disruption because of disability shows no significant relationship between the degree of family solidarity and rehabilitation response.[24] However, family support during rehabilitation has a significant effect on the patient's response to the program. The family consequently reexamines and probably reorients interpersonal relationships and readjusts living arrangements.

Employment, school attendance, or home responsibilities are insufficient measures of outcomes for many patients. A useful tool for assessing the level of rehabilitation in nonhospitalized patients by nonphysician raters is the Functional Life Scale.[35] It considers cognition, activities of daily living, home activities, activities outside the home, and social interaction. Regular use of such a tool could help nurses assess needs and evaluate outcomes in their efforts to improve the quality of life of patients with physical disabilities. Much more knowledge is needed in the area of evaluation of patient outcomes for persons with changes in body image.

REFERENCES AND SELECTED READINGS

1. Abramson, A. S., and Kutner, B.: A bill of rights for the disabled In Meislin, J.: Rehabilitation medicine and psychiatry, Springfield, Ill., 1976, Charles C Thomas, Publisher.
2. Berstein, N. R., and Cope, O.: Emotional care of the facially burned and disfigured, Boston, 1976, Little, Brown & Co.
3. Blaesing, S., and Brockhaus, J.: The development of body image in the child, Nurs. Clin. North Am. **7**:597-607, 1972.

3a. *Brown, M. S.: Distortions in body image in illness and disease. In Bower, F. L., editor: Wiley nursing concept modules, New York, 1977, John Wiley & Sons, Inc.

3b. *Brown, M. S.: Normal development of body image. In Bower, F. L., editor: Wiley nursing concept modules, New York, 1977, John Wiley & Sons, Inc.

4. Brundage, D. J.: Assessing rehabilitation in home dialysis patients. Paper presented at Thelma Ingles Scholarly Paper Presentation, Sigma Theta Tau, Beta Epsilon, 1976, Durham, N.C.
5. Brundage, D. J.: Physical disability: reactions and interventions, Durham, N.C., 1971 (unpublished teaching-learning resource unit).
6. Compton, C. Y.: War injury: identity crisis for young men, Nurs. Clin North Am. **8**:53-66, 1973.
7. Dempsey, M. O.: The development of body image in the adolescent, Nurs. Clin. North Am. **7**:609-615, 1972.
8. Engel, G. L.: Grief and grieving, Am. J. Nurs. **64**:93-98, 1964.
9. Engel, G. L.: Psychological development in health and disease, Philadelphia, 1962, W. B. Saunders Co.
10. Fisher, S.: Body experience in fantasy and behavior, New York, 1970, Appleton-Century-Crofts.
11. Fisher, S., and Cleveland, S. E.: Personality, body perception, and body image boundary. In Wapner, S., and Werner, H., editors: The body percept, New York, 1965, Random House, Inc.
12. Fujita, M. T.: The impact of illness or surgery on the body image of the child, Nurs. Clin. North Am. **7**:641-649, 1972.
13. Garrett, J. F., and Levine, E. S.: Rehabilitation practices with the physically disabled, New York, 1973, Columbia University Press.
14. Goffman, E.: Stigma: notes on the management of spoiled identity, Englewood Cliffs, N.J., 1963, Prentice-Hall, Inc.
15. Gorman, W.: Body image and the image of the brain, St. Louis, 1969, Warren H. Green, Inc.
16. Gruendemann, B. J.: Problems of physical self: loss. In Roy, S. C.: Introduction to nursing: an adaptation model, Englewood Cliffs, N.J., 1976, Prentice-Hall, Inc.
17. Gruendemann, B. J.: The impact of surgery on body image, Nurs. Clin. North Am. **10**:635-643, 1975.
18. Hirschfield, A. H., and Behan, R. C.: The accident process. 3. Disability: acceptable and unacceptable, J.A.M.A. **197**:85-89, 1966.
19. Hunt, P., editor: Stigma: the experience of disability, London, 1966, Geoffrey Chapman Publishers.
20. Kolb, L. C.: Disturbances of the body-image. In Arieta, S., editor: American Handbook of psychiatry, vol. 1, New York, 1959, Basic Books, Inc., Publishers.
21. Kutner, B., and Abramson, A. S.: Rehabilitation goals—myth or reality. In Meislin, J.: Rehabilitation medicine and psychiatry, Springfield, Ill., 1976, Charles C Thomas, Publisher.
22. Lee, J. M.: Emotional reactions to trauma, Nurs. Clin. North Am. **5**:557-587, 1970.
23. Leonard, B. J. Body image changes in chronic illness, Nurs. Clin. North Am. **7**:687-695, 1972.
24. Litman, T. J.: The family and physical rehabilitation, J. Chronic Dis. **19**:211-217, 1966.
25. MacGregor, F. C.: Psychosocial approach to patients with facial disfigurement. In Wood-Smith, D., and Porowski, P. C., editors: Nursing care of the plastic surgery patient, St. Louis, 1967, The C. V. Mosby Co.
26. McDaniel, J. W.: Physical disability and human behavior, New York, 1969, Pergamon Press, Inc.
27. Mital, M. A., and Pierce, D. S.: Amputees and their prostheses, Boston, 1971, Little, Brown & Co.
28. Murray, R. L. E.: Body image development in adulthood, Nurs. Clin. North Am. **7**:617-630, 1972.

*References preceded by an asterisk are particularly well suited for student reading.

29. Murray, R. L. E.: Principles of nursing intervention for the adult patient with body image changes, Nurs. Clin. North Am. **7**:697-707, 1972.
30. Norris, C. M.: The professional nurse and body image. In Carlson, C. E.: Behavioral concepts and nursing intervention, Philadelphia, 1970, J. B. Lippincott Co.
31. Riddle, I.: Nursing interventions to promote body image integrity in children, Nurs. Clin. North Am. **7**:651-661, 1972.
32. Rosillo, R. H., Welty, M. J., and Graham, W. P.: The patient with maxillofacial cancer. II. Psychologic aspects, Nurs. Clin. North Am. **8**:153-158, 1973.
33. Rubin, R.: Body image and self esteem, Nurs. Outlook **16**:20-23, 1968.
34. Salkin, J.: Body ego technique, Springfield, Ill., 1973, Charles C Thomas, Publisher.
35. Sarno, J. E., Sarno, M. T., and Levita, E.: The functional life scale, Arch. Phys. Med. Rehabil. **54**:216-220, 1973.
36. Schoenburg, B., Carr, A. C., Peretz, D., and Kutscher, A. H., editors: Loss and grief: psychological management in medical practice, New York, 1970, Columbia University Press.
37. Shontz, F. C.: Perceptual and cognitive aspects of body experience, New York, 1969, Academic Press, Inc.
38. Siller, J.: Psychosocial aspects of physical disability. In Meislin, J.: Rehabilitation medicine and psychiatry, Springfield, Ill., 1976, Charles C Thomas, Publisher.
39. Smith, C.: Body image changes after myocardial infarction, Nurs. Clin. North Am. **7**:663-688, 1972.
40. Tourkow, L. P.: Psychic consequences of loss and replacement of body parts, J. Am. Psychoanal. Assoc. **22**:170-181, 1974.
41. Wolanin, M. O.: Basic concepts of health: reactions to illness. In Moidel, H. C., Sorenson, G. E., Giblin, E. C., and Kaufman, M. A., editors: Nursing care of the patient with medical-surgical disorders, New York, 1970, McGraw-Hill Book Co.
42. Woods, N. F.: Altered levels of sexual function. In Boroch, R. M.: Elements of rehabilitation in nursing, St. Louis, 1976, The C. V. Mosby Co.
43. Wright, B. A.: Physical disability—a psychological approach, New York, 1960, Harper & Row, Publishers, Inc.

29

Chronic illness

PATRICIA BUERGIN

Prevention and control of chronic diseases is one of the major health problems in the United States today. The incidence and prevalence of and the mortality from chronic diseases has increased since the beginning of the nineteenth century, with the most rapid increase occurring in recent years. This increase has been brought about by a number of developments, one of the first of these being the general improvement in sanitation methods that led to reduction of many acute, often fatal infections such as typhoid fever. A further reduction in deaths caused by the acute communicable diseases came about as causative organisms were identified, immunizations against some of them were developed, and drugs to combat many others were discovered. In 1900 the leading causes of death were pneumonia, influenza, tuberculosis, and those diseases classified as gastritis. Today the leading causes of death are diseases of the *heart*, *malignant neoplasms*, and *vascular lesions* of the *central nervous system*.

There has been a tendency among health workers to equate chronic disease with old age. While it is true that many elderly people have one or more chronic diseases such as arteriosclerosis, osteoarthritis, and diabetes mellitus, chronic disease is also common in the younger age group. Because of strides made in pediatric medicine, children who 30 years ago would have died for lack of knowledge and treatment of diseases like cystic fibrosis are now living longer with those chronic diseases. Predictions of the number of persons who may be afflicted with chronic illness in the future must be based on predictions of population growth based on fertility rates. *Based on these predictions and present figures, it is estimated that by 1980 there will be 39.5 million more people than in 1965 who will have one or more chronic conditions, and that 24.4 million of these will be under 35 years of age.*[18]

DIFFERENCES BETWEEN ACUTE AND CHRONIC ILLNESS

An *acute illness* is one caused by a disease that produces symptoms and signs soon after exposure to the cause, that runs a short course, and from which there is usually a full recovery or an abrupt termination in death. Acute illnesses may become chronic. For example, a common cold may develop into chronic sinusitis. A *chronic illness* is one caused by disease that produces symptoms and signs within a variable period of time, that runs a long course, and from which there is only partial recovery. The symptoms and general reactions caused by chronic disease may subside with proper treatment and care. This period during which the disease is controlled and symptoms are not obvious is known as a *remission*. However, at a future time the disease becomes more active again with recurrence of pronounced symptoms. This is known as an *exacerbation* of the disease. A chronic disease is characterized by remissions and exacerbations and slowly progressive physical changes. Many emotional, social, and economic implications of chronic illness will be mentioned later in this chapter.

Acute exacerbations of chronic disease often cause the patient to seek medical attention and may lead to hospitalization. Distinction must be made between acute illness and an acute phase of a chronic illness. The needs of a patient who has an acute illness may be very different from those of the patient with an acute exacerbation of a chronic disease. For example, a young person may enter the hospital with complaints of fever, chest pain, shortness of breath, fatigue, and a productive cough. If the diagnosis is pneumonia, the patient usually can be assured of recovery after a period of rest and a course of antibiotic treatment. However, if the diagnosis is rheumatic heart disease, and if the patient is being admitted to the hospital for the third, fourth, or fifth time, the reassurance needed will not be so definite, clear-cut, or easy to give. In this instance it is necessary to begin planning care that will extend beyond the period of hospitalization, taking into consideration many aspects of the patient's total life situation. The concerns of the patient who has repeated attacks of illness will be very different from the concerns of the one who has a short-term illness.

Further, the needs of patients who are admitted to the hospital with an acute illness but who also have an underlying chronic condition must not be overlooked. For example, the elderly patient who enters the general hospital with pneumonia may receive treatment for the pneumonia and recover from his illness. However, he may still be hampered by the arteriosclerotic heart disease and arthritis that he has had for years. These two chronic conditions may have been aggravated by the acute infection, or the patient's return to his former activity may be hindered by joint stiffness resulting from enforced bed rest and inactivity. Consideration of the patient's several diagnoses can help in preventing new problems associated with his chronic illness.

■ CHRONIC ILLNESS AS A FORCE IN SOCIETY

□ Extent and effect of chronic illness

According to the National Health Survey, 73.8 million people have one or more chronic conditions. The National Health Survey list of chronic diseases includes asthma, allergy, tuberculosis, bronchitis, emphysema, sinusitis, rheumatic fever, arteriosclerosis, hypertension, heart disease, cerebral vascular accident and other vascular conditions, hemorrhoids, gallbladder or liver disease, diabetes mellitus, thyroid disease, epilepsy or convulsions, spinal disease, cancer, chronic dermatosis, and hernia.

In 1974 an estimated 29,292,000 persons, about 14.1% of the civilian, *noninstitutionalized* population of the United States, were reported to be limited to some extent in performing normal activities as a result of chronic disease or impairment. Of these, approximately 8% were under the age of 17 years; 24% were 17 to 44 years of age; 35% were 45 to 64 years of age; and the remaining 32% were 65 years and over.[31] Of the total 29.3 million persons who had activity limitations approximately 22 million (75%) were limited in their ability to carry on their major activity (work, keep house, go to school, engage in preschool activities). Those totally unable to carry on their major activity numbered 6.9 million (23.6%).[31] Research has further indicated that those persons with chronic illness who are limited in mobility as well as in ability to carry on their major activity are confined to bed more days per year than those who have only activity limitations.[33]

The inability to work or to move about influences greatly the kind of medical treatment and health supervision needed by persons who have chronic illness. Some persons need only periodic medical examination and perhaps continuing treatment with medications; others may require complete physical care. Some have a disease that progresses very slowly without remissions, while others may have episodes of acute illness and then seem comparatively well for a time. Each person requires a thorough assessment to determine the stage of his illness, the course his illness is likely to take, the type of care he will need, and the method by which that care will be delivered if he is to be helped appropriately.

□ Cost of disability

For the individual and his family, the costs of disability are temporal, emotional, and financial. The goal of maintaining the patient in the best possible condition relative to his illness must be the primary concern, since a good program of maintenance is the best way to help the patient avoid excessive financial drain caused by unnecessary or preventable complications. Meeting this goal, however, can require that extensive periods of time be spent on treatments, maintenance regimens, and follow-up appointments. Further, each chronically ill person and his family is subjected to great personal and emotional losses that must be dealt with—loss of self-esteem, loss of status within the family, loss of independence, feelings of rejection, and feelings of helplessness are only a few. These can be more devastating than economic deprivation.

The economic cost to the patient and his family is considerable. The cost of hospitalization rises yearly. Frequent or extended hospitalization and medical expenses can be ruinous if the patient is inadequately insured or if he is unable to qualify for insurance programs. Many are forced to seek public assistance merely to survive. Placement in quality nursing homes is frequently financially impossible for patients or their families to manage. The cost of medications to control or maintain a patient's health status may require a major portion of the family budget.

The ability of the individual family to pay its own way is determined in part by which member of the family becomes disabled. Studies show that if the wife is disabled, the family suffers less economic deprivation than if the husband is disabled. However, three fourths of the chronically ill persons unable to carry on their major activity are men.[31]

In considering the cost of disability to the community, it must be realized that most individuals who are unable to work must be supported by others, either from private or from public funds. There are 3 million adults between the ages of 18 and 64 years who are unable to work because of chronic disabilities. There are an additional 9.4 million who are partially limited in ability to work.[31] Many of the totally disabled persons are now receiving benefits under the *Social Security Administration's Old-Age, Survivors,* and *Disability Insurance* programs. An additional number receive public assistance from *Aid to the Permanently and Totally Disabled Program.*

The death rate of the disabled population is high. For

persons under 50 years of age, the death rate is ten times that of the total population between the ages of 25 and 49 years. The death rate for disabled persons between the ages of 50 and 54 years is higher than for all persons in the general population who are 75 to 84 years of age.

□ Chronically ill person and his family

The effects of chronic illness on individuals and their families are numerous and varied. The first impact of the disability may nearly immobilize them. Time must be provided for both to talk through their concerns and fears before either can be expected to begin coping with their new situation.

Marked changes often take place, and are often required to take place, in family living as a result of chronic illness. Some families may find themselves drawn closer together. For example, when it is suddenly learned that the mother has a heart condition, the husband and teenage children may rally to assist in household chores. All seem to work together with a special purpose in mind. Other families may drift apart, the individual members being incapable of helping one another. At times, chronic illness may threaten an individual's basic emotional stability, and the whole situation may be unbearable to others. Sometimes the individual's emotional needs may not have been apparent to the family early in the illness, but when such needs grow obvious, relatives feel inadequate in the situation. The length of illness, periodic hospitalization, and increased financial, emotional, and social burdens are stressors that threaten the family's integrity.

Many persons struggle on their own to assume the full financial burden and consequently expose other members of the family to lower standards of nutrition, housing, and care. Many times relatives move in with one another, arguments develop, and family ties are strained or broken. Public assistance may be accepted by some families, whereas others find it degrading.

Chronic illness imposes additional problems of learning how to cope with restrictions on activities of daily living (ADL), how to prevent or identify medical crises that occur, and how to carry out treatment regimens as delineated by the health care provider. Family members also need to learn about the restrictions, not only to be of assistance to the chronically ill person, but also because their own activity patterns may be disrupted by the patient's activites.

Since chronic illness has periods of exacerbation when symptoms become more acute and medical crises may occur, patients and family members need to know which symptoms must be reported to the health care provider as well as the time interval for reporting these symptoms. They also need to know how to contact the provider and what measures to take if a medical crisis occurs. For example, the person who has a history of myocardial infarction (heart attacks) and his significant others must know what to do if he should sustain severe chest pain. Should he be taken immediately to a hospital emergency room or should the physician be contacted first? Patient and family should thus plan in advance the sequence of actions to take during a medical crisis, depending on the nature and extent of the presenting symptoms.

Persons with chronic illness are often labeled as "compliant" or "noncompliant" in carrying out regimens prescribed for them. There are many factors that influence the person's ability or motivation to carry out the prescribed regimen. If the person does not carry out the regimen (noncompliant), it does not necessarily mean that he is refusing to do so deliberately, although this may sometimes occur. One reason for noncompliance may be lack of knowledge of the importance of doing what is required because learning never occurred. The person may have been "told" the reason for the regimen, but he may not have perceived it or have internalized it. In many situations, however, there are other more influential factors for noncompliance: (1) time-consuming activities, (2) difficult techniques to learn or carry out, (3) presence of side effects, (4) expense, (5) visibility to others, (6) inefficient as perceived by client, or (7) socially isolating.[42] Social and cultural patterns will also affect compliance. (For further information on sociocultural effects, see Chapter 3.) Conflicts occur within the family structure when one family member recognizes the importance of carrying out the prescribed regimen but another does not. For example, a wife may see the need for continuing checkups and medication for her husband's hypertension, whereas he may perceive this as a needless expense since he feels well and has no symptoms. Persons vary from time to time in the extent of compliance. The person in the noninstitutionalized setting is his own health care agent and he (or his significant others) determines the actions that he takes.

Both because they vary so greatly and because they are central to the life of the chronically ill person and his family, the coping mechanisms that have been developed should not be tampered with unless, based on thorough understanding of the situation, viable alternatives can be proposed. If the goal of maintaining the chronically ill person in his optimum state of health is being interfered with by the individual's or the family's attitudes or capacities, a change in those attitudes or capacities is necessary; but it must be a change that is mutually acceptable.

■ EARLY DETECTION OF CHRONIC ILLNESS

Relatively little is known about how to prevent chronic illness. Predisposing characteristics or habits that help to identify the person likely to develop a particular chronic disease have been studied extensively. By altering habits of eating, rest, activity, or smoking, the course of certain chronic illnesses such as emphysema, hypertension, or heart disease may be changed. Unfortunately, many chronic conditions begin without the individual's awareness of significant physiologic changes. An important step in prevention is early detection of these changes.

Screening programs and periodic health examinations are two methods that have helped to identify persons who are at "high risk" and considered more likely to develop certain chronic diseases. Simple tests are offered to all citizens of the community or to selected groups such as workers in industry, children at school, women, or men. Some of the more familiar screening tests are chest x-ray examinations to detect heart disease, cancer, or tuberculosis; urine or blood sugar tests to detect possible asymptomatic diabetes; blood pressure determinations to detect hypertension; and screening of school-age children for scoliosis.

Screening tests may be offered to apparently well persons who have no particular symptoms. Often in the course of interviews with persons coming to these screening programs, signs and symptoms of chronic illness are obvious to the interviewer although the person has either attached no meaning to them, ignored them, or attributed them to some other cause. Careful questioning about daily activities frequently uncovers discomforts such as joint pain, backache, swelling of the ankles, shortness of breath, and other signs that may indicate early and chronic disease.

The *interview* that accompanies a screening test can be as important in detection as the test itself. Those responsible for planning screening programs should try to ensure the inclusion of an interview as part of the program. In the hospital clinic or community agency, conferences scheduled with parents in order to discuss their children provide ideal circumstances and opportunity to offer counseling, health guidance, health appraisal, and appropriate referral for diagnosis.

Screening tests differ from diagnostic tests in that the latter are used either to establish the presence of disease or to rule it out. Nurses should know the diagnostic facilities available in their community and encourage the public to use them. Earlier medical treatment is now sought by families who carry medical hospitalization or group health insurance, but most persons need help in understanding the importance of early detection.

■ NURSING ASSESSMENT OF THE CHRONICALLY ILL PERSON

Before a plan of care can be devised for the chronically ill person, a thorough assessment of his needs and capabilities must be carried out. Included in such an assessment are the individual's physical, emotional, social, and financial status.

□ Physical status

Since medical diagnoses do not accurately reflect the *physical capacity* of the chronically ill person, the use of a *physical profile system* or assessment tool may be instituted as a guide for those working with the patient. One such tool[26] provides a guide for grading the patient in six different categories: (1) physical condition such as cardiovascular, pulmonary, gastrointestinal, genitourinary, endocrine, or cerebrovascular disorders; (2) upper extremities, including the shoulder girdle and cervical and upper dorsal spine; (3) lower extremities, including the pelvis and lower dorsal and lumbar sacral spine; (4) sensory components relating to speech, vision, and hearing; (5) excretory function, including the bowels and bladder; and (6) mental and emotional status. The completed assessment should indicate in what areas the patient has difficulty and the extent of that difficulty. Such a guide can be used in planning care, both immediate and long term, and will be useful in assisting the family to make realistic plans for the patient's care. Since a chronic condition is not static, reassessment should be carried out at regular intervals to indicate improvement or regression.

□ Emotional status

Assessment of the individual's emotional needs and capacities includes determining his attitudes and stage of adaptation to his illness,[7] his feelings concerning how his illness affects his family or significant others, and his own goals in regard to living with his illness. For example, a person who is almost totally helpless as a result of an accidental spinal cord injury may seem to have no interest in learning ways to help himself. His family may react in the same way and be of little help to him. At this time both the individual and his family need interest and support from professional persons.

□ Social and financial status

Social and financial status must be considered, as they relate specifically to the kind of support and resources available to the individual in meeting his goals. It would be unrealistic, for example, to plan for a hydraulic bathtub chair if the patient could not afford it, family members were unavailable to help operate it, or the patient's apartment manager would not permit it to be installed. Alternative methods of helping the patient to take a tub bath would have to be explored.

The data collected through the performance of this kind of thorough assessment should make it possible to devise a plan of care directed toward the accomplishment of attainable goals that are mutually acceptable to the patient, his family, and the care givers.

■ INTERVENTIONS FOR THE CHRONICALLY ILL PERSON

□ Physical considerations

The first focus in management of the chronically ill person is on *prevention and reduction of disability and on enabling the person to remain a socially functioning individual in every respect.* Some of the disability seen among the chronically ill might have been prevented if prompt, aggressive, suitable medical and nursing care had been available at the onset of the illness. Many of the difficulties that limit the chronically ill may not have been caused by the disease itself but may have developed because of immobility during the acute phase of the illness.

Keeping the patient's body in good alignment, maintaining joint range and strength, and preventing decubitus ulcers are physical measures that must constantly be borne in mind while working with any patient. (For further information see Chapter 41.) A careful plan of rest and activity helps preserve physical resources and makes the day purposeful. If assistance is needed, it should be given until the patient can manage the activity by himself or until an alternative method of management can be taught.

Second, recognizing what is meaningful to the patient is a primary step toward helping him to help himself. Personal needs become of paramount importance to the chronically ill person. Meeting these physical needs provides a way to convey to the patient an interest in his progress and welfare. Helping the patient to take his own bath, to attend to toilet needs, and to groom himself can give him some sense of accomplishment and help him to maintain his self-respect. Helping him to be dressed appropriately promotes a sense of wellness. Success in performing portions of his own self-care may be stimulating enough to strengthen the patient's motivation so that he and his family may make amazing strides in thinking through and working out future problems themselves. In order for their planning to be realistic and ultimately functional, all health care personnel must teach chronically ill persons the total physiologic ramifications of their disability as well as methods of coping with those ramifications.

Patients who are in their homes or in substitute homes should be encouraged to dress in regular, comfortable street clothing rather than in pajamas or gowns. Visitors coming into the home and members of the family who constantly see them dressed in bedclothes think of them as sick and are reminded of their illness. Seeing them dressed as they ordinarily would be helps to maintain normal attitudes, relationships, and expectations.

Activity with a purpose, no matter how small the activity may be, is desirable for the chronically ill person. One may hear him say to friends that he does not have time to visit because he has to take care of the plants, do personal laundry, or perform some other task that may seem unimportant to the casual observer. Actually, to him these jobs may be the most important in the world.

□ Psychosocial considerations

The care of chronically ill persons requires alertness of feeling, seeing, and hearing. Continued warmth and interest are necessary to the well-being of any chronically ill person. Very often it is a relationship based on an understanding of these requirements that helps the individual to become highly motivated. It may be taxing to listen to the same questions and to say the same things day after day, but the nature of chronic illness may require this attention, and the manner in which responses are given will convey warmth and interest. The world of a chronically ill person, whether he is in the hospital or elsewhere, becomes narrowed and circumscribed. He treasures and is interested in those things and those people who are close about him. His conversations may be largely about himself, his immediate environment, a few close objects, and the persons who are close to him. Although he may be confined to bed and to his room, others can keep him up-to-date on outside news. Depending on his level of adaptation to his illness, he may welcome hearing about outside events, or he may not be able to think beyond himself. When he reaches the stage of being able to look beyond himself, newspapers, magazines, radio, television, or creating something with his own hands (Fig. 29-1) may help to keep up his interest in others and in outside events.

Those who work with chronically ill persons need to be able to distinguish between their own values, standards, and goals and those of the patient. In day-to-day contact with an individual who is making little or no progress, it is tempting to make plans for his future because of a sincere interest in helping him. This is particularly true when the patient's age is similar to one's own. There may be a feeling that something must be done to speed progress. One may become frustrated by the feeling of wanting to do something or wanting to see some marked change. However, it must be recognized that management of the chronically ill person requires a slow-moving, persistent pace with possibly little or no change for a long time. His physical and mental condition must be maintained at its present level or improved, and effort must be made to further his progress and to encourage his and his family's adaptation to his condition. His eagerness and readiness to progress will be determining factors for his future. The "doing" in the care of the chronically ill person is not always an active, phys-

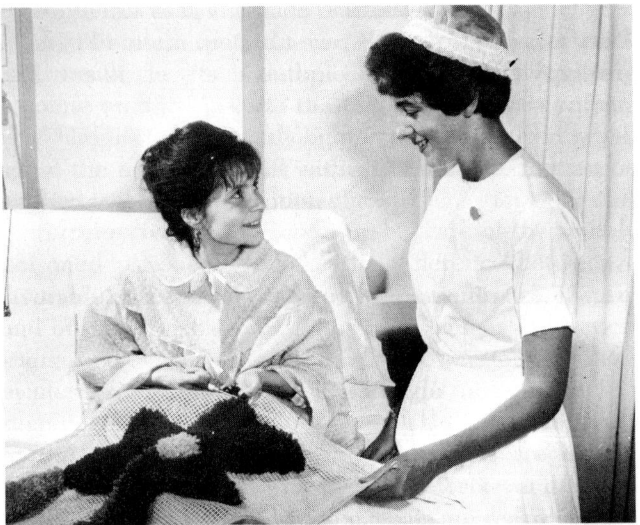

Fig. 29-1. Occupational therapy provides patient with purposeful activity. Interest shown by nurse encourages patient to complete project.

ical "doing" with the hands. Many times the maintenance of a positive approach and attitude and a demonstration of real interest are the greatest help to the patient. Teaching him to help himself in independently performing activities related to his own care, rather than performing those activities for him, is progress.

Health care personnel must also be prepared to provide care for those patients whose disease will follow a course of inexorably progressive disability, for example, multiple sclerosis or malignant rheumatoid arthritis. In these instances, goals of care must be modified to retard the downhill progression of disability rather than achieving maintenance or improvement of physical status. Helping the patient and his family cope with progressive deterioration, and in some cases eventual death, is a demanding task. Those who wish additional information relating to this aspect of care are referred to the literature treating this subject.[7,17,42]

□ Community activities

Some communities have organized "friendly visiting programs" in which volunteer workers go to the hospital or the home to provide companionship and to do errands for patients. Some evaluation of the advisability of such a plan as it relates to each patient should be carried out, since "visitors" are not advisable for all patients. Also, visitors should be selected carefully. Often nurses are called on to help the visitor give appropriate assistance to the patient.

In many communities, public libraries provide facilities for chronically ill or disabled persons. Ceiling projectors for books, books of current interest printed in large type, and recordings of books and music are often available on loan. Volunteer workers may act as readers both in hospitals and in homes (Fig. 29-2). Many libraries and other public buildings have elevators and ramps that make public facilities and activities available to the person who is unable to climb stairs or who is in a wheelchair. Institutions receiving federal funds are now required to make such aids to the handicapped available. Programs, facilities, and legislation of this nature reflect an increasing awareness on the part of the public of the difficulties that are faced by the chronically ill or disabled. That awareness is generating interest in providing further programs to assist these persons in assuming a more active role in their communities.

□ Rehabilitation—a patient care concept

Rehabilitation has been defined by many persons, and each definition seems to express the particular viewpoint of the person or organization offering it. "Rehabilitation is an adjustment to living"[28] is one simple definition. An expanded definition is as follows: "Rehabilitation is the process of assisting the individual with a handicap to realize his particular goals, physically, mentally, socially, and economically."[28] As such, "rehabilitation" is an *active* concept and must be clearly differentiated from the concept of "maintenance" care. Following a thorough assessment of a patient's disabilities and capabilities, assumptions can be made regarding his potential for improving his condition. If improvement can be made, the patient is a candidate for rehabilitation. If improvement cannot be made, care is directed toward maintaining his current condition, that is, preventing further disability. The process of rehabilitation can be viewed more appropriately as patient education rather that patient "care." It must be remembered, however, that the rehabilitation of every patient will reach an end point; that is, a point at which no further progress is possible. At that point the focus of care reverts to that of maintenance.

The purpose or extent of rehabilitation ranges from employment or reemployment for the handicapped person to the more limited achievement of developing the ability to give his own daily care. This latter accomplishment can be just as important to the individual as earning money and may represent his greatest life achievement. This might be true, for example, for a person who was born with a severe physical handicap such as cerebral palsy.

Success in learning to adjust to living with a disability will depend on the person's premorbid personality, total life experience, and premorbid family relationship, as well as the current behavior and motivation the person presents. Certainly some rehabilitation can occur in any

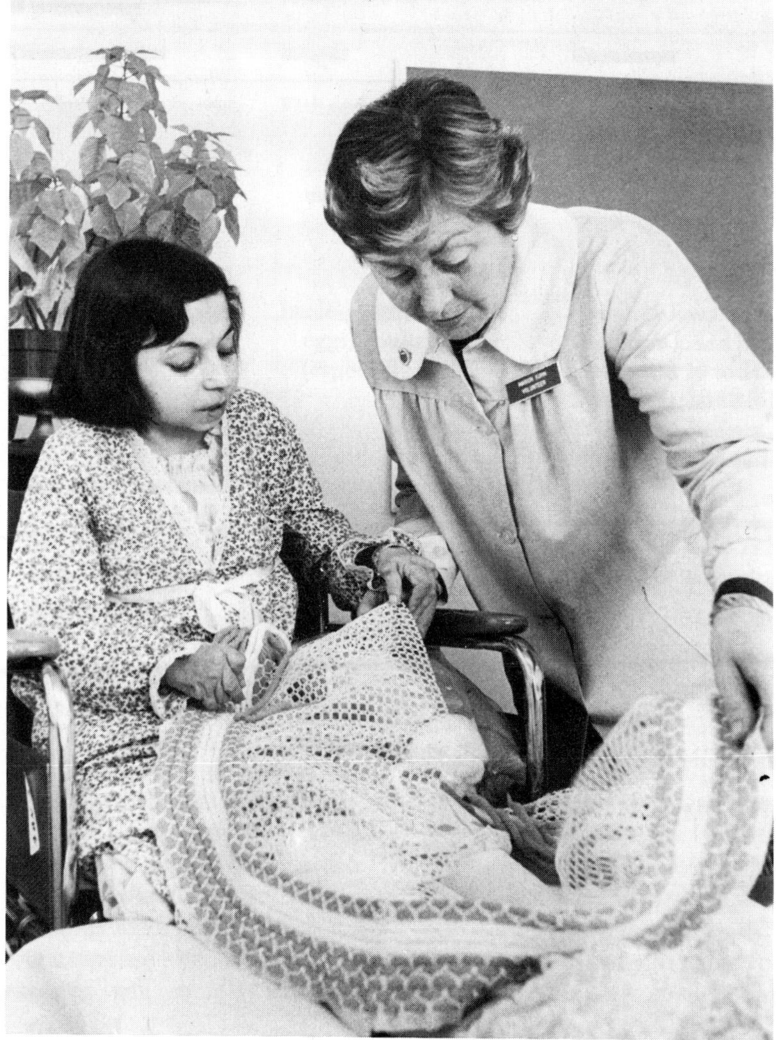

Fig. 29-2. Volunteer helping patient who has a chronic illness with some handwork.

health agency; nevertheless, the greater the number of rehabilitation disciplines that can be made available, as needed, to the individual, the greater is his chance of achieving his highest potential. The rehabilitative process, as any form of education, is involved as deeply in the motives and purposes of the teacher as those of the learner.[44]

The person with a disability, whether it is obvious to others or unrecognizable, should not be viewed from the standpoint of his disability alone. Usually his greatest need is for comprehensive health services and continuing care. *Comprehensive care* has been defined as "care that is provided to the patient according to his needs in an appropriate, continuous, and dynamic pattern."[35] Accommodating the plan of care to the needs and goals of the individual patient rather than to those of the providers of care is the essence of comprehensive care.

Teamwork and special services in rehabilitation

The number of professional people required to assist the patient and his family with rehabilitation will vary. Most often the patient, his family, the physician, and the nurse can work out a practical plan. If a patient's problems are complex, other members may be added to the team. Typically such a team consists of a physician, nurse, medical social worker, vocational counselor, psychologist, speech pathologist, occupational and physical therapists, and a caseworker from the patient's social agency. Teamwork requires that each member be able to use his special knowledge and skill and understand the value of his contribution to the patient's care. In addition, each team member needs some understanding of each of the other professional persons' functions and contributions. One of the cooperative efforts of the involved team members is to meet regularly to thoroughly

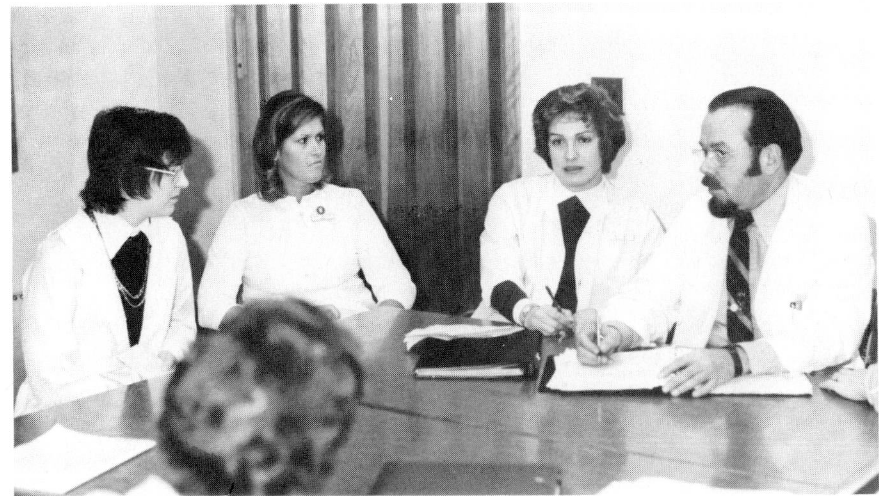

Fig. 29-3. Team approach to rehabilitation is essential. Here, physician, nurse, physical therapist, social worker, and occupational therapist review a patient's program and progress.

evaluate the patient and the abilities he has. Based on this assessment, the patient and the team devise a plan to help him readjust, compensate, and learn new ways of managing self-care and living. In Fig. 29-3 some of the members of a team review a patient's rehabilitation program.

Patients with very complex problems of rehabilitation may need to receive care at specialized centers for rehabilitation, or care at home may be combined with visits to a day rehabilitation center. The variety of specialized centers includes teaching and research centers (centers located in and operated by hospitals and medical schools), community centers wtih facilities for inpatients, community outpatient centers, insurance centers, and vocational rehabilitation centers. In addition to centers that provide multiple services for the physically disabled, there are specialized centers for rehabilitation of the blind, deaf, mentally ill, and mentally retarded. Most centers offer a wide range of services that usually fall into three areas:

Physical area

Physical and medical evaluation
Physical therapy
Occupation therapy
Speech therapy
Medical supervision of appropriate activities

Psychosocial area

Evaluation
Personal counseling
Social service
Psychometrics
Psychiatric service
Recreational therapy

Vocational area

Work evaluation
Vocational counseling
Prevocational experience
Industrial fitness of programs
Trial employment in sheltered workshops
Vocational training
Terminal employment in sheltered workshops
Placement

There are several advantages for patients participating in organized programs for rehabilitation. They have an opportunity to see and be with others who have similar or more extensive disabilities. Often they progress more rapidly when they realize that others have similar difficulties and are overcoming them. Group therapy often arouses a competitive spirit, and a formerly reluctant person may become willing and diligent. On the other hand, all personnel need to be alert to those patients who have had the opposite reaction. A patient who sees others advance in activity while he either does not improve or progresses very slowly may become so discouraged that he gives up trying.

On a rehabilitation unit, activities are scaled so that the individual can see his own progress in comparison with his beginning abilities. Patients may take an active interest in keeping their own scores. After a program of therapy has been planned and is scheduled as to time of day, the patient can help to keep himself on the schedule by having a copy of it at the bedside. He can then be helped to gradually assume more and more responsibility for getting himself ready for scheduled activities. In addition, a master plan of activities for all patients on the unit can be a useful device for nurses, physicians, and therapists. The plan can be kept in a central place on the unit and should list name, activity, and time of activity for each patient. This type of plan is helpful, too, when a patient's progress is to be reevaluated.

In the community a public program for vocational rehabilitation has been serving the nation since 1920 in a partnership between the state and the federal governments. Services for disabled persons are provided by state divisions of vocational rehabilitation. The federal government, through the Social and Rehabilitation Service (SRS), administers grants-in-aid and provides technical assistance and national leadership for the program. Opportunities and services are available in each of the 50 states, the District of Columbia, and Puerto Rico. All persons of working age with a substantial job handicap resulting from either physical or mental impairment are eligible for help or assistance. The purpose of this service is to preserve, develop, or restore the ability of disabled persons to earn their own living. The individual services offered are medical care, counseling and guidance, training, and job finding. Thirty-six states have separate rehabilitation programs for the blind. Application for such services can be made to the Social and Rehabilitation Service or to the agency in the state for serving the blind.

Nurse's role in rehabilitation

The concepts of comprehensive nursing management and rehabilitation can be considered synonymous. Helping the patient and his family to help themselves is an integral part of nursing care. Nurses who work with patients who have disabilities have two major responsibilities: (1) to see that disability from disease is limited as much as possible and (2) to see that a rehabilitation program is planned and implemented. Limitation of disability requires attention to the prevention of complications, to the early recognition of symptoms of exacerbations or complications, and to the prevention of deformity. For patients with chronic illnesses, the onset of exacerbations or complications is frequently subtle, marked by minute changes in functional ability or general performance or attitude. Nurses, working closely with such patients and understanding the pathophysiology of patient's diseases, are frequently the first to recognize initial signs of difficulty and make provision for appropriate intervention.

The second responsibility, planning and implementing a program of rehabilitation in accordance with the patient's goals, is a process in which nurses are intimately involved. Nursing personnel are likely to be in contact with a patient and his family for a greater period of time each day than are members of any other single discipline on the rehabilitation team. Both in the hospital and the home, nurses are in an excellent position to plan a reasonable care program with the patient, as well as to teach the patient, his family, and, if necessary, his employer about his limitations and rehabilitative expectations.

Much of the nursing activity in the rehabilitation process is no different than the nursing care given to all patients. Measures such as appropriate bowel and bladder programs, providing proper diet and fluid requirements, and implementing new methods of bathing and maintaining skin integrity fall within the domain of nursing concern and knowledge. Initially, nursing personnel may assume almost total responsibility for performing these activities for the patient. After assessing patient needs in these areas, nurses formulate, implement, and evaluate a teaching plan in much the same way as do therapists from other disciplines. The assistance nurses will be able to give the patient and his family will depend on an ability to understand self, personal feelings, and personal behavior as well as the behavior of the patient, his family, and other professional team members.

One of the most important aspects of giving continuing care to a patient with a disability is the nurse's own attitude, perseverance, and expectations. Improvement may be slow, and the patient may reach a "plateau" in his progress. Such a time can be critical for the patient because he may become discouraged and not wish to continue with his program of care. Realistic encouragement can often sustain the patient so that he will not regress in any respect until some improvement is noted.

Patients in a rehabilitation program must often learn and practice special physical techniques to strengthen muscles and to improve mobility. Such measures as physical exercise to improve walking, activities to improve self-care abilities, and the use of prostheses require the special knowledge and skills of physical and occupational therapists. To be effective in the rehabilitation process, nurses must have an understanding of the techniques used by the various therapists in order to be able to plan and work cooperatively with the therapist in caring for the patient and to be in a position to help the patient use these techniques in carrying out ADL.

Patient's role in rehabilitation

The most important contributions to the patient's rehabilitation are made by the patient himself. The patient, the nurse, the physician, the social worker, the occupational therapist (Fig. 29-4), and sometimes others planning together can arrive at the best goal for his future, but the patient's attitudes, acceptance, and direction of motivation are the most important considerations. If he cannot adjust to his disability, whatever it may be

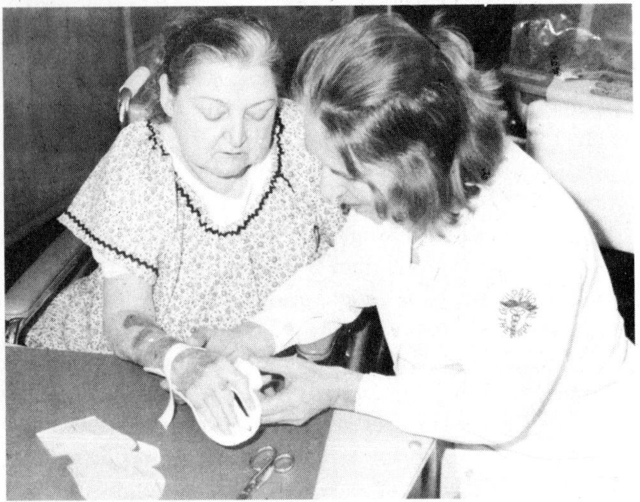

Fig. 29-4. Occupational therapist makes resting splint for patient whose hands are severely deformed by rheumatoid arthritis. Splint will be worn by patient in effort to prevent further deformity.

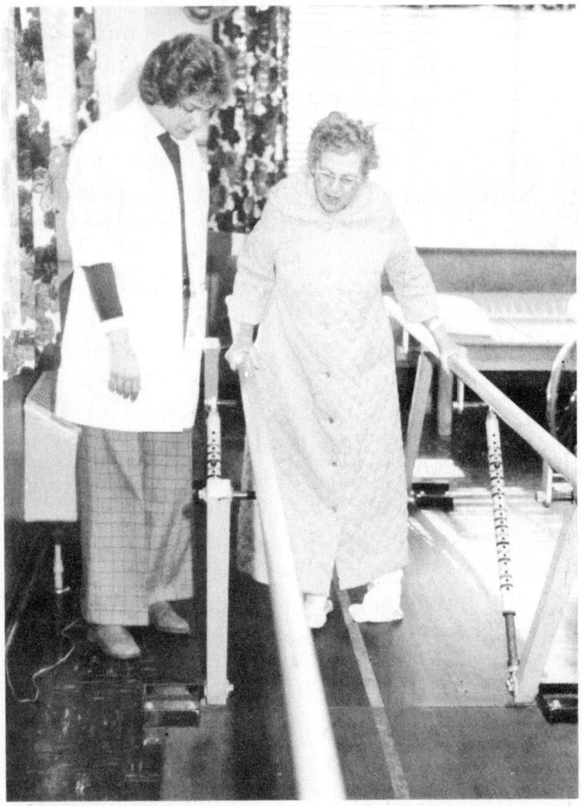

and however extensive it may be, attempts at rehabilitation usually are hindered. The patient is the person who really makes the decisions, and he changes within himself at his own pace. If he is agreeable to helpful suggestions but makes little or no effort to try them, one should question if he really has accepted them.

The patient's behavior from day to day in small ways can be the first indication of the direction of positive motivation. For example, if he makes every effort to resume normal daily activities such as feeding himself, bathing and dressing, one can be quite certain that he is a person with a sincere desire to be independent. As he becomes ready for more advanced activities such as ambulation and work in the occupational therapy shop, he needs continuing genuine interest and support (Figs. 29-5 and 29-6). As obstacles present themselves, he may

Fig. 29-5. Physical therapist begins patient's ambulation training by teaching her to walk with support of parallel bars. Patient's left foot is wrapped in a towel to remind her not to bear weight on it.

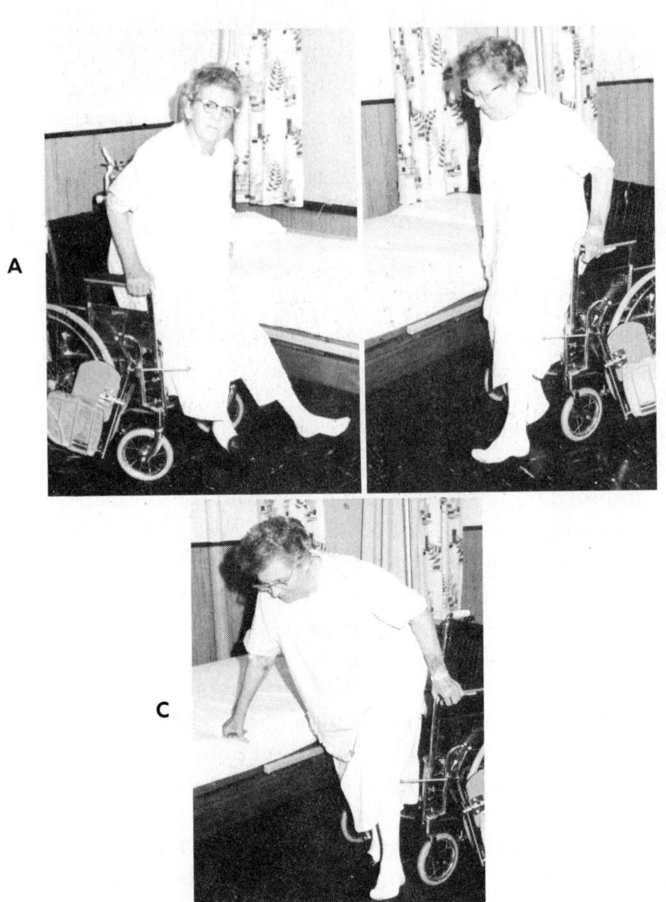

Fig. 29-6. A, Patient executes transfer from bed to chair. She is non-weight-bearing on her left leg; thus she moves toward her right, or strong side. **B,** Here, patient moves back into bed from wheelchair, again leading with her right, or strong side. She pushes up from chair, using arms of chair for support.

be able to accept them and eventually overcome them. Patients who are truly motivated toward helping themselves never seem to give up, finding ways of accomplishing activities that professional personnel might believe impossible. Each person working with the chronically ill has seen that many times life has meaning for the individual even though it may not be apparent to others. However, there are some patients who, when faced with an added burden, cannot accept it and give up trying. Guidance and support for the families of such patients become tremendously important. Health care personnel who understand these attitudes and behaviors can help make life more satisfying for the chronically ill person and can positively influence the behaviors of the family, professional co-workers, and the public.

☐ Considerations for ongoing care

Most persons with a chronic or long-term illness can be cared for at home, and actually prefer to be at home, where family and friends are close by and where they can still contribute something to family life. While they all require health care supervision, the arrangements that can be made vary greatly and depend on the needs of the individual and the facilities available. Many persons are ambulatory and, during remissions, are able to visit their local clinic. Others manage with visits from their personal physicians and with a periodic diagnostic workup done in the physician's office or with the assistance of a technician who goes into the home. Many chronically ill persons with disabilities also visit special rehabilitation units of hospitals or outpatient centers for daily or periodic instruction and practice in physical skills and job training.

Nurses from voluntary and official health agencies help the chronically ill in their homes. Nurses who visit the home to assist the individual or family members to accomplish daily care will need to understand the patient. The chronically ill person is very often misjudged by even the closest members of his family because of lack of understanding. The person's family needs to be helped to understand his limitations and his necessary restrictions. Hopefully this process will have begun while the patient was hospitalized, but will need to continue in the home setting.

Both the individual and his family may benefit from association with others who have had similar experiences. The chronically ill and their families often meet together in organized groups to share experiences. For example, there are organizations for persons who have an "ostomy" and for persons who have had a stroke. There has been a recent growth of such groups because of the increase in chronic illness and because people are reluctant to accept the isolation that chronic illness may impose.

■ PATTERNS AND FACILITIES FOR CONTINUING CARE

It is impossible to include here all of the many facilities that provide continuing care. Only those programs that have been developed or emphasized recently will be covered. It must also be noted that each of the programs that will be mentioned has its own criteria for acceptance of patients for the services it renders. *Before application for service is made, a determination of the individual patient's eligibility for that service must be carried out.*

☐ Ambulatory care

The term "ambulatory care" is used interchangeably with "outpatient care" and refers to health care facilities that provide care for ambulatory patients who return to their home at night. There has been a marked increase in the use of ambulatory care facilities because of the increase of chronic illness and the increase in cost of inpatient services. A good ambulatory care service constitutes one of the most important elements of the hospital's contribution to community health. There is a trend toward development of ambulatory care facilities in neighborhood health centers to assist the disabled, the aged, or the disadvantaged person to obtain needed health care. An ambulatory care center usually provides long-term follow-up care needed by the person with a chronic illness in addition to preventive health care, diasnostic workups, and treatment of acute illnesses for which hospitalization is unecessary.

☐ Home care

Prior to the 1940s the home was the place where medical treatment was given. Well-to-do persons rarely thought of going into a hospital, and they received the services of a private physician in their own home. The family was responsible for the day-to-day care. Poor families were among the first persons to use hospitals. The philosophy of home care can be traced as far back as 1796, when the Boston Dispensary provided medical care to the sick poor in their homes. One of the first institutions to study and demonstrate the advantages of continuous medical care for patients at home was University Hospital in Syracuse, New York, in 1940. By 1950, 16 New York City hospitals were offering this service, and by 1965 there were some 60 coordinated home care programs in the United States.

One of the most obvious reasons for the development of home care programs was to provide care to patients with long-term illnesses who did not need the around-the-clock services of an institution and yet might be too ill to go to an outpatient center. Caring for patients at home is what the individual and his family often want, and it also releases hospital beds for use by acutely ill patients.

In areas where they are available, coordinated home care programs provide comprehensive patient care for persons who otherwise might not receive it. The specification that the program is *coordinated* means that it is centrally administered and, through coordinated planning, evaluation, and follow-up procedures, provides physician-directed medical, nursing, social, and related services to selected persons at home. This program can be offered either by a hospital or by a community agency such as a local health department.

Most patients have been in the hospital before referral to home care and often have had short hospital stays for acute exacerbations or complicated treatments interspersed with periods at home. This service provides care that could not be equaled easily in institutional care. Not only does the patient have the security of knowing that he is counted as a part of the hospital census and will receive continuing care, but he also has the satisfaction of being cared for in his own environment by a group of professional people who know him, his family, and his total situation.

Home care is not the solution for all patients. For those living in smaller dwellings, adequate space for the patient and other members of the family may be at a premium. The choice of home care or institutional care will depend largely on the desires of the patient and his family. Despite many inconveniences, some families wish to have the patient with them. The family's understanding of the patient and his situation and their ability to assist one another will make a great difference. Not only may space be inadequate, but many times it is impossible to have a member of the family in attendance with the patient during the day. Members of the family who work cannot afford to sacrifice jobs to stay with the patient. However, many families find it easier financially to have the patient at home and are able to make satisfactory arrangements even though the facilities are limited.

Many communities now provide portable meals (Meals-on-Wheels) for homebound persons. Most programs provide one hot meal daily and unheated food for at least one other meal. The cost differs widely and depends on the services offered, such as special diets, and on the sponsorship of the plan. Volunteer groups frequently act as delivery messengers. The local public health nursing service usually participates actively in the plan by selecting suitable patients and by being a resource for the workers who encounter health problems on their "rounds." This service alone often makes it possible for a chronically ill person to remain at home.

□ Home health aide services

Home health aide services have developed with the increased use of home care plans and particularly since Medicare plans came into existence. The greater number of persons eligible for home health aide services under Medicare has spurred the growth of such services, not because the services were not needed before, but because the cost of such services would have been prohibitive for most of the persons who needed them. Patients meeting the eligibility requirements for acceptance into this program may be provided with up to 100 visits by a visiting nurse or home health aide. Home health aides, who provide actual physical care to the patient, are being trained in many states and are assigned to home care through a central office that coordinates plans of care, often in collaboration with public health nursing agencies. The public health nurse assists by evaluating the home situation and the patient's need for physical personal care. Consequently the public health nurse supervises the home health aide in the provision of continuing care.

□ Homemaker services

Homemaker services also have developed with the increased use of home care plans. These services are increasingly in demand in many communities and may be sponsored by a public or voluntary health or welfare agency. Homemakers provide service to families with children and to the person who is convalescing, aged, or acutely or chronically ill. Homemakers are trained to assist in homes where the responsible family manager is temporarily unable to perform his or her usual responsibilities because of illness or absence.

□ Day care centers

In a number of communities, some nursing homes are expanding their facilities and services to include day care centers. There are a great number of chronically ill persons who are able to live with their families, but who require 24-hour attendance. Often the caring persons in the family have to work 8 hours a day. Homemaker or home health aide services are generally not available 8 hours a day, 5 days a week. Day care centers fill this gap in care by providing a place where the chronically ill person can be looked after on a daily basis. Nursing services, physical and occupational therapy, recreational facilities, meals, and, in some instances, even transportation to and from the center are provided. This kind of service may very well allow a person to remain at home with his family rather than have to resort to full-time institutional care.

□ Institutional resources

Many patients and families have to resort to institutional care for the patient because their own facilities are not suitable, no member of the family can be in attendance during the day, community alternatives are not available, or the kind of care needed by the patient requires close professional supervision. A large or a limited selection of outside facilities may be available, depending on the community. These include chronic disease hospitals, skilled care facilities, convalescent homes, rest homes, homes for the aged, and nursing homes. The patient's potential for rehabilitation, his need for maintenance care, or the level of his physical disability are factors that will determine his eligibility for placement in any of these facilities.

□ Foster homes

Care in foster homes is a relatively new service that is now being widely used in many communities. Carefully selected families volunteer to take chronically ill persons into their own homes and provide the nonprofessional care that is needed. The family is paid either by the patient or his family, from public funds, or by some social agency. The plan is primarily for those patients who have no family and cannot live alone, but who neither desire nor need institutional care.

□ Nurse's role in continuing health care

A nurse may be involved in continuing health care in a number of ways: (1) as an independent nurse practioner assisting the person with chronic illness to cope with problems incurred by his illness; (2) as a public health nurse or visiting nurse involved in a primary rehabilitative program in the home; (3) as a supervisor of home health aides; or (4) as a nurse in a hospital concerned about the care a patient will be receiving after he leaves the hospital, particularly in situations where the patient's rehabilitation program is not completed or where rehabilitation is not possible. Nurses must know the community resources available to the patient in order to interpret to him and his family what resources he may be able to obtain, the types of services from which he may benefit, and what kinds of referrals he needs for obtaining those services. When care is to be continued beyond the hospital setting, the hospital nurse should clearly communicate (with the patient's permission) to the continuing care agency those data pertinent to the care of the patient in order to provide continuity in the transfer of services. Teamwork and continuity are the keys to successful rehabilitation and management services for patients, and they must be practiced at all stages of the patient's care if the patient is to realize his fullest potential.

OUTCOME CRITERIA

Discharge outcomes for specific chronic diseases are discussed in the chapters dealing with those diseases. However, it may be stated on a general basis that upon discharge from the hospital the patient with a chronic disease or his significant others should be able to:

1. Demonstrate or explain those measures that must be taken to avoid further preventable disability.
2. Demonstrate or explain those self-care activities of which he is capable.
3. Identify those activities for which help is needed.
4. Explain who will be available to help him with those activities and on what basis that help will be available.
5. Explain what community resources are available to him for help and how he may obtain that help.
6. Discuss in reasonable detail his plans for follow-up care and reevaluation.

REFERENCES AND SELECTED READINGS

1. Anderson, H. C.: Newton's geriatric nursing, ed. 5, St. Louis 1971, The C. V. Mosby Co.
2. Joint Committee of the Public Health Service: Areawide planning of facilities for rehabilitation services, U.S. Department of Health, Education, and Welfare, No. 930-B-2, 1963.
3. Christopherson, V. A.: Role modifications of the disabled male, Am. J. Nurs. **68**:290-293, 1968.
4. Cockerill, E., and Margolis, H. M.: The concept of disability, J. Chronic Dis. **3**:167-169, 1956.
5. Council on Medical Service, Committee on Aging: Report on conferences on aging and long-term care, Chicago, 1965, American Medical Association.
6. Cowdry, E. V., and Sternberg, F. U., editors: The care of the geriatric patient, ed. 4, St. Louis, 1971, The C. V. Mosby Co.
7. *Crate, M.: Nursing functions in adaptation to chronic illness, Am. J. Nurs. **65**:72-76, 1965.
8. Ford, A. B., Katz, S., Downs, T. D., et al.: Results of long-term home nursing: the influence of disability, J. Chronic Dis. **24**:591-596, 1971.
9. Garrett, J. F., and Levine, E. S.: Psychological practices with the physically disabled, New York, 1962, Columbia University Press.
10. *Goffman, E.: Stigma, Englewood Cliffs, N.J., 1963, Prentice-Hall, Inc.
11. Guidelines for the practice of nursing on the rehabilitation team, New York, 1965, American Nurses' Association.
12. *Hirschberg, G. G., et al.: Rehabilitation: a manual for the care of the physically disabled and elderly, ed. 2, Philadelphia, 1976, J. B. Lippincott Co.
13. *Hurd, G. G.: Teaching the hemiplegic self-care, Am. J. Nurs. **62**:64-68, 1962.
14. Katz, S., Ford, A. B., Moskowitz, R. W., et al.: Studies of illness in the aged. The index of ADL: a standardized measure of biological and psychosocial function. J.A.M.A. **185**:914-919, 1963.
15. Kolb, L. C.: Disturbances of body image. In Arieti, S., editor: American handbook of psychiatry, vol. 3, New York, 1966, Basic Books, Inc., Publishers.
16. *Kottke, F. J., and Anderson, E. M.: Deterioration of the bedfast patient: causes and effects and nursing care, Public Health Rep. **80**:437-451, 1965.
17. Kubler-Ross, E.: On death and dying, New York, 1969, The Macmillan Co.
18. Lilienfield, A. M., and Gifford, A. J., editors: Chronic disease and public health, Baltimore, 1966, The Johns Hopkins University Press.

---

*References preceded by an asterisk are particuarly well suited for student reading.

19. Litman, T. J.: An analysis of the sociological factors affecting the rehabilitation of physically handicapped patients, Arch. Phys. Med. Rehabil. **45**:9-16, 1964.
20. Littauer, D., Flance, I. J., and Wessen, A. F.: Home care, Hospital monograph series no. 9, Chicago, 1961, American Hospital Association.
21. *Madden, B. W., and Affeldt, J. E.: To prevent helplessness and deformities, Am. J. Nurs. **62**:59-61, 1962.
22. Martin, N., King, R., and Suchinski, J.: The nurse therapist in the rehabilitation setting, Am. J. Nurs. **70**:1694-1697, 1970.
23. Martinelli, R. P., and Dell Orto, A. E.: The psychological and social impact of physical disability, New York, 1977, Springer Publishing Co.
24. *Morris, E. M.: Choosing a nursing home, Am. J. Nurs. **61**:58-61 1961.
25. *Morrissey, A. B., and Zimmerman, M. E.: Helps for the handicapped, Am. J. Nurs. **53**:316-318 and 454-456, 1953.
26. *Moskowitz, E., and McCann, C. B.: Classification of disability in the chronically ill and aging, J. Chronic Dis. **5**:342-346, 1957.
27. Myers, J. S.: An orientation to chronic disease and disability, New York, 1965, Macmillan Publishing Co., Inc.
28. National Health Forum: Changing factors in staffing America's health services, New York, 1954, National Health Council.
29. *Olson, E. V., editor: The hazards of immobility, Am. J. Nurs. **67**:780-797, 1967.
30. Palmer, I. S., editor: Nursing in long-term illness, Nurs. Clin. North Am. **5**:1-84, 1970.
31. Public Health Service: Vital and health statistics—health characteristics of persons with chronic activity limitations (1974), U.S. Department of Health, Education, and Welfare, series 10, no. 112, Rockville, Md., Oct. 1976.
32. Public Health Service: Vital and health statistics—current estimates from the Health Interview Survey (1974), U.S. Department of Health, Education, and Welfare, series 10, no. 100, Rockville, Md., Sept. 1975.
33. Public Health Service: Vital and health statistics—bed disability among the chronically limited, National Health Survey, July 1957 to June 1961, U.S. Department of Health, Education, and Welfare, series 10, no. 12, Sept. 1964.
34. *Rifle, K. L., editor: The patient with long-term illness, Nurs. Clin. North Am. **8**:571-681, 1973.
35. Ryder, C. F.: The chronic disease era, J. Miss. State Med. Assoc. **4**:96-101, 1963.
36. Shapiro, L.: Rehabilitation stalemate, Arch. Gen. Psychiatry **15**:173-177, 1966.
37. *Sister M. Willa: Nursing in rehabilitation, J. Nurs. Educ. **4**:15-23, 1965.
38. *Skinner, G.: The nurse—key figure in preventive and restorative care, Hospitals **35**:52-56, 1961.
39. Skipper, J. D., Jr., Fink, S. L., and Hallenbeck, P. N.: Physical disability among married women: problems in the husband-wife relationship, J. Rehabil. **22**:16-19, 1968.
40. *Sorensen, K., and Amis, D. B.: Understanding the world of the chronically ill, Am. J. Nurs. **67**:811-817, 1967.
41. *Stoeckle, J. D., Noonan, B., Farrisey, R. M., and Sweatt, A.: Medical nursing clinic for the chronically ill, Am. J. Nurs. **63**:87-89, 1963.
42. *Strauss, A. L.: Chronic illness and the quality of life, St. Louis, 1975, C. V. Mosby Co.
43. Stryker, R.: Rehabilitative aspects of acute and chronic nursing care, Philadelphia, 1972, W. B. Saunders Co.
44. Talbot, H. S.: A concept of rehabilitation, Rehabil. Lit. **22**:358-359, 1961.
45. The expanding role of ambulatory services in hospitals and health departments, Bull. N.Y. Acad. Med. **41**:1-158, 1965.
46. Weeks, L. E., and Griffith, J. R., editors: Progressive patient care: an anthology, Ann Arbor, Mich., 1964, The University of Michigan Press.
47. Whitehouse, F. A.: The utilization of human resources: a philosophic approach, Chest **30**:606, 1956.
48. Williams, S. R.: Nutrition and diet therapy, ed. 3, St. Louis, 1977, The C. V. Mosby Co.
49. Wright, B. A.: Spread in adjustment to disability, Menninger Clin. **28**:198-208, 1964.
50. Wright, B. A.: Physical disability—a psychological approach, New York, 1960, Harper & Row, Publishers, Inc.

PART THREE

Clinical management of persons with medical-surgical problems

UNIT V

Failure of integrative mechanisms: regulatory problems

The effect of stress on the human body and the response of individuals to stressors are greatly affected by the status of the regulatory mechanisms of the body. Nurses assist persons to cope with deficiencies in regulatory mechanisms, to promote optimal functioning possible when deficiencies exist, and to decrease external stressors when the regulatory mechanisms are not at the optimal functioning level.

The integrative mechanisms were discussed in Chapter 13. The endocrine system and the liver are the focus of this unit for their role in regulating body functions. Chapter 30 identifies the parameters of *assessment of regulatory mechanisms.* Chapter 31 discusses interventions for persons during an acute phase of a *disturbance in some regulatory function* or during long-term care when learning to care for oneself. Specific problems and special nursing interventions for *dysfunctions of the endocrine system* and the *liver* are discussed in chapters 32 and 33.

30

Assessment of regulatory mechanisms

VIRGINIA CASSMEYER

The regulation of body mechanisms is controlled by the endocrine and hepatic systems. The hepatic system consists of the liver and gallbladder. Although the endocrine system consists of eight special glands—pituitary, thyroid, parathyroid, adrenals, pancreas, gonads, pineal, and thymus—only the first five will be considered in this chapter. The gonads are discussed in Chapter 60. The regulatory functions of the pineal and thymus glands are as yet poorly understood.

■ ANATOMIC LOCATIONS AND PHYSIOLOGIC CONCEPTS

□ Endocrine system

Location and function

The various endocrine glands are located throughout the body. The pituitary is approximately 1 cm in size and lies in the pituitary fossa of the sella turcica of the middle cranial fossa. The gland is connected to the hypothalamus by the hypophyseal stalk and by blood supply. The thyroid gland is located in the anterior aspect of the neck just below the larynx. It consists of two lobes connected by the isthmus that lies upon the upper part of the trachea. The parathyroid gland consists of four minute glands, two of which are located on the posterior aspect of each thyroid lobe. The adrenal gland is a retroperitoneal abdominal organ capping the upper pole of each kidney. The adrenal gland consists of two glands: the cortex and the medulla. The products of the medulla are associated with the integrative functions described in Chapter 13. The pancreas is both an exocrine and an endocrine gland. The islets of Langerhans are the cells that serve the endocrine function. These cells are located throughout the entire organ. The pancreas lies retroperitoneally behind the stomach, with its head and neck in the curve of the duodenum, its body extending horizontally across the posterior abdominal wall, and its tail touching the spleen.

The endocrine system functions in the regulation of multiple body mechanisms. The endocrine glands produce specific chemical compounds *(hormones)* that are synthesized in the glands under genetic control and then secreted into the blood. Hormones are continually lost either by excretion or metabolic inactivation.

The secretion of hormones varies. No hormone is secreted at a uniform rate; some seem to have rhythmic patterns (daily or periodic), such as adrenal cortisone or the female reproductive hormones. Others, such as insulin, glucagon, and aldosterone, are secreted in response to blood levels of specific substances. How hormonal production is stimulated or how the hormones act in the cell is not fully understood. No hormone is believed to initiate reactions in the cell de novo. The biochemical machinery of the cell responds to the presence of the hormone by increasing or decreasing the rate at which a reaction takes place, but all the equipment for the reaction is present in the cell.

It is hypothesized that many protein hormones exert their effect by activating the enzyme adenylcyclase. The hormones combine with receptors on the cell membrane, and this combination of the hormone and receptor activates the enzyme. Adenylcyclase causes the formation of 3′,5′-cyclic AMP from ATP. It is believed that 3′,5′-cyclic AMP acts as the intracellular mediator. Steroid hormones work directly inside the cell by binding two intracellular receptor proteins, which leads to the transcription of DNA. The specificity of the receptors on the cell membrane or inside the cell controls which hormones affect which cells.

Relationship between the hypothalamus and the endocrine glands

The anterior pituitary gland, often called the "master gland" because of its regulation of the production of other hormones, is under the control of the hypothalamus. The hypothalamus regulates anterior pituitary gland secretion by the release of *neurosecretory releasing* and *neurosecretory inhibitory factors.* The factors are presumably produced by neurons in the hypothalamus. The hypothalamus secretes growth hormone releasing factor (GRF), growth hormone inhibitory factor (GIF), thyrotropin releasing factor (TRF), corticotropin releasing factor (CRF), follicle-stimulating hormone releasing factor (FRF), luteinizing hormone releasing factor (LRF), prolactin releasing factor (PRF), and prolactin inhibiting factor (PIF).

Stimulation of the hypothalamus leads to the liberation of selected factors into the hypothalamic hypophyseal portal blood system, which carries them to the anterior pituitary gland to stimulate the release of appropriate hormones. The relationship between the hypothalamus, anterior pituitary gland, and target organs is summarized in Fig. 30-1.

The hormones of the posterior pituitary gland are produced by the paraventricular and supraoptic nuclei of the hypothalamus, are carried by neurons to the posterior pituitary gland, and are released from the posterior pituitary gland into the general circulation with appropriate stimulation.

The various endocrine glands, hormones, and the major known functions of the individual hormones are summarized in Table 30-1.

Control mechanisms

In a state of health the level of any one hormone is kept within very definite limits. The endocrine glands are regulated by a number of control mechanisms. The *closed-looped negative feedback system* is illustrated in Fig. 30-2. Gland A produces hormone X, which stimu-

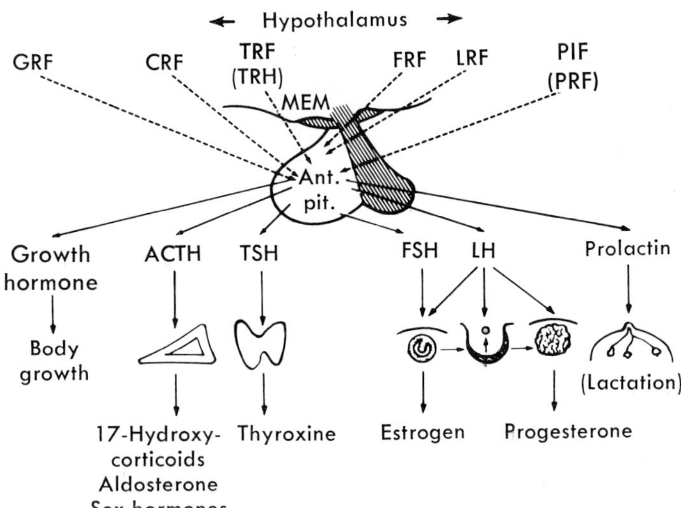

Fig. 30-1. Releasing factors that control output of hormones from anterior lobe of pituitary gland and ultimate hormone release from peripheral glands. *GRF*, Growth hormone releasing factor; *CRF*, corticotropin relasing factor; *TRF (TRH)*, thyrotropin releasing factor or hormone; *FRF*, follicle-stimulating hormone releasing factor; *LRF*, luteinizing hormone releasing factor; *PIF (PRF)*, prolactin inhibitory or releasing factor; and *MEM*, median eminence. Note that combination of FSH and LH produces maturation of follicle, ovulation, and corpus luteum formation. (From Mountcastle, V. B., editor: Medical physiology, vol. 1, ed. 13, St. Louis, 1974, The C. V. Mosby Co.; modified from Ganong.)

Table 30-1. Endocrine glands, hormones, and functions

Gland	Hormones	Functions
Pituitary anterior lobe	Growth hormone (GH; somatotropin)	Target organ: whole body Concerned with growth of bones, muscles, cells Affects carbohydrate, protein, and fat metabolism Insulin antagonist
	Thyroid-stimulating hormone (TSH)	Target organ: thyroid Necessary for growth and function of thyroid gland Controls release of thyroid hormone
	Adrenocorticotropic hormone (ACTH)	Target organ: adrenal cortex Necessary for growth of adrenal cortex Controls release of glucocorticoids and adrenal androgens Has minor role in release of aldosterone
	Gonadotropins Follicle-stimulating hormone (FSH)	Target organs: sexual organs Necessary for development of primary and secondary sex characteristics
	Luteinizing hormone (LH; also referred to as interstitial cell-stimulating hormone [ICSH] in males)	

Table 30-1. Endocrine glands, hormones, and functions—cont'd

Gland	Hormones	Functions
Pituitary—cont'd	Luteotropic hormone (LTH; prolactin)	Target organ: breast Necessary for development and lactation
Posterior pituitary	Antidiuretic hormone (ADH)	Target organ: kidney Necessary for maintenance of body fluid osmolarity by controlling water reabsorption in kidneys
	Oxytocin	Target organs: uterus and breast Causes "milk let-down" in lactating breast Causes contraction of pregnant uterus
Thyroid	Thyroxine (T_4) and triiodothyronine (T_3)	Regulates protein, fat and carbohydrate catabolism in all cells Regulates body heat production Insulin antagonist Maintains GH secretion, skeletal maturation Affects central nervous system development Necessary for muscle tone and vigor Maintains cardiac rate, force, and output
	Thyrocalcitonin	Lowers serum calcium and phosphorus levels
Adrenal medulla	Epinephrine and norepinephrine	Necessary for maintenance of integrative functions of body Elevates blood pressure, increases heart rate and vasoconstriction Stimulates conversion of glycogen to glucose for emergency fuel
Adrenal cortex	Glucocorticoids (cortisol)	Overall effect is to maintain blood glucose level by increasing gluconeogenesis, decrease rate of glucose utilization by cells Increases protein catabolism Promotes lipolysis Promotes sodium and water retention Antiinflammatory, decreases lymphocytes, decreases antibody formation Decreases scar tissue formation Increases RBC formation Increases gastric acid and pepsin production Maintains emotional stability
	Mineralocorticoids (aldosterone)	Major stimulus is renin-angiotensin system Primarily responsible for the maintenance of normovolemic state (sodium and water retention) Causes potassium excretion
	Androgens	Same functions as gonadal sex hormones
Parathyroid	Parathyroid hormone (PTH)	Increases serum calcium levels and decreases serum phosphorus levels by (1) increasing bone resorption, (2) increasing calcium absorption from GI tract (needs vitamin D), (3) decreasing urinary excretion of calcium, and (4) increasing urinary excretion of phosphorus.
Pancreas: islets of Langerhans Beta cells	Insulin	Overall, decreases blood glucose level Increases uptake and utilization of glucose by adipose and muscle cells and brain Increases glycogenesis Increases lipogenesis Increases amino acid incorporation into protein
Alpha cells	Glucagon	Actions contrary to insulin Increases blood glucose level

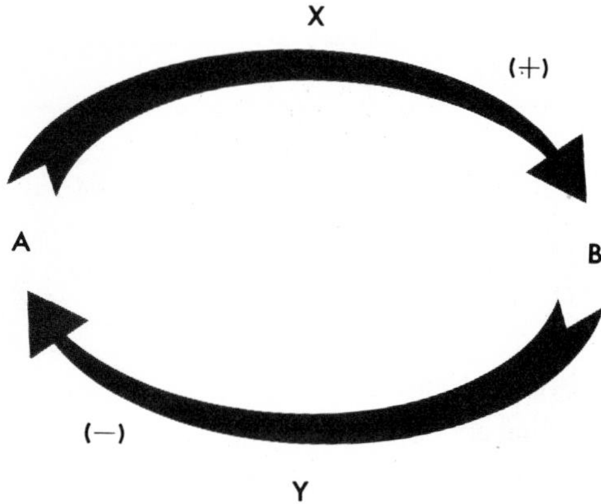

Fig. 30-2. Closed-loop negative feedback system. A principle of control that is applicable to all endocrine glands. (Redrawn from Harvey, A. M., et al.: The principles and practice of medicine, ed. 18, Englewood Cliffs, N.J., 1972, Prentice-Hall, Inc.)

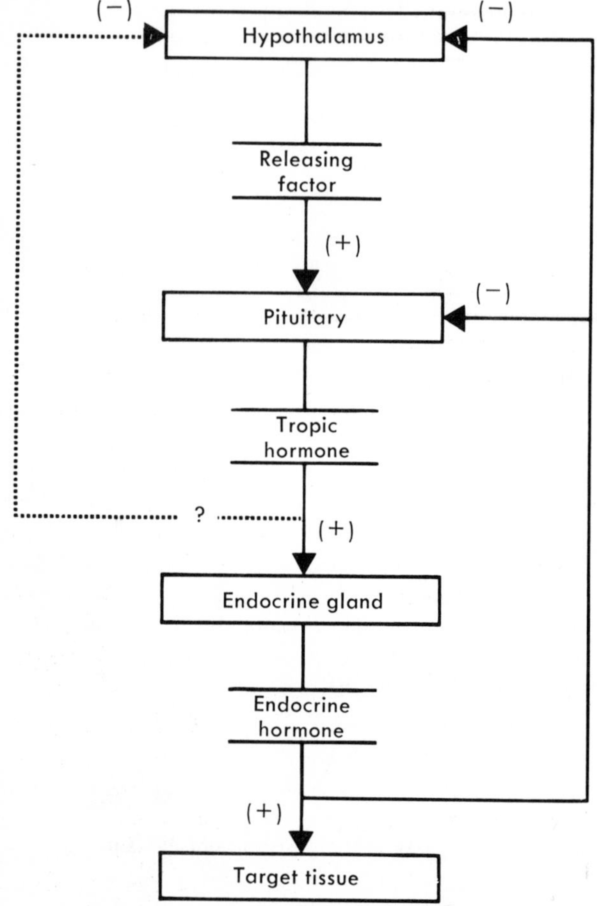

Fig. 30-3. Complex negative feedback loop system. Hypothalamus regulates this complex feedback system. (Redrawn from Harvey, A. M., et al.: The principles and practice of medicine, ed. 18, Englewood Cliffs, N.J., 1972, Prentice-Hall, Inc.)

lates organ B. In turn, organ B produces substance Y, which then inhibits secretion of gland A. A second feedback loop is regulated by the hypothalamus. Fig. 30-3 identifies *negative and positive feedback loops between the hypothalamus, pituitary gland, other endocrine glands, and the target organ.* A third regulating phenomenon is *internal rhythm.* The diurnal variations of ACTH and cortisol production provide examples. While a person is asleep at 2 AM, production of ACTH and cortisol is at the lowest level, but it rises sharply between 6 and 8 AM. The human menstrual cycle also illustrates this mechanism.

□ Hepatic system

The hepatic system is the other major system involved in regulation of body functions. The liver, which weighs 1.35 to 1.80 kg, is one of the largest organs of the body. It consists of two lobes and is located in the right upper quadrant of the abdomen under the diaphragm. It extends up under the ribs and is 4 to 8 cm in height in the midsternal line and 6 to 12 cm in height in the midclavicular line. The gallbladder lies under the inferior surface of the liver and serves as a storage place for bile produced by the liver.

The liver is made up of small liver lobules (Fig. 30-4) composed of hepatic cellular plates. Each hepatic cellular plate is usually two cells thick, and between these cells run bile canaliculi. Hepatic sinusoids, which receive blood from the portal vein and hepatic artery, lie on the opposite sides of the hepatic cells. After flowing through the hepatic sinusoids the blood is emptied into the central vein and from there flows into the hepatic vein. The hepatic sinusoids are lined with Kupffer cells. The Kupffer cells are reticuloendothelial cells that phagocytize bacteria and other foreign products.

The liver, as can be seen from this description, is ideally structured to receive large supplies of blood to carry out multiple functions. The major functions of the liver are (1) participation in various parts of fat, carbohydrate, and protein metabolism; (2) metabolism of bilirubin and production of bile; (3) detoxification of endogenous and exogenous substances. The liver cells contain many enyzmes to carry out these functions.

Fat, carbohydrate, and protein metabolism

The liver plays a major role in the metabolism of fats, carbohydrates, and proteins. Through various enzymatic activities the liver can oxidize fats, carbohydrates, and proteins for energy; use fat, carbohydrate, and protein products to produce compounds that can be stored for future use; or use fat, carbohydrate, and protein products to manufacture needed compounds. In fat metabolism the liver is responsible for the production of

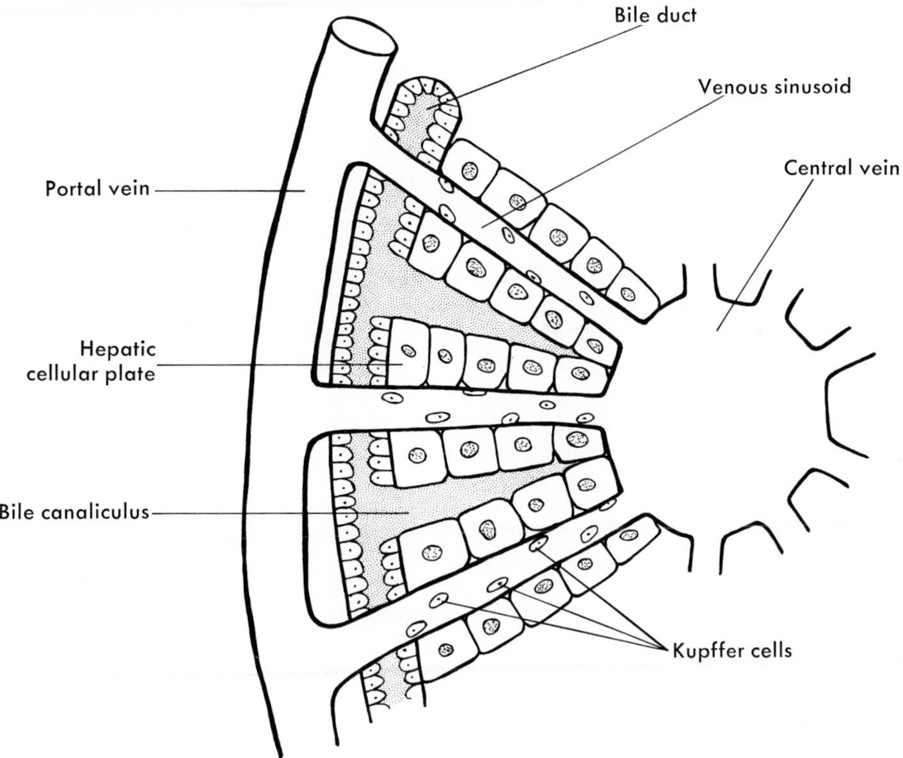

Fig. 30-4. Diagram of liver lobule. (Adapted from Guyton, A.: Textbook of medical physiology, ed. 4, Philadelphia, 1971, W. B. Saunders Co.)

phospholipids, lipoproteins, and cholesterol. It functions in protein metabolism by synthesizing essential proteins such as albumin, which is necessary for the maintenance of osmotic pressure, some globulin, blood-clotting factors such as fibrinogen and prothrombin, and converting the ammonia produced from the deamination of proteins to urea. In carbohydrate metabolism it is responsible for the production and storage of glycogen and is primarily responsible for the metabolism of galactose.

Bilirubin metabolism

Bilirubin is a by-product of the heme portion of red blood cells and is released when red blood cells are destroyed. The bilirubin released from the red blood cell is non-water-soluble (unconjugated) and is carried in the blood attached to protein. The liver is responsible for picking up this unconjugated bilirubin, combining it with glucuronide into a conjugated water soluble form, and secreting conjugated bilirubin into the bile. The bilirubin in bile is secreted into the duodenum and is broken down by bacteria into urobilinogen. Some of the urobilinogen is excreted with the feces, becoming stercobilin and giving the stool its brown color. Some is eliminated in the urine, and the remainder returns to the liver and is reconverted to bilirubin.

Detoxification

The liver has a prime role in detoxification of both exogenous and endogenous substances. It also has a major role in the detoxification of many drugs. All barbiturates (except phenobarbital and barbital) and many other sedatives are inactivated by the liver. The status of the liver plays an important role in the effectiveness or toxicity of these and other drugs. The liver also detoxifies corticosteroids, aldosterone, and estrogen. The inability of the liver to inactivate these hormones may account for prolonged and pathophysiologic levels of these hormones.

■ SUBJECTIVE DATA

Diseases of the hepatic and endocrine system lead to varied manifestations because of inadequate energy production, insufficient metabolism of nutrients and other products, water and electrolyte imbalance, abnormal growth and development, altered reproductive processes, and inadequate removal of toxic and waste products. Because of these varied manifestations, systematic assessment of numerous parameters is necessary to define the patient's total problems and needs. Since their anatomic locations for the most part preclude direct examination of the health of the various organs, assessment of the status of the regulatory mechanisms requires a thorough history from the patient or his significant others. Special attention should be paid to the patient's *energy level, nutritional intake, elimination patterns, subjective perception of changes in body characteristics,* and *tolerance to stress.*

☐ Energy level

Since the liver and the endocrine system are directly involved in the metabolism of nutrients for energy and the production of elements necessary for the formation of red blood cells to carry oxygen, diseases of these systems will change the patient's energy level. Many patients will complain of "not being able to do their normal things." It is important to assess the person's energy level and to use this as a guide for helping him plan activities of daily living. Some patients need help in adjusting their activities to allow for rest periods; they may need assistance in eliminating activities or in changing the ways to do activities to conserve energy.

Most hepatic and endocrine problems can be well controlled so that permanent changes in life style will not be necessary. Recovery may be slow, however, and the patient's physical status may be so damaged that although his energy level may be normal, additional time will be required for complete recovery.

☐ Nutritional intake

Problems of the hepatic and endocrine systems can lead to nausea and vomiting, anorexia, or polyphagia and may be associated with weight loss or weight gain. Qualitative and quantitative assessment of food intake is necessary to decide on the cause of weight changes. The preferences of the patient are important in assisting him to plan an adequate and pleasing diet. Dietary restrictions may be necessary for some conditions, and providing adequate dietary intake in cases of anorexia, nausea and vomiting, and dietary restrictions is a tremendous challenge. In some instances the restriction will be necessary for life, so it is very important to show the patient that the diet can be pleasing as well as therapeutic.

☐ Elimination pattern

Both the hepatic and endocrine systems are involved in maintenance of water and electrolyte balance. The history should include information on the frequency, approximate amount, and color of urinary elimination. The presence of nocturia or dysuria is also solicited. In liver disease a history of decreased output with a relative increase in weight may be elicited. In endocrine disease, depending on the cause, the client may give a history of increased output and increased thirst, or decreased output and increased weight. Some patients may be on diuretics, and their compliance with the therapy should be assessed. The frequency and color of bowel movements is also determined. Constipation or other changes in bowel habits that may be caused by changes in water balance, dietary intake, or sluggishness of the bowel may be elicited. Treatment of disease states may include changes in diet and fluid intake; the patient's previous pattern of intake will assist the nurse in teaching the patient about needed changes.

☐ Body characteristics

Changes in hair distribution, body proportions, voice, skin pigmentation, and facial appearance may accompany problems of the regulatory mechanisms. A description of changes by patients or their significant others is very important because the characteristics of persons vary so greatly, and changes may not be so great that observation alone will pick them up.

The collection of information regarding changes in body characteristics is not only important in helping to define the physiologic problem but also is very important in identifying potential or present emotional or psychologic problems. Some of the changes that occur with endocrine and hepatic problems are irreversible even when the physiologic problem is controlled. Body characteristics are part of the identity of the person, and the patient may have problems dealing with the changes. (See Chapter 28 for a detailed discussion of body image.)

☐ Tolerance to stressors

The regulatory mechanisms help to maintain the body's ability to respond to all types of physical and psychologic stressors. The patient or his significant others should be questioned in relation to the patient's ability (or change in ability) to tolerate stressors. Such things as intolerance to heat and cold, increased frequency of infections, increased irritation, euphoria, depression, increased crying, or increased anger may be elicited. Depending on the patient's ability to handle stressors, special environmental controls to decrease the chance of infection and to maintain an even emotional environment may be necessary.

■ OBJECTIVE DATA

The collection of objective data about the endocrine and hepatic system requires a thorough inspection and the use of the techniques of palpation and percussion. Most of the information that can be collected by physical examination is gathered by inspection.

☐ Inspection

Inspection should be used to assess the patient's body growth and developmental status. Such things as height, weight, body proportions, amount and distribution of muscle mass, fat distribution, skin pigmentation, and hair distribution should be assessed. A great variation in these parameters exists in the general population, and often the changes will not be obvious. Inspection of family members for like characteristics will provide information as to whether the characteristics seen in the patient are caused by hereditary or to pathophysiologic alterations. The patient's alertness and speech patterns can be assessed when the history is being collected.

The regulatory mechanisms play a major role in growth and development, metabolism of food products, and regulation of sex hormones. All of these functions, if affected, cause changes in body characteristics. Some examples of specific changes are (1) dwarfism caused by thyroid and pituitary problems, (2) jaundice caused by liver abnormalities (best seen in the sclera in dark-skinned persons), (3) changes in fat distribution, producing "buffalo hump" and "thickened girdle," from adrenal cortical excess, (4) presence of purplish striae instead of white striae because of adrenocortical excess, (5) muscle wasting with a wide variety of regulatory problems, and (6) change in sexual characteristics because of abnormalities of hormonal levels or hepatic problems. All of these changes can be identified during inspection.

Inspection along with palpation is used to check skin turgor, mucous membrane moisture, and the presence of edema. Abdominal girth should be measured. All of this data will give information about the fluid and electrolyte status of the patient.

Following are changes that may be found: The finger should slide over the mucous membrane easily. In states of fluid depletion the mucous membranes are sticky. Edema can be graded from 1+ to 4+ (see Chapter 20). Skin turgor can be checked on the forearm, forehead, or over the sternum (p. 1488).

□ Palpation and percussion

Of all the organs discussed, only the thyroid and liver will be routinely examined by use of palpation and percussion. In disease states, sometimes the pancreas and parathyroid gland can be palpated.

Examination of thyroid gland

The thyroid gland is usually examined along with examination of the head and neck. Palpation of the

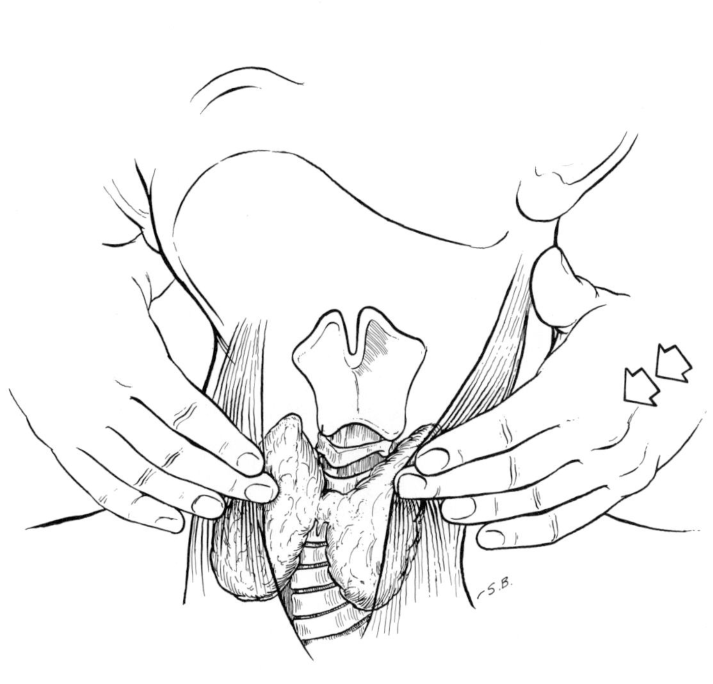

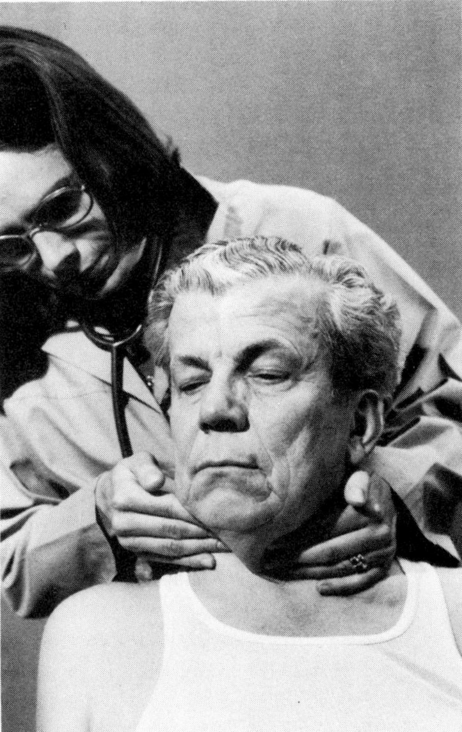

Fig. 30-5. Posterior approach to thyroid examination. In order to examine right lobe of thyroid gland, examiner displaces trachea slightly to right with fingers of left hand and palpates for right thyroid lobe with fingers of right hand. (From Malasanos, L., Barkauskas, V., Moss, M., and Stoltenberg-Allen, K.: Health assessment, St. Louis, 1977, The C. V. Mosby Co.)

thyroid provides information about the size, shape, and symmetry of the gland, and the presence of nodules or tenderness.

The first step in the examination is to inspect the neck for any visible thyroid tissue. Normally no tissue is visible. Palpation of the thyroid gland can be done from either the front or from behind the patient. Frequently the normal thyroid gland is not palpable and, if felt, is a layer of tissue that moves with swallowing. Normally each lobe is approximately 5 cm long and 2 cm thick. The right lobe is slightly larger than the left. A light rotary motion is used to delineate nodules and irregularities. Each step in the following description should be done before and while the patient swallows. Sips of water will assist the person to swallow.

Palpation from behind. Seat the person in a chair and stand behind him. Have the person lower his chin, place your thumbs on the back of his neck, and curve fingers anteriorly over the thyroid. Feel for the thyroid isthmus and anterior surface of the lobes. Second, have the patient flex his neck slightly forward and to the right. Displace the thyroid cartilage to the right with the fingers of your left hand. Palpate with your right hand, placing the right thumb behind the sternocleidomastoid and the index and middle finger in front of it. Reverse the procedure (Fig. 30-5).

Palpation from the front. Stand in front of the patient. With the second and third fingers, feel below the cricoid cartilage for the thyroid isthmus. Then move your fingers laterally and deep to the borders of the sternocleidomastoid muscle. Feel for each lateral lobe. Lastly, have the client flex his neck forward and to the right. Place your right thumb on the lower portion of the patient's thyroid cartilage and displace it to the client's right. Hook the tips of the second and third fingers of your left hand behind the sternocleidomastoid muscle while feeling in front of the muscle with your thumb. Reverse the procedure for the left side (Fig. 30-6).

Occasionally the thyroid gland is more easily palpated if the patient's neck is extended. The procedures described above can be repeated with the patient's neck extended. If an enlarged thyroid is felt, the thyroid should be auscultated for the presence of bruits. The increased vascular flow that occurs with hypertrophy of the gland can cause bruits.

Examination of the liver

Examination of the liver is done while examining the abdomen. The examination begins with inspection of the abdomen for striae, which may be caused by ascites; engorged veins, which may be caused by obstruction of portal flow; and abdominal distention, which also may be

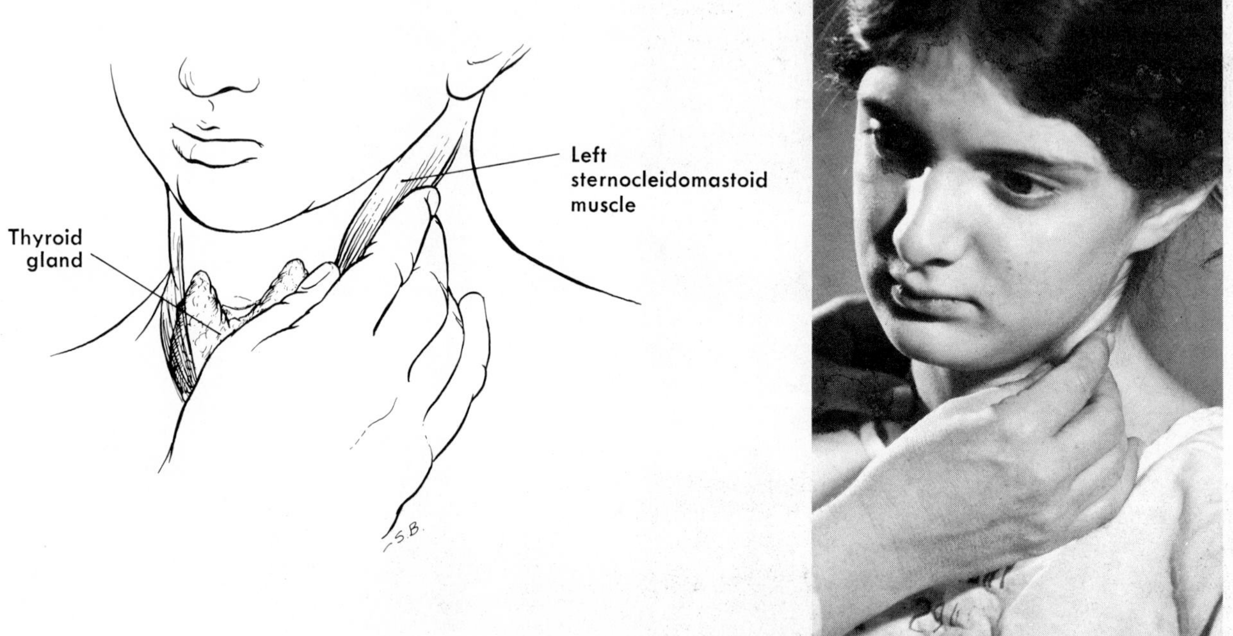

Fig. 30-6. Anterior approach to thyroid examination. Examiner grasps around left sternocleidomastoid muscle with right hand to palpate for enlarged left thyroid lobe. (From Malasanos, L., Barkauskas, V., Moss, M., and Stoltenberg-Allen, K.: Health assessment, St. Louis, 1977, The C. V. Mosby Co.)

caused by ascites. When auscultation of the abdomen is desired, it must be done prior to palpation and percussion of the abdomen.

Percussion. The technique of percussion is used to examine the liver. In percussion the fingers of one hand are placed over the organ to be examined. The fingers of the other hand are flexed and used to tap the fingers of the other hand (Fig. 8-5).

To percuss the liver, start at an area below the umbilicus in the midclavicular line and percuss upward until dullness is heard. Then start at about the third or fourth intercostal space, midclavicular line, and percuss downward until dullness is heard. Measure the vertical span of liver dullness. It should be approximately 6 to 12 cm in width. If this percussion reveals an enlarged liver, the liver can be percussed in the same manner at the

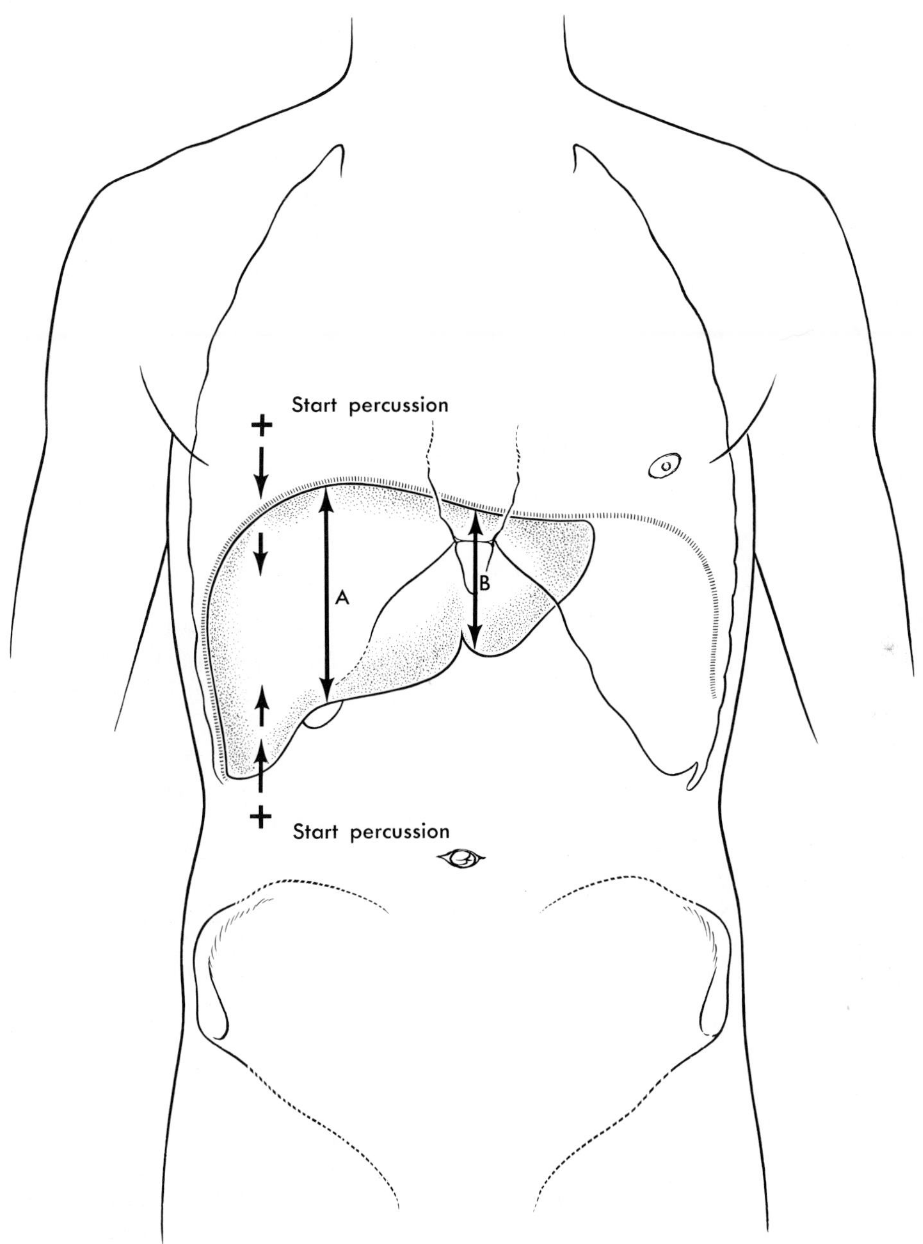

Fig. 30-7. Percussion of liver. Vertical span of liver dullness should measure approximately 6 to 12 cm at midclavicular line, *A*, and 4 to 8 cm at midsternal line, *B*.

midsternal line. At this point it normally is 4 to 8 cm in width (Fig. 30-7). Lung consolidation or right pleural effusion can obscure the upper border dullness, while gas in the colon can obscure the lower border dullness.

Percussion is also used to examine for the presence of ascites. Ascites causes bulging of flanks and dullness when the patient is supine. If the patient is turned to the side, the bulging is shifted to the dependent side, and the dullness is localized to that side.

Fluid wave. While the patient is lying supine, the abdomen can be examined for presence of a fluid wave. In performing this test, the left hand of the examiner is on the patient's right flank, and the ulnar edge of the hand of an assistant or the patient is placed over the upper middle abdomen as the examiner's right hand sharply strikes the left flank of the patient. A sharp wave will be felt by the examiner's left hand in the presence of a significantly large amount of fluid (ascites).

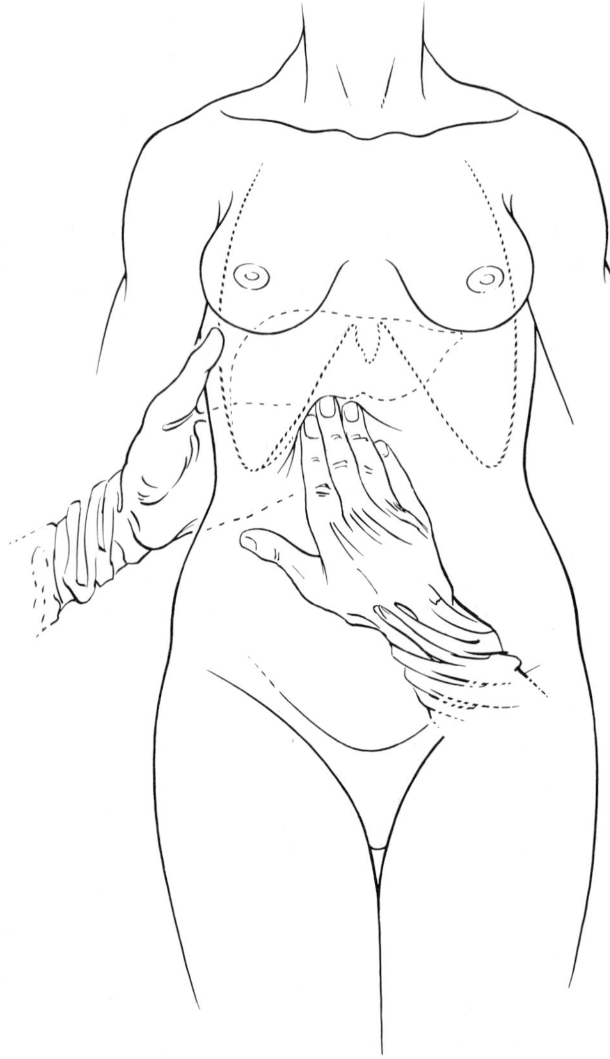

Palpation. Gently work the fingertips of the right hand deep into the right upper quadrant and place the left hand under the patient's back at the eleventh and twelfth rib to palpate the liver (Fig. 30-8). Instruct the patient to take a deep breath. The liver edge, if palpable, presents a firm, sharp, regular ridge with a smooth surface. When felt more than 1 cm below the costal margin, it is considered abnormal.

Fig. 30-8. Correct placement of hands for palpating liver.

■ DIAGNOSTIC EXAMINATIONS AND TESTS

Because of the multiple functions of the hepatic and endocrine systems, various tests are used to determine whether disease of these regulatory systems is present and, if so, to identify the cause of the patient's symptoms.

Many of the tests of regulatory function require taking samples of blood, other tests are more extensive and may cause discomfort, and many tests require the patient to fast. The nurse is responsible for preparing the patient appropriately. The routine physical preparation for any test will vary from institution to institution. Besides carrying out the physical preparation, the nurse prepares the patient for the test by explaining the purpose of the test, what can be expected prior to and during the test, and special care required after the test.

□ Liver function tests

Liver function tests include (1) blood, urine, and stool examination to determine amount and distribution of bile pigments; (2) blood tests that demonstrate the ability of the liver to carry out its metabolism functions; and (3) tests that determine its excretory functions. Other diagnostic procedures may be employed to determine causes of biliary and hepatic malfunction. Because the liver can be affected by processes outside of the hepatic system, the tests are of great importance in determining whether signs and symptoms are caused by disease of the hepatic cells themselves (hepatocellular) or to pathologic processes outside the hepatic system.

Laboratory tests

Multiple tests may be necessary to determine the extent and seriousness of hepatic disease. Many tests require serial reading to be of benefit. The test, procedure and special preparation, and interpretation of commonly used blood, stool, and urine studies for evaluation of liver function are summarized in Table 30-2.

Various other tests to measure different aspects of liver function are available and have been used in the past, but have been abandoned as more specific tests became available. These tests may be used in rare cases. A

Table 30-2. Laboratory tests of liver function

Function and test	Procedure and preparation	Interpretation
Fat metabolism		
Serum total cholesterol and cholesterol esters	Blood drawn. Fasting may be required.	Normal level is 140 to 220 mg/100 ml of blood. Approximately 70% is cholesterol ester. In hepatocellular disease, amount of total serum cholesterol and cholesterol ester may be decreased. In obstructive biliary tract disease, total serum cholesterol is increased, but amount of esterefied cholesterol is decreased. Normal cholesterol levels rise with age.
Serum phospholipids	Blood drawn. No special preparation.	Normal level is 150 to 250 mg/100 ml. Serum phospholipids tend to be low in severe hepatocellular disease and high in obstructive biliary tract disease.
Protein metabolism		
Total serum protein	Blood drawn. No special preparation.	Normal level is 6 to 8 g/100 ml. Measures all serum protein. May be normal in hepatocellular disease because an increase in serum globulin will replace decreased serum albumin.
Albumin	Blood drawn. No special preparation.	Normal level is 3.4 to 5 g/100 ml. Albumin made only in liver. In hepatocellular disease there may be decrease in serum albumin level.
Protein electrophoresis	Blood drawn. No special preparation. Protein fraction of blood will migrate in characteristic directions in an electrical field. After separation of fractions, specimen is stained and densitometer is used to measure amounts of various serum protein.	Normal fractions in relation to total serum protein (100%) are albumin, 52% to 68%; alpha globulins, 12% to 17%; beta globulins, 7% to 15%; and immune serum globulins (gamma globulins), 9% to 19%. In severe hepatocellular damage, amount of albumin may be decreased. Inflammatory processes of liver may produce increased amounts of alpha globulins, and some patients with obstructive biliary tract disease may have high levels of beta globulins.
Blood urea nitrogen (BUN)	Blood drawn. No special preparation.	Normal level is 10 to 20 mg/100 ml. In severe hepatocellular disease, if portal vein flow is obstructed, level may decrease. Varies with dietary protein intake and fluid volume.
Serum prothrombin time	Blood drawn. No special preparation. Reflects activity of prothrombin, fibrinogen, and factors V, VII, and IX.	Normal prothrombin time is 12 to 15 seconds or 100%, as compared to control level. Prothrombin time may be increased in hepatocellular disease because of inability of liver to produce clotting factors or in obstructive biliary tract disease because of malabsorption of vitamin K. Persistence of abnormal prothrombin time after parenteral administration of vitamin K is indicative of hepatocellular damage.
Blood ammonia levels	Blood drawn. May require fasting.	Normal level is less than 75 μg/100 ml. May be elevated in severe hepatocellular disease because of decreased urea production or obstruction of portal blood flow.
Bilirubin metabolism		
Total bilirubin Conjugated (direct) Unconjugated (indirect)	Blood drawn. No special preparation.	Total serum bilirubin measures both conjugated and unconjugated bilirubin. Normal values range from 0.1 to 1 mg/100 ml. Conjugated bilirubin acts directly with diazo- reagents. Unconjugated bilirubin requires addition of methyl alcohol. Thus

Continued.

Table 30-2. Laboratory tests of liver function—cont'd

Function and test	Procedure and preparation	Interpretation
Bilirubin metabolism—cont'd Total bilirubin—cont'd		the terms direct and indirect. Conjugated bilirubin is increased in the presence of hepatocellular and obstructive biliary tract disease. Unconjugated bilirubin is elevated with increased hemolysis of red blood cells or with hepatocellular disease.
Urine bilirubin	Spot urine specimen. No special preparation.	Normally no bilirubin is excreted in the urine. Urine with abnormal bilirubin is mahogany colored and has a yellow foam when shaken (foam test). Conjugated serum bilirubin levels greater than 0.4 mg/100 ml will lead to bilirubin being excreted in urine. This indicates hepatocellular or obstructive biliary tract disease. Bilirubinuria may be present before jaundice.
Urine urobilinogen	Twenty-four-hour urine collection or 2-hour afternoon collection.	Normally 0.2 to 1.2 units found in specimen. Fresh urine urobilinogen is colorless. Decreased amounts of urine urobilinogen found in obstructive biliary tract disease. Increased amounts found in hepatocellular disease. Alterations in intestinal flora by broad-spectrum antibiotics may change test.
Fecal urobilinogen	Stool specimen. No special preparation.	Normally 90 to 280 mg/day. Presence of urobilinogen gives stool brown color. Absence of urobilinogen causes stools to become clay to white colored. Increased amounts found in increased hemolysis of red blood cells. Absence of stercobilinogen indicates obstructive biliary tract disease.
Serum enzymes		
Serum glutamic-oxaloacetic transaminase (SGOT) Serum glutamic-pyruvic transaminase (SGPT) Lactic dehydrogenase (LDH)	Blood drawn. No special preparation.	Normal values vary depending on measurement used. These enzymes are present in hepatic cells, and with necrosis of hepatic cells, enzymes are released and elevated serum levels will be found. SGPT is primarily present in the liver. SGOT is also present in high levels in skeletal and heart muscle. LDH is also present in heart, kidneys, skeletal muscle, and erythrocytes. Therefore necrosis of other organs must be ruled out.
Alkaline phosphatase	Blood drawn. No special preparation.	Normal values vary depending on measurement used. This enzyme originates in liver, bone, intestines, and placenta. Alkaline phosphatase is slightly to moderately elevated in hepatocellular disease, but extremely elevated in obstructive biliary tract disease and bone disease.
Detoxification		
Hippuric acid test	Patient is given light breakfast of toast and coffee. One hour later, 6 g of sodium benzoate dissolved in 30 ml of water is given. An additional 100 ml of water may be given, and then the patient fasts. Patient is asked to void. This specimen is discarded. Patient then voids each hour for 4 hours. Specimens are labeled and num-	Normally 3 g of hippuric acid is excreted in 4-hour period following oral administration of sodium benzoate or 0.7 g or greater is excreted 1 hour after intravenous administration. Abnormal findings are found in hepatocellular disease.

Table 30-2. Laboratory tests of liver function—cont'd

Function and test	Procedure and preparation	Interpretation
Detoxification—cont'd Hippuric acid test—cont'd	bered. Hippuric acid may also be given intravenously. Patient voids, is given a glass of water by mouth, and 1.77 g of sodium benzoate is administered intravenously. One hour later one urine specimen is collected.	
Excretory function		
Bromsulphalein (BSP) excretion	Patient is weighed and BSP 5 mg/kg of body weight is injected intravenously. Blood sample is drawn from other arm 45 minutes later. Patient must be fasting.	Normally less than 5% of test dose is retained in serum after 45 minutes. Abnormal retention reflects presence of hepatic cell damage and inability of liver to remove dye and excrete it. Biliary tract obstruction may also cause retention. Extrahepatic conditions such as shock and congestive heart failure can cause retention of BSP. BSP dye causes necrosis of tissue if it extravasates during injection. Certain drugs (iopanoic acid) may cause retention; phenolsulfonphthalein test of kidney function should not be done for 24 hours after BSP test.

full description of other tests and their interpretation can be found in the identified references.[6,21]

Diagnostic examination

Roentgenologic and other diagnostic examinations are used to assist in identifying the cause and site of hepatic malfunction. Examination of the liver, portal system, gallbladder, and biliary duct is possible. Besides the examinations described below, the diagnostic examination of the patient with liver problems may include abdominal films, barium swallow (p. 1161), barium enema (p. 1161), and gastroscopy (p. 1162). The latter three tests assist in the detection of varices.

Cholecystography. A normal liver will remove radiopaque drugs such as iodoalphionic acid (Priodax), iopanoic acid (Telepaque), and iodipamide methylglucamine (Cholografin Meglumine) from the bloodstream and store and concentrate them in the gallbladder. Because the roentgen rays cannot penetrate the dye, the dye-filled gallbladder shows up as a dense shadow on x-ray examination *(cholecystogram, gallbladder series).* A satisfactory gallbladder shadow would indicate a functioning gallbladder. A total absence of opaque material in the gallbladder would suggest a nonfunctioning gallbladder. After ingestion of a fatty meal, a functioning gallbladder should contract and expel the radiopaque dye along with the bile through the common bile duct into the duodenum. X-ray examination at this point would outline the bile ducts. Stones, which are not radiopaque, show up as dark patches on the film. Visualization of the gallbladder depends on absorption of the dye through the intestinal tract, isolation of it by the liver, and a free passageway from the liver to the gallbladder. Therefore if the results show a nonfunctioning gallbladder, sometimes the test is repeated to be sure that failure to visualize the gallbladder by x-ray examination was not caused by insufficient dye.

On the evening before cholecystography is scheduled, the purpose of and preparation for the test is explained to the patient. The importance of following instructions regarding food restriction the morning of the test, as well as the need for the high-fat intake, which may cause nausea, should be discussed.

The average adult dose of both iodoalphionic acid and iopanoic acid is 3 g (45 grains) given orally following a low-fat evening meal, after which no food is given. The dose is calculated by body weight. An obese person would receive a larger dose than normal, and a very small person a smaller than normal dose. These drugs may cause nausea, vomiting, and diarrhea in some people. The nurse should check dosages accurately and watch carefully for toxic signs, which should be reported to the physician. If vomiting occurs soon after ingestion of the drug, the physician may ask that the tablets be repeated when nausea subsides, or the test may be delayed for several days. If the patient cannot tolerate the drug by mouth, a radiopaque substance such as iodipamide methylglucamine may be given intravenously by the physician in the radiology department. The radiopaque dyes are organic iodine compounds and may cause allergic reactions when given intravenously. Symptoms may include dyspnea, chills, diaphoresis, faintness, and tachycardia and are identical to symptoms that can occur when radiopaque substances containing iodine are injected intravenously for other tests such as pyelography or arteriography. (See discussion of intravenous pyelogram [IVP] for precaution and care.)

On the morning of the examination the patient may have only black coffee, tea, or water. One or more enemas may be given to help remove gas from the intestinal tract so that it will not interfere with a clear roentgenogram. The patient goes to the radiology department where two roentgenograms are taken during the morning. The first one is on a fasting stomach, and the second is taken after ingestion of a high-fat preparation. Ingestion of fat should stimulate flow of bile and emptying of the gallbladder. The dye is finally excreted in the urine, and some patients report slight temporary pain on urination following the test.

Cholangiography. Cholangiography is the x-ray examination of the bile ducts to demonstrate the presence of stones, strictures, or tumors. The radiopaque substance may be administered intravenously or injected directly into the common bile duct with a needle or catheter at the time of surgery. Following operations on the common bile duct, the radiopaque drug, usually iodipamide methylglucamine, may be instilled through a drainage tube such as the T tube to determine the patency of the duct before the tube is removed. This dye also may be injected through the skin and abdominal wall into a bile duct in the main substance of the liver *(percutaneous transhepatic cholangiography)*. This technique is useful in visualizing the location and extent of a pathologic process such as obstructive jaundice and permits decompression of the liver for improved function. The procedure helps the surgeon identify the location prior to surgery or may indicate that surgery is not necessary. The hazards of the examination occasionally may include bile leakage leading to bile peritonitis, or bleeding caused by accidental rupture of a blood vessel.[7]

Angiography. Catheterization of the hepatic artery, portal venous system (by various routes), and the hepatic vein allows the injection of a contrast media and the visualization of the vascular supply of the hepatic system. The patency of the system and the presence of tumors, abscesses, collateral circulation, varices, and bleeding may be determined by use of angiography.

Portal and hepatic vein pressure (wedged hepatic vein pressure [WHVP]) can be measured. These readings may be done in conjunction with angiography or as a separate study. These measurements help in determining the degree of portal hypertension.

The presence of allergy to contrast media must be ascertained prior to angiography. After both angiography and pressure readings, the site of insertion is observed for bleeding, and the patient's vital signs are checked frequently.

Radioisotope scanning. The liver may be outlined by radioisotope scanning techniques. Radioisotopes such as ^{131}I rose bengal, which is taken up by the hepatocytes, or colloidal technetium (^{99}Tc) or gallium citrate (^{67}Ga), which are taken up by the reticuloendothelial cells, are given intravenously. After the injection of the radioisotope, the patient is placed supine, and a scintillation detector is passed over the abdomen in the area of the liver. The radiation coming from the isotopes immediately beneath the probe of the scanner is detected, amplified, and recorded. Scanning helps to differentiate nonfunctioning areas from normal tissue and helps to identify hepatic tumors, cysts, and abscesses (Fig. 30-9). Usually a nonfunctioning area will appear as an area of decreased activity. However, ^{67}Ga is preferentially taken up by hepatocellular carcinomas and abscesses, and these areas will appear as areas of very heavy radioactivity. Untoward reactions to these radioisotopes are unusual, and the procedure is relatively safe. Discomfort is minimal and is related to the intravenous injection and the position on the x-ray table. Only small amounts of radioactive material are given, and radiation precautions are *not* necessary. Except for ^{67}Ga scanning, no special preparation is required. Gallium citrate is excreted by the gastrointestinal tract. To avoid absorption of the radioisotope by the gastrointestinal contents, the patient requires cleansing of the bowel with laxatives and enemas. The exact preparation will vary from institution to institution.

Ultrasound examination. In ultrasonic hepatography the liver is bombarded with sound waves and the reflected sound is recorded. The ability to portray an image is caused by the different sounds generated by solid tissue, air-filled cavities, and fluid-filled cavities. Air almost completely impedes transmission so that a 100% reflection occurs. The liver, predominantly a solid organ, provides no impedance; therefore no reflections occur. The vascular system and biliary ducts in the liver impede some transmissions, and small reflections occur from these areas. The presence of diffuse liver disease such as cirrhosis, the presence of cystic and solid tumors, and the presence of cavities cause the recording of different sound patterns.[21]

Ultrasound is a noninvasive procedure that can be used safely on most patients. Preparation for the test requires the bowel to be cleansed, since the presence of solid content in the gastrointestinal tract would cause changes in reflected sounds and distort the recording.

Endoscopy. The hepatic system and gallbladder can

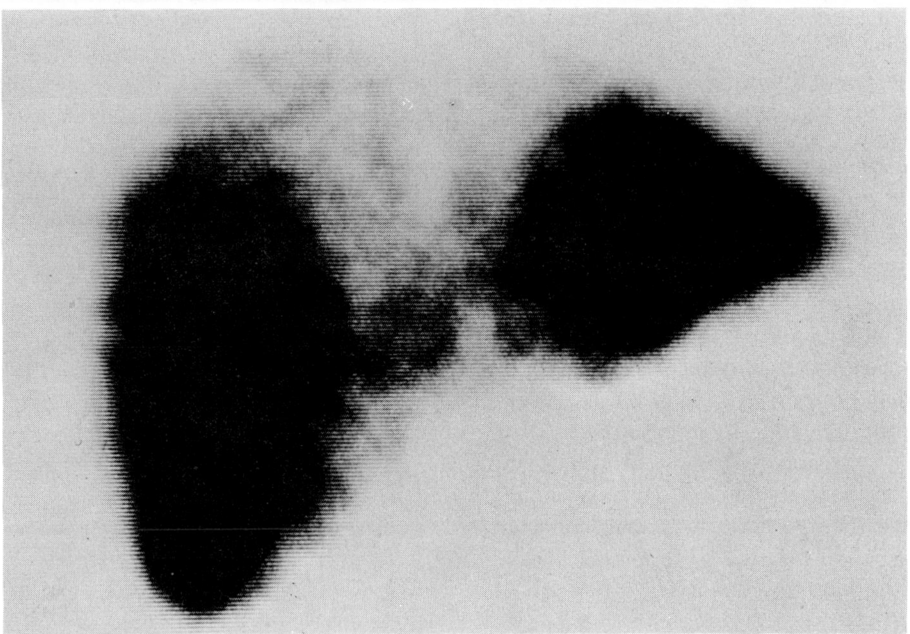

Fig. 30-9. Liver scan showing metastasis to liver (light area on right) of carcinoma of colon. (Courtesy Abbas M. Rejali, M.D., Department of Radiology, Case Western Reserve University, Cleveland, Ohio.)

be examined by endoscopy. Two types of endoscopy procedures can be done. The tube can be inserted through the peritoneum (peritoneoscopy), thus affording direct visualization of the abdominal organs and the taking of biopsies. Also the tube can be passed through the oral pharynx to the duodenum and into the biliary tract. Direct visualization is possible, dye can be injected through the scope, and biopsies can be taken.

Endoscopy is an invasive procedure that is not without risk and is used only when absolutely necessary. The patient is required to fast prior to the test and may be given a sedative before the procedure.

Biopsy of the liver. A biopsy of the liver may be used to aid in establishing the cause of liver disease. In this procedure a specially designed needle is inserted through the chest or abdominal wall into the liver, and a small piece of tissue is removed for study. This procedure is contraindicated if the patient has an infection of the right lower lobe of the lung, ascites, a blood dyscrasia, or is unable to cooperate by holding his breath. To avoid hemorrhage, vitamin K may be given parenterally for several days before and after the biopsy is taken. A biopsy may not be done if the prothrombin time is below 40%. The physician should explain the procedure to the patient; for example, the patient should know that he must hold his breath and remain absolutely still when the needle is introduced. Movement of the chest may cause the needle to slip and to tear the liver covering. Most hospitals require that the patient give written permission for the procedure to be done. Food and fluids may be withheld for several hours preceding the test, and a sedative usually is given about 30 minutes before the biopsy is to be taken.

The method is as follows: With the patient lying on his back, the skin over the area selected (usually the eighth or ninth intercostal space) is cleansed and anesthetized with procaine hydrochloride. A nick is made in the skin with a sharp scalpel blade. Then the patient is instructed to take several deep breaths and to hold his breath while the needle is introduced through the intercostal or subcostal tissues into the liver. The special needle assembly is rotated to separate a fragment of tissue and then is withdrawn. The specimen is placed into an appropriate container, which is then labeled and sent to the pathology laboratory. A simple dressing is placed over the wound.

The dangers of this procedure, which is done relatively "blind," are accidental penetration of blood vessels, causing hemorrhage, and accidental penetration of a biliary vessel, causing a chemical peritonitis from leakage of bile into the abdominal cavity. After the procedure the patient's pulse rate and blood pressure should be taken every 30 minutes for the first few hours and then hourly for at least 24 hours. The physician may order pressure applied to the biopsy site to help stop any bleeding. Pressure may be applied by having the patient lie on his right side with a small pillow or folded bath blanket placed under the costal margin for several hours after the biopsy. The patient remains on bed rest for 24 hours after the test.

□ Endocrine function testing

The suspicion that an endocrine disorder exists can be derived from information gained from the patient's history and physical examination. Since the endocrine system affects multiple body functions, all persons with suspected malfunction will have evaluations of the levels of normal blood constitutents. In this section specific diagnostic tests of endocrine function will be described. These tests are divided into two categories: direct measurement of various hormones or their by-products, and measurements of specialized body functions or particular blood and urine constituents known to be controlled by the hormone. The specific diagnostic tests will be discussed separately in relation to each gland.

Pituitary function testing

Pituitary gland malfunction can lead to a wide variety of symptoms, depending on which hormone is in excess or in deficit. The pituitary gland, as described previously, is interrelated with functions of the thyroid, and adrenal glands and the gonads. The tests for the function of the pituitary with regards to TSH, ACTH, and gonadotropins will be discussed when the diagnostic tests of each gland are discussed. Pituitary malfunction may be associated with pituitary tumors, and skull roentgenograms to assess the size of the pituitary gland will be carried out.

Somatotropin hormone. The absence or deficit of somatotropin (growth hormone) leads to dramatic changes in appearance. Diagnostic tests for somatotropin will include skeletal roentgenograms to assess changes in bone structure. Assay of the growth hormone is possible.

Antidiuretic hormone. Absence of ADH leads to a disease called *diabetes insipidus.* The major symptom of this problem is an output of large quantities of dilute urine (greater than 7 to 11 liters per day). Before diabetes insipidus can be conclusively diagnosed, the patient must be shown to have a deficit in ADH, and the patient's kidney must be able to respond to ADH. Exogenous sources of ADH have no effect if the patient's kidney cannot respond. Exogenous ADH will increase the osmolarity of the urine whether the dilute urine is caused by excess intake of water or by diabetes insipidus. The differentiation between these two conditions is made by demonstrating response or lack of response to osmolarity changes in the serum.

Water deprivation test. Water is withheld until 2% to 5% of body weight is lost. This may require up to 12 hours of deprivation. The patient who has no ability to produce ADH is susceptible to vascular collapse because the massive output of urine will continue unabated. Close monitoring for impending collapse during the test is required. The patient with *psychogenic polydipsia* may have extreme behavioral problems associated with the deprivation of water and will need emotional support during this long period of time.

Thyroid function testing

Testing for thyroid function can be made at the pituitary, thyroid, serum, or the peripheral tissue levels. The commonly used tests and procedures and preparations for and interpretations of them are presented in Table 30-3. Since many of the tests can be affected by the presence of iodine, in most instances a battery of tests will be done.

Parathyroid function testing

Since the maintenance of normal calcium and phosphorous metabolism involves multiple systems besides the parathyroid (skeletal, gastrointestinal, and urinary), when parathyroid function is being assessed, the patient will also have diagnostic tests of these other systems. This is necessary to determine whether the problem with calcium and phosphorous metabolism is caused by parathyroid metabolism or other disease states. In addition, because calcium has a very important role in the maintenance of normal neuromuscular irritability and because hypocalcemia can be lethal, when hypoparathyroidism is suspected, the patient will be assessed and continually monitored for the presence of Trousseau's and Chvostek's signs (see Chapter 20).

The specific tests of parathyroid function consist of serial lab determinations of serum calcium and phosphorous, urinary calcium and phosphorous, and serum alkaline phosphatase. In addition, two other commonly performed tests are the Ellsworth-Howard excretion test and the phosphate reabsorption test.

Ellsworth-Howard excretion test. This test provides for differentiation between normal parathyroid function and decreased parathyroid function. The test is done as follows: the patient fasts prior to the examination, 200 units of parathyroid extract are given intravenously, urine is collected on an hourly basis for 3 hours prior to the injection and 5 hours after the injection, and the urine is examined for the amount of phosphate excreted. Normally there will be a fivefold to sixfold increase in urinary excretion of phosphate. In hypoparathyroidism there is a tenfold increase in phosphate excretion.[30]

Phosphate reabsorption test. This test is used in the diagnosis of suspected hyperparathyroidism. It consists of collecting a urine sample for 4 to 24 hours, and a blood sample is collected at the beginning or end of

Table 30-3. Tests of thyroid function

Function test	Procedure and preparation	Interpretation
Pituitary level test		
TSH radio-immunoassay	Blood sample. No special preparation.	Directly measures TSH levels. Measurement aids in differentiating primary and secondary hypothyroidism. Values are elevated in primary hypothyroidism because of loss of negative feedback.
Thyroid-stimulating hormone (TSH) stimulation test	Baseline levels of radioactive iodine uptake (RAIU) and protein bound iodine (PBI) are taken. Patient is given injection of TSH and repeat levels of RAIU and PBI taken.	Assists in differentiating between primary and secondary hypothyroidism. In primary hypothyroidism, repeat level of RAIU and PBI stays the same. If they become normal, this indicates hypothyroidism caused by too little TSH (secondary).
Thyroid level test		
Radioactive iodine uptake (RAIU)	A tracer dose of radioactive iodine (^{131}I) is given by mouth. At 2, 6, and 24 hours following administration, scintillation detector is placed over neck in region of thyroid and amount of accumulated radioactive iodine is measured. Excess iodine in any foods, cough medicines, x-ray media, other medications, and enriched iodine foods affect the test by giving low readings. Diarrhea, causing decreased absorption of tracer dose, gives low readings. Renal failure, causing decreased excretion, can cause elevated readings. No radiation precautions are necessary.	Normal thyroid will take up 5% to 35% of tracer dose. Increased uptake occurs in hyperthyroidism. Excess tracer dose is excreted in urine and can be measured. Urine is collected for 24 hours. Decreased amounts in urine are indicative of hyperthyroid state.
Thyroid scan	Dose of ^{131}I is given, and scintillation scan is done. In this test, scanner is moved back and forth over thyroid gland, and a picture of distribution of radioactivity is recorded. No radiation precautions are necessary.	Size, shape, and anatomic function of gland is assessed. Areas of increased or decreased uptake are noted.
Thyroid suppression test	RAIU test done. Patient placed on thyroid hormone for 7 to 10 days and RAIU is repeated.	If euthyroid (normal), repeat RAIU would be low. Failure of hormone therapy to suppress RAIU is indicative of hyperthyroidism.
Tests related to serum levels of thyroid hormone		
Protein-bound iodine test (PBI)	Serum blood sample. Results of test are invalidated if patient has high exogenous sources of iodine. Cough syrups, x-ray media, estrogens, and enriched iodine foods may cause false high levels and should be avoided for 1 week before test. Mercury causes abnormally low readings.	Test indirectly measures circulating T_4 concentration. Normal range is 4 to 8 μg/100 ml of serum. A decreased PBI is indicative of hypothyroidism. An increased PBI is indicate of hyperthyroidism. This test is being used less frequently because of the availability of more specific tests.
Serum T_3 concentrations	Radioassay of blood sample. No special preparation.	Normal values are 100 to 170 ng/100 ml, and are elevated in T_3 thyrotoxicosis.

Continued.

Table 30-3. Tests of thyroid function—cont'd

Function test	Procedure and preparation	Interpretation
Triiodothyronine (T_3) resin or red cell uptake	Blood sample drawn. In laboratory, resin and radioactive T_3 are added to sample of blood. T_3 will bind to unoccupied sites of thyroid binding globulin (TBG). Radioactive counts are done on blood and resins to determine amount of T_3 (radioactive) that is bound to resin.	Normally 25% to 30% of radioactive T_3 will bind to resin. In hyperthyroidism where there are increased amounts of endogenous thyroid hormone, value will be increased; in hypothyroidism, T_3 resin uptake will be low. This is not a measure of the patient's endogenous T_3 level. Test is affected by total amount of TBG. In wasting diseases where amount of TBG may be decreased, reading may be falsely elevated. In conditions such as pregnancy and estrogen therapy, abnormal amounts of TBG may be available and a false low T_3 may be obtained. Dilantin and salicylates compete with thyroxine for TBG sites and may give false-negative T_3 resin uptake.
Serum T_4 concentration	Blood sample. Test determines ability of T_4 extracted from serum to displace radioactive T_4 from T_4-binding proteins. Not affected by iodides and dyes that elevate PBI and depress RAIU.	Measures circulating thyroxine that is bound to TGB. Normal 3 to 7 μg/100 ml.
Free T_4	Blood sample. Special laboratory procedures.	Measures unbound metabolically active T_4.
Thyroid antibodies	Blood sample. In laboratory, red cells are latex coated with thyroid globulin and mixed with blood.	Test may differentiate cause of thyroid enlargement. If antibodies present, agglutination occurs.
Test related to peripheral effects of thyroid hormone		
Basal metabolism role (BMR)	Patient at rest. Amount of oxygen used while at rest is calculated. Patient's oxygen utilization is compared with established norms for people of same sex, age, and size. Results expressed in percentage above or below normal. Patient receives nothing by mouth (npo) night before test, should have 8 hours sleep, and should stay in bed morning of test. No food or smoking is allowed. Anxiety will increase BMR, so patient needs explanation of what to expect.	Normal range is minus 15% to plus 15%. In hyperthyroidism, patient's BMR will be greater than plus 15%. In hypothyroidism, patient's BMR will be greater than minus 15%. BMR is less accurate, but may be used to follow patients on thyroid therapy.
Serum cholesterol level	Blood sample. Patient placed on npo list night before.	Normals vary from laboratory to laboratory. High levels found in hypothyroidism and low levels found in hyperthyroidism. Data augments other tests.
Achilles tendon reflex recording	Electrodes from recording drum attached to patient's ankle. While ankle tendon is tapped, recording is done.	Slow, sluggish jerk indicative of hypothyroidism. Rapid jerk indicative of hyperthyroidism.

the test. The amount of phosphate in the urine and blood is measured, and tubular reabsorption of phosphate is calculated. The normal tubular reabsorption of phosphate is 90% or greater. In hyperparathyroidism, values are less than 85%.[30] Although this is a relatively simple test, it is only valid if renal function is proven to be normal.

Adrenal function testing

The adrenal function tests can be divided into those designed to test *medullary* function and those designed to test *cortical* function.

Adrenal cortical function test. Since the adrenal cortex affects so many physiologic functions, tests that are diagnostic for many disorders may be ordered. Analysis of blood to ascertain electrolyte balance, a glucose tolerance test to determine the ability of the patient to utilize carbohydrates, and a test of the ability of the renal tubules to concentrate and dilute urine will probably be done. In addition, roentgenograms of the kidney area may be taken to ascertain the presence of adrenal tumors.

Diagnostic examination will include 24-hour urine collections, which are analyzed for 17-ketosteroids (17-KS), 17-ketogenic steroids (17-KGS), and 17-hydroxycorticosteroids (17-OHCS). These compounds are metabolites of the hormones produced by the adrenal gland. These 24 urine collections require special preservatives, and the nurse should know the institution's requirements and make sure the appropriate container is available. Blood levels of ACTH, cortisol, androgens, and aldosterone can be measured, although blood levels of aldosterone are infrequently measured.

In addition to the above studies, other definitive tests are available to determine whether hypofunction or hyperfunction of the adrenal cortex is present and to establish whether the malfunction is caused by a primary adrenal cortical problem or whether the malfunction is secondary to pituitary malfunction. These studies are described in Table 30-4.

Adrenal medulla function test. The function of the adrenal medulla can be assessed by the assay of catecholamines and their metabolites in the urine. A 24-hour urine collection is carried out, and the end product, 3-methoxy-4-hydroxymandelic acid, also called vanillylmandelic acid (VMA), is assayed.

Pressor tests to establish a diagnosis of *pheochromocytoma* (adrenal-medullary tumor) employ manipulation of the blood pressure. In one test, histamine 0.025 to 0.1 mg is given intravenously. A dramatic rise in blood pressure of at least 50 mm Hg higher than an elevation

Table 30-4. Tests of adrenal cortical function

Function test	Procedure and preparation	Interpretation
ACTH stimulation test (various tests are available); 3-hour intravenous ACTH test	Procedure and preparation: *Day one:* a 24-hour urine specimen for 17-KS, 17-OHCS, and 17-KGS is collected and patient is given dexamethasone 0.5 mg orally 3 times. *Day two:* ACTH 25 units in 500 ml of saline is given over 8 hours. Dexamethasone is continued. A second 24-hour urine specimen for 17-KS, 17-OHCS, and 17 KGS is collected.	Normally urinary levels of 17-KS, 17-OHCS, and 17-KGS will increase threefold to fivefold. In primary adrenal cortical insufficiency, urinary levels do not rise. In adrenal cortical insufficiency secondary to pituitary disease, urinary levels will rise slowly if test is repeated over several days. Slow rise is caused by adrenal atrophy that occurs with absence of ACTH. In adrenal cortical excess, urinary level may increase up to ten times normal because of adrenal cortical hyperplasia.
Plasma cortical response to ACTH	Fasting blood specimen for cortisol level is drawn. Twenty-five units of ACTH are administered; 30 minutes later second blood specimen is drawn.	Normally cortisol level will increase. If cortisol level fails to increase above 10 μg/100 ml, this is indicative of primary adrenal cortical insufficiency (Addison's disease).
Cortisone suppression test	Twenty-four-hour urine specimen for 17-OHCS is collected for baseline. Dexamethasone 0.5 mg is given every 6 hours for 2 days. Twenty-four-hour urine collection for these 2 days.	Dexamethasone suppresses pituitary secretion of ACTH but doesn't change steroid excretion. Normally by second day of dexamethasone, 24-hour urinary level of OHCS should drop more than 50% below baseline. Patients with adrenal cortical excess (primary) will show decrease in 24-hour urine levels. Patients with secondary adrenal cortical excess will have drop, but less than 50%.

Table 30-5. Diagnostic blood tests for pancreatic endocrine disease

Test	Procedure and preparation	Interpretation
Fasting blood sugar (FBS)	NPO after midnight.	Normal level at 80 to 120 mg/100 ml. Elevated level indicates a need for further study to rule out diabetes mellitus.
Two-hour post-prandial blood sugar	Blood sugar measured 2 hours after heavy meal or 2 hours after receiving loading dose of 100 g of sugar.	Blood sugar should be within normal limits. Levels above 120 mg/100 ml should be investigated further.
Glucose tolerance test (GTT)	NPO after midnight. Samples of blood and urine are collected at beginning of test. Patient is given mixture of glucose to drink. Blood and urine are collected at intervals of 1/2, 1, and 2 hours (2-hour GTT). Samples may be collected at 3-, 4-, and 5-hour intervals (5-hour GTT). Presence of gastrointestinal disorder that interferes with oral glucose absorption requires administration of intravenous glucose. Test is done in same manner as for oral GTT.	Interpretation of results differs according to source of blood, method of analysis, and critical levels established by various authorities. Patient with diabetes mellitus or hyperfunction of adrenal cortex will have high levels initially that remain higher than normal. Patients with hypoglycemia may have drop in blood sugar much below normal levels and must be monitored for signs of hypoglycemia.
Cortisone-glucose tolerance test	Performed similar to GTT except that cortisone is administered at start of test.	Used when GTT results are inconclusive. Cortisone causes an abnormal increase in blood glucose and decreased peripheral utilization of glucose in persons predisposed to diabetes. Blood glucose level of 140 mg/100 ml at end of 2 hours is considered positive test.
Tolbutamide test	NPO after midnight. FBS is drawn and sodium tolbutamide 1 g is given intravenously. Blood samples for glucose analysis are drawn at intervals of 15, 30, and 45 minutes and 1, 1 1/2, 2, 2 1/2, and 3 hours.	In normal persons, FBS level will fall by 30% within 30 minutes. In abnormal response, FBS fails to fall. In patients with insulin-producing tumors, blood sugar may drop drastically. Patient must be monitored for signs of hypoglycemia.

provoked by the immersion of the patient's hand in cold water will be seen if the patient has pheochromocytoma. Urine collection after the test will contain increased catecholamines. The patient needs to be monitored closely for hypertensive crisis, and intravenous antihypertensive agents should be readily available.

Another test employs phentolamine (Regitine). Phentolamine will cause a drop of at least 35 mm Hg in the systolic blood pressure and at least a 25 mm Hg drop in the diastolic blood pressure if the elevated pressure is caused by excess catecholamines. The patient can have a major hypotensive crisis during this test and needs very careful monitoring.

Pancreatic endocrine function testing

The pancreas has both exocrine and endocrine capabilities. The major endocrine disorder of the pancreas is caused by disturbance in production, action, or metabolic rate of utilization of insulin. The relative lack of insulin leads to elevated blood glucose levels and the presence of glucose in the urine. The majority of diagnostic tests of pancreatic endocrine function are based on assessment of urine and blood glucose levels. The hormone, insulin, can be measured by radioimmunoassay.

Urine tests. Urine testing is familiar to most of the public. Testing of urine for sugar is part of a complete urinalysis, and the urine of patients with known or suspected diabetes mellitus is tested frequently for sugar and acetone by one of the following methods. Patients with known diabetes mellitus may be asked to do the tests themselves at regular intervals as an indication of adequate control of the blood sugar level.

Clinitest is a copper reduction method of testing the urine for sugar. It comes in a compact kit and is convenient for use because it is small and easy to carry and store. The kit contains a test tube, a medicine dropper, caustic tablets, and a color chart. Either 2 or 5 drops of urine are placed in the test tube with 10 drops of water, and a Clinitest tablet is added. The tablet generates heat, and the color of the solution is graded by comparing it with the 2-drop or 5-drop color chart. Certain drugs can affect the accuracy of this testing product. Large amounts of vitamin C and cephalosporin preparations such as cephalothin (Keflin) can give false-positive readings.

Tes-Tape, Clinistix, and *Diastix* are strip tests for glucose. Since color charts vary for each product, caution must be exercised in interpreting results. Also, test results must be read at specified time intervals to be accurate. *Acetest* tablets may be used to test for acetone. Urine is dropped on the tablet. If acetone is present, varying shades of lavender will appear and can be compared with a color chart. *Ketostix* is a strip product that can also be used to detect the presence of ketones.

Increasingly, single specimens of urine are used to test the urine for the presence of sugar. If the physician desires to know the amount of sugar being excreted in the urine at a particular time, a *double-voided urine* is ordered. To obtain this type of specimen the patient is asked to void, then is given water to drink, and voids again in 30 minutes. The second specimen is tested by one of the methods described above. If the patients are taught to test their urine at home, usually the double-void technique is taught. *If insulin is being regulated on the basis of urine checks, double-voided specimens for testing are required.*

In some situations the physician may wish to find out what time of day the most sugar is excreted. To determine this, *fractional* or *group* urines may be collected. All the urine voided from before breakfast to just before lunch is collected, and a sample is tested for sugar. This is the first specimen; the second is collected from before lunch to just before dinner; the third, from dinner to before bedtime; and the fourth, from bedtime until the next morning.

Twenty-four-hour urine collections also may be obtained to determine the quantity of sugar excreted in a day. In this collection the first specimen of the morning is discarded. All urine excreted for the next 24 hours is collected in a gallon container and sent to the laboratory. It is important that the patient knows he must add the first urine voided the next morning to the specimen.

Blood tests. Common tests to assess blood glucose levels are described in Table 30-5.

REFERENCES AND SELECTED READINGS

1. Bates, B.: A guide to physical examination, Philadelphia, 1974. J. B. Lippincott Co.
2. *Berk, R. N.: Radiology of the gallbladder and bile ducts, Surg. Clin. North Am. **53**:973-1005, 1973.
3. *Black, M.: Diagnostic methods in liver disease, Med. Clin. North Am. **59**:1015-1023, 1975.

3a. Boyer, C. A., and Oehlberg, S. M.: Interpretation and clinical relevance of liver function tests, Nurs. Clin. North Am. **12**:275-290, 1977.

4. Chey, W. Y., Shay, H., and Nielsen, O. F.: Diagnosis of diseases of the pancreas and biliary tract, J.A.M.A. **198**:257-262, 1966.
5. Conn, H. O., and Simpson, J. A.: A rational program for the diagnosis and treatment of bleeding esophageal varices, Med. Clin. North Am. **52**:1457-1481, 1968.
6. Dworken, H.: The alimentary tract: basic principles and case problems, Philadelphia, 1974, W. B. Saunders Co.
7. Evans, J. A., and Mujahed, Z.: Percutaneous transhepatic cholangiography, Postgrad. Med. **53**:182-185, 1973.
8. Gorman, C. A.: Some problems in thyroid diagnosis, Med. Clin. North Am. **56**:841-847, 1972.
9. Guyton, A.: Textbook of medical physiology, ed. 5, Philadelphia, 1976, W. B. Saunders Co.
10. *Hallal, J.: Thyroid disorders, Am. J. Nurs. **77**:418-432, 1977.

*References preceded by an asterisk are particularly well suited for student reading.

11. Harvey, A. M., et al.: The principle and practice of medicine, ed. 18, Englewood Cliffs, N.J., 1972, Prentice-Hall, Inc.
12. Huang, S. H.: Nursing assessment in planning care for diabetic patients, Nurs. Clin. North Am. **6**:135-143, 1971.
13. Krueger, J. M., and Ray, J. C.: Endocrine problems in nursing, St. Louis, 1976, The C. V. Mosby Co.
14. *Leopold, G., and Sokoloff, J.: Ultrasonic scanning in the diagnosis of biliary disease, Surg. Clin. North Am. **53**:1043-1052, 1973.
15. Loeb, P. M.: Endoscopic pancreatocholangiography in the diagnosis of biliary tract disease, Surg. Clin. North Am. **53**:1007-1018, 1973.
16. Lomas, F.: Increased specificity of liver scanning with the use of ^{67}Ga citrate, N. Engl. J. Med. **286**:1323-1329, 1972.
17. Malasanos, L., Barkauskas, V., Moss, M., and Stoltenberg-Allen, K.: Health assessment, 1977, The C. V. Mosby Co.
18. Mountcastle, V. B., editor: Medical physiology, ed. 13, St. Louis, 1974, The C. V. Mosby Co.

18a. Pierce, L.: Anatomy and physiology of the liver in relation to clinical assessment, Nurs. Clin. North Am. **12**:259-273, 1977.

19. Sanders, T. P.: Liver scanning, Postgrad. Med. **53**:191-195, 1973.
20. Schein, C. J.: Influence of choledochoscopy on the choice of surgical procedure, Am. J. Surg. **130**:74-77, 1975.
21. Schiff, L., editor: Diseases of the liver, ed. 4, Philadelphia, 1975, J. B. Lippincott Co.
22. Schwartz, S. I., et al.: Principles of surgery, ed. 2, New York, 1974, McGraw-Hill Book Co.
23. Sherlock, S.: Diseases of the liver and the biliary system, ed. 5, Philadelphia, 1975, F. A. Davis Co.
24. Shore, J. M., Morgenstern, L., and Berci, G.: An improved rigid choledochoscope, Am. J. Surg. **122**:567-568, 1971.
25. Shultzev, G., Bogen, Y., and Sokolova, G.: Ultrasonic diagnoses of hepatic disorders, Am. J. Gastroenterol. **65**:432-436, 1976.
26. Small, D. M.: Gallstone diagnosis and treatment, Postgrad. Med. **51**:187-193, 1972.
27. Stauffer, M. H.: Needle biopsy of the liver, Surg. Clin. North Am. **47**:851-860, 1967.
28. Tepperman, J.: Metabolic and endocrine physiology, ed. 3, Chicago, 1973, Year Book Medical Publishers, Inc.
29. Vennes, J. A.: Endoscopic cholangiography for biliary system diagnosis, Ann. Intern. Med. **80**:61-64, 1974.
30. Widmann, F.: Goodall's clinical interpretation of laboratory tests, ed. 7, Philadelphia, 1973, F. A. Davis Co.
31. Williams, S. M.: Diabetic urine testing by hospital nursing personnel, Nurs. Res. **20**:444-447, 1971.
32. Wintrobe, M. M., et al., editors: Harrison's principles of internal medicine, ed. 7, New York, 1974, McGraw-Hill Book Co.

31

Management of persons with impaired regulatory mechanisms

VIRGINIA CASSMEYER

Persons with impairment of regulatory mechanisms will have some problems that are similar regardless of the particular site of pathology. This chapter will focus on the needs of these persons and measures to meet their needs. Desired patient outcomes to guide care are presented with each problem. Care of persons with specific problems is discussed in later chapters.

Persons with impairment of regulatory mechanisms will have a problem maintaining physiologic stability and integrity. Physiologic functions under the control of the hepatic and endocrine systems are diverse, and dysfunction may be reflected in many parts of the body. Because these functions are vital ones, disorders of any of the regulatory mechanisms may be extremely serious. A majority of the problems arising from dysfunction of these mechanisms are chronic in nature and require the individual to learn how to keep the problems under control. Regardless of cause, nursing management of these persons is centered on three areas: *prevention of the primary problem or complications, care during the acute episode, and preparation of the individual (and significant others) to care for himself on a long-term basis.*

■ PREVENTION

The public is becoming better informed about certain diseases of the regulatory mechanisms such as viral hepatitis and diabetes mellitus. This in turn may lead to better health habits in the future. At the same time many persons have friends or relatives who have died or have been handicapped by disease of the regulatory mechanisms; and this may cause fear and lead them to be hesitant in seeking help.

Certain diseases of the hepatic system can be prevented. For example, the spread of viral hepatitis can be halted if the public is taught to use good hygienic practices and proper sterilization techniques. Some degenerative diseases of the liver also can be prevented if the public is informed about precautions in the use of substances such as alcohol and carbon tetrachloride. Serious damage to the hepatic system can be avoided if early symptoms such as jaundice, light-colored stools, or dark-colored urine are recognized and the patient referred appropriately.

Some endocrine diseases can also be prevented. Simple goiter can occur because of a lack of iodine in the diet. Nurses also can do primary prevention of endocrine problems by working with the public on weight control. Obesity can lead to many health problems, including diabetes mellitus. Control of obesity is needed with all age groups, and nurses can be involved in teaching nutrition and weight control. Nurses need to be able to identify persons who are at high risk of developing diabetes and work with them to assure that they are checked for diabetes periodically and, if diabetes is diagnosed, that appropriate follow-up care is received.

As mentioned above, many of the diseases of the regulatory mechanisms are chronic in nature. The progression of many of them can be halted or slowed if the patient knows what he can do to control the disease process. Adequate control is dependent on knowledge and motivation to follow prescribed regimens. Nurses carry a major responsibility for teaching these patients and for supporting them in following the prescribed therapy.

■ MANAGEMENT

Nursing care for all types of regulatory problems is directed toward returning the body to a state of physiologic stability and maintaining that stability. There are common outcomes and interventions that are needed by many patients with diseases of the regulatory mechanisms and these are discussed next.

□ Care during acute phase

The care of the patient during the acute phase is guided by five desired outcomes.

Outcome: *The patient will have improvement in presenting signs and symptoms*

The most obvious signs and symptoms are the presence of fluid and electrolyte imbalance, lack of adequate nutrition for cell repair and growth, and lack of ability to handle waste products.

☐ Fluid and electrolytes will return to normal

The liver and the hormones of the endocrine system play a major role in maintaining adquate fluid and electrolyte balance. Depending on the abnormality, excessive amounts of fluid and electrolytes may be lost or retained. The patient may enter the hospital with any of a number of fluid and electrolyte problems. Specific therapy will depend on the fluid and electrolyte status, which is determined by history, physical examination, and diagnostic tests (Chapter 20). In most instances the identification of the particular pathology will provide data on which fluid and electrolyte problems will be present. Chapters 32 and 33 describe the problems that the nurse should anticipate when a particular problem is present. Replacement therapy for fluid or electrolyte deficits, or restriction of intake and therapy to rid the body of excess fluids or electrolytes, will be instituted as appropriate. In all instances the nurse needs to know the goals of medical therapy. The nurse functions in meeting this outcome by instituting the ordered therapy, adequately maintaining intake and output records, and recording losses by abnormal routes such as perspiration, vomiting, and diarrhea. Monitoring the patient's weight by careful weighing and recording is extremely important, since weight is used to determine adjustments in therapy. The patient with problems of regulatory mechanisms can easily and quickly move from a status of deficit to a status of excess, or from a status of excess to a status of deficit, so that the importance of careful monitoring cannot be overemphasized.

In addition, in all instances, whether there is a deficit or an excess, the status of the cardiovascular system needs to be assessed and monitored until fluid and electrolyte status is stable. The patient's cardiac reserve may be so limited that modifications in activities and independence may need to be made. With the addition of each new activity or increase in independence, monitoring of tolerance to these measures is necessary.

☐ Nutrition level will return to normal

Disturbances of regulatory mechanisms cause a deficit in nutrients for cell growth. The lack of nutrients may be caused by the inability of the cells to utilize the nutrients present, inadequate dietary intake of nutrients because of anorexia, nausea and vomiting, or abnormal loss of nutrients through vomiting and diarrhea. Early in the treatment the patient may have anorexia, nausea, and vomiting. In addition, some may require various food restrictions as part of the treatment of their underlying disease. All of this makes the food that the patient is allowed seem unappealing and unappetizing. Some foods may not be well tolerated, and the patient may be apprehensive about eating.

In recent years a great deal of attention has been given to diet and its relation to chronic degenerative disease of the liver. It is suspected that the liver's ability to excrete toxins and carry on its many other functions is seriously hampered by inadequate intake of protein and of vitamin B. If liver damage has occurred, the organ's ability to store glycogen and vitamins A, B complex, C, and D may also be decreased, and the patient may be in much greater need of regular intake of complete foods than before his illness. In the absence of bile salts, a major component of bile, the digestion and absorption of fats and the absorption of vitamin K are seriously hampered.

A diet high in calories, protein, and vitamins, fairly high in carbohydrates (unless weight reduction is desired), and with moderate amounts of fat is often ordered for patients with diseases of the liver. Many physicians believe that the patient who has liver damage should have 100 to 300 g of protein per day, but it is exceedingly difficult to have the patient eat this amount. Lean beef (broiled steak if it can be afforded), broiled chicken, and fish are some of the best high-protein foods. Egg white, gelatin, and cottage cheese provide large amounts of protein and can be prepared in a variety of ways. Yeast is particularly high in protein and in vitamin B. Dried skim milk is very useful for fortifying drinks taken between meals and can be added to muffins, sauces, and many other foods.

Diet therapy for persons with endocrine diseases may be directed toward increasing or decreasing calories and other nutrients. It is often exceedingly difficult to get patients to take the amount and type of food necessary.

Persons with anorexia need considerable support to eat some essential nutrients, and those who are nauseated require a carefully controlled environment conducive to retaining the food they ingest. (See Chapter 53 for more information.)

☐ Waste products will be eliminated

Drug therapy may be used to facilitate elimination of excess fluid, electrolytes, and waste products. The nurse assists in these functions by carrying out appropriate medical therapy and by monitoring for effectiveness of therapy and for side effects. Most important from the nurse's point of view is that restriction of certain products will be necessary to supplement the patient's inability to handle certain solutes. In addition, excess waste products from endogenous protein must be prevented from accumulating. Stress increases caloric needs and can lead to the breakdown of proteins for energy, thus adding more nitrogenous waste products. Also, the proteins in the diet will be used for caloric needs rather than to repair tissue, since catabolism is increased when the neuroendocrine response is triggered. Care to decrease stress in the environment and to prevent infection and other complications of bed rest that can initiate the neuroendocrine response is of primary importance and is a major responsibility of the nurse.

Outcome: *The patient will have energy to carry out activities that are necessary for well-being*

The patient will need constant monitoring, have many physical and preventive care needs, and may need to undergo many diagnostic tests. Careful planning and scheduling of activities are necessary to provide adequate rest and prevent fatigue. The nurse must set priorities on a day-to-day basis. Consultation with the physician in arranging diagnostic tests so that the patient does not receive unnecessary repeat preparation is very important. Not all hygiene needs may be met each day. The most important thing the nurse does to meet this second outcome is to make a total care plan so that important needs will not be missed.

Outcome: *The patient will be free of avoidable stressors*

The environment must be free of physiologic and psychologic stressors. Providing an environment that is restful and as anxiety free as possible may be one of the greatest challenges for the nurse. The emotional responses to hepatic and endocrine disease are often severe and require much support and understanding on the part of the nurse. Often these diseases are chronic, permanent changes in the individual's life style are usually required. Involving the patient and his significant others in developing a suitable plan of care for the hospital and at home will help reduce fear and anxiety and will also provide an opportunity for the nurse to explore the patient's fears about the disease with the patient and to determine where teaching emphasis needs to be placed.

The patient may be lethargic or extremely restless. It is important that family and friends be told that the change in behavior is caused by the disease. Otherwise they may become upset and add to the problem. Unexpected events and disturbing news usually are not well tolerated, and the patient must be spared from these. The effects of visitors on the patient must be assessed, and in some instances visitors may need to be restricted if they are upsetting the patient.

Planning with the patient the activities he finds restful and relaxing, modifying routines he finds upsetting, avoiding controversial topics, and remaining calm are important points in care.

Outcome: *The patient remains free of complications*

The major complications of impaired regulatory mechanisms are infection, hemorrhage, and those arising from immobility secondary to bed rest.

□ Free of infection

The person with pathology of regulatory mechanisms is a prime candidate for infection. This may be because of decreased phagocytosis, decreased ability to produce white blood cells and antibodies, masking of signs of infection, or a generalized decrease in resistance. Infections are acquired easily and may be difficult to cure. They increase catabolism and add stress. The patient needs to be protected from any kind of infection. This is accomplished by placing the person who is seriously ill in a private room, assuring that no one (staff or visitors) with an upper respiratory infection has contact with the patient, and observing strict technique in care of intravenous lines and drainage tubes and in changing dressings. Careful ongoing monitoring for early signs of infection is essential. The most common sites of infection are the respiratory, genitourinary, and gastrointestinal tracts and the skin.

□ Free of skin and foot problems

Because patients with problems of the regulatory mechanisms are more susceptible to infection and generally heal more slowly than other persons, special attention is given to skin care. A daily bath or shower is desirable. If this is not possible, emphasis is given to daily bathing of areas most likely to become infected. The back of the neck, the axillae, and the groin are prime sites for carbuncles to develop, and these areas should be bathed daily. Women who are obese need to give special care to areas under the breasts, since any place where two skin surfaces meet is a likely place for infection to develop. To prevent dry, cracked skin, a skin lubricant is helpful after bathing or showering. Areas between the toes are dried carefully after bathing as warm, moist areas are conducive to bacterial growth.

□ Free of hemorrhage

Hemorrhage may be a major problem in diseases of the hepatic system. Because the jaundiced person may have a low prothrombin level, the coagulation time of the blood may be prolonged and the person may bleed easily. For this reason the person is a poor surgical risk and may bleed profusely from minor procedures such as a venipuncture or an intramuscular injection. Normal production of prothrombin is dependent on four things: (1) ingestion of foods that can undergo synthesis in the intestine; (2) presence of bile in the intestine, thus enabling the intestine to produce vitamin K from food constituents; (3) absorption through the intestinal wall of the vitamin K produced; and (4) use of the vitamin K by the liver in the formation of prothrombin.

Since vitamin K depends on the presence of bile salts for its manufacture and absorption in the intestine, bile salts are often given by mouth to patients who are jaundiced. Vitamine K may be given both orally and parenterally in the hope that it will enable the liver to form more prothrombin. If vitamin K, which is not water soluble, is given by mouth, bile salts must be given as well. However, menadione sodium bisulfite (Hykinone), a water-soluble preparation of vitamin K, usually is ordered. The usual dose is 0.5 to 2 mg daily, given parenterally. If the jaundice is caused by obstruction in the biliary tract and not by liver disease, it can be treated satisfactorily. If the liver is severely diseased and unable to make use of the vitamin K provided, the prothrombin level will remain low despite the administration of bile salts and vitamin K. Fresh blood then may have to be given to provide the prothrombin essential for clotting.[2]

Since the jaundiced person may bleed more than usual from such minor procedures as drawing blood from a vein, plans should be made for samples of blood to be taken at the same time for several tests. If an infusion is ordered, it should be started at the time blood is drawn. When giving intramuscular and hypodermic injections, the nurse selects the smallest needle that can be used safely and is particularly careful that the needle is sharp and that, following an injection, firm pressure is exerted for longer than is normally necessary. The patient should be instructed to take special care when brushing his teeth. If prothrombin level is very low, a toothbrush is not used, but mouthwash or cotton swabs may be used instead to prevent bleeding gums. Urine and stools are checked for either old or fresh blood, and if bleeding is suspected, specimens are saved. Steady oozing of blood from hemorrhoids is not unusual in severe jaundice. Incisions heal more slowly when jaundice is present, and the nurse should inspect dressings frequently for bleeding. The patient's activity may be restricted until the wound has healed completely.

□ Free of injury

Persons with regulatory problems frequently have changes in sensorium secondary to an increase in toxic products, to a decrease in blood volume, or to inadequate brain perfusion. Precautions to prevent injury are necessary, and significant others require careful explanation of the reasons for the precautions.

□ Free of complications from bed rest

Because these persons may be treated with bed rest, have decreased nutrient levels for adequate cellular nutrition, may be dehydrated or have edema, leading to decreased perfusion to the periphery, and have decreased resistance to infection, they require care directed toward preventing skin breakdown, thrombophlebitis, and pneumonia. Frequent turning and good back care, range of motion exercises, and respiratory care must be part of the nursing care plan.

Outcome: *The client will be free of avoidable discomforts*

One of the major discomforts the person with disease of the hepatic system will have is pruritus caused by jaundice.

□ Jaundice

Jaundice is a symptom complex caused by a disturbance of the physiology of bile pigment and is present in many diseases of the hepatic and biliary system. There is an excess of bile pigment in the blood, which eventually is distributed to the skin, mucous membranes, and other body fluids and body tissues, giving them a yellow discoloration. Jaundice, caused by faulty live function due to disease of the hepatic cells, is described as *hepatocellular*. When jaundice results from intrahepatic or extrahepatic obstruction that interferes with the flow of bile, it is described as *obstructive*. *Hemolytic* jaundice presumably is caused by destruction of great numbers of blood cells, which results in the production of excessive amounts of bilirubin and the inability of the liver to excrete the bilirubin as rapidly as it is formed. The plasma concentration rises, the amount of urobilinogen in the intestines is greatly increased, and much of the urobilinogen is absorbed back into the blood and excreted in the urine. The results of these changes are summarized in Table 31-1.

□ Pruritus

The presence of bile pigment in the skin causes pruritus (itching) in about 20% to 25% of the patients who have jaundice. Pruritus was defined centuries ago as a disagreeable sensation that stimulates the urge to scratch. Actually, very little is known about the physiologic mechanism that causes pruritus. It is believed to be closely associated with the nerve mechanism that causes pain. The sensation arises in the nerve endings in the skin; it is unknown in lesions in which skin layers have been destroyed. Pruritus is known to be aggravated by dilation of capillaries, tissue anoxia such as occurs in venous stasis, and the presence of abnormal constituents such as bile pigment in the skin.

Pruritus can be exhausting and demoralizing. It is impossible for most people not to scratch the skin even

Table 31-1. Bile pigment metabolism: jaundice

Types of liver cell dysfunction	Serum bilirubin (conjugated)	Serum bilirubin (unconjugated)	Total serum bilirubin (conj. and unconj.)	Urine urobilinogen	Urine bilirubin	Stool	Jaundice (icterus)
Normal	<0.2 mg/100 ml	<0.2 mg/100 ml	+	±	0	Brown	0
Hemolytic	<0.2 mg/100 ml	>0.2 mg/100 ml	++	++++	0	Dark brown	Light reddish yellow
Familial	<0.2 mg/100 ml	>0.2 mg/100 ml	++	±	0	Brown (normal)	Reddish yellow
Hepatitis	+	>0.2 mg/100 ml	++	+++	++	Light brown	Deep reddish yellow
Cirrhosis	+	>0.2 mg/100 ml	++	+++	++	Light brown	Deep reddish yellow
Incomplete biliary obstruction	++	>0.2 mg/100 ml	+++	Variable and fluctuating	+++	Light	Light to deep greenish yellow
Complete biliary obstruction	+++	>0.2 mg/100 ml	++++	0	+++	Clay colored	Deep greenish

when told not to do so. Giving the person a soft cloth with which to rub the skin may help.

Medications such as an antihistamine or a tranquilizer may be prescribed to reduce the itching or to reduce the patient's response to the itching. Whenever possible, bed linens should be old and soft, since this will increase the patient's comfort. The patient's fingernails are kept short and hands are kept clean so that scratching is less likely to excoriate skin lesions that can become readily infected.

Cool, light, nonrestrictive clothing and bedclothes are desirable, and contact with wool is avoided, since it makes many persons itch. Because pruritus worsens when body temperature is increased, every attempt is made to keep the patient quiet and to avoid activities that increase metabolic needs.

Women with diabetes may develop pruritus vulvae, which will require special attention. They are taught to sponge the area after voiding and to pat the area dry. Some women find applying cornstarch to the vulvae is helpful. It is cheaper than talcum powder and is free of perfumes and other agents that may increase itching.

In general a warm, not hot, tub bath is more soothing than a shower and may relieve a great deal of discomfort. Colloidal baths using oatmeal or starch may be ordered. Medicated ointments or lotion to reduce itching also may be prescribed. Diversional activities may be helpful in reducing the patient's perception of pruritus.

A summary of the outcomes for the acute phase follows.

Outcome criteria for the person with impaired regulatory mechanism during the acute phase

The patient will:

1. Have improvement in signs and symptoms.
   a. Fluid and electrolytes will return to normal.
   b. Nutrition level will return to normal.
   c. Waste products will be eliminated.
2. Have sufficient energy to carry out activities that are necessary for well-being.
3. Be free of avoidable stressors.
4. Be free of complications such as infection, hemorrhage, injury, or complications from bed rest.
5. Be free of avoidable discomfort.

PREPARATION FOR DISCHARGE

Since many of the problems of regulatory mechanisms are chronic and often require the patient to take daily medications, adhere to a diet, learn measures to conserve energy, and prevent stress and infections, both children and adults are taught early to take care of these particular needs for themselves unless this is not possible for some reason. Children as young as 6 or 7 years of age can begin to learn to take care of their own needs. Patient outcomes should provide guidelines to meet these long-term needs. Family members should be included in the teaching even though they may not take an active part in carrying out procedures. Including them helps them to understand what is required of the patient. They can then encourage the patient to carry out instructions and can take over the care if this becomes necessary.

The teaching should be planned so that the patient is not rushed and has enough time for sufficient self-practice. If a significant other is to learn the care, arrangements must be made for this person to be taught at a time convenient for him.

Group teaching, in addition to individual teaching, is often desirable. Both the patient and significant others derive support and consolation from contact with persons with similar problems. In all of the teaching, emphasis is on the fact that the condition can be controlled and that the required restriction will help promote the physiologic and psychologic stability necessary to allow the patient to have energy to do the things he enjoys. Filmstrips, booklets, and other teaching aids are available from the U.S. Department of Health, Education, and Welfare; pharmaceutical companies; and voluntary agencies such as the American Diabetes Association. These materials should be reviewed before using them to assess their appropriateness for the individual or group being taught.

Outcome: *Patient or significant others can explain the replacement therapy planned for after discharge*

Persons with problems of the endocrine system may be on hormonal replacement therapy. Hormonal replacement therapy presents important implications for the patient whose prognosis depends on acceptance of drug therapy. The patient needs to learn the name, amount, and time of drug therapy, signs and symptoms indicating that the therapy is not effective, what to do if the therapy is not effective, and times when the amount of drug may need to be increased. Although hormonal replacement treatment may seem to restrict an individual's life, the person who has been helped to accept limitations and live within them is able to have a relatively normal life and is far less restricted than is a person with an uncontrollable problem. It is important for the individual to have the support of family members and for the family to understand the therapy and be willing to assume responsibility for it should this become necessary.

The patient must know that the treatment cannot be discontinued for a single day without specific direction from the physician and that the therapy does not usually provide for the excessive hormonal demands produced by unusually stressful physical or emotional situations. Because of this fact, stress-producing situations should be recognized and avoided. Sudden bouts of unaccustomed exercise, fasting, extremes of temperature, and fatigue are examples of undue stress. If any infection, no matter how minor, or any illness occurs, the person should seek medical advice. Pregnancy produces stresses, and therefore the physician should be consulted about family planning; additional hormones may be needed during the period of gestation and delivery. Because sudden, unexpected, stressful situations such as accidents or incapacitating illness may occur, the person on hormonal therapy should carry an identification card on which is noted the name of the physician, his or her address and telephone number, the prescribed hormone being taken, and the dosage to be used in event of an emergency.

Even in the absence of stressful situations, the normal person has changing needs for hormones. In replacement therapy, however, a specified amount of hormone must be given. It is not unusual, therefore, for the patient to develop symptoms of hypofunction or hyperfunction of the gland for which the hormone is being given. Both the patient and the family should be able to recognize symptoms of dysfunction of the gland and know what to do about them. If there is a means of compensating for too much or too little of the hormone, such as taking sugar for insulin reaction, the method should be taught. If this is not possible and the symptoms are acute, the patient must be taken at once to the physician or the emergency department of a hospital. Many times, if medical advice is sought at the first sign of even minor symptoms of dysfunction, the dosage of the hormone can be adjusted and further problems avoided.

A 2-month supply of the special drugs and equipment should be on hand so that an emergency does not interfere with obtaining supplies. As new supplies are bought, they should be kept in reserve and the old ones used. Continuous hormonal therapy is expensive, and the patient may require assistance from an appropriate social agency in the community. If the hormonal replacement therapy must be given by injection, the patient must be taught how to give the injection and how to maintain the necessary equipment (see p. 585).

□ Temporary replacement

The patient requiring only temporary replacement of hormones may be at home while taking them and, if so, must be taught the importance of taking the prescribed dosage regularly. Usually the dosage is reduced gradually and finally discontinued. While therapy is being tapered off, the person should be observed for symptoms of hypofunction of the gland that produces the hormone that has been given. The individual and the family should know the signs and symptoms of hormonal deficiency and should understand the need to seek immediate medical attention if these symptoms occur. They also should know that symptoms of hypofunction of the gland may occur even after the therapy has been discontinued. Regular medical follow-up should be continued until the physician determines that it is no longer needed.

Outcome: *The patient or significant others can explain dietary requirements*

The person with problems of the regulatory mechanisms will often require dietary modifications to assist in control of the problem. The patient and his significant others must be able to explain the type and amount of food needed and when needed, foods to be avoided or limited, how to measure foods, and foods that can be substituted for each other.

The nurse has an important role in helping the patient and his significant others understand dietary modifications. In all instances the patient's age, weight, activity level, medical problem, and nutritional state are considered when planning the dietary modification. Social and economic background and cultural preference should be accommodated, if possible. Dietary modifications may have to be adjusted for work, increased exercise, and other stressors.

The diet is part of the total treatment program and must be taken as ordered each day. In some cases, such as with diabetes mellitus, the diet is adjusted with the medications so that it becomes even more important that meals are not omitted or that unapproved changes are not made in meals. Sometimes patients may think that if they do not feel well, they can omit the meals and decrease the medications. This is not allowed. Clear liquids and full liquids in appropriate amounts can provide the essential amounts of nutrients for a short time. Directions on how to adjust the diet and how to prepare these foods should be given to patients and their families.

The restrictions in diet may require the elimination of certain foods or may require the measurement of food with kitchen equipment or with a scale. If the person is required to weigh food, he should learn how to estimate usual weighed amounts so that he can make adjustments when he eats out. The diet, whatever the restrictions, should be well balanced in selection of foods.

A clinical dietitian, if one is available, may initiate or participate in the diet teaching program. The nurse, however, often must give the diet instructions. If the dietitian does the teaching, the nurse and dietitian need to work closely together to assure adequate follow-up. A good time for teaching about diet is during mealtimes.

In planning the diet, written material on the type of diet being taught should be available. The material should explain foods that can be substituted for each other, foods that must be avoided, and foods that must be calculated. Sugar and salt substitutes can be purchased in most grocery stores.

If the nurse can help with menu planning on a weekly basis, patients can learn through demonstration how the diet can be varied and how they can have the food that they like even though restrictions are necessary. Most patients find it helpful to *see* food portions, especially such "unmeasurable" things as a small potato, an ounce of meat, or a slice of cheese. When possible, foods are measured using standard household measures such as an 8-ounce measuring cup, a teaspoon, or a tablespoon. All measurements are level, and cooked foods are measured after cooking. Persons on special diets do not need to buy special foods, but can select their diet from the same foods purchased for the rest of the family. Fruits may be fresh, dried, cooked, canned, or frozen as long as no ingredients that are restricted are added. Vegetables can be prepared with those for the rest of the family except that the patient's portion should be removed before ingredients that are restricted are added. Meats should be baked, broiled, or boiled. Any fat used must be accounted for in the measurements for the meal. Special cookbooks with recipes that can be used for patients as well as for other members of the family are available. They may help patients make meals more varied and appetizing. Special diet foods are expensive, and the patient should be reminded that they usually are not free of restricted items and must be counted in the daily dietary allowance.

Outcome: *The patient will have the energy necessary to carry out activities of daily living and social activities*

□ Conservation of energy

The regulatory mechanisms have a major role in the production of adequate energy. Most patients with problems of the regulatory mechanisms will complain of fatigue and weakness. Nursing care designed to assist them with this problem during the acute phase was presented earlier in this chapter. Some persons may continue to lack energy even after the problem is under control.

Reaching this outcome requires that the nurse know the patient's normal schedule and evaluate the things that the patient must do, things other persons can do, and the things the patient enjoys doing. The patient and nurse can plan how the significant others can be of most assistance without infringing on the patient's independence.

Activities of daily living can be spaced to allow rest periods. Some activities such as shaving or ironing can be carried out from a sitting rather than a standing position. Especially fatiguing activities are best scheduled at times of the day when there will be more opportunity to rest after completion of the activity. Rearranging the household might be indicated, since it can assist in preventing excess use of energy in walking stairs or reaching objects on high shelves. Significant others need to understand the patient's need for increased rest and their role in providing an environment that allows rest. Patients are often guided by how they feel and can use their feeling of well-being as a measure of what activities can be tolerated.

Outcome: *The patient or significant others can identify sressors in the environment, explain ways to cope with or limit stressors, and explain changes required in therapy when a stress situation is encountered*

Stressors are an everyday part of life but are increased at times. Each individual has unique ways in dealing with stressors. Stressors are often associated in peoples' minds with sad or depressing events, but they also may occur with happy or exciting events. The stressors in each person's life are different. The regulatory mechanisms play a role in how persons deal physiologically and psychologically with stressors. With dysfunction of the regulatory mechanisms, the person does not always have the ability to cope with additional stressors.

Reaching the above outcome requires that the nurse have good rapport with the patient so that he will feel free to discuss his stressors. Some stressors may concern very personal matters such as marital relationships and financial problems. The patient may need help from others in identifying ways to cope with identified stressors. If the patient is receiving hormonal replacement therapy, increased amounts may be necessary, since the daily therapy is only designed to meet normal requirements.

Outcome: *The patient or significant others can explain the recommended program for preventing infections*

The person with diseases of regulatory mechanisms has decreased ability to handle the stress of infection and has decreased resistance to infection.

To attain this outcome there must be appropriate ongoing monitoring for the presence of infection. Infections can cause serious problems, and the patient should know the signs and symptoms of common infections such as those of the respiratory tract and urinary tract. Patients also should be able to explain ways to decrease the chance of infections. They should recognize the need to avoid crowded places, areas with poor ventilation, and persons with upper respiratory infections. Because young children have frequent upper respiratory infections, contact with children may need to be limited.

In addition, patients with diabetes mellitus are especially prone to infections of the feet. All patients with this particular regulatory problem should know how to care for their feet properly and should see a podiatrist regularly (Fig. 31-1). The care of the feet is similiar to that for clients with diminished peripheral circulation described on p. 1021. Two pamphlets that are helpful in teaching clients are *Foot Care for the Diabetic Patient** and *Feet First.** Patients need to understand that the incidence of neuropathy is increased among diabetics and that neuropathy produces insensitivity to pain. As a result, blisters or cuts can become infected before they are noticed.

Finally, the patient and his significant others should be able to explain what to do if signs and symptoms of infection occur. Too frequently patients are taught signs and symptoms to monitor but are not told what to do should they occur. Since patients with problems of the regulatory mechanism have very poor resistance to infections, they must report any manifestations immediately. They also need to understand that infection is a stressor and may lead to a need for an increase in their replacement therapy.

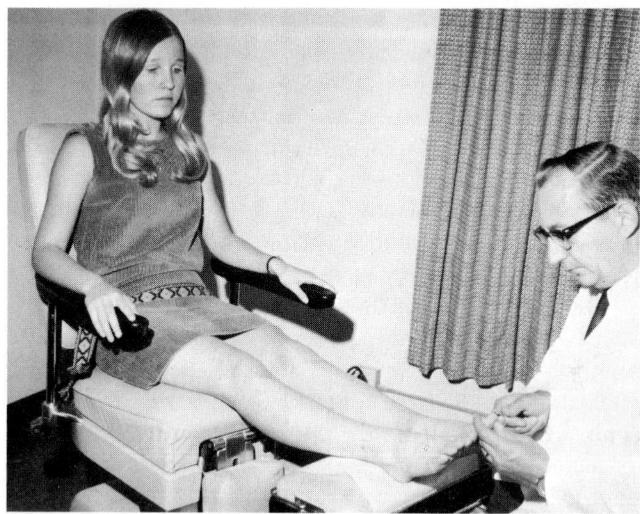

Fig. 31-1. Diabetic patients of all ages need special foot care and may receive it during visits to the clinic. Here the podiatrist cuts nails of patient.

The outcomes for care in the discharge phase are summarized below.

□ Outcome criteria for the person with impaired regulatory mechanism during the discharge phase

1. The patient will have the energy necessary to carry out activities of daily living and social activities.
2. The patient or significant others can:
   a. Explain replacement therapy to be maintained after discharge:
      (1) Name, amount, and time of therapy.
      (2) Signs and symptoms indicating when therapy is ineffective.
      (3) What to do if therapy is ineffective.
      (4) Times when therapy may need to be increased.
      (5) What to do if unable to take therapy.
   b. Explain dietary requirements:
      (1) Type and amount of food needed and when needed.
      (2) Foods to be avoided or limited.
      (3) Ways of measuring foods.
      (4) Foods that can be substituted for each other.

*Published by the Department of Health, Education, and Welfare, Public Health Service, Division of Chronic Diseases; available from the Superintendent of Documents, U.S. Government Printing Office, Washington, D.C., 20402.

(c) Identify stressors in the environment, explain ways to deal with or limit stressors, and explain changes in therapy when a stress situation is encountered.

d. Explain the recommended program for preventing and treating infection:
   (1) Avoid crowds.
   (2) Avoid persons with upper respiratory infection.
   (3) Notify the physician at the first sign of any infection, even a cold.
   (4) Follow prescribed therapy for an infection.

REFERENCES AND SELECTED READINGS

1. *Backsheider, J. E.: Self-care requirements, self-care capabilities and nursing systems in the diabetic nurse management clinic, Am. J. Public Health **64**:1138-1146, 1974.
2. Bergersen, B. S.: Pharmacology in nursing, ed. 13, St. Louis, 1976, The C. V. Mosby Co.
3. *Blout, M., and Kinney, A. B.: Chronic steroid therapy, Am. J. Nurs. **74**:1626-1632, 1974.
4. Burke, E. L.: Insulin injection: the site and the technique, Am. J. Nurs. **72**:2194-2196, 1972.
5. *Gabuzda, G. J.: Cirrhosis, ascites, and edema, Gastroenterology **58**:546-553, 1970.
6. *Garber, R.: The use of a standardized teaching program in diabetes education, Nurs. Clin. North Am. **12**:375-391, 1977.
7. Gartner, L. M., and Arias, I.: Formation, transport, metabolism and excretion of bilirubin, N. Engl. J. Med. **280**:1339-1345, 1969.
8. *Hallal, J. C.: Thyroid disease, Am. J. Nurs. **77**:417-433, 1977.
9. *Hayter, J.: Impaired liver function and related nursing care, Am. J. Nurs. **68**:2374-2379, 1968.
10. Kappas, A., and Alvares, A.: How the liver metabolizes foreign substances, Sci. Am. **232**:22-31, 1975.
11. Krysan, G. S.: How do we teach four million diabetics? Am. J. Nurs. **65**:105-107, 1965.
12. *Laugharne, E.: The role of the nurse in education of the diabetic, Diabetes Educator **1**:9-10, 1975.
13. Meltzer, L. E., Abdellah, F. G., and Kitchell, J. R.: Concepts and practices of intensive care for nurse specialists, ed. 2, Philadelphia, 1975, The Charles Press Publishers.
14. Mountcastle, V. B.: Medical physiology, ed. 13, St. Louis, 1974, The C. V. Mosby Co.
15. Nickerson, D.: Teaching the hospitalized diabetic, Am. J. Nurs. **72**:935-938, 1972.
16. Porter, A. L., McDonald, A., and Levine, M. E.: Giving diabetics control of their own lives, Nurs. 73 **3**:44-49, 1973.
17. Redman, B. K.: The process of patient teaching in nursing, ed. 3, St. Louis, 1976, The C. V. Mosby Co.
18. *Salzer, J. E.: Classes to improve diabetic self-care, Am. J. Nurs. **75**:1324-1326, 1975.
19. *Shea, K. M., O'Connor, C. P., Karefelis, E. G., et al.: Teaching a patient to live with adrenal insufficiency, Am. J. Nurs. **65**:80-85, 1965.
20. Sherar, L.: Ascites: pathogenesis and treatment, Postgrad. Med. **53**:165-170, 1973.

20a. Small, D.: A patient education program, Am. J. Nurs. **78**:889-890, 1978.

21. Strachan, C. B.: The diabetic's cookbook, Houston, 1969, Medical Arts Publishing Foundation.
22. *Suren, J.: Education of the culturally and educationally deprived diabetic, Nurs. Clin. North Am. **12**:427-437, 1977.
23. U.S. Department of Health, Education, and Welfare: Diabetes source book, Washington, D.C., 1969, U.S. Government Printing Office.
24. Williams, S. R.: Nutrition and diet therapy, ed. 3, St. Louis, 1977, The C. V. Mosby Co.
25. Williams, R.: Textbook of endocrinology, ed. 5, Philadelphia, 1974, W. B. Saunders Co.
26. Wintrobe, M. M., et al., editors: Harrison's principles of internal medicine, ed. 7, New York, 1974, McGraw-Hill Book Co.

*References preceded by an asterisk are particularly well suited for student reading.

32

Endocrine dysfunction

CAROL J. MITTEN
WILMA J. PHIPPS

Disturbance in the functioning of an endocrine gland may be caused by malfunction in the regulatory mechanism or by failure of the body processes to respond to regulation. Because the endocrine system is so closely interrelated and because the production of each hormone is dependent not only on other hormones but also on nervous stimulation, genetic controls, enzymatic action, and available energy and nutrients, it is obvious that endocrine dysfunction can arise from diverse causes. Dysfunction of one gland is likely to affect the function of one or more of the others. The structure and thus the function of an endocrine gland may be changed by abnormal embryonic development of the endocrine tissue, deprivation of blood supply to the gland, infection of the gland, tumor (benign or malignant) growths in it, overstimulation of it, or overgrowth of its tissues (hypertrophy and hyperplasia). In *hyperplasia* the size of the gland increases because it is continuously overstimulated, and there is a proliferation of active secreting cells. In *hypertrophy* there is an increase in the size of the gland caused by the increase in functional demands on it. Hypertrophy may or may not be accompanied by hyperplasia. *Hypoplasia* is a decrease in the amount of functioning tissue, and consequently there is a decrease in the amount of hormone produced. It may be caused by anything that inhibits tissue growth. It is believed that both the production of hormones and the effect of hormones on body cells can be affected by age, race, sex, season, climate, and disease.

Atrophy, or a decrease in the size of a gland, is caused by a decrease in functional demands. This could result from a failure of the gland to perform its function or from an exogenous supply of the hormone that makes the endogenous hormone produced by the gland unnecessary.

Disease of an endocrine gland usually causes a decrease or increase in the secretion of its hormones, and the symptoms are those of increased or decreased regulation of the processes normally controlled by it. Because of the diverse physiologic functions under hormonal control, symptoms of endocrine dysfunction may be reflected in many parts of the body, and because many of the functions controlled are vital ones, endocrine disorders may be extremely serious.

The specific treatment of endocrine diseases consists basically of decreasing the output of hormones from hyperactive glands and supplying or compensating for deficient hormones. Occasionally, in hypofunction, treatment may be designed to lessen the need for the hormone or to stimulate its production. Overproduction of a specific hormone often can be controlled by resecting part of the gland secreting the hormone or, if a tumor is stimulating the gland, by removing the tumor. However, the entire endocrine gland sometimes must be removed surgically or destroyed. Occasionally the pituitary gland may be removed or destroyed if it stimulates the secretions of the overactive gland. Sometimes radiation of either the specific endocrine gland or the pituitary gland destroys enough tissue to bring the symptoms under control. If endocrine glands are completely removed or destroyed, essential hormones must be supplied regularly for the remainder of the patient's life. Regular replacement also is necessary to control disease when there is hypofunction of the endocrine gland.

Only a few of the more common diseases of the endocrine system will be discussed in this chapter. Those occurring less often should be reviewed in appropriate specialized texts.

■ PITUITARY PROBLEMS

Because of the influence of the anterior pituitary hormones on other endocrine glands, dysfunction of the anterior pituitary gland may cause symptoms of malfunction in the target glands whose secretions are dependent on its tropic hormones (Chapter 30). In the same manner, secretion of the other glands can be deliberately reduced by irradiating or removing the pituitary gland.

□ Hyperpituitarism

The major cause of hypersecretion of the anterior lobe of the pituitary gland is a secreting tumor. There are three major types of secreting tumors resulting from an overgrowth of one of the basic cells in the anterior lobe: eosinophilic, basophilic, or chromophilic. Hypersecretion of the anterior pituitary results in a wide variety of signs and symptoms, depending on which hormones are being secreted in excess. If the hormone being secreted in excess is one of the tropic hormones, the signs and symptoms will be caused by hypersecretion of the target organ. If the growth hormone is being excreted in excess, the result will be either gigantism or acromegaly. Congenital hypersecretion of the growth hormone from the anterior pituitary gland causes excessive growth *(gigantism).* Hyperfunction of the anterior lobe in the adult results in *acromegaly* and usually is caused by a tumor in the eosinophil cells of the pituitary.

Clinical picture

The main symptoms or signs of both acromegaly and gigantism are those of excessive body growth. In gigantism, symptoms become apparent soon after birth, and since the child is in the growth period, the bones enlarge both in length and in width. In acromegaly, since epiphyseal lines have fused with completion of growth, bones enlarge transversely. The features become coarse and heavy, with the lower jaw becoming particularly large. Frontal sinuses are pronounced. Hands and feet become conspicuously wider, necessitating larger-sized gloves and shoes. Lips are heavier, and the tongue is enlarged. Striking changes in the patient's appearance may be noticed in comparing his present appearance with pictures of him taken before the onset of symptoms.

Intervention

Hyperfunction of the pituitary gland requires surgical removal or destruction of the gland by radiation. Various approaches are being used, such as external radiation, radiation implant, or surgery (hypophysectomy). Radiation is the treatment of choice for small tumors. The patient who has had external radiation may experience temporary or permanent impairment of pituitary function. If symptoms of tropic hormonal *hypofunction* develop as a result of therapy, replacement of the hormones of the target glands is necessary. The replacement of cortisone is crucial, however, since the individual cannot live any period of time without it. Following radiation implant, the patient may slowly develop symptoms of hormonal deficiency. Careful observation will be needed to determine whether hormonal replacement will be necessary.

A partial or total *hypophysectomy* (surgical removal of the pituitary gland) may be performed through a craniotomy or through the nose and sinuses (*transsphenoidal*). (See p. 588 for care of a patient with a craniotomy.) In the transsphenoidal approach there is no external incision. Newer microsurgery techniques have decreased the incidence of postoperative hemorrhage. A clear nasal drip that tests positive for protein content or constant swallowing by the patient may indicate a cerebral spinal fluid leak.

In the early postoperative period following a hypophysectomy, the patient is monitored closely for changes in vital signs, general appearance, emotional state, and mental alertness from thyroid and adrenal dysfunction. He is also observed for signs of thyroid crisis (p. 571) or addisonian crisis (p. 580). Corticosteroid drugs are started immediately after surgery because of the lack of ACTH, which is necessary for functioning of the adrenal cortex. Thyroid replacement is usually not given until the patient begins to show signs of hypothyroidism, as the stored thyroid hormone will serve the patient for several weeks.

Fluid and electrolyte changes may occur in the early postoperative period because of lack of antidiuretic hormone (ADH), as seen in *diabetes insipidus.* Urinary output is measured carefully and recorded every 2 hours for several days. A urine output of 300 ml or more in any 2-hour period or a low urine specific gravity is reported to the physician. Vasopressin, which is the principal pressor and antidiuretic of the posterior pituitary, is started early when signs of fluid imbalance occur. Weight loss may occur. The patient may experience thirst, and water intoxication may occur if water replacement is excessive.

Sterility occurs with the lack of gonadotropic hormones. Testosterone may be given for impotence in the male. Estrogen-progestin therapy may be helpful in stimulating ovulation in the female.

The patient who has had total hypophysectomy will need lifetime hormonal replacement therapy with frequent medical follow-up. The patient receiving steroid replacement must be aware that stress may increase the need for medication and that stress may seriously upset the hormonal balance.

Outcome criteria for the person who has had a hypophysectomy

The patient or significant others can:

1. Explain the prescribed medication program.

a. State awareness of lifelong need for replacement therapy.
b. Describe effect desired, name, dosage, frequency, and side effects of prescribed drugs.

2. Explain the effect of stress on hormonal balance, measures to decrease stress, and need for assistance of health professionals if severe stress occurs.
3. Describe need for ongoing medical follow-up.

□ Hypopituitarism

Hypofunction of the *anterior* lobe of the pituitary gland may result from compression of the gland by a tumor within the gland itself, tumors associated with contiguous structures, or from trauma or hemorrhage.

Clinical picture

If a tumor is present, the patient may have visual disturbances such as bitemporal hemianopia (p. 640) and loss of visual acuity caused by pressure on the optic nerve, severe headache caused by increased intracranial pressure, and symptoms associated with disturbance of the gland itself. These symptoms may vary according to which hormone insufficiency is manifested. (For discussion of the various hormones, see Chapter 30). One result of hypofunction is the effect on body growth. In the adolescent, sexual growth and development may be arrested. If TSH is decreased, symptoms of hypothyroidism may occur. If ACTH secretion is impaired, the person may have symptoms of adrenal insufficiency (Addison's disease). A combination of many endocrine deficiency diseases may be present. *Dwarfism* results from congenital deficiency of the growth hormone.

Intervention

Treatment of anterior pituitary hypofunction depends on the cause. Tumors causing pressure on the gland are removed surgically or irradiated.

□ Diabetes insipidus

Diabetes insipidus is a disease caused by failure of the *posterior* lobe of the pituitary gland to secrete ADH (p. 552). Primary diabetes insipidus is a rare disease, but its symptoms are seen fairly frequently, since they may occur when a tumor develops in the gland, following head trauma, or following hypophysectomy or irradiation of the pituitary gland.

Clinical picture

ADH increases reabsorption of water from the renal tubules, and in its absence a very large amount of urine is excreted—as much as 15 liters may be excreted daily. This causes fluid and electrolyte imbalance. Persons with diabetes insipidus also have insatiable thirst (polydipsia), anorexia, weight loss, and weakness.

Intervention

The goal of therapy is to provide adequate replacement of posterior pituitary hormone and correct the underlying pathology if possible. Surgical removal of a primary or secondary tumor may be necessary.

Vasopressin tannate (Pitressin Tannate) in oil, given intramuscularly, is usually recommended for immediate treatment to reduce urinary volume for 24 to 48 hours. Administration is easier if the vial is warmed first. Vigorous shaking of the vial is necessary before administration, since the active ingredient tends to precipitate out.

A synthetic lysine-vasopressing solution (Lypressin) can be used every 3 to 6 hours as a nasal spray or drops for ongoing therapy. The patient should watch for symptoms of rhinopharyngitis. He is taught to use the medication whenever he notices polyuria or polydipsia. In severe cases, Lypressin may be used as adjunct therapy between injections. The patient should carry an identification card that explains his condition and treatment program or should wear a Medic Alert bracelet in case an accident or injury should occur.

Outcome criteria for the person with diabetes insipidus

The patient or significant others can:

1. State dosage and side effects of prescribed medication.
2. Demonstrate how to use prescribed medication (nasal spray or drops).
3. State signs and symptoms that indicate the need to take prescribed medication (polyuria, polydipsia).
4. State when immediate medical follow-up is required (worsening of symptoms or symptoms not relieved by prescribed medication).
5. State plan for regular follow-up care.
6. Show the identification card that the person will carry at all times.

■ THYROID PROBLEMS

□ Simple goiter

Any enlargement of the thyroid gland is spoken of as a goiter. A goiter may be caused by various disorders, such as congenital metabolic defects that prevent synthesis of thyroid hormones or chronic thyroiditis. Simple goiter or hyperplasia results from impaired thyroid function. Inability to secrete sufficient quantities of necessary hormones results in increased secretion of TSH, which stimulates glandular growth. It frequently is seen in girls, appearing at puberty, when the metabolic rate is highest and the body need for thyroid hormones is greatest. It may diminish or disappear spontaneously after the age of 25 years. In temperate climates the greatest incidence of simple goiter occurs in late winter and in spring. The incidence of simple goiter in the United States is greatest in the Great Lakes Basin, Minnesota, the Dakotas, the Pacific Northwest, and the Upper Mississippi Valley because of the limited amount of iodine in the water and food supply of these regions. Iodine normally is found in seafood, and small amounts of iodine are found in green leafy vegetables that have been grown where iodine is present in the water and soil.

Prevention

The nurse can help to prevent simple goiter by teaching the importance of eating foods that contain iodine. The patient should be asked about the quantity of leafy vegetables and seafoods eaten and the kind of table salt used. Encouraging uses of iodized salt is important in parts of the country where there is a known deficiency of iodine in the natural water.

Clinical picture

Changes in the contour of the neck may give a clue to thyroid enlargement. Palpation may identify an enlarged thyroid (p. 543). A simple goiter may go unnoticed, or the person may ignore it unless it become nodular or symptomatic. Difficulty in breathing may occur as a result of pressure on the trachea.

Intervention

Large goiters may have to be removed surgically to relieve symptoms of pressure or for cosmetic improvement. More conservative methods include medication and diet therapy.

Medication therapy. In the early stages of simple goiter, one drop of saturated solution of potassium iodide (SSKI) a week usually provides enough extra iodine for the thyroid gland to use to produce thyroid hormones, and the hyperplasia will gradually decrease. If the goiter is moderately large, it may be necessary for the patient to take thyroid extract as well as iodine to decrease its size.

Diet therapy. Using iodized table salt is an easy and inexpensive way of assuring sufficient iodine intake, since the average adult can obtain more than twice the daily iodine requirement from the amount of salt normally used.

Outcome criteria for the person with simple goiter

The patient or significant others can:

1. Explain the medication program (effects, desired dosage, frequency, and side effects).
2. Explain the dietary changes required (use of iodized salt).
3. State plans for follow-up care.

□ Hyperthyroidism

Hyperthyroidism, or hyperactivity of the thyroid gland, may be called thyrotoxicosis, toxic goiter, or Graves' disease. The gland usually enlarges and always secretes excessive quantities of thyroid hormones, speeding up metabolic processes. It is more common in women than in men, and there is a higher incidence between 20 and 40 years of age. It often appears after emotional trauma, infection, or increased stress, and occurs frequently in persons who have had other endocrine disturbances.

Prevention

People with early signs of hyperthyroidism should be encouraged to seek medical attention, since the disease gradually becomes more serious and treatment is more effective if begun early. Hyperthyroidism is a serious disease that, if not checked, can lead to death from heart failure.

Clinical picture

The individual complains of being nervous, jittery, and tense. He appears overly alert and may give indications of being irritable. Reactions are often exaggerated, and the individual may weep or laugh out of proportion to the situation. Physical findings include a fine tremor of the hands and awkward and clumsy movements. Complaints include weakness, fatigue, and weight loss despite eating large amounts of food. The individual often states, "I'm ravenous all the time but I keep losing weight." Heat intolerance and increased perspiration are common. The palms of the hands are usually warm and moist. The skin is often described as being fine textured and velvety.

Palpitations and breathlessness can occur as a result of the increased metabolic rate. Gastrointestinal motility also is increased, and diarrhea is common. Usually the individual seeks treatment when the only obvious signs may be nervousness and weight loss.

Exophthalmos, abnormal protrusion of the eyeballs, is a characteristic, although not uniformly present, sign of hyperthyroidism. This condition, the cause of which is unknown, may become so severe that the eyes cannot be closed.

Thyroid storm or *thyroid crisis* may occur in persons with uncontrolled hyperthyroidism. Increased amounts of hormones are released into the bloodstream, and metabolism is markedly increased. It may be precipitated by infection, stress, or thyroid surgery undertaken on a patient who was not adequately prepared with antithyroid drugs. The onset often occurs spontaneously. The patient's temperature may rise to 41 C (106 F) as the body becomes unable to release the heat formed with increased metabolism. The pulse may be very rapid, and there is marked respiratory distress, apprehension, restlessness, irritability, and prostration. The patient may become delirious and finally comatose, with death resulting from heart failure.

Diagnostic studies to identify hyperactivity of the thyroid gland are described in Table 30-3.

Intervention

Therapy is directed toward reducing the output of thyroid hormone. Long-term antithyroid drug therapy to effect remission is usually the therapy of choice. Radioactive iodine treatment is commonly chosen over surgery for thyroid ablation. Antithyroid medications are usually used in treating adolescents, young adults, and pregnant women. Radioactive iodine is used to treat older persons with toxicity to the antithyroid medications or individuals who do not comply with the prescribed regimen. Surgery may be used in younger persons when antithyroid treatment has not been successful.

Drug therapy. *Propylthiouracil* and *methimazole* (Tapazole) are the most commonly used antithyroid drugs. The action of these drugs is slow, and it usually takes 2 to 4 weeks before improvement is noticeable. The patient usually is started on a relatively large dose of an antithyroid drug, and then the dosage is gradually reduced to a maintenance level. When antithyroid drugs are used as the primary therapy, they commonly are continued for 6 to 18 months or longer. It is important to give the drugs at regularly spaced intervals, since their blood levels are reduced in about 8 hours.

Patients are instructed to look for toxic signs of the drug, such as fever, sore throat, and skin eruptions, and to call their physician if these signs appear. If toxic reaction occurs, blood counts may show leukopenia. Continued use of antithyroid drugs may not be tolerated by some persons.

Preparations of iodine, such as *Lugol's solution*, also are used in the treatment of hyperthyroidism. These preparations can reduce the metabolic rate rapidly because their action is more rapid, although less sustained. They reduce glandular vascularity and help to prevent postoperative hemorrhage when a partial thyroidectomy is necessary. Lugol's solution is often prescribed after a course of propylthiouracil to prepare the patient for surgery. When Lugol's solution is ordered, it is more palatable given in milk or fruit juice. It should be taken through a straw because it may stain the teeth. A brassy taste in the mouth and sore teeth and gums are signs of toxicity, but this complication rarely occurs.

There are some disadvantages to the use of iodides, including (1) the patient cannot be treated for some time with radioactive iodine (RAI) because the thyroid gland is saturated with iodide and the RAI will not be taken up; (2) some persons develop an exacerbation of their disease when RAI is given following iodide treatment; and (3) if iodide is given before treatment with other antithyroid drugs, this also may result in an exacerbation of hyperthyroidism.[3]

Radioactive iodine therapy. Radiation can decrease thyroid activity. The most effective way is by the use of ^{131}I, a radioactive isotope of iodine. The isotope is given by mouth, is absorbed rapidly in the stomach, and becomes concentrated in the thyroid. Usually a single dose is given in a radioactive "cocktail." If an unusually large dose of radioactive iodine is given, hospitalization for several days may be necessary. Patients receiving usual amounts of the isotope may go directly home, and no special precautions are advised. It takes about 3 weeks for the symptoms of hyperthyroidism to subside, and over 2 months for thyroid function to become normal. Occasionally remission is not achieved with one dose, and the treatment is repeated after an interval of several months.

Patients who receive radioactive iodine for hyperthyroidism need to have the treatment explained to them with special care, and they usually need repeated reassurance that the radioactive properties are quickly dissipated. Since they often are more emotional than other persons, they sometimes think they are experiencing reactions to the drug long after this is possible.

Care of the eyes. Persons with exophthalmos need to have their eyes protected from irritation. Dark glasses will afford some protection from wind, sun, and dust, while soothing eye drops, such as methyl cellulose 0.5% to 1%, may provide comfort. For more severe protrusion, shields, tarsorrhaphy (suturing the eyelids together), or surgery for orbital decompression may be necessary.

Rest. Since the advent of the antithyroid drugs and the trend toward early treatment, most persons with hyperthyroidism can be cared for at home. Although those allowed to stay at home usually are not particularly overactive, they are likely to be very nervous and irritable. It is important that family and friends understand that extreme sensitivity and excessive irritability are part of the disease; otherwise they may become upset with the individual and aggravate the situation. Plans for maintaining a quiet environment should be made with the individual and the family. Assisting the individual to obtain sufficient rest is a real challenge. Quiet activities such as handicrafts that require gross motor movements like weaving or reading may provide rest. Family members should try to remain calm and avoid discussion of controversial subjects.

When the individual is nervous, he may drop articles or be clumsy in handling them. This usually is upsetting and may become a source of real frustration. It may be necessary, therefore, to do small things for the person that he may seem physically able to do for himself, and he needs to understand why he is being helped.

Diet. There is usually an increased need for food because of the increased metabolism. A high caloric diet with snacks between meals may be needed to maintain weight and meet energy requirements. Decaffeinated drinks are encouraged.

Complications. Therapy may be ineffective, causing thyroid crisis (p. 571), or may decrease thyroid activity to a point of hypothyroidism (p. 575). The goals of treatment and nursing care for thyroid crisis are to control the release of thyroid hormones and maintain vital functions. Treatment includes antithyroid drugs, oxygen and hypothermia blankets (to reduce fever) intravenous fluids, steroids, sedatives, and cardiac drugs as indicated.

Hypothyroidism may occur as a result of any of the prescribed treatment programs; however, it occurs more frequently after surgery or radiation. Significant decrease in pulse rate, rapid weight gain, mental dullness, or a change in tolerance to cold are some of the possible indications of hypothyroidism.

Relapse may occur in a number of patients treated for hyperthyroidism; therefore patients must be alert to return of former signs and symptoms and seek medical advice should they occur.

Outcome criteria for the person with hyperthyroidism

The patient or significant others can:

1. Explain the medication program (desired effects, dosage, frequency, toxic effects).
2. Describe plans for a quiet, restful environment.
3. Plan meals to meet energy requirements.
4. State plans for follow-up care.
   a. State symptoms necessitating immediate follow-up (signs of remission, thyroid crisis, hypothyroidism).
   b. State plans for regular medical appointments.
5. Describe eye care if exophthalmos is present.

Surgery of the thyroid

The patient usually is considered ready for surgery when thyroid function has returned to normal (euthyroid) and the patient has a consistent weight gain and a marked diminution of signs of thyrotoxicosis such as tachycardia. An ECG is made before surgery in order to detect evidence of heart damage. Patients with heart damage are preferably treated with radioactive iodine.

Part or all of the thyroid gland may be removed surgically, depending on the purpose for which the operation is done. In the case of a malignancy the gland may be removed completely *(total thyroidectomy)*, and the patient must then take thyroid hormones regularly for the remainder of his life. When antithyroid drugs do not correct the hyperthyroidism and treatment with radioactive iodine is contraindicated, hyperthyroidism may be treated surgically by removing approximately five-sixths of the gland *(subtotal thyroidectomy)*. In most cases this operation permanently alleviates symptoms, while the remaining thyroid tissue provides enough hormones for normal function.

Preoperative care

Because the patient who has a thyroidectomy must protect the suture line from strain while raising secretions and while repositioning in bed or ambulating, preoperative teaching includes this information. The patient is taught to support his neck by placing both his hands behind his head; this action avoids flexion and hyperextension during moving or coughing.

Postoperative care

The *complications* following thyroid operations are extremely serious, and if they are not recognized and treated at once, they can result in death. Complications that the nurse should be alert for are recurrent laryngeal nerve injury, hemorrhage, tetany, and respiratory obstruction. Since the thyroid gland partially surrounds the larynx and trachea, there is danger of respiratory obstruction from a variety of causes, and (a tracheostomy set should be kept readily available)

The dressing is observed for signs of *hemorrhage* for the first 12 to 24 hours postoperatively. Since blood may drain back under the patient's neck and shoulders, the nurse's hand should be slipped gently under the neck and shoulders each time the patient is observed to be certain that any bleeding will be detected early. A choking sensation, difficulty in coughing and swallowing, or tightening of the dressing usually means there is bleeding into the surrounding tissues, causing pressure on the trachea and epiglottis. If these symptoms occur, the dressing should be loosened at once and the surgeon notified. If loosening the dressing does not relieve the *respiratory difficulty* and medical assistance will not be immediately available, the surgeon may instruct the nurse to remove the clips or sutures from the wound to relieve pressure on the trachea. The procedure to follow

tetany: chara by muscle spasms & convulsions

until the surgeon arrives should be ascertained whenever the nurse is caring for a patient having a thyroidectomy. The surgeon may need to perform an emergency tracheostomy, and the patient often must be taken to the operating room for retying of the blood vessels and resuturing of the wound.

Although slight hoarseness is normal, the nurse observes the patient for any increase in it and for any respiratory difficulty accompanying it, since these conditions may be caused by injury to the recurrent laryngeal nerves, hemorrhage, or excessive edema about the vocal cords and larynx. The most common condition to suspect when the patient has difficulty in speaking or breathing is edema, but if the recurrent *laryngeal nerves* have been *injured* during an operation on the thyroid gland, the patient may have vocal cord spasm. If the nerve to one vocal cord only is injured, hoarseness may develop. If the nerves on both sides are injured, the vocal cords will become tight and close off the larynx, causing the patient to show signs of respiratory obstruction. As he attempts to pull air in through tightened vocal cords, a crowing sound is made and the tissues around the neck are retracted. To recognize early symptoms of recurrent laryngeal nerve injury, the patient is asked to speak as soon as he has reacted from anesthesia and at intervals of 30 to 60 minutes.

If one or both of the parathyroid glands have been removed or disturbed during thyroidectomy, symptoms of calcium deficiency, *tetany*, may develop (p. 312). This complication may appear from 1 to 7 days postoperatively. If not treated promptly, it can cause contraction of the glottis, respiratory obstruction, and death. Serum calcium levels are usually monitored, and hypocalcemia is treated by replacement of calcium intravenously.

Calcium gluconate is given intravenously as immediate treatment. Daily oral doses of calcium chloride are then started. If not all the glands were removed, the remainder hypertrophy, so that hypoparathyroidism is only temporary. If all were removed, the patient must have replacement therapy for the remainder of his life.

Diet. High-carbohydrate fluids by mouth and a soft diet are given as soon as tolerated. The throat is usually sore for several days, and this may make swallowing difficult. Analgesic throat lozenges or a narcotic may be ordered to be given as necessary. When possible, they are given about 30 minutes before meals to make swallowing easier. A humidifier may be used to decrease discomfort and to thin secretions, making them easier to raise.

Activity. Following surgery, any activity that does not put tension on the suture line is permitted. When the suture line has healed sufficiently, the patient begins gradually to practice full range of neck motion to prevent permanent limitation of head movements.

Outcome criteria for the patient who has had a thyroidectomy

The patient or significant others can:

1. Demonstrate neck exercises to be followed at home.
2. State plans for follow-up care.

□ Thyroiditis

There are three types of thyroiditis; acute, subacute, and chronic. *Chronic thyroiditis* occurs in two forms, one is a lymphocytic thyroiditis, also known as *Hashimoto's struma.* The other is *Riedel's struma* or ligneous thyroiditis, which is a rare disease that causes slowly progressive fibrosis of the thyroid.

Hashimoto's struma

In Hashimoto's struma the thyroid is infiltrated with lymphocytes and plasma cells. Since 1956, when antibodies were identified, it is believed to be an autoimmune disease. Positive titers have been found to thyroglobulin and thyroid cell cytoplasm, and in some individuals both titers are positive. The mechanisms for the autoimmunity is not understood, although there appears to be a strong hereditary link that is a dominant trait. Hashimoto's struma is associated with other possible autoimmune diseases such as pernicious anemia, rheumatoid arthritis, lupoid hepatitis, disseminated lupus erythematosus, and idiopathic adrenal insufficiency.

Some experts believe that hyperthyroidism (Graves' disease), Hashimoto's struma, and myxedema are variants of a common process.[1] It is not unusual to find family members with one of the three diseases.

Clinical picture. The incidence of Hashimoto's struma has tripled in the last three decades and is now similar to that of Graves' disease. It is 20 times more common in women than in men. It can occur in children but is most common in adults between 30 and 50 years old.[1]

There may be diffuse thyroid enlargement, and some persons complain of difficulty in swallowing or choking. Signs and symptoms of hypothyroidism may also be present.

The diagnosis is not always easy to establish, and several tests may be necessary to confirm the diagnosis. Antibody levels are determined and protein-bound iodine (PBI) and radioactive iodine uptake tests may be used. When the diagnosis is still inconclusive, a needle biopsy of the thyroid is indicated.

Intervention. The treatment depends on the clinical findings. Persons with signs of hypothyroidism are treated with thyroid hormone. The hormone is also used to treat some persons with an enlarged thyroid gland, others may receive no therapy unless they develop symptoms of hypothyroidism later on.

Acute thyroiditis occurs when there is an infection of the thyroid gland. It is not common and is treated symptomatically. Subacute thyroiditis may last weeks or months, but the majority of persons become asymptomatic and return to normal thyroid function in time.

□ Hypothyroidism

Hypothyroidism, a general slowing of the body's activities caused by decreased thyroid activity, may occur at any age. This condition is caused by reduction in the secretions of thyroid hormones because of atrophy of the thyroid gland, deprivation of stimulation from pituitary TSH, decreased influence of hypothalamic TRF, overtreatment for hyperthyroid states, or total removal of the gland. Congenital absence or atrophy of the gland in infancy leads to the condition known as *cretinism*, in which both physical and mental growth is stunted. Early recognition and treatment prevents retarded physical growth, but it does not seem to prevent mental retardation.

Clinical picture

Often the individual has no complaints but is urged to see a physician by his family because of weight gain, sluggishness, or sleepiness. Menorrhagia in younger women may be severe. In physical appearance the eyes are puffy and watery, the skin is dry and thickened, and the hair is sparse and dry. The tongue is thickened, speech is slurred, and there is intolerance to cold. About 12% of persons with hypothyroidism have pernicious anemia.

Other possible findings include slow pulse rate, an elevation of diastolic blood pressure, and there may be pericardial effusion. Pleural effusion also may be present, and some individuals have ascites. All body functions are slowed, and constipation is common. Deep tendon reflexes are diminished, and there may be joint stiffness, joint effusion, and arthritis or bursitis. Despite these marked changes, some individuals do not seem to be aware of the changes in their appearance and behavior.

The severest form of the disease is known as *myxedema*, in which there is nonpitting edema that is caused by accumulations of mucopolysaccharides in the tissues. Periorbital edema and puffy hands and feet are common at this stage.

Myxedema coma occurs as the myxedema worsens. The individual becomes less responsive and may go into coma from which he cannot be aroused. Sometimes an infection such as pneumonia, cellulitis, or pyelonephritis precipitates the coma. There is decreased blood flow to the brain. Hypotension, hypoglycemia, bradycardia, hypothermia, and hypoventilation resulting in carbon dioxide retention are common.

Table 32-1. Replacement therapy in hypothyroidism: approximate equivalents

Thyroid: combination of T_4 and T_3	Levothyroxine sodium: synthetic L-thyroxine (Synthroid, Letter, Levoid)	Liothyronine sodium: synsynthetic triiodothyronine (Cytomel, Trionine)	Liotrix: synthetic combination of T_4 and T_3 (Euthroid, Thyrolar)
30 mg	0.05 mg	12.5 μg	0.5
65 mg	0.1 mg	25 μg	1
130 mg	0.2 mg	50 μg	2
200 mg	0.3 mg	75 μg	3

Despite improvement in therapy, which is directed toward gradual reversal of the signs and symptoms, the mortality rate is still between 50% and 90%.[1]

Intervention

Treatment of hypothyroidism is by the administration of the deficient thyroid hormone. The drugs used to treat hypothyroidism are listed in Table 32-1. It is important that dosages be increased gradually because a sudden increase in metabolic rate can cause death from cardiac failure. The daily maintenance dose of thyroid hormones varies widely. The correct dose is determined by a remission in the symptoms of hypofunction. Adults with hypothyroidism respond quickly to the administration of thyroid hormones. Changes in appearance and physical symptoms occur within 2 to 3 days. Treatment must be continued throughout life, and the individual must be taught that failure to take the prescribed medication will result in an exacerbation of the disease. Medication dosage may need periodic adjustments to avoid symptoms of hyperthyroidism or hypothyroidism. A diet fairly high in protein and low in calories is often prescribed until weight returns to normal as a result of therapy.

Outcome criteria for the person with hypothyroidism

The patient or significant others can:

1. Explain the prescribed medication program.
   a. State reason for lifelong replacement therapy.
   b. State name, dosage, desired effects, frequency, and side effects of prescribed drugs.
2. Describe need for ongoing medical follow-up.
   a. State plans for regular medical follow-up.
   b. Describe signs or symptoms necessitating immediate medical care of (hypothyroidism or hyperthyroidism).

☐ Cancer of the thyroid

Cancer of the thyroid gland is less prevalent than other forms of cancer, and only a small percentage of thyroid lumps are found to be malignant. Encouraging persons to have yearly physical examinations can be very helpful in early detection.

This cancer is prevalent in all age groups and especially in those with a past history of irradiation to the neck structures. Recently there has been a concerted search in the United States for young adults who received irradiation of the thymus gland as children. These individuals are urged to seek medical attention so that they can be watched closely for the development of thyroid cancer. Chronic TSH stimulation has also been identified with the formation of thyroid carcinoma.[1] The cell type determines the rapidity with which the malignancy will advance and therefore influences the type of therapy required and the prognosis. Carcinomas that are well differentiated and encapsulated and can be completely surgically removed carry a good prognosis.

Clinical picture

Cancer of the thyroid is usually suspected from a painless nodule or by palpable lymph nodes along with thyroid enlargement. Surgical exploration may be necessary to confirm the diagnosis. Thyroid function tests are usually normal.

Intervention

Surgical removal of the lesion is the treatment of choice. Whether a subtotal or total thyroidectomy will be necessary depends on the findings at the time of surgery. In all cases, doses of thyroid hormone (large enough to suppress endogenous TSH) are given before and after surgery (because many of the tumors are TSH dependent). The parathyroid glands are preserved and may be transplanted if necessary.

Radioactive iodine (^{131}I) is used following surgery for patients with metastases or lymph node involvement. Thyroid hormone is discontinued while the radioactive iodine is being administered. Certain types of cancer of the thyroid (medullary) are treated by surgery and then by x-ray therapy of the neck because this tumor usually does not concentrate ^{131}I.

Recently bleomycin and doxorubicin (Adriamycin) have been used to treat thyroid cancer unresponsive to surgery, radioactive iodine, or x-ray therapy.[1]

Outcome criteria for the person with cancer of the thyroid

The patient or significant others can:

1. Explain the necessary follow-up therapy (x-ray, radioactive iodine).
2. List signs or symptoms requiring immediate medical attention.

■ PARATHYROID DYSFUNCTION

☐ Primary hyperparathyroidism

The most frequent causes of primary hyperfunction of the parathyroid glands are benign neoplasms, although malignant tumors and hyperplasia may occur. In about 80% of the cases there is a single adenoma.

Clinical picture

Parathyroid hormone regulates the level of calcium and phosphate ions in the body fluids (Table 30-1); therefore hypersecretions cause a disturbance in these ions. The serum calcium becomes elevated (hypercalcemia), and the phophorus level is decreased (hypophosphotemia). There is increased urinary excretion of both calcium and phosphorus, and renal calculi frequently develop. Other symptoms related to the electrolyte imbalance are anorexia, nausea, vomiting, weakness, fatigue, bone pain, polyuria, polydipsia, and constipation. Changes in behavior may also occur. If the calcium intake is not increased, calcium is removed from the bones and *osteoporosis* (a demineralization of the bones) results. Osteoporosis causes the bones to become fragile and to fracture easily. *Pathologic fractures* resulting from weight bearing or pressure often occur.

Intervention

Surgery *(parathyroidectomy)* is usually indicated in the treatment of primary hyperparathyroidism. Part or all of the gland may be removed, depending on the cause.

Prior to surgery, the fluid and electrolyte imbalance is treated. Phosphate is given by mouth, and intravenous saline and furosemide (Lasix) are used to treat the hypercalcemia, (since they aid in the renal clearance of calcium.) Surgery is undertaken as soon as possible.

Postoperative goals relate to prevention of complications. Following surgery the patient must be monitored for signs of tetany (p. 312). Significant and persistent hypocalcemia, accompanied by other signs and symptoms of tetany, indicate a need for intravenous calcium and vitamin D supplements by mouth.

Parathyroid function usually returns in 7 to 10 days. A high calcium diet (at least 1 g/day) supplemented with vitamin D is prescribed until parathyroid activity returns to normal. Until the bones have become recalcified, special care needs to be taken to prevent fractures.

☐ Hypoparathyroidism

The most common causes of hypoparathyroidism is mechanical injury or inadvertent removal of all or some of the parathyroid glands during thyroid surgery or other surgery in the neck region.

Clinical picture

In acute hypofunction of the parathyroid glands, serum phosphate is elevated (hyperphosphatemia), serum calcium is decreased (hypocalcemia), and neuromuscular symptoms appear. The individual may complain of numbness and tingling in the extremities and around the mouth. These complaints suggest tetany. Chvostek's and Trousseau's signs are present. (See Chapter 20 for description of these signs.) Carpal spasm, marked anxiety and apprehension, laryngeal stridor, dyspnea, and cyanosis may be present. Persons with chronic hypofunction may present with lethargy, personality changes, and cataracts. Some persons have epileptic-like seizures of the grand mal type.

Intervention

Care of the patient with tetany includes careful observation of beginning symptoms so that prompt treatment can be given and severe reactions such as convulsions can be prevented. Calcium gluconate, 10 to 30 ml of 10% solution in saline, is given intravenously for immediate replacement. Large daily doses (50,000 to 100,000 units) of vitamin D taken orally are also given. Calcium salts are started orally as soon as possible.

Maintenance doses of calcium salts and dihydrotachysterol (Hytakerol) or calciferol (vitamin D_2) will be prescribed. Vitamin D appears to be the principal regulator of the level of calcium ions in the body and therefore increases the absorption of calcium. A diet high in vitamin D will need to be followed. The amount of calcium and vitamin D is gradually reduced as the serum calcium level returns to normal.

Recognition of early symptoms of hyperparathyroidism, such as numbness or tingling of fingers or toes, is important so that further evaluation can be undertaken. Hypercalcemia is a continuous hazard, and serum and urinary calcium levels are evaluated at regular intervals.

Outcome criteria for the person with parathyroid dysfunction

The patient or significant others can:

1. Explain the prescribed drug therapy.
   a. State name, desired effect, dosage, frequency, and side effects of prescribed calcium salts.
   b. State reasons for lifelong calcium therapy if total parathyroid function is lost.
2. Plan a diet high in vitamin D.
3. Describe measures to prevent complications (renal calculi, fractures) if hyperparathyroidism is present.
4. Describe need for medical follow-up.
   a. List symptoms of tetany or hypercalcemia that necessitate immediate attention.
   b. State plans for ongoing follow-up care.

■ ADRENAL DYSFUNCTION

The *adrenal cortex* is essential to life. Without its hormones, cortisol and aldosterone, the body's metabolic processes respond inadequately to even minimal physical and emotional stresses, such as changes in temperature, exercise, or excitement. Severe stressors, such as those caused by serious infections or extreme anxiety, may result in shock and death.

The *adrenal medulla* is not essential to life because the sympathetic nervous system produces similar though slower and less extensive responses. Dysfunction of the adrenal gland can be manifested as an increased or decreased function of either the cortex or the medulla (Fig. 32-1).

□ Hyperfunction of the adrenal gland

Cushing's syndrome

In Cushing's syndrome there is an excessive secretion of the glucocorticoid cortisol. There are three causes

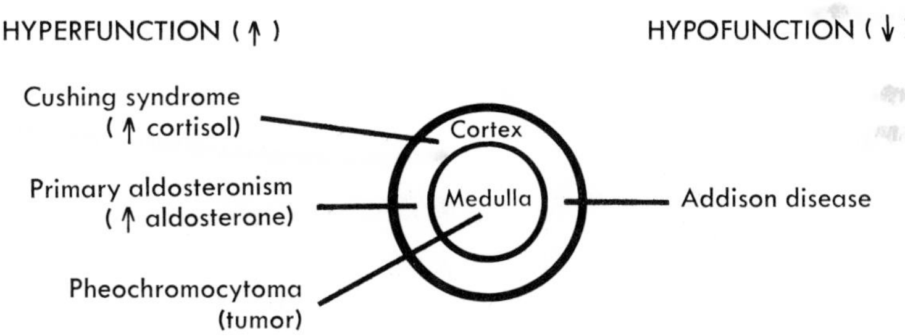

Fig. 32-1. Adrenal gland dysfunctions.

of this increase in secretion of cortisol: (1) adrenocortical tumors that result in hyperplasia of the gland and an increased production of the glucocorticoids; this occurs in about 1 out of 10,000 hospital admissions; the tumor may be adenoma or carcinoma; (2) a nonpituitary neoplasm that secretes ACTH, causing an increase in the secretion of the glucocorticoids by the target gland, the adrenals; this is also known as *ectopic ACTH syndrome;* and (3) a pituitary tumor, usually an adenoma, that occurs in about 1 out of 4,000 hospital admissions; in this situation the condition is referred to as *Cushing's disease.*[1] Manifestations of the oversecretion of cortisol have widespread effects: (1) protein wasting secondary to protein catabolism and an increase in hepatic uptake of amino acids; (2) capillary fragility occurs and ecchymoses are common; (3) adipose tissue accumulates along the trunk and purple striae appear; (4) resistance to infection is reduced; (5) sodium is retained and potassium is excreted, which results in hypertension secondary to sodium and water retention and ECG abnormalities and muscle weakness secondary to hypokalemia; and (6) congestive heart failure and strokes can occur.

Cortisol also interferes with the transfer of insulin across the cell membrane, resulting in hyperglycemia. There also are changes in the secondary sex characteristics.

Clinical picture. The person with Cushing's syndrome usually has a fat trunk with very slender arms and legs. There is muscle wasting and weakness. The distribution of fat is more noticeable in the face (moonface), neck (buffalo hump), and the abdomen. There are usually purple striae present on the trunk, and acne on the face is common. Women with Cushing's syndrome may show signs of masculinization, and menses often cease. Adolescent boys may have precocious sexual development. Osteoporosis is common and may result in pathologic fractures. Because of the hyperglycemia, diabetes mellitus is common, and there may be insulin resistance. Hypertension is usually present, and there is little resistance to infection. Because of these marked physiologic derangements and the drastic changes in their appearance, patients are usually irritable and depressed. They may have frequent mood swings related to the changes in cortisol blood levels.

Intervention. Treatment of Cushing's syndrome depends on the cause. If a tumor of the adrenal cortex is the cause, the tumor may be surgically resected. When there is a tumor of one of the adrenal glands, the increase in corticosteroids produced by that gland will cause suppression of ACTH (by negative feedback) and subsequent atrophy of the unaffected gland. In this situation the treatment of choice is the removal of the affected gland with replacement therapy given until the atrophic gland resumes normal functioning. If there is hyperplasia of both glands, then a bilateral total adrenalectomy is usually done. In this case the patient must be on *lifetime replacement therapy.* In nonpituitary neoplasms (ectopic ACTH syndrome), surgical removal of the neoplasm is the treatment of choice. However, it is often not possible to remove the tumor surgically. When this happens, the patient is treated with metyrapone, which inhibits the final step in cortisol synthesis.

In Cushing's disease the pituitary tumor can be ablated by irradiation. The results are not apparent for 1 to 4 months, and the patient may have severe physiologic problems in the interim, which are not easy to control. The pituitary gland may be removed surgically (hypophysectomy) by transsphenoidal microdissection, cryosurgery, or radioactive gold or yttrium may be implanted. These procedures are only available in major medical centers. For this reason the most common treatment of Cushing's disease is bilateral adrenalectomy with lifetime replacement therapy.[1]

The patient with Cushing's syndrome needs skilled nursing care and the utmost consideration. The patient usually is seriously ill and debilitated. Helping maintain adequate nutrition, some level of emotional balance, and an acceptance of the situation is a challenge. The patient, especially a woman, is greatly upset by the change in appearance. The moonface with acne, the buffalo hump on the back of the neck, the purple striae, and the obvious obesity of the trunk makes the patient look very unattractive. She usually is sensitive about her appearance, and may withdraw from others. The nurse needs to be aware of the patient's feelings and should protect the patient from upsetting situations. If the patient is to have surgery on either the adrenal glands or the pituitary gland, careful preparation is necessary. Patients who are untreated usually die of infection or from cerebrovascular accidents secondary to severe hypertension.

Many nurses may never see a patient with Cushing's syndrome from one of the tumors described above. However, most nurses come in contact with patients with *Cushing's syndrome medicamentous.* In this situation the patient is receiving large enough doses of the glucocorticosteroids to develop Cushing's syndrome. This condition is also referred to as iatrogenic Cushing's syndrome, since it is induced by the physician in the course of the treatment.

□ Primary aldosteronism

Primary aldosteronism is a rare disorder that is usually caused by an aldosterone-secreting adenoma (Conn's syndrome). It also can result from adrenal hyperplasia. Females are reported to have the condition twice as often as males.

Clinical picture

Hypersecretion of aldosterone increases the renal tubule exchange of sodium for potassium and hydrogen ions; hypernatremia, hypokalemia, and hypertension result. The hypertension is related to the increased sodium reabsorption, whereas severe muscle weakness and ECG abnormalities are the result of potassium depletion. The most definitive diagnostic tools are an abnormally high aldosterone secretion rate and abnormally low plasma resin activity.[1]

Intervention

The treatment goal is *surgical removal* of tumors or resection of hyperplastic glands. Successful surgery reverses the hypertension in about two-thirds of the patients. Early diagnosis and treatment are the goals, since patients who are untreated will in time develop the sequelae of hypertensive cardiovascular disease and renal insufficiency. In preparation for surgery, spironolactone, an aldosterone antagonist, is given daily in doses of 200 to 400 mg.

There is considerable controversy about the incidence of primary aldosteronism. Some experts believe that as many as 7% of the patients who appear to have essential hypertension may in fact have primary aldosteronism.[1] Persons who cannot be treated surgically are maintained on spironolactone, 100 to 400 mg daily, for life.

□ Pheochromocytoma

Pheochromocytoma is a catecholamine-producing tumor, usually benign, of the sympatheticoadrenal system, which causes hypertension. Although pheochromocytomas account for less than 1% of cases of hypertension, it is important that they be diagnosed, since they can be cured.

Clinical picture

Most of the persons diagnosed with pheochromocytoma are between the ages of 5 and 25. The diagnosis is often made during pregnancy when the blood pressure is taken more frequently. There is some belief that the pregnant uterus may produce pressure on the tumor. Some experts believe that the tendency to develop pheochromocytoma may be inherited along with other hereditary neuroectodermal disorders.[1]

The prominent sign is hypertension, which may be labile, depending on blood levels of the catecholamines, or may stay persistently elevated. Most persons have an elevated blood pressure reading at least 50% of the time.[1] Along with hypertension there may be palpitations, tachycardia, malaise, apprehension, and diaphoresis. A variety of other signs and symptoms have been described in the literature.

The diagnosis is confirmed by assays of catecholamines and their metabolites in the urine. In pheochromocytoma the levels of these compounds are increased. About 80% of the tumors are located in the adrenal glands, and more than 95% are situated in the abdominal and pelvic areas. Only a small percentage of the tumors are malignant.

Intervention

The usual treatment is *surgical excision* of the pheochromocytoma, which is successful in about 90% of the cases. This results in complete remission of the symptoms unless there is metastasis to another site. During surgery there may be excessive production of catecholamines as the tumor is manipulated. This causes very high blood pressure levels and cardiac arrhythmias. Administration of the alpha adrenergic blockers (trimethaphan camsylate and phentolamine) is common. Trimethaphan camsylate is given daily for 7 to 10 days prior to surgery and may be used to control preoperative hypertension and reduce these complications of surgery. Propranolol (Inderal), a beta sympathetic blocker, may be used when there is catecholamine-induced arrhythmias and tachycardia. It is given either by mouth or intravenously. The drug is used with caution, and patients receiving it must be carefully monitored.

Hypotension occurs as soon as the tumor is removed. This is best treated with plasma or a plasma substitute, preferably 5% albumin in normal saline. Volume expanders administered appropriately usually control the hypotension, and vasopressors are not necessary.[1]

On the first postoperative day, hypertensive episodes are common and are caused by the response to pain and the hypervolemia resulting from the treatment of hypotension following surgery. At this time the most effective therapy is with a rapidly acting diuretic such as furosemide (Lasix) or ethacrynic acid (Edecrin).

Persons with pheochromocytoma who cannot be treated surgically or who are not cured by surgery are treated with adrenergic blocking agents or alpha-methyl-tyrsine,[1] a research drug that reduces the production of norepinephrine about 75%.

□ Hypofunction of the adrenal gland

Addison's disease (primary adrenal cortical insufficiency)

In Addison's disease there is hypofunction of the adrenal cortex and an insufficient secretion of both the *mineralocorticoids* and the *glucocorticoids*. Since these hormones are essential for maintaining life, the person with Addison's disease will die unless he receives adequate exogenous replacement therapy. The disease is thought to be caused by granulomatous destruction or idiopathic atrophy of the adrenal cortex. The granulomatous destruction is usually secondary to tuberculosis or fungal infections. The idiopathic atrophy is believed to be an autoimmune process.[1] The disease develops insidiously and often is first manifested during a period of stress such as infection, trauma, or surgery.

Clinical picture. The symptoms of Addison's disease include asthenia, fatigue, and gastrointestinal complaints such as anorexia, nausea, vomiting, abdominal pain, and diarrhea. The patient with Addison's disease may also give a history of frequent hypoglycemic reactions with nervousness, headache, trembling, and diaphoresis. He is usually hypotensive, and frequently a chest roentgenogram will reveal a small heart. In addition, he usually has a severe deficiency of sodium and chloride *(hyponatremia* and *hypochloremia)* and an increase in serum potassium *(hyperkalemia)*. These imbalances in electrolytes are related to a deficiency in the *mineralocorticoids*, while a decrease in the *glucocorticoids* is responsible for the hypoglycemic reactions. Most persons with chronic Addison's disease develop a bronzelike pigmentation of the skin and mucous membrane. Thus they always appear to be tanned on those areas of the body that are exposed to the sun. They may also have hyperpigmentation of pressure points such as the knees and elbows and along the belt line.

Intervention. The treatment of Addison's disease consists of administration of a *glucocorticoid*, either cortisone or hydrocortisone, and a *mineralocorticoid*, usually 9-alpha-fluorohydrocortisone (fludrocortisone). The usual dose of cortisone is 37.5 mg daily, with 25 mg given on awakening and 12.5 mg given before 4 PM. Since cortisone is ulcerogenic for some patients, it should always be given after meals or with milk. Antacids may also be prescribed. The dose of fludrocortisone is 0.1 to 0.2 mg daily. Other forms of these drugs may be prescribed, but these are the most widely used ones at present.

The patient with Addison's disease should understand the serious nature of his disease and the importance of taking his replacement therapy daily as ordered (Fig. 32-2). He should also know that he should never omit a dose of the drug and that if he has a gastrointestinal disturbance and is unable to retain the drug, his physician should be notified at once. Since the prescribed replacement therapy is planned to meet normal requirements of daily living, the patient will require additional glucocorticoids and mineralocorticoids if he is subjected to increased stress such as that of infection, trauma, surgery, or emotional upset. For this reason the patient with chronic Addison's disease should carry an identification card with him at all times. It is recommended that the card state which of the adrenocortical hormones is to be given in case of illness or injury. In addition, it is recommended that patients with little or no function of the adrenal glands carry an emergency supply of cortisone, hydrocortisone, and desoxycorticosterone at all times.

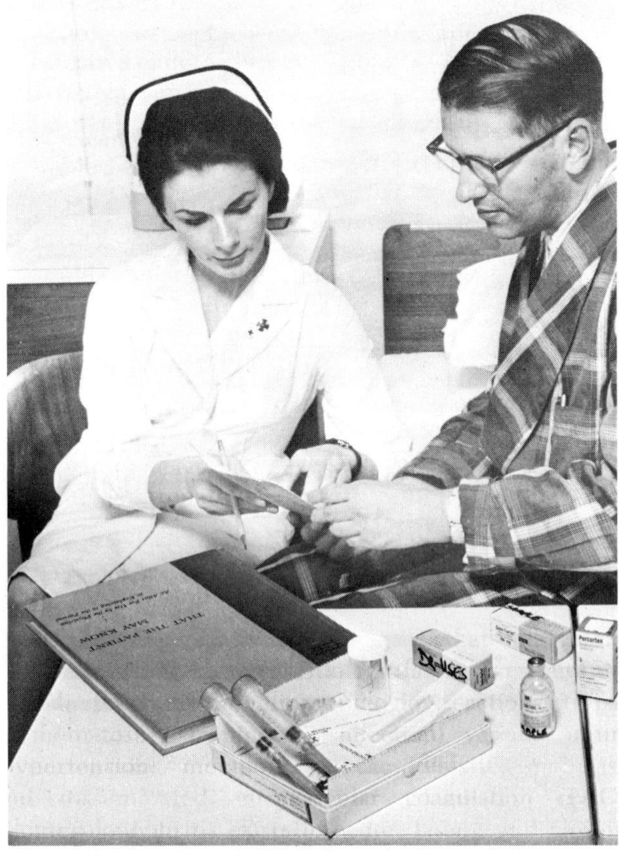

Fig. 32-2. Patients with Addison's disease should be taught about the disease, about the hormones they must take, and how they can live safely with the disease. (Reprinted with permission from Shea, K. M., et al.: Am. J. Nurs. **65:**80-85, 1965.)

The patient with Addison's disease who is on adequate replacement therapy can live a normal, productive life as long as he avoids undue stress.

Addisonian crisis. Addisonian, or adrenal, crisis is a severe exacerbation of Addison's disease. It is a very serious condition in which there is severe hypotension, shock, coma, and vasomotor collapse, and it quickly leads to death unless treated promptly. It may occur in any person with an insufficient amount of adrenocortical hormones, regardless of the cause, and may be precipitated by strenuous activity, infection or other stressful situations, or by failure to take prescribed steroids. (The latter is one of the most frequent causes of adrenal crisis.) It often is a complication of surgery or other treatment of the pituitary or adrenal glands. The signs of impending crisis are those of the disease in exaggerated form.

When addisonian crisis occurs, a large dose of hydrocortisone phosphate is given immediately by the intravenous route. A continuous and rapid infusion of normal saline solution is started immediately. Cortisone may be given intramuscularly also. The patient must do *absolutely nothing* for himself. If he is conscious, he is cautioned not to attempt to turn or otherwise help himself. The patient is *not moved* unless absolutely necessary and then only with physician consultation. It is essential that all forms of stimuli such as loud noises and bright lights be eliminated. Vital signs usually are taken every 15 minutes and temperature every hour. If hypotension is severe, a vasopressor drug such as phenylephrine (Neo-Synephrine) may be given. Whole blood and concentrated serum albumin are given if hypotension persists, since the protein in these fluids tends to hold fluid in the vascular compartment. The patient often complains of severe headache; an ice bag may be used to relieve it. The patient has an extremely low resistance to infection, and reverse isolation (p. 337) usually is used to protect the patient from exposure to infection. He must be protected from anyone, including members of his family and from hospital personnel, who has a cold or other infection. If the addisonian crisis was precipitated by an infection, appropriate antimicrobial therapy will be instituted.

SURGERY OF THE ADRENAL GLANDS

A bilateral adrenalectomy (surgical excision of the adrenal glands) is done most often for persons with cancer of the breast with metastasis, and occasionally for persons with cancer of the prostate gland with metastasis. Adrenalectomy may also be performed for the treatment of hypersecretion of the adrenal gland.

Preoperative care

When any surgery on the adrenal glands is planned, treatment with steroids usually is discontinued for several weeks preoperatively to prevent the danger of infection after surgery. This also allows postoperative control of blood levels of steroids to be regulated more accurately. If antihypertensive drugs are being used, they also are discontinued, since the surgery may cause a rather severe drop in blood pressure. Sedation may be given at this time.

Postoperative care

The immediate postoperative care for patients having any type of adrenocortical surgery is quite similar. Adrenocortical function is very labile when part of the adrenocortical tissue is removed, and, of course, it is labile when all the tissue is removed, since maintenance of the hormonal level then must be controlled completely by replacement therapy. The patient's special needs center around maintaining appropriate amounts of adrenocortical hormones in the blood.

Hormonal control and monitoring

Immediately after surgery, replacement of corticosteroids is started. Hydrocortisone is given continuously by intravenous drip, and dosage is adjusted at intervals according to the clinical findings. Since hormonal replacement is delicately regulated on the basis of continuous observations of electrolyte balance, blood sugar, and blood pressure determinations, the patient needs to be given constant nursing attention until hormonal stability is regained or a maintenance regimen established. Vasopressors may need to be given. Frequent blood pressure readings will be necessary to determine medication dosage needs.

The nurse should also observe the patient carefully for signs of *hypoglycemia*. This condition is most likely to occur if the patient had diabetes mellitus as a symptom, but it can occur in any patient who has adrenal gland surgery. Intravenous solutions containing glucose are usually ordered. If the patient is able to eat, the nurse should check to see that he has eaten the food served. Hypoglycemic reactions are most likely to occur in the early morning, and they may follow any unusual physical activity or any emotional upset. The nurse also should be alert for symptoms of *addisonian crisis*, (p. 580), which requires immediate treatment. *Markedly increased* urinary output may indicate the need for vasopressin (Pitressin) to control excessive diuresis.

Hypotension

Because of the instability of the vascular system following adrenalectomy, patients must be monitored closely for signs of hypotension. Blood pressure is taken every 15 minutes when the patient is first ambulated. If the blood pressure drops, the patient is assisted back to bed and the physician is consulted before ambulation is attempted again. Elastic stockings applied prior to ambulation may help to prevent hypotension.

Replacement therapy

The treatment for persons who have a bilateral adrenalectomy is the same as for patients with Addison's disease. They must be on replacement therapy for life and must understand the need to take their medication daily. They also need to know what to do when they are vomiting and cannot take the drug.

It is not unheard of for patients to be admitted in adrenal crisis because they did not understand the seriousness of not taking their medication as ordered.

Outcome criteria for the person with adrenal dysfunction

The patient or significant others can:

1. State why he is receiving medication daily for life.

2. Describe the effect of stress on his disease and measures to be taken to reduce stress.
3. Explain the home medication program.
   a. State name, dosage, frequency, and side effects of prescribed medications.
   b. State need for continued treatment if replacement therapy is necessary.
   c. State situations that will require an increase in the dose of medication.
4. Describe medical follow-up program.
   a. State symptoms indicating addisonian crisis and need for immediate medical attention.
   b. State need for continued medical follow-up.
   c. Show the card that the patient will carry at all times. The card will give the patient's name, address, and phone number; the name of the drug and its dose; and the physician's name and phone number.

■ PANCREATIC ENDOCRINE DYSFUNCTION

□ Diabetes mellitus

Etiology

Diabetes mellitus is a chronic metabolic disease involving a disorder of carbohydrate metabolism and subsequent derangement of protein and fat metabolism. Disturbance in the production, action, or metabolic rate of utilization of insulin, a hormone secreted by the islets of Langerhans in the pancreas, is involved in the disease.

Diabetes mellitus is found most frequently in persons over 40 years of age who are obese and who have a family history of diabetes, although the disease does occur in children and in young adults. It is more common in women than in men. The incidence increases steadily until the seventh decade of life. Elderly persons usually have a much less severe form of the disease than younger persons, although complications in the elderly may be severe.

According to the National Diabetes Commission, there are 6 million known diabetics in the United States and an additional 4 million with undiagnosed diabetes. In general, the increased incidence of diabetes can be attributed to a longer life span (with more people in the older age group), to a lower mortality rate among young people with diabetes mellitus since the discovery of insulin, to an increase in the number of persons with diabetes who now marry and have children, to the public's increased awareness of the disease, and to the availability of detection facilities. The specific causative factor or factors in diabetes continue to be explored while knowledge of related factors has increased.

Pathophysiology

Normally insulin speeds the oxidation of glucose in the cells and the conversion of glucose to glycogen, and facilitates the conversion of glucose to fat in adipose tissue. It is uncertain how insulin actually acts to accomplish these activities, but the most generally accepted theory is that it facilitates the transport of glucose across cell membranes. In diabetes mellitus there appears to be insufficient insulin available for use in carbohydrate metabolism.

The development of radioimmunoassay capabilities to measure circulating insulin has helped to distinguish between states of diminished insulin secretion and conditions of normal or above normal insulin secretion. Children are thought to have a primary insulin-producing deficiency, while obese adults may have a resistance to circulating insulin. In 85% of adults with diabetes mellitus, obesity precedes the disease.

Recent research suggests that glucagon plays a critical role in the pathophysiology of diabetes mellitus, while the theories regarding hereditary predisposition are being questioned. Juvenile onset diabetes may be caused by environmental factors such as a virus.

Prevention

Community efforts toward prevention of diabetes mellitus are directed toward (1) detection of diabetes and follow-up of suspected cases to confirm the diagnosis and to give treatment, (2) prevention or correction of obesity, (3) keeping patients with diabetes under medical supervision and their condition under control, (4) promotion of understanding of diabetes mellitus through education of professional groups, the patient, his family, and the community as a whole, and (5) mobilization of community resources such as medical, nursing, social, and nutrition groups to aid persons who have diabetes.

Multiphasic screening programs are being carried out to detect diabetes. To improve screening efficiency, it has been recommended that diabetic detection projects concentrate their efforts on the high-probability groups such as older persons, obese persons with a family history of diabetes, and persons with prior symptoms or an elevated blood sugar level. At the present time, some form of mass screening is being carried out in many states. These programs vary in scope, methods, and goals. Case-finding programs can be carried out in health department clinics, hospital outpatient clinics, physician's offices, industry, or the community (at health fairs or by mobile testing units). Selected groups or whole communities can avail themselves of these services. Follow-up of all positive findings is essential for a successful program. Public health nurses can help by making home visits if diabetes is definitely established, if retesting needs to be done, if individuals have indicated that they have no physician or are under no medical supervision, or if persons being tested request home visits by a nurse at the time of the first testing. Through the nurse's visits, misunderstandings about retesting can be clarified, and family reactions to the possibility of diabetes can be determined.

The passing of the National Diabetes Mellitus Research and Education Act in 1974 provided recognition of diabetes as a major health problem. In addition, the National Diabetes Advisory Board was created in 1976 to facilitate coordination of funds to provide several new diabetes research and training centers throughout the country.

The American Diabetes Association, Inc., furthers patient education, professional education, diabetes detection, public education, and research. It publishes both a professional journal, *Diabetes*,* that helps to keep health professionals informed and a bimonthly magazine, *Forecast*,* for persons with diabetes. Each year a National Diabetes Week is sponsored by the Association to stimulate early case finding in persons who do not know that they have diabetes and to educate the public about the disease. The Association has 50 local groups that work in their own areas. They sponsor camps for diabetic children and cooperate on nationwide projects.

The Juvenile Diabetes Foundation has also gained national prominence. This relatively new organization raises funds for research but also provides public education and counseling for juvenile diabetics and their families.

Health education. Preventive health education should be emphasized in high-risk groups. Much can be done by every nurse who is aware of the hereditary nature of the disease and its probable association with obesity. If diabetes is part of a family history, the nurse can explain to relatives of the patient the significance of periodic testing for detecting the disease early and can encourage all members of the family to maintain normal weight. Women who have had large babies also should be urged to avoid gaining weight and to have periodic tests for diabetes. Statistics show that diabetes develops later in life in 17% of mothers whose babies weighed over 9 pounds, and in 80% to 90% of those whose babies weighed over 13 pounds.

Studies of women with diabetes have shown that there is a high fetal and neonatal death rate, a high proportion of large babies with a high mortality rate, and a great tendency toward other abnormalities in pregnancy. Thus there is now greater emphasis on preventive intensive prenatal care. With improved monitoring devices available to determine placental function and fetal maturity, the pregnant woman with diabetes may be subjected to less risk to herself and the fetus.

In some sections of the country there are high-risk perinatal networks set up to provide specialized care to pregnant women with conditions such as diabetes, which put them and their fetus at risk. It has also been discovered that women who have repeated spontaneous abortions, although giving no signs of carbohydrate intolerance by a regular glucose tolerance test, often show evidence of a decreased insulin reserve when cortisone is given prior to the glucose tolerance test. A significantly large number of relatives of persons with diabetes also respond in this manner. Therefore it is suspected that these people may need close medical supervision during stress situations such as pregnancy, extensive surgery, or serious illness to determine a need for insulin or oral hypoglycemic agents. The nurse should look at the medical history of patients and watch those with family histories of diabetes mellitus closely for symptoms of the disease.

*American Diabetes Association, Inc., 18 East 48 St., New York, N.Y. 10017.

Clinical picture

The most common and characteristic symptoms of diabetes mellitus are increased appetite (polyphagia), increased thirst (polydipsia), and increased urine volume (polyuria). The signs and symptoms are directly related to faulty oxidation of carbohydrate and the chain of events that follows. Normally glucose is oxidized by the body to form carbon dioxide and water, with production of energy to meet body needs. Any excess is changed to glycogen in the liver and is stored in the liver and in the muscles, or it is converted to fat and stored. Insulin is needed for all these actions to occur.

In diabetes, glucose remains in the bloodstream and cannot be converted to glycogen because insulin is not present or is unusable. The amount of sugar in the blood increases (hyperglycemia), and some of it is eliminated in the urine (glycosuria). The glycosuria promotes polyuria because the increased glucose being filtered by the kidney acts as an osmotic diuretic and increases the volume of urine excreted. This eventually leads to dehydration and polydipsia as a consequence of losing large amounts of water and salt in the urine. Pruritus vulvae, caused by the irritating effect of the urine with its high sugar content, may occur in women.

Since the person with untreated diabetes mellitus is unable to utilize carbohydrates satisfactorily, essential carbohydrate starvation results, and the body attempts to compensate by an increased appetite (polyphagia). To provide energy for the body unable to utilize carbohydrates, large amounts of fat, including body fat, are oxidized. This utilization of fat depots may lead to weight loss. Fats, upon oxidation, form ketone bodies (fatty acids), which in normal amounts are neutralized with bases such as bicarbonate in the blood plasma to maintain the normal acid-base balance of the body. When excessive amounts of fat are burned, the bases in the blood plasma may become exhausted. Acidosis (ketosis) develops (p. 211), and acetone bodies are then excreted in the urine. Weakness and fatigue are common because of problems in meeting energy requirements.

The onset of symptoms in the young person often is rapid, but in the older, obese patient the onset usually is insidious. Complications often cause the elderly patient to seek medical care. Diabetes in children frequently is diagnosed when severe acidosis develops during the course of an acute infectious disease.

A fasting blood sugar (FBS) test for glucose level is used to diagnose diabetes. Because fasting blood sugar test results may be misleading, a 2-hour postprandial test is becoming the procedure of choice in screening for diabetes. These tests and the other blood tests useful in the diagnosis of diabetes mellitus are described in Table 30-5.

Intervention

Diabetes can be controlled to a large extent by regulating the diet and taking insulin or oral hypoglycemic agents. The controversy continues regarding the relationship between the degree of control and long-term complications. Some authorities believe that long-term problems are caused by an inherited defect and are not related to reduction of the blood sugar to close to normal levels; others feel that long-term complications are directly related to increased blood sugar levels and can be prevented by proper control. The degree of control should be the optimal level that can be reasonably maintained considering the life style of the person with diabetes. The degree to which the individual participates in control of the disease depends on how well he has adapted emotionally to having diabetes, his knowledge of the disease, and his motivation to pursue control measures.

The emotional response to a diagnosis of diabetes is often severe and is not easily dealt with. Part of this may result from fear of disability and eventual death. Since diabetes is so widespread, many people know of relatives and friends who have had the disease and who have eventually had an amputation or have become blind. Perhaps an even greater cause of emotional reaction is that diabetes affects the life pattern in regard to food. Food and eating have meaning beyond the actual meeting of nutritional needs, and changes in eating habits are extremely difficult for some persons to accept. Adolescents, perhaps more than any other age group, find restrictions almost intolerable and need much understanding in their adjustment to the disease.

Initiating a suitable plan of care for diabetes will often make a great difference in how the person continues with care. It can help him and his family avoid undue stress and concern that may make it difficult to control the diabetes. Since most persons with diabetes are now treated in a physician's office or a hospital clinic, the community health nurse may need to help them with the initial adjustment.

The majority of nursing interventions for the person with diabetes mellitus involve assisting him to learn about his condition, promoting self-care, and teaching measures for control of the disease and prevention of complications. Various teaching aids on diabetes are available for many sources, such as the American Diabetes Association, to supplement teaching programs.

Many diabetics are hospitalized for conditions other than their diabetes. In these situations the nurse identifies during the initial interview the diabetic regimen being followed at home. Whenever possible, the patient should continue this regimen in the hospital. This includes administering insulin, testing urine, and making personal food selections. Continuing to carry out their own regimen prevents the patient from becoming dependent on others. Sometimes it is appropriate for the patient to be dependent, however, and the nurse makes a judgment as to when and how much self-care should be assumed by the patient.

Diet. All persons with diabetes mellitus are placed on some type of a restricted diet. Some obese persons may be able to control diabetes by diet alone. In these persons the emphasis is on gradual weight reduction to a level that is considered normal or slightly below normal for their height and body build.

Most diabetic diets require the individual to use food exchange lists. The exchanges are divided into seven food groups. The first six groups that must be measured are milk, vegetables, fruits, bread, meat, and fats. The seventh group includes food with negligible calories that do not need to be measured. Examples are coffee, tea, bouillion, plain gelatin, mustard, lemon, rhubarb, spices, and vinegar. Nothing may be added to foods (e.g., cream, sugar) unless it is measured and counted as part of the allowed intake. Sugar substitutes are available despite the recent controversy about the possible carcinogenic effects of saccharin. Persons who go back to work after being on bed rest will find that they have to increase their caloric intake to meet their increased energy requirements. They also will need more food to offset the excess of insulin that occurs with an increase in exercise. When unusual exercise is being anticipated, the individual will have to adjust his food intake accordingly. Many persons with diabetes become very skillful at adjusting their food intake in accord with an increase or decrease in activity.

Although the use of the exchange lists may be taught by a dietitian or nutritionist, every nurse needs to know how to use the lists and how to teach others to use them. Often the patient does not know what he does not understand about the lists until he actually begins using them.

Table 32-2. Action of insulin preparations

Type of insulin	Time of onset	Peak of action	Duration of action
Rapid acting			
Crystalline zinc	Within 1 hour	2 to 4 hours	5 to 8 hours
Regular	Within 1 hour	2 to 4 hours	4 to 6 hours
Semilente	Within 1 hour	6 to 10 hours	12 to 16 hours
Intermediate acting			
Globin zinc	2 to 4 hours	6 to 10 hours	18 to 24 hours
NPH	2 to 4 hours	8 to 12 hours	28 to 32 hours
Lente	2 to 4 hours	8 to 12 hours	28 to 30 hours
Slow acting			
Ultralente	Within 8 hours	16 to 24 hours	36+ hours

Reinstruction and follow-up are indicated, and whenever a nurse encounters a diabetic patient, the patient's level of knowledge about his diet should be assessed even though the disease may have been diagnosed some time ago.

Medications

Insulin. Insulin is used in the treatment of 50% to 70% of persons with diabetes in the United States. There are now seven types of insulin in general use, and each is effective in lowering the blood sugar level by aiding in the metabolism of carbohydrates.

Insulins are classified as to their time of action as rapid, intermediate, and slow acting. Food should be taken within an hour after the injection of rapid-acting insulin to prevent an insulin reaction. *Regular* insulin is a clear liquid that begins to act approximately 45 minutes to an hour after injection. *Crystalline* insulin looks the same as regular insulin but is a more refined product. It remains effective 1 hour longer than regular insulin and is less likely to cause local reaction at the site of injection.

Five types of *modified* insulin are currently used, and all of these insulins contain substances that slow their action: globin zinc insulin, neutral protamine Hagedorn (NPH) insulin, and three lente insulins—lente, semilente, and ultralente. The time of onset, peak of action, and duration of action depend on whether the insulin is classified as rapid, intermediate, or slow in action (Table 32-2).

NPH insulin and lente insulins separate into layers on standing. To obtain an accurate dose of the active ingredient, the solution should be mixed by rotating the bottle between the palms of the hands and inverting the vial from end to end several times.

Each individual has his own particular insulin need, and suitable amounts as well as types are carefully selected by the physician. Persons receiving only rapid-acting insulin need more than one injection a day to enable them to metabolize the carbohydrates eaten. Many patients are given the slow-acting insulins because they eliminate the need for several doses during the day. Other patients may need a combination of regular insulin and a slower-acting insulin.

It is important that the nurse understand the type and the time of peak activity of each kind of insulin prescribed. Persons on rapid-acting insulin must have food soon after the insulin is given, while those on intermediate or slow-acting insulins will require a supplementary feeding in the midafternoon or a bedtime feeding or both. The between-meal snacks are timed to meet the peak action of the insulin being used.

U-100 INSULIN. This strength of insulin (100 units/ml) has been introduced to replace the 40 and 80 units/ml strengths of insulin. Hopefully this will eliminate dosage confusion and errors. This strength was recommended because it is compatible with the decimal system. The U-100 insulin is available in all types. All U-100 insulins are prepared in round vials with orange caps and black lettering. The U-100 syringes are available in glass and disposable forms (Fig. 32-3). Miniature syringes for measuring small doses are available, as well as 2 ml insulin syringes for unusually large doses.

To educate and assist persons in converting to U-100 insulin, nurses must have a thorough understanding of insulin concentration. U-100 insulin is a more concentrated insulin in less volume. The U-100 syringe makes the adjustment in volume; there is no need to calculate a conversion of the old insulin dose. For example, if the person's requirements are 24 units of U-80 insulin, then he will take 24 units of U-100 insulin. All diabetics must understand that U-100 insulin must be used with a U-100 syringe.

TEACHING THE PATIENT TO ADMINISTER AN INJECTION. The patient needs to learn about sterile technique, about the equipment to be used, and the proper sterilization of it unless disposable equipment is used (Fig. 32-4).

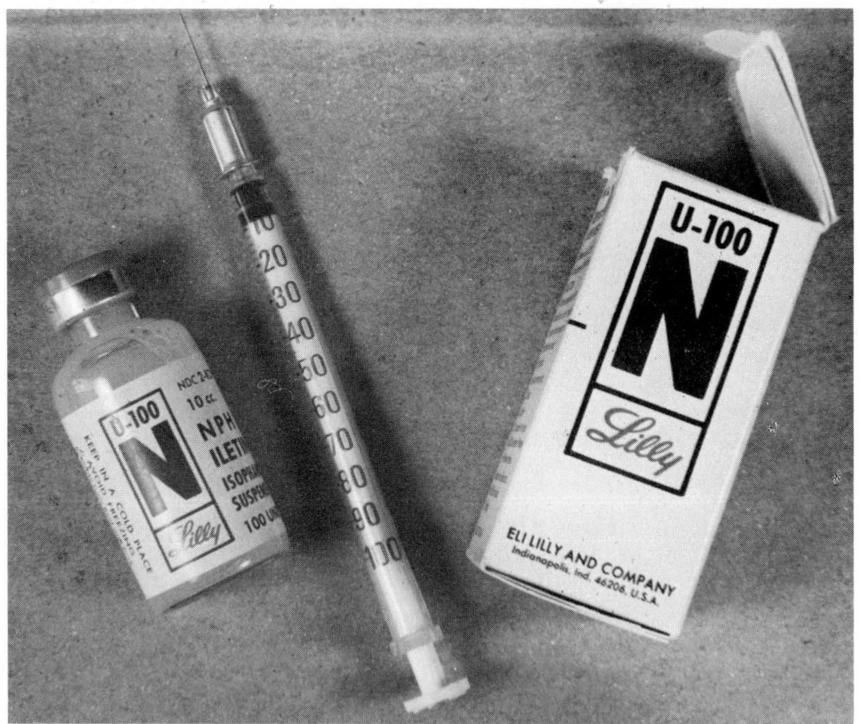

Fig. 32-3. U-100 insulin and disposable U-100 insulin syringe.

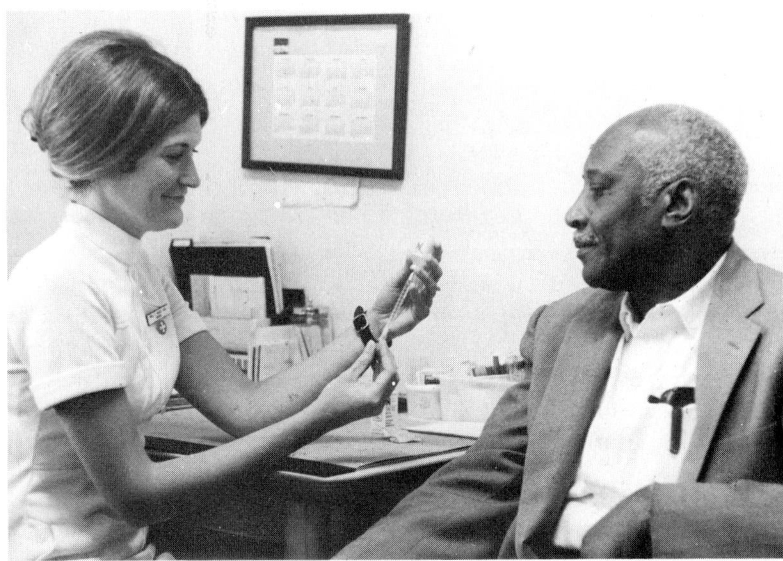

Fig. 32-4. Clinic nurse begins instruction in insulin administration by demonstrating procedure to patient.

Typical trays for the injection at home can be set up for use in demonstrations and for patients to use in practice. The nurse can discuss boxes or trays that can be set up at home to keep all equipment together. This should be stored on a shelf or closet out of reach of children and out of sight. Equipment needed for the injection includes a syringe (insulin syringe if insulin is to be used), hypodermic needles, a small jar for cotton or a box of roll cotton, and a bottle of alcohol. If the medication does not need to be refrigerated, it may be kept with the equipment. Insulin, however, must be refrigerated.

When repeated injections are necessary, as for insulin, the *site of injection, must be rotated* to assure proper absorption of medication (Fig. 32-5). Irritation from re-

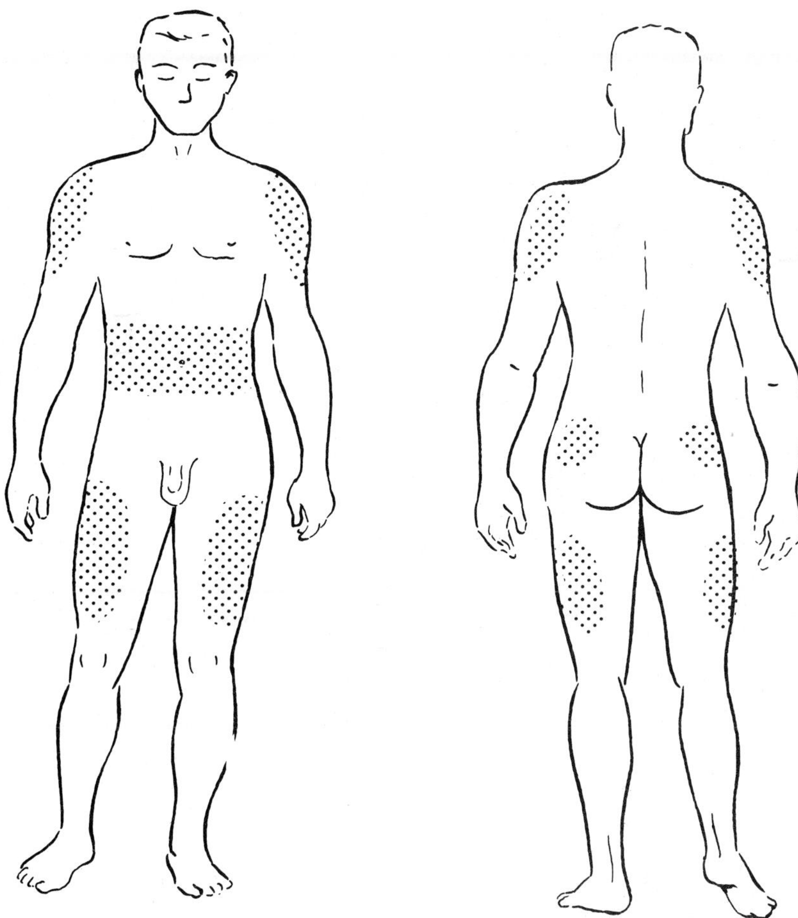

Fig. 32-5. Arms, legs, buttocks, and abdomen can be used for insulin injection. A different site should be used for each injection.

peated injections at the same site can cause induration of the tissue, so that the medication is absorbed too slowly or not at all. Injections should not be given in any one spot more often than every 2 weeks. A diagram of the possible sites can be made as a guide and the sites numbered so that they can be rotated according to the plan.

There are two different ways of sterilizing nondisposable equipment. The individual can choose between daily sterilization by boiling or soaking the syringe and needle in alcohol and boiling the equipment weekly. A strainer placed in a sauce pan makes it easier for the patient to drain and handle the equipment after boiling.

Because there are many things the patient and family must learn, this particular skill may be delayed until the patient feels more comfortable with other skills. Disposable equipment may be used at first, and then reusable equipment employed when the skill has been learned.

It may be necessary for a diabetic to take two types of insulin. If so, the nurse may teach him to *mix the two insulins* in the same syringe so that they may be given in one injection. A simple way of mixing insulins in the same syringe is to inject the correct amount of air into the second insulin bottle first. Then the correct amount of air is injected into the first insulin bottle and the insulin withdrawn. As a final step, the correct dose is withdrawn from the second insulin bottle. Regular insulin can be mixed with any other type of insulin. The lente insulins can also be mixed together. The syringe should be rotated gently to obtain a well-distributed solution. The injection is then given in the usual manner. The most important point to remember in mixing insulins in the same syringe is that regular (unmodified) insulin is always drawn into the syringe first, since if some of the regular insulin inadvertently enters the vial of modified insulin, it will not significantly change the action of the modified insulin.

At times *modification in methods of administration of insulin* may be necessary because of particular problems; for example, the person may be elderly, may have unsteady hands, or may have failing vision. In these instances, measurement of insulin as well as proper injection technique will require close attention. Adaptation of

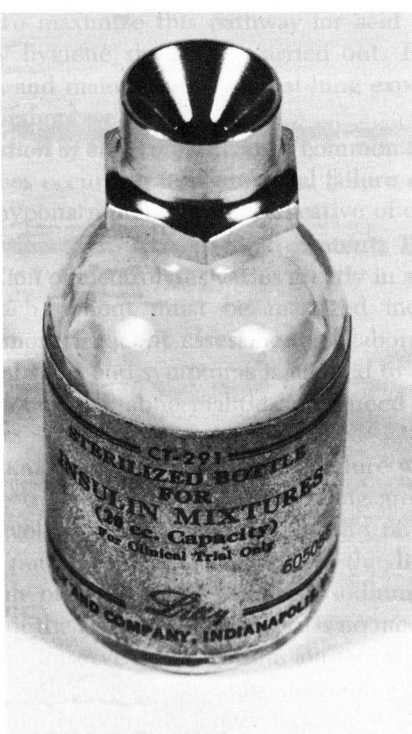

Fig. 32-6. Insulin needle guide that fits over top of insulin vial. Patient cleans stopper and guide with alcohol before placing guide on vial. Needle is laid in V of guide and vial is pushed toward it. (Courtesy American Foundation for the Blind, Inc., New York, N.Y.)

equipment may also be necessary. There are a number of aids available for the visually handicapped that are advertised in diabetic publications or are available from the American Foundation for the Blind.* Special syringes with plunger locks and attachable devices for locking the plunger can be purchased, as well as attachable needle guides and insulin bottle guides to facilitate entry of the needle into the bottle (Fig. 32-6). Persons who have failing vision may also use a small magnifying adapter that can be clipped to a syringe.

Persons with poor vision have the danger of drawing air instead of insulin into the syringe. They must be cautioned to invert the bottle completely and to insert the needle only a short distance. Often they are advised to use only about two-thirds of the bottle of insulin and to have on hand another full bottle. Some persons have a public health nurse or a friend withdraw the last doses in a bottle of insulin for them, or they go to a clinic for the last few injections.

An individual may not be able to prepare the insulin dose accurately because of motor and sensory handicaps. He may, however, be capable of giving his own injections. A family member or neighbor could be taught to prepare the correct dose of insulin, or a public health nurse could fill a week's supply of syringes and store them in the refrigerator. The syringe would need to be rotated gently before use to mix the insulin. In some instances a member of the family may have to give the insulin. A family member should always know how to do this in case impending coma or other illness makes it impossible for the individual to administer his own insulin.

Oral hypoglycemic agents. Several oral agents are now available for use in controlling blood sugar levels in persons with diabetes mellitus. These agents have proved effective in the treatment of many adults whose diabetes is stable. These drugs are not hormones, and it is a misnomer to refer to them as oral insulins.

As a result of a study conducted by the University Group Diabetes Program, the Food and Drug Administration now recommends that oral hypoglycemic agents be limited to persons with symptomatic adult onset nonketotic diabetes mellitus that cannot be adequately controlled by diet or weight loss alone, and in whom the addition of insulin is impractical or unacceptable. The oral hypoglycemic agents are most effective in the treatment of elderly persons; they are not used to treat diabetes in the young or in middle-aged or older persons whose blood sugar level fluctuates widely. They are useless in treating diabetic ketoacidosis.

Persons taking oral hypoglycemic medication instead of insulin need to be as careful about taking the prescribed dosage of the drug, following the prescribed diet, maintaining the usual amount of exercise, testing their urine for sugar, and taking general health precautions as do persons taking insulin.

The sulfonylurea compounds, which include acetohexamide (Dymelor), chlorpropamide (Diabinese), tolazamide (Tolinase), and tolbutamide (Orinase), are the oral agents prescribed. They are thought to act by increasing the ability of the islet cells of the pancreas to secrete insulin.

The dosages for these agents are presented in Table 32-3. In the University Group Diabetes Program Study, tolbutamide was the oral hypoglycemic agent investigated. The death rate from cardiovascular diseases was two and a half times higher in persons receiving tolbutamide as in those receiving a placebo. The Food and Drug Administration has therefore recommended that oral hypoglycemic drugs be used with caution and that emphasis be placed on diet and weight control for the management of adult-onset diabetes mellitus.

Phenformin (DBI), another oral hypoglycemic agent, has recently been banned because a significant number

*American Foundation for the Blind, Inc., 15 West Sixteenth St., New York, N.Y. 10011

Table 32-3. Oral hypoglycemic agents

Classification	Proprietary name	Usual daily dose	Divided dose per day
Sulfonylureas			
Acetohexamide	Dymelor	250 mg to 1.5 g	1 to 2
Chlorpropamide	Diabinese	100 to 500 mg	1
Tolazamide	Tolinase	100 mg to 1 g	1 to 2
Tolbutamide	Orinase	0.5 to 2 g	2 to 3 after meals

of deaths have been attributed to lactic acidosis, a side effect of this drug.

Hypoglycemic reaction. All diabetics may experience hypoglycemic reactions at times despite adherence to diet and medications. Severe reactions, however, are usually caused by too large a dose of insulin or antidiabetic drug, or too little food. It can occur when the individual does not eat all of his meals or skips between-meal or bedtime feedings. Sometimes the individual increases his insulin to cover excesses in eating, and the insulin dose may be greater than needed.

Vomiting, diarrhea, added exercise, or emotional stress may also precipitate an insulin reaction. Every person who has diabetes must carry a card that states that he is a diabetic and on which is recorded his name and address and the name and address of his physician. The insulin dose or oral antidiabetic drug dosage is also on the card. Some diabetics wear Medic Alert bracelets or necklaces that alert others to their diabetic status. This is very helpful if they faint or become unconscious when alone in a public place. Unconscious persons admitted to an emergency room of a hospital are always checked for such identification.

If for any reason the person who is on insulin or oral hypoglycemic therapy demonstrates signs of a hypoglycemic reaction (see boxed material), he should take or be given additional food. Many persons with diabetes carry lump sugar or hard candies to be eaten in such emergencies. If the person is at home, he should drink a glass of orange juice, other fruit juice, ginger ale, or any other readily available source of glucose. Sometimes the reaction comes on suddenly, and the person may not sense early signs. In such an instance a family member may have to give the orange juice or some other sweet fluid. One of the safest ways to administer sugar to a groggy person is to place a teaspoonful of corn syrup or honey in his mouth. This will be rapidly absorbed by the mucous membrane of the oral mucosa, and the person will usually arouse sufficiently to be able to drink a glass of juice or sweetened coffee or tea. If impending hypoglycemia is not treated immediately, the person becomes stuporous and unconscious. Because hypoglycemia interferes with the oxygen consumption of nervous tissue, there can be irreparable brain damage if sugar is not administered promptly.

EARLY SIGNS AND SYMPTOMS OF HYPOGLYCEMIA

Weakness	Palpitations
Shakiness	Tremors
Diaphoresis	Headache
Hunger	Blurring or double vision
Nervousness	Numbness of lips, tongue
Irritability	

NOTE: An easy way to remember the symptoms of hypoglycemia is to remember how you feel when you have not eaten in a long time.

The symptoms of insulin reaction vary both with the type of insulin used and with the individual. The pattern in a given person is usually the same, however, and he can generally tell when he is becoming hypoglycemic. If a question exists concerning the validity of the diabetic's feeling about an impending insulin reaction, blood should be drawn immediately for a blood sugar test and *sugar given at once.* The nurse should understand that when in doubt it is always safer to give sugar than to risk nervous system damage from hypoglycemia. Usually 20 to 25 g of carbohydrate will be sufficient to overcome hypoglycemia. This can be obtained from 8 ounces of fruit juice or sweetened soft drinks, four teaspoons of sugar, two tablespoons of syrup, or four pieces of hard candy. If the individual is already unconscious, 50% glucose will usually be given intravenously.

Glucagon, a pancreatic hormone that acts primarily by mobilizing hepatic glycogen, may be given to treat insulin reactions. The effects of this glycogen conversion last about 1½ hours, and therefore treatment with sugar will also be required to prevent a recurrence of the hypoglycemia. Glucagon is given intramuscularly, and some physicians instruct their patients to take it when an insulin reaction occurs. If the patient is unconscious, the family adminsters the drug and then seeks medical assistance.

Urine testing. Persons with diabetes mellitus need to know how to test their urine for sugar and acetone in order to monitor their control. The urine testing equipment used will depend on the stability of the disease, the degree of glycosuria anticipated, the life style of the person, his visual acuity, and his physical limitation. Different urine testing products can give 0.5%, 2%, or 5% maximum readings of glycosuria. Some require accurate timing or an ability to measure drops of urine. The individual may be able to distinguish shades of color more accurately on one specific color chart. (See p. 557 for urine testing techniques.)

What the person *does* if his test is abnormal depends entirely on the individual and the instructions he has received. Instructions should be in writing. The physician may, for example, instruct the patient to do nothing except repeat the test again during the same day and to keep a careful record of urine reactions, or may instruct the patient to increase or decrease his insulin or oral drug dosage, increase or decrease his food intake, or get in touch with the physician at once. Some physicians may want certain patients to show a trace or even 1% sugar in their urine once daily as evidence that the blood sugar is not going too low, whereas for other individuals this would not be considered good control. The age of the individual and the stability of his disease affect the physician's decision in advising a course of action. The nurse can assist the person in interpreting his urine test results and in understanding the rationale for his specific regimen.

Prevention of infection. Persons with diabetes are more susceptible to infection. The effectiveness of the skin as a first line of defense is diminished. Uncontrolled diabetes leads to loss of fat deposits under the skin, loss of glycogen, and catabolism of body proteins, which can hamper the inflammatory response and wound healing. Decreased circulation to the part can also delay healing. The skin must be kept supple and as free of pathogenic organisms as possible. This is especially true in warm moist areas that encourage growth of the organisms (i.e., between the toes, under the breasts, and in the axillae and groin). It is therefore very important that persons with diabetes carry out hygienic measures for prevention of infection, with special emphasis on good foot care (p. 566). They should also avoid persons with upper respiratory infections.

Some persons with diabetes may assume that medications for diabetes and food can be safely omitted if they have an upper respiratory infection or other minor ailment. They must understand that the contrary is true, that stress, such as a short-term illness, increases the body's need for insulin, and that even closer monitoring of the diabetes is essential. Liquid diets can provide essential food for a short time, but any person taking medication for diabetes who cannot eat or who is physically incapacitated should consult his physician without delay.

Exercise. All persons with diabetes need regular exercise, and this should be discussed with them as part of the overall treatment plan. Those receiving insulin or oral hypoglycemic agents should understand that the amount of medication prescribed by the physician is planned around their usual exercise pattern. Because an increase in activity will decrease the need for insulin or the hypoglycemic agents, patients should know that if they are going to exercise more than usual they should plan their dietary intake so that they eat a quick-acting form of glucose just before starting the activity. Also, many physicians will teach patients taking insulin how they may reduce their insulin dose or increase their food intake when they are planning more exercise than usual.

It may be helpful for young diabetics to know that several well-known athletes with diabetes have been able to perform at championship level in such sports as tennis, hockey, and professional baseball. In these cases they adjusted their insulin and food consumption to meet their athletic schedule.

Because an increase in exercise does decrease the need for insulin or hypoglycemic agents, an unusual amount of exercise can precipitate a hypoglycemic reaction. This can usually be handled by the person himself as long as he recognizes the symptoms and he carries some form of rapid-acting glucose such as sugar cubes or hard candy with him at all times.

Complications of diabetes

Diabetic ketoacidosis (DKA)

Etiology. The most common cause of diabetic ketoacidosis is an infection, such as of the upper respiratory or urinary tract or the skin, because infection increases the body's need for insulin. Other causes are failure to take prescribed insulin or an increased need for insulin such as occurs with surgery, trauma, or other stressors.

Pathophysiology. Diabetic ketoacidosis occurs when there is not sufficient insulin available to metabolize glucose. When this happens, as explained in the beginning of this section (p. 583), glucose is excreted in the urine, taking with it large amounts of water. Fats must then be burned for energy, and ketosis results. This increase in hydrogen ions in the blood calls on the alkali reserve of the body to combat the acidosis. Thus there is a loss of sodium, chloride, potassium, and more water. As the alkali reserve of the body is depleted, the pH of the blood goes down. At the same time the body attempts to rid itself of the increased acids by respiratory and renal means. Carbon dioxide is exhaled through the lungs in increasing amounts as the respirations become more deep and rapid (Kussmaul breathing). The kidneys attempt to excrete more of the acids in the urine, and even more water is lost. This results in hemoconcentration and, in time, in generalized hypoxia. In the presence of hypoxia, increased amounts of lactic acid are produced, which further increase the hydrogen ion concentration of the blood. If the process is allowed to continue, the patient will lapse into coma, since hypoxia and acidosis interfere with the function of the cerebral hemispheres.

Clinical picture. The signs and symptoms of diabetic ketoacidosis can be directly linked to the severe dehydration, loss of essential electrolytes, and acidosis. These signs and symptoms include weakness, dull headache, fatigue, general malaise, insatiable thirst, epigastric aching pain, and nausea and vomiting. Accompanying these signs and symptoms are the physical findings of one in severe dehydration and acidosis. The mucous membranes are dehydrated and there is loss of skin turgor, the eyeballs may be soft or sunken, the lips and tongue are red and parched, the face is usually flushed, and hyperpnea (Kussmaul breathing) is present. The temperature will be elevated at first, and then may go down with the resultant hypovolemia. Hypovolemic shock is common, and the systolic blood pressure may be as low as 60 to 70 mm Hg; in time the patient will become anuric, and circulatory collapse can occur.

Intervention. Diabetic ketoacidosis is a medical emergency that requires intensive care of the patient both by the physician and nurse. Therapy is directed toward correcting the acidosis, dehydration, electrolyte disturbances, and other factors such as infection that precipitated the ketoacidosis. It can be expected that all of these will be carried on simultaneously.

The severity of the patient's condition is determined by the level of ketones in the blood (ketonemia); therefore the patient's plasma is tested for a 4+ reaction for ketones. Dilutions of the patient's plasma are then made to determine the extent of the ketonemia. The greater the number of dilutions in which ketones remain 4+, the more severe the ketoacidosis. These dilutions are converted to an approximation of the acetone values per 100 ml of blood. Values over 50 mg/100 ml are considered severe ketosis, while those 80 mg or over are considered to be evidence of clinical coma.

The amount of insulin ordered for the patient is based on the initial level of ketonemia. The first doses of insulin may be given both intravenously and subcutaneously. The total amount of insulin needed to correct the ketoacidosis will depend on the patient's response to therapy. Some patients require as little as 200 or 300 units of regular insulin to correct ketoacidosis, while others may require 1,000 units or more.

To correct dehydration, normal saline solution or half-strength normal saline solution (0.45%) is given in large amounts—often 4 liters or more are required in the first 24 hours. If normal saline solution is not sufficient to replace the sodium loss, additional sodium is given either as sodium bicarbonate or sodium lactate. Potassium ordinarily is not given early in the treatment because patients with severe dehydration and hemoconcentration usually have hyperkalemia, which is caused by the movement of potassium from the intracellular to the extracellular fluid. As the dehydration is corrected, the potassium moves back into the cells, and hypokalemia may occur. Because of the effect of potassium on cardiac muscle, the patient should be carefully monitored by ECG tracings to determine the need for potassium (p. 921).

The nursing interventions planned for the patient depends on the severity of the ketoacidosis and the prescribed treatment. In addition to carefully monitoring vital signs and levels of consciousness, the nurse must see that blood and urine specimens are obtained as ordered and that necessary blood and urine tests are carried out. If the patient is in severe ketoacidosis, blood is drawn frequently to test for ketones, sugar, and electrolyte levels. If the patient is unconscious, an indwelling catheter is usually inserted.

As the patient's condition improves, the ketone levels in the blood can be expected to drop, and the blood sugar will return to more nearly normal levels. It is at this time that the patient should be watched most closely for signs of hypoglycemia. It should be remembered that blood levels of ketone and sugar will return to normal before urinary levels will. When the patient is able to take fluids by mouth, he will usually be given fruit juices, broth, cooked cereal, and milk. Solid foods are added as soon as possible to improve gastric tone and prevent further ileus.

As the patient recovers, the cause of his acidosis should be reviewed with him so that he understands how to avoid a recurrence.

The patient or his family should contact their physician at once if any signs or symptoms of acidosis occur. Carrying a card stating that he has diabetes helps to ensure prompt treatment in the event that coma develops while the patient is away from home. Such a card also helps prevent this condition from being mistaken for head injury, cerebrovascular accident, or drunkenness. A summary of the differences between insulin reaction and diabetic ketoacidosis is presented in Table 32-4.

Hyperglycemic, hyperosmolar, and nonketotic coma. This form of diabetic coma can develop in the diabetic who is ketosis resistant. It is more apt to occur

Table 32-4. Summary of differences between insulin reaction and diabetic ketoacidosis

Factors	Insulin reaction	Ketoacidosis
Onset	Rapid	Slow (days or weeks)
Precipitating factors		
Food	Insufficient	Excessive
Complications	None	Infection
Insulin	Excess	Too little
Exercise	Increased	Too little
Symptoms		
Thirst	Absent	Increased
Vomiting	Absent	Frequent
Hunger	Frequent	Absent
Abdominal pain	Absent	Frequent
Vision	Double	Dim
Signs		
Temperature	Normal or below	Elevated
Respirations	Normal	Hyperpnea (Kussmaul breathing), acetone odor to breath
Blood pressure	Normal or elevated	Lowered, may be in hypovolemic shock
Skin	Moist and pale	Hot, dry, and flushed
Dehydration	None	Loss of skin turgor, sunken eyeballs
Tremors	Frequent	Absent
Laboratory findings		
Urine		
Glycosuria	May be positive, but negative in second specimen	4+
Ketonuria	Negative	4+
Blood		
Sugar	Below normal	Elevated, usually above 200 mg/100 ml
Ketones	Normal	Elevated, usually 4+
Electrolytes	Normal	Decreased, except serum potassium

in the older person with mild diabetes, usually non-insulin-dependent, or in persons whose diabetes has been poorly controlled over a number of weeks or months. It is characterized by high concentrations of glucose in the blood with no acetone in the urine. The plasma hyperosmolality that develops creates the osmotic force that pulls water from the cells, particularly the cerebral cells. Coma is the end result.

The most important aspect of treatment is correction of dehydration with half-strength normal saline solution (0.45%) and insulin. The mortality rate from hyperosmolar coma is high, possibly because of the patient's advanced age and concomitant vascular diseases. On recovery, these patients often have the same teaching needs as those recovering from ketoacidosis.

Other complications of diabetes millitus. All diabetics have some changes in blood vessels that result in *vascular complications*. It is well known that diabetics are prone to develop atherosclerosis at an earlier age than nondiabetics. This appears to be related to the high levels of triglycerides found when diabetes is poorly controlled. In addition, diabetics have small vessel (microvascular) changes that are not seen in nondiabetics. These small vessel changes most commonly cause clinical effects in the kidneys, retinas, nervous system, and skin. The cause and rate of progression of these complications is controversial. Factors that may contribute to them include inadequate blood sugar control, diabetes of long standing, or a hereditary defect linked with diabetes that causes vascular difficulties in some diabetics.

Kimmelstiel-Wilson syndrome, a nephrotic syndrome with proteinuria, edema, and hypertension, has an unfavorable prognosis. Treatment is the same as for nephrotic syndrome from other causes. Pyelonephritis is treated with antibiotics.

Retinopathy occurs in time in about 70% of all diabetics. Some patients have some retinal changes at the time of diagnosis; however, it may be years before the patient complains of impairment of vision. Patients with retinopathy may have serious handicaps because failing vision makes it difficult, if not impossible, for them to inject insulin, test urine, prepare their own food, and give themselves general care. Helping them to accommodate to visual changes presents a great challenge to the nurse. (See discussion of diabetic retinopathy on p. 795.)

It is presumed that most diabetics have *asymptomatic polyneuropathy.* When disabling symptoms do occur, they are most likely to be manifested in the toes and feet and are symmetric. The most common symptoms are numbness, burning paresthesia, and stabbing pains. The person's limbs are very sensitive to touch and pressure, and the pain may be so severe that the patient cannot walk or wear shoes. Sometimes narcotics are required for pain relief.

Atherosclerosis can result in impaired circulation to the limbs, and serious infections of the toes and feet can result. Sometimes amputation is required to treat gangrene.

The nurse can help the patient to understand what he can do to help himself (proper foot care) and what the physician will check on the patient's visit. It can be reassuring to the patient if he realizes that the physician will be examining his urine for early signs of kidney complications and his eyes for any beginning changes. The nurse can also stress the need to be alert for any underlying problem such as an infection so that it can be promptly treated.

Outcome criteria for the person with diabetes mellitus and taking insulin

The patient or significant others can:

1. Explain the daily plan of care at home.
2. Test urine accurately.
3. Measure insulin accurately.
4. Use legs and abdomen as injection sites.
5. Use the food exchange lists in accord with written diet instructions.
6. Demonstrate proper foot care.
7. Describe daily program of exercise.
8. Explain the signs and symptoms of hyperglycemia and insulin reaction and tell what to do when they occur.
9. State plan for regular follow-up care.
10. Describe circumstances requiring immediate medical care.
11. Show the identification card the patient will carry at all times.

HYPOGLYCEMIC STATES

Hypoglycemia is a relatively common disorder characterized by blood sugar levels below 50 mg/100 ml. The blood sugar falls more rapidly than normal after eating and may drop to abnormally low levels several hours after a meal or after exercise. There is a sudden onset of faintness, hunger, weakness, and tremor. Headache and feelings of anxiety sometimes occur. In more severe cases, pallor, diaphoresis, rapid pulse, and even twitching, convulsions, and coma can occur. The symptoms may be intermittent, being relieved by food, or they may last for hours or for days.

Hypoglycemia is often functional, with no known cause demonstrable. It also may be caused by a pancreatic adenoma, causing extra insulin to be released; or by liver disease, causing inability to store glycogen; or by pituitary or adrenal dysfunction. If possible, the primary cause is treated.

A high-protein, high-fat, low-carbohydrate diet often relieves symptoms. Carbohydrates, especially simple sugars, are used quickly, but protein in excess of the normal body needs is converted gradually to glycogen, This helps to maintain the blood sugar at a more nearly normal and more stable level from meal to meal. The individual with this condition should eat meals that are spaced regularly. Many physicians advise their patients to carry lump sugar or candy with them at all times for immediate use if faintness occurs. Candy with nuts is best, since the nuts are a source of protein. The person must understand that he should not rely on these sugars as a substitute for regularly spaced meals, however, since *functional hypoglycemia is provoked by glucose stimulation, and more frequent attacks of hypoglycemia may occur.*

REFERENCES AND SELECTED READINGS

1. Beeson, P. B., and McDermott, W., editors: Textbook of medicine, ed. 14, Philadelphia, 1975, W. B. Saunders Co.
2. Beland, I. L. Rice, V. H., and Power, L.: Metabolic crises. In Meltzer, L. E., Abdellah, F. G., and Kitchell, J. R.: Concepts and practices of intensive care for nurse specialists, ed. 2, Philadelphia, 1976, The Charles Press Publishers.
3. Bergersen, B. S.: Pharmacology in nursing, ed. 13, St. Louis, 1975, The C. V. Mosby Co.

3.a *Bodhan, S. T., and Jans, K.: A new diabetic with complications, Nurs. Clin. North Am. **12**:393-406, 1977.

4. Bondy, P. K., and Rosenberg, L. E.: Duncan's diseases of metabolism, ed. 7, Philadelphia, 1974, W. B. Saunders Co.
5. *Boyles, V. A.: Injection aids for blind diabetic patients, Am. J. Nurs. **77**:1456-1458, 1977.
6. *Burke, E. L.: Insulin injection: the site and the technique, Am. J. Nurs. **72**:2194-2196, 1972.

6a. *Cataland, S.: Hypoglycemia: a spectrum of problems, Heart Lung **7**:459-462, 1978.

6b. *Cooperman, D., and Malarkey, W. B.: Pituitary apoplexy, Heart Lung **7**:450-454, 1978.

7. *Cranley, M. S., and Frazier, S. A.: Preventive intensive care of the diabetic mother and fetus, Nurs. Clin. North Am. **8**:489-499, 1973.

---

*References preceded by an asterisk are particularly well suited for student reading.

8. DeGroot, L. F., and Stanbury, J. B.: The thyroid and its diseases, ed. 4, New York, 1975, John Wiley and Sons, Inc.
9. Dillon, R. R.: Handbook of endocrinology, Philadelphia, 1973, Lea & Febiger.
10. Dolger, H., and Seeman, B.: How to live with diabetes, New York, 1965, W. W. Norton & Co., Inc.
11. *Elliott, D. D.: A self-instruction unit: adrenocortical insufficiency, Am. J. Nurs. **74**:1115-1130, 1974.
12. *Fletcher, H. P.: The oral antidiabetic drugs: pro and con, Am. J. Nurs. **76**:596-599, 1976.
13. *Friedland, G. M.: Learning behaviors of a preadolescent with diabetes, Am. J. Nurs. **76**:59-60, 1976.
14. Frohlich, E. D., editor: Pathophysiology, ed. 2, Philadelphia, 1976, W. B. Saunders Co.
15. *Fulton, M., Schweizer, D., Ruhland, F., et al.: vision, Am. J. Nurs. **74**:54-57, 1974.
15a. *Garber, R.: The use of a standardized teaching program in diabetes education, Nurs. Clin. North Am. **12**:372-391, 1977.
16. *Garofano, C.: Travel tips for the peripatetic diabetic, Nurs. 77 **7**:44-46, 1977.
17. Garofano, C.: Deliver facts to help diabetics plan parenthood, Nurs. 77 **7**:13-16, 1977.
18. *Gillies, D. A., and Alyn, I. B.: Caring for patients with thyroid disorders: how good are your skills?, Nurs. 77 **7**:71-80, 1977.
19. Gorman, C. A.: Some problems in thryoid diagnosis, Med. Clin. North Am. **56**:841-847, 1972.
20. *Gribbons, C. A., and Aliapoulios, M. A.: Treatment for advanced breast carcinoma, Am. J. Nurs. **72**:678-682, 1972.
21. *Grim, R. A.: Mr. Edward's triumph, Am. J. Nurs. **72**:480-481, 1972.
22. *Guthrie, D. W.: Exercise, diets and insulin for children with diabetes, Nurs. 77 **7**:48-54, 1977.
22a. *Guthrie, D. W., and Guthrie, R. A.: DKA: breaking a vicious cycle, Nurs. 78 **8**:54-57, 61, 1978.
23. *Guthrie, D. W., and Guthrie, R. A.: The infant of the diabetic mother, Am. J. Nurs. **74**:2008-2009, 1974.
24. *Guthrie, D. W., and Guthrie, R. A.: Coping with diabetic ketoacidosis, Nurs. 73 **3**:17-23, 1973.
25. *Hallal, J. C.: Thyroid disorders, Am. J. Nurs. **77**:417-432, 1977.
26. Harvey, A. A., et al.: The principles and practice of medicine, ed. 19, Englewood Cliffs, N.J., 1976, Prentice-Hall, Inc.
27. *Hayter, J.: Fine points in diabetic care, Am. J. Nurs. **76**:594-599, 1976.
28. *Huang, S. S.: Nursing assessment in planning care for a diabetic patient, Nurs. Clin. North Am. **6**:135-143, 1971.
29. *Isaf, J. J., and Alogna, M. T.: Better use of resources equals better health for diabetics, Am. J. Nurs. **77**:1792-1795, 1977.
30. *Kaufman, S. J.: In diabetic diets, realism gets results, Nurs. 76 **6**:75-77, 1976.
30a. *Keyes, M.: The somogyi phenomenon in insulin-dependent diabetes, Nurs. Clin. North Am. **12**:439-445, 1977.
31. Krueger, J. A., and Ray, J. C.: Endocrine problems in nursing, St. Louis, 1976, The C. V. Mosby Co.
32. *Krupp, M. A., and Chatton, M. J.: Current diagnosis and treatment, Los Altos, Calif., 1976, Lange Medical Publications.
33. *Lawrence, P. A.: U-100 insulin: let's make the transition trouble free, Am. J. Nurs. **13**:1539, 1973.
34. Martin, M.M.: Insulin reaction, Am. J. Nurs. **67**:328-331, 1967.
35. *McConnell, E. A.: Meeting the special needs of diabetics facing surgery, Nurs. 76 **6**:30-37, 1976.
36. Mountcastle, V. B., editor: Medical physiology, ed. 13, St. Louis, 1974, The C. V. Mosby Co.
37. Nickerson, D.: Teaching the hospitalized diabetic, Am. J. Nurs. **72**:935-938, 1972.
37a. *Petrokas, J.: Common sense guidelines for controlling diabetes during illness, Nurs. 78 **7**:36-37, 1978.
38. *Porter, A. L., et al.: Giving diabetics control of their own lives, Nurs. 73 **3**:44-49, 1973.
39. Rodman, M. J.: The pituitary hormones, RN **31**:55-67, 1968.
40. Rodman, M. J.: The thyroid and antithyroid drugs, RN **31**:52-59, 1968.
41. Schneeberg, N. G.: Essentials of clinical endrocrinology, St. Louis, 1970, The C. V. Mosby Co.
42. *Schulz, J. M., and Williams, M.: Encouragement breeds independence in the blind diabetic, Nurs. 76 **6**:19-20, 1976.
43. *Schumann, D.: Tips for improving urine testing techniques, Nurs. 76 **6**:23-27, 1976.
44. *Schumann, D.: Coping with the complex, dangerous, elusive problems of those insulin-induced hypoglycemic reactions, Nurs. 74 **4**:56-60, 1974.
45. *Schumann, D.: Assessing the diabetic, Nurs. 76 **6**:62-67, 1976.
46. Selenkow, H. A.: The normal and abnormal thyroid: an approach to diagnosis and therapy, New York, 1973, Medcom Books, Inc.
47. *Skillman, T. G.: Diabetic ketoacidosis, Heart Lung **7**:594-602, 1978.
47a. *Slater, N.: Insulin reactions vs. ketoacidosis: guidelines for diagnosis and interventions, Am. J. Nurs. **78**:875-877, 1978.
48. *Stowe, S. M.: Hypophysectomy for diabetic retinopathy, Am. J. Nurs. **73**:632-637, 1973.
49. *Suren, J. V.: Education of the culturally and educationally deprived, Nurs. Clin. North Am. **12**:427-437, 1977.
50. Sussman, K. E., and Metz, R. J. S.: Diabetes mellitus, ed. 4, New York, 1976, American Diabetes Association, Inc.
51. *Tribble, N. M., and Hollenberg, E. E.: The import of a quality assurance program on diabetic education, Nurs. Clin. North Am. **12**:365-373, 1977.
52. *Tzagournis, M.: Acute adrenal insufficiency, Heart Lung **7**:603-609, 1978.
53. Urbanic, R. C., and Mazzaferri, E. L.: Thyrotoxic crisis and myxedema coma, Heart Lung **7**:435-557, 1978.
53a. *Ventura, E.: Foot care for diabetics, Am. J. Nurs. **78**:886-888, 1978.
53b. *Walesky, M. E.: Diabetic ketoacidosis, Am. J. Nurs. **78**:872-874, 1978.
54. *Williams, S. R.: Nutrition and diet therapy, ed. 3, St. Louis, 1977, The C. V. Mosby Co.
55. Winter, C. C., and Morel, A.: Nursing care of patients with urologic diseases, ed. 4, St. Louis, 1977, The C. V. Mosby, Co.
56. Wintrobe, M. M., et al., editors: Harrison's principles of internal medicine, ed. 8, New York, 1977, McGraw-Hill Book Co.
57. *Wolfe, L.: Insulin: paving the way to a new life, Nurs. 77 **7**:38-41, 1977.

33

Dysfunction of liver and related structures

JUDITH L. GREIG

The liver and biliary system are affected by a variety of diseases that may present many nursing care challenges. Disorders that are encountered include not only those caused by infectious organisms but also abnormalities due to changes in structure and function that are essential to digestion and normal metabolic processes. In this chapter nursing care specific to general problems commonly seen in patients with hepatic, biliary, and pancreatic diseases is discussed.

■ DISORDERS OF THE LIVER

Disorders of the liver may be separated into several pathologic states. Hepatitis and cirrhosis and their sequelae are the most common problems and receive the most emphasis in this chapter. Other problems of the liver such as tumors, abscess, and trauma are presented briefly.

Regardless of the specific pathology, disorders of the liver present the patient with many problems. Inadequate nutrition and metabolism are common, as are fluid and electrolyte imbalances, coagulation problems, decreased resistance to infection, and inability to detoxify substances normally detoxified in the liver.

In many instances no specific curative therapy is available, and the treatment and care focus on providing physiologic and psychologic support until the liver heals itself. Emphasis is on assisting the individual to conserve energy and on health teaching related to preventing further liver damage.

Liver function studies, radiographic diagnostic procedures, and liver biopsy may be necessary to determine the exact disease process that is present and the extent of liver damage. Tests more frequently used are discussed in Chapter 30 along with a review of the normal physiologic mechanisms carried out by the hepatic system.

□ Hepatitis

Hepatitis may be defined as any acute inflammatory disease of the liver. Although the term *hepatitis* is most commonly used in conjunction with viral hepatitis, the disease can be caused by viruses, bacteria, or by toxic injury to the liver. Hepatotoxins include drugs (chlorpromazine, isoniazid, tetracycline, thiazide diuretics, thiouracils, and others), agents such as phosphorus, organic solvents (carbon tetrachloride and methylenedianiline [MDA][23]), plant poisons, and alcohol.

Although there are some differences in the pathologic and clinical phenomena of viral, bacterial, and toxic hepatitis, the clinical management of the person with hepatitis is quite similar. The particular aspects of care for viral hepatitis are discussed next. It should be pointed out that any form of hepatitis can result in postnecrotic cirrhosis unless the hepatitis responds to treatment.

Viral hepatitis

Viral hepatitis is by far the most important infection attacking the liver. Although the disease is not new, it assumed serious proportions during world War II when 50,000 men developed jaundice after receiving yellow fever vaccine containing human serum. Since that time it has become a major health problem in the United States as well as in many other countries and has been studied intensively. There are two types of viral hepatitis: type A (infectious hepatitis) and type B (serum homologous hepatitis).

Incidence. Viral hepatitis is a reportable disease in all states. The Center for Disease Control (CDC) statistics indicate that there has been some decline in the number of reported cases each year since 1971 when there were 69,000 cases of hepatitis in the United States. In 1976 the number of reported cases of viral hepatitis (A and B) was 48,261, and an additional 7,488 cases were unspecified as to type.[42] It is well accepted that the figures for any given year may be grossly underestimated, since carriers with subclinical manifestations are often not reported as having active disease. There are geographic differences in the number of cases of hepatitis, with the highest number of cases being reported in the Pacific area (Washington, Oregon, California, Alaska and Hawaii) and the lowest in the West North Central area (Minnesota, Iowa, Missouri, North Dakota, South Dakota, Nebraska, and Kansas).[42]

Most of the reported cases are of type A. The incidence of type B is felt to remain fairly constant, while the incidence of type A has a distinct pattern. It is more common in the fall and winter, peaks in the late winter and early spring, and falls to low levels in the summer. A high incidence of both type A and type B is noted in drug abusers. The increased rates are due to communal living under poor sanitary conditions (type A) and the sharing of unsterilized needles (type B) in parenteral drug use.

With type B hepatitis there is a somewhat higher mortality than with type A hepatitis, but it is thought that this higher rate may be due to the fact that many patients who are given plasma or blood transfusions are already quite ill. It is also believed that lowered host resistance, rather than a higher virulence of the virus, may be the cause of death.

Most persons recover from viral hepatitis within 3 to 4 months. Rarely the disease may run a mild but prolonged course, with enlargement of the liver and abnormal liver function studies persisting for 1 to 2 years. In approximately 5% of all persons with viral hepatitis there is exacerbation of the disease within 6 months of onset. In 15% to 45% of patients with postnecrotic cirrhosis, a history of hepatitis or symptomatology resembling viral hepatitis is given. More often the disease seems to be initiated by acute hepatitis that progresses to cirrhosis.[32]

One attack of viral hepatitis confers immunity for that strain of virus infection but does not protect against attack by the other virus. However, the disease can become chronic, with acute exacerbations occurring months after the first acute symptoms have subsided. Liver damage following attack by one virus naturally lessens the body's defenses if attack by the second virus should occur.

Viral hepatitis seems to be most prevalent in low-income areas where there is crowding and limited sanitation. Children's homes, schools, and housing projects with a high concentration of children produce optimum settings for spread by contact. Susceptibility to the disease is highest in persons between 6 and 25 years of age, but there is a trend toward an increased incidence in adults, particularly in the older age groups.[6] Recent studies show that pregnant women are highly susceptible to viral hepatitis during the second and third trimesters and that the mortality rate is extremely high in the last trimester.

Epidemiology. Until recently the viruses of hepatitis were not transmissible from humans to experimental animals, and study of the disease has been difficult. Recently tests have revealed the presence of circulating antigens (substances that induce formation of antibodies) in persons with acute viral hepatitis. One antigen previously referred to as Australia antigen and currently as hepatitis B surface antigen (HB_sAg) has been discovered in the serum of many patients with serum hepatitis. Tests demonstrate that the HB_sAg particles have the appearance of a virus, but to date researchers can only say it is a lipoprotein resembling an incomplete virus particle that is detectable in the blood of patients with the infection.

Viral hepatitis is caused by two distinct but similar viruses that produce almost identical symptoms but that vary in their incubation period and mode of transmission. These viruses are known as the "A" or IH virus (short-incubation virus), which causes infectious hepatitis, and the "B" or SH virus (long-incubation virus), which causes homologous serum hepatitis. The latter is associated exclusively with HB_sAg.

Some investigators prefer the older terminology of type A and type B in referring to infectious hepatitis and serum hepatitis, respectively. The reason given is the possibility that agents not yet discovered (type C, D, and so forth) may be responsible for some forms of hepatitis.[15] The incubation period of the IH virus is 10 to 40 days and for the SH virus probably 2 to 6 months. The source of the virus causing *infectious hepatitis* (HAV) is human blood and human feces. The infection is spread by the oral intake of food, milk, or water contaminated with the virus or by the parenteral introduction of the hepatitis virus through blood, blood products, or the equipment used for venipuncture or other procedures that require penetrating the skin. Biting insects, urine, and nasopharyngeal secretions also may be sources of the virus, but this possibility is still unproved. Viruses are excreted in the feces long before clinical symptoms appear, and they may remain for long periods of time in the feces of persons who have had the disease and in carriers. It is not known whether the carriers are natural carriers or whether they have had the disease in a less severe and unrecognized form. It is known that mild, *subclinical disease* that is not severe enough to cause jaundice can occur.

Causative agents. It has only been since the early 1940s that the true infectious nature of viral hepatitis has been recognized. One problem that has constantly thwarted researchers investigating virus hepatitis has been the lack of a suitable experimental animal host system for the transmission of the viral agents. Only recently has human viral hepatitis been transmitted to animals in the laboratory. The most significant breakthrough in the elucidation of the etiology of viral hepatitis came in 1965 when an antigen was demonstrated in the blood of an Australian aborigine and was shown to have some relationship to hepatitis. The antigen, initially called *Australia antigen,* was shown to be transiently but consistently present in the blood of several patients suffering from hepatitis type B infections. This antigen was first thought to be the hepatitis B virus (HBV), but researchers had no success in transmitting disease or getting the Australia antigen to propagate in tissue culture. In 1970, however, Dane and his co-workers[10] discovered a larger, more complex structure in the serum from infected individuals, which is known as the *Dane particle.* The Dane particle seems to be the free virus in the serum, and the Australia antigen (HB_sAg) represents an excess of viral coats free in the serum. Since these discoveries were made other immunologically distinct antigens and specific antibodies have been found in the serum of individuals suffering from hepatitis that further implicate the Dane particle as the causative virus. These discoveries were followed in 1973 by the identification of a similar viruslike particle in stool specimens from individuals with hepatitis type A (HAV).

Since the hepatitis viruses have only recently been identified, there is relatively little accumulated evidence on their physiochemical or biologic characteristics. On the basis of epidemiologic observations and some results obtained from human transmission studies, both HBV and HAV have been assumed to be extremely resistant to such antimicrobial measures as drying, chlorination, disinfectants, heat, ultraviolet radiation, and freezing. The viruses are especially refractive to such measures when protected by the presence of serum proteins. At boiling temperatures the viruses can survive for about 20 to 30 minutes. Autoclaving is the best method to ensure destruction of the viruses on contaminated articles.

The two viruses causing viral hepatitis are distinct but very similar in structure. The symptoms that they produce within the body are almost identical, but the course of the disease and the mode of transmission may vary somewhat depending on the causative agent. The older terminology used to indicate the type of hepatitis reflects these differences. Type A viral infections are still commonly called *infectious hepatitis, epidemic hepatitis,* or *short-incubation hepatitis;* type B infections are sometimes referred to as *serum hepatitis, homologous serum jaundice,* and *long-incubation hepatitis.*

Transmission. The incubation period for hepatitis A is usually about 30 days, with a range of 10 to 40 days from the time of exposure to the appearance of the initial prejaundice *(preicteric)* symptoms. The source of the virus is human feces and human blood. The disease is most often spread by the fecal-oral route. Fecally contaminated food, water, milk, shellfish, and objects can serve as potential sources of infection. If common sources such as communal wells, streams, or food supplies are contaminated with the virus due to the breakdown in sanitary safeguards, small or large epidemics may result. Often secondary epidemics may result due to close contact with infected persons; this is especially true of

Table 33-1. Characteristics of hepatitis A and hepatitis B infections

Features	Hepatitis A (infectious hepatitis)	Hepatitis B (serum hepatitis)
Sources	Contaminated food or water, contaminated needles or surgical instruments, asymptomatic carriers	Contaminated needles or surgical instruments, contaminated blood products, asymptomatic carriers
Route of infection	Fecal-oral, parenteral, or direct contact	Parenteral, oral, or direct contact
Incubation period	Short (10 to 40 days), 30 days average	Long (45 to 180 days), 60 days average
Onset of disease	Abrupt, often febrile	Insidious, seldom febrile
Viral antigens	Fecal antigens, liver antigens	HB_sAg in serum during incubation and acute phases
Diagnostic tests	Transaminase levels, liver biopsy	Transaminase levels, liver biopsy
Mortality	Low (1%)	High (50%)
Age group affected	Children, young adults, elderly persons	All age groups
Immunity	Recovery provides immunity to HAV but not HBV	Recovery provides immunity to HBV but not HAV
Immune globulin protection	Effective	Ineffective

transmission to members of the household of an infected individual. In addition to the fecal-oral route, parenteral introduction of HAV through blood products or contaminated parenteral equipment can occur, since the virus is found in the blood (viremia) during the latter half of the incubation period and the early acute phase of the infection. However, parenteral transmission is thought to be of only limited significance in the spread of HAV. The implication of a respiratory route of transmission has been suggested, but there is a little experimental or epidemiologic data to support this as an important mechanism of transmission.

The incubation period of HBV ranges from 45 to 180 days, with 60 days being about average. It is often difficult to assess the true length of the incubation period because by the time the symptoms appear the circumstances attendant to the exposure have been forgotten. The principal source of the virus is the blood of persons who have the virus or who are carriers of the virus. The virus is transmitted parenterally through blood, serum or plasma, or through equipment used for venipuncture or pricking the skin. The virus can also be spread by contact of mucous membranes of the mouth and respiratory tract or an open cut in the skin with contaminated blood. Those caring for or closely associating with the infected individual are highly vulnerable to infection. The disease can be transmitted from infected patients to medical, nursing, and other hospital personnel by accidental pricking of the skin with a needle contaminated by the patient's blood. Among those at highest risk are personnel in clinical laboratories, blood banks, dialysis units, and transplantation units. Since HBV can be transmitted by nonparenteral routes, other sources of spread have been identified but occur with much less frequency. A summary of the differences between type A and type B hepatitis are outlined in Table 33-1.

Pathophysiology. Viral hepatitis causes diffuse degeneration and necrosis of liver cells. Degeneration, regeneration, and inflammation may occur simultaneously, will distort the normal lobular pattern, and may create pressure within and about the portal vein areas. These change may be associated with elevated serum transaminase levels, prolonged prothrombin time, and slightly elevated serum alkaline phosphatase level. Because the pathologic process is usually distributed evenly throughout the liver, biopsy has been particularly useful in studying and diagnosing the disease. In most instances of nonfatal viral hepatitis, regeneration begins almost with the onset of the disease. The damaged cells and their contents eventually are removed by phagocytosis and enzymatic reaction, and the liver returns to normal. The outcome of viral hepatitis may be affected by such factors as the virulence of the virus, the amount of hepatic damage sustained during the patient's life before exposure to the virus, his natural barriers to damage and disease of the liver, and the supportive care he receives when symptoms appear. The disease may take several courses, and different terms describe each of them.

Fulminating viral hepatitis designates a sudden and severe degeneration and atrophy of the liver. This condition may follow acute poisoning, but it most often is associated with an overwhelming infection with the hepatitis virus that progresses rapidly to cause death unless corticosteroids are successful in arresting the process. The liver may shrink in size to as little as 600 g, in contrast to a weight of 1,500 g in a normal adult.

Subacute fatal viral hepatitis causes acute massive necrosis, which, even though it is not evenly distributed throughout the organ, finally destroys enough of the liver to cause death. This form of the disease may vary in duration from several weeks to several months, with apparent short remissions followed by exacerbations. In its late stages subacute fatal viral hepatitis is almost impossible to distinguish from cirrhosis of the liver by clinical manifestations and by liver function tests. However, history of exposure to viral hepatitis and symptoms of acute infection aid in diagnosis.

Chronic forms of the disease are still not well understood. Signs of chronicity may persist in biopsied liver tissue when liver function tests show no abnormality and when no clinical signs are evident. However, the opposite may also be true. Acute exacerbations of chronic viral hepatitis can progress to acute fatal liver necrosis.

Prevention. It is in the area of prevention that the nurse can make the greatest contribution to the control of viral hepatitis. Since there is no specific treatment for the disease and no adequate immunization, it is only by making use of what is known about the viruses that control can be accomplished.

Methods of destroying the viruses of hepatitis are limited. There is the possibility that undiagnosed hepatitis may be most infectious; therefore particular emphasis should be placed on *thorough washing of hands* with soap and running water after possible exposure. The staff must regard all feces, blood, and other body fluids as potentially infectious and not just those of patients with hepatitis or jaundice. The patient should be taught how to wash his hands thoroughly and should know why this is necessary, particularly after a bowel movement. Thorough washing of all equipment that might be contaminated lessens the danger to persons who must handle it and may help protect the next patient for whom the equipment is used. Since infectious hepatitis can be transmitted by infected stools and contaminated food and water, food handlers should be encouraged to pay careful attention to handwashing regulations.

At the present time dry heat and steam heat under pressure (autoclaving) are the only safe ways to sterilize needles and other equipment used to penetrate the skin. The adequate boiling time is still undetermined, and for this reason most hospitals use autoclave sterilization and sterile, disposable syringes and needles almost entirely. When boiling is the only way to sterilize needles and other equipment, the nurse should see that everything placed in the sterilizer is *covered completely and boiled for at least 30 minutes.*[14] (See fundamentals of nursing texts for the proper method of sterilizing equipment by boiling.)

Both hepatitis A and hepatitis B can be transmitted from one patient to another when multiple doses of a drug are put into one syringe and only the needle is changed between patients. This practice should be deplored! Regardless of the extra expense involved and the extra time and work entailed in preparation of materials for each injection, separate needles and syringes that have been autoclaved or disposable syringes and needles should be used. School immunization programs and practices in large outpatient clinics such as allergy clinics have been affected by recommendations in this regard. The nurse often must help explain the need for the extra cost to administrative personnel. The use of jet-spray guns to administer injections is safe, and they are especially helpful when immunizing a large number of persons.

Since individuals may be carriers of both type A and type B viruses, all needles and other equipment that have penetrated the skin of any patient should be handled with the greatest care. Type B hepatitis occurs quite frequently among hospital personnel. This is not surprising considering how often nurses, laboratory workers, or other members of the hospital staff may unwittingly prick themselves with needles that have been used for a wide variety of parenteral treatments. The safest way to handle any needle that is to be sterilized and reused is to rinse it carefully in cold water after use and place it in a puncture-resistant rigid container. Syringes and needles should be placed in a double bag and returned to central supply for decontamination and sterilization. Needles from infusion sets should be removed from the tubing immediately after an infusion is discontinued so that persons cleaning the equipment at a later time will not accidentally prick themselves. Special precautions should be used when disposing of disposable syringes and needles, both to protect refuse handlers from accidental infection and to keep them out of the hands of drug abusers. Used needles are not to be recapped or purposely bent; they are placed in a prominently labeled, impervious, puncture-resistant container designated for that purpose. Some hospitals use bright red cardboard containers labeled "Contaminated" for this purpose. Syringes are placed in an impervious bag. Both of these containers are incinerated or autoclaved before discarding.[44]

Because it is impossible on clinical grounds alone to determine which type of hepatitis is present, persons with hepatitislike symptoms are considered to have either type A or type B hepatitis until otherwise proved.

It is recommended that patients with hepatitis be placed on enteric and blood precautions. Children should be in a private room. Responsible adults need not be in a private room if all precautions are observed. The reasons for the precautions and how the patient can assist with them should be carefully explained to him. The greatest care should be taken in handling fecal matter and in performing treatments that involve contamination of the hands. Bedpans should be isolated and should be autoclaved following the patient's discharge from the hospital. Rubber gloves are often advised when handling urinals, bedpans, and commodes. In most localities feces need not be treated if proper sewage disposal is available. If there is any doubt, the local health department should be consulted.

To prevent spread of type A viruses by carriers, it is suggested that individual toilet paper packages, rather than rolls, be used in any public bathroom and that toilets be cleaned with 1% aqueous iodine. The use of disposable seatcovers and foot pedals for flushing the toilet would help to reduce the chances of spread of the infection.

All patients should have individual thermometers, and the thermometer used for a patient with infectious hepatitis should be disposed of on his discharge from the hospital. Since there is no really safe and satisfactory method of sterilizing a thermometer, discarding it is the only way to be certain that the disease is not spread by it. The cost of a thermometer is relatively small.

During hospitalization the thermometer is kept in 70% to 90% alcohol with 2% iodine. The solution is changed every 3 days. For the protection of the nursing personnel, the patient's temperature should be taken orally whenever possible. When small children must have their temperature taken rectally, gloves should be worn. Poor technique in carrying out temperature-taking procedures has been suspected as a cause of widespread infection from the type A virus in foundling homes and similar sheltered-care facilities for children.

Even though the virus of hepatitis A, unlike that of hepatitis B, has not been found in urine, special precautions should be taken in handling urine because of the possibility that urine may be contaminated with any of the potential hepatitis viruses as yet undiscovered.[15] Because both of the viruses may be transmitted by the oral route from contaminated hands and food, special care should be taken in handling nose and mouth secretions. The patient should be instructed to use tissues, which are then placed in an impervious paper or plastic bag and burned. Disposable dishes are preferred. Food waste should be burned and dishes boiled for 30 minutes or (ideally) autoclaved. If feasible, utensils may be washed in the patient's room, placed in an impervious plastic bag, labeled "Contaminated" or "Isolation,"[44] and autoclaved on his discharge. Rooms should be cleaned well and aired when the patient leaves the hospital. When the patient has hepatitis, utmost care must be given to syringes, needles and other instruments that are contaminated with the patient's serum. They should be autoclaved at 121 C (15 pounds pressure) for 15 minutes or dry-heat sterilized at 170 C for 2 hours. Use of disposable syringes and needles is recommended. Known or suspected carriers should not be blood donors. Patients should also be placed on stool precautions because of possible transmission by the fecal-oral route. If any doubt exists as to which of the virus diseases a patient has, it is safest to take the precautions necessary in the care of patients with type A hepatitis.

Anyone who has been exposed to viral hepatitis should be urged to report this fact to the physician. This is especially important for a woman in the second or third trimester of pregnancy. Although the role of transplacentally transmitted viral hepatitis in causing injury to the liver in newborn infants has not been determined, the disease is believed to increase the likelihood of abortion, stillbirth, and congenital abnormalities.[6] Immune serum globulin (ISG) offers some protection against type A hepatitis, but it does not protect against type B hepatitis. The routine use of ISG for hospital contacts of a patient with hepatitis is not recommended. It is given to some persons with known exposure to hepatitis A.[44] It is also recommended that persons planning to travel to areas where hepatitis is endemic receive immune serum globulin. The dose for an adult is approximately 2 ml (0.01 ml/lb body weight) intramuscularly.[15]

A simple test for bilirubinuria, the *Icotest*, has been developed. Since bilirubin is present in the urine of the person who has viral hepatitis before clinical signs appear, it has been suggested that as part of a disease detection program this test be done on anyone exposed to hepatitis A, all schoolchildren, hospital patients and employees, blood donors, employees in public institutions and industrial plants, and food handlers. Early recognition of the disease would make control of its spread easier. The test is done by placing 5 drops of urine on the Icotest reagent tablet.

Clinical picture. Collection of subjective and objective data through systematic assessment should be carried out paying particular attention to those parameters previously discussed (see Chapter 30). In addition the nurse should obtain information with regard to any recent exposure to possible hepatotoxic agents or persons who were jaundiced or any recent blood transfusions or injections. The clinical symptoms of viral hepatitis vary. Patients may be asymptomatic and show minimal laboratory evidence of liver disturbance. Some patients may have many symptoms of the disease but no jaundice. A few may have fulminating necrosis of the liver and die. In most instances, however, viral hepatitis is a mild disease, and complete recovery is the rule.

Symptoms of infectious hepatitis and serum hepatitis are not clinically distinctive from each other except that acute symptoms may be more severe in infectious hepatitis. Symptoms usually appear from 4 to 7 days before jaundice is apparent. Observations that the nurse may make to assist in determining a diagnosis include the presence of headache, elevated temperature, chills, nausea and vomiting, dyspepsia, anorexia, general malaise, arthralgia, and tenderness over the liver. Bleeding into the skin and mucous membranes may also occur due to a prolonged prothrombin time. Anorexia is one of the most frequent symptoms, and often the patient who smokes is repulsed by tobacco taste and smoke and other strong odors. This *preicteric stage* lasts for approximately 1 week and then subsides as jaundice occurs.

The *icteric stage* usually reaches its intensity in 2 weeks and may last from 1 to 2 weeks. Jaundice occurs when damaged liver cells are prevented from removing bilirubin from the blood, resulting in large amounts diffusing into the tissues. The patient may then be observed to have yellow sclera and skin. In addition the excess bilirubin may be excreted by the kidneys, producing dark amber urine and clay-colored stools. (For additional details about jaundice refer to p. 562.) Gastrointestinal tract symptoms may increase during the icteric stage, with the temperature elevation subsiding after the onset of jaundice. The liver frequently becomes more tender and swollen due to necrosis of the parenchymal cells.

The *posticteric* or *convalescent stage* begins with the disappearance of jaundice and may last from a few weeks to several months. Complete recovery is usually expected in 6 months. The disease may have relapsed during this stage, with recurrence of previous symptoms but to a milder degree. Children usually have a milder, nonicteric form of infectious hepatitis with symptoms predominantly those of an intestinal or respiratory tract illness.

Intervention. There is no specific medical treatment for viral hepatitis; therefore treatment is primarily aimed at providing sufficient rest and nutrition to allow the patient's body to tolerate the insult of the infection and to gradually return to a state of physiologic stability.

Acute phase

REST. Physical activity should be restricted and the patient usually is placed on bed rest. The amount of bed rest required will depend on the individual patient, but it will be longer in patients with severe disease and in the elderly. Extremely elevated serum enzyme levels may be indicative of hepatic cell damage and thus indicate the need for restricted activity. It is believed that activity and maintaining an upright position decrease hepatic blood flow, thus preventing optimum circulation to the already compromised liver cells.[32] Continued monitoring of these laboratory values can serve as an indicator for determining the amount of increased activity that the patient can tolerate. Relapses are frequently attributed to premature increases in activity.

During the first few days after the onset of symptoms the patient feels ill, and maintaining bed rest may not be difficult. However, bed rest should not be an irritating, uncomfortable experience. Changing the patient's position frequently along with the use of pillows for comfort may aid in promoting rest. A quiet environment is maintained, and necessary activities are carried out at one time so that the patient's rest is not interrupted. The nurse may also need to intervene if the patient is having prolonged visits or frequent visitors who interfere with adequate rest.

DIET. Fluids are encouraged by mouth if nausea is not a problem. The desirable fluid intake usually is considered to be at least 3,000 ml/day. If the patient's temperature is high and nausea and vomiting are severe, infusions containing glucose are given, and occasionally solutions containing other electrolytes and protein hydrolysates are ordered. Intake and output are monitored because some patients with severe viral hepatitis cannot excrete a normal amount of fluid. Occasionally a record of daily weight is instituted to assist in monitoring for fluid retention. If diarrhea occurs, the color, consistency, frequency, and amount of stool is carefully noted. Constipation is often present.

Even if nauseated the patient can usually tolerate some food by mouth. Fruit juices, carbonated beverages, and hard candy can sometimes be retained and are encouraged during the periods of anorexia. Antiemetics may be ordered one-half hour prior to meals and should be conscientiously administered if found to be of value in preventing nausea. No special diet is required, but usually one high in protein, calories, and carbohydrates is ordered. Fats may be poorly tolerated due to the lack of bile entering the gastrointestinal tract. General care, including attention to good oral hygiene, skin care, and elimination, is necessary. Special attention should be paid to protecting the patient from intercurrent infection.

MEDICATIONS. Therapy may include the administration of vitamin K if the prothrombin time is depressed. Vitamins B complex and C may be ordered as a dietary supplement. The use of corticosteroid therapy is not indicated unless the disease is particularly severe. If jaundice continues to increase after 3 weeks and nausea and vomiting remain uncontrolled, steroid therapy may be initiated. The nurse should observe for signs of sodium retention and potassium loss following steroid administration.

Convalescent phase. During the convalescent stage nursing care may become an even greater challenge. Although the patient's jaundice may be disappearing and he may be feeling well, this does not mean he is well, and there is a great need for caution against overexertion. When the patient begins to feel well, he becomes anxious to resume normal living and is irritated by the circumstances requiring enforced inactivity. His irritation may be expressed, for example, by complaining about the hospital menu, regardless of the quality of the food. The family should realize that in the home he may also be critical of food for the same reason. Wheeling the patient in his bed to the recreation area, where he may view television or converse with others, often helps him pass the day without boredom. Occupational therapy activities that can be brought to the bedside are useful in keeping the patient relatively content during the convalescent period.

There is a trend toward earlier ambulation of patients with viral hepatitis. When acute symptoms subside and the jaundice begins to recede, the patient may be permitted to walk about in his room with periods of rest after each meal. Activities are increased gradually, and if there are no adverse effects the patient may be permitted to convalesce at home under close medical supervision. Recurrence of anorexia, enlargement or tenderness of the liver, or lack of progress as shown by studies of hepatic function indicate a need to return to bed rest. Some patients are cared for at home from the onset of symptoms to complete recovery. With the assistance of a community health nurse, many families are able to care for the patient safely and adequately.

The nurse who cares for the patient in his own home should observe carefully for changes in the color of urine and stool and for jaundice and should report any changes to the physician.

Toxic hepatitis

Pathophysiology. The morphologic changes in the liver will depend on the toxic agent. For example, necrosis and fatty infiltrates are present when the causative agent is carbon tetrachloride, while cholestatsis with portal inflammation is seen when the toxic agent is chlorpromazine.[47] Microscopic examination of liver tissue obtained by biopsy helps to differentiate the causative agent. Two types of chemical hepatotoxicity occur: direct toxic and idiosyncratic. In *direct toxic* hepatitis the agent causes toxicity with predictable regularity. The occurrence of this form of hepatitis is dose dependent and usually occurs several hours to 2 days after exposure.[47]

The occurrence of *idiosyncratic toxic* hepatitis is infrequent and unpredictable, and the response is not dose dependent. Hepatitis may occur anytime, from during exposure to shortly after exposure to the toxic substance. Most cases of drug-induced toxic hepatitis are idiosyncratic reactions. It is thought that these idiosyncratic reactions may be due to unique host susceptibility or may be immunologically mediated, although immune-mediated hypersensitivity has not been proved.[47]

Prevention. The nurse can help in the prevention of toxic hepatitis by teaching the danger of injudicious use of materials that are known to be injurious to the liver and by emphasizing the need for a diet that is protective to the liver.

Since cleaning agents, solvents, and related substances sometimes contain products that are harmful to the liver, the public should read instructions on labels and should follow them explicitly. Dry-cleaning fluids may contain carbon tetrachloride, which can cause injury if warnings to avoid inhalation of the fumes and to keep windows open are not heeded. If people must use these agents inside the home, a good practice is to open the windows wide, use the cleaning materials as quickly as possible, and then vacate the room, the apartment, or the house for several hours, leaving the windows open.

Many solvents used to remove paint and plastic material and to stain and finish woodwork contain injurious substances and should be used outdoors and not even in the basement, since dangerous fumes may spread throughout the house. Cleaning agents and finishes for cars should be applied outdoors or in the garage with the door open. Nurses in industry have a responsibility to teach the importance of observing regulations to avoid industrial hazards. Nitrobenzene, tetrachlorethane, carbon disulfide, and dinitrotoluol are examples of injurious compounds used in industry.

Some drugs that are known to cause mild damage to the liver must be used therapeutically. However, the nurse should warn the public regarding the use of preparations that are available without prescription that may be injurious. Many drugs reach the market before dangers of their extensive use have been conclusively ruled out; for example, chlorpromazine, which was being widely used as a tranquilizer, is known to cause stasis in the canaliculi of the liver, which may lead to serious hepatic damage. A safe rule to follow is to avoid taking any medication except that specifically prescribed by a physician for a specific ailment.

Clinical picture. The symptoms of toxic hepatitis resemble those of viral hepatitis (p. 595). Liver function tests including serum transaminase levels are valuable in evaluating the severity of injury to liver cells.

Intervention. If the liver damage is from toxic agents, the treatment consists of identifying the toxic agent and removing or eliminating it. Gastric lavage and cleansing of the bowel may be indicated to remove the hepatotoxin from the intestinal tract. Antidotes such as BAL have been used with some degree of success in binding the agent for possible excretion by the kidneys. Patients with toxic hepatitis are placed on bed rest. Nursing measures include those for patients with any hepatic disease (see Chapter 31).

☒ Cirrhosis of the liver

Cirrhosis of the liver is a term applied by pathologists to several diseases that are characterized by diffuse inflammation and fibrosis of the liver resulting in drastic structural changes and significant loss of liver function. The basic processes leading to cirrhosis are liver cell death with scar tissue formation and regeneration of cell mass that causes distortion of the structure with a resultant change in circulation.

There are various types of cirrhosis. The following is a brief description of the four major types. *Biliary cirrhosis* refers to a disorder that occurs when there is chronic impairment of bile excretion. The liver shows morphologic evidence of liver destruction around the intrahepatic bile duct. It can result from chronic intrahepatic cholestasis or be secondary to blockage of the common bile duct. *Cardiac cirrhosis* is a form of chronic liver disease that results from severe right-sided congestive heart failure such as that found with valvular problems, constrictive pericarditis, and decompensated cor pulmonale. *Postnecrotic cirrhosis,* also called toxic cirrhosis, posthepatic cirrhosis, or multilobular cirrhosis, results from overall but unequal injury to liver cell due to toxic elements, usually viral hepatitis. This form of chronic liver disease is the most common type of cirrhosis worldwide. *Laennec's cirrhosis,* also called nutritional, fatty, alcoholic, and portal cirrhosis, is the most common type of cirrhosis in North America.

Epidemiology. In European and American studies of persons with Laennec's cirrhosis, chronic alcoholism was present from 50% to 80% of the time.[32] However, chronic alcoholism is by no means the only cause of Laennec's cirrhosis. Alcoholics often develop fatty degeneration of the liver that may lead to cirrhosis, but the same changes have been seen in persons who do not drink. Another major contributing cause of Laennec's cirrhosis is malnutrition, which is frequently found to exist simultaneously with chronic alcoholism, and the combined insult is particularly damaging to liver cells. There is evidence that alcohol alone can damage liver cells even in well-nourished persons.

Rare and nonspecific types of cirrhosis account for about 10% of deaths due to cirrhosis.[47] Nonspecific types of cirrhosis are associated with metabolic problems, infectious diseases, infiltrative disease, and gastrointestinal tract disorders. In the United States the number of deaths from cirrhosis continues to increase, and the incidence appears to parallel increases in alcohol ingestion. Cirrhosis as a cause of death in the United States now ranks fifth in persons between the ages of 45 and 64 years, with more men than women and more nonwhites than whites succumbing to the disease.

Pathophysiology. The morphologic changes in the liver will vary depending on the type of cirrhosis. In *biliary cirrhosis* there is a diffuse necrotizing and inflammatory process centered around the portal tract. The liver at first is enlarged and greenish yellow in appearance but evolves into a smaller, firmer, nodular organ as the disease progresses.

In *cardiac cirrhosis* the liver is swollen, tense, and dark colored with a thickened capsule. The liver may become nodular as the cirrhosis progresses.

In *postnecrotic cirrhosis* the liver is small and grossly distorted in shape and composed of many nodules of regenerated liver cells separated by broad areas of fibrous tissue. In Laennec's cirrhosis the liver is large, yellow, greasy, and firm. As the fatty infiltrate resolves, the liver shrinks and acquires a nodular appearance.

The symptoms seen in cirrhosis are similar regardless

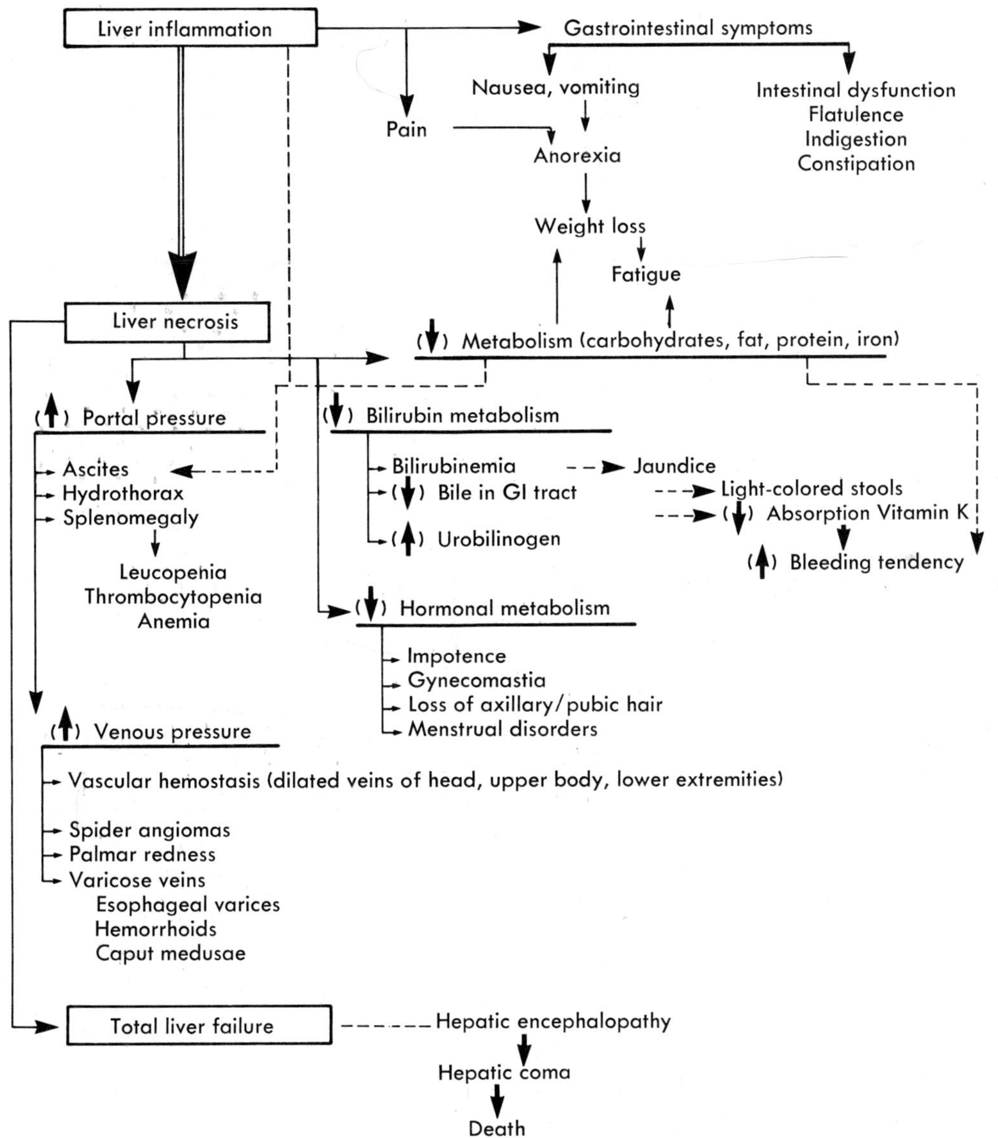

Fig. 33-1. Progression of liver cell failure. Pathophysiology of symptoms that occur in liver disease. NOTE: Process can be arrested if adequate liver regeneration occurs. Regeneration is rarely complete, and there is always some liver cell deficiency.

of the cause of the cirrhosis. The symptoms are due to progressive destruction of hepatic cells and the resultant regeneration and proliferation of interstitial tissue with fibrous tissue causing obstruction of the portal vein (Fig. 33-1). The body attempts to circumvent the obstruction to portal vein flow by establishing collateral circulation.

Ascites, or fluid in the peritoneal cavity, usually follows obstruction of the portal vein and occasionally is one of the first signs of cirrhosis, although it usually does not occur until the disease is quite far advanced and jaundice has become marked.

Once the disease is established, it usually advances slowly to cause death. Many people, however, can be helped to live for years if they follow instructions. The liver has remarkable powers of regeneration. Sometimes sufficient collateral circulation can be established and sufficient repair of hepatic tissue can be accomplished so that symptoms subside for long periods. At other times the person appears to be doing fairly well when he suddenly goes into coma and may die within a few days.

Prevention. In the United States programs aimed at the prevention of portal cirrhosis are designed primarily to control the ingestion of alcohol. The loss of time from work related to alcoholism is estimated to cost billions of dollars annually. Many large corporations have or are organizing incentive programs to assist employees in controlling their alcoholic intake.

Clinical picture. Biopsy is believed to be essential for a definitive diagnosis. Assessment and eventual diagnosis of cirrhosis involves a thorough analysis of history and physical examinations, liver function tests, and radiographic examination (see Chapter 30). The patient with cirrhosis may have a long history of failing health with vague symptoms typical of many gastrointestinal disorders. Initial complaints may include weight loss, anorexia, indigestion, nausea, vomiting, flatulence, and abnormal bowel function. These symptoms are probably due to metabolic dysfunctions of the damaged liver but also may be due to alcoholism. Abdominal pain is variable in character and may be dull, mild, sharp, steady, or wavelike. Pain may be confined to the liver or referred to the lower abdomen and is attributed to several factors: spasm of the biliary ducts, intermittent vascular spasm, swelling of the liver capsule, and inflammation of the peritoneum.

Later symptoms, which occur gradually, include ascites, edema, and jaundice. Peripheral edema may occur prior to ascites or the two may develop concomitantly. Hydrothorax may also be present in patients with ascites and is usually found in the right pleural space. Jaundice may range from being barely visible in the sclera of the eyes to deep yellowing of the skin. The severity is usually proportional to the amount of liver damage. Venules on the head and upper body becomes markedly distended, and spider angiomas (tiny, bright red, pulsating arterioles that disappear on pressure) frequently appear. Veins may become more prominent in the lower extremities as the patient loses weight. Palmar redness that blanches with pressure may also occur. This is sometimes referred to as *liver palm* (palmar erythematosus). As circulation in the portal system becomes impaired due to structural changes in the liver, portal hypertension occurs, producing splenomegaly and increasing edema of the lower extremities. As pressure increases in the portal veins, collateral circulation will occur, resulting in hemorrhoids, esophageal varices, or a ring of varicosities surrounding the umbilicus *(caput medusae)*. It has been estimated that roughly 30% of patients with Laennec's cirrhosis die from bleeding esophageal varices. The patient is carefully monitored for hematemesis, which indicates the presence of varices.

Since hormones of the adrenal cortex, testes, and ovaries are normally metabolized and inactivated by the liver, cirrhosis may cause a variety of endocrine disturbances. These include impotence, gynecomastia, loss of axillary and pubic hair, menstrual disorders, and fluid and electrolyte imbalance. As the disease advances, typical signs of severe anemia, including malaise and memory loss, may occur. Other hematologic changes that occur include coagulation defects, leukopenia, and thrombocytopenia. Increased erythrocyte destruction may also occur within the enlarged spleen. These changes may result in the development of bleeding tendencies with symptoms such as purpura, hematuria, gingival bleeding, and epistaxis.

As the cirrhotic process continues, the patient is prone to developing many life-threatening complications. Death may occur from total liver failure, bleeding esophageal varices, hepatic coma, or renal failure. Severe ascites and jaundice, neurologic symptoms, and decreased prothrombin, albumin, and sodium levels indicate a poor prognosis. Assessment and interventions utilized to treat these complications are discussed later in this chapter.

Intervention. There is no specific treatment for cirrhosis of the liver; the emphasis is on preventing further damage to the liver and on supportive care of the patient. Thus an adequate diet compatible with the ability of the patient's liver to handle protein will be ordered. Rest, moderate exercise, avoidance of exposure to infections, and protection from toxic agents of any kind are emphasized. Alcohol is forbidden. The patient is often disinterested in food and needs constant encouragement to eat the prescribed diet. As the disease progresses, increasing effort must be made to compensate for the failure of the several functions of the liver. Vitamins may be given to compensate for the organ's lost ability to store vitamins A, B complex, D, and K. Bile salts are usually given if the patient is jaundiced to facilitate absorption of fat-soluble vitamin A and synthesis of vitamin K.

Because alcohol is thought to interfere with the hepatic conversion of folic acid to its active metabolites, many persons with cirrhosis have a folic acid deficiency anemia that usually responds well to treatment with oral doses of folic acid.[3]

To achieve a remission of threatened hepatic failure in cirrhosis may take a long time. There may be setbacks and periods when there is no improvement. The person and his family often become discouraged and require support from the physician and nurse. On discharge from the hospital, visits from the community health nurse may be requested to give whatever care, supervision, and support seem necessary. The person must be taught to avoid substances potentially toxic to the liver such as alcohol and drugs that require detoxification in the liver (p. 541).

☐ Tumors of the liver

Tumors of the liver may be malignant or benign. Benign lesions include hemangiomas, hamartomas, cysts, and rarely adenomas. These benign tumors occasionally enlarge enough to become symptomatic and can present problems in differentiation from a malignant tumor. If the latter occurs, surgical intervention may be required.

Epidemiology. Malignant tumors of the liver may be primary, (originating in the liver) or secondary (as a result of metastasis). Primary hepatic carcinomas (hepatomas) are very rare and are estimated to account for only 2.5% of all malignancies in the United States. They are more common in males than females and also represent the most frequent malignant tumor found in children during the first 2 years of life. A malignant tumor appearing in a cirrhotic liver is usually of primary origin. More commonly the liver is the site of metastatic disease, since it receives and filters large amounts of blood from the gastrointestinal tract and pelvis. The liver most commonly receives metastatic cells from the breast, lung, kidney, ovary, or testes or may receive direct invasion from the gallbladder, colon, pancreas, or stomach.[26]

Pathophysiology. Primary tumors may arise from either liver cells or bile ducts or from both. The lesions may be multiple or singular, diffuse or nodular, and may spread to only a lobe or to the entire liver. The cancerous cells appear to compress the surrounding normal liver cells and to spread quickly by invading the portal vein branches. Some cells infiltrate the gallbladder, mesentery, peritoneum, and diaphragm by direct extension. Primary cancers also tend to cause hemorrhage and necrosis. The most common site for metastasis of the primary liver lesion is the lung, but it may also be found in the adrenal glands, spleen, vertebrae, kidney, ovary, or pancreas. Primary lesions tend to grow rapidly, sometimes without signs or symptoms, and the patient may live only a short time after their onset.[26]

It is estimated that approximately 30% of all patients with carcinoma demonstrate some liver metastasis; this occurs less frequently with sarcomas. Secondary carcinoma of the liver varies from a few small nodules to large nodes. Adjacent nodes may eventually grow together and compress the surrounding liver tissue. Usually different parts of the liver are uniformly involved so that liver biopsy may be a useful diagnostic aid.

Clinical picture. In the early stages tumors of the liver are difficult to differentiate from the symptoms of cirrhosis. Symptoms may be absent, acute, or referred to other areas if metastasis occurs. Metastasis to the liver should always be suspected when a patient with a history of carcinoma develops anorexia, weakness, loss of weight, secondary anemia, pain in the right upper quadrant, and general ill health. Jaundice and ascites are signs that the process is quite far advanced, and the patient may live only a short time after their onset. Unexplained temperature elevations accompany about 15% of carcinomas of the liver. Extreme weakness is also usually an outstanding symptom. The major physical sign is an enlarged liver. Ascites occurs secondary to compression of the portal vein. Gastrointestinal bleeding may also be present and may confuse the diagnosis.

Death occurs because of difficulty in making an early diagnosis and because it is usually impossible to remove the entire tumor once diagnosed. Liver biopsy is necessary for definitive diagnosis. Laboratory data usually show an increased sedimentation rate, anemia, decreased blood sugar, and elevated alkaline phosphatase, SGOT, and SGPT (see p. 548).

Intervention

Surgery. Until recently there was no treatment for carcinoma of the liver beyond symptomatic medical and nursing care. Now, provided that the growth is limited to a single lobe and there is no evidence of metastases elsewhere, a *hepatic lobectomy* may be done to remove metastatic as well as primary carcinoma. The remarkable regenerative capacity of the liver permits resection of 70% to 80% of the organ. *Preoperatively* the patient is given massive doses of vitamin K, blood volume is ascertained and necessary blood given, and preparation of the bowel is done as for intestinal surgery. *Postoperative* care may include the care given a patient who has had chest or abdominal surgery plus the general care needed by any patient with dysfunction of the liver. A nasogastric tube usually is inserted and attached to suction. Nothing is given by mouth for several days. Cortisone may be given to prevent fibrosis and enhance liver regeneration. The patient is acutely ill following surgery and must be attended constantly, with the most careful attention given to changes in vital signs. Hemorrhage is the complication most feared, and myocardial infarction is not uncommon.

Following surgery of the liver the patient may be out of bed by the third postoperative day, but he must be attended constantly, and his pulse, blood pressure, and respiratory rate are monitored before, during, and after any exertion, since complications such as hemorrhage may occur.

Chemotherapy. If the growth has spread throughout the liver, irradiated yttrium or radioactive gold (^{198}Au) may be injected into the metastatic tumor masses through the abdominal wall (percutaneous route). Continuous infusions of antitumor agents such as methotrexate or 5-fluorouracil (5-FU) into the liver through a catheter inserted into the hepatic artery also may cause regression of the tumor and alleviate symptoms (p. 476).

□ Liver abscess

A liver abscess may be caused by a variety of pyogenic organisms, the two most common being *Escherichia coli* and *Staphylocccus aureus.* Pyogenic liver abscess is a localized bacterial infection resulting in the formation of a pus-filled cavity in the liver. Bacteria may reach the liver from adjacent structures or from remote structures by way of the hepatic artery, biliary tract, or portal vein. Disease processes such as appendicitis, pneumonia, cholecystitis, peritonitis, and bacterial endocarditis may be the cause of liver abscesses.

A highly specific and sensitive indirect hemagglutination test now provides over 95% accuracy in the diagnosis of amebic liver abscesses. A liver scan and a hepatic arteriogram may be used in establishing the diagnosis.

Nausea, vomiting, and jaundice are frequent symptoms of abscesses of the liver. Chills and diaphoresis are common and are followed by temperature elevation, malaise, and dull, constant pain in the right upper quadrant. Treatment is usually by surgical incision and drainage and antibiotic therapy. The antibiotic used will depend on the causative organism. If the abscess ruptures causing peritonitis, the condition may be fatal. Emetine hydrochloride and chloroquine are used in the treatment of the amebic hepatic abscess, followed by aspiration or drainage as indicated.

□ Trauma to the liver

Because of its location and size, the liver is frequently subjected to trauma, which may be either penetrating (stab wounds) or blunt (automobile accidents or falls). If the injury is severe, rupture of the liver may occur with severe internal hemorrhage.

Pathophysiology. Small lacerations or ruptures, except for temporary peritoneal irritations from blood oozing into the peritoneal cavity, usually heal leaving a subcapsular scar. In some instances the hematoma may become infected and abscess formation complicates the healing process. Hepatic cysts may also develop. Rare complications include arterial aneurysms or portal vein thrombosis. Trauma that causes severe contusions may result in subsequent degeneration of the injured hepatic cells. The prognosis depends on the amount of tissue damaged, and the final outcome for the patient may not be known for many years after the initial injury.

Severe lacerations or rupture of the liver have a mortality estimated to be between 27% and 30%. Death that occurs shortly after the injury is due to uncontrollable hepatic hemorrhage. This happens in part because the walls of the hepatic veins are thin, the liver is very vascular, and the bile mixing with the blood interferes with clotting. Deaths occurring later after injury may be due to biliary peritonitis, shock, or infections.

Clinical picture. If the injury has not penetrated the abdomen, there may be no external evidence of injury. If conscious the patient may complain of pain. Symptoms of shock (pallor, tachycardia, hypotension) may develop depending on the rapidity of the bleeding. Needle aspiration of the abdominal cavity may show the presence of blood.

Intervention. Blood volume replacement is usually required. Emergency surgery may be needed to suture the ruptured liver and apply local pressure to stop the bleeding. Removal of necrotic tissue may also be indicated as well as drainage of any bile that may be leaking from the liver surface. Nursing care is the same as that for any patient requiring abdominal surgery due to trauma. The type of monitoring required will depend on the extent of the patient's injuries.

□ Sequelae of chronic liver disease

Any person with liver disease must be monitored for the presence of fluid and electrolyte changes, bleeding tendencies, portal hypertension, esophageal varices, and hepatic encephalopathy. Even though the liver disease may be minimal, there is the possibility that any or all of these alterations may occur. Most often severe alterations will occur only when liver disease is longstanding, chronic in nature, and subject to progressive worsening such as occurs with cirrhosis.

Fluid and electrolyte changes

Pathophysiology. Retention of sodium and water by persons with liver disease is attributable to both local and systemic factors. The sequence of these mechanisms and how they interact to intensify ascites is not well established.[32] The factors that are believed to contribute to the development of ascites include (1) decreased hepatic synthesis of albumin necessary for plasma osmotic pressure, (2) increased portal vein pressure creating transudation from the intestines and mesentery, (3) increased serum aldosterone level due to impaired degradation by the liver, and (4) transudation from the liver due to obstruction of hepatic lymph outflow. Fig. 33-1 summarizes the changes that occur. The diminished serum albumin level, which is osmotically the most potent fraction, reduces the colloidal osmotic pressure in the blood. This leads to an increase in filtration through the capillary wall, while the reabsorption of the escaped fluid is impaired. In addition the increased portal vein pressure facilitates the escape of fluid. A vicious cycle is established as the albumin lost into the peritoneal cavity further decreases the patient's serum albumin level.

Hydrothorax and ankle and presacral edema may accompany the ascites. The patient with cirrhosis frequently retains abnormal amount of water and sodium. The sodium retention appears to be related to excessive aldosterone activity. It has been postulated that water is retained by excessive secretion of antidiuretic hormone, possibly caused by the liver dysfunction.[6]

Renal function is also believed to affect fluid and electrolyte balance in patients with liver disease. Alterations in renal function may occur because of decreased blood volume secondary to vasodilation and portal hypertension. Thus patients with liver disease are monitored for signs of increased urea and decreased sodium. They are also monitored for hypokalemia, which can result from diuretic therapy, diarrhea, vomiting, and sodium retention.

Intervention. Ascites is treated in several ways. Restriction of sodium aids greatly in limiting the formation of ascitic fluid. The amount of dietary restriction necessary to reduce sodium and water retention may initially be based on a 24-hour urine collection to determine sodium loss.

The lack of salt in food makes it less palatable, and the patient may not consume adequate protein and total calories (see Chapter 20). The nurse should report the patient's food intake to the physician and dietitian, as adjustments may need to be made in the sodium restriction. Salt substitutes such as potassium gluconate may be permitted.

Many physicians try to control edema and fluid accumulation in the abdomen by giving diuretic agents. Removal of fluid through the kidneys has the advantage of usually not removing essential body protein, which is contained in fluid removed from the abdominal cavity. Since a single diuretic usually is not successful, a combination is used. Thiazide diuretics such as chlorothiazide (Diuril), which inhibits the reabsorption of sodium in the proximal tubules, and spironolactone A (Aldactone A), which prevents the reabsorption of sodium in the distal tubules, may be given. Occasionally one of the glucocorticoids such as prednisone may be added. Complications of diuretic therapy are discussed on p. 1009.

Fluid and electrolyte levels must be carefully monitored during the initial administration of diuretic therapy. An extremely rapid diuresis can precipitate oliguria and uremia due to the rapidly diminished blood volume. Additional mechanisms involved in fluid and electrolyte imbalance are discussed in Chapter 20.

In order to evaluate further the effectiveness of therapy, daily weights are required. Measurements of abdominal girth will also assist in determining the gross amount of abdominal swelling. Patients need to be taught the importance of monitoring and reporting weight gain or rapid increase in abdominal girth after discharge.

Patients with ascites may also experience dyspnea due to pressure being exerted upward on the diaphragm. A high Fowler's position may assist respiratory efforts. Skin care may present another problem as these patients are often emaciated despite edema.

The patient confined to bed is turned frequently to help prevent pressure areas from developing over the sacrum leading to skin breakdown. The use of alternating pressure mattresses and flotation pads may be helpful. When edema is severe, the skin may "weep" as the accumulation of fluid seeps through the pores. Frequent change of bed linen will be necessary.

If diet restrictions and diuretic therapy fail to diminish fluid accumulations or if renal function is impaired, the patient may be given albumin intravenously or paracentesis may be performed. The administration of salt-poor albumin expands the blood volume and should cause diuresis. After administration the patient is carefully monitored for signs of pulmonary edema.

Although once a standard therapy, paracentesis is used with caution and usually only as a last resort in patients with severe and chronic liver disease, since it may precipitate hepatic coma. If the abdomen is tight with fluid and is producing dyspnea and anorexia, paracentesis may be necessary. In general only small amounts of fluid are removed; this decreases the risk of rapid fluid shifts and additional protein loss. Dangers of paracentesis include shock and hypovolemia, which occur as the fluid from the general circulation shifts to the peritoneal cavity as the ascitic fluid is withdrawn. One liter of ascitic fluid contains as much protein as 200 ml of whole blood. Salt-poor human blood albumin may be administered following this procedure to counteract the loss of fluid and protein. (For details of paracentesis and the nursing care involved, see texts on fundamentals of nursing.)

Increased bleeding tendency

Pathophysiology. Bleeding tendencies may occur in persons with advanced hepatitis, cirrhosis, and biliary duct obstruction. These tendencies are due to deficiencies in the formation of clotting factors, leukopenia, and thrombocytopenia. Normally vitamin K is utilized by the liver cells in synthesizing various clotting factors. In patients with obstructive jaundice and liver disease, this synthesis is impaired. If the patient's bile duct is obstructed, absorption of fat and fat-soluble vitamins (vitamin K) is reduced. On the other hand, even if vitamin D is absorbed, severely damaged liver cells cannot synthesize adequate amounts of these factors, especially prothrombin.

The patient with liver disease may also develop an enlarged spleen due to portal hypertension. This is believed to be responsible for the resulting leukopenia and thrombocytopenia. In advanced liver cell destruction it has been suggested that a toxic effect on the bone marrow may take place causing hematologic changes.

Vitamin deficiencies due to inadequate intake, decreased absorption of fat-soluble vitamins, and the inability to store vitamins also occur. The person with cirrhosis will be deficient in vitamins A, B complex, D, and K.

Anemia is a common problem. Various factors contribute to the anemia, including increased blood loss due to gastrointestinal bleeding, decreased red blood cell production secondary to folic acid deficiency and poor protein intake, and increased destruction of red blood cells due to hypersplenism. In addition alcohol has a direct toxic effect on bone marrow.

Intervention. Therapy is aimed at the restoration of clotting factors. If a decreased prothrombin level is identified, the patient will be given vitamin K parenterally. This will not help if liver cell damage is the cause of the reduced prothrombin formation. If this is the case, whole blood or plasma may be given to replace clotting factors at least temporarily. If the patient has a reduced platelet level, he may be given platelet transfusions. Vitamin supplements of B complex, particularly thiamine, will be given. In addition bile salts to assist in the absorption of fat-soluble vitamins may be prescribed. Anemia is treated by measures that control blood loss, a high-caloric, high-protein diet (if ammonium can be handled by the liver), and avoidance of alcohol. Anemia usually responds well to these measures. For nursing interventions see Chapter 31.

Portal hypertension

Pathophysiology. A rise in portal venous pressure (portal hypertension) occurs when peripheral resistance is increased due to damage of vessels within the liver, there is an excessive flow of arterial blood from the splenic or hepatic artery to the liver, or there is increased tone of vessels due to control by hormonal and nervous factors. Whatever the cause, an obstruction of portal blood flow through the liver causes a backup of bloodflow into the veins that empty into the portal vein. These veins in turn develop collateral channels of circulation in order to bypass the obstruction. Collateral channels are most likely to occur in the paraumbilical veins, in the hemorrhoidal veins, and at the cardia of the stomach extending into the esophagus.

Intervention. The only way to achieve permanent lowering of portal pressure is by *surgical treatment* to reduce blood flow through the portion of the portal system that is obstructed. Depending on the location of the obstruction, various elective operative procedures may be employed. If the splenic vein is blocked, a *splenectomy* may be done. If the block is intrahepatic, a *portacaval anastomosis* (portacaval shunt) may be done. The portal vein is anastomosed to the inferior vena cava so that the blood from the portal system bypasses the liver (Fig. 33-2). This may be achieved by an end-to-side or side-to-side anastomosis. For more effective portal decompression the end-to-side anastomosis is preferred and is considered to be technically easier. With the side-to-side shunt the total portal blood flow to the liver is not diverted. When the portal vein is blocked the splenic vein is anastomosed to the left renal vein. This procedure is called a *splenorenal shunt* and relieves pressure on the portal vein, since approximately 30% of the blood in the portal vein comes from the splenic vein.[30] If there is no portal hypertension, the varicosed vessels may be ligated through a thoracotomy incision.

Careful *preoperative* preparation is necessary, since it must be remembered that the patient with liver damage severe enough to cause bleeding varices is not a good operative risk. Preoperative criteria for a portacaval shunt include at least one hemorrhage from esophageal varices, absence of ascites and hepatic coma, a bilirubin level below 1.5 mg, and an albumin level above 3 g/100

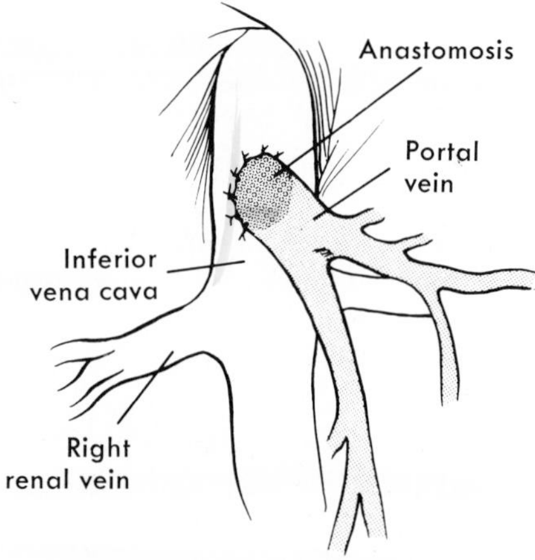

Fig. 33-2. Portacaval shunt. Anastomosis of portal vein to inferior vena cava by end-to-side insertion.

ml. It is generally felt that a *prophylactic* shunt is not usually justified. The patient is usually apprehensive about the recommended operation, yet in *selected* cases it is known that the operative risk is much less than the risk from recurring hemorrhage. Vitamin K, antibiotics, and transfusions are usually given preoperatively.

Postoperatively the patient needs close observation and often constant nursing attention. Narcotics should be given for severe pain, but sedative drugs usually are avoided because of their toxic effects on the diseased liver. Generally narcotics are given in guarded amounts and infrequently in the presence of liver disease. When they are given the patient must be observed carefully for impending hepatic coma. The patient must be encouraged to breathe deeply and to cough hourly. Fluid intake and output must be recorded accurately, and lessening of output must be reported, since renal function sometimes decreases for a time following this operation.

Hemorrhage may occur, since prothrombin levels may be lowered. Hepatic coma may also be a postoperative complication. The nurse can recognize impending hepatic coma by beginning signs of mental confusion, slowness in response, and generally inappropriate behavior.

Some surgeons do not pass a nasogastric tube because of danger of injury to the varices. Others pass a nasogastric tube and attach it to suction postoperatively, since it is believed that postoperative distention may predispose to thrombosis of the portal vein. In either instance the patient is fed intravenously and given nothing by mouth until signs of active peristalsis are apparent. The patient is observed closely for pain, distention, fever, and nausea, which may be signs of thrombosis at the site of anastomosis. *Regional heparinization* may be employed to prevent thrombus formation at surgery. A fine polyethylene catheter is inserted into the right gastroepiploic vein, brought out through the wound, and attached to a continuous drip of heparin and saline solution. The surgeon determines the rate of flow. The catheter may be left for 5 to 7 days and during this time the nurse must see that it is not obstructed or subjected to tension in any way. During heparinization the patient remains in bed or sits by the bedside. Particular attention should be paid, therefore, to exercising the lower extremities in an attempt to prevent development of thrombi.

Some surgeons prefer to keep the patient flat in bed for several days until the anastomosis is healed. Others have their patients get out of bed on the day after the operation. Leg and arm exercises are begun on the day after surgery. The lower extremities must be observed carefully for signs of edema, which may follow the sudden increase of blood flow into the inferior vena cava. Elevation of the lower extremities may be ordered, and the length of time the patient spends standing and walking should be medically prescribed.

After some shunting procedures none of the venous blood passes through the liver, and protein end products are not completely detoxified. For this reason the patient is usually placed on a low-protein diet. Neomycin or chlortetracycline (Aureomycin), both of which destroy the bacteria in the intestine, may be given so that fewer bacteria remain in the bowel to break down protein and increase the production of ammonia.

Esophageal varices

Pathophysiology. Esophageal varices occur in approximately 30% of all patients with cirrhosis of the liver.[30] The branches of the azygos and vena cava veins become distended where they join the smaller vessels of the esophagus. This occurs because of the greater volume of blood, which is under higher pressure as a result of portal hypertension. These small vessels become tortuous and fragile and may also be affected by mechanical trauma from ingestion of coarse food and acid pepsin erosion, which may result in bleeding.[37] Bleeding may also occur as a result of coughing, vomiting, sneezing, or any physical exertion that increases abdominal venous pressure or straining at stool (Valsalva maneuver). Bleeding is frequently abrupt and without pain. Severe hematemesis and resultant shock may follow, requiring emergency treatment.

Clinical picture. Along with routine liver function tests, esophagoscopy most clearly determines the diagnosis. There is danger of initiating hemorrhage while carrying out this procedure, however, and the risks should be carefully weighed depending on the patient's situation. Portal vein pressure readings may also be carried out as well as other specialized radiographic procedures. Hemorrhaging is a true medical emergency and requires prompt medical and nursing action.

Intervention

Control of bleeding. Management of bleeding esophageal varices consists of restoring blood volume and controlling the bleeding. Measures that may *control the hemorrhage* include gastric lavage with ice water, local gastric hypothermia using an esophagogastric balloon, or intravenous injection of vasopressin (Pitressin), which reduces portal pressure and blood flow by constricting the splanchnic arterioles. Since vasopressin also decreases the blood supply to the liver, it should be used with caution. Esophagogastric tamponade (with a Blakemore-Sengstaken tube) may be used to control massive hemorrhage. In selected persons, emergency surgical procedures such as direct ligation of the varices, esophagogastric resection, or splenorenal or portacaval anastomosis may be performed.

The esophagogastric tube (Blakemore-Sengstaken) is

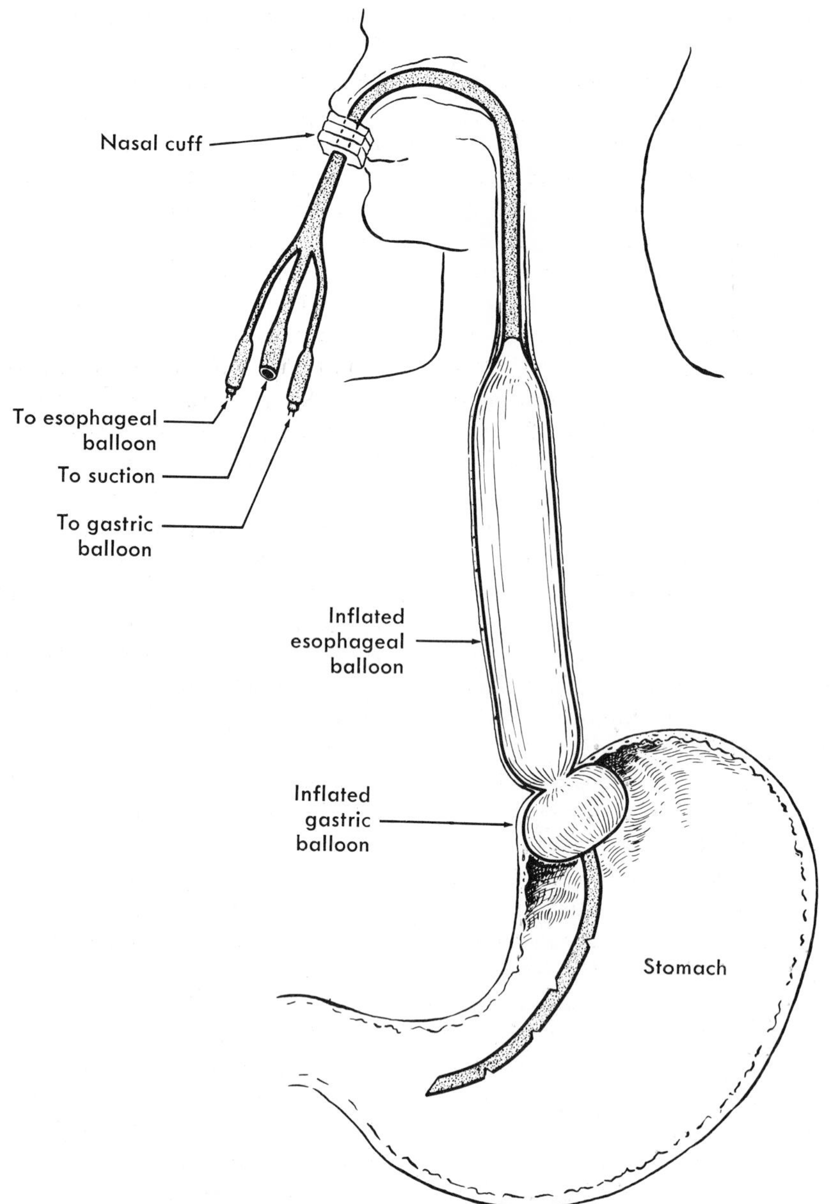

Fig. 33-3. Blakemore-Sengstaken tube with esophageal and gastric balloons inflated. (Redrawn from Rubber appliances in surgery and therapeutics, Providence, R.I., 1955, Davol, Inc.)

a three-lumen tube with two balloon attachments. One lumen serves as a nasogastric suction tube, the second is used to inflate the gastric balloon, and the third is used to inflate the esophageal balloon (Fig. 33-3). The tube is passed through the nose into the stomach with the balloons deflated. When the tube is in the stomach, the gastric balloon is inflated with 100 to 300 ml of air and the lumen is clamped; the tube is then pulled out slowly so that the balloon is held tightly against the cardioesophageal junction. A cube of foam rubber called a nasal cuff is placed between the tube and the nares, and the tube is secured to the face with pressure-sensitive tape. The cube of foam rubber absorbs excess nasal secretions and reduces trauma to the nostril. It also provides traction, which maintains the tube in the proper position. If after the gastric balloon is inflated there is further hematemesis or if bloody fluid is returned on aspiration, one can assume that the bleeding is from the esophagus, and the esophageal balloon should be inflated (Fig. 33-3). The esophageal lumen is connected by a Y tube to a manometer and the balloon is inflated with 20 to 45 mm Hg and clamped. In order to stop bleeding, the pressure must be greater than the patient's portal venous pressure. If bleeding is from esophageal varices, blood will no longer be aspirated from the stomach. If there is still blood present, the stomach may be lavaged with a small amount of ice water or a solution of iced alcohol and water may be circulated through the balloon to provide vasoconstriction as well as pressure. The nasogastric lumen is usually connected to intermittent gastric suction, which permits easy appraisal of whether bleeding has ceased and also serves to keep the stomach empty. It is important to remove all blood from the stomach because the presence of it may precipitate hepatic coma.

The person who is being treated for esophageal varices is very ill and may be disoriented. He requires constant attention, and if there is any chance he will pull on the tube, his arms should be restrained. The nurse must be constantly alert to the pressure in the balloons. If the gastric balloon should collapse or rupture, the entire tube may move up and obstruct the patient's airway. Should the gastric balloon rupture, the esophageal balloon is deflated at once and the entire tube is removed.

The esophageal balloon can be left inflated up to 48 hours without tissue damage or severe discomfort for the patient. The fully inflated gastric balloon with traction exerted on it, however, compresses the stomach wall between the balloon and the diaphragm, causing ulceration of the gastric mucosa, and is severely uncomfortable for the patient. To offset the possibility of necrosis, the physician may release the traction and balloon pressures periodically. A second tube should be in the patient unit ready for immediate use in case of damage to the one being used (the tubes are not reused). Before the tube is inserted, the balloon should be tested. The tubes have the date of manufacture stamped on them, and those over a year old should be discarded because of deterioration of the rubber. Before removal of the tube, the balloons are deflated gradually, and the tube is gently withdrawn by the physician. The patient then is observed closely for any indications of renewed bleeding.

Shock. As soon as the balloons are in place and bleeding has been controlled, transfusions of *fresh* whole blood are given to combat hypovolemic shock. Fresh blood is used for several reasons: (1) hepatic coma can be precipitated by blood that is only 3 to 4 days old because whole blood develops as increasing concentration of ammonia due to hydrolysis of various unstable compounds; (2) the damaged liver may be unable to metabolize citrate from the sodium citrate used to preserve stored blood, and citric intoxication can result; (3) patients with cirrhosis excrete sodium poorly; and (4) refrigerated blood is virtually devoid of prothrombin and coagulation factors essential for clotting.

Oxygen is usually administered to increase the oxygen available to the blood. A saline cathartic such as magnesium sulfate may be given through the nasogastric tube to hasten the expulsion of blood that has passed from the stomach to the intestine, and enemas may also be given in an effort to lessen bacterial action of the blood in the intestinal tract. This action produces ammonia, which passes to the bloodstream and in turn puts a burden on the liver, which must detoxify it to form urea. An antibiotic that destroys intestinal bacteria, such as neomycin, also may be given to lessen their activity in the decomposition of protein in the intestine. Antacids are commonly prescribed to reduce stomach acidity and to prevent a reflux of acid into the esophagus. They are given through the nasogastric lumen of the tube.

Emotional support. The patient with bleeding esophageal varices is acutely ill and extremely apprehensive. Discomfort from the tamponade tube and the potential onset of encephalopathy must be considered in the patient's behavior. He must be attended constantly, given reassurance, and kept absolutely quiet. All procedures and his part in them should be quietly and calmly explained to him and carried out with the minimum of activity. The family generally is very frightened and should be given as much information as necessary to relieve their concern. Some member of the family should be permitted to see the patient or to stay with him for a short time.

Monitoring. The nurse is responsible for checking the vital signs, which may be observed as often as every 15 minutes until there are signs that hemorrhage is controlled. The blood pressure cuff is left on the arm deflated, and care is taken to inflate it only a few degrees above the anticipated level. In this way many patients may sleep through the taking of blood pressure. Care also is taken to see that the transfusion and the infusions are running. The patient in shock may feel cold and must be kept warm but not perspiring. If iced solutions are used in the balloons, chills may occur. They should be reported to the physician, who may order a warming blanket.

When an esophagogastric tube is in use the nurse must also check the manometer attached to the tube. If the pressure rises or falls below the prescribed level, the amount of air or solution in the balloon must be adjusted. Often this adjustment is made by the physician, but it may be made by the nurse if there are orders to that effect.

Mouth care. Because the inflated esophageal balloon occludes the esophagus, the patient cannot take anything by mouth or even swallow his saliva. He should be provided with cleansing tissues and an emesis basin. The patient needs frequent mouth care, and all blood in his mouth should be removed. If he is very weak or if he is not permitted to move at all, gentle suctioning of the mouth and throat may be needed to prevent aspiration of saliva. The nostrils are kept clean, lubricated, and protected so that tissues do not sustain injury because of pressure from the tube. Care must be taken not to disturb the tube, and the physician is consulted as to how much movement the patient is permitted. Passive moving of extremities usually is allowed.

Hepatic coma (hepatic encephalopathy)

Pathophysiology. Hepatic coma (hepatic encephalopathy) is metabolic encephalopathy of the brain associated with liver failure. Dysfunctions of the central nervous system are thought to be precipitated by elevated ammonia concentrations, hypoxia, changes in electrolyte concentrations with disturbances of acid-base balance, infections, and depressant drugs. Many patients with hepatic coma have an increase in blood ammonia concentration. Normally ammonia, which is formed in the intestines from the breakdown of protein by intestinal bacteria, is converted to urea through the Krebs-Henseleit cycle in the liver. When liver failure occurs, ammonia is not converted into urea and ammonia concentration in the circulating blood is increased. The factors that may cause depression of liver function or an increase in the level of ammonia in the blood and thus may precipitate hepatic coma are summarized in the box below.

Clinical picture. The manifestations of hepatic coma vary and may occur quickly or gradually over the course of a few days. At least daily observation and interviewing of the patient are carried out and recorded in order to ascertain subtle personality and behavioral changes indicative of impending coma. Early signs may be missed if someone does not know the patient well or if a detailed assessment was not obtained initially. Manifestations may include impaired attention span, poor ability to concentrate, delayed rate of response, yawning, twitching, irritability, apathy, insomnia and restlessness, and loss of interest in the environment. Speech patterns and the ability to write should be evaluated for change. As the condition worsens, speech usually becomes slurred, confusion is more apparent, and the level of consciousness is gradually depressed. A characteristic flapping tremor (*asterixis*, or liver flap) may be elicited when the patient is asked to dorsiflex his hand while the rest of the arm is extended resting on the bed. A peculiar sweetish odor can frequently be detected on the breath (*fetor hepaticus*). Soon the patient cannot be aroused except by painful stimuli, and as the coma deepens there may be no response to pain and reflexes may be completely absent. At this point the patient's temperature may rise markedly and there may be alterations in pulse and respiratory rate.

The patient's consciousness level commonly fluc-

FACTORS COMMONLY PRECIPITATING HEPATIC COMA

Factors depressing liver function

Hypoxia
- Secondary to hemorrhage and hypovolemic shock
- Secondary to morphine and other sedatives

Intercurrent infection

Exercise
- In patients with chronic liver disease who are in impending coma
- In patients with acute hepatitis

Acute hepatitis during pregnancy, especially during last trimester

Abdominal paracentesis
- Secondary to reduction of plasma volume
- Patients may also have hyponatremia, especially if natriuretic diuretics were being administered before paracentesis

Factors increasing level of ammonia

Gastrointestinal ammonia (old blood in bowel from gastrointestinal hemorrhage)

High-protein intake

Transfusions, especially with stored blood

Thiazide diuretics and acetazolamide (Diamox)

Hypokalemia
- Secondary to thiazide diuretics
- Secondary to potassium loss from the bowel

Shunting of blood into systemic circulation without passing through hepatic sinusoids
- Natural collateral bypass of liver
- Surgical bypass of liver

Alkalosis secondary to hyperventilation and hypokalemia

Hyperbilirubinemia (serum bilirubin level greater than 35 mg/100 ml)

tuates, and if possible the same nurse should be assigned to the patient over time in order to document accurately changes in mental functioning. Early detection of symptoms allows for more rapid treatment and consequently improves the patient's chance of recovery. Progress notes should describe actual behavioral observations as opposed to generalizations that are vague and allow for various interpretations. In the assessment of the patient's ongoing clinical state, the nurse monitors for any changes in the rate or depth of respiration, the development of cardiac arrhythmias (cardiac monitors are usually used), evidence of rapid changes in peripheral edema or ascites, and neurologic changes.

Intervention. Treatment of hepatic coma centers around finding and treating the precipitating cause, general supportive measures, and avoidance of additional trauma to the liver. This is accomplished by completely eliminating protein from the diet for several days, giving carbohydrates by mouth or nasogastric feedings, and administering antibiotics such as neomycin that destroy bacteria in the intestine and subsequently reduce the amount of ammonia formed. Enemas and carthartics such as magnesium sulfate may be given to empty the bowel and prevent further ammonia formation. Some physicians prefer to rely on cathartics and on the use of cation exchange resins to help remove toxic substances from the bowel rather than to give antibiotics. Antibiotics destroy bacteria, which are active in the manufacture of vitamin K, and the absence of bacteria causes diarrhea and other symptoms. Lactulose is being used in an attempt to decrease the production of ammonia. Lactulose, which is given orally, is a synthetic disaccharide that cannot be utilized in the small intestine. It produces diarrhea, lowers the pH level, alters the bacterial flora of the colon, thereby decreasing the production of nitrogenous substances.

In some patients large doses of the adrenocortical steroids are effective in reversing hepatic coma, providing that hepatic cell destruction has not been overwhelming.

Many patients in hepatic coma die of renal failure secondary to an inadequate circulating blood volume (hypovolemia). In some patients renal function progressively deteriorates without any apparent cause. The treatment of hepatic coma requires a careful balancing of fluid administration to maintain adequate perfusion of the kidney without creating an excessive load on the cardiovascular system. Therefore when intravenous solutions are being administered, the desired flow rate and signs of cardiovascular overload are monitored very closely. In order to adequately monitor renal function, an indwelling catheter is often inserted, especially if the patient is being maintained on intravenous fluids. Central venous pressure (CVP) monitoring (p. 924) is also commonly used. The nurse is alert to changes in the CVP readings suggestive of either hypervolemia or hypovolemia. The supportive nursing care required by any patient with hepatic disease as well as by any unconscious patient should be given.

Tracheostomy may be performed as a prophylactic measure. Intermittent positive pressure breathing with oxygen may also be used to improve oxygenation (see pp. 947 and 953). Since most narcotics and sedatives must be detoxified by the the liver, they are contraindicated in patients with impaired liver function. If a sedative must be used, drugs such as chlordiazepoxide (Librium), barbital, or phenobarbital, which are excreted by the kidney, are prescribed.

Exchange transfusions have been used to combat hepatic coma on the premise that toxic substances are both diluted and removed from the blood. In selected patients a colon-bypass operation may be performed to stop function of the colon and prevent absorption of material from the intestines. Attempts have been made to replace nonfunctioning livers with those of recent cadavers. To date these transplants have not been successful because immunosuppressive therapy is inadequate and the transplanted organs have been rejected by the recipient's body.

The patient in hepatic coma is very ill and is vulnerable to any increase in stress. He should receive the meticulous nursing care necessary for any patient who is unconscious. Particular care should be taken to protect the patient from infection. If the patient survives, long-term care as discussed for the patient with cirrhosis of the liver should be planned. The patient who has had definite or threatened hepatic coma may be kept indefinitely on a diet low in protein. When protein is added to the diet, it is added gradually and often does not exceed 40 g daily (normal intake is 70 to 80 g daily). In addition the patient may receive neomycin, 2 to 3 g daily. Patients with chronic liver disease may go in and out of coma; therefore they are monitored for any change in behavior that would indicate early coma. The patient and his family should also be taught to be alert to subtle changes in his behavior and to seek medical assistance when this occurs.

□ Outcome criteria for patients with chronic liver disease

The patient or significant others can:

1. Explain the dietary plan to be followed after discharge:
   a. List daily food and fluid requirements (such as amount of protein allowed).
   b. List foods and fluids not allowed in diet (such as sodium restriction, elimination of alcohol).
   c. Explain plans for meeting nutritional needs.

2. Explain medications to be taken at home and precautions related to them:
   a. State name, dosage, expected effects, and side effects for each medication.
   b. State the untoward effects of medication that need to be reported to the health care provider at once.
   c. State reason for not using over-the-counter drugs.
3. Explain program to prevent complications:
   a. Explain the basic health problem.
   b. State how the prescribed treatment is helping.
   c. List daily schedule including rest periods.
   d. List ways to avoid bleeding episodes (such as using soft toothbrush, blowing nose gently, taking antacids as ordered).
   e. List ways to avoid infections.
   f. Explain plans for follow-up care.
4. Describe possible complications of illness and state what to do if they occur:
   a. State health care monitoring to be done daily (weight, abdominal girth, temperature, checking for bleeding).
   b. List signs and symptoms requiring immediate medical attention (e.g., weight gain, increase in abdominal girth, elevated temperature, bleeding from any orifice, frank blood in urine or stool, tar-colored stools, changes in behavior or memory).
   c. Has name and phone number of health care provider to be called in case of emergency.
   d. State plans for follow-up care.

DISEASES OF THE BILIARY SYSTEM

The biliary system consists of the gallbladder and its associated ductal system. The ductal system provides a pathway for the bile that is formed in the liver to reach the intestine and also functions to regulate bile flow. The liver produces up to 1 liter of bile per day. As it is formed, bile is excreted into the hepatic duct where it passes into the cystic duct to be stored in the gallbladder. After reaching the gallbladder, bile is altered to a concentrated form. When needed the gallbladder releases bile into the cystic duct where it goes into the common bile duct and then into the duodenum. On reaching the intestine, bile functions to emulsify undigested fat, facilitate the absorption of fat-soluble vitamins, iron, and calcium, and activate the release of pancreatic and intestinal enzymes. (See Chapter 30 for a discussion of laboratory and diagnostic tests used to assist in identifying the cause and site of biliary malfunction.)

There are no specific means to prevent disease of the biliary system. However, since disease of this system occurs much more often in obese persons, it is reasonable to suppose that control of obesity may contribute to its prevention. Women are more often affected than men, and the description "fair, fat, and forty" is fairly accurate. In all health education the nurse stresses the importance of avoiding excess weight. Patients with biliary tract disease are usually advised to keep fat intake to a fairly low level for the remainder of their lives, although no rigid dietary regulations are needed. Patients who tend to form stones in the ducts are usually advised to be careful of their fat intake and to drink generous amounts of fluids.

Most of the problems of the gallbladder are treated surgically. The following section describes the common problems and presents surgical care and management.

Cholecystitis

Epidemiology. Cholecystitis is inflammation of the gallbladder. The condition may be acute or chronic and usually is associated with gallstones or other obstructions of bile passage.

A large variety of organisms may contribute to acute disease of the gallbladder. Colon bacilli, staphylococci, streptococci, salmonellae, typhoid bacilli, and many other organisms have been found. Infection may reach the gallbladder through the bloodstream, the lymph system, or the bile ducts. Cholecystitis is more common in women than in men, the ratio being 2.5:1. Sedentary, obese persons are affected most often, and the incidence is highest in the fifth and sixth decades of life. The incidence of cholecystitis and mortality are high in the elderly.[31]

Pathophysiology. In acute cholecystitis the gallbladder is usually very enlarged, resembling a distended sac. The gallbladder wall becomes thickened and edematous. Inflammation may be confined to the mucous membrane lining, or the entire wall of the gallbladder may be involved. Sometimes damage to the wall of the gallbladder results from distention caused by obstruction of bile flow and from contractions of the smooth muscle as it attempts to dislodge a stone occluding the lumen of one of the bile ducts.

Chronic cholecystitis may produce a variety of structural changes whether or not stones are present. This is not the result of an infectious process but is related to a diseased gallbladder wall with inefficient emptying. It is believed that chronic cholecystitis is due to chemical or mechanical irritation from stones causing pressure on the mucosa or biliary stasis. The gallbladder walls are usually thickened and fibrous and it may be shrunken or distended. Eventually, due to destruction of the mucosa, outpouchings of the epithelium may form. Bacteria and other irritants may become trapped in them, which may help maintain a chronic inflammatory process.[26]

Clinical picture. Persons experiencing an acute attack of cholecystitis may be very ill. Acute cholecystitis is usually abrupt in onset; however, the individual often has a history of intolerance of fatty foods and general indigestion. Nausea and vomiting usually occur, and there is severe pain in the right upper quadrant of the abdomen. The pulse rate and respiratory rate are increased, and the temperature and white blood count are elevated. This acute phase may subside with medical treatment or it may require emergency surgery.

The chronic form of the disease is usually preceded by several acute attacks of moderate severity, and the individual gives a history of having learned to avoid fried foods and certain other foods such as nuts that are high in fat. Pain is usually located in the right upper quadrant but may be referred to the back. Nausea and vomiting and flatulence may also occur. Persons with chronic cholecystitis may not be as ill as those with acute disease and therefore may not seek medical attention until they experience pain from a biliary obstruction or develop jaundice.

Intervention. The treatment of choice for most patients with cholecystitis is surgery. The decision as to when to operate depends largely on the age and condition of the patient and the way he responds to treatment. Although some surgeons favor conservative treatment until the acute infection has subsided, others believe that the danger of rupture and subsequent peritonitis is so great that immediate surgery to drain the gallbladder is advisable *(cholecystostomy)*. All recommend removing the gallbladder *(cholecystectomy)* when the acute condition has subsided. Infection may spread to the hepatic duct and liver, causing inflammation of the ducts *(cholangitis)* with subsequent strictures that may cause obstruction of bile flow and are exceedingly difficult to correct surgically.

When medical treatment is prescribed it includes the administration of antibiotics and infusions of glucose and appropriate electrolytes. Food is withheld until acute symptoms subside. If vomiting persists, a nasogastric tube is passed and attached to suction. Meperidine hydrochloride (Demerol) may be given for pain, although it is thought by some authorities to increase spasm of the biliary sphincter. The inhalation of amyl nitrite may diminish intestinal and biliary spasms.

When food is tolerated, a reducing diet and careful avoidance of too much fat usually are recommended. Persons who have had acute attacks are more strongly motivated to follow dietary instructions, and the nurse may be of real help to them in planning attractive meals that are low in fat and total calories.

Cholelithiasis

Epidemiology. Cholelithiasis is the presence of stones in the biliary tract. The stones are composed largely of cholesterol, bile pigment, and calcium. Cholelithiasis may occur in either sex at any age, but it is more common in middle-aged women. The incidence increases gradually thereafter, and one out of every three persons who reach the age of 75 years will have gallstones.[30] It is not known why stones form in the gallbladder and in the hepatic duct. They may be present for years and cause no inflammation. Sometimes they appear to be preceded or followed by chronic cholecystitis. Chronic cholelithiasis is aggravated by pregnancy, perhaps because of the increased pressure in the abdomen.

Pathophysiology. Three specific factors appear to contribute to the formation of gallstones: metabolic factors, stasis, and inflammation. An increased concentration of one of the three substances present in bile (bile acids, bile pigments, and cholesterol) may result in their subsequent precipitation giving rise to the formation of stones. An increased serum cholesterol level is a *metabolic* disorder occurring in obesity, pregnancy, diabetes, and hypothyroidism. Ninety percent of gallstones in Western cultures are cholesterol stones. The remaining 10% consist of bilirubin pigment stones in persons with hemolytic disease.[3] Cholesterol stones are firm and radiolucent, but pure ones are uncommon. Bilirubin stones are small and soft and are found mostly in the ducts. Calcium salts usually contribute to the composition of both types of stones and make them radiopaque.[26]

Biliary *stasis* leading to stagnation of bile in the gallbladder leads to excessive absorption of water. This allows the salts to precipitate easily and leads to the formation of mixed stones. These stones may be quite variable in size and are sometimes small enough to have a gravellike appearance on gallbladder radiographs.

The third contributing factor to stone formation is *inflammation* of the biliary system. This condition causes the bile constituents to become altered, and the inflammed gallbladder mucosa absorbs more of the bile acids with a resultant reduction of the solubility of cholesterol.

Stones may lodge anywhere along the biliary tract where they may cause an obstruction which, if unrelieved, leads to jaundice, or they may cause pressure and subsequent necrosis and infection of the walls of the biliary ducts (Fig. 33-4). Occasionally a stone, because of its location, blocks the entrance of pancreatic fluid and bile into the duodenum at the ampulla of Vater. This condition is difficult to differentiate from obstruction caused by malignancy.

Clinical picture. There may be no signs of cholelithiasis until a stone becomes lodged in a biliary duct, although a history of indigestion after consuming rich, fatty foods, occasional discomfort in the right upper quadrant of the abdomen, and more trouble than the normal person with gaseous eructations after eating is common. Gaseous eructations in cholelithiasis charac-

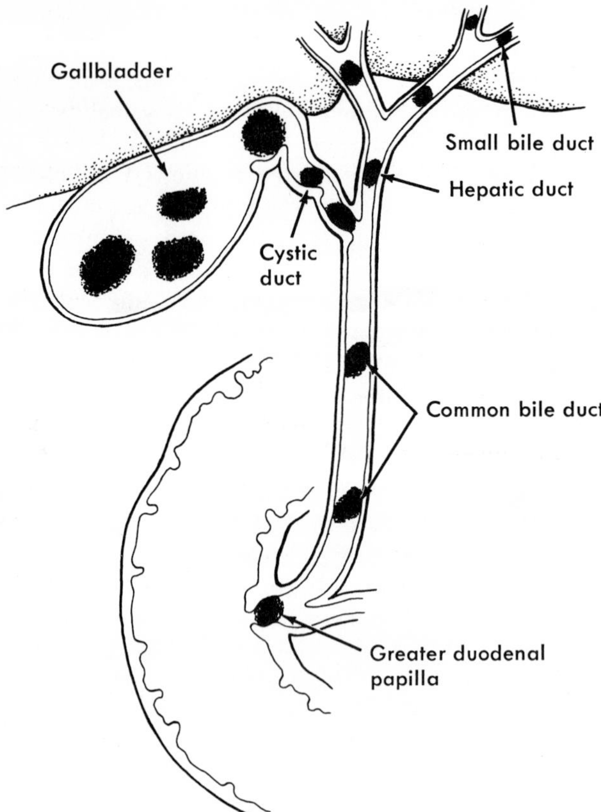

Fig. 33-4. Common sites of gallstones.

teristically occur almost immediately following meals, in contrast to those associated with gastric ulcer, which occur when the stomach is empty (usually several hours after a meal).

Gallstone colic, or *biliary colic,* can cause what is probably the most severe pain that can be experienced. The pain may come on suddenly and is probably caused by spasm of the ducts as they attempt to dislodge the stone. There is severe pain in the right upper quadrant of the abdomen, and it radiates through to the back under the scapula and to the right shoulder. Pain may be so severe that the patient writhes in agony despite large doses of analgesic drugs. Morphine sulfate and meperidine hydrochloride are avoided if possible because they are thought to increase spasm of the biliary sphincters and increase pressure, which can cause further trauma to the walls of the biliary passages. Nitroglycerin or inhalations of amyl nitrite are sometimes lpful, and papaverine hydrochloride, atropine, and ium gluconate often are given to help produce relaxa- f the biliary ducts. The patient usually has nausea iting, profuse diaphoresis, tachycardia, and oc- complete prostration. A nasogastric tube attached to suction often helps to relieve distention in the upper gastrointestinal tract and thereby lessens the pain. Occasionally following an acute attack of biliary colic the stools are saved to determine whether a stone has passed into the intestines. The stools may be sent to the laboratory, or they may be strained for examination on the patient unit.

Intervention. Because there is no suitable method at present to dissolve stones, the treatment of cholelithiasis is surgical removal of the gallbladder and exploration of the common bile duct. The physician must decide whether to treat the patient medically and wait until the acute attack has subsided or to carry out the surgery immediately. Supportive medical treatment includes relief of pain and control of nausea and vomiting. If the patient becomes dehydrated, intravenous therapy may be necessary along with the replacement of fat-soluble vitamins, which are not absorbed due to absence of bile. If surgery is further delayed, the patient is placed on a low-fat diet and given antispasmodics and anticholinergics to prevent smooth-muscle contraction. Surgery is carried out when the patient's condition has stabilized and after correction of any decrease in prothrombin level.

□ Carcinoma of the biliary system

Carcinoma can occur anywhere in the biliary system, and unfortunately at present there is no way of diagnosing early carcinoma in the abdominal viscera. Jaundice may be the first sign and indicates that the lesion has developed sufficiently to obstruct bile passage at some point. Carcinoma rarely develops in a normal gallbladder. Associated stones are present in a very high percentage of these patients, which suggests removal of all gallbladders with stones.

The treatment for carcinoma of the biliary system is surgical, and an operation is performed as soon as the patient's condition warrants it in the hope that complete surgical removal of the lesion is possible. Patients often benefit from surgery even when cure of the carcinoma is impossible, since various operations that help to restore the flow of bile into the gastrointestinal tract produce remarkable relief of symptoms, and the patient may feel relatively well for a time.

□ Biliary atresia

Biliary atresia is a condition in which there is a congenital absence or obliteration of the bile ducts. There is no known cause. Jaundice appears about 2 to 3 weeks after birth and progresses until the infant is a greenish bronze color. Tears and saliva may be pigmented, the urine is dark, and the stools are white or clay colored. The child may not be alert and may move slowly, but he usually has a good appetite. The treatment consists of an operation to establish a pathway for bile into the intestines. As surgery is possible for only a small percentage of these infants, the prognosis is poor.

☐ Surgical care and management of the patient with biliary disease

Terminology

The terminology used to indicate specific biliary tract surgery sounds somewhat complicated but actually is self-explanatory once common terms are understood. *Cholecyst-* refers to the gallbladder, *-docho-* refers to the common bile duct, and *litho-* refers to a stone.

Cholecystectomy is the removal of the gallbladder, whereas *cholecystostomy* refers to the creation of an opening into the gallbladder for decompression and drainage. *Choledochotomy* is a surgical incision into the common bile duct, usually for removal of a stone (*choledocholithotomy*). When carcinoma has been found or when strictures in the ducts make other methods of treatment unsatisfactory, *choledochoduodenostomy* and *choledochojejunostomy*, which refer to anastomoses between the bile duct and the duodenum and between the bile duct and the jejunum, respectively, also may be done. *Cholecystogastrostomy* is the surgical formation of an anastomosis between the gallbladder and the stomach.

Preoperative management

A general medical examination is done prior to biliary surgery, including a radiograph of the chest, x-ray study of the gallbladder, and examination of the urine and stools. Usually an electrocardiogram is ordered. Various tests of hepatic function may be made if disease of the liver is suspected, and if the patient is jaundiced, tests are done to determine the cause. The prothrombin level usually is determined.

If there is jaundice the prothrombin level usually is low, and vitamin K preparations such as phytonadione (vitamin K_1, Mephyton) may be given preoperatively. Occasionally when the prothrombin level is very low, yet surgery is imperative, transfusions of whole blood may be given immediately preoperatively to provide prothrombin, which is essential for blood clotting. If the patient is taking food by mouth poorly, infusions containing glucose and protein hydrolysates may be given in an effort to protect the liver from potential damage and to ensure wound healing. Signs of upper respiratory tract disease should be reported at once, since upper respiratory tract infections can lead to serious complications following surgery of the upper abdomen. A nasogastric tube may be inserted before the patient is taken to the operating room.

Preoperative preparation of the patient with biliary disease is the same as that carried out for any patient having abdominal surgery (Chapter 23). Emphasis is placed on teaching the patient how to deep breathe and cough postoperatively. This is particularly important because of the high abdominal incision, which makes these activities very painful. An explanation of the types of drainage tubes that may be in place postoperatively may also be helpful.

Postoperative management

Immediate care. On recovery from anesthesia the patient is usually placed in a low Fowler's position. Because breathing is painful the patient may hold his breath and take shallow breaths in order to splint the incision and lessen pain. Analgesic medications for pain should be given fairly liberally during the first 48 to 72 hours, and the patient must be urged to cough and to breathe deeply at regular intervals. He must also be helped and encouraged to change position and to move about in bed frequently. If a nasogastric tube is in use, it is attached to suction. Because essential electrolytes as well as gas are removed by this procedure, it is discontinued as soon as possible, usually within 24 hours. As with other postoperative patients, infusion of 5% glucose in distilled water usually is administered. Sometimes solution containing electrolytes and protein hydrolysates is ordered. When the nasogastric tube is removed the patient is given clear fluids by mouth. Sweet, effervescent drinks such as ginger ale usually are tolerated best at first. Within a few days the patient usually is able to eat a soft low-fat diet. Appetite will probably remain poor if bile is not flowing into the duodenum.

Dressings are checked as often as every 15 minutes for the first few hours postoperatively because, although hemorrhage from the wound is rare, it can occur. Occasionally internal hemorrhage follows surgery of the gallbladder and bile ducts, particulary when the inflamed gallbladder was adherent to the liver and was difficult to remove. Decrease in blood pressure, increase in pulse rate, and other signs of hemorrhage are reported to the surgeon at once.

Wound care. If the gallbladder is removed, the cystic duct is ligated and a drain usually is inserted near its stump and brought out through a stab wound. This tube drains bile and small amounts of blood and other serous fluid or exudates onto the dressings. It usually is removed with 5 to 6 days when drainage has largely subsided.

If a cholecystostomy has been performed, a self-retaining catheter is inserted through an opening in the gallbladder and is attached to straight drainage. Bile will drain out through this tube until it is removed, usually between 6 weeks and 6 months.

If exploration of the common duct has been done, a T tube, with the short ends placed into the common duct,

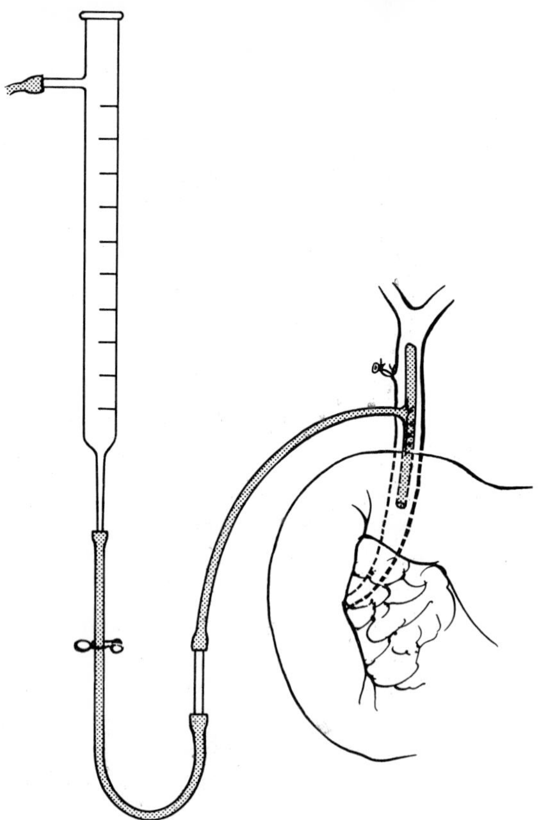

Fig. 33-5. T tube placed in common bile duct and attached to manometer for burette test. Common bile duct has been brought from its normal position for better visualization of T tube.

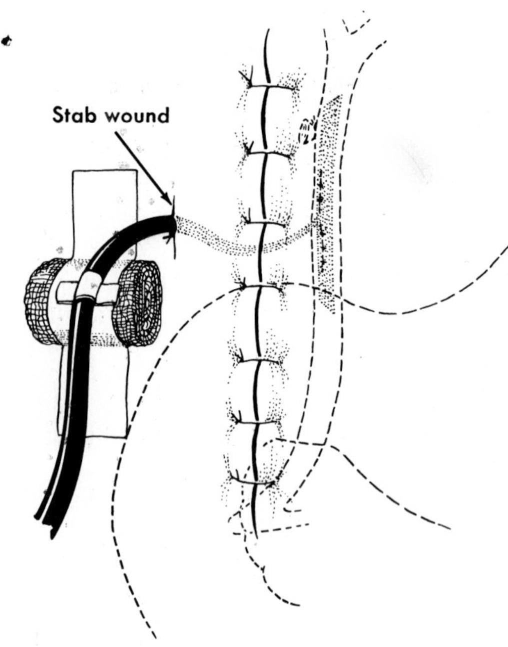

Fig. 33-6. Section of T tube emerging from stab wound may be placed over roll of gauze anchored to skin with adhesive tape to prevent its lumen from being occluded by pressure.

will probably be used (Fig. 33-5). The long end of this soft rubber tube is brought through the wound and sutured to the skin. The section of the T tube emerging from the stab wound may be placed over a roll of gauze anchored to the skin with adhesive tape to prevent it from occluding (Fig. 33-6). The T tube is inserted to preserve patency of the common duct and to ensure drainage of bile out of the body until edema in the common duct has subsided enough for bile to drain into the duodenum normally. If the T tube was clamped while the patient was being transported from the recovery room, it must be released *immediately* on arrival in his room. The nurse should check the operative sheet carefully and seek clarification if directions are not clear. The tube usually is connected to closed gravity drainage similar to that used to drain the urinary bladder. Sufficient tubing should be attached so that the patient can move without restriction. The purpose of the tube should be explained to the patient, and he should be told why it must not be kinked, clamped, or pulled. The drainage should be checked for color and amount at least every 2 hours on the operative day. The tube may drain some blood and blood-stained fluid during the first few hours, but drainage of more than a small amount of blood should be reported to the physician. After this the amount is measured and recorded each day. At first the entire output of bile (normally 500 to 1,000 ml daily) may flow through the tube, but within 10 days most of the bile should be flowing into the duodenum.

Usually the T tube is removed in 10 days to 2 weeks. Before this is done the patency of the common bile duct must be assessed. The tube is clamped for variable intervals and the patient monitored for sign of distress. If distress occurs the tube is unclamped immediately and the physician informed. Otherwise a *burette test*, similar to that performed prior to removing a nephrostomy tube, is done to determine the patency of the biliary system (Fig. 33-5). If the common bile duct is patent the pressure readings will fluctuate very little from the initial reading unless the patient is moving, coughing, talking, or laughing just prior to the reading. If the common bile duct is still obstructed, the level of bile will rise in the burette beyond the set point, usually 15 cm above the level of the common bile duct. If this happens the physician should be notified. A cholangiogram usually is done to confirm the patency of the duct before the tube is removed (p. 550). Following the removal of the T tube the patient may have chills and fever, but they usually subside within 24 hours. They are caused by edema and a local reaction to the bile. Occasionally flow of bile into the abdominal cavity causes peritonitis, and therefore any abdominal pain should be reported at once.

Postoperatively the bile should either drain out through the drainage tubes or flow into the intestine. If it does not do so, it can be assumed that the flow of bile is obstructed and that bile is being forced back into the liver and into the bloodstream. The nurse should observe the patient closely for jaundice, particularly in the sclerae. Urine should be examined for the brown color that is indicative of bile pigment. A specimen should be saved for the physician's inspection when bile pigment is observed in the urine. The nurse may observe the patient's progress by noting the stools: a light color is usual if all the bile is flowing out through the drainage tubes (unless bile salts are being given by mouth), but the normal brown color should gradually reappear as drainage diminishes and finally disappears.

The patient should be told about any drainage tubes that have been used. He should know if much bile is expected on the dressings so that he will not become alarmed by soiling of dressings, his gown, or bedclothes. Outer dressings usually should be changed frequently when there is excessive drainage, since the drainage is irritating to the skin and wet dressings interfere with the patient's comfort and rest. Soap and water will remove bile from the skin. Montgomery straps make the changing of dressings much easier.

Activity. The patient usually is permitted out of bed the day after the operation. If a T tube or a cholecystostomy tube is present, it may be attached to a small drainage bottle to permit greater freedom of movement. It may be placed in a pocket of the patient's bathrobe or attached to his robe below the level of the common duct. The patient may need help and encouragement because dressings are uncomfortable and he fears spilling the drainage when he moves about. He may still be receiving infusions, and transporting the infusion bottle is necessary. He often benefits from a regular schedule of getting up and sitting in a chair or walking with assistance.

Diet. Special diets are seldom prescribed by the physician following billary tract surgery, but the patient is advised to avoid excessive fats. The nurse should help to teach the patient the essentials of good nutrition, with emphasis on foods that are low in fat.

Occasionally if excessive drainage through the T tube or cholecystostomy tube continues for a long time, the bile collected in the drainage bottle is administered to the patient through a nasogastric tube to improve digestion. If this is done the funnel or Asepto syringe should be covered and the bile should be in a receptacle so that the patient does not see it. Sometimes the bile may be diluted with grape or other juices to disguise its appearance. The patient generally is not told that he is receiving bile.

Usually from 10 days to 2 weeks of hospitalization are required following biliary tract surgery when no complications occur. The length of convalescence depends on the individual patient, but usually at least a month is needed before normal activities can be resumed safely. The nurse should emphasize to the patient the importance of keeping medical appointments as scheduled.

□ Outcome criteria for patients with chronic disease of the biliary system

The patient or significant others can:

1. Explain dietary changes required:
   a. List foods to be avoided or limited (patient is frequently placed on low-fat diet).
   b. Discuss type and amount of food and calories needed and plans for achieving.
2. Explain any medications to be taken at home:
   a. State dosage of medications (such as, may require vitamin A, D, E, and K supplements and is aware of their importance to prevent recurrence of symptoms)
   b. State how and when to use medications such as anticholinergics and antispasmotics.
   c. State untoward effects of medications that need to be reported immediately.
3. Explain therapeutic follow-up necessary:
   a. Explain basic health problem and how the planned treatments will help.
   b. State signs and symptoms that should be reported to the health care provider (pain, fever, jaundice, dark urine, pale stools, pruritus).
   c. State plans for follow-up care.

■ DISEASES OF THE PANCREAS

The pancreas has both endocrine and exocrine functions. The endocrine functions along with diagnostic tests used to evaluate them are discussed in Chapter 30. A brief review of the exocrine functions to assist the reader in understanding the major disorders encountered follows.

As an exocrine organ the pancreas produces enzymes that are vital to normal digestion. The primary enzymes produced include *trypsin* and *chymotrypsin*, which digest protein; *pancreatic lipase* for fat digestion; and *amylase*, which digests carbohydrate. These enzymes do not become activated until they enter the duodenum. This is a particularly significant protective mechanism, since if trypsin were active in the pancreas it would digest pancreatic tissue. Through a complex interplay of neural, hormonal, and chemical interactions, the pancreas is activated by the ingestion of food to release the appropriate enzymes for digestion.

☐ Pancreatitis

Epidemiology. The three most important causes of acute pancreatitis are gallstones, alcohol, and "idiopathic" processes.[3] The amount of pancreatitis caused by biliary tract disease ranges from 10% to 95%. The percentage depends on the amount of alcoholism present in the population being studied. The association between biliary disease and pancreatitis is obscure.[3] For the reasons stated above, the percentage of persons with pancreatitis related to alcoholism ranges from 8% to 75%, depending on the socioeconomic status of the population served. The relationship between alcoholism and pancreatitis also is not well understood although several mechanisms have been postulated. It is possible that alcohol has a direct toxic effect on the pancreas. Animal studies indicate that there are pathologic changes with high ethanol intake. These same findings have not as yet been substantiated in humans. Other possible factors include the fact that increased alcohol intake stimulates gastric acid secretion by direct stimulation of parietal cells. The presence of acid in the duodenum stimulates the secretion of secretin and pancreozymin, which augments pancreatic secretion.

Chronic relapsing pancreatitis may be caused by a variety of mechanisms. The most common is chronic alcoholism, and a less frequent cause is untreated biliary tract disease. The disease tends to recur, and for this reason some experts suggest that an autoimmune mechanism or hypersensitivity reaction may be involved.[3] This has not been substantiated.

Pathophysiology. Pancreatitis is an inflammation of the pancreas. Most experts agree that it is associated with a number of causative mechanisms. In summarizing these mechanisms it would appear that the following commonly occur: (1) obstruction of pancreatic outflow due to duodenitis with resulting pancreatic edema; (2) vomiting, which may cause rupture of the ducts and acute hemorrhagic pancreatitis; and (3) dietary deficiencies that may make the pancreas more susceptible to the first two mechanisms. Obstruction of the pancreatic duct may be due to stones, tumors, or inflammatory strictures that prevent the free flow of pancreatic secretions into the duodenum. Regurgitation of bile through the pancreatic duct and activation of proteolytic enzymes in the pancreatic juice may also occur. It appears that the pancreas is particularly susceptible to protein deficiencies, perhaps because of its protein requirement to synthesize enzymes.

Regardless of the specific etiology, it appears that the release of trypsin takes place within the gland itself, causing activation of the enzymes. There may be edema of the tissues, suppuration and abscess formation, necrosis, or hemorrhage, depending on the cause and the severity of the disease. Consequently the disease process gradually destroys the pancreas, replacing it with fibrous tissue and calcification. The disease process may be localized or spread throughout the entire gland. The extent and severity of an acute attack depend on the amount of obstruction of the pancreatic flow, how much surrounding tissue is destroyed, and the amount of interruption of blood supply.

Clinical picture. The most outstanding symptoms of *acute hemorrhagic pancreatitis* are pain and shock; in *acute edematous pancreatitis* and *chronic relapsing pancreatitis* pain and metabolic disturbances are common. All three symptoms—pain, shock, and metabolic disturbances—may be absent in *painless pancreatitis.*[3]

Pancreatitis usually occurs suddenly, and the pain is severe, widespread, and constant. The pain may be experienced in the epigastrium and other parts of the abdomen and may radiate to the back, flanks, and substernal area. The pain may be more intense when the individual is lying supine. In addition to pain there is often fever and tachycardia. In more severe attacks cyanosis, cold clammy skin, rapid and feeble pulse, and subnormal temperature indicative of shock are seen.[3] On physical examination of the abdomen, tenderness is present and there may be a moderate degree of muscular rigidity.

When shock occurs death may ensue within a few hours. Several factors are felt to be responsible for the shock and include an increase in serum proteolytic activity; release of kallikrein, which forms kinins that stimulate smooth muscles, dilate blood vessels, and lower blood pressure; exudation of blood and plasma into the peritoneal cavity resulting in decrease in blood volume sometimes as great as 30%; acute coronary insufficiency caused by thrombosis and electrolyte disturbances; pulmonary embolus; and intravascular coagulability.[3]

Other metabolic disturbances that can occur are lowering of serum calcium, potassium, and sodium levels. There may be an increase in circulating levels of glucagon, injury to the beta cells, and increase release of glucocorticoids, all of which can result in hyperglycemia, glycosuria, and impaired glucose tolerance, which occurs in about 50% of patients.[3] Coma may occur in acute pancreatitis and sometimes may be confused with diabetic coma because of the elevated blood sugar and glycosuria.

Diagnostic tests of the greatest value in establishing a diagnosis are enzyme levels. A *serum amylase* level of greater than 300 Somogyi units in the presence of the symptoms outlined above usually establishes the diagnosis of acute pancreatitis. *Serum amylase* levels usually become elevated within 24 to 48 hours and may range from 300 to 800 units. Some clinicians have reported levels as high as 12,000 units.[3] There is no apparent relationship between the severity of the disease and the height of the enzyme levels.

Serum lipase also rises in pancreatitis and reaches its peak in 72 to 96 hours. When elevations in SGOT, alkaline phosphatase, and leucine aminopeptides occur there is usually obstruction of the common bile duct or liver disease.

Urinary amylase levels may also be used to diagnose acute pancreatitis is absence of kidney failure. Other laboratory findings include leukocytosis, elevated blood urea nitrogen, glycosuria, hyperglycemia, and decreased levels of calcium, potassium, and sodium. See Table 33-2 for tests used in evaluating pancreatic disease. After repeated attacks the enzyme levels may be normal or low due to reduction of functioning gland tissue.

Advances in fiberoptic techniques have made it possible to visualize the pancreatic duct by cannulation of the ampulla of Vater. It is possible to use this technique to determine an accurate diagnosis of obstructive biliary tract disease or chronic versus acute pancreatitis. This is a highly specialized test and at present is only carried out by very experienced endoscopists.[4]

Pancreatitis can become chronic with calcification and fibrous replacement of normal duct tissue. Nausea, persistent pain, and occasionally jaundice occur. Loss of weight also occurs although excessive amounts of food are ingested as the patient develops "intestinal malabsorption" syndrome. A problem that can occur with chronic fibrous changes is damage to the islet cells causing diabetes mellitus. In addition danger of addiction to narcotics becomes a problem with patients who have chronic pancreatitis, particularly alcoholics.

Intervention

Control of pain. Meperidine hydrochloride (Demerol), 75 to 100 mg every 4 to 6 hours, may be necessary to reduce pain. Morphine and codeine are not used because of their spasmogenic effects. Some patients find that the pain is decreased if they assume a sitting position with the trunk flexed, or with their knees drawn up to the abdomen in a side-lying knee-chest position. Sympathetic nerve blocks and epidural anesthesia can

Table 33-2. Laboratory tests used for evaluating pancreatic disease

Test	Sample	Interpretation
Amylase	Serum or whole blood	Normal serum amylase is 80 to 150 Somogyi units. In acute pancreatic cellular damage the serum amylase level may rise to 600 Somogyi units within 4 hours of onset reaching levels up to 2,000 units in a short time. The decrease also occurs rapidly, and values may return to normal within 48 to 72 hours. Chronic pancreatitis produces variable elevations that are less marked, and carcinoma of the pancreas does not usually affect amylase levels.
	Urine (single specimen)	Normal value is 2 to 50 Wohlgemuth units/ml.
	Urine (24-hr specimen	Normal value is 6 to 30 Wohlgemuth units/ml and up to 5,000 Somogyi units/24 hr. As amylase is excreted in the urine, the elevation level is dependent on the serum level, and if the serum level has already declined, the urine level may be diagnostically useful as it may remain elevated up to 7 days after an acute attack.
Lipase	Serum	Normal serum lipase is 0 to 1.5 units. In acute pancreatitis, lipase levels usually parallel serum amylase levels. The level rises somewhat slower (24 to 48 hr after attack) but may remain elevated for 5 to 7 days.
Calcium	Serum	Normal serum calcium is 4.5 to 5.75 mEq/liter (9.0 to 11.5 mg/100 ml). In severe cases of pancreatitis and steatorrhea, serum calcium may be low because calcium soaps are formed due to sequestration of calcium by fat necrosis.
Proteins (total)	Serum	Normal total serum protein is 6 to 8 g/100 ml. May be decreased in acute pancreatitis due to vascular colloid loss.
Glucose	Whole blood	Normal serum glucose is 90 to 120 mg/100 ml. In pancreatic disease serum glucose level may be elevated due to beta cell destruction causing decreased insulin production.

NOTE: Serum bilirubin and alkaline phosphatase levels may be elevated due to biliary tract or liver involvement.)

be used if pain is persistent and not relieved by meperidine.[3]

Treatment of shock. Shock is treated with whole blood. Central venous pressure and intake and output are carefully monitored. Volume expanders such as albumin, plasma, and low-molecular-weight dextran may be used. Isoproterenol hydrochloride (Isuprel), 1:500,000, may also be used if shock does not respond to fluid replacement alone.

Inhibition of pancreatic activity. Several measures are taken to rest the injured pancreas. These include absence of oral intake, continuous nasogastric suction, and use of drugs such as propantheline bromide (Pro-Banthine) or methantheline bromide (Banthine) to inhibit pancreatic secretion. These drugs are contraindicated in the presence of paralytic ileus and shock, and there is some question as to their efficacy in treating pancreatitis.

Fluids and electrolytes. Because of the lack of oral intake and continuous gastric suction, fluid and electrolytic replacement is necessary. Between 3 and 6 liters of normal saline with supplemental potassium may be given daily. The amount is carefully monitored to avoid fluid overload. When a diabetic state secondary to acute pancreatitis is present and there is severe hyperglycemia and glycosuria, small doses of insulin are given.[3]

Other measures. If paralytic ileus is present, a long intestinal tube such as a *Miller-Abbott* tube may be inserted. *Peritoneal* dialysis may be used for patients who are unresponsive to other therapy and whose condition is deteriorating.

An exploratory laparotomy may be performed in acute pancreatitis when a diagnosis cannot be established and the possibility of general peritonitis, perforation of an organ, or a bowel obstruction cannot be excluded. If cholecystitis or cholelithiasis is present, an operation may be performed when the patient can tolerate surgery. An operation also is sometimes done in an attempt to divert or increase bile flow at the sphincter of Oddi (entrance to the duodenum) and thereby reduce regurgitation of bile into the pancreatic duct.

After an acute attack, management is aimed at preventing further attacks. Patients are told to avoid alcohol and are generally placed on low-fat, bland diets distributed over 5 to 6 small feedings per day. Rich foods must sometimes be avoided to keep pancreatic secretions at a minimum. The dietician may need to work with the patient to help plan an appropriate diet. Patients may also require replacement enzymes to correct deficiencies that prevent adequate absorption of food. These substances are available in tablet or capsule form and contain amylase, lipase, and trypsin. Bile salts may also be given to facilitate the absorption of fat-soluble vitamins and to prevent further loss of fat. Calcium supplements may be necessary also. The stools are checked for steatorrhea, bleeding, or evidence of biliary obstruction. If diabetes is present, appropriate therapy is instituted.

□ Outcome criteria for patients with chronic disease of the pancreas

The patient or significant others can:

1. Explain necessary dietary changes required after discharge:
   a. Explain the relationship of attacks to ingestion of foods.
   b. List specific foods to be avoided (such as alcoholic beverages, excessive use of coffee, spicy or rich foods, and heavy meals).
2. Explain medications to be taken at home and their relationship to the condition present:
   a. Explain dosage and expected effects of medications (such as pancreatic enzyme replacements, oral hypoglycemics or insulin, bile salts, vitamin supplements).
   b. Explain any untoward effects of medications that need to be reported to the health care provider.
   c. Explain how and when to use medications such as antacids, anticholinergics, and analgesics.
3. Explain health maintenance necessary to assist in preventing further attacks or indicate need for therapeutic follow-up:
   a. Explain the need to avoid irritants and infectious agents and identify sources of these in the environment. (These may differ slightly depending on the precipitating cause of the illness.)
   b. List signs and symptoms indicative of an attack such as pain, nausea, vomiting, distention, and low-grade fever.
   c. Explain what steatorrhea is, how to monitor for it, and what it means.
   d. State whom to contact if the above signs and symptoms occur.
   e. Explain signs of diabetes such as polydipsia, polyuria, polyphagia, weakness, or weight loss and know that these must be reported to the health care provider immediately.
4. Explain need to identify, limit, and learn to cope with emotional stressors in the environment.
5. Explain how to obtain community resources if necessary:
   a. If alcoholic, is aware of available assistance programs in the community (Alcoholics Anonymous and other groups).
6. Explain plans for follow-up care.

□ Tumors of the pancreas

Epidemiology. Tumors of the pancreas may be malignant or benign. Benign tumors include islet cell tumors, cystadenomas, and duct cell adenomas. Malignant tumors occur more frequently and are most often found in the head of the pancreas. Men are affected far more often than women, and tumors usually occur after middle age. Sarcomas of the pancreas may be found in infants and young adults but are very rare.

Pathophysiology. Most malignant tumors of the pancreas appear to begin in the ductal areas, causing eventual blockage and resulting in chronic pancreatitis. Direct extension of the lesion may cause its spread to the posterior wall of the stomach, the duodenal wall, the colon, and the common bile duct. The tumor may be diffusely spread over the entire gland, or it may be a well-defined growth. It commonly grows in a rapid manner, is highly invasive, and vascular, lymphatic, and perineural metastases frequently occur. Many patients live only 3 to 6 months after diagnosis is confirmed.

Clinical picture. Symptoms of pancreatic malignancies are not usually detectable until late in the course of the disease. Pain occurs in about 85% of the patients. This may be preceded by vague anorexia, nausea, and weight loss over a period of months. Jaundice frequently occurs due to common duct obstruction but is seldom a primary sign. Changes in stools may occur if the pancreatic ducts are obstructed. Pain may be colicky or intermittent and often radiates to the back, abdomen, and chest.

Definitive diagnosis prior to surgery is difficult. Diagnostic studies include duodenal cytology, pancreatic scans, and arteriography. About half of these patients develop diabetes mellitus.

Intervention. Surgical treatment is most effective, although the prognosis is usually poor. If the tumor is operable, a pancreaticoduodenal resection (Whipple procedure), which includes removal of the head of the pancreas, the lower end of the common bile duct, the duodenum, and the distal portion of the stomach, may be done. The common bile duct and the remaining portions of the pancreas and stomach are then anastomosed to the jejunum. If the tumor is not resectable, a palliative operation such as a cholecystojejunostomy, a choledochojejunostomy, or a palliative gastrojejunostomy may be done to help restore temporarily a normal flow of bile and some pancreatic enzyme to the intestinal tract. The type of procedure performed depends on the involvement found at operation. Palliation of the symptoms also may be achieved by the administration of chemotherapeutic agents such as 5-fluorouracil.[31]

In addition to routine postoperative care following abdominal surgery, the patient who has had pancreatic surgery must be watched for signs of peritonitis, gastrointestinal obstruction, and jaundice until sufficient time for healing has elapsed and until it is determined that all the anastomoses are secure and patent.

Hypotension is a common occurrence after pancreatic surgery, and good baseline data should be obtained preoperatively. The patient may require the administration of vasopressor drugs for 24 to 48 hours postoperatively. Patients with extensive pancreatic resections may not be ambulated as soon as other patients with abdominal surgery and may be prone to developing pulmonary complications if excellent pulmonary hygiene is not encouraged and persistently carried out.

Stools should be observed, and frothy, light-colored stools containing conspicuously undigested fat are reported. If most of the pancreas was removed, the patient may have to take pancreatic enzymes in tablet form by mouth to aid the digestion of fat. The patient is watched for signs and symptoms of diabetes mellitus following this procedure, although it rarely occurs unless the entire pancreas has been removed. If hypoinsulinism occurs, treatment with insulin will be necessary for the remainder of the patient's life (p. 585). The average duration of life after the Whipple procedure is about a year.

Occasionally a patient may have an islet cell tumor of the pancreas. It is a benign lesion in the tail of the pancreas and results in overproduction of insulin, causing symptoms of hypoglycemia (p. 593). Surgical removal of the tumor relieves symptoms.

REFERENCES AND SELECTED READINGS

1. Altshuler, A., and Hilden, D.: The patient with hypertension, Nurs. Clin. North Am. **12**:317-329, 1977.
2. Anderson, W. A. D., and Scotti, T. M.: Synopsis of pathology, ed. 9, St. Louis, 1976, The C. V. Mosby Co.
3. Beeson, P. B., and McDermott, W., editors: Textbook of medicine, ed. 14, Philadelphia, 1975, W. B. Saunders Co.
4. Belinsky, S.: Visualizing the pancreatic and biliary ducts, Am. J. Nurs. **76**:936-937, 1976.
5. Bergersen, B. S., and Goth, A.: Pharmacology in nursing, ed. 14, St. Louis, 1979, The C. V. Mosby Co.
6. Bockus, H. L.: Gastroenterology, vol. 3, ed. 3, Philadelphia, 1974, W. B. Saunders Co.
7. Bossone, M. C. M.: The liver: a pharmacologic perspective, Nurs. Clin. North Am. **12**:291-303, 1977.
8. Boyer, C. A., and Oehlberg, S. M.: Interpretation and clinical relevance of liver function tests, Nurs. Clin. North Am. **12**:275-290, 1977.
9. Carey, L. C., editor: The pancreas, St. Louis, 1973, The C. V. Mosby Co.
10. Dane, D. S., Cameron, C. H., and Briggs, M.: Virus-like particles in serum of patients with Australia-antigen-associated hepatitis, Lancet **1**:695-698, 1970.
11. Daniel, E.: Chronic problems in rehabilitation of patients with Laennec's cirrhosis, Nurs. Clin. North Am. **12**:345-356, 1977.
12. Foster, J. H., Lawler, M. R., Jr., Welborn, M. B., Jr., et al.: Recent experience with major hepatic resection, Ann. Surg. **167**:651-668, 1968.
13. French, R. M.: Nurses guide to diagnostic procedures, ed. 4, New York, 1975, Mc Graw-Hill Book Co.
14. Fuerst, E. V., and Wolff, L. V.: Fundamentals of nursing, ed. 5, Philadelphia, 1974, J. B. Lippincott Co.
15. Gocke, D. J.: New faces of viral hepatitis, DM 1-32, Jan. 1973.

16. *Hayter, J.: Impaired liver function and related nursing care, Am. J. Nurs. **68**:2374-2379, 1968.
17. Host, W. R., Serlin, O., and Rush, B. F.: Hyperalimentation in cirrhotic patients, Am. J. Surg. **123**:57-62, 1972.
18. Howard, J. M.: Pancreatico-duodenectomy: forty-one consecutive Whipple resections without an operative mortality, Ann. Surg. **168**:629-640, 1968.
19. Jones, P. N., and Capps, R. B.: The management of hepatic coma, Med. Clin. North Am. **48**:37-51, 1964.
20. Linton, R.: The treatment of esophageal varices, Surg. Clin. North Am. **46**:485-598, 1966.
21. Mahood, W. H., Dill, J. E., and Dill, R. P.: Hepatic failure. In Meltzer, L. E., Abdellah, F. G., and Kitchell, J. R.: Concepts and practices of intensive care for nurse specialists, ed. 2, Bowie, Md., 1976, The Charles Press Publishers, Inc.
22. McElroy, D. B.: Nursing care of patients with viral hepatitis, Nurs. Clin. North Am. **12**:305-315, 1977.
23. McGill, D. B., and Motto, J. D.: An industrial outbreak of toxic hepatitis due to methylenedianiline, N. Engl. J. Med. **291**:278-282, 1974.
24. Nadkarni, S. V.: Amebic abscess of the liver, Int. Surg. **58**:112-115, 1973.
25. Nelson, W. E., Vaughn, V. C., and McKay, R. J.: Textbook of pediatrics, ed. 10, Philadelphia, 1975, W. B. Saunders Co.
26. Netter, F.: The Ciba collection of medical illustrations, Part III. Digestive system, vol. 3, Summit, N.J., 1964, Ciba Pharmaceutical Co.
27. Pierce, L.: Anatomy and physiology of the liver in relation to clinical assessment, Nurs. Clin. North Am. **12**:259-273, 1977.
28. Popper, H., and Schaffner, F., editors: Progress in liver diseases, vol. 3, New York, 1970, Grune & Stratton, Inc.
29. Rutherdale, J. A., Medline, A., Sinclair, J. C., et al.: Hepatitis in drug users, Am. J. Gastroenterol. **58**:275-287, 1972.
30. Sabiston, D. C., editor: Davis-Christopher textbook of surgery, ed. 11, Philadelphia, 1977, W. B. Saunders Co.
31. *Schaffner, F., et al.: Symposium: liver disease, J.A.M.A. **191**:466-486, 1965.

*References preceded with an asterisk are particularly well suited for student reading.

32. Schiff, L.: Diseases of the liver, ed. 3, Philadelphia, 1972, J. B. Lippincott Co.
33. Schweitzer, I. L., Dunn, A. E., Peters, R. L., et al.: Viral hepatitis B in neonates and infants, Am. J. Med. **55**:762-771, 1973.
34. Shahinpour, N.: The adult patient with bleeding esophageal varices, Nurs. Clin. North Am. **12**:331-343, 1977.
35. Sherar, L.: Ascites: pathogenesis and treatment, Postgrad. Med. **53**:165-170, 1973.
36. Sherlock, S.: Diseases of the liver and the biliary system, ed. 5, Philadelphia, 1975, F. A. Davis Co.
37. *Simmons, S., and Givens, B.: Acute pancreatitis, Am. J. Nurs. **71**:934-939, 1971.
38. Small, D. M.: Gallstones: diagnosis and treatment, Postgrad. Med. **51**:187-193, 1972.
39. Syndman, D. R., Bryan, J. A., and Dixon, R. E.: Prevention of nosocomial viral hepatitis, type B (hepatitis B), Ann. Int. Med. **83**:838-845, 1975.
40. Statement on hepatitis B antigen carriers, Hospitals **48**:95-98, 1974.
41. *Taylor, K., Commons, N., and Jack, M. S.: Liver transplant, Am. J. Nurs. **68**:1895-1899, 1968.
42. U.S. Department of Health, Education and Welfare, Public Health Service, Center for Disease Control: Reported morbidity and mortality in the United States 1976, vol. 25, no. 53, 1977.
43. U.S. Department of Health, Education and Welfare, Public Health Service, Center for Disease Control: Immune globulins for protection against viral hepatitis, vol. 26, no. 52, 1977.
44. U.S. Department of Health, Education and Welfare, Public Health Service, Center for Disease Control: Isolation techniques for use in hospitals, ed 2, 1975.
45. Wenzel, R. P., Adams, J. F., and Smith, E. P.: Patterns of illicit drug use in viral hepatitis patients, Milit. Med. **138**:345-350, 1973.
46. Williams, S. R.: Nutrition and diet therapy, ed. 3, St. Louis, 1977, The C. V. Mosby Co.
47. Wintrobe, M. M., et al.: Harrison's principles of internal medicine, ed. 8, New York, 1977, McGraw-Hill Book Co.

UNIT VI

Sensorimotor problems

Survival through the ages has depended on the ability to sense dangers in the environment and to be ready for flight or fight. The senses are used in many ways: for protection from injury, for aid in activities of daily living, and for enjoyment of the arts and music. The senses are part of the neurologic system that also has motor function. Nerves transmit messages to and from the muscles that permit a person to move about, to carry out daily activities, to work, and to play. Thus activity, which is one of the basic physiologic needs, depends on an intact nervous system and an intact musculoskeletal system. Problems with either of these systems will affect a person's ability to function in the environment and may require coping with permanent changes in life style.

Because both the neurologic and musculoskeletal systems are involved in the ability to be active, they have been grouped together in this unit. Three major topics are considered: *the neurologic system* itself, the *special senses (eye and ear)*, and the *musculoskeletal system*. Each section consists of a chapter on assessment, a chapter that reviews general management of persons experiencing problems with the system, and a chapter that examines specific problems. The special senses have been dealt with separate from the overall neurologic system because of the specific needs of persons who have impairment of sight and hearing.

34

Neurologic assessment

MARJORIE KINNEY

The reader should distinguish between neurologic assessment as performed by the medical specialist or neurologist and directed toward the localization of a neurologic lesion or disease and neurologic examination as carried out by the generalist to screen for neurologic symptoms. The assessment carried out by the specialist is more detailed, exact, and comprehensive; the assessment carried out by the generalist may be one part of a gross physical examination. It should be recognized that many systemic diseases, or diseases of organ systems other than the nervous system, have neurologic overtones. For this reason the person with neurologic symptoms may be referred by the generalist to a neurologist for definitive neurologic assessment or diagnosis.

ROLE OF NURSE IN NEUROLOGIC ASSESSMENT

The independent role of the nurse in neurologic assessment includes systematic and continuous assessment. The assessment by the nurse is performed primarily to define patient problems or to make nursing diagnoses as a basis for planning nurse interventions or actions. Neurologic assessment is only one part of the total assessment process. Collection of data by the nurse does not purposely duplicate the more detailed and complete assessment performed by the neurologist, and the nurse interdependently utilizes data collected by other professionals as one part of the total data base. At the same time, initial and ongoing data collected by the nurse supplement data collected by the neurologist and other professionals. The baseline information collected by the nurse upon admission is important for later comparative purposes. It is essential that the neurologic assessment performed by the nurse include a detailed appraisal of the functional status of the individual in relation to ability to perform self-care activities that may be limited by sensory, motor, and mental deficits.

The purposes of this chapter are to review selected neuroanatomy and physiology, to discuss aspects of history taking, to present the components and methods of and the observations to be made during the neurologic examination, and to discuss selected tests and procedures used to assist in the diagnosis of neurologic problems.

NEUROPHYSIOLOGIC AND NEUROANATOMIC CONCEPTS

Neurologic assessment is dependent on the examiner's knowledge of normal neurophysiology and neuroanatomy and ability to interpret the degree of change in status from what is considered to be normal. The attainment of a logical diagnosis (nursing or medical) begins with a recognition of abnormality followed by grouping of the data, analysis of data, and conclusions about what the data mean in terms of a diagnosis.

The complexity of the nervous system limits what can be presented here. Only selected concepts relevant to neurologic assessment are included. The reader is referred to current texts for a more detailed and comprehensive coverage.[4,10,21] Emphasis is placed on key concepts including the *neuron*, *motor system pathways*, *sensory system pathways*, and *effector organs*.

Functionally the nervous system, like an electrical conductance system, coordinates and controls all activities of the body. Broadly, the nervous system carries out four general kinds of functions as related to informational processes:

1. Receives stimuli or information from the internal and external environments over varied afferent or sensory pathways.
2. Communicates information between distant parts of the body (periphery) to the central nervous system
3. Computes or processes the information received at various *reflex* (spinal cord) and *conscious* (higher brain) levels to determine responses appropriate to existing situations
4. Transmits information rapidly over varied efferent or motor pathways to effector organs for body action control or modifications

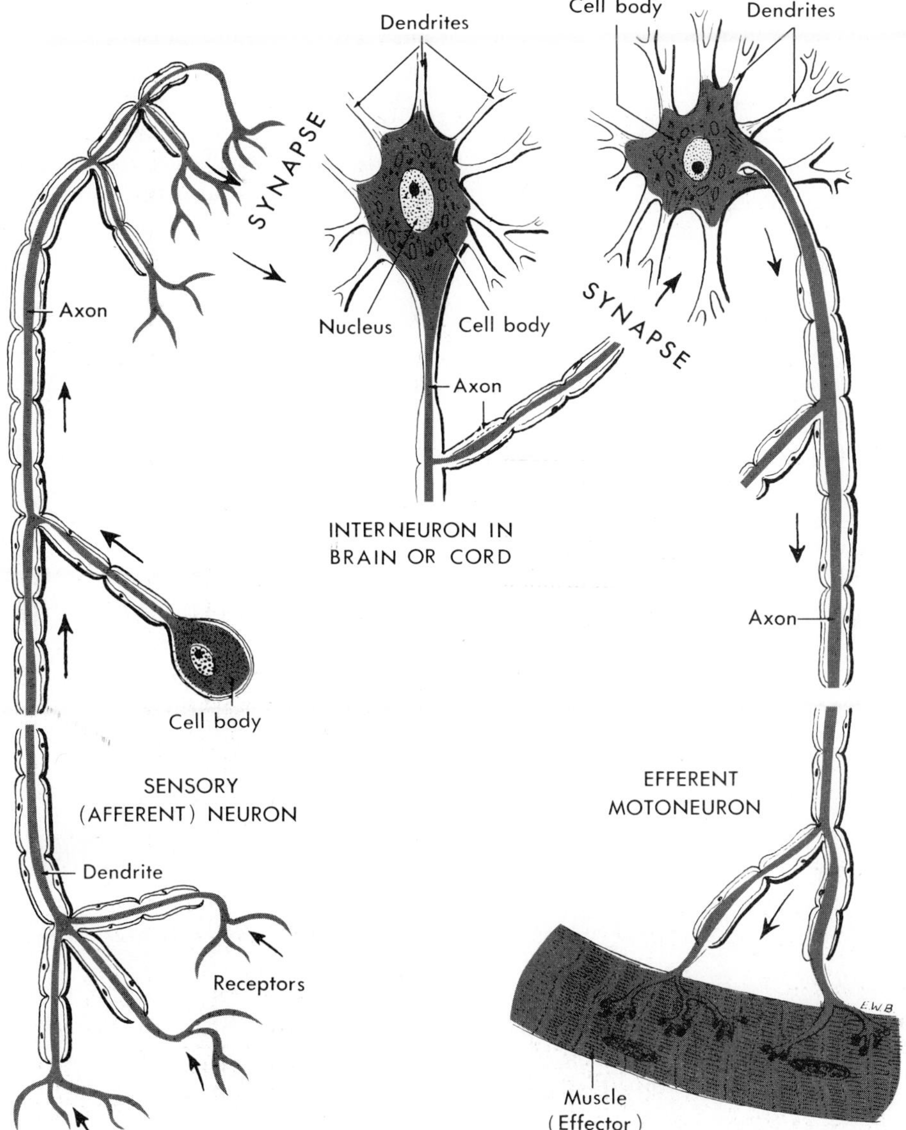

Fig. 34-1. Diagram of structure of three kinds of neurons. Note that each neuron has three parts: a cell body and two types of extensions, dendrite(s) and an axon. Arrows indicate direction of impulse conduction. (From Anthony, C. P., and Thibodeau, G. A.: Textbook of anatomy and physiology, ed. 10, St. Louis, 1979, The C. V. Mosby Co.)

Neuron

The single *neuron* is the basic structural and functional unit of the nervous system. It shares all of the basic biologic and biochemical properties of other body cells. It is also a highly specialized and differentiated cell. The single neuron acts as a miniature nervous system and has properties specialized for its electrical function.

Microscopically the neuron consists of a cell body, or *soma*, with two extensions that project from it: a *dendritic tree* and an elongated *cylindrical axon*. A *cell membrane* encloses the outer boundary of the soma, dendrites, and axon, thus separating the inside and outside of the cell. The presence of a large proportion of cell membrane makes it suitable to receive a large number of synaptic contacts at one time (Fig. 34-1). The *axon* is specialized for the transmission of information along its extension *away from* the cell body to adjacent neurons; the *dendrite(s)* is specialized for receiving information from the axon terminals at special sites called *synapses.* It should be noted that the word *axon* is used in various ways. It may be used to describe the extension of one cell or the extension of several cells comprising a nerve.

Many of the most important *functional* properties of the neuron lie within the *cell membrane* itself. Structurally the membrane is made up of lipids and proteins. Proteins are attached to both the inside and outside of the membrane and play an important functional role. The membrane has the property of translocating materials across itself. The membrane exhibits *differential permeability*, being permeable to oxygen, carbon dioxide, and certain inorganic ions and impermeable to organic compounds (proteins) and other inorganic ions. This differential permeability results in a characteristic ionic distribution. The inside of the neuron contains a high concentration of proteins (which are impermeable) and potassium (K+), while the outside of the cell is high in sodium (Na+). This unequal distribution, or gradient, of K+ and Na+ established across the membrane is due in part to differential permeability and to the presence of an active *sodium-potassium pump* within the membrane. The pump requires metabolic energy for rapid movement of sodium and potassium across the membrane. An electrical potential difference, or charge, is thus produced between the inside and the outside of the cell. The magnitude of the potential difference is a function of the ratio of charged particles on opposite sides of the membrane. This potential is called the *resting membrane potential* (resting potential). All cells exhibit this property of resting potential. It essentially remains constant over time. Thus in the resting state all neurons possess a potential for action and are said to be *polarized* (a difference in voltage charge between inner and outer cell membrane or surface). This resting potential is quite small, −60 mV with the inside of the cell electronically negative to the outside of the cell.[21]

Additionally the neuron exhibits the *unique* property of "*excitability*" along with muscle and certain gland

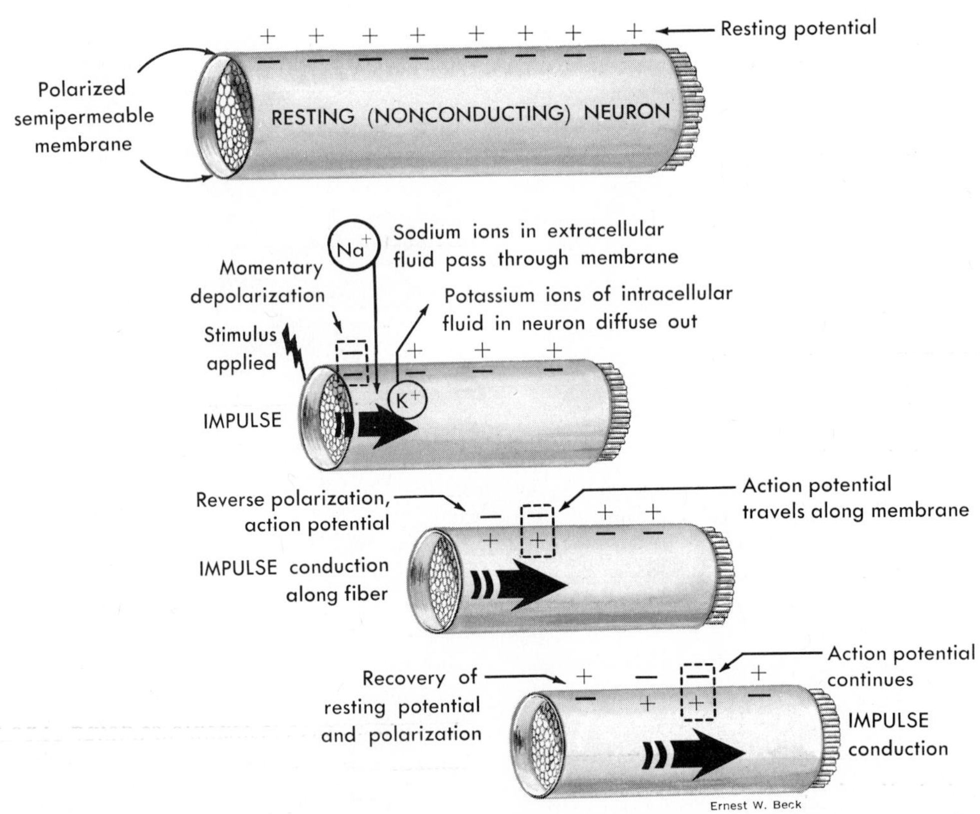

Fig. 34-2. Upper diagram represents polarized state of membrane of nerve fiber when it is not conducting impulses. Lower diagrams represent nerve impulse conduction: a self-propagating wave of negativity or action potential travels along membrane. (From Anthony, C. P., and Thibodeau, G. A.: Textbook of anatomy and physiology, ed. 10, St. Louis, 1979, The C. V. Mosby Co.)

cells. The resting potential of the neuron is unstable under certain conditions. It is capable of generating action potentials. When the neuron is stimulated internally or externally, the resting potential changes abruptly toward the cell's threshold or *depolarizes* and then quickly returns to its resting potential value *(repolarizes)*. This results in a brief change in the inside-outside voltage charge (Fig. 34-2). The resting potential changes or depolarizes abruptly from −60 to −40 mV toward zero, or its threshold. The membrane becomes momentarily more positive with a decrease in the inside-outside potential difference, and then it quickly changes back to −60 mV. This process of depolarization and repolarization is termed an *action potential*. It is unique to excitable cells and is the basic phenomenon underlying all nervous system function. These terms have their origin in the fact that the axon is normally polarized; that is, the axon has a resting potential value, and any alteration in resting membrane potential that decreases this resting polarization is called *depolarization*, any increase in the polarization is called *hyperpolarization*, and the return to resting potential is called *repolarization*. The action potential occurs within 1 to 2 msec.

When an action potential reaches a threshold value, it proceeds *automatically to completion* independent of the property of the stimulus that initiated the depolarization; that is, a strong stimulus does not give rise to a large action potential but does cause it to proceed to completion. This occurs in an all-or-none fashion. The action potential is also spread, or propagated, over its entire membrane without a decrease in its velocity. The propagation velocity is related to the size of the axon. The larger the diameter the higher the velocity. For a brief period the cell membrane is *refractory* and cannot generate another action potential. In review, the single neuron with its property of excitability when stimulated has the ability to react, spread, and subsequently stimulate the entire cell membrane.

Many action potentials of neurons originate in a receptor neuron where internal and external stimuli are normally received. A receptor is like a transducer and can change one form of energy into another form. A receptor, however, responds or depolarizes to *only one* type of stimulus. For example, the retina of the eye responds only to the stimulus of light, which is converted to electrical energy and travels over the optic nerves to the visual cortices for perception. In this way the receptor neuron may initiate the depolarization. It does, however, limit what the neuron responds to, although the receptor neuron does obey the all-or-none theory; a strong stimulus does make the receptor neuron fire more action potentials *per unit of time* within its time limitations than does a weak stimulus.

Neurons make functional contact with one another at specialized sites called *synapses*. Whenever an action potential is generated in one neuron that invades a synapse site, a sequence of processes results in the action potential affecting the second neuron. Transmission across a synapse is essentially a *chemical process*. The end of the axon contains a chemical substance located within its vesicles. When an action potential reaches the vesicle, it releases a transmitter substance, which then diffuses across the synapse to the adjacent neuronal cell membrane. *Synaptic transmission* is both *excitatory* and *inhibitory* in nature. Each neuron, however, only acts when its membrane is *depolarized to threshold*. Whether it fires depends on the sum of excitatory and inhibitory inputs.

In summary, the single neuron has all the structural and functional building elements of an electrical conductance system that also makes interconnections with adjacent neurons at synapses. Collectively neurons are in turn organized into larger and larger units of function that serve to coordinate all body activities. All neurons function basically in the same way. There is, however, a major difference in the functions carried out by the sensory and motor neurons.

In neurologic assessment it should be appreciated by the examiner that any disruption in the conductance system results in dysfunction distal to the break. The degree of change in status of a particular function(s) depends on the location and nature of the stressor or lesion causing the disruption.

□ Division of the nervous system

Macroscopically the nervous system is divided into two major divisions: the central nervous system and the peripheral nervous system.

Central nervous system

The central nervous system (CNS) is made up of collections of neurons and their connections organized into the brain and spinal cord areas. All of the basic informational processes as summarized on p. 626 occur within the CNS. Areas of the brain and spinal cord are distinguished where cell bodies are concentrated into *nuclei* and groups of axons running in *tracts* that interconnect the parts. Collections of neurons are connected in complex ways. The *connections* determine what each collection of neurons is capable of doing. The neurons are organized into circuits, some of which are simple and made up of relatively few neurons and others that are very complex. A single neuron may be a component of a number of different neuronal circuits and thus play a role in different functions.

Structurally the brain and spinal cord are continuous (Fig. 34-3). They are protectively housed within the skull and vertebral column, respectively. When injured, cen-

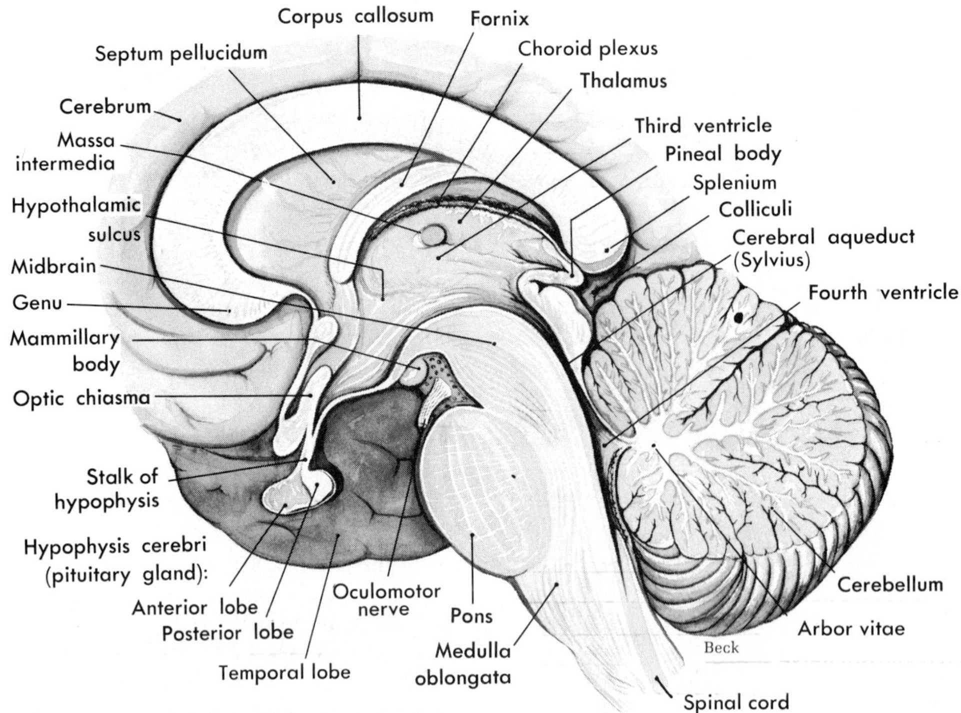

Fig. 34-3. Ventral surface of brain showing continuity of brain and spinal cord. (From Anthony, C. P., and Thibodeau, G. A.: Textbook of anatomy and physiology, ed. 10, St. Louis, 1979, The C. V. Mosby Co.)

trally located neurons are unable to reproduce themselves. The brain (encephalon) is grossly divided rostrally to caudally into three main areas: the *cerebrum*, *brainstem* (diencephalon, midbrain, pons, and medulla), and *cerebellum*. Each circuit or area carries out unique functions.

The *cerebrum* of each hemisphere (right and left) is further organized into four major lobes (frontal, parietal, temporal, and occipital). The cortex of the cerebrum receives and analyzes all impulses, controls voluntary movements, and stores knowledge of all impulses received. Each cerebral lobe is named from overlying cranial bones and carries out one or more of the following functions: general sensation perception (pain, touch, temperature, and pressure), special senses perception (hearing, vision, smell, taste), and speech. The brainstem is placed deeply in the center of the hemispheres and is not visible when viewing the intact brain. It includes a series of parts making connections with the spinal cord at the level of the medulla (Fig. 34-3), and it carries all nerve fibers passing between the hemispheres and the cord. All cranial nerves except the olfactory nerve (I) arise from it (Fig. 34-4). The *cerebellum* is attached to the lower portion of the brainstem. It generally aids in coordination of voluntary muscle movement.

The *spinal cord* structurally includes H-shaped central gray matter (nerve cell bodies) surrounded by white matter composed of ascending and descending tracts (Fig. 34-5). Functionally the spinal cord serves primarily as a passageway for conducting information over sensory, or afferent, tracts to the brain and over motor, or efferent, tracts from the brain.

The spinal cord is also the site of reflex pathways. Reflexes are an example of the simplest neuronal circuit. They do *not* require relay to the brain level for action. A reflex action consists of a *specific stereotyped motor response to an adequate sensory stimulus.* The response may involve movement or glandular secretion. It may involve only two neurons as in a simple monosynaptic reflex arc such as occurs with the myotactic knee jerk reflex. In the knee jerk reflex, a brisk tap over a partially stretched knee tendon stimulates sensory nerve endings within the tendons, and the stimulus travels over a sensory nerve fiber within a peripheral nerve toward the spinal cord where it synapses with a central motor neuron (anterior horn cell). Following stimulation across the synapse the impulse is transmitted down the motor nerve (over anterior nerve root of the spinal nerve or peripheral nerve). It is then transmitted across the neuromuscular junction to stimulate the muscle to con-

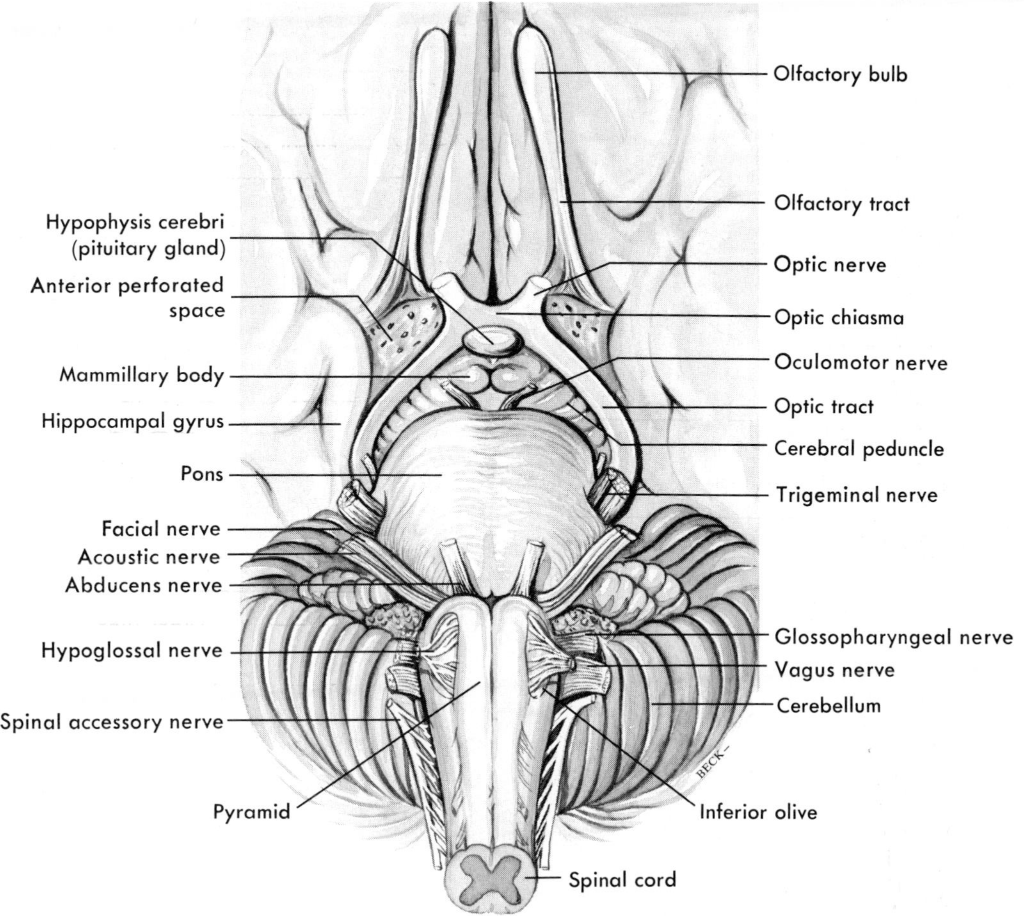

Fig. 34-4. Sagittal section through midline of brain showing structures around third ventricle and individual cranial nerves arising from midbrain. (From Anthony, C. P., and Thibodeau, G. A.: Textbook of anatomy and physiology, ed. 10, St. Louis, 1979, The C. V. Mosby Co.)

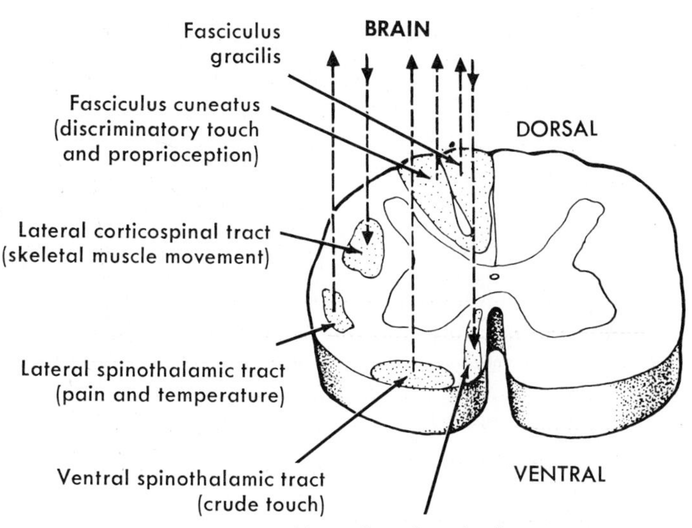

Fig. 34-5. Some nerve pathways between spinal cord and brain that arise from white matter of cord. Note H-shaped gray matter of cord.

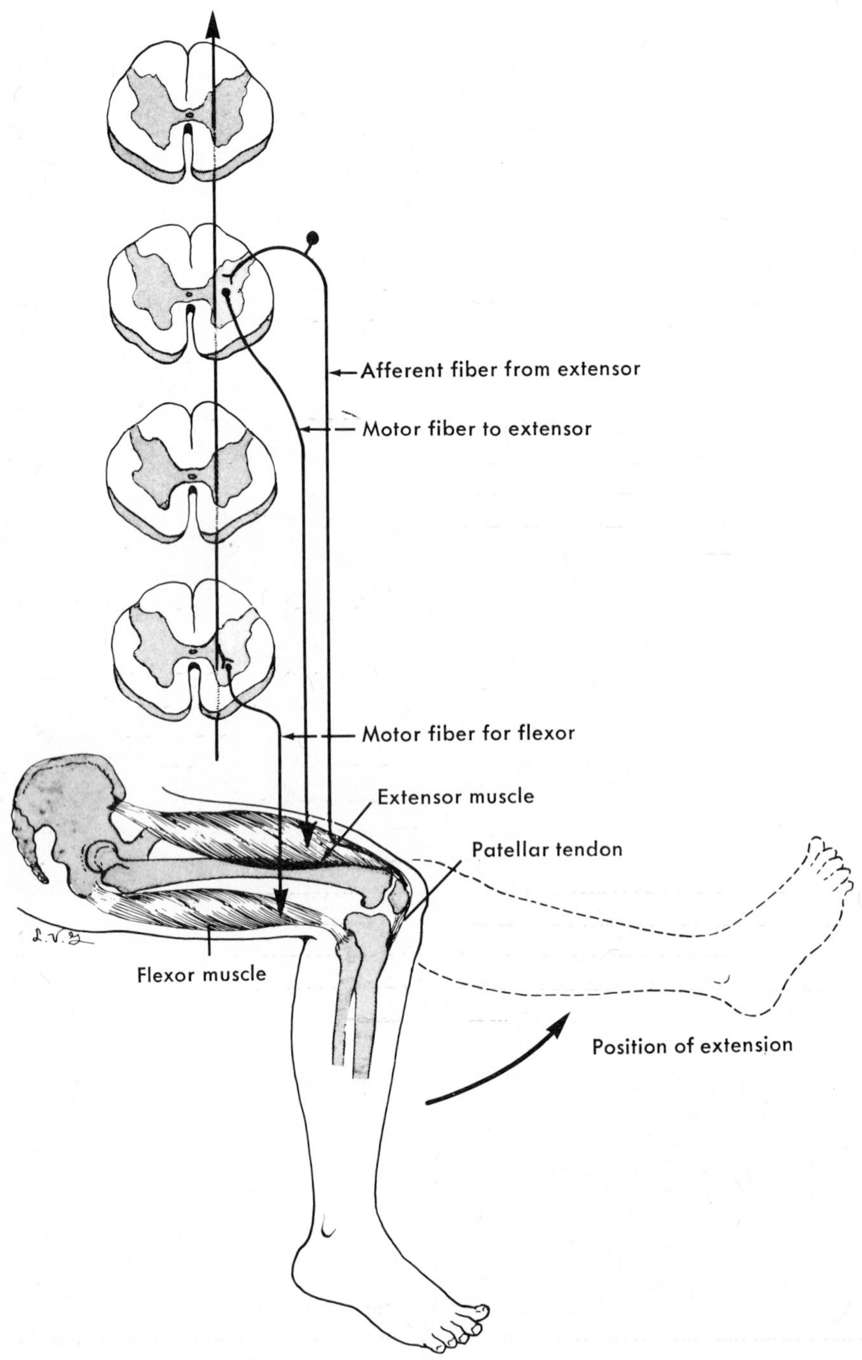

Fig. 34-6. Deep-tendon reflex (knee jerk or patellar tendon reflex) representative of reflex arc. Note that patellar tendon of extensor muscle is attached to tibia below knee. (From Schottelius, B. A., and Schottelius, D. D.: Textbook of physiology, ed. 18, St. Louis, 1978, The C. V. Mosby Co.)

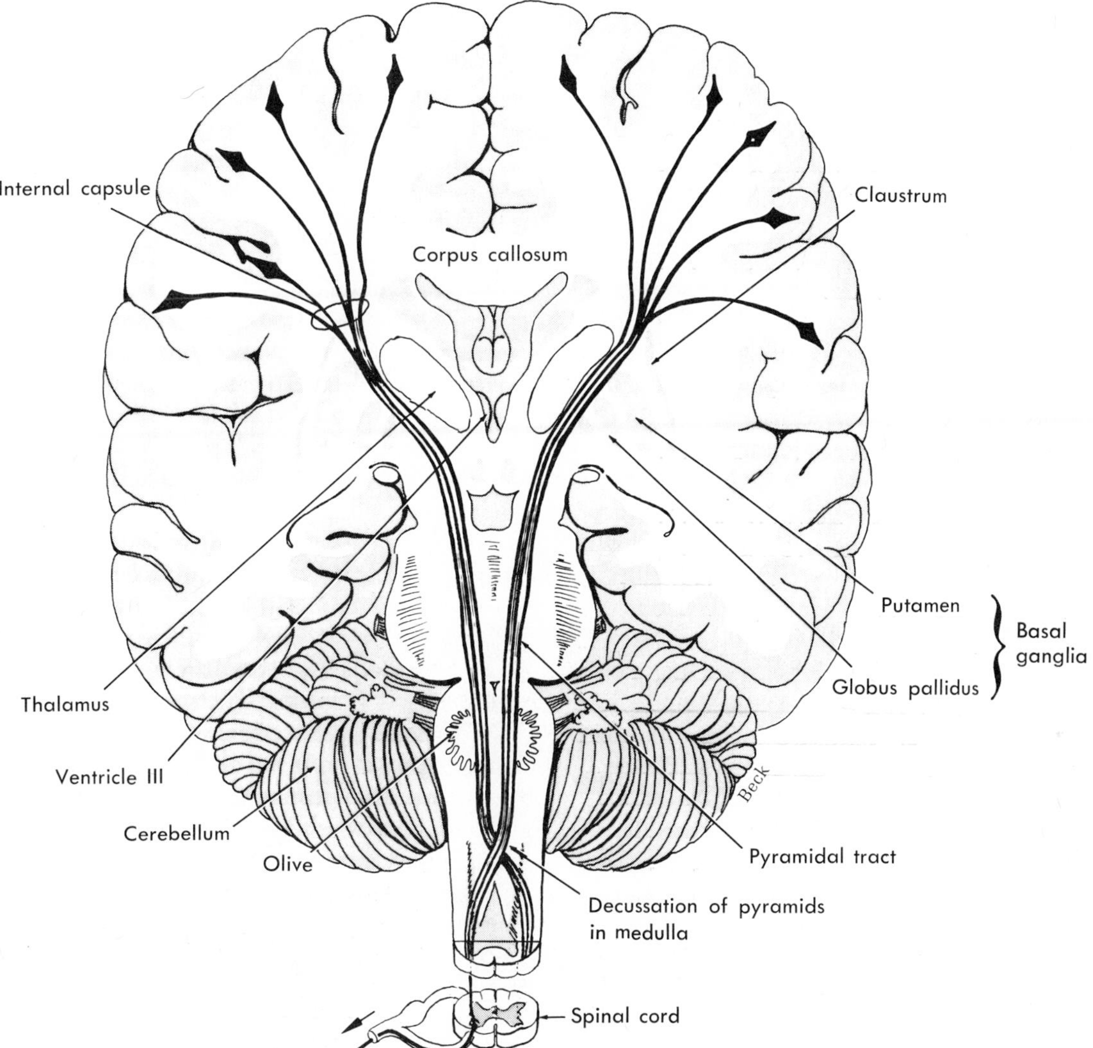

Fig. 34-7. Crossed corticospinal (pyramidal) tracts. Axons that compose pyramidal tracts (corticospinal) come from neuron cell bodies in cerebral cortex. After they descend through internal capsule of cerebrum and white matter of brainstem, about three fourths of fibers decussate (cross over from one side to the other) in medulla, as shown. Then they continue downward in lateral corticospinal tract on opposite side of cord. Each crossed corticospinal tract therefore conducts motor impulses from one side of brain to interneurons or anterior horn motoneurons on opposite side of cord. Therefore impulses from one side of cerebrum cause movements of opposite side of body. (From Anthony, C. P., and Thibodeau, G. A.: Textbook of anatomy and physiology, ed. 10, St. Louis, 1979, The C. V. Mosby Co.)

tract. Fig. 34-6 shows the reflex arc. In summary, a reflex arc is dependent on an intact sensory nerve, a functional synapse with a central neuron within the spinal cord, an intact motor nerve fiber, a neuromuscular junction, and a competent muscle.

A reflex may involve only one spinal cord level as in the knee jerk reflex, or it may involve one or a few spinal cord levels *(segmental reflexes)*, or it may involve structures in the brain that influence the spinal cord *(supraspinal* reflexes).

Peripheral nervous system

The peripheral nervous system (PNS) is basically a set of communication channels located outside the central nervous system. Peripheral nerves are bundles of individual nerves that are either sensory, motor, or mixed nerves. Structurally the PNS consist of 12 pairs of cranial nerves and 31 pairs of spinal nerves. The cranial nerves carry impulses to and from the brain; spinal nerves carry impulses to and from the spinal cord (Fig. 34-4).

Functionally the *autonomic nervous system* includes those peripheral nerves (both cranial and spinal) that regulate those functions occurring automatically in the body (cardiovascular, respiratory, endocrine, and other functional systems). The autonomic system is further subdivided into a *sympathetic nervous system*, which generally accelerates some body functions, and a *parasympathetic system*, which balances the action of the sympathetic system.

In summary, the function of nerves may be categorized generally as follows. Fibers that innervate the body wall are designated as *somatic;* those that innervate the viscera are termed *visceral.* Peripheral nerves that transmit information toward the CNS are *afferent* or *sensory* in nature, while peripheral nerves that transmit information away from the CNS are *efferent*, or *motor*, in nature. Peripherally the sensory and motor nerves usually travel together; however, they become separated centrally at the cord level into a *posterior* or sensory *root* and an *anterior* or motor *root*, respectively.

Injury to an individual peripheral nerve is followed by paralysis with loss of movement and sensation limited to those muscles and skin areas supplied by nerves distal to the lesion. Recognition of peripheral nerve losses is based on knowledge of the gross anatomy of the course and distribution of these nerves.

□ Motor system pathways

Descending motor pathways from the brain include the corticospinal tract, or the pyramidal system, the extrapyramidal system, and the cerebellar system.

Corticospinal tract fibers arise from neurons located in the primary motor area of the cerebral cortex in the precentral gyrus of the frontal lobe, premotor cortex, and the parietal lobe. This system is primarily concerned with skilled skeletal muscle movements of the distal extremities and in particular with the alpha and gamma motor neurons that innervate distal flexor musculature.

After fibers leave the cerebral cortex, they descend through the posterior limb of the internal capsule, middle of the cerebral cerebri, break up into bundles in the basilar portion of the pons, and then collect into discrete bundles within the pyramids of the medulla. In the medulla the majority of the fibers cross over, or *decussate*, to the opposite side of the medulla and become the *lateral* corticospinal tract, which then passes to all spinal cord levels in the lateral funiculus and terminally synapse in the lateral aspect of laminae IV through VIII (Fig. 34-7). The remaining fibers descend directly from the medulla (do not decussate) and synapse directly with alpha and gamma neurons in lamina IX of the spinal cord. The latter is known as the *anterior corticospinal tract.* The *left* cerebral motor strip of the primary motor area controls the muscular movement of the right side of the body.

Skeletal muscle activity is the result of the net influence on the alpha and gamma motor neurons of the spinal cord and on the motor components of the cranial nerve nuclei. Collectively these are the neurons that provide the final direct link with muscles through myoneural junctions at motor end-plates. Such neurons are referred to as lower motor neurons (pp. 674-676 for more complete discussion of upper and lower motor neurons).

The *extrapyramidal tracts* are complex and provide separate pathways between the cortex, the basal ganglia, the brainstem, and the cord. In general these include all descending motor pathways *other than* the corticospinal tract (indicating that they do not pass through the pyramids of the medulla). In general these tracts are named from point of origin to termination. The extrapyramidal tracts collectively assist in maintaining muscle tonus and the control of gross skeletal muscle movements. Some tracts tend to facilitate extensor activity and inhibit flexor activity (lateral vestigulospinal tract and pontine reticulospinal tract), while others facilitate flexor activity and inhibit extensor activity (lateral corticospinal tract and rubrospinal tract).

The *cerebellar system* is responsible for muscle synergy throughout the body. The cerebellum coordinates the action of muscle groups and controls their contractions so that movements are performed smoothly and accurately. Voluntary movements can proceed without the cerebellum, but movements would be clumsy and incoordinated *(asynergia* and *cerebellar ataxia).* The cerebellum receives both *sensory* and *motor inputs.* There are feedback circuits with all the descending

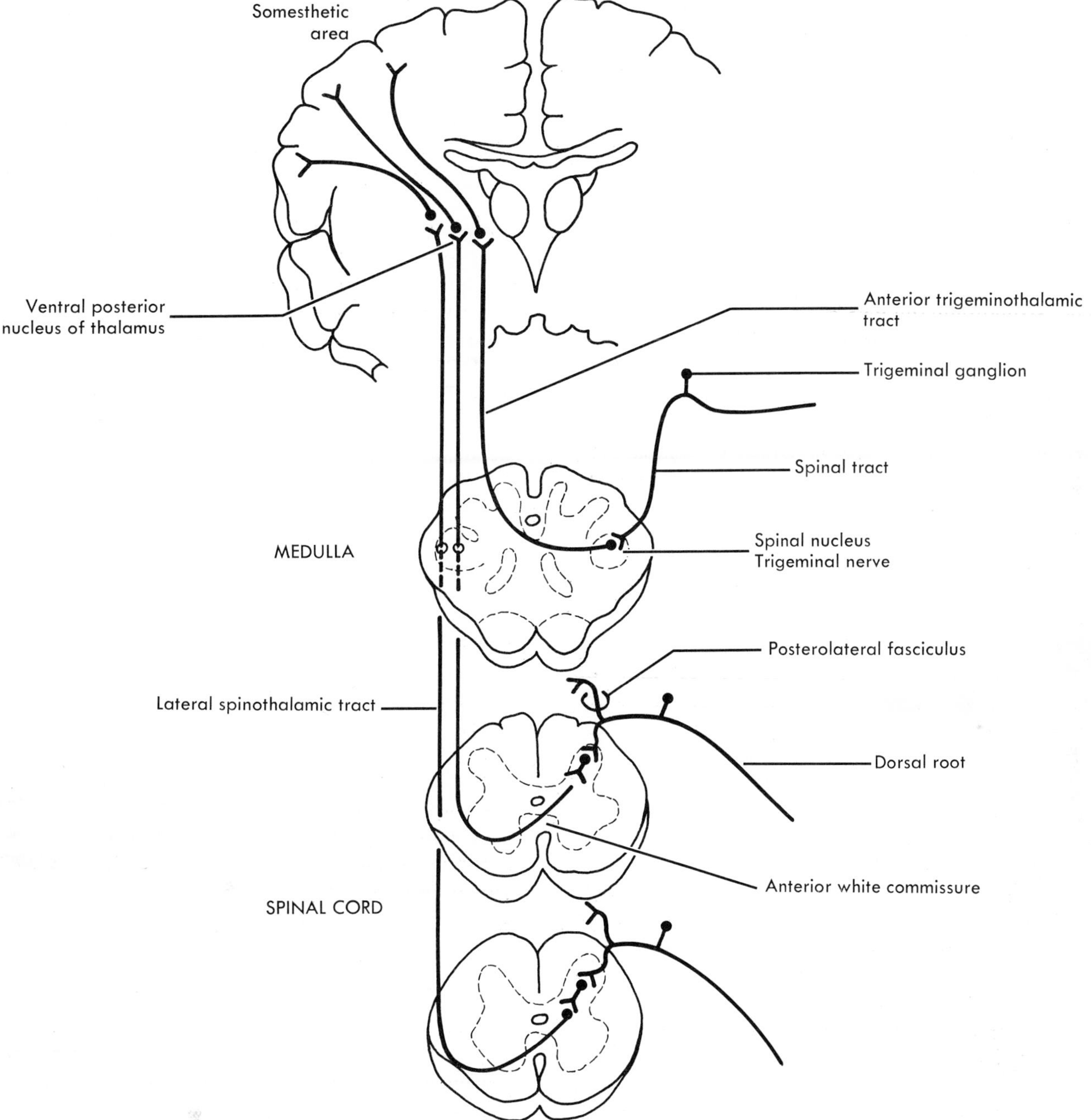

Fig. 34-8. Pain and temperature sensory pathway. Note how stimuli entering through dorsal root (posterior) cross over to opposite side to lateral spinothalamic tract and then ascend to thalamus and end in somesthetic area, where perception occurs.

motor pathways as discussed previously. All sensory modalities, including tactile, auditory, and visual, also feed impulses to the cerebellum. The general scheme of cerebellar operation allows nerve impulses to be returned to or fed back to, the same region from which they originated. These circuits can be compared with modern automatic control devices, or servomechanisms. The cerebellar cortex, similar to a computer, can detect any errors in muscle synergy and return the proper messages to adjust muscular control within the body.

Visceral efferent motor pathways from the spinal cord mediate the action of *involuntary*, or *smooth, muscles* located within walls of tubes, hollow organs, the heart, and the glands. Most viscera are supplied by both excitatory and inhibiting fibers.

☐ Sensory system pathways

Sensation as perceived by the person is initiated by stimulation of receptor neurons located throughout the body. The general sensory system pathways include (1) receptor neurons responsive to special stimuli from both the internal and external environments, (2) the posterior roots of the peripheral or afferent sensory nerves carrying action potential (nerve impulses) toward the central nervous system, (3) ascending or sensory tracts located within the spinal cord and upper brain centers, and (4) sensory areas of the cerebral cortex where stimuli are perceived and localized.

After entry into the spinal cord, sensory nerve impulses can proceed along one or two courses: the spinothalamic tract or the posterior columns. The pathway followed is specific to the sensation. For example, nerve fibers conducting the sensations of *pain* and *temperature* pass into the posterior horn of the spinal cord within a few spinal segments from entry and synapse with a secondary sensory neuron. From this neuron nerve impulses pass immediately to the *contralateral*, or opposite, side of the cord and then pass upward in the spinothalamic tract through the remaining pathways to the thalamus and then synapse with a third sensory neuron before termination in the sensory cortex (Fig. 34-8). Sensations of *fine touch, position,* and *vibration*, on the other hand, are conducted directly over the posterior columns to the level of the medulla before synapsing with a second neuron. The impulse then passes over to the opposite side to join the spinothalamic tract, continues on to the thalamus, and finally synapses with a third sensory neuron before termination at the sensory cortex. The general quality of sensation is perceived at the thalamic level. Full discrimination of senses is only made at *sensory cortex levels*.

It is the role of the receptor neuron to provide vital information to the body about the condition and composition of the internal environment, the position and action of the body, the status of internal viscera, and information from the external environment (through the eye, ear, nose, skin, and tongue).

Lesions at different points within the sensory pathways produce different types of sensory losses. Patterns of sensory loss such as to pain, temperature, touch, position, and vibration, along with motor findings, are helpful in localizing lesions. These may be shown as related to dermatomes as shown in Fig. 34-9. It should be understood that there is considerable variability and overlap of dermatomes.

Special sensory losses as related to the sensations of smell, vision, taste, and hearing follow unique sensory pathways and are relevant to the cranial nerve involved. Disruption of impulses from the receptor to any one part of the sensory pathway leads to a limitation of input and subsequent sensory loss.

☐ Effectors

Effectors may be thought of as the cells of the body that "do something." They in turn interact with the internal and external environments in some way and carry out the commands of the nervous system. The two classes of effectors are muscles and glands. They are both transducers and are capable of converting one form of energy into another form of energy. Effectors, like nerve tissue, are excitable tissues and are able to generate action potentials. The nervous system controls muscles and glands by directly turning them on or by altering their level of spontaneous activity through a neuron-to-effector chemical communication system.

■ NEUROLOGIC ASSESSMENT

Complete neurologic assessment is usually done in phases and is dependent on the condition of the person and the urgency in collecting the necessary data. It includes a *history, neurologic examination,* and *special neurodiagnostic procedures*. A discussion directed primarily to a description of the components of the neurologic examination follows.

☐ History

As in other specialties, a careful history precedes physical examination of the nervous sytem. In the course of the history taking, the person's chief complaints are elicited through an interview. The person is asked to give a timewise account of his illness in his own words. The onset and progression of the condition as well as the nature of symptoms should be determined. Special inquiry should be made in regard to common neurologic conditions or manifestations such as headache, convulsive seizures, and pain. Ongoing collection of psychosociocultural data is of special importance. Information is collected about family members and their relation-

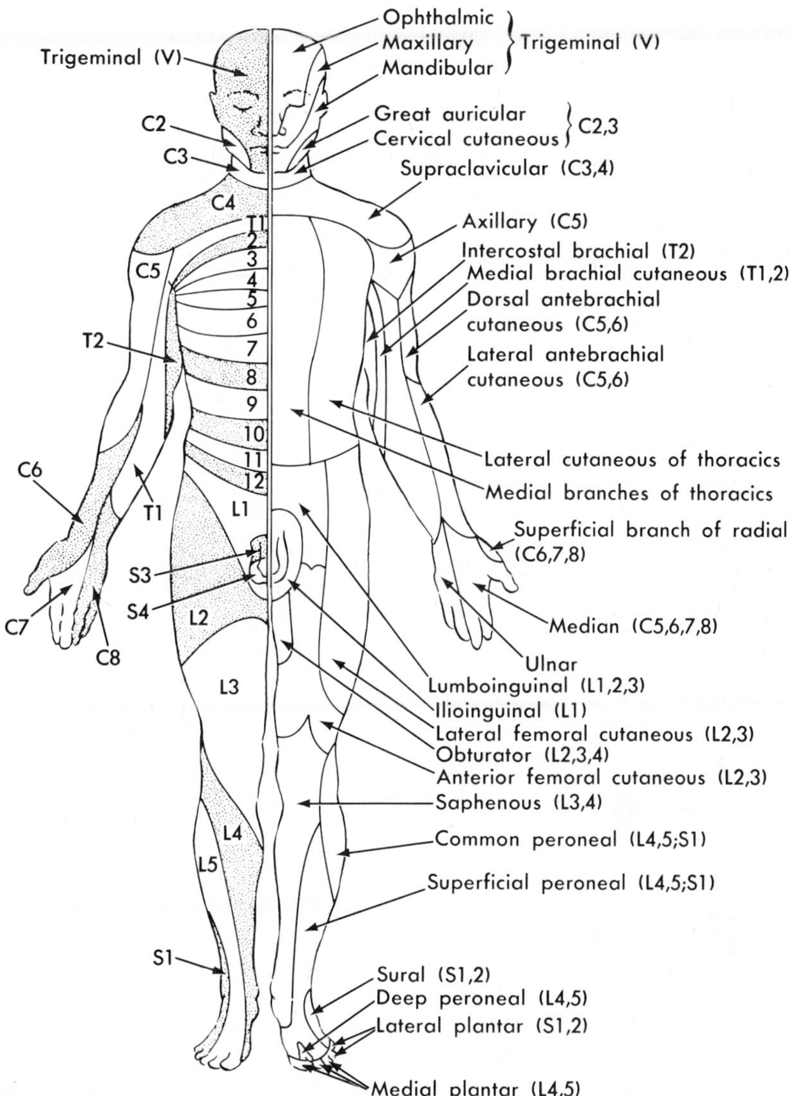

Fig. 34-9. Peripheral distribution of sensory nerve fibers. Anterior view. *Right,* distribution of cutaneous nerves. *Left,* dermatomes *(shaded)* or segmental distribution of cutaneous nerves. (Redrawn from House, E. L.: Neuroanatomy, ed. 2, New York, 1967, McGraw-Hill Book Co.)

ships and interactions, ethnic background, housing, recreational interests, occupation, education, coping pattern to stressors, dependence-independence characteristics, and usual activities of daily living and how they are correctly managed by the person. A family health history and developmental history is also included. During the course of the neurologic or physical examination, some of the observations made during the history may be confirmed. A skillfully taken history with accurate analysis and interpretation of the collected data often holds the key to diagnosis. Some observations made during the history that are validated during the examination will require further study through special neurodiagnostic procedures.

□ Neurologic examination

Neurologic examination of the conscious adult includes physical examination of the following components: *cranial nerves, mental status* (level of consciousness, orientation, mood and behavior, knowledge, vocabulary, memory), *sensory status* (touch, pain, temperature, proprioception), *language and speech, meninges,* and *motor status* (gait and stance, muscle strength, muscle tonus, coordination, involuntary movements, muscle

EQUIPMENT NEEDED TO PERFORM A NEUROLOGIC EXAMINATION

Compass
Cotton applicators
Diagram of dermatomes
Dynamometer
Flashlight
Miscellaneous items of varied shapes and sizes (coin, key, marble)
Ophthalmoscope
Otoscope
Colored pencil
Pins with sharp and blunt ends
Printed page
Reflex hammer
Tape measure
Tongue depressors
Tuning fork
Snellen chart
Stoppered vials containing:
1. Peppermint, oil of cloves, coffee, soap (smell)
2. Sugar, salt, vinegar, quinine (taste)
3. Cold and hot water (temperature)
Watch with second hand

stretch reflexes). The ongoing sequential discussion of each of these components provides the nurse with a framework for the kind of information that should be collected in order to make decisions about nursing care and to assist the physician in making a medical diagnosis.

The sequence in performing the neurologic examination varies with the examiner, but it should be one that ensures completeness and thoroughness without exhausting the person being examined. Throughout the examination the examiner attempts to localize the site of any abnormality. Using knowledge of normal neuroanatomy and neurophysiology, combined with a series of tests, the abnormal findings with reference to their *distribution* and *symmetry* of both sides of the body are noted by the examiner.

The examination depends largely on inspection and palpation and only occasionally on percussion. Auscultation may be used to detect related vascular abnormalities. Varied instruments are utilized. Initially, functions may be tested grossly, followed by definitive testing should an abnormality be identified.

Equipment required to perform a neurologic examination (in addition to materials used for a general physical examination) is often assembled for convenience on a neurologic tray (see box above).

Cranial nerve examination

A general description of cranial nerve testing is included at this point, since study of these nerves is essential to a complete study of the nervous system. Details as to techniques in the testing of each cranial nerve can be found in references 2, 7, and 11. It is further suggested in the study of the cranial nerves that it is helpful to recall from anatomy the number of the nerve (the sequence of the nerve along the rostrocaudal axis of the brain) and the name (explains the function or distribution). It is also helpful to be able to express in a few words the function(s) of each cranial nerve so that it has practical meaning. Knowledge of the brainstem anatomy assists in relating the cranial nerve locations (Fig. 34-4).

The 12 cranial nerves may be tested in numbered sequence as presented on the following pages. Some nurses prefer to test at the same time those cranial nerves that have similarity of function, such as voluntary motor function and visceral motor function and special sensory and general sensory functions. It should be recalled, however, that some cranial nerves have both motor and sensory functions, while others are purely motor or sensory. It also should be recognized by the examiner that data collected from sensory testing is subjective. To counteract this, the person should be retested several times and in a random order to avoid memorization by the examinee. Effort should be made to be as objective as possible and to collect valid data.

Cranial nerve I (olfactory). The function of this purely *sensory* nerve is smell. Special receptors located within the superior or uppermost part of each nasal chamber, when stimulated by odors, transmit neural impulses over the olfactory bulbs to the olfactory nerves terminating in the area of the central cortex concerned with olfaction. This nerve is tested with the examinee's eyes closed or blindfolded at all times. A nonpungent, familiar substance is held under each nostril. Each nostril is tested separately and with multiple substances, such as coffee, soap, tobacco, and peppermint, in a random pattern. The substance may be placed on an applicator or the person may be asked to sniff the substance from an open vial. First it is determined if an odor is perceived. If so, then identification of the specific odor is requested by name. Data is collected in relation to the ability to perceive odor and identify substances by their odor. The ability to be aware of an odor must be differentiated from the ability to name a specific substance. *Anosmia,* or the loss of sense of smell, is caused by varied lesions involving any part of the olfactory pathways. Neoplasia at the base of the frontal lobe and trauma are the common causes of neurogenic anosmia. Intranasal disease affecting the epithelium containing the receptors should be excluded before a diagnosis is made.

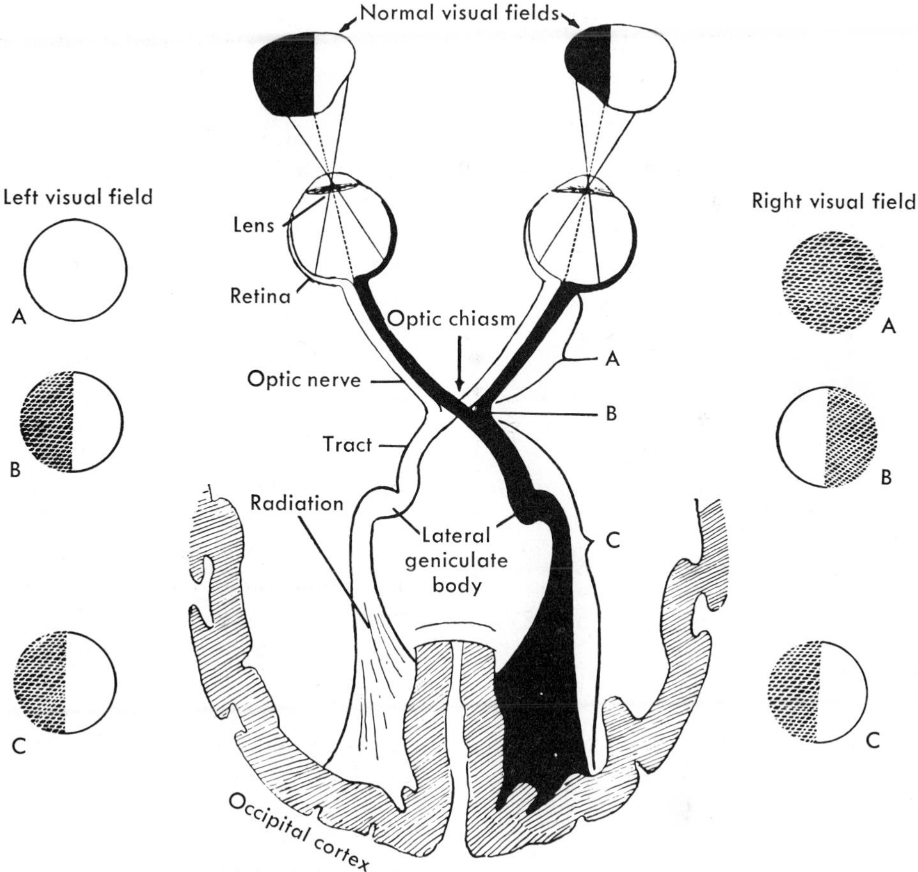

Fig. 34-10. Visual pathways showing partial decussation at optic chiasm and their radiation to end station of occipital cortex. Normal visual fields show reversal of light rays, through action of lens, from nasal and temporal sides to receptors in retina. Pathologic visual fields are illustrated. **A,** Loss of vision in right field resulting from complete lesion of right optic nerve; left field is normal. **B,** Loss of vision in temporal half of right and left fields caused by lesion involving optic chiasm (bitemporal hemianopia). **C,** Loss of vision in nasal field of right eye and in temporal field of left eye caused by lesion of right optic tract or radiation (homonymous hemianopia). Pathologic fields are lettered corresponding to sites of causative lesions. (From Conway, B. L.: Carini and Owens' neurological and neurosurgical nursing, ed. 7, St. Louis, 1978, The C. V. Mosby Co.)

Cranial nerve II (optic). The function of this purely *sensory* nerve is sight, or vision. Rods and cones, the special receptors sensitive to light, are located with the retina of the eye. When the retina is stimulated, nerve impulses are transmitted over the optic nerves (extend from the optic disc to the chiasm), over the optic tracts with the radiations terminating in the visual cortex of the occipital lobes. It should be noted, as shown in Fig. 34-10, that the medial (nasal) fibers of each optic nerve cross at the chiasm to the opposite side of the brain, while the lateral (temporal) fibers remain uncrossed. Thus fibers of the *left optic tract* contain only fibers from the left half of each retina and carry impulses to the left occipital lobe; fibers of the right optic tract contain only fibers from the right half of each retina and carry impulses to the right occipital lobe. Vision is dependent on the intactness of the visual pathways described above. Optic nerve function is assessed in relation to visual acuity, visual fields, and the appearance of the fundus (inner eye posterior to the lens). Each eye is tested separately.

Visual acuity. Central vision is grossly tested by reading fine newspaper print. Distant visual acuity is assessed through the use of the Snellen chart (p. 739).

Individuals with vision less than 20/20 are tested to determine light perception (LP), hand movement (HM), and finger count (FC).

Visual fields. Field of vision is defined as that portion of space in which objects are visible during the fixation of vision in *one* direction. The field of vision thus relates to peripheral vision, or indirect vision. As in visual acuity, normality is dependent on the intactness of all parts of the visual pathway of the eye. The receptors for peripheral fields are the rod neurons of the retina. These are efficient for detection of form and movement but are poor for vision and color. Visual acuity and color are functions of the central field. The visual fields are tested grossly by *confrontation techniques.* As the name implies, the examiner faces or confronts the person directly from a distance of 2 to 3 feet. Various methods are used; only one is discussed here. The individual is instructed to cover one eye and to focus steadily at a point directly ahead. Initially a small object such as a pencil or the examiner's finger is placed peripherally beyond the person's field of vision and then advanced centripetally until the examinee first indicates that the object is seen. Normally the individual should see about 60° nasalward, 50° upward, 90° temporally, and 70° downward. The eye should be tested in equally spaced meridians including the upper and lower nasal and temporal quadrants of each eye.

More accurate and discriminating study of the visual fields is performed through perimetry. With the aid of an arc marked in 90° sections it can be turned in any meridian.

Visual fields may be altered in a variety of central nervous system diseases such as neoplasia and vascular disease. Ocular disease such as glaucoma is a major cause. Damage to one optic nerve anterior to the chiasm affects only the field of the involved eye. Lesions at the chiasm or posterior to it produce bilateral visual field defects of a wide variety. For example, a pituitary gland tumor compressing the optic chiasm damages the crossing fibers from the nasal retina and classically causes bitemporal hemianopia, or the loss of vision in the temporal halves of each eye. Loss of vision in the corresponding halves of both visual fields produces *homonymous hemianopia* and can be further designated as right or left. Patients with right cerebrovascular accidents often experience hemianopsia.

Ocular fundus. The fundus is examined through the use of an instrument called an *ophthalmoscope.* The oscular fundus is defined as that portion of the interior of the eyeball that lies posterior to the lens. It includes the optic disc, blood vessels, retina, and macula.

The electric ophthalmoscope permits the examiner to see into the pupil through a lens and with a light along the viewer's line of sight. The latter is achieved by the light projected through a prism, which bends the light rays at a 90° angle. A number of different lenses arranged on a wheel can be dialed by a number on the instrument. A lens labeled with a red numeral assists in focusing farther away; a lens labeled with a black numeral assists in focusing nearer. The shape and color of the light beam can also be adjusted by the examiner; the light must always enter the pupil. Errors of refraction in the eyes of the examiner or examinee can be corrected by the use of lenses in the ophthalmoscope; as a rule glasses need not be worn by the examinee unless there is a high degree of astigmatism. The room is darkened so that the pupil dilates. Adequate funduscopic examination requires the use of mydriatic drugs such as phenylephrine (10%) to produce dilation of the pupil.

Examination, although painless in the normal eye, does require cooperation from the person being examined, who is asked to keep both eyes open and to focus on a distant object or on an imaginary point straight ahead. Care is taken that the person does *not focus* on the light from the instrument. Each eye is examined separately. The examiner stands or sits directly in front of the examineee. To avoid misalignment the instrument rests firmly against the nose or cheek of the examiner so that the lens of the instrument is directly in front of the pupil of the eye being examined.

The right hand and right eye are used to examine the person's right eye, the left hand and left eye to examine the left eye. The examiner's index finger rests on the lens dial to facilitate interchange of dials during examination. The position of the instrument is usually not moved, but the head of the examiner moves in closer to the examinee and in varying positions in order to better view the inner anatomic structures. Initially the focus is directly on the pupil; *a red glow or reflex* can be noted as directed. When the fundus is examined, the examiner is at a 15° angle temporal to the person's line of vision. The lens focus is then adjusted.

The entire fundus is not visualized at one time. The examiner *systematically* scans the fundus, examining each part in *detail* beginning with the optic disc. The optic disc, blood vessels, periphery, and macula are examined in sequence. The neurologist's primary interest in ophthalmoscopy is in determining whether abnormalities of the optic disc and retina or vascular diseases associated with neurologic diseases are present. Discussion here is limited to these aspects. The reader is referred to Chapter 38 for further discussion of ophthalmoscopy as related to diagnosing other diseases involving the eye.

Examination and interpretation of ophthalmoscopic findings. The optic disc (papilla) is normally the most prominent structure visible; *it is the center of observation from which the funduscopic* examination proceeds.

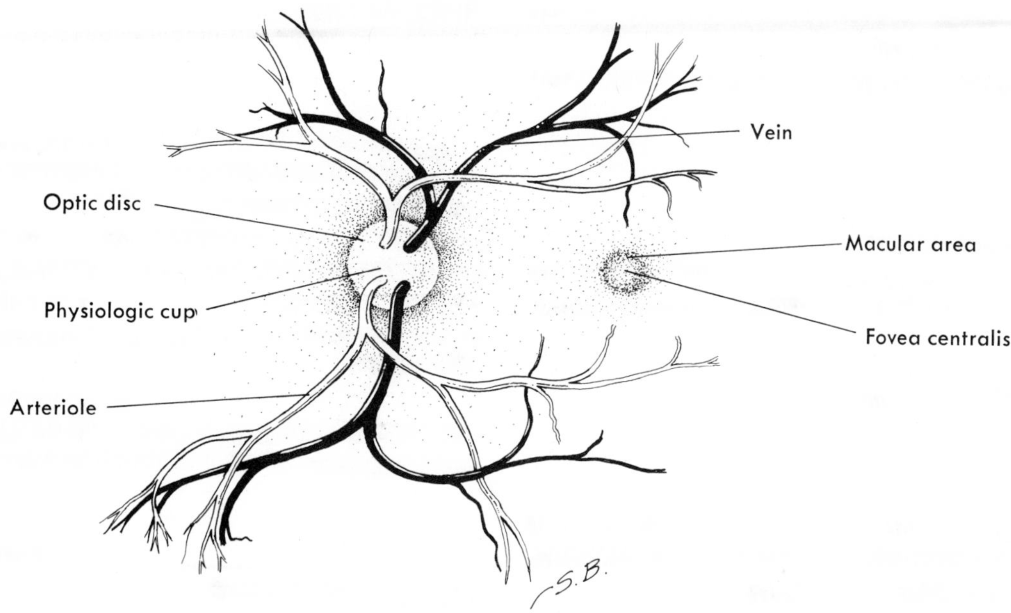

Fig. 34-11. Funduscopic structures of left eye. (From Malasanos, L., Barkauskas, V., Moss, M., and Stoltenberg-Allen, K.: Health assessment, St. Louis, 1977, The C. V. Mosby Co.)

It is the area where the blood vessels and nerve fibers enter and exit from the eyeball (Fig. 34-11). The normal characteristics of the optic disc are presented in the box at right.

The disc is examined in detail as to normality of size, shape, margins, and color. There can be excessive pallor or redness. Swelling of the optic disc, or *papilledema*, may be due to active inflammation or passive congestion. Papilledema due to passive congestion and edema from increased intracranial pressure is called *choked* disc (see Chapter 38). The neurologist is most interested in differentiating between early and late papilledema. *Optic atrophy* indicates partial or complete destruction of the optic nerve. It is associated with decreased visual acuity and with change in color of the disc to a lighter pink or gray. The recognition of advanced papilledema is relatively easy, but differentiation of physiologic variations is difficult.

The largest blood vessels just visible in the fundus, the central retinal artery and central retinal vein, branch throughout the retina. Each vessel is carefully examined along its length from the disc to the periphery. The arterioles of the retina diverge from the disc, and the veins converge toward the disc. The retina is the only site in the human body where microcirculation can be viewed directly. In examination of the blood vessels the arteries normally appear lighter in color and narrower than the veins, and they intertwine. Veins pulsate. Examination is made relative to size, color, or fullness. Normally arteries do not indent or displace veins. *Periphery* is the area adjacent to the disc, outside the disc and between the large vessels.

NORMAL CHARACTERISTICS OF THE OPTIC DISC

Size	1.5 mm
Shape	Flat round or vertically oval
Margins	Sharply defined
Color	Creamy red with a small whitish depression in the center (physiologic cup)

The macula is situated temporal to the optic disc. It is 1 DD (disc diameter) in size and is vascular. A glistening spot of reflected light seen in the macula represents a pinpoint depression and is the *fovea centralis* (region of retina with highest visual acuity). For this reason a small macular lesion may be more disabling than a considerably larger peripheral lesion and results in a greater decrease in visual acuity. Last, the direction of light beam is adjusted to view the extreme periphery (examinee's eyes follow the light beam).

Cranial nerve III (oculomotor), cranial nerve IV (trochlear), and cranial nerve VI (abducens). These three *motor nerves* arise from the brainstem and innervate the six extraocular muscles attached to the eyeball.

These muscles function as a group in the coordinated movement of each eyeball in the six cardinal fields of gaze (straight, up, and down on both nasal and temporal sides). The oculomotor nerves in addition send parasympathetic autonomic fibers to the constrictor muscles of the iris and to the levator palpebrae muscles of the upper eyelids.

Extraocular movements. Individual eye movements are tested by covering one eye and following the examiner's finger in all fields of gaze with the uncovered eye while keeping the head stationary. Limitations of movement in all directions are observed as well as actual paralysis *(ophthalmoplegia).* If one of the extraocular muscles is paralyzed by damage to the nerve, the eye is unable to deviate fully into the corresponding field of gaze.

Conjugate movements of the eyes are also tested by asking the person to look with both eyes as far possible to either side and then up and down. The examiner observes for parallel movements of the eyes in each direction or any deviation from normal.

Double vision *(diplopia),* squint *(strabismus),* and involuntary rhythmic movements of the eyeballs *(nystagmus)* may indicate weakness of some of the extraocular muscles due to deficits of these motor nerves. These nerves may be involved singly or in unison in some neurologic diseases. *Ptosis,* or drooping of the upper eyelid over the globe, may be caused by damage to the oculomotor nerve. Normally the upper lid minimally overlaps the iris as the examinee moves the eyes downward. The person with ptosis is unable to raise the lid voluntarily.

Pupils. Each pupil should be inspected first as to size then as to shape and equality. *Argyll Robertson* pupils, for example, are constricted and do not react to light, although they react to accommodation for near objects (p. 713). Pupil inequality, or *anisocoria,* may assist in diagnosis of some neurologic diseases. The pupil is normally round, centrally placed, regular in outline, and equal in size to the other pupil.

Pupillary reflex. The examiner darkens the room before examination. A small beam of light is focused directly into each eye in turn. The examiner avoids shining the light into both eyes simultaneously and instructs the person not to focus on the light beam, thus producing an accommodation reaction. Normally the pupil constricts quickly when a light is focused on the homolateral retina. After a head injury, for example, a *dilated, fixed* pupil may be observed on the side of the cranial injury. A slow or sluggish pupil occurs as the pupil contracts slowly or imperfectly and relaxes immediately.

Consensual light reflex. Observations include inspection for constriction of the pupil *opposite* to the one directly stimulated. As a result of the decussation (crossing) of nerve fibers both in the optic chiasm and in the pretectal area, the homolateral as well as the contralateral pupil normally react to light.

Cranial nerve V (trigeminal nerve). This is a *mixed* nerve, with motor and sensory components. It is the largest cranial nerve. The motor part innervates the temporal and masseter muscles; the sensory part supplies the cornea, face, head, and mucous membrane. The motor component is tested by asking the person to bite on a tongue blade and to resist its being removed as the examiner pulls on it and attempts to push it to the opposite side. The masseter, temporalis, and pterygoid muscles are palpated by the examiner at the same time to determine their size and strength. In muscle weakness the opened jaw tends to deviate to the opposite side of the weakened muscles. The sensory components supplying the face are tested for touch, pain, and temperature and for any deficits noted as to distribution. (See discussion of sensory status as to the technique of examination).

Cranial nerve VII (facial nerve). This *mixed nerve* has to do with facial movement and the sensation of taste. The motor part is tested by asking the person to perform specific facial movements while the examiner observes for muscle weakness. The inability to smile, close both eyes tightly, look upward and wrinkle the forehead, show the teeth, purse the lips, and blow out the cheeks constitutes weakness or paralysis of facial muscles innervated by this nerve. Distinction must be made between central and peripheral neurologic involvement. Special attention in examination is given to asymmetry. Peripheral involvement as in *Bell's palsy* is caused by compression of this cranial nerve and is a common *lower motor neuron* type of facial paralysis. Lesions affecting the facial nerve produce paralysis of half of the entire face including the eyelids, forehead, and lips. Forehead function, by contrast, remains intact in *central* or *upper motor neuron* lesions. The sensation of taste is tested by placing, in turn, salty, sweet, bitter, and sour substances on the side of the protruded tongue for identification. A loss of taste over the anterior two thirds of the tongue is present when the nerve is diseased, as in mastoid canal lesions.

Cranial nerve VIII (acoustic nerve). This nerve is composed of a *cochlear* division related to hearing and a *vestibular* division related to equilibrium. The cochlear portion is tested grossly by having the examinee listen and identify whispered words or the ticking of a watch. A more complete examination including bone and air conduction of sound includes testing with a tuning fork (p. 752) and audiometric testing (p. 749). The vestibular portion of the acoustic nerve may be tested in a variety of ways. In the *past-pointing test*, the examinee is asked to raise his arms and to bring the index finger down on the examiner's finger with the arm outstretched, first with the eyes open, then with eyes closed. Normally the examinee's finger touches the examiner's without difficulty. In vestibular disease the finger points to one side or the other consistently. The vestibular portion is also tested by looking for the presence of *nystagmus*, "to-and-fro" movements of the eyeballs on horizontal and vertical planes, as the examinee looks to one side and upward. True nystagmus is characterized by sustained movement of the eyeball including a fast jerk to the side of the deviation and a slow jerk back to the midline. Additional tests can include caloric tests and electronystagmography (p. 752). Nerve deafness is usually the result of disease of the peripheral nerve but may also occur from central lesions involving acoustic nerves and nerve pathways in the brainstem and their termination within the temporal lobe. The vestibular portion is frequently affected in diseases of the central nervous system, and the most prominent symptom is vertigo.

Normal hearing. Disease of the *cochlea* is characterized by nerve deafness (perception deafness). There is loss or impairment of hearing. Nerve deafness is usually the result of disease of the peripheral nerve. It may also occur from central lesions involving *acoustic nerves and nerve pathways* in the brainstem and their *termination within the temporal lobe.*

Cranial nerve IX (glossopharyngeal) and cranial nerve X (vagus). These nerves are tested together. The chief function of cranial nerve IX is *sensory* to the pharynx and taste to the posterior third of the tongue. Both nerves supply the posterior pharyngeal wall, and normally when the wall is touched there is prompt contraction of these muscles on both sides, with or without gagging. This test is thus unreliable in regard to either nerve alone. Since cranial nerve X is the chief *motor nerve* to the soft palatal, pharyngeal, and laryngeal muscles, the detection of abnormalities is made through testing of voice sounds and cough sounds. In unilateral involvement of the motor portion of the vagus nerve there is harshness and nasality of the voice. When the person says "ah" the soft palate does not stay in the midline but deviates to the intact side. Bilateral involvement produces more severe effects in speech; there is also difficulty in swallowing *(dysphagia)*, and fluids regurgitate through the nose because of palatal and pharyngeal involvement. Sensory function is not usually tested in the vagus nerve.

Cranial nerve XI (spinal accessory nerve). This nerve is tested by having the person rotate his head against resistance while any weakness of the sternocleidomastoid muscle on the opposite side is observed and palpated by the examiner. The ability of the person to shrug his shoulder is also tested. Weakness or paralysis of these muscles constitutes abnormality of this nerve.

Cranial nerve XII (hypoglossal nerve). This nerve is tested by having the person stick out his tongue and move it from side to side. When this nerve is involved, there is deviation of the tongue toward the side of the lesion. Atrophy of the tongue is shown through wrinkling and loss of substance on the affected side. In an upper motor neuron lesion there is involvement of the tongue on the side opposite (contralateral) the lesion.

Mental status

Specific abnormalities of higher cerebral function are particularly significant in determining the presence of organic brain disease; therefore clinical observation of mental function is important.

A determination of the level of consciousness of the person (awareness of self and environment) is necessary (see Chapter 27 for a more detailed discussion). Although many metabolic and toxic states produce changes in consciousness, destructive lesions of the brain do so directly. With destructive lesions there also may be elevation of consciousness as evidenced by insomnia, agitation, mania, and delirium.

The patient is also tested as to orientation to time (day, month, week), place, and person. Disorientation to place and person indicates a more profound cerebral disorder. It is helpful to remember that orientation depends on the ongoing sensory impressions.

The identification of mood and behavior is also included in a mental examination, since a particular mood may be associated with a specific disease. For example, emotional lability is often seen in bilateral (diffuse) brain disease, where the mood shifts easily and quickly from one extreme to the other. Euphoria is a superficial elevation of mood accompanied by unconcern even in the presence of threatening events. It needs to be determined if the person's mood is appropriate to the topic of conversation. Personality changes with the appearance of violent temper and aggressive behavior may occur with destructive lesions of the inferior frontal parts of the limbic system.

The individual's knowledge and vocabulary are tested in reference to common knowledge of current events. The ability to think abstractly may be tested by asking the person to explain the meaning of a proverb. Calculation is tested by examining the ability to subtract serially 7 from 100. *Dyscalculia* is the inability to solve simple problems. Recent memory loss is more common in brain disease than is remote memory loss. The findings of these gross tests may indicate the need for more definitive tests of mental function.

Sensory status

General sensory function of the trunk and extremities is tested for both superficial and deep sensations (the face is omitted if sensory status was tested during examination of cranial nerve V). Areas of sensory loss or abnormality are mapped out on a body diagram with a red pencil according to the distribution of the *spinal dermatomes* and peripheral nerves (Fig. 34-9). A dermatome, or skin segment, may be thought of as the area of skin supplied by one dorsal root of a cutaneous nerve. Light touch, pain, and temperature are used to test superficial sensation. Each dermatome is tested in turn with appropriate stimuli. The examiner determines the extent to which the individual senses touch (cotton), pain (pin prick), and temperature (hot and cold water) in the sites mentioned. An area in which sensory loss is absent *(anesthesia)* is differentiated from areas in which a sensation is intensified *(hyperesthesia)* or lessened *(hypesthesia)*. *Paresthesia* is an abnormal sensation that is perceived as burning, prickly, or itching.

Proprioception. The proprioceptive fibers transmit sensory impulses from muscles, tendons, ligaments, and joints. Normally they give one awareness of the position of the limbs and their movements. This is often referred to as kinesthetic sense. Proprioception is tested by the examiner grasping the sides of the examinee's thumb or great toe and passively moving it up and down. With both eyes closed the examinee is asked to identify the direction of movements. Recognition of the initiation of movement is also sought.

Deep pain sense is determined by compression of deep structures such as the Achilles tendon and calf muscles, noting *extremes* in responses to the pressure.

Vibration sense is tested by placing a vibrating tuning fork over the elbow, wrist, ankle, and shin. With eyes closed the examinee is asked to identify the sensation.

Stereognosis is tested by asking the person with eyes closed to identify the size, weight, and form of objects placed in his hand.

Since stereognosis is based on normal reception of touch stimuli, it is included at this point; it is also related to the recognition and interpretation of that which is perceived by other cortical senses.

The ability to recognize objects through any of the special senses is known as *gnosia*. Sensations require a high degree of cortical integration or a great degree of "knowing" or interpretation. The elaboration of sensation as to its ultimate meaning in the individual depends on certain association areas in the cortex. *Agnosia* is not knowing a specific sensation; if the sense of touch is affected, it is called *astereognosia;* if sight and sound are involved, it is termed relative to the sensation deficit. Thus *agraphognosia* means a loss of graphic or writing sense; *agnosognosia* refers to a lack of disease awareness or body parts. Lesions involving a specific association area produce a specific type of agnosia.

Language and speech

Gross assessment of these functions is made by the examiner while the history is being taken. When a problem is apparent, referral may be made to a speech pathologist for a definitive diagnosis and suggestions as to treatment. It is important to recall from neuroanatomy that language as such is not represented in one area of the brain but is concentrated in a cortical field that is inclusive of parts of the temporal lobe (superior and lateral), the temporoparietal-occipital junction, and the frontal lobe (opercular region). Also language is a function of the dominant hemisphere, which is the left one for most people. Lesions or injury in any of the language areas will produce some type (or combination) of impairment in the use of language (motor) or in the understanding of language (sensory). The general term for impairment of language function is *aphasia*. The specific type of aphasia must be diagnosed. Deficits in language are not usually limited to one area of the brain and may be mild or severe. Aphasia with reduced output (motor) may be caused by lesions in the Broca area; aphasia with fluent output but difficulty in reception may be caused by lesions in the Wernicke area. *Global aphasia* is almost a complete loss of language functions. (See p. 684 for discussion of nursing care of patients with language deficits.)

The ability to produce speech is tested through the detection of weakness or incoordination of muscles used in articulating speech. Limitations are observed during cranial nerve testing and particularly in reference to cranial nerves V, VII, IX, X, and XII. As previously discussed, involvement of the motor component of these nerves may produce alterations in phonation, resonance, and articulation. The examiner asks the individual to produce different speech sounds in order to localize the problem. Disorders of speech *(dysarthria)* may be manifested by a single alteration or a variety of alterations. There are characteristic changes in particular diseases. For example, in cerebellar disease speech is often thick and explosive with a prolongation of speech sounds occurring at intervals (scanning). In parkinsonism speech is referred to as being hyperkinetic and is characterized by a decrease in loudness and in vocal emphasis patterns that makes sounds seem monotonous to the listener.

Apractic speech is a rare, yet interesting, disorder in which there is difficulty in the production of speech volitionally in the absence of motor programming through cortical integration. (Apraxia is a general term and relates to motor acts other than speech).

Meninges

To test for meningeal irritation, or stiff neck, the head is passively flexed sharply toward the chest while the person is in a recumbent position. In the presence of meningeal irritation there is marked resistance to flexion, accompanied by rigidity of the neck (nucha), spasm, and pain. There is also resistance to extension and rotary movements of the neck. *Brudzinski's sign*, indicating meningeal irritation, is also elicited by passive neck flexion. When the neck is flexed, the hips and legs flex involuntarily. *Kernig's sign* is a classic test used in the diagnosis of meningitis. In this test the examiner flexes one of the patient's thighs to a right angle and then attempts to extend the leg on the thigh (there are many variations of this test). A positive Kernig's sign is present when there is spasm of the hamstring muscles with resistance to extension of the leg and with neck and head pain.

Motor status

Function of the motor system is assessed as to gait and stance, muscle strength, muscle tonus, coordination, involuntary movements, and muscle stretch reflexes.

Gait and stance should be recognized as complex activities that require muscle strength, coordination, balance, proprioception, and vision. Gait, or walking, and associated movements give considerable information about motor status. Changes in gait may be characteristic of a specific neurologic disease. In evaluation of gait the person is asked to walk freely and naturally. A request may be made to walk *heel to toe* in a straight line, since this exaggerates any abnormalities. To evaluate stance, the person is asked to stand with his feet close together, first with eyes open and then closed *(Romberg's sign)*. Patients with problems of proprioception have difficulty maintaining balance with their eyes closed; patients with cerebellar disease have difficulty even with their eyes open, and they walk with a wide-based, *staggering gait*. The *hemiparetic gait* seen in upper motor neuron disease is characterized by circumduction of the affected leg and inversion of the foot. Persons with Parkinson's disease walk with a slow, shuffling gait, and as they start walking there is an increase in rapidity until they are almost running (propulsive). They also have difficulty stopping, and deviation in the center of gravity causes retropulsion or lateropulsion. In addition there is loss of associated movements of the arms in walking. *Ataxia* is a general term meaning lack of coordination in performing a planned, purposeful motion such as walking. It can be caused by disturbance of position sense or by cerebellar or other diseases. It is important to recognize and describe gait disturbances and to interpret the cause only after all studies have been completed.

Muscle strength, or power, is assessed systematically, including trunk and extremity muscles. During manual testing of each muscle group the examinee attempts to resist the examiner in moving his muscles when placed in fixed positions. Weakness of a specific muscle is identified by the examiner as to distribution and degree of muscle weaknesses. *Akinesia* is loss of volitional muscle power. Evaluation may include all major muscles. At other times testing may be made only through gross tests of the extremities such as hand grip or foot strength or the ability to move all extremities. *Hemiplegia* is complete paralysis of one half of the body (linear), whereas *hemiparesis* is weakness or incomplete paralysis in the same distribution. *Paraplegia* is paralysis of the lower extremities, and *quadriplegia* is paralysis of the four extremities. The reader should note the distribution of peripheral motor nerves to skeletal muscles. (The distribution varies from that of sensory nerve distributions.)

Muscle tonus is tested by the examiner passively moving the examinee's limbs through a full range of motion. An increase *(hypertonia)* or a decrease *(hypotonia)* can be differentiated by the skilled examiner. Overextension and overflexion are found in hypertonia; resistance to passive movement increases rapidly and then suddenly gives way to pyramidal spasticity, or *clasp-knife rigidity*. A steady, passive resistance throughout the full range of motion is characteristic of *parkinsonism rigidity;* the combination of passive resistance and parkinsonism tremor with small regular jerks is called *cog-wheel rigidity*. In *decorticate rigidity* the upper limbs are flexed and pronated and the lower limbs are extended. In *decerebrate rigidity*, on the other hand, the upper limbs are extended and pronated and the lower limbs are extended. In hypertonia extremities tend to stay in fixed positions and feel firm; in hypotonia the extremities assume a position governed by gravity.

Coordination of muscle movements or the ability to perform skilled motor acts may be impaired at any level of the motor system. However, the cerebellum is primarily responsible for control, so that movements take place in a smooth and precise manner. Disturbance in cerebellar function may result in ataxia (as discussed relative to gait), difficulty in controlling the range of muscular movement *(dysmetria)*, and an inability to alternate rapid opposite and successive movements *(adiadochokinesia)*. Simple motor activities are evaluated on command of the examiner to perform rapid and rhythmic movements. For example, the nose-finger-nose test requires the individual to alternately touch his nose and the tip of the examiner's finger with variation in rate and level. Other tests include the knee pat (pronation-supination) and heel-knee or shin test, during which the examinee slides his heel over the shin toward the dorsum of the foot. There are many such tests, often modified by the examiner.

Involuntary movements also need to be observed and described during neurologic examination. Description of abnormal movements *(hyperkinesia)* is difficult but necessary. Observation of the presence or absence of the following is helpful: location of muscles involved, amplitude of movement, speed of onset, duration of contraction and relaxation, and rhythm. The effects of posture, rest, sleep, diversion of attention, voluntary movements, and emotional stress on involuntary movement is determined. Involuntary movements are usually increased by emotional stress and may subside during sleep. Involuntary movements can be the result of organic disease or may be psychosomatic in origin. A few of the more common types of involuntary movements are considered next. *Tremor* consists of rhythmic to-and-fro movements that are usually of small amplitude. They are due to alternate contractions of opposing groups of muscles; they are continuous while the patient is awake and may or may not be present during sleep. *Chorea* consists of short, sharp, rapid movements, usually of small excursion and irregular; movements occur in different parts of the body and persist during sleep. *Hemiballismus* is a variation of chorea in which movement is confined to one side of the body and affects the limbs to a great extent. *Athetosis* consists of slow, sinuous, and more sustained movements that may be of considerable amplitude; movements occur within the neck and trunk as well as the extremities and may be called *torsion spasms. Myoclonus* consists of irregular, abrupt, and arrhythmic contractions of a muscle or a group of muscles. Myoclonus may involve the extremities, the trunk, or the face and may be consistent in site.

Although all muscles can be made to contract reflexly, only a few reflexes are tested clinically. The *muscle stretch reflexes* (MSRs) (also called myotactic and deep-tendon reflexes) that are tested more routinely include the biceps, triceps, brachioradialis, quadriceps, and gastrocnemius and soleus muscles. (Superficial reflexes are omitted in this discussion.) Since the muscle reflexes are simply monosynaptic reflexes, they may be diminished in normal response *(hyporeflexia)* or lost completely *(areflexia)* because of interruption of afferent sensory fiber transmission or extensive destruction of efferent motor fibers of the anterior horn cells. On the other hand, release of the monosynaptic reflex from the influence of suprasegmental fibers (pyramidal and supplementary motor systems) produces an increased muscular response *(hyperreflexia)*. The general method for testing muscle stretch reflexes is through mechanical stimulation of the muscle spindles through stretching and by tapping a tendon or a bone or by depressing the distal phalanx and allowing it to flip up sharply (Hoffmann's sign). The degree of response, above or below normal, is noted and graded on a scale. The most important feature of any reflex pattern is not the absolute value on the scale but the difference between one side of the body and the other (asymmetry). Stick figures are commonly used to record the bilateral values (scale may range from 0 to 4+). See Table 34-1 for one example of how reflexes are graded on a scale. Since the threshold for muscle stretch reflexes has a normal range of variability, some individuals with generalized hypo or hyperreflexia will not have pathologic conditions but will rank at the end of the normal range. On the other hand, areflexia is usually a pathologic condition.

Table 34-1. Grading of muscle stretch reflexes (MSR)

Scale	Interpretation
0	Areflexia
±	Hyporeflexia
1+ to 3+	Normal
3+ to 4+	Hyperreflexia

One reflex often referred to clinically is the plantar reflex. This reflex when present in adults results in extension of the great toe (moves toward dorsum) with fanning (abduction) of the other toes when pressure is applied to the plantar surface of the foot laterally from the heel toward the toes. This response is known as the *Babinski's sign* and is associated with upper motor neuron disease.

Other reflexes may be classified as pathologic. These are reflexes that are present in infancy for variable periods. They are thought to be released in adults by acquired diseases of the cerebrum. Examples include the sucking, pouting, and grasp reflexes.

A reflex when present may assist in localizing a lesion, as does the presence of a unilateral Babinski's sign. Reflex findings, however, are only used in relation to total assessment data and are not used alone. (Refer to neurology texts for techniques on eliciting specific reflexes.) Variations of grading-scale values used should be noted. It also should be recognized that grading is somewhat subjective.

SPECIAL NEURODIAGNOSTIC TESTS AND PROCEDURES

Special neurodiagnostic procedures of the nervous system include examination of the cerebrospinal fluid by lumbar puncture, radioisotope brain scan, neuroradiologic studies of the spinal cord, and brain and electrodiagnostic studies to measure the electrical activity of the brain and muscles. Each is discussed generally as to use, methodology, data determined by the test, and nursing management. Some studies are invasive and carry a certain risk; they also are uncomfortable. Other studies are noninvasive and involve little risk. The reader is alerted to the fact that neurology tests give a variability of norms when interpreting laboratory findings. Tests related to specific neurologic problems are discussed in Chapter 36.

NORMAL VALUES OF CEREBROSPINAL FLUID (CSF)

Pressure	75 to 180 mm H_2O
Glucose	50 to 80 mg/100 ml
Chloride	118 to 132 mEq/liter
Protein	20 to 50 mg/100 ml
Gamma globulin	3% to 9%
Lymphocytes	0 to 8/ml

□ Lumbar puncture

Use

Lumbar puncture is used to obtain cerebrospinal fluid (CSF) for examination and to detect spinal subarachnoid block. The cerebrospinal fluid is examined for increase or decrease of its normal constituents; it is also examined for foreign substances such as pathogenic organisms and blood. Cerebrospinal fluid normally is a clear fluid that is formed in the lateral ventricles of the brain. It passes through the third ventricle, the aqueduct of Sylvius, the fourth ventricle, and finally into the cisterna magna at the base of the brain. From this location between the arachnoid space and the dura mater, the fluid bathes the entire brain surface and passes down to surround the spinal cord. The main purpose of the spinal fluid is to provide mechanical protection for the brain and spinal cord. The exact manner of its production and absorption is not entirely clear, nor is the rate of its production clearly determined. It is thought that approximately 150 to 200 ml of spinal fluid circulate within the system.

Interpretation

Spinal fluid normally is under slight positive pressure; 80 to 180 mm of water is considered normal. It is measured on a manometer when a spinal puncture is done. When a brain tumor or other space-occupying lesion is within the cranium, the spinal fluid pressure usually is greatly increased. For this reason a lumbar puncture is not performed in the presence of a choked disc or when a brain tumor is suspected, lest the quick reduction in pressure produced by removal of spinal fluid cause the brain structures to herniate into the foramen magnum, which would put pressure on vital centers in the medulla and might cause sudden death. The neurologist often writes "No spinal tap" on the patient's chart to be certain that no other medical staff member attempts this procedure.

Normally each milliliter of spinal fluid contains 0 to 8 lymphocytes. An increase in the number of cells may indicate an infection. Tuberculosis and viral infections may cause an increase in lymphocytes, while pyogenic infections may cause increase in polymorphonuclear leukocytes, which may be in large enough numbers to make the fluid cloudy. Bacterial infections such as tuberculous meningitis often lower the blood sugar levels. They may also reduce the chloride level. In the presence of degenerative diseases and when a brain tumor is present, the spinal fluid protein is usually increased. (See box above for normal values in spinal fluid.) The colloidal gold test is particularly helpful in diagnosing neurosyphilis or multiple sclerosis. Study of the spinal fluid may occasionally reveal the actual organism causing disease. Results of the serologic test for syphilis may be positive in spinal fluid even when the blood serologic test result is negative.

Blood in the spinal fluid indicates hemorrhage from somewhere into the ventricular system. It may be caused by a fracture at the base of the skull that has torn blood vessels, or it may be caused by the rupture of a blood vessel, which may occur, for example, with a congenital aneurysm. Occasionally the first specimen of spinal fluid contains blood from slight bleeding at the point of the puncture. For this reason the specimens of fluid are numbered, and the first one is not used to determine the cell count.

Method

Strict aseptic technique is mandatory in all procedures in which the cerebrospinal fluid system is entered. The nurse is responsible for seeing that all equipment is sterile and that safe technique is used throughout the procedure. Details of the *lumbar (spinal) puncture procedure* and a list of the equipment needed are given in texts on fundamentals of nursing.

The physician or nurse will explain to the patient that the needle is inserted below the level of the spinal cord (Fig. 34-12) so that there is little danger of injury. The patient will be positioned with both his knees and his head flexed at an acute angle so that there is a maximal lumbar flexion and separation of interspinous spaces. He should have constant nursing attention during the procedure. Even when a local anesthetic is used (usually procaine, 1%), the patient should be prepared to feel slight pain and pressure as the dura matter is entered. He should be reminded not to move suddenly and may

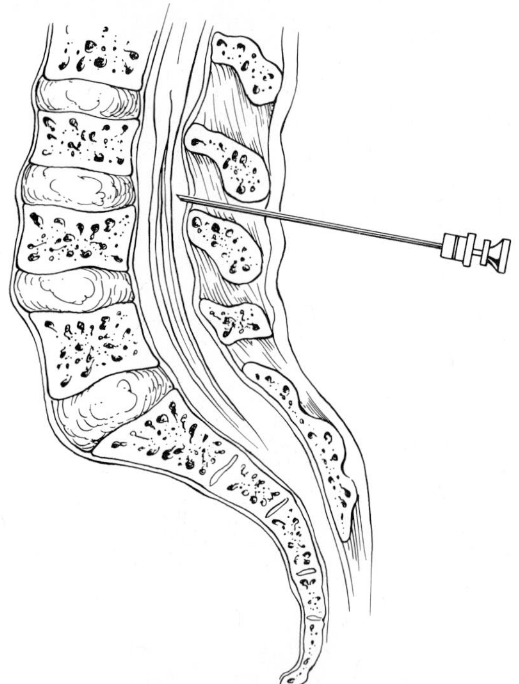

Fig. 34-12. Position and angle of needle when lumbar puncture is performed. Note that needle is in fourth lumbar interspace below level of spinal cord.

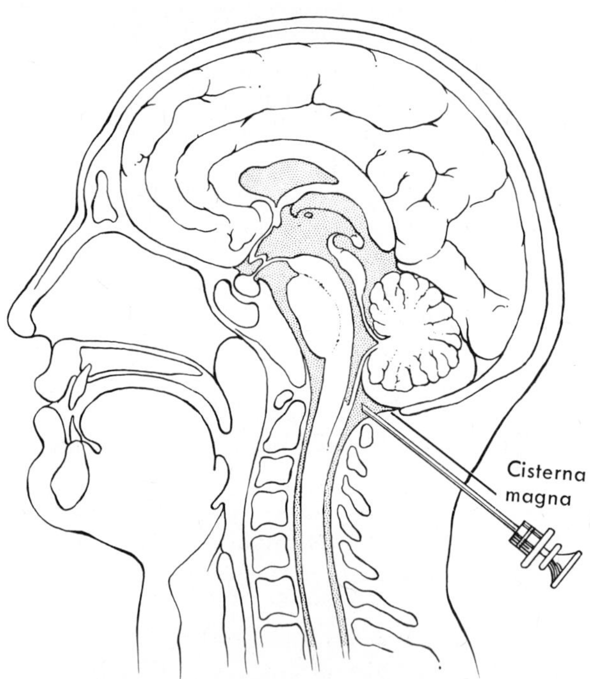

Fig. 34-13. Position of needle when cisternal puncture is performed. Note needle length and short bevel.

be told that he may experience a sharp shooting pain down one leg. This pain is caused by the needle's coming close to a nerve and is similar to hitting one's "funny bone"; however, the nerve actually is floating in fluid and is safe from injury.

The nurse prepares the equipment, assists the physician, assures sterility, monitors the patient during and immediately following the procedure, and arranges for suitable labeling and disposition of specimens. The nurse also assists during dynamic examination of CSF as detected through manometer readings. The level of the fluid column within the manometer is measured after needle entry into the subarachnoid space and after it is stabilized. The manometer is held by the nurse or another assistant above the point where the physician's hands need to come in contact with the instrument. When a subarachnoid block is suspected, a *Queckenstedt* test is performed. The nurse or another assistant compresses the jugular veins for 10 seconds, first on one side, then on the other side, and finally on both sides simultaneously. Pressure is exerted with the fingers flat against the patient's neck, avoiding the trachea.

Headache is fairly common following a lumbar puncture. Although its exact cause is unknown, it is thought to be due to loss of spinal fluid through the dura mater. It is currently believed that the smaller the needle used, the less likely that there will be fluid leak and headache. The sharpness and size of the needle used, the skill of the physician, and the emotional state of the patient are probably the determining factors in whether a headache will develop. If one does develop, it is treated with bed rest, an ice cap to the head, and an analgesic. Most headaches from this cause disappear within 24 hours.

Lumbar punctures are often performed on patients who are ambulatory and who go home immediately after the procedure is completed. It has been found that they suffer no more from headaches than do those who are treated more conservatively with bed rest and no elevation of the head.

In a *cisternal puncture* the cerebrospinal fluid is tapped by inserting a short-beveled needle immediately below the occipital bone into the cisterna magna (Fig. 34-13). This procedure may be more frightening to the patient than a lumbar puncture, since the approach is closer to the brain. The patient should have a detailed explanation by the physician before any head preparation is done or before he is placed in the required position. A permit for surgery is usually required. The back of the patient's neck may be shaved, and he is placed on

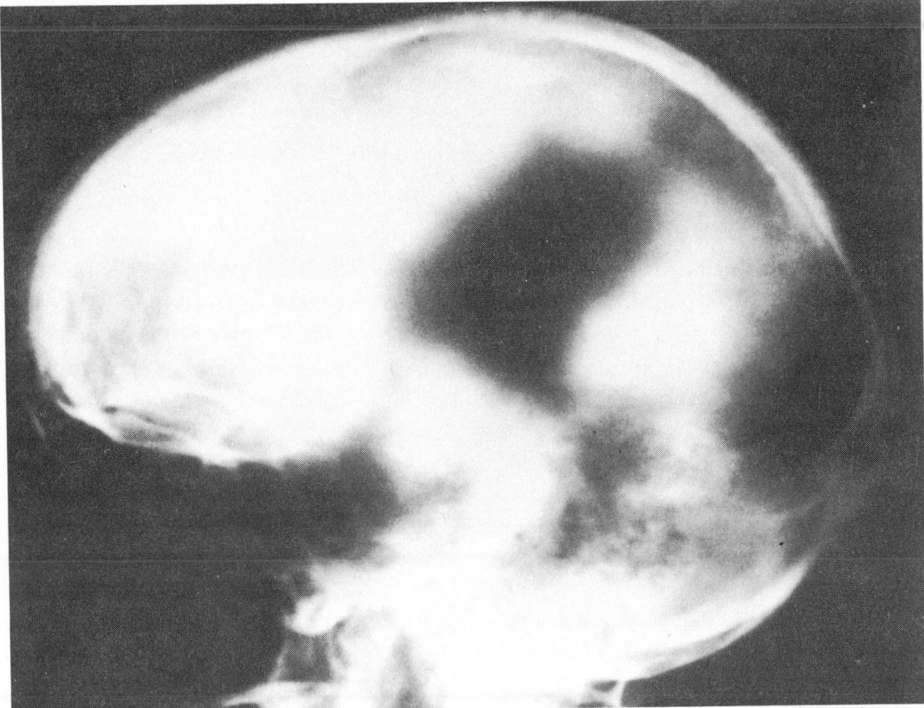

Fig. 34-14. Radioisotope brain scan. Intracranial mass (brain tumor) is seen in two dark areas (parietal and occipital) of scan where abnormal uptake of ^{197}Hg-tagged chlormerodrin accumulated. (Courtesy Abbas M. Rejali, M.D., Department of Radiology, Case Western Reserve University, Cleveland.)

his side at the edge of the bed or on a treatment table, with his head bent forward and held firmly by the nurse or another assistant. The patient is observed immediately following the procedure for dyspnea, apnea, and cyanosis, but these complications seldom occur. A cisternal puncture is often performed on children. In some outpatient departments it is more commonly performed than a lumbar puncture because it is less likely to be followed by headache.

□ Radioisotope brain scan

Radioactive isotopes are used with a scanner to detect brain lesions. This procedure is particularly successful in the detection of cerebral neoplasia and infarcts. A positive brain scan does not, however, provide histologic information about the kind of lesion, but it does provide information similar to that provided by other screening procedures such as electroencephalography. It is used adjunctively with neurologic examination and radiologic studies.

It is known that abnormal brain tissue selectively concentrates radioactive isotopes to a greater extent than does the normal brain tissue that is peripheral to a lesion. The procedure for the brain scan is a relatively simple one and consists of no physical preparation other than the intravenous administration of a radioactive isotope indicator such as mercury. This is followed by scanning of the patient's scalp with a special sensing device to pick up the concentrated areas of uptake. Serial scans and the structural features of the isotope uptake may suggest a particular pattern that is indicative of a specific lesion, but this is not reliable for a differential diagnosis. When mercury is used as the isotope indicator, a mercurial diuretic, meralluride (Mercuhydrin), is administered several hours prior to the procedure. This permits a greater concentration of radioactive mercury to be circulated to the brain tissue, since meralluride minimizes the uptake of mercury by the kidneys. Areas of concentration show up as very dark areas (Fig. 34-14). Sodium pertechnetate Tc 99m (^{99m}Tc) is also becoming widely used for brain scans.

□ Neuroradiologic studies

There are multiple radiologic procedures of the brain and spinal cord that are best carried out and interpreted by a neuroradiologist. These include plain radiographs and special contrast studies of the ventricular system (including the cisternal and subarachnoid space) and the cerebral vessels and the new computerized axial tomography.

Routine or plain radiographs

Routine or plain radiographs of the brain and spinal cord are usually taken first, using varied projections to detect any developmental, traumatic, or degenerative bone abnormalities.

Computerized transverse axial tomography (CAT scan)

One of the most significant of recent technologic advances in radiographic equipment is the EMI scanner, which is capable of providing up to 100% more information than conventional radiographic techniques. The EMI scanner is also referred to as CAT, CT scan, computerized tomography, and computerized assisted tomography. This technique offers increased versatility, efficiency, and enhanced image detail. It is becoming more available in the United States but is still limited by expense to larger hospitals and university medical centers. The EMI scanner is based on a technique of scanning the brain without isotopes in which series of images using the principles of tomography are x-rayed and where each of the images is derived from a specific layer of brain tissue. The brain is thus scanned in successive layers by a very narrow beam of x-rays. The total system includes a scanning unit that houses the x-ray tube, two scintillation detectors, an x-ray control unit, a computer and magnetic disk unit, viewing unit, a line printer, and a teletyper. Data is thus collected in x-ray form and printout form, and information is also stored for future use.[19]

As the patient's head is scanned in two planes simultaneously and at various angles, the computer calculates tissue absorption in contiguous tissues and displays on a printout the numerical values and a visualization of the tissue density. By comparing the tissue densities with norms, abnormalities can be detected. Tumor masses, infarctions, displacement of bone, and ventricles can be accurately detected. It is particularly efficient in the detection of brain neoplasia and cerebrovascular lesions.

The EMI scanner is noninvasive and does not carry the risk and discomfort of other procedures such as air contrast studies and cerebral angiography. For this reason it has largely replaced such studies when the scanner is available. The person lies supine with his head positioned within a rubber bag so that there is no air gap between it and the scalp. The cap does not cause any discomfort and assures more accuracy, since patient movement during scanning produces blurred images resulting in a poor examination. The procedure does not require hospitalization.

The nurse should stress the following points in preparation of the person who is to experience the EMI scan:

1. It is a noninvasive procedure and requires no special preparation prior to scanning.
2. It is painless and a safe method of x-ray examination.
3. The person should remain very still during examination to permit accuracy.
4. Most scans take about 30 to 40 minutes.

Pneumoencephalography

Pneumoencephalography (air encephalography) is a special contrast study of the ventricular and cisternal systems that permits accurate localization of brain lesions. It is known to provide greater visualization of the posterior fossa than ventriculography. This technically difficult and uncomfortable procedure combines a spinal or a cisternal puncture with an x-ray examination. Air or oxygen, used as a contrast medium, is injected (25 to 30 ml) and rises to the ventricles where its presence can be noted on x-ray examination. Abnormal shape, size, or position of the ventricles or failure of the ventricles to fill with the gas is diagnostically significant. See Fig. 34-15 for examples of normal and abnormal findings. The procedure usually is performed with the patient under local anesthesia, but a general inhalation, rectal, or intravenous anesthetic may be used for nervous or unstable patients. Headache is usually severe during and following encephalography. Nausea and vomiting are not uncommon. A nurse must be in constant attendance to observe the patient while a second person assists the physician.

The patient who is to have a pneumoencephalogram may be prepared as for surgery: no food or fluids by mouth for 6 hours before the procedure and a sedative the evening before and 1/2 hour prior to the procedure. A permit must be signed and dentures removed (p. 376).

The procedure may be started in the patient's room or in the treatment room. The patient is then taken to a special room in the x-ray department or operating room. The equipment needed is the same as that for a spinal puncture with the addition of a three-way stopcock, a 20-ml syringe with which to withdraw spinal fluid and inject air, a calibrated glass to measure any fluid that is removed, and an ampule of caffeine and sodium benzoate and an ampule of epinephrine (Adrenalin) for use in case of respiratory distress. Emergency oxygen equipment is also often requested.

The pressure of the spinal fluid is taken as soon as the needle is inserted into the lumbar spine arachnoid space. As the procedure is carried out, the patient is watched carefully for headache, nausea, and vomiting and his vital signs and color are noted and recorded. The head of the bed or table is gradually raised, and some physicians prefer to have the patient's head gently rotated after the air has been injected in the belief that this gives better filling of the lateral ventricles.

On his return from the x-ray department or the

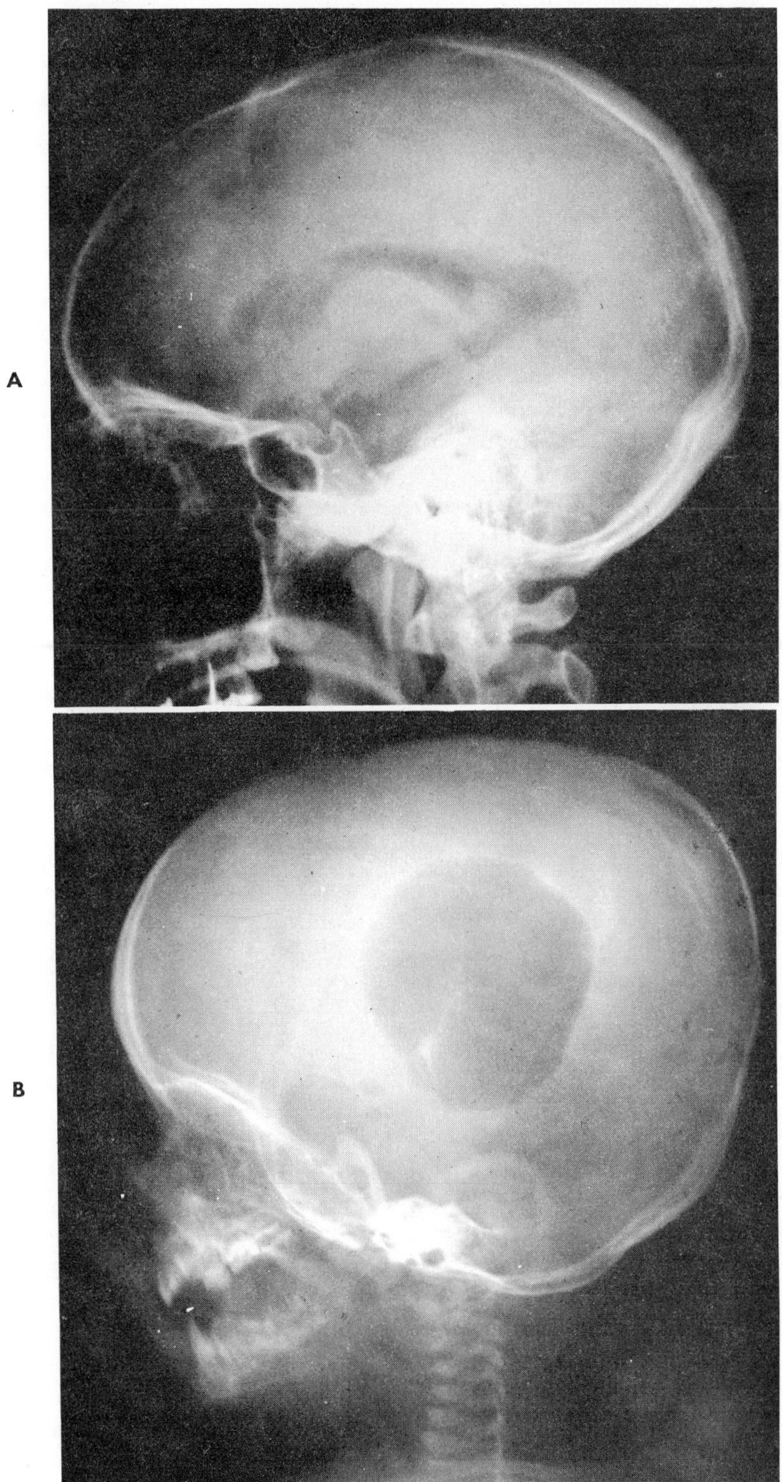

Fig. 34-15. Pneumoencephalogram. **A,** Lateral view showing outline of normal ventricle. **B,** Lateral view showing marked distention of ventricle with cerebrospinal fluid due to hydrocephalus.

operating room, the patient is placed in bed with his head flat. Usually he is more comfortable without a pillow. If a general anesthetic has been administered, he is kept on his side with head flat and constantly attended until awake. Vital signs are taken every 15 minutes for the first hour, then every 1/2 hour, and every hour for several hours or until they become stabilized. They are then taken every 4 hours. The level of consciousness is also noted. Any changes should be reported at once. The patient usually has a severe headache and may benefit from an ice cap applied to the head. Acetylsalicylic acid (aspirin), dextropropoxyphene hydrochloride (Darvon), or other nonnarcotic analgesics are given for severe headache. If the patient complains of noises in his head he should be assured that they are temporary, since they are caused by gas in the ventricles and will disappear when the gas is absorbed. If the patient has a history of convulsions or unpredictable behavior, side rails should be up and convulsion precautions taken. An emergency tracheostomy set may be kept on the unit for 48 hours following this procedure.

Infrequently reactions to pneumoencephalography are severe and include continued vomiting, convulsions, shock, and signs of increased intracranial pressure with respiratory difficulty. A severe prolonged headache may also follow this diagnostic procedure, although the headache usually disappears in 24 to 48 hours. For the first 24 to 48 hours the patient remains quiet in bed. After 48 hours the patient may be out of bed gradually. If headache and nausea increase when he is upright, they will be relieved by his lying flat until the symptoms gradually subside.

Pneumoencephalography is not done as frequently as formerly because of the availability of the EMI scanner in major medical centers. It is contraindicated when there is increased intracranial pressure because of the danger of herniation of the temporal uncus and cerebellar tonsils resulting in compression of the brainstem and death.

Craniotomy should be performed promptly when a tumor is detected during the procedure to prevent brainstem compression.

Ventriculography

Ventriculography is similar to pneumoencephalography except that air is introduced directly into the lateral ventricles through trephine openings (burr holes) into the skull. This procedure is always performed in the operating room. It may be used when the suspected diagnosis is such that a spinal or lumbar puncture is contraindicated because of the extreme pressure within the skull or because the spinal canal is blocked. The preparation is similar to that for encephalography except that the top or the back of the head must be partially shaved, depending on the physician's orders. An intravenous or general anesthetic is commonly used, and the patient may go directly from the x-ray department to the operating room for attempted removal of a tumor or for other brain surgery. If the radiography is normal, the patient is cared for in a manner similar to that following encephalography. Tissue and skin over the burr holes are sutured and the wounds covered with a collodion dressing.

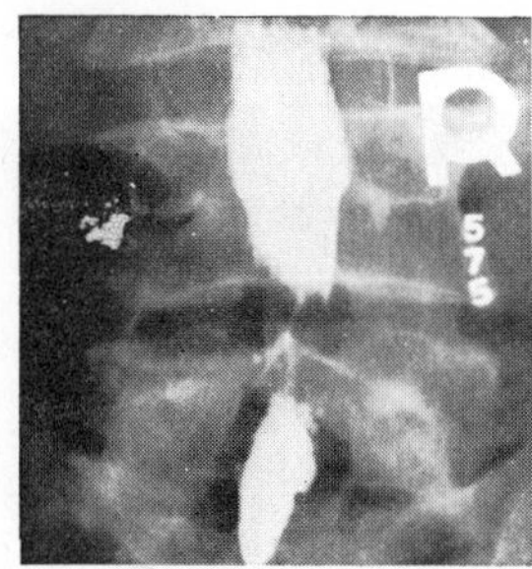

Fig. 34-16. Myelogram showing almost complete block of interspace between fourth and fifth lumbar vertebrae. (From Moseley, H. F., editor: Textbook of surgery, ed. 3, St. Louis, 1959, The C. V. Mosby Co.)

Myelography

In myelography either gas or a radiopaque liquid is injected into the spinal subarachnoid space by way of lumbar or cisternal puncture, and radiographs are taken. It is useful in the identification of lesions in the intradural or extradural compartments of the spinal canal. Observation of the flow of the radiopaque dye fluoroscopically through the subarachnoid space provides valuable information. Lesions in the spinal cord or in the subarachnoid space produce a blocking at some point (Fig. 34-16).

The blockage may be complete or incomplete. The exact configuration of the defect causing the block may be helpful in determining whether the lesion is intramedullary or extramedullary. Turning the patient in varied positions throughout the examination assists in securing a more complete visualization.

This procedure is thus similar to that for a spinal puncture except that after the air or the radiopaque substance is injected, the patient's head is elevated on two pillows and he is taken to the x-ray department. After the fluoroscopic examination and radiographs are completed, the dye is removed by lumbar puncture because it can cause serious irritation to the meninges. If some of it remains, care is taken to keep the patient's head elevated, and repeated attempts to remove the dye are made under fluoroscopy. One disadvantage of this test is the irritating quality of the available dyes. Therefore the

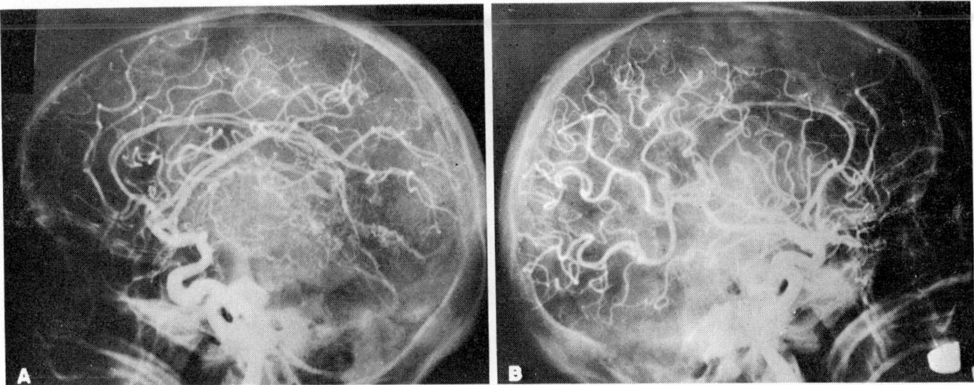

Fig. 34-17. A, Cerebral arteriogram showing elevation of middle cerebral arteries by glioblastoma multiforme containing abnormal vascular network. **B,** Arteriogram showing opposite normal side for comparison. (From Moseley, H. F., editor: Textbook of surgery, ed. 3, St. Louis, 1959, The C. V. Mosby Co.)

test is not performed when relatively certain diagnosis can be made by other means, and air is often used in preference to the dye.

Cerebral arteriography

Cerebral arteriography is a method of radiologic visualization of the cerebral arterial system during the injection of radiopaque material. The carotid or vertebral vessels in the neck are used directly. Four-vessel study in which a catheter is introduced percutaneously into the femoral artery and then directed into the innominate, carotid, and vertebral vessels under fluoroscopic control is also done. Each vessel is then injected with the contrast dye as serial radiographs are taken. The selection of needle puncture site is determined by the clinical problem under study. When injections of dye are made directly into the neck vessels the neck will be painful. The patient should be made aware that pain will be experienced with this procedure and that it will limit mobility; the indirect method is less traumatic. Arterial aneurysms, vessel anomalies, ruptured vessels, and displacements by mass lesions are often detected by this procedure. The large blood vessels of the circle of Willis at the base of the brain and the larger vessels penetrating the cerebrum can often be seen by this means (Fig. 34-17). Before the test is performed, a permit is signed by the patient or a responsible relative. Usually a sedative is given the night before, and scopolamine, atropine sulfate and sodium phenobarbital, or meperidine (Demerol) is given ½ hour before the procedure is performed. Occasionally, when the patient is confused or extremely restless, a general anesthetic is given. If this is necessary the procedure is usually performed in the operating room. If the dye can be injected directly into the carotid vessel without surgical exposure of the artery and if general anesthesia is not necessary, the procedure is usually performed in the x-ray department.

Following the test the patient is watched for changes in vital signs. The injection site is observed carefully for hematoma formation. The site will be swollen and painful. An ice cap may lessen swelling and pain and prevent bleeding. The artery may be blocked at the site because of hematoma or thrombus formation.

Occasionally neurologic deficits result or intensify following this procedure. Decreased hand grip on plantar pressure and facial weakness on the side opposite the injection site are significant. Convulsive seizures or aphasia may occur. Occasionally a delayed allergic reaction to the dye occurs, and this reaction may be serious (p. 195). An ice collar applied to the neck helps to prevent bleeding from the vessel and local edema, which might cause respiratory difficulty because of a carotid artery hematoma. Usually, however, the patient experiences little, if any, discomfort and can resume his usual activities within a few hours.

□ Electrodiagnostic examination

The electrodiagnostic examinations include electroencephalography and electromyography.

Electroencephalography

An *electroencephalograph* measures the electrical impulses of the brain; the *electroencephalogram* (EEG) is a pictured recording of the electrical activity of the brain amplified many times and recorded in a manner similar to that of the electrocardiogram. The recording represents the synthesis of collective neurons. Certain characteristic patterns in the record are normal, and by

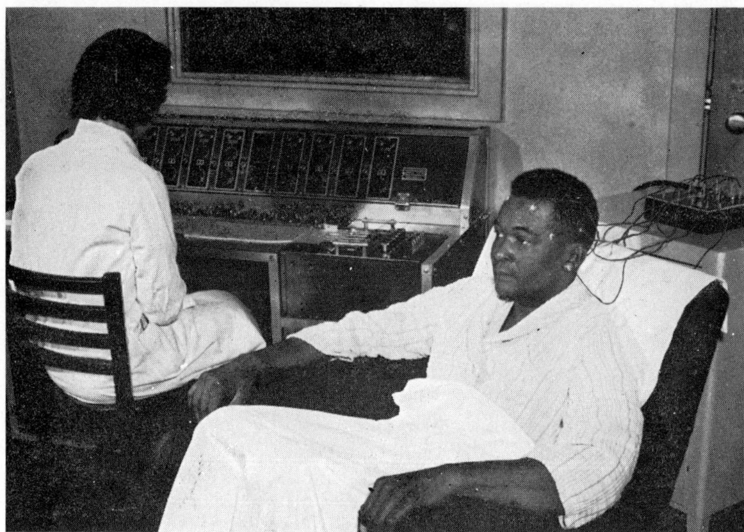

Fig. 34-18. Patient ready to have electroencephalogram. (From Conway, B. L.: Carini and Owens' neurological and neurosurgical nursing, ed. 7, St. Louis, 1978, The C. V. Mosby Co.)

study of the recordings of brain action, areas of abnormal action can sometimes be detected. This test is nonspecific and is only an adjunct to other diagnostic tests, but it may be helpful in locating the site of a lesion. Before the examination the patient should be quiet, and the procedure should be explained to him so that no undue excitement occurs. The scalp should be clean but no other local preparation is necessary. The hair need not be cut, which is often reassuring to the patient. The procedure involves the application of electrodes to the scalp to record cortical electrical activity. Sixteen or more tiny electrodes are fixed to the scalp with collodion. They are placed in a set pattern to cover all scalp areas (frontal, parietal, temporal, and occipital) (Fig. 34-18). Occasionally the electrodes used are tiny pins that are stuck into the scalp. The patient should know that this procedure will not be painful because there are very few nerve endings in the scalp. The examination is done in a special room where outside electrical activity is eliminated. The person usually sits in a comfortable chair or lies on a stretcher or table with his eyes closed. The basic resting rhythm is affected by opening the eyes or by alteration in attention. Cutaneous sensory stimulation or the induction of motor activity does not alter the scalp record. The test may last for 1 hour or more. Recordings may be made during sleep or when deprived of sleep and provide valuable information. Anticonvulsive drugs may be discontinued in patients with known convulsive disorders prior to the EEG. In general the EEG is used to provide evidence of focal or diffuse disturbances of increased brain function produced by organic lesions. The EEG has been particularly helpful in the diagnosis of epilepsy, in the differential diagnosis of convulsive disorders, and in locating lesions of the cerebrum.

Electromyography

The *electromyograph* measures the electrical activity of muscles; the *electromyogram* (EMG) is a recording of the variations of electric potentials (voltage) detected by a needle electrode inserted into skeletal muscle. The electrical activity can be heard over a loudspeaker and viewed on an oscilloscope and on a graph at the same time. No electrical activity can be detected in normal muscles at rest, but during volitional movement action potentials can be detected. However, in motor disease electrical activity of various types and abnormal patterns appear in resting muscles. An EMG provides direct evidence of motor dysfunction and can be used to some extent to detect a dysfunction located in the motor neuron, the neuromuscular junction, or muscle fibers. Thus it is particularly helpful in the diagnosis of lower motor neuron disease, primary muscle disease, and defects in the transmission of electrical impulses at the neuromuscular junction such as in myasthenia gravis. There is no special preparation for this procedure. The patient may be fearful that electrode needles will electrocute him and should be assured that there is no danger. (See p. 831 for discussion of EMG related to primary muscle problems.)

□ Echoencephalography

Echoencephalography is a rapid and simple diagnostic procedure that has become popular. Information provided is supplementary to an EEG and complementary to radiologic studies as to the nature and location of brain lesions.

Ultrasonic pulses (capable of reflection or refraction at cerebrospinal fluid and brain tissue surfaces) are delivered to the head in such a way that the beam intersects the site under study at a perpendicular angle, traverses the area, and is then reflected back. The returning echoes are then converted back to electrical impulses and recorded on a screen. For example, when a transducer is placed on the right temporal bone and directed toward the opposite temporal bone, the sound beams traverses the third ventricle area (which has two parallel walls) and is reflected back. This procedure provides a right, left, and lower trace, or picture, that gives reliable information as to position of the midline of the brain. Shifts from the midline, as caused by right or left hemispheric brain masses, can be inferred. Estimation of ventricular size can also be made from the traces.

REFERENCES AND SELECTED READINGS

1. Alpers, B. J., and Mancall, E. L.: Essentials of the neurological examination, Philadelphia, 1971, F. A. Davis Co.
2. Bates, B.: A guide to physical examination, Philadelphia, 1974, J. B. Lippincott Co.
3. Bickerstaff, E. R.: Neurology for nurses, ed. 2, London, 1971, English University Press.
4. Chusid, J. C.: Correlative neuroanatomy and functional neurology, Los Altos, Calif., 1973, Lange Medical Publications.
5. Clark, R. G.: Manter and Gatz's essentials of clinical neuroanatomy and neurophysiology, ed. 5, Philadelphia, 1975, F. A. Davis Co.
6. Conway, B. L.: Carini and Owens' Neurological and neurosurgical nursing, ed. 7, St. Louis, 1978, The C. V. Mosby Co.
7. DeMyer, W.: Technique of the neurologic examination, ed. 1, New York, 1969, McGraw-Hill Book Co.
8. Francis, G. M., and Munjas, B. A.: Manual of social psychologic assessment, New York, 1976, Appleton-Century-Crofts.
9. Fuerst, E. V., and Wolff, L.: Fundamentals of nursing, Philadelphia, 1974, J. B. Lippincott Co.
10. House, E. L., and Pansky, B.: A functional approach to neuroanatomy, ed. 2, New York, 1967, McGraw-Hill Book Co.
11. Judge, R. D., and Zuidema, G. D.: Methods of clinical examination: a physiologic approach, ed. 3, Boston, 1974, Little, Brown and Co.
12. Liechty, R. D., and Soper, R. T.: Synopsis of surgery, ed. 3, St. Louis, 1976, The C. V. Mosby Co.
13. *Malasanos, L., Barkauskas, V., Moss, M., and Allen, K. S.: Health assessment, St. Louis, 1977, The C. V. Mosby Co.
14. Mayo clinic and Mayo Foundation: Clinical examination in neurology, Philadelphia, 1971, W. B. Saunders Co.
15. *Michael, J. A.: Physiology of the nervous system: from the molecular to the behavioral, Nurs. Digest **4**:20-24, 1976.
16. *Patient assessment: neurological examination, part I, Am. J. Nurs. **75**:1511-1535, 1975.
17. *Patient assessment: neurological examination, part II, Am. J. Nurs., **75**:2037-2057, 1975.
18. *Patient assessment: neurological examination, part III, Am. J. Nurs. **76**:609-633, 1976.
19. *Patient assessment: examination of the eye, Am. J. Nurs. **74**:2039-2059, 1974.
20. Seeram, E.: The emi brain scanner, Can. Nurse **72**:40-42, 1976.
21. Selkurt, E. E.: Basic physiology for the health sciences, Boston, 1975, Little, Brown and Co.

*References preceded by an asterisk are particularly well suited for student reading.

35

Management of the person with common neurologic manifestations

MARJORIE KINNEY

Neurology as a field of nursing practice and study is concerned with problems of the nervous system that have an organic and physical cause. Many persons with neurologic conditions have serious emotional and even psychiatric disturbances that can be related in part to the organic nature of the problem. Because of this, neurology and psychiatry are often confused as fields of practice and require differentiation. Psychiatry is concerned with functional disorders of the mind, or psyche, and no organic cause can be demonstrated. It should be recognized that much about the physical basis of the psyche is unknown and that it is difficult to demonstrate the organic nature of psychologic manifestations in many instances. For this reason the nurse practicing in neurology should have knowledge that the psyche and soma (body) are one in the *person* and that often there can be no clear-cut distinction.

The nervous system as the coordinator and regulator of all body activities collects sensory information from the internal and external environments, communicates it to distant parts of the body, processes it to determine appropriate response patterns, and then generates control signals to the effector muscles and glands for action. Because of the nature of the function and structures of the nervous system when organic lesions or trauma occur at a particular site, the resulting clinical manifestations are related to the site affected regardless of the underlying pathologic findings. The clinical signs and symptoms manifested thus depend on the site, the extent, and the nature of the findings. When disease or injury affects a part of the nervous system, some neurons are destroyed and will not regenerate; some are partially damaged and may later recover; some are irritated into abnormal activity; others are undamaged. Manifestations reflect a complete loss or an alteration in normal function or body activity as a consequence of the degree of damage to the neurons at a particular site. Normal function and activities may thus be ablated, decreased, or increased.

Other clinical manifestations are an expression not of the damaged site itself but of other parts of the nervous system, the actions of which become unopposed after the involved part becomes nonfunctional, that is, a resultant lack of control or regulation of the part. Other manifestations are caused by pathologic findings of nonneuronal tissues such as cerebral blood vessels, muscles, and other supporting tissues within the nervous system. When manifestations are longstanding and the pathologic condition and its consequences are irreversible and progressive, the person is required to make necessary changes in life style. These changes can cause social and psychologic problems for the person.

Nursing management of the person with a clinical manifestation resulting from alterations in neurologic function and structure that are common to many types of pathologic conditions is discussed in this chapter. Discussion focuses on selected manifestations and their related pathophysiology and nursing management including prevention, intervention, and expected client outcomes.

■ HEADACHE (CEPHALGIA)

Headache, or head pain, is a common symptom experienced by many persons. As a symptom of an underlying disease, it varies in degree of severity from that of relative unimportance and transience to that of very serious prognosis. It is clear that this symptom may have its source in many different pathologic processes. *The source of recurring headache should be determined through careful physical examination and neurologic testing.* Persons have been known to self-treat headache for months in the belief that it was due to a sinus infection, only to learn later that it was caused by a more serious problem such as a brain tumor or hypertension.

Headache from a neurologic perspective may be due to an expanding cranial mass such as a neoplasm, to intracranial bleeding as in an aneurysm, to inflammation of the meninges as in meningitis and other cerebral infections, or to head trauma, cerebral hypoxia, or dilation of cerebral blood vessels. It is also important to recognize that psychologic factors may be involved in the cause of headache. Head pain is also commonly caused by systemic disease or by eye, ear, and sinus problems. Headache may be described by the person in terms of location (either diffuse or local) or as to the quality or nature of the pain.

The pathophysiology of head pain is not fully known. The skull and brain tissues from a neurophysiologic standpoint are not capable of sensing pain. Rather, the pain arises from the scalp and its blood vessels and muscles, from the dura mater and its venous sinuses, and from the blood vessels at the base of the brain. All of these structures have pain receptors. Pain most commonly originates in muscles (face, neck, head), blood vessels, and the dura mater. The blood vessels dilate and become congested with blood extracranially and intracranially. The pain is also thought to be the result of tension in or stretching of these tissues. For these reasons, headaches can be divided into three categories: vascular, muscular contraction (tension), or a combination of the two.[26]

□ Types of headaches

Discussion here is limited to migraine, cluster, and tension headaches and their treatment.

Migraine headache

Broadly defined, migraine is a recurring vascular headache. Exactly what causes an attack is not known, and there may be multiple causes. Chemical changes in and around the cranial blood vessel walls appear to play a role in causation. It is believed that the symptoms are produced by spasm of vessels inside the skull and dilation of vessels outside the skull; the latter is related to the head pain. Hereditary incidence is high, and migraine is more common in women than in men. Prodromal signs and symptoms *(aura)* occurring before the acute attack may include visual field defects, confusion, paresthesia, and even paralysis. The usual signs and symptoms occurring at the time of the attack may include nausea, vomiting, chilliness, fatigue, irritability, sweating, edema, and other autonomic signs. The acute symptoms are severe and vary in intensity and duration. The pain is usually severe and starts gradually. The headache is often present on awakening, and one side of the head usually is more affected than the other. Pain may be most severe over the temporal area but may occur anywhere in the head including the face. The associated symptoms may also be severe. The person is often forced to seek isolation in a dark room. The acute attack may last from several hours to many days. It concludes with a feeling of relaxation and need for sleep. Dull head and neck pain (probably due to tension during the attack) may persist for some time.

Specific treatment for migraine includes medications to relieve pain and psychotherapy. Acetylsalicylic acid (aspirin) is seldom effective for classic or common migraine but may be helpful after the headache has developed. Ergotamine tartrate preparations taken early in the attack may prevent the headache from developing. These drugs are the treatment of choice in migraine, and their efficacy in relieving the headache is often considered diagnostic of migraine. Ergotamine tartrate preparations act by constricting cerebral blood vessel walls, thus reducing cerebral blood flow. Ergotamine tartrate may be administered orally, sublingually, or rectally in 2- to 4-mg dosages. It is also available for injection in 0.25- to 0.5-mg. dosages. Ergot preparations are also available in combination with other drugs such as caffeine, phenobarbital, and belladonna. Pregnant women cannot take ergot preparations because they stimulate uterine smooth muscles, and other medications need to be substituted. Ergot preparations have the side effects of nausea, vomiting, numbness and tingling, muscle pain, and changes in heart rate and may not be tolerated by some persons. Other drugs that may be substituted include nonnarcotic analgesics, such as phenacetin, acetaminophen, or propoxyphene (Darvon), as well as narcotics such as codeine.

Other treatment includes cold packs applied to the forehead or the base of the brain; this may either relieve or aggravate the condition. Pressure applied to the temporal and carotid arteries may or may not be helpful. Psychotherapy may be helpful depending on the precipitating cause. Treatment between attacks includes efforts to reduce the frequency and severity of the headaches and in establishing definitive causes for the headache if unknown. It is particularly important to teach the person to initiate treatment early in the onset of headache.

Cluster headache

The onset of cluster headaches is usually in early adulthood. In this type of vascular headache pain episodes are clustered or spaced together in quick succession for a few days or weeks and with relatively long remissions that last for months. The frequency of the attacks is a unique characteristic. The duration of the pain is usually for a few minutes to a few hours. The pain is very intense, throbbing, and deep. It is abrupt in onset, and also stops abruptly. Prodromal signs are uncommon. Associated signs may include flushing, lacrimation (tearing), nasal stuffiness, sweating, and swelling of temporal vessels.

Tension headache (muscle contraction)

This common type of headache is associated with tension or anxiety and results from sustained contraction of extracranial skeletal muscles around the face, scalp, neck, and cervical areas. The headaches are episodic, vary in frequency and duration, and are related to stress. There is no aura. The pain is usually constant and bandlike; it is usually bilateral and involves the back of the head, neck, and shoulders. It may spread to all parts of the head and may be poorly defined. Treatment usually consists of analgesics and muscle relaxants. Modification of the environment with the reduction of sensory stimulation may be helpful. Psychotherapy may be indicated depending on the underlying stressors. See p. 730 for discussion of headache as a symptom of brain tumor.

□ Assessment

Information collected in the history should include the onset of the headache and any association with a life crisis, frequency, specific pain characteristics, location, prodromal signs if any (such as an aura, visual disturbances, and paresthesia), associated symptoms occurring at the same time as the headache, family history of headache (this is important in migraine), possible causes as ascribed by the person, and how the headache is usually treated by the person.

Identification of the triggering factors of severe recurring headaches will need to be made through ongoing assessment of personality, habits, and activities of daily living. The nurse seeks to determine what purpose if any the headache serves for the person. Internal conflicts lead to anxiety, and this may be manifested by headache. The headache may hide a serious emotional disorder or serve purposes of secondary gain. Clues may be learned from seeking information about goals and aspirations of the person, work habits, family relationships, coping mechanisms, and relaxation patterns. The person may be asked to keep a diary of activities of daily living and the occurrence of the headaches as well as their nature and treatment. Triggering factors may include fatigue, alcohol, stress, climatic changes, hunger, and menstruation. The nurse may be involved in assisting with special tests to determine the underlying cause of severe recurring headaches. These may include brain scans and an arteriogram to detect cerebral lesions.[26] In some instances no triggering factors may be identified.

Ongoing assessment by the nurse of patient responses to diagnostic tests and treatment is important. It is necessary to record pain descriptors in the person's own words, recognizing that headache is subjective. Any inferences made should be carefully validated.

□ Intervention

Treatment varies depending on the type of headache. Teaching is carried out concerning the treatment methods prescribed for the person. The person should learn about dosage, action, and side effects of prescribed medications. The nurse should counsel against the widespread use of aspirin for persistent headache. Prolonged and excessive use of aspirin has caused gastric bleeding and agranulocytosis in some individuals. The dangers of over-the-counter drugs should be explained. In teaching it is important to stress that persistent headache should be treated adequately and early. Persistent headaches (in which organic causes have been ruled out) indicate a need for the individual to examine his life style and make necessary adjustments. The nurse can sometimes be supportive to individuals who are trying to sort out possible causes of their headaches. Relaxation techniques can be demonstrated and supervised until the individual has mastered them.

Prevention of headache may be possible once the specific cause has been determined or the triggering factors have been isolated by the health professional or by the individual. Health teaching includes removal of the cause if known (and possible), the avoidance of triggering factors, and the importance of early treatment if *not* preventable. Early treatment lessens the more acute, prolonged, and incapacitating attacks such as occur in migraine.

□ Outcome criteria for the person with headache

The person or significant others can:

1. Explain prescribed medications:
   a. List and explain each prescribed medication as to dosage, action, side effects, and frequency.
   b. Explain how to use drugs as needed when headache recurs.
   c. Explain the reason for adequate and early treatment with prescribed drugs.
2. Explain the dangers of continued use of unprescribed drugs for chronic recurring headache.
3. Explain the importance of continued medical supervision for chronic recurring headache, whether the cause is known or unknown:
   a. State plans for follow-up care.
   b. Explain the dangers of undiagnosed headache.
   c. Recognize headache as a serious symptom.
4. Demonstrate prescribed relaxation techniques:
   a. Demonstrate the relaxation technique to the nurse.
   b. Explain in own words the values of adjustment of life style to lessen stress.
5. Identify factors that trigger the onset of headache:
   a. Discuss the factors that trigger the headache.
   b. State plan to avoid these factors.

■ SEIZURES

□ Etiology

Seizures may be defined as transitory disturbances in consciousness or in motor, sensory, or autonomic function caused by uncontrolled electrical discharges in the brain. All seizure activity in this sense is not visible. Seizures as a sign and symptom are of particular significance in neurologic diseases. They occur in many childhood and adult illnesses. Seizures may result from cerebral anoxia, hypoglycemia, disturbances of calcium balance, electrolyte imbalances, hydration, ingestion of drugs and poisons with convulsive activity, infections that produce high temperature elevations, and numerous metabolic disorders. In the majority of individuals with seizures a *localized* organic lesion serves as the focus for the abnormal neuronal discharges from the damaged brain tissues. This includes neoplasms, inflamed areas or abscesses, vascular formations or hematomas, congential malformation, trauma, or other space-occupying lesions. Quite often the lesion is microscopic in size and is related to the trauma of birth or scars from infantile or childhood infections. Seizure activity may be termed *acute seizures* or *epilepsy* when related to metabolic disorders. In *chronic epilepsy* the seizure activity recurs and the primary defect is in the brain itself, as described above. Seizures may also be caused by *generalized* inflammatory and degenerative brain diseases. Seizures that may be hysterical in origin are not considered true seizure disorders.

Seizures are most frequently associated with epilepsy, which may be considered a disease in itself. Epilepsy, however, is only a symptom and *not* a diagnosis. The word "convulsion" is frequently used interchangeably with the words "seizure," and "attack," and "fits." A *convulsion* by definition is more specific and refers to violent or abrupt involuntary contraction of muscles. Seizure connotes the abruptness or spasmlike character of the event or attack. In this sense *seizure* and *attack* relate to the whole event. Attack is the best term to use in conversation with laity; the term *fits* has unpleasant connotations and is avoided. The words seizure and convulsion each label the condition correctly.

□ Pathophysiology

Convulsions or seizures are brief "cerebral storms." They result from episodic, excessive, simultaneous, and disorderly ganglionic discharges. The patterns or forms of seizures vary and are dependent on the area of the brain from which the seizure arises. The pattern is stereotyped in the individual, although variations may occur with progression of the cerebral lesion. Seizures can involve essentially all parts of the brain at once, as in the generalized type, or only a minute focal spot. In the former the excessive neuronal discharges are thought to originate in the brainstem portion of the reticular activating system; these then spread throughout the central nervous system including the cortex and the deeper parts of the brain. This process may last from a few seconds to as long as 3 to 5 minutes, or the process may stop immediately as in a *petit mal* seizure. It is not known what stops the seizure at a given time, but it is believed to result from fatigue of the neurons involved in precipitating the seizure or inhibition by certain structures within the brain. Focally the excessive neuronal discharges may result in *tonic convulsions*, with the contraction of all muscles at once, or in *clonic convulsions*, with alternate contraction and relaxation of opposing muscle groups with characteristic jerking movements of the body. The seizure, regardless of origin or type, is always inappropriate to the immediate situation. It is followed by an inhibition of cerebral function; this period may last longer than the seizure itself. The inhibition of function is often incomplete and is dependent on the area of the brain from which the seizure arises.

□ Epilepsy

Epilepsy is one of the oldest diseases known. It was described in detail by Hippocrates. The term *epilepsy* means seizure, or "state." At one time it was thought to be of a divine origin and perhaps for this reason has been linked in the public mind with the occult, the strange, and the unmentionable. No disease has been more carefully concealed within families, and many attitudes toward the disease have persisted from early times to the present. Attitudes may also be affected by the frightening experience of having seen a person during a severe seizure, by the belief that mental deterioration always occurs in epilepsy, and by the fact that the tendency to develop epilepsy may be inherited.

Because of the emotional overtones associated with epilepsy and seizure disorders, it is often exceedingly difficult for parents to believe that their child might have such a condition. Sometimes they give an inadequate report to their family physician and receive the sought-for assurance that the child will probably outgrow the disorder. Many children would be spared severely traumatizing experiences at school and elsewhere if parents could only be convinced that the advice of a specialist is needed.

Epilepsy is a disease of unknown cause. When neurologic assessment and special procedures do not determine a cause for the seizure activity it is called *idiopathic epilepsy*. The use of this term is declining. The disease is not directly inherited, although abnormal brain waves, as shown on the EEG, are found in many relatives of persons having seizures, and it is likely that a predisposition to the disease is inherited. It is believed that some alteration of chemical balance touches off the seizure in susceptible persons. No accurate figures are available, but it is believed that more than 1 million persons in the United States are subject to recurring seizures.[1] Epilepsy is largely a disease of younger people; approximately three fourths of sufferers have seizures before the age of 20 years. The life expectancy of persons with epilepsy is less than that for the population as a whole, primarily because the person often dies of an accident incurred during a seizure.

□ Assessment

Types of seizures

There are numerous ways to classify seizures, and this makes more confusion. They may be classified broadly into generalized and focal types or as a combination of the two. *Status epilepticus* is the term used when the patient goes from one seizure to another without regaining consciousness; in this sense it is not a distinct type. Each major seizure type is discussed briefly. Generalized seizures include grand mal, petit mal, myoclonic, and akinetic.

The *grand mal seizure* is by far the most common type. It is the most dramatic and is often the final common event in convulsive disorders. Grand mal is generalized and is characterized by a loss of consciousness for several minutes (variable) and tonic and clonic convulsions (motor activity). The clinical course or sequence is the *aura, cry, loss of consciousness, the fall, tonic and clonic convulsions, and incontinence.* The symptoms that occur during the prodrome are called an *aura.* Prodromal symptoms occur in about 50% of all patients and usually include a change in sensation, or a change in affect. There may be numbness, flashing lights, dizziness, tingling of the arm, smells, or spots before the eyes. The patient may find it difficult to describe the aura precisely, but it gives conclusive warning of an impending seizure. The specific warning serves a useful purpose in that it enables the individual to seek safety and privacy before the onset of the seizure. Occasionally it occurs as much as a day before the seizure, so that the individual who works can remain at home and fellow workers may not know of the attacks. Grand mal is heralded by a sharp cry as air is rapidly inhaled. Following this there is a loss of consciousness, which is variable in duration and usually persists for several minutes. The individual slumps or falls, depending on the position at the time. This is followed by bilateral tonic contraction of all muscles; the legs are extended and the arms are flexed; jaws are clenched and the tongue is frequently caught between the teeth; the eyes roll upward and pupils dilate and become fixed. There is cessation of respiration, and cyanosis occurs. As the tonic phase ends, it is replaced by a series of clonic contractions. Breathing returns and is shallow and irregular at first. There is often frothing at the mouth, which may be streaked with blood if the tongue and lips have been bitten during the convulsion. Fecal or urinary incontinence often occurs during the clonic phase or earlier. As the clonic phase subsides within a few minutes, there is relaxation of muscles. Partial consciousness is regained and color improves.

During the *postictal* (postseizure) *period* the individual appears groggy and confused. He often complains of headache or muscular pain and usually falls into a deep sleep. During this phase the pupils may remain dilated and there may be abnormal plantar reflexes. After a variable period of time the patient awakens and is frequently unaware of the occurrence of the seizure. A dull headache and depression are common. It is possible that the depression is caused in part by knowledge that a seizure has occurred. Seizures occur during sleep in some individuals. In such instances the occurrence of the seizure is known on awakening by the presence of blood on the pillow or by soiled linen from fecal or urinary incontinence.

Petit mal seizures are characterized by an abrupt loss of consciousness that occurs without warning. This loss of consciousness, with arrest of all voluntary activity, is very brief and usually lasts about 10 to 20 seconds. In the classic petit mal seizure there is a sudden vacant facial expression, a stopping of all motor activity, except perhaps a slight symmetrical twitching of the face and arms, or a loss of muscle tone. Consciousness returns as quickly as it left, and the individual may resume speaking at the point interrupted, unaware that the seizure occurred. The individual may learn to recognize when he has lost a few seconds of time. Petit mal seizures usually occur many times a day and have no aura, falling, or tonic and clonic phases. In some instances the loss of consciousness may be accompanied by an exaggerated loss of muscle tone so that the patient falls; this is termed *akinetic. Myoclonus* may also occasionally be found in some petit mal seizures with the characteristic sudden, involuntary, jerking contractures of the neck or upper extremity muscles; the trunk may flex. Petit mal seizures occur most frequently in children and adolescents, particularly at the time of puberty. Although they do not represent the dramatic and frightening aspects of the grand mal seizure, they are disconcerting to the individual of any age. Also since this type of seizure is not preceded by an aura, the momentary loss of consciousness presents safety problems.

Focal or partial motor or sensory seizures are those that arise initially in the motor or sensory areas of the brain adjacent to the rolandic fissure or any localized part of the cerebral cortex. The clinical manifestations seen in this type of seizure are thus dependent on the site of the focus and differ from the generalized motor seizure (grand mal). If, for example, the abnormal neuronal discharge is initiated in the *precentral* or *motor region* of the cortex for the thumb, the individual will experience a tonic contracture of the thumb muscles. If the abnormal neuronal discharge spreads to adjacent parts of the motor strip, there is progressive involvement of associated musculature with a progression (march) of movements from thumb to hand, arm, face, and so forth. The discharge may or may not progress. The localized seizure that does spread progressively to other muscles following initiation is known as a *jacksonian seizure*. Focal motor seizures commonly begin in the hand, face, and foot but may arise in any part of the motor strip. The seizure may end in a shower of clonic movements, or it may end in a generalized convulsion. When abnormal neuronal discharges arise in the lower part of the motor strip, which controls salivation and mastication, seizures are then manifested by chewing, smacking of the lips, and swallowing movements. Salivation may be profuse. Other seizures may begin with a forced turning of the head and eyes. Such attacks are termed *adversive* and originate in the eye-turning fields of the brain; the head turns away from the side of the lesion, or focus. When the abnormal neuronal discharges arise in the *postcentral*, or *sensory strip*, of the cortex the seizure is initiated with complaints of disturbed sensations such as a numbness, tingling, prickling, or crawling feeling, and as in a focal motor seizure a march of sensations may or may not occur. The neuronal discharge may also spread from the sensory area to the motor area.

Psychomotor seizures

Variously known as psychic equivalents or automatisms, manifestations are characterized by the performance of automatic activities, impairment of consciousness, and psychic symptoms. No apparent convulsions occur. Consciousness may be lost, or amnesia may occur. During the attack the individual may appear drowsy, intoxicated, or violent, behave abnormally, and engage in antisocial activity. Activities such as driving a car, typing, eating, or going to the bathroom may continue at an automatic level. The individual is unable to make decisions and is not open to reason during the attack. No concern is given to the usual social amenities. States of furor may occur during attacks, and crimes have been committed. For this reason the diagnosis of this type of seizure is of interest to lawyers and judges as well as physicians. Psychic symptoms may occur with visual and auditory illusions and hallucinations, a sense of unreality and *déjà vu* (a sense that a new experience has occurred in all details some time before). Psychomotor seizures may, in addition, include visceral symptoms with autonomic complaints such as chest pain, respiratory arrest, tachycardia, urinary incontinence, and gastrointestinal tract discomforts. There may be abnormal sensations of taste and smell (uncinate). This type of seizure is often associated with the temporal lobe and may be labeled temporal lobe epilepsy.

□ Intervention

The treatment of persons with seizures is based on a careful study of the person to detect any remedial lesion or metabolic cause. When these have been eliminated or treated, care is then directed toward the prevention of seizures. Only rarely will the elimination of causative factors result in the complete disappearance of seizures. Some authorities believe that the only prevention of epilepsy is genetic counseling, since the predisposition to develop the disease appears to be inherited. There is no known cure for idiopathic epilepsy, although seizures can be controlled by anticonvulsive drugs and the regulation of mental and physical hygiene. The period of treatment is years or a lifetime for the majority of patients.

The nurse has responsibilities in the diagnostic, therapeutic, and instructional programs of persons with known seizures. The community health nurse and the clinic nurse will follow selected persons with seizures for extended periods. The person and family need to learn what to do during and after a seizure, to assume responsibility for drug therapy, and to recognize the need to seek assistance when side effects and toxic effects occur.

Care during a seizure

The primary goals of the nurse and family caring for a person having a seizure are protection from injury and observation and recording of the seizure activity. The person should never be left alone. If the person is in an upright position when a generalized motor seizure begins, he is lowered to the floor or a bed and adjacent articles and equipment are moved away to prevent injury during uncontrolled body movements. Constricting clothing is loosened, especially about the neck. The head should be supported and turned to the side to allow the tongue to fall forward so that it does not occlude the airway. *No effort should be made to restrain the person either manually or with restraints.* Attempting to resist body movements of a person in grand mal seizure may result in injury to bones and soft tissues. It is best to permit the person as much range of motion as possible without injury to self. Padded side rails are helpful for the person confined to bed and for individuals who have a pattern of seizures during sleep. Pillows should not be used for padding, since there is some danger from suffocation. *If the jaws are not already clenched* at the time when first observed, a padded tongue blade or rubber wedge may be inserted between the back teeth to prevent injury to the tongue and mouth tissues. At the same time care must be taken to avoid pushing the tongue back and occluding the airway. In many instances the jaws and teeth are already clenched and efforts to insert a tongue blade or any nearby substitute may damage the teeth and gums. The idea that one should pry the mouth open and insert a tongue blade or other object has been overemphasized. A judgment needs to be made about whether it is better to insert something, depending on the phase of the seizure and the condition of the person. It is the policy of many hospital nursing services that a padded tongue blade be kept at the patient's bedside when seizures are anticipated. It is less disturbing to the patient if the tongue blade is placed in the drawer of the bedside cabinet rather than being taped to the bed. A single oral airway may also be kept at the bedside along with other emergency equipment, dependent on the severity of seizures and the condition of the patient.

Accurate observation of the seizure (see box below) from the beginning, when possible, is important because it provides needed information that may assist the physician in locating the site of a cerebral lesion, or focus. It is more important to describe the seizure activity, sequence, and where it started than it is to name or classify the seizure. There is a tendency for nurses and others to forget the variations of seizure types and to relate more to the grand mal seizure.

OBSERVATIONS TO BE MADE ABOUT A PERSON HAVING A SEIZURE

Aura	Presence or absence, nature if present, ability of patient to describe it (somatic, visceral, psychic)
Cry	Presence or absence
Onset	Site of initial body movements, deviation of head and eyes, chewing and salivation, posture of body, sensory changes.
Tonic and clonic phases	Movements of body as to progression, skin color and airway, pupillary changes, incontinence, duration of each phase
Relaxation (sleep)	Duration and behavior
Postictal phase	Duration, general behavior, ability to remember anything about the seizure, orientation, pupillary changes, headache, injuries present
Duration of entire seizure	
Level of consciousness	Length of unconsciousness if present

When a person with known seizure activity is admitted to the hospital for diagnosis or reevaluation, it is important for the nurse to obtain a history of the pattern of seizure activity, the frequency and time of day, whether an aura is present, any precipitating factors, and any seizure characteristics. In this way nursing interventions can be planned more specifically. Admission of a person with known seizures who is undergoing treatment provides the nurse an opportunity to evaluate the person's understanding of the cause of the seizures and the prescribed therapy.

Mental health

From the standpoint of mental hygiene, the individual with seizures should use all resources to cope with feelings of self-consciousness and inferiority resulting from attacks. Adults should be encouraged to lead normal productive lives. Children should be kept in school unless the frequency of attacks disturbs the activities of the classroom. Family members need to be assisted to discuss their attitudes and feelings about the individual's illness. Excessive attention to the overprotection of the person with seizures is to be avoided. The family needs to understand the problems resulting from seizures and the prescribed therapy but should not make a chronic invalid of the person.

Activities of daily living

The physical activity of the person under treatment for seizures should be regulated so that eating, sleeping, and exercise schedules occur at about the same time daily. Exercises should be moderate and should not include competitive sports that are exhausting. No special diet is necessary, but alcohol should be avoided. When necessary, bowel movements should be regulated by training, diet, and the judicious use of mild laxatives. A regular time for retiring and arising should be established, and the person should not be allowed to stay in bed excessively. Swimming, horseback riding, and other dangerous sports are allowed with the proper safeguards. Activities that endanger the lives of others such as driving dangerous machinery and cars should be prohibited *when seizures are not under control* (despite treatment).

Drug therapy

Success in the prevention of seizures in persons under treatment is to a great extent dependent on the skill of the neurologist in selecting the type of anticonvulsant drug to be used and the regulation of dosage. The choice of medications to be used depends on the type of seizure. The person and family must understand

Table 35-1. Anticonvulsants used to prevent seizures

Drug	Use related to seizure type	Average daily dose	Toxic effects
Phenytoin sodium (Dilantin)	Grand mal, focal, psychomotor	0.4 to 0.6 g (divided dose)	Ataxia, vomiting, nystagmus, drowsiness, rash, fever, gum hypertrophy, lymphadenopathy
Phenobarbital (Luminal)	Grand mal, focal, psychomotor (adjunctive)	0.1 to 0.4 g (divided dose)	Drowsiness, rash
Primidone (Mysoline)	Grand mal, focal, psychomotor	0.5 to 2.0 g	Drowsiness, ataxia
Mephenytoin (Mesantoin)	Grand mal, focal, psychomotor	0.3 to 0.5 g	Ataxia, nystagmus, pancytopenia, rash
Ethosuximide (Zarontin)	Petit mal, psychomotor, myoclonic, akinetic	750 to 1,500 mg	Drowsiness, nausea, agranulocytosis
Trimethadione (Tridione)	Petit mal	0.3 to 2.0 g (divided dose)	Rash, photophobia, agranulocytosis, nephrosis
Diazepam (Valium)	Status epilepticus, mixed	8 to 30 mg	Drowsiness, ataxia
Carbamazepine (Tegretol)	Grand mal, psychomotor	0.3 to 2.0 g	Rash, drowsiness, ataxia

the importance of taking the prescribed drugs on schedule and in the correct dosage. Anticonvulsant drugs act generally on the cerebral cortex and are not selective in acting on the part of the brain involved in abnormal neuronal discharges.

There are currently many drugs that can be used to prevent the occurrence of grand mal and petit mal seizures and to a lesser extent psychomotor seizures in a high percentage of individuals. Selected commonly used anticonvulsant drugs as related to seizure types are listed in Table 35-1 along with average daily dose and toxic effects. Drugs may be used singly or in combinations based on the response of the person. Highly refractory seizures may require several drugs in full therapeutic dosages. Phenytoin sodium (Dilantin) has the highest therapeutic index and is the drug of choice for grand mal seizures. When the seizure fails to respond to phenytoin sodium alone, either phenobarbital or primidone (Mysoline) or related drugs may be added; in refractory seizures all three drugs may be utilized. The same three drugs are also often used in combination with psychomotor seizures, but the seizures are not so readily controlled as are grand mal seizures. Carbamazepine (Tegretol) appears to hold some promise in controlling psychomotor seizures. Ethosuximide (Zarontin) and trimethadione (Tridione) are the drugs of choice in petit mal seizures. The dosages of anticonvulsant drugs are difficult to establish and regulate due to the high incidence of side effects and the toxicity of the drugs. The drug of choice is introduced in average therapeutic dosage and is increased in dosage until control is reached; if toxicity is reached before control of the seizures, the dosage is decreased to the previous nontoxic or tolerated dosage. Additional secondary drugs are usually introduced at this point and increased similarly until control is obtained. It is important that convenient dosage schedules are established for the individual; dosage may be divided, with a smaller dose taken during the day and a larger dose taken during the evening.

Corticosteroids are used occasionally to treat myoclonus. Bromides are used less frequently than in the past and have been replaced to a great extent by the anticonvulsant drugs. Occasionally a ketogenic diet may be prescribed for patients with petit mal seizures. The diet is not easy to follow, and the effectiveness of ethosuximide has led to decline in its use.

Failure to take the prescribed medication or take an adequate dosage are frequent causes of failure in treatment. Some medical centers have facilities to determine the level of drugs in the blood. This is helpful in providing an accurate check on the therapeutic and toxic levels of the medications taken by the patient. Unfortunately most medications that help to control seizures produce toxic effects. It should be recognized that effects on the kidneys and bone marrow can be serious. The individual must remain under medical supervision in order to regulate the medications and to make changes as necessary. Persons with seizures often engage in wishful thinking once control is reached and believe that they have outgrown their disease. They often think that they can omit the prescribed medication, since they have gone for some time without a seizure.[28]

Status epilepticus

When recurrent generalized seizure activity occurs at such frequency that full consciousness is not regained between seizures, it is referred to as *status epilepticus* Although this condition is relatively rare, it can lead to death from brain damage secondary to prolonged hypoxia and exhaustion. Status epilepticus is a medical emergency requiring intensive medical and nursing care.

The person with status epilepticus is often in a coma for a period of 12 to 24 hours or longer, during which time there are recurring seizures. The seizures may cease spontaneously and consciousness return, or death may result from the repeated attacks. The attack usually is related to failure to take prescribed medication. Vigorous therapy is thus directed toward arrest of the seizures. The first priority is assuring an adequate airway, which may be compromised by the seizure and complication of certain drug therapy. Endotracheal tubes, a laryngoscope, aspirating equipment, and oxygen should be in the patient unit prior to administration of medications. This is important because the large drug dosages and the type of drugs used often lead to pulmonary complications. Drug therapy is given intravenously. Medications commonly used include sodium phenobarbital, diazepam (Valium), and paraldehyde. Results appear to be best from large or full (not divided) therapeutic dosages. Medications are stopped if respiratory depression occurs or if the seizure abates. At times it may be necessary to give a general anesthetic. Oxygen may be used to counter the effects of cerebral anoxia. Solutions of glucose may be ordered to treat dehydration.

Constant monitoring of vital signs of respiratory depression and cardiac changes is necessary. The responsibilities pertaining to the observation and recording of seizure activity are the same as described on p. 662. It may not be possible to note the separate seizure phases because of the frequency of them. A safe, quiet, and nonstimulating environment is essential. The head of the bed should be lowered and the patient turned to a side-lying position to lessen the danger of aspiration during seizures; padded side rails should be in place.

Home care of the person with seizures

Members of the family must learn to care for the person during and following a convulsion. A mouth gag should be on hand at all times, and family members should know how and when it should be inserted. They should also be alert for accident hazards. One of the most important things for the family to learn is the need to be calm and accepting of the family member's seizures. They should attempt to prevent the person from engaging in activity that may be dangerous and keep him from exposure to curious persons during convulsions, but they should not contribute to the person's feelings that he is different from others.

Public attitudes

One of the most important aspects in epilepsy therapy is changing the public's attitude toward the disease. The individual subject to seizures and the public must view seizures not as bizarre castrophies but as relatively normal events that can be dealt with rationally. Many persons with epilepsy lead normal productive lives. Indeed, many outstanding figures in world history had seizures (Julius Caesar, Lord Byron, and Napoleon). Studies do not bear out the popular assumption that mental deterioration occurs with epilepsy. Cognitive abilities vary among persons with epilepsy as with the population generally. Nor is there any evidence that personality changes are the result of pathologic processes; when they occur they are probably the result of society's attitude toward the person with epilepsy. For example, some people who are found to have epilepsy are immediately suspended from their work even when they are not dangerous to themselves or others. Some employers refuse to hire a person with known epilepsy, yet at least 80% of all persons with epilepsy are employable. The person is haunted by fear of being seen during a seizure, fear of being found to have seizures, fear of losing his job, and fear of losing the companionship of others. The Epilepsy Foundation of America has been active in trying to improve state laws regarding employment of persons with epilepsy. Children with epilepsy have been segregated to separate schools, and only recently have some major cities passed laws ensuring children with epilepsy the right to attend the public schools if they are under adequate medical care. In many schools children are barred from the classroom according to the inclination of the teacher. Limitation of environment and of education opportunity often limits the child's knowledge, but this does not mean that learning capacity is poor.

Interest in epilepsy and in the problems of the epileptic person has been increased by various organizations such as the National Association to Control Epilepsy, Inc.,* National Epilepsy League, Inc.,†

*Headquarters: 22 East 67th St., New York, N.Y. 10021.
†Headquarters: 203 Wabash St., Chicago, Ill. 60604.

Epilepsy Foundation of America,* and United Epilepsy Association.†

☐ Outcome criteria for the person with known epilepsy or seizures

The patient or significant others can:

1. Explain any medications to be taken or treatment program to be carried out at home:
   a. Explain the action, side effects, toxic effects, and dosage schedule of each anticonvulsant drug prescribed.
   b. Explain the importance of taking the prescribed anticonvulsants regularly according to schedule even though seizures are controlled.
   c. Explain the need to seek medical assistance when side effects or toxic effects occur.
   d. Explain the incompatibility of anticonvulsant drugs with alcohol and drugs that counteract the anticonvulsants.
2. Explain activities of daily living to be followed:
   a. Explain the need to structure a balance between rest and activity.
   b. Explain the need to avoid excessive exercise, fatigue, and stress.
   c. Explain the importance of continuing usual activities within the above limitations when seizures are under control.
3. Explain how to secure professional and community resources necessary to structure a satisfactory home and work environment:
   a. List agencies that can be contacted.
   b. Explain how to secure legal counsel relative to state laws.
   c. State plans for follow-up care.

The significant others can:

1. Demonstrate seizure precautions to be followed during and after an attack or seizure:
   a. Demonstrate how to maintain an open airway so that aspiration and blockage of the airway by the tongue is prevented.
   b. Explain the importance of staying with the person during the attack for protection and to make observations.
   c. Demonstrate how to loosen clothing around the neck and waist.
   d. Explain the need to provide rest and to make observations after a seizure.

■ NEUROLOGIC PAIN

Pain other than headache is one of the most common symptoms seen in neurology. It is difficult to distinguish between pain produced by lesions within the nervous system that cause objective sensory abnormalities and peripherally produced somatic pain in a distant organ. The neurologist and the neurophysiologist view pain from the standpoint of neural transmission. Neurologic pain may arise from lesions involving peripheral cutaneous nerves, the sensory nerve roots (posterior), the thalamus, and the central pain tract (spinothalamic) at some level (see sensory pathways, Fig. 34-8).

☐ Assessment

As in other types of pain, the quality of pain and its distribution are important for the nurse to assess. The quality of neurologic pain or *paresthesia* (abnormal sensation) may vary from mild to excruciating. The sensation of pain may be increased *(hyperalgesia)*, decreased *(hypalgesia)*, or blocked *(analgesia)*. The nurse may find that in some types of pain it is difficult for the person to describe the pain accurately. It is perceived variously as "burning," "pins and needles," or "numbness." The constancy of the pain makes it difficult for the person to bear.

Peripheral cutaneous nerves are particularly vulnerable to trauma and vascular effects. The pain resulting from peripheral nerve lesions is usually limited to the anatomic area supplied by the affected nerve or nerves. Thus the location or distribution may be compared with charts showing the distribution of peripheral sensory fibers (see Fig. 34-9). For example, a lesion involving the lateral femoral cutaneous nerve of the thigh produces pain limited to the area of the skin supplied by this nerve. Pain of this type is often described as a burning sensation. It should be recalled that all peripheral nerves are mixed nerves (sensory and motor). Each nerve has a definite area of skin from which to carry sensation and a definite muscle or muscle group to supply. Damage to a nerve at its periphery results in both loss of sensation and muscle function. An occasional sequela of peripheral nerve injury is *causalgia*, that is, intense and continuous burning type of pain. An attack may arise spontaneously, or in response to touch, or even as a result of emotions and stress. The quantity and quality of pain is disproportionate to sensory intake.

Root pain, or *radicular pain*, is limited to the dermatomes supplied by the affected sensory nerve roots (see Fig. 34-9). However, pain from lesions arising from deep somatic and visceral structures may radiate beyond the dermatomes. When assessing root pain the nurse should understand that it is often aggravated by anything that causes direct or indirect movement of the spinal cord. Such actions as sneezing, coughing, or straining increase intrathoracic and intraabdominal pressure and indirectly produce distention of veins in the epidural space, thus affecting the dura mater surrounding the

*Headquarters: 1828 L St., N.W., Washington, D.C. 20036.
†Headquarters: 113 West 57th St., New York, N.Y. 10019.

nerve roots. Pain occurring with the above events is of diagnostic value. It should be remembered that sensory (posterior) nerve roots are fixed directly to the cord, and lesions in this area may extend to include the motor (anterior) nerve roots and in addition cause motor signs and symptoms. Because of this anatomic fact, the person with this type of pain should not lie in a horizontal plane for long periods as this causes tension or traction on the thoracic and sacral nerve roots. Sitting up may help to relieve tension on the nerve roots. When moving a person with root pain, sharp flexion of the neck and leg extension should be avoided as much as possible, since this intensifies the pain by causing more direct movement of the meninges and roots.

Pain resulting from *central lesions within the thalamus* is confined to the contralateral side of the body, since the thalamus receives sensory pain impulses from the opposite side of the body. In massive thalamic lesions only contiguous portions of the body may be affected. This type of pain is described by patients as "burning," "pulling," and "swelling." It is often aggravated by emotional stress and fatigue and is influenced by cutaneous stimulations. The nurse may find it difficult to care for the person, both physically and emotionally. It is most important that the nurse understand the physiologic basis of this kind of discomfort, the factors that aggravate it, and why the person has persistent complaints.

Lesions involving the *central spinothalamic tracts* (see Fig. 34-8) produce pain sensation distributed to the level of the tract involved. Hemisection of the spinal cord involving the spinothalamic tract produces loss of pain and temperature perception on the contralateral side at a level one or two segments below the injury. Tract pain is similar to thalamic pain but may be less distressing.

□ Intervention

Providing relief from discomfort and pain from lesions arising from within the nervous system is challenging. It requires the ability to try varied methods to find the one that provides the most relief. Ongoing assessment includes the location, distribution, and site of origin of the pain. Observation of associated symptoms such as muscle weakness, vasomotor response, and the presence of abnormal sensations is equally important. The emotional and cultural aspects of pain and how it is perceived by the person are necessary data for planning care (see Chapter 22). Since environmental stimuli often initiate or intensify pain, these are significant data in planning specific interventions. Analgesics are prescribed to obtain the most effective relief of pain; alternate drugs are usually tried until the one providing the best result is determined.

Intractable pain

Unbearable pain that does not respond to definitive treatment of the causative lesion is classified as intractable. The pain is chronic and often disabling. The individual's degree of disability and suffering (despite the physiologic basis for the pain) must also be related to psychologic and personality factors. It is difficult to evaluate objectively a patient's complaints of pain. The chronic complainer of pain is often stereotyped by the nurse as a difficult patient. It is possible to alleviate intractable pain surgically through deafferentation at varied sites such as by *neurectomy*, *rhizotomy*, and *cordotomy*. These neurosurgical procedures are discussed briefly. Discussion is related to pain generally and is not limited to pain of neurologic origin.

Neurectomy. When pain is localized to one part of the body it can be relieved by interruption of the peripheral or cranial nerves supplying the area. The nerve fibers to the affected area are severed from the cord (cell body) in an operation known as neurectomy. The nerve may also be effectively destroyed by injecting it with absolute alcohol, but the results are unpredictable. Not only pain fibers are interrupted by these procedures but also fibers controlling movement and position sense. Therefore this type of treatment cannot be used to control pain in the extremities. A neurectomy probably is most often performed to relieve the pain of persons with trigeminal neuralgia, in which case it is referred to as a *fifth-nerve resection*. A neurectomy may also be performed to control incapacitating dysmenorrhea and is called a *presacral neurectomy*.

Rhizotomy. Resection of a posterior nerve root just before it enters the spinal cord is known as a rhizotomy. This procedure frequently is useful in controlling severe pain in the upper trunk such as that caused by carcinoma of the lung. It is also done to relieve severe spasticity in persons with paraplegia. However, it cannot be used to relieve pain in the extremities, since position sense is lost. The incision is made high in the thoracic or low in the cervical area and involves a laminectomy. The postoperative observations and care are similar to that necessary for any patient who has had a laminectomy, except that the patient who has had a rhizotomy is usually a poorer operative risk and may be suffering from a severe debilitating disease and therefore develops complications such as decubiti more easily. It is important for both the patient and the nurse to realize that this operation will not prevent pain at the level of the incision because the resected nerves affect only the area below the incision.

Cordotomy. A cordotomy is an operation performed to relieve intractable pain in the lower trunk and legs and is most often performed on patients with extensive carcinoma of the pelvis. The incision is made high in the

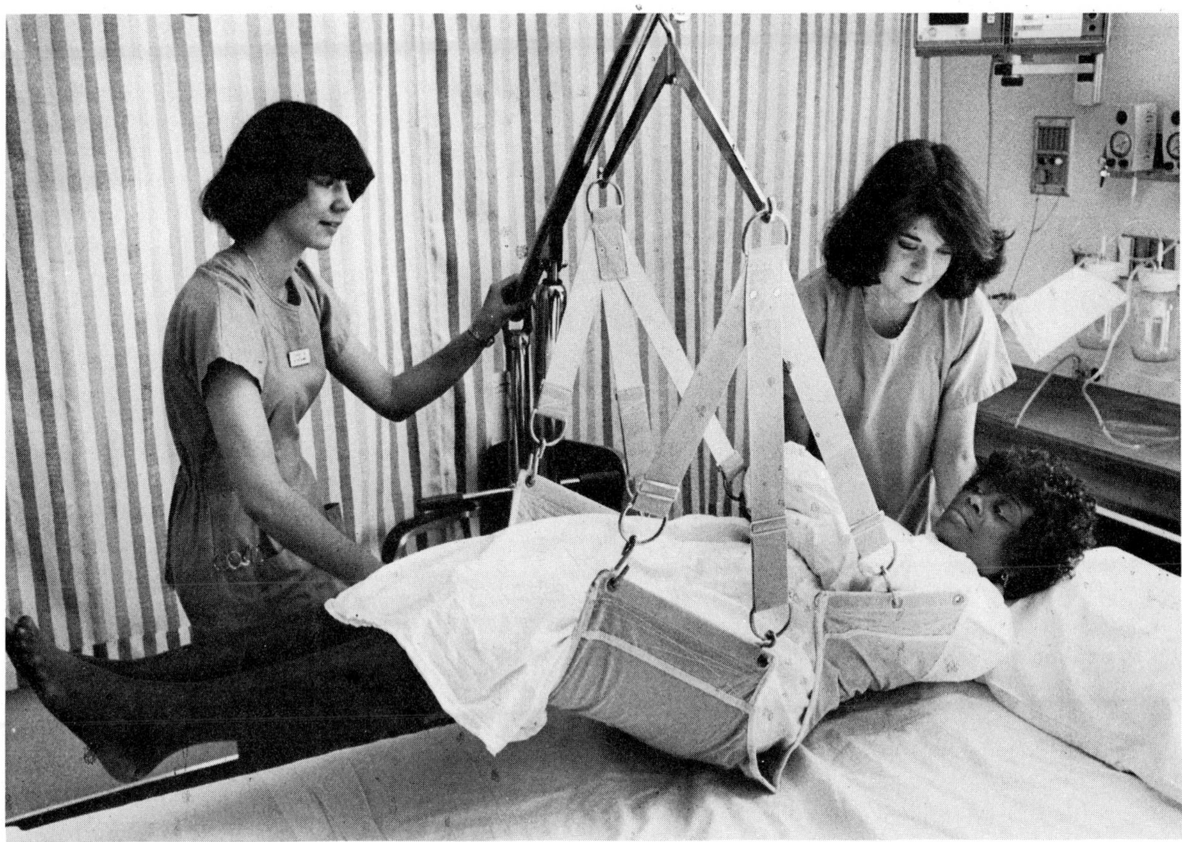

Fig. 35-1. Hydraulic lift can be used to move paralyzed patient from bed to chair.

thoracic area, two laminae are removed, and the pain pathways in the spinothalamic tract (anterior and lateral aspect of the cord) on the side opposite the pain are severed (see Fig. 34-5). If the pain is in the midline, the interruption must be made bilaterally. However, the two operations must be performed separately to avoid extensive damage to the cord from edema.

Following surgery, nursing care is similar to that given a patient who has had a cervical laminectomy for removal of a protruded nucleus pulposus. Frequently temporary paralysis, or at least leg weakness, and loss of bowel and bladder control follow a cordotomy; these result from edema of the cord and will gradually disappear in about 2 weeks. During the period of paralysis the patient may be helped out of bed by using a hydraulic lift (Fig. 35-1). Back care with special attention to pressure points should be given every 2 or 3 hours, since position sense is lessened and the patient is often debilitated. It is advisable to use an alternating-air-pressure mattress until the patient is allowed out of bed. Sometimes a Foster bed or a Stryker frame enables the nurse to give the patient better care. Because of the decreased position sense, special attention needs to be given to placing the patient in proper body alignment by using foot blocks. If quadriceps-setting exercises are begun in the early postoperative period, retraining in walking will be less difficult for the patient. It usually is easier for the patient to use a walker when he first begins to walk, but he should progress to a cane. Many patients will always feel more secure with a cane. Occupational therapy may be designed to strengthen the leg muscles, such as riding a stationary bicycle, which provides for hip and knee flexion and extension. Therapy can be started as soon as the patient can be out of bed comfortably for at least 2 hours at a time.

Because temperature sensation is permanently lost, the nurse must be careful to avoid burning or otherwise injuring the patient's lower trunk and legs and must teach the patient and family how to avoid injury. The lower portion of the body, especially the feet, is inspected routinely for any breaks in the skin or unnoticed infection.

Currently *percutaneous cordotomy* is the preferred surgical technique. It permits more precise control of the size and site of the surgical lesion than does the direct thoracic approach described previously. It is also less traumatic surgically for the debilitated person who has often been on continuous analgesic therapy for long periods.

The procedure consists of inserting a spinal lumbar puncture needle laterally between the cervical (C1 and C2) level. A wire electrode is then inserted into the anterior cord and a lesion is made at a designated site, under radiologic and stereotactic control, in order to destroy the ascending pain fibers. The procedure is performed with the patient under local anesthesia, and a sensation of tingling in the corresponding body area will be noticed when the electrode is stimulated minimally. This assists the surgeon in locating the exact site for the surgical lesion.

Preoperatively the patient is evaluated carefully as to his candidacy for this type of surgery and to establish baseline data. It is important to identify and exclude the individual whose pain is more functionally based. Cordotomy in this instance would not be successful in relief of the pain. Pulmonary function is also carefully evaluated. Regional anesthetic blocks (with an epidural catheter) are often evaluated prior to surgery for a 24-hour period or longer in order to test the benefits to the person. Placebo blocks with normal saline solution are also done and the results compared with the anesthetic block. The patient is carefully monitored by the nurse during the regional blocks as to hypalgesia and analgesia responses.

Postoperatively the patient is observed closely for postural hypotension when initially ambulated. The sympathetic fibers in the cord controlling blood pressure lie in close proximity to the surgical site, and blood pressure may be affected for a period of time. Temperature sensation is also expected to be lost after this type of surgery. Bladder function and motor function may also be affected and should be observed carefully by the nurse following surgery. Usually such deficits do not increase following unilateral cordotomy but may after bilateral cordotomy. The value of accurate presurgical baseline data of all components is particularly necessary for good postsurgical care of the patient with a cordotomy.

Trigeminal neuralgia

Trigeminal neuralgia (tic douloureux) is characterized by excruciating, burning pain that radiates along one or more of the three divisions of the fifth cranial nerve (Fig. 35-2). The pain typically extends only to the midline of the face and head, since this is the extent of the tissue supplied by the offending nerve. There are areas along the course of the nerve known as "trigger points," and the slightest stimulation of these areas may initiate pain. Persons with trigeminal neuralgia try desperately to avoid "triggering" the pain. It is not unusual to see them lying in bed with the covers over their heads in an effort to avoid drafts. They frequently have been

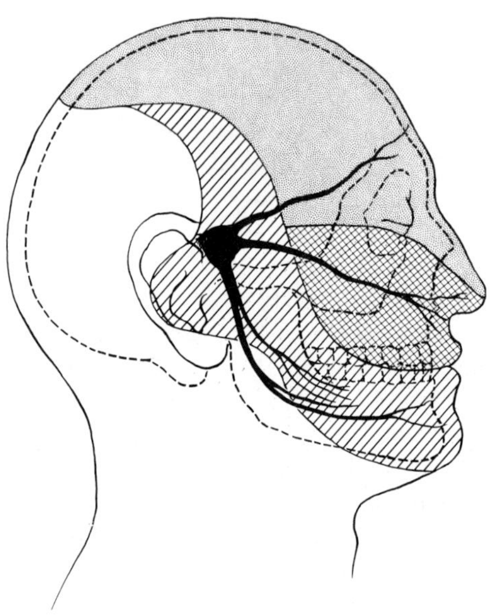

Fig. 35-2. Pathway of trigeminal nerve and facial areas innervated by each of three main divisions of this nerve.

unable to eat properly for some time, since chewing causes pain. They may therefore be undernourished and dehydrated. They may have slept poorly and not washed, shaved, or combed their hair for some time. Oral hygiene may often be neglected because of pain.

The person is usually treated medically first before attempting surgery. In caring for the person with trigeminal neuralgia *preoperatively* or in caring for the patient who is being treated medically, it is important that members of the nursing staff be sympathetic toward the person's behavior. Every effect should be made to avoid placing the bed in a draft and to avoid walking swiftly to the bed, because the slight motion of air may be enough to cause pain. The bed should not be jarred or the bedclothes fanned. It is unwise to urge the person to wash or shave the affected area or to comb his hair, since he may either become upset in feeling that it is required or he may comply and set off another siege of pain. The person will probably prefer to avoid self-care that involves touching the face. Some will do their own mouth care if applicators and a lukewarm mouthwash are provided. Often pureed foods or lukewarm fluids taken through a straw are the only diet that can be tolerated.

Carbamazepine (Tegretol) currently is the drug of choice for the treatment of the pain (also used for convulsions). The inhalation of trichloroethylene (10 to 15 drops on cotton) has been tried with variable success for relieving pain. Drugs such as nicotinic acid, thiamine chloride, cobra venom, and analgesics have all been tried, but usually they offer the person little if any relief. Sedatives are given for sleep.[10]

The peripheral branches of the trigeminal nerve may be injected with absolute alcohol. This provides relief for weeks or months, and the procedure may be repeated as necessary. Permanent relief can only be obtained by surgery that consists of dividing the sensory root of the trigeminal nerve intracranially. If not all of the nerve is involved, a partial resection is performed.

Postoperatively it is important to know what branches of the nerve have been cut in order to provide the necessary protection. If the *upper branch* is completely severed, the corneal reflex on that side will be lost. Usually an attempt is made to preserve a few of the fibers of the first division of the fifth nerve, since even a few intact fibers seem to preserve this vital function. Until the physician has tested the corneal reflex and verified its presence, an eye shield is used to prevent dust or lint from getting onto the cornea and causing injury.

The patient is instructed not to touch or rub his eye but to blink it often, since blinking helps to lubricate the eye. If the reflex is completely absent, each eye should be bathed at least every 4 hours and more often if necessary. The best solution for bathing the eye is normal saline solution. A solution of methylcellulose ("artificial tears"), 0.5% to 2% may be prescribed to help keep the cornea moist. Some experts recommend that 1 to 2 drops of mineral oil be instilled in each eye following eye irrigation; however, no medication should be instilled in the eye without an order from the physician. The lids should not be dried, since any material such as cotton, gauze, tissue, or toweling may leave lint. The patient should be taught eye care before discharge. Any contact with the eye should be carefully avoided when washing the face. The eye is inspected several times a day, and medical attention should be sought if it becomes inflamed. Persons are safer outdoors if they wear glasses, which will protect the eyes from dust and other flying particles. Contact lenses should never be worn because the lenses are too irritating.

When the *lower branch* of the fifth cranial nerve is interrupted hot foods will need to be avoided, since the person will not be aware if the mucous membrane is burned. There may be difficulty chewing and swallowing at first, and the person is instructed to place the food in the unaffected side of the mouth. Since food may be retained in the mouth on the affected side, mouth care should be given immediately following meals. Dental caries on the affected side will not cause pain; therefore there is need for a routine dental check every 6 months. The dentist should be informed that the person has had a fifth-nerve resection so that trauma is avoided. Care must be taken in shaving to avoid nicking the insensitive skin.

Within 24 hours after a fifth nerve resection, many patients develop herpes simplex (cold sores) about the lips. Phenol and camphor (Campho-Phenique) applied frequently seems to give more relief than any other treatment. Usually the lesions heal in about a week.

An operating microscope is used during surgery on the trigeminal nerve. Microsurgery permits greater precision in selective cutting of fibers; also, the sensation of touch and the corneal reflex are preserved.[10] More recently a new method to sever the nerve inside the skull is being utilized. A thin electrode needle is inserted through the cheek and into the nerve. This avoids a surgical procedure and may provide permanent relief of pain.[10]

Other cranial nerve surgery

Other cranial nerves may be surgically interrupted as necessary. It is sometimes necessary to resect both the fifth and the ninth nerves to relieve severe pain caused by carcinoma of the sinuses. The nursing problems in each instance are related to the areas that have been desensitized and the resulting handicaps. Often there is temporary and sometimes permanent loss or a change of facial expression after resection of these nerves, which may cause severe psychic problems. When any nerve is resected, whether it is peripheral or cranial, the patient must understand that all sensation in this area is lost and that he will therefore need to avoid injury, especially from heat, cold, and trauma.

□ Outcome criteria for the person with neurologic pain

The patient or significant others can:

1. Explain methods to control discomfort and pain:
   a. Explain the prescribed analgesics or alternates as to action, side effects, and dosage schedules.
   b. Demonstrate physical measures that can be safely used for pain control.
   c. Explain the advantages and disadvantages of available surgical interventions used to control intractable pain.
   d. Describe positioning methods and their relationships to the occurrence of pain.
2. Explain general health practices:
   a. Explain how to maintain sleep and rest patterns.
   b. Explain the relationship between pain and emotional upsets.
   c. State plans for follow-up care.

■ INCREASED INTRACRANIAL PRESSURE

Increased intracranial pressure (ICP) is a complex manifestation that is the consequence of multiple neurologic conditions and often requires surgical intervention.

The cranial contents, including the brain tissues, vascular tissues, and cerebrospinal fluid, are contained within a bony vault for protection. Any increase in the volume of any of the cranial contents, singly or in combination, results in increased intracranial pressure, since the cranial vault is rigid, closed, and nonexpandable. Several neurologic lesions, either by their nature or by inciting cerebral edema, increase the volume of tissue within the cranium. Any lesion that increases tissue volume is known as a space-occupying lesion. Common examples include cerebral contusions, hematomas, infarcts, abscesses, and other inflammations of brain tissues. Intracranial tumors arising from all types of brain tissues increase cell mass and as a consequence increase intracranial pressure. An increase in the production of cerebrospinal fluid, blockage of the ventricular system, or a decreased absorption of cerebrospinal fluid can likewise increase tissue fluid volume. According to the *box theory of the brain*, an increase in any one of the contents of the cranium is usually accompanied by a *reciprocal change* in the volume of one of the others. Brain tissue cannot expand without serious effects on the flow and amount of CSF and cerebral circulation. Space-occupying lesions must of necessity displace and distort the brain and vascular tissues as pressure increases. Pressure may build up slowly (days or months) or rapidly (minutes or hours), depending on the cause. At first one hemisphere will be more involved, depending on the lesion site, but eventually both hemispheres may become involved if the pressure continues to increase.

As pressure increases within the cranial cavity, it is at first compensated through venous compression and cerebrospinal fluid displacement. When the pressure within the cavity exceeds the compensatory mechanisms in the adult, the only escape for the swollen and displaced brain hemisphere is caudally or by downward herniation. The falx cerebri oppose medial shift of the hemispheres and the tentorium cerebelli oppose downward shift to some extent. Structures that allow internal herniation are the cingulate gyrus, which permits medial subfalcial herniation (under the falx); the uncus, which permits downward transtentorial herniation (across free edge of tentorium); and the cerebellar tonsil, which permits transforaminal herniation (through the foramen magnum) (see Fig. 35-3 for identification of these structures with internal herniations and shifting of the hemisphere). As a consequence of the herniation, the brainstem is compressed at variable levels, which in turn compresses the vasomotor center, posterior cerebral artery, oculomotor nerve, corticospinal nerve pathways, and fibers of the *ascending reticular activating system* (ARAS). Internal herniation in this way represents the critical state of decompensation. The life-sustaining mechanisms for consciousness, blood pressure, pulse, respiration, and temperature regulation fail.

□ Assessment

The detection of increased intracranial pressure ideally occurs *early,* when it is reversible and before the stage of decompensation. *The ability to make accurate observations, to interpret observations intelligently, and to record observations carefully is without question the most important part of nursing care of patients with increased intracranial pressure.* The nurse must know when to notify the physician relative to changes in the patient's condition. The nurse must be capable of implementing nursing, medical, and surgical measures appropriately. Because of the need to understand the neurophysiologic basis of observations, selected signs relative to increased intracranial pressure are discussed from a nursing standpoint.

Level of consciousness (LOC)

The mesencephalon and diencephalon, which act as way stations to the ascending reticular activating system (ARAS), become compressed following herniation of the brainstem. Nerve impulses are interrupted through the

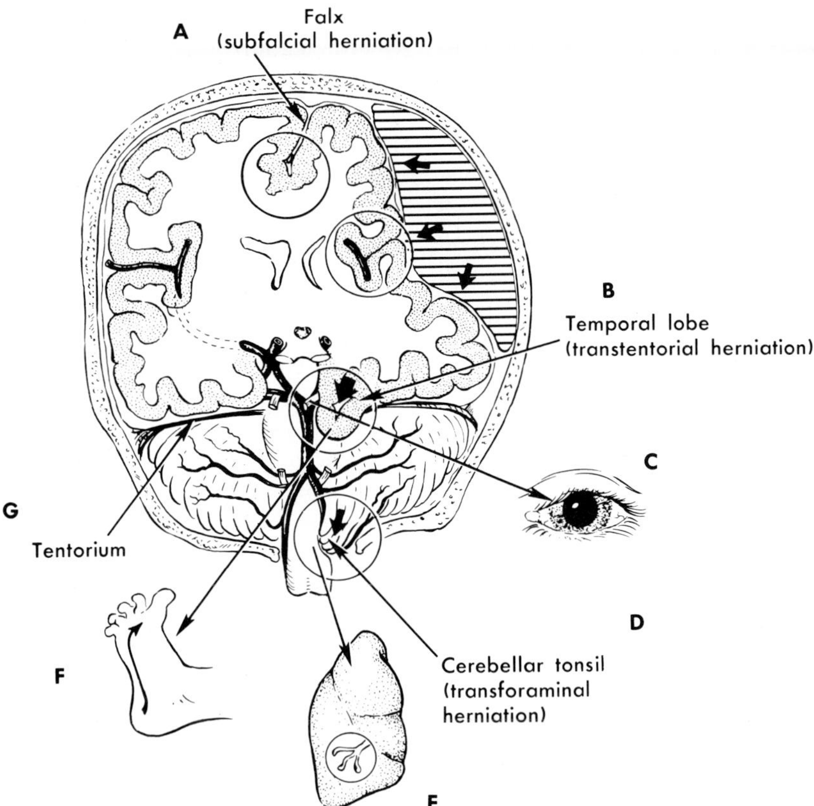

Fig. 35-3. Consequences of increased intracranial pressure. Expanding temporoparietal epidural hematoma with medial and downward pressure has produced subfalcial, transtentorial, and transforaminal internal herniations. Note distortion of falx, **A,** bulging of medial temporal lobe at tentorial edge, **B,** and herniation of cerebellar tonsil with descending pressure on brainstem, **D.** Also note how major blood vessels are collapsed in encircled areas. Some consequential effects of continuing or expanding pressure on neural structures with alterations in body functions are detailed. **C,** Homolateral dilation and fixation of pupil with ptosis of eyelid. **E,** Life-threatening respiratory centers in brainstem. **F,** Contralateral Babinski's sign showing extension of great toe and fanning of other toes following plantar stimulation. Coronal view of head, ventral view of brainstem. (Modified from original painting by Frank H. Netter, M.D.; from Clinical Symposia, Copyright by Ciba Pharmaceutical Co., Division of Ciba-Geigy Corp. All rights reserved.)

ARAS, which is considered to be the seat of the consciousness. There is hypoxia of tissue cells of the ARAS. A decreasing level of consciousness is an early sign of internal herniation. *Any change in the level of consciousness is one of the most important observations for the nurse to make, report, and record.* Level of consciousness is one of the earliest and most sensitive indicators of increased cranial pressure. (For further information on assessment of LOC, see p. 502.)

Pupillary signs

Pupillary responses are controlled by the oculomotor nerve (cranial nerve III). The oculomotor nerve is compressed by the herniating tissue and specifically by the downward displaced posterior cerebral artery. The pupilloconstrictor fibers of the oculomotor nerve run in a group in the top part of this nerve and are the first to be compressed. As a consequence the ipsilateral pupil (when the lesion is in one hemisphere) remains dilated and is incapable of constricting. The pupil appears larger than in the other eye and does not react to light. Eventually as cerebral pressure increases and both hemispheres are affected, there is bilateral pupil dilation and fixation. Inequality of the pupils may appear earlier than fixation when the nerve is only stretched. The pupil may respond to light slowly rather than with the usual brisk normal response. In examining the pupils the nurse should note the size and equality first and then test the reaction of each pupil to light in a darkened room.

Blood pressure and pulse

The effect of cerebral pressure on blood pressure and pulse is variable. Compensatory changes occur in the cerebral vasculature relative to hypoxia or diminished blood flow. As cerebral pressure rises, the blood pressure rises in response to the hypoxic stimulus in the vasomotor center. The rise in blood pressure may be sudden or gradual. As cerebral pressure rises, the blood pressure rises to a point or until terminal collapse. Blood pressure readings should be taken in the same arm for comparative purposes. The pulse slows reflexly as the blood pressure rises. *Slowing of the pulse rate in conjunction with a rising systolic blood pressure is a significant observation to be made and reported.* The pulse should be taken for a full minute and described as to its character.

Respiration

Herniation produces respiratory dysrhythmias that are variable and are related to the level of brainstem compression or failure. The breathing pattern may be deep and stertorous, or Cheyne-Stokes (periodic); terminally there is respiratory paralysis. The beginning of periodic breathing is significant. The usual picture is one of slowing of respiration, along with a slow pulse and a rising systolic blood pressure. The nurse should learn to look for variability in vital signs and detect trends as they occur. It is important to remember that the patient with a decreasing level of consciousness will require assistance in keeping the airway clear. Consequently respiration difficulty is further aggravated by this problem.

Temperature regulation

Failure of the thermoregulatory center due to compression occurs later and gives rise to high uncontrolled temperatures. It is important to understand that hyperthermia needs to be controlled, since it increases the metabolic needs of the brain tissues. Temperatures are taken rectally unless otherwise ordered.

Focal motor signs

Compression of upper motor neuron pathways (corticospinal tract) interrupts the transmission of impulses to lower motor neurons, and progressive muscle weakness results. For example, a contralateral weakened hand grasp may progress to hemiparesis and hemiplegia. The presence of the Babinski's sign, hyperreflexia, and rigidity are additional motor signs that provide evidence of decreasing motor function from upper motor neuron involvement. Transtentorial herniation of the upper or rostral part of the brainstem produces decerebrate rigidity. The motor inhibitory fibers are blocked, and the person involuntarily assumes a fixed posture with arms, legs, and trunk extended and with flexion of the palmar and plantar joints; seizures may also be present. The nurse should use gross tests or more definitive tests to determine motor changes. *The worsening in existing motor deficits is significant.*

Visual acuity and papilledema

The blind spot of the retina measures the size and shape of the optic papilla, or optic disc. As venous congestion and intracranial pressure increase, the resulting pressure is transmitted to the eyes through the cerebrospinal fluid and to the optic disc (choked disc). Since the meninges of the brain reflect out around the eyeball, they permit the direct transmission of pressure along the subarachnoid space through the cerebrospinal fluid. As the optic disc swells, the retina adjacent to it is also compressed. The damaged retina cannot detect light rays. As the size of the blind spot enlarges, visual acuity is lessened. The ability of the nurse to detect papilledema is dependent on skill in examination of the fundi. Decreasing visual acuity can be detected through the confrontation technique (p. 640). Papilledema is an early sign of increased intracranial pressure; loss of vision is a late sign.

Headache

Headache may occur as an early symptom. It is thought to result from venous congestion and the tension on the intracranial blood vessels as the cerebral pressure rises. The onset of the headache should be noted along with its location and duration. It increases in intensity with cough, straining, and stooping.

Vomiting

The occurrence of vomiting that is projectile is often associated with increased intracranial pressure. Its frequency and character should be noted. The significance of vomiting and headache needs to be associated with other clinical signs such as papilledema and vital signs. In summary, papilledema, headache, nausea, and vomiting are the cardinal signs of increased intracranial pressure.

□ Observation

The frequency of "neurologic checks" of the patient is often ordered by the physician. However, with significant deteriorating changes in the aforementioned signs, the nurse should decide when more frequent assessments and recordings are indicated. Based on the results obtained from observations and the medical history of the patient, the nurse will need to make a decision as to frequency of monitoring. Young reports that alterations in consciousness, blood pressure, pulse, pupillary responses, movement of extremities, temperature, and respiration provide the best guide for the nurse to estimate intracranial pressure.[42] A special craniocerebral nursing record has been developed based on these categories.[42] The patient's condition is regularly compared with an established baseline through continuous monitoring. In some medical centers electronic monitoring devices are being used to provide a continuous measure of intracranial pressure.

A method of direct measurement of ICP has been devised in which a hollow screw is placed through the skull into the subarachnoid space. The screw is attached to a Luer-Lok, which is connected to a transducer and oscilloscope for continued monitoring.[18] The transducer is fastened to the head of the bed and must be level with the screw for accurate monitoring. Direction for use of this measurement device can be found in the literature.[18]

□ Intervention

The *prevention* of increased ICP may not be possible, but prevention of *further rise* of ICP and resulting damage to brain tissues is crucial. The detection of *early signs* is important to prevent irreversible effects.

The medical treatment of patients with increased ICP depends on the underlying cause for the pressure increase. For example, if it is due to an intracranial tumor, the tumor is removed surgically. When surgery is not possible (or indicated), efforts are made to reduce the pressure through the use of drug therapy or direct physical measures.

Rapidly rising intracranial pressure must be relieved directly by mechanical decompression. This may be accomplished by a variety of procedures including (1) ventricular puncture with the withdrawal of CSF by needle or cannula, (2) continuous ventricular drainage with a special device that maintains the pressure at a set rate and level, and (3) removal of a piece of skull (craniotomy) to provide room for the cranial contents to expand. Each of these measures requires careful monitoring by the nurse for signs of increased ICP and the maintenance of asepsis at the entrance site into the skull.

Medications commonly ordered to promote rapid osmotic diuresis and the reduction of brain volume include the intravenous administration of urea (Urevert), mannitol, and hypertonic solutions of glucose (25% to 50%). Corticosteroids such as dexamethasone (Decadron) may also be ordered to lessen cerebral edema. The corticosteroids act more slowly, but their effect is more sustained. All these drugs cause dehydration and promote the movement of excess fluid from the brain tissues into the blood so that it can be eliminated. Narcotics and other drugs that cause respiratory depression are avoided. Phenytoin sodium (Dilantin) may be prescribed to prevent seizures.

Conservative measures to reduce venous volume may be implemented. The person is positioned to promote venous drainage; the head of the bed is elevated 15° to 30° so that the head is higher than the heart level and there is no neck flexure. Fluid intake may also be restricted so that there is a less total intake than is normally desired. Urine output with the administration of osmotic diuretics must be monitored carefully through an indwelling catheter and a urimeter. The patient's use of the Valsalva maneuver is eliminated to the extent possible, since it causes increased intrathoracic pressure that indirectly increases ICP. During the treatment phases the nurse makes ongoing, systematic assessment of neurologic status to detect *even slight changes in status.* In summary, medical and nursing interventions are directed toward achievement of the following treatment goals:

1. Reduction of cerebral edema and CSF excess
2. Prevention of cerebral hypoxia by maintaining a clear airway and reducing cerebral pressure
3. Reduction of activities that increase ICP
4. Limitation of fluid intake
5. Monitoring of intake and output so that the results of therapy can be evaluated

□ Outcome criteria for the person with increased intracranial pressure

The person or significant others can:

1. State signs or symptoms that indicate need for immediate medical assistance.
2. State plans for follow-up care.

■ MOTOR PARALYSIS OF UPPER AND LOWER MOTOR NEURONS

Disturbances of motor function probably surpass all other clinical neurologic symptoms in frequency and in importance. Since the nervous system is designed primarily for movement of the body in space and of the various parts in relation to each other, damages to it often causes serious problems in mobility. The term *paralysis* refers to a loss of function, either motor or sensory. When applied to motor function as below, it means loss of voluntary movement due to interruption of the descending motor pathways. A lesser degree of paralysis is called *paresis.* Damage to sensory pathways that are intimately concerned with motor function may occur concomitantly with the loss of motor function. Loss of sensory function is discussed on p. 685.

□ Assessment

Injury or disease of motor neurons and their extensions at any level results in alterations of muscle strength, tone, and reflex activity. The specific clinical manifestations differ according to whether the lesion in-

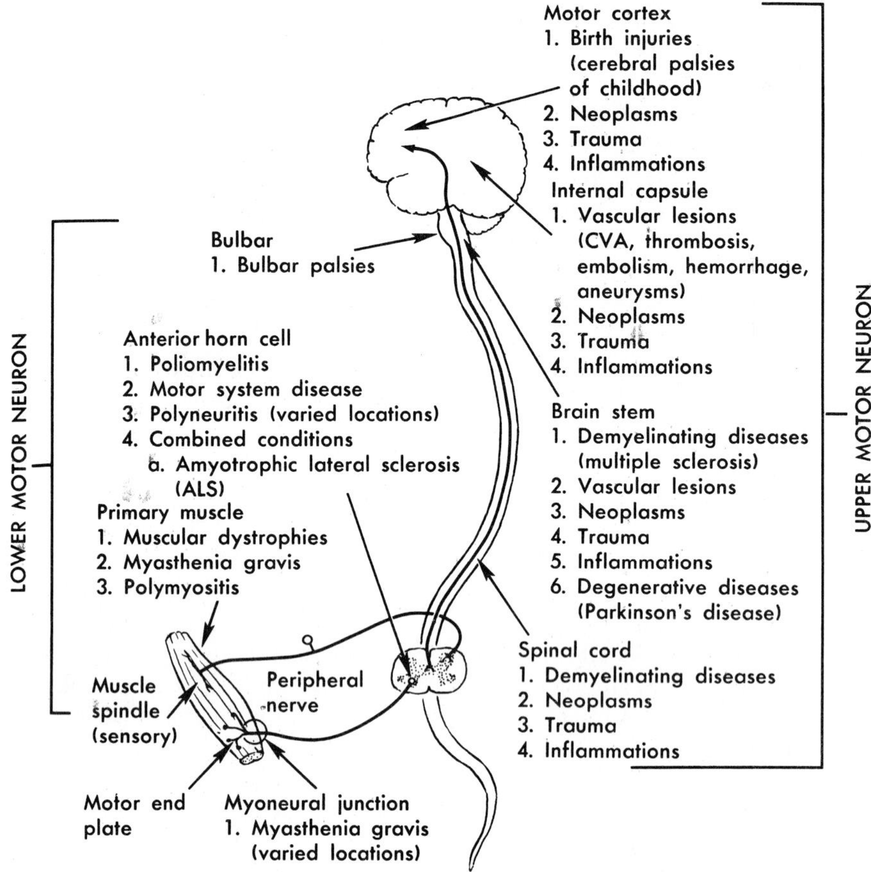

Fig. 35-4. Disturbances in motor function are classified pathologically along upper and lower motor neuron structures. It should be noted that same pathologic condition occurs at more than one site in upper motor neuron shown on right. A few pathologic conditions involve both upper and lower motor neuron structures, as in amyotrophic lateral sclerosis, for example. Other lesion sites include myoneural junction and primary muscle, making it possible to classify conditions as neuromuscular and muscular respectively. (Modified from Chusid, J. G.: Correlative neuroanatomy and functional neurology, ed. 15, Los Altos, Calif., 1970, Lange Medical Publications.)

volves an *upper motor neuron* or a *lower motor neuron*. In addition extension of lesions to the extrapyramidal and cerebellar tracts further alters normal motor activity. Diseases associated with disturbances in motor function are classified in Fig. 35-4.

An important concept in neurologic examination and diagnosis by the neurologist rests on identifying the abnormalities of motor function that result from disease or of injury to upper and lower motor neurons. The ability to differentiate between upper and lower motor neurons lesions is the first step in the localization of the site of a neural lesion that manifests itself by disturbances in normal motor function. When the site of the neural lesion has been decided, the neurologist can then consider the cause.

Lower motor neuron signs

It is necessary to recall that *lower motor neurons* (LMNs) consist of the large anterior horn cells in the spinal cord as well as the motor cranial nuclei in the brainstem and all of their respective axons that innervate striated muscle (Fig. 35-5). Although many fiber systems initiate and modify muscular action in some way, it is the LMN that achieve, or effect, the muscle action. This is also known as the *final common pathway* (Fig. 35-6). When a lesion selectively involves the LMN in some part (cell body, motor root, isolated peripheral nerve), it characteristically results in flaccid muscle weakness or paralysis, loss of reflex activity, loss of muscle tone, and atrophy confined to the involved muscle(s). Each effect is discussed briefly at this point and com-

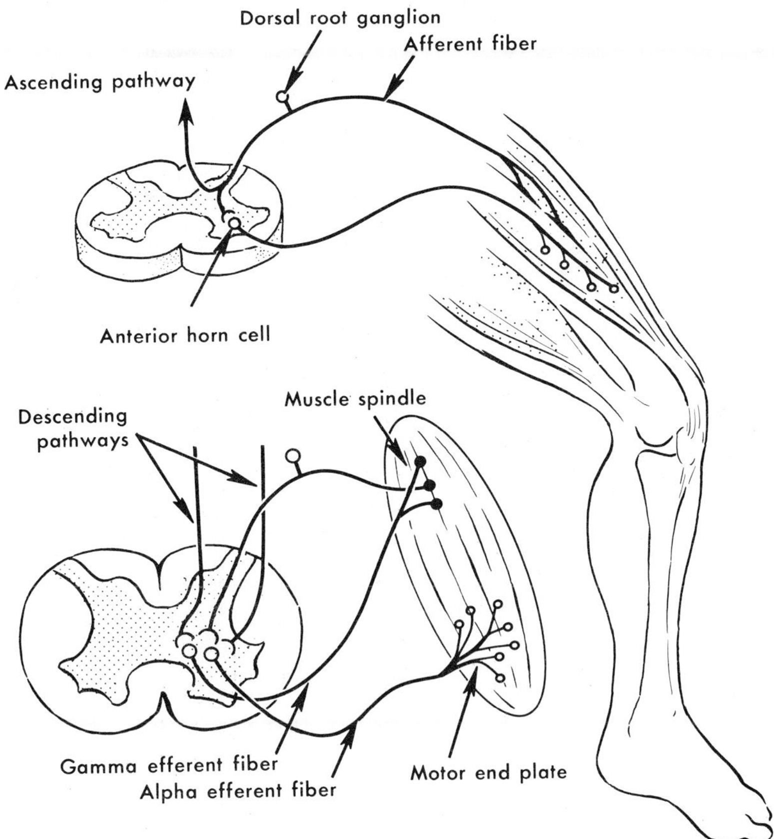

Fig. 35-5. Structures comprising lower motor neuron including motor (efferent) and sensory (afferent) elements. Shown on right is anterior horn cell in anterior gray column of spinal cord and its axon terminating in motor end plate as it innervates extrafusal muscle fibers in quadriceps muscle. Detailed in enlargement on left are sensory and motor elements of gamma loop system. Gamma efferent fiber is shown innervating polar or end region of muscle spindle (sensory receptor of skeletal muscle). Contraction of muscle spindle fibers stretch central portion of spindle and cause afferent spindle fiber to transmit impulse centrally to cord. Muscle spindle afferent fibers in turn synapse on anterior horn cell and are transmitted by way of alpha efferent fibers to skeletal (extrafusal) muscle, causing it to contract. Muscle spindle discharge is interrupted by active contraction of extrafusal muscle fibers. (Adapted from Truex, R. C., and Carpenter, M. B.: Human neuroanatomy, ed. 6, Baltimore, 1969, The Williams & Wilkins Co.)

pared later with upper motor neuron effects on muscle.

The *degree* of muscle weakness occurring in the involved muscle(s) in an LMN lesion bears a direct relationship to the extent and severity of the lesion. Since the anterior horn cells and their neurons, which innervate a single muscle, extend longitudinally through several spinal segments, and since several anterior horn cell columns exist at each spinal level, a lesion confined to one spinal segment will thus cause muscle weakness *(paresis)* rather than paralysis of the muscle. Some motor neurons are thus preserved. Complete paralysis occurs in LMN lesions only when the lesion involves the column or anterior horn cells in several spinal segments that innervate a particular muscle or the ventral roots arising from these cells. A lesion in a single motor nerve root will cause varying degrees of muscle weakness in several muscles. If *all* or practically all peripheral motor fibers supplying a muscle are destroyed, all voluntary postural and reflex movements are lost. The muscle becomes lax and soft, a condition known as *flaccidity.*

Muscle weakness itself cannot be classified as either lower or upper motor neuron, since it is common to both. It is the *distribution* of the muscle weakness that is important to distinguish. In summary, an LMN lesion

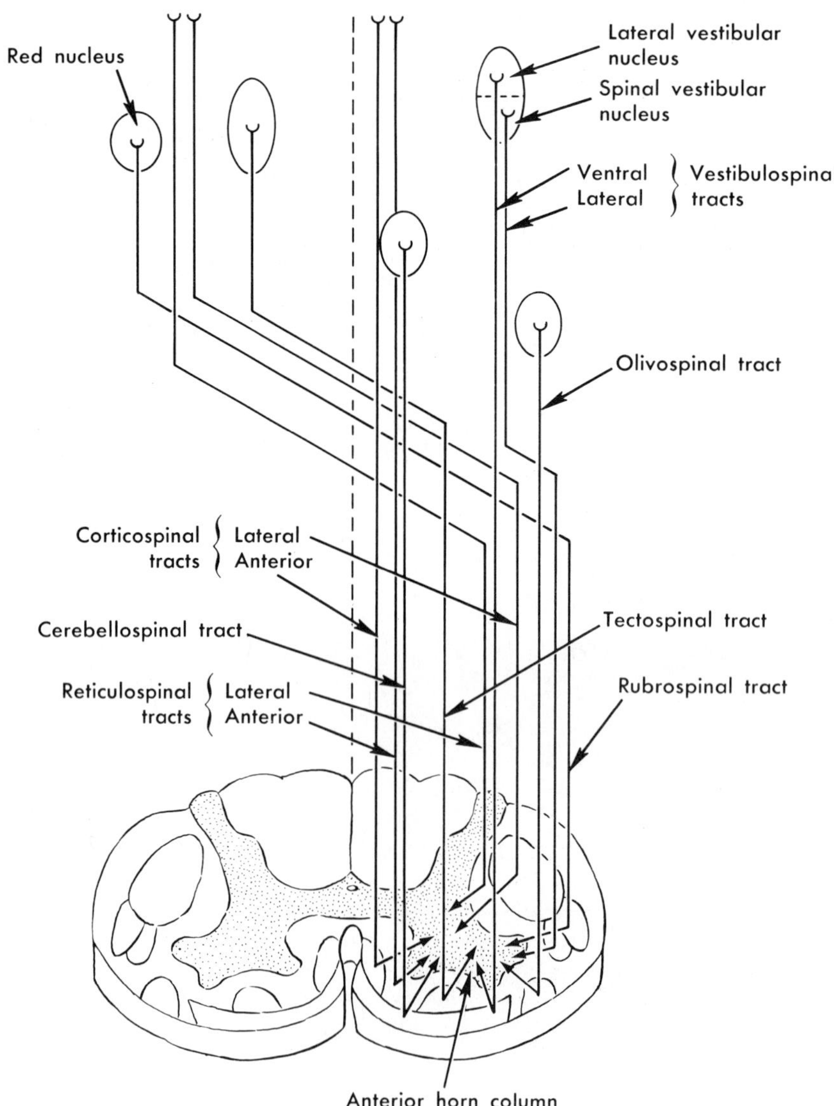

Fig. 35-6. Principle of final common pathway. Numerous nuclei and their respective pathways or tracts are shown descending and terminating around lower motor neuron of ventral column of spinal cord, where they exert combined influence on motor activity. (Redrawn from House, E. L., and Pansky, R.: A functional approach to neuroanatomy, ed. 2, New York, 1967, McGraw-Hill Book Co.)

weakens or paralyzes individual muscles or sets of muscles in the root or peripheral nerve distribution (based on knowledge of individual nerve distribution and in segmental distributions as in dermatomes).

The involved muscle(s) is flaccid due to the absence of normal muscle stretch reflexes (areflexia) or reduced reflexes (hyporeflexia), since there has been interruption of the reflex activity at the involved site. Flaccidity of the muscle is further evidenced by hypotonia with reduced or absent electrical impulses to the muscle. Localized muscle atrophy, or wasting, is apparent on inspection and corresponds to the spinal segment distribution of muscle involvement. This develops more slowly than the other muscle manifestations and is thought to be due to denervation (blocking).

Atrophy also increases with nonuse of the muscle. In some LMN lesions the affected muscle bundle or unit exhibits small localized, spontaneous, and involuntary contractions known as *fasciculations*. These are visible through the skin and should not be confused with fibrillation. The fasciculations are thought to represent the discharge of isolated muscle fibers arising from a single lower motor unit. They are coarse in large motor units but may be fine in smaller motor units, as in the hands.

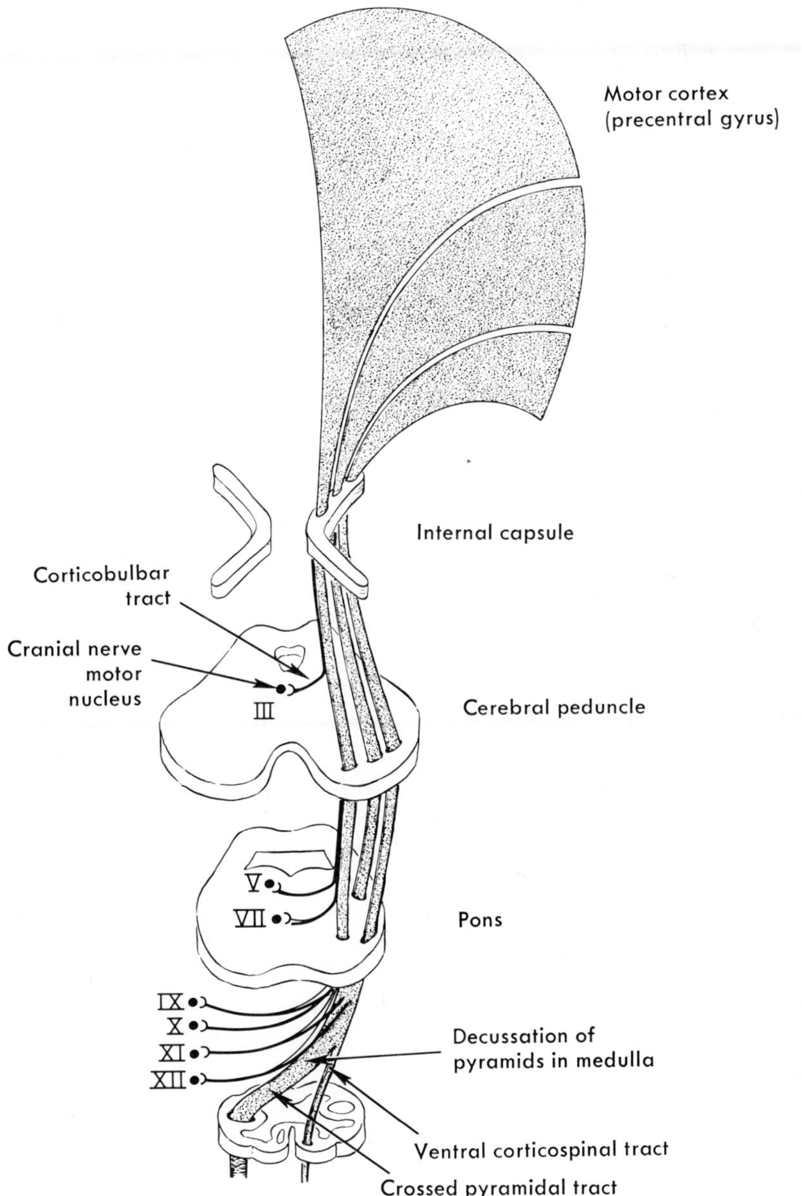

Fig. 35-7. Structures comprising upper motor neuron, or pyramidal system. Pyramidal system fibers are shown to originate primarily in cells in precentral gyrus of motor cortex; converge at internal capsule; descend to form central third of cerebral peduncle; descend further through pons, where small fibers are given off to cranial nerve motor nuclei along the way; form pyramids at medulla, where majority of fibers decussate; and then continue to descend in lateral column of white matter of spinal cord, where they synapse with anterior horn cells at all segments of cord. A few fibers descend without crossing at medulla level. (Adapted from original painting by Frank H. Netter, M.D.; from Ciba Collection of Medical Illustrations. Copyright by Ciba Pharmaceutical Co., Division of Ciba-Geigy Corp. All rights reserved.)

The criteria for an LMN lesion site or disease includes segmental or localized muscle weakness and atrophy in the same distribution, with absent or decreased muscle stretch reflexes in the affected muscles.

Upper motor neuron signs

The *upper motor neurons* (UMNs) arise from the motor cortex of the cerebrum (precentral gyrus), descend through long projection pathways by way of the pyramidal system (corticospinal and corticobulbar), and eventually synapse with the LMNs (Fig. 35-7). Some clinicians equate the UMNs only with the descending pyramidal system; other clinicians include in addition the rubrospinal, vestibulospinal, and reticulospinal descending fiber systems that can also influence the LMN's. When neural impulses are transmitted through all descending fiber systems to lower spinal segments, muscle tone, reflex activity, and somatic motor activity are maintained, mediated, or controlled in some way. It is believed that the pyramidal system is primarily responsible for the initiation and stimulation of muscle activity required for precise and fine voluntary muscle movements. Thus all descending systems collectively combine their influences on the LMNs so that volitional neural impulses are modified to result in fine, orderly, and smooth movements.

When lesions involve the UMNs at a wide variety of locations, characteristically *after a period of time* there is paresis of muscle movements, increased muscle tonus, and increased reflex activity. Since cerebrovascular accident (stroke) is the most common UMN lesion seen clinically, discussion is directed primarily to it. Trauma, neoplasia, and degenerative disease produce similar findings when located in UMN sites.

The *distribution* of paralysis or paresis is also significant in UMN lesions. The degree of muscle paralysis or paresis, however, does not bear such a direct relationship to the size of the lesion or the extent of involvement of the pyramidal system. It is important to realize that the paralysis is not that of individual muscle distribution but paralysis of movements in *hemiplegic* (and *paraplegic* and *quadriplegic*) distributions. Hemiplegia, or paralysis of both the upper and lower extremity on the same side, is the common distribution in stroke. Unilateral lesions of the motor cortex and the brainstem always produce paralysis of movement contralateral to the lesion if is it rostral to the decussation of the pyramids; ipsilateral paralysis of movement occurs if the lesion is caudal to the pyramids. The distribution or degree of paralysis is not always equal or the same within the hemiplegic distribution. For example, the face and arm may be weak or the weakness may involve the leg alone, depending on the part of the motor cortex involved. The following may be considered *UMN signs:* weakness of the mouth muscle associated with eye muscle weakness (forehead muscle is intact), weakness of forearm and wrist extensors, and weakness of the hip flexors and foot dorsiflexors. These muscle weaknesses result in the characteristic gait and appearance of the patient with a stroke. There is circumduction of the affected leg with inversion of the foot that drags. The arm is held semiflexed at the elbow and wrist. The facial muscles around the eye and mouth droop.

For a variable period of time the muscles on the involved side are usually flaccid, with hypotonia and hyporeflexia. Gradually the muscles become spastic, with hypertonia and exaggerated hyperreflexia. The spasticity is characterized by increased resistance to passive movement, hyperreflexia, clasp-knife phenomenon, and *clonus*. The latter is related to the hyperreflexia, in which the contraction of one muscle group is sufficient to stretch the antagonistic muscles and perpetuate the contractions. A unilateral Babinski sign is present on the hemiparetic side. Atrophy of the muscle results from disuse and occurs late.

UMN lesions within the brainstem also produce the characteristic motor manifestations as just described and, in addition, involvement of the cranial nerve nuclei and sensory pathways that are near the midbrain lesion site.

A complete transection of the spinal cord immediately produces loss of motor function, muscle tone, and reflex activity as well as somatic and visceral sensations below the level of the injury. Usually, when examined after a year, the same motor losses are present along with extensor spasticity and clonus. A bilateral positive Babinski's sign is also present. The problem of localizing the site of an UMN brainstem lesion is made more difficult by the close proximity of the descending fiber systems and cranial motor nuclei in the brainstem area. Table 35-2 summarizes and compares the charac-

Table 35-2. Clinical syndromes of upper motor neuron (UMN) and lower motor neuron (LMN) lesions

Motor component	UMN characteristics	LMN characteristics
Reflex	Hyperreflexia, extensor toe sign (Babinski's sign)	Hyporeflexia or areflexia
Muscle tonus	Hypertonia, clasp-knife spasticity, clonus	Hypotonia, flaccidity
Muscle movement	Paralysis or paresis of movements in hemiplegic distribution, etc.	Paralysis or paresis of individual muscles in peripheral nerve distribution
Muscle wasting	Late atrophy from disuse	Early atrophy of denervation
Muscle fasciculations	Not present	Present

teristic clinical syndromes as seen in UMN and LMN lesions.

Intervention

An ongoing assessment of basic needs and the ability of the paralyzed person to carry out movements in bed, range of motion, and activities of daily living provides the nurse with data necessary to plan the care of the paralyzed person. Successful intervention lies in prevention of joint contractures and decubitus ulcers and in development of the person's optimal level of functioning.

Safety needs

Patients who are paralyzed need to be protected from falling. Thus the person with hemiplegia needs to have the side rail raised on the affected side when he is unattended. If he is permitted up in a chair, a chair restraint is used.

The *eye on the affected side* should be protected if the lid remains open and there is no blink reflex. Otherwise damage to the cornea can lead to corneal ulcers and blindness. Irrigations with physiologic solution of sodium chloride, followed by drops of sterile mineral oil, sterile castor oil, sterile petroleum jelly, or artificial tears solution (methylcellulose), are sometimes used. After the lid is gently closed an eye pad may be taped over the affected eye. If a pad is used it must be changed daily and the eye cleansed and carefully examined for signs of inflammation or drying of the cornea. Eye shields are preferable to pads because they lessen the danger of lint entering the eye.

The *skin* over bony prominences needs to be inspected regularly for pressure signs (p. 817). There is decreased circulation to the tissues because of nonuse of the muscles; this is especially true the first few hours after spinal cord injury when vasomotor responses are lost. In monoplegic, hemiplegic, and quadriplegic distributions there are successively larger surfaces of skin to be protected (see p. 834 for interventions to prevent decubiti). The person with a lesser degree of paralysis is taught to turn himself in bed and to reposition himself depending on his condition. Persons with paraplegia who are confined to wheelchairs are taught to change position every 15 minutes by elevating themselves with their strong upper extremities. No external heat such as that from a hot-water bottle should be used if the person has loss of sensation, since the heat will not be felt and a burn could result. Care should also be taken to be sure that bathwater is not too hot, and paralyzed areas should be inspected daily for any signs of skin irritation.

Activity needs

The limbs of a person with acute hemiplegia, as with the person with paraplegia, are often flaccid at first. Spasticity with a tendency to muscle contracture develops gradually. The joints then become flexed and fixed in useless positions with deformity *unless preventive measures are taken by the nurse*. There is a shortening of joint capsules and ligaments around the immobile joint, and the limb may be drawn into flexure or extensor contracture with or without muscle spasm.

Through assessment the nurse determines the specific joints that are vulnerable to contracture and deformity formation as related to the existing degree and type of paralysis. For example, there will be a greater contracture vulnerability with quadriplegia than with paraplegia or hemiplegia, since the amount of muscle and joint involvement is greater. Assessment includes free range of motion (ROM) to determine the level of motion in all joints (p. 818). Based on assessment, the nurse carefully positions the flaccid limbs in normal anatomic positions in order to prevent deformity. By having knowledge of the distribution patterns of paralysis in UMN or LMN lesions, *counterpositioning* can also be initiated. In hemiplegia, for example, the neglected upper limb is pulled inward at the shoulder joint and the wrist drops; in the lower limb the knee flexes and the foot drops. In counterpositioning the nurse plans for the shoulder and upper arm to be in abduction, the elbow slightly flexed, the wrist in dorsiflexion, the knee in neutral position, and the foot in dorsiflexion. If the person is supine, a pillow can be placed between the upper arm and body to hold the arm in abduction. A roll made of one or two washcloths serves as a good support to prevent flexion of the fingers, and a splint made from a padded tongue blade may be used to ensure straightening of the thumb or other fingers for periods during the day. Dayhoff questions the common use of soft devices to prevent hand deformity and believes that there should be experimentation with hard devices to improve hand functioning following an UMN lesion such as a cerebral vascular accident.[12]

A firm box at the foot of the bed holds the feet at right angles and prevents contractures in the drop-foot position. Some physical therapists believe that footboards used in the prevention of foot drop contribute to increased spasticity and that their use should *not* be a routine practice for persons with UMN lesions.

Positioning is equally important as related to paraplegic and quadriplegic distributions. Knee flexion and foot drop are severe complications that can be prevented. The development of a flexion contracture at the knee joint interferes with the ability of the person to bear weight later in an upright position and to transfer unaided from one place to another. As a consequence the level of self-care and independence of the person may be greatly diminished when a joint deformity occurs.

Subluxation of a shoulder joint in a person with

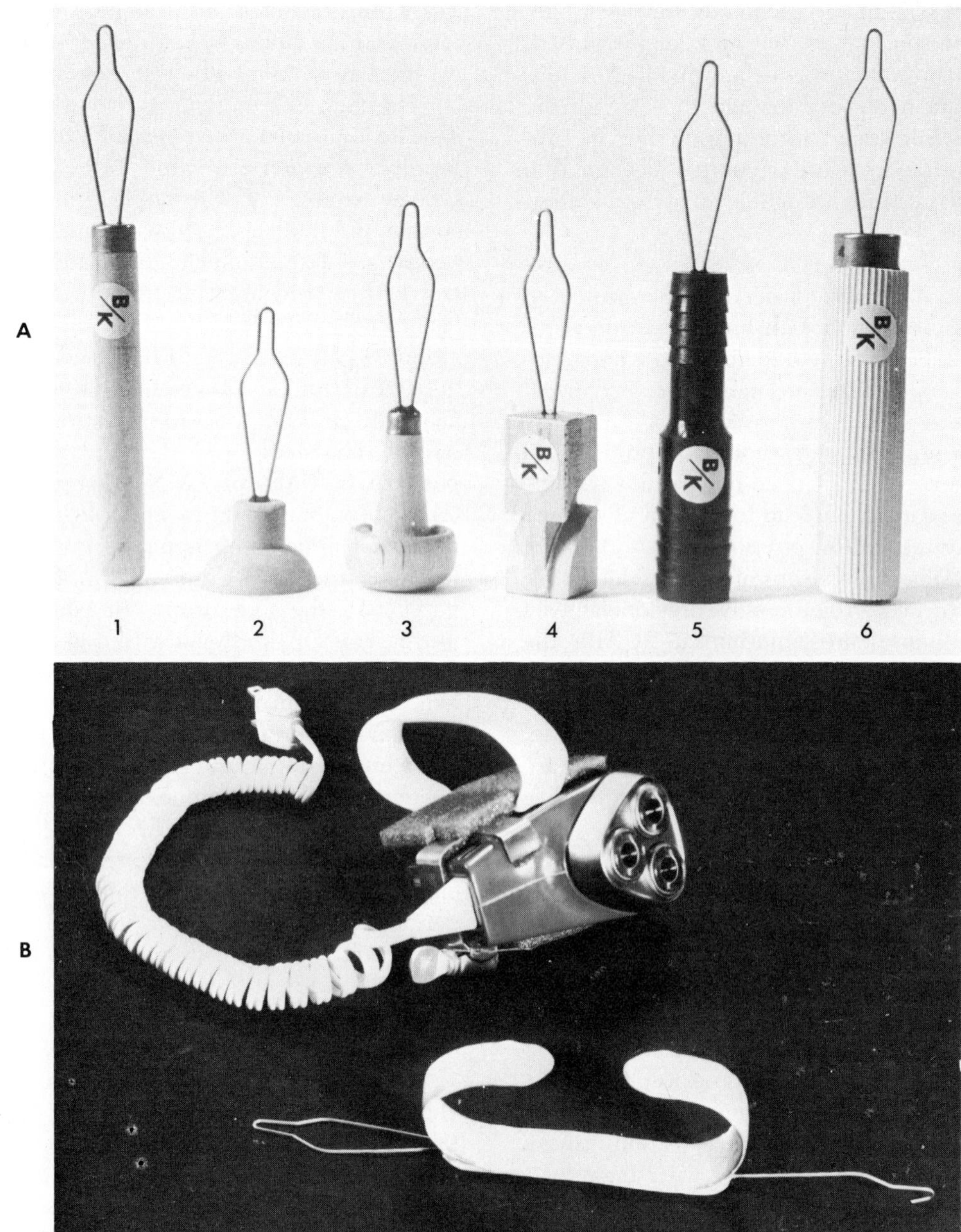

Fig. 35-8. Self-help or assistive devices. **A,** Variety of button hooks are available. Hooks are designed to meet needs of patients with *1,* hemiplegia or quadriplegia; *2,* hemiplegia (especially CVA) or upper extremity amputation; *3,* hemiplegia; *4,* upper extremity amputation and hook prosthesis (note handle is cut to be gripped by hook); *5* and *6,* hemiplegia or quadriplegia. **B,** Electric razor with universal cuff and combination button hook and zipper pull. These are designed to be used by quadraplegic patient. (Courtesy Fred Sammons, O.T.R., Chicago, Ill.)

hemiplegia, related to inadequate support of the joint when in an upright position, causes pain and limits therapy of the limb. In addition, keeping the paralyzed person in a semiupright position for long periods, whether in or out of bed, results in hip deformities. Positioning in the prone position helps to counteract the formation of this type of deformity. In summary, most joint deformities in a paralyzed person are *preventable* with early and continuing nursing interventions.

In addition to positioning, interventions for the person with paralysis includes range-of-motion exercises in all joints (p. 819). Passive ROM is indicated *twice daily* for all joints that the person cannot voluntarily move. Active ROM of the unaffected joints is carried out by the individual. The regularity of ROM is most important so that limitations do not develop.

The muscles of an unaffected leg need to remain strong in the person with hemiplegia as this leg must bear the person's weight when ambulation is begun. Quadriceps drills and isometric exercises are begun with the unaffected leg as soon as possible (p. 373).

During the rehabilitative phase the person with paralysis is taught how to carry out ADL to the extent of his capabilities. A variety of self-help devices are available (Fig. 35-8, *A* and *B*). Diversional activity should be started to keep the person constructively occupied, and an occupational therapist can help in selecting appropriate activities. The person may do any light handiwork that is enjoyable, feasible, and within physical capabilities. A radio, television, and reading material may help to pass the time. If the patient's neck is hyperextended, books that can be projected on the ceiling are useful if they do not cause eyestrain. Volunteers are very helpful in reading to patients.

Nutritional needs

Patience and persistence are necessary in giving food and fluids to the paralyzed person. The nurse must make him feel that the problem is not discouraging and that time taken to assist him in eating is well spent. He may encounter so much difficulty in getting food and fluids beyond his partially paralyzed mouth and throat that the effort may not seem worthwhile. Therefore each small step in improvement should be brought to the attention

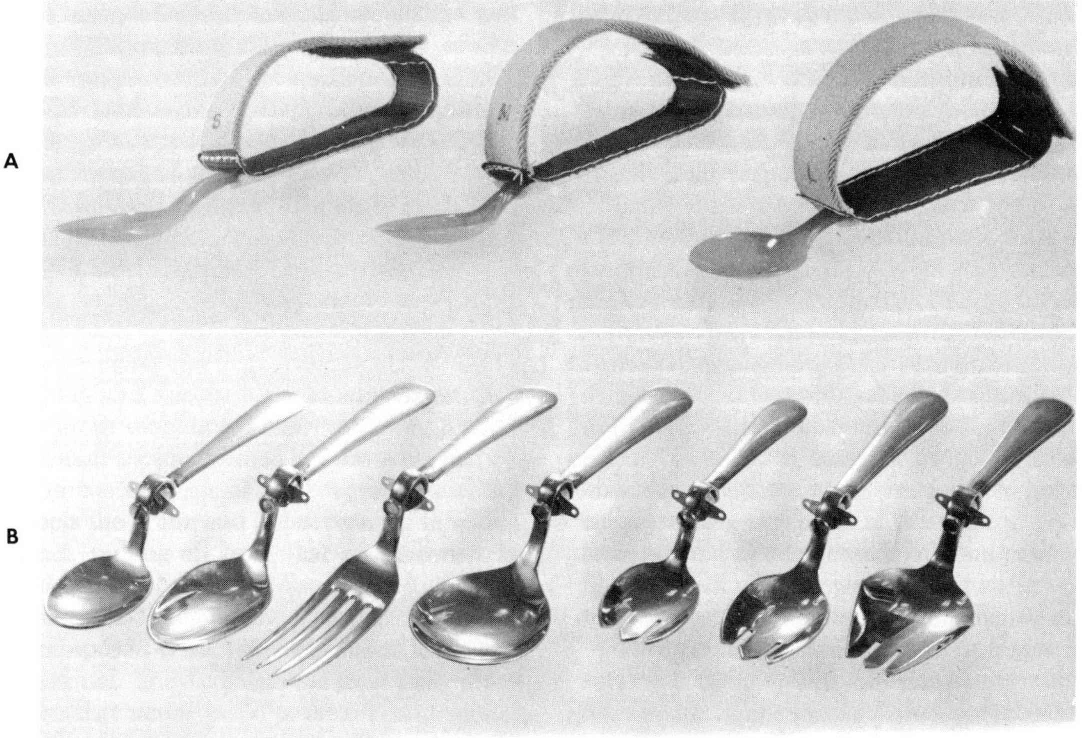

Fig. 35-9. Self-help devices for quadriplegic. **A,** Spoons with small, medium, and large universal cuff attachments that fit over hand. **B,** Swivel spoons, forks, and sporks (combination spoon and fork, last three on right), which are used with universal cuff. (Courtesy Fred Sammons, O.T.R., Chicago, Ill.)

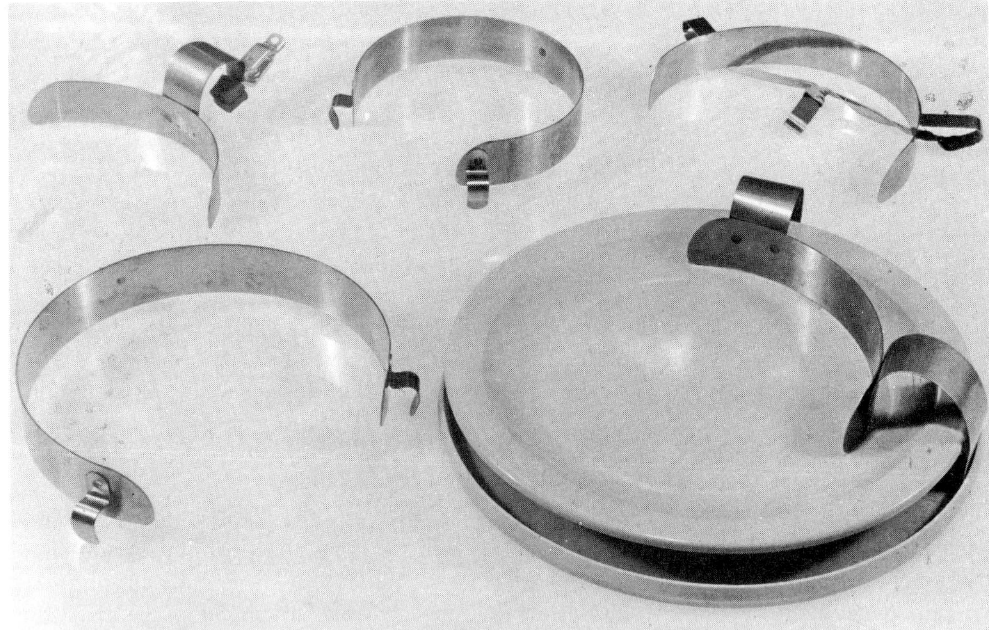

Fig. 35-10. Variety of food guards. Lower right-hand corner, food guard attached to plate. Food is pushed against guard to help get it onto utensil and to prevent it from being pushed off plate. (Courtesy Fred Sammons, O.T.R., Chicago, Ill.)

of the person. Turning him to his back or to the unaffected side may spare him the annoyance and embarrassment of having food spill from the affected side of the mouth. Foods that may cause choking, such as mashed potatoes, stringy meats, and semicooked vegetables, must be avoided. Since food may collect in the affected side of the mouth, it must be irrigated after eating to prevent accumulation of food and subsequent poor mouth hygiene.

The person should assist in feeding himself as soon as possible, since the helplessness of having to be fed by others is detrimental to emotional health. Self-help devices are available (Figs. 35-9 and 35-10). Food such as meats must be cut up. A covered plastic cup is available with a small center opening through which a straw can be introduced, or one can be improvised by using a straw and a covered plastic food container. This cup is useful for the person who can draw through a straw but whose hands are unsteady. If the person can swallow but cannot draw through a straw, an Asepto syringe with a piece of rubber tubing on the end or a pitcher must be used. Turning to the unaffected side before introducing fluids into the mouth often helps the person to control the mouthful of fluid and to swallow it successfully. If the person with dentures is able to keep them in the mouth, they should be placed in the mouth as soon as possible, since wearing dentures improves morale and increases interest in eating.

Elimination needs

The person with paralysis from an UMN or LMN lesion will experience problems with bladder and bowel control. The reader is referred to p. 1270 for a discussion of these problems.

Psychologic adjustment

The person with paralysis will need assistance in adjusting to this change in his body. The ability to move about at will and to control one's actions is a high priority for every human being. Regardless of the speed of its occurrence, the loss of ability to function independently when paralyzed is psychologically traumatizing. There may also be fears of rejection by loved ones, concerns about the future, and loss of self-esteem. Persons faced with such a major loss of body function also experience a grief reaction much like that experienced by one in mourning. In addition the person's image of himself, his body image, undergoes change. At times a person may relate to the paralyzed portion of the body as though it were unrelated to him. Interventions to assist the person to cope with losses and changes in body image are discussed in Chapters 19 and 28.

☐ Outcome criteria for the person recovering from paralysis

The patient or significant others can:

1. Describe dosage, function, side effects, and toxic effects of prescribed medications.
2. Demonstrate measures to prevent muscle or joint deformities.
3. Describe measures to prevent decubitus ulcers.
4. List signs of skin breakdown requiring professional intervention.
5. Demonstrate ADL that can be done alone and those that require assistance.
6. Discuss plans for bowel and bladder control.
7. State plans for follow-up care.

■ ALTERATIONS IN MOVEMENT AND POSTURE

Various neurologic lesions of the extrapyramidal motor system result in alterations of movement and posture. Clinically this is seen most commonly in paralysis agitans or parkinsonism. In this condition there is degeneration of various parts of the basal ganglia. The nuclear masses comprising the basal ganglia lie deep in the center of the cerebral hemispheres to either side of the midline and are a part of the extrapyramidal system. The motor pathways between the basal ganglia interconnect with both the cerebral motor strip and the cerebellum and affect lower motor neuron activity as related to the mediations of posture and coordination of movement.

☐ Assessment

In contrast to upper motor neuron syndrome with the loss of volitional movement and spasticity, in extrapyramidal lesions there is characteristic muscle rigidity, involuntary movements, and akinesia without loss of voluntary movement. Muscle rigidity, or *hypertonus,* is present in all muscle groups, both flexor and extensor, but appears to be more prominent in those muscles that maintain a flexed posture. The smaller muscles of the face, tongue, and even the larynx become involved with consequent difficulty in chewing, swallowing, and speech. The muscles remain continuously or intermittently firm and tense. Hypertonus is present even when the person is relaxed. There is an even or uniform quality to the hypertonus throughout the range of passive movement of a limb. The rigidity is often described as plastic.

Strength of muscle is not significantly decreased in akinesia or bradykinesia. Instead there is an extreme poverty of movement. The semiautomatic or habitual movements observed in the normal state such as putting the hands to the face, folding the arms, or crossing the legs are absent or greatly reduced. In looking to the side the eyes move but not the head. In arising from a chair the necessary adjustments such as putting the feet back and the hands on the arm of the chair are not made, although the person can do it with effort or will. The muscle is not paralyzed or apraxic. *Bradykinesia,* or *hypokinesia,* refers to slowness of movement rather than lack of movement *(akinesia);* the actual time in carrying out a movement is longer than normal. Formerly akinesia and bradykinesia were attributed to rigidity, which does hinder movement, but akinesia and rigidity are now considered separate phenomena. There are a variety of involuntary movements such as static tremor or pill rolling of the fingers, as seen in parkinsonism; these diminish at rest and go away during sleep. In all basal ganglia disorders, stress and nervous tension worsen motor performance; relaxation improves it.

☐ Intervention

Muscle rigidity may be relieved by physical therapy. It is important that the person remain physically active in order to prevent the complications of immobility (p. 834). It requires much patience and understanding on the part of the family not to take over physical activities for the person that he can only perform slowly and with much effort. Nursing interventions are planned to assist with feeding problems related to swallowing, ambulation, and speech. Often the person with parkinsonism is viewed as unintelligent because of dysarthria produced by the rigid and akinesic muscles of articulation and phonation. Education of the patient and family is a nursing priority. They need to understand the need to reduce stress and nervous tension in order to improve rigidity.

☐ Outcome criteria for the person with basal ganglia or extrapyramidal problems

The patient or significant others can:

1. Demonstrate how activities will be carried out at home:
   a. Explain the need to remain physically active despite difficulty and slowness in performance of activities.
   b. Demonstrate prescribed treatments (exercise, speech).
   c. Explain the need to prevent the complications of immobility (joint contractures, decubiti).
   d. Explain the dosage, side effects, and toxic effects of prescribed medications.
2. Plan for safety in performance of activities:
   a. Relate safety factors in ambulation related to gait.
   b. Demonstrate techniques in eating to prevent aspiration of food.
3. Explain the need for relaxation and freedom from stress to improve motor performance.
   a. Demonstrate relaxation techniques.
4. State plans for follow-up care.

■ APHASIA AND DYSPHASIA

Aphasia is a disorder of language caused by damage to the speech-controlling areas of the brain. *Aphasia* is a general term used to describe organic disturbances in language. It includes all areas of language, including speech, reading, writing, and understanding. *Dysphasia* implies a lesser degree of disability in language function.

Cerebral hemorrhage and cerebral thrombosis are the most common causes of cortical damage, but tumors, multiple sclerosis, and trauma may also lead to aphasia. Aphasia caused by cerebral edema following trauma is usually temporary. Occasionally a person cannot speak following a cerebrovascular accident because motor function of the vocal cords is affected, not because of damage to cortical speech centers. Defective innervation of the muscles of speech articulation such as vocal cords, tongue, cheeks, and palate results in dysarthria, which is not the same as aphasia. *Jargon aphasia* is the use of known words but in an illogical manner and with unawareness that the word sequence is senseless. *Automatic speech* is uncontrolled verbalization such as singing, counting, or overuse of common phrases.

A variety of abnormalities in communicaton can occur. The patient may be unable to comprehend the spoken word *(sensory aphasia)* or may comprehend and yet be unable to use the symbols of speech *(motor aphasia)*. He may also have both disorders at the same time *(global)*. He may be able to write but not speak; he may be able to speak but may use the wrong words or have a selective loss of words; or he may be able to read but be unable to speak or to write. Sensory aphasia is much more difficult to deal with than motor involvement. Explanations are difficult, and it is hard to reassure the person, who may become completely confused and undirected in his efforts to speak.

Each person reacts to language difficulty differently, depending on his pattern of adjustment to life's problems. Most persons with aphasia become tense and anxious. They may be irritable and emotionally upset because they are unable to evoke the words they need, and they become discouraged easily in their efforts to speak. Some may quickly refuse to attempt to communicate; others feel ashamed and withdraw from people, including their family and close friends. Yet desire to communicate and persistence in efforts to do so are the essential ingredients in speech rehabilitation.

□ Assessment

A history of the person's background pertaining to language, including education and languages spoken, should be secured from significant others. Assessment of sensory problems of vision and hearing is made as well as problems in speech articulation. Assessment of the person's communication efforts, however, is only possible by listening to and observing him.

Gross tests must be performed to determine what specific language abilities have been lost. In some hospitals a trained speech pathologist may be available to make an initial evaluation and to guide members of the nursing staff in making appropriate plans concerning the patient's speech problems. Sometimes, however, this assistance is not available, and the nurse must carry out simple tests that have been ordered by the physician or, more often, devise her own tests. They may be conducted as follows. Spread several familiar objects such as keys, a pencil, a book of matches, a penny, and scissors before the patient: (1) ask him to name each object; (2) as you name each object, ask him to point to it; (3) ask him to write the name of each object as you point to it; (4) ask him to write the name of each object as you say the word; (5) show him a card containing the printed name of each object and ask him to read the word orally and point to the object. It may be too fatiguing for the patient to take all the tests at one time, and they can be phased in gradually.

□ Intervention

Care is directed toward decreasing tension and should be started as soon as aphasia occurs in order to help the patient make a satisfactory adjustment to his limitation and to make later rehabilitative efforts less difficult. The nurse should anticipate the patient's needs so that he will not have to make repeated attempts to ask for things.

The environment of the aphasic patient should be relatively free of excessive stimuli. The patient is not deaf, and the voice does not need to be raised when speaking to him. Although he cannot respond, he should be talked to and have procedures explained in the same manner used with any patient. Recreational activities should be soothing and nonstimulating. Music is often relaxing, and the patient may enjoy listening to the radio. If a patient is able to read and comprehend the written captions on television, watching television may be particularly gratifying. Some patients may be made irritable by radio music they do not enjoy or television programs they do not like or cannot follow. Watching the patient's facial expression usually gives a clue as to the satisfaction derived from these activities.

The patient should be helped to understand that he may relearn speech and that in the interim there are other means by which he can communicate with others such as by gestures and writing. The most successful approach found to communicate with him will need to be shared with all who interact with him, including family and health workers. Amusement at the patient's attempts to communicate is avoided. Calmness and patience on the part of the nurse are essential to the patient's acceptance of his difficult program of practicing relearned words and patterns of speech.

Although the nurse does not initiate the formal speech therapy program with the patient, the nurse's cooperation is needed to reinforce the program. It is important that the nurse or family member articulate clearly in simple language. The patient's responses will indicate the best way to communicate with him. If he can only read, one should give him cards with the words and phrases needed in asking for the most common daily necessities. If the patient is unable to recognize the written word, he may be able to recognize pictures of objects. If he can write or draw a picture of his needs, he should be given a pad and pencil or magic slate with which to do so.

As the nurse cares for the patient, common objects should be named and the patient encouraged to handle them, to speak their names, and to write or copy their names. The patient should be helped to relearn the names of members of his family and friends. The family can supply these words and others that are particularly important for the patient. Speech retraining should be done for short periods of time because it is exceedingly trying, and fatigue tends to increase difficulty in speaking. Praising the patient for each small improvement and encouraging him to take his mistakes good-naturedly help to make this difficult problem more bearable. The patient's progress in language retraining will depend on his level of intelligence, his age (older patients have more difficulty), the severity of the damage, and whether the brain lesion is progressive. Complete language rehabilitation may require months of painstaking work on the part of skilled pathologists.* *A Guide to Clinical Services in Speech Pathology and Audiology*† lists clinics in the United States where speech and hearing services are available. Some of these clinics offer specialized help to persons with aphasia and dysphasia.

☐ Outcome criteria for the person with aphasia

The patient or significant others can:

1. Explain the recommended communication approach of the speech pathologist:
   a. Demonstrate the approach in communication to be used.
   b. Explain the need to provide an atmosphere conducive to communcation relearning.
   c. Explain the need to practice communication regularly but not to the point of frustration.
   d. Explain how to communicate basic needs associated with ADL.
2. The family or significant others shall have information about effective communication techniques and can:
   a. Explain alternate communication techniques (e.g., gesture, writing, and communication board) for the person with expressive aphasia.
   b. Explain the need to encourage the person in communication efforts.
   c. Explain the need to avoid the use of complex and long sentences in communication.
   d. Explain the need to articulate clearly in communication and not to speak loudly.
   e. Explain the need to listen carefully to what the person is communicating.
   f. Distinguish between communication and speaking.
   g. Explain the need to be realistic and honest with the person in his communication efforts.
   h. Explain the need to treat the person with aphasia as a person and not talk to others about him in his presence.
   i. Explain the need to prevent isolation of the person by socialization.
   j. State plans for follow-up care in relation to speech.

■ GENERAL SENSORY DYSFUNCTION

The presence of a lesion anywhere within the sensory system pathways, from the receptor to the sensory cortex, alters the transmission or perception of sensory information. The parietal lobe cortex is of major importance for interpretation of sensation with the exception of sight, hearing, smell, taste, and thermoregulation. A loss, decrease, or increase in the sensation of pain, temperature, touch, and proprioception, singly or in combination, results in difficult problems in daily living for the person. Since these sensations normally help the person to be aware of and discriminate relative to the internal and external environments, any alteration in sensibility lessens the ability to be completely and accurately protected. As a consequence there is a need to adapt to the alteration and plan for safety and comfort. For example, a lesion in the parietal sensory cortex can produce various sensory alterations on the contralateral side of the body including hypesthesia, hypoalgesia, and loss of proprioception. Fig. 35-11 shows common patterns of sensory alteration. The loss of proprioception, or the ability to know the position of the body and its parts without looking directly at the part, is a serious loss that

*Some institutions that specialize in working with patients who have aphasia are ICD Rehabilitation and Research Center, New York, N.Y.; The Institute of Logopedics, Wichita, Kan.; and Vanderbilt University Hospital Clinic, Nashville, Tenn.

†American Speech and Hearing Association, 9030 Old Georgetown Rd., Washington, D.C. 20014.

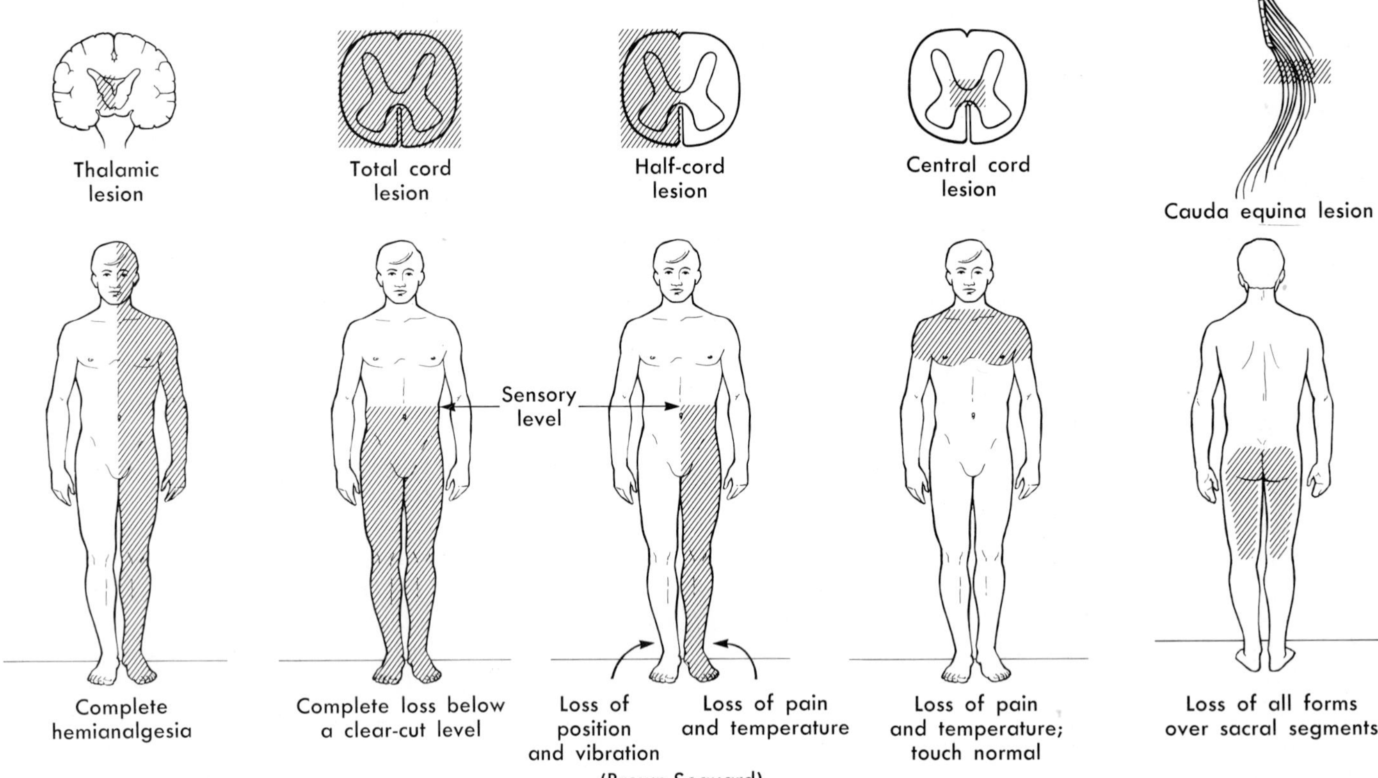

Fig. 35-11. Common patterns of sensory abnormality. Upper diagrams show site of lesion; lower diagrams show distribution of corresponding sensory loss. (Adapted from Bickerstaff, E. R.: Neurology for nurses, ed. 2, London, 1971, English Universities Press Ltd., and Hodder & Stoughton Ltd.)

requires considerable adaptation. Lack of control of body temperature, or hyperthermia, occurs due to malfunction of the thermoregulatory center in the brain, such as occurs following brain surgery near the hypothalamus, head injury, brain tumors, and other cranial conditions. It is believed that this failure in temperature regulation occurs as a result of hypoxia of the thermoregulatory center. Individuals quite often have complaints of *dysesthesia* or *paresthesia* that have reference to the abnormal sensation of touch. They are most commonly associated with peripheral neuropathies.

□ Assessment

The specific sensory alterations present in the person need to assessed as a basis for planning self-care. The nurse should recognize that sensory examination is the most difficult part of a neurologic examination. The detail in which a specific sensation is tested is determined by the clinical situation. The specific complaint of the person is thoroughly checked out by the examiner. Methods for sensory examination of each of these sensations are discussed in Chapter 34.

□ Intervention

The most important nursing intervention, once the alteration has been clearly identified, is teaching the person (and family) how to protect himself in relation to the sensory deficit or alteration. Teaching the person to utilize the noninvolved senses to an increased extent helps to avoid injuries. For example, teaching the person with hypoesthesia (lessened touch) to visually inspect his hands or involved body parts regularly will help to prevent injuries. Some nursing interventions will be more complex, such as in hyperthermia, and require lifesaving measures.

□ Outcome criteria for the person with alteration of one or more sensations

The patient or significant others can:

1. Demonstrate how to substitute for each sensation deficit or loss.
2. Explain safety factors needed in ADL to protect from injury:
   a. Demonstrate how to provide protection relative to the specific deficit.

   b. Demonstrate how to inspect the affected body parts for injury.
3. State signs or symptoms that would indicate worsening of the condition and the need to seek medical assistance immediately.
4. State plans for follow-up care.

APRAXIA AND AGNOSIA

Apraxia and agnosia are both fairly common perceptual deficits that occur in neurologic conditions. They may occur in association with each other or separately. Research concerning perceptual problems is still in the early stages. Even though the perceptual deficits and their corresponding lesion sites have been described in the literature, there is still much concern by the clinician as to how to rehabilitate the person.

Apraxia

Apraxia is the inability to perform certain skilled purposeful movements in the absence or loss of motor power, sensation, or coordination. Seldom is the word apraxia used without a qualifying descriptor as to the area in which the *praxia* deficit is present. It is a common occurrence following cerebrovascular accident in one or both cerebral hemispheres. Apraxia takes many different forms, and some may occur together. For example, *ideomotor apraxia* is the inability to imitate gestures or to perform a purposeful motor task on command even though the person fully understands the concept or idea of the task, such as tying a shoelace, that had been done automatically before his illness. A contrasting form is *ideational apraxia,* which is the inability to carry out activities on command because the person no longer understands the concept of the act.

Assessment of the specific form or forms of apraxia present in the person needs to be carried out first. Because of the nature of apraxia it is difficult to intervene in a way that assists the apraxic person to act. Some persons may be able to respond to verbal cues from the nurse and others from visual cues. Also, it is not always possible to determine if the person understands the instruction given. Collaboration with occupational therapists and speech therapists is necessary in order that information from definitive tests and treatment administered by them be shared.

Agnosia

Agnosia is the inability to recognize familiar objects perceived by the senses. This occurs frequently in stroke patients. It may be a disturbance in one or all of the following sensory modes—visual, tactile, proprioceptive, and auditory—or it may involve additional problems in body scheme, such as somatognosia or anosognosia. The form of agnosia can be related to the perceptual site of the brain involved; that is, *visual agnosia* is caused by a disturbance in the association area of the occipital cortex. In this deficit the person is unable to recognize objects visually although pathways for visual acuity and recognition of objects by touch are intact. The person will be unable to recognize his relatives or possessions. In other forms of visual agnosia there is difficulty in recognition of color, size of objects, and spatial relationships of objects viewed. Tactile and auditory agnosias are common.

As in other perceptual alterations, assessment of the specific form is carried out first. Treatment measures are directed toward repeated experiences in trial recognition of objects through other senses as well as the one where the deficit is present. If the deficit is severe the person will have to learn to discriminate through other senses. It is important that the person have an opportunity to practice tests with family members prior to discharge to the home environment.

Outcome criteria for the person with apraxia or agnosia

The patient or significant others can:

1. Explain the nature of the specific disorder.
2. Explain treatment methods to be carried out at home:
   a. Demonstrate prescribed treatment methods.
   b. Explain safety factors to be observed.
   c. State plans for follow-up care with the occupational therapist, speech pathologist, or both.

RESPIRATORY FAILURE

When there is dysfunction of respiratory muscles or the nerves innervating these muscles, serious problems in breathing ensue. This often necessitates the use of a respirator to assist or control breathing. Although tank and chest respirators are used infrequently today, when they are used it is most often in the care of patients with neurologic conditions; therefore the nursing care needed is included here.

A few neurologic conditions produce paralysis of intercostal muscles, the diaphragm, or both, such as acute polyneuritis, poliomyelitis, toxic encephalitis, myasthenia gravis, and fractures of the skull. Paralysis of respiratory muscles may be accompanied by paralysis of the palate and pharynx when the brainstem is involved and create increased difficulty in respiration. There is resultant difficulty in swallowing, coughing, breathing, and speech. When this occurs the person should be positioned so that secretions can be drained, or suctioned when a tracheostomy is present.

Respirators are mechanical devices used to substitute for normal respiratory action by creating negative pressure outside the chest wall. This pressure causes air to enter the respiratory passages. A mechanical device is a poor substitute for normal respiration and therefore is usually used as a last resort. For example, the rate of inhalation and rate of exhalation are the same when a respirator is used, whereas in normal respiration the time for inhalation is less than that for exhalation.

There are two main types of respirators and several manufacturers of each. The *tank respirator* encases the entire body except the head. Modern tank respirators are hinged at the foot to facilitate placement of the patient and include large portholes. The *chest respirator* encloses only the chest. Chest respirators permit the patient much greater freedom and simplify nursing care. They cannot, however, be used for long periods of time, since they may not provide adequate aeration of the lungs. Several variations of equipment are available to aid breathing. Some of these respirators employ the use of a mask over the face and do not encase the body; more frequently respirators are attached to a tracheostomy tube (p. 943). Other aspects of acute respiratory care are discussed in Chapter 46.

□ Intervention

If the patient is conscious it is imperative that the procedure of placing him into the respirator and the purpose of this treatment be explained to him. Usually he is told that the respirator has been ordered so that he can relax and breathe more easily and thus get necessary rest and sleep. Often the patient is so exhausted from having to remain awake and consciously use his accessory muscles of respiration in an effort to breathe that he welcomes use of the respirator. Occasionally he becomes panicky and "fights" the machine so that adjustment to it is extremely difficult. A nurse must always remain with the patient and help him to breathe with the machine until he becomes accustomed to it.

The patient in a respirator must never, under any circumstances, be left unattended. Patients have been known to die because an electric cord was inadvertently disconnected or because some other mechanical failure occurred.

■ ALTERED LEVEL OF CONSCIOUSNESS RELATED TO NEURAL CAUSES

In the practice of neurologic nursing the clinical assessment of unresponsive and comatose patients becomes a practical necessity. Patients are frequently admitted in coma as a result of direct trauma to the head, cerebrovascular problems, epilepsy, intracranial tumors, or increased intracranial pressure. Unconsciousness occurs when there is depression of transmission of impulses between the reticular activating system and the cerebral hemispheres. Level of consciousness is a reliable indicator of neurologic status. The assessment parameters for the unconscious patient are described in detail in Chapter 27.

■ ALTERATIONS IN COGNITION AND PERSONALITY

Cognitive behavioral changes are common in neurologic disease. Their slow development in the person may be the initial and only sign of a serious neurologic disorder. Assessment of cognition and personality should be made and reported accurately. Also, structural changes and loss of function caused by neurologic disease will affect self-concept and cause behavioral changes. Frustration resulting from restrictions and from attempts to get about, anxiety from increasing helplessness, and the feeling of powerlessness produce changes in personality. Cognition changes with resulting alteration in judgment, decision making, memory, and attention may become so serious that restrictions on the person's freedom by family and health professionals are necessary. Such situations are extremely difficult to manage because strong emotional reactions may follow curtailment of the person's freedom. The problem is usually dealt with by the family, the physician, and the social worker. When caring for such persons the nurse does not communicate to the patient knowledge of measures taken to prevent the consequences of errors in judgment.

■ INTRACRANIAL SURGERY

Intracranial surgery is commonly done for all types of pathologic conditions of the brain, including repair of aneurysm, evacuation of hematoma, relief of increased intracranial pressure, repair of fracture, and drainage of infections.

A surgical opening through the skull is known as a craniotomy. It is a basic preparatory procedure for intracranial surgery. A series of burr holes (trephine) is made first, and then the bone between the holes is cut with a special saw (Gigli) to permit removal of the bone. Bone is then removed in such a way that it can be replaced. The opening depends on the lesion site. Brain surgery may be done under hypothermia to lessen bleeding during the procedure. Drugs for hypotension may be used such as levarterenol bitartrate (Levophed). Fluorescein sodium, a dye, may be administered intravenously 1 hour preoperatively to help localize a tumor during surgery. Tumor tissue tends to retain the dye, which can be seen under ultraviolet light. The dye will cause the skin and the scleras to appear jaundiced for several days. The nursing staff, the patient, and his family should be aware of this.

When the brain lesion is in the *supratentorium* (above the tentorium or in the cerebrum), the incision is usually made behind the hairline. When the incision is into the *infratentorium* (below the tentorium or in the brainstem and cerebellum), it is made slightly above the nape of neck. Neither of these incisions is apparent when the hair has regrown.

Following craniotomy and removal of the bone, an incision is made into the meninges and the tumor is removed or other cranial surgery performed. The removed bone is carefully saved or preserved. Following brain surgery, *the bone may be replaced immediately (as in bone flap with muscle attachment) or when there are no evidences of infection or increased intracranial pressure.* Not infrequently the bone is left out for variable periods to prevent pressure from cerebral edema postoperatively or to permit expansion of an inoperable tumor. The preserved bone, in this instance, is used as a mold for a bone prosthesis, which is inserted with wire at a later date, or the bone is reinserted. Sterile acrylic is the material presently used to make the bone prosthesis. The acrylic can be molded directly into the skull opening after covering the dura mater with a thin plastic sheet at the time of surgery, or it can be molded from the preserved bone at a later time. The removal of part of the skull without replacement is called *craniectomy.* When a tumor cannot be removed because of its location and nature, a subtemporal decompression is made by leaving an opening in the dura and skull. *Cranioplasty* is the repair of a cranial defect through use of substitute bone materials.

Limitation of some functions may necessarily follow complete removal of brain tumors occurring in cerebral hemispheres. Portions of the frontal lobe are removed in some instances with little residual damage. Patients with tumors located where they are readily accessible to removal, such as meningiomas and tumors of outer cerebrum, have the best prognosis.

Although neurosurgery is most frequently performed in the treatment of brain tumors, it may be used in the treatment of hematoma or a brain abscess. It may also be employed to repair a cerebral aneurysm. Surgical procedures, in addition, are performed to produce destructive brain lesions in selected sites, as in the treatment of Parkinson's disease and in the control of intractable pain.

□ Preoperative care

Baseline data of neurologic and physiologic status should be recorded by the nurse prior to surgery. Written permission for surgery on the brain must be given by the nearest relative unless the patient himself is able to sign a permit. Even then close relatives are usually consulted, and the neurosurgeon obtains their consent before surgery. The patient and his family are usually very threatened by the prospect of brain surgery and should be encouraged to express their fears. Specific fears may be related to those of a permanent change in appearance, dependency, or death. Psychologic support of patient and family is a priority intervention. The nursing staff should provide time for this as part of essential nursing care of the patient. The patient may also wish to have his spiritual advisor visit him prior to surgery.

Treatments and procedures should be explained to the patient even though he *may not* seem to understand fully. Enemas may not be given prior to surgery because of the danger of increasing intracranial pressure further by exertion and by the absorption of fluid. Narcotics, excepting codeine, are rarely ordered preoperatively, since they may cause further depression of cerebral function. Any order for their use should be carefully verified by the nurse. If the head is to be shaved, the procedure may be delayed until the patient is in the operating room. Long hair should not be discarded but should be returned to the patient unit because the patient may wish to have it made into a wig. The availability and popularity of synthetic wigs also helps in the solution of the feeling associated with the loss of hair. It is rarely necessary to shave the entire head, and some surgeons order only a small area shaved. Hair along the front hairline can often be left so that after the operation it can be drawn backward to cover the scar. The hair is shampooed, and the condition of the scalp is noted.

□ Postoperative care

Immediate postoperative care

Whether in the patient unit or in the recovery room, the nurse should be certain that the following are readily available: side rails for the bed, suction machine or wall suction with disposable suction catheters, an airway, a padded tongue blade, a lumbar puncture set, and an emergency medication tray (cardiac and respiratory stimulants, amobarbital sodium [Amytal], anticonvulsive drugs), syringes, intravenous and hypodermic needles, and a tourniquet. An emergency tracheostomy tray should also be readily available on the unit.

The patient is *observed* regularly during the early postoperative period for signs of increased intracranial pressure (see p. 670 for a complete discussion of increased ICP). Specific observations are usually made and results recorded every 30 minutes for 6 hours, every hour for at least a day, and every 3 to 4 hours until the third or fourth postoperative day. *Frequency* of making and recording specific observations *depends on the patient's condition.* Temperature is usually taken every hour for 4 hours and then at least every 4 hours for 24 hours. If the lesion was in the infratentorium, the temperature may be taken every 2 hours for 2 or 3 days because edema of the brainstem might occur and upset the temperature control center in the hypothalamus.

Any change in the patient's *vital signs, state of consciousness, pupillary response, or ability to use muscles* is reported at once. Restlessness forewarns of hemorrhage or of irritation to the brain. Irregular or fixed pupils indicate pressure or disturbance that may be due to hemorrhage. In a patient who has intracranial bleeding the blood pressure rises and the pulse rate drops as the intracranial pressure increases. This process continues until the pressure becomes so great that all regulating control is lost, and the blood pressure drops and the pulse rises just before death.

Position

Immediately after surgery the patient is placed on his side to provide an adequate airway. To facilitate change of head dressings and other treatments following surgery, the patient may be placed in bed "head to foot." If a large brain tumor has been removed, he must not be turned on the affected side, since this position may cause displacement of brain structures by gravity. Otherwise he may be turned to either side. The primary objective is to eliminate pressure at the operative site. Handling of the brain tissues and surgical trauma causes cerebral edema, which contributes to increased intracranial pressure.

If there has been *supratentorial* surgery (above the cerebellum), *the head of the bed is elevated at least 45°, and a large pillow is placed under the patient's head and shoulders.* This position should lessen the possibility of hemorrhage, provide for better circulation of the cerebrospinal fluid, and promote venous return. All of these

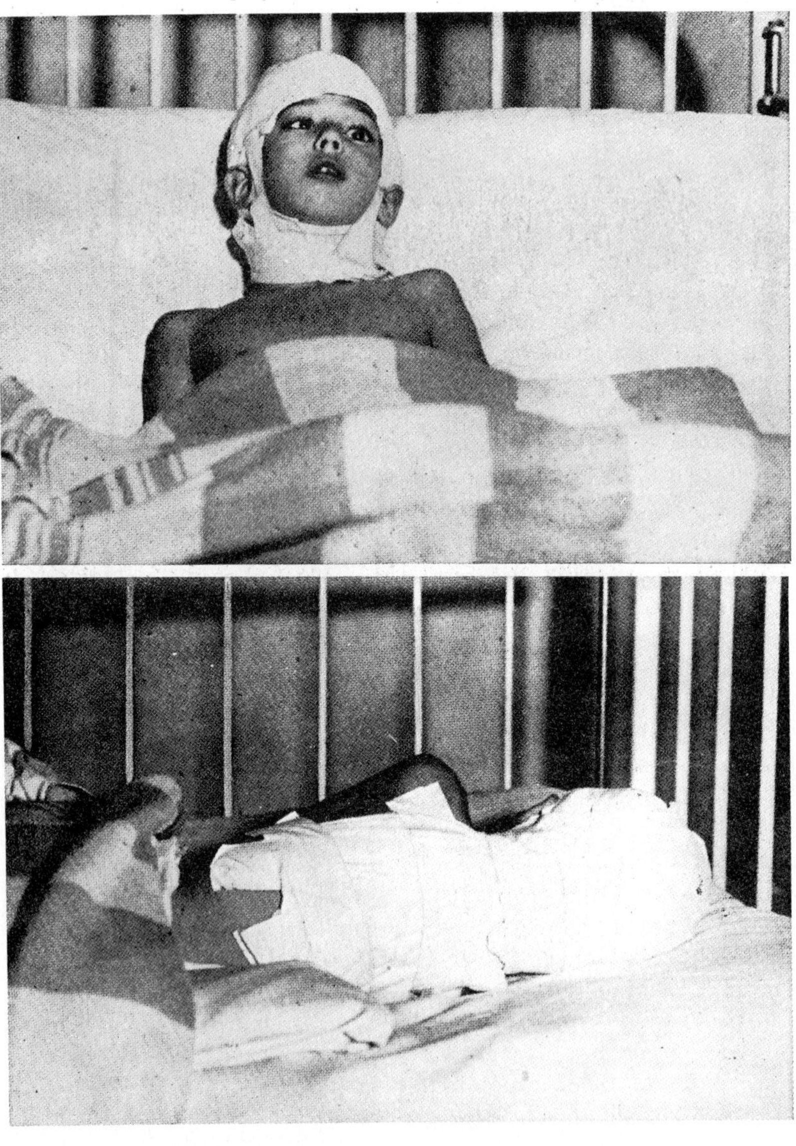

Fig. 35-12. Patient with infratentorial craniotomy dressing. Note that adhesive straps extend down back to prevent patient from flexing neck. (From Sachs, E.: Diagnosis and treatment of brain tumors and care of neurosurgical patient, ed. 2, St. Louis, 1949, The C. V. Mosby Co.)

measures assist in decreasing cerebral edema and in preventing increased intracranial pressure. Internal bleeding would also contribute to a rise in intracranial pressure. If an *infratentorial* tumor has been removed, *the bed should be kept flat with only a small pillow under the nape of the neck and the patient turned to either side.* The head dressing may extend down to the shoulders to support the neck and hold the head in slight hyperextension (massive dressings are used less frequently by some neurosurgeons). Fig. 35-12 shows one type of infratentorial head dressing. Any *flexion* of the neck should be *avoided,* either midline or laterally. Since infratentorial incisions are made adjacent to the medulla, vital centers, and cranial nerves IX and X, there is more danger of respiratory complications and brainstem compression.

Coughing and *vomiting* are to be avoided, since these increase ICP. Suctioning, if permitted, should be done gently and cautiously to avoid initiating coughing. Suctioning through the nose is also avoided (p. 693). Deep-breathing exercises should not be followed by coughing.

During the early postoperative period oral fluids are not usually given. The head *dressing* is inspected regularly for amount and type of drainage. Serosanguineous drainage on the dressings should be measured and marked, as is done with other dressings, so that it can be accurately checked for an increase in amount. Yellowish drainage should be reported immediately to the physician because it probably indicates loss of spinal fluid. If the head dressing appears to be soaked with drainage, it should be reinforced with sterile gauze sponges and covered with a sterile towel held in place with adhesive tape. Every half hour the towel should be removed and the dressing checked and reinforced with sterile towels if necessary. An unprotected wet dressing may cause the wound to become infected, which might lead to meningitis. Sometimes the neurosurgeon may need to change the entire dressing.

Family during the postoperative period

The family should be prepared to see the patient. They should know that he will return from the recovery room with a helmetlike head dressing and that edema may distort his features. If he is unconscious or has any noticeable limitation such as aphasia, they should be so informed before entering his room. If he is alert, members of the family should be advised to sit quietly at the bedside, since talking will tire the patient. If a supratentorial incision has been made, the family should be warned that when they see him on the day following surgery he may be unable to open one or both eyes, may have generalized facial edema, and may have discoloration of the skin about the eyes (ecchymosis). Periocular edema is caused by postoperative cerebral edema. It usually improves in 3 or 4 days. Ice compresses to the eyes may make the patient more comfortable.

Protective measures

Sometimes the patient must be protected from self-injury after a brain operation. If he pulls at dressings or a catheter or if he scratches or hits himself, he should be attended constantly, and occasionally some kind of hand restraint such as a large mitten made of dressings, bandages, and stockinette fastened at the wrist with adhesive tape may be used. Mittens usually upset the patient less than arm restraints, since with mittens he can move his arm freely. The fingers should be separated with gauze to prevent skin irritation and should be curled around a large bandage roll in the palm to prevent hyperextension of the fingers. The hand is then well covered with dressings held in place with a bandage. A piece of stockinette is closed at one end and everted so that the tied end cannot cause injury to the eye. It is then slipped over the bandaged hand and fastened securely at the wrist with adhesive tape. The wrist should be shaved and the skin protected with tincture of benzoin before adhesive is used. At least every other day the mitten must be removed, the hand washed in warm water, and passive exercise given to the fingers before the mitten is reapplied.

Ventricular drainage

Occasionally a catheter is placed in a ventricle of the brain to drain excess spinal fluid and prevent increased intracranial pressure. The catheter is usually attached to a drainage system on a level with the ventricle. The collection bottle is frequently attached to the bed. The tubing and drainage receptacle should be sterile, and care must be taken to prevent kinking of the tubing. If drainage seems to stop, the neurosurgeon should be notified. The catheter is usually left in place for 24 to 48 hours and is then removed by the surgeon.

Head dressings

Usually the wound is covered with gauze dressings, and a special head dressing (neurosurgical roll) is then applied in a recurrent fashion from the back to the front of the head and anchored (Fig. 35-13). If a drain has been used, the head dressing is changed in 24 to 48 hours. Otherwise it is not disturbed until the sutures can be removed. They are usually removed on the third postoperative day following a supratentorial incision and on the fifth postoperative day following an infratentorial incision.

Fluids and food

Fluid intake and output should be accurately recorded. If there is no special medical order to the con-

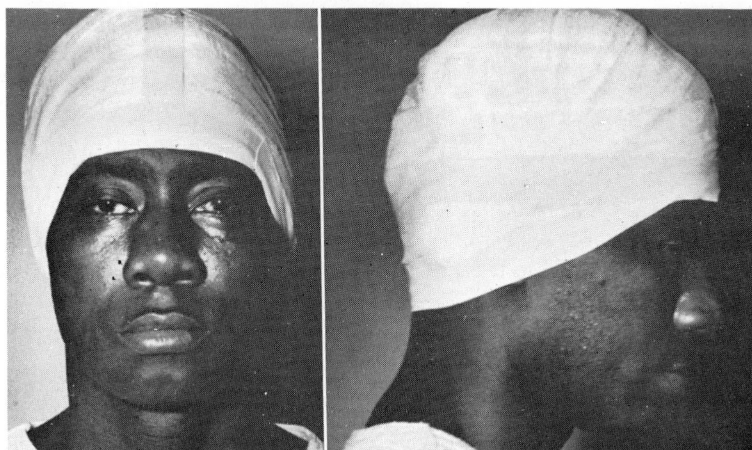

Fig. 35-13. Typical head dressing for patient who has had supratentorial craniotomy. (From Conway, B. L.: Carini and Owens' neurological and neurosurgical nursing, ed. 7, St. Louis, 1978, The C. V. Mosby Co.

trary, 2,500 to 3,000 ml of fluid should be given each day. Some neurosurgeons routinely restrict fluids to 1,500 ml/day for the first 3 days after a craniotomy.[45]

Since the gag and swallowing reflexes may be depressed or absent after *infratentorial* brain surgery, fluids by mouth are usually withheld for at least a day and intravenous fluids are substituted. They should be run very slowly to prevent increased intracranial pressure. If reflexes are present, water is carefully given by mouth. The patient should be placed on his side or in a semisitting position. Fluid is most easily given by placing a plastic Asepto syringe into the patient's mouth and allowing him to suck through it. Fluid should not be injected into his mouth. If he coughs or cannot swallow, the fluid should be discontinued.

A regular diet is usually given as soon as it is tolerated. After *supratentorial* surgery the regular diet may be given on the second postoperative day. Any patient who has had a craniotomy, however, should be fed for at least 48 hours to prevent undue fatigue. He may need to be fed for a longer time to ensure adequate food and fluid intake. If the patient is unable to take food and fluid by mouth, liquid foods by nasogastric tube are started 48 hours postoperatively.

Elimination

Care must be taken to see that the patient voids sufficiently. Urinary output must be carefully recorded, and sometimes an indwelling catheter may be used for a few days following surgery. A decrease in output must be reported, since it may indicate the onset of a metabolic disorder of central nervous system origin. Because straining increases intracranial pressure (Valsalva maneuver), the patient is urged not to try to have a bowel movement until the third postoperative day. On the second and third postoperative days the patient may be given a laxative or stool softener if indicated. He should be instructed not to strain. Bowel function is monitored by the nurse. If an impaction should develop, feces must be removed manually.

Comfort

Patients who are conscious after intracranial surgery may complain of severe *headache* for 24 to 48 hours. Central nervous system depressants, such as opiates and sedatives, are avoided, although codeine sulfate may be ordered parenterally in small doses if headache is severe. Acetylsalicylic acid (aspirin) may be given by rectum, or by mouth if fluids can be swallowed. An ice cap may be placed on the head, and sudden movement and jarring are avoided. The patient should be protected from loud noises and bright lights. Even if the patient is conscious, he should be turned with a turning sheet (p. 835) for the first 48 hours, since the effort needed to move himself may tire him excessively and cause further headache, increased intracranial pressure, or hemorrhage. The turning sheet should be placed well above the level of the patient's head to assure that the patient's body is turned as a unit.

Ambulation

The patient who has had surgery for a *supratentorial* lesion usually is allowed out of bed on the third to fifth postoperative day or earlier. Activity is increased gradually, and he is watched carefully for signs of increased intracranial pressure. First the head of the bed should be elevated to a high Fowler position, and then the patient should sit on the edge of the bed with his feet dangling over the side. If he tolerates this position, 4 to 6 hours later, with the help of two persons, he may be assisted to a chair and usually may sit up for a half hour. He then progresses to normal activity as quickly as he desires and is able. The patient who has had surgery for an *infratentorial* lesion usually may not be permitted up until the tenth postoperative day. The trend is toward getting up earlier, depending on the patient's condition. Initial progress may be slower, since patients who have been kept flat in bed for some time may be dizzy and experience orthostatic hypotension when arising until the circulatory system readjusts to the change in position.

Head care after wound healing

When the final dressings are removed, the scalp can be gently cleansed with hydrogen peroxide to remove dried blood. Crusts can be loosened with mineral oil. The head may then be shampooed with care taken not to rub the operative area or put traction on the healed suture line. A head covering is usually worn to protect the wound, to help remind the patient not to scratch, and for cosmetic reasons until the hair has grown back. A cap can be made by tying one end of a 10-inch piece of tubular stockinette. Head scarves or wigs are usually preferred by women, and wigs can also be worn by men. The patient who has had a piece of bone left out will have a depression in the scalp, and he should be warned of the danger of bumping his head in this area.

□ Complications

Meningitis is a relatively rare complication of brain surgery; it can follow infection during the operation or thereafter. Following supratentorial surgery, the nurse should watch for any clear, watery drainage from the nose. This drainage may be present if there has been a tear in the meninges, which causes subsequent loss of cerebrospinal fluid. The treatment consists of keeping the patient very quiet, avoiding any suctioning or blowing of the nose, and administering antibiotic drugs. The leakage usually subsides spontaneously. Because of the danger of causing damage that might be followed by the drainage of cerebrospinal fluid through the nose, many surgeons request that the nose never be suctioned when supratentorial surgery has been performed. A sign with this caution may be placed at the head of the bed.

Respiratory collapse may follow infratentorial surgery. It is caused by edema of the brainstem or edema above the brainstem that causes herniation of the brainstem into the foramen magnum and pressure on the respiratory center. Any irregularity of respiration, dyspnea, or cyanosis should be reported at once. Equipment should be ready for administering oxygen, doing a ventricular tap, and inserting an endotracheal tube if one is not already present. (For details of nursing care of the patient with an endotracheal tube, see p. 942). Occasionally a respirator is used (p. 955).

Convulsions are not unusual after a craniotomy, and therefore a padded tongue blade should be at the bedside and side rails should be used even if the patient is unconscious and it is believed that he cannot move. Phenytoin sodium (Dilantin) may be ordered prophylactically to prevent convulsions. The drug may be given intramuscularly or, infrequently, by rectum until the patient is able to take it orally. If the patient has a history of seizures before the operation or if convulsions occurred in the postoperative period, he may be given this drug for several months.

Loss of the corneal reflex may follow brain tumors or brain surgery. If the eye appears inflamed or if the patient does not seem to blink when objects approach the open eye, the neurosurgeon should be notified. Special eye care such as that given to patients who have had cerebrovascular accidents or who have had surgery for trigeminal neuralgia may be necessary (p. 669).

The patient may complain of *diplopia* after brain surgery. This condition is often temporary, and the patient should know that it will probably improve. It can be relieved by placing an opaque eye shield over one eye. The eye covered usually is alternated each day to prevent atrophy of eye muscles through disuse.

■ PLANNING WITH THE PATIENT'S FAMILY

Few illnesses tax the entire physical and emotional resources of the patient's family as do the chronic neurologic diseases. It is imperative that the family participate in long-term plans for the patient. Members of the family may have severe emotional reactions and difficulties in adjustment that may require the assistance of specially trained persons such as a psychiatrist. Both the patient and his family need time to work through their feelings. Sometimes the enormity of the significance of the diagnosis cannot be grasped for weeks or even months by either the patient or his family. Toxic polyneuritis in a young husband and father and multiple sclerosis in a young mother are examples of problems of such magnitude that long-term plans cannot be made quickly.

If the patient with neurologic disease has marked personality changes, aphasia, or convulsions, the family may even be afraid of him. Because the family is unaware that the patient may fully understand what is being said, they may make tactless remarks in his presence. When the patient is admitted to the hospital, it is often desirable to have him escorted directly to his room and then to take the family aside to ascertain their insight into the situation. This interview provides an opportunity to help interpret the patient's actions and responses so that his family may not inadvertently upset him. See Chapter 29 for more information about general care of persons with prolonged illness.

REFERENCES AND SELECTED READINGS

1. Adams, R. D., and Victor, M.: Principles of neurology, New York, 1977, McGraw-Hill Book Co.
2. *Belt, L. H.: Working with dysphasic patients, Am. J. Nurs. **74:**1320-1322, 1974.
3. Benson, V. M., McLaurin, R. L., Foulkes, E. C., et al.: Traumatic cerebral edema, Arch. Neurol. **23:**179-186, 1970.
4. Bergersen, B. S., and Goth, A.: Pharmacology in nursing, ed. 13, St. Louis, 1976, The C. V. Mosby Co.
5. Bickerstaff, E. R.: Neurology for nurses, ed 2, London, 1973, The English Universities Press.
6. Blinderman, E. E., Graf, C. J., and Fitzpatrick, T.: Basic studies in cerebral edema, J. Neurosurg. **19:**319-324, 1962.
7. *Blount, M., and Kinney, A. B.: Neurological and neurosurgical nursing, Nurs. Clin. North Am. **9:**591-772, 1974.
8. Boroch, R. M.: Elements of rehabilitation in nursing: an introduction, St. Louis, 1976, The C. V. Mosby Co.
9. *Bruya, M. A., and Bolin, R. H.: Epilepsy: a controllable disease, Am. J. Nurs. **76:**388-398, 1976.
10. *Conway, B. L.: Carini and Owens' neurological and neurosurgical Nursing, ed. 7, St. Louis, 1978, The C. V. Mosby Co.
11. Dalessio, D. J., editor: Wolff's headache and other pain, ed. 3, New York, 1972, Oxford University Press.
12. *Dayhoff, N.: Rethinking stroke: soft or hard devices to position hands, Am. J. Nurs. **75:**1142-1144, 1975.
13. DeJong, R. N., et al.: Essentials of neurological examination, New York, 1967, Hoeber Co.
14. *Delehanty, L., and Stravino, V.: Achieving bladder control, Am. J. Nurs. **70:**312-316, 1970.
15. Diamond, S., and Baltes, B. J.: Clinical clues to different types of headache, Hosp. Med. **9:**56, 1973.
16. Epilepsy Foundation of America: The legal rights of persons with epilepsy, ed. 4, Washington, D.C., 1976, The Foundation.
17. Jasper, H. H., et al.: Basic mechanisms of the epilepsies, Boston, 1969, Little, Brown and Co.
18. *Jimm, L. R.: Nursing assessment of patients for increased intracranial pressure, Nurs. Digest **3:**5-8, 1976.
19. *Johnson, M., and Quinn, J.: The subarachnoid screw, Am. J. Nurs. **77:**448-450, 1977.
20. *Kealy, S. L.: Respiratory care in Guillain-Barré syndrome, Am. J. Nurs. **77:**58-61, 1977.
21. *Keith, R. L.: Caring for the aphasic patient, Nurs. Digest **4:**37-39, 1976.
22. *King, I. M., guest editor: Symposium on neurologic and neurosurgical nursing, Nurs. Clin. North Am. **4:**199-283, 1969.
23. *Loetterle, B. C., Rogers, M., Valdner, T., et al.: Cerebellar stimulation: pacing the brain, Am. J. Nurs. **75:**958-969, 1975.
24. Lutz, E. H.: Treatment of tic doulourex with carbamazepine, Dis. Nurv. Syst. **27:**600-603, 1966.
25. *Harkness, L.: Bringing epilepsy out of the closet, Am. J. Nurs. **74:**875-876, 1974.
26. *Hoskins, L. M.: Vascular and tension headaches, Am. J. Nurs. **74:**846-851, 1974.
27. *Hughes, M. T.: Neuroradiology: a subspecialty, J. Neurosurg. Nurs. **4:**83-85, 1972.
28. Merritt, H. H.: A textbook of neurology, ed. 4, Philadelphia, 1973, Lea & Febiger.
29. Moos, R. H., editor: Coping with physical illness, New York, 1977, Plenum Medical Book Co.
30. *Mullan, J. F., and Van Shoick, M. R.: Intractable pain, Am. J. Nurs. **58:**228-230, 1958.
31. *Ostrow, L. S.: New hope for patients with trigeminal neuralgia, Am. J. Nurs. **76:**1301-1303, 1976.
32. Plum, F., and Posner, J. B.: The diagnosis of stupor and coma, ed. 2, Philadelphia, 1972, F. A. Davis Co.
33. Schmidt, R. P., and Wilder, J.: Epilepsy: a clinical textbook, Philadelphia, 1968, F. A. Davis Co.
34. Siev, E., and Freishat, B.: Perceptual dysfunction in the adult stroke patient, New York, 1976, Charles B. Slack, Inc.
35. Silverstein, A.: Arteriography of stroke, Arch. Neurol. **12:**387-389, 1965.
36. *Stoicheff, M. L.: Communicating with the aphasic patient, Nurs. Digest **3:**18-20, 1975.
37. *Stryker, R. P.: Rehabilitative aspects of acute and chronic nursing care, New York, 1977, W. B. Saunders Co.

37a. Swift, N., and Mabel, R. M.: Manual of neurological nursing, Boston, 1978, Little, Brown and Co.

38. Williams, A.: A study of factors contributing to skin breakdown, Nurs. Res. **21:**238-343, 1972.
39. Wintrobe, M. M., editor: Harrison's principles of internal medicine, ed. 8, New York, 1977, McGraw-Hill Book Co.
40. Wolff, H. G.: Headache and other head pain, New York, 1963, Oxford University Press.
41. Wright, G. N.: Epilepsy rehabilitation, Boston, 1975, Little, Brown and Co.
42. *Young, J. F.: Recognition, significance and recording of the signs of increased intracranial pressure, Nurs. Clin. North Am. **4:**223-236, 1969.

*References preceded by an asterisk are particularly well suited for student reading.

36

Problems of the nervous system

MARJORIE KINNEY

The neurologic problems selected for inclusion in this chapter are the ones most closely associated with the common clinical neurologic manifestations as presented in Chapter 35. The problems are categorized for discussion both from a broad pathologic standpoint and from the standpoint of the anatomic site of the neural lesion.

Discussion of each problem includes pathophysiologic explanation and the assessment, interventive, and evaluative aspects of patient care specific to the problem.

■ DEGENERATIVE DISEASES

The phrase *degenerative diseases* as used here refers to those neurologic diseases in which there is a premature senescence of nerve cells, when there is a known or suspected metabolic disturbance, or when the cause is unknown. (See Table 36-1 for a comparison of these degenerative neurologic diseases).

□ Multiple sclerosis (disseminated sclerosis)

Epidemiology

Multiple sclerosis is a common neurologic disease in northern climates. The exact prevalence of this disease is not known, since in many instances the diagnosis is not made, but probably at least 500,000 persons in the United States are known to have multiple sclerosis.[29] The onset of symptoms usually occurs between 20 and 40 years of age. The course of the disease is estimated to be 12 to 25 years. Multiple sclerosis has serious implications for family life, since it affects both men and women equally in the active productive years when their responsibilities are greatest.

During the past decade there have been major advances in the knowledge of the etiology, pathology, diagnosis, and treatment of multiple sclerosis. The etiology, however, remains unknown despite new findings and the numerous hypotheses that have been advanced as to cause. Mineral deficiency, toxic substances, disturbance of blood clotting mechanism, viruses, and autoimmunity are a few of the causes studied. The latter two are currently the most favored. Experimental allergic encephalomyelitis has been produced in animals by the injection of the basic protein from a homologous neuron sheath.[67] Despite the resemblance to multiple sclerosis, it is not yet clear to what extent this disease represents a human model for multiple sclerosis. The recent discovery of slow viruses (those with a long latent period) in association with the frequent findings of an increase of gamma globulin and immunoglobulin (IgG) in the spinal fluid of patients with multiple sclerosis gives support to these theories. What constitutes an elevation of gamma globulin or of IgG is not clear. Whether the gamma globulin and IgG get into the spinal fluid by transudation or by increased permeability of the blood-brain barrier is still controversial.

Pathophysiology

Multiple foci of demyelination are distributed randomly in the white matter of the brain stem, spinal cord, optic nerves, and cerebrum. During the demyelination process (primary degeneration) the myelin sheath and the sheath cells are destroyed, but there is early sparing of the axon cylinder. The outer myelin sheath in the spinal cord neuronal pathways is often compared to the insulation on an electric wire. Its destruction causes interruption or distortion of the impulse so that it is *slowed* or *blocked.* This type of demyelination differs from that of *wallerian degeneration* (p. 726) in that damage is always primary to the myelin sheath or sheath cells. There is evidence of partial healing in areas of degeneration, which accounts for the transitory nature of early symptoms. In late stages the degeneration may extend to gray areas of the cord and limit healing.

Because of the wide distribution of areas of degeneration, *there is a greater variety of signs and symptoms in multiple sclerosis than in other neurologic diseases.* The scarring that occurs at the degenerative lesions as well as the increasing sites provides the name "disseminated sclerosis."

Multiple sclerosis is a *chronic, remitting,* and *relapsing disease.* The majority of people recover from their

Table 36-1. Comparison of neurologic degenerative diseases

Disease	Pathology	Effect
Multiple sclerosis	Multiple foci (patches) of nerve degeneration throughout brain and spinal cord	Demyelination causes nerve impulse to be interrupted (blocked) or distorted (slowed)
Myasthenia gravis	Decreased secretion of acetylcholine or an increase of cholinesterase enzyme at myoneural junction	Interference of nerve impulse across myoneural junction
Amyotrophic lateral sclerosis	Destruction of myelin sheath of motor neurons of lateral tracts of spinal cord and brain	Demyelination causes nerve impulse to be interrupted (blocked) or distorted (slowed)
Parkinsonism	Destruction of nerve cells of basal ganglia of brain	Decreased dopamine (neurotransmitter substance with anticholinergic effect)
Syringomyelia	Destruction of gray then white matter of spinal cord by development of "syrinx" (cysts filled with CSF)	Destruction of nerve pathways in spinal cord—interruption of nerve impulses
Muscular dystrophy	*Not a neurologic disease:* atrophy of voluntary muscles	Effect is a wasting away of the voluntary muscles—no nerve effect

early episodes. Usually there are acute exacerbations and remissions that may last for a year or more, although eventually exacerbations will recur. There is no record of any patients having recovered from the disease, although many have lived for 20 years or more and have died from other causes. Exacerbations may be aggravated or precipitated by fatigue, chilling, and emotional disturbances.

Clinical picture

Early symptoms are usually transitory and may include double vision *(diplopia)*, spots before the eyes *(scotomas), blindness, tremor, weakness* or *numbness of a part of the body such as the hand, fatigue, susceptibility to upper respiratory infections, and emotional instability.* Many persons with early multiple sclerosis may be considered neurotic by their associates and sometimes by their physicians because of the wide variety and temporary nature of symptoms and because of their emotional instability. As the disease progresses, symptoms may include *nystagmus, disorders of speech (scanning), urinary frequency and urgency, constipation, and changes in muscular coordination and gait.* Late symptoms may include urinary incontinence, difficulty in swallowing, severe muscle spasm and contractures, and spastic ataxic gait.

A sense of optimism and well-being (euphoria) also seems to be characteristic of persons with multiple sclerosis, especially during remissions. It is suspected that this reaction is due largely to the patient's attempts to reassure himself that his condition is not so serious as is supposed. This response is helpful to the patient in many ways, but sometimes it may lead him to overdo, and thus increase symptoms.

Motor signs have upper motor neuron characteristics. Pain is not a common symptom of multiple sclerosis except when there is severe muscle spasm. Death may be caused by infection, usually developing in the respiratory or genitourinary system.

In the hospital the nurse may care for the patient for short periods when he is admitted for diagnosis or for some other condition or when he is terminally ill with advanced disease. Many patients are never hospitalized and will be cared for in their homes by public health nurses.

The fact that multiple sclerosis involves multiple parts of the nervous system is often characterized by exacerbations and remissions, and frequently includes transient and bizarre signs and symptoms, makes it difficult to diagnose with certainty. Because there is *no specific diagnostic test,* diagnosis is often a clinical judgment. The determination of cerebrospinal fluid gamma globulin by chemical or electrophoretic methods or of cerebrospinal fluid IgG by electroimmunodiffusion, when used with the history and neurologic examination, appears to be the most valuable single laboratory test.[60]

Intervention

Drug therapy. At the present time there is no specific treatment for multiple sclerosis. Many physicians get favorable results from symptomatic treatments and the judicious use of ACTH and the corticosteroids, psychotherapy, social rehabilitation, physical therapy, patient education, and a great deal of compassion. Although ACTH and the steroids are widely used, their efficacy remains controversial. These drugs have been shown to prevent experimental allergic encephalomyelitis. Currently some clinicians prefer oral prednisone; others prefer intramuscular ACTH; still others prefer intravenous ACTH. Dexamethasone (Decadron), administered intramuscularly or orally, has become popular. Its demonstrated antiedema effect may explain the favorable results in acute attacks of multiple sclerosis. The effects of ACTH and the steroids on the demyelinating activity per se are not known. It is known from testing that there is nothing to be gained from long-term treatment with either steroids or ACTH, and second, that there is possibly some gain from taking high doses of steroids at the start of a fresh episode, since the episode tends to resolve itself more rapidly if patients are treated with intensive courses of these drugs. The mood-elevating drugs are used to relieve depression, which is often present in multiple sclerosis.

Activity and rest. The person with multiple sclerosis should have a daily routine for rest and activity and should adhere to it strictly. Rest must be balanced with adequate exercise. The person is usually advised to exercise regularly but never to the point of extreme fatigue. Because he almost always feels tired, he must look for some special sign that tells him he has exercised enough. If he does more, he may suffer ill effects. For example, a tight feeling in the chest may indicate that the person must rest or else have severe discomfort. After an exacerbation, it may be difficult to resume exercises, but it is usually best that an established schedule be returned to as soon as possible. There is a need to conserve energy for priority activities.

One side of the body is usually affected more than the other, and the person may learn to stabilize his gait by leaning toward his uninvolved side. The annoyance of having the foot slap forward in taking a step may sometimes be overcome by putting the heel down in a pronounced fashion and rolling the weight forward on the side of the foot.

Effort is made to maintain activity and work for as long as possible, and many persons have worked for 5 to 10 years and even longer after the onset of the first symptoms. Women at home can be helped to plan their shopping, housework, and other duties so that they may continue to function as wives and mothers even when the disease is advanced.

Comfort. Diplopia can be relieved by an eye patch. Peripheral neurectomies, rhizotomies, and cordotomies are often used for the relief of spasticity, pain, and paresthesias. Relief from severe spasticity is often obtained from intrathecal injections of phenol.

Elimination. Urinary frequency and urgency, often the source of social disability, may respond to timed doses of propantheline bromide (Pro-Banthine). Prevention of urinary tract infection remains a problem, and such infections are a major cause of death. Cholinergic drugs such as bethanechol (Urecholine) may be of help in the patient with an atonic bladder. Cystometrographic study is important to detect the specific bladder problem.

Teaching needs. Good general health and hygiene are necessary for the person with multiple sclerosis. Hot baths should be avoided. It is essential that the person and the family understand the importance of checking the skin routinely and take measures to relieve tissue pressure in order to prevent the development of pressure sores secondary to immobilization and sensory loss (see Chapter 35).

Since association with others is good for physical and mental health, the individual with multiple sclerosis must be encouraged and helped to remain an active, participating member of his family and his community for as long as possible. Personal cleanliness adds to a feeling of acceptance and well-being; consequently, these persons should be encouraged to pay careful attention to personal appearance even though they may sometimes feel too tired to put forth the effort. The person should be encouraged to develop interests and hobbies that will help make up for things he should not do, such as driving a vehicle, and that will help to fill the time when physical activity becomes more difficult. Music, writing, reading, and question games are good hobbies to develop. Interest in politics and in world affairs, which may be followed on the radio if sight is lost, may stand the person in good stead.

The National Multiple Sclerosis Society* is a national voluntary, nonprofit organization founded in 1946. Its functions are to encourage and finance research, to gather statistics, and to act as an information center for patients and for the public. A recent development is the Multiple Sclerosis Home Care course planned by the Society in conjunction with the American Red Cross on a national basis to teach relatives and friends of MS patients how to provide better care at home. Some local chapters also supply equipment to patients. Membership is open to health and welfare workers and to patients and their families. Local organizations can be found in many large cities.

A well-balanced diet with plenty of high-vitamin foods and fluids is important. Obesity must be avoided because it is more difficult for the obese person to maneuver and detracts from his appearance. Fresh air and sunshine are helpful, but chilling and overheating must be avoided because they may aggravate symptoms or bring on exacerbations. A good night's sleep is important, and a rest period after lunch is recommended.

Adaptation. The decision as to whether the patient is told his diagnosis rests with the physician, and there is not full agreement among physicians as to the proper

*257 Park Ave. South, New York, NY 10010.

course of action. Usually the decision is made on an individual basis and depends on the person's emotional makeup and on the family's ability to cope with the economic, social, and emotional problems that a condition of this kind presents.

Persons with multiple sclerosis need a peaceful, relaxed environment. They should never be hurried and should not be expected to respond quickly either physically or mentally. They may have slowness in speech and slowness in ability to respond, and this difficulty should be ignored by persons around them. Members of the family and friends need help in understanding this problem and in meeting it calmly. The person may have sudden explosive emotional outbursts of crying or laughing brought on by such simple acts as putting something hot into the mouth. Close members of the family must protect both the patient and visitors from the embarrassment of prolonged emotional outbursts. Reminding the patient of something sad may stop him from laughing, and holding the mouth open will sometimes stop the crying.

Outcome criteria for the patient with multiple sclerosis

The patient or significant others can:

1. Explain the prevention of urinary-bladder infection and discomfort.
   a. Explain need for adequate or increased fluid intake during the day.
   b. Relate the need for a well-balanced diet for the prevention of infection generally.
   c. Explain home medications (actions and effects on the urinary system, dosage, and side effects of urinary antiinfective drugs).
   d. Explain need to consult with physician when there are urinary problems.
   e. State methods to keep the urine acid.
   f. Explain the need and method of perineal cleanliness.
2. Explain general health maintenance practices.
   a. Make a plan to balance rest and work activities at home.
   b. State how to conserve energy for priority activites.
   c. Explain plan for a balanced diet.
   d. Explain the need to avoid hurry in the performance of activities.
   e. Plan for the inclusion of hobbies and interests as related to mental health.
   f. Explain the occurrence of euphoria and other reaction to multiple sclerosis.
3. Explain safety factors related to the condition.
   a. Explain the relationship of gait patterns to the need for safety.
   b. Explain the relationship of sensory deficits to safety.
   c. State where to secure safety equipment.
4. Explain exercise program to be followed at home.
   a. Demonstrate physical and occupational therapy exercises prescribed for continuing care.
   b. Explain the need for exercise for the preservation of muscle strength.
5. Explain how to secure human and material resources.
   a. Explain how to contact community health nurses.
   b. Explain the availability of ambulatory clinics.
   c. Explain the services that are obtained from the local multiple sclerosis chapter.
   d. List the visual and adaptive equipment available and where purchase or loan can be made.
6. State plans for follow-up care.

☐ Paralysis agitans (Parkinson's disease, parkinsonism)

Parkinson's disease is one of the major causes of neurologic disability in the United States, especially in individuals over 60 years of age. Its prevalence is not known for sure. It has variously been estimated to have a prevalence rate of 100 to 150/100,000 population.[1] We can expect to see an increasing frequency because of the increased number of older people in our population.

Parkinson's disease is a slowly progressive degenerative disease of unknown cause in which there is destruction of nerve cells in the basal ganglia of the brain. It may follow acute encephalitis and occasionally occurs following carbon monoxide, metallic, or other poisoning. The disease, sometimes termed idiopathic parkinsonism, usually affects older persons. Sometimes it is associated with arteriosclerosis, but in many cases signs of arteriosclerosis are absent.

Advances in knowledge of the regional biochemistry of the brain, particularly of the biogenic amines, have made possible a new understanding of Parkinson's disease and have established a more rational basis for therapy. Parkinson's disease can now be defined as a dopamine deficiency condition with injury or disease of the dopaminergic neuronal system. Most neuropathologists agree that the loss of pigmented neurons occurs particularly in the substantia nigra. It has been demonstrated that dopamine, a *neurotransmitter substance,* is found in high concentrations in the neostriatum (caudate nucleus, putamen, pallidum). In Parkinson's disease it is selectively depleted in these structures. This depletion can be correlated with the degree of degeneration of the substantia nigra in experimental animals. The greater the cell loss in the substantia nigra, the lower the concentration of dopamine in the striatum. The physiologic role of dopamine appears to be the inhibiting modulation of the striatum that it produces by counterbalancing the excitatory cholinergic activity in this area. Acetylcholine, the excitatory neurotransmitter, is in abundant supply in the striatum. Thus there is an imbalance between the depleted dopamine and the acetylcholine. Therapy is now directed toward administering a precursor of dopamine, levodopa, which passes the blood-brain barrier, or anticholinergic drugs that act againt the acetylcholine.

Clinical picture

Parkinson's disease begins with a faint tremor and progresses so slowly that the person is seldom able to recall its onset. There is not true paralysis and no loss of sensation. Tremor (pill rolling of the fingers or resting tremor) are the two outstanding signs of the disease. Parkinson's disease has some characteristics of upper motor neuron signs (see p. 676). It is essentially a problem in motion. Muscle rigidity seems to prevent normal response in commonly performed acts and leads to characteristic changes that make the diagnosis almost unmistakable to persons who have observed patients with the disease. There is a masklike appearance to the face and slowed, monotonous speech. Drooling may occur because of the difficulty of swallowing saliva. This may cause skin irritation that is best prevented or treated by frequent sponging followed by protecting the skin with an emollient such as cold cream. There is a characteristic shuffling gait in which the patient tends to walk on his toes. The trunk is bent forward, and the arms fall rigidly to the sides and do not swing as in normal rhythmic gait. Neuromuscular control may be altered so that the patient is unable to stop his propulsive gait until he meets an obstruction; finally he may become unable to walk at all. The patient usually has a moist, oily skin. Defects in judgment and emotional instability may occur, but intelligence is not impaired. The appetite may be increased and there is heat intolerance. All signs and symptoms increase with fatigue, excitement, and frustration.

Intervention

Drug therapy. Treatment for Parkinson's disease is palliative and symptomatic and depends on the pharmacologic manipulation of the pathophysiologic state. The severity of symptoms and presence of associated disease processes determine the drugs to be used. Anticholinergic alkaloids such as scopolamine hydrobromide and related drugs (hyoscyamine) have been used for more than a century. They act against cholinergic excitatory effects and are more effective in lessening muscle rigidity than in controlling tremor. Many synthetic anticholinergic drugs of varied chemical structure are also available. There is little to recommend one over the other, aside from personal preference, but each has some degree of central nervous system anticholinergic action. However, they are incapable of restoring striatal balance. The preferred anticholinergic agents are trihexyphenidyl (Artane), benztropine mesylate (Cogentin), procyclidine (Kemandrin), and biperiden (Akineton).[67] These drugs have some selectivity of action in that they have greater central than peripheral anticholinergic activity. Optimal results from these drugs depend on a dosage that provides a compromise between the limited symptomatic improvement given by these drugs and the disagreeable symptoms of central and peripheral cholinergic blockade (blurring of vision, dryness of mouth and throat, constipation, urinary urgency or retention, ataxia, dysarthria, mental disturbances). Antihistaminic drugs such as diphenhydramine (Benadryl), which are not primarily anticholinergic, exert mild central anticholinergic properties when used alone or in combination with other drugs.

Some patients with severe Parkinson's disease have experienced dramatic benefits from levodopa not experienced from anticholinergic drugs. Levodopa assists in restoring striatal dopamine deficiency, since it is a precursor of dopamine. This drug does not affect the underlying process of parkinsonism.[13] In this way, levodopa is more like a replacement drug than a cure. Once benefits are obtained from levodopa, they are likely to be sustained. After prolonged periods of treatment, there may be an increased appearance of side effects. Levodopa (Larodopa, Dopar) is introduced slowly over a period of weeks or months. Usually patients remain on anticholinergic drugs or they may be added as an adjunct. Most individuals experience side effects from levodopa, such as nausea and vomiting, orthostatic hypotension, insomnia, agitation, and mental confusion, but these lessen with continued medication and dosage modification.

There have been some cases of kidney and liver damage. Candidates for levodopa should be selected carefully.[13] Amantadine hydrochloride (Symmetrel), an antiviral agent, is known to have antiparkinson activity by blocking the reuptake and storage of catecholamines and allowing the accumulation of dopamine in extracellular or synaptic sites. This drug may not sustain its effectiveness for more than 3 months in some patients. Side effects, although infrequent, include mental confusion, visual disturbances, and seizures.

Carbidopa-levodopa (Sinemet) is a drug that is more recently utilized in neurologic practice. It is a combination of levodopa with an inhibitor of the enzyme dopa decarboxylase, which limits the metabolism of levodopa peripherally. It thus reduces some of the side effects of levodopa seen with higher dosages.

Surgery. A surgical procedure has been used with some success in the treatment of selected patients with Parkinson's disease. Descriptions of successful operations in popular magazines have led some patients and their families to believe that a cure for all patients has been found. The nurse should refer those asking questions to a qualified neurologist. Many patients cannot be treated surgically. Results seem to be best in younger patients who have unilateral involvement following other disease and who have marked tremor and rigidity. Treatment consists of destroying portions of the globus pallidus (relieves rigidity) or the thalamus (relieves tremor) in the brain by stereotatic methods through the use of cautery, removal, or injection of alcohol. Operative techniques involving cooling or freezing with liquid nitrogen (cryogenic surgery) have been attempted with good results in selected cases and with fewer complications than when cautery or alcohol was used. Medications used to control rigidity and tremor are discontinued several days preoperatively so that patients' symptoms will be at their maximum during the operation.[40] Nursing care *preoperatively* includes seeing that nutrition is adequate as well as other general preoperative care.

Postoperative care includes the most careful attention to the vital signs, use of side rails to prevent accidents in the event of convulsions, disorientation, or temporary hemiplegia, and frequent turning and moving to prevent respiratory and circulatory complications. Excessive salivation and difficulty in blinking the eye on the operated side may be problems requiring nursing attention.

Activity. Special attention should be paid to *posture.* Lying on a firm bed without a pillow during rest periods may help to prevent the spine from bending forward, and lying in the prone position also helps. Holding the hands folded behind the back when walking may help to keep the spine erect and prevent the annoyance of the arms falling stiffly at the sides. The tremor often is less apparent when the person is sitting in an armchair, since he can grip the arms of the chair and partially control the tremor in his hands and arms. The reader is referred to Chapter 35 for discussion of alterations of movement and posture.

Feeding the patient becomes a real problem when the disease is far advanced because of the danger of choking in attempts to swallow; eventually, aspiration pneumonia may terminate the patient's life. Unless the patient is well controlled by medication, drooling can be a real problem and increases with general excitement. A bib can be used to protect the clothing during napping hours. When the patient is dressed, a garment with generous pockets well supplied with soft tissues will help him be less conspicuous and more comfortable.

The patient with Parkinson's disease should continue to work as long as possible. Most physicians advise this unless the occupation is such that continued work is dangerous. The patient should reduce his regular work gradually while developing hobbies and interests in which he may *engage when the disease* becomes more advanced.

Teaching needs. The progress of Parkinson's disease, a condition that often lasts for years, may be slowed by good nutrition, sufficient rest, moderate exercise in fresh air, and other measures that improve general health. Patient and family education is a primary nursing intervention. Instruction should include general health maintenance practices, prevention of the complications of poor posture and immobility, and drug therapy. The nurse needs to assist the patient and family in communication techniques. Speech exercises directed toward relaxation of speech muscles and improvement of voice volume has assisted some persons.[18]

Relatives need complete understanding of the circumstances so that they may intelligently assist in the adjustments that will eventually be necessary. Such problems as accidents, personality changes, and progressive helplessness must be anticipated. While drooling and difficulty in swallowing often limit the important social outlet of eating at group gatherings, the patient should have his meals at home with the family as long as possible.

Outcome criteria for the person with Parkinson's disease

The patient or significant others can:

1. Explain each home medication prescribed for the relief of parkinsonism.
   a. Explain use, action, dosage, frequency, and side effects of each medication.
   b. Explain that dosage may require modification until side effects are stabilized.
   c. Explain how to take medications for best results in the relief of signs and symptoms and side effects.
   d. Explain the value of taking medications regularly.
2. Explain the importance of adherence to general health practices.
   a. Make a plan of activities of daily living (ADL) that is balanced as to rest, physical activities, and socialization.
   b. Recognize emotional responses to illness and the effects of fatigue and stress.
3. Describe potential safety factors related to parkinsonism.
   a. Respiratory infection related to rigidity of respiratory muscles.
   b. Aspiration of food caused by difficulty in swallowing.

   c. Social isolation related to embarrassment about speech and physical appearance.
   d. Accidents related to difficulty in gait.
4. State plans for follow-up care.

□ Myasthenia gravis

Myasthenia gravis is a relatively rare disease of unknown cause. It usually occurs in young adults. Nerve impulses fail to pass to muscles at the myoneural junction. It is not known specifically why the motor nerve impulses fail to pass to the muscle and cause it not to contract. It is believed variously to be caused by the inability of the motor end plate to secrete adequate acetylcholine, excessive quantities of the cholinesterase enzyme at the nerve ending, or a nonresponse of the muscle fibers to acetylcholine. Relative to the third theory, myasthenia gravis may be considered a primary muscle disease; relative to the first two theories it is a neuromuscular disease with lower motor neuron characteristics. Myasthenia gravis is considered a grave disorder, since the respiratory muscles and the bulbar cranial nerves may be involved. During periods of exacerbation or lack of drug control, the patient may be cared for in a respiratory intensive care unit.

Clinical picture

The outstanding symptoms are muscle weakness and severe generalized fatigue that come on quickly and, in the early stages of the disease, disappear quickly with rest. Weakness of arm and hand muscles may be first noticed when shaving or combing the hair. Facial muscles innervated by the cranial nerves are often affected, and it may not be possible for the person to hold his eyelids open (ptosis), to keep his mouth closed, or to chew or swallow. Diplopia (double vision) is also common. Muscle weakness may become so severe that the person cannot breathe without assistance. Exacerbations of the disease may be initiated by upper respiratory infections, emotional tension, and menstruation.

Intervention

There is no known cure for myasthenia gravis. There is, however, a very marked improvement following the use of neostigmine (Prostigmin) or pyridostigmine (Mestinon). These drugs block the action of cholinesterase at the myoneural junction and allow the action of acetylcholine, a chemical necessary for transmission of impulses to the muscles. Treatment is planned so that the patient may be maintained on the amount of drug that he can tolerate without side effects and yet carry out activities essential for normal living. Usually the patient is permitted to adjust his own dosage. *The nurse should teach the importance of taking medications at the time prescribed.* If the drug is delayed, dyspnea may result followed by severe respiratory distress, which if untreated can cause death.

It is important also to teach that (1) dosage is individually determined and related to the activity of the person, (2) dosage needs to be adjusted to maintain muscle strength, and (3) the effects of drugs need to be monitored. The nurse and family must understand that it is often difficult to distinguish between myasthenic crisis (too little drug) and cholinergic crisis (too much drug). Drugs to be avoided are muscle relaxants, morphine, barbiturates, tranquilizers, and neomycin.

The patient with myasthenia gravis should take particular care of his health, and it is preferable that the patient not live alone. Upper respiratory infections may be serious because the person may not have the energy to cough effectively and may develop pneumonia or airway obstruction. Because of weakness in swallowing, food may be aspirated. The patient who is living at home may feel more secure if there is a tracheal suction apparatus and other airway and ventilatory equipment available and if a member of the family knows how to use it if an emergency arises.

During acute episodes of the disease a tracheostomy set is kept in the patient's room ready for immediate use. Often it is necessary to suction the patient before he eats. If swallowing is too dangerous, a nasogastric tube is used, and great care must be taken to be certain that the tube is in the stomach before fluid is introduced, since the patient cannot cough to indicate its presence in the trachea. When caring for the patient with severe symptoms of myasthenia gravis, the nurse should remember that he is too weak to do anything for himself. Therefore the patient may not take a drink and may not turn over in bed unless the nurse thinks to help him.

Persons with myasthenia gravis must often change their method of earning a living. The nurse can help the patient and family plan so that a minimum of energy is used in activities that are essential to remaining relatively self-sufficient.

Outcome criteria for the person with myasthenia gravis

The person or significant others can:

1. Explain each prescribed anticholinesterase or cholinergic drug.
   a. Explain the action, effects, side effects, and toxic effects.
   b. Explain the reason for taking the medication at the exact time scheduled.
   c. Explain the need to monitor the effect of the medication particularly on respiration, swallowing, and general muscle strength.
   d. List the drugs that act on the neuromuscular junction and that are contraindicated.

2. Describe measures to prevent respiratory infection.
3. Demonstrate use of airway and ventilatory equipment.
4. Explain the need to avoid overexertion and emotional tension.

□ Amyotrophic lateral sclerosis

Amyotrophic lateral sclerosis (ALS) is a motor neuron disease that affects upper or lower motor neurons lying within the brain or spinal cord or a combination of the two. There is direct involvement of the lateral tracts of the spinal cord with possible eventual involvement of the medulla and the ventral tracts. Myelin sheaths are destroyed and are replaced by scar tissue. The nerve impulses are distorted or blocked. Symptoms depend on which motor neurons are affected.[8]

Clinical picture

Early symptoms include fatigue and awkwardness of fine finger movements and muscle wasting. There is *progressive muscle weakness, atrophy,* and *fasciculations.* Spasticity of flexor muscles is commonly present. With involvement of the brainstem and medulla there is dysphagia, dysarthria, jaw clonus, tongue fasciculations, and respiratory difficulty. As the disease progresses, there is disability relative to both upper and lower limbs, and one side of the body becomes more involved than the other. The person remains alert.

Intervention

Treatment is directed toward relieving the symptoms with medications. Nursing interventions include assistance with activities of daily living as limb deficits increase and much *emotional support.* Prostheses are often applied to support the weakened muscles. The person is always afraid as the disease progresses and respirations are affected. At this time constant nursing attention is required. Most patients live about 3 years after diagnosis; occasionally there are periods of spontaneous arrest.

Outcome criteria for the person with amyotrophic lateral sclerosis

The person with ALS is evaluated based on the outcome criteria described relative to upper and lower motor neuron paralysis (p. 683) and bulbar respiratory failure (p. 687).

□ Syringomyelia

Syringomyelia is a chronic, slowly progressive, and rare condition. It involves the spinal cord or the lower brainstem (syringobulbia). There is some tendency for it to occur in families.

Syringomyelia is the name given because of small tubelike cavities or cysts called "syrinx" that form and progressively destroy the cord from the inside out, involving first the gray matter near the central canal and then the white matter. The syrinxes become inflated with cerebrospinal fluid and communicate with each other and with ventricular fluid pathways, causing distention. The widest parts of the cord (cervical and lumbar) become inflated with fluid first, and early symptoms can be related to cord damage at the cervical or upper arm level. There is blockage of nerve impulse transmission. At first there is involvement of the spinothalamic sensory pathway and later involvement of motor neuron pathways. As the cord inflates with fluid, the spinothalamic pathway becomes *vulnerable to destruction first because the nerve cell fibers from the cell bodies in the gray matter cross the cord to the opposite side* and then travel to the brain in the spinothalamic tract. The cell bodies lie within the posterior horn, and the fibers run across the cord. The causes for the development of the initial syrinx are variable, including glioma and failure of the ventricular system to circulate cerebrospinal fluid properly within its normal channels.

Clinical picture

The precise clinical picture depends on the cross-sectional and vertical extent of cord destruction, but certain clinical signs and symptoms are usual. An early finding is segmental loss of pain and temperature sense and preservation of the sense of touch with losses over the arms, shoulders, and neck areas in a capelike distribution. This dissociated sensory loss is explained by the cervical cord involvement and distention as discussed above. There is also weakness and atrophy of the hands and arms and loss of tendon reflexes. As the lesions continue to extend within the cord, the anterior horn cells of the gray matter become affected, producing lower motor neuron paralysis with flaccidity and loss of reflexes. Later, as cavitation of the cord widens, the corticospinal tracts become compressed with upper motor neuron involvement (spasticity and hyperreflexia). If lesions extend upward, the upper end of the cord or bulb then becomes involved. In the latter there is numbness of the face, wasting of the tongue, difficulty in swallowing, coughing, or difficulty in breathing. The early analgesia and thermoanesthesia account for the painless infections, skin ulceration, injuries, and burns seen in patients with this condition. Lumbar puncture, myelography, and air encephalography are the diagnostic procedures most helpful.

Intervention

There is no specific treatment for syringomyelia. Surgical treatment is attempted in carefully selected cases, depending on the cause. Decompression of a distended syrinx may temporarily relieve symptoms of local compression of ascending and descending spinal tracts. Unroofing the spinal cord by removing the posterior rim of the foramen magnum and the cerebellar tonsils has relieved neurologic symptoms in some persons. Shunt operations to relieve blocked cerebrospinal fluid and to provide a different drainage system have been successfully attempted. Nursing interventions are directed toward prevention of injury caused by sensory losses. When the brainstem is affected, respiratory care takes priority, as does the utilization of feeding techniques to prevent aspiration.

Outcome criteria for the person with syringomyelia

The person with syringomyelia is evaluated by the same outcome criteria as for the person with the general sensory dysfunction (p. 686), upper and lower motor paralysis (p. 683), and respiratory failure (p. 1134), as related to the presenting clinical symptoms and signs.

■ VASCULAR DISEASE

□ Cerebrovascular accident

Cerebrovascular accident (CVA) is the most common disease of the nervous system and is the third highest cause of death in the United States. The condition is often associated with vascular disease of the heart, kidneys, other organs, and peripheral blood vessels. It is a major cause of chronic disability.

Usually the vessel involved in a cerebrovascular accident is a relatively large one and affects one side of the brain, which leads to partial or complete paralysis of the opposite side of the body (hemiplegia). *Shock, hemiplegia,* and *stroke* are other terms used in referring to cerebrovascular accidents. *The term "stroke" clinically refers to the sudden and dramatic development of focal neurologic deficits.* Hemiplegia is one neurologic deficit that commonly occurs. If a small blood vessel is involved, there may be symptoms of short duration or that are less severe as described later in this section. The extent of neurologic deficits is directly related to the specific blood vessels occluded and the area of the brain supplied by the vessels.

The "stroke prone" person often has a history of previous transient cerebral ischemia attacks (TIA) that last for minutes to almost 24 hours. Early identification and treatment of underlying conditions may prevent a CVA in these persons. When a TIA lasts for several days and resolves, leaving minimal residual evidence, it is known as TIA-IR (incomplete recovery). When the ischemic attack is characterized by a marked and persistent neurologic deficit, the diagnosis of completed stroke (CS) is made.[21]

Vascular lesions of the brain are often categorized as caused by embolus, hemorrhage, or thrombosis. Cerebral embolism is usually caused by a mass breaking away from a thrombosed blood vessel elsewhere in the body. This condition has been less frequent since patients with bacterial endocarditis have been treated with antibiotic drugs.

□ Cerebral thrombosis and cerebral hemorrhage

Cerebral thrombosis is by far the most common cause and accounts for approximately 90% of all cerebrovascular accidents in persons over 65 years of age. It is caused by the formation of a thrombus, or clot, in a blood vessel of the brain.

Cerebral hemorrhage is caused either by the rupture of a congenital aneurysm or by the rupture of a sclerosed blood vessel in persons who have high blood pressure. Although the symptoms of rupture of an aneurysm and of hemorrhage caused by arteriosclerosis and high blood pressure may be similar, the treatment is different. Therefore the nursing care will be considered separately. Cerebral thrombosis and cerebral hemorrhage may occur at any time, although thrombosis is more likely to occur when the patient is sleeping, and the hemorrhage is more likely to occur when physical or emotional stress is encountered. The prognosis for the patient who has had a cerebrovascular accident is poor, particularly during the first few days. The mortality rate is somewhat higher in cerebral hemorrhage than in cerebral thrombosis.

Clinical picture

Cerebral *hemorrhage* may be preceded by headache, vertigo, flushing of the face, momentary loss of consciousness, nausea and vomiting, and a foreboding that something is wrong. If a large artery ruptures, a sizable portion of the brain may be deprived of its blood supply and the onset may be sudden. If a smaller vessel ruptures, only a small portion of the brain may be affected, and symptoms may become pronounced only when enough blood has flowed into the brain tissue to produce pressure. Symptoms of cerebral *thrombosis* are most likely to be obvious on the person's awakening, but they usually vary in degree. There may be only a slight difficulty in speech, in walking, or in recalling events of the day before. The effects of the thrombosis may become progressively worse over a 24-hour period, and the person may awake to find one side of his body paralyzed. If the thrombosis is massive or develops quickly, death may occur during sleep.

Following a cerebral hemorrhage or a cerebral thrombosis, the person may fall and lapse into total unconsciousness, and convulsions may occur immediately following the accident. Loss of consciousness may come on slowly or quickly and may last for a few minutes or many days until slow recovery occurs, or it may continue until death, which usually does not occur for several days. The pulse is rapid and bounding, the respirations are labored or stertorous, and the blood pressure is elevated; vomiting may also occur. The pupils may not react normally to light, and one side of the body may appear limp. If the paralysis is on the right side of the body, the person may not be able to speak even if consciousness returns, because the speech center in most right-handed persons is located on the left side of the brain along with the cortical sensory and motor areas for the right side of the body. If the patient is hospitalized, a spinal puncture is usually performed. It may reveal blood in the spinal fluid if hemorrhage has occurred in an intracerebral artery that communicates with the spinal fluid system.

Intervention

Emergency care. A cerebrovascular accident may occur when the person is at work or elsewhere outside his home and may be confused with convulsive seizures, diabetic coma, or drunkenness. Emergency care at the scene of the episode consists of turning the person carefully on to his affected side (determined by the puffiness of the cheek on this side) and elevating the head without tilting the neck forward, since tilting may constrict blood vessels and in turn cause congestion of blood within the cerebrum. Turning to the affected side permits saliva to drain out of the mouth and lessens the danger of aspiration into the lungs. Elevation of the head may help to prevent edema of the brain. Clothing should be loosened about the throat to further aid in preventing engorgement of blood vessels in the head, which may lead to cerebral edema. The person should be kept quiet, moved as little as possible, and protected from chilling. Medical assistance is sought at once.

Initial phase. Nursing intervention during the initial phase does not differ whether the person is in the hospital or in his own home, although oxygen is more likely to be given in the hospital. In an attempt to prevent further thrombosis, bishydroxycoumarin (Dicumarol) and heparin may be given in the hospital if it is certain that the cause is cerebral thrombosis and not cerebral hemorrhage. The use of anticoagulants is controversial.

Goals are directed toward survival needs and preventing further brain damage. Care by the nurse is directed toward the unconscious state if present (see Chapter 27). Neurologic assessment is done at regular intervals to detect changes in status and complications. The vital signs should be carefully checked, and the nurse should observe for such things as a rise in temperature within the first day or two, slowing of pulse and respiration, and deepening of the coma, all of which indicate pressure on the vital centers and a poor prognosis.

Acute phase. Since a cerebrovascular accident frequently results in some paralysis, the reader is referred to Chapter 35, p. 679, for a discussion of the care of the paralyzed person.

Food and fluids. Fluids may be restricted for the first few days after a cerebrovascular accident in an effort to prevent edema of the brain. Then patients will be fed intravenous fluids, or the physician may insert a nasogastric tube and order tube feedings. When the patient is no longer comatose, small amounts of fluid, 5 to 10 ml, can be given several times daily to determine the patient's ability to swallow and to help him regain this function. Returning as soon as possible to a regular diet and a normal fluid intake is desirable.

Activity. Rest and quiet are important even if the accident has not been serious enough to cause complete loss of consciousness. Some neurologists may prescribe that the head of the bed be kept flat for several days. This is believed to assist cerebral perfusion. No attempt should be made to rouse the patient from coma, although respiratory and circulatory stimulants may be prescribed by the physician.

The length of time the patient remains in bed depends entirely on the type of cerebrovascular accident suffered and the judgment of the physician in regard to early mobilization. Some physicians prescribe fairly long periods of rest following cerebrovascular accidents, whereas others believe that early mobilization is best. However, the trend is toward early mobilization of the patient with cerebral thrombosis, and mobilization sometimes begins a day or two after the accident has occurred.

Prevention of joint deformity (p. 840) is initiated during the acute stage. This includes positioning of affected limbs in anatomic position and range of motion exercises. There should be a regular schedule for turning the patient to avoid the danger of circulatory stasis, hypostatic pneumonia, and decubitus ulcer.

Elimination. Urinary output should be noted carefully and recorded for several days after a cerebrovascular accident. Retention of urine may occur, but it is more likely that the patient will be incontinent. If urinary incontinence occurs, the patient may be told that his control of excretory function probably will improve day by day. Offering a bedpan or a urinal immediately after meals and at other regular intervals helps to overcome incontinence. A retention catheter may be used for the first few days for women patients.

Fecal incontinence is fairly common following a cerebrovascular accident, and again the patient must be reassured that as general improvement occurs, this condition will be overcome. Some patients develop constipation, and impactions develop readily. Elimination must be noted carefully, since diarrhea may develop in the presence of an impaction, thus causing it to go unnoticed for several days. Suppositories such as bisacodyl (Dulcolax) are generally prescribed to be given daily or every other day. However, some physicians order laxatives or enemas. Massage to the abdomen may be helpful in starting peristalsis, but it is done only when ordered by a physician. Warm oil-retention enemas are sometimes given regularly in an attempt to prevent impactions and when impactions occur. Milk of magnesia by mouth is often given, since straining in the act of defecation must be avoided. The patient must be cautioned not to strain and must be assured that the suppositories can easily be repeated if no results are obtained. He usually needs assistance in getting on and off the bedpan. Side rails that he can hold on in turning himself or a trapeze that he can reach with his unaffected hand is useful if he is permitted this exertion.

Emotional support. If the patient survives the first few days, he may begin to regain consciousness, and some of the paralysis may disappear. It is then that the greatest understanding is needed by persons attending him. He may realize that he cannot talk, that he drools, that he cannot move a hand or a leg, or if he can move the limbs, that the motions are shaky and uncertain. The patient's condition is a terrible shock to him, and it is at this point that the nurse's active part in rehabilitation begins. By quiet assurance a nurse can help the patient feel that his progress toward recovery and self-sufficiency has begun and will continue. The nurse can help by telling the person what is going to be done even though he cannot answer. If the patient is right-handed and cannot speak, he has the added difficulty of having to learn to write with his left hand in addition to being partially speechless. The nurse should try to anticipate the patient's needs and should make every effort to understand his indistinct speech, since repeated attempts to make himself understood only augment his misery and frustration. Usually, if partial speech is present at the time of return to consciousness, there is likelihood that speech will improve, and the patient is heartened by the knowledge of this fact. Speech may also be affected because of involvement of the tongue, mouth, and throat muscles.

The patient who has sustained a cerebrovascular accident may be overly emotional, and this reaction, combined with his fear and frustration on becoming aware of his condition, is upsetting to his family. Crying is common, and sometimes family members believe that they are responsible for this sadness when this is usually not true. Family, staff, and other patients need reassurance that they are not the cause of the reaction.

Following a stroke, the person may have difficulty relating to himself and to his environment. After the acute stage a multibed environment is advocated, as the sensory input from others is helpful. In the initial stage, bringing familiar articles into the patient's environment can be a very helpful stimulus. Examples are a clock, watch, family picture, or a Bible. *Hemianopia,* or decreased visual field, occurs rather commonly. Approaching the patient from the side of intact vision and teaching him to scan will not only make him more aware of stimuli but can help prevent injury. Diminished awareness or denial of his affected side (anosognosia) can occur and could be a safety hazard. This possibility should be considered when the patient runs into objects with the wheelchair or allows the affected arm or leg to drag behind him when transferring from chair to bed.[20]

The nurse's observations regarding the mental status of the patient are important. The patient may be disoriented and have decreased judgment or poor memory. A constant environment and routine are quite helpful in improving orientation and the ability to function. Poor judgment and impulsiveness can be major safety hazards. Such behavior is brought to the attention of the physician. The family also will have to be aware of this if they are to care for the patient at home.

Rehabilitation phase. The greatest challenge for the nurse in care of the patient who has had a cerebrovascular accident comes after the patient is past the point of danger, for then he must face the long, slow process of learning to use whatever abilities that remain or can be relearned, and he must adjust to his limitations if he and his family are to be reasonably happy for the remainder of his life.

As a member of the rehabilitation team, the nurse must be capable of exercising initiative and judgment in making a nursing diagnosis and in planning and implementing care to meet rehabilitation goals. Three basic goals are (1) prevention of further impairment, (2) maintenance of existing abilities, and (3) restoration of as much function as possible. Knowledge of the physical arrangements of the setting where the patient will go after discharge should be a priority in planning and implementing care.

If there is ability to use the arm, there is reason to believe that the leg function will return sufficiently for the patient to walk. Return of motor impulses and subsequent return of function are evidenced by a tightening and spasticity of the affected part. This may appear from the second day to the second week after the cerebrovascular accident. Return of motor impulses is significant for the future use of the affected part, but presents new problems for the patient, nurse, and all others who may care for him. Muscles that draw the limbs toward the midline become very active, and the arm may be held tightly adducted against the body. The affected lower limb may be held inward and adducted to, or even beyond, the midline. Muscles that draw the limbs into flexion are also stimulated, with the result that the heel is lifted off the ground, the heel cord shortens, and the knee becomes bent. In the upper limb, flexor muscles draw the elbow into the bent position, the wrist is flexed, and fingers are curled in palmar flexion. This is often seen following a cerebrovascular accident because the adductor and flexor muscles are stronger than the opposing muscles.

Persistent nursing efforts must be directed toward prevention of further impairment and keeping any part of the body from remaining in a position of flexion long enough for the occurrence of muscle shortening and joint changes that might interfere with free joint action. If a physical therapist is not available, the total responsibility for preventive measures may rest with the nurse. *Every minute counts in prevention, and the nurse must not miss one opportunity to move the patient's adducted or flexed limbs back to the correct position. Passive exercise* stimulates circulation and may help to reestablish neuromuscular pathways. No difficulty is encountered with these procedures until tightening of the muscles begins to appear, then other physical measures are needed, and at this point, if not earlier, the patient's treatment should be under the direction of a physical therapist.

Active exercise of the affected side also may be started early. It is ordered by the physician and, in the hospital, may be directed by the physical therapist. Under the guidance of the physical therapist the nurse checks the exercises while the patient is in the hospital, and the nurse or the physical therapist may teach the exercises to the family in preparation for the patient's return home.

Since the patient will depend a good deal on his unaffected arm and leg when he begins to move about, the unaffected part of the body needs attention to prevent contractures and preserve muscle strength. Even while he is in bed, the patient should exercise his unaffected arm and use it in all normal positions. The unaffected leg should be in a position of slight *internal rotation* most of the time while the patient is in bed, and the knee should be bent several times each day. Exercise to strengthen the quadriceps muscle should be done because the quadriceps is the most important muscle in providing stability to the knee joint needed for walking (p. 373).

Early *ambulation* facilitates vasomotor tone and has positive psychologic effects on the patient and family members. Ambulation is started by the physical therapist by having the person walk between parallel bars. Transfer techniques are also taught to the patient and family members (p. 849).

When the patient begins to move about and to try to help himself, he may have several problems that can alter his ability to proceed. He may have loss of position sense, so that it is awkward for him to handle his body normally even when he has the muscular coordination to do so. He may have dizziness, spatial-perceptual deficits, diplopia, and alteration of skin sensation. He may also have to work harder than other persons to receive a normal amount of air on inhalation, since the involved side of the chest does not expand easily. This difficulty may lead to excessive fatigue unless those caring for the patient plan activities so that the patient's effort is not wasted.

Before standing or walking, the patient may practice raising himself up in bed and may sit on the side of the bed while holding firmly to an overbed table or to a strap with his good hand and pressing his feet on a chair or stool. The patient benefits from wearing shoes, since it is good for his morale and keeps his paralyzed foot in good position.

If preparation for walking has been adequate, the patient usually needs only one crutch when he begins to walk, and then he progresses to the use of a cane. When he first begins to walk, the nurse must remain close to him to allay his fear of falling. He may practice balancing himself by standing between parallel bars or by leaning on the backs of two chairs (provided the chairs are heavy enough to support weight safely). Good walking patterns must be established early because incorrect patterns are difficult and sometimes impossible to change. A sideward shuffle should be watched for and avoided. The patient should begin by leaning rather heavily on his crutch or cane and lifting his body sufficiently to bring the leg and foot forward so that the toes point straight ahead and not inward. The cane or single crutch is held in the hand opposite the paralyzed or weakened side of the body.

The patient is evaluated on ability to carry out his usual *activities of daily living* and is assisted by the occupational therapist or nurse in becoming independent in each activity to the extent possible. Rehabilitation in this way is essentially a teaching-learning process in which the patient is actively involved. Motivation is absolutely essential to rehabilitation. Most patients who have suffered a cerebral thrombosis are motivated and desire deeply to help themselves, even though some are so overcome with the enormity of their limitations that they are very quiet and are misunderstood by those around them. *If there is return of hand function in 2 to 3 weeks, fecal incontinence has disappeared, and no contractures, decubiti, or other complications have developed, there is reason to believe that the patient can learn to care for himself.*

The patient needs preparation for each new step in learning to move and care for himself. He must be shown each new activity as it will apply to him, and he then needs practice under supervision and recognition of each accomplishment. Careful and detailed instructions on how to hold and support himself will save him much embarrassment and confusion. By using his unaffected hand, he may, for example, straighten out the flexed fingers on the affected side and move his affected arm to a position where, with the weight of gravity, the elbow will be straightened. Most patients can relearn to do activities of daily living such as those pertaining to personal hygiene and dressing.

Long-range plans. General care and the pattern of living that should be followed after a cerebrovascular accident vary for each patient and are determined by his own circumstances, the amount of recovery he has, and the guidance he received in the early stages of his illness. Despite all effort he may, for example, never be able to negotiate stairs. The social worker and the community health nurse are indispensable in helping to arrange the patient's home so that the greatest possible degree of self-sufficiency and independence is possible. Members of the family often need help in assisting the person to accept limitations, both physical and emotional. The family must also make adjustments to actual circumstances. Almost all persons who have cerebrovascular accidents need health supervision for the rest of their lives. Whether the patient will be able to return to his own home or must go to a nursing home will depend a great deal on his family's understanding and acceptance of the patient and his limitations when maximum rehabilitation may have been achieved.

While it is not uncommon for cerebrovascular accidents to recur, the person may go for years with no further difficulty and eventually die of some other cause. The physician usually explains the prognosis to the person and to the family. The nurse should know what explanation has been given by the physician and must sometimes help in interpreting it to the family. Some persons must curtail activity to such a point that they have little enjoyment in living and still have recurrences, whereas others may be active and escape further cerebrovascular episodes for many years.

The person who has sustained a cerebrovascular accident and who has high blood pressure is usually advised to take his antihypertensive medications religiously and to get sufficient rest and to avoid strain and excitement. Persons involved in strenuous work may be advised to reduce their work schedule and take more frequent vacations. Those who are overweight are advised to bring their weight within normal limits, and those who smoke are advised of the hazards of vasoconstriction caused by nicotine in tobacco. Activities of daily living may be modified; sitting while shaving or doing other like activities helps conserve energy. When there is imminent danger of cerebral hemorrhage, activities that promote dilation of cerebral blood vessels such as vigorous exercises, hot or cold baths or showers, violent coughing or laughing, straining at defecation (Valsalva maneuver), and sexual activity are to be avoided. Occasionally retirement at an early age is necessary. Relocation in a warmer climate or in a more rural area is helpful to some people, provided they can afford it and it does not upset their relationships with significant others who are support figures.

Prior to discharge to the home or to another health care setting, certain outcomes should be achieved. The major emphasis is on maintaining structural and body integrity consistent with pathologic involvement. The parameters involved in achieving this are an intact skin, normal range of joint motion with no contractures, loss of muscle tone confined to that which is consistent with pathology, and maintenance of bladder and bowel function. When these outcomes are achieved at the highest degree possible, the person is ready for discharge. Obviously some persons' pathology will limit their ability to become completely sufficient in activities of daily living and some persons will benefit from long-term rehabilitation either by hospitalization in a rehabilitation hospital or through outpatient follow-up care on a regular basis.

Outcome criteria for the person with a cerebrovascular accident

1. The patient shall have made progress toward independence in activities of daily living consistent with neurologic deficits and can:
   a. Feed self independently with or without adaptive equipment.
   b. Bathe self independently with or without adaptive equipment.
   c. Groom self independently with or without adaptive equipment.
   d. Dress self independently with or without adaptive clothing or devices.
   e. Toilet self independently with or without adaptive equipment.
   f. Ambulate independently with or without adaptive equipment (cane, crutch, brace, walker).
   g. Transfer independently from one surface to another (bed to chair, toilet, car, and so on).
   h. Safely compensate for visual field/cuts, perceptual, motor, and sensory losses.
2. The patient or significant others can:
   a. Explain each prescribed therapy to be followed at home.
   b. Accurately demonstrate each exercise to physical therapist, occupational therapist, or nurse.
   c. Explain method, rationale, and daily schedule for each exercise.
   d. Explain schedule for return visits to evaluate progress.
   e. Relate need for daily, regular therapy.

3. The patient or significant others can explain long-term goals set mutually and with the rehabilitation team and can:
   a. State need to be independent in activities of daily living despite effort and time involved in doing so.
   b. Rationally explain present motor, sensory, proprioceptive, and perceptual status in relation to activities of daily living goals.
4. The patient and significant others are able to communicate with each other within pathologic limits and can:
   a. Demonstrate the ability to communicate utilizing verbal, written, and or gestural approaches.
   b. Explain the methods to be followed as recommended by the speech pathologist.
5. The patient or significant others know about professional and community resources necessary to achieve long-term goals and can:
   a. State how to contact agencies (vocational counselor, rehabilitation counselor, community health nurse).
   b. State how to secure equipment.
   c. State plans for follow-up care.

□ Cerebral aneurysm

A cerebral aneurysm is a weakening and outpouching of the wall of a cerebral artery and is usually secondary to a congenital weakness in the vessel wall. It is caused by an absence of the media or muscle layer of the vessel wall. As a result, the elastic layer develops a berrylike sac that becomes the aneurysm. The aneurysm usually forms where the vessel bifurcates. The most common sites are the internal carotid, the posterior communicating, the middle cerebral, and the vertebral and basilar arterial systems.[57] The internal carotid artery comes from the common carotid artery and branches to form the ophthalmic, the anterior, and the middle cerebral arteries. The posterior communicating artery comes from the posterior cerebral artery. The vertebral and basilar arteries come from the subclavian artery; each of these arteries sends communicating branches to the internal carotid branches (anterior and middle cerebral arteries) to form the circle of Willis at the base of the brain. Hemorrhage occurs when the aneurysm ruptures and the blood seeps into the subarachnoid spaces. This condition accounts for the sudden death of young people from "strokes" during strenuous exercise or excitement that causes the blood pressure to rise. The aneurysm commonly ruptures in persons between the ages of 20 and 40 years.

Clinical picture

Symptoms of a cerebral aneurysm include sudden explosive headache, photophobia, neck rigidity, nausea and vomiting, loss of consciousness, shock, convulsions, a full, bounding pulse, and noisy, labored respirations.

The following system of grading has been developed to classify the clinical state of the patient by level of consciousness and neurologic deficit.

Grade I Minimal bleeding, alert, no neurologic deficit

Grade II Mild bleeding, alert, minimal neurologic deficit such as third nerve palsy and stiff neck

Grade III Moderate bleeding, drowsy or confused, stiff neck with or without neurologic deficit

Grade IV Moderate or severe bleeding, semicoma with or without neurologic deficit

Grade V Severe bleeding, coma, decerebrate movement

Additional grades are also added for patients over 50 years of age and those with major heart, lung, kidney, and liver conditions that increase risk for procedures.[69]

Intervention

The immediate treatment for *subarachnoid hemorrhage* is to keep the person absolutely quiet to prevent additional bleeding. An antifibrinolytic agent (Amicar) may be used to seal the clot. The person should be very gently moved to bed, and sometimes it is not advisable to move him to a hospital. He is kept flat in bed in a darkened room and attended constantly to be sure that he does not raise his head. Blood pressure may be taken as often as every 15 minutes. This procedure is best accomplished and is less disturbing to the patient if the cuff is left (deflated) about the arm. If he is conscious, he is given small amounts of water by mouth, but the water must be given through a straw so that his head is not elevated. Intravenous fluids may be given by slow drip so that blood pressure is not increased, and often an indwelling catheter is inserted to avoid the exertion of voiding.

Bowel elimination is usually ignored for several days, and then oil-retention enemas or small doses of bulk laxatives may be given. Under no circumstances should the patient be permitted to strain, cough, sneeze, or otherwise exert himself because these activities increase intracranial pressure. Visitors must be carefully prepared so that they will not upset the patient, and no mail should be given to him unless it is certain that it contains no disturbing information. Hypothermia may be used to lessen the need of the brain for oxygen and thereby decrease the danger of damage to vital brain tissues (p. 384).

About 50% of patients with rupture of an aneurysm recover from the initial episode, but at least 50% of these persons will have recurrences of hemorrhage if untreated. Recurrence may occur within 2 weeks, and the danger of death increases with each recurrence. If the aneurysm is not obliterated by surgery, the patient may die eventually from recurrent hemorrhage.

If the aneurysm cannot be successfully treated, however, the family needs to be aware that there is always the danger of sudden death. The patient must be protected from strenuous activity and excitement.

Surgery. The only satisfactory treatment for congenital aneurysm is surgery. Before surgery can be performed, however, the location of the aneurysm must be determined by arteriography (angiography), as described on p. 653. The time after the acute rupture when arteriograms are taken and when surgery is performed varies with the person, his age, the intensity and kind of symptoms present, and the judgment of the surgeon. Since angiography may increase symptoms, it may be followed by immediate surgery. Lumbar puncture is also performed initially to verify the presence of blood in the cerebrospinal fluid.

Before surgical treatment of an aneurysm is attempted, the surgeon usually explains the hope for cure and the risks involved to the patient's family. The nurse must appreciate how distressing the situation is for the family and should realize that the time spent waiting to know whether the outcome will be favorable seems interminable to them. The nursing care the patient will receive postoperatively should be explained to them if they are to be with the patient. For example, it is important that both the patient and his family know that blood pressure, pulse rate, respiratory rate, and other pertinent observations will be taken frequently, since these procedures can be most upsetting if their purpose and the need to check them so frequently is not understood.

Surgery consists of a *craniotomy* and *location of the aneurysm*. When found, the aneurysm may be obliterated by ligation at its neck with the application of a silver clip. If the base of the aneurysm is too large for ligation to be practical, it may be coated with a liquid, adherent, plastic substance that hardens to form a firm support about the weakened vessel wall and thereby prevents rupture. If the aneurysm has not ruptured but has produced symptoms, attempts may be made to produce thrombosis within the aneurysm by use of an electric current and other means.[57] Both before and after surgery the nurse should observe for signs of increased intracranial pressure (p. 670). Common causes of increased intracranial pressure in aneurysm include the local pressure from the aneurysm and the presence of blood or hematoma from the ruptured aneurysm.

If the surgery is successful, the patient will be cured, although usually he will be advised to avoid strenuous exercise and emotional stress for the rest of his life. Occasionally he may have a severe physical or mental handicap resulting from damage to brain tissue during surgery.

Other procedures. Not all aneurysms can be treated surgically at the site of the lesion. If surgery is not feasible, in order to reduce the chances of hemorrhage the common carotid artery in the neck may be completely or partially obliterated to lessen the flow of blood to the site of the aneurysm, *provided* enough blood can be supplied from collateral vessels to preserve vital brain function. The procedure usually is done in stages of several days. A clamp (Silverstone or Salibi clamp) that has a detachable screw stem and can be tightened gradually is used.[57] Usually the surgeon adjusts it each day, and the nurse who attends the patient watches him closely and is instructed to release the clamp at once if there is evidence of inadequate blood supply. Neurologic checks are done regularly by the nurse relative to placement of the clamp in the dominant or nondominant hemisphere. Any signs of muscle weakness in the face or in either extremity on the side opposite the incision or any changes in the level of consciousness, vital signs, or sensory or muscular coordination or control should be reported to the neurosurgeon at once. Immediate removal of the clamps may prevent irreversible complications such as hemiplegia, aphasia, and loss of consciousness. If symptoms of inadequate blood supply appear, further surgical treatment cannot be done safely, although the clamp may be left indefinitely to partially obliterate the vessel. If complete occlusion can be tolerated, the vessel may be permanently ligated. Thrombus formation with resultant cerebral embolism may complicate the patient's postoperative course following any surgery for a cerebral aneurysm. It is a feared and often fatal complication.

□ Cerebral arteriosclerosis and multiple small thrombi

Cerebral arteriosclerosis may lead to deterioration of brain tissue, even though cerebrovascular accidents do not occur. This condition, which usually is associated with high blood pressure, may occur in people in their fifties, although it is usually considered a disease of old age.

Multiple small thrombi may occur in persons whose blood pressure is normal or even below normal if atheromatous changes have occurred in the lining of arteries. This condition causes frequent small and barely perceptible strokes. Both cerebral arteriosclerosis and multiple small strokes from thrombi may produce personality changes. The person who has arteriosclerosis is likely to have a more consistent downward course, whereas the one suffering from multiple small thrombi may have periods of apparently normal physical and mental response between episodes of confusion.

Both cerebral arteriosclerosis and multiple small thrombi cause slowly progressive changes that are particularly distressing to members of the person's family. Complete brain deterioration may occur. The person may feel irritable and unhappy with apparently little cause, and no amount of reassurance can make him feel better. The family must be prepared for gradual deterioration of the person's condition and should make provision for his safety and for the results of the poor judgment he may demonstrate; for example, he may forget to dress appropriately, may give away family possessions, and may enter into unwise business dealings. The family needs help in learning how to treat the patient as an adult and yet deal with his limitations. The physician, the social caseworker, and the nurse can help family members care for the patient in such a way that their own lives are not completely disrupted and yet that they are not plagued by guilt feelings when the patient dies. Institutional care is sometimes necessary, and the family needs encouragement and help in arriving at joint decisions that serve the best interests of all its members.

□ Atherosclerosis of carotid system

Atherosclerosis of the extracranial carotid system has been considered important in the etiology of some strokes. This atherosclerosis most commonly involves the common carotid artery at or distal to its bifurcation into the internal and external carotid arteries. Narrowing (stenosis) of the internal carotid artery reduces blood flow to the corresponding side of the brain and is thought by many to be the source of small particles of blood clot that dislodge from the area of stenosis and embolize to the smaller blood vessels of the brain to cause strokes. Complete occlusion of the internal carotid may occur from this process with or without stroke manifestations.

Carotid endarterectomy essentially involves the reaming out of these diseased vessels. Postoperative care of these patients should include close attention to neurologic signs (changes in strength, mentation, speech, and level of consciousness). (See p. 973 for a discussion of cardiovascular surgery.)

■ INFECTIONS

The nervous system may be attacked by a variety of organisms and viruses and may suffer from toxic reactions to bacterial and viral disease. Sometimes the infection becomes walled off and causes an abscess; sometimes the meninges, or coverings of the brain and spinal cord, are involved; and sometimes the brain itself is affected most. Organisms and viruses may reach the nervous system by a variety of routes. Untreated chronic otitis media and mastoiditis, chronic sinusitis, and fracture in any bone adjacent to the meninges may be the source of infection. Some organisms such as the tubercle bacillus and probably the pneumococcus reach the nervous system by means of the blood or the lymph system. The exact route by which some infective agents, such as the meningococcus in epidemic meningitis and the viruses that cause encephalitis, reach the central nervous system is not known.

Meningococcal meningitis (epidemic) and poliomyelitis are reportable communicable diseases. Because they are becoming less common and because they are discussed in specialized texts, they will be mentioned only briefly here.

□ Meningitis

Meningitis is an acute infection of the meninges usually caused by pneumococci, meningococci (epidemic), staphylococci, streptococci, or aseptic agents (usually viral). Any other pathogenic organism, such as the tubercle bacillus, that gains access to the subarachnoid spaces can cause meningitis. Mild forms of the disease do occur and may be referred to as *meningism.* They may be caused by viruses. A common form of the disease is lymphocytic meningitis, believed in many instances to be associated with a virus.

The incidence of bacterial meningitis is higher in fall and winter when upper respiratory infections are common. Children are more often affected than adults because of frequent colds and ear infections. Disease caused by the enteroviruses is more common in the summer and early fall than in other seasons of the year.

Clinical picture

Meningitis is a medical emergency. The onset (except when caused by tubercle bacilli) is usually sudden and characterized by severe headache, stiffness of the neck, irritability, malaise, and restlessness. Nausea, vomiting, delirium, and complete disorientation may develop quickly. Temperature, pulse rate, and respirations are increased. The diagnosis is usually confirmed by examination of spinal fluid obtained from a lumbar puncture. Usually the offending organism can be isolated from the spinal fluid, and if a pyogenic organism is the cause, the fluid is cloudy.

Intervention

Treatment consists of massive doses of the antibiotic specific for the causative organism. Culture and sensitivity studies determine the most effective antibiotic. The antibiotic may be given directly into the spinal canal (intrathecally) as well as by other routes.

Respiratory isolation is required until the pathogen can no longer be cultured from the nasopharynx. This is usually accomplished after 24 hours of effective antimicrobial therapy. Therapy is continued until the patient has been afebrile for 5 days or after 7 days of therapy (whichever is longer). The patient should be in a private room, and masks are worn for the 24-hour period described above. Discharges from nose, throat, and mouth are discarded in impervious plastic or paper bags, which are closed securely and placed in a second impervious bag before incinerated. Nursing care for the patient with meningitis includes the general care given a critically ill patient who may be irritable, confused, and unable to take fluids and yet who is dehydrated because of elevation of temperature. The room is kept darkened, noise is kept at a minimum, and care is taken not to jar the bed, since any increase in sensory stimulation can cause a seizure. The patient must be observed very carefully and must be constantly attended if he is disoriented. Padded side rails should be placed on the bed.

Residual damage from meningitis includes deafness, blindness, paralysis, and mental retardation. However, these complications are now rare because the infection is effectively treated with antibiotics before permanent damage to the nervous system occurs.

□ Encephalitis

Encephalitis is inflammation of the brain tissues and its coverings. Occasionally the meninges of the spinal cord are also involved. Encephalitis can have a variety of causes. A generalized inflammation of the brain can be caused by syphilis, and encephalitis can follow exogenous poisoning such as that which follows the ingestion of lead or arsenic or the inhalation of carbon monoxide. It can be caused by reaction to toxins produced by infections such as typhoid fever, measles, and chickenpox, and occasionally it follows vaccination.

Encephalitis caused by a virus and occurring in epidemic form was first described by von Economo in Austria, and the name von Economo disease is still used to identify the widespread epidemic in the United States that followed the influenza epidemic in 1918. This form of the disease has not recurred since 1926. Von Economo disease was also called encephalitis lethargica and sleeping sickness, a term still used by laymen. The demonstration that viruses can affect the central nervous system after a prolonged incubation period has resulted in considerable search for viral agents in many chronic neurologic diseases.

The death rate from encephalitis varies with epidemics but is generally fairly high. The most common and most serious sequela for patients who do recover from the acute disease is paralysis agitans, which may come on suddenly or develop slowly. Other residual neurologic symptoms may also occur and occasionally incapacitate the patient completely.

Acute viral encephalitis

Viral encephalitis appears to be caused by a number of viruses, some of which may be interrelated. Acute viral encephalitis can be classified as epidemic and sporadic forms. The primary causes of acute epidemic encephalitis are members of the *arbovirus* (those transferred by a biting arthropod to humans) or togavirus group (named after properties of the virus). There are

Table 36-2. Arbovirus infections of the central nervous system occurring in the Western Hemisphere*

Disease	Causal agent	Where found	Incubation period (days)	Clinical manifestation
California encephalitis	Arbovirus of California virus (mosquito-borne)	United States, Canada, Alaska, and Yukon	5 to 15	Aseptic meningitis, encephalitis
Eastern equine	Eastern equine encephalomyelitis virus (mosquito-borne)	Eastern seaboard and Gulf states, Caribbean	5 to 15	Severe encephalitis (usually infants and children)
Pawassan encephalitis	Pawassan virus (tick-borne)	Canada, Northeastern and North Central Central United States	4 to 8	Encephalitis
St. Louis encephalitis	St. Louis encephalitis virus (mosquito-borne)	Western and Central United States, Florida, Caribbean	4 to 21	Encephalitis, aseptic meningitis
Venezuelan equine encephalomyelitis	Venezuelan equine encephalomyelitis virus (mosquito-borne)	Texas, Florida, Mexico, Central and South America	2 to 5	Fever, headache, myalgia, malaise, cough, encephalitis
Western equine encephalomyelitis	Western equine encephalomyelitis virus	Western United States and Canada, Central and South America	5 to 10	Encephalitis (infants), fever, aseptic meningitis

*Adapted from Report of the Committee on Infectious Diseases, American Academy of Pediatrics, 1974.

about 80 viruses of the arbovirus group that cause disease in humans. Six of the viruses cause infections of the central nervous system (Table 36-2).

Clinical picture. Clinical features of *acute epidemic encephalitis*, caused by the arboviruses that infect humans, are similar. The eastern equine form is more severe than the western form. The onset is abrupt, with a *high fever, headache, meningeal signs, nuchal rigidity, and vomiting. Drowsiness or coma and focal or generalized convulsions develop within 24 to 48 hours after onset.* Focal neurologic signs develop, such as hemiplegia and cranial nerve palsies. There are typical findings in the cerebrospinal fluid. Fatality rates may be as high as 60%. Those who survive usually have no sequelae.[3]

Intervention. Nursing care consists mainly of symptomatic or supportive care and careful observation. Any change in appearance or behavior must be reported at once, since the progress of this disease sometimes is extremely rapid. The patient is kept in bed, and side rails are used if disorientation develops. The patient must be constantly attended to prevent injury. During the period when the temperature is high, sponging or other hypothermia measures may be ordered. Frequent changes of linen may be necessary if perspiration is excessive. There is no specific medical treatment for this disease. No isolation is necessary, since encephalitis is not transmitted from person to person. Prevention of arboviral infections consists of eradication of the mosquito or tick vector, including destruction of larvae and elimination of breeding places. Control is by avoiding bites of the mosquito or tick vectors.

Acute encephalitis (nonepidemic)

Acute encephalitis occurs sporadically and is caused by the herpes simplex virus (HSV). It occurs at any age, but over half of the cases are in persons at least 15 years of age. Upper respiratory complaints often precede the onset of neurologic symptoms by at least 24 hours or longer. Headache and focal or major convulsions are the common early signs of cerebral involvement. A persistent high fever and coma are common. Spinal fluid proteins may be moderately elevated, and red blood cells are often present when spinal fluid is examined. Herpetic skin lesions are not common. Treatment is supportive with anticonvulsant drugs and steroids to reduce cerebral edema.[35]

□ Poliomyelitis

Poliomyelitis is an acute febrile disease caused by poliovirus types 1, 2, and 3; paralysis is more common with type 1. With discovery of the Salk vaccine, its wide use since 1956, and the availability of a safe "live virus" vaccine (Sabin vaccine), this disease, which had been a serious crippler of children and young adults, has become quite rare. In 1976 there were only 14 cases reported in the United States.[11]

The incubation period for poliomyelitis is from 7 to 21 days. The virus attacks the anterior horn cells of the spinal cord where the motor pathways are located and may cause motor paralysis. Sensory perception is not affected since posterior horn cells are not attacked. Poliomyelitis sometimes takes a somewhat different form and attacks primarily the medulla and basal structures of the brain, including the cranial nerves; the term *bulbar* poliomyelitis is used for this form.

An important responsibility of the nurse is to help prevent poliomyelitis by encouraging immunization. In the United States there is a concerted effort to have all children immunized, since the number of immunizations have decreased in recent years.

□ Guillain-Barré-Strohl syndrome (polyneuritis)

This disease, known variously as acute inflammatory polyradiculoneuropathy, postinfectious polyneuritis, and Guillain-Barré-Strohl syndrome, is often serious because of the extent to which the nervous system may be affected. This condition has become better known to the public since it was identified as a sequela of swine flu immunization. There is patchy demyelination found in nerve roots, root ganglia, and spinal and peripheral nerves. It may be classified for this reason as a neuritis. Axons are generally spared to that recovery may occur early; in severe forms, *wallerian degeneration* (p. 726) occurs with involvement of the axons, making recovery slow. In the severe forms there is an elevation of the protein in the cerebrospinal fluid. It is probably caused by a virus. The disease is most common in persons 30 to 50 years of age and is seen equally in men and women. If the seventh, ninth, and tenth cranial nerves are involved, the patient may have varying degrees of difficulty in swallowing, speaking, and breathing. The vital centers in the medulla oblongata may be affected, and the patient may die of respiratory failure. Patients with less severe involvement may recover fully, although a year or more may transpire before the patient is completely well.

Clinical picture

There is *rapid* occurrence of symmetrical muscle weakness of lower motor paralysis characteristics (flaccidity). The paralysis often starts in the lower extremities, but it may ascend upward to include the thorax, upper extremities, and face. Selected cranial nerves may also be affected, as previously mentioned. Other symptoms that may be assessed clinically are paresthesias and sensory alteration as the sensory roots and nerves also become involved. Respiratory failure may occur as intercostal muscles are affected, and without mechanical ventilation there is a 10% to 20% mortality rate.[4]

Intervention

A priority goal for nurse and patient is the maintenance of respiratory function. Close observation of respiratory function is necessary. Urinary retention occurs in about 5% of patients. Patients who develop respiratory failure require mechanical ventilation and are usually placed in an intensive care unit. Nursing care of patients with respiratory failure is discussed on p. 1134. Adrenocortical steroids are used empirically to treat symptoms. Convalescence may require several months.

□ Neurosyphilis

In the late or chronic stage of syphilis, infection may involve the brain and spinal cord. Neurosyphilis is becoming less common with improved treatment of syphilis as a communicable disease. The oculomotor nerves may be involved, causing inability of the pupil to react to light (Argyll Robertson pupil). *Tabes dorsalis* is the name given to the involvement of the posterior columns of the spinal cord and the posterior nerve roots. Since the sensory nerves are primarily involved, sensory symptoms predominate. The patient may have severe paroxysmal pain anywhere in the body, although perhaps the most common location is in the stomach. This condition, known as *gastric crisis*, may be confused with ruptured peptic ulcer or other acute conditions of the stomach or gallbladder. There may be areas of severe paresthesia. A common finding in tabes dorsalis is loss of position sense in the feet and legs. The patient is unable to sense where he places his feet, and as a result there is a slapping gait that is highly characteristic of the disease. There is increased difficulty walking in the dark because the person relies on vision in placing his feet. Visual loss or even total blindness also occurs. Tabes dorsalis can cause trophic changes in the limbs and changes in the joints so that stability is lost (Charcot's joint).

General paresis is the term used to designate another late manifestation of syphilis in which there is degeneration of the brain with deterioration of mental function and varying evidences of other neurologic disease. More specific information can be found in neurology texts.

□ Outcome criteria for the person with an infection of the nervous system

The patient or significant others can:

1. Explain the nature of the infection, infectious agent, and method of transmission.
2. Explain any neurologic deficits resulting from the infection.
3. Explain how to prevent further infection.
4. State plans for follow-up care.

■ TRAUMATIC LESIONS

Part of the nervous system commonly subjected to trauma include the crainocerebrum, spinal cord, and the peripheral nerves. With the exception of the peripheral nerves, each is protected by a bony covering. The phrase *traumatic lesions*, as used here, includes lesions resulting from direct physical force and injuries that result from sustained compression. Attention is directed primarily to the former in the following discussion.

□ Craniocerebral trauma

Craniocerebral trauma, or head injury, causes death and serious disability in people of all ages. In the United States, head injuries result in about 77,000 deaths yearly. Primary traumatic lesions result from industrial, motor vehicle, and military accidents. Head injury is the second most common cause of major neurologic deficits, and the major cause of death between ages 1 and 35.[4] It is estimated that 70% of motor accidents result in head injury. Brain injury causes more deaths than does injury to any other organ.

Craniocerebral trauma may result in injury to the scalp, skull, and brain tissues, either singly or collectively. Some of the variables that may modify the extent of the injury to the head include the location and direction of the impact, rate of the energy transfer, the surface area of energy transfer, and the status of the head at the time of the impact. Injuries vary from minor scalp wounds to concussions and open fractures of the skull with severe damage to the brain. The amount of obvious damage is not indicative of the seriousness of the trouble.

Contusions, abrasions, and lacerations of the scalp may occur. Lacerations of the scalp bleed profusely because of its large blood supply. A patient may bleed to death quickly if the external bleeding is not controlled. Most bleeding, however, is minor and controlled readily. An internal hematoma of the scalp may form and resemble a depressed fracture. Infection of the scalp may result from the presence of foreign debris. It should be stressed that the absence of external scalp injury does not preclude serious craniocerebral damage.

The skull indents and deforms when a physical impact occurs. Fractures commonly result, and they are classified as in other parts of the body (p. 903). Skull x-ray films may detect the fractures; a negative x-ray film does not exclude the presence of a fracture such as a hairline fracture. Fractures can occur distal to the point of impact. A compound and depressed fracture causes serious complications. *The presence of a skull fracture does not necessarily indicate that brain injury has occurred.* There is often a reverse correlation between skull damage and brain damage. Complications of skull damage may include injury to cranial nerves, epidural hemorrhage, and brain contusion.

Types of lesions

Damage to the brain tissues per se may include concussion, contusion, or laceration. Each is discussed briefly to differentiate them as to degree of damage and significance. The dura may remain intact in brain damage and is thought of as a *closed injury*, or the dura may be opened from a direct blow or from penetrating objects such as bone fragments or knives and is then classified as an open injury. A *concussion* is characterized by immediate and transitory impairment of neurologic function caused by the mechanical force. There is no demonstrable structural alteration. There may be loss of consciousness that is instant or delayed and is usually recovered. The effect of a blow on the cranium to the soft brain tissues contained within the closed cavity is one of sudden and continuing movement. This effect can be likened to what happens as one stops suddenly when moving quickly with an open dish of fluid—some of the fluid spills. The only difference is that instead of spilling in the closed cavity, the brain tissues strike the bony coverings forcibly. The sustained damage is variable in degree. There is damage to the brainstem centers and cerebral hemispheres. There can be loss of consciousness, the cause of which is not clearly understood. Any person exhibiting an alteration in consciousness following a blow on the head should be under constant observation for a period of time, since damage is not always immediately apparent.

A *contusion* is a structural alteration characterized by extravasation of blood cells. It can be likened to bruising without tearing of the tissues. The contusion may be at the site of the impact or on the opposite side. A concussion or contusion site may be classified as a *coup* (at the site), *contrecoup* (opposite the site), or *intermediate*. Contusions often damage the cortex. *Laceration* of the brain tissues and blood vessels is a tearing of the tissues that may be caused by a sharp fragment or object or a shearing force. It is obvious that hemorrhage may be a serious complication.

In summary, when the head receives a direct blow or injury, the brain moves in the skull and suffers varying degrees of damage. In addition, the brain swells to a great extent. It is unfortunate that the capacity of the brain to swell far exceeds the capacity of the closed cranial cavity to expand. Most deaths from head injury are from the brain swelling rather than from the actual primary destruction of vital centers. Brain edema is thus a major cause of increased intracranial pressure and its consequences as previously discussed on p. 670). Local and systemic disturbances in circulation occur with resulting anoxia. The brain damage may be minor or severe. There is often a great disparity between functional neurologic derangement and structural damage that can be demonstrated.

Assessment of head injury

Most patients with head injuries will be examined in the emergency department where beginning treatment is instituted. The airway is assessed first, and if necessary, an endotracheal tube will be inserted. A careful neurologic examination is done. The patient's responsiveness is determined and is described in terms of his behavior.[5] Pupils are checked for inequality. If a unilaterally enlarged pupil is present, this is indication for immediate surgery. Blood is drawn for baseline tests.

Since many persons with head injury have sustained other injuries, especially those involved in automobile accidents, the intrathoracic and intraabdominal areas are checked carefully and the limbs are examined for fractures or injury to nerves or arteries.

Diagnostic procedures are performed as necessary and most commonly include skull roentgenograms and cerebral angiography. Cerebral angiography requires 30 to 60 minutes to complete, and if the patient's condition is deteriorating, this luxury of time cannot be afforded.[5] When a hematoma is suspected, a trephine of the skull (burr holes) is performed, and the dura at the frontal, posterior, and temporal locations is opened bilaterally.

While the patient's emergency needs are being met, a history is obtained from family members or other witnesses. Details are collected about the accident and especially about the duration of unconsciousness, since this is a rough index of the severity of the injury.[4] If the patient regained consciousness and then slipped out of contact, it is presumed on this fact alone that an expanding intracranial hematoma is present.

Neurologic examination is repeated at frequent intervals to determine changes in consciousness, respiration, pupils, motor strength, speech, and vision. Changes in any of these may indicate an expanding intracranial mass. Vital signs are also checked frequently, and intracranial pressure may be monitored continuously by a ventricular catheter.

Lumbar puncture is usually not performed in the presence of head injury because the sudden withdrawal of fluid can precipitate transtentorial or foramen magnum herniation when there is cerebral edema or an intracranial clot.

Hemorrhage resulting from craniocerebral trauma may occur at the following sites: scalp, epidural, subdural, subarachnoid, intracerebral, and intraventricular. Epidural and subdural hematomas are discussed because of the need for careful and continuing observations by the nurse. An *epidural hematoma* forms as blood collects between the dura and the skull. Since bleeding in this area is commonly caused by laceration of the middle meningeal artery, it is capable of producing rapid clot formation. *If lethargy or unconsciousness develops after regaining consciousness,* an epidural hematoma may be suspected. Bleeding needs to be controlled promptly and the blood evacuated. Common sites for bleeding include basal and temporal skull fractures. The nurse should be alert for potential epidural hematomas when it is known that fractures exist in these sites. A *subdural hematoma* forms as venous blood collects below the dural surface. Since the bleeding is under venous pressure, the hematoma formation is relatively slow. However, the clot formation will cause pressure on the brain surface and may eventually displace brain tissue. If this expanding clot is not evacuated, it can contribute to a rise in intracranial pressure and its sequelae. Thus a subdural hematoma can become serious because of its location and compression of vital areas. If a patient who has been conscious for several weeks or months after a head injury becomes unconscious and develops neurologic symptoms, a subdural hematoma should be suspected. *Nurses need to be aware of the delayed signs of head injury as well as the immediate and more obvious ones. The focal neurologic signs from clot formation can be related to the site of the clot.*

Fractures of the *base of the skull* are usually serious because of their site. When one is sustained, *vital centers, cranial nerves, and nerve pathways may be permanently damaged.* Trauma and the resulting edema may obstruct cerebrospinal fluid flow directly or indirectly with resultant increased intracranial pressure. If the injury has caused a direct communication between the cranial cavity and the middle ear or the sinuses, meningitis or a brain abscess may develop. Bleeding from the nose and the ears is suggestive of a basal fracture. Serosanguineous drainage from these orifices may contain cerebrospinal fluid and should be noted.

Intervention. The saving of life and preservation of neurologic function is dependent on understanding the pathophysiology involved. The ability of the nurse to follow the prescribed therapy and to make nursing decisions based on this understanding is essential. The immediate care is directed toward lifesaving measures and the maintenance of normal body functions until the time when recovery is assured. With appropriate continuing care and rehabilitation, even the severely injured may regain consciousness, recover to some extent, and return to an active life.

The patient who has a skull fracture or other serious head injury must be attended constantly. The major aims of medical and nursing management are (1) to be constantly alert for changes in the patient's condition, especially changes that indicate any increase in intracranial pressure; (2) to sustain the patient's vital function until he has recovered sufficiently to resume them on his own; and (3) to minimize complications that will be life threatening or interfere with full recovery. (See p. 670 for a discussion of the components of increased intracranial pressure.)

Many neurosurgeons feel that alert and intelligent nursing care is often the decisive factor in determining the outcome of the patient. Side rails should always be on the bed, and a padded tongue blade or an airway to protect the tongue should be kept at the bedside, since restlessness may come on suddenly and convulsions may occur. Usually the bed is kept flat, although some neurosurgeons believe that the danger of edema to the brain may be reduced by slight elevation of the head of the bed.[51]

Rest and control of convulsions. The patient should be kept absolutely quiet. No vigorous effort should be made to "clean the patient up" during the first few hours after an accident. Rest and constant observation are much more important. Sudden noises, flashes of light, and the clatter of equipment can increase the patient's restlessness and should be avoided. Portable equipment may be used to take roentgenograms. The nurse must remain in the room with the patient to help him move and to protect him from exertion. Restlessness may be caused by the need for a slight change of position, the relaxation of a limb, or the need to empty the bladder. If nursing measures fail to allay extreme restlessness, the physician may order sodium amytal intramuscularly or paraldehyde. Morphine is not given to relieve pain because it will depress the patient's responsiveness and cause pupillary constriction, thus interfering with the necessary observation of pupillary change. Codeine or other mild analgesics may be necessary, however.

Twitching or convulsive movement of a body part is recorded in detail and reported at once. In some medical centers, anticonvulsants are given prophylactically when seizures are anticipated; they are always given once seizures occur.

Vital signs and temperature control. Usually the blood pressure, pulse, and respiratory rate are taken and recorded every 15 minutes until they become stabilized and remain within safe limits. Leaving the deflated blood pressure cuff on the arm helps to prevent disturbing the patient unduly when the pressure must be taken often. Developing the habit of not forcing the mercury column much above the expected reading also sometimes enables the nurse to take the blood pressure and yet barely disturb the patient. The eyes are observed for inequality of the pupils and the lips and fingernails for cyanosis. A sudden sharp rise in temperature, which may go to 42 C (106 F) or higher, and a sudden drop in blood pressure indicate that the regulatory mechanisms have lost control and the prognosis is poor. When there is elevation in temperature, measures will need to be instituted to reduce the temperature to normal. Although hypothermia has been used in the treatment of patients with severe brain contusions, it is being used less often because of some of the undesirable side effects. Instead, the nursing measures usually employed to reduce temperature such as the administration of aspirin, tepid sponges, ice bags to the groin and axillae, and reduction of the temperature in the patient's room are used. Electrically controlled cooling mattresses are also frequently used.

Respiratory insufficiency. One of the most common complications of severe head injury is respiratory insufficiency. Cerebral anoxia, which is a sequela of respiratory insufficiency, is a leading cause of death in these patients.[64] The patient who has respiratory insufficiency may have hypoxia, hypercarbia, hypotension, and dyspnea. Most generally these patients will have a tracheostomy performed and will receive respiratory assistance with one of the mechanical respirators (p. 955). Arterial blood gas levels and pH are checked frequently to determine whether respiratory exchange is adequate. The patient will have to be suctioned as necessary to maintain a patent airway. (See p. 947 for further nursing care of the patient with a tracheostomy.)

Drainage from ears and nose. The patient's ears and nose are observed carefully for signs of blood and for serous drainage, which may indicate that the meninges have been torn (common in basal skull fractures) and that spinal fluid is escaping. No attempt should be made to clean out these orifices. Loose sterile cotton may be placed in the outer openings only. This procedure must be done with caution so that the cotton does not in any way act as a plug to interfere with free flow of fluid. The cotton should be changed as soon as it becomes moistened. Usually the flow of fluid subsides spontaneously. Antibiotics usually are given when a basal fracture has been sustained. Suction is never used to remove nasal secretions in any patient who has a head injury or who has undergone brain surgery because of the danger of causing further damage. *Meningitis is a possible complication when communication with the nose and ears occurs.* If there is evidence of drainage of spinal fluid from the nose, the patient should not cough, sneeze, or blow his nose. These activities may, in addition to contributing to the development of meningitis, enable air to enter the cranial cavity, where it may increase symptoms of intracranial pressure. Sometimes it is difficult to determine whether drainage from the nose is mucus or cerebrospinal fluid. A Tes-Tape will give a positive sugar reaction to spinal fluid and a negative reaction to mucus.[5]

Control of cerebral edema. Cerebral edema and increased intracranial pressure are common problems in patients with head injuries. Osmotic diuretics that penetrate the brain slowly, such as 30% solution of urea in 10% invert sugar or 20% mannitol, may be given intravenously for several days.[4] When the patient's condition is deteriorating because of cerebral edema, dexamethasone is usually administered intravenously. The usual dose is 10 mg initially, followed by 4 mg intramuscularly every 6 hours thereafter. The steroids are also useful in combating shock associated with head injury. Usually they are employed only during the acute phase because of their associated side effects (p. 850).

Electrolyte balance. Careful monitoring of electrolytes is necessary. Several types of sodium imbalance are known to occur in head injury. *Natriuresis*, or increased urinary excretion of sodium, is common. More recently this has been attributed to the inappropriate ADH syndrome (with an increased plasma level of ADH, serum hyponatremia, and hypotonicity). This aggravates cerebral edema. Hypernatremia, or cerebral sodium retention, may also occur. No specific variations in potassium or chlorides have been noted. Plasma cortisol levels are also elevated in acute head injury. Plasma, BUN, pH, electrolytes, and urinary electrolyte levels are checked frequently.

Elimination. The patient's intake and output should be carefully measured and recorded. The specific gravity of the urine is also measured and recorded. These measures may be performed hourly when the patient's condition is acute.

Fluid intake may be restricted to 1,500 to 2,500 ml daily, and it is the nurse's responsibility to see that this is spread over the 24-hour period. Fluids may be given parenterally, by nasogastric tube, or by mouth, depending on the condition of the patient. The nurse must use caution in administering fluids orally, since the patient may have difficulty with vomiting and aspiration. The urinary output should be approximately 0.6 to 1 ml/kg of body weight per hour. This means that a person weighing 175 lb (79 kg) should eliminate between 45 and 80 ml/hour, and if osmotic diuretics have been given, this amount may be greater. If necessary, an indwelling catheter will be inserted. The presence of an indwelling catheter increases the risk of urinary tract infection, and efforts are taken to prevent this from occurring (p. 1260).

Bowel function is not encouraged for several days following a head injury. Mild bulk laxatives, bisacodyl (Dulcolax) suppositories, and oil-retention enemas may be prescribed. The patient is cautioned repeatedly not to strain in an effort to defecate, since straining increases intracranial pressure. When the patient is receiving steroids, it is important to check stool guaiac frequently to determine the presence of occult blood. Some patients develop diarrhea secondary to antibiotic therapy.

Complications of head injury

Patients with severe head injuries are candidates for several complications, some of which will be discussed in this section. As with any other patient who is seriously ill, the patient may develop atelectasis, pneumonia, or a urinary tract infection (secondary to an indwelling catheter). These infections are treated with a suitable antibiotic. *Stress ulcers* of the stomach and duodenum are also common after a head injury and are apparently caused by autonomic imbalances associated with the injury.

Prolonged unconsciousness. General nursing care as described in Chapter 27 is necessary for the patient with a head injury who remains unconscious for some time. Patients may be unconscious for as long as a month or more and yet finally make a satisfactory recovery, provided good supportive care has been given.

Extradural hematoma. Because of the danger of extradural hematoma, as discussed previously, many physicians believe that any patient who has sustained any injury to the head with loss of consciousness should be hospitalized for at least 24 hours. If he is asleep during this time, he should be awakened hourly to determine his state of consciousness. Some physicians believe that fluids should be restricted to 1,000 to 1,500 ml for the first day or two and that an osmotic diuretic should be given. If the patient does remain at home, the family should be told to watch him closely for signs of increased intracranial pressure, to awaken him hourly during the night after injury, and to bring him to a hospital at once if drowsiness, stupor, paralysis, convulsions, or inequality of the pupil size occur. The surgical treatment for extradural hematoma consists of making a burr hole through the temporal bone to relieve the pressure caused by the bleeding and to attempt to control the bleeding; sometimes a craniotomy, removal of a large bony window, is performed. Occasionally the patient has so much damage to the soft tissue of the brain that he dies despite relief of pressure caused by the bleeding. Usually such a patient is unconscious after the accident and is taken to a hospital at once.

Convalescence. The length of convalescence will depend entirely on how much damage has been done and how rapid recovery has been. Patients are usually urged to resume normal activity as soon as possible. Headache and occasional dizziness may be present for some time following a head injury. These difficulties should disappear within 3 to 4 months. Loss of memory and loss of initiative may also persist for a time. Occasionally convulsions develop because of the formation of scar tissue in injured brain substance or in its coverings. Such scar tissue may often be surgically removed to effect the complete cure. Loss of hearing and strabismus (cross-eye) sometimes complicate basal skull fractures and require a long period of rehabilitation. Sometimes corrective surgery can be performed for the strabismus.

Some persons require intensive rehabilitation in a rehabilitation center. Recovery from head injury is most likely in those under age 20. Persons between the ages of 20 and 50 who remain in a coma longer than 2 weeks rarely recover.[4]

□ Spinal cord trauma

Spinal cord injury (SCI) from accidents is a frequent and increasing cause of serious disability and death in the United States. It has been estimated that there are more than 100,000 individuals with serious spinal cord injury in the United States today and approximately 6,000 to 8,000 new cases occur annually.[38]

Violent accidents are occurring more frequently, and the patients are living longer. Automobile, diving, and other athletic accidents are the major causes in civilian life, and war injuries are a major cause among military personnel.

Neuroanatomy

There are important variations in the neuroanatomy of the vertebral column at the cervical, thoracic, and lumbar areas as well as important segmental variations in the spinal cord itself. In the cervical area the vertebrae are unstable (to permit movement of the neck), and the cord at this level houses the most important neural structures in a copious dural tube. The anterior horn cells innervating the diaphragm (above C4) and the upper extremities are located in the cervical cord segments as well as the long motor tracts to the remainder of the body. In the thoracic area, by contrast, there is a stable bony column supported by the rib structures. The thoracic spinal cord fills the subarachnoid space almost completely, and injuries in this area produce bony malalignments and are often associated with serious neurologic deficits. Finally, in the lumbar area the vertebrae are heavier and are supported by massive lumbar paraspinal muscles. The lumbar vertebrae thus have more stability than the cervical vertebrae but less than the thoracic vertebrae. The lumbar spine is more apt to be injured at the junction between the thoracic and lumbar area. The cauda equina, rather than the spinal cord, is housed below L1. The tip of the spinal cord, or the conus, houses the micturition center.

Types of lesions

The spinal cord may be damaged by lesions arising outside the cord or by intramedullary lesions. The latter is a less common cause and is usually the result of intramedullary tumors (p. 732). Variable types of lesions arising *outside* the cord eventually cause damage within it. (The word "lesion" as used here is inclusive of both disease and injury.) For example, there may be direct extension of an extramedullary vertebral tumor to the cord, the protrusion of a ruptured intervertebral disc into the spinal canal (p. 882), or a fracture of the spine

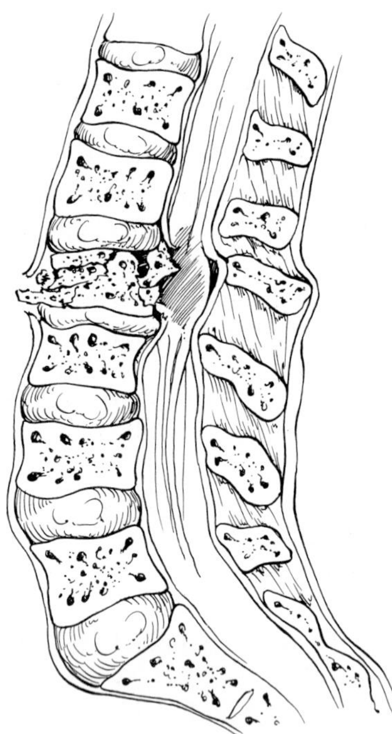

Fig. 36-1. Damage to spinal cord and distortion of adjacent structures that may occur in traumatic injuries to spine.

Table 36-3. Muscle function after spinal cord injury

Spinal cord injury	Muscle function remaining	Muscle function lost
Cervical		
Above C4	None	All, including respiration
C5	Neck Scapular elevation	Arms Chest All below chest
C6-C7	Neck Some chest movement Some arm movement	Some arm, fingers Some chest All below chest
Thoracic	Neck Arms (full) Some chest	Trunk All below chest
Lumbosacral	Neck Arms Chest Trunk	Legs

from direct trauma with resultant tearing of the spinal cord. (Fig. 36-1). All such lesions may produce compression of the cord. The anatomy and size of the spinal cord subjects the cord to compression with even minimal inward encroachment by extramedullary lesions. Edema then forms and contributes even more to cord compression. With damage to any part of the vertebral column, the cord itself becomes more vulnerable to damage. Recognition of the function of the spinal cord as the only conducting system of nerve impulses to and from the brain makes one realize the seriousness of spinal cord damage from any cause.

Severe traumatic lesions of the spinal cord, as from accident, may result in total *transection* of the spinal cord or a tearing of the cord from side to side at a particular level. This represents the most serious damage to the cord, with a complete loss of spinal cord functions. A partial transection or *cross section* is serious and disabling. Because of the suddenness of a transection and the extensiveness of the tear, this results in a state known as *spinal* or *neural* shock. It is transitory and refers more to the areflexic state of the body than to cardiogenic shock. Following the injury, afferent impulses are unable to ascend from below the injured site to the brain, and efferent impulses are unable to descend to points below the site. Because transection represents an acute form of spinal cord damage, it is used as an example to relate and discuss the symptoms of spinal cord damage. *There is considerable variability in the extent to which signs and symptoms are manifest in the individual patient.*

Clinical picture

The signs and symptoms of cord transection and of lesser cord lesions depend on the level at which the lesion occurs and the degree of the damage (Table 36-3). In the *immediate stage* of a *transection* there is a complete loss or deficit of motor and sensory functions as well as somatic and visceral sensations below the level of the tear (areflexia). The individual has flaccid paralysis, areflexia, and hypotonia caused by the disruption of nerve impulses as related to the injured level. Within hours, days, or weeks the involved muscles gradually become spastic and *hyperreflexic* with the characteristic signs of an upper motor neuron lesion. These changes are thought to represent the release of the muscle stretch reflexes from the inhibitory influence of the damaged pyramidal tract, resulting in hyperactive responses. Another theory is that damage of the extrapyramidal descending fibers, in close proximity to the pyramidal fibers, permits unmodified excitatory impulses to reach the lower motor neurons via the muscle spindles. There is thus an increased sensitivity of the lower motor neurons to afferent stimulation from the muscle spindles. Nurses need to be able to explain spinal shock to patients and their families so that involuntary movements are not confused with voluntary movements.

Damage at the cervical cord level is the most critical level for an injury to occur. It causes paralysis of all four extremities and the trunk *(quadriplegia).* The sparing of any one muscle movement of the shoulder, arms, and fingers is dependent on the specific cervical level of the injury. At the C5 level, for example, there would remain scapular elevation movements only. All other muscle movements in the arms, chest, trunk, and legs are lost. In the immediate stage, muscles of internal organs such as the bladder and bowel are atonic. Perspiration is diminished, as is touch sensation. Since the diaphragm and intercostal muscles are affected, respiratory failure and death may result unless the patient receives adequate respiratory assistance. A pulmotor is sometimes necessary during transportation of the patient to the hospital where equipment to aid respiration is available. Pain is not usually an early problem.

At the thoracic level, injury results in chest, trunk, bowel, bladder, and lower extremity muscle losses. The amount of remaining function varies in this area relative to the specific level. Fortunately the individual has use of his upper extremities; the lower extremities are not functional *(paraplegia).*

Injury at the lumbar and sacral levels results in paralysis of the lower extremities. The center for micturition is located in the conus medullaris (S2 to S4) and is linked to the detrusor muscle of the bladder by parasympathetic sensory and motor fibers that run in the pelvic nerves; together they form the reflex arc. Sympathetic motor fibers (T11 and L2) control the trigone of the bladder. Somatic lower motor neuron fibers travel through the pudendal nerves to the external urethral sphincter and external anal sphincter and the perineal muscles. Impulses descend via the pyramidal system and synapse with the anterior horn cells at the sacral level and thus provide central control over micturition. *Lesions above the conus result in a bladder that is capable of emptying itself reflexly or involuntarily after the spinal shock phase. The bladder is hypertonic, and it is variously know as an "upper motor neuron bladder" and "automatic bladder."* The emptying occurs spontaneously or automatically. The patient has no control over the act of micturition. Voiding may occur at intervals of 3 to 4 hours; there may be frequency, urgency, and incontinence. The reflex arc of micturition is intact in this type of bladder. *When the cord lesion is at, or below, the micturition center, there is destruction of the center or the sacral nerve roots; the reflex arc is no longer intact. This type of bladder is known as a "lower motor neuron bladder" or an "autonomous bladder."* Any contractions of the bladder muscle are the result of impulses transmitted through an intrinsic nervous mechanism that is within the bladder wall. The contractions, however, are not of sufficient strength or duration to empty the bladder. This can be done only by abdominal straining or by manual compression. Since the bladder musculature is hypotonic or flaccid, retention of urine and infection are common complications.

When injury occurs in the lower sacral area and the cauda equina nerve roots, away from the cord, the signs are variable and less severe. Often there is paraparesis and scattered lower motor neuron signs.

In the past 5 years, nursing literature has placed increased emphasis on the problems and care of the paraplegic and quadraplegic with decreased sexual functioning.[12,22,24,67] In most instances men experience impotence, decreased sensation, or difficulties with ejaculation. Impairment of fertility is common. Little research evidence is available regarding sexual function in SCI women; however, the interferences with perception of sexual pleasure are likely to be troublesome to the female patient as well as the male. Some suggestions for assisting the spinal cord injury patient to adjust to changes in sexual function are discussed later in this chapter (p. 725).

Diagnosis of spinal cord injury or compression from accidents

Diagnosis is made from the history of the trauma, neurologic examination, and selected studies. It is most important to first detect if there has been any cervical vertebra fracture or displacement and concomitant spinal cord damage. Roentgenograms are always taken to detect fracture dislocations of the vertebrae or their parts. Roentgenograms are often taken while the injured patient is still on the stretcher in the emergency room. This lessens movement of the spinal column at a critical period. Myelograms or lumbar puncture may be done to detect subarachnoid blockage. Myelography can be carried out with ease and without moving the patient when contrast material is introduced through a lateral puncture at the junction between the first cervical vertebra and the base of the skull. In this way the contrast material flows downward across the site of a cervical fracture dislocation to demonstrate the presence or absence of subarachnoid block. Further diagnostic measures are often delayed until there has been correction of any cervical fractures as established by roentgenograms. The thoracic and lumbar spine areas rarely justify priority diagnosis and treatment. There is, however, a need to determine the presence of spinal compression in these areas. Both the lumbar and cervical spines are prone to flexion and extension movements that result from severe trauma.

Intervention

The therapeutic and rehabilitative measures are discussed briefly relative to the *immediate, intermediate,* and *late stages of care.* It should be made clear that a tremendous variation in therapy is required for the individual patient, as related to variations in levels of injuries and in combinations of injuries to the spine and the cord.

Immediate stage. During the stage immediately following the injury the cervical area is given priority in treatment because of the neuroanatomic and physiologic features of the *cervical* vertebrae and cord. Therapy is directed first to realignment of the cervical bony column in the presence of demonstrated fractures, dislocations, or other cervical lesions. Any concomitant damage sustained by the cervical cord (or other levels) can be worsened *by continuing bony instability.* Therapeutic measures necessary to protect the cervical cord may include simple mobilization, skeletal traction, or surgery for spinal decompression through varied operative techniques. Stabilization of cervical vertebrae is usually accomplished by skeletal traction through the application of Crutchfield tongs (p. 902) or Vinke tongs. Once skeletal traction for the bony cervical abnormality has been established, further diagnostic and therapeutic measures are considered. The neurologist or neurosurgeon is also guided by the presenting neurologic deficits through continued monitoring of neurologic or spinal cord function.

With the introduction of the anterior surgical approach to the cervical spinal column, early surgical intervention is now more frequently attempted, since sometimes, despite skeletal traction, extruded cervical disc materials produce continued compression of the cord. The primary advantage of the anterior surgical approach (or anterior laminectomy) is that it provides immediate stabilization of the spinal column by techniques of interbody cervical fusion and the direct removal of any extruded disc materials. Surgery, however, may be delayed by some neurosurgeons for several weeks after the injury, irrespective of the absence or presence of neurologic deficits, and when spontaneous healing of the fracture site provides a more stable cervical area. If evidences of spinal cord compression are demonstrated early, surgery may be warranted by the anterior approach.

Tracheostomy and respiratory assistance with a ventilator is required in the immediate stage following upper cervical cord injury. Careful monitoring of blood gases and regular pulmonary toilet is essential. For this reason the patient may be admitted to a pulmonary intensive care unit. He is placed on a Stryker or a Foster frame with skeletal traction attachments.

Less immediate attention to *thoracic* fracture immobilization is necessary for the patient *with limited neurologic* deficits. He is often treated later with simple bed rest, hyperextension, and bracing (p. 724). Diagnosis is necessary, however, to determine the presence or absence of spinal cord compression at this level. Patients who show subarachnoid blockage and have associated neurologic deficits are treated through early surgical decompression. The onset of instantaneous paraplegia following direct thoracic trauma is often reversible through spinal decompression.

An early to an intermediate laminectomy may be performed in the presence of even severe *lumbar* neurologic deficits. Stabilization of the spine is done at the time of the primary surgical intervention or delayed until later in the posttraumatic period. Long delays in lumbar laminectomies or exploration in patients who show early partial recovery are reported to be beneficial for recovery of some neurologic function.

Also threatening to the life of the individual is the extent and effects of paralysis. Immediately, during the areflexic period, medical attention is directed toward the prevention of complications that occur as a result of the loss of motor function. In addition to the more obvious effects apparent in the involved skeletal muscles, there may be loss of vasomotor tone, bladder tone, and bowel peristalsis. The prevention of bladder and bowel distention must be avoided, since they may result in mass reflex or autonomic hyperreflexia (p. 722).

There has been increased interest in the early treatment of the spinal cord injury. This interest was stimulated by demonstrations that experimentally produced cord injuries in animals are reversible if treated early. Some forms of early treatment such as localized spinal cord cooling and myelotomy are undergoing experimentation in some university centers.[2,16] It is too early to assess their value at this time. *Continued research in the immediate care at the time of injury is crucial to progress in treatment.* Also, care received during transportation requires study and control, since poor first-aid care negates the effects of optimal care given during the later stages.

The use of adrenal corticosteroids for the prevention and alleviation of spinal cord edema has gained more acceptance. The efficacy of steroids in the reestablishment of membrane stability and in the control of central nervous tissue edema has been documented clinically. Methylprednisolone (Solu-Medrol) at a dosage level of 60 to 80 mg/day (or equivalent dosage of other corticosteroids) may be utilized for the first week or longer following injury.

Throughout all stages of hospitalization of the SCI person, nursing and medical interventions are directed toward restoration of structural or body integrity consistent with the pathology present. This means that all efforts are taken to assure that the skin is intact, that con-

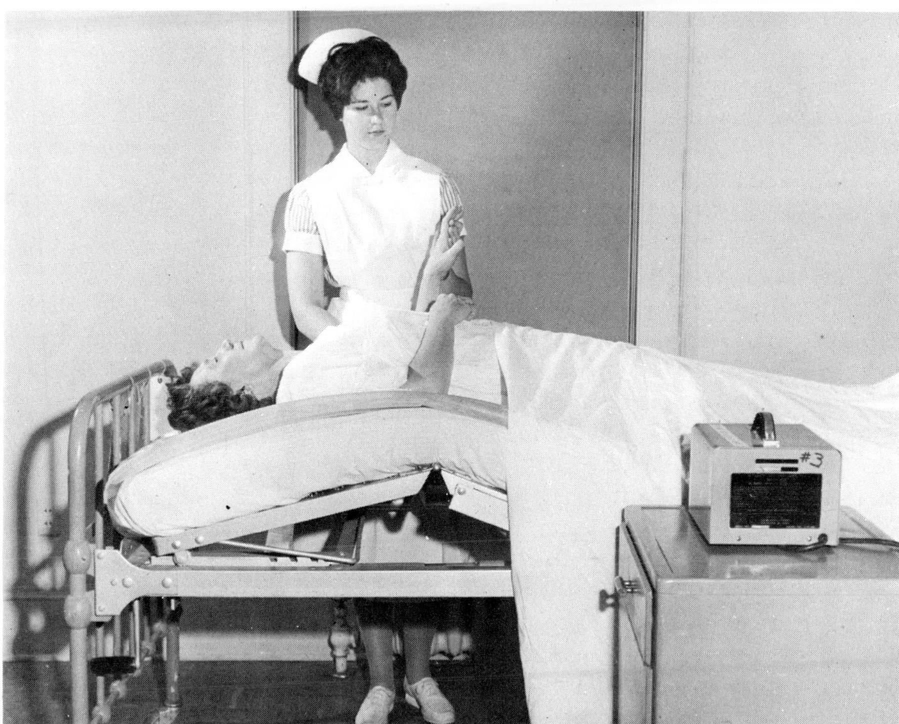

Fig. 36-2. Hyperextension for thoracolumbar spinal fracture can be accomplished by gatching bed with patient head to foot in bed. Patient is placed so that highest point is directly under fracture. Alternating-air-pressure mattress is often used on bed to prevent pressure sores. Patient must be observed carefully for changes in sensation or use of extremities.

tractures do not develop, that range of motion is maintained to the greatest degree possible, that muscle tone is consistent with pathology, and that bladder and bowel functions are maintained. The following section discusses specific interventions to achieve these outcomes.

Position and movement. Before moving a patient with acute spinal cord injury onto a bed from the stretcher on which he is admitted, the physician should be consulted about the type of bed he wishes used. The selection will depend on the physician's preference, the type of injury, the size of the patient, and the equipment available. If a regular bed is to be used, a full-length fracture board should be placed on top of the bedspring under the mattress. This board prevents sagging of the mattress and motion of the spine. If the bed is to be gatched, the board must be hinged, or two or more boards with correctly placed breaks can be used. Mattresses containing springs should not be used. Instead of springs and one mattress, some physicians prefer two hair mattresses placed on top of the fracture board. Some use the knee gatch to provide hyperextension to the spine in selected thoracic and lumbar fractures (Fig. 36-2); the bed must then be made up "head to foot." Sponge rubber mattresses are widely recommended and, when available, are commonly used when there is the possibility that for some time the patient will be moved very little and with extreme difficulty. If available, an alternating air-pressure mattress often is used. Since it may be dangerous to move the patient for some time and since he may have loss of sensation and paralysis of part of the body, pressure areas develop easily. The mattress and entire bed foundation must be well protected with plastic sheeting so that incontinence will not cause damage.

To prevent injury when moving the patient, the bed foundation should be completely adjusted, with gatches raised as ordered, bolsters placed in the desired positions, and a turning sheet available so that a minimum of motion will be necessary. Three to five people are needed to move the patient from the stretcher to the bed, depending on his size and the location of the spinal injury. The physician may supervise moving the patient. The body should be supported in proper alignment, and if necessary, a manual hyperextension should be applied to the spine as the patient is moved (p. 439).

Observations. The nurse must carefully observe the patient with a spinal fracture, a cord tumor, or a ruptured intervertebral disc for signs of cord compression. The motion, strength, and sensation in the extremities should be tested at least four times a day and more frequently if specifically ordered. Any change in motion or sensation should be reported at once as related to level, since immediate surgery may be needed to relieve pressure on the cord. Some of the laminae may be removed to prevent pressure from edema.

Maintenance of function. If cord damage has occurred, nursing care will depend on the level of the injury. Patients with cervical lesions, for instance, will be unable to do anything for themselves. Meticulous skin care, maintenance of correct body alignment, preservation of range of joint motion, and attempts to preserve muscle tone are imperative nursing measures as in the care of any paralyzed person. (See Chapter 35, p. 679, for a discussion of the care of the person with paralysis.)

Elimination. The patient may have urinary retention because of injury to lumbar and sacral spinal nerves. Since he may have no sensation of needing to void, *the nurse should check carefully for voiding and for distention of the bladder.* A Foley catheter may be inserted into the bladder, or a cystostomy may be performed. Later, if the injury is not in the lumbar area, automatic bladder function may be established (p. 1273). The presence of an indwelling catheter makes the patient highly susceptible to urinary infection. The best means of preventing infection is maintenance of fluid intake (3 to 4 liters daily) and meticulous aseptic technique in changing and irrigating catheters. The patient *must* know the signs of infection and *must* have a genitourinary checkup once a year or more frequently. Following an acute injury to the spinal cord, the patient often has abdominal distention. A rectal tube may be used, and neostigmine may be administered hypodermically to stimulate peristalsis. A nasogastric tube or a Miller-Abbott or Cantor tube attached to suction may be tried.

Stool softeners, adequate fluids, prune juice, and suppositories are recommended to obtain bowel function. Long-term use of laxatives and enemas is discouraged, although they may be necessary during spinal shock. If it is necessary to give an enema, 200 ml should be sufficient; no more than 500 ml should be used. There may be fecal incontinence caused by loss of sphincter control (see p. 1276 for care of the incontinent person.)

Pain. Patients with spinal injuries often have a great deal of pain at the level of the injury that radiates along the spinal nerves. A thoracic injury causes chest or back pain, whereas a lumbar injury causes pain in the legs. Analgesics such as acetylsalicylic acid (aspirin) or other nonnarcotic analgesics are ordered. Narcotics may be given for a short time, but are contraindicated for long-term use because the patient's problem may be chronic and addiction is possible. Psychologic assistance is often recommended to help the patient learn to cope with pain. If the patient has a high cervical injury, no narcotics should be administered because respirations may be further depressed. Sometimes the paravertebral nerves are injected with 95% alcohol to relieve thoracic pain. This measure may provide relief for several weeks or even months.

Complications. Autonomic hyperreflexia (mass reflex) occurs in patients with cord lesions above the sixth thoracic vertebra; most commonly it occurs in cervical injuries. The clinical signs are bradycardia, paroxysmal hypertension, sweating, and severe headache. The hypertension can be profound and may result in death if not treated immediately.

The most common causes are visceral distention (distended bladder, impacted rectum). If the patient complains of these symptoms, the patency of the catheter should be checked and a new catheter inserted *immediately* if the catheter is plugged. This should result in reversal of symptoms. In addition, a ganglionic blocking agent such as hexamethonium chloride, 12.5 mg intravenously, may be administered.[56] The patient must be made aware of the symptoms of autonomic hyperreflexia and call the nurse or physician immediately if they occur.

Respiratory complications are common following injury of the spinal cord. Persons who have injury at the cervical level may need respiratory assistance to prevent respiratory arrest. Persons who have injury at the thoracic level tend to splint their chests and have shallow breathing; therefore measures to facilitate deep breathing and aeration of the alveoli are carried out (see Chapter 45). Since coughing can increase spinal pressure, the physician should be consulted before urging the patient to cough.

Intermediate stage. During this stage of treatment, rehabilitation and nursing care measures are focused on mobilization and patient-family education. Quadriplegics and paraplegics need to learn to live with the sequelae of paralysis. The goal of rehabilitation is to minimize the disability and assist the patient toward independence to the extent possible. Rehabilitation depends on the extent and level of the cord injury, the emotional reactions of the patient, his age, and other factors.

Early mobilization of the patient is important regardless of the level of injury. At first, mobilization includes active or passive turning movements and range of motion exercises to prevent pressure sores and contractures and

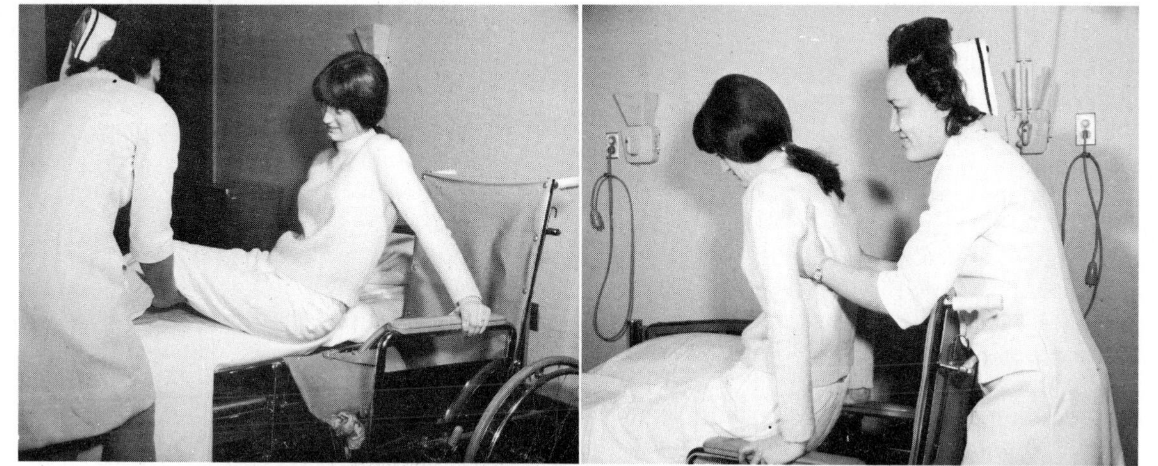

Fig. 36-3. Two methods of transferring patient with paraplegia from bed to wheelchair. In both methods patient pushes up with arms to lift buttocks from bed to chair. **A,** Patient moves sideways into chair as nurse transfers patient's legs. Note that wheelchair is placed next to bed and that right armrest has been removed. **B,** Patient moves backward into wheelchair. Paralyzed legs rest on bed and must be lifted down. Patients with spinal tumors or injuries are often paraplegic. (Courtesy Neuropsychiatric Institute, University of Illinois Hospitals at Medical Center, Chicago, Ill.)

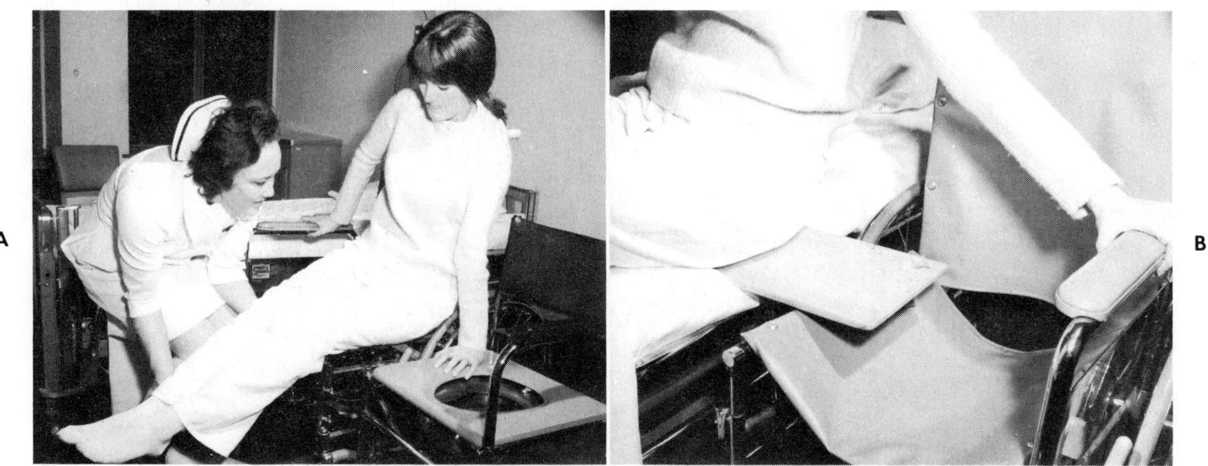

Fig. 36-4. Teaching paraplegic patient methods of transfer. **A,** Moving from wheelchair to commode requires same techniques as moving from bed to chair. Note that adjacent arms of both chairs have been removed. **B,** Sliding board may also be used to provide firm surface on which to move from bed to chair. (Courtesy Neuropsychiatric Institute, University of Illinois Hospitals at Medical Center, Chicago, Ill.)

to develop independence in bed activities. Later, mobilization is progressively effected through crutch walking or bracing or wheelchair activities. Mat exercises and resistive exercises are initiated to increase muscle strength and endurance in remaining muscles. The patient with paraplegia and his family are taught proper methods of transfer from bed to wheelchair or commode (Figs. 36-3 and 36-4). Physical therapy activities facilitate learning to transfer and ambulate.

Before the patient is permitted to be up following a spinal injury, a brace may be prescribed. A *Taylor back brace,* made of padded and covered metal bars to support the back, is often used. It has sturdy straps that come forward to be fastened over a muslin "apron." All braces and corsets must be custom made and are quite expensive. The cost of a back brace varies according to the materials used in construction. The brace or corset should be applied before the patient gets out of bed, and he will need help in getting into it. The patient should wear a thin knitted undershirt next to the skin to keep the brace clean and to protect the skin. Correct use so that the brace fits contours of the buttocks and chest as designed makes a great deal of difference in the patient's comfort. Care should be taken that the apron is smooth and that tapes are not twisted. The patient's emotional reaction to wearing a brace or a corset is important, since it vitally affects ultimate rehabilitation. Attention to small details that help in initial acceptance of this somewhat uncomfortable and unfamiliar piece of "clothing" is important. The patient should practice putting the brace on while he is in the hospital if he must wear it for some time. A close member of his family may visit the hospital and learn to assist him. Patients who live alone and who are unable to care for their braces themselves may need to have a public health nurse help them in the home or teach someone else to assist. The patient wearing a brace should be especially careful in crossing streets and in engaging in activities such as walking down stairs, since he is limited in his ability to shift his balance quickly to prevent an accident.

In addition to instruction about mobilization techniques, the patient is trained to be *functional in activities of daily living,* with or without equipment and as related to his life style. The patient needs to know how to obtain bowel and bladder automaticity (p. 1274), and he needs to know how to prevent bladder infection. It is essential to understand how to prevent decubitus ulcers when one sits in a wheelchair most of the day, and it is important to know how to manage the wheelchair itself. *The patient's family is included in instruction, since many quadriplegic patients may require some supervision or assistance in activities of daily living following discharge from the hospital.* The reaction of family members to spinal cord injury is often great. The family as well as patient needs help in coping. In addition to medical and physical rehabilitation measures, there is equal need for psychologic, emotional, sociologic, and vocational rehabilitation. The trauma of spinal cord injury also results in numerous interpersonal problems and makes adjustment to one's environment difficult.

Late stage. Education, continued psychologic support for patient and family, and medical and surgical follow-up are continued through the late stage as related to the rehabilitation goals of the individual patient. There may be need for surgical treatment of spasticity or mass reflex, with denervation procedures.

Orthoptics, or the application of external appliances to support a paralyzed muscle or to promote a specific motion required in activities of daily living, may require further follow-up care. Patients who have a ruptured cervical disc may need to use a neck brace, and the *Thomas collar* (Fig. 36-5) is often used. The collar is usually anchored at the side with wide adhesive tape and must never be removed without specific orders from the surgeon. The collar extends well up under the chin and

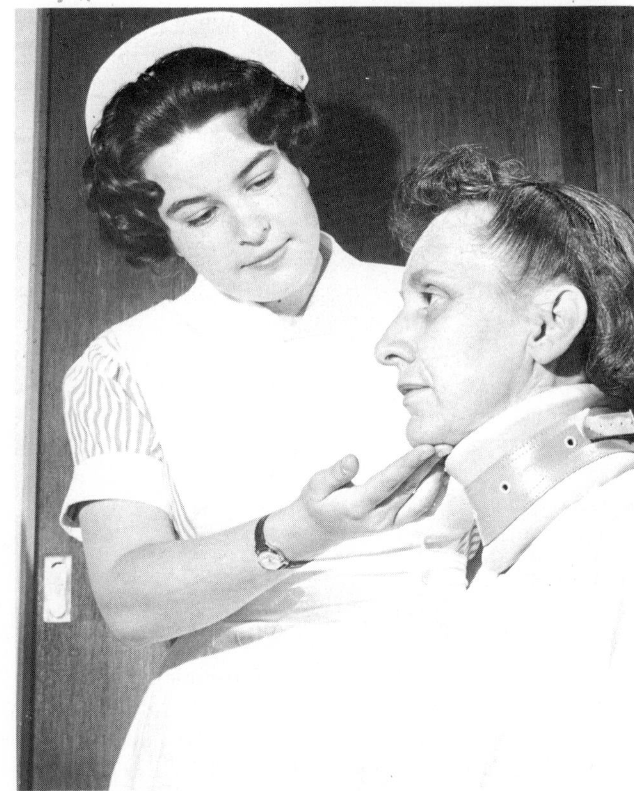

Fig. 36-5. Patient has been fitted with neck brace following cervical fracture or ruptured cervical disc. As patient becomes accustomed to brace, nurse checks to see that skin irritation does not occur.

prevents flexion of the neck. Leg braces may be ordered for the paraplegic.

Sexual needs. Persons with cord injuries need assistance in learning about the effects of their injury on sexual functioning. Men with cord injuries usually cannot achieve an erection, and even when they can achieve one, they are unable to ejaculate.[17] Some SCI men are able to achieve a psychogenic erection. In this type of erection, messages are passed down the spinal cord from the brain to the sacral area. The messages sent by the brain are in response to stimuli received through sight, sound, and smell, or through imagination and memory. In some SCI men the message from the brain bypasses the injured portion of the cord via the autonomic nervous system.[17] A reflexogenic erection may also be achieved by some SCI men. This occurs secondary to direct stimulation of the genital area. For men unable to achieve an erection, techniques such as "stuffing" described in Chapter 64 may be helpful.

Cord injured women can conceive as long as they continue to menstruate. Some SCI women never stop menstruating, while others find that menstruation returns within 6 months of injury.[17]

The nurse can be supportive and helpful to cord injured patients by making it comfortable for them to discuss sexual matters. Nurses not prepared to do sexual counseling need to be aware of resources available in the community to help the SCI person. Some general suggestions that may be helpful to any cord injured persons are (1) sex has many meanings, and for persons with no genital function, alternate ways of expression are available; (2) it will take time for a partner to adjust to the situation; openness in communication is helpful; and (3) it is sometimes difficult for a partner who routinely provides bladder and bowel care to view the person as sexually desirable; it may be helpful in this situation if this care can be provided by a community nurse or part-time attendant.[17]

Research

Research data on spinal cord injuries continues to be gathered.[38] It is of interest that electrostimulation of muscles of the bladder through remote control to regain micturition control in the paraplegic patient has been tested clinically. Success of this electronic spinal neuroprosthesis will assist in preventing urinary complications that are often a cause of death. Functional intramuscular electrostimulation of paralyzed upper extremities muscles is also currently being tested.[42] Since there is little or no external splinting required in the latter orthosis, it will be cosmetically appealing to the quadriplegic if successful.

In summary, although most of the complications of paralysis are now preventable, it is regrettable that complications do occur during and after hospitalization. Under optimal conditions a spinal cord injury person would be evacuated by a knowledgeable first-aid team from the site of the accident to a regional spinal cord center. At the center a team of specialists would supervise treatment while planning a long-term rehabilitation program. Rehabilitation begun in the center eventually would be carried out consistently until patient discharge. Thereafter the center would provide a continuity in management throughout the residual stages.

Outcome criteria for the person with spinal cord injury (paraplegia, quadriplegia)

1. The patient shall have made progress toward functional independence in ADL, consistent with level of cord injury and can:
   a. Feed self independently with or without adaptive equipment.
   b. Bathe self independently with or without adaptive equipment.
   c. Groom self independently with or without adaptive equipment.
   d. Toilet self independently with or without adaptive equipment.
   e. Dress self independently with or without adaptive clothing and devices.
   f. Transfer independently with or without adaptive equipment.
   g. Ambulate independently with or without ambulation aids (braces, crutches, wheelchair).
   h. Utilize communication aids independently (telephone, typewriter).
2. The patient or significant others can explain skin care measures and can:
   a. Inspect skin through use of mirror.
   b. List areas of skin vulnerable to breakdown.
   c. Demonstrate how to relieve pressure on skin surfaces when in bed or wheelchair.
   d. Explain how to avoid irritation and abrasion to skin surfaces during transfer activities.
3. The patient or significant others can explain bowel training program to be followed at home and can:
   a. Demonstrate recommended method.
   b. Explain alternate methods for bowel evacuation.
   c. Relate diet and fluid intake to bowel activity.
   d. Demonstrate digital stimulation.
   e. Relate bowel incontinence to skin breakdown.
4. The patient or significant others can explain bladder training program and can:
   a. Demonstrate recommended method to be followed at home.

   b. Explain alternate methods for emptying bladder.
   c. State the amount and type of fluids to be taken daily to prevent bladder infection.
   d. Demonstrate how to perform intermittent catheterization using clean technique.
   e. Relate bladder incontinence to skin breakdown.
   f. Explain the need to regularly observe amount and color of urine.
5. The patient or significant others can explain prescribed therapies to be followed at home and can:
   a. Accurately demonstrate each prescribed therapy to physical therapist, occupational therapist, speech therapist, nurse.
   b. Explain method, rationale, and daily schedule for each therapy.
   c. Explain time of scheduled return visit to outpatient therapy for reevaluation.
   d. Relate need for regular daily therapy.
6. The patient can effectively utilize the wheelchair in ADL and can:
   a. Explain the parts of the wheelchair and how to maintain it.
   b. Explain the importance of safety checks.
7. The patient or significant others can explain how to obtain professional and community resources and can:
   a. State how to contact agencies.
   b. State how to secure equipment.
   c. State how to join social clubs for paraplegics and quadraplegics.
   d. State financial resources available to the disabled.
8. The patient or significant others can:
   a. Explain long-term goals.
   b. Relate need to be independent in ADL despite time and effort required.
   c. Explain motor and sensory status in relation to goal setting.
   d. State signs or symptoms that require immediate attention.
   e. State plans for follow-up care.

□ Peripheral nerve trauma

The peripheral nerves that lie outside the brain and spinal cord include the cranial and spinal nerves and their branches and plexuses. The disorders involving the peripheral nerves are similar to those that affect the central nervous system and are the result of traumatic, degenerative, vascular, inflammatory, neoplastic, and metabolic causes. *Neuropathies,* noninflammatory disorders, may involve one peripheral nerve (mononeuropathy) or involve multiple nerves (polyneuropathies). *Neuritis* refers to an inflammatory disorder, while *neuralgia* means a painful nerve disorder. Although discussion in this section is limited to neuropathies caused by trauma, it should be clear that regardless of cause, the resulting nerve dysfunction will be similar and will be related to the site of the lesion. Some of the more common neuropathies (other than trauma) include nutritional, alcoholic, diabetic, lead, arsenic, hereditary, and infectious neuropathies.

Traumatic causes of peripheral nerve injury commonly include gunshot and knife wounds, fragmented fracture wounds, and surgical transections, as in denervation surgery and amputations. They variously result in stretching, laceration, and compression of the peripheral nerve; there also is much variation in the degree of injury. Fortunately the axons of peripheral nerves are capable of regeneration under favorable conditions.

Pathophysiology

Following trauma (or disease), the axon undergoes *secondary* or *wallerian degeneration* distal to the lesion (that is distal to the cells of origin) and for several segments proximal. The axon and the myelin sheath (secondary) degenerate and immediately undergo fragmentation; the fragmented particles are completely ingested within several weeks; the axis cylinder remains. Schwann cells and fibroblasts begin to proliferate along the degenerated fibers. (Myelin in *peripheral fibers* is formed by the Schwann cells.) During the regenerative phase, new axoplasm forms at the proximal edge of the injury and the regenerating fibers now grow distally and enter the empty neurolemmal sheath, which has in the meantime proliferated. Myelin then forms around the regenerated axon. When a nerve has been severely damaged and fibrous tissue is abundant, regeneration is interfered with by a tangled mass known as a *traumatic neuroma;* this may have to be removed surgically.

Clinical picture

The clinical signs and symptoms resulting from peripheral nerve lesions depend on the exact location of the lesion and the specific function of the involved nerve or nerves. Since peripheral nerves contain both sensory and motor components, there may be deficits in both components distal to the site. There will be alterations in pain, touch, temperature, proprioception, and stereognosis. Motor alterations include lower motor neuron signs such as flaccid paralysis and muscle wasting in those muscles innervated by the affected nerves.

Intervention

Nursing care is specific to the areas of the body affected by the sensory and motor deficits. Plans for care are based on the nurse's understanding of the distribution and function of the involved peripheral nerves. The flaccid muscles demand attention to prevent deformities. Because of the atonia or hypotonia of the paralyzed muscles, they will be pulled excessively by the muscles that normally oppose them into abnormal or contracted positions. When associated tendons shorten, the contracture is permanent. Positioning of extremities in neutral or counterpositions will help in preventing joint deformities. Those areas of the body in which there is a loss of sensation need to be protected from injury. The patient needs to be taught *protective measures* such as not staying in one position too long, since he cannot sense that damage is occurring in an area served by a damaged nerve. When positional sense is lost, there is also need to teach the patient to protect himself in walking and in other activities. Pain is usually localized, and there may be more paresthesia than pain. The painful areas need to be protected from external stimulation when present. Following surgical intervention, careful positioning of the operative area, as prescribed, is important. Finally, the promotion of general health measures assists in the creation of conditions favorable to nerve regeneration.

■ NEOPLASMS OF THE CENTRAL NERVOUS SYSTEM

Neoplasms of the central nervous system include those arising from cells of structures within the cranium as well as those arising within or outside the spinal cord. In general, they occur in great variety; produce neurologic symptoms because of size, location, and invasive qualities; usually destroy the tissues in which they are situated and displace those around them; and are a frequent cause of increased intracranial pressure.

□ Intracranial tumors

Primary *intracranial* tumors, or *neoplasms*, arise from the intrinsic cells of brain tissues and the pituitary and pineal glands. *Secondary* or *metastatic* tumors are also a frequent contributing type of intracranial tumor. Intracranial tumors are only one example of intracranial lesions. Variable intracranial lesions occur, such as hemorrhage, abscess, and trauma, and cause similar signs and symptoms as a neoplasm dependent on the site of the lesion.

With the development of newer diagnostic techniques, modern surgical and roentgenologic methods, chemotherapeutic agents, and an increased understanding of functional anatomy of the cerebrum, the prognosis for patients with intracranial tumors is more favorable today than in the past. The prognosis, however, is dependent on early diagnosis and treatment, since as the tumor grows within the cranial cavity, it exerts lethal pressure on vital brain centers and causes irreparable brain damage and death. Although approximately one-half of all primary brain tumors are benign, they may cause death by exerting lethal pressure on vital centers of the brain. It is important to remember that although cells of the central nervous system can regain function, even after cerebral edema, dead cells cannot regenerate. Early treatment is thus necessary in order to preserve cerebral functions. Early treatment also becomes important as newer techniques have been developed that improve operative risks and postoperative prospects for patients with intracranial tumors. These techniques include hypothermia (p. 384), the establishment of controlled hypotensive states during surgery by means of sympathetic blocking agents such as trimethaphan camphorsulfonate (Arfonad), and dehydration of cerebral tissues by administering osmotic diuretics such as urea compounds or mannitol before, during, and after surgery. Because the attitude of the nurse about the treatment of brain tumors cannot help but be communicated to the patient and his family, the nurse should make an effort to communicate a hopeful attitude while stressing the importance of early diagnosis and treatment of intracranial tumors.

Types

Brain tumors are named for the tissues from which they arise. The more frequently encountered ones include gliomas, meningiomas, pituitary adenomas, and acoustic neuromas; the brain, in addition, is a frequent site for secondary tumors from other organs.

Gliomas account for about one-half of all brain tumors. They arise in any part of the brain connective tissue. As a rule, in adults they infiltrate primarily the cerebral hemisphere tissues and are not so well outlined that they can be completely excised surgically. They grow rapidly, and most persons do not live longer than a year after diagnosis.[4] The less malignant gliomas are the *astrocytomas* and the *oligodendrogliomas*. *Ependymomas* arise from the walls of the ventricular system. They cause death in about 3 years.[4] The most malignant and rapid growing forms are the *glioblastoma multiforme* and *medulloblastoma*. Gliomas not infrequently start as one type and develop into more malignant forms if untreated.

The *meningiomas*, which account for 13% to 18% of all primary tumors in the intracranial cavity, arise from the meningeal coverings of the brain. They occur most frequently in the meninges over the cerebral hemispheres in the parasagittal region along the ridge of the sphenoid bone and in the anterior fossa in relation to the olfactory groove or the sella turcica. When located in the posterior fossa, they arise from the cerebellopontine angle, from the tentorium, or rarely in the region of the foramen magnum. Meningiomas vary widely as to size and histologic findings. They are usually benign but may undergo malignant changes. The neurologic signs and symptoms produced by meningiomas relative to these sites may include anosmia, optic atrophy, extraocular palsies, visual defects, papilledema, pituitary disturbances, and cerebellar dysfunction. Meningiomas frequently cause seizures and involvement of the limbs as related to their presence in the convexity of a cerebral hemisphere.

Acoustic neuromas constitute about 8% of all primary intracranial tumors. Neuromas may arise from any cranial nerve. The tumor affecting the acoustic nerve usually arises from its sheath but usually extends to affect the nerve fibers. The signs and symptoms resulting from these slow-growing tumors are related to compression of adjacent cranial nerves (trigeminal and facial), cerebellum, and the brainstem.[66]

Metastatic tumors that arise primarily in the lung, kidney, breast, colon, and other organs account for about one-fifth of all intracranial tumors. Primary brain tumors, conversely, rarely metastasize to other organs.

Pathophysiology

The symptoms of intracranial tumors result from both local and general effects of the tumor. Locally, the effects are from infiltration, invasion, and destruction of brain tissues at a particular site. There is also direct pressure on nerve structures, causing degeneration and interference with local circulation. Local edema develops, and if it is long-standing, it is often sufficient to interfere with the function of nerve tissues. A brain tumor of any type situated anywhere in the cranial cavity may cause an increase in intracranial pressure. The increased intracranial pressure is then transmitted throughout the brain and the ventricular system. Eventually the ventricular system is distorted and displaced sufficiently to cause partial ventricular obstruction at some site, even though the tumor is some distance from the ventricular system. A tumor may directly obstruct a particular ventricle early when it grows adjacent to the ventricle. A tumor of the cerebrum can distort the lateral ventricles (Fig. 36-6). A tumor pressing on the third ventricle, the aqueduct of Sylvius, or the fourth ventricle can result in obstruction of cerebrospinal fluid flow into the central canal of the spinal cord. Cerebral edema forms even at some distance from the tumor and generally adds to the increasing pressure. Papilledema results from the general effects of the increased intracranial pressure. Death is usually from brainstem compression resulting from herniation. The mechanism for the occasional acute focal symptoms that occur is thought to be caused by rapidly increasing cerebral edema or by functional decompensation of edematous tissues.[66]

Common clinical circumstances in which intracranial tumors present, or are likely to be found, include those persons with (1) general impairment of cerebral function or a seizure, (2) evidence of increased intracranial pressure, and (3) specific or focal intracranial tumor syndrome.

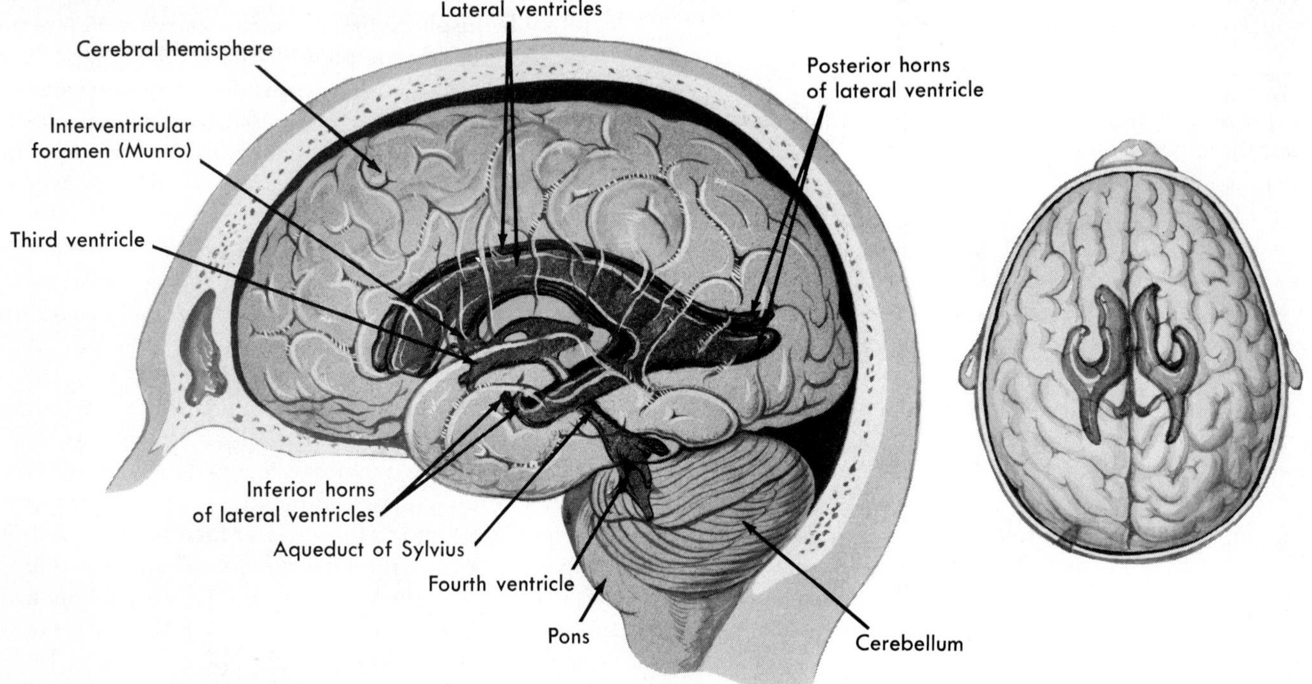

Fig. 36-6. Cerebral ventricles projected upon lateral surface of cerebrum. Smaller drawing shows ventricles from above. (From Anthony, C. P., and Thibodeau, G. A.: Textbook of anatomy and physiology, ed. 10, St. Louis, 1979, The C. V. Mosby Co.)

Radiation therapy is given to many patients following surgery for brain tumors. (See p. 467 for discussion of nursing the patient receiving radiation.)

Long-term care

Some patients who have had cranial surgery will have residual physical and mental limitations. The patient may have hemiplegia, aphasia, and personality changes, including severe depression. The rehabilitative care and planning both for the patient and for his family are the same as for other patients with chronic and permanent neurologic disease. Specific rehabilitation for patients with hemiplegia and aphasia from this cause is similar to that following a cerebrovascular accident. Preventive exercises should be started as soon as possible postoperatively. Regardless of the eventual prognosis, each patient should be helped to be as independent as possible for as long as possible.

The patient who has had intracranial surgery may need the same protection from injury as do other patients with neurologic disease when judgment defect, disorientation, or locomotor difficulties make it unsafe for him to move about without assistance.

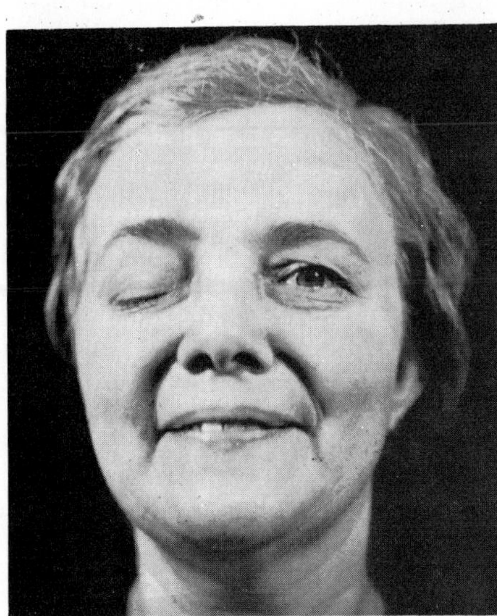

Fig. 36-7. Patient with marked ptosis of right eyelid. (From Davis, L.: The principles of neurological surgery, Philadelphia, 1942, Lea & Febiger.)

Assessment

Every nurse should recognize the early and progressive symptoms of intracranial tumors. The presenting symptoms and the rapidity of their progression depends on the location of the tumor as well as on the type of brain tissue involved. The onset of symptoms begins either with evidences of neurologic dysfunction, which may be generalized or focal, or with symptoms of increased intracranial pressure. Progressive involvement of the brain occurs in either a stepwise or linear manner regardless of the type of onset. Subsequently both types of symptoms are present if the tumor is untreated.

Focal and generalized signs and symptoms of neurologic dysfunction as a rule are referable to a specific area of the brain. Occasionally the concomitant occurrence of focalizing signs and symptoms and the symptoms of increased intracranial pressure produce false focalizing signs that are difficult for the neurologist to interpret. Localizing signs usually appear slowly and increase in severity over time. Such signs are rarely abrupt in appearance, but their appearance may vary from a few weeks with highly malignant tumors to years with a be-

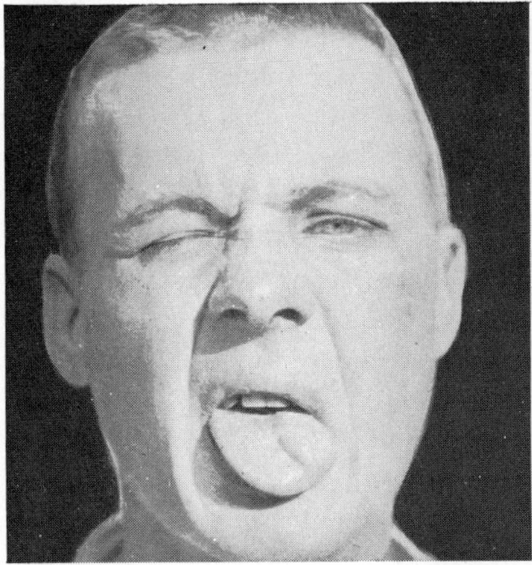

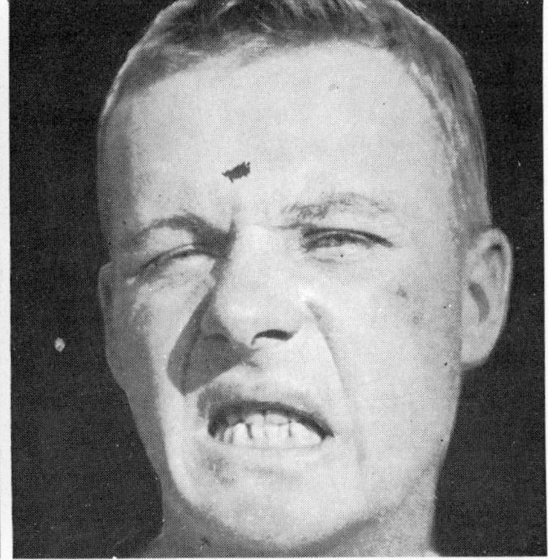

Fig. 36-8. Patient with muscle weakness caused by left facial nerve and hypoglossal palsy. Note deviation of tongue and drooping of mouth on left side when patient clenches teeth. (From Davis, L.: The principles of neurological surgery, Philadelphia, 1942, Lea & Febiger.)

nign tumor. Some benign tumors may, however, produce acute signs. In many instances, especially if the tumor is infiltrating brain tissue, an alert observer may recognize subtle changes that may suggest the need for neurologic examination before the signs and symptoms of increased pressure appear.

Clinical picture

The first noticeable symptom may be a change in personality or judgment. If motor areas of the cerebrum are involved, there may be weakness of the eyelid and facial muscles, as illustrated in Figs. 36-7 and 36-8, respectively. Sometimes the patient complains of paresthesia or anesthesia of a part of the body. He may complain of unpleasant odors, a sensation that often accompanies tumors of the temporal lobe. If the speech centers are involved, the patient may be unable to use words correctly, or he may be unable to understand the written or spoken word. The patient may complain of loss of visual acuity or of double vision. These signs are indicative of pressure on the optic nerve or on one or both abducent nerves. Unexplained loss of hearing in one ear is suggestive of a brain tumor, although there are other causes to be ruled out. Other localized signs may include a staggering, wide-based gait that is suggestive of a cerebellar tumor. Convulsions occurring for the first time after middle age are suggestive of a brain tumor in the cerebrum or its coverings.

Intracranial tumors occurring within the cerebral lobes present disturbances that can be related to the different lobes (Fig. 36-9). A person with a tumor of the *frontal* lobe may demonstrate personality disturbances that range from subtle personality changes to frank psychotic behavior. There may be indifference to bodily functions such as urinary elimination and inappropriate affect with lack of concern.[68] Persons with tumors in the area of the *precentral gyrus* may develop convulsive seizures of the Jacksonian type (involuntary clonic movements with retention of consciousness). Tumors of the *occiptal* lobe result in visual disturbances preceding convulsions. Persons with tumors in the *temporal* lobe may have olfactory, visual, or gustatory hallucinations or psychomotor seizures during which automatic behavioral patterns are carried out.[68] Observations of such disturbances by the nurse assists in location of brain tumors. The signs and symptoms often develop gradually, although at times the onset may be sudden.

Signs and symptoms of increased intracranial pressure resulting from intracranial tumors usually occur after localized signs and symptoms have been present for varying time periods. However, signs and symptoms of intracranial pressure may occur first when a brain tumor is located within or near a ventricle, as previously shown in Fig. 36-6. The signs of increased intracranial pressure are the same as those discussed on p. 670. Headache at first is transitory and later becomes more constant; it increases in intensity with straining, coughing, stooping, and change of position. Nausea and vomiting usually occur as headache increases. Alteration in mental responses also occurs as the tumor grows and the pressure increases.

Headache associated with brain neoplasia. Headache is an early symptom in about one-third of patients with brain tumors and is variable in nature. The pain can be either slight or severe, dull or sharp, and transitory or intermittent. Possible characteristics of the headache is its nocturnal occurrence or its presence on first awaking and its deep nonpulsatile quality; however, these are not specific attributes, since they occur in headaches from other causes. The person may not complain of headache but may betray its presence by placing his hands on his forehead and looking distressed. The mechanism for the headache is not known. In the majority of patients, the intracranial pressure is normal for the first weeks when headache is present. It may be caused by local swelling of tissues and to distortion of blood vessels in and around the tumor. Later, headache seems to be related to increased intracranial pressure. Tumors above the tentorium cause headache on the side and in the vicinity of the tumor; those on the posterior fossae usually cause ipsilateral, retroauricular, or occipital headache. With elevated intracranial pressure, the headache becomes bilateral regardless of location.[1]

Tests. No one diagnostic procedure is entirely diagnostic in brain tumors, and if the patient's condition is stable, electroencephalography, brain scan, or echoencephalography will be used to determine the exact site and nature of the tumor. Patients with increased intracranial pressure but with no evidences of specific neurologic deficits are evaluated as rapidly as possible. In emergency situations, arteriography or ventriculography may be used to locate the tumor.

A lumbar puncture may be helpful in assessment of patients with potential brain tumors; as mentioned previously, it is not carried out in patients with symptoms of increased intracranial pressure except in special circumstances (p. 714).

Brain scans are particularly useful in screening patients for suspected brain tumors by demonstrating the size and site of the tumor. A negative brain scan does not, however, exclude a tumor, since a small tumor may not be visualized. Conversely, a positive scan may be caused by a cranial lesion other than a tumor. Electroencephalography is particularly useful in the detection of abnormal brain waves, generally or focally, within the cerebral hemispheres or their coverings. The echoencephalogram is helpful in identifying displacement of the ventricular system and the pineal gland from their normal midline positions. Displacement to the right of the midline or to the left may be indicative of a tumor within the respective hemisphere. Radiographic studies of the skull are carried out initially and may reveal increased intracranial pressure and abnormal calcifications.

Intervention

The general methods of treatment for intracranial tumors include *surgical removal* when feasible, *radiotherapy*, and *chemotherapy*. Therapy choice is related to the tumor type and specific site of the tumor. A combination of methods is often necessary.

When gliomas are located in areas that are not critical to vital function, they are usually removed surgically. However, because gliomas infiltrate and some forms are malignant, they are difficult to completely excise and treat. Surgery is often combined with radiotherapy and chemotherapy. When the tumor is located in a more critical area, the tumor is biopsied, if possible, and the patient treated with radiotherapy or chemotherapy (with nitrosureas).

Meningiomas are commonly treated by complete excision of the tumor (and overlying bone if infiltrated), since they are usually located in areas that permit removal.

Acoustic tumors are usually treated surgically, with an effort to preserve the facial nerves and their functions. (The care of the person who has had intracranial surgery is discussed in Chapter 35.)

Outcome criteria for the person with an intracranial neoplasm

The patient or significant others can:

1. Explain the outcome of therapy(ies) implemented.
   a. Explain each therapy implemented and the desired outcome.
   b. Explain prognosis.
   c. State symptoms to be observed and reported (intracranial pressure).
   d. Explain neurologic deficits.
2. Explain any home medication or treatment program.
   a. State name, dosage, expected action, and side effects of each prescribed medication.
   b. Explain when to use medications ordered on a prn basis (analgesics, steroids).
   c. Explain exercise program.
   d. Explain care of the skin in relation to radiation and surgical incision.
3. Explain the patient's follow-up program.
   a. State symptoms that require immediate medical attention.
   b. State plans for ongoing care.

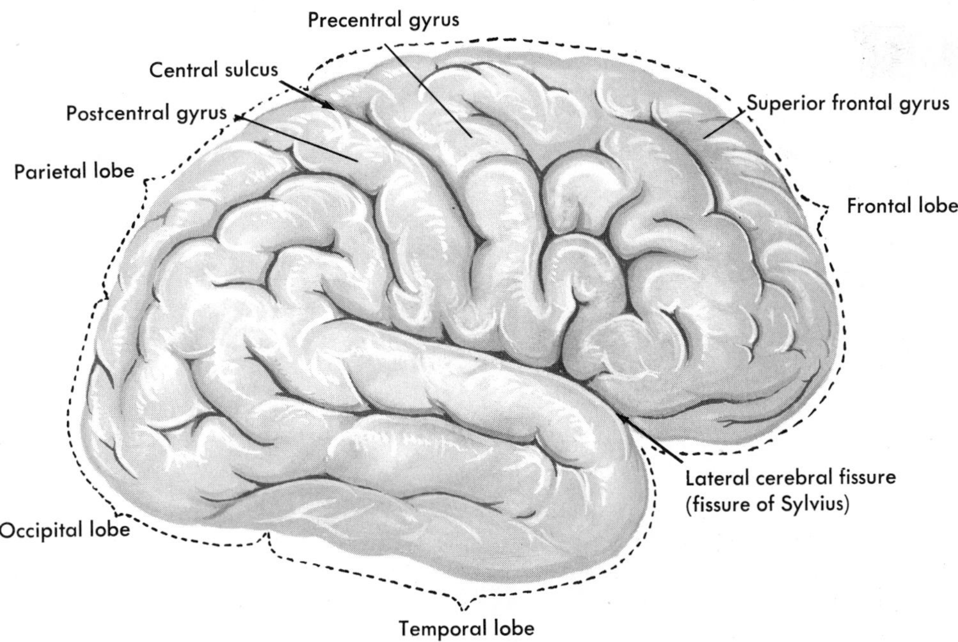

Fig. 36-9. Right hemisphere of cerebrum, lateral surface. Note location of each lobe. (From Anthony, C. P., and Thibodeau, G. A.: Textbook of anatomy and physiology, ed. 10, St. Louis, 1979, The C. V. Mosby Co.)

□ Intravertebral (intraspinal) tumors

Primary intravertebral tumors, or neoplasms, occur either as extramedullary (involving tissues outside the cord substance) or intramedullary (involving tissue cells within the cord substance). *Secondary* or metastatic tumors may also involve the spinal cord, its coverings, and the vertebrae.

Clinical picture

Extramedullary tumors of the intradural type may at first cause subjective nerve root pain. Subsequently, with tumor growth, this will include motor and sensory deficits relating to the level of root and spinal cord involvement. As the tumor enlarges, it compresses the cord. The nurse can learn to relate the initial signs and symptoms to the segmental level of involvement. A cervical lesion will cause pain and motor and sensory deficits in the arms in relation to segmental level. A thoracic lesion causes pain in the chest, and a lumbar lesion causes pain in the legs. Foot and hand pain are rare, but there may be tingling and numbness in the extremities. Eventually the patient loses all motor and sensory function below the level of the tumor.

An *intramedullary* tumor, beginning with the spinal cord substance, presents a different clinical picture. A central cord syndrome includes segmental loss of pain and temperature function. In addition, there is often loss of anterior horn cell function, especially in the hands. Most of the central long tracts next to the gray matter become dysfunctional. There is a gradual, progressive, and descending loss of pain and temperature sensations and motor weakness that is pronounced in the arms when the tumor begins in the cervical area. Caudal motor and sensory functions are the last to be lost, including loss of bowel and bladder control.

In summary, intravertebral tumors, depending on the site, can produce both upper and lower motor neuron signs as well as sensory deficits. This is also true of other intravertebral lesions such as disc herniation and syringomyelia (cavitation of the spinal medulla) and ependymoma (growths involving the central canal of the cord and ventricles).

Intervention

It is obvious that tumors involving the meninges are more likely to be removed successfully than other types. Even when complete removal is not considered possible, surgery is often performed to remove part of the tumor or to remove part of the bone surrounding the spinal column and thus reduce the obstruction for a time; this is called *spinal decompression*. It can be done at any level of the vertebral column and may include several vertebrae. The operation is sometimes palliative for malignant and nonremovable tumors. Radiation therapy is helpful in the treatment of inoperable intramedullary tumors.

Nursing care for a patient with a tumor of the spinal cord is the same as that for a spinal cord injury. The care given after a decompression operation is similar to that given the patient who has had excision of a ruptured nucleus pulposus, except that recovery is much slower (p. 883). The patient who has severe pain requires narcotics.

Convalescent care and rehabilitation depend entirely on the type of tumor and whether it has been successfully removed. Even if it cannot be removed, the decompression operation may give relief of symptoms for months and sometimes for years. If the tumor is a slow-growing one, radiation therapy may be given while the patient is recovering in the hospital and continued after his discharge. The family often needs help in caring for the patient and in meeting his continuing problems. The patient often knows or guesses his prognosis (if little can be done for him medically) because he does not have the mental dulling that so often accompanies brain tumors.

Outcome criteria for the person with an intravertebral tumor

The outcome criteria for the person with an intravertebral tumor is the same as that for the person having intravertebral surgery (p. 903).

REFERENCES AND SELECTED READINGS

1. Adams, R. D., and Victor, M.: Principles of neurology, New York, 1977, McGraw-Hill Book Co.
2. Albin, M. S., White, R. J., Yashon, D., et al.: Effects of localized cooling on spinal cord trauma, J. Trauma **9**:1000-1008, 1969.
3. American Academy of Pediatrics: Report of the Committee on Infectious Diseases, ed. 17, Evanston, Ill. 1974, The Academy.
4. Beeson, P. B., and McDermott, W.: Textbook of medicine, ed. 14, Philadelphia, 1975, W. B. Saunders Co.
5. *Bell, M., Karb, V. B., and Nulsen, F. E.: Head injuries and craniotomies. In Meltzer, L. E., Abdellah, F. G., and Kitchell, J. R., editors: Concepts and practices of intensive care for nurse specialists, ed. 2, Bowie, Md., 1976, The Charles Press Publishers, Inc.
6. Benenson, A. S.: Control of communicable diseases in man, ed. 12, Washington, 1975, The American Public Health Association.
7. Boroch, R. M.: Elements of rehabilitation in nursing, St. Louis, 1976, The C. V. Mosby Co.
8. *Boyle, M. A., and Cluca, R. L.: Amyotrophic lateral sclerosis, Am. J. Nurs. **76**:66-68, 1976.
9. Brunnstrom, S.: Movement therapy in hemiplegia, New York, 1970, Harper & Row, Publishers, Inc.
10. Burch, G. E., and DePasquale, N. P.: Axioms on cerebrovascular disease, Hosp. Med. **11**:8-10, 1975.
11. Center for Disease Control: Reported morbidity and mortality in the United States: 1976, Atlanta, 1977, U.S. Department of Health, Education, and Welfare.
12. *Comarr, A. E., and Gunderson, B. B.: Sexual function in paraplegia and quadriplegia, Am. J. Nurs. **75**:250-255, 1975.

*References preceded by an asterick are particularly well suited for student reading.

13. Cotzias, G. C., and McDowell, F. H., editors: Developments in the treatment for Parkinson's disease, New York, 1973, Medam Press.
14. *Dayhoff, N.: Rethinking stroke: soft or hard devices to position hands, Am. J. Nurs. **75**:1142-1144, 1975.
15. *Delehanty, L., and Stravino, V.: Achieving bladder control, Am. J. Nurs. **70**:312-316, 1970.
16. *Dohrmann, G. J., and Wick, K. M.: Research in experimental cord trauma: past and present, a brief review, J. Neurol. Nurs. **4**:115-124, 1972.
17. Eisenberg, M. G., and Rustard, L. C.: Sex and the spinal cord injured: some questions and answers, ed. 2, Washington, 1975, U.S. Government Printing Office.
18. *Erb, E.: Improving speech in Parkinson's disease, Am. J. Nurs. **73**:1910-1911, 1973.
19. *Feldman, J. L., and Schultz, M.: Rehabilitation after stroke, Nurs. Digest **4**:63-66, 1976.
20. *Fowler, R. S., and Fordyce, W. J.: Adapting care for the brain damaged patient, Am. J. Nurs. **72**:1832-1835 and **72**:2056-2059, 1972.
21. Haas, W. K.: Occlusive cerebrovascular disease, Med. Clin. North Am. **56**:1281-1925, 1972.
22. Hardy, A. G., and Elson, R.: Practical management of spinal injuries, ed. 2, London, 1976, Churchill Livingstone.
23. *Hinkhouse, A.: Craniocerebral trauma, Am. J. Nurs. **73**:1719-1722, 1973.
24. Hohmann, G. W.: Consideration in the management of psychosexual adjustment in the cord injured male, Rehabil. Psychol. **19**:50-59, 1972.
25. *Hurd, G. G.: Teaching the hemiplegic self-care, Am. J. Nurs. **65**:64-68, 1965.
26. *Jackson, R.: Sexual rehabilitation after cord injury, Paraplegia, **10**:50-55, 1972.
27. *Jacobansky, A. M.: Stroke, Am. J. Nurs. **72**:1260-1263, 1972.
28. *Kelly, R.: Management of MS, Nurs. Mirror **143**(6):48-49, 1976.
29. Kingdon-Ward, W.: Helping the stroke patient speak, London, 1969, J. & A. Churchill Co.
30. Kintzel, K. C., editor: Nursing interventions for the patient with CNS dysfunction in advanced concepts in clinical nursing, Philadelphia, 1971, J. B. Lippincott Co.
30a. *Larrabee, J. H.: The person with a spinal cord injury: physical care during early recovery, Am. J. Nurs. **77**:1320-1329, 1977.
31. Loetterle, B. C., Rogers, M., Valdner, T., et al.: Cerebellar stimulation: pacing the brain, Am. J. Nurs. **75**:958-960, 1975.
32. Maddox, M.: Subarachnoid hemorrhage, Am. J. Nurs. **74**:2199-2201, 1974.
33. Melnick, J. L.: Classification and nomenclature of viruses, Prog. Med. Virol. **14**:321-332, 1972.
34. Merritt, H. H.: A textbook of neurology, ed. 4, Philadelphia, 1973, Lea & Febiger.
35. Miller, J. D., and Ross, C. A. C.: Encephalitis: a four year survey, Lancet **1**:1121-1126, 1968.
36. National Multiple Sclerosis Society: 1976 Annual Report, New York, 1976, The Society.
37. National Multiple Sclerosis Society: MS messenger, New York, 1976, The Society.
38. National Spinal Cord Injury Data Research Center Hospital Data Base Syllabus, 1975, Phoenix, Ariz.
39. *Norsworthy, E.: Nursing rehabilitation after severe head trauma, Am. J. Nurs. **74**:1246-1250, 1974.
40. Olson, C. K., and Tollefsrud, V. E.: Chemosurgery for parkinsonism and when the patient has chemosurgery, Am. J. Nurs. **59**:1411-1416, 1959.
41. Olson, E. V., et al.: The hazards of immobility, Am. J. Nurs. **67**:779-797, 1967.
42. Peckham, P. H., et al.: Intramuscular stimulation: applications to upper extremity orthotics. In Proceedings of the fourth annual meeting of the Biomedical Engineering Society, Los Angeles, 1973.
42a. *Pepper, G. A.: The person with spinal cord injury: psychological care, Am. J. Nurs. **77**:1330-1335, 1977.
43. *Pfaudler, M.: Motor skill rehabilitation for hemiplegic patients, Am. J. Nurs. **73**:1892-1896, 1973.
44. *Pfaudler, M.: Flotation therapy: flotation, displacement and decubitus ulcers, Am. J. Nurs. **68**:2351-2355, 1968.
45. Quesenbury, J. N.: Nursing action—not reaction—for a stroke patient's rehabilitation. In Bergersen, B. S., Anderson, E. H., Duffey, M., Lohr, M., and Rose, M. H.: Current concepts in clinical nursing, vol. 2, St. Louis, 1969, The C. V. Mosby Co.
46. Rhodes, M., Gruendemann, B. J., and Ballinger, W. F.: Alexander's care of the patient in surgery, ed. 6, St. Louis, 1978, The C. V. Mosby Co.
47. *Robinson, M. B.: Levodopa and parkinsonism, Am. J. Nurs. **74**:656-661, 1974.
48. Rocklin, R.: The Guillain-Barre syndrome and multiple sclerosis, N. Engl. J. Med. **284**:803-808, 1971.
49. Romano, M.: Sexuality and the disabled female, Accent on Living, Winter 1973, pp. 26-34.
50. Ruge, D., editor: Spinal cord injuries, Springfield, Ill., 1969, Charles C Thomas, Publisher.
51. Sabiston, D. E., editor: Davis-Christopher textbook of surgery, ed. 11, Philadelphia, 1977, W. B. Saunders Co.
52. Sarno, J., and Sarno, M. T.: Stroke: the condition and the patient, New York, 1969, McGraw-Hill Book Co.
53. Schontz, F. C.: The psychological aspects of physical illness and disability, New York, 1975, MacMillan Publishing Co., Inc.
54. *Skelly, M.: Rethinking stroke: aphasic patients talk back, Am. J. Nurs. **75**:1140-1142, 1975.
55. *Stackhouse, J.: Myasthenia gravis, Am. J. Nurs. **73**:1544-1547, 1973.
56. Stryker, R. P.: Rehabilitation aspects of acute and chronic nursing care, ed. 2, Philadelphia, 1977, W. B. Saunders Co.
57. Taren, J. A., and Martin, M. A.: Cerebral aneurysm and care of the patient with a cerebral aneurysm, Am. J. Nurs. **65**:90-95, 1965.
58. *Taylor, J. W.: Measuring the outcomes of nursing care, Nurs. Clin. North Am. **9**:337-340, 1974.
59. *The person with spinal cord injury: self-study program, Am. J. Nurs. **77**:1319-1342, 1977.
60. Tourtelotte, W. W.: Cerebrospinal fluid in multiple sclerosis. In Vinken, P. J., and Bruyn, G. W., editors: Handbook of clinical neurology, Amsterdam, 1970, North Holland Publishing Co.
61. *Ullman, M.: Disorders of body image after stroke, Am. J. Nurs. **64**:89-91, 1964.
62. U.S. Department of Health, Education, and Welfare: Isolation techniques for use in hospitals, ed. 2, Washington, 1975, U.S. Government Printing Office.
63. *Wheeler, P.: Care of the patient with a cerebellar tumor, Am. J. Nurs. **77**:263-266, 1977.
64. Wintrobe, M. M., et al., editors: Harrison's principles of internal medicine, ed. 7, New York, 1974, McGraw-Hill Book Co.
65. *Woods, N. F., and Woods, J. S.: Human sexuality in health and illness, St. Louis, 1975, The C. V. Mosby Co.
66. Yahr, M. D.: Brain tumors, Hosp. Med. **9**:8-35, 1973.
67. Yahr, M. D., editor: Symposium on clinical neurology, Med. Clin. North Am. **56**:1225-1418, 1972.
68. Yase, Y.: Amyotrophic lateral sclerosis, Arch. Neurol. **27**:118-128, 1972.
69. *Young, J. F., and Reid, M.: Care in the surgical management of

intracranial aneurysms, J. Neurosurg. Nurs. 4:21-31, 1972.
70. Zankel, H. T.: Stroke rehabilitation, Springfield, Ill., 1971, Charles C Thomas, Publisher.

AUDIOVISUAL RESOURCES

1. Ambulation training for the Parkinson patient (motion picture), National Medical Audiovisual Center, Atlanta, National Audiovisual Center, Washington, 1965.
   The purpose of this presentation is to describe and demonstrate methods used in ambulation training for Parkinson patients. The importance of practice by the patient after treatment is stressed.
2. A new approach to physical therapy in parkinsonism (motion picture), Norwich, N.Y., 1971, Eaton.
   The purpose of this program is to demonstrate the use of group physical therapy in parkinsonism.
3. Epileptic children (motion picture), New York, National Educational Television, Bloomington, Ind., Indiana University Audio-Visual Center, 1959.
   Oriented primarily toward the layman, this program focuses on the social relationships of children with epilepsy in the hope of helping children with this condition find a better and more wholesome relationship. An interview with an individual who has epilepsy and is seeking a job with an individual who is prejudiced against epilepsy is presented to show the need for a good attitude toward epilepsy on the part of society. The film concludes with an interview with a pediatrician who discusses the role of heredity in epilepsy.
4. Care of the patient with a head injury (filmstrip), Garden Grove, Calif., Trainex.
   The purpose of this teaching presentation is to describe and demonstrate the nursing care of the patient with a head injury. Observations and the recording of vital signs and reflexes are described and demonstrated in detail.
5. The quadraparetic patient: changing position and sitting up in bed (motion picture), New York University Medical Center, Institute of Rehabilitation Medicine, produced by the National Medical Audiovisual Center, for sale by National Audiovisual Center, Washington, 1968.
   The purpose of this presentation is to demonstrate step-by-step the movements made by the quadraparetic patient to change position and sit up in bed.
6. The quadraparetic patient: sitting balance in bed (motion picture), New York University Medical Center, Institute of Rehabilitation Medicine, produced by National Medical Audiovisual Center, 1968.
   This program describes and demonstrates with a therapist and quadraparetic patient the techniques for moving the extremities and trunk while sitting in bed.
7. The quadraparetic patient: transfer from wheelchair to car and reverse using sliding board (motion picture), New York University Medical Center, Institute of Rehabilitation Medicine, produced by National Medical Audiovisual Center, 1969.
   The purpose of this presentation is to demonstrate step-by-step the transfer of a quadraparetic patient from the wheelchair to the car and reverse using a sliding board.
8. Driving (motion picture), Rehabilitation-Education Center, University of Illinois, Urbana-Champaign, Ill., produced by Motion Picture Production Center, 1974.
   The purpose of this program is to demonstrate functional skills necessary and equipment available to assist the quadriplegic patient in driving a car. Several types of vans are demonstrated to illustrate equipment that is available to the quadriplegic.
9. Showering and grooming (motion picture), Rehabilitation-Education Center, University of Illinois, Urbana-Champaign, Ill., produced by Motion Picture Production Center, 1974.
   The purpose of this presentation is to describe and demonstrate several techniques developed by quadriplegic patients for showering and grooming.
10. Dressing (motion picture), Rehabilitation-Education Center, University of Illinois, Urbana-Champaign, Ill.
    The purpose of this presentation is to demonstrate functional skills and techniques used in dressing, which the quadriplegic has developed through rehabilitation training to achieve independence.
11. Initial parallel bar exercises for the paraplegic patient (motion picture), Institute of Rehabilitation Medicine, New York University Medical Center, produced by Public Health Service Audiovisual Facility.
    The purpose of this presentation is to describe and demonstrate the initial parallel bar exercises the paraplegic patient must master to begin crutch walking.
12. Wheelchair transfers for the paraplegic patient (motion picture), Institute of Rehabilitation Medicine, New York University Medical Center, produced by Public Health Service Audiovisual Facility, 1967.
    This presentation demonstrates three wheelchair transfer techniques for the paraplegic patient with the aid of an adult male paraplegic patient and a female physical therapist.
13. An active future (motion picture), American Rehabilitation Foundation, Minneapolis, Minn., 1969.
    The purpose of this patient education program is to describe and demonstrate to the paraplegic patient the fact that despite a spinal cord injury which has resulted in paralysis, he can still have an active future. The effects of activity on various body functions are also discussed.
14. Walking with braces and crutches (motion picture), American Rehabilitation Foundation, Minneapolis, Minn., 1969.
    The purpose of this patient education program is to discuss and demonstrate the preparation and training necessary for the paraplegic patient to achieve independent ambulation using crutches and braces.
15. Planning your bowel program (motion picture), American Rehabilitation Foundation, Minneapolis, Minn., 1969.
    The purpose of this paraplegic patient education program is to discuss the important of planning a bowel program based on scheduling, diet, and stimulation.
16. Bowel and bladder techniques (motion picture), Rehabilitation-Education Center, University of Illinois, Urbana-Champaign, Ill., 1974.
    The purpose of this program is to present some of the methods that may be utilized by the quadriplegic patient in the management of bowel and bladder functions.
17. Moving in and out of your wheelchair (motion picture), American Rehabilitation Foundation, Minneapolis, Minn., 1969.
    The purpose of this patient education program is to demonstrate the independent transfer of a paraplegic patient into and out of a wheelchair.
18. The paraplegic patient: in and out of car (motion picture), New York University Medical Center, Institute of Rehabilitation Medicine, The University of New York, 1969.
    This program describes and demonstrates with the help of an adult male paraplegic patient and a therapist a technique for getting in and out of a car.
19. Activities in your new life (motion picture), American Rehabilitation Foundation, Minneapolis, Minn., 1969.
    This program is oriented toward paraplegic patients and is aimed

at showing them that they can make a happy and satisfactory adjustment to their condition. The main focus of the program is on the degree of enjoyment of life the paraplegic person can attain.

20. The paraplegic patient (motion picture), Institute of Rehabilitation Medicine, New York University Medical Center, The University of New York, 1968.
    The purpose of this presentation is to demonstrate step-by-step the method used by a paraplegic patient to remove his body brace.
21. Prevention of disability from stroke (motion picture), National Heart and Lung Institute, Chronic Disease Section, Bethesda, Md., 1960.
    The purpose of this presentation is to describe and demonstrate some modern techniques used to prevent disability from stroke. The importance of proper positioning of the patient while in bed is stressed.
22. The causes and effects of stroke and acute care (filmstrip), Concept Media in cooperation with Department of Medical Education, Memorial Hospital of Long Beach, Costa Mesa, Calif., 1969.
    This presentation describes the causes and effects of stroke and discusses the nursing care of the patient in the acute phase with the aid of male and female clinical subjects, drawings, and diagrams.
23. Molbilization of the stroke patient (slides), University of Michigan Medical Center, Ann Arbor, Mich., 1975.
    This program describes and demonstrates useful therapeutic approaches in the mobilization of the stroke patient. This objective is achieved with the aid of clinical subjects, hospital personnel, drawings, and diagrams.
24. Deficits and emotional reactions (filmstrip), Concept Media in cooperation with Department of Medical Education, Memorial Hospital of Long Beach, Costa Mesa, Calif., 1969.
    The purpose of this presentation is to describe the common deficits and emotional reactions of stroke patients and to discuss nursing measures that may help to minimize the effects of these deficits. Part two of this presentation explores the emotional reactions of the stroke patient.
25. Post critical care and discharge planning (filmstrip), Concept Media in cooperation with Department of Medical Education, Memorial Hospital of Long Beach, Costa Mesa, Calif., 1969.
    The purpose of this presentation is to describe the role of the members of the team in determining the total needs of patients and developing a treatment plan to meet these needs. The primary goal of the health care team at this time is to ensure as smooth a transition from hospital to home as possible.

37

Assessment of special senses: eye and ear

LYNN CHENOWETH McWILLIAMS
LINDA ANNE BROSEMAN

Sensations in general orient people to themselves and their environment. We learn about our world and about ourselves through sensations. Sensations contribute meaning and pleasure to the human experience. A world without the sounds and sights of children playing or the aesthetic pleasure of museums and symphonies may be bleak indeed. Besides pleasures, sensations provide necessary data for our safety and well-being. A fire alarm or a flashing red light provides clues to danger in our environment. We learn as infants to distinguish between what is "us" and what is the world by our senses. Our sensations directly contribute to our self-concept and feelings of personal worth and well-being.

Sensory impairment is often not the initial problem or major diagnosis but is often present in patients for whom the nurse is providing care for other medical or surgical conditions. Health workers need to be able to assess all patients in relation to sensory capabilities and plan their care accordingly.

Nursing assessment is focused on the degree to which the sensory loss affects the person's ability to carry out activities of daily living, the support systems available to him, and the coping skills that he has successfully utilized in the past. Nursing interventions are designed to help people meet their basic needs as they are affected by hospitalization or illness, to strengthen existing support systems, and to encourage the use of successful coping mechanisms.

Two major senses, vision and hearing, are considered in the next three chapters. Further information on other sensory alterations can be found in the discussion of management of neurologic manifestations (see Chapter 35).

Many aspects of assessment of the eyes, including visual acuity, and the ears, including hearing, may be carried out by different professionals or trained auxiliary personnel, as described in the text. The extent of the nurse's activities in assessment of the eye and ear depends on the level of preparation and place of employment.

■ ASSESSMENT OF EYES AND VISION

The eye is an extremely complicated structure but very accessible for examination. See Fig. 37-1 for the landmarks of the eye. Assessment of the eye's structure and functioning is done by physicians, nurses, optometrists, and some paraprofessional health workers. Assessment includes inspection of the external structures and gross measures of visual acuity. Lay persons are trained by the National Society to Prevent Blindness to conduct vision screening tests with preschool children. The more complex eye examinations such as electrophysiologic studies of the retina and other fundus examinations are done by physicians or specially trained nurses or technicians.

The nurse's exact activities in assessment of the eye and vision depend on that nurse's particular place of em-

BASIC ASSESSMENT OF THE EYE AND VISION

Facial and ocular expression	Prominence of eyes, alert or dull expression
Eyelids	Symmetry, presence of edema, ptosis, itching, redness, discharges, blinking equality
Iris and pupils	Irregularities in color, shape, size
Pupillary reflex	Constriction of pupil in response to light in that eye (direct light reaction), equal amount of constriction in other eye (consensual light reaction)
Lens	Transparent or opaque
Peripheral vision	Ability to see movements and objects well on both sides of field of vision
Acuity with and without glasses	Ability to read newsprint, clocks on wall, and namepins, to recognize faces at bedside and at door
Supportive aids	Glasses, contact lenses, false eye

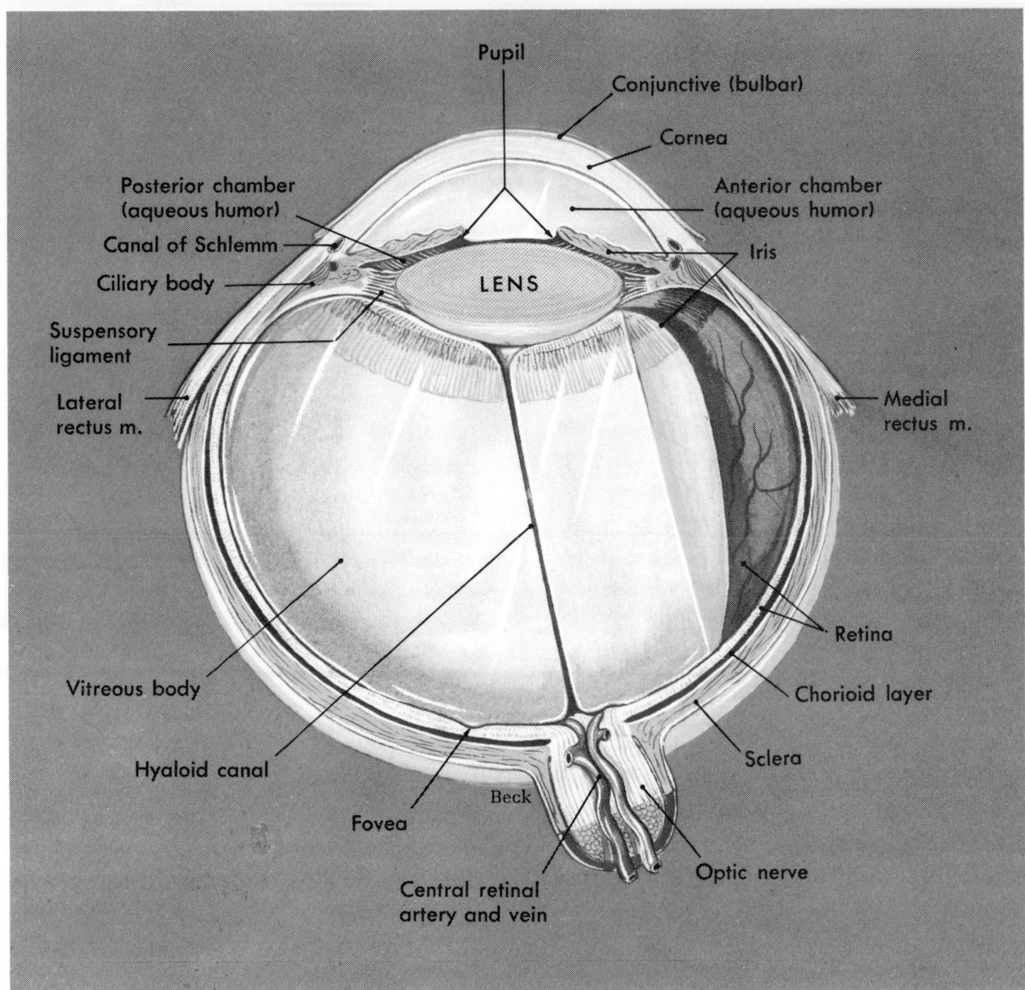

Fig. 37-1. Horizontal section through left eyeball. (From Anthony, C. P., and Thibodeau, G. A.: Textbook of anatomy and physiology, ed. 10, St. Louis, 1979, The C. V. Mosby Co.)

ployment, education, interests, and the patient's age and health. For instance, a nurse working in a community health agency may have the need and opportunity to do more extensive eye assessment than a nurse in a teaching hospital where physicians abound. Every nurse should at least be able to carry out a basic assessment of the eye and vision as described in the box below. For information on more detailed eye assessment see references 1, 10, 13, and 21.

OCULAR EXAMINATION

Assessment of visual acuity
Assessment of ocular movement
Inspection of external structures
Inspection of internal structures
Estimation of intraocular pressure

A complete ocular assessment consists of subjective data elicited by means of an interview with the individual and objective data obtained by inspecting external structures and functions of the eye and some internal parts of the eye (see box).

☐ Subjective data: history

Because many eye disorders can be inherited, a family history is necessary. The individual's previous eye problems, diagnoses, and treatment are recorded as well as the presence of any systemic disease. The interviewer determines if the individual perceives any of the following: changes in visual acuity; abnormal signs and symptoms such as burning, tearing, or blurred vision; and events surrounding onset of symptoms, duration of symptoms, and sources of relief.[21]

☐ Objective data

Measurement of visual acuity

When light passes through the eye, the bending of the light rays and the location of the image depend on the shape and condition of ocular structures. Ocular *refraction* is a procedure that reveals the degree to which the various light-transmitting portions of the eye bring light rays into correct focus on the retina. When the image is not clearly focused on the retina, *refractive error* is present. Refractive errors account for the largest number of impairments of good vision. The refractive error is tested by means of trial lenses and the Snellen chart. Suitable corrective lenses are prescribed if needed. In situations where formal acuity testing equipment is not available, estimates of refractive error can be made. For instance, the person can be asked to read print or identify pictures at varying distances. The person's visual acuity can be compared with that of the examiner's.

Some specific terminology must be understood before refractive studies can be meaningful. *Emmetropia* refers to a normal eye, whereas *ametropia* indicates that a refractive error is present. *Accommodation* is the ability to adjust vision from far to near objects. This is normally accomplished by the ciliary muscles, which by means of contraction or relaxation can cause the lens to flatten or thicken as the need arises. *Myopia*, or nearsightedness, is caused by an abnormally long anteroposterior dimension of the eyeball resulting in light rays being focused in front of the retina. *Hyperopia*, or farsightedness, is caused when the anteroposterior dimension is too short resulting in light rays being focused behind the retina. *Astigmatism* is a condition caused by asymmetry, or irregular curvature, of the cornea so that rays in the horizontal and vertical planes do not focus at the same point. In *presbyopia*, which occurs in all persons past 40 years of age, the lens becomes more firm and responds less to the need for accommodation in viewing near objects. Blurring of near objects results, and those who require different lenses for distant and for close vision must obtain bifocal lenses or separate pairs of glasses.

Before refraction is tested, a cycloplegic drug is instilled into the eyes to dilate the pupils and temporarily paralyze the ciliary muscles. Cyclopentolate (Cyclogyl), 1% or 2%, is usually used, since it is effective in 30 minutes and the effect generally wears off completely by the end of 6 hours. The duration of effect will vary, however, lasting longer than 6 hours in persons with a light blue iris. A blue-eyed person's iris will dilate more rapidly and remain dilated longer than that of a brown-eyed person because more of the drug is absorbed into the iris with less pigmentation.

When the appointment is made for an eye examination with the use of a cycloplegic drug, the person is told that blurred vision will be present after the examination. It should be explained that he will not be able to drive or read until the effect of the drug subsides. In some cases a miotic drug, pilocarpine, is instilled after the examination to constrict the pupil and reduce the uncomfortable glare from lights. Homatropine occasionally is used for adults and atropine for children to dilate the pupils for refraction, but both of these drugs require longer to take effect, and their effects persist longer. Atropine must be instilled at intervals for 3 days prior to examination and persists in its action for at least 10 days with some residual effect for up to 3 to 4 weeks.

Distance vision is usually determined by use of a *Snellen* chart (Fig. 37-2, *A*). Examination is done with the person standing 20 feet from the chart. The chart consists of rows of letters, numbers, or other characters arranged with the large ones at the top and the small ones at the bottom. The upper-most letter on the chart is scaled so that it can be read by the normal eye at 200 feet, and the successive rows are scaled so that they can be read at 100, 70, 50, 40, 30, 20, 15, and 10 feet, respectively. Visual acuity is expressed as a fraction, and a reading of 20/20 is considered normal. The upper figure refers to the distance of the person from the chart, and the lower figure indicates the distance at which a normal eye can read the line. For example, the person who is able to read at 20 feet only the line that should be readable at 70 feet has 20/70 vision in that eye. A score of 20/30 means that the person is 20 feet from the chart and can read the line that a normal eye should see at 30 feet.[7] The distance from the chart to where the individual stands must be carefully measured. The examiner usually stands beside the chart and points to the line to be read so that no mistake occurs. Each eye is tested separately, and its performance is carefully recorded. The person is tested with and without his distance lenses. When testing vision a piece of stiff paper or a plastic occluder is placed over one eye while the other eye is tested.

For preschool children and others unable to read the English alphabet, a modified Snellen chart is used (Fig. 37-2, *B*). In this chart a block E is shown in varying positions and the individual is asked to indicate in which direction the "legs" or "fingers" of the E point.

Near vision can be tested with use of a Jaeger chart or newsprint. The Jaeger chart is a card containing varying size print, which is held 35 cm (14 in) from the eye. The score attained can be expressed in Snellen, metric, and percentage figures.[21]

Any person with vision less than 20/30 OD (right eye)

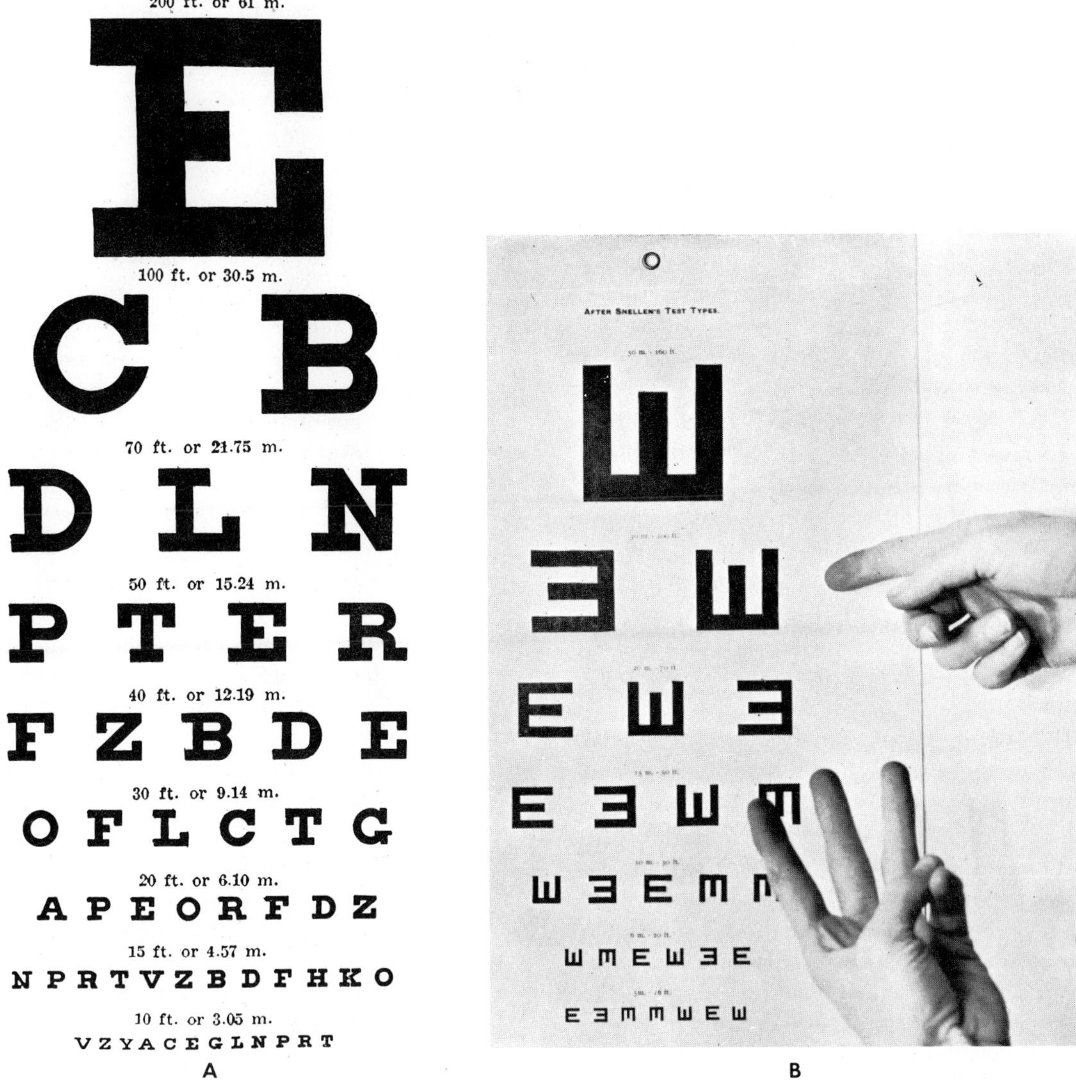

Fig. 37-2. A, Snellen chart used in testing vision. **B,** Modified Snellen chart, called "E" game, for testing vision of small children and persons unfamiliar with English alphabet.

or OS (left eye) or with a two-line difference between eyes should be referred to an ophthalmologist for further testing and treatment.[21] The Snellen, block E, or Jaeger chart examinations provide only basic screening test data. Additional detailed procedures must be done to test for nearsightedness, astigmatism, color blindness, and many other abnormalities. The nurse who works in a clinic, in an ophthalmologist's office, or in schools must know how to do vision screening tests and how to teach others to do them.

Assessment of ocular movements

Ocular movements are evaluated to determine whether the eyes are moving together in a synchronous manner. Muscle imbalances and cranial nerve damage also can be detected.

To test ocular muscles the examiner and person being tested are seated facing each other. While the person looks straight ahead at a target, a penlight is shined on the cornea. The corneal light reflex should be in exactly the same position on each pupil. The examiner then covers one of the person's eyes while he looks at the light. When the cover is quickly removed, the examiner notes whether that eye moves to regain fixation on the light. Movement may indicate a drift of the eye behind the cover, which can indicate muscle imbalances.[10]

To evaluate possible weaknesses of individual extraocular muscles, muscle balance testing can be done in eight positions of gaze as well as straight ahead. The reader is referred to texts on physical appraisal for more detailed information about assessment of ocular movements.[1,10,12,21]

Inspection of external structures

The general appearance of the face and eyes is observed for the type of expression (dull or alert) and prominence of the eyes. When there is an abnormal protrusion or bulging of an eye, the condition is called exophthalmia or exophthalmos.

The appearance of the *eyelids* is noted in relation to color, texture, mobility, and position. The lids should be able to close completely to prevent drying of the conjunctiva and cornea. Any swelling, redness, or discharge is noted. If one upper lid seems to be in a position lower than the other, or "droops," the condition may be *ptosis* of the eyelid. When there is ptosis in both eyes, the upper lids will be observed to be in an abnormally low position covering the upper portion or more of the iris. Ptosis of the upper lids may be due to extreme debility or to neuromuscular disease.[10] Extreme ptosis can interfere with vision by covering the pupil.

The *conjunctiva* is a transparent membrane that lines the inside of the eyelids and covers the exposed portion of the eyeball except for the cornea. The conjunctiva of the lower lid is examined by pulling downward on the lid as the individual looks upward. In order to examine the conjunctiva of the upper lid, the lid must be everted. To evert the eyelid the individual looks down; the examiner grasps the eyelashes and pulls gently down and forward while pushing down on the upper lid border with an applicator or tongue blade. When the lid is everted it is held in position by the fingers holding the lashes to the brow.

Small blood vessels are normally visible in the conjunctiva. The *sclera,* or white covering of the eye, shows through the conjunctiva and has a shiny porcelainlike appearance. Dilation of blood vessels of the conjunctiva may indicate disease of the cornea or disease within the eye. Spontaneous small hemorrhages may occur beneath the conjunctiva in the normal eye. A yellow discoloration of the sclera indicates jaundice. The *lacrimal gland* may be observed in the inner canthus and may be palpated for patency of the lacrimal puncta.

The *cornea,* which is normally invisible except for surface reflections, must be smooth and transparent for good vision. It should look shiny and bright when examined with a penlight. Moving the light and directing it from the side, the examiner looks for abrasions and opacities.

The *iris* of each eye is compared for color, pattern, and shape. When looking through the pupillary opening, the examiner is also inspecting the *lens,* which is normally transparent. An opaque lens is termed a *cataract.*

Pupillary reflexes

While approaching from the side, the examiner quickly shines a light into one eye causing constriction of the pupil in that eye (direct light reaction). The pupil of the other eye should also constrict the same amount (consensual light reaction, p. 642). The other eye is then tested in the same manner.

A light shined into a blind eye will not produce a pupillary response; however, a light shined into a normal eye will produce a pupillary response in the blind eye by consensual reaction if the oculomotor nerve is intact.[1]

Another test of pupillary reflex is to have the person focus on an object that is moved directly toward his nose. When focusing on the near object, the pupils of both eyes should constrict (near reaction, reaction in accommodation). The examiner looks for the presence of a response and whether the response is equal in both eyes. Loss of pupillary reflexes when sight is present is due to neurologic disease (p. 642).

Visual fields

The visual field for an individual is that portion of the world that his eye can perceive. Lesions of the retina, optic pathways, and central nervous system affect sections of the field of vision (p. 640). The location of visual field loss indicates the location of the lesion. For instance, glaucoma decreases peripheral vision, indicating damage to the optic nerve at its head or the optic disc.

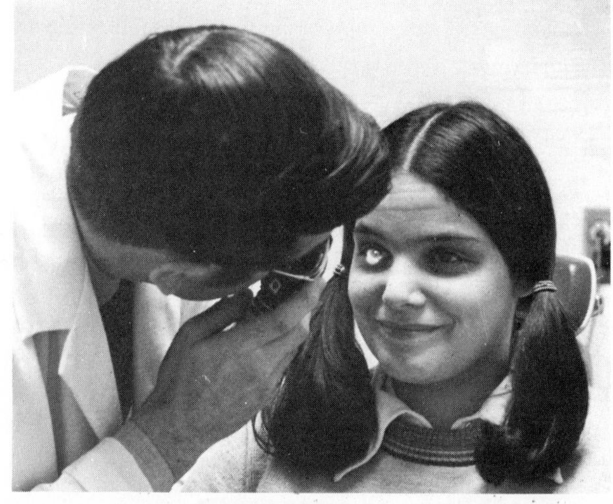

Fig. 37-3. Direct method of opthalmoscopic examination. Ophthalmoscope is used to examine optic disc, blood vessels, macula lutea, and fovea centralis of retina.

A rough measurement of the visual fields can be made by using the confrontation test (p. 000). If there appears to be any abnormality in the field of vision, more precise testing should be done with precision instruments by an ophthalmologist or a specially trained technician.

Evaluation of ocular fundus

The fundus, or back portion of the interior of the eye, is examined with an ophthalmoscope. The ophthalmoscope magnifies the view of the back of the eye so that the optic nerve, retina, blood vessels, and nerves can be seen through the pupil. The examiner may use either the direct (Fig. 37-3) or the indirect (Fig. 37-4) method of ophthalmoscopic examination. When examined with the indirect ophthalmoscope, the person may experience a great deal of light sensitivity. The direct method is the more commonly used approach. The entire retina is not visualized at one time, so the examiner moves the ophthalmoscope until the entire fundus is visualized. (For further discussion on the use of the ophthalmoscope, see p. 640).

Difficulty in perceiving the fundus may be due to interference with the light penetrating the eye as a result of intraocular inflammation, corneal scarring, or cataract. Data obtained from visualization of the fundus may indicate eye disease (cupping of the disc in glaucoma) or systemic disease (arteriosclerosis, hypertension). Hemorrhages in deep retinal layers occur in advanced hypertension, severe renal disease, certain collagen diseases, advanced diabetes, and blood dyscrasias.

Estimation of intraocular pressure

An instrument known as a *tonometer* is used to measure ocular tension and is helpful in detecting early glaucoma. Some ophthalmologists suggest that tonometric readings be taken by the medical internist or the family physician as part of a regular annual physical examination. The most common indentation tonometer in clinical use is that of Schiøtz. The procedure is performed with the individual lying down and looking upward at some fixed point. The eye may be anesthetized with one or two drops of proparacaine hydrochloride (Ophthaine), 0.5%, after which the tonometer is placed on the cornea (Fig. 37-5). While the weight of the tonometer is supported by the cornea, the amount of indentation that the plunger of the instrument makes in the cornea is measured on the attached scale. This reading is used to determine the pressure within the eye. Readings over 24 mm Hg (Schiøtz) may suggest glaucoma, but tests usually are repeated because temporary increases sometimes may be caused by such things as emotional stress.

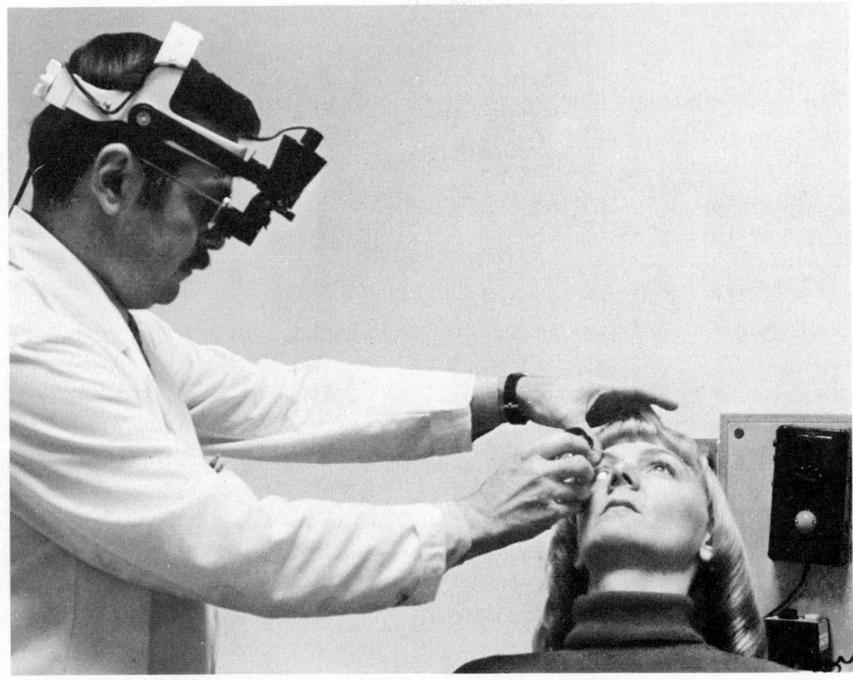

Fig. 37-4. Indirect method of ophthalmoscopic examination. Indirect ophthalmoscope provides binocular view of fundus and allows excellent observation of extreme periphery of retina.

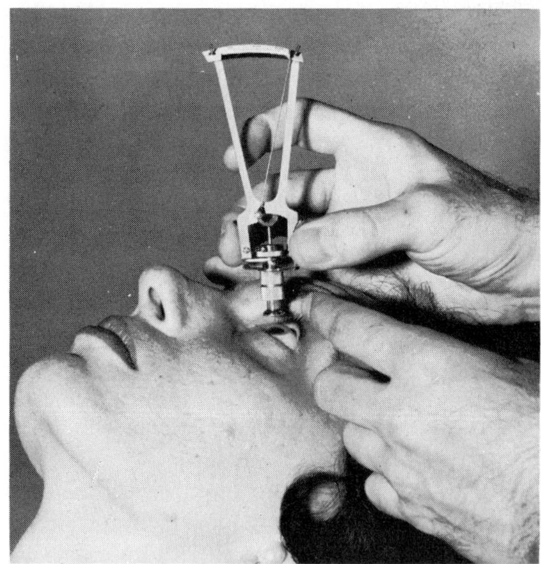

Fig. 37-5. Measurement of intraocular pressure with Schiøtz tonometer. (From Havener, W. H., Saunders, B. A., Keith, C. F., and Prescott, A. W.: Nursing care in eye, ear, nose, and throat disorders, ed. 3, St. Louis, 1974, The C. V. Mosby Co.)

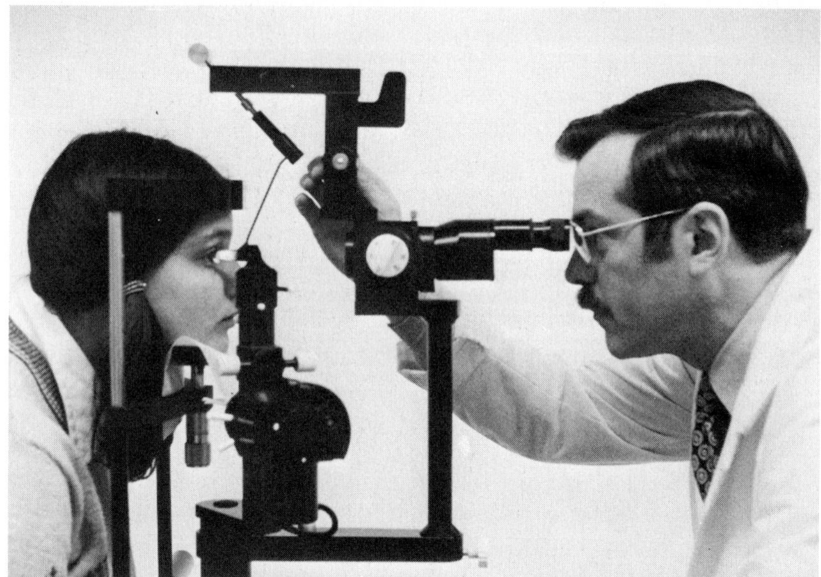

Fig. 37-6. Measurement of ocular tension with Goldmann applanation tonometer.

The applanation tonometer (Goldmann) is more accurate in estimating intraocular pressure (Fig. 37-6). The applanation tonometer is attached to the slit lamp. Instead of indenting the eye, a small area of the cornea is flattened to counterbalance a spring-loaded measuring device, and the pressure is measured directly. Newer means of tonometry include the air tonometer, the scleral and air indentation types, and the electronic tonometer.

■ ASSESSMENT OF EARS AND HEARING

Assessment of the ear and its functioning is done by physicians, nurses, audiologists, and occasionally by some paraprofessional health workers. Lay persons can be trained to conduct hearing screening tests for preschool-aged and school-aged children. Assessments of the ear structures and sophisticated assessment of ear functioning are done by physicians, nurses, and audiologists.

The nurse's exact activities in assessment depend on the nurse's education and focus of care. All nurses, however, should be prepared to carry out an inspection of the outer ear and at least a gross assessment of hearing ability for all persons entering a health care setting regardless of the presenting problem. Gross assessment of hearing may be accomplished by evaluating the logical sequences of replies during the admission history. One method is to turn one's head away from the individual when asking a simple question that cannot be answered by a yes or no response.

A complete hearing assessment consists of subjective data from the history relating to the person's perceived difficulties with hearing or a family history of hearing loss and objective data obtained by inspection of the external structures of the ear and audiometric testing of hearing. Additional objective data include behavioral signs indicating the need for more complete hearing assessment.

For clarity of discussion the ear and its structures are presented in three parts: the outer ear, the middle ear and mastoid process, and the inner ear.

□ Early identification of hearing loss

The detection of persons with hearing impairment is an important nursing responsibility. Often the nurse is the first member of the health team to be approached by persons seeking help regarding hearing problems. Community screening programs for detecting children with possible hearing losses are helpful in limiting the handicap by getting the child under medical care. Identification of persons who are having difficulty hearing and helping them and other family members in understanding the problem and improving their communication is important.

Behavioral clues useful in assessing hearing difficulties are listed by age group in the box at right. The person who seems to be inattentive or who has a strained facial expression, particularly when conversing or listening to others, may be hard of hearing. An early indication of loss of hearing is difficulty communicating in noisy environments as compared with quiet ones. Persons with faulty articulation in speech may be deaf; this may result from not being able to hear themselves speak. The person who habitually fails to respond when spoken to or who makes mistakes in carrying out directions should be encouraged to have his hearing tested. The repetition of, "What did you say?" or "Uh huh" with a quizzical expression is often a symptom of hearing loss. Persons who exhibit any of these behavioral clues should be encouraged to have their hearing tested and are referred to the otolaryngologist in the event that the hearing loss is caused by more serious disease.

The nurse can help find and direct the person with a hearing loss and his family to the appropriate agencies for assistance (p. 777). There may be ways of improving hearing through medical or surgical therapy. If the loss is irreversible, aural rehabilitation may make it possible for the person with hearing loss to understand and communicate with others so that he can lead a useful, mean-

BEHAVIORAL CLUES INDICATING DIFFICULTY IN HEARING

Infant
- Decreased or absent babbling
- Failure to produce syllables with distinct consonants (e.g., mama, dada)
- Difficult to awaken without touching
- Comforted only when held
- Decreased response to speech, musical toys, noisemakers

Toddler, preschooler
- Delayed speech and language development
- Communicates wants through gesturing
- Emotionally immature, demanding, fearful, tantrums
- Responds to vibration and touch more than speech or noise
- Ignores telephone and doorbell

Schoolchild
- Scholastic performance below level of apparent ability
- Truancy problem
- May be labeled as slow learner or behavior problem
- Asks to have things repeated
- Inattention, daydreaming
- Irrelevant answers
- Hears better when watching speaker's face
- Withdrawn, bored, or disinterested in activities involving conversation
- Deviations in speech, mispronounces or omits some sounds
- Monotonous voice tone
- Interrupts without being aware of it
- Hears better in noisy environment where people shout
- Undue tension and fatigue with normal activities
- Seems to hear better at some times than others
- Fails to follow directions or does so incorrectly
- Turns up volume and sits close to television
- Has frequent respiratory infections or earaches with subsequent changes in behavior

Adult
- Irritability, hostility, hypersensitivity in interpersonal relations
- Difficulty in hearing upper-frequency consonants
- Complains about people mumbling
- Turns up volume on television
- Asks for frequent repetition and answers questions inappropriately
- Loses sense of humor, becomes grim
- Leans forward to hear better, face serious and strained
- Shuns large and small group audience situations
- May appear aloof and "stuck up"
- Complains of ringing in the ears
- Voice may be unusually soft or loud

ingful life. Rehabilitation is more difficult if loss of vision is present in addition to loss of hearing.

□ Assessment of external ear

Anatomy and physiology

The external ear has two parts: the *auricle*, or pinna, and the *ear canal* (Fig. 37-7). The auricle is generally made up of cartilage and skin with little subcutaneous fat except for the lobule. The blood and lymphatic supply to the auricle is excellent. The nerve supply to the external ear is chiefly from the trigeminal (fifth cranial) nerve and a branch of the vagus (tenth cranial) nerve going to the posterior part of the ear canal, and from the cervical nerves. The external ear and auditory canal provide a channel along which sound travels to the tympanic membrane. The outer third of the canal is lined with skin containing wax and sweat glands. The inner part of the canal is lined with squamous epithelium.

Physical assessment

The assessment of the external ear begins with inspection of the auricle and surrounding tissues for deformities, lumps, or skin lesions. The normal auricle varies considerably from person to person. Observations include the placement of the ears on the head; the normal ear is set so that the upper tip of the pinna is on a line with the corner of the eye and occipital protuberance at the back of the head. Abnormalities in the height of the ear can indicate the presence of some congenital defects such as Down's syndrome and trisomy.[21] Normally the ear is attached vertically to the head; attachments with deviation more than 10° from vertical are abnormal and should be referred to an otolaryngologist.[1]

Shape, size, and degree of protrusion of the ears from the head are also noted in addition to redness or scratches, particularly in the crevices behind the ear. Some common nodules bound in and around the ear include furuncles, palpable lymph nodes anterior to the tragus or overlying the mastoid process, sebaceous cysts especially behind the ear, tophi (deposits of uric acid crystals characteristic of gout), and chondrodermatitis helcis (a small, chronic, painful, tender nodule in the superior helix). Since the latter may be confused with skin cancer, biopsy is important.

If ear pain, discharge, or inflammation is present, the ear is checked for tenderness by moving the auricle and

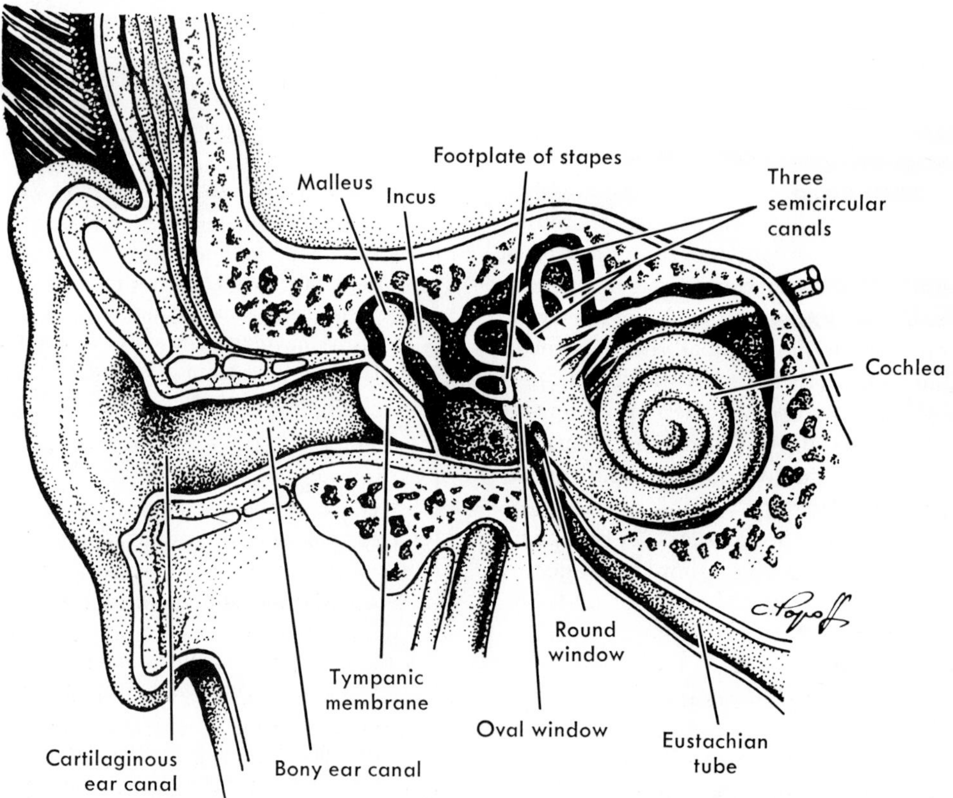

Fig. 37-7. External auditory canal, middle ear, and inner ear. (From Malasanos, L., Barkauskas, V., Moss, M., and Stoltenberg-Allen, K.: Health assessment, St. Louis, 1977, The C. V. Mosby Co.)

pressing on the tragus and mastoid process. Pain on movement of the auricle and tragus is a symptom of acute external otitis (p. 798) and distinguishes it from otitis media (p. 800). Tenderness of the mastoid process suggests mastoiditis (p. 801).

For inspection of the ear canal the adult is instructed to tip his head slightly to the opposite side while the examiner pulls the auricle up, back, and out. The auricle of an infant or small child is held down and out. A penlight may be used for inspection, although a good practice in assessing and in treating the ear canal is to use an adjustable light such as a standing gooseneck lamp that does not need to be held. The ear canal is examined for the presence of wax, discharge, or foreign bodies and for redness or swelling, which may indicate acute external otitis.

The use of an otoscope may be necessary to dilate and straighten the ear canal for easier examination (Fig. 37-8). The largest speculum that the ear will accommodate is used. The speculum is inserted slightly down and forward. The ear canal often has to be cleansed of cerumen (wax), desquamated epithelium, and other accumulations with a cotton wick, cotton-tipped applicator, cerumen spoon, or "loop" before the eardrum can be seen.

□ Assessment of middle ear

Anatomy and physiology

The external ear is separated from the middle ear by the tympanic membrane (eardrum) (Fig. 37-7). It is a fairly tough membrane that serves to protect the middle ear and also vibrates with incoming sound waves for hearing. The middle ear, which lies directly behind the eardrum, is a small air-filled space in the tympanic portion of the temporal bone. It contains the three small bones (ossicles): *malleus, incus, and stapes.* The footplate of the stapes fits into the oval window, which is a small opening in the wall between the middle ear and the inner ear. The ossicles amplify sound waves received by the tympanic membrane and transmit them through the membrane in the oval window to the fluid in the inner ear. Also communicating with the middle ear is the *eustachian tube*, which allows air into the middle ear, thus equalizing pressure on both sides of the eardrum. The middle ear communicates posteriorly with mastoid air cells. The *chorda tympani* of the seventh cranial (facial) nerve is also located in the middle ear.

Physical assessment

The tympanic membrane is inspected by using the otoscope with the largest speculum that the ear will accommodate (Fig. 37-8). The tympanic membrane is positioned at a slant with the upper edge nearer the front; therefore care is needed when inserting the speculum so as not to push against the membrane. Young children who have difficulty remaining still may have to be restrained for examination of the eardrum. An otoscope with a magnifying lens commonly is used to supplement the examination with a speculum, particularly for small children. The ear may require examination under a binocular microscope, which provides depth perception as well as increased magnification (Fig. 37-9). Sometimes the view of the tympanic membrane may be obstructed by cerumen, which must be removed, and an ear irrigation (p. 770) may be necessary. If a perforated tympanic membrane is suspected, irrigation is not done because of the possibility of enlarging the perforation or of allowing contaminated fluid to enter the middle ear. *Pneumatic otoscopy*, in which air is compressed into the ear canal, exerting pressure against the drumhead, may be performed (Fig. 37-10, *A* and *B*). It is particularly useful in detecting pinhole perforations that otherwise might not be found, since middle ear secretions are drawn through them by the suction.

The eardrum is important in physical assessment of the middle ear because it serves as a translucent window through which disease processes in the middle ear may be inferred. The normal tympanic membrane is pearly gray and presents certain landmarks (Fig. 37-11). The prominent short process of the *malleus* (the first of the ossicles) stands out like a tiny knot. Extending downward from the short process is the *manubrium* with the *umbo* at the end. The tympanic membrane is shaped like a cone and thus reflects light in the shape of a triangle. The triangular reflection is called the light reflex. The membrane is stretched tight except for the part above the manubrium, which is flaccid and is called the *pars flaccida.*

Abnormal findings on physical assessment include inflammation, blue or black (hemorrhage) coloring of the membrane, and bulging of the tympanic membrane. Purulent material such as might be present from acute otitis media[2] (p. 800) may be seen through the thin membrane and may be white or amber. When the eardrum perforates, the fluid behind the membrane bursts out into the auditory canal and results in a discharge, which is examined for odor and color and then cultured. Because mastoiditis is a complication of otitis media (p. 801), the mastoid bone should be firmly pressed. If pain is elicited when pressure is applied to the bone, *mastoiditis* should be suspected. Sensation of pressure or blockage of the middle ear unrelieved by yawning or swallowing may indicate *otitis media.* Crackling in the ear may also be associated with otitis media, probably as the result of dried debris or fluid in the middle ear. Insufflation of the eustachian tubes may or may not be performed during physical assessment of the middle ear. Insufflation may be performed either to test the patency of

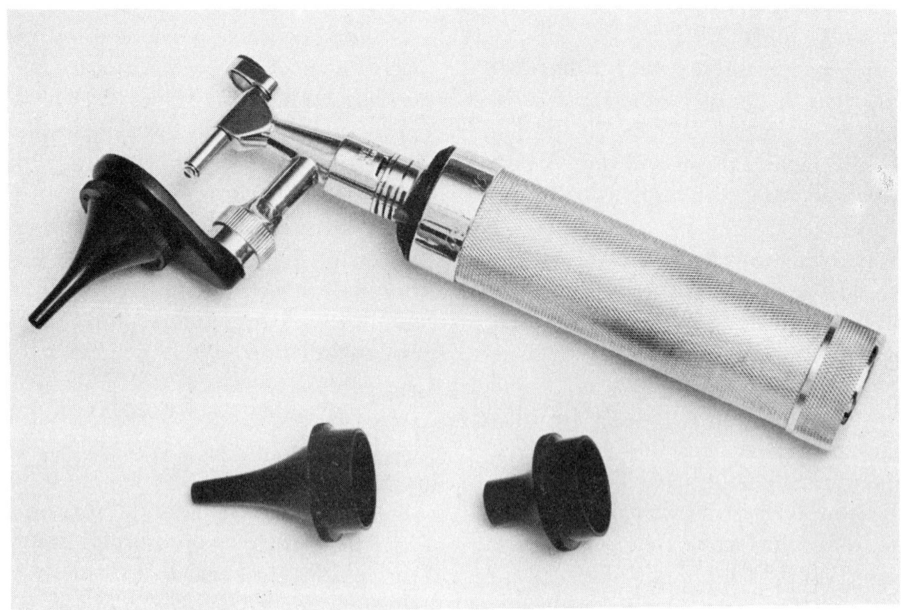

Fig. 37-8. Otoscope.

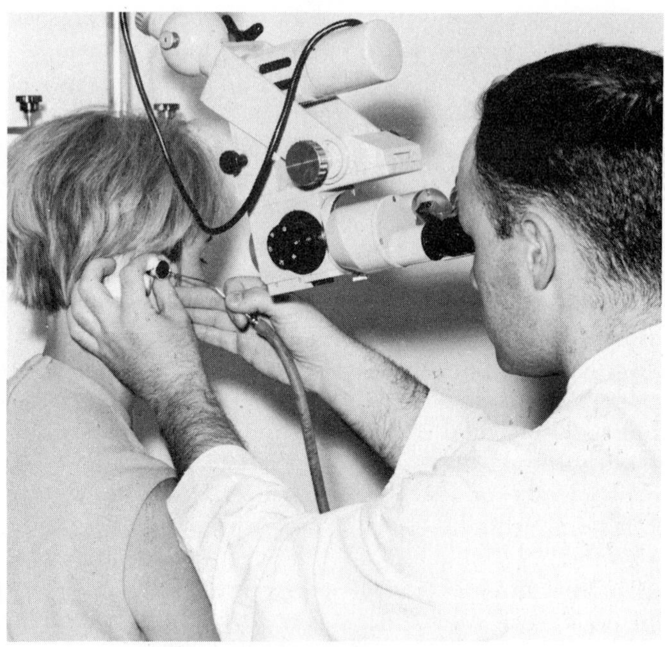

Fig. 37-9. Operating microscope used as diagnostic instrument. Small aural suction tip aspirates serum or pus from ear canal or middle ear. (From DeWeese, D. D., and Saunders, W. H.: Textbook of otolaryngology, ed. 5, St. Louis, 1977, The C. V. Mosby Co.)

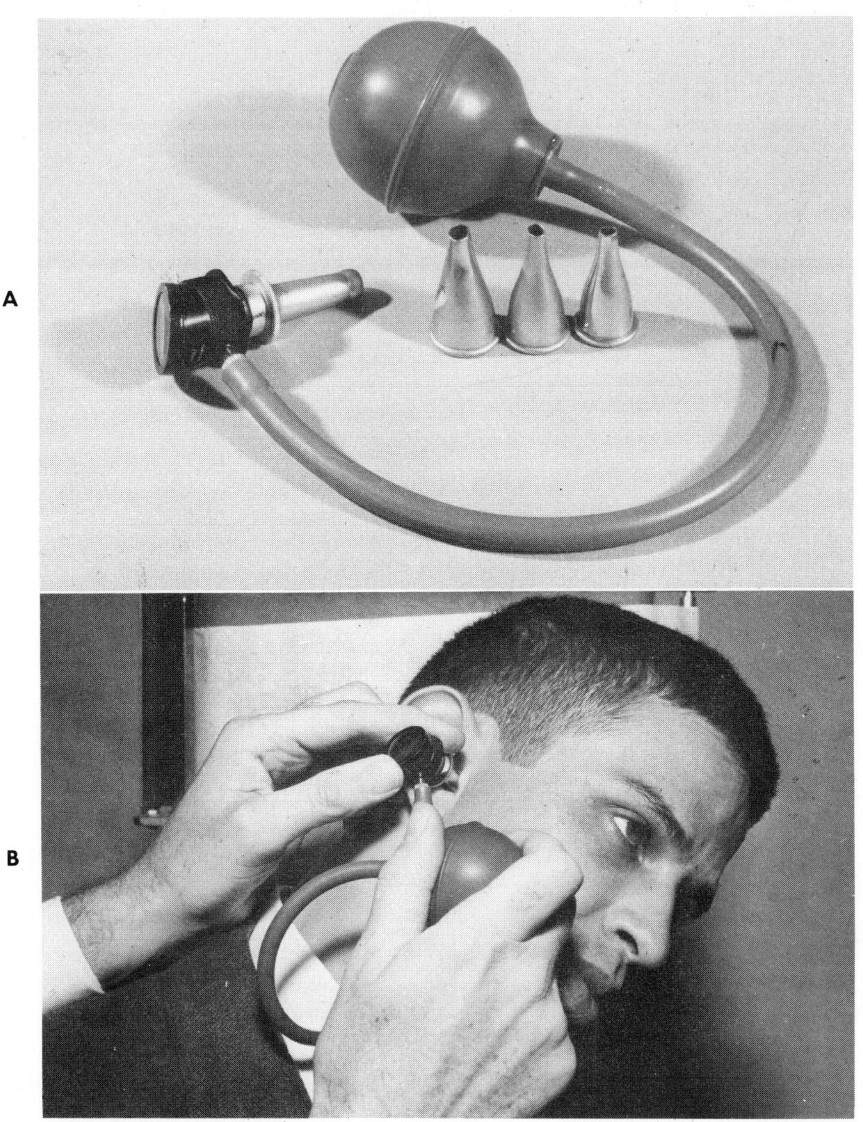

Fig. 37-10. A, Siegle pneumatic otoscope. Speculum that fits otoscope is attached. Magnifying lens also may be used with usual type of speculum if magnification only is desired. **B,** Pneumatic otoscope in use. (From DeWeese, D. D., and Saunders, W. H.: Textbook of otolaryngology, ed. 4, St. Louis, 1973, The C. V. Mosby Co.)

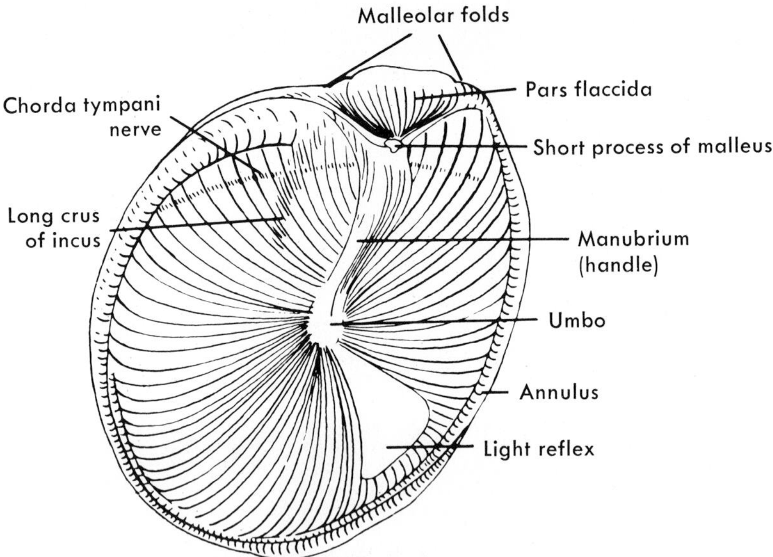

Fig. 37-11. Right tympanic membrane. (From Prior, J. A., and Silberstein, J. S.: Physical diagnosis: the history and examination of the patient, ed. 5, St. Louis, 1977, The C. V. Mosby Co.)

the eustachian tubes or to mechanically force them open. Insufflation of the eustachian tube is accomplished by having the patient compress his nose with his thumb and forefinger, close his mouth, and blow both cheeks out (modified Valsalva maneuver).

□ Assessment of inner ear

Anatomy and physiology

The inner ear or *labyrinth* contains both the organ of hearing, the cochlea, and the organ of balance, the vestibule (Fig. 37-7). The labyrinth, made up of delicate nerve tissue, will not recover if damaged. The inner ear is protected from damage by being situated deep in the head in the petrous bone. Two separate fluids, the perilymph and the endolymph, are found in tiny channels in the labyrinth. The endolymph is contained in a membranous tube, which is then surrounded by the perilymph, which cushions the tube. The endolymph is in a contained closed system, while the perilymphatic spaces connect with the subarachnoid space and its cerebrospinal fluid.

The end organ for hearing, the organ of Corti, has thousands of tiny "hair cells" that project from its neuroepithelium. Sound waves enter the cochlea and mechnically bend the hair cells. At this time sound, which had been a mechanical force, is converted into an electrochemical impulse. The impulse travels along the acoustic nerve to the temporal cortex of the brain and is interpreted as meaningful sound. The hair cells are the most fragile elements in the ear and are crucial to hearing; as long as a person has normal hair cells he may have some hearing. In some instances persons with normal hair cells are unable to hear because of destruction of the eighth cranial nerve by a tumor.

Normal hearing process

Functional examination of the inner ear may be better understood by a short review of the normal hearing process (Fig. 37-12). Sound is a form of energy generated by a vibrating source. Pure tones such as those generated by a tuning fork are simple sound waves. The human voice, however, produces more complex sound waves. *Intensity* of sound is actually the pressure exerted by a sound and is measured in decibels (dB). *Loudness* is not quite the same as intensity but refers to the sensation experienced by a person to the intensity of sound. Speech that is comfortably loud to a person with normal hearing ranges in intensity from approximately 40 to 65 dB.

Frequency refers to the number of sound waves emanating from a source per second and is expressed in hertz (Hz). *Pitch* relates to frequency and describes a sensation experienced by a person rather than a physical measurement. A sound with a low frequency is perceived as a tone low in pitch, whereas a sound with high frequency is perceived as a high-pitched tone. A child or

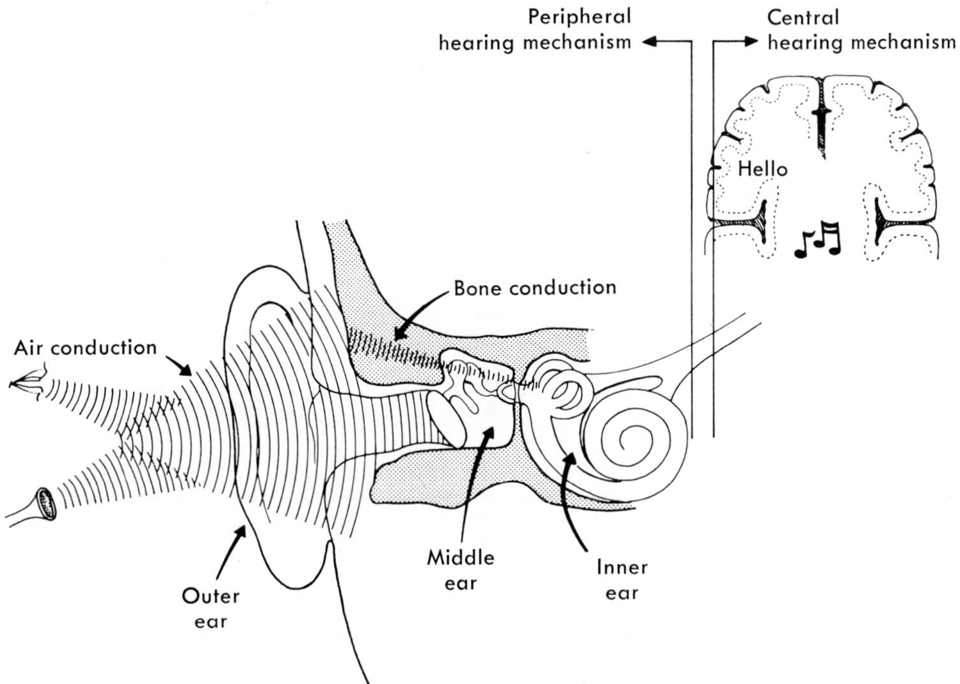

Fig. 37-12. Schema depicting functions of hearing mechanism as it translates sound waves into meaningful sensations. (From Havener, W. H., Saunders, W. H., Keith, C. F., and Prescott, A. W.: Nursing care in eye, ear, nose, and throat disorders, ed. 3, St. Louis, 1974, The C. V. Mosby Co.)

young adult with normal hearing can often hear frequencies ranging from 20 to 20,000 Hz. Hearing is most sensitive for frequencies of 500 to 4,000 Hz.

Sound reaches the inner ear by one of two ways: air conduction or bone conduction. Air conduction is the more sensitive. In air conduction sound waves pass through the ear canal to the ossicular chain to the inner ear. In bone conduction hearing is caused by sound being transmitted through the bones of the skull to the inner ear. Sound energy is transformed in the inner ear into neural energy and is then "decoded" and interpreted by the brain as sound.

Testing

The inner ear cannot be examined visually. Functional examination is done by testing hearing by audiometry and by testing function of the semicircular canals by the caloric examination (p. 752) or electronystagmography (p. 752). Complete examination of the ear must include a hearing examination.

A child's acquisition of speech is critically dependent on proper hearing. It is imperative that if a hearing loss is suspected by the parent or health professional the child be referred to an otologist for a medical examination and to an audiologist for proper testing. Until the child is 4 to 5 years of age, he may be difficult to test by conventional methods. Impedance audiometry is very useful for testing young children. Special testing procedures utilize rewards for correct responses and aid in conditioning the child to behave in an expected manner if he hears the sound. Audiology is presently at a very sophisticated level and yields much information as to the child's hearing status, although definitive statements about hearing often cannot be made. All statements referring to hearing capabilities of very young children should be guarded and interpreted with care.[10] It should be remembered, however, that given the proper testing facilities and setting, it is possible for the audiologist to make a gross assessment of the hearing of a child or infant of any age. Proper management and counseling can only be initiated once bearing loss is suspected and the child is properly evaluated.

Audiometry. Functional examination for sensitivity (ability to hear sounds) and for speech discrimination (ability to distinguish different speech sounds) is done by audiometry. The graph of the hearing levels of both

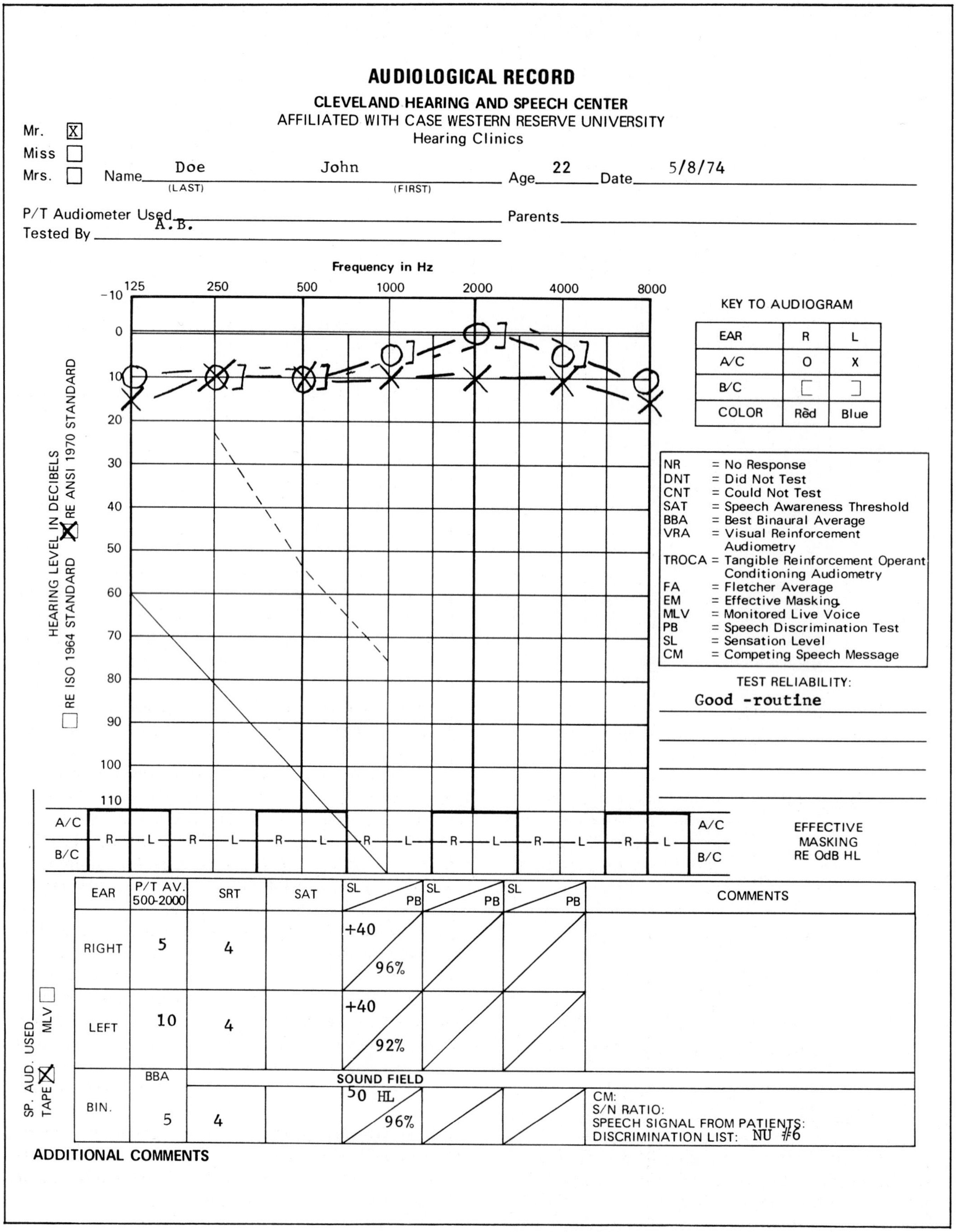

AUDIOLOGICAL RECORD

CLEVELAND HEARING AND SPEECH CENTER
AFFILIATED WITH CASE WESTERN RESERVE UNIVERSITY
Hearing Clinics

Mr. [X]
Miss [ ]
Mrs. [ ] Name Doe (LAST) John (FIRST) Age 22 Date 5/8/74

P/T Audiometer Used ______ Parents ______
Tested By A.B.

Frequency in Hz

125 250 500 1000 2000 4000 8000

HEARING LEVEL IN DECIBELS [ ] RE ISO 1964 STANDARD [X] RE ANSI 1970 STANDARD

-10 0 10 20 30 40 50 60 70 80 90 100 110

A/C — R — L — R — L — R — L — R — L — R — L — R — L — R — L — A/C
B/C B/C

KEY TO AUDIOGRAM

EAR	R	L
A/C	O	X
B/C	[	]
COLOR	Red	Blue

NR = No Response
DNT = Did Not Test
CNT = Could Not Test
SAT = Speech Awareness Threshold
BBA = Best Binaural Average
VRA = Visual Reinforcement Audiometry
TROCA = Tangible Reinforcement Operant Conditioning Audiometry
FA = Fletcher Average
EM = Effective Masking
MLV = Monitored Live Voice
PB = Speech Discrimination Test
SL = Sensation Level
CM = Competing Speech Message

TEST RELIABILITY:
Good -routine

EFFECTIVE MASKING RE OdB HL

SP. AUD. USED TAPE [X] MLV [ ]

EAR	P/T AV. 500-2000	SRT	SAT	SL / PB	SL / PB	SL / PB	COMMENTS
RIGHT	5	4		+40 / 96%			
LEFT	10	4		+40 / 92%			
	BBA			SOUND FIELD			
BIN.	5	4		50 HL / 96%			CM: S/N RATIO: SPEECH SIGNAL FROM PATIENTS: DISCRIMINATION LIST: NU #6

ADDITIONAL COMMENTS

Fig. 37-13. Normal audiogram. (Courtesy Cleveland Hearing and Speech Center, Cleveland, Ohio.)

of these is called an audiogram (Fig. 37-13). *Hearing threshold* is defined as the lowest intensity of sound at which an auditory stimulus can be heard. Speech considered comfortably loud to a person with normal hearing ranges from 40 to 65 dB. Fig. 37-14 lists the decibel level of various environmental sounds and situations.

In recent years audiologists (specialists in administering hearing tests) have developed some very useful audiometric tests such as pure tone audiometry to determine not only whether a hearing loss is present but also the frequency of the loss, how well the person can understand speech, and whether the problem site is in the middle ear (conductive loss), inner ear, or auditory nerve system (sensorineural loss). (See pp., 768 and 769 for further discussion of the types of hearing loss.) Pure tone audiometry must be performed in a specially constructed soundproof booth for best results. Group screening examinations such as are done in schools are only helpful in detecting children who need individual examination.

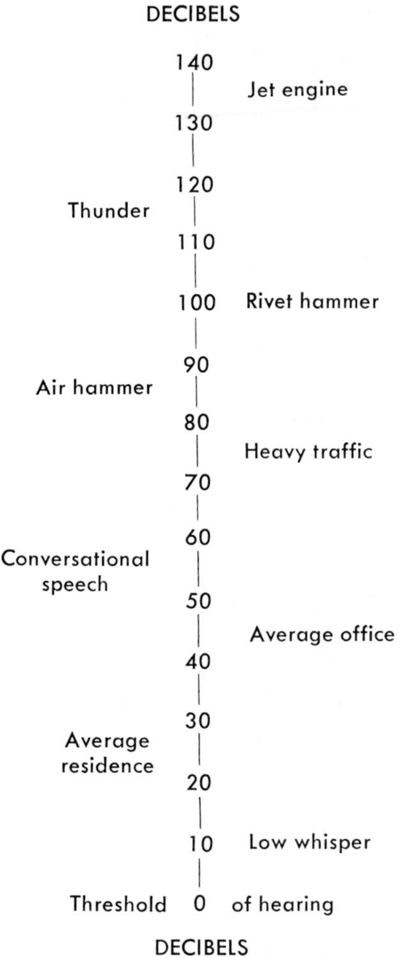

Fig. 37-14. Intensity range of human hearing. Intensity levels of various environmental sounds and situations. (From Havener, W. H., Saunders, W. H., Keith, C. F., and Prescott, A. W.: Nursing care in eye, ear, nose, and throat disorders, ed. 3, St. Louis, 1974, The C. V. Mosby Co.)

To test the sound intensity by air conduction, the person wears earphones and is instructed to signal with his finger when he first hears the tone and when he no longer hears it. The middle frequencies are tested first, and the operator alternately increases and decreases the intensity of sound until he or she finds the dial setting at which the person being tested can just perceive sound (threshold). In audiometric testing the frequencies 125, 250, 500, 1,000, 2,000, 4,000 and 8,000 Hz are commonly employed to assess the hearing sensitivity of an individual. Hearing loss is identified as the number of decibels reached before the person hears the sound for each specific frequency. Zero loudness is calibrated for that sound barely heard by a person with normal hearing. A range of O- to 20-dB loss for a tested frequency is considered to be within the normal range. Mild hearing loss ranges between 20 and 50 dB; moderate loss, 50 to 69 dB; severe loss, 70 to 89 dB; and profound hearing loss, above 90 dB.

Impedance audiometry is a technique that was developed because of the limitation of pure tone audiometry.[9,22] It provides a rapid and reliable means of assessing the presence or absence of abnormality of the conductive mechanism of the middle ear. It is an objective test in that it does not require a response from the individual and is therefore very valuable in assessing a child's hearing. The examinee sits with a headset on, and a mushroom-shaped plastic eartip is placed on a probe. This probe is inserted into the ear canal, an airtight seal is secured, and middle ear pressure measurements are obtained. The data consist of muscle reflex measurements in response to sound.

Speech audiometry is used to determine how well the person can hear and understand speech. There are two primary tests included in speech audiometry: the speech reception threshold (SRT) test and a speech discrimination test. The SRT is simply the lowest intensity level in decibels at which the person can correctly repeat specially selected bisyllabic words 50% of the time. Usually the SRT closely corresponds to the air conduction thresholds. Speech discrimination tests require the person to repeat 50 monosyllabic words common to the English language. These words are usually presented at an intensity level easily heard by the person (25 to 40 dB above the threshold). The number of correctly repeated words is converted to a percentage score. Individuals with normal hearing generally score 90% to 100% on this test.

Electrocochleography evoked response audiometry are also tests to assess hearing. EEG- type leads are attached, and clicks are played to the ear. Subsequent changes on the EEG recording are noted.

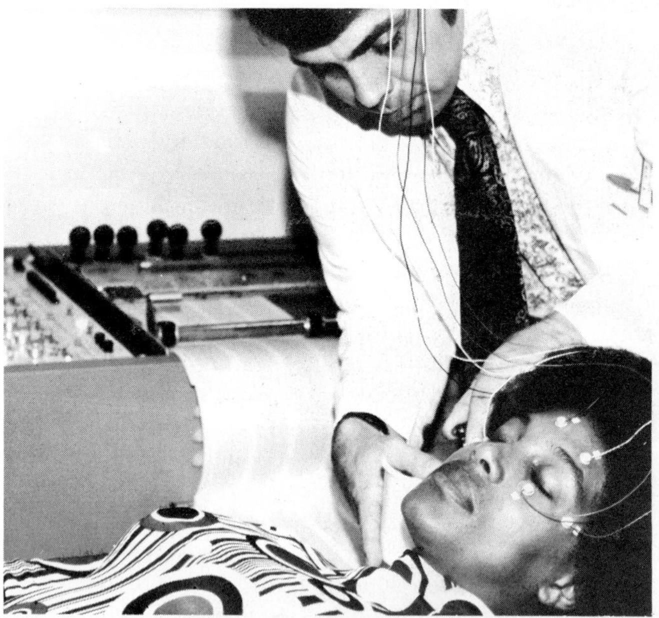

Fig. 37-15. Electronystagmography. Patient undergoing caloric stimulation as nystagmus is recorded on graph. (From DeWeese, D. D., and Saunders, W. H.: Textbook of otolaryngology, ed. 4, St. Louis, 1973, The C. V. Mosby Co.)

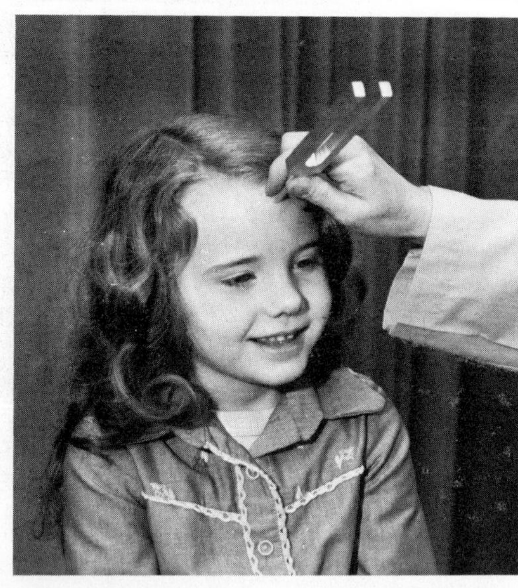

Fig. 37-16. Weber test. (From Malasanos, L., Barkauskas, V., Moss, M., and Allen, K. S.: Health assessment, St. Louis, 1977, The C. V. Mosby Co.)

Electronystagmography. Electronystagmography (ENG) is a test that records the position and movement of the eyeball by recording the changes in the electrical field around the eye when there is a change in position of the eye (Fig. 37-15). A graph is made of the amplitude, direction, and speed of *nystagmus,* which is an abnormal rhythmic jerking movement of the eyeball. ENG is useful in diagnosing vestibular disease and is an important test in evaluating persons with symptoms of vertigo, hearing loss, and tinnitus.

Both spontaneous nystagmus and induced nystagmus can be tested. Nystagmus occurs in normal persons after stimulation of the active vestibular labyrinth with cold or warm water (caloric test). In the caloric examination, cold or warm water is douched into the external auditory canal for 25 seconds (10 seconds for ice water). As the labyrinth is stimulated the person starts to become dizzy, and if stimulation is excessive some persons may vomit. Dizziness and nausea are accompanied by nystagmus.

Persons with no labyrinthine function have no reaction; persons with partial function have a hypoactive response. Persons with diseases of the central nervous system (such as acoustic neuroma) will have no reaction to the test or the nystagmus experienced will be abnormal; that is, nystagmus will be vertical rather than horizontal. Persons with Meniere's disease usually have a hypoactive reaction to caloric stimulation, sometimes unilaterally but often bilaterally.

Tests for hearing acuity. Gross examination of hearing acuity may be made by assessing the person's ability to hear a whispered or spoken voice or to hear a ticking watch. The ticking of a watch normally produces high-pitched tones and may be useful in testing persons for high-frequency sounds. Since hearing loss is often insidious in onset, all adults entering the health care system should have at least a gross examination of hearing.

Tuning fork tests are useful in testing hearing acuity and especially for discriminating conductive and sensorineural hearing losses. In the *Weber* test a tuning fork is placed in the center of the forehead or on the maxillary incisors (Fig. 37-16). Normally the sound is heard equally in both ears. If a person has *conductive* hearing loss, the hearing is *better* in the *affected* ear. This happens because the ordinary room noise tends to mask hearing in the normal ear; the ear with conductive hearing loss does not hear the room noise but receives sound waves by bone conduction. When *sensorineural* loss is present in one ear, the sound from the fork is louder in the *normal* ear.[7]

In the *Rinne* test bone conduction is compared with air conduction. The activated tuning fork is alternately placed opposite one external ear and on the adjacent mastoid bone (Fig. 37-17). In the person with normal

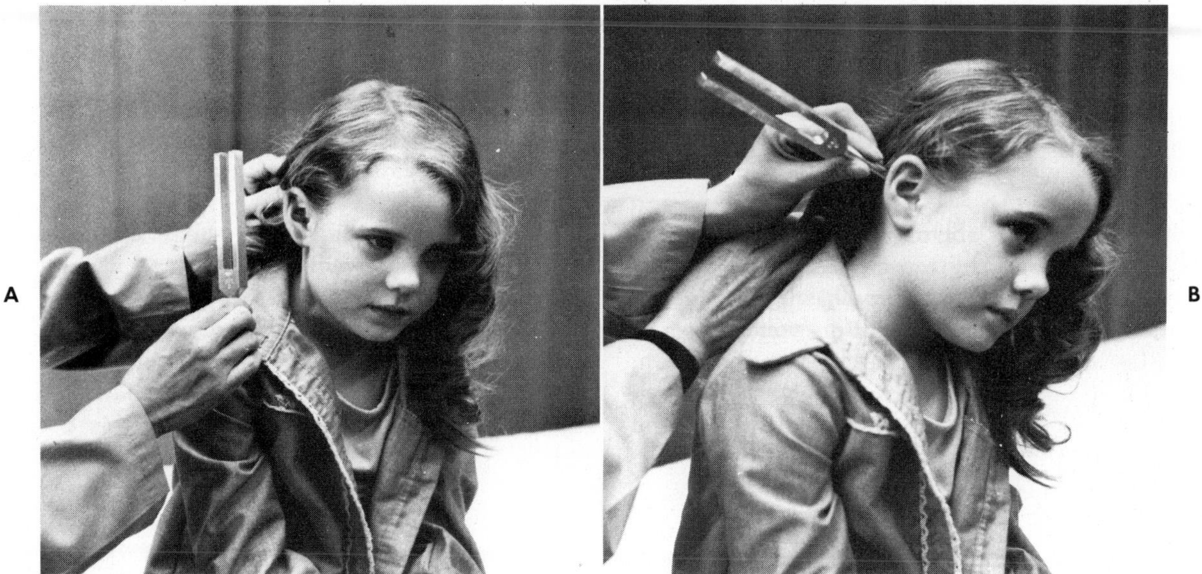

Fig. 37-17. Rinne test. **A,** Air conduction. **B,** Bone conduction. (From Malasanos, L., Barkauskas, V., Moss, M., and Allen, K. S.: Health assessment, St. Louis, 1977, The C. V. Mosby Co.)

hearing the vibrations are twice as long by air as by bone conduction. With conductive hearing loss the ratio alters in favor of bone conduction. In persons with sensorineural loss the ratio remains about the same, but both air and bone conduction are reduced.[7]

In the *Schwabach* test the hearing by bone conduction of the person being examined is compared with the bone conduction hearing (normal) of the examiner. The activated tuning fork is alternately placed on the individual's and the examiner's mastoid processes. Persons with normal hearing will hear the tone for the same length of time as the examiner. Persons with conductive losses will hear the tone longer than the examiner because the examiner's hearing will be masked by background noises. Persons with sensorineural loss will not hear the tone for as long as the examiner.

REFERENCES AND SELECTED READINGS

1. *Bates, B.: A guide to physical examination, Philadelphia, 1974, J. B. Lippincott Co.
2. Bergstrom, L., et al.: A high risk registry to find congenital deafness, Otolaryngol. Clin. North Am. **4:**369-379, 1971.
3. Dodds, J.: Testing hearing ability in the under fives, Nurs. Times **71:**1791-1792, 1975.
4. Downs, M. P.: Audiological evaluation of the congenitally deaf infant, Otolaryngol. Clin. North Am. **4:**347-357, 1971.
5. Downs, M. P., and Sterritt, G. M.: A guide to newborn and infant hearing screening programs, Arch. Otolaryngol. **85:**15-22, 1967.
6. Galloway, N. R.: Ophthalmic electrodiagnosis, Philadelphia, 1975, W. B. Saunders Co.
7. Havener, W. H., Saunders, W. H., Keith, C. F., and Prescott, A. W.: Nursing care in eye, ear, nose and throat disorders, ed. 3, St. Louis, 1974, The C. V. Mosby Co.
8. Hersch, L. B., and Amon, C.: A child has a hearing loss; reporting the diagnosis of handicaps in children and its impact on parents, Am. Ann. Deaf **120:**568-571, 1975.
9. Jerger, J.: Modern developments in audiology, New York, 1975, Academic Press, Inc.
10. *Judge, R. D., and Zuidema, G. D.: Physical diagnosis: a physiological approach to the clinical examination, ed. 2, Boston, 1968, Little, Brown and Co.
11. Lowenfels, A. B.: Letter: obtaining a history from hard-of-hearing patient, J.A.M.A. **233:**953, 1975.
12. *Malasanos, L., Barkauskas, V., Moss, M., and Allen, K. S.: Health assessment, St. Louis, 1977, The C. V. Mosby Co.
13. *Mechner, F., and Saffiati, L. J.: Patient assessment: examination of the eye, Am. J. Nurs. **74:**2039-2068, 1974.
14. Moller, A.: Basic mechanisms in hearing, New York, 1973, Academic Press, Inc.
15. Moore, M. V.: Diagnosis: deafness, Am. J. Nurs. **69:**297-300, 1969.
16. Norris, T. W.: Electronystagmography, New York, 1974, Medcom, Inc.
17. Programmed instruction: Patient assessment: examination of the ear, Am. J. Nurs. **75:**457-476, 1975.

*References preceded by an asterisk are particularly well suited for student reading.

18. Programmed instruction: Patient assessment: examination of the eye, part I, Am. J. Nurs. **74**:Suppl., Nov. 1974.
19. Programmed Instruction: Patient assessment: examination of the eye, part II, Am. J. Nurs. **75**:Supple., Jan. 1975.
20. Rubin, W.: Electronystagmography and its value in the diagram of vertigo. In Wolfson, R. J., editor: The Otolaryngologic Clinics of North America, Symposium on vertigo, Philadelphia, 1973, W. B. Saunders Co.
21. Sana, J. M., and Judge, R. D.: Physical appraisal methods in nursing practice, Boston, 1975, Little, Brown and Co.
22. Symposium on sensorineural hearing loss in children: early detection and intervention, Otolaryngol. Clin. North Am. 8(1), Feb. 1975.
23. Weinstock, F. J.: Tonometry screening, Am. J. Nurs. **73**:656-657, 1973.

AUDIOVISUAL RESOURCES

1. Physical diagnosis: examination of the eye, Cleveland, 1962. School of Medicine, Case Western Reserve University, Film (Edward Feil, producer), 25 min., sound, color, 16 mm.
2. Anatomy of the human eye series, 1972. Teaching films, 15 min. each. sound, color, super 8 mm.
3. Physical assessment of the eye and ear, Concept Media, 1500 Adams Ave., Costa Mesa, Calif. 92626, 1977. Slide-tape.
4. The ear, Department of Anatomy, University of Texas Medical School, San Antonio, Texas, 1971. Videotape, 20 min., color.
5. The ears, National Medical Audiovisual Center, Washington, D.C., 1970. Film, 16 mm. color.
6. The otorhinolaryngic examination, Brooke Army Medical Center, Fort Sam Houston, Texas, 1971. Videotape, color.
7. Child development: testing hearing in the pre-school child, National Medical Audiovisual Center, Washington, D.C., 1970. Motion picture, 16 mm, color.

38

Management of persons with special sensory problems: eye and ear

LYNN CHENOWETH McWILLIAMS
LINDA ANNE BROSEMAN

Reactions of health professionals and the general public to the blind or deaf person tend to be rather negative. There appears to be a general feeling that persons with sensory impairment are inferior, socially unacceptable, too difficult to deal with, and generally to be avoided. The person with normal sight and hearing may feel embarrassed, helpless, hostile, aggressive, and generally uncomfortable in dealing with people with impaired senses. Nurses can help co-workers and the general public become more informed about the nature of blindness and deafness and ways in which to relate to persons with sensory disabilities.

■ IMPACT OF SENSORY LOSS

The loss of a sense, be it hearing or sight, should be viewed in terms of a multiple handicap. In general a loss or a severe impairment of a sense can cause disequilibrium in a person's feelings of psychologic security. He may have a decrease in self-confidence, self-concept, or feelings of well-being. The physical integrity of the person has been breached, and confidence in the adequacy of the remaining senses may diminish. Some environmental stimuli are no longer perceived or are perceived differently.

Communication with others is also affected. If one cannot hear conversation or see others with whom one interacts, the desire or ability to retain contacts with others is impaired and the person may experience a feeling of isolation. Depending on the age at which the handicap occurs, written or spoken communication can be severely compromised. As mentioned previously, aesthetic enjoyment of that which is pleasurable or beautiful is diminished and the ability to share the human experience is decreased.

Loss or impairment of one of the senses may affect a person's activity. His mobility or ability to carry out activities of daily living may be restricted or at least modified. The ability or opportunity to carry out usual sexual roles or activities may also be affected. Career options, job opportunities, and financial security may be decreased. A sensory loss may influence the person's ability to remain independent, to feel socially adequate, or to feel that he is an esteemed contributing member of society.

■ COPING WITH SENSORY LOSS

Persons with sensory handicaps experience varying degrees of stress, isolation, and behavior changes depending on the extent and duration of the handicap, the age at which the handicap occurs, and how the person has successfully coped with stressors in the past. Other factors that influence the ability to cope include the support systems available to the person and the extent to which the handicap affects financial security and the ability to meet societal and familial role expectations.

Over a period of time people with a sensory loss appear to be able to compensate for their deficit by an increase in sensitivity in the other senses. For example, some people who are blind compensate for their deficit by increasing auditory acuity, tactile acuity, sense of smell, or kinesthetic awareness. People who are deaf tend to become keen observers.[62]

■ MANAGEMENT OF PERSONS WITH IMPAIRED VISION AND EYE PROBLEMS

Vision, one of a person's most priceless possessions, is essential to most employment and necessary in countless experiences that make life enjoyable and meaningful. Yet in the United States there are an estimated 475,000 legally blind persons.[8] Approximately 1.5 million Americans are so visually handicapped that they cannot read ordinary newsprint even with the aid of corrective lenses.[22] In underdeveloped countries of the world there is a high incidence of blindness from preventable causes such as malnutrition and eye infections. Although there has been a reduction of blindness in the United States from infections and certain diseases and injuries, there has been an increase in blindness resulting from diseases that occur most frequently among older persons. These include diabetic retinopathy, glaucoma, cataract, and retinal degeneration (see Chapter 39). It is likely that the incidence of blindness will increase in the future due to the steady growth in the number of persons aged 65 and older in the population.

□ Implications of impaired vision

Vision enables persons to experience pleasure and safety in the world about them. Of all the senses, the capacity to see is the most highly developed, critically needed, and cherished. In an opinion poll Americans indicated that they fear blindness more than any other physical problem with the exception of cancer.

Persons experiencing severe vision impairment or blindness have difficulty meeting basic human needs such as security, self-esteem, safety, nutrition, or activity, among others. Impaired vision interferes with learning, communication, mobility, and enjoyment of the environment.

□ Definition of impaired vision

Vision impairment ranges from refractive errors correctable with lenses to total blindness in which the person may not even be able to perceive light. For legal purposes blindness is defined very precisely in order to determine eligibility for assistance of various kinds. Although many nonseeing persons now prefer to be called "visually handicapped," the term "blindness" is still in common usage. See box below for the legal criteria of blindness.

□ Adjusting to impaired vision

The physician who is certain that blindness will occur or is irreversible will usually consider it best to be completely honest with the person and his family. When a person has been told that he will become blind, there is a normal reaction described by psychiatrists as a period of mourning for the "dead" eyes. Grief and mourning over the loss of vision cause emotional reactions such as denial, anger, guilt, resentment, loneliness, and depression. These strong emotional feelings interfere with the blind person's ability to plan for new ways of living. It is the responsibility of the nurse working with other members of the health team to help the individual and his family adjust to the condition of blindness or severe vision impairment.

Nurses can listen to the person talk of what blindness means to him; they can observe exaggerated reactions that might indicate thoughts of self-destruction; they can direct the person's thinking gradually along positive, constructive lines; and they can help to make available to him the resources that he will need.

The child who has never known sight adjusts well and is happy provided that he is treated as a normal child and is neither overprotected nor rejected. It is chiefly the parents who must adjust to and accept the child's handicap and be willing to use the resources available in the community to develop his independence and enable him to face problems of living. Both the parents and the child need special consultation and training in order to achieve this end.

It is important for the health worker to provide explanations and support to family members also, so that the family can provide the help and acceptance needed by the blind person.

LEGAL CRITERIA OF BLINDNESS*

A person is considered legally blind when either of the following conditions exist:

1. Visual field no greater than 20 degrees.
2. Central distance vision in better eye is 20/200 or worse with use of corrective lenses. This means the person can see at 20 feet what the person with normal vision can see at 200 feet.

*Report of the National Advisory Eye Council, U.S. Department of Health, Education and Welfare, No. (NIH) 75-664.

□ Prevention

Because nurses have contact with persons in all age groups and stages of development, they have the opportunity to be involved in many aspects of health care for the eye. These aspects include health education, care of the healthy eye, safety measures, and eye examination.

Health education in care of eyes

The nurse can explain the complex structure of the eye, teach people to care for their eyesight, and direct them to the proper specialist. A nurse also should recognize signs suggestive of eye disease and teach them to others. Knowledge of ophthalmic drugs, first aid for eye trauma, corrective lenses, eye patching, surgical procedures, and other modalities of assessment and treatment should be understood by the nurse. Nursing activities regarding protection of sight are outlined as follows and are described in succeeding paragraphs:

1. Protection of sight from impairment or further impairment:
   a. Teaching and providing safety measures and first aid

b. Promoting regular eye examination by an eye specialist
c. Detecting evidence of disease or impaired acuity
d. Explaining and administering treatments used to improve sight or prevent further loss (medications, surgery, eye patching)
2. Adjustment of the individual to impaired vision
a. Identifying basic human needs that have been affected
b. Understanding the effects on adaptation of different degrees of impairment (whether one or both eyes affected, partial or complete loss, acquired or congenital loss)
c. Assisting the newly blinded person through stages of psychologic adaptation to blindness
d. Assisting persons to cope with unmet needs for physical and emotional security, socialization, enhancement of self-esteem, and role identification
e. Using available community resources to help persons with impaired vision to cope more successfully (e.g., hospital, Lion's Club, school facilities, National Society for the Prevention of Blindness)

Care of healthy eyes

Normal healthy eyes do not need special local treatment. The secretions of the conjunctiva are protective and should not be removed by frequent bathing with unprescribed solutions. Boric acid solution and numerous trade preparations recommended to cleanse the eyes are usually unnecessary. Although these preparations are generally harmless, some proprietary solutions contain substances that may cause allergic reactions in sensitive persons.

People frequently treat eye ailments with proprietary remedies or with eyedrops and other medication that they or others have used at some time in the past. Self-treatment of the eyes is not only dangerous but may also lead to loss of much valuable time for treatment. There are many disorders that can affect the eyes for which many different drugs are used, each of which has a specific purpose. Two drugs may have completely opposite effects. Since liquids evaporate and drugs deteriorate or become contaminated with bacteria or fungus, use of preparations that a person or his friends have on hand can contribute to actual damage.

Boric acid solution, like other ophthalmic solutions, may present the problem of drug crystals precipitating on the tip of the dropper and then irritating the eye. Preparations containing phenylephrine hydrochloride, 0.8%, have been reported to produce sufficient mydriasis (dilation of pupil) to cause an attack of narrow-angle glaucoma in susceptible persons.[88] Contamination of ophthalmic solutions may also be a problem. It is best to *discard* any ophthalmic solution that is cloudy, discolored, has been opened for 3 months, or contains particles.

Many people believe erroneously that eyestrain causes permanent eye damage. Eyestrain actually refers to strain of the ciliary muscles when there is difficulty in accommodation. It causes a sense of fatigue but does not produce serious damage to the eyes. To avoid eyestrain a good light should be used when reading and doing work that requires careful visual focus, and extremely fine work should not be done for long periods of time without giving the eye muscles periodic rest. Looking at distant objects for a few minutes helps to rest the eyes after close work.

Care should be taken not to irritate the eyes or introduce bacteria into the eyes by rubbing them. Rubbing the eyes may be a natural response of many persons who are nervous, fatigued, or wear contact lenses. It also may be due to eczematous scaling, infection of the lids, or occasionally to louse attachment on the lashes. The cause of severe or chronic irritation should be investigated.

While adequate nutrition is as important for eye health as it is for maintaining other body functions, persons with nutritionally caused eye disorders are rarely found in the United States. Vitamin deficiencies can cause night blindness (vitamin A), corneal damage (vitamin A), optic neuritis (vitamin B), and other disorders. Although a sufficient vitamin intake is necessary, an excessive amount is wasted and may actually do more harm then good. For example, too much vitamin A can damage the optic nerve.[37] Some elderly persons and teenagers eat a diet consisting mainly of carbohydrates, which does not supply the protein, vitamins, and minerals needed for body growth and cell replacement. When assessing a person's nutritional status the nurse can learn if the person needs some assistance in meeting his need for adequate quantity and quality of nutrients (p. 1145).

Safety measures

Prevention of accidental injury to the eyes should be stressed in child and parent education. Slingshots, BB guns, and even seemingly harmless rubber bands and paper wads can be dangerous. The nurse can help physical education teachers and others to be alert to hazards to the eyes in gymnasiums and on playgrounds.

Protective goggles and break-resistant corrective lenses are available for persons engaging in very active physical exertion such as sports and selected occupations (see section on lenses, p. 758). The eyes should be protected by goggles or special dark glasses from prolonged exposure to very bright light such as sunlight over snow. They also need special protection from sudden flashes of light and heat that occur in some industrial occupations. Nurses may be asked the effect of television on the eyes.

There is no evidence that prolonged watching of television will damage eyesight.

First-aid measures necessary in the event of eye injury should be known by everyone; these measures can be taught in schools and in industry (p. 782). The sight of many persons could be saved each year if everyone understood the need for immediate copious flushing of the eye with water when an acid, alkali, or other irritating substance has been accidentally introduced. Much damage is done by the layman's well-intentioned efforts to remove foreign bodies from the eye and by not obeying the important rule of always washing the hands before attempting to examine the eye or to remove a foreign body.

It is essential to know that a person who has a foreign object lodged on the cornea must be referred to a physician; the layman should never attempt to remove it. The eye should be closed to prevent further irritation and the lids gently shut and loosely covered with a dressing or patch anchored with a piece of cellophane or adhesive tape. The person is advised not to squeeze the eye and is taken to an ophthalmologist at once.

Regular eye examinations

The eyes should be examined by an ophthalmologist at regular intervals throughout life. Many authorities believe the child should have his eyes examined at birth, at age 3 or 4 years, at approximately age 10, and in early adolescence. The young adult should consult an ophthalmologist at least every 5 years. After the age of 40 years the lens become firmer and less resilient (presbyopia). The individual begins to hold written material at a distance for better vision, and close vision may become blurred. Medical specialists recommend an eye examination every 2 years after the age of 35.

Since the eyes are often profoundly affected by conditions within the rest of the body, they cannot be considered alone. In fact, nearly all diseases cause some eye change that is diagnostically important. The nurse who is teaching eye health must be aware of *total health*. When apparently minor disease or abnormality of the eyes occurs, the nurse must be particularly alert for other signs of illness. Many serious medical conditions such as diabetes, renal disease, neurologic disease, and generalized arteriosclerosis may be diagnosed through early recognition of eye symptoms and examination of the eyes by an ophthalmologist.

There is widespread confusion and misunderstanding on the part of the public as to the proper specialist to consult about visual problems (see box above). People who demand the best care when other medical and surgical problems arise may fail to seek help from an ophthalmologist when they have eye difficulties.

In their search for help some people may purchase glasses from stores or use glasses originally prescribed for friends or relatives. Nurses can explain that eye conditions cannot always be remedied simply by the purchase of a pair of glasses or a change of lenses. A serious disease process such as glaucoma or cataract formation could be the cause of the problem.

PERSONS WHO SPECIALIZE IN EYE PROBLEMS OR IN VISUAL PROSTHESES

Ophthalmologist	Physician who specializes in the diagnosis and treatment of eye diseases; may also prescribe lenses
Oculist	Same as ophthalmologist
Optometrist	Professional person with special preparation in assessment of vision and in treatment of visual problems (e.g., prescribes lenses, visual training, or orthoptic exercises); is not a physician and does not treat eye diseases
Optician	Person who grinds and fits lenses according to prescriptions written by ophthalmologists or optometrists

Lenses

Eyeglasses. Acceptance of glasses seems to be influenced by the improvement in vision that they afford, the personality of the wearer, and the current fashion trends. To some persons, however, glasses may appear as a cosmetic blemish. Because there may be some stigma attached to wearing glasses, the young child will have a period of adjustment after receiving glasses. While the preschool child may reject glasses, he almost always accepts them on entering school when he realizes that without them he cannot see the blackboard. The vogue for attractive frames makes the wearing of glasses more acceptable to teenagers and adults. All persons should be encouraged to wear their glasses as prescribed and to have periodic examinations of their eyes by an ophthalmologist. Instructions for persons who wear glasses include how to clean their glasses, how to protect them from being scratched or broken, and how to care for them when they are removed.

Federal law now requires that all prescription glasses be made with impact-resistant lenses. Each finished lens must pass an impact test before it is dispensed. *Plastic* lenses weigh less than half of equivalent glass lenses but cost more and scratch more easily. They are useful for persons who wear thick lenses that are heavy when made of glass and for those who are active in sports. *Hardened* lenses have been exposed to a tempering process that makes them extremely hard and resistant to impact and breakage. *Safety* lenses are similar to hardened lenses but are 1 mm thicker. They are used in goggles worn by workmen whose eyes may be injured by such articles as chips of metal or glass.

Bifocal lenses consists of an upper portion of one focus used for distance and a lower part of another focus used for reading and close work. They make constant changing from distance to reading glasses unnecessary. *Trifocal* lenses are divided into three focuses to give correction for distance, intermediate, and near vision. *Sunglasses* should be carefully ground, large enough to exclude bright light around their edges, and dark enough to exclude about 30% of the light. The amount of light filtered can be varied according to the needs of the person.

Contact lenses. Contact lenses are thin shells of transparent, ground plastic material designed to be worn over the cornea (microlenses) or the cornea and sclera (scleral type) to replace eyeglasses. Although expensive, they may be used by persons who engage in sports because they do not fog or break easily, or they may be worn for cosmetic reasons. They are sometimes prescribed for persons who have a cone-shaped deformity of the cornea (keratoconus), which may prevent satisfactory fitting with conventional glasses. Elderly persons who have lenses removed because of cataracts benefit from wearing contact lenses but may have difficulty adapting to their use. Some industrial occupations prohibit the use of contact lenses because of irritation of the cornea from dirt or dust, which can become trapped under the lens.

Persons interested in wearing contact lenses are encouraged to consult an ophthalmologist who will make recommendations regarding their use. The person who dispenses the contact lenses may be an ophthalmologist, optometrist, or technician supervised by the former. "Hard" lenses are usually tinted, cover the cornea, and are the most frequently used type of contact lens. "Soft," or hydrophilic, lenses are flexible when in contact with the cornea and have been used successfully by many persons who cannot tolerate the hydrophobic hard lens. The disadvantages of the soft lens include a higher initial cost and need for more frequent replacement. They also are more difficult to clean and maintain. Newer types of lenses that have the optical qualities of the hard lens and the comfort of the soft lens are being explored. Scleral lenses are much larger than the other types and are less frequently used.

Contact lenses are inserted after being cleaned thoroughly and immersed in a wetting agent such as methylcellulose. Conjunctival secretions provide the lubrication needed for the lenses to be worn in comfort, and the lenses are held in place by capillary attraction and by the upper lid. Although some people wear the lenses continuously, a few can never physiologically or psychologically tolerate the constant presence of a foreign object in the eye. Contact lenses should not remain in the eyes for long periods of time as the epithelium of the cornea can be damaged through lack of oxygen.[29] If the patient is unconscious, the nurse removes the contact lenses (see box above) and stores them in a suitable container filled with saline solution or distilled water.[29]

REMOVAL OF CONTACT LENSES

Hard lens

Method 1:

1. Place finger at outer canthus of patient's eye.
2. Pull skin obliquely upward, then straight down.
3. Lens will appear on lower lashes as the upper lid moves downward.

Method 2:

1. Place finger or thumb of each hand at base of eyelashes.
2. Bring eyelids together, trapping the lens (the lens will eject).

Soft lens

1. Pull up upper lid with one thumb.
2. Grasp lens between thumb or forefinger of other hand and lift.

Scleral lens

1. Spread eyelids with both thumbs.
2. Exert slight downward pressure on upper lid (the lower edge of the lens will lift above the lid margin).
3. Slide thumbs to outer canthus to eject lens.

NOTE: A small suction device shaped like a miniature "plumber's helper" is available for removal of a contact lens.

Environment

The person who has loss of vision in both eyes depends on sound and tactile sensation to maintain his feeling of security and kinship with those around him. He must be spoken to frequently in a quiet and reassuring voice. This is particularly important when he is in a strange hospital environment and awaiting diagnostic procedures and perhaps surgery. It is upsetting for the person who cannot see to be touched without first being addressed; such an occurrence can be irritating and humiliating as well as actually dangerous. The nurse must teach all persons who attend the patient the importance of making their nearness known before touching him. They should introduce themselves and explain why they are there. On leaving the room they should inform him so that he is spared the embarrassment of talking to someone who is not there. A small bell often is given to a patient with visual loss instead of a call signal. It gives the patient who can hear the assurance that his request has been made. The person who is also deaf presents a real problem. If one cannot direct conversation into his ear and have it heard, there is no alternative but to touch him gently to make one's presence known. If he is to remain in contact with his environment, frequent physical contact must be made with him. Elderly persons who use hearing aids are urged to bring them to the hospital.

Most persons with eye conditions are more comfortable when the lighting is dimmed. Screens or curtains can be arranged so that bright light does not enter the room. Bright artificial lighting should be shaded. The patient in the hospital is usually happiest in a room with other patients, especially if both eyes are covered or if he is unable to see. The sound of voices and normal activity around him tends to relieve the feeling of isolation that the blinded person experiences. He benefits from having others around him who may, for example, share newspaper headlines with him. Some patients may prefer to be alone. Radios help the patient to keep up with everyday events. Recordings of entire books are also available.

Accidents present a real hazard when eye disease occurs, especially if an eye is covered or there is loss of vision. It is estimated that 20% of the field of vision is lost if one eye is covered or removed. If the onset of visual loss is slow, the person and his family may have sufficient time to eliminate common household hazards such as stairs without banisters. The partially blinded person who receives care on an ambulatory basis is taught to have someone accompany him to the physician's office or clinic because he may need additional help for a short time after certain treatments. In the hospital, special measures to prevent accidents are necessary. Side rails may be used, but low beds are safer, particularly for older patients who may forget that they are in a hospital bed. Particular effort should be made to have the space around the patient's bed and chair uncluttered; for example, bedside lamps must have short cords that do not fall to the floor. Furniture should be firmly anchored with casters locked. Rails along hallways and in bathrooms are also helpful.

Life for the person who has both eyes covered should be made as normal as possible. If he is used to smoking, he may be permitted to smoke, although someone must be in attendance to prevent a fire. Visitors should be allowed, though sometimes they need assistance in learning how to conduct themselves when they are with the patient who cannot see. They should be as natural as possible; for example, they should not make a conspicuous attempt to avoid such common phrases in speech as "see what I mean." Common sense dictates that gifts should appeal to other senses than vision. Scented colognes and soaps or a small bouquet of highly scented favorite flowers may be brought if the patient is not allergic to these items.

Restraints are sometimes necessary to prevent the patient from disturbing his dressings during sleep. They can be psychologically traumatizing even if carefully explained to the patient. The patient should be told that the restraints are used only to prevent him from accidentally disrupting his dressings. The use of side rails should also be explained. They are primarily to assist the patient in carefully shifting his position and to remind him not to get out of bed. They are not used to keep him in bed forcibly except in the case of patients with delirium tremens or acute brain syndrome.

□ Intervention
Medications

Accuracy in the administration of medications and treatments is essential. Irreparable damage can follow instillation of unprescribed or deteriorated preparations into the eyes. All medication bottles must be checked frequently for smearing or obliteration of labels. Solutions that have changed in color, are cloudy, contain sediment, or whose expiration date has passed are never used. Eye medications in the home are discarded when

Table 38-1. Mydriatic and cycloplegic drugs

Drug	Form and concentration	Duration of effect
Mydriatics		
Phenylephrine (Neo-Synephrine)	Eyedrops, 1% to 10%	12 hours
Epinephrine (Epitrate)	Eyedrops, 1% to 2%	12 hours
Cycloplegics		
Atropine sulfate	Eyedrops, 1% to 3% Ointment, 1%	2 to 4 weeks
Scopolamine (hyoscine)	Eyedrops, 0.25% to 0.5%	1 to 3 weeks
Homatropine hydrobromide	Eyedrops, 0.5% to 3% Ointment, 1% to 3%	1 to 2 days
Cyclopentolate hydrochloride (Cyclogyl)	Eyedrops, 0.5% to 1%	4 to 12 hours
Tropicamide (Mydriacyl)	Eyedrops, 0.5% to 1%	2 to 8 hours

Table 38-2. Drugs used in treatment of glaucoma

Drug	Form	Dose
Cholinergic drugs (miotics)		
Pilocarpine	0.5% to 3% solution	1 drop q6h
Carbachol (Carcholin)	0.25% to 3% solution	1 drop q6h to q8h
Cholinesterase inhibitors (miotics)		
Physostigmine (Eserine)	0.25% to 1% solution	1 drop q6h to q8h
Isoflurophate (DFP) (Floropryl)	0.01% to 0.1% solution	1 drop q24h to q48h
Demecarium bromide (Humorsol)	0.125% to 0.25% solution	1 drop q12h to q24h
Echothiophate iodide (Phospholine)	0.06% to 0.125% solution	1 drop q12h to q24h
Adrenergic agents		
Epinephryl borate (Eppy)	1% solution	1 drop q12h, often used with a miotic such as a cholinesterase inhibitor
Epinephrine hydrochloride (Glaucon)	2% solution	
Epinephrine bitartrate (Epitrate)	2% solution	
Carbonic anhydrase inhibitors		
Acetazolamide (Diamox)	250-mg tablets 500-mg tablets 500-mg vials for IM or IV use	
		1 tablet q6h to q8h
Ethoxzolamide (Cardrase)	125-mg tablets	1 tablet q12h
Dichlorphenamide (Daranide)	50-mg tablets	250 to 500 mg in
Methazolamide (Neptazane)	50-mg tablets	ml diluent
Osmotic agents		1 tablet q6h to q8h 1 tablet q6h to q8h
Glycerin	Mix with equal amount of orange juice	1 tablet q6h to q8h
Mannitol (Osmitrol)	10% to 20% solution for IV use	
Urea (Ureaphil)	30% solution for IV use	1 to 1.5 ml/kg body wt
		1 to 1.5 g/kg body wt 1 to 1.5 g/kg body wt

Table 38-3. Other ophthalmic drugs

Drug	Form	Dose
Antibiotics and antiviral drugs		
Polymyxin B, bacitracin (Polysporin)	Ointment or eyedrops, 0.1% to 1% solution	
Polymyxin B, neomycin, bacitracin (Neosporin)	Eyedrops or ointment	
Bacitracin	Ointment, 500 units/g	
Idoxuridine (IDU) (Herplex, Stoxil, Dendrid)	Eyedrops, 0.1% solution; ointment, 0.5%	
Steroids		
Prednisone	Topical, 0.25% to 0.5% suspension; oral, 5 to 15 mg	1 tablet q6h
Prednisolone	Topical ointment, 0.1% to 0.25%; oral, 5 to 15 mg	1 tablet q6h
Methylprednisolone (Depo-Medrol)	Subconjunctival, 0.5 mg; IM 4 mg	q 2 to 4 weeks
Triamcinolone (Aristocort)	Solution or ointment, 1%	
Dexamethasone (Decadron)	Solution or ointment, 0.1%	
Anesthetics		
Proparacaine (Ophthaine, Ophthetic)	Eyedrops, 0.5% solution	1 drop
Lidocaine (Xylocaine)	Local infiltration, 2% to 4% solution	4 ml
Lubricants and tear substitutes		
Methylcellulose, gonioscopic	Eyedrops, 1% solution	
Methylcellulose	Eyedrops, 0.1% solution	

the course of the treatment is completed. The nurse must know the usual dosage and strength of medications being used as well as signs of toxicity. For example, osmotic agents that reduce intraocular pressure by increasing plasma osmolarity are contraindicated in patients with poor kidney function. Steroids may cause an exacerbation of an already existing herpes corneal ulcer or increase the intraocular pressure.[32] Children and elderly persons are particularly susceptible to side effects of medications.

Ophthalmic drugs. A large variety of drugs are used for treatment of eye diseases (Tables 38-1 to 38-3). Most of the drugs are applied as drops, irrigations, or ointments.

Mydriatics are drugs that dilate the pupil. Mydriasis is necessary for thorough examination of the back of the interior of the eye (fundus). Examples are phenylephrine (Neo-Synephrine) and hydroxyamphetamine (Paredrine).

Cycloplegics are drugs that not only dilate the pupil but also block accommodation by paralyzing the ciliary muscles. These drugs are used to keep the pupil dilated as part of the treatment for diseases of the cornea and for inflammatory diseases of the iris and ciliary body, after certain operations, and for eye examination. Commonly used cycloplegics are cyclopentolate (Cyclogyl), tropicamide (Mydriacyl), and atropine. Cycloplegic and mydriatric drugs should not be instilled in the eyes of a person with glaucoma as this prevents drainage of the aqueous humor, thus increasing intraocular pressure to levels where eye damage can occur.

Miotics are drugs that contract the pupil, permitting the aqueous humor to flow our more readily and thus reduce intraocular pressure. Miotics such as pilocarpine are most often used in the treatment of glaucoma. *Osmotic agents* may also be used to reduce intraocular pressure. These drugs, for example, urea and mannitol, are given intravenously in the treatment of acute glaucoma or to reduce intraocular pressure during eye surgery.

Secretory inhibitors decrease intraocular pressure by reducing aqueous humor production. Drugs in this classification inactivate the enzyme carbonic anhydrase, which is necessary for the production of aqueous humor. These drugs are given orally and include acetazolamide (Diamox). Local *topical anesthetics* such as tetracaine (Pontocaine) are used frequently for treatments and operations on the eye. Epinephrine (Adrenalin), 1:50,000 or 1:100,000, may be used in combination with local anesthetics to prolong the duration of anesthetics by constricting blood vessels so that the drug remains longer in the injected area and its absorption is delayed. Hyaluronidase (Wydase), which makes cell membranes more permeable, often is mixed with local anesthetic solutions to increase the diffusion of the anesthetic through the tissues.

Ophthalmologists may employ uncommonly used *antibiotics* such as bacitracin, polymyxin B, gentamicin, and neomycin for ocular instillation because bacteria are less likely to be resistant to them. Because penicillin causes ocular allergy in about 5% of adult patients, it is not often used.[17]

If the patient is being treated for an active infection, individual medicine bottles, droppers, tubes of ointment, and other equipment are mandatory. This precaution is also necessary when an infected eye is being treated with an antibacterial drug such as bacitracin and the same medication is ordered prophylactically for the other eye.

A *lubricant* such as methylcellulose may be used for dryness of the cornea and conjunctiva caused by deficiency in production of tears or faulty lid closure due to nerve involvement or unconsciousness.

Antiinflammatory drugs such as prednisone, cortisone, and hydrocortisone as drops and in ointment, 0.1% to 2.5%, are used to control inflammatory and allergic reactions postoperatively as well as for a variety of conditions involving the eyelids, the conjunctiva, and the cornea. Steroids also may be given systemically for the treatment of acute or subacute infections such as those of the iris and choroid.

Astringents such as zinc sulfate preparations are often useful in treating chronic conjunctivitis. The *dye* fluorescein is used to stain and thereby outline superficial injuries and infections of the external globe of the eye, to check for proper fit of contact lenses, and for applanation tonometry. Strips of filter paper impregnated with the dry dye are used in place of prepared solutions as the solution is easily contaminated by *Pseudomonas aeruginosa*.[8]

Systemic effects. Drugs applied topically to the eye can be absorbed and may cause systemic side effects. Systemic reactions may occur when anticholinergic drugs are instilled into the eye to produce mydriasis. Atropine is the anticholinergic drug that most frequently causes systemic reactions. Signs and symptoms of systemic atropine toxicity include flushing, dryness of mouth and skin, fever, rash, tachycardia, confusion, and rarely progression to coma and death.

Topically instilled miotic drugs can also cause unwanted systemic effects, most frequently with the long-acting anticholinesterase drugs such as echothiophate. Signs and symptoms include hypersalivation, sweating, gastrointestinal tract disturbances, decrease in heart rate and blood pressure, and bronchoconstriction. These drugs should be used with caution in patients with intestinal obstruction or bronchial asthma.

To avoid undesired systemic reactions, care should

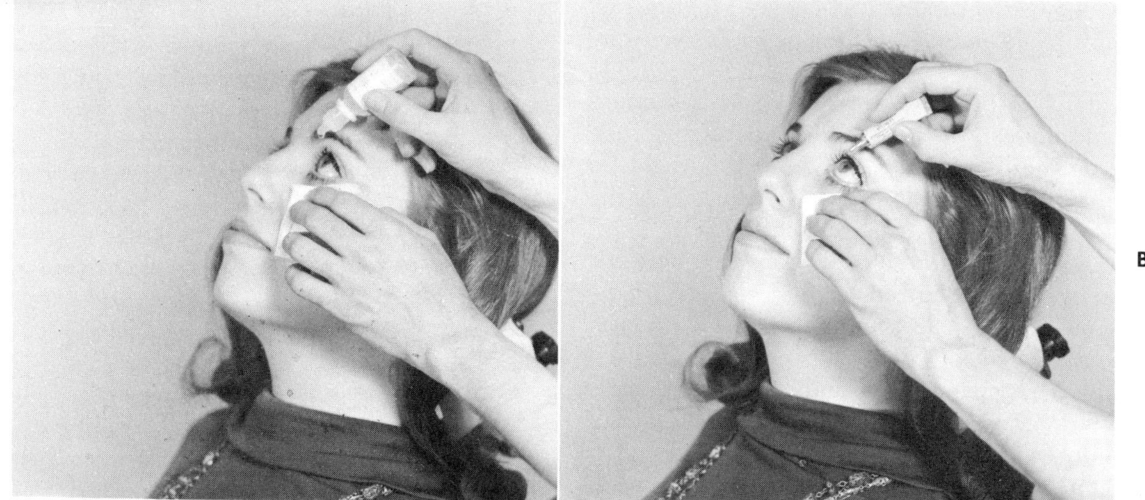

Fig. 38-1. To instill ophthalmic solution **(A)** or ointment **(B)** tilt patient's head backward supported by chairback or headrest. Use absorbent tissue pad under forefinger to depress lower lid to form conjunctival sac. Introduce medication into sac, never directly at or into eye. (Courtesy Eye and Ear Infirmary, University of Illinois Hospitals, Chicago.)

be taken with topically applied medications to give exactly what is ordered and no more. It may also be helpful to apply pressure at the inner canthus after instillation to minimize drainage into the nose and throat.

Instillation of medications. *Solutions* as eyedrops are the most commonly used preparations in the local treatment of eye disease. Advantages of solutions are that they (1) are easily instilled, (2) do not interfere with vision, (3) cause few skin reactions, and (4) do not interfere with the mitosis of the corneal epithelium. The major disadvantage of eyedrops is that they do not remain in contact with the eye very long.

Approximately 90% of aqueous solutions are eliminated from the eye within the first minute of application. It is sometimes necessary therefore to instill the solution at frequent intervals to achieve therapeutic results.

Eyedrops and eyedroppers must be sterile. Each patient should have his own bottle of medication. If the bottle is small it may be warmed slightly by holding it in the hands for a few moments. Blunt-edged eyedroppers are available and are used for children. The dropper is held downward so that medication does not flow into the rubber bulb, since foreign material from the bulb can contaminate the solution. Most eyedrops are packaged in small plastic bottles with a dropper attached.

When eyedrops are instilled the patient is asked to tilt his head back and look toward the ceiling. The lower lid is pulled gently outward, and the dropper should approach the patient's eye from the side and not directly from the front (Fig. 38-1, *A*). Drops are placed on the lower conjunctiva. Care must be taken not to touch the eyelids, the conjunctiva, or the eyeball with the dropper. The eyelids should then be closed. The person should be reminded not to squeeze the eye shut as this causes the medication to escape. Absorbent tissue or cotton held against the cheek will prevent the drops from running down the cheek.

Ointments remain in contact with the eye much longer, providing a prolonged effect. They usually do not cause discomfort when instilled. There is less absorption into lacrimal passages. Ointments, particularly those containing antibiotics, are more stable than solutions. Disadvantages are that ointments (1) produce a film in front of the eye, which may obstruct vision, (2) cause contact dermatitis reaction more frequently, and (3) may inhibit mitosis of the corneal epithelial cells.

To instill ointment the nurse asks the person to tilt his head back and to look toward the ceiling. The lower lid is gently pulled down, and the ointment is expressed directly onto the exposed conjunctiva from a small, individual tube (Fig. 38-1, *B*). Care is taken not to touch the tissues with the tube. A small sterile glass spatula may also be used to apply ointment to the eye.

Treatments

Gentleness is extremely important in performing all treatments. The natural sensitivity of the eye and the reluctance of the normal person to have anything done to his eyes are increased by pain, discomfort, and fear. Nature's powers of repair may be retarded by trauma resulting from pressure on the irritated or inflamed tissues. Hands must be washed thoroughly before giving any eye treatment, and all materials placed in the eyes must be sterile.

A good light is necessary when giving treatments, but care must be taken to protect the patient's eyes from direct light.

Eye pads. Eye pads are worn to absorb secretions and blood, to limit movement of the eyes after certain operations or injuries, to protect the eye from light, to eliminate double vision, or to conceal a deformity of the eye. The use of an eye pad is contraindicated in the presence of an eye infection because it enhances bacterial growth. An eye pad is secured with two pieces of tape placed diagonally from cheek to forehead, one on each side of the pad. The new plastic and paper tapes are used because they are easy to remove and do not cause allergic reactions. If an eye closes poorly, a drop of a lubricant such as methylcellulose may be ordered to be placed in the eye before it is covered with a dry pad to prevent scratching the cornea. After an operation on the anterior portion of the eye, a metal eye shield may be worn over the dressing to protect the eye from injury until it heals.

Compresses. Warm moist compresses are used in the treatment of surface infections of the cornea, conjunctiva, or eyelid and after many types of eye surgery to help relieve pain, promote healing, and help cleanse the eye, which is normally cleansed by tears. Compresses may be sterile or unsterile, depending on the eye condition, and should be large enough to cover the entire orbit. If both eyes are involved and the condition is infectious, separate trays must be prepared and the hands carefully washed between treatment of each eye. The temperature of the solution used for compresses should not be over 49 C (120 F), and the treatment usually lasts for 10 to 20 minutes and is repeated hourly or several times a day. Great care must be taken not to exert pressure on the eyeball when applying compresses. If there is evidence of irritation of the skin about the eyes from the hot water, a small amount of sterile petrolatum can be used, but it should not be allowed to enter the eyes. Moist heat may be applied to the eye by using a clean washcloth soaked in hot water and squeezed free of excess moisture. When the cloth cools, the process is repeated.

Cold moist saline compresses often are ordered to help control bleeding immediately following eye injury, to prevent or control edema in allergic conditions, and to control severe itching. A small basin of sterile solution may be placed in a bowl of chipped ice at the bedside. Sterile forceps are used to wring out and apply the compress. If the compress does not need to be sterile, a washcloth or compress may be placed on pieces of ice in a basin at the patient's bedside. A rubber glove or small plastic bag packed with finely chipped ice may be applied to the eye and necessitates fewer changes of compresses. A piece of plastic material loosely filled and secured with a rubber band is effective also.

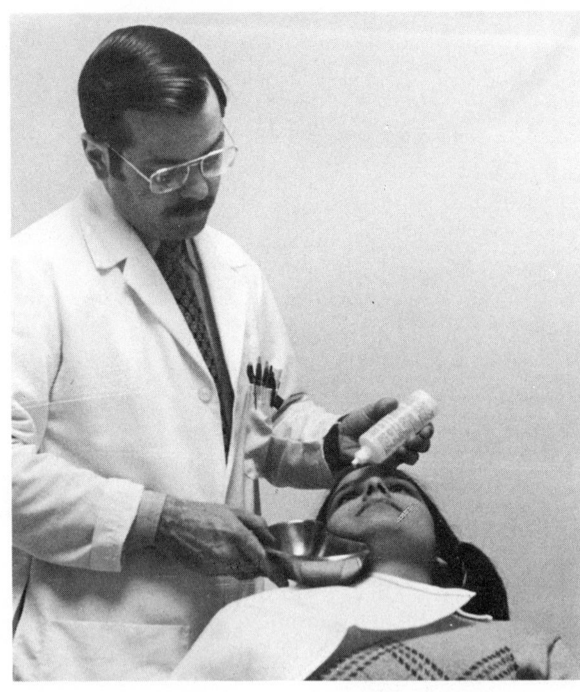

Fig. 38-2. When irrigating eye, ophthalmologist directs fluid along conjunctiva and over eyeball from inner to outer canthus.

Eye irrigations. Eye irrigations are used to remove secretions, foreign bodies, and chemical irritants and to cleanse the eye preoperatively. Irrigations are done with the patient lying comfortably toward one side so that fluid cannot flow into the other eye. A plastic squeeze bottle is commonly used unless a very large amount of fluid is needed (Fig. 38-2). If only a small amount of fluid is needed, sterile cotton balls may be used. Physiologic solution of sodium chloride or lactated Ringer's solution is most often used as an irrigating solution. These solutions are isotonic and do not remove the electrolytes necessary for normal action of the eyes. Irrigating fluid is directed along the conjuctiva and over the eyeball from the inner to the outer canthus. Care is taken to avoid directing a forceful stream onto the eyeball and to avoid touching any eye structures with the irrigating equipment. If there is drainage from the eye, a piece of gauze may be wrapped about the index finger to raise the lid and ensure thorough cleansing.

Surgical care

Preoperative care. Routines for preoperative treatment and care vary with the institution and the eye surgeon. When the patient is admitted, his general condition and reaction to the anticipated surgery are assessed. If both eyes are to be patched following surgery, the patient is introduced to all persons who will be interacting with him postoperatively. While it is unusual for both eyes to be covered at once, the patient needs to be prepared if this is to be the case. He can become well oriented to his immediate surroundings prior to surgery. Preoperative counseling also includes explaining routines necessary for his care following his return from the operating room. The patient appreciates knowing what he can expect in relation to discomfort, treatments, dressing, tubes, and other equipment. The patient often benefits from meeting and talking to another patient who has successfully recovered from a surgical treatment such as he is to receive. The child should practice having his eyes covered so that he will not be too frightened or restless postoperatively. If possible the child's mother should be permitted to stay with him before the operation and to sleep in his room.

The preparation of the patient on the evening before surgery is similar to that described on p. 373. If the patient has both eyes covered, it is *essential* that his call light be available. Since the older patient frequently becomes disoriented with his eyes covered, he should be visited frequently. The child may become frightened and will need to be comforted if his mother is not with him.

The preparation of the eye on the day of surgery may include the instillation of a combination of drugs such as atropine sulfate, 1%, cyclopentolate (Cyclogyl), 1%, and phenylephrine (Neo-Synephrine), 10%, into the eye at various intervals to dilate the pupil. The medications *must* be given at the prescribed times so that the eye is prepared at the time of surgery. If anesthetizing drops are instilled before the patient goes to the operating room, the patient is asked to close his eye, and a pad is applied to protect the insensitive eye from injury due to rubbing, dryness, or dirt and dust. If only one eye is to be operated on, a mark may be placed on the forehead over that eye so that it can be identified easily in the operating room. It is vital to carefully check the patient's records so that the surgeon knows which eye is to be operated on.

If a local anesthetic is to be used, chloral hydrate, pentobarbital sodium (Nembutal), or meperidine hydrochloride (Demerol) may be given preoperatively. Atropine sulfate may be included if a general anesthetic is to be administered. When possible, general anesthesia is avoided because the patient may be restless on reacting and disturb the eye dressing and the strain of vomiting may increase the tension on the suture line. Children, however, require general anesthesia and must be supervised closely until they have recovered fully from its effects.

If the eyelashes are cut, the surgeon uses straight, sharp scissors with fairly short blades that have been lubricated with petrolatum to help prevent the cut lashes from entering the eye. After the skin preparation has been completed and the eye has been irrigated, if local anesthesia is being used, additional anesthetic drugs such as lidocaine (Xylocaine), 2%, may be injected into the operative area at this time.

Postoperative care. Specific routines for postoperative care following eye surgery vary and change rapidly as new techniques are developed. However, general goals of postoperative care are to *prevent* (1) increased intraocular pressure, (2) stress on the suture line, (3) hemorrhage into the anterior chamber, and (4) infection. A few general principles of postoperative care are included here.

Immediately after the operation the patient must keep his head still and try to avoid coughing, vomiting, sneezing, or moving suddenly. He should lie on the unoperated side to prevent pressure on the operated eye and to prevent possible contamination of the dressing with vomitus. A pillow placed along his back will help keep the patient on his side. The patient may turn from his back to the unoperated side, but he may not lie on his stomach or on the operated side.

Postoperative confusion is a problem, particularly in elderly persons and in persons who have had both eyes covered. If confusion does occur, the surgeon may decide that the danger of activity due to confusion is worse than activity resulting from having one eye uncovered. For this reason few surgeons cover the unoperated eye.

Side rails are placed on the bed immediately postoperatively and are kept on while both eyes are covered, if the patient cannot see, or as long as necessary for his protection. The bedside table should be placed on the side of the unoperated eye so that the patient can see it without excessive movement of his head.

Care should be taken that the *dressing* is not loosened or removed. If the patient is not reliable he should be attended constantly. Restraints may occasionally need to be applied if the patient does not understand or cannot cooperate and if it is not possible to have him attended constantly. If the dressings are removed, they are replaced and the surgeon is notified. It is usual for some bleeding and serous drainage to occur, but these should be minimal. The lid is edematous, but this condition subsides with 3 or 4 days. Mild pain and pressure can be normal in the postoperative course. However, sensation of pressure within the eye may suggest hemorrhage; sharp pain is suggestive of infection or hemorrhage. These symptoms should be quickly reported to the surgeon.

Postoperative *ambulation* depends on the type of operation, the general condition of the patient, and the surgeon's preference. The patient may be up on the first postoperative day, or he may be in bed 5 or 6 days after surgery. Whatever the regimen, supervision and assistance are given by the nurse to be sure that the patient is

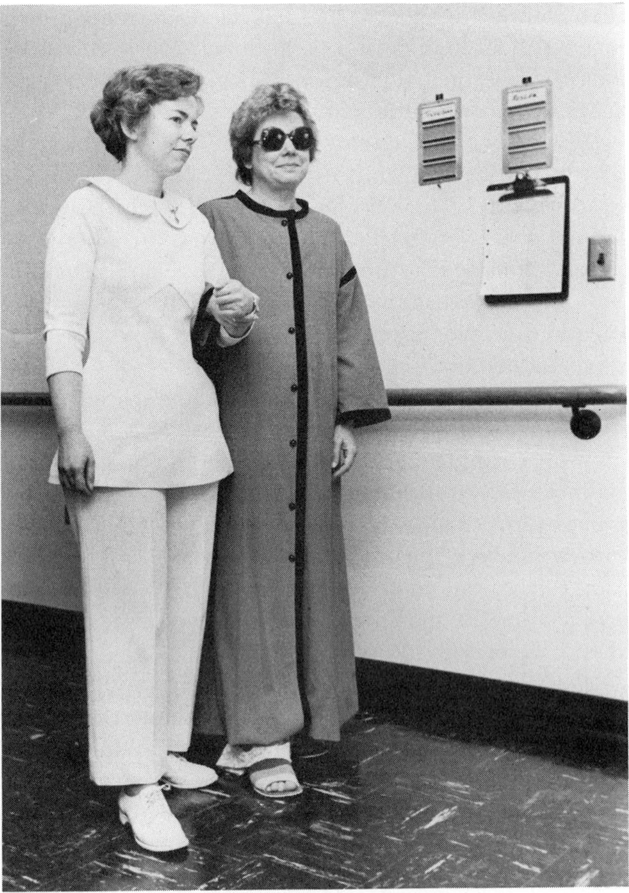

Fig. 38-3. Ambulation of patient who cannot see. Note that patient holds onto nurse's arm and is led without being held.

able to walk without sustaining injury. Because he cannot see out of the covered eye, he must try to avoid bumping into things and jarring the operative site. To avoid falls he should not sit down until he has located both arms of the chair with his hands. He usually is advised not to bend or stoop or to lift objects for several weeks after the operation in order to prevent increasing intraocular pressure, which might nullify the surgery. Slippers or shoes that he can slip into without tying or buckling are preferable during this time. Patients who have both eyes covered should be assisted to their destinations (Fig. 38-3). They should be informed of obstacles in their path, alerted when to turn before the turn appears, and told when to move to *their* right or left.

Because increased intraocular pressure may result from the Valsalva maneuver, a stool softener or milk of magnesia often are given postoperatively to lessen difficulty in having bowel movements.

Discomfort in the eye ususally is relieved by acetylsalicylic acid (aspirin), 0.6 g, meperidine (Demerol), 25 to 75 mg, or dextropropoxyphene hydrochloride (Darvon), 32 to 67 mg.

The amount of vision a person has and his general condition determine whether assistance in eating is necessary. When helping the patient who cannot see, it is important to identify the kind of food he is to receive. The nurse must not allow feeding a patient to become a routine procedure and should not appear hurried. If the patient is to have visual limitation for some time, he must be helped to learn to feed himself. Very exact descriptions of the kind and location of food and equipment and guiding the patient's hands so that he may feel the outline and placement of dishes helps. It is important that, if possible, the bed patient have the bed raised so that he may sit in a somewhat normal position for eating. Having him go through the motions a few times with an empty utensil helps to give him a correct feeling for distance. The patient should have privacy while eating meals until he learns to handle food in a fairly normal way.

Surgery may not cure the patient's eye condition; it may never be cured but only improved. The patient should be informed of this possibility by the physician. It should also be explained preoperatively that it may take weeks and even months for him to become accustomed to the type of glasses he may need to wear.

Outcome criteria for the person having eye surgery

1. The patient does not sustain injury to his eye or himself during hospitalization.
2. The patient is as independent as possible in his activities of daily living.
3. The patient or significant others can:
   a. State precautions necessary after surgery.
   b. State the dosage, method of administration, and side effects of medications to be taken at home.
   c. State how to use special lenses or eyeglasses as prescribed.
   d. Describe the rationale for and demonstrate actions that prevent increased intraocular pressure.
   e. Describe symptoms requiring medical attention and the need for medical follow-up.

□ Community services

Many federal, state, and local agencies provide services to persons with severe visual impairment. The health professional can refer these persons and their families to a social worker who is familiar with services and facilities available in their home area. Community health nurses often have this information readily available. Services to the sight impaired include mobility training, personal counseling, vocational rehabilitation,

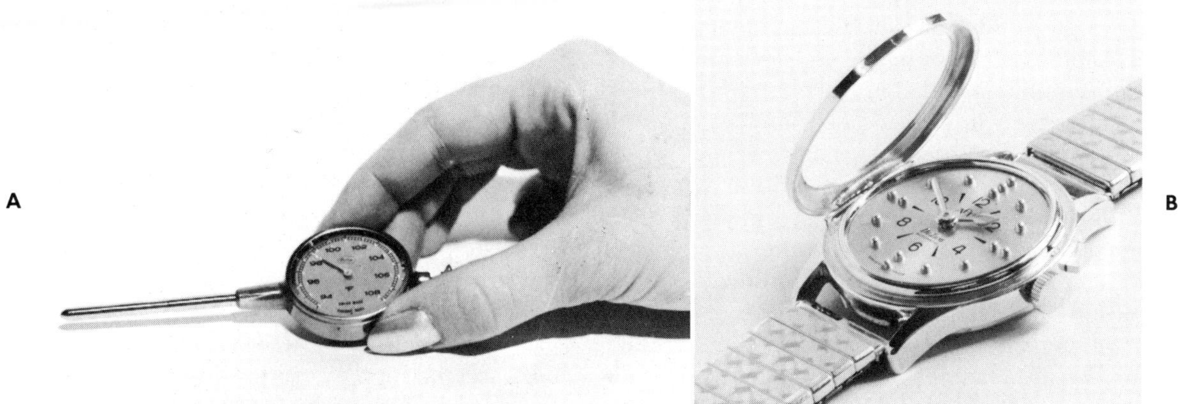

Fig. 38-4. A, Dial-type clinical thermometer with unbreakable stem. Braille (raised) dots mark scale, one dot at odd numbers and two at even numbers. Raised line is at 98.6 F. Button is pushed to register temperature, which remains set until button is released. Needle then returns to zero. **B,** One of many models of watches available in both braille and inkprint. (Courtesy American Foundation for the Blind, New York.)

relearning independent self-care, special education, and financial compensation in some instances.

National voluntary organizations

Two national voluntary health agencies concerned with blindness and the prevention of blindness are the American Foundation for the Blind* and the National Society for the Prevention of Blindness.† Both organizations have literature that is available to nurses and patients on request. The American Foundation for the Blind distributes a free catalog, *Aids and Appliances* (also available to the blind in braille, free of charge), which contains a list of devices for the visually handicapped. The catalog includes sewing and kitchen utensils as well as various kinds of tools and instruments (Fig. 38-4). Medical appliances such as special syringes and aids for the person who must give himself insulin (see Fig. 32-1) or other parenteral medication can also be obtained. Founded in 1908, the National Society for the Prevention of Blindness, Inc., is engaged in the prevention of blindness through a comprehensive program of community services, public and professional education, and research. Publications, films, lecture, charts, and advisory service are available on request. The quarterly publication of this voluntary organization, *The Sight-Saving Review*, covers many aspects of sight conservation and eye health.

Recording for the Blind, Inc.,‡ is a national, nonprofit voluntary organization that provides recorded educational books free on loan to anyone who cannot read normal printed material because of visual or physical handicaps. "Talking books" produced by this organization are fundamental aids to high school and college students and persons who require educational or specialized material in the pursuit of their occupations. These recordings also may be obtained from many local and state libraries. Talking-book machines are loaned free to persons who are legally blind. Information can be obtained from public libraries or organizations for the blind.

*15 West 16th Street, New York 10011.
†79 Madison Ave., New York 10016.
‡215 East 58th St., New York 10022.

Government assistance

Legal blindness entiles a person to certain federal assistance. A 1952 amendment to the Social Security Act made provision for assistance to the blind, and now all 50 states and all territories have approved plans for such aid. Assistance through this program is based on need. The Internal Revenue Act of 1948 permits blinded persons an extra deduction ($750) in reporting income. In 1943 the federal government established a counseling and placement service for the blind in the Vocational Rehabilitation Administration. This agency is now called the Social and Rehabilitation Service (SRS). It shares cost of rehabilitation with the states. The Veterans Administration provides a substantial pension for the single veteran who has enucleation of both eyes.

Schools

Progress has been made in improving educational opportunities for the blind. It is believed now that the blind child, like any other handicapped child, does best when he is accepted and is in as normal an environment as possible. Blind children of school age are being educated in regular public or religious schools, where special provisions for their individual needs are being met, or they attend special residential schools. Schools emphasize the use of auditory instruction and the development of reading skills through touch perception by the braille system. The child needs to encounter as much of his environment as is practical in order to develop concepts that other children acquire by sight. Many states have legislated funds to provide higher education for the blind and to provide readers for them, and many blind students go on to college and compete successfully with their sighted peers.

■ MANAGEMENT OF PERSONS WITH IMPAIRED HEARING AND EAR PROBLEMS

□ Meaning of hearing

More than 13 million people in the United States have some kind of hearing impairment. Six million of these persons are serioulу handicapped, and more than 1.7 million are totally deaf.[64]

Hearing is as important as speech in our daily lives. Sound helps keep us in touch with reality and our environment; it adds aesthetic pleasure as well as warnings of danger to our world. People with normal hearing are always perceiving sound both consciously and unconsciously. One hears background noises, a clock ticking, or family conversations without concentrating on them; these sounds help us to be alert to our world. Other sounds such as fire alarms or a child crying signal us so that we consciously hear them and take action depending on our interpretation of the sound. This preconscious level of hearing is not perceived by the person who is hard of hearing and causes them to perceive the world as being "dead" about them. The sense of hearing is critical to normal development and maintenance of speech. Infants learn to speak by emulating sounds from others. They listen to the sounds they make in relationship to the sounds of others, a skill necessary in the formulation of adequate speaking skills. Congenitally deaf individuals lack aural stimulation, which affects their development of speech and conceptual ability. This severe handicap can affect both personality development and responses on intelligence tests. People with lesser degrees of hearing loss who have learned speech normally also may have behavioral changes not necessarily proportional to the degree of hearing loss.[74]

The meaning of the loss of aesthetic experiences such as listening to music may vary from individual to individual depending on the person's previous life style. As hearing diminishes, the impact of not understanding others and of not being understood may make the person withdraw from social situations, and he may become anxious and insecure. His fear of inadequacy and inferiority may make him suspicious and depressed. When hearing is completely gone the person may find his silent world almost intolerable. Loneliness and isolation eventually may lead to disorientation or the lack of desire to live.

People who are hard of hearing or deaf are not easily recognized by others; they appear quite normal. When they fail to respond or respond inappropriately to oral communication, their actions are interpreted as slow or odd, and the speaker may withdraw. This withdrawal response of others may be perceived as rejection by the aurally handicapped and may further increase isolation and withdrawal. The person who is hard of hearing or deaf may experience varying degrees of stress depending on his personality, the extent and type of loss, the age of onset of loss, and his support system's (family and friends) reaction to loss.

Nursing activities regarding protection of the ears and prevention of hearing loss are outlined as follows and are described in succeeding paragraphs:

1. Protection of the ears from impairment or further impairment
   a. Teaching proper care of the ear
   b. Preventing hearing impairment from environmental forces including infection, noise pollution, and injury
   c. Working with people who evidence ear disease or impaired hearing
   d. Explaining and administering treatment to improve or prevent further hearing loss
2. Adjustment of the individual to impaired hearing
   a. Identifying those basic needs that have been affected by loss of hearing
   b. Understanding the effects on adaptation related to the different degrees and types of hearing loss
   c. Assisting the individual to cope with unmet needs of security (physiologic and psychologic), self-esteem, and love and belonging
   d. Directing individuals in using available community resources

□ Classification of hearing loss

Hearing loss may be classified in several ways; one approach is according to type (conductive, sensorineural), another is according to severity.

Conductive hearing loss

Any interference with the conduction of sound impulses through the external auditory canal, the eardrum, or the middle ear produces a conductive hearing loss.

The inner ear is not involved, and sound directed to it is heard clearly. Amplifying sound by use of hearing aids or raising the voice may be useful so that sound will reach the inner ear. Conductive hearing loss may be due to impacted cerumen or a foreign body in the external auditory canal; a thickening, retracting, scarring, or perforation of the eardrum; pathologic changes in the middle ear that prevent movement of one or more of the ossicles; or fixing of the stapes due to otosclerosis. At the present time the conductive type of hearing loss is more effectively treated by surgery than the sensorineural type (p. 804).

Sensorineural hearing loss

Sensorineural hearing loss results from disease or trauma of the inner ear or its neural pathways. Some of the causes include arteriosclerosis; infectious diseases such as mumps, measles, and meningitis; ototoxic drugs (see box below); neuromas of the eighth cranial nerve; blows to the head or the ears; or degeneration of the organ of Corti due to exposure to noise of high intensity. Treatment usually is not effective for sensorineural loss because the damage has been done by the time the individual sees the physician, and the process is irreversible. Some surgical procedures have been developed to aid in restoring this type of loss (p. 807). Amplifying sounds by shouting causes distortion of the sound and may increase the hearing problem.

Severity

Hearing loss is also classified according to severity, that is, slight loss or severe loss. Persons who have only slight hearing loss often are unaware of it or try to minimize it. Listening becomes a strain; difficulties arise in communication causing embarrassment or irritation. Exhaustion can occur, and social contacts are avoided. The recognition of the defect in hearing by the individual is necessary before corrective or rehabilitative steps can be taken.

People with *slight to moderate* hearing loss are found often in the aged population. Their hearing loss is most often sensorineural loss compounded at times by conductive loss. Typically these persons have decreased ability to hear or discern higher pitched sounds; increasing the loudness of the voice only increases the distortion of sound and compounds hearing problems.

People with *severe* hearing loss usually seek help because of the problems they have in functioning. Because they no longer hear themselves speak, their speech may become slurred or too loud. Severe hearing loss is exemplified by the congenitally deaf who may be severely limited in their psychologic and mental development. Deafness alters the individual's awareness of self. Early case finding of congenitally deaf children is necessary so that corrective measures can be taken early to facilitate their learning.

SELECTED OTOTOXIC DRUGS

These drugs may affect the cochlea, vestibule of the ear, or the eighth cranial nerve.

Antibiotics	Streptomycin Dihydrostreptomycin Neomycin Kanamycin Viomycin Vancomycin Polymyxin B/Colistin Chloramphenicol (Chloromycetin) Capreomycin
Diuretics	Ethacrynic acid (Edecrin) Furosemide (Lasix) Acetazolamide (Diamox)
Salicylates	Acetylsalicylic acid (aspirin)
Other drugs	Quinine Chloroquine Nitrogen mustard Bleomycin Quinidine

□ Prevention

Hearing difficulties may begin at any age. Understanding of the many causes of hearing loss is important for all health team members in all settings. Because nurses occupy a unique position in the health care system, they have the opportunity to be involved in many aspects of health care of the ear.

Care of healthy ears

The ear should be cleaned only with a wet washcloth over the tip of a finger. Nothing should be inserted into the ear beyond the extent of vision. A certain amount of cerumen (ear wax) in the ear canal is normal, and persons who have no wax have itching and scaling in the ear canal. Usually it is not necessary to clean the ears to remove wax. Occasionally when the cerumen becomes impacted and causes pain or temporary deafness it must be removed by the physician, nurse, or member of the person's family who has been instructed in the procedure. The person is usually asked to instill several drops of a warm sweet oil (mineral oil, glycerin) or hydrogen peroxide or peroxide in glyceryl (Debrox) into the auditory canal for several days to soften the wax. Directions for instillation of ear drops are as follows:

1. Wash hands before and after the procedure.
2. Check the eardropper if glass or plastic to make sure it is not rough.
3. Warm the solution to body temperature (no more than 38C [100F]); vertigo may result from high or low temperatures. The bottle of solution may be warmed by holding it in the hand for a minute or two.
4. Have patient tilt his head so that the ear to be treated is uppermost.
5. Cleanse the external ear with a clean washcloth.
6. Straighten ear canal by pulling up and back in adults, down and back in children.
7. Instill the drops so that they run along the wall of the canal and do not entrap air.
8. Have the patient hold his head position for 5 to 10 minutes.
9. Gently insert a piece of cotton moistened with the eardrop solution into the external auditory canal to keep the drops from running out of the ear.
10. Dry the external ear thoroughly to prevent skin irritation.

To *irrigate* the ear canal, a solution of tap water or normal saline with hydrogen peroxide added to help dislodge the wax is used. The person sits with his head inclined slightly forward and toward the affected side (Fig. 38-5). His clothes are protected and a basin placed below his ear to catch excess solution. The auricle is pulled upward and backward and the solution directed along the upper wall of the meatus. If irrigation does not remove the wax easily, removal with a cerumen spoon by the physician may be necessary. It is usually necessary to dry the ear canal gently with a cotton wick or applicator. Teaching the individual or a member of his family to irrigate the ear should include the above steps in addition to the following guidelines:

1. The procedure should not be undertaken without the approval of a qualified member of the health team.
2. Wash hands before and after the procedure.
3. Always warm the solution to be used to body temperature to prevent vestibular stimulation and consequent vertigo.
4. Never try to irrigate the ear canal to remove foreign objects of vegetable material; the moisture will cause the object to swell.
5. Irrigations are rarely used if the eardrum is punctured, since this can cause further infection.
6. Use a steady stream of solution against the roof of the auditory canal; if directed downward, the plugging material will be forced further into the canal.
7. Do not use excessive force, and make sure the syringe used has no rough edges.
8. Air should be expelled from the bulb syringe prior to instilling solution, and the tip of the syringe should be directed either toward the roof or toward the floor of the canal but not straight inward.
9. The canal should not be completely obstructed by the syringe, since this will keep solution from flowing back and will cause pressure against the eardrun.
10. The person should lie on the affected side for several minutes to assure complete drainage of irrigation fluid.
11. The external ear should then be dried throughly to prevent excoriation of the skin.

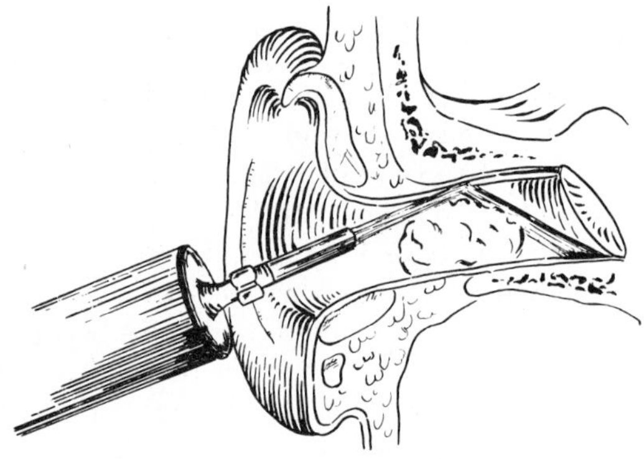

Fig. 38-5. Irrigation of external auditory canal with warm tap water. (From Havener, W. H., Saunders, W. H., Keith, C. F., and Prescott, A. W.: Nursing care in eye, ear, nose, and throat disorders, ed. 3, St. Louis, 1974, The C. V. Mosby Co.)

Early adequate treatment of childhood diseases

Prevention of hearing loss involves teaching persons the necessity for adequate treatment of childhood diseases. Since viral diseases (especially measles) can cause a hearing impairment in the fetus, immunization programs and treatment of the pregnant woman who contracts the disease can prevent hearing loss in the child. Other high-risk infants who may develop hearing impairments are those who are premature or who have experienced anoxia postnatally. Good prenatal care can help prevent hearing loss in high-risk infants.

Hearing loss may also begin later in childhood. Before the advent of antibiotics, hearing loss was a frequent sequella of middle ear and mastoid process infections. Adequate treatment of upper respiratory tract and particularly of ear infections can prevent this loss. Persons need to taught to blow the nose gently with both nostrils open (not sniffing) to avoid contamination of the eustachian tubes with mucus, especially during an upper respiratory tract infection. Individuals with upper respiratory tract infections should be encouraged to seek medical attention if they experience (1) increasing pain in the ear or increasing headache even after application of heat, (2) any reddish fluid oozing from the ear (this may indicate rupture of the eardrum), (3) temperature higher than 39C (102F), (4) any convulsive twitching of the facial muscles, or (5) dizziness. Medical attention should be sought if a child less than 3 years of age has any symptoms related to the ear.

Prevention of trauma

Children should be taught to avoid inserting hard articles deep into the ear canal, obstructing the ear canal with any objects, inserting unclean articles or solutions into the ear, or swimming in stagnant water or in water identified as being polluted. These practices can lead to damage of the tympanic membrane or to ear infections. Adults often insert hard articles into the outer ear in an attempt to remove cerumen.

Monitoring side effects of ototoxic drugs

Persons taking ototoxic drugs (see box on p. 769) need to know the signs and symptoms of side effects of these drugs in order to prevent loss of hearing from developing. If these symptoms (dizziness, decreased hearing acuity, tinnitus) occur, the next dose of the drug is omitted and the physician is consulted. Audiometric testing may be necessary.

Monitoring noise pollution

Hearing loss caused by loud noise is the most common type of occupational hearing loss. Exposure to industrial noise levels greater than 85 to 90 dB for months or years causes cochlear damage. Health team members in industry can help prevent deafness due to noise of high intensity by teaching employees why they should wear earplugs. The nurse in industry faces a task calling for special knowledge and training. Industrial noise and occupational or noise-induced hearing loss are primary causes of hearing loss in our society. Some 9 million workers are exposed daily to noise levels on the job that are potentially hazardous to hearing.[16,56,60,79] This occupational hearing loss is preventable, and the nurse must be familiar with both the causes and the possible means of prevention of such loss. Courses are available to familiarize nurses with industrial hearing conservation requirements.

Concern with noise pollution as well as with other occupational hazards prompted the passage of the *Williams-Steiger Occupational Safety and Health Act* (OSHA) in 1970. The provisions regarding noise protection are too complex to include in detail, but in general, exposure to noise levels in excess of 90 dB over an 8-hour day are considered excessive and should be avoided (Table 38-4). The requirement means that no worker should be exposed *unprotected* for over 8 hours to levels of 90 dBA or higher. The term *dBA* relates to one of three possible scales or networks found on most sound-level meters. These scales essentially respond differently to different frequencies or wavelengths in noise. The A network, like the human ear, is not responsive to (does not measure) low-frequency sound and thus is used in many situations such as the OSHA regulation or in specifying the annoyance of humans to noise. The B network is used for certain engineering applications, and the C scale measures the entire spectrum. A copy of the Occupational Safety and Health Act may be obtained from local offices or the Occupational Safety and Health Agency, which is part of the U.S. Department of Labor.

Other causes of noise-induced hearing loss include firearms and high-intensity music such as rock music. With an M-16 rifle or sports rifle, hearing loss tends to be greater in the ear opposite the dominant hand (that is, left ear hearing loss in a right-handed person). With revolvers, hearing loss is equal in both ears. If a person firing guns notices tinnitus, sensation of fullness in the ear, or temporary hearing loss he should stop firing guns or a least wear suitable ear protectors. Sound in front of a rock band can reach up to 120 dB, and hearing losses up to 50 dB have been measured in some rock group band members. In the early stage there is loss of hearing at or near frequencies of 4,000 Hz. Later the damage extends to both higher and lower tones, with the lower tones affected least. If proximity to the high noise level cannot be avoided, ear protectors or plugs should be worn. The plugs are inserted into the external auditory canal and

Table 38-4. Permissible noise exposures

Duration per day (hours)	Sound level (dBA, slow)
8	90
6	92
4	95
3	97
2	100
1½	102
1	105
½	110
¼	115

From U.S. Department of Labor, Occupational Safety and Health Administration: Noise: the environmental problem, a guide to OSHA standards, Washington, D.C., 1973, U.S. Government Printing Office.

can reduce the noise reaching the middle ear by 10 to 30 dB. Usually standard plugs are effective, but custom-made plugs molded to the individual's ear canal may be obtained. If the noise level is extremely high (sound levels may reach 140 dB or higher), individuals are not adequately protected with earplugs alone and must wear muffs over their ears, and at times a shield must be worn over the entire head.

□ Intervention

Local treatment of ear problems

Often treatment of external ear infections includes local application of medicated ointments or powders, hot compresses to soften crusts, or cool applications to lessen inflammation and relieve discomfort.

To apply *ointment* to the ear canal, an applicator with a tufted end is used (Fig. 38-6); a Q-Tip or other commercially prepared cotton applicator is usually too thick. The tufted end of the applicator is inserted deep into the canal, and ointment is applied to the outer surface of the eardrum as well as to the ear canal. Care must be taken to prevent damage to the eardrum. A new applicator is used each time the canal is entered. The person is cautioned not to move his head during the procedure.

When *compresses* are used, the pillow is protected and a loose gauze plug is placed in the outer ear canal. This plug can be moistened with solution if the outer ear canal is also involved or may be used dry to prevent spread of the infection to the inner part of the canal. Compresses of single-thickness gauze fit the contours of the outer ear best. They should be moist but not dripping. Since ice bags are too heavy to use on the sensitive external ear, a cold application can be made by placing about 2 cupfuls of crushed ice in a small sealed plastic bag or glove. In caring for patients with infections of the external ear it is important to avoid further infection; thus handwashing is important and all equipment and material used must be sterile.

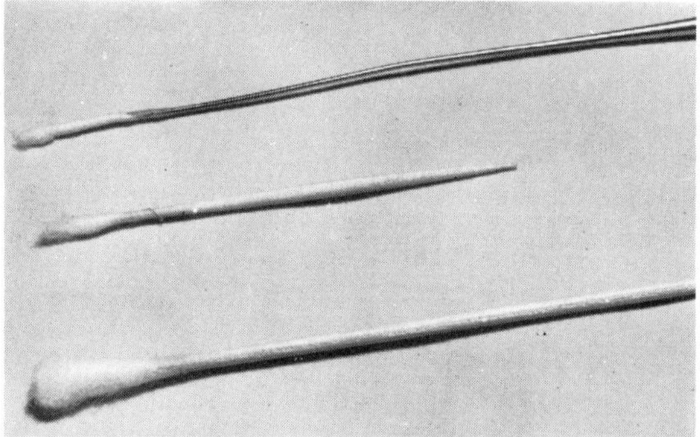

Fig. 38-6. *Top:* Physician's cotton applicator. Note tuft at end. *Middle:* Toothpick with cotton. *Bottom:* Usual commercial applicator (too thick). (From Havener, W. H., Saunders, W. H., Keith, C. F., and Prescott, A. W.: Nursing care in eye, ear, nose, and throat disorders, ed. 3, St. Louis, 1974, The C. V. Mosby Co.)

Earwicks or *drains* may be used to encourage passage of exudate from the ear canal. Sterile wicks may be made by twisting a single layer of sterile gauze that has been picked up at its center. The wick is inserted gently only as far as the eye can see with the loose end extending outside the ear canal. Wicks must be changed often and never allowed to become hardened with exudate because this interferes with the flow of drainage. Commercially prepared earwicks, such as the Pope earwick (Xomed Co.) or Merocel earwick (Codman Co.) are essentially expanding cellulose sponges that are harder than a gauze wick but which serve as excellent vehicles for medicating the ear canal. A wick saturated with a medicated solution may be used both as a drain and as a local compress. A wick also may be inserted after eardrops have been given to distribute the medication and help retain it in the ear canal.

Nursing management for persons having ear surgery

Most persons having ear surgery have short hospitalizations. The different types of ear surgery are described in detail in Chapter 39. With any operative procedure on the middle ear, patients may experience *vertigo* for a few days postoperatively, probably related to the stimulation of the inner ear. Patients usually require assistance or supervision when ambulating for the first 2 or 3 days to protect them from falling. Some persons who are quite dizzy will also exhibit nystagmus resulting from labyrinthine stimulation. Keeping the patient from moving his head may help lessen vertigo. Nausea can accompany vertigo, and often both may be relieved by antimotion drugs such as dimenhydrinate (Dramamine), diazepam (Valium), or promethazine (Phenergan).

Fluids may be tolerated orally if given in small amounts with the patient keeping his head still. Pain is not usually a major problem for patients with ear surgery but may be present, and if so it may be relieved by analgesics.

Small amounts of serosanguineous drainage on ear dressings is expected, but signs of bright blood on outer dressings are reported to the physician. Signs of facial paralysis such as inability to smile or to wrinkle the forehead are assessed immediately postoperatively in the recovery room and again when the patient returns to the clinical unit. Patients are cautioned not to blow their noses for a time postoperatively so as not to increase air pressure in the eustachian tube.

Careful handwashing before and after contact with

the patient is an effective way to prevent infection. Handling contaminated dressings appropriately also helps to prevent infection. Often antibiotics are given prophylactically. Patients often are cautioned against swimming, washing their hair, or getting the affected ear wet in any way for a limited amount of time (about 2 weeks). Once healing is complete, most persons may resume all normal activities. Since persons often are concerned about apparent lack of immediate improvement in hearing, especially following stapedectomy (p. 804), careful explanations about hearing restoration are necessary.

Outcome criteria for persons having ear surgery

The patient or significant others can:

1. State the rationale and desired outcome of the procedure.
2. Describe the rationale for the following safety precautions:
   a. Side rails or assistance during early ambulation.
   b. No nose blowing postoperatively.
   c. Keeping the ear dry postoperatively.
   d. Handwashing and dressing procedures.
3. State the symptoms requiring medical attention and need for follow-up care.

□ Aural rehabilitation

If hearing loss is irreversible and not amenable to surgical intervention, aural rehabilitation may make it possible for the individual to understand and communicate with others again. The purpose of aural rehabilitation is to maximize the hearing-impaired person's communication skills. Because the auditory sense is our primary mode of communication, it is imperative that hearing-impaired individuals be given the opportunity to utilize their hearing for this purpose. When a person exhibits irreversible hearing loss, his ability to hear conversational speech may be improved through the use of an appropriate hearing aid.

The hearing-impaired person must be helped to understand the implications of hearing loss for communication purposes. There are potential social and psychologic implications of hearing impairment, and it is most helpful for the individual to gain insight into his specific communication problems. This can be accomplished through discussions pertaining to daily communicative interactions at home, at work, or at play. The presence of a family member in such discussions is often most helpful in determining how the individual's hearing impairment may have affected others. These insight are extremely important in planning appropriate rehabilitative strategies.

Formal aural rehabilitative training may be necessary to improve an individual's communication skills. Many hearing-impaired persons do not utilize their residual hearing. *Auditory training* is a process by which the person is helped to make maximum use of his residual hearing. *Speech reading* is taught to supplement the hearing function and includes lipreading and the study of facial expressions, gestures, and body movements used in communication. *Speech therapy* is given to develop, conserve, or correct speech.

The person's acceptance of the fact that he has a hearing impairment, his desire to seek help, and his use of the facilities available, coupled with motivation, perseverance and patience, contribute to the success of aural rehabilitation. Rehabilitation is affected by age and severity of impairment. Infants and children with hearing disorders require assistance from specialists to help them learn and communicate. For people who, although hard of hearing, have normally acquired communication skill, efforts are geared toward correcting, restoring, complementing, and maintaining those skills. For the deaf who have not developed communication skills, efforts are made to teach language and speech skills by special methods.

Hearing aids

Hearing aids (Fig. 38-7) are commonly used by both hard of hearing individuals and deaf persons. Hearing aids are instruments through which sounds are amplified in a controlled manner. Generally an aid consists of a microphone to receive and convert speech and other sounds into electric signals, an amplifier to increase the strength of the sound, a receiver to convert electric signals back to sound, and a battery to supply the electric power. Hearing aids are used to increase the intensity of the sound reaching the ear of the person with hearing loss. They do not improve the ability to hear, but they make the sound louder. They are usually recommended when the person has difficulty in understanding speech in his everyday conversations.

When the person has difficulty with speech discrimination, benefits from an aid are more restricted. Persons with a conductive hearing loss benefit most from wearing a hearing aid because their ability to understand speech is usually not impaired if the speech is loud enough. They will not hear as well as they did with normal hearing, but they will be able to hear speech in the frequencies at which most ordinary conversations occur. Persons with sensorineural hearing losses often exhibit problems with amplification such as an intolerance for loud speech and noise and difficulty understanding speech even if loud enough. It should be noted, however, that this is the most common type of hearing loss and affects the majority of individuals successfully wearing hearing aids. Appropriate aural rehabilitation will ensure a successful adjustment to amplification in most instances.

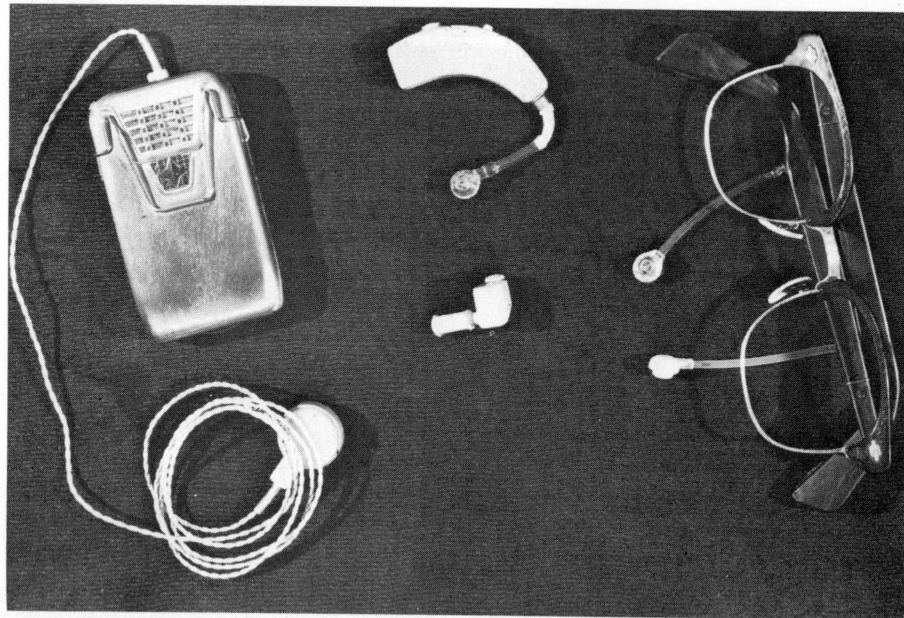

Fig. 38-7. Body and headborne hearing aids. *Left:* Body-type aid. Button receiver is coupled to ear with insert, and component housing is either clipped to clothing or worn on body in harnessed cloth pouch. *Top center:* Behind-ear aid. *Center:* In-ear aid. *Right:* Eyeglass aid. (From Havener, W. H., Saunders, W. H., Keith, C. F., and Prescott, A. W.: Nursing care in eye, ear, nose, and throat disorders, ed. 3, St. Louis, 1974, The C. V. Mosby Co.)

Elderly persons often have difficulty adjusting to the use of a hearing aid, partially because their hearing loss usually is of sensorineural origin. Their problems also may be due to a lack of patience, concentration, or the mental energy needed to learn to use a hearing aid. Small children with a hearing loss should be fitted with a hearing aid as soon as a hearing deficit is diagnosed, usually at several months of age, because reinforcement from auditory feedback is paramount for appropriate linguistic development.

If a person's hearing problem indicates need for a hearing aid, he should be seen both by an otologist and an audiologist. The audiologist can perform various tests and help determine if a hearing aid will benefit the person and what specific type of hearing aid will be the best for him. The otologist can determine the medical nature of the problem and decide whether there is any medical reason why a hearing aid cannot be worn. Federal Drug Administration (FDA) regulations restrict the sale of hearing aids to those individuals who have received a medical evaluation, with the provision that any person over 18 years of age, or any parent or guardian, can be permitted to waive the medical evaluation requirement, provided they do not have any one of seven designated otologic conditions: (1) a visible congenital or traumatic deformity of the ear, (2) a history of active drainage from the ear within the last 90 days, (3) a history of sudden progressive hearing loss within the last 90 days, (4) a history of acute or chronic dizziness, (5) unilateral hearing loss of sudden or recent onset, (6) an audiometric air-bone gap equal to or greater than 15 dB at 500, 1,000, and 2,000 Hz, or (7) visible evidence of cerumen or a foreign body in the ear canal. The waiver privilege has been allowed in those instances where it would be very inconvenient to have a medical evaluation, for example, in rural areas, and for those instances where religious beliefs forbid medical evaluation but do not forbid the wearing of hearing aids.

The retail prices of hearing aids range from $200 to $900, and over 1,200 different models of hearing aids are available. They may be worn on the body, built into the temple bow of eyeglasses, or worn as individual units behind the ear (Fig. 38-8, *A* and *B*) or in the ear canal. Aids worn on the body are the most powerful and are generally fitted to people with moderate to severe hearing losses. Aids worn in eyeglasses or behind the ear are generally equivalent to each other in amplifying power.

Implanting of hearing aids is under consideration, although it has not been demonstrated, as yet, that speech discrimination is superior with implantation than with conventional aids.[99]

The person should be instructed in the care of his

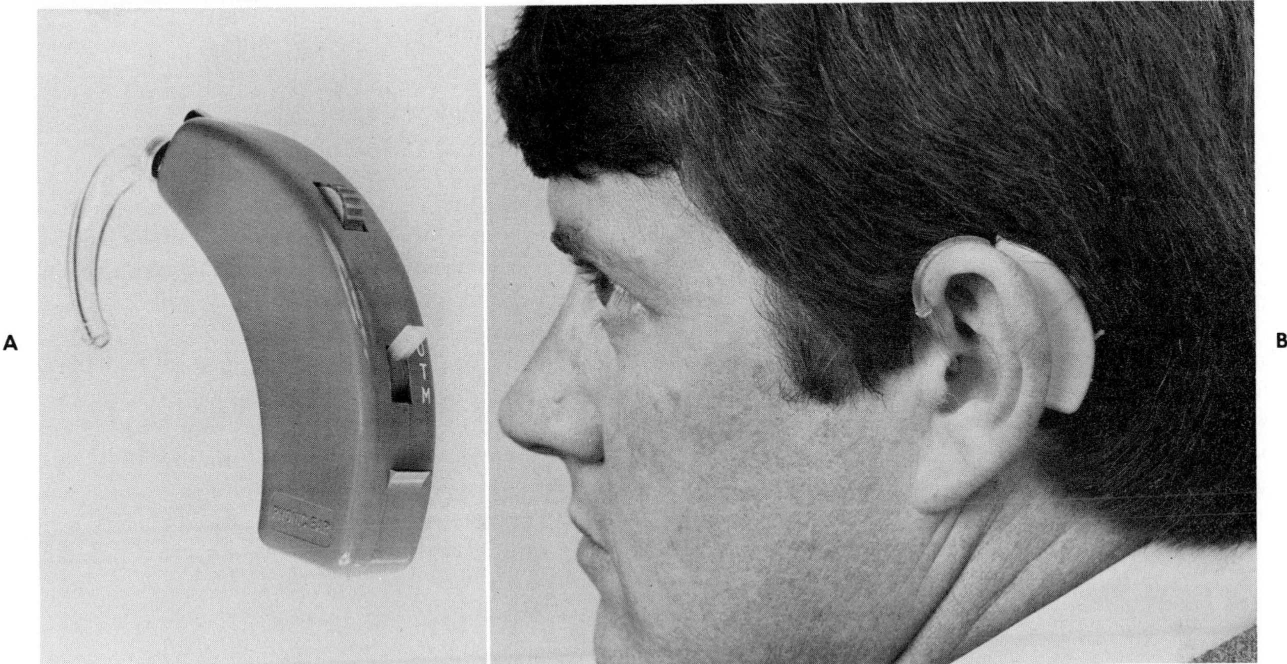

Fig. 38-8. A, Hearing aid. **B,** Hearing aid in place. (Courtesy HC Electronics, Inc. [Phonic Ear], Mill Valley, Calif.)

hearing aid. The earmold or plug may be washed daily in mild soap and water using a pipe cleaner to cleanse the cannula. It should be thoroughly dried before being reconnected to the receiver. If a hearing aid is worn on the body, the microphone should face the speaker and should not be covered by heavy clothing. Men often wear the transmitter in their shirt or upper pocket. Women may fit it into a special pocket sewn on the outside of their underclothing. Children often wear it on a fabric harness placed over their undergarments. The person who uses a hearing aid should carry an extra battery and cord at all times.

Hearing aids have adjustable tone and volume controls, and several adjustments may have to be made before the aid is correctly set for the individual's needs. Since a hearing aid is not selective when amplifying sounds, often the amplified background sounds can be annoying to the individual. Persons who wear hearing aids should know what to do if the aid fails to work:

1. Check the on-off switch.
2. Inspect cleanliness of earmold.
3. Examine battery for tightness or leaks.
4. Examine cord plug for tightness of insertion.
5. Examine cord plug for breaks.
6. Replace battery, cord, or both.
7. Take hearing aid to local service agency if above steps fail to correct problem.

Persons who are reluctant to wear their hearing aids (usually for cosmetic reasons) need counseling about the benefits of wearing the aid and the improvements in their ability to communicate. The aid may also serve to notify others to speak more distinctly. When a person with a hearing aid is hospitalized, it is important to encourage use of the aid during the hospitalization and its safe storage when not in use.

Outcome criteria for persons with hearing aids

The person or significant others can:

1. Explain the rationale for using the hearing aid.
2. Demonstrate the proper care of the aid.
3. Explain what to do if the aid does not work.
4. Explain what the aid can and cannot do.

Auditory training

Auditory training is used to encourage those who are hard of hearing to use their residual hearing more effectively. The training consists of helping the affected individual to develop his listening skills. It helps the hard of hearing to (1) establish attitudes of critical listening, (2) develop an awareness of the kinds of listening errors that are most likely to be made in view of the nature of the hearing impairment, (3) compensate for these errors by using other special clues that are still heard correctly, and (4) improve listening habits and skills in general.

Speech reading

Speech reading (commonly known as lipreading) is taught to supplement the hearing function. It includes lipreading, the study of facial expressions, and the study of gestures and body movements used in speech. It also uses environmental clues that help supplement the hearing function in communication.

Speech training

Speech training in given to conserve speech skills, to prevent deterioration of skills, or to develop speech skills. Hearing is necessary not only for the development of speech but also for the monitoring of loudness, clearness, pitch, quality, and rate. Hearing loss reduces the reliability of the monitoring system, which may cause the speech to deteriorate.

Special interventions for the congenitally deaf child

Development of speech and language skills require special attention for those born deaf or who become deaf in early childhood because these persons do not develop language and speech normally. Not only is it medically important to detect deafness or hearing impairment in the young child, but also, for an educational standpoint, it is imperative that remedial measures be taken during the early years (between the ages of 2 and 5 years) when language and speech skills are most easily acquired (Fig. 38-9). The child who has never heard speech is unable to imitate it. He is educable, but his education requires more time than that of the child with normal hearing. Since a period of about 3 years is required for a child to learn sufficient language to begin the first grade, he should start receiving formal training as soon as a hearing loss is detected. He may then attend classes with children who have normal hearing or go to a public or pri-

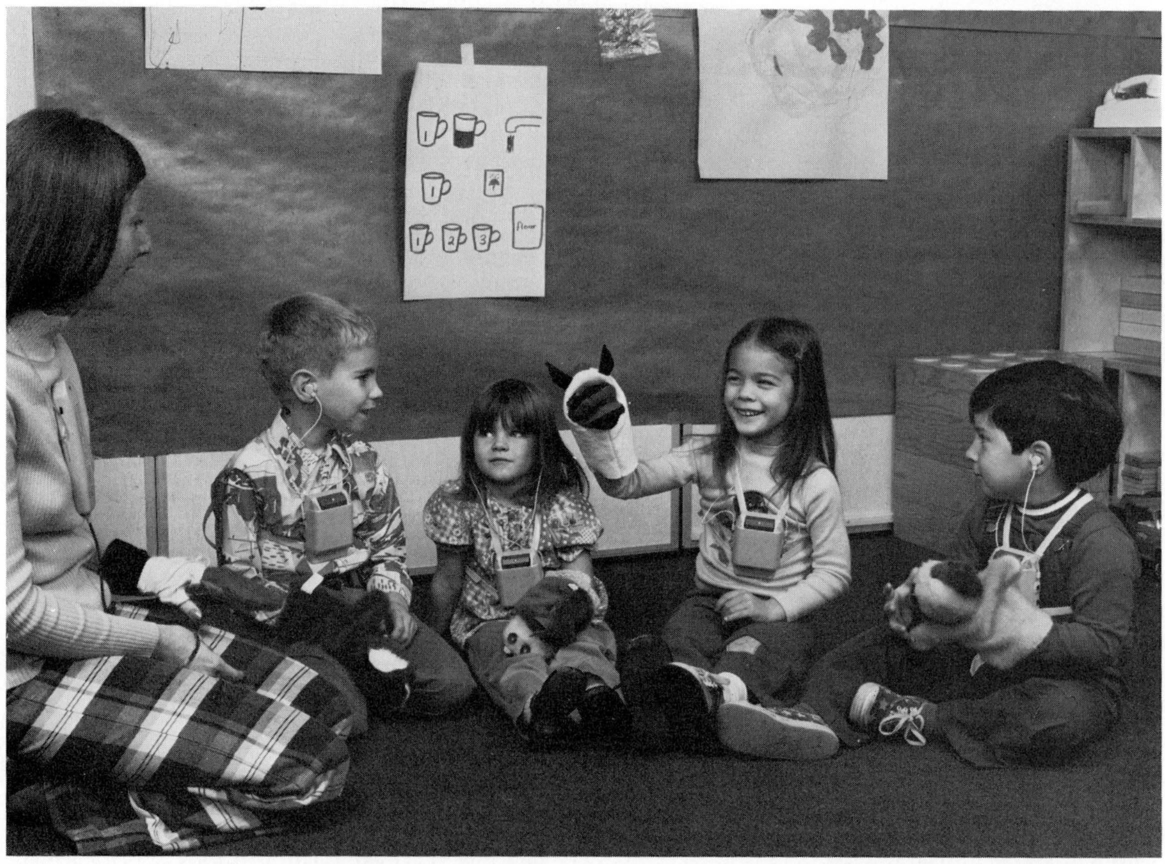

Fig. 38-9. Preschool children with hearing difficulties attend special classes to develop communication skills. (Courtesy HC Electronics, Inc. [Phonic Ear], Mill Valley, Calif.)

vate school for the deaf. The John Tracy Clinic (see box below) provides information and has correspondence classes for parents who have preschool children with severe hearing impairment or deafness.

Recent research has indicated that deaf children's learning abilities can be greatly enhanced by employing the language of signs. In these cases it appears that the "total communication" approach that includes speech reading, auditory training, and sign language is most advantageous. There is a great need for programs that focus on finding these individuals and providing services to help them learn the necessary skills for developing a sense of self-worth.

Hospitalization of the hearing-impaired person

Hospital settings require identification of patients with difficulty with hearing. If a deaf or hard of hearing person is hospitalized, the new environment and unfamiliar faces may accentuate his loneliness and isolation, and anxiety may reduce hearing even further.[15] The following are some specific points to facilitate speech reading or hearing for persons with impaired hearing:

1. Get the person's attention by raising an arm or hand.
2. Start with the light on your face; this will help the person speech read.
3. Talk directly to the person, facing him.
4. Speak clearly but do not overaccentuate words.
5. Speak in a normal tone; do not shout. Shouting overemploys normal speaking movements and may cause distortion and be too loud for the person with sensorineural damage. If the person has conductive loss only, sometimes making the voice louder without shouting is helpful.
6. If the person does not seem to understand what is said, express it differently. Some words are difficult to "see" in speech reading, such as white and red.
7. Move closer to the person and toward the better ear if he does not hear you.
8. Write out proper names or any statement that you are not sure was understood.
9. Do not smile, chew gum, or cover the mouth when talking to a person with limited hearing.
10. Inattention may indicate tiredness or lack of understanding.
11. Use phrases to convey meaning rather than one-word answers. State the major topic of the discussion first and then give details.
12. Do not show annoyance by careless facial expression. Persons who are hard of hearing depend more on usual clues for acceptance.
13. Encourage the use of a hearing aid if the person has one; allow him to adjust it before speaking.
14. If in a group, repeat important statements and avoid asides to others in the group.
15. Avoid the use of the intercommunication system as this may distort sound and cause poor communication.
16. Do not avoid conversation with a person who has hearing loss. It has been said that to live in a silent world is much more devastating than to live in darkness, and persons with hearing loss appear, by and large, to have more emotional difficulties than those who are blind.*

Persons who are hard of hearing depend on their other senses to provide information about changes in their environment. The patient is helped to use visual clues by placing him in a bed where he can observe activity and anticipate others approaching him. He will be easily startled if people suddenly enter his unit if his vision is obscured. Many patients feel less isolated if the nurse touches them lightly on the arm to gain their attention and wakes them by touching them on the arm.

AGENCIES THAT PROVIDE ASSISTANCE FOR THE HEARING IMPAIRED

American Annals of the Deaf, 5034 Wisconsin Ave., N.W., Washington, D.C. 20016. The April issue every year lists a directory of programs and services for the deaf available by state, including information about the type of facilities.

American Federation of the Physically Handicapped, Inc., 1370 National Press Building, Washington, D.C. 20004. Provides counseling and information.

American Speech and Hearing Association, 9030 Old Georgetown Rd., Washington D.C. 20014. Membership is composed of professional persons who teach individuals who have hearing and speech problems.

Gallaudet College, Washington, D.C. The only liberal arts college in the world for the deaf.

The John Tracy Clinic, 806 West Adams Blvd., Los Angeles, Calif. 90007. Provides information and correspondence classes for parents with deaf children.

National Association of Hearing and Speech Agencies, 919 18th St. N.W., Washington, D.C. 20006. Provides counseling and information.

State Office of Vocational Rehabilitation (in each state). Provides vocational training and placement services.

Veterans Administration. Provides audiology clinics and rehabilitative services for veterans.

*Adapted from Conover, M., and Cober, J.: Understanding and caring for the hearing-impaired, Nurs. Clin. North Am. 5:497, 1970.

Because hearing-impaired people are often sensitive to light changes, they can easily be awakened by turning on a light. Special effort must be made to communicate information about the hospital routine to the deaf or hard of hearing patient and to prepare him for special tests.

Acupuncture

Recently there has been a resurgence of interest in acupuncture for the treatment of hearing loss. Audiometric testing of large groups of persons with hearing loss who underwent acupuncture demonstrate that hearing loss is not improved.[20,21] For more information on acupuncture, see p. 356.

Community services

Selected agencies exist for helping the hearing impaired person. The telephone company can provide information with regard to special amplifiers or flashing lights that can be placed on doorbells or telephones. Services for persons with a hearing loss are offered by audiology clinics sponsored by universities, hospitals, community programs, local or state departments of health and education, or the Veterans Administration. National organizations are available to give information and counseling (box, p. 777).

For the person whose vision and hearing both are severely impaired, a catalog distributed by the American Foundation for the Blind includes a vibrator attachment to be used with a timer or clock. The vibrator is placed under the bed mattress, and its vibrations act as an alarm to wake the occupant. (For further information about the catalog, see p. 767).

REFERENCES AND SELECTED READINGS

1. American Foundation for the Blind: Directory of agencies serving the visually handicapped in the United States, ed. 8, New York, 1973, The William Byrd Press.
2. American Institute of Public Opinion Poll, commissioned by Research to Prevent Blindness, Inc., Oct. 1965.
3. American Medical Association drug evaluation, ed. 2, Acton, Mass., 1973, Publishing Sciences Group Inc.
4. American Public Health Association: Services for children with eye problems, New York, 1967, The Association.
5. Beaver, R.: Hearing loss in the elderly: a community health perspective, Publ. Health **88:**19-25, 1973.
6. Beeson, P. B., and McDermott, W., editors: Cecil-Loeb textbook of medicine, ed. 14, Philadelphia, 1975, W. B. Saunders Co.
7. *Bender, R. E.: Communication with the deaf, Am. J. Nurs. **66:**757-760, 1966.
8. Bergeson, B. S., and Goth, A.: Pharmacology in nursing, ed. 13, St. Louis, 1976, The C. V. Mosby Co.
9. Bitonte, J. L., and Keates, R. H., editors: Symposium on the flexible lens, St. Louis, 1972, The C. V. Mosby Co.

*References preceded by an asterisk are particularly well suited for student reading.

9a. Boyles, V. A.: Injection aids for blind diabetic patients, Am. J. Nurs. **77:**1456-1458, 1977.
10. Brown, R. A.: Noise and urban man, Am. J. Publ. Health **58:** 2060-2066, 1968.
11. Bumbold, J., and Seidel, M.: Identifying and serving a multiplying handicapped population. Nurs. Clin. North Am. **10:**341-352, 1975.
12. Carroll, F. J.: Blindness, Boston, 1961, Little, Brown and Co.
13. Carty, R.: Patients who cannot hear, Nurs. Forum **11:**290-299, 1972.
14. Chial, M. R.: Hearing aid evaluation methods, J. Speech Hearing Disord. **39:**270-279, 1974.
15. *Conover, M., and Cober, J.: Understanding and caring for the hearing impaired, Nurs. Clin. North Am. **5:**497-506, 1970.
16. Craig, W. N., and Craig, H. B.: Directory of programs and services for the deaf in the United States, Am. Ann. Deaf, April 1977. (New updating published every year in the April issue.)
17. Cullin, I. C.: Techniques for teaching patients with sensory defects, Nurs. Clin. North Am. **5:**527-538, 1970.
18. Davis, H., and Silverman, S. R.: Hearing and deafness, New York, 1970, Holt, Rinehart, and Winston, Inc.
19. DeWeese, D. D., and Saunders, W. H,: Textbook of otolaryngology, ed. 5, St. Louis, 1977, The C. V. Mosby Co.
20. Downs, M. P.: The deafness management quotient, Hearing Speech News **42:**8, 1974.
21. Downs, M. P.: Overview of the management of the congenitally deaf child, Otolaryngol. Clin. North Am. **4:**223-226, 1971.
22. Downs, M. P.: Audiological evaluation of the congenitally deaf infant, Otolaryngol. Clin. North Am. **4:**347-357, 1971.
23. Editorial, Sight Sav. Rev. **43:**66-67, 1973.
24. Ellis, P. P.: Ocular therapeutics and pharmacology, ed. 5, St. Louis, 1977, The C. V. Mosby Co.
25. Fuerst, E. V., et al.: Fundamentals of nursing, ed. 5, Philadelphia, 1974, J. B. Lippincott Co.
26. Gellis, S. S., and Kagan, B. M.: Current pediatric therapy, ed. 6, Philadelphia, 1973, W. B. Saunders Co.
27. Goetzinger, C. P.: The psychology of hearing impairment. In Katz, J., editor: Handbook of clinical audiology, Baltimore, 1972, The Williams & Wilkins Co.
28. Gordon, R. D.: Experience with a visually disabled mother, Am. J. Nurs. **68:**1943-1945, 1968.
29. *Gould, H.: How to remove contact lenses from comatose patients, Am. J. Nurs. **76:**1483-1485, 1976.
30. Graham, A. B.: Sensorineural hearing processes and disorders, Boston, 1967, Little, Brown and Co.
31. Griffith, J.: Persons with hearing loss, Springfield, Ill., 1969, Charles C Thomas, Publisher.
32. *Haddad, H. M. Drugs for ophthalmologic use, Am. J. Nurs. **68:**324-327, 1968.
33. Hanson, D. R., and Fearn, R. W.: Hearing acuity in young people exposed to pop music and other noise, Lancet **2:**203-205, 1975.
34. Hardy, B. P.: Assessment and instruction: don't push the hard-of-hearing child into the pit!, Am. Ann. Deaf **120:**555-557, 1975.
35. Hatfield, E. M.: Why are they blind? Sight Sav. Rev. **45:**3-22, 1975.
36. Hatfield, E. M.: Estimates of blindness in the United States, Sight Sav. Rev. **43:**69-80, 1973.
37. Havener, W. H.: Ocular pharmacology, ed. 4, St. Louis, 1978, The C. V. Mosby Co.
38. *Havener, W. H., Saunders, W. H., Keith, C. F., and Prescott, A. W.: Nursing care in eye, ear, nose and throat disorders, ed. 3, St. Louis, 1974, The C. V. Mosby Co.
39. Havighurst, R.: Optometry: education for the profession, Re-

port of the National Study of the Optometric Education, Washington, D. C., 1973, National Commission on Accrediting.
40. Hearing aids and the older American, hearings before the Subcommittee on Consumer Interests, Washington, D.C., 1974, Government Printing Office.
41. Hemingway, W. G., and Bergstrom, L.: Symposium on congenital deafness, Otolaryngol. Clin. North Am. 4(2):369-399, 1971.
42. Hersch, L. B., and Amon, C.: A child has a hearing loss: reporting the diagnosis of handicaps in children and its impact on parents, Am. Ann. Deaf **120**:568-571, 1975.
43. Hughes, R. L.: Special devices for the hearing-handicapped patient, Arch. Otolaryngol. **86**:522-527, 1967.
44. Jaffe, B. F.: Sudden deafness: an otologic emergency, Arch. Otolaryngol. **86**:55-60, 1967.
45. Jeffers, J., and Bailey, M.: Speechreading, Springfield, Ill., 1971, Charles C Thomas, Publisher.
45a. Jensen, D.: The silent minority, Nursing '76 **6**:15, October 1976.
46. Journal of American Speech and Hearing Association **1**:29, 1973.
47. Kabins, S. A.: Interactions among antibiotics and other drugs, J.A.M.A. **219**:206-212, 1972.
48. Kannapill, B. M., Hamilton, L. B., and Bornstein, H.: Signs for instructional purposes, Washington, D. C., 1969, Gallaudet College Press.
49. Katz, J.: Handbook of clinical audiology, Baltimore, 1972, The Williams & Wilkins Co.
50. Koetting, R. A.: Contact lenses and the athlete, J. Sch. Health **41**:75-77, 1971.
51. Konopa, V. O., et al.: Noise: the challenge of the future, J. Sch. Health **42**:172-175, 1972.
52. Kornzweig, A. L.: The eye in old age, Am. J. Ophthalmol. **60**:835-843, 1965.
53. Kravitz, H., Neyhus, A. I., Dale, D. O., Laker, H. I., Gomberg, R. M., and Korach A.: The cotton-tipped swab: a major cause of ear injury and hearing loss, Clin. Ped. Phil. **13**:965-970, 1974.
54. Kurtland, L. T., et al.: Epidemiology of neurologic and sense organ disorders, Cambridge, Mass, 1973, Harvard University Press.
55. Linnell, C., and Long, Sr. V.: The hearing-impaired infant: diagnosis and rehabilitation, Nurs. Clin. North Am. **5**:507-515, 1970.
56. Lucente, F. E.: Psychological problems in otolaryngology, Laryngoscope **83**:1684-1689, 1973.
57. Maloney, W. H.: Otolaryngology, New York, 1974, Harper & Row, Publishers.
58. Mamaril, A. P.: Sudden deafness, Am. J. Nurs. **76**:1992-1994, 1976.
59. Marlow, D. R.: Textbook of pediatric nursing, ed. 5, Philadelphia, 1977, W. B. Saunders Co.
60. McConnell, F., and Ward, P.: Deafness in childhood, Nashville, 1967, Vanderbilt University Press.
61. Meadow, K. P.: Self-image, family climate, and deafness, Soc. Forces **47**:428-433, 1969.
62. Mitchell, P. H.: Concepts basic to nursing, New York, 1973, McGraw Hill Book Co.
63. Morrison, A.: Management of sensorineural deafness, Reading, Mass., 1975, Butterworth (Publishers) Inc.
64. Muhooney, J.: A special concern to me: deaf patient care, RN **39**:69-70, 1976.
65. Nelson, W. E.: Textbook of pediatrics, ed. 10, Philadelphia, 1975, W. B. Saunders Co.
66. Niemyer, W.: Psychological aspects of hearing aid fitting, J. Audiol. Tech. **12**:70, 1973.
67. Nilo, E. R.: Needs of the hearing impaired, Am. J. Nurs. **69**:114-116, 1969.
68. Northern, J.: Hearing disorders, Boston, 1976, Little, Brown and Co.
69. Northern, J.: The current status of implantable hearing aids, Hearing Aid J. **26**:15, 1973.
70. Northern, J., and Downs, M.: Hearing in children. Baltimore, 1974, The Williams & Wilkins Co.
71. Occupational Safety and Health Administration, U.S. Department of Labor: Williams-Steiger Occupational Safety and Health Act of 1970, Fed. Reg. **36**:105, 1971; rev. April, 1977.
72. Ohno, M. I.: The eye-patched patient, Am. J. Nurs. **71**:271-274, 1971.
73. Paparella, M. M., and Shumrick, D. A., editors: Otolaryngology, Philadelphia, 1973, W. B. Saunders Co.
74. Quick, C. A.: Chemical and drug effects on the inner ear. In Paparella, M. M., and Shumrick, D. A., editors: Otolaryngology, Philadelphia, 1973, W. B. Saunders Co.
75. Research to Prevent Blindness, Inc.: Annual Report, New York, 1976, Research to Prevent Blindness, Inc.
76. Registry of interpreters for the deaf, P.O. Box 1339, Washington, D.C.
77. Riffenburgh, R. S.: The blind patient, Arch. Ophthalmol. **79**:361-365, 1968
78. Riffenburgh, R. S.: The psychology of blindness, Geriatrics **22**:127-130, 1967.
79. Rose, M.: Coping behavior of physically handicapped children, Nurs. Clin. North Am. **10**:329-339, 1975.
80. Ross, M.: Aural rehabilitation, Indianapolis, 1972, The Bobbs-Merrill Co., Inc.
81. Ruben, M.: Contact lens practice, Baltimore, 1975, The Williams & Wilkins Co.
82. Ruben, M.: Contact lenses, shells and prosthetics, Nurs. Times **68**:133-136, 1972.
83. *Sabatino, L.: Do's and dont's of deaf patient care, RN **39**:64-68, 1976.
84. Sataloff, J.: Preventing hearing loss due to excessive noise exposure, J. Occup. Med. **16**:470-471, 1974.
85. Shein, J.: The deaf population of the United States, Silver Spring, Md, 1975, National Association of Deaf.
86. Siegelaub, A. B., Friedman, G. D., Adour, K., and Seltzer, C. C.: Hearing loss in adults: relation to age, sex, exposure to loud noise, and cigarette smoking, Arch. Environ. Health **29**:107-109, 1974.
87. Simmons, F. B.: Acupuncture and hearing loss. In Northern, J.: Hearing disorders, Boston, 1976, Little, Brown and Co.
88. Smith, M. B.: Handbook of ocular toxicity, Acton, Mass., 1976, Publication Sciences Group, Inc.
89. Spar, H. J.: The deaf-blind. In Garrett, J. F., and Levine, E. S., editors: Rehabilitation practives with the physically disabled, ed. 2, New York, 1973, Columbia University Press.
90. Support for vision research: interim report of the National Advisory Eye Council, U.S. Department of Health, Education and Welfare, No. (NIH) 76-1098, 1976.
91. Symposium on sensorineural hearing loss in children: early detection and intervention, Otolaryngol. Clin. North Am. 8(1), Feb. 1975.
92. Taub, H.: Acupuncture and sensorineural hearing loss, J. Speech Hear. Dis. **40**:427-433, 1975.
93. Taylor, I. G., Hine, W. B., Brasier, V. J., Chiveralls, K., and Morris, T.: A study of the causes of hearing loss in a population of deaf children with special references to genetic factors, J. Laryngol. Otol. **89**:899-914, 1975.

94. The eye in nursing literature 1968-1973: a bibliography, A.O.R.N. J. **18**:1013-1014, 1973.
95. Thompson, I. S., and Willis, L. C.: A prospective study of children "at risk" for deafness, J. Laryngol. Otol. **90**:167-172, 1972.
96. Vernon, J., Mahoney, T., and Schlming, A.: Implantable hearing aids. In Northern, J.: Hearing disorders, Boston, 1976, Little, Brown and Co.
97. Vernon, M.: Major current trends in rehabilitation and education of the deaf and hard of hearing, Rehab. Lit. **36**:102-107, 1975.
98. Vernon, M.: Early profound deafness. In Garrett, J. F., and Levine, E. S., editors: Rehabilitation practices with the physically disabled, ed. 2, New York, 1973, Columbia University Press.
99. Vision research program planning, U.S. Department of Health, Education and Welfare, No. (NIH) 75-664, vol. 1, 1975.
100. Ward, W. D.: Proceedings of the International Congress on Noise as a Public Health Problem, USEPA document 550-9-73-006, Washington, D.C., 1974, U.S. Government Printing Office.
101. What if your patient is also deaf, RN **39**:59-70, 1976.
101a. Wolf, E. M.: Communicating with deaf surgical patients, A.O.R.N. J. **26**:39-47, July 1977.
102. Wright, J.: Deaf but not mute, Am. J. Nurs. **76**:795-800, 1976.
103. Yates, J. I.: Rehabilitation of hearing impaired adults, J. Rehabil. **39**:20-22, 1973.

AUDIOVISUAL RESOURCES

1. Nursing techniques for the care of patients with impaired vision, Ohio State University, Columbus, Ohio. Series of eight films.
2. Where old age begins, Video Nursing, Evanston, Ill., 1970. Film, 16mm, black and white.
3. Silent world, muffled world, Deafness Research Foundation, National Audiovisual Center, Washington D.C., 1966. Film, 16 mm, color.
4. The ear and hearing, Wayne State University, College of Medicine, Detroit; available through Ciba Pharmaceutical Co., 1959. Film, 16 mm, color.
5. With these hands, WKYC, Cleveland, August 5, 1976, Videotape.

39

Problems of special senses: eye and ear

LYNN CHENOWETH McWILLIAMS
LINDA ANNE BROSEMAN

■ PROBLEMS OF THE EYE

The major disorders of the eye that can affect vision are trauma and infection in persons of all ages; strabismus in children; and cataract, glaucoma, retinal detachment and diabetic retinopathy in adults, primarily older persons. Information on assessment of the eye, prevention of visual impairment, general therapeutic intervention, and services for visually impaired persons is given in Chapter 37 and 38.

In order to decrease the problem of vision impairment, health workers need to focus on prevention of eye disease and injury, early detection of disease and injury, and adequate treatment. As participants in planning, providing, and evaluating health care, the nurse assumes responsibilities in all these areas.

□ Eye manifestations of systemic diseases

Diseases and infections that affect other parts of the body also affect the eye. The eye has been described as the most important square inch of body surface, both diagnostically and functionally.[28] By examining the back portion of the interior of the eyeball (fundus) with an ophthalmoscope, the practitioner can recognize many major diseases. Some of the diseases and pathologic states that can be identified through their typical fundus picture and other eye assessment include metabolic diseases, vascular and hematologic disorders, neurologic problems, and nutritional deficiencies. Assessment of the eye often will indicate the severity of the disease.

Metabolic diseases

Of the metabolic diseases affecting the eye, diabetes is the most common. Diabetes may affect any of the structures of the eye. Senile cataracts occur earlier in persons who have diabetes and progress more rapidly than in most elderly people. Diabetic retinopathy produces characteristic changes in the retina that can cause severe visual damage and eventually result in blindness. Diabetes also causes the growth of new blood vessels on the surface of the retina and optic disc that later extend into the vitreous humor (*retinitis proliferans*). This condition often causes blindness due to recurrent vitreous hemorrhages and retinal detachment (see p 795, diabetic retinopathy).

Vascular and hematologic disorders

Vascular disorders, such as persistent systemic hypertension, will eventually produce changes in the retina (hemorrhage, edema, and exudates), which may result in the loss of sight. If the cause of the elevated blood pressure is eclampsia of pregnancy and is of short duration, the *retinopathy* (any disorder of the retina) usually subsides when the pregnancy is terminated. Retinopathy due to hypertension resulting from renal arteriosclerosis or diffuse glomerulonephritis is usually progressive and irreversible. The severity of the hypertension causes narrowing of the retinal arteries, and the blood flow through the retina and choroid is diminished resulting in degenerative changes in the retina and loss of vision.

Visual loss may follow vascular accidents to vessels anywhere in the eye or in the main blood vessels outside the eye. A cerebrovascular accident may cause hemianopia (blindness for one half of the field of vision in one or both eyes) or total blindness, depending on its location. Arteriosclerosis and atheromatosis, particularly involving the carotid and cranial arteries, may release emboli that lead to occlusion of the retinal vessels.

Hematologic disorders cause characteristic retinal hemorrhages or neovascularization as in the case of sickle cell disease.

Neurologic problems

Neurologic disorders include a wide range of problems. Eye examination aids in evaluation of seven of the 12 cranial nerves (II through VIII) and provides information about the sympathetic and parasympathetic pathways (see Chapter 34). Demyelinating disorders such as multiple sclerosis and infections such as syphilis cause typical nerve damage to the eye. Increased intracranial pressure causes swelling of the optic disc (papilledema). Through eye examination (perimetry studies) lesions of the brain can be attributed to a specific lobe in the brain (temporal, parietal, or occipital). Unilateral dilation of the pupil helps diagnose severity and location of head injury.

Nutritional deficiencies

Nutritional deficiencies can cause pathologic changes in the eye. There seems to be direct relationship between good nutrition and eye health. A lack of vitamins A and B in the diet can cause changes in the conjunctiva, corneal epithelium, and retina. Tears are reduced, and eyes and lid margins become reddened and inflamed. Sensitivity to light is often present, and some loss of visual acuity is noticed at night. Significant difficulty is called night blindness *(nyctalopia).* When nutritionally caused, night blindness may respond favorably to ingestion of a nutritious diet and vitamin A. On the other hand *excessive* amounts of vitamin A can damage the retina. Vitamin B deficiency may cause bilateral optic neuritis, especially in individuals who drink large quantities of alcohol. When damage to the optic nerve has been severe and prolonged, a diet high in vitamin B and other essential nutrients can accomplish only partial recovery. Fortunately eye problems from nutritional deficiency are rarely found in the developed countries.

□ Trauma

Prevention

Although the eye is vulnerable to trauma, natural protective mechanisms can prevent or minimize injury (Table 39-1).

In addition to the body's natural defenses against injury, *protective equipment* such as goggles, shields, and shatterproof safety lenses are advised for certain occupations, sports activities, and the like. Knowledge of safety precautions and first-aid techniques are valuable in preventing serious damage from trauma.

Prompt and appropriate care of the injured eye may prevent serious vision impairment or loss of the eye (Table 39-2). The two major categories of trauma are *burns* and *contact (mechanical) trauma.*

Burns

Chemical burns such as those caused by acid or alkali must be treated immediately to prevent the possibility of permanent visual impairment from damage to the cornea. For chemical trauma of any nature prompt immediate irrigation is the essential action that may result in salvaging an otherwise irrevocably lost eye. Irrigation after chemical trauma should be performed immediately after the injury and carried on for a prolonged period of time, a minimum of 15 minutes. While cool tap water is excellent for irrigation, any nontoxic solution can be used. After irrigation, and *only after* irrigation, is the patient transported to a physician.

Ultraviolet burns of the cornea may occur from exposure under a sunlamp. The individual becomes aware of painful eyes several hours after exposure. Treatment consists of cold compresses, analgesics such as aspirin or codeine, and topical ophthalmic anesthetics. Topical antibiotics may also be used to prevent infection. Most pa-

Table 39-1. Protective mechanisms of the eye

Protective feature	Function
Bony orbital rim	Prevents many mechanical injuries
Orbital fluids and tissues	Cushion direct blows
Eyelashes and eyelids	Quickly close reflexly from visual or mechanical stimuli
Bell phenomenon	Eyes reflexly rotate upward with lid closing to protect cornea
Lacrimal secretions	Can flush away chemicals or foreign bodies

Table 39-2. First aid for eye injuries

Injury	Interventions
Burns: chemical, flame	Flush eye immediately for 15 minutes with cool water or any available nontoxic liquid. Seek medical assistance.
Loose substance on conjunctiva: dirt, insects	Lift upper lid over lower lid to dislodge substance and produce tearing; irrigate eye with water if necessary. Do not rub eye. Obtain medical assistance if above interventions fail.
Contact injury: contusion, ecchymosis, laceration	Apply cold compresses if no laceration present; cover eye if laceration present. Seek medical assistance.
Penetrating objects	Do not remove object. Place protective shield over eye (e.g., paper cup); cover uninjured eye to prevent excess movement of injured eye. Seek medical assistance.

tients are comfortable within 24 hours after treatment begins. Rarely is the cornea scarred permanently.[62] Ultraviolet burns may also occur from the use of germicidal lamps, electric flashes, and arc welding.

Thermal burns of the eyelids can cause lid contracture. Skin grafting may be necessary to prevent severe contractures and exposure of the eye. Full-thickness grafts can be taken from the uninjured eyelid, the inner aspect of the forearm, or behind the ear.[62]

Contact trauma

Lacerations of the eyelid require treatment by an eye specialist because there is danger of scar formation as healing occurs. Even though lid lacerations may bleed freely, pressure against the lid to stop bleeding can cause damage to the eye beneath. Cuts or tears in the eyelid may need to be sutured after the bleeding is controlled and any foreign material is removed. Antitetanus serum usually is given to all patients who sustain eye wounds.

Injuries to the ciliary body and sclera and injuries involving the orbit are critical because adjacent tissues usually are injured also and there may be escape of contents of the eyeball and possible infection of the interior of the eye. If these injuries result in wounds that are small and clean, treatment consists of bed rest, antibiotics given systemically and topically, suturing the wound, instilling atropine to put the iris and the ciliary body at rest, and a firm dressing. If the injury is extensive and if sight is lost, enucleation (removal of the eyeball) may be necessary.

Persons with *ecchymosis* of the eyelid and surrounding tissues (black eye) should be examined to rule out coexisting skull fractures and intraocular bleeding or other eye damage. Initially, cold compresses will help to control the bleeding. Subsequent hot compresses after 48 hours will speed up the reabsorption of blood from the tissues. The discoloration, which will last about 2 weeks, can be covered to some extent with cosmetics.

Penetrating injury of the eye requires medical care as soon as possible. The most important goal is to prevent further damage before reaching the ophthalmologist. It is very easy to convert a minor corneal laceration without iris prolapse into the loss of an eye when applying even gentle pressure on the eye during transportation of the patient. To protect the eye against pressure, a shield can be used. A cardboard cone or a paper cup can be taped securely over the patient's eye to prevent anyone or anything from touching it. Tears, blood, and other discharges cannot be wiped away without risking dangerous pressure changes. Covering the uninjured eye will prevent excessive movement of the injured eye. While the patient may walk or be transported sitting up in an automobile, unnecessary exertion such as bending over or carrying heavy objects should be avoided. These activities could increase the intraocular pressure and cause more damage to the eye.

Corneal injuries are serious because resistance to infection is low in the cornea, and scarring can impair vision. It has been estimated that foreign bodies on the surface of the cornea constitute about 25% of ocular injuries.[48] Tearing, photophobia, and a sensation of "something in the eye" warn a person that a foreign body is present if his neuromuscular networks are functioning properly. If an abrasion of the cornea occurs there may be considerable pain. For those persons with impaired sensorimotor function, the nurse must observe for damage to the cornea.

A dreaded sequela to eye injury is *sympathetic ophthalmia*. This complication is a serious inflammation of the uveal tract (ciliary body, iris, and choroid) in the uninjured eye that follows a penetrating injury to the other eye. While the cause of this condition is unknown, it may be due to an allergic reaction to the uveal pigment that is set free in the bloodstream at the time of the injury. Children are especially susceptible; however, it may occur at any age. The uninjured eye becomes inflamed; photophobia, lacrimation, dimness of vision, and pain in the eye may be experienced. Sympathetic ophthalmia may appear 3 to 8 weeks after the eye injury or months or years later. The injured eye may be removed soon after the injury in an attempt to prevent the developmentof sympathetic ophthalmia.

Because of increased medical skill in treating perforating wounds and the administration of cortisone at the earliest suggestion of inflammation, sympathetic ophthalmia has become a rare disease in recent years.

□ Infections and inflammation

Infections and inflammation can occur in any of the eye structures and may be caused by microorganisms, mechanical irritation, or sensitivity to some substance. Inflammation of the eye accounts for more than one half of the total incidence of acute disease conditions, with an estimated 1,180,000 cases per year. Conjunctivitis represents about two thirds of the total.[70]

Styes

Styes (hordeola) are relatively mild but extremely common infections of the follicle of an eyelash or the small lubricating glands of the lid margins. Staphylococci are often the infecting organisms. Patients should be taught not to squeeze styes because the infection may spread and cause cellulitis of the lids. If warm moist compresses are used, styes usually open and drain without surgery. These infections tend to occur in crops because the infecting organism spreads from one hair follicle to another. Poor hygiene and excessive use of cosmetics may be contributing causes.

Chalazion

A chalazion is a cyst caused by an obstruction in the ducts of the sebaceous glands (meibomian glands) located in the connective tissue in the free edges of the eyelids. The cysts present a hard, shiny, lumpy appearance as viewed from the inner side of the lid. They may cause pressure on the cornea. Small chalazions may disappear after massage and hot compresses. If they are large or become infected, they ususally require surgical incision and curettage. When an antibiotic is needed, the systemic route is used because topically applied antibiotics will not penetrate into the substance of the eyelids. Chalazions usually are removed in the physician's office or in the clinic with the patient under local anesthesia. An antibacterial ointment such as neomycin sulfate may be applied to the conjuctiva, and an eyepad is worn for a few days.

Conjunctivitis and blepharitis

Conjunctivitis (inflammation of conjunctiva) and blepharitis (inflammation of the eyelids) are common infections that can occur from a variety of causes. They may result from mechanical trauma such as that caused by sunburn or infection with organisms such as staphylococci, viruses, streptococci, or gonococci. Inflammation is often due to allergic reactions within the body or to outside irritants such as poison ivy or cosmetics. Two of the viral agents that cause conjunctivitis are trachoma and herpes simplex. Although rare in the United States, approximately 15% of the world's population suffer from trachoma.

Acute bacterial conjunctivitis is often called "pinkeye." Common in school children, pinkeye is highly infectious. Conjunctival redness and crusting discharge deposited on the lashes and corners of the eye are the characteristic findings. Treatment includes cleansing of the lids and lashes, use of topical antibiotics, and precautions to prevent the spread to others. Firm adherent crusts may be softened by use of hot moist compresses. Because the material is infectious it should be disposed of in a sanitary way. A topical antibiotic such as neomycin is instilled in the eyes every 1 or 2 hours while the patient is awake.[28] Fortunately acute bacterial conjunctivitis is usually self-limited, leaving no permanent scars.

Seborrheic blepharitis, often occurring in children, involves both upper and lower lids. The lid margins are reddened with scales attached to the base of the lashes. Some degree of conjunctivitis is present. Application of local antibiotics and local steroids is helpful. The condition can be kept under control if treated effectively before any serious eye involvement (such as keratitis) develops.

Keratitis

Inflammation of the cornea is called keratitis. It may be acute or chronic and superficial or deep (interstitial). Acute epithelial keratitis commonly occurs in association with bacterial conjunctivitis caused by staphylococci, pneumococci, and *Haemophilus aegyptius.* Viruses such as herpes simplex may also cause a type of keratitis. Keratitis may be associated with a corneal ulcer or be caused by diseases such as tuberculosis and syphilis. Allergic reactions, vitamin A deficiency, or viral diseases such as mumps, measles, and herpes simplex may contribute to its development in children.

Assessment. Keratitis causes severe pain in the eye, photophobia (sensitivity to light), tearing, and blepharospasm (spasm of the eyelids). Uncontrolled keratitis can result in loss of vision due to impairment of corneal transparency or destruction of the eye by corneal perforation.

Intervention. If possible the systemic cause is found and treated. Cortisone may be used cautiously to control the inflammation; antibiotics are given to treat the infection. Atropine sulfate, which blurs visions for at least 1 week, will keep the iris and ciliary body at rest; hot compresses will help promote healing. Idoxuridine (IDU) applied locally is effective in helping to clear keratitis caused by herpes simplex in 80% of cases. The eyes may be covered to limit eye movements, and the person may be placed on bed rest.

When the cornea is so damaged that severe vision impairment occurs, *corneal grafting (keratoplasty)* may be done. Loss of vision caused by an opaque or destroyed cornea may be restored by replacing the damaged layers with a corresponding corneal graft obtained from a new cadaver or from an eye freshly removed by operation. For best results the donor cornea must be removed within 6 hours of death and ideally should be used within 24 hours. Transplants preserved for longer periods may be used for lamellar grafts. The present practice is to keep a waiting list of persons who need grafts, since eye banks are not able to keep up with the demand. Eye Bank for Sight Restoration, Inc.,* is a nonprofit organization that collects and distributes donated eyes throughout the country. Donors or their relatives usually make arrangements before death for donating the eyes.

Corneal transplantation cannot be done if there is any infection. The kind of corneal graft used depends on the depth and size of the damaged part that must be replaced (Fig. 39-1). Corneal transplants, or grafts, may

*210 East 64th Street, New York 10021.

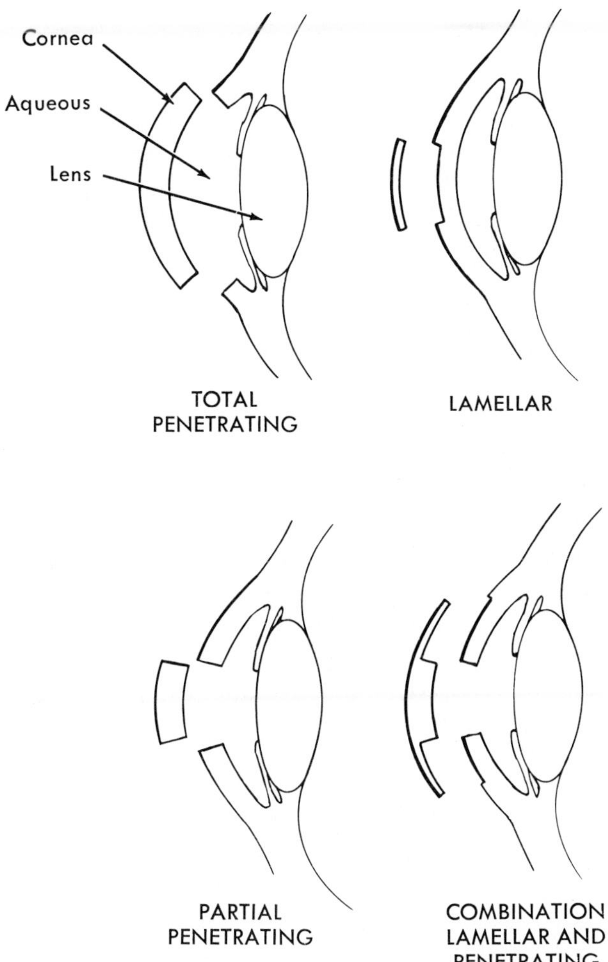

Fig. 39-1. Types of corneal grafts now being used. Note that in lamellar graft, defect does not penetrate entire thickness of cornea.

involve the entire thickness of the cornea (total penetrating), only part of the depth of the cornea (lamellar), or a combination of these, in which a small part of the graft involves the entire thickness of the cornea (partial penetrating). Obviously the penetrating graft is the more difficult to establish and requires the more definitive care postoperatively. For the penetrating graft the eye surgeon seldom uses a donor eye that is over 48 hours old.

Because a large amount of tissue is removed and replaced, the patient who has had a penetrating graft transplant usually remains in bed with both eyes bandaged for 1 to 2 days so as not to disturb the graft. The patient who has had a mixed or partial penetrating graft usually has both eyes bandaged and is kept very quiet for at least 24 hours, whereas the patient who has had a lamellar graft only may not have the unaffected eye covered at all and may be out of bed and able to feed himself on the day of the operation. Corneal grafts heal very slowly because of the lack of blood vessels in the cornea and require from 3 weeks to 6 months to heal firmly. The patient is advised to avoid sudden, quick movement, jarring, bending, or lifting during this period in order to avoid disturbing the healing process. Success also depends on the basic disease process.

Complications of corneal transplant operations include blood vessels that grow into the new cornea (compensatory neovascularization), so that clarity may be lost, or clouding of the new cornea for no apparent reason. While the operation can usually be repeated, performing a second operation depends on the condition of the patient's eye.

Corneal ulcer

Because of its location the cornea is vulnerable to trauma and contamination with microorganisms. Infections of the cornea are not common occurrences. When present, however, they can lead to scarring, perforation, extensive intraocular infection, and loss of the eye. The ulcer may be caused by trauma, by contact lenses, or by infections of the conjunctiva that have spread to the cornea. Prompt treatment of ocular injuries can usually prevent the complication of infection. Persons with a low resistance to infection may develop ulcers from little apparent cause (for example, the individual who has diabetes mellitus).

Assessment. The shape, size, and depth of the ulcer can be outlined by instilling sterile fluorescein, a yellow-green harmless dye. Because fluorescein harbors the growth of microorganisms such as *Pseudomonas*, only a new unopened bottle should be used. Also available are single-use fluorescein-impregnated paper strips that are gently touched to the inside of the lower lid.

Assessment of a corneal ulcer is accomplished by the use of a bright movable light such as a small flashlight. Details are seen more clearly with oblique illumination directed from the side rather than from straight ahead. Since the cornea has many pain-transmitting fibers, damage to its epithelium is easily recognized when pain is present on blinking. If pain and blepharospasm interfere with examination, a drop of anesthetic such as 0.5% proparacaine can be used.

Intervention. The ulcer may be self-limiting, it may spread across the cornea, or it may penetrate into its deeper layers. Nonpenetrating ulcers such as those caused by fingernail scratches heal readily unless infected. Antibiotic drops may be instilled to prevent infection, and a protective dressing may be worn for a few days. Ulcers that penetrate to the deep layers of the cornea are serious because the central cornea is an avascular area. Deep ulcers may be cleansed with an antiseptic solution, cauterized, treated with antibiotics locally and systemically, and covered with a firm dressisng. Atropine sulfate may be instilled to keep the pupil dilated and to put the ciliary body and iris at rest, thus reducing pain. Hot compresses may be applied to help clear the infection, and cortisone may be administered cautiously to control the inflammation. The corneal ulcer is a form of keratitis. When the corneal ulcer causes impaired vision, corneal transplant may be done (see p. 784).

Uveitis

The uvea or uveal tract is a vascular and pigmented layer of the eye that includes the choroid, the ciliary body, and the iris. Inflammation of the area is referred to as uveitis.

Inflammatory lesions of the uvea are caused by a wide variety of factors and infectious agents, which may involve one portion or all three simultaneously. Etiologic classification includes infection, allergy, trauma, toxic agents, noninfective systemic diseases (such as diabetes), and unknown factors. The specific cause of most cases of uveitis cannot be diagnosed.[62]

Assessment. Uveitis produces pain in the eyeball radiating to the forehead and temple, photophobia (sensitivity to light), lacrimation, and interference with vision. There is edema of the upper lid, the iris is swollen because of congestion and exudation of cells and fibrin, and the pupil is contracted and irregular as a result of the formation of adhesions.

Intervention. The instillation of 1% atropine sulfate or 0.2% scopolamine into the eye puts the iris and ciliary body at rest, relieves pain and photophobia, and diminishes congestion. By keeping the pupil dilated, these cycloplegic drugs prevent adhesions from forming between the anterior capsule of the lens and the iris and tend to cause those already formed to regress. Moist warm compresses may be applied several times each day to help diminish pain and inflammation. The eyes usually are covered, and in the convalescent period dark glasses are ordered to be worn. The patient is on bed rest during the acute stages. Although acetylsalicylic acid (aspirin) may be helpful for relieving pain, sometimes morphine sulfate is necessary. Cortisone preparations are of great value in controlling the inflammation in many patients, but the inflammation in other patients resists almost all forms of treatment. If a systemic cause cannot be found and treated, the injection of a foreign protein (fever therapy) such as the typhoid H antigen into the body to stimulate its defense mechanism may be used. Complications of these infections of the uvea include the formation of adhesions, keratitis, secondary glaucoma, and the loss of vision.

Outcome criteria for the person with inflammation of the eye

The patient or significant other can:

1. State name, dosage, and frequency of eye medication to be taken and the need to destroy unused ophthalmic antibiotics after therapy.
2. Describe method and frequency of eye compresses to be used.
3. Describe measures to prevent spread of infection to the uninvolved eye.
4. Describe the activity and movements that are to be avoided after corneal grafting.
5. Describe measures to prevent spread of eye infection to others in the household.

□ Strabismus

Strabismus (squint, cross-eye, walleye) is characterized by misalignment of the visual axes. Normally when both eyes look at the same object, the image of the object is fused by the brain into a single picture (fusion). When there is fusion of the two images perceived by the eyes, binocular vision is present, providing stereoscopic (three-dimensional) vision for the individual.

Etiology. Strabismus may be paralytic or nonparalytic. *Paralytic* strabismus (inability to move the eye) is caused by loss of function of the ocular muscles resulting from damage to the muscles or the cranial nerves (III, IV, or VI) by tumor, infection, or brain or eye injuries. Its main symptom in addition to the strabismus is double vision (diplopia).

Nonparalytic strabismus affects 1% of the population. The child may look straight with either the right eye or the left eye but not with both simultaneously. If he fixes (looks straight ahead) with one eye and then the other, he has alternating strabismus. If he prefers to use one eye to the exclusion of the other and always uses the preferred eye, he has monocular strabismus.

Prevention. Any child who does not have straight eyes at birth or shortly after should be considered to have strabismus and be examined promptly. While loss of sight from strabismus is *preventable,* it is the most common cause of partial blindness in one eye in children. It usually can be treated successfully before the child is 6 years of age. The younger the child the easier he is to treat. The public health nurse and the school nurse should be particularly alert to children who show signs of strabismus and should direct them to medical care. The establishment of free preschool vision screening programs for children in the 3- to 5-year-old age group has been extremely helpful in getting the child with strabismus referred for treatment early enough to be treated satisfactorily. A health teaching packet, including an attractive story booklet designed by two nurses, has been developed to encourage mothers to seek eye testing for their children.* There is no cheaper, easier, or more rewarding way to restore vision to an otherwise legally blind eye than by simply patching the eye of a young child with strabismus. It is extremely important the these children by identified, referred, and properly treated.

Assessment. Evaluation of strabismus includes physical examination to rule out major cerebral and ocular disease, refraction with use of a cycloplegic drug to discover errors of refraction, and orthoptic evaluation to measure the angle of strabismus. During examination, when the child with strabismus looks straight ahead with one eye, the other deviates. A light source directed straight into normal eyes forms a reflected spot image symmetrically located in each pupil; in strabismus the image is off center in one eye compared with its location in the other eye. The crossing may be slight or very noticeable. If the eye is turned inward toward the nose, it is called convergent strabismus *(esotropia).* If the eye is turned outward, it is called divergent strabismus *(exotropia)* (Fig. 39-2). If the child never uses the crossed eye, impaired vision may result. This type of defective vision is called *amblyopia.*

When the two eyes are not coordinated and send two different mental images to the brain, fusion cannot occur. Inability to obtain fusion causes diplopia or suppression. *Diplopia* is referred to as double vision. It is possible for normal healthy persons to experience transient diplopia when they are tired or have ingested too much alcohol. These are cases of temporary failure of fusion mechanisms in the brain. In *suppression* the mental image from one eye is ignored. Suppression of the image from one eye occurs as a normal cerebral phenomenon when a monocular microscope is used. With both eyes open the viewer is able to see the magnified field and to

*Lazy Eye, Ltd., P.O. Box 161, Eau Claire, Wis. 54701.

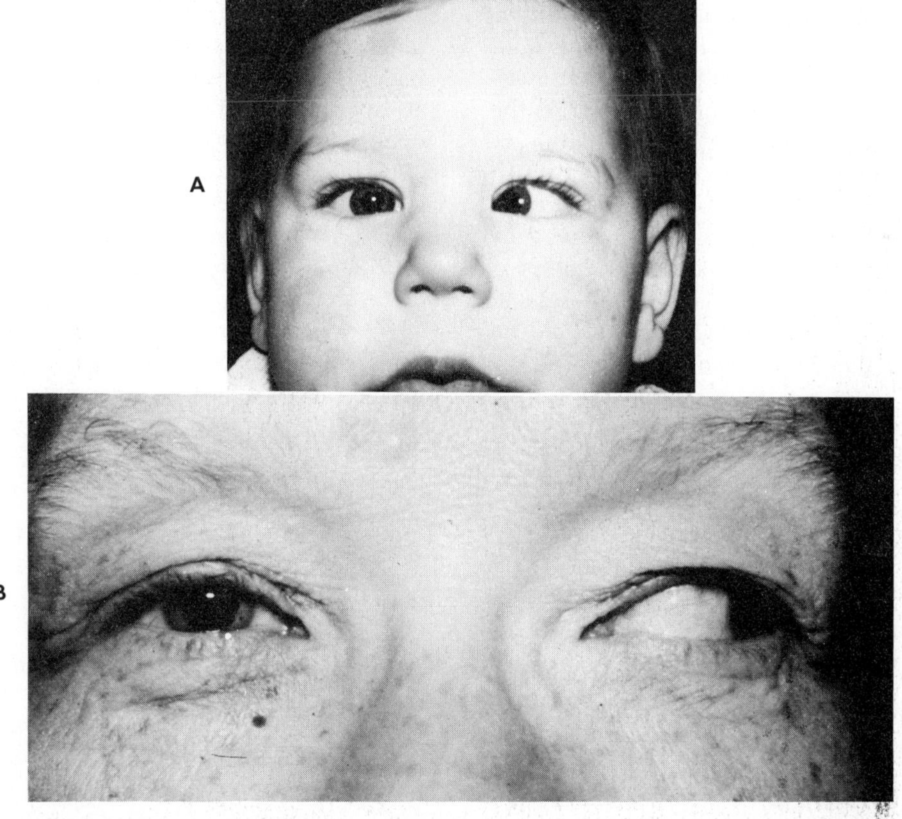

Fig. 39-2. A, Esotropia with right eye fixing and left eye deviating. There is slight epicanthus bilaterally. **B,** Comitant exotropia. (From Newell, F. W., and Ernest, J. T.: Ophthalmology: principles and concepts, St. Louis, 1974, The C. V. Mosby Co.)

disregard the picture of the table top perceived by the other eye. In strabismus, however, suppression of vision in one eye may lead to irreversible vision impairment called *suppression* (strabismic) *amblyopia*.

In amblyopia vision is reduced in an eye that appears normal on examination. Suppression amblyopia refers to cerebral blocking of vision in an eye that either is deviated (crossed, strabismic) or has a refractive error more marked than that of the "good" eye.

Intervention. Early medical attention is important in strabismus, both to save vision and to prevent the emotional trauma that is always associated with crossed eyes. Treatment should begin as soon as the diagnosis is made. During early childhood *occlusion* is used to improve vision. The "good" eye is covered with a patch, bandage, or attachment to the glasses, forcing the child to use the weaker eye. The length of time necessary for occlusion might be as short as 1 or 2 days in a 6-month-old child, 1 or 2 months in a 6-year-old child, and 1 or 2 years in an 8-year-old child. *Orthoptics* is nonsurgical treatment of strabismus in which prisms, glasses, and exercises are used to train the child to use the two eyes together. Orthoptics is used as an adjunct to other methods of treating strabismus.

Strabismus in children who are farsighted and who accommodate excessively may be corrected by constantly wearing glasses. Glasses with harness frames can be safely worn by children 5 to 6 months of age. As the child becomes more independent it is sometimes very difficult to get him to wear glasses consistently. When the glasses are removed the eyes tend to cross. Long-acting miotics such as isoflurophate (DFP) instilled daily potentiates constriction of the ciliary muscle and helps to diminish the esotropia. Sometimes the use of glasses and the use of drugs are combined. A recent article on strabismus describes the nature and treatment of the condition.[30]

Surgery to correct strabismus may be performed very early (by 6 months of age) in an attempt to prevent the loss of fusion potential (binocularity). In most patients, particularly esotropic patients, the younger the child when surgery is performed the more the likelihood of restoring binocular vision. After the age of 6 years, surgery may achieve only cosmetic improvement and may not restore fusion, particularly in esotropic patients. Surgery consists of shortening or lengthening the muscle to straighten the eye. The child may wear a dressing over the eye for a few days and is permitted to move about freely. Surgery may be followed by the prescription of corrective glasses and eye exercises, depending on the individual patient. The child's family should understand that the operation may need to be repeated. Parents should be encouraged to continue with medical treatment for as long as recommended. If they believe that the condition is completely cured and neglect medical attention until a conspicuous squint again appears, damage to vision may have occurred.

□ Cataract

A cataract is a clouding, or opacity, of the lens that leads to gradual, painless blurring of vision and eventual loss of sight (Fig. 39-3). A cataract is *not* a growth on the eye. The opacity is due to chemical changes in the protein of the lens caused by slow degeneration (age), injury, poison, or intraocular infection. Cataracts can occur at any time of life and may be associated with iritis, uveitis, and other conditions such as diabetes.

Etiology. In general, cataracts are classified as *senile*, those associated with aging; *traumatic*, those associated with injury; *congenital*, those that occur at birth; or *secondary*, those that occur following other eye diseases.

Acquired cataracts resulting from aging, trauma, and disease usually develop gradually. Symptoms may be hazy vision and difficulty seeing at night. However, patients with cataract development in the center portion of

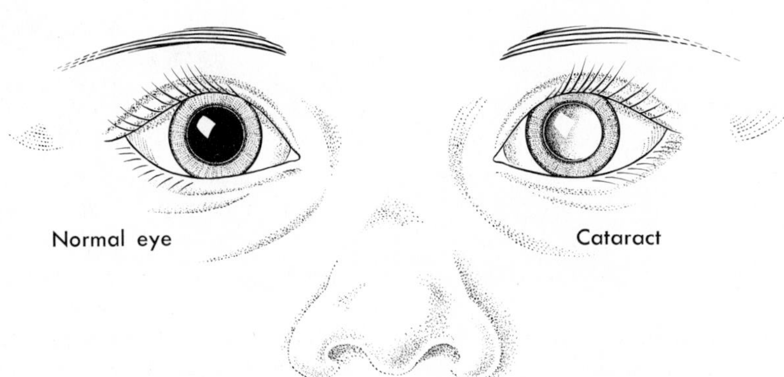

Fig. 39-3. Cataract visible in left eye as white opacity of lens seen through pupil.

the lens can generally see better in dim light when the pupil is dilated. The ophthalmoscope and the slit lamp are used to examine the lens through a dilated pupil.

Cataracts occur so often in the elderly that the term *senile cataract* is used. At 80 years of age about 85% of all persons have some clouding of the lens. Senile cataracts are listed as the most common cause of blindness in older persons, yet the response of the condition to surgery often is excellent. Unlike most other damaging diseases of the eye, vision loss from cataract can be restored by surgical removal of the cataract. Even patients who are in their nineties can often be operated on with good results.

After aging, the next most common cause of cataract is injury to the eye.[28] The transparency of the lens may be destroyed by either a penetrating wound or a contusion. Cataracts may result from the ingestion of injurious substances such as dinitrophenol or nephthalene.

While most cataracts occurring at birth (congenital) are hereditary, they may be caused by virus infections such as German measles that the mother had during the first trimester of pregnancy. Cataracts account for 11.5% of blindness in preschool children.[31] When assessing a child's eyes, the cataract may be obvious and appear as a white pupil. Cataracts also be may present in a child with strabismus, decreased visual acuity, family history of the disease, and other ocular or systemic defects. Treatment of cataracts in children depends on the degree of visual impairment and associated anomalies.

Intervention. Operative treatment is the only method for treating cataracts. From 90% to 95% of all cataract operations are successful.[70] The decision as to when to remove the cataract depends largely on the general health of the patient and the use he makes of his eyes. Surgery is advised when the cataract interferes with a person's visual needs or when the cataract may lead to other eye complications such as glaucoma.

Because surgery is usually indicated only for advanced cataracts, an elderly person may believe he should wait until his vision loss is far advanced before seeing an ophthalmologist. Delaying medical examination of the eye can lead to permanent vision loss if the problem is not cataracts but glaucoma or a combination of the two.

It is the nurse's responsibility to explain the disease, refer the person with a suspected cataract to an ophthalmologist, and encourage him to accept treatment as recommended. Informational material designed to educate patients about cataracts may be found in *Synopsis of Ophthalmology.*[28]

Cataracts usually are removed with the patient under local anesthesia. Removal has been simplified in many cases by the use of the enzyme alpha-chymotrypsin, which weakens the zonular fibers that hold the lens in position. Cataracts may be removed within their capsule *(intracapsular technique)*, or an opening may be made in the capsule and the lens lifted out without disturbing the membrane *(extracapsular technique)*.

To remove the lens and its capsule, instruments such as a forceps or vacuum cup are used. Another method is *cryoextraction*. In this case the cataract is lifted from the eye by a small probe, cooled to a temperature below zero, that adheres to the wet surface of the cataract. All these procedures usually are preceded by an iridectomy, performed to create an opening for the flow of aqueous humor, which may become blocked postoperatively when the vitreous humor moves forward.

Congenital cataracts are never removed intracapsularly because the capsule is adherent to the vitreous face. The method used to remove a congenital cataract depends on the size of the eye and the size of the pupil. Children may be operated on for cataract removal as early as 6 months of age.

A new method of cataract removal is called *phacoemulsification*. This procedure breaks up the lens and flushes it out in tiny pieces. The phacoemulsification method requires an incision just large enough to insert a needle probe that vibrates 40,000 times per second to break up the lens. As the lens is broken up, the area is flushed with fluid, and pieces of the lens are carried from the eye by a tiny suction unit. Only one stitch is needed to close the incision. Healing and convalescence are considerably quicker than for patients who have had cryosurgical removal previously described. The size and shape of the eye are factors in determining if this method is suitable for a particular patient.

Postoperative care. For general care after eye surgery, see p. 765. Following any cataract operation a dressing is applied to the eye and covered with a metal shield to protect if from injury. During the hospital stay of 2 or 3 days, the surgeon changes the dressing daily; at home the patient or his family also may change the dressing daily. After 7 to 10 days all dressings are removed. During the first month, protection of the operated eye with a metal shield at night is important. Eyedrops and moist warm compresses also may be ordered. Postoperative resumption of normal activities is much more rapid than in earlier years due to advancements in techniques of lens extraction and suturing.

If vision in the unoperated eye is not good, the patient will need considerable assistance and supervision to meet his safety needs. Temporary glasses may be prescribed 1 to 4 weeks after surgery, depending on the rate of healing and the amount of vision in the other eye. Usually after 6 to 12 weeks healing has been sufficient for the fitting of permanent glasses or contact lenses. Soft contact lenses, made from a porous flexible plastic, are now often used in place of the older hard lenses (p. 759).

The elderly patient sometimes finds it difficult to adjust to removal of a cataract. The little remaining ability to accommodate the eye is lost when the lens is removed, and the patient must wear corrective lenses at all times.

Cataract glasses. While cataract glasses do restore sight, there are some problems inherent in strong glasses that cannot be avoided. The health care worker needs to be familiar with the characteristics of cataract glasses so that the patient can be helped to adjust [28]:

1. *Cataract lenses magnify.* Everything appears about one fourth closer than it is. For example, the patient may reach for his coffee cup but grasp in front of it and knock it over. This distortion of distance also causes problems in climbing stairs and many other activities.
2. *Cataract lenses distort peripheral images.* Because clear vision is only possible through the center of the lens, the wearer must learn to turn his head farther and more frequently to ensure his safety.
3. *Thick lenses are heavy.* Pressure sores on the nose and ears can be troublesome. Lighter weight plastic lenses are now being made, which are much more comfortable than the glass lenses and create less peripheral distortion.
4. *Colors may be distorted.* The colors of objects seen with the eye from which the lens has been removed are slightly different.
5. *Inaccurate positioning causes distortion.* Accurate positioning of cataract glasses is important to prevent distortion. If the glasses are dropped or bumped, they should be readjusted so that they are at the correct angle and distance from the eye.

Contact lenses. Younger persons and some older persons prefer to use contact lenses after cataract surgery. On the other hand some elderly persons may have difficulty inserting the lenses or may reject the idea without trying them. The advantages of contact lenses include improved visual correction and better cosmetic appearance. Use of contact lenses is especially recommended when only one lens is removed. Unilateral removal of a lens causes a difference in the size of the optical images perceived by the brain. This causes difficulty with binocular vision, and the person can effectively use only one eye at a time.

Lens implant. An alternative to cataract glasses and contact lenses is an artificial lens implant (intraocular lens). The lens, which is made of polymethylmethacrylate, is implanted at the time of cataract extraction. It may be held in position either by a suture to the iris (iris fixation) or by implanting it into the capsular sac. Advantages of the implanted lens include better binocular vision. When the lens is implanted without sutures, miotic agents (pilocarpine) are needed to prevent the iris from dilating too widely and causing the lens to slip.[34] While cataract glasses produce about 24% larger images on the retina than the normal eye and contact lenses produce 8%, the implanted lens produces only 2%.[50]

Now becoming more widespread in the United States, implantation of intraocular lenses was first used in England in 1953. Several patients who underwent the procedure in 1953 have retained highly satisfactory results. Currently the implantation procedure is generally restricted to the physically handicapped and the elderly, those not likely to succeed with a contact lens, and is restricted to one eye. The surgeon must be very skilled and well trained in this procedure. Studies are currently being conducted to establish additional guidelines for selection of likely patients and for improved surgical techniques that will keep complications at a minimum.

Outcome criteria for the person with cataract extraction

The patient or significant other can:

1. Demonstrate method of changing the eye dressing.
2. State name, dosage, and frequency of any eyedrops to be given.
3. Describe extent of activity to be permitted:
   a. Avoidance of bending over.
   b. Avoidance of Valsalva maneuver.
4. Describe expected changes in vision with and without lenses.
5. State need for follow-up by ophthalmologist.

□ Glaucoma

The term *glaucoma* designates eye disease characterized by increased intraocular pressure associated with progressive loss of peripheral visual fields. Glaucoma is responsible for 12% to 15% of all blindness in the United States today.[28,62] About 2% of persons over the age of 40 years have glaucoma. It has been estimated that nearly 1 million persons in the United States have glaucoma that has not been diagnosed. It is important to detect and treat this disease because the permanent vision loss it causes is preventable.

The increase in pressure usually is caused by an obstruction to the circulation of aqueous humor through the meshwork at the angle of the anterior chamber of the eye where the peripheral iris and the cornea meet (Fig. 39-4). The blockage may be secondary to an infection or injury. More commonly it is caused by a hereditary predisposition to thickening of the meshwork (chronic simple glaucoma). Most rarely glaucoma results from an abnormal placement of the iris against the angle of the anterior chamber (acute glaucoma).

In either chronic or acute glaucoma early diagnosis and treatment are mandatory to prevent destruction of

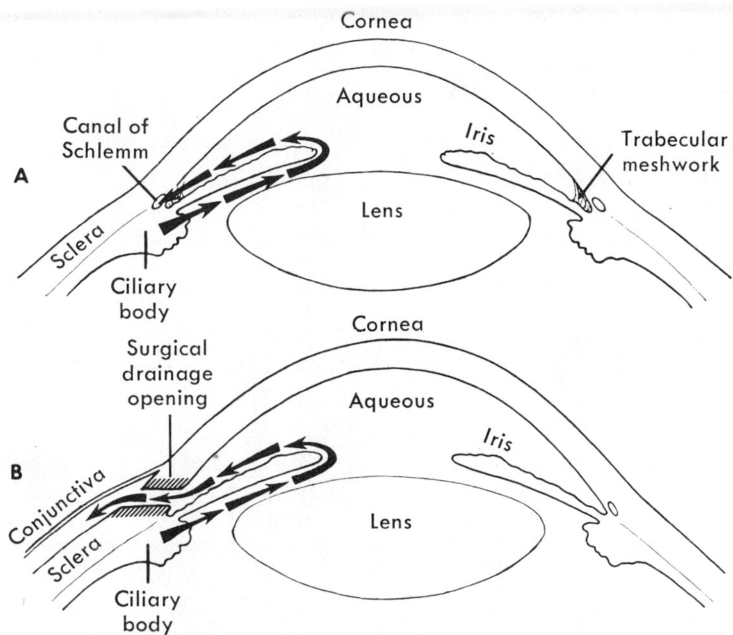

Fig. 39-4. A, Originating from ciliary processes, aqueous flows through pupil into anterior chamber and normally leaves eye by way of the canal of Schlemm. **B,** In glaucoma, normal aqueous outflow is blocked. Purpose of glaucoma surgery is to create new channel through which aqueous can leave eye. (From Havener, W. H.: Synopsis of ophthalmology, ed. 4, St. Louis, 1975, The C. V. Mosby Co.)

nerve fibers on the optic disc due to increased intraocular pressure. Mass screening programs are important in detecting possible glaucoma in persons who do not have periodic medical eye examinations. The incidence of glaucoma is increasing as the number of older persons in our population rises. While it is seldom seen in persons under 35 years of age, it does occur in infancy. Glaucoma is the greatest threat to vision in older persons.

Chronic simple glaucoma

Assessment. The most common type of glaucoma is chronic simple glaucoma, also known as *wide-angle* or *open-angle* glaucoma. At first symptoms may be absent. Progression of the disease is slow and insidious. Permanent vision loss may occur before the individual is aware he has the disease.

Chronic glaucoma gives one characteristic sign that is important: before central vision becomes affected, the peripheral visual fields are impaired so that objects to the side are not seen (Fig. 39-5). Limitation of vision may not be so apparent as in other eye diseases, and much damage can occur before medical assistance is sought. The patient may bump into other persons in the street or fail to see passing vehicles, yet not realize that the fault lies in his own vision. A diminished field of vision may cause the driver of an automobile to have an accident. The loss of peripheral vision ("tunnel vision") can progress until the patient is legally blind, yet he may be able to see well straight ahead. The community nurse who recognizes this difficulty may be most helpful in early case finding and in promptly referring patients to an ophthalmologist. Because vision loss due to glaucoma is irreversible, early diagnosis is mandatory.

Chronic glaucoma usually begins in one eye, although if it is left untreated both eyes often become affected. Symptoms are most apparent in the morning, when a persistent dull eye pain may develop. Frequent changes of glasses, difficulty in adjusting to darkness, failure to accurately detect changes in color, and slight blurring of vision are fairly early signs of open-angle glaucoma. Then follows a steamy appearance of the cornea and further blurring of vision. Tearing, misty vision, blurred appearance of the iris (which becomes fixed and dilated), headache, pain behind the eyeball, nausea, and vomiting can then occur. Halos, resembling streetlights seen through a steamy windshield, may be seen about lights.

Intervention. Treatment of chronic simple glaucoma is designed to reduce intraocular pressure and keep it at a safe level. Miotics such as pilocarpine are

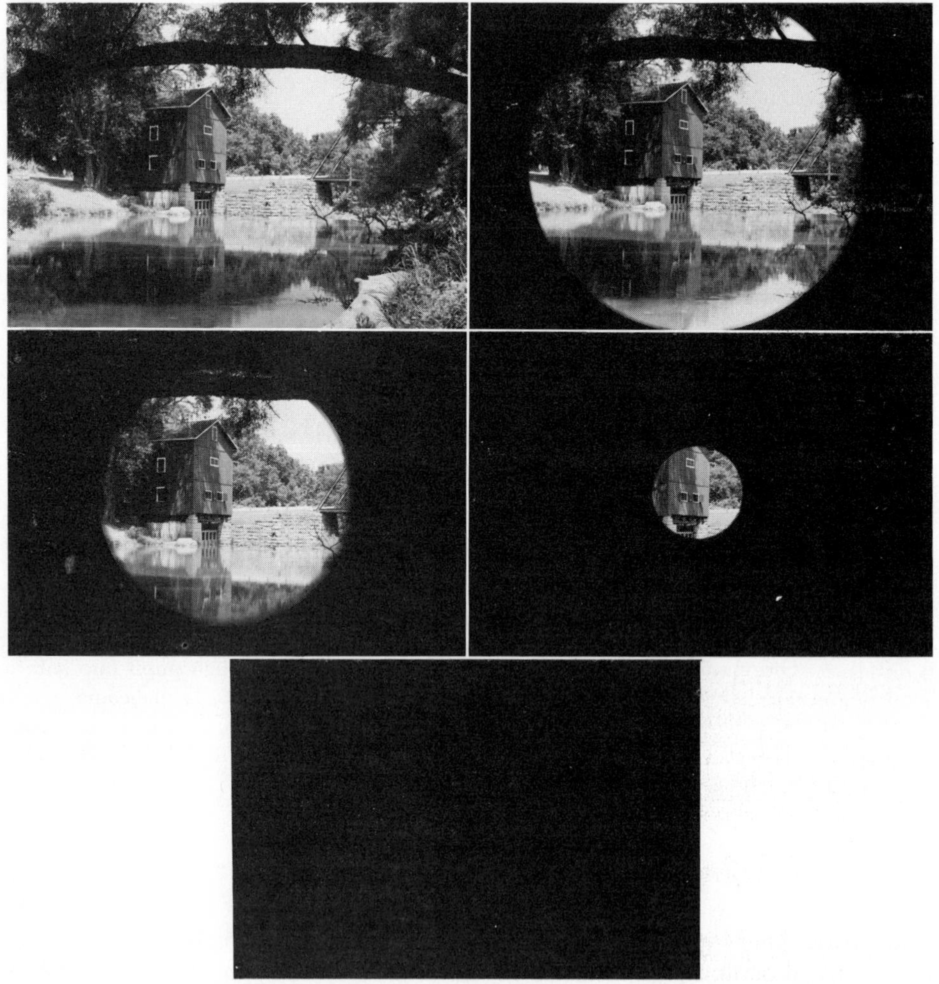

Fig. 39-5. Gradual loss of sight from glaucoma so insidiously destroys vision that person is unaware of impending blindness until extensive and irreversible damage is already present. (From Havener, W. H., Saunders, W. H., Keith, C. F., and Prescott, A. W.: Nursing care in eye, ear, nose, and throat disorders, ed. 3, St. Louis, 1974, The C. V. Mosby Co.)

used to constrict the pupil and to draw the smooth muscle of the iris away from the canal of Schlemm to permit aqueous humor to drain out at this point. Acetazolamide (Diamox), a drug that tends to reduce the formation of aqueous humor, is used successfully in some types of chronic glaucoma.

Surgery may be performed to produce a permanent filtration pathway for aqueous fluid. Filtering procedures such as *trabeculectomy*, *sclerotomy*, *iridencleisis*, and *trephine* operations provide a permanent fistula from the anterior chamber to the subconjunctival space. In selected cases the production of aqueous fluid may be decreased by destroying part of the ciliary body. This may be accomplished by diathermy or cryosurgery. Following surgery the patient usually is allowed out of bed at once, although one or both eyes may be bandaged for several days. Postoperative management of patients having eye surgery is discussed on p. 765.

Acute-angle closure glaucoma (narrow-angle glaucoma)

Assessment. Acute glaucoma has been described as one of the most dramatic and rapidly destructive diseases of the eye.[28] Characteristically there is severe eye pain, which may radiate to any part of the head. Because nausea, vomiting, and abdominal pain also commonly occur, the primary problem is sometimes thought to be abdominal. Additional signs and symptoms include blurred vision, colored halos around lights, dilated pupil, reddened appearance of the eye, and increased intraocular pressure. Since a marked increase in intraocular pressure for 24 to 36 hours may lead to complete and permanent blindness, immediate treatment is necessary.

A relatively rare disease, acute glaucoma occurs when the iris blocks the outflow of aqueous humor. In an eye with a narrowed peripheral angle of the anterior chamber, dilation of the pupil caused by darkness, excitement, or a mydriatic drug may cause blockage of the outflow mechanism.

Intervention. Treatment consists of lowering intraocular pressure by increasing the outflow of aqueous humor and by decreasing the rate of its production. Miotics are given to constrict the pupil. Carbonic anhydrase inhibitors (Diamox) may be given orally or intravenously to reduce the production of aqueous humor. Osmotic agents such as glycerol also act to reduce the pressure of acute glaucoma. When the pressure is reduced and the eye is less inflamed, a portion of the peripheral iris is surgically excised (iridectomy). (See Table 38-2 for drugs used in glaucoma.) Prophylactic surgery on the fellow eye may be performed.

Other types of glaucoma

Congenital glaucoma, which is very rare, may be present at birth or may develop in the first few months of life. Surgery is necessary to correct the abnormal development of the filtration angle and allow normal aqueous flow.

Secondary glaucoma occurs when the rise in intraocular pressure is due to some other eye condition such as uveitis, trauma, or a postoperative complication.

Absolute glaucoma is the end result of uncontrolled glaucoma. The eye is hard, sightless, and may be painful. Enucleation is often recommended to relieve the discomfort.

Long-term care

The person with glaucoma needs assistance in understanding and learning to live with the disease. Despite explanations from his physician, he frequently hopes that an operation will cure his condition, that no further treatment will be necessary, and perhaps that the sight he has lost will be restored. It should be explained that the vision lost cannot be restored but that further loss can usually be prevented and his life can be quite normal if he continues under medical care. There usually is no restriction on the use of the eyes. Fluid intake generally is not curtailed, and exercise is permitted. Bright lights or darkness are not harmful to the eyes of the patient with glaucoma. There is apparently no relationship between vascular hypertension and ocular hypertension.[28]

The person with glaucoma should be under medical care for the rest of his life, receiving either drug or surgical therapy or both. Following the operation he should return regularly to the surgeon, since one operation does not necessarily mean that drainage will be continued. Any obstruction or closing of the artificial pathway will result in reappearance of symptoms and further visual damage. The patient and his family should know specifically what to do if essential eyedrops are accidentally spilled; for example, they should know which local drugstore is open at night and on holidays. The patient often is advised to have an extra bottle of medication in his home and to carry one with him if he works away from home. It is advisable also for the patient to carry a card or other information to identify him as having glaucoma in case an accident occurs.

Nurses and other health care workers must determine whether their patient has been treated for glaucoma so that mydriatics are not administered and prescribed glaucoma medications are not omitted.

Outcome criteria for the person with glaucoma

The patient or significant others can:

1. Describe effects of surgery or medication on visual acuity.
2. State name, dosage, frequency, and side effects of eye medications.
3. State recognition of lifetime need to continue use of eye medications.
4. Describe preventive measures:
   a. Have reserve bottle of eyedrops at home.
   b. Carry eyedrops when away from home.
   c. Carry card identitying that he has glaucoma and the eyedrop solution prescribed.
5. List signs indicating need to report immediately to the ophthalmologist.
6. Describe purpose of regular lifetime medical follow-up.

□ Detachment of the retina

The retina is the part of the eye that perceives light; it coordinates and transmits impulses from receptor nerve cells to the optic nerve. There are two primitive retinal layers: the outer pigment epithelium and an inner sensory layer. Retinal detachment occurs when a separation of the two primitive layers of the retina occurs due to accumulation of fluid between them or an elevation of both retinal layers away from the choroid occurs due to a tumor (Fig. 39-6). As the detachment extends and becomes complete, blindness results. Myopic degeneration, trauma, and aphakia (absence of the crystalline lens) are the most frequent causes of retinal detachment in children and adults. It may also result from hemorrhage, tumor, or exudates that occur in front of or behind

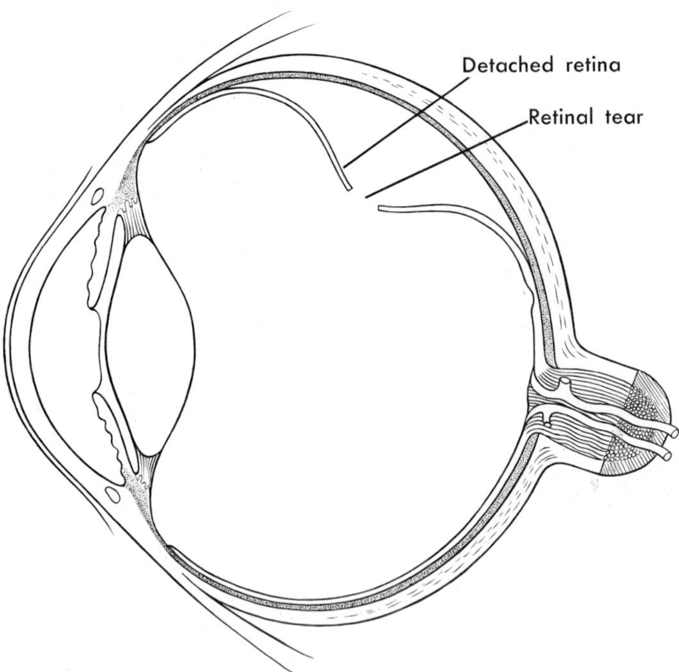

Fig. 39-6. Retinal detachment.

the retina. Detachment of the retina may follow sudden severe physical exertion, especially in persons who are debilitated. Most often, however, there is no apparent cause.

Assessment. Retinal detachment may occur suddenly or may develop slowly. Symptoms include floating spots or opacities before the eyes, flashes of light, and progressive constriction of vision in one area. The floating spots are blood and retinal cells that are freed at the time of the tear and cast shadows on the retina as they seem to drift about the eye. The diagnosis of retinal separation is based on the ophthalmoscopic appearance of the retina. The area of visual loss depends entirely on the location of the detachment. Usually there is a superior retinal detachment with inferior visual loss. When the detachment is extensive and occurs quickly, the patient may have the sensation that a curtain has been drawn before his eyes or that of looking over a fence.

Intervention. Immediate care for detachment of the retina includes keeping the patient quiet in bed with his eyes covered to try to prevent further detachment. His head is positioned so that the retinal hole is in the lowest part of the eye. Because extended conservative treatment for detachment of the retina has not been successful, early surgery is now the approved method of treatment.

Surgical procedure. The surgery may be performed with the patient under either local or general anesthesia. Cyclopentolate or phenylephrine is used to keep the pupils widely dilated so that tears in the retina may be identified during the operation. The surgical procedure may include draining the fluid from the subretinal space so that the retina returns to its normal position, thereby closing the opening in the retina. To drain the fluid from the subretinal space, the sclera and choroid are perforated at the time of the operation.

The retinal breaks are sealed off by various methods that produce an inflammatory reaction *(chorioretinitis)* in the area of the tear so that adhesions will form between the edges of the break and the underlying choroid to obliterate the opening. When the tears are small or of recent origin, diathermy may be applied through the sclera with needlepoint electrodes to produce the inflammatory process. An intense beam of visible light directed to the area by means of an elaborate ophthalmoscope may be used to close retinal tears when the retina is not elevated *(photocoagulation).* The *laser* beam is used by some surgeons as a source of intense energy to produce chorioretinitis. Subfreezing temperatures (−40 C to −60 C) may be applied to the surface of the sclera in the area of the hole to produce the inflammatory reaction *(retinal cryopexy).* Nitrous oxide or carbon dioxide under pressure flowing through a tube attached to a delicate instrument is used to produce these low temperatures.

For most retinal detachments, including those previ-

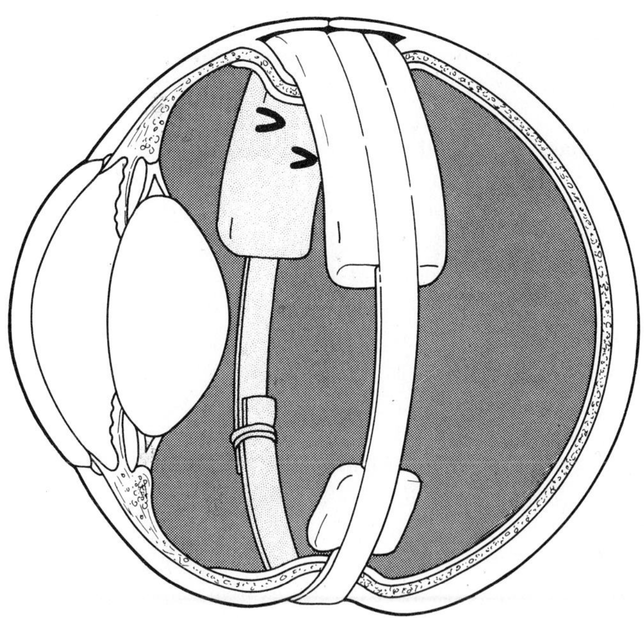

Fig. 39-7. Scleral buckle.

ously considered inoperable, *scleral buckling* procedures are used. A scleral buckle serves as a splint to hold the retina and choroid together until the choroidal scar can form to permanently seal the hole or tear. The retinal break or tear is closed by the following procedure. The area overlying the treated tear is indented, or "buckled," inward toward the vitreous cavity (Fig. 39-7). To create the buckle a fold is taken in the treated sclera and choroid and sutured into place, or a segment of the sclera is resected and shortened. This procedure may be combined with the implantation of a foreign material such as various shaped pieces of silicone or with an eye-bank sclera to cause further indentation of the choroid. By these procedures the choroid is pushed into contact with the retinal tear during healing, and vitreous adhesions that have exerted traction, or pull, on the retinal break are relaxed as the size of the scleral shell is decreased.

Postoperative care. The patient's postoperative position in bed will depend on the extent and location of the retinal detachment. Because postoperative routines vary a great deal, the nurse must be certain that orders for bed position and for ambulation have been written by the surgeon and that the patient understands exactly how much activity he may undertake. (For general discussion of the postoperative care of a patient having eye surgery see p. 765). Dressings are usually changed daily, but it is about a week before the eye can be fully examined and a determination made as to whether the operation has been successful. It may be possible to reoperate when surgery has not been successful, although a second operation usually is delayed for at least 1 or 2 weeks. Hemorrhage is a common complication of an operation for detachment of the retina. It may result from cryosurgery, diathermy, or puncture of the choroid to obtain release of subretinal fluids at the time of operation. When dressings are removed, the patient is usually allowed to ambulate progressively over the next several days.

Resumption of sedentary duties may be permitted 3 weeks after surgery, while activities or occupations requiring heavy physical exertion may not be permitted for 6 weeks or more. Restoration of sight will depend on the extent and duration of the detachment prior to surgery as well as the degree of success of the treatment. Some ophthalmologists advise their patients to avoid contact sports for the rest of their lives.

Outcome criteria for the person with retinal detachment

The patient or significant other can:

1. State signs and symptoms indicating further retinal detachment.
2. State need for medical follow-up should further symptoms occur.
3. Describe the extent of limitations on activity.

□ Diabetic retinopathy

The quality of health and life expectancy of the person with diabetes have improved due to the use of insulin and regulated exercise and diet. Because of the longer life span, however, some of the complications associated with diabetes such as pathologic conditions of the retina have increased.

Diabetic retinopathy is a disorder of the blood vessels of the retina, the light-sensitive tissue at the back of the eye that transmits visual impulses by way of the optic nerve to the brain. Diabetic retinopathy is responsible for approximately 10% of all new blindness reported each year in the United States. Among those 45 to 74 years of age the disease accounts for about 20% of all new blindness.[69] At this time there is no known way of preventing diabetic retinopathy. Keeping the blood sugar level under strict control may delay the onset. The incidence of diabetic retinopathy seems to depend mainly on the duration of the diabetes.

Assessment. Diabetic retinopathy produces characteristic changes in the retina: capillary microaneurysms, neovascularization, hemorrhage, arteriolar and venous changes, exudates, and new connective tissue. Hemorrhage is the chief cause of visual loss of diabetic retinopathy. In mild forms of diabetic retinopathy, hemorrhage in the retina may be absorbed spontaneously, restoring vision without treatment.

Intervention. Several methods of treatment are currently being used and studied for effectiveness.

Sponsored by the National Eye Institute, *photocoagulation* of the retina is being studied in 16 participating medical centers involving more than 1,700 patients. Both the argon laser and xenon arc are being evaluated. In this therapy an intense beam of light is directed into the eye and focused on a small spot on the retina. The light energy is transformed into heat energy, coagulating the new vessels and preventing hemorrhage into the vitreous.

After severe hemorrhage into the vitreous has occurred due to proliferative diabetic retinopathy, the vitreous can become permanently opaque, and vision is lost. The vitreous is the clear, jell-like fluid that fills the center of the eye. Bleeding into the vitreous blocks the transmission of light and can damage the retina. During the last 5 years researchers have developed new instruments for surgically removing the diseased vitreous, a very difficult procedure. Removal of the vitreous *(vitrectomy)* is now being intensively studied in 14 medical centers across the United States.

Hypophysectomy (surgical removal of the pituitary gland) is another surgical procedure sometimes performed to treat diabetic retinopathy (p. 569). This procedure decreases or prevents the secretion of hormones that act to raise the level of blood sugar making diabetes easier to control. This action is designed to slow or halt the progression of diabetic retinopathy.

Because of the limitations of surgical methods to preserve vision in diabetic retinopathy, efforts are continually being made to find medical means of preventing the condition from developing.

□ Retrolental fibroplasia

Retrolental fibroplasia, or retinopathy of prematurity, is a disease of premature infants in which a dense, opaque, fibrous membrane forms in the anterior vitreous behind the lens, causing blindness. An abnormality involving both eyes, retrolental fibroplasia is caused by high oxygen levels administered to premature infants in the hospital. In premature infants with incomplete vascularization of the eye, high oxygen levels cause vasoconstriction and destruction of blood vessels that supply the retina. Incomplete retrolental fibroplasia may lead to gradual deterioration of the eye in adolescence.

Premature infants suffering from respiratory distress syndrome require excessively high oxygen levels to raise the arterial Po_2 to that of a normal infant. These children need careful monitoring of arterial blood gas levels and of the retinal blood vessels.

□ Tumors

Both benign and malignant tumors may occur in the eye or related structures such as the eyelid. Neoplasms may originate in the retina or the uveal tract or metastasize to the eye from a primary site. Orbital neoplasms include benign hemangiomas, pseudotumors, lymphomas, mucoceles from the sinuses, malignant melanomas, retinoblastomas, and others. When tumors are malignant, both vision and life are endangered. Tumors within the eyeball are often silent except for a bloodshot appearance of the eye. As in all malignant tumors, the prognosis depends on early diagnosis and prompt treatment.

The eyelids are subject to the usual tumors of the skin such as nevi and verrucae (warts). Carcinoma of the lids is a common type of ocular malignancy. Any warty growth in the eyelids should be removed for histologic examination. Treatment consists of surgical excision of the growth.

Retinoblastoma is an inherited, highly malignant congenital neoplasm that arises from the retina. The most frequent ocular malignancy in childhood, it occurs in one of every 23,000 to 34,000 births.[62] The diagnosis is made in 90% of patients by the age of 4 years. Signs and symptoms may include decreased vision, strabismus, retinal detachment, white pupillary reflex, and secondary glaucoma. In about one third of the patients the tumors invade both eyes. Retinoblastomas grow rapidly and spread backward along the optic nerve to invade the brain. Retinoblastomas can also metastasize to distant sites by way of the bloodstream and lymphatics.

Treatment of retinoblastoma consists of enucleation with removal of as much of the optic nerve as possible. Frequent examination of the remaining eye is recommended. When the tumor is bilateral, the most involved eye is removed. An attempt is made to save the other eye by using radiation, chemotherapy, or both. If the tumor is very advanced, removal of both eyes may be necessary to save the child's life. When the tumor is unilateral and diagnosed and treated early, there is a 90% survival rate.

When normal parents have one child with retinoblastoma, there is a likelihood of less than 4% that a subsequent child will have such a tumor. There is a 50% chance that children of the individual who has survived a proved hereditary retinoblastoma will also be so affected. Persons who survive the tumors should receive genetic counseling to alert them to the danger of transmissions to their offspring.

Malignant melanomas are neoplasms that occur in the choroid and iris of adults. They grow slowly, but due to the vascularity of the choroid they metastasize early to the liver and lungs.

Medical treatment of tumors of the eye may include

enucleation, radiation treatment, use of chemotherapeutic agents, and plastic surgery.

The emotional response to a tumor of the eye is perhaps even greater than to malignancies elsewhere. The surgeon may advise immediate enucleation of the eye in the hope of saving life. Both the patient and his family need to be encouraged to talk about their feelings and concerns and helped to readjust their lives when confronted by this serious situation.

□ Removal of an eye

Surgical procedure. An eye, with or without its supportive structures, may be removed for four reasons: (1) in an attempt to save a life when a malignant tumor has developed, (2) to save sight in the other eye when sympathetic ophthalmia is feared or threatens, (3) to control pain in an eye blinded by disease such as chronic glaucoma or chronic infection, or (4) for cosmetic reasons following blindness from trauma or disease.

Three types of surgery may be performed. *Enucleation* is surgical removal of the entire eye including the sclera. *Evisceration* is removal of the contents of the eye with retention of the sclera. *Exenteration* involves removal of the entire eye and all other soft tissues in the bony orbit.

If feasible the eyeball alone is removed, leaving the surrounding layers of fascia (Tenon capsule) and the muscle attachments. A silicone, plastic, or tantalum implant is inserted into the eye socket, the cut ends of the muscle attachments are overlapped and sutured around it, and the Tenon capsule and the conjunctiva are closed. This procedure provides a stump that supplies both support and motion for an artificial eye and therefore gives the patient whose eye has been removed a more normal appearance. The ball-shaped implant is left in place permanently.

Postoperative care. Hemorrhage, thrombosis of blood vessels, and infection are possible complications following enucleation, exenteration, or evisceration of an eye. Pressure dressings are used for 1 or 2 days to help control possible hemorrhage. Headaches or pain in the side of the head operated on should be reported at once, since meningitis occasionally occurs as a complication following thrombosis of adjacent veins. The patient is usually allowed out of bed the day following surgery.

When a person has lost one eye the preservation of sight in the other eye becomes crucial. Wearing impact-resistant glasses provides some protection from injury. Because binocular vision is gone when there is only one functioning eye, depth perception is affected. The individual needs to be taught about the adjustments necessary in learning to carry out normal activities with one eye and of the potential safety hazards. Driving a car, for example, is dangerous for the person who suddenly must use only one eye and is not accustomed to the alteration in depth perception. With patience and practice, however, almost all normal activities are possible; surgeons who have had an eye removed have even been able to operate successfully.

Artificial eye. An artificial eye can be used as soon as healing is complete and edema has disappeared, usually 6 to 8 weeks after surgery, although many patients begin to wear an artificial eye after only 3 weeks. Artificial eyes are made of glass or plastic materials. Glass eyes last longer if not broken, but they are heavier. Plastic ones are more expensive and may need to be replaced in a few years because they become more easily scratched or roughened around the edges, causing irritation to the conjunctiva. Plastic prostheses are more popular than those made of glass.

There are two kinds of artificial eyes: the shell-shaped and the hollow artificial eye. The choice of the individual patient depends on which operation has been done. Artificial eyes may be bought in shades that closely match the normal eye or they may be specially made. Most artificial eyes are plastic shells fitted and then painted by an artist. The cost varies from $100 to $250 or more. The life expectancy of the prosthesis is as great as 5 years with good care. Despite care taken to match shape and color, the pupil of the artificial eye remains fixed, which is apparent to close observers.

Even young children can be taught to care for their own artificial eyes. A well-fitting prosthesis may not need to be removed for 30 days. When removed, however, the prosthesis should be cleansed immediately. Care should be taken not to scratch its surface. The artificial eye is removed by gently pressing upward on the lower lid, being certain that the cupped hand is held against the cheek so that the eye does not fall to the floor and break or become lost. It is inserted by gently everting the lower lid, being certain that the narrower end of the eye is placed next to the inner angle of the orifice. Then, by grasping the upper lashes and gently raising the upper lid, the eyes is easily slipped into place (Fig. 39-8).

■ PROBLEMS OF THE EAR

Disorders of hearing and vestibular function are common and can occur at any age. Prevention, detection, and treatment of these disorders are highly diversified. Professional nursing has the responsibility of teaching preventive methods to help persons avoid damage to ear structure, including noise-induced damage, encouraging persons with aural disorders to seek appropriate medical care, caring for patients hospitalized with hearing disorders, and case finding and rehabilitation of persons with hearing disorders. The possible serious complications following infections of the ear and re-

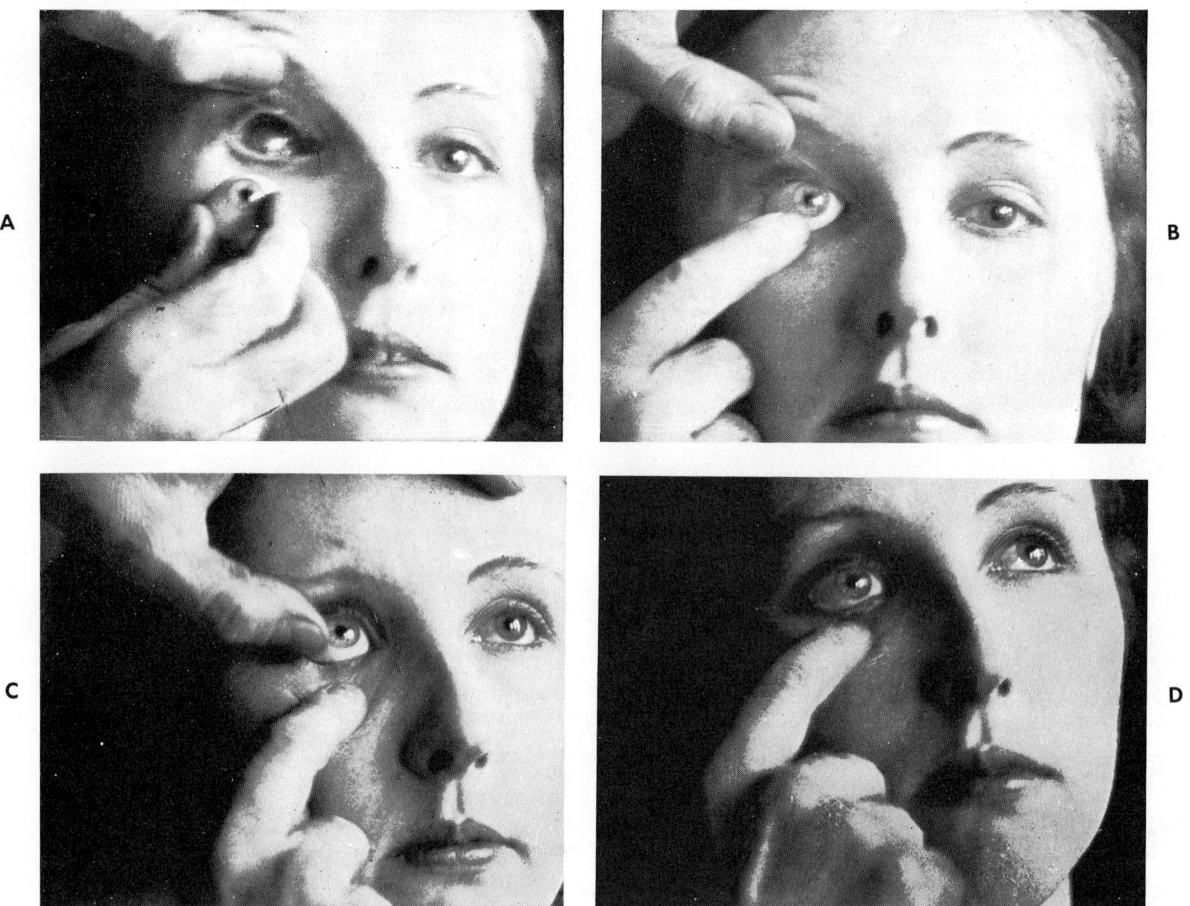

Fig. 39-8. Steps in inserting artificial eye. (From Parkinson, R. H.: Eye, ear, nose, and throat manual for nurses, ed. 8, St. Louis, 1959, The C. V. Mosby Co.)

lated structure make prompt appropriate medical care important.

For clarity in presentation, discussion of the ear and its structures is divided into three parts: the outer ear, the middle ear and mastoid process, and the inner ear. Specific prevention and management are considered separately for each part in this chapter. Assessment of the ear, general management of hearing disorders, and general care of the person with ear problems are discussed in Chapters 37 and 38.

□ External ear

External otitis

Infections of the external ear are generally called external otitis. They are usually more common in the summer than in the winter. The external ear may be affected by acute and chronic forms of such conditions as eczematous dermatitis, diffuse dermatitis, and fungal and bacterial infections. These conditions may be associated with systemic diseases; with diseases of the skin of the adjacent face, neck, and scalp; or with diseases of the middle ear. They may be caused by trauma or may be the result of a primary invasion by organisms.

Assessment. Pain is the chief symptom of acute external otitis, although any symptoms of redness, scaling, itching, swelling, watery discharge, or crusting should be referred to the otolaryngologist. If these infections are not treated, chronic changes may result causing thickening of the skin and stenosis of the external canal. There may be partial hearing loss and a blocked sensation in the affected ear. Pain increases with movement of the auricle and tragus. In chronic external otitis the chief symptom usually is itching.

Intervention. As described in Chapter 38, local treatment of both chronic and acute external otitis may include analgesics, application of medicated ointments or powders, hot compresses to soften crusts or supply medication, or cool applications to lessen inflammation and relieve discomfort. Usually ointments are avoided with acute external otitis. Burow's solution (aluminum acetate solution) often is used for its astringent action, which has a cooling and soothing effect. Antibiotic preparations such as those containing bacitracin, neomycin, and polymyxin and the corticosteroids may be prescribed to be applied locally as eardrops (p. 770). In caring for persons with either chronic or acute external otitis, it is important to avoid further infection; thus handwashing is important, and all equipment or material used should be sterile.

Foreign bodies in the ear canal

Children and mentally disturbed adults occasionally insert foreign bodies such as beans, peas, paper, erasers, crayons, chalk, or buttons in their ears. Depending on how loosely the foreign body fits the ear canal, removal may be by irrigation (p. 770), forceps, or cerumen loop. Irrigation should be avoided with any foreign bodies of vegetable matter because they may increase in size if moistened and become impacted. Insects occasionally lodge in the ear canal; their movements cause pain and noise. A few drops of mineral oil, alcohol, or olive oil instilled into the ear canal will suffocate or immobilize the insect, and it may then be removed with forceps or irrigation. Nursing responsibilities include teaching parents or guardians of children or mentally disturbed adults never to poke in the ears with small or sharp objects such as cotton-tipped applicators, hairpins, matchsticks, or toothpicks. The ear should be cleaned only with a wet washcloth over the tip of a finger. *Nothing should be inserted into the ear beyond the point of vision.*

Congenital defects and deformities

Absence of the auricle is unusual; more common is a partial deformity of the ear. Often the latter is associated with absence of the external auditory meatus and at times with deformity of the middle ear and consequent deafness. Attempts have been made to surgically reconstruct the auricle with limited success. The external ear can also be deformed by trauma (cauliflower ear), which may be amenable to reconstruction surgery. Sometimes having the person wear his hair covering the area is the best solution.[29] An artificial prosthesis may also be designed.

Furunculosis of the external auditory canal

Furuncles, or boils, usually are confined to the external auditory meatus and most often are caused by *Staphylococcus aureus*. They cause severe pain because there is little expansile tissue in the area, and as they enlarge the skin becomes taut and is under great pressure. The swelling may occlude the auditory canal, causing temporary deafness. The administration of antibiotics systemically may resolve the condition, an incision and drainage may be necessary, or wicks (p. 772) treated with antibiotics or drugs such as Burow's solution may be inserted.

Malignancies of the external ear

Cancer of the external ear is usually either a basal cell or squamous cell carcinoma.[14,51] It is not uncommon and usually appears as an ulcer on the auricle that fails to heal. Treatment is usually by surgical excision. Squamous cell carcinomas may metastasize to the neck or other parts of the body, although they usually remain localized for a long time. Basal cell carcinomas usually do not metastasize. The cure rate is reasonably good except when the osseous portion of the canal is invaded. Once this happens, temporal bone resection and deep irradiation therapy are employed.

Outcome criteria for the person experiencing problems of the external ear

The patient or significant others can:

1. Describe safety precautions related to the ear:
   a. Handwashing techniques in the presence of ear infection.
   b. Dangers of foreign bodies in the ear.
   c. Methods for cleaning the ear.
2. Demonstrate correct technique in the application of compresses, eardrops, ointment, or ear irrigations.
3. State symptoms requiring medical attention.

□ Middle ear

Serous otitis media

Serous (catarrhal) otitis media is a condition in which sterile serum is present in the middle ear, which interferes with hearing.[15] Normally the nasopharyngeal end of the eustachian tubes opens periodically to permit the passage of air up into the middle ear as swallowing or yawning occurs. This air helps to maintain the pressure within the middle ear equal to that of the external ear. When the opening of the eustachian tube is blocked by nasopharyngeal infections or enlarged adenoids, or when its lumen is swollen by allergic reactions, air cannot enter. The remaining air eventually is absorbed by the mucous membrane lining, and negative pressure is created, which draws fluid from the surrounding tissues into the middle ear. A sudden change in atmospheric pressure such as that which occurs in flying can also produce this condition. Ascending from a high atmospheric pressure to a low atmospheric pressure moves air from the middle ear out through the eustachian tube, but as the person descends, air may be unable to pass through the eustachian tube back into the middle ear. Chewing gum or swallowing helps to open the tube, thus permitting air to enter the middle ear.

Assessment. Serous otitis media may be acute or chronic. It may last for a few days or persist for years. The person may complain of a sense of fullness or blockage in the ear, hearing loss, a low-pitched tinnitus, and an earache. The eardrum usually appears retracted on examination.

Intervention. Serous otitis media resolves as the cause of the eustachian obstruction is removed. Gentle inflation of the eustachian tube may bring relief. Aspiration of the fluid with a needle or through a myringotomy incision may be necessary in some instances. Polyethylene, Teflon, or stainless steel ventilation tubes can be inserted through an opening in the eardrum to equalize pressure and to speed the absorption of the fluid. The use of these tubes seemingly has reduced the incidence of otitis media especially in children. Treatment in children may be aided by adenoidectomy (p. 1097).

Early and adequate treatment of nasopharyngeal infections and allergic conditions can usually prevent chronic serous otitis media from developing. Since this disease is a cause of conduction deafness in children, the nurse should urge mothers of children who complain of persistent earache to seek medical advice. Any person who complains of tinnitus or who seems to have loss of hearing should be advised to seek medical attention promptly.

Acute purulent otitis media

Most of the diseases that affect the middle ear and mastoid process are caused by infection.[52] Acute purulent otitis media is an acute inflammatory process in the middle ear. It is common in infants because their eustachian tubes are short and straight, and thus almost any infection in the nasopharynx has direct access to the middle ear. This disease most often follows the common cold or tonsillitis but may be a complication of measles or scarlet fever. It may also be caused by the forcing of contaminated water into the middle ear through the eustachian tube while swimming or by blowing the nose improperly. People should be urged to avoid swimming in uninspected pools and in stagnant water, and they should be taught to blow the nose gently, lest infected material be forced into the middle ear. The offending organisms usually are streptococci or staphylococci, which reach the middle ear by way of the eustachian tube. In children under 6 years of age, however, the most common offending organisms are the pneumococci and *Haemophilus influenzae*.

Assessment. The infection usually begins with local engorgement of the blood vessels, which causes swelling of the mucous membrane lining of the eustachian tubes and middle ear. The exudate becomes serosanguineous and later mucopurulent. The pressure of the exudate may cause the eardrum to rupture. The fluid may drain into the external auditory canal or it may be forced back into the mastoid cells.

In the early stages the child may complain of a sensation of fullness in the ear. As infection progresses, the eardrum bulges and pain becomes severe and throbbing. The pain may cause the child to tug on his ear, or the infant may roll his head from side to side, cry constantly, and refuse to eat. There may be decreased hearing in the affected ear, tinnitus, and fever, which in a child may range as high as 40 C to 41 C (104 F to 106 F).

Intervention. Since antibiotics have been used to treat tonsillitis, pharyngitis, rhinitis, and sinusitis (p. 1085), otitis media is no longer a common complication of these conditions. When otitis media does develop, however, antibiotics are given at once, and the infection usually subsides before acute, painful symptoms occur. Treatment also may include bed rest, administration of acetylsalicylic acid or codeine for pain, instillation of warm eardrops such as Auralgan (antipyrine and benzocaine in glycerin) to relieve discomfort, administration of nasal vasoconstrictors to open blocked eustachian tubes, application of dry heat such as hot-water bottle, and forcing of fluids. Eardrops such as Auralgan are contraindicated if the eardrum is perforated because they cause a brisk mucositis of the middle ear and can damage the middle ear. Instead, antibiotic steroid drops such as Cortisporin, Colymycin, Pyocidin, or VoSol are prescribed. Lidosporin is an analgesic type of eardrop which also contains an antibiotic and is effective in treating these patients.

A *myringotomy* (incision into the tympanic membrane) may be performed to relieve pressure and remove pus in the middle ear during acute otitis media. An older procedure, it is still performed, although less frequently since the advent of antibiotic therapy.[29,64] Once a purulent process is established, myringotomy is performed to prevent spontaneous rupture of the eardrum, since scar tissue that will impair hearing will develop if the membrane is allowed to rupture spontaneously. A popular misconception regarding myringotomy is that by incising the eardrum hearing is lost. This is not true; usually a myringotomy heals rapidly with only slight scarring and does not affect hearing. The procedure is usually performed in an ambulatory setting. The physician requires a good light, a head mirror, an aural speculum, and a very sharp myringotomy knife. If necessary a short-acting anesthetic such as nitrous oxide or an injected anesthetic such as lidocaine may be used. A single incision is made, usually posteriorly and inferiorly in the eardrum to avoid injuring the medial wall of the middle ear (Fig. 39-9). A suction tip may be used to remove fluids from the middle ear after the incision is made, and cultures may be taken.

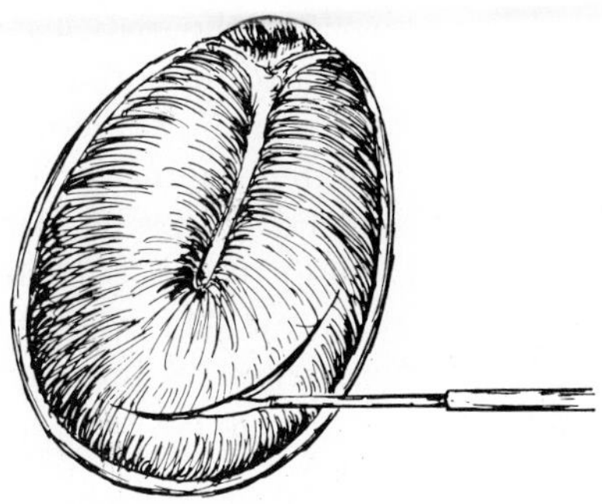

Fig. 39-9. Myringotomy incision made through posteroinferior part of eardrum to release pus in acute otitis media. (From Havener, W. H., Saunders, W. H., Keith, C. F., and Prescott, A. W.: Nursing care in eye, ear, nose, and throat disorders, ed. 3, St. Louis, 1974, The C. V. Mosby Co.)

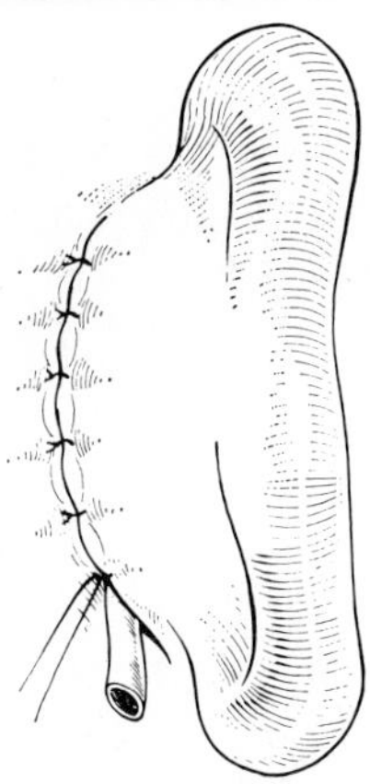

Fig. 39-10. Postauricular incision is sutured, and one Penrose drain is brought out of lower part of wound. Such incision now is commonly used for any type of mastoidectomy and often for tympanoplasty. (From Havener, W. H., Saunders, W. H., Keith, C. F., and Prescott, A. W.: Nursing care in eye, ear, nose, and throat disorders, ed. 3, St. Louis, 1974, The C. V. Mosby Co.)

Free drainage must be maintained so that no pressure is put on the mastoid cells. Cotton may be placed loosely (not stuffed) in the outer ear to collect drainage. Sometimes eardrops may be ordered to maintain drainage but are used with caution. The external ear is kept clean and dry. The cotton is replaced when it becomes moist to minimize the possibility of secondary infection. Dry wipes may be used to remove excess drainage. Petrolatum may be placed around the outer ear to prevent it from becoming excoriated from the drainage. It is important to prevent secondary infection through contamination of the wound; therefore parents and patients should know that the discharge may be infectious and that the hands should be washed before and after changing cotton plugs or cleaning the ear. Elbow restraints may be necessary to keep the young child from touching his ear and the drainage. Antibiotics are continued for several days after the discharge has stopped. If the patient has a rise in temperature, complains of headache, or becomes drowsy, irritable, or disoriented, the physician must be notified at once. These signs may indicate that the eardrum needs to be reopened, that mastoid cells are involved, or that a brain abscess or meningitis is developing.

Usually otitis media is treated on an ambulatory basis, and parents of the infant or young child need careful instruction in his care. In order to prevent otitis media, all parents should be taught to seek medical attention for a child with an earache. The importance of taking prescribed antibiotics for the number of days ordered, even though symptoms have subsided, is stressed.

Acute mastoiditis

An acute infection of the middle ear usually is accompanied by some inflammatory reaction in the mucosa of the adjacent mastoid process. If the middle-ear infection is not treated early or adequately, or if the infection is particularly virulent, or if the person is very debilitated, acute mastoiditis may occur. Streptococci, pneumonocci, staphylococci, or *Haemophilus influenzae* may be the causative organisms. The inflammatory reaction proceeds from edema of the tissues to the formation of exudate and pus that fills the mastoid cells. Pressure on the blood supply causes necrosis to develop and an abscess to form. There may be pain in the ear, mastoid tenderness, fever, headache, and a profuse discharge from the affected ear.

Intervention. Intervention consists of the use of antibiotics, antihistamines, decongestants, bed rest, and the forcing of fluids. If an abscess forms or if the symptoms persist or become worse and cause an elevation of temperature, vertigo, or facial paralysis, surgery is necessary. A simple mastoidectomy may be performed.

There are three types of mastoidectomy: simple, radical, and modified radical.[67,69] Simple mastoidectomy was developed in the nineteenth century. In the past, patients who developed acute mastoiditis from a middle-ear infection were in danger of their lives because of the proximity of the mastoid process to the vital structures of the brain. Today antibiotics are used to control acute infections of the mastoid process, and surgery is seldom necessary. However, in some underdeveloped countries, acute mastoiditis is common, and in the presence of complications surgery may still be necessary. In a *simple mastoidectomy* an incision is made in front of or behind the ear (Fig. 39-10), the necrotic mastoid cells

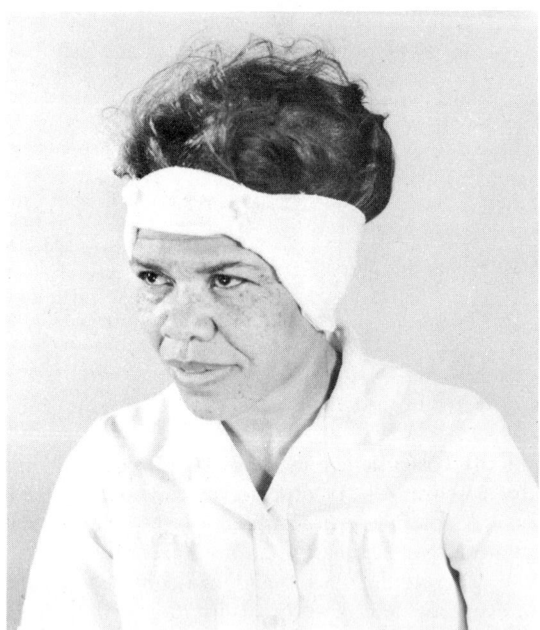

Fig. 39-11. Cling-type 3-inch roller bandage and forehead ties ensure secure and comfortable head dressing. (Courtesy Eye and Ear Infirmary, University of Illinois Hospitals, Chicago.)

are removed, a small rubber drain is inserted, and the wound is closed. The middle ear is left intact, and hearing is not affected. Preoperative preparation for a simple mastoidectomy is similar to that for any operative procedure. If the earache is severe, an ice bag may be used, and acetaminophen or codeine sulfate may be ordered.

Postoperatively a tight bulky dressing is applied to provide some hemostasis and to absorb drainage (Fig. 39-11). The dressing may be reinforced as necessary, but it is not changed by the nurse; the surgeon usually changes it every other day. There may be a small amount of serosanguineous drainage apparent on the dressing, but signs of bright blood on the outer dressing should be reported at once. If a drain has been inserted it is usually removed in 72 hours. Sutures are removed on the fifth or sixth postoperative day. As with any ear surgery, any signs of facial paralysis such as inability to smile or to wrinkle the forehead should be reported. Headache, vomiting, stiff neck, dizziness, irritability, or disorientation may forewarm of a septic thrombosis of the lateral sinus in the brain, meningitis, or a brain abscess. Chronic purulent otitis media also occasionally follows this operation, necessitating more radical mastoid surgery. The patient is usually allowed out of bed within 24 to 48 hours. Fluids are forced throughout the postoperative course.

Radical mastoidectomy consists of a simple mastoidectomy plus removal of the ossicles (except the stapes), remnants of the eardrum, and all of the middle ear mucosa. The facial nerve is preserved. The stapes is left in position to protect the entrance to the inner ear. The middle ear and mastoid process become one large cavity. The radical mastoid cavity may be left to gradually reline with epithelium, or skin or muscle graft may be performed (musculoplasty). Sterile packing is placed in the wound to keep the graft in position, to hold the external meatus open, and to provide hemostasis. The packing is removed gradually through the external ear. The ungrafted radical mastoid cavity usually is healed 2 to 3 months after the operation. It is very important that sterile technique be observed at all times and that the external ear be kept scrupulously clean. Radical mastoidectomy is used for the patient with chronic infection of the mastoid process. Unlike simple mastoidectomy, radical mastoidectomy *does* affect hearing. In actual practice, however, radical mastoidectomy ordinarily does not diminish hearing appreciably because by the time the patient has the operation hearing has already been affected; many persons, even after a radical mastoidectomy, have enough hearing left to manage without a hearing aid.

A *modified radical mastoidectomy* is a more commonly used procedure because it preserves as much of the eardrum as possible. Hearing is better following the modified radical than the radical mastoidectomy. Nursing care for the patient with a radical mastoidectomy is similar to that given the patient with a simple mastoidectomy.

Chronic otitis media

Chronic purulent otitis media is characterized by chronic purulent discharge from the middle ear. It is a sequela of acute otitis media and involves both the middle ear and the mastoid cells. The mastoid bone cells become thickened, and polyps may develop from the mucous membrane of the middle ear.

Assessment. The patient's main complaint may be deafness, occasional pain, or dizziness. If chronic purulent otitis media is permitted to progress unchecked, labyrinthitis, meningitis, brain abscess, or facial paralysis may eventually occur because the infection gradually erodes the surrounding bone. Usually more than one bacterial organism is found on culture; streptococci, staphylococci, *Proteus*, and *Pseudomonas* organisms are most common.

Another complication of chronic purulent otitis media is cholesteatoma (cystic mass).[29] It often occurs when the eardrum has been ruptured and the ear has drained for some time. Skin cells from the ear canal grow into the middle ear (excrescence), where they combine with mucus and purulent exudate to form a mass that becomes firm and erodes the tissue surrounding it. This mass must be removed surgically.

Intervention. The best treatment for chronic purulent otitis media is prevention by early treatment of the acute disease. If the chronic condition does occur, it should be treated as soon as it is recognized. Because the infection is walled off, systemic antibiotics alone are not effective. They may be effective, however, following meticulous local debridement with suctioning and application of topical antibiotics. Antibiotic eardrops may also be prescribed. When this treatment is not indicated or is not effective, a radical mastoidectomy or modified radical mastoidectomy is performed. An effort is made to reconstruct the sound-conducting mechanism by either myringoplasty or tympanoplasty. Persons who have chronic otitis media should not swim or allow water to enter the ear. When showering they must keep their ears covered.

Perforation of the eardrum

The eardrum may be perforated as the result of infection (acute or chronic purulent otitis media) or trauma (skull fracture, puncture). Usually accidental perforations heal spontaneously. Often the patient is given prophylactic antibiotics. Patients with perforated eardrums should not dive, swim, or allow water to enter the ear while showering because of the danger of infection. Eardrops are avoided if the eardrum is perforated. (For further discussion on eardrops see p. 770.) Because of the increased possibility of infection with a perforated eardrum and the possibility of conductive hearing loss, surgical repair often is necessary.

Tympanoplasty is a general name given to a group of operative procedures designed to restore hearing in patients with middle ear or conductive hearing loss. It is used for people who have perforation of the tympanic membrane or necrosis of one of the ossicles due to a middle ear infection, otosclerosis, stenosis, or dislocation of the incus following trauma. By reconstructing or preserving the middle ear conductive mechanism, hearing may be improved or maintained. Closing the tympanic membrane seals the middle ear and protects it from infection. The ear should preferably be free of infection before tympanoplasty is performed. Tympanoplasty differs basically from mastoidectomy in that it seeks to correct hearing loss, while mastoidectomy seeks to correct infection even at the sacrifice of hearing. Tympanoplasty has been performed for about 25 years. Reconstructive procedures of the ear are highly individualized for each patient and depend on the extent of mechanical derangement noted. Eustachian tube functions are necessary if reconstruction of the drum or middle ear space is contemplated. If the eustachian tube does not function properly the reconstruction procedure will fail because of a lack of a proper air-containing environment in the middle ear. Usual surgical approaches are postauricular or endaural. If the ear is not free of infection, the operation includes removal of all infected tissue to make sure that the grafts and prosthesis used do not become infected.

Myringoplasty is used to close a perforation in the eardrum causing conductive hearing loss secondary to trauma or infection. Myringoplasty is performed by surgically enlarging the opening in the eardrum and placing a piece of skin, vein, or fascia over the opening. An absorbable gelatin sponge (Gelfoam) or clotted blood may be used to fill the middle ear space to support the graft, and sterile packing is placed in the external ear to help keep the graft in position. If the graft takes, a considerable degree of tympanic function will return. Patients are typically given antibiotics to prevent infections and antihistamine medications to prevent sneezing. The patient should avoid sneezing and blowing the nose postoperatively so as not to disturb the graft. If the patient must sneeze, he should open his mouth and not cover his nose to prevent pressure building up in a closed space. Eardrops are not used. Occasionally patients with small tympanic perforations who exhibit no signs of infection of the middle ear may be treated successfully by trichloracetic acid microcauterization and placement of material for a graft to the area. The procedure is usually performed in an ambulatory setting and generally must be repeated many times. The postoperative precautions described above also apply to these patients. These procedures are usually not performed on children who are highly susceptible to infections because the infection would reach the middle ear by way of the eustachian tubes and infect the graft.

In addition to repairing a perforation of the eardrum, tympanoplasty may include examination and, if necessary, removal of any scar tissue that interferes with the function of the ossicles, replacement of diseased ossicles with plastic or metal prostheses or homograft ossicles, and reconstruction of the eardrum. Homograft or autograft ossicles are being used more frequently with a high rate of success. Some intact tympanic membranes with intact ossicles from cadavers are being used. One type of tympanoplasty changes the normal route of sound transmission across the middle ear. Usually the normal route has been disrupted by disease; therefore in this type of surgery the eardrum or graft is made to touch the head of the stapes so that sound will pass directly from eardrum to stapes. As with any operative procedure on the middle ear, patients with tympanoplasty may have problems with vertigo.

Tumors of the middle ear and mastoid process

Tumors in this region are rare and when present are squamous cell carcinomas.[51] Symptoms are usually aural discharge, loss of hearing, deep-seated pain, and eventual facial paralysis. Radical resection of the temporal bone may be necessary, and the prognosis is poor. Glomus tympanium and glomus jugulare are rare tumors; they grow slowly, rarely metastasize, and in the case of glomus tympanium are relatively easy to remove.

Otosclerosis

Otosclerosis is a progressive condition in which the normal bone of the bony labyrinth is replaced by highly vascular spongy bone. It produces loss of hearing by fixing or immobilizing the footplate of the stapes in the oval window. The new growth about the stapes blocks its movement so that it is no longer free to vibrate effectively in response to sound pressure. The cause of otosclerosis is not known, but it tends to run in families and is more common in women than in men. In some women pregnancy may be a precipitating factor. Hearing loss is gradual and usually becomes noticeable between puberty and age 30. Usually both ears are affected, one more than the other, and tinnitus is a troublesome symptom. Hearing loss may be solely of the conductive variety due to the fixation of the stapes or of the sensorineural variety due to the direct effect on the inner ear. Audiometric testing (p. 749) is used to diagnose otosclerosis. A tuning fork demonstrates that bone conduction is superior to air conduction (p. 752).

Intervention. The treatment for hearing loss due to otosclerosis is surgical, most commonly a *stapedectomy*. Surgery consists of removal of the stapes and replacing it with some type of prosthesis. Stapedectomy is performed on only one ear at a time, usually the poorer ear. Local anesthetic is administered, and an incision is made deep in the ear canal close to the eardrum, without cutting the eardrum itself, so that the drum can be turned back and the middle ear exposed. Working through an electron microscope, the surgeon frees and removes the stapes and the attached footplate, leaving an opening in the oval window. The patient can usually hear as soon as this step is completed. The opening in the oval window is closed with a plug of fat, vein graft, or absorbable gelatin sponge (Gelfoam), which the body eventually replaces with mucous membrane cells. A steel wire, polyethylene prosthesis, or a Teflon piston is inserted to replace the stapes and is attached at one end to the incus and at the other to the graft or plug to transmit sound to the inner ear. As soon as the connection is made with the incus, the patient's hearing is improved.

When the eardrum is replaced, the patient hears even better. Later in the operative day, blood forms in the middle ear and in the ear canal so that hearing is reduced temporarily. Postoperative edema and packing placed in the ear will also diminish hearing. The reasons for diminished hearing should be explained to the patient preoperatively to relieve worry about diminished hearing after surgery compared with the hearing regained initially in the operating room. Full effects of the operation cannot be evaluated immediately postoperatively.

Postoperative routines differ in various centers. Some surgeons prefer that the patient lie with the operative ear uppermost to prevent displacement of the graft, while others prefer the patient to lie on the operative ear to facilitate drainage. Some physicians permit the patient to lie on whichever side is most comfortable and does not cause vertigo. If postoperative pain occurs, it is usually relieved by codeine sulfate, 60 mg, or meperidine hydrochloride (Demerol), 100 mg. Postoperative trauma and edema may cause vertigo for a few days, and dimenhydrinate (Dramamine), 50 mg, may be given every 6 hours to relieve it. The patient is cautioned against rapid turning, since this may cause vertigo. To prevent falls, side rails should be raised when the patient is in bed, and the patient needs supervision and assistance when getting out of bed and walking. Antibiotics are given to help prevent postoperative infection or meningitis, and the patient is instructed not to blow his nose for a week to prevent air and organisms from being forced up the eustachian tube. Sneezing should also be avoided, but if a sneeze appears imminent, the patient is advised to open his mouth wide and to sneeze as lightly as possible. He should not lift heavy objects or bend over until such activity is approved by the surgeon. He usually is advised not to wash his hair for 2 weeks and not to get water into his ear for 6 weeks. The hospital stay is 4 to 5 days. The packing usually is removed in the surgeon's office or in the clinic about the sixth day, and most patients are allowed to return to work in 2 weeks. During the first week the patient may be advised to wear cotton in the ear when outdoors. The cotton should be placed loosely in the meatus (not into the ear canal) and should be changed once or twice daily. Persons with colds should be avoided because of the danger of middle ear infections. Flying should be avoided for 6 months after the operation, especially if an upper respiratory tract infection is present, so as to prevent the prosthesis from moving out of place. With these exceptions usual activities are permitted once the ear has healed.[46] After stapedectomy, hearing improves permanently in the great majority of cases. Completely normal hearing may be restored, but occasionally hearing may become worse.

Fenestration is a surgical procedure for the treatment of otosclerosis in which the fixed stapes is bypassed and a new window is created in the inner ear. Sound then enters the new window, and hearing is partially restored. Fenestration is rarely performed today. Some persons have developed reduced hearing 6 to 12 months postoperatively when sterile labyrinthitis developed, closing the new window with fibrous or bony growth. Postoperatively patients are usually placed on their back or operative side to facilitate drainage. Severe vertigo is often present as well as nausea and pain on moving the jaws.

Stapes mobilization, like fenestration, is a surgical procedure that was once popular but is now used less often. The stapes is broken loose and the middle ear left as normal as possible. Unfortunately in about one half of the successful cases refixation of the stapes developed, either by healing of the fractured footplate or by new otosclerotic growth. Stapes mobilization is performed with the patient under local anesthesia; it requires briefer hospitalization than fenestration and little postoperative care. It may produce immediate dramatic hearing improvement.

Outcome criteria for the person who has had surgery of the middle ear

The patient or significant others can:

1. Describe measures to prevent infections of the middle ear until the incision is healed:
   a. Blow nose with both nostrils open.
   b. Open mouth when sneezing.
   c. Avoid getting water in the affected ear when showering or bathing.
   d. Avoid exposure to persons with upper respiratory tract infection.
   e. Avoid flying for 6 months.
2. State plans for medical follow-up until the incision is healed.

Outcome criteria for patients experiencing problems of the middle ear not requiring surgery

The patient or significant others can:

1. State preventive measures:
   a. Adequate and early treatment of upper respiratory tract infections and allergic conditions.
   b. Adequate treatment of acute purulent otitis media if necessary.
   c. Prevention of complications following a perforated eardrum, such as not swimming in contaminated water.
   d. Adequate antibiotic therapy continued for prescribed number of days even when symptoms disappear.
2. Describe symptoms indicating need for medical attention (persistant earache, tinnitus, loss of hearing).

□ Inner ear

Presbycusis

Presbycusis is the term given to the hearing loss associated with the aging process. Some of the degenerative change probably is the result of atrophy of the ganglion cells in the cochlea. Presbycusis is characterized by bilateral gradual loss of hearing beginning with a loss of high-frequency tones. It typically cannot be completely improved with hearing aids or surgery.

Meniere's disease

The cause of Meniere's disease is unknown, but it seems to be related to dysfunction of the autonomic nervous system producing a constriction of blood vessels supplying the inner ear.[32,54] Hypertension of the endolymphatic fluid circulation in the cochlea due to either increased production or decreased absorption of the endolymph is present. Meniere's disease most typically occurs in women 50 to 60 years old. Usually there are several attacks during each year. The attacks may disappear without treatment or they may continue until the person is completely deaf in the affected ear. The disease may become quiescent without further attacks and with stable but severe hearing loss; there is no evidence that the acoustic nerve is in any way involved. The disease process appears to affect the hair cells of the inner ear.

Assessment. Meniere's disease is characterized by recurrent episodes of vertigo accompanied by progressive deafness and tinnitus in the affected ear. The vertigo comes in attacks at irregular intervals of days, months, or years. The onset of the attack is sudden and without warning. During an attack any sudden motion of the head or eyes tends to precipitate nausea and vomiting. There may be profuse perspiration and nystagmus. If it is of otologic origin the nystagmus will consist of involuntary horizontal jerking movements of the eyeball. Vertigo may be so severe that persons with Meniere's disease are unable to cross a room without falling. They describe their surroundings as whirling wildly about them. Usually they must sit down to keep from falling and must hold their head very still. Persons with Meniere's disease remain vertiginous for several hours or all day but do not have vertigo between attacks.

Hearing loss is also present and is of the sensorineural type. Usually the hearing loss is unilateral (in about 90% of the cases) although a lesser degree of hearing loss in the opposite ear is not uncommon. Patients with Meniere's disease often complain of a sensation of fullness in the ear.

Tinnitus or ringing is present in one ear most of the time. Like the hearing loss, it may worsen during a life crisis but usually is present all the time. Meniere's disease is a chronic disease; while temporary or complete remissions of the attacks of vertigo may occur, the tinnitus and hearing loss are usually permanent.

Diagnosis is made chiefly from the patient's history. Audiometry reveals low-tone sensorineural loss. The caloric test (p. 752) is still performed although it is now considered to be of limited value in establishing the diagnosis. Electronystagmography (ENG) is becoming more widely used (p. 752).

If the patient has syncope or significant pain, a neurologic consultation is usually obtained to rule out neurologic disease. Other systemic diseases such as syphilis, and lipid disorders may mimic Meniere's symptomatology and need to be investigated.

Intervention. No medical treatment for Meniere's disease has proved entirely successful. In order to reduce endolymphatic hypertension, the patient's fluid intake may be restricted and he may be placed on a salt-free or low-sodium diet. Diuretics such as chlorothiazide, (Diuril), or acetazolamide (Diamox) may be ordered. Other medications that may be used between attacks include histamine subcutaneously (in desensitizing doses) and antivertiginous medications such as dimenhydrinate (Dramamine), nicotinyl alcohol-trimenthobenzamide hydrochloride (Tigacol), meclizine nicotinic acid (Antivert), and nicotinic acid. Medications are changed if relief is not rapid. If a patient suffers a severe attack, diphenhydramine (Benadryl) or dimenhydrinate (Dramamine) is given parenterally. Also an attack may be terminated in 15 to 20 minutes with a high dose of atropine sulfate, 0.06 mg subcutaneously, intramuscularly, or intravenously. Atropine acts by abolishing impulses from the autonomic system that may have precipitated the attack. Mild sedatives and tranquilizers may be prescribed. Emotional support and reassurance are important. Some patients are advised to discontinue smoking to avoid vasospasm and vasoconstriction.

About 10% of patients with Meniere's disease require surgery if medical therapy does not adequately control the vertiginous episodes. There are several surgical procedures. The initial procedure is usually one to conserve hearing, such as endolymphatic sac decompression. If the patient's hearing level is very poor or if this conservative procedure fails, a more destructive procedure may be employed. Labyrinthectomy destroys the membranous labyrinth and sacrifices the balance and hearing end organs. Relief from vertigo may not occur for several weeks in some cases. Ultrasonic labyrinthectomy is also used especially for patients who have symptoms of vertigo but still have worthwhile hearing that should be preserved. A pencil-sized probe of the ultrasonic generator is applied directly to the bone of the horizontal canal through a mastoidectomy incision, and energy is directed into the labyrinth. Cryosurgical labyrinthectomy is also used for some patients. It is performed similarly to the ultrasonic surgery except that it is done through the ear canal without mastoidectomy.[55]

Caring for the patient hospitalized with Meniere's disease requires understanding of the frustrating, incapacitating, and uncomfortable acute attacks the patient suffers.[59,64] Because sudden movement or jarring aggravates vertigo, the person usually prefers to move at his own rate and to take care of himself. If one stands directly in front of the person when talking, so that he does not have to turn his head or his eyes, he will experience less dizziness. Although movement increases the symptoms, the patient should be encouraged to move about in bed occasionally and to permit gentle back care to preserve good skin tone. Lying quietly on the unaffected side with eyes turned toward the direction of the affected ear sometimes is recommended to relieve an acute attack. The patient should not try to read, and bright glaring lights are avoided. Side rails should be on the bed at all times, and the patient should not attempt to get up and walk without assistance. Because it is usually very difficult to get the patient with Meniere's disease to take food or fluids, efforts should be made to obtain something that the patient will eat or drink. Patients should be encouraged to call the nurse at the first indication of an attack so that medication may be given.

Labyrinthitis

Labyrinthitis is an infection of the inner ear of unknown cause although it often follows a head cold and occasionally a middle ear infection. If labyrinthitis progresses to a suppurative stage, hearing loss will be profound and permanent. Damage to the vestibilar system is compensated for by central mechanisms, and the dizziness subsides. Meningitis may develop from labyrinthitis as well as the reverse, in which case the labyrinthitis is usually bilateral. A special form of localized labyrinthitis tends to follow infection and involves the balance mechanisms only. Since the inner ear also helps maintain equilibrium, problems there produce loss of hearing and disturb the function of the semicircular canals.

Typical symptoms include severe sudden vertigo, nausea, vomiting, sudden disturbances of equilibrium, and nystagmus. If nystagmus is of an otologic origin, there is involuntary horizontal jerking movements of the eyeball. During the attack the patient is kept in bed in a darkened room lying quietly without turning his head; he is usually photophobic, has a headache, has an ataxic gait, and refuses food. No specific treatment exists. Antibiotics are usually given in high doses. To relieve vertigo the patient may be given dimenhydrinate (Dramamine) or pronethazine. If vomiting persists, fluids must be given parenterally. However, fluids given orally are usually retained if taken in small amounts with the patient keeping his head perfectly still. Because of the severe vertigo, side rails should be kept up and the patient is assisted when walking. If the patient prefers, his room may be kept darkened at all times. Generally after a period of several days or weeks vertigo diminishes. At times surgery such as a radical mastoidectomy is performed to remove the source of infection.

Nursing care is similar to that for a patient with Meniere's disease.

Outcome criteria for persons with Meniere disease or labyrinthitis

The patient or significant others can:

1. Describe circumstances that may precipitate an attack and what to do when an attack occurs.
2. Describe symptoms requiring medical intervention.
3. State rationale for safety precautions such as walking with assistance and use of side rails during a vertiginous attack.
4. Describe dosage and side effects of prescribed medications.

Fluctuant hearing loss

Fluctuant hearing loss is a form of sensorineural hearing loss that is now thought to be more common than Meniere's disease.[65] It is characterized by a triad of symptoms that includes fullness, roaring tinnitus, and fluctuating hearing loss. Vertigo may or may not be present. Hearing may return to normal and the fullness and roaring disappear after the first attack, but this is unusual. Recovery is usually not complete and becomes worse after each attack. Fluctuant hearing loss is thought to be caused by excessive production of endolymph or a reduction in the absorption of endolymph. Some conditions that contribute to the occurrence of fluctuant hearing loss include poor circulation, diabetes mellitus, hyperlipoprotinemia, high salt intake, allergies, smoking, and syphilis. Results of electronystagmography are positive about 20% of the time. Treatment is similar to the treatment for Meniere's disease; a low-sodium diet and diuretics are often helpful. Patients are usually told to refrain from tobacco. Often antihistamines are administered either intravenously or orally. Diazepam (Valium) is sometimes prescribed for both its tranquilizing and antivestibular effects. Treatment of any contributing medical condition such as diabetes mellitus is indicated.[45]

Cochlear implantation or stimulation

Cochlear implantation or stimulation are operations designed to benefit persons who have severe sensorineural hearing loss who do not benefit from hearing aids.[7,33] Through the procedures an attempt is made to replace a function of the cochlea, that is, the function of transducing the mechanical energy of sound vibrations to electrical energy, which directly stimulates the auditory nerve. An electrode with a single wire of either platinum, iridium, or titanium is placed in the scala tympani (the central portion of the cochlear cavity). The wire is connected with a ground wire in the area of the temporal muscle. The leads are connected to an induction cord containing a small-amplitude modulation radio, which is imbedded in the bone of the mastoid process. The radio receiver is driven by an external antenna placed over it. Externally applied sound waves generate an audioelectrical field within the cochlea. Presently with this technique speech discrimination is still not possible, but some hearing does take place such as hearing the horn of an approaching automobile. Cochlear stimulation also imparts a rhythm to speech, which is helpful in speech reading. Cochlear stimulation may be helpful for at least two thirds of persons with sensorineural loss. Research and experimentation are being carried out on brainstem and cortical stimulation, which may prove helpful for the other third of people with sensorineural loss.

REFERENCES AND SELECTED READINGS

1. Allen, J. H.: May's manual of the diseases of the eye, Baltimore, 1968, The Williams & Wilkins Co.
2. *Ammon, L. L.: Surviving enucleation, Am. J. Nurs. **72:**1817-1821, 1972.
3. Ballenger, J.: Diseases of the nose, throat, and ear, ed. 11, Philadelphia, 1969, Lea & Febiger.
4. Beeson, P. B., and McDermott, W., editors: Cecil-Loeb textbook of medicine, ed. 14, Philadelphia, 1975, W. B. Saunders Co.
5. Blancher, G.: My trip through the semicircular canals, Am. J. Nurs. **74:**1842-1844, 1974.
6. Booth, J. B.: Tympanoplasty, Nurs. Mirror **140:**48-49, 1975.

6a. Boyd-Monk, H.: Helping the corneal transplant patient to see again, Nursing '78 **8:**47-51, Feb. 1978.

7. Brackman, D., and House, W.: Direct stimulation of the auditory nerve in hearing disorders. In Northern, J.: Hearing disorders, Boston, 1976, Little, Brown and Co.
8. Bull, T., and Cook, J.: Speech therapy and ENT surgery, London, 1976, Blackwell Scientific Publications.
9. Chadwick, D. L.: Treatment of ENT conditions, Nurs. Times **70:**424-425, 1974.
10. Chadwick, D. L.: Advances in the treatment of diseases of the ear, nose and throat, Practitioner **209:**460-473, 1972.
11. Condl, E. D., et al.: Ophthalmic nursing, Nurs. Clin. North Am. **5:**449-496, 1970.
12. Cooke, E. T.: Chronic suppurative otitis media, Nurs. Times **70:**1846-1847, 1974.
13. Delaney, R. E.: Stapedectomy, Am. J. Nurs. **69:**2406-2409, 1969.
14. DeWeese, D. D., and Saunders, W. H.: Textbook of otolaryngology, ed. 5, St. Louis, 1977, The C. V. Mosby Co.
15. *Elkington, A. R.: Intraocular foreign bodies, Nurs. Times **69:**1638-1639, 1973.
16. *Elkington, A. R.: Non-perforating wounds, Nurs. Times **69:**1562-1563, 1973.
17. *Elkington, A. R.: Perforating wounds, Nurs. Times **69:**1597-1598, 1973.
18. English, G. M., Northern, J. L., and Fria, T. J.: Chronic otitis media as a cause of sensorineural hearing loss, Arch. Otolaryngol. **98:**17-20, 1973.
19. *Fersberger, W.: Early diagnosis of acute angle-closure glaucoma, Am. J. Nurs. **75:**1154-1155, 1975.

*References preceded by an asterisk are particularly well suited for student reading.

20. Fulton, M. K., Schweizer, D., Ruhland, F., et al.: Helping diabetics adapt to failing vision, Am. J. Nurs. **74**:54-57, 1974.
21. Gellis, S. S., and Kagan, B. M.: Current pediatric therapy, ed. 6, Philadelphia, 1973, W. B. Saunders Co.
22. Girard, L. J.: Cryotherapy in ophthalmology, Sight Sav. Rev. **35**:87-90, 1965.
23. Girard, L. J.: Ultrasonic aspiration-irrigation of cataracts and the vitreous. In Emery, J. M., and Paton, D.: Current concepts in cataract surgery, St. Louis, 1974, The C. V. Mosby Co.
24. Glorig, A., and Gerwin, K. S.: Otitis media, Springfield, Ill., 1972, Charles C Thomas, Publisher.
25. Gordon, D. M.: The inflammed eye, Am. J. Nurs. **64**:113-117, 1964.
26. Hall, I. S., and Colman, B.: Diseases of the nose, throat, and ear, New York, 1975, Churchill-Livingston.
27. Hammond, V.: A symposium on the surgery of deafness: Stapedectomy, Nurs. Mirror **140**:45-48, 1975.
28. Havener, W. H.: Synopsis of ophthalmology, ed. 4, St. Louis, 1975, The C. V. Mosby Co.
29. Havener, W. H., Saunders, W. H., Keith, C. F., and Prescott, A. W.: Nursing care in eye, ear, nose and throat disorders, ed. 3, St. Louis, 1974, The C. V. Mosby Co.
30. Hiles, D. A.: Strabismus, Am. J. Nurs. **74**:1082-1089, 1974.
31. Hiles, D. A.: Results of the first year's experience with phacoemulsification, Am. J. Ophthalmol. **75**:474-477, 1973.
32. House, W. F.: Meniere's disease: management and theory, Otolaryngol Clin. North Am. **8**:515-535, 1975.
33. House, W. F., and Urban, J.: Long term results of electrode implantation and electronic stimulation of the cochlea in man, Ann. Otol. Rhinol. Laryngol. **82**:504-517, 1973.
34. *Jennings, B.: Intraocular lens for cataracts, A.O.R.N.J. **23**:664-672, 1976.
35. Kelman, C. D.: Symposium: phaco-emulsification and aspiration of senile cataracts, Trans. Am. Acad. Ophthalmol. Otolaryngol. **78**:7-9, 1974.
36. Levenson, L., and Levenson, J.: Corneal transplantation, Am. J. Nurs. **77**:1160-1163, 1977.
37. Lucente, F. E.: The dying patient in otolaryngology, Laryngoscope **83**:292-298, 1973.
38. Maolone, W. H.: Otolaryngology, New York, 1974, Harper & Row, Publishers.
39. Marlow, D. R.: Textbook of pediatric nursing, ed. 5, Philadelphia, 1977, W. B. Saunders Co.
40. Mausolf, F. A.: The eye and systemic disease, St. Louis, 1975, The C. V. Mosby Co.
41. Mawson, S. R.: Management of complications of stapedectomy, J. Laryngol. Otol. **89**:145-149, 1975.
42. McKenzie, W.: Vertigo, Nurs. Mirror **139**:56-57, 1974.
43. Michalson, R., et al.: Cochlear implant, J. Speech Hear. Disord. 1975.
44. Moody, E.: Amblyopia. In Harley, R.: Pediatric ophthalmology, Philadelphia, 1975, W. B. Saunders Co.
45. Naftalin, L.: The medical treatment of fluctuant hearing loss, Otolaryngol. Clin. North Am. **8**:475-482, 1975.
46. Nelson, W. E.: Textbook of pediatrics, ed. 10, Philadelphia, 1975, W. B. Saunders Co.
47. Newell, F. W.: Ophthalmology: principles and concepts, ed. 4, St. Louis, 1978, The C. V. Mosby Co.
48. Newell, F. W.: Strabismus and amblyopia, Acton, Mass., 1975, Publishing Sciences Group Inc.
49. Nordlohne, M. E.: The intraocular implant lens development and results, with special reference to the Binkhorst lens, ed. 2, Baltimore, 1975, Williams & Wilkins Co.
50. Norton, E.: Symposium: intraocular lenses, Trans. Am. Acad. Ophthalmol. Otolaryngol. **81**:64-137, 1976.
51. Paparella, M. M., and Shumick, D. A., editors: Otolaryngology, Philadelphia, 1973, W. B. Saunders Co.
52. Pereira, P.: Screening for glaucoma, Nurs. Times **68**:771-774, 1972.
53. *Pilgrim, M., and Sigler, B.: Phaco-emulsification of cataracts, Am. J. Nurs. **75**:976-977, 1975.
54. Public, J. L.: Meniere's disease: etiology, natural history, and results of treatment, Otolaryngol. Clin. North Am. **6**:25-28, 1973.
55. Quimby, M. A.: Care of patients with labyrinthine dysfunction, Am. J. Nurs. **60**:1780-1781, 1960.
56. Reinecke, R. D., Stein, H. A., and Slatt, B. J.: Introductory manual for the ophthalmic assistant: a programmed text, St. Louis, 1972, The C. V. Mosby Co.
57. Robinson, M.: A four-year study of the stainless steel stapes, Arch. Otolaryngol. **82**:217-235, 1965.
58. Rosborough, J. F.: Hosp. Med. **7**:46-49, 1971.
59. Rowe, D. S.: Acute suppurative otitis media, Pediatrics **56**:285-294, 1975.
60. Rubenstein, K.: Ophthalmic cryosurgery, Nurs. Times **63**:1640-1642, 1967.
61. Sabiston, D. C., editor: Davis-Christopher's textbook of surgery, ed. 11, Philadelphia, 1977, W. B. Saunders Co.
62. Scheie, H. G., and Albert, D. M.: Adler's textbook of ophthalmology, Philadelphia, 1969, W. B. Saunders Co.
63. *Schultz, J. M., and Williams, M.: The blind diabetic, Nurs. '76, **6**:19-20, 1976.
64. Shambaugh, G. E.: Surgery of the ear, Philadelphia, 1967, W. B. Saunders Co.
65. Shea, J.: Fluctuant hearing loss, Otolaryngol. Clin. North Am. **8**:263-267, June 1975.
66. Sheehy, J. L.: Ossicular problems in tympanoplasty, Arch. Otolaryngol. **81**:115-122, 1965.
67. Shuknecht, H. F.: Stapedectomy, Boston, 1971, Little, Brown and Co.
68. Smith, J. F., and Machazel, D. P.: Retinal detachment, Am. J. Nurs. **73**:1530-1535, 1973.
69. U.S. Department of Health, Education and Welfare: Diabetic retinopathy, No. (NIH) 75-406, National Eye Institute, 1975.
70. U.S. Department of Health, Education and Welfare: Support for vision research: interim report of the National Advisory Eye Council, No. (NIH) 76-1098, 1976.
71. Walloch, R. A., and Cowden, D. A.: Placement of electrodes for the excitation of the eighth nerve, Arch. Otolaryngol. **100**:19-23, 1974.
72. *Weinstock, F. J.: Emergency treatment of eye injuries, Am. J. Nurs. **71**:1929-1931, 1971.
73. White, N.: OR nursing in otomicrosurgery, A.O.R.N. J. **22**:889-897, 1975.
74. Williams, S. R.: Nutrition and diet therapy, Ed. 3, St. Louis, 1977, The C. V. Mosby Co.
75. Wood, C.: Medications for vertigo and motion sickness, Am. J. Nurs. **66**:1764-1767, 1966.
76. Zweng, H. C., Little, H. L., and Peabody, R. R.: Argon laser photocoagulation of diabetic retinopathy, Arch. Ophthalmol. **86**:395-400, 1971.

AUDIOVISUAL RESOURCES

1. Pediatric ophthalmology, Part 1 and Part 2, New York, MEDCOM, 1972. Slides, (105, 2x2), color.
2. *Emergency eye care, 1971, Trainex Corp. Filmstrip.
3. Surgical management of chronic ear diseases; videotape, Digest, Inc., Cincinnati, 1970. Motion picture, 16-mm, color, audiocassette or super 8-mm sound cartridge.

40

Musculoskeletal system assessment

PATRICIA BUERGIN

The eagle that cannot fly will starve to death. The deer that cannot run becomes the easy prey of its enemies. And if humans had to rely solely on themselves for their food, shelter, and protection, without the ability to move, they too would surely die. This is the importance of the musculoskeletal system. Yet there are many illnesses and disorders that deprive individuals of their ability to move about freely.

In order to plan appropriate interventions for individuals who have locomotor disabilities, the disabilities and the individual's reaction to them require careful assessment. Such assessment is based on knowledge and understanding of the anatomy and physiology of the musculoskeletal system, and understanding of the laboratory studies involved and what the results of these studies mean. In this chapter the anatomy and physiology of the musculoskeletal system, methods for obtaining subjective and objective data about the patients and their disabilites, and the pertinence of selected laboratory studies are discussed.

■ ANATOMY AND PHYSIOLOGY

□ Bones

If you can imagine a human body without bones, you can define the three mechanical functions of bones: (1) *support* as provided by the skeletal framework itself; (2) *protection*, as in the example of the bony casing of the skull that protects the brain; and (3) *movement*, in which muscles contract, pulling on bone that act as levers to provide motion for the body. Bone also has a physiologic function as a storehouse of calcium.

Bones are composed of both living cells and nonliving intracellular material. They are derived from embryonic hyaline cartilage that undergoes a process known as *osteogenesis* or *endochondral ossification* to become bone. This process is accomplished through the synthesis of mucopolysaccharides and collagen by cells called *osteoblasts*. These two substances comprise the material known as *bone matrix*. Calcium salts are deposited in the bone matrix, giving it the "hard" quality by which bone is characterized.

There are four types of bones according to their shape: long (femur, humerus), short (carpals), flat (skull), and irregular (vertebrae). Each bone is composed of *cancellous* (spongy) and *compact* (dense) bone. In the long bones the cancellous portions are found in the ends of the bones, while the compact bone is located in the shaft. The short and irregular bones have an inner core of cancellous bone with an outer layer of compact bone. The flat bones have two outer plates of compact bone with an inner layer of cancellous bone.

Cancellous and compact bone are differentiated from one another by the arrangement of the *lamellae* within them. Lamellae are concentric cylindrical layers of calcified matrix. At the center of this arrangement of concentric rings is a canal, called the *haversian canal*. This canal contains a capillary. Some canals may also contain a small a.teriole, venule, and lymphatics. Small spaces between the rings of the lamellae, called *lacunae*, are occupied by bone cells (osteocytes). Lacunae are connected with the haversian canal, and therefore the nutrient supply, by very small canals called *canaliculi*. The lamella with its haversian canal, lacunae, and canaliculi is called a haversian unit (Fig. 40-1). Haversian units fit closely together in compact bone. In cancellous bone, however, there are many open spaces between thin interconnecting processes of bone called trabeculae. This arrangement of fine threads of bone resembles the fine filigree work of the jeweler. Such an arrangement provides strength to the bone while reducing its weight.

A typical long bone is covered, except on its articular surfaces, by a white, fibrous membrane called the *periosteum*. The articular surfaces are covered with resilient *hyaline cartilage*. The periosteum provides a place for muscle fibers to attach, and its inner layers contain osteoblasts. Because of the presence of osteoblasts, the periosteum is considered an organ of growth and repair. The ends of the bone are called *epiphyses*, and the shaft

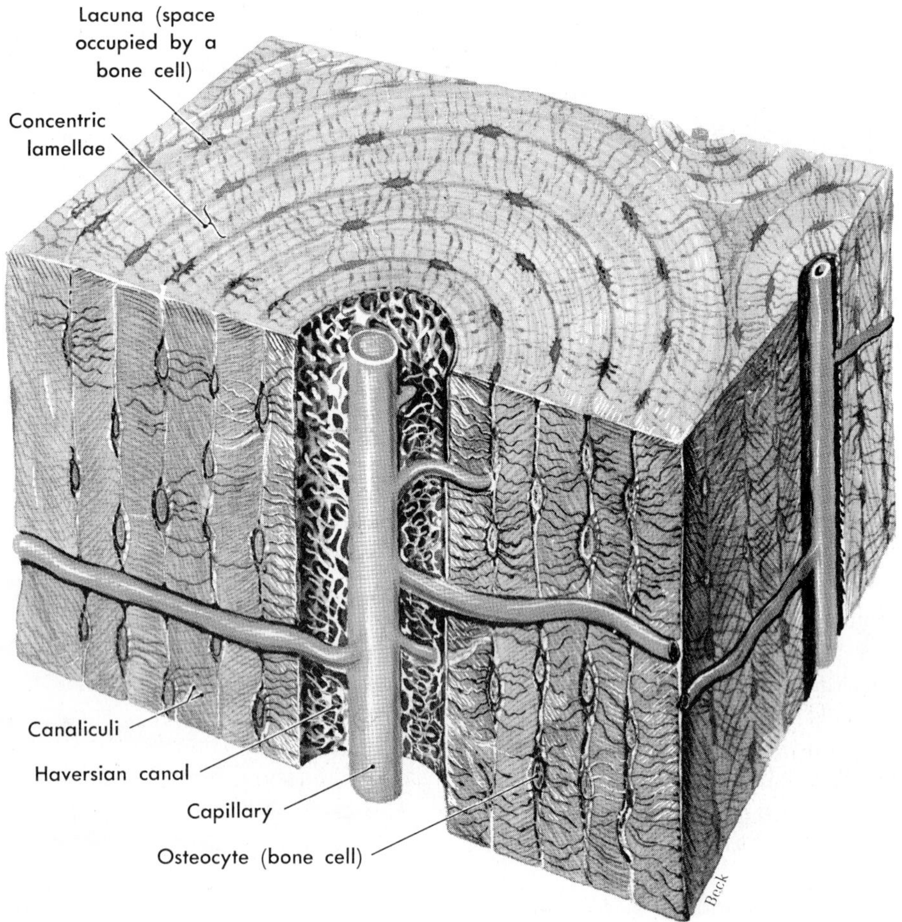

Fig. 40-1. Section of compact bone showing details of haversian system. (From Anthony, C. P., and Thibodeau, G. A.: Textbook of anatomy and physiology, ed. 10, St. Louis, 1979, The C. V. Mosby Co.)

is known as the *diaphysis.* The membranous *endosteum* lines the marrow-filled *medullary cavity* and the haversian canals (Fig. 40-2). The endosteum contains some osteoblasts.

Longitudinal growth of the long bones emanates from the epiphyseal cartilage, located between the diaphyseal and epiphyseal centers of ossification. This epiphyseal cartilage thickens because of rapid proliferation of the cartilage cells, and this additional cartilage undergoes ossification. Growth in the diameter of the bone is accomplished as osteoclasts (bone-destroying cells) enlarge the medullary cavity while osteoblasts in the periosteum produce new bone at the outside of the bone (membranous ossification). In older people or in people who are quite inactive, degeneration and reabsorption of bone occurs more rapidly than growth of new bone. This leads to a condition called *osteoporosis.* In this condition bone becomes porous and fragile. Bone will reshape itself in response to alterations of its mechanical function. Such a response is in accordance with *Wolff's law:* "Every change in the form and function of bones or their function alone is followed by certain definite changes in their external configuration in accordance with mathematical laws."[9]

Blood is supplied to the bone by three routes: (1) through the arterioles in the haversian canals; (2) through vessels located in the periosteum that penetrate the bone through structures known as *Volkmann's canals,* which connect with the vessels of the haversian canals; and (3) through vessels in the marrow and the ends of the bone. Therefore damage to a nutrient artery, to the periosteum, or to the bone itself, resulting in separation of the broken ends of the bone, causes an interruption of the blood supply to the bone.

Further, bones are supplied with a network of sensory nerves that connect with the central nervous sys-

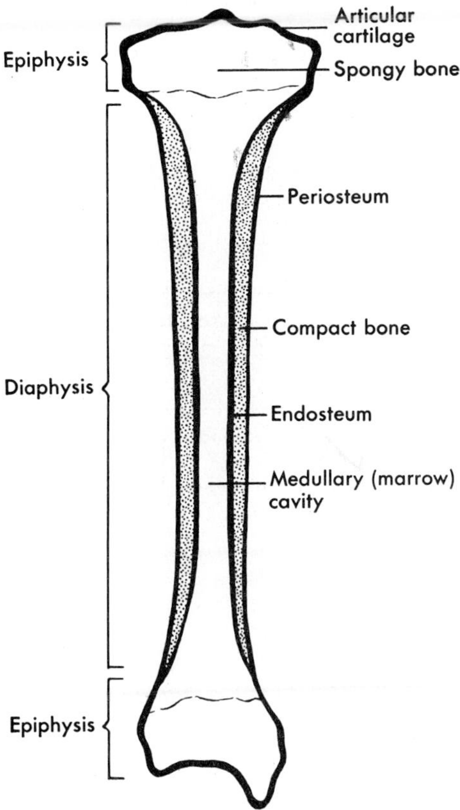

Fig. 40-2. Structure of long bone as seen in longitudinal section. (From Anthony, C. P., and Thibodeau, G. A.: Textbook of anatomy and physiology, ed. 10, St. Louis, 1979, The C. V. Mosby Co.)

tem. Thus if there is damage to a bone (fracture, infection, or other lesions), pain will result.

□ Muscles

Muscles are divided into three major groups: skeletal (striated, voluntary), visceral (smooth, involuntary), and cardiac. Visceral muscle, as in the stomach and intestines, is innervated by the autonomic nervous system and therefore is not under the control of the will. Skeletal muscle, however, is innervated by nerve fibers from the cerebrospinal system and is under control of the will. Skeletal muscle provides controlled movement, one of the three major functions of muscles. The other two functions are maintenance of posture and production of heat.

Skeletal muscle cells are long and narrow. This lends to their being called *fibers* rather than cells. They are composed of a *sarcolemma*, or cell membrane, and *sarcoplasm*, or cytoplasm. Small, closely packed fibers within the sarcoplasm, called *myofibrils*, that alternate light and dark horizontal stripes, give the striated appearance that gives this type of muscle its name. The dark stripes are "A bands," and the light stripes are "I bands." Light bands crossing the middle of the dark stripes are called the "H zone," and dark lines crossing the middle of the light stripes are called "Z lines." Myofibrils consist of several sections called *sarcomeres*. Each sarcomere is a section that extends from one Z line of a myofibril to the next.[1] Bundles of muscle fibers (cells) comprise the muscle itself.

It is the function of muscles to contract. This is accomplished by a complex process triggered by nerve impulses arriving at the muscle fiber. Calcium ions are released when the impulse is received and bind to troponin (an inhibitor of the molecular myosin-actin interaction). Once troponin is bound, the myosin-actin interaction takes place and the sarcomeres of the myofibrils contract. The energy for muscle contraction is supplied by the breakdown of ATP (adenosine triphosphate), which the muscle cells produce by combining ADP (adenosine diphosphate) with creatine phosphate. Relaxation of the muscle occurs when the calcium separates from the troponin[1] (Fig. 40-3). Muscle cells obey the "all-or-none" law; that is, they contract fully or not at all. This does *not* mean that the entire muscle contracts fully, but just those individual cells that have received the nerve impulse. Muscle fibers that are adequately oxygenated will contract more forcefully than when they are not adequately oxygenated.

Skeletal muscles are organs; they vary in size and shape from long and thin to broad and flat, or they may form bulky masses. The arrangement of the fibers within the muscle determines the capacity of the forceful contraction of the muscle. Skeletal muscles contract only if they are stimulated. There are several types of contractions: (1) *tonic*, or a continual partial contraction that is vital in the maintenance of posture; (2) *isotonic*, where the tension within the muscle is unchanged but the length of the muscle changes (shortens); (3) *isometric*, where the tension increases but the muscle does not shorten; (4) the *twitch* or jerky reaction to a single stimulus; (5) *tetanic*, a more sustained contraction than the twitch and produced by a series of stimuli in rapid succession; (6) *Treppe*, stronger twitch contractions in response to regularly repeated constant strength stimuli; (7) *fibrillation*, asynchronous contraction of individual fibers; and (8) *convulsion*, or abnormal uncoordinated tetanic contractions occurring in varying groups of muscles.[1]

Movements of the body are produced by muscles pulling on bones, with bones serving as levers, and joints serving as fulcrums for the levers. Most movements depend on several muscles acting in a coordinated manner. *Prime movers* produce the movement; *antagonists* relax while the prime movers contract, thereby permitting

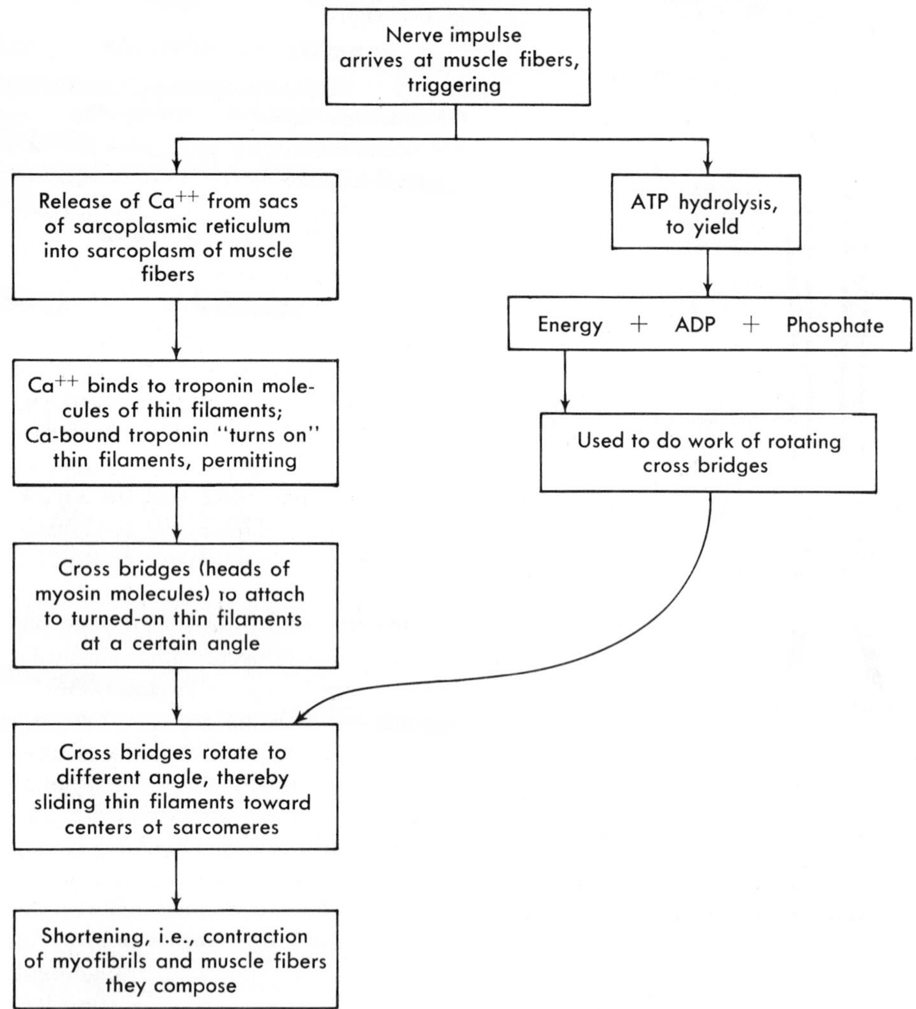

Fig. 40-3. Mechanism of skeletal muscle contraction. (From Anthony, C. P., and Thibodeau, G. A.: Textbook of anatomy and physiology, ed. 10, St. Louis, 1979, The C. V. Mosby Co.)

movement; and *synergists* contract at the same time as the prime movers to produce movement or to stabilize a part so the contraction of the prime movers is more efficient.[1]

Skeletal muscle is highly vascular. Waste products (lactic acid) resulting from the chemical changes that occur during muscle contraction must be transported to the liver to be resynthesized, and oxygen must be transported to the muscle fibers if those fibers are to perform their work. Muscle fatigue and pain result when lactic acid cannot be adequately carried off. Conditions such as anemia, in which the amount of hemoglobin available to carry oxygen is reduced, or trauma, which interrupts circulation to the muscle fibers, will result in poor muscle work, since contractions depend on an adequate oxygen supply.

Adequate muscle contractions also depend on effective innervation. It is the cerebellum that is primarily responsible for control of muscle movements (Chapter 34). Every muscle cell is supplied with the axon of a nerve cell. Nerve cells that transmit impulses to skeletal muscles are known as *somatic motoneurons.* The neuron and the muscle cells it activates are called a *motor unit.* The axon of one somatic motoneuron may be divided into any number of branches and therefore innervate a like number of muscle cells. The fewer muscle cells innervated, the more precise (or fine) are the resultant movements. The actual contraction of the muscle is set off by the release of acetylcholine, a chemical contained in small vesicles in the axon terminal. When acetylcholine contacts the sarcolemma, it stimulates the contraction. This reaction takes place across a structure known as the *motor end plate* or *neuromuscular junction* where the muscle and the nerve are in contact. Damage to the nervous system at the cerebrospinal level or at any point in the course of the nerve through the local motoneuron level will result in muscular dysfunction.

□ Cartilage

Cartilage is a material composed of fibers imbedded in a firm gel. It is a strong but flexible material, and it is avascular. Nutrients must reach the cartilage cells by the process of diffusion through the gel from capillaries located in the *perichondrium* (fibrous covering of the cartilage), or in the case of articular cartilage, through the synovial fluid. The number of collagenous fibers found in the cartilage will determine its type: *fibrous*, *hyaline*, or *elastic*. Fibrous (or fibrocartilage) has the greatest number of fibers and therefore the greatest tensile strength. Fibrocartilage composes the intervertebral discs. Articular (hyaline) cartilage—smooth, white, shiny, and resilient—covers the articular surfaces of the bone and serves as a cushion. Elastic cartilage has fewest fibers and may be found in areas such as the external ear.

□ Ligaments

Ligaments are bands of dense fibrous connective tissue that are flexible and tough. These structures connect the articular ends of bones and provide stability. Examples are the medial and lateral collateral ligaments of the knee that provide mediolateral stability to the knee joint, and the anterior and posterior cruciate ligaments within the joint capsule of the knee that provide anteroposterior stability. Ligaments may also attach to soft tissue to suspend structures. An example of this is the suspensory ligament of the ovary that passes from the tubal end of the ovary to the peritoneum.

□ Tendons

Tendons are bands of dense fibrous tissue that form the termination of a muscle and serve to attach it to a bone. The tendon is an extension of the fibrous sheath that envelops each muscle and is continuous with the periosteum at its other end. *Tendon sheaths* are tubular structures of connective tissue that enclose certain tendons, especially in the wrist and ankle. These sheaths are lined with synovial membrane that provides the lubrication for the easy movement of the tendon.

□ Fascia

Fascia is a sheet of loose connective tissue that may be found directly under the skin as *superficial fascia*, or as a sheet of dense, fibrous connective tissue comprising the sheath of muscles, nerves, and blood vessels. The latter is known as *deep fascia*.

□ Bursae

Bursae are small sacs of connective tissue located wherever pressure is exerted over moving parts. They may, for example, occur between skin and bone, tendons and bone, or between muscles. These structures are lined with synovial membrane and contain synovial fluid. They serve as cushions between moving parts. Such a bursa, the olecranon bursa, is located between the olecranon process and the skin.

□ Joints

Movement would not be possible unless some flexibility were provided within the skeletal framework. This flexibility is provided by the joints, or places where the bones come together. The shape of the joint will determine the amount of movement that is possible, and the classification of joints is based on the amount of movement they allow.

Classification

There are three major classifications of joints: (1) *synarthroses* (or fibrous joints) such as the sutures of the skull that do not allow movement; (2) *amphiarthroses* (or cartilaginous joints) such as the intervertebral joints that allow little movement (The synarthroses and the amphiarthroses may be classified together as synarthroses, designating that they have no joint cavity but rather tissue [fibrous, cartilage, or bone] growing between their articular surfaces.); and (3) *diarthrodial* or *synovial joints* that allow free movement. This type of joint includes the hip, knee, shoulder, and elbow. Since diarthrodial joints are the joints that permit movement, they are discussed in the most detail.

Each diarthrodial joint contains a small space or *joint cavity* between the articulating surfaces of the bones that comprise the joint. Articular hyaline cartilage covers the articulating surfaces of both bones. Additionally, a *joint capsule* or sleeve of fibrous tissue encases the joint. This capsule is lined with synovial membrane that secretes *synovial fluid*, which serves to lubricate the joint (Fig. 40-4). Additionally, ligaments may be present between the bones (as with the cruciate ligaments of the knee) to provide internal stability to the joint. Small pieces of dense cartilage may also be interposed between the articulating surfaces. These are crescent-shaped or half-moon-shaped structures that serve to provide additional cushioning for the joint. Examples are the semilunar cartilages or *menisci* of the knee joint.

Diarthrodial joints are further classified by the shape of their surfaces and the type of movement they permit. Specialized texts should be consulted for discussion of these subtypes. However, it may be generally stated that the diarthrodial joints permit one or more of the follow-

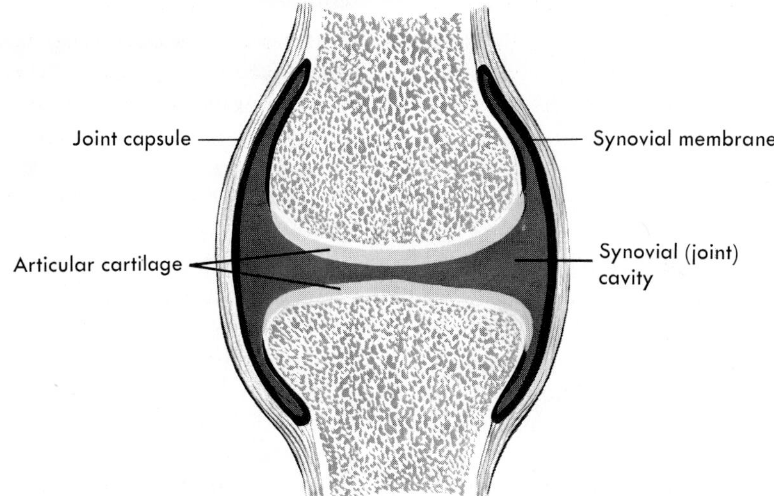

Fig. 40-4. Structure of diarthrotic joint. (From Anthony, C. P., and Thibodeau, G. A.: Textbook of anatomy and physiology, ed. 10, St. Louis, 1979, The C. V. Mosby Co.)

ing movements: flexion, extension, adduction, abduction, rotation, circumduction, supination, pronation, inversion, eversion, protraction, or retraction. The latter six movements are considered special movements (Figs. 40-10 and 40-11).

□ Pathology in the musculoskeletal system

As discussed in the anatomy and physiology of the musculoskeletal system, the musculoskeletal and nervous systems are interrelated. The muscles, bones, joints, supportive structures, and sensory and motor nerves all work together to provide controlled movement. However, any problem that causes interference or disturbance at any level—innervation, contractility, articulation, or support—of this well-integrated system results a musculoskeletal dysfunction. Problems can occur when there is interruption of blood supply to the involved structures; disease affecting the contour of bones or joints; disease that affects the nerves that innervate the musculoskeletal system; and trauma, of whatever origin, that interrupts the integrity of any of the involved structures.

■ ASSESSMENT OF THE PERSON

As with any other type of illness, plans for the care of the person and eventual discharge arrangements are based on a systematic assessment of needs, capabilities, and resources. Many persons with musculoskeletal problems will have additional problems such as cardiovascular or respiratory disorders, and assessment of these disorders can be found in the chapters dealing with those specific disorders. Only data that has particular relevance to musculoskeletal problems will be discussed here.

□ Subjective data

Collection of subjective data usually begins with questions related to the history of the patient's present illness or dysfunction. The second area of questioning relates to pain or discomfort. Some determination should be made as to the nature, location, and duration of the patient's pain or discomfort. There should also be an attempt to determine what measures the patient has taken to relieve his pain or discomfort and whether these measures were effective. A list of the patient's current medications is obtained, along with a list of any allergies he may have, particularly drug allergies. The third area, and one of major importance, relates to questions about activities of daily living (ADL), since dysfunction of the musculoskeletal system often leads to a loss of independence in ADL. The major functions included in *personal* ADL are feeding, bathing, toileting, dressing, transfer, ambulation, and sleep. Pertinent questions include: Is assistance needed from other people to perform any of these functions? Are assistive devices used to help perform these functions independently? Does pain or other symptoms interfere with sleep? *Social* ADL functions include household activities, work activities, recreational activities, and sexual activities. Have these activities been curtailed or modified because of symptoms? How successful have the modifications been?

If the person needs assistance to perform any activities, who provides the assistance? Is that person able to provide adequate assistance? What modifications have been made in his environment? How well do these modifications work?

Some individuals with musculoskeletal disorders are highly imaginative, inventive, or are well informed regarding the variety of assistive devices that are available. These individuals are often able to determine methods of dealing with their dysfunctions in clever ways, often managing to maintain their independence despite a significant degree of pathology. Others, not so clever or so well informed and with less pathology, may find themselves markedly handicapped because they are not aware of alterations that could be made in ADL or the environment to enhance their functional ability.

Person's perception of the problem

During the course of the interview the person will give information relating to how his disease has affected his life style; to what degree he has been able to accept his problem and make necessary adaptations; and how he complies with his program of treatment. Much of this information is put forth as he discusses his ADL abilities. Some individuals perceive that they are minimally affected by their disorder, others may be at their wit's end to know how to cope, and others fall somewhere in between these two extremes. How the person perceives the manner in which his illness has affected him may influence how he feels about his current therapy and what expectations he holds for future therapy. If he is unable to function as he would like while on his current therapy, he may either be overly confident in his expectations of future therapy or he may believe that nothing further will help him. If he is satisfied with his current therapy, he may not perceive a need for further therapy. In any of these instances, where there is a need for the individual to learn about his disease, its treatment, or adaptations that can be helpful to him, his perception of his current status is a significant clue as to the type of teaching approach that should be utilized by those concerned with his care.

Family's perception of the patient's problem

An individual's illness generally has some effect on the other people who are intimately associated with that individual. Therefore it is important to determine the effects of the person's illness on those who are close to him. The individual may see himself as a burden, an embarrassment, or an object of pity. On the other hand, if the significant others are supportive, the individual may feel well accepted, respected, and loved, even though the role relationships with others have been altered.

Frequently, when a person has a disabling chronic musculoskeletal illness, family roles are changed. Not infrequently, these changes in roles and status are resented, not only by the family, but by the person who may feel worthless or inadequate. When these conditions prevail, some intervention by health personnel (physician, nurse, social worker, or psychiatrist) may be necessary in an attempt to assist the person and the family to work through these feelings and to provide support.

Listening to what the person and the family have to say about the illness, the treatment, the long-term outcomes of the illness, and their feelings about the changes the illness has necessitated in their lives will give clues as to interventions that might be tried to alleviate existing problems.

□ Objective data

Behavior

Assessment of the person's behavior includes making observations related to the patient's mental status: his orientation to time, place, and person; his ability to understand directions; his capacity to retain information; and his span of attention. (See Chapter 34 for more information.) The person's *ability to relate to others*—is he withdrawn, quiet, talkative, tense, nervous, guarded, hostile—as seen in his responses, affect, and behavior must also be considered. Interventions, if they are to be successful, must be based on the person's ability to understand and willingness to accept those interventions.

General appearance

General appearance is a second area to be assessed. The person's age and sex may bear a relationship to the specific disorder and can well have a bearing on his attitude toward his disorder. Posture can sometimes give clues to the nature of the problem such as the severe kyphotic posture in ankylosing spondylitis (Fig. 40-5). The person may be stooped and unable to straighten up or may hold himself in a tense attitude to guard against pain from a severe whiplash.

Nutritional status—well nourished, overweight, or underweight—is also important. Obesity may be the result of general lack of activity in persons who have musculoskeletal disorders, since they do not perform enough activity to utilize the calories taken in. Extra pounds will also tax a diseased musculoskeletal system, making it more difficult for the person to perform ADL. Severe thinness may be an indication of the individual's inability to secure and prepare nutritional meals or to adequately feed himself; or it may be related to a specific systemic condition that causes nausea and vomiting or malabsorption of food. The person can usually given an accurate account of why he is overweight or underweight.

Deformity

Many musculoskeletal problems are marked by deformity of one or more extremities or joints. Deformities

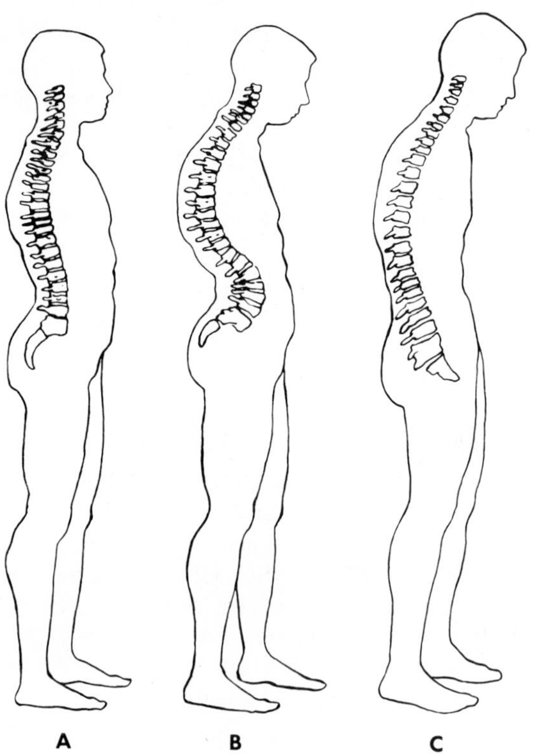

Fig. 40-5. A, Curves of spine in good posture. **B,** Curves of spine in slump posture. **C,** Obliteration of spinal curves as in early spondylitis. (From Larson, C. B., and Gould, M.: Orthopedic nursing, ed. 8, St. Louis, 1974, The C. V. Mosby Co.)

should be specifically noted and described, and some evaluation is made of the extent to which the deformity curtails normal function. For example, the person who has severe "swan-neck" deformities of the fingers, ulnar deviation of the hand, and subluxation (incomplete dislocation) of the wrist may well be restricted in both fine and gross motor functions of the hand. Deformity can be thought of as a change in size, shape, or position of a body part. Following are some of the more common deformities as related to position:

1. *Swan-neck deformity,* a flexion contracture of the metacarpophalangeal joint, hyperextension of the proximal interphalangeal joint, and flexion of the distal interphalangeal joint (Fig. 40-6).
2. *Ulnar deviation,* or drift, with the fingers deviating at the metacarpophalangeal joints toward the ulnar aspect of the hand.
3. *Valgus* deformities (away from the midline of the body) may be present in a number of joints. In *hallux valgus* the great toe turns toward the other toes. In *genu valgum* (Fig. 42-11) the knees are "knock-kneed." In *talipes valgus* the foot is everted.
4. *Varus* deformities (toward the midline of the body) may also be present in a number of joints. *Genu varum* (Fig. 42-10) denotes a bowing of the knees, and *talipes varus* denotes inversion of the foot.
5. *Scoliosis* is a lateral curvature of the spine.
6. *Kyphosis* is also a curvature of the spine, but the convexity of the curve is posterior, usually in the thoracic area.
7. *Atrophy* (reduction in size of an organ) may lead to

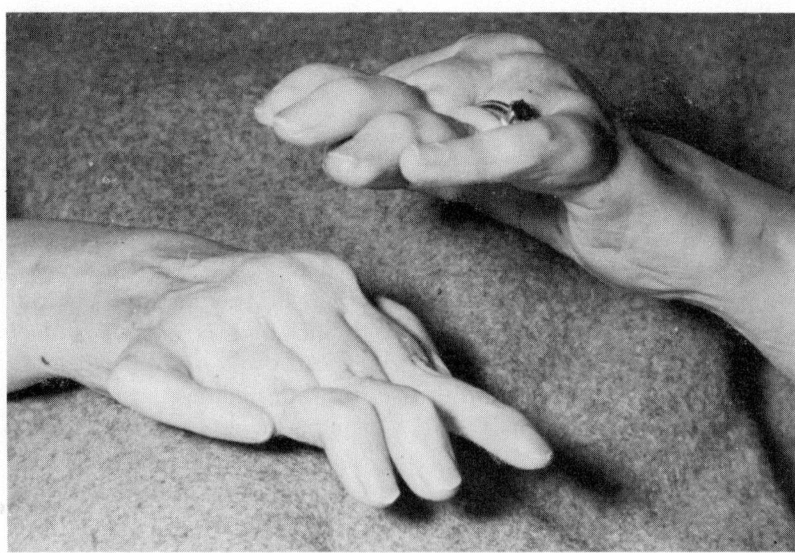

Fig. 40-6. Swan-neck deformities of fingers in rheumatoid arthritis. (From Flatt, A. E.: Care of the rheumatoid hand, ed. 3, St. Louis, 1974, The C. V. Mosby Co.)

a difference in the appearance of an extremity or other body part. Atrophy of muscles is characterized by a wasting of the muscles so that in appearance they lack the bulk of normal muscle. This can result from disuse or from a disease process such as polymyositis. Atrophied muscle will be weaker than normal muscle.

8. *Hypertrophy* is abnormal enlargement of an organ. In reference to the musculoskeletal system, hypertrophy is generally used to describe enlargement of muscle caused by a disease process. In pseudohypertrophic muscular dystrophy, for example, there is enlargement of the muscles of the calf of the leg. There is limitation of function associated with this enlargement.

Skin, nails, and hair

A third area of assessment is the condition of the skin and nails. The first areas to be assessed are *turgor* (fullness) and *texture* (feel). Many individuals, particularly those who are in late middle age and who have been taking steroid preparations for a prolonged period of time, will have a wasted appearance to their skin. It is dry and papery, almost having a transparent quality to it. This type of skin is easily broken. Individuals with scleroderma, on the other hand, will have patches of hard, nonelastic, leathery skin, often over the forearms, hands, chest, and face. This type of skin restricts movement of the structures underlying it.

The *integrity* of the skin must also be considered. Are there breaks in the skin, ulcerations, or reddened areas? Individuals with limited mobility are subject to skin breakdown. Pressure being exerted over skin areas and interfering with circulation to these areas may cause necrosis and breakdown of the skin, resulting in what are commonly known as pressure sores or *decubitus ulcers* (p. 834). In addition, individuals who do not move well are subject to greater sheering forces against sheets, chair surfaces, bedpans, and other objects over which they move or are moved. Such shearing can irritate, abrade, or tear the skin. The complications that can arise from skin breakdown can last months or years longer than the acute process that brought the person to the hospital initially. Accurate assessment (which includes a determination of the status of the circulation in the extremities) of the potential for skin breakdown is vital in planning care that will help to prevent breakdown.

Assessing the *temperature* of the skin over painful joints (by palpating the skin) can help to determine the presence and degree of an inflammatory or an infectious process within the joint. *Erythema* of the skin may be present over acutely inflamed joints. Increased warmth is a positive indication of the presence of inflammation and of the need for keeping the joint at rest.

Skin *rash* may be present in psoriasis, scleroderma, rheumatic fever, dermatomyositis, and a number of other musculoskeletal disorders. A description of the nature (smooth, scaly, red, dusky) and location (over limbs,

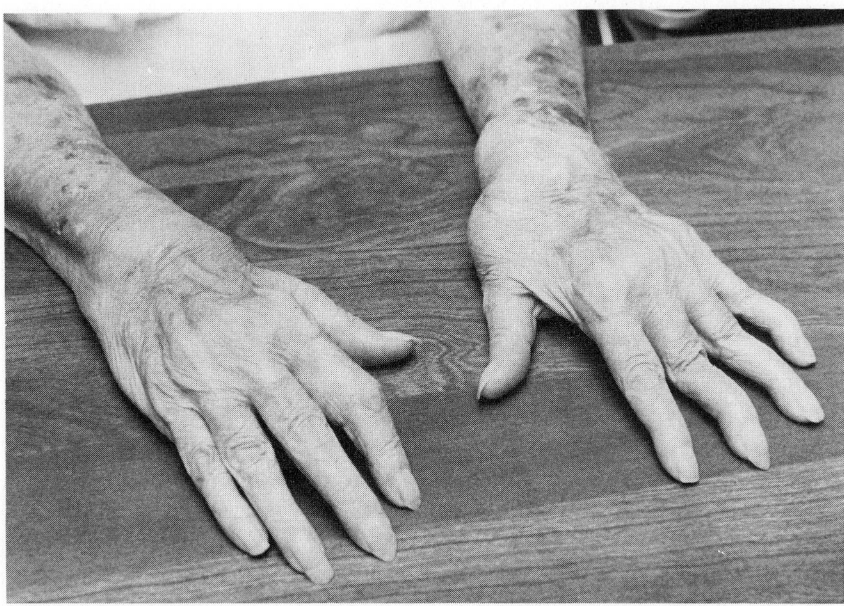

Fig. 40-7. Hands and forearms of woman with advanced rheumatoid arthritis. Note areas of bruising on forearms. Such ecchymoses are not uncommon in individuals who have rheumatoid arthritis and who take steroids in treatment. Handling of such individuals must be extremely gentle, both to avoid bruising and potential sloughing of these areas.

joints, face, trunk) of the rash provides a useful baseline in later determining the effectiveness of treatment.

A number of individuals with connective tissue diseases may demonstrate *color changes* in the skin on their hands when they are exposed to cold. The characteristic color change is from white (resulting from arteriolar spasm) to blue (cyanosis caused by stagnation of blood) to red (caused by warming and reactive vasodilation).[14] These changes are known as *Raynaud's phenomenon*, and the presence of this phenomenon requires specific management consideration (p. 1031).

Bruising (ecchymosis) of the skin often occurs in individuals with connective tissue disease, particularly when they have had long-term treatment with corticosteroids (Fig. 40-7). Such areas of bruising may slough, become ulcerated, and at times become infected. Bruising will also be present in the soft tissue adjacent to and overlying areas that have been traumatized, as in persons who have suffered fractures or crushing injuries. The presence of bruising and skin fragility should be well established in order to plan for precautions in the management and physical handling of the patient.

Areas of *swelling*, either of the extremities or of specific joints, must be noted and the degree of swelling described. Peripheral edema may be present because of prolonged dependent position of the extremity, lack of activity, circulatory disturbances, or renal involvement. Joints may be swollen as part of the inflammatory process (p. 178). The presence of serous, purulent, or bloody fluid in the joint capsule is termed *effusion* and is visible as a marked swelling of the joint. Inflamed synovium feels boggy and full on palpation. *Bony enlargements*, such as Heberden's nodes in osteoarthritis (Fig. 42-2), may be felt as hard, irregular swellings over the distal interphalangeal joints of the hands. *Subcutaneous nodules*, found in rheumatoid arthritis, are hard, most often mobile swellings found commonly in the subolecranon area. *Bursal swelling* is noted as a soft, palpable swelling over the bursa. Swelling may also be noted in the presence of a *synovial cyst*, such as a Baker's cyst, which is characterized by swelling in the popliteal area, often extending into the calf. *Tophaceous deposits*, indicative of gout, are hard, translucent swellings that may be noted in cartilage such as that of the ear.

Tenderness may be elicited by direct pressure to a joint and may be grossly graded by the amount of pressure required to produce discomfort. Sometimes joints are not tender to palpation but are painful on active or passive range of motion. The degree of tenderness is usually in direct proportion to the severity of joint inflammation. Following trauma, tenderness is also present in the injured soft tissue and overlying areas of fractures.

Nails and hair are often a problem. Individuals with severe joint involvement, weakness, or paralysis may literally not be able to reach their toes or the top of their head or have the strength to cut their fingernails or toenails or comb their hair. Some diseases like psoriasis cause changes in the structure of the nails (p. 1489) and a scaling condition of the scalp. Poorly cared for or diseased toenails can even prevent the person from wearing shoes or walking well. In individuals with some connective tissue diseases, alopecia (loss of hair) may occur. In most instances plans must be made for the proper care of fingernails, toenails, and hair.

Finally, during the examination of the skin there is opportunity to assess the person's *hygiene* status. Individuals with musculoskeletal disorders often cannot tend to their own hygiene needs effectively, but they may not want to admit it. If evidence is found that hygiene needs are not being adequately met, plans can be made to introduce self-help devices or to assist the person in ways that will not cause embarrassment.

Strength and range of motion

Assessment of strength and range of motion are, in effect, measurements of the person's functional capacity. In discussing this area, there must first be some definition of terms:

Strength can be simply defined as the capacity to perform work.

Range of motion is the normal arc of movement that is provided for by the structure of a joint.

Active range of motion is the movement of a joint that can be accomplished by the person without assistance.

Passive range of motion is the movement of a joint through its normal range by someone other than the person.

Active assisted range of motion is active range of motion by the person with assistance to perform that motion. Active assisted range of motion can be employed with the person who has polymyositis and who has the strength to move the joint through only part of its normal range and may need assistance to complete the movement.

Dexterity refers to the coordination and agility with which movements are performed.

An extremity may be *flaccid*, having defective or absent muscle tone; *paralyzed*, having loss of function, especially loss of sensation or voluntary motion; or *paretic*, having incomplete loss of muscle power or partial paralysis. The suffix *-plegia* is used to describe paralysis. Involvement of one extremity is referred to as a *mono*plegia or monoparesis; of both extremities on one side of the body, *hemi*plegia; and of all four extremities, *quadri*plegia.

Prior to any testing of muscle strength or range of motion of a joint, there must be some assessment of the

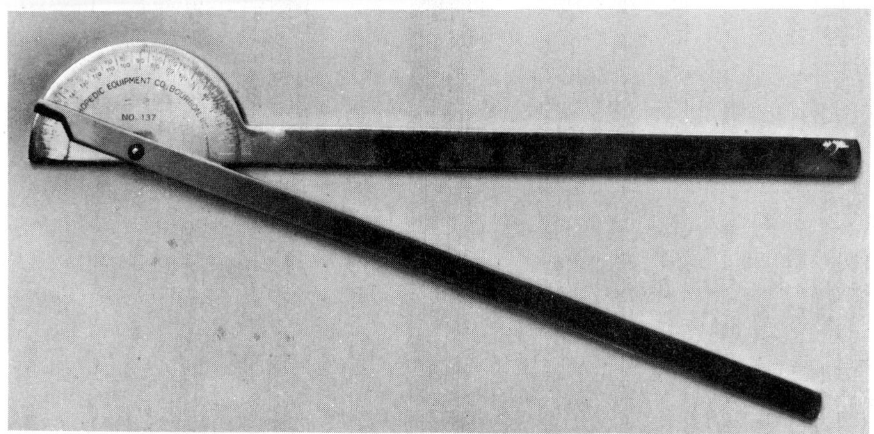

Fig. 40-8. Goniometer for measuring joint motion. (From Larson, C. B., and Gould, M.: Orthopedic nursing, ed. 9, St. Louis, 1978, The C. V. Mosby Co.)

position of the person's extremities. Positions that vary from normal and that have an acute onset may be indications of fractures, dislocations, or ruptures of supporting structures. Typical of this kind of sudden change is the marked external rotation and shortening of the leg following a hip fracture; the inability to extend a "dropped" finger following rupture of an extensor tendon in the hand; or the postoperative "drop foot," a complication that may occur following surgical procedures to the back or hip because of stretching of the sciatic nerve.

Subluxation, or partial dislocation of a joint, should also be noted. This is often a chronic problem, as in the shoulder of the hemiplegic or in the wrist of the arthritic; but its presence is usually accompanied by some loss of function or need for support. Subluxation of the shoulder may be detected by feeling a space between the head of the humerus and the glenoid cavity of the scapula.

Loss of strength or limitation of joint motion will result in some degree of loss of function. Such a loss of strength or joint range of motion may be the result of a neurologic, skeletal, muscular, or traumatic disorder. Detailed tests of strength and joint range of motion require instruments such as the *dynamometer,* which measures grip strength in the hand, and the *goniometer* (an instrument resembling a protractor), which is useful in measuring joint motion (Fig. 40-8).

Gross testing of strength, however, may be done very simply. To test the upper extremities, apply moderate pressure with your hand against the person's upper arm to resist his movement, then have him flex, extend, and abduct the shoulder; with resistance at the forearm, flex and extend the elbow; and at the wrist, flex and extend the hand. Hand grip strength may be tested by having the person squeeze your hand as hard as possible. The same maneuvers can be performed with the lower extremities. Applying moderate pressure with your hand against the person's foot to resist his movement, have him invert and evert his foot, dorsiflex and plantar flex his ankle; with resistance at the lower leg, flex and extend his knee; and with resistance at the thigh, raise and lower his leg. In all these instances the area proximal to the joint being moved is stabilized by one of the examiner's hands, while moderate resistance to movement distal to the joint being moved is provided by the other hand. Trunk strength may be tested by having the person attempt to sit up from the supine position.

Gross muscle testing will provide very useful data for determining the amount of assistance the person needs. More specific testing can be done by a physical therapist and is useful to the physician in diagnosis and to the therapist in planning a program of muscle-strengthening exercises (p. 832).

Coordination of the upper extremities can be tested by having the person extend his arm, touch one of the examiner's fingers with one of his, then touch his nose, then the examiner's finger, and so on. This ability to pick up small objects, like a coin or a pen, from a smooth, hard surface will provide some indication of the person's manual dexterity.

Range of motion is tested by having the person *actively* perform with each joint those motions that joint is capable of performing (Figs. 40-9 to 40-11). In some instances where the person cannot actively move a joint, as with the person where paralysis has previously been diagnosed, the joint may be passively moved. (Refer to Chapter 41 for discussion of passive range of motion and joint instability). When passive range of motion is being performed, support must be given proximal to the joint moved (Fig. 40-12). Comparing the limitation of movement or instability that is present in one joint with its similar opposite joint is helpful in differentiating normal from abnormal findings.

Text continued on p. 824.

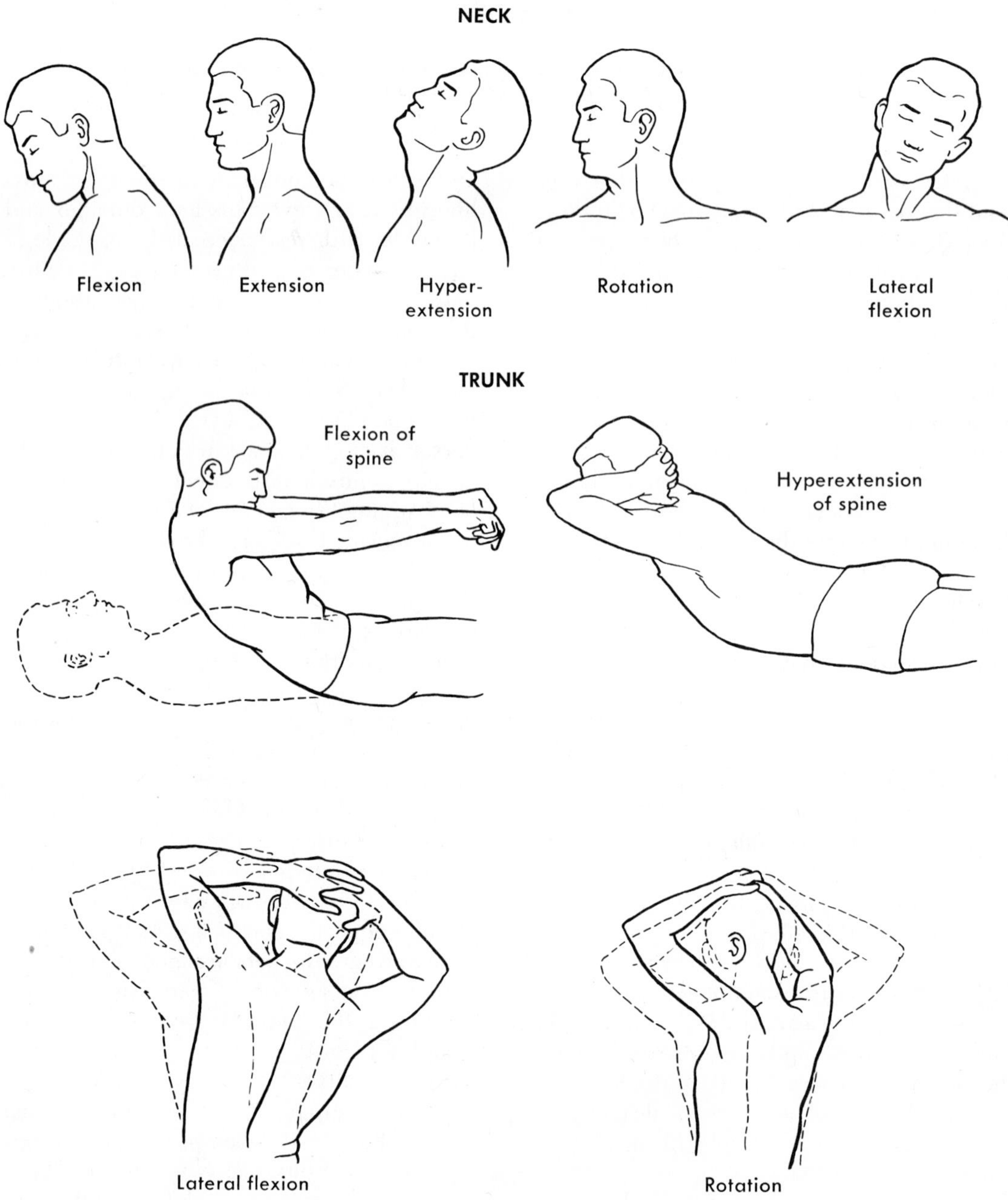

Fig. 40-9. Range of joint motion for neck and trunk.

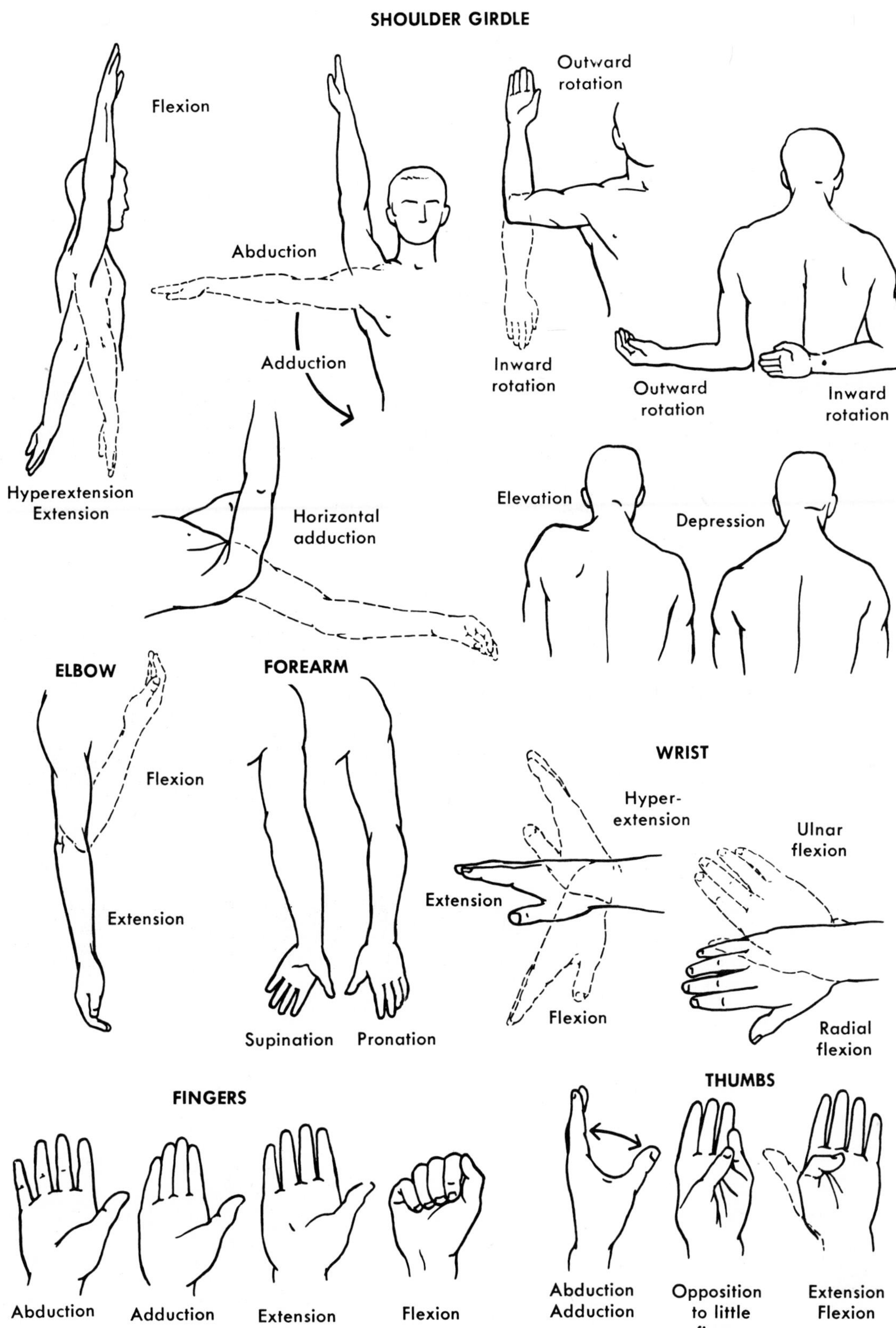

Fig. 40-10. Range of joint motion for shoulder and shoulder girdle, elbow, wrist, forearm, and hand.

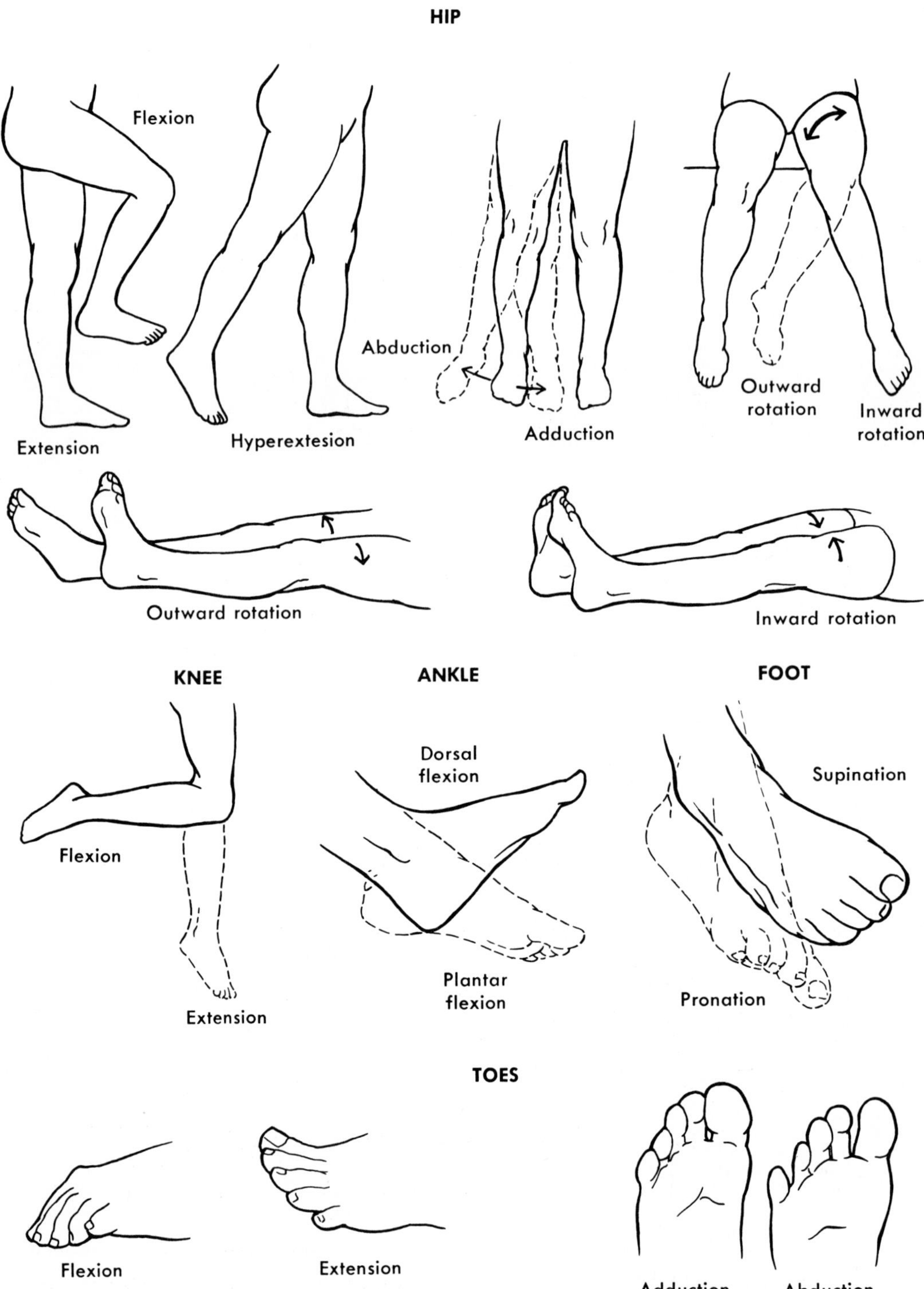

Fig. 40-11. Range of joint motion for hip, knee, ankle, foot, and toes.

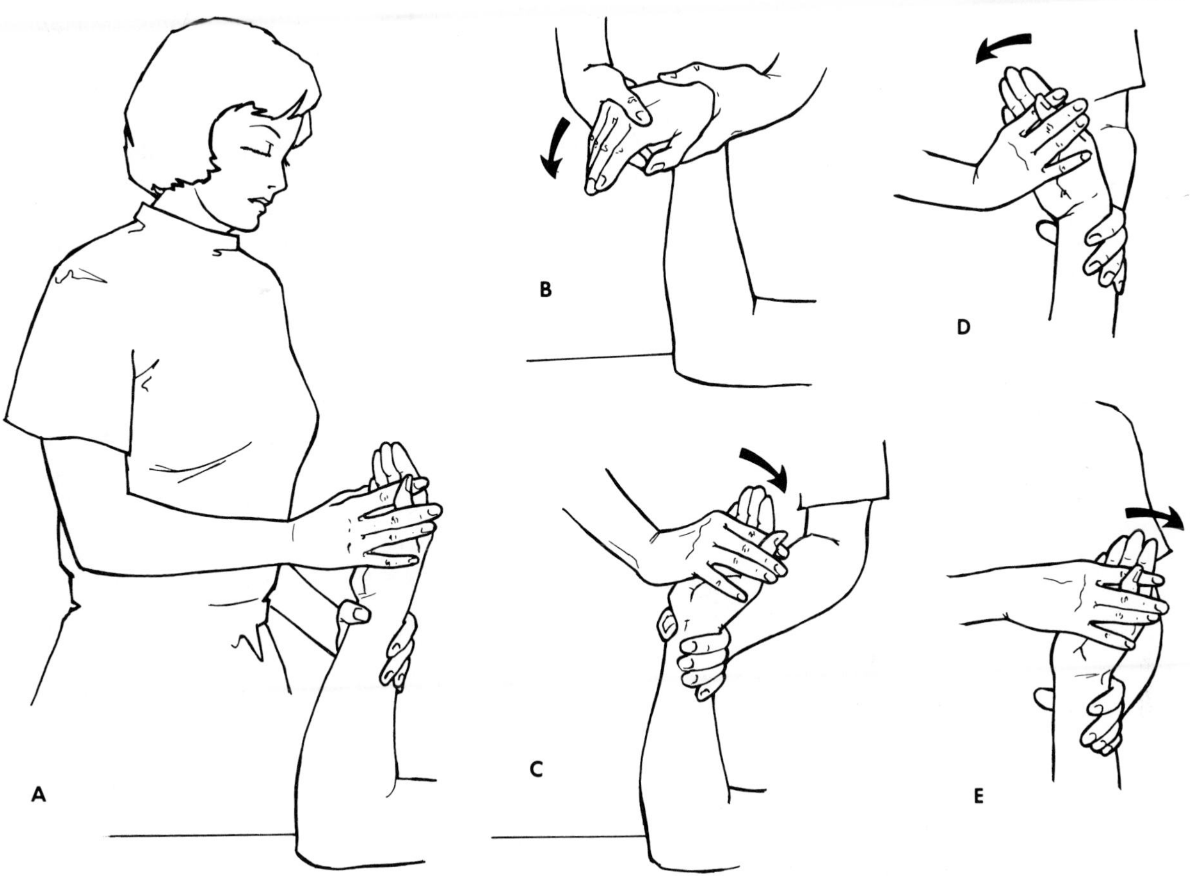

Fig. 40-12. With patient in supine position, upper arm is supported on bed. **A,** Forearm is supported with nurse's hand; hand is supported with nurse's other hand. **B,** Wrist is then flexed forward. **C,** Extended. **D,** Moved to ulnar side. **E,** Moved to radial side. (Modified from Larson, C. B., and Gould, M.: Orthopedic nursing, ed. 8, St. Louis, 1974, The C. V. Mosby Co.)

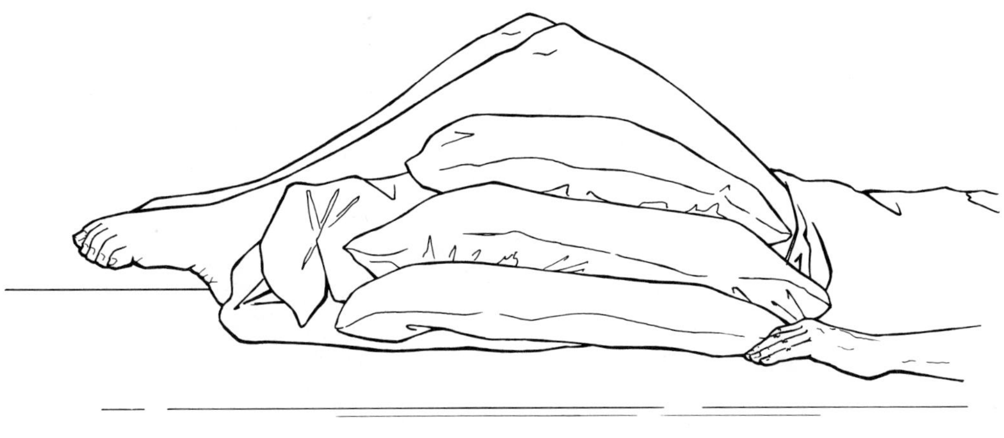

Fig. 40-13. Contractures of hips and knees in patient with rheumatoid arthritis caused by continuous use of pillows to support knees in flexed position. (Modified from Larson, C. B., and Gould, M.: Orthopedic nursing, ed. 8, St. Louis, 1974, The C. V. Mosby Co.)

If a joint cannot be moved beyond a certain point in its range (a knee that does not extend beyond 30° of flexion), it is said that the joint is contracted, or that a *contracture* is present. Contractures may exist because of soft tissue limitation (following a fracture with immobilization) or because of bony limitation (Fig. 40-13). The location and nature of contractures can be a significant indication of functional limitation. For example, a person with only 15° of knee flexion in one knee will be able to climb steps only one at a time.

Crepitus, or a crunching or grating sound when the joint is actively or passively moved, is a significant indicator of the presence of pathology within the joint. This sound will also be heard if the two broken ends of a bone move against one another. *In the presence of a possible fracture, no attempt should be made to elicit crepitus.* At times, grating within a joint may be felt, rather than heard, by placing a hand over the joint as it moves.

The foregoing tests of strength, dexterity, and range of motion are simple to perform; however, it must be noted that the person's ability to perform the movements described may be limited by pain rather than weakness, lack of coordination, or joint limitation. It is often difficult to differentiate these factors, and while quantitatively the effect of the pain is the same as the effect of the weakness or limitation—that is, diminished function—qualitatively it makes a difference, since treatment measures will be geared to relief of pain rather than to muscle strengthening. To further confuse the situation, the

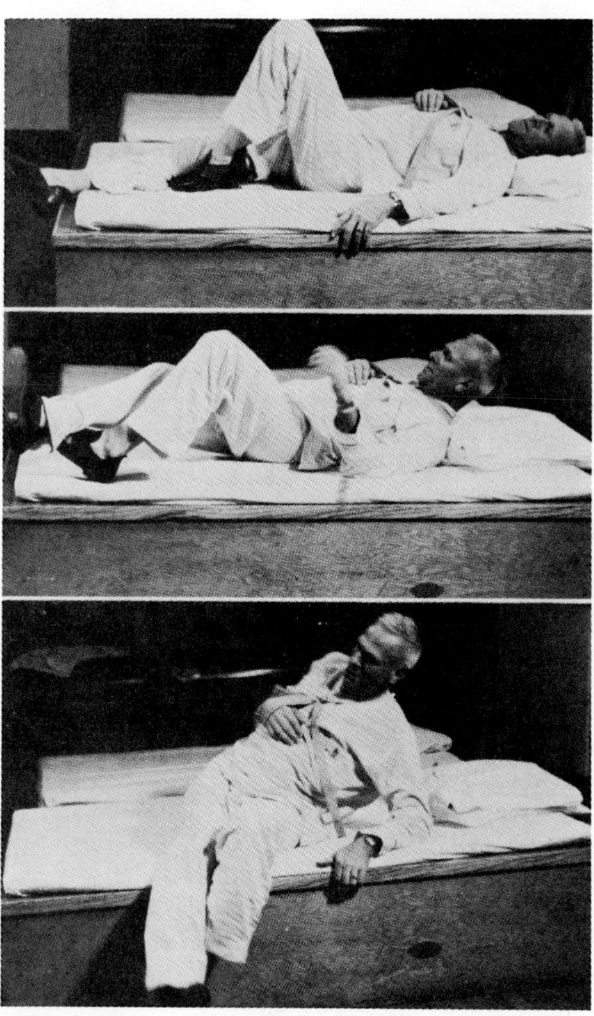

Fig. 40-14. When patient wishes to transfer from mat (bed) to wheelchair, chair is placed as illustrated near patient's uninvolved side. Patient uses his normal arm and leg to help him assume sitting position on bedside and then to transfer to chair. For this patient to transfer from wheelchair to bed, position of chair would be reversed. (From Larson, C. B., and Gould, M.: Orthopedic nursing, ed. 8, St. Louis, 1974, The C. V. Mosby Co.)

person with pain may have actual concomitant muscle weakness on the basis of long-standing pain and consequent disuse of muscles. It must be remembered, however, that in performing this kind of testing the person *must not be moved beyond the point of pain.* Pain is an indication that something is wrong. Injudicious testing techniques can produce untoward results; for example, the fracture of an osteoporotic bone. The desired result of such testing is the establishment of a baseline of strength, motion, and dexterity from which interventions to assist the person to gain strength, regain lost motion, and increase functional capacity may be planned and evaluated.

Transfer

The next area to be assessed is the ability of the person to transfer or to move from one surface to another: from bed to chair, to toilet, to bed again (Fig. 40-14). The person may have no difficulty with such a movement, or he may have made some modification in his environment to enable him to accomplish it, or he may need the assistance of someone else.

The knowledge required to make an assessment of the person's transfer ability is a basic understanding of the principles of transfer techniques (p. 849). The first step in making an assessment of transfer ability is to correlate some of the data already obtained in order to anticipate problems he may experience during the transfer. If, for example, the patient is a bilateral amputee or paraparetic, the assessor would know that a transfer board may be necessary for transfers rather than a standing transfer.

Second, input from the person concerning any modifications made in order to transfer safely (having a grab bar on the bathroom wall, raising the surface of the bed or chair or toilet, using chairs with arms to facilitate pushing up from the seat) is helpful information in determining the extent of the person's limitation. Similar modifications in the patient's hospital environment usually can be arranged.

Balance is a third consideration in assessing ability to transfer. Inability to maintain balance, a problem seen in a variety of conditions, may severely limit transfer ability. Balance can be easily tested by having the person sit on the side of the bed without using his hands to support himself once he is in the sitting position.

Other considerations that will influence the person's ability to transfer are ability to follow instructions, attention span, and fear of pain on movement. Obviously transfer will not be evaluated in those persons who are not permitted to be out of bed, such as the patient who is in traction.

The results of transfer assessment should reflect how much, if any, assistance will be required, what modifica-

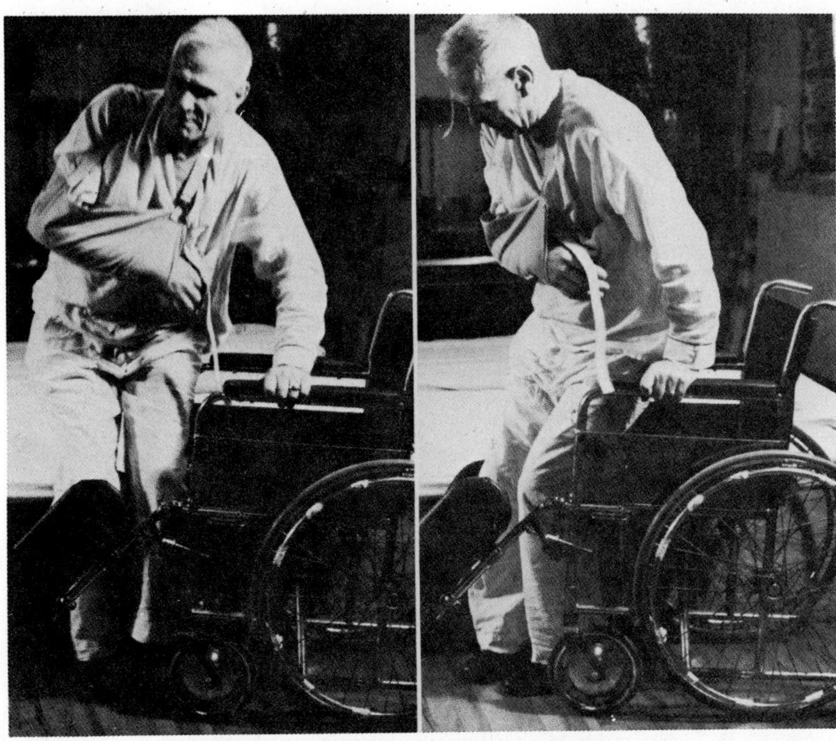

Fig. 40-14, cont'd. For legend see opposite page.

tions had to be made in the environment, and whether the transfer was performed safely.

Ambulation

Assessment of ambulatory ability follows assessment of transfer ability. Some individuals will not be able to ambulate because of pain, contractures, immobilization, fracture, weakness, or balance problems. Others may be able to walk only with assistive devices such as a cane, crutches, or walker. These devices are often used improperly. For example, a patient may use a cane on the wrong side of his body or support his weight on his axillae when using axillary crutches. Note should be taken of this kind of problem, and interventions that will correct it should be planned.

Nursing assessment of ambulatory ability can usually be accomplished with the person walking only a short distance (20 to 25 ft). Observations should be made regarding the use of assistive devices, balance, and gait pattern. If the unsupported sitting balance is very poor, no attempt should be made to ambulate the person without assistance of another person.

Gait is the manner or style of walking. An altered *gait pattern* is indicative of the presence of a pathologic process (Fig. 40-15). The normal *gait cycle* consists of two phases: *stance phase*, beginning with heel strike and ending with toe off, and *swing phase*, beginning with toe off and continuing through heel strike. The brief period when both feet are on the ground is called the period of *double support*. These phases are usually rhythmic and symmetric. When they are markedly asymmetric, the alteration in gait is called a *limp*.

While ambulation is being observed, note should be taken of the presence and type of limp displayed, the joints in which there is complaint of pain, the degree to which there is reliance on assistance for weight bearing (either on devices or on a person), balance, and the degree of deformity in the lower extremities. Deformity of the lower extremities (genu valgum, genu varum, genu talipes, and so on) may not be as apparent when the joint is examined at rest as when weight-bearing forces are exerted across the joint. Further, in persons who have significant upper extremity involvement, some consideration must be given both to the amount of weight bearing that might be expected from the arms and hands and to the type of assistive device that would be appropriate

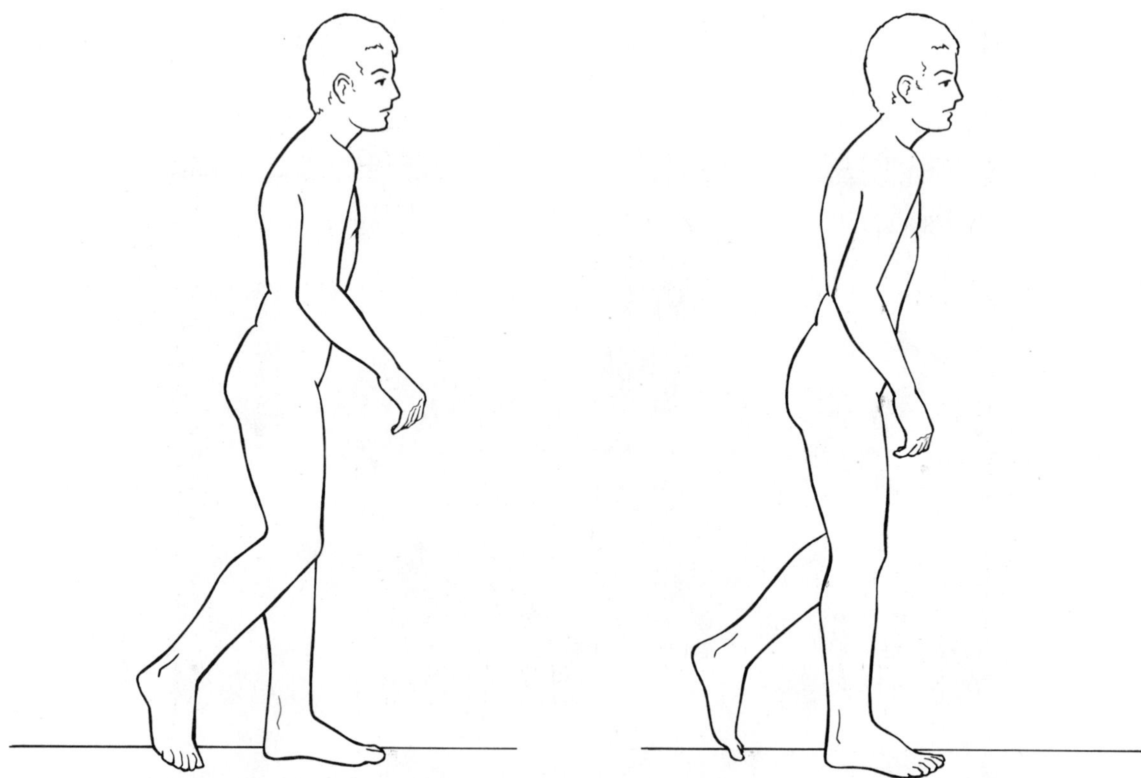

Fig. 40-15. Altered gait pattern caused by bilateral stiff hips. Angle of flexion at hips is constant, requiring that knees and ankles control leg length adjustment and propulsion. (Modified from Larson, C. B., and Gould, M.: Orthopedic nursing, ed. 8, St. Louis, 1974, The C. V. Mosby Co.)

for the person to use. For example, an individual with severe rheumatoid involvement of the hands might have to use a device that would permit weight bearing on the forearms.

Other problems such as cardiovascular disease, respiratory impairment, or anemia may also affect ambulatory ability and must be taken into consideration during the assessment of ambulation. Assessment of transfer ability and ambulatory ability will help to determine a suitable level of activity for the person.

Other ADL assessment

The ability to dress and undress, bathe and the style of bathing employed (tub, shower, sponge), and the management of toileting needs should be assessed as soon as possible. If a physical problem has been longstanding, the individual may have devised ways of managing these activities despite physical limitations that may appear prohibitive. On the other hand, if the problem is one of acute onset, methods of dealing with these activities may need to be taught. In the hospitalized patient, assessment and evaluation of ADL abilities is an ongoing process throughout the hospital stay.

Mention must also be made of toileting needs. When activity level is far below normal, there may be trouble with chronic constipation. Also, individuals with profound muscle weakness or neurologic problems such as stroke may have lost control of bowel and bladder functions. The presence of these problems must be known and management programs established as soon as possible (p. 1274). The person who experiences great difficulty in getting to a bathroom may limit fluid intake to avoid having to make trips to the bathroom. Such individuals are often troubled with chronic bladder infections. Plans must be made to make toileting facilities easily available to the patient, and fluid intake should be encouraged.

Pain or the lack of ability to move freely often interferes with sleep. Observations regarding the person's comfort and ability to rest and sleep should be made. If problems exist in these areas, appropriate interventions must be planned.

Observations of the interactions of the patient with hospital staff, his family, and his friends will often verify what the patient and his family have said about his reaction to and acceptance of his problem and the significance the problem has in their relationships. Assess-

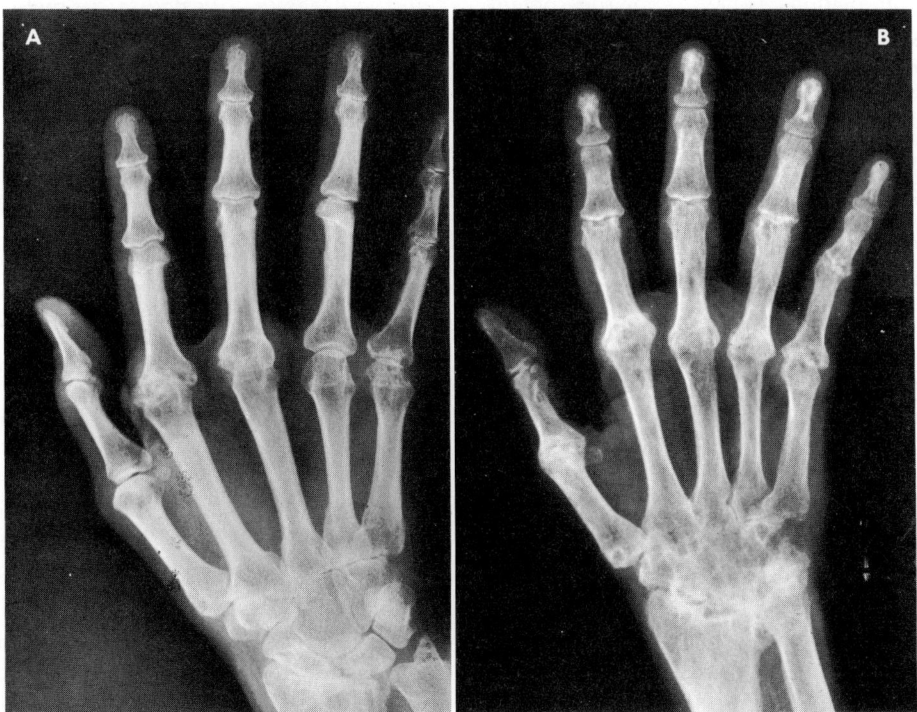

Fig. 40-16. Roentgenograms of rheumatoid arthritis in hand and wrist. **A,** Moderate changes ranging from atrophic bone areas and narrowed cartilage spaces to subluxation of second and third metacarpophalangeal joints. **B,** More advanced case with severe destructive changes including multiple subluxations in digits and ankyloses in carpus. (From Raney, R., and Brashear, H.: Shand's handbook of orthopaedic surgery, ed. 8, St. Louis, 1971, The C. V. Mosby Co.)

ment of these interactions should take place throughout the patient's hospital stay. The data gathered will be helpful in planning with the patient and his family for the patient's eventual discharge and in devising teaching approaches for both the patient and the family.

DIAGNOSTIC TESTS

As with other illnesses, diagnostic tests are employed to provide information to assist in diagnosing a patient's illness and to aid in devising a treatment program for the patient. Elements of the patient's care may be dependent on the outcomes of diagnostic studies. Some of the principal studies that may be performed on the person who has a musculoskeletal problem are discussed below.

Roentgenologic examinations

Bones and joints

Roentgenologic examination of bones and joints is imperative in the identification and treatment of fractures. Roentgenograms are also most helpful in determining not only the presence of disease, such as rheumatoid arthritis, spondylitis, avascular necrosis, and tumors, but also the progress and effects of treatment on these disorders (Fig. 40-16). Specialized texts should be consulted for reference to the variety of views that are obtained in such examinations as well as for the specific findings that are present in the various disorders. However, it is important to remember that many patients are not able to lie on x-ray tables for long periods of time. Persons with arthritis in particular develop joint stiffness and pain if their ability to move about is restricted. Since roentgenologic examinations for individuals with rheumatic diseases are often quite extensive, careful thought should be given to the scheduling of these examinations. Very few of these patients can tolerate having all the required views of all the involved joints taken at one session. A day or even 2 days of rest between sessions may be required by patients with severe joint involvement. Analgesics or local heat applications for relief of joint pain may be necessary for some patients following their return from the radiology department.

Systemic roentgenologic studies

Systemic roentgenologic studies such as the barium enema, upper gastrointestinal series, esophagogram, and intravenous pyelogram are helpful in determining the extent of involvement of various internal organs (bowel, kidneys) when the patient has a systemic rheumatic disease. Discussion of these examinations will be found on pp. 1161 and 1238.

Myelography

As discussed in Chapter 34, myelography is useful in identifying lesions, such as a herniated nucleus pulposus, that are blocking the subarachnoid space. Discussion of this procedure and the precautions that must be exercised in caring for the patient after the procedure are discussed on p. 652.

Arthrography

Arthrography permits visualization of components within the joint that are not normally seen on routine x-ray films. The joint cavity is injected with radiopaque dye, air, or both. The latter is called a double-contrast arthrogram. The dye or air serves as a contrast medium against which the outlines of soft tissue components of the joint may be seen. Tears of the menisci, internal derangements of the joint, and synovial cysts may be diagnosed with the aid of arthrograms. Prior to the study, it must be determined whether the patient has a history of an allergy to the radiopaque dye. No other special preparation is required.

Radioistope scans

Radioisotope *bone scans* are performed primarily to demonstrate the presence of metastatic disease. Intravenously injected sodium pertechnetate Tc 99m is the isotope most frequently used in this study. The ^{99m}Tc will concentrate in areas of osteoblastic activity involved in the exchange of calcium. In malignancies this activity is accelerated. Lesions may be visualized on bone scans as early as 6 months before there is evidence of the lesions on routine roentgenograms.[8]

Technetium Tc 99m scans are also of some use in determining the degree of *parotid gland* involvement in Sjögren's syndrome. The uptake, concentration, and excretion of the isotope by the major salivary glands is measured by a technique called sequential scintiphotography.[14]

Persons being prepared for these procedures should know that the procedures will not cause them pain, that the isotopes will not harm them, but that they will, however, have to remain in one position quietly for up to 1 hour or more.

Serologic tests

Serum muscle enzymes

The serum muscle enzymes, SGOT (serum glutamic-oxaloacetic transaminase), aldolase, and CPK (creatine phosphokinase), are elevated in the presence of primary myopathic (muscle) diseases. The SGOT is the least sensitive indicator of muscle involvement and the CPK the most sensitive. The SGOT is also elevated in patients who have myocardial or hepatic disease. The CPK is elevated in myocardial conditions or in the patient who has had frequent intramuscular injections. Elevated serum levels of these enzymes may occur as a result of the degeneration of muscle fibers or may result from diffusion of the enzymes through a muscle membrane that has increased permeability. The levels of these enzymes may be followed as an index of both the progress of the myopathic disorder and the effectiveness of treatment. If treatment is adequate, the serum enzyme levels will decrease. In patients in whom these enzyme levels are being monitored, intramuscular injections should be avoided.[14]

STS and FTA-ABS

The serologic test for syphilis (STS) is of some value in the diagnosis of connective tissue disease as 10% to 15% of persons with these diseases will have a *false-positive* STS result. In these persons the presence of syphilis may be excluded by the more sensitive fluorescent treponemal antibody absorption test (FTA-ABS).

Rheumatoid factor (latex fixation)

Abnormal proteins classified as antibodies are found in the sera of individuals with rheumatoid arthritis. These antibodies are called rheumatoid factors, and they will react with IgG (7S) gamma globulin. The test to determine the presence of these factors is called a *latex fixation test*. Latex particles are coated with denatured IgG. The serum from the patient is heated and then added to the suspension of coated latex particles. If the serum contains the rheumatoid factor, the rheumatoid factor will react with the IgG and cause the latex particles to agglutinate. Titrated solutions of latex particles are used, and the rheumatoid factor is considered to be present if the particles agglutinate in dilutions of 1:40 or higher. It should be noted, however, that rheumatoid factor is present in a significant number of other conditions in addition to rheumatoid arthritis: aging, scleroderma, acute pulmonary tuberculosis, parenteral narcotic addiction, systemic lupus erythematosus, and others.

Antinuclear antibodies and LE cell reaction

Circulating antibodies (protein material) that react with nuclei and various individual constituents of nuclei are known as *antinuclear antibodies*. These antibodies can be identified by fluorescent techniques utilizing antihuman gamma globulin labeled with fluorescein. Test serum from a patient is applied to a section of tissue that contains nucleated cells. Antinuclear antibodies, if they are present in the serum, bind to the nuclei of the cells. When the antihuman gamma globulin is applied to these cells, it reacts with the antinuclear antibodies and the nuclei become fluorescent when examined under ultraviolet light. Tests for antinuclear antibodies are helpful in diagnosing Sjögren's syndrome, scleroderma, and systemic lupus erythematosus. The pattern of nuclear staining varies with the different diseases.[14]

The test for LE cells is based on the interaction of antinuclear antibodies, nuclear material, and phagocytic white blood cells. The *LE cell factor* (an antinuclear antibody) reacts with nuclear material from damaged white blood cells. This interaction results in an alteration of the nuclear material. The nuclear material is then called a *hematoxylin body*. The hematoxylin body typically stains red-purple with Wright's stain and has the appearance of "ground glass." The hematoxylin body attracts polymorphonuclear leukocytes. These leukocytes surround the hematoxylin body in the form of rosettes. When one of the leukocytes ingests the nuclear material (hematoxylin body), the nuclear material is then known as an *inclusion body*.[14]

The cell with the inclusion body is known as an *LE cell*. LE cells are seen in 80% to 85% of patients with systemic lupus erythematosus during acute disease activity.[14]

Complement

The complement studies relate to a system of protein substances (at least nine) that are found in the serum and in synovial fluid. These proteins are related both to the immune and the inflammatory mechanisms. Low serum and synovial complement levels often occur in systemic lupus erythematosus and rheumatoid arthritis.

Erythrocyte sedimentation rate

The erythrocyte sedimentation rate (ESR) is the most important index of the presence of inflammation. The test is a measurement of the rate of settling of erythrocytes, an increased rate of settling indicating the presence of inflammation.[11] There are two major methods of determining the ESR: the Westergren method and the Wintrobe method. The Westergren method is considered by some experts to be the most dependable. Normal values for men are a fall of 1 to 3 mm per hour; for women, 4 to 7 mm per hour.[11]

Hematocrit

The hematocrit is a measure of the size, capacity, and number of cells present in a person's blood. A blood sample is centrifuged to separate the cells from the plasma. The results of the test are expressed as cubic milliliters of packed cells per deciliter of blood or in volumes per deciliter of blood. The normal range for men is 45 to 50 vol/dl; for women, 40 to 45 vol/dl. Individuals who have hematocrits *below* normal levels are considered to be *anemic*.[8]

Patients with systemic connective tissue diseases or notable rheumatoid arthritis are very often anemic. The red blood cells in this particular form of anemia are normal (normocytic) and carry a normal amount of iron (normochromic), and the anemia exists in the absence of any abnormal bleeding. In contrast, individuals who suffer trauma with subsequent blood loss or who undergo major surgery with intraoperative and postoperative bleeding will have an acute drop in hematocrit. When the hematocrit drops rapidly, symptoms of anemia—extreme tiredness, fatigue, and weakness—are more likely to be experienced. A chronically low hematocrit that develops gradually allows a person to become used to functioning at lower hematocrit levels, and there may be no acute symptoms.

□ Urinary tests

Creatine-creatinine ratios

Creatine-creatinine values derived from studies of 24-hour urine collections are helpful in diagnosing and evaluating the progress of treatment in primary myopathies. Creatine is a substance that is formed in the liver and converted into creatinine by muscle. When muscle disease is present, the ability of the muscle to convert creatine is decreased; therefore the amount of creatine that is excreted by the kidneys is increased, and the ratio of urinary creatine to creatinine is increased. A carefully collected 24-hour urine specimen is first tested for the amount of creatinine it contains. Then the creatine in the specimen is converted to creatinine, and the creatinine content is redetermined. The first value subtracted from the second value yields the amount of creatine that was contained in the specimen. *Percent creatinuria* is determined by dividing the amount of creatine by the total amount of creatine plus creatinine. Normal values for percent creatinuria should not exceed 6% in men and women.[14]

To ensure the accuracy of this test, two consecutive 24-hour urine specimens are obtained. If there is a variance of more than 10% in the two values obtained, the urine collections are considered inadequate and must be repeated. The person needs to be carefully taught how to collect these urine specimens.

Urinary uric acid levels

Not all individuals who have gout overexcrete uric acid. However, urinary uric acid levels, determined from 24-hour urine collections, can be helpful in establishing a diagnosis of gout. Daily uric acid excretion for individuals on a normal diet should not exceed 900 mg. Individuals with higher levels of urinary uric acid who also have only slightly elevated or high normal serum uric acid levels probably have gout.[14] Treatment decisions as to whether to give uricosuric agents that increase urinary uric acid output and therefore increase the hazard of kidney stone formation may be guided by determination of the amount of uric acid excretion. The accuracy of the collection is important in establishing the diagnosis and in determining an appropriate treatment program.

□ Joint aspiration

Joint aspiration is performed to obtain samples of the synovial fluid from within the joint cavity. This procedure (performed by introducing a needle into the joint cavity and withdrawing fluid) will aid in determining the presence of an aseptic inflammatory process, such as rheumatoid arthritis, or a septic process, such as bacterial arthritis. Samples of synovial fluid are cultured and are examined both microscopically and chemically.

The synovial fluid is normally straw-colored and clear. Its viscosity resembles that of motor oil. In the presence of inflammation it becomes turbid and more watery. The *mucin clot test* is performed by mixing synovial fluid with glacial acetic acid. Normal synovial fluid will form a white, ropy mucin clot. When inflammation is present, the clot breaks apart easily and becomes flaky (flocculent). The degree of flocculence increases with the degree of inflammation. Also, when inflammation is present, the number of white blood cells, the protein content, and the number of polymorphonuclear cells in the synovial fluid are increased; glucose content is decreased.[14]

Strict asepsis is observed in the procedure. A local anesthetic is usually administered before the procedure. After the procedure the joint is often wrapped in a small compression (Ace) dressing. The joint may be rested for 8 to 24 hours. If infection is present in the joint and there is drainage from the joint following the aspiration, precautions should be observed in dressing the wound and in handling the contaminated dressings.

□ Arthroscopy

Arthroscopy is a procedure performed in the operating room. A specially designed endoscope (arthroscope) is inserted through a small incision into the joint cavity, enabling the physician to visualize the structure and contents of the joint. The usefulness of this procedure is limited chiefly to the knee.[10] The procedure permits biopsy of the synovium or cartilage, is useful in the diagnosis of torn meniscus, and in some instances permits the removal of loose bodies from the joint space. The patient is treated in much the same manner as following a synovial biopsy; however, the period of time that the joint is rested is determined by the extent of the procedure. The surgeon should be consulted to determine how long the patient's activity is to be restricted.

□ Biopsy

Skin biopsy

Skin biopsy may be performed to aid in the diagnosis of such rheumatic diseases as scleroderma, systemic

lupus erythematosus, or psoriatic arthritis. Generally a small "punch" biopsy is taken with a punch biopsy needle at a site where a clinical rash is evident. This skin specimen may be studied for histopathologic evidence of disease, or may be subjected to *immunofluorescent staining*. This is done by washing the specimen, which has been placed on a glass slide, with a solution of fluorescein-labeled antihuman gamma globulin antibody. A positive reaction, indicating the presence of disease, is the appearance of a band of immunofluorescence at the epidermal-dermal junction.[14]

The biopsy site will appear as a punched-out lesion approximately 0.625 cm in diameter on the patient's skin. This area should be kept clean and may be covered with a small adhesive bandage until an eschar develops. Hydrogen peroxide (3%) may be used to cleanse the open area if necessary, particularly when healing takes more then 3 to 4 days. Generally only very mild discomfort is experienced after this procedure.

Muscle biopsy

Muscle biopsy is performed to aid in the diagnosis of specific myopathic disorders. The muscle to be biopsied is determined by prior gross muscle testing by the physical therapist and by EMG (electromyography) studies. In early disease, a muscle that is found to be "weak" is most likely to provide histopathologic evidence of disease. Histochemical staining of muscle tissue may reveal features of lower motor neuron disease (such as atrophy of groups of fibers innervated by single motor units), or it may reveal degeneration, inflammatory reactions, or involvement of specific fibers that would indicate primary myopathic disease.

A muscle biopsy is an operative procedure usually performed by the general surgeon. The patient may be given either a local or a general anesthetic. Following the procedure, the patient will experience minor to moderate discomfort, depending on the location of the muscle biopsied. The discomfort may be in the form of stiffness or pain at or around the operative site. In most instances, if the muscle biopsied is in the lower extremity (one of the gluteals or quadriceps), the patient is encouraged to resume ambulation within 24 hours of the procedure to avoid undue stiffness.

Synovial biopsy

Synovial biopsy is helpful in differentiating various forms of arthritis. It may be performed as a closed biopsy with a special synovial biopsy needle (such as the Parker-Pearson) or as an open biopsy. The latter is performed in the operating room. If a closed biopsy is being performed, the patient is given a local anesthetic. The specimen of synovium obtained is examined histologically for evidence of inflammation; and a specimen of synovial fluid, obtained at the same time, is sent for culture and other studies.

A closed biopsy of the synovium is performed with strict attention to aseptic technique to avoid introducing infectious agents into the joint. A small compression dressing, usually an Ace wrap, is placed around the joint involved, and the patient is generally asked to rest the joint for 24 hours to prevent hemorrhage or effusion.

Buccal biopsy

Biopsy of the buccal mucosa is performed to aid in defining the presence of Sjögren's syndrome. A small punch biopsy is taken from the lower lip, and the tissue is examined for evidence of lymphoid involvement of the minor salivary glands located in that area. The procedure causes minor discomfort, and the mucosa heals quickly. However, the diet may have to be altered slightly until healing takes place, since rough foods or hot fluids may irritate the biopsy site.

Temporal artery biopsy

Temporal artery biopsy is an operative procedure performed to definitely establish the presence of temporal arteritis (inflammation of the temporal arteries with tenderness and swelling over the temples, headaches, and visual disturbances). Histologic examination reveals stenosis and dilatation of segments of the artery in the presence of the disease. Generally there is only minor discomfort at the biopsy site. A small compression dressing is applied over the area and should be checked frequently during the first 24 hours for evidence of bleeding.

□ Electromyography

Electromyography measures the electrical activity of muscles; and *electromyogram* (EMG) is a recording of the variations of electrical potentials (voltage) detected by a needle electrode inserted into skeletal muscle. The electrical activity can be heard over a loud speaker and viewed on an oscilloscope and on a graph at the same time. No electrical activity can be detected in normal muscles at rest, but during volitional movement, action potentials can be detected. In both primary myopathic and neuropathic disorders there are specific variations in the size of individual motor unit potentials. In neurogenic atrophy there may be fibrillations in the resting muscle. An EMG provides direct evidence of motor dysfunction and can be used to some extent to detect a dysfunction located in the motor neuron, the neuromuscular junction, or the muscle fibers. Thus it is particularly helpful in the diagnosis of lower motor neuron disease, primary muscle disease, and defects in the transmission of electrical impulses at the neuromuscular junction such as myasthenia gravis. However, electromyography cannot be used to differentiate *specific* disease entities in either the myopathic or neuropathic categories. There is no special preparation for this procedure. The patient may be fearful that electrode needles will cause an electric shock and should be assured that there is no danger.

□ Manual muscle test

Manual muscle tests are used in an attempt to determine the degree of muscular weakness resulting from disease, injury, or disuse. The muscle test rates the strength of muscles by their performance in relation to gravity and manually applied resistance and is usually performed by a physical therapist. Factors such as gravity, stabilization of the tested part, proper positioning, amounts of resistance, range of the joint, pain, and abnormal muscle tone must be considered in the performance of this test and can influence the test's objectivity. There are several grading systems used such as 0 to 5 and the percentage system. The Lovett scale is probably the system most frequently used by physical therapists. This scale employs a grading system that allows muscle strength to be rated on a scale from "zero" (no contraction seen or felt) through "trace," "poor," "fair," and "good" to "normal" (the muscle contracts to overcome greater resistance than a "good" muscle).[6]

Muscle testing is particularly helpful in determining which muscle should be biopsied when confirmation of diagnosis of myopathic disorders is required. Further, the initial test is used as a baseline examination against which later test results can be compared to demonstrate progress or lack of progress in the treatment of myopathic and other musculoskeletal diseases. When muscle-strengthening exercises are indicated, the test will indicate the group of muscles that require the most therapy.

□ Schirmer test

The Schirmer test is a simple test used to determine the presence of lacrimal gland involvement in suspected Sjögren's syndrome. A strip of filter paper is folded and placed in the lower conjunctival sac of both eyes. In the normal individual, the portion of the paper that becomes moistened measures 15 mm or greater; in the individual with Sjögren's syndrome the moistened area measures 5 mm or less.[14] This test is painless, and no special preparation is necessary.

REFERENCES AND SELECTED READINGS

1. *Anthony, C. P., and Thibodeau, G. A.: Textbook of anatomy and physiology, ed. 10, St. Louis, 1979, The C. V. Mosby Co.
2. *Arthritis Foundation: Primer on the rheumatic diseases, ed. 7, New York, 1973, The Foundation. (Prepared by a committee of the American Rheumatism Association Section of the Arthritis Foundation. Reprinted from J.A.M.A. **224**:Suppl., April 30, 1973.)
3. Beetham, W. P., et al. Physical examination of the joints, Philadelphia, 1965, W. B. Saunders Co.
4. *Brunner, N. A.: Orthopedic nursing: a programmed approach, ed. 2, St. Louis, 1975, The C. V. Mosby Co.
5. *Committee on Trauma of The American College of Surgeons: An outline of the treatment of fractures, ed. 8, Philadelphia, 1965, W. B. Saunders Co.
6. Daniels, L., et al. Muscle testing, ed. 3, Philadelphia, 1972, W. B. Saunders Co.
7. Flatt, A. E.: The care of the rheumatoid hand, ed. 3, St. Louis, 1974, The C. V. Mosby Co.
8. *French, R. M.: Guide to diagnostic procedures, ed. 4, New York, 1975, McGraw-Hill Book Co.
9. *Gartland, J. J.: Fundamentals of orthopedics, ed. 2, Philadelphia, 1974, W. B. Saunders Co.
10. Helfet, A.: Disorders of the knee, Philadelphia, 1974, J. B. Lippincott Co.
11. Hollander, J. L., and McCarty, D. J., editors: Arthritis and allied conditions, ed. 8, Philadelphia, 1972, Lea & Febiger.
12. *Larson, C. B., and Gould, M.: Orthopedic nursing, ed. 9, St. Louis, 1978, The C. V. Mosby Co.
13. Malasanos, L., Barkauskas, V., Moss, M., and Allen, K. S.: Health assessment, St. Louis, 1977, The C. V. Mosby Co.
14. *Moskowitz, R. W.: Clinical rheumatology, Philadelphia, 1975, Lea & Febiger.
15. *Salter, R. B.: Textbook of disorders and injuries of the musculoskeletal system: an introduction to orthopaedics, rheumatology, metabolic bone disease, rehabilitation and fracture, Baltimore, 1970, The Williams & Wilkins Co.
16. Siegel, M., and Seelentreuna, M.: Racial and social factors in systemic lupus erythematosus, J.A.M.A. **191**:77-80, 1965.
17. Webb, K. J.: Early assessment of orthopedic injuries, Am. J. Nurs. **74**:1048-1052, 1974.

*References preceded by an asterisk are particularly well suited for student reading.

41

Management of the person with motor problems

PATRICIA BUERGIN

The essence of nursing individuals with musculoskeletal problems lies in assisting the individual to make the physiologic and psychosocial adaptations necessary to minimize his temporary or permanent disability. It is the purpose of this chapter to define some of the common problems (both physiologic or functional, and psychosocial) experienced by individuals with motor disabilities, and to discuss specific methods that may be employed in managing these problems.

■ PHYSIOLOGIC OR FUNCTIONAL DISABILITIES

Six major problems must be considered in the area of physiologic disability: pain, stiffness, loss of strength, loss of dexterity, loss of locomotor ability, and complications common to immobility. Most patients with a motor disability will have one or more of these problems.

□ Pain

Pain is a problem common to many musculoskeletal disorders. When it exists, it ranks as the priority problem that must be dealt with in planning care for the person. Regardless of its intensity, unrelieved pain can become so all-consuming a concern of the person that has entire attention is focused on relieving it. Pain prevents activity, predisposes the patient to the complications of immobility, and dulls receptiveness to care and to teaching. In the extreme, it can affect the individual's attitude toward life. Therefore pain must be relieved to the greatest extent possible before other needed interventions can be implemented.

□ Stiffness

Stiffness (decreased flexibility) can be a result of pain or of disuse (as in the case of persons who are immobilized), or it can be a result of pathophysiologic changes (as in scleroderma or degenerative joint disease). Stiffness cannot be defined as pain; however, pain may well result as an attempt is made to use an extremity that is stiff. Stiffness may discourage the person from activity, thereby affecting him in much the same manner as pain.

□ Decrease in muscle strength

Decrease in muscle strength is sometimes a primary problem, as with some myopathic and neuropathic disorders; or it can result from prolonged bed rest or immobility. Interventions designed to improve strength (such as increasing mobility or exercises) can be implemented when some progress is made with treatment of the primary problem.

When it is not possible for the person to regain muscle strength, some means of modifying activities in order to maintain function must be provided.

□ Loss of dexterity

Loss of dexterity (skillful use of the hands or body) is a problem again encountered either as a result of a primary pathophysiologic process (such as rheumatoid arthritis or ataxic neurologic disorders) or as a result of pain, stiffness, or enforced immobility. And again the primary problem must be treated before measures to improve dexterity can be implemented. If the primary problem cannot be controlled, measures can be taken to provide alternative methods of performing activities so that function can be maintained. Examples of such interventions would include specially built utensils and other assisting devices as discussed on p. 842.

□ Loss of locomotor ability

Perhaps the most threatening component of many musculoskeletal disorders is the temporary or complete loss (or potential for loss) of the ability to move freely from one place to another. Consider what it must be like not to be able to reach for a glass of water, not have the means to escape a potentially threatening situation such as a fire, or having to be dependent on others for all of one's personal requirements. While some problems present only short-term immobility, others such as spinal cord damage can cause lifelong disability.

Various groups of handicapped persons throughout the United States have in the past several years been active socially and politically to inform the general public of the architectural barriers encountered by individuals with limited mobility. It is now a federal requirement that public facilities be equipped to accommodate the handicapped individual. All new public buildings must have wheelchair ramps, special toilet facilities, and easy-access parking spaces.

The concern of those caring for hospitalized persons with activity or motor restrictions is directed toward preventing complications such as contractures that would further restrict mobility; helping the person to work through his feelings about his restricted mobility; assisting him to adapt to having his mobility restricted (regardless of whether this is a short-term or a long-term problem); when possible, providing the patient with and teaching him how to use alternative means for moving about (wheelchair, crutches) or extending himself (long-handled reachers); and helping him plan for adaptations that he will have to make in his home environment and in his life style.

□ Complications of immobility

Immobility may be accompanied by a number of complications that can involve any or all of the major systems of the body. It is of the utmost importance that those caring for the patient whose mobility is impaired be aware of these potential complications and be skilled in interventions designed to help prevent them. Perhaps the most effective method of reviewing these complications is to consider them system by system in terms of the person who is most severely immobilized—the patient on bed rest.

Cardiovascular system

The three major problems associated with the cardiovascular system in the patient who is on bed rest are (1) a decreased ability to adapt to an erect posture, (2) an increased incidence of deep vein thrombosis and pulmonary embolus, and (3) an increased work load on the heart. Failure of the vessels in the legs to assume or maintain a state of vasoconstriction results in the pooling of venous blood, decreased venous return, and a diminished cardiac output. This may result in postural hypotension on assuming an erect position. While the heart beats more slowly when the patient is first placed on bed rest, the rate gradually increases. This results in decreased tolerance to exercise or activity when activity is begun. Active or passive range of motion, isometric exercises of the legs, frequent turning, and slow mobilization all may help to offset or prevent these complications. Following trauma, both prothrombin time and platelet adhesiveness are increased, thereby increasing clotting potential. Improper positioning, with pressure being exerted over major vessels, may enhance the possibility of thrombus formations.

Respiratory system

When the patient is on bed rest, decreased movement, decreased stimulus to cough, and decreased depth of ventilation all contribute to the pooling of secretions in the bronchi and bronchioles. Unabated, this will lead to hypostatic pneumonia. Turning, active range of motion, encouragement to deep breathe and cough, and encouraging the patient to move as much as he is able will help to prevent this problem.

Skin integrity

Loss of skin integrity (abrasions, decubitus ulcers) is caused by friction, pressure, or shearing forces (two or more tissue layers sliding on each other).[27] Pressure exerted over an area for a period of time will restrict the circulation of blood to that area and result in tissue destruction by the process of ischemic necrosis. Infection, trauma, obesity, sweating, increased age, and a poor nutritional state tend to hasten this process. Body weight and infections, other than genitourinary, have been found to have the highest correlation with decubitus formation.[62] Moisture from any cause, as from urinary and fecal incontinence, leads to skin breakdown and infection.

Prevention. The prevention of skin breakdown is vital in the care of any patient and especially in those with limited mobility. A person in traction is forced to lie supine for a period of time; a person with a neurologic problem producing immobility, such as quadriplegia (p. 719), is unable to move himself. In extreme situations, such as with the severely debilitated person with diabetes or quadriplegia, large areas of ulceration can be life threatening. Measures must be taken by others to prevent decubitus formation. Nurses play a major role in prevention.

The skin is inspected regularly for pressure signs (erythema, induration). Areas of the skin where bone is more superficial, such as the sacrum, elbows, and heels, are most vulnerable to breakdown and require careful inspection. The frequency of inspection depends on the presence of risk factors, but should be carried out at least once every 8 hours.

As has been noted on p. 817, turning the patient (changing points of pressure) at frequent intervals is one of the most effective methods of preventing the development of skin breakdown. Turning the patient with a turning sheet can help in preventing trauma to the skin by pressure and shearing forces (Fig. 41-1). When per-

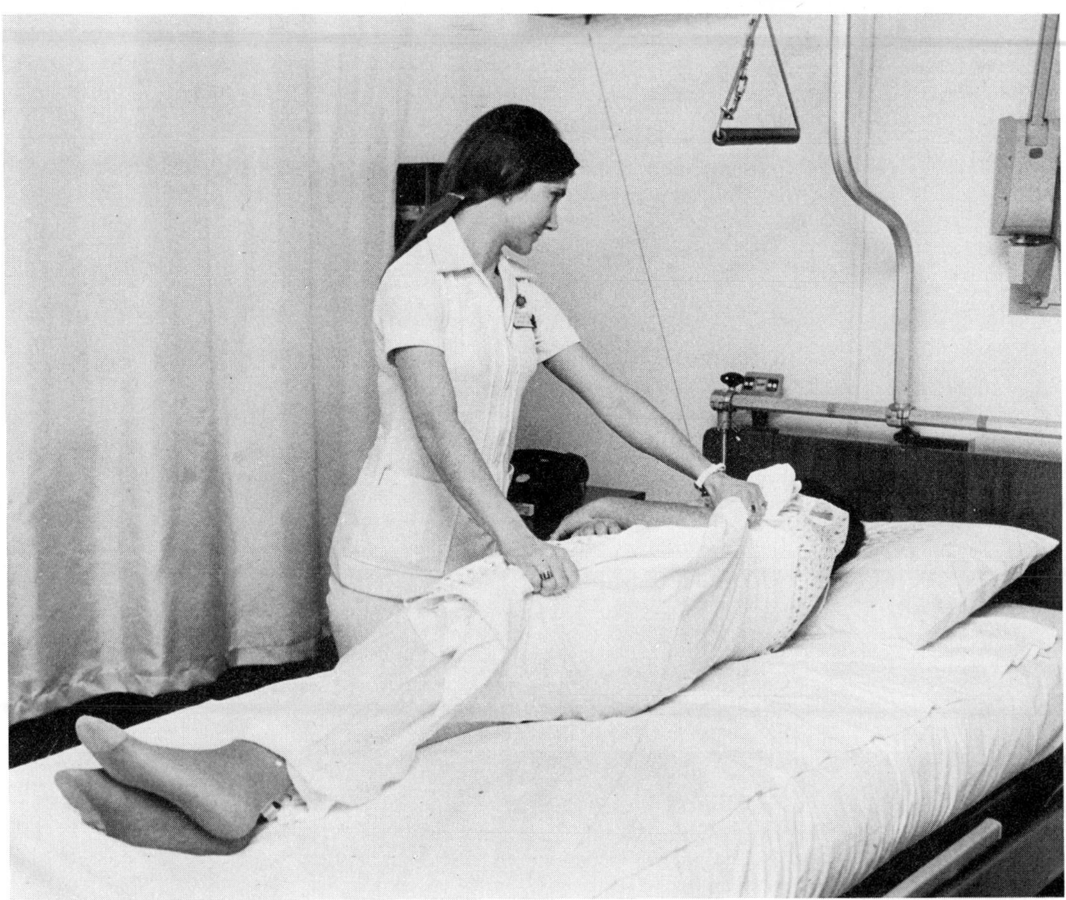

Fig. 41-1. Use of turning sheet. Sheet is held taut with one hand at level of patient's shoulder and other hand below patient's buttocks, thus providing patient with a sense of support and control.

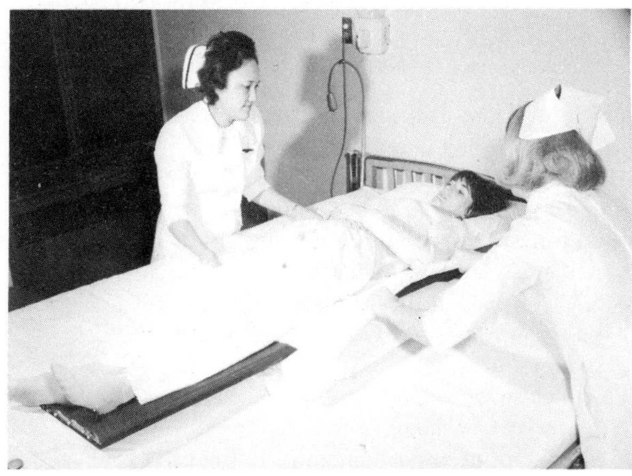

Fig. 41-2. Nurses using roller board to move patient from bed to cart. (Courtesy Neuropsychiatric Institute, University of Illinois Hospitals at the Medical Center, Chicago, Ill.)

sons who cannot move themselves are moved to another surface, such as to a cart, pull sheets or roller boards (Fig. 41-2) should be used to avoid friction against the surface of the bed or cart. Rolling the patient to his side or lifting him to place him on a bedpan will prevent friction against the surface of the pan.

Some patients cannot be fully turned because of traction apparatus or other limiting factors. For these persons especially, other methods such as air pressure mattresses, sheepskin pads, flotation pads, elbow and heel pads, and elevation of the heels may be helpful in preventing circulatory compromise to a skin area. Flotation pads distribute pressure equally over large skin areas, thereby decreasing pressure on any one site. Air pressure mattresses alternate pressures on the skin. Sheepskin decreases friction, distributes pressure, reduces moisture, and must be changed if dampness occurs.

Special beds may be used to turn the immobile pa-

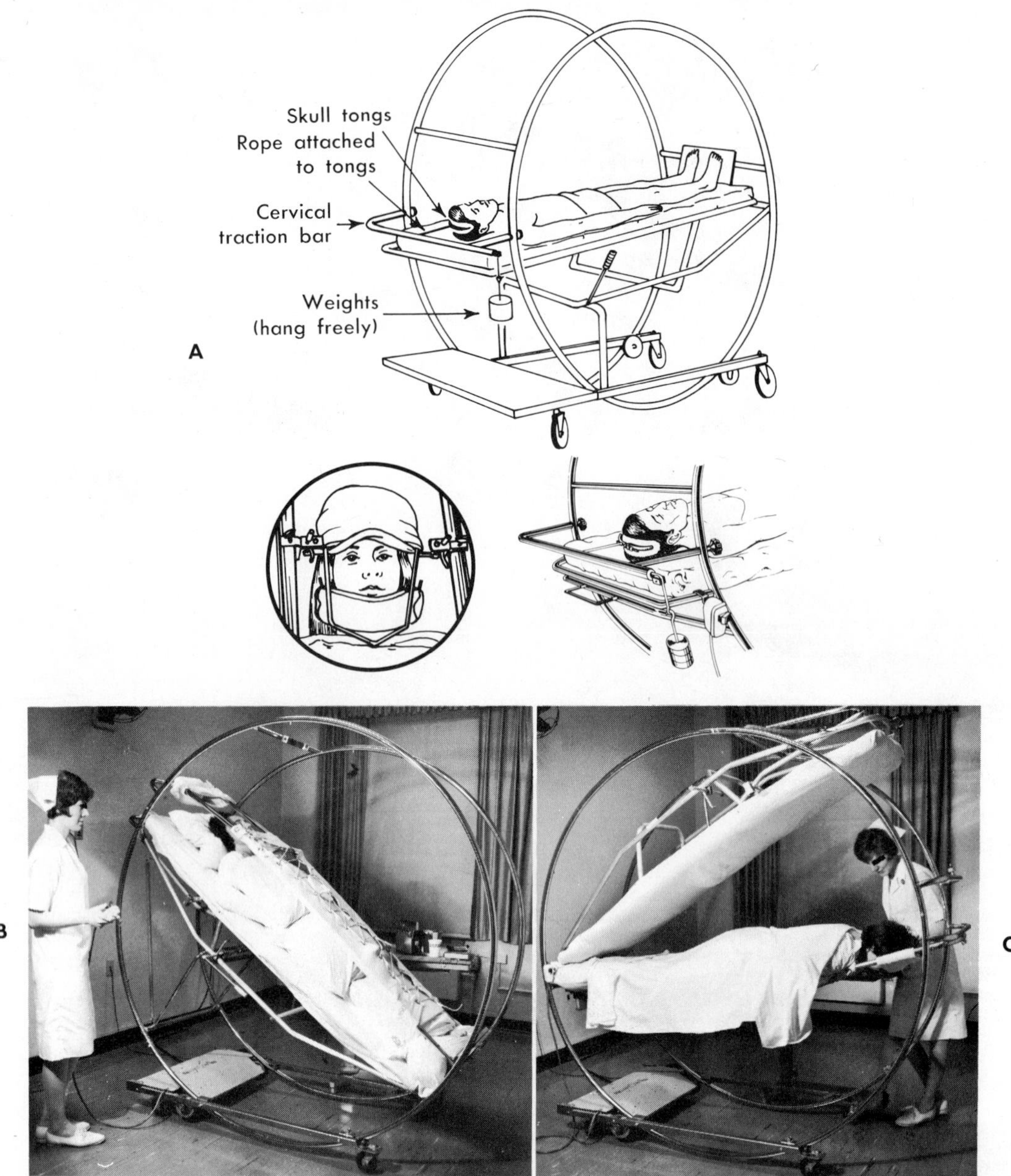

Fig. 41-3. CircOlectric bed consists of anterior and posterior frame and provides for vertical turning as opposed to lateral turning of patient. Thus standing, Trendelenburg, and sitting positions also may be utilized. Since bed is operated with an electric motor, even the very helpless patient may be able to adjust his position and assume a greater degree of independence. The many benefits (physiologic and psychologic) derived from frequent position changes and from self-dependence may be augmented with use of this bed. In addition to hospital use, the CircOlectric bed can be used advantageously in the home to facilitate care of the disabled person. **A,** Use of CircOlectric bed for patient with skull tongs (cervical traction). Arrangement of traction apparatus provides for maintenance of continuous traction as patient is turned vertically from supine to prone position or vice versa. Note close view of adjustable face piece. Support for head in either prone or supine position is an important factor in maintaining desired position of cervical vertebrae. **B,** Anterior frame has been put in position and turning of patient is started. **C,** Prone position, with posterior frame in elevated position. (**A** from Orthopedic nursing procedure manual, University of Iowa Hospitals and Clinics, The University of Iowa, Iowa City, Iowa; **B** and **C** from Larson, C. B., and Gould, M.: Orthopedic nursing, ed. 9, St. Louis, 1978, The C. V. Mosby Co.)

tient from supine to prone positions. The Stryker or Foster frame permits movement in a horizontal direction to only two positions: supine and prone. The CircOlectric bed (Fig. 41-3) permits many more position changes; movement is vertical and can be stopped at any angle while good body alignment is being maintained.

Intervention for decubitus ulcers. If a decubitus ulcer does develop, treatment consists of prevention of further extension of the ulcer through vigorous application of the preventive measures listed above and in the promotion of wound healing (p. 401). The ulcer must be kept clean if healing is to occur. There are numerous topical agents that have been used over the years; the large numbers attest to the fact that no one best method has yet been found. However, when a method of treatment is decided upon, it should be consistently carried out for several days. Failure to be consistent with treatment is one reason why there is little data available as to whether one method may be more efficacious than another.

The ulcer can be debrided mechanically or by the use of a fibrinolytic enzyme. If the enzyme is used, the wound is cleaned first with water, peroxide, or saline, and dried gently before the enzyme is applied. The ulcer is covered by a nonadhering dressing. This procedure is repeated two to three times daily. If skin erosion only is present, positioning to relieve pressure and application of heat may encourage healing. With very large deep ulcers, packing and irrigations are necessary, and excision and reconstructive surgery may be indicated. To reiterate, the most effective intervention for skin breakdown is *prevention*.

Gastrointestinal system

Constipation is perhaps the most frequent complication of immobility. The change in normal dietary habits and fluid intake, lack of activity, and having to use a bedpan are contributing factors. Turning, movement, elevation of the head of the bed, increased fluid intake, good dietary intake, use of stool-softening agents or laxatives, or suppositories to which the person is accustomed, and use of a commode, if possible, will help to alleviate this problem. (See Chapter 57 for further information.)

Muscular system

Disuse, atrophy, and weakness affect the muscles within a relatively short period of time. Efforts made to actively exercise the muscles within the restrictions imposed by the cause of the immobility can help reduce this effect.

Joints

Contractures secondary to muscle shortening, fibrosis, or bony ankylosis around the joints can develop quickly and take months to correct. Use of active and passive range of motion, isometric exercises, encouraging the person to perform all activities not retricted by the cause of his immobility, and attention to positioning can help prevent this loss of joint motion.

Skeletal system

Immobility disrupts the balance of osteoblastic (bone growth) and osteoclastic (bone destruction) activity. Osteoclastic (destructive) activity takes precedence with the result that bone matrix is destroyed and calcium is released. The end result is osteoporosis. Exercises (active, to whatever extent possible, and isometric) may be helpful in reducing the effects of this complication.

Urinary system

Increased calcium from bone destruction, increased urine pH (alkaline), increased citric acid (which causes the precipitation of calcium salts), stasis of urine in the bladder, and infection can all cause urinary problems. An increased fluid intake, decreased calcium intake (milk), and use of the commode (instead of the bedpan), whenever possible, are recommended to help reduce the potential for bladder infection and the formation of renal stones.

Neurologic system

Prolonged bed rest deprives a person of usual intellectual and social mobility. The older person in particular may respond to loss of stimuli by becoming disoriented or incapable of retaining information. Frequent contact by staff, provision of diversionary material such as magazines, radio, or television, and orienting mechanisms such as clocks or calendars can help to offset these complications.

In summary, those caring for the patient must understand the reason for the patient's immobility, how that immobility must be maintained to obtain maximum healing benefits, and what systems or organs are to be rested and to what extent. Organs or systems that need not be immobilized must be identified, and provision must be made for their continued use and development within the prescribed limits of rest.[17]

■ PSYCHOSOCIAL PROBLEMS

□ Reaction to disfigurement or disability

A major problem faced by many individuals who have problems that lead to motor impairment is that the disease itself can be disfiguring. Not only must the person adapt to functional disability, but he may have to adapt to "looking different" than other people. Severe deformities such as occur with rheumatoid arthritis (Fig. 42-1) or amputation, or uncontrolled movements that occur with Huntington's chorea are all problems that affect the person's self-image. (For further information on body image see Chapter 28.) For some individuals the problem may not be so much with disfigurement but rather with loss of alteration of function (such as ambulatory ability), or the need to use an assistive device or prosthesis. In such a situation the person views himself as different from others.

Depending on the nature and pressures of family, social, or work situation, or the person's self-image, he may try to cover up his disability, fearing the loss of support and esteem of friends, or even his job. If the disability cannot be covered up, the person may become withdrawn—limiting his contact with others. An example of such a situation would be the middle-aged woman with hip disease who, though in pain, will not use a cane to assist her in ambulation for fear of being thought "old." As walking becomes more and more difficult, she limits her social contacts and even necessary functions such as shopping to avoid having others see her.

It takes a great deal of patience and time to help individuals affected in this manner to accept that hiding their disability is not a reasonable method of dealing with it. Treatment that can restore function may be available (medical therapy or corrective surgery). If not, the hospital staff can often set the tone for a patient to adapt to his altered appearance or function by their understanding and accepting attitude. Helping the person to recover a sense of self-worth by encouraging his participation in activities, referring to his disability or disfigurement in a very matter-of-fact manner, helping him to be neatly groomed, or encouraging him when he tries new activities or demonstrates an improvement in ability can often improve the person's motivation.

□ Dependence, independence, and interdependence

Most people want to be able to live their lives independently. In the sense of this discussion, independence would mean freedom from having to make demands on others for personal and social activities of daily living. However, individuals with musculoskeletal problems may be unable to manage one or more activities of daily living for themselves. If help from another person is needed to perform a certain function, such as buttoning buttons, the individual is dependent in that area. If an assistive device (button hook, Velcro closures) can be made available and the individual can master the use of the device, he can again be independent in that function.

The major objectives in caring for an individual who has motor impairment are to allow the person to do what he can for himself, to devise ways to help him achieve independent function in impaired areas, and lastly to assist him to the extent necessary in areas where independent function cannot be achieved. If the patient is not allowed to perform the functions that he can perform, he can quickly become angry, discouraged, and lose motivation. Loss of the desire to be independent, subjecting oneself to a state of dependence, can be the most destructive element of a musculoskeletal disorder.

Interdependence is the third area for consideration. Very few people live truly independent lives. As a society, we depend on the farmer to grow our food, the lawyer to attend to our legal affairs, the mechanic to repair our automobile. Families also are structured around interdependent functions. The person with a motor disability may at some time be faced with losing his interdependent role; that is, he may no longer believe that he is useful or needed by anyone else. Counseling, by members of the health team, of the patient and his family concerning the nature of the disability, and discussing the patient's areas of independence and dependence may be helpful in assisting the patient and his family to define new roles for themselves—roles in which the patient can have an active part in the family's life and concerns.

Goals of care in relation to these entities (dependence, independence, and interdependence) are (1) to assist the patient to maintain or achieve a state of independence consistent with his physical capabilities, (2) to define and share with his family or significant others the areas in which he is dependent, and (3) to return him to his living situation able to resume an interdependent role with his family.

□ Adaptation to assistive, supportive, and corrective devices

Walkers, canes, crutches, splints, braces, and feeding aids often have a negative connotation in our society. A major problem in caring for the patient with a motor disability can be that of helping the patient to overcome his aversion to such devices and to accept them as a means of maintaining his independence and safe functioning. On the more optimistic side, many patients are quite happy to learn that there are aids that can improve or extend their abilities. Sometimes all that is necessary is to demonstrate the effectiveness of the device in alleviating pain or eliminating dependence in a certain area of functioning. However, some patients may need constant encouragement before they will accept the device; and some may never accept it. Family members or significant others may be enlisted to provide encouragement, and it is often their support that will produce the desired result.

□ Socioeconomic impact

Many disorders that affect motor function occur at an age when wage earning, childrearing, and other functions can be seriously impaired. Loss of income and self-esteem, the inability to maintain one's standard of living, and increased stress on the family can all result. There are agencies available to help with employment problems (bureaus of vocational guidance, vocational guidance and rehabilitation centers, sheltered workshops). Often there is an opportunity for hospital staff to advise the patient of the availability of such services and to make the appropriate referrals.

By no means, however, is motor impairment less of a problem for the older patient. Living alone or on a fixed income and faced with the possibility of not being able to maintain independence, the patient can become very frightened, depressed, or withdrawn. Nursing homes are costly, as are persons who are hired to help in the home, if they are even available in a community. The idea of giving up one's home and way of life can be very threatening and demoralizing.

It is important, then, to identify the socioeconomic problems facing any patient with motor impairment. Often the patient can be helped to work through some of his physical limitations with modifications that will not cost a great deal and that will allow him to continue living in his present circumstances. For example, applying a levering device to a garage door could help the individual with limited lifting ability and would be less expensive than an automatic garage door opener. For those who cannot sit in a bathtub, bathing while sitting on a chair in the tub and using a shower hose extension on the faucet would be a less expensive arrangement than purchasing a hydraulic tub seat, and would be more satisfying than a sponge bath. Referrals to community resources such as the Visiting Nurse Association or arranging for Meals on Wheels can sometimes be all the support that is needed to keep an individual in his own home and out of a dependent setting.

In working with individuals who have motor impairment, one must be inventive and innovative and should possess a working knowledge of community resources available to help the individual maintain satisfactory functioning in a setting that he can afford.

□ Family relationships

Reference has already been made to the fact that family roles and relationships (social and economic) may be changed, owing to a patient's restricted motor function and areas of dependency. It is important that those caring for the patient recognize when those relationships are destructive and help the patient and his family obtain appropriate guidance. Sometimes psychiatric counseling is necessary. Whenever it is possible, support should be given to "healthy," caring relationships that are identified in the situation.

■ PREVENTION

□ Factors affecting the alteration

Whatever the nature of the musculoskeletal disability, there are factors of prevention and teaching that must be considered.

Nonpreventable factors

Many of the diseases that affect the musculoskeletal system have at this time an unknown cause. Rheumatoid arthritis and the systemic connective tissue diseases are but a few examples. While these diseases are not now preventable, there are complications of the diseases that are preventable—contractures, atrophy, skin breakdown, and others. In these instances, prevention depends on teaching the patient to understand his disease process and to employ preventive measures (pp. 875 and 877).

Preventable factors

Polio vaccine, screening of school-age children for scoliosis, and screening tests for streptococcal infections with early treatment of the infection to prevent rheumatic fever are examples of preventive measures that can be employed on a community-wide basis in combating illnesses that cause musculoskeletal disability. Early attention to posture, good dietary habits, genetic counseling for individuals with sickle cell anemia and hemophilia, teaching of good body mechanics for individuals whose jobs entail lifting or carrying heavy objects, and concern and attention to the recommendations of the National Safety Council to help avoid accidents at home, on the job, and on the road are all examples of preventive measures that may be employed to decrease musculoskeletal disability within the general population.

□ Promotion of safety

For those individuals who have limitations of motion or mobility, there are a variety of precautions and protective or safety devices that can be employed in the hospital or in the home. Examples would be grab bars that can be mounted on a wall near a tub or toilet, safety arms that fit around a toilet, and rails that fasten onto the side of a bathtub. These devices provide the patient with both a stable place to hold onto and a point of leverage for assuming a standing or a sitting position. Throw rugs and obstacles should be removed from areas used by individuals with ambulatory difficulties, and floors should not be highly waxed. Wheelchairs should have adequate locking devices, and patients who must use wheelchairs should be taught how to lock and unlock the chair.

While some of these measures may seem to be common knowledge, patients are frequently not aware of them or their need for them. One of the most important functions nurses can perform—and because of their 24-hour contact with the patient they are in a unique position to do so—is to assess the safety requirements of their patients and then to teach the patient or his family what steps are necessary to ensure safety. It is helpful if nurses know where in the community needed equipment can be obtained. Often the hospital social worker or physical therapist provides this information and assists the patient or his family in obtaining the equipment. By the time the patient is to be discharged from the hospital, arrangements should be made for him to have the equipment and instruction that he requires for safe functioning at home.

☐ Prevention of muscle and joint complications

Maintenance of joint mobility

For the individual with limited motion or mobility, range of motion exercises should be carried out to prevent joint stiffness or contractures from disuse. (Techniques of range of motion are discussed in Chapter 40.) Whenever it is possible, except in conditions where there is acute joint inflammation, range of motion should be performed several times a day. *Active range of motion* is most beneficial for the patient. Encouraging the patient to do as much of his own care as he is able to do within the restrictions of his disability will often satisfy active range of motion requirements.

Several precautions should be mentioned. *Passive range of motion* should not be performed past the point of the complaint of pain. Particularly in individuals with skeletal pathology (gross deformity, osteoporosis), fractures can result if a joint is forced through "normal" range of motion. Also, acutely inflamed, painful, or septic joints should be rested, since harm can be done by moving the joint before inflammation has subsided. The person who has pain is also likely to resist movement in order to avoid further pain.

Maintenance of posture

Although maintenance of good posture is important for all persons, it is especially important for the patient with chronic arthritic disease. Poor posture exerts further strain on already damaged joints and not only may cause pain and fatigue but predisposes to increased deformity.

The patient who must remain in bed for a long period of time in traction or in a cast should be in a bed with a firm mattress, and a bed board should be placed under the mattress. A firm bed lessens pain by preventing motion and consequent pull on painful joints, and helps to keep the spine in good alignment. Boards should be long enough and wide enough to rest firmly on the main side and end rails of the bed, not on the bedsprings. The person with arthritis should either use no pillow or should use one small pillow that fits well down under the shoulders so that forward flexion of the cervical spine is not encouraged. Knees should not be flexed on pillows, and all patients who must be confined to bed most of the day should lie prone with a pillow under the abdomen for a part of each day to relieve supine pressure areas (inferior scapular areas and the ischial tuberosities) (Fig. 41-4).

Careful positioning with trochanter rolls (rolled towels or bath blankets to brace an extremity in the desired position), supportive pillows, attention to avoiding extreme flexion of joints, and care to avoid compressing nerves or arteries (the result of which can be neurologic or circulatory compromise) are all important considerations for both skin care and general maintenance of the patient.

The unaffected foot (or feet) should rest against a

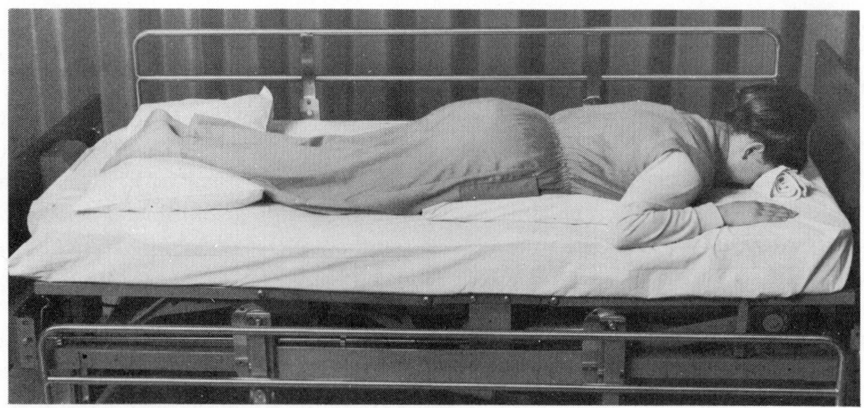

Fig. 41-4. Good body alignment in prone position. Lower legs are elevated off bed to avoid forcing feet into plantar flexed position. (From Rantz, M., and Courtial, D.: Lifting, moving and transferring patients, St. Louis, 1977, The C. V. Mosby Co.)

footboard at least part of the day. This helps to maintain the foot in a neutral position for a more normal walking position, prevents the weight of bed clothes from contributing to foot drop, and provides a firm surface against which the person can do resistive foot exercises. The patient should be taught to check the position of his lower limb when at rest. If his problem is nonneurologic, he should "toe in" to prevent external rotation contracture of the hip and pronation of the foot. These complications cause serious difficulty when walking is resumed.

For the general public, it should be remembered that poor posture throughout life may contribute to hypertrophic arthritis. The child should be taught to stand correctly so that strain caused by prolonged hyperextension does not occur in points such as the knee joints. Molding the pelvis correctly with a posterior pelvic tilt will help prevent increased curvature of the lower back with its resultant strain on muscles and joints. Holding the head up with the chin in takes a great deal of strain from the joints of the upper spine. It is surprising how many older persons can benefit from posture improvement even though damage may date from childhood.[33] (For more complete discussion of posture, see specialized texts.)

Attention should also be paid to correct mechanical use of the body. Techniques such as stooping with knees and hips flexed (Fig. 42-6), rather than bending over, prevent muscle strain that may pull a joint out of alignment just enough for osteoarthritic changes to develop or to cause symptoms. Techniques for lifting, using the strong muscles of the legs rather than the weak back muscles, should be taught particularly to individuals whose work involves heavy lifting and to hospitalized patients who have suffered back injuries. Nurses are frequently in an excellent position to teach patients good body mechanics because of the work they do, and it is important that they serve as positive role models by exhibiting good body mechanics in their work.

In regard to sitting posture, furniture should be such that good posture can be maintained during working and recreational hours with a minimum of drain on vital energy resources. There are five criteria for a good chair: (1) the seat should be deep enough to support the thighs but not so deep that circulation in the popliteal spaces is hampered; (2) the seat should be high enough so that the feet rest firmly on the floor and do not dangle, placing increased pressure on the posterior thighs; (3) the seat should be level or tilted slightly forward so that flexion of the knees and hips is at a minimum and not at more than a right angle; (4) the chair should have arms so that arm and shoulder muscles can provide leverage to help in moving from the chair, the arms of the chair at a level such that with the patient's arms at right angles, the shoulders are neither too high nor too low; and (5) the rungs must be such that one foot can be placed partially under the chair in preparation for rising so that the person is better able to stabilize his center of gravity as he assumes an erect position. Chairs with seats a little higher than is usually considered comfortable provide better leverage when arising. Sometimes adding an inch or two to the height of the person's favorite chair will increase his comfort while sitting and make it easier to arise from. This is particularly true for persons with hip girdle weakness or hip or knee joint involvement. If the patient is to spend much time with the feet elevated, a small stool on which to comfortably rest the feet should be available. Occasionally it is also necessary to build up the toilet seat. Devices to be placed over the seat to provide height can be improvised, or they can be purchased from hospital supply stores. A rail beside the toilet seat is as necessary as arms on any chair the patient uses if the arms must be used to arise from the seat safely.

■ INTERVENTION

□ Conservative intervention

The interventions that will be discussed in this section are those that are used primarily for individuals with joint and muscle diseases. They can be restorative, preventive, or analgesic in nature.

Activity

Because motor problems are essentially problems of activity limitation, many of the appropriate interventions are directed toward improving activity.

Rest, activity, and joint protection. Rest is a therapeutic measure employed in many inflammatory and in some traumatic (back injuries) conditions. However, it cannot be overemphasized that too much rest can at times be as detrimental as too much activity. Absolute rest of a particular limb, joint, or the entire body in acute inflammatory conditions helps to prevent further tissue destruction and pain. Resting a joint of the lower extremity may mean placing that joint on a non-weight-bearing status by having the person "unload" it through the use of crutches or a walker. The usefulness of resting splints in controlling muscle spasm is discussed on p. 847. As symptoms subside, activity will be gradually increased to the limits that can be tolerated without pain or fatigue. The patient must strike a balance of rest and activity to maintain function and to prevent further disability.

The physician is usually the one to determine when activity is to begin, but the nurse can be very instrumental in helping the patient recognize when activity should be stopped in favor of rest. Clues include increase in pain, tiredness, and progressive loss of dexterity in the use of the involved part. As the condition that requires rest improves, the patient should be assisted to develop a plan for his daily activities that provides for both a gradual increase in activity and adequate periods of rest. The patient should be encouraged to do as much as he is able without becoming overtired.

Patients who have chronic conditions that will continue to require rest periods should try, while in the hospital, to work out a schedule for themselves approximating the activity schedule that meets their rest and activity requirements at home or work. This is often difficult to do. Many times persons will have to be helped to work through their feelings about not being able to attend to all the activities they believe are necessary or desired. They need support from both the hospital staff and their families to come to terms with their limitations.

Patients with joint involvement must be made aware of techniques they can use to protect their joints from overuse, misuse, and stress. Joint protection techniques should be implemented in all possible activities of daily living (ADL) situations, and the improper use of joints should be pointed out to patients as they are observed. Learning to function in different but still effective ways is difficult for most people, but the most frequent indicator that they have overused or misused their joints is an increase in pain or fatigue. Individuals need to learn to recognize these symptoms and need to be assisted to take steps to modify the offending activity.

Splinting and bracing to protect joints is discussed on p. 847. Another form of joint protection is modification of activities that can stress or harm joints. Joint protection techniques are particularly beneficial in chronic inflammatory joint diseases such as rheumatoid arthritis. These techniques involve the person's learning to find easier ways of accomplishing what he *needs* to do. These techniques can be broken down into several categories.

The first category is *energy conservation techniques*. Examples are sliding rather than lifting objects and moving dishes, utensils, or equipment from one room to another on a wheeled cart rather than carrying them.

The second category is *avoiding positions of possible deformity*. Flexor muscles are generally stronger than extensor muscles, and joints tend to become deformed in a position of flexion. External pressures that put stress on joints in the wrong direction and internal pressures from muscle forces can produce deformities in joints that have been affected by chronic inflammatory processes. Sitting for long periods, keeping the knees or elbows bent to avoid pain, and twisting motions such as turning a doorknob or removing a jar lid are examples of stressful or harmful activities that can result in joint deformity or contracture. Performing active range of motion, varying sitting and standing activities at frequent intervals, turning sideways to a doorknob, and using wrist motion rather than finger motion to turn it are examples of how harmful positions can be avoided.

The third approach is *learning to avoid holding muscles or joints in one position for a long time*. Varying activities as mentioned above and learning to stop activity before it becomes painful will help prevent fatigue and possible joint damage.

The fourth technique is *learning to use the strongest joints for all activities*. A good example of this is using the knees, not the back, when lifting objects, or pushing a door open with the shoulder, not the hand. Joints should be used in their best position. This means using good standing and sitting posture, working at a comfortable height, and not reaching or bending when another approach would do as well.

For the patient to learn these techniques he must be introduced to them and be afforded the opportunity to practice them. The occupational therapist is instrumental in this teaching, but in areas where occupational therapists are not available, nurses are often the resource persons for teaching joint protection. Nurses are also in a position to observe the patient's follow-through on the techniques he has been taught, and they can provide encouragement and reminding as necessary.[44]

Assistive, supportive, and safety devices. There are many *assistive devices* available for persons who have impairment of upper and lower extremity function; some examples of these devices are described in Table 41-1. Although the occupational therapist is generally the person who evaluates the patient's disability, recommends specific assistive devices, and teaches the patient how to use them, the nurse is often the person who recognizes the need for referral to the occupational therapist.

Table 41-1. Some assistive devices for persons with motor impairments

Assistive device	Patient limitation
Utensil with built-up handle (Fig. 41-5)	Cannot adequately close hand
Utensil with cuffed handle (Fig. 35-9)	Loss of opposition of thumb
Combination knife-fork (Fig. 41-6)	Use of only one hand
Mug with special handle	Unable to grasp regular cup handle
Long-handle shoe horn (Fig. 41-7)	Unable to bend to reach feet
Long-handle reacher (to reach for or pick up objects) (Fig. 41-8)	Unable to stoop or reach
Long-handle comb, fork, spoon (Figs. 41-9 and 41-10)	Limited shoulder or elbow motion
Stocking guide (Fig. 41-11)	Inability to reach feet

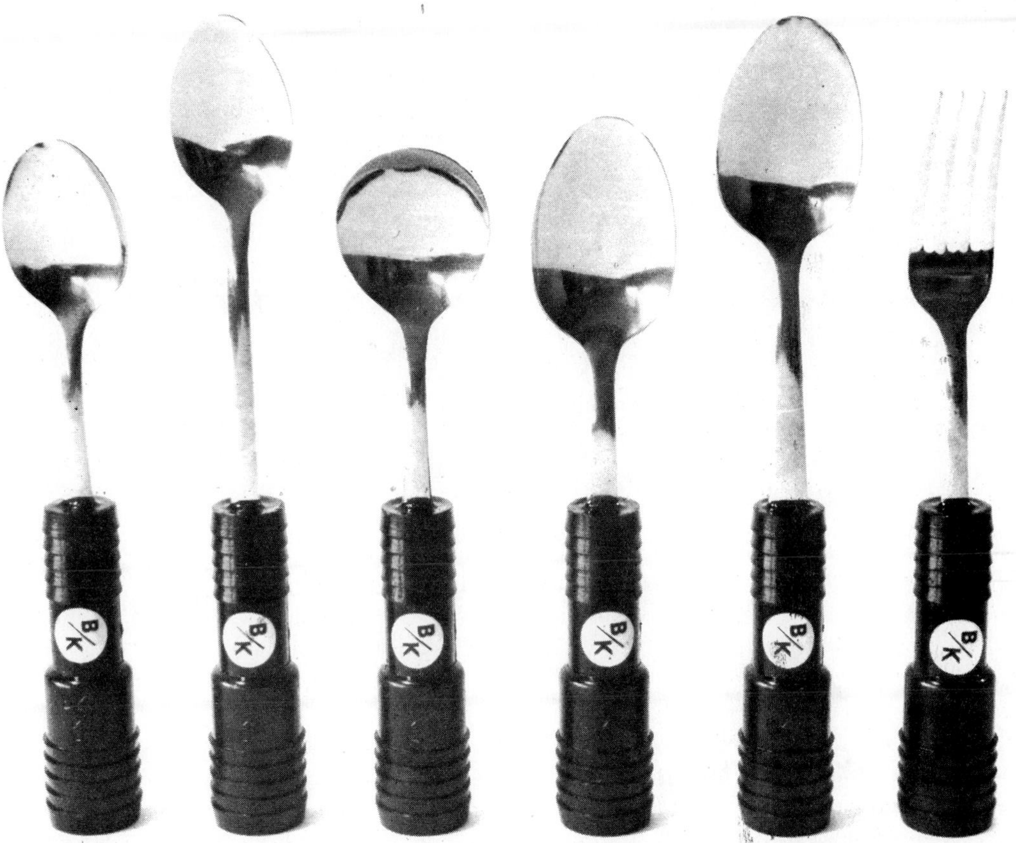

Fig. 41-5. Several different utensils with built-up handles are available. They are used to improve grasp of hand. (Courtesy Fred Sammons, O.T.R., Chicago, Ill.)

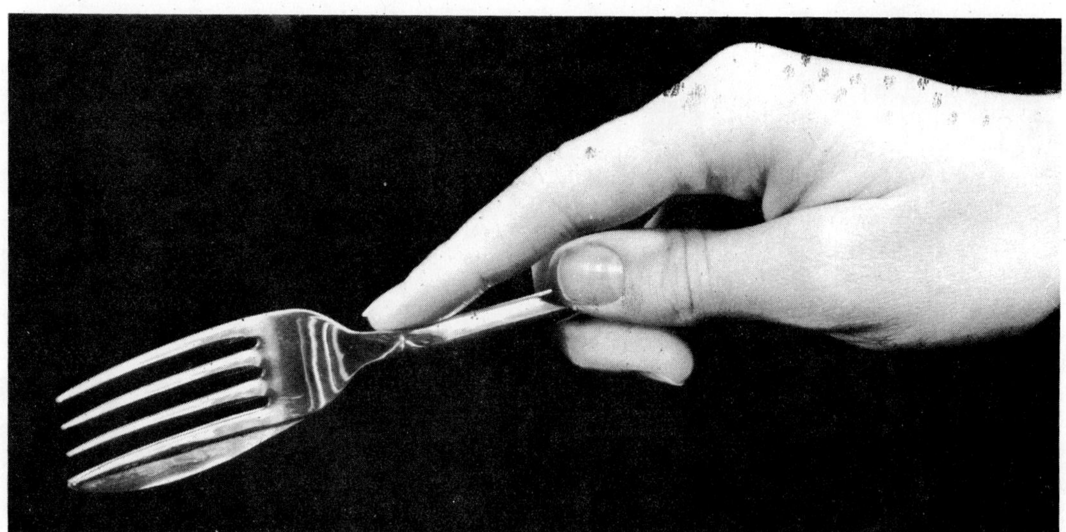

Fig. 41-6. Side-cutter fork for use by person with one functioning hand. (Courtesy Fred Sammons, O.T.R., Chicago, Ill.)

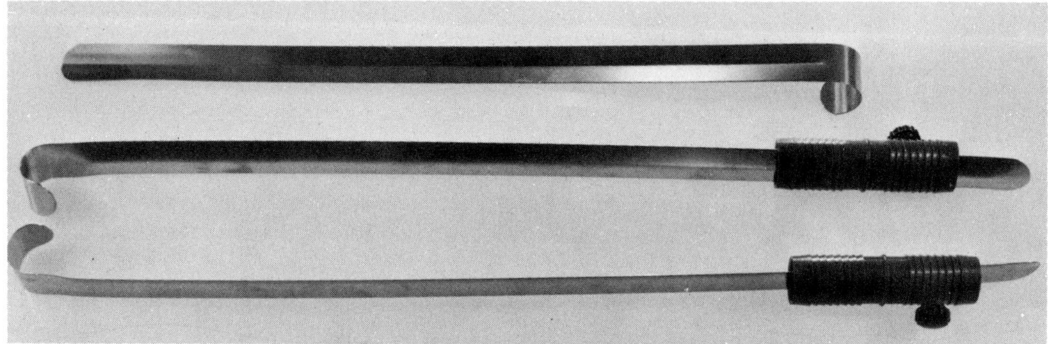

Fig. 41-7. Long-handled shoe horn and dressing aids. (Courtesy Fred Sammons, O.T.R., Chicago, Ill.)

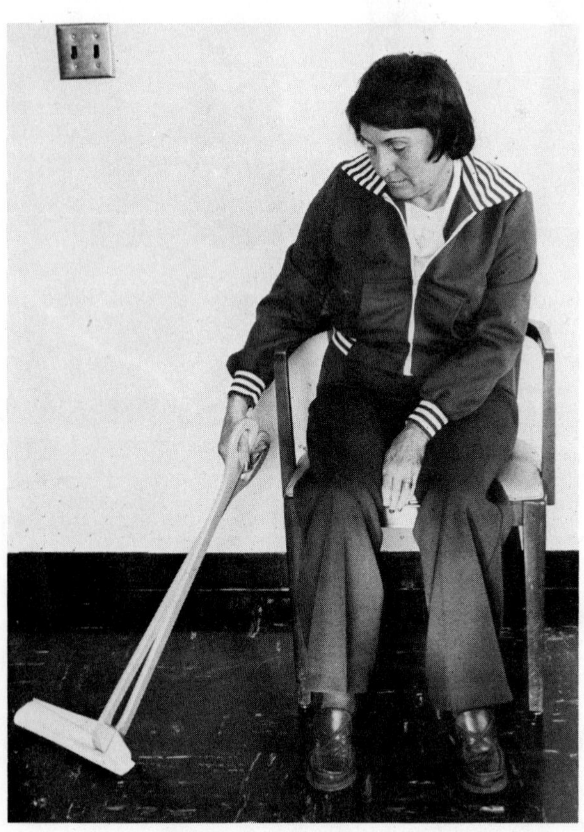

Fig. 41-8. Long-handled reachers are handy for picking things up off floor if person is not to bend or stoop.

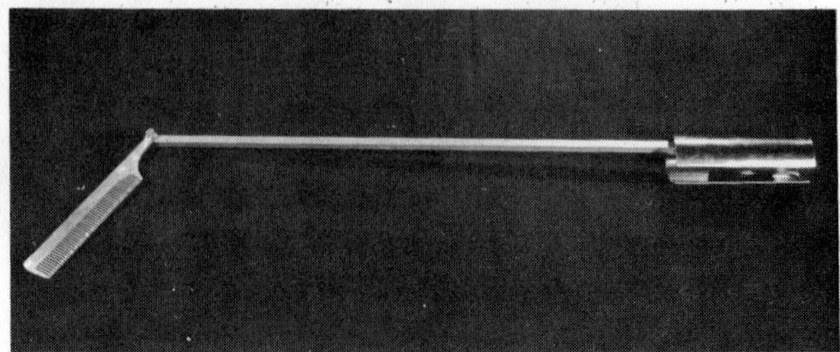

Fig. 41-9. Long-handled comb for use by persons with limited shoulder motion. (Courtesy Fred Sammons, O.T.R., Chicago, Ill.)

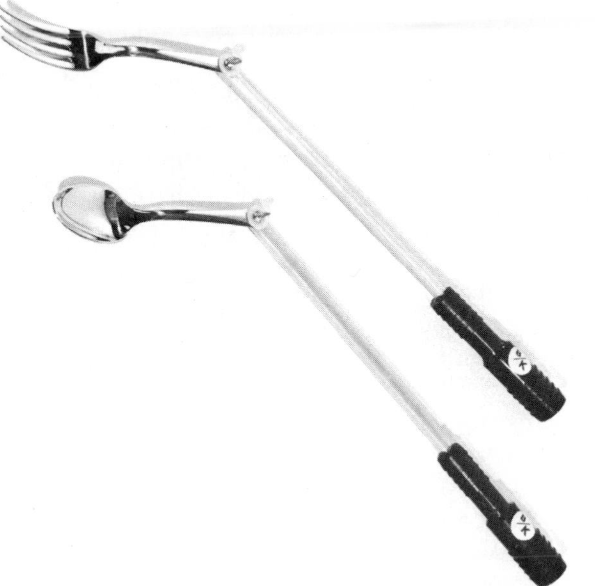

Fig. 41-10. Extension utensils are useful to persons with limited range of motion at elbow or shoulder. (Courtesy Fred Sammons, O.T.R., Chicago, Ill.)

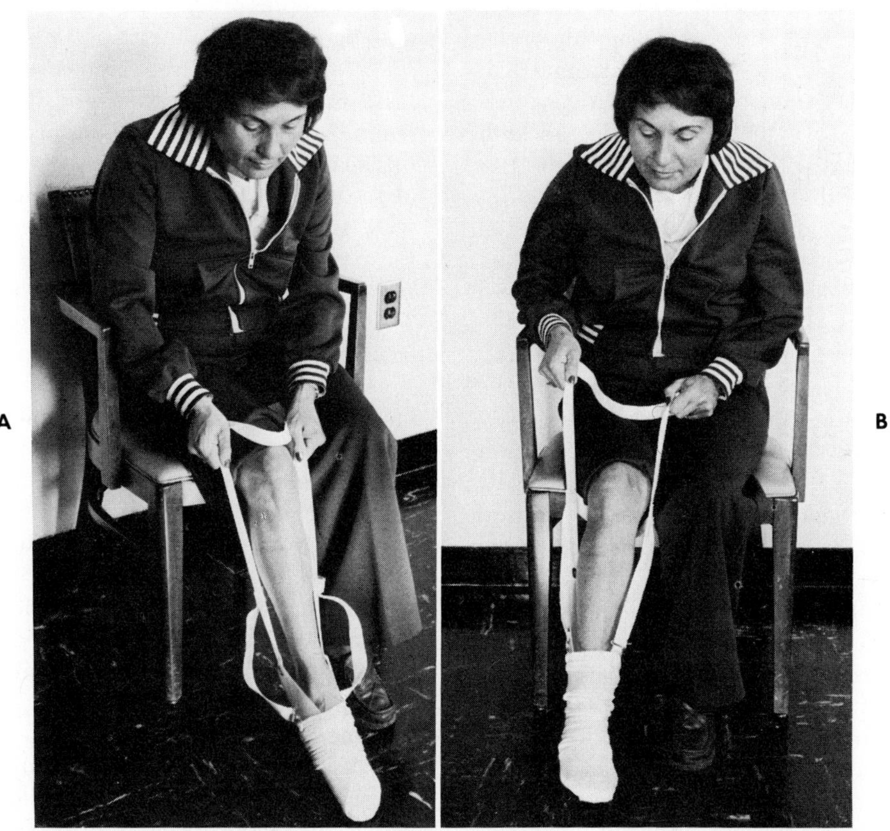

Fig. 41-11. A, Using stocking aid. Stocking has been placed over plastic guide; garter clips at ends of strap have been attached to top of stocking. Woman then places her foot into stocking. **B,** Straps are used to pull stocking over foot and up leg; when top of stocking is at knee, patient can release garters. This apparatus is useful for persons who cannot bend over to reach feet.

Nurses need to be aware of what self-help devices the person has, and should encourage him to use them in activities in the hospital or in the home. For example, it is nontherapeutic and time consuming to feed a person who can feed himself independently with aids that can be provided.

Supportive devices or ambulatory aids (walkers, canes, crutches) are usually recommended for persons who cannot bear weight on one or more joints of the lower extremities. These devices permit part of the person's ambulatory weight to be transferred to the upper extremities. Some other indications for their use are instability, poor balance, or pain on weight bearing.

The physical therapist evaluates the patient to determine the specific device that will match the patient's needs and abilities. Axillary crutches require that the person be fairly dexterous and have a good sense of balance, especially if no weight bearing is permitted on one leg; however, crutches permit faster ambulation and can be used on stairs as well as on level surfaces (Fig. 47-7). Walkers provide a more solid support than crutches and in most instances are more useful for individuals with problems of balance and dexterity. Ambulation with a walker is slower than with crutches, and it is hazardous on stairs and uneven ground outdoors. Canes allow the person greater mobility and are less cumbersome than either crutches or walkers, but with a single cane the person cannot unload his weight from the affected limb as effectively as he could with a walker or crutches. A number of variations of the three basic ambulatory devices are available, depending on the person's special needs (special handles on canes, forearm supports on crutches, reciprocal walkers, elevated walkers, and others).

Physical therapists generally select and teach the person how to use ambulatory devices. However, nurses may at times be called on to do this teaching and they must, in any case, know how to supervise the person who uses ambulatory aids. The most common gait pattern is the *three-point gait.* This pattern may be used with a walker, cane, or crutches. Regardless of the appliance used, the appliance is placed forward first, then the affected leg, then the unaffected leg (Fig. 47-8). The *two-point gait,* used with crutches or bilateral canes, most nearly resembles a normal walking pattern: one crutch and the opposite leg are moved simultaneously, then the other crutch and its opposite leg. The *four-point gait* (Fig. 47-9, *A*) is also used with two crutches or two canes, is somewhat more difficult to learn, but is useful when partial weight bearing is permitted on the affected leg or legs. One crutch is advanced, then the opposite leg, then the other crutch, then the other leg. If verbal directions were being given, they would sound like this: "Right arm, left leg, left arm, right leg."

The person learning how to use ambulatory aids will need close supervision or assistance until he feels steady and confident. The person doing the supervision should walk along with the patient on the patient's *affected* side, slightly to the patient's rear and about one-half step behind the patient, keeping in step with him so that both the patient and person supervising have the same balance point at any given time. The hand closest to the patient should be positioned at the patient's unaffected hip, and the hand farthest from the patient should be positioned to hold the patient's shoulder on his affected side. In this fashion the patient can be prevented from falling forward, backward, or to either side. Likewise the person assisting will not obstruct the patient's movement of the ambulatory aid. As the patient develops more skill, assistance and supervision is gradually withdrawn.

Persons using ambulatory aids should have instruction by the physical therapist. When possible, they should practice with the device prior to discharge from the hospital. Proper instruction, adjustment of, and practice with the device may prevent accidents after discharge.

Points of safety have already been discussed on p. 839. Examples of *safety devices* commonly employed are grab bars around toilets, tubs, or showers; elevated toilet seats; skidproof mats or adhesive strips on tub floors; hand rails along staircases; and nonskid wax applied to floors. Areas in which the patient is unsafe or potentially unsafe can only be identified through careful observation of the patient and through testing him in a variety of ADL situations. Only those devices that are appropriate for a particular patient should be recommended. This requires some familiarity with the various aids available. That familiarity can be easily obtained by examining a catalogue from the orthopedic supply house.

Heat and cold. Heat and cold have a variety of uses for individuals with musculoskeletal problems. Heat, particularly moist heat, is often used for relaxation of muscles and for its sedative and analgesic effects. It is particularly useful in relieving stiffness. Heat treatments early in the morning may make it possible for an individual to move into his day more comfortably and more quickly than if he waited for stiffness to resolve without treatment. Cold is often used to reduce or prevent swelling after trauma, and some patients find that it reduces pain and stiffness better than heat.

One of the most effective means of delivering moist heat is through warm, moist compresses or hot packs. These packs contain a chemical filler that expands in hot water and retains heat. They are heated to 80 C (174 F) in water-filled machines, and are then wrapped in toweling before application. At least six to eight layers of thick toweling should separate the pack from the patient's skin. Other forms of heating devices (Aqua-K pads and electric heating pads) provide a dry or less conductive heat to the affected part. When any form of heat application is being used, the patient's skin is checked for evidence of burning a few minutes after application. If the application is too hot, it should either be removed or additional protective toweling applied.

Moist compresses should be left on (if not contraindicated) from 15 to 20 minutes to achieve maximum effect. Dry heat can be left on for considerably longer times if there is a control device to regulate the heat at a low level. It should be noted, however, that head is not to be used on *joints* that are or may be infected (p. 890).

Ice packs must also be wrapped in toweling prior to application to the patient's skin, since cold "burns" can result if the skin is unprotected. Continuous applications of ice may be required to reduce swelling following trauma to a body part; however, the skin should be checked frequently to determine if there are any signs of tissue damage.

Any person with decreased sensation must have heat or cold applied with caution, since that person will not be able to determine if damage is occurring. If the patient is to use heat or cold in the treatment of his problem at home, he should be taught what safety precautions to observe. For individuals with sensory deficits, this often means that someone else must be taught how to perform the treatment for them.

Traction. In addition to the use of traction in acute trauma and postoperative orthopedic situations (p. 860), *intermittent* traction can be used to assist in reducing contractures or to relieve pain in the presence of muscle spasm. The principles of maintaining the patient's comfort and safety while in traction are the same as discussed on p. 863. However, the patient who is in intermittent traction (as with acute low back injuries) should have the traction disconnected when the traction itself causes discomfort. It can be reapplied when the patient believes he can tolerate it.

Splinting and bracing. Splints and braces (orthoses) are used to stabilize or support a joint to protect it from improper use or external trauma. Braces are also used to mechanically correct dysfunction such as foot drop by supporting a joint in its functional position. Splints and braces are used in arthritic conditions (rheumatoid arthritis, Charcot's joints), orthopedic situations (scoliosis), and in neurologic conditions (peripheral nerve lesions such as foot drop). The need for splints or braces is determined by the physician or the physical therapist.

Spring-loaded braces are designed to oppose the action of unparalyzed muscles and to act as partial functional substitutes for the paralyzed muscles[51] (Fig. 41-12). *Resting splints* are designed to maintain a limb or joint in a functional position while permitting the muscles around the joint to relax. They are frequently used for the patient with rheumatoid arthritis to decrease muscle spasms that contribute to joint deformity. *Functional splints* maintain the joint or limb in a usable posi-

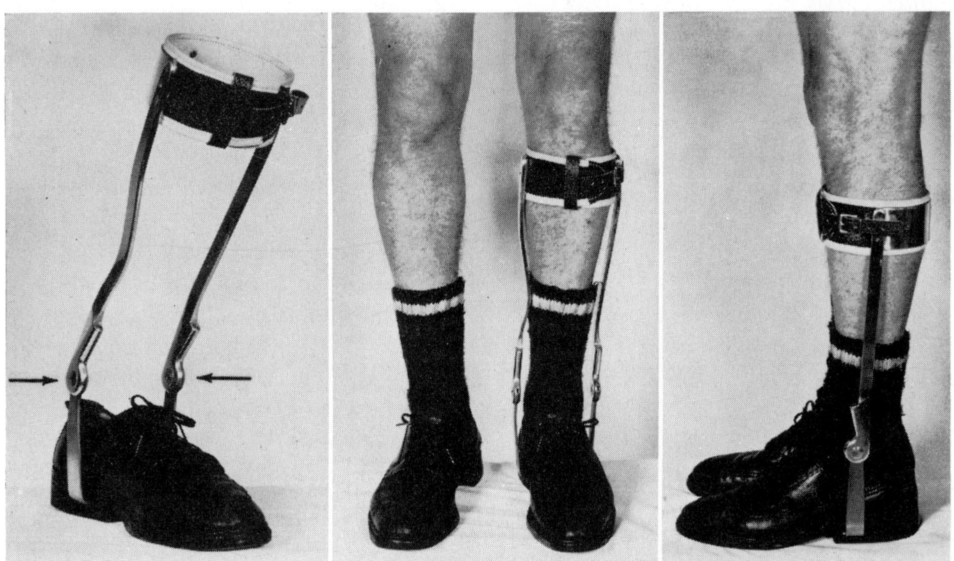

Fig. 41-12. Spring footdrop brace. When weak dorsiflexor muscles are overbalanced by stronger plantar flexors, adjustable spring at ankle hinge of each upright (Klenzak joint, Pope Foundation, Inc.) is used to supply passive dorsiflexion and thus prevent footdrop and an equinus limp. (From Raney, R., and Brashear, H.: Shand's handbook of orthopaedic surgery, ed. 8, St. Louis, 1971, The C. V. Mosby Co.)

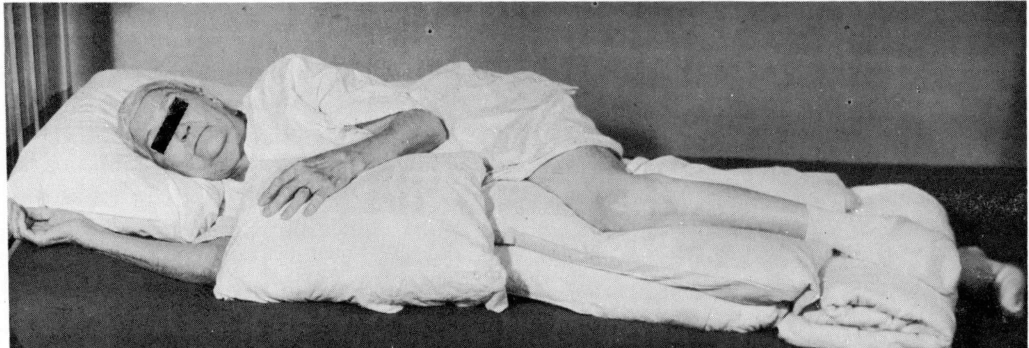

Fig. 41-13. Good side-lying position for patient who has had internal fixation of hip fracture. Upper leg is supported with pillows its entire length, maintaining hip and knee in same plane. Pressure on lower leg is prevented by bringing upper leg forward with flexion at hip and knee. (From Larson, C. B., and Gould, M.: Orthopedic nursing, ed. 8, St. Louis, 1974, The C. V. Mosby Co.)

tion. For example, if the patient has a drop wrist, a splint will support the wrist in a "cock-up" position so that the patient can use his hand for feeding or other functions.[51] (For a complete discussion of splints and braces, see specialized texts.)

Splints and braces are designed to be as lightweight and cosmetically acceptable as possible. Advances have been made in this area by *orthotists* (brace makers) who have developed plastic molded braces made out of lightweight materials that are custom-fit to the patient. In some instances these have replaced the cumbersome metal and leather braces that are often obvious, even though worn under loose-fitting clothing.

Shoes may be modified, or the physician may prescribe corrective shoes to provide special support for the feet. For reasons of safety as well as support, sturdy, preferably lacing shoes of an oxford type should be worn by patients for ambulation. not soft bedroom slippers.

Observations of the patient's skin should be made after an orthosis has been worn for a short period of time (several hours) to make certain that it has caused no skin irritation. The skin must be checked for areas of redness or abrasion. If the patient complains of discomfort or has evidence of skin irritation after wearing the brace, it will need to be checked and perhaps readjusted by the orthotist.

Nurses are frequently instrumental in helping the patient make the psychologic adjustment to wearing such appliances, as well as in helping the patient learn to apply and care for them.

The patient is taught how to apply and remove his own brace or splint and how to care for it. Metal braces should be stored upright. Splints fabricated of molded materials should be stored away from sources of heat. Leather materials should be treated occasionally with Neatsfoot Compounds or another leather preservative to prevent their drying and cracking. Additionally, if the patient gains or loses weight after the orthosis is made for him, it may no longer fit. The patient should understand this problem and the need to have the brace adjusted if there is a change in his weight.

Positioning. Principles of positioning (Fig. 41-13) can be found in most fundamental nursing texts. Special considerations for positioning of patients with specific musculoskeletal problems are discussed in Chapter 42. Posture and the specifications for a "good" chair are discussed on p. 841. Wheelchairs are another kind of device that should be mentioned briefly.

Wheelchairs come in a great variety of shapes and sizes and may be equipped with custom features. If a patient is to use a wheelchair as his mode of moving about, the chair should be fitted to him. Familiarity with the equipment available will aid in making the decision as to what chair the patient should use. No wheelchair should be purchased for permanent use by a patient unless someone knowledgeable about wheelchairs, preferably a physical therapist, has evaluated the patient and determined what special equipment is needed. Chairs poorly fitted to the patient's needs can be unsafe, encourage poor posture, and are an unsound financial investment.

Because pain accompanies nearly all musculoskeletal diseases, it must be taken into consideration when positioning the patient. Pain may be exquisite in acute stages of diseases such as rheumatic fever, atrophic arthritis, gout, and diseases of the muscles and tendons. The patient requires the greatest care and gentleness when he must be moved. Fear of pain often causes irritability and can lead to muscular resistance, which worsens the pain. Care must be taken not to jar the bed. Heavy bedclothes may cause added pain. If cradles are used, caution must be taken not to accidentally bump an involved part of the body when adjusting or removing the cradle. Footboards help to relieve the pressure of covers, provided the patient can be kept warm enough during their use. Patients with rheumatoid arthritis must be encouraged to change position frequently, since their general nutrition is often poor and pressure sores and contractures can develop readily. Sometimes a very painful joint such as a wrist, elbow, or ankle can be placed on a pillow, and the pillow and the limb can be moved together when the patient must turn over or otherwise adjust his position. Frequently patients prefer to *move themselves* rather than risk pain from having someone else move them. When that is the patient's preference, *it should be permitted.*

Transfer. Moving patients from one surface to another is termed *transfer.* A number of references are available regarding proper transfer techniques. Those wishing specific information should consult one or more of those references.[35,50] Following are a few basic guidelines:

1. If one side of the body is stronger than the other, *the patient should always be moved toward the strong side.* This guideline correlates with the principle that it is easier to move objects by pulling them than by pushing them. If the patient moves toward his strong side, he is using his strong side to pull his weak side through the required movement. The person assisting with the move should *support the strong side* to make it more effective.
2. If there is any question regarding the patient's ability to cooperate with the transfer, a second person should be standing by for assistance if needed.
3. If the person helping with the transfer has any doubt about his ability to accomplish the transfer safely for himself and the patient, he should obtain help before attempting it.
4. The transfer should be accomplished using the strong muscles of the legs rather than the weak muscles of the back.
5. If lifting is required, there should be adequate help available. If adequate help is not available, the transfer should not be attempted at that time.
6. Whenever possible, pull sheets should be used to move the patient rather than trying to slide him (such as from bed to cart).

Therapeutic exercise. Exercise is a prescribed form of activity designed most often to preserve joint mobility or to strengthen specific muscle groups. These can be simple maintenance exercises (passive range of motion or isometric), or they can be active or resistive exercises (performed against resistance provided by another person or weights). Heat is frequently used to relax muscles and adjoining tissue prior to exercise; however, some patients respond well to cold applications. *Exercise is contraindicated in the presence of acute joint or muscle inflammation* until the inflammatory process subsides.

The patient's exercise program should be tailored to his specific needs and capabilities. The physician or physical therapist generally outlines the program of exercise to be performed and instructs the patient; however, nurses should be aware of the specific exercise program the patient is following in order to support him in performing it or to provide the assistance he needs. They should also be prepared to refer problems to the physician or the physical therapist if further instruction or closer follow-up is necessary. Whatever exercises are prescribed, the patient should be instructed about the purpose, technique, frequency, and duration of performing them, and he should be supervised in the performance of his exercise program until he can do it independently.

Job retraining. As soon as it becomes apparent to the health team that a patient will be unable to return to his former job, the situation should be discussed with him and the types of jobs that he could handle should be explored. Not infrequently, employers will permit a patient to move to another job within the same company, as for example, from a walking job to a desk job, and will undertake the necessary retraining themselves. Others, however, may have to seek a new job. Referrals to vocational guidance and rehabilitation services and job retraining centers (p. 528) are appropriate at this time. Social workers should be made available to such patients for discussion of these services when their use is indicated.

Medication

Although a number of medications are utilized in the treatment of various musculoskeletal problems, the emphasis here will be on those used in the treatment of the various rheumatic diseases.

Salicylates. Salicylates are specific in their antiinflammatory and analgesic effect and are generally considered the *drug of choice* in the treatment of rheumatoid and other forms of arthritis. Because aspirin is a "common" drug, many patients find it difficult to believe that it will be effective in a serious problem like arthritis. Considerable teaching may be necessary to assure the patient that aspirin, taken as ordered, will help relieve his pain, and further, by reducing inflammation, help to prevent joint deformities and other sequelae of acute joint inflammation.

It is not unusual for as many as 12 to 16 tablets (gr v or 320 mg per tablet) of acetylsalicylic acid per day, given in divided doses, to be prescribed for the treatment of arthritic conditions. Blood salicylate levels of 20% to 30% are recommended for the drug to be clinically effective in rheumatoid arthritis.[45] Large doses of acetylsalicylic acid may cause local irritation to the stomach mucosa (gastritis). Consequently, unbuffered aspirin is nearly always given with milk or with meals, or is followed in 1 hour by antacids. Enteric-coated aspirin may be prescribed to help offset the problem of gastritis and the development of ulcers. Other forms of salicylates, such as liquid choline salicylate or salicylsalicylic acid, do not seem to have this pronounced effect and may be prescribed instead of acetylsalicylic acid if the patient demonstrates gastric intolerance.[45]

The signs of salicylate poisoning—ringing in the ears (tinnitus), nausea, vomiting, tachycardia, and hepatic abnormalities—should be watched for, although aspirin usually can be taken over a long period of time without the occurrence of toxicity or the acquisition of tolerance. If tinnitus occurs, the drug is usually discontinued until the symptoms subside, then restarted at a lower dosage level. Aspirin is also known to prolong bleeding time. This is thought to be because of its effect on platelet adhesiveness. For this reason, acetylsalicylic acid is sometimes discontinued 2 weeks prior to elective surgery. Further, because of its effect on bleeding time, aspirin is being used prophylactically as an anticoagulant drug following some forms of major surgery, such as total hip arthroplasty.

Persons with rheumatoid arthritis who are taking aspirin tend to perspire a great deal. When they are on bed rest, they will require frequent bathing and frequent linen changes for comfort and skin protection.

Other nonnarcotic, antiinflammatory, and analgesic agents. There are other antiinflammatory and analgesic agents that can be used in the treatment of various rheumatic diseases. Propoxyphene hydrochloride (Darvon) and acetaminophen (Tylenol) may be used as helpful analgesic adjuncts to acetylsalicylic acid (ASA) therapy. Indomethacin (Indocin), an antiinflammatory agent, may be effective for patients who do not respond to aspirin, but side effects (occipital headaches, gastrointestinal disturbances) are common. Phenylbutazone (Butazolidin), a potent antiinflammatory agent, is very effective in the treatment of acute inflammatory episodes, but because of its potential to produce gastric irritation and bone marrow depression, is generally confined to short-term (7 to 10 days) use.[45] Ibuprofen (Mortin), tolmetin sodium (Tolectin), and fenoprofen calcium (Nalfon) are all relatively new nonsteroidal antiinflammatory agents that are now being used to treat rheumatoid arthritis and degenerative joint disease. While these drugs are now receiving wide attention, it will be some time before their usefulness can be fully determined.

Antimalarials. Antimalarial drugs, hydroxychloroquine (Plaquenil) and quinacrine (Atabrine), are used to help control inflammatory joint disease when salicylate therapy alone is insufficient. Because response is slow, hydroxychloroquine is given on a trial basis in doses of 200 mg twice a day for a period of 3 to 6 months. If improvement occurs, the dose is adjusted to 200 mg once daily. If there is no favorable response, the drug is discontinued.[45] Toxic reactions include gastrointestinal upset, rash, headaches, and retinal changes. The latter problem is of the most concern. Patients who are placed on hydroxychloroquine therapy should have baseline eye examinations when treatment is begun and every 6 months thereafter. If retinal changes are detected early, they are reversible, providing the drug is discontinued. If not detected until later, changes resulting in visual loss may not be reversible. Patients who are begun on hydroxychloroquine therapy should be advised of this toxic effect and be encouraged to have regular eye examinations.

Quinacrine, used in the treatment of arthritis and the skin rash of systemic lupus erythematosus, will cause yellowing of the skin. This yellowing can be controlled if the drug is periodically discontinued.[45] Patients are generally advised of this side effect before treatment is begun.

Corticosteroids. The corticosteroid drugs have a potent antiinflammatory effect. They are used in chronic connective tissue diseases (rheumatoid arthritis, systemic lupus erythematosus, progressive systemic sclerosis, polymyositis, and the various forms of necrotizing vasculitis) to control inflammation and reduce pain. They also inhibit other effects of inflammation such as the overgrowth of fibrous tissue. *In most instances, steroid drugs are not used if other, less toxic forms of treatment will be effective.* A major objective in treating patients with corticosteroids is to control symptoms at dosage levels that will cause the fewest side effects and complications. Depending on the severity of the disease being treated, the dosage may range anywhere from the equivalent of 1 mg of prednisone (Deltasone) to 200 mg of prednisone per day.[45] The latter doses, equivalent to 800 mg of hydrocortisone, are not considered excessive in the treatment of such problems as severe lupus vasculitis. Steroids may be administered orally, intramuscularly, intraarticularly (to treat inflammation in a particular joint), intravenously, or topically (in the form of creams and ointments to treat skin rashes or lesions).

Side effects and toxic effects are dose related; the higher the dose, the more likely complications are to occur. Side effects include an increased susceptibility to infection and decreased healing potential caused by suppression of the inflammatory responses; osteoporosis; psychologic disturbances (euphoria, depression, manic-depressive psychoses), particularly when dosages *per day* reach or exceed the equivalent of 40 mg of prednisone; gastrointestinal irritation and ulceration; diabetes mellitus; myopathy; hypokalemia; and hypertension. These problems are generally reversible if steroid therapy is discontinued. If treatment of the disease demands that steroid therapy be continued, some of these problems are amenable to treatment; for example, diabetes may be treated with insulin, and hypertension with sodium restriction and antihypertensive drugs.[8]

Another major problem to be considered in the management of persons who are being treated with steroids is that *prolonged steroid therapy suppresses adrenal cortical activity;* therefore the body is incapable of mounting its own response in times of severe stress. If the steroids are suddenly withdrawn, or if the person is subjected to physical trauma such as accident or surgery, he may suffer adrenocortical insufficiency. (For further information on adrenal insufficiency, see p. 579.) Persons taking steroid drugs for musculoskeletal problems should observe the same precautions as carried out by persons taking steroids as a hormonal replacement (p. 580).

Gold therapy. Treatment with gold salts is effective in inducing partial or complete remission in many patients with rheumatoid arthritis and in some patients with psoriatic arthritis.[45] Aurothioglucose (Solganal) and gold sodium thiomalate (Myochrysine) are the two forms of gold most frequently used. The usual dose is 10 mg given intramuscularly as a test dose. If no ill effects such as *nitritoid vasomotor reaction* (flushing, lightheadedness, syncope) or other evidences of clinical or laboratory toxicity are encountered, a second dose of 25 mg is given. Then 50 mg are administered at weekly intervals until the patient has received a total of 750 to 1,000 mg. A maintenance dose of 25 to 50 mg is then given every 3 to 4 weeks to maintain remission. Steroids, dimercaprol (BAL), or d-penicillamine (Cuprimine) may be needed to treat untoward reactions.[45]

While gold salts control the symptoms of rheumatoid arthritis in some patients, they may cause serious reactions. Gold toxicity may cause severe renal and hepatic damage, and gold may be deposited in the cornea of the eye. Dermatitis is a common side effect. Before gold is administered, the patient is checked for sore mouth, a metallic taste in the mouth, skin rash or itching of the skin, and diarrhea. Blood and urine studies are done prior to each of the first 15 to 20 injections and every second or third injection thereafter. Evidence of toxicity includes a decreased platelet count, leukopenia, eosinophilia, or proteinuria.[45] Mild toxicity is treated by stopping the gold therapy, while more severe reactions may be treated with corticosteroids.[45]

Immunosuppressive agents. Immunosuppressive agents—azathioprine (Imuran), cyclophosphamide (Cytoxan), and chlorambucil (Leukeran)—have been used on an *investigational basis* in the past several years for patients with severe diseases, such as lupus vasculitis and "malignant" rheumatoid arthritis, which do not respond to treatment, or for patients who have toxic reactions to other forms of therapy.[45] *They are used only with great care because of their severe side effects and the attendant risks of the development of neoplasms.*

Narcotic analgesics. The use of narcotic analgesics (morphine sulphate, codeine phosphate, meperidine [Demerol]) is generally discouraged in patients with chronic arthritic conditions, as their effect is only temporary, they are not antiinflammatory, and the patient can develop a tolerance to them. Narcotic agents do have their place in the treatment of acute injuries to the musculoskeletal system and are a vital adjunct to the management of the patient following orthopedic surgery. They should, however, be withdrawn in favor of nonnarcotic agents when the patient's pain level permits.

Diet

The essentials of good nutrition, including fruits, vegetables, proteins, and vitamins, are as important for individuals with musculoskeletal problems as for anyone else. Special diets are usually not recommended except in instances where the patient is overweight or has some metabolic problem such as gout (p. 890).

The patient should be urged to eat regular meals and should be given plenty of time to eat. Even if the patient has marked limitation of movement, he should be urged to feed himself (Fig. 41-14). This may require that food be prepared beforehand, for example, cut up, or that the patient be provided with special feeding utensils (p. 842). Foods should be attractively served.

Patients who have restricted mobility may have difficulty with constipation. Foods high in roughage or fiber should be available to help relieve this problem. The diet for a patient who has had a fracture needs to be high in protein, iron, and vitamins if bone repair is to progress normally.

During immobility, catabolic activity is accelerated, producing a rapid breakdown of cellular materials. This leads to protein deficiency and negative nitrogen balance. Decalcification and demineralization of bone takes place *during immobility* regardless of the quantity of calcium intake. Increasing calcium in the diet above normal requirements is *not* recommended for the immobile patient because it cannot be used. A diet high in protein is indicated, however, in order to overcome protein deficiency and return the body to a state of *positive nitrogen balance.* At times 150 to 300 g of protein are required daily to achieve this.

Weight gain should be avoided if at all possible. Added weight increases the patient's energy consumption and causes weight-bearing joints to be abnormally stressed. For the individual who has joint problems such as with degenerative joint disease or rheumatoid arthritis, every movement can be made a task because of

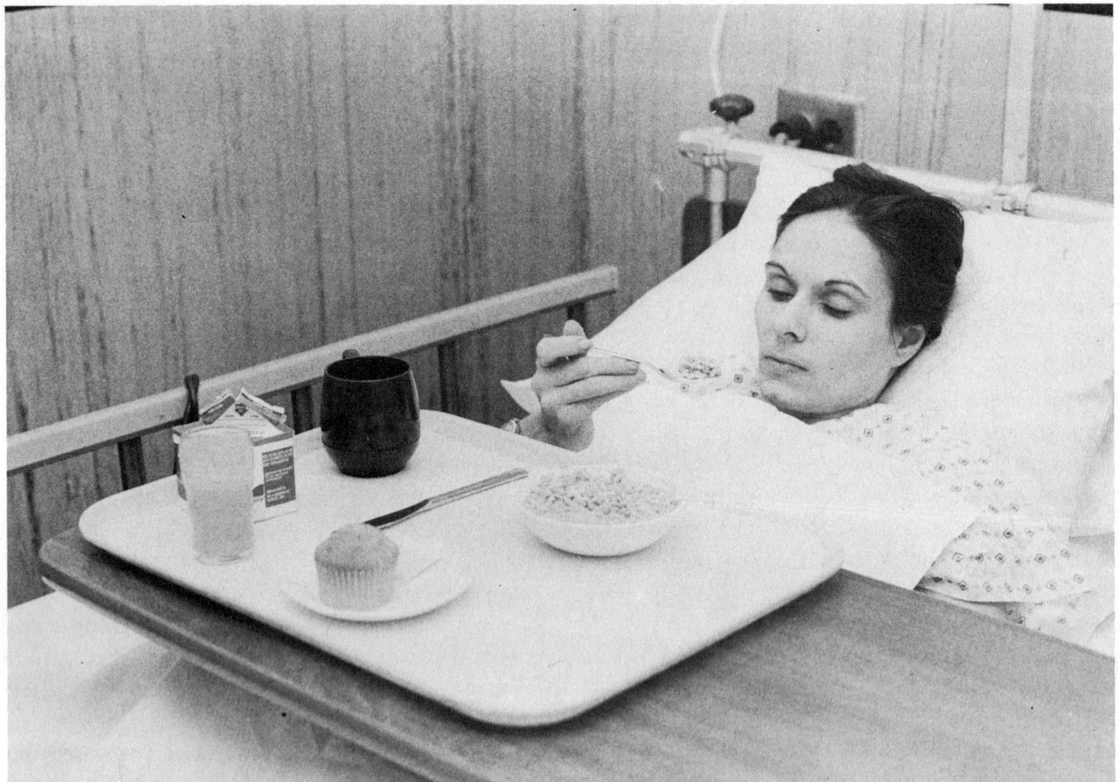

Fig. 41-14. Patient who can neither sit up nor lie on one side to eat meals can still be made comfortable with some elevation of head and shoulders on pillows. Additional means of elevating patient to a more upright position is to put frame of bed in reverse Trendelenburg position.

excessive weight. For many individuals with mobility problems, the problem of weight and movement becomes a vicious circle. Mobility is impaired, therefore activity is limited, calories are not used in activity, more weight is added, and further immobility results as the individual finds it harder to move the weight he must carry. Weight restricts mobility, and weight gain may be inevitable if mobility is decreased. The cycle must be broken, and it must be broken by weight loss.

Psychologic and social support

The importance of family support for patients with musculoskeletal problems, especially chronic problems, is discussed in Chapter 40. When problems are serious enough to require that the patient change his lifestyle and limit his activities, family members must be given the same opportunity to cope as the patient. Social workers and other members of the health team are very often instrumental in assisting the patient and family to define new roles and responsibilities that each can assume with the least disruption in family continuity.

The idea of trying to help the patient "accept" his disability is generally not workable. Most musculoskeletal disabilities have a visible form, and patients know that they look, walk, use their hands, or sometimes even talk differently than "normal" people. They know that they are physically limited and that they cannot do all the things they would like or even need to do. As the physical problems become more pronounced and more limiting, it can be expected that the patient will go through a period of depression and grieving for his lost abilities. Sometimes it is necessary for the patient to have psychiatric counseling before he can move into a phase of adapting to his illness. *Adaptation* is a more functional term than "acceptance." The patient may never accept his illness, but he may *adapt* to it very well by changing his life style and adjusting his level of activity.

It is the process of adaptation and the individual's capacity to make adaptations that must be tapped by those caring for patients with musculoskeletal problems. Helping the patient to see that there are ways of doing things in spite of limitations on motor ability, that he can lead an active life in spite of activity limitation, and that there are measures that can be taken toward pain relief and preservation of remaining function are all interventions appropriate and necessary in the care of these patients.

Outcome criteria for persons with motor problems requiring conservative interventions

The patient or significant others can:

1. Explain the ADL program.
   a. Demonstrate competence and independence in all ADL that are within his physical capabilities.
   b. Explain in what areas, if any, help is necessary.
   c. Explain what provisions have been made for obtaining that help.
   d. Explain limitations of ADL that must be observed and for what period of time.
2. Explain medication regimen.
   a. Explain the expected effect, dosage, administration times, side effects, and toxic effects of each of the prescribed medications.
   b. Demonstrate safe, competent practice in administering each medication.
   c. Explain what is to be done if toxic effects occur.
   d. Explain the nature and rationale for any special precautions that must be taken in relation to the prescribed drugs (such as with antacids, regular eye examination, special laboratory studies).
3. Explain pain relief.
   a. Explain the use of pain-relieving agents.
   b. Explain and demonstrate the value of moderating activity and rest.
   c. Explain and demonstrate various positioning techniques that will relieve pain.
   d. Demonstrate the safe use of heat and cold applications to relieve pain and stiffness.
   e. Demonstrate the application, use, removal, and proper care of various splinting or bracing devices.
4. Explain exercise program.
   a. Explain the rationale for and demonstrate correct performance of prescribed exercise program.
5. Explain use of assistive and supportive devices.
   a. Demonstrate correct use of feeding, bathing, and dressing utensils.
   b. Demonstrate safe and proper use of prescribed ambulatory or locomotor device on level surfaces (and when appropriate, stairs).
   c. Explain weight-bearing limitations.
6. Explain safety precautions.
   a. Describe the safety devices to be obtained for use at home and how and where they will be obtained.
   b. Describe and demonstrate how these safety devices and precautions will be used at home.
   c. Describe what alterations must be made in the home environment to render it safe.
7. Explain preventive measures or techniques.
   a. Demonstrate proper positioning techniques in the prevention of contractures and atrophy.
   b. Demonstrate joint-protection techniques to prevent stress or damage to joints.
   c. Demonstrate proper body mechanics in ADL.
   d. Explain the use of bracing or splinting techniques in preventing damage to the extremities.
   e. Explain the value of maintaining an "ideal" weight to prevent joint stress and fatigue.
8. Explain diet.
   a. Explain the importance of maintaining an "ideal" weight.
   b. Demonstrate knowledge of prescribed dietary restrictions through ability to select foods that are within the dietary restrictions.
9. Explain follow-up care.
   a. Explain plans for follow-up care.
   b. Explain what he will do if he runs short of medication or experiences some complication.

□ Surgical intervention

Patients admitted to hospitals for orthopedic procedures usually fall into one of two categories: persons who have suffered trauma such as a fracture, or persons who require an elective orthopedic procedure for the correction of deformity, relief of pain, or the restoration of musculoskeletal function. There are four major objectives of orthopedic treatment: (1) *restoration or maintenance of function of a body part,* (2) *prevention of deformity,* (3) *correction of deformity* if it already exists, and (4) *development of the patient's powers of compensation and adaptation* if loss of function or permanent deformity is not preventable.[51]

Prior to performing surgery, the orthopedist considers what procedure is best suited to achieve the objectives for the individual patient. There will usually be a discussion with the patient or the patient's family concerning the outcomes that may be expected following the recommended procedure. It is important that those caring for the patient in both the preoperative and postoperative periods know and understand what the expected outcomes are so that care may be adapted to achieving them. To illustrate, the expected outcomes following a total knee replacement will not be the same for a 75-year-old woman with multiple joint involvement from rheumatoid arthritis as they would be for a 50-year-old man with degenerative joint disease in only one knee. Orthopedic care is highly individualized to the patient being treated, and those who work with orthopedic patients must not lose sight of the practical aspects of the treatment rationale.

Trauma

Initial care. Patients who are admitted to orthopedic units following trauma are usually seen because of fractures, and the management of patients with fractures will be discussed next.

Treatment of the acute fracture is usually carried out in the hospital's emergency room or in the operating room prior to the patient's admission to the general hospital unit. The patient will have had little or no opportunity to become oriented to the hospital or to the care that he will be receiving. Additionally, he will most likely be frightened or overwhelmed by what has happened to him, groggy from pain medications or anesthesia, and in pain. He will need careful and often repeated explanation and direction regarding positioning, skin care routines, the need for him to perform adequate deep breathing and coughing, and measures for pain relief. Direction, explanation, and physical handling must be accomplished gently but efficiently during the initial stages of hospitalization. The patient must be given time to adjust to the situation before he can begin to understand how he can cooperate in his care.

During the initial 24- to 48-hour period there are many observations of the patient that must be carried out. Circulation and sensation in the involved extremity must be checked on an hourly basis. Evidence of impaired circulation (coolness, cyanosis, poor capillary refill) or impaired sensation (diminished sensation, parasthesias, intense pain) must be reported to the physician immediately, as these signs can indicate damage to arteries or nerves. Some swelling of an injured extremity may be expected and is most often well controlled by elevating the extremity. However, unrelieved swelling of an extremity that is in a cast or a compression dressing can result in tissue damage and neurologic impairment. Unusual swelling, and the pain that usually accompanies it, must also be quickly reported to the physician so that measures may be taken to relieve pressure and reduce the swelling.

Fractures of the hip and spine may be complicated by paralytic ileus (p. 1293), and pulmonary embolus or fat embolus (pp. 1130 and 905) are not infrequent complications of fractures of the extremities. The patient must be observed carefully for signs and symptoms of these complications.

As with any postanesthesia patient, the patient who has been operatively treated for a fracture should have supervised pulmonary toileting, frequent turning, and leg exercises. Positioning of the patient must be carried out with careful attention to avoid altering the alignment of the fracture, changing the direction of the pull of the traction, compromising the integrity of the cast, or placing undue stress on the internal fixation device. It is of the utmost importance that, before any changes in position are undertaken, there be an understanding of where the fracture is, the nature of the fracture, the method used to reduce the fracture, and the tolerances of that particular method. This information, as well as any special precautions that are to be observed, should be obtained from the orthopedist.

Skin care, with attention to turning, petalling rough edges of casts (p. 858), proper cleansing of pin sites (p. 869), and maintenance of good hygiene, must be conscientiously carried out, particularly when treatment of a fracture demands that the patient be confined to bed for a period of time.

Objectives in the treatment and care of fractures include reduction of the fracture, maintenance of the fragments in the correct position while healing takes place, and prevention of excessive loss of joint mobility and muscle tone. Care must also be taken to prevent complications and maintain good general health so that after healing takes place the patient can continue activity as before his accident or injury.

Reduction of fractures. *Reduction* is the term used for the return of bone fragments to their normal position. This may be accomplished by closed manipulation, traction, or surgery.

Closed manipulation. When closed manipulation is used to reduce a fracture, the patient is often given a general anesthetic. The physician reduces the fracture by pulling on the distal fragment (manual traction) while he or someone else applies countertraction to the proximal fragment until the bone fragments engage or fall into their normal alignment. The physician may also apply direct pressure over the site of the fracture to correct angulation or lateral displacement of a fragment. Usually when this type of reduction is performed, a cast is applied to hold the fragments in the desired position while healing occurs.

Traction. Continuous traction (pull on the affected extremity) for a period of days or even weeks may be necessary to reduce fractures of the femur or humerus because the large muscles draw the bone fragments out of normal alignment, making immediate reduction by manual traction impossible. Continuous traction may also be used to reduce fractures when there is very extensive tissue damage and when the physical condition of the patient is such that anesthesia cannot be safely given. Thus traction may be used for immobilizing the limb while soft tissue healing takes place, for reducing the fracture, and for maintaining correct position of fragments during bone healing.

Open reduction. Open reduction may be necessary if closed manipulation or traction is unsuccessful. Open reduction has the advantage of allowing visualization of the fracture and surrounding tissues. The bone fragments can be arranged and held by internal fixation if necessary. This method is indicated when there is soft tissue caught between bone fragments or when there is known damage to nerves or blood vessels. The disadvantages of open reduction are the need for anesthesia and the possibility of introducing organisms into the fracture site at the time of surgery. In certain fractures, open reduction is the treatment of choice. Even then it may not be used if closed reduction or traction will suffice.

Healing of the fracture (Chapter 42) following reduction occurs over a period of time, depending on the location and severity of the fracture, blood supply to the body part, and the age and general physical condition of the patient. Evidence of callus formation (p. 906) on x-ray films indicates the healing has begun. Eventually callus is replaced by true bone that grows from beneath the periosteum of each fragment to meet and fuse across the defect. *Delayed healing* or *delayed union* is said to occur when the fracture has not healed within the usual time for the particular bone involved. Delayed healing will occur if the space between the two bones is such that neither the callus nor bone cells can bridge the gap, if the callus is broken or torn apart by too much activity, if muscle or fascia is caught between the fragments, if an infection develops, or if there is poor blood supply to the part or marked dietary deficiency. Occasionally delayed union occurs with no obvious cause. Open reduction and more complete immobilization may be necessary.

Nonunion is the term used when healing does not take place even in much longer time than is usually required. Congenital conditions and obscure medical diseases occasionally account for this, and nonunion may occur in the aged. When it occurs, the patient may have to wear a brace to support the limb. If the fracture is in the lower extremity, crutches may have to be used indefinitely. Surgery may be performed and an attempt made to unite the fragments with a bone graft. Nonunion occurs most often in the middle of the humerus, the neck of the femur in older people, the lower third of the tibia, and the carpal bones of the wrist.

It should be noted that *impacted fractures* do not need to be reduced. However, some form of immobilization, such as a sling in the case of an impacted fracture of the humerus, may be used to prevent movement or use of the affected extremity that could lead to displacement of the bone fragments.

Immobilization of the reduced fracture. The purpose of immobilization is to hold the bone fragments in contact with each other until healing takes place. All activity of the part that might cause separation of the fragments is restricted, and the fractured bone is kept in position by immobilizing the entire limb. Usually immobilization includes the joints immediately proximal to and distal to the fractured bone. Devices for external immobilization include bandages, adhesive tape, plaster-of-Paris casts, splints, braces, cast-braces, and traction. Internal immobilization (or internal fixation) may be accomplished by such devices as metal pins, screws, plates, and nails. These devices, made of stainless steel or vitallium, are used to hold the bone fragments together when an open reduction is done. A plaster-of-Paris cast may be used to provide extra protection in instances when a comminuted fracture has occurred.

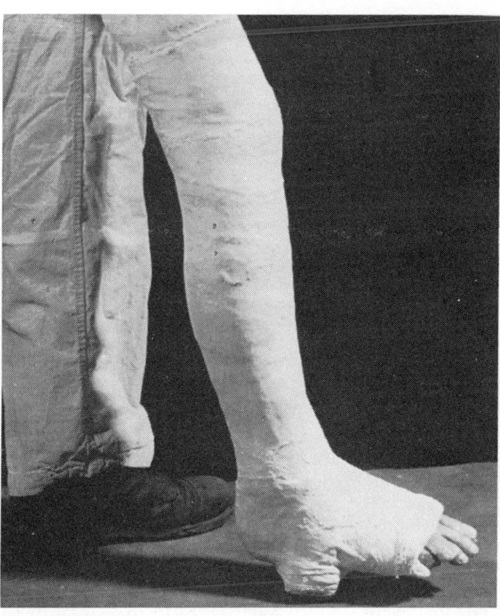

Fig. 41-15. Long leg walking cast. A wooden or hard rubber block or metal iron may be incorporated into plantar surface of cast to provide stable surface for weight bearing when weight bearing is permitted. (From Larson, C. B., and Gould, M.: Orthopedic nursing, ed. 8, St. Louis, 1974, The C. V. Mosby Co.)

Plaster casts. Plaster-of-Paris casts have been used for many years and are still widely employed in the treatment of fractures. Unless a cast has been applied to the entire trunk and legs, the person who is treated with a plaster-of-Paris cast can usually move about and carry on most activities of daily living (Fig. 41-15). Often the person may return to school or to work and participate in many activities without damage to the site of injury. Use of casts shortens hospitalization, and many persons with simple fractures can be treated in a physician's office, the emergency room, or the outpatient department of a hospital. After a short period of observation, they can be discharged and treatment continued under close medical or nursing supervision.

Plaster-of-Paris casts can, however, restrict activities because of their weight and their inflexibility. A cast can cause complications because of interference with normal physiologic functions and can cause actual physical injury if incorrectly applied and improperly cared for. A cast

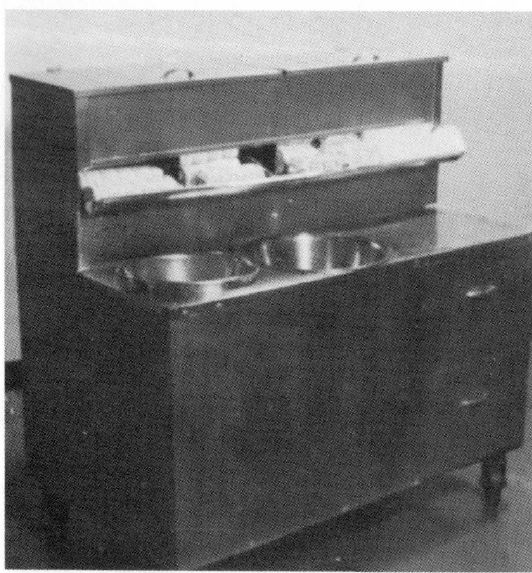

Fig. 41-16. Portable plaster cart contains all supplies necessary to apply or repair cast at patient's bedside. (From Larson, C. B., and Gould, M.: Orthopedic nursing, ed. 8, St. Louis, 1974, The C. V. Mosby Co.)

applied to the arm or shoulder may limit the kind of clothing worn and may interfere with eating, writing, or other uses of the arm. If applied to the leg, a cast may change body alignment, putting strain on the opposite leg, and limit locomotion.

Those caring for the person must know not only how to maintain the integrity of the cast, but must understand how the person is affected by it. The person must be helped to be as independent as possible. Care is designed to help prevent complications, and the patient is monitored for early signs of complications. Developing complications are reported to the physician promptly.

APPLICATION OF THE CAST. Most hospitals have a specially equipped cast room where casts are applied. Some hospitals also have a cart equipped with plaster and other cast material that can be taken to the bedside (Fig. 41-16).

Plaster-of-Paris bandages come in various widths (5 to 20 cm). Each roll is wrapped in waxed paper to prevent sifting of the plaster from the bandage and to prevent deterioration from exposure to moisture. The bandage itself is made of crinoline into which plaster-of-Paris (gypsum or calcium sulfate dihydrate) has been rubbed. When water is added, the gypsum assumes its crystalline state and the wet plaster bandage can be molded to fit the shape of a body part or wrapped about a limb. When the water evaporates, the cast becomes firm and is able to withstand considerable stress and strain. The number of layers of plaster used determines the strength of the cast.

After reduction has been accomplished and before the cast is applied, the skin is usually protected with sheet wadding (a thick, nonabsorbent cotton web covered with starch to hold it together), and felt or sponge rubber is used over bony prominences to protect them from pressure. Tubular stockinette, from 5 to 45 cm wide, is used as lining for the cast and is applied so that it will extend over the edge to cover the round edges of the plaster. The excess stockinette and sheet wadding are usually folded back over the cast after it has been applied and bound down with a final roll of plaster.

If the cast is applied elsewhere than in a special plaster room, the floor and table should be protected from wet plaster. When the person who will apply the cast is ready, the bandage is placed in a bucket of water at 21 to 24 C (70 to 75 F) for 5 seconds. The bandage should be carefully removed from the water so that none of the plaster is lost. It should be held horizontally with an end in the palm of each hand and gently compressed to remove excess water. It should then be quickly handed to the person applying the cast so that it can be used before it begins to set. Only a few bandages should be placed in the water at a time. The bucket containing the water should be lined with a cloth or paper to collect waste plaster. When the procedure has been completed, the cloth or paper containing waste plaster can be removed and discarded into a garbage can. The water from the bucket, if it contains no loose plaster, can be emptied into the sink. Plaster-of-Paris will clog ordinary plumbing and should never be emptied into ordinary drains.

CARE OF THE CAST. Plaster bandages are fast setting (3 to 7 min). Thin casts may dry completely in several hours, but thick casts may require several days to dry completely. The cast can be cracked or broken by inadequate support or by unwise handling before it is dry. A wrinkle in the plaster and indentations caused by the fingertips can alter the inner shape of the cast and cause pressure on the body part encased in the plaster. Wet casts should always be handled with the flat of the hand, not with the fingers.

A firm mattress and, if necessary, a bedboard should be used to prevent uneven weight on the fresh plaster cast. To protect the new cast and ensure its efficiency, the patient is carefully transferred from the stretcher onto his bed. If he is conscious, he can move onto the bed with the assistance of one nurse, while another person supports the wet cast at the areas of greatest strain—usually at the joints. If the patient is asleep or is in a body cast, three or four people should lift him onto the bed. The entire cast as well as the patient's head and his extremities must be fully supported.

The wet cast should not lie unsupported on the hard bed because it may become flattened over bony prominences and weight bearing areas such as the back of the heel, buttocks, and shoulders. This can cause pressure. The wet cast should always be fully supported on a pillow or pillows that are protected with waterproof material to prevent their becoming damp. Although the pillows must be protected with a waterproof material, they should also be covered with cloth so that the waterproof material is not directly in contact with the cast. Some heat is given off as the cast hardens. If the cast is completely surrounded with a waterproof material, not only will it not dry but a burn may result. The patient should be in proper body alignment, and there should not be any break in the support provided by the pillows to cause weakening of the cast. If the patient has a cast on the leg, the foot should extend over the edge of the pillow or the bed to avoid pressure on the heel.

In order for the cast to dry, there must be provision for evaporation by exposure to circulating air. A hair dryer or cast dryer can be used to provide warm *(not hot)* moving air; this is particularly helpful when wet, humid weather delays drying. Heat from radiant lamps is not advocated because it can cause severe burns beneath the cast. Cradles equipped with electric bulbs are not recommended unless there is also provision for free circulation of air; moisture-laden air becomes trapped under the cradle and delays the drying process. The cast should not be covered with bed linen until it is dry. Therefore the bed must be made in such a way that the cast is exposed but the patient kept warm and free from drafts. Blankets may be used to protect body parts not encased in plaster.

The patient in a body cast should be turned every 2 hours to ensure uniform drying of the cast, to prevent continuous pressure on any one area while the cast is drying, and to make him more comfortable. Sufficient personnel should be used in turning the patient to ensure support of the patient and the cast. Patients are usually more comfortable turned toward the uninjured side. Whether the patient in a cast may be turned toward the affected side depends on the type of injury sustained.

To protect body and long leg casts from becoming soiled or wet, waterproof material should be applied around the perineal area. Continuous dampening will soften the cast and impair its effectiveness, and a soiled cast lining will irritate the patient's skin and cause an offensive odor. The area can be covered with plastic material, oiled silk, or waxed paper. These materials can be anchored with adhesive or cellophane tape and changed as necessary.

If the cast become soiled, scouring powder on a damp cloth will usually remove surface stains. The area must be allowed to thoroughly dry again. Baking soda rubbed onto the surface of the cast will help to reduce odors emanating from soiled areas. However, there is no way to clean a badly soiled cast; therefore it is essential that preventive measures be used to keep it clean.

People often like to decorate their casts; however, casts should never be covered with paint, varnish, or shellac. Plaster-of-Paris is porous and allows circulation of air to the skin. When the plaster cast is covered with a substance that decreases the porosity, the skin underneath the cast may become macerated.

CARE OF THE PATIENT IN THE CAST. After the patient has been carefully transferred into bed and his cast is supported on pillows, his general condition is checked. After fracture reduction and immmobilization, observations are made for signs of delayed shock such as sudden faintness, dizziness, pallor, diaphoresis, or change in pulse rate. Drainage through a cast is a poor indicator of actual blood loss. The wet plaster acts as a wick to spread the drainage, often making it appear that the patient is losing large amounts of blood when he is not. For this reason the time-honored practice of circling areas of drainage on casts to estimate drainage is now generally considered a useless activity. Monitoring of the patient's systemic signs and symptoms, urinary output, and hematocrit levels are much more accurate indicators of blood loss.

Medication is given as ordered for general pain. Bone pain is one of the most severe types of pain and medications may have to be given as often as every 3 to 4 hours in order to keep the patient comfortable.

The affected extremity is elevated on pillows to aid in preventing edema. Most swelling occurs within the first 24 to 48 hours. Complaints of pressure are often relieved either by elevation or by a change in position. *Continuous pressure, pain, or swelling that is not relieved by change in position or elevation must be reported to the physician at once as this often represents neurologic or circulatory impairment in the affected area.* Neurocirculatory impairment is usually caused by a tight cast or by edema, although it occasionally may be caused by bruising of a blood vessel or by stretching or bruising of a nerve during manipulation or surgery.

Areas of pressure are usually over bony prominences or places where bones lie in close proximity to the skin (the instep, lateral border of the foot, heel, malleoli, iliac crests, and sacrum). The skin distal to the cast is inspected frequently and routinely for signs of vascular impairment. Changes in skin color or temperature (cyanosis or coldness), swelling, and slow return of color (delayed capillary refill) after pressure has been applied to the fingers or toes below the cast indicate that pressure may be restricting circulation.

Signs and symptoms of neurologic impairment include complaints of tightness of the cast, numbness or tingling of the fingers or toes, and loss of motion at the free joints distal to the cast. These sensorimotor distur-

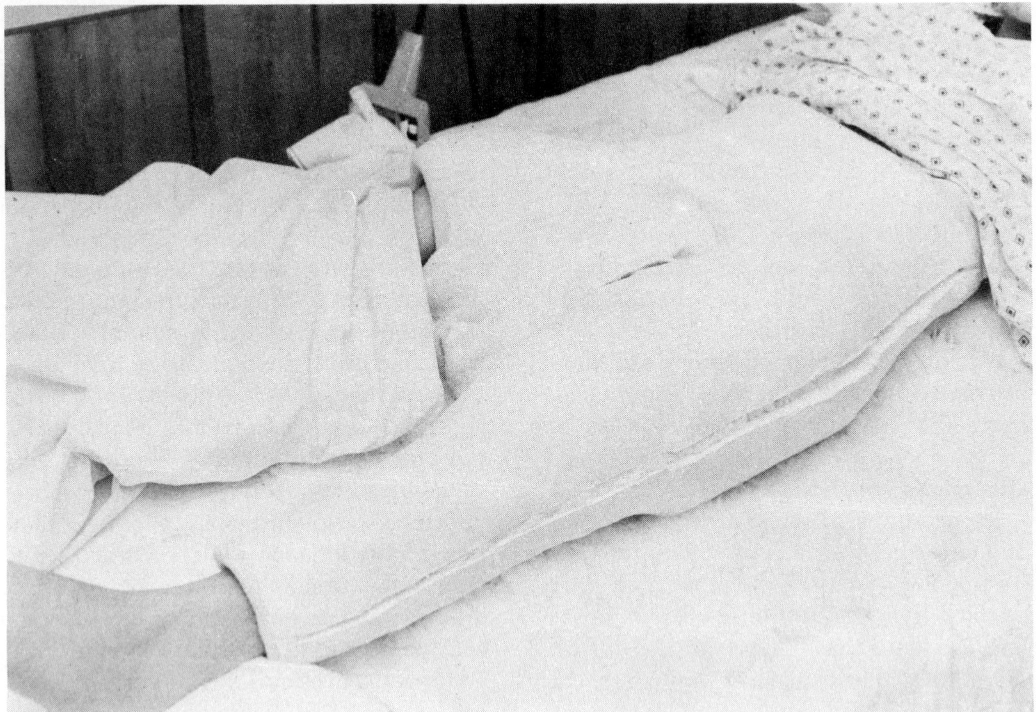

Fig. 41-17. Hip spica cast. Cast was applied to provide immobilization of left femoral fracture. Note that cast was bivalved when patient developed severe pain and swelling of left leg several hours after cast was applied. Ace bandages wrapped over cast to provide support have been removed for purposes of this picture.

bances are indications of nerve compression. The nerve in the lower extremity most often affected is the peroneal nerve, located below the head of the fibula on the lateral aspect of the leg. Continuous pressure on this superficial nerve by a leg cast or by the patient lying with his leg in extreme external rotation may result in paralysis with a loss of the ability to dorsiflex the foot or to extend the toes (drop foot). Any complaint of pressure on the lateral side of the leg, numbness or tingling of the foot, or burning pain in the area covered by, or distal to, the cast may be an indication of nerve compression.

When there is evidence of neurologic or circulatory impairment, the pressure must be relieved at once. Failure to do so can result in nerve paralysis or lack of circulation to the part with resultant necrosis. The ultimate consequence of unrelieved pressure can be the loss of the extremity. Pressure is relieved by splitting the cast and the padding underneath it. If the cast is bivalved (cut in two) (Fig. 41-17), it can be held in place by bandages. This will provide adequate temporary immobilization for the part while relieving the pressure of the cast on the nerve or that caused by edema. A cast cutter should be readily available, and the nurse must know how to bivalve a cast should it be necessary to do so. A new cast will be applied when the swelling is reduced.

Skin care for the patient with a cast must be thorough. Plaster on the skin should be removed with plain water. The skin around and directly under the cast edges should be washed and then massaged with alcohol to prevent skin irritation. Creams and lotions may be used with caution. They tend to soften the skin under the cast and also may cause the skin to stick against the cast lining. In addition, continuous use of excessive lotions dampens the inside of the cast. The skin should also be inspected for pressure areas and signs of irritation from rough plaster edges. Petal-shaped strips of adhesive tape or moleskin may be applied to the exterior surface of the cast, over the rough edges of the cast, and anchored smoothly to the interior surface of the cast to prevent irritation or abrasion. This process is called *petaling*. As the patient remains in the cast, his elbows may become irritated from bracing himself to move about in bed. Frequent massage and protective pads will help to prevent this. An orthopedic bed frame with a trapeze will assist the patient to move about in bed.

If the patient is in a body cast or a long leg cast, the

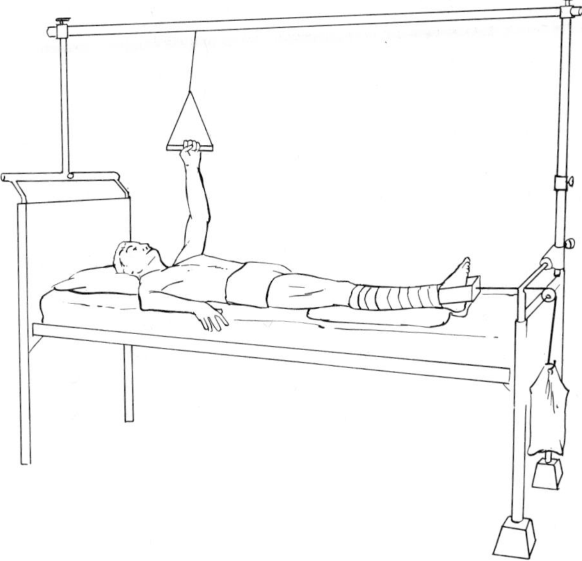

Fig. 41-18. Buck's extension. Note that limb is not raised, but lies parallel with bed. Note also blocks to raise foot of bed to provide countertraction and to help keep patient from moving to foot of bed.

head of the bed should be elevated when a bedpan is used. This helps to keep urine or stool from running back and under the cast. If the cast is new and still damp, it is better to elevate the head of the bed on shock blocks (or use the reverse Trendelenburg position with electric beds) instead of using the gatch, as the gatch will put a strain on the cast and may cause it to crack. A pillow should be placed against the small of the back, and a cotton pad protected with plastic material may be tucked under the sacral area to protect the cast from soiling. The leg in the cast should be supported with pillows so that the patient does not feel insecure in this position. An overhanging trapeze (Fig. 41-18) will permit him to help lift himself as the nurse places the bedpan under him. Side rails also assist the patient to turn and give him protection from falling out of bed.

If abdominal distention is troublesome, a "window" or opening may be cut in the cast over the abdomen. The edges of this opening must also be petaled. Such a window is useful in checking for distention of the bladder.

For the person in a cast, turning from side to back to side to abdomen is seldom restricted by any consideration other than the person's discomfort. The injured part is immobilized and protected from twisting or pulling by the cast.

Many persons are discharged after the cast is dry if there is no evidence of circulatory or nerve impairment. They should be taught never to insert a sharp object (coat hanger, pencil) under the cast, since abrasions by such objects can easily become infected. Small objects (coins) lost in casts become sources of pressure. If a cast is applied to the arm, a sling should be worn to support the full weight of the cast, and the hand should be supported to prevent the development of wrist drop. The ends of the sling should be secured with two pins instead of being tied at the back of the neck. If the sling is to be worn for some time, sling ties may be lengthened with bandage or muslin so that they can be crossed in the back and brought around and tied in the front of the body. This helps to prevent forward and downward pull on the neck that may cause a postural defect and fatigue.

Depending on the injury, the person may or may not be permitted to bear weight on his cast. If weight bearing is permitted, a leg cast is usually fitted with a rubber heel or walking iron that prevents wear on the plaster. Cast shoes having a thick, styrofoam-like, one-piece flat sole and heel, open vinyl sides, and adjustable Velcro closures are also available. (However, weight bearing on a cast is never permitted until the cast is completely dry.) If the cast is a cylinder cast that does not enclose the foot (such as the cast applied following a tibial osteotomy), the person's own shoes can be worn.

CAST REMOVAL. The cast is usually removed when roentgenograms show that union is sufficient to allow safe removal. This is often done in the physician's office or in the hospital cast room or emergency department. The cast is bivalved with manual or electric plaster cutters. While the procedure is not painful, some pressure or vibration may be felt. The skin is usually dry and scaly and is washed as soon as possible with mild soap and water and lubricated with mineral oil. Since there is usually some stiffness of the joints, the limb should be moved very gently. The individual is usually encouraged to move the limb as much as he is able within limits of pain or stiffness. Exercises for the stiff joint are usually started. After a leg cast is removed, swelling and edema occur for some time when the leg is placed in the dependent position. The limb should be elevated during sleep and at intervals during the day. Elastic bandages or stockings may be prescribed to help reduce dependent edema.

PLASTER JACKET. A plaster jacket that extends from the shoulders to below the hips is sometimes used to immobilize the spine of the patient who has a fractured vertebra below the cervical area or another lumbodorsal disorder. Care of the patient in a plaster jacket is the same as care for the patient in a body cast except that in many instances the patient is permitted to ambulate. Once the cast is dry, transferring the patient in and out of bed should be done following the guidelines for transferring the patient who has had a laminectomy or spinal fusion (p. 901).

Traction. Continuous traction, or pull, is used to reduce and immobilize fractures, to overcome muscle spasm, to stretch adhesions, and to correct certain deformities.

SKIN TRACTION. Skin traction is achieved by applying wide bands of moleskin, adhesive, or commercially available devices such as the Richards foam rubber Buck's extension splint directly to the skin and attaching weights to these. The pull of the weights is transmitted indirectly to the involved bone. Buck's extension, Bryant's traction, and Russell traction are the three most common forms of skin traction used for injury to the lower extremities.

Buck's extension is the simplest form of skin traction and provides for straight pull on the affected extremity (Fig. 41-18). It is often used to relieve muscle spasm and to immobilize a limb temporarily, such as the leg when a hip fracture has been sustained by an elderly person and internal fixation is to be done within a short time. The skin of the leg is usually shaved, and tincture of benzoin is applied to protect it if adhesive substances are to be used. (If strips of the commercially available foam rubber Fas-Trac strips, which are wrapped on with Ace bandages, or the Richards splint, which fastens on itself with Velcro, are to be used, shaving and benzoin are not needed.) Adhesive tape or moleskin is placed on the lateral and medial aspects of the leg and secured with a circular gauze or elastic bandage. The tape should not cover the malleoli, as skin breakdown is certain to occur over these bony prominences. The tapes are attached to a spreader bar. The spreader bar should be sufficiently wide to pull the tapes away from the malleoli. Rope is attached to the spreader, passed through a pulley on a crossbar at the foot of the bed, and suspended with weights. The maximum weight that should be applied by skin traction is 3.6 kg (8 lb). Greater amounts of weight will cause skin damage.

Not everyone will be able to be placed in Buck's extension. Contraindications include stasis dermatitis, arteriosclerosis, allergy to adhesive tape, severe varicosities or varicose ulcers, diabetic gangrene, and marked overriding of bone fragments that would require 4.5 kg (10 lb) or more of weight to reduce the deformity.

Russell traction is widely used because it permits the patient to move about in bed somewhat freely and permits bending of the knee joint (Fig. 41-19). This is skin traction in which four pulleys are used. A Balkan frame must be attached to the bed before the procedure is started. Moleskin or adhesive is then applied to the leg as in Buck's extension. The knee is suspended in a hammock or sling to which a rope is attached. This rope is directed upward to a pulley that has been placed on the Balkan frame at a point located over the tubercle of the tibia of the affected extremity. The rope is then passed downward through a pulley on a crossbar at the foot of the bed, back through a pulley on the footplate, back again to another pulley on the crossbar, and then sus-

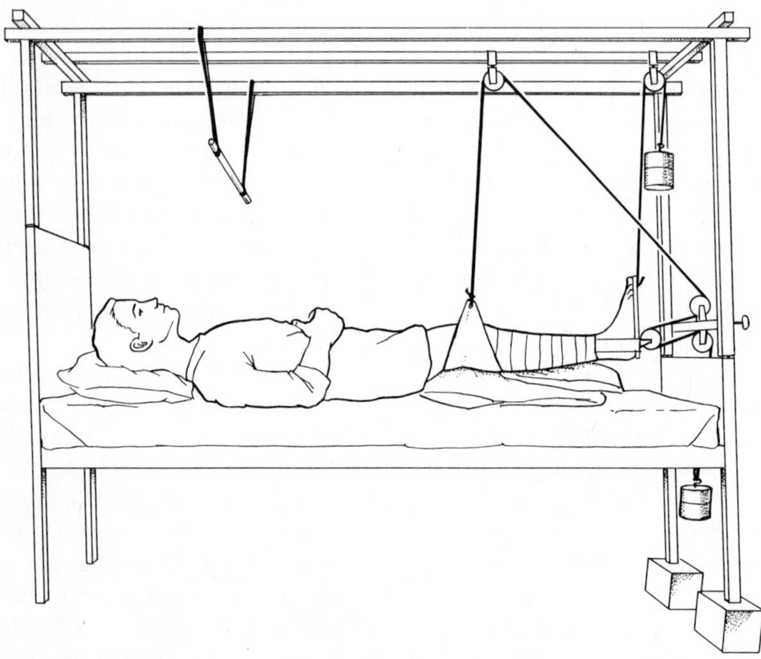

Fig. 41-19. Russell traction. Note that Balkan frame is attached to bed, that leg is supported on pillows, and that heel extends beyond pillow.

pended with weights. Because there is double pull from the crossbar to the footplate, the traction is equal to approximately double the weight used. Since there is upward pull from the hammock, skin under the popliteal space should be protected with a piece of felt or sponge rubber and should be inspected regularly. The patient's heel should just clear the bed so that there is no weight or pressure on the heel. Usually a pillow is placed lengthwise under the thigh, and a second pillow is placed under the leg. This traction results in slight flexion of the hip. The angle between the thigh and the bed should be approximately 20°. Usually the foot of the bed is elevated on blocks (or in the Trendelenburg position for electric beds) to provide countertraction.

Any complaints of pain or discomfort should be reported to the physician at once. Occasionally thrombophlebitis develops from inactivity or from pressure on the popliteal vessels. Often the patient is permitted to have the head of the bed elevated slightly, but as elevation of the head of the bed does reduce the amount of the traction, the physician should be consulted about the amount of elevation permitted. Russell traction is used in the treatment of intertrochanteric fracture of the femur when surgery is contraindicated, especially in the aged. Bilateral Russell or Buck's traction may be used to treat back pain, since it immobilizes the patient and reduces muscle spasm.

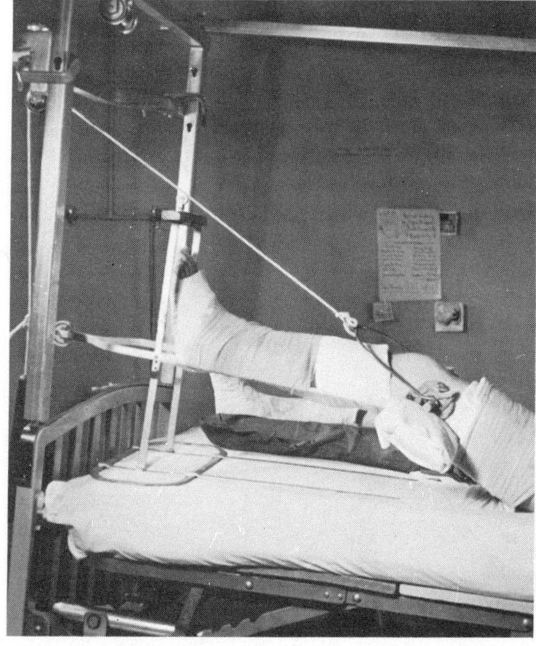

Fig. 41-20. Skeletal traction. Pin has been inserted through distal femur. Sharp ends of pin are covered with cork, and small dressing occludes pin sites. Pin and traction rope are attached to spreader. In this case, entire limb is supported by Braun-Böhler inclined plane splint. (From Larson, C. B., and Gould, M.: Orthopedic nursing, ed. 8, St. Louis, 1974, The C. V. Mosby Co.)

SKELETAL TRACTION. Skeletal traction is traction applied directly to bone. Under general or local anesthesia a Kirschner wire or Steinmann pin is inserted distal to the fracture (the site of insertion varies with the type of fracture) (Fig. 41-20). For a fractured femur, the pin is often inserted through the tibia. The pin protrudes through the skin on both sides, and the ends are covered with corks or metal protectors. Small sterile dressings are usually placed over the entry and exit sites of the pin. The utmost care must be taken to guard against infection at the pin site, as infection on the surface can proceed to the bone along the pin tract. This may result in osteomyelitis (p. 905). A metal U-shaped spreader or bow is attached to the pin. The rope for the traction is attached to the spreader. Skeletal traction can be used for fractures of the tibia, femur, humerus, and neck or cervical spine. Skeletal traction to the cervical spine is achieved by use of tongs applied to the skull (p. 902).

BALANCED TRACTION. When a balanced or suspension apparatus (Fig. 41-21) is used in conjunction with skin or skeletal traction, the patient is able to move about in bed more freely without disturbing the line of traction. The extremity is balanced with countertraction, and any slack in the traction caused by the patient's movement is taken up by the suspension apparatus. The use of a balancing apparatus also facilitates nursing measures such as bathing the patient, caring for his skin, and placing the bedpan correctly.

A full or half-ring *Thomas* or *Hodgen splint* is used for balanced tractions. (Prior to application, these splints should be checked to see that they are the proper size for the patients who will be using them.) Straps of canvas, muslin, or synthetic "lamb's wool" are placed over the splint and secured to provide a support for the leg. The areas under the popliteal space and heel are left open to prevent pressure on these parts. If it is desirable to have the knee flexed and to permit movement of the lower leg, a *Pearson attachment* is clamped or fixed to the Thomas splint at the level of the knee. The attachment is also covered with a soft, strong material to support the lower leg. The leg is put through the ring and placed on the canvas support. The ring is placed firmly against the ischium. When a half-ring splint is used, the ring is placed on the anterior aspect of the thigh (Fig. 41-22). Rope is attached to the ring or to the frame on either side of the ring and to the end of the Thomas splint, directed upward to pulleys on the frame, and then suspended with weights. Rope is also attached to the end of the Pearson attachment, directed upward to a pulley on the overbed frame, and suspended with weights. A foot support may be fastened to the Pearson attachment to pre-

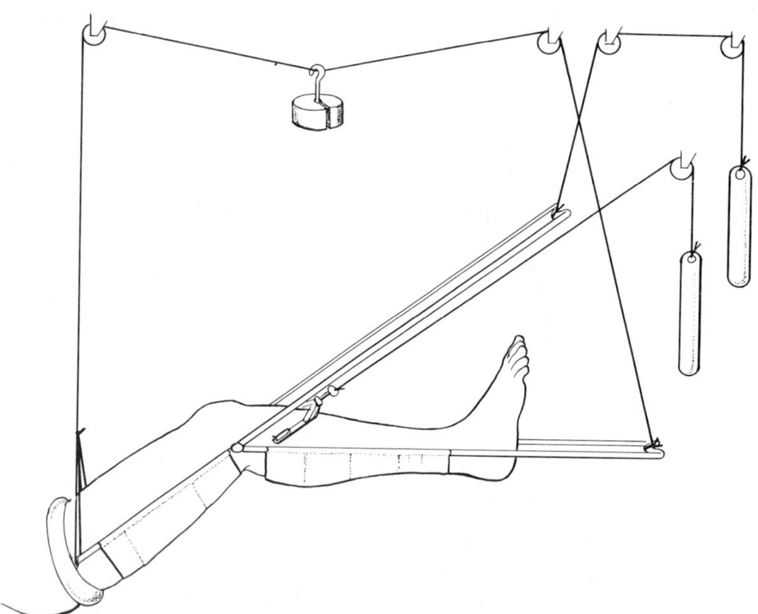

Fig. 41-21. Balanced suspension used in conjunction with skeletal traction.

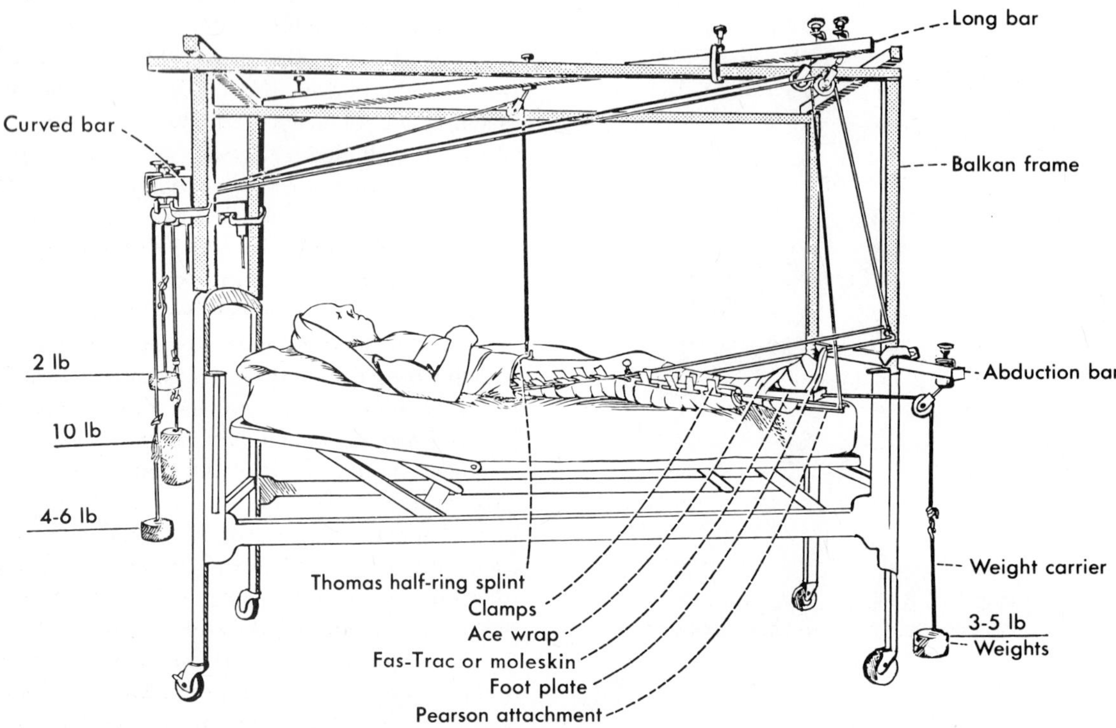

Fig. 41-22. Suspension in Thomas half-ring splint in conjunction with skin traction to lower extremity. Note that in this illustration suspension of splint is arranged at head of bed. (From Larson, C. B., and Gould, M.: Orthopedic nursing, ed. 8, St. Louis, 1974, The C. V. Mosby Co.)

vent foot drop, or the foot may be left free so that the patient can exercise it more fully. Skin or skeletal traction can be added as described earlier.

The ring is made of smooth, soft, moisture-resistant plastic material or of leather. It is not necessary to wrap the ring with padding. The padding cannot be changed after it is applied, and inevitably it gets damp from perspiration, bedpan accidents, and bathing the skin. The padding holds moisture against the skin and causes skin irritation. When the patient is bathed, the skin beneath the ring must be moved back and forth so that all areas are washed, dried thoroughly, and powdered. The patient may be turned toward the leg in the splint.

NURSING INTERVENTION FOR THE PATIENT IN TRACTION. Before the nurse attempts to give care to a patient in traction, the patient's problem and what is to be achieved by the use of traction must be clearly understood. For example, the patient with arthritis who is in skin traction to help release flexion contractures of his knees may be permitted to be out of traction for periods of time, whereas the patient with a recent fracture of the femur would be harmed if the traction were released.

In order for traction to be effective, the patient must lie on his back. Turning onto the side or sitting up changes body alignment, and the pull (traction) is lost or becomes less effective. However, patients in traction to the leg can usually be turned *slightly* from side to side to relieve skin pressure. The motion allowed depends on the injury and kind of traction used. Those caring for the patient must consult with the physician to determine what the limitations of motion are so that appropriate care can be planned. The patient will be extremely limited in activity. Limitations should be explained to the patient, and he should be helped to be as comfortable as possible while remaining in the correct position. The patient who must lie flat often feels handicapped and helpless because he cannot readily see what is going on about him. Ceiling mirrors and prism glasses may be used to help the patient feel less isolated. Television sets are sometimes placed on high wall shelves or suspended from the ceiling so that they can be seen by patients who must lie flat in bed.

Traction weight must hang free with no obstruction to interfere with straight, even, continuous pull. Traction should be inspected frequently. For example, when traction is being applied to the lower limb, bedclothes must not press on the rope or against the footplate. The footplate must never push against the foot of the bed or the pulley, since this will completely negate traction. There should be no knots in the rope, since these may become caught in the pulley and interfere with traction. The rope should be long enough so that weight will not be hampered by the pulley as the patient pulls himself up in bed, yet not long enough to rest on the floor if he slips down to the foot of the bed. The rope must be strong enough so that it will not break if more weights are added. The weights must be securely fastened so that they will not drop off if they are disturbed accidentally, and the equipment should be visible so that it is not jarred, swung inadvertently, or present a hazard to persons moving past the bed. If sandbags are used for weights, they are tied to the rope. When regular scale weights are used, they should be fastened with adhesive tape so that they will not slip off. Jarring the bed and swinging the weights may cause pain and upset the patient. Any extremity in traction must be checked frequently for adequate circulation. Patients in Buck's extension or Russell traction should be checked for inability to dorsiflex and invert the foot on the affected side. The inability to perform these motions would be indicative of peroneal nerve damage (p. 858).

An important concept in the care of the patient in traction is that the patient should not suffer from lack of any kind of nursing care because of his immobilization. At first glance it might sometimes appear that good back care, for example, is impossible. This is not true. The patient in traction should be on a firm bed and should have an orthopedic frame or overhead attachment with trapeze bar so that he can help to lift himself and take some weight off his back for short periods. Usually he can be moved enough for good back care to be given and for linen to be changed. This is accomplished by having the patient raise himself straight up in bed with the help of the trapeze while care is given and the bed linen slid under him. Depending on the site and the extent of the fracture, the patient may be permitted to turn toward the side of the fracture enough for back care to be given. It is a good practice for a second nurse or an attendant to steady the traction and even increase the pull slightly as the patient carefully and steadily turns or raises himself. The same principles are followed when the patient has the bedpan placed under him. A very small, flat bedpan (fracture pan) should be used, and the back above the pan should be supported by a small pillow or a bath blanket folded to the height of the pan.

The patient who is in traction needs the same attention to nutrition, elimination, exercise of noninvolved extremities, prevention of postural defects, and skin care as any other patient who is immobilized. Particular attention must be given to the skin that comes into contact with any traction apparatus. For example, the skin over the bony hip prominences may become reddened and painful if a pelvic band is being used, adhesive tape may work downward so that straps may rub against the ankle when skin traction is used on the lower limb, and a *Thomas splint* may cause injury to the skin of the groin. Skin irritation of this kind must be reported to the physician, who may alter the amount of weight used or take other action. Nursing measures to relieve skin irritation are initiated.

Internal fixation. Depending on the location and type of fracture, *open reduction with internal fixation* may be necessary. Open reduction with internal fixation is used only when other methods of reduction are not suitable. Although this method allows direct visualization of the injury, it also carries the risk of infection; consequently, it is performed under the most vigorous aseptic conditions.

Internal fixation is achieved by using a metal device (Fig. 41-23). There are a wide variety of metal pins, wires, intramedullary rods, compression plates, nails, and so on available. Each has its particular advantage and indications for use. The care of the patient who has internal fixation of a fracture depends on the site of the fracture and the device used for stabilization. The major aim of care is to protect the part until healing takes place. Metal that can fatigue and break cannot be expected to substitute for intact bone. If the fixation device breaks, healing of the fracture will be disrupted. Depending on the fracture, protection may be achieved by using a cast, by limiting stressful forces on the metal by restricting positioning, or by placing the patient on limited weight bearing until healing occurs. For examples of care of patients following open reduction with internal fixation, see pp. 906 and 910.

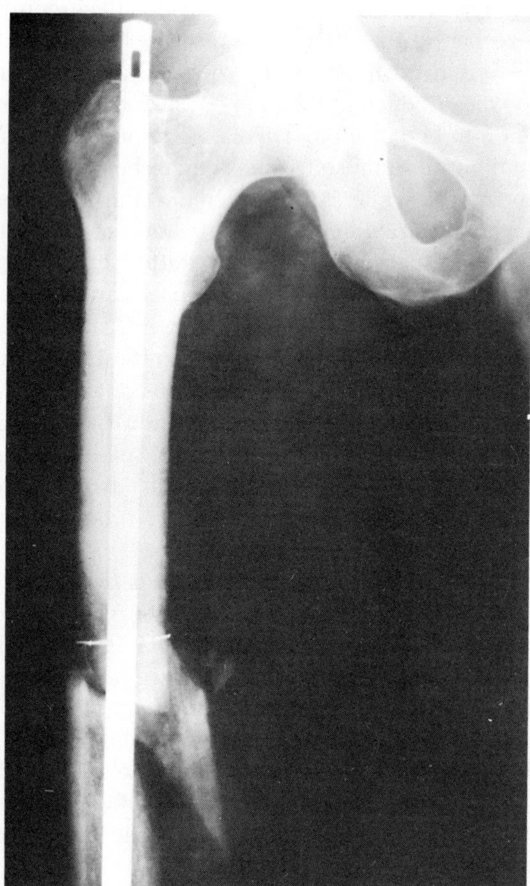

Fig. 41-23. Internal fixation of fracture of middle third of femur by means of intramedullary nail (Kirschner nail).

Cast braces. The cast brace is used in the treatment of patients with femoral shaft fractures. It has three components: (1) a plaster-of-Paris cast (or thigh cuff) that encloses the patient's thigh, (2) two metal or high-density polyethylene hinges, one on either side of the knee, and (3) a short leg plaster-of-Paris walking cast that extends from just below the knee to and enclosing the foot. The proximal ends of the hinges are imbedded in the plaster of the thigh cuff; the distal ends are imbedded in the short leg cast. The thigh cuff compresses the thigh muscles, thus providing immobilization of the fracture fragments. The hinges allow flexion and extension of the free knee joint. The walking cast provides support for the thigh cuff and prevents the thigh cuff from slipping distally.

The advantages of using this apparatus are that the period of time required for fracture healing is shortened and the hip and knee joints can be mobilized. The cast brace is applied after the fracture has been aligned in skeletal traction for 2 to 6 weeks. The patient progresses to fairly normal ambulation with crutches and may even be permitted to return home within a week of the cast brace application.[23]

The care of the patient in a cast brace and the care of the cast are essentially the same as have been outlined on pp. 856 to 859. Particular attention must be paid to checking for neurocirculatory compromise in the affected leg throughout the hospitalization. Some swelling of the knee and foot may be experienced when the leg is in a dependent position during ambulation. This swelling can usually be relieved by prompt elevation of the extremity, but if it is not, the pressure of the cast must be relieved. If knee swelling is present, the knee should be carefully checked to determine if the skin is rubbing against the hinges. Friction from the hinges will quickly abrade the skin.

Halo cast. The halo cast is another apparatus that employs both a plaster-of-Paris cast and a metal frame. It is used to immobilize the cervical spine (or the entire spine) following cervical spinal fusion. It provides for greater stability than a neck brace and has an advantage over cervical tongs because the patient can be ambulatory. A plaster cast, extending from the axillae to the iliac crests, houses a metal frame (Fig. 41-24,*A*). The struts of the frame extend to the skull at the parietal areas. These struts attach to a round metal (halolike) device. The halo itself is fixed to the skull by screws inserted in the same

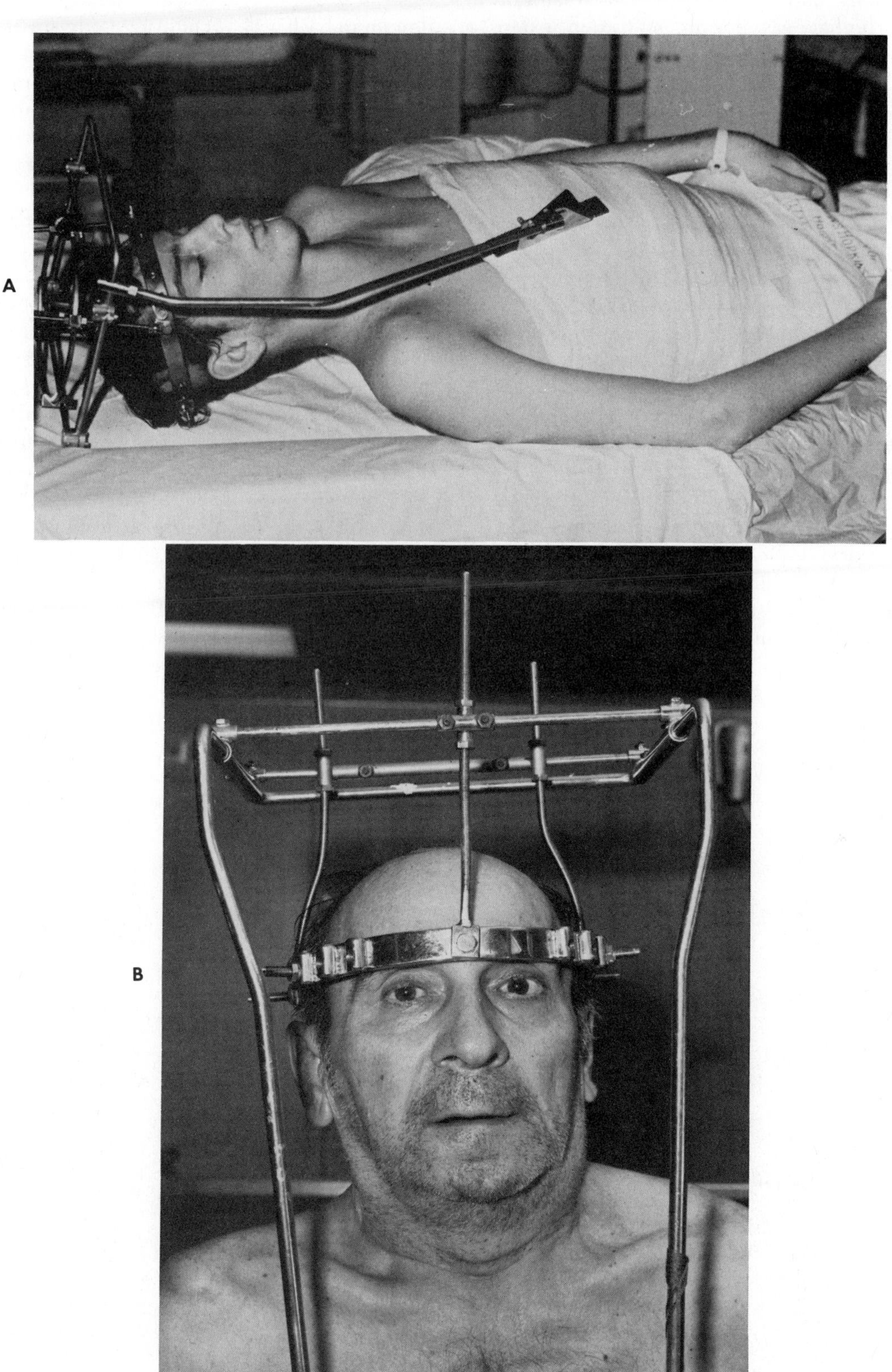
A

B

Fig. 41-24. A, Halo attached to body cast. **B,** Metal ring, or halo, that attaches to skull.

fashion as tongs (p. 902). There are four screws: two located anterolaterally and two located posterolaterally (Fig. 41-24, *B*). The halo cast permits no flexion, extension, or rotational movements of the neck, thus completely immobilizing the site of the fusion to prevent displacement of the grafts.

It is helpful if the patient who is to wear this apparatus has the opportunity to see it and have its function explained to him before it is applied. The cast and the frame are cumbersome, and the idea of having something screwed into the skull frightens most people. It is not reasonable to assure the patient that the frame will not give him discomfort, as some persons do complain of headaches. The patient in a halo cast can be taught to transfer and ambulate, but he will need help to do this in the initial postoperative period, as the weight of the cast and frame will make him feel "top-heavy."

The care of the patient in a halo cast is essentially the same as for the patient in a plaster jacket (p. 859). Additionally, the screws to the skull and the screws that hold the upper portion of the frame together must be checked several times per day *throughout the time that the patient is in the frame* to be certain that they are tight. If any part of the frame is allowed to come apart, the position of the patient's head can change and the fusion can be displaced.

Stryker frame and Foster bed. For the patient with an injury that allows him to be placed flat in bed but who is not allowed to turn, a Stryker frame or a Foster bed may be used (Figs. 41-25 to 41-27). These devices are used for patients with some types of spinal injury. They make it possible to change a person's position from abdomen to back without altering body alignment. Usually the patient on one of these beds is turned every 2 to 4 hours. Traction, particularly cervical traction, can be used on a frame; however, the frame cannot be used for very obese patients because space between the top and bottom frames is inadequate and cannot be adjusted sufficiently.

The beds have two metal frames to which canvas covers are attached. The canvas used for the back-lying position has an opening under the buttocks to allow for use of a bedpan, and the canvas used for the prone-lying position can be cut out so that the male patient can void. When the patient is in the prone position, the canvas should extend from below the shoulders to the ankles, and a narrow head strap should be used to support the forehead. In the prone position the patient can eat, read, and do light activities with his hands. The canvas may be covered with thin sponge rubber mattresses cut the same size as the canvas and covered with bed linen. To turn the patient, the linen, mattress, and opposite canvas and frame are placed in that order over the patient. The frame is then fastened by bolting it securely in place to the metal attachment at the head and foot. Safety straps are placed around both frames; then two people release pivot pins at either end of the frame and slowly turn the patient on the frame from his abdomen to his back or vice versa. The pins are reinserted and the upper frame, canvas, and mattress are removed. The bed has

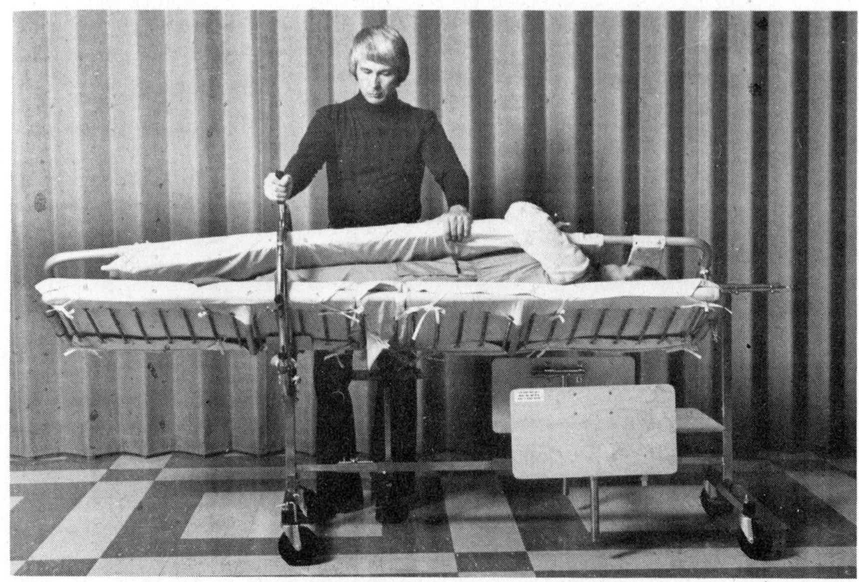

Fig. 41-25. Patient is in supine position on Foster bed. Anterior frame is fastened in place and additionally secured by turning straps prior to turning patient. (From Rantz, M., and Courtial, D.: Lifting, moving and transferring patients, St. Louis, 1977, The C. V. Mosby Co.)

armboard and footboard attachments to use, if desired, for permissible activity or for good alignment. The patient may be quite apprehensive about being placed on this bed, and if possible, a demonstration of turning should be given to him before he is moved onto it. Another advantage of these beds is that they wheel easily so that the patient may be taken to the operating room, radiology department, or to a recreational area for a change of surrounding. This type of bed is unsafe for a very restless or disoriented patient, although the safety straps may be used to give some security and protection.

Another type of turning frame, the CircOlectric bed (Fig. 41-3), also allows patients to be turned without changing their alignment. However, since this bed rotates the patient by turning him through the standing position rather than through the sidelying position, it is often not used for patients who are not permitted weight bearing. This includes patients with unresolved spinal injuries, as the standing position does load (puts weight through) the spine.[9]

Wounds. The assessment of wounds in patients who have had orthopedic surgery is often complicated by the fact that the wound is covered by a cast or other occlusive dressing, sometimes for a period of several weeks. In instances where the wound cannot be visualized, those caring for the patient may have to rely on their

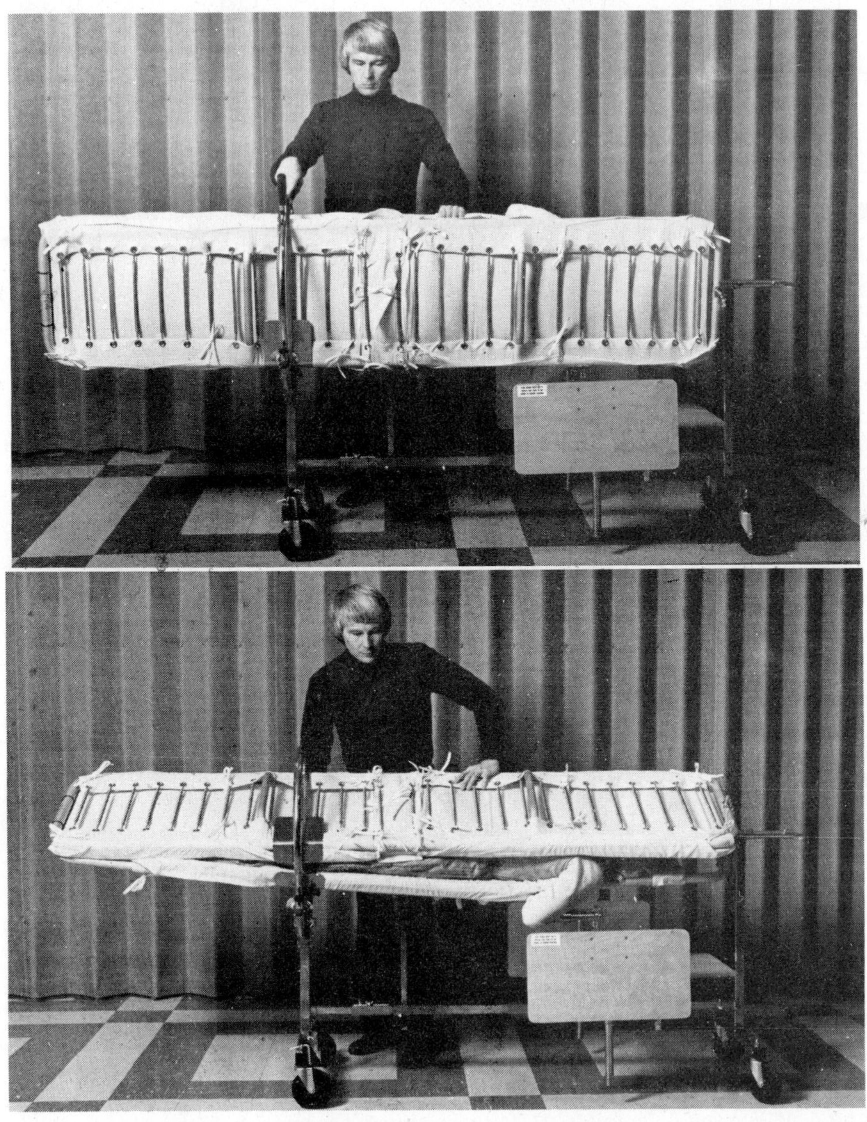

Fig. 41-26. Turning process is started. Narrow canvas strip is placed across forehead to support head when in prone position. (From Rantz, M., and Courtial, D.: Lifting, moving and transferring patients, St. Louis, 1977, The C. V. Mosby Co.)

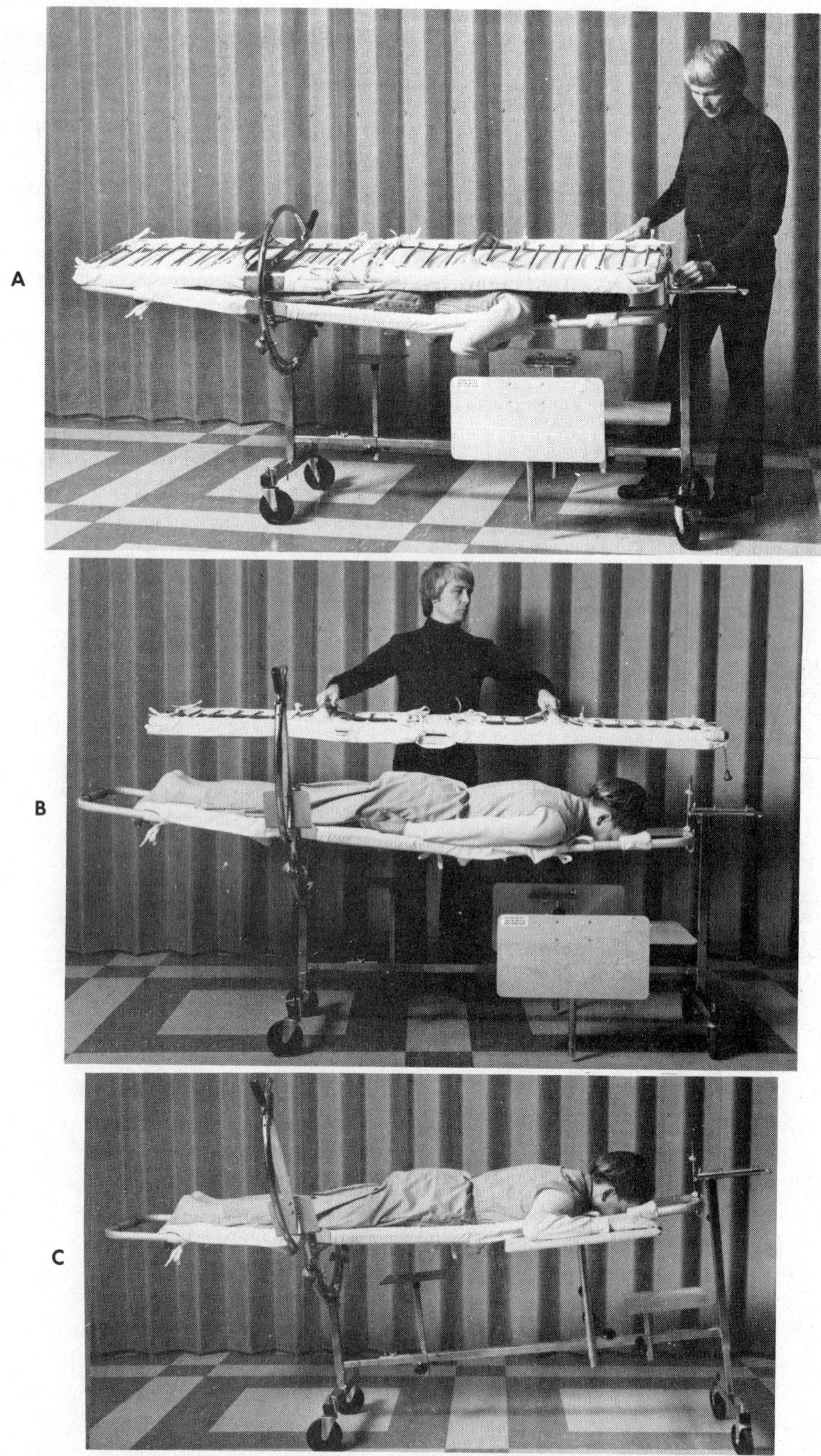

Fig. 41-27. A, Turning is complete. **B,** Posterior frame has been removed. **C,** Adjustable arm boards have been replaced for support. Lower shelf may be used to hold reading material or diet tray. (From Rantz, M., and Courtial, D.: Lifting, moving and transferring patients, St. Louis, 1977, The C. V. Mosby Co.)

sense of smell to alert them to potential problems. Foul odors emanating from under occlusive material, particularly in the presence of a temperature elevation or other systemic evidence of infection, should be called to the attention of the physician and investigated. Casts and other dressings can be cut (windowed) at the site of the incision and the condition of the wound assessed. If a cast is windowed, it is necessary to replace the portion of the plaster removed—either by taping or replastering it—to prevent swelling (window edema) in the area that would no longer be contained by the cast. If necessary, irrigations, soaks, or dressing changes can be carried out by removing the window at regular intervals and replacing it when the treatment is finished. If irrigations or soaks are done, care must be taken to line the surrounding portions of the cast with moisture-resistant material to prevent the cast from becoming wet.

Initial dressings are changed as necessary to prevent drainage from coming in contact with potential sources of contamination. After the initial dressing is changed, subsequent dressings are changed as necessary using aseptic technique to keep the wound clean and dry. It has already been noted that the plaster-of-Paris cast acts as a wick to promote drainage away from the wound. Compressive-type dressings, composed of many layers of cotton wadding and wrapped on the outside with Ace bandages, will also promote drainage away from the wound.

Depending on the type of surgery and the location of the surgery, some form of wound drainage may be employed. This may be in the nature of a Penrose drain (as in surgery to the hand), a self-contained vacuum suction device such as Porto-Vac (Fig. 23-10), or polyethylene tubing attached to electric suction. These types of drainage prevent hematoma formation at the operative site, and the latter two collect drainage so it can be measured accurately. It should also be noted that, because of its density, a compressive dressing can contain very large amounts of drainage before drainage becomes visible. Frequent checks of vital signs will aid in early detection of excessive blood loss by the patient who has this type dressing.

It has also been noted that infection may proceed from the surface of the skin along pin tracts (in patients who are in skeletal traction) to the bone (p. 861). Collodion dressings are sometimes applied to the entry and exit sites of pins immediately after the pins are inserted. If the wounds are not so occluded, and *if the surgeon requests care to the pin site,* drainage may be gently removed from around the wounds with hydrogen peroxide applied with cotton swabs. Dry sterile dressings may be applied to the wounds, and the wounds should be checked frequently for any signs or symptoms of infection (erythema, swelling, warmth, tenderness, unusual drainage). Movement of the pins may also carry infection along the pin tract and irritate the bone the pin traverses. Therefore care is taken to avoid manipulating or putting undue stress on the pins themselves. If it is noted that a pin is moving in and out of its tract, it should be reported to the surgeon as soon as possible.

Prevention of postoperative complications. Patients having orthopedic surgery for the treatment of a fracture have many of the same needs as any other surgical patient. Whenever possible, they should have preoperative teaching regarding postanesthesia care. Since these patients are very likely to be relatively immobile, they especially need to understand the importance of good pulmonary toilet. Movement of all uninvolved extremities should be encouraged in order to maintain muscle tone and prevent circulatory stasis. Full plantar flexion and dorsiflexion of the feet, isometric quadriceps-setting and gluteal-setting can be encouraged to these ends (Fig. 23-3). Quadriceps-setting is contraindicated until specifically ordered by the surgeon for patients who have patellar or patellar tendon surgery, or when surgical drains are in the parapatellar area. These exercises are generally done five times every hour initially, and the number can be increased up to 20 times every hour as the patient can tolerate them.

Limitation on positioning, movement, and ambulation will be determined by the body part involved, the nature of the surgical procedure, the type of fixation device used, or the type of immobilization device used (traction, cast, and so on). This means that those caring for the patient must be familiar with the patient's problem and the method of treatment used in order to avoid giving improper care that can lead to the displacement of fracture fragments.

Because of the complex arrangement of muscle attachments and because of muscle action, the surgeon should be consulted before attempts are made to assist or encourage the patient to exercise the involved limb. A safe rule is never under any circumstances have the patient move or use the joint either immediately distal or immediately proximal to the fracture before consulting the physician. For example, if the fracture is in the radius, the wrist and elbow joints should not be moved without an order; however, the shoulder can and should be protected from muscle weakness, muscle shortening, and joint changes by regular motion and exercise. The legs, trunk, and unaffected upper limb should be checked regularly (at least daily) to be certain that the patient is doing some systematic, routine exercises. The patient is mobilized as soon as possible.

Prevention of infection is discussed under wound care. The complications of fat embolus and osteomyelitis and their treatment are discussed in Chapter 42. Other interventions relating to the prevention of complications of immobility are discussed on p. 834.

Pain relief. The person who has sustained a fracture will most often have severe pain at and around the site of the fracture. Extensive soft tissue injury may be present adjacent to the fracture, edema is present, and there may be considerable spasm of muscles in the fracture area. In the initial stages of treatment, narcotic analgesics are effective in relieving pain and should be used as needed to help the patient obtain satisfactory relief. Continued pain and the muscle spasm accompanying it can put undue stress on the fracture fragments and retard efforts both to reduce and to maintain reduction of the fracture. Further, the patient who is in severe pain will resist efforts to assist him to cough and deep breathe and other measures designed to prevent complications. If the fracture is repaired by open reduction and internal fixation, the patient will have operative pain. If muscle spasm is a continuing problem, an agent such as diazepam (Valium) can be employed to reduce the spasm. It will not, however, relieve operative pain.

As healing progresses, the strength and frequency of analgesics can be decreased. It is important, however, to try to strike a balance in the use of analgesics; that is, the patient should be helped to be comfortable enough to perform required exercises and other acitivities, but not so heavily medicated that he is unaware of potential damage that he might do to himself by overextending his activity. Many times, simple changes in position, within the restrictions of the prescribed treatment, are enough to relieve the patient's discomfort without having to use analgesics.

Patient education. Prior to leaving the hospital, the patient who has been treated for a fracture must be aware of any activity restrictions or limitations that he must observe, how long he must observe them, how he is to use his ambulatory or other assistive devices (if needed), what kind of assistance he may need to perform his activities of daily living, and who will be available to help him. If necessary, referral can be made to a community nurse or other community agency for assistance.

The easiest and most effective way to teach the patient how to handle these problems is to have him function to the point of his limitations with whatever assistive aids he needs while he is still in the hospital. His functioning and abilities should be assessed and he should be helped to correct problems such as incorrect gait with crutches while he is still in a supervised situation. Whenever possible, it is best to have the patient perform all of his ADL as independently as he possibly can so that problem areas can be identified and satisfactory solutions worked out so that he will not be confronted with the problem when professional guidance is no longer available.

Reconstructive surgery

In addition to treatment for traumatic injuries, orthopedic interventions are also carried out for patients who require correction of a deformity, relief of pain, or restoration of musculoskeletal function. These are termed reconstructive (or palliative) surgeries. Surgeries of this nature include osteotomies (p. 897), arthrodeses (p. 898), arthroplasties (p. 892), arthrotomies (p. 892), synovectomies (p. 897), tendon transplants (p. 897), and the various spinal surgeries (p. 898). Those procedures that involve structures inside the joint capsule are termed *intraarticular* procedures; those outside the joint capsule are *extraarticular* procedures.

Patient education. One of the major advantages in caring for the patient who is to have a reconstructive surgery as opposed to the patient who has sustained a fracture is that there is more time to teach the patient preoperatively about the care that he will receive and how he can participate in that care in the postoperative period. This preoperative teaching should include information on positioning, activity limitation, exercises he will be required to perform, the necessity of and techniques of pulmonary toileting, and in some cases, transfer and ambulation techniques. Patients are often frightened by the prospect of surgery, and their fears are increased if they are confronted with procedures or techniques that they do not understand, or for which no rationale has been presented, or that they do not know how to perform. A few patients may be comfortable knowing as little as possible about what is going to happen to them, but most want to know as much as they can be told. For some, this will even include information about intravenous therapy and drainage devices.

The patient who accepts and understands what will be required of him in the postoperative period is more likely to follow through with exercises, activity limitation, and other requirements than the patient who is poorly prepared. The least that can be said for preoperative teaching is that it involves the patient in his care. If he accepts and learns the information that is given, his postoperative course may be facilitated. If he does not accept the information, that fact in itself provides cues for postoperative management.

Positioning. For the patient who has had an extraarticular procedure, positioning will be dependent on the type of immobilization device that is used. If the patient has had an intraarticular procedure, positioning will be limited both by the immobilizing device (most often a bulky compression dressing) and the tolerances of any prosthetic implant. An example of a prosthetic implant is the total hip prosthesis discussed on p. 893. Elevation of the extremity to aid in preventing edema should be maintained for the first 24 to 48 hours for the patient who has had either an extraarticular or an intraarticular pro-

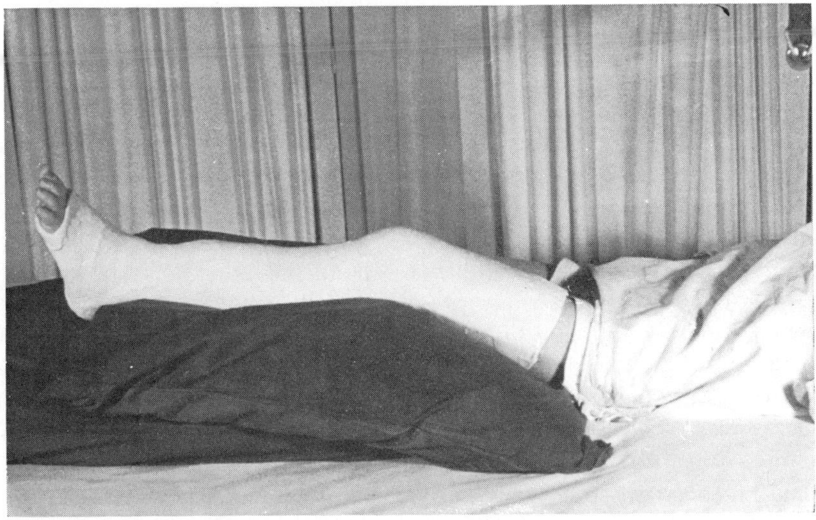

Fig. 41-28. One method of providing elevation to an extremity is to support it on pillows. Note that two pillows are wedged to provide support for entire extremity while still providing elevation for distal portion of extremity. (From Larson, C. B., and Gould, M.: Orthopedic nursing, ed. 8, St. Louis, 1974, The C. V. Mosby Co.)

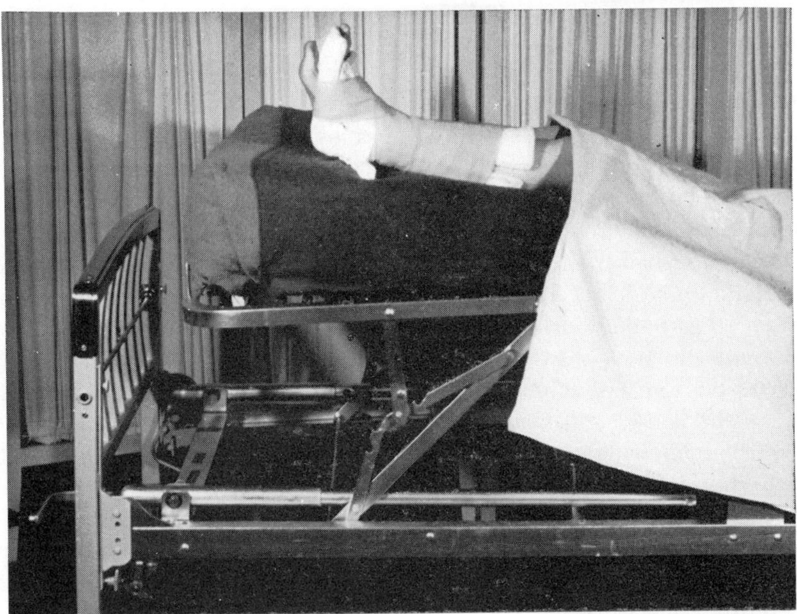

Fig. 41-29. Another method of elevating patient's foot is to gatch knee, then raise lower portion of springs. (From Larson, C. B., and Gould, M.: Orthopedic nursing, ed. 8, St. Louis, 1974, The C. V. Mosby Co.)

cedure (Figs. 41-28 and 41-29). In the lower extremities, some form of skin traction may be used in the initial postoperative period to help maintain position and to reduce muscle spasm, but it is generally removed after 2 to 5 days. The physician should be consulted to determine if there is any position that the patient should avoid, as is necessary with a total hip arthroplasty. (See also Chapter 39 for a discussion of positioning restrictions for patients having spinal surgeries.) Otherwise, the patient should be turned every 2 hours while in bed, and begin sitting in a chair or ambulating as soon as possible. When he is sitting (or, in the case of upper extremity surgery, standing) elevation of the operated extremity should be maintained. If the joint operated on is the knee, pillows should never be put under the knee in such a way that the knee will be allowed to flex. Full knee extension must be maintained to prevent the formation of knee flexion contracture or laxity of the knee after the immobilizing device is removed. Further, the patient who has had knee surgery should not be allowed to position his leg in extreme external rotation (p. 858), thus putting pressure on the peroneal nerve.

Skin care. Care of the skin for the patient who has had a reconstructive surgery is the same as for any patient who is immobilized or who is confined by a cast or traction (p. 858).

Prevention of postoperative complications. The measures pertaining to prevention of postoperative complications discussed on p. 869 are equally applicable for the patient who has had a reconstructive surgery. The bulky compression dressing, usually applied following an intraarticular procedure to prevent edema and joint effusion, can contain a large amount of drainage before that drainage becomes visible; therefore systemic signs and symptoms of excessive blood loss must be frequently and carefully monitored for the first 48 hours after surgery. The compression dressing can also be as constricting as a cast if swelling does occur. Neurocirculatory checks must be carefully performed every 1 to 2 hours until the danger of excessive swelling is over. Evidence of neurocirculatory compromise should be reported to the physician immediately so that the dressing can be split and the pressure relieved.

Immobilization. Immobilization of the operated extremity is carried out by plaster-of-Paris casts, bulky compression dressings, traction, braces, or bed rest. The major difference between the patient who is immobilized for a fracture and the patient who is immobilized following a reconstructive procedure is that the period of immobilization and non-weight-bearing are usually shorter. Immobilization following an intraarticular procedure is necessarily shorter (2 to 7 days, depending on the joint operated and the procedure performed), since prolonged immobilization will lead to the development of adhesions that will prevent joint motion. If adhesions develop, they often have to be broken (the joint flexed) with the patient under anesthesia.

Wounds. Wound care considerations are the same as discussed on p. 867. Additionally, patients who have had reconstructive surgeries are often elderly, have chronic underlying diseases such as rheumatoid arthritis, or may be taking medications that will retard wound healing. If wound healing is slow, continued attention to strict asepsis in dressing techniques is required. It is also not unusual for blisters to develop adjacent to the surgical incision or, particularly with hand surgery, on the operated extremity as a result of excessive edema. Such blisters should be kept intact and allowed to resolve on their own. If they do break, however, they can be covered with a piece of sterile petrolatum gauze cut to size and allowed to remain on the area until healing takes place.

Mobilization. Patients who have had reconstructive procedures are mobilized as soon as possible. For example, the patient who has had a knee procedure may usually be up in a wheel chair with his leg elevated the first postoperative day. The patient who has had a wrist or hand procedure may be out of bed with the hand elevated on the operative evening, depending on his recovery from anesthesia and the type of anesthesia used. The weight-bearing status of the patient will be determined by the procedure that is performed. Some weight-bearing restrictions that will require the patient to use ambulatory aids are generally enforced for those patients having lower extremity surgery.

In most instances, patients who have had intraarticular procedures will begin gentle *active* range of motion exercises to the involved joints as soon as the danger of joint effusion is past and the restrictive dressing is removed. These exercises will cause pain. However, if the joint is not moved, adhesions will develop. Whenever possible, pain medication should be given prior to the exercise period to help the patient relax to achieve the greatest range of motion possible. Local heat applied to the joint prior to exercising will also aid the involved muscles to relax. Application of ice following the exercise period can help retard swelling that results from exercising.

It must be stressed that these range of motion exercises must be done *actively* by the patient. *Under no circumstances should passive exercises be performed by another person.* If attempts are made to passively exercise the joint, the patient will most probably respond by resisting the exercise that is causing him pain and no movement will be achieved. If the joint is moved for the patient, and if that movement does cause him great pain, he may resist further attempts to actively move it. Most importantly, if the patient has osteoporosis, passive movement beyond the point of pain may result in pathologic fracture. Splints (or Buck's traction for the knees) may be used to rest the joint during periods between exercising. Balanced suspension traction or a system of slings and pulleys can be set up for the patient to perform active-assisted exercises. Special "dynamic" splints are fabricated by the occupational therapist to help the patient exercise his fingers following arthroplasties of the metacarpophalangeal joints of the hand. With these splints, individual slings for each finger are suspended by rubber bands from a heavy wire hoop that extends over the dorsal surface of the hand. The slings hold the fingers in extension, and the patient is required to flex his fingers against the gentle resistance provided by the rubber bands.

Pain relief. General measures for pain relief are discussed on p. 870. Many patients who undergo orthopedic procedures for the relief of pain (such as the patient who has a total hip replacement) often consider the operative pain minor compared to the pain they had prior to the surgery. It is not unusual for these patients to require minimal analgesia postoperatively.

Adaptation to change in function. The person who has undergone a surgical procedure to correct deformity, relieve pain, or to improve musculoskeletal function usually has a positive attitude toward the outcome of his surgery. One problem that can be encountered is that the patient expects much more of the surgery than the surgery is designed to provide. He may tend to overdo and perhaps cause himself some damage. This is another good reason for providing preoperative instruction for the patient. Informing the patient before he has the surgery about the limitations that he must observe may help him adjust to those limitations after the surgery.

A second problem that can be encountered is that the hospital staff or the patient's family can hold unrealistic expectations for the outcomes of a particular procedure on an individual patient. If it is not clearly defined prior to surgery that the outcomes for an individual patient will be limited by other conditions (such as multiple joint problems), there may be pressure on the patient to achieve the same as other patients who do not have his limitation.

Happily, most patients do have their functional abilities extended or improved by the surgeries that are performed. However, depending on how long standing the situation was that precipitated the surgery, the patient will have to be given time to adjust to his new abilities. Patterns of dependence may have to be broken down gradually as the patient discovers that "I now can do it myself." The patient's family may have to be reassured that the patient can now manage activities that formerly they carried out. These kinds of adjustments will begin in the hospital setting, and they will continue for some time after discharge. If it is anticipated that the patient will have adjustment problems in his home situation, it may be advisable to make a referral to the Visiting Nurse Association or another community resource so that the patient can have continuing support after discharge.

Outcome criteria for persons requiring surgical intervention

The patient or significant others can explain or demonstrate the following components of care:

1. Care of wound.
   a. Demonstrate the care of the wound, including dressing changes, that will be required until healing occurs.
   b. Explain the care of the cast (if applicable).
   c. Explain what to do if the nature or character of wound drainage changes.
   d. Explain the rationale and use of antibiotics (if prescribed).
2. Restriction or limitation of activity.
   a. Explain the limitations of activity to be observed and for what length of time.
   b. Explain the nature of and rationale for prescribed weight-bearing restrictions and limitations of joint movement.
   c. Demonstrate the appropriate, safe use of assistive and supportive devices.
   d. Demonstrate safe performance of ADL within the prescribed limitations or restrictions of activity, weight bearing, or joint movement.
3. Use of medication. State dosage of medications, when to take them, and possible side and toxic effects.
4. Safety measures.
   a. Describe the safety devices to be obtained for use at home and how and where they will be obtained.
   b. Describe and demonstrate how safety devices and precautions will be used at home.
   c. Describe what alterations must be made in the home environment to render it safe.
5. Techniques for the prevention of complications.
   a. Demonstrate the techniques appropriate to the prevention of infection, cardiorespiratory problems, skin breakdown, swelling, and neurocirculatory impairment.
   b. Demonstrate the uses, application and removal, and care of splints or braces.
   c. Demonstrate proper posture, body mechanics, and other specific joint protection techniques.
6. Infection.
   a. Demonstrate care of the wound.
   b. Explain and demonstrate the proper care of wires or pins used for fixation (if applicable).
   c. Explain what measures are to be taken if there is a change in the nature or character of drainage.
7. Follow-up care.
   a. Explain plans for follow-up care.
   b. Explain measures to take when a complication arises.

REFERENCES AND SELECTED READINGS

1. Adams, J. C.: Outline of fractures, ed. 5, Edinburgh & London, 1969, E. & S. Livingstone, Ltd.
2. *Alba, I. M., and Papeika, J.: The nurse's role in preventing circulatory complications in the patient with a fractured hip, Nurs. Clin. North Am. 1:57-61, 1966.
3. *American Heart Association: Prevention of rheumatic fever, New York, 1968, The Association.

*References preceded by an asterisk are particularly well suited for student reading.

4. Ansell, B. M., and Bywaters, E. G. L.: Rheumatoid arthritis (Still's disease), Pediatr. Clin. North Am. **10**:921-939, 1963.
5. *Arthritis Foundation: Primer on the rheumatic diseases, ed. 7, New York, 1973, The Foundation. (Prepared by a committee of the American Rheumatism Association Section of the Arthritis Foundation. Reprinted from J.A.M.A. 224:suppl., April 30, 1973.)
6. *Beetham, W. P., Jr.: The management of the collagen diseases, GP **31**:113-123, 1965.
7. Bergersen, B. S.: Pharmacology in nursing, ed. 13, St. Louis, 1976, The C. V. Mosby Co.
8. *Blount, M., and Kinney, A.: Chronic steroid therapy, Am. J. Nurs. **74**:1626-1631, 1974.
9. Bohlman, H.: Personal communications, Dec. 1976 and Sept. 1978.
10. *Bray, A. P., and Thomas, J. R.: Severe fat embolism syndrome following multiple fractures, Nurs. Times **65**:109-110, 1969.
11. *Brewer, E. J., Jr.: Rheumatoid arthritis in childhood, Am. J. Nurs. **65**:66-71, 1965.
12 *Browse, N. L.: Physiology and pathology of bed rest, Springfield, Ill., 1965, Charles C Thomas, Publisher.
13 *Brunner, N. A.: Orthopedic nursing: a programmed approach, ed. 2, St. Louis, 1975, The C. V. Mosby Co.
14. Brunnstrom, S.: Clinical kinesiology, ed. 3, Philadelphia, 1972, F. A. Davis Co.
15. *Buck, B. I.: Hip replacement, Sup. Nurse **3**:75-78, 1972.
16. *Campbell, E. B., Hogsed, C. M., and Bogdonoff, M.: Lupus erythematosus, Am. J. Nurs. **62**:74-77, 1962.
17. Canda, K.: The hazards of bedrest, unpublished paper, Cleveland, Ohio, December 1, 1972. (Written in fulfillment of requirements for master's degree, Case Western Reserve University.)
18. *Covalt, N. K.: Bed exercises for convalescent patients, Springfield, Ill., 1968, Charles C Thomas, Publisher.
19. Crenshaw, A. H., editor: Campbell's operative orthopedics, ed. 5, St. Louis, 1971, The C. V. Mosby Co.
20. Eaton, P., and Heller, F.: Therapeutic nursing care of orthopedic patients, Nurs. Clin. North Am. **2**:429-435, 1967.
21. Ehrlich, G. E., editor: Total management of the arthritic patient, Philadelphia, 1973, J. B. Lippincott Co.
22. *Farrell, J.: Illustrated guide to orthopedic nursing, Philadelphia, 1977, J. B. Lippincott Co.
23. *Farrell, J.: Nursing care of the patient in a cast brace, Nurs. Clin. North Am. **11**:717-724, 1976.
24. *Francis, Sister M.: Nursing the patient with internal hip fixation, Am. J. Nurs. **64**:111-112, 1964.
25. *Freyberg, R.: Rheumatoid arthritis, the natural history, diagnosis, prognosis and management, Med. Times **95**:742-752, 1967.
26. *Gartland, J. J.: Fundamentals of orthopedics, ed. 2, Philadelphia, 1974, W. B. Saunders Co.
27. *Gruis, M. L., and Innes, B.: Assessment: essential to prevent pressure sores, Am. J. Nurs. **76**:1762-1764, 1976.
28. Hollander, J. L., and McCarty, D. J., editors: Arthritis and allied conditions, ed. 8, Philadelphia, 1972, Lea & Febiger.
29. *Kelly, M. M.: Exercises for bedfast patients, Am. J. Nurs. **66**:2209-2213, 1966.
30. Kerr, A.: Orthopedic nursing procedures, ed. 2, New York, 1969, Springer Publishing Co., Inc.
31. *Kirk, J. A., and Kersley, G. D.: Heat and cold in the physical treatment of rheumatoid arthritis of the knee, Ann. Phys. Med. **9**:270-274, 1968.
32. *Knocke, L.: Crutch walking, Am. J. Nurs. **61**:70-73, 1961.
33. *Larson, C. B., and Gould, M. L.: Orthopedic nursing, ed. 9, St. Louis, 1978, The C. V. Mosby Co.
34. *Larson, C. B., and Gould, M. L.: Fractures of the hip and nursing care of the patient with a fractured hip, Am. J. Nurs. **58**:1558-1563, 1958.
35. *Long, B., and Buergin, P.: The pivot transfer, Am. J. Nurs. **77**:980-982, 1977.
36. Lowman, E. W.: Clinical management of disability due to rheumatoid arthritis, Arch. Phys. Med. Rehabil. **48**:136-141, 1967.
37. Lowman, E. W.: Rehabilitation of the patient with chronic rheumatoid arthritis, J. Chron. Dis. **1**:628-637, 1955.
38. Lutwak, L.: Calcium and nitrogen balance studies during Gemini VII flight, Lectures in aerospace medicine, Brooks Air Force Base, Texas, 1967.
39. MacGinnis, O.: Rheumatoid arthritis—my tutor, Am. J. Nurs. **68**:1699-1701, 1968.
40. *Madden, B. W., and Affeldt, J. E.: To prevent helplessness and deformities, Am. J. Nurs. **62**:59-61, 1962.
41. Martin, D. S.: The necessity for combined modalities in cancer therapy, Hosp. Pract. **8**:129-136, 1973.
42. *Mayer, J.: Nutrition and gout, Postgrad. Med. **45**:277-278, 1969.
43. *Mayo, R. A., and Hughes, J. M.: Intramedullary nailing of long bone fractures and nursing care after intramedullary nailing, Am. J. Nurs. **59**:236-240, 1959.
44. Melvin, J. L.: Rheumatic disease: occupational therapy and rehabilitation, Philadelphia, 1977, F. A. Davis Co.
45. *Moskowitz, R. W.: Clinical rheumatology, Philadelphia, 1975, Lea & Febiger.
46. *Nuefeld, A.: Surgical treatment of hip injuries, Am. J. Nurs. **65**:80-83, 1965.
47. *Olsen, E. V.: Hazards of immobility, Am. J. Nurs. **67**:779-797, 1967.
48. *Peers, J.: The care and handling of orthopedic implants, RN **28**:66-71, 1965.
49. Pendleton, T., and Grassman, B. J.: Rehabilitating children with inflammatory joint disease, Am. J. Nurs. **74**:2223-2225, 1974.
50. *Rantz, M. J., and Courtial, D.: Lifting, moving and transferring patients: a manual, St. Louis, 1977, The C. V. Mosby Co.
51. *Roaf, R., and Hodkinson, L. J.: Textbook of orthopaedic nursing, Oxford, 1971, Blackwell Scientific Publications.
52. Ryan, J.: Compression in bone healing, Am. J. Nurs. **74**:1998-1999, 1974.
53. *Salter, R. B.: Textbook of disorders and injuries of the musculoskeletal system: an introduction to orthopaedics, rheumatology, metabolic bone disease, rehabilitation and fracture, Baltimore, 1970, The Williams & Wilkins Co.
54. Schmeisser, G. J.: A clinical manual of orthopedic traction techniques, Philadelphia, 1963, W. B. Saunders Co.
55. *Schneider, F. R.: Handbook for the orthopaedic assistant, ed. 2, St. Louis, 1976, The C. V. Mosby Co.
56. Synnestvedt, N.: The do's and don'ts of traction care, Nurs. 74 **3**:35-41, 1974.
57. *Talbott, J. H.: Gout and gouty arthritis, Nurs. Outlook **2**:540-543, 1954.
58. Townley, C., and Hill, L.: Total knee replacement, Am. J. Nurs. **74**:1612-1617, 1974.
59. Turek, S. L.: Orthopaedics: principles and their application, ed. 2, Philadelphia, 1967, J. B. Lippincott Co.
60. *Walike, B. C., et al.: Rheumatoid arthritis, Am. J. Nurs. **67**:1420-1433, 1967.
61. Wiebe, A. N.: Orthopedics in nursing, Philadelphia, 1961, W. B. Saunders Co.
62. Williams, A.: A study of factors contributing to skin breakdown, Nurs. Res. **21**:238-343, 1972.
63. Williams, S. R.: Nutrition and diet therapy, ed. 3, St. Louis, 1977, The C. V. Mosby Co.

42

Musculoskeletal problems

PATRICIA BUERGIN

The disorders and injuries of the musculoskeletal system are vast in scope. They range from those that cause the patient only minor discomfort and inconvenience to those that are life threatening. The purpose of this chapter is to discuss those specific musculoskeletal conditions that commonly necessitate the adult individual's hospitalization and need for specific nursing care. Included are both the rheumatic diseases and conditions that require orthopedic surgical intervention. Some clinical conditions present localized signs and symptoms, while others present systemic signs and symptoms. Assessment of the patient with musculoskeletal signs and symptoms is discussed in Chapter 40, and general management considerations for such patients are discussed in Chapter 41. The epidemiology, pathophysiology, and clinical manifestations of specific disorders will be discussed in this chapter. In instances where specific management techniques pertain, those techniques will be discussed; otherwise the reader will be referred to the discussion in Chapter 41. This will also apply to discussion of outcome criteria.

Rheumatic diseases include a wide range of clinical conditions that cause pain and stiffness in the musculoskeletal system. The American Rheumatism Association has classified rheumatic diseases into the following 13 categories:

1. Polyarthritis of unknown cause
2. Connective tissue disorders (acquired)
3. Rheumatic fever
4. Degenerative joint disease (osteoarthritis, osteoarthrosis)
5. Nonarticular rheumatism
6. Diseases with which arthritis is frequently associated
7. Disorders associated with known infectious agents
8. Traumatic or neurogenic disorders
9. Disorders associated with known or strongly suspected biochemical or endocrine abnormalities
10. Neoplasms
11. Allergy and drug reactions
12. Inherited and congenital disorders
13. Miscellaneous disorders[5]

There are some commonalities shared by a number of these disorders; however, their differences will be emphasized. It may also be noted that many of these disorders require corrective surgical intervention at some point in their course. Surgery is more and more a vital adjunct to the management of individuals with rheumatic diseases. Nurses caring for patients with these diseases must have an appreciation for and an understanding of both the medical and the surgical approaches that will be employed in treatment.

The term *arthritis* means inflammation of a joint. Arthritis is a condition that exists in a number of specific rheumatic diseases. However, like the term rheumatism, it is often used by the public to apply to any pain or stiffness of the musculoskeletal system whether or not the cause is an inflammatory process. It is estimated that 20 million people in the United States are suffering from arthritis or arthritis-like conditions.[44] As such, it may be anticipated that a significant proportion of the patients with whom a nurse has contact will have some discomfort or disability caused by musculoskeletal disorders.

■ RHEUMATIC DISEASES

□ Systemic connective tissue diseases

Rheumatoid arthritis

Epidemiology. Rheumatoid arthritis is a chronic *systemic* disease. The disease process, while most prominent as a nonsuppurative inflammation in the diarthrodial joints, may also be manifested by lesions of the vasculature, nervous system, and other major organs of the body.

Rheumatoid arthritis is more prevalent in women than men by a ratio of 2:1 or 3:1. Usually it appears during the productive years of life when career and family responsibilities are greatest. While the cause of this disease is unknown, there are several theories of causation under investigation. Areas of study include (1) immune mechanisms, such as the interaction of the IgG class of immunoglobins with the rheumatoid factor that appears to play a role in perpetuating rheumatoid inflammation[5]; (2) metabolic factors; and (3) infection, with particular attention to viruses.

Pathophysiology. The disease process within the joints (intraarticular) begins as an inflammation of the synovium with edema, vascular congestion, fibrin exudate, and cellular infiltrate.[5] The amount of synovial fluid increases while the fluid itself becomes turbid and has a decreased viscosity. Continued inflammation leads to thickening of the synovium, particularly where it joins the articular cartilage. At these junctures, granulation tissue forms a *pannus* or mantle that covers the surface of the cartilage. The pannus also invades subchondral bone. As the amount of granulation tissue from inflammation increases, it interferes with normal nutrition of the articular cartilage. The cartilage becomes necrotic. The degree of erosion of the articular cartilage will determine the amount of articular disability. If large areas of cartilage are destroyed, adhesions form between the joint surfaces and fibrous or bony union (ankylosis) develops between what were previously articulating surfaces. Destruction of cartilage and bone, in addition to some weakening of tendons and ligaments, may lead to subluxation or dislocation of joints. Invasion of the subchondral bone may cause eventual regional osteoporosis.

Clinical picture. The early manifestations of the disease may include fever, weight loss, fatigue, and generalized aching. Early morning stiffness lasting a few minutes to an hour or more is characteristic. The patient may describe the location of aching and stiffness in general terms, such as "in my arms," "in my hands," or "in my legs," as opposed to naming specific joints. This kind of discomfort, commonly referred to as fibrositis, is *poorly localized.* Such discomfort is often seen in rheumatoid arthritis and may be the patient's earliest complaint. This symptom picture may be present for some period of time before it is followed by more specific, or localized, problems—frank articular inflammation with joint swelling, pain, redness, warmth, and tenderness. In other patients, fibrositis and joint inflammation occur together at the onset.[44]

The proximal interphalangeal and metacarpophalangeal joints of the hands and the metatarsophalangeal joints of the feet are often affected early. As the disease progresses, the fingers develop a characteristic tapering appearance with a classic ulnar deviation of the hand. Virtually all joints can become involved—hips, knees, wrists, elbows, shoulders, and jaw. Joint involvement most often occurs in a *bilaterally symmetrical* pattern with involvement of the same joints on both sides of the body. (*Asymmetrical distribution* is the term used to indicate a scattered type of involvement.) Even such small structures as the cricoarytenoid joints of the larynx can be affected. Laryngeal involvement, if severe, may result in hoarseness or voice changes, dysphagia, and dyspnea on exertion.[32] Fortunately it causes symptomatic problems in relatively few patients.

Inflammation of the tendon sheaths, particularly in the wrist, may occur. There is spasm of the muscles attached to the involved joints. Such spasm is believed to contribute to deformity of the involved joints, and since the patient will tend to guard painful joints, there may be some atrophy of muscles from disuse (Fig. 42-1). Subcutaneous nodules may develop near joints, over bony prominences, or along extensor surfaces.

The course of rheumatoid arthritis varies greatly from patient to patient. It is marked by periods of exacerbation and remission. Some individuals have been known to recover from a first attack and never suffer a recurrence. For others, particularly those in whom the rheumatoid factor is found (seropositive rheumatoid disease), the disease tends to be chronically progressive.[32] In a small number of individuals the disease may be rapidly progressive, marked by unremitting joint destruction and diffuse vasculitis. This form of the disease is referred to as malignant rheumatoid disease.[5] The length of time between exacerbations varies greatly with individuals. There is some evidence that exacerbations can be triggered by mental stress such as worry or grief,[32] by overexertion, and at times by physical trauma such as surgery. The likelihood that the patient will enter a complete remission after 3 years of sustained disease activity is very slight.[32]

If it is not treated, rheumatoid arthritis has a tendency to relapse and to recur in more severe form. Continued competent medical care is of the utmost importance for anyone who has rheumatoid arthritis. Some individuals, when experiencing a remission of their symptoms, believe they are cured and discontinue their therapy, only to have a later and more severe exacerbation of the disease. Even with careful management, approximately 10% of patients with rheumatoid arthritis progress to a crippling state of complete incapacity.[32]

Laboratory findings usually include an elevated erythrocyte sedimentation rate and mild leukocytosis. A positive rheumatoid factor (latex fixation test, p. 829) is seen in 50% to 90% of patients, depending on disease duration and severity.[44] Roentgenographic examination may reveal narrowing of the joint spaces and erosion of the articular surfaces. Synovial biopsy and examination of synovial tissue can establish the presence of inflammatory changes in the synovium, and synovial fluid obtained by needle aspiration will have increased turbidity and decreased viscosity.

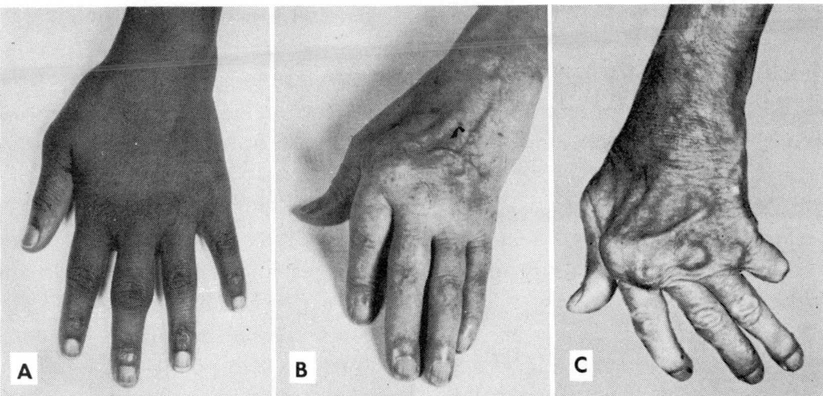

Fig. 42-1. Rheumatoid arthritis of hand. **A,** Early stage. Note fusiform swelling of proximal interphalangeal joints, especially that of middle finger. **B,** Moderate involvement. Note swelling from chronic synovitis of metacarpophalangeal joints and early ulnar drift. **C,** Advanced stage. Note marked ulnar drift and subluxation of metacarpophalangeal joints with extension of proximal interphalangeal joints and flexion of distal joints. Note also deformed position of thumb. (From Raney, R., and Brashear, H.: Shand's handbook of orthopaedic surgery, ed. 8, St. Louis, 1971, The C. V. Mosby Co.)

Intervention. The basic principles of management of rheumatoid arthritis are (1) rest, (2) relief of pain, (3) maintenance of joint function, (4) prevention and correction of deformities by application of orthopedic principles, and (5) correction of other health factors. These principles, as well as the specific medications used in the treatment of rheumatoid arthritis, are discussed in Chapter 41.

One special consideration in dealing with the rheumatoid patient requires further discussion. Depending on the disease condition, the patient's disability may increase in spite of all efforts, including his own. The patient and his family often become very discouraged. The person who is discouraged and in pain is very vulnerable to promises of a "cure." Millions of dollars (estimates range as high as $400 million) are spent each year by persons who can ill afford the expense on gadgets, programs, and "medicines" that allegedly are able to "cure." While the ultimate decision to try a program rests with the individual, the health care team can provide guidance to the patient and his family. Teaching the patient about his care and seeing that he is referred to reputable resources for additional assistance and information is one of the most valuable services that can be rendered to him. The local chapter of the Arthritis Foundation can be of great assistance to the patient and his family. The Arthritis Foundation is also keenly aware of the relative merit or lack of merit of resources available in the community.

The Arthritis Foundation* has prepared the following material, all of which is helpful to nurses working with person who have arthritis: *Home care programs in arthritis; Arthritis and related disorders: a manual for nurses, physical therapists, and social workers; Arthritis: the basic facts; Rheumatoid arthritis; Osteoarthritis;* and *Gout.* The last four of these references are written in such a way that many patients can understand and learn from them. After appropriate consultation with the physician to determine which particular books will be most helpful to the individual patient, those planning to teach the patient about his disease and his treatment will find these books are helpful teaching aids to share with the patient.

Outcome criteria for the person with rheumatoid arthritis. The patient or significant others can:

1. Explain the basic nature of rheumatoid arthritis.
2. Demonstrate the prescribed methods of joint protection.
3. Explain how medications are to be taken (dose, what times, side effects, toxic effects).
4. Demonstrate prescribed exercise program.
5. Demonstrate how to use moist heat applications to relieve pain in joints.
6. Demonstrate how to apply and explain when to use splinting devices.
7. Explain plans for follow-up care.

Systemic lupus erythematosus

Epidemiology. Systemic lupus erythematosus (SLE) is a chronic inflammatory disease of unknown cause. It affects women, particularly adolescents and young

*3400 Peachtree Drive NE, Atlanta, GA 30326.

adults, four times more often than it affects men. The disease was named after its characteristic rash, the erosive nature of the rash being "likened to the damage wrought by a hungry wolf."[5] Once thought to be relatively rare and always fatal, better techniques for recognition of the disease have demonstrated it to be fairly common, and its course can be controlled by corticosteroids. Some patients do, however, die as a result of lesions affecting major organs or from secondary infections.

Pathophysiology. The pathology of the disease includes severe vasculitis with necrosis of the walls of the small arteries, renal involvement with thickening of the basement membrane of the glomerular tuft and necrosis of the glomerular capillaries, lymph node necrosis, synovial involvement as a fibrous villous synovitis, lesions of the nervous system, and the development of small white spots in the retina called *cytoid bodies.* Two major areas are being investigated as possible causes of this disease. One possibility is that an aberration of the immune system causes immune complexes containing antibodies to be deposited in tissue, thereby causing tissue damage; the second possibility is the presence of a viral infection caused by or resulting from some immunologic abnormality. A third possibility is that both of these factors combine to produce the disease. Some drugs, notably procainamide (Pronestyl), isonicotinic acid hydrazide (INH, Isoniazid), and penicillin are known to induce lupus-like syndromes.

Clinical picture. The initial manifestation of SLE is often arthritis. In many instances the joint symptoms are transient and respond to treatment. Weakness, fatigue, and weight loss may be present. The patient may complain of sensitivity to the sun, developing rash and at times fever or arthritis on exposure to sunlight. Erythema, usually in a butterfly pattern, appears over the cheeks and bridge of the nose. The margins of the lesions are bright red, and the lesions may extend beyond the hairline with partial alopecia (loss of hair) above the ears. Lesions may also occur on the exposed part of the neck. The lesions spread slowly to the mucous membranes and other tissues of the body, or they may originate there. The lesions do not ulcerate, but cause degeneration and atrophy of tissues.

Depending on the organs involved, the patient may have findings of glomerulonephritis, pleuritis, pericarditis, peritonitis, neuritis, or anemia. Renal and neurologic manifestations are among the more serious manifestations of the disease.

Laboratory findings may be specific to the organs involved, as with proteinuria, abnormal cerebrospinal fluid, or roentgenographic evidence of pleural reactions. A positive LE cell reaction and immunoflourescent studies to identify the antibody responsible for LE cell reaction are helpful in making the diagnosis of the disease (p. 829).

Intervention. Adrenocorticosteroid therapy is used to control active manifestations of SLE. In the presence of lupus nephritis, steroids are frequently given in very high doses (60 mg or more of prednisone per day). The management considerations in caring for patients on high doses of steroids as discussed in Chapter 41 should be well understood in these instances (p. 850). Joint pains are often treated with salicylates. Antimalarial drugs may be helpful in treating the cutaneous lesions; however, the possibility of serious retinal damage with prolonged use must be carefully checked (p. 850). If skin lesions are present or if there is exacerbation of symptoms on sun exposure, exposure to the sun is to be avoided.

Outcome criteria for the person with SLE. The patient or significant others can:

1. Explain how medications are to be taken (dosage, what times, side effects, toxic effects).
2. Explain the reason for immediate medical consultation if for any reason he cannot take the prescribed steroids.
3. Explain reason for carrying an identification card stating name of prescribed steroid, dose, and name and phone number of physician.
4. Describe the clothing to be worn when out in the sun (all body surfaces covered, wide-brimmed hat).
5. Explain plans for follow-up care.

Polymyositis (dermatomyositis)

Epidemiology. Polymyositis (dermatomyositis) is an inflammatory disease involving striated (voluntary) muscle. Polymyositis occurs two times more frequently in women than men, and it may occur at any age. It is estimated that the disease occurs in one of every 200,000 of the population per year.[5] The cause of the disease is unknown; however, it is thought that some reaction of the autoimmune system is involved.

Pathophysiology. Pathologic findings on histologic studies of biopsied muscle are variable, but the alterations found, in order of their frequency, are the following: (1) primary degeneration of muscle fibers, either focal or extensive; (2) basophilia of some fibers with central migration of the sarcolemmal nuclei; (3) necrosis of parts or of entire groups of muscle fibers; (4) lymphocytic and plasma cell infiltrates near or surrounding blood vessels or between individual muscle fibers; (5) interstitial fibrosis varying in severity with the duration and to some extent the type of disease; (6) variation in the cross-sectional diameter of fibers.[5,32]

Clinical picture. Polymyositis, which usually runs a course of exacerbations and remissions, is usually first noted in proximal muscles, in particular the pelvic and shoulder girdles. Climbing stairs, arising from a chair, and other activities that involve lifting the body become increasingly difficult or impossible. Lifting of the arms becomes progressively more difficult. Hair combing may be impossible. Other muscles—neck flexors, the muscles of swallowing—may also become involved. Muscle pain or tenderness is present in some instances in the early stages, but not necessarily. Involvement of the skin in the form of a rash marks the disease as *dermatomyositis.* A dusky red lesion may be found in the periobital region, along with periorbital edema. This dusky red rash may extend over the face, forehead, neck, upper shoulders, chest, and upper back. Lesions on the arms and legs commonly affect the extensor surfaces. These patches are sometimes slightly scaly.[44]

The weakness of myositis, if it persists, can lead to contractures and atrophy. The individual with the dermatomyositis form of the disease, particularly if he is over 40 years of age, has a 40% to 50% greater chance of having evidence of a malignant neoplasm found during the first 5 years of illness than the population at large. Some physicians believe that routine yearly examinations should be performed to define or exclude the presence of neoplasms in these patients during that 5-year period.

The physical therapist is helpful in delineating which specific muscles are involved (or are weak) by performing a manual muscle test (p. 832). An electromyogram (p. 831) is useful in diagnosis, as it can delineate a specific pattern of findings that helps to differentiate polymyositis (dermatomyositis) from other types of muscle disease. Muscle biopsy (p. 831) results may define the specific pathologic changes within the involved muscle. Serum enzymes—SGOT, CPK, and aldolase (p. 828)—are elevated in the presence of active polymyositis or dermatomyositis. Close monitoring of these enzyme values will give indications of the progress of the disease or the effects of treatment. Twenty-four-hour urine collections for the creatine-creatinine ratio (indicating the amount of muscle disease that is present) are also obtained on a frequent basis (p. 830).

Intervention. Polymyositis (dermatomyositis) responds to corticosteroid therapy. Prednisone is often given in high (50 mg or more per day) doses. Those management principles relating to rest, positioning, assisted transfer and locomotion, prevention of skin breakdown, and care of the individual receiving high doses of corticosteroids (p. 850) are all relevant in caring for the patient who has myositis.

Outcome criteria for the person with polymyositis or dermatomyositis. The patient or significant others can:

1. Describe how to balance rest and activity.
2. Demonstrate ability to safely perform ADL or explain how these needs will be met if unable to do for self.
3. Explain how medications are to be taken (dosage, what times, side effects, toxic effects).
4. Explain the reason for immediate medical consultation if for any reason he cannot take the prescribed steroids.
5. Demonstrate prescribed program of exercises.
6. Demonstrate proper positioning in bed.
7. State symptoms that would indicate need for immediate medical assistance.
8. Explain reason for carrying identification card stating name of prescribed steroid, dose, and name and phone number of physician.
9. Explain plans for follow-up care.

Progressive systemic sclerosis (PSS, scleroderma)

Epidemiology. Progressive systemic sclerosis involves the connective tissue throughout the body. It affects women three times more often than men, usually in the 30- to 50-year age group. The cause of PSS is unknown. Some aberration of the immune system may be involved.

Pathophysiology. As this disease runs its course, involved tissue becomes fibrotic. These changes may be accompanied by vascular lesions, and the tissue involved may be the skin (scleroderma), synovium, esophagus, intestinal tract, heart, lungs, or kidneys. The disease may exist in a mild chronic form or, depending on the organs involved, may progress to rapid death.

Clinical picture. The word "scleroderma" means "hard skin," and that accurately describes the skin manifestations that are present. Usually local areas such as the face and fingers are affected first with gradual thickening and tightening of the skin. The skin may first appear slightly edematous, then turn pale, become steadily more firm, and finally become fixed to underlying tissue. The skin may also appear mildly pigmented. *Telangiectases* (elevated dark red spots formed by the dilatation of groups of capillaries) appear on the lips, tongue, fingers, and face. Normal skin folds are lost as the skin hardens, and as a result, the facies appear "pinched."[44] This is sometimes referred to as "birdlike" facies. Articular symptoms—pain and stiffness—are present in about one-third of the patients as an initial symptom. Raynaud's phenomenon (p. 818) may be pronounced. Muscle weakness (sclerodermatomyositis) may be present. In the presence of pain on joint motion, skin, and muscle contractures develop to produce deformity of the joint.

As the face becomes masklike, the ability to chew food may be impaired. The patient may have difficulty swallowing. Chest expansion may be impaired by the firming of the skin so that respiratory failure threatens. If the disease progresses to its end stage, all body motion becomes so restricted that the patient has the appearance of a living mummy. Tissues of essential organs such as the heart, kidneys, and liver may be affected in a similar manner, and fatal impairment of their function may result.

Laboratory and other diagnostic tests are helpful in defining the extent of the disease. For example, a barium swallow will help to define the presence of reflux esophagitis; upper gastrointestinal studies may demonstrate decreased peristalsis in the small intestine; pulmonary function studies may indicate impaired gas exchange, decreased vital capacity, and total lung capacity (p. 935); and antinuclear antibody studies may show a speckled pattern on nucleolar immunofluorescence (p. 829).

Intervention. There is no cure for PSS. Treatment with corticosteroids is generally limited to those patients who have evidence of myositis. Salicylates and mild analgesics are used for joint pain. Physical therapy, while only partially effective in preventing contractures, should be ordered to help preserve muscle strength. Frequent small feedings and the use of antacids, along with elevation of the head of the bed, may be helpful in relieving reflux esophagitis.[5] Meticulous hygiene (including frequent mouth care), assisting the patient while eating to prevent choking, and skin care directed to the prevention of decubiti, as well as emotional support are important.

Outcome criteria for the person with PSS. The patient or significant others can:

1. Demonstrate prescribed exercises.
2. Explain precautions that must be taken while eating when experiencing difficulty chewing or swallowing. Pureeing of foods and so on may be necessary.
3. Explain skin care precautions.
4. Demonstrate ability to safely perform ADL or explain how these needs will be met by others.
5. Explain how medications are to be taken (dosage, what times, side effects, toxic effects).
6. State symptoms that indicate need for immediate medical care.
7. Explain plans for follow-up care.

Necrotizing arteritis and other forms of vasculitis

Necrotizing arteritis and other forms of vasculitis comprise a group of syndromes in which inflammation of blood vessels is seen. This group of syndromes includes the vasculitis found in rheumatoid arthritis, systemic lupus erythematosus, progressive systemic sclerosis, and polyarteritis nodosa.

Inflammation of the arterial wall is associated with necrosis. The body's natural attempts to repair the necrosed area result in fibrosis of the arterial wall or rapid growth of the intima (inner coat of the artery). Intimal proliferation may partially or completely occlude the vessel, thus causing infarction. If only a portion of the circumference of a vessel is involved, *aneurysms* (dilatations of the wall of the artery) can develop. Such aneurysms may rupture.[5]

Clinical picture. Vessels in any part of the body—heart, lungs, kidneys, or nerves, either centrally or peripherally—may be involved. The result of such involvement can be angina, myocardial infarction, hypertension, peripheral neuropathy, or focal central nervous system involvement. *Temporal arteritis,* which usually presents with intractable headaches (p. 666), can result in blindness caused by occlusion of the central retinal artery.

Laboratory tests may reveal leukocytosis and elevated erythrocyte sedimentation rate, or may be specific to certain organs as, for example, with proteinuria in renal involvement. Angiography will often demonstrate aneurysmal dilatation of the involved vessels.

Intervention. Corticosteroids administered in high doses in the initial phases of these diseases may prompt remission. Rest is generally prescribed until there is a remission of symptoms. The sections dealing with rest (p. 841) and steroid treatment (p. 850) in Chapter 41 should be consulted for additional information.

Outcome criteria for the person with vasculitis. The patient or significant others can:

1. Describe the program of rest that should be adhered to until symptoms are in remission.
2. Explain how medications are to be taken (dosage, what times, side effects, toxic effects).
3. Explain the reason for immediate medical consultation if for any reason the prescribed steroids cannot be taken.
4. Explain reason for carrying identification card stating name of prescribed steroid, dose, and name and phone number of physician.
5. Describe symptoms that require immediate medical attention.
6. Explain plans for follow-up care.

Sjögren's syndrome

Epidemiology. Sjögren's syndrome is a chronic inflammatory disorder affecting the lacrimal and parotid glands. The disease occurs dramatically more often in women than in men, the ratio being about 9:1. One-half of the patients who display this syndrome are people who have rheumatoid arthritis, systemic lupus erythematosus, or progressive systemic sclerosis. There is diminished lacrimal and salivary secretions, and this is known as the *sicca complex*.

salivary gland

Pathophysiology. The disorder is associated with lymphocytic and plasma cell infiltration of the lacrimal and parotid glands, causing a decrease in the production and flow of tears and saliva. The parotid involvement *(xerostomia)* occurs more slowly than the lacrimal *(keratoconjunctivitis sicca)*.[5]

Clinical picture. Patients complain of a dry or gritty sensation in the eye, redness, itching, or a filmy sensation that interferes with vision. When parotid involvement is present, there may be difficulty chewing and swallowing, and some persons experience some difficulty with speech. While the symptoms of this syndrome are distressing, the complications can be even more severe. Corneal ulceration, ulcers of the tongue and lips, and dental caries may occur. In some instances the parotid glands become enlarged.

Lacrimal gland involvement can be measured by a Schirmer test (p. 832), while parotid gland function can be measured by a technetium Tc 99m uptake scan (p. 828). A biopsy of the inside lower lip, where minor salivary glands are located, may demonstrate lymphoid involvement.

Intervention. Treatment is symptomatic. It includes the use of methylcellulose eyedrops on an as needed basis to alleviate the discomfort of dry eyes. Some patients may find it necessary to use these drops as often as every hour. Fluids should be readily available to help keep the mouth moist. Some patients are able to alleviate the dry mouth by sucking on sour candy, as this stimulates the secretion of saliva. It is also vital to remember that the majority of patients with this syndrome have a systemic connective tissue disease as well. If they have dysfunction of their hands caused by pain, deformity, or contracture, they may not be able to administer their own eyedrops or handle a glass in order to drink fluids. Provision must be made for these complications when planning patients' care or discharge from the hospital. Mouth care is especially important; and if there is difficulty chewing, a change in the texture of the diet is indicated. Junior foods or baby foods may be helpful to some patients.

Outcome criteria for the person with Sjögren's syndrome. The patient or significant others can:

1. Explain the basic nature of this syndrome.
2. Demonstrate the administration of prescribed eyedrops.
3. Demonstrate how adequate fluid intake will be maintained.
4. Explain how the texture of the diet can be changed (chopping, pureeing, junior and baby foods).
5. Describe how to facilitate chewing and swallowing by increasing fluid intake with meals.
6. Explain plans for follow-up care.

□ Degenerative joint disease

Epidemiology

Degenerative joint disease (DJD), also known as osteoarthritis, hypertrophic arthritis, osteoarthrosis, or senescent arthritis, is an extremely common disease that is probably as old as civilization. Almost everyone past 40 years of age has hypertrophic changes in the joints. While symptomatic degenerative joint disease is usually noted in the 50- to 70-year age group, it has been observed as early as age 20. On the basis of one study, it is estimated that 40 million Americans have degenerative changes of the hands and feet, and estimates are that 175,000 Americans 65 years old and over have been incapacitated by DJD of the hip.[5]

Pathophysiology

Degenerative joint disease is a disease of the articular cartilage. It is thought to accompany aging, but may develop as a result of trauma, congenital problems (such as hip dislocations), or childhood diseases such as Legg-Calvé-Perthes disease. The articular cartilage, normally dense, white, translucent, and smooth, becomes yellow and opaque. Areas of the cartilage may become soft and the surface becomes roughened, frayed, and cracked. Eventually this cartilage may be destroyed, and the underlying subchondral bone goes through a remodeling process (p. 810). *Osteophytes* or spurs of new bone that appear at the joint margins and at the sites of attachment of supporting structures may break off and appear in the joint cavity as "joint mice." While the cause of the degeneration of articular cartilage is unknown, several theories of causation include digestion of the cartilage by enzymes and alteration of the nutrition of the cartilage. Individuals affected with degenerative joint disease may be predisposed to the disease by excessive "wear and tear" of the affected joints. Obesity, metabolic disturbances (e.g., acromegaly), repeated joint hemorrhages, trauma, or a genetic predisposition are examples of contributing factors. Also, certain occupations such as coal mining and boxing tend to be associated with osteoarthritis.

Clinical picture

The individual with degenerative joint disease experiences pain in the movable joints, particularly on weight bearing. Inflammation is usually not present, and tenderness is mild; however, the joints may become enlarged. Crepitation may be present, and there may be changes in the alignment of the extremity. The patient may experience stiffness after periods of rest.

Characteristic changes occur in certain joints. Bony protuberances on the dorsal surface of the distal interphalangeal joints of the fingers, known as *Heberden's*

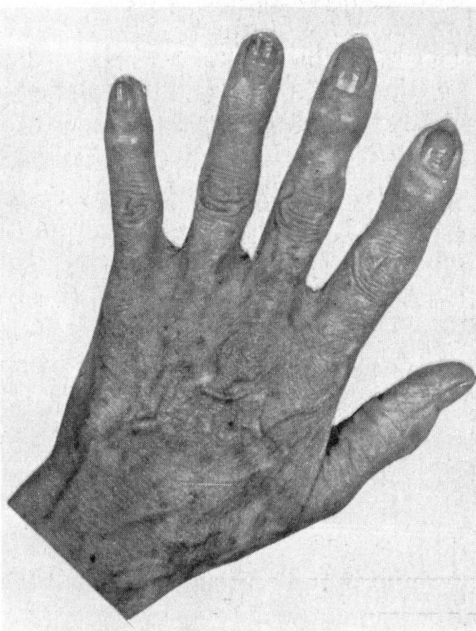

Fig. 42-2. Osteoarthritis of hand. Note enlargement of distal joints of index, middle, and little fingers. (Heberden's nodes). (From Raney, R., and Brashear, H.: Shand's handbook of orthopaedic surgery, ed. 8, St. Louis, 1971, The C. V. Mosby Co.)

nodes, may appear (Fig. 42-2). *Bouchard's nodes* on the proximal interphalangeal joints of the fingers are not uncommon. *Coxarthrosis* (degenerative joint disease of the hip) presents with pain in the hip on weight bearing and may progress to include pain in the groin and along the medial side of the knee. Range of motion of the hip becomes markedly limited. When the knee is involved, there is loss of motion, crepitus, and flexion deformity.

Serologic and synovial fluid examinations will be essentially normal. Roentgenographic examinations may reveal narrowing of the joint space, osteophyte formation, and *eburnation* (sclerosis) of subchondral bone.

Intervention

The major objectives of treatment of degenerative joint disease are relief of pain, restoration of joint function, and prevention of disability or further progression of the disease. Attention to posture, loss of unnecessary weight, unloading the painful joints by using ambulatory aids such as canes, crutches, or walkers, altering activities of daily living to avoid particularly painful activities, and the use of external measures such as local heat, prescribed exercises, or traction (p. 847) can be helpful in achieving these objectives. Salicylates, used in combination with these physical measures, seem to be the most useful pharmacologic agents in the relief of the pain of degenerative joint disease. When these measures are not reasonably successful, surgery may be employed both to relieve pain and to correct deformity. Specific procedures available are (1) debridement, (2) arthrodesis, (3) arthroplasty, (4) osteotomy, and (5) total joint replacement. Principles related to the conservative management measures noted above are discussed in Chapter 41; the surgical measures are discussed on p. 892.

Outcome criteria for the person with degenerative joint disease

The patient or significant others can:

1. Explain the alterations that must be made in ADL to avoid excessive use of affected joints.
2. Explain the importance of losing excessive weight.
3. Review plans for reduction diet.
4. Explain the basic nature of degenerative joint disease.
5. Demonstrate safe use of ambulatory assistive devices.
6. Demonstrate ability to safely perform ADL or explain how ADL needs will be met.
7. Demonstrate how to safely apply moist heat to painful joints.
8. Explain how medications are to be taken (dosage, what times, side effects, toxic effects).
9. Explain plans for follow-up care.

□ Degenerative joint disease of the spine

Pathophysiology

Degenerative joint disease of the spine is a common but difficult problem that merits special consideration. The spine has 23 intervertebral disc joints and 46 posterior facet joints, all of which are subjected to stresses and strains in holding the human body upright and moving it about. The vertebrae in the spinal column are articulated in a series of "couplets" that are able to move through an intervertebral disc joint and two posterior facet joints. The intervertebral discs are composed of an outer layer of cartilage called the *anulus fibrosus* and an inner layer of cartilage called the *nucleus pulposus*. The degeneration and dehydration of this cartilage results in a loss of elasticity. The disc normally functions as a shock absorber. As it loses its resiliency, a strong force exerted across the disc can result in herniation of the nucleus through the anulus either posteriorly or laterally. This results in compression of a spinal nerve root and subsequent pain (Fig. 42-3). The facet joints that stabilize the spine are synovial joints, and their articular surfaces are covered with articular cartilage. This means that these joints can be affected by rheumatoid arthritis as well as degenerative joint disease (Fig. 42-4). Osteophytes developing along the vertebral column can fuse and cause a limitation of motion, usually in the lumbodorsal region. The intervertebral foramina in the cer-

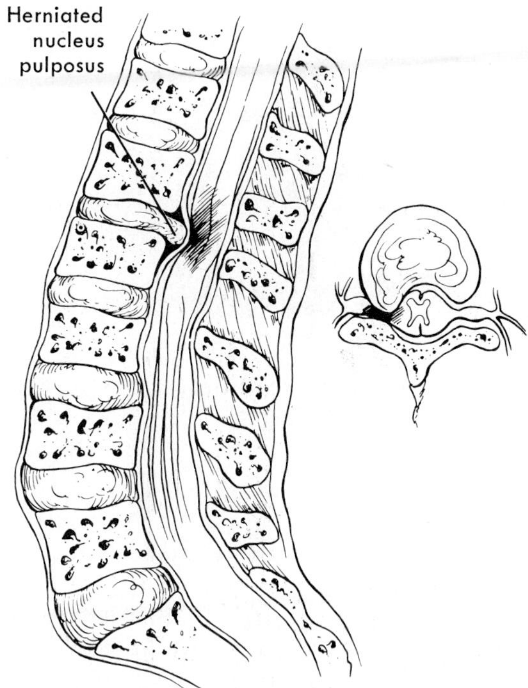

Fig. 42-3. Note compression of spinal cord caused by herniation of nucleus pulposus into spinal canal. *Inset,* Pressure on nerves as they leave spinal cord.

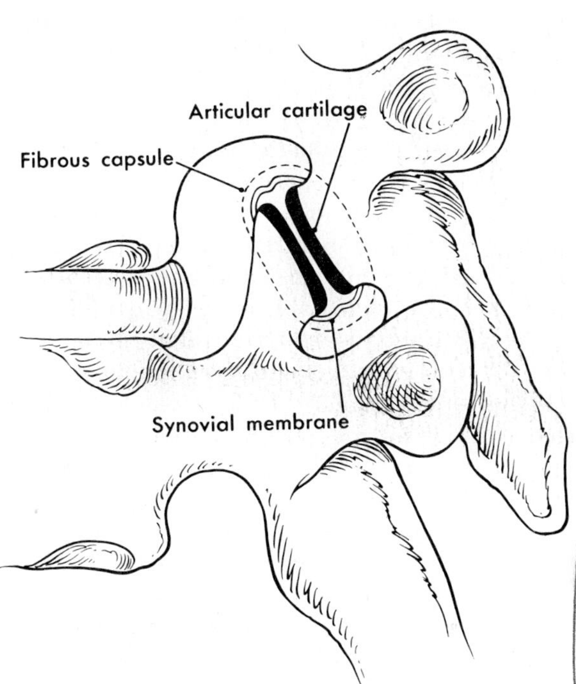

Fig. 42-4. Normal posterior facet joint.

vical spine (C2-3 through C6-7) can become narrowed by spurs, thus creating pressure on the nerve roots in this area and resulting in neurologic symptoms.

Clinical picture

The diagnosis of a herniated disc is usually made on the basis of the history and physical examination. The history of low back pain that is relieved by recumbency and aggravated by flexion of the trunk, coughing, or sneezing is typical. The patient will often complain of sciatic pain radiating down his leg. Some patients, after the initial injury, will have sciatic pain but no pain in their back. Deep pressure over the interspace will usually elicit pain. Straight leg raising with the hip flexed and the knee extended (a positive Laseque sign) will produce the sciatic pain. Neurologic signs and symptoms help in determining the level of the disc involved. The sensory and motor changes depend on the nerve root involved.

If the back problem has been long-standing, the patient may have some muscle atrophy in the affected leg. Roentgenography of the spine is performed. Myelography may be performed if necessary to confirm the physical findings prior to surgery, or to exclude conditions such as tumors. The most common sites of lumbar herniation are L3-4, L4-5, and L5-S1.

Intervention

Unless there are major neurologic deficits indicating a need for immediate surgery, the patient is usually managed conservatively. (This course of treatment may have been attempted at home prior to admission.) The patient is placed on bed rest in a bed with a firm mattress and bed boards. The patient with a herniated disc is usually most comfortable when supine with his head elevated a few degrees and his knees flexed (Fig. 42-5). This decreases the lordosis of the lumbar spine and relieves the pressure on the nerve roots. The bed should be flat when the patient is on his side, and he will probably be most comfortable with pillows between his legs. The pillows should support the upper leg and therefore lessen the pull on the back. The patient should be taught to turn himself in a logrolling fashion: to cross his arms over his chest, bend the uppermost knee to the side to which he wishes to turn, and then to roll over. This position helps him to maintain good spinal alignment.

If there is any motor nerve loss, a footboard or splint should be used to prevent footdrop. The patient may complain of a burning sensation in his feet because of paresthesia, and a footboard helps by keeping the bedclothes off the feet. If the patient has a sensory nerve loss, hot water bottles or heating pads should not be used on the feet or legs, and other precautions (protection from trauma, avoidance of prolonged pressure to skin

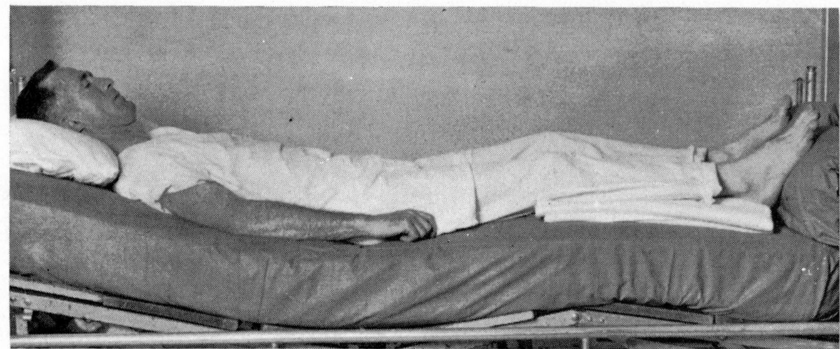

Fig. 42-5. Elevating head of bed 20° to 30° and flexing knees slightly provides comfortable position for patients with acute back pain. (From Larson, C. B., and Gould, M. L.: Orthopedic nursing, ed. 9, St. Louis, 1978, The C. V. Mosby Co.)

surfaces, proper handling during positioning) should be taken to prevent further injury.

A small bedpan should be used with a small towel roll placed directly behind it to support the arch of the lower back. The patient should roll onto the bedpan instead of lifting his hips. Straining to defecate is avoided, since straining will increase pain. Constipation is a common problem. The patient is urged to increase the amount of roughage eaten; bran and fresh fruits are helpful. At least 3,000 ml of fluid should be taken daily, and a regular time for defecation should be established. A mild laxative such as one of the bulk laxatives may be ordered.

Many patients with a ruptured lumbar intervertebral disc suffer from severe muscle spasm in the lower back. A heating pad may relieve it, although analgesic drugs are often necessary. Antispasmodics such as diazepam (Valium) may be used in conjunction with analgesics. Physical therapy in the form of heat, massage, and active and passive muscle exercises carried out in warm water may also be tried to help relieve the muscle spasm. Exercises are more easily performed in water, and the heat helps to relax muscles. The patient should be transferred to the physical therapy department by stretcher, and extra covers, such as a towel to wrap around the head if the hair becomes wet, should be sent with him to avoid chilling after treatment.

Traction may be ordered to relieve muscle spasm. This is usually accomplished by bilateral Buck's extension (p. 860) or pelvic traction. The patient may begin with short periods in traction and gradually increase his tolerance until he remains in traction most of the time.

Patients with a ruptured disc may be discouraged by the prospects of a long period of bed rest and possible surgery. If they have motor or sensory losses, they worry that they may be unable to walk. To some people, spinal surgery is synonymous with paralysis. Worries about family relationships, finances, loss of a job, and about collecting compensation if the injury was sustained at work are common. Nurses, other health care providers, and the patient's spiritual adviser may all be involved in helping to alleviate the patient's fears and anxieties.

If improvement is shown on bed rest, as occurs with 90% of the patients for whom this is the first occurrence, a brace or corset may be ordered to provide external support for the spine. This support may be needed for several months or until the patient is asymptomatic. The external supports are discarded as soon as possible, since prolonged use fosters muscle weakness, which then increases the load on the vertebral column.

The principles of body mechanics should be taught and demonstrated to the patient, since particular care will need to be taken in lifting. Some patients may have to change their type of work. Movements and positions that cause poor alignment of the spinal column and put a strain on the injured nerves should be avoided. A firm, straight chair should be used instead of an overstuffed one. (See p. 841 for a description of an ideal chair.) The knees should not be crossed or the feet or legs elevated on a footstool. It is inadvisable for the patient to drive a car, since this activity would necessitate stretching the legs. Stairs should be climbed as infrequently as possible, and great care should be taken in walking over rough ground or in stepping off curbs to avoid sudden twisting of the back. If a tub bath must be taken, the knees should be kept flexed. However, getting in and out of the tub may aggravate the symptoms, and showers are preferable. A warm shower before bed and on arising often helps to reduce discomfort. In picking things up off the floor, the patient should assume a squatting posture with the knees bent and the back held straight (Fig. 42-6). Anything weighting more than 2.25 kg (5 lb) should not be carried.

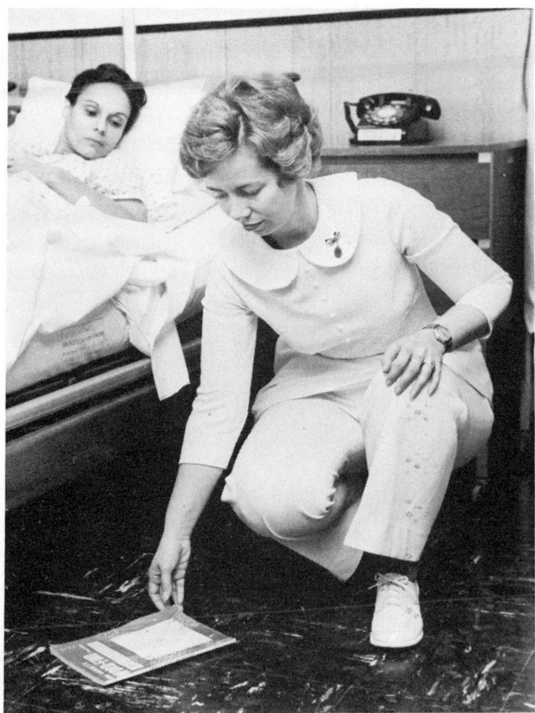

Fig. 42-6. Good body mechanics being used to pick up object from floor. Note that nurse's back is straight while her knees and hips are flexed sharply.

When the acute episode has subsided, the physician may prescribe exercises designed to strengthen the back and abdominal muscles to decrease the load carried by the vertebral column.

Outcome criteria for the person with degenerative joint disease of the spine or a herniated disc

The patient or significant others can:

1. Explain the basic nature of his disorder.
2. Explain the alterations that must be made in ADL to avoid activities and positions that will cause pain or further damage to the back (bending at the waist, straight leg raising, lifting).
3. Demonstrate how to put on and take off the prescribed brace or corset.
4. Demonstrate exercise program (if prescribed).
5. Demonstrate how traction will be set up at home (if prescribed).
6. Explain how medications are to be taken (dosages, what times, side effects, toxic effects).
7. State symptoms that would indicate the need for immediate medical consultation.
8. Explain plans for follow-up care.

□ Traumatic or neurogenic disorders

Neuropathic arthropathy

Epidemiology. Neuropathic arthropathy (Charcot's joints) is a chronic, progressive degeneration of joints resulting from a disturbance in sensory innervation of the joints. Men over 40 years of age are most commonly affected.

Pathophysiology. The primary neurologic disorder (tabes dorsalis, diabetic neuropathy, meningomyelocele) causes loss of proprioception at the joint. As a result, the supporting structures around the joint relax and the joint becomes unstable. The patient, having lost the ability to protect the joint, overuses or misuses it while remaining relatively unaware of pain. Joints most often affected are the knees, tarsal areas, and lower vertebrae. The primary neurologic disorder will determine the specific joints that are involved.

Clinical picture. The first symptoms that may be noticed are enlargement or instability of the joint. While there may be some pain, the pain is much less than would be expected when compared to the extent of the joint effusion and destruction. Swelling, warmth, and tenderness may be present, and the joint is hypermobile. As loss of cartilage, overgrowth of bone, and formation of loose bodies in the joint progress, enlargement of the joint increases and crepitation will be present.

Intervention. Management usually includes bracing or splinting to afford support for the affected joint through immobilization. Further support and protection may be achieved by limiting weight bearing through the use of assistive ambulatory devices such as crutches. (See Chapter 41 for discussion of bracing and other forms of join protection.)

Outcome criteria for the person with neuropathic arthropathy. The patient or significant others can:

1. Explain the basic nature of the joint disorder.
2. Demonstrate appropriate joint protection techniques.
3. Demonstrate how to apply, take off, and care for the prescribed brace.
4. Explain plans for follow-up care.

□ Polyarthritis of unknown cause

For discussion of rheumatoid arthritis, see p. 875.

Juvenile rheumatoid arthritis

Epidemiology. Juvenile rheumatoid arthritis is generally considered to be rheumatoid arthritis that occurs before the age of 16. As with rheumatoid arthritis, the incidence of this disease is greater among girls than boys. Onset of the disease can occur as early as 6 weeks of age, but more typically it occurs between the ages of 2 to 5 years and 9 to 12 years.[5]

Pathophysiology. Juvenile rheumatoid arthritis

may be a more severe systemic disease than adult rheumatoid arthritis. An acute febrile illness and polyarthralgia (pain in many joints) may precede the onset of frank arthritis. When the presence of arthritis is preceded or accompanied by fever, hepatosplenomegaly, lymphadenopathy, a maculopapular erythematous rash, pleuritis, pericarditis, and pronounced leukocytosis, the disease is called *Still's disease.*[5] In juvenile rheumatoid arthritis, joint involvement may vary from all joints to one joint, often the knee.

Clinical picture. Premature closure of the epiphyses, failure of development of the cervical vertebrae and jaw, widening of the phalanges, and impaired development of the head of the femur and acetabulum are common manifestations of the disease. As a result, normal growth and development are impaired. The deformities that result can be quite severe and seriously impair normal function.

Intervention. General management considerations, rest, relief of pain, and so on are the same as for adults (p. 841). Specific attention must be paid to proper positioning, splinting, an individually prescribed program of exercise, and avoidance of highly active and contact sports. Additionally, the child's family must have an understanding of the disease. Their expectations of the child to move, perform his activities of daily living, and cooperate with the treatment program should be neither too great nor too small. Particularly when the child experiences pain, concerned parents may not insist on the child following the treatment regimen. Results of such lapses may result in the development of contractures, loss of function in some joints, and becoming overdependent on the parents. Such problems are difficult, if not impossible, to overcome. Therefore the family needs as much support and attention from the health care team as the patient.

Salicylates are the drug of choice in the treatment of juvenile rheumatoid arthritis. The corticosteroids are reserved for patients who have severe disease that has not responded to salicylates alone, or for those patients who have evidence of systemic involvement (myocarditis or vasculitis). Iridocyclitis (inflammation of the iris and ciliary body) is a serious complication of juvenile rheumatoid arthritis that, if untreated, may lead to serious impairment of vision. This problem is amenable to treatment with corticosteroids.

Outcome criteria for the person with juvenile rheumatoid arthritis. The discharge outcomes for the person with juvenile rheumatoid arthritis are the same as those for any patient with rheumatoid arthritis (p. 877).

Ankylosing spondylitis

Epidemiology. Ankylosing spondylitis is a chronic progressive disorder that occurs nine times more frequently in men than women. It usually occurs between the ages of 10 and 30. The cause is unknown, and the progression of the disease cannot be stopped by any treatment now known.

Clinical picture. The major joints involved are the hips and the sacroiliac joints. A chronic synovitis followed by fibrosis then ankylosis is the pattern of involvement. The patient's initial symptoms are aching and stiffness. This gives way to pain and restricted motion of the back. Pain may be intermittent. Fusion of the sacroiliac joints and spine up through the cervical vertebrae may occur over a period of 10 to 20 years; and as a result, the patient may develop either a "poker-back" deformity or a kyphosis at the cervicodorsal junction (Fig. 42-7).

Roentgenograms are most helpful in delineating this condition, as the findings are usually specific. Bony growths, called *syndesmophytes*, that bridge the adjacent vertebrae give the appearance of a "bamboo spine."

Intervention. Management of patients with ankylosing spondylitis includes attention to the principles of rest, proper positioning and posture, postural exercises, heat application, and in some instances external support through splinting or bracing. Spinal osteotomy

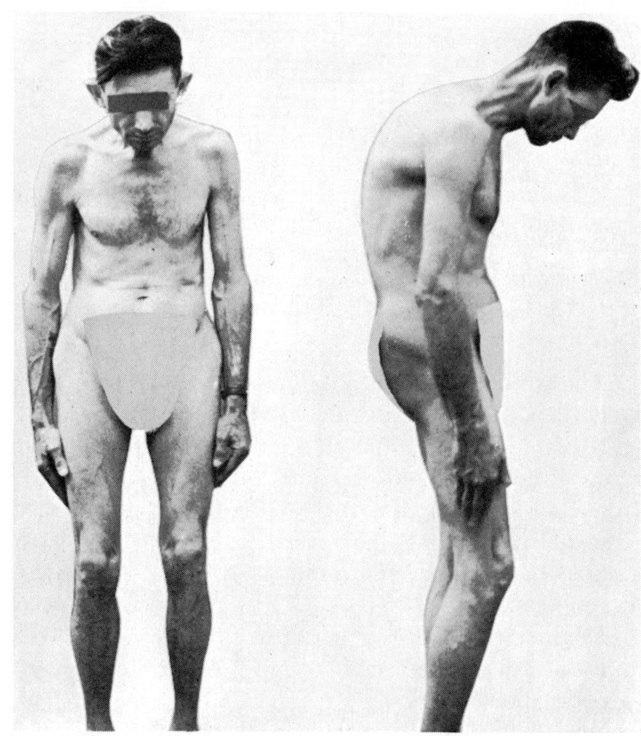

Fig. 42-7. Ankylosing spondylitis in 46-year-old man with ankylosis of entire spine in faulty position. (From Raney, R., and Brashear, H.: Shand's handbook of orthopaedic surgery, ed. 8, St. Louis, 1971, The C. V. Mosby Co.)

or hip arthroplasty might be necessary for patients with severe symptoms. Salicylates are used to decrease inflammation, and in some instances where stronger antiinflammatory agents are needed, phenylbutazone (Butazolidin) or indomethacin (Indocin) may be tried. The objectives of treatment are to relieve pain, achieve and maintain the best possible alignment of the spine, strengthen the paraspinal muscles, and prevent interference with breathing capacity.[5] See Chapter 41 for full discussion of these management considerations.

Outcome criteria for the person with ankylosing spondylitis. The patient or significant others can:

1. Explain the basic nature of the disease.
2. Demonstrate the prescribed program of exercises.
3. Demonstrate how to apply heat to back and hips.
4. Explain how medications are to be taken (dosage, what times, side effects, toxic effects).
5. Describe signs or symptoms that would indicate need for immediate medical consultation.
6. Explain plans for follow-up care.

Psoriatic arthritis

Epidemiology. Psoriatic arthritis is a complicated problem. As many as 3% to 4% of patients with psoriasis (p. 1531) have some inflammatory joint disease. However, the epidemiology of the disease is unclear, as psoriatic arthritis can exist for a time in the absence of skin lesions.

Clinical picture. The interphalangeal and metatarsophalangeal joints of the feet and the distal interphalangeal joints of the fingers are commonly involved, usually in an asymmetric pattern, frequently only two or three joints at a time. Spine and sacroiliac joint involvement as spondylitis is common.[44] The activity of the joint disease may vary with that of the skin disease, and involvement of the nails is common. The nails become discolored, pitted, thickened, and begin to loosen from their beds. This loosening process (oncholysis) begins at the free edge of the nail and progresses gradually back to the root of the nail.[44] When other joints are involved (knee, ankle, and so on), the involvement is consistent with that of rheumatoid arthritis.

Patients with psoriatic arthritis usually can be grouped into one of several distinct categories: (1) those with asymmetric peripheral polyarthritis, usually with involvement of the distal interphalangeal joints of the fingers or the interphalangeal joints of the toes; (2) those with *arthritis mutilans;* (3) those with a pattern of involvement that cannot be distinguished from rheumatoid arthritis except that the swelling of the small joints in psoriatic arthritis appears sausage-shaped; (4) those with symptoms of spondylitis; (5) those who have skin and nail changes preceding or occurring simultaneously with articular disease; and (6) those whose joint manifestations precede skin and nail changes by months or years.[44] With arthritis mutilans, areas of or whole bones (usually the phalanges) may be destroyed, causing a "telescoping" of the digit.

Intervention. Management measures for patients with psoriatic arthritis are limited generally to the physical measures available for the management of other forms of arthritis: rest, local heat, and splinting (Chapter 41). Nonsteroidal antiinflammatory drugs such as aspirin or indomethacin (Indocin) are helpful. Antimalarials are specifically avoided as they may aggravate the psoriatic rash. The skin lesions can be treated with local applications of coal tar or steroid creams. Ultraviolet light is helpful.[44]

Outcome criteria for the person with psoriatic arthritis. The discharge outcomes for the person with psoriatic arthritis are essentially the same as for the patient with rheumatoid arthritis (p. 877). Additionally, the patient or significant others need to be able to explain the use of the various topical medications he is to use in controlling his psoriatic lesions.

Reiter's syndrome

Epidemiology. Reiter's syndrome mainly affects young adult men. Its cause is unknown, but its occurrence usually follows exposure to venereal disease. Since it has also been associated with the occurrence of bacillary dysentery, there is some thought that it may be caused by an inflammation of the prostate or the bowel.[5]

Clinical picture. Symptoms usually include urethritis, conjunctivitis, and arthritis. The arthritis is generally asymmetrical and mainly involves the large joints, for example, the knee joints. When the sacroiliac joints are involved, a form of spondylitis may result. A skin condition known as *keratodermia blennorrhagicum* may be present, with lesions resembling psoriatic pustules appearing chiefly over the palms of the hand and soles of the feet. Small lesions of the glans penis (circinata balanitis) may also be present.

While the disease runs its course in 6 weeks to 6 months, it recurs in about 50% of patients. Joint deformities may occur when the disease runs a recurrent course, and spondylitis may remain active for many years.

Intervention. Management techniques are designed to provide relief of pain and inflammation in involved joints. (See Chapter 41 for specific measures.) Antiinflammatory agents such as salicylates can be used. Severe inflammation may require the use of phenylbutazone (Butazolidin), indomethacin (Indocin), or systemic corticosteroids. Local applications of steroid creams can be used to clear skin lesions.[44]

Outcome criteria for the person with Reiter's syndrome. The patient or significant others can:

1. Explain the basic nature of the disease.
2. Describe the program of rest to be observed until the disease has run its course.
3. Explain the dose, side effects, and toxic effects of the prescribed medications.
4. Explain plans for follow-up care.

□ Rheumatic fever

Rheumatic fever is a systemic disease that is a sequela of infection by group A hemolytic streptococcus. It is most common in children between the ages of 5 and 15, though it may occur at any age. The incidence is highest among those members of the population who are most susceptible to any infection. Thus the incidence is highest among the lower economic groups who live in substandard, overcrowded housing and who are poorly nourished. There seems to be some evidence that the incidence of rheumatic fever in the United States is declining. One possible explanation for this decline is the widespread use of antimicrobial agents to treat childhood infections.

Clinical picture

The inflammatory lesions of the disease occur throughout the body, especially in connective tissue. The attack of rheumatic fever occurs several weeks following a streptococcal infection. The patient often does not remember having had an infection, but careful questioning may reveal a history of sore throat a few weeks previously. The symptoms of rheumatic fever—elevation in temperature, inflamed and painful joints, and cardiac symptoms—are believed to be caused by antibodies produced in response to the *Streptococcus* organism.

The disease varies in its severity, but most commonly the patient has migratory joint pains accompanied by heat, redness, and swelling. In addition, he may have the usual systemic symptoms found in most infections: anorexia, fatigue, and weight loss. The joint manifestations of rheumatic fever are not permanent, and no deformity occurs. However, the patient is at risk of dying from cardiac complications during the acute phase of the disease, and rheumatic heart disease may develop as a complication if the patient survives the acute disease. It is common for an individual to have more than one attack of rheumatic fever. Each succeeding attack is usually more severe and more likely to result in cardiac involvement.

Intervention

Management considerations for the arthritis of rheumatic fever (rest, proper positioning, and other supportive measures) are discussed in Chapter 41. In addition, although not all medical authorities would agree on the need for *absolute* bed rest, it is generally accepted that the patient should be on bed rest until the acute symptoms subside and longer if there is evidence of cardiac involvement.

Salicylates are most effective in reducing fever and reducing joint pain. These are given in high doses—100 mg/kg of body weight[44]—or in sufficient doses to achieve blood levels of 25 mg/100 ml.[34] Corticosteroids may be used, particularly when active cardiac involvement is present, and in some patients in whom salicylates fail to control the disease.[5,44] Penicillin is ordered once or twice daily for 10 days, or a long-acting form of the drug may be given intramuscularly. Oral penicillin or monthly injections of long-acting penicillin may also be prescribed for long-term prophylactic follow-up of the patient to prevent recurrent streptococcal infection. If there is any doubt that the patient will adhere to the regimen of daily oral penicillin, the long-acting parenteral form should be given. Sulfonamides (sulfadiazine, sulfisoxazole) may also be used for continuous prophylaxis. They are most commonly prescribed for individuals allergic to penicillin.

Observations and care considerations for patients receiving high doses of salicylates should be adhered to (p. 849). In the presence of the febrile condition, fluids are usually given in large amounts (3 to 4 liters daily). Further, since these patients often become very bored and restless, espcially when confined to bed for long periods of time, those caring for them may be taxed to develop diversional activities for them in accord with their physical limitations. The American Heart Association publishes many booklets that are helpful in understanding rheumatic fever. One of the most useful is *Home care of the child with rheumatic fever*.

Outcome criteria for the person with rheumatic fever

The patient or significant others can:

1. Explain the program of rest to be observed until the acute symptoms have subsided.
2. Explain the importance of continuing prophylactic antiobiotic therapy for life.
3. Explain the doses, side effects, and toxic effects of prescribed medications.
4. Describe signs and symptoms that would indicate need for immediate medical consultation (fever, joint pain, any new symptom).
5. Explain the plans for regular follow-up care, including when and how to receive the supply of oral penicillin or intramuscular injection of penicillin.

□ Nonarticular rheumatism

Nonarticular rheumatic diseases include those disorders in which the supportive structures and structures located near the joints are involved, but the joints themselves are not involved, except by the limitations imposed by the supportive structures.

Fibrositis

Fibrositis, or fibromyositis, is a common symptom complex. Its cause is unknown and its course seems self-limited. Pain and stiffness in the neck, shoulder girdle, and extremities worsen with activity and subside with rest. Occasionally there are specific areas of tenderness and ill-defined nodules. Psychogenic factors, particularly a chronic tension state, may be important to some patients.[32]

Management is generally related to the specific symptoms. Rest, analgesics, and physical therapy may be utilized (see Chapter 41).

Outcome criteria for the person with fibrositis. The patient or significant others can:

1. Explain the program of rest to be observed until acute symptoms have subsided.
2. Explain the doses, side effects, and toxic effects of prescribed medications.
3. Explain exercise program (if prescribed).
4. Explain plans for follow-up care.

Tenosynovitis

Tenosynovitis tends to be self-limiting. Symptomatic relief may be obtained through rest, splinting, and anti-around the wrists, ankles, or shoulders. Symptoms may vary from local tenderness to inability to move the joint because of pain. The tendon sheath may become thickened and may even prevent free motion of the joint. This disorder, the cause of which is not known, is generally idiopathic but may be found in association with rheumatoid arthritis. When it is associated with rheumatoid arthritis, granulation tissue invades the tendon as well as the tendon sheath and weakens the tendon. The tendon may rupture, requiring surgical intervention.

Tenosynovitis tends to be self-limiting. Symptomatic relief may be obtained through rest, splinting, and anti-inflammatory agents such as indomethacin (Indocin) or phenylbutazone (Butazolidin) (p. 850). Steroid injections into affected joints are very helpful in quickly relieving symptoms.

Outcome criteria for the person with tenosynovitis. The patient or significant others can:

1. Explain the program of rest to be observed until his acute symptoms have subsided.
2. Demonstrate how to use prescribed splinting device.
3. Explain the doses, side effects, and toxic effects of prescribed medications.
4. Explain plans for follow-up care.

Bursitis

Bursitis, or inflammation of the bursa, may be acute or chronic. It usually is caused by trauma, strain, and overuse of the joint with which the bursa is associated. The shoulder bursa is most often affected and may be exceedingly troublesome. Severe pain can occur, especially on movement of the joint.

Management of patients with bursitis includes rest for the involved area. Antiinflammatory agents such as salicylates or phenylbutazone can be utilized to decrease symptoms; local steroid injections may be utilized. Application of cold during the early acute phase may help to relieve discomfort. Much of the discomfort at this time is caused by the presence of additional fluid in the bursa; therefore heat is avoided as this increases the fluid exudate during the early inflammatory period. Occasionally, large calcium deposits are present, and these can be surgically removed. Care of patients receiving these forms of treatment are discussed in Chapter 41.

Outcome criteria for the person with bursitis. The patient or significant others can:

1. Explain the program of rest to be observed until acute symptoms have subsided.
2. Explain modifications in ADL to avoid overuse of the joint associated with the inflamed bursa.
3. Explain the doses, side effects, and toxic effects of the prescribed medications.
4. Explain plans for follow-up care.

Carpal tunnel syndrome

Carpal tunnel syndrome is caused by pressure being exerted on the median nerve at the wrist. The median nerve passes through a tunnel bounded by the carpal bones dorsally and the transverse carpal ligament volarly. Flexor tendons run through the tunnel parallel to the median nerve. The pressure on the nerve may derive from trauma, swelling of the tendon sheaths caused by other processes like rheumatoid arthritis, or it may be associated with systemic disorders such as myxedema (p. 575).

The patient will complain of paresthesia or pain in the first three fingers of the hand, singly or in combination. These complaints will usually increase when there has been forced flexion of the hand for long periods, as in knitting. The symptoms can be elicited by tapping the median nerve at the wrist (Tinel's sign). Atrophy of the thenar eminence (the padded area of the palm below the base of the thumb) may be present in late disease.[44]

Rest, splinting of the wrist, local steroid injections, or, finally, surgery (release of the transverse carpal ligament to decompress the median nerve) are treatment measures that can be employed. Often the conservative measures are all that are needed. Rest, splinting, and steroid injections are discussed in Chapter 41. If surgery is performed, active use of the hand is encouraged as soon as possible following the surgery.

Outcome criteria for the person with carpal tunnel syndrome. The patient or significant others can:
1. Explain the program of rest to be observed until acute symptoms subside.
2. Demonstrate how to apply and take off splint (if prescribed).
3. Demonstrate range of motion of wrist (if surgery has been performed.)
4. Demonstrate care of the surgical wound (if surgery has been performed).
5. Explain plans for follow-up care.

□ Rheumatic diseases associated with known infectious agents

Bacterial arthritis

Epidemiology. Bacterial arthritis is the result of invasion of the synovial membrane by microorganisms, most often gonococci, meningococci, staphylococci, coliforms, salmonellae, and *Haemophilus influenzae.* Factors that predispose to such infections are a high degree of susceptibility on the part of the patient, recent joint surgery or trauma, intraarticular injections, and rheumatoid arthritis.

Clinical picture. The synovial tissues respond to bacterial invasion by becoming inflamed. The joint cavity may become involved, and pus will be present in the synovial membrane and the synovial fluid. If allowed to progress, the infection will cause abscesses in the synovium and subchondral bone and will destroy cartilage. Ankylosis of the joint may result. The patient will complain of pain, swelling, and tenderness of the joint.

Joint aspirations are helpful in making a diagnosis if the presence of organisms can be demonstrated in the synovial fluid. Joint fluid white cell counts will be high, and glucose content of synovial fluid may be reduced. Roentgenograms taken days to weeks after onset of the infection may reveal loss of joint space and lytic changes in bone.

Intervention. Untreated joint infections can result in damage to contiguous bone and in osteomyelitis. Antibiotic therapy will be specific to the organism that is present. Rest or immobilization of the joint is necessary in the initial stages of the infection and may help control pain or prevent deformity, but the patient should begin to move the joint regularly when he can tolerate motion in order to prevent contracture. Local heat is *not* generally used in the presence of infection, as it may increase the inflammatory process.[44] Surgical drainage or a system of irrigation and drainage may be employed if the infection does not respond to antibiotic therapy or if osteomyelitis is present. Death, though rare, can result if there is dissemination of the infection. The patient is usually hospitalized until the infection is cleared, and active range of motion of the involved joint can be resumed.

Outcome criteria for the person with bacterial arthritis. The patient or significant others can:
1. Demonstrate exercises (if prescribed).
2. Demonstrate how to safely use ambulatory assistive devices (if prescribed).
3. Explain the dosages and side effects of antibiotics (if prescribed).
4. State how long antibiotic therapy is to be continued (if prescribed).
5. Explain plans for follow-up care.

□ Rheumatic diseases associated with known or strongly suspected biochemical or endocrine abnormalities

Gout

Epidemiology. Gout or gouty arthritis is a metabolic disorder that affects men eight to nine times more frequently than women. It can occur at any age, the peak age of onset occurring in the fifth decade.[32] Eighty-five percent of all patients with gout have a familial tendency to develop the disease.

Clinical picture. Prolonged hyperuricemia (elevated serum uric acid levels) caused by a metabolic problem in synthesizing purines or by poor renal excretion of uric acid leads to the formation of urate crystals in the synovial tissue. The inflammatory process that results is extremely rapid, occurring over a few hours. Gout is a chronic diathesis, but patients who have it will have acute symptoms of pain, swelling, and erythema in the involved joints. Typically the great toe is involved (the first metatarsophalangeal joint), but other joints, such as the ankles and knees, may also be affected. The pain is so severe that the patient may not tolerate even the weight of a sheet over the joint. Renal damage may occur, especially if recurrent uric stones have been present. Between attacks of gout, the patient may be asymptomatic, but repeated attacks can occur with gradually increased frequency if the disease is untreated. Patients with gouty symptoms may develop *tophi,* or deposits of monosodium urate in their tissues. These consist of a core of monosodium urate with a surrounding inflammatory reaction. Patients with tophaceous deposits tend to have more frequent and more severe episodes of gouty arthritis (Fig. 42-8).

Laboratory studies will indicate an elevated serum uric acid, normal or increased urinary uric acid over a 24-hour period, and the presence of monosodium urate monohydrate crystals in the synovial fluid and in the tophi.

Intervention. The management of patients is directed toward control of acute attacks and prevention of

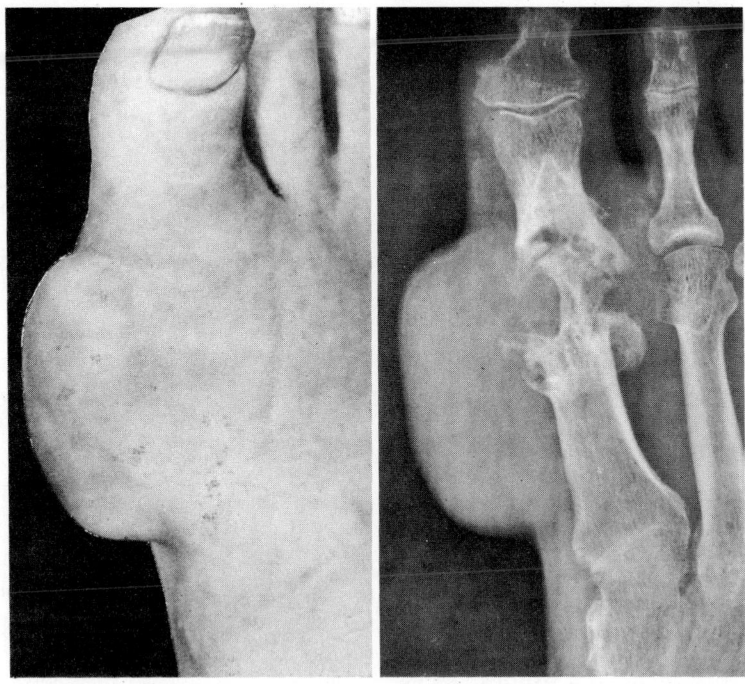

Fig. 42-8. Gout of long duration. Tophaceous mass at base of great toe, as well as destructive bone and joint changes shown in roentgenogram, are associated with extensive urate deposits. (From Raney, R., and Brashear, H.: Shand's handbook of orthopaedic surgery, ed. 8, St. Louis, 1971, The C. V. Mosby Co.)

recurrent attacks and tophaceous deposits (interval therapy). In an *acute attack*, treatment consists of pain relief and rest of the affected limb. Medications such as colchicine, phenylbutazone (Butazolidin), indomethacin (Indocin), corticosteroids, or corticotropin (ACTH gel) are used to reduce pain. Colchicine is the standard drug used in the treatment of acute gout. When an acute attack of gout is imminent, the usual treatment is oral administration of 0.6 mg of this drug each hour until nausea, vomiting, or diarrhea develops, or until joint pain is relieved. Usually not more than 8 tablets are given. Camphorated tincture of opium (paregoric) is sometimes given as treatment for the gastrointestinal irritation caused by the colchicine.[44]

Interval therapy to prevent the chronic manifestations of gout is directed toward reducing the body pool of urates and serum uric acid. The presence of tophi, recurrent acute gouty arthritis, or significant asymptomatic hyperuricemia (over 9 mg/100 ml) are indications for such a preventive program.[44] Because they are likely to develop renal stones, patients who overexcrete uric acid will also be treated with an interval program. The medications used in an interval program are uricosuric agents such as probenecid (Benemid) and sulfinpyrazone (Anturane), and agents that decrease uric acid formation such as allopurinol (Zyloprim). Dietary regulation in the form of a low purine diet and increased fluid intake (3 to 4 liters per day) may also be helpful.[44]

The usual dosage of probenecid is an oral dose of 0.5 g daily for 1 week, then increased by 0.5 g weekly until the serum uric acid is brought into a normal range.[44] This drug may cause gastric distress and is best tolerated if taken with meals. For those patients who do not tolerate probenecid, sulfinpyrazone may be used. One hundred milligrams of sulfinpyrazone are approximately equivalent to 0.5 g of probenecid. Patients who are being treated with either probenecid or sulfinpyrazone should not use compounds that contain salicylates, as the salicylate will nullify the uricosuric action of the drugs. Allopurinol is the drug of choice for patients who have an allergy to the usual uricosuric agents, have a history of uric acid stones, have renal impairment, or who overexcrete urinary uric acid.[44] The initial dose is 100 mg twice a day, and the dose is increased by 100 mg every 2 to 4 weeks until the serum uric acid level is normal. Sodium bicarbonate, 5 to 7.5 g daily, may be given to help prevent the formation of renal stones by making the urine more alkaline.

Patients with gout who are able to maintain normal uric acid blood levels with prescribed medication do not need to be on a restricted diet unless they have other health problems. If overweight, the patient is advised to lose weight, since excess weight will aggravate the joint symptoms. However, an alkaline-ash diet, high in fruits and vegetables with lower amounts of meat proteins, may be prescribed to increase the alkalinity of the urine, thereby decreasing the possibility of urate crystal formation. In either case, a high fluid intake is advisable to minimize uric acid precipitation. The daily urine *output* for the patient should be 2,000 to 3,000 ml per day.

Outcome criteria for the person with gout. The patient or significant others can:

1. Explain the basic nature of the disease.
2. Explain the dietary restrictions to be observed (if any).
3. Explain the dosage and side effects of the prescribed medication.
4. Explain the amount of fluid to be taken each day and the plan to achieve this.
5. Explain plans for follow-up care.

□ Miscellaneous rheumatic disorders

Avascular necrosis of bone

Avascular necrosis of bone, or bone death caused by inadequate blood supply, is a problem resulting from a variety of conditions. It can be a complication of bone fractures, connective tissue diseases such as rheumatoid arthritis or systemic lupus erythematosus, irradiation, alcoholism, and sickle cell anemia. Patients who have received prolonged corticosteroid therapy have an increased incidence of avascular necrosis.

Unlike some other forms of connective tissue, bone has a highly developed vascular system and will die without an adequate blood supply. There is a well-developed collateral blood supply to most bone so that infarction from vascular interruption is infrequent. Several areas of bone, however, have a rather precarious blood supply. One such area is the femoral head. Hence avascular necrosis of the femoral head is a common late complication of a fracture of the femoral neck, since the blood supply to the head comes up through the neck and has been interrupted by the trauma.

The pain is insidious in its onset and gradually increases. There may be development of flexion contractures of the affected joint. Later, pain at rest, restricted motion, and gait disturbances are characteristic. Reducing the work of the joint through rest may help, as may assisted weight bearing through the use of ambulatory aids. Analgesics may help. However, where destruction is severe, surgery, particularly of the hip in the form of total joint replacement, is performed to alleviate pain and increase motion.

Outcome criteria for the person with avascular necrosis of bone who has undergone a conservative program of treatment. The patient or significant others can:

1. Explain how to alter ADL to avoid stressing the affected joint.
2. Demonstrate how to safely use ambulatory assistive aids.
3. Explain the dosage and side effects of the prescribed medications.
4. Explain plans for follow-up care.

■ SURGICAL INTERVENTION

Surgery is being used increasingly to correct deformity and to improve function of the musculoskeletal system. Surgery may also be performed as an adjunct to medical management in certain instances such as synovectomy to arrest the course of rheumatoid arthritis in a particular joint. Frequently, surgery is indicated when other measures designed to relieve pain or prevent deformity are ineffective. Advances in other fields such as bioengineering have made reconstructive surgery possible in patients for whom there were formerly very limited means of treatment available. The following discussion will be limited to commonly used operative orthopedic procedures of bone and joint.

□ Intraarticular surgical intervention

Arthrotomy

Arthrotomy is simply the opening of a joint. This procedure is usually done for exploration of the joint to determine the presence of a disease process, for drainage, or for removal of damaged tissue or foreign bodies within the joint. While any joint may be so opened, it is frequently the knee joint that is involved, often to remove a torn meniscus, foreign bodies, or calcium deposits.

Following an arthrotomy, the joint must be protected until healing takes place. After an arthrotomy of the knee, the patient is often placed in a Robert-Jones compression dressing. Depending on the procedure, the surgeon may order straight leg raising exercises to be done postoperatively. Active flexion exercises may usually be started when the compression dressing is removed. Limited weight bearing will be ordered on that leg, and crutches will be utilized for a prescribed period of time.

Arthroplasty

An arthroplasty is the reconstruction of a joint that has been destroyed by injury or disease. The purpose of the procedure is to restore motion to the joint, relieve pain, and correct deformity.

Interposition arthroplasty. There are several types of arthroplasties. One type involves replacement of part of a joint with a prosthesis made of metal or other material. An example of this type of arthroplasty is the

D-shaped McIntosh prosthesis designed to fit on the tibial plateau of the knee joint. This prosthesis on one or both tibial plateaus enables the surgeon to correct either genu varum or genu valgum in addition to providing a smooth articulating surface.

Another common interposition arthroplasty is the "cup" or "mold" arthroplasty of the hip joint. The usual indication for this procedure is osteoarthritis of the hip. In this procedure both the acetabulum and the femoral head are reshaped, and a Vitallium cup is interposed between the head of the femur and the acetabulum. In the immediate period following a mold arthroplasty, the patient is placed in some form of traction with an apparatus to allow him to begin prescribed exercises. The period of hospitalization is usually 5 to 6 weeks, during which the patient will undergo an extensive program of physical therapy. The patient will not be permitted full weight bearing for at least 6 months. Therefore crutches are necessary. An exercise program to be performed at home will be prescribed and followed for several years. The cup arthroplasty provides relief of pain, increases motion in the hip, and corrects deformity. To achieve these results a patient must be highly motivated and committed to the long-term exercise program.

A second type of interposition arthroplasty involves surgical reshaping of the bones of the joint that are then covered by soft tissue used as an interposition device. An example of this is an elbow fascial arthroplasty for either degenerative joint disease or rheumatoid arthritis. This surgery involves removing bone from the lower end of the humerus and the trochlear notch of the ulna, excising the head of the radius, and covering the raw bone ends with a sheet of fascia lata form the thigh. The elbow is immobilized in 90° of flexion for 3 weeks, then active exercises are begun.

Replacement arthroplasty. A third type of arthroplasty is the *total joint replacement,* where both sides of the joint are replaced by metal or plastic implants. These implants are held into the bone by a groutlike material called polymethylmethacrylate. The replacement arthroplasty is one of the most rapidly expanding areas of orthopedic surgery. The results are quickly apparent and very dramatic. Partially for these reasons this type of surgery has received wide coverage in the lay press. Many patients with diseased joints seek out an orthopedic surgeon with the expressed hope that they might benefit from joint replacement. However, not all persons with diseased joints are candidates for joint replacement. Joint replacement is still a relatively new procedure and is usually considered when there is no other operative procedure that would be effective for the individual. A yet unknown problem in the use of joint replacements is the life expectancy of the prosthesis with respect to wear. All artificial joints have a finite life and are used most frequently in the older person. Replacement arthroplasties are considered for individuals who have significant pain, limitation of motion, and deformity in the affected joint. The causes of these problems include osteoarthritis, rheumatoid arthritis, avascular necrosis, congenital deformities or dislocations, and numerous systemic diseases.

Replacement arthroplasties are available for the shoulder, elbow, the phalangeal joints of the fingers (in the form of silicone or Silastic implants), the hip, knee, and the ankle. The hip and knee are most commonly replaced, and this discussion will be limited to those two joints.

Total hip replacement. The hip prosthesis consists of an acetabular portion (cup) and a femoral component. There are numerous types of total hip replacements in use (Fig. 42-9). Some prostheses (McKee-Farrar, Ring) are made entirely of metal (Vitallium or stainless steel). Other prostheses (Charnley, Charnley-Müller, Trapezoidal-28) have a metal femoral component and a high-density polyethylene acetabular component (Fig. 42-9). The metal component moving within a polyethylene cup is expected to cause less friction and therefore should wear at a slower rate. The designs of the different prostheses vary in size of the femoral head, shape and length of the femoral neck, and shape of the acetabular component. Each type of prosthesis has its own mechanical advantages and disadvantages of design, and each prosthesis is inserted by a particular operative technique. The relative merits of the design and operative techniques are discussed at great length in the orthopedic literature. As in any new and expanding field, changes are constantly being made. For this reason *it is essential that the nurse caring for a patient with a total hip replacement become familiar with the literature pertaining to the prosthesis and the procedure being used for each patient.*

INTERVENTION. The postoperative positioning of the total hip patient is directly dependent on the design of the prosthesis and the method of insertion. Positioning is generally directed at keeping the patient's operative leg in *abduction* and in limiting excessive flexion of that hip. To plan care for the patient the nurse must have the following information:

1. What degree of flexion in the operative hip is permitted and for how long?
2. In what rotation is the leg to be held?
3. How much weight bearing is allowed on the operative leg?
4. What exercises, if any, are to be done?

The care of the patient with a *Charnley total hip replacement* will serve as an example of a partial care plan regarding positioning and ambulating. The Charnley prosthesis has a small (22.5 mm) head that, once healing has taken place, can be flexed to 90° without dislocating it. In the Charnley procedure the greater trochanter is detached with all its muscles still in place. After placement of the prosthesis, the trochanter is wired back into place. Until bony union takes place (6 to 8 weeks), pull on the abductor muscles attached to the trochanter must be avoided. However, protected weight bearing on the operative leg is permitted with the use of crutches.

During surgery, drains are placed in the wound to prevent formation of a hematoma. The drains are connected to constant suction and are usually the self-contained vacuum type such as the Porto-Vac (Fig. 23-10). It is imperative that the system remain closed and that sterility be maintained. Because the drains are inserted deep in the wound, contamination of the tubing would provide a portal of entry for bacteria. The drainage is emptied as necessary to maintain an accurate record of output from the wound, and the suction device should be recompressed every few hours to maintain suction. Aseptic technique is required for these procedures.

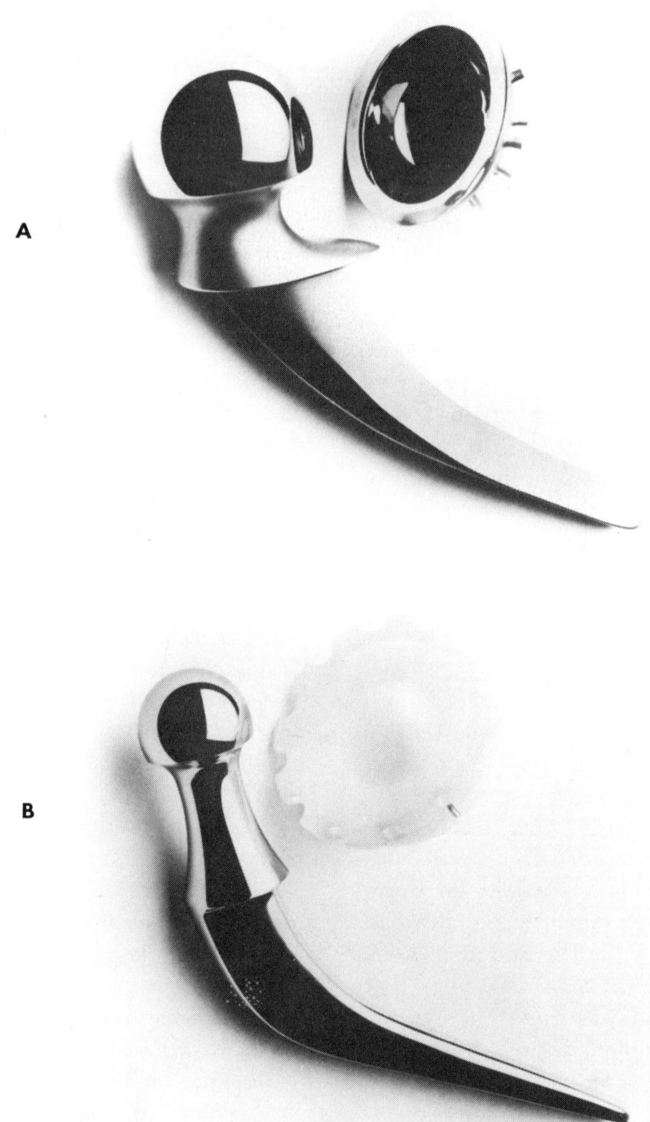

Fig. 42-9. A, McKee-Farrar prosthesis. **B,** Charnley prosthesis. **C,** Charnley-Müller prosthesis. **D,** Trapezoidal-28 prosthesis. (Courtesy Zimmer USA, Warsaw, Ind.)

Since the patient remains in bed for at least 3 postoperative days, care is directed at keeping him as active as possible within the specified restrictions. The head of the bed may be elevated for comfort (usually about 60°) for short periods of time. The patient is encouraged to spend some time flat with his operated hip in full extension. He is instructed in the use of the overbed trapeze and how to shift his weight using his unoperated leg and the trapeze. The operated leg is maintained in abduction with an abduction block, and the patient is turned only slightly side to side. Plantar flexion and dorsiflexion of the feet as well as quadriceps and gluteal-setting exercises are encouraged to promote venous return and prevent thrombi. These exercises are taught preoperatively (Chapter 23).

Because of the increased risk of thromboembolic phenomena in hip surgery, prophylactic anticoagulant treatment is often prescribed. The various methods of treatment are debated in the literature. While there is not general agreement on which method is preferable, three types of treatment are most common: acetylsalicylic acid (aspirin), usually 600 mg four times a day; low molecular weight dextran, which increases microcirculation and decreases platelet cohesiveness; and small dosages of heparin. Each method has its particular advantages and hazards with which the nurse must be familiar. (Refer to specialized texts for further details.)

Ambulation begins on the third to fourth postoperative day. Nursing personnel and the physical therapist assist the patient to stand without flexing his operative hip more than 60°. The amount of walking, using a walker for support, that is permitted is variable and depends on the patient's progress. The patient is usually discharged 3 weeks after surgery. He must use crutches and limit his hip flexion to 90° for 2 months.

The nurse, physical therapist, and occupational therapist evaluate the patient's ability to carry out activities of daily living throughout his postoperative course, and necessary equipment is secured. A raised toilet seat extension must be used for at least 2 months to protect against the extreme hip flexion needed to rise from a standard toilet seat. Long-handled shoe horns and devices to pick up dropped items (reachers) are also necessary.

Some surgeons, depending on the prosthesis used and their personal preference, will place the patient in

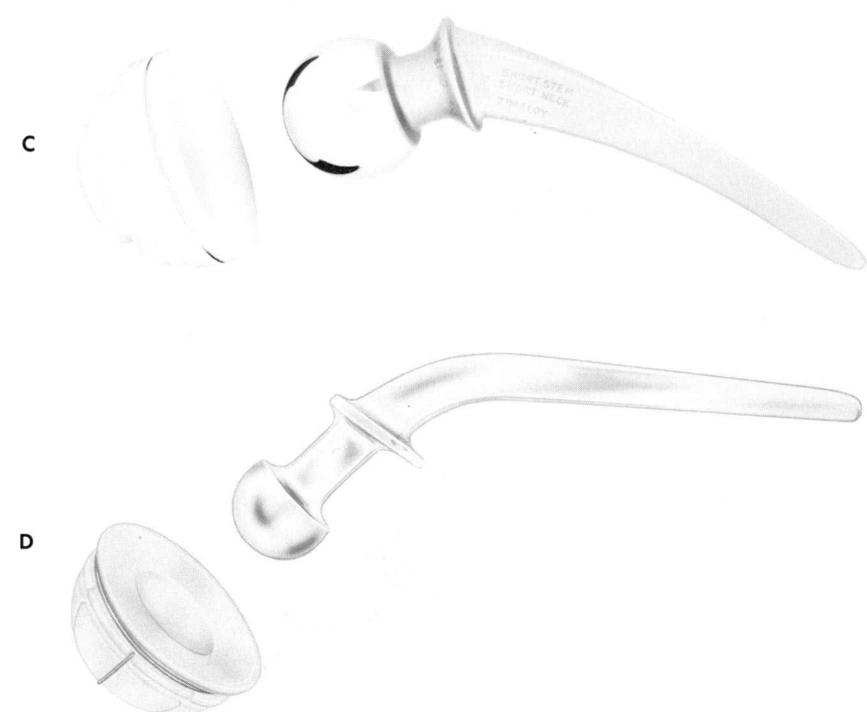

Fig. 42-9, cont'd. For legend see opposite page.

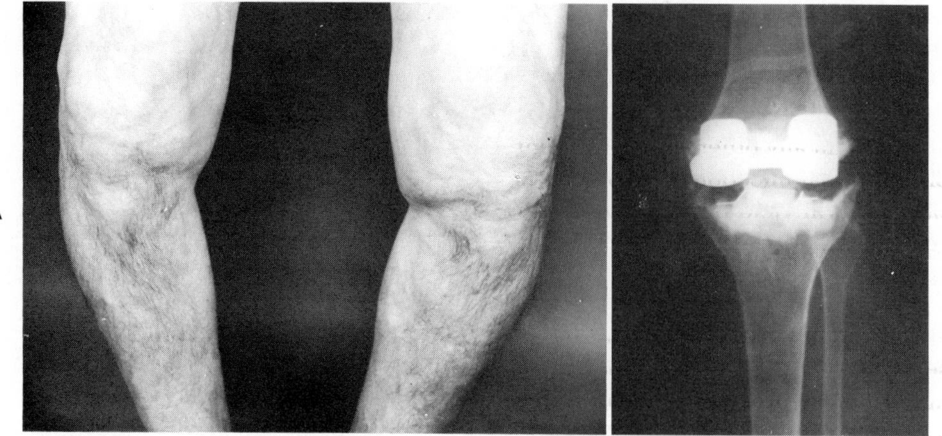

Fig. 42-10. A, Marked varus deformity in both knees. **B,** Varus deformity corrected by proper insertion and alignment of total knee replacement. Prosthesis provides joint surface for both motion and weight bearing. (From Larson, C. B., and Gould, M. L.: Orthopedic nursing, ed. 9, St. Louis, 1978, The C. V. Mosby Co.)

various slings or traction devices to facilitate motion of the hip while maintaining the desired position. It is important for the nurse as well as the entire health team to understand what will be required of the patient in the postoperative period so that the necessary preoperative teaching can be provided.

Total knee replacement. A replacement arthroplasty of the knee is also used. Once again there are numerous prosthetic designs, each with its distinct mechanical advantage (Fig. 42-10). Care of the patient with a total knee replacement is not usually as complex as that for a patient with a total hip replacement. The postoperative course follows that of most intraarticular procedures performed on the knee; however, there is more emphasis on active exercising. While the bulky compression dressing is still in place, usually about 5 days, the patient is strongly urged to do quadriceps-setting exercises and to attempt straight leg raising. When the dressing is removed, *active* flexion exercises are begun. These exercises may increase discomfort greatly. The patient will need considerable encouragement as well as prescribed medication and other comfort measures. Once the patient is able to do independent straight leg raising and actively flex the knee to 45°, ambulation with partial weight bearing using a walker or crutches may begin. The walker or crutches will continue to be used for 2 months. If the patient is not able to achieve active knee flexion to 70° within a period of time determined by the surgeon, the knee may be manipulated (flexed) under anesthesia to break adhesions that are preventing flexion.

Total elbow and ankle replacement. Total replacement of both the *elbow* and the *ankle* is available. A complication associated with both of these procedures is poor wound healing caused by the proximity of the joint to the skin. Silastic implants are used to replace *metacarpophalangeal* and *proximal interphalangeal joints* in persons with severe rheumatoid arthritis. While these implants restore cosmetic appearance and reasonable function, there can sometimes be some loss of hand strength postoperatively. Specialized texts should be consulted for information related to these procedures.

Wound infections. Any general discussion of total joint replacement must include reference to the dreaded complication of *infection.* Many total prostheses are held in place by polymethylmethacrylate. This material is a filling or grouting agent that gives off heat as it solidifies. The temperature is high enough to cause minimal local tissue necrosis. Because necrotic tissue is a good culture medium for bacterial growth and because of the presence of a large foreign body, there is an increased risk of infection. Although any bone infection is serious, it has especially grave consequences for a patient having a joint replacement. Infection at the site of the prosthesis results in total failure of the surgery. The prosthesis must be removed and cannot be replaced except under unusual circumstances. When the prosthesis is removed, the patient is left (after healing) with a pain-free but unstable hip and must use crutches or other ambulatory aids for the rest of his life. If the knee is the joint involved, the joint can be fused. This may result in some shortening of the leg, and the patient will not be able to flex the knee; however, the knee will be stable and pain free. Because of the possibility of infection, utmost care must be taken in preparing the operative site preoperatively. Each hospital will have its own procedure for preoperative preparation, but the goal is the same—keeping the patient and his environment as free as possible from potential sources of contamination. Once the joint is replaced and the wound closed, the patient has no more risk of infection than any other surgical patient, but it must be emphasized that infection occurring in the operated joint *at any time* will yield the same disastrous results. Precautions necessary to guard against infection should be explained to the patient prior to his discharge from the hospital.

A relatively new system of wound irrigation[26] has offered some promise in the treatment of wound infections and may be attempted before prostheses are removed. This system involves a set-up of polyethylene tubing utilizing crisscross tubes that allow for reversal of the flow of irrigation fluid and effluent. It is a completely closed system. The effluent is drawn off by an electric suction pump such as a Gomco or an Emerson. When an Emerson pump is used, the suction is adjustable. As the flow of irrigation fluid and effluent can be reversed, the system is self-irrigating and need not be opened. Irrigation rates are generally maintained fast enough to keep the system patent (often 200 to 300 ml per hour), and suction is maintained at a level that will draw off the effluent at the same rate as the flow of the irrigation fluid. Careful *running totals* of intake and output must be maintained to aid in determining if the system is patent or if fluid is being retained in the tissue surrounding the wound. Leakage of fluid out through the dressings covering the wound will indicate that the system is no longer functioning as it should. Clamping the system for longer than 60 seconds can result in loss of patency; therefore changes of irrigation fluid bottles and bottles used for the collection of the effluent must be accomplished quickly and with strict attention to asepsis. Cultures of the effluent will be obtained on a regular basis, and the irrigation will be discontinued when the surgeon is satisfied that there is no longer evidence of infection (often 2 weeks or more). The patient is maintained on appropriate intravenous antibiotics throughout the period that the irrigation apparatus is in place, and sometimes antibiotics may be added to the irrigating solution. After the irrigation is stopped, the patient is maintained on oral antibiotics for a prolonged period.

Outcome criteria for the person having had an arthroplasty. The patient or significant others can:

1. Demonstrate the prescribed program of exercise.
2. Explain the limitations on motion or restrictions on activity and for how long these are to be observed.
3. Demonstrate the safe use of ambulatory assistive devices (if prescribed).
4. Demonstrate how to perform or modify ADL to be within the limitations on motion.
5. Explain precautions to be observed to avoid infection in the operated joint (if a total joint replacement), for example, dental work, future surgery.
6. Explain plans for follow-up care.

Synovectomy

Synovectomy (removal of the synovial membrane) is often performed in the early stages of rheumatoid arthritis when little or no destruction of joint surfaces has occurred. Joints commonly subjected to this procedure are the knee and the wrist. It should be noted that this is not a curative procedure. The synovium will grow back and the disease process can begin again; however, the patient does experience relief of discomfort in the operated joint for a prolonged period.

When the joint operated on is the knee, a bulky compression dressing is applied for approximately 72 hours postoperatively. While the dressing is still in place, the patient usually begins isometric quadriceps exercises prescribed by the physician. As pain decreases, the patient is encouraged to exercise more actively. Active flexion is begun after the compression dressing is removed, usually 3 to 5 days after surgery. Ambulation is begun on the parallel bars and progresses, as the patient is able, to crutches. Partial weight bearing on the operative leg is begun when the patient is able to demonstrate active straight leg raising and active flexion to 45° (Chapter 41).

Outcome criteria for the person having had a synovectomy. The discharge outcomes for the patient having had a synovectomy are the same as those for the patient having had an arthroplasty.

□ Extraarticular surgical interventions

Osteotomy

An osteotomy is a frequently used orthopedic procedure that involves cutting a bone to change alignment, thereby correcting deformity in the bone or adjacent joint. This procedure may be used to correct angulation or rotational deformities, or to alter the weight-bearing surface in a diseased joint. An osteotomy may be thought of as an intentional fracture (Fig. 42-11). Postoperatively the involved extremity is immobilized in some manner, and the care of the patient is the same as that of a patient who has had a fracture in that area. Likewise, the time that weight bearing may begin and the amount of weight bearing that will be allowed will be dependent on the specific area of the surgery (Chapter 41).

Tendon transplants

Transplanting a tendon from its usual position to another position is a technique that can be utilized to substitute one tendon for another that is not working or for realignment of tendon function. An example of this type of procedure is the transplanting of the insertion of

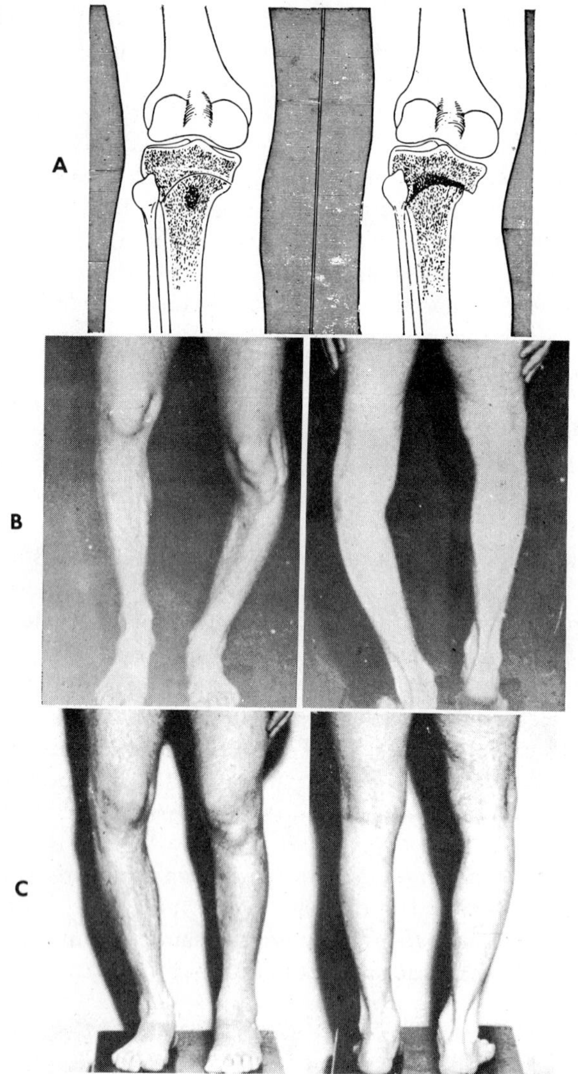

Fig. 42-11. A, Tibial osteotomy for correction of genu valgum (bowing) deformity of knee. **B,** Anterior and posterior views of left knee demonstrating severe valgus deformity of tibia. **C,** Same patient after corrective osteotomy of proximal tibia, left leg. (From Larson, C. B., and Gould, M. L.: Orthopedic nursing, ed. 9, St. Louis, The C. V. Mosby Co.)

the patellar tendon to correct recurrent dislocation of the patella. Dislocation may occur as a result of trauma or may occur repeatedly because of postural or congenital factors. It is the latter condition that is referred to as recurrent dislocation.

In individuals in whom recurrent dislocation of the patella occurs, the patellar tendon may be more laterally placed than usual so that when the quadriceps contracts, the patella is pulled to the outside and dislocates to the lateral side of the knee. Surgery involves moving the tendon from its insertion on the tibial tubercle to a point more medial and distal to the preoperative insertion. Postoperatively the leg is protected with splints, and a bulky compression dressing is used to aid in preventing edema. Once the danger of postoperative swelling is past, a cylinder cast is applied to immobilize the knee to permit healing; however, weight bearing is permitted. After about 6 weeks the cast may be bivalved, and active flexion exercises are begun. Postoperative management considerations are discussed in Chapter 41.

Outcome criteria for the person who has had extraarticular surgery

The patient or significant others can:

1. Describe the limitations of activity.
2. Explain how long these limitations are to be observed.
3. Demonstrate how to perform or modify ADL to be within the prescribe limitations of activity.
4. Explain how to care for the cast.
5. Explain plans for follow-up care.

□ Arthrodesis

An arthrodesis (fusion) is a form of surgery designed to cause the bones of a joint to grow firmly together. The procedure involves removal of the articular hyaline cartilage and, usually, the addition of bone grafts across the joint surface. Metallic internal fixation devices are sometimes used to help effect the fusion (Fig. 42-12).[25] Postoperatively the joint that has been fused must be immobilized until bone healing has occurred. Immobilization is usually accomplished by a plaster cast. The permanent immobilization of the joint accomplished by this procedure provides for a stiff but stable, pain-free joint.

Arthrodesis of the knee or wrist, for example, may be an end-stage procedure for rheumatoid arthritis or other destructive processes when other treatment measures have failed. A triple arthrodesis of the ankle is often done to stabilize the foot when there is inadequate or absent neuromuscular control. The three joints involved in the triple arthrodesis are the subastragalar, the astragaloscaphoid, and the calcaneocuboid joints. The patient who has had a triple arthrodesis will be held in a leg cast with no weight bearing for 6 weeks. The non-weight-bearing period for the patient who has had a fusion of the knee may be shorter. Postoperative management considerations are discussed in Chapter 41.

□ Spinal surgery

Problems precipitating surgery

Two of the most common reasons for performing surgery on the spine are spinal fractures and herniation of a disc. Spinal fractures may occur as the result of trauma or they may be pathologic. Pathologic fractures occur most often as a complication of cancer, osteo-

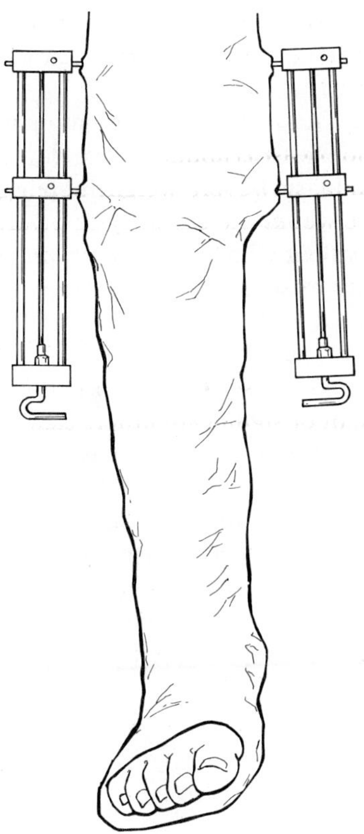

Fig. 42-12. Arthrodesis of knee with compression apparatus. Pins are placed through proximal tibia and distal femur. Compression is maintained by adjusting hand screws, bringing bone wires closer together.

porosis of the vertebrae, and other metabolic problems. Fractures in the thoracolumbar area are usually compression fractures wherein the vertebral body collapses. Other types of fractures involve the transverse processes or the spinous processes of the vertebrae. Generally these fractures are not complicated by spinal cord or nerve root compression and heal with bed rest as the only treatment. However, if there is displacement of the fracture and if spinal cord or nerve root compression is present, surgery may be necessary.

The structure of the intervertebral disc, the causes of herniation of a disc, and conservative management of the patient with a herniated disc have been discussed (p. 883). When the patient's symptoms fail to respond to conservative management, when there is progressive neurologic impairment, or when the patient has repeated episodes of herniation when he attempts to resume activity, surgical intervention is usually indicated.

A third problem that precipitates spinal surgery is subluxation of the vertebrae. Rheumatoid arthritis is often a factor leading to subluxation of vertebrae in the cervical spine. As has been noted on p. 886, the cervical spine is very frequently involved in juvenile rheumatoid arthritis. In adults the inflammatory process of the disease may erode bone. The atlantoaxial area is commonly involved, and there may be complete or partial destruction of the odontoid process.[44] Occipital headaches, compression of vascular and neurologic structures, and upper extremity weakness may be present. When subluxation of vertebrae in the cervical spine is causing neurologic symptoms, surgery is generally indicated.

Types of spinal surgery

Three major types of spinal surgery will be discussed: discectomy, laminectomy, and spinal fusion. *Discectomy* and *laminectomy* are procedures classified as decompression procedures; that is, they are procedures designed to relieve pressure on the spinal cord or spinal nerve roots caused by herniated nuclear material. *Discectomy* is removal of that portion of the disc that is impinging on the nerve or spinal cord, and it is most often performed through a posterior approach in which a portion of the lamina is removed *(laminectomy)*. These procedures are generally unilateral and do not create any instability of the spine. However, removal of the disc can cause increased stress on the posterior articulations of the spine, which then may develop degenerative changes. Therefore, depending on the extent of the pathology and the type of activities the patient usually engages in, the surgeon may elect to perform a *spinal fusion*. A spinal fusion may also be performed when there is anatomic reason for instability of the spine. Unstable fractures of the spine may be treated by fusion. There are numerous techniques for spinal fusion, details of which may be found in orthopedic texts. Most commonly, lumbar fusion is performed through a posterior incision, with the bone for the graft being taken from the iliac crest. The approach for a cervical fusion may be either anterior (through the front of the neck) or posterior (through the back of the neck).

Postoperative care

Care of a patient who has had a *discectomy* or *laminectomy* is similar to that needed in conservative management (p. 883). In addition, the patient needs that care indicated for any postanesthesia patient. The patient should be told preoperatively that he may have much the same pain in the initial postoperative period as he did prior to surgery. Although the pressure from the disc has been removed, there is pressure from edema at the operative site, which causes pain.

Postoperative care must include routine checking of the patient's motion and sensation in the lower extremities along with vital signs. Prescribed analgesics should be given as necessary to control postoperative pain. The patient is encouraged to move his legs and continue plantar flexion and dorsiflexion of his feet. Bowel and bladder dysfunction may be present for several days. Urinary retention and ileus are the most common complications. A Foley catheter may be used during the first few days postoperatively or until postoperative edema is sufficiently reduced to allow normal bladder function. Rectal tubes, suppositories, or enemas are used as needed to relieve abdominal distention. It is advisable to limit oral intake in the immediate postoperative period until the danger of ileus is past; however, if ileus occurs, a nasogastric tube will probably be required. When the patient is able to take oral medications, it is very beneficial if a stool softener is prescribed.

Surgeons vary in their postoperative management of a patient who has had a laminectomy. Generally the patient is allowed a position of comfort in bed. The dressing should be inspected frequently for signs of bleeding or leakage of spinal fluid. Any evidence of either is reported at once. If the patient is having increased drainage, he may be placed on his back to put pressure on the operative site. As with any dressing, it should be kept dry to prevent contamination.

Following the surgery, the patient may be ambulated anytime after the first postoperative day. Orders to ambulate depend largely on the general postoperative condition and the surgeon's preference.

For the patient who has had a *lumbar fusion* through a posterior approach, the bed is kept absolutely flat. Raising the head of the bed would increase the lordosis in the lumbar spine, putting strain on and possibly dislodging the graft. The patient is usually kept flat for 10 days to 2 weeks.

Any twisting motion of the trunk must be avoided. The patient should be logrolled (Fig. 42-13) from side to side (p. 883). The technique is taught preoperatively but the patient is expected to assist with it for several days postoperatively. Patients anticipate pain with turning and tend to be very tense. Giving a patient medications for pain before turning is beneficial. Having the patient

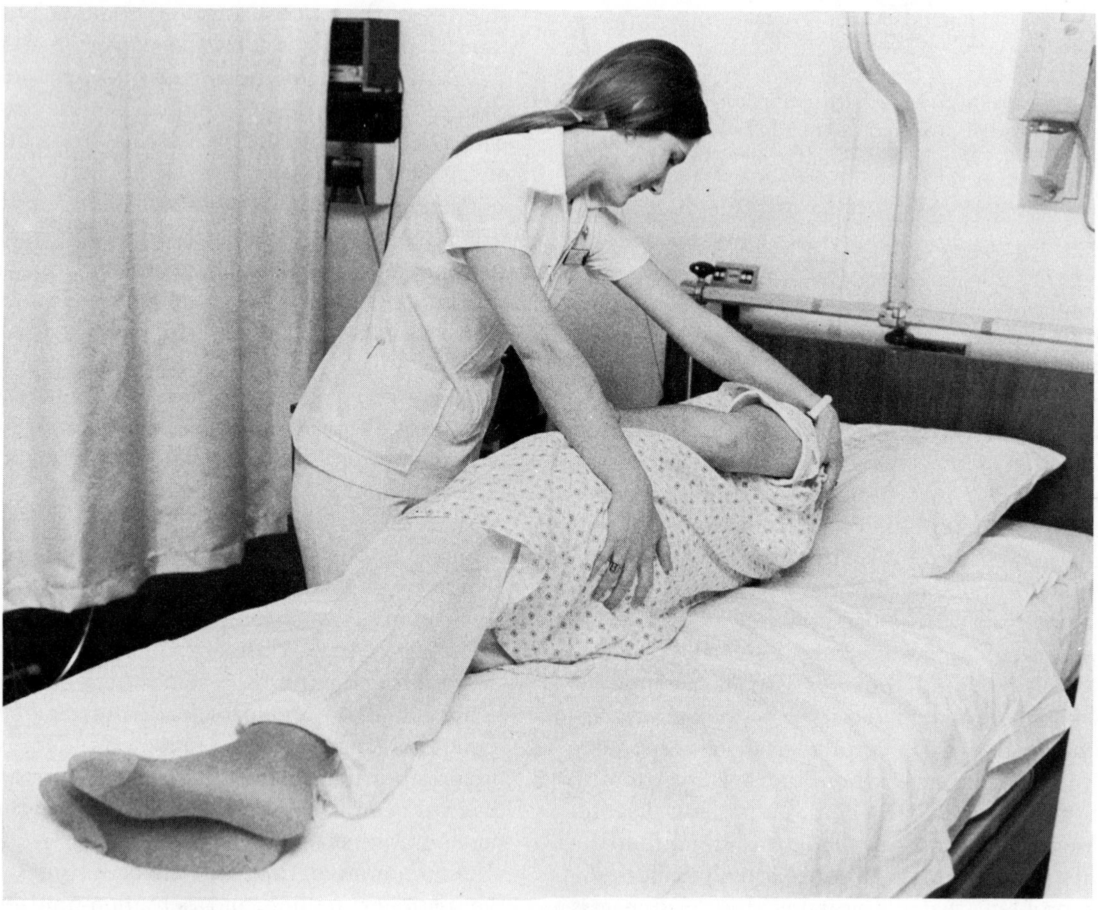

Fig. 42-13. Logrolling of patient. Patient crosses arms over chest, holds legs in extension and feet together. Nurse supports patient at level of shoulders and buttocks.

fold his arms across his chest lessens the possibility of his reaching out and twisting as he is turned. A turning sheet, although not essential, makes it easier to turn the patient while keeping the trunk in good alignment. When the patient is on his side, pillows between his legs are needed to maintain proper alignment, as described on p. 883. A pillow behind his back will lend support. Multiple small adjustments are usually necessary to get the patient in a position of comfort. Although for several days the patient will have a great deal of discomfort for which pain medication will be necessary, positioning is often the key factor in providing comfort. If the patient must be transferred from bed to cart, a sheet or roller board should be used along with adequate personnel to maintain proper alignment of the patient's body during transfer.

Some surgeons prefer that patients who have had fusions remain flat on their backs for several hours. This is to provide additional pressure on the operative site and increase hemostasis. The patient who has had a spinal fusion is more likely to develop a hematoma than is the person who has had a laminectomy. A pressure dressing is applied and should be checked frequently for drainage. Also, the contour of the area around the dressing should be noted as the patient is turned. A change in contour may indicate that a hematoma is developing. The patient may also complain of a feeling of pressure at the site. When the bone graft is taken from the iliac crest, the patient may be very uncomfortable when positioned on that side. It is not unusual for the patient to complain of intense discomfort at the graft site.

Bowel and bladder considerations are the same as for the patient who has had a laminectomy.

Depending on the type of fusion that was done and the preference of the surgeon, the patient may have to wear a brace when ambulation is begun. If a brace is to be worn, it is obtained for use when the patient first begins getting out of bed. It is put on while the patient is lying in the bed. Transfer, which is to be accomplished without placing the patient in a sitting position, begins with the patient moving from a side-lying position in the bed. At least two people should be present the first time this is done. Having been horizontal for an extended period of time, the patient may very likely have postural hypotension on assuming an upright position. He is moved to the very edge of the bed and then turned on his side. He is then instructed to push up with his elbow as one person lifts his shoulders and the other person guides his legs to the floor. The weight of the lower extremities moving to the floor assists in pivoting the trunk upwards when the patient is on his side. After several days of getting out of bed in this manner, the patient will need the assistance of only one person. As postoperative pain decreases, he will be able to do this unassisted. A walker will be a useful source of support when he begins ambulating.

When the patient is able to ambulate without problems, bathroom privileges for bowel movements are usually allowed. A raised toilet seat results in less discomfort. The patient may not be permitted to actually sit for several weeks. When sitting is permitted, a firm, straight-backed chair with arms is provided so that sitting is bolt upright. Sitting will be the least comfortable position for the patient because of the load that this places on the lumbar spine. Although surgery may have corrected the initial disorder, the patient who has had a back problem is very vulnerable to further trauma. The teaching of good body mechanics to avoid putting unnecessary stress on his back is mandatory.

Cervical spine involvement presents some different problems. Cervical disc degeneration, degenerative arthritis of the cervical spine, herniated cervical disc, trauma to the neck with subluxation of or fracture of vertebrae, or metabolic and other disease conditions leading to destruction of the vertebrae are all conditions that can require interventions designed to relieve pain, promote stability, or decompress the spinal cord or nerve roots in the cervical region. The cervical vertebrae are designed to permit more mobility than are the thoracic or lumbar vertebrae. Consequently, support and immobilization are of vital importance in situations (such as displaced fractures) that can result in spinal cord or nerve root compression. Paralysis results from spinal cord or nerve root damage at the cervical level, and at the C1-2 level, respiratory failure can occur.

In non-life-threatening situations or in instances where paralysis does not threaten, symptoms of pain, muscle spasm, or mild neurologic symptoms such as tingling or paresthesias of the hands and arms can often be relieved by resting the neck. A soft cervical collar or Thomas collar worn around the neck provides a degree of immobility by preventing flexion and hyperextension movements. Cervical traction, either continuous or intermittent, may also aid relaxing muscles. These physical measures are often used in conjunction with mild analgesic or muscle-relaxing agents. (See Chapter 41 for management of patients in splints and traction.)

For patients whose symptoms do not respond to conservative management or who are threatened with severe spinal cord or nerve root damage, surgery, usually in the form of spinal fusion, is indicated. The surgical approach for cervical fusion may be either anterior or posterior, depending on the preference of the surgeon and the location of the area to be fused. (See specialized texts for detailed descriptions of techniques.)

Prior to fusion, the neck is immobilized with the spine in proper alignment. This may be done with a hard collar, brace, a halo cast (p. 864), or with traction. If trac-

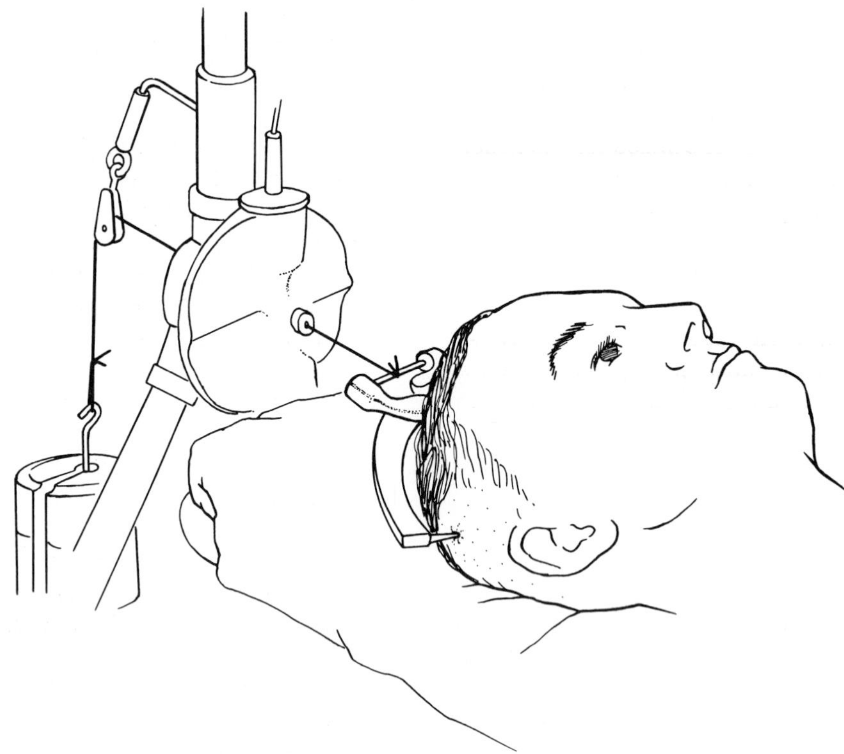

Fig. 42-14. Patient with Crutchfield tongs inserted into skull to hyperextend head and neck.

tion is used, it is most often achieved with the use of tongs (usually Vinke or Crutchfield). Small bur holes are drilled in the outer portion of the skull over each parietal region. The tongs are then inserted into the holes, the skin around the tongs is sutured, and a collodion dressing is applied. From 4.5 to 9 kg (10 to 20 lb) of weight are attached to a rope coming from the center of the tongs and extending over a pulley attached to the head of the bed (Fig. 42-14). Sandbags may be placed above the patient's shoulders to help prevent his slipping toward the head of the bed. Occasionally the head of the bed may be elevated by placing the bed on blocks to give counter traction and to prevent the patient from slipping toward the head of the bed. However, as such countertraction increases the traction, it is not done without first consulting the physician.

Use of the halo cast, which is also a form of skeletal traction, or the use of the hard collar or brace permits the patient to be ambulatory. The patient who is in tong traction is obviously confined to bed. Individuals so immobilized may develop pneumonia. Movement is difficult, and if there is paralysis, movement is impossible. Measures to prevent respiratory and thromboembolic complications must be taken. Skin care must be exquisite. The patient can be "logrolled" off his back periodically (p. 883). In doing so, his head must be held firmly and maintained in proper alignment with the body. Extreme care must be taken in feeding any patient who is in extension and lying on his back, since it is difficult to swallow in this position. Obviously, if the patient chokes, he cannot turn or raise forward. Suction equipment should always be on hand for immediate use in case of aspiration of food into the trachea. Some attention must be given to the texture of the patient's diet to provide foods that are easy to swallow.

The patient may be immobilized in this fashion for some time, often weeks, before surgery is performed. When surgery is performed, the tongs or the halo cast remain in place to maintain alignment. If the patient has been wearing a collar, he will probably be placed in tongs in the operating room. Postoperatively the surgeon may elect to use a neck brace to maintain position rather than skeletal traction. If this is the case, the brace will have been made preoperatively and will be sent to the operating room with the patient for immediate application postoperatively. The brace will allow for early, safe mobilization of the patient. This is also true of the halo cast. Braces must be checked frequently to assure that there is no loosening of the adjustment screws or straps. Such loosening would permit the patient movement that could result in slippage or nonunion of the fusion.

When the anterior approach is utilized for the fusion, postoperative edema in the soft tissues of the neck makes it difficult initially for the patient to swallow and cough. Mucous secretions are thick and difficult for the patient to manage. Edema may progress to a point that the patient experiences difficulty with respirations. For these reasons, suction equipment and a tracheotomy set should be readily available until postoperative edema begins to subside. Diet should be confined to fluids until there is no longer difficulty experienced in swallowing or clearing secretions from the throat. If the patient is allowed to sit up, he should be assisted to do so, since often less pressure is felt over the throat in the sitting position. If a brace is in place, the patient may be mobilized as early as the evening of surgery; however, this depends on the desires of the surgeon.

As for lumbar fusions, bone grafts for cervical fusions are usually taken from the iliac crest. Pain over the iliac crest is to be expected, and it is often greater than at the site of the fusion.

Outcome criteria for the person who has had spinal surgery

The patient or significant others can:

1. Explain the nature of the surgery that has been performed.
2. Explain the limitations of motion and restrictions of activity that must be observed.
3. Explain how long limitations and restrictions are to be observed.
4. Demonstrate how to apply and remove the brace (if it may be taken off).
5. Demonstrate how to perform or modify ADL within the limitations of activity and motion to be observed.
6. Explain plans for follow-up care.

■ TRAUMA

The patient who has suffered trauma to the musculoskeletal system, like the postoperative patient, has had an interruption in the integrity of the locomotor system. Trauma as seen in fractures—and to a lesser extent, trauma that involves tendons, ligaments, and muscles—will be considered here. When sufficient force is applied to bone it breaks. As it breaks, the original force is dissipated through the soft tissue. Small fragments of bone may become embedded in the soft tissue such as muscle, blood vessels, and nerves. It is because of the potential injury to soft tissue that an extremity that has sustained a fracture must be carefully checked for neurocirculatory impairment.

□ Fractures

Definitions and terminology

A bone is said to be fractured or broken when there is an interruption in its continuity. This is usually caused by a blow or injury sustained in a fall or other accident. A fracture may also occur during normal activity or following a minimal injury when the bone is weakneed by disease such as cancer or *osteoporosis*. This is called a *pathologic fracture* and causes collapse of the bone. A bone may fracture when the muscles involved are unable to absorb energy as they usually do. This type of fracture, a *fatigue fracture*, has been seen in persons who have been on long foot marches and the muscles have become fatigued.

There are several types of fractures. A fracture is *complete* when there is complete separation of the bone, producing two fragments. It is *incomplete* when only part of the bone is broken. The part of the bone nearest to the body is referred to as a *proximal* fragment, whereas the one most distant from the body is called the *distal* fragment. The proximal is also called the uncontrollable fragment because its location and muscle attachments prevent it from being moved or manipulated when attempting to bring the separate fragments into correct alignment. The distal is referred to as the controllable fragment because it can usually be moved and manipulated to bring it into the correct relationship to the proximal fragment. Fractures in long bones are designated as being in the proximal, middle, or distal third of the bone.

If the skin is intact, the fracture is classified as *simple* or closed. A fracture is classified as *compound* when there is a direct communication between the skin wound and the fracture site. An open or compound fracture has a high risk of contamination, and this is an important factor in its treatment. When the two bone fragments are in good alignment with no change from the normal position despite the break in continuity of bone, the fracture is referred to as a *fracture without displacement*. If the bone fragments have separated at the point of fracture, it is referred to as a *fracture with displacement*. This may be slight, moderate, or marked.

The line of fracture as revealed by x-ray examination or fluoroscopy is usually classified as to type. It may be *greenstick*, with splintering on one side of the bone (this occurs most often in young children with soft bones); *transverse*, with a break straight across the bone; *oblique*, with the line of fracture at an oblique angle to the bone shaft; or *spiral*, with the fracture lines partially encircling the bone. The fracture may be referred to as *telescoped* if a bone fragment is forcibly pushed against and into the adjacent fragment. If there are several fragments, the fracture is referred to as *comminuted* (Fig. 42-15).

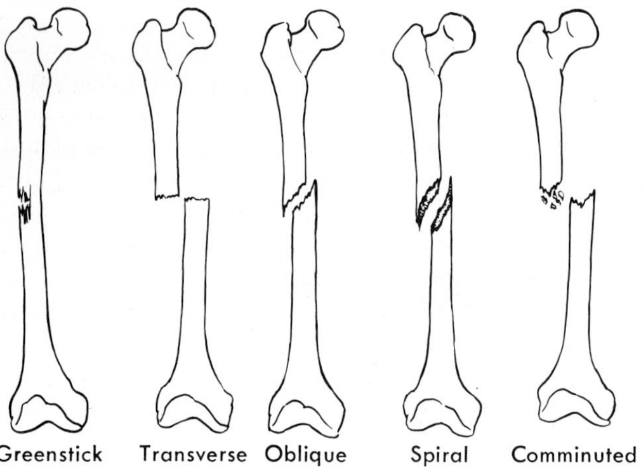

Fig. 42-15. Types of fractures.

Symptoms of fracture and related injury

The signs and symptoms of fracture vary according to the location and function of the involved bone, the strength of its muscle attachments, the type of fracture sustained, and the amount of related damage.

Pain is usually immediate and severe following a fracture. It may continue and is aggravated by attempted motion of any kind and by pressure at the site of injury. *Loss of function* is another characteristic sign. If the person attempts to use the injured part, he may be unable to do so. If there has been marked displacement of fragments, there will be obvious gross deformity, and there may be motion where motion does not usually occur. When the fractured limb is moved gently, there may be a characteristic grating sound (crepitus) as the bone fragments come in contact with each other. *No attempt should ever be made to elicit this sign when fracture is suspected, since it may cause further damage and increase pain.* It is possible, though unusual, for a fracture to occur with no displacement of fragments, little or no swelling, and pain only when direct pressure is applied to the site of fracture or on use of the limb or body part. Fractures of this kind might be missed if x-ray examinations were not routinely ordered when there was reason to suspect that a fracture may have occurred.

Since the bones are firmer than their surrounding structures, any injury severe enough to cause bone fracture will also cause injury to muscles, nerves, connective tissue, and blood vessels that may be evident by hemorrhage externally or into surrounding tissues. Bleeding may not be fully apparent for several hours, and discoloration of the skin (ecchymosis) may not be apparent until several days after injury. Edema may follow extravasation of blood into the tissues and localization of serous fluid at the site of injury, and paralysis or other evidence of nerve injury may develop. Occasionally a large nerve becomes locked between two bone fragments, causing immediate paralysis. The patient who has a fracture usually has signs and symptoms of injury of both bone and surrounding tissues. He may go quickly into shock from severe tissue injury, blood loss, or intense pain.

Immediate management

Perhaps the most important basic principle in the care of a patient with any fracture is to provide some kind of splint before moving him. This is emphasized in the emergency care of patients at the scene of accidents (p. 423). It is equally important for the nurse to remember to preserve body alignment when caring for patients who are in traction or some other mechanical apparatus.

Since it is known that edema will occur following a fracture, the injured part usually is elevated. One or more protected pillows are used, and these can support the extremity if moving must be done. If a temporary splint has been applied, this is not removed without orders from the physician no matter how crude or soiled it may be. The limb encased in the splint can be elevated.

The injured part should be observed at frequent intervals for local changes in color, sensation, or temperature. Care should be taken that emergency splinting bandages do not cause constriction as edema develops. Tingling, numbness, or burning pain may indicate nerve injury. Coldness, blanching, or cyanosis usually indicates interference with circulation. Increased warmth and swelling may indicate infection or may relate to the body's reaction to the fracture itself. The patient should be observed for early signs of shock, especially if the injury is severe. Vital signs should be taken every 15 minutes until the patient's condition has stabilized.

It should be anticipated that the physician may order local cold applications during the first 24 hours following a fracture, since these help to reduce hemorrhage and edema and contribute to the patient's comfort. Ice bags are often used and must be covered and moved at regular intervals to prevent skin damage.

When a patient with a compound fracture is admitted to the hospital, his wounds will be surgically cleansed to remove dirt and foreign material; surgically debrided to remove devitalized tissue and detached pieces of bone; cultured; and if the wound was extremely dirty or if there was a delay in treatment, it will be packed open. Closure of the wound will be accomplished in a few days if there is no sign of infection. The patient is treated with appropriate antibiotics intraoperatively and postoperatively. Following care to the wound, the fracture is appropriately reduced and immobilized.[25] Osteomyelitis, tetanus, and gas gangrene are three major complications in grossly contaminated compound fractures. Antibiotics are used in conjunction with cleansing and debridement to prevent osteomyelitis, tetanus immunization is generally given when a compound fracture has been sustained, and the patient should be carefully observed for signs of gas bacillus infection—sudden increase in edema and pain associated with darkening of the tissues. These signs should be reported to the physician at once.

Pain is usually relieved in the first few hours by giving acetylsalicylic acid (aspirin) or narcotics. Adjustment to sudden immobilization is difficult for the patient, and those caring for him must appreciate what it means to him to be unable to move about freely. Even a fracture of an arm bone may make the patient quite helpless at first. He may be unable to move or use the rest of his body without severe pain. Sometimes treatment of the fractured bone makes it physically impossible for him to care for some of his most basic physical needs. The patient usually needs a sedative such as secobarbital (Seconal) to help him sleep the first few nights after he has sustained a fracture.

Complications

Fat embolism is a serious complication that may follow a fracture, especially a comminuted fracture of a long bone. One source of the emboli is thought to be the fat of the bone marrow. There is evidence of a change in lipid metabolism after a fracture, and the metabolic influence on the development of fat emboli is also under investigation. The signs of a fat embolus are similar to the signs of other kinds of emboli and consist of sudden severe pain in the chest, pallor, dyspnea, prostration, and collapse. The development of these signs and symptoms constitutes a medical emergency, and the physician should be called at once. In some instances signs are less dramatic, consisting of subtle changes in the patient's behavior.

Petechial hemorrhages of the skin and conjunctivae are a classic sign of systemic fat embolism. These usually appear on the second or third day after injury and are commonly found in the conjunctivae, skin of the neck, shoulders, and axillary folds.

There is no specific treatment for systemic fat embolism. Treatment is geared to supportive measures. The patient can usually breathe best in high Fowler's position and will require oxygen therapy. Blood transfusion may be necessary to relieve hypovolemic shock and maintain an adequate hemoglobin level. If the patient has heart failure, he will be digitalized. He should be kept as quiet as possible and subjected to no unnecessary movement. Some experts feel that proper immobilization and careful handling of patients with bone injuries *may* help prevent the occurrence of fat emboli.

Ischemic paralysis (contracture) is a somewhat rare complication of a fracture and develops when an artery is injured by trauma or pressure so that arterial flow is interrupted. *Volkmann's contracture* is a complication of fractures about the elbow caused by circulatory impairment due to pressure from a cast, constricting bandages, or injury to the radial artery. The muscles of the forearm atrophy, and the fingers and forearm are permanently flexed (clawhand). Signs of coldness, pallor, cyanosis, pain, and swelling of the part below the cast must be watched for and reported promptly so that pressure may be relieved by either loosening the bandage or removing the cast in order that circulation may be restored before damage can develop.

Osteomyelitis refers to an infection of bone by pyogenic bacteria. Such an infection can occur as a result of a compound fracture, or it can occur as a complication of surgery. The infection involves the marrow spaces, the haversian canals, and the subsperiosteal space. The bone is involved secondarily. It is destroyed by proteolytic enzymes, and interference with the blood supply causes necrosis. *Acute osteomyelitis* may be caused by introduction of bacteria through a wound, but the most common route of infection is *hematogenous spread* from a preexisting focus such as a boil.

There is initially a small focus of inflammation with hyperemia and edema. Since bone is a rigid material, this edema causes increased pressure and pain. The pus that forms further increases the pressure, which compromises local circulation and results in necrosis of the bone.

The initial treatment of *acute osteomyelitis* involves rest and large doses of appropriate antibiotics prescribed following culture and sensitivity testing. If dramatic improvement is not seen within 24 hours, the involved bone is usually surgically decomposed to relieve the pressure and provide for drainage. Inadequate treatment leads to *chronic osteomyelitis,* which is extremely difficult to eradicate. After a relatively long period of being symptom free, the patient may again present with an acute episode. The infected dead bone separates from the living bone and becomes a *sequestrum.* The infection cannot be permanently cleared until the sequestrum is removed. This is usually done surgically, although it will sometimes happen by a natural process.

Osteomyelitis is extremely difficult to treat and often means years of recurrent episodes of disability for a patient. It can result in failure of surgical procedures such as arthroplasty. A major nursing role in osteomyelitis is in its prevention. Aseptic technique is always indicated when caring for an open wound, and the nurse working with the orthopedic patient must be acutely aware that this is one means by which osteomyelitis can be prevented.

Physiology of healing of fractures

Immobilization of a bone that is fractured is necessary for bone healing. Such immobilization may take place in any of three ways. The first is *physiologic splintage*. This form of splintage will occur naturally, since guarding, avoidance of use, and muscle spasm will occur as a result of pain in the affected limb. Further, there will be a desire to rest the whole body until some repair has occurred. The second method is *external orthopedic splintage* with devices such as plaster casts. The third method is *internal fixation* wherein the opposing ends of the fracture are held in place by screws, plates, or rods.

Once immobilization is accomplished, the bone heals by a process known as *callus formation*. New growth of bone is called a *callus*. Callus formation proceeds in three general stages. First, bone being highly vascular, there is bleeding at both broken ends of the injured bone. The blood collects in the periosteal sheath or adjacent tissues and fastens the broken ends together. This blood forms into a firm clot or *hematoma*. Second, the hematoma becomes organized, thus uniting the broken ends of the bone by fibrous soft tissue. Third, osteoblasts invade the fibrous union, converting it into hard bone as they deposit mineral salts in it and shape it. Factors that will impede good callus formation are inefficient immobilization, infection at the site of injury, anemia or other systemic conditions, endocrine imbalance, and poor dietary intake.[51] If callus formation does not occur normally and efficiently, the resulting lack of repair is termed *nonunion*, or an *ununited fracture*.

Methods of treatment

The usual methods of treatment—reduction, immobilization, traction, and internal fixation—and their management are discussed at length in Chapter 41.

Fractures of the hip

Patients with fractured hips are frequently seen in the hospital, so these fractures will be discussed in more detail. The hip joint is a ball-and-socket joint and is formed by the acetabulum, a deep round cavity in the innominate bone, and the upper portion of the femur. The upper part of the femur is composed of a head, neck, greater and lesser trochanter, and shaft. The distal part of the femur ends in two condyles. The head of the femur fits into the acetabulum. The hip joint is surrounded by a capsule, ligaments, and muscles. The greater trochanter serves as a point of insertion for the abductor and short rotator muscles of the hip, whereas the lesser trochanter serves as a point of insertion for the iliopsoas muscle.

The blood supply to the femoral head is of paramount importance in fractures in or about the hip joint. The blood supply to the femoral head varies with age. The chief source of blood supply to the femoral head in adults is the posterior retinacular arteries (Fig. 42-16). The nutrient and periosteal vessels of the femoral shaft extend into the trochanteric region and lower part of the neck.

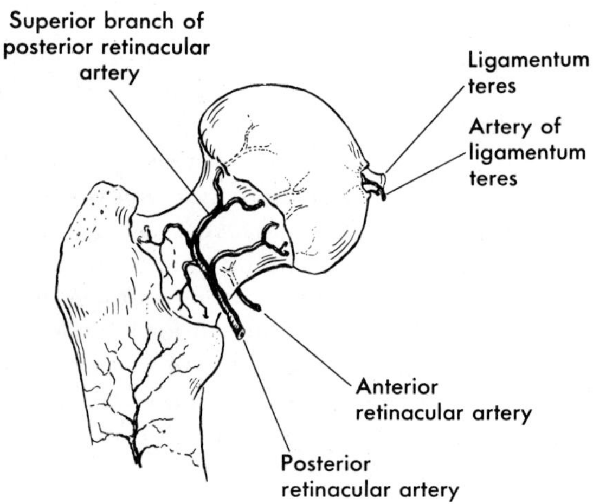

Fig. 42-16. Posterior view of blood supply to head of femur.

Fractured hips occur more frequently in women than in men. Some factors explaining this are (1) women have a wider pelvis with a tendency to coxa vara; (2) women experience postmenopausal hormonal changes often accompanied by an increased incidence of osteoporosis; and (3) women's life expectancy is greater than that of men.

Fractures of the hip may be classified in two general categories: intracapsular and extracapsular fractures. The patient with a fractured hip will present with pain in the hip. The affected leg will be shorter and externally rotated.

Intracapsular fractures of the hip are those occurring within the hip joint and capsule. These include *subcapital, transcervical*, and basal neck fractures. *Extracapsular* fractures occur outside of the capsule to an area 5 cm (2 inches) below the lesser trochanter (Fig. 42-17).

Impacted intracapsular fractures may be treated by bed rest without internal fixation. *Other intracapsular fractures* of the hip may be treated by the use of nails or pins. The choice of device depends on the location of the fracture and the personal preference of the surgeon. Since the blood supply to the head of the femur comes up through the neck, it is often disrupted in an intracapsular fracture (Fig. 42-17). When the blood supply is interrupted, there may be eventual avascular necrosis of the femoral head (p. 892). This complication occurs in a significant percentage of patients following intracapsular fracture of the hip. For this reason, particularly in the elderly patient, the physician may elect to remove the head of the femur and insert a prosthesis such as the Austin-Moore type (Fig. 42-18).

The care of the patient following insertion of a hip prosthesis is directed toward preventing dislocation. The patient may be placed in a spica cast, in traction, or left

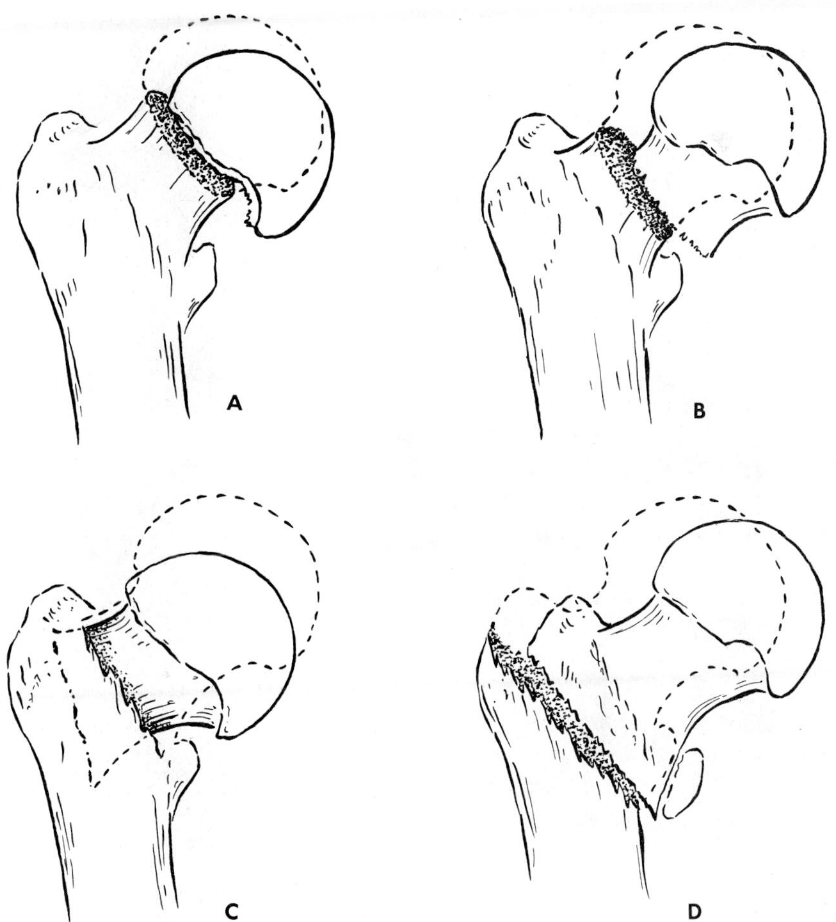

Fig. 42-17. Fractures of hip. **A,** Subcapital fracture. **B,** Transcervical fracture. **C,** Impacted fracture of base of neck. **D,** Intertrochanteric fracture.

free in bed. The type of traction and length of immobilization may vary from 10 days to 3 weeks, depending on the wishes of the orthopedic surgeon. Types of traction used include Buck's extension (Fig. 41-18) and Russell traction (Fig. 41-19). The postoperative position is dependent on the surgical approach. With a *posterior approach* the incision is similar to the one used for the neck of the femur, and one end of the incision is carried upward from the trochanteric area toward the posterosuperior iliac spine. When the capsule of the hip is opened posteriorly and the prosthesis is inserted, the leg must be placed in slight external rotation with slight abduction. The head of the bed must be relatively flat. Acute flexion of the hip, adduction, and internal rotation must be avoided to prevent dislocation of the hip prosthesis before complete healing has occurred. With an *anterior approach,* the upper end of the incision is carried forward to the anterior spine of the ilium. The position of the operated leg is abducted or neutral with internal rotation.

Since adduction must be avoided, if the patient does not have traction or a cast, turning to the unaffected side may be done only on the physician's order. The nurse supports the leg in adduction while the patient turns the rest of his body (Fig. 42-19). Several pillows are placed between the thighs and staggered forward to the foot to avoid adduction. The leg must not slip off the pillows (Fig. 42-20). Sandbags may be used to help maintain this position. Careful instruction must be given to the patient.

Complete soft tissue healing occurs within 3 weeks, and partial weight bearing may be ordered at this time. Management of a patient with a hip prosthesis will depend on the surgical approach and the type of immobilization used. The physician's orders should be checked carefully for the amount of movement and position in bed. Movement of all uninvolved extremities should be encouraged in order to maintain muscle tone and prevent circulatory stasis.

Abduction exercises may be started 2 to 3 weeks fol-

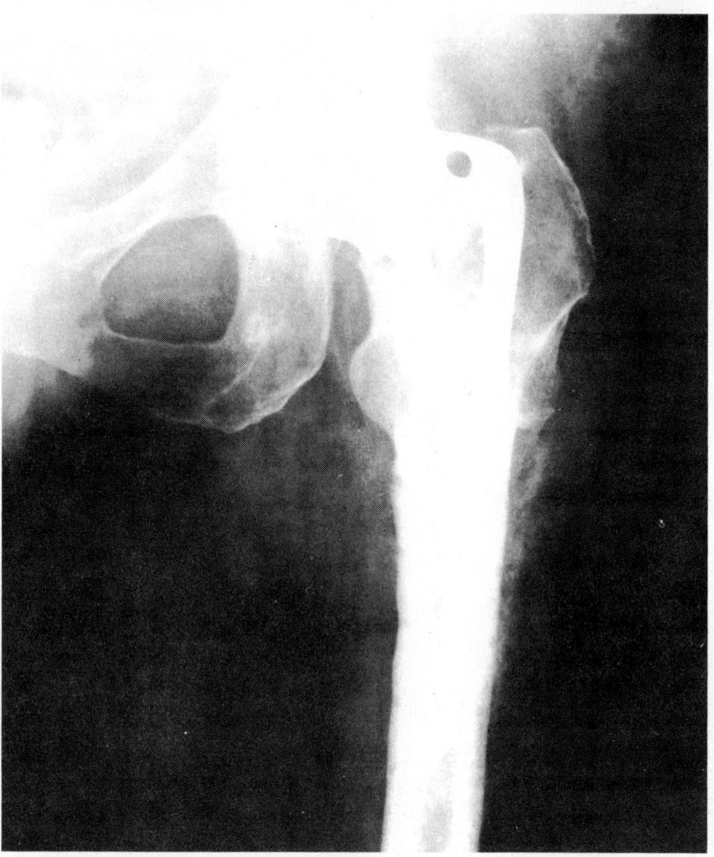

Fig. 42-18. Roentgenogram showing Austin-Moore prosthesis in place. Tracts of nails and screws of recently removed Smith-Peterson nail and plate are still visible in remaining bone. (Courtesy The University Hospitals of Cleveland, Cleveland, Ohio.)

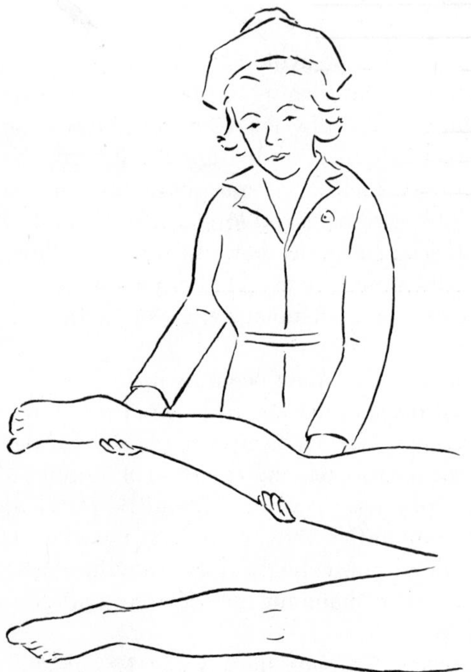

Fig. 42-19. Maintaining abduction position while turning patient. (Redrawn from Wiebe, A.: Orthopedics in nursing, Philadelphia, 1961, W. B. Saunders Co.)

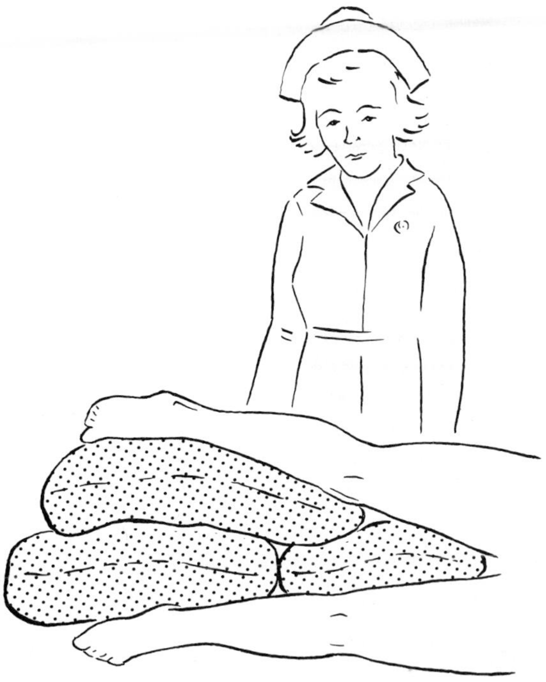

Fig. 42-20. Staggering pillows to avoid adduction of leg. Pillows must be placed so that leg does not slip off of them. (Redrawn from Wiebe, A.: Orthopedics in nursing, Philadelphia, 1961, W. B. Saunders Co.)

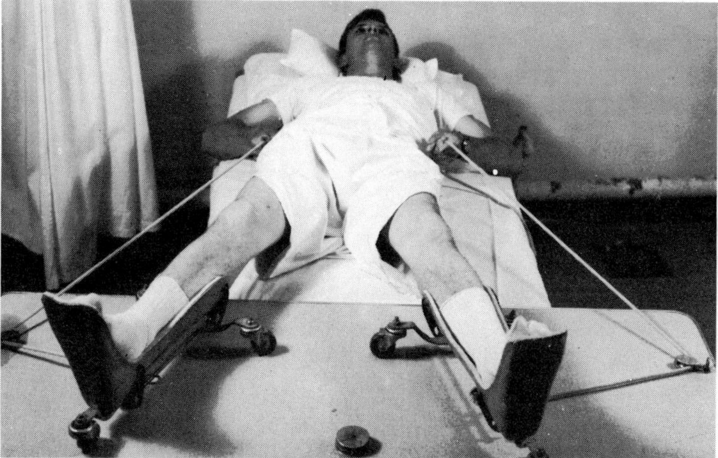

Fig. 42-21. Skates and board used to facilitate abduction exercise of lower extremity. With rope arrangement, patient can passively increase amount of abduction obtained. (From Larson, C. B., and Gould, M. L.: Orthopedic nursing, ed. 7, St. Louis, 1970, The C. V. Mosby Co.)

lowing surgery or when the patient has been taken out of traction. This may be accomplished by the use of roller skating board exercises. The shoe with a skate is placed on the patient's foot. A board with a slight elevation is used with an attached pulley and rope. The patient pulls the rope to abduct the operated extremity. The patient returns the affected leg to the midline. (Fig. 42-21). The patient may need assistance to hold the opposite hip to prevent compensatory adduction when the affected hip is pulled into abduction.

Progressive ambulation begins about 2 to 4 weeks postoperatively. When able, the patient advances to crutches with a three-point, partial-weight-bearing gait. Before total weight bearing is resumed, he may progress to using canes.

Extracapsular fractures are usually caused by direct

violence, by a fall directly onto the trochanter, or by a twisting of the leg. The leg will be externally rotated. The shaft fragment tends to shorten, producing an acute angle between the shaft and the neck of the femur. Shortening occurs because of the fracture itself and the angulation. Such fractures may be *comminuted.* If the fracture is not treated, the leg will be externally rotated and adducted. The intertrochanteric region has a rich blood supply, and union usually occurs without difficulty. A common complication is the *varus deformity.* A varus deformity occurs when the angle of the femoral shaft to the neck is less than the normal 120°.

Extracapsular fractures of the hip are reduced under general or spinal anesthesia. The objectives of treatment include (1) overcoming the shortening by traction or pull; (2) correcting the external rotation so that the leg is rotated while forward pressure is applied to lift the greater trochanter out of the buttock; (3) swinging the leg in abduction; and (4) maintaining the reduction by pinning or support. A lateral incision is made from the greater trochanter down along the outer side of the thigh for 15 or 17.5 cm (6 or 7 inches). The incision is placed toward the posterior surface of the shaft of the femur to produce easier access to the femur's lateral surface. After reduction, the fracture may be immobilized by a *three-flanged Smith-Petersen nail,* a *Jewett nail,* a *Sarmiento nail,* or other similar metallic device that keeps the fractured ends of the bone in good approximation (Fig. 42-22). Internal fixation permits more mobility for the patient, thereby reducing systemic complications common in the aged. Complications associated with some methods of internal fixation include displacement of fragments, causing deformities that may require further and more extensive surgery, including bone grafts.

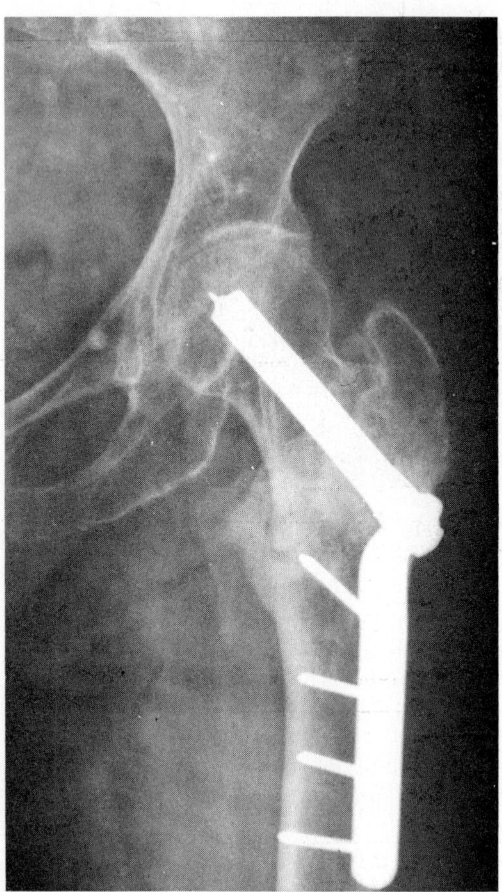

Fig. 42-22. Roentgenogram showing internal fixation of intertrochanteric fracture with McLaughlin plate and pins.

Outcome criteria for the person who has sustained a fracture

The patient or significant others can:

1. Explain the nature of the injury and the treatment.
2. Explain the limitations of motion and restrictions of activity to be observed and how long they must continue.
3. Demonstrate how to perform or modify ADL within the limitations of activity and motion that must be observed.
4. Explain how to care for the cast (if applied).
5. Demonstrate how to safely use an ambulatory assistive device (if necessary).
6. Explain plans for follow-up care.

□ Soft tissue injuries

Twisting of joints may result in damage to ligaments, muscles, or tendons. Damage to ligaments and tendons may also be secondary to degenerative changes in the tissue comprising these structures. *Sprain* usually refers to damage to ligaments, while *strain* refers to muscle damage. All three structures—ligaments, muscles, and tendons—may rupture. If stretching is the only damage sustained, the usual treatment is rest for the involved area. Cold applications may be used immediately to help retard swelling and ease discomfort. A soft support such as an Ace wrap may be used in less serious injuries, whereas more severe injuries may require immobilization in a plaster cast (as with rupture of the Achilles tendon). The most severe injuries are those that involve laceration or rupture. These are treated surgically by suturing the torn ends of the structure together. Depending on the location of the surgery, immobilization of the involved part may be accomplished with a plaster cast or with an internal fixation wire (as in tendons of the finger).

Outcome criteria for the person who has sustained a sprain

The patient or significant others can:

1. Explain the limitations of motion and restrictions of activity that must be observed and for how long.

2. Demonstrate how to perform or modify ADL within the limitations of activity and motion that must be observed.
3. Explain how to care for the cast (if applied).
4. Explain plans for follow-up care.

REFERENCES AND SELECTED READINGS

1. Adams, J. C.: Outline of fractures, London, 1969, E. & S. Livingstone.
2. American Heart Association: Prevention of rheumatic fever, New York, 1968, The Association.
3. Ansell, B. M., and Bywaters, E. G. L.: Rheumatoid arthritis (Still's disease), Pediatr. Clin. North Am. **10**:921-939, 1963.
4. *Anthony, C. P., and Thibodeau, G. A.: Textbook of anatomy and physiology, ed. 10, St. Louis, 1979, The C. V. Mosby Co.
5. *Arthritis Foundation: Primer on the rheumatic diseases, ed. 7, New York, 1973, The Foundation. (Prepared by a committee of the American Rheumatism Association Section of the Arthritis Foundation. Reprinted from J.A.M.A. **224**:suppl., April 30, 1973.)
6. *Barnes, R.: Salvage procedures, failed treatment of fractured neck of the femur. In Anderson, W. F., editor: Current achievement in geriatrics, London, 1964, Cassell & Co.
7. *Beetham, W. P., Jr.: The management of the collagen diseases, GP **31**:113-123, 1965.
8. Bergersen, B. S.: Pharmacology in nursing, ed. 13, St. Louis, 1976, The C. V. Mosby Co.
9. Braidwood, R. J.: Prehistoric man, no. 37, Chicago, 1966, Chicago Natural History Museum Popular Series Anthropology.
10. *Bray, A. P., and Thomas, J. R.: Severe fat embolism syndrome following multiple fractures, Nurs. Times **65**(4):109-110, 1969.
11. *Brewer, E. J., Jr.: Rheumatoid arthritis in childhood, Am. J. Nurs. **65**:66-71, 1965.
12. Bryan, R. S., and Lowell, F. A. P.: The quest for the replacement knee, Orthop. Clin. North Am. **2**:715-728, 1971.
13. *Buck, B. I.: Hip replacement, Sup. Nurse **3**:75-78, 1972.
14. *Campbell, E. B., Hogsed, C. M., and Bogdonoff, M.: Lupus erythematosus, Am. J. Nurs. **62**:74-77, 1962.
15. *Clissold, G. K.: The body's response to trauma: fractures, New York, 1973, Springer Publishing Co., Inc.
16. Cockin, J.: Osteotomy of the hip, Orthop. Clin. North Am. **2**:59-74, 1974.
17. *Committee on Trauma of The American College of Surgeons: An outline of the treatment of fractures, ed. 8, Philadelphia, 1965, W. B. Saunders Co.
18. *Compere, E. L.: Orthopaedic surgery, Chicago, 1974, Year Book Medical Publishers, Inc.
19. Crenshaw, A. H., editor: Campbell's operative orthopaedics, vol. 2, ed. 5, St. Louis, 1971, The C. V. Mosby Co.

19a. *Darst, B. J.: I have a new hip, Am. J. Nurs. **78**:1489-1490, 1978.

20. Dee, R.: Total replacement arthroplasty of the elbow for rheumatoid arthritis, J. Bone Joint Surg. (Br.) **54**:88-95, 1972.
21. Ehrlich, G. E., editor: Total management of the arthritic patient, Philadelphia, 1973, J. B. Lippincott Co.
22. Evarts, C. M., and Kendrick, J. I.: Cup arthroplasty, Orthop. Clin. North Am. **2**:93-111, 1971.
23. *Francis, Sr. M.: Nursing the patient with internal hip fixation, Am. J. Nurs. **64**:111-112, 1964.
24. Freyberg, R.: Rheumatoid arthritis, the natural history, diagnosis, prognosis and management, Med. Times **95**:742-752, 1967.
25. *Gartland, J. J.: Fundamentals of orthopedics, ed. 2, Philadelphia, 1974, W. B. Saunders Co.
26. Goldner, J. L., McCollum, D. E., and Urbaniak, J. R.: Anterior disc excision and interbody spine fusion for chronic low back pain. In American Academy of Orthopedic Surgeons: Symposium on the spine, St. Louis, 1969, The C. V. Mosby Co.
27. Harvey, A. M.: Diseases of the connective tissue (the "collagen" diseases). In Beeson, P. D., and McDermott, W., editors: Cecil-Loeb textbook of medicine, ed. 12, Philadelphia, 1967, W. B. Saunders Co.
28. Helfet, A.: Disorders of the knee, Philadelphia, 1974, J. B. Lippincott Co.
29. Henkind, P.: Iatrogenic eye manifestations in rheumatic disease, Geriatrics **20**:12-19, 1965.
30. Herbert, J. J., and Alain, H.: A new total knee prosthesis, Clin. Orthop. **94**:202-210, 1973.
31. Hoaglund, F. T.: Osteoarthritis, Orthop. Clin. North Am. **2**:3-18, 1971.
32. Hollander, J. L., and McCarty, D. J., editors: Arthritis and allied conditions, ed. 8, Philadelphia, 1972, Lea & Febiger.
33. Hubbard, M. J. S.: One treatment of femoral shaft fractures on the elderly, J. Bone Joint Surg. (Br.) **56**:96-101, 1974.
34. Krause, R. M.: Rheumatic fever. In Beeson, P. D., and McDermott, W., editors: Cecil-Loeb textbook of medicine, ed. 13, Philadelphia, 1971, W. B. Saunders Co.
35. *Lamont-Havers, R. W.: Arthritis quackery, Am. J. Nurs. **63**:92-95, 1963.
36. *Larson, C. B., and Gould, M. L.: Orthopedic nursing, ed. 9, St. Louis, 1978, The C. V. Mosby Co.
37. *Larson, C. B., and Gould, M. L.: Fractures of the hip and nursing care of the patient with a fractured hip, Am. J. Nurs. **58**:1558-1563, 1958.
38. Lonergan, R. C.: Osteoporosis of the spine, Am. J. Nurs. **61**:79-81, 1961.
39. *Mayer, J.: Nutrition and gout, Postgrad. Med. **45**:277-278, 1969.
40. *Mayo, R. A., and Hughes, J. M.: Intramedullary nailing of long bone fractures and nursing care after intramedullary nailing, Am. J. Nurs. **59**:236-240, 1959.

40a. *Meyers, M. H., McNell, D. B., and Nelson, K.: Total hip replacement—a team effort, Am. J. Nurs. **78**:1485-1488, 1978.

41. Miescher, P. A., and Mueller-Eberhard, E. H. J.: Textbook of immunopathology (2 vols.), New York, 1969, Grune & Stratton, Inc.
42. *Monteirio, L. A.: Hip fracture—a sociologist's viewpoint, Am. J. Nurs. **67**:1207-1210, 1967.
43. Morris, J. M.: Biomechanical aspects of the hip joint, Orthop. Clin. North Am. **2**:33-54, 1971.
44. *Moskowitz, R. W.: Clinical rheumatology, Philadelphia, 1975, Lea & Febiger.
45. Murray, D. G., and Racz, G. B.: Fat embolism, the role of respiratory failure and its treatment, J. Bone Joint Surg. (Am.) **56**:1327-1337, 1974.
46. *Nuefeld, A.: Surgical treatment of hip injuries, Am. J. Nurs. **65**:80-83, 1965.
47. Peers, J.: The care and handling of orthopedic implants, RN **28**:66-71, 1965.
48. Pendleton, T., and Grassman, B. J.: Rehabilitating children with inflammatory joint disease, Am. J. Nurs. **74**:2223-2225, 1974.
49. *Peszczynski, M.: Why old people fall, Am. J. Nurs. **65**:86-88, 1965.
50. Rabb, S.: Bunion surgery, Am. J. Nurs. **74**:2185-2187, 1974.
51. *Roaf, R., and Hodkinson, L. J.: Textbook of orthopaedic nursing, Oxford, 1971, Blackwell Scientific Publications.

*References preceded by an asterisk are particularly well suited for student reading.

52. Robinson, W. D.: Diseases of joints. In Beeson, P. B., and McDermott, W., editors: Textbook of medicine, ed. 13, Philadelphia, 1971, W. B. Saunders Co.
53. Ryan, J.: Compression in bone healing, Am. J. Nurs. **74**:1998-1999, 1974.
54. *Salter, R. B.: Textbook of disorders and injuries of the musculoskeletal system: an introduction to orthopaedics, rheumatology, metabolic bone disease, rehabilitation and fracture, Baltimore, 1970, The Williams & Wilkins Co.
55. Schmeisser, G. J.: A clinical manual of orthopedic traction techniques, Philadelphia, 1963, W. B. Saunders Co.
56. *Schneider, F. R.: Handbook for the orthopaedic assistant, ed. 2, St. Louis, 1976, The C. V. Mosby Co.
57. *Seegmiller, J. E.: Goals in gout, Postgrad. Med. **45**:99-103, 1969.
58. Shaw, B. L.: The nursing challenge of lupus: the uncertain killer, RN **31**:32-35, 1968.
59. Siegel, M., and Seelentreuna, M.: Racial and social factors in systemic lupus erythematosus, J.A.M.A. **191**:77-80, 1965.
60. Stiles, P. J.: Internal fixation of fractures in patients with diffuse malignant disease, Nurs. Mirror **125**:i-iv, 1967.
61. Talbott, J. M.: Gout, ed. 3, New York, 1967, Grune & Stratton, Inc.
62. *Talbott, J. H.: Gout and gouty arthritis, Nurs. Outlook **2**:540-543, 1954.
63. Thomas, J. E., and Ayyar, D. R.: Systemic fat embolism, Arch. Neurol. **26**:517-523, 1972.
64. Thomas, S.: Fat embolism—a hazard of trauma, Nurs. Times **65**(4):105-108, 1969.
65. Townley, C., and Hill, L.: Total knee replacement, Am. J. Nurs. **74**:1612-1617, 1974.
66. Turek, S. L.: Orthopaedics: principles and their application, ed. 2, Philadelphia, 1967, J. B. Lippincott Co.
67. Walike, B. C., et al. Rheumatoid arthritis, Am. J. Nurs. **67**:1420-1433, 1967.
68. Webb, K. J.: Early assessment of orthopedic injuries, Am. J. Nurs. **74**:1048-1052, 1972.
69. Wiebe, A. N.: Orthopedics in nursing, Philadelphia, 1961, W. B. Saunders Co.
70. Wilde, A. H.: Synovectomy of the knee, Orthop. Clin. North Am. **2**:191-205, 1971.
71. Williams, J. M.: Fractured neck of femur and subsequent gas gangrene, Nurs. Mirror **124**:63-64, 1967.
72. Williams, S. R.: Nutrition and diet therapy, ed. 3, St. Louis, 1977, The C. V. Mosby Co.

UNIT VII

Gas transport problems

The ability to take in oxygen, transport the oxygen to the cells for utilization, and carry carbon dioxide and other waste products to organs of elimination is vital for survival. Failure of any part of the respiratory or cardiovascular systems to carry out these functions is inimicable with survival. The airway must be patent; gasses must be able to diffuse across the alveolar capillary membranes; the blood must have the capacity to transport the gasses; the heart must provide adequate pumping to move the blood to the tissues; and the vascular system must ensure a free passageway for the blood to reach the tissues.

Because of the interrelationship of the respiratory and cardiovascular systems to meet the body's basic need for oxygen and elimination of carbon dioxide, the care of persons experiencing problems with both systems is considered in this unit. Assessment has been subdivided into two chapters, *cardiovascular assessment* and *respiratory assessment,* for easier retrieval of information. Chapter 45 discusses *general nursing care requirements* of persons who have some form of impairment with getting the oxygen to the tissues or removing the carbon dioxide. The last five chapters examine problems at different phases of getting the gases to and from the tissues. Thus these chapters deal with *problems of the heart and major blood vessels, problems of the peripheral circulation, problems of the blood and blood-forming tissues,* and *problems of the upper airway* and *lower airway.*

43

Cardiovascular assessment

FRANCES R. BROWN

More persons in the United States are directly or indirectly affected by cardiovascular alterations than by any other illness. When the heart is affected by disease or structural alterations, it can no longer function efficiently as a pump, which then causes disruption of the balance between movement of nutrients to the cells and of wastes away from the cells.

■ ANATOMY

□ Structure

The human heart is a relatively small organ located in the mediastinum between the lungs. It is about the size of an adult fist and must pump continuously during periods of stress as well as during basal metabolic conditions. The heart has a series of chambers and valves, an electrical system, three tissue layers, and a protective covering (Fig. 43-1). This covering, the pericardium, loosely surrounds the heart and is made up of several layers. The outer layer, or *fibrous pericardium*, is attached to the great vessels. The inner layer, or *serous pericardium*, is composed of two additional layers, an outer or *parietal* layer, which is in contact with the fibrous pericardium, and an inner or *visceral* layer, which adheres to the heart itself. Between the parietal and visceral layers is the *pericardial space*, which is filled with fluid to lubricate the heart surfaces.

The three layers of cardiac tissue are the *epicardium*, the *myocardium*, and the *endocardium*. The outer layer, the epicardium, is structurally the same as the visceral pericardium. The middle layer, the myocardium, is composed of striated muscle fibers and is responsible for the heart's contractile force. The inner layer of the heart, the endocardium, consists of endothelial tissue and lines the inside of the heart chambers and thinner structures.

□ Chambers

The heart is divided into two halves by a muscular wall (septum). Each half has an upper chamber *(atrium)* and a lower chamber *(ventricle)*. Both ventricles contain papillary muscles that are fingerlike projections attached to fibrous cords (chordae tendineae) that control movement of the atrioventricular valves.

Oxygen-poor venous blood from the peripheral circulation enters the *right* atrium, flows by gravity into the right ventricle when the tricuspid valve is opened, and is then pumped to the lungs when the ventricle contracts. Oxygen-rich blood returns to the *left* atrium, enters the left ventricle when the mitral valve opens, and is pumped throughout the body when the ventricle contracts.

□ Valves

The cardiac valves that control blood flow in and out of the heart chambers can be classified into two types: atrioventricular (AV) valves and semilunar valves. The semilunar valves are the *aortic valve*, located between the aorta and left ventricle, and the *pulmonic valve*, located between the pulmonary artery and the right ventricle. These valves are open during ventricular systole (contraction) to permit blood flow into the aorta and pulmonary artery. They are closed during diastole (relaxation) to prevent leakage of blood out of the ventricles while these chambers fill.

The atrioventricular valves are the *tricuspid valve*, located between the right atrium and right ventricle, and the *bicuspid* or *mitral valve*, located between the left atrium and left ventricle. The tricuspid and mitral valves open when blood in the atria has filled these chambers and close during ventricular systole to prevent leakage of blood back into the atria.

□ Conduction system

In order for the heart to maintain life support it must beat continuously. The heart's electrical system must stimulate the heart to contract, forcing blood throughout the body, and must permit the cardiac muscle to relax to permit filling of cardiac chambers. The sinoatrial or SA *node* is the main pacemaker of the heart and is located in the upper right atrium near the superior vena cava (Fig. 43-2). It usually generates 60 to 100 impulses per minute in the adult, and faster in infants and children. This property is known as automaticity or rhythmicity. If the SA node is not functioning because of disease or other alteration, the atrioventricular (AV) node or a focus in the His-Purkinje system may take over. If this happens, impulses at the rate of 40 to 60 per minute (AV node) or 20 to 40 per minute (His-Purkinje system) will usually be generated.

Electrical impulses generated in the SA node pass through the atria along muscle fibers and through three internodal tracts terminating in the *AV node*, located in the lower right atrium near the interatrial and atrioventricular septums. The impulses continue moving through the *bundle of His* (which is directly attached to the AV node), across the penetrating portion of the atrioventricular system, and into the branching portion. The right bundle branch is a long, thin neuromuscular structure that primarily innervates the right ventricle and terminates in Purkinje fibers. The left bundle branch is a short neuromuscular structure that further divides

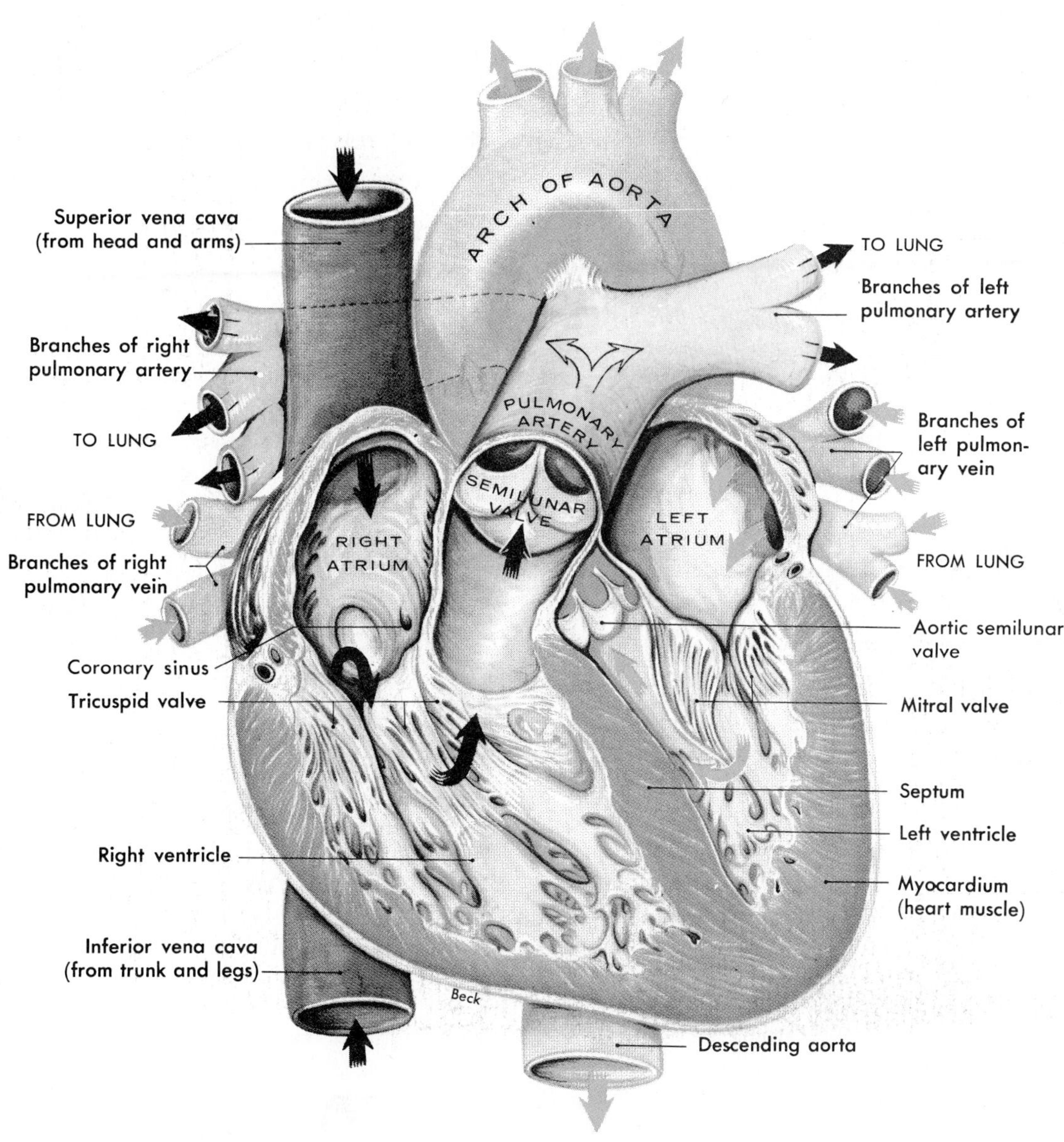

Fig. 43-1. Frontal section of heart showing four chambers, valves, openings, and major vessels. Arrows indicate direction of blood flow. Black arrows represent unoxygenated blood; gray arrows represent oxygenated blood. Two branches of right pulmonary vein extend from right lung behind heart to enter left atrium. (From Anthony, C. P., and Thibodeau, G. A.: Textbook of anatomy and physiology, ed. 10, St. Louis, 1979, The C. V. Mosby Co.)

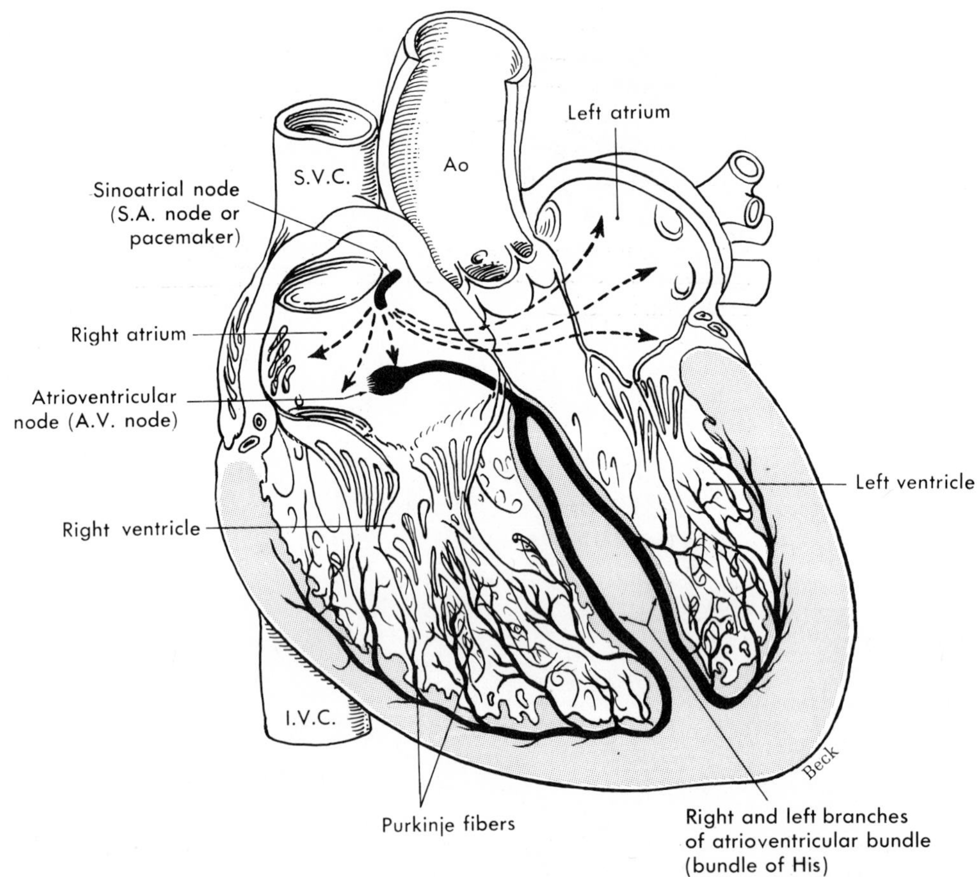

Fig. 43-2. Conduction system of heart. Sinoatrial node in wall of right atrium sets basic pace of heart rhythm, so it is called the "pacemaker." (From Anthony, C. P., and Thibodeau, G. A.: Textbook of anatomy and physiology, ed. 10, St. Louis, 1979, The C. V. Mosby Co.)

into the left anterior division and the left posterior division before terminating in Purkinje fibers.[21]

PURPOSE OF CARDIAC ASSESSMENT

Systematic cardiac assessment provides the nurse with data useful for identifying nursing problems and for evaluating desired patient outcomes. In addition, the nurse is in a unique position of constant or frequent patient monitoring. Thus action can be taken immediately when signs indicating alteration of cardiac function occur, since they can result in severe disequilibrium in other body functions and be a threat to life itself.

SUBJECTIVE DATA

Subjective data obtained by means of a brief history from the individual includes previous health problems, family history of heart disease, hypertension, or diabetes, and usual coping behaviors. This information is helpful in determining dominant cardiac risk factors and for understanding psychologic responses exhibited by patient and family. Additional data collected includes (1) chest discomfort of any kind (precipitating factors, character of discomfort, and methods of relief), (2) leg cramps related to exercise such as walking, (3) smoking habits, (4) intake of alcohol, (5) headache (precipitating factors, character of pain, methods of relief), (6) fatigue, and (7) shortness of breath related to activity.

Information about *chest discomfort* is useful in determining patterns of *angina pectoris*, in identifying the relationship of dietary intake to chest discomfort, and in identifying specific activities that cause pain or that have been eliminated because of pain. This data is very important in planning nursing care. For instance, if angina usually develops after eating or drinking very hot or very cold foods, after walking 30 feet or more at a moderate pace, or when climbing stairs, the nurse can consult with the dietician, talk with the family about rearranging the household so that the patient will not have to climb stairs or walk far, and so on.

If a patient experiences *leg cramps* with walking, this

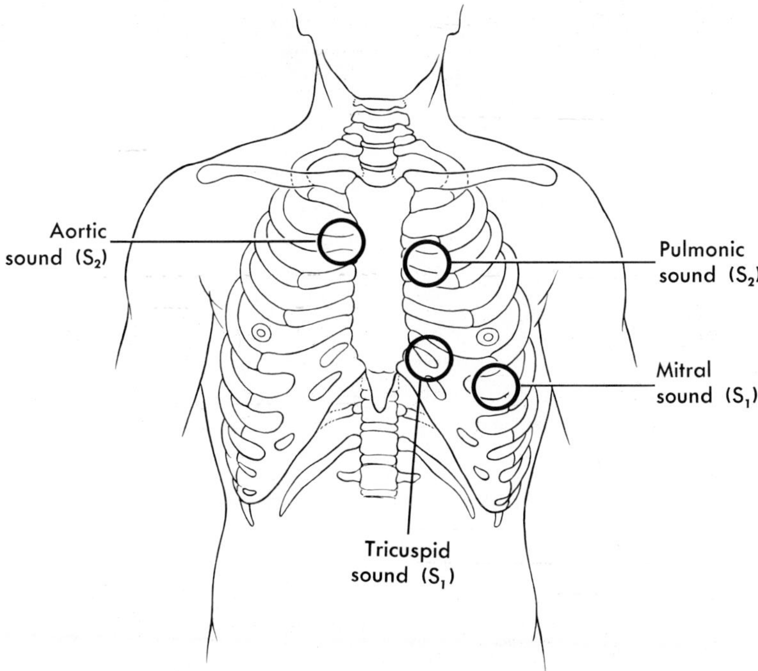

Fig. 43-3. Auscultation of heart sounds.

may be a sign that peripheral atherosclerosis with decreased circulation is present. Prevention of mechanical or thermal injury would be essential (p. 1023). Determining a person's *smoking habits* is important not only for identifying teaching needs relative to heart disease and smoking but also for identifying possible peripheral vascular and pulmonary manifestations. Information about *headaches* is helpful in screening for hypertension, especially when used with data obtained from serial blood pressure measurements. Finally, a history of *fatigue* and *shortness of breath* related to activity may indicate the presence of cardiac disease secondary to the myocardium losing some of its compensatory mechanisms.

■ OBJECTIVE DATA: PHYSICAL ASSESSMENT

□ Cardiac auscultation

Auscultation of heart sounds enables a nurse to establish baseline data for identifying current and future cardiac problems that require nursing intervention. Cardiac auscultation also assists the nurse in evaluating a patient's progress (for example, effect of activity on heart rate) or to monitor responses to medications such as quinidine or digitalis preparations.

Cardiac auscultation always should be carried out systematically, either from the base of the heart to the apex or from the apex to the base (Fig. 43-3). The apex of the heart is found by palpating the left anterior chest at the level of the fifth intercostal space starting at the left sternal border, until a pulsation is felt. The base of the heart is approximately in the area of the second intercostal space. Intercostal spaces are located as follows: With the index finger, start at the suprasternal notch and move downward until a ridge is felt (angle of Louis). Move the finger either to the right or left of the sternum. The space felt is the second intercostal space. With the index finger still on the second intercostal space, place the next finger on the next space below and so forth, ending with the little finger, which is in the fifth intercostal space.

When using the apex-to-base system of auscultation, the listener uses the following technique, listening first with the diaphragm and then with the bell of the stethoscope. (The first and second heart sounds are best heard with the diaphragm, and if present, the third and fourth heart sounds are best heard with the bell). Starting at the apex of the heart, the listener should be able to identify the first and second heart sounds. The first heart sound (S_1) is caused by closure of the mitral and tricuspid valves with the mitral component heard loudest at the apex of the heart and the tricuspid component heard loudest at the left fourth intercostal space at the sternal border. The listener next moves the stethoscope across the sterum to the right sternal border and listens carefully before slowly moving upward. The second heart sound (S_2), caused by closure of the aortic and pulmonic valves, is heard best over the second intercostal space, with the aortic component being loudest on the right side and the pulmonic component being loudest on the left side of the sternum. After the listener has auscultated the base of the heart, the rest of the left sternal border is auscultated.

Intensity of normal heart sounds is determined by direction of blood flow with sound being carried in the direction of blood flow. Thus the first heart sound is best heard near the apex because blood is flowing toward the stethoscope and the second heart sound is diminished because blood is flowing away from the stethoscope. The reverse is true when one listens to the base of the heart. The first and second heart sounds are heard as the familiar "lub-dub." Often other heart sounds are also present and may make identification of the first and second sounds difficult. To compensate for this the listener can palpate an arterial pulse, since this coincides with the first heart sound. If the carotid artery is used, very gentle pressure is exerted, since pressure on the carotid artery of an elderly person or someone with severe atherosclerosis could impede cerebral circulation.

Even the normal heart sounds of S_1 and S_2 can have variations called *split sounds*. This occurs when either or both the S_1 and S_2 have two components and is caused by asynchronous closure of the valves. For instance, the S_1 may be split in persons who have right bundle branch block, left-sided mechanical defects such as mitral stenosis, or tricuspid valve dysfunction associated with pulmonary hypertension. A split S_2 is more common than a split S_1 and can occur with normal inspiration as well as with septal defects, pulmonic stenosis, and other mechanical problems.

Abnormal heart sounds include murmurs which are caused by turbulent blood flow and the third and fourth heart sounds. The third heart sound (S_3) is heard best at the apex of the heart by the bell of a stethoscope. It is caused by vibrations resulting from ventricular filling. Often this sound is called a *ventricular gallop* or *diastolic gallop*. The S_3 may be normal in children, young adults, or very thin adults, or it may be a sign of problems such as congestive heart failure or hypertension causing left ventricular failure. When auscultated, the S_3 comes after the second heart sound and is heard best at the beginning of expiration. The fourth heart sound (S_4) also is heard best at the apex of the heart by the bell of a stethoscope. This sound often is called an atrial or presystolic gallop and is caused by vibrations of the atria following atrial contraction. An S_4 usually is considered abnormal and may be caused by problems such as myocardial infarction or impending heart failure from some other cause. When auscultated, the fourth sound occurs just *before* the S_1 and is heard best during expiration.

The nurse uses cardiac auscultation in determining the effects of rest and activity on a person's heart rate and rhythm as well as in identifying changes in the person's clinical status. For example, an irregular heart rhythm (identified by irregular "lub-dubs") could mean that a patient who had a myocardial infarction was experiencing premature ventricular beats with activity or it might be normal for a person who has mitral valve disease. The appearance of an S_3 in a cardiac patient who previously had none could mean that congestive heart failure was developing. The occurrence of *tachycardia* (heart rate over 100) can mean many things. Fever, anxiousness, or physical inability to carry out activities of daily living (ADL) can all cause tachycardia. The nursing care plan would have to be altered and cardiovascular assessment repeated at selected intervals. Another example would be the occurrence of a *bradycardia* (heart rate less than 60). It could mean that a patient had developed heart block, digitalis toxicity, or increased intracranial pressure. Whatever the situation, the nurse would have to assess the change, intervene appropriately, and then monitor the situation to evaluate the effectiveness of the intervention.

□ Vascular auscultation

Vascular auscultation usually means measurement of arterial blood pressure. This is done with a sphygmomanometer and stethoscope. Initial blood pressure measurements should be taken on both arms, and all measurement should be recorded according to the sounds of *Korotkoff;* that is, the first, fourth, and fifth phases of sound are included in the reading (e.g., 120/80/74). The first phase of the Korotkoff sounds is a tapping sound caused by an initial spurt of blood into the collapsed artery as deflation of the cuff is begun. This sound is considered the measurement of *systolic blood pressure*. As the cuff is deflated, more blood rushes into the artery, causing a murmur that is known as the second phase of the Korotkoff sounds. The third phase occurs when the murmur changes to a tapping sound again; the fourth phase begins when the tapping of the third phase becomes muffled; and the fifth phase occurs when sound disappears entirely. It is felt that true *diastolic pressure* is between the fourth and fifth phases. In order to accurately identify the Korotkoff sounds, the nurse should rapidly pump up the blood pressure cuff and then slowly deflate it at a rate of approximately 2 mm Hg per minute.

Deviation from the normal sounds of Korotkoff can indicate cardiac or vascular abnormalities. Because of this, the technique used for measuring blood pressure is very important. Of significance is the false low reading obtained because of an *auscultatory gap* (no second phase or murmur) being present. The listener hears just one tapping sound that becomes muffled and then disappears. To avoid missing the true systolic reading, the nurse should first measure the systolic blood pressure by palpation and then auscultate it by pumping up the cuff at least 10 mm Hg above the palpated pressure.

Another important factor in accurate measurement of blood pressure is use of a properly fitting cuff. Children and very thin adults require use of small cuffs, while very large or obese persons may require an extra large cuff commonly called a leg cuff. Even though the upper extremities are most commonly used to measure blood pressure, the lower extremities may also be used if necessary. In addition, with an obese patient the nurse can wrap the blood pressure cuff around a patient's forearm, just below the elbow, and place the stethoscope over the radial artery to obtain a blood pressure.

Vascular auscultation also means listening for *bruits*, especially over the carotid arteries. These sounds are murmurs caused by turbulent blood flow due to narrowing of the arteries.

□ Peripheral arterial palpation

Peripheral arterial pulses, which indicate circulation to body parts, are palpated systematically, usually from head to foot in the following sequence: carotid, brachial, radial, femoral, popliteal, posterior tibial, and dorsalis pedis. Palpation should be gentle, especially in patients who have diminished circulation to an area and in the elderly, so that circulation is not further compromised. Pulses on both sides of the body should not be palpated simultaneously but should be compared as to presence and equality of strength.

Usually a radial artery is used to obtain detailed information about the patient's pulse. The character and rate of the pulse are important. A patient's pulse may be abnormally rapid or unusually slow. It may be very irregular or there may be an irregularity that recurs in the same pattern. The apical and radial pulse may not be the same, since sometimes the heart contracts weakly and little blood is pushed out into the arteries.

□ Capillary filling

Capillary filling, commonly called blanching, is an indicator of peripheral circulation to the fingers and toes and can be tested in all nail beds. This is done by pressing the thumbnail against the edge of a patient's fingernail or toenail and then quickly releasing it. The normal response is whitening (blanching) of the area when pressure is applied and return of color quickly when pressure is released. Lack of the blanching response may indicate lack of circulation to the finger(s) or toe(s) because of arterial insufficiency secondary to atherosclerosis or spasm. It could also be a reflection of severe vasoconstriction.

□ Color

A further indication of cardiovascular status is the patient's color. This information is obtained through inspection of the skin, lips, oral mucosa, conjunctiva, and nail beds. A person's "normal" color depends on race, ethnic background, and life style, and is an indication of adequate cardiac output and circulation. Pallor may indicate anemia, hypoxia, or peripheral vasoconstriction. Cyanosis appearing in oral mucosa and conjunctiva is an indication that arterial oxygen saturation of the blood is low due to many causes, including inadequate ventilation or shunting of blood past a portion of the lung. Cyanosis appearing in areas such as the skin and nail beds indicates sluggish blood flow caused by inadequate cardiac output such as occurs in shock, severe congestive heart failure, or in conditions such as polycythemia when blood viscosity is increased. (For further information on skin color see Chapter 64.)

□ Edema

A very important indicator of cardiovascular function is the presence or absence of peripheral edema, especially in the feet, ankles, and legs. Edema that disappears upon elevation of the body part or extremity may be caused simply by gravity flow or interruption of venous return to the heart by constricting clothing or pressure on the veins of the lower extremities. Pitting edema, on the other hand, does not disappear with elevation of the extremity or body part and may be an indication of fluid overload in the body or pathology such as congestive heart failure when cardiac pumping efficiency is impaired.

Edema is identified by inspection and palpation. Pitting edema is present if an indentation is left in the skin after a thumb or finger has been used to apply gentle pressure (Chapter 46).

■ DIAGNOSTIC TESTS

Heart diseases usually are diagnosed from clinical signs and symptoms. Laboratory tests and x-ray examinations are helpful in confirming the diagnosis, indicating complications, showing residual effects, and predicting results of treatment. The nurse may be directly or indirectly involved in these tests and examinations and should know why a particular test or observation is being made and what it will contribute to the patient's diagnosis. This information will help the nurse in explaining tests to the patient and in observing and recording signs and symptoms while caring for the patient.

□ Blood tests

Blood count

A complete blood count is made on all patients with heart disease. In bacterial endocarditis an anemia persists as long as inflammation is active. The blood count therefore guides the physician in determining when the patient's physical activity can be increased. The red blood cell count and the hemoglobin level are observed carefully in patients with heart disease that involves intracardiac shunts, since the test results enable the physician to determine how well the blood is being oxygenated. Adequate oxygenation of the blood is a major problem in cardiac disease, since the diseased heart may not be able to adequately circulate the blood through the lungs. If there has been a myocardial infarction, which causes death of a portion of the heart muscle, the white blood cell count is usually elevated, since the presence of necrotic tissue anywhere in the body causes leukocytosis.

Coagulation or clotting time

Though not very specific for analyzing coagulation factors, a clotting time is still used by some physicians for monitoring patients receiving heparin therapy. This test measures the time required for venous coagulation; the normal range is generally 9 to 12 minutes.

Partial thromboplastin time (PTT)

In recent years this test, also done with venous blood, has been used. More specific than the coagulation time, the PTT is prolonged by factors such as fibrinogen or fibrin, split products, and heparin. The normal PTT usually ranges from 50 to 90 seconds.

Activated partial thromboplastin time (APTT)

Even more sensitive to screening coagulation factors is the APTT, which is determined from platelet-poor plasma.[25] This test now is being used in many hospitals to monitor patients receiving heparin therapy. The normal APTT is approximately 29 to 34 seconds.

Blood sedimentation rate

The blood sedimentation rate is a nonspecific test that measures the rate at which red blood cells settle in a glass test tube. It is used to follow the course of inflammation and infection. It is often used to monitor the progress of patients who have rheumatic heart disease or some other inflammatory condition of the heart. A decrease in the sedimentation rate usually indicates that the condition of a patient with an infection is improving.

Prothrombin time (PT)

A prothrombin time determination is a blood test that indicates the rapidity of blood clotting. This test is done routinely on persons receiving anticoagulant therapy with drugs such as bishydroxycoumarin (Dicumarol), warfarin sodium (Coumadin, Prothromadin), or a combination of heparin and one of these drugs. A daily prothrombin time is usually performed to determine the dosage of the anticoagulant that is necessary to bring the prothrombin time to the desired level. The coumarin derivatives affect the formation of prothrombin as well as other coagulation factors. With decreased prothrombin activity, the prothrombin time will be prolonged. The nurse should be sure that the blood for the prothrombin time is drawn and that the results are available. Often the physician will attempt to increase the prothrombin time to two or two and one-half times the normal range of 11 to 18 seconds or about 20% to 30% of normal activity.

Blood urea nitrogen

A blood urea nitrogen (BUN) test, used to determine kidney function, is usually ordered to learn whether kidney function is disturbed as a result of impaired cardiac output or as a result of other causes. The normal range is 9 to 17 mg/100 ml of blood.

Serum cholesterol

Serum cholesterol tests are used to determine the cholesterol level in the blood. Persons with a high cholesterol level are known to have a higher incidence of coronary artery disease. Considerable research is being done on the relationship between elevated cholesterol levels and coronary artery disease. The normal levels are considered to be between 150 and 280 mg/100 ml of blood.[5]

Serum triglycerides

Serum triglycerides are another component of blood fat and may be associated with an increased incidence of coronary artery disease. They must be measured when the patient is fasting, since triglycerides may be elevated by carbohydrate ingestion. Normal blood levels range from 50 to 150 mg/100 ml.[2]

Serum enzymes

Enzyme level measurements are helpful in determining the existence of damage to cardiac muscle as in myocardial infarction. When the muscle cells are damaged or destroyed by the disease process, these enzymes are released into the blood. The transaminases are present in many tissues throughout the body (as are all the other enzymes mentioned), but serum glutamic-oxaloacetic transaminase (SGOT) is somewhat more predominant in the heart, and serum glutamic-pyruvic transaminase (SGPT) occurs in greater quantities in the liver. The normal SGOT range is 10 to 40 units, but in an acute myocardial infarction the level may increase to 50 to 500 units within 24 hours. Another enzyme present in cardiac muscle is lactic dehydrogenase (LDH). This enzyme has five isozymes of which LDH-5 occurs in greater quantities in the heart. The other isozymes of LDH (1,2,3,4) occur more predominantly in the liver, spleen, lung and pancreas, and kidney, respectively.[13] LDH levels peak about 12 hours after an infarction. The normal level ranges from 165 to 300 units, but in an infarction the level may rise from 2 to 10 times normal. Creatinine phosphokinase (CPK) levels are also frequently used in diagnosing a myocardial infarction, since they show an increase within 2 to 5 hours of the infarction.

□ Urinalysis

A routine urinalysis is done on all patients with heart disease. This test includes a description of the color, pH, specific gravity, protein content, glucose content, and sediment of the specimen. It is used to determine the effects of cardiac disease on kidney function and to determine the existence of concurrent renal or systemic diseases such as glomerulonephritis, hypertension, or diabetes mellitus.

□ Electrocardiogram

An electrocardiogram (ECG) is a record of the electrical activity of the heart. Certain medications such as digitalis and quinidine as well as exercise and anxiety produce changes in the ECG similar to those seen in disease. Therefore if the patient is receiving such a medication or if the patient is anxious, the cardiologist should be so informed.

Electrodes, or leads, are placed against the patient's skin on the extremities and the thorax and then connected by wires to a recording galvanometer. They are usually placed on both forearms, on both lower legs, and over the precordial area, but many variations may be ordered.[14] A special electrode jelly is rubbed onto the portion of the skin on which the electrode, a small strip of metal, is strapped. The patient lies down or sits and should be relaxed while the ECG is recorded. An explanation of the procedure should be given. If the patient is hospitalized, a technician may come to the bedside to do this procedure. The recording machine may be brought to the bedside, and in some institutions the wires are plugged into special wall outlets that transmit recordings to a central location or "heart station."

The nurse needs to understand what creates the ECG and how it is recorded in order to be able to explain the procedure to the patient and understand the significance of the tracings (Fig. 43-4). An ECG is simply a graphic representation of electrical impulses generated by and conducted through the heart, that is, the cardiac cycle (p. 922).

For purposes of assessment, recording, and reporting, the deflections appearing on an ECG, which represent electrical activity generated during the cardiac cycle, have been designated *P,Q,R,S,* and *T waves, PR interval,* and *ST segment.* They are recorded by using electrodes placed on the surface of the body and connected to an ECG machine, or cardiac monitor. Because the flow of electrical forces (vector) spreads in several directions, the ECG must be recorded in different planes. When a cardiac monitor is used, recording is done from only one plane or lead, usually equivalent to lead II or V_1 (Fig. 43-4).

The graph paper used for recording is divided by horizontal lines that measure voltage in millivolts, and vertical lines that measure time in seconds. Thus the *P wave* represents the electrical impulses initiated in the SA node and the spread through the atria. If these waves are normal in size and shape (Fig. 43-5), one can assume that the impulse began at the SA node. If the waves are absent or unusual in shape, the impulse began outside of the SA node.

The *PR segment* is designated as the interval between the end of the P wave and the beginning of the QRS complex. It represents normal delay of the impulse in the AV junction (AV node and bundle of His).

The *PR interval* is designated as the period between the start of the P wave and the beginning of the QRS complex (P wave and PR segment) (Fig. 43-5). It indicates the time it takes for the original impulse to reach the ventricles. This may be referred to as *depolariza-*

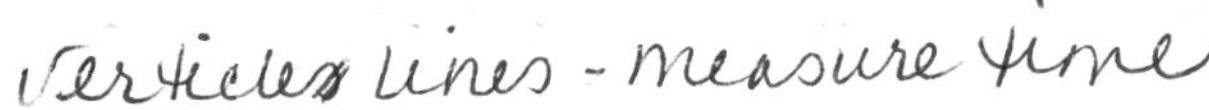

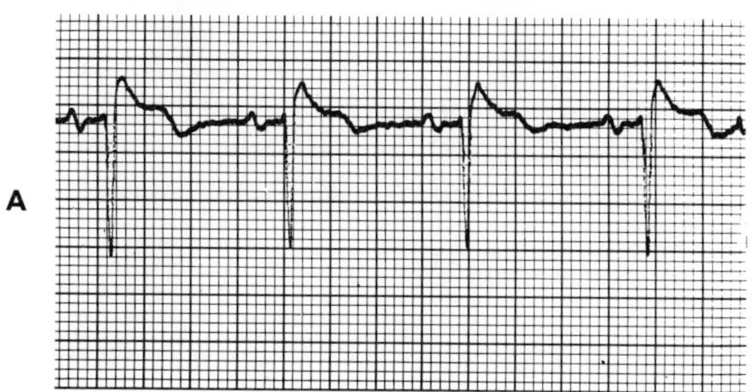

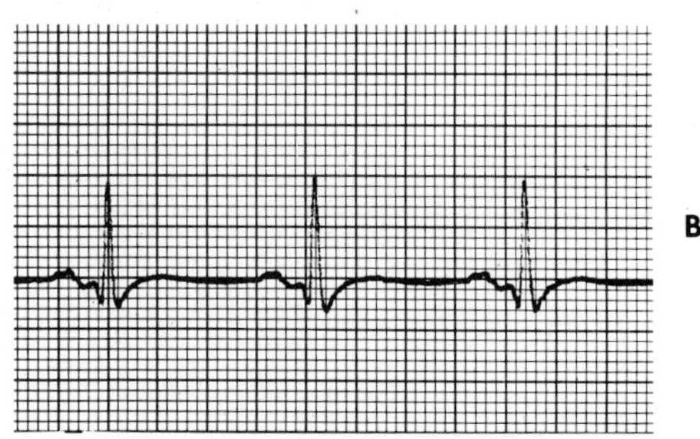

Fig. 43-4. Electrocardiogram tracings. **A,** Lead V_1, **B,** Lead II.

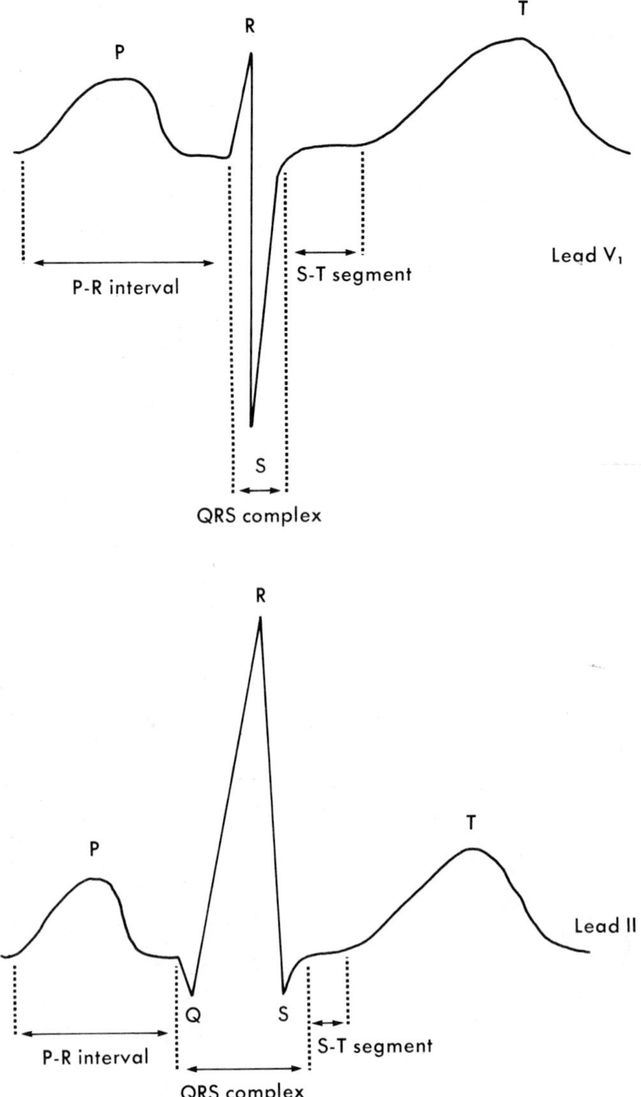

Fig. 43-5. Components of cardiac cycle as shown on lead V_1 and lead II of electrocardiogram.

tion. During this time (usually not exceeding 0.20 second) the impulse has passed through the atria and the AV junction. If the time exceeds 0.20 second, a conduction delay is considered to have occurred in the AV junction. If the PR interval is shorter than 0.12 second, the impulse may have reached the ventricles through a shorter-than-normal path.

The *QRS complex* in lead II generally consists of three waves, an initial downward deflection (Q wave), an upward deflection (R wave), and a second downward deflection (S wave). This complex reflects the time necessary for the impulse to spread through the bundle of His and its branches and initiate contraction. This impulse usually takes less than 0.12 second. An increased amount of time indicates that the ventricles have been stimulated in a delayed, abnormal manner, such as occurs in a bundle branch block.

The *ST segment* is the time interval between completion of depolarization and beginning of repolarization (recovery) of the ventricular muscles. If there is injury to the muscle, as in myocardial infarction, the ST segment may be elevated or depressed, while the T wave may be inverted and shortened or prolonged. The *T wave* is the recovery phase after contraction (repolarization).

The resting ECG shows electrical forces of the heart that may or may not be disturbed by a pathologic process. It does not show the actual physical state of the heart or its function. The most important diagnostic use of the resting ECG is the identification of abnormal cardiac rhythms. Since the rhythm may be normal even in the presence of serious heart disease, a single ECG often is not significant, and repeated tracings may be necessary before evidence of disease can be detected. ECGs also are done at intervals to follow the course of disease. These repeated examinations may be upsetting to the patient unless the purpose of the repeated tracing is explained.

The exercise ECG (stress test) usually is recorded while a person walks a treadmill or pedals a stationary bicycle. This test is important in the diagnosis of coronary artery disease and other diseases of the heart because ECG changes may appear with exercise which were absent during rest.

☐ Direct pressure measurements

Venous pressure

Venous pressure is the pressure exerted by the circulating blood against the venous walls. It is elevated in congestive heart failure, in acute or chronic constrictive pericarditis, and in venous obstruction caused by a clot in a vein or external pressure against a vein, as when the jugular vein is manually compressed. The measurement of venous pressure is particularly helpful after open heart surgery in detecting hypervolemia, hypovolemia, congestive failure, and cardiac tamponade.

Venous pressure may be determined in several ways. The easiest of these is examination of the neck veins. Normally these veins are collapsed above the level of the suprasternal notch when the client is sitting with his head elevated 30° to 45°. With increased venous pressure the veins are distended in this position. The veins on the dorsum of the hand also provide a ready source of information about venous pressure. While the person is sitting, the hand is held below the level of the heart, and the veins become distended. Normally, as the hand is raised to the level of the sternal notch, the veins collapse. With increased venous pressure the veins will remain distended even if the hand is raised above the notch.

Central venous pressure

To obtain an accurate central venous pressure (CVP) reading, particularly useful in the patient with heart disease, a catheter is inserted into a major vein and threaded through the superior vena cava into the right atrium. The catheter is attached by a three-way stopcock to an intravenous infusion and a water manometer (Fig. 43-6). The intravenous solution (usually 5% glucose in water) is allowed to drip slowly into the vein to keep the vein open. When a reading is to be taken, the stopcock is opened to the manometer and the manometer is filled with the intravenous solution. Then the stopcock is turned to the venous opening. The fluid level in the manometer should fluctuate with each respiration. The fluid is allowed to stabilize before a reading is taken, and the highest level of the fluid column is then used for the reading. As soon as the reading is taken, the stopcock is turned to the solution position, and the infusion is continued.

For the CVP reading to be accurate the patient must be relaxed, and the *zero point of the manometer must always be at the level of the right atrium,* which in most people is level with the midaxillary line. If the patient cannot be flat in bed, the zero point on the manometer is adjusted to the level of the right atrium in a sitting position. Any change in the patient's position requires that the zero point be reset. The initial CVP reading and the position that the patient was in when it was taken should be recorded, as these will serve as a baseline for comparison with subsequent readings. For each reading the patient should be placed in the same position, since even a slight change in position alters the CVP. The physician should be informed promptly if there is a significant change in the reading. A high or rising reading usually indicates that the contractility of the heart is impaired; congestive failure and pulmonary edema may occur. A low or falling reading indicates inadequate blood volume (hypovolemia); fluid replacement may be necessary. The normal range for CVP is from 4 to 10 cm of water. The catheter insertion site should be kept scrupulously clean to minimize the possibility of phlebitis. Changing the dressing daily after cleansing and application of a bactericidal ointment are helpful. Patient movement is not restricted as long as the catheter and tubing are secured adequately and intravenous flow maintained.

Peripheral venous pressure can also be measured, and the normal peripheral pressure ranges from 60 to 120 mm of water. This procedure is used much less than formerly, and the reader is referred to hospital procedure manuals for details.

Pulmonary artery and pulmonary capillary wedge pressures

To obtain information about left ventricular function, a balloon-tip catheter (Swan-Ganz catheter) may be introduced into the pulmonary artery (Fig. 43-7). A small incision usually is made over the antecubital or brachial vein and the catheter is threaded into the vein, through the superior vena cava, the tricuspid valve, and into the pulmonary artery. One lumen of the Swan-Ganz catheter is attached to a pressure transducer which, in turn, is attached to a monitor that usually presents a numerical reading as well as a display of waveforms indicating location of the catheter-capillary bed, pulmonary artery, or right ventricle. The balloon then is inflated so that it wedges the catheter in the pulmonary capillary bed. This wedge pressure, in turn, reflects pressures in the left

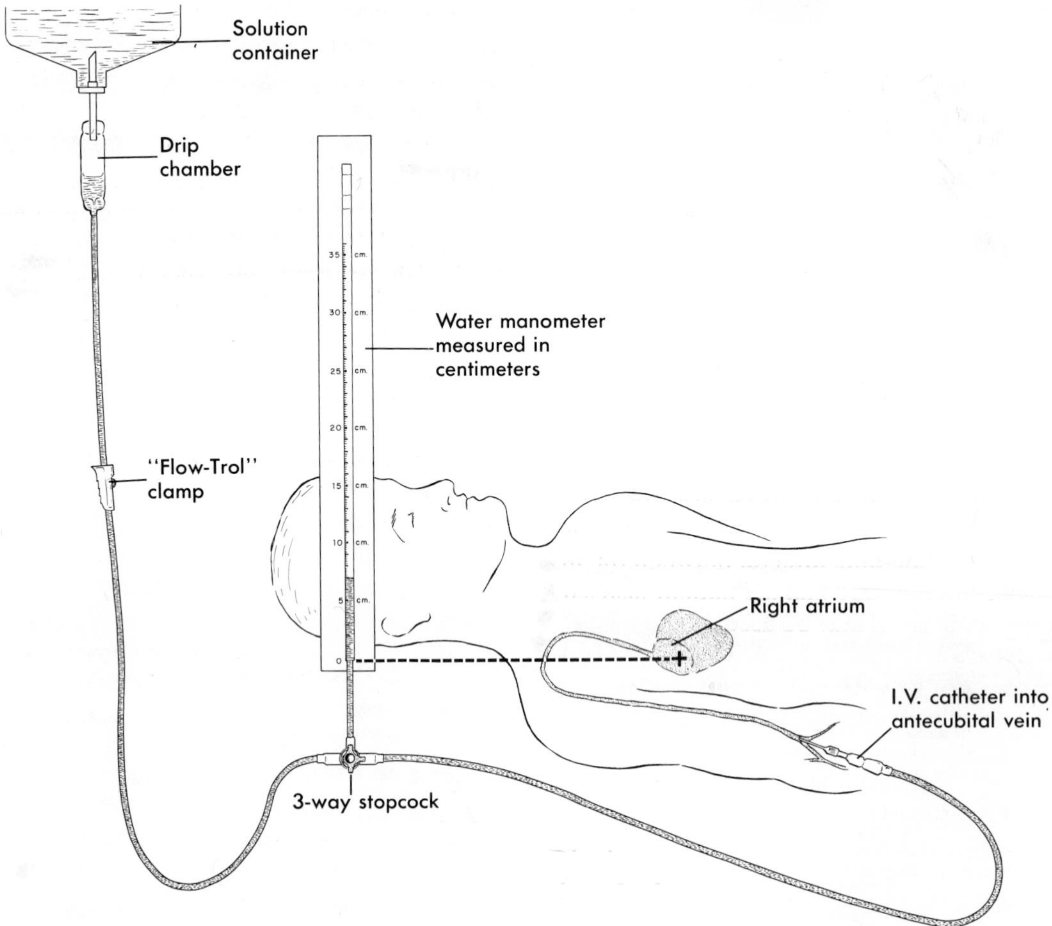

Fig. 43-6. Measurement of central venous pressure using water manometer. Zero point on manometer is at level of midright atrium, and CVP reading is 7 cm of water.

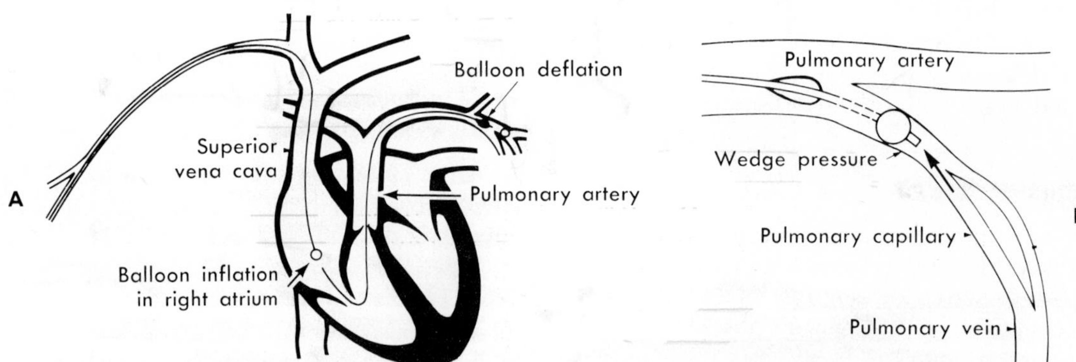

Fig. 43-7. A, Flow-directed, balloon-tipped catheter showing inflation of balloon in right atrium and consequent "floating" of catheter through right ventricle and out to distal PA branch. Balloon is deflated, advanced slightly, and reinflated slightly to obtain PCW pressure. **B,** During initial positioning of balloon-tipped catheter in pulmonary artery, balloon is deflated. Catheter is then advanced, and balloon is reinflated just enough to obtain PCW pressure. (From Schroeder, J., and Daily, L.: Techniques in bedside hemodynamic monitoring, St. Louis, 1976, The C. V. Mosby Co.)

atrium and left ventricle. The balloon must be deflated quickly and never left inflated for more than a few seconds so that damage to pulmonary circulation does not occur.

Circulation time

Circulation time is determined by the amount of time it takes a patient to taste a substance such as sodium dehydrocholate (Decholin sodium) injected intravenously. The normal arm-to-tongue time is 15 seconds or less. Circulation time is prolonged in congestive heart failure. To do this test the following equipment is necessary: a stopwatch, a sterile 5 ml syringe, a no. 19 needle, a tourniquet, an ampule of sodium dehydrocholate, sucrose, or calcium chloride, a solution such as benzalkonium chloride or 7.0% alcohol, and sponges to cleanse the skin. The nurse explains the test carefully to the patient and may be asked to record the time interval between the injection of the drug and the time that the patient tastes it. Special variations on this test may be used.

Cardiac catheterization

Cardiac catheterization is the procedure of passing a catheter into the heart to study heart function. Cardiac catheterization, once limited to the study of the right side of the heart, has been improved and is now used to study the left side of the heart also. *Right cardiac catheterization* is done when congenital heart disease is suspected, but it may also be used to evaluate certain acquired heart conditions such as tricuspid stenosis and valvular incompetence. Blood samples and blood pressure readings are taken, ECG studies are done, and radiographs of the right heart chambers and the pulmonary arterial circulation are made. The physician who obtains the patient's written permission should explain the procedure to the patient. The nurse reinforces this explanation, and to do so the nurse needs to know what the physician told the patient. Even with careful explanation most patients are apprehensive. The meal prior to the procedure is withheld. A sedative is given the evening before and the morning of the procedure, and an anti-

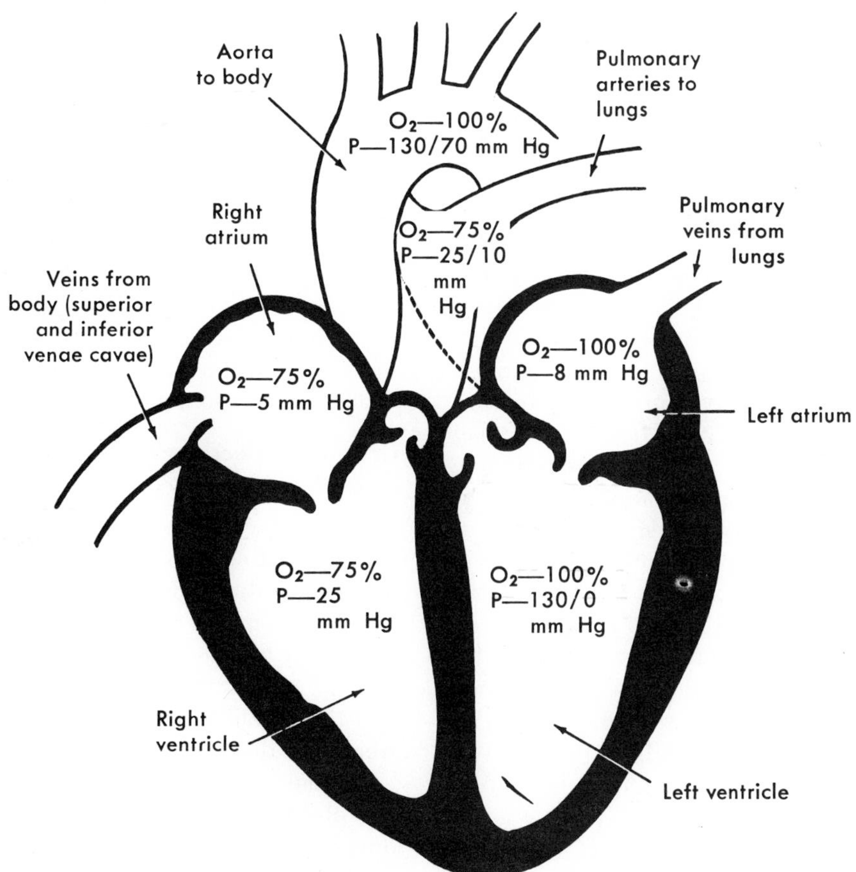

Fig. 43-8. Pressure readings and concentration (percentage of saturation) of oxygen in chambers of heart, and major blood vessels entering and leaving heart.

biotic such as penicillin may be given the day before, the day of, and the day following the procedure as a prophylactic measure. Young children may be given a general anesthetic. For adults a local anesthetic is injected over the vein to be used. A cutdown similar to that for an angiocardiogram is done, usually using the antecubital vein.

A sterile radiopaque catheter similar to a ureteral catheter, but 100 to 125 cm in length, is passed into the incision in the vein and through the vein into the superior vena cava, through the right atrium and the right ventricle, and into the pulmonary artery. The course of the catheter is followed by fluoroscopy, and radiographs may be taken at any point. An ECG is monitored on an oscillograph, and pressures can be checked regularly. As the catheter is passed through the various vessels and heart chambers, samples of blood are taken to study the oxygen content and blood pressures are recorded (Fig. 43-8). Normal blood pressures in the heart vary among the chambers. The pressure is highest in the left ventricle because of the stronger ventricular contractions. Normally the pulmonary artery pressure is about 25/10 or roughly one-fifth of systemic blood pressure. When there is an interatrial septal defect, the oxygen content is higher in the blood of the right atrium than in the superior or inferior vena cava. In certain heart conditions, such as pulmonary or mitral stenosis, the pressure readings within the heart may be elevated three to four times above normal.

The patient has no pain during a right cardiac catheterization, and usually he is alert and anxious. As the catheter is passed along the vein, the patient may complain of a feeling of warmth and of a fluttering sensation around the heart. There is also a tendency to cough as the catheter is passed up the pulmonary artery. The examination takes from 1 to 3 hours and is very tiring. Following the procedure, most patients like to rest or sleep but may resume usual activity as desired. The patient's pulse on the operative side and blood pressure (on the opposite side) are taken every 15 minutes for 1 hour and then every 30 minutes for 3 hours. Tachycardia or other arrhythmia should be reported to the physician immediately. The temperature may be slightly elevated for 4 to 6 hours after the procedure, and the patient may complain of some discomfort at the site of cutdown, which is inspected hourly for several hours to note any bleeding or inflammation. If bleeding occurs, firm pressure is applied at the cutdown site and the physician is notified. If a local thrombophlebitis occurs, it is treated with warm, moist compresses.

In *left cardiac catheterization* a catheter is passed through the aorta from either the brachial or femoral artery using fluoroscopic visualization. After the catheter reaches the aorta, it then is passed around the aortic arch, down the ascending aorta, and through the aortic valve into the left ventricle. Care of the patient is the same as that for a patient having selective arteriography.

In addition to study of the left side of the heart, study of the coronary arteries also is done by fluoroscopy with passage of a peripheral arterial catheter. After the catheter is passed into the aorta, it then is guided into the left and right coronary arteries. Once the catheter has been placed in the artery, dye is injected to outline coronary circulation. Care of the patient having this procedure also is the same as that for a patient having selective arteriography.

Risks during cardiac catheterization are slight, although complications can occur. Cardiac arrhythmias, thrombophlebitis, and local infection are the most common complications. Right cardiac catheterization may be performed in the radiology department, but left cardiac catheterization and coronary arteriography usually are performed in a specially equipped laboratory.

The time required for the catheterization may distress the patient. The patient's tension is increased by lying rather still for several hours while procedures are done, by instructions given back and forth among physicians and technicians, by changes in voice tones of personnel, and by equipment noises. Encouraging patients to verbalize their reactions to the procedure usually is helpful.

To reduce stress on the patient, many cardiac catheterization laboratories allow patients to wear their glasses, dentures, and watches. They also provide piped-in music or may allow patients to bring a radio or favorite records with them. Children especially are encouraged to bring a favorite toy or stuffed animal. Many times someone from the cardiac catheterization laboratory will visit the patient before and after the procedure to answer questions and offer emotional support.

□ Graphic procedures

Selective arteriography

Selective visualization of the aorta and its major arterial systems enables the physician to study a particular vessel closely. For example, in a person with renal hypertension, the renal arteries, including the very fine intrarenal branches, can be studied. The physician can study the pathologic anatomy of the coronary arteries and their branches and by this means plan a course of treatment that is best for the individual.

Initial preparation of the patient usually is done by the physician, who gives an explanation of the procedure. The nurse reinforces this explanation and assists the patient to express feelings and concerns. Simple diagrams of the heart and coronary arteries (right coronary artery [RCA], left coronary artery [LCA] and its branches, left anterior descending artery [LAD], circumflex coronary artery [CCA]) usually are helpful in teaching the patient. On the day the procedure is to be performed the patient receives nothing by mouth. A sedative is given to help relieve anxiety. Local anesthesia is used, and the patient is placed on a special fluoroscopic table that tilts from side to side.

Usually the femoral artery, aorta, or the brachial artery is used. The site of puncture is infiltrated with procaine hydrochloride. The technique of entry to the artery is known as the *percutaneous catheter placement technique*. A special needle is inserted, and a long, flexible spring guide is passed through the needle for about 15 cm. At this point the needle is removed, and an arterial catheter is threaded over the spring guide into the artery. The guide and the catheter are advanced until the desired position is reached, and then the guide is withdrawn. A few milliliters of a radiopaque substance are injected through the catheter so that the tip of the catheter can be seen under the fluoroscope, and at the same time the patient is observed for signs of sensitivity to the radiopaque substance, such as chills, tremor, or shortness of breath. Since the radiopaque substance is eliminated very quickly by the kidneys, rapid films are taken by means of a special camera that makes it possible to take four to six pictures per second. This type of film is known as a *cinefluorogram*.

On completion of the films the catheter is withdrawn, and manual pressure is applied over the puncture site for about 5 minutes. A pressure bandage is applied before the patient is returned to the hospital division. Usually the pressure bandage is removed in approximately 30 minutes, and an Ace bandage is applied firmly. After 48 hours this bandage may be removed and a small strip of adhesive tape used. Patients who have no local or systemic reactions to the examination may be up and about within several hours of returning to their room.

After the patient is back on the division, blood pressure readings are taken (on the opposite arm if the brachial artery has been used) every 15 minutes for 2 hours, and the puncture site is inspected frequently for bleeding. Findings are recorded and reported. Chance of hemorrhage from the puncture site is much greater than would be the case if a vein had been opened. If bleeding does occur, pressure is applied firmly 2.5 cm (1 inch) above the site of bleeding and the physician is notified immediately.

Echocardiogram

In echocardiography the heart is bombarded with high-frequency ultrasonic energy. This technique of ultrasound makes it possible to determine the presence or absence of certain kinds of heart pathology in a noninvasive manner. In this regard it is safer than cardiac catheterization; thus whenever possible, echocardiography is carried out first and then followed with cardiac catheterization as necessary. There is no special preparation for the test, but the individual must be able to cooperate and to lie quietly. The position assumed for the test is lying supine turned slightly onto the left side with the head elevated about 15°. The echocardiogram takes about 30 minutes to complete as it must be carried out very precisely. The data obtained appear as lines and spaces on an oscilloscope. These lines and spaces represent bone, cardiac chambers and valves, the septum, and muscle. The oscilloscope findings are photographed and become a permanent graphic record of findings.

Echocardiography is most valuable in determining (1) the presence of pericardial effusion, (2) the function of cardiac valves, especially the mitral valve, (3) the presence of cardiac tumors, (4) left ventricular function, and (5) the presence of congenital heart disease.

Ballistocardiogram

A ballistocardiogram is a record of the headward-footward movement of the body of a person during systolic ejection of the blood from the heart into the aorta and pulmonary arteries. When a ballistocardiogram is ordered, the patient is placed on a special table that is so delicately balanced that any vibration of the body can be recorded by a machine attached to the table. There is no special preparation for this test other than explaining the procedure to the client. The individual simply lies quietly on the table and may be aware of the vibrations and may be startled by them. The ballistocardiograph is thought to be more sensitive in some instances than an electrocardiograph. It may be used to measure cardiac output as well as to study the force of contraction of the heart.

Other graphic procedures

Many other tests have been and are being developed. Two new tests are *phonocardiography*, which produces an electrical record of the heart sounds, and *electrokymography*, which produces a record of the border movements of the heart.

Radiography. A radiograph of the chest may be taken to determine the size and shape of the heart and the aorta. Calcifications in the pericardium, heart muscle, valves, or large blood vessels also can be visualized in such an x-ray film, which is sometimes called a *cardiovascular film*. Chest radiographs will also reveal any lung congestion associated with cardiac disease.

Cardiac fluoroscopy. Cardiac fluoroscopy enables observation of the size of the heart borders and pulsations of the pulmonary artery and aorta. Calcifications in the heart are identified more easily, and motility of the mediastinum and diaphragm can be observed. Exposure to radiation also is reduced when cardiac fluoroscopy is used to study the heart and related structures in the chest.[16]

Angiocardiogram. An angiocardiogram is a radiograph of the heart and its vessels made after the intravenous injection of a radiopaque substance. It outlines the chambers of the heart and the large blood vessels and enables the physician to see how these chambers function. The meal preceding the x-ray procedure is omitted, and the patient is given a sedative to relieve apprehension about 30 minutes before going to the radiology department. After injecting a local anesthetic, the physician makes a skin incision over the antecubital vein and then inserts a no. 19 needle, attached to a syringe, into the vein. The dye is forced rapidly into the vein, and a series of radiographs is taken as the solution flows through the heart, pulmonary vessels, and aorta (Fig. 43-8).

Some persons are sensitive to substances containing iodine, such as sodium acetrizoate (Urokon sodium) and iodopyracet (Diodrast), which may be used as the radiopaque substance. Nausea is a frequent untoward reaction, and urticaria, shortness of breath, or severe anaphylactic reaction may occur. If the person has a history of asthma or other allergic reactions, this test is seldom done. Any systemic reaction to the dye usually occurs immediately, and an antihistaminic drug such as diphenhydramine hydrochloride (Benadryl), tripelennamine hydrochloride (Pyribenzamine), epinephrine (Adrenalin), and oxygen should be readily available.

Leakage of the dye outside the vein may cause irritation and sloughing of tissue. Thrombosis of the vein at the site of the injection may occasionally occur.

When the patient returns from the radiology department, nursing action includes inspection of incision for bleeding and irritation and recording of findings. Succeeding assessments include inspection and palpation of the arm to detect phlebitis or thrombosis of the vein. If this occurs, warm, moist compresses usually are applied. The vein normally is tender, and the patient may have difficulty bending that arm. This condition is temporary and probably will disappear within 24 hours.

REFERENCES AND SELECTED READINGS

1. American Heart Association: Examination of the heart, parts 1-4, New York, 1970, The Association.
2. Andreoli, K. G., Hunn, V. K., Zipes, D. P., and Wallace, A. G.: Comprehensive cardiac care: a text for nurses, physicians, and other health practitioners, ed. 3, St. Louis, 1975, The C. V. Mosby Co.
3. Anthony, C. P., and Thibodeau, G. A.: Textbook of anatomy and physiology, ed. 10, St. Louis, 1979, The C. V. Mosby Co.
4. Bates, B.: A guide to physical examination, Philadelphia, 1974, J. B. Lippincott Co.
5. Beeson, P. B., and McDermott, W., editors: Cecil-Loeb textbook of medicine, ed. 14, Philadelphia, 1975, W. B. Saunders Co.
6. Bergerson, B. S.: Pharmacology in nursing, ed. 13, St. Louis, 1976, The C. V. Mosby Co.
7. *Betson, C., and Ude, L.: Central venous pressure, Am. J. Nurs. **69**:1466-1468, 1969.
8. Castellanos, A., Jr., Lemberg, L., Berkovits, B., et al.: Didactic vectorcardiography: general concepts, Heart Lung **4**:697-723, 1975.
9. Cogen, R.: Cardiac catheterization: preparing the adult, Am. J. Nurs. **73**:77-79, 1973.
10. Dietschy, J. M., and Weis, H. J.: Cholesterol synthesis by the gastrointestinal tract, Am. J. Clin. Nutr. **24**:70-76, 1971.
11. Fredrickson, D. S., and Lees, R. S.: Familial hyperlipoproteinemia. In Stanbury, J. B., Wyngaarden, J. B., and Fredrickson, D. S., editors: The metabolic basis of inherited disease, New York, 1966, McGraw-Hill Book Co.
12. Friedberg, C. K.: Diseases of the heart, ed. 3, Philadelphia, 1966, W. B. Saunders Co.
13. French, R. M.: Nurse's guide to diagnostic procedures, ed. 3, New York, 1971, McGraw-Hill Book Co.
14. Goldman, M. J.: Principles of electrocardiography, ed. 8, Los Altos, Calif., 1973, Lange Medical Publications.
15. Hudak, C., Lohr, T., and Gallo, B.: Critical care nursing, ed. 2, Philadelphia, 1977, J. B. Lippincott Co.
16. Hurst, J. W., et al.: The heart—arteries and veins, ed. 3, New York, 1974, McGraw-Hill Book Co.
17. *Kelly, A. E., and Goffredo, G. G.: Coronary arteriography and left-heart studies, Heart Lung, **4**:85-98, 1975.
18. *Lamberton, M. M.: Cardiac catheterization: anticipatory nursing care, Am. J. Nurs. **71**:1718-1721, 1971.
19. Lawson, B.: Clinical assessment of cardiac patients in acute care facilities, Nurs. Clin. North Am. **7**:431-444, 1972.
20. Malasanos, L., Barkauskas, V., Moss, M., and Allen, K. S.: Health assessment, St. Louis, 1977, The C. V. Mosby Co.
21. Rosenbaum, M., Elizari, M., and Lazzari, J.: The hemiblocks, Oldsmar, Fla., 1970, Tampa Tracings.
22. Ross, J., and O'Rourke, R.: Understanding the heart and its diseases, New York, 1976, McGraw-Hill Book Co.
23. Schroeder, J. S., and Fitzgerald, J. W.: Indications and techniques for ambulatory electrocardiogram monitoring, Heart Lung, 4:540-545, 1975.
24. Swan, H. J.: Complications of cardiac catheterization, Cardiovasc. Nurs. **4**:27-30, 1968.

24a. Tilkian, S. M., and Conover, M. H.: Clinical implications of laboratory tests, St. Louis, 1975, The C. V. Mosby Co.

25. Williams, W. J., et al.: Hematology, New York, 1972, McGraw-Hill Book Co.

*References preceded by an asterisk are particularly well suited for student reading.

44

Respiratory assessment

BARBARA J. DALY
ALICE NORMAN

Assessment of the lungs requires knowledge of the airways that conduct air to and from the lungs, the lungs themselves, and the surrounding structures and landmarks. A brief review of these will be provided, with emphasis upon the significant characteristics and functions of each.

The upper airway consists of the nose and nasopharynx, mouth and oropharynx, and the larynx. The lower airway is comprised of the trachea, mainstem bronchi, bronchioles, and alveolar ducts, which lead to the alveoli themselves (Fig. 44-1). The airway, in addition to providing a passageway for air, serves three functions: filtering, warming, and humidifying air.

Air inspired through an intact respiratory tree is cleansed before reaching the alveolus of all particles larger than 2 μm in diameter. The removal of this particulate matter, such as dust and bacteria, preserves the sterility of the alveolus. Foreign material is filtered through several mechanisms. *Goblet cells* in the epithelial layer of the airways secrete copious amounts of a thick mucopolysaccharide substance, mucus, which coats the airways and entraps particles. *Cilia,* which are found as far into the respiratory tree as the bronchi, then propel the mucus and foreign material up into the pharynx where it can be propelled by coughing or sneezing.

The warming and humidifying functions are made possible by the rich capillary blood supply in the submucosal layer of the airways. During inspiration, air is heated to body temperature, and up to 1,000 ml of water is utilized per day to raise the humidity of the air to at least 80%. On expiration some of this water is reabsorbed, thus conserving fluid; an average of 300 ml per day is lost in normal respiration.

The basic gas exchange unit of the respiratory system is the alveolus. Alveoli, which number over 300 million in the healthy adult, are minute sacs that arise from alveolar ducts. The ducts are composed of smooth muscle that is capable of expanding and contracting; the alveolus itself is composed of a single layer of squamous epithelium and an elastic basement membrane. These two layers, in addition to the endothelial and basement layers of the adjacent capillary, form the *alveolar-capillary* membrane or interface. It is across this membrane, a distance of less than 1 μm, that gas exchange takes place.

The lungs themselves are subdivided into lobes. The right lung has three lobes: upper, middle, and lower. The left lung has only two lobes: upper and lower. Air is conducted to each lobe through lobar bronchi that branch off of the mainstem bronchus. An important difference between the right and left lungs is the size of the airways leading to them. The right bronchus is significantly wider, shorter, and extends at a straighter angle from the trachea, making it the more likely site of aspirated material. The left bronchus is narrower and extends at more of a right angle off of the trachea, making it more difficult to suction secretions from the left lung.

The thoracic cavity is lined with pleura. The pleura is a continuous *serous* membrane, one surface of which lines the inside of the rib cage (parietal pleura) while the other surface (visceral pleura) covers the lungs. The space between the two surfaces is known as a *potential space.* It normally contains a few milliliters of serous fluid that prevents friction rub when the two surfaces come together.

Control of respiration is primarily dependent upon the activity of the respiratory center in the *medulla oblongata.* This center responds to the CO_2 and hydrogen ion content of the cerebrospinal fluid by increasing or decreasing the respiratory rate. However, there are actually several complex mechanisms that operate to ensure appropriate respiratory rate, depth, and regularity. The reader is referred to a text on pulmonary physiology for a more detailed explanation.

Inspiration is an active process requiring energy and

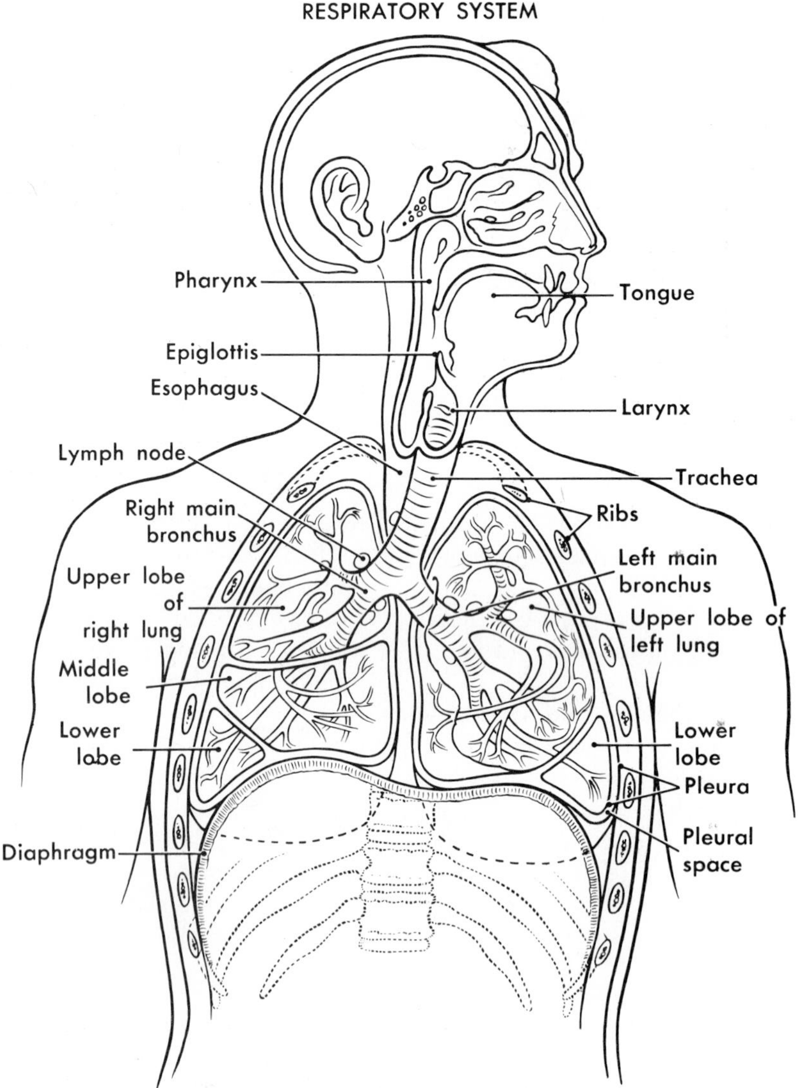

Fig. 44-1. Anatomy of thorax and lungs.

muscular contraction. Expiration is normally a passive process that results from the elastic recoil of the lungs and thoracic muscles. The muscles that are involved in normal, easy inspiration are the diaphragm, which shortens and flattens to increase the longitudinal diameter of the lung, and the external intercostals, which pull the ribs up and out, increasing the anteroposterior diameter of the lung. The accessory muscles (scalene, sternocleidomastoid, trapezius, and pectoralis) are active only in labored respiration.

The lungs lie in and are protected by the thoracic cavity. This bony cage is composed of the sternum and ribs anteriorly and the ribs, scapulae, and vertebral column posteriorly. On the anterior surface the apices of the lungs lie just above the scapula posteriorly and extend to the eleventh or twelfth rib. Figs. 44-2 and 44-3 illustrate the borders of each lobe and placement of the stethoscope for auscultation.

■ PHYSICAL ASSESSMENT

Prior to performing the physical examination, the nursing history is obtained. The nurse reviews with the individual the development of symptoms, precipitating events, and previous respiratory problems. In assessing the person's current status, the nurse specifically inquires about diet and fluid intake, activity tolerance, sputum production, use of medications (both prescription and nonprescription substances such as deconges-

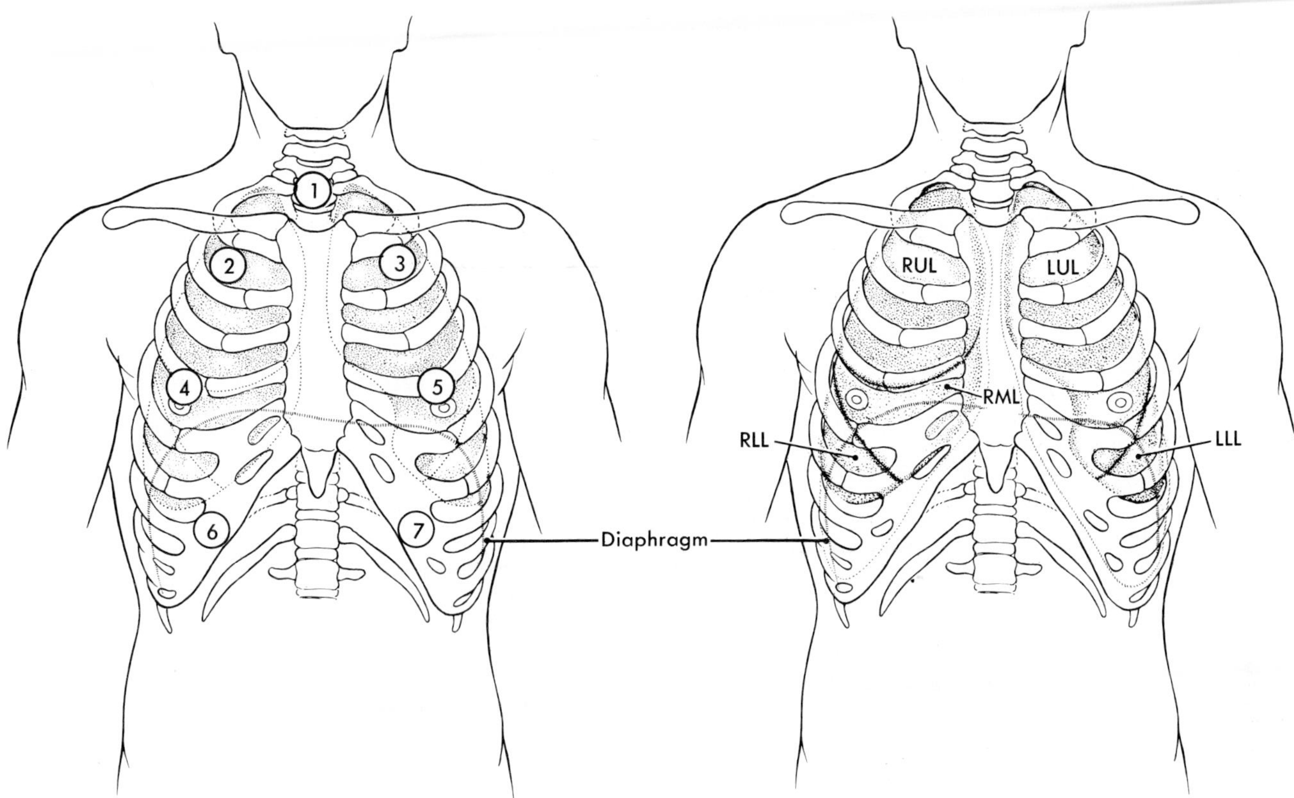

Fig. 44-2. Anterior thorax showing placement of stethoscope when listening to breath sounds and position of lobes of lung.

tants and allergy preparations), and exposure to known allergens.

Risk factors are particularly relevant. Smoking habits and the presence of other diseases should be established. The role that environmental pollutants have played in the patient's illness may be investigated through inquiries about the individual's occupation and knowledge of the pollution level in the geographic area at that time. Exposure to others with respiratory infection may also be a precipitating event.

□ Physical examination

The methods for physical examination are described below. The techniques are used in the order listed.

Inspection

If possible, the individual should be sitting upright. The examiner first observes the person's general appearance before inspecting the thorax itself. Color of the skin is not a very reliable indicator of oxygenation, but should be obtained as part of the baseline data. Central cyanosis of the tongue and mucous membranes more accurately reflects respiratory status than does peripheral cyanosis, which may be caused by vascular disease. The ease with which the person can talk in complete sentences without stopping to catch his breath often yields a clue to respiratory function. Posture and any variations from normal structure of the thorax, such as scoliosis, kyphosis, funnel or barrel chest, and pigeon breast are observed.

The quality of respirations is assessed next; this includes rate, rhythm and depth of respiratory excursions, and uniform expansion of the chest wall. Diminished chest expansion may occur with pulmonary embolus, pneumonia, pleural effusion, pneumothorax, or the pain caused by fractured ribs. The examiner compares respiratory excursion of both sides of the posterior thorax by placing the hands so that the thumbs meet at the midline as the hands extend over the chest wall. The entire thorax should move as one unit as the thumbs move away from each other; expect 7.5 cm (3 inches) expansion.

Abnormalities that may be observed in the presence of disease include the use of accessory muscles or the presence of nasal flaring, both present with labored respirations. The trachea may also be deviated from the

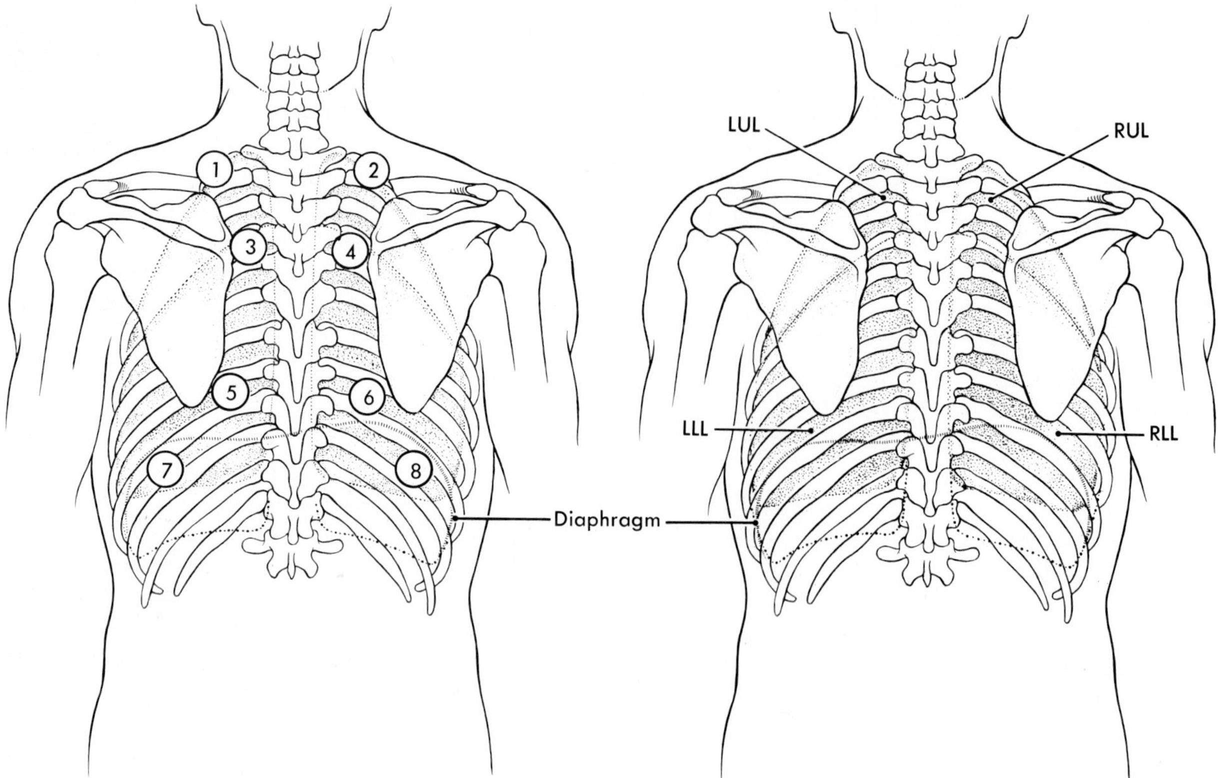

Fig. 44-3. Posterior thorax showing placement of stethoscope when listening to breath sounds and position of lobes of lungs.

midline. Deviation occurs in pleural effusion, pneumothorax with mediastinal shift, and atelectasis.

Palpation

Palpation of the chest is performed with the palmar surface of the hand flat against the posterior chest to determine the presence of tactile fremitus when the patient is asked to say "ninety-nine." Normally a vibration is felt over the exterior chest wall when the patient speaks. The examiner uses the same hand to palpate all areas of the chest. Diminished or absent fremitus may occur with pleural effusion, pneumothorax, and atelectasis. One may also detect areas of pain or masses of the thorax with this examining technique.

Percussion

Percussion of the chest is performed by placing the middle finger flat against the chest at an interspace and striking the knuckle sharply with the end of the middle finger of the other hand. Percussion is done from apex to base with the patient in the supine position for examination of the anterior thorax and in a sitting position for examination of the posterior thorax. Normally percussion elicits a resonant sound. The examiner compares the sound of each area with the sound of the opposite side as percussion proceeds. During percussion of the posterior bases the individual is asked to hold his breath at the end of inspiration and then at the end of an expiration. This maneuver allows the examiner to determine the amount of diaphragmatic descent during inspiration. Normally the diaphragm moves downward 5 to 6 cm.

Dull or flat percussion is heard in the presence of atelectasis, pneumonia, pleural effusion, or a tumor mass. The same dull sound is heard over the heart and liver. Hyperresonance occurs when there is air trapped in the lungs or chest, as with pulmonary emphysema or pneumothorax.

Auscultation

Auscultation consists of listening to the chest to determine the presence of normal breath and voice sounds and to detect the presence of any abnormal sounds. If possible, the patient should be sitting upright. With the diaphragm of the stethoscope, the examiner begins auscultation of the anterior and posterior thorax at the position shown in Figs. 44-2 and 44-3. The patient is in-

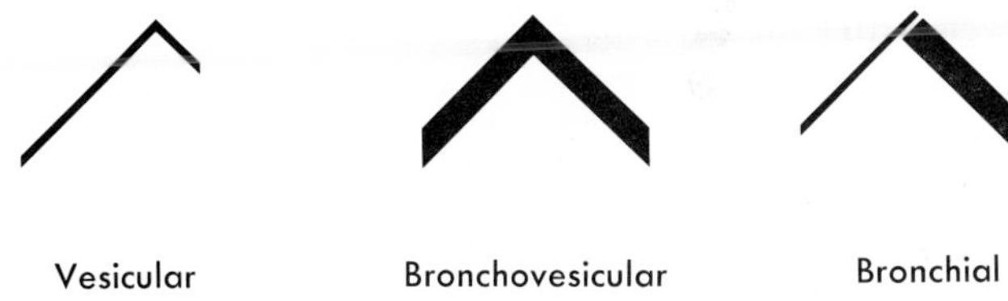

Fig. 44-4. Schematic representation of three types of breath sounds.

structed to take slow, deep breaths through the mouth. When listening to the posterior chest, the examiner has the patient bring the shoulder forward to abduct the scapula so that a greater lung surface can be auscultated. The examiner auscultates the anterior and posterior thorax from apices to bases, comparing one side with the other.

It is particularly important when examining the patient who is on bed rest to have the patient sit up in bed or turn onto the side while you listen to the posterior aspect in order to detect pooled secretions.

Breath sounds. The three types of breath sounds are vesicular, bronchial, and bronchovesicular (Fig. 44-4). *Vesicular breath sounds* are heard in the periphery of the lungs, are of a low pitch, and have a soft rustling or swishing quality (Fig. 44-2, *4* to *7*). The sound of the inspiratory phase is longer and higher in pitch than that of the expiratory phase, which is a short, soft, low-pitched, almost inaudible sound. *Bronchial breath sounds* are heard over the trachea and the main bronchi and are the opposite of the vesicular breath sounds (Fig. 44-2, *1*). Bronchial sounds are high pitched and loud; during the expiratory phase they increase in duration, pitch, and intensity. Bronchial breath sounds heard in other areas of the lung indicate the presence of consolidation from pneumonia, pleural effusion, or compression of the lung. *Bronchovesicular breath sounds* may be heard in the major airways of the lungs such as the anterior second interspaces (Fig. 44-2, *2* and *3*) and in the posterior interscapular area (Fig. 44-3, *3* and *4*). Inspiration and expiration are loud and nearly equal in duration and intensity.

Voice sounds. Auscultation for voice sounds aids in detecting changes indicating such conditions as atelectasis and consolidation. Whispers, normally indistinct, are heard over areas of compression or consolidation. In the presence of bronchial breathing in an area of consolidation, other changes occur. They are egophony and whispered pectoriloquy. *Egophony* is an "E" to "A" change in which the patient says "E" and the examiner hears "A". *Whispered pectoriloquy* is the loud transmission of the patient's whispered voice. These changes are heard when there is consolidation or compression of the alveoli or replacement of air by fluid in the alveoli.

Abnormal sounds or extra sounds. These sounds are superimposed on the normal breath sounds and include rales, rhonchi, wheezes, and friction rub. The term *adventitious sounds* is sometimes used to refer to these. *Rales* are divided into fine, medium, and coarse. Fine rales produced in the small airways, as in pneumonia or heart failure, are heard at the end of inspiration and likened to the sounds of several hairs rubbed together between the fingertips. Medium rales produced in the medium airways occur in the later stages of pneumonia, heart failure, and pulmonary edema. The medium rales have been compared to the fizzling of a carbonated drink. They are heard about midway through the inspiratory phase. Coarse rales are heard at the beginning of inspiration and produce a rough, gurgling sound; they often can be cleared with a cough, as they are produced by secretions in the larger airways. *Rhonchi* and *wheezes* are continuous sounds, although they may be more prominent in expiration. Some authors use the terms coarse rales and rhonchi synonymously. Rales and wheezes are produced by air flowing through passages narrowed by secretions, mucosal swelling, tumors, or other obstructions; like coarse rales, they may be cleared with coughing. They are classified as *high-pitched, sibilant rhonchi,* which have a musical quality and originate in smaller air passages, and *low-pitched, sonorous rhonchi,* which originate in larger air passages and have a snoring sound. *Friction rubs* are crackling, grating sounds that originate in inflamed pleura. They are usually, but not always, heard on both inspiration and expiration and are not affected by coughing. Rubs are heard most easily over the anterolateral area where the greatest expansion occurs.

■ DIAGNOSTIC EXAMINATIONS AND RELATED NURSING CARE

□ Roentgenologic examination of the chest

Roentgenologic examination is probably familiar to most patients and the general public. Roentgenology has had extensive use as a screening test and as a diagnostic measure. Some persons are concerned about the radiation hazards associated with x-rays and may need reassurance that the knowledge gained from the examination outweighs the risks.

When chest disease is suspected, a roentgenogram is almost always ordered to help identify the disease and to visualize the extent of the disease process. Various types of roentgenograms may be ordered. For survey purposes a minifilm may be used. If the history and physical examination or survey film indicate possible pulmonary pathology, full-size chest films are obtained. These include posteroanterior and lateral views.

When the patient goes to the radiology department,

the nurse should be sure that an open-backed gown is worn and that all metal objects above the waist have or will be removed, since metal restricts passage of the x-rays and will cause a shadow on the film. Care should be taken that such articles are not misplaced or lost. If the patient is acutely ill, a portable x-ray machine is brought to his bedside, and the nurse assists the patient into correct position. The x-ray plate is covered and then placed flat on the bed. If the patient can sit up, the plate is put in place, the patient leans back on it, and the head of the bed is lowered as far as can be tolerated; or the patient may sit on the side of the bed, holding the x-ray plate against the anterior chest, resting it on a pillow. When the roentgenogram is taken, the nurse should step out of the room to avoid being exposed to unnecessary radiation. If the patient requires nursing assistance during the procedure, the nurse should wear a lead-lined apron.

□ Fluoroscopic examination

For certain types of information in which visualization of thoracic contents in a dynamic rather than static manner is helpful (such as diaphragmatic movement and size and contour of the heart), fluoroscopy is the preferred examination.

Whether fluoroscopic examination is performed in the physician's office or in the hospital, the patient must go to a room where the fluoroscope is installed. Assistance may be required in rising to a sitting or standing position or in remaining still during the examination. If the patient is in a wheelchair, a stool in front of the machine will be used to sit on. Prior to the examination the physician wears dark red goggles to aid adaptation to the darkened fluoroscopy room. During the examination the physician wears a protective lead apron and gloves. Fluoroscopic examination is performed with the lights off, and the machine is operated with a foot pedal. Patients need a careful explanation of the procedure and should be told that they will be in darkness and that they may be asked to hold their breath for a few seconds during the examination. They should be assured that there will be no discomfort.

□ Special roentgenologic examinations

Special views of the lungs may be obtained by placing the patient in various positions. The most common are the *right* and *left anterior obliques*, The *recumbent lateral (decubitus)*, and the *lordotic*. The oblique positions allow better visualization of the mediastinum and areas of the lung often hidden or obscured by normal thoracic structures in the posteroanterior position. The decubitus film is used to locate fluid in the pleural space and the lordotic to better visualize the apices. *Laminography (tomography, planography)* is a technique whereby the level of the lung that is in focus changes. It is used to study cavities, neoplasms, and densities of the lung.

□ Examination of sputum

Examinations of sputum are usually required when chest disease is suspected. The mucous membrane of the respiratory tract responds to inflammation by an increased flow of secretions that often contain causative organisms. Volume, consistency, color, and odor of the sputum are recorded. These observations are helpful both in diagnosis and evaluation of therapy. For example, thick, tenacious mucoid sputum is characteristic of asthma; green, musty-smelling sputum, *Pseudomonas* pneumonia; and rusty sputum, pneumococcal pneumonia. A *smear of sputum* gives information about the morphology and staining characteristics of organisms. The presence of neutrophils and eosinophils is also noted. A *culture of the sputum* is also ordered. On culture the specific organism can be identified. *Sensitivity studies* done on the culture serve as a guide to the selection of antimicrobial therapy. A *cytologic* examination of the sputum is ordered if carcinoma is suspected.

Tests to be done on sputum are explained to the patient so that a suitable specimen will be obtained. The patient is instructed to collect only sputum that has come from deep in the lungs. When instructed inadequately, patients often expectorate saliva rather than sputum. They are likely to exhaust themselves unnecessarily by shallow, frequent coughing that yields no sputum suitable for study and that affords them little relief from discomfort. *The first sputum raised in the morning is usually the most productive of organisms.* During the night, secretions accumulate in the bronchi, and just a few deep coughs will bring them to the back of the throat. If the patients do not know this fact, on awakening they may almost unconsciously cough, clear their throat, and swallow or expectorate before attempting to produce the specimen.

The patient should be supplied with a widemouthed container and instructed to expectorate directly into it. Because the sight of sputum is often objectionable to the patient and to others, the outside of a glass container is covered with paper or other suitable covering. Usually 4 ml of sputum is sufficient for necessary laboratory tests and examinations. Initial specimens for culture and sensitivity are usually collected before antibiotic therapy is started. Occasionally, however, all sputum collected over a period of 24 to 72 hours is needed. If there is any delay in sending the specimen to the laboratory, it should be placed in the refrigerator.

Sputum collection using saline inhalation

Inhalation of a heated saline solution is used to help some persons raise sputum for specimens. A 10% solution of saline in distilled water is placed in a heated nebulizer, and a fine spray is produced by attaching the nebulizer to compressed air or oxygen. When inhaled, the heated vapor condenses on the surface of the tracheobronchial mucosa and stimulates production of secretions.

Patients who have difficulty raising sputum for specimens can learn this procedure readily. The patient is taught how to deep breathe and cough before the procedure. The mouth is placed over, but not sealed around, the nebulizer before inhaling. Inhalation of the vapor is repeated for a few minutes or until coughing is stimulated. Some patients begin to cough after the first inhalation. The patient should have a supply of tissues to cover the cough and should expectorate sputum into the collection container.

It is important to encourage patients to rest for a few seconds between periods of inhaling and coughing so that they do not become overtired. If the patient complains of lightheadedness or dizziness caused by hyperventilation, sitting quietly and breathing slowly normally for a few minutes will bring relief. If nausea occurs, the inhalations should be discontinued. The patient usually feels nauseated for only a few minutes, and it may be associated with factors other than inhalation. The advantage of this method of raising sputum is that the patient can do the procedure at any time of the day and needs no special preparation.

If the patient is suspected of having tuberculosis and specimens are being collected for screening purposes, the hospital or outpatient personnel use appropriate precautions. The room should be well ventilated so that there are frequent changes of air. If the patient is known to have sputum positive for tubercle bacilli, the extra precaution of wearing a high-filtration mask may be taken. Special ultraviolet lights may be installed to rid the rising circulating air of infectious droplets. They are installed high enough to protect the patient and the personnel from direct exposure to the light.

Gastric washings

Gastric aspiration is occasionally used to collect gastric contents, which may contain swallowed sputum. It is usually done when the diagnosis or suspected diagnosis is tuberculosis. Since most patients swallow sputum when coughing in the morning and during sleep, an examination of gastric contents may reveal causative organisms. Breakfast is withheld for gastric aspiration. (The procedure for passing the nasogastric tube is the same as that discussed on p. 1164.) Once the tube is passed, a large syringe is attached to the end, and by gentle suction a specimen of stomach contents is withdrawn. The specimen is placed in a covered bottle, and the tube is withdrawn. The specimen is examined microscopically on slides, and culture media are inoculated as is done with other sputum samples. For the patient the disadvantages of this method of sputum collection are the discomforts of going without food and the passage of the nasogastric tube.

□ Pulmonary function measurements and arterial blood gases

Physiologic tests of pulmonary function are performed in order to provide information regarding abnormalities in function, progression or improvement in clinical status, effects of medication, and degree of disability present. The tests themselves cannot be used alone to diagnose specific diseases, but are an integral part of the diagnostic process.

There are two general kinds of respiratory function tests. One measures the bellows action of the chest and lungs, or the ability to move air in and out of the alveoli. This aspect of respiration is referred to as *ventilation;* the other measures are *diffusion*, the movement of the gas across the alveolar-capillary membrane, and *perfusion*, the supply of blood to the lungs.

In order for the lung to perform gas exchange efficiently, the ventilation-perfusion ratio ($\dot{V}/\dot{Q}$ ratio) must be balanced. That is, areas that receive ventilation should be well perfused with blood, and areas that receive blood flow should be capable of ventilation. Although in the normal lung with its many millions of gas exchange units some imbalance in ventilation and perfusion exists, this has little effect on overall gas exchange function. In fact, adaptive mechansims appear to exist that divert blood flow to the best ventilated regions of the lungs or redirect ventilation away from nonperfused areas in order to maintain a normal ratio in the range of 0.8 to 1.0.[4] However, even though overall amounts for each of these two values (ventilation and perfusion) may be adequate, normal exchange of oxygen and carbon dioxide will not occur if areas of the lung that are well ventilated are not also well perfused. The reverse situation, in which well-perfused areas are underventilated, will also result in impairment of respiratory function with inadequate gas exchange caused by changes in the $\dot{V}/\dot{Q}$ ratio. In fact, $\dot{V}/\dot{Q}$ mismatch, or alteration in ventilation-perfusion relationships, is largely responsible for the *hypoxemia* and *hypercapnia* seen in clinical practice. (For a more detailed explanation, see specialized texts.[4,25]) The nurse should be familiar with the tests to be able to explain them to the patient.

Measurement of pulmonary volumes and capacities

To determine the functional capacity of the lungs, basic ventilation studies are performed by using a spirometer. Some measurements such as the *residual volume* cannot be measured directly and are calculated mathematically. The total gas content of the lungs can be subdivided into volumes and capacities as defined below.

Definitions of lung volumes

Tidal volume (TV)	Volume of gas inspired and expired with a normal breath
Inspiratory reserve volume (IRV)	Maximal volume that can be inspired from the end of a normal inspiration
Expiratory reserve volume (ERV)	Maximal volume that can be exhaled by forced expiration after a normal expiration
Residual volume (RV)	Volume of gas left in lung after maximal expiration
Minute volume (MV)	Volume inspired and expired in 1 minute of normal breathing

Definitions of lung capacities

Vital capacity (VC)	Maximal amount of air that can be expired after a maximal inspiration (TV + IRV + ERV)
Forced vital capacity (FVC)	Maximal amount of air that can be expelled with a maximal effort after a maximal inspiration
Maximal midexpiratory flow (MMEF)	Average rate of flow during middle half of forced vital capacity
Forced expiratory volume in 1 second (FEV_1)	Amount of air expelled in the first second of the forced vital capacity maneuver
FEV_1/VC ratio	Amount of air forcefully expelled in 1 second compared to total amount forcefully expelled
Maximal voluntary ventilation (MVV), also termed maximal breathing capacity (MBC)	Amount of air exchanged per minute with maximal rate and depth of respiration
Inspiratory capacity (IC)	Maximal amount of air that can be inspired after a normal expiration (TV + IRV)
Functional residual capacity (FRC)	Amount of air left in lungs after a normal expiration (ERV + RV)
Total lung capacity (TLC)	Total amount of air in lungs after after maximal inspiration (TV + IRV + ERV + RV)

A spirogram showing the normal volumes and lung capacities is shown in Fig. 44-5. These volumes and capacities vary with age, sex, weight, and height. Two ventilatory studies are of particular clinical significance. They are the *forced expiratory volume* (FEV), or *timed vital capacity*, and the *maximal voluntary ventilation* (MVV), or *maximum breathing capacity* (MBC). The FEV measures the volume expired forcefully at 1,2, and 3 seconds after a full inspiration. The FEV at *1 second* is the most useful of the three values, particularly when it is compared with the vital capacity (FEV_1/VC ratio). The MVV measures the volume of air exchanged per minute with maximal rate and depth of respiration. Other tests and techniques of studying pulmonary function are described in specialized texts.[4,12,18,25]

The patient is usually instructed in how to participate in the tests by the physician or the technician in the testing laboratory. For all these tests the patient must breathe only through the mouth. A recording device and a spirometer are used. When the patient breathes through the mouthpiece and connecting tube, a noseclip is usually used so that the patient cannot breathe through the nose. Although a noseclip may seem like a small, harmless piece of equipment, the patient often becomes apprehensive about it. Time should be allowed for the patient to adjust to the clip. Fear of cutting off the air supply, particularly when a person has a breathing limitation, may cause anxiety. Because these tests are dependent on patient effort and can also be very exhausting to a patient with respiratory disease, rest both before and after the testing is carried out. If the patient is receiving regular bronchodilator treatments, these are withheld for 4 hours prior to testing if a part of the examination is to include measurements taken before and after the use of nebulized bronchodilators. Nurses can allay some of the patient's apprehension by giving clear and confident explanations.

Blood gas studies

Arterial blood gas studies have become a common tool to aid in physiologic diagnosis and therapeutic management of patients. These studies determine blood pH, carbon dioxide tension (Pco_2), oxygen tension (Po_2), and percent of oxyhemoglobin saturation (Sao_2). Gas tensions refer to partial pressure, or that part of the total pressure exerted by a specific gas. For example, pressure exerted by the atmosphere at sea level is 760 mm Hg. The amount of oxygen in air at sea level is 21%; that is, 21% of the total pressure is exerted by oxygen. Since 21% of 760 is approximately 159, the Po_2 of air at sea level is 159 mm Hg. Definitions of gas exchange functions and their normal values are as follows:

Definitions and normal values of gas exchange functions

pH	Acidity of blood	7.38 to 7.42
Pco_2	Partial pressure of carbon dioxide in blood	38 to 42 mm Hg
Po_2	Partial pressure of oxygen in blood	80 to 100 mm Hg
Sao_2	Percentage of available hemoglobin saturated with oxygen	95% to 98%

The measurement of oxygen values includes both the

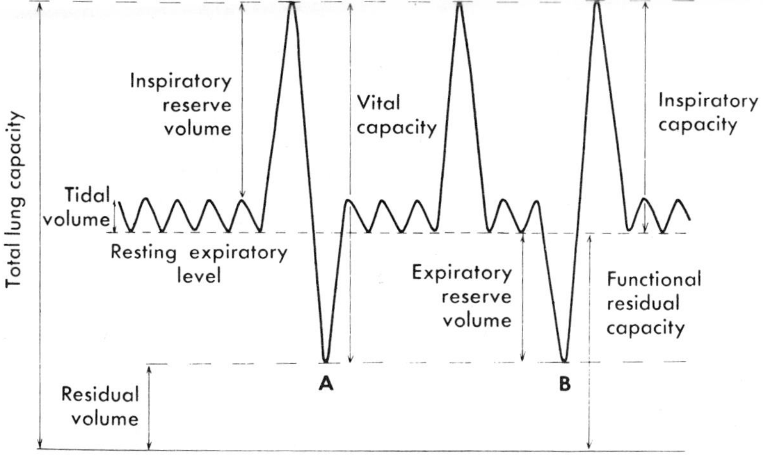

Fig. 44-5. Lung volumes and their subdivisions illustrated by spirograph tracing. *A*, Inspiratory vital capacity. *B*, More common expiratory vital capacity. (From Wade, J. F.: Respiratory nursing care, ed. 2. St. Louis, 1977, The C. V. Mosby Co.)

Po_2 and Sao_2. The Po_2 measures oxygen dissolved in the blood; however, the amount of oxygen carried in the blood in this form is small, as most oxygen is transported in chemical combination with hemoglobin. Oxyhemoglobin saturation refers to that percentage of the hemoglobin that is combined with oxygen. More than 90% of the oxygen-carrying capacity of blood is accounted for by oxyhemoglobin, with the partial pressure of oxygen acting as the driving force for this chemical combination. Therefore both Po_2 and Sao_2 levels must be examined in order to determine the adequacy of oxygenation of the tissues.

It is particularly important to understand the relationship of the Po_2 to oxyhemoglobin saturation in order to assess adequacy of tissue oxygenation. This relationship is not directly linear; many factors affect the affinity of the heme molecule for oxygen. A sigmoid curve (Fig. 44-6) represents the saturation percentages that occur at various Po_2 levels. Most significant of the factors that affect the ability of the blood to carry oxygen is the partial pressure of the oxygen itself in the blood. As can be seen in the oxyhemoglobin dissociation curve (Fig. 44-6), in the upper portion of the curve, hemoglobin has an increased affinity for oxygen, so that large changes in Po_2 levels can be tolerated without significantly changing the saturation. For example, at a Po_2 of 100 mm Hg, hemoglobin saturation is almost total, 97%; even if the Po_2 should fall to 70 mm Hg the saturation would only decrease to 94%. This serves as a protective mechanism that assures adequate tissue oxygenation even when there is mild hypoxemia. It should be noted, however, that once the Po_2 level falls below 60 mm Hg, saturation begins to decrease sharply, thus reducing the ability of the hemoglobin to transport oxygen.

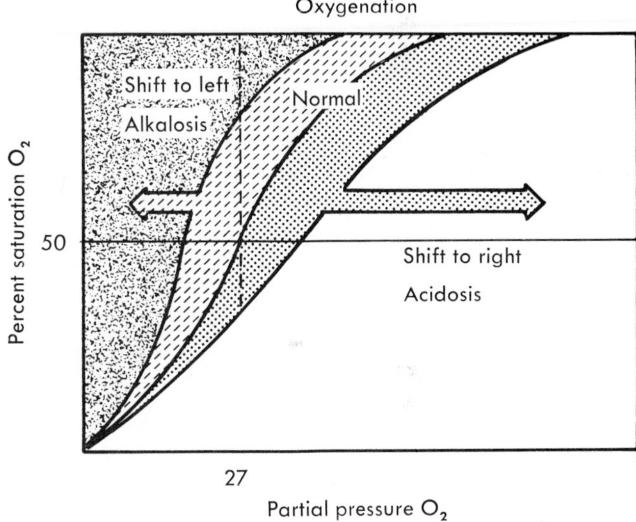

Fig. 44-6. Oxyhemoglobin dissociation curve. Shift to right indicates acidosis. Shift to left indicates alkalosis.

Other factors that influence the oxygen affinity of hemoglobin are temperature, pH, and Po_2. At higher temperatures, increased levels of Pco_2 (hypercapnia), and acidosis, the curve shifts to the right. This means that at any given Po_2 the hemoglobin has less affinity for oxygen and lower saturations will result. The converse of this is also true; with decreased temperature, decreased Pco_2, and alkalosis, higher saturations occur with any given Po_2.

The Pco_2 is utilized as a measurement to determine the adequacy of ventilation and is dependent on the amount of carbon dioxide produced by the body and the ability of the lungs to eliminate it. *Hypoventilation* therefore is shown by an elevated P_{CO_2}, while *hyperventilation* is indicated by a decrease in P_{CO_2} below normal levels.

The pH refers to the acidity of the blood and is an expression of the hydrogen ion concentration. Because pH is expressed as a negative logarithm, as hydrogen ion concentration increases and blood becomes more acid, the pH value falls. When hydrogen ion concentration decreases, the blood becomes more alkaline and the pH value rises.

The P_{CO_2} is related to the pH because of the chemical reaction of carbon dioxide and water in the blood, which results in the formation of carbonic acid. Carbonic acid, in turn, dissociates to form hydrogen and bicarbonate ions, as illustrated in the following equation:

$$CO_2 + H_2O \rightleftarrows H_2CO_3 \rightleftarrows HCO_3^- + H^+$$

The maintenance of a normal pH is dependent on a ratio of 20 bicarbonate ions to 1 hydrogen ion. It can be seen from the equation that the presence of an elevated P_{CO_2} will result in an excess of hydrogen ions. When this occurs, the pH falls and the patient is said to be in *respiratory acidosis.* Conversely, when P_{CO_2} is decreased, the pH increases and the result is termed *respiratory alkalosis.* (For a more detailed explanation, see references 4 and 25.)

Bronchospirometry

Bronchospirometry measures the ventilation and oxygen consumption of each lung separately. For this procedure a specially constructed double-lumen catheter with two ballons is used. Whe the catheter is in place, one balloon is inflated to seal off the contralateral lung. After measuring the ventilation of one lung, that balloon is deflated; the other balloon is inflated, and the procedure is repeated on the opposite side. This test aids the surgeon in determining whether the ventilatory capacity of the unaffected lung is sufficient to maintain the patient after pulmonary resection. This determination is most crucial prior to pneumonectomy.

□ Bronchography and bronchoscopy

Examinations by bronchography and bronchoscopy are somewhat complicated diagnostic procedures that may be ordered. A thorough explanation of what will happen during these examinations can do much to allay anxiety. Since instruments are passed through one nostril or the mouth and pharynx, the patient may be apprehensive about being able to breathe. It is helpful to teach the patient to breathe in and out of the nose with the mouth open. Practice in relaxing the shoulders and hands while lying on the back also helps.

A *bronchogram* enables the physician to visualize the bronchial tree by x-ray film after the introduction of an iodized radiopaque liquid. To lessen the number of bacteria introduced from the mouth into the bronchi, the patient should pay particular attention to oral hygiene on the night before and on the morning of the procedure. No food or fluids are allowed for 8 hours preceding the examination. Since, if the smaller bronchi contain secretions, the radiopaque liquid will not reach them, postural drainage may be ordered for the morning the bronchogram is made (Fig. 45-9). The patient should be asked about any loose or capped teeth or dental bridges. Dental prostheses should be removed, and loose teeth should be brought to the physician's attention. Bronchograms are *contraindicated* during acute infections and in individuals sensitive to iodine.

Approximately 1 hour before the examination the patient is given a short-acting barbiturate to minimize the stimulating effects of the anesthetic agent and to sedate him. To lessen the patient's discomfort during the procedure, a local topical anesthetic agent is administered. Usually 0.5% tetracaine (Pontocaine) or cocaine is used. These drugs can cause toxic reactions in some patients. Thus the client is observed closely for signs of central nervous system stimulation. Rapid pulse rate, excitation, headache, and palpitation are some of the signs of toxicity. When these occur, the physician is notified at once. Usually a short-acting barbiturate such as secobarbital (Seconal) is given intravenously. Oxygen may also be administered. If the patient is not treated promptly, the central nervous system can become depressed and the patient may die from respiratory failure.

The pharynx, larynx, and major bronchi are anesthetized immediately before the radiopaque substance is introduced. The patient is informed that the local anesthetic will taste bitter and that it should not be swallowed but expectorated into tissues or an emesis basin, which will be provided. When the gag reflex disappears, a metal laryngeal cannula is passed into the trachea, and then a catheter is passed through the nose into the cannula and into the trachea. The radiopaque substance is then introduced, and the patient is tilted into various positions to distribute it to the bronchi and bronchioles. These positions are the reverse of those used in postural drainage. A series of radiographs is then taken. Following this procedure, postural drainage is usually ordered to help remove the radiopaque substance from the lungs. Follow-up films may also be taken to ascertain how much dye remains in the tracheobronchial tree. No permanent damage results, however, if some of it remains for an indefinite period. Food and fluid should be withheld until the gag reflex returns, which can be tested by gently tickling the posterior pharynx with a cotton swab.

A *bronchoscopic examination* is performed by pas-

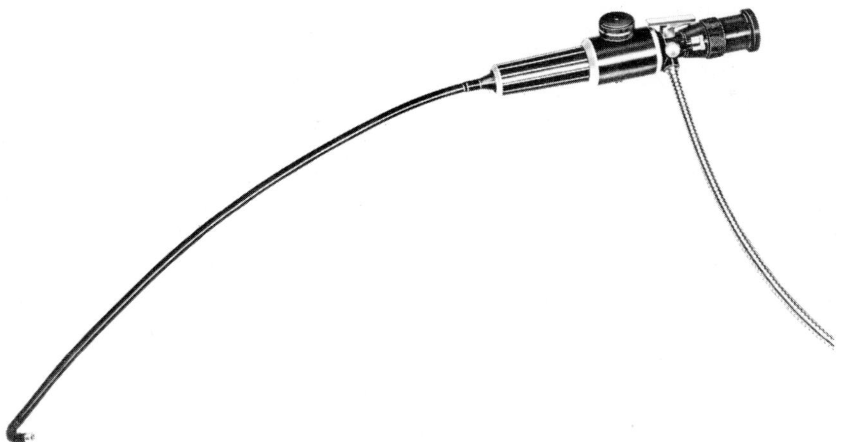

Fig. 44-7. Fiberoptic bronchoscope. Because of its flexibility, it allows better visualization of bronchi. (Courtesy American Cystoscope Makers, Inc., Pelham, N.Y.)

sing a bronchoscope into the trachea and bronchi. Preparation of the client for a bronchoscopic examination is similar to that for bronchography except that postural drainage is less often ordered. In addition to a spray anesthetic, cocaine may be applied locally by holding small cotton pledgets soaked in solution in the posterior fossa of the pharynx. If the patient is very apprehensive or if a sponge biopsy (abrasion of the lesion with a sponge) is to be done or a tissue biopsy obtained, intravenous anesthesia may be used. A bronchoscope is a long, rigid, slender, hollow instrument through which light can be reflected and visual examination of the trachea and major bronchi with their branchings can be made. In recent years the *fiberoptic bronchoscope,* which is a flexible instrument allowing greater visualization with passage into segmental and subsegmental bronchi, has been employed with increasing frequency particularly for diagnostic examination (Fig. 44-7). The use of this instrument is also associated with less discomfort for the patient as compared to the rigid metal bronchoscope. Bronchoscopy may be done to remove a foreign body, to facilitate free air passage by removal of mucus plugs with suction, to obtain a biopsy and samples of secretions for examination, and to observe the air passages for signs of disease.

Following bronchoscopy the patient is given no food or fluids until the gag reflex returns. Some physicians prefer that the patient lie flat after this procedure, while others prefer a semi-Fowler's position. Unless intravenous anesthesia is used, the patient is awake and conscious, although drowsy from sedation. Lying on the side facilitates removal of secretions into disposable tissues or a small emesis basin. The patient usually produces large amounts of sputum. All sputum is saved for culture and cytologic studies because the postbronchoscopy specimens are often positive diagnostically. However, if the patient has had bronchograms, the sputum is often not helpful for cytologic examination, as the base of the dye makes fixation of the cells difficult.

The patient frequently complains of a sore throat and may have hoarseness after the procedure. Lidocaine (Xylocaine) is often helpful in reducing discomfort. In some instances, laryngeal edema follows bronchoscopy and can cause airway obstruction. After this procedure, there frequently is a shortness of breath and laryngeal stridor. If laryngeal edema occurs, the physician should be notified immediately. Cool mist is often given prophylactically to prevent the development of this complication. When cocaine is used for local anesthesia, the patient is watched for the signs of central nervous system stimulation described previously.

If a biopsy is taken during bronchoscopy, the patient is kept under close surveillance until clotting occurs—usually in 5 to 7 minutes. Sputum should be observed carefully for a few hours after the procedure for signs of hemorrhage. The patient should not smoke for several hours because smoking may cause coughing and start bleeding. Although normally the sputum may be streaked with blood for a few days after a biopsy, any pronounced bleeding is reported at once to the physician.

□ Mediastinoscopy

In this examination a *mediastinoscope,* which is an instrument much like a bronchoscope, is inserted through a small incision in the suprasternal notch and advanced into the mediastinum where inspection and biopsy of the lymph nodes can then be carried out. Consult the article by Klause[16] for further information.

☐ Lung scan (pulmonary scintiphotography)

Lung scan procedures involve the use of a scanning device that records the pattern of pulmonary radioactivity after the inhalation or intravenous injection of gamma ray–emitting radionuclides, thus providing a visual image of the distribution of ventilation or blood flow in the lungs. These studies provide valuable information regarding *ventilation-perfusion patterns* and aid in the diagnosis of parenchymal lung diseases and vascular disorders such as pulmonary embolism.

☐ Pulmonary angiography

Pulmonary angiography is used to detect pulmonary emboli and a variety of congenital and acquired lesions of the pulmonary vessels. A radiopaque material is injected via a catheter into a systemic vein, the right chambers of the heart, or the pulmonary artery, and the distribution of this material is recorded on film. Following this procedure the nurse observes the site of insertion of the catheter and reports any adverse signs and symptoms such as inflammation, formation of a hematoma, absence of peripheral pulses, or complaint of numbness, tingling or pain in the extremity involved.

☐ Thoracentesis

Thoracentesis involves the insertion of a needle into the pleural space and aspiration of fluid for either diagnostic or therapeutic purposes. Biopsy specimens of the pleura may also be obtained by the use of needles specially constructed with a cutting edge and a mechanism for retaining the biopsy specimen. When thoracentesis is done for diagnostic purposes, the fluid may be examined for specific gravity, white blood cell count, differential cell count, red blood cell count, protein, glucose, and amylase concentrations. The fluid may also be cultured and checked for the presence of abnormal or malignant cells. The gross appearance of the fluid, the quantity obtained, and the location of the site of the thoracentesis should be recorded.

When a thoracentesis is to be done, the procedure should be explained to the patient. It is necessary that the patient understand the importance of not moving when the needle is inserted to avoid damage to the lung or pleura. Usually a local anesthetic such as procaine or lidocaine is used to eliminate pain at the site of insertion of the needle. However, when the pleura is entered, a sensation of pain or pressure may occur. Whenever possible, the patient should be in an upright position, either sitting on the side of the bed with the feet supported and arms and head on a padded overbed table or straddling a chair with the arms and head resting on the back of the chair. This position with arms and shoulders raised elevates the ribs and makes it easier to carry out the procedure. Patients who cannot sit up are turned onto the affected side so that the side to be tapped is uppermost.

Vital signs (pulse, respiration, and blood pressure) are taken several times during the procedure, and the patient is monitored for changes in color and character of respirations and the presence of diaphoresis. The needle and syringe should be carefully checked to see that they fit snugly so that no air is permitted to enter the pleural space. Fluid may be aspirated directly into the syringe, or a three-way adaptor may be used with one end attached to tubing leading to a receptacle into which the fluid is drained. Specimens are placed in the appropriate containers and labeled according to the examinations ordered by the physician. Following a thoracentesis the patient is watched for signs of coughing or expectoration of blood, since these signs might indicate that the lung was traumatized inadvertently. (For details on the equipment needed, see texts on fundamentals of nursing.)

REFERENCES AND SELECTED REFERENCES

1. Alexander, M. M., and Brown, M. S.: Physical examination. Pt. 12. Chest and Lungs, Nursing (Jenkintown) **5**:44-48, 1975.
2. *American Lung Association: Introduction to lung diseases, New York, 1973, The Association.
3. Bates, B.: A guide to physical examination, Philadelphia, 1974. J. B. Lippincott Co.
4. Bendixen, H. H., Egbert, L. D., Hedley-Whyte, J., Laver, M. B., and Pontoppidan, H.: Respiratory care, St. Louis, 1965. The C. V. Mosby Co.
5. Blood-gas and acid-base concepts in respiratory care: programmed instruction, Am. J. Nurs. **76**:1-30, 1976.
6. Bouhuys, A.: The physiology of breathing, New York, 1977, Grune & Stratton, Inc.
7. *Broughton, J.: Chest physical diagnosis for nurses and respiratory therapists, Heart Lung **2**:200-206, 1972.
8. Comroe, J. H.: Physiology of respiration, ed. 2, Chicago, 1974, Year Book Medical Publishers, Inc.
9. Delaney, M. T.: Examining the chest. Pt. I. The lungs, Nursing (Jenkintown) **5**:12-14, 1975.
10. Demers, R. R., and Saklad, M.: Fundamentals of blood gas interpretation, Respir. Care **18**:153-159, 1973.
11. Finch, C., and Lenfant, C.: Oxygen transport in man, N. Engl. J. Med. **286**:407-415, 1972.
12. *Foley, M. F.: Pulmonary function testing, Am. J. Nurs. **71**:1134-1139, 1971.
13. Hudak, C. M., Gallo, B. M., and Lohr, T., editors: Critical care nursing, Philadelphia, 1973, J. B. Lippincott Co.
14. Keyes, J. L.: Blood-gas analysis and the assessment of acid-base status, Heart Lung **5**:247-255, 1976.
15. Keyes, J. L.: Blood-gases and blood gas transport, Heart Lung **3**:945-954, 1974.
16. Klause, M. L.: Mediastinoscopy, AORN J. **15**:55-59, 1972.

*References preceded by an asterisk are particulary well suited for student reading.

17. Malasanos, L., Barkauskas, V., Moss, M., and Allen, K. S.: Health assessment, St. Louis, 1977, The C. V. Mosby Co.
18. *Phipps, W. J., Barker, W. L., and Daly, B. J.: Respiratory insufficiency and failure. In Meltzer, L. E., Abdellah, F. G., and Kitchell, J. F.: Concepts and practices of intensive care for nurse specialists, ed. 2, Philadelphia, 1975, The Charles Press Publishers.
19. Shapiro, B. A., Harrison, R. A., and Trout, C. A.: Clinical application of respiratory care, Chicago, 1975, Year Book Medical Publishers, Inc.
20. Simmons, D. H.: Evaluation of acid-base status. In American Thoracic Society: Basics of RD, New York, 1974, The Society.
21. Slonim, N. B., and Hamilton, L. H.: Respiratory physiology, ed. 3, St. Louis, 1976, The C. V. Mosby Co.
22. Tinker, J. H.: Understanding chest x-rays, Am. J. Nurs. **76**:54-58, 1976.
23. Traver, G.: The nurses' role in clinical testing of lung function, Nurs. Clin. North Am. **9**:101-110, 1974.
24. *Traver, G.: Assessment of thorax and lungs, Am. J. Nurs. **73**:466-471, 1973.
25. Wade, J. F.: Respiratory nursing care: physiology and technique, ed. 2, St. Louis, 1977, The C. V. Mosby Co.
26. Winslow, E. H.: Visual inspection of the patient with cardiopulmonary disease, Heart Lung **4**:421-429, 1975.

45

Management of the person with impaired oxygen–carbon dioxide exchange

BARBARA J. DALY
WILMA J. PHIPPS
FRANCES R. BROWN

In order for oxygen–carbon dioxide exchange to take place normally several factors are necessary: (1) an adequate supply of oxygen in the environment, (2) a patent airway, (3) normal functioning bellows motion of the chest wall and diaphragm, (4) an adequate number of functioning alveoli and capillaries that together form a terminal respiratory unit (TRU), (5) an adequate amount of hemoglobin to carry oxygen to the cells, (6) an intact circulatory system and an effective heart pump, and (7) a functioning respiratory center. Problems in one or more of the above can result in inadequate exchange of oxygen and carbon dioxide and, if severe enough, can cause death. Table 45-1 lists some of the conditions that can lead to inadequate oxygen–carbon dioxide exchange.

■ PREVENTION

Prevention of conditions that impair oxygen–carbon dioxide exchange requires that health care providers be aware of the factors that cause problems and try to prevent their occurrence. Prevention involves teaching of the public about certain hazards such as the need to become acclimated to high altitudes before engaging in other than minimal activities, and working with parents and others having contact with toddlers to emphasize the need to keep the environment free of small objects that could be aspirated by curious youngsters who have a tendency to put everything in their mouths.

Because of the deleterious effects of cigarette smoking on the cardiopulmonary systems, a concerted effort is indicated to teach persons about the hazards of smoking. In addition, the prevention of pulmonary infections requires that all persons understand how pulmonary infections are spread and what they can do to prevent themselves from acquiring frequent infections.

Many conditions that affect oxygen–carbon dioxide exchange may be difficult to prevent, but the nurse has a major role to play in preventing the airway of an unconscious person from becoming obstructed and in recognizing complications, such as atelectasis, congestive heart failure, pulmonary edema, and cardiac or pulmonary arrest, that require immediate intervention if adequate oxygenation is to be provided.

The interventions necessary to maintain adequate tissue oxygenation are discussed in detail in the following sections.

■ INTERVENTIONS

The first objective in providing care for the person with impaired oxygen exchange is to ensure a patent airway. Several measures may be used, depending upon the degree of impairment.

The most basic measure involves simply positioning the person in such a way as to prevent obstruction of the airway. This is most relevant in resuscitations or in caring for an unconscious person. The position of choice is supine or side-lying with the neck hyperextended. Persons who are unconscious or very lethargic may suffer airway obstruction if the tongue is allowed to fall back and cover the glottis; the side-lying position prevents this from happening (Fig. 23-9).

□ Maintaining a patent airway

Types of artificial airways

When a person has a mechanical obstruction of the airway and is expected to be unconscious for some time, it may be necessary to use an artificial airway. An endotracheal tube is usually chosen initially as a means of providing the airway; tracheostomy is only performed if airway maintenance is necessary for a prolonged period of time or if trauma to the airway prevents the use of an endotracheal tube. Although the tracheostomy has the *disadvantage* of a higher risk of infection, it is often elected

Table 45-1. Factors interfering with normal oxygen–carbon dioxide exchange

Necessary component	Interference
Adequate supply of oxygen	Smoke inhalation Carbon monoxide poisoning High altitudes = low O_2 concentration
Patent airway	Foreign bodies in treacheobronchial tree Children (aspiration of objects such as pennies, pins, jacks) Unconscious adults (tongue obstructing airway, aspirated vomitus, loose dentures) Mucus plug resulting in atelectasis Allergic reactions resulting in bronchoconstriction, increased mucus secretions, and increased capillary permeability
Normally functioning bellows	Trauma to chest wall with possible sequelae of paradoxical breathing, pneumothorax, mediastinal shift Muscle or nerve trauma or impairment (quadriplegia, paraplegia, poliomyelitis, myasthenia gravis, Guillain-Barré-Strohl syndrome, Landry ascending paralysis, muscular dystrophy)
Adequate functioning alveoli and capillaries (TRU)	Pulmonary edema Adult respiratory disease syndrome (interstitial edema) Physiologic shunts Damage to alveolar-capillary membrane secondary to conditions such as pulmonary emphysema
Adequate amount of hemoglobin	Severe anemia Carbon monoxide poisoning Methemoglobinemia
Intact circulatory system and pump	Congestive heart failure (CHF) Hemorrhage
Functioning respiratory center	Depression of respiratory center by drugs (heroin, morphine, barbiturates, alcohol or a combination of alcohol with a tranquilizer or barbiturates) Increased intracranial pressure (head injury or disease such as meningitis)

for airway management because it is much more comfortable than an endotracheal tube and allows the person to eat.

In endotracheal intubation a tube is passed through either the nose or mouth into the trachea, while in a tracheostomy an artificial opening is made in the trachea into which a tube is inserted (Fig. 45-1). These procedures are used (1) to establish and maintain a patent airway; (2) to prevent aspiration by sealing off the trachea from the digestive tract in the unconscious or paralyzed person; (3) to permit removal of tracheobronchial secretions in the person who cannot cough adequately; and (4) to treat the patient who requires positive pressure ventilation that cannot be given effectively by mask.[71] Whether an intubation or a tracheostomy is performed initially depends on the facilities available and the wishes of the physician. Most physicians now consider it safer to do an emergency endotracheal intubation and then perform a tracheostomy as a nonemergency procedure in the operating room if prolonged support of the airway is needed. In this instance the endotracheal tube is not removed until after the tracheostomy opening is made.

A tracheostomy is necessary when an endotracheal tube cannot be inserted or when it is contraindicated, as in severe burns or laryngeal obstruction caused by tumor, infection, or vocal cord paralysis.[71] Tracheostomy may also be required when a patient is conscious and cannot tolerate an endotracheal tube. Once the airway is secured either by intubation or by tracheostomy, secretions are aspirated and well-humidified oxygen is usually given. If the patient is unable to sustain respiration, a mechanical ventilator (such as a Bennett or a Bird ventilator) is attached to either the endotracheal tube or the tracheostomy tube. When mechanical ventilation is required, a cuffed tube is used. Usually an endotracheal tube is not left in place longer than 5 to 7 days. If the patient is unable to maintain a free airway after this period of time, a tracheostomy is performed.

The endotracheal tube may be made of either plastic or rubber with an inflatable cuff so that a closed system with the ventilator may be maintained (Fig. 45-2). The tube is inserted via the mouth or nose through the larynx into the trachea. If an oral endotracheal tube is used, a rubber airway or bite block is often necessary to prevent

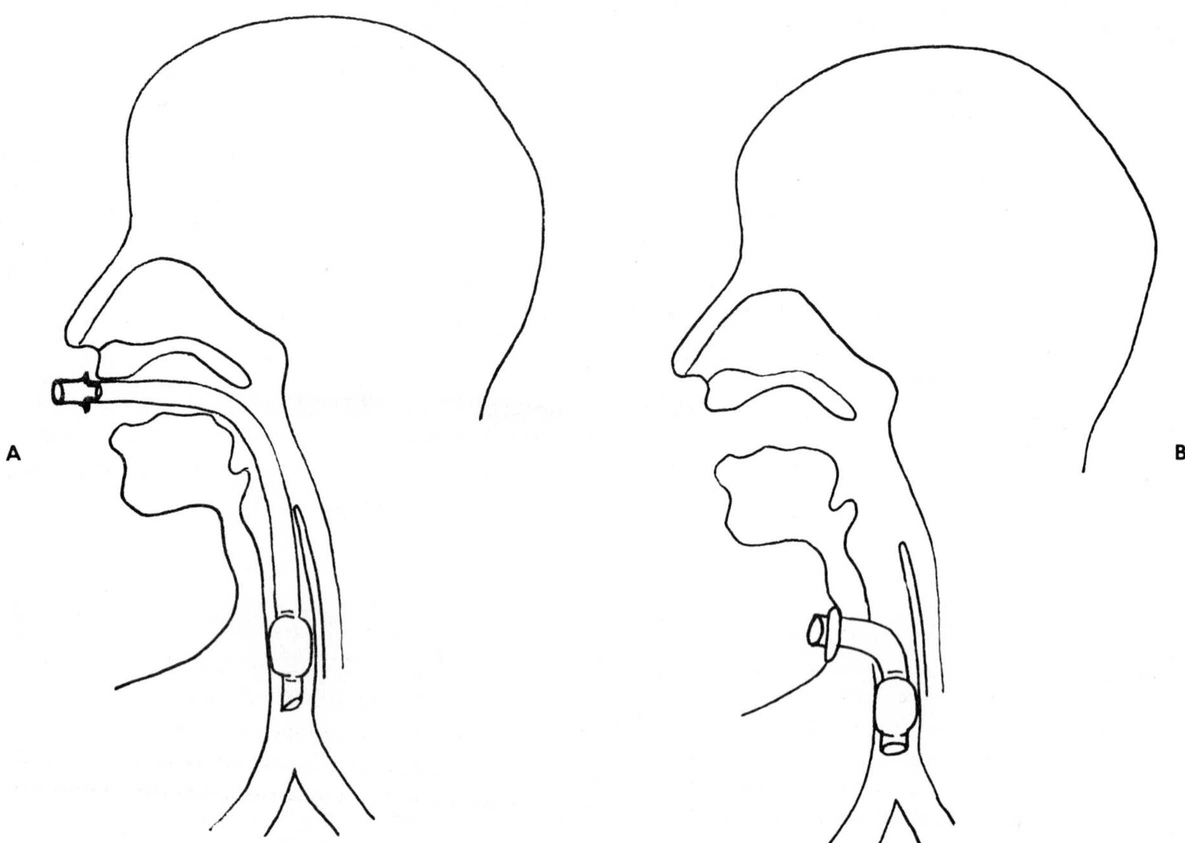

Fig. 45-1. A, Position of endotracheal tube. **B,** Position of tracheostomy tube.

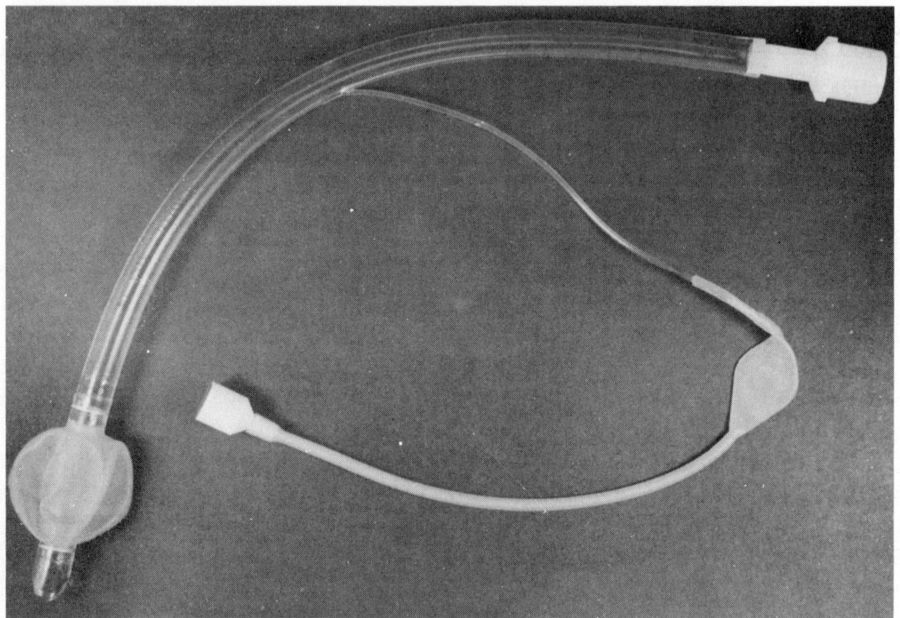

Fig. 45-2. Forregar high-volume, low-pressure cuffed endotracheal tube. Cuff shown here is not inflated. Low-pressure cuff is preferred because it is less likely to cause tracheal damage.

the patient from biting down on the tube and obstructing the airway.

The tracheostomy tube is usually made of plastic, silver, or nylon. It may be either a single-lumen or double-lumen (Jackson) type (Fig. 45-3). Both types of tubes may be cuffed, and the newer plastic tubes come with high-volume, low-pressure cuffs that are less likely to cause damage to the trachea (Fig. 45-4). Single-lumen tubes must be changed about every 72 hours, since they are more difficult to clean and more likely to become plugged than are double-lumen tubes.

Twill tapes attached to either side of the tube (Fig. 45-3) are tied securely behind the neck to prevent the tube from becoming dislodged when the patient coughs or moves about.

Should the tube be coughed out, the opening may close and the patient will be unable to breathe. Therefore a tracheal dilator or curved hemostat is always kept at the bedside so that the opening can be held open if the tube is dislodged. Some surgeons prefer to place a retention suture on each side of the tracheostomy opening and tape the end of the suture to the skin. If the opening shows signs of closing, tension can be placed on the sutures to widen the opening. Silver tubes are commonly available in sizes nos. 00 to 8 (no. 00 is used for the premature or newborn infant, while a no. 6 or 7 is used for most adults). The silver tracheostomy tube consists of two parts, an inner and an outer cannula. The outer cannula is removed only by the physician, while the inner cannula is removed regularly by the nurse for cleaning. The silver tracheostomy tube has a lock that must be turned in order to remove the inner cannula. The lock should be secured when the inner cannula is reinserted after cleaning.

The operative wound may be sealed with a plastic spray, or a small dressing may be placed around the tracheostomy tube. Although drainage should be minimal, the wound is inspected frequently for bleeding during the immediate postoperative period. The dressings are changed as they become soiled with drainage of mucus. Occasionally young children require elbow restraints to prevent them from removing the tube or putting objects into it.

Immediately after insertion of the endotracheal tube and periodically thereafter the chest is auscultated to ensure that there are breath sounds on both sides. If a cuffed tube is inserted too far, it will slip into one of the mainstem bronchi (usually the right) and occlude the opposite bronchus and lung, resulting in atelectasis on the obstructed side. Even if the tube is still in the trachea, airway obstruction will result if the end of the tube is located on the carina (area at lower end of trachea at point of bifurcation of mainstem bronchi). This will result in dry secretions that obstruct both bronchi. Although these complications are more common with the use of an endotracheal tube, they can occur with a tracheostomy tube, especially in a small person with a short neck. In either case the tube is pulled back until it is positioned below the larynx and above the carina. The tube is then fastened securely in place. A replacement tube of the same size should always be kept at the bedside in the event that it is needed.

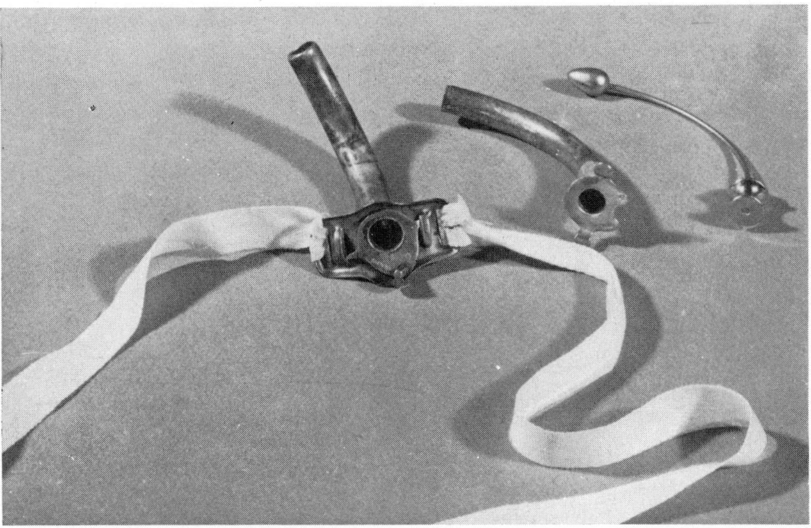

Fig. 45-3. Parts of silver tracheostomy tube: outer tube with ties attached, inner tube, and pilot. (From DeWeese, D. D., and Saunders, W. H.: Textbook of otolaryngology, ed. 5, St. Louis, 1977, The C. V. Mosby Co.)

Depending on the patient's condition, a tracheostomy can be either temporary or permanent; the person who has a laryngectomy will have a permanent tracheostomy. Any patient who has had a tracheostomy is apprehensive and is often fearful of choking. Thus when feasible, the procedure is thoroughly explained to the patient before surgery. Both patient and family need to understand that the patient will be unable to speak and that constant attendance will be provided until the patient can give self-care safely. The nurse should plan with the patient for some means of communication after the surgery. Hand signs such as the OK sign or a raised finger might be used as a means of expressing, for example, the need to void. The patient may want to write on a pad or a Magic Slate, or a word or picture chart can be used. The patient's ideas about means of communication should be considered. Patients should have their bell cords within reach, and a tap bell is reassuring to some patients.

Nursing care of a person with a cuffed tube

The use of a cuffed endotracheal or tracheostomy tube has several implications for nursing care. Although the advent of low-pressure cuffs has significantly lowered the incidence of tracheal erosion and necrosis from pressure on the wall of the trachea, there are still some hazards inherent in the use of artificial airways.

The cuff on the tube is used to maintain a closed system (Fig. 45-4) that will permit positive pressure ventilation. It is also used to prevent aspiration of secretions by the unconscious person. Sometimes the cuff is used to exert pressure on bleeding sites in patients who have undergone throat or neck surgery, such as a radical neck dissection. If none of these considerations apply, the cuff does not need to be inflated.

If the patient is being mechanically ventilated, the cuff should be inflated during the positive pressure phase (inspiration) of the ventilator. Two different methods may be used to inflate the cuff, depending on the patient's condition and the preference of those responsible for care. In the first method, air is injected into the cuff until a full seal is attained. At this point a pressure-cycled respirator will turn off and no air will escape around the tube or through the nose and mouth. The tubing leading to the cuff is then clamped. In the other method, air is injected until a full seal is attained, and then 0.5 ml of air is withdrawn and the tubing clamped. This latter method creates a partial leak for which the respirator can be set to compensate. The nurse should note the amount of air needed to inflate the cuff and use the smallest amount required to attain a seal. Overinflation of the cuff is extremely dangerous because it can lead to the development of tracheomalacia, tracheal stenosis, tracheoesophageal fistula, or erosion through a major blood vessel.

In the past it had been recommended that the cuff be routinely deflated for several minutes each hour in order to prevent tracheal necrosis. This is not necessary with low-pressure cuffs. It is sufficient to deflate the cuff and reinflate it once every 8 hours. This is necessary to ensure that the cuff is not overinflated and to check for tracheal dilatation, indicated by the requirement of pro-

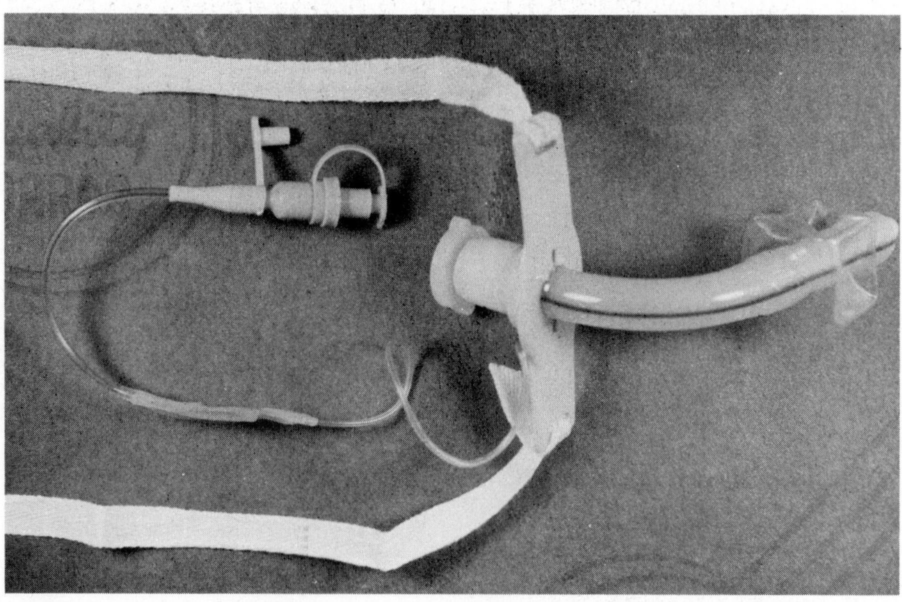

Fig. 45-4. Portex high-volume, low-pressure cuffed tracheostomy tube.

gressively larger amounts of air in order to obtain a seal.

It is important to remember that speaking is impossible with a cuffed tube in place because air does not pass directly through the larynx. The person is informed that speech will be normal when the tube is removed. Persons who are not informed of the change in function may believe that they have permanently lost their ability to speak.

Often the person with a tracheostomy tube can speak when the cuff is not fully inflated. Speech is still difficult as air must be forced around the tube and up through the larynx. For those who can tolerate it, it is often helpful to obstruct the opening of the tracheostomy tube while the cuff is deflated. This allows the person to breathe through the upper airway. See p. 946 for discussion of means of communication provided for the patient who cannot speak.

Suctioning the tube. All persons with tubes require suctioning and should be suctioned as often as necessary. The frequency of suctioning is a nursing judgment. Many patients in respiratory failure have an infection and accumulation of secretions before intubation or tracheostomy is performed. Once the patient is intubated, the tube produces a natural route for introduction of bacteria into the lower airway, increasing the risk of infection. Much of the ability to produce an effective cough is lost, as it is impossible for the person to build up the pressure needed to create an expulsive cough. Because the patient has difficulty moving secretions up the tracheobronchial tree, it is important to suction as deeply as possible. The depth to which a catheter can be inserted through an *endotracheal tube* in an adult is approximately 18 to 22 inches. Postural drainage with percussion and vibration (p. 957) is extremely helpful in moving secretions up to a point where they can be suctioned.

If the catheter cannot be inserted as far as usual, a mucus plug may be obstructing passage of the catheter. Saline irrigation (approximately 5 to 10 ml) will often liquefy the obstructing secretions so they can be aspirated. When plastic suction catheters and plastic tubes are used, it is not uncommon for the surface of the catheter and tube to stick to each other, inhibiting passage of the catheter. Instilling 1 to 2 ml of sterile saline solution during insertion of the catheter usually prevents this problem.

Nursing care of the person with a tracheostomy

Analgesics and sedatives are given judiciously so as not to depress the respiratory center. The patient is suctioned as often as necessary, possibly every 5 minutes during the first few postoperative hours. The need for suctioning can be determined by the sound of the air coming from the tracheostomy tube, especially after the patient takes a deep breath. When respirations are noisy and pulse and respiratory rates are increased, the patient needs to be suctioned. Patients who are conscious can usually indicate when they need to be suctioned. With any sign of respiratory distress, the tube should be suctioned. If mucus is blocking the inner cannula of a silver tube and cannot be removed by suction, the inner cannula is removed to open the airway. When the mucus is thick, the inner cannula should be cleaned and replaced at once because the outer tube may also become blocked. If, despite these measures, the patient becomes cyanotic, the physician should be summoned at once. A patient who is able to cough up secretions probably will require suctioning less frequently. The amount of mucus subsides gradually and the patient eventually may go for several hours without being suctioned. However, even when secretions are minimal, the patient is apprehensive and needs constant attendance.

Suctioning technique needs to be carefully performed in order to prevent damage to the tracheobronchial mucosa. Some of the problems associated with suctioning are discussed in more detail in various sources.[46,51,71,78] The purpose of the following section is to provide detailed guidelines about how to suction the tracheostomy tube efficiently and safely.

Suctioning the tracheostomy tube. The aim in suctioning is to remove all secretions that have accumulated in the tracheobronchial tree since the last suctioning. In general, suctioning techniques are the same no matter what type of tracheostomy tube is in use. However, silver tubes have both an inner and an outer cannula, while plastic tubes have only one cannula. Physicians vary in their preference as to the type of tube used. Some otolaryngologists prefer that only metal tubes with an inner cannula be used because they believe that they are safer. When a double-lumen tube is used, the inner cannula can readily be removed for suctioning and cleaning, whereas tubes without an inner cannula may have to be completely removed and replaced should they become plugged with secretions. This can usually be prevented, however, by adequate humidification and frequent suctioning. The following guidelines apply to the suctioning of any type of tracheostomy tube.

1. Sterile technique is recommended; sterile gloves or forceps and a sterile catheter are used for suctioning. In some hospitals, clean rather than sterile technique is believed to be sufficient when suctioning patients with a *permanent tracheostomy* who will be caring for their own tube after they go home (Fig. 45-5). In the clean technique the hands are washed well with soap or pHisoHex before suctioning.

2. The catheter must be of a small enough size that it does not occlude the cannula (one-half to two-thirds the diameter of the tube). Commonly, when a silver tube

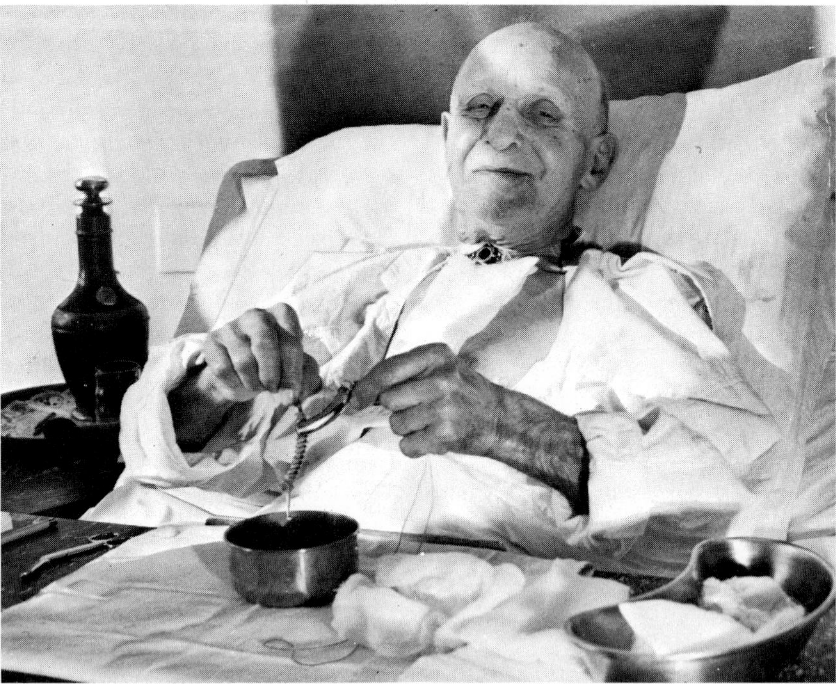

Fig. 45-5. This 82-year-old man cares for his own tracheostomy tube. He is about to clean inner tube with small tube brush. (From Anderson, H. C.: Newton's geriatric nursing, ed. 5, St. Louis, 1971, The C. V. Mosby Co.)

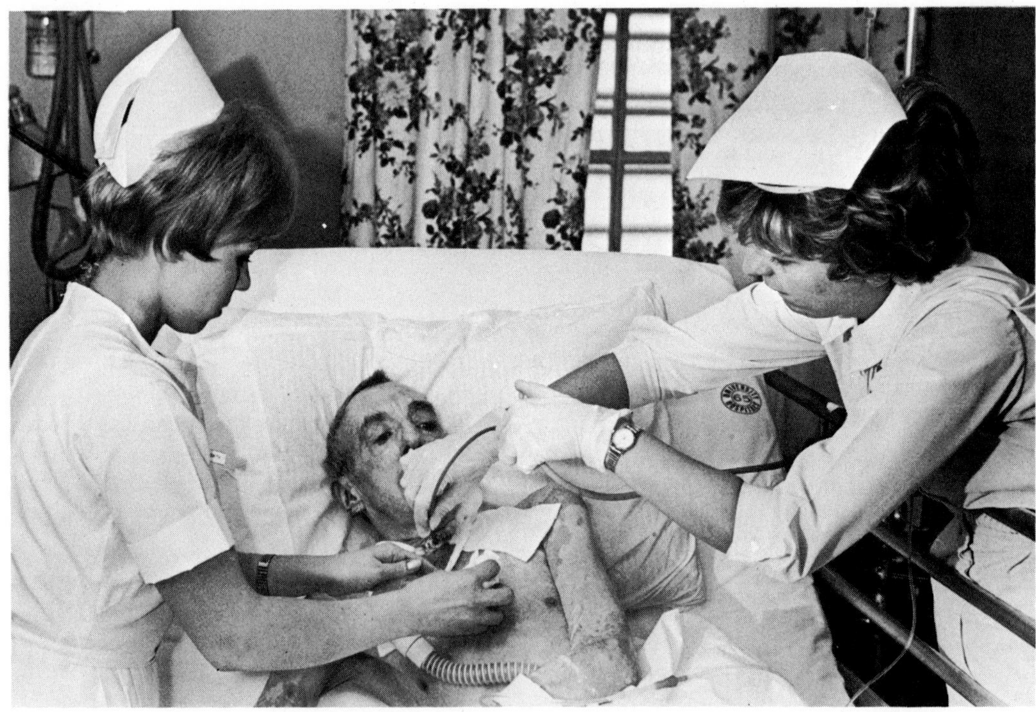

Fig. 45-6. Nurse is wearing sterile gloves and using Y tube attachment to suction patient's tracheostomy tube. (Courtesy Medical-World News.)

is suctioned, a no. 8 or 10 catheter is used for children, and a no. 14 or 16 for adults.

3. A sterile catheter is used each time the tube is suctioned.

4. Before suctioning, the patient is usually given a few breaths of oxygen to assure that hypoxia will be minimized during suctioning. Unless contraindicated, 100% oxygen is used for this preoxygenation.

5. A fenestrated catheter with a whistle tip is attached to the suction machine. If a nonfenestrated catheter is used, it is connected to the suction machine with a Y tube. The catheter is always inserted without suction. Once the catheter is in place, suction is applied by placing the thumb over the fenestration in the catheter or over the open end of the Y tube (Fig. 45-6).

6. The suction catheter is lubricated with normal saline solution and inserted deep enough into the bronchus to stimulate coughing. Unless otherwise ordered, the recommended depth through the tracheostomy tube is 20 to 30 cm (8 to 12 inches) as this permits removal of secretions lying beyond the tip of the cannula (Fig. 45-7). If the patient coughs, the catheter is removed because its presence obstructs the trachea and the patient must exert extra pressure to cough around it. As coughing occurs, the nurse or the patient should have tissues ready to receive mucus, which may be ejected with force. When the patient coughs, the tracheostomy tube is held in place, since it could come out with vigorous coughing.

7. If mucus is tenacious and difficult to remove, sterile saline solution may be instilled into the tube just prior to suctioning. From 5 to 15 ml is commonly ordered.

8. To aspirate the right bronchus, the patient's head is turned to the left and the chest is tilted to the right. This procedure is reversed to suction the left bronchus (Fig. 45-7). The catheter is always rotated 360° as it is withdrawn, with suction on.

9. To prevent hypoxia, the patient must *not* be suctioned longer than 10 to 15 seconds at a time, should rest 3 minutes between aspirations, and 100% oxygen should be administered. If secretions are interfering with breathing, suctioning may have to be more frequent.

10. The inner cannula of a silver tube is removed for cleaning every 2 to 8 hours, depending on the amount and consistency of secretions. If mucus collects and partially obstructs the lumen, it may be necessary to clean the inner cannula even more often than every 2 hours. Sterile water, detergent solution, pipe cleaners, and a small test-tube brush are used for cleaning. Hot water is not used because it coagulates mucus. The tube may be soaked in a solution of half-strength hydrogen peroxide to soften congealed secretions. The tube is inspected to see that all mucus has been removed. Gauze can be threaded through it to extract excess secretions and solution. Before reinserting the inner tube, the outer tube is suctioned.

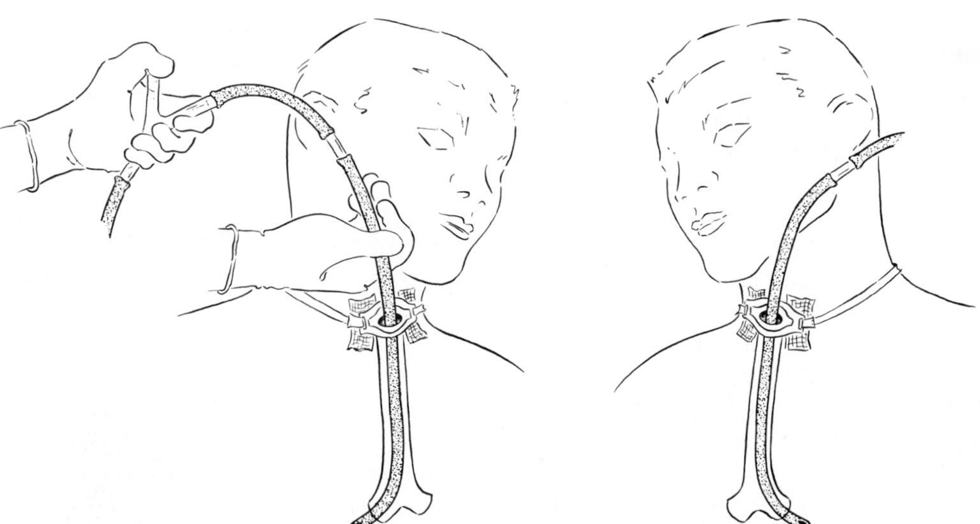

Fig. 45-7. Suction catheter is guided into either mainstem bronchus by turning patient's head away from side to be suctioned. Note that Y tube is being used to apply suction after catheter is in place.

Air humidification. Because the insertion of the endotracheal or tracheostomy tube creates a bypass of the upper airway, the patient's ability to humidify and warm inspired air is lost. Therefore whether the patient is on or off the respirator, the inspired air should be heated and humidified to prevent mucosal irritation and drying of secretions. *Large-bore* tubing is needed to provide this mist, as water particles will condense in *small-bore* tubing. A noticeable difference in the viscosity of secretions is evident in patients who do not receive mist for even as short a period as 30 minutes. Other important nursing care measures and observations vary with the route of intubation—via the larynx or from below the larynx. The patient who has an endotracheal tube in place usually has an increased volume of oropharyngeal secretions because of irritation from the tube. The patient also has great difficulty in swallowing (especially if an oral tube is used), necessitating frequent oropharyngeal suctioning.

Nourishment. The patient with an endotracheal tube is allowed nothing by mouth. Nourishment will be given intravenously or by nasogastric tube feedings. The patient with a tracheostomy tube in place is usually able to swallow and have a normal oral intake. Some experts prefer that the cuff on the tracheostomy tube be inflated while the patient is eating to prevent aspiration. Others believe that the inflated cuff bulges into the esophagus and makes swallowing more difficult, and they therefore prefer the cuff to be deflated. Nursing assessment will determine which technique to use. In determining if the patient aspirates food, it is often helpful to feed the patient red gelatin. The consistency of gelatin makes it easier to swallow than water, and the red color makes it easy to detect if aspirated into the lower airway.

Complications. Both a tracheostomy tube and an endotracheal tube have a direct effect on the airway, but the potential damage of an endotracheal tube is more extensive than that of the tracheostomy tube. Movement with rubbing of the endotracheal tube may produce laryngeal erosion and damage to the vocal cords. There is also the danger of laryngeal edema when the tube is removed. The nurse must be alert to signs of laryngeal stridor and upper airway obstruction. Mist given by mask or tent immediately after extubation helps to prevent this complication. If upper airway obstruction occurs, reintubation or tracheostomy is necessary. With both endotracheal and tracheostomy tubes, tracheal stenosis may result from irritation and scarring at the cuff site. Conscientious nursing care can often prevent this complication.

An additional consideration after the removal of a tracheostomy tube is assisting the patient to cough effectively. When an endotracheal tube is removed, the normal airway is restored and the patient is usually able to cough without difficulty. However, when a tracheostomy tube is removed, there is an air leak at the incision site. This air leak prevents the buildup of intrathoracic pressures high enough to produce an effective cough until the incision is healed. The patient can be taught to place two or three fingers firmly over the dressing that covers the tracheostomy site to reduce the air leak. If this is not successful in helping to generate a cough that clears the airway, the stoma can be suctioned. Frequent use of the stoma for suctioning, however, can delay closure and healing of the tracheostomy incision.

Persons discharged with a tracheostomy. Persons to be discharged with a tube in place are taught to care for and change the tube while in the hospital. A mirror will be necessary to do this procedure, which may be begun a few days after surgery (Fig. 45-4).

Patients who go home with the tracheostomy tube still in place must be provided with necessary supplies or with instructions as to where to secure them and with knowledge of how to care for themselves. They should have suction equipment. Suction machines can be rented for home use or obtained in many communities through the local chapter of the American Cancer Society. Suction can be provided by attaching a suction hose to a water faucet. Many hardware stores carry the necessary equipment. The amount of suction is controlled by the stream of water.

Persons who have a permanent tracheostomy must take some special precautions. They must not go swimming and must be careful while bathing or taking a shower that water is not aspirated through the opening into the lungs. They are advised to wear a scarf or a shirt with a closed collar that covers the opening, yet is of porous material. This material substitutes for some functions normally assumed by nasal passages, such as the warming of air and the screening out of dust and other irritating substances.

□ Maintaining adequate aeration of the alveoli

The individual with pulmonary disease may have impaired ability to aerate alveoli. This impairment may be related to an inability to move adequate amounts of air, or may be caused by an interference in alveolar expansion secondary to accumulation of secretions and alveolar collapse (atelectasis), or may be caused by a restriction to lung expansion by the presence of air (pneumothorax) or fluid (pleural effusion) in the pleural space.

The person with pulmonary disease may have very slight or severe difficulty in breathing (dyspnea). There may be obstruction of the free passage of air through the bronchi, or damage to lung tissue itself, or both may be present. If so, more effort is required for breathing, and the person is very conscious of breathing. This is tiring and unpleasant. With increased difficulty in breathing, most persons become apprehensive and even panicky. A nurse who understands this can be a great comfort to the patient. The presence of another person often helps to control fear and eases breathing efforts. The person with chronic obstructive pulmonary disease has often discovered ways to minimize these breathing difficulties. The nurse needs to assess the person's wishes about position, exercise, and so on, and should utilize these in planning nursing care.

Position

The most comfortable position for more relaxed breathing is a semiupright or upright sitting position. In these positions the lungs and respiratory muscles are not cramped and thus are not working against resistance. A pillow placed lengthwise at the patient's back provides support and keeps the thorax thrust slightly forward, allowing freer use of the diaphragm, and increases the ability to breathe deeply. For those persons who must be upright to breathe, the overbed table with a pillow on top can be used as a support and a resting place for the head and arms (Fig. 45-8). If the patient has marked breathing difficulty and is not sufficiently alert or is alert and fearful, side rails can provide additional security. They also may be used to assist patients to pull themselves up into a higher sitting position. At home, some persons may prefer to sit up in a large chair that supports them well and to lean on a smaller chair placed in front of them. This chair should be blocked to prevent it from slipping.

Since the diaphragm becomes flattened and less active in persons with chronically overinflated lungs secondary to an increase in residual volume, some patients find breathing is helped by wearing an elasticized abdominal support. The support is often made of material similar to that used in elasticized girdles. Men may need to be persuaded to wear this kind of support but, on trial, learn how much the support adds to the comfort and accept it quite readily. Pressure from the girdle must be from below the umbilicus upward so that the flattened diaphragm is forced up into the thorax.

Environment

Proper ventilation, humidity, and temperature of the room will help the patient to breathe more easily. Irritants such as tobacco smoke from cigarettes, cigars, and pipes should be excluded. Patients may have preferences as to room temperature and amount of fresh air, and the nurse assesses and responds to those preferences. In general, most patients breathe more easily if the air is cool and not too humid. An air-conditioned room may make breathing easier.

Persons with nose, throat, and bronchial irritation may benefit from warm, moist air produced by a *humidifier* or *vaporizer*. A vaporizer can be used to humidify the air throughout the room, or it can be placed close so

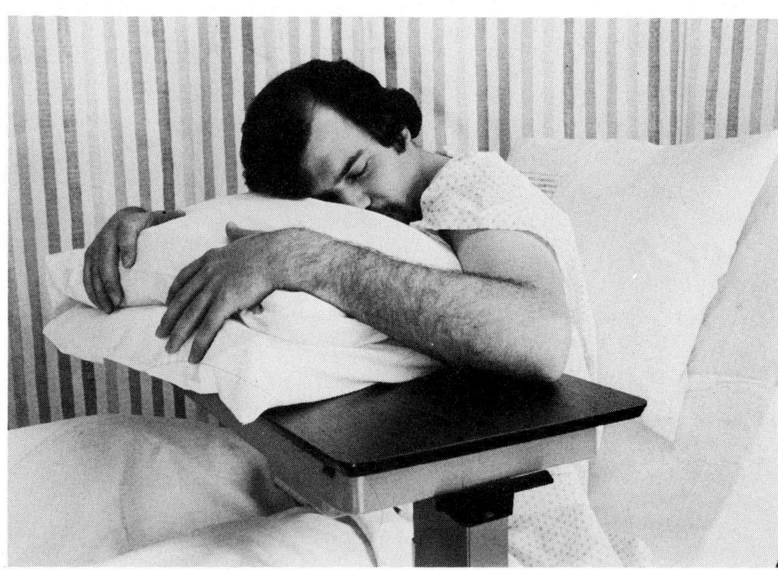

Fig. 45-8. Pillows placed on overbed table provide comfortable support for patient who must sleep in sitting position.

that steam is inhaled as it is released. The large electrically operated vaporizers used in hospitals serve to moisten the air in the entire room. Water flowing from a gallon-sized jar is heated to form steam that is then directed out through a long, flexible spout. Inhalation of plain steam or of an aromatic medication such as tincture of benzoin or menthol is often ordered.

Small electric vaporizers can be purchased at most local drugstores. However, when the person cannot afford to purchase one, the nurse can assist in improvising equipment for inhalation and for proper humidity. An empty coffee can or a shallow pie tin can be filled with water and placed on an electric plate in the person's room to increase humidity. If the inhalation is to be directed, an ordinary steam kettle or a kettle with a longer improvised paper spout may be used. The paper should be changed frequently. A few drops of menthol or oil of eucalyptus can be put into the water. Benzoin will cause corrosion in the kettle, which is exceedingly difficult to remove. The kettle and electric plate should be placed a safe distance from the face so that the medicated steam can be breathed freely, and yet the person will not be burned by accidentally tipping the kettle or by touching the hot plate. After the 25- to 30-minute treatment, equipment should be removed from the bedside.

Continued uncorrected difficulty in breathing may result in carbon dioxide being accumulated in the blood. This is the result of inadequate exchange of oxygen and carbon dioxide and is termed *carbon dioxide narcosis.* It causes flushing of the skin and a slow, deep respiratory pattern. The nurse notifies the physician at once if this occurs. (See p. 1135 for a discussion of the use of low-flow oxygen and the danger of oxygen administration in the person with chronic obstructive lung disease.)

Breathing exercises

The person who has difficulty in breathing may be taught how to increase the efficiency of his breathing pattern. Breathing exercises are usually a part of pulmonary physiotherapy, which may also include segmental postural drainage, clapping, and vibrating. Although pulmonary physiotherapy activities may be performed by a

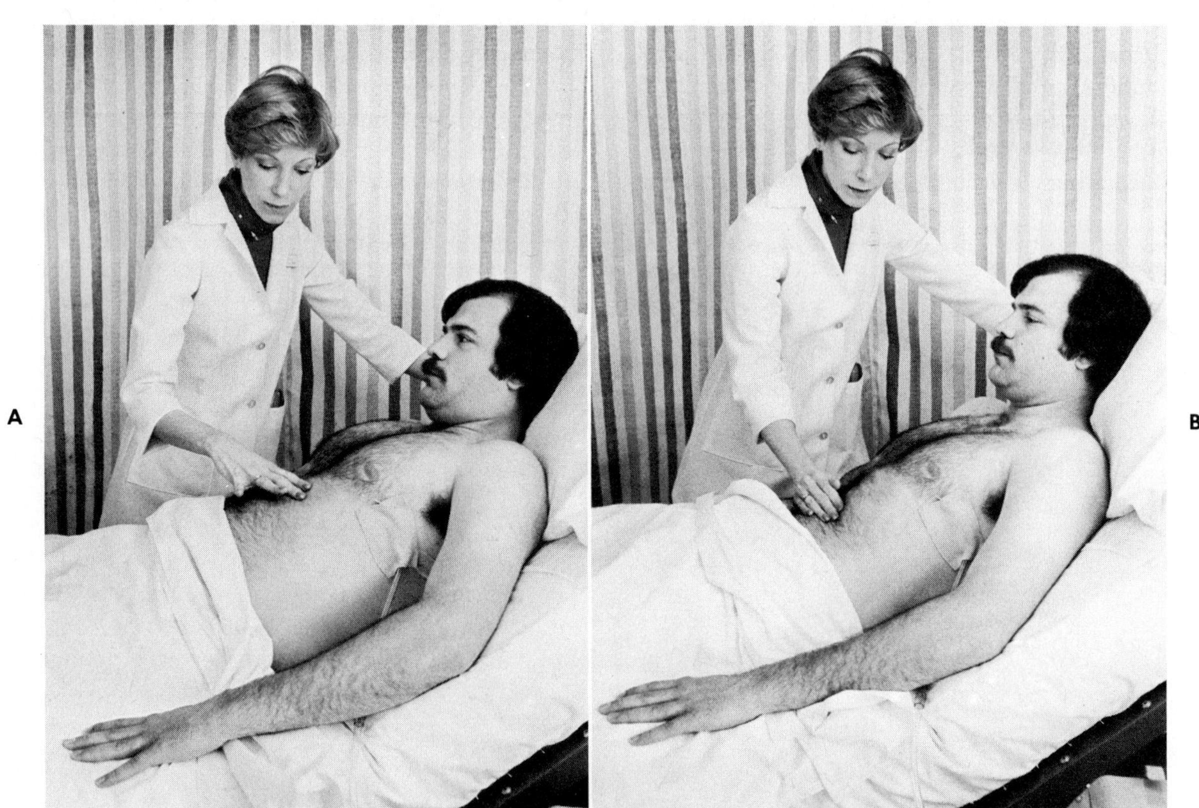

Fig. 45-9. A, Physical therapist assists patient in learning augmented abdominal breathing. Patient is instructed to breathe in through nose, using abdominal muscles and concentrating on moving lower ribs under therapist's hand. This exercise improves ventilation of bases of lungs. **B,** Therapist places hand on upper abdomen in assisting patient to exhale fully.

physical therapist, they are often part of a nurse's responsibility. Regardless of where the primary responsibility lies, nurses must be familiar with the techniques so that they can demonstrate and reinforce them and be sure that the individual is doing them correctly. Also, the need for pulmonary physiotherapy may occur at a time when the physical therapist is not available to the patient.

Persons who have a restriction to chest expansion, such as those who have had thoracic surgery, and patients with chronic obstructive lung disease (COPD) are taught to use an augmented abdominal breathing (diaphragmatic pattern). In teaching, exhalation is stressed rather than inspiration. The person is taught to exhale slowly and fully through *pursed lips* while contracting the abdominal muscles. Manual pressure on the upper abdomen during expiration facilitates this maneuver (Fig. 45-9). On inhalation through the nose, the abdominal muscles are relaxed. This technique will slow the respiratory rate, encourage deep breathing, and facilitate expiration. This "controlled" breathing pattern is to be used while performing various activities of daily living—from sitting, standing, walking, and climbing stairs to more complex activities. As this pattern becomes natural, it will be used automatically during periods of increased shortness of breath. Persons who do not know how to use controlled breathing tend to increase their respiratory rate and their work of breathing when they are short of breath. As a result, physiologic obstruction increases, oxygen requirements increase, and effective ventilation decreases. Changing a person's respiratory pattern requires a great deal of effort by both the individual and those providing care.

This same method of teaching augmented abdominal (diaphragmatic) breathing can be used to teach the patient to cough. The difference is that expiration is forced down to residual volume. This maneuver often stimulates the cough reflex. If it does not, the person is taught to actively cough at the end of full expiration. Physiologically, forced expiration simulates the effects of a cough and is therefore more effective than telling the patient to take a deep breath and then cough.

Respiratory assistive devices

A variety of devices may be used to help the patient to breathe more easily and more effectively and to assist in raising secretions. These devices may be directed at either improving the inspiratory or the expiratory phase of respiration.

Blow-bottles. The most commonly used expiratory device is a set of blow-bottles. Blow-bottles consist of two bottles half-filled with water and connected by tubing. The person is instructed to move the water from one bottle to another by blowing into a short tube in the first bottle, thus increasing the pressure in the bottle and displacing the water with air. In doing so the person creates an increase in alveolar pressure through prolonged expiration against resistance; this is believed to aid in reexpanding collapsed alveoli thus preventing atelectasis.

Initially many persons cannot move the entire contents of one bottle into the other with one breath, especially if they have had recent chest surgery. They can be encouraged to work toward increasing the amount of fluid moved with each use. If the person understands the reason for the use of blow-bottles, the therapy will be carried out more faithfully and will be treated more seriously.

Use of blow-bottles increases intrathoracic pressure, creating pressure on the vena cava similar to that of the Valsalva maneuver. Pulse rate will increase when the pressure is relieved with the surge of blood return to the heart. Blow-bottles should therefore be used cautiously by persons with any signs of cardiac failure.

IPPB. Intermittent positive pressure breathing (IPPB) is the most commonly used method for improving the inspiratory phase of ventilation. The IPPB machine delivers air or oxygen under pressure until a preset pressure limit is reached. It is cycled and controlled by the patient's own respiratory rate. Positive pressure breathing improves the inspiratory phase of ventilation and enhances the flow of air to the alveoli, since much of the work of breathing is done by the machine rather than the patient. However, this relief from the work of breathing lasts only the length of the treatment—usually 15 to 20 minutes three or four times a day. Also, the use of IPPB has become a controversial issue in recent years. Studies have shown that IPPB as a means for promoting increased alveolar ventilation, delivering aerosols, and removing secretions is no more, and possibly less, effective than other methods in patients who are able to deep breathe effectively by their own effort.[7,87] In those who are unable to do this, however, IPPB continues to be a useful method of treatment.[7,87]

When used for intermittent treatments, IPPB is usually ordered at 15 to 20 cm water pressure for 15 minutes three to four times a day. In acute situations, treatment may be ordered every hour. Many persons are at first unable to tolerate this high level of pressure. Initial treatments therefore may be begun at a lower pressure, for example 5 cm of water, which is then gradually increased to the most effective level as the person learns to use the machine correctly.

During use of the IPPB the patient is taught to maintain a slow respiratory rate using a diaphragmatic respiratory pattern. It is important that expiration be prolonged, with the latter part of exhalation being active. Every several breaths the patient should deep breathe

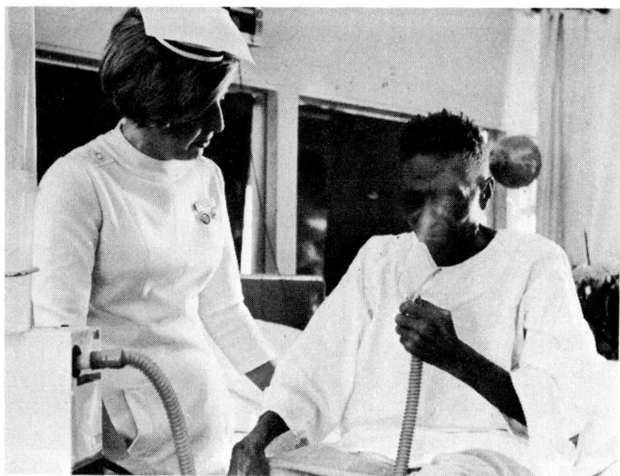

Fig. 45-10. Nurse specialist instructs patient in use of ultrasonic mist therapy. (Courtesy University Hospitals of Cleveland, Cleveland, Ohio.)

Table 45-2. Side effects of mist therapy

Cause	Effect
↑ H_2O content of inspired air	↑ Volume of secretions Shortness of breath Feeling of suffocation Bronchospasm
Tight-fitting mask, mist, or tent with ultrasonic nebulizer	Feeling of suffocation
Heavily misted tent	Feeling of isolation

and exhale as fully as possible. Correct positioning, with the patient sitting upright unless contraindicated, is necessary to achieve the most beneficial effects. In addition, if clearance of secretions is an objective, the person must be taught to cough effectively and should do this several times during the treatment and at the end.

Precautions to be taken when using IPPB equipment include those to protect the patient from cross contamination. Medication or water left in the tubing or nebulizer serves as a medium for bacterial growth, particularly of *Pseudomonas.* Use of individual tubing, nebulizer, and mask or mouthpiece as well as proper cleaning techniques and filters are recommended to prevent such cross contamination. Other possible complications of IPPB are dizziness resulting from hyperventilation, which lowers P_{CO_2} levels; toxic reactions to prescribed medications; gastric distention; exacerbation of hemoptysis; and ruptured alveoli. IPPB administered sooner than approximately 1 hour following meals may cause nausea and vomiting.

Mist therapy. Inhalation therapy also includes mist therapy. There are various ways to administer mist. A small particle size is preferred because large particles of mist are filtered out in the upper airway and never reach the lower airway where secretions collect. If an extremely small particle size is desired (one that can reach the smaller airways and alveoli), ultrasonic mist is used (Fig. 45-10). Nebulizers that are heated can produce a gas flow with a higher water vapor content than can those that are cold. Mist therapy is administered by mask, tent, or IPPB units. Individuals vary in their ability to tolerate therapy and in the amount or type of mist necessary to produce therapeutic effects. The high water content of air often makes persons who are already short of breath and anxious feel that they are suffocating. This is especially common with a tight-fitting mask or when a mist tent with an ultrasonic nebulizer is used. In a heavily misted tent the person is unable to see out and therefore feels cut off from those in the environment. Claustrophobia is another common complaint.

Ultrasonic mist temporarily increases the volume of secretions because of the added volume of water. The patient may therefore complain of increased shortness of breath until the secretions are expectorated. It may also induce bronchospasm; therefore treatment may be preceded by inhalation of a bronchodilating agent and the volume of mist carefully adjusted to avoid this complication.

The nurse must closely observe both the physiologic and psychologic response so as to assure optimal therapeutic effects of the treatment without worsening the patient's condition. The patient is encouraged to cough during and after the treatment. Because mist therapy is so effective in liquefying secretions, it is helpful before postural drainage. Controversy exists as to whether mist should precede or follow IPPB when both treatments are being used. Some experts believe that IPPB facilitates removal of secretions and therefore should be used after mist therapy has loosened secretions; other experts believe that IPPB given before mist will help to establish effective breathing patterns so that moisture will better penetrate the respiratory tract and, particularly if bronchodilators are being used, afford a degree of bronchodilation that will increase the effectiveness of the mist therapy and prevent bronchospasm. The side effects of mist therapy are outlined in Table 45-2.

Some of the bronchodilators and mucolytic agents are administered in aerosol form via nebulizers. Several types of nebulizers may be used. Some medications come in commercial metered-dose hand nebulizers, or the medication may be diluted with water or saline solution and administered via a hand bulb nebulizer. Another method is to connect a nebulizer by rubber tubing to a source of compressed gas (air or oxygen). Midway in the rubber tubing connection a Y tube is inserted. The air is turned on after the medication is placed in the nebulizer. Usually 4 to 6 liters of gas per minute are sufficient. The nurse should test the amount of spray briefly by placing a finger over the open end of the Y tube. If fine spray cannot be seen, the equipment is not working properly. With all methods the person needs to be taught how to self-administer prescribed medications. Following are steps to be followed in teaching a person to use a hand nebulizer:

1. Exhale fully
2. Position nebulizer in mouth *without* sealing lips around it
3. Take a deep breath through the mouth while squeezing the bulb of the nebulizer *once*
4. Hold breath for 3 to 4 seconds at full inspiration
5. Exhale slowly through pursed lips
6. Usually one inhalation is sufficient
7. Several inhalations of a bronchodilator may cause medication overdosage and result in side effects (tachycardia, palpitation, nervousness)

Mechanical ventilation. If, despite the use of the techniques and devices mentioned, the patient is still unable to ventilate well enough to maintain desired levels of oxygen and carbon dioxide in his blood, mechanical ventilation by a respirator is indicated. This requires the use of a cuffed endotracheal or tracheostomy tube.

Many different kinds of respirators are available. In general, there are two kinds, pressure cycled and volume cycled. The Bird and Bennett (PR series) are pressure-limited ventilators while the Möerch, Emerson, Engstrom, Air Shields, Bennett MA-1, and Ohio 560 are volume-limited machines. Both types of machines can be used intermittently or continuously to assist or to control respiration.

When a *pressure-cycled* ventilator is used, the machine is set to deliver a predetermined amount of pressure (usually 15 to 25 cm of water) with each breath. When this pressure is reached, the machine turns off and normal exhalation begins. The volume of gas delivered to the patient is not necessarily constant because it depends on the resistance of the entire system, including the patient's lungs. For this reason the expired tidal volume must be monitored frequently and adjustments made in the respirator controls as needed.

With a *volume-controlled* machine a constant volume of air is delivered with each breath. The volume is preset and is delivered to the patient at whatever pressure is necessary to attain that volume. A volume-cycled machine should have a pressure cutoff valve. Such a mechanism allows a pressure limit to be set. If the pressure required to deliver the set volume exceeds the pressure limit, the machine will turn off before the entire volume is delivered. The pressure limit on a volume-cycled machine usually has an audible alarm. The nurse can set the limit slightly above (approximately 5 cm of water) the pressure required to ventilate the patient. The alarm will then go off if the patient coughs, accumulates secretion, or starts to resist the machine.

Regardless of which type ventilator is used, mechanisms for various regulations are necessary if the machine is to be adjusted to each patient. It is preferable to have a respirator that can be used to assist or control the patient's breathing. "Assist" means that the patient's own inspiratory effort trips (turns on) the machine. Most respirators have a *sensitivity control knob* that can be adjusted to respond to weak inspiratory efforts. "Control" implies the use of automatic cycling. The patient may be apneic and the machine set at the desired rate; the patient's own respiratory rate may be too slow and the automatic cycling can be used to force an increase in the rate; or the patient's own respiratory efforts can be ignored and an automatic rate used to ventilate the patient. (Some machines with automatic cycling do not allow for the latter adjustment.) It is also helpful to be able to regulate the flow rates at which the gas is delivered to the patient. For example, patients breathing at rapid rates and high volumes need faster flow rates than those breathing slowly and at moderate volumes. A final necessity is the ability to regulate the inspired concentration of oxygen from 20% (room air) to 100%.

All respirators used for mechanical ventilation must

1. Provide for the heating and humidification of inspired air
2. Provide a means for measurement of expired volumes
3. Be dependable for long periods of use
4. Be easily cleaned

Any patient on continuous mechanical ventilation should be "sighed" (given a deep breath) several times an hour. Some respirators automatically "sigh" the patient, while with others the patient is "sighed" manually using a self-inflating (Ambu) or anesthesia bag. This periodic deep breathing is necessary to prevent alveolar collapse and resultant atelectasis.

A negative-pressure respirator such as the tank respirator (iron lung) may also be available. This type of respirator is usually used for patients with neuromuscular problems without intrinsic lung disease. The tank respirator creates subatmospheric pressure around the chest. Since there is atmospheric pressure at the mouth and nose, air enters the lungs. This type of ventilator does not require tracheal intubation and is usually not used in patients with increased airway resistance.

Weaning from the ventilator. The nurse plays an important role in weaning the patient from the ventilator. Both physiologic studies (blood gases, tidal volume) and clinical status determine the patient's readiness to breathe without mechanical assistance. Prior to weaning, the person should have been taught breathing exercises. Removal from the respirator is very frightening to most patients. Ideally a nurse with whom the patient has developed rapport is present when the respirator is removed. It is also helpful if the environment around the patient is calm. Much of the success of weaning is dependent on the interrelationship between the person's physiologic and psychologic responses. Those who become very anxious and take rapid, shallow breaths often will not tolerate being off the respirator. If a pattern of controlled breathing can be maintained, success is much more likely. Weaning is usually begun with short periods off the respirator. The amount of time off the respirator is increased according to the patient's tolerance. The nurse must carefully assess the adequacy of ventilation while the patient is off the respirator. If, in the nurse's judgment, the patient cannot tolerate breathing on his own because of inadequate tidal volume, cyanosis, tachycardia, diaphoresis, or restlessness, mechanical assistance should be reinstituted.

Throughout the treatment of the patient in respiratory failure, ventilation should be carefully monitored by blood gas studies and simple spirometry (tidal volume, vital capacity). Alert nursing observation of the patient can determine the adequacy of ventilation. Meticulous attention is given to maintaining a patent airway, which is the prime nursing responsibility. (See specialized material for further details.[66,71,90])

Removal of secretions

Coughing. Two of the most troublesome symptoms of respiratory disease are the increase in mucous secretions secondary to mucous membrane inflammation or allergic response and the stimulation of coughing caused by irritation of the respiratory tract. If coughing is productive, the person needs to be encouraged to cough effectively in order to keep air passages clear and allow sufficient oxygen to reach the alveoli. Periodic changes in position will help to prevent pooling of secretions in the lungs and will stimulate coughing. The patient is instructed to breathe as deeply as possible to loosen secretions and to stimulate productive coughing. For an effective cough, the patient should take a deep inspiration, force it down to residual volume, contract the diaphragm and intercostal muscles, and exhale forcefully. Any sputum raised should always be expectorated, not swallowed. When a patient cannot cough forcefully enough to raise sputum and when respirations are very shallow or sound very moist, extra fluids or a liquifying agent to thin the secretions may be given. The liquefying agent is often given as a nebulized aerosol so that it reaches deep into the tracheobronchial tree.

Many patients with obvious, noisy respirations caused by accumulated sputum hesitate to cough because coughing causes pain. To assist such a patient the nurse's hands can be placed on the front and back of the chest to give support as the patient coughs (Fig. 45-16). A towel placed around the chest and held snugly as the patient coughs may also be used.

Although coughing is a physiologic protective reflex, constant nonproductive coughing and hacking can lead to exhaustion. Medications therefore are often prescribed for problems related to cough. The type prescribed depends on the nature of the cough and the type of secretions. The purposes of various cough medications are to increase secretions, to decrease secretions, to thin secretions so that they can be raised and expectorated more easily, or to *depress* the cough reflex. Some of these medications are summarized in Table 45-3.

Sedative expectorants increase secretions, protect ir-

Table 45-3. Medications used to treat cough

Desired effect	Medications prescribed
↑ Secretions	Expectorants Ammonium chloride Ammonium carbonate Sodium iodide Potassium iodide (saturated solution; SSKI) Ipecac Terpin hydrate
↓ Secretions	Anticholinergic agents Atropine
Thin secretions	Mucolytic agents Acetylcysteine (Mucomyst) Deoxyribonuclease (Dornavac)
Depress cough reflex	Antitussives Narcotic Codeine Nonnarcotic agents Benzonatate (Tessalon) Noscapine (Nectadon) Dextromethorphan hydrobromide (Romilar Carbetapentane citrate (Toclase) Levopropoxyphene napsylate (Novrad) Chlophedianol hydrochloride (Ulo)

ritated membranes, and lessen the amount of coughing. Increased secretions may result in a productive cough and make paroxysms of coughing less frequent. For this purpose, ammonium chloride in wild cherry or orange syrup is often ordered, and other mixtures such as iodide solutions or ipecac syrup are sometimes used. Aerosolized normal or half-normal saline solution is also effective in thinning secretions. The mucolytic enzyme pancreatic dornase (Dornavac) is useful if the secretions are purulent. Stimulating expectorants such as terpin hydrate diminish secretions and promote repair and healing of the mucous membrane.

When the main objective of treatment is to suppress coughing, drugs depressing the cough center in the medulla are ordered. Codeine is frequently used and may be added to elixir of terpin hydrate, but there is danger of addiction with its prolonged use. Some nonnarcotic drugs with actions similar to codeine have been prescribed widely. Among them are dextromethorphan (Romilar) and noscapine (Nectadon).

When respiratory difficulty is severe, secretions are present, coughing is unproductive, and intratracheal suctioning and occasionally bronchoscopy are necessary. By means of bronchoscopy, mucus plugs may be loosened or removed and intratracheal suctioning made more effective. Equipment for emergency bronchoscopy may be kept in the patient's room. When this procedure is ordered, the nurse must see that electrical outlets are adequate and that the necessary equipment is assembled in one place and ready for immediate use. (See p. 938 for care of the patient during bronchoscopy.)

Postural drainage. *Segmental postural drainage* with clapping and vibration is a technique used to combine the force of gravity with the natural ciliary activity of the small bronchial airways to move secretions upward toward the main bronchi and the trachea. From this point the patient can cough them up, or they can be suctioned. In the treatment of chronic obstructive pulmonary disease, drainage of all segments is usually accomplished by placing patients in various postural drainage positions (Fig. 45-11). Treatment may also be directed at draining specific areas of the lung. While the patient is in each position, *clapping* with a cupped hand is done over the area being drained. This maneuver

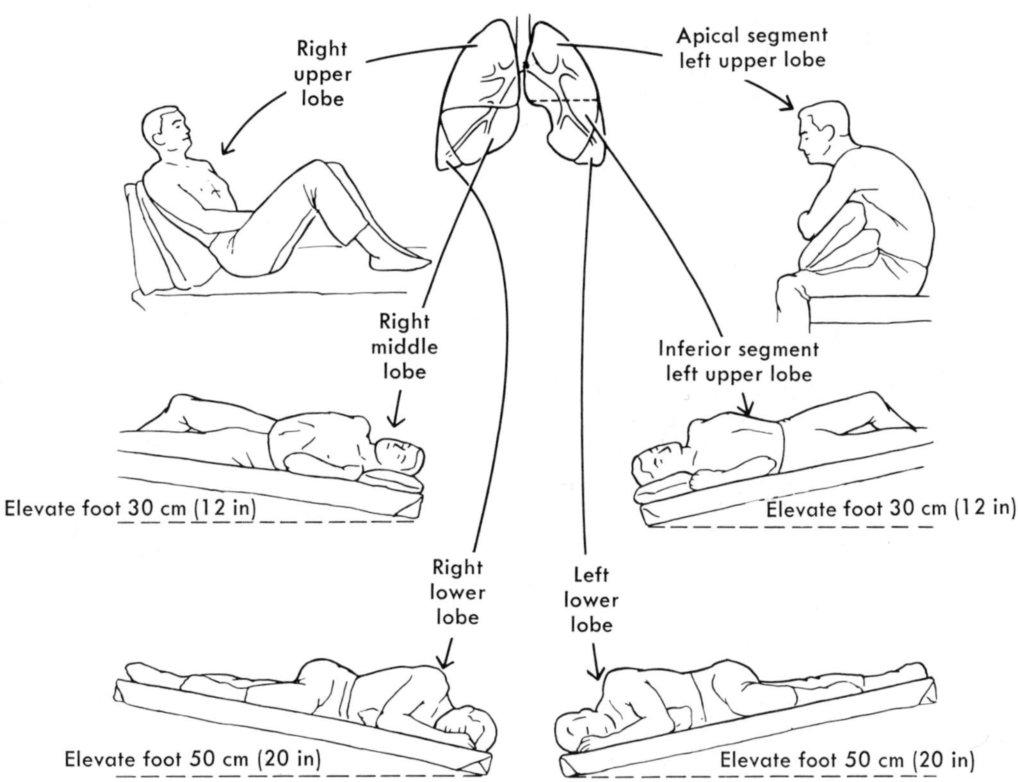

Fig. 45-11. Postural drainage requires that patient assume various positions to facilitate flow of secretions from various portions of lung into bronchi, trachea, and throat so that they can be raised and expectorated more easily. Drawing shows correct positions to drain various portions of lung.

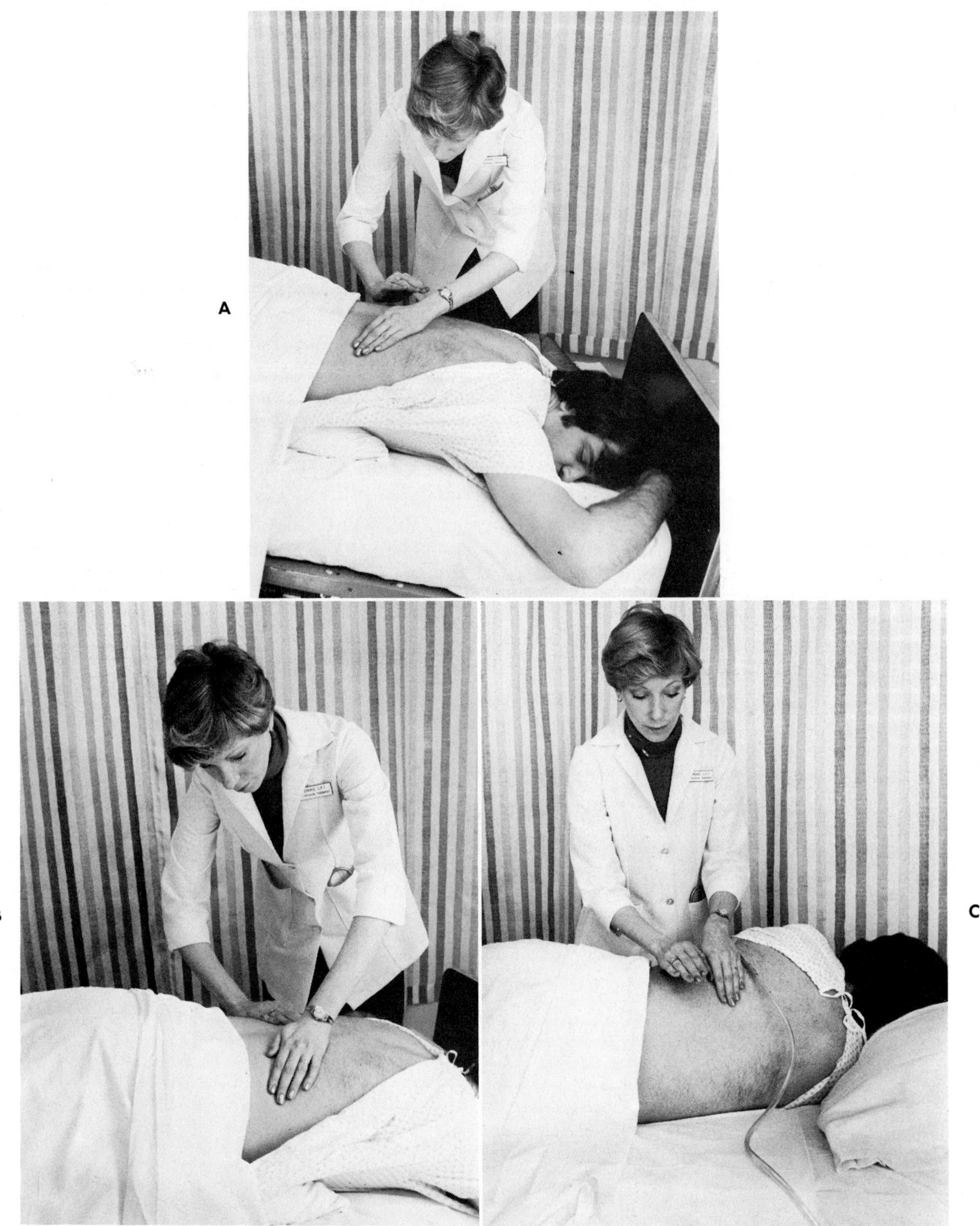

Fig. 45-12. A, Patient is in supine position with head down at 15° angle for postural drainage of lower lobes. Note cupped position of therapist's hands as she claps patient. Patient's gown is pulled aside for purposes of illustration; ordinarily clapping is never done on bare skin. **B,** Therapist follows clapping with vibrating, applying pressure during expiration. **C,** Even when patient cannot tolerate head-down position, such as after thoracic surgery, patient can still receive chest physiotherapy in modified positions.

helps to loosen secretions and stimulate coughing (Fig. 45-12, *A*). After clapping of the area for approximately 1 minute, the patient is instructed to breathe deeply. *Vibrating* (pressure applied with a vibrating movement of the hand on the chest) is performed during the expiratory phase of the deep breath (Fig. 45-12, *B*). This assists the patient to exhale more fully. The procedure is repeated as necessary. When the patient cannot tolerate a head-down position, a modified position is used (Fig. 45-12, *C*).

Positions that provide gravity drainage of the lungs can be achieved in several ways, and the procedure selected usually depends on the age and general condition of the person as well as the lobe or lobes of the lungs where secretions have accumulated. A young person usually can tolerate greater lowering of the head than an elderly person whose vascular system adapts less quickly to change of position. A severely debilitated patient may only be able to tolerate slight changes in position.

Postural drainage achieved merely by putting blocks under the casters at the foot of the bed sometimes produces excellent results. The foot of the bed may also be supported on the seat of a firm chair to provide a position in which the head is lowered. Tilt boards (special tables that can be raised or lowered to any angle) or Stryker frames are sometimes used, but many physicians prefer raising the foot of the bed, since this entails much less exertion on the part of the patient.

The nurse needs to know the part of the lung affected and how to position the patient to drain that portion of the lung (Fig. 45-11). For example, if the right middle lobe of the lung is affected, drainage will be accomplished best by way of the right middle bronchus. The patient should lie supine with the body turned at approximately a 45° angle. The angle can be maintained by pillow supports placed under the right side from the shoulders to the hips. The foot of the bed is raised about 30 cm (12 inches). This position can be maintained fairly comfortably by most patients for half an hour at a time. On the other hand, if the lower posterior area of the lung is affected, the foot of the bed can be raised 45 to 50 cm (18 to 20 inches) with the patient assuming a prone position for drainage. A summary of the positions for segmental postural drainage is given in Table 45-4.

Postural drainage and percussion should be planned so as to achieve maximum benefit. The best time is generally in the morning soon after arising and at night prior to retiring. Frequency of treatments will depend on each

Table 45-4. Positions for segmental postural drainage, clapping, and vibrating

Area of lung	Position of patient	Area to be clapped or vibrated
Upper lobe		
Apical bronchus	Semi-Fowler's position, leaning to right, then left, then forward	Over area of shoulder blades with fingers extending over clavicles
Posterior bronchus	Upright at 45° angle, rolled forward against a pillow at 45° on left and then right side	Over shoulder blade on each side
Anterior bronchus	Supine with pillow under knees	Over anterior chest just below clavicles
Middle lobe (lateral and medial bronchus)	Trendelenburg position at 30° angle or with foot of bed elevated 14 to 16 inches, turned slightly to left	Anterior and lateral right chest from axillary fold to midanterior chest
Lingula (superior and inferior bronchus)	Trendelenburg position at 30° angle or with foot of bed elevated 14 to 16 inches, turned slightly to right	Left axillary fold to midanterior chest
Lower lobes		
Apical bronchus	Prone with pillow under hips	Lower third of posterior rib cage on both sides
Medial bronchus	Trendelenburg position at 45° angle or with foot of bed raised 18 to 20 inches, on right side	Lower third on left posterior rib cage
Lateral bronchus	Trendelenburg position at 45° angle or with foot of bed raised 18 to 20 inches, on left side	Lower third of right posterior rib cage
Posterior bronchus	Prone Trendelenburg position at 45° angle with pillow under hips	Lower third of posterior rib cage on both sides

person's needs, but care should be taken to avoid exhaustion, which will result in shallow ventilation and negates the positive effects of the treatment.

Patients having postural drainage of any kind are encouraged to breathe deeply and to cough forcefully to help dislodge thick sputum and exudate that is pooled in distended bronchioles, particularly after inactivity. Humidity, bronchodilators, or liquefying agents often are given 15 to 20 minutes before postural drainage is started, since they facilitate the removal of secretions. The patient may find that sputum can best be raised on resuming an upright position even though no drainage appeared while lying down with the head and chest lowered.

Since some patients complain of dizziness when assuming positions for postural drainage, the nurse stays with the patient during the first few times and reports any persistent dizziness or unusual discomfort to the physician. Postural drainage may be contraindicated in some persons because of heart disease, hypertension, increased intracranial pressure, extreme dyspnea, or age. However, most people can be taught to assume the positions for postural drainage and can proceed without help after being supervised once or twice.

Chest percussion (clapping) is contraindicated in the case of pulmonary emboli, hemorrhage, exacerbation of bronchospasms, severe pain, and over areas of resectable carcinoma. Often patients with a chronic pulmonary problem need to be taught to do postural drainage independently so that they can continue at home. The position usually is maintained for 10 minutes at first, and the period of time is gradually lengthened to 15 to 20 or even 30 minutes as the patient becomes accustomed to the position. At first, elderly persons usually are able to tolerate these positions only for a few minutes. They need more assistance than most other patients during the procedure and immediately thereafter. They should be assisted to a normal position in bed and requested to lie flat for a few minutes before sitting up or getting out of bed. This helps to prevent dizziness and reduces the danger of accidents.

The patient may feel nauseated because of the odor and taste of sputum. Therefore the procedure should be timed so that it comes at least 1 hour before meals. A short rest period following the treatment often improves the appetite. The patient needs mouth care following postural drainage. Aromatic mouthwashes should be available for frequent use by any patient who is expectorating sputum freely.

Care of sputum. Since the causative organisms may not be known early in the respiratory disease, the nurse should use caution in the disposal of sputum and should instruct the patient how to protect others. Patients who are coughing or clearing their throat forcefully should be instructed to cover their mouth and nose with several thicknesses of disposable tissues to prevent possible spread of infectious organisms. Used tissue should be crumpled and placed in a paper bag or flushed directly down the toilet. If a bag is used, it is closed securely and preferably burned. Used tissues should be collected from the bedfast patient at frequent intervals, and whoever handles the bags should wash his or her hands thoroughly to avoid transfer of infection to others.

Patients who have a copious amount of sputum are instructed in the use of a sputum container.

When patients cannot care for and dispose of their own sputum, assistance must be provided. Tissues may be placed in the patient's hand, and a paper bag may be placed on each side of the bed so that the patient does not have to turn to dispose of the soiled tissues. The bedfast patient should be offered soap and water for handwashing before meals.

Suctioning

Nasotracheal suctioning. If the patient is unable to clear secretions effectively by coughing, suctioning of the tracheobronchial tree may be necessary to maintain a patent airway and achieve adequate oxygenation. Suctioning is uncomfortable and is used only when the patient is too tired or weak to raise secretions through coughing. The procedure is carried out as follows:

1. The patient is prepared for suctioning by a thorough explanation of what is to be done. If coughing is painful, as with the postthoracotomy patient, for example, analgesic medication is administered 30 minutes prior to the procedure. Suctioning is not done immediately before or after meals.
2. Proper positioning of the patient will assist with suctioning. The patient should be in a sitting position, with the head of the bed elevated. A pillow under the shoulders will help hyperextend the neck, which facilitates entry of the catheter into the trachea. It may also be helpful to elevate each shoulder in turn, while having the patient turn the head to the opposite side in an attempt to direct the catheter first into the right and then into left mainstem bronchi.
3. Nasotracheal suctioning is a *sterile procedure;* each piece of equipment, catheter, glove, water, lubricant, basin, is used only once. A suction source that is capable of creating a vacuum of −80 cm H_2O is necessary. For adults, a size 14 French catheter, 35 cm (14 inches) in length, is usually used. A water-soluble lubricant should be applied to the outside of the catheter. The sequence of steps of the procedure is as follows:
   a. Preoxygenate the patient with a few breaths of

a high concentration of oxygen (80% to 100%) from an anesthesia or Ambu bag. This helps prevent hypoxia during suctioning.

b. Insert the lubricated catheter, without applying suction, through the nares. When the catheter reaches the posterior pharynx (a distance of about 10 to 12.5 cm [4 to 5 inches]), the patient is asked to cough in order to facilitate entry into the trachea. If the tongue is obstructing passage of the catheter, have the patient stick his tongue out while coughing or have another person pull the tongue forward.

c. Continue to insert the catheter until meeting resistance. At this point suction is applied intermittently while removing the catheter, rotating the catheter 360° at the same time.

d. Administer oxygen as in *a* above.

Endotracheal suctioning. The procedure for suctioning a patient who has an endotracheal or tracheostomy tube is described on p. 947. The principles underlying the procedure are the same; it is much easier in the patient who has an endotracheal tube, however, since the pathway to the trachea is assured. Because the patient who has an endotracheal tube cannot clear this artificial airway by coughing, suctioning is performed routinely and the frequency of suctioning depends on the amount of secretions.

Maintaining intrathoracic pressure

As described earlier, the lungs are surrounded by the pleura. Under normal conditions a negative pressure exists within the pleural space. This vacuum keeps the lung adherent to the chest wall so that as the thorax expands with inspiration the lung also expands. If the intactness of the pleural membranes is disrupted, as by penetrating trauma to the chest wall, by thoracic surgery, or by an open communication with alveoli (as with a ruptured emphysematous bleb), air (positive pressure) enters the pleural space and the negative pressure is lost. The lung then collapses. The presence of excessive

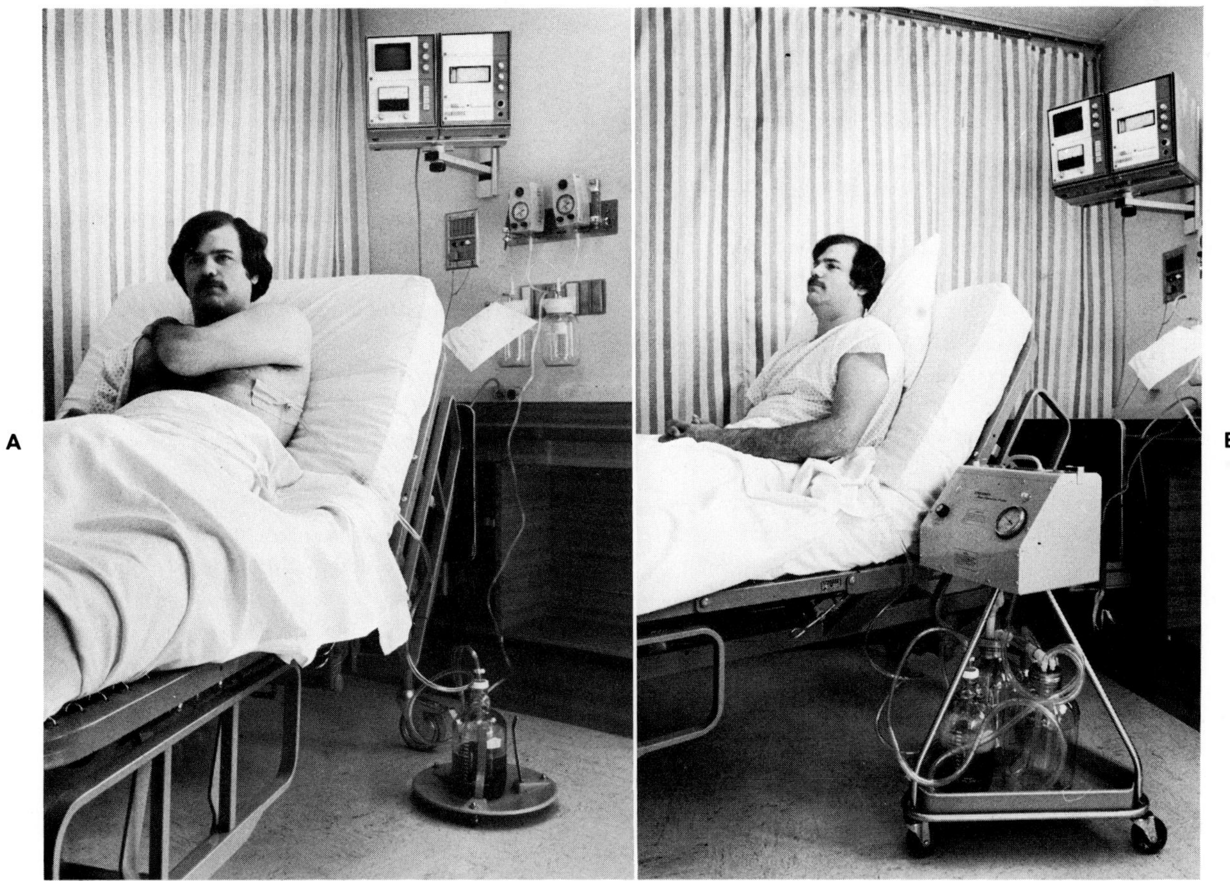

Fig. 45-13. Chest tube with water-seal suction. **A,** Wall outlet provides source of suction; note holder used to secure bottle in upright position. **B,** Emerson suction machine as source of vacuum.

fluid (pleural effusion) or blood (hemothorax) in the pleural space will also restrict lung expansion. The degree of compromise depends upon the amount of air or fluid in the pleural space and the extent of lung collapse. Correction of the condition and reexpansion of the lung is accomplished by the insertion of a chest tube connected to water-seal drainage.

The chest tube may be connected to a water-seal bottle alone or may have additional suction applied (Fig. 45-13, *A*). With a water-seal system the chest tube is connected to tubing that extends below the level of water in a bottle. A second tube in the bottle, above the water level, opens to the air. In this system, as the patient inspires and expands his lung, air and fluid in the pleural space is forced out through the chest tube. As he exhales, the pressure of the water on the tube in the bottle prevents air from reentering the pleural space, and the lung gradually reexpands.

If there is a large leak in the pleural space or if more rapid reexpansion of the lung is desired, suction may be applied to the end of the short tube that is above the water level. If an exact amount of suction is to be used, an additional bottle that functions as a "breaker" can be added (see p. 971 for an explanation of this system).

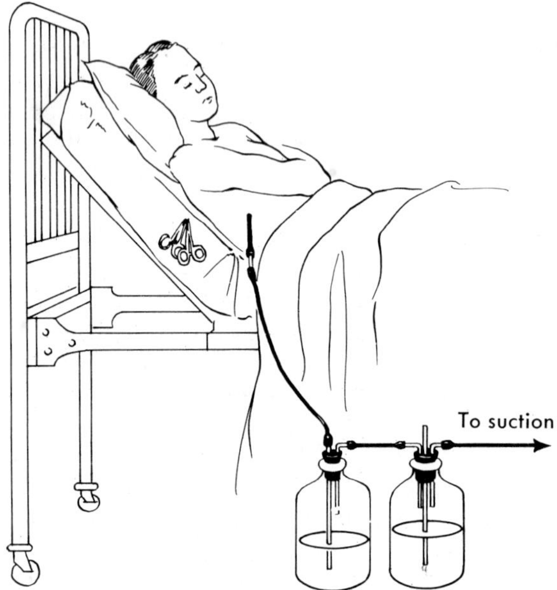

Fig. 45-14. Chest catheter in place. Chest catheter is attached to closed drainage system. Note that glass tube in drainage bottle connected to tubing of chest catheter is below level of water. Bottle to right of drainage bottle is "breaker bottle" and regulates amount of suction transmitted to drainage bottle, chest catheter, and pleural cavity. Two hemostats attached to bed are available should bottle break or water-seal system be otherwise interrupted.

Regardless of whether suction is to be applied to the water-seal drainage system, several precautions are necessary. The first of these relates to the proper setup of the system itself.

Initiating chest tube drainage. When initiating chest tube drainage, a 2 liter clear glass bottle is usually used, although other commercial devices, such as the Pleuravac system, are available. Approximately 300 ml of sterile water, or enough to fill the bottle 1 to 2 cm from the bottom, is then added. The tubing is fastened to the bed so that there are no dependent loops between the bottles and the bed (Fig. 45-14). The tip of the tube should be kept from 1 to 2 cm under water so that if the bottle accidentally tips over, the tube will remain under water. The water level in the bottle is marked by placing an adhesive strip at the water line. The date and hour are written on the tape, which gaves a ready indication as to the amount of drainage. If considerable drainage accumulates in the bottle, this will increase the amount of subatmospheric (negative) pressure in the system, and it will be more difficult for the patient to expel air and fluid through it. In this instance the glass rod may be pulled up so less of it is under water or the surgeon may order that the drainage bottle be changed. In this case a sterile setup is prepared. When the bottle with sterile water and tubing are ready, the chest tube is clamped as close to the patient's chest as possible. The chest tube is then disconnected from the drainage tubing, the new setup is connected, and the chest tube is unclamped. The drainage should be measured and may be sent to the laboratory for examination.

As the patient breathes, there will be movement of fluid in the glass tube that is under water. This is known as fluctuation or oscillation, and the column will move up when the patient inhales or coughs, and it will fall when the patient is exhaling. The tubes should be checked for fluctuation frequently, and they should be "milked" or "stripped" every hour to prevent formation of clots that could plug the tubes. If the column of water is not fluctuating, the nurse should be sure that the patient is not lying on the tubes or that they are not blocked by a clot. Asking the patient to cough or to change position often restores visible fluctuation. If fluctuation still does not occur, this should be reported.

Two hemostats should be kept at the bedside at all times (Fig. 45-14). These are to be used to clamp the tube if the water-seal bottle is accidentally broken. For this reason the patient and all personnel should know what to do if a bottle is broken. When a bottle is broken, the chest catheter should be clamped and then reconnected to a sterile setup as soon as possible. Sterile water should be used in the bottle. As soon as the system is reconnected with the tip of the tube under water, the clamp should be removed. Except in case of emergency such as broken bottle, most physicians prefer that tubes not be clamped, and a specific order is written if clamping is desired. The reason for this is that when the tubes are clamped, air (positive pressure) may leak from the pleural surface and further collapse the lung. Therefore if the patient is being transported from one place to another, such as to the radiology department, tubes should not be clamped unless it is for a very few minutes. In general, water-seal bottles are changed only when broken or on specific order of the physician. If the nurse is expected to change the bottles routinely, the procedure outlined at the beginning of this section should be employed using strict asepsis.

Water-seal bottles should never be lifted above the level of the patient's chest, since this would allow the water in the bottle to be pulled into the pleural space. The bottle should be placed on the floor so that they will not be broken by a lowered side rail. When Hi-Lo bed is being used, care must be taken not to lower the bed onto the bottles.

Ambulation. There is no contraindication to ambulating with a chest tube in place. As long as the water-seal bottle remains below the level of the chest, the patient may assume any position of comfort in bed, or may be out of bed in a chair.

Removal of the chest tube. Chest tubes are removed when there is no fluctuation of fluid in the tubing and when roentgenograms confirm the full reexpansion of the lung. The patient should be medicated for pain 30 minutes prior to removal of the tube. Physicians vary in the exact procedure used to remove the tube, but generally a sterile scissors, 4×4-inch gauze squares, and adhesive tape are required. The suture holding the tube in place is cut, the patient is asked to exhale deeply, and the tube is removed. If a purse-string suture was used, it is retied and a dry sterile dressing is placed over the site. Some physicians cover the site with a Telfa dressing or a layer of petrolatum gauze to ensure an airtight dressing. The dressing is covered securely by three strips of 2-inch adhesive tape.

Fluid and electrolyte management

Persons with respiratory disease often have a tenuous fluid balance. The older person, whose respiratory disease may be complicated by the existence of congestive heart failure or cor pulmonale, may be on diuretic therapy in order to avoid overloading of the vascular system. The person with chronic lung disease often has inadequate food and fluid intake because of anorexia and fatigue.

Accurate assessment of fluid balance, as indicated by daily weights, is of utmost importance. Excessive fluid administration may lead to pulmonary edema in a patient whose cardiopulmonary system is already compromised. Dehydration, on the other hand, will result in thick, tenacious secretions. The best liquefying agent is water, and it is preferable to adequately hydrate the patient rather than attempt to loosen secretions by administering mist therapy. Providing the patient does not have cardiovascular disease requiring fluid restriction, a fluid intake of 3 to 4 liters per day should be provided.

□ Promoting adequate oxygenation of tissues

In order to provide sufficient oxygen for tissue metabolism, the previously mentioned two needs—a patent airway and aeration of alveoli—must be accomplished first. While interventions are directed at achieving these, it may be necessary to provide supplemental oxygen therapy before the underlying disease condition is corrected. It is also necessary to provide for adequate transportation of oxygen to the cells and to decrease the demand for oxygen.

Maintaining transportation of oxygen

In order to transport oxygen to the cells there must be (1) an adequate heart pump and (2) a vascular system capable of maintaining the blood pressure necessary to perfuse distant tissues. When blood pressure falls (hypotension), there is inadequate oxygenation of vital organs and of skeletal muscles. The sequelae of hypotension can be manifested in many ways (p. 215). Anginal pain may occur, since the coronary vessels that normally extract almost the maximum amount of oxygen from the blood cannot significantly increase oxygen uptake to meet their needs. Changes in sensorium and behavior become evident with hypotension secondary to cerebral anoxia. Most importantly, all the effects of hypotension will be exacerbated when hypoxemia is also present.

Hypotension must be corrected either by removing the underlying cause or by administering vasopressor agents if adequate oxygen transport is to be achieved. Failure to maintain adequate oxygenation of tissues can result in respiratory or cardiac arrest, and cardiopulmonary resuscitation must be instituted.

Cardiopulmonary resuscitation

The American Heart Association estimates that 52% of all deaths in the United States are caused by cardiovascular disease. Many of these deaths are the result of cardiac arrest. Cardiac arrest requires immediate intervention and is potentially reversible if resuscitation is begun within 3 to 6 minutes of cessation of circulation.

Clinical picture. The person who has suffered a cardiac arrest appears clinically dead. Unresponsiveness, cessation of respirations, development of pallor and cyanosis, absence of heart sounds, absence of blood pressure, loss of palpable pulse, and dilation of pupils are present. Pupillary response may be misleading, however, if the person is receiving medications such as atropine or has pathology involving the cornea or lens of the eye. If a hospitalized patient is being monitored by means of a cardiac monitor or ECG machine, the pattern of ventricular fibrillation (p. 1001) or, less commonly, ventricular asystole (p. 1003) will appear. Frequently seizure activity is present at the onset of cardiac arrest.

Unresponsiveness, loss of pulse, and cessation of respirations are the main criteria for determining that a cardiac arrest has occurred. Unresponsiveness is assessed by shaking the shoulders and calling the person's name. A carotid or femoral artery is palpated to determine loss of pulse. The carotid artery usually can be found more quickly; this is accomplished by placing the index and second fingers of one hand on the "Adam's apple" and then moving these fingers to one side. The carotid pulse can then be felt next to the trachea.

Cessation of respirations is determined in several steps. First, if no head or neck injuries are present, the person's airway should be opened by hyperextending the neck (placing one of the rescuer's hands under the neck and the other hand on the person's forehead [head-tilt]). Next, respirations are assessed by looking for movements of the chest wall, listening for the sound of air escaping from the mouth and feeling for the movement of air against the rescuer's cheek. Looking, listening, and feeling for respiration are all equally important, since movement of the chest wall does not mean that the person is breathing.

The purpose of performing cardiopulmonary resuscitation (CPR) is to provide oxygenated blood to the brain and other vital organs. The nurse can determine effectiveness of CPR by noting return of color, spontaneous movement, and pulses in the carotid or femoral artery. Other indicators that CPR is effective are occasional respirations, constriction of pupils, and return of normal heart rhythm (when patient is monitored).

Intervention. Any person who has received special preparation in CPR may save a life by taking immediate action. If nothing is done for the person until the physician arrives, it may be too late to save the person's life, or extensive brain damage may have occurred. Skill in cardiopulmonary resuscitation is now an accepted part of nursing, and all nursing personnel should be properly prepared.

Many hospitals have a prepared team of personnel, including physicians, nurses, anesthesiologists, and technicians who can be called on to give immediate and complete care when cardiac arrest occurs. Most hospital units are equipped with a cardiac arrest tray or have access to a specially equipped cart on which all necessary items are available. Equipment needed includes an electrocardiograph, a defibrillator, an airway and Ambu bag or other breathing bag, a laryngoscope, a variety of endotracheal tubes, a venous cutdown set, fluids for intravenous use, a suction machine, oxygen, and a tracheotomy set. The medications usually given are epinephrine (1:1,000) for direct intracardiac injection, sodium bicarbonate (44 mEq) to combat acidosis, and calcium chloride (10% solution) to improve myocardial tone.

The nurse keeps the immediate area clear of persons not directly involved in the resuscitation effort. Usually two nurses working together can keep medications ready and assist in the observation of blood pressure and femoral pulse as well as direct others to obtain any additional equipment required.

External cardiac massage. External cardiac massage is the rhythmic compression of the heart between the lower half of the sternum and the thoracic vertebral column. As pressure is applied, blood is forced out into the systemic and pulmonary circulation. With relaxation, the heart fills with venous blood. The rescuer either kneels or stands to one side of the patient and applies pressure with the heel of the hand to avoid pressing on a large area of the chest wall and to minimize rib damage (Fig. 45-15). The rate of compression and relaxation is usually 60 to 80 times per minute. The patient's body should be supported by a firm mattress or board (floor when necessary) to provide proper resistance when pressure is being applied to the sternum. While cardiac massage is being done, mouth-to-mouth breathing must also be maintained in order to oxygenate the blood being pumped through the circulatory system.

Mouth-to-mouth breathing. Mouth-to-mouth breathing is performed by hyperextending the individual's neck, making a seal over the victim's mouth with the rescuer's mouth while pinching the nostrils shut, and then blowing into the person's mouth. Exhalation is accomplished by letting the person exhale naturally. It is important for the rescuer to breathe between giving artificial respirations. When performing resuscitation by oneself, the victim is given two breaths after every 15 compressions of the chest. If there are two rescuers, one breath is interposed *between every fifth and sixth* compressions.

The most common complication of external cardiac massage is fracture of the ribs. If medications are injected into the heart, signs of pneumothorax or pericardial tamponade should be watched for carefully. Signs include labored respirations, paradoxical pulse (an exaggerated drop in blood pressure with inspiration), muffling of heart sounds, loss of breath sounds, pneumothorax, and drop in blood pressure. Other possible complications are hepatic hematoma or rupture and fracture of the sternum.

Open cardiac massage. In this seldom used method of cardiac massage the chest cavity is surgically incised

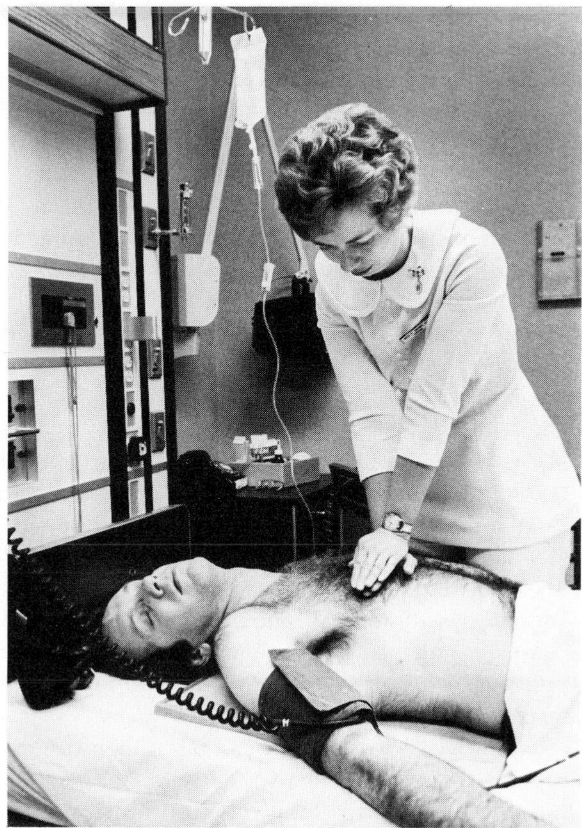

Fig. 45-15. Registered nurse performing external cardiac massage. Note position of hands on lower half of sternum with fingers extended away from ribs. Elbows should be straight and shoulders directly above patient's sternum. Cardiac board is under patient's chest.

directly over the heart, the ribs are spread apart, and the heart is massaged with the hands or stimulated with an electric current. A 100-volt alternating current with an amperage of 1.5 is used. An electrically operated defibrillator and pacemaker may be used; the defibrillator stops the irregular heartbeat, and the pacemaker then restarts heart action. Occasionally a patient is saved by the use of open cardiac massage, but it must be employed within 3 minutes after the cessation of cardiac function.[42]

Providing rest

Rest is frequently prescribed as a regimen for persons who have some impairment of tissue oxygenation. The cause may be a respiratory problem interfering with oxygen reaching the blood, a cardiac problem interfering with oxygen being pumped to the tissues, or a red blood cell (hemoglobin) deficiency interfering with the oxygen carrying capacity of the blood. Any excess demand on the body for oxygen, resulting from increased need by the muscles during increased activity, places a severe burden on the already compromised lungs or heart. Dyspnea or hyperventilation may occur as the person attempts to increase oxygen intake, and the pulse rate increases as the heart works harder to send more oxygen to the muscles. Fatigue occurs as products of anaerobic metabolism build up in the muscles. The person with impairment of tissue oxygenation may require periods of decreased activity at regular intervals in order to provide decreased cellular demand for oxygen.

Physical rest implies a state of minimal functional and metabolic activities. The term "rest," however, is interpreted by people in different ways and may vary from complete immobility to fairly strenuous activity that achieves a sense of peace and relaxation after the activity is completed. If rest is prescribed as a regimen for the person with impairment of tissue oxygenation, the extent of permissible activities must be clarified by health personnel and the patient.

The person with severe cardiac impairment may be placed on "absolute" bed rest to decrease the cardiac work load. In this situation the person is bathed, shaved, and assisted in most activities. Self-feeding may or may not be permitted. Many persons react to this routine with tension, anxiety, and resentment, and explanations of the basis of the therapy should be given. The person needs to be encouraged to ventilate feelings of frustration about the imposed restrictions. Since anxiety increases pulse rate and muscle activity, some degree of self-activity may be permitted.

"Armchair care" may be prescribed for some persons with severe cardiac impairment. The rationale behind this treatment is that the work load on the heart is lessened by an upright or semiupright position in a comfortable chair. A larger blood volume tends to "pool" in the pulmonary vessels when the person is in a recumbent position, and it is believed that this position may increase strain on the heart that may be relieved by permitting more blood to flow into the lower extremities, as when the person sits up.

The provision of armchair care does not imply that rest is less important or that activity is permitted. Since getting out of bed has been found to be an activity that requires a large expenditure of energy under normal circumstances, the person receiving armchair care is lifted out of bed into the chair. When in the chair, the person must be protected from chilling and is observed closely for changes in vital signs that would indicate increased cardiac work load. Sometimes a low footstool is used to elevate the feet slightly, and some persons are more secure and comfortable with a light restraint, such as a loose drawsheet, across the front of the chair to give them security when they relax and sleep.

Physical rest is difficult to achieve if the person is

restless or anxious. Persons having respiratory problems or who know they have an acute cardiac disease may be extremely apprehensive. Explanations about what is occurring, and a calm, confident manner on the part of the nurse, help to decrease the anxiety. Close family members or other significant persons are usually permitted to visit the acutely ill hospitalized person, but other visitors should be restricted. Family members and significant others should be kept informed about the person's condition and therapy to decrease their anxiety and gain their cooperation. Calmness on their part will contribute to the patient's rest. Members of the family should be encouraged not to worry the person, but mention of daily problems should *not* be avoided, since the person may suspect that information is being withheld, and the worry will interfere with achieving rest.

Adequate rest is important in combating respiratory disease. During respiratory illness, however, normal sleep may be interrupted for a number of reasons. The patient may be plagued with frequent coughing, and breathing may be difficult. Airways may become blocked with secretions, and the patient may be awakened by shortness of breath.

The nurse should be alert for signs of what irritates the patient, precipitates cough, and therefore prevents rest. For example, excessive talking, smoking, or laughing or sitting in a draft or in a dry, overheated room may predispose to coughing. Cough medications given before the hour of sleep and when rest is disturbed by coughing are often helpful. However, when noisy breathing occurs and it is obvious that secretions are present in the respiratory tract, the person should be encouraged to cough deeply and to expectorate until the airway is free of obstruction before cough medication is given. A suitable position in bed and changes in position also help the patient to rest more quietly. Room temperature and ventilation should be kept at the level most comfortable for the patient.

As the person's condition improves and a greater number of activites are permitted, the person needs to guard against overexertion as evidenced by dyspnea, fatigue, or chest pain. Periods of more strenuous activity should be interspersed with periods of decreased physical activity. The amount of rest required will depend on the severity of the underlying problem and the extent of presenting symptoms.

Providing proper environmental temperature and humidity

Considerations related to environmental temperature are relevant in the care of the person with a cardiac or respiratory problem in two ways. First, the vasoconstriction that is associated with breathing cold air further compromises oxygen delivery to tissues. Second, cold air contains less moisture than warm air. Consequently, in addition to using calories to heat the inspired air, moisture is taken from the tracheobronchial tree. The nurse needs to be alert to environmental temperature and humidity and its physiologic effects on the patients. Patients in air-conditioned rooms may require closer monitoring. Prior to discharge, precautions related to being out on a cold day without adequate covering over the face should be discussed with the patient. Many persons with chronic heart and lung problems wear some type of face mask when they must be out in cold weather.

Providing adequate nutrition

The person with hypoxia often experiences anorexia, nausea and vomiting from decreased gastrointestinal motility, fluid and electrolyte imbalances, dyspnea, or fatigue. The odor and taste in the mouth caused by frequent raising of sputum may seriously affect appetite and may impair nutrition. Provision should be made for oral hygiene before meals—washing of hands is encouraged, and sputum containers should be removed before meals are served.

Frequently persons with breathing difficulties tolerate regular-sized meals poorly, and smaller and more frequent feedings provide for better nutrition. Gas-forming foods should be avoided. Large meals increase cardiac work load to provide increased blood flow to the stomach and increase dyspnea; therefore small frequent meals are more desirable for persons with cardiac disease. For the person with respiratory problems who does not have a fluid restriction, taking adequate amounts of fluids helps to liquefy the secretions so that they may be coughed up more easily.

If generalized edema is present due to inadequate pumping by the heart, sodium may be restricted in the diet (p. 1006). Following is a list of the types of foods to be avoided on restricted sodium diets:

1. *No-added-salt diet* (2 to 3 g sodium). Avoid salting food at table, highly salted foods such as potato chips, luncheon meats, pickled foods, and seasoning such as catsup and mustard.
2. *Moderate low-sodium diet* (1 g sodium). Avoid (in addition to above) milk and cheese; canned fruits, vegetables, or soups; products containing baking powder or baking soda; commercial salad dressings; carbonated beverages; and antacids

Persons may need help in planning diets to meet prescribed sodium restrictions. Special foods need not be prepared for the person on a restricted sodium diet. The simplest method is to cook the food for the entire family without salt, set aside the one portion, then season the remainder.

Promoting adequate venous return

Decreased venous return occurs when (1) the heart pumps ineffectively as in cardiac failure (p. 1003), (2) the veins are diseased as in varicose veins (p. 1035), or (3) the veins are partially obstructed as in thrombophlebitis (p. 1033). Decreased venous blood flow can interfere with tissue oxygenation by the formation of peripheral edema interfering with diffusion of oxygen from the capillary to the cells. The cells are pushed away from the capillaries as the intracellular spaces become filled with fluid, resulting in a greater distance for the oxygen to travel to reach the cells.

There are a number of activities that can lead to venous stasis and should therefore be avoided. Pressure on the popliteal area from sitting or from crossing the legs can obstruct venous return from the lower leg. All persons should avoid wearing tight constricting bands on the legs such as tight sock tops or garters. Sitting for long periods of time with the legs in a dependent position, such as on long airplane trips, causes increased venous pressure and subsequent edema from increased hydrostatic pressure. Isometric exercises can utilize the muscle pumps to aid in venous return. Persons who are at high risk for decreased venous return should elevate the legs when sitting to decrease the hydrostatic pressure. These persons should also wear elastic stockings if they will be standing for long periods to time. Isometric exercises can also be carried out while standing to increase venous return.

Exercise. Correction of the underlying pathology is the primary therapy for promotion of adequate venous return. Exercise is also of primary importance. Blood return to the heart can be promoted through muscle activity of the legs, either by ambulation or by leg exercises in the bedfast or sedentary person. When the leg muscles contract, pressure is exerted on the veins, forcing the blood forward. The blood does not flow backward when the pressure is relieved because of the valves present in the veins.

Elastic bandages and stockings. Another method of encouraging venous blood flow is by the application of elastic bandages (Ace) or elastic stockings (TED). The elastic wraps apply pressure, forcing the bloodflow from the superficial veins into the deeper veins for return to the heart. Counterpressure also increases pressure outside the capillaries to counteract the increased fluid pressure occurring with venous stasis, thus decreasing edema formation.

Elastic stockings are easier to apply and produce more even pressure on the veins than do the elastic bandages. Elastic stockings that reach above the knee are often less than effective, as they tend to slip down and bunch up around the knee, which applies excessive pressure that collapses the veins and thus increases rather than decreases venous pressure. If elastic wraps are desired to reach a mid-thigh level, either elastic bandages are used over the entire leg or a below-the-knee stocking is used with an elastic bandage applied at the top of the stocking.

The two most important principles in the application of elastic wraps are that there *must be even pressure* applied and that the leg *must be elevated* during application of the elastic wrap. Uneven pressure may result in (1) excessive pressure on some areas, which occludes the veins, or (2) pushing of edema fluid to areas of lesser pressure, thus causing decreased tissue oxygenation and pain. Elevating the leg decreases hydrostatic pressure and prevents trapping of venous blood in the lower legs and feet. Stockings and bandages should be snug and free of wrinkles. A stocking should not be folded back on itself, as this causes increased pressure. The person's calf is measured according to the manufacturer's directions; the correct-sized stocking is selected for the person in order to apply the desired amount of pressure.

Elastic bandages must be wrapped with an even, moderate amount of stretch. Bandages applied too tightly will occlude veins and cause pain; bandages applied too loosely will slip and not provide the desired effect. The person can often verify the degree of comfort as the bandages are applied. The bandage is wrapped with *even overlapping* in order to apply even pressure. A well-wrapped elastic bandage will have two layers of bandage at any site on the leg. This can be achieved by overlapping each row by one-half the width of the bandage. A poorly wrapped elastic bandage would have one, two, or three layers of bandage along the length of the leg, applying uneven pressure. The toes are checked for warmth and color, indicating adequate tissue oxygenation.

Elastic bandages or stockings that are applied with the goal of promoting venous return are removed at least twice a day, preferably every 8 hours in the hospitalized patient, as they tend to wrinkle or slip down. They are also removed so that the leg may be washed and inspected.

■ MANAGEMENT OF THE PERSON REQUIRING THORACIC SURGERY

Intelligent nursing care of patients undergoing thoracic surgery depends on knowledge of the anatomy and physiology of the chest, of the surgery performed, and of procedures and practices that assist the patient to recover from the operation. When endotracheal anesthesia became possible, surgery of the chest was given a great impetus. Before that time it had not been possible, except in the rarest of circumstances, to operate on the lung without causing collapse of the good lung and death. By means of endotracheal anesthesia, it is possible to keep the good lung expanded and functioning even when it is subjected to atmospheric pressure. Endotracheal anesthesia is used for surgery involving the lungs and for most chest surgery in which the pleural space is entered.

□ Principles of resectional surgery

In order to understand resectional surgery and the purpose of chest tubes and water-seal drainage, it is important to review a few points about the anatomy of the lung. The pleura, which lines the chest wall and covers the lung, is one continuous serous membrane. The portion that covers the lung is the *visceral pleura*, and that covering the inside of the chest wall is the *parietal pleura*. Together they form a *potential space*, which normally contains a few milliliters of serous fluid that lubricates the surfaces and prevents friction rub during respiration. The pressure in the pleural space is subatmospheric (less than 760 mm Hg) and is referred to as being negative. This pressure is usually 756 mm Hg and goes down to about 751 mm Hg prior to inspiration. It is this change in pressure that allows air (atmospheric pressure) to enter and expand the lungs. The pressure within the lung itself *(intrapulmonic)* always remains near 760 (758 to 762) mm Hg.

When the pleura is entered surgically or by trauma to the chest, atmospheric pressure (positive pressure) enters the pleural space and the lung collapses. Thus after resection of the lung (except pneumonectomy) two drainage tubes are inserted into the pleural space and each tube is connected to a water-seal drainage bottle. As long as the tip of the tube in the chest bottle is 1 to 2 cm under water and all connections between it and the patient's chest tube are secure, the system is "sealed" (Fig. 45-14); that is, air and fluid can escape from the pleural space into the drainage bottles and no air (positive pressure) or fluid can reenter.

In all resectional surgery (except pneumonectomy) the remaining portions of the operated lung must overexpand and fill the space that is left by the removal of the resected portion. *Thus the primary purpose of chest tubes and water-seal drainage is to (1) aid in the expansion of the remaining portions of the lung and (2) reestablish negative pressure in the pleural space.* This is accomplished as air and fluid are removed from the pleural space. Nursing actions necessary to maintain the integrity of this system are discussed on p. 961.

□ Operative procedures

Exploratory thoracotomy. An exploratory thoracotomy is an operation done to confirm a suspected diagnosis of lung or chest disease. The usual approach is by a posterolateral parascapular incision through the fourth, fifth, sixth, or seventh intercostal space. Occasionally an anterior approach is used. The ribs are spread to give the best possible exposure of the lung and hemithorax. The pleura is entered and the lung examined, a biopsy usually is taken, and the chest closed. This procedure may also be used to detect bleeding in the chest or other injury following trauma to the chest. Since the pleural space was entered, a chest tube and water-seal drainage are necessary.

Pneumonectomy. A pneumonectomy, the removal of an entire lung, is most commonly done to treat bronchogenic carcinoma (Fig. 50-4). It may also be used to treat tuberculosis, bronchiectasis, or lung abscess. However, a pneumonectomy is only done in those instances when a lobectomy or segmental resection will not remove all the diseased tissue. A thoracotomy incision is made in either the posterior or anterior chest using the method described under exploratory thoracotomy. Before the lung can be removed, the pulmonary artery and vein are ligated and then cut. The mainstem bronchus leading to the lung is clamped, divided, and sutured, usually with black silk. To assure an airtight closure of the bronchus, a pleural flap is placed over it and sutured into place. The phrenic nerve on the operative side is crushed, causing the diaphragm on that side to rise and reduce the size of the remaining space. Because there is no lung left to reexpand, drainage tubes are not used. Ideally the pressure in the closed chest is slightly negative. This pressure is taken postoperatively using a pneumothorax machine, and air can be removed or added to attain the desired pressure. The fluid left in the space will consolidate in time, preventing the remaining lung and heart from shifting toward the operative side (mediastinal shift).

Lobectomy. In a lobectomy one lobe of the lung is removed (Fig. 50-4). It is used to treat bronchiectasis, bronchogenic carcinoma, emphysematous blebs or bullae, lung abscess, benign tumors, fungal infections, and tuberculosis. For a lobectomy to be successful the disease must be confined to one lobe and the remaining lung tissue must be capable of expanding to fill up the space. Two chest tubes are connected to water-seal bottles for postoperative drainage.

Segmental resection (segmentectomy). In a segmental resection one or more segments of the lung are removed. This operation is used in an attempt to preserve as much functioning lung tissue as possible. It is a very taxing operation for the surgeon, since the dissection between segments must be done very carefully and slowly, and the identification of the segmental pulmonary artery and vein and bronchus is more difficult than when a lobe is involved. Since there are ten segments in each lung, only a portion of a lobe may need to be removed. The most common indication for segmentectomy is bronchiectasis. It is also used to treat tuberculosis.

Chest tubes and water-seal drainage are necessary postoperatively. Because of air leaks from the segmental surface, the remaining lung may take longer to reexpand.

Wedge resection. In a wedge resection a well-circumscribed diseased portion is removed without regard to the segmental planes. The area to be removed is clamped, dissected, and sutured. Chest tubes and water-seal drainage are used postoperatively.

Decortication. In a decortication a fibrinous peel is removed from the visceral pleura, allowing the encased lung to reexpand and obliterate the pleural space. This procedure is discussed further under the treatment of empyema (p. 1134). Chest tubes and chest suction are used to facilitate the reexpansion of the lung. If the lung has been encased for a long time, it may be incapable of reexpanding following decortication. In this situation thoracoplasty may be necessary.

Thoracoplasty. A thoracoplasty is an extrapleural procedure involving the removal of ribs. By removing ribs it is possible to reduce the size of the chest cavity. Prior to the widespread use of resectional surgery, thoracoplasty was the basic surgical treatment for tuberculosis. Today thoracoplasty is used (infrequently) primarily to prevent or treat the complications of resectional surgery. When it is felt that a patient's lung may not be able to expand sufficiently after a resection to fill the space, a thoracoplasty is done 2 or 3 weeks prior to the resection. It also may be done prior to pneumonectomy, since this will reduce the chance of mediastinal shift after surgery. This type of thoracoplasty is often called a *preresection* or *tailoring* thoracoplasty; that is, the chest wall is tailored to reduce its size.

If the remaining portions of the lung fail to reexpand sufficiently after resection or if another complication such as empyema occurs, a thoracoplasty is done. In general it is employed when there is a space in the chest that cannot be obliterated by other means. Usually no more than three ribs are removed, and therefore paradoxical motion following thoracoplasty is seldom seen anymore. Paradoxical motion is discussed under chest injuries (p. 1132).

□ Preoperative period

Evaluation. In addition to the screening tests that are run on all preoperative patients, special tests are usually required for persons having chest surgery. These may include chest radiography, including laminography (p. 934), pulmonary function tests, electrocardiography, blood gas studies, bronchospirometry, bronchoscopy, and, in some instances, bronchography. If the patient is scheduled for a pneumonectomy, the evaluation will be even more precise and often includes a cardiac catheterization. Since the tests may be done on an outpatient basis, the office nurse or clinic nurse must be sure that the patient understands what tests are to be performed and the preparation for them. The person's significant others also are kept informed.

Teaching. The operation is discussed with both the patient and family. The preoperative nursing care is similar to that discussed on p. 372. The patient should be told that oxygen usually by mask or nasal prongs is given postoperatively to all patients undergoing thoracic surgery. The patient also needs to know that frequent turning and coughing every 1 to 2 hours postoperatively will be necessary to maintain a clear airway and to aid in the reexpansion of the remaining portions of the lung.

The nurse teaches the patient how to cough prior to surgery. Patients who practice coughing preoperatively usually will cough more effectively postoperatively. Exercises to preserve symmetric body alignment, full range of motion of the shoulder, and maximum pulmonary function are usually started during the preoperative period and continued postoperatively. In some hospitals the physical therapist instructs the patient. The nurse, however, provides follow-up instructions and is responsible for seeing that the patient carries out the instructions properly. Many times the nurse must take the responsibility for teaching the exercises. If so, the nurse should find out which exercises the surgeon believes should be used and, if possible, should obtain assistance from a physical therapist in how best to provide each specific exercise.

If a catheter is to be used for drainage of the chest, the patient can be told that it will be used to drain fluid and air that normally accumulates after a chest operation. The patient should also be told to expect to have pain for some time postoperatively because intercostal nerves are severed, but that medication can be given for this pain and that pain cannot interfere with the need to cough as directed. The patient should also understand that it is all right to ask whether pain medication can be given. The patient should also know that the physician may start an intravenous infusion in a vein in the arm or leg before going to the operating room.

□ Postoperative period

Immediate care. Usually the patient is kept flat in bed until vital signs are stabilized. After vital signs are stable, frequent turning is instituted, with care being taken that the patient is not lying on the tubes so that drainage is occluded. Oxygen is usually administered and continued until the patient has fully reacted from anesthesia.

Vital signs are taken every 15 minutes for 2 hours and then every hour for several hours. It is not unusual for blood pressure to fluctuate during the first 24 to 36 hours, and close monitoring of the patient is essential.

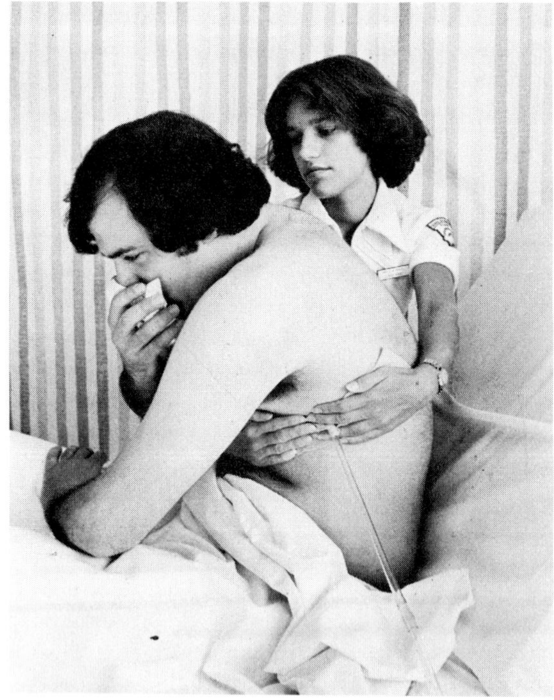

Fig. 45-16. Nurse assists patient to cough by splinting incision with firm support from hands. This lessens muscle pull and pain as patient coughs. Note that nurse stands behind patient while he coughs, and patient uses tissue to cover mouth.

Bleeding on chest dressings is unusual, and should it occur, it should be reported at once.

When fully reacted the patient can usually breathe best in a semi-Fowler's position. Patients are most comfortable if a pillow is placed under the head and neck but not under the shoulder and back. When assisting the patient to and from a sitting position, the nurse should use the arm on the patient's unoperated side. The back of the neck should also be supported. When the patient lies back down, the head and neck are supported until they are on the pillow. The patient should be assisted to cough as soon as conscious. If the blood pressure is stable, the patient is assisted to a sitting position and the incision is supported anteriorly and posteriorly by the nurse's hands. Firm, even pressure over the incision with the open palm of the hands is a most effective method. The nurse's head should be behind the patient when he coughs (Fig. 45-16). The patient is encouraged to breathe deeply and then cough. Sips of fluids, especially warm ones such as tea or coffee, often facilitate coughing. *Coughing keeps the airway patent, prevents atelectasis, and facilitates reexpansion of the lung.* The patient should cough every hour for the first 24 hours and then every 2 to 4 hours. The patient should cough until the chest sounds clear. Otherwise secretions will accumulate in the tracheobronchial tree. If the patient is unable to cough effectively, tracheal suctioning may be necessary. The patient can cough most effectively 20 to 30 minutes after receiving pain medication, and this should be capitalized on by the nursing staff. Mist therapy or IPPB treatment with drugs such as isoproterenol also may be used postoperatively to loosen secretions and to make coughing more effective.

Pain. Morphine or meperidine hydrochloride is usually ordered for pain. Medication for pain should be given as needed and may be required as often as every 3 to 4 hours during the first few postoperative days. The patient is extremely uncomfortable and will not be able to cough or turn unless there is relief from pain. In some instances the dosage of the narcotic is decreased so that it may be given oftener and yet not depress respirations. The tubes in the chest cause pain, and the patient may attempt rapid, shallow breathing to splint the lower chest and avoid motion of the catheters. This impairs ventilation, makes coughing ineffective, and causes secretions to be retained. Thus it is a nursing responsibility to do all that is possible to make the patient comfortable, as this facilitates deep breathing and coughing. If, despite all efforts, the patient's discomfort is interfering with adequate chest excursion, an intercostal nerve block may be performed.

The patient is encouraged to take fluids postoperatively, and to progress to a general diet as soon as it is tolerated. Forcing fluids helps to liquefy secretions and makes them easier to expectorate. Usually fluids by mouth and mist therapy are all that are needed to thin and loosen secretions.

Exercises. Abdominal breathing exercises such as those described on p. 952 are a valuable adjunct to the care of the patient with chest surgery because they improve ventilation without increasing pain and assist him to cough more effectively. The exercises should be taught preoperatively so that the patient has time to practice them before surgery.

Passive arm exercises are usually started the evening of surgery. The purpose in putting the patient's arm through range of motion is to prevent restriction of function. Most patients are reluctant to move the arm on the operative side, but with proper preoperative instruction and postoperative follow-through they do so readily. It is important for both the patient and nurse to understand that the longer the arm is unexercised, the stiffer it will become. The patient should put both arms through active range of motion two or three times a day within a few days. The recommended exercises are similar to those done following mastectomy (p. 1465). The exercises are best done when the patient is upright or when lying on the abdomen. Exercises such as elevating the scapula and clavicle, "hunching the shoulders," bringing the

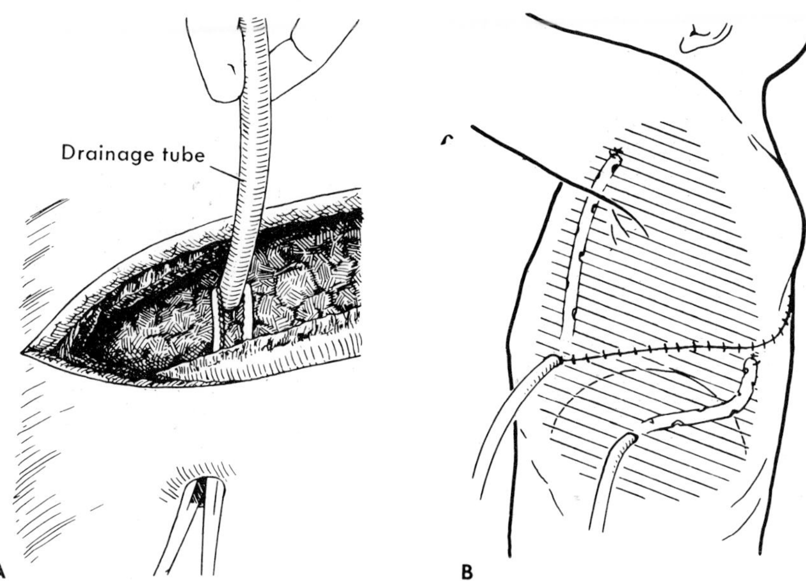

Fig. 45-17. A, Drainage tube being inserted into pleural space. **B,** Note that upper and lower tubes are placed well into pleural space. (From Johnson, J., MacVaugh, H. III, and Waldhausen, J. A.: Surgery of the chest, a handbook of operative surgery, 4th edition. Copyright © 1970 by Year Book Medical Publishers, Inc., Chicago. Used by permission.)

scapulae as close together as possible, and hyperextending the arm can only be done in these positions. Since lying on the abdomen may not be possible at first, these exercises are done when the patient is sitting on the edge of the bed or standing.

Chest tubes. Care of the chest tubes and water-seal drainage system was discussed on p. 961. All patients who have had thoracic surgery, except pneumonectomy patients, will require drainage of the pleural space by chest tube. Usually two tubes are used. One catheter is inserted through the anterior chest wall above the resected area. This is referred to as the *anterior* or *upper tube*. It is used to remove air from the pleural space. The second tube is inserted through the posterior chest and is referred to as the *posterior* or *lower tube*. It is primarily for the drainage of *serosanguineous* fluid that accumulates as the result of the operative procedure. The lower tube may be of a larger diameter than the upper tube to prevent it from becoming plugged with clots. Fig. 45-17 shows the placement of tubes within the pleural space.

As the patient breathes, there will be movement of fluid in the glass tube that is under water. This is known as fluctuation or oscillation, and the column will move up as the patient inhales or coughs, and it will fall when the patient exhales. The tubes should be checked for fluctuation frequently and they should be "milked" or "stripped" every hour to prevent formation of clots that could plug the tubes. If the column of water is not fluctuating, the nurse should be sure that the patient is not lying on the tubes or that they are not blocked by a clot. Changing the patient's position or coughing often restores visible fluctuation. If fluctuation still does not occur, this should be reported.

Suction is usually used to speed reexpansion of the lung after surgery, using either wall suction or an Emerson suction machine (Fig. 45-13 *B*). Most often −30 cm of suction is applied, but this varies according to the surgeon's preference. When it is particularly important to regulate the exact amount of suction used, a "breaker" bottle may be added to the system between the suction source and the patient's drainage bottle. The use of a breaker bottle provides for control of the amount of suction that is applied to the water-seal bottle and thus to the patient's pleural space. The stopper in the control bottle has three openings. One is connected to the water-seal bottle, one is connected to the suction source, and the third contains a glass rod that is under water and open to the outside (Fig. 45-14). The amount of suction produced will be determined by the distance between the surface of the water and the tip of this tube. When the suction source is turned on, the level of water in the open tube will sink in proportion to the amount of negative pressure in the system. Thus if there is 15 cm of water between the surface of the water and the tip of the tube, the amount of negative pressure in the system will be 15 cm of water pressure. Since the water will be at the bottom of the tube when this amount of pressure is reached, any increase in negative pressure will cause air to be drawn in from the outside, *breaking* the suction at this level. Therefore it can be expected that the water in the breaker bottle will bubble almost continuously. If it fails to bubble at all, the desired level of suction is not being attained. When the water in the breaker bottle is not bubbling, the tubing should be checked for air leaks. If there are no leaks and bubbling still does not occur, the surgeon should be notified at once since the air leak in the pleura may be so great that the amount of negative pressure is not sufficient to overcome it. In this instance water will be added to the breaker bottle to increase the distance between the surface of the water and the tip of the tube, thereby increasing the amount of negative pressure being exerted on the pleural space.

The distance the tube is placed under water in the breaker bottle is determined by the surgeon. A breaker bottle and suction may be attached to one or both tubes. Most commonly it is attached to the upper tube, since this is where air is most likely to be leaking from the pleural surface. A small empty trap bottle is usually attached by tubing between the breaker bottle and the suction source. The purpose of this bottle is to protect the suction motor from becoming wet should the breaker bottle overflow. (Further information about other kinds of chest suction devices in common use can be found in other sources.[27,34,52,88])

□ Complications of resectional surgery

The most common complications of resectional surgery include a persistent air space that is not filled by the remaining lung, bronchopleural fistula, and empyema. A thoracoplasty may be necessary eventually to correct any of these complications.

□ Special care following pneumonectomy

Generally the patient is permitted to be only on his back or his operated side, since some surgeons fear that the sutured bronchus may not stay closed. If it should open while the patient is lying with the operative side uppermost, fluid in the operative side would drain into the good lung and drown the patient. Although the chances of this occurring are small, this precaution is usually observed. Another reason for not allowing the patient to lie on the unoperated side is that this compresses the remaining lung and restricts lung excursion and ventilation. The patient is watched immediately post-operatively for cardiac overload and CVP monitoring (p. 923) is common. The patient should also be watched closely for mediastinal shift. If pressure builds up within the operated side, it can cause the mediastinum to shift toward the unoperated side. Conversely, the unoperated lung may shift toward the empty space left after a pneumonectomy. For this reason the surgeon will palpate the patient's trachea at least daily to be sure that it is in midline. If a shift occurs toward the good lung, it is treated by removing air (positive pressure) from the empty space. If the shift is toward the empty space, air may be instilled into the space to increase the pressure and cause the mediastinum to shift back. If the mediastinum persists in shifting toward the empty side, a thoracoplasty may be necessary. This will reduce the size of the space and keep the mediastinum in midline. A patient with mediastinal shift resembles the patient in congestive heart failure. Neck veins are distended, the trachea is displaced to one side, pulse and respirations are increased, and dyspnea is present.

Patients who have had a lung removed may have a lowered vital capacity, and exercise and activity should be limited to that which can be done without dyspnea. Since the body must be given time to adjust to getting along with only one lung, the patient's return to work may be delayed. If the diagnosis is cancer, radiation therapy is usually given, and it may be started before the patient leaves the hospital. (See p. 467 for further discussion of nursing care for patients receiving radiation therapy.) The patient who has had a pneumonectomy for cancer is urged to report to the physician at once if he has hoarseness, dyspnea, pain on swallowing, or localized chest pain, since these difficulties may be signs of complications.

□ Special care following thoracoplasty

Since thoracoplasty is an extrapleural procedure, chest tubes are not necessary unless the pleura is inadvertently entered during surgery. Because portions of several ribs (usually three or four) have been removed, the patient may have considerable pain. Drainage on the dressings may also occur. Although paradoxical motion is rarely seen unless more than three ribs are removed, the patient's breathing pattern should be watched closely. (See p. 1132 for description of paradoxical motion.)

Since thoracoplasty is done either prior to or after resectional surgery, the patient is faced with more than one surgical procedure. Therefore the patient may require additional emotional support in accepting the need for two operations.

□ Outcome criteria for the person who has had thoracic surgery

The person or significant others can:

1. Explain recommended home ADL program.
   a. Which usual activities to limit and for how long.
   b. Exercise program.
2. Explain any changes required in life style (reason and plans for changes in occupation and habits such as smoking, activity level, and so on).

3. State name, dosage, action, and side effects of medications ordered.
   a. How and when to use prn medications.
   b. Schedule for other medications and how to take them.
4. Describe professional and community resources necessary for structuring an environment compatible with convalescence.
   a. Plans for obtaining assistance of agencies such as VNA.
   b. Plans for necessary modifications of home.
5. Describe plans for follow-up care.
   a. Signs or symptoms requiring immediate medical assistance.
   b. State plans for ongoing medical care.

MANAGEMENT OF THE PERSON REQUIRING HEART SURGERY

Some heart diseases can be successfully treated by surgery. The majority of the operations on the heart are being performed with full visualization *(open technique)*. The heart is opened and the defect is inspected and repaired. Openings in the atrial or ventricular septa may be sutured or patched with plastic material. Valves may be opened or reconstructed, or they may be replaced with artificial cusps or ball valves. When the *closed technique* is used, the defect is not seen by the surgeon, who inserts a finger into the heart through a small incision and explores the obstructed valve digitally (Fig. 46-1, *D*). The surgeon may be able to open the obstructed valve with the finger, or a special knife or instrument may be guided into the area to release the adhesions. The closed technique is used most often to treat uncomplicated mitral stenosis. While the risks during and after surgery are greater with open heart surgery, the results generally are better than can be obtained using the closed technique. Operations such as repair of some congenital and acquired defects of the heart could not be performed unless direct visualization was possible.

The open heart approach can be used only if extracorporeal circulation is maintained by means of a heart-lung apparatus (pump oxygenator). In addition, hypothermia may be used to reduce the metabolic rate. This permits tissue tolerance of the somewhat lower blood flow rates with extracorporeal circulation (p. 974) and longer periods of total cardiac standstill than are tolerable at normal body temperatures. Increased atmospheric pressure in special chambers is occasionally used as a supplement to either hypothermia or extracorporeal circulation. The tissues appear to become so saturated with oxygen that they withstand temporary ischemia very well. An adequate amount of oxygen can be carried dissolved in the blood, with no need for hemoglobin.

Preoperative period

Evaluation. Before heart surgery is scheduled, the person's general health and the status of the heart are evaluated very carefully. Arrhythmias and cardiac failure should be controlled, and the person should be in fluid and electrolyte balance. The severity of signs and symptoms such as edema, fatigue, and pain, and progressive changes in these signs and symptoms assist the surgeon and cardiologist to decide when or whether heart surgery is indicated. Laboratory tests that are important sources of data in making the decision include chest roentgenogram, cardiac catheterization, coronary angiography, echocardiography, serum enzyme levels, and electrocardiogram.

Even if persons have been hospitalized many times for their heart conditions, they still need explanations of tests and procedures so that they can be involved in making decisions about their care and can rationally consider the possibility of surgery.

When it has been decided that benefit can be derived from an operation, the physician or surgeon discusses the procedure with the person and the family. They are told why the operation must be done, what the surgeon hopes to accomplish, and what the surgery will entail. If the patient is a child, the parents should explain the admission to the hospital and the operation to the child as simply as possible.

In some instances patients or parents have read or heard about heart operations and have come to the surgeon and asked to have the procedure done. Some men and women, faced with increasing invalidism, decide that they would like to risk an operation in the hope of being able to live normally.

Teaching. Although the surgeon has talked with the person about the operation and the person is emotionally prepared to some degree, anxiety and apprehension are normal, and a great deal of reinforcement and emotional support from the nurse is necessary. Surgery on the heart carries a risk. The individual realizes that there is no substitute for the heart and that life without it is impossible. Provision should be made for the patient and family to visit on the morning of surgery. Some persons may also desire to see their clergyman before surgery. Many persons may wish to prepare a will. The anesthesiologist's preoperative visit may also provide some reassurance.

One of the most important contributions to the care of children can be made by the nurse through support, understanding, and teaching of the child's parents. Helping them to obtain the necessary examinations for the child and explaining required procedures can be helpful in reducing the parents' worry and concern.

Accepting the fact that the child has a defect in the heart is sometimes the most difficult problem. Parents

extracorporeal - outside of the body. Blood passes thru mechanical pump which connects to the body.

react in a variety of ways, but most wish to have all possible help given to the child. Helping parents to accept a "guarded" prognosis or a poor prognosis when operative procedures are recommended requires patient, careful guidance by physician, nurse, and social worker.

The preoperative care is similar to that discussed on p. 373. Most cardiac patients are very apprehensive about the surgery, and the nurse should learn to know the patient as well as possible in order to ascertain how to plan the preoperative teaching. For example, an explanation of chest drainage is welcomed by some persons but greatly upsets others. Preoperatively the nurse should determine and record the amount of activity the person is able to engage in without becoming tired, as this will serve as a guide in determining the postoperative condition.

A sedative such as flurazepam (Dalmane) or diazepam (Valium) is usually ordered on the preoperative night so that the person will sleep. If necessary, the medication usually can be repeated. A narcotic often is ordered on the day of surgery; frequently morphine sulfate (8 to 10 mg) and secobarbital (dosage based on body weight) are given a few minutes before the person is taken to the operating room.

□ Intraoperative period

During open heart surgery the pump oxygenator is used as a temporary substitute for the person's heart and lungs *(extracorporeal circulation)*. The heart and lungs are bypassed so that the surgeon can work in a relatively bloodless field and can see the cardiac defect more clearly. Maintenance of body circulation by this artificial means also allows more time in which to correct the defect (Fig. 45-18).

Several extracorporeal oxygenator systems are available. The most widely used are the bubble method and the screen or rotating disk types. Immediately before the operation the machine is prepared or primed for use by filling it with 2.5 liters (5 pints) of fresh blood that must match that of the patient. Donors are asked to report the morning of the operation to ensure freshness of the blood. Heparin is added to the blood to prevent clotting. Another method is to prime the pump oxygenator with glucose or lactated Ringer's solution. While amounts vary, one medical center primes the unit with 16 to 20 ml of fluid/kg body weight. Two-thirds of the fluid consists of 5% dextrose in water and one-third of 10% dextran 40 (Rheomacrodex) in saline solution. The use of solutions other than blood leads to a significant decrease in complications and also is much less costly. Also, an

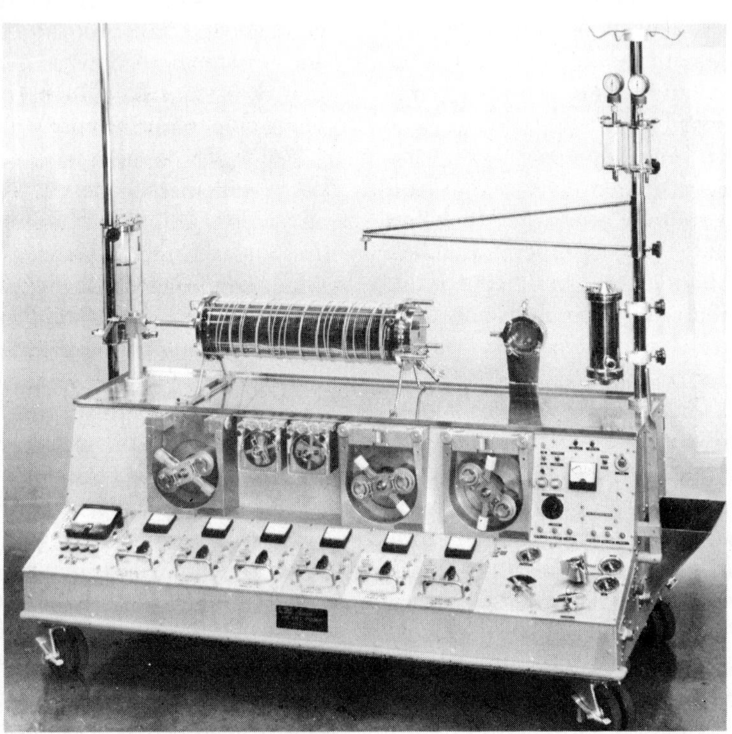

Fig. 45-18. Pump oxygenator used during open heart surgery. (Courtesy PEMCO, Inc., Cleveland, Ohio.)

oxygenator primed with glucose can be used on short notice. This is not possible with blood priming.

The patient receives a general anesthetic via an endotracheal tube. The surgeon then makes a midline sternal splitting or lateral intercostal incision and enters the pericardium. Heparin is given intravenously, and catheters are inserted into the superior and inferior venae cavae. By means of a Y connecting tube, these catheters are attached to the machine, and through them will pass the venous flow of blood. Another catheter is inserted into the common femoral artery and attached to the pump, and through this catheter, blood that has been oxygenated will be returned to the systemic circulation.

When all catheters are inserted and attached, the machine is set into operation, the venae cavae are occluded, and correction of the defect is undertaken. Blood is returned to the patient's body at the rate of 50 to 60 ml/kg of body weight per minute to maintain adequate peripheral blood pressure. Blood return does not determine rate, which will be slowed if hypothermia is used. A heating unit within the machine keeps the blood the same temperature at which the body is being maintained. Oxygenation of blood is accomplished by means of an oxygen inlet within the machine, and carbon dioxide is removed by a chemical bath process. Throughout the surgical procedure, heart action, brain action, and blood pressure are monitored. These recordings allow the anesthesiologist and the surgeon to keep a constant check on the adequacy of circulation being provided to the patient.

After the defect has been corrected, heart action is stabilized, air is vented from the heart chambers, the venae cavae are unclamped, the venous catheter sites are closed, and the pump is discontinued. Protamine sulfate is given to counteract the heparin and to restore the coagulation time of the blood to normal. At least one chest catheter is inserted near the incision to prevent formation of a hematoma.

□ Postoperative period

Postoperative unit. Some medical centers have special units (cardiac recovery rooms or surgical intensive care units) set aside to care for persons who have had heart surgery. Patients usually remain in these units 24 to 48 hours.

In preparation for receiving the patient from the operating room, oxygen equipment is prepared. Other inhalation therapy equipment such as ultrasonic nebulizers and intermittent positive pressure machines may be used, depending on the practice of the individual surgeons. Chest suction apparatus should be ready to attach, and a thoracentesis set, equipment for cardiac massage, and emergency stimulants should be readily available in the event that air or fluid must be withdrawn from the chest cavity or cardiac massage done as emergency measures. Infusion poles, a sphygmomanometer, and a stethoscope should also be at the bedside. Suction apparatus should be available, since suctioning may be necessary to maintain a patent airway. If the heart surgery was done while the temperature of the body was lowered (hypothermia), equipment to apply external heat or to maintain hypothermia will be needed (p. 384).

Immediate care. The person who has undergone heart surgery under either the closed or the open technique requires constant nursing care for 24 to 72 hours. The nurse must be alert for signs of hemorrhage, hypotension, ventricular fibrillation, other arrhythmias, sudden chest pain, and pulmonary edema. Mortality is highest within the first 48 hours.

After open heart surgery the patient may be maintained on continuous respiratory support for the first few hours. To accomplish this a respirator is connected to the endotracheal tube. Oxygen is administered to increase the efficiency of breathing and to minimize complications of hypoxia such as cardiac arrhythmias. The person may be placed with his head elevated to facilitate movement of the diaphragm. A cardiac monitor will be connected to provide a continuous ECG. Central venuous pressure and vital signs will be monitored frequently. As soon as the blood pressure is stable, the patient is turned from the back to the operated side at least every 2 hours. Chest tubes are attached to closed drainage and to chest suction apparatus (Fig. 45-13) to drain air and fluid from the pleural space. The amount and color of the drainage should be checked at least hourly and the time and amount recorded. There will be some bleeding during the first 48 hours, and provision should be made for blood replacement. The dressings are inspected frequently for blood and the chest tubes for patency. Because of the large amounts of heparin used with the pump oxygenator, bleeding may occur. Preparations of vitamin K and protamine sulfate are given to counteract the bleeding tendency caused by the heparin. The patient is observed for any signs of shock, hemorrhage, spontaneous pneumothorax, mediastinal shift, cardiac arrhythmias, or congestive heart failure. Sudden hypotension with sharp pain would indicate a coronary occlusion. Blood-tinged or frothy sputum usually indicates pulmonary edema. As soon as the patient is awake from anesthesia and can follow directions, deep breathing is encouraged. Intermittent positive pressure may be used to facilitate deep breathing and coughing.

Monitoring vital signs. Blood pressure and pulse rate measurements are taken every 15 minutes, and the frequency is decreased gradually as the patient's condition stabilizes. The pulse needs to be checked carefully for rhythm, strength, and rapidity of beat; it may also be monitored electronically. The patient may be aware of palpitation. Since this is frightening, the patient should be told that it can be expected and controlled. When atrial fibrillation occurs, it is usually controlled by medication such as digoxin or propranolol. If the person has been on digitalis, antiarrhythmic preparations, or diuretics preoperatively, these medications may be resumed.

Cardiac monitors may be used continuously for the first few days. The nurse observes the readings closely and reports abnormal rhythms to the physician at once. Roentgenograms of the chest taken with a portable machine and ECGs are made daily to evaluate lung expansion and heart function.

Fluid and electrolyte balance. Although clear fluids are usually allowed as soon as tolerated, supplementary intravenous fluids are given for 2 or 3 days to ensure prescribed intake and an intravenous route for medication. Depending on the postoperative cardiac condition, the physician determines the amount of fluids the person may take. Usually from 1.5 to 1.8 liters are permitted per day. The patient, the nurse, and members of the nursing staff should be aware of this restriction and keep accurate measurement of the fluid intake, including that used to swallow oral medications. Intravenous fluids need to be administered slowly to prevent overloading the circulatory system, thus placing additional load on the heart. The prescribed diet usually does not exceed 2 or 3 g of sodium, and some restriction may be continued indefinitely to prevent fluid retention.

A self-retaining (Foley) catheter is commonly inserted into the bladder and remains in place for several days; urine is collected every hour and checked for specific gravity, color, and amount. Hourly urine volume should not be less than 15 to 30 ml. Frequent observation of urine output helps detect signs of hypovolemia, hemolysis, and kidney shutdown or failure. Disturbance of electrolyte balance with development of acidosis can occur following open heart surgery, particularly following a shunt repair. The nurse should anticipate that blood chemistries will be ordered and should have the needed equipment available.

Relief of pain. A narcotic such as meperidine hydrochloride (Demerol) or morphine sulfate may be prescribed to relieve pain. Some surgeons order small doses given frequently because the pain is severe and larger doses may depress respirations. Severe pain usually persists for 2 or 3 days, caused in part by severance of the intercostal nerves and retraction of the ribs and sternum. The chest catheters may also irritate the pleura and cause pain. If pain in the incision persists over a long period of time, the physician may infiltrate the area above and below the incision with procaine. Since the pain is often made more severe by coughing, the patient may refuse to cough or take deep breaths unless pain medication is given on a regular basis. Most patients can cough best about 30 minutes after a narcotic is given. For care of the person with a chest tube, see p. 962.

Many patients have profuse diaphoresis after heart surgery, and it may be more pronounced at night. The exact reason is not known. The person should be kept dry and comfortable and should be reassured that it is a fairly common occurrence and that it will gradually subside. The temperature may rise markedly and remain elevated for several days. In the immediate postoperative period this is attributed to postperfusion syndrome, a transfusion reaction, or atelectasis.

Some persons experience a period of depression or even disorientation after heart surgery, although this reaction does not generally last very long.[41] The person may become very excited and fearful or may have hallucinations (false visual perceptions). Other persons exhibit varying degrees of depression. This reaction often occurs about 3 days postoperatively. The cause is unknown, but it is thought that it may be caused by medication, fear, sleep loss, or sensory monotony. Panic may develop. The nurse should be alert for these changes in behavior and should reassure the person and family that these are common reactions and that the person is not "losing his mind." The person needs a calm environment, orientation as to time and place, and much support and understanding. Because sleep loss and sensory monotony are more likely to occur when the person is kept in an intensive care unit, some heart surgeons are transferring their patients out of these units as early as 24 hours after surgery. This is only possible when the patients can be closely monitored on a general care unit.

Activity. Passive arm exercises are started shortly after surgery (p. 849), followed by active exercises as the person gains strength. Mobilization of the person depends on the operation and the status of the heart. In general, persons who have had surgery for a coarctation of the aorta or any other surgery on the aorta are kept flat in bed for several days to prevent unnecessary strain on the vessel (the blood pressure is lower when the patient is flat). Some surgeons do not permit the patient to be turned for several days. Before getting out of bed, the person must gradually become accustomed to having the head of the bed elevated. When this procedure is first attempted, dizziness and faintness may be experienced; the person is returned to a flat position, and elevation is attempted again later. Persons who have had surgery for patent ductus arteriosus and mitral stenosis may be kept in Fowler's position postoperatively and are encouraged to move their arms and legs. Backache from lying flat on the back is common.

The time of ambulation for each patient depends on his progress and condition, but (other than the above exceptions) it usually proceeds as follows: The first day the feet are dangled over the side of the bed for 15 minutes in the morning and afternoon. The second day the person is allowed to sit in a chair at the side of the bed for 15 minutes in the morning and afternoon. Walking around the room is permitted on the third day. The fourth day the patient is allowed to walk around the room and to sit in the chair for gradually increasing periods of time. By the fifth day, walking longer distances is encouraged. During ambulation, close supervision is necessary, and activity that causes excessive fatigue, dyspnea, or an increased pulse or respiratory rate should be discontinued. If any of these symptoms appear, the patient is returned to bed, and the physician is consulted before further activity is attempted.

Definite instructions are left by the physician regarding when the person may attempt to climb stairs. The activity should be done slowly. Only two or three steps should be attempted the first time, after which the number of steps is gradually increased, depending on the surgeon's evaluation of the patient's condition. The patient should rest two or three times while climbing one flight of stairs. For further information and explanations concerning postoperative cardiac care, the reader is referred to specialized articles and texts.[20,24,41,93]

Long-term care. The person and the family need to be told that no marked improvement will be noticed immediately after the operation—that it will be at least 3 to 6 months before the full result of the surgery can be ascertained. It is essential that all persons be given this information so that they will not be depressed by dyspnea or pain that may still be present postoperatively.

In preparation for discharge from the hospital, the person is asked to make a list of activities usually carried out at home. This list is discussed with the physician to ascertain the activities that are appropriate. Sexual activity usually is permitted within 3 to 4 weeks postoperatively. Patients are usually advised to start activities slowly and progress gradually to more energy-consuming tasks. The physician will want a patient to return for frequent medical follow-up examinations, at which time advice will be given regarding additional activities. The person is allowed to do anything that does not cause fatigue, but must be kept from attempting too much too soon.

The family should be aware of how much the person may be encouraged to do. Since the patient may have been an invalid preoperatively, the family may be as fearful as is the person about an increase in activity.

□ Outcome criteria for the person who has had open heart surgery

The person or significant others can:

1. Describe extent of permissible activity.
   a. Describe plans for progressive return to physical activity as recommended by the physician.
   b. State awareness of when sexual activity may be resumed (3 to 4 weeks).
   c. Describe criteria to use as a guide in determining if overexertion occurs (fatigue, dyspnea).
   d. Describe plans to return to work if employed.
2. Plan meals incorporating a balanced diet with any prescribed modifications (no added salt, low cholesterol).
3. State name, dosage, action, and side effects of medications ordered.
   a. How and when to use prn medications.
   b. Schedule for other medications and how to take them.
4. Describe plans for follow-up health care.
   a. Explain basis of any symptoms that may persist (dyspnea, pain, night sweats).
   b. Describe signs or symptoms requiring immediate medical attention (fever, increasing dyspnea, or chest pain with minimal exertion).
   c. State plans for ongoing medical care.

REFERENCES AND SELECTED READINGS

1. Agle, D. P., Baum, G. L., Chester, E. H., et al.: Multidiscipline treatment of chronic pulmonary insufficiency. I. Psychologic aspects of rehabilitation, Psychosom. Med. **35**:41-49, 1973.
2. American Heart Association: 1975 Heart Facts, Dallas, 1975, The Association.
3. *American Lung Association: Introduction to lung diseases, New York, 1973, The Association.
4. American Thoracic Society: Guidelines for work for patients with tuberculosis, Am. Rev. Respir. Dis. **108**:160, 1973.
5. Andreoli, K. G., Hunn, V. K., Zipes, D. P., and Wallace, A. G.: Comprehensive cardiac care: a text for nurses, physicans, and other health practitioners, ed. 3, St. Louis, 1975, The C. V. Mosby Co.
6. Barstow, R. E.: Coping with emphysema, Nurs. Clin. North Am. **9**:137-145, 1974.
7. Barlett, R. H., Gazzaniga, A. B., and Geraghty, R. T.: Respiratory maneuvers to prevent postoperative pulmonary complications: a critical review, J.A.M.A. **224**:1017-1021, 1973.
8. Bates, B.: A guide to physical examination, Philadelphia, 1974, J. B. Lippincott Co.
9. Bates, D., Macklem, P. T., and Christie, R. V.: Respiratory function in disease, ed. 2, Philadelphia, 1971, W. B. Saunders Co.
10. Beeson, P. B., and McDermott, W., editors: Cecil-Loeb textbook of medicine, ed. 14, Philadelphia, 1975, W. B. Saunders Co.
11. Bendixen, H. H., Egbert, L. D., Hedley-White, J., Laver, M. B., and Pontoppidon, H.: Respiratory care, St. Louis, 1965, The C. V. Mosby Co.
12. Bergersen, B. S.: Pharmacology in nursing, ed. 13, St. Louis, 1976, The C. V. Mosby Co.

*References preceded by an asterisk are particularly well suited for student reading.

13. Berne, R. M., and Levy, M. N.: Cardiovascular physiology, ed. 3, St. Louis, 1977, The C. V. Mosby Co.
14. *Bloomfield, D. A.: The recognition and management of massive pulmonary embolism, Heart Lung **3**:241-246, 1974.
15. Boyd, D. R.: Monitoring patients with post-traumatic pulmonary insufficiency, Surg. Clin. North Am. **52**:31-46, 1972.
16. Brannin, P.: Oxygen therapy and measures of bronchial hygiene, Nurs. Clin. North Am. **9**:111-121, 1974.
17. *Brooks, W.: Replacing ritual with reason in tuberculosis isolation, Am. J. Nurs. **69**:2410-2411, 1969.
18. *Broughton, J.: Chest physical diagnosis for nurses and respiratory therapists, Heart Lung **2**:200-206, 1972.
19. Bureau of the Census: Statistical abstract of the United States, ed. 98, Washington, D.C., 1977., U.S. Department of Commerce.
20. *Calhoun, P. S., and Bozorgi, S.: Postoperative care following coronary surgery, Heart Lung **3**:912-915, 1974.
21. Callard, G., and Jude, J.: Cardiopulmonary resuscitation in the cardiac care unit, Nurs. Clin. North Am. **7**:573-585, 1972.
22. *Closed-chest method of cardiopulmonary resuscitation, Am. J. Nurs. 65:105, 1965.
23. Collart, M. E., and Brenneman, J. K.: Prevention of postoperative atelectasis, Am. J. Nurs. **71**:1982-1987, 1971.
24. *Collins, J. J., and Morgan, A. P.: Automated management of postoperative cardiac surgical care, Heart Lung **3**:929-932, 1974.
25. Comroe, J. H.: Physiology of respiration, ed. 2, Chicago, 1974, Year Book Medical Publishers, Inc.
26. Crosby, L., and Parsons, L. C.: Measurements of lateral wall pressures exerted by tracheostomy and endotracheal tube cuffs, Heart Lung **3**:797-803, 1974.
27. Daly, B. J., Gorenshek, N., and Mendelsohn, H.: Chest surgery. In Meltzer, L., et al., editors: Intensive care for nurse specialists, ed. 2, Philadelphia, 1975, Charles Press Publishers.
28. Downs, J. B., Block, A. J., and Vennum, K. B.: Intermittent mandatory ventilation: a new approach to weaning patients from mechanical ventilators, Chest **64**:311-335, 1973.
29. *Dyer, E., and Peterson, D.: Safe care of IPPB machines, Am. J. Nurs. **71**:2163-2166, 1971.
30. Edwards, P. Q., and Ogasaware, F. R.: Phasing out the child-centered TB program, NTRDA Bull., Nov. 1971, pp. 12-13.
31. Egan, D. F.: Fundamentals of respiratory therapy, ed. 2, St. Louis, 1973, The C. V. Mosby Co.
32. Eliot, R. S., editor: The acute cardiac emergency: diagnosis and management, Mount Disco, N.Y., 1972, Futura Publishing Co. Inc.
33. *Ellis, R.: Unusual sensory and thought disturbances after cardiac surgery, Am. J. Nurs. **72**:2021-2025, 1972.
34. *Enerson, D. M., and McIntyre, J.: A comparative study of the physiology and physics of pleural drainage systems, J. Thorac. Cardiovasc. Surg. **52**:40-46, 1966.
35. Farer, L. S.: Infectiousness of tuberculosis patients, Am. Rev. Respir. Dis. **108**:152, 1973.
36. Farer, L. S.: Preventive treatment of tuberculosis. In American Thoracic Society: Basics of RD, New York, 1973, The Society.
37. Fayerhaugh, S. Y.: Getting around with emphysema, Am. J. Nurs. **73**:94-99, 1973.
38. Finch, C., and Lenfant, C.: Oxygen transport in man, N. Engl. J. Med. **286**:407-415, 1972.
39. *Fitzgerald, L. M.: Mechanical ventilation, Heart Lung **5**:939-949, 1976.
40. *Foley, M. F.: Pulmonary function testing, Am. J. Nurs. **71**:1134-1139, 1971.
41. Frater, R. W. M.: Postoperative care in the pediatric cardiac patient, Heart Lung **3**:903-911, 1974.
42. Gordon, A. S., editor: Cardiopulmonary resuscitation conference proceedings, National Research Council, Washington, D.C., 1967, National Academy of Sciences.
43. *Graham, L. E.: Patient's perceptions in the CCU, Am. J. Nurs. **69**:1921-1922, 1969.
44. *Haas, A.: Essentials of living with pulmonary emphysema: a guide for patients and their families, patient publ. no. 4, New York, 1963, The Institute of Physical Medicine and Rehabilitation.
45. Haberman, P. B., Green, J. P., Archibald, C., et al.: Determinants of successful selective tracheobronchial suctioning, N. Engl. J. Med. **289**:1060-1062, 1973.
46. Hardy, K. L.: Tracheostomy: indications, technics, and tubes: a reappraisal, Am. J. Surg. **126**:300-310, 1973.
47. Hargreaves, A. G.: Emotional problems of patients with respiratory disease, Nurs. Clin. North Am. **3**:479-487, 1968.
48. *Helming, M. G., editor: Symposium on nursing in respiratory diseases, Nurs. Clin. North Am. **3**:381-487, 1968.
49. Hohle, B. M.: The atypical mycobacteria: patient care at home, Am. J. Nurs. **67**:1033-1036, 1967.
50. Hunt, W. J., and Bespalec, D. A.: An evaluation of current methods of modifying smoking behavior, J. Clin. Psychol. **30**:431-438, 1974.
51. *Jacquette, G.: To reduce hazards of tracheal suctioning, Am. J. Nurs. **71**:2362-2364, 1971.
52. Johnson, J., et al.: Surgery of the chest, ed. 4, Chicago, 1970, Year Book Medical Publishers, Inc.
53. Jude, J. R., Kouwenhoven, W. B., and Knickerbocker, G. G.: Cardiac arrest, J.A.M.A. **178**:1063-1070, 1961.
54. Karetzky, M. S., and Khan, A. U.: Review of current concepts in aspiration pneumonia, Heart Lung **6**:321-326, 1977.
55. Kersten, L.: Chest tube drainage system—indications and principles of operation, Heart Lung **3**:97-101, 1974.
56. Klause, M. L.: Mediastinoscopy, AORN J. **15**:55-59, 1972.
57. Kudia, M. S.: The care of the patient with respiratory insufficiency, Nurs. Clin. North Am. **8**:183-190, 1973.
58. *Kurihara, M.: Postural drainage, clapping and vibrating, Am. J. Nurs. **65**:76-79, 1965.
59. Lagerson, J.: Nursing care of patients with chronic pulmonary insufficiency, Nurs. Clin. North Am. **9**:165-179, 1974.
60. *Lewis, E., and Browning, M., editors: Nursing in respiratory disease, New York, 1972, The American Journal of Nursing Co.
61. Malkus, B.: Respiratory care at home, Am. J. Nurs. **76**:1789-1791, 1976.
62. McCormick. K. A., and Brinbaum, M. L.: Acute ventilatory failure following thoracic trauma, Nurs. Clin. North Am. **9**:181-194, 1974.
63. Modell, W.: Drugs of choice: 1974-1975, St. Louis, 1974, The C. V. Mosby Co.
64. *Moddy, L. E.: Primer for pulmonary hygiene, Am. J. Nurs. **77**:104-106, 1977.
65. Moody, L. E.: Nursing care of patients with asthma, Nurs. Clin. North Am. **9**:195-207, 1974.
66. Nett, L.: The use of mechanical ventilators, Nurs. Clin. North Am. **9**:123-136, 1974.
67. Nett, L., and Petty, T. I.: Oxygen toxicity, Am. J. Nurs. **73**:1556-1558, 1973.
68. Niewoehner, D. E., Kleinerman, J., and Rice, D. B.: Pathologic changes in peripheral airways of young cigarette smokers, N. Engl. J. Med. **291**:755-758, 1974.
69. Obley, F. A., and Preiser, F. M.: Comprehensive outpatient respiratory care: a program conducted in a suburban private practice, J. Am. Geriatr. Soc. **22**:521-524, 1974.
70. Petty, T. L.: Intensive and rehabilitative respiratory care, ed. 2, Philadelphia, 1974, Lea & Febiger.
71. *Phipps, W. J., Barker, W. L., and Daly, B. J.: Respiratory in-

sufficiency and failure. In Meltzer, L. E., Abdellah, F. G., and Kitchell, J. R.: Concepts and practices of intensive care for nurse specialists, ed. 2, Philadelphia, 1975, The Charles Press Publishers.

72. Powaser, M. M.: The effectiveness of hourly cuff deflation in minimizing tracheal damage, Heart Lung **5**:734-741, 1976.
73. Rie, M. W.: Physical therapy in the nursing care of respiratory disease patients, Nurs. Clin. North Am. **3**:463-478, 1968.
74. *Sackner, M. A.: Pathogenesis and prevention of tracheobronchial damage with suction procedures, Chest **64**:284-290, 1973.
75. Scheuer, R.: Cardiopulmonary resuscitation in seven community hospitals, Heart Lung **1**:810-817, 1972.
76. Schrogie, J. J.: Cardiopulmonary resuscitation in practice, Public Health Rep. **81**:128-132, 1966.
77. Sedlock, S. A.: Detection of chronic pulmonary disease, Am. J. Nurs. **72**:1407-1411, 1972.
78. *Selecky, P. A.: Tracheostomy: a review of present day indications, complications, and care, Heart Lung **3**:272-283, 1974.
79. *Shapiro, B. A., Harrison, R. A., and Trout, C. A.: Clinical application of respiratory care, Chicago, 1975, Year Book Medical Publishers, Inc.
80. Simmons, D. H.: Evaluation of acid-base status. In American Thoracic Society: Basics of RD, New York, 1974, The Society.
81. Sitzman, J.: Nursing management of the acutely ill respiratory patient, Heart Lung **1**:207-215, 1972.
82. Slonim, N. B., and Hamilton, L. H.: Respiratory physiology, ed. 3, St. Louis, 1976, The C. V. Mosby Co.
83. *Sorensen, K. M., and Amis, D. B.: Understanding the world of the chronically ill, Am. J. Nurs. **67**:811-817, 1967.
84. Standards for cardiopulmonary resuscitation (CRP) and emergency cardiac care (ECC), J.A.M.A. **227**(suppl.):7, 1974.
85. Traver, G.: The nurse's role in clinical testing of lung function, Nurs. Clin. North Am. **9**:101-110, 1974.
86. *Traver, G.: Assessment of thorax and lungs, Am. J. Nurs. **73**:466-471, 1973.
87. *Traver, G. A.: Effect of intermittent positive pressure breathing and use of rebreathing tube upon tidal volume and cough, Nurs. Res. **17**:100-103, 1968.
88. U.S. Public Health Service: Closed drainage of the chest: a programmed course for nurses, publ. no. 1337, Washington, D.C., 1965, U.S. Department of Health, Education, and Welfare.
89. Vaughan, V. C. III: The place of drug therapy in childhood asthma, Am. J. Nurs. **66**:1049-1052, 1966.
90. Wade, J. F.: Respiratory nursing care: physiology and technique, ed. 2, St. Louis, 1977, The C. V. Mosby Co.
91. *Wagner, M. M.: Assessment of patients with multiple injuries, Am. J. Nurs. **72**:1822-1827, 1972.
92. White, H.: Tracheostomy care with a cuffed tube, Am. J. Nurs. **72**:75-77, 1972.
93. *Wolfer, J., and Davis, C. E.: Assessment of surgical patients' preoperative emotional condition and postoperative welfare, Nurs. Res. **19**:402-414, 1970.

46

Problems of the heart and major blood vessels

FRANCES R. BROWN

It is difficult to determine the exact prevalence of cardiac disease (and associated vascular conditions such as cerebrovascular and peripheral vascular disease) in a community or in the entire country. Diagnostic techniques have not yet been developed that can be used in mass screening for all types of cardiovascular disease. Many persons do not know that they have heart disease until severe symptoms develop.

EPIDEMIOLOGY

Cardiovascular diseases cause more deaths than all other diseases combined. In 1978 almost 52% of deaths in the United States were caused by cardiovascular diseases.[98] Thus at the present time it can be safely predicted that unless some remarkable events occur to change the present trend, at least one out of every two persons alive in the country today will die of cardiovascular disease.

Deaths caused by cardiac disease vary with age. Congenital malformations of the heart and closely related vascular system are the cause of over 90% of the deaths from these causes in children under 5 years of age and of more than 33.3% in persons 5 to 24 years of age. By far the most common cause of death from heart disease after the age of 25 years is ischemic heart disease (coronary artery disease), which accounted for 642,519 deaths in 1975.[98]

Despite some advances in prevention and treatment, the incidence of heart disease continues to be high. Approximately 10 million persons in the United States, including 500,000 children, have heart disease. Most of the advances in treatment deal with amelioration of heart disease and not with removal of its causes.[98] Research efforts continue in attempts to find effective medications, but results from use of the medications now available have not always been beneficial over long periods of time. For example, widespread use of antibiotics has produced drug-resistant strains of bacteria and drug-resistant persons. Medications used to lower the cholesterol level in the blood and perhaps reduce the incidence of coronary artery thrombosis are not wholly satisfactory, and some new drugs that produce vasodilation in animal studies have not proved helpful to humans. Heart surgery is publicized widely and is a valuable treatment at times, but at present it is practicable for less than 1% of all patients with heart disease.

Although the causes of many types of heart disease are not yet known, extensive epidemiologic studies and research are being carried on currently in an attempt to determine preventive measures. Organizations such as the American Heart Association are financing research to uncover further information on the causes of heart disease and to develop new methods for its treatment. As part of the National Institutes of Health, supported by the federal government and under the United States Public Health Service, the National Heart Institute is conducting an intensive study on the cause, control, and treatment of heart disease. Vital statistics are being studied carefully in an attempt to discover whether such factors as sex, occupation, constitutional makeup, ethnologic background, or dietary patterns are associated with certain types of heart disease. Grants have been made to study the effects of new drugs on the heart, to perfect techniques that will make cardiac surgery possible for more patients, and to study the mechanisms by which heart diseases affect the tissues. Future studies of many people in their own home and community settings, to learn how diet, living practices, regular exercise, and many other aspects of living affect heart disease, will require the help of nurses who are particularly skilled in working with people.

In recent years there has been increasing concern about the gap between medical research and new knowledge and its application to patient care. Congress passed a bill in October 1965 establishing Regional Medical Programs for Heart Disease, Cancer, Stroke and Related Diseases. The Regional Medical Programs had many objectives, all of which were designed to improve the knowledge of physicians and nurses and thereby improve patient care. These programs have been phased out, but many health professionals have benefited from programs sponsored by them.

CLASSIFICATION OF HEART DISEASE

Heart diseases may be divided into two general groups: those that are *congenital* and those that are *acquired* (after birth). Congenital heart disease follows an abnormality of structure caused by error in embryologic development of the heart. Acquired disease may affect the heart either suddenly or gradually. There may be damage to the heart from bacteria, chemical agents, or diminished blood supply. For example, inflammation may cause scarring of heart valves, muscle, or outer coverings that may impair the heart's function. Any changes in the coronary vessels supplying the heart muscle may decrease its efficiency.

Heart disease may also be classified according to a specific cause such as rheumatic fever, bacterial endocarditis, or hypertension. It is also classified according to anatomic change such as valvular scarring or according to a physiologic abnormality such as arrhythmia.

Despite the varied methods of classification, progression of any of these diseases may lead to cardiac arrhythmias or cardiac failure. Varying degrees of cardiac arrhythmia and cardiac failure are the cause of many of the symptoms commonly associated with the various cardiac diseases, but with early diagnosis and treatment these complications may be prevented.

CONGENITAL HEART DISEASE

Congenital heart disease is discussed in detail in pediatric nursing texts and is only reviewed briefly here. Congenital heart disease occurs in about six of every 1,000 live births and accounts for about 28% of deaths caused by congenital defects in the first year of life.[98] Heart defects may be caused by heredity (defects inherent in the genes) or by a viral infection such as German measles in the first trimester of pregnancy. For the majority of cases, however, the cause is unknown or is associated with other defects such as Down's syndrome.

Congenital heart diseases usually are classified as (1) those that cause cyanosis such as tetralogy of Fallot or transposition of the great vessels and (2) those that do not cause cyanosis such as coarctation of the aorta, aortic stenosis, patent ductus arteriosus, interatrial septal defects, interventricular septal defects, and pulmonary stenosis (Fig. 46-1). *Tetralogy of Fallot* consists of four defects: a ventricular septal defect, pulmonary stenosis, right ventricular hypertrophy, and overriding aorta. This combination produces cyanosis, and the infant is often referred to as a "blue baby." In *transposition of the great vessels* the aorta arises from the right ventricle and the pulmonary artery arises from the left ventricle. Thus two separate, parallel circuits exist and the blood is not oxygenated. A communication between the right and left side of the heart must remain open after birth to maintain life. Usually the foramen ovale or ductus arteriosus remains patent.

A *coarctation of the aorta* is a localized stricture just below the origin of the left subclavian artery. It causes the pressure in the blood vessels above the constriction to become elevated and the pressure below the constriction to become lower than the pressure above the

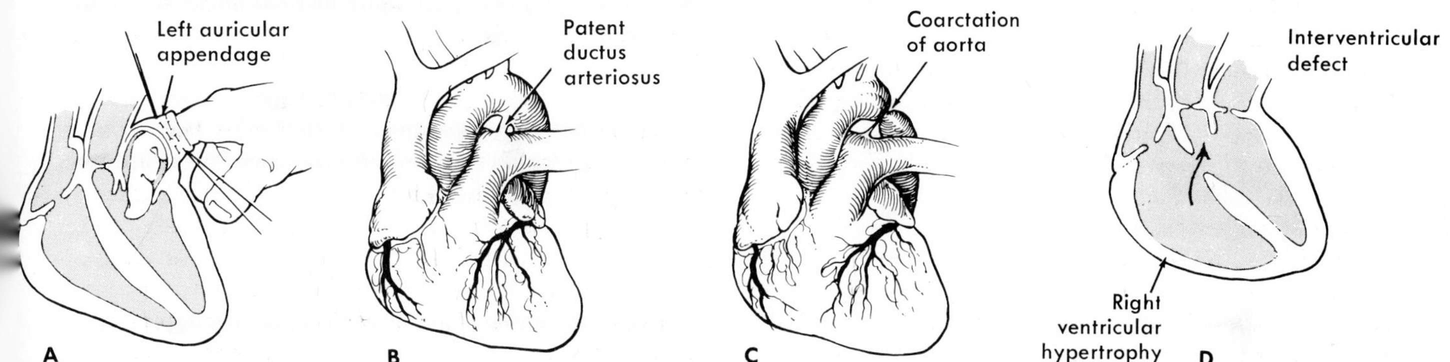

Fig. 46-1. A, Technique used in mitral commissurotomy for adhesions of mitral valve. **B,** Communication between aorta and pulmonary artery found in patients with patent ductus arteriosus. **C,** Abnormality found in coarctation of aorta. Note engorgement above constriction. **D,** Abnormal opening between right and left ventricles that exists when ventricular septal defect is present.

constriction. Pulses in the lower extremities are weak or absent. *Aortic stenosis* is a fusing of the commissures of the aortic valve or narrowing of the valve, which obstructs the flow of blood from the left ventricle. A *patent ductus arteriosus* permits the shunting of oxygenated blood from the aorta back to the pulmonary artery. In *interatrial septal defects* the foramen ovale, or normal opening in the atrial septum, fails to close as it should shortly after birth, and blood returning from the lungs to the left atrium shunts over to the right atrium. An *interventricular septal defect* is an abnormal opening between the right and left ventricles through which blood from the left ventricle is shunted into the right ventricle and is recirculated through the pulmonary artery and lungs. *Pulmonary stenosis* is a narrowing of the pulmonary valve, which decreases the amount of blood flowing into the lungs.

Prevention

Rubella infection can cause disruption of embryonic cardiac development in the fetus during the first trimester of pregnancy. Because school-aged children are the major source of rubella infection in the community, the best method for preventing this infection in pregnant women is to vaccinate these children.

Clinical picture

Nurses can be instrumental in the detection of congenital heart disease. Signs and symptoms of congenital heart disease may include abnormal heart murmurs, varying degrees of cyanosis, clubbing of fingers and toes, shortness of breath, and generalized poor development. A child may have no symptoms, such as may occur with an interatrial septal defect, but a heart murmur may be discovered during routine physical assessment. Infants with severe congenital heart disease become symptomatic shortly after birth and require medical or surgical intervention. Because more accurate early diagnosis and evaluation of cardiac defects are now possible (such as by means of cardiac catheterization, angiography, or echocardiography) parents of children with suspected anomalies of the heart should be urged to seek early medical care.

Intervention

Recent advances in anesthesiology and surgical techniques have made correction or palliation of most congenital cardiac defects possible. Most children will undergo elective cardiac surgery to repair the defect in early childhood. Operative mortality is low, and results are favorable after most of the procedures. The child should continue to have periodic medical supervision following the surgical correction.

Parents of children who have congenital heart defects are urged to treat their children as normal. In most situations the child's activity need not be restricted, since a child who has a significant congenital heart defect usually limits physical activity automatically. Antibiotic prophylaxis still is recommended prior to dental and surgical procedures to prevent bacterial endocarditis.

■ INFLAMMATORY HEART DISEASES

□ Pericarditis

Pericarditis is an inflammatory process of the pericardium. It may be an isolated event; however, it usually is a manifestation of disease elsewhere in the body. It occurs primarily in adults. Pericarditis may be acute or chronic.

Acute pericarditis

Acute pericarditis may be caused by viral or bacterial infections, chemical changes, connective tissue diseases, neoplastic processes, myocardial infarction, or trauma such as cardiac surgery. The inflammatory process may be associated with accumulation of serous, purulent, or hemorrhagic fluid in the pericardial sac (pericardial effusion).

Clinical picture. A predominant clinical manifestation of acute pericarditis is a pericardial friction rub along with precordial chest pain, which may closely resemble that of acute myocardial infarction. Arrhythmias such as atrial tachycardia and atrial flutter-fibrillation as well as sinus tachycardia are common,[20] as are fever, chills, and fatigue. If pericardial effusion occurs, either rapidly or gradually, the pressure of the fluid will exert counterpressure on the heart *(cardiac tamponade)* with resulting decreased cardiac output and symptoms such as syncope. Signs of tamponade may include tachycardia, hypotension, distended neck veins, and *pulsus paradoxus* (an abnormal fall in systolic blood pressure with inspiration), as well as an enlarged heart shadow on chest radiographs. The heart shadow often is referred to as a "water bottle" heart.

Intervention. General treatment for acute pericarditis consists in providing the patient with rest (usually bed rest) to reduce fatigue and treating infections with appropriate antibiotics. Aspirin often is an effective analgesic, although narcotics may be required to relieve severe precordial pain. Steroids also may be used to diminish the inflammatory process.[20]

Specific therapy includes *pericardiocentesis* (aspiration of fluid from the pericardial sac) when periocardial effusion is present, either to reduce tamponade or to obtain fluid for diagnostic purposes, and use of antiarrhythmic medications such as digitalis preparations.[20] It is important to distinguish between acute pericarditis and acute myocardial infarction. If anticoagulants are given in acute pericarditis, there may be bleeding into the pericardial sac resulting in fatal cardiac tamponade.

Chronic pericarditis

As inflammation of the pericardium becomes chronic, the thin pericardial membrane becomes thickened and fibrotic, interfering with movement of blood during systole and diastole *(constrictive pericarditis).*

Clinical picture. Signs and symptoms of chronic pericarditis include all those of congestive heart failure (p. 1003), making it difficult for the physician to make an accurate diagnosis.[6]

Intervention. If chronic pericarditis causes severe constriction, a *pericardectomy* is performed. During this procedure scar tissue and pericardium that adhere to the heart are removed, relieving many of the symptoms almost immediately. A chest catheter is usually inserted for drainage postoperatively. The nursing care of persons undergoing a pericardectomy is similar to that of those having other cardiac surgery (p. 973). Preoperative and postoperative medical management of persons with constrictive chronic pericarditis includes digitalization, sodium restriction, and cautious use of diuretics.[20] Overdiuresis can reduce central venous pressure to levels below those required (15 cm H_2O or more) to maintain cardiac output.[20] Provision for rest, analgesics, and steroid therapy are the same as for acute pericarditis.

☐ Myocarditis

Myocarditis is an inflammatory disease of the myocardium and may occur with a wide variety of systemic diseases including viral and bacterial infections and allergic and hypersensitivity reactions. Myocarditis also may occur in conjunction with acute endocarditis or pericarditis.

Symptoms of myocarditis often are vague. The person may experience precordial discomfort and sometimes shortness of breath. Frequently arrhythmias such as tachycardias or premature beats occur and occasionally there is an increase in the SGOT level. Anorexia, fever, and fatigue also may be present.

Persons with myocarditis often are treated with bed rest and digitalis to prevent heart failure and cardiogenic shock. Medical therapy also involves treatment of the underlying disease with antibiotics and steroids as well as management of arrhythmias.

☐ Subacute bacterial endocarditis

Subacute bacterial endocarditis (SBE) is a serious complication of heart disease. Organisms in the bloodstream invade the heart. The valves are most often involved, being covered with vegetations or products of bacterial degeneration. During healing after active infection the cardiac valves may become scarred, resulting in functional difficulty and eventual heart failure, although the infection itself is cured. The most common organisms affecting the heart are *Streptococcus viridans* (30% to 40%), enterococci (10%), other streptococci (20% to 30%), and *Staphylococcus aureus* (9% to 27%).

Congenital cardiac anomalies that cause turbulent blood flow are more likely to be associated with SBE and include ventricular septal defects, coarctation of the aorta, aortic stenosis, and mitral insufficiency.[20] SBE also occurs with artificial heart valves. Young adults (aged 20 to 40) are more prone to SBE, but the incidence is increasing in the older adult population. In addition persons who "mainline" street drugs are at high risk because of the possibility of bacteremia from contaminated needles and syringes.

Prevention

Prevention of bacterial endocarditis should include correction of any underlying cardiac defect, if possible, as well as utilization of measures to prevent bacteremia. Early and vigorous treatment of infections, maintenance of oral hygiene, avoidance of intraarterial or intravenous catheters, and prophylactic use of antibiotics when a person undergoes dental treatment or a surgical procedure are important.[20]

Clinical picture

The person usually has recurring bouts of fever and malaise, often dating from an attack of "flu." There may be petechiae (small capillary hemorrhages) in the conjunctiva, in the mouth, and on the legs, and the fingers may be clubbed if the infection occurs in the presence of congenital heart anomaly. If the disease is untreated it progresses rapidly to heart failure from valvular inefficiency or injury to the myocardium. Death may follow within 1 or 2 months of onset as a result of emboli to the lungs, kidneys, brain, or spleen or as a result of heart failure.

Intervention

Therapy for SBE is based on identification of the specific organism and then administering antibiotics that are effective against that organism. For this reason serial blood cultures are essential. Generally persons are hospitalized for 2 to 6 weeks, although strict bed rest usually is not enforced. Fever is treated with analgesics such as aspirin and fluids, and good nutrition is encouraged.

☐ Rheumatic heart disease

Acute rheumatic heart disease is an acute inflammatory reaction. It may involve (1) the lining of the heart, or endocardium, including the valves, resulting in scarring, distortion, and stenosis of the valves, (2) all muscle of the heart, or myocardium, where small areas of necrosis develop and heal, leaving scars (Aschoff bodies), or (3) the outer covering of the heart, or pericardium, where it may cause adhesions to surrounding tissues. The development of symptoms of chronic rheumatic heart disease in later life depends on the location and severity of the damage and other factors. Probably somewhat less than 10% of persons with rheumatic fever develop rheumatic heart disease, and about one half of those with rheumatic heart disease have mitral stenosis[24] (p. 985). It is possible for rheumatic fever and rheumatic heart disease with mild symptoms to go undiagnosed, or the disease may be subclinical with no noticeable symptoms. Thus the discovery of rheumatic heart disease is made years later. Careful recall of illness in childhood may include a recollection of "growing pains," confirming the likelihood that the patient had rheumatic fever during childhood.

About 20% to 40% of persons who have acute rheumatic heart disease are disabled or have life shortened from this cause. The nurse should understand rheumatic fever, its origin and its consequences, in order to help to prevent the rheumatic infection or to prevent the development of the complications of heart disease.

Children who have rheumatic heart disease are usually advised by the physician to lead a relatively normal, unrestricted life in which only vigorous, competitive athletics are prohibited. The recommendations are specific for the individual person and his particular situation, and they vary a great deal. If heart damage has been severe and permanent damage is likely, the nurse should help the child's parents to direct the child's interest toward activities that can become satisfying and rewarding and yet are not strenuous. For example, artistic interests developed from childhood might lead to skills that earn recognition and a livelihood or to a variety of other satisfying occupations that are within the person's physical capacity.

Overprotection by parents is sometimes a serious problem. The nurse needs to be understanding and accepting of the parents' fears and concerns and provide sufficient time to allow discussion of them. The parents may also be referred to a medical social worker, if one is available, or work with the physician in seeking psychiatric consultation.

□ Cardiovascular syphilis

Cardiovascular syphilis usually occurs from 15 to 20 years after the primary syphilitic infection. Since the highest incidence of primary syphilis is among persons in their early twenties, persons with symptoms of cardiovascular syphilis are usually over 35 years of age. If the primary infection is not treated, approximately 10% of persons affected will develop syphilitic aortitis or aneurysm.[6]

Prevention

It is the aim of health organizations and medical personnel to treat all persons with syphilis before they develop cardiovascular disease or any of the other complications of late syphilis. Primary syphilis can be arrested; however, once syphilis has affected the aorta and the valves of the heart, little can be done except to treat the patient symptomatically.

Clinical picture

In cardiovascular syphilis the spirochetes attack the aorta, the aortic valve, and the heart muscle. The portion of the aorta nearest the heart is usually affected, and the elastic wall of the aorta becomes weakened and bulges. This bulge is known as an *aneurysm*. As the aneurysm grows it may press on neighboring structures such as the intercostal nerves and cause pain. Aneurysms may also be present without symptoms. Evidence may be discovered on radiographic examination. There is a possibility that the aneurysm may rupture as it increases in size, and the person is encouraged to avoid strenuous activities that might cause a sudden increase in the pressure exerted against the bulging vessel. Surgical resection of the aneurysm sometimes is possible (p. 1012).

Syphilis may also attack the aorta more diffusely causing aortitis. The aorta becomes dilated, and small plaques containing calcium are laid down. There may be complaints of substernal pain associated with exertion due to constriction at the orifices of the coronary arteries. Thrombi may develop along the aorta, and emboli may occur resulting in severe complications such as myocardial infarction or cerebral emboli.

Spirochetes may also attack the aortic valve causing it to become scarred. This causes aortic insufficiency, and the person may have a bounding pulse and a high systolic blood pressure because of the extra effort demanded of the ventricles to pump blood into the systemic circulation. Heart failure eventually occurs.

Intervention

The use of penicillin in the treatment of the patient with cardiovascular syphilis is thought to possibly prolong life, since penicillin destroys any active organisms and permits healing to occur. Treatment at this stage, however, will not restore damaged aortic tissue or damaged aortic valves, and extensive scarring may occur. The person with cardiovascular syphilis should be given guidance in planning his activities of daily living and in selecting work that places the least possible burden on the damaged heart and aorta. In certain cases of aortic insufficiency, surgery is possible.

□ Outcome criteria for the person with inflammatory heart disease

The person or significant others can:

1. Describe the rationale for the degree of rest and activity prescribed and plan activities within the established prescription.
2. Demonstrate ways to carry out activities of daily living to conserve energy.
3. Plan a diet to include adequate nutrients and fluids and avoidance of sodium if so prescribed.
4. Describe the medication program:
   a. State name, dosage, frequency, and side effects of prescribed medications (antibiotics, analgesics, digitalis, or steroids).
   b. Describe activities (dental therapy, surgery) that require prophylactic antibiotics.
   c. State plans to follow through on prescribed antibiotic therapy even after symptoms abate.
5. State plans for regular follow-up care.

■ VALVULAR HEART DISEASE

Valvular heart disease, particularly mitral stenosis and mitral regurgitation, may develop from rheumatic endocarditis. Other causes of valvular incompetence include bacterial endocarditis, syphilis, congenital malformation of the valves, and rupture of the chordae tendineae. With valvular dysfunction there are pressure changes within the heart as well as pulmonary and peripheral circulatory changes. The dysfunction may eventually lead to cardiac failure, cardiac arrhythmias, and cardiogenic shock.

About one half of the persons with rheumatic heart disease have mitral stenosis.[24] After repeated attacks of rheumatic fever, rheumatic nodules grow on the mitral valve at the line where the valves meet. The valves thicken and fuse together, the chordae tendineae shorten and thicken, and the valve opening narrows from 4 to 6 cm sq to 1 cm sq or less.[24] There is increased pressure in the left atrium, which is reflected to the pulmonary vessels and the right ventricle, and the load on the right ventricle may lead to right-sided heart failure (p. 1004).

Aortic stenosis and insufficiency usually are caused by rheumatic fever. The disease attacks the valve cusps, which become stiff and calcified and obstruct blood flow, or the infection may cause degeneration of the valve, leading to valvular incompetence. There is an elevation of left ventricular pressure and low cardiac output.

Clinical picture

Signs and symptoms of *mitral stenosis* and *insufficiency* include shortness of breath on exertion, progressing to orthopnea, pulmonary edema, and hemoptysis. The person usually becomes incapacitated, and without treatment death usually occurs between 30 and 50 years of age.

The person with *aortic stenosis* may have few clinical symptoms for some time, even though the obstruction may be substantial. Symptoms of *aortic insufficiency* usually occur sooner. Some persons complain of fatigue, faintness, and angina, and radiographs may show a heart either of normal size or with slight enlargement of the left ventricle. Untreated aortic valvular disease will contribute to and often finally cause congestive heart failure. ECG changes may be the only evidence of the severity of the stenosis.

Intervention

Mitral valve. The goals of therapy are a decrease in the shortness of breath, edema, arrhythmias, and cough. Treatment for mitral stenosis varies with the degree of severity of the disease. Conservative treatment includes limitation of activity to decrease the work load on the heart, sodium restriction, use of diuretics, and digitalis. Surgical treatment is used when the symptoms limit the person's activity. Mitral commissurotomy is often the first step. *Mitral commissurotomy* is the fracturing (breaking apart) of the stenosed leaves (commissures) of the mitral valve which is located between the left atrium and the left ventricle. At the present time most surgeons operate on the person who has simple mitral stenosis by the closed technique. In this operation the thorax usually is entered through a left anterolateral incision. The fourth rib may be partially resected to give adequate ex-

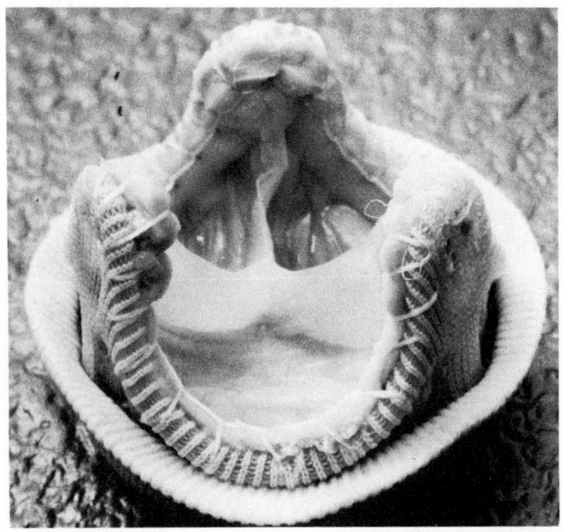

Fig. 46-2. Porcine aortic valve prosthesis; a natural-tissue valve. Note that valve leaflets are sutured to Dacron-covered fabric frame. Outer ring is sutured into heart.

posure, and then the heart is entered through the left auricular appendage. The surgeon inserts a finger through the incision into the atrium and through the mitral valve (Fig. 46-1, *A*). Several attempts are made to release the leaves of the mitral valve either with a finger, with a special knife, or with a transventricular dilator.[24] At this point the surgeon will know whether the operation can be expected to relieve the person's symptoms. Sometimes it is impossible to release the stenosed valve because of excessive calcium deposits around it or because of other pathologic conditions. If any clots are found, they are removed to prevent their escape into the general circulation.

If the operation has been successful there will be a decline in the pulmonary pressure, reduction of the heart size, and a gradual diminishing of the symptoms previously experienced. Many persons who have been semiinvalids are able to return to a relatively normal life. In some persons, however, the stenosis may recur after varying periods of time and the symptoms may become

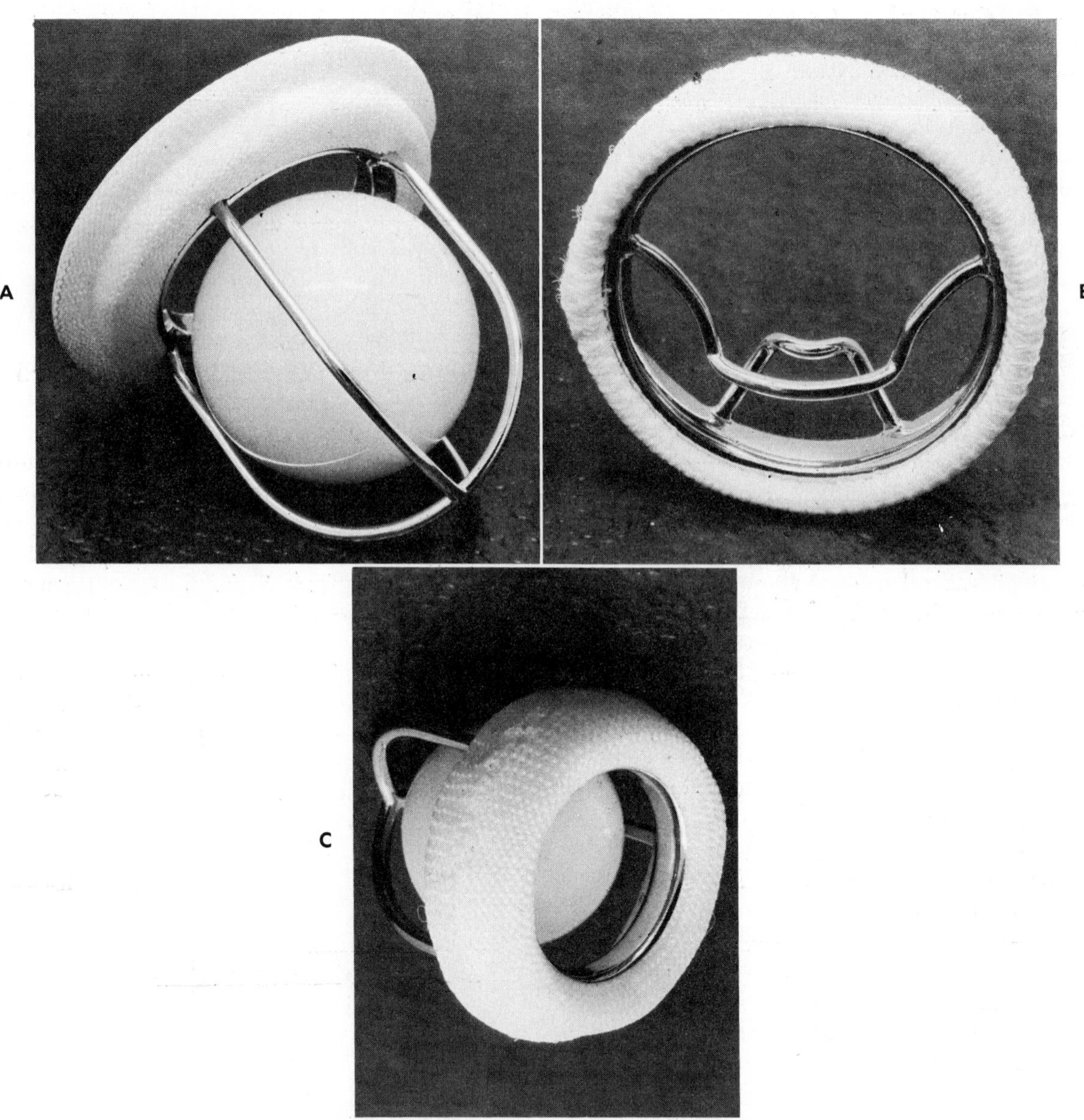

Fig. 46-3. A, Starr-Edwards mitral valve prosthesis, "ball-in-cage" mechanical valve. **B,** Bjork/Shiley mitral valve prosthesis, "tilting disk" mechanical valve. In this picture the disk has been omitted to show metal supports that hold disk in place. **C,** Starr-Edwards aortic valve prosthesis, "ball-in-cage" valve.

worse than preoperatively. The surgeon then may attempt to relieve the stenosis by doing open heart surgery.

If the mitral valve is mainly insufficient (not closing tightly and allowing blood to escape from the left ventricle back into the left atrium) a *valvuloplasty* (repair) may be performed. If the valve is severely diseased or is markedly stenotic, replacement may be necessary. Replacement of the mitral valve is done by direct visualization (open heart surgery). The type of valve used often depends on the size of the person's own valve and the preference of the surgeon. Currently mitral valves being used for valve replacement are composed either of a natural tissue (porcine valve from a pig's heart, Fig. 46-2) or of synthetic material such as silicone, stainless steel, or Dacron or Teflon. The artificial (mechanical) valves (Fig. 46-3) usually are either ball-in-cage devices or flat disk devices.

A person receiving a mechanical mitral valve is placed on long-term anticoagulant therapy postoperatively; when a porcine valve is used, anticoagulant therapy continues only for several months. Anticoagulants are used with persons who have artificial cardiac valves to prevent thrombus formation caused by turbulent blood flow around or through the valve itself or by red cell adhesion to the synthetic materials. Porcine valves, however, are made of natural tissue attached to a relatively small Dacron ring, and blood flow through them is similar to blood flow through a human valve.

Aortic valve. As symptoms of aortic valve stenosis-insufficiency become progressively worse, the person usually will need surgical correction. Surgery for aortic stenosis-insufficiency is done with the use of extracorporeal circulation (Fig. 45-18), which permits full visualization of the operative area. The aortic valve may be repaired by one of three methods: (1) calcium may be removed and the fused commissures may be opened, (2) the valve may be reconstructed by removing one cusp and rebuilding a valve consisting of only two cusps, or (3) the valve may be removed and a valve similar to one used for mitral valve replacement may be used.

Tricuspid valve. Rheumatic heart disease may involve the tricuspid valve in addition to involvement of the mitral and aortic valves. The severity of the tricuspid valve involvement and associated signs and symptoms determine whether tricuspid valve repair will be sufficient or whether replacement will be necessary. Tricuspid valve surgery may be performed by itself or in conjunction with surgery on other heart valves. A valvuloplasty may be done or the valve may be replaced, as with the mitral and aortic valves.

The care of the person undergoing valvular heart surgery is similar to that of those having other cardiac surgery (p. 973).

□ Outcome criteria for the person with valvular heart disease

The person or significant others can:

1. Explain required dietary changes including any sodium restrictions.
2. State name, purpose, dosage, frequency, and side effects of any medication therapy (digitalis, diuretics).
3. Describe a work, rest, and activity program to conserve energy.
4. Describe the rationale for and the type of surgery to be performed, if surgery is indicated.
5. State plans for medical follow-up including ongoing laboratory tests if required.

■ HYPERTENSIVE HEART DISEASE

Hypertensive heart disease refers to changes in the heart from prolonged sustained hypertension (p. 1048). The heart enlarges (seen on radiographic examination) as a result of the increased cardiac work load. If the underlying hypertension is untreated, cardiac failure (p. 1003) results.

■ ISCHEMIC HEART DISEASE

□ Epidemiology

Ischemic heart disease is the primary health problem of our times. Deaths from ischemic heart disease appear to be higher in the United States than in certain other countries, and it is believed that lesions leading to ischemic heart disease are developing at an earlier age. Ninety percent of the persons who develop symptoms of ischemic heart disease are between the ages of 40 and 70 years. The incidence is much higher in men than in women until the menopause is reached, when women quickly lose their immunity.

Although an enormous amount of research (both epidemiologic and in the laboratory) is being conducted in order to learn the cause of ischemic heart disease, at the present time the cause is unknown. Certain characteristics, however, have been singled out as being common in persons who have or who will develop coronary atherosclerosis:

1. Familial history of coronary artery disease
2. Elevated serum lipoproteins
3. Hypertension
4. Excessive cigarette smoking
5. Diabetes
6. Sedentary life pattern
7. Stressful, competitive life style
8. Elevated serum uric acid levels

Individuals who have most of these conditions are considered to be at high risk of coronary heart disease. These characteristics of the high-risk group have been studied intensively.

One of the most comprehensive studies conducted

(in Framingham, Mass., under the sponsorship of the National Heart Institute) attempted to outline the observations and determinations by which risk of heart attacks can be expected. These findings consider age, the level of serum cholesterol, blood pressure, ECG abnormalities, vital capacity, and cigarette smoking. The study showed the following. A man in his fifties has four times the risk of attack as a man in his thirties. A man with a serum cholesterol level above 240 mg/ml of blood has more than three times the risk of a man with a serum cholesterol level below 200 mg. An individual with systolic blood pressure greater than 160 has four times the risk of one with systolic pressure of less than 120. An individual with an ECG abnormality has two and one-half times the risk of one with a normal ECG. An individual with a low vital capacity has approximately twice the risk of one with a high vital capacity; and one who smokes has almost twice the risk of the nonsmoker.

□ Role of the nurse in detection

The nurse is often in a position to assess patients and to observe symptoms that may be significant in the detection of heart disease or may pick up clues of significant symptoms from details of family history. Frequently it is the alert nurse who can help persons with undiagnosed heart disease to obtain medical attention.

A fatalistic attitude about heart disease and a conviction that nothing can be done about heart attacks, which "just happen," prevent many persons from reporting early signs of heart disease to their physicians. Since early medical treatment could often prevent or delay progress of the condition, this is doubly unfortunate. Persons who are unfamiliar with the symptoms often ignore them or attribute them to some other cause. Many elderly persons hesitate to report symptoms because they believe that nothing can be done for them because of their age. Again this idea is very seldom accurate. A friendly interest on the part of the nurse and assurance that medical care can be helpful will often lead them to seek medical treatment.

□ Fear of ischemic heart disease

One of the biggest problems to be met in educating the public about heart disease is overcoming fear. Awareness of the fact that the heart is necessary to life makes most people view heart disease differently from diseases of other organs. Much of the publicizing of heart disease in magazine articles, television programs, and films depicts the fatality more than the control of the disease. Although public education measures are intended to motivate people to have physical examinations and to use discretion in eating, exercising, resting, not smoking, and checking symptoms with their physician, they create threats for some people. Some persons who are told that their symptoms are suggestive of heart disease often continue to worry when diagnostic tests prove nothing, and they cannot accept the fact that nothing is wrong. The person who has had one heart attack may live in fear of another and be prevented from resuming his place as a useful member of society. Others cannot find work because employers are afraid to hire them. Heart associations, health departments, and insurance companies spend large sums of money each year for educational publications on heart disease in an attempt to overcome these problems.

The nurse needs to face realistically any personal fear about heart disease before assistance can be given to patients and families. Helping others see the positive side of the picture, such as the fact that many who have heart attacks recover almost completely and are able to live relatively normal lives, also helps the nurse. The nurse should try to gain patients' cooperation in following medical advice, helping them to see how they themselves can participate in keeping well. Much of this ability stems from the nurse's own confidence in and a realistic approach to treatment of heart disease.

□ Prevention

Many of the risk factors of ischemic heart disease (p. 987) are preventable but involve habits or patterns of behavior that were developed in the younger years and persist during a lifetime. Poor habits well established are difficult to change, and coronary artery disease may be advanced when adulthood is reached. Prevention of ischemic heart disease therefore involves health education starting with young children and continuing into adulthood.

Diet

To date it has not been definitely proved that *any* food has *any* effect on the development of arteriosclerosis, atherosclerosis, and coronary artery disease. There are some facts or circumstances, however, that appear to indicate that there may be some relationship between diet and coronary artery disease: (1) the national dietary average for fat consumption is still very high in the United States, with approximately 50% of our dietary calories being derived from fats, (2) studies show that populations that consume low-fat diets generally have been found to have lower blood serum cholesterol levels than those consuming high-fat diets, and there seems to be a strong correlation between high-fat consumption and mortality from coronary heart disease, and (3) it is known that the atheromatous lesions of atherosclerosis contain free cholesterol, that certain dietary constituents have been found to increase the concentration of blood cholesterol, that blood cholesterol level is lowered when fats containing a high proportion of polyunsaturated fatty acids (especially linoleic acid) are substituted for the more saturated fats, and that a high-fat meal induces hypercoagulability of the blood for several hours.

Cholesterol in the body comes from two sources: it can be taken into the body directly in food or it can be manufactured by the liver and intestine. Approximately 0.8 g of cholesterol is manufactured by the liver each day. Cholesterol is involved in lipid transport and excreted with bile salts into the intestine to participate in the digestion and absorption of fats. The complex process by which cholesterol is manufactured, distributed, and eliminated is not very well understood, although it is widely believed that the inherited endocrine system plays a definite part because of its effect on the metabolic processes. Studies have shown that when a large amount of saturated fat is eaten, the cholesterol level in the blood tends to rise. When the saturated fats are replaced by polyunsaturated fats, the blood cholesterol level tends to fall. Some sources of polyunsaturated fat are corn, cottonseed, soy, and safflower oils and margarines incorporating these oils in liquid form. Oils that have been hydrogenated contain more saturated fat, as do coconut oil, butterfat, and animal fats.

Coronary risk is related to the plasma concentration of β-lipoproteins, which carry about two thirds of the total plasma cholesterol, and possibly to the concentration of pre-β-lipoproteins. The hyperlipoproteinemias have been classified on the basis of clinical and laboratory data into five types with recommendations for therapy.[35,60] The conditions may be primary (familial) or secondary to some other condition or process. The goal of therapy for the majority of patients is reduction of the rate of development of atherosclerosis. Some clinicians are urging that blood lipid testing be done periodically and that preventive therapy begin early in childhood.

The American Heart Association has endorsed a policy recommending some modification in diet for everyone: reducing the fat content of the diet from 40% to 50% of calories to about 35%; substituting polyunsaturated fat for saturated fat; and maintaining body weight at normal levels. Rigorous changes in diet are not recommended, and not all clinicians agree on the need for change on the basis of current evidence.

Smoking

Persons who smoke need to learn about the increased risk of ischemic heart disease in addition to the more well-known relationship to lung cancer. Health education should be aimed primarily at the preteen and teenager. If teenagers and young adults can be convinced not to smoke or to stop smoking, their risk will be lessened, and they would help by setting a good example for younger children. Nurses need to remember that they serve as role models for health to the general public.

Exercise

There is increasing evidence that exercise is important in the prevention of coronary artery disease and there is general agreement that regular moderate exercise contributes to good general health and better functioning of many body systems. Yet many people in the United States do not exercise at all. Teenagers should plan to obtain in young adulthood a somewhat modified form of the exercise they receive in the usual school activities. Our present way of life, in which we ride to work in automobiles, spend working hours sitting down in many cases, and then spend evenings sitting in front of a television set, may need modification to allow for more exercise.

Early medical attention

Nurses can help to prevent the development of serious heart disease by teaching the public the early signs of possible heart disease and by urging prompt referral to physicians when they occur. For example, attacks of shortness of breath or unexpected dyspnea on exertion, feelings of pressure in the chest, awakening in the night with consciousness of heart action or distress, and discomfort resembling indigestion that is relieved by sitting up are reasons to see a physician even though the cause may be found to be trivial. Most persons have read magazine articles about anginal attacks with pain. They should be taught that pain is *not* a common sign of coronary artery disease. Dyspnea and signs of cardiac decompensation occur much more often.

Some families in which a member has heart disease live in fear of a repeated heart attack, particularly because they realize that they do not know what to do in such an emergency. Some families find little consolation in being told to call an ambulance or the police or fire department, but if they also know the position in which to place the person and how to administer medication, they will react better in an actual emergency and possibly prevent additional cardiac damage.

□ Coronary artery disease

Coronary artery disease is caused by a narrowing or obstruction of the coronary arteries resulting in a reduction of blood supply to the myocardium. In most instances atherosclerosis and general arteriosclerosis cause the narrowing or obstruction in the coronary arteries. As atherosclerosis (p. 1028) develops, yellowish fatty material composed largely of cholesterol is gradually deposited as plaque along the walls of the arteries, causing them to become fibrotic, thick, calcified, and narrowed in their lumen. This condition may cause a temporary anoxia of the myocardium such as occurs in angina pectoris, or it may cause a complete obstruction of the blood supply to a portion of the myocardium such as occurs in myocardial infarction. The resultant damage to the heart muscle may cause severe cardiac complications such as congestive heart failure and arrhythmias, or it may cause cardiac standstill and immediate death. If the obstruction is only slight, the blood supply may not be reduced significantly and the disease may be asymptomatic. Autopsies on persons who died from other causes frequently show some obstruction in their coronary arteries.

Clinical picture

The major clinical manifestation of coronary artery disease is *angina pectoris*. Angina pectoris is a serious cardiac disorder. Although it is usually caused by atherosclerosis of the coronary vessels, the incidence of angina pectoris is high in persons with hypertension, diabetes mellitus, thromboangiitis obliterans, polycythemia vera, periarteritis nodosa, and aortic regurgitation due to syphilis or rheumatic heart disease. It is characterized by paroxysmal retrosternal or substernal pain, often radiating down the inner aspect of the left arm. The pain is often associated with exertion and is relieved through vasodilation of the coronary arteries by means of medication or by rest. It is believed to be caused by a temporary inadequacy of the blood supply in meeting the needs of the heart muscle. The location and severity of the pain vary greatly, but the same pattern recurs repeatedly in a given individual. The frequency and severity of the attacks usually increase over a period of years, and less and less exertion may cause pain. No matter how mild the attacks, they may be complicated at any time by acute myocardial infarction, cardiac standstill, or death. The diagnosis of angina pectoris may be confirmed by ECGs taken at rest, after exercise, or preferably during an attack. Cardiac catheterization also may be done.

Intervention

Treatment of the person with angina pectoris is based on the symptoms and is individualized for each patient. The success of the treatment in achieving a comfortable and worthwhile existence depends on education to live within limitations, being guided by the pain. The nurse as well as the physician should participate in the teaching program. Since the person often is not hospitalized, nurses outside of the hospital carry the major nursing responsibility for helping the person with angina pectoris. The individual is taught to cease effort immediately on experiencing pain and to rest for several minutes after the pain has subsided.

Medication. Nitroglycerine tablets placed under the tongue and allowed to dissolve in the saliva often relieve the pain by causing vasodilation of the coronary arteries. Usually tablets containing 0.4 mg (1/150 grain) of the drug are prescribed. Effects should be noticed in 2 or 3 minutes, but if pain persists the dose may be repeated two or three times at 5-minute intervals. Some persons use nitroglycerine prophylactically when they have no choice but to undertake some activity that usually causes pain. The action lasts for about 1/2 hour.

Other nitrate preparations are available, but most persons prefer nitroglycerine because it is less expensive and causes fewer side effects. Perles of *amyl nitrite* come in 3-ml doses and are preferred by some persons because the action is immediate. The perle is crushed into a handkerchief, and it should be inhaled no more than three times. Pentaerythritol tetranitrate (Peritrate) is a long-acting preparation that is taken twice daily. One tablet is taken on arising and another 12 hours later. Isosorbide dinitrate (Isordil) is another nitrite prescribed and is available in sustained-release tablets, which last 12 hours. Nitrate preparations cause flushing of the skin because of capillary dilation. The pulse and respirations increase, and the blood pressure may fall slightly. Many persons develop severe headaches from the use of nitrates. This difficulty can usually be overcome by decreasing the dosage.

The person with angina pectoris should always carry a nitrate preparation with him. He may use it freely, since the effects do not decrease with usage and it is not habit forming. Many individuals are reluctant to use the medication for various reasons and must be encouraged to do so by careful discussion of their objections to it.

Diet. Frequently a low-cholesterol diet is prescribed. If the person is overweight, a low-caloric diet may be prescribed. The physician may suggest that the person drink 15 to 30 ml (1/2 to 1 oz) of brandy or whiskey several times a day to dilate the blood vessels. Physicians usually advise the avoidance of smoking since nicotine has a vasoconstrictive effect. If the attacks of anginal pain are precipitated by eating, six small meals taken at evenly spaced intervals, rather than three average meals, may give relief.

Activity. Most persons with angina pectoris can tolerate mild exercise such as walking and playing golf, but exertion such as running, climbing hills or stairs rapidly, and lifting heavy objects causes pain. The pain is likely to be evoked more easily in cold weather, since the vessels normally constrict to conserve body heat. When the person with angina pectoris must be exposed to the cold, he should err on the side of being too warmly clothed. It is unwise to sleep in a cold room, and walking against the wind and uphill should be avoided because these activities increase the work load of the heart and cause pain.

Emotional adjustment. Since excessive emotional strain also causes vasoconstriction by releasing epinephrine into the circulation, emotional outbursts, worry, and tension should be minimized. The person may need continuing help in accepting situations as he finds them. The family, the spiritual adviser, business associates, and friends can sometimes help. An optimistic outlook helps to relieve the work of the heart. Many persons who learn to live within their limitations live out their expected life span in spite of the disease. Helping a person adjust to living with this disease can be most rewarding for the individual, the family, the physician, and the nurse. Fear of impending catastrophe is almost a characteristic of anginal pain, and many persons believe each episode of pain is a "heart attack"; therefore reassurance and education are extremely important.

Surgery. If cardiac catheterization has been performed and severe narrowing of one or more branches of the coronary arteries exists, coronary artery bypass surgery may be recommended as a prophylactic measure. The purpose of coronary artery bypass (jump graft) surgery is to increase blood flow to the myocardium (myocardial revascularization). Many persons show marked improvement after this surgery and usually do not require nitrates to maintain relief of symptoms.

The surgical technique varies somewhat among surgeons, and some surgeons routinely use extracorporeal circulation during the operation, while others do not. When the saphenous vein is used for the graft, one end is sutured to the aorta and the other end is sutured to the coronary artery distal to the occlusion (Fig. 46-4). When an internal mammary artery is used, the distal end of this vessel is freed from the anterior chest wall and sutured in place distal to the occlusion in the coronary artery (Fig. 46-5). Coronary bypass surgery is performed on the right coronary artery (RCA), the left anterior descending (LAD) artery, and the circumflex coronary artery (CCA) and their major branches. The care of the person undergoing coronary artery surgery is similar to that of those having other cardiac surgery (Chapter 45, p. 973).

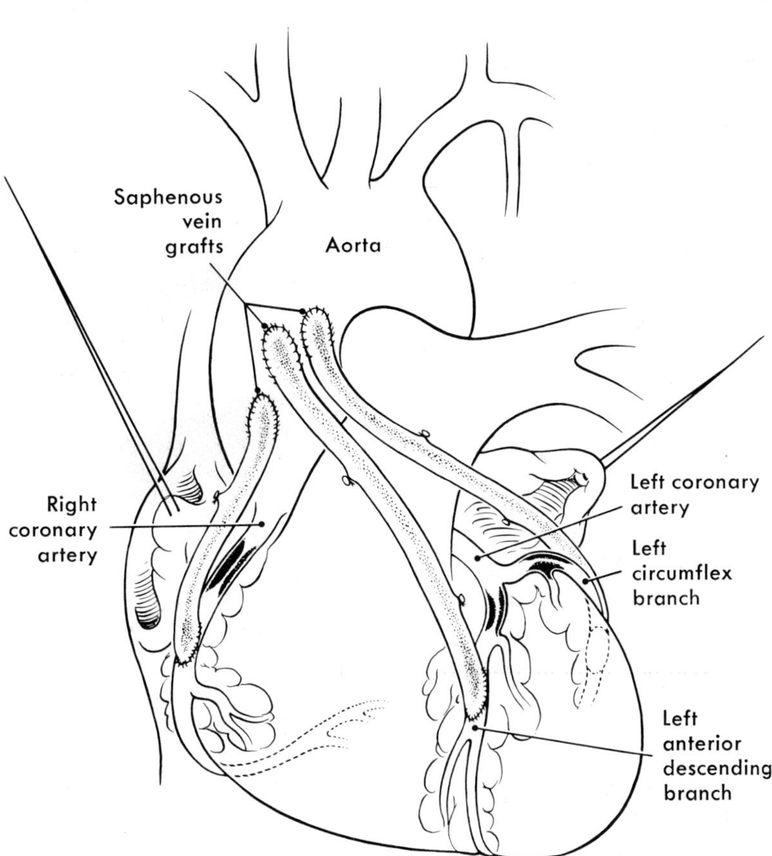

Fig. 46-4. Triple coronary bypass in which all grafts were from saphenous veins. (Many surgeons use combination of internal mammary artery and saphenous vein grafts when performing double or triple bypass procedures.)

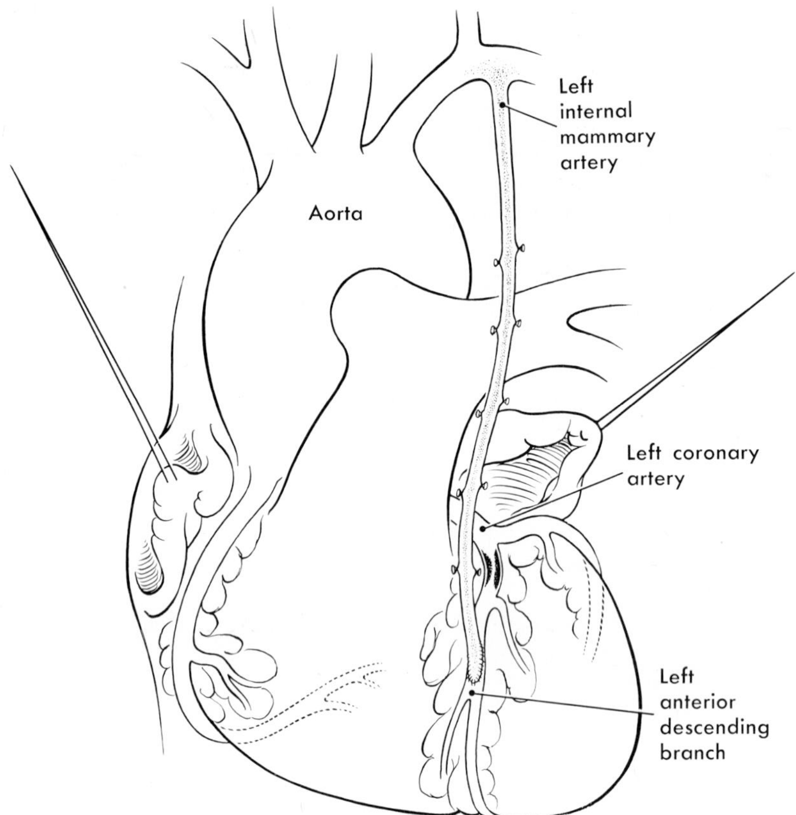

Fig. 46-5. Single coronary bypass in which left internal mammary artery has been used to bypass obstruction. Saphenous vein also may be used.

□ Myocardial infarction

Acute myocardial infarction is caused by sudden blockage of one of the branches of a coronary artery. It may be extensive enough to interfere with cardiac function and cause immediate death, or it may cause necrosis of a portion of the myocardium with subsequent healing by scar formation or fibrosis. *Coronary occlusion* is a general term for blockage of a coronary artery. The blockage may be due to formation of a thrombus in the coronary artery *(coronary thrombosis)*, sudden progression of atherosclerotic changes, or prolonged constriction of the arteries.

Of the 738,171 deaths from heart disease in 1974, 45% were attributed to acute myocardial infarction.[123] There are indications that the death rate from myocardial infarction may be leveling off in white men. From 1968 to 1972 the death rate dropped 8.7%, from 441 deaths per 100,000 persons to 427 deaths per 100,000 persons. The rates also appear to be declining for black men. Although the reason for this decrease has not been proved, some clinicians believe that it is related to a decrease in smoking by American men since the 1950s.

Acute myocardial infarction is the most common cardiac emergency. The mortality for a first attack is about 20%, although this percentage is decreased to 15% or less when patients are cared for in well-run coronary care units that are equipped to handle the slightest change in the patient's condition.[6]

The prognosis of a patient who has had an acute myocardial infarction is always guarded until about 4 weeks after the attack. There is a danger of such complications as pulmonary or systemic embolism, cardiac rupture, cardiac standstill, ventricular fibrillation, irreversible shock, and acute pulmonary edema. The first 2 weeks are considered the most dangerous, and patients who survive the third week usually recover from the attack.[6] The degree of residual disability cannot be predicted, however, and some patients are permanently incapacitated with severe angina pectoris or congestive heart failure. Many patients may return to normal or near normal activity, and perhaps 60% to 80% of patients who have recovered can return to some employment. The convalescent period for most persons following a coronary occlusion is 2 to 3 months.

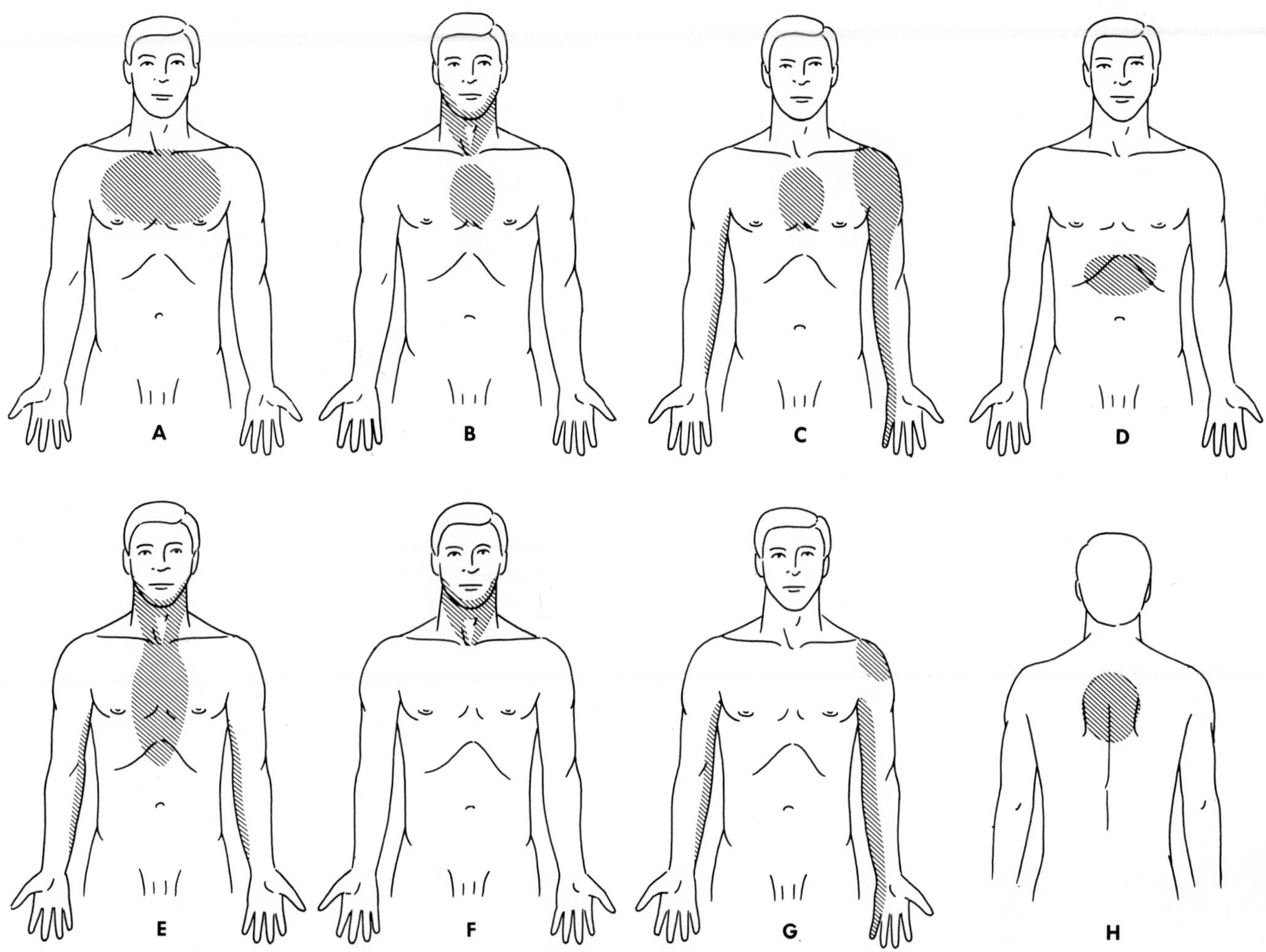

Fig. 46-6. Sites where ischemic myocardial pain may be referred. **A,** Upper chest. **B,** Beneath sternum radiating to neck and jaw. **C,** Beneath sternum radiating down left arm. **D,** Epigastric. **E,** Epigastric radiating to neck and jaw. **F,** Neck and jaw. **G,** Left shoulder, inner aspect of both arms. **H,** Intrascapular.

Clinical picture

The individual typically complains of sudden, severe, crushing or viselike pain in the substernal region. This pain may radiate into the left and sometimes the right arm and up the sides of the neck (Fig. 46-6). At other times it may simulate indigestion or a gallbladder attack with abdominal pain. The person often becomes restless, gets up and paces about the room, throws open the windows, or has a sudden urge to have a bowel movement. He often feels that he is dying, and his skin becomes ashen and clammy. He may become short of breath and cyanotic and show signs of severe shock. The pulse is usually rapid, and it may be barely perceptible. The blood pressure usually falls, and the patient may collapse. The symptoms of cardiogenic shock occur as a result of inadequate cardiac output from inadequate pumping.

To confirm the diagnosis, the blood sedimentation rate and the enzyme levels (SGOT, SGPT, LDH, CPK) of the blood serum are determined, and an ECG is made. The ECG may show no changes for several days but then usually shows changes indicative of a myocardial infarction. These changes include the appearance of large Q waves, elevated S-T segments, and inverted T waves. The blood sedimentation rate and enzyme levels are elevated, and the blood cholesterol level often is elevated.

In the acute period, nursing assessment includes data obtained through *inspection* (identification of cyanosis), *palpation* (determination of peripheral pulses and edema), and *auscultation* (identification of clearly audible breath sounds, apical pulse, and blood pressure). Nursing assessment also includes identification of normal and abnormal cardiac rhythms on the cardiac monitor (p. 995). All of the data obtained are then recorded and reported for use by all members of the health team. Within the first 24 hours the temperature may become slightly elevated, and leukocytosis occurs. It is unusual for the temperature to be over 38.5 C (101 F), and any further elevation should be reported to the physician because it may be caused by a complication such as a pulmonary infarction. The fever and leukocytosis are normal reactions to tissue necrosis.

Intervention

Acute phase. The outcomes of therapy during the acute phase of myocardial infarction include relief of chest pain or discomfort and relief of dyspnea. This is accomplished by providing the person with physical and mental rest and preventing complications such as arrhythmias, cardiac rupture, congestive heart failure, and shock. Currently most persons with acute myocardial infarction are admitted to a coronary care unit (CCU) for at least the first 48 to 72 hours where they can be closely monitored. The damaged heart may be able to maintain basal activity, but additional strain may cause it to fail and cardiopulmonary resuscitation (CPR) (p. 963) may be necessary. Measures are instituted to prevent shock.

Physical and mental rest. Usually the person is bathed, shaved, and assisted in most activities. Many persons react to this routine with tension, anxiety, and resentment. Explanations as to the reasons for this care as well as explanations of procedures are helpful in gaining the person's cooperation, relieving anxiety, and providing rest. A calm, unhurried atmosphere should be provided. "Armchair care" (p. 965) may be ordered. The length of time the person is kept on bed rest varies. Some physicians order strict bed rest for a week or more, while others allow their patients up for commode privileges within a few days. If the patient has no complications, he may gradually resume normal activities. During this period collateral circulation has had a chance to develop, and the necrotic tissue in the myocardium has healed, forming a fibrotic scar.

Since the person who has a myocardial infarction is quite likely to be in the prime of life and to have become suddenly ill, it can be anticipated that the person may have many worries and concerns related to the work situation and to the family. It is often better for the person to be allowed to make some arrangements or at least be told what arrangements are being made. The family, a business associate, or the social service worker may be able to give help needed so that the person can be more relaxed. The decision in this regard, however, is the physician's, who sometimes orders sedation for the person who seems exceedingly upset over business or personal matters.

Medications. The physician usually orders morphine sulfate or meperidine hydrochloride (Demerol) to be given at frequent intervals until the pain is relieved. If the patient complains of dyspnea, is cyanotic, or has severe pain, oxygen usually is given. If pain continues, the physician may order theophylline ethylenediamine (aminophylline) or papaverine hydrochloride. Since both of these drugs relax smooth muscle, they help to dilate the coronary vessels. Positioning the patient to relieve pain and facilitate breathing (semi-Fowler's position) may also be helpful.

To decrease the possibility either of further extension of the thrombus or of embolic complications, the person who has had a myocardial infarction may be given an anticoagulant such as bishydroxycoumarin (Dicumarol) for 3 or 4 weeks. While the person is receiving anticoagulants the physician will order a periodic prothrombin time determination. The dosage of the anticoagulant is based on this determination. The prothrombin time is maintained at approximately 30 seconds, or 10% of normal.[6] If the prothrombin time should drop below 10%, there is danger that the person will bleed profusely from minor cuts such as shaving nicks or from gum injuries sustained while brushing his teeth. Hematuria may also occur. Any signs of excessive or unusual bleeding are reported to the physician. If bleeding should occur, the patient may be given vitamin K preparations or a small blood transfusion. Other medications with anticoagulant properties such as aspirin should not be taken by the person without physician approval.

Recovery phase. The myocardial necrosis usually heals within 6 weeks; therefore the person may be told to remain on limited activity for the duration of this period. The program varies with each person. Hill and stair climbing are usually among the last activities permitted because they add to the work load of the heart substantially. Walking is considered a desirable exercise, and increased distances can be walked daily. This activity also helps to combat the weakness and fatigue that result from muscle disuse. However, a person may be allowed to do too much for himself and to return to activity too quickly because he appears to be quite well. His appearance may also make it more difficult for the family to comprehend fully the seriousness of the situation and the very real possibility of repeated attacks or death for the person who does not respect his condition and live in moderation both physically and emotionally. A person recovering from an acute myocardial infarction may also needlessly be made an invalid for the rest of his life. Since there is evidence that exercise is beneficial in myocardial disease, return to work may be much better for the person than a long period of enforced inactivity and leisure. It has been found that more myocardial infarctions occur during leisure hours than at work.[21]

The person and his family should be instructed before discharge concerning appropriate activities, how to follow a pattern of living in moderation, and how to recognize when activity or emotional strain is too great. Sexual activity also should be discussed, and persons need to know that gradual return to their usual sexual activity is encouraged. The person should know that if any further symptoms occur rest is of prime importance and that the physician should be contacted at once. The person should remain under close medical supervision.

☐ Outcome criteria for the person with ischemic heart disease

The patient or significant others can:

1. Identify changes required in physical activity:
   a. Describe limitations recommended by physician.
   b. Describe plans for resumption of permitted activities.
   c. Perform activities of daily living in a manner that conserves energy.
2. Identify necessary dietary requirements:
   a. Describe own nutritional habits.
   b. Plan modified-cholesterol menus.
   c. State name, purpose, dosage, frequency, and side effects of medication (nitrates, anticoagulants).
   d. State plans for follow-up care including signs and symptoms indicating need for immediate care.

■ CARDIAC ARRHYTHMIAS

The rhythm of the heartbeat is usually regular but may vary under certain circumstances. These variations may be a normal physiologic response, may have no clinical importance, or may be a symptom or a complication of organic heart disease (Table 46-1). Although some arrhythmias do not cause hemodynamic consequences, many produce noticeable sensations, which may cause apprehension. The person may describe a "flutter" in the chest or a "turning over," "pounding," or "palpitation" of the heart. Some persons feel that their hearts have "skipped a beat." The pulse may be very rapid, irregular, or very slow. The above sensations are less likely to occur with slow pulse rates.

Persons with abnormal heart rates or rhythms should be urged to seek medical attention. If after thorough examination the physician finds nothing organically wrong, the person should be urged to live normally.

Cardiac irregularities in persons hospitalized with organic heart disease should be reported to the physician immediately, since they may become incompatible with life. The pulse rate of a hospitalized patient with cardiac disease should be noted for any marked increase or decrease in the rate, the presence of alternating strong and weak beats *(pulsus alternans)*, coupling of beats (two together followed by a pause), or other irregularities in the rhythm. Abnormal rates and rhythm in a person with heart disease often mean that the left ventricle is not pumping adequate blood into the systemic circulation to take care of body needs. Congestive heart failure may then occur.

Desired outcomes of therapy for persons experiencing a cardiac arrhythmia include improvement in signs and symptoms and a regular resting heart rate between 60 and 100 beats per minute.

☐ Cardiac monitors

It is becoming more common that nurses in general hospitals encounter cardiac monitors. As intensive cardiac care units are established, this equipment becomes concentrated in one area staffed by specialized personnel; however, a staff nurse on a general patient unit may be expected to care for a patient on a cardiac monitor. It is therefore necessary for the nurse to know the purpose of the monitor and how to recognize the various cardiac rhythms displayed on the screen. This section will deal *briefly* with the common arrhythmias. Since the care of persons with cardiac arrhythmias is complex, the general review that follows is not sufficient for persons with primary responsibility for monitored patients in an intensive care setting. For further study the reader is referred to more specialized texts.[3]

As described in Chapter 43, an ECG tracing usually consists of five major wave deflections: P, Q, R, S, and T. These deflections are recorded on graph paper, with the vertical lines measuring time (Fig. 43-4). On the time axis each small square represents 0.04 second; the time between the heavy lines is 0.20 second. On the voltage axis each small square represents 0.1 mV.

In interpreting an ECG tracing it is helpful to approach each tracing systematically. One suggested approach is to determine in the following order the (1) rate, (2) rhythm, (3) occurrence of a P wave, (4) PR interval, (5) QRS interval, (6) relationship of QRS to P wave, and (7) QT interval. A normal sinus rhythm (Fig. 43-4) has a rate of 60 to 100, a regular rhythm (regular RR intervals) with P waves before each QRS, a PR interval of 0.12 to 0.2 second, and a QRS interval of 0.06 to 0.1 second. There are several methods of determining the rate:

1. Count the number of beats in a 6-inch ECG strip (a 6-second interval); multiply by 10. This method is used for a regular heart rhythm.
2. Count the number of *small* squares between two heart beats (RR interval); divide 1,500 by this number.
3. Count the number of *large* squares between two

Table 46-1. Comparison of cardiac arrhythmias

Arrhythmia	Description	Etiology	Symptoms/consequences	Treatment
Sinus tachycardia	P waves present followed by QRS Rhythm regular Heart rate 100 to 150	Increased metabolic demands Decreased oxygen delivery: CHF, shock, hemorrhage, anemia	May produce palpitations Prolonged episodes may lead to decreased cardiac output	Treat underlying cause Occasionally sedatives
Sinus bradycardia	P waves present Rhythm regular Heart rate less than 60	Physical fitness Parasympathetic stimulation (sleep) Brain lesions Digitalis excess	Very low rates may cause decreased cardiac output; light-headedness, faintness, chest pain	Atropine if cardiac output is decreased Pacemaker
Complete heart block	Atria and ventricles beat independently P waves have no relation to QRS Heart rate 20 to 40	Digitalis toxicity Infectious disease Coronary artery disease Myocardial infarction	Very low rates may cause decreased cardiac output: light-headedness, faintness, chest pain	Pacemaker Isoproterenol to increase heart rate
Premature atrial beats	Early P wave followed by normal QRS Rhythm irregular	Stress, ischemia, atrial enlargement, caffeine, nicotine	May produce palpitations Frequent episodes may decrease cardiac output Is sign of chamber irritability	Sedation Quinidine
Premature ventricular beats	Early wide bizarre QRS, not associated with a P wave Rhythm irregular	Stress, acidosis, ventricular enlargement Electrolyte imbalance Drug toxicity (digitalis, quinidine) Hypoxemia, hypercapnia	Same as PAB	Procainamide (Pronestyl) Lidocaine Oxygen Sodium bicarbonate Potassium Treat CHF
Atrial fibrillation	Rapid, irregular waves (over 350/min) Ventricular rhythm irregularly irregular Heart rate varies, may be increased to 150 to 170/min	Rheumatic heart disease Mitral stenosis Atrial infarction	Pulse deficit Decreased cardiac output if rate is rapid Promotes thrombus formation in atria	Digitalis Quinidine Cardioversion
Ventricular fibrillation	Chaotic electrical activity No recognizable QRS complex	Myocardial infarction Electrocution Freshwater drowning Drug toxicity	No cardiac output Absent pulse or respiration Cardiac arrest	Defibrillation Epinephrine Sodium bicarbonate
Ventricular standstill	Can only be distinguished from ventricular fibrillation by ECG P waves *may* be present No QRS "Straight line"	Myocardial infarction Chronic diseases of conducting system	Same as ventricular fibrillation	CPR Pacemaker Intracardiac epinephrine

heart beats (RR interval); divide 300 by this number.

When there are differences in the RR interval, the rhythm is irregular. Analysis of the other parameters may indicate the mechanism of this irregularity.

When the patient is being monitored, the nurse is responsible for regular patient care, attention to the patterns on the monitor, and special care of the electrode areas on the patient's chest to provide clear monitor patterns and to prevent skin irritation. The electrodes should be removed and the areas washed and dried at least once every 24 hours or as recommended by the manufacturer. The electrode paste and electrodes can then be reapplied (Fig. 46-7) and the patient reattached to the monitor. The electrode site usually is changed daily to avoid skin irritation.

□ Sinus tachycardia

Sinus tachycardia is the most common cardiac rhythm disturbance of the heart (Fig. 46-8). It is a normal physiologic reaction to exercise, fever, fear, excitement or any other condition in which the basal metabolism is increased, thus necessitating a greater supply of blood.

Clinical picture

The heart rate in sinus tachycardia is greater than 100 beats per minute, usually in the 101 to 150 range. This arrhythmia is common in patients with anemia, rheumatic fever, hyperthyroidism, congestive heart failure, and hemorrhage. The person may be unaware of the accelerated heart rate or may complain of palpitations.

Usual ECG manifestations of sinus tachycardia include a heart rate greater than 100 with normal P wave, PR interval, and QRS duration. The ST segment and T wave may or may not be normal.

Intervention

The physician may order sedatives to relieve annoying symptoms. When the underlying cause is corrected, the heart rate returns to normal. If this condition is allowed to persist, heart failure may result.

□ Sinus bradycardia

A slow heart rate is common in young adult men and in trained athletes. Bradycardia also normally occurs during sleep. It may also occur in patients with brain lesions and in patients receiving digitalis because of the drug's action in slowing the heart rate.

Clinical picture

In sinus bradycardia (Fig. 46-9) the heart rate falls below 60 beats per minute. Patients may complain of fatigue or light-headedness. The ECG should show a normal tracing except for heart rate.

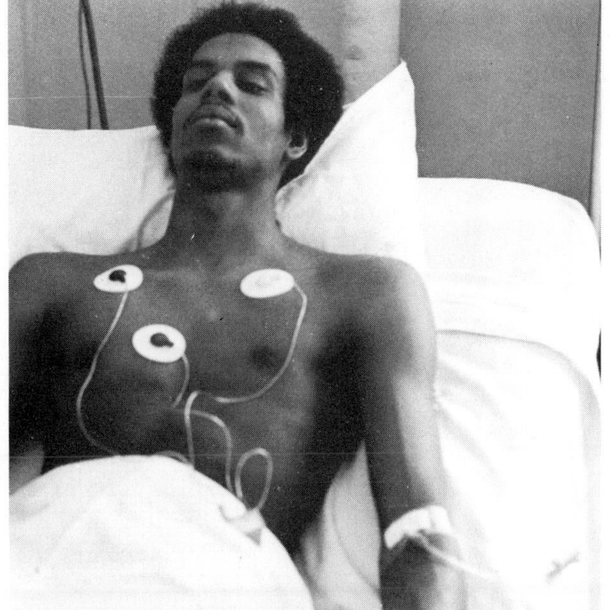
A

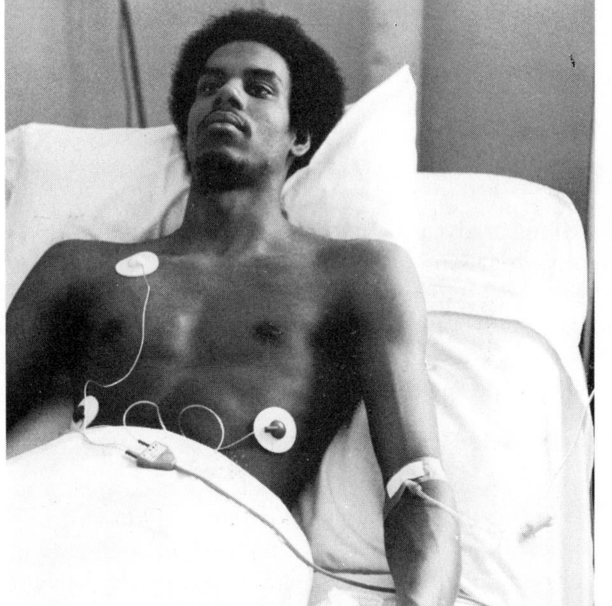
B

Fig. 46-7. A, Placement of ECG electrodes on anterior chest wall for lead V_1. Grounding electrode is on upper right chest, negative electrode on upper left chest (midclavicular line), and positive electrode on right fourth intercostal space (sternal border). **B,** Placement of ECG electrodes on anterior chest wall for lead II. Grounding electrode is on lower right chest, positive electrode on lower left chest (anterior axillary lines), and negative electrode on upper right chest (midclavicular line).

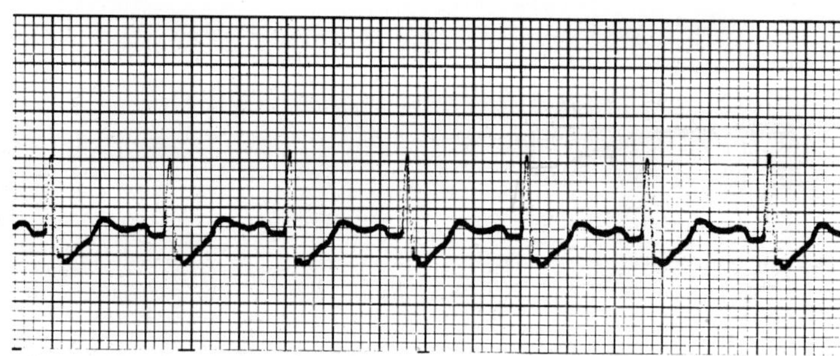

Fig. 46-8. Sinus tachycardia. Lead II showing heart rate of 115, regular rhythm, normal PR interval, and normal QRS duration.

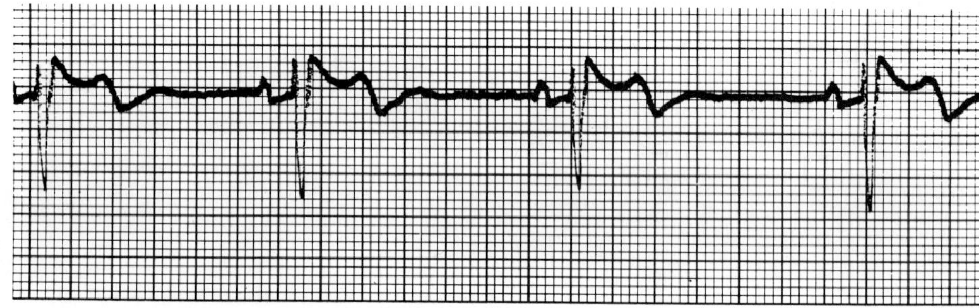

Fig. 46-9. Sinus bradycardia. Lead V_1 showing heart rate of approximately 44, regular rhythm, normal PR interval, and normal QRS duration.

Intervention

Sinus bradycardia may not require treatment. If a patient is receiving a digitalis preparation, withdrawal of the medication should allow the heart rate to return to normal. Other methods of therapy include treating the underlying cause, giving medication such as atropine, or artificially pacing the patient's heart.

□ Heart block - see chart p 996

In atrioventricular (AV) heart block, normal stimuli arise in the sinoatrial node, but they are blocked or delayed on their way through the AV junction. This may occur occasionally without evidence of organic heart disease or in digitalis toxicity, infectious diseases, coronary artery disease, and myocardial infarction.

The passage of a stimulus from its point of initiation in the right atrium to the ventricles normally takes less than 0.2 second. If there is any interference in its passage, the ventricles are not stimulated when expected, and thus a heart block has occurred. It may be only partial or it may be complete.

Clinical picture

The person with complete AV heart block may have no symptoms once the block is established because, although no impulses from the atria reach the ventricles, the ventricles have adjusted by setting up their own rate. However, this rate is usually very slow (20 to 40 beats per min), and the person may become dyspneic or light-headed from even minimal exertion.

Intervention

This syndrome may be treated by giving isoproterenol hydrochloride (Isuprel) tablets, 10 to 15 mg, administered sublingually. Isoproterenol has a stimulating effect on the heart, resulting in an increased ventricular rate and improvement of blood circulation. When the block is due to an acute inflammatory disorder as in acute rheumatic fever, steroids may be given. There is some evidence that steroids given intravenously may promote normal conduction in persons with acute myocardial infarction who develop heart block. Heart block in a person with arteriosclerosis or a myocardial infarction is indicative of progressive heart damage.[6]

Often a person with heart block will require use of a pacemaker to increase the heart rate. The artificial pacemaker is an electrically operated mechanical device that electronically stimulates atrial or ventricular heart action, but is used most often in the ventricles.[46] It can be adjusted to stimulate the ventricular contractions

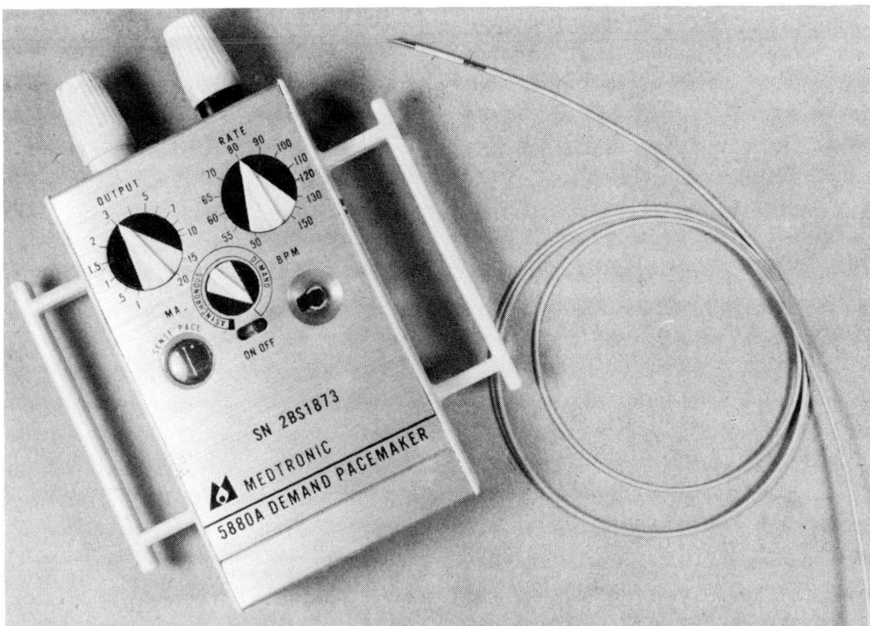

Fig. 46-10. Temporary (external) pacemaker. Pulse generator is battery powered. Electrode is passed into heart before being attached to pulse generator.

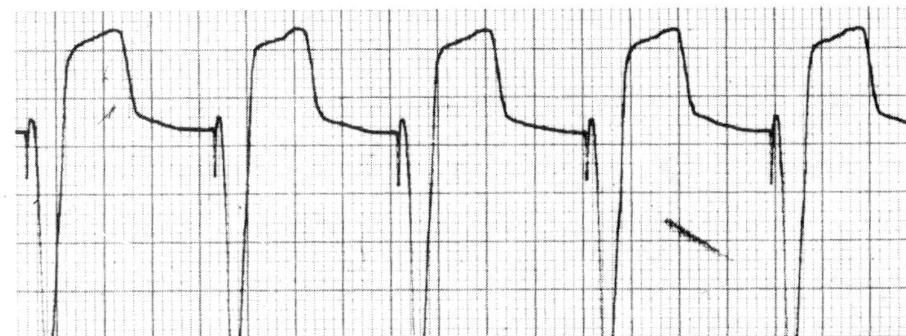

Fig. 46-11. Pacemaker ECG (lead V_1). Rate is 78, rhythm regular, QRS complex wide, no P waves visible, pacing stimulus (spike) precedes each QRS.

either constantly and at a normal rate or only when normal impulses are not forthcoming or fall below a rate set by the physician. There are both temporary and permanent pacemakers. In temporary pacing the pulse generator is usually located externally in a self-contained battery (Fig. 46-10). In permanent pacing the pulse generator is implanted subcutaneously. The pacemaker may be used as an emergency measure in event of sudden heart block, as a safety measure following cardiac surgery, or in medical illness when it is suspected that heart block may occur.

In temporary pacing there are several methods of placing an electrode in the heart. Usually an electrode catheter is inserted through an antecubital, external jugular, or subclavian vein and passed into the superior vena cava, the right atrium, the tricuspid valve, and then the right ventricle. The electrodes or pacing catheter then are connected to the external pulse generator.

Pacing wires also may be placed in the myocardium at the time of surgery and connected by wires brought out through the skin to the external pacemaker. The ECG of a patient with a pacemaker will show the pacing stimulus (Fig. 46-11).

The maintenance and operation of the external pacemaker is the responsibility of the physician, but the nurse must understand its use and be able to care for the patient when it is used. In addition to providing general nursing care, the nurse must continually assess functioning of the pacemaker and safety of the patient and prevent avoidable complications. Assessment includes inspecting the catheter insertion site for irritation or infection, inspecting the pulse generator and electrode ter-

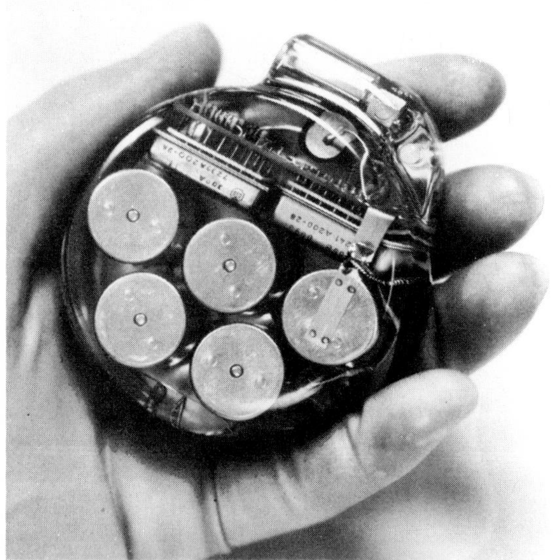

Fig. 46-12. Implantable pacemaker (pulse generator). Unit is implanted subcutaneously and then attached to electrode in contact with myocardium. (Courtesy Cordis Corp., Miami, Fla.)

minals to be certain that insulation is intact, identifying that the pulse generator is attached to the patient so as to prevent disconnection of the electrodes, and identifying the pacing stimulus on the cardiac monitor and ECG. Prevention of avoidable complications includes support of the extremity (if the pulse generator is attached there) to prevent external rotation that can displace the electrode, prevention of infection, and identification and immediate reporting of any pacemaker malfunction. The nurse also should reinforce information given by the physician as well as provide emotional support to the patient.

External pacemakers are unsatisfactory for long-term use because infection will ascend along the electrode wires. Several types of implantable (internal) pacemakers are available. One type uses mercury cells as its source of power and is estimated to last 5 years.[24] Another type of implantable pacemaker is a tiny, self-contained, transistorized unit measuring 6 cm in diameter and 1.5 cm in thickness (Fig. 46-12).

A transvenous approach is now common for the insertion of a permanent pacemaker. A catheter (wire) is inserted into the external jugular vein and advanced under fluoroscopy to the right ventricle where it is wedged in place. The distal end of the wire is connected to the subclavicular pacemaker (pulse generator) by means of a subcutaneous tunnel. Generally pacemakers deliver from 2 to 9 V to the heart muscle at regular intervals and may last for as long as 5 years. Batteries or cells can be replaced without disturbing the electodes by making a small surgical opening in the tissue directly over the pacemaker.

Any person who uses an internal pacemaker should have careful medical and nursing supervision. If the person returns home, referral to the community health nursing agency is often needed. Many persons do surprisingly well with this seemingly complicated form of treatment; however, any part of the equipment may act as a foreign body and cause local or systemic reaction. The person who develops any pain or tenderness at the point of insertion or of attachment of any piece of the equipment, or who develops an elevation of temperature or any other general symptoms should be advised to contact the physician at once.

Outcome criteria for the person with an internal pacemaker

The person or significant others can:

1. Describe the purpose and function of the pacemaker.
2. Describe plans for resuming normal life activities.
3. Carry an identification card with the type of pacemaker, rate, milliamperage, manufacturer, model number, and physician's telephone number.
4. Describe plans for follow-up care:
   a. State need for regular medical visits.
   b. Describe signs requiring immediate medical attention (pain or tenderness at point of insertion, fever, pulse rate below or double the preset rate).

□ Ventricular and atrial premature beats

When an atrial or ventricular beat occurs before the next expected excitation, it is called a premature beat (Fig. 46-13). The irregularity in rhythm of both the atria and the ventricles gives similar symptoms, but atrial premature beats occur more often in young persons, whereas ventricular premature beats occur more often in older persons. The person is often aware of the irregularity, complaining of palpitation and "flutter." This premature beat may occur only occasionally, it may occur in a regular pattern, or there may be several beats in sequence. Atrial and ventricular arrhythmias may be of no significance, or they may be associated with organic heart diseases such as mitral stenosis and coronary artery disease. Isolated premature atrial beats (PABs) may occur in normal persons. Frequent PABs indicate atrial irritability and may forewarn of a more serious arrhythmia such as atrial tachycardia or atrial fibrillation.

Occasional premature ventricular beats (PVBs) are usually not clinically significant. Frequent PVBs indicate irritability of the myocardium and must be treated to avoid ventricular tachycardia or fibrillation, which may

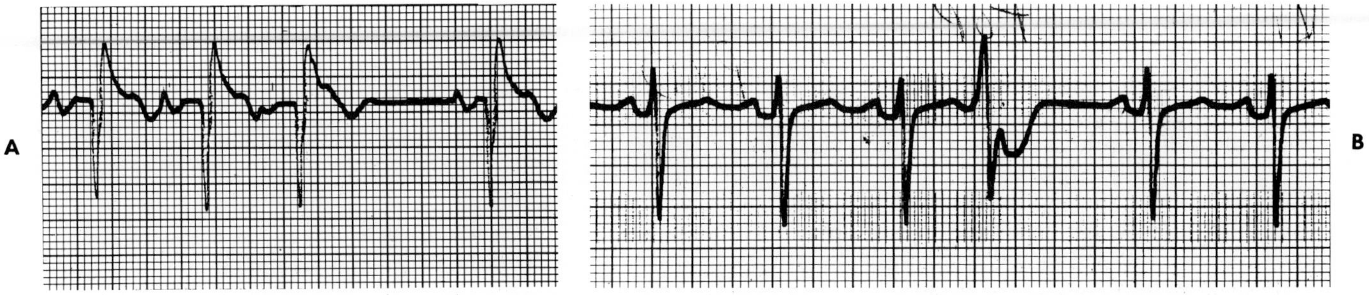

Fig. 46-13. A, Premature atrial beat. Lead V_1 showing third beat is premature atrial beat with abnormal, early P wave followed by normal QRS complex. **B,** Premature ventricular beat. Lead V_1 showing fourth beat is premature ventricular beat with wide, early QRS complex, no P wave associated with beat, and ST segment T wave going in opposite direction of main part of QRS.

lead to cardiogenic shock and death from inadequate cardiac output.

Irregularities seen in ECG tracings are depicted in Fig. 46-13, *A* and *B*.

Intervention

The treatment of PABs may include sedation along with quinidine or procainamide (Pronestyl). Treatment may also include the use of quinidine, procainamide, and lidocaine (Xylocaine) to decrease myocardial irritability in addition to correcting the underlying cause.

□ Paroxysmal tachycardia

Paroxysmal tachycardia may be either atrial or ventricular in origin. Atrial paroxysmal tachycardia is seen more frequently in young people, and ventricular paroxysmal tachycardia, a more serious problem, is seen more frequently in older persons. An attack of atrial tachycardia may be precipitated by stress; the consumption of large amounts of alcohol, caffeine, or nicotine; hyperthyroidism; or enlargement of the atrial chamber. Ventricular tachycardia is more likely to be associated with underlying organic heart disease or drug toxicity.

Clinical picture

Paroxysmal tachycardias are characterized by a sudden onset of rapid, regular heartbeats. The rate frequently increases to over 150 beats per minute. The person complains of palpitations and flutter of the heart, feels weak and faint, and is short of breath and apprehensive.

Intervention

Persons often arrest attacks of atrial paroxysmal tachycardia by holding their breath, bending forward, or pressing on the carotid sinuses. The latter is dangerous and should be done with caution. If the attack persists over an extended period of time, the person is put to bed, and the physician may order digitalization and sedation. The treatment of ventricular paroxysmal tachycardia is lidocaine administered intravenously. If ineffective, procainamide hydrochloride (Pronestyl), which also decreases the irritability of the ventricular myocardium, may be given. If given intravenously it must be given very slowly, and the blood pressure must be taken as it is administered. If hypotension occurs, the rate of administration must be slowed down. If drug treatment fails, conversion of this arrhythmia by electrical means must be considered, particularly if the person exhibits signs of decreased cardiac output. If untreated this condition can lead to ventricular fibrillation and death.

□ Fibrillation

Atrial fibrillation is a common irregularity of cardiac rhythm (Fig. 46-14). It usually is associated with organic heart diseases such as rheumatic heart disease and mitral stenosis. The sinus node no longer controls the rhythm of the heart, the atria no longer contract in coordination, and there is a complete irregularity of the ventricular beats. The atria may initiate as many as 400 to 600 stimuli per minute, but the ventricles rarely contract more than 130 to 150 times per minute, since not all the stimuli are carried through the AV junction and the ventricles do not respond to all the impulses that are sent through. When the ventricle contracts, various amounts of blood are pumped into the aorta. At times there is a small cardiac output, and not enough blood is pumped into the aorta with each beat to produce radial pulsation. This produces a *pulse deficit* (the difference between the apical pulse and the radial pulse). The pulse deficit represents wasted cardiac energy.

In *ventricular fibrillation* the coordinated contrac-

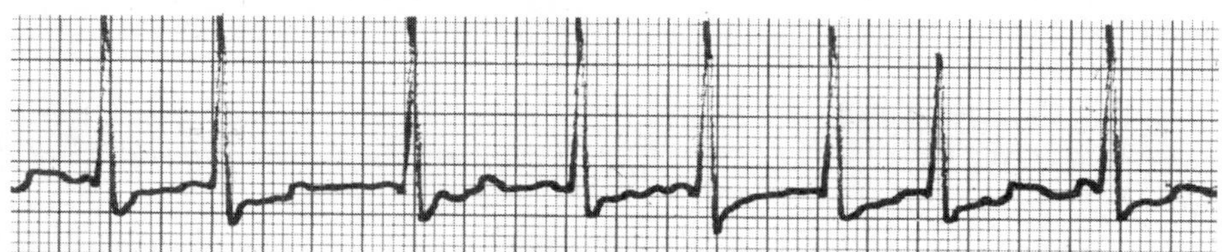

Fig. 46-14. Atrial fibrillation (lead II). Atrial rate is rapid with varying conduction to ventricles, rhythm irregular, QRS complex normal, no definite P waves visible, PR interval not measurable.

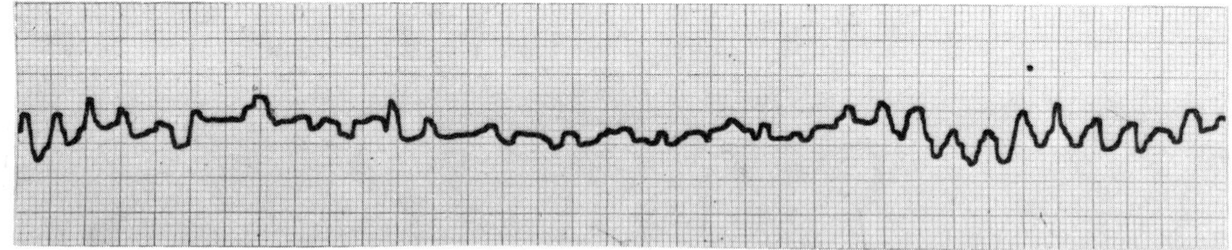

Fig. 46-15. Ventricular fibrillation (lead II). Rate is rapid, rhythm irregular, no QRS complexes, no definite P waves visible. Tracing shows electrical chaos in myocardium.

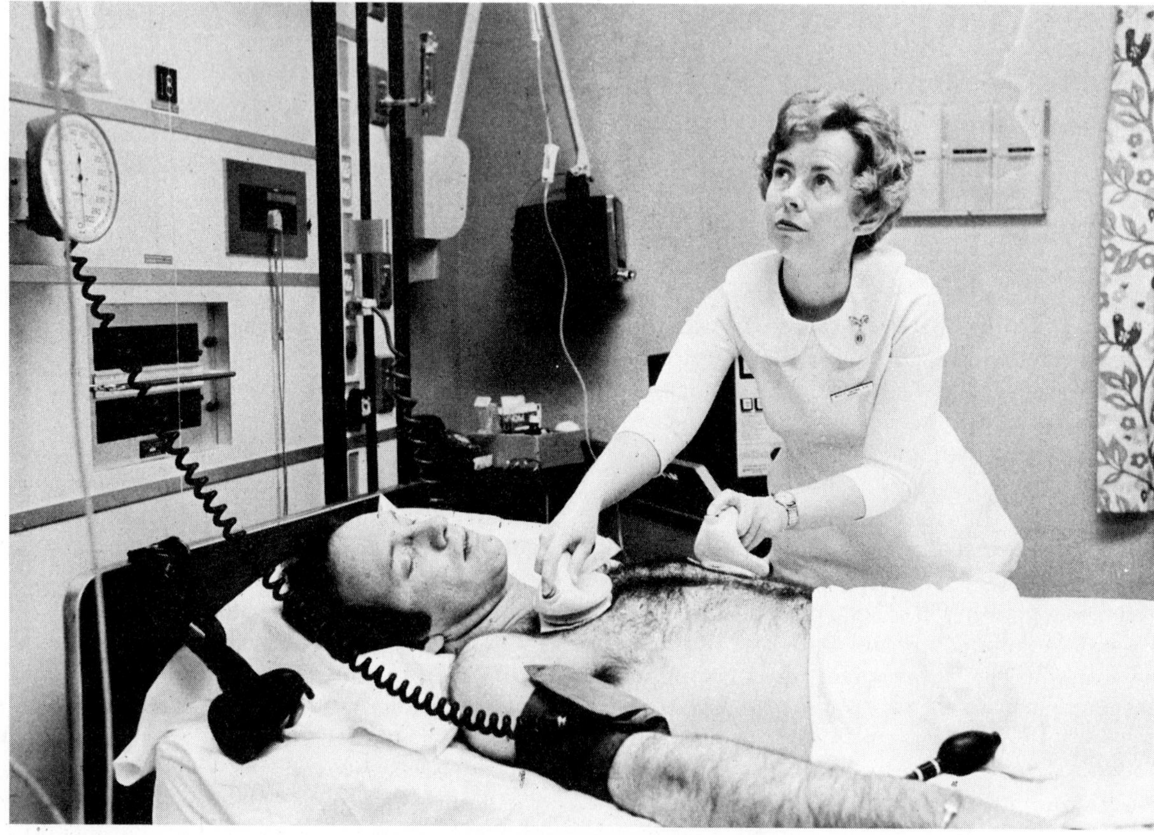

Fig. 46-16. Nurse defibrillating patient.

tion of the ventricles is replaced by rapid irregular twitching of the ventricular muscles (Fig. 46-15). Ventricular fibrillation is one of the mechanisms of sudden cardiac death. This condition is known as *cardiac arrest* and requires immediate emergency measures (p. 963).

Changes in ECG tracings are depicted in Figs. 46-14 and 46-15.

Intervention

The person whose heart is in atrial fibrillation may be given digitalis and quinidine sulfate. Digitalis acts by blocking the impulses that pass from the atria to the ventricles, increasing the interval between the heartbeats so that the ventricles will contain more blood before they contract. Quinidine sulfate restores the normal rhythm by increasing the rest period of the atrial muscles. The usual dose of quinidine is 0.2 to 0.4 g by mouth. It may be repeated every 4 hours for 2 to 3 days. When quinidine is first given the patient should be watched carefully for toxic signs, since many persons are allergic to it. If the person becomes flushed, complains of ringing in the ears, or becomes nauseated or faint, or if the pulse rate increases, the medication should be withheld until the physician is consulted. In the person with a diseased heart there is also the danger that the sudden return to a regular atrial heartbeat may cause emboli to break away from the atrial walls. Thrombi are likely to have formed there while the blood has been pumped inadequately.

The treatment of ventricular fibrillation is defibrillation. The physician or specially trained nurse applies electrical precordial shock to stop the fibrillation (Fig. 46-16). If the first attempt at defibrillation is unsuccessful, cardiopulmonary resuscitation (CPR) may be instituted until a second defibrillation attempt can be made.

Another mechanism of sudden cardiac death is *ventricular asystole*. Cardiopulmonary resuscitation is begun and is continued until a transvenous pacemaker can be inserted. Intracardiac epinephrine may be given to stimulate electrical activity.

■ CONGESTIVE HEART FAILURE

Heart failure is a state in which the heart is no longer able to pump an adequate supply of blood.[47] Failure may occur when there is inadequate ventricular filling (as in mitral stenosis, cardiac tamponade, pericarditis, or a shortened diastole in high ventricular rates), an increased blood volume, or a disease of the myocardium (including degenerative diseases, myocardial infarction, or arrhythmias). In these states the heart will initially try to compensate with an increased rate, dilation, and hypertrophy. When this fails, the blood supply becomes inadequate and decompensation exists. With decreased cardiac output, homeostatic compensatory mechanisms come into play and the kidney works to retain salt and water. With continued low cardiac output, cardiogenic shock occurs. If allowed to persist, these conditions will lead to death. The amount of blood the heart pumps to all parts of the body varies with body activities. Under normal conditions the heart and blood vessels adjust the flow of blood to body needs, and usually the heart is not worked to capacity. Moderate activity such as sitting, standing, or walking places only nominal demand on the heart. However, when the pumping action of the heart is decreased because of some impairment, the heart may have to work to capacity to meet even modest demands.

In congestive heart failure (CHF) the heart is unable to receive its normal flow of blood from the venous system and to pump out the required amount through the arterial circulation. The left ventricle does not empty completely into the aorta, and the blood that would normally enter the right atrium from the superior and inferior venae cavae cannot do so. Pressure rises in the venous circulation and the organs and tissues that are normally drained by the veins become congested with the blood that is flowing slowly against increased pressure. The left ventricle, meanwhile, tries to do extra work to pump this blood, and it becomes enlarged. This process is usually a gradual one, occurring over a period of months or years. Congestive heart failure is also known as *cardiac decompensation*, *cardiac insufficiency*, *heart failure*, and *cardiac incompetence*.

Congestive heart failure is often classified as right-sided or left-sided, according to the side of the heart at fault. Most often it begins in the left ventricle and later becomes a combination of left-sided and right-sided failure. Heart failure may temporarily disappear as soon as the mechanisms causing it are rectified. It may be present for the rest of the person's life and require continuous care and medication, or despite treatment it may quickly become worse and cause death.

Clinical picture

The most common symptoms of heart failure are edema and dyspnea (shortness of breath). These symptoms are caused by the accumulation of fluid throughout the body and by an inadequate blood flow to body tissues. *Edema*, which is an excessive amount of fluid in the extracellular tissues and body cavities, is a common symptom of congestive failure. It may occur in the legs, the liver, the abdominal cavity, the lungs, the pleural spaces, or other parts of the body. When the heart becomes an inefficient pump, venous stasis occurs and venous pressure increases. Because of this, fluid remains in the venous system rather than circulating normally to the kidneys where the excess sodium would be excreted. The decreased renal blood flow resulting from the decreased cardiac output stimulates the production of aldosterone (p. 209), which results in sodium reabsorption. The decreased renal blood flow also stimulates the production of antidiuretic hormone (ADH) leading to water retention. If the person consumes more sodium in his diet than can be excreted, the excess is stored in the body. Sodium is a water-fixing ion; that is, it holds water to prevent body fluids from becoming too salty. Therefore the more salt in the body, the more water will be retained. Some of this fluid passes into the interstitial spaces and causes generalized edema (p. 303).

In *right-sided heart failure* the right ventricle hypertrophies in response to an increase in pulmonary artery pressure and cannot effectively propel into the lungs the blood returning to it from the inferior and superior vena cavae through the right atrium. This causes the blood to dam back into the veins of the systemic circulation and leads to edema in the lower extremities. This edema is of the pitting type (can be depressed by pressure) and is nontender. It is known as dependent edema because it occurs in dependent parts of the body such as the legs. It almost always disappears at night when the legs are at the same level as the rest of the body. As the edema becomes more pronounced it progresses up the legs into the thighs, external genitalia, and lower trunk. If the tissues become too engorged the skin may crack, and fluid may "weep" from the tissues.

The liver may also become engorged with blood, causing it to enlarge and producing tenderness in the right upper quadrant of the abdomen. As the venous stasis increases, increased pressure within the portal system often forces fluid through the blood vessels into the abdominal cavity. This is known as *ascites*. As much as 8,000 to 10,000 ml (8 to 10 liters) or more of serous fluid may accumulate in the abdominal cavity. The accumulation may cause severe respiratory distress as a result of elevation of the diaphragm, and paracentesis may be necessary.

Distended neck veins can be observed when the person with right-sided heart failure is in a sitting position. This results from the increased systemic venous pressure.

In *left-sided heart failure* the weakened left ventricle of the heart cannot effectively pump into the arterial circulation the oxygenated blood coming from the lungs through the pulmonary veins into the left atrium. A third heart sound may be ascultated producing a cadence of sounds resembling galloping horses. This gallop rhythm results from increased end-diastolic pressure caused by the weakened left ventricle. The ineffective pumping causes the blood to dam back into the pulmonary vessels so that serous fluid is pushed out into the pulmonary tissues, causing *pulmonary edema* and *pleural effusion*. The fluid may be present in the lower interstitial tissues of the lungs, in the alveoli of the lungs, in the bronchioles, or in the pleural space. *Dyspnea*, or shortness of breath, is an early symptom of left-sided heart failure. It is caused by interference with gas exchange because of the fluid in the alveoli. Dyspnea may occur or may become worse only on physical exertion such as climbing stairs, walking up an incline, or walking against the wind, since these activities require increased amounts of oxygen. Sometimes dyspnea occurs on lying down. This type is called *orthopnea*. When the patient is lying flat on his back, there is decrease in ventilation and the blood volume to the pulmonary vessels is increased. Persons with orthopnea often must sleep propped up in bed or in a chair. Although orthopnea may occur immediately after lying down, it often does not occur until several hours later, when it causes the person to wake up with severe dyspnea and coughing. This condition is known as *paroxysmal nocturnal dyspnea*. It is caused by an accumulation of fluid in the lungs, which occurs as the person slips down in bed. The person usually feels like he is suffocating and often awakens in a panic. Signs and symptoms include a cold sweat, pale skin, tachycardia, and gallop rhythm.[6]

In cardiac failure the patient may have alternating periods of *apnea* and *hyperpnea* (Cheyne-Stokes respirations). Often because of respiratory insufficiency, an insufficient amount of oxygen is carried by the blood to the brain. Oxygen insufficiency makes the respiratory center in the brain insensitive to the normal amounts of carbon dioxide in the arterial blood, and respiration ceases until either the carbon dioxide content in the arterial blood increases enough to stimulate the respiratory center or until the oxygen level in the blood drops to a level that is low enough to stimulate the respiratory center. The carbon dioxide content of the arterial blood is also decreased by the periods of overbreathing. Periodic overbreathing often begins as the patient goes to sleep and decreases as sleep deepens and ventilation decreases.[6] Morphine sulfate may relieve Cheyne-Stokes respirations because it slows the respiratory rate. Usually the physician does not prescribe high concentrations of oxygen for this condition because this would prevent the reflex stimulus caused by low oxygen content in the blood, which is actually what stimulates the patient to start breathing again.

Pulmonary edema caused by left-sided heart failure may be very severe, and moist rales (moist breath sounds) sometimes may be heard across the room. This condition is known as *acute pulmonary edema*. The patient is extremely dyspneic, is apprehensive and struggles for breath, has a persistent cough and may expectorate frothy or even blood-tinged sputum, is usually cyanotic, and his heart pounds rapidly. Acute pulmonary edema is a medical emergency, since if it is not immediately treated the patient may "drown" in his own secretions. Treatment is discussed more fully on p. 1009.

A persistent hacking cough and expectoration of mucoid material are frequent symptoms of left-sided heart failure. They are usually caused by the congestion of the lungs and bronchi. Cardiac pain is not common in congestive heart failure, although some persons develop discomfort in the chest on lying down. This discomfort is often described as a "heavy feeling" or a "feeling of pressure." It arises in persons with a diseased heart that is sensitive to a deficiency in the oxygen content in the coronary circulation because the blood is less completely oxygenated when the person is lying flat than when sitting, standing, or even walking.

Fatigue is also a common sign of congestive heart failure and is one of the earliest signs to develop. The person notices tiredness following activities that ordinarily are not tiring. This fatigue results from the impaired circulation of blood to the tissues and from the consequent lack of sufficient oxygen and nutrients for the needs of the cells. The reduction in oxygen decreases the aerobic production of adenosine triphosphate (ATP), which is the immediate source of energy required for muscular contraction. In addition the inadequate blood supply does not carry off wastes with sufficient speed to permit optimum muscle function.

Because of the edema, weight loss may not be noticed in persons with congestive heart failure. Often 5 to 10 kg of fluid may be retained. The muscle tissue may have been lost, however, because of inadequate nutrition, and on reduction of the edema the person may appear as emaciated as a person with an advanced malignancy.[6]

Intervention

In many hospitals the person with acute congestive heart failure is admitted to a medical or cardiac intensive care unit if the institution has such special facilities. In other instances the physician or nurse may elect to place the patient in the usual patient room accommodations where the environment is less stressful and where family members may remain with him. The decision is made on the basis of degree of failure and specific response by the individual to the acute situation.

The principles of treatment for congestive heart failure are to bring back into balance the supply and demand for blood and to remove and thereafter to prevent the accumulation of excess fluid and excess blood volume when the output of the heart cannot be made to meet normal requirements of the body. The desired outcome of therapy is improvement in signs and symptoms: (1) breathing is easier, (2) edema is absent or markedly reduced, and (3) respiratory rate is normal without the use of supplemental oxygen. These objectives are accomplished by reducing requirements of the body for oxygen, by increasing cardiac output, and by eliminating excess fluid.

Oxygen. In cardiac failure the oxygen content of the bloodstream may be markedly reduced because of the less effective oxygenation of the blood as it passes through the congested lungs. The person may be more comfortable and rest better when receiving oxygen, since it helps to relieve the dyspnea and fatigue. The oxygen is usually administered by nasal cannula at 2 to 6 liters/minute. If acute pulmonary edema occurs, oxygen may be given under pressure by means of an intermittent positive pressure breathing (IPPB) machine. This helps prevent additional filling of alveoli with fluid by increasing alveolar pressure.

Rest-activity. Reducing the requirements of the body for oxygen can best be effected by providing the person with the degree of activity that does not compromise myocardial function, as demonstrated by the presence of symptoms. If the degree of cardiac failure is mild, with only edema of the legs or minimal signs of pulmonary edema, the person may be treated on an ambulatory basis with only a regimen of less strenous activity and more rest than usual.

If the degree of cardiac failure is severe a program of bed rest or "armchair rest" (p. 965) may be maintained until symptoms abate. The amount of activity permitted each person depends on the extent of symptoms, for example, dyspnea or fatigue. A careful assessment must be made each day to determine to what extent the person can feed, turn, or bathe himself. Most persons prefer to be as independent as possible, and this can be encouraged within the given limitations.

Sedatives are used judiciously for the person with cardiac failure as oversedation may mask symptoms of increasing failure. In addition immobility increases the risk of venous thrombosis or embolus. Cardiac patients are likely to be apprehensive and may have difficulty relaxing, and diazepam (Valium) 2 to 10 mg three times a day may be prescribed. Chloral hydrate or flurazepam hydrochloride (Dalmane) may be used if the person is unable to sleep despite nursing measures that promote physical or mental rest.

Position in bed. Most persons with congestive heart failure are more comfortable and can breathe more easily with the head of the bed elevated in a high Fowler's position. A pillow may be placed lengthwise behind the shoulders and back in such a manner that full expansion of the rib cage is possible (Fig. 46-17). A footblock is useful in preventing the person from slipping toward the foot of the bed. Persons who must be in a high Fowler's position are usually more comfortable and have less pull on their shoulder muscles if both arms are supported by pillows. If the person must remain upright all the time,

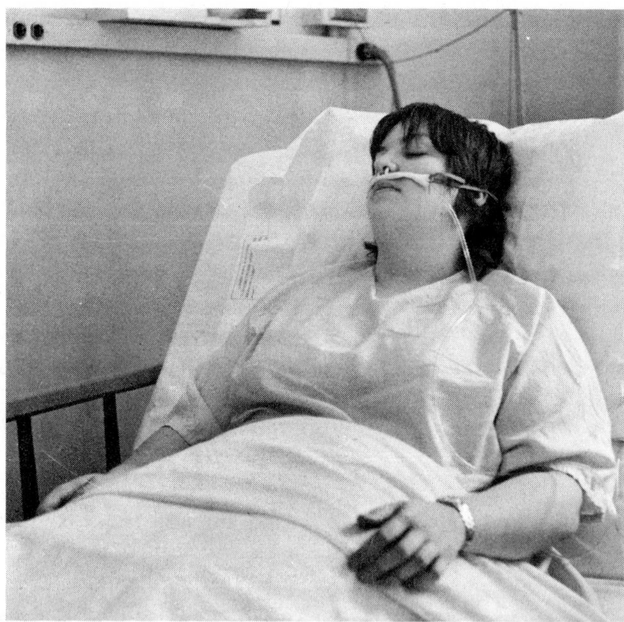

Fig. 46-17. Pillow placed under patient's head and shoulders with head of bed in Fowler's position provides comfort and support for patient with congestive heart failure. Pillows under arms may provide additional comfort and place less strain on shoulder girdle.

an overbed table may be pulled up close to the person to allow resting of the head and arms on pillows placed on the table (Fig. 45-8). Both the pillows and the table may need to be tied to prevent slipping. Side rails provide something firm for the person to hold during changes of position and to prevent accidents.

Ambulation. Ambulation is started slowly to avoid overload on the heart and to determine how much activity the heart can tolerate without again showing signs of failure. The regimen varies depending on patient response. For the person who has been on restricted bed rest, activities progress slowly through the stages of dangling, sitting up in a chair, then walking increased distances under close supervision. The person is assessed for signs indicating that the activity cannot be tolerated, including dyspnea, fatigue, and increased pulse rate that does not stabilize readily. If these signs or symptoms occur, the person is returned to bed. If dyspnea is present, the head of the bed is elevated and oxygen is administered at a low flow of 1 to 3 liters/minute. The physician is consulted before further ambulation is attempted. The plan for increased activity is explained to the person and family. They should understand that if activity tires the person excessively, it may be curtailed. Overactivity can produce physical and mental setbacks that delay ultimate recovery. In the early stage of ambulation it is important to begin stressing the importance of *rate* of activity; that is, the demand on the heart is decreased when a normal activity is performed more slowly than before.

Daily weights. Although careful records of intake and output are kept on most persons with cardiac failure, the best method to estimate progress and response to prescribed diet, medications, or other forms of treatment is monitoring the person's weight. Weight gain indicates fluid retention. The person's weight is carefully recorded on admission and frequently thereafter, usually at least once a day depending on the degree of failure and presence of edema. The person with severe cardiac failure is weighed on a litter scale, which contains a stretcher so that the person may be weighed with the minimum of exertion. If the armchair regimen is being used, a chair scale will be more comfortable and less fatiguing for the person. No matter what type of scale is used, the most important principle is that the person be weighed at the same time each day with the same amount of clothing on.

Skin care. Edematous skin is poorly nourished and very susceptible to skin breakdown. Edema of the sacrum is prevalent in the person restricted to bed because of its dependent position, and decubiti can develop quickly. Measures to prevent decubiti are instituted early (p. 834). The elbows are also observed closely and a lubricant applied to the skin since irritation often occurs if the person must be kept in high Fowler's position.

Nutrition. During the acute stage of congestive heart failure the diet should be soft or liquid and easily digested foods should be served. Anorexia is often present due to edema in the gastrointestinal tract, dyspnea, fatigue, and effect of medications. Frequent small feedings minimize exertion; the work of the heart is increased during digestion, since blood is needed by the digestive tract for its function.

Sodium. Edema is often effectively controlled in persons with heart failure by restriction of sodium intake. The degree of restriction depends on the severity of the failure and the extent of diuretic therapy. The severely restricted sodium diet is rarely prescribed, since the diet is unpalatable and expensive and the degree of patient compliance is low.

The amount of sodium in the normal diet is 3 to 10 g/day. If the person is receiving diuretics, sodium may *not* be limited below 3 to 5 g/day because of the danger of hyponatremia (p. 307). In mild cardiac failure sodium may be restricted to 1 to 2 g/day, a no-added-salt (NAS) diet. This diet is essentially normal except that no extra salt is added to prepared foods and obviously salted foods such as potato chips are omitted (p. 966). For moderate or severe cardiac failure the amount of sodium permitted is prescribed. Vitamin supplements are usually required when severely restricted sodium diets are prescribed.

Fluids. Fluid restriction is less commonly instituted than in the past as long as the person is on a sodium-controlled diet and is receiving diuretics and digitalis. The ingested fluids can act as a diuretic in helping to remove fluid from the tissues. If fluids are restricted, the amount of fluid permitted is prescribed by the physician and a plan is made, in conjunction with the patient if possible, to space the fluids over the day depending on patient desires. Usually one half of the fluids are planned for meals and the other half for between meals. If thirst is present, frequent mouth care may add to patient comfort.

Nutrition education of person and family. The reason for diet and fluid restrictions are explained to both the person and the family so that the person does not become unduly upset and so that the family does not bring food or fluids that are unacceptable. The patient needs to learn early about the food and fluid restrictions to be followed after discharge from the hospital. The ambulatory person may need frequent interactions with the dietitian or nurse before being able to follow the diet adequately.

Elimination. It is advisable for the person with cardiac disease to avoid straining at defecation since it places an extra burden on the heart. The feces are kept soft by giving daily a mild cathartic such as milk of magnesia, a mild bulk cathartic such as psyllium (Metamucil), or a stool-softening agent such as dioctyl sodium sulfosuccinate (Colace). If an oil enema is necessary, it should be given with a small rectal tibe inserted only 3 to 4 inches. Most persons dislike using the bedpan, and the effort required to get onto the pan and to maintain a satisfactory position on it often puts a real strain on the heart. Some physicians prefer that the patient slide off the bed onto the commode to have a bowel evacuation. The desirability of using a commode depends on the size of the person and his condition. Commodes raised to bed height, so that little moving is necessary to get the patient onto them, are now available. The person with cardiac disease should not be left alone when on the commode or a bedpan, although the nurse or attendant may leave the room or step outside the curtain to give privacy. The patient should never be made to feel hurried.

Digitalization. Digitalis is the major therapeutic approach in the treatment of congestive heart failure. Digitalis and its derivatives usually are effective in improving myocardial function in persons with congestive heart failure. The positive inotropic action of digitalis preparations enhances mechanical performance by strengthening the force of myocardial contraction.[7] This leads to increased cardiac output and increased blood flow to the kidneys. Digitalis preparations also decrease heart rate (automaticity) and cardiac conduction velocity which permits the ventricles to relax more in order to allow time for better filling of the ventricles with blood.

SIGNS AND SYMPTOMS OF DIGITALIS TOXICITY

- Cardiovascular effects
  - Bradycardia
  - Tachycardia
  - Bigeminy
  - Ectopic beats
  - Pulse deficit
- Gastrointestinal effects
  - Anorexia
  - Nausea and vomiting
  - Abdominal pain
  - Diarrhea
- Neurologic effects
  - Headache
  - Double vision
  - Blurred or colored vision
  - Drowsiness, confusion
  - Restlessness, irritability
  - Muscle weakness

When acute congestive heart failure occurs, the physician usually orders an *optimum therapeutic dose* of a digitalis preparation to slow the ventricular rate and decrease symptoms. This larger dose given over a short period of time, usually 24 to 48 hours, is called a *digitalizing* dose. In some instances the dose may approach the toxic level, and the person is observed carefully for signs and symptoms of toxicity (see box above). The full effect of the digitalizing drug is realized when the heart and circulation return to normal under treatment, and the symptoms of toxicity are more evident at this time. Since digitalis preparations have a *cumulative effect* and are slowly eliminated, early recognition of toxic symptoms and discontinuance of the drug will decrease their severity and duration. After the optimum therapeutic dose has been determined, the person is placed on a daily maintenance dose of digitalis.

Several factors predispose the person to digitalis toxicity. One of the most common is hypokalemia, which potentiates the effects of digitalis. When potassium is depleted in the body or myocardium, the heart becomes more excitable and arrhythmias may occur.[7] Decrease in potassium levels below the normal range of 4.0 to 5.4 mEq/liter can occur whenever excess potassium is lost from the body such as occurs in vomiting and diarrhea or induced diuresis. Most of the diuretics used to treat congestive heart failure result in the loss of potassium along with sodium and water. Therefore the nurse must be alert to changes in the patient's serum potassium blood levels. In order to replace the potassium loss through diuresis, persons are often placed on a supplemental form of potassium such as potassium chloride. Some diuretics have potassium added to them, but many physicians prefer to order the diuretics and potassium separately. In addition foods such as orange juice or bananas, which are high in potassium and low in sodium content should be encouraged.

Other predisposing factors to digitalis toxicity include severe liver and kidney disease since the liver inactivates the drug and the kidney excretes it and primary myocardial disease, which makes the myocardium more sensitive to the drug. Increased toxicity also occurs with alkalosis, hypercalcemia, hypomagnesemia, and hypothyroidism. If digitalis toxicity occurs, the medication is stopped at once and other therapy instituted as necessary. This often includes administration of procainamide and potassium chloride.

Numerous types of digitalis preparations may be used (Table 46-2). For rapid digitalization in emergency situations, deslanoside (Cedilanid-D) or G-strophanthin (Ouabain) are usually selected. Digoxin or digitoxin are the most commonly used drugs for maintenance therapy. Digoxin has a more rapid effect than digitoxin, yet has sufficient duration for adequate maintenance therapy. If given intramuscularly, digoxin should be injected deeply and the area massaged after injection because the drug is a tissue irritant. Powdered digitalis is highly toxic and is therefore rarely used.

Before a digitalis preparation is given, the apical pulse rate is taken. If this rate is below 60, the medication should be withheld until the physician has been consulted. The pulse rate of persons with irregular rhythm should always be taken for a full minute for accuracy. Response to digitalis is evaluated on the basis of relief of symptoms, that is, decreased edema, loss of weight, fluid output greater than fluid intake, and no dyspnea or cyanosis.

Diuretic therapy. Diuretic therapy is not a substitute for digitalis therapy, which has a direct action on the

Table 46-2. Digitalis preparations

Generic name	Trade name	Digitalizing dose (time)	Maintenance dose	Route	Onset	Duration
Purple foxglove (*Digitalis purpurea*)						
Powdered digitalis	Digifortis Digiglusin	1 to 2 g (24 to 48 hr)	100 to 200 mg	Oral	Slow	Long
Digitoxin	Crystodigin Purodigin Digitaline Nativelle Unidigin	1.5 mg (24 to 48 hr)	100 to 200 mg	Oral IV	Slow	Long
Gitalin	Gitaligin	4 to 6 mg (3 to 4 days)	0.5 mg	Oral	Fast	Moderate
White foxglove (*Digitalis lanata*)						
Digoxin	Lanoxin	1.5 mg 1.0 mg (12 to 24 hr)	0.125 to 0.50 mg	Oral IV IM	Fast	Moderate
Deslanoside	Cedilanid-D	1.6 mg (12 hr)	0.25 to 0.5 mg	IV IM	Fast	Short
Lanatoside C	Cedilanid	10 mg (4 days)	0.5 mg	Oral	Variable	Short
Acetyldigitoxin	Acylanid	1.6 to 2.2 mg (24 hr)	0.1 to 0.2 mg	Oral	Moderate	Short
Strophanthus gratus						
G-strophanthin	Ouabain	0.25 to 0.5 mg (12 to 24 hr)	—	IV	Fast	Short

myocardium. The purpose of diuretic therapy is to decrease the extracellular fluid volume and thus decrease symptoms of fluid retention. Diuretic therapy is usually initiated when a program of digitalis, restriction of strenuous physical activity, and a no-added-salt diet have not controlled the symptoms.

Diuretics are drugs that increase the urine output primarily by inhibiting the reabsorption of sodium in the proximal tubule (mercurial diuretics), ascending loop of Henle (furosemide, ethacrynic acid), distal tubule (thiazides, triamterene), or collecting duct (spironolactone). (The reader is referred to Table 47-1 for a listing of these diuretics including dosages and side effects.)

The development of the newer more potent oral diuretics in the late 1950s has enhanced the success of relieving symptoms of excessive fluid retention in persons with severe congestive heart failure. Prior to that time, mercurial diuretics were given intramuscularly and in combination with several other drugs such as acidifying chlorides (ammonium chloride), carbonic anhydrase inhibitors (Diamox), and aminophylline in order to achieve potent diuresis. Mercurial diuretics are still used for certain patients.

The *thiazides* are the diuretics of choice when diuretic therapy is initiated for congestive heart failure. The thiazides are inexpensive, easy to take, and effective when taken over a period of time. Although they are potent drugs that can cause electrolyte imbalance, the toxicity can be effectively controlled. The major complication is hypokalemia that can be prevented by the intake of foods high in potassium or by potassium supplements.

If thiazides are ineffective, an oral *aldosterone antagonist* such as spironolactone (Aldactone) or triamterene (Dyrenium) is given with the thiazide. Since the effect of these two drugs is to block certain effects of aldosterone, potassium is retained when the sodium is excreted (potassium-sparing diuretics). The aldosterone antagonists potentiate the action of the thiazides.

The *most potent* diuretics, furosemide (Lasix) or ethacrynic acid (Edecrine), are given when CHF is severe and the thiazides and aldosterone antagonists are unable to control the fluid retention. Therapy is best initiated in the hospital setting so that electrolyte and acid-base balance may be monitored. Diuresis begins within an hour after oral ingestion and lasts about 6 to 8 hours. The action is more rapid with parenteral administration (5 minutes for intravenous injection, lasting for 2 hours).

Acute pulmonary edema

Acute pulmonary edema is a medical emergency in persons with heart disease. It is caused by additional or prolonged strain on an already damaged heart, with resultant failure. Either physical or emotional stress can precipitate pulmonary edema. Cardiac output is decreased, and serous fluid under pressure is pushed back through the pulmonary capillaries into the alveoli. Fluid rapidly reaches the bronchioles and bronchi, and the person begins to drown in his own secretions. Acute pulmonary edema also may follow such conditions as inhalation of irritating gases; cerebrovascular accident; fractures of the skull; too rapid administration of plasma, serum albumin, whole blood, or other intravenous fluids; and barbiturate or opiate poisoning. Severe dyspnea, cyanosis, and restlessness are usual symptoms.

The goals in the treatment of acute pulmonary edema include physical and mental relaxation, relief of hypoxemia, retardation of venous return, and improvement of cardiovascular function. The patient with acute pulmonary edema should be placed in bed in a high Fowler's position, and the physician should be summoned immediately. Morphine sulfate, 15 mg (1/4 grain), is usually ordered to be given at once to quiet breathing and to allay apprehension. It may be given intravenously, since circulatory collapse may hinder its absorption from the tissues.

To relieve hypoxemia the physician may order intermittent positive pressure breathing (IPPB) with oxygen and humidification and an airway pressure of 15 to 30 cm of water. IPPB creates counterpressure on the alveolar capillaries to decrease transudation of fluid into the alveoli. IPPB also increases pleural pressure, thus decreasing venous return to the heart. If the person is not already receiving digitalis therapy, it will be instituted and a potent fast-acting diuretic such as furosemide or ethacrynic acid may be given intravenously. Aminophylline, a bronchodilator and diuretic, may also be given intravenously.

Good results are often obtained with the regimen previously described. More radical treatment such as phlebotomy or rotating tourniquets is used less frequently than in the past as the treatment may be worse than the effect of the pulmonary edema if the patient's condition is poor.[6] The purpose of *phlebotomy* is to decrease the amount of circulating blood to decrease pulmonary engorgement; however, this removes hemoglobin that may further contribute to hypoxemia and also removes electrolytes contributing to electrolyte imbalances.

The purpose of *rotating tourniquets* is to pool blood in the extremities, thus reducing the amount of blood that must be circulated by the overtaxed heart. The tourniquets are placed on three extremities at one time (Fig. 46-18). Every 15 minutes in clockwise or counterclockwise order, one tourniquet is placed on the extremity that has no tourniquet and one tourniquet is removed. Thus each extremity is occluded for 45 minutes at a time. A rotating touniquet machine (Fig. 46-19) uses

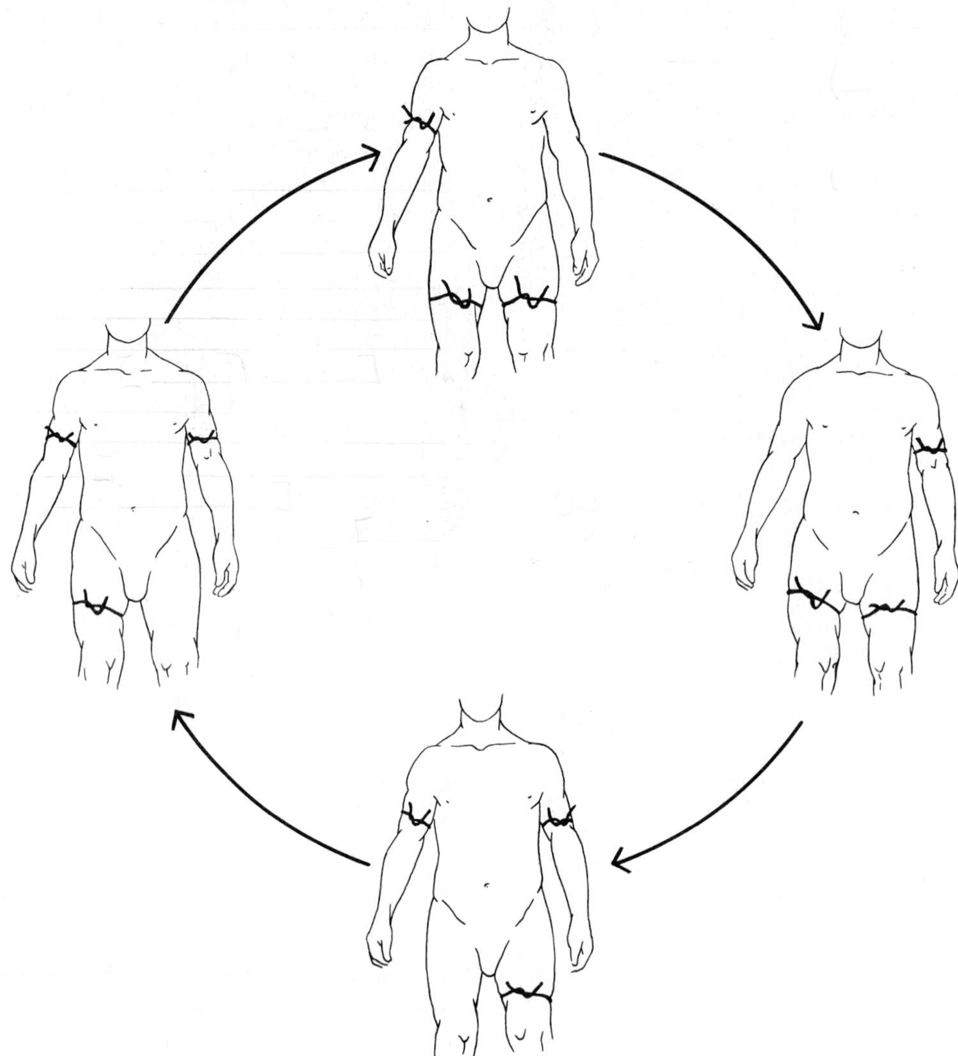

Fig. 46-18. Clockwise method of removing and applying rotating tourniquets.

blood pressure cuffs as tourniquets and automatically pumps and deflates the cuffs to obtain the desired effect. The purpose of the therapy is to occlude *venous* blood; therefore the tourniquets should not obliterate arterial pulses in the extremity. If an extremity does not return readily to normal color on release of a tourniquet, the physician is informed. When the procedure is terminated the tourniquets are released, one every 15 minutes to prevent a sudden increase in venous return and recurrence of pulmonary edema.

Long-term care

The person with congestive heart failure needs to know the reasons for symptoms and the rationale for the therapies, especially those that will be carried out on a long-term basis. Digitalis and diuretic medications are often prescribed for long periods of time, and it is often difficult for persons to remember when to take each medication. Often some method must be worked out so that the person can carry out the routine correctly. It is also important that the individual know about the action and side effects of the prescribed medications so that he does not "double up" on a dose if one dose was missed. Teaching should also be directed at prevention of overexertion or prevention of complications such as hypokalemia. If diet or fluid restrictions have been prescribed, the nurse can be very helpful in assisting the person to incorporate any changes in a plan that has the greatest chance of being carried out. Ongoing health management of persons who have had congestive heart

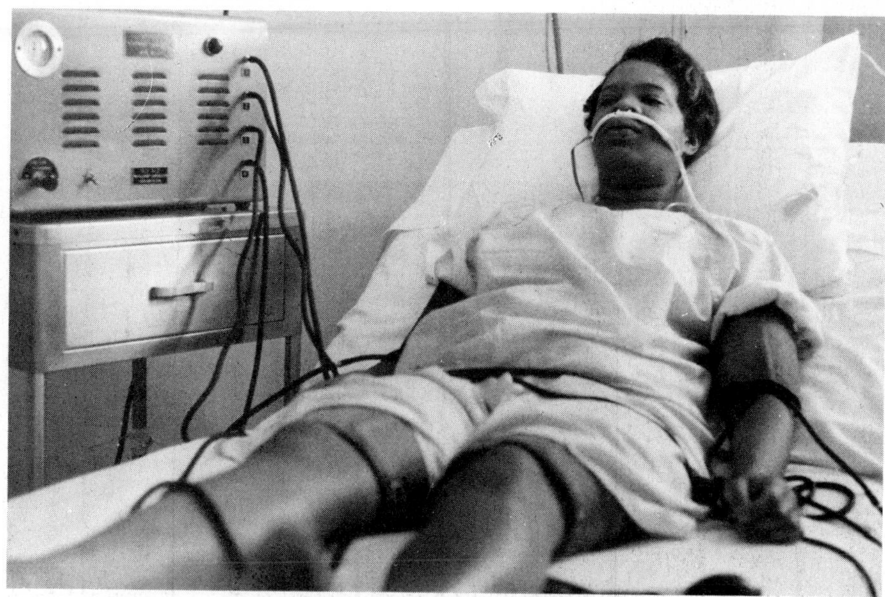

Fig. 46-19. Patient in acute pulmonary edema; rotating tourniquet machine is being used. Note that intravenous infusion is in subclavian vein.

failure and whose condition has been stabilized is one area in which nurses are assuming a more active role.

Outcome criteria for the person with congestive heart failure

The person or significant others can:

1. Describe a plan for activity (ADL, work, recreation) that will avoid fatigue or dyspnea.
2. Plan a diet incorporating any prescribed sodium or fluid restrictions.
3. Explain the medication therapy:
   a. State name, purpose, dosage, frequency, and side effects of prescribed medications (digitalis, diuretics).
   b. Describe a method for remembering to take prescribed medications as directed.
   c. State what to do if a medication has been omitted.
4. State plans for follow-up care:
   a. State signs and symptoms requiring health care follow-up (dyspnea, rapid weight gain or weight gain in absence of increased food intake, edema).
   b. State plans for ongoing care with a health professional.

■ ANEURYSMS

An aneurysm is a localized or diffuse enlargement of an artery at some point along its course. Aneurysms occur when the vessel wall becomes weakened due to trauma, congenital vascular disease, infection, and atherosclerosis. Syphilitic aneurysms of the arch of the aorta still occur, but the vast majority of aneurysms, regardless of location, are due to atherosclerosis.

Although the pathologic processes involved in the formation of an aneurysm are varied, certain factors are common to all. Once an aneurysm develops and the arterial tunica media (the middle coat composed of layers of smooth muscle and elastic tissue) is damaged, there is a tendency toward progressive dilation, degeneration, and a risk of rupture. Aneurysms may develop in any blood vessel, but the most common site is the aorta.

□ Types of aneurysms

A *saccular* aneurysm involves only part of the circumference of the artery. It takes the form of a sac or pouchlike dilation attached to the side of the artery. A *fusiform* aneurysm is spindle shaped and involves the entire circumference of the arterial wall (Fig. 46-20). A *dissecting* aneurysm involves hemorrhage into a vessel wall, which splits and dissects the wall causing a widening of the vessel. Dissecting aneurysms are caused by a degenerative defect in the tunica media, probably as a result of the great hemodynamic stresses to which it is subjected.

Clinical picture

The most common site for the formation of an aortic aneurysm is the abdominal aorta below the renal arteries. The person may be asymptomatic and the condition evident only as a pulsatile abdominal mass which

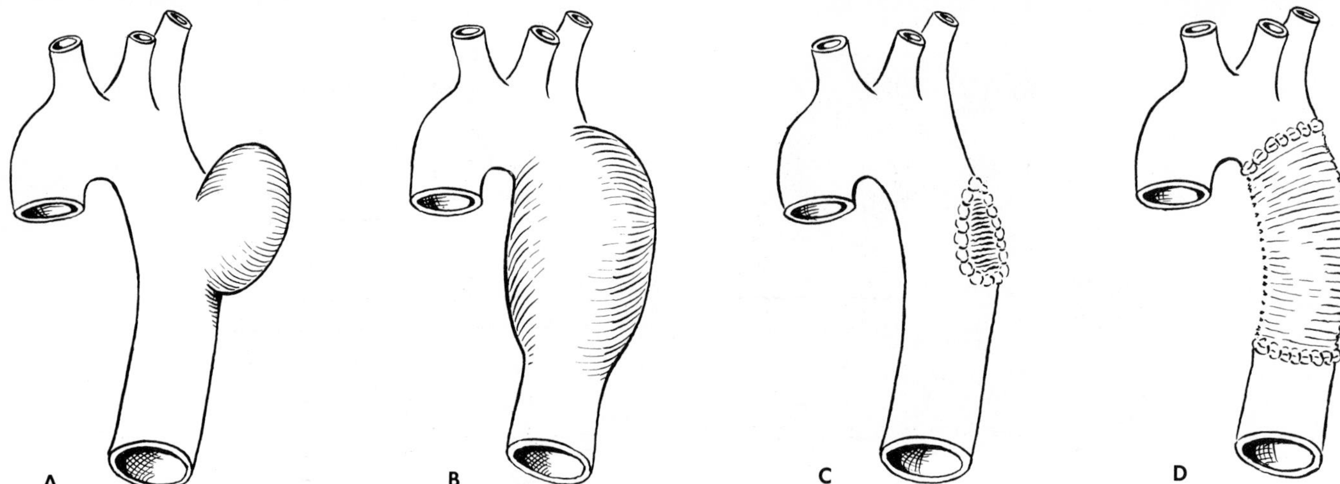

Fig. 46-20. Aneurysms of thoracic artery. **A,** Saccular aneurysm. **B,** Fusiform aneurysm. **C,** Patch-graft repair of saccular aneurysm. **D,** Replacement graft for fusiform aneurysm. (Redrawn from Bloodwell, R. D., et al.: Surg. Clin. North Am. **46:**901-911, 1966).

may be found on a routine physical examination. At other times the person may have pain or tenderness in the mid- or upper abdomen. Aneurysm of the abdominal aorta is a serious disease entity, and the mortality is high with rupture. A dissecting aneurysm of the aorta may develop slowly with few symptoms or may be acute with severe chest pain that may be mistaken for a myocardial infarction.

Routine chest and abdominal radiographs have proved to be very helpful in case finding and preliminary diagnosis of aortic aneurysms. Such studies frequently reveal a ring of calcification outlining the aneurysm and displacement of surrounding structures. Angiographic studies are usually conducted to provide the surgeon with a definite diagnosis, accurate location, and delineation of the lesion. Numerous techniques are used for these studies, and selection of the particular angiographic procedure (p. 1019) depends on a number of factors including the clinical condition of the person and the location of the lesion.

Intervention

If the aneurysm is a small chronic aneurysm with no worsening of symptoms, the person may be treated medically with antihypertensives, pain medication, and negative inotropic agents that decrease the force of muscular contractions (Inderal).

Surgery. Surgical treatment and nursing care differ depending on the location of the aneurysm.

Surgical treatment of aneurysms that involve the ascending, transverse, and descending *thoracic aorta* is considered comparable to open-heart surgery. Operative mortality is highest in those persons who have an acute onset of symptoms and in whom a dissecting aneurysm begins in the ascending aortic arch and causes insufficiency of the aortic valve. A form of total cardiopulmonary bypass (p. 974) is needed to maintain tissue oxygenation when the aorta is clamped. Hypothermia may be used to decrease the need of tissues for oxygen and thus decrease metabolic waste production (see p. 384). After the chest is opened, the aneurysm exposed, and an extracorporeal bypass instituted to produce a satisfactory flow of oxygenated blood, cross clamps are applied proximal and distal to the lesion (Fig. 46-21). The aneurysm is then resected and replaced with a Teflon or Dacron prosthesis. (See p. 975 for care of the person after open heart surgery.)

Treatment of an *abdominal aneurysm* is resection of the lesion and replacement with a graft. Extracorporeal perfusion (heart-lung bypass) is *not* necessary because arterial flow to the lower extremities can be interrupted safely for the time needed to complete the operation. The aneurysm is opened, the clots and debris are removed, the graft replacement is inserted, and the remaining arterial wall is closed over the graft (Fig. 46-22).

Immediate postoperative management of the person who has had an *abdominal* aortic prosthesis replacement includes constant nursing observation in the recovery room and intensive care unit. Continual reassessment and monitoring of all parameters are essential in the first 24 to 48 hours. The blood pressure, pulse (radial and apical), and respirations are taken every 15 minutes until stabilized. The central venous pressure is also monitored to evaluate the adequacy of total blood volume. Of most

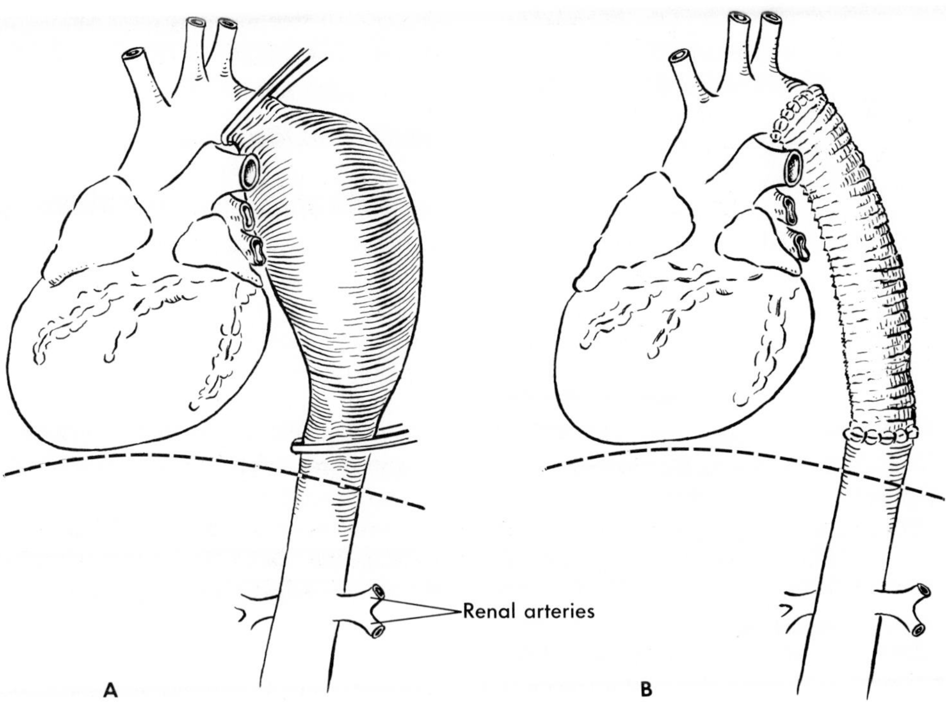

Fig. 46-21. Aneurysm of descending thoracic artery. **A,** Resection of thoracic aorta with cardiovascular clamps in place. **B,** Permanent replacement graft after resection of aneurysm. (Redrawn from Bloodwell, R. D., et al.: Surg. Clin. North Am. **46:**901-911, 1966.)

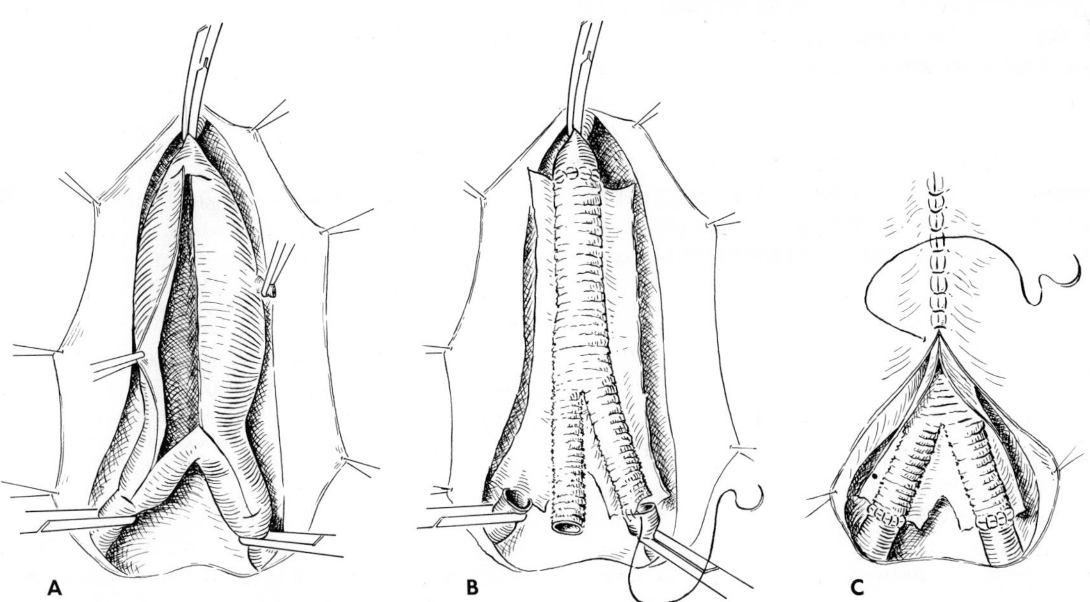

Fig. 46-22. Abdominal aneurysm. **A,** Aneurysm of aorta and iliac arteries. **B,** Bifurcation graft used to replace excised aneurysm. **C,** Closure of posterior peritoneum over graft and suture line. (Redrawn from Crawford, E. S., et al.: Surg. Clin. North Am. **46:**963-978, 1966.)

concern would be a rising CVP, which would indicate overload of the venous circulation due to administration of too much blood or fluid replacement, inadequate cardiac function, or both (p. 923). The pulses of the distal arterial vessels of the extremities are taken hourly, as is done with peripheral arterial bypass grafts. These include the posterior tibial and dorsalis pedis pulses. Initial spasm or trapping of air bubbles may cause these pulses to be absent on the person's return from the operating room.

If pulses continue to be absent for more than 6 to 12 hours (even less if a prosthetic failure has occurred), it generally indicates an arterial occlusion. Signs of *poor* peripheral perfusion include a drop in blood pressure and a weak and thready pulse. The person may feel cool to the touch and be perspiring. Signs of *advanced occlusion* distal to the thrombus are pain, cramping, or numbness in one or both of the extremities. The leg or legs may be blanched (white) or blue in appearance and be cool or cold to the touch. The person may appear anxious, and the elderly patient may even be disoriented. These signs and symptoms are reported to the surgeon immediately. The person who has had an abdominal aneurysm resected must be observed for complaints of back pain, which may indicate a retroperitoneal hemorrhage or a thrombus at the graft site.

Renal failure may be a complication of abdominal aortic aneurysm resection. Maintenance of adequate urine output is essential. Accurate *hourly* intake and output records must be maintained. Anuria deserves immediate attention and must be reported to the physician. Oliguria (less than 30 to 50 ml/hour) may indicate poor hydration and also should be reported.

The patient usually is placed flat in bed, and sharp flexion of the hip is avoided because it causes pressure on the femoral artery. Flexion of the knee also is avoided because it causes pressure on the popliteal artery. The person is moved gently from side to side and should dorsiflex and extend the feet at regular intervals to prevent congestion of venous blood in the lower legs. Because the incision is long and pain may be pronounced, the person is able to breathe more deeply, cough productively, and move more easily if a firm abdominal binder is used and if instructions are given to support the incision while coughing or moving. The nurse often needs to help the patient. Narcotics are given fairly liberally for pain during the first few days postoperatively.

Since some handling of the viscera must occur during surgery, postoperative ileus and distention is sometimes a problem. Aspiration of flatus from the stomach with a nasogastric tube may be necessary. On about the second postoperative day the person usually is permitted out of bed for a short time. Persons having abdominal aortic surgery are at high risk of developing thrombophlebitis, and preventive measures are carried out such as the use of elastic stockings, encouragement of ambulation, and avoidance of leg massage.

□ Ventricular aneurysm

Aneurysms of the ventricular myocardium can occur as a complication of myocardial infarction (p. 992). After an acute myocardial infarction, healing occurs and a scar is formed. Occasionally this scar causes weakening of the myocardial wall, which results in an outward bulging of the scar as the ventricle contracts. Blood may collect in the pouch and constitute a potential source of emboli. The wall usually does not rupture. The presence of a ventricular aneurysm may be suspected when a person develops recurrent ventricular arrhythmias or is refractory to usual treatment with antiarrhythmics such as procainamide or quinidine after myocardial infarction. The diagnosis can be confirmed by routine chest x-ray examination and cardiac catheterization. Occasionally if the aneurysm is very small, medication such as propranolol, procainamide, or digoxin may be sufficient. Usually, however, the treatment for a ventricular aneurysm is surgical removal of the scar. Postoperative care is the same as for persons having other types of heart surgery (p. 975).

REFERENCES AND SELECTED READINGS

1. Abdellah, F.: The physician-nurse team approach to coronary care, Nurs. Clin. North Am. **7**:423-430, 1972.
2. American Academy of Pediatrics: Report of the Committee on Infectious Diseases, ed. 18, Evanston, Ill., 1977, The Academy.
3. Andreoli, K. G.: The cardiac monitor, Am. J. Nurs. **69**:1238-1243, 1969.
4. Baden, C.: Teaching the coronary patient and his family, Nurs. Clin. North Am. **7**:563-571, 1972.
5. Barstow, R.: Nursing care of patients with pacemakers, Cardiovasc. Nurs. **8**:7-10, 1972.
6. Beeson, P. B., and McDermott, W. editors: Textbook of medicine, ed. 14, Philadelphia, 1975, W. B. Saunders Co.
7. Bergersen, B. S., and Goth, A.: Pharmacology in nursing, ed. 14, St. Louis, 1979, The C. V. Mosby Co.
8. Berne, R. M., and Levy, M. N.: Cardiovascular physiology, ed. 3, St. Louis, 1977, The C. V. Mosby Co.
9. Bielski, M.: Continuity of care for the patient with coronary heart disease, Nurs. Clin. North Am. **7**:413-421, 1972.
10. Blake, F. G.: Open heart surgery in children: a study of nursing care, Children's Bureau, Washington, D.C., 1964, U.S. Department of Health, Education and Welfare.
11. Blakeslee, A., and Stamler, J.: Your heart has nine lives, New York, 1966, Pocket Books.
12. *Bozorgi, S.: Postoperative care of the cardiac surgical patient, Heart Lung **3**:891-892, 1974.
13. Brener, E.: Surgery for coronary artery disease, Am. J. Nurs. **72**:469-473, 1972.

*References preceded by an asterisk are particularly well suited for student reading.

14. Brest, A., editor: Cardiovascular clinics: arrhythmias, II, Philadelphia, 1970, F. A. Davis Co.
15. Brest, A. N., Onesti, G., Swartz, C., et al.: Mechanisms of antihypertensive drug therapy, J.A.M.A. **211**:480-484, 1970.
16. *Brogan, M.: Nursing care of the patient experiencing cardiac surgery for coronary artery disease, Nurs. Clin. North Am. **7**:517-527, 1972.
17. *Calhoun, P. L., and Bozorgi, S.: Postoperative care following coronary surgery, Heart Lung **3**:912-915, 1974.
18. Chow, R.: Postoperative cardiac nursing research: a method for identifying and categorizing nursing action, Nurs. Res. **18**:4-13, 1969.
19. *Collins, J. J., and Morgan, A. P.: Automated management of postoperative cardiac surgical care, Heart Lung **3**:929-932, 1974.
20. Conn, H. F.: Current therapy, Philadelphia, 1978, W. B. Saunders Co.
21. *Cross, C. J.: Back to work after myocardial infarction, Am. J. Nurs. **62**:58-61, 1962.
22. *Culbert P., and Kos, B.: Teaching patients about pacemakers, Am. J. Nurs. **71**:523-527, 1971.
23. Curtin, B. C., and Reick, K. L.: Effects of bodily position on the systolic blood pressure response to Valsalva's maneuver, Nurs. Res. **18**:119-123, 1969.
24. Davis, L., editor: Christopher's textbook of surgery, ed. 11, Philadelphia, 1977, W. B. Saunders Co.
25. Dawber, T. R., and Thomas, H. E.: Risk factors in coronary heart disease, Cardiovasc. Nurs. **6**:29, 1970.
26. DeBakey, M. E., Jordan, G. L., Jr., Beall, A. C., Jr., et al.: Basic biologic reactions to vascular grafts and prostheses, Surg. Clin. North Am. **45**:477-497, 1965.
27. *DeMeyer, J. A.: The environment of the intensive care unit, Nurs. Forum **6**:262-272, 1967.
28. Dietschy, J. M., and Weis, H. J.: Cholesterol synthesis by the gastrointestinal tract, Am. J. Clin. Nutr. **24**:70-76, 1971.
29. *Ellis, R.: Unusual sensory and thought disturbances after cardiac surgery, Am. J. Nurs. **72**:2021-2025, 1972.
30. Escher, D. J. W.: Types of pacemakers and their complications, Circulation **47**:1119-1130, 1973.
31. Flores, A. M., and Zohman, L. R.: Energy cost of bedmaking to the cardiac patient and the nurse, Am. J. Nurs. **70**:1264-1267, 1970.
32. *Foster, S.: Pump failure, Am. J. Nurs. **74**:1830-1834, 1974.
33. *Foster, S., and Andreoli, K.: The postcoronary patient: behavior following acute myocardial infarction, Am. J. Nurs. **70**:2344-2352, 1970.
34. Frater, R. W. M.: Postoperative care in the pediatric cardiac patient, Heart Lung **3**:903-911, 1974.
35. Fredrickson, D. S., Goldstein, J. L., and Brown, M. S.: The familial hyperlipoproteinemias, In Stanbury, J. B., Wyngaarden, J. B., and Fredrickson, D. S., editors: The metabolic basis of inherited disease, ed. 4, New York, 1978, McGraw-Hill Book Co.
36. Friedberg, C. K.: Diseases of the heart, ed. 3, Philadelphia, 1966, W. B. Saunders Co.
37. Gentry, W. B., and Haney, T.: Emotional and behavioral reaction to acute myocardial infarction, Heart Lung **4**:738-745, 1975.
38. Grace, W. J., Gregory, J. J., Kennedy, R. J., et al.: Use of the permanent subcutaneous transvenous pacemaker in Adams-Stokes syndrome, Am. J. Cardiol. **18**:888-891, 1966.
39. *Graham, L. E.: Patient's perceptions in the CCU, Am. J. Nurs. **69**:1921-1922, 1969.
40. Griffith, G. C.: Sexuality and the cardiac patient, Heart Lung **2**:70-73, 1973.
41. *Hanchett, E. S., and Johnson, R. A.: Early signs of congestive heart failure, Am. J. Nurs. **68**:1456-1461, 1968.
42. *Harken, D. E.: Postoperative care following heart-valve surgery, Heart Lung **3**:893-902, 1974.
43. Harrison, T. R., et al., editors: Principles of internal medicine, ed. 8, New York, 1977, Blakiston Division, McGraw-Hill Book Co.
44. Harper, H.: A review of physiological chemistry, ed. 16, Los Altos, Calif., 1977, Lange Medical Publications.
45. Hodges, L.: Systems and nursing care of the cardiac surgical patient, Nurs. Clin. North Am. **6**:415-524, 1971.
46. *Hunn, V. K.: Cardiac pacemakers, Am. J. Nurs. **69**:749-754, 1969.
47. Hurst, J. W. editor: The heart, arteries and veins, ed. 3, New York, 1974, McGraw-Hill Book Co.
48. *Jarvis, D.: Open heart surgery: patients' perceptions of care, Am. J. Nurs. **70**:2591-2593, 1970.
49. Jenkins, A. C.: Successful cardiac monitoring, Nurs. Clin. North Am. **1**:537-547, 1966.
50. *Jenkins, A. C., et al.: Symposium on care of the cardiac patient, Nurs. Clin. North Am. **1**:561-649, 1969.
51. *Johnson, J., and Kirby, C. K.: Surgery of the chest, ed. 4, Chicago, 1970, Year Book Medical Publishers, Inc.
52. *Jones, B.: Inside the coronary care unit: the patient and his responses, Am. J. Nurs. **67**:2313-2320, 1967.
53. Joyce, P.: The effectiveness of coronary-care units in reducing the mortality of acute myocardial infarction, Heart Lung **1**:487-489, 1972.
54. Julian, O. C.: Cardiac pacemakers, Surg. Clin. North Am. **48**:155-162, 1968.
55. Kannel, W., and Dawber, T.: Contributors to coronary risk implications for prevention and public health: the Framingham study, Heart Lung **1**:797-809, 1972.
56. *Kennedy, M. J.: Coping with emotional stress in the patient awaiting heart surgery, Nurs. Clin. North Am. **1**:3, 1966.
57. *Lamberton, M. N.: Cardiac catheterization: anticipatory nursing care, Am. J. Nurs. **71**:1718-1721, 1971.
58. Lane, C.: Intra-aortic phase-shift balloon pumping in cardiogenic shock, Am. J. Nurs. **69**:1654-1659, 1969.
59. *Lasater, K. L., and Grisanti, D. J.: Postcardiotomy psychosis: indications and interventions, Heart Lung **4**:724-729, 1975.
60. *Lees, R. S., and Wilson, D. E.: The treatment of hyperlipidemia, N. Engl. J. Med. **284**:186-195, 1971.
61. LeMaitre, G. D., and Finnegan, J. M.: The patient in surgery: a guide for nurses, ed. 3, Philadelphia, 1975, W. B. Saunders Co.
62. *Long, B.: Sleep, Am. J. Nurs. **69**:1896-1899, 1969.
63. *Maclean, D. M., and Fowler, E. A.: Heart transplant: early postoperative care, Am. J. Nurs. **68**:2124-2127, 1968.
64. Malmros, H.: Dietary prevention of atherosclerosis (letter to editor), Lancet **1**:94-95, 1970.
65. Mansour, K. A., Dorney, E. R., Tyras, D. H., et al.: Cardiac pacemakers: comparing epicardial and pervenous pacing, Geriatrics **28**:151-155, 1973.
66. Marriott, H. J. L.: Practical electrocardiography, ed. 6, Baltimore, 1977, The Williams & Wilkins Co.
67. Meltzer. L. E., Pinneo, R., and Kitchell, J. R.: Acute myocardial infarction. In Meltzer, L. E., Abdellah, F. G., and Kitchell, J. R., editors; Concepts and practices of intensive care for nurse specialists, ed. 2, Philadelphia, 1976, The Charles Press, Publishers.
68. Merkel, R., and Sovie, M. D.: Electrocution hazards with transvenous pacemaker electrodes, Am. J. Nurs. **68**:2560-2563, 1968.
69. Meserko, V.: Preoperative classes for cardiac patients, Am. J. Nurs. **73**:665-669, 1973.

70. Modell, W., and others: Handbook of cardiology for nurses, ed. 5, New York, 1966, Springer Publishing Co.
71. Moffitt, E. A., Sessler, A. D., and Kirklin, J. W.: Postoperative care in open heart surgery, J.A.M.A. **199**:161-163, 1967.
72. Moss, A. J., Adams, F. H., and Emmanovilides, G. C.: Heart disease in infants, children and adolescents, ed. 2, Baltimore, 1977, The Williams and Wilkins Co.
73. Nadas, A. S., and Fyler, D. C.: Pediatric cardiology, ed. 3, Philadelphia, 1972, W. B. Saunders Co.
74. Nelson, W. E., et al.: Textbook of pediatrics, ed. 10, Philadelphia, 1975, W. B. Saunders Co.
75. Norman, J. C., editor: Cardiac surgery, ed. 2, New York, 1972, Appleton-Century-Crofts.
76. *Nye, A. W., Yorio, M., and Karlskind, M. L.: Sixteen patients: postoperative nursing experience with heart transplantation, Am. J. Nurs. **69**:2630-2634, 1969.
77. Ochsner, J. S.: Surgery for myocardial revascularization, Postgrad. Med. **49**:127-130, 1971.
78. Perloff, J. K.: The cardiomyopathies: current perspectives, Circulation **44**:942-950, 1971.
79. *Pinneo, R.: Cardiac monitoring, Nurs. Clin. North Am. **7**:457-467, 1972.
80. *Pitorak, E.: Open-ended care for the open heart patient, Nurs. Clin. North Am. J. Nurs. **67**:1452-1457, 1967.
81. *Pitorak, E., et al.: Nurses' guide to cardiac surgery and nursing care, New York, 1969, McGraw-Hill Book Co.
82. *Puksta, N. S.: All about sex . . . after a coronary, Am. J. Nurs. **77**:602-605, 1977.
83. *Roberts, S. L.: The patient's adaptation to the coronary care unit, Nurs. Forum **9**:56-63, 1970.
84. Rosenberg, H. S., and Muldar, D. G.: Dissecting thoracic aneurysms, Arch. Surg. **105**:19-20, 1972.
85. Sanderson, R. G.: The cardiac patient, Philadelphia, 1972, W. B. Saunders Co.
86. Scalzi, C. C.: Nursing management of behavioral responses following an acute myocardial infarction, Heart Lung **2**:62-69, 1973.
87. Schamroth, L.: Some basic principles governing the electrophysiology and the diagnosis of heart rhythms, Heart Lung **1**:45-50, 1972.
88. Schamroth, L., and Jaspan, J.: Variant angina pectoris: a typical Prinzmetal's angina pectoris, Heart Lung **2**:431-433, 1973.
89. *Schmitt, Y., Hood, W. B., Jr., and Lown, B.: Armchair treatment in the coronary care unit: effect on blood pressure and pulse, Nurs. Res. **18**:114-118, 1969.
90. *Shor, V.: Congenital cardiac defects: assessment and care finding, Am. J. Nurs. **78**:256-261, 1978.
91. Sirak, H. D.: Operable heart disease, St. Louis, 1966, The C. V. Mosby Co.
92. *Smith, C. A.: Body image changes after myocardial infarction, Nurs. Clin. North Am. **7**:663-667, 1972.
93. Sovie, M., and Fruehan, C.: Protecting the patient from electrical hazards, Nurs. Clin. North Am. **7**:469-480, 1972.
94. Spandau, M.: Insertion of temporary cardiac pacemakers without fluoroscopy, Am. J. Nurs. **70**:1011-1013, 1970.
95. Traught, E.: Equipment hazards, Am. J. Nurs. **73**:858-862, 1973.
96. Turpeinen, O.: Diet and coronary events, J. Am. Diet. Assoc. **52**:209-213, 1968.
97. *Twerski, A. J.: Psychological considerations on the coronary care unit, Cardiovasc. Nurs. **7**:65-68, 1971.
98. U.S. Department of Health, Education and Welfare, National Center for Health Statistics: Vital statistics of the United States, 1974, vol. 2, part B, 1976.
99. *Varvaro, F. F.: Teaching the patient about open heart surgery, Am. J. Nurs. **65**:111-115, 1965.
100. *Vinsant, M., et al.: Pacemakers in 1972, Heart Lung **1**:362-373, 1972.
101. Waechter, E. H., and Blake, F. G.: Nursing care of children, Philadelphia, 1976, J. B. Lippincott Co.
102. *Weiler, Sister M. Cashel: Postoperative patients evaluate preoperative instruction, Am. J. Nurs. **68**:1465-1467, 1968.
103. Whipple, G., et al.: Acute coronary care, Boston, 1972, Little, Brown and Co.
104. *Williams, C.: The CCU nurse has a pacemaker, Am. J. Nurs. **72**:900-902, 1972.
105. Williams, S. R.: Nutrition and diet therapy, ed. 3, St. Louis, 1977, The C. V. Mosby Co.
106. Willis, F. N., and Dunsmore, N. M.: Work orientation health attitudes and compliance with therapeutic advice, Nurs. Res. **16**:22-25, 1967.
107. Wilson, S.: Aortocoronary saphenous vein bypass: a review of the literature, Heart Lung **2**:90-103, 1973.
108. *Winslow, E. H., editor: Teaching and rehabilitating the cardiac patient, Nurs. Clin. North Am. **11**:2, 1976.
109. *Wolfer, J., and Davis, C. E.: Assessment of surgical patients' preoperative emotional condition and postoperative welfare, Nurs. Res. **19**:402-414, 1970.
110. Yokes, J. A.: The influence of bioengineering on the nurse and the cardiac patient. In Bergersen, B. S., Anderson, E. H., Duffey, M., Lohr, M., and Rose, M. H., editors: Current concepts in clinical nursing, vol. 1, St. Louis, 1967, The C. V. Mosby Co.
111. Yokes, J. A., and Reed, W. A.: Heart surgery. In Meltzer, L. E., Abdellah, F. G., and Kitchell, J. R., editors: Concepts and practices of intensive care for nurse specialists, ed. 2, Philadelphia, 1976, The Charles Press, Publishers.
112. *Yudkin, J., and Morland, J.: Sugar intake and myocardial infarction, Am. J. Clin. Nutr. **20**:503-506, 1967.

47

Problems of peripheral circulation

BARBARA J. DALY

Peripheral vascular disease refers to a number of disease entities that may affect any part of the vascular system. Diseases of the heart and coronary arteries are *not* usually included in this classification, although the pathophysiologic changes may be identical. The term peripheral vascular disease also refers to the pathologic sequelae such as disease changes that result from any interruption in the normal circulatory mechanics.

This chapter also discusses lower limb amputation as one of the surgical interventions for vascular disease. Techniques of treatment and management are similar to those used for the patient who has had an amputation following trauma, although rehabilitation of the latter usually is less difficult because the amputation is less likely to accompany a chronic medical disease.

Hypertension, one of the major etiologic factors in peripheral vascular disease, is discussed as a separate entity. It may exist without the presence of significant arterial or venous disease, or it may be a complicating factor.

All of the clinical conditions included under peripheral vascular disease manifest signs and symptoms in the individual because of some type of interference in normal blood supply to the tissues. The interference may be of an obstructive nature, as with the presence of a thrombus or fatty plaque on the wall of the vessel, or an interruption due to anatomic abnormalities, such as is the case with varicose veins and arteriovenous fistulas.

Several general factors lead to the development of peripheral vascular disease. The most common of these are pathologic processes occurring in the vessels themselves, such as occurs in atherosclerosis and the inflammation of lymphedema. Changes in blood hemodynamics such as hypertension, states of hypercoagulability, and stasis may be the significant factor leading to circulatory interference in some disorders. External damage to vessels, as with phlebitis associated with intravenous therapy, may also be implicated in peripheral vascular disease. In addition, in some individuals an inherent weakness in the vessel may lead to the development of an abnormality such as an aneurysm.

Regardless of the specific disorder or primary cause, many factors significantly influence both the occurrence of the disease and its course once symptoms are manifested. The overall aim of intervention is to enhance those factors that promote good circulation and to eliminate or reduce factors that further inhibit circulation. Common nursing interventions for the individual with peripheral vascular disease are discussed. Specific disorders, pathophysiology, and interventions are then considered.

■ PREVENTION

Health teaching about the factors influencing peripheral vascular disease should be done by the nurse working in any clinical setting. With advancing age, arterial walls lose elasticity and undergo a thickening of the intima; this predisposes to vascular problems, and all individuals will benefit from education about this as they grow older. All hospitalized patients with restricted activity, regardless of their primary disease, need to be taught measures to reduce the stasis associated with immobility. Intervention in areas of everyday life such as diet and activity of the nonhospitalized individual may prevent or at least slow the development of acute disease. This is one of the most important disease groups with which the nurse works and one in which the rewards of early interventions are greatest.

■ ASSESSMENT

Because peripheral vascular disease affects so many individuals, particularly in later life, the nurse should incorporate assessment for signs and symptoms of diminished circulation in working with all patients regardless of the primary problem. Assessment of patients with known peripheral vascular disease is, of course, much more thorough.

□ Subjective data

A *history of pain* is of prime significance. Pain is one of the most common symptoms of diminished circulation to an extremity, and the type of pain may help differentiate between embolic phenomena and arteriosclerosis. The length of time since pain first occurred is a guide to how far the disease has progressed. Other areas to investigate include when the pain occurs, what factors initiate pain, and what relieves the pain.

The presence of *intermittent claudication* is especially significant. This is pain in the muscles caused by inadequate arterial circulation to the contracting muscles and occurs primarily in the calf. Except in rare instances it is brought on only by continuous exercise and is relieved at once by resting. Knowing the amount of exercise that can be performed before claudication occurs helps determine the severity of the condition. The presence of rest pain, or pain that occurs without any activity, is indicative of severe disease.

In advanced disease, and occasionally in early stages, the individual may notice a change in functional ability. Persistent diminished circulation will cause atrophy of muscles of the extremity, and occlusion of the aortic and femoral trunks may result in impotence. Prior to a change in function the individual may note a change in appearance in an extremity.

Information should also be sought about healing. Has the patient had any abrasions or cuts recently? If so, how quickly or slowly did they heal? Was treatment required or obtained?

Diet information includes the caloric intake, type of fats predominantly used, amount of carbohydrates, and general nutritional adequacy of the diet.

The patient's life style and daily habits often significantly influence the course of his illness. If he smokes, the nurse determines how long he has smoked and how much he smokes. Although occupation itself has not been linked with peripheral vascular disease, knowing the patient's occupation assists in judging the level of physical activity and may also point out the need for counseling in other areas. For example, if the patient is involved in physical labor on his job, he may need to take special precautions to avoid trauma to his hands or feet. The same information can be partly elicited by asking about leisure-time activities.

As part of the nursing history, the nurse learns about how the patient's life style affects his ability to comply with the prescribed therapy. For example, does the patient have to walk a long distance or climb several flights of stairs to bring groceries home? Climbing may cause severe pain in the legs because of inadequate oxygenation of the tissues. Some arrangements therefore must be made to assist the patient with this task. If he lives alone it should be determined whether someone in the building or neighborhood can shop for him. A thorough nursing history might reveal that the young mother with a stubborn ulcer that complicated phlebitis before delivery is so harassed with feeding the baby or with getting other children off to school that she neglects her own breakfast and lunch. The nurse may discover that the elderly man with arteriosclerosis develops intermittent claudication when he walks from his rooming house to the nearest restaurant, causing him to skip one or two meals each day. The assistance of the family or social worker may be needed to solve such problems.

□ Objective data

The first part of the physical assessment usually involves checking all peripheral pulses for the presence or absence of pulses, their quality or strength, and also the comparison of pulses in each extremity with those of the other. The pulses that should routinely be checked with each assessment include the *radial, ulnar, posterior tibial, dorsalis pedis, popliteal,* and *femoral.*

Inspection of the skin yields valuable information about the adequacy of circulation. Poorly oxygenated skin has a pale, bluish, or mottled appearance, and the affected arm or leg will be cooler than the other extremity. There is often a loss of hair in the affected area, and the skin has a tight, shiny look to it. Nails may be thickened and black or brownish. The entire extremity should be inspected to determine how far from the tips of the fingers or toes the circulatory impairment extends.

Neurologic deficits also serve as indications of the extent of disease. Absent or diminished sensation, tingling, or reduced sense of temperature may all result from insufficient oxygen supply to the nerves.

□ Tests and examinations

Several specific procedures help in diagnosis of vascular disease and determine the progress in treatment. Most tests are relatively simple and require no specific preparations. The patient, however, usually is in pain and fears any procedure that he believes may even temporarily increase his pain. Nervousness sometimes causes spasm of blood vessels and sensations of chilliness that may interfere with the accuracy of a test by diminishing pulsations and altering circulation. The patient should be told that the tests are painless, and the nurse should explain to him what is to be done if the physician has not already done so.

The room in which the tests are done should be kept warm, and if the patient has to be transported to another area for the tests the nurse should check to see that he has sufficient covering to prevent chilling.

Oscillometric readings

Oscillometric readings help determine the effectiveness of the larger arteries. (Collateral vessels cannot be measured with an oscillometer.) Oscillometric readings are more useful in demonstrating relative differences between the deep pulses of two contralateral limbs than in measuring absolute deviations from normal. The change in the volume of the limb measured when arterial flow is occluded with a cuff, then released, serves as an indicator of the rate of arterial inflow.

Skin temperature studies

Attempts are made to record the skin temperature as a gauge of the effectiveness of the circulation to an extremity. These tests are not performed often because to be accurate they must be carried out in an environment with carefully controlled temperature and humidity. Normal skin temperature can be recorded by applying a thermocouple (a device for measuring skin temperature) to the skin. The temperature then is recorded on a potentiometer. With a humidity of 40%, the surface temperature of the skin usually varies from 24 C to 35 C (73 F to 93 F). Normal persons have a wide range of temperature difference in various parts of the body. For example, the forehead and the thorax are usually 5 to 8 degrees warmer than the toes. People with arterial disease may have even greater temperature variations between the extremities and the rest of the body. Skin temperature readings are considered as only suggestive because many factors (for example, a rise in metabolic rate) increase the temperature of the skin surface. The patient who is excited or upset by the anticipated test may have an increase in skin temperature. The test is usually scheduled several hours after a meal, since eating alters the skin temperature. Smoking also affects the accuracy of the readings.

A test for the efficiency of vasodilation in the extremities consists of immersing one of the limbs in water heated to 42 C to 44 C (107.6 F to 112 F) and then recording the skin temperature of the opposite limb. In the normal person with no vascular disease the temperature of the unimmersed limb will rise to a minimum of 34 C (93 F) within 35 minutes. A person with arterial disease may have little elevation in the skin temperature. An accurate bath thermometer is needed to measure the water temperature, and sufficient blankets should be used to protect the patient from chilling during and after the test.

Arterial disease can be confirmed by the *cold pressure test.* The patient's blood pressure and pulse pressure are determined under normal conditions. He then immerses his hand in ice water, and his blood pressure and pulse pressure are taken again. Normal subjects have an average blood pressure increase of 25 mm Hg with no change in pulse pressure; patients with internal occlusive disease have an average increase in blood pressure of 45 mm Hg with an increase in pulse pressure of 20 mm Hg.

Angiography

Angiography is an x-ray procedure that permits visualization of the internal anatomy of the heart and blood vessels through the intravascular injection of radiopaque contrast material. By this method calcification and other anomalies of the arteries may be demonstrated. Calcified atherosclerotic plaques at the site of an occlusion may be visualized, and calcification can sometimes be traced distally throughout the entire length of an artery and can even be seen as far away as the great toe. The information revealed by such an examination is not of itself evidence of arterial insufficiency, because some patients who have extensive calcification of the small arteries evidently have sufficient collateral circulation to permit good blood supply and thus have no symptoms of arterial insufficiency.

Radiopaque substances such as Hypaque or Renografin are injected into an artery, and serial radiographs are taken during the last few seconds of the injection and immediately thereafter. Usually this test is done in the radiology department. A cutdown on the vessel may be required in order to inject the dye. When visualization of the arteries of a lower extremity is desired, the dye is injected into the femoral artery.

The radiopaque substances used contain iodide, and the patient may have a severe allergic reaction to the dye, with dyspnea, nausea, vomiting, numbness of the extremities, diaphoresis, and tachycardia. Any signs of a reaction should be reported at once. Occasionally a delayed reaction occurs after the patient returns to his room. Antihistaminic drugs, epinephrine, and oxygen are used to treat these hypersensitivity reactions to the dye. The site of injection of the dye must be monitored for signs of irritation or local thrombosis, which may occur if any of the irritating dye gets into the surrounding tissue. The area may have to be treated with massive warm moist packs.

The procedure is uncomfortable for the patient because even without a reaction to the dye he feels a flushing and burning sensation. One or more injections into deep arteries are made, and he must remain on the x-ray table for an hour or more. Afterward he needs to be given water in generous amounts to hasten the excretion of the dye through the kidneys. He usually needs a backrub to relieve pressure areas resulting from lying on the hard x-ray table.

Of utmost importance after arteriography is assessment of the involved limb. The injection site must be closely observed for excessive bleeding. The patient will return from having the arteriogram with just a small dressing over the site, and a 1- or 2-pound sandbag should be placed over the dressing for 3 or 4 hours. Peripheral pulses distal to the injection site are checked every hour for the first 4 to 8 hours after angiography.

Venography

Radioactive isotopes may be used to confirm the presence or absence of deep-vein thrombosis. A substance that will become incorporated into the thrombus, such as *fibrinogen* or *urokinase*, is administered intravenously, and the area is scanned by x-ray. An increased uptake of the radioactive material indicates the presence of a thrombus.

Plethysmography

Sometimes *plethysmography* may also be used as an aid to diagnosis. This is a graphic device that measures variations in the electrical resistance associated with changes in blood volume. It involves applying electrodes that are connected to a recorder to the extremity. Venous flow is occluded with a cuff, and changes in resistance are measured as blood pools in the extremity. *Oculoplethysmography* refers to detection of changes in the blood volume of the eye and is used in detection of carotid lesions.

Capillary fragility test

A test for capillary fragility is sometimes ordered for patients with peripheral vascular disease. Since it is more often ordered for patients with suspected disease of the blood or blood-forming organs, it is described in Chapter 48.

Lumbar sympathetic block

Paravertebral injection of the sympathetic rami or sympathetic ganglia may be used to diagnose peripheral vascular disease. Evidence of vasodilation following the block indicates that the circulation to the limbs may be improved by subsequent injections of procaine or by sympathectomy.

With the patient in a prone or semiprone position, a needle is inserted at the level of the second or third lumbar vertebra into the sympathetic tract within the spinal canal, and 10 to 20 ml of a 1% solution of procaine hydrochloride, is injected. If the procedure is successful the sympathetic tracts will be blocked causing a definite warming and drying of the skin surface of the limb on the same side as the injection. This response may be grossly measured by touch, or skin temperature studies may be done.

The patient should be told that there will be little pain associated with the test beyond the first needle prick and that there may be a sensation of tingling and warmth in the legs for several hours following the test. He is observed carefully during and immediately following the procedure for signs of shock, which may result from the sudden shifting of so much blood into the peripheral circulation that the blood volume in the heart and vital vessels is depleted.

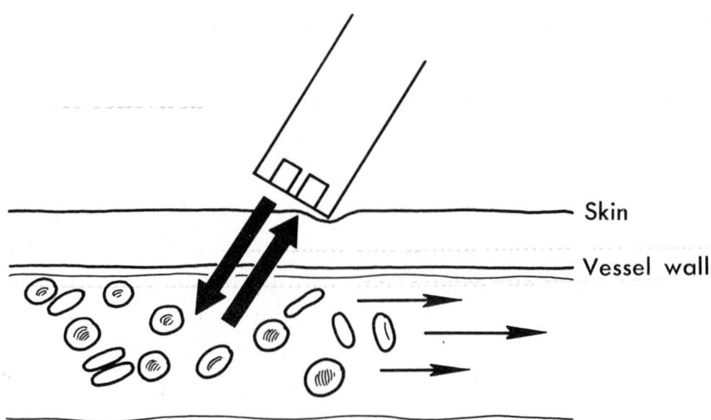

Fig. 47-1. Doppler effect showing red blood cells reflecting sound.

Ultrasound

Ultrasound is used to detect aneurysms and to measure flow through vessels. This technique involves directing an ultrasound beam at the involved area; the beam is reflected off of red cells moving through the vessel. The reflection varies according to the velocity of flow in the vessel. This change in the frequency of reflected sound according to velocity is referred to as the Doppler effect[18] (Fig. 47-1).

Simple, portable Doppler devices are often used both to diagnose arterial disease and to ascertain the effectiveness of corrective procedures. They may also be used to measure blood pressure in low-flow states.

■ GENERAL INTERVENTION FOR PERSONS WITH PERIPHERAL VASCULAR DISEASE

□ Activity

Because of our upright posture, the danger of peripheral vascular disease is greatest in the lower extremities, where adequate circulation is most difficult to maintain. Both the arteries and veins are subject to hydrostatic change; for example, when a person rises from a lying to a standing position the pressure in the dorsalis pedis artery rises from 120/80 to 215/175.[46] The activity level and exercise habits of the individual may have either deleterious or beneficial effects on his circulation.

Intervention in this area may be quite informal but often involves a good deal of ingenuity on the part of the nurse. In industry the nurse who helps the employees find chairs of a suitable height in order to prevent sharp knee flexion is contributing to prevention of disease. Sitting for long hours with the knees bent causes pressure on the arteries and veins of the legs resulting in slight swelling and discomfort. The nurse may plan with supervisors in industry to provide short rest periods at frequent intervals for persons who must stand still or sit with knees bent while they work. Since walking and moving about improve circulation, such activities should be encouraged during rest periods.

The nurse making an antepartal home visit is contributing to prevention of vascular disease when questioning the woman about her posture and the kind of girdle and shoes she wears. The woman is also reminded to take regular exercise such as walking and to rest periodically with her legs elevated above heart level. A careful balance of rest and activity is essential for any person with progressive peripheral vascular disease.

Exercise improves arterial circulation by promoting alternate muscle contraction and relaxation, thereby causing blood vessels to contract and dilate. Exercise not only improves return of venous blood from the extremities to the heart but also is one of the most important stimuli for the development of collateral circulation. Too much exercise, however, increases metabolism, thereby increasing the demands placed on the circulation to take nutrients to the tissues and to remove the products of metabolism. Complete rest may be necessary in the presence of associated medical conditions such as heart disease, thrombophlebitis, or gangrene. The nurse should plan with the physician so that proper instruction can be given regarding achieving a balance between rest and activity. In regard to posture the following is a safe guide for all persons, especially those with peripheral vascular disease: do not remain in *any* one position too long; this is particularly important for the elderly person, who often has both arterial and venous disease.

Much emphasis has been placed on *elevation of the feet*, and many persons believe that this is beneficial. However, elevation of the feet may cause damage when the patient has *arterial* insufficiency because it interferes with adequate circulation through arteries in the lower extremities. The nurse must *clearly understand* the patient's condition and the physician's orders before giving instructions in this regard. The effect of position on circulation can be best understood by relating direction of blood flow to the effects of gravity. Arteries take oxygenated blood away from the heart; elevating the extremities tends to deliver blood back to the heart, hence it tends to hamper arterial function. Long periods of standing may result in venous congestion as the effect of gravity increases the work of the veins as they return deoxygenated blood to the heart. It is safe to assume that, unless otherwise ordered, the flat position is best for circulation over an extended period.

Long periods of standing still should be avoided by persons with either venous or arterial disease, and short periods should be alternated with exercise such as walking. Persons who have venous disease should alternate standing and walking with elevation of the affected limbs.

The importance of *posture* must be stressed in the care and teaching of patients with peripheral vascular disease. The person should sleep on a firm mattress. A soft mattress may allow enough flexion of the trunk at the hips to impede circulation to the lower extremities. It may also permit the lower limbs to be higher than the heart, which is undesirable in arterial disease. The height of a chair should be such that the knees are not bent at more than a 90° angle, and the depth of the seat should permit two fingers between the chair seat and the popliteal spaces. Both of these provisions will help to prevent pressure on the popliteal vessels, which would obstruct arterial flow to the limbs and interfere with venous return. Furthermore the person should never cross his legs at the knee because this also causes pressure on the popliteal vessels. He should develop the habit of rotating his foot at the ankle, bending the foot up and down, and straightening the knee at intervals. The person should be taught to do these exercises while traveling. The importance of frequent stops if traveling by automobile or getting out of one's seat and walking in the aisle for a few moments if traveling by airplane, bus, or train should be emphasized. Attendance at movies or other sedentary diversions may be made safe and comfortable for persons with imparied circulation by the use of the above measures to improve circulation.

Specific exercises *(Buerger-Allen)* to empty blood vessels and stimulate collateral circulation are rarely used today. Instead, moderate exercise is recommended. One of the best exercises for stimulating the flow of blood to the legs is walking. The patient may be able to build up tolerance so that he can walk a mile or more a day. He should be instructed to stop and rest if pain develops and then to continue walking after it disappears. Some physicians also recommend the use of a rocking chair because it helps to stimulate the muscles in the legs to contract and relax as the person rocks.

□ Compromise of circulation

The patient with peripheral vascular disease must not wear anything that constricts. Rolled garters, socks with thin tight bands, and girdles or support pantyhose that cause constriction should be avoided. Some physicians believe that tight waistbands also should not be worn. Men may be advised to wear suspenders instead of belts. Shoelaces should be tied loosely. If edema of the feet occurs at the end of the day, the shoelaces should be loosened and relaced several times each day. Some persons who have a moderate amount of edema of the feet or ankles prefer to use elastic shoelaces. As mentioned before, any activity, posture, or position that impedes circulation is to be avoided.

It must be remembered that exposure of any part of the body to cold can cause chilling of the entire body. This in turn causes vasoconstriction and lessens circulation in a diseased extremity. In cold weather the person with peripheral vascular disease should wear warm clothing such as thermal underwear, fleece-lined shoes or boots, hats with ear flaps or earmuffs, scarves, and warm coats, suits, or dresses. Several layers of lightweight clothing are preferable to heavy bulky garments. If chilling has been experienced, the individual should drink something hot and get to a warm room as soon as possible.

The patient should be in a warm environment whenever possible. The temperature of the room should be at least 21 C (70 F), and hospitalized patients may need even more warmth for maximum comfort. The patient should be able to sense that he is rather warm but should not be warm enough to perspire more than usual.

□ Diet

Diet affects the development and course of peripheral vascular disease in two ways. First, the presence of obesity places an added burden on the heart and blood vessels. Not only must the heart pump more forcefully to circulate blood effectively in the obese individual, but the excess fat tissue tends to compromise vessels and increase venous congestion. Obesity is often associated with physical inactivity.

The second way in which diet contributes to peripheral vascular disease is related to the level of serum lipids. All lipids, or fats, in plasma are transported as constituents of lipoproteins; elevations in serum lipids are classified according to the specific lipoprotein that is elevated. Levels of *cholesterol* and *triglycerides* have been implicated for some time in the development of atherogenic disease and its sequelae such as stroke and myocardial infarction. For more detailed discussion see p. 989.

Dietary counseling is an especially important area for nursing intervention because obesity and hyperlipidemia are contributing factors to disease and an attempt should be made to eliminate them if possible. The nurse and dietitian, in consultation with each other, may provide the patient not only with the necessary teaching but also with the emotional support and encouragement required to change lifetime eating habits.

When a reduction diet has been prescribed the nurse can be of assistance in helping to plan meals that are satisfying to the individual and yet within caloric restrictions and financial means. Because protein helps to prevent breakdown of tissues, a diet high in protein but low in saturated fats is usually advised. If a lesion such as a varicose ulcer is present, a diet high in protein should help to promote healing. The diet should include foods high in B complex vitamins, which are important in maintaining tonicity of smooth muscle of blood vessels, and vitamin C, which is essential to healing and the prevention of both internal and external hemorrhage.

It is generally recommended that persons with peripheral vascular disease take more fluids than the normal person. As many as 15 to 20 glasses of water or equivalent fluids are often recommended. This amount may improve the quality of the limited blood supply to the limbs by increasing the elimination of waste products. It is also believed that it may lessen the viscosity of the blood and thus help to prevent the formation of thrombi.

□ Smoking

Nursing intervention in teaching the individual about the hazards associated with smoking and assisting him to stop smoking are essential, since smoking is one of the greatest risk factors in the development of peripheral vascular disease. Both the incidence and mortality of myocardial infarction, cerebral infarction, aortic aneurysm, intermittent claudication, and thromboangiitis obliterans are increased in the smoker.[67] Smoking exerts an influence on circulation in two ways.

First, nicotine causes vasoconstriction and spasm of the peripheral arteries; therefore smoking is contraindicated in all vascular diseases. Damage results from inhaling smoke; there is no evidence that chewing tobacco or using snuff contributes to vasospasm. The relationship between arteriospasm and smoking is so definite that many physicians feel it is useless to try to treat the patient unless he gives up smoking. Smoking should be discontinued immediately in any kind of arterial vascular disease and is also contraindicated in venous disease because the arteries surrounding a thrombosed vein often develop spasms. Nicotine also increases the heart rate, causing further stress on the circulatory system.

Second, the carbon monoxide inhaled in cigarette smoke raises the carboxyhemoglobin level and reduces the oxygen carrying capacity of the blood.[67] Thus in addition to causing vasoconstriction, smoking lowers the oxygen available in the blood for tissue demands.

Although difficult for some nonsmokers to understand, the giving up of cigarettes is almost impossible for some people. In some individuals the dependency on cigarettes can be almost as strong as a dependency on narcotics. Many persons continue to smoke even after they have lost a toe or a foot as a result of vascular disease and are informed that the incidence of amputation decreases when smoking is stopped.[33] Even if the individual has smoked for many years, stopping smoking lessens their risk. The reduction in mortality is related to the length of time that they have not smoked and the amount previously smoked.[67] The heavier the smoker, the longer it takes before there is a significant reduction in risk. Because of this and because smoking causes immediate and consistent vasconstriction, assisting the individual to stop smoking is of highest priority for the nurse.

Again, teaching of the effects of smoking is the first step, coupled with support of the person's efforts to stop. Although there is no sure way to help the individual give up smoking, there are some measures that may be helpful. Chewing gum or engaging in distracting activities sometimes helps. Some persons find that cutting down to fewer and fewer cigarettes each day is easier than stopping suddenly. Constant reminders and strict discipline often do more harm than good. Patience, understanding, and reiteration of faith in the person's ability to stop smoking are more helpful than disapproval of lapses. The essential factor is that the person wants to stop smoking. Group support and behavior modification are other methods being used to help people try to stop smoking. The nurse needs to be aware of resources available in the community to assist persons who wish to quit smoking.

□ Preventing skin breakdown

Because resistance to infection is low when tissues are inadequately nourished and oxygenated, the risk of infection is high in persons with peripheral vascular disease. A great deal of teaching is required in order for patients to know which activities will help maintain skin integrity and which may contribute to skin breakdown and secondary infection.

Use of heat

Warmth is advised for most patients with peripheral vascular disease because it causes vasodilation and thereby improves circulation to the affected part. However, warmth in the form of direct heat is seldom if ever applied to the affected part because it results in an increased demand for blood in the extremity already suffering from depleted circulation. Another reason for not applying local heat is that many patients with peripheral vascular disease also have peripheral nerve degeneration, which lessens sensitivity to heat, thus predisposing to burns. A safe rule to follow is never, under any circumstances, apply hot-water bottles, heating pads, or other forms of local heat to the legs or feet of persons with peripheral vascular disease without a specific medical order. Soaking the feet in hot or even very warm water is seldom advised. The temperature of the water into which the individual places his feet should always be tested; it should not exceed 32 C (90 F). The patient must be cautioned not to attempt to warm his feet by placing them on a warm radiator, too close to a fire in the fireplace, or in an open oven. Warmth to the extremities can be increased by placing a hot-water bottle or heating pad on the abdomen. This causes reflex dilation of the blood vessels of the legs. Immersing the entire body in a warm bath also warms the extremities. Loose woolen bed socks can be worn at night.

Care of feet

All persons with vascular disease need instruction in the care of their feet. A daily bath is recommended except for the elderly, for whom two or three baths a week are sufficient. The person should be advised to check the temperature of the bathwater carefully with his elbow before stepping into the tub because sensation in his feet may be diminished. This simple practice would prevent many persons from being burned. A small amount of a superfatted soap should be used. The skin should be dried by gentle patting; vigorous rubbing should be avoided.

While bathing, the person should look for any skin changes on his legs and feet. A dry scaling over the tibia may be the beginning of "bath itch," common in older people who have dry skin and who bathe too often and use regular soaps. If dry scales appear, fewer baths should be taken, superfatted soap should be used, and the skin should be lubricated with lanolin or a moisturizing agent after bathing and between baths. Blueness or swelling around varicosities, and hard, reddened, or painful areas, which may indicate phlebitis, should be reported to a physician at once. Tropic changes such as dryness, cracking, hardness, thickening, and brownish discolorations of the toenails indicate impairment of blood supply and should also be called to the physician's attention.

If the individual does not bathe each day, he should wash his feet in tepid water, dry them thoroughly, being particularly careful to dry between the toes, and inspect them for calluses, blisters, or any other abnormalities. If he is old and has failing vision, a member of the family should inspect his feet periodically. In the daily routine care of the feet, the skin and base of the nails should be gently massaged with lubricants or moisturizing agents. Alcohol is drying to the skin and should not be used. Each toe should be gently massaged from the distal end proximally to stimulate circulation. Powder may be used between the toes, with care being taken that it does not cake and that it is thoroughly removed at the next washing. Authorities maintain that epidermophytosis (athlete's foot), which is often a precursor of infection, ulceration, and gangrene in the feet of persons with arterial insufficiency, will seldom develop if the toes and feet are kept dry at all times. The individual who perspires profusely should powder between his toes more than once a day and should change his socks at least daily. Over-the-counter preparations available in drugstores should not be used, since they are usually too strong for feet with impaired circulation. Foot powders should only be used if prescribed. Directions should always be read carefully. Small pieces of lamb's wool or cotton can be placed between the toes to absorb perspiration.

To avoid fungal infections of the feet, socks or stockings should be washed daily. If they are wool or have a tendency to shrink, they should be stretched over a dryer; otherwise they may constrict circulation. Sock frames can be purchased at most notion counters, or a simple, inexpensive dryer can be made from a metal coat hanger.

To prevent ingrown toenails the nails should be cut carefully at regular intervals. Before the nails are cut the feet should be soaked in tepid water. The nails should be cut straight across and slightly rounded at the sides with a file. They must never be cut down to the level of the tissue. Pocketknives, razor blades, or scissors should never be used. The patient should equip himself with a pair of toenail clippers. Nail files are usually considered safe; however, tissues can be traumatized by emery boards and files, particularly when the patient lacks normal sensation in the toes. Elderly persons with poor vision should not cut their own toenails; a member of the family or a podiatrist should do it for them.

With daily care a toenail that has a tendency to "curl under" at the side of the toe can be trained to grow more normally, but no effort should be made to "straighten" the nail by vigorous treatment. With the rounded end of an ordinary toothpick, a small wisp of cotton may be inserted gently under the edge of the nail. The cotton must be changed daily. Although it may be weeks before any improvement is seen, with patience and persistence most nails that tend to grow under can be made to grow more normally unless there is aggravation by a condition such as pressure from shoes. Nails that are thickened or deformed should not be cut or filed but should be treated only by a podiatrist or physician who knows of the individual's circulatory impairment.

Medical care should be sought for blisters and for corns, calluses, and areas of thickened skin that cannot be rubbed away with a washcloth and an emergy board following soaking. Soap poultices made of any soft soap such as shaving cream may be used to soften corns and calluses before rubbing is attempted. The patient with circulatory disease of any kind should seek medical advice before going to a podiatrist.

Protection from trauma and pressure

The person should be warned to avoid injury to his feet and legs and to watch carefully for infection following trauma. He should not walk barefoot for fear of splinters causing injury. It also is dangerous for him to scratch any minor skin lesions. Many stubborn ulcers of the leg have followed the vigorous scratching of mosquito or other insect bites. Venous stasis may cause itching that can be most annoying. This itching usually follows long periods of standing and will subside if the person rests with the feet elevated for a few minutes every hour or two. The warning not to scratch the skin is hard to heed at times. Calamine lotion is sometimes suggested when pruritus is troublesome. Any minor infection of the legs or the feet should be viewed as a major one by a person with peripheral vascular disease. He should never attempt self-treatment when any signs of infection develop.

The individual should have at least two pairs of shoes and should wear them on alternate days, thus giving each pair a chance to air. If shoes become wet, they should be dried slowly on shoe trees to help preserve their shape. New shoes should be broken in gradually. Leather shoes are best because they give good support to the feet. Canvas, linen, or perforated nylon shoes provide ventilation, are comfortable in warm weather, and are safe if they have leather soles. *Rubber-soled shoes are not advised for persons who have any kind of vascular disease because they retard evaporation and thus may contribute to the development of fungal infection.* Shoes should be carefully fitted by experienced persons. They should extend about 1/2 inch beyond the longest toe and should be wide enough to avoid pressure anywhere on the foot and to allow fairly free movement of the toes within the shoe. The inner last of the shoe should be straight, and the longitudinal arch of the shoe should support that of the foot. Shoes that afford little or no support are not recommended for persons with peripheral vascular disease, although there is no objection to women wearing pumps with moderately high heels. In fact, pumps are good because the feet can be readily slipped out of the shoes and the toes wiggled at intervals; however, the shoes should be roomy enough so that they can be put on again easily.

When sleeping, the person with peripheral vascular disease should have lightweight covers that are loose and do not cause any pressure on the toes, which often burn and are painful. He can be taught how to improvise a board at the foot of the bed to keep the weight of covers from his feet. During hospitalization the patient is provided with a padded board or box at the foot of the bed. These devices are preferable to a cradle, which may hamper freedom of movement and against which the patient may accidentally strike his foot. If a cradle must be used, it should be padded, and bath blankets should be placed over the cradle and tucked securely under the mattress to prevent drafts on the feet.

Care of ulcers

Despite many precautions some patients with peripheral vascular disease still develop areas of ulceration secondary to trauma or pressure. Even the smallest of cuts can rapidly develop into a deep ulcer when the tissue is inadequately nourished; the ball of the foot, the ankle, and the lower calf are the most commonly involved areas.

Ulcers occurring in any person with vascular disease require meticulous care to prevent infection or to prevent further infection with new organisms. Since local tissue resistance to infection is lessened and the rate of healing is slowed because of impaired circulation to the area, a long period of healing must be anticipated. Wet-to-dry dressings are often used for debridement. These dressings are applied wet, using sterile saline solution, allowed to dry, and then removed, taking away necrotic and sloughed tissue that adheres to the dried dressing. Foot soaks may be used, although this procedure cannot be sterile because it is impossible to cleanse the entire foot properly.

Preventing infection is one of the two most difficult problems confronting the nurse in caring for patients with ulcers. The second is providing for comfort. Although there is often diminished sensation in superficial tissue, there may be considerable pain when deep tissue layers are involved, and the patient may suffer a great deal of pain during dressing changes and wound soaks. Administering pain medication 15 to 30 minutes prior to wound care is of major importance.

The patient with an ulcer on his foot usually is urged to keep off his feet, although there is not complete agreement on the value of this restriction. Some physicians believe that, provided there is no direct weight bearing on the wound, the arterial circulation and healing are improved by a moderate amount of moving about and by keeping the limb in a dependent position for part of the day at least.

Cradles with lights are seldom used, but occasionally the physician may feel that dry warmth will improve healing of the ulcer. Using extreme caution, the nurse then leaves the wound exposed and places a cradle with a light in it over the ulcerated part. The bulb should never be larger than 25 W, and there should be a definite order from the physician as to how long it should be left on and how far from the limb it should be placed. Too much heat will increase the metabolic needs of the tissues and thus will be injurious.

A wide variety of agents are used in the local treatment of ulcers. These include castor oil and zinc oxide, nitrofurazone (Furacin), and scarlet red ointment. The effects of antibiotic and antibacterial topical agents such as penicillin, nitrofurazone, bacitracin, and neomycin need to be carefully monitored, since local allergic reactions are common. Streptokinase-streptodornase (Varidase) may be applied locally. Deep ulcers that do not heal properly often require skin grafting. (For special treatment of ulcers occurring in conjunction with varicose veins see p. 1037.)

Since many persons who have chronic ulcers of the legs and feet are not hospitalized, they must be taught how to bathe and otherwise care for themselves without contaminating the ulcer. Many elderly persons have lived with a chronic ulcer for so long that they become careless about their technique in changing soiled or loosened dressings. A periodic visit from a community health nurse, who can reemphasize essentials of care both to the person and to members of the family, is often beneficial.

□ Medications

Patients being treated with medications for peripheral vascular disease must have an understanding of the purpose of the medication and the way in which it is to be taken. Four general types of agents are used: anticoagulants, vasodilators, fibrinolytics, and plasma expanders.

Anticoagulants

Two of the commonly used anticoagulant drugs are *heparin* and *bishydroxycoumarin* (Dicumarol), although many other prothrombin depressants are now available. These drugs are used widely in the treatment of both venous and arterial thrombosis and are used prophylactically for persons with threatened thrombosis or threatened recurrence of a condition such as thrombophlebitis. They act therapeutically by prolonging the clotting time of the blood. They will not dissolve clots already formed but will prevent extension of a clot and inhibit formation of new clots.

Heparin antagonizes the activation of prothrombin to thrombin and in this way prolongs the clotting time of blood. It can be given only parenterally because it is destroyed by the gastric secretions of the stomach. Its effect is almost immediate, but its action ceases after 3 to 4 hours. Heparin dosage is expressed in units or milligrams and is calculated individually for each patient; 5,000 units (50 mg) is an average dose and is administered through an intravenous line every 3 to 4 hours. This drug is often used to lower the prothrombin time until an oral anticoagulant that acts more slowly can take effect; frequent clotting time determination must be done.

In order to achieve uniform blood levels over a period of time, heparin is sometimes administered as a continuous intravenous drip. It may be administered prophylactically in this form to patients on prolonged bed rest before overt signs and symptoms of clot formation are evident. For prophylactic purposes it may also be administered subcutaneously in dosages of 5,000 units every 12 hours. Planning of nursing care must emphasize the increased tendency for bleeding to occur in these patients. Nursing responsibilities are discussed below.

Bishydroxycoumarin acts by suppressing the activity of the liver in its formation of prothrombin. It takes 12 to 24 hours to take effect, and its action persists for 24 to 72 hours after the drug is discontinued. The usual maintenance dosage is 25 to 100 mg/day administered orally.[11] Frequent determinations of the prothrombin level must be obtained and the dose regulated accordingly. Daily prothrombin levels are important while the dose is being regulated. Most physicians believe that the prothrombin level should be kept between 10% and 30% of normal.

Warfarin sodium (Coumadin, Panwarfin, Prothromadin) is now widely used. Ethyl biscoumacetate (Tromexan) is another synthetic drug that has an action similar to that of bishydroxycoumarin, although it acts more quickly and its effect lasts for a shorter time.

Any anticoagulant drug requires very careful regulation as to amount and continuity of dosage. If the dosage is too large, the increased tendency to bleed reaches dangerous levels, and if given in combination with other drugs predisposing to bleeding such as acetylsalicylic acid preparations (aspirin) the problem becomes aggravated. If the dosage is too small the patient may have no relief from symptoms of thrombosis and may even have additional thrombus formation.

If bleeding results from too much heparin, protamine sulfate, a heparin antagonist, is given. Protamine acts almost immediately, and its effect persists for about 2 hours. The physician slowly injects a 1% solution intravenously. The total amount given depends on the amount of heparin that was given and on the patient's symptoms. If a patient taking bishydroxycoumarin should bleed from any body orifice such as the nose, mouth, or urinary tract, the physician should be notified before another dose is given. Usually the drug is discontinued, and vitamin K (menadione sodium bisulfite) or vitamin K_1 (phytonadione) is given intravenously or orally. If the hemorrhage is excessive, transfusions are given. Nursing care includes reassurance of the patient and careful observation for signs of further hemorrhage.

Anticoagulant therapy has prolonged the lives of many persons and enabled them to live quite satisfactorily and productively. The person who must remain on this drug indefinitely, however, needs encouragement and supportive medical and nursing care. Unfortunately the vein must be punctured at regular intervals to obtain blood for prothrombin determination. If large doses are needed, this procedure must be done at least two to three times a week and sometimes daily. When smaller doses of anticoagulant are given over long periods, a prothrombin determination is done every 1 to 4 weeks. This experience is unpleasant for the patient, and its continuance over weeks and months may place restraint on his activities. Vacations, for example, present problems, and even short trips must be carefully planned.

Teaching is one of the most important nursing measures in caring for the patient receiving anticoagulants. The patient must be taught to recognize the signs of bleeding from any site and to report them immediately. He should carry an identification card stating that he takes anticoagulant drugs so that in the event of accident persons who give him emergency care will have this information. The identification card should also contain the name and telephone number of the physician prescribing the drug.

Patients should also be taught not to take any other medications while taking anticoagulants without first consulting a physician. Aspirin and steroid preparations can be particularly dangerous in conjunction with heparin and warfarin (Coumadin). Other anticoagulants still being investigated are those that decrease fibrinogen levels, such as snake venom derivatives and staphylcoagulase.

Vasodilators

The second type of medications used to treat peripheral vascular diseases are vasodilators. Vasodilators are given to lessen vasospasm in the arterioles of the lower extremities when arteriosclerosis has caused narrowing of the lumen of the vessel or neighboring vessels, or when a thrombus has formed and caused partial or total obstruction. If a clot is adherent to a blood vessel, an anticoagulant drug may be given with the vasodilator to prevent further clot formation. While several drugs are useful for vasodilation, the excellent vasodilatory effects of warm baths, heat to the abdomen, and hot fluids taken orally should not be overlooked.

Papaverine, a non-habit-forming alkaloid of opium, has long been known to have a relaxing effect on the smooth muscle of the blood vessels, especially when spasm occurs. The usual dose is 300 mg orally once a day. This drug may be used in the treatment of acute arterial occlusion associated with arteriosclerosis obliterans.

Tolazoline hydrochloride (Priscoline), 25 to 50 mg ($^3/_8$ to $^3/_4$ grain), given orally three to four times a day, is an adrenergic blocking agent (sympatholytic drug). It also may be given intravenously. It prevents the transmission of impulses from the ends of the vasoconstrictor sympathetic fibers to the smooth muscle of the arterioles and thus produces vasodilation. Other drugs that have a similar effect and are prescribed for vasodilation in peripheral vascular diseases are *azapetine phosphate* (Ilidar), *dibenzyl-B-chlorethylamine* (Dibenamine), and *phenoxybenzamine hydrochloride* (Dibenzyline). Toxic reactions to these drugs include palpitation, tachycardia, nausea and vomiting, pruritus and abnormal skin sensations, and drop in blood pressure. Toxic signs should be carefully watched for in any patient receiving these drugs and are reported to the physician at once. The patient who cannot tolerate one of these drugs may be able to take another without untoward effects.

Besides the adrenergic blocking agents there are other drugs that are used for their beneficial effect in peripheral vascular disease. *Isoxsuprine* (Vasodilan) and *nylidrin hydrochloride* (Arlidin) are sympathomimetic amines chemically similar to epinephrine. They possess vasodilating effects, particularly in the vessels in skeletal muscles. Favorable results have been reported with the use of these agents in the treatment of intermittent claudication. Isoxsuprine is usually given orally (10 to 20 mg four times a day); an intramuscular form is also available. Nylidrin is administered orally (6 to 12 mg three times a day) or intramuscularly (5 mg once daily). Side effects include nervousness, palpitation, and nausea and vomiting. *Cyclandelate* (Cyclospasmol) and *nicotinyl tartrate* (Roniacol) produce direct vasodilation of the smooth muscle of the peripheral blood vessels. The usual dosage of cyclandelate is 100 to 200 mg four times daily; the dose of nicotinyl is 50 to 150 mg three times daily after meals. Both can produce dizziness, flushing, and nausea and vomiting. The latter is more likely to occur with nicotinyl because it acts like nicotinic acid.

Alcohol is a very useful drug in dilating the blood vessels. The usual dosage is 30 to 60 ml three to four times a day. The alcohol preparation often ordered is whiskey and soda, but any of the common beverages containing alcohol can be used. Some physicians order a double dose at bedtime to produce maximum effect during the hours when muscle action is not assisting the flow of blood to the legs. *Caffeine* (contained in tea and coffee) and *theobromine* (found in chocolate) also are peripheral vasodilators, but these drugs are seldom given for their vasodilating effect. However, because they have this effect there usually is no need to eliminate tea, coffee, and chocolate from the diet of the person with peripheral vascular disease.

Fibrinolytics

The third type of medication that may be ordered is a fibrinolytic drug. Unlike heparin and warfarin, these drugs will dissolve fibrinous material through direct enzyme action. They are generally available in topical forms or for systemic use.

Streptokinase-streptodornase (Varidase), purified *trypsin crystalline* (Tryptar), and *fibrinuclease* (Elase) are ointment forms that will dissolve fibrinous material and purulent accumulations. They are valuable in removing necrotic tissue for debridement. These enzymes are frequently ordered in treatment of ulcers on the legs, which may occur as a complication of peripheral vascular disease resulting from inadequate circulation. The enzymes used in conjunction with antibiotics seem to promote more rapid healing. The drugs are usually applied topically in the form of wet dressings.

Purified streptokinase and urokinase may be used for systemic therapy in treating thrombosis. Streptokinase is extremely antigenic and is not used often because of the incidence of allergic reactions. Urokinase, although expensive, has been used both intraarterially and intravenously.

Plasma expanders

Drugs that affect the surface factors of blood constituents comprise the fourth category. *Dextran* is administered intravenously for its ability to prevent thrombus propagation and hasten resolution of the thrombus. The hazard associated with the drug is that of fluid overload. It is generally administered as 500 ml of a 6% solution of sodium chloride and may expand plasma volume to such a degree that circulatory overload develops.

□ Prevention of complications

The person with peripheral vascular disease has a chronic, potentially disabling process and is subject to periods of exacerbation. The single most important treatment is prevention. The person must be assisted and encouraged to become knowledgeable about all facets of his disease, particularly those that indicate a worsening condition. Prompt medical attention can often preclude complications such as infection or even amputation.

The most serious change in condition that warrants contacting a physician is an area of skin breakdown that does not heal rapidly. Once the integrity of the skin is broken, the diminished circulation often cannot supply the area with sufficient oxygen, nutrients, and leukocytes to protect against infection, and once begun, small infections readily become worse.

Persons with any vascular disease are prone to thrombosis, and any *sudden* change in circulation to an extremity must be promptly evaluated. This would include any change in sensation, color, or temperature in the extremity.

Pain that grows progressively worse over time may also indicate a worsening condition. The patient's physician must be kept aware of changes of this nature in order to evaluate therapy and make necessary alterations.

Peripheral vascular disease has no single cure, and the patient must be knowledgeable about his disease as it affects and is affected by his life style and daily habits. This same knowledge guides the nurse in providing care in the hospital setting. For example, when the patient is hospitalized for treatment of a leg ulcer, he must be provided with a warm environment to prevent chills and vasoconstriction and with a diet high in protein to facilitate healing. A sheepskin or flotation pad may be needed to prevent further skin breakdown.

Persons with peripheral vascular disease often have many hospitalizations or frequent ambulatory care visits. It is essential that the patient's record reflect what teaching has been accomplished and how the patient responded to it so that subsequent teaching can build on his knowledge and level of understanding.

□ Emotional support

Emotional support of the person with peripheral vascular disease warrants special consideration because the disease is chronic, affects the person throughout his life, and often requires changes in lifetime habits. It may be difficult for the person to perceive how much control over the disease process he can exert, although this perception is essential in eliciting his active involvement in the treatment program. Improvements in circulation are often slow, and the person needs constant encouragement to maintain the therapeutic regimen. What may seem like minor external changes, such as a better color of nailbeds, can be pointed to as signs of significant internal improvement in the change of the vasculature. Again, the person needs to be taught what to observe.

The pain associated with peripheral vascular disease can also be quite discouraging The more the nurse can learn about the person's pain, how it affects him, and how he copes with it, the better the nurse will be able to plan with him measures to alleviate his discomfort. Interest in the individual, recognition of the difficulty in coping with persistent pain, and willingness to listen are often the first steps in helping.

The problems that peripheral vascular disease presents often complicate the adjustments involved in the aging process. Additional physical limitation may be imposed when the individual is already attempting to cope with a less active life style. Dependency-independency conflicts may be aggravated by the older individual's need for health care at home. For further information on assisting the individual with a chronic disease, see Chapter 29.

□ Outcome criteria for the person with peripheral vascular disease

The patient or significant others can:

1. Explain restrictions on activity or prescribed exercise routines.
2. Explain the prescribed diet and plan appropriate meals.
3. Explain the hazards of smoking.
4. Demonstrate measures to prevent skin breakdown.
5. Explain how to avoid external factors that compromise circulation (not cross legs, avoid binding clothing such as garters, etc.).
6. Explain medication and treatment program:
   a. State dosage, action, frequency, and side effects of prescribed medications.
   b. If taking anticoagulants, can state precautions to be observed (attention to bleeding, prevention of bleeding, carrying an identification card).
   c. Describe how and when to apply any topical medication or dressings.
7. Explain health maintenance program:
   a. State symptoms that indicate the need for obtaining medical attention (bleeding, pain, skin breakdown).
   b. State plans for follow-up care.

■ ARTERIAL DISEASE

The function of the arteries is to transport blood from the heart to the tissues, utilizing the pressure pulses generated by the heart. Any disturbance in the structure of the arteries interferes with this function, resulting in diminished blood and decreased oxygen supply to the tissues. The symptoms of arterial disease are not caused by the degree of obstruction or narrowing but by the degree to which the involved body part is deprived of circulation. This in turn is affected by such factors as blood pressure and presence or absence of collateral circulation. For example, 50% occlusion of one artery may cause severe symptoms, while 50% occlusion of another artery will cause no symptoms if collateral circulation is sufficient to provide oxygenation.

The arteries are comprised of three layers: the *intima*, consisting of a single endothelium; the *media*, containing smooth muscle cells and elastic fibers; and the *adventitia*, the outermost layer of connective tissue. The proportion of elastic tissue and muscle tissue varies with location in the body and age.

□ Arteriosclerosis

Arteriosclerosis is a general term that literally means hardening of the arteries. It primarily affects the medial layer and occurs as the result of senile changes and calcification. Over time the arteries become less distensible and lose their elastic properties. The cerebral arteries and arteries of the lower extremities are the most commonly affected.

Atherosclerosis is generally viewed as a type of arteriosclerosis or as part of the aging process that also results in arteriosclerosis. Atherosclerosis refers to the development of lesions on the intimal wall. Three types of lesions have been identified: (1) fatty streaks, which consist of smooth-muscle cells, and lipid depositions, which are present in the aorta of all individuals by age 10 years but which do not necessarily progress to produce disease; (2) fibrous plaques, which involve a thickening of the intima and are surrounded by lipids, collagen, and elastic fibers; and (3) the complicated lesion associated with disease, which is a large mass consisting of lipids and extracellular and intracellular debris, ulceration, hemorrhage, and thrombus formation.

The exact pathogenesis of atherosclerosis is not clearly understood. Endothelial cell injury, smooth-muscle cell proliferation, and lipid and cell debris accumulation are among the factors that seem to be inherent in the development of lesions. The exact sequence of events, the mechanism for transport of lipids into the arterial wall, and the factors that promote cell proliferation are unknown.

The lesions of atherosclerosis tend to be focal rather than diffuse, increase with age, and involve primarily the larger arteries, particularly the lower portion of the aorta. Persons who develop myocardial infarctions or cerebral infarctions are usually found to have atherosclerotic involvement in many other sites.[33]

The risk factor that has gained the most attention is relationship to atherosclerosis is the level of serum lipids. Of all risk factors, hyperlipidemia has the highest correlation with coronary heart disease. Lipoproteins may be elevated due to dietary excesses alone; may be genetically determined, as in type II hyperlipoproteinemia; or may be a combination of excessive intake of saturated fats in combination with inborn errors of carbohydrate metabolism, as in type IV hyperlipoproteinemia. Although all types are associated with increased incidence of coronary artery disease, types II and III carry the greatest risk.

Other variables associated with atherosclerosis include diabetes, hypertension, and sex. Coronary and peripheral atherosclerosis is two to three times more prevalent in the diabetic, regardless of serum lipid levels. Hypertension is believed to accentuate the process of lesion formation, perhaps by producing mechanical stress. The incidence is also greater in men than in women.

□ Arteriosclerosis obliterans

Arteriosclerosis obliterans is an obstructive, degenerative arterial disorder representing a late stage of atherosclerosis and involving both the medial and intimal layers. It is characterized by partial or complete occlusion of arteries by atheromas on the intima, segmental in nature, but with changes evident distal and proximal to the stenosis. The media gradually loses elasticity as the disease progresses, and the development of thrombi are common.

As a result the artery gradually becomes unable to transport the required amount of blood to the affected part. Symptoms appear when the blood vessels can no longer provide enough blood to supply oxygen and nutrients to the limbs and to remove the waste products of metabolism.

Arteriosclerosis obliterans is the most common form of obstructive disease after 30 years of age. The femoral artery is the most commonly involved, although the carotid artery may also be involved. The disease affects men more often than women, and the greatest incidence is between 50 and 70 years of age. It is associated with diabetes and with cigarette smoking.

Clinical picture

Early signs and symptoms of arteriosclerosis obliterans may include skin temperature changes, differences in color and size of lower limbs, altered arterial pulsations, and the presence of *bruits* (sounds heard over the artery on auscultation). Intermittent claudication (p. 1018) is the most common symptom. Later the patient may complain of pain in the affected part even at rest. Pain at rest indicates that the artery cannot supply sufficient circulation to meet even minimal metabolic demands. The pain often occurs at night, and the patient may report that it subsides with movement and particularly with walking. Very elderly patients may be awakened by excruciating cramplike pains in the muscles of the calf and the thighs that are believed to be due to lack of oxygen to the tissue *(ischemia)*. Tingling and numbness of the toes may be mentioned by the patient, and a very common complaint is difficulty in keeping the feet and hands warm enough for comfort. Occasionally the first sign of limited circulation is necrosis following mild trauma such as cutting the skin when trimming the nails; ulcers and gangrene may develop.

The disease is usually present to some extent in both limbs, although symptoms may be grossly apparent in only one. Occlusion of a fairly large artery by a thrombus will cause numbness, marked coldness, and a chalk-white appearance to the part of the limb supplied by the obstructed vessel. An essential nursing function when caring for patients with peripheral vascular disease is the checking of the arterial pulses. Symptoms of cerebrovascular insufficiency may result from blockage of flow through one or both carotid arteries. The first overt physical sign may be a frank stroke, transient ischemic attacks (TIAs), or asymptomatic bruits.

Medical intervention

Medical treatment for arteriosclerosis obliterans includes provision for general warmth, use of drugs to produce vasodilation, specific exercises to stimulate collateral circulation, carefully prescribed general exercise to maintain circulation and yet not tax the arterial system, encouragement, and instruction in avoiding injury, preventing infection, and maintaining nutrition. Pain at rest may be treated by having the patient sleep with the head of the bed elevated on blocks 7.5 to 15 cm (3 to 6 in) in height to aid gravity in carrying arterial blood to the legs and feet. The patient should be advised not to walk about during the night unless he is warmly clothed and to avoid sitting with his legs over the side of the bed because he may become chilled and knee flexion further hampers circulation. He should not rub the extremity because of the danger of trauma and of releasing an embolus into the circulation. *Vigorous massage is always contraindicated in any patient with vascular disease.* A graduated program of exercise may be prescribed.

Nursing intervention is directed toward helping the person to live within his limitations and encouraging him and his family to carry out medical instructions so that the disease may be held in check for an indefinite time. All nursing measures discussed earlier in this chapter under general interventions may be necessary in caring for the persons. If the condition cannot be checked, gangrene of the extremity eventually may occur, making amputation necessary.

Surgical intervention

If the disease is rapidly progressive and the patient is in reasonably good health otherwise, surgery to correct the obstruction may be indicated. The most common procedure is a bypass of the obstructed arterial segment, using saphenous vein grafts or grafts made of synthetic materials such as Teflon or Dacron. The bypass may involve the aorta itself, as with an aortofemoral bypass, or more distal vessels such as the femoral-popliteal (Fig. 47-2).

Procedures that may be performed either in conjunction with a bypass or by themselves include *patch grafting* (replacing a damaged segment of the arterial wall with a vein patch), *profundoplasty* (widening of the origin of the femoral artery with a vein patch), and *endarterectomy* (stripping arteriosclerotic plaques from the intima and inner media using balloon catheters or other instruments). Carotid endarterectomy has become more frequently used as diagnostic methods have improved. Patency rate of the artery following surgery has averaged 95%, with a mortality of 0.5% to 3%.[33]

Postoperative nursing intervention for patients undergoing arterial reconstructive surgery centers around assessment of circulation to the involved extremities.

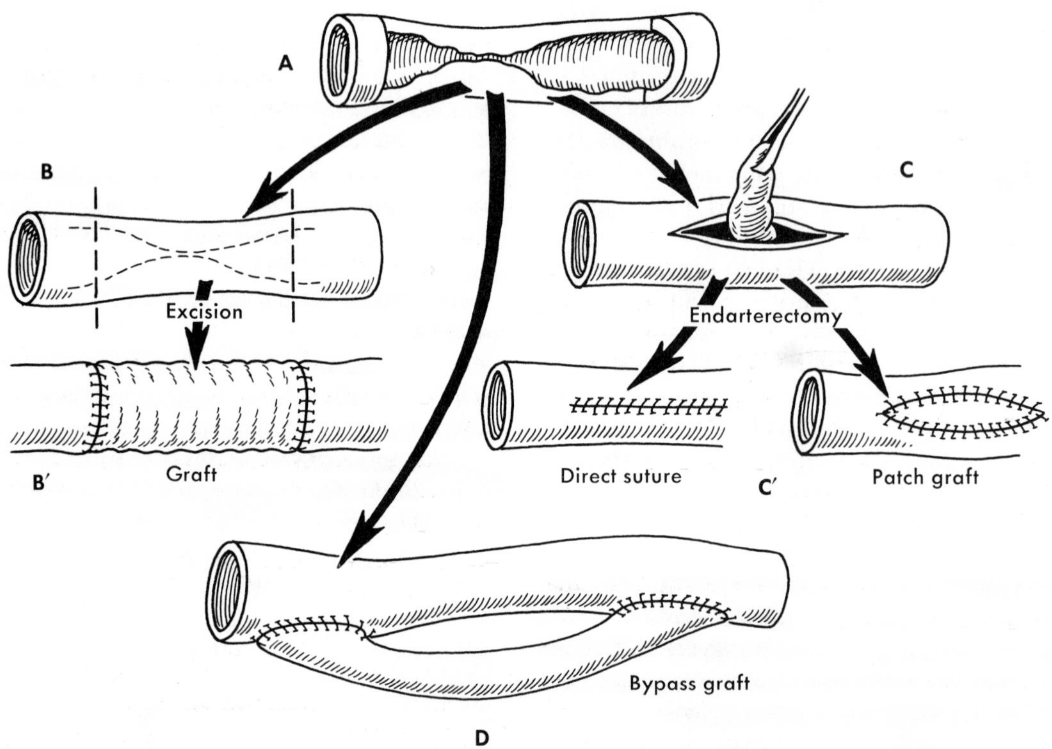

Fig. 47-2. A, Obstructed artery. Methods of restoring arterial blood flow include **B,** excision; **B′,** graft; **C,** endarterectomy; **C′,** direct suture and patch graft reconstruction; and **D,** bypass graft. (Redrawn from Fairbairn, J. F., Jurgens, J. L., and Spittell, J. A.: Peripheral vascular disease, Philadelphia, 1972, W. B. Saunders Co.)

The nurse needs to be aware of the preoperative condition of the extremities in order to make meaningful postoperative comparisons. The color, temperature, sensation, and quality of pulses in the extremity must be checked hourly for the first 8 hours. Initially vasospasm may make it difficult or impossible to palpate the pedal or posterior tibial pulses, and a Doppler machine may be used (p. 1020). When adequate circulation has been restored it will be evident from the color and temperature of the limb, which often will be warmer than its counterpart. Obstruction is indicated by a marked coldness, sudden disappearance of a pulse that was palpable the previous hour, or a progressive whitening, later changing to cyanosis, of the toes and foot. The surgeon is notified immediately if these changes occur.

Patients are usually kept flat in bed for the first 12 to 24 hours and then are allowed out of bed but must *avoid sharp flexion in the areas of the grafts.* The success of the surgery is dependent on the general health of the patient and the size of the vessels involved. The larger the vessel the more effective the surgery, with aortic-iliac grafts having the highest success rate (90%).[6] The nurse must be alert to any sign of infection in the incisional area (redness, swelling, or purulent drainage). Infection of a prosthetic graft, although occurring rarely, invariably means failure of the graft.

□ Thromboangiitis obliterans

Thromboangiitis obliterans (Buerger's disease) is an idiopathic disease in which there is inflammation of the walls of the blood vessels, thrombus formation, fibrous thickening and scarring, and eventual occlusion of the vessels. Superficial veins may be affected early in the disease, but it primarily involves small- and medium-sized arteries. Arteriolar spasm is common, aggravating the fibrous constriction. Although the feet usually are affected first, vascular changes may occur in the hands and eventually throughout the entire body. The disease rarely occurs in those who do not smoke, and cigarettes are being investigated as the causative factor. Hypercoagulability of the blood is also thought to play a role. The outcome of acute exacerbations depends on the size of the area deprived of normal blood supply and the amount of collateral circulation that can be established. Collateral vessels attempt to keep pace with the destruction, but over a period of years they usually cannot do so, and ulceration and gangrene are common. This disease is most common in men aged 25 to 40 years. It is slightly more prevalent in persons who are Jewish. It rarely occurs in females or in blacks.

Clinical picture

The signs and symptoms of thromboangiitis obliterans are caused by peripheral ischemia. The most common complaint is persistent coldness of one or both lower extremities. Arterial pulses are reduced or absent. Numbness, tingling, and aching pain also may be present. General chilling and exposure of the hands and feet to cold aggravate the symptoms. There may be hardened, red, and painful areas along the affected vessels, and the person often reports that there is a burning or boring pain that is aggravated by chilling, smoking, and nervous tension. There is often edema about the areas of inflammation, and the entire limb, except where there is acute inflammation, may be cooler to the touch and whiter than normal. Cyanosis may occur when the feet are lowered.

Intervention

It is often possible to arrest thromboangiitis obliterans completely and indefinitely by merely having the patient stop smoking. This restriction is considered the most important aspect of treatment. Smoking must be given up immediately, completely, and forever. Other measures prescribed to foster circulation and to help make use of limited resources include warmth, use of vasodilating drugs such as alcohol and tolazoline (Priscoline), moderate exercise, use of an oscillating bed, and instruction to prevent infection and to avoid trauma and exposure to cold. Some physicians believe that *bilateral preganglionic sympathectomy* is helpful when the lower extremities are involved because it produces permanent vasodilation of the blood vessels. Sympathetic impulses may also be blocked by paravertebral injection of alcohol. Although pain may be severe, narcotics are rarely prescribed because of the obvious danger of drug addiction in young persons with a chronic disease such as thromboangiitis obliterans.

The nurse can often help by emphasizing to the patient the precautions he should take to prevent the onset of acute symptoms including pain. He should be encouraged not to smoke, and he should be advised to wear warm gloves and footwear in cold weather. Both of these measures prevent extensive vasoconstriction. He should be taught to avoid any injury to his feet, especially when cutting toenails. Wounds heal slowly, and gangrene may develop.

□ Raynaud's disease

Raynaud's disease is a condition of unknown cause characterized by arterial spasm of the extremities, most often the hands. Cold and emotional stress are the usual precipitating factors. Pallor and cyanosis occur during the spasm, followed by rubor resulting from vasodilation. Although the exact mechanism is unknown, abnormal sympathetic innervation, or hypersusceptibility to certain stimuli, is thought to be a possible cause. When spasm is not occurring, circulation is usually adequate, although gangrene of the fingertips may occur in severe cases.

Raynaud's disease occurs almost exclusively in women, and symptoms are usually evident before the age of 40 years. Patients often respond well to a sympathectomy in which the nerve control of blood vessels to the hands is removed, leaving the blood vessels permanently dilated. Patients in whom the condition is mild may be treated with drugs such as dibenzylchlorethamine (Dibenamine), which inhibits sympathetic nervous system activity. The patient is advised to avoid smoking and to keep the hands and the rest of the body warm.

Raynaud's phenomenon refers to any condition involving vasospasm that produces local functional changes in the peripheral circulation associated with other factors or conditions. This would include the vasospasm that occurs with scleroderma and rheumatoid arthritis or that associated with mechanical trauma such as occurs in those whose occupation involves the use of the pneumatic air hammer.

□ Embolism

Emboli are blood clots floating in the circulating blood. These clots most commonly originate in the heart. They may be a fragment of an arteriosclerotic plaque loosened from the aorta or a thrombus released when inefficient heart pumping is suddenly corrected by digitalization. Emboli usually lodge at the bifurcations, or divisions, of the arteries because of the diminishing caliber of the vessels beyond these points. An embolus lodging at the bifurcation of any artery is called a *saddle embolus*. As soon as an embolus lodges, thrombi (propagated emboli) form in the involved vessel.

The signs of sudden lodging or formation of a large thrombus in an artery are dramatic and vary with the part of the arterial system and associated organ system involved. There is severe pain at the site of the thrombus formation. Fainting, nausea, vomiting, and signs of pronounced shock may appear. Almost immediately areas supplied by the vessel may become white, cold, and blotched, and they may tingle and feel numb. Cyanosis, followed by even greater darkening and gangrene, occurs if the blood supply is completely obstructed and collateral circulation is inadequate. Vasodilating drugs are given to improve the collateral circulation, warmth is applied to the body, and a sympathetic block of the lumbar ganglia may be performed in an attempt to produce vasodilation of other vessels. Oxygen may be administered to alleviate hypoxemia and dyspnea. Vasopressors may be necessary if shock ensues. Heparin and bishydroxycoumarin may be administered to help prevent further thrombus formation. The patient who is suspected of having or who has an acute embolic obstruction of a larger artery needs constant nursing supervision. Pain is severe, and fear is pronounced.

If the patient does not respond to the medical treatment within a few hours, surgery may be performed. Surgical procedures that may be done include opening the vessel and removing the clot *(embolectomy)*, removing the clot and also removing adherent substances and part of the lining of the vessel (*endarterectomy*, or "reaming"), arterial resection with removal of the clot and the adherent diseased artery surrounding it with subsequent grafting, and bypassing the diseased portion of the vessel with a graft as is sometimes done for an aneurysm. Embolectomy is usually the treatment of choice for aortic embolus and for an embolus of the common iliac artery.

Nursing care following embolectomy is similar to that for the patient who has had surgery for an aneurysm. Blood pressure must be carefully recorded preoperatively so that suitable comparisons can be made postoperatively. It is important that the blood pressure not vary too much from what it was preoperatively because variation will predispose to thrombus formation. A complication that must be carefully watched for is hemorrhage. Small arteries that may have been useless while the embolus was in the artery may not bleed freely during surgery and may therefore be missed when bleeding vessels are tied off. They may resume normal function after the operation and cause hemorrhage.

□ Aneurysm of the extremity and arteriovenous fistula

Aneurysms of the arteries of the lower extremities, particularly in the popliteal area, are quite common in persons over 60 years of age who have pronounced arteriosclerosis (Fig. 47-3). These aneurysms often are easily palpable. Thrombi form at the site of an aneurysm, and emboli may travel to obstruct more distal portions of the artery. This type of aneurysm is sometimes confused with an arteriovenous fistula, which is an abnormal communication between an artery and a vein caused either by a congenital anomaly or by trauma. In arteriovenous fistulas the blood in the artery bypasses the capillary bed, which has a strong resistance to flow, and flows instead directly into the vein. Both lesions produce a characteristic sound called a *bruit*, which is heard on auscultation. If the cause is an aneurysm the bruit may be interspersed with the arterial pulsations, whereas the bruit caused by a fistula is often a constant soft, purring sound. Both conditions impair the supply of blood to the portion of the limb supplied by the vessel, and various signs of poor blood supply such as atrophy, cyanosis, tropic changes, or even gangrene may occur.

Closure of the fistula or removal of a portion of the aneurysm is the preferred treatment. When one of these

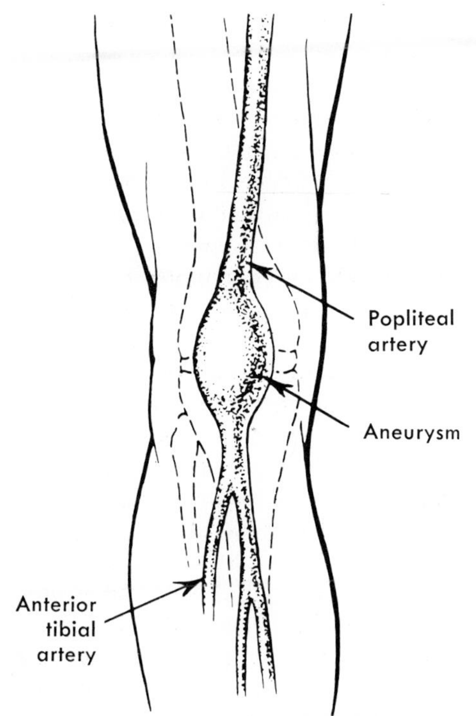

Fig. 47-3. Posterior view of knee with aneurysm of popliteal artery. (From Anderson, H. C.: Newton's geriatric nursing, ed. 5, St. Louis, 1971, The C. V. Mosby Co.)

measures is not possible, the vessel may be ligated unless ligation is incompatible with the life of tissues distal to the lesion. Homografts (a section of the patient's vein) or Teflon or Dacron grafts can be used in larger blood vessels of the extremities either to replace portions of the artery that contain the aneurysm or to bypass the abnormality. In addition to general postoperative care, the patient who has had this surgical procedure may be treated with any or all of the medications and other means described in this chapter to augment circulation when arterial supply is limited or when thrombosis threatens.

■ VENOUS DISEASE

□ Thrombophlebitis

Thrombophlebitis, or venous thrombois, is characterized by inflammation of a vein and by clot formation. Although much is known about some mechanisms producing inflammatory changes and thrombus production, the incidence of this condition continues to increase,[1] and the exact interrelationship of the factors is not clearly understood. In some cases the thrombosis appears to be the primary event, and in others inflammation of the vein endothelium is thought to precede the development of the thrombus.

Many factors are associated with thrombophlebitis. Venous stasis, damage to the endothelium, and hypercoagulability of the blood are all significant etiologic mechanisms. Stasis may result from relatively simple circumstances such as taking a long trip during which hours were spent sitting with the knees flexed. Pregnancy is often complicated by thrombophlebitis due to interference with venous return in the lower abdomen. Before the days of early ambulation and emphasis on exercises postoperatively, thrombophlebitis was a frequent complication of surgery. It remains a dreaded complication of any illness that requires immobilization for any length of time, and the use of low-dose heparin prophylactically is becoming more common.

Trauma to venous walls may result from the irritating effects of certain drugs or hypertonic solutions. The presence of intravenous catheters, particularly when left in place longer than 48 hours, has been associated with increased thrombosis. Damage to the veins may accompany trauma such as fractures and has been known to follow unusual physical exertion and muscle strain.

States of hypercoagulability, such as occurs with hematologic diseases such as polycythemia and severe anemia, also predispose to the development of thrombophlebitis. Thrombosis is known to occur to some degree in all types of systemic infections, and this may reflect hypercoagulability caused by endotoxins. It is believed that the use of oral contraceptives is correlated with increased intravascular clotting, but the exact mechanism responsible for this association is not yet known.

Clinical picture

Thrombophlebitis of superficial veins is readily apparent. On palpation the veins appear hard and thready and are sensitive to pressure. The entire limb may be swollen, pale, and cold, and the area along the vein may be reddened and feel warm to the touch. Deep veins in the legs may be affected, and the pain they cause when the patient dorsiflexes his foot or walks is known as *Homan's sign.* Thrombophlebitis may be accompanied by reflected pain in the entire limb. Systemic reaction to the infection, which may occur in any blood vessel when free flow of blood is interrupted, may rarely cause symptoms such as headache, malaise, and elevation of temperature. Of utmost importance in the assessment of patients is the knowledge that thrombophlebitis is a common condition, occurring in at least 5% of all surgical patients and going unrecognized in half of these. Embolization of the thrombus to lungs, heart, or brain may be a fatal complication and at the very least results in prolonged hospitalization and increased cost to the patient.

Intervention

Superficial thrombophlebitis is usually treated by rest; however, physicians differ in regard to the amount of activity the patient is allowed. Some believe that the clot is sufficiently adherent to the vein wall to make its release unlikely and that moving about helps to improve general circulation and to prevent further congestion of blood in the veins. Others believe that complete immobilization is necessary to prevent a part of the thrombus from breaking away and becoming an embolus. The patient who has thrombophlebitis of large and deep vessels, however, usually is kept quiet. Care must be taken that the patient is not frightened by being kept quiet; explanations from both the physician and the nurse will be helpful in reassuring the patient. Occasionally the vein is ligated above the involvement (usually at the femoral junction) to decrease the danger of embolism, but this procedure is not possible unless there is adequate collateral circulation. The period of immobilization depends entirely on the response of the patient to treatment.

Continuous applications of warm moist heat are often used for both deep and superficial thrombophlebitis. Some physicians feel, however, that heat increases the risk that emboli will be released because it induces vasodilation, and they order ice packs for their patients, especially for those with deep venous thrombosis. When warm packs are used they are usually ordered to cover the entire extremity.[10] Heating pads permanently set on "low" may be used to keep the packs at a consistently safe temperature.

Many physicians prefer that the affected limb be elevated slightly to reduce edema and to prevent stasis distal to the thrombus. It may also relieve pain. Some physicians believe, however, that the danger of an embolus being released is greater if the limb is elevated. Therefore the nurse will need to check on the procedure to be followed in the care of each patient.

Heparin and bishydroxycoumarin are used for patients with thrombophlebitis, and sometimes patients must remain on prophylactic doses of bishydroxycoumarin for an indefinite period to prevent recurrences of the disease. Vasodilating drugs are given to combat the arterial vessel spasm that occurs at the site of a venous thrombus and to improve general circulation, thus increasing the rate of absorption of the thrombus.

All persons with thrombophlebitis are observed closely for any signs of embolism, which must be reported at once. Pulmonary embolism (p. 1130) is the most common type, but emboli may also lodge in the coronary vessels (p. 992) or elsewhere.

Following thrombophlebitis in a lower limb that is severe enough to require hospitalization or bed rest, the patient usually needs to wear an elastic stocking or elastic bandage when walking. The stocking or bandage is also often ordered for patients who have superficial thrombophlebitis, which tends to recur. After 4 to 6 weeks, if the patient is progressing favorably, the stocking or bandage may be removed for periods of 1/2 to 1 hour and the results noted. If there is no evidence of edema or discomfort, it may be removed for longer and longer periods until its use may be discontinued completely. Many patients wear the stockings indefinitely when their work necessitates standing for long periods or sitting with the knees bent. Two stockings or bandages are necessary for each affected limb so that they can be laundered as necessary.

The *elastic stocking*, accurately fitted to the patient's measurements, must be obtained before the patient gets out of bed for the first time. The stocking is used to compress superficial veins, increase flow through the deep veins, and prevent venous pooling. Stockings of various sizes and lengths are usually stocked by hospital supply stores, and many large department stores also carry them. The measurements that must be taken are printed on the box or can be obtained by calling the store. The most satisfactory length is 2.5 cm (1 in) below the bend of the knee joint. The patient must be taught how to put on the stocking. It should be rolled on evenly before he gets out of bed in the morning. It should be removed once during the day for a few moments and the skin very gently stroked and powdered as necessary. The stocking need not be worn during sleeping hours.

Elastic bandages may be used instead of an elastic stocking, but they are more conspicuous and are difficult to apply evenly. They may be used for short periods following surgery and are sometimes ordered for use on

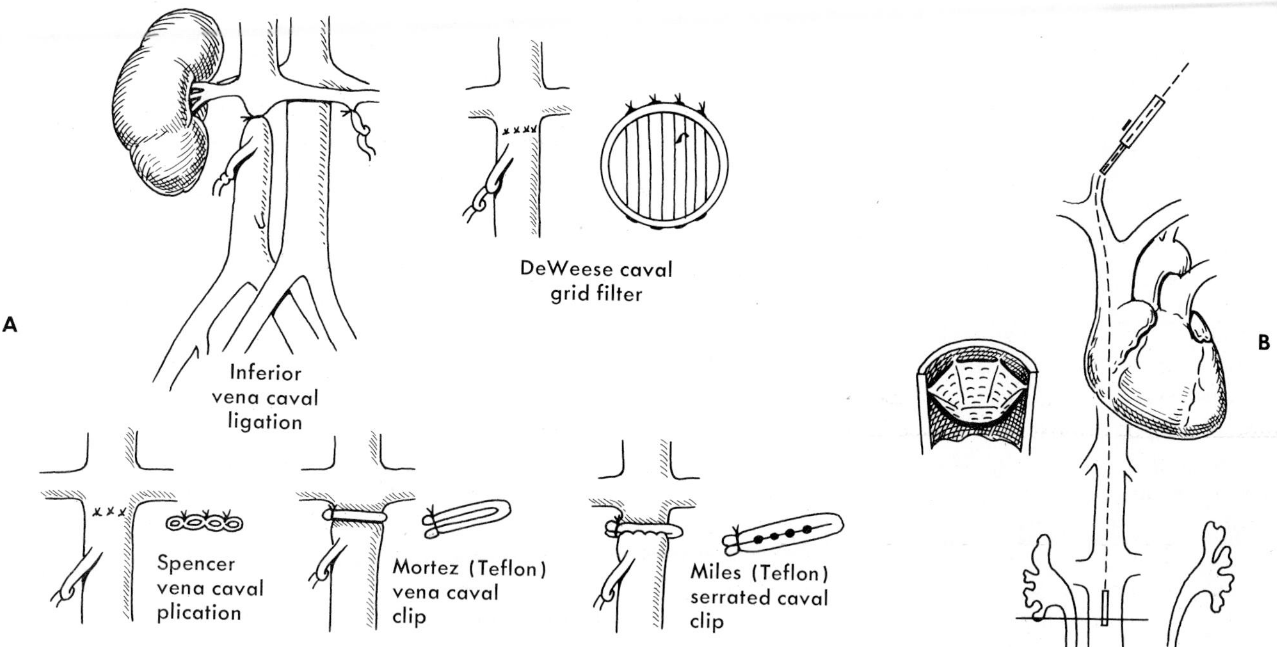

Fig. 47-4. A, Various surgical techniques for preventing embolism from pelvic and lower extremity veins. **B,** Transvenous method of vena caval interruption using caval prosthesis of umbrella design. Insert illustrates open umbrella. (Redrawn from Fairbairn, J. F., Jurgens, J. L., and Spittell, J. A.: Peripheral vascular disease, Philadelphia, 1972, W. B. Saunders Co.)

those occasions when the person will be lifting heavy objects or standing still for a period of time. When a bandage has been ordered for continuous use it should be applied before the person gets out of bed in the morning. The bandage is applied with equal pressure and overlap from the foot upward. Usually the entire foot, including the heel, is wrapped. The bandage will extend either to just below the knee or to the groin, depending on the physician's orders. It should be smooth and snug but must not be so tight that it interferes with circulation.

Swimming and wading in water are among the best activities for prevention of recurrences of thrombophlebitis of the lower extremities and are highly recommended for persons with other venous diseases as well. Water, which is denser than air, exerts a smooth, even pressure on the skin, and wading is especially beneficial because the greater pressure (the deeper water) surrounds the distal portion of the extremity and helps in the return flow of venous blood.

If conservative measures such as bed rest and anticoagulation are not successful, if the thrombosis is extensive and recurrent, or if embolization is recurrent, surgical treatment may be necessary. The peripheral vein involved, such as the superficial femoral vein, may be ligated or the vena cava interrupted by ligation or placement of a vena caval umbrella or grid to impede blood flow.

Caval ligation and plication are major surgical procedures requiring general anesthesia. In addition to the usual postoperative nursing interventions, the nurse must focus on assessing all parameters of circulation. Postoperative bleeding and hematoma formation occasionally occur, especially if anticoagulants are continued. Collateral circulation should be sufficient to prevent pooling of blood in the extremities, but stasis and edema may be noted in the late postoperative period. The caval umbrella can be inserted with instruments transvenously while the patient is under local anesthetic and is much more commonly used (Fig. 47-4). Postoperative nursing care is similar to that for the patient who has had a cardiac catheterization (p. 925).

□ Varicose veins

Varicose veins are abnormally dilated veins with incompetent valves, occurring most often in the lower extremities and the lower trunk. In the lower limbs the great and small saphenous veins are most often involved. At least 20% of the total population is affected by varicose veins. The highest incidence is in the third, fourth, and fifth decades of life. Factors that predispose a person to the development of varicosities include congenitally defective valves, hereditary weakness of the vein walls, and prolonged standing, which places strain on the valves because muscle action is not helping to return the blood. Our upright position further aggravates the problem, and poor posture with sagging of abdominal organs causes additional pressure. Pregnancy and abdominal tumors that cause pressure on the large veins of the lower abdomen and interfere with good venous drainage predispose a person to the development of varicose veins. Chronic systemic disease such as heart disease and cirrhosis of the liver may interfere with adequate return of blood to the heart and contribute to varicosities. Infections and trauma to the veins with resultant thrombophlebitis may also lead to varicose veins, since the valves are destroyed as the acute inflammation subsides.

Clinical picture

Varicosities of superficial veins are often quite apparent through the skin even before they cause symptoms. They appear as darkened, tortuous, raised blood vessels that become more prominent on standing and when positions that cause congestion such as sitting with the knees crossed are assumed. Sometimes the sclerosed valves can be seen as nodular protrusions. The varicosity is more pronounced just above the valve that has become ineffective. Pain, fatigue, feeling of heaviness in the legs, and muscular cramps may occur. Discomfort is worse during hot weather and when there is a change from a low to a high altitude. It is greatly increased by prolonged standing.

The simplest test for varicose veins is known as the *Trendelenburg* test. The patient lies down with the leg raised until the vein empties completely. He then stands, and the vein is observed as it fills. A normal vein fills from below; a varicose vein fills from above because the valve fails to retain the blood that has drained into the portion of the vessel above (Fig. 47-5).

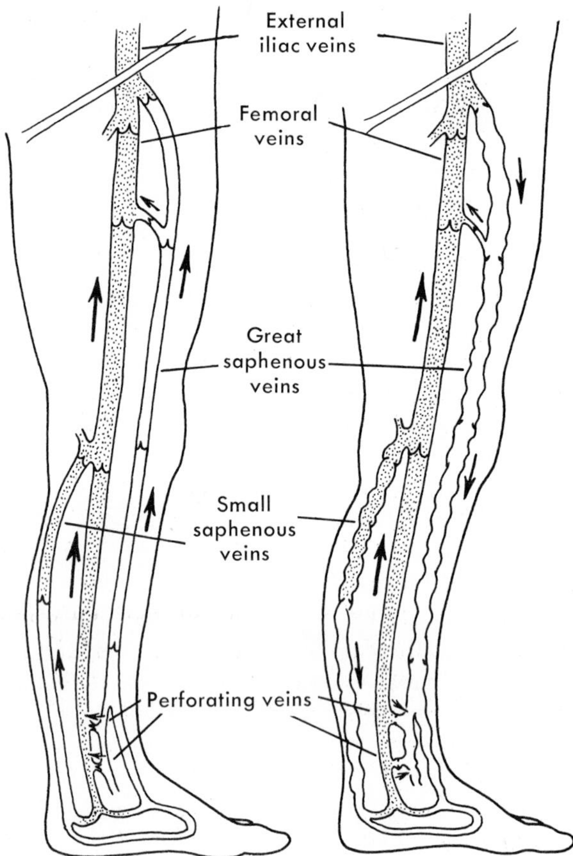

Fig. 47-5. *Left,* venous flow in normal veins. *Right,* venous flow in varicose veins. (Redrawn from Fairbairn, J. F., Jurgens, J. L., and Spittell, J. A.: Peripheral vascular disease, Philadelphia, 1972, W. B. Saunders Co.)

Intervention

Conservative management. Mild discomfort from varicose veins may be treated conservatively by advising the patient to elevate his feet for a few minutes at regular 2- to 3-hour intervals throughout the day, to avoid constrictions about the legs, to avoid standing for long periods of time, and to wear an elastic stocking or elastic bandage. All of these measures help to reduce venous pooling and increase venous return. Improvement in posture sometimes helps to prevent further development of the varicosities, and the patient may be advised by his physician to lose weight.

Ligation and stripping of veins. Surgical treatment for varicosities consists of ligation of the vein above the varicosity and removal of the varicosed vein distal to the ligation, provided that the deep veins are able to return the venous blood satisfactorily (Fig. 47-5). The great saphenous vein is ligated close to the femoral junction if possible, and the great and small saphenous veins are then stripped out through small incisions at the groin, above and below the knee, and at the ankle. Sterile dressings are placed over the incisions, and an elastic bandage extending from the foot to the groin is applied firmly.

General anesthesia is usual, since the procedure is very tiresome and painful. To prevent the development of thrombi in other veins, the patient usually walks about on the day of the operation and at frequent intervals during his remaining 2 to 3 days in the hospital. Unless the patient is elderly and also has arterial insufficiency, the foot of the bed is usually elevated on blocks for the first 24 hours to help in venous return of blood. Moving, walking, and bending the leg are extremely difficult for the patient, and he may have more pain and discomfort following this surgical procedure than following much more serious surgery. Analgesic drugs may be necessary for the first 24 to 48 hours.

Although the operation is considered a relatively

minor one and the patient is out of bed at once, nursing care is important. The patient should be assisted when he walks on the first day and thereafter if he is receiving an analgesic. Throughout hospitalization the patient is encouraged and assisted as necessary. He may have difficulty walking because of the firm binding around his knees; therefore care is taken to prevent accidents. The elastic bandage and the dressings are checked several times a day because they may become loosened with walking and the incisions may become exposed. Hemorrhage may occur and should be watched for, especially on the operative day. If bleeding does occur, the leg is elevated, pressure is applied over the wound, and the surgeon is notified.

A patient who has had surgery for varicose veins should know that the condition may recur, since large superficial collateral vessels may develop and in turn become varicosed. Therefore he should take the general precautions of any patient with varicosities, since the operation cures the acute symptoms but does not remove the tendency to develop varicose veins. Weight reduction, posture improvement, avoidance of pressure on blood vessels, and elevation of the lower limbs should be practiced postoperatively exactly as is recommended for the patient with mild varicosities who is receiving conservative treatment only. The booklet *Varicose Veins,* which can be obtained from the American Heart Association, is useful in teaching patients.

Treatment by sclerosis. Sclerosing solutions are occasionally used in the treatment of very small varicosities. The solutions cause an irritation within the vessel, development of a thrombus, and eventual occlusion of the lumen of the vein. This treatment is used rarely anymore because of the frequency of allergic reactions, the need for repeated treatments, and the danger of tissue sloughing if the solution touches healthy tissue. Sodium tetradecyl sulfate (Sotradecol) and monoethaline oleate (Monolate) are two of the solutions commonly used.

The injection of sclerosing solutions is usually performed in the clinic or in the physician's office. The nurse assumes responsibility for seeing that emergency equipment for treating allergic reactions is available and for preventing accidents to patients. Many patients are elderly, and some tend to become faint while standing for the treatment. Footstools can be equipped with side attachments and handlebars on which the patient may lean for comfort and security. The site of injection is covered with a small dressing. The patient is urged not to scratch the skin over the site of injection because scratching may lead to an infected excoriation and eventual ulceration. He also should be cautioned about bruising or otherwise traumatizing the veins, which also may lead to ulceration. He is usually instructed to walk about immediately, and elastic stockings or bandages may be ordered.

Management of varicose ulcers. Stasis of blood in tissues around marked varicosities, particularly when deep veins are also involved, leads to changes in normal tissue. The tissue becomes pigmented and edematous as fluid and the waste products of metabolism are inadequately cleared. There is often severe pruritus and discomfort. Small arteriovenous fistulas may develop as a result of the increased pressure in the thrombosed venous system, and tissue hypoxia occurs around the capillary bed when the blood is diverted into the venous system. As a result of these changes, stasis ulcers develop following small bruises or scratches or may develop spontaneously.

As part of the treatment of a stasis ulcer, ligation of varicose veins may be necessary because the ulcer will not heal while marked varicosities persist in the vessels above it. Besides the general measures already mentioned for any ulcers of vascular origin, treatment of *varicose ulcers* includes grafting of skin to cover the wound and the use of pressure bandages. Grafting may not be successful if the arterial supply is also affected because poor circulation to the fibrotic tissue surrounding the ulcer causes healing to be slow. (See p. 1505 for care of a graft.)

Medical treatment of ulcers consists of bed rest, protection of the area from trauma and infection, and promotion of healing. If the ulcerated area is small and the patient is able to remain ambulatory, a semirigid boot may be applied. The boot protects the ulcer and provides constant, even support to the area. An Unna paste boot is a commercial preparation containing gelatin, glycerin, and zinc oxide. It is not used often because the mixture must be melted and brushed on in several coats and is somewhat inconvenient and cumbersome to apply. Instead an elastic bandage (Elastoplast) over a layer of foam rubber and dry sterile gauze or gauze impregnated with medication may be prescribed. The boot is generally left on for 10 days to 2 weeks, although it may be changed sooner if there is copious drainage from the ulcer.

■ LYMPHEDEMA

Lymphedema is a swelling of soft tissue that occurs as a result of an increase in the quantity of lymph. It may be a primary disorder or secondary to other diseases. It always involves either inflammation or obstruction of the normal lymph channels. It primarily affects females. Primary lymphedema may be congenital or may occur at puberty (lymphedema praecox) and is thought to result from hypoplastic development of lymph vessels.

Secondary lymphedema may follow mastectomy and surgical removal of lymph channels (p. 1468). It is also seen when malignant tumors cause mechanical obstruction to lymph drainage and with repeated infections and cellulitis as occurs with filiarisis and malaria. Repeated, severe attacks of lymphedema may result in eventual fibrosis and hyperplasia of lymph vessels; the progressive, severe enlargement of the extremity led to the term *elephantiasis* being used for this condition.

Clinical picture

Lymphedema of the lower extremities begins with mild swelling on the dorsum of the foot, usually at the end of the day, which gradually extends to involve the entire limb. It is aggravated by prolonged standing, pregnancy, obesity, warm weather, and the menstrual period.

Intervention

There is no cure for lymphedema, although there are measures to control the progression of the disease. Treatment is conservative, and use is made of basic physiologic principles to improve the lymph drainage. Because gravity helps to drain lymph from the extremities, the person may be advised to sleep with the foot of the bed elevated 10 to 20 cm (4 to 8 in). Very light massage in the direction of the lymph flow is recommended,[33] and the patient is advised to wear elastic stockings or an elastic sleeve and to take moderate exercise regularly. Constricting clothing must not be worn, and avoiding salty or spicy foods that increase thirst and predispose to edema may be helpful. Thiazide diuretics are often prescribed to minimize fluid accumulation. Surgery may be performed to remove hypertrophied lymph channels and hypertrophied, disfiguring tissue.

One of the greatest problem in lymphedema is the emotional reaction of patients to disfigurement. Patients often attribute difficulties encountered in working in their chosen field or social rebuffs to their disfigurement and tend to become withdrawn and depressed. The emphasis on women's legs in our culture adds to the difficulties. One leg only may be involved, accentuating the abnormality even in fairly mild cases. The patient needs help and encouragement in learning to live with an exasperating chronic condition.

■ SPECIAL SURGICAL PROCEDURES

□ Sympathectomy

Vasospasm often accompanies arterial diseases, and a sympathectomy often is performed in an attempt to relieve it, although there is not full agreement as to its value. Occasionally the operation, which helps dilate the blood vessels, is performed as an emergency when there is severe vasospasm from poisons such as ergot, when a limb has been frozen, or when an arterial embolism has lodged in a major vessel supplying the limb. Usually, however, before a sympathectomy is performed the ganglia are injected with procaine to determine whether the treatment will be of value for the particular patient (p. 1020).

A *lumbar sympathectomy* deprives the leg and foot of sympathetic innervation and thereby dilates the vessels in the lower extremity. It is accomplished by making a small incision in the lower lateral aspect of the abdomen. The peritoneal cavity is not opened, but the sympathetic ganglia supplying the lumbar region are removed and their fibers are cut. This operation may be unilateral or bilateral, depending on whether dilation of vessels in both legs is desired.

After a lumbar sympathectomy the patient should be placed on his side. Blood pressure must be taken every 15 minutes until it is stable. Pulse rate and respiratory rate are also checked, and the patient is watched closely for signs of shock, which may result from the sudden reallocation of the blood in the dilated vessels of the lower abdomen and legs. Distention may be troublesome after a lumbar sympathectomy, and a rectal tube or rectal irrigations may be used to expel the flatus. Hourly turning should be insisted upon, and deep breathing is to be encouraged. Following a lumbar sympathectomy the patient may notice a new feeling of warmth in his feet and legs. Very occasionally this warmth causes a slight discomfort and a feeling of fullness, which is relieved by wearing an elastic stocking.

To relieve vasospasm in the arms and hands, the thoracic ganglia of the sympathetic chain may be resected *(cervicothoracic sympathectomy).* Because the ribs must be resected in this operation, nursing care is similar to that for any patient having chest surgery (p. 962). The problem of postoperative shock encountered in the patient with a lumbar sympathectomy also is present. In addition the patient may become quite dizzy on assuming an upright position. Dizziness gradually subsides as the circulation becomes readjusted, but in the meantime the patient must be assisted while he is up. Elastic bandages may be ordered to prevent pooling of blood in the legs and thus lessen the circulatory problem.

□ Amputation

Although partial or complete amputations of either the legs or the arms may be necessary as a result of sarcoma or trauma, the majority are necessitated by arteriosclerosis obliterans. The presence of diabetes and superimposed infection in an extremity increases the likelihood of amputation in this condition.

It is believed that the number of amputations will increase each year because of the longer life span and the consequent increase in the number of elderly people in whom peripheral vascular disease is likely to develop.

An amputation is a serious operation and usually is

performed as a lifesaving measure; it may be necessary at any age. Occasionally a deformed leg or arm is amputated because it is believed that the patient will do better with a prosthesis than with the deformed limb. Only simple amputations of the lower limb are considered here. The reader is referred to selected reading pertinent to amputations of the arms.[59]

Preoperative preparation

Because of the seriousness of amputation and its impact on the patient, preoperative nursing care is of major importance. The two areas of greatest significance are the patient's emotional readiness for the amputation and physical readiness for rehabilitation.

The first goal of nursing intervention is for the patient and his family to be in accord with and able to state the goals of the procedure. Throughout the hospitalization it is essential that all care be coordinated among the patient, nurse, physician, physical therapist, and prosthetist.

The initial response on learning of the need for amputation is usually distress, anger, or grief. The patient has already undergone a period of hospitalization during which conservative treatment was attempted. The failure of this treatment may generate feelings of anger and discouragement. It is not unusual for the patient to refuse the amputation initially. The patient and family need to have factual information about the consequences of the decision to amputate or not amputate, about the rehabilitative program, and what to expect. The timing of the presentation of this information is important in determining whether the patient will agree to the amputation.

Loss of the power of locomotion means loss of the power of flight, which is one of the instinctive means of self-preservation. It may be for this reason that loss of a leg depresses the patient more than loss of an arm, even though the latter is a much greater handicap. Something about the loss of power to move about at will casts a shadow on the patient's spirit that can be relieved only by the most thoughtful and sensitive care. Even the patient who has suffered for a long time with a chronic disease that has hampered his freedom of motion feels the anticipated loss keenly. Perhaps this is because there is such finality in an amputation. As long as the limb is there, imperfect though it may be, the patient usually retains the hope that normal or near-normal function will be restored. If amputation is necessary because of an accident, the suddenness of the change in the patient's image of himself may produce real shock.

Whether the amputation is sudden or planned, it will have an impact on the individual's body image. The individual facing an amputation is confronted with the task of incorporating a major change in his body into his perception of himself and then dealing with the meaning of this. The feedback or information he receives from others concerning the impact of this body change is a major determinant of the success of his efforts and his resultant attitude. The nurse must therefore not only be sensitive to the patient's needs and questions but must help the family work through them so they can support the patient.

Other emotional reactions to amputation are more tangible and more easily understood. The handicap is obvious (or at least the patient believes that it is), and he fears that he will be pitied. Young children, although they adjust to the physical limitations readily, may be taunted by their playmates for being different. Older children and adolescents may be handicapped in their social life and may develop serious emotional problems. To the wage earner an amputation may mean learning a new occupation. To the older person it may mean dependence on children or on the community.

Emotional reactions to an amputation have an enormous effect on the patient's rehabilitation. The reactions depend on the patient's emotional makeup and his response to other life crises as well as on circumstances leading to the amputation and the care he receives. The most perfect surgical operation and the best-fitting prosthesis are useless if the patient remains a complete invalid and a burden to himself, his family, and the community. The nurse must think of the long-range plans for the patient from the time that it is learned that an amputation is necessary. It is at this time, when emotional reactions to the amputation and the idea of using a prosthesis are forming, that the nurse can make the greatest contribution to the patient's rehabilitation by helping him to realize that his problems are not insurmountable and by utilizing other members of the health team in planning for his care and rehabilitation.

The second goal of preoperative intervention focuses on exercises that will prepare that patient for the activities he must perform in the postoperative period. The time available before surgery may limit what can be accomplished, but the nurse can at least explain postoperative routines and demonstrate these to the patient. He should be told that he will be repositioned frequently after surgery and that he must lie on his abdomen at intervals. Depending on the type of amputation to be performed, the patient can be shown exercises that strengthen the thigh muscles and prevent knee and hip contractures.

When time permits, the patient is assisted to do exercises that strengthen his arms. This will facilitate teaching transfer techniques postoperatively. Push-ups and weight lifting are excellent for improving muscle tone and strength in the arms and shoulders. If the patient is able to be ambulatory, instructions in crutch walking may be started. The more fully the postoperative routine can be explained, demonstrated, and practiced by the patient preoperatively, the smoother will be rehabilitation.

The amputation

The choice of anesthetic depends on the surgeon and the condition of the patient. General anesthetic (intravenous and inhalation) is the most frequently used. However, an amputation can be done with the patient under spinal anesthesia or with only the leg being cooled (refrigeration anesthesia), but the procedure is then very distressing to the patient, since the sawing of bone can be heard despite large doses of sedation.

In amputating a limb the surgeon attempts to remove all diseased tissue yet leave a stump that permits satisfactory use of a prosthesis. Many factors determine the level of amputation. Transmetatarsal and toe amputations are occasionally done when the disease is very limited but are rare compared with the incidence of above- and below-the-knee amputations.

Below-the-knee (BK) amputations comprise about 60% of all amputations for peripheral vascular disease.[1] This amputation is usually done in the middle third of the leg, leaving a stump at 12.5 to 17.5 cm (5 to 7 in) below the knee. This type of amputation is preferable for younger persons who will remain physically active because preservation of knee function permits a more natural gait. Also, the lower the level of amputation the less energy and balance will be required for walking.

Above-the-knee amputations (AK) are frequently necessary because of the extent of disease. The most important factor in determining the level of amputation is the adequacy of arterial blood supply, and although the BK amputation is preferred for rehabilitation, the AK procedure has been found to require reamputation less frequently, and it heals more successfully. The AK amputation is usually performed between the lower third to the middle of the thigh.

For the best function of the limb, the stump should be long enough to permit sufficient leverage to move the artificial limb but not long enough to interfere with the movement of the joint distal to the amputation. The end of the bone should be covered with skin and subcutaneous tissue and with muscle that is not adherent to the bone end. The stump should be healthy and firm without creases, folds, or flabby parts. It should be painless with no nerve endings remaining in the scar, and the scar should not fall over the weight-bearing end of the bone. The stump should have a smooth, conical contour and should be freely movable by the patient in any normal range of motion.

There are two common types of amputations. One, the *guillotine, circular,* or *open-flap amputation,* is used when there has been serious trauma, when gas bacilli are present in the wound, or when the patient cannot tolerate a long operative procedure. The disadvantage of this amputation is that another operation is necessary. The blood vessels and nerves are ligated, but the wound is left open and a secondary closure is necessary in 3 to 7 days. Because the wound is not sutured there may be muscle and skin retraction, which makes the fitting of a prosthesis difficult or impossible unless the stump is operated on again. After final healing the resultant stump is as adequate for prosthetic fitting as in other types of amputation.

The *flap* type of amputation is by far the more satisfactory if it can be done. In this operation a long flap of full-thickness skin is loosened from the anterior portion of the limb about to be amputated. Following the amputation the end of the flap is sutured to the skin edges of the stump so that the stump is covered and the suture line is along the back of the stump. This wound usually heals completely within 2 weeks.

Postoperative care

Amputation of a lower extremity is a major surgical procedure with a 10% mortality.[1] The most common complication occurring in the postoperative period is pulmonary embolus, and the nurse must be alert to the signs and symptoms of this (p. 1130).

When the patient returns from the operating room or the recovery room, vital signs are monitored and the stump dressing observed for signs of hemorrhage. If there is bright red drainage, an outline of the stain should be marked on the outside of the dressing with pencil so that the rate of bleeding can be determined easily.

The stump is usually elevated on a plastic-covered pillow for 12 to 24 hours immediately after surgery to lessen edema and bleeding or serous oozing from the wound. However, *the pillow must be removed after 24 hours* to prevent hip and knee contractures.

When the guillotine procedure has been used, the patient usually returns to his room with traction applied to the stump to prevent retraction of skin and muscle away from the surgical incision. Wide bands of adhesive tape are placed on the skin above the wound and attached to a metal spreader bar placed below the stump. Weights are attached to provide traction (see skin traction, p. 860). Traction pulleys at the foot of the bed should be placed toward the center so that the patient can turn onto his abdomen. A Thomas splint sometimes is used for traction so that the patient can be moved more easily and can be out of bed without the traction being released (see p. 863 for care of the patient in traction).

If the amputation is below the knee, the stump may be firmly bandaged on a padded board to prevent contracture at the knee joint. The nurse must check the padding carefully because muscle spasm that results in pulling of the limb against the board may be so great that a pressure sore develops. If spasm seems severe, a piece of sponge rubber can sometimes be slipped between the bandaged stump end and the padded board for additional protection. The surgeon may remove the limb from the board for part of the day.

Immediate postsurgical fitting. Some surgeons utilize the techniques of rigid plaster dressings or immediate postsurgical fitting (IPSF). This procedure is also referred to as immediate postoperative prosthesis (IPOP). After surgery, while the patient is still in the operating room, a plaster bandage is applied to the dressing over the stump. Embedded in the base of the cast is a metal socket to which a metal pylon can be attached when the patient is to bear weight. This plaster mold or cast reduces postoperative edema, hastens desired stump shrinkage, and if a foot attachment is to be used, allows for early standing and ambulation. In fact, the plaster mold becomes the patient's first or temporary prosthesis; the permanent prosthesis can usually be fitted in 3 to 4 weeks. IPOP procedures may also be used for upper extremity amputees.

For the plaster mold to be effective it must remain tight and snug. If the cast slips on the stump or comes completely off, the physician and prosthetist must be notified immediately so that a new cast can be applied. A heavy strap, attached proximally and on the anterior surface of the cast, is fastened to a waistband to help secure the cast and prevent it from slipping. This strap is loosened to a slight degree when the patient is in bed and tightened when he is out of bed. The site of any drainage coming through the cast is marked (including the time) with indelible pencil. Hemovac drainage or a Penrose drain will have been inserted before the plaster is applied, so drainage should not be great. In 48 hours a window may be cut in the cast to permit removal of the drain. The opening in the plaster is then closed. This rigid dressing is kept in place for approximately 2 weeks, when it is taken off for removal of sutures. A new cast is then applied. As the stump shrinks in size, the cast becomes too large and will have to be replaced by a tighter one. Usually after the application of the third plaster cast, the cast can be removed daily for stump hygiene and inspection for pressure areas.

Usually a foot-ankle attachment with a shoe is attached to the pylon when the patient is to stand. In this case the prosthetist will mark on the pylon the place where the attachment is to be placed. Most often the physician will be in attendance when the patient first bears weight. No weight is to be placed on the stump until the cast is completely dry. The exact amount of weight the patient should bear on the amputated side will be specifically ordered by the physician. Unless otherwise ordered, the prosthetic foot should always be removed when the patient is in bed because the tension produced by the twisting of the prosthesis can be harmful to remaining muscle and bone (for example, the anterior tibial crest in the below-the-knee amputee).

In IPOP, as with any cast prohibiting full view of the involved area, the nurse must be alert to the patient's complaints of pain under the cast, elevated temperature, or foul odor coming from the cast. Such signs or symptoms are reported to the physician at once. Continued observation will be necessary to determine whether the cast is sufficiently snug.

Exercises. To prevent flexion contracture of the hip, unless there is a medical order to the contrary, the patient who has had a lower limb amputation is turned on his abdomen for a short time the day following surgery. Thereafter he should lie on his abdomen for some time at least three times each day. Even the patient who has a limb in traction can turn on his abdomen with assistance. If the leg has been amputated below the knee, the patient can begin at once to hyperextend his thigh and leg as he lies on his abdomen. This exercise strengthens muscles in preparation for walking. If the amputation is above the knee, a medical order should be obtained before the patient hyperextends the thigh because this exercise may cause strain on the suture line. While on his abdomen the patient can practice the push-up exercises he started before the operation, strengthening his arm and shoulder muscles in preparation for crutch walking.

While on his back the patient with a recent midthigh amputation should be kept flat or in a low Fowler's position except for short periods such as for meals. A firm trochanter roll (a sheet or bath blanket firmly rolled) should be placed along the outer side of the affected limb to prevent its outward rotation. If permitted the patient should lie on the side of the amputation part of the time.

The patient with a below-the-knee amputation can be in a mid- or high Fowler's position if he wishes, but special care must be taken to prevent flexion contracture of the knee. Usually the physician orders the stump removed from the padded board or splint several times a day and has the patient sit on the edge of the bed. While sitting, he should practice extending his knee and lower limb. The nurse may be asked to press slightly against the lower limb to provide resistance.

The patient with either type of amputation should practice lifting the stump and buttocks off the bed while he is lying flat on his back. This exercise helps develop the abdominal muscles, which are necessary for stabilizing the pelvis when the patient stoops or bends.

If the amputation involves only one limb, the nurse must not become so occupied with the affected side that he or she neglects the other leg and foot. Supervision of regular exercises to strengthen leg muscles and prevention of drop foot and pronation deformities are nursing responsibilities. The patient should have a firm board or block of wood at the foot of the bed against which he can push the involved leg and thereby receive essential active exercise.

When the patient is permitted out of bed, he is taught self-care activities such as rising from a chair. To preserve his center of gravity and balance, the patient should keep his remaining leg well under him before he shifts his weight, as when rising from a chair. If available, a physical therapist should be consulted regarding exercise.

The patient who has had an amputation because of vascular disease must be reminded to take particular care of his remaining foot and leg. Exercises and other measures to keep the arterial supply as adequate as possible must be carried out while the patient is in the hospital, and he must be urged to follow his physician's instructions carefully when he leaves the hospital.

Stump care. If a prosthesis is to be worn comfortably, a healthy stump is necessary. Teaching the patient how to care for his stump is a nursing responsibility that is carried out both in the hospital and in the patient's home. The patient may be discharged from the hospital within a few weeks but may not be fitted for a prosthesis for 6 weeks to 6 months after surgery, depending on the condition of the stump.

When the wound is completely healed, the patient is taught to wash the stump daily. Most surgeons advise their patients not to soak the stump because soaking may cause maceration of the skin. The skin should be massaged gently, directing the motion toward the suture line. The use of oils or creams should be avoided as these agents only increase the possibility of skin maceration; lanolin may be used sparingly. Usually the patient is instructed to push forcefully over the bone to toughen the

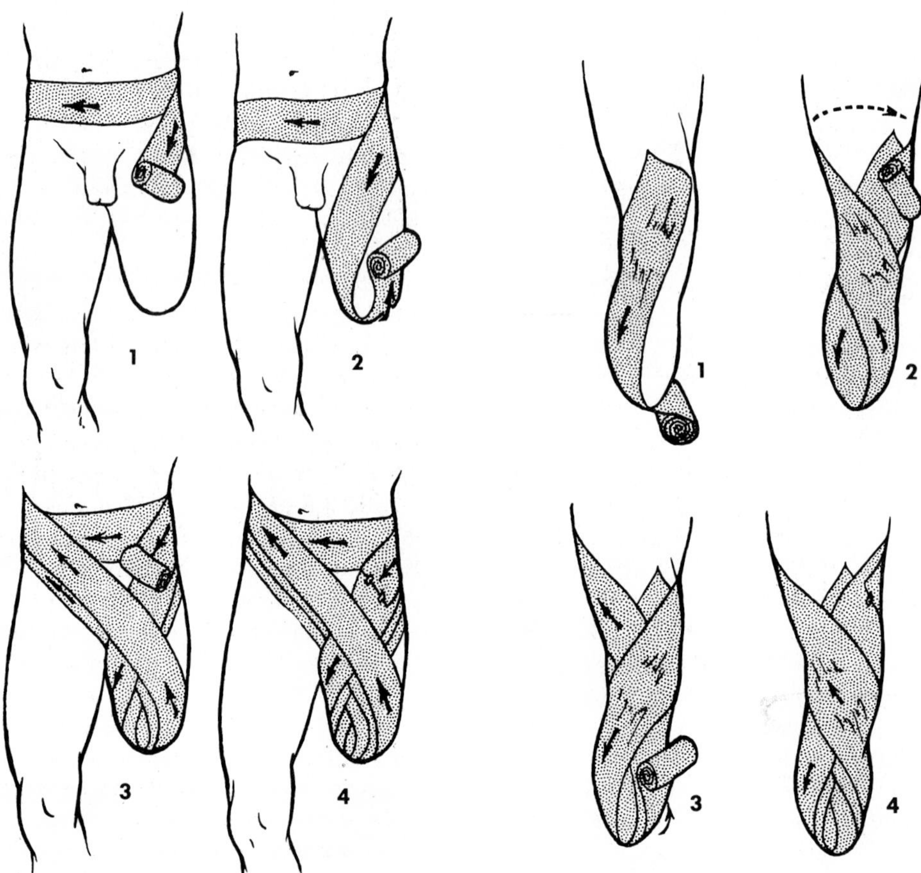

Fig. 47-6. *Left,* correct method for bandaging midthigh amputation stump. Note that bandage must be anchored around patient's waist. *Right,* correct method for bandaging midcalf amputation stump. Note that bandage need not be anchored about waist.

limb for weight bearing. Sometimes this process is begun by placing a pillow on a footstool, chair, or high stool (depending on the site of operation) and having the patient bear some weight on the stump while steadying himself on the bed or against the wall.

There should be no tenderness, redness, or other signs of skin irritation or abrasion at the end of the stump. The skin and underlying tissue should be firm and without flabbiness and should be without tautness over the bony end of the limb.

For 2 to 3 weeks postoperatively the stump is kept bandaged at all times in order to reduce swelling and shape the stump. Some patients are taught to bandage the stump themselves. However, they need careful instruction and supervision (Fig. 47-6). The bandage must not be so tight as to cause pain or numbness from hampered circulation, and if it is too loose it will defeat its purpose. If the patient is unable to apply a firm, even bandage, a member of his family may help him. The bandage should be removed and reapplied at least twice daily, and the skin should be washed, dried, powdered, and exposed to the air for a short time before the bandage is reapplied. The patient should have at least two bandages so that one may be washed daily; they should be laid flat to dry so as not to stretch.

When a leather prosthesis is used, the patient should have several pairs of stump socks of the right size. They should be made of cotton and wool and should be washed daily after use and dried over a mold to prevent shrinkage. Usually the patient wears out one sock a month when he begins to use a prosthesis. A worn sock should not be mended because it may cause irritation to the stump. Routine care of the stump, including bathing, massage, and inspection, should be continued. If the weather is warm and the skin perspires freely, the limb should be removed from the prothesis socket and bathed and exposed to the air more often than during cooler weather. The person who works may take an extra stump sock with him so that he can change it during the day in hot weather. To prevent tension on the sock as the limb is placed in the socket, a string may be attached to the end of the sock and brought through a hole that is usually left in the prosthesis below the level of the stump. The patient should be instructed to report calluses or any abnormalities on the stump to his physician at once.

Phantom limb sensation. Phantom limb sensation is an unpleasant complication that sometimes follows amputation and is difficult to treat. It is a sensation that the limb is still present. The sensation may disappear if the patient looks at the stump and recalls that the limb has been amputated. *Phantom limb pain* also occurs. The patient may have the sensation, for example, that something is burning his foot or that there is pressure on it, or the pain may be identical to that experienced before surgery. The cause is not fully understood, but it is thought possibly to result from stimulation of afferent nerves severed in surgery. Phantom limb pain may disappear of its own accord, it may lessen for a time and then recur with severity. When it is really troublesome to the patient, the nerve endings may be injected with alcohol to give temporary relief. Occasionally when pain persists, an operation is performed to remove the nerve ends that may have developed to form a tuft on the weight-bearing part of the stump. A few patients are troubled with phantom limb pain for an indefinite time following amputation, and it may interfere seriously with their rehabilitation. Reamputation is sometimes done, but even this procedure does not always bring relief, since the same sensations may be experienced at the end of the new stump.

Ambulation. Teaching the patient who has had an amputation to walk with crutches, with crutches and prosthesis, and then with the prosthesis alone is a complicated task that lies within the responsibility of physical medicine and nursing. In the past, teaching the patient to walk with a prosthesis often was left to the limb maker. However, learning to walk well with an artificial limb requires instruction by a skilled physical therapist. It is the responsibility of nurses working with the surgeon, the social worker, the physical therapist, the prosthetist, and other members of the professional health team to see that the patient receives continuous care, teaching, and encouragement until he is able to manage on his own.

Crutch walking. The nurse has the responsibility to prepare every patient for crutch walking and may have to teach the patient to use crutches, especially if a physical therapist is not available. Therefore every nurse should know the essentials about using crutches and something about the gaits that can be used. Preparation for the use of crutches should include exercises to strengthen the triceps muscles, which are used to extend the elbows and are therefore most important in the satisfactory use of crutches. These exercises can be started before the operation by teaching the patient to lie on his abdomen and to do push-up exercises (p. 1039). When lying on his back he can hold bags of sand or other weights on his palms and straighten his elbows. In another exercise that strengthens the triceps muscles, the patient sits on the edge of the bed with his foot in a chair and, while pressing his palms against the mattress, lifts his hips off the bed. This procedure provides good exercise in extension of the elbow and helps the patient become accustomed to resting his weight on his hands. Use of an overbed trapeze bar postoperatively is helpful as it enables the patient to handle himself much more independently than would otherwise be possible. Its use, however, strengthens primarily the biceps muscles, which are less essential in crutch walking than are the triceps muscles. Further preparation includes prevention of contractures and deformities that will interfere with the use of crutches and with the use of a prosthesis. Exercises to prevent hip and knee contractures and to maintain the muscle tone and strength in the unaffected leg are described on p. 1041. Even before the stump is healed enough to permit use of a prosthesis, the patient can learn to do a good deal to help himself.

Crutches should be measured for each patient. In *method 1,* the patient lies on his back with his arms at his sides. The measurement is taken from the axilla to a point 15 cm (6 in) out from the side of the heel. This is the length of the crutch minus 1.9 cm (3/4 in) for crutch tips. In *method 2,* the patient is measured from 5 cm (2 in) below the level of the axilla to the base of the heel. In *method 3,* 40 cm (16 in) are subtracted from the patient's total height. Even with careful measurement, alterations may have to be made after the crutches are used. Posture, for example, may change, altering the length needed. The crutches should not cause pressure on the axillae, and the patient is taught not to rest his weight on the axillary bars more than a few minutes at a time. Pressure on the axillae causes pressure on the brachial plexus, which can lead to severe and sometimes permanent paralysis of the arms ("crutch paralysis"). The patient is taught that weight should be borne on the palms of the hands.

Before the patient attempts to walk with crutches, he should be assisted out of bed and should stand with help by the bed to get the feel of normal balance. He may then use a walker or parallel bars until he is relatively secure. At this time he should begin to practice correct standing posture with head up, chest up, abdomen in, pelvis tilted inward, a 5° angle in the knee joint, and the foot straight (Fig. 47-7). Practice in front of a mirror is very helpful. The patient is encouraged not to look toward his foot. Next the patient should practice standing while supported by his crutches so that he can get the "feel" of them. The nurse should be sure that he begins at this time to bear his weight on his palms and not his axillae. Before the patient begins to try to use crutches,

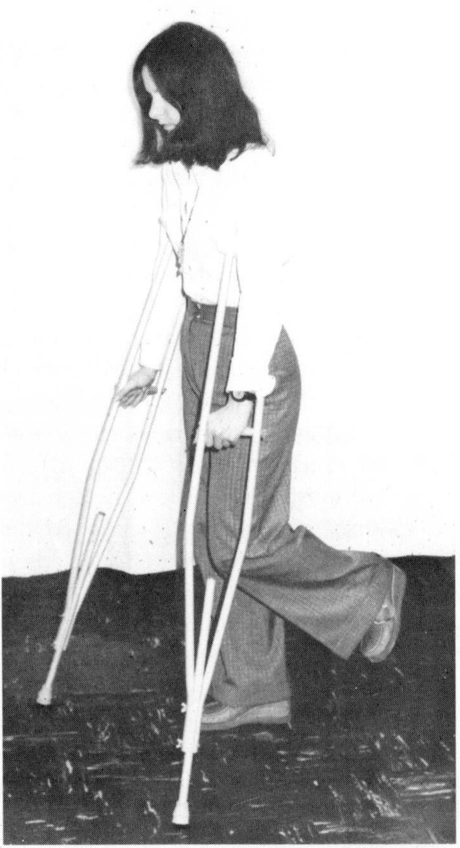

Fig. 47-7. Axillary crutches are ambulatory aids best used by young persons or persons with good motor ability, particularly if patient is non-weight-bearing on one leg. Here patient has good balance and erect posture.

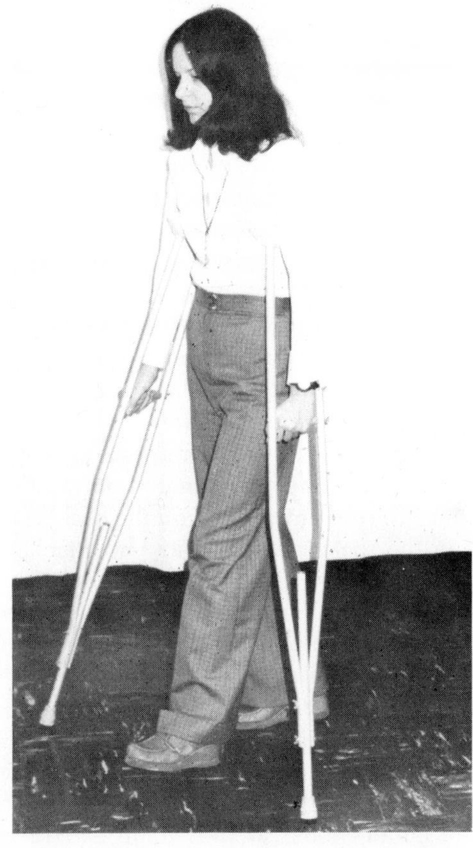

Fig. 47-8. Three-point gait is more stable crutch gait and can be used by most patients who can use walker. It provides for greater mobility than walker so patient may also negotiate stairs.

he should be shown the proper hand and arm position and the gait he will use. This not only helps him to understand what he must do but, if he is worried about whether the crutches will support him, may increase his confidence (Fig. 47-8). In all crutch walking the patient is taught to concentrate on a normal rhythmic gait.

The first gait that he will use is the *swing-through* (Fig. 47-9, *A*) or *swing-to gait* (Fig. 47-9, *B*), which require no carefully guided instruction provided the patient knows how to bear his weight and has been taught to check posture, balance, and rhythm. In this gait the amputated limb and the crutches both advance either to or beyond the level of the normal limb and are followed by the normal leg. This is a simple fast gait that gives little leg exercise but is useful for rapid maneuvers such as are needed in crossing streets. The patient may use this gait when he begins to walk with one prosthesis, in which case both crutches and the prosthesis move forward, followed by the normal leg.

When the patient with double amputations has been fitted with prostheses, he may be taught the *four-point gait* (Fig. 47-9, *C*). This gait is taught to the count of four as follows: right crutch, left foot, left crutch, right foot. Some patients with bilateral amputations must always use this gait (which is also widely used by those with involved neuromuscular disabilities and poor balance). It is

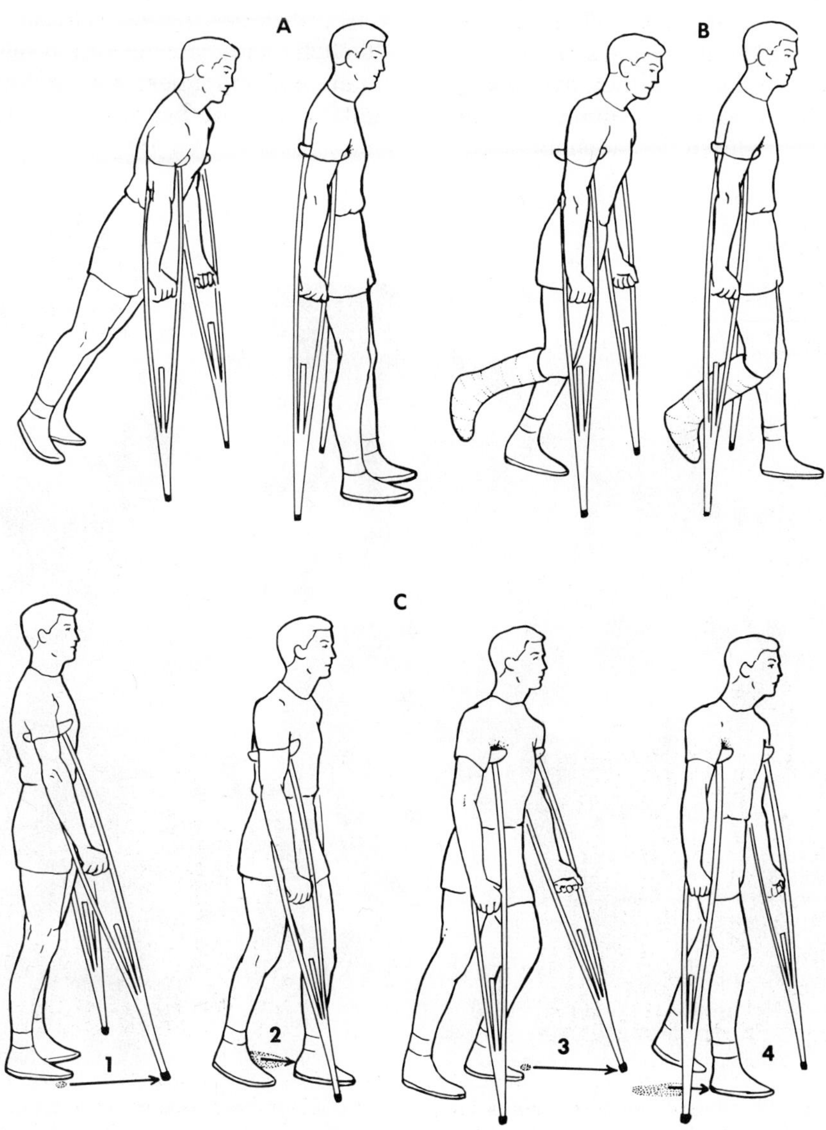

Fig. 47-9. A, Swing-through gait. **B,** Swing-to gait. **C,** Four-point gait.

a safe gait because the patient always has three points of contact with the ground at any time. Most patients progress to the *two-point gait*, in which the foot and the opposite crutch move together and then the prosthesis and the opposite crutch. It is often taught to the count of two as follows: left crutch and right foot (one) and right crutch and left foot (two). The two-point gait is much faster and is easier to maintain in a rhythmic pattern than the four-point gait.

The patient with one prosthesis may progress to one crutch and then to a cane, which should be abandoned eventually. The crutch or cane should be held in the hand on the side *opposite* the prosthesis because, as the patient normally walks, the arm on the opposite side of the body alternately swings forward. Holding the cane or crutch on the same side as the prosthesis results in an awkward, unrhythmic gait.

It is important for the nurse to know which gait the physical therapist is teaching the patient so that he may be reminded if, on leaving the physical therapy department, he reverts to a swing-to gait, for example. It is to be expected that the patient with a double amputation will learn to manage himself much more slowly than if only one limb were gone. Persons with an above-the-knee (AK) amputation also take much longer to learn to walk and otherwise manage their movements than do persons with below-the-knee (BK) amputations.

The prosthesis

The physician prescribes the type of prosthesis that is best for the patient and usually refers him to a limb maker. After the limb is made, the patient returns to the amputee clinic, hospital department of physical medicine, physician's office, or rehabilitation center to learn the best use of the artificial limb (Fig. 47-10). The community health nurse, particularly if also trained in physical therapy, often gives care and supervision to the person in his home.

The type of prosthesis is selected for the individual. Most prostheses are made of well-seasoned willow wood, although some are made of metal (Duralumin and aluminum) and fiber materials. Metal prostheses are lighter in weight than wooden ones, but they tend to be noisy. Usually the below-the-knee prosthesis weighs

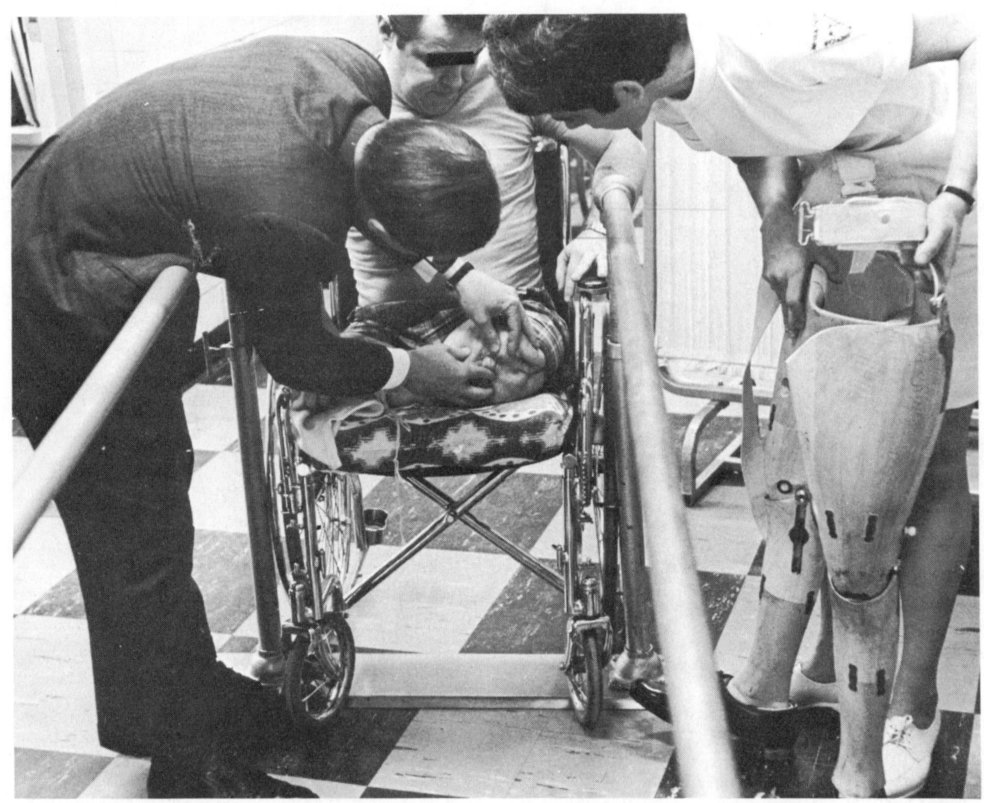

Fig. 47-10. Physician examining stump of patient with bilateral above-knee amputation while physical therapist holds prosthesis. (Courtesy Rehabilitation Institute of Chicago, Chicago, Ill.; photograph by Edwin Bonk.)

about 2.25 kg (5 lb) and the midthigh prosthesis about 2.67 kg (7½ lb), although the weight of the prosthesis is adapted to the size and weight of the individual and his kind of work.

The prosthesis has a socket, or "bucket," into which the limb fits. In the past the socket was usually made of leather, but plastic materials are now widely used as they are lighter, easier to keep clean, and odorless. The socket has a one-way valve that allows air to escape but not reenter as the stump is inserted. It eliminates the need for a stump sock but does require a good fit between stump and prosthesis. Shrinkage of the stump may interfere with obtaining a good fit. It is usually greater after amputation of the foreleg than after amputation of the thigh. Suction is now quite generally used to hold the stump in the socket and obviate wearing a heavy, laced belt about the waist, although persons with high, above-the-knee amputations may wear a pelvic band (Fig. 47-11). The patient needs constant encouragement to use the prosthesis, particularly in the beginning when he is adjusting to all features of the device. He should start to use the prosthesis as soon as his stump has healed.

The nurse should determine whether the person is using his prosthesis when at home. If he is not, the reason should be identified and reported to the physician. Often the nurse can help make the arrangements for more instruction. It is important that there be no delay, because the longer the person puts off using the prosthesis the less likely he is to use it satisfactorily. If crutches are used for too long and if the person depends on other forms of getting about such as a wheelchair, he may have considerable difficulty in developing a normal rhythmic gait.

Care of the prosthesis should be reviewed with the patient. He should be taught to fasten the cuff above the stump from the bottom up, even though this method may seem more difficult at first. The cuff should be snug but not uncomfortable. If the cuff is leather, care should be taken that the stump sock is long enough to protect the cuff from perspiration, and it should be rubbed with saddle soap at least weekly. The inside of the stump socket should be washed frequently to ensure cleanliness. Shoes should be kept in good repair and should have rubber heels. Broken shoelaces should be replaced

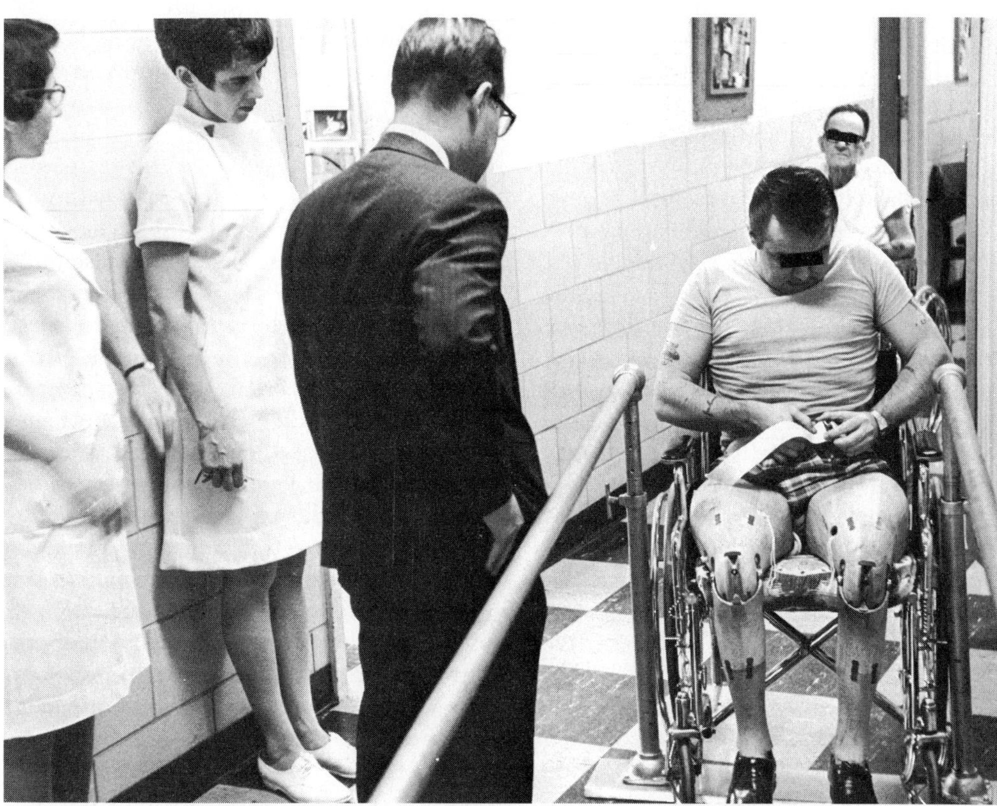

Fig. 47-11. Physician and physical therapist observing patient with bilateral above-knee amputation fastening pelvic belt to secure prosthesis. (Courtesy Rehabilitation Institute of Chicago, Chicago, Ill.; photograph by Edwin Bonk.)

at once. If the prosthesis has a joint, the person should be taught to keep this free from lint and dust, to oil the joints and locks every few weeks, and to keep screws tightened. If he feels adjustments are needed, he should return to the limb maker.

The person should be told that his artificial limb is a tool and that it will be most useful to him when he has mastered its use. With good care it will last him 3 to 10 years. Its value will depend on how well he can learn to balance himself, how much muscle strength he develops, and how smooth and rhythmic a gait he learns. Above all, its value will depend on his attitude toward the challenge that its use presents.

Long-term care

Most persons who have an amputation must remain under medical supervison for a long time, and it is safe to assume that any person with an amputation needs nursing care and supervision long after the wound has healed. It must be remembered that although the amputation has removed a diseased segment of the vasculature, the person still has peripheral vascular disease. If possible, a community health nurse should visit the patient's home before he leaves the hospital and help the family make any structural changes necessary for facilitating the person's ambulation. If it should happen that a person is equipped with an artificial limb but is not taught how to use it, the community health nurse should initiate steps toward his rehabilitation. Occasionally the limb maker believes that the hospital clinic personnel are taking responsibility for teaching the patient to walk, and the physician or the hospital clinic personnel believe that the limb maker is taking the responsibility. The person may become discouraged and, after months of what appears to be a good adjustment, may lay the limb aside and return to a wheelchair or crutches. Sometimes he reports that the prosthesis is not comfortable and that he is reluctant to go back to the limb maker because of costs. If so, the nurse can help to find agencies in the community that can give appropriate assistance. It may be, however, that this statement is made to conceal a much more important and deep-seated rejection of his difficulties. When the nurse suspects that the patient is not accepting his prosthesis, consultation with the physician and other health professionals may be necessary to determine the appropriate step to be taken to assist the person to work through his feelings.

Occasionally a patient, especially an elderly one, can use neither a prosthesis or crutches but must be confined to a wheelchair. The nurse should give special attention to the rehabilitation of this patient in an effort to make him as self-sufficient as possible. Many patients can be taught to move themselves from the bed to the wheelchair, from the chair to the toilet, and even in and out of a car. The patient and family often need help in arranging facilities at home, and plans should be made with the family to let the patient do useful chores such as fixing vegatables, mending, or doing small repairs. He also should be encouraged to become interested in some hobby or pastime.

There are many rehabilitation centers in the United States, but most of them are located in the larger cities. The division of vocational rehabilitation of the department of education in every state is, however, available to all patients. Most communities, counties, and states have voluntary programs that are designed to help the physically handicapped, including the amputee. The nurse should consult the local health department for information on the resources available in the person's own community.

Outcome criteria for the person who has had an amputation

1. The patient achieves the established goal in relation to ambulation.
2. The patient or significant others can:
   a. State the plan for obtaining a permanent prosthesis.
   b. Explain how to care for the prosthesis and stump.
   c. Demonstrate the prescribed program of exercise and activity.
   d. State plans for follow-up care.

■ HYPERTENSION

As discussed earlier in this chapter, hypertension is often considered in conjunction with peripheral vascular disease for several reasons: both are disorders of the circulation, the courses of both diseases are affected by similar factors, and hypertension is a major risk factor in atherosclerosis, the largest single cause of peripheral vascular disease.

The blood pressure level in a given individual is determined by many variables such as age, activity, emotional state, presence of other diseases, pumping effectiveness of the heart, amount of circulating blood, and the state of the vasculature. Although 120/80 is commonly given as the "normal" level, many individuals such as infants, most adults while sleeping, and athletes have very adequate circulation at lower levels. Conversely, older persons, individuals under emotional stress, and obese individuals often demonstrate levels above this with no adverse consequences.

Because of these variables, statistics describing the prevalence of this disease are quite varied. When hypertension is defined as a consistent systolic level above 150 mm Hg or diastolic level above 90 mm Hg, the incidence is 15% among men in their thirties and 20% among men in their fifties. According to this common definition 20 million Americans suffer from hypertension. It has also been estimated that of this number hypertension is undiagnosed in one half, and of those in whom the disease has been diagnosed, one half are receiving no or inadequate treatment.[101]

The incidence of hypertension varies considerably among different groups in the population. Hypertension occurs more often in men than in women and is twice as prevalent among blacks than among whites. When present the degree of hypertension is also more severe in blacks than whites. In all groups the incidence of this disease increases with age.

Hypertension may be classified into three groups: hypertension from a known cause, essential hypertension and malignant hypertension. In only a small percentage of cases is the cause known. Examples of these are coarctation of the aorta, which may be corrected surgically; pheochromocytoma, a catecholamine-secreting tumor; Cushing's disease and other disorders of the adrenal gland; toxemia of pregnancy; and thyrotoxicosis, which causes increased stroke volume of the heart. Chronic glomerulonephritis is the most common known cause. In the majority of cases the exact cause of hypertension is unknown; this is classified as *essential hypertension*.

Malignant hypertension (accelerated hypertension) refers to hypertension that is severe and rapidly progressive, resulting in fibrinoid necrosis, especially of the heart, kidneys, brain, and eyes. The patient often has papilledema and retinal exudates and hemorrhages. The eye changes are rated according to severity from 1+ to 4+. Unless medical treatment is successful, the course is rapidly fatal and most persons do not survive longer than 2 years. Causes of death in malignant hypertension are secondary to the fibrinoid necrosis of the kidney, heart, and brain. Thus the patient may succumb to uremia, myocardial infarction, congestive failure, or a cerebral vascular accident. Malignant hypertension is seen most often in blacks, especially men under age 40 years.

□ Pathophysiology

Blood pressure is determined by two factors: flow and resistance. Blood flow is in turn determined by cardiac output (strength, rate, rhythm of heart beat, and blood volume). The resistance to flow is primarily determined by the diameter of blood vessels and, to a lesser degree, by the vicosity of the blood. Elevation of peripheral resistance due to narrowing of the arterioles is the single most common characteristic in hypertension. Dilation and constriction of peripheral arterioles may be controlled by several mechanisms.

Stimulation of the sympathetic nervous system causes the release of the catecholamines epinephrine and norepinephrine. This stimulation can be the result of environmental stressors, adrenal hormones, or autonomic nervous system activity (such as impulses from the cartoid sinus). Epinephrine is an inotropic agent that increases the force of cardiac contraction, thus increasing cardiac output; norepinephrine primarily causes vasoconstriction, which increases peripheral resistance. Stress therefore increases the force while narrowing the passageway, causing the blood presssure to increase. Parasympathetic stimulation has the opposite effect, causing relaxation of the smooth muscle of the vessels.

With prolonged hypertension the elastic tissue in arterioles is replaced by fibrous collagen tissue. The thickened arteriole wall then becomes less distensible, offering even greater resistance to the flow of blood. The left ventricle then must exert more force in order to empty completely; it becomes more distended as it fails to eject a normal stroke volume, and the muscle fibers stretch (hypertrophy) in an attempt to increase the strength of contraction. Inadequate blood supply through the coronary arteries may cause angina pectoris, or a myocardial infarction may occur. Eventually the hypertrophy of the left ventricle results in congestive heart failure.

Outside of the heart itself, the changes in the arteriolar walls may result in permanent damage to organs. The kidney is especially susceptible, and when fibrinoid necrosis occurs in the afferent arteriole, the glomerulus is deprived of its blood supply; permanent kidney damage and possible renal failure result. Cerebral vessels are also frequently affected; neurologic changes or frank stroke may result either from hemorrhage from a leaky vessel or from thrombosis.

□ Etiology

Although no single causative mechanism has been identified in *essential hypertension*, several risk factors are known. As mentioned earlier, many of the factors influencing the course of other peripheral vascular diseases also influence hypertension and the likelihood of the development of pathologic sequelae. In attempting to predict the occurence of hypertension, it has been found that both a positive family history and the occurrence of episodes of elevated blood pressure in youth correlate highly with the eventual development of adult hypertension.

Diet is also of significance in the course of this disease. Obesity, increased serum sodium levels, and hypercholesteremia all increase the risks of hypertension, as does smoking. In men aged 30 to 59 years, the death rate of those with hypertension is twice as high as those without hypertension; this rate is trebled in the presence of either hypercholesteremia or smoking and five times higher if both risk factors exist.[101] Hypertension is also thought to increase the problems of arteriosclerosis by favoring hyperplasia of connective tissue in the intima of arteries.

Prevention

Because of the alarming statistics regarding this disease, national attention has been focused on the task of detecting persons with hypertension and assuring that they receive treatment. The National Institutes of Health, part of the Department of Health, Education and Welfare, has created and coordinated the National High Blood Pressure Education Program, including a Task Force on Nursing in High Blood Pressure Control. In addition other organizations such as the American Heart Association, the National Heart Institute, and the Public Health Service have all been involved in this effort to identify and treat persons with hypertension.

One of the most problematic aspects of this disease is that it is asymptomatic until pathologic and sometimes fatal sequelae occur. Although it has been shown that proper treatment can greatly reduce the incidence of these sequelae, it has required a program of this magnitude to educate both the lay public and health professionals as to the importance of obtaining early treatment and follow-up for all persons with hypertension.

There have been three general approaches to this problem. First, efforts have been directed at public awareness, informing them and making available educational materials explaining hypertension and its treatment. Second, screening programs in schools and shopping centers have been organized in order to identify the hypertensive population. Third, there has been an attempt to develop innovative techniques to motivate hypertensive individuals to obtain and continue treatment. For example, persons have been taught to check their own blood pressure at home in order to monitor more closely their response to treatment without requiring frequent trips to the physician's office, and many insurance companies offer reduced premiums to persons with hypertension who maintain treatment regimens.

The National Task Force on Nursing in High Blood Pressure Control has confirmed that nurses are an invaluable resource in dealing with this major health problem. Although a complete report is not yet available, some of their recommendations can be implemented now. Industrial nurses can set up formal and informal screening programs in their work settings. Individual nurses can become involved in community screening and education programs. Community health nurses can ensure that blood pressure checks of every family member are part of every initial visit. Fig. 47-12 gives recommended steps in the screening program. In addition the nursing profession has a unique contribution to make in the identification of methods that ensure patient compliance and research into those factors that hamper patient compliance.

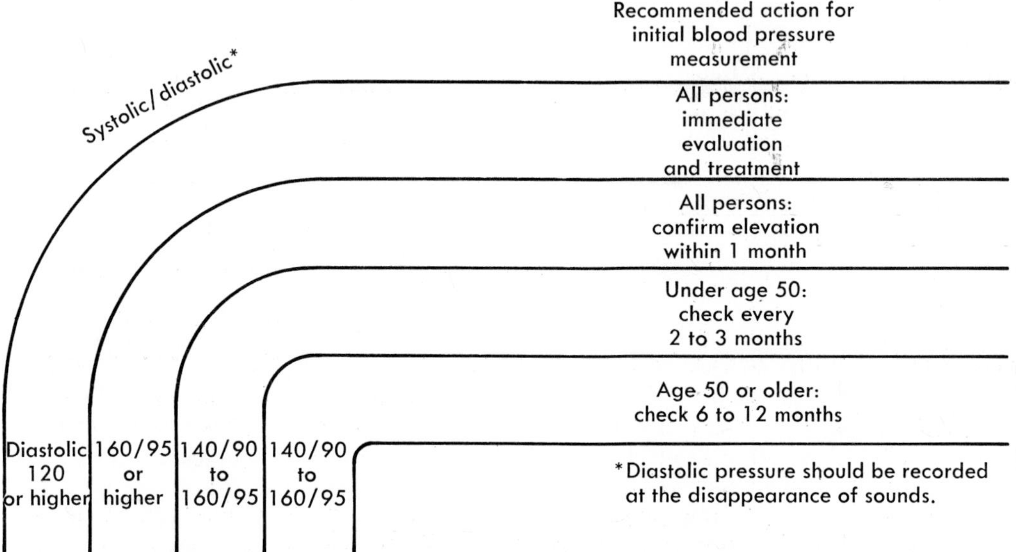

Fig. 47-12. Detection and confirmation of high blood pressure. Anyone measuring blood pressure should have resources available for confirmation and follow-up. (From U.S. National High Blood Pressure Education Programs, Recommendations of the Joint National Committee on Detection, Diagnosis, and Treatment of High Blood Pressure, Bethesda, Md., 1973, National Institutes of Health.)

Intervention

Diet

In addition to the restrictions in caloric intake and specific prescription of the type of fat intake, a low-sodium diet is frequently ordered. Very often the nurse, together with the dietitian, can be helpful in assisting the client in determining how to stay within dietary limits without exceeding financial resources.

Modification of stress

The person with hypertension needs to avoid external factors that compromise circulation; this means a reduction in stress-producing activity or events. Helping the patient achieve this outcome requires an extremely individualistic approach on the part of the nurse. For some patients a mild tranquilizer such as diazepam (Valium) may be indicated, while for others it might mean enlisting the help of family members in freeing the home environment of tension-creating situations.

Medications

Drug therapy is currently the only successful means of treating hypertension, with the exception of hypertension that is secondary to a cause such as coarctation of the aorta. It is essential that the individual be knowledgeable about his medications. The person with hypertension is often in the position of being told he must take medication, which may have unpleasant side effects, for a condition of which he was unaware and which is producing no symptoms! A thorough comprehensive teaching program is necessary if patient cooperation is to be enlisted (Fig. 47-13).

Medications commonly used in the treatment of hypertension fall into several categories, including sympathetic nervous system depressants, such as the alkaloids of rauwolfia; selective sympathetic nervous system inhibitors such as guanethidine (Ismelin) and methyldopa (Aldomet); drugs acting on smooth muscle to cause vasodilation such as hydralazine hydrochloride (Apresoline) and prazosin (Minipres); ganglionic blocking agents such as pentolinium tartrate (Ansolysen); and the thiazides (Diuril, Hydroduiril, Esidrix), which reduce the amount of water, sodium, and chloride in the body and may augment the effect of other antihypertensive preparations.[7] (See Table 47-1 for a summary of the most commonly used preparations.)

The physician makes a very careful selection of medications to treat hypertension. Fig. 47-14 outlines the regimen recommended by the Joint National Committee on Detection, Diagnosis, and Treatment of High Blood Pressure.[105] Caution is necessary not only because of the particular stage of the person's illness but also be-

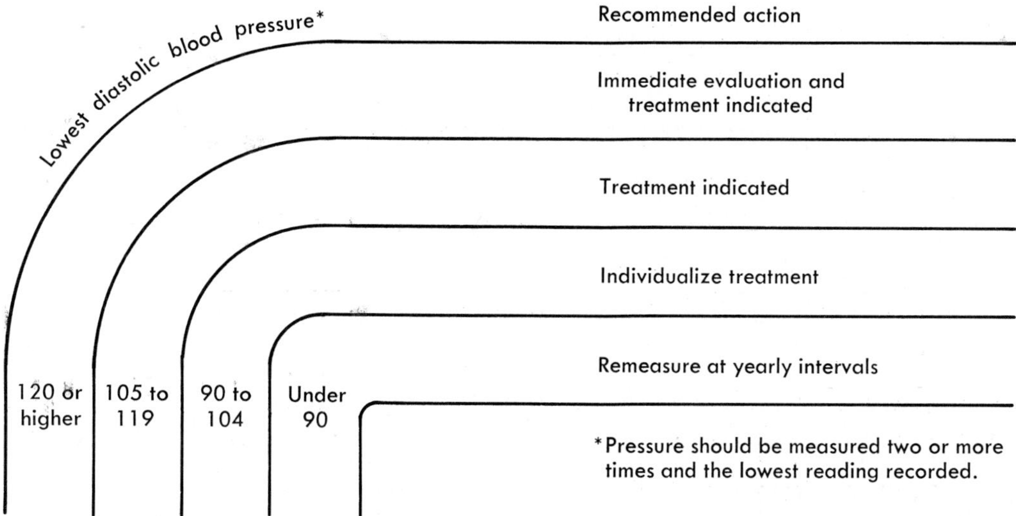

Fig. 47-13. Follow-up recommendations for persons with high blood pressure. Patient education begins when blood pressure is measured initially. Without alarming patient, person taking pressure should inform patient of blood pressure reading and carefully communicate importance of following recommended action. Patients not requiring evaluation or treatment are to be reassured and importance of annual blood pressure measurement strongly emphasized. (From U.S. National High Blood Pressure Education Programs, Recommendations of the Joint National Committee on Detection, Diagnosis, and Treatment of High Blood Pressure, Bethesda, Md., 1973, National Institutes of Health.)

Table 47-1. Oral drugs used in hypertension

Drug	Trade name	Dosage (mg/day)	Mode of action	Side effects
Diuretics				
Thiazide derivatives				
Chlorothiazide	Diuril	500 to 1500	Block sodium reabsorption in cortical portion of ascending tubule; water is excreted with sodium, producing decreased blood volume	↑ BUN ↑ Uric acid ↓ Potassium ↑ Blood glucose ↑ Calcium Less common: sensitivity reactions, gastrointestinal tract irritation, rashes, anemia, thrombocytopenia, purpura, pancreatitis NOTE: Thiazides are ineffective in renal failure
Hydrochlorothiazide	Hydrodiuril	50 to 150		
	Esidrix	50 to 150		
	Oretic	50 to 150		
Trichlormethazide	Naqua	4 to 8		
	Metahydrin	4 to 8		
Methylchlothiazide	Enduron	10 to 15		
Benzthiazide	Exna	100 to 150		
	Aquatag	100 to 150		
Polythiazide	Renese	2 to 8		
Cyclothiazide	Anhydron	2 to 6		
Furosemide	Lasix	40 to 160	Block sodium reabsorption in medullary portion of ascending tubule; same action as thiazides	Same as for thiazides; more likely to result in hypovolemia and dehydration
Ethacrynic acid	Edecrin	50 to 200		
Chlorthalidone	Hygroton	50 to 100	Same action as thiazides	Same as for thiazides; more likely to result in hypovolemia and dehydration
Quinethazone	Hydromox	100 to 150		
Potassium sparing				
Spironolactone	Aldactone	100 to 400	Antagonizes the effect of aldosterone on the tubular cells; sodium is excreted in exchange for potassium	Hyperkalemia, gynecomastia, hirsutism, irregular menses, rash, drowsiness, confusion
Triamterene	Dyrenium	100 to 300	Acts directly on sodium pump to excrete sodium in exchange for potassium	Hyperkalemia, diarrhea, nausea, vomiting, rash, photosensitivity
Combination drug				
Spironolactone-hydrochlorothiazide	Aldactaside			
Drugs acting on central nervous system				
Rauwolfia compounds				
Reserpine	Sandril Serpasil Reserpoid	0.1 to 0.25	Depletion of catecholamines in sympathetic postganglionic fibers	Drowsiness, lethargy, nasal congestion, bradycardia, depression, gastric hyperacidity

Table 47-1. Oral drugs used in hypertension—cont'd

Drug	Trade name	Dosage (mg/day)	Mode of action	Side effects
Drugs acting on central nervous system—cont'd				
Rauwolfa compounds—cont'd				
Whole root	Raudixin	50 to 100		
Alseroxylon fraction	Rauwiloid	2 to 4		
Deserpidine	Harmonyl	0.25		
Guanethidine	Ismelin	10 to 150	Blocks norepinephrine release from adrenergic nerve endings	Orthostatic hypotension (very common), diarrhea, impotence or loss of ejaculation NOTE: Poor, inconsistent absorption from GI tract
Methyldopa	Aldomet	500 to 2,500	Metabolized into a false neurotransmitter displacing norepinephrine from its receptor sites; sympathetic activity reduced	Orthostatic hypotension, drowsiness, fever, liver damage, anemia, impotence NOTE: Drug of choice in presence of renal disease
Propranolol	Inderal	80 to 320	Beta-adrenergic blocker at peripheral autonomic site	GI tract disturbance, thrombocytopenia, rash, CHF, aggravation of asthma, fever
Phenoxybenzamine	Dibenzyline	20 to 80	Alpha-adrenergic blocker at peripheral autonomic site	Nasal congestion, blurred vision, tachycardia, GI tract disturbance
Other mechanisms				
Ganglionic blockers				
Pentolinium	Ansolysen	40 to no limit	Block both parasympathetic and sympathetic nerve transmission at the ganglia	Orthostatic hypotension, dry mouth, blurred vision, constipation, urinary retention
Mecamylamine	Inversine	5 to no limit		
Control in sympathetic release				
Clonidine	Catapres	0.1	Stimulation of alpha-adrenergic receptor in brain; causes inhibition of sympathetic vasoconstriction	Orthostatic hypotention, dry mouth, sedation, headache, constipation, fatigue
Vasodilators				
Hydralazine	Apresoline	50 to 250	Direct relaxation of arteriolar smooth muscle causing vasodilation	Headache, tachycardia, nausea, weakness, angina, rash, dizziness, fever
Prazosin	Minipres	3 to 20		

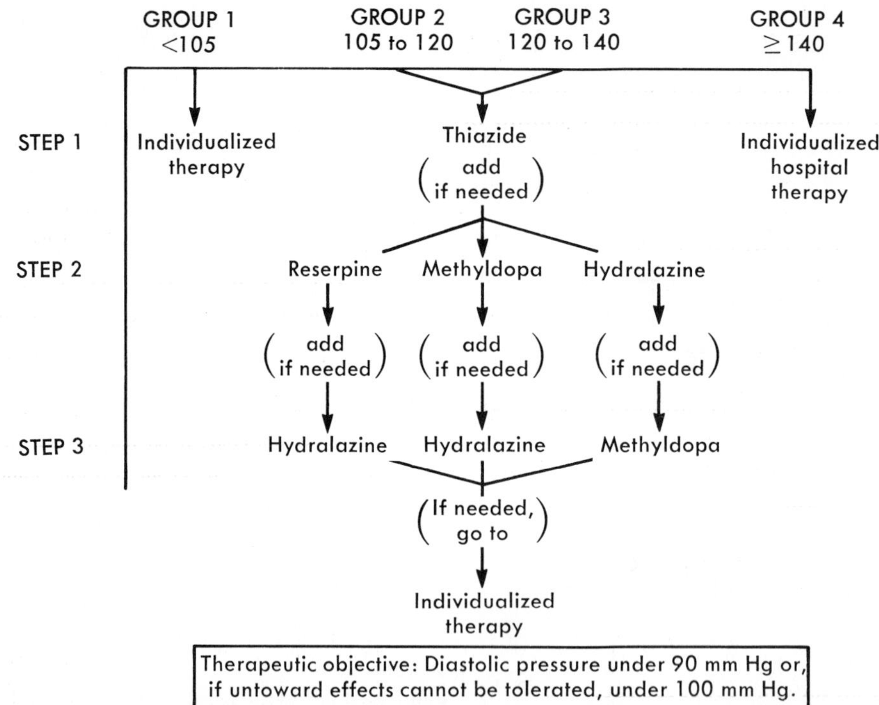

Fig. 47-14. Outline of recommended antihypertensive regimens for groups with varying degrees of severe hypertension as indicated by diastolic pressure in mm Hg. (From U.S. National High Blood Pressure Education Programs, Report of Task Force 1, Data Base, Bethesda, Md., 1973, National Institutes of Health.)

cause of the possible side effects of some of the medications. An ideal antihypertensive preparation should decrease the resistance of the arterioles and lower the blood pressure. It should not decrease the output of the heart, and unpleasant side effects should be minimal.

In general there are two aspects of drug therapy on which the nurse focuses attention. First, the patient must know how and when to take the medication. Some medications that are taken only once a day can be taken at bedtime so that the patient is asleep during the peak action of the drug when side effects will be greatest. Diuretics are generally taken early in the day so the patient will not be awakened with the need to void at night.

Second, the patient must be informed of possible side effects. Many of the untoward effects, such as the depression associated with reserpine or impotence associated with methyldopa (Aldomet) and guanethidine (Ismelin), are such that the individual does not automatically associate them with his anithypertensive medication and may be hesitant about discussing them. By informing him when the medication is started that these effects occur in a small percentage of people, that they are transient, and that he should inform his physician if they do occur in order that the medication can be changed, there is a greater chance that he will continue his therapy. The patient must also know the hazard of sudden cessation; for example, hypertensive crisis can follow withdrawal of clonidine (Catapres), and when this medication is withdrawn careful supervision by the physician is required. All aspects of the patient education program require careful coordination of the efforts of the nurse and physician.

All individuals with hypertension require close medical supervision. The blood pressure of some persons tends to be quite labile, and frequent adjustment in the dosage of their medications may be necessary. With certain drugs, response varies according to other variables such as the variability of guanethidine associated with shifts in extracellular fluid. Tolerance to the prescribed drug may also occur, and persons need to know what symptoms indicate the need to contact their physician.

If the blood pressure becomes very high some symptoms may occur. The most common symptom of high blood pressure is headache. The headache is usually occipital and is commonly present in the early morning. Sometimes the headache may be severe enough to waken the patient from sleep. Flushing of the face may be noted, and occasionally the nose bleeds. If the patient is older or has some degree of congestive heart failure, he may experience fatigue or shortness of breath on exertion; angina pectoris may occur. The patient should be aware that if any of these symptoms occur he should contact his physician immediately. Since the blood pressure can increase substantially without symptoms, the person should also be aware that he will probably need supervision by health professionals for the rest of his life.

□ Outcome criteria for the person with hypertension

The patient or significant others can:

1. Explain dietary modifications including decreased sodium intake.
2. Describe how to avoid external factors such as stress that compromise circulation.
3. Describe the medication and treatment program:
   a. State name, dosage frequency, and side effects of prescribed medication; state how to avoid side effects such as postural hypotension.
   b. Demonstrate awareness of probable need to continue medication for the rest of his life.
   c. Demonstrate ability to take blood pressure correctly (if applicable).
4. Explain health maintenance program:
   a. State symptoms that necessitate immediate medical attention.
   b. State plans for follow-up care by health professionals for the rest of his life.

REFERENCES AND SELECTED READINGS

1. Abramson, D. I.: Vascular disorders of the extremities, ed. 2, New York, 1974, Harper & Row, Publishers.
2. Alderman, D. B.: Surgery—and schlerotherapy—for varicose veins, RN **39**:OR-1, OR-4, OR-6, 1976.
3. Alderman, M. H., editor: Hypertension: the nurse's role in ambulatory care, New York, 1977, Springer Publishing Co., Inc.
4. Alderman, M. H., and Schoenbaum, E. E.: Detection and treatment of hypertension at the work site, N. Engl. J. Med. **293**:65-68, 1975.
5. Baird, R. N., and Abbott, W. M.: Vein grafts: an historical perspective, Am. J. Surg. **134**:293-296, 1977.
6. Barker, W. F.: Peripheral arterial disease, ed. 2, Philadelphia, 1975, W. B. Saunders Co.
7. Batterman, B., Stegman, M. R., and Fitz, A.: Hypertension. Part I. Detection and evaluation, Cardiovasc. Nurs. **11**:35-40, 1975.
8. Batterman, B., Stegman, M. R., and Fitz, A.: Hypertension. Part II. Treatment and nursing responsibilities, Cardiovasc. Nurs. **11**:41-44, 1975.
9. Beeson, P. B., and McDermott, W., editors: Textbook of medicine, ed. 14, Philadelphia, 1975, W. B. Saunders Co.
10. Bergan, J. J., and DeBoer, A.: Venous thrombosis and pulmonary embolism; total care, Surg. Clin. North Am. **50**:173-192, 1970.
11. Bergersen, B. S., and Goth, A.: Pharmacology in nursing, ed. 13, St. Louis, 1976, The C. V. Mosby Co.
12. Bibliography on hypertension therapy, Postgrad. Med. **56**:95-97, 1974.
13. *Bosanko, L. A.: Immediate postoperative prosthesis, Am. J. Nurs. **71**:280-283, 1971.
14. Brown, D. F.: Blood lipids and lipoproteins in atherogenesis, Am. J. Med. **46**:691-704, 1969.
15. *Buck, B., and Lee, A. D.: Amputation: two views, Nurs. Clin. North Am. **11**:641-657, 1976.
16. Burgess, E., et al.: Immediate postsurgical prosthetics in the management of lower extremity amputees, Department of Medicine and Surgery, Veterans Administration, Washington, D.C., 1967.
17. *Clark, A. B., and Dunn, M.: A nurse clinician's role in the management of hypertension, Arch. Intern. Med. **136**:903-904, 1976.
18. *Cobey, J. C., and Cobey, J. H.: Chronic leg ulcers, Am. J. Nurs. **74**:258-259, 1974.
19. Coffman, J. D.: Vasodilator drugs in peripheral vascular disease, J. Maine Med. Assoc. **66**:262-268, 1975.
20. Collins, G. J., et al.: Chronic abnormalities in patients with arterial, venous, and combined arterial and venous thrombosis, Arch. Surg. **112**:1347-1351, 1977.
21. Davies, M.: Streptokinase therapy for deep vein thrombosis, Nurs. Times **69**:211-212, 1973.
22. Dean, R. H., and Yao, J. S.: Hemodynamic measurements in peripheral vascular disease, Curr. Probl. Surg. **13**:1-76, 1976.
23. del Bueno, D. J.: The renal humoral system: a cause of hypertension? RN **38**:109-110, 1975.
24. DePalma, R.: Surgical therapy for venous stasis, Surgery **76**:910-917, 1974.
25. *deTornyay, R., and Doswell, W. M.: Nursing decisions. 8. Experiences in clinical problem solving: Nora L., a disturbed patient with hypertension, RN **39**:39-45, 1976.
26. *Dhar, S. K., and Freedman, P.: Clinical management of hypertensive emergencies, Heart Lung **5**:571-575, 1976.
27. Draye, M. A., and Robin, N.: Management of the hypertensive patient, Nurs. Pract. **1**:98-101, 1976.
28. *Eddy, M. E.: Teaching patients with peripheral vascular disease, Nurs. Clin. North Am. **12**:151-159, 1977.
29. Ellis, H.: Arteriosclerotic disease of the lower limbs, Nurs. Times **69**:698-700, 1973.
30. *Engstrand, J. L.: Rehabilitation of the patient with a lower extremity amputation, Nurs. Clin. North Am. **11**:659-669, 1976.
31. Executive summary of the task force reports to the Hypertension Information and Education Advisory Committee, U.S. Department of Health, Education and Welfare, No. (NIH) 74-592, 1973.
32. *Fagin-Dubin, L.: Atherosclerosis: a major cause of peripheral vascular disease, Nurs. Clin. North Am. **12**:101-108, 1977.
33. Fairbairn, J. F., Juergens, J. L., and Spittell, J. A., editors: Peripheral vascular disease, Philadelphia, 1972, W. B. Saunders Co.
34. *Fenn, J. E.: Reconstructive arterial surgery for ischemic lower extremities, Nurs. Clin. North Am. **12**:129-142, 1977.
35. Finnerty, F. A., Jr.: Hypertension as a clinical problem: the hospital based population, Prev. Med. **3**:323-327, 1974.
36. *Finnerty, F. A. Jr.: Aggressive drug therapy in accelerated hypertension, Am. J. Nurs. **74**:2176-2180, 1974.
37. *Freis, E. D.: Introduction to the nature and management of hypertension, Bowie, Md., 1974, Robert J. Brody Co.
38. *Garrett, J. F., and Levine, E. S., editors: Psychological practices with the physically disabled, New York, 1962, Columbia University Press.

*References preceded by an asterisk are particularly well suited for student reading.

39. Getz, G. S., Vesselinovitch, D., and Wissler, R. W.: A dynamic pathology of atherosclerosis, Am. J. Med. **46**:657-673, 1969.
40. *Gordon, T., and Kennel, W. B.: Predisposition to atherosclerosis in the head, heart, and legs: the Framingham study, J.A.M.A. **221**:661-666, 1972.
41. Greep, J. M., Aleman, P. J., Jarrett, F., et al.: A combined technique for arterial embolectomy, Arch. Surg. **105**:869-874, 1972.
42. Gross, F.: Drug therapy of hypertension: what we have, what we need, what we expect, Am. J. Cardiol. **34**:471-475, 1974.
43. Haimovici, H.: Vascular surgery: principles and techniques, ed. 2, New York, 1976, McGraw-Hill Book Co.
44. *Hirschberg, G. G., et al.: Rehabilitation: a manual for the care of the elderly and disabled, ed. 2, Philadelphia, 1976, J. B. Lippincott Co.
45. Hobbs, J. T., editor: The treatment of venous disorders: a comprehensive review of current practice in the treatment of varicose veins and the post-thrombotic syndrome, Philadelphia, 1977, J. B. Lippincott Co.
46. Holling, H. E.: Peripheral vascular diseases: diagnosis and management, Philadelphia, 1972, J. B. Lippincott Co.
47. Hull, P., and Thomas, E.: Nursing regimen in the care of the amputee with contracture, A.N.A. Clinical Sessions, Dallas, Texas, 1968, American Nurses' Association.
48. *Ingelfinger, J. A., and Goldman, P.: Therapy for hypertension. How much of what drug for whom? J.A.M.A. **238**:1369-1370, 1977.
49. *Jackson, B.S.: Chronic peripheral arterial disease, Am. J. Nurs. **72**:928-934, 1972.
50. *Jones, L. N.: Hypertension: medical and nursing implications, Nurs. Clin. North Am. **11**:283-295, 1976.
51. Juergens, J. L., and Payne, W. S.: Obstructive disease of the veins. In Fairbairn, J. F., Juergens, J. L., and Spittell, J. A.: Peripheral vascular surgery, Philadelphia, 1972, W. B. Saunders Co.
52. Kerstein, M. D., Zimmer, H., Dugdale, F. E., et al.: Amputations of the lower extremity: a study of 194 cases, Arch. Phys. Med. Rehabil. **55**:454-459, 1974.
53. Kessro, B.: Peripheral arterial insufficiency: postoperative care, Nurs. Clin. North Am. **12**:143-149, 1977.
54. Larson, C. B., and Gould, M. L.: Orthopedic nursing, ed. 9, St. Louis, 1978, The C. V. Mosby Co.
55. Laughlin, E., Stanford, J., and Phelps, M.: Immediate postsurgical prosthetics fitting of a bilateral, below-elbow amputee: a report, Artif. Limbs **12**:17-19, 1968.
56. Lofgren, K. A.: Varicose veins. In Fairbairn, J. F., Juergens, J. L., and Spittell, J. A.: Peripheral vascular surgery, Philadelphia, 1972, W. B. Saunders Co.
57. *Long, M. L., Winslow, E. H., Scheuhing, M. A., et al.: Hypertension: what patients need to know, Am. J. Nurs. **76**:765-770, 1976.
58. Mannick, J. A., and Coffman, J. D.: Ischemic limbs: surgical approach and physiological principles, New York, 1973, Grune & Stratton, Inc.
59. *Martin, N.: Rehabilitation of the upper extremity amputee, Nurs. Outlook **18**:50-51, 1970.
60. McClinton, V. S.: Nursing of the upper extremity amputee and preparation for prosthetic training, Nurs. Clin. North Am. **11**:671-677, 1976.
61. *Mitchell, E. S.: Protocol for teaching hypertensive patients, Am. J. Nurs. **77**:808-809, 1977
62. Modell, W., editor: Drugs of choice 1978-1979, St. Louis, 1978, The C. V. Mosby Co.
63. *Moore, W. S., Hall, A. D., and Lim, R. C., Jr.: Below the knee amputation for ischemic gangrene, Am. J. Surg. **124**:127-134, 1972.
64. Moser, M., editor: Hypertension: a practical approach, Boston, 1975, Little, Brown and Co.
65. Murphy, B. S.: Management of hyperlipidemia, J.A.M.A. 230:1683-1691, 1974.
66. National Health Education Committee, Comp.: The killers and the cripplers: Facts on the major diseases in the United States today, ed. 11, New York, 1976, David McKay Co., Inc.
67. National Heart and Lung Institute task force on arteriosclerosis: Arteriosclerosis, vol. II, U. S. Department of Health, Education and Welfare, No. (NIH) 72-219, 1971.
68. National High Blood Pressure Education Program: Guidelines for the evaluation and management of the hypertensive patient, High Blood Pressure Information Center, National Institutes of Health, U.S. Department of Health, Education, and Welfare, No. (NIH) 76-744, 1976.
69. Nicholas, G. G., and DeMuth, W. E.: Evaluation of the use of the rigid dressing in amputation of the lower extremity, Surg. Gynecol. Obstet. **143**:398-400, 1976.
70. O'Neill, M. F.: Patients with hypertension: a study of manifest needs with self-actualization, Nurs. Res. **25**:349-351, 1976.
71. O'Reilly, R. A., and Aggeler, P. M.: Determinants of the response to oral anticoagulant drugs in man, Pharmacol. Rev. **22**:35-96, 1970.
72. *Pasnau, R. O., and Pfefferbaum, B.: Psychologic aspects of post-amputation pain, Nurs. Clin. North Am. **11**:679-685, 1976.
73. Perloff, D., editor: Symposium on hypertension, Med. Clin. North Am. **61**:463-700, 1977
74. Perloff, D.: Diagnostic assessment of the patient with hypertension, Geriatrics **31**:77-83, 1976.
75. Pfefferbaum, B., and Pasnau, R. O.: Post-amputation grief, Nurs. Clin. North Am. **11**:687-690, 1976.
76. *Pierce, P. F.: Gains and losses of vascular surgery patients, Nurs. Clin. North Am. **12**:119-127, 1977.
77. *Plaisted, L. M., and Friz, B. R.: The nurse on the amputee clinic team, Nurs. Outlook **16**:34-37, 1968.
78. Pratt, G. H.: Vascular surgery: a guide and handbook, St. Louis, 1976, Warren H. Green, Inc.
79. Proceedings of the symposium on venous surgery in the lower extremity, Walter Reed Army Medical Center, 1973, St. Louis, 1975, Warren H. Green, Inc.
80. *Ram, C. V.: Newer antihypertensive drugs, Heart Lung **6**:679-684, 1977.
81. Reis, R. L., and Hannah, H.: Management of patients with severe, coexistent coronary artery and peripheral vascular disease, J. Thorac. Cardiovasc. Surg. **73**:909-918, 1977.
82. Richardson, D. W.: Can physicians effect persistent control of blood pressure? Arch. Intern. Med. **137**:1598-1599, 1977.
83. *Robinson, A. M.: Detection and control of hypertension: challenge to all nurses, Am. J. Nurs. **76**:778-780, 1976.
84. Rodman, M. J.: Thromboembolic disorders. Part I. Venous thrombosis, RN **39**:81-82, 85-86, 1976.
85. Rodman, M. J.: Thromboembolic disorders, Part II. Arterial thrombosis and embolism, RN **39**:61-66, 1976.
86. Roon, A. J., Moore, W. S., and Goldstone, J.: Below-knee amputation: a modern approach, Am. J. Surg. **134**:153-158, 1977.
87. *Rose, M. A.: Home care after peripheral vascular surgery, Am. J. Nurs. **74**:260-262, 1974.
88. Rosen, A. J., DePalma, R. G., and Victor, Y.: Risk factors in peripheral atherosclerosis, Arch. Surg. **107**:303-308, 1973.
89. Ross, R., and Glomset, J.: The pathogenesis of artherosclerosis. Part I, N. Engl. J. Med. **295**:369-377, 1976.

90. Ross, R., and Glomset, J.: The pathogenesis of atherosclerosis. Part II, N. Engl. J. Med. **295**:420-425, 1976.
91. Royster, T. S., Mulcare, R. J., and Marks, R. A.: Peripheral arterial disease: recognizing the need for surgery, Postgrad. Med. **62**:153-159, 1977.
92. Rutherford, R. B., editor: Vascular surgery, Philadelphia, 1977, W. B. Saunders Co.
93. Ryzewski, J.: Factors in the rehabilitation of patients with peripheral vascular disease, Nurs. Clin. North Am. **12**:161-168, 1977.
94. Sabiston, D. C., Jr., editor: Christopher's textbook of surgery: the biological basis of modern surgical practice, ed. 11, Philadelphia, 1977, W. B. Saunders Co.
95. Sarmiento, A., et al.: Immediate postsurgical prosthetics fitting in the management of upper-extremity amputees, Artif. Limbs **12**:14-16, 1968.
96. *Sexton, D. L.: The patient with peripheral arterial occlusive disease, Nurs. Clin. North Am. **12**:89-99, 1977.
97. *Shank, L. F., and Ludewig, J.: Hypertension, Nurs. Clin. North Am. **9**:677-692, 1974.
98. Simpson, F. O., editor: Symposium on hypertension: drugs, **11**(Suppl. 1):2-5, 1976.
99. *Sister Mary Elizabeth: Occlusion of the peripheral arteries: nursing observations and symptomatic care, Am. J. Nurs. **67**:562-564, 1967.
100. Stahl, S. M., Lawrie, T., Neill, P., et al.: Motivational interventions in community hypertension screening, Am. J. Publ. Health **67**:345-352, 1977.
101. Stamler, J., et al.: Hypertension: the problem and the challenge. In The hypertension handbook, West Point, Pa., 1974, Merck Sharp & Dohme.
102. Stubbins, J., editor: Social and psychological aspects of disability: a handbook for practitioners, Baltimore, 1977, University Park Press.
103. Tarazi, R. C., Dustan, H. P., and Brayd, E. L.: Haemodynamic effects of propranolol in hypertension: a review, Postgrad. Med. J. **52**(Suppl. 4):92-100, 1976.
104. *Task Force on the Role of Nursing in High Blood Pressure Control: Nursing education in high blood pressure control: report, National Institutes of Health, U.S. Department of Health, Education and Welfare, No. (NIH) 76-1052, 1976.
105. U.S. National High Blood Pressure Education Program: Report to the Hypertension Information and Education Advisory Committee: task force reports, Bethesda, Md., 1973, National Institutes of Health.
106. U.S. National High Blood Pressure Education Program: Directory of community high blood pressure control activities. Prepared by the National High Blood Pressure Education Program with the assistance of Merck Sharp & Dohme, ed. 2, National Institutes of Health, U.S. Department of Health, Education, and Welfare, No. (NIH) 77-1243, 1977.
107. Warren, R.: Procedures in vascular surgery, ed. 2, Boston, 1976, Little, Brown and Co.
108. Weinstein, M.C., and Stason, M. C.: Hypertension: a policy perspective, Cambridge, Mass., 1976, Harvard University Press.
109. Wilhelmsen, L., and Berglund, G.: Prevalence of primary and secondary hypertension, Am. Heart J. **94**:543-546, 1977.
110. Wintrobe, M. M., et al., editors: Harrison's principles of internal medicine, ed. 7, New York, 1974, McGraw-Hill Book Co.

48

Problems of the blood and blood-forming organs

DEANNA MELTON XISTRIS

The hematopoietic system is comprised of the blood and blood-forming organs. In the normal adult, production of hematopoietic cells is limited to the bone marrow of the sternum, vertebrae, ribs, and the proximal epiphyses of the femur and humerus. In disease states the sites of blood cell production may expand to include other areas of the bone marrow and the widespread lymphatic system, predominately the spleen.

Hematopoiesis (blood cell production) is a self-renewal process that involves cellular proliferation, the division of immature cells (hematopoietic stem cells), and subsequent differentiation of the stem cells into mature cell forms. This differentiation from stem cell to blood cells with both morphologic and functional maturity is shown in Fig. 48-1.

Blood cells (erythrocytes, platelets, neutrophils, lymphocytes, monocytes, eosinophils, and basophils) are constantly being lost and replaced. Homeostasis is maintained through a balance between the rate of production of blood cells and the rate of destruction. Disorders of the blood are manifested when this balance is lost. An imbalance occurs when there is a decrease in the rate of blood cell production, an increase in cell destruction at a rate that exceeds cell production, or when the production of a single type accelerates at a rate disproportionate to that of other blood cells.

To understand the disease processes of the hematopoietic system, some knowledge of each of the blood components is necessary. Discussion of the blood components is presented in this chapter along with related disease processes.

■ ASSESSMENT

A wide variety of disorders affect the hematopoietic system. In addition to primary hematologic disorders, secondary effects from disease of another body system may manifest themselves in abnormal hematologic findings. For example, the anemia associated with azotemia is the consequence of disease outside of the hematopoietic system.

The cause of any hematologic abnormality must be assiduously pursued. The importance of accurate diagnosis combined with the very diverse and frequently nonspecific signs and symptoms makes it likely that the person will become involved in an arduous diagnostic process. At the time of initial contact the patient is already experiencing the stress of sudden onset of illness or the gnawing fear or suspicion that all is not well. The explanations that are offered and the time allowed for verbalization and questions are means of providing a positive foundation for the long-term care that may follow.

□ Subjective data

A thorough history includes detailed information about the person's symptoms and a thorough review of systems. In the history taking of a person with suspected hematologic disease, other key points to include are family history, drug history, exposure to chemicals, and general nonspecific complaints offered by the patient.

Family history

The existence of inherited hematologic disorders necessitates a detailed family history. Questions regarding disease or presence of symptoms among relatives should include reference to parents, siblings, grandfathers, uncles, and nephews. Questions should explore instances of severe or prolonged bleeding in relation to minor trauma, dental extractions, or surgery. The occurrence of jaundice or anemia in relatives should also be ascertained.

Drugs and chemicals

Drugs may induce or potentiate hematologic disease. Most notable are the hematologic effects of the cytotoxic

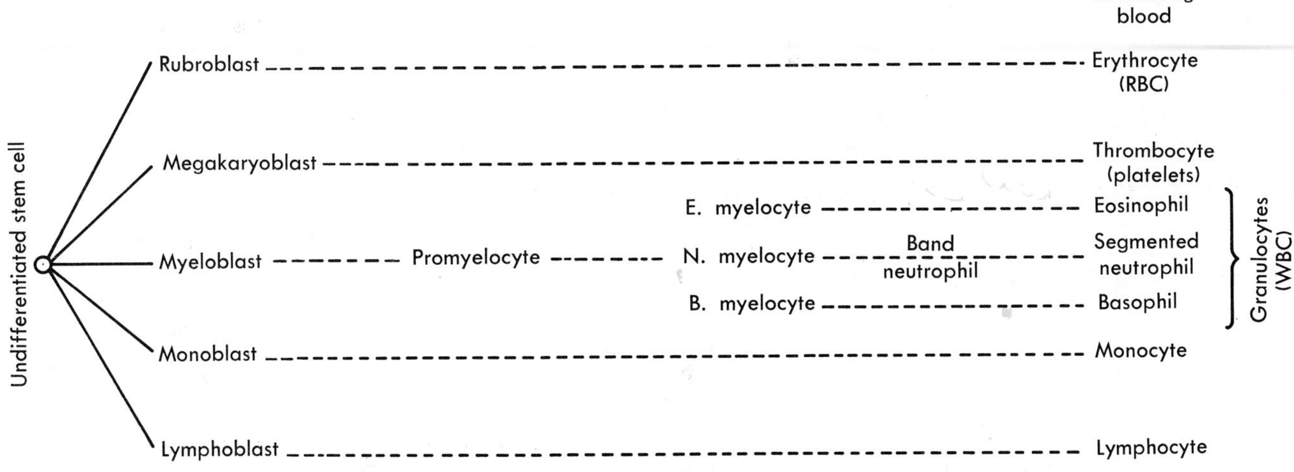

Fig. 48-1. Maturation of hematopoietic tissue. Precursor of final cell form is specialized blast cell that arises from undifferentiated stem cell.

drugs used in cancer chemotherapy and the neutropenia associated with chloramphenicol. A thorough history of drugs ingested by a person is a crucial part of assessment. Many persons regularly ingest "something to help me sleep," "something to calm me down," or "just aspirin." Analgesics, tranquilizers, laxatives, and sedatives are often overlooked by persons when asked about drugs. Specific, often rephrased questioning is necessary to obtain a complete drug history.

Chemicals are generally viewed as potentially harmful agents that may exert an effect on the hematopoietic system. Recently benzene as a harmful agent has been the focus of much research. To obtain a history of exposure to chemicals, an occupational history is useful. In addition such common practices as the use of hair dye should also be explored.

Weight loss

Weight loss may be associated with primary hematologic disorders. Commonly weight loss is mild or absent. Marked weight loss suggests disease other than a primary hematologic disorder.

Fever

Fever is a common manifestation of many of the hematologic disorders and is an important question to be asked during the history. Fever is a common manifestation in lymphoma, primarily Hodgkin's disease and leukemia. Severe chills may accompany hemolytic disorders. Night sweats are frequently associated with both lymphoma and leukemia.

Fatigue and malaise

Fatigue and malaise are difficult symptoms to evaluate, since they frequently accompany many physical and emotional disorders. These symptoms may also be seen in association with anemia and hematologic malignancies. Information regarding the occurrence of these symptoms should be included in the history. In addition to being of diagnostic value, the person's subjective description of such symptoms lends some insight into perception of the illness, the extent to which the illness is affecting daily living, and the ability to adapt.

□ Objective data

A thorough physical examination is performed in the assessment of a person with a hematologic disorder. It is useful to recognize target organs and alterations that may be reflective of hematologic disease.

Skin

Skin manifestations of hematologic disease are often readily visible. *Petechiae* and *ecchymoses* are associated with decreased platelets (thrombocytopenia) and other bleeding disorders. *Jaundice,* when observed, may be associated with pernicious anemia or hemolytic disease. *Pallor* is commonly associated by the lay person with disorders of the blood. Pallor as a criteria for assessment may be deceptive, since many healthy persons have pale complexions, while some severely anemic patients may have ruddy complexions.

Changes in skin texture may also be observed. Except in severe cases it will most likely be the person who observes such changes. With iron deficiency the person may notice dry skin, dry hair, and brittle nails. Severe itching is commonly associated with Hodgkin's disease and may also occur with polycythemia vera, especially after bathing. In persons with leukemia and lymphoma, infiltrative lesions of the skin may be observed on any portion of the body.

Head and neck

The sclerae of the eyes are examined for jaundice and the conjunctivae for pallor. Since retinal hemorrhages may occur in persons with severe anemia and thrombocytopenia, ophthalmoscopic examination must be included. Questions may also elicit a history of visual disturbances.

The oral mucosa is observed for pallor, bleeding tendency, and ulceration. The tongue may be markedly smooth in association with both pernicious anemia and nutritional deficiencies.

The neck is observed primarily for evaluation of lymph nodes. Nodes may be so large as to be visible. A "lump" on the neck is often the reason for seeking medical attention.

Chest

Firm pressure with the fingertips is exerted along the sternum and ribs to elicit any tenderness that may be present. Such tenderness may reflect a leukemic process or multiple myeloma.

Abdomen

The abdomen is percussed and palpated with special attention to the liver and spleen. Both organs are prone to enlarge in association with hematologic disease.

Back and extremities

The skeletal system is evaluated primarily for pain, joint deformity, and arthritis. Bone pain is frequently associated with hematologic malignancies. In persons with hemolytic processes and some hematologic malignancies, there is increased uric acid production and a corresponding increase in the incidence of gout. Joint deformities are associated with bleeding disorders. Leg ulcers are frequently seen with sickle cell anemia.

Lymph nodes

Lymph nodes are widely distributed in the body and are routinely examined by palpation of the body part being examined. In the healthy adult the only palpable nodes are in the inguinal region and less commonly in the axilla. With disease the cervical and supraclavicular nodes may become palpable. Further evaluation of lymph nodes requires radiographic examination and lymphangiography. It is important to recognize that any enlarged lymph node may reflect a disease process and should be evaluated thoroughly.

Nervous system

Many neurologic abnormalities may be manifested in persons with hematologic disorders. The catastrophic complications are caused by bleeding or infection within the central nervous system. Infiltration of malignant leukemic or lymphomatous cells may produce signs and symptoms of cerebral tumor. In addition some of the lymphomas, especially Hodgkin's disease, may produce a dementia as a remote effect. Initial physical examination should therefore include assessment of mental status, cranial nerve function, sensory function (pain, touch, position, and vibratory sensation), and motor function (strength, reflexes, and plantar response).

□ Diagnostic studies

Extensive blood examinations are performed as part of the diagnostic workup of a person suspected of having a hematologic disorder. The most common laboratory tests are listed in Table 48-1. The information obtained from such studies provides important clues as to the pathology of the disorder. In addition to their diagnostic value, blood studies are used to monitor an individual's progress and response to treatment.

Because of the necessity for frequent blood tests the person needs to learn the rationale for the tests. Even with an intellectual understanding of why frequent venipunctures are necessary, it is easy for an individual to become discouraged. Recognizing the unpleasantness of having blood samples taken, giving a word of encouragement, and being with the person during the procedure are nursing activities that may bolster the person's spirits.

The final diagnosis of a hematologic disease is often dependent on an examination of a peripheral blood smear and the bone marrow.

Peripheral blood smear

Each blood cell possesses microscopic features that identify and set the cell apart from other cell types. Examination of the peripheral blood smear allows for the determination of the morphology of the cells (type, origin), the extent of cell maturity, and the ratio of the various cell types to each other. Often this information, when combined with the data from the history, physical examination, and other laboratory tests, determines the medical diagnosis.

Bone marrow examination

An adjunct to the peripheral blood smear is the bone marrow examination. Generally the bone marrow is examined in those instances in which the diagnosis is not

Table 48-1. Laboratory tests for hematologic assessment

Blood cell	Function	Diagnostic test
Erythrocytes (RBC)	Mediate the exchange of O_2 and CO_2 between the lungs and the tissue	RBC, hemoglobin, hematocrit, reticulocyte count Blood indices: Mean corpuscular hemoglobin concentration (MCHC), mean cell volume (MCV), mean corpuscular hemoglobin (MCH) Red cell fragility Morphologic description in stained smear
Platelets	Platelet plug; promotion of thrombin production	Platelet aggregation Platelet count Bleeding time
Leukocytes (WBC)		WBC WBC with differential
Granulocytes		
Neutrophils	Phagocytosis	
Eosinophils		
Basophils	Allergic and immunologic responses	
Lymphocytes	Formation of immunoglobulins	
Monocytes	Phagocytosis	

clearly established from the peripheral blood smear or when further information is needed. A bone marrow specimen is obtained by bone marrow aspiration or bone marrow biopsy.

Bone marrow aspiration. Aspiration is the most common procedure for obtaining a bone marrow sample. The procedure is possible because normal bone marrow is soft and semifluid and can therefore be removed by aspiration through a needle. Bone marrow aspiration is most likely to be performed in persons with marked anemia, neutropenia (decreased number of white blood cells), acute leukemia, thrombocytopenia (decreased number of platelets), or immunoglobulin disorders.

When persons are informed ahead of time and prepared accordingly, few require sedation. Should an individual express extreme fear or apprehension, the physician is notified so that the person's fears and questions may be further addressed and sedation ordered if it is indicated.

The bone marrow aspiration is usually performed in the patient's room. The skin surrounding the puncture site is shaved, if necessary, and cleansed with an antiseptic such as povidone-iodine complex (Betadine). Sterile towels are placed around the site. The skin and periosteum are anesthetized to avoid severe pain. First, the most superficial layer of the skin is infiltrated with procaine. After a few seconds the needle is further advanced until bone is touched. Procaine is then injected to anesthetize the periosteum.

The marrow aspiration needle is inserted into the sternum between the second and third ribs. Other sites such as the iliac crest may also be used (Fig. 48-2). When the marrow cavity is entered, the marrow stylet is removed from the needle and a sterile syringe is attached. The syringe plunger is drawn back until marrow appears in the syringe. As the plunger is drawn back the person will experience a brief, sharp pain. The pain is caused by

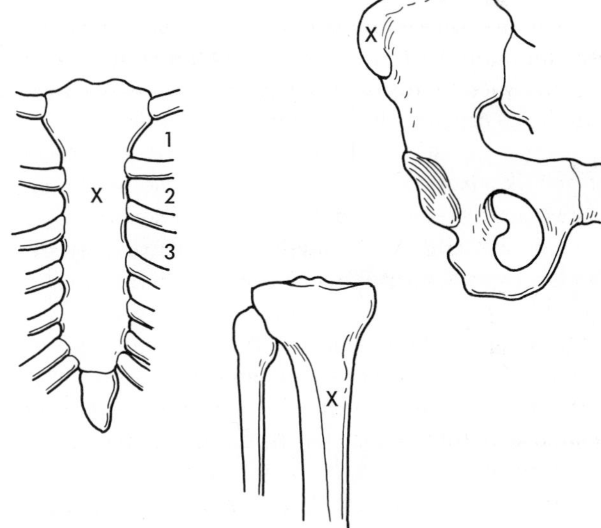

Fig. 48-2. Sites for bone marrow aspiration: sternum, iliac crest, tibia.

the suction exerted as the plunger is pulled back. The nurse's hands placed gently on the person's shoulder and a calm warning coupled with a reminder to lie still serve well to prevent a sudden jerk or movement by the person.

After the needle is removed, pressure is applied briefly over the aspiration site to arrest the scant bleeding that occurs. An adhesive bandage placed over the site is usually sufficient. Marked bleeding following bone marrow aspiration is rare but may occur in those persons with a bleeding disorder. If marked bleeding does occur, a pressure dressing is applied and the aspiration site and the vital signs are monitored frequently to assess the severity of bleeding.

Some persons may complain of tenderness at the aspiration site for a few days. Analgesics may be prescribed to alleviate the discomfort. Other persons experience no pain or discomfort following the procedure.

Bone marrow biopsy. A bone marrow biopsy is indicated when a large sample of bone marrow is needed. Persons most likely to undergo a bone marrow biopsy are those with pancytopenia (more than one altered cell type), myelofibrosis, metastatic tumor, lymphoma, and multiple myeloma. The most common site for bone marrow biopsy is the posterosuperior iliac spine. The initial steps in the biopsy procedure are similar to those outlined for bone marrow aspiration. At the point where the cavity is entered, in this case the medullary cavity, cutting blades are inserted through the cannula. The cutting blades are pressed into the medullary bone. The outer cannula is advanced over the cutting blades, the specimen is secured, and the entire unit is removed.

A pressure dressing is applied over the biopsy site for about 1 hour. During this time the person may be required to remain in bed in a recumbent position.

Following a bone marrow biopsy, patients are assessed for bleeding from the biopsy site and for pain. They may or may not require analgesics. Some other comfort measures such as assisting the person to freshen up are often needed to help the person relax and rest comfortably.

■ DISEASES ASSOCIATED WITH RED BLOOD CELLS (ERYTHROCYTES)

In the normal adult, red cell production (erythropoiesis) occurs in the bone marrow of the axial skeleton and proximal long bones. The normal erythrocyte circulates in the blood 120 days, at which time it is destroyed by the macrophages of the reticuloendothelial system. The spleen plays the predominant role in the normal destruction of senescent (aged) red cells, although other reticuloendothelial organs, predominantly the liver, are able to assume this role. The primary functions of the circulating erythrocyte are transportation of hemoglobin (Hb), and the mediation of the exchange of oxygen and carbon dioxide between the lungs and peripheral tissue.

□ Polycythemia vera

In polycythemia vera there is excessive production of red blood cells, white blood cells, and platelets. The red blood count may rise to 7 to 12 million. The hemoglobin is increased, and the patient characteristically has a reddish purple complexion, with reddening of the hands and feet. Headache, weakness, dyspnea, itching, and lacrimation may be other complaints. There may be bleeding from the skin and from the mucous membranes. This disease usually occurs in persons over 50 years of age, and the average age at death is approximately 60 years. Death is usually from thrombosis, progression to bone marrow fibrosis, or acute leukemia.

Phlebotomy is the main treatment, and it may be necessary every 6 months or more often. Radioactive phosphorus, busulfan (Myleran), or triethylenemelamine (TEM) can often control the disease. The patient should have a diet not excessively high in iron, and the nurse can help him with the selection of foods. Other nursing care during an exacerbation consists of supportive care, with special attention to hemorrhage.

□ Anemia

Etiology. Anemia is defined as a lower than normal number of circulating erythrocytes. The anemic state may be the result of (1) acute or chronic blood loss, (2) bone marrow dysfunction, (3) immaturity of erythrocytes due to absence of an essential factor, or (4) increased rate of destruction of erythrocytes.[30]

Assessment. The decreased ability of the blood to mediate the exchange of oxygen and carbon dioxide results in the classic signs of anemia: weakness, dyspnea on exertion, and fatigue. The significance of an anemia is evaluated through the person's symptoms and the determination of the underlying pathologic cause of the anemia.

The history for a person with anemia must include detailed information about exposure to chemicals and drugs, menstrual history, and dietary habits. The person is asked about the occurrence of blood in stool, either frank red blood or black, tarry stools. Occurrence of headache, faintness, muscular weakness, fatigability, irritability, and tinnitus are also elicited during the history taking.

Few manifestations of anemia are apparent by physical examination alone. A thorough physical examination is indicated to determine the severity of the anemia and to identify any source of blood loss that may exist. Particular attention is given to evaluation of the pulse and blood pressure with the patient in both the lying and standing positions (postural signs). A drop in blood pressure with an increase in pulse when the standing position is assumed is indicative of severe hypovolemia or marked anemia. The conjunctiva of the eye is observed for pallor. Rectal examination is performed to assess for blood loss from the gastrointestinal tract and from hemorrhoids.

Laboratory tests used to evaluate anemia include red blood cell count, reticulocyte count, hemoglobin, red blood cell indices, total bilirubin, and a serum iron determination.

□ Anemia secondary to blood loss

The anemia associated with *acute* blood loss is the direct result of the marked decrease in circulating red blood cells. The adult of average build has a total blood volume of approximately 6,000 ml. Usually an adult can lose 500 ml without serious or lasting effects. If the loss reaches 1,000 ml or more, serious consequences may result, and 1 to 2 months may be required for the hemoglobin concentration of the blood to return to normal.

The body has remarkable adaptive powers and may adjust fairly well to a marked reduction in red blood cells and hemoglobin, provided the condition develops gradually. An individual may remain asymptomatic even though the total red cell count may drop to almost half of its normal figure of between 4.5 and 5 million/cu mm. *Chronic*, unrecognized blood loss may occur in the presence of an unsuspected gastrointestinal tract malignancy, a slowly bleeding peptic ulcer, or hemorrhoids that bleed without the person's awareness. When blood loss is continuous and moderate in amount, the bone marrow may be able to keep up with the losses by increasing the production of red blood cells. Eventually if the cause of chronic blood loss is not found and corrected, the bone marrow will not be able to keep pace with the loss, and symptoms of anemia appear.

Clinical picture. The patient with anemia secondary to acute loss of blood from hemorrhage has signs and symptoms of hypovolemia and hypoxemia. Weakness, stupor, irritability, and cool moist skin are all symptoms that may be observed. Vital signs will demonstrate hypotension and tachycardia. The severity of the patient's symptoms correlates with the severity of blood loss.

Intervention. Treatment for anemia secondary to blood loss is dependent on identification of the source of blood loss so that the cause may be corrected. For persons who are hypovolemic, whole-blood transfusions are given to supplement both the intravascular volume and the numbers of circulating red blood cells. Persons with slow, chronic blood loss may receive whole-blood transfusions or packed cells.

□ Anemia secondary to bone marrow dysfunction

Aplastic anemia

Aplastic anemia is characterized by depression or cessation of activity of all blood-producing elements. There is a decrease in white blood cells (leukopenia), a decrease in platelets (thrombocytopenia), and a decrease in formation of red blood cells.

Etiology. The cause of aplastic anemia is complex and somewhat uncertain. In approximately one half of the cases of aplastic anemia in the United States, no etiologic agent is identifiable. Predictable bone marrow depression occurs with antineoplastic drugs, particularly the alkylating agents and the vinca alkaloids and immunosuppressive drugs. Frequently the occurrence of aplastic anemia follows exposure to drugs such as chloramphenicol, sulfonamides, phenylbutazone (Butazolidin), anticonvulsants such as mephenytoin (Mesantoin), and thiazide diuretics. Exposure to insecticides, such as DDT, and chemicals, particularly benzene, are also thought to cause aplastic anemia through some influence on the bone marrow. It is thought that aplastic anemia is due to injury or destruction of a common stem cell (Fig. 48-1) affecting all subsequent cell populations.

Clinical picture. Symptoms of aplastic anemia may appear suddenly but usually develop gradually over a period of weeks and months. Symptoms include pallor, weakness, dyspnea, anorexia, headache, fever, and bleeding of the mucous membranes, often first noticed in the mouth or the nose. Laboratory tests reveal pancytopenia (a marked decrease in the numbers of all cell types). Attempts at bone marrow aspiration may yield a "dry tap" (due to hypocellularity and a decrease in active marrow), and bone marrow biopsy is often necessary.

Intervention. The most immediate treatment for aplastic anemia is the removal of the causative agent, if it is known. Once this is done the person may recover spontaneously. For those persons with marked aplasia, diligent medical care and nursing care are required. Because all of the blood cells are decreased, the individual is prone to severe and life-threatening complications, primarily infection and bleeding. (The nursing care of persons with decreased white blood count and platelets is discussed on pp. 1069 and 1075.) Intensive supportive care through transfusion of the specific components that are lacking (red blood cells, platelets, white blood cells) is frequently necessary to maintain life. In recent years bone marrow transplantation has emerged as a treatment for persons with aplastic anemia.

Aplastic anemia is a severe and life-threatening condition. Persons and their significant others are under severe stress because of the severity of the illness. Frequently "not knowing the cause" is an additional stress. Talking with family members and explaining the rationale for procedures such as reverse (protective) isolation are helpful ways to convey a caring concern.

☐ Anemia due to absence of an essential factor

Iron-deficiency anemia

Iron-deficiency anemia is the most common form of anemia. Approximately 20% of women, 50% of pregnant women, and 3% of men are iron deficient.[45]

Iron is normally obtained through the food we eat. Absorption occurs in the duodenum and upper portion of the small intestine. In addition to the iron that is ingested, the body's supply of iron is augmented by the iron derived from the breakdown of hemoglobin. Factors that contribute to or cause an iron-deficient state include inadequate iron from dietary intake, impaired iron absorption commonly following gastric and intestinal tract surgery, and blood loss. In the United States blood loss is the most common cause of iron-deficiency anemia.[45]

Clinical picture. Many iron-deficient persons are asymptomatic. Iron deficiency may be an incidental finding during a routine physical examination. When symptoms do occur, they are the symptoms common to all anemias: fatigue, headache, dyspnea on exertion, tachycardia, and pallor. The progression of symptoms is so gradual that when the person does see the physician the iron deficiency is usually quite severe. Physical findings are frequently normal; however, special attention should be given to the neuromuscular system. There may be neuralgic pains, vasomotor disturbances, and most commonly numbness and tingling.[45]

Intervention. The treatment of iron-deficiency anemia is to determine and correct the cause. Repletion of iron stores in the body is then accomplished by the administration of iron. Oral iron supplement is usually given in the form of ferrous sulfate. If the person is to take the medication at home, patient instruction is necessary. Because it is irritating to the gastrointestinal tract, ferrous sulfate should be taken after meals. The person should also be told that stools will be black and to report to the physician any symptoms of diarrhea or nausea. When the individual cannot tolerate oral preparations of iron, parenteral iron therapy is used. Parenteral therapy is also indicated when the person is unable to absorb iron from the gastrointestinal tract, either because of disease or the presence of a colostomy.

Occasionally poor diet is the cause of iron-deficiency anemia, but more often it is only a contributing factor. All persons with iron-deficiency anemia must be assessed for their knowledge of a well-balanced diet and their ability and willingness to provide themselves with such a diet. When indicated, follow-up through a clinic, home visits by a dietitian, and such community resources as "meals on wheels" can be effective ways of assuring the person of a well-balanced diet.

Pernicious anemia

Pernicious anemia was first described by Thomas Addison in London in 1849, and the term "addisonian anemia" is still sometimes used. The fundamental defect in pernicious anemia is the absence of intrinsic factor, which is normally produced by the parietal cells of the stomach mucosa, with the resulting inability of the body to absorb vitamin B_{12}. The deficiency of vitamin B_{12} is then reflected in altered red blood cell maturation, resulting in abnormally large (megaloblastic) cells.

Adult pernicious anemia occurs most often after the age of 40, affecting both sexes equally. The cause of pernicious anemia remains unclear. Congenital pernicious anemia occurs most often in children under 2 years of age. There is a high incidence of pernicious anemia in the parents and siblings of children with congenital pernicious anemia; therefore it is suspected that congenital pernicious anemia is inherited through an autosomal-recessive pattern.

The cause of adult pernicious anemia is even less certain; however, there does appear to be a hereditary predisposition toward development of the disease. There is a familial tendency (several members of the same family may have the disease.) Persons with pernicious anemia have common characteristics. Many are of the Nordic race and have broad faces, blond hair that grays early, and wide-set blue eyes. Because of the late onset of the disease, environmental influences are thought to play a role in the occurrence of pernicious anemia. Pernicious anemia may also follow total gastrectomy, since the body is no longer able to produce intrinsic factor. Any disorder that compromises the absorptive capacity of the distal ileum may also lead to vitamin B_{12} deficiency.

Clinical picture. The onset of pernicious anemia is slow. Although the anemia may be quite severe at the time of diagnosis, it is likely that the individual has been able to compensate quite well. The classic signs of pernicious anemia are generalized weakness, soreness and burning sensation of the tongue (glossitis), and numbness and tingling (paresthesia) of the extremities. Other findings may include smooth tongue (due to absence of papillae), yellowish skin color, slight icterus of the sclera, tachycardia, and a palpable spleen and liver. Neurologic assessment may reveal a loss of vibratory sense in the lower extremities, loss of coordination of the lower extremities, and loss of fine hand movements. More severe signs of neurologic involvement include presence of Babinski reflex (dorsiflexed toe), disturbed position sense, spasticity, increased or decreased reflexes, and mental disturbances (irritability, memory loss, and mild depression).

Laboratory evaluation of the blood reveals anemia that may be mild or severe. The reticulocyte count is decreased, as are the platelets and white blood cells.

Peripheral blood smear is routinely done for persons with pernicious anemia and reveals red cells, bizarre in shape and abnormally large. Bone marrow aspiration is done and shows signs of hyperplasia (crowding with cells). The increased cell production is a compensatory attempt by the body to keep up with the increased destruction of the faulty red cells.

A diagnostic test used specifically when pernicious anemia is suspected is the Schilling test. The person is given 2 μg of radioactive vitamin B_{12} by mouth, followed 2 hours later by the parenteral administration of 100 μg of unlabeled (nonradioactive) vitamin B_{12}. If the individual is able to absorb vitamin B_{12}, radioactivity will appear in the urine within 48 hours after ingestion. Persons with pernicious anemia excrete less than 5% of the dosage given. Further testing is done with the individual being given simultaneous doses of intrinsic factor and radioactive vitamin B_{12}. Persons with pernicious anemia show an increased excretion of vitamin B_{12}, reflecting the increased ability to absorb vitamin B_{12} when intrinsic factor is supplied.

Intervention. There is no cure for pernicious anemia, since at the present time there is no way to help the stomach lining regain its capacity to produce intrinsic factor. Fortunately, however, the anemia can be corrected by supplying cyanocobalamin (vitamin B_{12}), which is given only by the parenteral route. The preparation of vitamin B_{12} is extremely potent, and daily intramuscular injections of as little as 1 μg will cause production of normal blood cells. An initial dose of 50 to 100 μg is given and is repeated every day for 7 to 10 days. Dosage is then usually reduced to 15 to 30 μg once or twice a week, and after a few weeks the individual can often be maintained on a dosage of 50 to 100 μg at monthly intervals. Sometimes adequate treatment is maintained with injections given as infrequently as every 6 months.

Nursing care for the person with pernicious anemia depends on the symptoms present at the time of treatment. Irritability, impatience, and apprehension should be expected and should be dealt with by showing the individual particular attention and by giving medications and other treatments on time and with as little confusion as possible. The person may need extra warmth, special mouth care, and a carefully selected diet until severe symptoms subside, usually within 1 to 2 weeks after initiation of treatment. Neurologic symptoms may be more persistent and may be irreversible despite intensive treatment with vitamin B_{12} and physical therapy. The person may be discouraged when the neurologic symptoms do not disappear quickly. In the presence of permanent neurologic deficit, patience and persistence are tremendous assets in learning to meet the demands of the illness and to continue in the activities of daily living. The person may be reassured that although some neurologic damage may not be completely reversible, there will be no serious increase in symptoms provided treatment is continued.

The most common cause of relapse in persons with pernicious anemia is their reluctance to continue therapy for life. Patient teaching is a focus of nursing care and discharge planning. The individual must be assisted to understand the nature of the illness and the absolute necessity of continued treatment for life.

The prospect of needing intramuscular injections at monthly intervals for the rest of one's life is not a happy one. The person may need to be encouraged that, although injections must certainly be continued, they may be needed less often when symptoms subside. If medication must be given frequently, the physician may wish the person or a family member to learn to give the injections. Most persons receiving vitamin B_{12}, however, return to the physician's office or clinic for injections or may make arrangements through the physician to have the community health nurse give them. Community health nurse visits to the home are also a means of the providing ongoing assessment and the much needed encouragement to continue therapy.

Folic-acid-deficiency anemia

Persons who have a deficiency in folic acid develop macrocytic anemia associated with megaloblastic arrest in red blood cell production. The body can store only small amounts of folic acid, and without adequate dietary intake this supply will be depleted within 3 to 4 months. The symptoms of folic-acid-deficiency anemia are similar to those of pernicious anemia. However, persons with folic-acid-deficiency anemia will not respond adequately to treatment with vitamin B_{12}.

Folic-acid deficiency accompanies malnutrition such as occurs in the chronically malnourished, in alcoholic cirrhosis, in the last trimester of pregnancy when metabolic needs are increased, in intestinal tract malabsorption, and in infants who are fed exclusively a milk diet. Most persons respond promptly to oral doses of 0.1 to 0.2 mg of folic acid daily for 1 to 2 weeks along with a well-balanced diet. Women in whom anemia developed during pregnancy should be treated for several months after delivery. Most persons can remain well as long as they are on a normal diet adequate in meats and vegetables. Foods high in B complex vitamins are also good sources of folic acid.

Discharge planning and follow-up care is aimed at assisting the person to understand the components of a well-balanced diet and determining with the person how such diet is to be provided within his or her economic and cultural environment. Return visits to nurse clinics and community health nurse home visits are frequently

HEMOLYTIC DISORDERS

Congenital hemolytic anemias
- Hereditary spherocytosis
- Glucose-6-phosphate dehydrogenase (G6PD) deficiency
- Sickle cell anemia
- Thalassemia

Acquired hemolytic anemias
- Transfusion of incompatible blood
- Thrombotic thrombocytopenia purpura (TTP)
- Disseminated intravascular clotting (DIC)
- Spur cell anemia in liver disease

Modified from Wintrobe, M., et al.: Clinical hematology, ed. 8, Philadelphia, 1977, Lea & Febiger.

needed to assist the person in incorporating a well-balanced diet into a daily life.

☐ Anemia secondary to increased erythrocyte destruction

Hemolytic anemia is not a single disease entity but rather a category of diseases in which there is an increase in the rate of erythrocyte destruction. Though the causes of hemolysis in the hemolytic anemias vary, the clinical manifestations demonstrated are quite similar. The anemia results because the red cells are destroyed at such a rapid rate that the bone marrow is unable to compensate for the loss. The severity of the anemia manifested is determined by the degree of lag between the rate of erythrocyte destruction (hemolysis) and the rate of bone marrow production of new red blood cells (erythropoiesis).

Diagnosis of a hemolytic anemia is made when there is laboratory evidence of an increased rate of erythrocyte destruction and a corresponding compensatory effort of the bone marrow to increase the rate of erythropoiesis.

The hemolytic anemias can be divided into two main categories: congenital hemolytic anemia and acquired hemolytic anemia. Some of the specific diseases contained within each category are listed in the box above.

Congenital hemolytic anemia

Though present at birth, many congenital hemolytic anemias go undiagnosed until the affected individual is well into adulthood because many of these persons are asymptomatic or have only subclinical symptoms. Usually the anemia is mild because the shortened life span of the erythrocyte is at least partially compensated for by increased erythropoiesis by bone marrow. The individual rarely notices symptoms associated with anemia, such as fatigue or dyspnea, because the cardiovascular system has also had ample time to adjust.

Clinical manifestations that may be present on physical examination include jaundice, scleral icterus, splenomegaly, and symptoms of cholelithiasis. Questions during the history taking may reveal episodes of jaundice associated with infection. When present the jaundice is a direct result of the increased bilirubin from hemolysis. It is interesting that the bilirubin is not excreted in excess by the urine and that the usual pruritus associated with jaundice is not present with the jaundice secondary to hemolytic disease. The occurrence of cholelithiasis is associated with the excessive bilirubin load presented to the gallbladder.[44] Splenomegaly results because it is predominantly the spleen that removes defective and abnormal erythrocytes from the circulation.

The *crisis* associated with congenital hemolytic anemia is a sudden episode of increased hemolysis. Symptoms manifested by individuals during such an episode are acute anemia, jaundice, and icterus. The immediate cause of a crisis episode is unclear, although such episodes are frequently precipitated by an infection, particularly of the upper respiratory tract.[45] Folate deficiency may also precipitate an episode of hemolysis. In addition to reduced numbers of circulating erythrocytes, concomitant leukopenia (decreased WBC) and thrombocytopenia (decreased platelets) are common during a crisis phase of chronic hemolytic anemia.

Acquired hemolytic anemia

Acquired hemolytic anemia may be caused by burns, snake venom, certain heavy metals, a number of different drugs (i.e., sulfonamides, para-aminosalicylate, phenol derivatives, phenacetin), and antibodies directed against the red blood cells. The use of incompatible blood for transfusions causes severe hemolysis of the red blood cells. Hemolysis can be associated with infections with *Plasmodium* (malaria), *Clostridium, Toxoplasma, Bartonella* (Oroya fever), the organism of primary atypical pneumonia, and *Streptococcus*. Hemolytic anemia may also be caused by pathologic processes involving the spleen, causing it to destroy red blood cells excessively. Acquired hemolytic anemia may have either an insidious onset or present as an acute life-threatening event.

When the hemolytic process has been gradual in onset (weeks to months) the affected individual has had time to adjust and, like the person with congenital hemolytic anemia, experiences few symptoms. Findings that may be present on physical examination are pallor, scleral icterus, and slight jaundice.

An acute episode of hemolytic anemia, with rapid destruction of red blood cells, usually causes chills and fever, headache, irritability, precordial spasm, and pain.

There may be abdominal pain and nausea, vomiting, diarrhea, blood in the urine, and marked jaundice. Urinary output may be diminished. Shock and prostration may occur.

Intervention. Aggressive treatment is indicated both for the person with congenital hemolytic anemia who is in crisis and the individual with an acute episode of acquired hemolytic anemia. Treatment is directed toward eliminating the cause of the anemia while maintaining renal function and fluid and electrolyte balance.

When blood cell destruction is rapid, blood is given as supportive therapy. Presence of antibodies makes matching of blood difficult, and blood transfusions must be used with caution in persons with hemolytic anemia. Even with careful matching of the blood, destruction of the transfused blood increases the burden on excretory organs and the person is prone to thromboses.[45] Transfusion may also accelerate hemolysis. Any time a person with hemolytic anemia is receiving a blood transfusion, careful monitoring is of the utmost importance. Should marked accelerated hemolysis occur, exchange transfusions may become necessary.

Splenectomy as a form of treatment for hemolytic anemia is controversial among physicians. The rationale for a splenectomy is that the spleen is a major site of red cell destruction in hemolytic disorders. Removal of the spleen may therefore bring about improvement in hemolytic disease. The spleen removes mildly damaged red cells from circulation, while the more severely damaged red cells are destroyed by other parts of the reticuloendothelial system, particularly by the liver. Therefore persons with diseases associated with mild red cell defects are most likely to have a positive response following splenectomy.[45] Corticosteroids are of significant benefit to many persons in whom hemolytic anemia has an autoimmune basis. Folic-acid therapy (0.15 to 0.3 mg/day) is sometimes used in the treatment of the chronic hemolytic disorders to prevent crisis episodes.

Nursing care of persons with hemolytic disorders is planned in response to the individual's symptoms. Principles of nursing care of persons in shock (p. 274) and those receiving transfusions (p. 1543) apply to the person with hemolytic anemia.

In addition persons with chronic forms of hemolytic disorders need assistance in understanding the nature of the disease and in identifying those factors that predispose to episodes of hemolytic crisis.

Sickle cell anemia

Etiology. Sickle cell anemia is one of the inherited types of hemolytic anemias. It has its highest incidence in the United States among blacks, Puerto Ricans, and persons of Spanish, French, Italian, Greek, Turkish, North African, Middle Eastern, and Indian origin. The disease is attributed to a chemical defect within the hemoglobin of red blood cells. The characteristic sickle shape of red blood cells is due to a mutant gene that is responsible for the synthesis of hemoglobin that is different from normal hemoglobin.

Pathophysiology. The basic abnormality lies within the globin (protein) fraction of the hemoglobin, where a single amino acid is substituted for another in one of the polypeptide chains. This single amino acid substitution profoundly alters the properties of the hemoglobin molecule, changing its electric charge and making it less soluble and more prone to precipitate. Crystallization within the red blood cells distorts their shape, and they take on the characteristic appearance of sickles. As a consequence of the intermolecular rearrangement, hemoglobin S is formed instead of normal hemoglobin (A). The tendency toward sickling is dependent on both the relative quantity of hemoglobin S in the red blood cells and the levels of oxygen tension within the tissues of the body.

The sickling phenomenon is seen in persons with sickle trait (SA), homozygous sickle cell disease (SS), sickle cell–hemoglobin C disease, and sickle cell thalassemia.

Sickle cell trait is present in those who are heterozygous for sickling and represents a combination of sickle hemoglobin (SA) and normal hemoglobin (AA). The red cells of such persons contain from 20% to 40% hemoglobin S but are not misshapen under normal conditions. The sickle cell trait produces no clinical disorder and is compatible with a normal life span. The person may, however, suffer sickling if exposed to conditions causing hypoxia such as flying at high altitudes in nonpressurized airplanes, respiratory depression of deep anesthesia, or severe respiratory disease with extreme oxygen unsaturation. It is reported that 8% to 12% of the black population has sickle cell trait.

Unfortunately the most common form of sickle cell disease is *homozygous sickle cell disease* (SS), which occurs in a ratio of 1:400 to 1:500 in the black population in the United States. Persons with this variant have inherited sickling genes from both parents and cannot form normal hemoglobin. The average age of onset of symptoms is 2 years. Sickling is present at all times, and minor reductions in blood oxygen levels induce sickling crises. These individuals have full-blown anemia, and their red blood cells contain 80% to 100% hemoglobin S. Few persons live beyond 40 years of age. Intercurrent infections, multiple pulmonary emboli, or thrombosis of a vessel to a vital organ may cause death.

Some persons inherit more than one genetic mutation and produce not only hemoglobin S but hemoglobin C, D, or one of the other abnormal hemoglobins. *Sickle cell–hemoglobin C disease* is second in occurrence among black Americans. It is caused by the presence of the gene for sickle hemoglobin and the gene for hemoglobin C. Although the symptoms and course of the disease are milder than in homozygous sickle cell disease (SS), it nonetheless can cause marked discomfort and occasionally painful crises.

Sickle cell thalassemia is a combination of sickle cell trait and beta-thalassemia trait. The defect in this variant is in the beta chain of the globin that produces defective hemoglobin. This disease is also known as Mediterranean anemia and occurs in most cases of sickle cell disease in nonblacks, particularly those persons of Greek or Italian ancestry. The clinical course and symptoms are less severe than in other forms of the disease, and crises are not as common.

Persons with sickling disorders may experience increased sickling during the stress of pregnancy or surgery or as a consequence of infection, dehydration, or trauma. Acidosis and conditions that lead to fluid and electrolyte imbalance such as vomiting, fever, or disturbed renal flow may promote sickling of the person's red blood cells. The distorted shape of the cells, the changes in red cell membrane, and the presence of cells that will not unsickle even when oxygenated lead to thickening of the blood and predispose to sludging in the microcirculation. These disturbances can cause impaired blood flow and produce ischemic obstruction and infarction of vital organs. Because sickled cells are fragile, they are less able to survive the mechanical trauma caused by circulating in the blood. When they are released into the free circulation, hemolysis occurs, and repeated episodes lead to severe anemia. The clinical manifestations then are due to anemia, thrombosis, and infarction.[17]

Sickle cell crisis. The sudden exacerbation of sickling can bring about a condition known as "crisis," which is serious and life threatening. Crises are divided into three types: painful or thrombotic, aplastic, and hemolytic.[17]

Painful crisis is the most common type and is due to occlusion of small arterioles and venules by the abnormally shaped cells. The pain is usually severe and may be confined to the abdomen, musculoskeletal system, brain, lung, or heart. The person will generally require pain medication including narcotics to obtain relief from pain. In the treatment of painful crises it is important that dehydration and acidosis be corrected, since they in themselves induce further sickling. Appropriate cultures and sensitivity studies are obtained and antibiotics administered when there is indication of infection. An attempt may be made to reverse sickling by the use of rapidly infused isotonic saline solution or with the phenothiazines, corticosteroids, or low-molecular-weight dextran. Limited exchange transfusion (replacing the person's blood with packed red cells, unit for unit, until the concentration of sickle cells is below 50% concentration of erythrocytes) may be used to reduce the number of circulating sickle cells. Urea and potassium cyanate have been used experimentally to impair the sickling process, but to date researchers remain cautious about the use of these two substances.[17]

Aplastic crisis occurs when the mechanism for erythroblast division or maturation is depressed, and a profound anemia results. Infection or drugs known to be toxic to hematopoiesis (for example, chloramphenicol) may be the cause. The diagnosis of aplastic sickle crisis is made after bone marrow analysis. Since the anemia may progress rapidly, transfusions using packed cells may be used daily in volumes sufficient to maintain vital signs and function until erythropoiesis resumes.

Hemolytic crisis involves a rapid decrease in hematocrit, and this too may be due to infection or drug-induced destruction of red blood cells. Symptoms are those due primarily to increasing anemia together with severe jaundice. It is treated with infusion of packed red cells.

Intervention. Since there is no cure for sickle cell disease, treatment is geared to alleviating symptoms and keeping the person comfortable. Nursing, care of the person in crisis involves managing the person's activity, monitoring vital signs and infusion, observing the individual's reaction to medication and transfusion, interpreting the plan of care to the person, his family, and appropriate nursing personnel, and coordinating laboratory and treatment regimens. The person or the family may need counseling to help them work through the many anxieties and fears associated with a chronic disease. The nurse needs to assess the person's response to the disease and provide appropriate emotional support and teaching.

Much more attention has been directed toward this disease in the past few years, and educational campaigns are being directed at helping those at high risk to seek genetic counseling.

Outcome criteria for the person with anemia

The person or significant others can:

1. Explain the basis for the anemia.
2. Describe dietary modifications:
   a. Describe components of a well-balanced diet.
   b. Plan menus based on inclusion of deficient substances (iron, vitamin B_{12}, B complex vitamins, folic acid).
3. State name, dosage, frequency, desired actions, and side effects of prescribed medications.
4. Demonstrate accurate technique for administration of intramuscular injections of vitamin B_{12}, if pertinent.

5. State plans for follow-up health care:
   a. State need for avoidance and early treatment of infections.
   b. State need for adequate hydration (sickle cell anemia).
   c. State need for avoidance of cold environment or constricting clothing (sickle cell anemia).
   d. Describe hereditary factors and plans to seek genetic counseling, if appropriate.
   e. Describe early signs of deficiency requiring medical attention.

■ DISORDERS ASSOCIATED WITH PLATELETS

Platelets are formed in the bone marrow. In the normal adult approximately 80% of the platelets are in free circulation and 20% are stored in the spleen. It is estimated that the normal life span of a platelet is 7 to 14 days. The senescent platelets are removed from circulation primarily by the spleen, although the liver may also assume this role. Platelet function is responsible for the formation of the platelet plug and the initiation of thrombin production.

Hematologic disorders associated with platelets may be the result of diminished numbers of platelets (thrombocytopenia), increased number of platelets (thrombocytosis), or an abnormality in platelet function.

□ Thrombocytopenia

Thrombocytopenia is defined as a lower than normal number of circulating platelets. Laboratory values for a normal adult platelet count range from 150,000/cu mm to 400,000/cu mm.[30] Thrombocytopenia may occur when there is deficient platelet production, accelerated platelet destruction, or an abnormal pooling of platelets within the body.

A *decreased production* of platelets is often secondary to exposure to toxic agents (drugs, chemicals, radiation). In such individuals complete recovery usually follows the removal of the causative agent. Bone marrow production of platelets (thrombopoiesis) may be interfered with by such processes as a leukemic or carcinomatous infiltration of the bone marrow.

Numbers of circulating platelets are rapidly diminished with the occurrence of *abnormal platelet destruction*. Examples of abnormal platelet destruction include the antibodies against the platelets that are associated with massive transfusions and drug therapy (quinidine, quinine, sulfonamides), which lead to increased platelet destruction and thrombocytopenia.

Abnormal pooling of platelets results in diminished numbers of circulating platelets. With disease, and particularly with splenomegaly, 80% of the platelets may be located in the spleen. Such an abnormal distribution of platelets caused by the increased platelet uptake (sequestration) by the spleen may result in marked thrombocytopenia.

Idiopathic thrombocytopenia purpura (ITP) is a syndrome in which thrombocytopenia occurs spontaneously and cannot be associated with etiologic factors or underlying disease. The cause of ITP is not well established, although indirect evidence shows ITP to be due to platelet destruction as the result of an immunologic process.[45]

The course of ITP may be acute or chronic. The acute form of the disease occurs most often in young children but is also seen in adults. An acute bleeding episode is the most common clinical manifestation of acute ITP. Chronic ITP occurs most often in women between 20 and 40 years of age. Onset is usually gradual, and long periods of remission (months to years) are common.[44]

Clinical picture. The major symptoms of thrombocytopenia observable through physical examination are those that reflect a bleeding tendency. Petechiae and ecchymoses are hallmarks of decreased platelets and are most commonly present on the arms, legs, and upper chest. The person may give a history of menorrhagia, epistaxis, and gingival bleeding. An individual with thrombocytopenia should be questioned for a history of recent viral infection, since this may produce a transient failure of platelet production. A detailed history of drug and alcohol use also should be obtained. Alcohol, thiazide diuretics, and estrogens may produce thrombocytopenia by a direct toxic effect on the marrow.[30]

Complete laboratory studies are done to ascertain the status of all blood components. The most commonly used tests for assessment of platelets are platelet count, peripheral blood smear, and bleeding time. In addition a bone marrow examination (aspiration or biopsy) is routinely performed to determine the presence or absence of megakaryocytes (precursors of platelets normally present in the bone marrow). Their presence suggests that the thrombocytopenia is due to peripheral platelet destruction, and their absence suggests a failure of thrombopoiesis. Examination of the bone marrow also reveals the presence or absence of primary bone marrow abnormalities such as neoplastic invasion, aplastic anemia, and fibrosis.

Intervention. A marked decrease in platelets renders the individual vulnerable to bleeding and requires prompt medical determination of the precipitating cause of the thrombocytopenia. A primary concern in the nursing care of persons with decreased numbers of platelets is the concomitant *bleeding tendency*. Bleeding associated with trauma is likely with a platelet count less than 100,000/cu mm. Spontaneous hemorrhage looms as a life-threatening possibility in individuals with a platelet count of less than 20,000/cu mm.

Ongoing nursing assessment of the patient is essential and includes alertness to increased ecchymoses, petechiae, and any change in mental status. The need for avoidance of trauma is obvious. For persons with a platelet count of 20,000/cu mm or less, bleeding precautions should be instituted. Routinely such precautions should include:

Guaiac test of all urine and stools
No rectal temperatures taken
No intramuscular injections given
All venipuncture sites held with pressure over the site for 5 minutes
All arterial puncture sites held for 10 minutes

Platelet transfusions in ITP and drug-induced thrombocytopenia are used in life-threatening situations (as supportive therapy during hemorrhage). However, the benefit is only transitory because the transfused platelets are destroyed by the same mechanism and as rapidly (often in only a few hours) as the person's own platelets.

If the individual is to be discharged to home with maintenance doses of immunosuppressive drugs, explicit patient education is needed. The individual must have knowledge of the importance of not omitting doses and the danger inherent in suddenly stopping the medication.

Prior to discharge from the hospital, individuals should be able to describe the signs of decreased platelets (bleeding gums, petechiae, ecchymoses) and the corresponding risk of a bleeding tendency. The person and significant others should be advised to continue under medical supervision and to report any signs of bleeding to the primary physician at once.

□ Thrombocytosis

Thrombocytosis is defined as the presence of an abnormally high number of platelets in the circulating blood.[45] Thrombocytosis rarely occurs as a single entity but is seen in association with polycythemia vera and myelofibrosis. A transitory increase in the numbers of circulating platelets may be seen as rebound effect following splenectomy and in association with infectious and inflammatory disease processes. In such instances treatment is aimed at the underlying disease process. Should the thrombocytosis be marked, the individual is at risk for thrombosis and hemorrhage. Medical and nursing care are similar to that described for anticoagulation (p. 1025).

Therapy is also aimed at lowering the platelet count. Certain chemotherapeutic agents may be used for this purpose. Intermittent drug therapy with the alkylating agents melphalan and busulfan is the regimen most commonly used. Nursing care is the same as that described for patients receiving chemotherapy (p. 481).

□ Disorders of platelet function

Disorders of platelet function have clinical manifestations and patient care needs similar to those of thrombocytopenia. Symptoms include petechiae, epistaxis, and prolonged bleeding time. Disorders in platelet function may follow infection and a variety of systemic diseases. In addition there are many congenital platelet disorders. Most of the congenital defects involve platelet aggregation.

Acquired disorders of platelet function include injury due to drugs, the most common being aspirin and phenylbutazone. Aspirin inhibits the release of intrinsic platelet ADP and produces a defect in platelet aggregation. The defect remains for the life span of the platelet. This alteration in platelet function is the reason why the ingestion of a therapeutic dose of aspirin by a healthy person may prolong the bleeding time for 2 or 3 days.

□ Disorders of coagulation

The clotting mechanism is a complex system involving numerous extrinsic and intrinsic factors (Fig. 48-3). Disorders of coagulation may result from interferences in one or more components of the clotting system.

Disorders of coagulation may be congenital or acquired. The *acquired* disorders of coagulation are much more common and include liver disease, decreased vitamin K, and systemic disease such as nephrotic syndrome. The most notable of the acquired disorders of coagulation is disseminated intravascular coagulation (DIC). Of the *congenital* disorders of coagulation, the most common are hemophilia A, a deficiency of factor VIII, and hemophilia B, a deficiency of factor IX.

Disseminated intravascular coagulation

Disseminated intravascular coagulation (DIC) is a recently recognized pathophysiologic response of the body's hemostatic mechanisms to disease or injury. DIC is a complicated and potentially fatal process that is characterized initially by clotting and secondarily by hemorrhage. It always occurs in response to a primary disease.

Etiology. DIC is essentially an imbalance between the processes of coagulation and anticoagulation. Many diseases states may alter the normal balance of clotting factors and fibrinolytic factors, which under normal conditions prevent bleeding while maintaining the fluidity of the blood. DIC may be initiated by diseases that involve the introduction of a foreign substance into the bloodstream such as endotoxins, snake venom, or placental matter from abruptio placentae. This syndrome may also be triggered by conditions associated with thrombus formation such as hypotensive states. The third group of diseases that may lead to DIC are those in

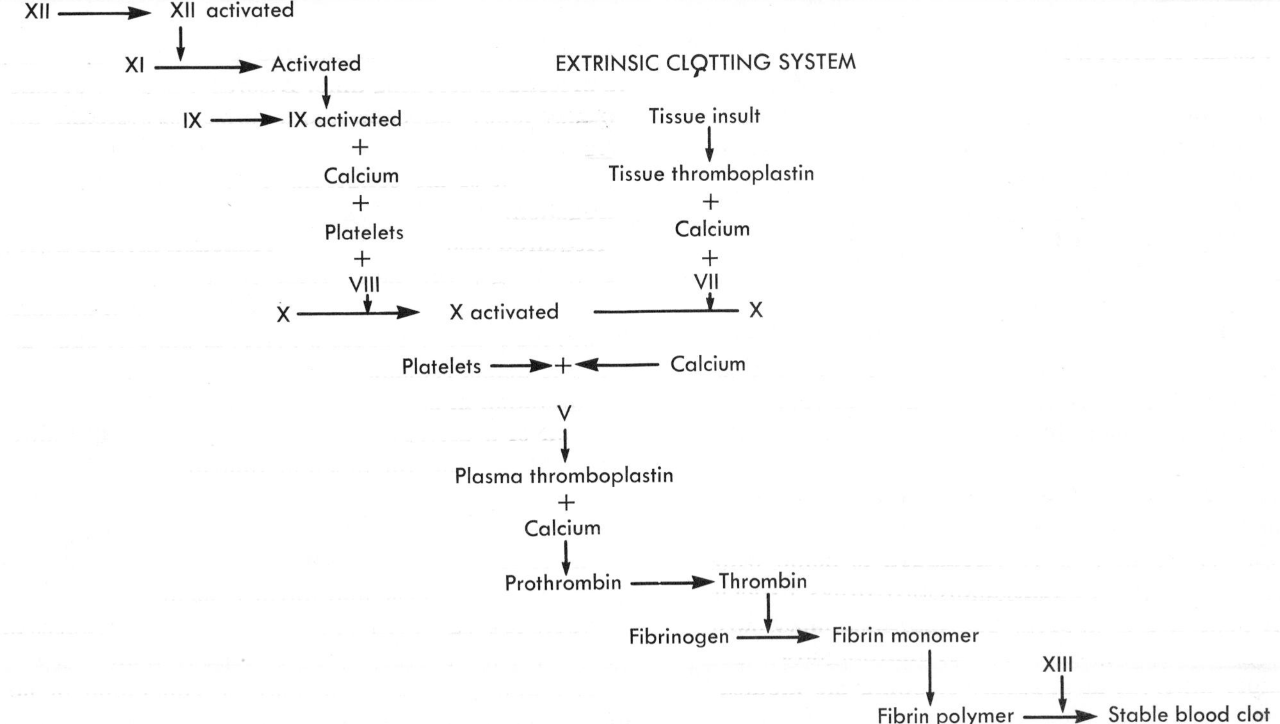

Fig. 48-3. Mechanism of clot formation illustrating relationship of intrinsic and extrinsic clotting factors.

which there is massive tissue damage such as blunt trauma or neoplasms.

Pathophysiology. The primary disease causes the initiation of the clotting process. This response is generalized and occurs throughout the vascular system, creating a state of *hypercoagulability*. The fibrinolytic processes, which normally operate to limit clot extension and dissolve clots, are then stimulated. As clotting factors are depleted and fibrinolysis continues, a state of *hypocoagulability* develops.

The first phase of DIC, then, is characterized by the appearance of free thrombin in the blood, fibrin deposition, and the aggregation of platelets. Microthrombi are formed, which obstruct circulation to various organs, and the fibrin deposits cause red cell damage. Ischemic renal failure, respiratory failure, and adrenal insufficiency are common sequelae. Often the first sign of DIC is the widespread appearance of purpura over the chest and abdomen, the result of numerous fibrin deposits in the capillary bed.

The second phase of DIC is one of hemorrhage. This paradox is caused by the depletion of clotting factors II, V, VIII, IX, X, and XII and platelets in the first phase and by the production of fibrin degradation products (FDP) through fibrinolysis. The thrombin that initially accelerated coagulation also converts plasminogen into plasmin, which then breaks fibrin and fibrinogen into fibrin degradation products. The fibrin degradation products act as anticoagulants, and bleeding from many sites ensues.

Clinical picture. Laboratory determinations that confirm the diagnosis of DIC are the presence of thrombocytopenia, low levels of fibrinogen, and prolonged prothrombin and partial thromboplastin times. In addition low levels of factors VII and V are present, and abnormal red blood cells are found on peripheral smear.

Intervention. The management of DIC must always begin with treatment of the primary disease. Once this has been initiated, the goal is to control the bleeding and restore normal levels of clotting factors. Heparin may be administered to inhibit the formation of thrombin and allow fibrinogen and platelet levels to increase; blood products such as platelet packs, cryoprecipitate, and fresh whole blood may be given to replace the depleted factors. Heparin, however, may increase bleeding while preventing clotting and therefore is not always used with surgical patients. The third aspect of management involves treatment of the sequelae such as hemodialysis for renal failure.

Nursing intervention in the care of the patient with DIC is extremely challenging. The person who develops DIC is critically ill and frequently has numerous sites of bleeding before DIC becomes evident. Identification of the early signs may be made first by the observant nurse. The amount and nature of drainage from chest and nasogastric tubes, oozing from surgical incisions, or progressive discoloration of the skin should be noted and recorded.

Continual observation for new bleeding sites and for an increase or decrease in bleeding is an integral part of the nursing plan, especially if heparin therapy is being employed. The susceptibility of these persons to bleeding presents special problems; medications should be given intravenously if at all possible and small-gauge needles used when other injections are necessary. Toothbrushes must be used with caution, and soft swabs are often more effective for mouth care. If scabs have formed over small bleeding sites they should not be removed as this will only initiate fresh bleeding. When bleeding occurs, pressure should be applied to both arterial and venous puncture sites for a minimum of 15 minutes.

Maintaining fluid balance is another aspect of nursing care that assumes great importance. Persons with DIC usually lose large quantities of blood and receive frequent transfusions and other fluid replacement. In addition to carefully monitoring blood infusion rates, the nurse must be alert to signs of fluid overload such as increasing pulse rate and central venous pressure. Hourly urine output should be recorded not only as another indication of cardiac function but also because of the possibility of renal thrombi formation and subsequent renal failure.

Emotional support of the person with DIC and his family is essential. Bleeding into joints may cause a great deal of pain, and the frequent venous and arterial punctures necessary for laboratory tests also may cause much distress. Frequently the patient is comatose, and the presence of purpura, numerous intravenous lines, and drainage tubes makes his appearance especially upsetting to the family. Most of the primary conditions associated with DIC are of a sudden nature, and the family requires help in understanding this catastrophic occurrence and support during the long period of treatment.

Hemophilia

Hemophilia is a hereditary coagulation disorder. Both hemophilia A (factor VIII deficiency) and hemophilia B (factor IX deficiency) are inherited as sex-linked recessive disorders and are therefore almost exclusively limited to males. An example of the inheritance pattern of hemophilia is shown in Fig. 48-4.

Clinical picture. The diagnosis of hemophilia may be made in infancy or early childhood. The clinical history is one of lifelong bleeding tendency. A history of excessive bleeding following circumcision or dental extractions is frequently obtained. Individuals with hemophilia may give a history of bleeding into any part of the body, spontaneously or following trauma.

A diagnosis of hemophilia is made by specific assays for factors VIII and IX. The partial thromboplastin time, which reflects the intrinsic pathway of coagulation, is prolonged in both hemophilia A and B. The platelet count and prothrombin time are normal.

Complications associated with hemophilia are the direct result of the bleeding tendency. Frequently the individual experiences repeated episodes of spontaneous bleeding into the joints resulting in several joint deformities. Bleeding that is life threatening involves retroperitoneal, intracranial, and paratracheal soft-tissue hemorrhages.

Intervention. Treatment consists of replacement of the deficient coagulation factor when bleeding episodes do not respond to local treatment (ice bags, manual pressure or dressings, immobilization, elevation, and topical coagulants such as fibrin foam and thrombin). Because the deficient factors are contained in plasma, the treatment used for many years was fresh plasma and blood or fresh frozen plasma. In major hemorrhages, adequate blood levels were difficult to maintain without overloading the person's circulation with large volumes of blood and plasma. The discovery of cryoprecipitate in 1964 led the way to the development of commercially prepared concentrated preparations such as fibrinogen, factor VIII, and a concentrate containing the four vitamin K–dependent factors (prothrombin and factors VII, IX, and X). Concentrates avoid the problem of circulatory overload and produce fewer adverse effects in some patients (urticarial or febrile reactions). High cost and contamination with the virus of serum hepatitis are drawbacks, however, to the use of concentrates.

In classic hemophilia the treatment of choice for an acute bleeding episode is infusion of cryoprecipitated antihemophilic factor (factor VIII). This concentrate is made by slowly thawing previously frozen plasma at refrigerator temperature. Most of the factor VIII remains as a gel and can be separated from the rest of the plasma by centrifugation. The gel is reconstituted by the addition of saline solution. After the antihemophilic factor is extracted, the remaining plasma may be used for other purposes. This process results in a concentration of factor VIII as much as 15 to 40 times that of normal plasma. It can be produced and stored in any well-equipped blood bank at a cost well below that of other concen-

Defective gene is found on X chromosome.
When faulty X chromosome is present in a male,
the male will be a hemophiliac.

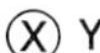

When faulty X chromosome is present in a female,
she will be a carrier of hemophilia.

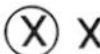

In conception between a normal male and a carrier
female, four possibilities arise:

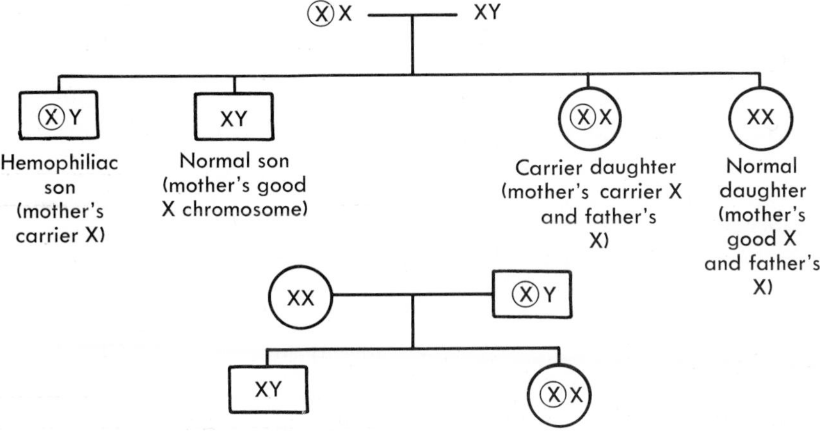

In conception between a hemophiliac male and a normal female,
son will be normal but daughter will be carrier.

Fig. 48-4. Pattern of inheritance of hemophilia.

trates. Treatment with cryoprecipitate is being given in outpatient departments and clinics. Home infusion programs have gained interest and are seen as a way of more quickly controlling bleeding episodes, thereby decreasing the need for hospitalization and long absence from school or work.

Giving an injection requires that particular care be taken to use a small needle, to apply pressure at the site of injection, and to inspect it for bleeding frequency for some time thereafter. The person should have a diet high in iron. One of nature's compensations for this condition is a remarkable capacity to regenerate red blood cells when bleeding has caused their loss. The person who has hemophilia should carry a card on his person that includes his name, blood type, physician's name, and the fact that he has hemophilia so that medical treatment will not be delayed if he should accidentally sustain injury and lose consciousness.

It is estimated that the average person with hemophilia has between 10 and 18 bleeding episodes a year and will require 13 to 24 bags of frozen factor VIII (cryoprecipitate) to stop each episode. The cost of treatment is estimated at $4,000 to $5,000 a year. Such medical costs place a tremendous burden on an individual and family members.

The National Hemophilia Foundation* is an organization established for persons with hemophilia and their families. There are 51 chapters scattered across the United States. The basic function of the national organization is hemophilia research. In addition it establishes standards for chapters, publishes literature, produces films, and promotes health care legislation in Washington. Local chapter services include special camps for children with hemophilia; parent, child, and adult counseling; group therapy sessions for parents; and a newsletter that reports on advances in hemophilic care. A chapter may function as a liaison agent between hospitals and families with insurmountable bills for blood.

The outlook for the person with hemophilia has been greatly improved by the availability of transfusion therapy. In the past many persons with factor VIII deficiency died in infancy or in the first 5 years of life.

*25 West 39th St., New York 10018.

Today persons with moderate or mild hemophilia may live normal, productive lives.

Adults with hemophilia are generally very knowledgeable about their disease. They must be aware of the possibility of hemorrhage after dental extraction, injury, or surgery. Pain control and the threat of spontaneous bleeding episodes are ongoing stresses the individual must confront. Those individuals who are able to meet the demands of their illness and adapt their life styles accordingly are able to live productive lives as individuals, spouses, parents, and employees. Genetic counseling, aimed at explaining the pattern of inheritance of hemophilia, may be of great value to adults contemplating parenthood. Such counseling can serve to assist potential parents to evaluate realistically their ability to raise a child afflicted with hemophilia and to anticipate ways to meet the demands placed on both them and the child.

Outcome criteria for the person with a platelet disorder

The person or significant others can:

1. Explain the medication program:
   a. State name, dosage, frequency, action, and side effects of prescribed medication.
   b. State awareness of not stopping immunosuppressive medications suddenly.
   c. State need for avoidance of aspirin.
2. State need for genetic counseling, if appropriate (hemophilia).
3. Explain plans for health care follow-up:
   a. Describe signs and symptoms requiring *immediate* medical intervention (excessive bleeding, hematuria, melena, pain or swelling in joint or muscle, head trauma, abdominal pain, swelling in neck).
   b. Describe signs of decreased platelets (bleeding gums, petechiae, ecchymosis).
   c. State plans for continued medical follow-up.
   d. State plans to obtain Medic-Alert identification if he does not already possess this.

■ DISORDERS ASSOCIATED WITH WHITE BLOOD CELLS

□ Types of white blood cells

The white blood cell (WBC) system is comprised of granulocytes (neutrophils, eosinophils, basophils), agranulocytes (lymphocytes, monocytes), and plasma cells. The primary function of the WBC is to provide for humoral and cellular response to infection and foreign materials. Blood disorders affecting any of the white blood cells render the individual highly susceptible to infection and decreased host response to foreign matter.

Granulocytes

The process of granulocytopoiesis (WBC production) consists of cellular proliferation and maturation within the bone marrow. The life span of the granulocyte is short, estimated at ½ to 6 hours.[30] The major function of the granulocytes is phagocytosis.

Agranulocytes

Lymphocytes originate in the bone marrow. Two lymphocyte populations have been differentiated: (1) those that originate in the bone marrow (B cells) and are not exposed to the thymus gland and (2) those that leave the bone marrow and migrate to and are exposed to the thymus gland (T cells) (p. 184). Both B and T cells circulate through the blood, lymph nodes, spleen, and other tissue. It is estimated that the lymphocyte life span ranges from several months to years.[30] The major function of the lymphocyte is the immunologic response.

Monocytes

Monocytes are produced in the bone marrow. Final differentiation may not occur until after the cells are released into the circulation. The monocytes complete their differentiation at specific tissue sites, acquiring characteristics specific to a particular site. The functions of the monocytes are phagocytosis and bactericidal action. The estimated life span of the monocyte is 12 to 24 hours.

□ Pathophysiology

Neutrophilia

Neutrophilia is defined as a neutrophil count greater than 10,000/cu mm.[44] Such an increase is a normal healthy response to infections, primarily bacterial infections. Prolonged elevation of the neutrophil count, especially in the absence of an apparent cause, is reason for a diligent search for the underlying pathology. Persistent elevated neutrophil counts are associated with leukemia, polycythemia vera, myeloid metaplasia, and a variety of systemic and inflammatory disorders. Each WBC may become elevated as a response to a disease process. Lymphocytosis, monocytosis, and eosinophilia simply describe an increase in the numbers of specific circulating cells.

Neutropenia

Neutropenia is defined as a neutrophil count of less than 2,000/cu mm.[44] Neutropenia may occur as a primary hematologic disorder. Most often it is seen in association with other disorders (malignancies, agranulocytosis, infectious mononucleosis, and the nutritional deficiencies). Each WBC may be abnormally reduced. Lymphocytopenia and monocytopenia simply describe a decrease in the specific cell unit. Individuals with neutropenia are at risk of contracting a life-threatening infection. The degree of increased susceptibility to infection is in direct proportion to the degree of neutropenia.

Agranulocytosis

Agranulocytosis is a disease in which production of white blood cells is depressed and the total number of white blood cells may be reduced to between 200 and 500/cu mm. Severe neutropenia occurs as a reaction to a variety of drugs and chemicals. Sulfonamides, coal-tar analgesics, tripelennamine (Pyribenzamine), thiouracil, chloramphenicol, and heavy metals such as gold are examples. The nurse has an important role in the prevention of this disease. In the community the nurse has frequent opportunity to advise against use of medications not therapeutically prescribed. In the hospital as well as in the home the nurse must constantly be aware of the possible toxic effects of various drugs. Many times nursing care can reduce the period of necessary treatment with drugs. Also nurses must be constantly alert for toxic signs of the drugs they administer. On the community level, nursing input in governmental and environmental programs is valuable in influencing local antipollution laws in addition to providing consumer education.

Treatment consists of removing the offending agent. Sometimes the cause is difficult to determine, and a careful history is essential. With such a low white blood cell count, precautions must be taken to control infections. The first signs of the disease may be the onset of an acute infection with chills, fever, sore throat, and prostration. There may be enlargement of cervical lymph nodes. Infection may occur anywhere in the body. The mortality in agranulocytosis is high, although antibiotics have been found extremely helpful in controlling the infection until the cause can be found and corrected.

Nursing care of persons with WBC disorders. An individual with a compromised white blood cell system is highly susceptible to life-threatening infections. Nursing care is directed toward protecting the patient from potential sources of infection and assiduous monitoring to detect the earliest signs of infection so that prompt therapy may be instituted. Meticulous washing of the hands by medical and nursing personnel and strict asepsis are mandatory. The environment should be kept scrupulously clean and dustless, and no person with any type of infection should be allowed in contact with the patient. Family members and hospital personnel need frequent reminders of this. Slight colds and respiratory tract infections, taken for granted in daily life, are serious threats to patients with decreased WBCs.

Patients should be in private rooms. When this is not possible, cautious screening of other patients for a potential source of infection is mandatory. Occasionally isolation technique (reverse precautions) is ordered to protect the patient from hospital personnel and visitors (p. 337).

Since steroids and antibiotics may mask fever as a symptom of infection, the nurse needs to be particularly alert for any sign of infection such as local redness, cough, increased malaise, or anorexia. Any slight change or seemingly unimportant symptom should be called to the physician's attention.

□ Leukemias

Approximately 21,000 new cases of leukemia are diagnosed and 15,000 deaths related to the disease are reported each year in the United States. Leukemia occurs in all age groups. There is a peak incidence among children between 3 and 4 years of age. The incidence of leukemia then declines until 35 years of age, at which point there is a steady increase with each sucessive year of life.

The cause of leukemia remains unclear. It is known that leukemia can occur as a result of exposure to ionizing radiation and to some chemicals that are toxic to the bone marrow.

Leukemia is a disease of the blood-forming tissue (bone marrow, spleen, and lymph nodes). The disease is characterized by an abnormal and uncontrolled proliferation of immature and mature forms of the white blood cells (granulocytes, lymphocytes, monocytes). The leukemias are classified according to the prominent cell type (lymphocytic, myelocytic or granulocytic, and monocytic). The disease is further defined as acute or chronic. Historically the terms reflected the expected duration of the illness and life. With the advent of chemotherapy the terms "acute" and "chronic" are now used to describe the maturity of the cells involved. *Acute* leukemia refers to the disease with a preponderance of immature and poorly differentiated cells (blasts). *Chronic* leukemia refers to the proliferative process of more mature and well-differentiated WBC. A common classification of leukemias identifies four main types:

Acute lymphocytic leukemia (ALL)
Acute myelogenous leukemia (AML)
Chronic lymphocytic leukemia (CLL)
Chronic myelogenous leukemia (CML)

Acute lymphocytic leukemia (ALL)

ALL results from the proliferation of an abnormal leukocyte in the blood-forming tissue and the subsequent displacement of normal blood-forming elements. ALL is primarily a childhood illness; 80% of persons with ALL are children. Tremendous gains have been made in the treatment of this disease and ALL now carries the best prognosis among leukemias. Although the life span of a child with ALL is only 3 months without treatment, chemotherapy has brought an 80% to 90%

remission rate. Five years after diagnosis and initial treatment, 30% to 40% of persons are still in remission, and of those 10% are considered cured.

Acute myelogenous leukemia (AML)

AML occurs equally throughout all decades of life. The disease affects both sexes equally. There is, however, a slight increased incidence in men over the age of 40 years.

The defect in AML is twofold: the inability of the WBC to mature, and defective or abnormal growth of the WBC that do mature. As a result of this defect there is an increase in the total leukocyte count with a predominance of immature cells (blasts). If left untreated, AML will lead to death within 3 to 4 months. With aggressive chemotherapy the mean survival span is 2 years. Chemotherapeutic agents used in the treatment of AML include daunomycin, prednisone, vincristine, and cytosine arabinoside (p. 476). Intensive supportive therapy is often necessary to maintain an individual during the prescribed chemotherapy regimen.

Chronic myelogenous leukemia (CML)

CML is uncommon before the age of 20 years and increases in frequency with each succeeding decade of life.

The prime defect in CML is an abnormal stem cell leading to an abnormal proliferation of the granulocytic cells. As a result of this proliferation there is a marked increase in the number of circulating granulocytes.

The median survival time for an individual diagnosed as having CML is 3.5 years. Chemotherapy has not increased the life span for persons with CML but has influenced the quality of life. With treatment the person has prolonged periods of being asymptomatic and is able to enjoy and participate fully in the activities of daily living.

Chronic lymphocytic leukemia (CLL)

CLL occurs most commonly after 35 years of age, with an increased incidence with each successive decade of life. The prime hematologic defect associated with CLL is an increased proliferation of lymphoid cells within the bone marrow, liver, spleen, and lymph nodes. There is a marked increase in the number of both leukocytes and mature lymphocytes. At the time of diagnosis the bone marrow is often filled by lymphocytic infiltration.

The median survival time of persons with CLL without treatment is 4.5 to 5.5 years. As a general rule persons are treated only when symptoms appear, particularly anemia, thrombocytopenia, or enlarged lymph nodes and spleen. Chemotherapeutic agents used in the treatment of CLL are most often one of the alkylating agents such as chlorambucil and glucocorticoids (p. 476).

Clinical picture

The leukemic process of uncontrolled growth of one cell type causes a crowding out of other normal blood cell components. Because of the impaired production of all cell types, anemia and thrombocytopenia occur and are often the initial symptoms of a leukemia. Abnormalities are reflected in laboratory data. In addition to the marked elevation in the white blood cells, marked anemia and decreased platelets, an abnormal alkaline phosphatase level, an elevated BUN, and decreased clotting factors may also be present. The actual diagnosis of leukemia can only be made through detailed morphologic study of the bone marrow samples obtained through bone marrow aspiration and biopsy.

Symptoms of persons with leukemia vary greatly. In general, assessment includes an astute alertness to symptoms associated with anemia, neutropenia, and thrombocytopenia. In addition arthralgia and bone pain may occur as a result of the expansion of the bone marrow due to rapidly proliferating cells.

Nursing care of persons with leukemia

Leukemia, by its nature, is a diverse illness. The varied courses and response or lack of response to treatment also add to the diversity.

In acute phases of the disease and during aggressive chemotherapy, nursing care is aimed toward the prevention of complications and supportive therapy. Decreased WBC and decreased platelet counts render the individual vulnerable to severe infections and bleeding episodes. Frequent transfusions of both whole blood and component therapy (platelets, WBC) are often necessary.

There are many foci of nursing care beyond those found in the life-threatening situations. Each individual with leukemia responds in a different way. It cannot be predicted for certain if an individual will respond to a prescribed treatment or how long a remission will last. Likewise, how the individual incorporates the illness into life is also unique to each person. Nursing has a key role in patient education. Prior to discharge from the hospital, the person should possess basic knowledge of the disease process and the importance of continued medical follow-up. Knowledge of specific drug therapy and anticipated side effects is also a component of the teaching plan. Of utmost importance in learning is the ability of the person to identify the body's signals that blood abnormalities exist. Petechiae, ecchymoses, and gingival bleeding are again the hallmarks to seek prompt medical attention. Bone pain, often severe, may signal blast crisis (acute proliferation of immature cells).

Individuals whose illness runs the course of several months to years often become very knowledgeable about blood components' related symptoms and specific chemotherapeutic drugs. These persons often discuss their progress in terms of changes in their blood counts. Over time many individuals become attuned to how such changes affect them. For example, they often can predict their platelet count by how they feel. Many such persons respond well to being included in their plan of care during hospitalization and in preparation for discharge.

Time set aside for patient teaching also allows for a sharing time with the individual. This time may provide the foundation for an honest nurse-patient relationship from which emotional support may be given the person as attempts are made to adapt to the many stresses associated with leukemia.

Outcome criteria for the person with leukemia

The person or significant others can:

1. Explain the nature of the disease process.
2. State name, dosage, frequency, action, and side effects of prescribed medication.
3. State plans for follow-up care:
   a. Describe symptoms requiring medical attention (petechiae, ecchymosis, gingival bleeding, bone pain).
   b. State plans for continued medical care.

■ DISORDERS ASSOCIATED WITH LYMPH SYSTEM

Lymph node

The normal lymph node consists of connective tissue encapsulating a fine mesh of reticular cells. The reticuloendothelial cells function chiefly in the phagocytosis of cellular debris. The chief function of lymphocytes, which are the main cells comprising the lymph nodes, is to provide an immune response to antigens presented to the node from the structure being drained by the node.

Lymphadenopathy

Lymph node enlargement results from an increase in the number and size of lymphoid follicles with proliferation of lymphocytes and reticuloendothelial cells. Lymphadenopathy may also occur when the node is invaded by cells normally not present (leukemic cells, cancer cells). In the lymphomas the actual nodal structure is destroyed by the malignant cells.[6]

Assessment of lymph nodes

Normally lymph nodes are not palpable. With disease and the consequent increase in size, the nodes become palpable. In the course of a routine physical examination the lymph nodes are examined by palpation.

Lymphangiography is a radiologic technique used for evaluation of lymph nodes to detect the presence of disease. This procedure is especially valuable in the assessment of those nodes that are anatomically too deep to allow for evaluation by palpation (mediastinal, paraaortic). For this procedure a small incision is made on the dorsal surface of each foot so that the small lymph glands are made accessible. The glands are then cannulated, and a dye is slowly instilled over a few hours. All lymph chains and nodes fill with dye and are then visible on radiographs. Radiographs are usually done immediately after the dye is absorbed and again at intervals of 24 and 48 hours after the procedure.

□ Lymphomas

Lymphoma is a classification of disorders arising from within the lymph system. The lymphomas are malignant in nature and comprise approximately 3% of all forms of cancer. There is a slightly higher incidence of the disease in men.[6] Over the past several decades the incidence of lymphoma has remained stable.[6] Approximately 21,900 new cases of lymphoma are diagnosed annually. Hodgkin's disease comprises approximately 50% of all lymphomas, and the highest incidence is in young adults between the second and fourth decades of life. The non-Hodgkin's lymphomas (reticulum cell sarcoma and lymphosarcoma) occur later in life. The cause of the lymphomas remains unknown.

Hodgkin's disease

Hodgkin's disease is a malignant disorder that produces painless enlargement of the lymph nodes. The first nodes to be involved are those in the cervical region. Less commonly axillary, inguinal, or mediastinal nodes are the first lymph nodes to show enlargement.

Clinical picture. A thorough diagnostic workup is indicated if Hodgkin's disease is suspected. Such an extensive workup is often arduous and difficult for the patient. Explanations of the many facets of the diagnostic procedures helps provide the emotional support so often needed during this time.

Systemic symptoms associated with Hodgkin's disease are a prolonged low-grade fever, night sweats, weight loss, generalized pruritus, and pain in the lymph nodes after the ingestion of alcohol. Physical examination may show enlargement of the peripheral lymph node chain, liver, and spleen. A chest x-ray may identify the presence of a mediastinal mass. Complete blood work is done including CBC, platelet count, alkaline phosphatase, and sedimentation rate. A decreased CBC and platelet count is usually indicative of bone marrow and splenic involvement. A bone marrow biopsy may be done. Tuberculin tests (PPD) may be done to assess the person's immune response. The liver and spleen are evaluated by scanning for the presence of a disease process. Bilateral lymphangiograms are done for evalua-

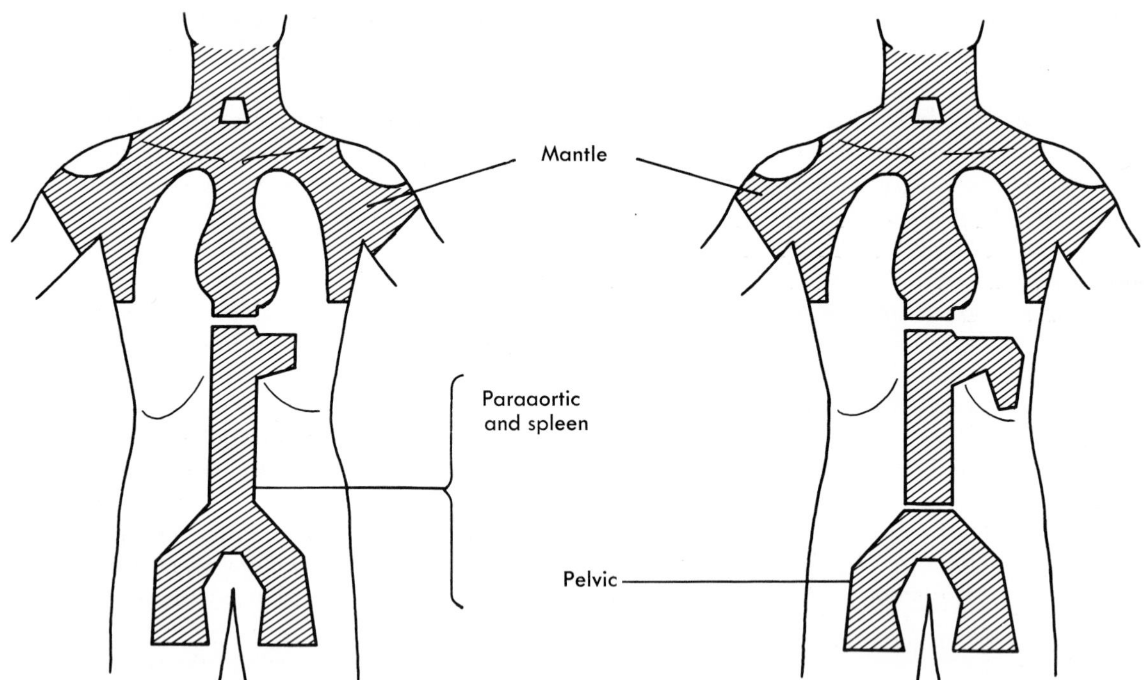

Fig. 48-5. Diagram of mantle and inverted Y fields used in total lymphoid radiotherapy of Hodgkin's disease. (From Rosenberg, S. A., and Kaplan, H. S.: Calif. Med. **113:**23, 1970.)

tion of the entire lymph chain and all lymph nodes. The giant Reed-Sternberg cell characteristic of Hodgkin's lymphoma is identified through lymph node biopsy. An exploratory laparotomy determines the extent of involvement of the lymph system. The information obtained from the exploratory surgery coupled with the presence or absence of systemic symptoms provides the information needed for final diagnosis and staging. The classification into stages allows for comparison of persons with similar disease involvement and their response to a given treatment regimen. Over time such comparison has identified the treatment course most appropriate for a described disease involvement. The Ann Arbor staging classification, the most commonly used classification for Hodgkin's disease, is shown in the box on p. 1079.

Intervention. Radiation therapy is generally used for stages IA, IB, IIA, IIB, and IIIA. The specific x-ray field used in radiation treatment for stage I and II encompasses the involved lymph nodes and adjacent lymphatic sites and is achieved by means of a covering mantle (Fig. 48-5). Total nodal irradiation is used for stage IIIA. Patient outcomes and nursing interventions are those associated with persons receiving radiation therapy (see Chapter 25). Chemotherapy is the treatment of choice for stage IIIB and stage IV Hodgkin's disease. Single-agent therapy is seldom used except for the very nonaggressive histologic types of Hodgkin's disease. The most widely used combination chemotherapy is the MOPP regimen (box, p. 1079). Individuals receiving chemotherapy have many needs to be met through nursing intervention (see Chapter 25).

Hodgkin's disease is perhaps one of the most optimistic frontiers in the oncologic field. With more precise staging and the effectiveness of both radiation therapy and combination chemotherapy, increased survival rates and cure rates are striking. There are many individuals with Hodgkin's disease who are alive well beyond the 5-year mark. The nurse has a crucial role in assisting such individuals in developing a realistic approach to the illness. Like persons with leukemia, an individual with Hodgkin's disease is likely to have periods of remission and regression. Such peaks and valleys are stressful and disruptive. Support systems must be available to the individual. The health care team can provide some of this needed emotional support and guidance as the individual learns to incorporate the illness into daily life.

Lymphosarcoma

Lymphosarcoma is classified according to cell type: giant follicular lymphoma, follicular lymphosarcoma, and diffuse lymphosarcoma (the most common and representative of the disease). The abnormal lymphocytes diffuse throughout the involved tissue causing disruption of function. Specific complaints vary with the location of the lesion. Mediastinal and retroperitoneal lymph node enlargement may cause pressure on adjacent organs; gas-

CLINICAL STAGING CLASSIFICATION

Stage	Definition
I	Involvement of a single lymph node region (I) or of a single extralymphatic organ or site (I_E)
II	Involvement of two or more lymph node regions on the same side of the diaphragm (II) or localized involvement of an extralymphatic organ or site and of one or more lymph node regions on the same side of the diaphragm (II_E)
III	Involvement of lymph node regions on both sides of the diaphragm (III), which may also be accompanied by involvement of the spleen (III_S) or by localized involvement of an extralymphatic organ or site (III_E) or both (III_{SE})
IV	Diffuse or disseminated involvement of one or more extralymphatic organs or tissues, with or without associated lymph node involvement

The presence or absence of fever, night sweats, or unexplained loss of 10% or more of body weight in the 6 months preceding admission are denoted by the suffix letters B and A, respectively. Biopsy-documented involvement of stage IV sites is also denoted by letter suffixes: M, marrow; L, lung; H, liver; P, pleura; O, bone; D, skin and subcutaneous tissue.

COMBINATION CHEMOTHERAPY: MOPP REGIMEN

Nitrogen mustard	6 mg/sq m, IV, days 1 and 8
Vincristine	1.0 to 1.4 mg/sq m, IV, days 1 and 8
Procarbazine	100 mg/sq m/day, PO, days 1 through 14
Prednisone	40 mg/sq m/day, PO, days 1 through 14

tric and intestinal masses may simulate gastrointestinal tract carcinoma; and large, hard lymph nodes may be adherent to the skin. Fever, diaphoresis, weight loss, and weakness are common symptoms. Treatment with radiation therapy and chemotherapy may be very effective. Individuals with localized disease may experience remission after radiation therapy. Although not as effective as in the treatment of Hodgkin's lymphoma, combination chemotherapy may provide periods of extended remission in lymphosarcoma.

Reticulum cell sarcoma

Reticulum cell sarcoma may involve any part of the body. Normal tissue is replaced by the abnormally high numbers of reticulum cells.[6] Reticulum cell sarcoma is the most aggressive and invasive of the malignant lymphomas. The treatment regimen is the same as for the other lymphomas.

■ INFECTIOUS MONONUCLEOSIS

Infectious mononucleosis is an acute disease thought to be caused by a herpeslike virus, the Epstein-Barr virus. The disease is not new, having been described many years ago as acute "glandular fever" because of the enlargement of the lymph glands. Infectious mononucleosis is more common in young persons, the highest incidence occurring in persons between 15 and 30 years of age. It sometimes occurs in more or less epidemic form among closely associated groups or may also be sporadic in occurrence. Hospital personnel seem to be affected often by the disease, although this higher incidence is thought to be due to better reporting. The infection is believed to be transmitted from one person to another by means of secretions of the mouth and throat, although repeated efforts to transmit the disease to humans in this fashion have failed. The incubation period has not been definitely established, but it is believed that it may be several weeks in length.

Clinical picture. Signs and symptoms of infectious mononucleosis are varied. Usually it is a benign disease with a good prognosis. Malaise is a frequent early complaint, and it is often accompanied by an elevation of temperature, enlargement of the lymph nodes, sore throat, headache, increased nasal secretions, aches and pains resembling those of influenza, and moderate enlargement of the liver and spleen. Jaundice, rupture of the spleen, encephalitis, and even death may occur. Diagnosis is established by the heterophil agglutination blood test. This test is based on the fact that a certain substance that is present in the person's blood causes clumping, or agglutination, of the washed erythrocytes (antigen) of another animal (in this case, sheep cells are used). The test is almost always positive at the end of 10 to 14 days of the illness. Another conclusive laboratory finding is a marked increase in the number of mononuclear leukocytes, which lends the name to the disease. At the height of the disease the white blood cell count usually ranges between 10,000 and 20,000 cells/cu mm. At this time antibiotic therapy is not effective in treating infectious mononucleosis, and no immunization is available.

Intervention. Nursing care of the patient with infectious mononucleosis is purely symptomatic. If sore throat is severe, warm gargles may be ordered; glucose solutions often give greater relief than saline solution.

Liquid and soft foods may have to constitute the person's entire menu. Acetylsalicylic acid is usually given for headache and generalized discomfort, and the person is encouraged to remain in bed. If allowed up, the person is advised to stay indoors and engage in little activity. The disease usually disappears within 2 weeks, but it may continue in a chronic form for several weeks and even months. For this reason patient education regarding the nature of the disease is indicated. Relapses do occur, and this explains the need for rest at the time of acute illness even though the person does not feel ill and may resent the time spent away from work and regular activities.

Outcome criteria for the person with infectious mononucleosis

The person or significant others can:

1. Describe the nature of the disease and the need for avoidance of fatigue.
2. Describe a plan for rest until the temperature returns to normal.
3. Describe measures to relieve discomfort (aspirin, warm gargles).
4. Describe measures to prevent spread of infection by the oral route.
5. State plans for follow-up care:
   a. Describe symptoms requiring further medical attention (continued fever, malaise, anorexia).
   b. State plans for medical follow-up.

REFERENCES AND SELECTED READINGS

1. Aledort, L.: The management of hemophilia: a perspective, Drug Ther. **1**:55-59, 1971.
2. Alexander, M. M.: Physical examination. IV. The lymph system, Nursing '73 **3**:49-52, Oct. 1973.
3. Alsop, S.: Stay of execution: a sort of memoir, Philadelphia, 1973, J. B. Lippincott Co.
4. American Cancer Society, Inc.: 1977 Cancer facts and figures, New York, 1976, The Society.
5. Arnold, P.: Total-body irradiation and marrow transplantation, Am. J. Nurs. **63**:83-88, 1963.
6. Baldy, C. M.: The lymphomas: concepts and current therapies, Nurs. Clin. North Am. **7**:763-775, 1972.
7. Bolin, R. H., and Auld, M. E.: Hodgkin's disease, Am. J. Nurs. **74**:1982-1986, 1974.
8. Bouchard, R., and Owens, N. F.: Nursing care of the cancer patient, ed. 3, St. Louis, 1976, The C. V. Mosby Co.
9. Brenner, P.: Transfusions: what blood component does your patient really need? Nurs. Update **4**:1-10, 1973.
10. Cohn, H. D.: Hemostasis and blood coagulation, Am. J. Nurs. **65**:116-119, 1965.
11. Devita, V., et al.: New hope for the Hodgkin's patient, Nurs. Update **4**:1-12, July 1973.
12. Donovan, M. and Pierce, S.: Cancer care nursing, New York, 1976, Appleton-Century Crofts.
13. Eisenhauer, L. A.: Drug-induced blood dyscrasias, Nurs. Clin. North Am. **7**:799-808, 1972.
14. Ferrer, T.: Counseling patients with genetic abnormalities, Nurs. Clin. North Am. **10**:293-305, 1975.
15. Franklin, F. I., et al.: The many facets of hemophilia, J.A.M.A. **228**:85-92, 1974.
16. Gorst, D. W.: Sickle cell disease, Nurs. Times **72**:1436-1438, 1976.
17. Guy, R. B., and Rothenberg, S. P.: Sickle cell crisis, Med. Clin. North Am. **57**:1591-1598, 1973.
18. Hynes, J. F., and Jansson, E. B.: Hodgkin's disease, Am. J. Nurs. **58**:371-372, 1958.
19. Isler, C.: Blood: the age of components, RN **36**:31-41, June 1973.
20. Jackson, D. E.: Sickle cell disease: meeting a need, Nurs. Clin. North Am. **7**:727-741, 1972.
21. Kaplan, H.: Hodgkin's disease, Cambridge, Mass., 1972, Harvard University Press.
22. Kraveny, E., and Wiley, L.: Hodgkin's disease. . . the curable cancer, Nursing '75 **5**:48-55, March 1975.
23. Lamberg, L.: Genetic screening: learning what you never wanted to know, Today's Health **54**:28-31, 53-54, March 1976.
24. Lazerson, J.: The prophylactic approach to hemophilia A, Hosp. Practice **16**:99-102, 106-109, 1971.
25. Lund, D.: Eric, Philadelphia, 1974, J. B. Lippincott Co.
26. Massie, R., and Massie, S.: Journey, New York, 1976, Warner Books.
27. Miller, A.:. Systems of life. Part 7. Blood, Nurs. Times **71**: center pages, 1975.
28. Patterson, P. C.:. Hemophilia: the new look, Nurs. Clin. North Am. **7**:777-785, 1972.
29. Prosnitz, L. R.: Radiation therapy, RN **34**:42-51, March 1971.
30. Refkind, R., Bank, A., Marks, P., and Nossel, H.: Fundamentals of hematology, Chicago, 1976, Year Book Medical Publishers, Inc.
31. Rogers, J.: Hodgkin's disease: hope is the key to nursing care, Nursing '75 **5**:55-58, March 1975.
32. Rossman, M., Slavin, R., and Taft, E.: Phoresis therapy: patient care, Am. J. Nurs. **77**:1135-1141, 1977.
33. Schumann, D., and Patterson, P. C.: The adult with acute leukemia, Nurs. Clin. North Am. **7**:734-761, 1972.
34. Sergis, E., and Hilgartner, M. W.: Hemophilia, Am. J. Nurs. **72**:2011-2017, 1972.
35. Showferty, M. P.: The ordeal of Hodgkin's disease, Am. J. Nurs. **74**:1987-1991, 1974.
36. Snell, P.: Acute myeloblastic leukemia, Nurs. Times **71**:693-695, 1975.
37. Tenczynski, J.: Leukaphoresis: the process, Am. J. Nurs. **77**:1133-1134, 1977.
38. Thorn, G. W.: Harrison's principles of internal medicine, ed. 8, New York, 1977, McGraw-Hill Book Co.
39. Timmons, A. L.: Is it so awful? Am. J. Nurs. **75**:988, 1975.
40. Whitehouse, J. M.: The leukemias. Part 2. Chronic leukemia, Nurs. Times **68**:737-738, 1972.
41. Williams, S. R.: Nutrition and diet therapy, ed. 3, St. Louis, 1977, The C. V. Mosby Co.
42. Williams, W. J., et al.: Hemotology, ed. 2, New York, 1977, McGraw-Hill Book Co.
43. Wilson, P.: Iron-deficiency anemia, Am. J. Nurs **72**:502-504, 1972.
44. Wintrobe, M. M., et al: Harrison's principles of internal medicine, ed. 8, New York, 1977, McGraw-Hill Book Co.
45. Wintrobe, M. M., et al.: Clinical hematology, ed. 7, Philadelphia, 1974, Lea & Febiger.
46. Vaz, D. D. S.: The common anemias: nursing approaches, Nurs. Clin. North Am. **7**:711-725, 1972.

49

Problems of the upper airway

LINDA ANNE BROSEMAN

Disorders of the upper airway are very common, and nurses in particular are often asked to give advice about these problems. To be effective, nurses need a basic understanding of the structure and function of the organs of the upper airway, as well as the knowledge of the medical and nursing regimens for problems affecting these organs. For clarity, this chapter will be divided into three sections; problems of the nose and sinuses, problems with the upper throat (pharynx and tonsils), and problems of the lower throat (larynx). For problems of the mouth and parotid gland, see Chapter 54.

PROBLEMS OF THE NOSE AND SINUSES

The nose is supported by the nasal bones, the nasal processes of the maxillary bones, the cartilaginous and bony parts of the septum, and the upper and lower nasal cartilages. Air enters the nose through the two nostrils (nares), which are separated by the septum. The septum, which is usually straight and thin in the child, is rarely straight in adults because it is subject to injury.[25]

The nasal cavities are located between the roof of the mouth and the frontal, ethmoid, and sphenoid bones. Three projections, lined with mucous membrane, called the turbinate bones are located on the walls of each nasal cavity (Fig. 49-1). Their purpose is to increase the mucous membrane surface over which air passes as it travels to the nasopharynx.

The vestibule of the nose is the anterior part of the nose. The vestibule extends posteriorly a short distance where its lining changes from skin to mucous membrane.

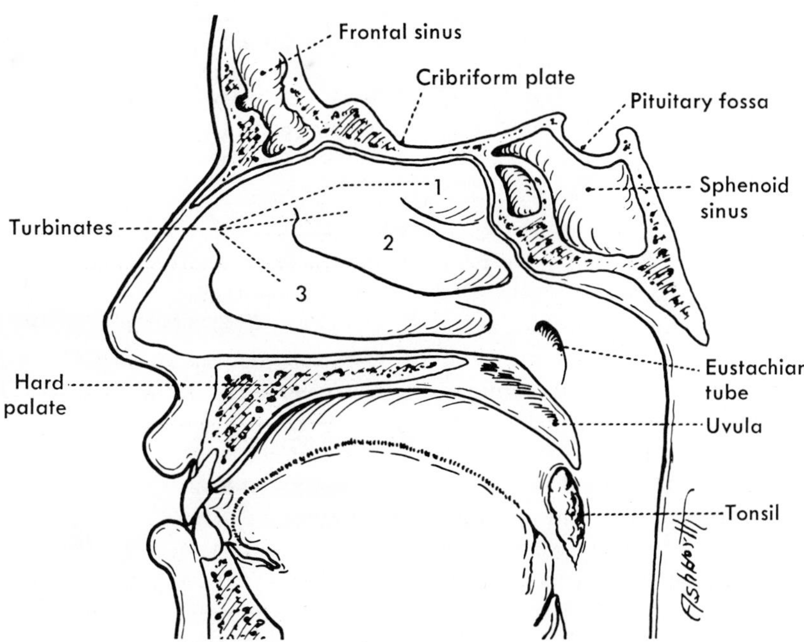

Fig. 49-1. Turbinates of nose: *1*, superior; *2*, middle; *3*, inferior. (From DeWeese, D. D., and Saunders, W. H.: Textbook of otolaryngology, ed. 5, St. Louis, 1977, The C. V. Mosby Co.)

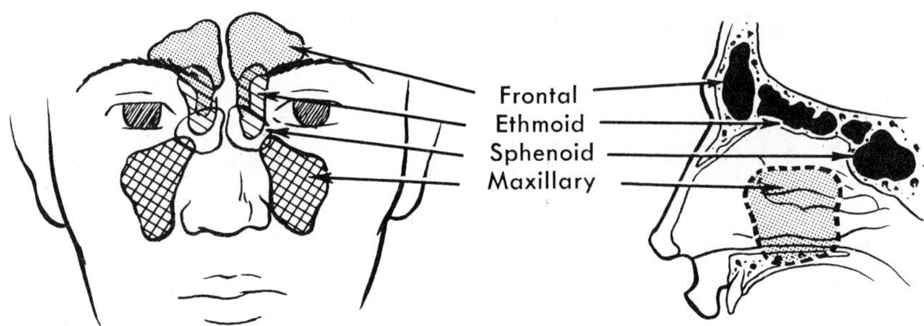

Fig. 49-2. Location of sinuses.

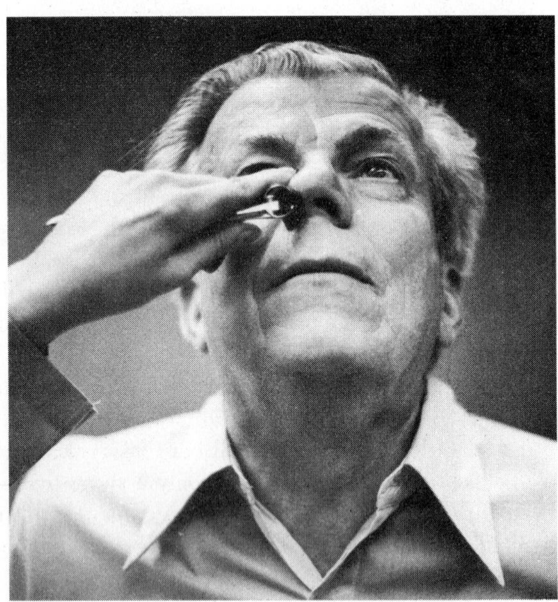

Fig. 49-3. Proper position for insertion of nasal speculum with index finger on side of nose. (From Malasanos, L., Barkauskas, V., Moss, M., and Stoltenberg-Allen, K.: Health assessment, St. Louis, 1977, The C. V. Mosby Co.)

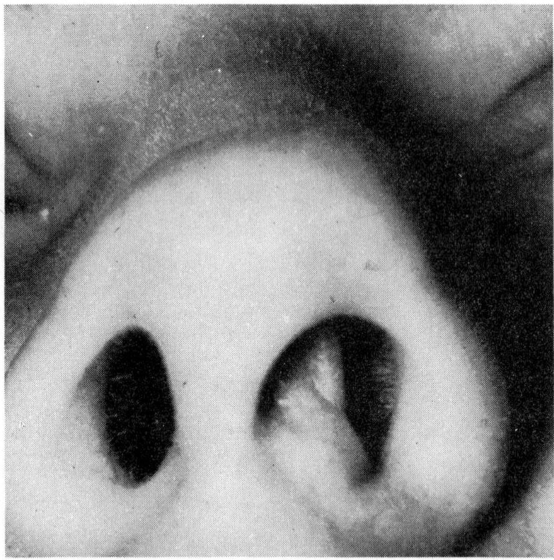

Fig. 49-4. Septal deviation. Anterior end of septal cartilage is dislocated and projects into nasal vestibule. (From Havener, W. H., Saunders, W. H., Keith, C. F., and Prescott, A. W.: Nursing care in eye, ear, nose, and throat disorders, ed. 3, St. Louis, 1974, The C. V. Mosby Co.)

This mucous membrane contains cilia that beat in a constant wavelike motion to carry mucus into the nasopharynx. The olfactory epithelium is located in a small area superiorly and provides the end organ of smell. The lateral walls of the nose contain the openings for the paranasal sinuses and the nasolacrimal ducts. These openings provide a means of aeration of and mucus drainage from the sinuses. The blood supply to the nose comes from both the external and internal carotid systems.

There are four sets of paranasal sinuses located on either side of the head (Fig. 49-2). These sinuses are air-filled spaces in the skull that serve to lighten the head. They drain into the nasal cavities through the openings behind the turbinates. The maxillary sinuses are the largest and most accessible. The sinuses are lined with mucous membrane that is continuous with that of the nose. The chief functions of the nose include providing an airway to warm and moisten air in preparation for the lungs and as the organ of smell.

□ Assessment

Inspection of the nose includes looking for deformities, asymmetry, and inflammation.[5] To visualize the nose a nasal speculum or an otoscope fitted with a nasal speculum is inserted about 1 cm into the vestibule, avoiding the nasal septum (Fig. 49-3). The lower portion of the nose is inspected first using a light source such as a pen light. The person then tilts his head back so that the upper portions of the nose can be visualized.

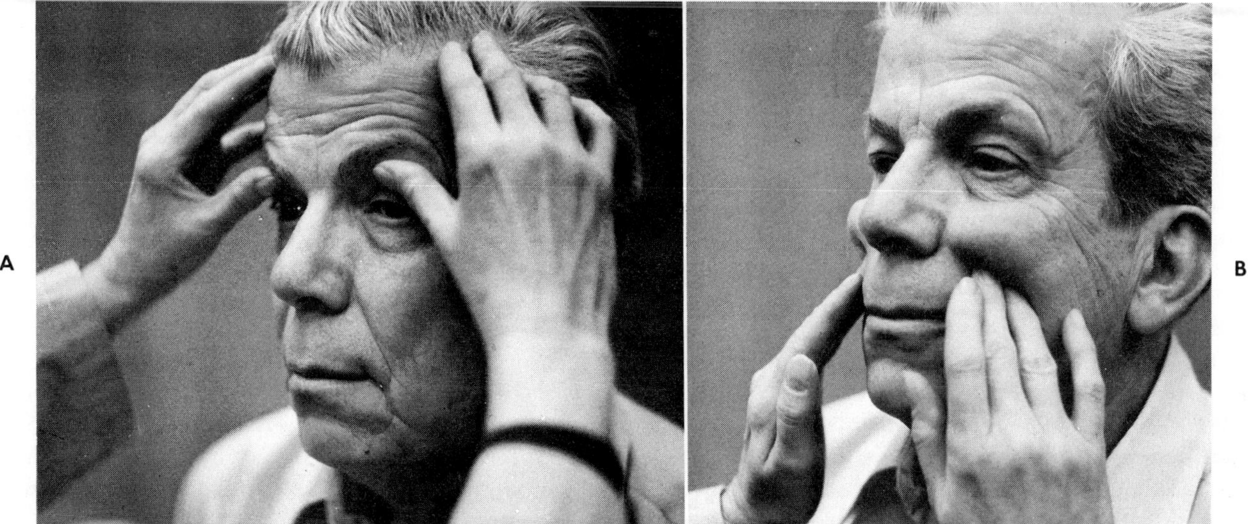

Fig. 49-5. Palpation of frontal, **A,** and maxillary, **B,** sinuses. (From Malasanos, L., Barkauskas, V., Moss, M., and Stoltenberg-Allen, K.: Health assessment, St. Louis, 1977, The C. V. Mosby Co.)

Nasal mucosa is normally redder in appearance than oral mucosa. Excessive redness, edema, exudate, or bleeding is noted as is the presence of any furuncles. The nasal septum is observed for deviation, bleeding, or perforation. The inferior and middle turbinates are observed for color, edema, exudate, or polyps. Red, swollen nasal mucous membranes accompanied by watery to mucopurulent nasal discharge indicates acute rhinitis. Nasal mucosa that is swollen, pale, boggy, and usually gray or dull red is seen in persons with allergic rhinitis. Soft, pale gray mobile structures found in the middle meatus are polyps that may develop in persons with allergic rhinitis. Some septal deviation (Fig. 49-4) is common in most adults and is usually asymptomatic, although it may produce nasal obstruction. The sinuses are palpated for signs of tenderness of the frontal and maxillary areas when inspecting the nose (Fig. 49-5).

To visualize the nasal mucosa clearly a vasoconstrictor such as phenylephrine (Neo-Synephrine) may be applied to shrink the mucous membrane. The throat often is examined superficially with a tongue depressor and flashlight at this time. For a more extensive examination of the posterior nares and the throat, a nasopharyngeal mirror is warmed with hot water or in a flame from an alcohol lamp to prevent fogginess and failure to reflect. Because this examination may make the person gag, he is instructed to breathe through his mouth while the mirror is being directed toward the pharynx.

The normal frontal and maxillary sinuses can be visualized by illuminating them in a dark room with a specially shaped, lighted bulb or a lighted transillumination tip. This examination is referred to as transillumination. If disease is present, the light will not penetrate the sinuses, or it will reveal fluid levels indicative of obstruction to drainage of the sinuses. Roentgenograms of the sinuses may be ordered to help establish the diagnosis of sinusitis. No physical preparation is necessary and usually no contrast medium is used since the normal sinus is filled with air, which in itself casts a shadow in contrast to surrounding structures.

Anosmia

Anosmia is the loss of the sense of smell. It may be the result of (1) nasal obstruction, which prevents air currents from reaching the olfactory epithelium; (2) skull fracture across the cribiform plate at the roof of the nose where the part of the olfactory nerve enters the nose; (3) viral infections, which affect the olfactory nerve; or (4) some meningiomas, which may form in the olfactory area. A perverted sense of smell called *parosmia* may also be present during sinusitis or an upper respiratory infection.

□ Infections of the nose and sinuses

Rhinitis

Rhinitis refers to inflammation of the mucous membrane of the nose. Rhinitis may be acute or chronic.

Acute rhinitis. Simple, acute rhinitis (coryza, common cold) is an inflammatory condition of the mucous membranes of the nose and accessory sinuses caused by a filtrable virus. It affects almost everyone at some time in his life and occurs most often in the cold winter months. It is generally believed that the infecting agent is present in the nose and sinuses at all times and that fatigue and chilling are among many factors influencing susceptibility. Some of the known agents causing the common cold are more than 30 identified rhinoviruses, adenovirus, Echovirus, influenza and parainfluenza viruses, and coxsackievirus. The common cold is spread by droplet nuclei from sneezing. The condition is contagious for the first 2 to 3 days.

Prevention. The best prevention is to avoid exposure. Since this is not possible, adequate diet, rest, and exercise presumably help to maintain resistance to a cold. Persons with colds should avoid crowded places where the cold can be easily transmitted to many others and should avoid infants or very young children, the elderly, or persons with chronic lung diseases. Frequent washing of hands, covering of coughs and sneezes, and careful disposal of waste tissue are protective health measures that are advisable for everyone.

Clinical picture. The person usually complains of dryness of the nose, eyes, and soft palate, general malaise, chilliness, and headache. These symptoms are followed in 12 to 24 hours by obstruction to nasal breathing caused by swelling of the mucous membrane and a profuse, watery nasal discharge. Sneezing, tearing of the eyes, and nasal irritation also occur, and the postnatal discharge may cause pharyngitis, laryngitis, or bronchitis, although a sore throat is not always associated with a cold. If uncomplicated, the cold is usually self-limiting and lasts for about 6 to 7 days.

Intervention. Most people with colds do not go to their physician unless symptoms persist or make them very uncomfortable. Medical therapy, if sought, usually consists of rest, fluids, moist inhalations, and antihistamines and decongestants. The antihistamines do not cure the cold but are helpful in alleviating symptoms such as sneezing and tearing of the eyes during the initial inflammatory phase only. Since the antihistamines cause drowsiness in most persons, they should not be used when driving a car or working near moving machinery.

People with acute rhinitis are instructed not to blow their nose too hard or unnecessarily. The mouth should be open slightly when blowing the nose and both nostrils should be open to prevent any infected matter from being forced into the eustachian tube. Nose drops are sometimes recommended for infrequent use (every 4 hours for a few days) if there is some nasal obstruction. Many otolaryngologists now believe that the frequent use of nose drops results in rhinitis medicamentosa (p. 1085), an "addiction" of the nasal mucosa to their use.[12,25] Some physicians believe that the obstruction of the nose may be a protective device that prevents the spread of infection to other parts of the body.

When *nose drops* are ordered, the individual is taught how to use them correctly as follows:

1. Sit in a chair and tip head well backwards, *or* lie down with head extended over edge of bed, *or* lie down with a pillow placed under shoulders and head tipped backwards.
2. Place no more than 3 drops of solution into each nostril at one time (unless ordered otherwise).
3. Remain in position with head tilted backwards for 5 minutes to permit solution to reach posterior nares.

If after 10 minutes following insertion of nose drops marked congestion is still present, another drop or two of solution may be administered. The mucous membrane of the anterior nares by this time should have become constricted so that the solution may reach the posterior nares more easily. Some physicians feel that the instillation of nose drops is too upsetting for children and thus order nasal decongestants such as pseudoephedrine, 30 mg every 3 to 4 hours, and steam inhalations. A rubber bulb ear syringe may be used to *aspirate* the mucus discharge from the nose of infants so that they can breathe and be able to take their feedings. Nasal decongestants may also be administered by means of an atomizer or inhalator as follows:

1. Sit upright with head tilted backward.
2. Place inhalator or atomizer in nostril.
3. Occlude the opposite nostril with finger pressure to prevent entrance of air (allows medication to penetrate further).
4. Administer no more than three sprays of solution into each nostril.

Secondary invasion by bacteria may complicate the cold, causing symptoms to persist and become worse. If the nasal discharge persists for more than about 7 to 10 days or if the person develops an elevation of temperature, medical attention should be obtained. Possible *complications* include pneumonia, bronchitis, sinusitis, and otitis media. Infants and young children are particularly susceptible to colds and the complication of otitis media (p. 799). They should be isolated from persons with colds, and if they develop a cold, they should be observed carefully for symptoms suggesting otitis media. If a high temperature occurs or if the infant becomes restless, rolls his head from side to side in bed, or pulls at his ear, medical attention should be sought.

Persons who have *recurrent* colds should seek medical attention because nasal deformity such as enlarged turbinates or a deviated septum and chronic sinusitis may cause the repeated attacks. Repeated colds eventually may lead to chronic rhinitis.

Allergic rhinitis. Allergic rhinitis (hay fever) can be acute and seasonal when caused by the pollens of grasses and flowers, or it may be chronic and perennial when associated with numerous allergens such as dust, animal dander, wool, and certain foods. Common symptoms include sneezing, nasal obstruction, tearing, recurrent thin watery nasal discharge, frontal headache, and itching of the eyes and nose. Typically on physical examination the turbinates are pale and edematous.

The best intervention for any kind of allergy is to separate the person from the allergens to which he is sensitive. If that is not feasible, then attempts are made to desensitize the individual. For some persons a series of injections for desensitization given in anticipation of the hayfever season (late summer) works well. Antihistamines are helpful in alleviating symptoms.

If nasal obstruction persists, surgery such as submucous resection or septoplasty may be performed. Often people with allergic rhinitis develop polyps, which are pale, soft edematous outpouchings of nasal or sinal mucosa. Polyps are usually bilateral and may cause obstruction of the airway. Multiple polyps may cause severe nasal obstruction as well as anosmia. Polypectomy (p. 1090) is the surgical procedure used to remove polyps.

Chronic rhinitis. Chronic rhinitis is a chronic inflammation of the mucous membrane caused by repeated, acute infections, by an allergy, or by vasomotor rhinitis. The cause of *vasomotor rhinitis* is unclear, but may result from an instability of the autonomic nervous system resulting from stress, tension, or some endocrine disorder. Often it is mistaken for nasal allergy, but the allergen cannot be identified. There is an increased formation of nasal mucus.

Clinical picture. Regardless of cause of chronic rhinitis, the symptoms are similar. Nasal obstruction accompanied by a feeling of stuffiness and pressure in the nose is the chief complaint. A nasal discharge is always present and may be serous, mucopurulent, or purulent, depending on the amount of secondary infection present. Polyp formation may occur, and the turbinates may enlarge as a result of the chronic irritation. Complaints of frontal headache, vertigo, and sneezing are common.

Intervention. Antibiotics may be used to treat the secondary infection. If the cause is allergy related, the offending allergen is removed or the person is desensitized to it. Antihistamines are helpful in alleviating symptoms. Polyps or hyperplastic tissues may require surgical removal.

Nasal irrigations are no longer used frequently in the treatment of chronic rhinitis. Details of this procedure are described in texts on fundamentals of nursing or in textbooks on otolaryngology.[12,17,46] Care should be taken to assure that both nostrils are open and that the pressure in the nostrils is not excessive (the irrigating container should not be higher than 12 to 15 inches above the level of the nose). Excess pressure may force infected material into the sinuses or the middle ear. This procedure should not be performed on a child who is crying or struggling to avoid it.

Rhinitis medicamentosa. Rhinitis medicamentosa is a common condition caused by the overuse of nose drops.[12,25] A rebound phenomenon occurs after the immediate effect of the nose drops with return to congestion. Treatment consists of stopping the use of all nose drops completely. Usually within a week or two the person can breathe through the nose again. Orally administered decongestants may often help.

Outcome criteria for the person with rhinitis. The person or significant others can:

1. Describe ways to prevent future attacks (e.g., avoiding persons with colds, avoiding allergens to which the person is sensitive).
2. List allergens to which the person is sensitive and describe how to avoid them (e.g., environmentally controlled room [p. 1541], electrostatic filter, air conditioning, face masks).
3. Demonstrate procedure for instilling nose drops or nasal spray.
4. State name, dosage, frequency, and side effects of medications being used, and state danger of using over-the-counter preparations.
5. Describe symptoms requiring medical intervention.
6. State plans for follow-up care.

Sinusitis

The sinuses are air-filled cavities lined with mucous membrane. Any inflammation of the mucous membranes of the sinuses is referred to as sinusitis. This is still a frequent disorder, although it is less common since the advent of antibiotics. Often persons who complain of sinusitis do not have sinus trouble but actually have other disorders. When an otolaryngologist refers to sinusitis, a bacterial invasion of the mucous membrane is implied. This can be either an acute or a chronic condition.

Acute sinusitis. The most common cause of acute sinusitis is the obstruction of the paranasal sinuses that blocks the egress of secretions of the sinuses. These secretions become infected, giving rise to acute sinusitis. Sinusitis may follow acute or allergic rhinitis or other respiratory diseases such as pneumonia or influenza. Streptococci, staphylocci, pneumococci, or anaerobes are the infecting organisms. Abscessed teeth or tooth extraction are increasingly important causes of acute maxillary sinusitis, since the apices of many of the upper teeth roots are in close contact with the mucosal lining of these sinuses.

Clinical picture. The person with acute sinusitis often complains of a constant, severe headache and of pain over the infected sinuses. Maxillary sinusitis will cause pain under the eyes, whereas frontal sinusitis often

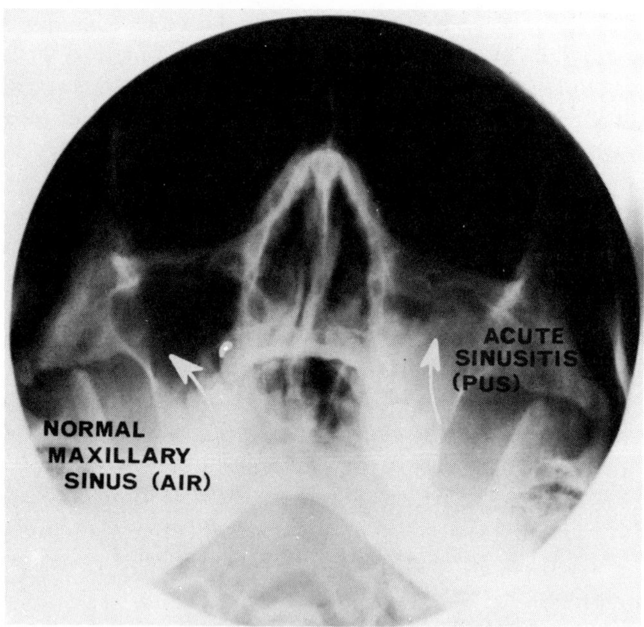

Fig. 49-6. Roentgenogram of maxillary sinus showing normal sinus on left and acute sinusitis on right. (From Havener, W. H., Saunders, W. H., Keith, C. F., and Prescott, A. W.: Nursing care in eye, ear, nose, and throat disorders, ed. 3, St. Louis, 1974, The C. V. Mosby Co.)

causes pain over the eyebrows. The person may have the sensation of "pain in the bone" with even slight pressure over the affected sinus.[5] Pain from the ethmoid and sphenoid sinuses usually is referred and is felt at the top of the head. Occasionally there may be noticeable swelling over the maxillary or frontal sinuses, or there may be orbital edema. The person may have nausea, purulent discharge from the nose if the duct is not closed, obstruction to nasal breathing, fever, and general malaise. Fever is proportional to the amount of obstruction present and the virulence of the infection. If the sinus is completely obstructed, the temperature may be as high as 40 C (104 F). The throat may be sore from irritation caused by postnasal drainage.

Medical evaluation usually consists of sinus roentgenograms, which are useful in determining the presence and extent of disease and indicate involvement of the bony walls (Fig. 49-6). When infection is present, the film appears cloudy. Complications of severe untreated sinusitis include osteomyelitis in the adjacent bone, an abscess that may involve the brain, venous sinus thrombosis, orbital cellulitis, orbital abscess, and septicemia.

Intervention. Treatment is directed at relieving pain, establishing drainage of the sinuses, and controlling the infection.[3] Broad-spectrum antibiotics such as penicillin, especially ampicillin, tetracycline, or erythromycin, are given systemically for their specific action on the causative organism. Medications such as phenylephrine (Neo-Synephrine) 0.25%, and ephedrine sulfate 0.25% to 3%, which constrict the blood vessels and thus reduce hyperemia and improve drainage, may be given as nose drops or by inhalation. Forced air pressure of the atomizer breaks the large droplets of fluid into a fine mist. If a nebulizer is used, the solution is usually forced through the apparatus by a current of oxygen or compressed air. In addition to these, cocaine pledgets may be placed in the nasal cavity to exert a direct effect on the nasal mucosa.

Pain may be relieved by the administration of various analgesics. Because aspirin may be associated with nasal polyposis, it is usually avoided as a pain medication. Acetaminophen (Tylenol) is a good substitute for the aspirin, and occasionally codeine or even morphine sulfate or meperidine may be necessary to relieve the pain. Heat over the sinuses also gives some relief from pain. Warm, wet dressings or a heat lamp may be used. Moist steam in the room may help to facilitate drainage by liquefying the secretions. The room temperature should be kept constant, since changes in room temperature aggravate sinusitis.

If conservative measures do not cure an acute sinus infection, the physician may irrigate the maxillary sinuses by means of an *antrum puncture.* The nasal mucosa is usually anesthetized with cocaine, and the maxillary sinus (the antrum) is perforated with a trocar and cannula. The patient is urged to breathe through the mouth during the procedure. The person's head is supported while the treatment is given, since a sensation of pressure is felt that, although not painful, may produce dizziness and nausea. Saline rather than air is used, as deaths caused by air embolism have been reported.

Persons with symptoms of acute sinusitis are urged to seek medical attention, since early treatment of acute sinusitis is more successful than treatment after the condition becomes chronic.

Chronic sinusitis. In chronic sinusitis the mucous membrane lining or sinus becomes thickened from prolonged or repeated irritation and infection. The person usually has a chronic purulent nasal discharge, a chronic cough caused by a postnasal drainage, and chronic dull sinus headache that is present on awakening and subsides during the day. The varied positions and movement of the head during the day help the sinus to drain, diminishing the headache. As passage of air through the nose becomes blocked, there may be loss of ability to smell. Roentgenograms, which indicate thickening in the mucous membrane as well as diffuse cloudiness, are useful in establishing the diagnosis.

Treatment of chronic sinusitis may be surgical. Removal of nasal deformities such as a deviated nasal septum, hypertrophied turbinated bones, or nasal polyps that are obstructing the sinus openings may give relief. Sinus irrigations may be done to ensure better drainage. If the condition is caused by an allergy, it responds to general treatment of the allergy. In general, antibiotics are not very helpful in treating chronic sinusitis.

The person with chronic sinusitis should avoid chilling and cold, damp atmospheres. Change to a warm, dry climate, though helpful to some people, is not necessarily helpful to all. The person is advised not to smoke because smoking further irritates the damaged mucous membranes. Air conditioning often causes discomfort, particularly if the outside air is warm and moist. The person with chronic sinusitis often sleeps poorly and lacks pep and vigor in his living and in his work. Persistent postnasal discharge is believed to contribute to bronchiectasis, a chronic lung disease, as the person grows older.

Outcome criteria for the person with sinusitis. The person or significant others can:

1. State factors that contribute to development of sinusitis and how to prevent future attacks.
2. Explain medication program.
   a. State name, dosage, frequency, route of administration, and side effects of prescribed medications.
   b. State rationale for full course of antibiotics even when obvious symptoms have subsided.
3. State plans for follow-up health care.
   a. Describe symptoms of secondary infections that require further medical attention.
   b. State plans for stopping smoking, if appropriate.
   c. State plans for controlling environmental temperature.
   d. State plans for seeking medical attention for acute episodes.

Infections of external tissues about the nose

The skin around the external nose is easily irritated during acute attacks of rhinitis or sinusitis. Furunculosis and cellulitis (inflammation of connective tissue) occasionally develop. (See p. 1527 for discussion and treatment of furunculosis.) Infections about the nose are extremely dangerous, since the venous supply from this area drains directly into the cerebral venous sinuses. Septicemia therefore can occur easily. No pimple or lesion in the area should ever be squeezed or "picked"; hot packs may be used. If any infection in or about the nose persists or shows even the slightest tendency to spread or increase in severity, medical aid should be sought.

□ Nasal obstructions

Nasal obstruction is a common condition caused by a number of complaints. Physical inspection of the nose is necessary for identification of the cause of obstruction.

Deviated septum

Deviated septum is a common cause of nasal obstruction. The septum, which is normally thin and straight, may be deviated from the midline and protrude more to one side of the nasal passage than to the other. The deviation may cause a nasal obstruction that increases when infection or allergic reaction occurs. If the obstruction is marked, noisy and difficult breathing will result. There may be a postnasal drip, or the mucosa may become dry so that crusts form. This deformity of the septum is common in older children and adults. It may be congenital but usually is the result of an injury. The person with trauma to the nose should be encouraged to seek medical attention, since a broken nose can lead to chronic sinusitis if not treated, even though it may cause no immediate problem. If the deformity causes nasal obstruction, a submucous resection or septoplasty (reconstruction of the septum) may be performed (p. 1091).

Hypertrophy of the turbinates

The inferior turbinates are sometimes the cause of considerable nasal obstruction. Hypertrophied turbinates may be medically treated by the use of aerosols containing corticosteroids such as dexamethasone (Decadron Turbinaire).[26] These aerosols are used for their antiinflammatory response and have proven to be effective for allergic and inflammatory nasal conditions as well as for treatment of nasal polyps. Although not employed as often since the advent of the corticosteroid aerosol, local surgery on the turbinates such as electric fulguration may still be used to restore the airway.

Nasal polyps

Nasal polyps are grapelike growths of mucous membrane and loose connective tissue. They are usually bilateral and may be caused by irritation to mucous membranes of the nose or sinuses from an allergy or by chronic sinusitis. Nasal polyps in children may be caused by cystic fibrosis. Polyps also cause anosmia by preventing air from reaching the olfactory mucosa high in the nose. Since they may obstruct breathing or may bleed, nasal polyps are removed (polypectomy, p. 1090). Aerosol sprays such as the ones discussed for hypertrophied turbinates have also proven effective for the treatment of nasal polyps. Since the sinus mucosa may also be involved in the polypoid process, surgery on the sinuses such as an ethmoidectomy may be necessary (p. 1092).

Foreign bodies

Foreign bodies of the nose are suspected when a child has unilateral nasal obstruction and discharge. It is usually necessary to use a vasoconstrictor such as ephedrine or Neo-Synephrine 1% topically to provide shrinkage of the intranasal membranes and to make it easier for extraction of the foreign body. Usually it is necessary to restrain the arms of the child during the procedure.

Tumors

Tumors both benign and malignant can produce nasal obstruction either unilaterally or bilaterally. Nasopharyngeal carcinomas obstruct the nose at first on one side and then on both sides. These tumors metastasize early to the neck. Carcinomas of the maxillary or ethmoid sinuses may erode through the adjacent nasal walls. They often bleed easily.[23,44]

□ Nose trauma

Fractures of the nasal bones and septum

Fractures of the nasal bones and septum commonly occur from relatively minor injuries such as falls or from more severe injuries such as automobile accidents or fights. If there is no displacement of the bone, no obstruction to the airway, nor any cosmetic deformity, treatment is not needed. When airway obstruction or bone displacement occurs (Fig. 49-7), then simple reduction is performed. Most simple nasal fractures can be reduced by applying firm pressure on the convex side of the nose. Fractures that cannot be reduced by this technique are reduced surgically under local anesthesia.

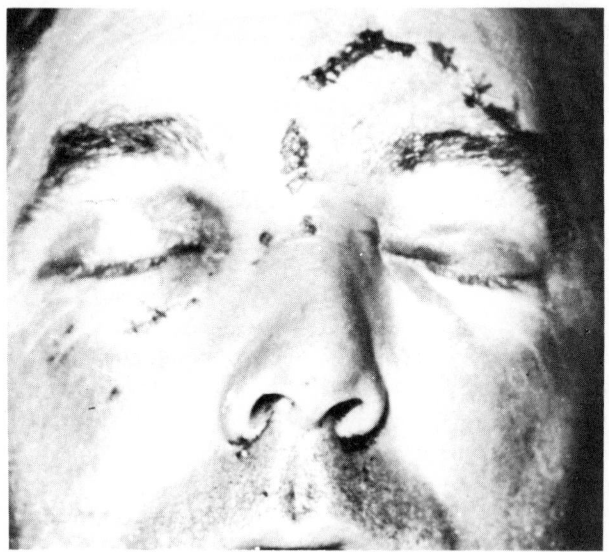

Fig. 49-7. Laterally displaced fracture of nose secondary to trauma. Pressure on convex side will restore alignment. (From Havener, W. H., Saunders, W. H., Keith, C. F., and Prescott, A. W.: Nursing care in eye, ear, nose, and throat disorders, ed. 3, St. Louis, 1974, The C. V. Mosby Co.)

Fractures of the maxillary and zygomatic bones

Fractures of the maxillary and zygomatic bones are seen after automobile accidents and fights. These fractures are generally reduced under anesthesia. Patients may also have some teeth wired together with all the attendant problems of that procedure (see p. 1194 for nursing interventions for patients with fractured jaws).

□ Epistaxis

Epistaxis, or nosebleed, may be caused by local irritation of mucous membranes, chronic infection, lack of humidity in the air that is breathed, violent sneezing or nose blowing, or trauma to the nose resulting in damage to or rupture of superficial blood vessels. One of the most common causes of nosebleeds is picking of the nose. General or systemic causes may be hypertension and arterial blood vessel changes, blood dyscrasias such as leukemia, or a deficiency of vitamin K. In adulthood, nosebleeds are more common in men than in women. They are most frequent in early childhood and puberty. Persons who have frequent nosebleeds should have a complete medical examination to determine the cause.

Most nosebleeds come from the tiny blood vessels in the anterior part of the nasal septum. This bleeding usually can be controlled at least temporarily by compressing the soft tissues of the nose against the septum with a finger. Firm pressure should be maintained for at least 5 to 10 minutes, and it may be necessary for as long as 30 minutes. The person should breathe through the mouth during this time. Ice compresses may be applied over the nose; however, the primary benefit of the application of ice is that it requires the patient to remain still. Bleeding may be controlled by placing a cotton ball soaked in a topical vasoconstrictor such as Neo-Synephrine into the nose and applying pressure. Other first-aid measures include having the person sit quietly with the head up and inclined slightly forward to prevent blood from entering the pharynx and causing gagging or swallowing of blood. The person is instructed not to blow the nose for several hours after a nosebleed.

If the above measures do not control bleeding, the help of a physician should be sought. In order to treat a nosebleed effectively, the physician must first determine the site of the bleeding. This is done best with the person seated in a chair facing the physician. Both should wear gowns to protect their clothing. An angulated suction tip is used to suck clots from the nose. If suction is not available, the person is instructed to blow the nose to remove the clot. The physician will then use a bright light (either head mirror or lamp) to inspect the anterior nares. After anesthetizing the nasal mucosa with topical lidocaine (Xylocaine), the bleeding point is cauterized with a silver nitrate stick or electrode cautery.

Bleeding from the posterior part of the nasal septum is more common in the elderly person and is more likely to be severe. If the bleeding point cannot be seen and treated as described above, a postnasal pack may be inserted (Fig. 49-8). Because this procedure is extremely painful and sometimes causes faintness, patients usually are admitted to the hospital. The pack is left in place 2 to 5 days and then removed very gently. If bleeding has been severe, a transfusion may be necessary. Severe bleeding results in a drop in blood pressure, which will cause the bleeding to stop. Therefore exsanguination from the usual nosebleed is not possible. Sedation may be ordered, since bleeding tends to be increased by apprehension and restlessness. To prevent recurrent hemorrhage, the person is warned not to blow the nose vigorously and to avoid dryness of the nose. This can be accomplished by using saline or nasal lubricants.

Nosebleeds can cause severe apprehension, since bleeding may be profuse not only from the nose but also flowing into the throat. The patient is usually kept in Fowler's position and is urged not to swallow blood because it may cause nausea and vomiting. Adequate oxygenation with humidification is important with persons who have posterior packing in place. Pain medication, antibiotic therapy, and sedation may also be ordered for a person with posterior packing. The position of a postnasal pack must be checked frequently, since it may slip out of place and cause airway obstruction. Nasal packs make eating and swallowing difficult. A liquid diet may be ordered. Persistent or recurrent profuse epistaxis, especially posterior epistaxis, may require surgical ligation of the external carotid artery, the ethmoid artery, or the internal maxillary artery, which supply blood to the nose.

Outcome criteria for the person with epistaxis

The person or significant others can:

1. Describe dangers inherent in picking of nose and violent nose blowing.

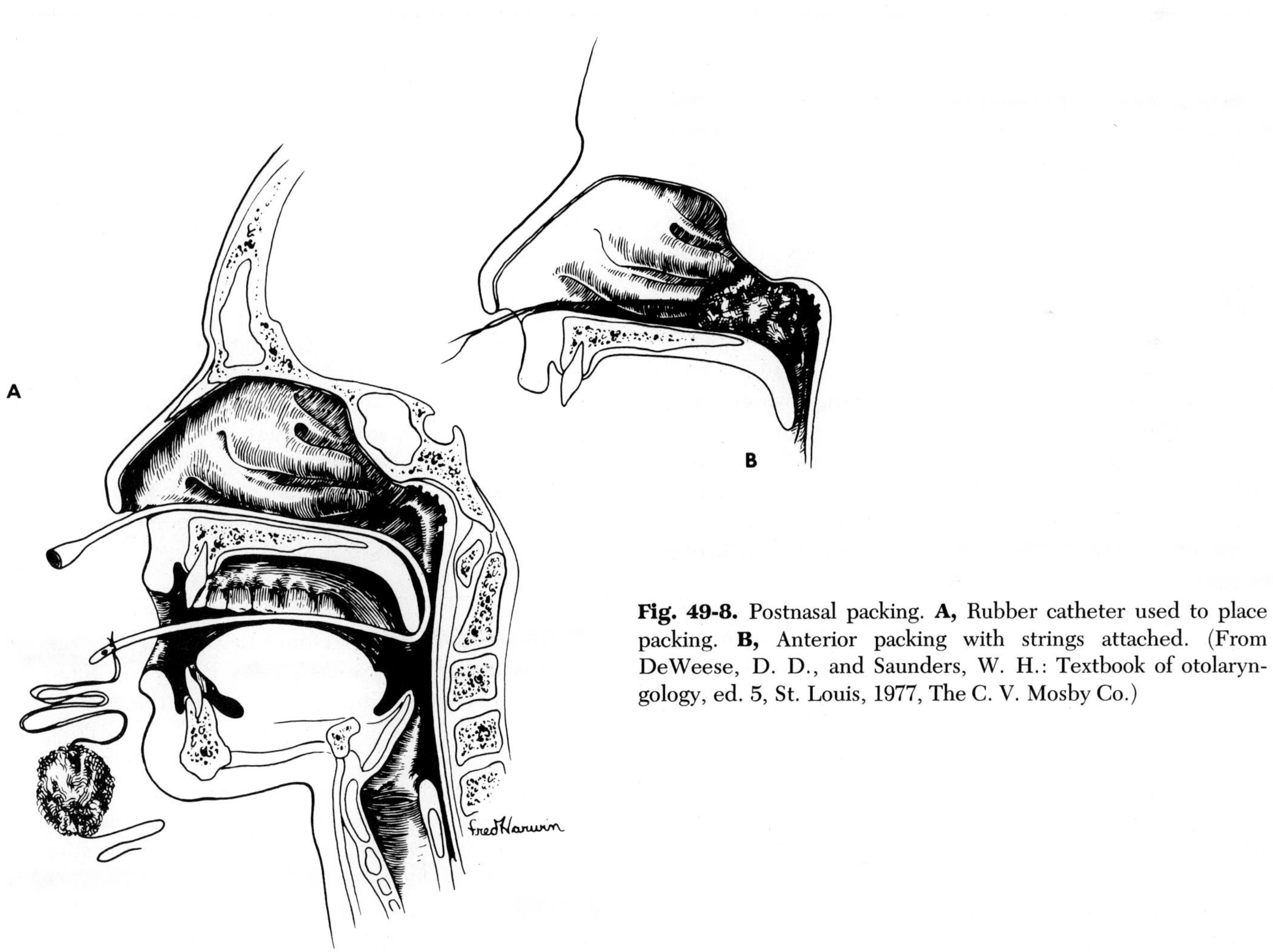

Fig. 49-8. Postnasal packing. **A,** Rubber catheter used to place packing. **B,** Anterior packing with strings attached. (From DeWeese, D. D., and Saunders, W. H.: Textbook of otolaryngology, ed. 5, St. Louis, 1977, The C. V. Mosby Co.)

2. State rationale for medical examination if nosebleeds are frequent.
3. Describe simple first aid for nosebleeds.
4. Describe when simple first aid is not adequate and medical attention is required.

□ Carcinoma of the maxillary and ethmoid sinuses

Carcinoma of the paranasal sinus is relatively uncommon. Carcinoma of the maxillary sinus presents no early symptoms. The first complaints usually are dental in origin, either the person complains of loosening of the upper teeth, or if a denture is worn, of the upper plate no longer fitting.[23] Other symptoms may include nasal obstruction caused by the tumor eroding into the nose, nosebleeds, and displacement of the eye. Carcinoma of the ethmoid sinus presents no oral or dental symptoms. The tumor causes outward displacement of the eye, disturbance of the sense of smell, and nosebleeds. Often, tearing of the eye or diplopia occurs. Treatment usually consists of irridiation therapy and surgery.

□ Surgery of the nose and sinuses

Management of the person requiring nasal surgery

Most nasal surgery on adults is done under local anesthesia. The person should not be given anything orally for 6 hours preoperatively, since he may become nauseated during the operation. A sedative and a narcotic are usually given preoperatively. Children require general anesthesia and may be given a medication such as atropine to reduce secretions. The nose is usually packed with ½-inch gauze at the conclusion of the operation. Commonly used packs are petrolatum-impregnated gauze, Adaptic gauze, iodoform gauze with chlortetracycline (Aureomycin), and Cortisporin-impregnated gauze. The latter is particularly effective in reducing the odor of the nasal pack. If the packing should slip back into the throat, the surgeon is notified immediately. The pack is usually removed and replaced as necessary.

Following nasal surgery there is danger of hemorrhage. Blood may be evident on the external dressing that is applied under the nose, or the person may expectorate or vomit bright red blood. The back of the throat should be examined to see if blood is running down into it. The patient's pulse may be rapid, or he may swallow repeatedly. Some oozing on the dressing is expected, but if it becomes pronounced or if any other symptoms appear, the surgeon is notified, and material for repacking the nose is prepared. This material consists of a hemostatic tray containing gauze packing, umbilical tape for posterior packing, a few small gauze sponges, a small rubber catheter (used for inserting a postnasal plug), a packing forceps, tongue blades, and scissors. A head mirror, a good light, epinephrine 1:1,000 or some other vasoconstrictor, applicators, a nasal speculum, suction, and metal Frazer tip aspirators should be available.

If the dressing under the nose becomes soiled, it may be changed as necessary. This is very important from an aesthetic standpoint. Sedation and encouragement are necessary because of general discomfort and apprehension caused by having the nasal passages packed and having to breathe through the mouth. Antihistamines may be administered to reduce nasal secretions.

Frequent oral care is given, and fluids are given freely. Since packing blocks the passage of air through the nose, a partial vacuum is created when the person swallows, and he may complain of a sucking action when attempting to drink. Postnasal drainage, the presence of old blood in the mouth, and the loss of the ability to smell lessen the person's appetite. Because it is difficult to eat while the nose is packed, most persons prefer a liquid diet until the packing is removed, but they can have whatever food is tolerated.

In some persons, packing may remain in the nares as long as 1 week, while in others it is removed in 48 hours. After the nasal packing has been removed, the person is asked not to blow the nose for 48 hours because blowing may start bleeding. Fever is reported to the surgeon because it may be caused by infection. Since the person has swallowed blood, it is normal for the stools to be tarry for a day or two. Because the *Valsalva maneuver* can initiate bleeding, the person is instructed not to bear down, and milk of magnesia or prune juice is usually ordered to be given as necessary. The person is also cautioned about coughing too vigorously.

Following external nasal surgery the person frequently has discoloration about the eyes and can be told preoperatively that this will occur. To decrease local edema, the person is kept in a mid-Fowler's position. Ice compresses can be used over the nose for 24 hours to lessen discoloration, bleeding, and discomfort. If a bowl of ice and several wet 4×4-inch gauze sponges are left within easy reach at the bedside, the person can apply the ice compresses himself.

Specific surgical procedures on the nose

Polypectomy. Polypectomy is usually performed in the hospital under local anesthesia. Polyps are removed with a small snare or biting forceps, and the nostrils are packed.[52] Packing is left in place several days. Polypectomy would give lasting relief except that nasal polyps tend to recur and often affect the sinus mucosa, thus requiring ethmoidectomy for more complete removal.

Submucous resection. Submucous resection is used for relief of nasal obstruction related to septal deformities. This surgery is performed under local anesthesia. An internal incision is made on one side of the nasal septum from top to bottom. The mucous membrane is elevated away from the bone, the obstructive parts of the cartilage and bone are removed, and the mucous membrane is sutured back into place. Packing is placed in both nostrils to prevent bleeding and to splint the operative area. *Nasoseptoplasty* is becoming more widely used to treat a deviated nasal septum. Plastic reconstruction (septoplasty) may be necessary if a large part of the septum must be removed.

Rhinoplasty. Reconstruction of the external nose is called rhinoplasty; it is often done for cosmetic reasons and is often combined with septoplasty. Rhinoplasty is an operation that may improve nasal function and will improve appearance. The operation is usually done under local anesthesia, and the nasal bones or cartilaginous framework of the nose are altered. A protective plaster-of-Paris splint, or a dressing of adhesive tape, or a plastic mold usually is placed over the nose after a plastic procedure on the nasal bones and also after a reduction of a fractured nasal septum. When plaster of Paris is used, care must be taken to keep droplets of plaster out of the patient's eyes. If the person has a fractured nose, however, the surgeon usually removes the protective dressing daily to manually mold the broken parts. Firm healing develops about the tenth day. If a splint is used, the skin adjacent to the splint is observed for signs of pressure areas. Usually only the surgeon changes a rhinoplasty dressing. Immediately postoperatively the patient is placed in Fowler's position to minimize oozing. Discoloration about the eyes is common. To avoid disappointment, the person should know that the cosmetic result of the operation cannot be evaluated for several weeks.

Outcome criteria for persons having nasal surgery

The person or significant others can:

1. Describe measures to prevent complications (not blowing nose for 48 hours after packing removed, avoidance of Valsalva maneuver until healing occurs).
2. Describe comfort measures (ice packs, frequent oral care).
3. Describe signs indicating complications (fever, excessive bleeding).
4. State reasons why discoloration of eyes is present.
5. State reasons for not judging cosmetic effect of rhinoplasty until several weeks after surgery.
6. Describe plans for follow-up care.

Management of the person requiring sinus surgery

If the person has recurrent attacks of sinusitis, it may be necessary to provide better drainage by permanently enlarging the sinus openings or by making a new opening and removing the diseased mucous membrane.[53] Surgery usually is performed during the subacute stage of infection. Surgery on the sinuses is done under general as well as under local anesthesia. To prevent swallowing or aspiration of bloody drainage from the nose and throat postoperatively, the patient who has had a general anesthetic is turned well to the side. On recovery from the anesthesia or following local anesthesia, the patient may be in a mid-Fowler's position, which will help decrease edema at the operative site and promote drainage. Ice compresses are usually applied over the nose, or an ice bag is placed directly over the maxillary or frontal sinuses. Ice constricts blood vessels, decreasing oozing and edema, and relieves pain. The patient should be watched carefully for hemorrhage. The nasal drip pad may be changed when it becomes soiled. Excessive bleeding should be called to the surgeon's attention. Repeated swallowing by the patient who is recovering from anesthesia may indicate hemorrhage.

Gauze packing is usually inserted into the nares and usually remains there for 48 hours. Consequently the person breathes through the mouth, and the lips and mouth become dry and need frequent care. Aromatic solutions are refreshing, and petrolatum helps to prevent dryness of the lips. Warm or cool vapor inhalations often are ordered. The person should be reminded not to blow the nose, since this procedure may cause trauma to the operative site and can cause an increase in local blood pressure and cause bleeding.

A gross check of the person's visual acuity is advisable after sinus surgery to be sure that there is no damage to the optic nerve. A check for diplopia is advisable to determine any damage to the nerves or muscles at the globe of the eye. Fever or complaints of tenderness or pain over the involved sinus is reported to the physician, since they may indicate postoperative infection or inadequate drainage. Antibiotics may be given prophylactically. For a week or two postoperatively there may be swelling or ecchymosis of the area. Fluids should be given liberally to all patients following surgery of the sinuses. If there is an oral incision, mouth care is given before meals to improve appetite and after eating to decrease the danger of infection.

Specific surgical procedures on the sinuses

Caldwell-Luc surgery. The Caldwell-Luc operation is surgery of the maxillary sinus through an incision under the upper lip (Fig. 49-9), and is indicated as partial treatment for repeated sinusitis. An opening is made in the anterior wall of the sinus, and the infected contents of the sinus are stripped out. A larger opening in the nose is created to promote better aeration and drainage. The sinus is packed with petrolatum or antibiotic-impregnated gauze for about 48 hours. Numbness of the upper lip and upper teeth may be present for several

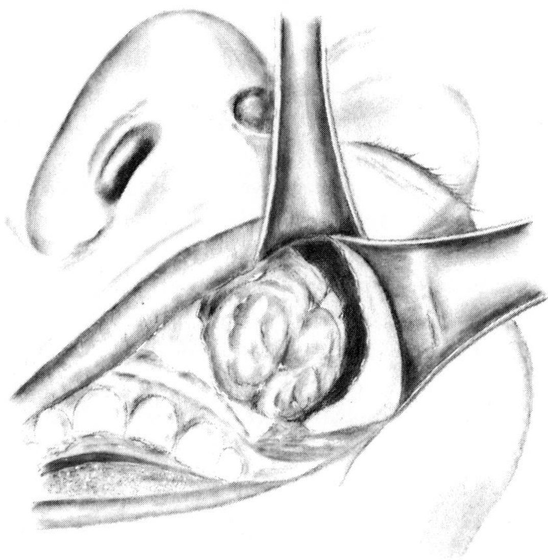

Fig. 49-9. Caldwell-Luc incision under upper lip to expose maxillary sinus. (From Havener, W. H., Saunders, W. H., Keith, C. F., and Prescott, A. W.: Nursing care in eye, ear, nose, and throat disorders, ed. 3, St. Louis, 1974, The C. V. Mosby Co.)

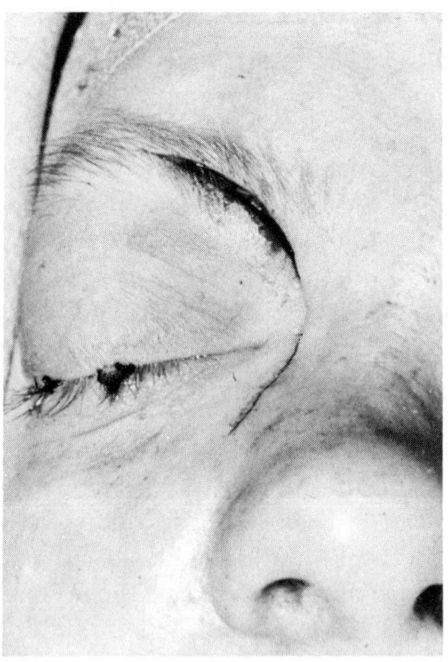

Fig. 49-10. Incision in inner half of eyebrow to expose ethmoid and frontal sinuses. Almost no visible scar results. (From DeWeese, D. D., and Saunders, W. H.: Textbook of otolaryngology, ed. 5, St. Louis, 1977, The C. V. Mosby Co.)

months after a Caldwell-Luc operation because some nerves to these structures pass through the site of the incision.

After Caldwell-Luc surgery, the patient usually is given only liquids for at least 24 hours and a soft diet for several days. The person should not chew on the affected side and should avoid wearing upper dentures for about 10 days, since the plate will rub on the suture line. Oral hygiene is important after Caldwell-Luc surgery, but the person must be careful not to abrade the incision about the teeth. Blowing the nose should be avoided for about 2 weeks after the packing is removed. The Caldwell-Luc operation is usually not performed on children because they may have unerupted teeth near the site of the incision.

Ethmoidectomy. The *ethmoid* sinuses can be surgically approached either intranasally or externally through an incision made in the inner half of the eyebrow downward along the side of the nose[52] (Fig. 49-10). The latter is usually preferred as visualization is better. Ethmoidectomy is performed for ethmoiditis and for correction of nasal polyps, since nasal polyps frequently originate in the ethmoid cells. The *frontal* sinuses are approached by a similar incision as for ethmoidectomy. The *sphenoid* sinuses are approached either intranasally or externally through the eyebrow incision. Sometimes all four sinuses on one side are operated upon together.

Outcome criteria for the person having sinus surgery

The person or significant others can:

1. Describe rationale for frequent oral care.
2. Describe rationale for not blowing the nose until healing occurs.
3. Describe signs of possible complications (fever, sinus pain).
4. State plans for follow-up care.

Surgery for carcinoma of the maxillary or ethmoid sinuses

Surgery for sinal malignancy often consists of removal of the entire upper jaw (maxillectomy) and one eye (orbital exenteration). Split-thickness skin grafts (p. 1049) are usually applied to the operative area. Postoperatively the deformity of the jaw is managed with a dental prosthesis which closes off the defect in the mouth (Fig. 49-11). Radical surgery is required because of the danger of recurrence. Postoperatively the patient must be watched for the complication of meningitis; usually antibiotics are given prophylactically. A nasogastric tube is usually inserted to ensure adequate liquid and caloric intake, since eating is difficult until the prosthesis is fitted. Several different prostheses may be needed before a final one fits because of shrinking of the cavity as healing progresses. All patients are uncomfortable and

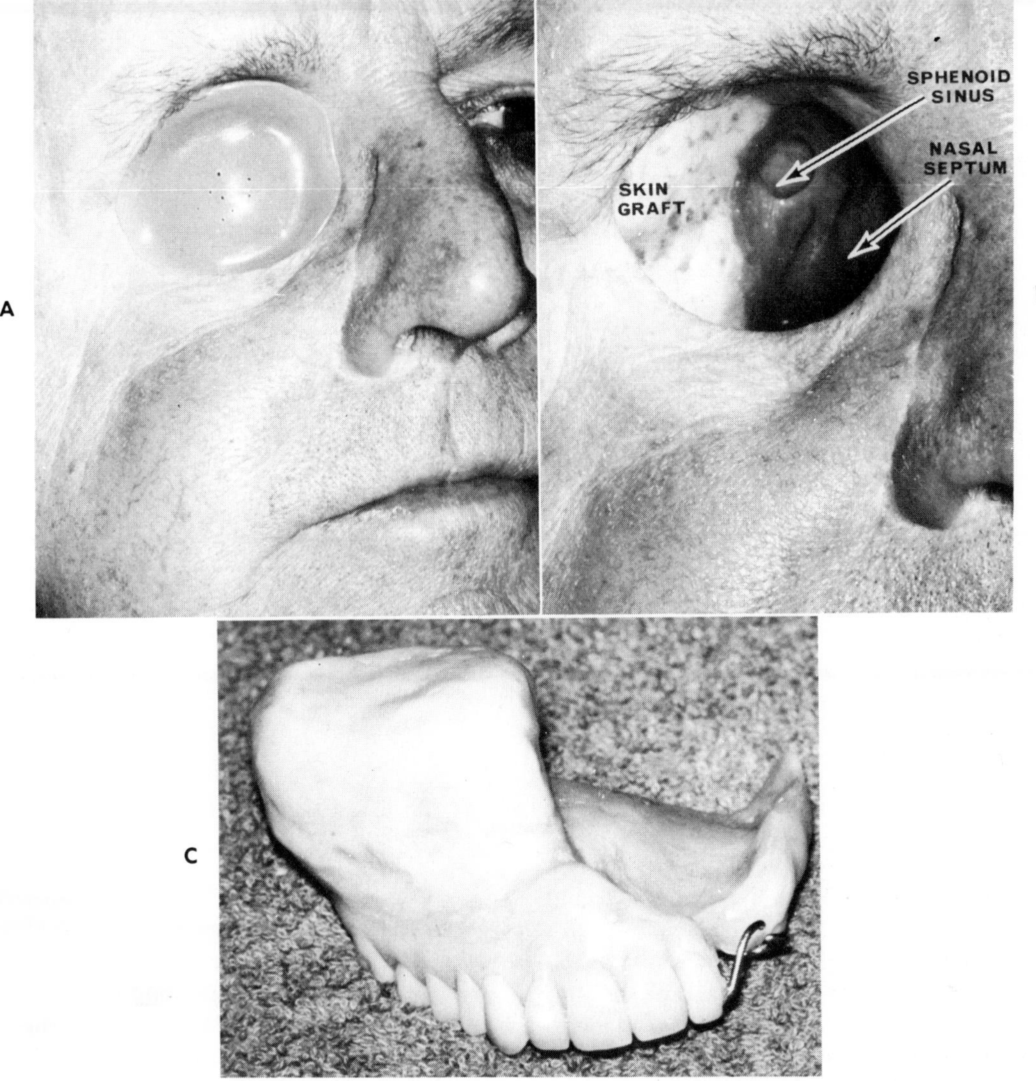

Fig. 49-11. Patient after maxillectomy and orbital exenteration. **A,** Orbital prosthesis in place. Eyeglasses worn over this further improves appearance. **B,** Defect in orbit with skin graft lining upper and lateral wall of orbital-maxillary cavity. **C,** Upper denture worn with large obturator to fill in defect created by maxillectomy. (From Havener, W. H., Saunders, W. H., Keith, C. F., and Prescott, A. W.: Nursing care in eye, ear, nose, and throat disorders, ed. 3, St. Louis, 1974, The C. V. Mosby Co.)

require analgesics following the procedure. Early ambulation is desirable. Maintenance of an airway is critical for these patients.[22,41,44] Often tracheostomy is performed (see p. 947 for care of a patient with tracheostomy).

Mouth care for patients with this type of surgery is important.[41,58,59] Sometimes a gentle spray or oral irrigation using saline with hydrogen peroxide, weak sodium bicarbonate, or antibiotic solution may be used. Because the person may have difficulty swallowing, it may be necessary to aspirate the irrigating solution from the mouth; care must be taken to prevent trauma to the sutures by the suction tip. Management of saliva may also be a problem because of the swallowing difficulty (dysphagia).

Persons who undergo radical surgery of this type have a number of emotional adjustments to make.[31,57,62] The alteration in their physical appearance is readily visible; the person feels conspicuous and different. In addition to disfigurement, the person has all the normal fears of surgery and of cancer. Fear, anger, and grief are normal reactions to the situation. Fear is focused on con-

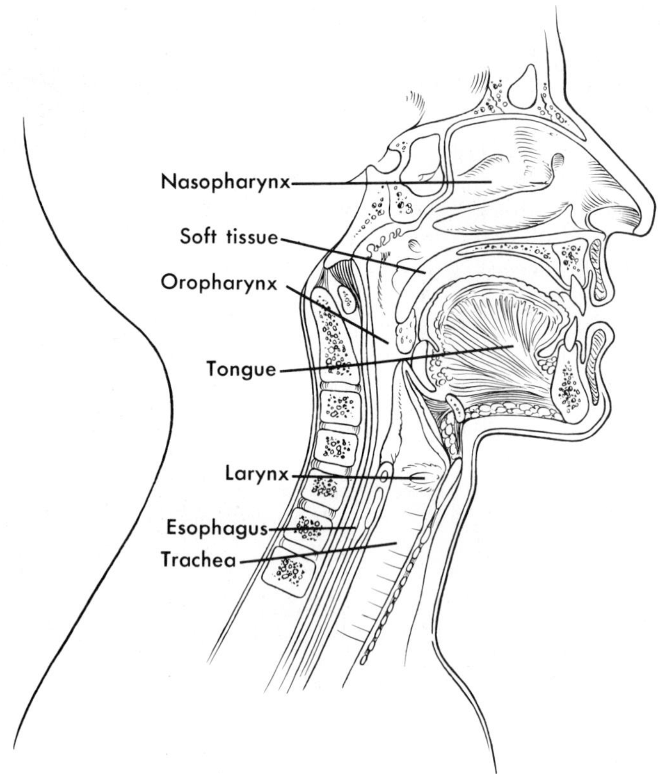

Fig. 49-12. Sagittal section of head showing pharynx and larynx.

cerns about the future, the ability to live normally, and also of being rejected. Anger and grief are common responses to the loss and the helplessness to control the loss. Oral communication also may be a problem immediately following surgery, and every effort is made to allow the person to express needs and feelings by writing if necessary. Conveying compassion and concern to the person is important.

Outcome criteria for the person having radical surgery of the sinuses

The person or significant others can:

1. State plan for achieving adequate nutritional meals.
2. Demonstrate proper care of prosthesis.
3. Demonstrate procedure to be used for maintaining oral hygiene.
4. Describe rationale for not blowing the nose until healing occurs.
5. Describe plans for socialization.
6. State plans for follow-up care.

■ PROBLEMS OF THE UPPER THROAT (PHARYNX AND TONSILS)

□ Anatomy and physiology

The pharynx is the space behind the oral cavity that extends from the base of the skull to the larynx. The pharynx can be considered in three parts: the nasopharynx, the oropharynx, and the hypopharynx (Fig. 49-12). It is lined with mucous membrane. The pharynx contains the adenoids (pharyngeal tonsils), the palatine tonsils, and the lingual tonsils, which are all lymphoid tissue.

□ Inspection

To inspect the pharynx the examiner asks the person to open the mouth without protruding the tongue.[5] A tongue blade is pressed firmly down on the midpoint of the arched tongue; pressing farther back may cause gagging (Fig. 49-13). The person then says "ah" while breathing through the mouth to prevent gagging.

The oropharynx, that portion of the pharynx directly posterior to the oral cavity bounded by the nasopharynx above and laryngopharynx below, is examined with a tongue blade and a mirror. The anterior and posterior pillars, the uvula, tonsils, and posterior pharynx are inspected for color, symmetry, evidence of exudate, edema, ulceration, and tonsillar enlargement. Redness and swelling of the tonsils, pillars, and uvula with white or yellow exudate on the tonsils may indicate streptococcal infection. Tonsils may be enlarged without being infected.

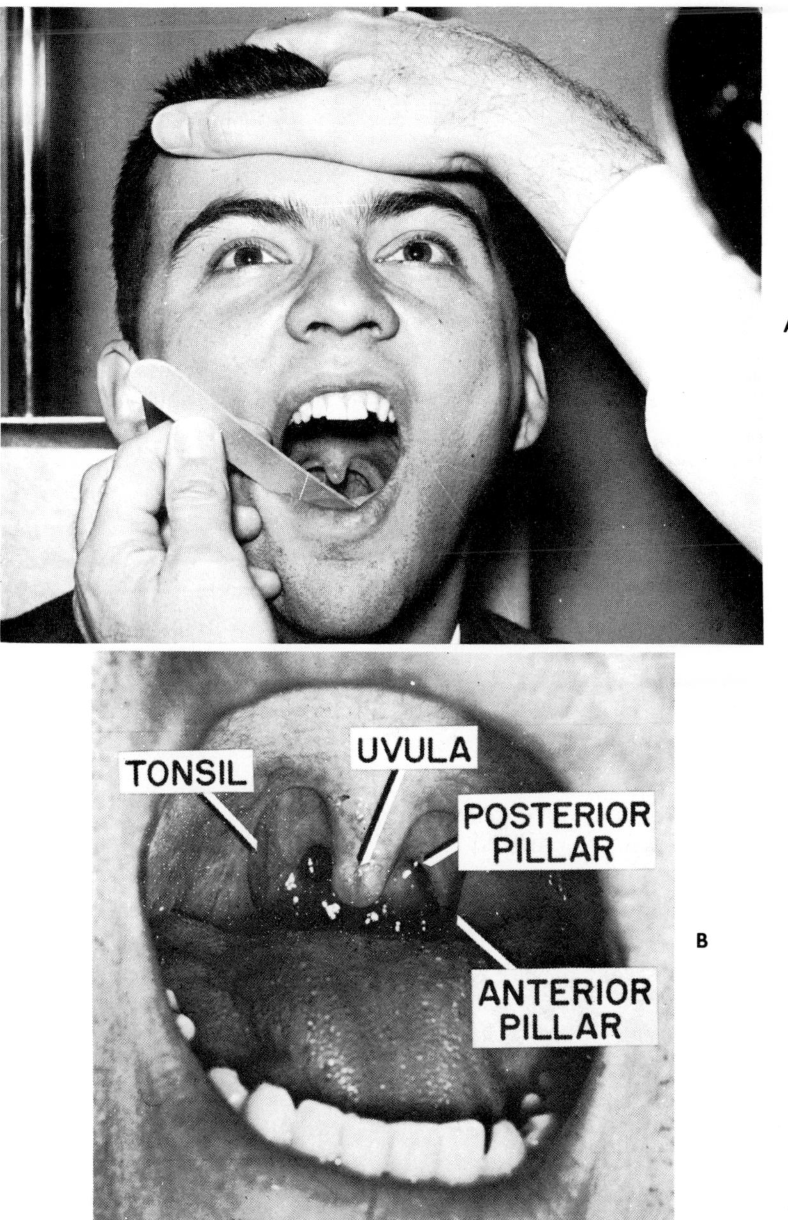

Fig. 49-13. A, Depressing of tongue. Tongue blade is held in left hand, which leaves right hand free for positioning of head and use of other instruments. Hand is braced on patient's cheek as tongue is depressed and scooped forward. **B,** Landmarks of pharynx. (**A** from Saunders, W. H.: Ears, nose, and throat. In Prior, J. A., and Silberstein, J. S.: Physical diagnosis, ed. 5, St. Louis, 1977, The C. V. Mosby Co.; **B** from Havener, W. H., Saunders, W. H., Keith, C. F., and Prescott, A. W.: Nursing care in eye, ear, nose, and throat disorders, ed. 3, St. Louis, 1974, The C. V. Mosby Co.)

□ Specific problems

Chronic enlargement of the tonsils and adenoids

Tonsils and adenoids are lymphoid structures located in the oropharynx and the nasopharynx. They reach their full size in childhood and begin to atrophy during puberty. When adenoids enlarge, usually as a result of chronic infections but sometimes for no known reason, they cause nasal obstruction. The person breathes through the mouth, may have a dull facial expression, and may have a reduced appetite, since the blocked nasopharynx can interfere with swallowing. In children, enlarged adenoids may block openings to the eustachian tubes in the nasopharynx, predisposing to middle ear infections and hearing impairment. Hypertrophy of the tonsils does not usually block the oropharynx but may affect speech and swallowing and cause mouth breathing. Occasionally adenotonsillar hypertrophy in children may so restrict breathing as to precipitate pulmonary hypertension and cor pulmonale. The condition is reversed by surgical removal of the tonsils and adenoids.

Infections

Acute pharyngitis. Acute pharyngitis is the most common throat inflammation. It may be caused by hemolytic streptococci, staphylococci, or other bacteria or filtrable viruses. There is increased evidence of gonococcal pharyngitis. A severe form of acute pharyngitis often is referred to as "strep throat" because of the frequency of streptococci as the causative organisms. Dryness of the throat is a common complaint. The throat appears red, and soreness may range from slight scratchiness to severe pain with difficulty in swallowing. A hacking cough may be present. Children often develop a very high fever, while adults may have only a mild elevation of temperature. Symptoms usually precede or occur simultaneously with the onset of acute rhinitis or acute sinusitis. Pharyngitis can occur after the tonsils have been removed, since the remaining mucous membrane can become infected.[37] Pharyngitis is also a common manifestation of infectious mononucleosis (p. 1079).

Acute pharyngitis usually is relieved by hot saline throat gargles. An ice collar may make the person feel more comfortable. The physician may prescribe acetylsalicylic acid administered orally as a gargle or in Aspergum. Lozenges containing a mild anesthetic may help relieve the local soreness. Moist inhalations may help relieve the dryness of the throat. A liquid diet usually is more easily tolerated, and fluids to at least 2.5 liters per day are encouraged. Oral hygiene may prevent drying and cracking of the lips and usually refreshes the mouth. If the temperature is elevated, the person should remain in bed, and even if he is ambulatory and has no fever, he should have extra rest. Occasionally antibiotics such as penicillin or erythromycin are used to treat severe infections, or they are prescribed prophylactically to prevent superimposed infections, particularly in persons who have a history of rheumatic fever or bacterial endocarditis (see discussion of rheumatic fever, p. 985). Most pharyngitis in children is caused by viruses; therefore antibiotics should not be used for treatment, since antibiotics are not effective against viruses.

Acute follicular tonsillitis. Acute follicular tonsillitis is an acute inflammation of the tonsils and their crypts. It is usually caused by the *Streptococcus* organism. It is more likely to occur when the person's resistance is low and is very common in children. The onset is almost always sudden, and symptoms include sore throat, pain on swallowing, fever, chills, general muscle aching, and malaise. In children the temperature may rise suddenly to 40.5 C (105 F). These symptoms often last for 2 or 3 days. The pharynx and the tonsils appear red, and the peritonsillar tissues are swollen. Sometimes a yellowish exudate drains from crypts in the tonsils. A throat culture usually is taken to identify the offending organism. The person with acute tonsillitis is encouraged to rest and take generous amounts of fluids orally. Warm saline throat irrigation may be ordered, and antibiotics are usually given. Acetylsalicylic acid and sometimes codeine sulfate may be ordered for pain and discomfort. An ice collar may be applied to the neck, and if the temperature remains above 39 C (102 F), an alcohol sponge bath may be given. Until the temperature subsides and the sore throat improves, a bland diet is given. Complications of untreated tonsillitis include heart and kidney damage, chorea, and pneumonia. Incidence of these complications is decreasing with the widespread use of penicillin and early diagnosis. Most physicians believe that persons who have recurrent attacks of tonsillitis should have a tonsillectomy. This procedure is usually performed from 4 to 6 weeks after an acute attack has subsided.

Since the person with acute tonsillitis is usually cared for at home,[13] the nurse should help in teaching the general public the care that is needed. The office nurse, the clinic nurse, the nurse in industry, the school nurse, and the community health nurse have many opportunities to do this teaching.

Outcome criteria for the person with pharyngitis or tonsillitis. The person or significant others can:

1. Describe measures for relief of discomfort (hot gargles, ice collar, moist inhalations, mouth care).
2. State rationale for prophylactic antibiotic therapy for pharyngitis in persons with a history of rheumatic fever or bacterial endocarditis.
3. State plans for drinking at least 2.5 liters of fluid per day (adults).
4. Describe symptoms indicating need for medical supervision (recurrence, prolonged fever, excessive pain, presence of pus, dysphagia).
5. State plans for follow-up care, if appropriate.

Peritonsillar abscess. A peritonsillar abscess, or quinsy, is an uncommon, local complication of acute follicular tonsillitis in which infection extends from the tonsil to form an abscess in the surrounding tissues. The presence of pus behind the tonsil causes difficulty in swallowing, talking, and opening the mouth, and the person may be unable to swallow. Pain is severe and may extend to the ear on the affected side. If antibiotics to which the offending organism is sensitive are administered early, infection subsides. It is felt that some cases of peritonsillar abscess are caused by anaerobic organisms. In these instances, hydrogen peroxide (an oxidizing agent) in the form of a mouthwash may help relieve symptoms. Acute streptococcal or staphylococcal tonsillitis may also cause a peritonsillar abscess to form. If an abscess forms, incision and drainage are necessary. During the operation the patient's head usually is lowered and suction is applied as soon as the incision is made to prevent the patient from aspirating the drainage. Warm saline irrigations, an ice collar, or narcotics may help relieve discomfort. If acute follicular tonsillitis is treated adequately, peritonsillar abscess is unlikely to occur.

Diphtheria. Diphtheria is a serious disease of the throat that most often affects children. It is caused by the bacillus *Corynebacterium diphtheriae.* It is highly contagious and is transmitted by droplet nuclei. There are also "carriers," that is, healthy people who carry the illness even though they are not ill. The incidence of diphtheria has rapidly decreased because of effective immunization programs. Occasional infections do occur, which increases the importance of preventive measures. Parents should be strongly encouraged to have their children immunized with the DPT (diphtheria, pertussis, tetanus) immunizations. Three separate injections are given, 1 month apart, beginning when the infant is about 2 months old.

Malignancy of the tonsils

Malignancy of the tonsils is second only to malignancy of the larynx in malignancies of the upper respiratory tract. The malignancy can be one of three types: carcinoma, lymphoepithelioma, or lymphosarcoma. Carcinomas are more common in men, possibly related to the increased incidence of smoking among men. The carcinomas spread upward into the soft palate and usually metastasize early to the neck. Local ulceration and otalgia (earache) are early symptoms. Lymphoepitheliomas often remain small and do not ulcerate, but neck metastasis occurs early. Lymphosarcomas produce large tonsils, usually without ulceration or pain, and metastasize early to the neck. Medical intervention for all tonsillar malignancies includes irradiation, which usually produces a good initial response. Recurrence often occurs locally or with distant metastasis.[23]

□ Surgical procedures

Tonsillectomy and adenoidectomy

The tonsils and adenoids are removed when the adenoids become enlarged and cause symptoms of obstruction, when they are chronically infected, when the person has repeated attacks of tonsillitis, or after peritonsillar abcess. Chronic infections of these structures usually do not respond to antibiotics, and they may become foci of infection, spreading organisms to other parts of the body such as the heart. If a child's tonsils must be removed, the adenoids, even if they are not infected or enlarged, usually are removed also as a prophylactic measure. If possible, the removal of the tonsils is postponed until the child is about 6 years of age, but obstructing adenoids may be removed earlier. The former practice of routinely removing tonsils and adenoids for recurrent upper respiratory infections is no longer advocated.

Preoperative care. The patient who is to have a tonsillectomy and adenoidectomy usually is admitted to the hospital on the morning of the operation. Some physicians prefer that the child be admitted the evening before surgery so that he can become accustomed to the hospital and have special laboratory tests. These tests would include a partial thromboplastin time test and for black children a sickle cell preparation test. Children should be carefully prepared for surgery by their parents and the professional staff who care for them.

The complete examination is carried out in the physician's office, but the general physical condition, urine, blood count, and bleeding and clotting times are rechecked before surgery. In children the operation is performed under general anesthesia, while in adults the tonsillectomy may be done under either general or local anesthesia. In the operating room, after the tonsils are removed, pressure is applied to stop superficial bleeding. Occasionally bleeding vessels are tied off with sutures, or an electrocoagulation current is used.

Postoperative care. Postoperatively the person who has had a tonsillectomy may have a small amount of dark, bloody drainage from the operative area and may vomit blood that has been swallowed. The person is placed on the side or abdomen with a pillow under the chest until fully reacted from the anesthesia (Fig. 49-14). When the patient is awake, he is permitted to sit up in a mid-Fowler's position. Sometimes an ice collar is applied about the throat for comfort and to lessen the chance of hemorrhage. Young children usually resist the application of an ice collar, and therefore it is not used.

Bleeding. Following a tonsillectomy or an adenoidectomy the patient should be watched carefully for signs of hemorrhage. The person is urged not to cough or attempt to clear the throat immediately after surgery and thereafter, since these actions may initiate bleeding. Efforts are made to prevent the small child from crying lustily, and if he has fully responded from anesthesia, he may be rocked. If the person swallows frequently, hemorrhage should be suspected, and the throat is inspected, since any signs of hemorrhage must be reported to the surgeon at once. Vomitus containing bright red

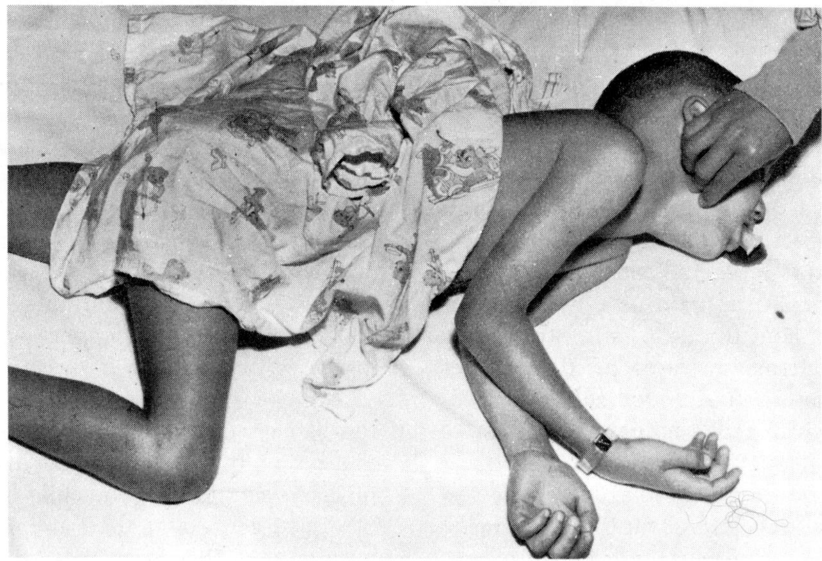

Fig. 49-14. Child is in recovery room after tonsillectomy. Note that he is propped on his side. Oral airway is in place. Nurse is supporting jaw to assist airway. (From Havener, W. H., Saunders, W. H., Keith, C. F., and Prescott, A. W.: Nursing care in eye, ear, nose, and throat disorders, ed. 3, St. Louis, 1974, The C. V. Mosby Co.)

blood is reported, and the specimen is saved for the surgeon's inspection. It is especially important to observe the sleeping patient for signs of hemorrhage, since he may swallow blood and lose a very large amount of it without any external evidence of bleeding. The pulse rate is taken every 15 minutes for the first hour and every 30 minutes for several hours thereafter.

The physician may be able to control minor postoperative bleeding by applying a sponge soaked in a solution of epinephrine to the site. The person who is bleeding excessively often is returned to the operating room for surgical treatment to stop the hemorrhage. This may be done by ligating or by cauterizing the bleeding vessel. If sutures must be used, the person will have more pain and discomfort than he would have following a simple tonsillectomy. He may be unable to take solid foods until the sutures have been absorbed. Some otolaryngologists no longer prescribe acetylsalicylic acid for pain after tonsillectomy, since it increases the tendency to bleed. Acetaminophen or another aspirin substitute is usually ordered.

Diet. When vomiting has ceased, fluids and bland nourishment are offered. While the person usually will only take small amounts because of pain, he is urged to take large swallows because they hurt less and because more fluid can thus be taken. Drinking through a straw is not advisable because of the danger of physical trauma and because the suction on the throat may cause bleeding. Ice cold fluids are most acceptable and are given frequently. Ice cream usually is well tolerated, and ginger ale, cold milk, and cold custard often are offered next, followed by cream soups and bland juices such as pear juice. The morning after surgery the person is usually offered foods such as refined cereal and soft-cooked or poached eggs. When he goes home, he is advised to avoid citrus fruit juices, hot fluids, rough foods such as raw vegetables and crackers, and highly seasoned foods for at least 1 week because these foods irritate the operative area.

Discharge teaching. Most persons are discharged from the hospital the day after surgery; some are permitted to return home the night of the operation, and if so, the child's parents are instructed to watch for bleeding and to report it to the physician at once. The child is usually kept indoors for 3 days. Usually the person is told to avoid vigorous exercise, coughing, sneezing, clearing of the throat, and vigorous blowing of the nose, since these actions can cause bleeding. If bleeding occurs at any time, the physician should be contacted immediately. The tough, yellow fibrous membrane that forms over the operative site begins to break away between the fourth and eighth postoperative days, and hemorrhage may occur. The separation of the membrane accounts for the throat being more painful at this time. Pink granulation tissues soon become apparent, and by the end of the third postoperative week the area is covered with mucous membrane of normal appearance.

The adult patient or the parents of a young child are

given specific instructions for home care, and most hospitals and otolaryngologists have these in written form. Acceptable foods and fluids are outlined, and the diet can be increased as tolerated. The person should continue to drink sufficient fluids (2 to 3 liters daily) to help relieve the objectionable mouth odor common after any oral surgery. The stool may be black or dark for a few days because blood has been swallowed during surgery.

A temperature of 37.5 to 38.5 C (99 to 101 F) may occur after tonsillectomy, but a persistent temperature elevation is reported to the physician. Discomfort in the ears may also occur and should be reported if it persists. The person usually reports to the surgeon for a follow-up examination about 1 week after the operation.

Outcome criteria for the person who has had a tonsillectomy and adenoidectomy. The person or significant others can:

1. Describe rationale for not coughing, clearing throat, and blowing nose until healing occurs.
2. State plans to avoid citrus juices and hot, rough, or spicy foods.
3. Demonstrate procedure for gargling if ordered.
4. State plans for restricting activity for 2 to 3 days after discharge.
5. Describe signs that indicate possible complications (excessive bleeding, persistent fever).
6. State plans for follow-up care.

■ PROBLEMS OF THE LOWER THROAT (LARYNX)

□ Anatomy and physiology

The larynx forms the upper extremity of the trachea. The framework of the larynx is made up of several cartilages held together by muscle and ligaments. The cartilaginous framework of the larynx protects the vocal cords and affords a stiffness that permits an airway. The thyroid cartilage, the "Adam's apple," is the largest cartilaginous element in the larynx and serves to protect the inner structures. The hyoid bone lies just above the thyroid cartilage and forms an attachment for the larynx and tongue. The cricoid cartilage lies just below the thyroid cartilage and articulates with the arytenoid cartilages, which swing in and out to open and close the vocal cords, opening and closing the glottis. The larynx is lined with mucosa continuous with that of the hypopharynx and trachea. The vagus nerve innervates the larynx by means of the recurrent laryngeal nerve.

The chief function of the larynx is to serve as an airway between the pharynx and trachea. Because the glottis opens and closes, aspiration of food or fluids is prevented during swallowing. The closing of the glottis also allows for an increase of intrathoracic pressure, which is needed, for example, in coughing or lifting. This increased pressure gives added advantage to the use of the muscles of the shoulder and thorax. In addition to these, a most important function of the larynx is *phonation.* The larynx creates sounds as a result of vocal cord vibrations that are formed into speech patterns by the movement of the pharynx, palate, tongue, teeth, and lips.

□ Assessment

The larynx may be examined by an indirect laryngoscopy; the patient sits in a chair with the head tilted back and is asked to stick out the tongue. The examiner then grasps it with a gauze sponge and pulls it forward and downward. A warmed laryngeal mirror is introduced into the back of the throat until the larynx is visualized. It is examined at rest and during attempts to speak (phonation). If the gag reflex is very sensitive, the pharyngeal wall may be sprayed with a topical anesthetic such as 2% cocaine or 2% pontocaine. Pontocaine is preferred by some physicians because it is less toxic than cocaine. A direct laryngoscopy is performed on children, on adults who are unable to cooperate for an indirect examination, and on all persons with suspicious lesions of the larynx.[12] Direct laryngoscopy is usually performed under local anesthesia with 10% cocaine or under general anesthesia. A sedative such as secobarbital, meperidine, or other narcotic and atropine sulfate is given 1 hour before the examination. Atropine is essential prior to both local and general anesthesia because it reduces the volume of secretions. For direct laryngoscopy the person is placed in a reclining position, with the head in a head holder. If no head holder is available, the person's head is extended over the edge of the table and manually supported by a physician or nurse. In some cases a suspension device may be applied to the laryngoscope so that the physician's hands are free for instrumentation or manipulation of the focus of the microscope.

The laryngoscope, a hollow, metal tube with a handle at the proximal end and a light at the distal end, is introduced by a physician through the mouth into the hypopharynx, elevating the epiglottis, and making the interior of the larynx easily visible. Minor surgical procedures such as a biopsy or the removal of a small benign tumor may be performed through this instrument.

After a laryngoscopy under local anesthesia, the person should not eat or drink anything until the gag reflex returns, usually within 2 hours. The gag reflex can be tested by "tickling" the throat with a tongue blade or applicator. After the gag reflex returns the person should try first to drink water, since if it is accidentally aspirated into the trachea or lungs, it is the fluid least likely to cause aspiration pneumonia.

Microlaryngoscopy using an operating microscope is becoming more widely used (Fig. 49-15). This method provides magnification and binocular vision.

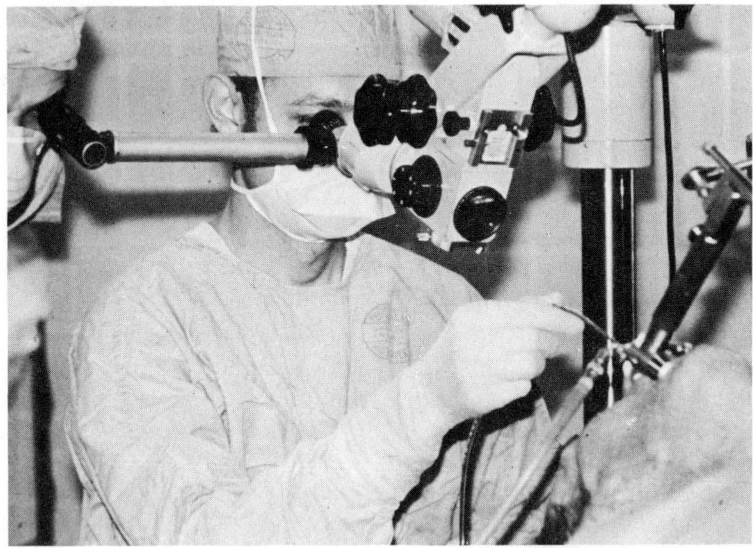

Fig. 49-15. Laryngoscopy using operating microscope to provide both illumination and magnification. Laryngoscope is self-retaining. (From DeWeese, D. D., and Saunders, W. H.: Textbook of otolaryngology, ed. 5, St. Louis, 1977, The C. V. Mosby Co.)

The interior of the larynx may also be visualized by radiographs. Radiopaque contrast material is instilled into the larynx (as in a bronchogram.) These radiographs are less commonly used than laryngoscopy. Xerography is also used to evaluate the larynx.

□ Problems

Laryngitis

Simple acute laryngitis. Simple acute laryngitis is an inflammation of the mucous membrane lining the larynx accompanied by edema of the vocal cords. It may be caused by a cold, by sudden changes in temperature, or by irritating fumes. Symptoms vary from a slight huskiness to a complete loss of voice. The throat may be painful and feel scratchy, and a cough may be present. Laryngitis usually requires only symptomatic treatment. The person is advised to remain indoors in an even temperature and to avoid talking for several days or weeks, depending on the severity of the inflammation. Steam inhalations with aromatic vapors such as tincture of benzoin, oil of pine, and menthol may be soothing. Cough syrups or home remedies for coughs provide relief to some persons. Smoking or being where others are smoking should be avoided.

Acute laryngitis may cause acute respiratory distress and prostration in children under 5 years of age. Because the larynx of the infant and young child is relatively small and is susceptible to spasm when irritated or infected, it easily becomes partially or totally obstructed. After exposure to cold air or as a result of an upper respiratory infection, the child may develop a hoarse, barking cough and an inspiratory stridor (a form of *croup*). He may become restless, the muscles about the clavicle may be visibly retracted as he attempts to get more air, and his nostrils may flare. The child may sit up and grasp his throat as he tries to breathe. He may be completely well before and after the attack, which may last 30 minutes to 3 hours. The usual treatment is the administration of copious amounts of vaporized cool mist. Some children's hospitals have "croup rooms" where a continuous "fog" of cool mist is generated into the room. If cool mist is not available, warm steam inhalations may be used to provide humidity and liquefy secretions. In the home an improvised steam room can be created by running a hot shower.

A second and more deadly form of croup syndrome in young children between 2 and 12 years of age is *acute epiglottitis.*[50] The child rapidly develops fever, inspiratory stridor, and progressive toxicity. The symptoms are caused by inflammatory edema of the epiglottis from the *Haemophilus hemolyticus* organism.

The treatment of acute laryngitis is intravenous antibiotics (usually ampicillin), intravenous steroids, and other supportive measures. The steroid therapy appears to prevent the necessity of tracheostomy or endotracheal intubation.

The airway must remain patent to prevent suffocation, and an artificial airway, however, may be necessary. In certain emergency situations, when endotracheal intubation or tracheostomy equipment are not available, the most expedient method of establishing an airway to avoid asphyxia and death is to perform a "mini-tracheotomy" or cricothyroid stab. A large-bore intravenous needle may be inserted into the cricothyroid space.[43] The needle is inserted slightly downward and backward. Another method of maintaining an airway during an acute attack of epiglottitis is by using a breathing bag attached to a mask and performing positive pressure ventilation. This method seems to be most helpful when the medical treatment has already been started but has not yet been effective, or when the patient must be transferred to another unit and tracheostomy is to be avoided if possible.[27]

The child with croup will be less frightened if he is held or if someone stays with him during the attack. Ordinarily, sedatives will not be ordered, since they tend to depress the person's limited respiratory effort. For severe attacks not relieved by conservative treatment, corticosteroids in high doses are usually administered parentally. If the person's condition becomes worse despite treatment, a tracheostomy may be necessary.

Chronic laryngitis. Some people who use their voices excessively, who smoke a great deal, or who work continuously where there are irritating fumes develop a chronic laryngitis. Hoarseness usually is worse in the early morning and in the evening. There may be a dry, harsh cough and a persistent need to clear the throat. Treatment may consist of removal of irritants, voice rest, correction of faulty voice habits, steam inhalations, and cough medications. The physician may order spraying of the throat with an astringent antiseptic solution such as hexylresorcinol (S.T. 37). To carry out this procedure properly the person must use a spray tip that turns down at the end so that the medication reaches vocal cords and is not dissipated in the posterior pharynx. The spray tip is placed in the back of the throat with the bent portion behind the tongue. The person should then take one or two deep breaths and spray the medication on inhalation. This procedure may cause temporary coughing and gagging. Many medications used as throat sprays are now sold in plastic squeeze bottles with tube and spray tip attached.

Laryngeal paralysis

Laryngeal paralysis may result from disease or injury of either the laryngeal nerves or the vagus nerve. Some causes of this include aortic aneurysm, mitral stenosis, bronchial carcinoma, neck injuries, and severing or stretching of the recurrent laryngeal nerve during thyroidectomy. Hoarseness may be present, but the only diagnostic method is laryngoscopy. Either one or both vocal cords may be paralyzed. If only one cord is affected, the airway is adequate and only the voice may be affected.[12] Efforts to improve the voice in persons with unilateral cord paralysis have been accomplished by injecting a small quantity of Teflon into the paralyzed cord. This swells the cord and pushes it toward the midline where the other cord can approximate it better during phonation. With bilateral paralysis the voice is weak. Bilateral paralysis causes a poor airway that results in incapacitating dyspnea and stridor upon exertion. Treatment of bilateral cord paralysis is aimed at restoration of the airway, not at improvement of the voice. An arytenoidectomy may be performed, which consists of resection of one of the arytenoid cartilages, thus increasing the diameter of the posterior portion of the glottis sufficiently to improve breathing. If both cords are paralyzed and the airway is inadequate, a tracheostomy will be necessary to restore the airway.

Laryngeal edema

Acute laryngeal edema is a potential medical emergency and may be caused by anaphylaxis, urticaria, acute laryngitis, serious inflammatory disease of the throat, and edema following intubation.[25] Acute laryngeal edema causes the airway to narrow or close and requires restoration of the airway. Treatment of acute laryngeal edema consists of administration of an adrenal corticosteroid or epinephrine. A tracheostomy or intubation may be necessary. Edema of the larynx may be chronic because of irradiation treatment of the larynx or tumors of the neck, thus requiring a tracheostomy.

Carcinoma

Squamous cell carcinoma of the larynx is increasing in frequency. It is estimated that in the United States there were over 9,000 new cases in 1976.[2] Cancer of the larynx limited to the true vocal cords grows slowly because of the limited lymphatic supply. Elsewhere in the larynx, such as the epiglottis, false vocal cords, and pyriform sinuses, lymph vessels are abundant, and cancer of these tissues often spreads rapidly and metastasizes early to the deep lymph nodes of the neck.

Cancer of the larynx is eight times more common in men than in women, and it occurs most often in persons over 60 years of age. There appears to be some relationship between cancer of the larynx and heavy smoking, alcohol, chronic laryngitis, vocal abuse, and family predisposition to cancer. Because of the increase in the number of women who are heavy smokers, some specialists believe that the incidence of carcinoma of the larynx among this group will increase. Any person who becomes progressively hoarse or is hoarse for longer than 2 weeks should be urged to seek medical attention at once. Hoarseness is an early symptom of cancer of the vocal cords. If treatment is given when hoarseness appears (caused by the tumor's preventing the complete approximation of the vocal cord), a cure usually is possible. Signs of metastases of cancer to other parts of the larynx include a sensation of a lump in the throat, pain in the Adam's apple that radiates to the ear, dyspnea, dysphagia, enlarged cervical nodes, and cough. The diagnosis of cancer of the larynx is made from the history, from visual examination of the larynx with a laryngoscope, and from a biopsy and microscopic study of the lesion.

Surgical procedures

Partial laryngectomy

If the tumor has not involved the muscles, a partial laryngectomy may effect a cure in early carcinoma of the vocal cords. Recent studies have indicated that mobility of the cord does not necessarily have to be normal in order to perform a partial laryngectomy.[25] The most common technique for partial laryngectomy is to make an opening into the larynx through the thyroid cartilage (laryngofissure) and remove the involved cord and tumor. As healing takes place, scar tissue fills the defect where the diseased cord was removed and becomes a vibrating surface within the larynx. This tissue permits husky but acceptable speech. A tracheostomy tube is inserted at the time of operation but is removed when edema in the surrounding tissues subsides. For 48 hours postoperatively, nutrients may be supplied intravenously or by a nasogastric tube. Fluids and soft foods may then be taken orally. Soft foods may be easier for the pharyngeal musculature to handle than fluids. Foods usually well tolerated include scrambled eggs, cottage cheese, and baked potatoes. Other care is similar to that given any patient having a tracheostomy.

A hemilaryngectomy, which removes one-half or more of the larynx, is performed for more extensive lesions involving one side of the larynx that are too extensive for a laryngofissure and cordectomy. A supraglottic partial laryngectomy is performed for lesions that involve laryngeal structures above the vocal cords. The postoperative rehabilitation of persons with these two procedures is more arduous than those with a laryngofissure.

The person who has had a partial laryngectomy usually is not on absolute voice rest but is not permitted to use his voice until the surgeon gives specific approval (usually 3 days postoperatively). He should then only whisper until healing is complete, after which time he usually adjusts quite readily to his relatively minor limitation of speech. The main problems encountered by patients undergoing partial laryngectomy are those of swallowing and aspiration.

Total laryngectomy

When cancer of the larynx is advanced, a total laryngectomy may be performed. This includes removal of the epiglottis, thyroid cartilage, hyoid bone, cricoid cartilage, and two or three rings of the trachea. The pharyngeal opening to the trachea is closed, the anterior wall of the esophagus is reinforced, and the remaining trachea is brought out to the neck wound and sutured to the skin. It forms an opening (permanent tracheostomy) through which the patient breathes (Fig. 49-16).

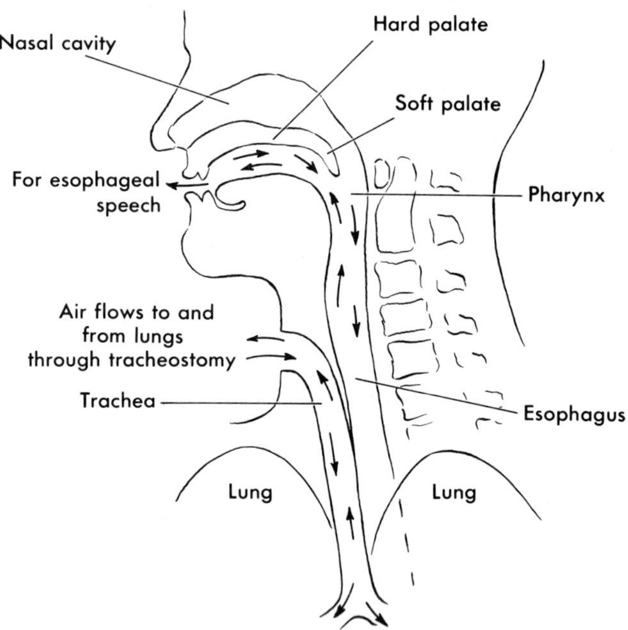

Fig. 49-16. Permanent opening in trachea following total laryngectomy. Note that nose is not used for breathing and that all air enters through tracheostomy opening. Air swallowed through mouth is used to produce laryngeal speech. (Redrawn from Havener, W. H., Saunders, W. H., Keith, C. F., and Prescott, A. W.: Nursing care in eye, ear, nose, and throat disorders, ed. 3, St. Louis, 1974, The C. V. Mosby Co.)

The sense of smell is often affected after laryngectomy. The presence of an opening in the trachea has a deleterious effect on the sense of smell; this may be a result of simply not breathing through the nose so that the patient does not get olfactory sensations or of airflow patterns that do not stimulate the trigeminal nerve and therefore olfaction is not evident.

The person who is to have a laryngectomy is told by the physician that he will breathe through a special opening made in his neck and that he no longer will have normal speech. He is often depressed by this, as it threatens his economic status as well as his life. In some instances it is helpful for him to be visited by another person who has made a good recovery from laryngectomy and who has undergone rehabilitation successfully. In other instances this visit may depress the patient further. Careful assessment must be made of each person to determine if he will benefit from such a visit and

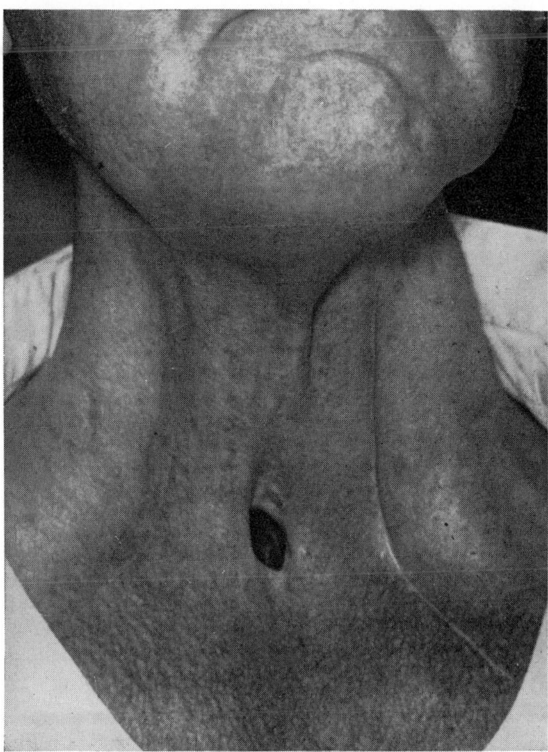

Fig. 49-17. After laryngectomy. Note scars of bilateral radical neck dissections. (From DeWeese, D. D., and Saunders, W. H.: Textbook of otolaryngology, ed. 5, St. Louis, 1977, The C. V. Mosby Co.)

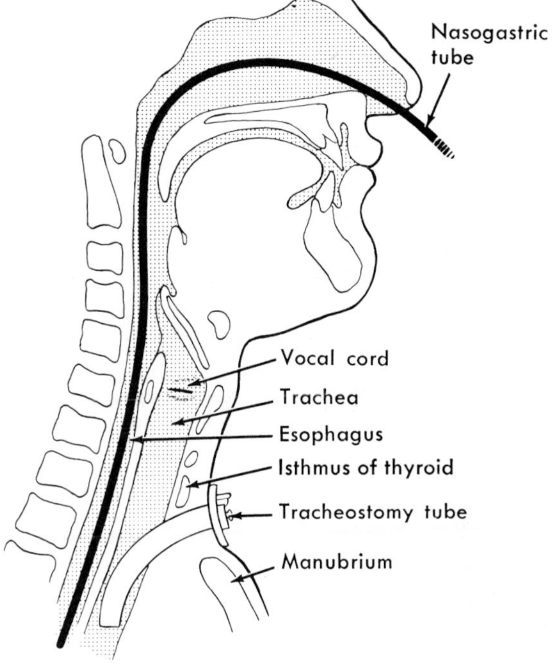

Fig. 49-18. Position of tracheostomy tube and nasogastric tube if both are used.

whether the visit should be made preoperatively, immediately after surgery, or later in the recovery period. Often no one else can give a person the reassurance that he can regain speech as well as a fellow patient. Many large cities have a "Lost Chord Club" or a "New Voice Club," and the members are willing to visit hospitalized patients. Information regarding these clubs may be obtained by writing to the International Association of Laryngectomees.* Local speech rehabilitation centers may supply instructive films and other resources. The local chapter of the American Cancer Society and the local health department also have information available. If possible, the family also should learn about the method of esophageal speech that the person will learn to use.

Preoperative and postoperative care of the person is essentially the same as that described for tracheostomy (p. 947) except that these persons will have a laryngectomy tube in place, a tube that is shorter and wider in diameter than a tracheostomy tube. Some patients may not have a tube in the stoma after the operation because the stoma is a permanent one kept open initially by the sutures and because their surgeon believes that there is less tissue reaction and a better stoma if no tube is used. Most otolaryngologists believe that a laryngectomy tube is better than a tracheostomy tube because it is shorter and there is less danger that it will obstruct the left mainstem bronchus. The tube will remain until the wound is healed and a permanent fistula has formed, usually in 2 or 3 weeks (Fig. 49-17). Frequent suctioning is necessary in the early postoperative period to keep the trachea free of secretions.

A nasogastric tube may be inserted during the surgical procedure for the instillation of food and fluids at regular intervals postoperatively (Fig. 49-18). The use of the tube to give food is thought to minimize contamination of the pharyngeal and esophageal suture lines and to prevent fluid from leaking through the wound into the trachea before healing occurs. Some surgeons feel that, with modern suturing and drainage techniques, tube feedings are not necessary, and they permit the patient to take food and fluids orally after the second postoperative day. If the nasogastric tube is used, it is removed as soon as the person can safely swallow. The person then needs careful attention in his first attempts to swallow. He may feel that he is choking and may have severe

*219 East 42nd St., New York, NY 10017.

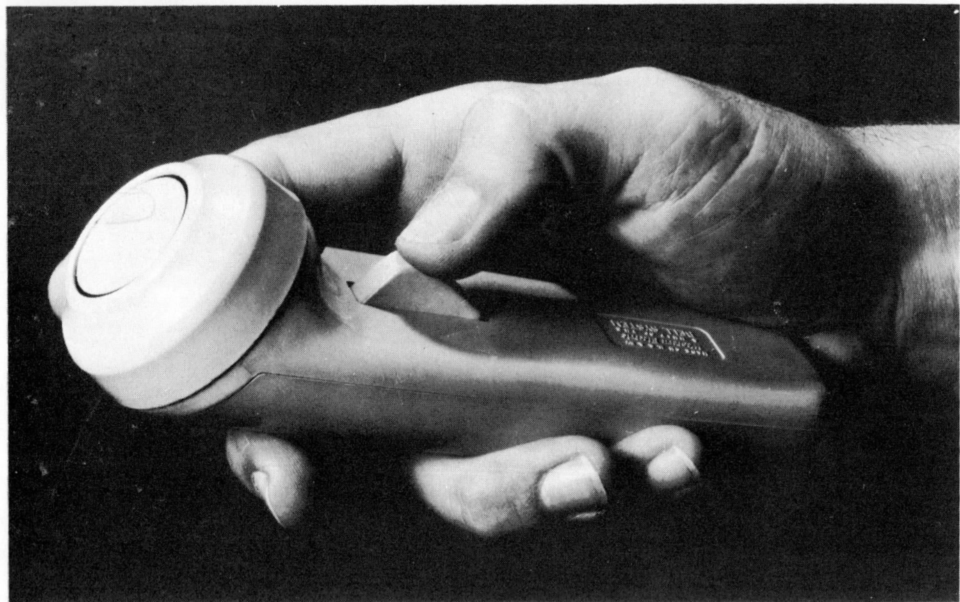

Fig. 49-19. Battery-powered electronic artificial larynx for patient who has total laryngectomy and cannot learn esophageal speech. (Courtesy Illinois Bell Telephone Co.)

coughing that is frightening and painful. Aspiration cannot occur because the trachea no longer communicates with the esophagus.

Speech rehabilitation may be started as soon as the esophageal suture line is healed. In addition to the International Association of Laryngectomees and the local chapter of the American Cancer Society (p. 1103), information on laryngeal speech can be obtained from the American Speech and Hearing Association.* Most persons learn esophageal speech best at a special clinic. Although some persons may need to go to a nearby city for this instruction, they usually must remain away from home for only 1 or 2 weeks. Motivation and persistant effort are essential in learning this kind of speech; encouragement and support from the professional staff and the person's significant others are important to the person's morale. About 75% of all persons who have their larynx removed master some sort of speech, and the average person can return to work 1 or 2 months after leaving the hospital.

To learn *esophageal speech* the person must first practice burping. This provides the moving column of air needed for sound, while folds of tissue at the opening of the esophagus act as the vibrating surface. The person must learn to coordinate his articulation with esophageal vocalization made possible by aspirating air into the esophagus. His new voice sounds are natural although somewhat hoarse. The qualities of speech provided by the use of the nasopharynx are still present, however. The client may have digestive difficulty during the time he is learning to speak, which is caused by swallowing air as he practices, by unusual strain on abdominal muscles, and by nervous tension. The individual should be told that digestive difficulty may occur but that it is not cause for alarm. It abates with proficiency in speaking. See references 1, 8, 36, 45, and 54 for more information.

If a person is unable to learn esophageal speech in 60 to 90 days after surgery, a speech aid such as a vibrator or an electronic artificial larynx (Fig. 49-19) may be prescribed for him. An individual who has a hiatal hernia may not be able to accomplish esophageal speech and will have to use another method for speech. Various mechanical devices are available, and the new ones permit a natural type of speech, providing pitch inflections and volume control. The local chapter of the American Cancer Society or the local telephone company can provide information about the purchase of these devices.

Several other surgical and prosthetic techniques are being tested. Most have not been widely used because of technical complications, and for most patients esophageal speech is still the best method of communication. A summary of some of these procedures can be found in the literature.[14,15,29]

Persons with laryngectomies must take some special precautions. They must be careful while bathing or taking a shower that water is not aspirated through the

*9030 Old Georgetown Rd., Washington, DC 20014.

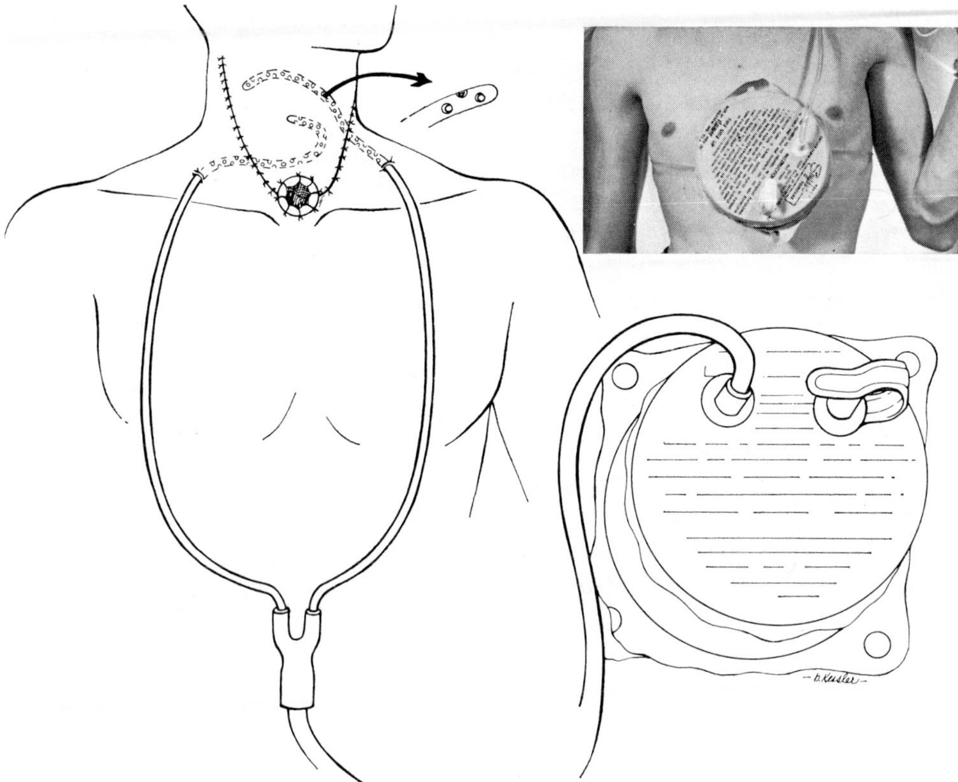

Fig. 49-20. Hemovac apparatus for constant closed suction. In this system of wound drainage, suction is maintained by plastic container with spring inside that tries to force apart lids and thereby produces suction that is transmitted through plastic tubing. Neck skin is pulled down tight, and no external dressing is required. Container serves as both suction source and receptacle for blood. It is emptied as required, and drainage tubes are left in neck for 3 days. (From DeWeese, D. D., and Saunders, W. H.: Textbook of otolaryngology, ed. 5, St. Louis, 1977, The C. V. Mosby Co.)

opening into the lungs. Some otolaryngologists caution their patients not to go swimming or take boat trips; others state that as long as the person is careful, these activities are permitted. A snorkle device to fit over the stoma is available to laryngectomized persons so that swimming can be permitted. Persons with laryngectomies are advised to wear a scarf or a shirt with a closed collar that covers the opening, yet is of porous material. This material substitutes for the nasal passages to warm the air and screen out dust and other irritating substances.

Usually by the time of discharge persons with laryngectomies do not need to be suctioned but can cough up secretions. If suctioning is deemed necessary, the person or his family needs to be provided with necessary supplies or with instructions as to where to secure the necessary suction equipment and of how to care for themselves. Suction equipment can be rented for home use or obtained in many communities through the local chapter of the American Cancer Society. Suction can be provided by attaching a suction hose to a water faucet. Many hardware stores carry the necessary equipment. The amount of suction is controlled by the stream of water.

Radical neck dissection

Radical neck dissection often accompanies total laryngectomy because of the possibility of metastases to the neck from carcinoma of the larynx. It is always indicated when cervical nodes are palpable at the time of surgery. The surgery is aimed primarily at removing the cervical lymph nodes. To do that the sternocleidomastoid muscle, the internal jugular vein, and the spinal accessory nerve have to be sacrificed. These resections cause atrophy of the trapezius muscle, and the shoulder drops on one side.

Persons can be taught to do exercises to gradually replace the function of the lost muscles with that of other muscles. A person may have some difficulty lifting his head, and he can assist himself by placing his hands behind his head. The person is more comfortable and can breathe better when placed in a mid-Fowler's position. Pressure dressings are best avoided in radical neck dissection because they compromise the blood supply to the skin flaps protecting the vital neck structures. The Hemovac (Fig. 49-20) is currently the best device available to keep constant drainage from the neck wound without pressure on the flaps. The Hemovac must be checked to see that it is working properly and that there is no edema, which might indicate hematoma.

There is some readily visible alteration of appearance that may cause the person to feel somewhat conspicuous. Anger, grief, or denial may be part of the person's normal response to the change in body image. (For further information on body image, refer to Chapter 28.)

Radical neck dissection can be performed without laryngectomy for persons whose primary malignant lesion is in the tongue, tonsil, lip, nasopharynx, or thyroid. Often the procedure accompanies other procedures and is termed a *composite* resection. Composite resections may include radical neck dissection along with either the removal of the mandible, removal of mandible and resection of the floor of the mouth, or removal of mandible, floor of the mouth, and tongue. The nursing care for these patients is similar to the care given for maxillectomy and orbital exenteration (p. 1092). Emotional reactions to this type of radical surgery may be profound. Disfigurement is readily visible, and reactions to the change in body image are marked. In addition to the usual fears of surgery and cancer, the person having a composite resection may have fears of rejection and fears concerning the future.

Outcome criteria for the person having a laryngectomy or radical neck dissection. The patient or significant others can:

1. Verbalize feelings about the surgery and changes in life style.
2. Discuss plans for speech rehabilitation, including community resources available (e.g., laryngectomee clubs, American Cancer Society).
3. State reasons for wearing a scarf or other porous material over stoma.
4. Demonstrate suctioning if this is to be necessary after discharge.
5. Identify persons who can provide needed emotional support.
6. State plans for follow-up care:
   a. Time of next medical appointment.
   b. Signs or symptoms indicating need for immediate medical attention (e.g., respiratory infection, bleeding).

REFERENCES AND SELECTED READINGS

1. Adler, S.: Speech after laryngectomy, Am. J. Nurs. **69:**2138-2142, 1969
2. American Cancer Society: 1977 cancer facts and figures, New York, 1977, The Society.
3. Bailey, B. J.: Management of sinus infections, Am. Fam. Phys. **8:**100-107, 1973.
4. Ballenger, J.: Diseases of the nose, throat, and ear, Philadelphia, 1969, Lea & Febiger.
5. Bates, B.: A guide to physical examination, Philadelphia, 1974, J. B. Lippincott Co.
6. Beattie, E. J., and Economou, S. G.: The current state of radical laryngectomy, Nurs. Clin. North Am. **3:**515-519, 1968.
7. Beeson, P. B., and McDermott, W., editors: Textbook of medicine, ed. 14, Philadelphia, 1975, W. B. Saunders Co.
8. Bull, T., and Cook, J.: Speech therapy and ENT surgery, London, 1976, Blackwell Scientific Publications.
9. Chadwick, D. L.: Advances in the treatment of diseases of the ear, nose, and throat, Practitioner **209:**460-467, 1972.
10. Chiang, T. M., Sukis, A. E., and Ross, D. E.: Tonsillectomy performed on an outpatient basis, Arch. Otolaryngol. **88:**307-310, 1968
11. *Davison, F. W.: Hyperplastic rhinosinusitis: a twenty year review, Ann. Otol. Rhinol. Laryngol. **82:**703-708, 1973.
12. DeWeese, D. D., and Saunders, W. H.: Textbook of otolaryngology, ed. 5, St. Louis, 1977, The C. V. Mosby Co.
13. Dison, N.: Tonsillectomy: mother's view, Am. J. Nurs. **69:**1024-1027, 1969.
14. Ewing, D.: Electronic larynx for aphonic patients, Am. J. Nurs. **75:**2153-2157, 1975.
15. Flowers, A. M.: Electronic mechanical aids for the laryngectomized patient, Nurs. Clin. North Am. **3:**529-532, 1968.
16. Frederick, J., and Braude, A. I.: Anaerobic infections of the paranasal sinuses, N. Engl. J. Med. **290:**135-137, 1974.
17. Fuerst, E. V., and Wolff, L.: Fundamentals of nursing, ed. 5, Philadelphia, 1974, J. B. Lippincott Co.
18. *Gardner, W. H.: Adjustment problems of laryngectomized women, Arch. Otolaryngol. **83:**31-42, 1966.
19. Gellis, S. S., and Kagan, B. M.: Current pediatric therapy, ed. 7, Philadelphia, 1976, W. B. Saunders Co.
20. Goodyear, A.: A symposium on laryngectomy: the team approach. The nurse's role, Nurs. Mirror, **141:**51-52, 1975.
21. Hall, I. S., and Colman, B.: Diseases of the nose, throat, and ear, New York, 1975, Churchill-Livingston.
22. *Harmon, W. G.: Nursing care in surgery of the head and neck, Nurs. Clin. North Am. **2:**475-581, 1967.
23. Harrison, D. P.: The natural history of some cancers affecting the head and neck, J. Laryngol. Otol. **86:**1189-1202, 1972.
24. Harvey, T. J.: Diagnosis and surgical management of laryngectomy, Nurs. Mirror, **141:**48-50, 1975.
25. Havener, W. H., Saunders, W. H., Keith, C. F., and Prescott, A. W.: Nursing care in the eye, ear, nose, and throat disorders, ed. 3, St. Louis, 1974, The C. V. Mosby Co.
26. Hoshaw, T. C., and Nickman, N. J.: Sinusitis and otitis in children, Arch. Otolaryngol. **100:**194-195, 1974.
27. Isler, C.: This technique may make tracheostomy unnecessary, RN **40:**32-33, 1977.
28. Keough, G., and Niebal, H.: Oral cancer detection, Am. J. Nurs. **73:**684-686, 1973.
29. Komon, R. M.: Laryngectomy and surgical vocal rehabilitation, AORN J. **17:**73-79, 1973.

---

*References preceded by an asterisk are particularly well suited for student reading.

30. Lederer, F. J., et al.: Medical problems related to diseases of the larynx, Otolaryngol. Clin. North Am. **3**:599-608, 1970.
31. Lucente, F. E.: Psychological problems in otolaryngology, Laryngoscope **83**:1684-1689, 1973.
32. Lucente, F. E.: The dying patient in otolaryngology, Laryngoscope **83**:292-298, 1973.
33. Malasanos, L., Barkauskas, V., Moss, M., and Stoltenberg-Allen, K.: Health assessment, St. Louis, 1977, The C. V. Mosby Co.
34. Maloney, W. H.: Otolaryngology, Hagerstown, Md., 1974, Harper & Row, Publishers, Inc.
35. Marlow, D. R.: Textbook of pediatric nursing, ed. 5, Philadelphia, 1977, W. B. Saunders Co.
36. Matalon, V.: Rehabilitation of head and neck cancer patients, Cancer Bull. **24**:82-85, 1972.
36a. *McConnell, E. A.: How to truly help the patient with radical neck dissection, Nurs. 76 **6**:58-65, 1976.
37. Merenstein, J. H., and Rogers, K. D.: Streptococcal pharyngitis: early treatment and management by nurse practitioners, J.A.M.A. **227**:1278-1282, 1974.
37a. *Millspaugh, D.: I was mad at God, Nurs. 77 **7**:136, 1977.
38. Montgomery, W. W., and Toohill, R. J.: Voice rehabilitation after laryngectomy, Arch. Otolaryngol. **88**:499-506, 1968.
39. Murillo, G.: The popinjay club, Nurs. Mirror **141**:55-56, 1975.
40. Nelson, W. E.: Textbook of pediatrics, ed. 10, Philadelphia, 1975, W. B. Saunders Co.
41. *Newcombe, B.: Care of the patient with head and neck cancer, Nurs. Clin. north Am. **2**:599-607, 1967.
42. *Nicholson, E.: Personal notes of a laryngectomee, Am. J. Nurs. **75**:2157-2158, 1975.
43. O'Dell, A.: Emergency care in establishing an effective airway, Nurs. Clin. North Am. **3**:413-424, 1973.
44. Oliver, P.: Cancer of the nose and paranasal sinuses, Surg. Clin. North Am. **47**:595-599, 1967.
45. Owlett, A.: A symposium on laryngectomy: the team approach. Speech rehabilitation, Nurs. Mirror **141**:53-54, 1975.
46. Paparella, M. M., and Shumrick, D. A., editors: Otolaryngology, Philadelphia, 1973, W. B. Saunders Co.
47. Parvulescu, N. F.: Care of the surgically speechless patient, Nurs, Clin. North Am. **5**:517-525, 1970.
48. Pilgrim, M. C., and Sands, D.: Reconstructive nasal surgery, Am. J. Nurs. **73**:451-456, 1973.
49. Pitorak, E.: Laryngectomy, Am. J. Nurs. **68**:780-781, 1968.
50. Reeves, K. R.: Acute epiglottis—pediatric emergency, Am. J. Nurs. **71**:1539-1541, 1971.
51. Russell, J.: The patient voice: starting from scratch, Nurs. Mirror **141**:56-57, 1975.
52. Sabiston, D. C., editor: Davis-Christopher's textbook of surgery, ed. 11, Philadelphia, 1977, W. B. Saunders Co.
53. Saunders, W. H., Havener, W. H., Fair, C. J., and Hickey, J. T.: Nursing care in eye, ear, nose, and throat disorders, ed. 2, St. Louis, 1968, The C. V. Mosby Co.
54. *Searcy, L.: Nursing care of the laryngectomy patient, RN **35**:35-41, 1972.
55. Smith, C.: Infections of the mouth and pharynx, Nurs. Times **68**:566, 1972.
56. *Stanley, L. M.: Meeting the psychologic needs of the laryngectomy patient, Nurs. Clin. North Am. **3**:519-527, 1968.
57. *Tierney, E.: Accepting disfigurement when death is the alternative, Am. J. Nurs. **75**:2149-2150, 1975.
58. *Trowbridge, J.: Caring for patients with facial or intraoral reconstruction, Am. J. Nurs. **73**:1930-1935, 1973.
59. *Trowbridge, J., and Williams, C.: Oral care of the patient having head and neck irritation, Am. J. Nurs. **75**:2146-2149, 1975.
60. Williams, S. R.: Nutrition and diet therapy, ed. 3, St. Louis, 1977, The C. V. Mosby Co.
60a. Wong, R.: Sore throat, Am. J. Nurs. **77**:1796-1798, 1977.
61. Yonkers, A. J.: Diagnosing and treating common disorders of the larynx, Geriatrics **28**:150-155, 1973.
62. *Zavertnick, J.: Emotional aspects of patients with head and neck surgery, Nurs. Clin. North Am. **2**:503-505, 1967.

AUDIOVISUAL RESOURCE

The otorhinolaryngic examination, Brooke Army Medical Center, Fort Sam Houston, Texas, 1971, color (videotape).

50

Problems of the lower airway

WILMA J. PHIPPS
BARBARA J. DALY

There are numerous diseases that affect the respiratory system. They include both acute (short-term) and chronic (long-term) diseases. Substantial changes in the relative incidence of diseases affecting the respiratory system have occurred in the past few decades. While chronic infectious disorders such as tuberculosis, lung abscess, and bronchiectasis have decreased, persons with chronic bronchitis and emphysema now survive longer and constitute an increasing number of persons with chronic respiratory disease, along with those with environmental lung disease. In addition, modern intercontinental travel has increased the incidence of parasitic lung infestations in the western world, and the reduction of immunologic competence that occurs in the treatment of persons with various malignancies and following organ transplantation has resulted in an increasing incidence of opportunistic infections of the lungs with a variety of microorganisms rarely pathogenic in the past.

Since most diseases of the respiratory tract are not reportable, the full extent of both acute and chronic illness is difficult to estimate. The mortality rates for chronic conditions, bronchitis, emphysema, asthma, and tuberculosis have all decreased in recent years; however, they are still leading causes of disability. Influenza and pneumonia rank fifth as a cause of death; emphysema ranks twelfth.[5] Those known facts concerning the incidence of disability and death caused by respiratory disease indicate clearly that they are a serious health problem and that they cause tremendous loss in the nation's productivity.

The objectives of health education in relation to pulmonary diseases are the same as for other diseases. Prevention, early diagnosis, prompt and often continued treatment, limitation of disability, and rehabilitation should be emphasized for all persons. Early symptoms of respiratory diseases are probably those most often ignored by the general population. Perhaps this is because, with the exception of influenza and some types of pneumonia such as that caused by Friedländer's bacillus, respiratory diseases often develop slowly and progress without the individual's awareness. Nurses should encourage individuals and families to seek proper medical attention if they have symptoms such as cough, difficulty in breathing, production of sputum, shortness of breath, and nose and throat irritation that does not subside within 2 weeks. These symptoms are suggestive of respiratory disease and should be investigated.

With increased study and new knowledge about respiratory diseases, methods of treating patients with these diseases are changing rapidly. The American Thoracic Society, the medical section of the American Lung Association (ALA), publishes a journal* that is an excellent source of current information on all acute and chronic respiratory diseases. The ALA also publishes the *Bulletin*, many booklets and pamphlets, and newsletters that are useful to nurses in education of the public and in teaching patients.

■ INFECTIOUS DISEASES OF THE PULMONARY TRACT

□ Viral infections

Many respiratory diseases are probably caused by viral infections. Presently, over 30 have been found to be directly related to viral infections, and there are probably many more. Some diseases may be caused by one virus, or different viruses may cause the same symptoms.

If specific signs are not evident, the clinical illness is termed a common cold, viral infection, fever of unknown origin, or acute respiratory illness. The most common specific respiratory diseases caused by the various viruses are epidemic pleurodynia (Bornholm's disease), acute laryngotracheobronchitis, viral pneumonia, and influenza. Most adults have developed antibodies for the more common viruses, and most viral infections are

---

**American Review of Respiratory Diseases*, published by the American Lung Association, 1740 Broadway, New York, N.Y.

relatively mild. However, they are frequently complicated by secondary bacterial infections. When new strains of the influenza virus develop, severe epidemics may ensue, and many people may die from secondary infections such as pneumonia.

Common cold

Few persons escape having a "cold." The average among the general population is three colds per person each year.[14] Respiratory diseases, primarily virus infections, are responsible for 30% to 50 % of time lost from work by adults and from 60% to 80% of time lost by children from school. The frequency of their occurrence, the number of people affected, the resulting economic loss, and the possibility that a cold may lead to more serious disease are reasons why colds merit serious attention.

Since persons with colds are rarely hospitalized, nurses will encounter them at work, in public places, or in their homes. It is important to note the symptoms at the onset of the cold. Many other more serious diseases begin with a cold or with symptoms resembling those of the common cold. Because a cold is considered a minor but bothersome condition and because the person has possibly had many colds, the person, rather than a physician, makes the diagnosis. Helping persons to realize the importance of an illness that may appear slight but that may have serious consequences is an integral part of the nurse's role.

Although the specific agent causing the common cold is unknown, it can be stated that it is a syndrome that is produced by a variety of viral infections. Viral studies do not yield the causative agent, nor is there usually any immunologic evidence of infection.

Prevention. The common cold is a communicable disease spread by droplet nuclei. The only known way to prevent spread of a cold from one individual to another is to isolate the infected person, and this is extremely difficult in our society. However, there are measures that help to prevent the development of a cold, its complications, and transfer to other person. Good general hygiene, adequate rest, adequate diet, sufficient exercise, and fresh air presumably help maintain resistance to colds. Most persons can go through the usual course of a common cold without difficulty if they obtain enough rest.

There are several ways to minimize the spread of infection. Crowded places such as theaters should be avoided by persons with colds. The individual should particularly avoid contact with, and therefore exposing, infants and young children, persons who have chronic lung diseases such as bronchitis and emphysema, those who have recently had an anesthetic, and elderly people. Covering the nose and mouth when sneezing and coughing prevents the contamination of the air breathed by others. Frequent washing of hands, covering of coughs and sneezes, and careful disposal of waste tissue are protective health measured that are advisable for everyone, but they become increasingly important when known respiratory infection exists. Since the common cold is a communicable disease, the principles for protection of oneself as well as others should be practiced.

Clinical picture. Symptoms of a cold usually appear suddenly, and the infection may be full-blown within 48 hours. The acute inflammation usually begins in the pharynx, and there is a sensation of dryness or soreness of the throat. This is followed by nasal discharge and frequent sneezing. The eyes may water, the voice may become husky, breathing may be obstructed, and ability to smell and taste may diminish. Often a cough develops, and it may become productive of sputum.

The person with a cold may have various complaints. Lethargy and vague, aching pains in the back and limbs may be experienced. Most adults are afebrile, but those with a tendency toward developing complications, such as persons with chronic illness and lowered resistance, may have a temperature elevation. The course of the cold is variable, but ordinarily it lasts from 7 to 14 days. It is difficult to determine when the cold ends and when complications appear. Laryngitis and tracheitis may be part of the cold, while tracheobronchitis is a complication usually caused by secondary bacterial infection. Acute sinusitis and otitis media may also follow the common cold.

Intervention. All treatment of colds is directed toward relief of symptoms and control of complications. If the person has an elevated temperature and complains of headache and muscular aching, the advice of a physician should be sought. Acetylsalicylic acid may be prescribed for mild aches and discomfort. Salicylates, however, do not influence the course of the common cold and lack specific action in this disorder.

If the patient has *nasal congestion*, the physician may recommend nose drops. Ephedrine, 0.5% to 2% aqueous solution, with isotonic sodium chloride solution, is used frequently. (See p. 1084 for method of administration.) This medication shrinks swollen nasal tissues and allows for free passage of air. Many physicians advise against the use of nose drops, maintaining that constriction of blood supply to the tissues lowers resistance. In general, oily solutions are not recommended because of the danger of inhaling oil droplets, which might cause lipid pneumonia. Nasal sprays containing antihistamine may be ordered. They should be given with the person sitting upright. The nurse should emphasize to patients and their families the importance of using only prescribed solutions and only those that are fresh, since old solutions frequently become more concentrated. Nose drops should be prescribed by a physician, and only the specified amount should be used; excessive use may aggravate symptoms. Many persons prefer a medicated nasal inhaler, since it can be carried easily in a pocket and is more pleasant to use. Benzedrex containing propylhexedrine is one that is widely used. Propylhexedrine is a volatile drug with a minimum stimulating effect on the central nervous system.[15] Soft disposable paper tissues should help to prevent dryness, redness, and irritation about the nose. Some dryness can be prevented by treating the skin early with mild, soothing creams such as cold cream.

The *dryness, cough,* and *"tickling sensation"* in the throat so often associated with a cold can be relieved in a variety of ways. There are many cough drops and lozenges on the market. Lozenges relieve irritation and are pleasant to use. Persons should be advised not to use them just before dozing off to sleep, since they may be accidentally aspirated into the trachea during sleep. A mixture of honey and lemon may be preferred to cough medications by some persons. This mixture increases mucous secretions and thereby softens exudate and facilitates its expectoration. It also relieves dryness that predisposes to coughing. Some people report that undiluted lemon or orange juice is helpful. A section of the fruit with the rind may be placed at the bedside for easy accessibility during the night. Hot fluids often relieve coughing. The person may be advised to keep a small vacuum bottle of hot water or other liquid at the bedside. If cough medication has been taken, it should not be followed by water because the effect will be dissipated. If the cough associated with a common cold persists or does not yield to the simple home remedies mentioned or to specific medication that may have been ordered, the patient should be urged to consult the physician.

Acute bronchitis

Bronchitis can be acute or chronic. Acute bronchitis is an inflammation of the bronchi and sometimes the trachea (tracheobronchitis). It is often caused by an extension of an upper respiratory tract infection such as the common cold and is therefore communicable. It also may be caused by physical or chemical agents such as dust, smoke, or volatile fumes. As air pollution increases, the incidence of acute bronchitis increases.

The person with acute bronchitis usually complains of chilliness, malaise, muscular aches, headaches, a dry, scratchy throat, hoarseness, and a cough. The temperature may be elevated and the person may be confined to bed at home or in the hospital. In either case, exposure to others should be kept to a minimum. Early in the disease the complaints are the dry, irritating cough and the feeling of tightness and soreness in the chest that follows coughing. The person may obtain relief by the same means as those described for the common cold. Cough may be relieved by cough mixtures or aerosolized medications. Humidifying the air eases breathing and lessens irritation. Tincture of benzoin, menthol, or oil of eucalyptus may be ordered for the steam vaporizor for its soothing and aromatic effect. Some physicians prefer that cool humidification be used; this is particularly true of children, whose smaller-sized airways can be further occluded by the administration of warm mist. As the disease progresses, secretions usually increase. Congestion and dryness of the bronchial mucous membrane are then relieved.

Treatment of acute tracheobronchitis is usually conservative in an attempt to prevent extension of infection to the smaller bronchi, the bronchioles, and the alveoli of the lungs. Measures that maintain good drainage of tracheobronchial secretions are prescribed. (See details in discussion on chronic obstructive pulmonary disease.) The patient should be protected from chilling and should take from 3 to 4 liters of fluid daily. A simple bland diet is usually most easily eaten. Antibiotics are commonly prescribed for an elevation in temperature.

Most persons need a period of convalescence following an attack of acute bronchitis because of weakness and fatigue. The person should not return to work without medical approval. Extra rest, a well-balanced diet, and avoiding exposure to further infection are recommended. Chronic bronchitis is discussed later in this chapter.

□ Bacterial infections

Pneumonia

Acute pneumonias are responsible for 10% of hospital admissions in the United States.[84] Pneumonia can occur in any season, but is most common during winter and early spring. Persons of any age are susceptible, but pneumonia is more common among infants and the elderly. Pneumonia is often caused by aspiration of infected materials into the distal bronchioles and alveoli. Certain individuals are especially susceptible. This includes persons whose normal respiratory defense mechanisms are damaged or altered (those with chronic obstructive pulmonary disease, influenza, and tracheostomy, and those who have recently had anesthesia); persons who have a disease affecting antibody response (those with multiple myeloma, hypogammaglobulinemia, and so on); and alcoholics in whom there is increased danger of aspiration and persons with delayed white blood cell response to infection. Pneumonia is a communicable disease; the mode of transmission is dependent on the infecting organism. Pneumonia is classified according to the offending organism rather than the anatomic location (lobar or bronchial) as was the practice a few years ago.

Most persons with *pneumococcal pneumonia* complain of an upper respiratory infection several days before involvement of the lower respiratory tract. The spread of infection to the lower respiratory tract is usually very acute and is often what causes the individual to seek health care.

Staphylococcal and *gram-negative pneumonias* are not diseases of otherwise healthy individuals, but they occur as complications of other diseases. They are therefore seen frequently in hospitalized patients and are often caused by organisms that are resistant to commonly used antibiotics. Many times a person has been on antibiotics prior to the development of pneumonia. Antibiotic therapy destroys the normal flora of the respiratory tract, and an infection caused by a resistant organism develops. *Pseudomonas pneumonia* is often caused by contaminated aerosols that pass upper airway defenses. Culture and sensitivity studies of sputum are done to determine the causative agent and to select appropriate antimicrobial therapy.

Prevention. Pneumonia can often be prevented in susceptible patients by meticulous nursing care. Frequent turning or changing position of persons confined to bed will lessen the possibility of pulmonary stasis. Prompt suctioning of secretions in patients who cannot cough and expectorate forcibly will reduce the chances of aspiration and atelectasis. These persons need special attention when they are being given medication, food, drink by mouth. Apprehensive patients with swallowing difficulties need time to learn to swallow with expiration. These persons need constant encouragement to relax while swallowing.

Recently it has been demonstrated that many persons may develop aspiration pneumonia without any clear evidence of having vomited, and that as many as one out of every ten hospitalized patients may aspirate gastric contents. The consequences of aspiration include not only infection, but also the presence of acid gastric contents in the lung may result in hemorrhagic pneumonitis, interstitial edema, and severe hypoxemia. These are all elements of a potentially fatal disorder, the *adult respiratory distress syndrome* (ARDS) (p. 1135). Because of the serious consequences of this event, it is imperative that nurses identify those patients at risk of aspirating—the elderly, those with impaired levels of consciousness such as the postanesthesia patient or the alcoholic, the debilitated, and those with swallowing difficulties. These persons should be given food and fluids with caution, with the nurse in constant attendance.

Strict medical asepsis will decrease transmission of organisms from one patient to another via the nurse. Nursing personnel who have colds should not be in direct contact with patients. Good ventilation systems (transfer with fresh air rather than recirculated air) will decrease transmission of airborne infections between patients. The best way to prevent airborne transmission is to be sure that infected individuals cover the mouth and nose when coughing or sneezing.

Clinical picture. The signs and symptoms of bacterial pneumonia usually appear suddenly. The person is febrile, has chills, anorexia, and malaise. The white blood cell count is high (leukocytosis).

Chest pain in pneumonia is caused by inflammation of the pleura and usually is confined to the affected side. Involvement of the pleura and empyema often complicate staphylococcal pneumonia.[14,84] Pain may be severe and stabbing in nature and may be exaggerated by coughing and by deep breathing. Respirations are often described as "grunting." Close observation of the chest may show that there is limitation of movement of the affected side. The patient may use accessory muscles to aid in breathing instead of expanding the lower chest fully. Decreased breath sounds and a pleuritic friction rub may be auscultated over the affected areas. Percussion may elicit dullness of sound.

Initially a dry hacking *cough* will be experienced. As the inflammatory process progresses, the cough will become increasingly productive. Thick purulent sputum is common in *staphylococcal* pneumonia, while blood-tinged (rusty) sputum is characteristic of *pneumococcal* pneumonia.

Since the treatment and prognosis of pneumonia depend on the causative organism, sputum smears are examined and cultures obtained *before* administration of an antibiotic is started. Blood cultures may also be drawn. If antibiotic therapy is begun before cultures can be collected, it may be impossible to grow out the causative organism. Diagnosis is confirmed by roentgenographic examination and by positive blood cultures.

Intervention. Bacterial pneumonia is treated with antibiotics that are ordered by the physician based on the sputum or blood culture and sensitivity tests. Response to therapy usually occurs within 24 to 48 hours, the temperature decreases, and the pulse rate returns to normal. During the period of hyperthermia, the person requires rest, fluids, mouth care, and control of environmental factors similar to those of any person with a fever.

Hypoventilation results from decreased chest expansion caused by chest pain and secretions that block passage of oxygen in the airway, or exudations that fill the alveoli. The surface area available for gas exchange becomes decreased. Oxygen may be ordered if the person is very dyspneic. Low-flow oxygen is used with caution if the pneumonia is superimposed on chronic obstructive pulmonary disease (p. 1135).

Chest expansion should be encouraged to increase ventilation through deep-breathing exercises. Analgesics may be ordered for chest pain that restricts deep breathing. Narcotics inhibit the cough reflex but may be required if pain is severe; codeine is less likely to inhibit productive coughing than are stronger narcotics. The person with severe chest pain often requires help and encouragement to move about in bed and to cough productively in order to mobilize and expectorate the secretions. Measures to splint the chest (p. 970) may be helpful. The person is encouraged to cough *deeply* to produce sputum from the lungs and not expand needless energy in raising secretions from the upper trachea and posterior pharynx only.

Prevention of complications. With the advent of antibiotics and better diagnostic measures such as x-ray procedures, complications during or following pneumonia are rare in otherwise normal persons. Atelectasis, delayed resolution, lung abcess, pleural effusion, empyema, pericarditis, meningitis, and relapse are complications that were common in the past. The fact that pneumonia and influenza rank fifth as a cause of death in the United States is an impressive reason for strict adherence to the prescribed medical treatment. Careful and accurate observation as well as sufficient time for convalescence will also help to ensure the average patient a smooth recovery. Aged persons and those with a chronic illness are likely to have a relatively long course of convalescence from pneumonia, and there is a greater possibility of their developing complications. There has been an increase in the incidence of staphylococcal pneumonia subsequent to influenza. Consolidation of lung tissue, pleural effusion, and empyema frequently occur soon after the onset of this type of pneumonia and may cause death.

Tuberculosis

Epidemiology. In 1900 tuberculosis was the leading cause of death in the United States. It remained a major cause of death until the introduction of antituberculosis drug therapy in the late 1940s and early 1950s. The most effective of these agents is isoniazid, which first became available clinically in 1952. The use of isoniazid in combination with two agents introduced earlier, streptomycin and para-aminosalicylic acid, resulted in a striking decrease in tuberculosis death rates. It also made it possible for patients with tuberculosis to be treated on an outpatient basis. However, some patients still have to be hospitalized at some time in their illness, and most all nurses will care for a patient with tuberculosis at some time in their careers. At one time patients with tuberculosis were hospitalized in specialized hospitals called sanitoria. Today these sanatoria are being used for patients with other illnesses, and the patient with tuberculosis is being admitted to the general hospital. Because many persons in our society, including medical personnel, are afraid of tuberculosis, it is important that nurses learn as much as possible about the disease so that they can give effective care to the person with tuberculosis. Unfortunately some persons still associate tuberculosis

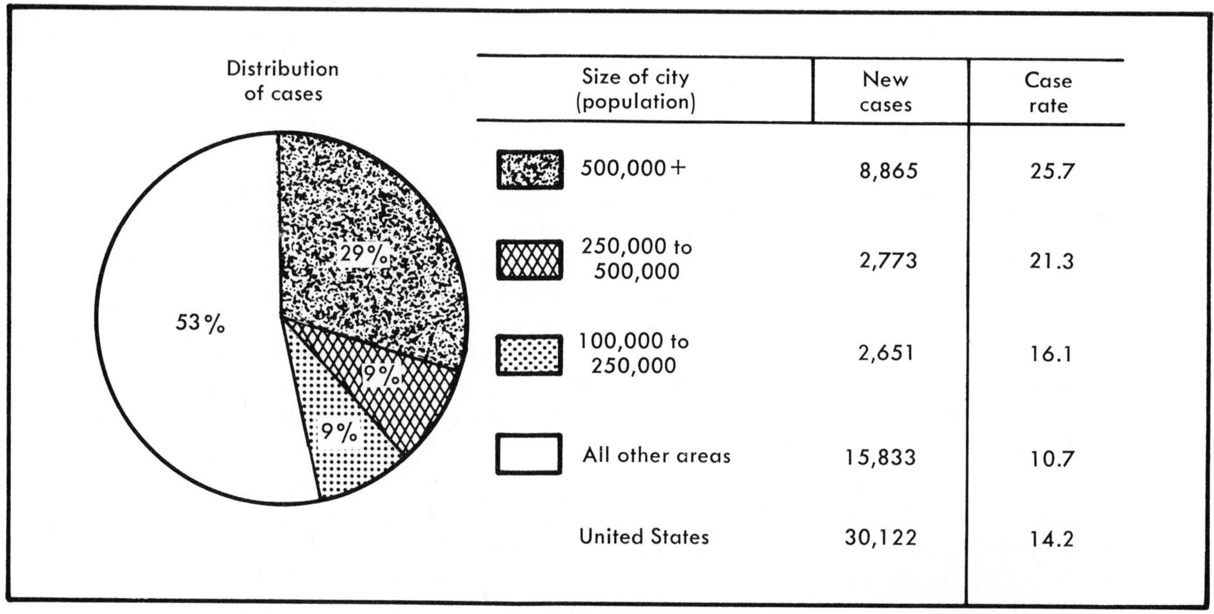

Size of city (population)	New cases	Case rate
500,000+	8,865	25.7
250,000 to 500,000	2,773	21.3
100,000 to 250,000	2,651	16.1
All other areas	15,833	10.7
United States	30,122	14.2

Fig. 50-1. Tuberculosis cases in large cities of United States in 1974. (From Department of Health, Education, and Welfare, Public Health Service: Tuberculosis in the United States, Atlanta, 1976, Center for Disease Control.)

with lack of cleanliness and careless living. This may make both the individual and family unwilling to speak openly about the disease, making treatment of the disease difficult.

Although tuberculosis is now considered a preventable and curable disease, it still is a disease requiring public health attention. In 1976 there were 22,105 new active cases of tuberculosis reported in the United States. This was 1,884 fewer cases than the 23,989 cases reported in 1975.[68] These new cases were not evenly distributed throughout the population, however, and some differences bear mentioning.

In the past few years the greatest numbers of tuberculosis have been found in the counties with the largest populations, especially when the county encompasses a major city. Nearly one-half of the tuberculosis cases are found in cities (Fig. 50-1), and rates are highest in the largest metropolitan areas.[68] Other regions where the case rates are higher than the average are counties close to the Mexican border and a few areas where there is a large population of American Indians. Tuberculosis rates are also higher than the average in areas of the United States where there are large numbers of immigrants from countries where tuberculosis is far more prevalent than in this country. For example, in Hawaii, which had the highest case rate in the United States in 1976, a large portion of the new cases is among persons who have lived in Hawaii for 1 year or less. Other places where similar situations are reported are San Francisco, Dade County, Florida, and Boston. Canada reports a similar finding. These figures point out that with a few exceptions most countries of the world have much higher tuberculosis morbidity and mortality rates than does the United States. In general, Latin America, Africa, Asia, and Oceania have considerably higher case rates than do the United States and the English-speaking and Western European countries. Thus Americans residing for prolonged periods of time in countries where the tuberculosis rates are very high run an increased risk of becoming infected with tubercle bacilli.

As had been true for several years the new active case rate for men is double than for women. The nonwhite population has a case rate over four times as high as that of the white population (Fig. 50-2), but almost half of all new active cases occurred among white men. In both white men and women the greatest number of cases are found in those age 65 and over. In other races the greatest number of cases also occur in men age 65 and over

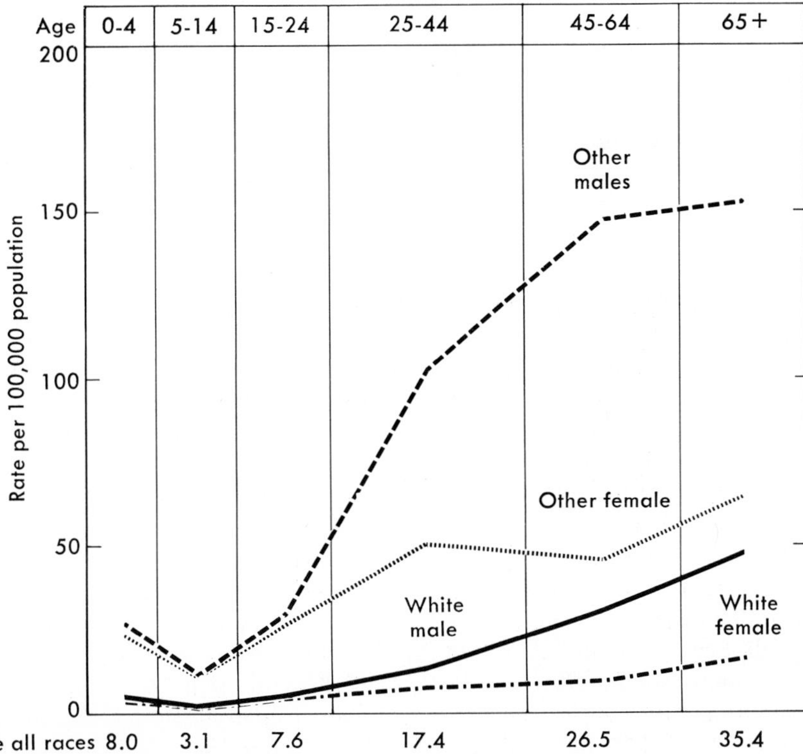

Fig. 50-2. New active tuberculosis case rates by age, race, and sex in United States. (From Department of Health, Education, and Welfare, Public Health Service: Tuberculosis in the United States, Atlanta, 1976, Center for Disease Control.)

and in women between age 25 and 44 and over age 65. The case rates for children under age 5 and those age 5 to 14 have shown a decline every year since 1964.

As was pointed out earlier, there has been a steady decline in deaths caused by tuberculosis in the United States since the introduction of effective chemotherapeutic agents. Today the tuberculosis death rate is around 2.0/100,000 people. However, the tuberculosis death rate for males is more than double that for females, and the death rate for nonwhites is three times that for the white population.

In an attempt to eliminate tuberculosis from the United States, concerted effort must be made to prevent persons from becoming infected with the tubercle bacillus. Measures to do this are discussed under prevention on p. 1115.

Etiology. Tuberculosis is caused by a bacillus, the *Mycobacterium tuberculosis*, or tubercle bacillus, a gram-positive and acid-fast organism. If microscopic study of a slide prepared from the sputum of an individual reveals tubercle bacilli, the individual is said to have positive sputum, and this confirms the diagnosis of tuberculosis. Some persons with tuberculosis will not have positive sputum on smear, however, and a positive sputum culture will be necessary to confirm the diagnosis. Patients who have a positive culture and negative smear are less infectious than are those with both a positive smear and culture.

Transmission. When a person with tuberculosis coughs, sneezes, or laughs, minute droplets fall to the ground, while the smaller ones evaporate, leaving *droplet nuclei* that remain suspended indefinitely in the air and are carried on air currents. Droplet nuclei are 1 to 5 μm in size and are small enough to be inhaled into the alveoli. Thus it is by inhalation of tubercle-laden droplet nuclei that tuberculosis is transmitted.

When an individual with no previous exposure to tuberculosis (negative tuberculin reactor) inhales a sufficient number of tubercle bacilli into the alveoli, tuberculosis *infection* occurs. The body's reaction to the tubercle bacilli depends on the susceptibility of the individual, the size of the dose, and the virulence of the organisms. Inflammation occurs within the alveoli (parenchyma) of the lungs, and natural body defenses attempt to counteract the infection. Lymph nodes in the hilar region of the lung may be involved as they filter drainage from the infected site. The inflammatory process and cellular reaction produce a small, firm, white nodule called the *primary tubercle.* The center of the nodule contains tubercle bacilli. Cells gather around the center, and usually the outer portion becomes fibrosed. Thus blood vessels are compressed, nutrition of the tubercle is interfered with, and necrosis occurs at the center. The area becomes walled off by fibrotic tissue around the outside, and the center gradually becomes soft and cheesy in consistency. This latter process is known as *caseation.* This material may become calcified (calcium deposits), or it may liquefy. The first infection is usually successfully overcome, and the calcified nodule is known as the *Ghon tubercle.* The evidence on x-ray film of enlarged hilar lymph nodes and Ghon tubercle is sometimes referred to as the *primary complex.*

Persons who have been exposed to the tubercle bacillus become sensitized to it, and this is confirmed by a positive tuberculin test. Sensitization, once developed, usually remains throughout life. Recent evidence suggests that about 50% of tuberculin reactors who take isoniazid for 1 year convert back to negative test results. A positive tuberculin test does not mean that one has tuberculosis, however, and nurses should explain this fact to persons who are having the test.

Tuberculosis infection is unlike other infections. Usually other infections disappear completely when overcome by the body's defenses and leave no living organisms and generally no signs of infection. However, a person who has been infected with tubercle bacilli harbors the organism for the remainder of his life. Fig. 50-3 illustrates the number of infected persons in the United States by age groups. Tubercle bacilli remain in the lungs in a dormant, walled-off, or so-called resting stage. When a person is under physical or emotional stress, these bacilli may become active and begin to multiply. If body defenses are low, active tuberculosis may develop. Most persons who have active tuberculosis developed it in this manner. However, it is generally accepted that only 1 out of 20 persons with a positive tuberculin test will ever develop active tuberculosis, and the incidence is expected to be much lower among those who receive preventive therapy with isoniazid.

Classification. Following is the classification used by states and territories of the United States when reporting morbidity statistics to the Center for Disease Control (CDC) of the Public Health Service. The four basic classifications cover the total child and adult population, those unexposed to tuberculosis, those uninfected even though exposed, those with evidence of tuberculosis infection without disease, and those infected with disease:

Category 0: No tuberculosis exposure, not infected. No therapy necessary.

Category I: Tuberculosis exposure, no evidence of infection. Persons who may be in the process of converting their tuberculin test from negative to positive may be given "primary prophylaxis." Household contacts should be considered for such therapy. Primary prophylaxis is standard for all children, and most especially for those under 5 years of age. It is absolutely essential for neonates.

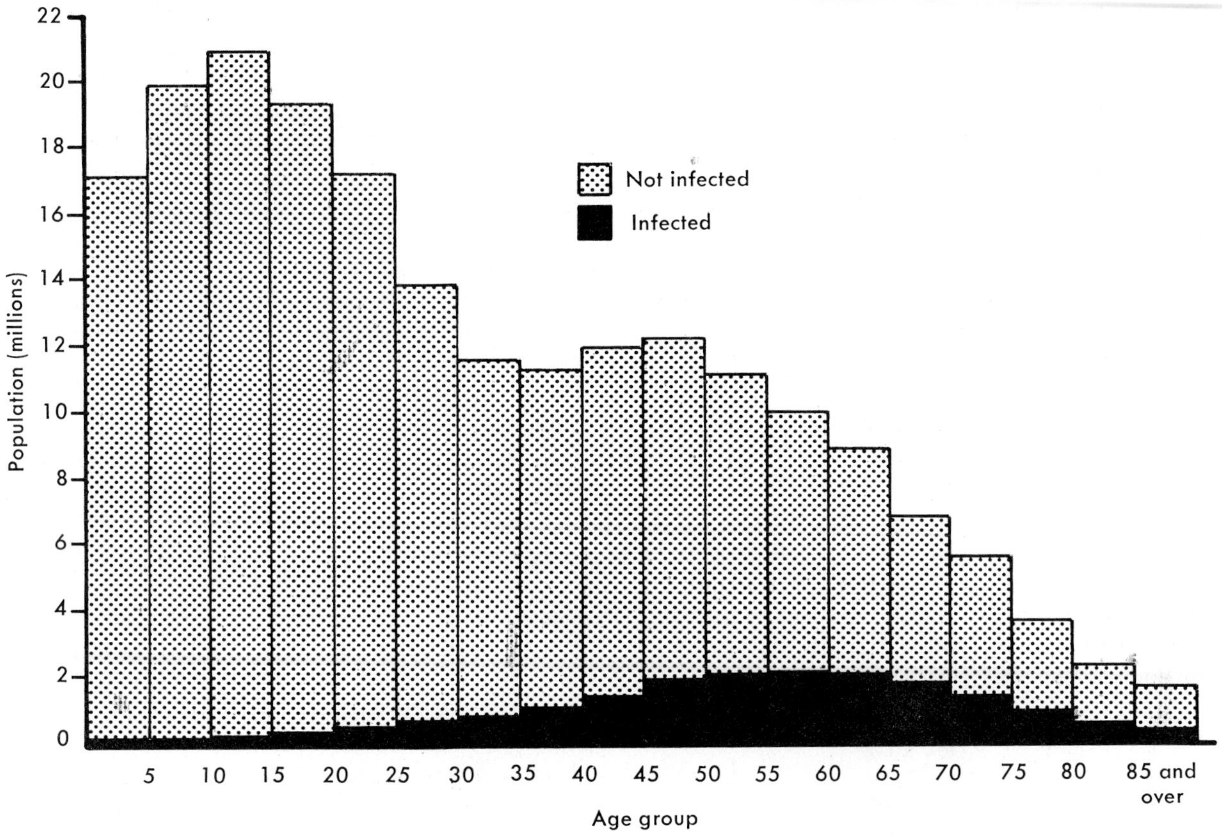

Fig. 50-3. Numbers of persons infected with tuberculosis in United States by age groups. (From Department of Health, Education, and Welfare, Public Health Service: Tuberculosis in the United States, Atlanta, 1976, Center for Disease Control.)

Category II: Tuberculosis infection, without disease. Positive reactors under 35 years of age are considered candidates for "primary prophylaxis." Persons who are over 35 years of age who are at risk should also be treated. This would include persons receiving corticosteroid or immunosuppressive therapy or who have a disease state where the immune response is impaired.

Category III: Tuberculosis infection, with disease.

1. *Past tuberculosis previously untreated.* This group includes those who were not treated adequately with chemotherapy and persons with positive tuberculin (Tbn) skin test and x-ray findings of scarring. Recommended therapy is isoniazid for 1 year.
2. *Current tuberculosis.* Treatment with at least two of the first-line or primary drugs (isoniazid, ethambutol, rifampin, or streptomycin). Administration of isoniazid and ethambutol for 18 months is the most commonly prescribed therapy today. Many combinations of the drugs, including triple-drug therapy, may be prescribed.

   If a woman is also pregnant, the preferred drug combination is isoniazid and ethambutol.
3. *Disease caused by drug-resistant bacilli.* When the person's organisms are resistant to the first-line drugs, second-line drugs are prescribed (Table 50-1). At least two drugs and preferably three are prescribed when resistant organisms are present. The ones used will depend on the findings of sensitivity studies. All these drugs are more toxic, and viomycin, capreomycin, kanamycin, and streptomycin are usually not given together because of their toxic effect on the eighth cranial nerve and the kidneys. Some persons with resistant-organisms may require more than 18 months of therapy.

Prevention. In order to eliminate tuberculosis, the organism must be prevented from being transmitted from one person to another. Preventive measures are directed toward the recommendations described under classification. Preventive therapy emphasis is on (1) finding all persons who have tuberculosis and getting

Table 50-1. Treatment of mycobacterial disease in adults and children*

Drugs	Dosage: Daily	Dosage: Twice weekly	Most common side effects	Tests for side effects	Remarks
First-line drugs					
Isoniazid	5 to 10 mg/kg up to 300 mg PO or IM	15 mg/kg PO or IM	Peripheral neuritis, hepatitis, hypersensitivity	SGOT/SGPT (not as a routine)	Bactericidal; pyridoxine 10 mg as prophylaxis for neuritis; 50 to 100 mg as treatment
Ethambutol	15 to 25 mg/kg PO	50 mg/kg PO	Optic neuritis (reversible with discontinuation of drug; very rare at 15 mg/kg), skin rash	Red-green color discrimination and visual acuity	Use with caution with renal disease or when eye testing is not feasible
Rifampin	10 to 20 mg/kg up to 600 mg PO	Not recommended	Hepatitis, febrile reaction purpura (rare)	SGOT/SGPT (not as a routine)	Bactericidal; orange-urine color; negates effect of birth control pills
Streptomycin	15 to 20 mg/kg up to 1 g IM	25 to 30 mg/kg	Eighth cranial nerve damage, nephrotoxicity	Vestibular function, audiograms; BUN and creatinine	Use with caution in older patients or those with renal disease
Second-line drugs					
Viomycin	15 to 30 mg/kg up to 1 g IM		Auditory toxicity, nephrotoxicity, vestibular toxicity (rare)	Vestibular function, audiograms; BUN and creatinine	Use with caution in older patients; rarely used with renal disease
Capreomycin	15 to 30 mg/kg up to 1 g IM		Eighth cranial nerve damage, nephrotoxicity	Vestibular function, audiograms; BUN and creatinine and creatinine	Use with caution in older patients; rarely used with renal disease
Kanamycin	15 to 30 mg/kg up to 1 g IM		Auditory toxicity, nephrotoxicity, vestibular toxicity (rare)	Vestibular function, audiograms; BUN and creatinine	Use with caution in older patients; rarely used with renal disease
Ethionamide	15 to 30 mg/kg up to 1 g PO		GI disturbance, hepatotoxicity, hypersensitivity	SGOT/SGPT	Divided dose may help GI side effects
Pyrazinamide	15 to 30 mg/kg up to 2 g PO		Hyperuricemia, hepatotoxicity	Uric acid, SGOT/SGPT	Combination with an aminoglycoside is bactericidal
Para-aminosalicylic acid (aminosalicylic acid)	150 mg/kg up to 12 g PO		GI disturbance, hypersensitivity, hepatotoxicity, sodium load	SGOT/SGPT	GI side effects very frequent, making cooperation difficult
Cycloserine	10 to 20 mg/kg up to 1 g PO		Psychosis, personality changes, convulsions, rash	Psychologic testing	Very difficult drug to use; side effects may be blocked by pyridoxine, ataractic agents, or anticonvulsant drugs

*Adapted from American Thoracic Society: Treatment of mycobacterial disease, Am. Rev. Respir. Dis. **115**:185-187, 1977.

them under adequate treatment, (2) identifying persons who should be on "primary prophylaxis" and getting them under treatment, and (3) locating persons who had tuberculosis in the past who did not receive adequate treatment with chemotherapy.

Following is a listing of persons who should be considered for "primary prophylaxis":

1. Persons known to be exposed to tuberculosis who may be in the process of converting their tuberculin test (recent convertors under 35 years of age)
2. Household contacts of persons diagnosed as having tuberculosis, especially children under age 5
3. Positive reactors to the tuberculin test under age 35
4. Positive reactors over age 35 who are at special risk
   a. Those on corticosteroid therapy
   b. Those on immunosuppressive therapy
   c. Those having a disease that impairs the immune response

Vaccination. Efforts continue in search of a more satisfactory tuberculosis vaccine. Presently, BCG (bacillus Calmette-Guèrin) vaccine is in use in some parts of the United States and in many countries throughout the world. This vaccine contains attenuated tubercle bacilli that have lost their ability to produce disease. The vaccine should be given only by persons who have had careful instruction in the proper technique. A multiple-puncture disk is used. When there is a positive reaction to skin testing with tuberculin, when acute infectious disease is present, or when there is any skin disease, BCG vaccine is not given. Possible complications following vaccination are local ulcers, which occur in a relatively high percentage of persons vaccinated, and abscesses or suppuration of lymph nodes, which occur in a small percentage.

In countries where living conditions are such that transmission of the disease is to be expected, BCG vaccine is given early in life and then repeated after 12 to 15 years. The intradermal method is used to administer the vaccine so that a uniform controlled dose can be given. BCG vaccine is not generally recommended for use in the United States, although some highly susceptible groups such as migrant workers may be immunized.

Assessment

Tuberculin skin testing. Tuberculin skin testing provides evidence of whether the individual tested has been infected by tubercle bacilli. A negative tuberculin skin test usually rules out disease and past infection. A positive test indicates that infection has occurred.

Two substances are used in tuberculin skin testing: OT (old tuberculin), which is prepared from dead tubercle bacilli and contains their related impurities, and PPD (purified protein derivative), which is a highly purified product containing protein from the tubercle bacilli.

The tuberculin test that gives the most accurate results is the *Mantoux test*, or intracutaneous injection of either PPD or OT. A tuberculin syringe and a short (½-inch), sharp, 24- to 26-gauge needle are used. With the skin (usually the inner forearm is used) held taut, the injection of 0.1 ml of PPD or OT is made into the superficial layers, and it produces a sharply raised white wheal. Weak dilutions are used first. If the reaction is negative, stronger dilutions are used. This precaution prevents severe local reactions that might occur in highly sensitive individuals if the higher dilutions were used initially. If old tuberculin is used, tests are begun with a dilution of 1:10,000 or 0.001 mg of OT. If this test is negative, successive tests with stronger dilutions are made. The most frequently used strength of PPD is an intermediate strength of 0.0001 mg/dose, or 5 tuberculin units (5 Tu). PPD is also available in first- and second-strength dilutions. For broad-screening and case-finding purposes, a single test of intermediate strength is recommended. Interpretations of the test are made after 48 hours. A positive reaction may begin after 12 to 24 hours with an area of redness and a central area of induration, but it reaches its peak in 48 hours. The area of induration (not the erythema) indicates how positive the test is. Induration should be examined in a good light and palpated gently. Tuberculin reactions should always be measured and recorded in millimeters at the largest diameter of the induration. When successive dilutions are being used, it is advisable to have tests read by the same person so that individual variation in interpretation can be prevented. If the test is negative, there may be no visible reaction or there may be only slight redness with no induration.

One of the most important steps in tuberculin testing is the accurate measurement of reaction. A reaction is considered to be positive when it is 10 mm or more in diameter. Reactions between 5 and 9 mm are considered to be doubtful reactions and are more likely to indicate infection with atypical acid-fast bacilli (p. 1121) than with *M. tuberculosis.* A reaction of 4 mm or less is considered to be a negative reaction.

Other diagnostic studies. Results of roentgenograms and sputum examinations will either rule out the possibility or confirm a diagnosis of tuberculosis. Both tests have been described (pp. 933 and 934). Bacteriologic confirmation of the presence of *M. tuberculosis* is necessary to establish the diagnosis of tuberculosis. Because it is impossible to differentiate between typical and atypical acid-fast bacilli by a sputum smear, cultures are obtained on all persons. Cultures are also used for antimicrobial susceptibility (sensitivity) studies. *Despite the introduction of improved culture media, the tubercle bacillus grows slowly on artificial media, and culture reports will not be available for 3 to 6 weeks.*

Blood-streaked sputum in the absence of pronounced coughing may be the first indication to the person that anything is wrong. Pathologic changes may have occurred in the lungs, but sputum examination may not show tubercle bacilli. However, if the nodules produced in the parenchyma of the lung become soft in the center and then caseated and liquefied, the liquefied material may break through and empty into the bronchi and be raised as sputum. Cavities in the lung may appear on x-ray film and may be present in more than one lobe of the lung.

Intervention. Once the diagnosis of "tuberculosis: infection, with disease" is made, steps are taken to prevent the patient from contaminating the air with tubercle bacilli. This is accomplished by (1) *treatment of the patient with antituberculosis drugs* and (2) *preventing contamination of air with tubercle bacilli.* Each of these measures will be discussed in detail.

Preventing transmission: chemotherapy. Whether the patient with tuberculosis is being treated at home or in the hospital, the same drugs are given. Isoniazid (INH), streptomycin, ethambutol, and rifampin are the drugs in common use. These four drugs are considered to be the "first-line," or *primary,* medications in the treatment of tuberculosis. If they prove to be ineffective or if the patient develops resistant tubercle bacilli, the "second-line," or secondary, drugs are used—cycloserine (Seromycin), pyrazinoic acid amide (Pyrazinamide), viomycin (Viocin), kanamycin (Kantrex), ethionamide (Trecator), para-aminosalicylic acid (PAS), and capreomycin (Capastat). (See Table 50-1 for additional information.)

Previously untreated pulmonary tuberculosis can nearly always be controlled bacteriologically with drugs alone. Most failures of antimicrobial therapy are caused by errors in choice of drug, inadequate dosage, or failure of the patient to take the drugs regularly as prescribed.[44] Choices of drugs are made with the objective of both effective treatment of disease and minimizing the development of drug-resistant organisms.

SUSCEPTIBILITY TESTING. Prescriptions for antituberculosis drugs are made according to the susceptibility of the organisms isolated from the patient's sputum to the primary drugs. Susceptibility testing indicates the effectiveness of a specific drug in inhibiting the growth of the organism or the organism's resistance to the drug. Until testing can be completed, the physician will start the patients on the drugs to which it is believed the bacilli are most likely to be susceptible.

Testing is done by growing cultures of the organisms in special media. The culture plate is divided into sections so that the organisms, if present in the patient's sputum, will grow on one section. Each of the other sections contains a medium plus one of the primary drugs. Thus if the organisms multiply on one section of medium but do not appear on other sections of the medium, the organisms are susceptible to those drugs that inhibit their growth. Testing usually takes about 3 weeks, about half the time formerly required to grow cultures of tubercle bacilli.

Although it is the physician's responsibility to make susceptibility tests, the nurse should understand the basis on which drugs are prescribed and help the patient understand the drugs that are prescribed.

In the last few years it has been recognized that there are naturally occurring drug-resistant tubercle bacilli. It is estimated that in every group of 100,000 bacilli there is one naturally occurring isoniazid-resistant organism, while for each group of 1 million bacilli there is one streptomycin-resistant organism.[31] Therefore antituberculosis drugs are always given in combination. Usually two of the drugs are combined, but patients with far-advanced cavitary disease often receive three drugs.

DRUGS FREQUENTLY USED. The peripheral neuritis associated with isoniazid therapy is more common in persons who are malnourished or who are receiving large doses of the drug. To prevent neuritis, the physician usually orders pyridoxine, 50 to 100 mg daily. Occasionally isoniazid may affect memory and the ability to concentrate, and rarely it may cause psychosis.

Streptomycin is often given as part of an initial program of *triple drug therapy.* It is given intramuscularly in 1 g doses daily or twice a week for 6 to 12 weeks or more, depending on the patient's improvement. Smaller doses may be prescribed for elderly patients or for patients who have hearing impairment or renal damage. The most important untoward reaction to streptomycin is labyrinth damage with resulting vertigo and staggering. Skin rash, itching, and fever can occur. Although renal damage is uncommon, urinalyses and blood urea nitrogen determinations usually are ordered at periodic intervals.

PATIENTS' PROBLEMS WITH CHEMOTHERAPY. It is *imperative* that the patient who has tuberculosis *take the prescribed medications regularly and without interruption.* Because patients usually must take drugs daily for 18 to 24 months, some persons become discouraged and stop taking the drugs. If symptoms of intolerance to a drug such as those produced by PAS occur, the patient may simply stop taking the one drug and continue with the other. The patient may feel quite well, work regularly, yet must continue the therapy. Because most patients feel well, they may be tempted to discontinue the drugs altogether or perhaps take the one drug that bothers them the least. *All patients must be taught that the discontinuance of even one drug will allow drug-*

resistant organisms to flourish and will make the disease more difficult to treat. The nurse should help all patients develop a daily routine for taking the drugs. For those who have difficulty remembering to take their medications, pill calendars that have each day's medications in a plastic bag stapled to a large cardboard calendar may be helpful.

Some persons stop taking drugs and then restart them. Because they may feel guilty about this interruption in therapy, they do not tell the physician or nurse, and it may not be evident until their condition fails to improve. The nurse can help by allowing time for patients to talk about themselves, their families, and their treatment. This may be done when the patient visits a health department clinic to receive a new supply of drugs, when the person comes for periodic medical examination, or when the nurse visits in the home. Patients may be asked to collect a urine specimen periodically for examination. Since the metabolic products of some of the drugs are excreted in the urine, a urinalysis will indicate whether the patient is following the therapy. The best indication, of course, is the progress of the patient. If there is improvement, therapy is effective and the medications probably have been taken as prescribed.

Preventing transmission: preventing contamination of the air. As soon as the diagnosis of tuberculosis is established, the person is taught to cover the nose and mouth with disposable tissues when coughing, sneezing, or laughing. This stops the organisms at the source and prevents them from becoming droplet nuclei capable of transmitting disease (p. 1114). Soiled tissues are collected in a paper bag for subsequent burning, or they may be discarded in the toilet. The patient should wash the hands after expectorating or handling the sputum container.

The most effective way to kill the tubercle bacillus in moist sputum is by burning. All tissues and disposable receptacles for collection of sputum should be burned. Direct sunlight destroys the bacillus in 1 to 2 hours. Five minutes at boiling temperature and 30 minutes at pasteurizing temperature (61.7 C, 143 F) kill the bacillus. Autoclaving also destroys the bacillus. Disposable articles may be used if desired.

The natural movement of air in a room carries droplet nuclei containing the tubercle bacillus, and if windows are kept open or air is circulated mechanically, changes of air dilute the contaminated air below the level where infection can take place. If patients who have positive sputum have been taught to cover coughs and sneezes, air contamination in the room is even lower.

Tubercle bacilli in droplet nuclei are highly susceptible to sterilization by sunlight. *Ultraviolet light* also kills tubercle bacilli in droplet nuclei. Ultraviolet lights installed in air ducts through which room air passes or mounted high on side walls of the room are effective.

It is important that nurses understand how tubercle bacilli are transmitted through air so that they can teach the patient how to protect others and also allay fears that family members and others may have about contracting the disease. It has been well documented that patients taking antituberculosis drugs are not likely to transmit the infection even when their organisms are resistant to treatment. *Because only droplet nuclei are capable of transmitting tubercle bacilli, there is no need for those caring for the patient with active tuberculosis to wear either a mask or a gown. Droplet nuclei are so small (1 to 5 μm) that they readily pass through conventional masks or are breathed in around the edges of them.* Chemotherapeutic treatment of the patient and adequate air changes in the patient's room offer all the protection that is needed. In a situation in which the patient is unable to cover the mouth when coughing, it is more effective for the patient to wear a mask than for personnel to do so. *Newer-type high-filtration masks such as the Ultra-Filter have proved to be effective filters. If a mask is deemed necessary, this type should be used.*

Since many people with active tuberculosis are cared for in their homes, the nurse should help them and their families to understand the communicability of tuberculosis and the precautions that must be taken. Family members and friends may be frightened at the thought of contact with the patient and with articles the person has touched. On the other hand, they have often had long, intimate contact with the patient without developing the disease. Careful observation of the family will help the nurse determine how many and what kind of explanations are needed regarding spread of infection. If the family is overly cautious in handling the patient's personal articles, the nurse may need to advise against discarding articles that are costly to replace. In contrast, if the family is too casual about spread of the disease, the nurse should urge more caution in care of sputum and in exposure to the patient's cough. If possible, the patient should occupy a room alone, but usually the patient does not need to be strictly isolated from the rest of the family. Careful planning with the family often helps ensure that the patient will not infect others yet can be part of the family. The susceptibility of infants and very young children must be emphasized in all teaching.

Acceptance of the diagnosis. Acceptance of a diagnosis of tuberculosis and of its many implications for the future is difficult for anyone. The patient or the patient's family should be referred to a community health nurse immediately after the diagnosis of tuberculosis is made so that initial explanations can be given and essential teaching begun. It is important that any problems that might interfere with acceptance of the disease and the need to take antituberculosis drug therapy be identified early, since the earlier efforts are made to solve them, the less difficulty they may be to overcome.

Real acceptance of the disease, however, may come only after months of illness and after steady help and support from the family, the physician, the social workers, and the nurse. The acceptance of facts and realities varies according to each patient's basic personality and lifelong pattern of behavior in stress situations. The nurse should realize that for some time after the diagnosis is made, patients may deny having tuberculosis or may be very angry that it has happened to them. Some persons may become depressed and may have periods of withdrawal as they work through their feelings about the diagnosis. Many of their feelings about the diagnosis are more emotionally than intellectually determined. Even though persons having tuberculosis understand that the disease is not caused by being "unclean" or "sinful," there may still be a carry-over of these kinds of feelings from things they heard when they were a child, since these are common feelings expressed by some persons with tuberculosis.

There is a high incidence of alcoholism among patients with tuberculosis, probably because of the increased possibility of alcoholics coming into contact with tubercle bacilli during drinking bouts and because of their decreased resistance to infection. Some of these patients have been committed to the hospital by legal action after refusal to obtain treatment, even though their disease is a threat to the health of their family and community. They present the dual problem of the patient with alcoholism and the patient with tuberculosis who cannot accept the disease.

Increased attention needs to be given to patients who refuse treatment and thus stand in the way of eradication of tuberculosis. The nurse often is the member of the health team called on to work with these patients. Patience and understanding as well as flexibility in trying new approaches are essential in working with them. Although the patient needs explanations as to the need for treatment and time to make decisions regarding means of obtaining it, delaying tactics should be discouraged by setting limits. Avoidance of questions that permit categorical refusal is wise. It is often helpful to discover the person for whose judgment the patient has the greatest respect and to seek his or her help in encouraging treatment. This person may be a physician, a clergyman, a family member, or a close friend. Persons who have completed treatment for tuberculosis and are well again often are helpful in answering specific questions the person may have and may thus relieve many of the patient's anxieties. Every effort should be made to help the person feel there is sincere concern for his welfare. In spite of all efforts, some patients will not consent to treatment. Sometimes, if they become suddenly worse, they may then be receptive to treatment, and the opportunity to work with them and help them at this time should not be missed.

Nurses working with patients having tuberculosis must be able to accept the diagnosis if they are to help the patient. Nurses who have a fear of tuberculosis show it in their behavior. Most patients with tuberculosis are extremely sensitive to ways in which various health workers approach them. If personnel are obvious about precautions in giving care, this may make the patient feel rejected. Nurses may be fearful of the disease for various reasons. If the nurse is aware of being fearful, talking it over with an experienced person who is unafraid of tuberculosis may prove helpful. Reassurance that tuberculosis is not highly communicable is usually very helpful to the nurse who has not previously cared for a patient with tuberculosis.

The majority of patients with tuberculosis are able to assume responsibility for their own care. The nurse's major responsibility is to help patients learn what they should do and why and to give encouragement and supervision in the simple but essential elements of good care. Group teaching often is a very productive method of instructing both patients and family members, since they often learn from each other and give each other emotional support.

Activity. Although tuberculosis previously was treated with bed rest, restriction of activity is no longer ordered except as warranted by the patient's general physical condition. Persons who are febrile are usually kept in bed until the fever subsides.

Surgical treatment. When medical treatment has failed to check and heal the disease process, surgical treatment for tuberculosis may be necessary. Surgical treatment for tuberculosis includes pneumonectomy, lobectomy, segmental lobe resection, and wedge resection. Usually parts of the lungs with active disease are resected, and as much unaffected lung tissue as possible is preserved. The nursing care and descriptions of operative procedures are explained on p. 968.

Extrapulmonary tuberculosis. Tuberculosis may affect other parts of the body besides the lungs, such as the larynx, gastrointestinal tract, lymph nodes, skin, skeletal system, nervous system, and urinary and reproductive systems.

Tuberculous meningitis. The onset of symptoms of tuberculous meningitis usually is sudden. The patient has marked constipation, an elevation of temperature, chills, headache, convulsions, and sometimes loss of consciousness. The disease is most common in infants and young children who most often contract the disease from an adult with an undiagnosed case of pulmonary tuberculosis. If untreated, this disease causes death, but with the use of antituberculosis drugs it is usually controllable. A 12-month course of chemotherapy is essential, however, and the nurse must help the patient and family realize that it is absolutely necessary. Ethambutol, streptomycin, and isoniazid are given concurrently. Corticosteroids are usually ordered to reduce neurologic complications.[78] Nursing care is the same as that for any other type of meningitis.

Skeletal tuberculosis. Since the advent of antituberculosis drugs, better case-finding methods, pasteurization of milk, and tuberculin testing of cattle, skeletal tuberculosis is less common. It is most common in children, but adults also are sometimes affected. Although tubercle bacilli may attack any bone or joint in the body, the spine, hips, and knees are most often involved. Deformities occur as a result of bone destruction. Tuberculosis of the spine is now rare in the United States. The "hunchback" deformity it causes can still be seen in some people, particularly in those who have come from countries where standards for pasteurization of milk and tuberculin testing of cattle were not rigid. (For nursing care of patients having tuberculosis of the spine, see specialized texts on orthopedic nursing.)

Outcome criteria for a person having tuberculosis. The person or significant others can:

1. Explain how tuberculosis is spread and those measures necessary to prevent spread (maintain persons on chemotherapy, cover mouth and nose when coughing or sneezing).
2. Explain basic food groups and how a nutrionally adequate diet will be achieved.
3. State name, dosage, actions, and side effects of prescribed medications.
4. State why at least two chemotherapy agents must be taken uninterruptedly.
   a. Explain drug-resistant organisms and relate this to the need to take chemotherapy uninterruptedly.
   b. Explain why the health care provider should be notified immediately if for any reason (such as side effects) chemotherapy cannot be taken.
5. State where to receive new supply of chemotherapy and date it is to be obtained.
6. State plans for follow-up care.
   a. List signs and symptoms that indicate need for immediate medical care (increased cough, hemoptysis, unexplained weight loss, fever, night sweats).
   b. State when next sputum test or roentgenogram is to be taken and where.
   c. State plans for ongoing follow-up care.

Infection with atypical acid-fast bacilli

Pulmonary disease that is indistinguishable from tuberculosis can be produced by a number of species of mycobacteria other than *M. tuberculosis.* These organisms are strongly acid-fast, but differ from *M. tuberculosis* on culture. Four groups have been classified by Runyon: group I, *M. kansasii* (photochromogens); group II, scotochromogens, which are commonly found in soil and water; group III, Battey bacilli (nonchromogens), which are found mainly in Georgia; and group IV, *M. fortuitum* (rapid growers).[7] These atypical organisms are found in various geographic locations. Group I is the most widely distributed, and many organisms have been identified in the Midwest. Group III is found more in the southeastern portion of the United States. The pulmonary disease caused by atypical bacilli closely resembles tuberculosis. The disease often causes lung cavities, responds poorly to antituberculosis drugs, and quite often requires surgery. It occurs most commonly in persons in high socioeconomic groups—especially those residing in suburban areas of large cities. As is true with tuberculosis, the disease is three to four times more common in men than in women. Most of those infected are middle-aged or older, and men with emphysema seem to be particularly susceptible. Atypical bacilli are not believed to be airborne; thus isolation is not required. Because of the seriousness of the pulmonary disease caused by these organisms, patients are usually given chemotherapy for at least 2 years and should have careful medical follow-up after discharge from the hospital. It is possible for persons to be infected with both tubercle bacilli and atypical bacilli at the same time.

Lung abscess

A lung abscess is an area of localized suppuration within the lung. It usually is caused by bacteria that reach the lung through aspiration. The infected material lodges in the small bronchi and produces inflammation. Partial obstruction of the bronchus results in the retention of secretions beyond the obstruction and the eventual necrosis of tissue. Before the advent of antibiotics and specific chemotherapy, lung abscess was a fairly frequent complication following pneumonia. When a lung abscess forms, various organisms are found. Lung abscess may follow bronchial obstruction caused by a tumor, a foreign body, or a stenosis of the bronchus. Children particularly may aspirate foreign material such as a peanut, and a lung abscess results. Metastatic spread of cancer cells to the lung parenchyma may also cause an abscess, and occasionally the infection appears to have been borne by the bloodstream. In recent years the incidence of lung abscess caused by infection has decreased, and secondary lung abscess following bronchogenic carcinoma has increased. Bronchoscopy is used to identify the infected segment and to obtain specimens for culture.

Clinical picture. Symptoms of lung abscess include cough, elevation of temperature, loss of appetite, and malaise. Unless the abscess is walled off so that there is no access to the bronchi, the patient usually raises sputum. There may be hemoptysis, and often the patient raises dark brown ("chocolate-colored") sputum that contains both blood and pus.

Intervention. The course of lung abscess is influenced by the cause of the abscess and by the kind of drainage that can be established. If the purulent material drains easily, the patient may respond well to segmental postural drainage, antibiotic therapy, and good general supportive care. When obstruction interferes with drainage into the bronchi, bronchoscopic procedures should be employed not only to improve drainage but to rule out obstructing foreign bodies or neoplasms.[36] Today, surgical treatment to establish drainage has become increasingly less necessary, but if after several weeks of medical treatment a cavity persists, a segmentectomy or lobectomy may be performed.

Medical treatment cannot cause a walled-off abscess to disappear, and surgery may be necessary. If surgery is done, the portion of lung containing the abscess is removed. If the abscess is caused by carcinoma, the surgery may be much more extensive.

□ Fungus infection

Histoplasmosis

Histoplasmosis is a fungus disease that affects the lungs. Its incidence is quite high in the United States, and it is especially common in certain areas of the central and eastern part of the country. Endemic areas are found in Missouri, Kentucky, Tennessee, Southern Illinois, Indiana, and Ohio. It is not communicable from human to human. Organisms are transmitted to humans by inhaling spores that thrive in moist, dark, protected soil. The disease masquerades as either influenza or chronic tuberculosis with cavities. Chest films demonstrate a nodular infiltrate. Special stains are required to see *Histoplasma capsulatum* on sputum smears. Skin tests for histoplasmosis are available, but if active disease is suspected, a serum complement fixation test should be obtained rather than using the skin test. Skin testing with histoplasmin is helpful in screening programs. In endemic areas, between 90% and 95% of young adults have positive test results.

Nurses working in areas where this disease is prevalent have an important role in helping to locate sources of infection and in teaching the public to prevent inhalation of potentially infected material. Since the disease can be fatal and children appear to be particularly susceptible, the nurse should point out potential danger to rural families when it is known that the soil is contaminated.

Clinical picture. The signs and symptoms of histoplasmosis show a variable range from those of a slight self-limited infection to fatal disseminated disease. Severe infections are characterized by acute onset, fever, chest pain, dyspnea, prostration, weight loss, widespread pulmonary infiltrates, hepatomegaly, and splenomegaly. Some infected persons may have only a benign acute pneumonitis lasting a week or less, while others may be symptom free.

Intervention. Histoplasmosis responds to treatment with an antibiotic drug, *amphotericin B.* Since it must be given intravenously and causes toxic reactions such as gastrointestinal symptoms, headache, cough, and decreased renal clearances, the patient is hospitalized and observed closely during treatment. The infusion containing the drug is given over a 4- or 6-hour period. It is administered every other day for about 8 weeks. Fever and chills are common with the first five to ten doses. Acetylsalicylic acid and an antiemetic are often given 30 minutes before the infusion is started and repeated as necessary. Hydrocortisone may be given to reduce the side effects. A blood urea nitrogen test or nonprotein nitrogen determination is usually taken every 2 to 3 days during treatment because amphotericin may cause kidney damage. Any symptoms of potassium deficiency or anemia should be reported to the physician at once. The general nursing care is similar to that for the patient with noninfectious tuberculosis.

■ CHRONIC LUNG DISEASES

□ Chronic obstructive pulmonary disease

Chronic obstructive pulmonary disease (COPD) refers to diseases that produce obstruction of airflow and includes *asthma, chronic bronchitis,* and *pulmonary emphysema.* The disease spectrum associated with this diagnosis ranges from pure obstructive airway disease with the presence of bronchitis but no emphysema, through various combinations, to severe emphysema without bronchitis. The pathophysiologic processes that cause these changes are neither static nor are they necessarily progressive. Thus all stages are possible, from reversible abnormalities to relentlessly progressive cardiopulmonary insufficiency. There has been much confusion concerning the clinical usage of the terms "chronic bronchitis," "emphysema," and "asthma"; therefore the term "chronic obstructive pulmonary disease" is now frequently seen rather than a designation of the specific disease. However, as more is being learned regarding the pathophysiology involved in these diseases, the trend is once again to define each specific abnormality more precisely.[65] These diseases often begin insidiously and progress slowly. Early symptoms may be only a slight morning cough and slight shortness of breath on exertion that is not noticed because the person has gradually reduced activities to compensate for shortness of breath. By the time medical attention is sought, pathologic changes have occurred and symptoms are often moderately severe.

The incidence of chronic obstructive pulmonary disease has increased spectacularly in recent years. Between 1950 and 1966 the number of deaths from emphysema and chronic bronchitis increased 800%. By the early 1970s over 30,000 deaths were attributed to these diseases, and in 50,000 other deaths, chronic bronchitis or emphysema was listed as a contributory cause. These diseases are more prevalent among men than women, but death rates for asthma and emphysema are now showing a higher percentage rate of increase in women than in men. This is believed to be directly related to the increase in smoking among women.

Chronic bronchitis and emphysema

Chronic bronchitis and emphysema are discussed together for a number of reasons: they are difficult to differentiate clinically; they often co-exist in the same individual; and many of the medical and nursing care measures are similar. In specifying the differences that do exist, however, it is helpful to examine the effect that each disease has on the individual.

Chronic bronchitis is defined as follows:

> . . . a clinical disorder characterized by excessive mucous secretion in the bronchial tree. It is manifested by chronic or recurrent cough. . . . Thus, the diagnosis of chronic bronchitis can be made only by excluding other bronchopulmonary or cardiac disorders as the sole cause of the symptoms.[8]

Pulmonary function studies demonstrate reduced expiratory flow rates, reduced vital capacity, and increased residual volume, but the total lung capacity is frequently within normal limits. As the disease progresses, hypoventilation occurs and arterial blood gases usually show a low *resting* PO_2 and, if the obstruction is severe, an elevated PCO_2. During exercise the PCO_2 increases and the PO_2 may also rise, perhaps because of an improvement in ventilation-perfusion relationships. Cor pulmonale (right ventricular hypertrophy, which develops as the result of increased pulmonary vascular resistance in response to hypoxemia and hypercapnia), right-sided heart failure, and respiratory failure are also frequent complications of chronic bronchitis. The patient is short of breath; he uses accessory muscles of respiration and complains of chronic cough and sputum production. His color is dusky to cyanotic and he is often stout to overweight in body build. Such patients are often termed "blue bloaters" because of their color, frequent hypoxia, and right-sided heart failure.[82]

Emphysema is defined in morphologic terms as follows:

> . . . an anatomic alteration of the lungs characterized by an abnormal enlargement of the air spaces distal to the terminal non-respiratory bronchioles, accompanied by destructive changes of the alveolar walls.[8]

This destruction of tissue leads to physiologic obstruction by collapse of the airways on expiration. As a result, full exhalation is difficult and air trapping ensues. Pulmonary function studies demonstrate decreased expiratory flow rates, particularly forced expiratory volume and maximal midexpiratory flow, increased total lung capacity, and increased residual volume (p. 935). The vital capacity may be normal or only slightly reduced until late stages of the disease; thus the FEV_1/VC ratio is changed. Arterial blood gas tests of persons with emphysema usually show a normal PCO_2 and a PO_2 that is normal or only slightly low *at rest* but falls during exercise. Late in the course of the disease the PCO_2 is elevated, and cor pulmonale and respiratory failure may arise as complications.[82]

Clinically, cough and sputum production are not striking symptoms unless there is a superimposed infection. Because of the increased total lung capacity, the diaphragm becomes relatively fixed in a flattened position. Many patients use abdominal muscles as well as other accessory muscles to aid breathing. Pursed-lip breathing is often used naturally by the patient as this aids exhalation. (Pursed-lip breathing on exhalation slows the expiratory flow rates and results in less of an increase in intrathoracic pressure that "pushes in" on the airways.) Patients with emphysema are often not as cyanotic as patients with bronchitis; they are usually thin and often have a barrel chest. Because *resting* hypoxemia is absent and ventilation is high, these patients maintain a normal PCO_2 despite abnormal gas exchange function, and are frequently termed "pink puffers."[82]

The specific etiology of these two diseases is not known, but their development has been related to inhaled irritants, especially cigarette smoke, and chronic infection. The only exception is the discovery of the relationship of familial emphysema to alpha-1 antitrypsin deficiency. Persons who have this deficiency may develop severe, disabling emphysema early in life, usually of the bullous type. (Bullae, large air spaces, are formed by the destruction of many alveoli.) The finding of low levels of alpha-1 antitrypsin in patients with emphysema indicates a need to screen relatives and provide counseling regarding the use of preventive measures.[37,41] The only way to prevent the development of emphysema is to avoid inhalation of irritants, especially cigarette smoke, and to seek prompt treatment of any respiratory infection.

Intervention. The goals in the treatment of chronic bronchitis and emphysema are to improve ventilation and to overcome hypoxemia. There is a variety of means by which these goals can be met, and most of them are dependent on skilled nursing care if full benefit is to be derived.

In order to improve ventilation the patient must avoid respiratory irritants. Since the single most important cause of respiratory irritation is cigarette smoke, the patient is urged to give up smoking. Persons whose jobs involve inhaling dust or fumes may have to change occupations. They should also avoid breathing cold air and may benefit from a move to a warm, dry climate. Respiratory allergens to which the patient is sensitive should be avoided (p. 1541).

Bronchodilators. Since most patients have a bronchospastic component to their disease, they are treated with bronchodilators. Both direct and indirect bronchodilators are used. *Direct bronchodilators* act on the smooth muscle of the bronchi to relieve spasm. These include aminophylline, isoproterenol (Isuprel), isoetharine (Bronkosol), and ephedrine preparations. Aminophylline is usually given as a rectal suppository or, in the acute situation, intravenously. The usual dose is 250 to 500 mg (3³/4 to 7¹/2 grains). Isoproterenol is administered as an aerosol. Since it is an adrenergic agent, its side effects include tachycardia, tremor, and vasoconstriction. It should be used in small doses; usually 8 to 10 drops diluted in 4 ml of saline solution are given. Bronkosol has less effect on cardiostimulating receptors, and therefore the incidence of tachycardia associated with its use is less, although it may occur. The usual dose is 0.25 to to 0.5 ml in 4 ml of saline solution. Commercially prepared pressurized cartridges containing these drugs are available. The usual dose is two deep inhalations of the medication three to four times a day. The patient should be instructed to reduce the frequency of administration if side effects occur. The person also should be cautioned not to use them too often, since high frequent doses may result in resistance to the bronchodilating effect.

Indirect bronchodilators include the *adrenocortical steroids* and *antibiotics*. Because infections increase mucus production and further limit ventilation, antibiotic therapy is instituted at the first sign of infection. Since organisms causing respiratory infections are usually sensitive to broad-spectrum antibiotics, tetracycline is often initiated before culture and sensitivity studies are available. Some physicians prescribe antibiotics prophylactically either intermittently or continuously, and patients are instructed in the schedule to be followed. Persons with chronic obstructive pulmonary disease should receive flu vaccine (attentuated preparations of the current infecting strains) each fall to protect them from influenza. Because adrenocortical steroids reduce the inflammatory response seen in chronic bronchitis, they may also be prescribed. Prednisone in small doses is frequently used. If the person has a positive tuberculin test, isoniazid will be given prophylactically along with the steroids. Occasionally a person with bullous emphysema that is confined to one area of the lung may be treated by surgical resection of the involved area.

Other therapy. Oxygen may also be used. For patients with carbon dioxide retention, flow rates are adjusted so that the inhaled concentration of oxygen is not greater than approximately 30% (low flow rate). (See section on respiratory failure.) Some patients have to receive supplementary oxygen at home in order to maintain function. They may use oxygen continuously or only with exercise. Others may use it only at night when sleep and a supine position reduce ventilation. Portable units with liquid oxygen are now available so that the patient's activity is not limited by the length of tubing connecting him to the oxygen source.

Other treatments may include measures to liquefy secretions, use of intermittent positive pressure breathing (IPPB), and pulmonary physiotherapy, all of which are discussed in Chapter 45.

Rehabilitation

It is now recognized that patients with chronic obstructive pulmonary disease can maintain a much higher level of functioning for longer periods than was once thought possible. The patient is no longer told, "You have emphysema—there is nothing we can do to help you. Go home and don't overexert yourself." Many communities now have programs in pulmonary rehabilitation. Some of these programs are sponsored by the local Christmas Seal agencies, which are affiliates of the American Lung Association (ALA), and others are part of a hospital program.

Pulmonary rehabilitation programs stress the attainment and maintenance of optimal functioning for the individual patient. Emphasis is placed on bronchial hygiene, using all the measures described previously as well as physical retraining. Specific exercise programs vary, but all attempt to rebuild muscle strength so that the patient can undertake activity at a smaller oxygen cost to himself.* The psychosocial aspect of care is also stressed in these programs, which utilize a multidisciplinary approach whenever possible. Therapy is structured according to the individual's medical stability, physiologic need, stamina, personality, and life style.

*Details about breathing exercises can be found in Bendixen, H. H., Egbert, L. D., Hedley-White, J., Laver, M. B., and Pontoppidan, H.: Respiratory care, St. Louis, 1965, The C. V. Mosby Co.; and Hass, A.: Essentials of living with pulmonary emphysema, a guide for patients and their families, patient publ. no. 4, New York, 1963, The Institute of Physical Medicine and Rehabilitation.

Studies have shown that while overall lung function may not improve and the course of the disease is not halted, the patient and his family can be helped to cope with the symptoms of his disease and therefore to lead a more satisfying life.

Although it is difficult to measure the physiologic effects of these programs, hospitalization of patients who have participated in them is less frequent, and most patients state that they feel better.[2] The patient is seen regularly by the physician, and it is extremely helpful if both the hospital and community health nurses are able to be involved in the long-term care of the patient. In some centers, clinical nurse specialists follow the patients and refer them to the physician when problems requiring medical consultation arise.

Outcome criteria for the person with chronic bronchitis or pulmonary emphysema. The person or significant others can:

1. Explain dietary changes required after discharge.
   a. Explain food and fluid requirements and plan for meeting them.
   b. List specific foods to be avoided.
   c. Explain plan for frequent, small feedings that are soft and that do not require much chewing, and the need for increased time required for eating if indicated.
2. Explain any home medication or treatment program.
   a. State name, dosage, action, and side effects of each home medication.
   b. Explain how and when to use medications ordered on a prn basis (e.g., bronchodilators, antibiotics, steroids, antacids).
   c. Demonstrate techniques necessary for follow-up care (segmental postural drainage, clapping and vibrating, inhalation therapy treatments [IPPB], and so on).
3. Explain exercise program to be followed at home.
   a. Demonstrate effective methods of coughing.
   b. Demonstrate efficient breathing patterns with emphasis on increasing time of exhalation in relation to inhalation (e.g., use of diaphragm, expansion of lower thoracic cage, use of abdominal muscles, use of pursed-lip breathing).
4. Explain health maintenance or therapeutic follow-up program.
   a. Explain basic pathology and overall treatment for his medical problem in own words.
   b. Explain need to avoid respiratory irritants and infectious agents and identify sources of these in environment (e.g., tobacco smoke, industrial pollutants, allergens, persons with upper respiratory infections).
   c. List signs or symptoms requiring institution of specific therapy or contact with physician (change in amount, color, or consistency of sputum; increased cough, hemoptysis, drowsiness, changes in behavior, increasing fatigue, weight gain, increase in peripheral edema, change in color of stool, and so on).
5. Explain how to obtain professional and community resources necessary to structure a satisfactory environment at home.
   a. State how to contact other agencies (vocational counselor, VNA and so on).
   b. Describe how to obtain and maintain any needed equipment or supplies (oxygen, nebulizers, humidifiers, mistometers, IPPB, syringes, medications, and so on).
6. State plans for ongoing follow-up care.

□ Asthma

Asthma is discussed separately from bronchitis and emphysema because it results in intermittent rather than continuous airway obstruction. Its onset is sudden as opposed to the slow indisious progression of symptoms seen in bronchitis and emphysema. In differentiating asthma from other chronic obstructive pulmonary disease, the American Thoracic Society has described it as follows:

> . . . a disease characterized by an increased responsiveness of the trachea and bronchi to various stimuli and manifested by a widespread narrowing of the airways that changes in severity either spontaneously or as a result of therapy.[8]

The specific cause of asthma is as yet unknown. It may be classified as extrinsic (allergic or atopic) or intrinsic (nonallergenic); in some individuals it may be both. In one-third of asthmatics no allergic component can be demonstrated, and in many individuals no obvious cause for an attack can be identified. In individuals with allergic asthma, levels of immunoglobulins (IgE) are higher than normal, although there is no direct correlation between changed serum levels and the severity of an asthmatic attack.[63] Atopic allergy is discussed more fully in Chapter 69.

In those whose asthma is caused by allergy, attacks are precipitated by contact with the allergen to which they are sensitive. This type of asthma is seen most often in children and young adults.

Intrinsic asthma usually develops in adults over 35 years of age. Attacks are most frequently triggered by an infection in the sinuses or bronchial tree. Asthma may also be classified as *mixed* asthma. In this type of asthma, attacks are initiated by viral or bacterial infections or by allergens. At different times attacks may be precipitated by different factors.

In any type of asthma the airway is in a state of easy

provocation, and attacks may be precipitated by a variety of factors including changes in temperature and humidity, irritating fumes and smoke, strong odors, physical exertion, and emotional stress. Some allergists refer to asthma in children as the "Christmas and birthday disease," because the excitement and stress related to these special days often precipitate an asthmatic attack.

Hypoxemia, hypercapnia, and the overuse of bronchodilators may also lead to an acute asthmatic attack.[13,34,51]

Pulmonary function studies done during nonsymptomatic periods may show no significant changes. During periods of airway obstruction, however, FEV_1, FEV, and MVV are decreased, while FRC is increased. Hypoxemia may be present, the degree depending on the severity of the obstruction and the resultant changes in the $\dot{V}/\dot{Q}$ ratio (p. 935). Pulmonary function studies for asthmatic patients include measurements before and after the use of a bronchodilator to determine therapeutic response.

Persons who have asthmatic attacks usually seek medical care because the attacks are both incapacitating and frightening. The individual must often make an attempt to reduce emotional stress and to control physical exertion, since these factors are less amenable to management than are specific allergens. If the underlying cause of an allergy is obscure, if it is resistant to treatment, or if the person has nonallergenic asthma, the recognition and control of secondary factors may be the main approach to treatment. *It is imperative to understand that even though psychologic factors may precipitate an attack, the response to it is physiologic and requires the same treatment as that prescribed for an attack precipitated by an allergen or any other factor.*

There is perhaps no disease in which knowing the patient well is more important than in asthma. Since sensitivity tests can be done with only a very small fraction of the substances with which the patient is in contact, the physician usually makes the diagnosis on the basis of a careful history. Knowing about the person's life style such as the type of work, leisure-time activities, and even food preferences may give useful clues as to what precipitates the asthmatic attack. Although the allergist urges persons to report seemingly trivial and insignificant details, they often hesitate to do so, since they are accustomed to reporting only physical changes within themselves. The alert nurse can be of real help in learning the cause of an allergic reaction. It is often the nurse who may learn that a relative has just visited in the home and was accompanied by a cat or dog. This information would be of great importance because animal dander is one of the most common allergens for individuals with atopic asthma.

The nurse may make observations regarding emotional stresses that appear to aggravate the patient's condition. Careful observation of relationships between the person and his significant others may give clues to sources of emotional stress. Some patients remain in the hospital during an acute episode and return home relieved of serious symptoms. However, unless life circumstances can be altered, family relationships and general socioeconomic conditions that cause stress may send the patient back to the hospital with another attack.

Patients with chronic asthma may gain a sense of security while in the hospital and may be reluctant to return home. Asthmatic attacks can be precipitated by plans for discharge, and the patient's stay may thus be prolonged. Patients with severe emotional problems may benefit from psychotherapy.

Clinical picture. Asthmatic attacks often occur at night. The person awakens with a feeling of choking, since there is difficulty moving air in and out of the lungs. The bronchioles react with swelling of the mucosa, muscle spasm (bronchospasm), and increased amount of thick secretions. The patient's breathing has a characteristic wheezing sound as air moves through the constricted and obstructed airways. Cyanosis may develop. When an attack starts, the patient should sit upright and be given something on which to lean forward such as an overbed table (Fig. 45-8). During an acute attack the patient uses the accessory muscles of respiration in an effort to get enough air, and leaning forward helps to use them more effectively. During an acute attack the person's major concern is breathing. Medication for relief of the attack should be given as soon as possible, and the patient should be constantly attended until acute symptoms subside. The attack usually ends with the patient coughing up large quantities of thick, tenacious sputum. Most attacks subside in 30 minutes to 1 hour, although repeated asthmatic attacks associated with infection may continue for days or weeks. The person is usually exhausted and should rest quietly after the attack. Diaphoresis is common because of the expenditure of energy, and linen changes may be necessary.

Persons who are severely affected with asthma and who have attacks that are difficult to control with the usual medications may develop *status asthmaticus*. In this case the symptoms of an acute attack continue despite measures to relieve them. The patient is acutely ill. When admitted to the hospital, emergency treatment is begun. Aminophylline, 500 mg in an intravenous drip, is given over a 20-minute period. A prolonged attack causes exhaustion, and death from heart failure may occur. Oxygen is administered, and positive pressure may be used intermittently. Blood gases are carefully monitored, and intravenous steroids are frequently given. During an acute attack the alveoli progressively distend as in emphysema; actually acute emphysema exists. Unless relaxation of the bronchioles can be accomplished, insufficient oxygen passes through the alveolar membrane into the bloodstream (hypoxemia), and the person becomes progressively more cyanotic. Intubation and assisted ventilation may also be necessary. The person needs constant observation and support, and should have everything done for him. Repeated attacks of status asthmaticus may cause irreversible emphysema, resulting in a permanent decrease in total breathing capacity.

Some persons have *chronic mild asthma.* Symptoms are not noticeable when the person is at rest. However, after exertion such as laughing, singing, vigorous exercise, or emotional excitement, dyspnea and wheezing develop rapidly. These attacks are controlled with medications, and patients usually can continue their usual mode of living with a few modifications and no serious lung changes. They are not hospitalized, but they sometimes come to outpatient clinics for medical supervision.

Intervention. The management of asthma is directed toward symptomatic relief of attacks, control of specific causative factors, and general care for maintenance of optimum health. The chief aim of various medications is to afford the patient immediate and progressive bronchial relaxation. Following are some approaches to therapy*:

1. Acute asthma
   a. Moderate severity: treated safely on an outpatient basis.
      (1) Nasal oxygen.
      (2) IV aminophylline or subcutaneous terbutaline or both may be given simultaneously.
      (3) Monitor FEV and symptoms; when they improve, begin oral therapy.
      (4) Follow carefully for 48 hours and monitor for signs of relapse.
   b. Severe attack with one or more danger signs: vital capacity < 1.0 liter, $FEV_1 < 0.5$ liter, Po_2 under 50 mm, increase in Pco_2, exhaustion, disturbed consciousness.
      (1) Hospitalize. Give supplemental oxygen. Intubate if necessary.
      (2) Administer IV steroids (100 mg Solu-Cortef or equivalent every 6 hours for four doses). Begin prednisone 60 to 80 mg every 24 hours until FEV_1 nears best previous value. Then reduce dose over next 2 to 3 weeks. Begin use of beclomethasone inhaler.
      (3) Aminophylline IV in a loading dose and then in maintenance dose for 48 to 72 hours. Monitor aminophylline blood levels.
      (4) Administer beta-2 adrenergic agents (terbutaline or epinephrine initially).
      (5) IPPB may be used to deliver adrenergic agents.
2. Chronic asthma
   a. Mild to moderate, or recurring
      (1) Theophylline compounds; cromolyn sodium may be tried; adrenergic inhaler prn.
      (2) Oral beta-2 adrenergic agents added in divided doses if above not effective.
   b. Moderately severe: add beclomethasone inhaler to *1* and *2* above.
   c. Severe asthma causing interferences with work: oral steroids every day in addition to *1*, *2*, and *3* above; keep steroids to minimal effective dose.

In an asthmatic attack, the beta receptors are blocked, causing bronchoconstriction. For this reason a beta adrenergic agent is administered to relax the bronchi. Some of the most commonly prescribed ones are epinephrine, ephedrine, isoproterenol (Isuprel), isoetharine (Bronkosol), and terbutaline (Bricanyl).

Epinephrine is usually administered during an acute attack. The usual dose is 0.3 to 0.5 ml of a 1:1,000 solution. If relief is not obtained within a few minutes, a repeat dose may be ordered. *Ephedrine* is a longer-acting agent and therefore is not effective during an acute attack. It is believed that ephedrine produces bronchodilatation by stimulating the production of cyclic 3,5 AMP (adenosine monophosphate), thus producing bronchodilatation. The usual dose is 25 to 50 mg every 4 to 6 hours. Many persons with asthma take this medication regularly. One of its side effects is cerebral agitation, and for this reason a barbiturate such as phenobarbital, 8 to 15 mg, may also be prescribed to be taken at the same time as the ephedrine. Combined medications are also available. Most contain theophylline (aminophylline), ephedrine, and phenobarbital. Tedral and Bronkotabs are examples of agents containing all three medications.

Isoproterenol (Isuprel) and *isoetharine* (Bronkosol) are widely used inhaled bronchodilators. These medications come in metered dose cartridges and should not be used more than two inhalations at a time and not over three times a day to avoid dependence. Sudden death during status asthmaticus has been attributed to overuse of these gas-propelled inhalants.

Terbutaline is a new bronchodilator that works at beta-2 receptors in smooth muscle (bronchi, blood vessels). A dose of 2.5 mg of terbutaline is equivalent to 25 mg ephedrine orally. Frequent side effects include increased heart rate (average 30 beats per minute) and tremors. Less frequent side effects are palpitations, sweating, headache, and cramps in hands and feet. Terbutaline is almost four times as expensive as ephed-

*Adapted from Jenne, J. W.: The clinical pharmacology of bronchodilators, Basics RD **6**:1-6, Sept. 1977.

rine, and since the effects of the two drugs are comparable, cost may be a factor considered in determining which of the two drugs will be prescribed, especially for persons on chronic maintenance therapy.

Cromolyn sodium (Arane, Intal) was first released for use in the United States in 1973. It is used to prevent asthmatic attacks and is of no benefit in the treatment of an acute attack. The usual dose is 20 mg four times a day. Cromolyn sodium is believed to interfere with the release of the chemical mediator (histamine) that causes the symptoms seen in an asthmatic attack.

Another new drug being used in treating persons with asthma is *beclomethasone*. It is a synthetic corticosteroid closely related to prednisolone in structure. It possesses potent antiinflammatory activity (500 times that of dexamethasone) but very weak systemic corticoid effects. For this reason it may be preferable to other corticosteroids in treating persons with asthma. Beclomethasone is available as an aerosol inhalant. For adults the dose is two inhalations (100 μg) three to four times a day. Sometimes a smaller dose is instituted first and then the dose is adjusted according to the response of the patient.

Beclomethasone is being prescribed as a substitute for systemic corticosteroids by some physicians. When this is done, care has to be taken to withdraw the systemic corticosteroids slowly so as not to precipitate symptoms of adrenal insufficiency. Patients should be advised to resume or increase their systemic corticosteroids during increased stress if their asthma symptoms worsen or if symptoms of adrenal insufficiency occur.

Beclomethasone is not prescribed alone for an acute asthmatic attack, as it does not work that rapidly, and in acute asthma systemic corticosteroids should be given.

Sedatives are used with caution during an asthmatic attack to avoid depressing the respiratory center. During an acute attack the patient is usually very frightened and much reassurance is necessary—the patient is never left alone. Intubated patients who are receiving assisted ventilation may be sedated, and frequently morphine is prescribed.

One of the main nursing measures is to provide frequent care to remove secretions from the airway before they become impacted. Mucous plugs are commonly a problem, and liquefying agents and humidification are indicated.

When an infection is present, appropriate antibiotic therapy is prescribed.

Outcome criteria for the person with chronic asthma

The person or significant others can:

1. State the factors most likely to precipitate an asthmatic attack (stress, allergens, infections, and so on).
2. If the cause is allergic, state how to prepare an environmentally controlled bedroom (p. 1541).
3. Explain any home medication program.
   a. Give name, dosage, action, and side effects of each medication.
   b. State conditions under which medications might be increased (infection—start or increase antibiotics; increased stress or worsening of symptoms—increase corticosteroids).
4. Demonstrate how to take inhaled medications.
5. Describe what to do when an acute attack occurs (take medication, be quiet).
6. State signs and symptoms that indicate need for immediate medical attention (asthmatic attack unrelieved by usual treatment).
7. If on corticosteroid therapy, show card to be carried at all times giving data about the drug, dosage, and name of physician. Alternate would be to wear a Medic Alert bracelet.
8. State plans for ongoing follow-up care including plans for desensitization if appropriate.

□ Bronchiectasis

Bronchiectasis means dilation of the bronchus or bronchi. When infection attacks the bronchial lining, inflammation occurs and an exudate forms. The progressive accumulation of secretions obstructs the bronchioles. The obstructed bronchioles then break down and enlarge, appearing saccular and cylindric in shape (saccular bronchiectasis). Their expulsive force is diminished, and they may remain filled with exudate. Only forceful coughing and postural drainage will empty them. Bronchiectasis may involve any part of the lung parenchyma, but it usually occurs in the dependent portions or lobules. Prior to the widespread use of antibiotics in treating persons with respiratory infections, this disease began to develop in young people, with many showing symptoms in childhood or by age 20. Although the incidence of childhood bronchiectasis is decreasing, it is increasing in individuals with cystic fibrosis, immune-deficiency diseases, or atopic asthma in which repeated respiratory infections have been successfully treated with antibiotics. These persons now survive the acute episodes of bacterial infection that complicate their underlying disease but not infrequently develop bronchiectasis as a sequela. If the disease is widespread, it may resemble other forms of chronic obstructive lung disease, with generalized wheezing and eventual progression to cor pulmonale.[82] A contributing factor in bronchiectasis may be a congenital weakness in the structure of the bronchi that results in impairment of elasticity. Bronchiectasis may occur without previous pulmonary disease, but it usually follows such diseases as bronchopneumonia, lung abscess, tuberculosis, or asthma.

Clinical picture. Symptoms of bronchiectasis vary with the severity of the condition. Complaints of fatigue, weakness, and loss of weight are common. Appetite can be affected by the fetid sputum. The condition may develop so gradually that the person in often unable to tell when symptoms first began. Clubbing of the fingers is common, as it is in other chronic respiratory disease. The chief complaint in bronchiectasis is severe coughing (brought on by changing position) that is productive of large amounts of blood-tinged sputum and causes dyspnea. Paroxysms of coughing when arising in the morning and again when lying down are common.

Intervention. Treatment of bronchiectasis is not very satisfactory. Surgical removal of a portion of the lung is the only cure (p. 968). Therefore patients who have bronchiectasis that involves both lungs are not candidates for surgery and do not have a good prognosis. The life expectancy usually is considered to be no more than 20 years. Many patients develop cardiac complications (cor pulmonale) resulting from the extra strain on the heart caused by inability of the lungs to oxygenate the blood adequately.

Postural drainage at least twice a day helps to remove secretions and thus helps to prevent coughing (p. 957). During severe episodes of coughing the patient should not be left alone, since a large plug of thick secretion may block a large bronchiole and cause severe dyspnea and cyanosis. Occasionally a bronchoscopy may be done to remove the plug of mucus or to break adhesions that may be interfering with postural drainage by blocking passage to the main bronchi. Antibiotics may be used in the treatment of bronchiectasis. Although they do not cure the condition, they may prevent further infection and are often used prior to surgery. If the involvement of the lung is widespread, oxygen may be used. Nursing care should stress good general hygiene, which may contribute to relief of symptoms. Adequate diet, rest, exercise, and diversional activity are important, and avoiding superimposed infections such as colds should be emphasized. Frequent mouth care is essential, and cleansing the mouth with an aromatic solution before meals often makes food more acceptable.

□ Pulmonary fibrosis

Pulmonary fibrosis is a diffuse interstitial disease of the lung. It is seen in a wide variety of diseases, but the specific cause and etiology are often unknown. Pulmonary fibrosis may develop as a reaction to noxious gas inhalation, to silicosis, or to radiation; it may develop in collagen disease, extensive tuberculosis, and many other diseases. Hamman-Rich disease is a syndrome of pulmonary fibrosis of unknown cause.

The patient with pulmonary fibrosis is short of breath because of his "small lung" and problems with gas exchange. Blood gas findings demonstrate hypoxemia and often hypercapnia. Clubbing of the fingers is also a common sign. Cardiac complications may follow, since heart rate must be increased to make up for respiratory impairment. There is no cure and no specific treatment for pulmonary fibrosis, but adrenocortical steroids are often helpful in reducing pulmonary dysfunction and in relieving symptoms. The patient is cautioned to avoid strenuous exercise that will tax the respiratory and cardiac systems and, above all, to guard against exposure to upper respiratory infection.

□ Sarcoidosis

Sarcoidosis is a systemic disease of unknown cause. Any organ system may be involved, but pulmonary manifestations are the most common. Sarcoidosis is most prevalent in American blacks and in northern European whites and occurs most often between the ages of 20 and 40.

Clinical picture. The central pathologic event involves the growth of granulomas and proliferation of lymph tissue. It commonly presents on chest x-ray films as enlarged lymph nodes in the hilar area. The patient with sarcoidosis may initially complain only of vague symptoms of malaise, fever, aching in the joints, or weakness. In addition to mediastinal lymph node enlargement, ocular manifestations, such as uveitis and conjunctivitis, and dermatologic changes, such as erythema nodosum, are commonly found.

Diagnosis of sarcoidosis is based on roentgenographic findings, organ biopsy, and positive skin test. The Kveim-Siltzback test involves the injection of sarcoid tissue; if the reaction is positive, a visible, palpable nodule develops at the site 3 to 6 weeks after the antigen is injected. The nodule must then be biopsied to confirm the presence of granulomatous tissue. The Kveim test is not always performed as part of the diagnostic process, however, because it is difficult to obtain the active antigen and because the test is associated with frequent false-negative results. Organ biopsy yields the most conclusive evidence of sarcoidosis and is most helpful in differentiating it from Hodgkin's disease and tuberculosis.

Intervention. In most cases sarcoidosis is a benign, self-limiting process that resolves with no residual damage within 2 years of diagnosis. However, about 10% of patients do have the chronic form of sarcoidosis. In this form the disease proceeds to nodular granulomatous depositions in lung tissue and eventual pulmonary fibrosis. In severe cases this will advance to pulmonary hypertension and right ventricular failure (cor pulmonale). The only treatment available at this time is the administration of corticosteroids. Nursing care is similar to that of the patient with pulmonary fibrosis and includes teaching the patient about the use of the corticosteroids.

PULMONARY EMBOLISM AND PULMONARY INFARCTION

Pulmonary embolism is the lodgment of a clot or other foreign matter in a pulmonary arterial vessel, and pulmonary infarction is the hemorrhagic necrosis of a part of the lung parenchyma caused by interruption of its blood supply, usually as a result of embolism.[14]

The source of the embolism may be thrombi originating in the iliac, femoral, or pelvic veins; the prostatic venous plexus; the vena cava; and the right atrium. They are common in older persons who are confined to bed. Postoperative embolism usually comes from a thrombosed vein in the pelvis or the lower extremities. It may cause symptoms before any signs of venous thrombosis appear at its place of origin.

The size of the pulmonary artery in which the clot lodges and the number of emboli determine the severity of symptoms and the prognosis. If the embolus blocks the pulmonary artery or one of its main branches, immediate death may occur, and it is often mistaken for a coronary occlusion. The actual incidence of pulmonary emboli is difficult to determine; many small emboli remain undiagnosed. Depending upon the population studied, the occurrence in hospitalized patients may be as high as 14%.[83]

Clinical picture. If the embolus blocks a smaller vessel, the person may complain of sudden sharp upper abdominal or thoracic pain, become dyspneic, cough violently, and have hemoptysis; shock may develop rapidly. If the area of infarction is small, the symptoms are much milder. The patient may have cough, pleuritic chest pain, slight hemoptysis, and elevation of temperature with an increase of leukocyte count in the blood. An area of dullness can be detected on listening to the patient's breath sounds.

The diagnosis of pulmonary embolism is made by the clinical history, by changes in blood chemistries, and by chest films. Lung scans and pulmonary angiography are also done; pulmonary angiography is a definitive diagnostic tool if a sharp cut-off is seen. As recannulization often takes place rapidly, the procedure must be done in the acute phase, or else it may be negative. The diagnosis of pulmonary embolism is often, of necessity, based on clinical criteria alone.

Intervention. If the person survives a severe pulmonary infarction, immediate medical attention is required. While awaiting the physician, the person should be kept in bed and as quiet as possible. A high Fowler's position usually helps breathing. The subsequent medical and nursing care are similar to that needed by the person who has an acute myocardial infarction (p. 992). If the infarction is a mild one, the treatment is more conservative and resembles that provided for the patient with pneumonia. In either case an immediate attempt is made to locate the original source of the embolus and to treat the thrombosis with anticoagulants. (See references 38 and 59 for a detailed discussion of therapy.)

The development of techniques to provide extra corporeal circulation (p. 974) has made it possible to remove emboli from the pulmonary arteries—a major step forward, since pulmonary emboli cause many deaths. At present this surgery is done quite rarely. The nursing care following pulmonary artery surgery combines that needed after any operation on major blood vessels and the postoperative care of patients having thoracic surgery as well as the care of the patient being treated medically for pulmonary embolism.

The best treatment for pulmonary embolism is prevention. Prevention of thrombophlebitis in patients undergoing surgery is discussed on p. 405. The same nursing measures should be used to prevent emboli in medical patients, especially when the patient is elderly and has chronic vascular or heart disease.

CARCINOMA

During the last 40 years there has been a startling increase in the incidence of carcinoma of the lung. There were nearly 80,000 deaths from carcinoma of the lung in 1974.[5] It is the leading cause of cancer deaths in men, the rate being 14 times greater than 40 years ago. The death rate in women, although lower than in men, is increasing at a much faster rate. The mortality rate of lung cancer is primarily dependent upon the specific type of cancer and the size of the tumor when detected. Squamous cell carcinoma is the most common, followed by adenocarcinoma; undifferentiated small cell (oat cell) is the least common and has the lowest 5-year survival rate (less than 1%). If the tumor is of the squamous cell type and is detected while still small and localized (less than 3 cm), the 5-year survival rate is as high as 40%.[30] Most people who develop the disease are over 50 years of age. Some of the factors believed to be involved in the increased incidence of carcinoma of the lung include an increase in smoking among women, more accurate diagnosis, and a tendency to name the lung as the primary site.

Carcinoma of the lung may be either metastatic or primary. Metastatic tumors may follow malignancy anywhere in the body. Metastasis from the colon and kidney is common. Metastasis to the lung may be discovered before the primary lesion is known, and sometimes the location of the primary lesion is not determined during the person's life.

Prevention. The cause of carcinoma of the lung is closely related to cigarette smoking. Table 50-2 shows

Table 50-2. Deaths caused by lung cancer, according to smoking habits*

	Deaths per 100,000 population
Nonsmokers	3.4
10 to 20 cigarettes per day	54.3
20 to 40 (1 to 2 packs) per day	143.9
> 40 (2 packs) per day	217.3

*From American Cancer Society: Cancer facts and figures, New York, 1976, The Society.

the extreme increase in mortality due to lung cancer in those who smoke. Prevention is the best protection against carcinoma of the lung because early detection of the disease if difficult, and at the present time only about 1 person in 10 (10%) is "cured" (living at the end of 5 years). From available research data it seems evident that curtailing smoking is a primary preventive measure. The nurse should be active in teaching the dangers in smoking and should set a positive health example in this regard. It is especially important that teenagers be given specific facts concerning the dangers involved in cigarette smoking because they are not likely to be habitual smokers at that age. Recent studies indicate that the incidence of smoking among teenagers is on the increase. People who are already habitual smokers should also be urged to stop smoking, even though it may be very difficult for them to do so. Various types of programs to assist persons to stop smoking are available. See reference 29 for more information. Since air pollution affects the lungs and may predispose to the development of carcinoma, the nurse should encourage and actively support community programs to decrease the amount of air pollution. Industrial exposure, particularly to asbestos, is also associated with an increased risk of carcinoma and has received increased attention recently.

Clinical picture. Since most new growths in the lungs arise from the bronchi, the term *bronchogenic* carcinoma is widely used. The symptoms that a patient has will depend on whether the neoplasm is located peripherally or centrally. Peripheral lesions may not cause any symptoms and be discovered only on routine chest roentgenograms. If peripheral lesions perforate into the pleural space, there will be *pleural effusion* (fluid in the pleural space), and direct invasion of the ribs and vertebral bodies may follow. If this occurs, the pain may be severe.

Centrally located lesions arise from one of the larger branches of the bronchial tree. They cause obstruction and ulceration of the bronchus with subsequent distal suppuration. Symptoms include cough, hemoptysis, dyspnea, chills, and fever. Unilateral wheezing may be heard on auscultation.

In the later stage of the disease, weight loss and debility usually indicate metastases, especially to the liver. Carcinoma of the lung may metastasize to nearby structures such as the prescalene lymph nodes, the walls of the esophagus, the pericardium or the heart, or to distant areas such as the brain, liver, or skeleton.

Intervention. Time is very important in the treatment of lung cancer. If carcinoma is detected while it is still confined to a local area, immediate surgery, with removal of all or part of a lung (pneumonectomy or lobectomy), may be successful. The nursing care of the patient following surgery of the lung is discussed on p. 969.

Palliative treatment (irradiation, chemotherapy, or both) may be used for those persons who cannot be treated surgically, particularly when there is obstruction of an airway, obstruction of major vessels, severe pain, or recurrent pleural effusion. Chemotherapy using numerous combinations of drugs is presently being tested. Experimental studies with immunotherapy as an adjuvant to surgery and radiotherapy are also under way.

Efforts to detect malignant lesions of the lung early while curative treatment may be possible must be continued. The nurse should urge all persons, particularly men over 40 years of age, to have an x-ray examination of the chest periodically in addition to a yearly physical examination. As a result of various public education media, many people have become more conscious of early signs of pulmonary cancer, but there is still a great need for them to learn about diagnostic tests that are available, including x-ray examinations, bronchoscopic examinations, and cytologic studies of sputum. The nurse should know of available cancer detection clinics in the community and should assist patients to secure proper medical supervision (Chapter 25).

■ PROBLEMS OF THE THORAX

□ Chest trauma

Trauma to the chest is a major problem most often seen first in the emergency department. The injuries to the chest range from a few fractured ribs to major trauma to the chest wall, sternum, lungs, heart, and major blood vessels. Injuries to the chest are broadly classified into two groups—blunt and penetrating. *Blunt* or nonpenetrating injuries include fractures of the ribs in which there is no damage to the pleura and lung. These injuries occur most commonly as the result of automobile accidents, falls, or blast injuries. Automobile accidents in the United States kill approximately 45,000 persons each year. Of this number, 40% have a major thoracic injury.[47] The injury is most often sustained when striking the steering wheel or being hurled from the car.

Fractures of the ribs

The fourth, fifth, sixth, seventh, and eighth ribs are most commonly fractured. Fractures of the ribs are caused by blows, crushing injuries, or strain caused by severe coughing or sneezing spells. If the rib is splintered or the fracture displaced, sharp fragments may penetrate the pleura and the lung. Persons with possible rib fractures should have an x-ray examination of the chest and should be observed carefully for signs of pneumothorax or hemothorax. The person with a rib fracture complains of pain at the site of the injury that increases on inspiration. The area is very tender to the touch, and the individual splints his chest and takes shallow breaths. Unless the lung has been penetrated, the usual treatment for rib fracture is conservative and includes strapping the chest with adhesive tape from the affected side to the unaffected side or applying a circular strapping, using an Ace bandage. A chest binder also may be used. If adhesive tape is used, the skin may be shaved and painted with tincture of benzoin to prevent blistering and other irritation. When the pain is severe and is not relieved by strapping and analgesic medications, the physician may do a regional nerve block. This procedure consists of infiltrating the intercostal spaces above and below the fractured rib with 1% procaine. If the lung has been penetrated, the person may raise bright red sputum.

Paradoxical breathing. When ribs are fractured in more than one place, the chest wall on that side becomes unstable and the result is a *flail chest.* Thus the chest wall no longer provides the rigid bony support that is necessary to maintain the bellows function required for normal ventilation. This causes paradoxical breathing. In *paradoxical breathing* the portion of the lung underlying the unstable chest wall moves opposite to the remainder of the lung. On inspiration that portion of the lung sucks in while the remaining lung expands. On expiration it balloons out as the remaining lung contracts. This results in a vicious cycle of events leading to *hypoxia.* The treatment of paradoxical motion is to *stabilize the chest wall.* The treatment may either be by internal or external stabilization of the chest wall.

Internal stabilization is the treatment of choice and is best obtained by use of a *volume-controlled* ventilator attached to a cuffed tracheostomy tube (p. 946). The ventilator is set to automatically control the patient's respirations. The patient who is breathing against the ventilator will need to be sedated. Narcotics, sedatives, and even muscle relaxants may have to be given. When the patient also has a head injury, narcotics are contraindicated and muscle relaxants will be used until ventilatory control is achieved. Once the person is quieted down and is no longer resisting the ventilator, hyperventilation can be used to depress the respiratory center so that ventilatory control is maintained.[47] The patient will require meticulous tracheostomy care in order to maintain a clear airway and to prevent infection. The patient may have to be on the ventilator for as long as 8 to 14 days. During this time the attention of experienced respiratory therapists, frequent blood gas studies, and constant care by skilled nursing personnel will be required. Culture and sensitivity studies of tracheal aspirations should be repeated at least every 4 to 5 days. These can be obtained by collecting the tracheal aspiration in a Luken's tube.

External stabilization was widely used before the development of modern mechanical ventilators and still may be used occasionally. Under local anesthesia a small incision is made, and stainless steel wire is attached to the ribs or sternum to pull the chest wall outward. The wire is connected to a rope and pulley with about 2.25 kg (5 lb) of weight. Usually in 14 to 21 days the chest wall becomes rigid enough to permit removal of the traction.

Penetrating wounds of the chest

When a knife, bullet, or other flying missile enters the chest, a penetrating wound occurs. The major problem in penetrating injury is not injury to the chest wall but injury to the structures within the chest cavity. Penetration of the lung is associated with leakage of air from the lung into the pleural cavity (pneumothorax) (Fig. 50-4). Blood may also leak into the pleural cavity (hemothorax). As the air or fluid accumulates in the pleural cavity, it builds up positive pressure, which causes the lung to collapse and may even cause a mediastinal shift, thus compressing the opposite lung and interfering with cardiac action. The person then has serious difficulty in breathing and may go into shock. The pulse may become weak and rapid and the skin cold and clammy, and blood pressure falls rapidly.

Emergency treatment is directed toward sustaining oxygen exchange and correcting circulatory failure. Usually the patient is intubated with an endotracheal tube and then is checked for air or blood in the pleural cavity. An emergency thoracentesis is done, and air and fluid are removed by syringe. Usually a catheter is inserted into the pleural space and connected to water-seal drainage (p. 971). If the lung fails to reexpand with this treatment or there is evidence of internal bleeding, surgical exploration may be necessary and will be done as soon as shock and other complications are under control.

In order to monitor the patient for hypovolemia, a central venous pressure (CVP) line is inserted (p. 923). This line can also be used to administer intravenous fluids and blood as necessary. If it is suspected that cardiac injury and tamponade may be present, a *pericardicentesis* will be done. The CVP is a very effective way to monitor for tamponade. A pressure above 15 cm of water or a rising CVP in a patient in shock with penetrating trauma in the region of the heart often indicates cardiac tamponade.[47]

If an open sucking wound of the chest has been sustained, it should be covered immediately to prevent air from entering the pleural cavity and causing a pneumothorax. Several thicknesses of nonporous material may be used, and these are anchored with wide adhesive tape, or the wound edges may be taped tightly together. If an object such as a knife is still in the wound, it must never be removed until a physician arrives. Its presence may prevent the entry of air into the pleural cavity, and its removal may cause further damage. The person who has sustained a penetrating wound of the chest should be placed in an upright position and taken to the nearest emergency room.

□ Pneumothorax

Pneumothorax is a condition in which there is air in the pleural space between the lung and the chest wall (Fig 50-4). It usually results from the rupture of an emphysematous bleb on the surface of the lung, but it may also follow severe bouts of coughing in persons who suffer from a chronic chest disease such as asthma. It also occurs when wounds have penetrated the chest wall and perforated the pleura. Rather frequently it occurs as a single or recurrent episode in otherwise healthy young people. As atmospheric pressure builds up in the pleural space, the lung on the affected side collapses and the heart and mediastinum shift toward the unaffected lung. If untreated, the person may die.

Clinical picture. A *spontaneous pneumothorax* occurs without warning. The person has a sudden sharp pain in the chest, accompanied by dyspnea, anxiety, increased diaphoresis, weak and rapid pulse, fall in blood pressure, and cessation of normal chest movement on the affected side. Roentgenograms are always ordered to determine the amount of air in the pleural space and the amount of collapse of the lung as well as the degree of mediastinal shift. When roentgenograms are taken, the patient needs help to prevent overexertion.

Intervention. When a spontaneous pneumothorax is suspected, a physician should be summoned immediately. The patient should not be left alone and should be reassured and urged to be quiet and not to exert himself. Oxygen and equipment for a thoracentesis should be assembled at once. Air is immediately aspirated from the affected pleural space, and the intra-

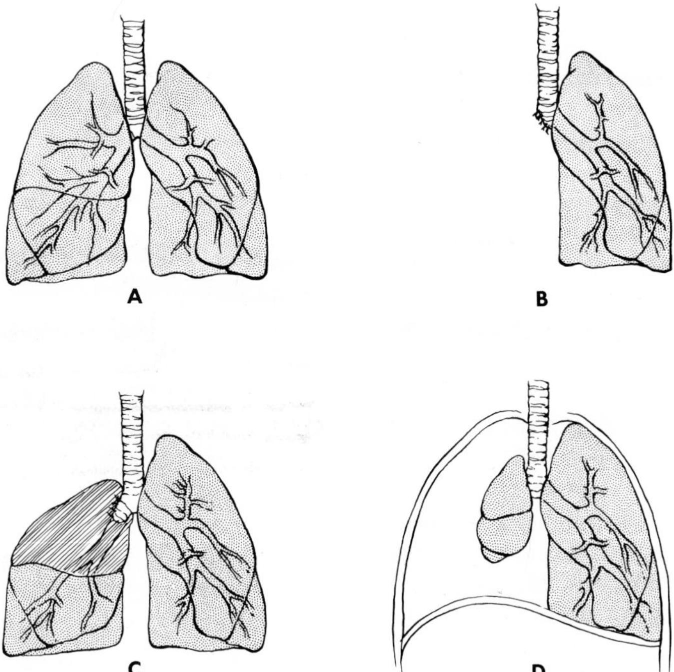

Fig. 50-4. A, Normal expanded lungs. **B,** Surgical absence of right lung following pneumonectomy. **C,** Surgical absence of right upper lobe following lobectomy. **D,** Complete collapse of right lung caused by air in pleural cavity (pneumothorax).

pleural pressure is brought to normal if possible. If air continues to flow into the pleural space, a chest tube will be inserted and connected to water-seal drainage. If the cause of the condition is trauma, the immediate treatment is to seal the chest wound and then to aspirate air from the pleural space.

The person who has had a spontaneous pneumothorax is usually most comfortable in a sitting position. Physical activity is kept at a minimum for at least 24 hours. The patient is asked to remain as quiet as possible and to avoid stretching, reaching, or moving suddenly. Breathing should be normal, and the breath should not be held. Pulse rate and respirations must be checked frequently.

When air no longer is expelled from the pleural space through the underwater drainage system and a roentgenogram reveals that the lung has completely reexpanded, the chest tube is removed and the person is allowed out of bed. Strenuous exertion, which increases rate and depth of respirations for a time, should be avoided, but relatively normal activity may be resumed rather quickly. If there are frequent recurring episodes, some physicians instill silver nitrate into the pleural space to cause adhesions between the visceral and parietal pleurae. If this procedure is unsuccessful, the portion containing the defect may be resected from the lung and the parietal pleura abraded so that it will adhere to the visceral pleura.

□ Empyema

Empyema means pus within a body cavity. It usually applies to the pleural cavity. Empyema occurs as a result of, or in association with, other respiratory disease such as pneumonia, lung abscess, tuberculosis, and fungous infections of the lung and also following thoracic surgery or chest trauma. It is now occurring fairly often as a complication of staphylococcal pneumonia.

Clinical picture. The patient with any kind of lung infection or chest injury should be observed closely for signs of empyema, which include cough, dyspnea, unilateral chest pain, elevation of temperature, malaise, poor appetite, and unequal chest expansion. The condition may develop several weeks after an apparently minor respiratory infection. The diagnosis can usually be made from the signs and symptoms and the medical history, but it is confirmed by a chest roentgenogram that demonstrates the presence of a pleural exudate. A thoracentesis is done to obtain a sample of the pus for culture and sensitivity studies and to relieve the patient's respiratory symptoms.

Intervention. The aim in the treatment of empyema is to drain the empyema cavity completely and thus obliterate the pleural space. This can be accomplished in several ways. Initially the cavity may be aspirated daily and antibiotics instilled in it in an attempt to sterilize this space. If the cavity cannot be evacuated within a few days of if the lung fails to reexpand so as to obliterate the space, surgical treatment is necessary. Depending on the situation, either closed or open chest drainage may be employed. In closed chest drainage a trocar is inserted between the ribs at the base of the empyema cavity. A chest catheter is then threaded through the trocar, the trocar is removed, and the tube is connected to water-seal drainage (p. 971). This allows the pus to drain from the cavity into the water-seal bottle. It will only be effective, however, if the pus in thin and easily removed and if the visceral pleura is capable of moving out to the parietal pleura to eliminate the space. When empyema is chronic and the lung is adherent to the chest wall, rib resection with open drainage is often employed. In this procedure a portion of one or two ribs is removed. A large tube is inserted into the cavity and allowed to drain into a chest dressing. The tube is changed weekly. If this method of treatment is successful, the empyema cavity will gradually be eliminated. In some instances of chronic empyema a fibrinous peel forms on the visceral pleura, keeping the lung from reexpanding and filling the space left after the empyema cavity was drained. In this situation a *decortication* is performed. In decortication the fibrinous peel is removed from the lung by blunt dissection, freeing the lung so that it can expand and fill the pleural space. In order to assure that expansion will occur, chest tubes are inserted into the pleural space and connected to water-seal drainage and suction. When there is evidence that the lung has reexpanded, the tubes are removed. (See p. 971 for further discussion of chest drainage.) If none of these methods are successful in closing the pleural space, a thoracoplasty (removal of ribs) may be necessary.

■ RESPIRATORY INSUFFICIENCY AND RESPIRATORY FAILURE

The term *respiratory insufficiency* is usually used to indicate that the exchange of oxygen and carbon dioxide is not adequate to meet the needs of the body during normal activities. Respiratory failure is said to occur when ventilation is not sufficient to achieve gas exchange

CRITERIA FOR DIAGNOSIS OF RESPIRATORY FAILURE

$P_{O_2} < 50$ mm Hg when breathing room air
$P_{CO_2} > 50$ mm Hg
Vital capacity < 15 ml/kg
Respiratory rate > 30/min or below 8/min

Table 50-3. Disorders associated with respiratory insufficiency and failure

Pulmonary disorders	Nonpulmonary disorders
Severe infection Pulmonary edema Pulmonary embolus COPD Adult respiratory distress syndrome Cancer Chest trauma Severe atelectasis Airway compromise secondary to trauma, infection, or surgery	CNS disturbance secondary to drug overdose, anesthesia, head injury Neuromuscular disorders (e.g., Guillain-Barré, myasthenia gravis, multiple sclerosis, poliomyelitis, muscular dystrophy, spinal cord injury) Postoperative reduction in ventilation following thoracic and abdominal surgery Prolonged mechanical ventilation

even at rest. Many disorders can lead to or are associated with both respiratory insufficiency and failure; these are listed in Table 50-3.

The diagnosis of respiratory insufficiency or failure is based on arterial blood gas studies, pulmonary function testing, and the clinical status of the patient. The criteria in the boxed material on p. 1134 are generally used in defining a state of failure. However, it cannot be overemphasized that these parameters are only *guidelines* and must be applied in light of the individual's history, age, and overall condition.

Regardless of the underlying condition, the resultant events or processes that occur in respiratory failure are the same. With inadequate ventilation, the arterial PO_2 falls and tissue cells become hypoxic. The PCO_2 accumulates, leading to a fall in pH, and the patient becomes acidotic. The reader must keep in mind, in working with the patient with COPD who has developed respiratory failure, that this patient normally exists in a compensated state with decreased PO_2 levels and elevated PCO_2 levels. Thus the parameters in the boxed material are not applicable; the pH, however, is a useful guide in assessing the degree of insufficiency. When the pH begins to fall below 7.3, it is an indication that the patient is no longer able to compensate for the elevated PCO_2 level.

□ Adult respiratory distress syndrome

Respiratory insufficiency and failure can result from a worsening in the condition of the patient with any of the disorders already mentioned. The adult respiratory distress syndrome (ARDS), however, always involves a degree of respiratory failure that requires special mechanical ventilatory techniques.

ARDS refers to a syndrome of pathophysiologic changes in lung tissue that may be secondary to a number of events, including cardiopulmonary bypass, multiple blood transfusions, aspiration, gram-negative sepsis, and oxygen toxicity. In the past it was believed that these were separate clinical entities, and terms such as shock lung, postperfusion lung, wet-lung syndrome, and stiff-lung syndrome were used to describe each. It is now believed that each of these describe the same pathophysiologic reaction to varying stressors.

The changes that occur in the patient with ARDS are presented in Fig. 50-5. In general, two events produce the changes that lead to the necessity for mechanical ventilation. First, there is usually some degree of capillary membrane damage. This leads to hemorrhage and the leaking of fluid from the capillary. The damage and presence of interstitial edema impairs gas exchange between the alveoli and blood stream, and ventilation-perfusion abnormalities result (p. 935). In addition, disturbances in surfactant production lead to alveolar collapse. As areas of the lung become atelectatic, it is more difficult to inflate them with each breath, compliance decreases, and the work of breathing increases. The atelectasis also further increases the ventilation-perfusion disparity. The end result of these processes, hypoxemia, and inability to adequately ventilate, necessitate mechanical ventilation in almost all cases and the use of positive end expiratory pressure (PEEP), which is discussed under mechanical ventilation.

□ Intervention

Interventions for the patient who has respiratory insufficiency or failure always begin with a recognition of the underlying disease state or cause of the disturbance in ventilation. Therapy is first directed at improving the underlying condition, such as sepsis, or removing the cause, such as fluid overload.

The goals of intervention are to improve oxygenation and ventilation in order to restore the person's normal PO_2 and PCO_2 levels. The initial medical management can often be conservative if the diagnosis is made early enough. All of the intervention measures discussed in Chapter 45 may be used.

Oxygen. Particular care is needed in working with the patient who has chronic lung disease. As mentioned earlier, individuals with COPD normally exist with elevated PCO_2 levels and have lost the usual respiratory drive, carbon dioxide stimulation. They no longer respond to increased carbon dioxide levels by increasing their rate and depth of respiration; rather, the elevated PCO_2 depresses the respiratory center. Their respiratory drive is now derived from their low PO_2 levels.

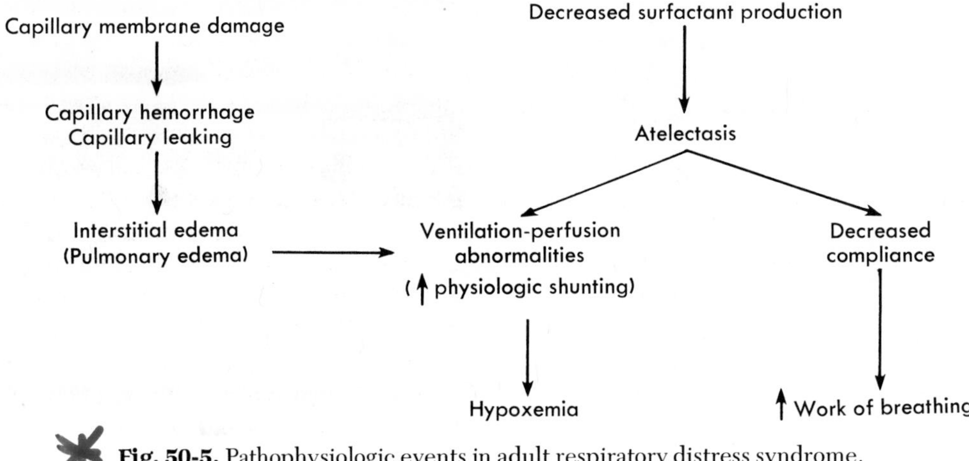

Fig. 50-5. Pathophysiologic events in adult respiratory distress syndrome.

Therefore even though these persons lack oxygen, it is extremely dangerous to raise their Po_2 to normal levels. If the arterial Po_2 is normal and there is retention of carbon dioxide *(hypercapnia)*, the person will have no respiratory drive. Hypoventilation becomes more severe and Pco_2 continues to rise. This situation results in *carbon dioxide narcosis*, a markedly elevated carbon dioxide level that causes coma or semicoma. Persons with COPD are therefore treated with low flow or controlled flow oxygen; that is, inspired oxygen concentrations of 24% to 30%. These concentrations can easily be obtained by using a Venti-mask or a two-pronged nasal cannula with a 1 to 2 liter oxygen flow. This amount of oxygen can significantly increase the amount of oxygen carried by hemoglobin without a significant increase in arterial Po_2. Therefore the patient's blood carries much more oxygen even though hypoxemia is still present. The person continues to have respiratory drive, and the Pco_2 does not rise. These patients also receive frequent (every 1 to 2 hours) IPPB therapy to aid ventilation and reduce CO_2 levels. Because the IPPB machines deliver 60% to 80% oxygen (not 40%) when set on oxygen with air dilution, the equipment must be modified to administer low flow oxygen. Low concentrations of oxygen are obtained by using compressed air for the driving force and adding 1 liter per minute of oxygen through the nebulizer. By the use of low flow oxygen the amount of oxygen carried in the patient's blood can often be increased enough to maintain basic body function without further reduction of ventilation. Persons who do not have COPD, who have a normal Pco_2, but who are hypoxic are usually able to tolerate high flow rates of oxygen (5 to 10 liters per minute). Oxygen is an integral part of the therapy of patients with respiratory insufficiency and failure; however, some hazards are associated with prolonged use.

Oxygen toxicity is the term used to describe the damage to lung tissue that results from prolonged exposure to high concentrations. Although the exact effects of oxygen in any one individual may be dependent upon the person's underlying pathology, it is believed that exposure to greater than 60% oxygen for a period of more than 36 hours, or exposure to 100% oxygen for a period of more than 6 hours, will result in atelectasis and alveolar collapse. Breathing very high concentrations of oxygen (80% to 100%) for prolonged periods (24 hours or more) is often associated with the development of ARDS.[61,75] Thus it is a firm general principle that the lowest amount of oxygen that will achieve an acceptable Po_2 is the amount that should be used.

Rest. In addition to providing supplemental oxygen, care of the person with respiratory insufficiency usually also includes aggressive airway management and attempts to improve ventilation. Thus suctioning, IPPB, ultrasonic mist therapy, and postural drainage with clapping and vibrating are all employed in an attempt to halt the progression of insufficiency. The patient who is subjected to many treatments can become excessively fatigued, further compromising ventilatory capacity. Frequent rest periods must be interspersed with treatments, and it is the nurse's responsibility to see that the patient is provided with a quiet environment and is not disturbed by unnecessary interruptions at rest times. Unfortunately, persons who have severe insufficiency must have frequent treatments and interventions; it is *not* appropriate, even though the person may be quite tired, to allow the patient to sleep through the night and omit treatments. This will inevitably lead to a worsened status.

Although persons with respiratory insufficiency are often anxious and frightened, sedation is contraindicated because it depresses respiration. Therefore it is especially important that the nurse be supportive of the patient and be skillful in assisting with effective breathing. The patient can be extremely demanding, and the nurse must understand the fear and anxiety that is often the basis for the patient's behavior.

Monitoring. Aggressive, constant nursing care is essential for these patients. The nurse must be continually alert to clinical changes that represent changes in the patient's ventilation. Increasing confusion and behavioral changes often indicate an elevated P_{CO_2}. The behavioral changes may range from pugnacious, combative behavior to lethargy. Other clinical signs of *hypercapnia* are flushed skin color caused by reflex vasodilation, muscle twitching, and headache. Signs commonly seen in *hypoxia* include tachycardia, increased pulse rate, cyanosis, changes in blood pressure, and changes in behavior. In *early* stages of hypoxia, the blood pressure is elevated as a result of vasoconstriction and increased peripheral resistance. In *later* stages the blood pressure falls to hypotensive levels, and circulatory arrest can occur. It is important to point out that cyanosis is not an early sign of hypoxia, since it does not occur until arterial oxygen saturation is less than 85%. Thus the nurse needs to be alert to earlier signs of hypoxia.

Mechanical ventilation. If, despite all the measures discussed, the person is unable to maintain ventilation, as indicated by a rising arterial P_{CO_2}, mechanical ventilation is necessary. The basic use of respirators, endotracheal and tracheostomy tubes, and the suctioning procedure used with an artificial airway are discussed in Chapter 45.

Positive end expiratory pressure (PEEP), is a ventilator mode that has recently been shown to increase the effectiveness of mechanical ventilation in certain patients. PEEP involves the maintenance of positive pressure, usually between 5 and 15 cm water pressure, at the end of expiration, rather than allowing airway pressure to return to normal (atmospheric) as usually occurs. By maintaining positive pressure, alveoli that would otherwise collapse on expiration are held open, thus increasing the opportunity for gas exchange across the alveolar-capillary membrane. This effect, which is equivalent to increasing the functional residual capacity, decreases physiologic shunting and makes it possible to achieve a higher level of P_{O_2}, with lower concentrations of delivered oxygen (F_1O_2). PEEP has its greatest use in the treatment of ARDS, but is also used in any patient who would otherwise require unacceptably high concentrations of oxygen.

The hazards of PEEP are related to the increase in intrathoracic pressure. Most serious of the dangers related to this technique is the increased incidence of pneumothorax, particularly in those with friable lung tissue, as seen in persons with emphysema or lung cancer. The sudden disappearance of breath sounds on one side, in conjunction with signs of respiratory distress, in the patient being ventilated with PEEP *must be taken as an indication of a pneumothorax.* This can develop into a life-threatening episode if the pneumothorax is large, and the physician must be called immediately. Another less serious consequence of PEEP may be a reduction in venous return, which is impeded by the increased intrathoracic pressure, and a subsequent fall in cardiac output. This effect seems to be particularly common in patients who are relatively dehydrated and can sometimes be avoided by careful fluid administration.

Weaning from the ventilator. The nurse plays an important role in weaning the patient from the ventilator. Both physiologic studies (blood gases, tidal volume) and clinical status determine the patient's readiness to breathe without mechanical assistance. Prior to weaning, the patient should have been taught breathing exercises. When the patient is taken off the respirator, a nurse in whom the patient has confidence should remain with him. It is also helpful if the environment around the patient is calm. Much of the success of weaning is dependent on the interrelationship between the patient's physiologic and psychologic responses. If the patient becomes very anxious and takes rapid, shallow breaths, being off the respirator will be poorly tolerated. If a pattern of controlled breathing can be maintained, success is much more likely. Weaning is usually begun with short periods off the respirator. The amount of time off the respirator is increased according to the patient's tolerance. The nurse must carefully assess the adequacy of the patient's ventilation during the time off the respirator. If, in the nurse's judgment, the patient cannot tolerate breathing on his own because of inadequate tidal volume, cyanosis, tachycardia, diaphoresis, or restlessness, mechanical assistance should be reinstituted.

A more recent technique of weaning is the use of *intermittent mandatory ventilation (IMV).* This involves the addition of an oxygen reservoir with a one-way valve to the respirator circuit. The rate on the ventilator is reduced below the patient's normal rate. The ventilator then delivers the set minimum, and the patient spontaneously breathes several breaths in addition to this from the oxygen reservoir. For example, if the patient's natural respiratory rate is 16, the ventilator might be set to deliver 10 breaths per minute. The patient will then take an additional six breaths independently. In this way the patient can gradually build up strength and gain respiratory independence without having to be taken completely off the ventilator for periods of time.

Throughout the treatment of the patient in respiratory failure, ventilation should be carefully monitored by blood gas studies and simple spirometry (tidal volume, vital capacity). Alert nursing observation of the patient can determine the adequacy of ventilation. Meticulous attention is given to maintaining a patent airway, which is the prime nursing responsibility. (See specialized material for further detail.[45,54,75])

REFERENCES AND SELECTED READINGS

1. Abraham, A. S.: The management of patients with chronic bronchitis and cor pulmonale, Heart Lung **6**:104-108, 1977.
2. Agle, D. P., and Baum, G. L.: Psychological aspects of chronic obstructive pulmonary disease, Med. Clin. North Am. **61**:749-758, 1977.
3. Agle, D. P., Baum, G. L., Chester, E. H., et al.: Multidiscipline treatment of chronic pulmonary insufficiency. I. Psychologic aspects of rehabilitation, Psychosom. Med. **35**:41-49, 1973.
4. American Academy of Pediatrics: Report of the Committee on Infectious Diseases, ed. 17, Evanston, Ill., 1974, The Academy.
5. American Cancer Society: Cancer facts and figures, New York, 1976, The Society.
6. American College of Chest Physicians: A report of the Committee on Emphysema: recommendations for continuous oxygen therapy in chronic obstructive lung disease, Chest **64**:505-507, 1973.
7. *American Lung Association: Diagnostic standards and classification of tuberculosis, ed. 13, New York, 1974, The Association.
8. American Lung Association: Chronic obstructive pulmonary disease, a manual for physicians, New York, 1972, The Association.
9. American Thoracic Society: Treatment of mycobacterial disease, Am. Rev. Respir. Dis. **115**:185-187, 1977.
10. American Thoracic Society: Guidelines for the investigation and management of tuberculosis contacts, Am. Rev. Respir. Dis. **114**:459-463, 1976.
11. American Thoracic Society: Guidelines for long-term institutional care of tuberculosis patients, Am. Rev. Respir. Dis. **113**:253-254, 1976.
12. American Thoracic Society: Intermittent chemotherapy for adults with tuberculosis, Am. Rev. Respir. Dis. **110**:374-376, 1974.
13. Bates, D., Macklem, P. T., and Christie, R. V.: Respiratory function in disease, ed. 2, Philadelphia, 1971, W. B. Saunders Co.
14. Beeson, P. B., and McDermott, W., editors: Cecil-Loeb textbook of medicine, ed. 14, Philadelphia, 1975, W. B. Saunders Co.
15. Bergersen, B. S.: Pharmacology in nursing, ed. 13, St. Louis, 1976, The C. V. Mosby Co.

15a. Carr, D. T., and Rosenow, E. C.: Bronchogenic carcinoma, Basics RD **5**:1-6, May 1977.

16. Cimprich, B., Gaydos, D., and Langan, R.: A preoperative teaching program for the thoracotomy patient, Cancer Nurs. **1**:35-39, 1978.
17. Cushing, R.: Pulmonary infections, Heart Lung **5**:611-613, 1976.
18. Dunn, C. R., Dunn, D. L., and Moser, K. M.: Determinants of tracheal injury by cuffed tracheostomy tubes, Chest **65**:128-135, 1974.
19. Eickhoff, T. C.: The current status of BCG immunization against tuberculosis, Ann. Rev. Med. **28**:411-423, 1977.
20. Fergus, L. C., and Cordasco, E. M.: Pulmonary rehabilitation of the patient with COPD, Postgrad. Med. **62**:141-144, 1977.
21. *Fitzgerald, L. M.: Mechanical ventilation, Heart Lung **5**:939-949, 1976.
22. *Fitzmaurice, J. B., and Saskara, A. A.: Current concepts of pulmonary embolism: implications for nursing practice, Heart Lung **3**:209-218, 1974.
23. *Fuhs, M. F., and Stein, A. M.: Better ways to cope with COPD, Nurs. 76 **6**:28-38, 1976.
24. Gracey, D. R.: Home oxygen therapy for the COPD patient, Heart Lung **4**:792-794, 1975.
25. Gracey, D. R.: Adult respiratory distress syndrome, Heart Lung **4**:280-283, 1975.
26. *Grimes, O. F.: Neuromuscular syndromes in patients with lung cancer, Am. J. Nurs. **71**:752-755, 1971.
27. Herxheimer, H.: A guide to bronchial asthma, New York, 1975, Academic Press, Inc.
28. Hinshaw, H. C.: Diseases of the chest, ed. 3, Boston, 1969, Little, Brown & Co.
29. Hunt, W. J., and Bespalec, D. A.: An evaluation of current methods of modifying smoking behavior, J. Clin. Psychol. **30**:431-438, 1974.

29a. Israel, H. L., and Atkinson, G. W.: Sarcoidosis, Basics RD **7**: 1-6, Sept. 1978.

30. Israel, L., and Chahinian, A.: Lung cancer—natural history, prognosis, and therapy, New York, 1976, Academic Press, Inc.
31. Johnston, R. F., and Wildrick, K. H.: State of the art review: the impact of chemotherapy on the care of patients with tuberculosis, Am. Rev. Respir. Dis. **109**:636-664, 1974.

31a. Jones, R. W., and Weill, H.: Occupational lung disease, Basics RD **6**:1-6, Jan. 1978.

32. Karetzky, M. S., and Khan, A. U.: Review of current concepts in aspiration pneumonia, Heart Lung **6**:321-326, 1977.
33. Keim, L. W., Schuldt, S., and Bedell, G. N.: Tuberculosis in the intensive care unit, Heart Lung **6**:624-634, 1977.
34. Kopetzky, M.: Normal and asthmatic lungs: how they work. In Essays in medicine: asthma, New York, 1972, Medcom Books, Inc.
35. Lance, E., and Sweetwood, H.: Chest trauma, Nurs. 78 **8**:28-33, 1978.
36. Langston, H. T., and Barker, W. S.: The adult thoracic surgical patient. In Neville, W. E., editor: Care of the surgical cardiopulmonary patient, Chicago, 1971, Year Book Medical Publishers, Inc.
37. Larson, R. K., Barman, M. L., Kueppers, F., et al.: Genetic and environmental determinants of chronic obstructive pulmonary disease, Ann. Intern. Med. **72**:627-632, 1970.
38. Le Quense, D. M.: Relation between deep vein thrombosis and pulmonary embolism in surgical patients. N. Engl. J. Med. **291**:1202-1204, 1974.
39. Lowell, A. M.: Tuberculosis in the world: trends in tuberculosis incidence, prevalence, and mortality at the beginning of the third decade of the chemotherapeutic era, HEW publ. no. CDC 76-8317, Atlanta, 1976, U.S. Center for Disease Control.
40. Martini, N.: Lung cancer—an overview, Cancer Nurs. **1**:31-33, 1978.
41. Mittman, C.: Chronic obstructive lung disease: the result of the interaction of genetic and environmental factors, Heart Lung **2**:222-226, 1973.
42. Moody, L. E.: Primer for pulmonary hygiene, Am. J. Nurs. **77**:104-106, 1977.
43. *Moody, L. E.: Asthma, physiology and patient care, Am. J. Nurs. **73**:1212-1217, 1973.
44. National League for Nursing: Patient care in tuberculosis, ed. 2, New York, 1973, The League.
45. Nett, L.: The use of mechanical ventilators, Nurs. Clin. North Am. **9**:123-136, 1974.
46. Nett, L., and Petty, T. I.: Oxygen toxicity, Am. J. Nurs. **73**:1556-1558, 1973.

*References preceded by an asterisk are particularly well suited for student reading.

47. *Neville, W. E.: Care of the surgical cardiopulmonary patient, Chicago, 1971, Year Book Medical Publishers, Inc.
48. Niewoehner, D. E., Kleinerman, J., and Rice, D. B.: Pathologic changes in peripheral airways of young cigarette smokers, N. Engl. J. Med. **291**:755-758, 1974.
49. Perry, P. A.: A perspective on chronic obstructive pulmonary disease. In Andersen, E. H., Bergersen, B. S., Duffey, M., and Rose, M. H., editors: Current concepts in clinical nursing, vol. 4, St. Louis, 1973, The C. V. Mosby Co.
50. Peterson, L. D., and Green, J. H.: Nurse-managed tuberculosis clinic, Am. J. Nurs. **77**:433-435, 1977.
51. *Petty, T. L.: A chest physician's perspective on asthma, Heart Lung **1**:611-620, 1972.
52. *Petty, T. L.: Respiratory failure and the heart, Heart Lung **1**:84, 1972.
53. Petty, T. L. et al.: The adult respiratory distress syndrome, Chest **60**:233-242, 1971.
54. *Phipps, W. J., Barker, W. L., and Daly, B. J.: Respiratory insufficiency and failure. In Meltzer, L. E., Abdellah, F. G., and Kitchell, J. R.: Concepts and practices of intensive care for nurse specialists, ed. 2, Philadelphia, 1975, The Charles Press, Publishers.
55. Pontoppidan, H., Geffin, F., and Lowenstein, E.: Acute respiratory failure in the adult, N. Engl. J. Med. **27**:690-698, 743-752, 799-806, 1972.
56. *Rassmussen, D. L.: Black lung in southern Appalachia, Am. J. Nurs. **70**:509-511, 1970.
57. *Riley, R. L.: Air-borne infections, Am. J. Nurs. **60**:1246-1248, 1960.
58. Robinson, A. M.: Pulmonary TB: not quite a disease of the past, RN **38**:77-80, 82, 1975.
59. Sasahara, A. A.: Therapy for pulmonary embolism, J.A.M.A. **329**:1795-1798, 1974.
60. *Scott, B. H.: Tensions linked with emphysema, Am. J. Nurs. **69**:538-540, 1969.
61. *Shapiro, B. A., Harrison, R. A., and Trout, C. A.: Clinical application of respiratory care, Chicago, 1975, Year Book Medical Publishers, Inc.
62. *Sladin, A.: Pathogenesis of the shock lung, RN **34**:1-12, 1971.
63. Stechschulte, D. J.: Asthma and immunology. In Essays in medicine, New York, 1972, Medcom Books, Inc.
64. Sweetwood, H.: Acute respiratory insufficiency, Nurs. 77 **7**:24-31, 1977.
65. Thurlbeck, W. M.: Chronic bronchitis and emphysema—the pathophysiology of chronic lung disease. In American Thoracic Society: Basics of RD, New York, 1974, The Society.
66. Tomashefski, J. F., editor: Chronic obstructive pulmonary disease: a perplexing and challenging spectrum: core curriculum symposium (pulmonary disease) Postgrad. Med. **62**:87-151, 1977.
67. Traver, G. A.: Living with chronic respiratory disease, Am. J. Nurs. **75**:1777-1781, 1794, 1975.
68. U.S. Center for Disease Control, Tuberculosis Branch: Tuberculosis statistics: cities and and states—1976, Atlanta, 1977, The Center.
69. U.S. Center for Disease Control, Tuberculosis Control Division: Tuberculosis in the United States, 1976, HEW publ. no. CDC-76-8322, Atlanta, 1976, The Center.
70. U.S. Department of Commerce, Bureau of the Census: Statistical abstract of the United States, ed. 98, Washington, D.C., 1977, U.S. Government Printing Office.
71. U.S. Department of Health, Education, and Welfare: Guidelines for prevention of TB transmission in hospitals, Atlanta, 1975, U.S. Center for Disease Control.
72. U.S. Department of Health, Education, and Welfare: Current trends. Isoniazid-associated hepatitis: summary of the report of the tuberculosis advisory committee and special consultants to the director, U.S. Center for Disease Control, Morbid. Mortal. **23**:97-98, 1974.
73. U.S. Department of Health, Education, and Welfare: Recommendation of the public health service advisory committee on immunization practices—BCG vaccines, U.S. Center for Disease Control, Morbid. Mortal. **24**:69-80, 1975.
74. VanArsdel, P. P., Jr., and Glennon, G. H.: Drug therapy in the management of asthma, Ann. Intern. Med. **87**:68-74, 1977.
75. Wade, J. F.: Respiratory nursing care: physiology and technique, ed. 2, St. Louis, 1977, The C. V. Mosby Co.
76. *Wagner, M. M.: Assessment of patients with multiple injuries, Am. J. Nurs. **72**:1822-1827, 1972.
77. Ward, J.: Cromolyn sodium: a new approach to treatment of asthma, Heart Lung **4**:415-419, 1975.
78. Weg, J. G.: Tuberculosis and other mycobacterial diseases, American Lung Association, 1976.
79. *Weg, J. G.: Tuberculosis and the generation gap, Am. J. Nurs. **71**:495-500, 1971.
80. West, J. B.: Causes of carbon dioxide retention in lung disease, N. Engl. J. Med. **284**:1232-1236, 1971.
80a. West, J. B.: Pulmonary pathophysiology—the essentials, Baltimore, 1977, The Williams & Wilkins Co.
80b. West, J. B.: Respiratory physiology—the essentials, Baltimore, 1974, The Williams & Wilkins Co.
81. Wilson, R. F., and Sibbald, W. J.: Acute respiratory failure, Crit. Care Med. **4**:79-89, 1976.
82. Wintrobe, M. M., et al., editors: Harrison's principles of internal medicine, ed. 7, New York, 1974, McGraw-Hill Book Co.
83. *Wyper, M. A.: Pulmonary embolism: fighting the silent killer, Nurs. 75 **5**:31-38, 1975.
84. Ziskind, M. M.: The acute bacterial pneumonias in the adult. In American Thoracic Society: Basics of RD, New York, 1974, The Society.

AUDIOVISUAL RESOURCES

1. Care of the patient with pulmonary emphysema, Garden Grove, Calif., 1971, Trainex (cassette tape, filmstrip, instructor's guide and script).
2. Chronic obstructive pulmonary disease: breathing patterns, Washington, D. C., 1974, National Medical Audiovisual Center (movie, 16 mm).
3. Chronic obstructive pulmonary disease: diaphragmatic pattern, Washington, D. C., 1975, National Medical Audiovisual Center (movie, 16 mm).
4. Postural drainage: patient positioning, Washington, D.C., 1976, National Medical Audiovisual Center (movie, 16 mm).
5. The pathophysiology of emphysema, Garden Grove, Calif., 1971, Trainex (cassette tape, filmstrip, instructor's guide and script).

UNIT VIII

Problems of nutrition

Without food, human beings cannot survive. A person must be able to take in food and swallow it (ingestion) and to dilute and process the food in such a manner that nutrients are available to be transmitted to cells (digestion). Problems with structure or function of the upper gastrointestinal system or with amount or quality of food being processed can affect life itself. Problems with nutrition also affect other organs of the body, rendering them more susceptible to infections or other diseases. Maintenance of health therefore requires an intact and functioning gastrointestinal system and practices leading to the ingestion of adequate amount and quality of nutrients.

This unit consists of four chapters. The first two chapters discuss *assessment of nutritional status and of the upper gastrointestinal system* (mouth, throat, and stomach). This is followed by a discussion of *problems of malnutrition.* The last chapter deals with *specific problems of the mouth, throat, and stomach.*

51

Assessment of nutritional status

JANICE NEVILLE

National attention has been focused on nutrition since the White House Conference of 1969. The Conference stimulated public, political, and professional examination of nutritional care within medical and health care delivery systems in addition to publicizing hunger, malnutrition, and food concerns of the American public.[30] Malnutrition has been indicted as a major problem in hospitalized patients.[7] Nurses, physicians, and dietitians have been challenged to identify the nutritional needs of patients and to improve the quality of care.* The patient also has responsibilities,[25] whether hospitalized or at home, but should be able to expect nutritional care as an integral component of health care.

Many persons enter the hospital in poor nutritional status, and the nutritional status may deteriorate during hospitalization.[5,6,27,54] Studies of general populations in the United States have identified very few cases of frank deficiency disease, but a significant proportion of the population is either malnourished or at significant risk of developing nutritional problems.[9,51] Obesity is a major health problem in the United States and is present in the population at all age levels. Adolescents have the highest prevalence of unsatisfactory nutritional status, and many persons over 60 years of age present evidence of poor status. People are adopting new eating styles that may increase nutritional risk,[12,14,20,36] and eating patterns have been identified as a critical public health concern and national dietary goals have been proposed.[45]

Individuals with good nutritional status are less likely to get sick and generally are less seriously ill when sickness does occur. They also are better able to withstand trauma and stress. Recovery is significantly affected and can be enhanced by appropriate nutrition therapy.

Good nursing care has always included attention to the patient's food needs. Maintenance of good nutrition is a major nursing objective. Nutritional evaluation is an important part of total patient assessment and provides essential information for differential diagnosis and for planning appropriate interventions. An awareness of nutritional deficits, excesses, or imbalances that may exist can be of particular importance in determining management of the person. Monitoring the nutritional well-being of the person throughout hospitalization or on an ongoing basis to assure maintenance of or improvement in status is as important as the initial assessment.

*References 8, 13, 24, 41, 46.

Nutrition needs

Good nutritional status exists when protein, fat, carbohydrate, minerals, vitamins, and water are consumed in sufficient amounts and are used appropriately by the body to meet needs regardless of age, sex, life style, or state of health. All persons need the same nutrients throughout life (box below). The amounts required vary in predictable patterns. Growth, basal metabolic needs,

NUTRIENTS REQUIRED BY THE HUMAN BODY

Water	Minerals	Vitamins
Protein	Calcium	Vitamin C
Total nitrogen	Chromium	Biotin
Isoleucine	Phosphorus	Folacin
Leucine	Copper	Niacin
Lysine	Fluorine	Pantothenic acid
Methionine (cystine)	Iron	
	Iodine	Riboflavin
Phenylalanine (tyrosine)	Magnesium	Thiamin
	Manganese	Vitamin B_6
Threonine	Molybdenum	Vitamin B_{12}
Tryptophan	Selenium	Vitamin A (carotene)
Valine	Zinc	
Histidine (infant)	Sodium	Vitamin D
	Potassium	Vitamin E
Carbohydrate	Chloride	Vitamin K
Starch, sugar, fiber		
Fat		
Linoleate (arachidonate)		

Table 51-1. Recommended daily dietary allowances[1]* (designed for maintenance of good nutrition of practically all

	Age (yr)	Weight kg	Weight lb	Height cm	Height in	Energy (kcal)[2]	Protein (g)	Fat-soluble vitamins: Vitamin A activity RE[3]	Vitamin A activity IU	Vitamin D (IU)	Vitamin E activity[5] (IU)	Ascorbic acid (mg)	Folacin[6] (μg)
Infants	0-1/2	6	14	60	24	kg × 117	kg × 2.2	420[4]	1,400	400	4	35	50
	1/2-1	9	20	71	28	kg × 108	kg × 2.0	400	2,000	400	5	35	50
Children	1-3	13	28	86	34	1,300	23	400	2,000	400	7	40	100
	4-6	20	44	110	44	1,800	30	500	2,500	400	9	40	200
	7-10	30	66	135	54	2,400	36	700	3,300	400	10	40	300
Males	11-14	44	97	158	63	2,800	44	1,000	5,000	400	12	45	400
	15-18	61	134	172	69	3,000	54	1,000	5,000	400	15	45	400
	19-22	67	147	172	69	3,000	54	1,000	5,000	400	15	45	400
	23-50	70	154	172	69	2,700	56	1,000	5,000		15	45	400
	51+	70	154	172	69	2,400	56	1,000	5,000		15	45	400
Females	11-14	44	97	155	62	2,400	44	800	4,000	400	10	45	400
	15-18	54	119	162	65	2,100	48	800	4,000	400	11	45	400
	19-22	58	128	162	65	2,100	46	800	4,000	400	12	45	400
	23-50	58	128	162	65	2,000	46	800	4,000		12	45	400
	51+	58	128	162	65	1,800	46	800	4,000		12	45	400
Pregnancy						+300	+30	1,000	5,000	400	15	60	800
Lactation						+500	+20	1,200	6,000	400	15	60	600

*From Recommended dietary allowance, ed. 7 (revised 1973), Publication no. 1694, Washington, D.C., 1968, National Academy of Sciences–
[1]The allowances are intended to provide for individual variations among most normal persons as they live in the United States under usual
have been less well defined.
[2]Kilojoules (KJ) = 4.2 × kcal.
[3]Retinol equivalents.
[4]Assumed to be all as retinol in milk during the first 6 months of life. All subsequent intakes are assumed to be one half as retinol and one half as
[5]Total vitamin E activity estimated to be 80% as α-tocopherol and 20% other tocopherols.
[6]The folacin allowances refer to dietary sources as determined by *Lactobacillus casei* assay. Pure forms of folacin may be effective in doses less
[7]Although allowances are expressed as niacin, it is recognized that on the average 1 mg of niacin is derived from each 60 mg of dietary tryptophan.
[8]This increased requirement cannot be met by ordinary diets; therefore the use of supplemental iron is recommended.

and physical activity are the major factors responsible for changing nutrient needs. Disease, trauma, variations in metabolism (normal and abnormal), medications, and treatments can also affect needs.

Since 1940 the Food and Nutrition Board of the National Academy of Sciences has periodically reviewed existing nutrition knowledge and research to formulate recommendations for the amounts of the different nutrients to be used as a basis for planning nutritionally adequate diets.[33,39] Table 51-1 illustrates the changes in amounts of nutrients recommended from infancy throughout life. Not all of the nutrients identified in the box are listed in the table because it is assumed that when an appropriate variety and amount of ordinary foods are consumed to meet the levels of nutrients recommended the diet will supply the other nutrients as well. The level of iron intake recommended for women during the reproductive years is high because many young women do not include iron-rich foods in their diet and their iron stores are poor.

All nutrients are of equal importance although they are not required in equal amounts (Fig. 51-1). The nutrients providing energy (protein, fats, carbohydrates) and water are required in much larger quantities than vitamins that regulate body processes. The differences in the quantities of various nutrients required by an individual are much greater than the change in amounts of any one nutrient over the life cycle. Note in Table 51-1 that 0.3 μg of Vitamin B_{12} are recommended for the infant and 3.0 μg for the adult; 360 to 1,200 mg of calcium are recommended at different points in the life cycle. There is no overlapping of requirements. If a person healthy people in the United States)

Water-soluble vitamins					Minerals						
Niacin[7] (B_1) (mg)	**Riboflavin (B_2) (mg)**	**Thiamin (mg)**	**Vitamin B_6 (mg)**	**Vitamin B_{12} (μg)**	**Calcium (mg)**	**Phosphorus (mg)**	**Iodine (μg)**	**Iron (mg)**	**Magnesium (mg)**	**Zinc (mg)**
5	0.4	0.3	0.3	0.3	360	240	35	10	60	3
8	0.6	0.5	0.4	0.3	540	400	45	15	70	5
9	0.8	0.7	0.6	1.0	800	800	60	15	150	10
12	1.1	0.9	0.9	1.5	800	800	80	10	200	10
16	1.2	1.2	1.2	2.0	800	800	110	10	250	10
18	1.5	1.4	1.6	3.0	1,200	1,200	130	18	350	15
20	1.8	1.5	1.8	3.0	1,200	1,200	150	18	400	15
20	1.8	1.5	2.0	3.0	800	800	140	10	350	15
18	1.6	1.4	2.0	3.0	800	800	130	10	350	15
16	1.5	1.2	2.0	3.0	800	800	110	10	350	15
16	1.3	1.2	1.6	3.0	1,200	1,200	115	18	300	15
14	1.4	1.1	2.0	3.0	1,200	1,200	115	18	300	15
14	1.4	1.1	2.0	3.0	800	800	100	18	300	15
13	1.2	1.0	2.0	3.0	800	800	100	18	300	15
12	1.1	1.0	2.0	3.0	800	800	80	10	300	15
+2	+0.3	+0.3	2.5	4.0	1,200	1,200	125	18[+8]	450	20
+4	+0.5	+0.3	2.5	4.0	1,200	1,200	150	18	450	25

National Research Council.
environmental stresses. Diets should be based on a variety of common foods in order to provide other nutrients for which human requirements

β-carotene when calculated from international units. As retinol equivalents, three fourths are as retinol and one fourth as β-carotene.

than one fourth of the RDA.

consumed Vitamin A in the quantities recommended for calcium or phosphorus, toxicity would result.[35] When food is used as the source of nutrients, such imbalances are unlikely to occur; however, nutrients are available in concentrated forms as dietary supplements, over-the-counter preparations, and prescription drugs. Should these concentrated nutrients be prescribed for the person, the nurse handles them with the same care as any other medication. There is an unsupported intuitive feeling that nutrient supplements are essential. However, response to these supplements occurs only when persons have been relatively nutrition deficient, eating diets marginal in nutrient value, and when the supplement provides the specific nutrient(s) that is deficient. There is a point beyond which supplementation does not help the person and *may actually cause harm.* Continued intake of vitamins and minerals at levels from 10 to 100 times the recommended daily allowance (RDA) is associated with chronic toxicity.

■ NUTRITION PROCESS

Nutrition can be defined as the sum of the processes by which a living organism ingests, digests, absorbs, transports, uses, and excretes nutrients and their metabolites. With adequate supplies of the proper nutrients, the organism can grow, function, and reproduce. When supplies are limited, growth, function, or reproduction may be impaired. Since the body exists in a state of dynamic equilibrium, anabolism and catabolism are continuous. Muscle, organs, bone, fat, and the blood participate in the constant exchange of materials, with some tissues more active than others. There is some loss;

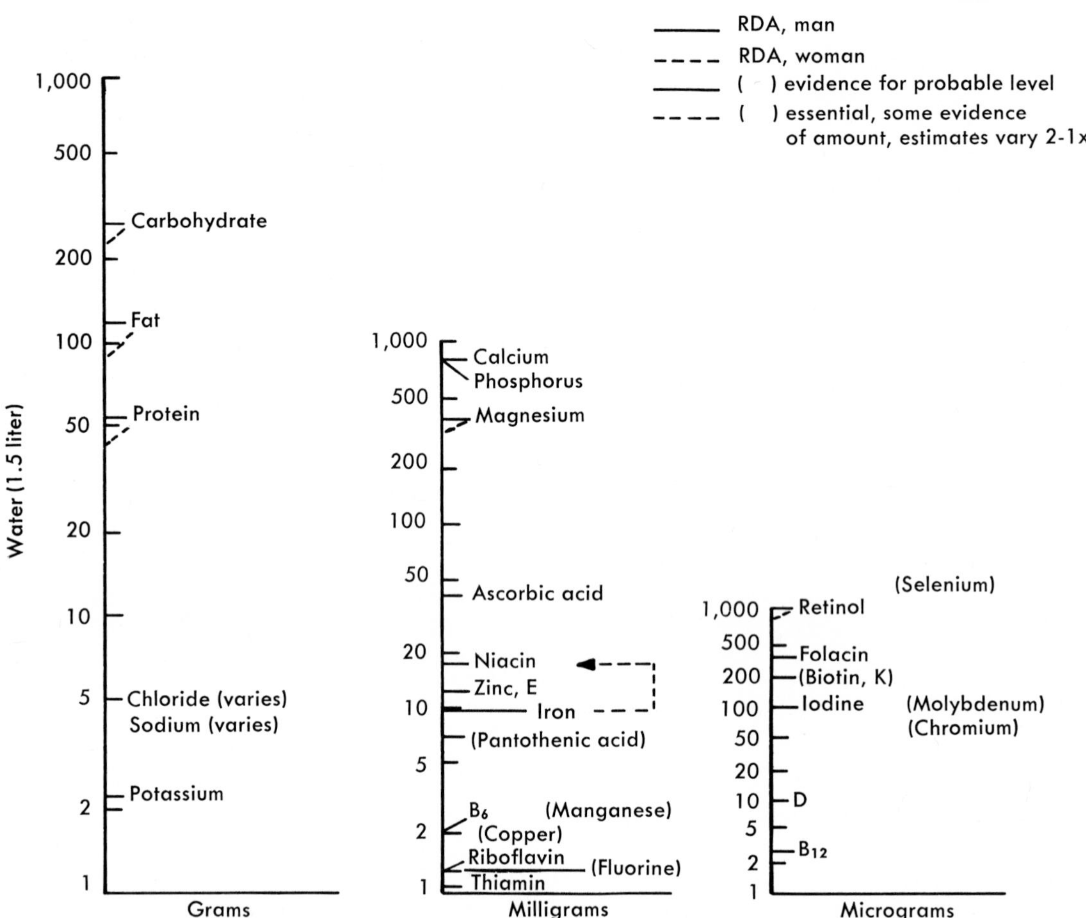

Fig. 51-1. Recommended dietary allowances, 1974, National Research Council, National Academy of Sciences. Energy: varies, U. S. adults sedentary. Carbohydrates and fat: vary with energy needs. Chloride: daily turnover in adults (intake-output) 85 to 250 mEq. Sodium: usual adult intake 100 to 300 mEq; need estimated at 500 mg but varies due to sweating, diarrhea, vomiting, and so forth. (Adapted from Kelvay, L. M.: Am. J. Clin. Nutr. **23:**1619-1641, 1970.)

therefore replacement from food is necessary throughout life. Periods of growth increase requirements for nutrients and energy.

Homeostatic mechanisms tend to protect the body against minor or temporary changes in nutrient status as nutrient reserves are mobilized to meet needs. With nutrient *deficits* adaptations occur to conserve body resources. For example, when energy supplies are limited, physical activity and then basal metabolism are reduced. Decreases in urinary excretion levels of certain nutrients can be measured, as can increased efficiency in the absorption of certain nutrients such as iron. Over time gradual tissue desaturation of the nutrients occurs. Reductions in enzyme activity and altered levels of metabolites develop.[26] If this process is permitted to continue long enough, anatomic lesions become evident.[16] The classical deficiency diseases such as scurvy, beriberi, and pellagra are results of depletions of Vitamin C, thiamin, B complex vitamins, and niacin that are continued long enough for identifiable lesions in skin, tongue, and organs to develop as clinical signs of malnutrition. If untreated, progressive depletion results in death.

Nutrition *excesses* can also produce malnutrition.[2,19,35,55] Mechanisms tend to protect the body by accumulating reserves or, for some nutrients, by increasing the rate of excretion from the body or decreasing efficiency of absorption. When excesses are large or prolonged over time, increased concentrations of nutrients and alterations in enzyme activities and levels of metabolites develop. Over time clinical signs and symptoms develop. The most common example of this type of malnutrition in the United States population is obesity. Consumption of energy-yielding compounds (protein, fat, carbohydrate, alcohol) in amounts greater than needed for energy expenditure result in storage of energy as body fat. Eventually the stores of body fat become large enough to affect body functioning, physical mobility, and health. Obese persons have greater risk of osteoarthritis, diabetes mellitus, cardiovascular disease, and hypertension.[28]

■ NUTRITIONAL STATUS

In order to assess nutritional status it is necessary to determine the nutrient supply to the body, availability for stores and metabolic processes, body size and composition, and physical signs. The basic principles are those used in general evaluation: (1) observing the person's general appearance and (2) obtaining careful medical and dietary histories, physical examination, and selected laboratory measurements. There is no one simple test of a person's nutritional state. Furthermore, long periods of time may elapse from the initial limitation of nutrient supply until malnutrition becomes clinically obvious. A person with good body stores of a nutrient due to consuming a nutritionally sound diet can tolerate relatively long periods of deprivation of that nutrient. The rate at which depletion progresses will be affected by the stores available and the rate of body utilization or excretion of the nutrient. The time elapsing between the insult to nutrient supply and the actual appearance of clinical signs obvious on physical examination can be as little as a week or as long as several years. For this reason it is important to remember that dietary, laboratory, and clinical data may appear to be poorly correlated. This lack of correlation has been interpreted by some persons as demonstrating the impossibility of making an assessment and by others as evidence that one type of data is superior or more reliable than another. Actually these data measure different points along a continuum of deprivation or excess. It is hoped that attention to the nutritional needs of the person, assessment, and appropriate interventions will protect the person and reduce the risk of impaired growth and body function. Prevention or alleviation of malnutrition requires identification of its degree and cause so that appropriate remedies may be instituted.

The nurse has the opportunity to incorporate questions and observations relevant to nutritional needs in the health assessment. Not only does this identify nutrition-related nursing diagnoses, it also identifies persons at risk who require more extensive evaluation. As stated previously, the person's nutritional well-being is a shared responsibility and frequently requires the knowledge and skills of nurse, dietitian, physician, and others. The initial assessment is important, but nursing responsibility does not end there, as the patient's condition may improve or regress, and changes need to be identified. The earlier problems are identified, the earlier appropriate interventions can be formulated and the person protected from serious sequelae.

■ ASSESSING NUTRIENT SUPPLY

□ Dietary history

Information about nutrient supply obtained during the initial assessment is necessarily subjective. It must be obtained from the patient or family by interview. Since both kinds and amounts of nutrients are important, intake data must be both qualitative and quantitative. Skill in interviewing is required, since biases can be introduced or "proper" answers supplied by leading questions. Consider the following questions one at a time:

When did you first have something to eat or drink yesterday?

Did you eat breakfast yesterday?

Did you have orange juice for breakfast yesterday?

Notice that the first question makes no assumptions. The second question reminds one that breakfast is desirable and tempts one to provide information about breakfast whether real or imaginary. The third question restricts freedom to answer even more and includes the interviewer's perception of an appropriate food choice. Further it implies that orange juice at breakfast is essential, in effect misinforming the patient.

Directing specific questions about food consumption to the day preceding the interview is a technique frequently used in nutrition surveys designed to assess the nutritional status of groups. It is simple and rapid, taking about 15 minutes. Although the 24-hour recall is useful as a device for continued monitoring, it should not be used for initial assessment. Food intake on a single day is a poor indicator of nutrient supply for an individual.[56] Not only does food intake vary over the week according to work, school, and family schedules, but intake immediately preceding hospitalization or appointments for care is often atypical.

It is more useful to ask the person to describe his or her *usual eating patterns,* including when, what, and how much foods or liquids are consumed, with gentle probing to obtain details about food preparation, use of seasonings, and so forth. Far too often the questions about diet provide a social rather than information exchange.

"Has the baby been eating well?" "Yes."

"How's your diet?" "Fine."

Unfortunately exchanges such as these may be charted as "Nutrition no problem" or "Patient well nourished." Any problems the patient may have are unidentified and are likely to remain so.

Questioning should elicit a picture of total food consumption for the day. Designation of meals and snacks is not really necessary and may bias answers by implying value judgments. The following approach is more likely to provide useful information:

> What usually is the first thing you eat or drink? When? How much? What else? You said you usually have 2 slices of toast; do you put anything on your toast? When do you eat or drink again? Let's review this now. You said you usually have a cup of soup for lunch at work; what do you have on the days when you're not working? What kind of milk do you buy?

The interviewer should make no assumptions. Some people put cream or milk or sugar in coffee or tea, and some do not. Some people put dressing on their salads, and some do not. Find out what the person does by asking.

Portion sizes are important and are difficult to estimate without some visual reference. A hamburger can vary from 42 g (1.5 oz) to 168 g (6 oz) or more, making a significant difference in determining whether nutrient supply is adequate. The glass used at home may hold 90, 240, 300, 360, or even 480 ml (3, 8, 10, 12, or 16 oz) of fluid. Dietitians frequently use food models, measuring cups, spoons, and other aids for obtaining intake data. For the hospitalized patient the equipment and portions on the tray can be used as a basis for comparison.

When the usual eating pattern has been determined, any *recent changes* from the pattern should be identified and described together with any explanations. Changes may be due to illness (anorexia, nausea, vomiting, diarrhea), self-imposed dietary regimens, or emotional or physical stress. Experience with special or prescribed diets should be recorded.

Since nutrient supply is affected by use of *supplements, medications,* and *drugs,* the person is asked about intake of these items whether prescribed by a physician or not. Whenever possible the product, content, and size of dose should be recorded.

Food and fluid *preferences* and *dislikes* should be identified. This information is most frequently asked in order to be sure a patient is satisfied with hospital meals. It is also useful in determining fluid intake, potential inadequacies or excesses, and food intolerances. If a person reports not eating a particular food, it is important to determine if taste, intolerance, or allergy is a determinant.

Information about *financial resources* for food, *facilities* for purchasing, storing, and preparing food, as well as occupation and *daily activities* provide information about nutritional needs and the ease with which needs are met.

The person should be invited to describe any *problems with diet.* These can include problems due to lack of information about a diet previously prescribed; concerns or fears about food, which may generate from the media or from ideas of others; and physical difficulties with sight, taste, chewing, movement, or pain, which may affect intake. Does the person need help with eating? What kind of help?

It is also useful to have the person describe *weight* and *nutrition status.* Does the person perceive body weight as normal, excessive, or low? Have there been major fluctuations in weight over the last year? Does the person consider diet or nutritional state a problem?

An important source of objective information about intake of the institutionalized patient is frequently ignored, that is, the choice of food the patient makes from menus and the food actually consumed from the tray, snack bar, and gifts, as well as from other modes of nutrient supply such as medications, intravenous or tube feedings, and fluids kept at the bedside. Not only can the patient be asked about these, but direct observations can be made. Unexpected or inappropriate response to nutrition therapy may be explained by the difference between plans and implementation if someone takes the time to observe what is happening and intervenes. For example, two women were admitted to the hospital for evaluation and treatment of heart disease. Both women had severe hypertension and were obese; both were prescribed 1,000-calorie, limited-sodium diets. After 1 week the physician noted that one patient was responding well, with significant weight loss recorded, while the other was gaining weight, both as body fat and increased edema, despite eating only half the food on the tray. The dietitian, when called, determined that the second patient was consuming a high-calorie, high-sodium diet consisting primarily of candy and other items brought daily by visitors at the patient's request.

The information gathered by the nurse about usual dietary patterns and changes provides basic data that can be evaluated rapidly to estimate adequacy of intake and to identify current and potential problems. For more complete and detailed study of intake and analysis, the dietitian can offer special expertise and assistance.

☐ Evaluating nutrient intake

The food guides that have been developed to help people choose the kinds and amounts of food to eat for health can be used for a rapid evaluation of adequacy of the diet eaten at home or food intake in the hospital. There are many different food guides, since to be effective they must be devised for a specific country or culture and feature the foods readily available and acceptable to the people being evaluated.

A guide used in the United States is shown in the box on p. 1147. The guide groups staple food items rich in protein, vitamins, and minerals into four major classes according to their major nutrient contributions. Recommendations are made for the number and size of servings

Table 51-2. Protein and calorie values of basic diet selected to meet recommendations outlined in food guide for an adult

Group and food chosen	Protein (g)	Calories
Milk, 1/2 liter (1 pint) Whole (skim)	18	330 (180)
Vegetable-fruit, 4 servings	6	190
Broccoli (1/2 cup)		
Potato, 1 medium		
Potato, 1 medium		
Lettuce, 1/6 head		
Apple, 6 cm (2 1/2-in) diameter		
Meat, 2 or more servings	56	341
Cheese, 30 g (1 oz)		
Beef, 75 g (2 1/2 oz)		
Poultry, 75 g (2 1/2 oz)		
Bread-cereal, 4 servings	8	290
Cornflakes, 30 g (1 oz)		
Bread, 3 slices		
	88	1,151 (1,001)

DAILY FOOD GUIDE

Food group	Servings recommended
A Milk:	
Fluid milk—whole, skim, cultured, evaporated; milk solids may be in beverage or mixtures fortified with vitamin D	Children: 3 to 4 glasses Teenagers: 4 glasses Adults: 2 or more glasses Pregnant women: 4 glasses
B Vegetables and fruit:	
Dark green or deep yellow (e.g., broccoli, kale, carrots, squash, turnip, mustard greens)	1 serving at least every other day (1/2 cup)
Citrus fruits and juices, cantaloupe, tomato, broccoli, cabbage, pepper, strawberries,	1 serving (1/2 cup or usual portion)
Other fruits and vegetables including potatoes	2 or more servings (1/2 cup or usual portion, i.e., medium potato or apple)
C Meat	
Meat, fish, poultry, eggs, dried beans and peas, nuts	2 or more servings (60 to 75 g [2 to 3 oz] meat, fish, poultry, liver; 2 eggs; 1 cup beans, peas, lentils; 4 tbsp peanut butter)
D Bread and cereal	4 or more servings (1 slice bread; 30 g [1 oz] dry cereal; 1/2 to 3/4 cup cooked cereal, rice, macaroni, noodles, spaghetti)

Amounts recommended for a preschool child are 1/2 liter (1 pint) of milk, 1/2 cup fruits or juices, 1/2 cup vegetables, 75 g (3 oz) meat and eggs, and 2 servings of bread and cereal.

to be selected from each food group. One can evaluate a diet quickly by checking to see if the recommended types of food and servings are included in the usual dietary pattern.

Since foods are mixtures of nutrients, the protein, vitamin, and mineral requirements are substantially met when the daily intake includes the recommended servings from each group. The calorie level of the basic diet is low (Table 51-2) but is approximately sufficient for adult basal metabolism. Adequacy of energy intake is best judged by evaluation of body weight. In this method of evaluation fats, oils, and sweets are not tabulated, since they provide primarily energy.

Each food grouping contributes particular nutrients to the total diet. The absence of any one food group from the diet or particular types of food should alert the nurse that the patient has a potential nutrition problem.

Milk and milk products are excellent sources of high-quality protein, as are foods from the meat group. In contrast to the meat group, milk provides calcium, phosphorus, and riboflavin abundantly as well as other minerals and vitamins. Milk is not a rich source of iron or vitamin C and should not be used as the sole protein food in the diet. There are many different types of milk: homogenized, 2%, skim milk, buttermilk, yogurt, and powdered, evaporated, and condensed milk. Use of milk fortified with vitamin D is desirable, especially for children, pregnant or lactating women, and persons with limited exposure to sunlight due to their life style. The person should be questioned, therefore, to determine if fortified milk is used. Skim milk may be fortified with vitamin A as well as D, since that fat-soluble vitamin is removed when milkfat is removed. Cheese is included in this group because of its calcium value. When evaluating the diet be sure to consider all milks and cheeses used. There is a tendency to consider only milk used as a beverage, but it is an important ingredient in soups, puddings, ice cream, and frozen desserts. Five level tablespoons of dried skim milk solids are equivalent to 240 ml (8 oz) of fluid milk. Two cups of cottage cheese, 40 g ($1^1/_2$ oz) of cheddar cheese, 1 cup of pudding, or $1^3/_4$ cups of ice cream yields calcium equivalent to 1 cup of fluid milk.

Vegetables and fruits are important primarily as sources of vitamins and minerals. They contribute some protein depending on their type, but the plant foods in the meat group and cereal grains contribute more. Fruits and vegetables are low in calories unless prepared with additional fats or sugars. They are high in nutritional value. Since vitamins C and A are not evenly distributed in all fruits and vegetables, the diet should be checked to be sure that a food rich in vitamin C is included daily and a food rich in vitamin A is included at least every other day. Foods rich in vitamin C include citrus fruits and juices, melons, berries, dark green leafy vegetables, broccoli, cabbage, green peppers, and tomatoes. Foods rich in vitamin A include dark green or deep yellow vegetables. As a general guide, foods with the deeper colors are richer sources of vitamins. Other fruits and vegetables may contribute varying amounts of vitamins C and A, but the choices described above are needed to assure adequate intake. In addition fruits and vegetables contribute a wide range of other vitamins including folacin (folic acid) and minerals including potassium. They are quite low in sodium unless salt is added in preparation. They also contribute fiber to the diet.

The *meat* group includes animal and plant products that are rich in protein. Meat, fish, poultry, and eggs contribute protein, fat, B complex vitamins including B_{12}, and minerals such as iron and copper. Nuts and seeds contribute protein and fat, while the legumes contribute protein and starch. The plant products also contribute vitamins and minerals except vitamin B_{12}. The meat-plant group described here is primarily important for protein content, trace minerals, thiamin, and niacin.

Bread and cereals should be whole-grain or enriched. They contribute some protein, but most of their energy value is supplied as complex carbohydrates. The whole-grain forms are important sources of fiber. These foods are important as sources of many vitamins and minerals, especially because they are inexpensive in comparison with most food items. In surveys it has been noted that these foods provide important amounts of iron in the diet for many people. They are not good sources of vitamins A and C, however, although they contribute valuable levels of thiamin, riboflavin, and niacin. Desserts (cookies, cake, doughnuts) are grain foods of high caloric value because of added fats and sugars.

The box on p. 1149 is an assessment of a diet history. The individual is a 45-year-old woman with obesity and hypertension; meals eaten at home.

When using the *Daily Food Guide* for rapid screening of nutrient supply, the nurse should remember that the food group system is not a complete diet but the foundation for meal planning. Additional servings from the groups as well as fats, oils, and sweets are used to meet energy and growth needs. Alcoholic beverages may be used by the person as well, thus increasing caloric intake with little contribution of protein, vitamins, or minerals. Levels of folacin and magnesium are likely to be low unless the diet includes green leafy vegetables. Levels of vitamin E might be low if vegetable oils are not used in food preparation or as salad dressings. The diet histories of girls and women should be checked to see if iron-rich foods are included because menstruation and child-bearing increase iron needs. Iron-rich foods include green leafy vegetables, meat, liver, seafood, egg yolks, nuts, legumes, and whole and enriched grains and cereals.

The *Daily Food Guide* can also be used for evaluating vegetarian diets. Many people are vegetarians, and their reasons vary (e.g., religion, food cost, philosophy[15]). The diets vary as well. Some persons eliminate only red meat such as beef, lamb, veal, and pork but do eat fish. Others eliminate all muscle meats including fish and poultry. Still others use animal products such as milk, cheese, and eggs. These last persons are called lacto-ovo-vegetarians. There are some who eliminate all foods of animal origin from the diet and some who choose from a very limited list of plant products. Some eat only cereal grains, others only fruits or seeds. Generally, the lacto-ovo-vegetarian diet is nutritionally sound when a variety of foods is included.[40,47] Persons on more restricted vegetarian (vegan) diets should be considered at nutritional risk and candidates for more detailed study. One potential problem is vitamin B_{12} insufficiency unless fortified cereal or a dietary supplement is taken. The young adult who has changed to a vegan diet may use body stores of B_{12} for a time (a 5-year store is possible) but is at potential risk especially if intake of folacin in vegetables is high, masking the signs of megaloblastic anemia.

Other dietary guides could be used in the same manner if the population served represents a particular ethnic or cultural group with a different pattern of food use. The pattern described here is applicable for the majority of the United States population. Hospital diet

ASSESSMENT OF A DIET HISTORY

45-year-old woman with obesity and hypertension; meals eaten at home

7:00 AM
1 cup cooked oatmeal
2 tsp sugar
1 cup skim milk (fortified)
3 cups coffee, plain

10:15 AM
2 cups coffee, plain

1:00 PM
Sandwich
 2 slices white bread, enriched
 1/2 tsp margarine
 1/2 tsp mayonnaise
 60 g (2 oz) meatloaf or luncheon meat
4 cookies (fig bars, gingersnaps)
3 cups coffee, plain

4:00 PM
7 cookies
1/2 cup unsweetened fruit (canned, frozen, or fresh)
2 cups tea, plain

10:00 PM
8 soda crackers
60 g (2 oz) American cheese
360 ml (12 oz) cola (sweet)
1/2 cup homemade bread-and-butter pickles

Midnight
2 aspirin
1 cup tea, plain

ASSESSMENT

Food group	Servings	Evaluation
Milk		Choice from the milk group adequate. Fruits and vegetable intake low, and choice of items rich in vitamin C or A happenstance. Meat intake low. Bread intake is six servings. Intake of sweets, particularly cookies, high. Use of pickles and soda crackers questionable, since patient reports that a low-sodium diet was prescribed for her several years ago.
Skim milk	1	
Cheese	1	
Fruits, vegetables		
Fruit	1	
Vegetable	1	Dietitian was asked to check caloric value. Intake is 1,500 to 1,600 calories per day with about 800 calories coming from basic food items and the rest from sweets and fat. Protein levels adequate, although source of protein could be improved.
Meat-protein		
Meatloaf	1	
Bread, cereal		
Oatmeal	2	
Bread, enriched	2	
Crackers	2	
Sweets		
Cookies	11	
Cola (360 ml [12 oz])		
Pickles, cucumber		
Fats		
Margarine		
Mayonnaise		

To the reader: Identify nutritional risks for this person. Identify appropriate interventions and behavioral goals for her.

manuals also provide food patterns that can be used as evaluation tools. In addition to describing regular or normal diet, the manuals provide patterns for modified diets prescribed as therapeutic regimens. When these patterns are used for evaulation, they provide a mechanism for separating quickly those persons who are most likely consuming an adequate nutrient supply from those who are not. When an individual's food intake does not adhere to a recommended pattern, he or she may or may not be obtaining adequate nutrients. The evaluation of the diet must be extended, and the evaluation becomes more arduous. Tables of food composition can be used and nutrient intake estimated through calculation of the nutrient value of each food.* Referral to the dietitian is appropriate.

■ ASSESSING NUTRITIONAL DEFICIENCY

At one time a great deal of emphasis was placed on looking for specific signs of nutritional deficiency as part of the clinical examination. This was based on the observation made of populations with classic deficiency diseases. One can find lists of the signs in most nutrition textbooks. One need not to be a physician to recognize major signs of nutritional deprivation. It is hoped that nutrition problems can be identified before major signs and symptoms appear.

Signs of malnutrition may be due to a nutrient lack or to nonnutritional factors such as poor hygiene (bleeding gums, bad teeth). They may be due to inadequate nutrient intake or to a disease or condition that interferes with the body's ability to digest, absorb, or metabolize nutrients. It is important to make these differentiations.

□ Subjective data

The patient's (or family's) description of the current illness, previous illness and surgery, pregnancy, weight, weight change, and growth, and use of prescribed and over-the-counter medications provide information, most of which can be checked by examination, measurements, and appropriate laboratory studies. The history provides data for determining likely problems and defining the priorties for testing.

□ Objective data

The World Health Organization (WHO) has published classifications of the physical signs most often associated with malnutrition, and these have been adapted for use in the United States.[10,23] Table 51-3 lists the signs associated with normal appearance and with malnutrition. Evaluation also includes height, weight, and growth patterns.

Height and weight

Height and weight are easily measured and are important data to obtain and use. Delayed growth and development in a child should be regarded as an important sign. This may be determined by comparing the child's measurements with normal values on growth charts. Even better, if available, are serial measurements over time so that deviations in growth rate may be identified for the specific child. There should be records of height and weight for children whether care is provided in office, clinic, or hospital.

Height and weight for adults is also easily measured, with weight and height compared with tables of recommended values as a guide. A useful item of historical information is the weight of the adult at age 25 and the person's perception of desirable body weight. The first provides data about a good weight for the person (if not obese at 25), and the second helps predict the person's response to attempts to change weight.

For all persons, periodic recording of weight changes can provide valuable data about health status and response to therapy and can serve as early warning of problems. Even in hospitals where weight is measured, the data usually are not used as they should be.

The nurse should review the methods for obtaining accurate measurements of height or length. Errors of up to 5 cm have been recorded in measurements made on the commonly used type of clinical scale with a measuring rod. The most reliable measurement of weight is made in the morning after voiding and before food or drink are taken.

Interpretation of weight requires some knowledge of body fluid compartments (p. 207). Very rapid fluctuations in weight (possibly as much as 5 kg in 24 hours) are usually due to body fluid changes and may signal difficulties with edema or dehydration. A steady downward course in weight may signal that the person is catabolizing body protein or possibly body fat. For some persons this weight loss represents significant deterioration and should be stopped if possible. If loss of fat is the goal, the record represents progress. In general loss of body fat is a slower process (about 0.5 to 1 kg/week), since fat is a concentrated source of energy.

Body fatness can be estimated from weight for height. Generally a weight of 15% to 20% above the standard tables represents excessive body fat, although some persons can be overweight but not overfat because of muscle development. The person's general appearance gives one a rapid estimate of overweight or underweight. Fatness can be checked with the use of calipers.

Mouth and teeth

Although all of the physical signs listed in Table 51-3 should be considered, evaluation of the mouth and teeth

*References 11, 34, 37, 48-50.

Table 51-3. Physical signs indicative or suggestive of malnutrition*

Body area	Normal appearance	Signs associated with malnutrition
Hair	Shiny, firm, not easily plucked	Lack of natural shine; hair dull and dry, thin and sparse; hair fine, silky, and straight; color changes (flag sign); can be easily plucked
Face	Skin color uniform; smooth, pink, healthy appearance; not swollen	Skin color loss (depigmentation); skin dark over cheeks and under eyes (malar and supraorbital pigmentation); lumpiness or flakiness of skin of nose and mouth; swollen face; enlarged parotid glands; scaling of skin around nostrils (nasolabial seborrhea)
Eyes	Bright, clear, shiny; no sores at corners of eyelids; membranes a healthy pink and moist. No prominent blood vessels or mound of tissue or sclera	Eye membranes are pale (pale conjunctivae); redness of membranes (conjunctival injection); Bitot spots; redness and fissuring of eyelid corners (angular palpebritis); dryness of eye membranes (conjunctival xerosis); cornea has dull appearance (corneal xerosis); cornea soft (keratomalacia); scar on cornea; ring of fine blood vessels around cornea (circumcorneal injection)
Lips	Smooth, not chapped or swollen	Redness and swelling of mouth or lips (cheilosis), especially at corners of mouth (angular fissures and scars)
Tongue	Deep red in appearance; not swollen or smooth	Swelling; scarlet and raw tongue; magenta (purplish color) tongue; smooth tongue; swollen sores; hyperemic and hypertrophic papillae; atrophic papillae
Teeth	No cavities; no pain; bright	May be missing or erupting abnormally; gray or black spots (fluorosis); cavities (caries)
Gums	Healthy; red; do not bleed; not swollen	"Spongy" and bleed easily; recession of gums
Glands	Face not swollen	Thyroid enlargement (front of neck); parotid enlargement (cheeks become swollen)
Skin	No signs of rashes, swellings, dark or light spots	Dryness of skin (xerosis); sandpaper feel of skin (follicular hyperkeratosis); flakiness of skin; skin swollen and dark; red swollen pigmentation of exposed areas (pellagrous dermatosis); excessive lightness or darkness of skin (dyspigmentation); black and blue marks due to skin bleeding (petechiae); lack of fat under skin
Nails	Firm, pink	Nails are spoon shaped (koilonychia); brittle, ridged nails
Muscular and skeletal systems	Good muscle tone; some fat under skin; can walk or run without pain	Muscles have "wasted" appearance; baby's skull bones are thin and soft (craniotabes); round swelling of front and side of head (frontal and parietal bossing); swelling of ends of bones (epiphyseal enlargement); small bumps on both sides of chest wall (on ribs), beading of ribs; baby's soft spot on head does not harden at proper time (persistently open anterior fontanelle); knock-knees or bow-legs; bleeding into muscle (musculoskeletal hemorrhages); person cannot get up or walk properly
Internal systems		
Cardiovascular	Normal heart rate and rhythm; no murmurs or abnormal rhythms; normal blood pressure for age	Rapid heart rate (above 100, tachycardia); enlarged heart; abnormal rhythm; elevated blood pressure
Gastrointestinal	No palpable organs or masses (in children, however, liver edge may be palpable)	Liver enlargement; enlargement of spleen (usually indicates other associated diseases)
Nervous	Psychologic stability; normal reflexes	Mental irritability and confusion; burning and tingling of hand and feet (paresthesia); loss of position and vibratory sense; weakness and tenderness of muscles (may result in inability to walk); decrease and loss of ankle and knee reflexes

*From Christakis, G.: Nutritional assessment in health programs, Am. J. Public Health **63:**(Suppl.) 1-82, 1973.

are especially important. Persons with missing or decayed teeth or dentures that are uncomfortable may have poor nutritional status because eating is painful and unpleasant. They may have problems with appropriate oral hygiene as well. Not only may these difficulties be present at the initial contact, but further problems may develop such as increased pain, bleeding, and infection. Identification of these problems and care directed toward them are essential to the person's well-being. The mouth is checked for cleanliness, odor, evidence of irritation or lesions, soreness, paralysis, and ability to chew. Although bleeding gums historically are associated with vitamin C deficiency, they are more frequently associated with poor oral hygiene and periodontal disease in the American population.

■ DIAGNOSTIC TESTS

The blood urine analyses routinely done for patients contain data useful in the evaluation of nutritional status. There are also special tests that can be used to confirm impressions obtained from evaluation of nutrient supply and the clinical examination.*

Urinalysis routinely includes tests of pH, protein, glucose, and acetone. Urine can also be tested for creatinine, thiamin, riboflavin, N'methylnicotinamide, and pantothenic acid. If these tests are ordered, a protocol for collecting and handling the specimens should be requested from the laboratory.

Blood is frequently tested for hemoglobin, hematocrit, serum protein, and cholesterol. The values will be influenced by recent blood loss, so one should determine whether the person was a recent blood donor as well as checking for loss from bleeding. The values may also be affected by blood transfusions or intravenous solutions, so timing of the sample is important.

Low levels of *hemoglobin* most frequently are associated with iron or protein deficiency; however, a variety of nutritional and nonnutritional factors may be involved. In the United States about 10% of the population is estimated to have some degree of anemia related to low *iron* intake.[9] Women and children are at risk because of menstruation and growth and often because intake of iron-rich foods is low. Hemoglobin levels are also affected by increased volume of blood in late pregnancy. Elevated hemoglobin levels are also seen with dehydration and polycythemia. Hematocrit values are indicative of anemias resulting from low intake of iron and are elevated in polycythemia. More specific evidence of iron deficiency is obtained from tests of serum iron and transferrin, which detect reduced stores before anemia develops. If these are normal, another explanation for the anemia must be sought.

Protein deficiency is uncommon in the United States but not necessarily in the hospitalized patient.[5] The patient's appearance, muscle mass, and body weight are indicative of protein status. The serum protein level, and especially albumin in relation to globulin, falls with protein deficiency but is not considered particularly sensitive or specific for protein. Serum protein levels may be maintained for some time even with limited protein intake. Nitrogen-creatinine ratios in the urine and ratios of specific amino acids in plasma have been used but are not standard procedures as yet for determination of protein deficiency.

Other blood tests are available to test nutritional status. Some tests measure the stores of a nutrient, some measure the circulating nutrient, and others measure the activity of enzymes dependent on the nutrient for activity. These are not routine tests and may be costly to the patient in terms of laboratory fees or discomfort. The decision to request such tests is based on the evaluation of the patient's nutrient intake and physical condition and identification of the possible nutrient problem and the proper test to verify it. For many nutrients, especially the trace elements, laboratory methods have not been standardized and criteria for interpretation of results have not been developed. When the information is essential for patient care, the knowledge and skills of nurse, physician, dietitian, and laboratory personnel are needed.

Although many persons in the United States consume diets that do not provide the recommended levels of *calcium*, there is no suitable method for documenting calcium lack by means of clinical or laboratory studies. Blood levels of calcium are used to test parathyroid function, not nutrient adequacy, as they are relatively constant over wide ranges of intake. Bone serves as a calcium reserve for the body, but there is no standard method as yet to determine degree of mineralization. Visualization by radiograph provides some information on mineralization, particularly for children. Unfortunately by the time problems are identified by radiograph, they are far advanced. Children and postmenopausal women appear to be at highest risk, and identification of risk relies heavily on evaluation of nutrient intake, particularly of calcium and vitamin D.

Serum *copper* levels and ceruloplasmin can be measured, as can *zinc* levels.[18,19] Hair has been proposed as a biopsy material for determination of trace mineral nutrition, but standardization and interpretation of results remain to be firmly established.[21]

Iodine evaluation relies principally on functional tests such as protein-bound iodine and other standard clinical tests for thyroid gland function.

Tests for levels of glucose, cholesterol, and triglycerides are often part of the regular series of studies.

---

*References 1, 10, 16, 23, 38, 44, 52.

These have implications for nutritional status and for health status, particularly as related to the development of diabetes mellitus and coronary heart disease. They are discussed in the chapters describing these diseases.

Vitamin C status can be checked by measuring the level of the vitamin in serum. The levels vary substantially with intake and thus can be interpreted to represent stores. Serum levels over 0.2 ml/100 ml are considered acceptable, providing sufficient vitamins to meet needs although the recommended levels of intake (Table 51-1) are set to provide higher serum levels. The blood sample should be a fasting sample for best results, as is true for all tests described here. If this is not possible and a casual sample is obtained, this should be recorded along with the person's food intake for at least 4 hours preceding the test.

Thiamin status can be checked by testing urine as mentioned previously or by a functional enzyme test. *Transketolase* is an enzyme in red blood cells that requires thiamin to function. Measurement of its activity before and after adding thiamin pyrophosphate to the sample is made. An increase in enzyme activity after the addition of cofactor in a ratio of more than 15% indicates thiamin lack. Thiamin content of the blood can be directly estimated with microbiologic assays.

Riboflavin status is most often tested by urinary excretion, with high levels of excretion denoting good intake, fasting, or protein depletion (thus dietary history is important in interpretation). Recently, functional enzyme tests have been developed using erythrocyte glutamic oxaloacetic transaminase (EGOT) or erythrocyte glutamic pyruvate transaminase (EGPT). The principle is similar to thiamin testing, with measurement of the increase in activity due to the addition of flavin adenine dinucleotide. Chemical and microbiologic methods are available to measure riboflavin concentration in blood as well as in urine. Since riboflavin is sensitive to ultravioliet light, handling of the sample is critical. In practice riboflavin status is rarely checked. Riboflavin lack is rarely a problem in persons consuming the equivalent of 480 ml (1 pint) or more of milk daily.

Niacin status has been of particular interest in the United States since pellagra was a major public health problem in the Southwest in the early 1900s. It is rare now, occurring occasionally in chronic alcoholics or persons on severly limited diets. This is due in part to enrichment of grain and bread products, but probably due more to the generous protein level of most American diets. In addition to obtaining preformed niacin found from food, the body can obtain the vitamin from the amino acid tryptophane. When evaluating intake one considers the protein content of the diet as well as the niacin content. Testing urine for end products of niacin metabolites is the most frequently used method, although microbiologic methods are available to test for circulating niacin.

Of all the vitamins, *folacin* is probably the most frequently tested in patients. This is because deficiency has been reported as common in pregnant women and in women taking estrogens. In addition megaloblastic anemia can be identified readily in standard clinical blood examinations. The concentration of folacin in serum or red blood cells can be determined by microbiologic methods. Another test measures the excretion of formiminoglutamic acid (FIGLU) in the urine, since increased excretion of this metabolite of histidine metabolism may occur with B_{12} deficiency and other causes. Serum folacin is a more specific test.

Vitamin B_{12} status can also be checked by measuring serum levels. Since B_{12} deficiency may be caused by inadequate intake or by an inability to absorb the vitamin from food (pernicious anemia), a series of tests is used by the physician for differential diagnosis. Megaloblastic anemia is a clinical sign of folacin or B_{12} inadequacy. When folacin intake is very high in relation to B_{12} supplies in the body, megaloblastic anemia may not be apparent, and the permanent damage to the body may occur if one waits until clinical signs appear. This can happen in persons whose diet appears adequate in B_{12} but who cannot absorb it. It may occur in persons on diets inadequate in B_{12} (such as vegans) whose folacin intake is high because of good intakes of foods such as green leafy vegetables or, more frequently, because of folic acid supplements that may be self-chosen.

Pantothenic acid and *biotin* usually are not nutrition problems. They are widely distributed in foodstuffs, and deficiencies have been rarely documented. Although the picture may change in the future, there is little evidence that these two vitamins pose problems for many people. Identification of growth retardation or of inadequate weight for height should warn of possible nutrition problems, and an evaluation of intake for all of the vitamins would help identify the specific problem. The few cases of biotin deficiency that have been identified have been associated with intake of excessive amounts of raw egg white, with otherwise limited diet, over a long period.[3] This can be identified from the dietary history.

Assessment of *vitamin A* nutriture is important for two reasons. Repeated studies of the American population show significant numbers of people with inadequate vitamin A intake and low vitamin reserves in the liver.[9] Persons with impaired fat absorption or other absorption problems such as gluten enteropathy will have impaired absorption of fat-soluble vitamins. In addition vitamin A is a popular dietary supplement for persons concerned about their skin or health, and they frequently take very large doses of the vitamin over long periods. Vitamin A is toxic when taken in excess and may result in either acute or chronic, hard-to-identify symptoms. Plasma levels of vitamin A and of the provitamin carotene can be measured. A individual may maintain acceptable levels (20 μg/100 ml) even with low intake if liver stores are available for mobilization. Plasma carotene levels reflect one form of vitamin intake: that from green leafy and yellow vegetables. A low plasma carotene level would be expected in persons not including these foods, just as a high level would be expected in persons eating generous amounts. The high intake of carotenes does not pose the same hazard of toxicity as does high intake of vitamin A.

Tests for *vitamin D* nutriture are not particularly satisfactory. The signs of rickets in children can be identified radiographically, but one does not wait for this condition to develop before correcting the problem. Elevated serum alkaline phosphatase levels have been associated with vitamin D deficiency, but they are not specific. With the identification of the forms of vitamin D in body processes, tests to measure compounds such as 1,25-dihydroxycholecalciferol have been developed. These tests are difficult and expensive and are not suitable for general determination of nutritional status.

Vitamin E status may be checked by determining plasma vitamin E concentrations. A plasma fragility test has been used also, since red blood cell fragility increases with vitamin E. Inadequate vitamin E status is not reported frequently. It does occur in infants (especially the premature), apparently because the absorption of the vitamin is limited in the immature gastrointestinal tract. Increased hemolysis has been noted in adults consuming diets high in polyunsaturated fatty acids, although this is not usual because the oils high in polyunsaturates are also good sources of vitamin E.

The test for *vitamin K* nutriture is the test for prothrombin time. Since vitamin K is present in many foods, including green leafy vegetables, and is synthesized by the flora of the intestinal tract, dietary dificiency is rare. One dose of the vitamin is given at birth to prevent hemorrhagic disease until the flora are established in the infant within a week or so. Vitamin K inadequacy is more often seen in patients who receive antibiotics for long periods, antibiotic enemas prior to surgery of the colon, or intravenous feedings without the vitamin. Since many patients are treated with anticoagulants as a component of therapy, the physician must be concerned with the relative supplies of vitamin K and the anticoagulant to maintain the prothrombin time desired for the particular patient.

The nurse, in accepting the responsibility of providing care for the person as an individual, accepts responsibility for aspects of nutritional care as well. The perceptive nurse identifies problems, seeks answers, and incorporates solutions in the nursing care plan. Identification of nutritional problems, current and potential, is the purpose of assessing nutritional status. Although medical, dietary, and laboratory personnel share responsibility, the nurse must be alert to the person's needs. Assessment should be made at the initial contact and at regular intervals to ensure the person's well-being. The nutrition assessment forms the basis for care plans and specific interventions.

REFERENCES AND SELECTED READINGS

1. Baker, H.: Clinical vitaminology: methods and interpretation, New York, 1968, Interscience Publishers.
2. Barness, L. A.: Safety considerations with high ascorbic acid dosage, Ann. N.Y. Acad. Sci. **258**:523-528, 1975.
3. Baugh, C. M., Malone, J. H., and Butterworth, C. E., Jr.: Human protein deficiency, Am. J. Clin. Nutr. **21**:173-182, 1968.
4. *Bing, F. C.: Dietary fiber—in historical perspective, J. Am. Diet. Assoc. **69**:498-505, 1976.
5. Bistrian, B. R.: Nutritional assessment and therapy of protein-calorie malnutrition in the hospital, J. Am. Diet. Assoc. **71**:393-397, 1977.
6. Bollet, A. J., and Owens, S.: Evaluation of nutritional status of selected hospitalized patients, Am. J. Clin. Nutr. **26**:931-938, 1973.
7. Butterworth, C. E., Jr., and Blackburn, G. L.: Hospital malnutrition, Nutr. Today **10**:8-18, March-April 1975.
8. Caly, J. C.: Helping people eat for health: assessing adults' nutrition, Am. J. Nurs. **77**:1605-1609, 1977.
9. Center for Disease Control, Health Services and Mental Health Administration: Ten-state nutrition survey 1968-1970, Department of Health Education and Welfare, Publication nos. (HSM) 72-8130, 72-8131, 72-8132, 72-8133, and 72-8134, Washington, D.C., 1972, U.S. Government Printing Office.
10. *Christakis, G.: Nutritional assessment in health programs, Am. J. Public Health **63** (Suppl.):1-82, Nov. 1973.
11. Church, C. F., and Church, H. M.: Food values of portions commonly used, ed. 12, Philadelphia, 1975, J. B. Lippincott Co.
12. Committee on Nutrition, American Academy of Pediatrics: Nutritional aspects of vegetarianism, health foods and fad diets, Pediatrics **59**:460-464, 1977.
13. Dansky, K. H.: Helping people eat for health: assessing children's nutrition, Am. J. Nurs. **77**:1610-1611, 1977.
14. Deutsch, R. M.: The new nuts among the berries, Palo Alto, Calif., 1977, Bull Publishing Co.
15. Dwyer, J. T., Kandel, R. F., Mayer, L. D., et al.: The "new" vegetarians: group affiliation and dietary structures related to attitudes and life style, J. Am. Diet. Assoc. **64**:376-382, 1974.
16. *Goldsmith, G. A.: Nutritional diagnosis, American Lecture Series, Publication No. 356, Springfield, Ill., 1959, Charles C Thomas, Publisher.
17. *Goodhart, R. S., and Shuls, M. E.: Modern nutrition in health and disease, ed. 5, Philadelphia, 1974, Lea & Febiger.
18. Halsted, J. A., Smith, J. C., Jr., and Irwin, M. I.: A conspectus of research on zinc requirements of man, J. Nutr. **104**:345-378, 1974.
19. Hambidge, K. M., Hambidge, C., Jacobs, M., et al.: Low levels of zinc in hair, anorexia, poor growth, and hypogeusia in children, Pediatr. Res. **6**:868-874, 1972.
20. Henderson, L. M.: Nutritional problems growing out of new pat-

*References preceded by an asterisk are particulary well suited for student reading.

terns of food consumption, Am. J. Public Health **62:**1194-1198, 1972.

21. Hilderbrand, D. C., and White, D. H.: Trace element analysis in hair: an evaluation, Clin. Chem. **20:**148-151, 1974.
22. *Howard, R. B., and Herbold, N. H.: Nutrition in clinical care, New York, 1978, McGraw-Hill Book Co.
23. Jelliffe, D. B.: The assessment of the nutritional status of the community, WHO Monograph No. 53, Geneva, 1966, World Health Organization.
24. Karp, R. J., Nuchpakdee, M., Fairorth, J., et al.: School health service as a means of entry into the inner-city family for the identification of malnourished children, Am. J. Clin. Nutr. **29:**216-218, 1976.
25. Knowles, J. H.: Responsibility for health, Science **198:**1103-1107, 1977.
26. Krehl, W. A.: The evaluation of nutritional status, Med. Clin. North Am. **48:**1129-1140, 1964.
27. Levy, C. M., et al.: Incidence and significance of hypovitaminosis in a randomly selected municipal hospital population, Am. J. Clin. Nutr. **17:**259-271, 1965.
28. Mann, G. V.: The influence of obesity on health, N. Engl. J. Med. **291:**178-185, 226-232, 1974.
29. *Marsh, A. G., et al.: About nutrition, Nashville, Tenn., 1971, Southern Publishers Association.
30. Mayer, J.: U.S. Nutrition policies in the seventies, San Francisco, 1973, W. H. Freeman and Co.
31. *McLaren, D. S.: Nutrition and its disorders, ed. 2, New York, 1976, Churchill Livingstone.
32. *Mitchell, H. S., et al.: Nutrition in health and disease, ed. 16, New York, 1976, J. B. Lippincott Co.
33. Munro, H. N.: How well recommended are the recommended dietary allowances? J. Am. Diet. Assoc. **71:**490-494, 1977.
34. Murphy, E. W., Willis, B. W., and Watt, B. K.: Provisional tables on the zinc content of food, J. Am. Diet Assoc. **66:**345-355, 1975.
35. *National Research Council, Committee on Food Protection, Food and Nutrition Board: Toxicants occurring naturally in foods, ed. 2, Washington, D. C., 1973, National Academy of Sciences.
36. Pearson, A. M.: Some factors that may alter consumption of animal products, J. Am. Diet. Assoc. **69:**522-530, 1976.
37. Perloff, B. P., and Butram, R. R.: Folacin in selected foods, J. Am. Diet. Assoc. **70:**161-179, 1977.
38. *Prasad, A. S.: Trace elements in human health and disease, Foundation Monograph Series; vol I, Zinc and copper; vol II, Essential and toxic elements, New York, 1976, Academic Press, Inc.
39. *Recommended dietary allowances, ed. 8, Washington. D.C., 1974, National Academy of Sciences, National Research Council.
40. Register, U. D., and Sonnenberg, L. M.: The vegetarian diet: scientific and practical considerations, J. Am. Diet. Assoc. **62:**253-261, 1973.
41. Rickard, K., Brady, M. S., Hempel, J., et al.: care of children with conditions characterized by high nutritional risks, J.A.M.A. **68:**546-549, 1976.
42. *Robinson, C., and Lawler, M.: Normal and therapeutic nutrition, ed. 15, New York, 1977, Macmillan, Inc.
43. *Roe, D. A.: Drug-induced nutritional deficiencies, Westport, Conn., 1976, AVI Publishing Co.
44. *Sauberlich, H. E., et al.: Laboratory tests for the assessment of nutritional status, Cleveland, 1974, CRC Press.
45. Select Committee on Nutrition and Human Needs, United States Senate: Dietary goals for the United States, ed. 2, Washington, D.C., 1977, U.S. Government Printing Office.
46. Schneider, H. A., Anderson, C. E., and Coursin, D. B.: Nutritional support of medical practice, New York, 1977, Harper & Row, Publishers.
47. Smith, E. B.: A guide to good eating the vegetarian way, J. Nutr. Ed. **7:**109-112, 1975.
48. U.S. Department of Agriculture, Agricultural Research Service: Nutritive value of foods: home and garden bulletin, No. 72, revised April 1977, Washington, D.C., 1977, U.S. Government Printing Office.
49. U.S. Department of Agriculture, Agricultural Research Service: Nutritive value of American foods in common units, Washington, D.C., 1975, U.S. Government Printing Office.
50. U.S. Department of Agriculture: Pantothenic acid, vitamin B-6 and vitamin B-12 in foods, Home Economics Research report no 36, Washington, D.C. 1969, U.S. Government Printing Office.
51. U.S. Department of Health, Education and Welfare, National Center for Health Statistics: Dietary intake findings, United States 1971-1974. Data from the National Health Survey, Health and Nutrition Examination Survey, Vital and Health statistics, series 11, number 202, DHEW No. (HRA) 77-1647, Hyattsville, Md., 1977, Public Health Service, Health Resources Administration.
52. Widmann, F. K.: Goodale's clinical interpretation of laboratory tests, Philadelphia, 1973, F. A. Davis Co.
53. *Williams, S. R.: Nutrition and diet therapy, ed. 3, St. Louis, 1977, The C. V. Mosby Co.
54. *Winick, M.: Nutritional disorders of American women, New York, 1977, John Wiley & Sons, Inc.
55. Winter, S.L., and Boyer, J. L.: Hepatic toxicity from large doses of vitamin B_3 (nicotinamide), N. Engl. J. Med. **289:**1180-1182, 1973.
56. Young, C. M., Hagan, G. C., Tucker, R. E., and Foster, W. D.: Comparison of dietary study methods: dietary history vs. seven-day record vs. 26-hr. recall, J. Am. Diet Assoc. **28:**218-221, 1952.

52

Assessment of upper gastrointestinal tract function

NANCY DURHAM

Maintenance of an adequate nutritional status requires a functioning upper gastrointestinal tract. Normally food and fluids are placed in the mouth, pushed to the pharynx by the tongue, and swallowed by automatic reflex activity down the esophagus into the stomach. Digestion starts in the mouth and terminates in the small intestine, although fluids continue to be reabsorbed in the colon. Abnormalities that interfere with passage of food will interfere with nutrition; therefore assessment of nutrition requires assessment of the gastrointestinal tract. (For assessment of the lower gastrointestinal tract, see Chapter 55.)

PHYSIOLOGY OF THE UPPER GASTROINTESTINAL TRACT

The subconscious or actively conscious thought of food initiates the physiologic responses of the body that are ultimately responsible for delivery of a particular nutrient to the individual cell. The hypothalamus is responsible for notifying the body that it is satiated or has received sufficient food substances to maintain proper homeostasis.

Salivation

The cortical thought regarding "food" initiates saliva production from the parotid, submaxillary, buccal, and sublingual glands. The salivary secretions are made up of *serous* secretion containing ptyalin for starch digestion (produced by the parotid and submaxillary glands) and *mucous* secretion for lubrication (produced by the buccal, sublingual, and submaxillary glands). These two secretions account for one-half of the upper gastrointestinal tract secretions.

Mastication

The teeth serve the function of initial food breakdown. No other part of the gastrointestinal tract can perform this function if the teeth are missing. Enzymes can act only on the exposed surfaces of the food particles. Very fine particulation prevents excoriation of the lining of the tract, and the rate of digestion is dependent on the total surface area of food particle exposed.[8] General health teaching for children and adults should stress the reason behind thorough mastication of all food substances that are ingested.

Deglutition

Swallowing (deglutition) must be accomplished without compromising respiration. It consists of two phases, a voluntary phase in which the tongue forces the bolus of food into the pharynx, and an involuntary (pharyngeal) phase in which the food moves into the upper esophagus. Food is prevented from passing into the trachea by the closing of the trachea and the opening of the esophagus.

The esophagus is a hollow tube whose upper one third is composed of skeletal muscle and the remainder of smooth muscle. It is lined with mucous membrane, which secretes a mucoid substance for protection. The bolus of food arrives at the cardiac sphincter of the stomach within 5 to 10 seconds of ingestion.[8]

The cardiac sphincter prevents reflux of stomach contents back into the lower esophagus. This area is heavily layered with mucoid glands. The secretions adhere to the food particles and prevent actual contact with the wall mucosa. The coated particles adhere to each other, forming a bolus for digestion. These secretions act as a protective mechanism for the sphincter zone as they themselves are strongly resistant to digestion.

Stomach function

The food bolus enters the stomach, the largest dilated portion of the tract. There is relatively little muscular tone, allowing for increased distention. Movement of food through the stomach and intestines is by *peristalsis*, alternate contraction and relaxation of the muscle fibers which propels the substance in a wavelike motion. The mucous membrane lining of the stomach is arranged in thick folds known as *rugae*. These rugae provide an increased surface area for exposure and contain the gastric pit openings from the fundic, pyloric, and cardiac glands. The gastric secretions are clear and colorless and contain water, salts, enzymes, and hydrochloric acid. The amount of enzymes produced is in direct proportion to that needed, and the actual food substance stimulates the release of a particular enzyme. The gastric mucosa releases gastrin, which stimulates the production of *pepsinogen* (the precursor of pepsin), *rennin*, and *lipase*. The activity of pepsin, which digests protein, depends on an acid media. Rennin also digests protein, and lipase splits fats. The production of hydrochloric acid (HCl) does not appear to be dependent on the presence of any particular food.

As the food moves toward the pyloric sphincter, peristaltic waves increase in force and intensity. The fluid mass now becomes known as *chyme*. Chyme is pumped through the pyloric sphincter into the duodenum. Emptying of stomach contents is regulated by two factors: *consistency* of the fluid chyme and the *receptiveness of the duodenum*.[8] The pyloric sphincter activity stops with vagal stimulation of the *enterogastric* reflex. This sphincter activity is also slowed when the chyme requires an increased time for digestion (fatty foods or high levels of protein). The production of gastric secretions decreases when the pH falls and as enterogasterone is released from the small intestine.

The stomach and remainder of the gastrointestinal tract are made up of five layers of smooth muscle. This smooth muscle has two types of contractions: (1) *tonus* contractions, which are continuous and which determine both the amount of steady pressure exerted within the area and the degree of resistance to the movement of food at the sphincter, and (2) *rhythmic* contractions, which may be either as slow as every 2 to 3 minutes or very rapid and are responsible for the mixing of the food and peristaltic propulsion of it.

The entire tract is innervated through the intramural plexus, which begins in the wall of the esophagus and extends through the anus. The plexus is composed of two layers, the *Auerbach* plexus and the *Meissner* plexus. Stimulation to the plexus increases the tonic contractions and the intensity and rate of rhythmic contractions.[8] Innervation is accomplished through the vagus nerve and comprises both sympathetic and parasympathetic fibers.

■ SUBJECTIVE DATA

General questions asked of the client or significant other may give clues to actual or potential problems of upper gastrointestinal tract function. Data to be gathered include the following:

- General data
  - Presence of dental prosthesis
  - Difficulty eating or digesting food
  - Nausea or vomiting
  - Weight loss
  - Pain
- Specific data if symptoms are present
  - Situations or events that affect symptoms
  - Onset, possible cause, location, duration, character of symptoms
  - Relationship of specific foods, smoking, or alcohol to severity of symptoms
  - How the problem was managed before seeking assistance of a health care provider

Pain may be reported in the mouth, throat, upper abdomen, or radiating from the abdomen to the back. It may interfere with chewing or swallowing food. Specific foods such as spicy foods or alcohol, very hot or cold foods, or smoking may initiate or aggravate the pain. Abdominal pain may have been self-treated with commercial antacids or by baking soda.

Nausea and *vomiting* may be due to a gastrointestinal problem such as gastritis or to a number of other factors unrelated to pathology of the upper gastrointestinal tract. These may include side effects of drugs, fluid and electrolyte imbalances, or radiation effects.

Weight loss may be due to a pathologic condition, nausea and vomiting, anorexia, or deliberate action on the part of the person to lose weight. Gradual weight loss and lack of appetite in the older person is not necessarily an abnormal finding but bears investigation.

All persons should be asked about the presence of *dental prostheses*. It is important to ascertain if the person has any artificial dentures (bridges, partial or full plates), if he is wearing the prosthesis, and if it fits and is comfortable. Chewing and digestion can be impaired if the person does not wear the prosthesis. If during the physical inspection of the mouth the teeth are noted to have caries, data are obtained concerning regularity of dental checkups for use in health teaching.

■ OBJECTIVE DATA

□ Mouth and pharynx

Physical examination of the mouth (Fig. 52-1) will provide data indicating ability to salivate, masticate, and swallow as well as signs of local or systemic disease that can interfere with nutrition. A tongue blade and flashlight are needed for the examination of the oral cavity. The person should be seated comfortably on a level with the examiner and should remove any dental appliances and makeup.

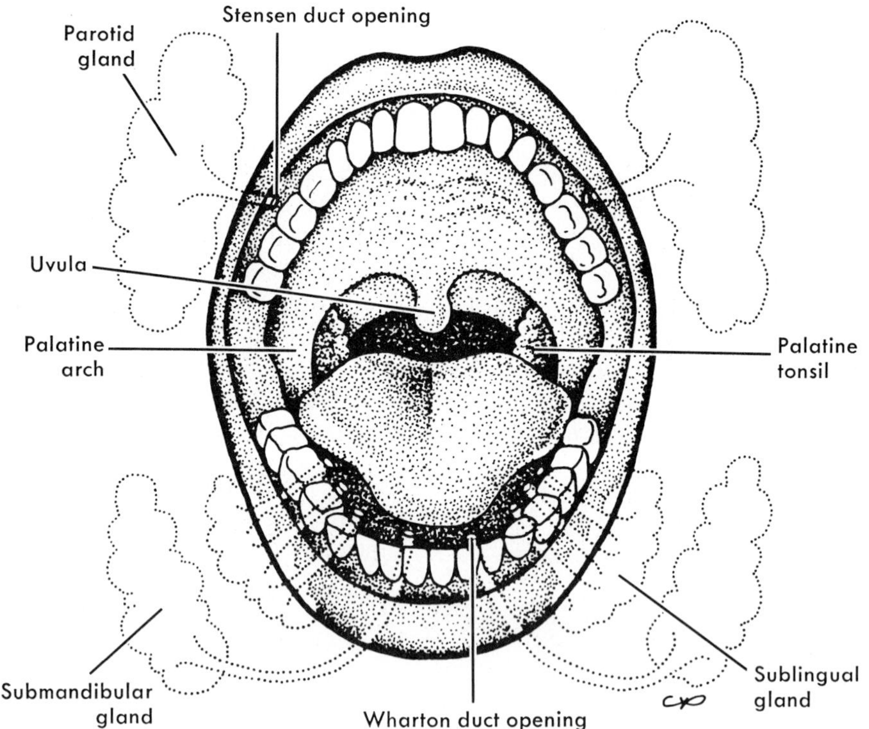

Fig. 52-1. Structures of mouth. (From Malasanos, L., Barkauskas, V., Moss, M., and Stoltenberg-Allen, K.: Health assessment, St. Louis, 1977, The C. V. Mosby Co.)

Lips

The person is asked to purse his lips, which are observed for symmetry in form and function and for color, moisture, swelling, cracks, or lesions (Fig. 52-2). Asymmetry is often accompanied by drooling and may be due to facial nerve paralysis from peripheral or central nervous system involvement.[9] If noted, the ability to masticate and swallow is assessed. A congenital malformation such as cleft lip may be observed, or signs of residual dysfunction if this condition has been surgically corrected.

The lips are normally reddish in color and are good indicators of pallor or cyanosis (p. 1487). Dryness may indicate dehydration. Swelling is usually due to edema of the inflammatory response such as with allergy. Cracks or fissures can occur with overdryness or exposure to cold or, if in the corners of the mouth *(angular stomatitis)*, from lack of dentures, poorly fitting dentures, or a riboflavin deficiency.

Lesions may be benign or malignant. A frequently encountered benign lesion is *herpes simplex* (cold sore, fever blister), which is caused by a virus and which can create enough discomfort to limit mastication. Any lesion on the lip that does not heal should be referred to the physician for tests for possible malignancy.

Teeth

A full set of teeth consists of 20 teeth in children and 32 teeth in adults. The enamel surface should be white but will darken with surface stains (tea, coffee, tobacco). Commonly found abnormalities include caries, loose teeth, absence of some or all teeth, failure of a tooth to erupt resulting in swelling and possible discomfort, and worn crown surfaces. These conditions may impair adequate mastication.

Gums

The gums, or *gingivae*, are normally pink in color, attach to the teeth, and fill the interdental surfaces. If the person is edentulous, the gingivae are examined for areas of redness caused by improperly fitting dentures. The person is then asked to insert the dentures to assess correct fit and comfort for adequate mastication. Recession of the gum line is not uncommon in the older individual. Bleeding of the gums may occur with improper teeth brushing, dental calculus, oral infections, or blood dyscrasias. Painful gums may interfere with mastication.

Mucosa

A tongue blade is inserted between the cheek pockets and tooth surfaces, and the buccal mucosa is illumi-

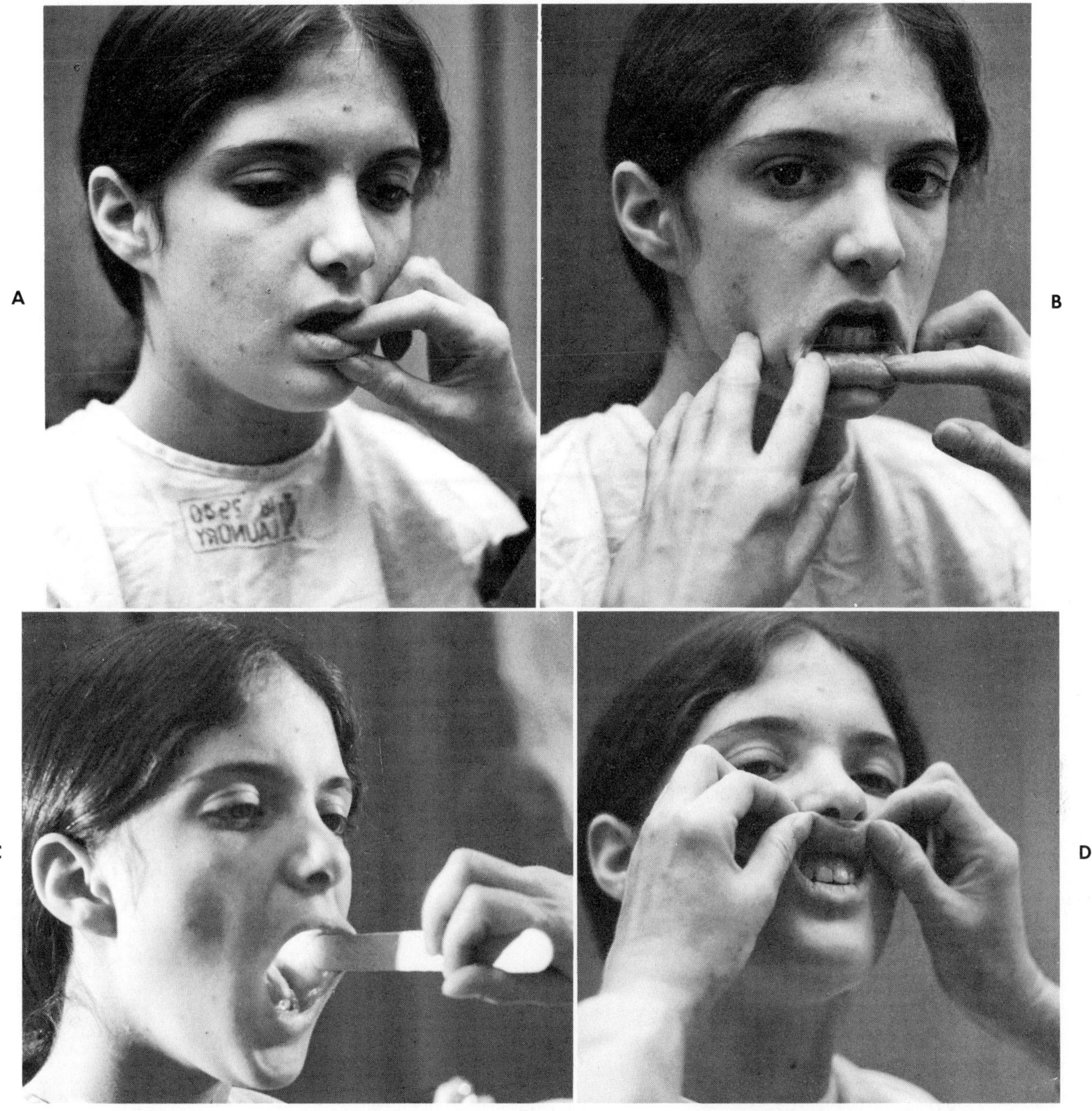

Fig. 52-2. Examination of lips and oral mucosa. **A,** Palpation of lips. **B,** Inspection of mucosa of lower anterior area. **C,** Inspection of mucosa of each cheek with identification of Stensen's duct opening. **D,** Inspection of mucosa of upper anterior area. (From Malasanos, L., Barkauskas, V., Moss, M., and Stoltenberg-Allen, K.: Health assessment, St. Louis, 1977, The C. V. Mosby Co.)

nated by a flashlight for inspection (Fig. 51-2, C). The mucosa is light pink in color, although patchy pigmentation is seen in blacks.[1] The mucosa is examined for moisture, white spots or patches, debris, areas of bleeding, or ulcers. Dryness and debris may indicate dehydration. White curdy patches, which are removable with some effort, may be due to *moniliasis* (thrush).[1] A round or oval white ulcer surrounded by an area of redness is indicative of an *aphthous ulcer* (canker sore). The orifice of the parotid gland can be observed on the buccal mucosa near the upper second molar; inflammation of the parotid gland occurs with mumps.

Pharynx

The uvula, soft palate, tonsils, and posterior pharynx are usually observed at this time while the examiner still has the tongue blade. The middle of the tongue is pressed down firmly while the client says "Ah." This raises the soft palate, and symmetry should be noted (necessary for effective swallowing). The areas are examined for signs of inflammation (redness, edema, ulceration, thick yellowish secretions), and the size of the uvula is noted. A swollen uvula can cause pain and can limit swallowing. Changes in signs are reported to the physician.

Tongue

Tongue mobility and function are essential to mastication, taste, and swallowing. Inspection of the tongue is accomplished in two steps. First, the person is asked to protrude his tongue and rotate it in all four directions. Normally there is no limitation in movement in any direction, but the tongue will deviate to the paralyzed side with paralysis of the twelfth cranial (hypoglossal) nerve. Second, the person is asked to protrude his tongue so that the dorsal surface can be observed and to elevate the tongue for inspection of the ventral surface and floor of the mouth. A thin white coating and the presence of large papillae on the dorsum are normal findings. A thick coating indicates poor oral hygiene, and a smooth red surface suggests a nutritional deficiency.[9] The ventral surface is examined for leukoplakia (a thickened white patch that is not removable), ulceration, or nodules, which may indicate malignancy.

Breath

Any distinctive odor of the breath is noted. A foul odor, *fetor oris,* may occur with poor oral hygiene or with dental or oral infections. Odors may occur after certain foods such as garlic or alcohol or with some systemic diseases (odor of acetone in diabetes, ammonia in liver disease).

□ Jaws

Examination for jaw articulation is generally performed last. The examiner places the fingertips of each hand at the angle of the temporomandibular joint (Fig. 52-3). The person is instructed to open and close his

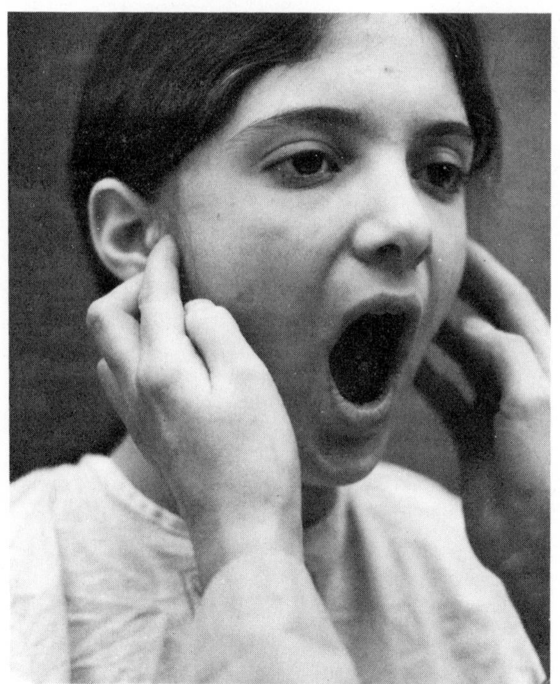

Fig. 52-3. Palpation of temporomandibular joint. (From Malasanos, L., Barkauskas, V., Moss, M., and Stoltenberg-Allen, K.: Health assessment, St. Louis, 1977, The C. V. Mosby Co.)

mouth slowly. Normally the mandible may be felt to slide forward and down with ease. A normal sound of "cracking" may be heard when the person opens the mouth widely. Limitation of motion will affect mastication.

☐ Stomach

Physical examination of the stomach is usually carried out in conjunction with assessment of the abdomen (p. 220). Since most of the stomach lies beneath the ribs and liver, it is not usually palpable. Percussion is also of limited value. Pain elicited from palpation of the epigastric region may represent referred pain such as from acute appendicitis or hiatal hernia.

■ DIAGNOSTIC TESTS

Many of the examinations and tests performed for diagnosis of problems of the upper gastrointestinal system are both time consuming and vaguely unpleasant. Several of the tests are intrusive procedures and as such may present added stress for the individual and family.

The individual may already be physically debilitated due to poor nutritional intake and may be vomiting and experiencing acute or chronic pain. This data is utilized to plan for thorough and complete explanation of the tests and examinations to be done so that the patient or significant other may offer the optimum cooperation.

In many institutions the responsibility for explaining the procedures to the patient has been assumed by representatives from the radiology department or laboratory. Prepared literature that explains the procedure is also available for the patient and family. This approach, however, does not relieve the nurse from the responsibility of understanding the rationale and technique for each procedure, assessing the patient's understanding, and answering questions that the patient or family may have. The various tests and procedures are scheduled so that the time expended by the patient is best utilized; for example, a gastric analysis should be scheduled prior to a barium swallow, since the stomach must be empty for the gastric analysis.

The person's ability to tolerate discomfort prior to and during the examination is assessed. Narcotics and many sedatives will depress gastric emptying; therefore a notation to the radiologist or physician is made if these drugs are given prior to diagnostic tests of the stomach. If the radiologist is aware that a narcotic has been given within 2 hours prior to the ingestion of barium, he or she would not necessarily attribute the decreased emptying time of the stomach to a definite pathologic problem. In this way inadvertent errors may be avoided as well as unnecessary repetition of time-consuming and expensive examinations.

☐ Radiographic studies

Dental radiographs

Dental x-ray examinations are most frequently carried out as part of routine dental hygiene. The person needs no specific preparation for the examination. He will be seated comfortably in the chair and asked to assist the dentist or hygienist by holding or supporting the radiographic films against the tooth surfaces. Radiographs are taken either of all the teeth (full-mouth) or of specific teeth.

The results of dental radiographs show the integrity of the enamel surface as well as the root shadow and alignment of the individual teeth in the bony structure. The most common abnormalities include caries within the internal tooth structure, pulp abnormalities from infection, abnormal alignment of the tooth and root structure, and the presence of nonerupted teeth. Dental radiographs may also be done for the hospitalized patient to determine the possible cause for dental pain and prior to dental extraction.

Facial bone radiographs

Facial bone x-ray examinations are most commonly used to determine alignment of the bone structure when trauma has occurred. The radiographs will be done soon after the initial trauma. The patient is usually experiencing pain; therefore gentleness in movement, proper administration of analgesics, and monitoring for adequacy of airway are guidelines to be implemented in the nursing care.

Gastrointestinal series

A gastrointestinal series consists of several radiographs of the stomach and intestinal tract and is used to detect tumors, ulcerations, or inflammation of the stomach and duodenum and to reveal any abnormal anatomy or malposition of these organs. As the person swallows barium (a radiopaque substance), the radiologist makes a fluoroscopic examination and then takes radiographs of the stomach and the duodenum. Since the barium tastes like chalk, it is often flavored to make it more palatable. After the person has drunk the barium, he is asked to assume various positions on the x-ray table, and the table may be tilted so that the barium will outline the stomach wall and flow by gravity into the intestinal loops as the radiologist, using the fluoroscope, watches the television monitor and takes the radiographs. Successive films are taken as the barium moves into the areas to be observed or into the large bowel, thus completing the visualization of the upper gastrointestinal tract, the ileum, or the small intestine. If the person has a spastic duodenal bulb or increased peristalsis in the duodenal area, atropine may be administered prior to the radiograph to slow down the action of the small intestine, permitting better visualization of the area. This procedure is called hypotonic duodenography.

In preparation for a gastrointestinal series the nurse explains the procedure to the person and tells him that he must not take food or fluids for 6 to 8 hours before the examination. The presence of food in the stomach prevents the barium from outlining all of the stomach wall, and the radiographs will be inconclusive and misleading. If the patient eats, the radiographic examination should be postponed until the next day. The patient can be assured that the test will not cause discomfort and that he may eat as soon as the nurse is notified by the radiologist department that the series is completed. However, breakfast will probably be omitted, and lunch may be delayed. After a gastrointestinal series a cathartic may be ordered to speed the elimination of barium from the intestines. Retained barium may become hard and cause obstruction in the intestine or an impaction in the rectum.

□ Endoscopy

Esophagoscopy and gastroscopy

Esophagoscopy and gastroscopy are procedures performed to visualize the esophageal and gastric mucosa. By these means a disease process may be located and inspected, and a specimen of tissue may be obtained for microscopic study.

The conventional gastroscope is a hollow, cylindrical metal tube that permits visualization of the inner surface of the stomach mucosa except the fundus, the greater curvature, and the pylorus. The *fiberscope*, a type of gastroscope, has a shaft made of rubber or plastic that allows for greater flexibility and permits visualization of the greater curvature, the antrum, the pylorus, and the duodenal bulb. Glass fibers incorporated into the shaft of the instrument transmit light to the mucosa and the image back to the examiner. Cameras may be attached to either instrument for the purpose of taking pictures of abnormalities of the gastric mucosa during the examination (Fig. 52-4).

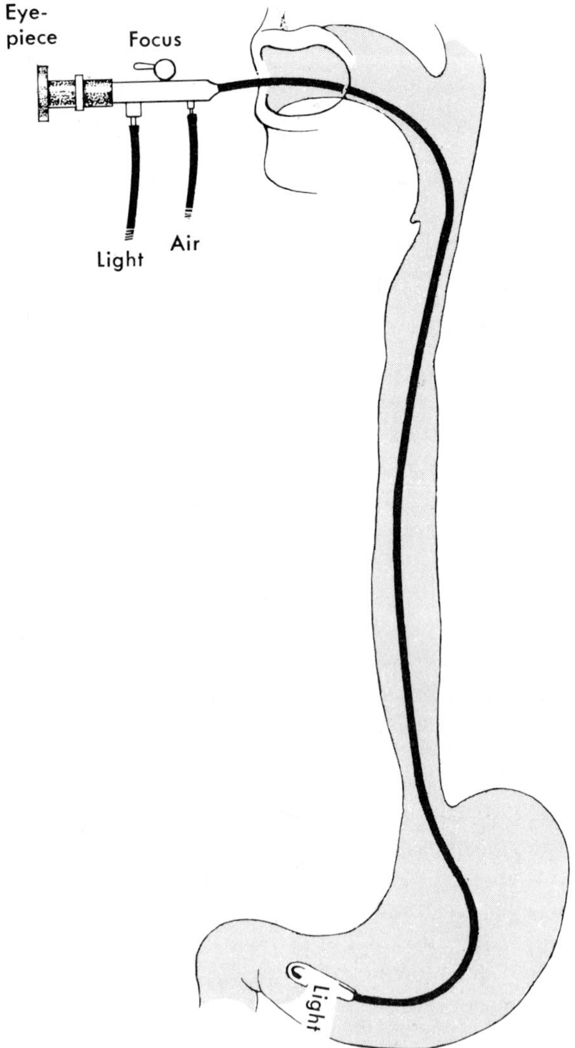

Fig. 52-4. Interior of stomach may be visualized by means of fiberscope.

Radiographs of the stomach and esophagus are taken prior to these examinations, since an obstruction of the esophagus might make passing an instrument dangerous. The physician will often use the radiographs to guide him in passing the gastroscope.

Although these procedures are not actually painful, patients find them extremely exhausting and uncomfortable. The nurse should explain the examination to the patient in simple terms, emphasizing that if he carefully follows the physician's instructions and remains quiet during the passing of the instrument, he can help make the procedure a short and successful one. Food and fluids are witheld for 6 to 8 hours before the examination so that the patient does not regurgitate as the tubular instrument is passed through the mouth into the esophagus and so that the lining of the stomach is visible. Occasionally an esophagoscopy or a gastroscopy must be performed as an emergency measure to remove a foreign object such as a bone or a pin. In such an emergency the stomach cannot be emptied, but suction should be available for use to prevent aspiration of regurgitated food or fluid. Eyeglasses and dentures are removed to prevent their being broken. The patient should void before the examination to prevent discomfort or embarrassment. Pajama bottoms should be worn to prevent inadvertant exposure during the procedure. The patient's written permission is obtained before this examination is performed.

The patient is given sedatives $1/2$ to 1 hour before the

examination or at the time of the examination to lessen apprehension and to make him less aware of the passage of the instrument. The premedication also decreases the possibility of toxic effects from the local anesthetic. A narcotic such as meperidine hydrochloride (Demerol) and a barbiturate such as soluble phenobarbital are ordinarily used for sedation. To decrease secretions, atropine sulfate may be administered. The patient should be observed carefully for possible reactions to these drugs, and he should be protected from injury while under their influence.

Before the examination begins, the physician explains the procedure to the patient and tries to gain his full understanding and cooperation. During the procedure, both the physician and the nurse should reassure the patient and tell him what is happening. The patient is unable to speak and may be very frustrated by his inability to communicate. The patient's posterior pharynx is then sprayed with cocaine or tetracaine (Pontocaine) to inactivate the gag reflex and to lessen local reaction to the instrument. In order to prevent the aspiration of medication, the patient is asked to hold his breath while the posterior pharynx is sprayed and not to swallow saliva but to expectorate it into an emesis basin that is provided. The nurse should watch the patient for any toxic reactions to the anesthetic. An emergency tray containing intravenous barbiturates should be readily available. (See p. 382 for the toxic reactions to cocaine and tetracaine.)

When the gag reflex has disappeared (usually within 5 to 10 minutes), the patient assumes a dorsal recumbent position on the treatment table for passage of the conventional gastroscope. For an esophageal examination his head and shoulders extend over the edge of the table, and for the passage of a gastroscope he lies on his side. The nurse supports the patient's head, and he is told again how important it is to remain perfectly still while the instrument is passed. Sudden movement at this time might cause the instrument to perforate the esophagus. Children and patients whose behavior is unpredictable should be firmly restrained if this procedure is attempted without the use of a general anesthetic. For passage of the fiberscope the patient sits or lies on the side of the bed or table facing the physician. If tissue is removed for pathologic examinations, it should be placed immediately into a specimen bottle and correctly labeled.

When the examination is finished, the patient is instructed not to eat or drink until the gag reflex returns, lest fluid be aspirated into the lungs. The gag reflex usually returns is about 4 hours. In the hospital the physician or the nurse tests for the return of the gag reflex by gentling tickling the back of the throat with a cotton swab or a tongue depressor. If the patient goes home, he should check by touching his throat with a swab or his finger before he attempts to eat or drink.

Following an esophagoscopy or a gastroscopy, the patient may be hoarse and complain of a sore throat. These symptoms should disappear within a few days. The patient should be so informed because he will not notice discomfort until the anesthesia wears off. Warm saline solution gargles may give some relief. These procedures are exhausting to the patient, and provision should be made for him to rest when they are completed.

□ Tests for malignancy

Exfoliative cytology

Exfoliative cytology is the study of the individual cells or clumps of cells to identify or to exclude the presence of malignancy. Because malignant cells tend to exfoliate (separate from the tumor), methods of accelerating exfoliation are used. This is accomplished by passing a Levin tube and lavaging the stomach vigorously with quantities of saline solution or by passing stomach tubes to which gastric brushes or abrasive balloons are attached to collect fragments of mucosa. *Chymotrypsin* may be administered to digest the overlying protective coat of mucus and thereby expose the mucosa to the irrigating solution or abrasive collecting agent. All the aspirated irrigating solution, cells, and bits of tissue obtained are sent to the laboratory for study.

Biopsy

A biopsy of the oral cavity or tongue may be done on any lesion or ulcerated area that requires a differential diagnosis. This procedure is most generally carried out with the patient under local anesthesia. Following the biopsy the biopsy site is assessed for bleeding. Planned oral hygiene utilizing a neutral mouthwash solution is implemented at least every 4 hours until drainage from the site has ceased and at least 3 times a day thereafter.

□ Tests of gastric function

Gastric analysis (with histamine)

Examination of the fasting contents of the stomach is helpful in establishing a diagnosis of gastric disease. For example, an unusual amount of gastric secretions containing food ingested the night before suggests pyloric obstruction. An absence of free hydrochloric acid in the stomach contents may indicate the presence of gastric malignancy or pernicious anemia, whereas an increased amount of free hydrochloric acid suggests a duodenal ulcer. In a gastric ulcer the amount of acid may be either decreased or normal in amount.

To obtain fasting stomach secretions, a nasogastric tube must be passed. The procedure must be explained to the patient, and food and fluids are withheld for 6 to 8 hours before the test is to be done. Anticholinergic drugs are omitted for 24 hours before the test. Smoking is prohibited the morning before the test, as smoking stimulates secretory action of gastric cells.

The procedure may be performed with the person seated comfortably in a secure chair and the head hyperextended for greater ease in inserting the tube. If the person is in bed, this position can be accomplished by raising the head of the bed to high Fowler position and arranging pillows under the shoulders, allowing the head to rest on the mattress. The head is then slightly flexed to a more normal position as the person swallows the tube. The person's clothing or gown is protected, with a towel or plastic apron, and he is provided with an emesis basin and paper tissues.

A nasogastric tube (Levin #12, #14, or #16) is used. The tip of the tube is lubricated with a water-soluble lubricant and inserted through the nose (or mouth) into the posterior pharynx. The person is asked to swallow hard and repeatedly, and he may be given sips of water as the tube is advanced quickly into the stomach. A syringe is then fitted onto the end of the tube, and all the stomach contents are aspirated and placed in a specimen bottle. The reactions of the aspirated secretions may be tested by using litmus paper. Blue litmus turns pink in the presence of acid. The tube is then secured to the nose and to the forehead with adhesive tape. Care should be taken that the tube does not pull or press against the nostril or cross in front of the eye. The end of the tube is closed with a clamp or with an elastic band to prevent leaking. Most patients are inclined to hold themselves very rigid while the tube is in the stomach, and they may be afraid to move. They are encouraged to assume any position that is most comfortable and instructed to expectorate saliva because it may act as a buffer and invalidate the examination.

After a fasting specimen has been collected, histamine phosphate, 0.25 to 0.5 mg of a 1:1,000 solution, or betazole hydrochloride (Histalog) is given subcutaneously. *Histamine is not given to persons with a history of allergy.* A skin test is carried out before the test in initiated if histamine is to be given. Betazole hydrochloride produces fewer side effects than histamine. Pulse and blood pressure are taken immediately after administration of histamine; normally the pulse is increased and the blood pressure is slightly lowered.[2] The person is told that he will look and feel flushed and warm and that he may develop a headache. These symptoms are caused by the vasodilating effects of histamine and will subside fairly rapidly. Vasogenic shock may occur; therefore vasoconstricting drugs such as epinephrine should be available.

After the histamine injection has been given, the stomach contents are aspirated every 10 to 20 minutes until three or more specimens of gastric secretions have been obtained. When histamine is administered to a person who has a peptic ulcer, there is a definite increase in the total output of gastric secretions and an increase in the amount of free hydrochloric acid in the stomach. The peak in hydrochloric acid secretion usually occurs about $^1/_2$ hour after the administration of histamine. A reduction in the amount of free acid or the absence of it may indicate that a malignancy is present. True achlorhydria (absence of hydrochloric acid even after the administration of histamine) is characteristic of pernicious anemia.

When the test is completed, the tube is clamped and quickly withdrawn. The person will need tissues to wipe away secretions from the eyes, nose, and throat that occur as the tube is withdrawn, and he may wish to rinse out his mouth. Food is permitted if nausea is not present.

Tubeless gastric analysis

This procedure is thought to be useful as a screening technique for detection of gastric achlorhydria. The test will indicate the presence or absence of free hydrochloric acid but cannot be used to determine the *amount* of free hydrochloric acid if it is present. Quantitative determinations must be done through aspiration of stomach contents.

For a tubeless gastric analysis, a gastric stimulant such as caffeine or histamine phosphate is given to the patient. One hour later he is given 2 g (30 grains) of a cation exchange resin containing 90 mg ($1^1/_2$ grains) of azure A (Azuresin, Diagnex Blue) with 240 ml of water orally on an empty stomach. If there is free hydrochloric acid in the stomach, on the introduction of this resin a substance will be released in the stomach that will be absorbed from the small intestine and excreted by the kidneys within 2 hours. Absence of detectable amounts of dye in the urine indicates that free hydrochloric acid probably was not secreted.

Insulin tolerance test

An insulin tolerance test is another test used to evaluate the secreting action of the gastric mucosa. The test is carried out in the same way as a gastric analysis, except that instead of histamine a specified amount of regular insulin is administered intravenously. The drop in blood sugar produced by the insulin stimulates the vagus nerve, and the flow of gastric secretions may be increased. A normal stomach responds only slightly to stimulation of the vagus nerve, and there will be no significant increase in the gastric secretions. In the patient with a peptic ulcer, however, there will be a marked increase in the total gastric output and in the amount of free hydrochloric acid. The insulin tolerance test may be used to determine the success of a resection of the vagus nerve in decreasing the hyperactivity of the stomach. It is therefore often performed before and after a vagotomy. In the event that symptoms of insulin reaction appear, orange or other fruit juice should be available as well as 50% glucose for intravenous injection.

REFERENCES AND SELECTED READINGS

1. *Bates, B.: A guide to physical examination, Philadelphia, 1974, J. B. Lippincott Co.
2. Bergersen, B. S., and Goth, A.: Pharmacology in nursing, ed. 14, St. Louis, 1979, The C. V. Mosby Co.
3. Bockus, H. L.: Gastroenterology, ed. 3, vol. 1, Philadelphia, 1974, W. B. Saunders Co.
4. Davidsohn, I., and Henry, J. B.: Todd-Sanford clinical diagnosis by laboratory methods, ed. 15, Philadelphia, 1974, W. B. Saunders Co.
5. DeGowin, E., and DeGowin, R.: Bedside diagnostic examination, ed. 2, London, 1965, Macmillan, Inc.
6. French, R.: Guide to diagnostic procedures, ed. 4, New York, 1975, McGraw Hill Book Co.
7. *Given, R., and Simmons, S.: Gastroenterology in clinical nursing, ed. 2, St. Louis, 1975, The C. V. Mosby Co.
8. Guyton, A.: Textbook of medical physiology, ed. 5, Philadelphia, 1977, W. B. Saunders Co.
9. Judge, R., and Zuidema, G.: Physical diagnosis: a physiological approach to the clinical examination, ed. 2, 1963, Little, Brown and Co.
10. Krupp, M., and Chatton, M.: Current medical diagnosis and treatment, Los Altos, Calif., 1974, Lange Medical Publications.
11. *Malasanos, L., Barkauskas, V., Moss, M., and Allen, K. S.: Health Assessment, St. Louis, 1977, The C. V. Mosby Co.
12. Sleisinger, M., and Fordtram, J.: Gastrointestinal disease; pathophysiology, diagnosis, management, Philadelphia, 1973, W. B. Saunders Co.
13. Sodeman, W., and Sodeman. W.: Pathologic physiology, ed. 4, Philadelphia, 1967, W. B. Saunders Co.
14. Spiro, H. M.: Clinical gastroenterology, New York, 1970, Macmillan, Inc.

*References preceded by an asterisk are particularly well suited for student reading.

53

Management of the person with impaired nutrition

JANICE NEVILLE

Nutritional impairment can be defined in broad terms as any situation in which an inadequate, excessive, or imbalanced supply of nutrients to the body results in impairment of growth or productivity, increased susceptibility to infection or chronic disease, or impairment in functioning in the day-to-day activities of life. A child consuming a diet with marginal levels of iron and zinc may grow and function at relatively normal rates until challenged by one of the common infectious diseases of childhood. The obese person pays a price for excessive energy intake in the large deposits of adipose tissue that create increased risks of diabetes mellitus, coronary artery disease, or gallbladder disease and that interfere with functioning of organs and with ordinary activities such as walking or running or with finding attractive clothing at reasonable price. The adolescent girl who has maintained a slim and attractive appearance by limiting caloric intake without considering the vitamin and mineral content of foods has set the stage for nutritional impairment both of herself and of the child she bears. The middle-aged woman whose diet is low in calcium and vitamin D due to diet or to lack of exposure to the sun has increased risk of osteoporosis and bone fracture, conditions for which postmenopausal women are already at considerable risk. The person who doses himself with protein or vitamin or mineral supplements can produce imbalances that may result in physical impairment, symptoms mimicking serious disease, impairment of growth (in children), or deficiencies of other nutrients.

Management of nutritional impairment requires assessment of the nutritional status of the individual (see Chapter 51) so that the nutritional needs of the person are identified and appropriate interventions to meet the needs are devised. This includes seeing that the hospitalized patient receives and eats the foods he needs, whether a regular or modified diet is prescribed, and that the person learns how to meet his nutritional needs at home. The nurse serves as a liason between the patient and other professional persons in interpreting the patient's nutritional and dietary problems. Interpretation to family and friends is often needed as well.

Nutrition science has identified the nutrients required by human beings, the quantities needed for optimum growth and function, and the effects of environment, metabolism, disease, and activity on these needs. Research continues in these areas with much effort devoted to defining the relationship between diet, disease, nutrition processes, and people. Foods have been analyzed so that their nutrient composition is known. The ability of the body to absorb and utilize nutrients has been and continues to be an important area of research. Although much remains to be learned, there is a significant body of knowledge to be applied in patient care.

The nurse in accepting responsibility for patient care accepts responsibility for applying principles of nutrition. This requires knowledge of the principles and appreciation of food composition, understanding of the role of food in the person's life, and appreciation of modifications of diet and food behavior as a part of the total therapeutic regimen. The patient may be nourished by food served in the traditional manner, by tube or intravenous feedings, by nutrients supplied as medication, or by blood transfusion. The person's perceptions of food or nutrient need may differ from reality. His acceptance of proposed interventions may be affected by sociocultural factors, difficulties with appetite or taste perception, pain, weakness, depression, or a myriad of other reasons. The perceptive nurse must identify these problems, seek answers, and incorporate solutions in the nursing care plan.

■ PROMOTING ADEQUATE INTAKE

The adequacy of the diet, in terms of quality and quantity, can be quickly estimated by comparing it with recommended patterns of food intake (see Chapter 51). A good, or balanced, diet consists of any combination of foodstuffs that yields needed nutrients in sufficient amounts to promote growth and metabolism. For most persons a good diet is one that is tasty, filling, refreshing, or desirable for some special reason important to that person. Persons may believe that a particular food or nutrient has special properties to improve or harm health.[9,11,26,49] The terms "normal," "usual," or "average" diet are ambiguous and uninformative.

Diagnoses of malnutrition are of five general types:

Quantity	Quality
Excessive	Satisfactory
Inadequate	Satisfactory
Satisfactory	Inadequate
Inadequate	Inadequate
Excessive	Inadequate

Quantity refers to volume of food, intake and particularly to the energy intake. Quality relates to the protein, vitamin, and mineral content.

□ Quantity of diet

Requirements

Energy needs can be predicted from patterns of growth and body size and from physical activity. There is a constant need for energy to maintain circulation, respiration, muscle tone, and body temperature. People of similar size have similar basal energy requirements, since the requirement is related to the amount of muscle tissue and can be predicted from body weight (excluding excess body fat, since adipose tissue is relatively inert). The total energy requirement may vary widely depending on physical activity (Table 53-1). Recommendations for caloric intake are based on the growth, activity, and life style of most Americans (Fig. 53-1). Since this is a sedentary life pattern, the levels recommended are moderate, particularly for the adult. The best method for determining the adequacy of energy intake for the person is to evaluate weight for height (and rate of growth for children) in relation to energy intake assessed from dietary information.

Problems of inadequate quantity of food often are not given the attention they deserve, possibly because Americans are so conditioned to regard obesity as a national problem that loss of weight seems benign. For many patients, loss of weight impedes recovery at best and well may be life threatening. Interference with growth due to inadequate energy intake may impose a burden on a child for his lifetime.

Table 53-1. Comparison of calories used in 1 hour for different types of physical activity by a woman weighing 121 lb and a man weighing 143 lb (exclusive of basal energy needs)

Activity	Calories expended per hour	
	Woman	Man
Lying quietly	6	7
Sitting	22	26
Standing	28	32
Ironing, dishwashing, driving car	55	65
Office work, painting furniture	82	98
Walking, waltzing, bicycling	138	162
More active walking, skating, foxtrot	220	260
Running, climbing stairs, sawing wood	358	422
High-speed walking, swimming	468	552

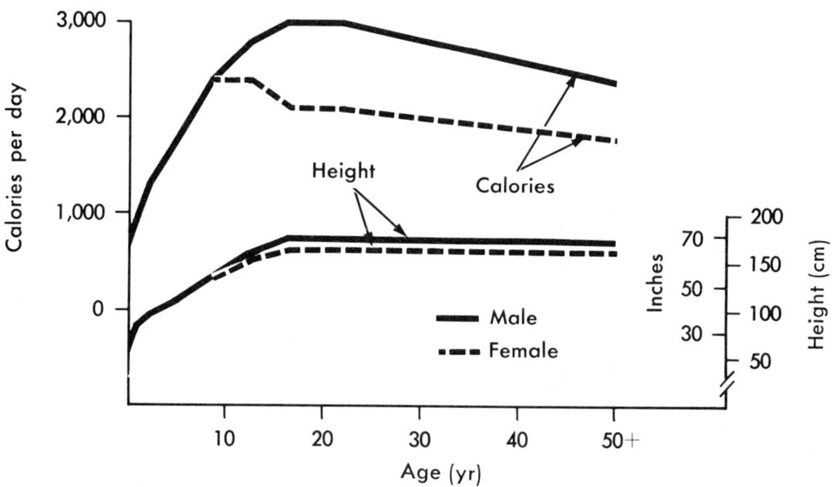

Fig. 53-1. Recommended daily dietary allowances for calories over life cycle.

Methods of promoting adequate intake

How can the nurse assure the patient's intake of adequate quantities of food? In the hospital setting there are some very simple and practical measures that can be taken. Make sure the patient gets the right tray, that the food on it is acceptable to him, that enough food is available, that the environment is pleasant, and that he is fed if necessary.

Regardless of the diet prescribed (regular "house diet" or a modified diet), adjustments can be made to fit the patient's likes and dislikes for particular food items. Most hospitals offer selective menus for regular and many modified diets. This system provides the patient an opportunity to choose foods he likes. No institutional food will match individual tastes in methods of preparation or seasoning, and the patient's taste perception can also be altered by illness or medications. Nevertheless flexibility is built into the food service system to permit menu changes to meet patient requests. The nurse can request assistance from the dietitian if necessary. Should nothing be satisfactory to the patient except food from home, food from home should be permitted. It is necessary to be sure that food provided by family and friends meets any constraints imposed by prescribed dietary modifications. Special dietary desires such as kosher foods or vegetarian meals require consultation with the dietitian.

Is the person getting enough to eat? If not, larger portions of food at regular meals may be the answer. More frequent meals of moderate size might be better, or the person might be able to handle smaller portions of food of greater caloric density.

Environment and appearance are important. The food (and tray) should be neat and attractive in appearance, and utensils should be clean. Lukewarm soup, melted ice cream, soggy toast, and tepid tea are not likely to appeal to anyone and especially not to someone who is not feeling well or who has loss of appetite. Is the room pleasant? Unpleasant smells and sights abound in hospitals and can reduce an already finicky appetite. Visitors or other patients may help by providing social ease. Guest trays can be provided in most institutions.

Is the patient comfortable? A clean face and hands are refreshing. Are the patient's dentures in? Is his mouth clean and free of foul odors? Is the patient free of pain? Position is also important. Eating is most comfortable when one is sitting up. If the patient is unable to sit in a chair or sit upright on the bed with feet dangling, the bed should be adjusted and the patient assisted up in the bed to a comfortable position. If the head cannot be raised, the patient should be helped to lie on his side and the food placed for easy access. Delivery of food to the mouth is difficult for the recumbent person, and there is increased risk of choking. Fear, discomfort, embarrassment, and possibly distaste for clothing or linen spotted with food may keep a patient from eating.

Is the patient able to get the food to his mouth and swallow it? Arranging food on the tray, opening the milk carton, or cutting meat into bite sized pieces may be needed. Each patient should be encouraged to do as much as possible for himself, and this is determined in the nursing assessment. If the patient cannot lift a spoon to his mouth, the nurse may make arrangements for someone else to feed him or may suggest that the diet be supplied as a liquid that can be drunk through a straw. Many devices are available to assist persons with physical weakness and disability to feed themselves.[20,37] These include plate guards, weighted dishes and cups, specially designed forks, knives, and spoons, and spouted cups (p. 682).

Fatigue can be a major problem for the patient or for the person feeding the patient. Rest periods before and during meals may be advisable. Often fatigue can be lessened by attention to details such as placement and height of table, tray, or chairs.[20,37]

General quantitative diet problems

Most problems of excessive quantity of food are problems of weight control. This is discussed separately. There are problems of excessive intake of vitamins and minerals that are associated with pharmaceutical products rather than food. Vitamins and minerals, alone and in various mixtures, are available to anyone who wishes to purchase them and are often prescribed for persons in and out of the hospital. The symptoms and signs of excessive intake are vague and difficult to determine. Therapeutic preparations contain concentrations far beyond daily needs and are meant to be used for a short period to meet an acute need and to replenish stores. Therapeutic levels of iron may cause severe gastrointestinal tract distress and eventually iron overload.

A person's daily energy requirements are large and measured in thousands of calories. In addition to the question of adequate but not excessive energy supply to meet patient needs is the question of the importance of the energy source. In the United States, from 10% to 12% of the fuel value of the diet is obtained from protein, about 44% from fat, and about 46% from carbohydrate. These figures reflect the variety of foods available and American food preferences. The relative contributions of protein, fat, and carbohydrate to the fuel value of the diet can be varied within wide limits without harm. Up to 80% of dietary calories may be supplied by carbohydrate in persons whose major food staple is grain. This pattern is seen in some persons, although it is not typical. The usual American food pattern includes generous use of animal foods (particularly beef), fats, oils, and sugars. As much as 25% of total calories may

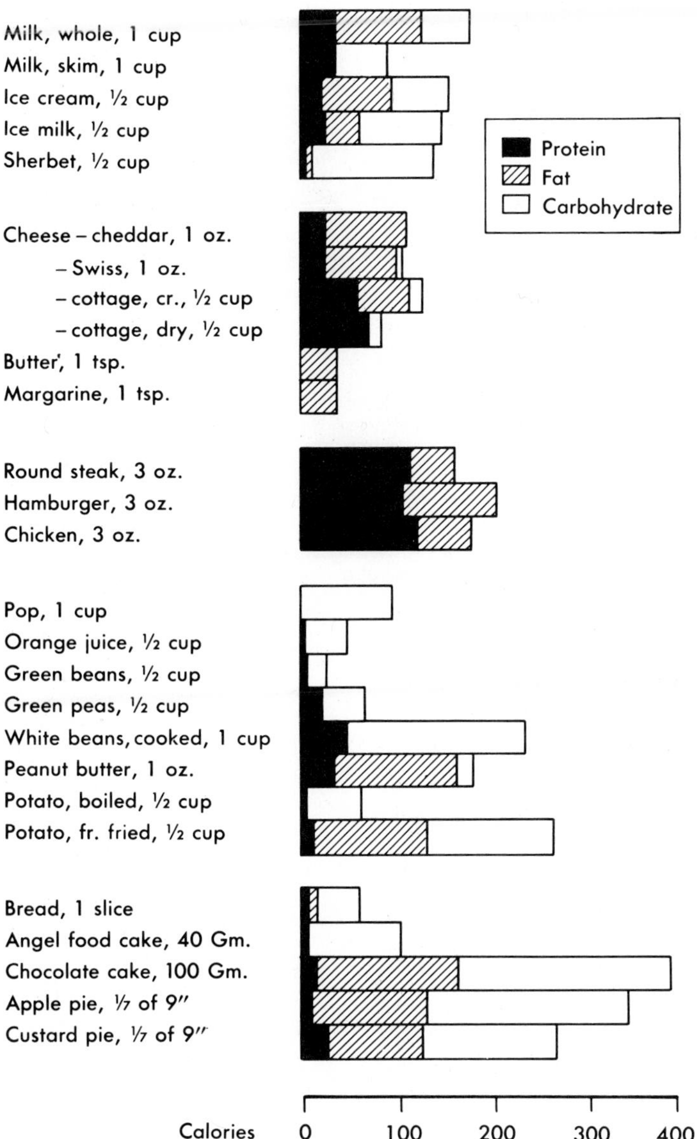

Fig. 53-2. Protein, fat, and carbohydrate concentrations in some common foods, presented as calories contributed by each and total calories in ordinary portions.

come from protein in self-selected diets. Levels above this are rare, since the diet becomes unpalatable and expensive. Provision of 10% of required calories as protein from a variety of foods (animal and plant) is generally sufficient to meet needs for protein of good quality, that is, containing the essential amino acids and sufficient nitrogen for body needs. Some fat in the diet is needed to provide the essential fatty acids and to ensure adequate supplies and efficient absorption of fat-soluble vitamins. Dietary fats are concentrated sources of energy and are useful in providing calories for persons unable to consume large volumes of food. There is a basic requirement for some carbohydrate in the diet as starch and sugar (to prevent ketosis) and as fiber. Most foods are mixtures of protein, fat, and carbohydrate (Fig. 53-2).

It is difficult to separate consideration of calories and protein. The recommended daily dietary allowances (RDA) for protein and the growth curve for the reference woman and man are illustrated in Fig. 53-3. The curves are similar, since protein needs vary with growth and with body size. For both men and women the RDA is 0.8 g/kg of body weight. The average man needs more protein per day than the average woman because of his larger body size. The pregnant woman should be supplied with extra protein for fetal growth. The child's diet should supply more protein per unit of weight than

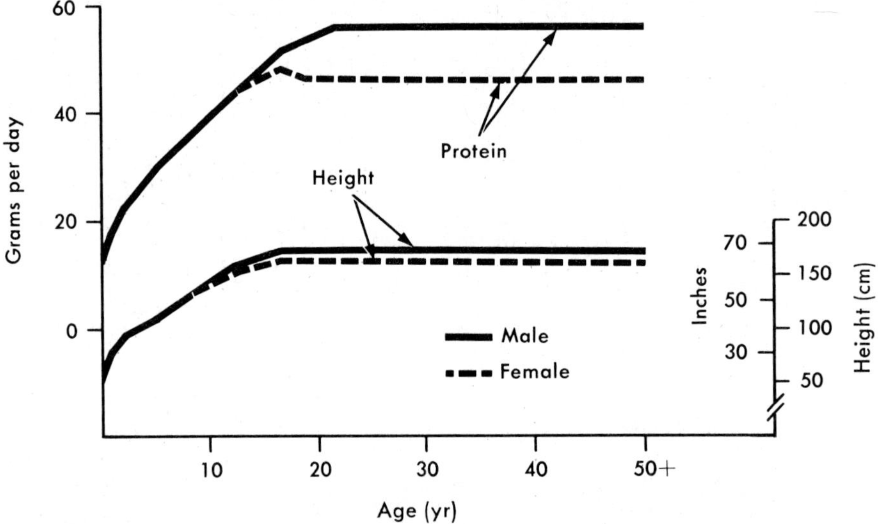

Fig. 53-3. Recommended daily dietary allowances for protein over life cycle.

the adult's diet to allow for growth (see Table 51-2). The recommendations exceed actual protein requirements for most persons. The protein not needed for synthesis is used as energy or converted to body fat. If energy intake is not sufficient to meet needs, protein may be used for fuel rather than for synthesis of new tissue. Schrimshaw has said:

> There is no doubt that good nutrition requires a balanced complement of protein and calories, and neither can be neglected in the diets of the underprivileged and the vulnerable. To the extent that the pendulum swung too far in emphasizing protein in the 1960s, and too far in emphasizing calories in the 1970s, it must come to a more appropriate intermediate position for the 1980s and beyond.[35]

This is true when considering nutritional needs of individuals as well as needs of populations. Severe limitations in protein supply (50% or less RDA) can stunt growth and reduce body protein content. Adequate protein supplies in a diet of insufficient fuel value help set the stage for protein-calorie malnutrition. Generous supplies of protein will not result in increased body protein or muscle mass without exercise or physical activity. Body protein (and body calcium) may be lost despite adequate dietary intake in the absence of physical activity. Early ambulation of patients, bed exercises, and physical therapy may contribute to improved nutritional status.

When there is doubt that the patient is obtaining sufficient food to meet quantitative needs, the nurse should check the patient's selection of foods from the menu and inspect the patient's tray to determine how much food has been eaten. Strategies are then devised with the patient, and the dietitian if necessary, to increase intake. For some patients a combination of food by mouth and by vein may be needed for a time.

Weight control

Obesity is malnutrition due to intake of foods in amounts exceeding body needs. *Underweight* and *emaciation* are malnutrition due to intake of foods in amounts insufficient to meet body needs. Weight control involves evaluation of gross body size and proportions of body fat, lean body mass, and body water in assessing the person's nutritional status. The goal of therapy is to promote optimal gross body size and distribution of weight in proper proportions of muscle, bone, fat, and water throughout the life cycle.

Obesity. Obesity is the most frequently encountered type of malnutrition in the general population. In practice the person's weight is compared with a standard table of weight for height to determine degree of overweight or underweight. Skin-fold measurements give a direct estimate of fat. Therapy goals are then stated in terms of the number of pounds of body weight to be lost. This is an oversimplification. Some persons may be normal in body weight but overfat. Others may be overweight but not overfat because of muscular development. In the first group reduction of body fat but not necessarily of body weight is indicated. Obese children belong in this group, since the goal is to promote normal growth and increase of muscle while reducing the proportion of body fat. In the second group weight is not a problem.

Therapy for the obese person should have three objectives: (1) reduction of the body fat compartment, (2)

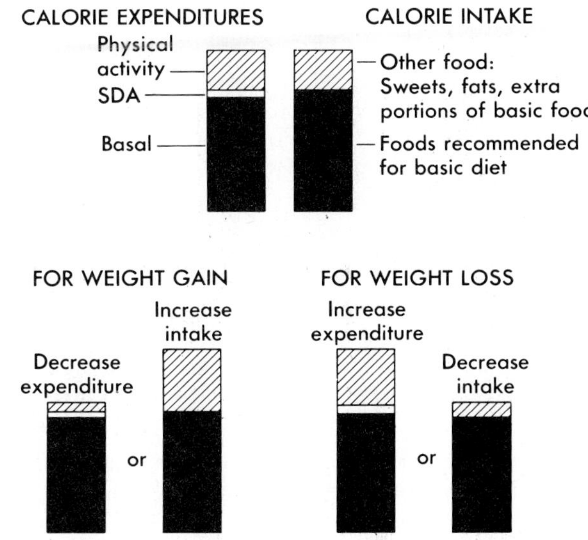

Fig. 53-4. Calorie balance in average adult.

reduction of total body weight when indicated, and (3) maintenance of desirable body size and composition. Far too often both patient and therapist look only at the pounds of weight lost or the rate of loss.[9,42] No differentiation is made as to whether the pounds represent water, muscle, or fat. Very rapid weight loss is satisfying to both patient and therapist, whether the loss is in body fat or water and whether the loss is permanent. Fasting regimens are popular because they induce rapid weight loss in a relatively easy way and are immensely satisfying to "scale watchers." Yet these regimens result in marked protein catabolism with losses of nitrogen, phosphorus, calcium, potassium, sodium, and water and may precipitate undesirable effects such as gout or orthostatic hypotension. The questions remain to be answered about the long-term effect of such losses on the health of the individual.

Weight reduction is not achieved simply by lowering the fuel value of the person's diet. A deficit must be produced between energy expenditure and fuel intake so that body stores of fuel will be mobilized. The deficit may be achieved by increasing energy expenditures or decreasing calorie intake as illustrated in Fig. 53-4. A pound of adipose tissue has an energy potential of 3,500 calories.[47] To lose 1 pound of adipose tissue/week, a calorie deficit of 500 calories/day must be induced. If a person requires only 1,500 calories to maintain his current weight, he should not be expected to lose more than 1 pound of body fat/week when adhering to a 1,000-calorie diet. Weight loss is more rapid when lean body tissue is catabolized, since lean tissue has an energy potential of about 1,850 calories. If a deficit of 500 calories/day were met by catabolizing lean tissue, the rate of loss would be about 2 pounds/week. Dehydration produces very rapid loss. Water has no calorie value per se, but 1 liter of water weighs approximately 1 kg.

Persons consuming high levels of calories prior to weight reduction therapy are likely to be successful in achieving rapid weight loss because the calorie deficit between need and the recommended diet is large. Men have a reputation for being more cooperative than women because they lose weight more rapidly. If both a man and a woman are instructed to adhere to a 1,000-calorie intake, the man should lose at a faster rate. This is not because he is more cooperative, but because his calorie deficit is larger. Although the average woman may need 2,000 calories to maintain weight, the patient may not. It is not inconceivable that a particular person needs only 1,400 calories to maintain excessive body weight. If she is told to consume a 1,500-calorie diet and she cooperates, she will gain weight despite the fact that an average woman on this regimen would be expected to lose weight. This person has a right to be upset or indignant when accused of "cheating" on the diet. (Terms such as "cheating" serve no useful purpose and may lead to silence when communication is essential). In one study, evaluation of food intakes of a large group of obese adults revealed that half of the women maintained obesity with intakes of 1,500 calories or less and half the men with intakes of 2,200 calories or less.* An obese person is not necessarily a glutton. Obesity is not a condition that develops suddenly. Body fat may accumulate slowly over years. A positive calorie balance of 100 calories/day could, in a year's time, result in 10 pounds of adipose tissue. A positive balance of only 10 calories/day could result in 1 pound of adipose tissue in 1 year, or 10 pounds in 10 years. A negative balance of 100 calories/day could result in a loss of 10 pounds in a year's time. Sudden weight changes, gain or loss, should alert the nurse to possible edema, diuresis, or dehydration.

A weight control regimen for women who are sedentary, obese, and edematous might include a restriction in dietary calories, an increase in physicial activity, control of sodium content in the diet, a diuretic, and other drugs. It should also include teaching the principles of good nutrition so that weight loss, when achieved, is maintained. The weight control regimen should be designed to meet the individual's nutritional, physical, and social needs. Many highly publicized dietary regimens for weight loss emphasize rapid loss at the expense of health. As can be seen in Table 51-2, the food guide used for evaluation provides a good pattern for weight control as well as for needed nutrients. Obese individuals have large fuel reserves but not necessarily large reserves of vitamins and minerals.

*From Neville, J.: Unpublished data, 1965.

Weight control for the obese person can be effective in improving health. In a study of overweight persons with uncomplicated hypertension, one group was placed on a weight-reduction program, one group on a weight-reduction program plus antihypertensive drug therapy, and one group received antihypertensive drug therapy but no dietary program. Salt intake was not restricted. The dietary program included individual planning to meet patient concerns and regular visits with the dietitian. The 81 persons who started the diet did not drop out. The majority (73) lost more than 5 kg, and all lost at least 3 kg, although practically none achieved ideal body weight. There was a significant drop in blood pressure in all groups. The authors noted, "Weight control seems to offer an efficient, low-cost means of blood pressure control that is free of side effects and often makes it possible to avoid or to institute a lower dose of medication."[30] Modest salt restriction is recommended by most authorities.[40] Weight control is also beneficial in the prevention and management of diabetes mellitus.[44]

Despite current emphasis in both the popular press and professional journals, weight reduction is not the goal of nutrition care or diet therapy for the obese person. Weight control throughout the life span is the goal. There are times when the physician may decide rapid weight loss is essential to the patient's physical or psychologic well-being. Fasting regimens, of which there are many types, may be used.[1,13] Close medical supervision is important, since risk may be high.[1] Unfortunately many people prescribe fasts or bizarre and unbalanced diet regimens for themselves without realizing the dangers. A balanced low-calorie diet can be useful.[49]

Weight loss. Weight loss and emaciation are major malnutrition problems in the hospitalized population. Weight loss is often the first sign of ill health. Loss may be mild or severe, insignificant or serious. It may be caused by inadequate calorie intake, by problems in digestion or absorption, by abnormalities in metabolism, or by excretion of nutrients before they can be utilized. Sometimes weight loss is a result of failure to increase calorie intake when physical activity is increased. Calorie levels sufficient for inpatient activities may not be enough for outpatient activities. Management will vary depending on the basic cause of weight loss.

Missed meals, blood loss, and anorexia contribute to emaciation in many patients. In every instance, however, the goal is to restore normal body composition, not just weight. A patient will derive no advantage from becoming obese. Restoration of muscle mass occurs slowly. Providing excessive amounts of dietary protein will not hasten this process. Since growth requires energy, calorie intake should exceed calorie expenditures for basal and physical activity. There are strong physiologic arguments for preventing obesity and debilitation rather than waiting to treat it after it occurs. Every child, ill or healthy, should be provided with the essentials for attaining his growth potential. As a result, weight control is a component of the health care program for any patient and includes ensuring that the person knows the principles of weight control and food choice.

Anorexia

Lack of appetite, or anorexia, needs to be differentiated from hunger. *Hunger* is a physiologic state that occurs when the lateral nuclei of the hypothalamus are stimulated. A satiety center in the ventromedial nuclei of the hypothalamus inhibits the hunger center. "Hunger pangs" are sensations experienced in the abdomen from contractions of the empty stomach. The mechanisms that regulate the amount of food eaten and provide for a rhythmic supply of food are not clear, but a number of theories have been postulated.[39] Low serum concentration of glucose and amino acids appear to stimulate hunger. It is also thought that sensory receptors of the mouth, throat, stomach, and intestine may meter the amount of food intake.

Anorexia is a mental state, a desire not to eat, whether hunger is or is not present. It is affected by feelings about the food, either because of present factors such as the appearance of the food or because of past experiences. Offensive sights and smells or unattractive food can decrease the desire to eat. A number of people will not eat food that is new to them or that is not a regular item in their usual dietary pattern. Eating is also related to the development in childhood of love and security, and a desire not to eat may develop when love and security are threatened at a later date. Severe stress may lead either to anorexia or to excessive eating.

A number of other factors may contribute to anorexia. Poor oral hygiene decreases the sense of smell and taste and leads to dryness of the mucous membranes, all of which reduce the desire to eat. Providing good oral hygiene is important, therefore, when trying to encourage a person to eat. Increased blood temperature from hot weather or fever, or the systemic effect of the inflammatory response as seen in acute infectious diseases or allergies contribute to anorexia. Decreased tonus as seen in chronic gastritis, constipation, failure of the detoxifying function of the liver, and distention of abdominal viscera are additional contributing factors to anorexia. Drugs such as the amphetamines may act directly to reduce appetite; other drugs contribute to decreased food intake due to the side effects of nausea and vomiting.

Motivating a person with anorexia to eat can be a challenge. Interventions that can correct the cause will lead to improved appetite. Persons with inadequate nutrition stores need encouragement to eat, although forced feeding may lead to frustration or nausea and vomiting. Determining the person's likes and dislikes, providing an environment conducive to eating (p. 1168), and providing several small meals rather than three large meals a day may facilitate an adequate nutrition intake.

Anorexia nervosa. A severe form of anorexia that leads to emaciation and death is termed anorexia nervosa. One group noted that "an effective therapy for this disorder is crucial, since it is one of the few psychiatric disorders that can result in death."[17] The typical patients are young and female. Diagnostic criteria include age of onset prior to 25 years; anorexia with weight loss of at least 25% of original body weight; a distorted implacable attitude toward food, eating, or weight that overrides hunger; no known medical illness to account for the loss of appetite and weight; and no other known psychiatric disorder. Amenorrhea occurs before dieting in at least 25% of the cases and concurrently with dieting and weight loss in others. Vande Wiele suggests that the condition be named "puberal starvation-amenorrhea" because the cause is in doubt. In the series of patients reported, spontaneous recovery occurred if there were early diagnosis and a policy of benign neglect. As weight loss continued, the patients' perception of body image became more distorted and weight goals became lower. This author suggests that distorted body image may lessen with weight gain and that weight loss is a cause rather than result of distortion. In the series of 42 persons studied, 32 improved, five were unchanged, two deteriorated, and three died.

An initial treatment regimen has been suggested that emphasizes a firm and open approach with high-calorie liquid feedings dispensed as medication by the nursing staff when the specified weight gain is not achieved daily. Once weight gain is achieved so that the threat to life is reduced, the patient is discharged with psychotherapy scheduled if needed.[24] In this approach weight gain is praised but failure to gain is not criticized. Behavior modification without drug therapy has been reported with positive reinforcements by means of granting of privileges tied to weight gain.[17] There is concern that behavior modification may be effective in the management of mild cases only.[6]

Dysphagia

Some patients have a problem with quantity of diet due to interference of difficulty with swallowing *(dysphagia)*. There are essentially three major causes of dysphagia: partial obstruction to the passage of food, paralysis of the muscles involved in swallowing, and inability to initiate and carry out the process of swallowing.

Obstruction to passage of food through the mouth or esophagus may be due to birth defects, trauma, inflammatory disease, or neoplastic disease. The person may not want to swallow because of pain in the mouth or throat. Fluids or semisoft foods are frequently easier for these persons to swallow. If the difficulty is in the mouth, the person may need to use a feeding syringe (asepto syringe with a short rubber tip) to deposit the feeding at the back of the throat.

Paralysis of swallowing may result from disease or trauma of cranial nerves, V, IX, or X; diseases such as poliomyelitis that can affect the swallowing center in the brainstem; and in muscle weakness diseases such as muscular dystrophy or myasthenia gravis. Some function may be present so that swallowing may occur with difficulty. Aspiration of feedings may occur. Assessment consists of eliciting the gag reflex and assessing the patient's ability to swallow by placing 1 to 2 ml of sterile water in the oropharynx and instructing the patient to swallow. A finger can be placed lightly over the larynx in order to identify movement during swallowing. Drooling at the corners of the mouth occurs with facial paralysis as seen in the patient with a cerebrovascular accident (stroke) or with Bell's palsy. If the ability to swallow is absent, the patient must be fed by tube. If partial paralysis is present, oral feeding can be attempted, but the patient must be closely supervised and suction equipment should be available. Soft foods may be easier to swallow than liquids. A feeding syringe may be helpful when facial paralysis is present. If a head-elevated position (the position of choice) is not possible, the patient should be positioned on the unaffected side.

In some situations, such as with upper motor neuron lesions (p. 676), the patient has the ability to swallow but has difficulty initiating and carrying out the function of swallowing. The patient may chew a mouthful for a period of time and then accept a second mouthful, unaware that swallowing has not occurred. Considerable amounts of food can collect between the cheek and gums. This patient needs to be taught how to swallow. Directions must be kept simple and extraneous conversation omitted so that the patient can concentrate on swallowing. He may need to be told to hold his breath when swallowing.

□ Quality of diet

Individuals need energy, nitrogen, essential amino acids, at least 17 mineral elements, and 13 vitamins. Foods are mixtures of these nutrients. No one food provides the full range of nutrients in proper proportions to meet needs. It is important to know whether the patient is consuming a sufficient variety of different foods to provide the full spectrum of nutrients. The system of food grouping (p. 1147) is based on analysis of foods to determine their nutrient concentration. The recommended numbers of servings from different classes of foods are

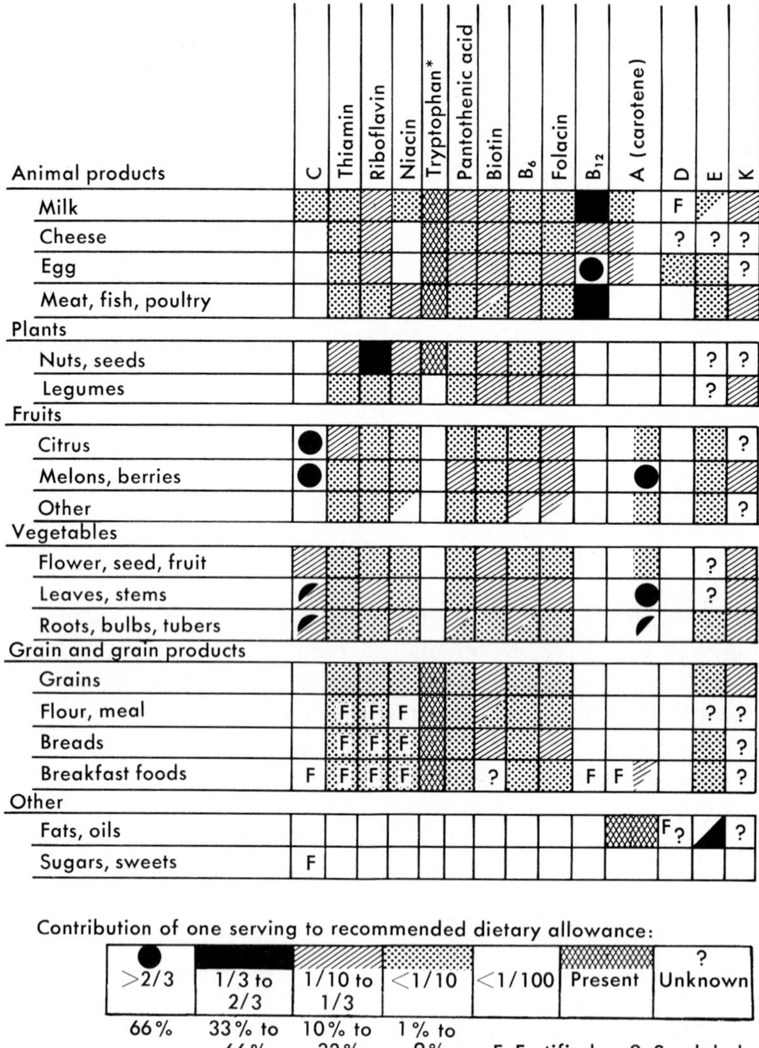

*Tryptophan can be converted to niacin in the body.

Fig. 53-5. Foods as sources of vitamins. Serving size is household portion.

designed to provide the range of nutrients needed in amounts relative to body needs. Persons who eliminate one or more types of food from the diet are likely to have diets of poor quality.

Fig. 53-5 illustrates the vitamin contributions of different types of foods. The standard is rigorous in that one serving (e.g., 240 ml [8 oz] of milk, two eggs, 1/2 cup of fruit) is modest in size and judged against the amount of the vitamin recommended for total intake (RDA, Table 51-1, Fig. 51-1). The food guide suggests two servings of milk or milk products, two servings of protein-rich meats, eggs, nuts or legumes, four servings of fruit and vegetables, and four servings of grain and grain products to make a total of at least 12 servings of food per day as a minimum. To interpret Fig. 53-5, one might judge any food that provides one tenth of the day's recommended vitamin intake as being an important source. Note that for the range of vitamins provided by each food, none provides 10% or more of each of the 13 vitamins. Milk comes closest in that all vitamins are provided. Of plant foods, vegetable leaves and stems are consistent in providing important quantities of many, but not all, vitamins. Milk also provides high-quality protein, significant calcium, and other minerals and is readily available at reasonable cost. It is a basic food in most hospital diets and is recommended in most nutrition education materials for that reason. The green leafy vegetables are superior sources of vitamins A and C and

Table 53-2. Nutrient densities of foods: Calcium and iron contributions of common foods yielding 1,000 calories*

Food	Amount	Calcium (mg)	Iron (mg)
Milk (regular, whole)	190 ml ($6\frac{1}{3}$ cups)	1,814	0.6
Milk (fluid, skim)	340 ml ($11\frac{1}{3}$ cups)	3,362	1.1
Cheese	220 g ($\frac{1}{2}$ lb)	1,701	2.3
Beef (lean, cooked)	450 g (1 lb)	54	15.9
Eggs (large)	12	324	14.4
Almonds	$1\frac{1}{4}$ cups	380	7.6
Kidney beans	$4\frac{2}{3}$ cups	327	20.5
Orange juice	9 cups	243	4.5
Lettuce	14 heads	1,512	37.8
Potatoes	1.35 kg (3 lbs [9 medium])	91	7.2
Bread, (white, enriched)	16 slices, standard	348	9.0
Oatmeal (cooked)	$7\frac{1}{2}$ cups	165	10.5
Honey	1 cup	17	1.7
Margarine	150 g (5 oz)	29	0
Beer	2.4 liters (80 oz [$6\frac{2}{3}$ bottles])	120	trace
Whiskey	450 ml (15 oz)	0	0
Apple pie	$\frac{2}{5}$ of pie	33	1.1
Chocolate cake with icing	$\frac{1}{3}$ of cake	216	3.1
Recommended dietary allowance for 1 day		800	10.0
Man		800	18.0
Woman			

*Based on data from United States Department of Agriculture, Agriculture Research Service: Nutritive value of American foods in common units, Agriculture handbook no. 456, Washington, D.C., 1975, U.S. Government Printing Office.

of iron as well as other minerals, thus complementing milk and improving the nutritional quality of the diet.

The vitamins are not equally distributed in foods. Note in the column for vitamin C in Fig. 53-5 that foods appear to be either rich sources of the vitamin or severely limited. This is also true for vitamin A, B_{12}, and D. Certain fruits or vegetables must be selected to assure adequate intake of vitamins C and A. Animal products contribute vitamins B_{12} and D, although some ready-to-eat breakfast cereals and some soy-milk products may be fortified with these vitamins. Sunshine provides additional vitamin D and our symbiotic relationship with intestinal flora appears to provide biotin and vitamin D. Deficiencies in these nutrients are rare, as are deficiencies in vitamin E. In contrast to vitamin C, thiamin is found in most foods, but no one food is superior in content. When persons substitute sugars and sweets (including honey) or alcohol for other foods, they obtain concentrated sources of energy that yield small levels of vitamins or minerals.

A similar illustration could be presented for many of the minerals, but complete analyses of food for all the mineral elements are not yet available. Table 53-2 illustrates the contributions of calcium and iron of various foods in relation to their energy value. The contributions of calcium from milk and green leafy vegetables are obvious. Calcium and iron are not evenly distributed in foods. Meat, vegetables, breads, and cereals are important contributors.

A warning is needed. This discussion of diet quality and the importance of careful choice in kinds and amounts of food might tempt one to conclude that it is simpler to rely on vitamin and mineral supplements. These drugs, when subjected to the same rigorous examination for the range of nutrients and amounts in relation to people's needs, are no panacea. One popular brand with an advertising campaign directed primarily at women provides three times the level of iron recommended, with none of the other minerals important for hemoglobin formation, and "some" vitamins. Many over-the-counter vitamin preparations provide excess amounts of vitamins relatively inexpensive to produce and minimal quantities of others. It is not an uncommon occurrence for a person to be carefully taking a diet supplement that does not provide the nutrient really needed. The pharmacist can provide information concerning content adequacy of the dosage, and potential toxicity of dietary supplements.[22]

The quality of the diet is most easily judged by determining whether the person is consuming the recommended amounts of the different types of foods. Intervention can be of two different types: (1) working with the person so that he includes the missing items in his intake or (2) finding an acceptable alternate food that provides the missing nutrients.

Protein is widely distributed in foods (Fig. 53-2). When these foods are consumed in quantities sufficient to provide adequate protein, the fats and carbohydrates are also provided to meet minimum needs. Energy needs have already been discussed. The question of the quality of protein remains. As a general rule, proteins of animal origin provide the essential amino acids in appropriate quantities. Plant proteins may be limited in one or more of the essential amino acids, but few persons limit their intake to only one protein source even if they eliminate meat. The quality of dietary protein is a function of the amino acid supply provided by the combination of foods eaten at one feeding. A mixture of plant-animal protein or of plant-plant protein can provide the full range of essential amino acids. The protein status of the patient is more often at risk because total food intake is limited in quantity than because of poor quality of protein. An exception to this is the patient being maintained too long on a clear-liquid diet or intravenous saline or dextrose as the sole source of nourishment. Problems incurred from imbalances of fluid and electrolytes are discussed in Chapter 20.

■ DIET MODIFICATIONS

The modification needed by the person may be simply assistance in changing his usual food intake pattern to the normal pattern recommended for health. It may involve adjustments to meet special dietary problems imposed by disease, trauma, or metabolic abnormalities. For this reason dietary modifications must be considered before determining intervention. Therapeutic diets should not be imposed on the person without good reason. Principles basic to prescribing diets are listed in the box below. A diet prescription is based on the determination of each patient's nutrient needs. When no constraints have been imposed by temporary or permanent alterations in nutritional processes (such as digestion or absorption) or body functioning by illness or trauma, the "normal" ("house") diet is prescribed. This is not considered a "modified diet," since "modified" is used to describe diets different in some way from normal. The nurse will find, however, that meeting the prescription for a "normal" diet does require modification of usual food behavior for persons whose food practices are poor. The diet prescrition may consist of one or many

PRINCIPLES OF THERAPEUTIC DIETS*

In deciding on the dietary management of a disease certain general principles should govern the prescription and formulation of any special diet.

1. The diet should provide all essential nutrients as generously as its special characteristics permit.
2. The special therapeutic regimen should be patterned as much as possible after a normal diet.
3. The special diet should be flexible; it should consider the patient's gustatory habits and preferences, his economic status, and any religious rules that may govern his food intake.
4. A diet should be adapted to the patient's habits with regard to work and exercise.
5. The foods that are included in the special diet must agree with the patient.
6. The diet should emphasize natural, commonly used foods that are readily available and easily prepared at home.
7. A simple and clear explanation of the purpose of the diet and reason for it should be given to the patient and to the members of his family who are responsible for the preparation of his meals.
8. Except for cases where a maintenance diet must be adhered to for life, patients should be taken off special diets as soon as possible. Practically anybody required to follow a therapeutic diet feels conspicuous and set apart; this is especially important in the case of young children, who are more impressionable and for whom a prolonged special diet may be the making of an emotional problem.
9. The diet must be absolutely justified and defensible. Hospitals, patients, and patients' families alike will benefit if the number of speical diets is reduced to those that are really necessary.
10. Feeding by mouth is always the method of choice; only when the patient is incapable or will not eat and drink enough should tube feeding or, if this is contraindicated, parenteral feeding be resorted to.

*From Human nutrition, ed. 3, by Benjamin and Burton. Copyright © 1976, McGraw-Hill Book Co. Used with permission of McGraw-Hill Book Co.

modifications to be followed for varying lengths of time—from 1 day to a lifetime. The person with chronic disease is often faced with the necessity for permanent changes in food habits. In some instances dietary modification does not necessitate change in food behavior, since the person's usual diet actually meets the prescribed modification. A brief discussion of diet modifications and possible applications is included here to illustrate the scope of diet therapy. Consult this text and suggested reading lists for details.

Protein may be increased to levels twice those usually recommended for persons with protein losses from tissue catabolism, bleeding, and exudates. On the other hand, protein may be decreased to levels one-half to one-third those recommended. In chronic renal failure, diet management involves providing sufficient protein to prevent tissue protein catabolism and yet avoid accumulations of urea. In hepatic coma, dietary protein is adjusted to individual tolerance. In some instances control of the amino acid content of the diet may be required. The child with phenylketonuria needs the same nutrients for growth as the healthy child. His diet must be modified, however, because he cannot convert phenylalanine to tyrosine and subsequent normal metabolites. The diet should provide sufficient phenylalanine for growth but not enough to raise serum levels to those causing central nervous system damage. Phenylalanine cannot be eliminated from the diet as it is an essential amino acid. Tyrosine becomes an essential amino acid for this child as his body cannot covert phenylalanine to tyrosine as normal children do. Specific proteins may be eliminated with gluten-induced enteropathy or allergies.

Fat modifications include increasing or decreasing total fat intake, altering the proportion of dietary calories obtained from fat, and altering the fatty acid composition of the diet. Total fat may be increased to provide essential calories in a concentrated form. Total fat may be decreased for patients with gallbladder disease to reduce pain and contraction of the gallbladder. Alterations in the proportion of dietary calories from fat may be used for patients with primary or secondary disorders of lipid metabolism or to induce ketosis. The prescription should specify the proportions desired for the patient: 10% to 15% of total calories ("low"); 25% to 30% of total calories ("moderate"); 40% to 45% of total calories ("usual"); 60% to 80% of total calories ("ketogenic"). Modifications may also be made in the kind of fat in the diet: short-chain, medium-chain, or long-chain triglycerides or saturated, monounsaturated, and polyunsaturated fatty acids. Modifications in chain length may be prescribed for patients with disorders of digestion and absorption. Modifications in saturated and unsaturated fatty acids may be prescribed to alter serum lipid levels.

Carbohydrate modifications include increasing or decreasing total carbohydrate intake altering the proportion of dietary calories obtained from carbohydrate, controlling the type of carbohydrate, and eliminating or reducing specific carbohydrate components. The dietary prescription for a patient with diabetes mellitus might include a decrease in total carbohydrates, a change in the ratio of simple to complex carbohydrates, and substitution of carbohydrate derivatives such as hexitols or dextrins for sucrose. Lactose may be eliminated from the diet of patients with lactase insufficiency and sucrose from the diet of patients with invertase insufficiency. Fructose and sucrose are excluded from the diet of persons with hereditary fructose intolerance and galactose and lactose from the diet of patients with galactosemia.

Modifications in *vitamin* concentrations are generally limited to increasing dosage or providing the vitamin in an alternate form to enhance absorption or utilization. Medicinal sources are frequently used. A diet low in vitamin A and carotene is prescribed for patients with vitamin A toxicity.

Often the *mineral* content of a diet must be controlled. Sodium restriction is one of the most common dietary modifications prescribed and is frequently combined with modifications in calories, sources of carbohydrate, and other minerals. Persons with hypertension, fluid retention, or kidney disease are usually expected to control the amount of sodium they eat. The term "control" is used here deliberately, since the goal is to balance sodium intake with sodium need, with the body's ability to handle sodium, and with the physiologic effects of drugs or medications. The level of sodium recommended may vary from 250 mg to 2 g or more per day. Elimination of sodium from the diet can precipitate dehydration.

Potassium levels may be specified for patients with kidney disease and for those with disorders of electrolyte imbalance. *Other mineral* modifications include diets low or high in calcium and diets low in copper. Medicinal sources of minerals are frequently prescribed.

Liquid (clear and full), *purêed*, and *soft* diets represent modifications in consistency. They may be used when the patient has difficulties in chewing or swallowing or when the patient has lesions of the gastrointestinal tract. They may be used serially for the postoperative patient. Modifications in fiber or residue content of the diet are often prescribed.

Meal size amd *frequency* may be modified for treatment of appetite disorders, diabetes mellitus, dumping syndrome, hypoglycemia, peptic ulcer, and other disorders. Modifications in the *method of feeding* include tube feeding, parenteral or intravenous infusions, and sterile food service.[44]

In some cases the prescription may specify *elimination of specific foods* or beverages from the diet. This approach is used in food allergy. Food elimination may lead to rather bizarre and unusual dietary patterns that should be checked closely for adequacy. Sometimes the diet order specifies foods thay may be served to the patient. This is usually a list of bland items such as gelatin, soft-cooked egg, farina, and mashed potato. The nurse may alleviate patient distress and boredom by asking the physician to change the order to "diet as tolerated."

Any diet modification, when imposed, should be justified. Theories of the appropriate nutritional therapy in some diseases vary depending on the interpretation of indirect evidence. Carefully controlled studies are needed to determine the efficacy of modifications, including some that have been used for years (such as the elimination of "gas-forming" or strong-flavored foods). At times it appears as though folklore rather than scientific method fathered some diet and food restrictions. In recent years there has been a trend toward liberal interpretation of dietary therapy. This has been due in part to a recognition that many restrictions were without basis in fact and that life lived according to these restrictions was so onerous that emotional well-being was lost without a compensating increase in physical well-being.

Various drugs and medications that a person is taking may affect body functions in such a way that diet modification is needed. The obvious illustration of this phenomenon is the treatment regimen for persons with diabetes mellitus: diet, exercise, insulin activity, and hypoglycemic drugs. Moderate to severe elevations in blood pressure may be experienced by patients taking monoamine oxidase inhibitors when they consume large quantities of foods such as aged cheedar cheese, herring, or wines. These foods are rich in tyramine, and metabolism of tyramine is dependent on monoamine oxidase. Some persons receiving penicillamine therapy may experience a subjective loss of taste for salt and sweet. The diarrhea commonly associated with high-dosage neomycin therapy reflects an induced malabsorption syndrome. Some persons being maintained on barbiturates or anticonvulsants may develop folic acid deficiency, and some taking large doses of isoniazid may show signs of vitamin B_6 deficiency. Thiazide diuretic therapy may deplete cellular potassium. Some medications or products may yield so much sodium as to negate any benefit from a sodium-controlled diet; some products contain lactose as a filler. Since new and more powerful drugs are constantly being developed, this list is certain to grow. A diet prescription must be translated into a diet plan or food pattern that will meet the person's physical needs and yet provide enough flexibility that the patient will enjoy his food. If a modification is required for only a short time, it may not be difficult to plan. However, if the modification is one to be followed at home after discharge from the hospital, such things as cost, availability, ease of preparation, and relationship to family food requirements must be taken into account.

An unwritten but essential part of each diet order is that the diet should provide all nutrients as generously as its special characteristics permit. If the modification is so restrictive that the food plan will not provide adequate supplies, the physician should be notified so that appropriate adjustments in diet or medication can be made. Clear-liquid diets, for example, supply important fluids, some calories, and some sodium and chloride, but they have little other nutrient value. When milk must be eliminated from the diet, it is necessary to identify and eliminate all food items containing milk and replace the calcium, phosphorus, riboflavin, and protein value of milk by incorporating other foods into the food plan. Alterations in the diet—changes in the proportions of calories from protein, fat, and carbohydrate—may in themselves change nutrient requirements. For example, increased polyunsaturated fat should be accompanied by increased dietary levels of vitamin E and increased protein accompanied by increased vitamin B_6. This is accomplished by including foods rich in the desired components in the patient's diet. For example, the polyunsaturated fat may be provided by corn oil or safflower oil which contain both the desired fat and vitamin E.

Vigorous therapeutic measures aimed at treating one condition may precipitate others when care is disease focused. For example, the traditional regimen for peptic ulcer emphasized maintaining the patient on a diet of milk, cream, and foods high in calories and fat for months or years. Gain in weight and particularly in body fat was not unusual. Ulcers are most prevalent in middle-aged men, the group most at risk from coronary artery disease.

Foods contain a variety of nutrients in varying proportions. The diet plan should guide selection of the kinds of foods in the amounts dictated by the diet prescription. Calorie, protein, fat, and carbohydrate concentrations of some common foods are shown in Fig. 53-2. Notice how many of the foods contain protein. Intake of all these foods would have to be limited if protein is restricted. Calorie needs would have to be supplied by foods consisting primarily of carbohydrate or fat.

Some dietary prescriptions can be met only be using different or unusual food items such as casein hydrolysate (low in phenylalanine or starches) made from wheat or corn or other plant sources. These cannot be handled in the same way as the foods they replace. New techniques and recipes must be developed. The final products differ in appearance, texture, and taste from those they replace. Patients whose diets require such products should have help in learning how to cook the products and use them in the diet. Since information about staple food items is the best available, food plans for diet modifications tend to emphasize staple foods and do not include many new and convenient items on the food market.

Interest in dietary fiber has been renewed,[41] although there is disagreement regarding the definition of fiber, conflicting data about the values of high- and low-fiber diets, and disagreements as to the relative merits of fiber from grains, vegetables, and fruits. Bran may be prescribed as an adjunct to diet together with increased use of foods containing complex carbohydrate. Sufficient fiber in the diet has been recommended for many years for proper elimination of waste products.

■ DIETARY COUNSELING

□ Assessment

The dietary history of a person serves as a useful screening device. The adequacy of the diet in terms of quality and quantity can be quickly estimated by comparing it with recommended patterns of food intake. It may also provide information about unusual or bizarre uses of food, which in turn may be a key factor in the health problem. Examples are hypokalemia associated with excessive intake of licorice or cathartics and fever associated with consumption of a gallon of coffee. These imbalances are rare. Identification of factors affecting nutrition status (such as faulty dietary habits, inadequate intake, poor absorption, decreased utilization, increased excretion, increased destruction, increased requirements) permits designing an effective treatment program. Treatment may require dietary modifications, medications, and changes in living patterns.

□ Planning

The goals for dietary counseling are determined by the results of the nutritional assessment (see Chapter 51) and the diet prescribed while the patient is hospitalized or to be followed at home.

The definition of "good" food is very personal and is a product of all the experiences associated with food over a lifetime. The major challenge in diet therapy can be summarized as providing "good" food for the person within the limits imposed by his health and nutrient needs. One basic principle of learning is that an individual learns by building on what he already knows. The individual knows what he is eating now, and he is much more likely to learn when he is taught how to make changes in his current pattern to meet the diet prescription. Too often a diet is imposed on the individual as though he had no previous experience with food. Instructions for diet modifications should begin with the person's current food habits and should stress the necessary changes to be made.

The person's history of usual food intake is compared with the appropriate guide for food choice (basic food pattern or therapeutic regimen as described in the diet manuals or nutrition texts). The patient's food consumption in the hospital is observed. Good food practices that should be continued, practices that are neither particularly valuable nor harmful, and practices that need to be changed are identified. Treatment and medications are checked to determine if these affect appetite, nutrient need, meal composition, or frequency. It is determined whether the diet to be followed at home is the same as or different from the current diet.

The special services the person requires need to be coordinated so that schedule conflicts are avoided. For example, some laboratory studies require that the patient fast; others require that he eat a special type of test meal. Coordination of laboratory, dietary, and nursing care schedules in such situations is essential to the accuracy of the results and to the patient's comfort. Quite often the need for consultation can be identified by the nurse early in the patient's hospital stay. The consultation can then be scheduled and provided before the day of discharge. The so-called discharge diet instruction is often omitted or rendered useless because it is left until the last minute when the patient's major interest is to get home as quickly as possible.

□ Intervention

The nurse serves as an interpreter to the patient by providing brief and easily understood explanations about his diet, any modifications in it, and the food selections on his tray. The nurse also serves as an interpreter by providing pertinent information about the patient to the physician, dietitian, or food service unit so that the diet prescription or food on the tray provides not only nutrients but also conforms insofar as possible to ethnic, religious, or personal preferences and provides eating pleasure.

One goal of patient education is to provide information so that the person can make informed choices. The final goal, however, is a change in behavior related to food so that the person is well nourished. Even small changes in food behavior can benefit the person. An obese person who reduces caloric intake from 3,000 to 2,500 calories per day has made a significant behavior change, although one cannot credit him with complying to a dietary prescription of 1,000 calories. The person with inadequate calcium intake may be willing to use milk instead of cream substitutes in coffee. The final goal of dietary adherence is more obtainable when changes are taken in small steps, one at a time. In part this is because the goal is realistic and progress can be measured. In addition the patient has been involved in setting the goals, and the patient, not the nurse, is the one who must implement the goal.

This approach to patient teaching is more efficient for the therapist and less frustrating for the patient. It is irritating to be lectured on the importance of including milk in the diet when milk and cheese are favorite foods. It can be boring to listen to a description of the evils of salt and calories in potato chips or french-fried potatoes when one never eats them. A patient can say, "Yes, I understand" aloud and in many instances truly understand but not accept the recommendations. Consideration must be given to social, cultural, and economic factors as well as to the person's knowledge of and beliefs about nutrition.

The convention of three meals a day is just that—a convention and a convenience. For many it is a fiction. Most people eat more often, while the economically deprived may eat only once a day. There may be some advantage to eating smaller meals at shorter intervals as long as total nutrient needs are met. Although physiologic evidence does not support a rigid pattern of three feedings a day, there is evidence that omitting breakfast impairs physiologic and mental efficiency. Except in special circumstances (insulin-dependent diabetes, for example), the number of feedings a day can be determined by the person's desires and life style. If no breakfast is eaten, however, consumption of some food at the beginning of the day should be considered as a desirable goal. Since breakfast is generally the meal most enjoyed by hospitalized patients, this can be a useful mechanism for initiating breakfast as a meal at home as well. Each feeding, whether called a meal or snack, should include a mixture of nutrients.

Food costs

Cost is an important factor in family food patterns.[33] The nurse, when attempting to teach a person about diet, is frequently challenged about food cost. Vague generalities such as "use cheaper cuts of meat" are not particularly helpful. Suggestions should be specific, based on the person's diet and income. They should provide enough information to serve as a basis of action. The price of an envelope of flavored sugar used by many low-income families to make a beverage is equivalent to the price of enough dried skim milk solids for 1 liter of milk. Which is the better buy? Where and how can a person get food stamps? The nurse with personal experience in managing food budgets, purchasing, cookery, and so forth, is in a position to offer practical advice. There are many useful materials available on food purchasing, storage, and preparation. The dietitian will be able to help select the materials that are best for the patient.

In most cases, money spent for food can be reduced and the nutritive value of the diet improved by (1) planning the menu at home, (2) listing kinds and amounts of food to be bought, (3) purchasing items on this list, and (4) controlling waste due to preparing more food than is needed or due to foods spoiling before use.

Food labeling

Food labels can be used as a basis for food choice. Currently many changes are being made in food-labeling practices and regulations governing the use of certain terms describing foods. These changes are designed to improve the nutrition information given on food labels and to provide meaningful information to the public. The nutrition-labeling program is voluntary for most foods; however, if a nutrient is added to any product or if a nutritional claim is made either on the label or in advertising, the product label must have full nutrition labeling. On food labels the levels of vitamins and minerals will be listed as a percentage of the US-RDA. To meet the regulations the label must include size of serving, number of servings per container, calories, protein, carbohydrate, fat, and the percentage of the US-RDA for vitamin A, vitamin C, thiamin, riboflavin, niacin, calcium, and iron. Another 12 vitamins and minerals may be listed at the option of the food producer. The US-RDA is based on the standard RDA but is condensed to four categories: infants, children under 4 years of age, adults and children over 4 years of age, and pregnant or lactating women. Consumer memos describing the regulations are available from the Food and Drug Administration. The regulation allows for a statement on the label of cholesterol, total fat, and polyunsaturated and saturated fat. This is helpful for persons on fat-modified diets.

The data in Table 53-3 were taken directly from food labels. One advantage to the system is that information on the label is based on the analysis of the specific brand so that differences in an item such as tuna packed by several different companies can be identified by comparing the labels. The labeling system may be changed, but the concept of nutrition labeling has apparently been accepted. The advantages to persons attempting to control energy intake or modifying protein, fat, or carbohydrate intake are obvious. For those concerned with cost, the attraction of getting more nutritional value for the money may provide motivation for reading labels.

Nutrition labeling does not include the listing of the ingredients. Lists of ingredients are not required on foods covered by "standards of identity" such as mayonnaise, ice cream, or peanut butter. Current regulations require that ingredients be listed in descending order by weight. This does help, although general terms such as "spices," "vegetable oil," or "starch" offer insufficient information for someone who must avoid a particular spice or choose food high in polyunsaturated fat.

Many new products are specifically designed by intent and advertising to replace staple items. Several breakfast drinks are being marketed that look and taste

Table 53-3. Nutrition label as a guide for choosing food

	Tuna packed in oil	Chocolate bar	Skim milk	Gelatin dessert
Serving	3¼ oz	1½ oz	1 cup	½ cup
Servings per container	2	1	4	4
Required				
Calories	230	230	90	80
Protein (g)	22.5	3	8	2†
Fat (g)	15	4	1	0
Carbohydrate (g)	0.5	12	11	18
US-RDA	%	%	%	%
Required listing				
Protein	100	4	20	*
Vitamin A	*	*	10	*
Vitamin C	*	*	4	*
Thiamin	2	2	6	*
Riboflavin	8	6	25	*
Niacin	120	*	*	*
Calcium	*	8	30	*
Iron	8	2	*	*
Optional listing				
Vitamin D			25	
Vitamin B_6	25		4	
Vitamin B_{12}	45		15	
Vitamin E	10			
Pantothenic acid			6	
Phosphorus			20	
Magnesium			8	
Zinc			4	

*Contains less than 2% of the U.S. Recommended Daily Allowances.
†Not a significant source of protein.

like orange juice and that have been enriched with ascorbic acid so that they may have as much or more ascorbic acid as orange juice. But these breakfast drinks are high in sodium and low in potassium, whereas orange juice is low in sodium and high in potassium. A wide variety of substitutes for coffee cream, sour cream, and whipped cream are on the market. They are convenient to use, easy to store, and acceptable in flavor to most people. Can they be used by persons on restricted diets? Many of these products are made from coconut oil, which is a highly saturated fat. Such products cannot be recommended as a source of polyunsaturated fat. They are excellent calorie sources, however.

Notice the difference in protein, fat, and carbohydrate in ice cream, ice milk, and sherbet in Fig. 53-2. The fat of ice cream is butterfat; that of ice milk is vegetable fat; sherbet is essentially fat free. All contain sucrose. "Diabetic" ice creams substitute other carbohydrates for sucrose and usually have a high-fat level to provide good texture. As a result the calorie content of "diabetic" ice creams is often higher than that of conventional ice cream.

Food additives

The public has become more interested in food and nutrition. The consumer movement has, among other things, focused attention on food processing and food additives.[8,16,21,28] Additives may be foods, derived from foods, or products created in the laboratory. The most widely used food additive is sucrose, ordinary table sugar. Sodium chloride, table salt, is the second. Monosodium glutamate, mustard, and black pepper are food additives used in large quantities also. Most of the current concern about food additives relates to safety. Excessive intake of sugar has been related to obesity, tooth decay, and coronary artery disease; excessive intake of salt has been related to hypertension. Questions have been raised about the safety of nonnutritive sweeteners, nitrates used in curing meats, and antioxidants such as BHT used to keep fat from becoming rancid. The food industry's use of additives is regulated by the Food and Drug Administration. In 1958 the food additives amendment to the Food, Drug, and Cosmetic Act of 1938 was passed; it requires proof of safety before a substance may be added to food. In 1960 the color additive amendment was enacted to control all color additives, natural and synthetic.

Generally recognized as safe (GRAS) substances have been classified by technical effect, and each group is being reviewed for use and safety. One such group is Technical Effect Code 16, leavening agents that include yeast and baking powder. The review for each group will be published as completed.

Concern with pesticide residues (as well as food additives) has caused some people to turn to a "natural" or "organic" diet. Some believe that the body can use only nutrients from a natural source despite evidence to the contrary. Others want food that has been grown without the use of chemical fertilizers or pesticides and processed without additives. Foods labeled "organic" or "natural" usually cost more. The terms are not defined by law, and values are being claimed for products without evidence to support them. Current concern with food additives and pesticides has obscured other issues of food safety. It is just as important to be sure that food is free of microbiologic and insect contamination. Foods themselves contain natural substances that can be harmful. Legislation cannot protect the individual from poor food choices nor ensure good food handling practices in the home.[4]

Dental care

Poor dental hygiene influences the adequacy of nutritional intake. Nutrition, on the other hand, affects the growth and quality of the teeth. Nutrients supply the calcium, protein, and vitamin D needed for growth of teeth. Fluorides help to prevent dental caries. One of the most effective means of altering plaque formation and the development of dental caries is the restriction in frequency and amount of sucrose intake. Lactic acid is produced by the action of bacteria on the sugars and can be destructive to tooth enamel within a very short time.

Teaching about care of the teeth is an important part of health education. In addition any misconceptions should be clarified. For example, there is no evidence that any general systemic disease is caused by decayed teeth. There is no evidence that calcium is removed from the mother's teeth during pregnancy and lactation regardless of how deficient in calcium her diet may be. There is, however, abundant evidence that a diet adequate in calcium, phosphorus, and other essential elements during pregnancy contributes to good tooth formation in the growing fetus and that a diet rich in these substances is essential during the years of life when the permanent teeth are being formed. Calcium is deposited in the buds of the permanent teeth almost immediately after birth. A high-calcium diet after teeth have erupted probably has no effect on their preservation.

Bacterial plaque is a soft, white mucoid material derived from the breakdown of saliva. Toxin-producing bacteria thrive in its matrix. Their enzymes and other products accumulate within the sulcus (crevice between the gingiva and the crown), causing inflammation and bleeding. Plaque that remains on the teeth for longer than 24 hours begins to mineralize or calcify, forming a hard, tenacious deposit known as calculus (tartar). Calculus has a consistency similar to sandpaper and causes abrasions and ulceration of the internal sulcus. It also has toxin-producing action.

Although plaque can be removed from the teeth by a procedure known as scaling, the most effective means of controlling its formation is by brushing the teeth. The nurse is frequently asked about the kind of tooth brush to use and about general care of the teeth. The points to be emphasized are the use of a proper toothbrush and the correct method and time of brushing.

There is general agreement among dental authorities that *toothbrushes* should be small enough to reach all tooth surfaces. Usually two or three rows of bristles are recommended, depending on how much space exists between the cheek and the outer tooth surface. Bristles should be soft and cut straight across the brushing surface. Soft bristles conform to the tooth surface by bending or flexing and cleanse more effectively. A dentifrice together with the soft, multitufted bristled brush forms a "matte effect," thereby increasing the amount of friction and the cleansing effect. While nylon bristles are durable, natural bristles are preferred because they are less abrasive. Toothbrushes should dry thoroughly between use to help keep the bristles firm and to prevent bacterial growth. Two brushes may be necessary (particularly if bristles are natural) and should be used alternately. The electric-powered toothbrush is easy to use and safe to operate. Its use may encourage children to brush their teeth more often and may help incapacitated person to clean their teeth more thoroughly. The individual, detachable brushes make it convenient for use in a family or hospital unit.

Dentifrices containing stannous fluoride help to prevent caries, and their value has been officially recognized by the American Dental Association. Other dentifrices simply make brushing the teeth more pleasant. It is estimated that the American public pays approximately $80 million each year for mouthwashes and cleansing agents for their teeth, whereas sodium bicarbonate and salt flavored with peppermint would cost only a fraction of that amount. Ammoniated dentifrices and those containing chlorophyll have been subject to much inquiry, but their benefits have not been proved.

Brushing the teeth should remove debris from between the teeth, stimulate the gums, and yet not traumatize the delicate gingival papillae between the teeth. Many people brush their teeth by passing the bristles quickly across the lateral surfaces of the teeth. This method damages the enamel, does not clean between the teeth, and may injure the gums. The brush should be placed along the gum line with the bristles toward the roots of the teeth. The bristles should then be brought down over the gum and teeth with a gentle sweep, using a downward and upward motion (Fig. 53-6). Although using a longer stroke is easier for the patient, it has a higher potential for traumatizing the gingiva or abrading tooth structure. Also, long strokes will generally pass over irregularly aligned teeth without cleansing adequately. Short strokes, on the other hand, may be more difficult for some patients to perform, since they require fine movements and coordination. They are more efficient in the cleansing process because the bristles bend or flex into malaligned or depressed areas. Crosswise motion should be reserved for the top grinding surfaces of the back teeth.

Some dentists recommend a slight vibrating motion over the gums with the brush for further stimulation before each downward and upward sweep of the brush, whereas others recommend massage of the gums following brushing. Massage is accomplished by gently rubbing of the gums with a finger, using very gentle pressure toward the biting surfaces of the teeth. Gum surfaces may be massaged for a few minutes two or three times a day.

A toothbrush will cleanse most surfaces of the teeth adequately except the proximal surface (near the gum line). For cleaning this area dentists suggest the use of rubber tips, floss, and water irrigation. The rubber tip not only removes plaque from the proximal surface of the teeth but also massages as it cleans. It should be used in every interdental space where there is room for it and inserted as far into the space as it will go without force. As the tip rests on the interdental tissue, the tip should be activated in a gentle rotary motion so it rubs against the gingiva and proximal surfaces of the teeth.

Dental floss is a useful adjunct for cleaning plaque from interdental spaces. Not matter how well instructed, when patients first use floss they tend to injure the gingiva as they pass the floss through tight contact areas. The tooth surface is cleansed by gently forcing the floss between the teeth with pressure exerted toward the side of the tooth and by moving the floss up and down the tooth surface for several seconds (Fig. 53-7). Water

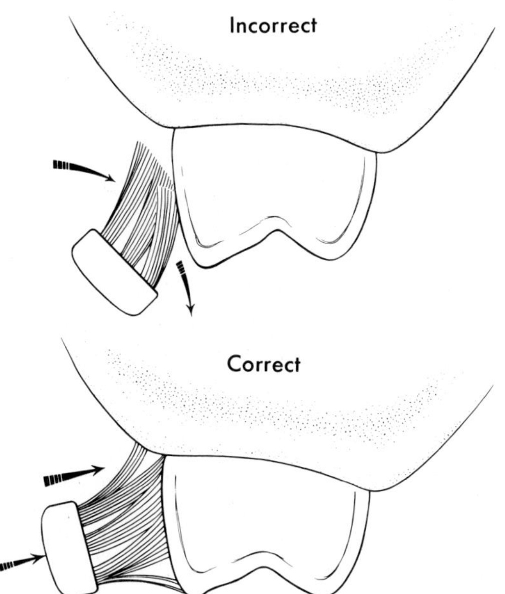

Fig. 53-6. Brushing teeth. Application of brush so that bristle ends slide gently under margin of gingiva.

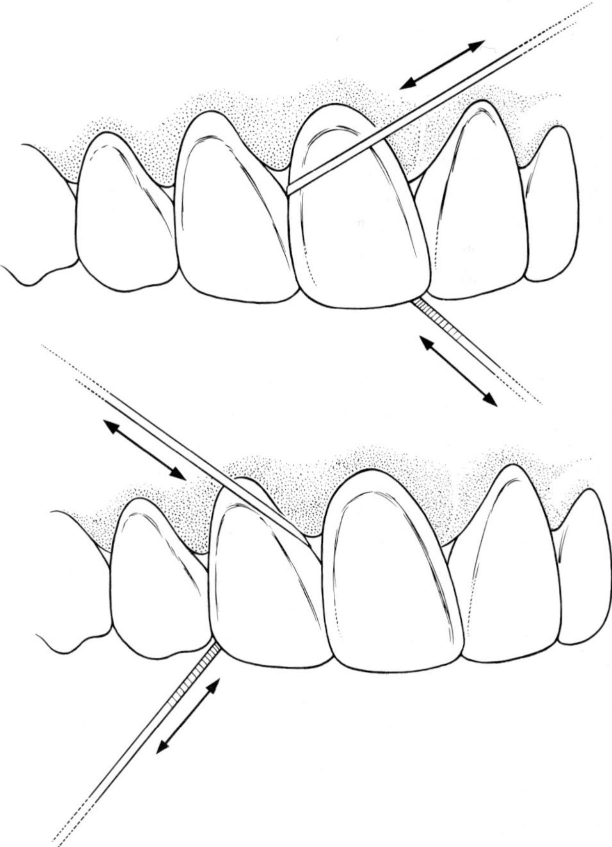

Fig. 53-7. Flossing. Proper placement of floss for effective interproximal cleaning.

irrigation by means of the Water Pik is a useful and recommended aid. It acts by flushing away the plaque, food, and debris that has been loosened by the brush, rubber tip, or floss.

Disclosants (vegetable dyes) are important for effective plaque removal, as teaching aids in the dentist's office, and for the person at home. They can be used before brushing to alert the person to the hard-to-clean areas. After brushing they act as a test of the effectiveness of the technique used. It is suggested that petroleum jelly be applied to the lips and gingiva prior to application of the disclosant to avoid staining of these areas.

Mouthwashes do not significantly inhibit bacterial growth in the mouth. They should not be used in an effort to treat an oral infection because they may be irritating to an infected mouth, and if used excessively they may be harmful to natural bacterial flora in the mouth. For the most part, however, they are harmless and are acceptable additions to oral hygiene if desired by the person and if he can afford them. Most dentists suggest warm water and salt to rinse the mouth if occasional bleeding of the gums occurs. Sodium perborate may be irritating to gum tissues and should not be used without special medical or dental instruction.

When a child has erupted teeth, it is important for the parent to begin brushing the child's teeth, using a small, soft brush. This practice not only provides for effective oral hygiene of the primary teeth but also begins teaching the child good oral hygiene practices. The child should be taken to the dentist at the age of 3 years, or perhaps earlier, and every 6 months thereafter.

■ ENTERAL AND PARENTERAL NUTRITION

Oral feeding is the method of choice; however, when patients cannot take food by mouth, alternative methods are employed. The time period may be short or long. The same considerations governing oral nourishment apply to nourishment by tube or vein. Are all of the nutrients being supplied? For short-term care, patient stores may provide missing nutrients. For long-term care or for persons without stores (infants, debilitated persons), adequacy of all nutrients should be checked, or deficiencies may occur.[29] Providing sufficient calories without unfavorable reactions may present a problem.

□ Tube feeding (gavage)

The type of feeding and route are usually determined by the physician. Nasogastric tubes may be used for short-term feeding. For long-term feeding a new opening (gastrostomy) may be made in the stomach (p. 1199). The nasogastric tube is left in place for adults and older children, but for infants it usually is passed and removed for each feeding (see p. 1164 for the technique of passing the tube).

No feeding should be introduced into a nasogastric tube until it has been ascertained that the tube is in the stomach. The most accurate method is aspiration of gastric contents. A *left* side-lying position facilitates aspiration of gastric contents as the tip of the tube will move toward the greater curvature of the stomach. If gastric contents are aspirated, they are returned to the stomach to prevent loss of electrolytes. Some physicians request that the tube feeding not be given if a specified large amount of gastric contents are aspirated. Alternative methods of checking the placement of the tube are (1) inserting approximately 5 ml of air in the tube and listening with a stethoscope over the left upper abdominal quadrant for the sound of air entering the stomach, (2) placing the end of the tube in water and observing a continual rhythmic flow of air bubbles indicating that the tip of the tube is in the upper air passages rather than the stomach, or (3) injecting 1 to 2 ml of sterile water into the tube and observing a forceful cough resulting from fluid in the upper respiratory tract.

A sitting position is best for the patient receiving a tube feeding. If this is not possible a *right* side-lying position facilitates movement of the fluid to the distal portion of the stomach and permits easier filling of the stomach.

The feeding should be nutritionally adequate, well tolerated (no vomiting, diarrhea, constipation, or distention), easily prepared, and reasonable in cost.[14,15] The tube feeding should be handled carefully with attention to sanitation. It is kept refrigerated until ready to use and may be given either at room temperature or cold depending on patient tolerance and preference.

The tube feedings used in an institution are usually described in the hospital diet manual. Three types of formulas are common: blended formulas, milk-based formulas, and elemental-diet formulas. *Blended* formulas are foods (baby food, ordinary foods from a normal diet) liquified with a high-speed blender. The formulas are similar to the usual adult diet and are generally well-tolerated and relatively inexpensive. *Milk-based* formulas may be mixtures of egg, milk, and sugar with skim milk powder and protein hydrolysates. Recipes for formulas to be made in the hospital or at home are available. Diarrhea may result from the high content of simple sugars such as lactose. *Elemental-diet* formulas are synthetic low-residue mixtures of amino acids, sugars, vitamins, and minerals that may be given orally or by the tube. They are expensive and require careful monitoring of blood glucose and electrolytes. Commercial formulas are available for tube feedings and are convenient although more costly.

The proportions of protein, carbohydrate, and fat

should approximate that of the normal diet. High-protein tube feedings have been associated with severe effects.[12] The concentration is important and is usually adjusted to about 1 kcal/ml. If the patient is very young, elderly, or severely debilitated the initial feeding should be more dilute, about 0.5 kcal/ml. Two liters every 24 hours is a customary volume. If the patient can tolerate 1,000 kcal over a 24-hour period, the concentration can gradually be increased. Rapid or forced feedings of large volumes or excessively concentrated mixtures, especially with insufficient water, increase danger of dehydration. The patient should be monitored for thirst, abdominal cramping, diarrhea, and low urine output. In patients with an inadequate swallowing reflex, vomiting should be avoided since aspiration of the vomitus may occur. Positioning of these patients to avoid aspiration is important, and suction equipment must be readily available at the bedside. A patient with a cuffed endotracheal or tracheostomy tube in place is never left alone while fluids are being given by gavage. Feedings should be given at a slow constant rate, either through a gavage drainage system or by an electric food pump. Water should be given in a small quantity before the feeding in the event that the tube is displaced and after the feeding to flush out the tube, in sufficient quantity to avoid dehydration and to permit excretion of urinary waste products.

☐ Parenteral feeding

An alternative route for nourishing patients who cannot be fed by mouth or through the digestive tract is by intravenous infusion. The nutrients and fluid may be delivered into a peripheral vein (intravenous feeding) or into the vena cava (total parenteral nutrition, TPN). (The reader is referred to Chapter 20 for a discussion of these two methods.) The supply of calories and amino acids that can be delivered by the intravenous route is limited. TPN has made it possible to deliver a slow, continuous infusion of hyperosmolar fluid without damage to the vein. The benefits of TPN, however, have their costs as well, such as complications related to the central venous catheter, electrolyte imbalance, metabolic disturbances, and occasionally allergic reactions following administration of protein hydrolysates. The composition of the infusate varies. Certain vitamins and minerals may be absent and others provided in concentrations high enough to produce overload if continued for long periods.[3,10,32] The ingestion of foods and fluids by way of the gastrointestinal tract is a far more efficient and effective method of meeting the body's nutrition needs.

REFERENCES AND SELECTED READINGS

1. After the "last chance" diet, Consumer Reports, Feb. 1978, pp. 92-95.
2. American Dietetic Association: Position paper on bland diet in the treatment of chronic duodenal disease, J. Am. Diet. Assoc. **59**:244-245, 1971.
3. Arakawa, T., Tamura, T., Igarashi, Y., et al.: Zinc deficiency in two infants during total parenteral alimentation for diarrhea, Am. J. Clin. Nutr. **29**:197-204, 1976.
4. Bradley, H., and Sundberg, C.: Keeping food safe, Garden City, N.Y., 1975, Doubleday & Co., Inc.
5. Bruch, H.: Perils of behavior modification in treatment of anorexia nervosa, J.A.M.A. **230**:1419-1422, 1974.
6. *Bruch, H.: Eating disorders: obesity, anorexia nervosa and the person within, New York, 1973, Basic Books, Inc., Publishers.
7. Coates, T. J., and Thorensen, C. E.: Treating obesity in children and adolescents: a review, Am. J. Public Health **68**:143-151, 1978.
8. DeRitter, E.: Stability characteristics of vitamins in processed foods, Food Technol. **30**:48-54, 1976.
9. Fineberg, S. K.: The realities of obesity and fad diets, Nutr. Today **7**:23-26, July-Aug. 1972.
10. Fleming, C. R., Hodges, R. E., and Hurley, L. S.: A prospective study of serum copper and zinc levels in patients receiving total parenteral nutrition, Am. J. Clin. Nutr. **29**:70-77, 1976.
11. Food and Drug Administration: Consumer nutrition knowledge survey, report II, 1975, U.S. Department of Health, Education and Welfare, No. (FDA) 76-2059, 1975.
12. Gault, M. H., Dixon, M. E., Doyle, M., et al.: Hypernatremia, azotemia and dehydration due to high-protein tube feeding, Ann. Int. Med. **68**:778-791, 1968.
13. Genuth, S. M., Castro, J. H., and Vertes, V.: Weight reduction in obesity by outpatient starvation, J.A.M.A. **230**:987-991, 1974.
14. Gormican, A., and Liddy, E.: Nasogastric tube feedings, Postgrad. Med. **53**:71-76, 1973.
15. Gormican, A., and Liddy, E., and Mrush, L. B.: Nutritional status of patients after extended tube feeding, J. Am. Diet. Assoc. **63**:247-251, 1973.
16. Hall, R. L.: Food additives, Nutr. Today **8**:20-28, July-Aug. 1973.
17. Halmi, K. A., Powers, P., and Cunningham, S: Treatment of anorexia nervosa with behavior modification effectiveness of formula feeding and isolation, Arch. Gen. Psychiatry **32**:93-96, 1975.
18. Hathcock, J. N.: Nutrition: toxicology and pharmacology, Nutr. Rev. **34**:65-70, 1976.
19. Heird, W. C., and Winters, R. W.: Parenteral nutrition: pediatrics. In Schneider, H. A., Anderson, C. E., and Coursin, D. B.: Nutritional support of medical practice, New York, 1977, Harper & Row, Publishers.
20. Institute of Rehabilitation Medicine, New York University Medical Center: Mealtime manual for the aged and handicapped, New York, 1977, Essandess Special Editions, Simon & Schuster, Inc.
21. Johnson, P. E.: Misuse in foods of useful chemicals, Nutr. Rev. **35**:225-229, 1977.
22. Jukes, R. H.: Megavitamin therapy, J.A.M.A. **233**:550-551, 1975.
23. Kark, R. M.: Liquid formulas and chemically defined diets, J. Am. Diet. Assoc. **64**:476-480, 1974.
24. Maxmen, J. S., Siberfarb, P. M., and Ferrell, R. B.: Anorexia nervosa: practical initial management in a general hospital, J.A.M.A. **229**:801-803, 1974.
25. Meng, H. C.: Parenteral nutrition: principles, nutrient requirements, techniques and clinical applications. In Schneider, H. A., Anderson, C. E., and Coursin, D. B., Nutritional support of medical practice, New York, 1977, Harper & Row, Publishers.

*References preceded by an asterisk are particularly well suited for student reading.

26. Nutritional misinformation and food faddism, Nutr. Rev. **32** (suppl.):1-73, July 1974.
27. *Ohlson, M. A.: Diet therapy in the U.S. in the past 200 years: a bicentennial study, J. Am. Diet. Assoc. **69**:400-497, 1976.
28. Packard, V. S., Jr.: Processed foods and the consumer: additives, labeling, standards and nutrition, Minneapolis, 1976, University of Minnesota Press.
29. Paulsrud, J. R., Pensler, L., Whitten, C. F., Stewart, S., and Holman, R. T.: Essential fatty acid deficiency in infants induced by fat-free intravenous feeding, Am. J. Clin. Nutr. **25**:897-904, 1972.
30. Reisin, E., et al.: Effect of weight loss without salt restriction on the reduction of blood pressure in overweight hypertensive patients, N. Engl. J. Med. **298**:1-6, 1978.
31. *Robertson, L., Flinders, C., and Godfrey, B: Laurel's kitchen: a handbook for vegetarian cookery and nutrition, Berkeley, Calif., Nilgiri Press.
32. Safety of hydrolysates in parenteral nutrition (Editorial), N. Engl. J. Med. **289**:426-427. 1973.
33. Schafer, R. B.: Factors affecting food behavior and the quality of husbands' and wives' diets, J. Am. Diet Assoc. **72**:138-143, 1978.
34. Schuman, B. M.: Tube feeding using a food pump, Am. Fam. Physician **5**:85-88, 1972.
35. Scrimshaw, N. S.: Through a glass darkly: discerning the practical implications of human dietary protein–energy interrelationships, Nutr. Rev. **35**:321-337, 1977
36. Shuls, M. E.: A program for total parenteral nutrition at home, Am. J. Clin. Nutr. **28**:1429-1433, 1975.
37. Smith, M. A.: Feeding the handicapped child, Memphis, 1970, Child Development Center, University of Tennessee.
38. Thiele, V. F.: Clinical nutrition, St. Louis, 1976, The C. V. Mosby Co.
39. *Theologides, A.: Why cancer patients have anorexia, Geriatrics **34**:69-71, June 1976.
40. Tobian, L.: Hypertension and obesity, N. Engl. J. Med. **298**:46-48, 1978.
41. Trowell, J.: Definition of dietary fiber and hypotheses that it is a protective factor in certain diseases, Am. J. Clin. Nutr. **29**:417-427, 1976.
42. Tullis, I. F.: Rational diet construction for mild and grand obesity, J. Am. Med. Assoc. **226**:70-71, 1973.
43. Vande Wiele, R. L.: Anorexia nervosa and the hypothalamus, Hosp. Practice **18**:45-51, Dec. 1977.
44. Watson, P., and Bodey, G. P.: Sterile food service for patients in protected environments, J. Am. Diet. Assoc. **56**:515-520, 1970.
45. West, K. M.: Prevention and therapy of diabetes mellitus, Nutr. Rev. **33**:193-198, 1975.
46. White, P. L., and Nagy, M. E., editors: Total parenteral nutrition, Acton, Mass., 1974, Publishing Sciences Group Inc.
47. Wilmore, D. W., and Dudrick, S.: Growth and development of an infant receiving all nutrients by vein, J.A.M.A. **203**:860-864, 1968.
48. Wishnofsky, M.: Caloric equivalents of gained or lost weight, Am. J. Clin. Nutr. **6**:542-546, 1958.
49. Wolff, R. J.: Who eats for health? Am. J. Clin. Nutr. **26**:438-445, 1973.
50. Worthington, B. S., and Taylor, L. F.: Balanced low-calories vs. high-protein–low-carbohydrate reducing diets. 1. Weight loss, nutrient intake and subjective evaluation; 2. Biochemical changes, J. Am. Diet. Assoc. **64**:47-51, 52-55, 1974.

AUDIOVISUAL RESOURCES

1. Guide to good eating, 1977, National Dairy Council, 6300 N. River Road, Rosemont, Ill. 60018. (Full-color poster, miniature posters in English and Spanish.)
2. Eat right to your heart's delight, 1976, International Producers Services, 3518 Cahuenga Blvd., West Hollywood, Calif. 90068. (Six 16-mm films or 8-mm videocassettes, color, sound 12 to 15 min. each: Meals in a half hour; Meatless menus; New ways with chicken; Modifying recipes to control saturated fats and calories; Low-fat meat preparation; Seafood specialities. Produced as part of the government-funded "Mr. Fit" programs. (For teenage and adult audiences, food demonstrations.)
3. Nutritional principles of nasogastric tube feeding, Ross Laboratories, Columbus, Ohio 43216. (Slides and audiocassettes.)
4. Dysphagia, Fairview General Hospital, Cleveland, Ohio 44111. (16-mm, color, sound film.)

54

Problems of the upper gastrointestinal tract

NANCY DURHAM

Disorders of the gastrointestinal tract, whether caused by psychologic or physiologic factors, interfere in some manner and to some degree with the normal maintenance of gastrointestinal tract function and hence the nutritional status of the individual. Interruptions of gastrointestinal tract functions can create acute as well as chronic health problems.

Complaints of gastrointestinal tract disturbances are common and numerous. The major ones include *dysphagia* (difficulty in swallowing), *dyspepsia* (heartburn), abdominal pain, hemorrhage, nausea and vomiting, diarrhea, and constipation. Most people have experienced the stomach upset and diarrhea that often accompany disorders such as influenza, dietary indiscretions, or emotional upsets. These experiences are frequently uncomfortable and contribute to temporary abnormalities of gastrointestinal tract motility and absorption. Too often conditions of the gastrointestinal tract are viewed as short term and functional in nature, and medical opinion is not sought until it may be too late to reverse the damage to the gastrointestinal tract.

■ ORAL AND DENTAL CONDITIONS

The mouth has special emotional significance for every individual, perhaps because it is associated in infancy with food, sucking, warmth, love, and security. It continues to be associated throughout life with survival through the intake of food and with pleasurable sensations related to love and companionship, acceptance and belonging. Therefore severe emotional reactions frequently occur when treatment involving the mouth is necessary. The patient may refuse to visit his dentist, may go into complete panic when the jaws must be wired and normal eating is impossible, and may refuse to accept the fact that a lesion of the mouth is any threat to health. An understanding of what may be some of the patient's unspoken and often unrealized fears will enable the nurse to give him better care. Patience in explaining tests and treatments often helps. Sometimes merely taking time to explain to the patient how he may be fed following oral surgery may make the difference between his acceptance or rejection of the procedure. Sometimes the patient needs time to accept the need for referral to an oral surgeon and to accept the suggested treatment.

□ Infections of the mouth

Etiology

The mouth is an excellent barometer of general health, reflecting general disease and debility as well as good health. Specific diseases of the mouth most often occur when general nutrition and oral hygiene are poor, when people neglect their teeth, when smoking is excessive, and when broken teeth irritate the tissues.

Infections can occur in the buccal mucosa or the salivary glands. *Stomatitis* is an inflammation of the buccal mucosa occurring as a result of pathogenic organisms (bacteria, viruses, fungi), mechanical trauma, irritants (tobacco, alcohol, excessively spicy foods), nutritional disorders (vitamin deficiencies), disease (liver, kidney, blood dyscrasias), or following chemotherapy.

Aphthous stomatitis or canker sore is usually caused by biting the cheek or by a recurrent virus, which can remain inactive in the mucosa for a period of years. The virus of *herpes simplex* can cause inflammation of the mouth with vesicle formation or may be limited to lips or nose (coldsore, fever blister). A combination of the *Bacillus fusiformis*, which resembles the spirochete of syphilis, and *Borrelia vincentii* cause *ulceromembranous stomatitis*, or Vincent's angina. During World War I this disease was so common that the name "trench mouth" was acquired. *Streptococcus* is the causative organism of Ludwig's angina, a rare deep and serious infection of the tissue of the floor of the mouth around the submaxillary gland. The fungus *Candida albicans* causes thrush. This is sometimes seen following treatment by antibiotics over a period of time. It is thought that the antibiotic eliminates the bacteria permitting existing fungus to flourish.

Parotitis is an inflammation of the parotid gland, a salivary gland. Acute communicable parotitis (epidemic mumps) is caused by a virus that is transmitted by direct contact with the saliva. Noncommunicable parotitis occurs in debilitated persons whose oral hygiene is poor, whose mouths have been permitted to become dry, and who have not chewed solid foods regularly. Elderly persons are more susceptible than younger ones. Usually the *Staphylococcus* organism is present.

Prevention

Infections of the mouth can be prevented in many instances by adequate nutrition, maintenance of moist mucous membranes, and good oral hygiene. Excessive use of tobacco or hot spicy foods is discouraged for persons who have increased risk of developing stomatitis. Prevention of nutritional deficiencies, especially vitamin deficiencies, will help prevent stomatitis, and emphasis on restoring nutritional balance of the debilitated patient will decrease the incidence of mouth infections.

In addition to maintaining the nutrition of the cells, the mucous membranes must be kept moist to prevent infection. Adequate hydration is therefore important. Patients who are not permitted to drink fluids should have frequent mouth care to keep the mouth clean and the mucous membranes moist. Persons whose normal habits include poor mouth or dental care need health teaching. It takes creative teaching to motivate changes of long-standing habits, and this is not usually accomplished in one session. Mouth breathers and persons receiving oxygen therapy may develop mouth infections because dry mucous membranes increases the risk of infection.

The importance of good mouth care cannot be overemphasized. If the patient is unable to do this for himself or if self-care is inadequate, the nurse must intervene. In situations where the mouth is in poor condition and a fetid odor is present, the task is disagreeable and thus unfortunately is often not carried out as frequently as is needed. Patients who are at high risk of developing infections need mouth care several times a day, and those whose mouths are in poor condition and who are on the verge of developing stomatitis may need attention to oral hygiene as often as every 1 to 2 hours while awake.

Assessment

In patients at high risk of developing infections the mouth is assessed daily for signs of developing or healing infection. Signs and symptoms may include mild erythema and edema of the mucous membranes, ulcerations, increased or decreased salivation, pain (especially when inflamed or ulcerated areas are touched by the teeth or foods), fetid odor to the breath, and a foul taste. Bleeding of the gums and a gray membrane over the gums may occur with Vincent's angina. Fever and edema, which may lead to obstruction of the throat, may occur with Ludwig's angina. Redness around the orifice of the parotid gland is seen with parotitis. Thrush is characterized by white patches (resembling milk curds) over the inflamed mucous membranes.

In addition to assessing the condition of the mouth, the nurse needs to assess the ability of the patient to carry out his own oral hygiene. Assessment includes the patient's level of consciousness, ability to open the mouth, presence of mouth breathing, and ability to feed self or drink fluids.[9]

Intervention

Maintenance of adequate nutrition and hydration is as important after mouth infections develop as it is in prevention. If the mouth is very sore and painful, eating may be difficult, and the patient may need considerable encouragement. Soft foods, including strained meats and fish, pureed vegetables and fruits, cooked cereals, soups, jello, and ice cream, are best tolerated. Hot spicy foods are to be avoided; cold drinks may be soothing. High-protein, high-caloric drinks such as eggnog serve both nutritional and fluid needs.

Thorough and frequent mouth care is a must. The frequency of mouth care and the effectiveness of agents in relation to therapeutic outcomes has not yet been thoroughly studied. It has been suggested that for mild stomatitis, mouth care at least every 4 hours around the clock is essential and at least every 2 hours for very severe cases.[9] If dentures are present and are increasing pain, they should be removed. Alkaline mouthwash solutions such as sodium bicarbonate or sodium perborate can be used. Hydrogen peroxide diluted with normal saline 1:4 is effective in treating anaerobic infections, since it is an oxidizing agent. It should be mixed immediately prior to use because it decomposes rapidly. If the tissues are not too painful, a soft toothbrush may be used. If pain is severe, one layer of gauze may be wrapped around a finger to gently wipe the gums and teeth. The mouth is then rinsed with the solution, followed by rinsing with tap water.

With severe Vincent's angina or with Ludwig's angina antibiotics are ordered and should be given on time to maintain blood levels. If the patient has difficulty swallowing tablets, they are crushed if possible or the antibiotic may be given intramuscularly.

Pain may be partially relieved by good oral hygiene. Smoking is contraindicated. Cold drinks or sucking on frozen popsicles may be soothing. Analgesic drugs may be necessary and lidocaine hydrochloride (Xylocaine) may be applied to provide topical anesthesia.

Outcome criteria for the person with a mouth infection

The patient or significant others can:

1. State the underlying cause of the infection.
2. Describe a specific plan to avoid future infections that includes:
   a. Maintenance of a balanced nutritional and fluid intake.
   b. Avoidance of causative factors.
   c. Good oral hygiene.
   d. Semiannual dental examinations.
3. State the action, dosage, and side effects of medications to be taken at home including the need to complete antibiotic therapy.
4. State signs or symptoms necessitating medical follow-up.

□ Diseases of teeth and gums

Dental caries

Tooth decay is probably the most common yet most neglected chronic ailment of modern times. Dental caries is a progressive disease of the teeth related to the consumption of refined carbohydrates. Within 30 minutes after eating, organisms in the mouth act on the refined sugars left on the teeth and may produce acids that eventually dissolve the enamel surface of the tooth. Decay, cavity formation, inflammation, infection, and loss of teeth follow. Malocclusion gradually develops as teeth are lost. Methods to control and prevent dental caries include good oral hygiene, dental examinations every 6 months, nutritional foods including avoidance of refined sugars, and the use of fluorides.

Brushing the teeth (Fig. 53-6) or even rinsing the mouth with plain water immediately after ingestion of refined carbohydrate foods helps prevent decay. The times when most people brush their teeth are entirely wrong from the standpoint of prevention of dental caries. It is during the first half hour after eating refined carbohydrate that the most harm is done. Immediate rinsing of the mouth with plain water is more helpful than is thorough brushing of the teeth hours afterward when the bacterial damage has been done.

The elimination or drastic *curtailment of refined carbohydrate foods* would reduce the prevalence of dental caries. In 1823 the average American consumed 8 pounds of sugar a year, whereas now he uses over 100 pounds a year. The consumption of lollipops, ice cream, hard candies, and soft drinks, which are so much a part of American culture, should be curtailed or, preferably, eliminated. The custom of concluding a meal with a sweet dessert or candies contributes to tooth decay. The European custom of ending the meal with fresh fruit is an excellent one, since fresh fruit sugars and unrefined starches contain properties that inhibit bacterial enzyme action in the mouth. In fact, eating a raw apple before retiring is an excellent way to clean one's teeth.

The use of *fluoride* has been shown conclusively to increase resistance of tooth enamel to bacterial action during the formative period of tooth growth in children. Fluoride may be added to drinking water, given by tablet, mixed in toothpaste, or applied topically to the teeth. Most urban communities in the United States fluoridate their water supplies. In areas where well water is used, fluoride should be taken in tablet form. The optimum dosage is 0.5 mg/day from birth to 3 years and 1 mg/day after the age of 3. Use of fluoridated toothpaste is highly recommended by the American Dental Association. Local application is less effective and more expensive than fluoridation of water. Some dentists recommend the local application of fluoride to the teeth in addition to the systemic ingestion of flouride as an extra protection against the development of caries.

Periapical abscess

A periapical abscess develops around the root of a tooth. It usually is an extension of an infection arising in the pulp caused by dental caries. The abscess may perforate along the gum margin, or it may travel medially to form an abscess over the palate or spread directly to the soft tissues, causing cellulitis and a severely swollen face.

Periapical abscess can cause severe local pain and systemic reactions, including malaise, nausea, and elevation of temperature. The treatment consists of drilling an opening into the pulp chamber of the tooth to establish drainage and to relieve pain. Penicillin may be administered, and warm saline mouthwashes usually are ordered several times a day. After the acute phase the tooth may be extracted, or root canal therapy may be started if a sound, permanent tooth is involved.

Periodontal disease

Periodontal disease is a disease of the tissues that support the teeth (the periodontium) and affects the gingivae, bone, cementum, and periodontal membrane (Fig. 54-1). Symptoms include infection, bleeding, recession of the gums, and loosening of the teeth. Deterioration of bone structure occurs, and teeth may eventually fall out or have to be extracted. After the age of 40 years more people lose their teeth from this cause than from dental caries. Periodontal disease is receiving much more attention than formerly, partly because of the recognition of the whole field of dental health as a major public health problem. The Public Health Service is cooperating in studies, and most states now have preventive dental health programs that include attention to other dental diseases besides caries.

Many factors contribute to the development of periodontal disease, among them malocclusion, accumu-

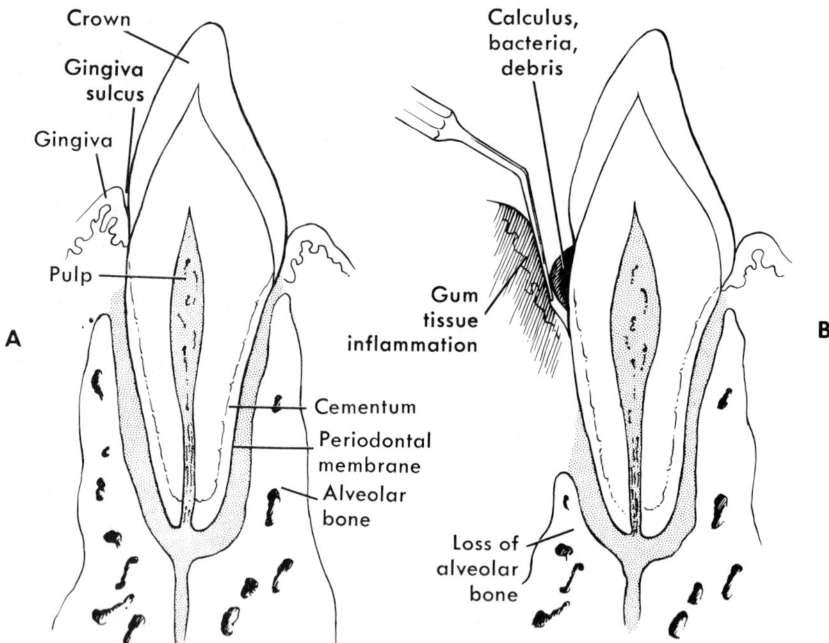

Fig. 54-1. A, Normal tooth with gum and root structure. **B,** Note presence of foreign materials along gum margin, which may lead to periodontal disease.

lation of tartar, poor nutrition including eating too much soft food instead of solid food that requires mastication, poor mouth hygiene, and improper brushing of the teeth. Certain systemic conditions may contribute to the development of periodontal disease. These include alcoholism, diabetes, thyroid imbalance, hormonal imbalance (menstruation and pregnancy), response to chemotherapy, and blood dyscrasias.[31] *Malocclusion* may result in a poor bite with unequal pressure on teeth. It leads to deterioration of bony supportive structures. Removal of teeth without proper replacements permits the teeth to drift backward and alters the bite, again producing unequal pressure on working surfaces of the teeth. Premature loss of deciduous teeth in children should be referred to a dentist. Nonmineralized plaque can form on the calculus surface and destroy the tiny tendrils holding the tooth in the socket. This situation eventually leads to unhealthy receding gums with lessened tooth support (Fig. 54-1). Poor nutrition, improper brushing of the teeth, and local infection may augment the destruction of gums and supportive gum structures to such a degree that they recede. The leverage of daily use then becomes too great on the teeth, and they loosen and finally have to be removed.

Treatment of periodontal disease includes maintenance of oral hygiene and nutrition, control of local irritations and infections by regular visits to the dentist, removal of accumulations of tartar on the teeth, replacement of lost teeth, and correction of malocclusion. Even if treatment has been delayed until there is already a good deal of damage, care by an *orthodontist* (one who specializes in straightening teeth) may be surprisingly helpful. Sometimes bridgework and other forms of splinting can be used so that further erosion of bone and supportive tissue can be halted even if teeth cannot be straightened and the actual bite improved.

Nutrition is so important for patients with periodontal disease that some periodontists have their patients keep weekly food-intake charts to determine what essentials of diet may be lacking. Intake should be evaluated carefully for inclusion of fresh citrus fruits and fresh vegetables, and protein consumption should be noted, since it is so important in gum healing and in gum health.

Artificial dentures

Artificial dentures and other dental prostheses are resisted by most people. Serious emotional reactions are manifested when the patient must give up all of his own teeth, no matter how unsatisfactory they may be. Dental prostheses need not be conspicuous. A proper fit can be obtained in almost all instances, and there is often cosmetic improvement. The patient should be urged to have patience in learning to use the new teeth. Many elderly people become discouraged easily and lay artificial teeth aside and then, because they are embarrassed by their appearance without teeth, avoid people.

Artificial dentures should be cleaned at least twice daily and preferably after each meal. Salt and sodium bicarbonate, a mild tasteless soap such as Ivory, or any good dentifrice can be used. Odor should not be a problem since plastic materials have largely replaced vulcanite materials, which sometimes retained odors. A few drops of ammonium hydroxide or a drop of chlorine household bleach, which is a good deodorant, added to the water used to wash the dentures may make the teeth feel and taste fresher. When artificial teeth are removed for cleansing, the patient should massage his gums thoroughly for a few minutes. Teeth that fit snugly naturally interfere with circulation to some extent. Some dentists encourage their patients to wear their teeth both during waking and sleeping hours, since facial contours may be preserved better by this means. Other dentists recommend that the dentures be removed at night to prevent irritation to underlying tissues. Dentures that fit properly should not cause discomfort after the general slight discomfort associated with their newness is overcome. The patient should be advised to report any persistent pressure or irritation to his dentist, since adjustment can usually be made. Any lesion in the mouth associated with the use of dental prostheses should be reported at once, since it may be an early malignancy.

Very occasionally there has been so much recession and atrophy of bone structures that it is extremely difficult to fit prostheses properly. A magnetic device has been perfected that can be embedded in the palate and that, by attraction to a magnetized dental plate, helps to hold the dentures in good position.

Outcome criteria for the person with a full-mouth extraction

The patient or significant others can:

1. Demonstrate good mouth care.
2. Demonstrate proper technique for brushing artificial dentures.
3. Demonstrate proper techniques for cleansing the gums.
4. Describe the importance of removing food particles from the dentures at least twice a day.
5. Determine which dentrifice, soaking solution, or adhesive is most acceptable for personal needs.
6. State a specific plan for dental follow-up:
   a. State where dental services will be obtained.
   b. State situations under which the fit of the prosthesis may need to be adjusted (weight gain or loss, pain or tenderness in the gum area, slippage of the plate).

□ Tumors of the mouth

Epidemiology

The lips, the oral cavity, and the tongue are prone to develop malignant lesions. The largest number of these tumors are squamous cell epitheliomas that grow rapidly and metastasize to adjacent structures more quickly than do most malignant tumors of the skin. In the United States oral cancer accounts for 5% of the cancers in males and 3% in females.[1] Recent investigation has revealed a higher incidence of cancers of the mouth and throat among persons who are heavy drinkers and smokers. The combination of high alcohol consumption and smoking causes an apparent breakdown in the body's defense mechanism, as evidenced by an increase in the levels of immunoglobulin A (IgA) in saliva.[25]

The cure rate for cancer of the lips is high because the lesion is easily apparent to the pateint and to others. Metastasis to regional lymph nodes has occurred in only 10% of persons when diagnosed. In some instances a lesion may spread rapidly and involve the mandible and the floor of the mouth by direct extension. Occasionally the tumor may be a basal cell lesion that starts in the skin and spreads to the lip.

Cancer of the anterior tongue and floor of the mouth may seem to occur together because their spread to adjacent tissues is so rapid. Metastasis to the neck has already occurred in over 60% of the patients when the diagnosis is made because of the tongue's abundant vascular and lymphatic drainage. The mortality is high. Lesions about the base of the tongue may go unnoticed by the patient and may be far advanced when treatment is started.

Tumors of the salivary glands occur primarily in the parotid gland and are usually benign. Tumors of the submaxillary gland have a high incidence of malignancy. The malignant tumor grows more rapidly and may be accompanied by pain and impaired facial function.

Prevention

Avoidance of predisposing factors may decrease the potential for developing cancer of the mouth. This includes avoidance of excess exposure to sun and wind on the lips, elimination of smoking or chewing tobacco or betel leaf, and maintenance of good oral and dental care. There is a high correlation between the incidence of cancer of the mouth and cirrhosis of the liver associated with alcohol intake. Early detection of oral cancer can help increase the patient's chance of survival. Any person with a mouth lesion that does not heal within 2 to 3 weeks is urged to seek immediate medical care.

Clinical picture

Malignant lesions of the mouth are usually asymptomatic. *Leukoplakia,* white patches on the tongue and buccal mucosa that are not easily removed, are not cancerous but often become malignant. Early malignant lesions are difficult to detect as there may be initial inflammatory response that frequently disappears leaving only a small ulcer or growth. Cancer of the lips usually occurs on the lower lip as a fissure or a painless, indurated ulcer with raised edges. Cancer of the anterior tongue and floor of the mouth occurs as hard plaquelike or ulcerated areas that do not heal. Lesions are usually unilateral, and multiple lesions may occur.

Parotid tumors occur as painless lumps that can be palpated anterior to or directly below the ear. Biopsy of the parotid gland is not recommended because of the potential for tumor seeding; therefore the entire gland is usually removed for examination. If diagnosed as a malignancy, more extensive surgery may be indicated.

Intervention

Treatment consists of one or more approaches depending on the location, type, extent, and size of the tumor. Modalities include surgery, radiotherapy, cryotherapy, and chemotherapy.

Cancer of the lip may require excision and reconstructive surgery of jaw and mandible if extension to these areas has occurred. A complete neck dissection may be done if the lymph nodes are involved (p. 1105).

Cancer of the anterior tongue and floor of the mouth may require partial or total surgical excision of the tongue *(hemiglossectomy, glossectomy)* or a radical neck dissection if lymph nodes are involved. Intraarterial perfusion of antimetabolites into the site may be instituted prior to surgery (p. 479). Radiation treatment may be used instead of surgery or following surgery.

Surgery for cancer of the parotid gland may include removal of large amounts of surrounding tissue and nodes, but radical neck resection is not routine.[50] Radiation is only instituted for palliative effect. Tumors of the submaxillary gland usually require complete excision of the gland and more radical surgery.

Preparation for therapy. The treatment for cancer of the mouth, whether by chemotherapy, surgery, or radiation, interferes with normal functions of the mouth. The patient and his family should be told about the changes that will occur and about the methods that will be used to help him communicate and take nourishment. For example, local excisions of the lip or tongue may affect speech to some degree, and the patient may have difficulty making himself understood. Patients having a hemiglossectomy will be unable to speak. The provision of a pad of paper with a pencil, a tiny blackboard with chalk, ar a Magic Slate will permit the patient to communicate with others. If a hemiglossectomy is done, taking food orally is impossible for a time, and the patient should know that he will be fed by other means. Because it may be difficult for patients with radon seeds in the tongue or for those who have local excisions of the mouth to eat, parenteral fluids, fluids through a catheter or nasogastric tube, or the administration of food through a feeding cup may be necessary. The patient who is to have a hemiglossectomy should be told that suction may be used to remove saliva.

If a radical neck dissection and tracheostomy are to be done at the same time as the treatment of the primary tumor, the patient's care after these procedures should be explained (pp. 1105 and 947). The patient and his family should be assured that he will be attended constantly until he is conscious and able to care for himself. The nurse should get to know the patient in order to judge how much he should be told about his treatment. For example, some patients who are to lose teeth and part of the jaw are relieved to know something about prosthetic devices that are available. Impressions sometimes are taken preoperatively to guide in making suitable prostheses following surgery. Other patients are so overwhelmed by the prospect of the operation itself that they are far from ready to think beyond the most immediate future.

Surgery. Preoperatively, oral prophylactic treatment usually is given, and antibiotics may be administered to decrease the number of bacteria present in the mouth at the time of surgery. The surgery may be performed with the patient under local or general anesthesia, depending on whether a radical neck dissection also is being performed. While recovering from general anesthesia, the patient may be placed in a prone position or on his side to facilitate drainage from the mouth. When he has reacted, he usually is more comfortable in Fowler's position. Bleeding and drainage from the suture line on the lip or tongue should be minimal.

Because of the vascularity of the tongue, patients who have had a wide resection of the tongue should be watched carefully for hemorrhage. If a hemiglossectomy has been performed, the patient will have difficulty in swallowing saliva or expectorating secretions, and the mouth may need to be suctioned frequently. Occasionally a suction device such as is used by dentists is employed to carry away saliva as it accumulates. A gauze wick may be used to direct saliva into an emesis basin. The patient should be provided with mouth wipes and a bag for disposing of them. If he is unable to swallow, the nurse should attend the patient constantly until such time as he is accustomed to the situation and can help to care for himself.

The seventh cranial (facial) nerve passes through the posterior portion of the parotid gland and may be affected by removal of this gland. Temporary facial paralysis frequently occurs, and permanent paralysis may result following radical surgery. Facial weakness is assessed daily by asking the patient to pucker his lips, smile, show his teeth, and raise his eyebrows.[50] If the patient cannot close his eye, the cornea must be protected by lubricating eyedrops and patches while sleeping.

Oral hygiene. Good mouth care is essential for comfort, prevention of infection, and promotion of healing. Teeth brushing is usually contraindicated because of discomfort and potential trauma. Uninvolved areas may be cleansed by using a cotton applicator moistened with hydrogen peroxide and saline. The mouth may be irrigated with sterile water, diluted hydrogen peroxide, normal saline, or a solution of sodium bicarbonate. Commercial mouthwashes are too astringent. Sterile equipment is used to prevent introduction of exogenous organisms.

A catheter may be inserted along the side of the mouth between the cheek and the teeth and solution injected with gentle pressure, or a spray may be used. Remaining fluid and mucus drains into an emesis basin or is removed with the suction apparatus. Dressings may be protected during this treatment by fitting a plastic sheet snugly over them. As soon as the patient is able to do so, he is encouraged to assist with this part of his care.

Eating. The method used to feed the patient will depend entirely on the extent and nature of his surgery. Most patients can suction and feed themselves a few days following mouth surgery and are happier doing so. An Asepto syringe with a catheter attached may be used, and from this apparatus the patient may progress to a feeding cup with a piece of rubber tubing attached. Through practice the patient will develop confidence in caring for himself, and he is often more adept than the nurse in placing the catheter or tube in a position where fluids can be received into the mouth and swallowed without difficulty. A mirror often helps. He needs privacy when he is experimenting with the method that is best for him. He should not be hurried and be observed very carefully to determine how much assistance he needs. As he begins to take liquids and then soft, pureed foods, he is taught to follow all meals with clear water to cleanse the mouth and foster good oral hygiene.

If the patient has had a hemiglossectomy, he may be fed through a nasogastric tube or through a soft catheter that is passed into the throat and beyond the operative site. (See p. 1184 for further information on tube feedings.) The patient must be watched carefully after the liquid diet is given, since nausea and vomiting must be avoided.

Speech. While the patient does experience some pain in the area of the incision, most of his difficulty arises from his inability to swallow and speak normally. Other persons should be alerted to his problem with oral communication. Conversation can be carried out so that the patient's responses can be limited to affirmative and negative gestures or to minimal written replies. If extensive resection of the tongue or palate has occurred, speech retraining may be necessary.

Socialization. Because of difficulties with eating or talking or with disfigurement in the event of radical surgery, some patients may hesitate to move among strangers. A two-bed room provides contact with others while still maintaining some privacy. The patient is supported and encouraged to mingle with others as soon as he evidences clues that he is ready. Men are encouraged to shave using an electric razor as soon as this is permitted. Members of the family are encouraged to visit.

Prosthetic devices are available following radical surgery but cannot be fitted until healing has taken place, but pictures of persons who are wearing such devices with resultant marked improvement in their appearance are often encouraging to the patient. Prostheses are individually designed to replace portions of the palate and jaw that have been resected and to make the use of dentures possible. Plastic surgery may be done to partially replace lost tissue. Meeting and talking to other patients who have had similar operations with good results and good adjustment are very helpful to the patient.

Radiation. Tumors of the mouth may be treated by radiation in various forms. Needles containing radium, radioactive cobalt, or other radioactive substances may be inserted and left in place for a prescribed time. Seeds containing emanations from radium or radioactive cobalt may be used and left in place indefinitely or else removed (see Fig. 25-7). External radiation treatment using x-rays or other radioactive substances may be prescribed.

Whatever the method of treatment chosen, it should be explained fully to the patient. If needles containing radioactive elements are used, he must know that the needles are fastened to string that must not be pulled lest the dosage or direction of radiation be altered or the needle lost. He must understand that talking with the needles in place will be difficult or impossible. Radioactive needles must be checked several times each day. Auxiliary personnel and all other persons in attendance should understand the need to watch all equipment carefully for needles that have been removed or dislodged (for example, when emptying an emesis basin), lest radioactive materials be unwittingly discarded.

Radiation therapy produces secondary effects in the mouth that include mucositis, xerostomia (dryness), dental decay, and trismus (tightening of the jaw muscle).[54] Some of the changes may be permanent. The initial reaction is an inflammation of the mucous membrane (mucositis). Sloughing of the tissues may occur and cause a fetid odor. Dentures are not tolerated for some time thereafter because of the sensitivity of the tissues. When dentures are worn they should be checked frequently for fit and removed at night. Good oral hygiene is essential.

Because smoke is irritating to the mucous membranes, the patient should not smoke. Hot and cold foods

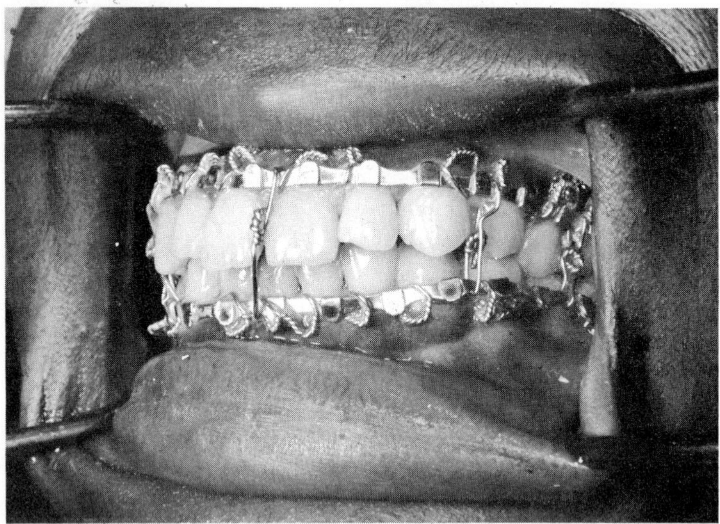

Fig. 54-2. One method of wiring jaw. (Courtesy Dr. Marsh Robinson.)

or fluids should be avoided because the injured mucous membranes are extremely sensitive to changes in temperature. Solutions of local anesthetics or lozenges may be prescribed by the physician if discomfort in the mouth caused by the local irritation seriously interferes with eating.

Dryness of the mouth begins 1 to 2 weeks after radiation is started and may persist throughout life.[54] The dryness makes the mouth feel uncomfortable and gives an unpleasant taste. Frequent drinks of water, saline-peroxide mouthwashes, and increased humidity in the room contribute to added moisture and comfort.

Decreased salivary secretion and altered pH of the saliva contributes to rapid dental decay, especially at the gingival margins. In the past all teeth were extracted prior to radiation of the mouth, but this is being done less commonly. An active control program is started before radiation therapy is initiated. Fluoride treatments to the teeth may be given and a conscientious teeth-brushing regimen using fluoride toothpaste, a soft toothbrush, and dental floss is instituted.

Persons who have had surgery in addition to radiation may be unable to open their mouth widely. This can interfere with talking, eating, or dental care.

Palliative care. Tissue necrosis and severe pain occur in advanced cancer of the mouth, either from failure of treatment or from death of tissue due to radiation. The patient is harassed by difficulty in swallowing, fear of choking, and the constant accumulation of foul-smelling secretions. The danger of severe, and even fatal, hemorrhage must always be considered. Nursing care of these patients include the most careful and thoughtful attention to certain details; for example, secretions left in emesis basins or in suction bottles can be most upsetting to the patient. It is exceedingly difficult to induce patients with advanced carcinoma of the mouth to take sufficient nourishing fluids, and the nurse can often help by finding out specifically what fluids or foods the patient likes and believes are easiest for him to take. Relatives may be permitted to prepare and bring special dishes to the hospital if the patient so desires. Sometimes a gastrostomy is done to permit direct introduction of food into the stomach (p. 1199). Most physicians prescribe analgesic drugs freely for patients whose disease has progressed beyond medical control.

If the patient is to be cared for at home, the family is taught how to feed, suction, and otherwise care for the patient. Assistance and support can be provided by a community health nurse.

□ Trauma

Fracture of the jaw

Fracture of the jaw occurs quite frequently as a result of vehicular accidents and of combative physical encounters with others. Treatment consists of bringing the separated fragments together and immobilizing them. This is accomplished with wires that are attached to the upper and lower rows of teeth and twisted together or with arch bars fastened by rubber bands or tie wires (Fig. 54-2). Rubber bands are used most often since they can be removed readily and the degree of fixation can be adjusted easily. If an open operation is necessary, interosseous wiring or plating may be done. Because of the excellent blood supply to the jaw, fractures usually heal rapidly (5 to 8 weeks). Tetanus prophylaxis and antibiotic therapy are usually started on admission.

Preoperatively the patient is told that he will be able

to breathe normally, to talk, and to swallow liquids, but that he will not be able to eat solid food. He should be assured, however, that he will be able to take sufficient food for health. Many times the patient with a fracture of the jaw can resume quite an active life during convalescence. Most patients are in the hospital a very short time or are treated on an ambulatory basis unless they have sustained other injuries.

Immediately following wiring of the teeth, the patient is watched for nausea and vomiting, which may be caused by emotional trauma, blood or other swallowed material, or anesthesia. Care must be taken to prevent aspiration of vomitus. Vomitus and secretions must be removed by suction, since the patient cannot expectorate them through the mouth. Usually a catheter can be inserted through the nasopharynx or into the mouth through a gap created by missing teeth or in the space behind the third molar. Scissors or a wire cutter should be at the bedside so that the wires can be cut or the elastic bands released if necessary. Specific orders should state the circumstances under which wires or rubber bands should be released.

Patients who have fixation by wiring need much the same care as is needed following surgery of the mouth. They must often subsist on liquids and must learn to take a high-caloric liquid diet through a catheter, an Asepto syringe, a feeding cup, or a straw. They need instruction about mouth hygiene, and they must be instructed to report any sudden swelling, pain, or other symptoms that may occur after dismissal from the hospital. Osteomyelitis is much less common now that antibiotics are available, but it can occur and is more likely to do so in the unusual cases of compound fracture in which bone fragments have penetrated either the outer skin or the inside of the mouth.

Outcome criteria for the person with immobilized jaws. The patient or significant others can:

1. Describe situations that may require the establishment of an immediate clear airway (vomiting, increased secretions).
2. Describe methods of releasing the wires and reestablishing an airway if the airway becomes obstructed.
3. Describe the necessary dietary modifications (types of feedings, methods of preparation, foods to avoid that might cause vomiting or obstruction) and method of feeding.
4. Explain how to contact community or professional persons who can assist him (counseling, vocational guidance).
5. State plans for follow-up care.

Injury to soft tissue

Injuries to soft tissues within the mouth usually are caused by pressure against teeth, direct trauma from a foreign object, or protrusion of bone through the buccal mucosa following fracture of the jaw. Breaks in the skin about the mouth often accompany these injuries. Treatment consists of thorough cleansing of the wounds. Usually an antibacterial solution is used and is followed by irrigation with sterile normal saline solution. Skin wounds are gently debrided and sutured with an extremely fine, nonabsorbable suture for best cosmetic results. Because of the vascularity of the scalp and face, infection is rare following traumatic injury to these areas.

Lacerations within the mouth are cleansed and sutured if their extent and location make these measures necessary. Hemorrhage must be watched for, especially if total injuries necessitate extensive dressing, which may hinder normal expectoration of blood and cause it to be swallowed. Edema may be pronounced following trauma to the mouth and may interfere with respirations. Usually the head of the bed is elevated in a semi-Fowler's position to aid in venous drainage from the area and thereby lessen edema. Tight dressings about the face must be checked carefully, since they may contribute to development of edema and may cause headache.

Patients who have sustained penetrating wounds of the mouth are usually given antibiotics and tetanus serum prophylactically. The nurse should question the patient about a history of sensitivity to serum before treatment of prevention of tetanus is given. Mouth care and feeding of patients with these injuries present problems similar to those encountered following surgery or a fracture.

Outcome criteria for the person with sutures in the oral cavity. The patient or significant others can:

1. Demonstrate techniques to keep the suture line clean (method, frequency, agents to avoid).
2. Describe any dietary modifications required during healing (soft, nonirritating foods).
3. State symptoms that require immediate medical supervision (increased temperature, swelling or redness of the suture line, drainage, loss of sutures).
4. State plans for follow-up care.

■ ESOPHAGEAL DISORDERS

□ Achalasia (cardiospasm, aperistalsis)

Achalasia is a condition in which there is an absence of peristalsis in the esophagus and the esophageal sphincter fails to relax following deglutition (swallowing). The cause is unknown, but the disorder is a direct result of disruption of the normal neuromuscular mechanism of the esophagus. Anxiety and tension seem to aggravate the symptoms and bring on exacerbations. The disease is most common in middle life and is the most common cause of dysphagia in women. Because the condition is found in older persons, cancer of the lower end of the esophagus must be ruled out by esophagoscopy.

In the early phases of achalasia there is no gross lesion, but as the disease persists, the portion of the esophagus about the constriction dilates and the muscular walls become hypertrophied. The dilated area becomes atonic, and esophageal peristalsis may be absent so that little or no food can enter the stomach. While varying degrees of the condition exist, in extreme cases the esophagus above the constriction may hold a liter or more of fluid.

Clinical picture

The person may first complain of substernal fullness following the hasty ingestion of bulky or cold foods. He may have to make a determined, conscious effort to pass food beyond the constricted area. He may have difficulty swallowing liquids and this may be the initial symptom. In time there is frank dysphagia with or without malnutrition. The person loses weight and may suffer from avitaminosis. He may also complain of chest pain similar to that of angina pectoris. As the condition progresses, there is regurgitation rather than vomiting of esophageal contents which do not contain gastric acid, onto the pillow or into the larynx during sleep. The diagnosis is confirmed by radiographs taken as the person swallows barium and by esophagoscopy.

Intervention

If the constriction is not severe, the person usually is advised to eat a bland diet, avoiding bulky foods. Meals should be eaten slowly, and drinking fluids with meals helps the food to pass through the narrowed opening. Frequent changes of position during eating may also help. The person should sleep with his head elevated to avoid the possibility of aspiration of esophageal residue.

If the patient cannot pass food beyond the constriction, forceful dilation of the narrowed opening with the specific purpose of tearing some of the muscle fibers in the area may be done. This procedure is accomplished by passing graduated mercury-tipped bougies, passing tubes with bags attached that can be inflated under pressure, or passing a mechanical (Starck) dilator. The generally accepted surgical procedure is a cardiomyotomy. The muscular layer is incised longitudinally down to but not through the mucosa. The incision is so done that two thirds of its length are in the esophagus and the remaining one third is in the stomach. This permits the mucosa to expand so that food can pass more easily into the stomach.

Postoperatively the nursing care is the same as the routine care given any patient who has had chest surgery (p. 969). A rare complication is accidental perforation of the esophageal mucosa so that leakage may contaminate the mediastinum. Regurgitation occasionally occurs after surgery but can usually be controlled by the administration of antacid medications. Since overflow may still occur at night, the patient is advised to refrain from food or fluid for several hours before retiring.

□ Esophageal diverticulum

An esophageal diverticulum is the bulging of the esophageal mucosa and submucosa through a weakened portion of the muscular layer of the esophagus. It is most often located at the pharyngoesophageal junction, in the lower end of the thoracic esophagus, or just above the diaphragm (epiphrenic diverticulum). As food is ingested, some of it may pass into the diverticulum. After a sufficient amount has accumulated in the pocket, it overflows into the esophagus and is regurgitated. There is always danger that some of the regurgitated material may be aspirated into the trachea and lungs during sleep or that the diverticulum may enlarge and cause esophageal obstruction.

Clinical picture

The patient may complain of pain on swallowing, of gurgling noises in the area, and of a cough due to tracheal irritation. His breath usually has a foul odor caused by decomposition of food in the diverticulum. The odor can be alleviated somewhat by frequent brushing of the teeth and the use of aromatic mouthwashes.

Intervention

If the symptoms become severe, surgery is performed. The herniated sac is excised, and the resultant esophageal opening is closed. These procedures are well tolerated, and the administration of antibiotics makes postoperative infections rare. If a supraclavicular approach has been used, fluid are usually permitted as soon as nausea subsides, and a bland diet is prescribed soon afterward. If a transthoracic approach is utilized, chest drainage may be used, and the patient usually is allowed nothing by mouth for several days.

□ Stricture of the esophagus

The deliberate or accidental swallowing of caustic materials such as lye may cause serious strictures in the esophagus as the mucosa heals. Unfortuantely many of the patients are small children, and they may suffer from the effects of such an accident for the remainder of their lives. Although the patient may be able to swallow fluids for a while after the accident, strictures develop as healing occurs, and sometimes no food can pass into the stomach.

Intervention

Careful attempts are made to dilate the stricture by passing bougies. Usually this is done under the fluoroscope so that danger of causing damage that would result in further stricture formation is lessened. If the destruction of the esophageal mucosa is extensive, a *gastrostomy* (permanent opening into the stomach) may be performed (p. 1199). Braided silk thread is then inserted through the mouth and esophagus into the stomach and brought out through the gastrostomy opening. The two ends of the thread are tied together to form a complete loop, and the thread is used for pulling bougies or beads tied to it through the esophagus to dilate it and to prevent complete closure of the lumen. Such treatment may be necessary for months or years after the ingesting of a caustic substance. If a satisfactory esophageal lumen cannot be maintained, surgery may be performed. The stricture may be resected or bypassed with a segment of jejunum or colon.

Outcome criteria for the person with esophageal disorders causing difficulty in swallowing

The patient or significant others can:

1. Explain any dietary changes required after discharge:
   a. List specific foods to be avoided.
   b. State a plan for frequent small feedings that are soft and easily swallowed and will maintain nutrition.
   c. Determine daily fluid requirement and state a plan regarding intake or fluids prior to, during, and after food ingestion.
2. State plans for follow-up care.

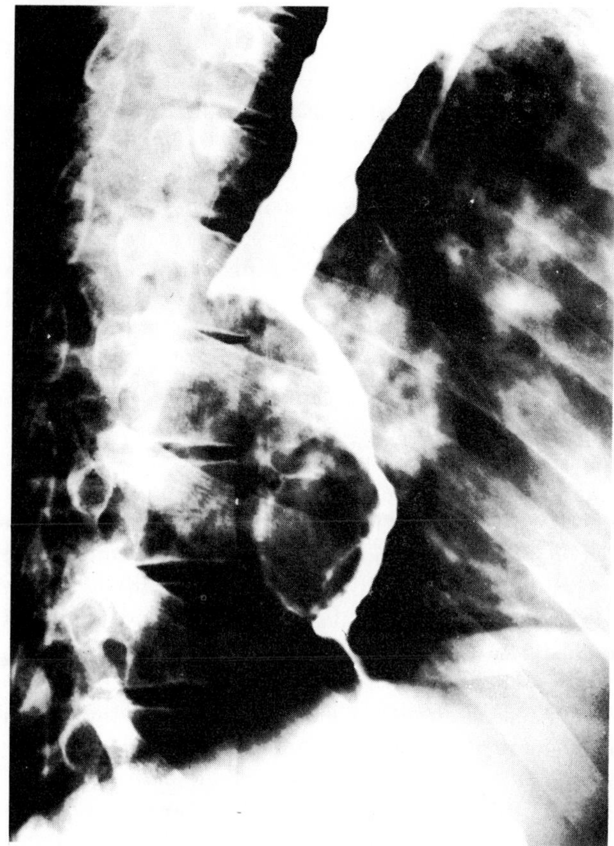

Fig. 54-3. Radiograph taken after patient had swallowed barium, showing location of lesion in esophagus as it approaches stomach.

□ Esophageal tumors

Carcinoma is the most common condition causing obstruction of the esophagus and accounts for about 2% of all deaths from cancer in the United States. The incidence is increasing in nonwhite females, in persons with achalasia or hiatus hernia, and among alcoholics.[13] The tumor may develop in any portion of the esophagus, but it is most common in the middle and lower thirds.

The only possible hope for successful treatment lies in very early diagnosis and surgical treatment. Any person who has difficulty in swallowing, no matter how trivial it may seem, should be urged, to seek medical advice at once. This applies particularly to persons over 40 years of age, since cancer of the esophagus occurs more often in middle and later life than at younger ages.

Clinical picture

The person who has cancer of the esophagus initially complains only of mild and intermittent dysphagia. Gradually he finds it extremely difficult to swallow solid food, and by the time he seeks medical attention he often has resorted to strained foods and liquids. He may regurgitate after eating and has gradual weight loss. Pain in the back may indicate that the growth has extended into surrounding structures. Unfortunately, even if the patient reports to a physician when the first symptoms appear, the disease is often already well established, has metastasized, and is incurable. Diagnosis is made by radiographs of the esophagus taken as the patient swallows barium (Fig. 54-3) or by examination of tumor cells obtained during esophagoscopy.

Intervention

Treatment for cancer of the esophagus is surgical. If obvious metastasis is present or if the patient's physical condition is poor, only palliative surgery may be attempted. If major surgery is performed, the type of surgery depends on the site of the lesion. Upper thoracic lesions are resected through a right thoracotomy or thoracic abdominal incision. An *esophagogastrostomy*

(p. 1199) may be performed or a segment of colon may be anastomosed to the resected areas of the esophagus and stomach. Lower esophageal lesions are removed through a left thoracotomy or thoracic abdominal incision. The operation includes an *esophagogastrectomy*, splenectomy, and wide resection of lymph nodes. A major portion of the acid-secreting portion of the stomach is removed to reduce the occurrence of reflux esophagitis.

If the patient cannot tolerate major surgery or if the lesion is inoperable, a *gastrostomy* may be performed. Radiation therapy is sometimes used to inhibit growth of tumor cells.

Since the malignant lesion is seldom completely removed, only a small percentage of persons live more than 5 years after the surgery, and many are chronic invalids during that time. Both the patient and his significant others should be told of the need for close medical supervision. Persons with upper respiratory infections should be carefully avoided, and medical help should be sought at once if signs of even minor indisposition occur.

Many patients with cancer of the esophagus receive terminal care at home. The nurse who visits the patient in the home can often give helpful suggestions regarding the preparation of suitable food and care of the mouth.

Some persons with cancer of the esophagus are not found to be suitable candidates for esophageal surgery. Their skin care, mouth care, and nutrition are similar to that described for the person being prepared for esophageal surgery. As mentioned previously, a gastrostomy may be done as a palliative procedure, and care as described on p. 1200 is indicated.

□ Hiatus hernia (esophageal or diaphragmatic hernia)

There are three variations of hiatus hernia, but the *sliding hiatus hernia* is by far the most common and is now known to be one of the most common pathologic conditions of the upper gastrointestinal tract[37] (Fig. 54-4). In this condition, part of the stomach "slides" or follows the normal path of the esophagus through an enlarged hiatal opening in the diaphragm into the thorax. The cause of this abnormal enlargement may be trauma, congenital weakness, relaxation of ligaments of skeletal muscles, or increased abdominal pressure. Hiatus herniation can occur at any age but is more often found in persons who are middle aged or elderly. The condition is often misdiagnosed or diagnosis is delayed. Sometimes the hernia is not apparent when swallowing barium unless the patient is placed in a Trendelenburg position.

When a hiatus hernia develops, the function of the cardioesophageal sphincter is lost, permitting a reflux of unneutralized gastric juices into the esophagus, which in turn produces inflammation of the lower esophagus. If

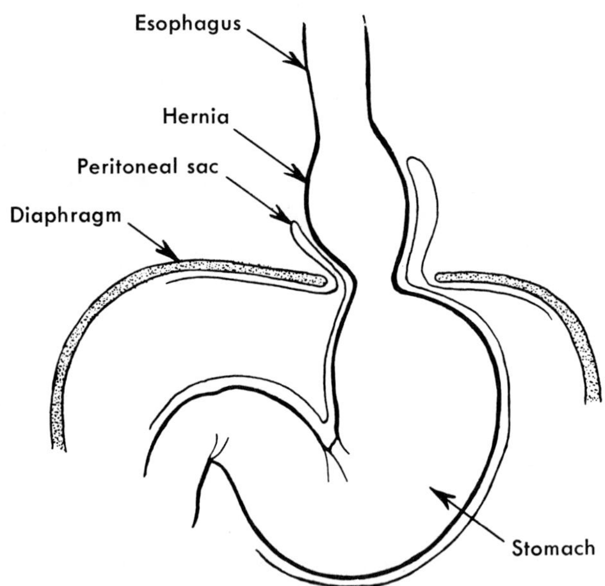

Fig. 54-4. Displacement of portion of cardia of stomach through normal hiatus into thoracic cavity (sliding hiatus hernia). (From Anderson, H. C.: Newton's geriatric nursing, ed. 5, St. Louis, 1971, The C. V. Mosby Co.)

this condition persists over weeks and months, ulceration occurs, accompanied by hemorrhage and formation of fibrous tissue. An occasional complication is incarceration of a portion of the stomach in the chest with constriction of the blood supply and possibly necrosis, causing peritonitis and mediastinitis. Another problem may be caused by regurgitation of gastric contents during sleep and subsequent aspiration into the lungs. The elderly person may visit his physician with signs of pneumonitis, since because his reflexes are less acute, he aspirates fluids into the lungs more easily than the younger person.

Clinical picture

Symptoms of hiatus hernia vary greatly. Some small hernias may cause no symptoms, whereas others cause the person serious difficulty. A frequent complaint is heartburn after meals and during the night. Heartburn and pain beneath the sternum may occur after meals, on physical exertion, particularly when bending forward is entailed, or on any sudden change of posture. Food may be regurgitated several hours after meals, and the patient may complain of the sensation of food "sticking" as he swallows (dysphagia).

Intervention

If the hiatus hernia causes no symptoms, treatment is usually not necessary. The treatment for hiatus hernia with symptoms may be either medical or surgical, depending on how well the hernia responds to medical treatment. Medical treatment of hiatus hernia includes a regular schedule of meals, avoiding highly seasoned foods, coffee, and fruit juices. The patient is instructed to eat slowly, to reduce weight if obese, and to avoid heavy weight lifting. He is advised to eat small meals, to avoid carbonated beverages, and to sit in an upright position during meals and for at least 2 hours thereafter. When the patient is in the hospital for other causes and there is no reason why he cannot sit upright, the head of the bed should be raised to an upright position for meals and left in this position for ½ hour following meals. Antacids such as aluminum hydroxide gel may be prescribed to be taken ½ hour after meals and at bedtime.

The problem of regurgitation of food during sleep can be minimized by elevating the head of the bed on 4- or 6-inch blocks and avoiding bedtime snacks. The patient is often advised to avoid wearing tight, constricting clothing about the waist. He should be taught to go about usual activities but give attention to changes in posture, particularly if they involve sharp forward bending. For example, in picking up an object from the floor, he should use proper body mechanics and stoop rather than bend from the waist. Kneeling rather than bending or even stooping may be better for some activities.

Hiatus hernia can be corrected surgically by repair that may involve entering the abdominal or the thoracic cavity to return the stomach to the abdominal cavity and to repair the diaphragm. Surgery is generally reserved for persons with unrelieved and persistent symptoms.

Outcome criteria for the person with a hiatus hernia

The patient or significant others can:

1. Describe any dietary changes required after discharge:
   a. Keep weight at normal level and if obese reduce weight.
   b. State the plan to be followed to assure adequate nutrition.
   c. Avoid foods that cause discomfort.
2. State body position and activity requirements (sitting position to aid in digestion; a method to provide elevation of the head of the bed while sleeping; and specific activities to be avoided such as heavy lifting, bending).
3. State the action, dosage, frequency, and possible side effects of medication (antacids) to be taken at home.
4. State symptoms to be reported to the physician (vomiting, substernal or thoracic pain, increasing dysphagia, increasing abdominal fullness).
5. State plans for follow-up care.

□ Surgery for esophageal disorders

When normal deglutition is descreased either by stricture, erosion, or tumor of the esophagus, maintenance of adequate nutrition is altered. The approach used to correct such problems is often a surgical resection, anastomosis, or a complete bypass of the affected part.

A *gastrostomy,* the insertion of a catheter through an abdominal incision into the stomach, will bypass the esophageal area and allow for feedings that are nutritionally sound. A gastrostomy is usually a permanent procedure but may be used temporarily for healing of the esophagus.

An *esophagectomy,* the removal of a section of or the entire esophagus with the insertion of a tissue or Dacron graft, allows the individual to return to near normal deglutition and subsequent nutrition.

An *esophagogastrostomy,* the resection of a portion of the esophagus with anastomosis, is generally performed for tumors of the lower one third of the esophagus. In some cases the stomach will be brought up into the chest cavity and the proximal end of the esophagus implanted into it. Other surgeons prefer to use a section of bowel as a tissue graft between the remaining esophagus and stomach. This procedure will allow for nearly normal deglutition and promote adequate nutrition.

An *esophagogastrectomy,* the removal of the lower esophagus and cardia of the stomach, is generally reserved for those individuals who have extensive malignant tumor infiltration. The remaining end of the esophagus and stomach are rejoined resulting in a smaller food reservoir although nearly normal deglutition remains.

Management of the patient requiring a gastrostomy

It is usually very difficult for the patient to accept the need for gastrostomy, probably partly because of the deep psychologic significance of food and eating. After a long period of vomiting, discomfort, and inability to eat, however, the patient may become so debilitated that both he and his family are willing for the surgery to be performed.

Surgery. The procedure is usually performed with the patient under local anesthesia. An opening is made into the stomach through a small upper left abdominal incision. The anterior wall of the stomach is exposed, drawn forward, and sutured to the anterior abdominal wall about the incision, thus preventing the stomach contents from entering the abdominal cavity. A small incision is then made into the stomach, and a catheter, tube, or special prosthesis such as the Barnes-Redo (Fig 54-5) is inserted into it. A Foley or mushroom catheter is

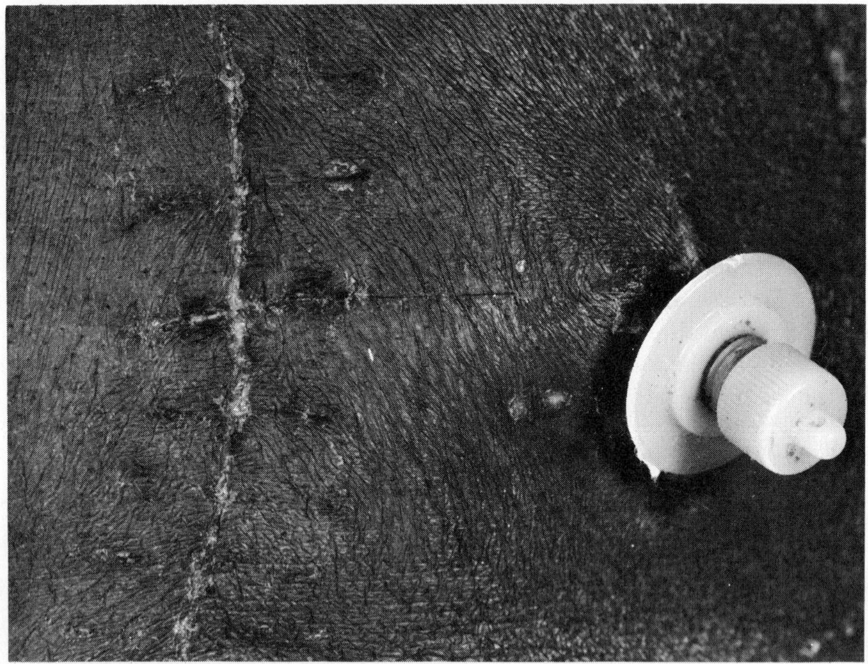

Fig. 54-5. Barnes-Redo prosthesis is sutured into gastrostomy opening. Cap can be unscrewed easily for tube feedings. (Courtesy Dr. William Barnes and Dr. Frank Redo.)

more often used. The opening is sutured tightly around the catheter so that leakage of stomach contents cannot occur, and the catheter is secured to the abdominal wall by a suture or adhesive tape to prevent its slipping out. A clamp is applied to the end of the catheter to prevent leakage of gastric secretions onto the skin. A small dressing covers the incision, and there should be very little bloody drainage postoperatively. Food can then be introduced directly into the stomach.

Postoperative care

Skin care. The skin around the gastrostomy is inspected frequently, because if there is leakage of gastric secretions around the tube, the skin will become irritated and excoriated from the action of the digestive enzymes. The skin is kept clean with frequent use of soap and water and is kept dry; a protective ointment such as zinc oxide or petrolatum gauze may be applied around the tube.

After 10 to 14 days the tube may be removed and reinserted only when food is given. The patient is taught to perform this procedure himself. The tube is kept clean by washing it with soap and water after each meal. It is inserted 10 to 15 cm (4 to 6 in). A catheter plug or rubber-tipped hemostat may be used to close the catheter and prevent leakage from the gastrostomy tube between meals. There is less likelihood of leakage if the patient relaxes for a short time after the meal and if the meals are not too large. If the Barnes-Redo prosthesis is used, a catheter is inserted into the shaft as far as it will go prior to giving the feeding.

Food and fluids. Soon after the operation, fluid nourishment may be given through the catheter. The initial meal, consisting of a small amount of tap water or glucose in water, is given followed by fluids every 4 hours. If there is no leakage of fluid around the tube and if the patient appears to tolerate the clear fluids, foods blended into a mixture may be added until a full diet is eventually given through the tube. The meal is warmed to room or body temperature before it is given and is diluted if too thick. It should be given with screens drawn about the patient for privacy if he does not occupy a single room. A funnel or syringe is used to introduce the liquid into the catheter. Before the meal is given, a small amount of water should be introduced through the tube to make sure it is patent. In order to prevent air from entering the stomach, the catheter should not be unplugged until the nurse is ready to give the feeding. The fluid should flow in by gravity. Sometimes a small amount of pressure from the bulb of the Asepto syringe or on the barrel of the syringe is necessary to pass thicker fluids through the tube. The usual amount of each meal is 200 to 500 ml and should take 10 to 15 minutes to flow through the tube. If the patient feels "full" or nauseated, meals may be decreased in amount and their frequency increased. A small amount of water is instilled to cleanse the tube at the end of the meal. In order to aid digestion the head of the bed should be elevated for at least ½ hour following a feeding.

The meals may be a special formula or regular food blended so that it will pass through the tube. The use of regular foods helps maintain the patient's nutritional state, prevents diarrhea that often accompanies the use of specially prepared tube feedings that are high in fat, and makes it easier for the patient and his family to prepare his food at home. Food that is normally cooked should be cooked until it is soft, and the juices from cooking should be included since they contain essential vitamins and minerals. Solid and liquid foods are blended into a mixture with a food blender, fork, potato masher, or egg beater and are strained. Water is given through the tube between feedings so that approximately 2,500 to 3,500 ml of fluids are received daily. If diarrhea occurs, camphorated tincture of opium (paregoric) may be ordered and given with the meal.

The patient should see, smell, taste, and chew small amounts of food before taking his feeding in order to stimulate the flow of gastric secretions and give him some of the satisfaction of normal eating. It is sometimes recommended that the patient chew his food normally and then deposit it into a funnel attached to the gastrostomy tube. If he can accept this sensible although somewhat unesthetic procedure, it is unquestionably beneficial because saliva is mixed with the food. The teeth and mouth also maintain better health. Privacy must, of course, be assured the patient who takes his meals in this way.

If the patient is not upset by sitting down to meals with his family when he cannot eat, he should be encouraged to do so, since this socializing usually helps his digestion and is good for his morale.

The psychologic trauma of not being able to eat normally is usually severe. The patient may become depressed, and he needs a great deal of encouragement. Most patients, however, as they become proficient in feeding themselves, gradually accept this method of obtaining nourishment as inevitable and adjust remarkably well.

Teaching. Both the patient and his family should learn how to care for the skin and the tube and how to prepare the liquid meals as well as how to insert the tube and instill the nourishment through it. They should be told of the need for close medical supervision, and they should be encouraged to consult the physician, the nurse, or the dietitian when problems arise. It may be desirable for a community health nurse to visit the patient at home to supervise the initial preparation of food and giving of the feeding and to answer any other questions in regard to the patient's care.

Outcome criteria for the person with a gastrostomy. The patient or significant others can:

1. Demonstrate how to prepare and introduce nutrients through the gastrostomy tube:
   a. Prepare food using the equipment that will be used in the home (blender).
   b. Prepare to receive the food by proper positioning.
   c. Introduce the nutrient into the tube without discomfort or irritation
   d. Clean the equipment and discuss how it will be stored at home.
2. Demonstrate how skin integrity around the tube will be maintained:
   a. Clamp tubes between feedings and state reason for this.
   b. Demonstrate how skin will be inspected daily.
   c. Discuss measures to be instituted if redness or soreness develops.
3. State how a nutritionally balanced diet and adequate fluid intake will be achieved:
   a. State amount of foods necessary to meet the dietary prescription (protein, carbohydrates, fats).
   b. List foods that may cause diarrhea or constipation.
   c. State when water will be given with feedings (before and after).
4. Discuss the emotional impact of the gastrostomy:
   a. Discuss plans for returning to activities of daily living.
   b. Discuss plans for joining others at mealtimes.
   c. State modifications that might be needed in clothing.
5. State plans for regular follow-up care:
   a. List symptoms requiring immediate medical assistance (dislodgement, occlusion, bleeding, or leakage of fluid around the opening).
   b. Identify community resources available to assist in care at home.

Management of the patient requiring esophageal surgery

Preoperative care

Food and fluids. If the nutritional status of the patient is poor, an attempt is made preoperatively to improve nutrition and to reestablish fluid and electrolyte balance. Glucose, amino acids, electrolytes, and vitamins usually are prescribed to be administered intravenously. Hyperalimentation (p. 321) may be necessary. An accurate record of the intake and output is mandatory, since this information is important in ordering fluids to be administered parenterally. If food and fluids can be taken orally, they should be high in protein and in total calories. Occasionally a temporary gastrostomy may be performed to supply food preoperatively. It is closed a few weeks after the esophageal resection if this operation has been successful in reestablishing a communication between the esophagus and the stomach.

Mouth care. Since the breath may be foul, special oral care should be given. The patient may raise a mixture of pus, blood, and decomposed food. He must be assured privacy when he is attempting to clear his throat and particularly when he is attempting to get food and fluids past the obstruction. The emesis basins should be changed often, and a cover should be provided. Mouthwashes are useful in making the mouth feel fresher and should be offered to the patient before he attempts to take food. They should be varied from time to time unless the patient has one he prefers, because sometimes the flavor of the solution becomes identified with the unpleasant throat secretions and becomes almost as distasteful as the secretions.

Preoperative teaching. Teaching includes instructions about chest drainage tubes, coughing and turning after the operation, postoperative exercises, restriction of oral fluids, oxygen, frequent observation of pulse and blood pressure, intravenous fluids, and the nasogastric tube.

Postoperative care. The immediate postoperative care for the patient who has had esophageal surgery centers about the maintenance of an airway, observation for circulatory or respiratory difficulties, protection from injury, care of the chest drainage system (p. 971), and care of the nasogastric tube (p. 1211).

Gastric drainage. Small amounts of bright red blood may drain from the nasogastric tube for a short time (6 to 12 hours). The color of the drainage should then become greenish yellow. Because esophageal tissue is very friable and because the anastomosis may be under tension, the tube is usually left in place until complete healing of the esophageal anastomosis has occurred.

Food and fluids. When the tube is removed, oral fluids are not usually permitted for several days. Fluids are given parenterally to meet fluid, electrolyte, and caloric needs. When fluids are permitted orally, a small amount of water (30 to 60 ml) is given hourly, and the patient is observed for signs of leakage of fluid into the mediastinum such as pain, a rise in temperature, and difficulty in breathing. If no untoward symptoms occur, foods are introduced and gradually increased until the patient is receiving several small meals of bland food daily. If an esophagogastrostomy has been performed, the patient may complain of a feeling of fullness in the chest or difficulty in breathing after eating. Smaller more frequent meals often help to relieve these problems.

When the cardia of the stomach has been removed, some patients complain of nausea and vomiting. This difficulty is usually caused by irritation of the esophageal mucosa by the gastric juices. After an esophagogastrostomy the gastric secretions flow readily into the esophagus when the patient lies flat. He should be advised to rest his head and shoulders on pillows when he lies down and to eat in an upright position.

Activity. Resumption of activity must be gradual. If the patient has had extensive surgery of the esophagus for cancer, he may require several months of convalescence.

Outcome criteria for the person with esophageal surgery. The patient or significant others can:

1. Determine a specific plan for dietary modification that maintains an adequate intake of nutrients and fluids.
2. State specific position and activity requirements (see outcome criteria for esophageal disorders, (p. 1197).
3. List name, dosage, frequency, action, and side effects of medications to be taken at home.
4. Demonstrate exercises to be done at home (exercises to be followed after thoracic surgery).
5. Discuss the emotional impact of the surgery and plan for the future.
6. State plans for follow-up care:
   a. State signs or symptoms requiring institution of specific therapy or contact with physician (respiratory infection, pain, hemoptysis, hematemesis, weight loss, increasing dysphagia).

■ GASTRIC DISORDERS

□ Gastritis

Gastritis is an inflammation of the gastric mucosa and is the most common pathologic condition of the stomach. It may be acute or chronic, based on histologic criteria. Acute gastritis may be caused by exogenous or endogenous factors. The exogenous factors include (1) bacterial infections, especially staphylococcal endotoxins; (2) drugs such as alcohol, salicylates, indomethacin, sulfonamides, and steroids; (3) ingestion of corrosive substances (acid and alkali); (4) irritating foods; and (5) thermal or mechanical injuries.[12] Endogenous factors include certain infectious diseases such as typhoid fever and viral hepatitis and allergic and systemic diseases that affect the cells of the gastric mucosa.

The diagnosis is made by histologic evidence obtained from gastric biopsy. The flexible, fiberoptic gastroscope makes repeated biopsies possible. In acute gastritis the gastric mucosa appears red, inflamed, congested, and edematous. Acute episodes may become chronic, and various pathologic changes occur depending on the site involved. In *atrophic gastritis* there is atrophy of gastric glands and the appearance of patches of thin, gray or greenish gray mucosa and red or blue blood vessels of the submucosa on the fundus and body of the stomach. The loss of gastric mucosa will result in eventual diminution of gastric secretion and the development of pernicious anemia. Persons with a positive Schilling test (p. 1065) will receive Vitamin B_{12} for about 3 months.[12]

Clinical picture

The symptoms depend on the cause of the gastritis and its severity. Some persons have only mild gastric discomfort or pain, while others have severe nausea and vomiting. In *acute hemorrhagic gastritis* the person complains of epigastric discomfort, nausea, hematemesis, and melena. There may be a severe drop in the hemoglobin and hematocrit levels. In *corrosive gastritis* caused by acid or lyes there will be bloody vomitus, bloody stools, and collapse. Death may occur secondary to blood loss or perforation of a viscus. Those who recover will have an obstruction later on.

Intervention

The treatment will depend on the cause of the gastritis and the initial symptoms. Mild gastritis requires only a carminative antacid and rest. Belching and defecation often relieve the symptoms.

When nausea and vomiting are present, the person is given nothing by mouth until symptoms subside. With severe vomiting fluids and electrolytes will be replaced intravenously and a sedative such as sodium phenobarbital or an antinauseant such as prochlorperazine (Compazine) or trimethobenzamide (Tigan) will be given parenterally or by suppository. When vomiting subsides tea, broth, and gingerale are given orally every hour. Bland feedings of custard, gelatin, and cream soups are usually tolerated after 12 to 24 hours, then other foods are added gradually. It may be 1 to 2 weeks before all symptoms subside and a normal diet can be resumed. Persons with epigastric discomfort will also receive antacids. When an infectious agent is the cause, appropriate antimicrobial therapy is prescribed.

Persons who develop chronic gastritis will usually respond to an ulcer regimen of a bland diet and antacids. They must avoid salicylates, caffeine, spices, and alcoholic beverages. Many will be advised to avoid smoking. If symptoms do not respond to this therapy, a vagotomy may be necessary. Persistent symptoms are monitored closely, and gastroscopy with biopsy is necessary to rule out malignancy.

Outcome criteria for the person with chronic gastritis. The patient or significant others can:

1. List substances that cause recurrence of the condition and should be avoided (alcohol, aspirin, spicy foods).
2. Discuss plans for a diet that meets nutritional requirements and is nonirritating:
   a. Plan for adquate protein, carbohydrate, fat, minerals, and vitamins.
   b. Plan for frequent feedings during times of added stress.
3. Describe the medication program to be followed at home:
   a. State dosage, action, and side effects of prescribed medications such as antacids.
   b. List over-the-counter medications that are to be avoided such as aspirin and aspirin-containing compounds such as Alka-Seltzer.
4. State plans for follow-up care:
   a. List community resources available to those with alcohol dependence if this is a problem.
   b. State signs and symptoms that indicate need for immediate medical assistance (recurrence of symptoms, especially nausea and vomiting, hematemesis, or bloody stools).

□ Peptic ulcer

Pathophysiology

A peptic ulcer is an ulceration involving the mucosa and deeper structure and is due in part to action of the acid gastric juices. The acid induces a chemical inflammation that lowers the pain threshold of the nerve endings in the margins and in the base of the ulcer. Vascular engorgement with or without acute inflammation further decreases the threshold for pain.

The site of the peptic ulcer may be the distal esophagus, stomach, upper duodenum, or the jejunum (Fig. 54-6). Peptic ulcers are described as gastric or duodenal depending on their location. An ulcer (usually of the jejunum) occurring near the site of anastomosis is termed a *marginal* ulcer. Most gastric ulcers occur on the lesser curvature of the stomach. Such ulcers tend to be larger and deeper than duodenal ulcers, and they

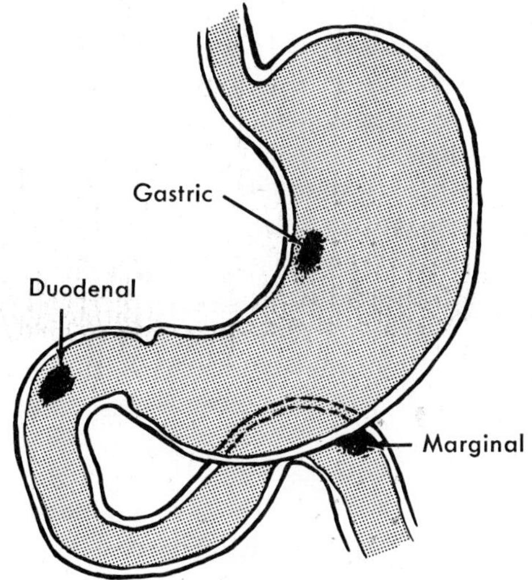

Fig. 54-6. Most common locations of peptic ulcers.

have a tendency to undergo malignant changes. Duodenal ulcers are not as well defined as gastric ulcers, but the pathology is the same. Most of them occur on the first part of the duodenum and are more common than gastric ulcers.

Gastric hyperacidity is common in persons with *duodenal* ulcers along with an increased emptying rate of the stomach. Protein is a food substance that normally acts as a buffer for gastric acid. When the stomach empties more rapidly, this buffering mechanism is decreased and more gastric acid moves into the duodenum. In *gastric* ulcers gastric hyperacidity is not necessarily a factor, and the stomach empties at a normal rate. Gastritis is a common finding, and reflux of duodenal contents back into the stomach may be a contributing factor.[22]

Acute ulcers are usually superficial, involving only the mucosal layer. In most cases they heal within a relatively short time, but they may bleed, perforate, or become chronic.

A chronic peptic ulcer is a deep crater with sharp edges and a "clean" base. It involves both the mucosa and the submucosa. If the ulcer penetrates the stomach wall and becomes adherent to an adjacent organ such as the pancreas, the organ may become the base of the ulcer.

Zollinger-Ellison syndrome, first described in 1955, refers to the peptic ulceration associated with a noninsulin-producing islet cell tumor of the pancreas.[49] The syndrome is characterized by one or more peptic ulcerations occurring in the lower end of the esophagus, stomach, duodenum, and jejunum and by enormous gastric hypersecretion and acidity and the presence of nonbeta islet cell adenomas of the pancreas. Frequently the syndrome is accompanied by diarrhea and steatorrhea. The latter is thought due to lack of pancreatic lipase needed for fat digestion, whereas the diarrhea may result from large quantities of acid passing into the duodenum. Diarrhea of long duration can cause serious loss of electrolytes (potassium and sodium in particular) and may prove fatal.

These tumors of the pancreas have been found to produce enormous quantities of gastrin or a gastrinlike substance that is responsible for the excessive stimulation of gastric acid and the subsequent ulcerations. Because of the repeated reappearance of the peptic ulcers and the multiple and aberrant locations, it is usually impossible to resect all areas involved.

Epidemiology

It is believed that 10% of the male population suffer from peptic ulcer sometime during their lifetime. Peptic ulcer occurs four times as commonly in men as in women, but the incidence in women seems to be increasing. At the present time peptic ulcer of the stomach and duodenum afflicts more than 10 million citizens of the United States and is most common in persons between 20 and 60 years of age. The incidence of peptic ulcer as well as the number of people who die of the disease are steadily increasing.

The cause of peptic ulcer is not known, but it is believed that there are three factors that greatly influence its development: a source of irritation such as an increase of hydrochloric acid with a decrease of alkaline mucus secreted by the surface cells; a breakdown of the local tissue resistance and defense mechanisms, and the influences of heredity, hormones, and personality. The hormones appear to have some effect on ulcer formation, since ulcers are more prevalent in men than in women. In Zollinger-Ellison syndrome a gastrinlike hormone released by the noninsulin-producing islet cell tumor of the pancreas is known to produce extreme gastric hypersecretion and hyperacidity and severe recurrent peptic ulceration.[15]

Certain so-called ulcerogenic drugs such as corticotropin and the adrenocorticosteroids, the salicylates, and phenylbutazone (Butazolidin) are known to contribute to the development of peptic ulcers in some patients. The mechanism of these ulcerogenic drugs is varied. With the antiinflammatory steroids, it involves mucosal injury secondary to increased gastric acid secretion and reduced gastric mucus secretion. The latter is due to the steroid antiprotein synthetic action. With aspirin there is an increased exfoliation of mucous cells and a decrease in mucus production.[24]

The tendency for ulcers runs in families. It has been demonstrated that emotional factors influence the function of the stomach and cause changes in the gastric mucosa. Persons who are under continuous pressure and who are nervous, tense, perfectionists, or unhappy may develop symptoms of peptic ulcers. It has not been proved, however, whether these symptoms truly follow or precede the development of the ulcer.

Stress ulcers

Persons who are undergoing major stress as from sepsis, severe trauma, burns, or other life-threatening conditions are prone to develop stress ulcers. Patients in intensive care units should be monitored closely for bleeding and hemorrhage, which commonly occur about 7 to 10 days after injury or surgery. The cause of stress ulcers is not well understood, although several factors such as ischemia of the bowel and hypoxia have been proposed.[5]

Clinical picture

The person who has a peptic ulcer usually complains of pain that is characteristic in its nature, intensity, radiation, location, and periodicity. Initial attacks of pain often occur in the spring and the fall, last for a few weeks, and then disappear. Each succeeding attack is more severe and more prolonged than the preceding one. The pain is described as gnawing, aching, or burning. It is usually located in the upper abdomen, near the midline, and it is usually confined to a small area. However, it may radiate around the costal border or to the back. Pain from a duodenal ulcer is usually located in the right epigastric area, whereas that from a gastric ulcer is usually located in the left epigastric area. Pain usually starts 1 to 2 hours after eating, when the stomach begins to empty, and it may disappear spontaneously, after the ingestion of food, or after the ingestion of an antacid medication such as aluminum hydroxide gel. If the ulcer is severe it may cause pain at night. It is not unusual for the person to awaken with pain during the night, when gastric secretion is at its peak.[51]

Although pain is felt at the site of the existing lesion, it is known that normal stomach mucosa does not have pain sensation. It is thought therefore that the inflamed mucosa around the ulcer must be sensitive to the gastric secretions because inflammation lowers the pain threshold.[5] Eructation is common in peptic ulcer but differs from that occurring in gallbladder disease in that it occurs more often when the stomach is empty and does not follow the ingestion of fatty foods. When edema around the lesion obstructs the pylorus, gastric retention with dilation of the stomach occurs causing nausea and vomiting. This occurrence, however, is not common in peptic ulcer.

The diagnosis of peptic ulcer is made from the patient's history, a gastrointestinal series, a gastric analysis, and stool examinations for occult (hidden) blood. Direct visualization of the ulcer by endoscopy differentiates gastric ulcer from gastric carcinoma. Development of the flexible fiberoptic panendoscope (p. 1162) has greatly improved the diagnosis and evaluation of healing of gastric ulcers. Selective angiography is becoming useful in the diagnosis and evaluation of treatment of gastric hemorrhage when it is combined with endoscopy.

Intervention

Treatment is directed toward relief of symptoms, healing of the ulcer, prevention of complications, and prevention of recurrence. The majority of peptic ulcers heal under medical treatment. Surgery is used most often following a second or third recurrence and in the treatment of complications.

Treatment consists in the use of antacids and anticholinergic medications to relieve pain, avoidance of known causative or irritating drugs and foods, and an attempt to decrease stress by rest and counseling. New medications are showing some promise by increasing the rate of healing.

Antacids. Drugs that decrease ulcer pain by lowering the acidity of gastric secretions have been used for many years. Antacids reduce gastric acidity by physical absorption or by chemical neutralization. They do not hasten healing, but do appear clinically to decrease pain. Antacids of choice are the nonsystemic antacids (Table 54-1), which are poorly absorbed from the stomach and therefore do not alter the pH of the blood or interfere with normal acid-base balance. Sodium bicarbonate is readily absorbed and therefore should be avoided as an antacid for relief of ulcer pain. Also the reaction of sodium bicarbonate and hydrochloric acid forms carbon dioxide, which may cause distention.

Antacids may be administered frequently, and if symptoms are severe it may be necessary to give them as often as every 30 to 60 minutes. When given in a fasting state, the buffering power is usually transitory. For maximum effectiveness antacids should be given *1 hour* after meals; this produces a buffering effect lasting approximately 3 to 4 hours.[22] Liquids are more effective than tablets. If tablets are used they should be chewed slowly to permit complete pulverization. Aluminum hydroxide becomes less reactive over time and should not be given with anticholinergic drugs or with tetracycline as it interferes with absorption of these drugs.

Anticholinergic drugs. Drugs used to decrease gastric motility are anticholinergic agents of the belladonna group. These drugs are very effective in relieving nocturnal pain. Most of the drugs presently used as antispasmodics are synthetic substitutes for atropine. Some of the more commonly used are methscopolamine bromide (Pamine Bromide), methantheline bromide (Banthine Bromide), propantheline bromide (Pro-Banthine Bromide), pipenzolate methylbromide (Piptal), and atropine sulfate–phenobarbital–hyoscyamine hydrobromide (Donnatol). Side effects include dryness of the mouth, blurred vision, headache, constipation, urinary retention, palpitation, and flushing and dryness of the skin. When given to relieve ulcer pain, anticholinergic drugs are usually prescribed in dosages that do produce some side effects such as a dry mouth. The physician may change the antispasmodic in order to produce the fewest untoward effects for the person. If anticholinergic drugs are given *30 minutes* before meals, the effect is longer lasting as gastric acid produced by the effect of the food is inhibited.

Histamine antagonist. *Cimetidine* is a new drug that decreases secretion of gastric acid by inhibiting the action of histamine at the histamine H_2 receptors of the parietal cells.[21] Cimetidine is not an antihistamine drug. It has been demonstrated to produce an increased healing effect on ulcers in addition to a decrease of symp-

Table 54-1. Commonly used antacids

Trade name	Drug composition	Comments
Maalox	Magnesium and aluminum hydroxide	Preferred antacid Good buffering effect Good taste Nonconstipating Low sodium content Can cause hypermagnesemia in persons with renal failure
Maalox Plus	Magnesium and aluminum hydroxide Simethicone	Same as above Antiflatus
Mylanta	Magnesium and aluminum hydroxide Simethicone	Same as Maalox Plus
Amphogel	Aluminum hydroxide gel	Constipating Can interfere with absorption of anticholinergic drugs Contains sodium Decreases absorption of phosphate Good antacid effect Give with water so that medication reaches stomach Can be given by continuous drip (1 part amphogel to 2 or 3 parts water)
Gelusil	Magnesium trisilicate Magnesium and aluminum hydroxide	Slower buffering effect Gelatin effect in stomach to coat and protect the ulcer Nonconstipating
Riopan	Magaldrate (chemical combination of magnesium and aluminum hydroxide)	Rapid antacid action High acid-buffering effect No acid rebound Nonconstipating Low sodium content Can cause hypermagnesemia in persons with renal failure
Marblen	Magnesium and calcium carbonate Aluminum hydroxide Magnesium trisilicate	Neutralizes more acid than other antacids Nonconstipating Low sodium content
Alka-2	Calcium carbonate	Rapid neutralization of acid Constipating May cause hypercalcemia May cause acid rebound Not suitable for long-term therapy

toms. No effect on the recurrence of ulcers has been noted, but both day and night pain are decreased, thus decreasing the use of antacids. For persons with Zollinger-Ellison syndrome, diarrhea and anorexia are decreased. Cimetidine therapy may extend for 8 weeks. Side effects include muscle pain, transient diarrhea, dizziness, and rash. Cimetidine is given in dosages of 300 mg four times a day (with meals and at bedtime). The person should be encouraged to continue therapy for the prescribed period even when symptoms have abated.

Other drugs. *Carbenoxolene*, an extract of licorice, has been reported to hasten gastric healing by increasing the production and viscosity of gastric mucus. The drug is structurally similar to aldosterone, and side effects include hypertension, fluid retention, and hypokalemia. A thiazide diuretic may be given to counteract the side effects. *Prostaglandins* are also being studied for their effect on inhibition of acid secretion.

Diet. Over the years many theories and diet prescriptions have been suggested for the treatment of peptic ulcers. Modified *Sippy* diets are based on the acid-buffering power of food proteins. Constant dilution and neutralization of stomach contents are achieved by giving whole milk, skim milk, and half milk–half cream punctually every hour. Bland foods are then added at specified intervals. *Bland* diets (diets that exclude "irritating" foods) have also been used. The interpretation of what constitutes a bland diet differs from hospital to hospital and from one part of the country to another.

There is no experimental evidence that modifying the diet accelerates healing of an uncomplicated peptic ulcer.[5] Spices such as pepper or roughage foods such as bran have not been shown to be ulcerogenic, although they may not be tolerated by some persons. Substances that have been demonstrated to increase acid secretions are caffeine-containing beverages such as coffee, tea, and cola drinks. Individuals may find that certain foods increase ulcer pain; if so, these foods should be avoided. Eating frequent small feedings provides an acid neutralizing effect. Overdistention of the stomach should be avoided also as this predisposes to reflux.

If milk and antacids are given by continuous tube feeding for severe symptoms, the prescribed amount is spaced over the 24-hour period and must include sufficient water to supply the patient's daily needs. Only a small amount of milk is placed in the dispensing bag at one time to prevent the milk from becoming sour. A mechanical food pump may also be used.

Rest. Both physical and mental rest are necessary for the healing of a peptic ulcer. It may take the combined efforts of health professionals and significant others to help the person understand the need for complete rest and to secure his cooperation in achieving it. Since rest means different things to different people, the person is assisted in identifying those activities that specifically achieve mental and physical rest for him.

If the person has severe pain or complications that do not respond to treatment at home, hospitalization will be necessary. Nursing care that provides a regular, smooth routine is the goal. Meals, medications, and treatments need to be given at correctly spaced intervals and on time. Noise, rush, confusion, and impatience on the part of members of the staff are avoided.

Surgery. Treatment of recurrent ulcers is primarily surgical. The lowest rate of recurrence occurs following vagotomy with antrectomy. (See p. 1212 for further discussion of gastric surgery.)

Preventive health teaching. The person with an ulcer needs to understand about factors that contribute to the development of ulcers and about excesses in his life style that may cause the ulcer to become reactivated. If he cannot remove himself from stressful environmental influences, he must learn to accept the stressful situations without reactivating the ulcer. Occasionally the person is advised to obtain psychologic counseling so that he may understand his problems better and thus be better able to cope with them.

The person should practice moderation in diet and activities of work and play. Dietary teaching should include avoidance of situations that cause emotional stress before and during meals. Meals should be eaten slowly in a quiet environment. The work situation sometimes makes the selection and eating of suitable meals difficult. If the selection of food is limited, the person can take milk in a vacuum bottle to supplement the limited selection. If he becomes emotionally upset by situations at work or at home, he can eat frequent feedings and drink milk between meals. These measures may prevent a serious exacerbation of the ulcer. Alcohol should be avoided as much as possible as it tends to increase the secretion of acid and is irritating to the gastric mucosa, particularly if taken on an empty stomach. Some physicians allow their patients to take small amounts of alcohol with their meals.

There seems to be a relationship between smoking and irritation of a peptic ulcer; therefore most physicians believe that the person who has a peptic ulcer should give up smoking permanently. To do so is often very difficult, since often the person's life and work situations as well as his personality are such that a change of this sort is a major one. For some persons the stress of trying to give up smoking causes greater irritation of the ulcer than does the smoking. These persons are permitted to continue smoking, but moderation is strictly advised.

Ulcerogenic drugs such as salicylates, corticosteroids, and phenylbutazone are contraindicated for persons with history of peptic ulcer. Medication such as acetaminophen (Tylenol) and Ascriptin (aspirin and magnesium aluminum hydroxide) can be used safely for relief of mild pain.

If every consideration is given to adjusting the prescribed regimen to fit the physical, economic, and social pattern of the person with an ulcer, he will be better able to follow the treatment. Some individuals may not appear to benefit from the dietary modifications, medications, and counseling, and they return to the hospital or outpatient health center several times a year. These persons require the same careful attention as that given to the newly diagnosed patient so that any underlying feelings of staff rejection are avoided.

The person who has had a peptic ulcer must remain under medical supervision for about a year. He may have periodic x-ray examinations of the stomach to determine the extent to which the ulcer was healed. After that time, if healing is complete, he should be advised to report to his physician at once if symptoms reappear, since peptic ulcers can recur after the person has enjoyed several years of good health.

Complications

A peptic ulcer may perforate the stomach wall, cause an obstruction at the pyloric end of the stomach, or perforate a major blood vessel causing hemorrhage.

Perforation. Acute perforation of a peptic ulcer is a surgical emergency and is the most frequent cause of death in patients with peptic ulcer. Between 1% and 2% of all ulcers will perforate. After the perforation occurs, gastric contents pour into the peritoneal cavity, causing peritonitis. Both gastric and duodenal ulcers may perforate.

The patient who has a perforated ulcer has symptoms similar to those occurring when any abdominal organ or other part of the gastrointestinal tract perforates. The extremely irritating qualities of the gastric contents released into the abdominal cavity, however, may be quite overwhelming and lead to prostration and severe shock in a short time. There is a sudden sharp pain that spreads quickly over the abdomen. Characteristically, the patient bends over with pain and draws up his knees to prevent pull on the abdominal wall. He is reluctant to move, holds himself tense, and protests against having his abdomen touched. On palpation the abdomen is found to be boardlike and very tender. The patient usually perspires profusely, and his facial expression is one of agony and apprehension. Since his breathing is rapid and shallow to prevent pull on abdominal muscles, he may be cyanotic. The patient's temperature is usually normal or subnormal, and his pulse is usually rapid and weak. A positive diagnosis is made by taking a radiograph of the abdomen with the patient standing. If the ulcer has perforated, air under the diaphragm is visible on the film. It is important for the nurse to remember that patients taking corticosteroids may develop a peptic ulcer and perforation without exhibiting any of the usual symptoms.

Some perforations are minor and close within a short time or wall themselves off. However, most perforations require surgery and should be closed surgically as soon as possible. The longer the perforation exists, allowing the irritating (and infected) gastrointestinal secretions to pour into the abdominal cavity, the higher the mortality becomes.

Immediate therapy consists of passing a nasogastric tube connecting it to continuous suction to drain gastric contents. Following the initial emptying of the stomach, the suction is generally returned to the intermittent level. Nothing is given orally. Parenteral fluids are given to combat fluid and electrolyte imbalance, and antibiotics are administered. The patient is kept in a low Fowler's position so that the gastric contents that have escaped will collect in the pelvic cavity and will be more accessible surgically. The patient is very frightened and apprehensive and the nurse should stay with him to explain what is being done, what will be done in surgery, and to offer reassurance.

The operation used to close a perforation consists of suturing the opening and reinforcing the area with a omental graft; it is known as a *plicating* operation. The gastric contents that have escaped into the peritoneal cavity are aspirated by suction during the operation. A solution containing antibiotics may be placed in the abdominal cavity before the abdomen is closed. In selected patients, *gastric resection, vagotomy* and *antrectomy*, or *vagotomy* and *pyloroplasty* may be performed (p. 1212). Some physicians believe that early perforations seal rapidly if the stomach is kept empty by continuous gastric aspiration and if the patient is maintained on intravenous fluids and antibiotics.

Postoperatively the patient should be watched carefully for signs of continuing peritonitis and for abscess formation. Elevation of temperature, respiratory distress, continued abdominal pain, and signs of paralytic ileus such as distention, hyperactive or absent bowel sounds, and the inability to pass flatus or stool should be reported to the physician. The physician may also perform periodic rectal examinations to determine the presence of pelvic masses caused by abscess formation. Such an abscess may need to be incised and drained. The nurse should explain to the patient why the rectal examinations are necessary. (A full discussion of the complications of peritonitis is given on p. 1285.)

Pyloric obstruction. Pyloric obstruction may be caused by edema of tissues around an ulcer or by scar tissue from a healed ulcer located near the pylorus. It may be only partial and cause dilation of the stomach, or it may be complete. Persons with this complication may have severe projectile vomiting that may or may not be preceded by nausea. A positive diagnosis is made by gastrointestinal tract x-ray examination and gastric analysis. Obstruction caused by edema and spasm generally responds to medical management. A nasogastric tube is passed and connected to gastric suction or may be clamped and aspirated twice daily. Sometimes continuous-drip feedings of milk and cream are given to neutralize the stomach secretion and permit the running for several hours (commonly 8), the tube will be clamped for 15 to 30 minutes and the stomach contents aspirated to see how much of the feeding has passed through the pylorus. If the patient does not vomit during the continuous feeding it can be assumed that the feeding is passing through the pylorus and that the obstruction will respond to medical treatment. If the patient does vomit, the nasogastric tube will be attached to intermittent suction and fluids and electrolytes will be given intravenously.

When the obstruction is relieved and the patient's condition permits, surgery may be performed. The operation performed is usually a gastric resection involving the pylorus or the antrum section of the stomach with a part of the duodenum. Either a Billroth I or II procedure or a gastroenterostomy and vagotomy may be performed (p. 1212).

Hemorrhage. Peptic ulcers cause bleeding in about 15% to 20% of all persons who have the disease.[5] If the ulcer has perforated a major blood vessel, the patient may have a severe hemorrhage, vomiting large amounts of blood and passing tarry stools. Vomiting of blood usually occurs with a gastric ulcer, whereas tarry stools are more common with a bleeding duodenal ulcer. It must be remembered, however, that the color of the stool may depend more on the length of time the blood has been within the intestine than on the actual source of the hemorrhage. About 25% of patients with hemorrhage have never had recognizable symptoms of ulcer previously.[5]

The patient may also complain of feeling faint, dizzy, and thirsty. He may become dyspneic, apprehensive, and restless as the blood volume is reduced, the blood pressure drops, the pulse rate increases, and signs of shock become apparent. The systemic signs of hemorrhage may appear before (or without) hematemesis and before passage of blood or tarry stools.

The patient with a bleeding ulcer is placed on bed rest and is given a sedative such as phenobarbital sodium to alleviate restlessness and apprehension. Morphine sulfate may be used, since it aids rest and also helps to slow down intestinal peristalsis. Anticholinergic drugs are not given as they obscure signs of bleeding (hyperactive bowel sounds). The blood pressure, pulse rate, and respirations are checked and recorded frequently (as often as every 15 minutes when acute bleeding is suspected). Blood transfusions are often given slowly to avoid increasing the blood pressure and thereby increasing the bleeding. Vital signs and urinary output are monitored frequently to determine the body's response to fluid replacement and possible continuation of the hemorrhage.

If the patient is not vomiting and only a small amount of blood is being passed rectally, he is given milk every hour and antacids are prescribed. A full bland diet may be ordered because it maintains nutrition, neutralizes gastric acidity, reduces absorption of the formed clot, and slows peristalsis. If the patient is vomiting blood, however, he is given nothing orally. All bloody vomitus should be measured and described. The physician may wish it saved for inspection. A nasogastric tube may be passed and attached to suction to collect the blood so that it can be more accurately measured and replaced by transfusion. The fluid and electrolyte balance are maintained by infusions. Sometimes there is an order to irrigate the tube with iced physiologic saline solution or iced tap water or a combination of iced saline and water. If so, the irrigating fluid usually must be suctioned back, as the iced fluid caused blood to clot not only in the stomach but also within the tube. The pateint who is vomiting blood will need special mouth care. A weak solution of hydrogen peroxide may be used to more easily remove blood from the tongue, teeth, and gums.

The number of tarry (or currant jelly-like) stools should also be measured and recorded, and they may be saved for laboratory examination. Since the patient may be alarmed at the sight of blood, all evidence of bleeding is quickly removed from the bedside, and the linen is changed as needed without disturbing the patient any more than necessary. The patient should be told that he is receiving blood transfusions to replace the blood he has lost and that rest and quiet will help stop the bleeding. The sedative or narcotic should be given regularly to allay anxiety and apprehension. If large doses of sedative and narcotic drugs are given, attention must be taken to turning the patient hourly and encouraging him to breathe deeply to prevent the possibility of respiratory congestion.

The mortality from upper gastrointestinal tract hemorrhage is about 10% and is more common in those over 50 years of age. Bleeding gastric ulcers are more likely to result in a fatal outcome than are bleeding duodenal ulcers because those with gastric ulcers are usually older and the bleeding from gastric ulcers tends to be more severe.[5] Of those who survive hemorrhage, 30% to 50% will hemorrhage again.

The operations performed for continued or massive hemorrhage include partial gastric resection; excision of the ulcer, if possible, and ligation of the bleeding vessel; and vagotomy and pyloroplasty for bleeding duodenal ulcers in patients who are poor risks.

The general principles of nursing a patient after gastric surgery are applicable (p. 1214). The drainage from the nasogastric tube is usually dark red for 6 to 12 hours after surgery. It should turn greenish yellow within 24 hours. The patient may continue to pass tarry stools for several days postoperatively, but this is usually because the blood from the hemorrhage before surgery has not yet completely passed through the gastrointestinal tract.

Outcome criteria for the person with a peptic ulcer

The patient or significant others can:

1. Describe plans for dietary management (not going for long times without eating, avoiding irritating foods).

2. Explain the need to be relaxed while eating (not eating on the run).
3. Explain the need for planned rest periods following food ingestion.
4. Describe medication program to be followed at home:
   a. Describe dosage, action, and possible side effects of medications (antacids, antispamodics, tranquilizers).
   b. Discuss need to keep antacids at work or with them.
   c. State when the dosage and timing of the antacids may be safely and therapeutically increased (dietary indiscretion).
   d. List over-the-counter medications that are not used unless specifically ordered (aspirin products, scopolamine derivatives, bicarbonate of soda).
5. Discuss ways by which home and work environment can be structured so that stressors are kept at a reasonable level.
6. Describe how to obtain professional and community resources necessary to structure a satisfactory life style.
7. List symptoms requiring medical follow-up (return of previous symptoms, onset of symptoms suggesting perforation or bleeding).
8. State plans for health maintenance and follow-up care.

□ Cancer of the stomach

Cancer of the stomach is responsible for approximately 14,000 deaths each year in the United States, or a little less than 8% of the deaths from cancer. The incidence has continued to decrease in the United States over recent years, although the reason for this is unknown. There is a high incidence of stomach cancer in Japan, thought to be related to the high intake of smoked and dried salted fish or meats. Despite a decrease in the number of cases of stomach carcinoma in the United States, the overall outcome is not encouraging. Stomach cancer is inoperable in between 10% and 15% of persons by the time they are seen by a surgeon, and the overall 5-year survival rate for those who undergo surgery is only about 25%.[12]

Stomach cancer is found more often after the age of 45 years and is more common in men than in women. Hereditary factors are influential in its development, and chronic gastritis and chronic gastric ulcers are thought to be precursors.

Cancer may develop in any part of the stomach but is found most often in the distal third. It may spread directly through the stomach wall into adjacent tissues, to the lymphatics, to the regional lymph nodes of the stomach, to the esophagus, spleen, pancreas, and liver, or through the bloodstream to the bones. Involvement of regional lymph nodes occurs early and is found in about 60% to 75% of all patients in whom the cancer would seem to be curable at the time of surgery.

Cancer of the stomach occurs three times more frequently in persons who have pernicious anemia than in others. This is primarily due to achlorhydria associated with chronic gastritis and gastric atrophy.

Clinical picture

Unfortunately the person with cancer of the stomach usually has no symptoms until the growth spreads to adjacent organs. Symptoms may occur only after the disease has become incurable. Vague and persistent symptoms of gastric distress, flatulence, loss of appetite, nausea, gradual weight loss, and loss of strength may be the only complaints of the patient. These vague symptoms should never be ignored, and the person should be encouraged to seek immediate medical advice. However, since such symptoms are not necessarily symptoms of cancer, the person should not be unduly frightened. Pain does not appear usually until late in the disease, and the absence of this symptom is often the reason for the delay in seeking medical help. If the disease progresses untreated, marked cachexia develops, and eventually a palpable mass can often be felt in the region of the stomach. Often no early gastric symptoms appear, and fatigue and persistent anemia may be the only signs.

A positive diagnosis of gastric carcinoma is usually made by means of a gastrointestinal tract x-ray series. The tumor may not be evident in its early stages, and the x-ray examinations may have to be repeated at intervals. Gastroscopy is used to determine the type and site of the lesion. It also may identify small lesions not visible on x-ray film. An absence of free hydrochloric acid in stomach secretions obtained by gastric aspiration is suggestive of a gastric neoplasm. Gastric cytologic studies may demonstrate the presence of malignant cells in the stomach. Occult blood is frequently found in the stools.

Intervention

Preoperative preparation includes antibiotic bowel preparation (p. 1281) and decompression when there are symptoms of gastric outlet obstruction. The operative treatment for cancer of the stomach is either a subtotal gastrectomy or a total gastrectomy (p. 1212). Whichever procedure is used, the omentum and the spleen usually are also removed because of the common occurrence of metastasis to these areas. A total gastrectomy is never done when signs of metastasis to other abdominal organs such as the liver are evident. A palliative resection of the stomach is usually done for patients who have cancer of the stomach with metastases. Radiation therapy is sometimes used, but for cancer in this location it is of limited use. Chemotherapy usually is not effective in treating gastric carcinoma but may be helpful in controlling massive ascites.[12]

□ Pyloric stenosis

Pyloric stenosis in the adult is usually the result of previous duodenal ulceration or carcinoma. It is one of the most common conditions requiring surgery in infancy. It occurs most often in tense infants of tense, apprehensive parents and is seen most often in firstborn children. In children the cause is hypertrophy of the sphincter muscle of the pylorus, which often may be felt as a tumor mass in the right upper quadrant of the infant's abdomen.

Clinical picture

Pyloric stenosis causes vomiting that usually if forceful and occurs soon after eating. The copious vomiting requires urgent attention because fluid and electrolyte loss follows rapidly. As the condition persists and loss of weight occurs, peristaltic waves can be seen passing across the abdomen from right to left and reversing immediately prior to vomiting. Symptoms in infants usually appear in the second or third week of life and seldom develop after 3 or 4 months of age.

Intervention

Pyloric stenosis is treated medically before surgery is considered. If it is treated early before hypertrophy is pronounced and malnutrition is severe, surgery may be avoided. Medical treatment consists of administering small amounts of sedative drugs such as phenobarbital or the alkaloids of belladonna such as atropine or Banthine in regular doses several times a day, usually preceding meals, and modifying the diet. Smaller feedings may be given at more frequent intervals, and cereals may be substituted for some of the milk, since solid foods are less easily vomited. The infant needs a quiet, relaxed environment. In the hospital the nurse should see that all his needs such as a change of diapers or extra warmth are met at once so that he does not become upset. Very gentle rocking prior to and immediately following meals sometimes helps. If the infant is at home, the community health nurse can often help the family to ensure a more relaxed environment for the infant. Sometimes, for example, it appears that a mother's fears about whether she is properly caring for her baby contribute to the infant's difficulties.

Surgical treatment for pyloric stenosis is used when the condition does not respond to medical treatment alone. It consists of incision into the sphincter muscle of the pylorus (pylorotomy, Ramstedt operation), and the response to this treatment is almost uniformly good.

□ Decompression of the stomach

Cessation of peristalsis in the gastrointestinal tract (*ileus*) or a marked decrease in gastrointestinal tract motility may occur following anesthesia or manipulation of the viscera during abdominal surgery or as a result of gastrointestinal obstruction or peritonitis. Food cannot be propelled through the gastrointestinal tract; therefore digestion and absorption cannot take place. When peristalsis ceases, the stomach or small intestine (depending on the site of obstruction) becomes distended by large quantities of fluids and gas. The secreted fluid has a high electrolyte content and is acid if in the stomach or alkaline if in the small intestine. Gas in the stomach results primarily from swallowed air. Gas in the small intestine may result from swallowed air or from gas that has diffused from blood vessels of the gastrointestinal tract. As the fluid and gas collect, the resulting distention causes edema of tissues of the gut wall with subsequent impairment of circulation and, if severe, may cause rupture of the stomach or intestine. Shock occurs from excessive protein loss.

Gastric distention can be prevented by *gastric intubation* (passage of a nasogastric tube) for the purpose of decompression of the stomach (removal of the fluids and gas as they collect). Gastric intubation may also be performed when gastric hemorrhage occurs in order to remove and to measure accurately the blood loss for replacement therapy, and when perforation occurs to decrease the amount of gastrointestinal secretions leaking into the peritoneal cavity. A nasogastric tube may be inserted for the giving of tube feedings (p. 1184). Gastric intubation is performed less frequently than in the past for certain types of surgery such as gall bladder surgery because of newer surgical techniques that decrease excessive manipulation of abdominal viscera. (Passage of the nasogastric tube is described on p. 1164).

The nasogastric tube may be inserted prior to surgery and removed after normal peristalsis returns (usually in 48 to 78 hours), or it may be inserted only if signs of distention occur after surgery. Tubes used in conjunction with gastric or esophageal surgery are carefully placed by the surgeon during surgery so that the tube does not intrude on the suture line. These tubes are not manipulated lest injury result. If there is some question about the tube's position or function, the surgeon should be consulted. The length of time that the tube remains in the stomach depends on the reason for its use and the physician's opinion of the physiologic effects of intubation on electrolyte balance and the psychologic effects on the patient.

The need for continuous intubation should be explained to both the patient and his family. If the purpose of the tube is not fully understood, its use may cause apprehension and fear. Acceptance by the patient usually facilitates passage of the tube, and there is less possibility that he will pull it out. The presence of the tube in the nasopharynx causes local discomfort, and the patient may complain of a lump in his throat, difficulty in swallowing, a sore throat, hoarseness, earache, or irritation of the nostril. He may also expectorate and wish to blow his nose often because the irritation of the tube causes an increase in mucous secretions. Many patients report that discomfort from the tube far exceeds that from the incision. To lessen this discomfort, the tube should be secured so that there is no pressure against the nostril. Excess secretions from around the nares should be removed, and a *water-soluble* lubricant such as K-Y jelly should be applied to the tube and to the nostril to prevent crusting of secretions.

When the tube is in the nostril, the patient tends to breathe through his mouth, and his lips, mouth, and tongue may become dry and cracked. *Good mouth care is essential* (for further information on mouth care, see p. 1188). Fluids are usually restricted, but the patient may chew gum or suck sour-ball candies to increase salivation. This helps maintain moisture of the mucous membrane and prevent infection of the parotid gland. Although ice chips are sometimes permitted, they should be used sparingly as large amounts may result in ingestion of a hypotonic solution that may increase electrolyte loss through gastric drainage. Warm saline solution gargles may relieve dryness and soreness of the throat, and throat lozenges may be prescribed. Phenylephrine (Neo-Synephrine), 0.25%, nosedrops are sometimes helpful in relieving nasal stuffiness. Frequent changing of the patient's position helps to relieve pressure from the tube on any one area in the throat. Unless contraindicated, elevation of the bed to 30° helps to prevent esophageal reflux and subsequent esophagitis.

Nasogastric tubes usually are attached to suction to ensure drainage, since the stomach contents must flow against gravity. Intermittent suction is commonly ordered, since constant suction could damage the mucosal wall if a section of the wall were to be pulled continually against the drainage holes of the gastric tube. Intermittent suction permits the wall to drop away from the tube during periods when suction is not occurring. The tubing from the suction apparatus is attached by a connecting tube to the nasogastric tube, permitting observation of the fluid being removed from the stomach. A clamp, pin, or adhesive sling should be used to support the weight of the additional drainage tubing so that the patient can turn freely, and the device used to secure the tubing to the bed is placed so as not to obstruct the drainage or inhibit the patient's movement.

Mechanical failure of the suction apparatus or blockage of the drainage tubing or of the nasogastric tube itself may stop the suction, impeding drainage and causing distention, discomfort, and sometimes vomiting. The apparatus is checked frequently to minimize this possibility. The physician may wish the tube irrigated with small amounts (30 ml) of *normal saline solution* at specified intervals to keep the lumen of the tube open and free from mucus plugs or blood clots. Use of a hypotonic solution such as water would increase electrolyte loss through irrigation. After the fluid is inserted into the tube it should be aspirated if possible. Fluid that is instilled but not immediately withdrawn will be removed by suction. If the fluid does not flow easily into the tube or return by aspiration or suction, the physician should be consulted.

Gastric secretions collected in the drainage bottle should be measured every 24 hours. The amount of fluid instilled by irrigation but not immediately withdrawn is subtracted from the 24-hour total in order to determine the actual amount of gastric secretion lost through drainage. The total amount of fluid and electrolytes lost through drainage must be replaced by parenteral routes.

□ Surgery of the stomach

Emergency surgery is necessary when a peptic ulcer perforates and causes peritonitis or erodes a blood vessel causing severe hemorrhage. Elective surgery may be performed if the ulcer does not respond to the medical regimen and continues to produce symptoms, if it causes pyloric obstruction, or if a chronic recurring gastric ulcer is thought to be precancerous. Surgery may also be performed to remove a malignant tumor.

Types of gastric surgeries

Several different operations may be used in the treatment of chronic peptic ulcers (Fig. 54-7). The *Billroth II* operation or variations thereof (such as Polya and Hofmeister) consist of the removal of one half to two thirds of the stomach *(subtotal gastrectomy)*. In this type of gastric resection the ulcer and a large amount of acid-secreting mucosa are removed. The duodenal stump is closed, and the remaining segment of the stomach is anastomosed to a loop of jejunum *(gastrojejunostomy, gastroenterostomy)*. Gastric contents now will pass directly from the stomach to the jejunum. Since the distal end of the duodenum still connects the jejunum, bile now flows from it to the jejunum to mix with the food.

The *Billroth I* operation (or variations thereof) consists of the removal of the lower half to two thirds of the stomach. The remaining portion of the stomach is anastomosed to the duodenum *(gastroduodenostomy)*.

An *antrectomy* consists of the removal of the entire antrum (area between the fundus and the pylorus) of the stomach and the anastomosing of the remaining stomach to the duodenum *(gastroduodenostomy)*. A *vagotomy* is performed by resecting the vagus nerve branch to the

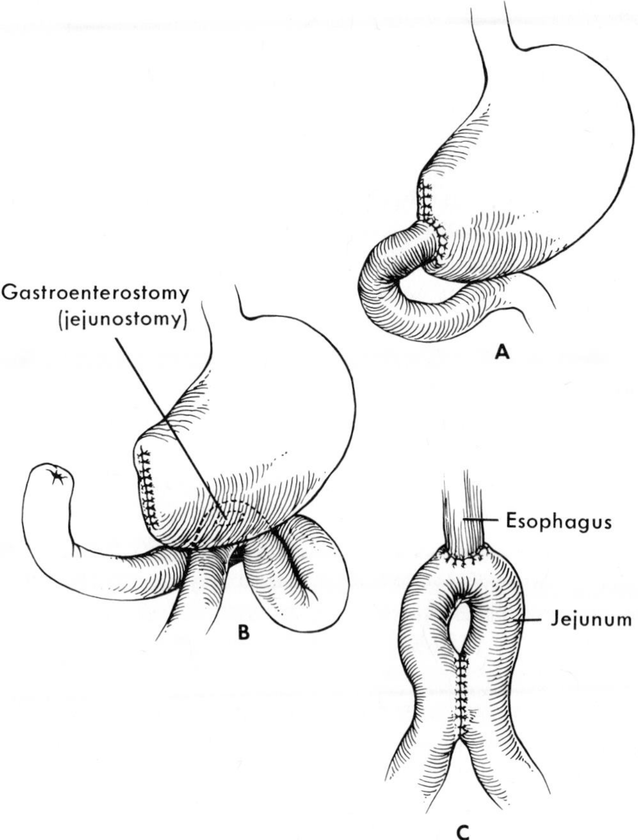

Fig. 54-7. Types of gastric resections and anastomoses. **A,** Gastric resection with anastomosis of remaining segment of stomach with duodenum (Billroth I). **B,** Gastric resection with closure of duodenum and anastomosis of remaining segment of stomach to jejunum (Billroth II). **C,** Total gastrectomy with anastomosis of esophagus to jejunum. Duodenum has been closed.

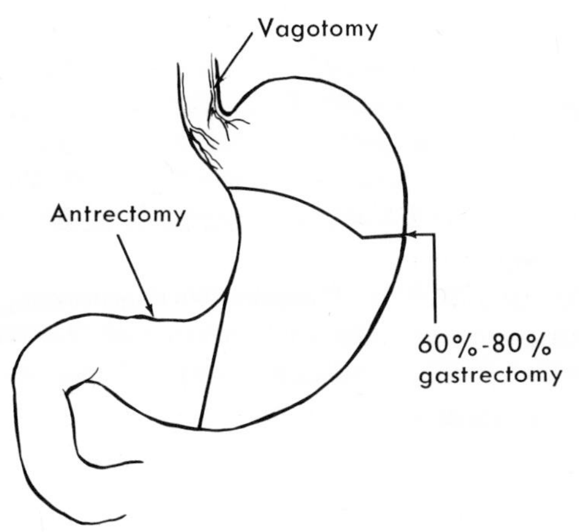

Fig. 54-8. Some surgical approaches used in treatment of peptic ulcer.

stomach 6 to 7 cm above the junction of the esophagus and the stomach. An antrectomy with a vagotomy may be performed. Theoretically, resecting the entire antrum of the stomach removes the source of the hormone gastrin, and the gastric hormonal phase of gastric hypersecretion is eliminated (Fig. 54-8). In addition, by eliminating the cerebral stimuli to the stomach by a vagotomy, the motility of the stomach muscle and the volume of gastric secretions are lessened. A *pyloroplasty* is a procedure performed to facilitate gastric emptying by enlarging the pyloric opening and eliminating its sphincteric action.[41] A *vagotomy* (by way of the parasympathetic system) causes considerable reduction in gastric secretion and greatly suppresses gastric motility. More than half of the persons who have a vagotomy alone will later require some procedure to enhance emptying of the stomach. The poor emptying of the stomach results in antral stasis and distention, causing release of the hormone gastrin from the gastric mucosa. The secretion of acid and pepsin is thus enhanced further through the response to gastrin.

A *gastrojejunostomy* (gastroenterostomy) or a vagotomy combined with a gastrojejunostomy may be the treatment of choice for elderly patients who cannot tolerate extensive surgery, for very young patients whose nutritional state suffers irreparably from removal of large amounts of stomach, or for patients with penetrating ulcers of the duodenum or with a deformed duodenum where a Billroth I type of anastomosis would be technically difficult to perform. In a gastrojejunostomy (gastroenterostomy), the jejunum is pulled up and anastomosed with the stomach. A new opening for the food to pass from the stomach is then made between the stomach and the jejunum without removal of any portion of the stomach.

In a *total gastrectomy* the entire stomach is removed, and continuity of the gastrointestinal tract is reestablished by anatomosis of a loop of the jejunum to the esophagus. The two portions of the jejunum meeting the esophagus are sometimes joined to form a reservoir for food.

Preoperative care

Except in emergencies all patients who are to have stomach surgery undergo extensive diagnostic studies before surgery is preformed. If the patient is to have surgery for an ulcer, he is maintained on a medical regimen during the preoperative period. If the surgery will involve a thoracic approach, special preoperative teaching given before any thoracic surgery is instituted. Since the incision will be high in the abdomen, special emphasis is placed on teaching the patient breathing exercises preoperatively. The patient should know that a nasogastric tube will be in place postoperatively and that he will be receiving fluids and nourishment intravenously for several days until peristalsis is reestablished.

Postoperative care

Comfort. Because of the high upper abdominal incision the patient is inclined to breath shallowly to limit incisional pain. The prescribed medications for pain should be given as necessary, and special attention should be given to encouraging the patient to turn every 2 hours, to breathe deeply, and to cough productively during the first few days. The patient is usually more comfortable in a modified Fowler's position. He is usually ambulated the day after surgery and his activity increased progressively thereafter.

Drainage. Drainage from the nasogastric tube after gastric surgery usually contains some blood for the first 12 hours, but bright red blood, large amounts of blood, or excessive bloody drainage should be watched for and its occurrence reported to the surgeon at once. If the nasogastric tube stops draining, the surgeon is notified immediately. As the level of gastric secretions increases, tension on the suture line may occur resulting in rupture or dislodgement of the sutures. It is the responsibility of the surgeon to adjust the placement of the nasogastric tube so that inadvertent dislodgement of the sutures is prevented.

After most gastric surgery, drainage on the dressing is minimal. If a total gastrectomy is performed, however, drains are usually inserted from the site of the anastomosis, and there may be serosanguineous drainage.

Food and fluids. While the nasogastric tube is used and until peristalsis resumes, fluids by mouth are restricted. Mouth care is therefore needed frequently to keep the mucous membranes of the throat and mouth moist and clean.

Until the tube is removed and until the patient is able to drink enough nutritious fluids, fluids are given parenterally. The average patient is given about 3,500 ml of fluids intravenously each day (2,500 ml for his normal body needs plus enough to replace fluids lost through the gastric drainage and vomitus). It is important that gastric drainage and urinary output be accurately measured and recorded.

Vitamins are usually prescribed until the patient is eating a full, well-balanced diet. Fluids by mouth are restricted for about 12 to 24 hours after the nasogastric tube is removed. Small amounts of fluid are then given frequently. If water is well tolerated, small amounts of bland food may be added until the patient is able to eat six small meals a day and to drink 120 ml of fluid every hour between meals. This dietary regimen must be adapted to the individual since some persons tolerate increasing amounts of food and fluids better than others.

Regurgitation after meals may be caused by eating too fast, by eating too much, or by postoperative edema about the suture line that prevents the food from passing into the intestines. If regurgitation occurs, the patient is encouraged to eat more slowly and the size of the meals is decreased temporarily. If the gastric retention continues, it is probably caused by edema about the suture line, and food and fluids by mouth are discontinued for a time. A nasogastric tube may be passed and attached to a suction apparatus, and fluids will be administered parenterally until the edema subsides.

After a gastric resection the *"dumping syndrome"* sometimes occurs. It may also occur in patients who had a vagotomy, antrectomy, or gastroenterostomy. Mild symptoms occur in approximately 50% of patients and usually disappear in a few months to a year. They remain troublesome in approximately 7% of all patients who undergo gastric resection.[5] The onset may occur during the meal or from 5 to 30 minutes after the meal. The duration of the attack may last 20 to 60 minutes[15] The patient complains of weakness, faintness, palpitations of the heart, and diaphoresis. A feeling of fullness, discomfort, and nausea often occurs, and diarrhea may also develop. These symptoms are thought to be due to the entrance of food directly into the jejunum without undergoing usual changes and dilution in the stomach. The food mixture, more hyperosmolar than the jejunal secretions, causes fluid to be drawn from the bloodstream to the jejunum. The reaction appears to be greater after the ingestion of sugar, since sugar is the most osmotically active food. The symptoms just described are also attributed to the sudden rise in blood sugar (hyperglycemia), with the entrance of glucose into the bloodstream, and the subsequent fall in the blood sugar level. Blood glucose falls to subnormal levels, producing the symptoms of hypoglycemia. The rapid gastric emptying and the propulsion of chyme into the small intestine is felt to initiate an intensive gastrocolic reflex and cause diarrhea and a feeling of fullness and discomfort.

Fear of symptoms makes the patient reluctant to eat, and he may lose weight. He should be advised to avoid concentrated carbohydrates such as heavily sweetened cereals and sweet desserts that are rapidly dissolved into a concentrated solution. A diet high in protein and high enough in fat to compensate for the carbohydrate restriction should be encouraged. The patient should lie down after eating, should eat frequent, small, dry meals, and should avoid drinking fluid with meals or for about 2 hours after eating. The dumping syndrome may be a serious postoperative complication, but it usually improves over time.

Discharge planning. Before discharge, radiographic studies may be done to observe functioning of the remaining portions of the stomach. The patient still may be eating six small meals a day, or he may tolerate three larger meals of bland food. He should be advised to eat slowly and to decrease the size of the meals if he is uncomfortable after eating. The remaining stomach gradually is able to accept larger amounts of food and fluids. Within 6 months to a year, the patient is usually able to eat three regular meals. He requires about 3 months to convalesce before he regains his strength completely and is able to resume full activity. After discharge he needs medical supervision and should be advised to keep appointments either in his physician's office or in the hospital clinic. During these visits the nurse can help to determine the patient's understanding of his condition. He may need to discuss problems about his diet with the dietitian.

Special needs after total gastrectomy. The nursing care of a patient who has had a total gastrectomy differs in some ways from that of patients undergoing other types of gastric surgery. Since the chest cavity must be entered, the patient will have a catheter for chest drainage, and the nursing care will be that of the patient who has had chest surgery (p. 969). There is little or no drainage from the nasogastric tube because there is no longer any reservoir in which secretions may collect, and there is no stomach mucosa left to secrete. When normal peristalsis returns, the nasogastric tube is removed. The patient is given clear fluids hourly, and if after 2 or 3 days there is no evidence of leakage through the anastomosis, the diet is increased to several small meals (usually six) of bland foods a day. An elevation of temperature of dyspnea should make one suspect leakage from the anastomosis, and all oral intake should be stopped until the physician has been consulted.

Following a total gastrectomy the maintenance of good nutrition is difficult because the patient can no longer eat regular meals and because the food that is taken is poorly digested and therefore poorly absorbed from the intestines. Since the patient also becomes anemic, ferrous sulfate, folate, and vitamin B_{12} are often prescribed. Patients who have had a total gastrectomy rarely regain normal strength. Most of them are semiinvalids as long as they live.

Outcome criteria for the person who has had gastric surgery

The patient or significant others can:

1. State a specific plan for dietary modifications following discharge:
   a. List specific types of fluids and foods to be avoided.
   b. Determine a specific plan for small frequent feedings that maintain optimal nutrition.
   c. Determine daily fluid requirements and state a plan for intake of fluids prior to, during, and after meals.
   d. Explain the need for planned rest periods following food ingestion.
2. Describe any medication or treatment program (antibiotics, iron and vitamins, antacids) to be followed at home.
3. State plans for follow-up care:
   a. Describe how the surgical procedure relates to the dietary and fluid modifications.
   b. List symptoms requiring medical follow-up (vomiting after meals, increasing feeling of abdominal fullness, increasing weakness, hematemesis, tarry stools, pain, increased temperature, persistent diarrhea).
4. Discuss the emotional impact of surgery:
   a. State a specific plan for returning to activities of daily living and work (as appropriate).
   b. State situations within the environment that may produce increased stress and determine a plan to cope effectively with these.
5. Describe how to obtain professional and community resources necessary to structure a satisfactory life style.

REFERENCES AND SELECTED READINGS

1. American Cancer Society, Inc., 1977 Cancer facts and figures, New York, 1977, The Society.
2. American Medical Association drug evaluations, ed. 3, Acton, Mass., 1977, Publishing Sciences Group, Inc.
3. Ayulo, J. A.: Hiatus hernia: a review, Am. J. Gastroenterol. **58:**579-593, 1972.
4. *Barnes, C. M.: Support of a mother in the care of a child with esophageal lye burns, Nurs. Clin. North Am. **4:**53-57, March 1969.
5. Beeson, P. B., and McDermott, W., editors: Textbook of medicine, ed. 14, Philadelphia, 1975, W. B. Saunders Co.
6. Bergersen, B. S., and Goth, A.: Pharmacology in nursing, ed. 14, St. Louis, 1979, The C. V. Mosby Co.
7. Bockus, H. L.: Gastroenterology, ed. 3, Philadelphia, 1974, W. B. Saunders Co.
8. Brown, M., and Alexander, F.: Improved intermaxillary wiring, Arch. Otolaryngol. **88:**193-195, 1968.
9. *Bruya, M., and Madeira, N.: Stomatitis after chemotherapy, Am. J. Nurs. **75:**1349-1452, 1975.
10. Bryant, L., Mobin-Uddin, K., Dillon, M. L., et al.: Comparison of ice water and ice saline solution for gastric lavage in gastroduodenal hemorrhage, Am. J. Surg. **124:**570-572, 1972.
11. Casey, D. E.: Treatment of fractures of the maxilla and mandible, Surg. Clin. North Am. **48:**191-200, 1968.
12. Conn, H. F.: Current therapy 1978, Philadelphia, 1978, W. B. Saunders Co.
13. Dodsworth, J. M., and Fisher, J. E.: Surgical therapy of chronic peptic ulcer, Surg. Clin. North Am. **54:**529-543, 1974.
14. Dworken, H. J.: The alimentary tract, Philadelphia, 1974, W. B. Saunders Co.
15. Egdahl, R. H., and Mannick, J. A.: Modern surgery, New York, 1970, Grune & Stratton, Inc.

---

*References preceded by an asterisk are particularly well suited for student reading.

16. Ellis, F. H., Jr.: Esophageal hiatal hernia, N. Engl. J. Med. **287**:646-649, 1972.
17. *Franks, A. S.: The mouth in old age, Nurs. Times **69**:1292-1293, 1973.
18. Gellis, S. S., and Kagen, B. M.: Current pediatric therapy, ed. 5, Philadelphia, 1973, W. B. Saunders Co.
19. Given, B., and Simmons, S.: Gastroenterology in clinical nursing, ed. 2, St. Louis, 1975, The C. V. Mosby Co.
20. Glickman, I.: Clinical periodontology, ed. 4, Philadelphia, 1972, W. B. Saunders Co.
21. Grafe, W. R., Loehr, W., and Thorbjarnarson, B.: Gasteroenterostomy and vagotomy in the treatment of duodenal ulcer disease, Ann. Surg. **168**:966-970, 1968.
22. *Grossman, M. I., Guth, P. H., Isenberg, J. I., et al.: A new look at peptic ulcer, Ann. Int. Med. **84**:57-67, 1976.
23. *Herter, R. P.: Preparation of the bowel for surgery, Surg. Clin. North Am. **52**:859-869, 1972.
24. Hunt, T. K.: Injury and repair in acute gastroduodenal ulceration, Am. J. Surg. **125**:12-18, 1973.
25. Ippoliti, A. F., Maxwell, V., and Isenberg, J. I.: The effect of various forms of milk on gastric acid secretions, Ann. Int. Med. **84**:286-289, 1976.
26. Ivey, K. J.: Anticholinergics: do they work in peptic ulcers, Gastroenterology **68**:154-158, 1975.
27. Jaffe, P. E.: Dental cleansing tape, N.Y. J. Dent. **43**:245-247, 1973.
28. *Keogh, G., and Niebel, H.: Oral cancer detection, a nursing responsibility, Am. J. Nurs. **73**:684-686, 1973.
29. Krupp, M., and Chatton, M.: Current medical diagnosis and treatment, Los Altos, Calif., 1974, Lange Medical Publications.
30. Lawton, D. M., Williams, J. I., and Martinello, B. P.: Determinants of dental care, Can. J. Public Health **64**:343-350, 1973.
31. *Less, W.: Mechanics of teaching plaque control, Dent. Clin. North Am. **16**:647-659, 1972.
32. *Levine, P., et al.: Safeguarding your patients against periodontal disease, R.N. **36**:38-41, 1973.
33. *Mandel, I. O.: New approaches to plaque prevention, Dent. Clin. North Am. **16**:661-670, 1972.
34. Mandel, M. A., Dvorak, K., and DeCosse, J. J.: Salivary immunoglobulins in patients with oropharyngeal and bronchopulmonary carcinoma, Cancer **31**:1408-1413, 1973.
35. McCredie, J. A.: Basic surgery, New York, 1977, Macmillan, Inc.
36. McDonald, R. E., and Avery, D. R.: Dentistry for the child and adolescent, ed. 3, St. Louis, 1978, The C. V. Mosby Co.
37. Nankin, P., et al.: Hiatus hernia, Surg. Clin. North Am. **51**:1347-1353, 1971.
38. Nelson, W. E.: Textbook of pediatrics, ed. 10, Philadelphia, 1975, W. B. Saunders Co.
39. Paparella, M. M., and Shumrich, D. A., editors: Otolaryngology, ed. 3, Philadelphia, 1973, W. B. Saunders Co.
40. Putt, A. M.: One experiment in nursing adults with peptic ulcers, Nurs. Res. **19**:484-494, 1970.
41. *Reitz, M., and Pope, W.: Mouth care, Am. J. Nurs. **73**:1728-1730, 1973.
42. Robinson, C.: Normal and therapeutic nutrition, ed. 15, New York, 1972, Macmillan, Inc.
43. Sabiston, D. C., editor: Davis-Christopher textbook of surgery, ed. 11, Philadelphia, 1977, W. B. Saunders Co.
44. Sandlow, L. J., and Spellberg, M. A.: Gastric hyperthermia for control of upper gastrointestinal bleeding, Am. J. Gastroenterol. **59**:307-314, 1973.
45. Schwartz, S. I., et al.: Principles of surgery, ed. 2, New York, 1974, McGraw-Hill Book Co.
46. Schultz, R. C.: The nature of facial injury emergencies, Surg. Clin. North Am. **52**:99-106, 1972.
47. Scopp, I. W.,Oral medicine, a clinical approach with basic science correlation, ed. 2., St. Louis, 1973, The C. V. Mosby Co.
48. Shklar, G., and Schwartz, S. M.: An approach to the diagnosis of disease of mouth and jaws, Dent. Clin. North Am. **18**:55-75, 1974.
49. Sleisinger, M., and Fortran, J.: Gastrointestinal disease: pathophysiology, diagnosis, management, Philadelphia, 1973, W. B. Saunders Co.
50. *Smith, M.: Parotidectomy, Am. J. Nurs. **76**:422-425, 1976.
51. Spiro, H. M.: Clinical gastroenterology, ed. 2, New York, 1977, Macmillan, Inc.
52. Spouge, J. D.: Oral pathology, St. Louis, 1973, The C. V. Mosby Co.
53. Stookey, G. K., and Katz, S.: Chairside procedures for using flourides for preventing dental caries, Dent. Clin. North Am. **16**:681-692, 1972.
54. *Trowbridge, J., and Carl, W.: Oral care of the patient having head and neck irradiation, Am. J. Nurs. **75**:2146-2149, 1975.
55. Welsh, J. D.: Diet therapy of peptic ulcer disease, Gastoenterol. **72**:740-745, 1977.
56. Williams, S. R.: Nutrition and diet therapy, ed. 3, St. Louis, 1977, The C. V. Mosby Co.
57. Wintrobe, M. M., et al.: Harrison's principles of internal medicine, ed. 8, New York, 1977, McGraw-Hill Book Co.
58. Zollinger, R. M.: Surgical management of the ulcerogenic syndrome, Hosp. Prac. **9**:72-79, 1974.

UNIT IX

Problems of elimination

Elimination of waste products is a basic physiologic need; a person cannot live long without the ability to get rid of waste products resulting from metabolic processes. There are several body systems involved with elimination, only two of which (urinary and bowel elimination) are discussed in this unit. The respiratory system eliminates carbon dioxide but is also involved with oxygen intake and is discussed in the unit of gas transportation. The skin is also an organ of elimination, but its primary function is that of protection from the environment, and it is therefore included in Unit XI.

Assessment of lower gastrointestinal (small and large intestines) *function* and of *urinary function* is discussed in separate chapters. *Management of persons with impaired elimination* involves preventing dysfunction of the system, facilitating an open system for elimination of urine and feces, promoting adaptation to drainage through unnatural openings (stoma), and promoting control of output (continence). The last two chapters deal with *specific problems of each of the systems,* and include a discussion of the care of the person experiencing kidney dialysis and kidney transplantation.

55

Assessment of lower gastrointestinal tract function

NANCY DURHAM

■ PHYSIOLOGY OF THE LOWER GASTROINTESTINAL TRACT

The primary function of the small and large intestine is to receive the partially digested food components from the stomach and move these components forward to facilitate proper absorption of water, nutrients, electrolytes, and bile salts. Secondary functions include secreting mucus, potassium, and bicarbonate, and serving as a storage area prior to waste discharge.

□ Movement

Contents of the small intestine *(chyme)* are propelled analward by peristaltic movement, wavelike forward movements produced by alternating contraction and relaxation of the muscles of the intestinal wall. This movement also mixes the intestinal contents. Chyme moves slowly and normally takes 3 to 10 hours to move from the stomach to the ileocecal valve which decreases the backward flow of fecal contents from the large to the small intestine.[6]

In the colon the fecal contents are pushed forward by mass movements occurring only a few times each day. These mass movements are stimulated by gastrocolic reflexes initiated when food enters the duodenum from the stomach, especially after the first meal of the day. This is therefore the most frequent time of the day for defecation to occur.

The *defecation* reflex occurs when feces enters the rectum. Afferent impulses are transmitted to the sacral segments of the spinal cord from which reflex impulses are transmitted back to the colon, sigmoid, and rectum, initiating relaxation of the internal anal sphincter.

□ Secretion

Gastrointestinal tract secretions are specific to the type of food that is present and the amount that is needed. These secretions are stimulated in part by autonomatic *sympathetic* innervation, *hormonal* regulation, and local *mechanical pressure*.

Mucus secretion throughout the tract increases food adhesion, prevents contact of the food with the wall of the mucosa, enhances free passage of the food, neutralizes the small amounts of acid or alkali, and makes some particles more resistant to digestion.

Secretions of the small intestines provide for the final digestion of food. As chyme enters the small intestine, gastric secretion of hydrochloric acid is slowed and *secretin, pancreozymin,* and *cholecystokinin* are released.

□ Absorption

Ninety percent of absorption occurs within the small intestine either by active transport or diffusion. Approximately 450 ml of chyme reaches the cecum per day. The transit time in the large bowel is slow, taking about 12 hours for material to reach the rectum. Reabsorption of water, electrolytes, and bile salts occurs predominantly in the ascending colon. The colon has the capacity to absorb six to eight times more fluid than is delivered to it daily. Approximately 100 ml of fluid contents remain to be mixed with the residue of feces. Normally this residue *(feces)* is evacuated on a fairly regular schedule. This schedule differs for each individual and may vary from daily evacuation to evacuation every 4 to 5 days.

□ Fluid and electrolyte balance

Pathologic alterations occur with the *loss* of particular segments of small or large bowel or when there is inability for proper reabsorption. The loss of small bowel contents precipitates metabolic acidosis and hypokalemia (p. 309). This problem may occur with drainage of small bowel contents through a suction tube or fistula, or with persistant vomiting of the intestinal contents. Losses from the large intestine comprise mainly loss of water, sodium, and to a lesser extent chloride, resulting in dehydration and hyponatremia. This occurs in conditions in which the rate of peristalsis is increased.

☐ Bacteria

In addition to its role in nutrition, the alimentary tract supports bacterial growth that enhances digestive processes and has a role in antibody formation. Within 4 weeks after birth the characteristic flora is established. The organisms are less in number in those portions of the bowel concerned with digestion and absorption. Certain disease conditions increase the breakdown of nonabsorbable carbohydrate, leading to the production of diarrhea. It is important to remember that whenever the motility of the bowel is depressed or interrupted, bacterial overgrowth will occur.

It is presently known that the gastrointestinal tract has a role in immunology. The thymus exerts control over lymphoid elements that are scattered throughout the tract. Of these elements, the plasma cells of the mucosa are believed to synthesize and secrete antibodies. The cells are relatively resistant to proteolytic digestion and may play a role in delayed hypersensitivity, graft and host relationships, and immunologic memory.

■ SUBJECTIVE DATA

Eliciting a health history regarding bowel habits of the patient is an area in which the nurse must provide a tactful, considerate, and matter-of-fact approach. Patterns of bowel evacuation have in most instances been established in early infancy or childhood, and the effect of this training lasts throughout life. The infant learns to "control" his bowel evacuation and is rewarded for this, therefore problems may be encountered when this function is altered or lost. The symptoms that the person may have are often varied, vague, and ill defined, and are frequently perceived by the individual to represent a loss of control of his bodily functions.

Because normal bowel evacuation is not usually a topic of general conversation within the family group or among strangers, the person may be hesitant about expressing data about elimination. Embarrassment on the part of either the person or the nurse may limit accurate or complete data taking. There will be situations in which the nurse must interview a significant other to obtain information regarding bowel functioning of the patient. Following is a listing of data obtained when eliciting a history of bowel function:

1. Normal pattern of bowel elimination
   a. Frequency and character of the stool
   b. Use of measures to encourage evacuation (specific food, laxatives, enemas)
2. Recent changes in normal pattern
   a. Changes in character of stool: constipation, diarrhea, or alternating constipation or diarrhea
   b. Changes in color of stool (if bleeding present: stool mixed or streaked with blood, amount, rectal bleeding after evacuation, menstruation present)
   c. Drugs or medications being taken, if changes in elimination are present
   d. Measures taken to relieve symptoms
3. Pain in rectal area or abdomen
   a. Onset, frequency, location, intensity
   b. Relationship of pain to activity or to foods
   c. Possible cause as perceived by person
   d. Measures taken for relief of pain; effectiveness of such measures

Normal patterns of evacuation vary greatly. Problems may exist without the person's awareness, therefore all persons are asked what their normal pattern is, if they take anything to maintain this pattern, and if they have noticed any changes in this pattern.

Constipation is identified by small hard stools passed with difficulty and usually at infrequent intervals, although a person may pass a constipated stool every day. Data concerning the frequency of bowel elimination is obtained on all hospitalized persons at the time of admission; this serves as a baseline against which subsequent elimination is compared. Continued assessment of frequency is also indicated on all persons who are inactive or who have fluid or diet restriction, as they have a high potential for developing constipation or fecal impaction (p. 1244). Information concerning measures used frequently by the person to help maintain normal bowel elimination will provide data for health teaching.

Changes in the normal pattern of bowel elimination may indicate a physiologic deviation, such as constipation, or a pathologic deviation, such as enteritis or cancer. Diarrhea and stools containing mucus, pus, and possible undigested food may indicate an enteritis (inflammation of the bowel) or invasion by a parasite. Alternation of diarrhea and constipation may occur as a result of cancer of the colon. Partial obstruction of the descending colon may produce small ribbon-shaped stools, whereas no stool will be passed if obstruction is complete. Diarrhea and constipation may also occur as a result of medical therapy or surgical intervention.

Bright red blood in the stool indicates lower gastrointestinal bleeding. Blood from the upper gastrointestinal tract is changed by digestive secretions, and the stool appears black and sticky (tarry). Blood in the stool (*melena*) may be a recent or a chronic symptom and may result from erosion of the mucosa, leading to perforation of the muscle wall or rupture of a blood vessel.

Pain may be experienced as a general sensation throughout the abdomen, may be specifically directed to one particular quadrant, or may be referred to another somatic or skeletal part that shares the same innervation.

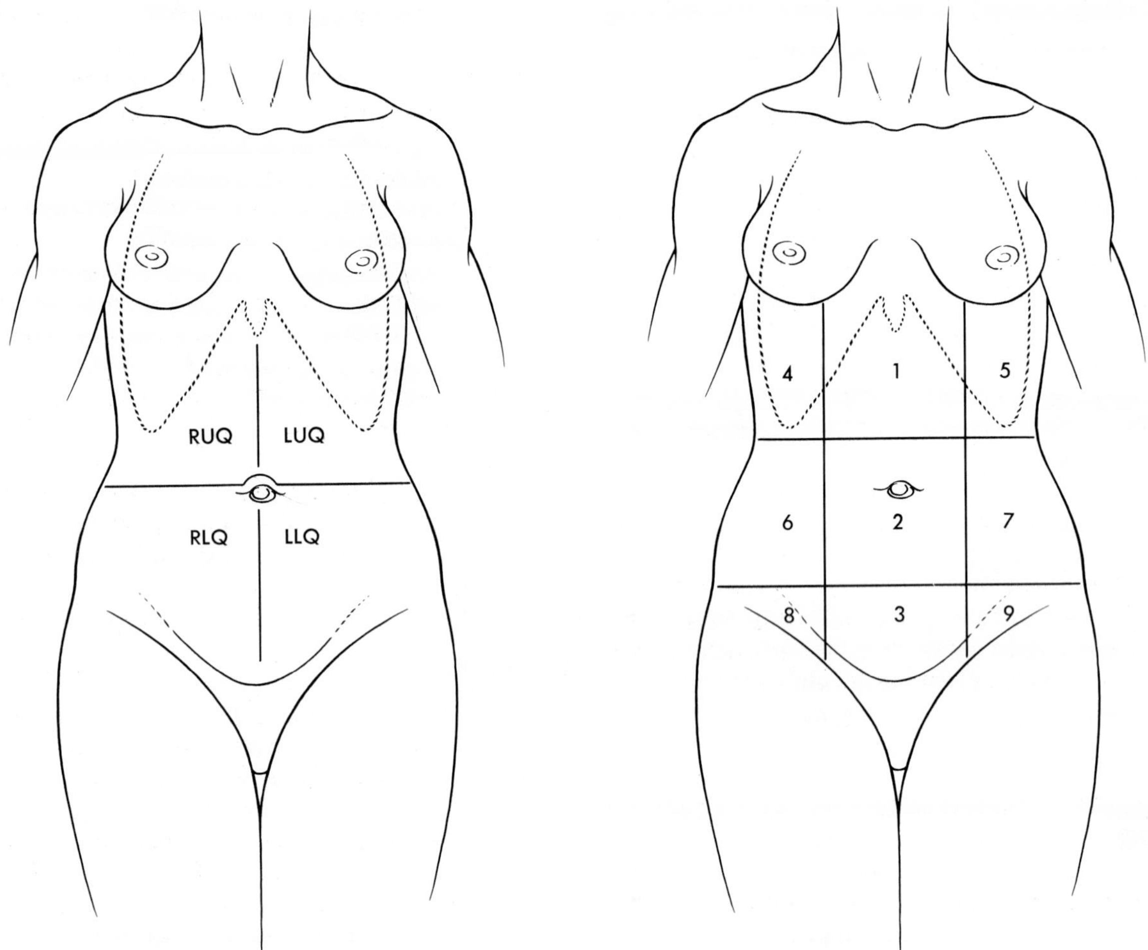

Fig. 55-1. Topographic division of abdomen commonly used to localize signs and symptoms, and anatomic location of viscera within abdomen. *1*, Epigastrium; *2*, umbilical; *3*, suprapubic (bladder and uterus); *4* and *5*, right and left hypochondrium; *6* and *7*, right and left lumbar or flank; *8* and *9*, right and left iliac or inguinal.

The pain sensation is thought to arise from the distention or sudden contraction of a hollow viscus; therefore local stretching or traction on pain-sensitive structures will elicit the pain stimulus. The painful area may demonstrate local muscle guarding, which serves as a protective mechanism as the overlying muscles contract. Pain is frequently the reason given when seeking medical attention, despite the fact that pain by itself is not an early or common symptom of gastrointestinal disease.

■ OBJECTIVE DATA

Examination of the abdomen may not follow a structured pattern, as signs are often found that require alteration in technique. The examination is supported by the attainment of a meaningful history describing the nature and site of pain and any alterations in bowel habits.

Examination will determine the presence or absence of (1) tenderness, (2) organ enlargement, (3) masses, (4) spasm or rigidity of the abdominal muscles, and (5) fluid or air in the abdominal cavity. During this part of the assessment the examiner will be locating the hollow viscera (small intestine, colon, and urinary bladder). These are not normally palpable.

Examination of the abdomen requires knowledge of the terms used to designate the divisions of the abdomen (Fig. 55-1) and the anatomic structures located therein (see box, p. 1221).

Normal findings are variable and will depend on general body build, the amount of abdominal fat, and the patient's ability to cooperate. Although the examination may be initiated in any quadrant, it is recommended that the lower quadrant be examined first, followed by upward movement toward the costal margins. The approach will need to be altered as necessary, with painful

ANATOMIC LOCATION OF VISCERA WITHIN EACH ABDOMINAL QUADRANT

Right upper quadrant (RUQ)	Left upper quadrant (LUQ)
Liver	Stomach
Gallbladder	Spleen
Duodenum	Left kidney
Right kidney	Pancreas
Heptatic flexure of colon	Splenic flexure of colon

Right lower quadrant (RLQ)	Left lower quadrant (LLQ)
Cecum	Sigmoid colon
Appendix	Left ovary and tube
Right ovary and tube	

areas being examined last. The examination is conducted in an unhurried manner. The methods for physical examination of the abdomen are performed in the following order: (1) inspection, (2) auscultation, (3) percussion, and (4) palpation.

□ Inspection

Arrange the illumination to shine across the abdomen and toward the examiner or have the light source lengthwise over the patient. Inspect the skin color and texture and observe for scars, engorged veins, visible peristalsis, masses, or abnormal contour.

Interpretation

Scars or striae	May be result of pregnancy, obesity, ascites, tumors, edema, surgical procedures, or healed burned areas
Engorged veins	May be caused by obstruction of vena cava or portal vein and circulation from abdomen
Skin	Observe for evidence of jaundice or pallor
Visible peristalsis	May be caused by pyloric or intestinal obstruction; normally peristalsis not visible except for slow waves in thin persons
Visible pulsations	Normally slight pulsation of aorta visible in epigastric region
Visible masses and altered contour	Observe for hernias, distention of ascites, and obesity; instructing patient to cough may bring out hernia "bulge" or elicit pain or discomfort in the abdomen

A normal finding is an *umbilical calculus*, which is an accumulated hard mass of debris and desquamated skin within the umbilicus, causing inflammation and resulting from poor hygiene. The integrity and turgor of the skin are reliable indicators of total body hydration. Measurement of abdominal girth provides a baseline for the evaluation of increase or decrease in size because of distention. A measuring tape is placed around the abdomen at the level of the umbilicus or 2.5 cm below, and the reading is taken. It is important that all subsequent measurements be taken at the same level for accurate evaluation.

Abdominal distention may be caused by air or fluid in the gastrointestinal tract or fluid in the peritoneal spaces (ascites). Air collects from the air that is swallowed, from gas formed by bacterial action, or from gas that has diffused from the blood.[6] Decreased peristalsis permits the air to collect in one portion of the gastrointestinal tract. Fluid accumulates in the tract as it become obstructed. Ascites usually results from increased portal hypertension secondary to liver or heart disease.

□ Auscultation

Auscultation is used primarily to determine the presence or absence of peristalsis and is done before percussion and palpation to avoid an increase or decrease of peristalsis secondary to disturbing the viscera and causing abnormal activity. Other sounds such as friction rubs or murmurs may be heard (Fig. 55-2). Using the diaphragm, the stethoscope is placed lightly over the abdominal wall. Most intestinal sounds occur at a rate of five or more per minute (although some may not be audible for up to 5 minutes) and are high pitched and gurgling in quality. A normal peristaltic wave produces audible sounds of air and fluid movement through the intestine. The stethoscope diaphragm is placed to the right and below the umbilicus where the sounds are the loudest.

Interpretation

Absence of sounds	Peritonitis, and paralytic ileus, pneumonia, and hypokalemia
Increased peristalsis	Repeated, high pitched, and occurring at frequent intervals; heard in early pyloric obstruction, early intestinal obstruction and diarrhea
Bruit	Presence of abnormal sounds (turbulence of blood flow through partially occluded or diseased artery of aorta or renal artery)
Hum and friction rub	Heard over liver and splenic areas, indicating peritoneal inflammation

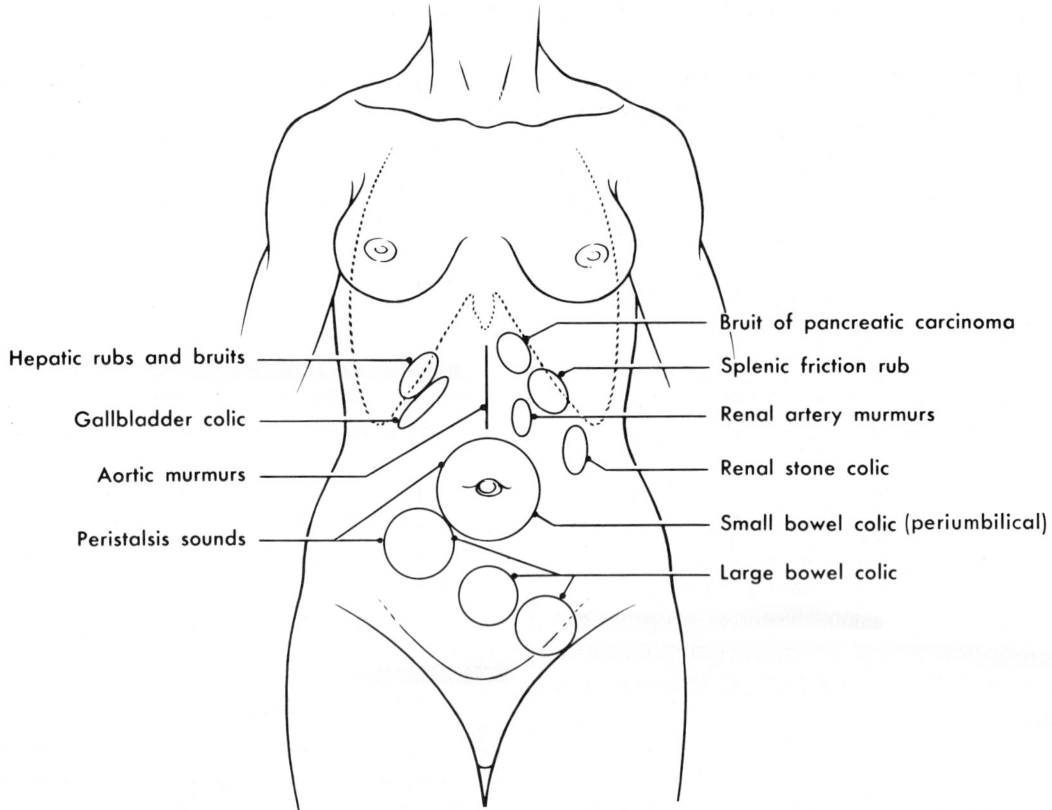

Fig. 55-2. Optimum areas for auscultation of various sounds in abdomen and localization of some types of pain. Note arrow from peristalsis sounds to small bowel and from large bowel colic to circle of ascending colon, which is the peristalsis sounds circle.

□ Percussion

Percussion of the abdomen (Fig. 8-4) has relatively limited value. It is used primarily to confirm the size of various organs and to determine the presence of excessive amounts of fluid or air. Normally, percussion over the abdomen is tympanic because of the presence of a small amount of swallowed air within the gastrointestinal tract. A dull or flat percussion note will be found over a solid structure such as a distended bladder or enlarged uterus and over the lower border of the liver in the seventh interspace. Tympanic sounds should be heard beginning at the ninth interspace in the left upper quadrant of the abdomen (Traube's space). Dullness or flatness of tone in this area may be caused by some enlargement of the spleen or the left kidney.

The four quadrants should be percussed beginning with the thorax area and moving downward systematically. The degree of soft to pronounced tympany determines gaseous bowel distention.

□ Palpation

Palpation is an important procedure that aids in confirming the findings of inspection and history data. Palpation is of value in determining the outlines of the liver, spleen, kidneys, uterus, and bladder when these organs are enlarged and in determining the presence and characteristics of abdominal masses and the degree of tenderness or muscle rigidity. This procedures will elicit subjective as well as objective findings.

The examiner begins palpation at the pubis and works upward towards the costal margins. When moving from one quadrant to another, the entire hand is moved, avoiding a dragging motion across the skin surface as this is generally an unpleasant or irritating feeling.[7] The entire palm and the extended fingers are placed lightly on the abdominal surface with the fingers approximated. With the palms and pads of the fingertips flat, pressure is applied gently to the depth of about 1 cm as each quadrant is palpated carefully. Normally no masses, swellings, or areas of tenderness will be encountered.

Abnormal findings may include (1) direct tenderness over an organ capsule, (2) rebound tenderness (Blumberg's sign), (3) muscular rigidity, or (4) masses that may be felt if they are sufficiently large enough or close enough to the surface. Distinction should be made between a distended abdomen that is firm to touch (indicating an active obstruction with fluid and gas accumulation) and an abdomen that is soft to touch (indicating a resolving obstruction or a normal occurrence).

□ Rectal examination

A thorough abdominal examination is not complete without a rectal examination. The examiner will need a rubber glove, water-soluble lubricating jelly, and a direct light source. A complete examination would include sigmoidoscopic examination, which is generally performed by the physician.

The patient is placed in the left lateral prone (Sims) position and draped. The examiner separates the buttocks and inspects the skin of the perineal and perianal region. The normal perineal skin and perianal area resembles the remainder of the body with no breaks in its integrity. Abnormal findings may include pruritus ani, coccygeal or pilonidal sinus tract openings, fistulas, fissures, external hemorrhoids, or rectal prolapse. Internal hemorrhoids may appear when the patient strains down.

The glove is placed on the examining hand and the perineum is palpated for any tenderness or swelling. The examiner lubricates the index finger well, and, placing the pad of the finger next to the anal opening, presses gently and slowly until the rectal sphincter relaxes and allows the curve of the pad to enter the anus. Normally the sphincter offers some resistance but should allow free passage of the examining finger. The walls should feel smooth with no areas of swelling or depressions. A normal occurrence is the presence of feces within the rectum. Possible pathology includes stricture of the sphincter, a fixed or movable mass, and coccygeal tenderness.

At the completion of the rectal examination the patient should have the perineal area cleansed and dried well.

■ DIAGNOSTIC TESTS

The examinations and procedures performed to rule out problems of the lower gastrointestinal tract are time-consuming for the patient and may also be viewed as intrusive procedures. Frequently the patient is elderly, debilitated, has some decrease in optimal motor function, or may have a chronic medical problem.

Preparations for the examinations (cathartics, suppositories, enemas, restriction of food and fluid) frequently result in a decreased circulating volume, leading to weakness. Safety needs of the person assume priority. For example, the person who is having extensive testing may bathe more safely at the bedside than in the shower, or he may need to be transported by wheelchair. Consideration given to these needs will enhance the comfort and cooperation of the person and provide a safe environment.

Table 55-1. Interpretation of feces color

Color	Interpretation
White	Barium
Gray, tan (clay)	Lack of bile; biliary obstruction
Red	Lower gastrointestinal bleeding
	Beets
Black	
Tarry	Upper gastrointestinal bleeding
Dry	Iron

□ Stool examination

Gross, microscopic, chemical, and bacterial examinations of the stool supply information that is helpful in establishing a diagnosis of gastrointestinal disease. Stools that are abnormal in color (Table 55-1), odor, amount, consistency, and number are significant. Abnormal stools should be accurately described and a specimen saved for examination by the physician. The physician may order further laboratory studies to be performed. Stool examinations are required for the complete evaluation of all patients with gastrointestinal complaints. A guaiac test for the presence of occult blood is performed whenever bleeding is suspected.

The nurse is responsible for seeing that specimens are collected. If the person is ambulatory, he may be given a specimen box and spatula and instructed in obtaining a specimen. Otherwise the specimen should be collected by the nursing personnel. The nurse should be familiar with and also inform auxiliary staff of any special techniques that are required to preserve stools for special examinations. For example, a specimen to be examined for amebae must be kept warm and taken immediately to the laboratory for examination. It can be kept warm by placing the specimen box in a pan of warm water or on a hot-water bottle. If an enema must be given to collect a stool specimen, it is important that plain tap water or normal saline solution be used, since soaps or hypertonic solutions may change the consistency of the stool and alter any abnormal contents.

At any time during hospitalization that any abnormality in the color of the stool is noted, a specimen is collected and retained for physician inspection. This applies to all patients irrespective of their primary medical diagnosis.

☐ Barium studies

A roentgenogram of the small intestine is most frequently performed in conjunction with the oral ingestion of contrast media to visualize the stomach (gastrointestinal series, p. 1161). The *barium enema* is performed after the gastrointestinal series, usually on the following day. A series of roentgenograms taken after a barium enema has been given is used to demonstrate the presence of polyps, tumors, and other lesions of the large intestine and to reveal any abnormal anatomy or malfunction of the bowel. As the barium is instilled through a rectal tube, the radiologist, using a fluoroscope and television monitoring screen, observes its passage into the large intestine. The person is asked to retain the barium while roentgenograms of the intestines are taken. He is then allowed to go to the bathroom to expel the barium. This may take as long as 30 minutes. After the barium is expelled another film is taken to see if any pockets of barium are retained. This procedure is commonly referred to as a lower GI (gastrointestinal) series.

The preparation for a barium enema includes an explanation of the x-ray procedure, of the importance of retaining the barium during the examination, and of the need for the preparatory regimen. For the barium to clearly outline the lumen of the bowel, the bowel must be empty. This is best accomplished by giving enemas, laxatives, or rectal suppositories as ordered. Food and fluids, including oral medications, are restricted after midnight. The person may wish to take reading material with him so that he may read while expelling the barium.

Barium that is retained in the bowel becomes hard and difficult to expel. To ensure complete evacuation of the barium from the intestinal tract after this procedure, the physician may order an oil retention enema or a laxative such as magnesium citrate. The debilitated patient is usually exhausted after a barium enema and the subsequent cleansing regimen; he should have rest. Petroleum jelly or, if ordered, a local analgesic ointment such as dibucaine (Nupercaine) may be applied to the anus to alleviate discomfort. If the patient is not too tired, a warm bath may also be soothing.

☐ Endoscopy: anoscopy, proctoscopy, and sigmoidoscopy

Anoscopy, proctoscopy, and sigmoidoscopy are procedures performed to visualize the mucosa of the anus, rectum, and sigmoid. Tumors, polyps, or ulcerations may be discovered, examined, and biopsied. An *anoscopy* is an examination of the anus; a *proctoscopy* is an examination of the anus and rectum; and a *sigmoidoscopy* is an examination of the anus, rectum, and sigmoid. Most often a sigmoidoscopy is done, and this examination is routinely performed before rectal surgery and as part of the physical examination of persons who complain of chronic constipation or hemorrhoids or have any other symptoms of lower intestinal disease such as bleeding. Many physicians recommend that a sigmoidoscopy be included in the annual physical examination of men over 40 because of the relatively high incidence of cancer of the rectum and sigmoid in this age group. The sigmoidoscopic examination permits inspection of a segment of the bowel that is particularly difficult to examine satisfactorily with contrast media. Approximately 75% of all polyps and tumors of the large bowel are within the visualization of the sigmoidoscope.

The preparation for endoscopic examination of the bowel varies in different hospitals and clinics, but the person should always receive an explanation of the procedure and of the preparation to be carried out. Usually he is instructed to eat a light evening meal prior to the examination. On the morning of the examination, enemas may be given until the return is clear, or a small hypertonic salt solution enema may be ordered. If ulcerative colitis is suspected, the physician will probably not order a hypertonic enema, since it would cause inflammation of the mucosa and confuse the findings of the examination. Cathartic rectal suppositories such as bisacodyl (Dulcolax) are also used. If enemas are to be taken at home, a Fleet enema is usually prescribed. More than one enema may be necessary. Visualization of the bowel mucosa is impossible unless all the fecal material is evacuated. Enema fluid should also be completely expelled before the examination is performed, since it too will obstruct visualization. Cathartics are seldom used in preparation for this examination because they may cause downward flow of material from the upper bowel when the test is being performed. A light breakfast is usually permitted on the day of the scheduled test.

Since the examination is upsetting to many persons, all possible preparations should be made before the patient is brought to the examining room to ensure a smooth-running and rapid procedure. The instrument must be checked to see that all the parts are functioning. The electric light bulb should be tested by attaching the instrument cord to the battery or to the electrical outlet. Besides the instrument, a draping sheet, gloves, lubricant, cotton swabs (12 inches in length), an emesis basin, toilet tissue, biopsy forceps, a suction machine with suction tip, and a paper bag are required.

Before the examination begins, the physician again explains the procedure to the patient. It is preferable for the person to assume a knee-chest position, and he is draped so that only the rectum is exposed. Because it may be difficult for an elderly or a very ill person to assume or maintain a knee-chest position, a side-lying (Sims) position occasionally may be used. The nurse should assist the patient in maintaining the correct position. He should be encouraged to remain still, to relax as much as possible, and to take deep breaths. He should also be watched carefully, lest he become faint. Since the lights are turned off during the examination, it is sometimes difficult to note the patient's color. If any doubt exists about his condition, his pulse rate should be taken.

The rectum is examined first with a gloved finger. The lubricated instrument is then inserted. After the instrument has been passed into the rectum, the solid, round-tipped inner portion (obturator) is removed. The intensity of light is reflected on the mucosa. If the sigmoidoscope is being used, the instrument is advanced slowly through the bowel for about 25 cm (10 inches). Forceful advancement of the instrument is to be avoided as perforation of the bowel may occur. The patient feels the instrument entering the rectum and sigmoid. This process may cause discomfort but should not cause any real pain. Most patients are surprised that so little discomfort is associated with the procedure. Air is sometimes pumped into the bowel through the sigmoidoscope to distend the lumen of the bowel, thus permitting better visualization. The air may cause severe "gas pains," and lower abdominal cramps may be experienced as the instrument is passed through the sacral promontory. If small amounts of fluid or stool are still present in the bowel, they are removed with the cotton swabs and by suctioning.

As the instrument is removed, a careful observation of all of the mucosa is made. Normal variations include (1) temporary hyperemia caused from the irritation of the enema solutions; (2) increased mucus production caused by inflammation, emotional disturbances, or sodium biphosphate found in commercial enema preparations; and (3) decreased mucus production resulting from habitual cathartic ingestion.

Common abnormalities noted include (1) local trauma caused by enema tips or instrumentation and enema solutions heated above 41 C (105 F); (2) diffuse hyperemia, edema, increased mucus, and a mucosa that bleeds easily (ulcerative colitis); (3) loss of valve edge sharpness, scars, strictures, and contractures (ulcerative colitis, pelvic irradiation); (4) discrete ulcers or polyps; and (5) evidence of an invasion by organisms or bacteria (tuberculosis, bacillary or amebic dysentery, eggs of *Schistosomiasis* or *Balantidium* organisms).

A proctoscopic procedure may be tiring, depending on the age and physical condition of the person. After the instrument is removed the person is given tissues to wipe excess lubricant from the anus or this is done for him. When indicated, the person is assisted back to bed and allowed to rest. The person who is examined in an outpatient setting may need to rest for an hour and have some food and fluid before leaving. This is especially important for the elderly or debilitated person.

□ Biopsy

Biopsy of tissue includes rectal biopsy and peroral small bowel biopsy. In both instances tissue samples are removed and sent to the laboratory for definitive diagnosis.

Rectal biopsy

Biopsy of lesions, polyps, or tumors of the lower sigmoid colon, rectum, and anal canal are generally taken at the time of the sigmoidoscopic examination. A knife

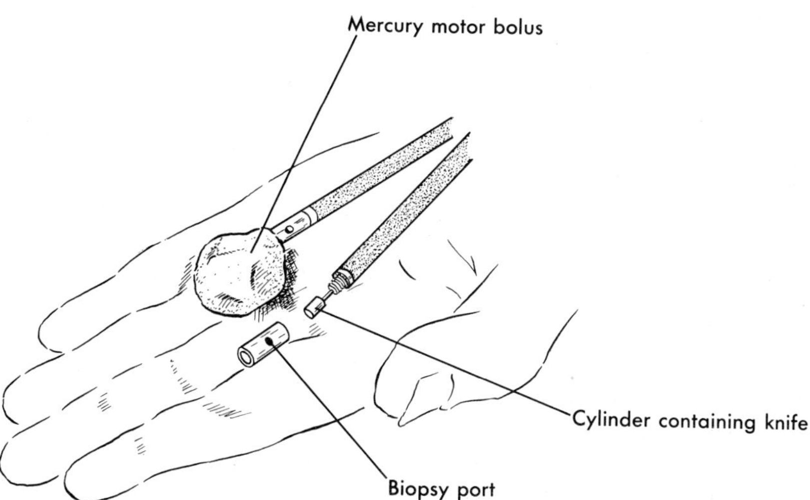

Fig. 55-3. Multipurpose biopsy tube. Biopsy tube assembled and disassembled to show location of its parts. Note small size of tube in relation to human hand.

blade or snare is used to obtain the tissue sample. The sample is placed on a slide or in a fixative solution and sent to the laboratory for analysis. The procedure is not generally painful although a feeling of pressure may be experienced. Bleeding from the site of the biopsy is uncommon. The person is instructed to report immediately any signs of rectal bleeding and to curtail physical activity until examined by a physician.

Peroral small bowel biopsy

Biopsy of the mucosa and of lesions of the small intestines is possible through the passage of a biopsy capsule. The capsule consists of inner and outer shells that are attached to the distal end of a Miller-Abbott tube or to special tubes constructed for this purpose. The inner shell encloses a cylindric cavity that contains a blade. The biopsy opening is located in the distal end of the capsule (Fig. 55-3). The tube with the capsule is swallowed, and by peristaltic activity it reaches the biopsy site as established by fluoroscopy. At this point the biopsy port is opened and the blade is operated by hydrostatic pressure and vacuum created by syringes attached to the double lumen openings at the other end of the tube. The specimen is guillotined off and collected in the capsule. After the tube is removed, the tissue is sent to the laboratory for study.

REFERENCES AND SELECTED READINGS

1. *Bates, B.: A guide to physical examination, Philadelphia, 1974, J. B. Lippincott Co.
2. Bockus, H. L.: Gastroenterology, ed. 3, vol. 1, Philadelphia, 1974, W. B. Saunders Co.
3. Davidsohn, I., and Henry, J. B.: Todd-Sanford clinical diagnosis by laboratory methods, ed. 15, Philadelphia, 1974, W. B. Saunders Co.
4. DeGowin, E., and DeGowin, R.: Bedside diagnostic examination, ed. 3, London, 1976, Macmillan Publishing Co., Inc.
5. French, R.: Guide to diagnostic procedures, ed. 4, New York, 1975, McGraw-Hill Book Co.
6. Guyton, A.: Textbook of medical physiology, ed. 5, Philadelphia, 1977, W. B. Saunders Co.
7. Judge, R., and Zuidema, G.: Physical diagnosis: a physiological approach to the clinical examination, ed. 2, Boston, 1963, Little, Brown & Co.
8. Krupp, M., and Chatton, M.: Current medical diagnosis and treatment, Los Altos, Calif., 1974, Lange Medical Publications.
9. *Malasanos, L., Barkauskas, V., Moss, M., and Allen, K. S.: Health assessment, St. Louis, 1977, The C. V. Mosby Co.
10. *Mansell, E., Stokes, S., and Adler, J.: Patient assessment: examination of the abdomen: programmed instruction, Am. J. Nurs. **74:**1679-1702, 1974.
11. Sleisinger, M., and Fortran, J.: Gastrointestinal disease: pathophysiology, diagnosis, management, ed. 2, Philadelphia, 1978, W. B. Saunders Co.
12. Sodeman, W., and Sodeman, W.: Pathologic physiology, ed. 5, Philadelphia 1974, W. B. Saunders Co.

*References preceded by an asterisk are particularly well suited for student reading.

56

Assessment of urinary function

PAULA LAMBRECHT MILLER

In maintaining an internal environment compatible with life, the body must be able to regulate fluid volume and electrolyte composition and maintain a means for excreting metabolic wastes. Primary effectors of these regulative functions are the organs and structures of the urinary system (Fig. 56-1). The kidneys control composition of body fluid, waste, and electrolytes and maintain these substances in the body within a narrow and critical range. The kidneys also are the primary organs responsible for maintaining the acid-base balance in the body and figure importantly in the following regulatory functions:

1. Regulation of volume and composition of body fluid
   a. Fluid volume control
   b. Electrolyte regulation
   c. Excretion of metabolic waste, toxins, and drugs
2. Regulation of acid-base balance
3. Regulation of body processes
   a. Blood pressure regulation
   b. Erythropoietin production
   c. Activation of vitamin D
   d. Synthesis of glucose

The ureters, bladder, and urethra serve as the mechanism whereby waste that is filtered and secreted by the kidneys is eliminated. In assessment of elimination from the urinary tract, both the upper urinary tract that produces the urine and the lower urinary tract that removes the urine need to be considered.

■ STRUCTURE AND FUNCTION OF THE URINARY SYSTEM

□ Kidneys

The kidneys are two bean-shaped organs that lie behind the parietal peritoneum at the costovertebral angle. The organs are comprised of nephrons, a vascular system, an interstitium, and the kidney pelvis. The *nephron* is the functional unit of the kidney, and each kidney contains approximately one million of these units. The reserve capacity of the kidneys to maintain the internal environment is quite remarkable; duirng progressive chronic illness where nephrons are destroyed gradually, the sheer number of nephrons and their capacity to hypertrophy allow the individual to maintain a fairly normal internal environment until 80% of all functional kidney tissue has been destroyed. The kidneys receive 25% of cardiac output, and renal blood flow approximates 600 ml/min. This blood supply to the kidneys is basic to the formation of glomerular filtrate, or beginning urine, and to the nutrition and respiration requirement of kidney cells. Severe and prolonged problems with maintaining cardiac output and renal perfusion will have profound effects on the formation of urine and the viability of the cells responsible for maintaining consistency in the internal environment.

After passing through a series of progressively smaller arteries, the blood enters the afferent arteriole that branches into the glomerular capillaries (Fig. 56-2). The glomerulus, located in Bowman's capsule, is the first functional portion of the nephron (Fig. 56-3). When blood enters the glomerular capillaries at a pressure not less than 60 to 70 mm Hg, an ultrafiltrate of plasma is formed. This ultrafiltrate (primitive urine) contains approximately the same concentration of the elements of plasma minus the proteins. This ultrafiltrate then passes through the remainder of the nephron for modification into actual urine. The structures of the nephron involved in the process of urine formation include the glomerulus and Bowman's capsule, the proximal convoluted tubule, the loop of Henle, the distal convoluted tubule, and the collecting tubule.

Regulation of fluid volume and composition

The ultrafiltrate arising from the glomerular capillaries approximates 180 liters per day. Were it not for some conserving mechanism in the kidneys, a person would be depleted of fluid and salts within 3 to 4 minutes. The proximal convoluted tubule reabsorbs up to 85% to 90% of water in the ultrafiltrate, up to 80% of

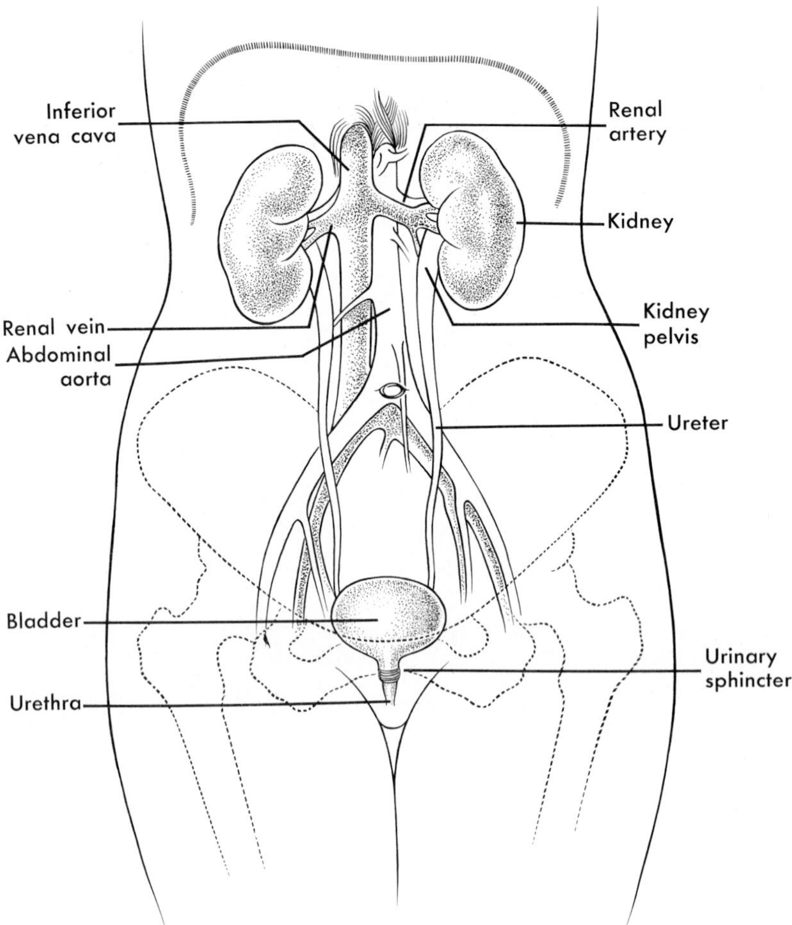

Fig. 56-1. Organs and structures of urinary system.

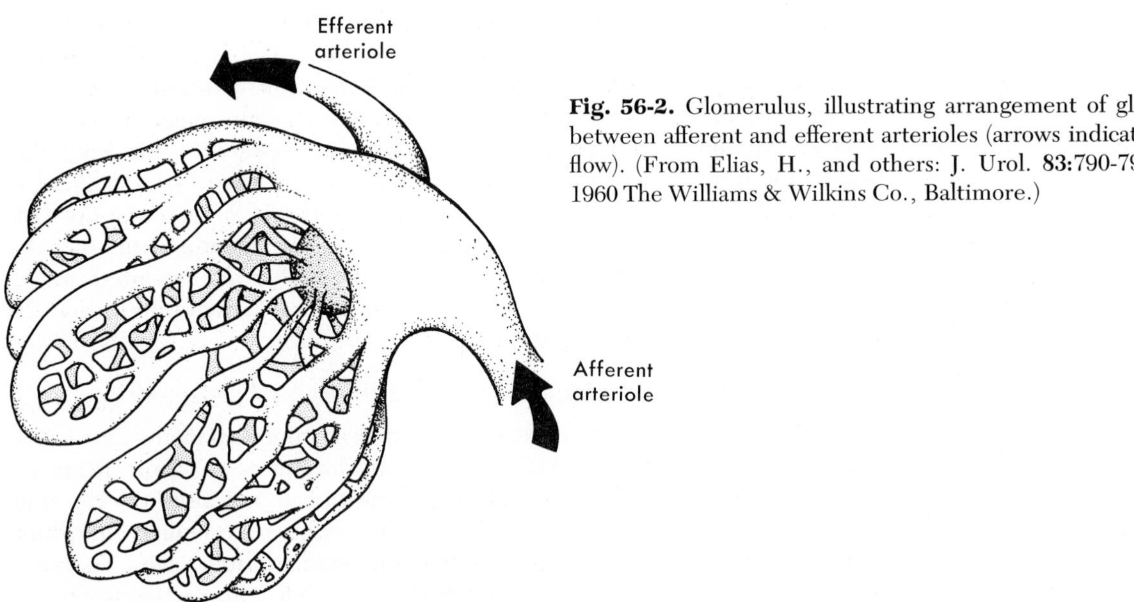

Fig. 56-2. Glomerulus, illustrating arrangement of glomerular capillaries between afferent and efferent arterioles (arrows indicate direction of blood flow). (From Elias, H., and others: J. Urol. **83:**790-798, 1960. Copyright 1960 The Williams & Wilkins Co., Baltimore.)

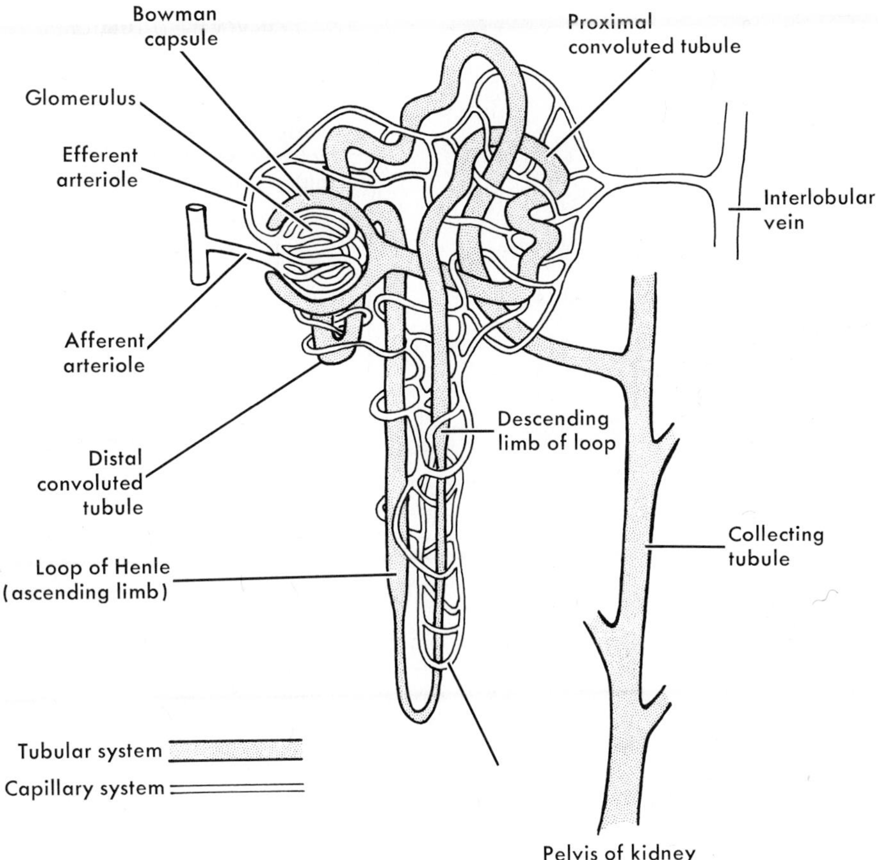

Fig. 56-3. Nephron. (From Groër, M. E., and Shekleton, M. E.: Basic pathophysiology: a conceptual approach, St. Louis, 1979, The C. V. Mosby Co.)

filtered sodium, and the majority of filtered potassium, bicarbonate, chloride, phosphate, glucose, and protein.

Dehydration would still occur if the body did not have an additional mechanism within the kidneys to conserve filtered water. This mechanism allows urine to be concentrated to less than 1% of the daily filtered volume. The kidneys can vary the amount of fluid excreted so precisely that ingestions over that required for normal fluid balance are excreted and ingestions under that required for normal fluid balance lead to further concentration of the urine. The mechanisms responsible for this increased urine concentrating ability and precision in excreting appropriate urine volume exist in the loop of Henle and the distal convoluted and collecting tubules (Fig. 56-4). The loop of Henle reaches into the medullary portion of the kidney, which is very hypertonic in comparison to the filtrate. In the descending portion of the loop, sodium diffuses into the filtrate as the tubule passes deeper into the medullary area, and water moves out of the primitive urine in response to the high sodium concentration. The result is a reduction in volume of the glomerular filtrate and a dramatic increase in its osmolarity. In the ascending limb of the loop of Henle, sodium is reabsorbed into the interstitium (Fig. 56-4), but the loop is impermeable to the movement of water either into or out of the tubule. The primitive urine now presented to the distal convoluted and collecting tubules is greatly reduced in volume, but hypotonic from the reabsorption of sodium. The influence of antidiuretic hormone (ADH) upon these last two segments of the tubule allows water to be reabsorbed into the interstitium in an amount compatible with maintenance of proper fluid balance. The reabsorption of water from the forming urine increases osmolarity and results in the excretion of a hypertonic urine.

Electrolyte balance is achieved mainly in the distal convoluted and collecting tubule portions of the nephron. As with fluid, the major conservation site for electrolytes is the proximal convoluted tubule where the vast majority of all filtered electrolytes are reabsorbed, thus preventing rapid depletion of these substances. The precise regulation of body electrolyte composition occurs in

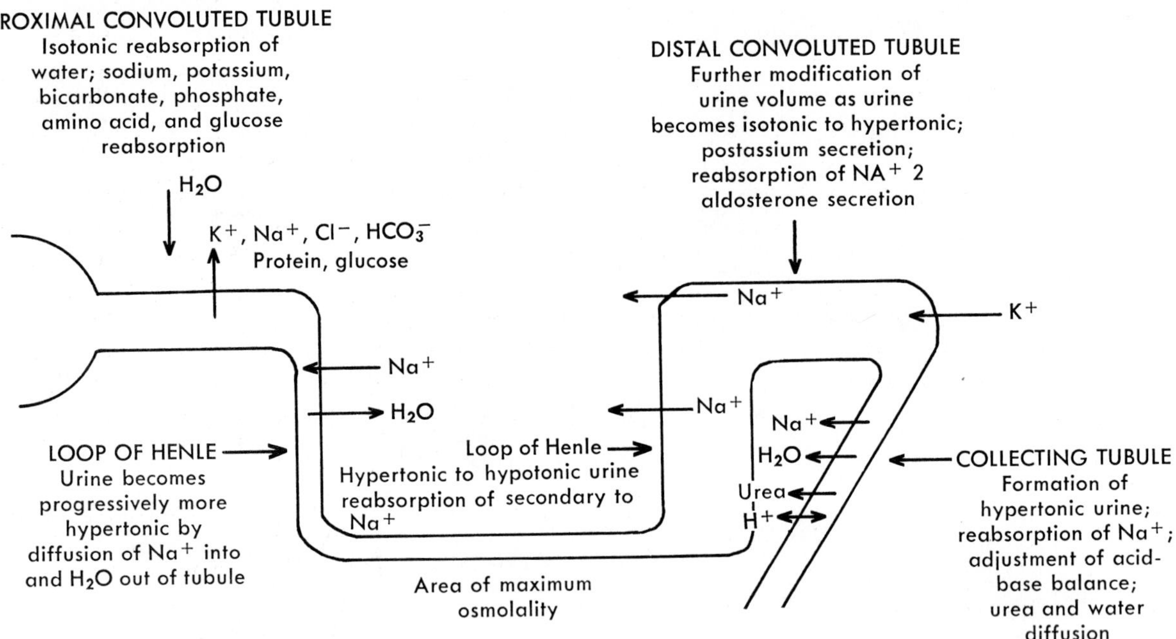

Fig. 56-4. Sites in nephron at which various changes occur in transforming primitive glomerular filtrate into definitive urine. (Adapted from Hamburger, J.: Structure and function of the kidney, Philadelphia, 1971, W. B. Saunders Co.)

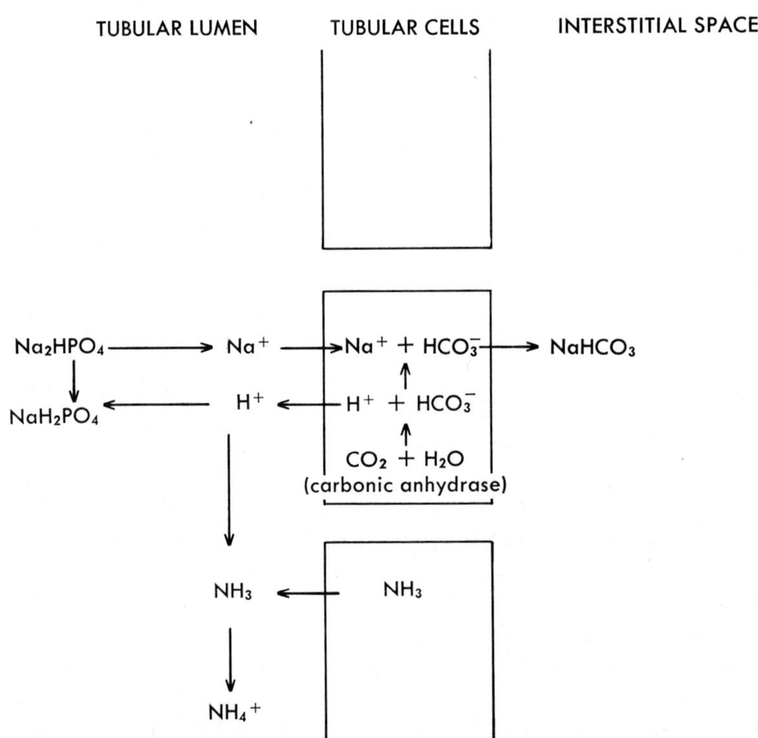

Fig. 56-5. Acid-base regulation in distal nephron. Combination of CO_2 and H_2O by enzyme carbonic anhydrase in tubular cells leads to formation of bicarbonate and free hydrogen ions. H^- ions are excreted in urine either by exchanging with sodium (Na_2PO_4 + H^-—NaH_2PO_4 + Na^-) or by combining with NH_3 to form NH_4. Bicarbonate combines with reabsorbed sodium and diffuses back into interstitial spaces. (Adapted from Hamburger, J.: Structure and function of the kidney, Philadelphia, 1971, W. B. Saunders Co.)

the distal tubular segments. Depending upon the concentrations of electrolytes presented to the tubular cells in the primitive urine and the concentrations of these substances in the interstitium, tubular cells secrete or further reabsorb electrolytes into the urine.

Acid-base balance is maintained partially through the reabsorption of bicarbonate in the proximal tubule. More precise control of acid-base status is achieved through the regeneration of bicarbonate and secretion of hydrogen ions into the urine during passage through the collecting tubule (Fig. 56-5). (The reader is referred to p. 211 for further information on acid-base balance.)

Metabolic wastes are excreted in the glomerular filtrate. Creatinine is little modified in its passage through the nephron; creatinine contained in the glomerular filtrate is excreted unchanged in the urine. Other wastes such as urea are contained in the glomerular filtrate but undergo reabsorption during passage through the nephron. The amount of waste material excreted in urine in such an instance is only a fraction of that originally contained in the glomerular filtrate.

Excretion of drugs by the kidneys occurs through both filtration at the glomerular level and secretion into the urine by distal tubular cells. Penicillin is an example of a drug secreted by tubular cells.

Additional kidney functions

Endocrine functions of the kidney include stimulation of red cell production, regulation of blood pressure, synthesis of glucose, and metabolism of calcium. Red cell *production* is influenced through secretion of erythropoietin. Though the exact nature of this factor is unknown, indirect evidence supports the presence of a kidney factor that stimulates bone marrow production of red cells. Serum hematocrit values of 20% to 30% (normal values are 42% to 47%) are commonly found in persons with chronic end-stage renal failure and are attributed in large part to a decrease in functional kidney tissue and subsequent secretion of erythropoietin.

Renal *regulation of blood pressure* is effected by three major mechanisms: (1) the control of fluid balance, which in some degree determines the circulating blood volume; (2) a hormone-mediated vasoconstrictor response; and (3) a hormone-mediated vasodilator influence. The renin-angiotensin system is responsible for renally mediated vasoconstriction. Renin is a hormone released in the juxtaglomerular apparatus in response to sodium depletion, reduction in renal arterial perfusion, and stimulation of renal nerves through the sympathetic pathways. Angiotensinogen, a protein produced by the liver, is activated in the presence of renin to angiotensin I, which is converted to angiotensin II in the lungs. Angiotensin II is a powerful vasoconstrictor and stimulates aldosterone secretion. Recent research has revealed the presence of vasodilator substances within the kidney. These substances are thought to be prostaglandins, though little more is known about the nature or mechanism of action of the substances.

The kidneys are capable of *gluconeogenesis*, although their significance in overall carbohydrate metabolism and maintenance of blood sugar is yet unknown. It has been estimated that the kidneys are capable of synthesizing glucose at an amount equal to 10% of that synthesized by the liver.[10] Through the activation of vitamin D, the kidneys influence the absorption of calcium from the gut and its deposition in bone matrix. The hydroxylation of vitamin D that occurs in the kidney is so important to the activity of this vitamin that in children with chronic renal failure of end-stage severity, the active vitamin form must be supplemented to produce growth.

□ Ureters, bladder, and urethra

The ureters arise as extensions of the kidney pelvices and empty into the bladder in an area called the trigone. These small tubes are comprised of smooth muscle; their function is to propel the urine from the kidneys into the bladder. Spasm and severe colic-type pain results from obstruction of the ureters. The bladder, situated behind the symphysis pubis, can retain urine until an appropriate time for urination arises. This voluntary control is based upon the learned inhibition of reflex pathway messages arising from the bladder walls. The urethral sphincter operating under voluntary control allows the urine to pass into the urethra for discharge from the body.

■ DATA COLLECTION

□ Lower urinary tract

Most disorders of the lower urinary tract relate to inability to void easily or to empty the bladder, inability to control voiding, or pain with urination.

Inability to void

Subjective data includes the person's description of his ability to void. Difficulty starting the stream or maintaining a flow of urine is usually indicative of partial obstruction at the bladder outlet or weakness of the bladder muscles. Persons who must use a bedpan or urinal when lying in bed may have difficulty initiating voiding because of the change from the usual posture for voiding. Those who have had an indwelling catheter removed may have temporary weakness of bladder muscles. Men with enlarged prostates may have partial obstruction of the prostatic urethra. Assessment should be made of the duration of the problem and the person's perceptions about it. Data about usual voiding patterns is obtained as a baseline for future reference. Observation of the urinary stream confirms the person's report of hesitancy and intermittent stream. Catheterization after voiding may reveal residual urine volume.

Bladder distention occurs with complete urethral obstruction or with inability to initiate the stream. Data includes the presence of a sensation of fullness in the lower abdomen with a desire to void although unable to do so. Restlessness can be observed. Palpation or percussion of the bladder above the symphysis pubis is a nonintrusive means to detect bladder distention.

Inability to control voiding

Incontinence is assessed by determining the specific nature of the problem: whether it occurs continually or only with stress, presence of sensation of fullness prior to voiding, the person's awareness of and feelings regarding the incontinence, and health conditions associated with the incontinence (spinal cord damage, central nervous system disease, urinary tract infection or obstruction). The method used by the person or family for controlling the incontinence must be identified. The skin is examined for areas of irritation or breakdown.

Pain with urination

Normal voiding is painless. *Dysuria*, or painful urination, is usually a sign of urinary tract infection. The most common description given by the person is *burning* with urination. *Frequency* of urination and a sense of *urgency* to void usually accompany the dysuria. Malaise, fatigue, and fever may also be present. The frequency of symptoms, the person's current physical condition, and his plans for managing the symptoms are assessed. On examination, the urine may appear clear, cloudy, or purulent.

Obstruction of the ureters produces pain along the course of the ureter radiating down to the groin, which is not associated with voiding per se. The pain is intermittent and severe, and vomiting may occur in association with the pain.

Toileting ability

Patients who are admitted to a hospital or other nursing care facility should have their toileting ability assessed. This includes the person's level of consciousness in order to be able to initiate toileting in addition to the ability to carry out toileting independently.

■ UPPER URINARY TRACT

□ Renal disease

Health problems that arise for persons with renal disease are varied in number and extent and depend on both the type and severity of the underlying disease. Some persons may appear well and have little or no physiologic dysfunction while others with advanced renal disease will reflect changes in every organ system and in all aspects of their daily living.

The following data is useful in making a nursing assessment of a person with renal disease:

1. Person's perception of illness
   a. Factors leading person to the seeking of health care
   b. Knowledge of health status and care needs
   c. Expectations regarding current health care
   d. Knowledge of significant others about person's health status
2. Previous or concurrent illness
   a. Other chronic health problems
   b. Medications currently taken
3. Social needs
   a. Resources for assistance as needed
   b. Current occupation; capacity to continue present work
4. Fluid balance
   a. Subjective
      (1) Shortness of breath (relate to position of comfort; activity tolerance)
      (2) Visual changes
      (3) Headaches
   b. Objective
      (1) Apprehension
      (2) Blood pressure (related to normal levels for the person; postural blood pressure)
      (3) Central venous pressure
      (4) Respirations (rate; depth)
      (5) Breath sounds
      (6) Pulse irregularities
      (7) Pericardial friction rub
      (8) Peripheral edema (location and extent)
      (9) Weight (direction of change; rate and extent of change)
      (10) Output (amount per hour; amount per day; related to intake)
      (11) Urine specific gravity
5. Electrolyte balance
   a. Subjective
      (1) Lethargy
      (2) Memory function
      (3) Parasthesias
      (4) Vague muscle weakness
   b. Objective
      (1) Behavior (observe for changes)
      (2) Level of alertness and orientation
      (3) Kussmaul respirations
      (4) Blood pH
      (5) Serum electrolytes
      (6) ECG pattern
6. Nutrition
   a. Subjective

(1) Anorexia, nausea, or vomiting
(2) Aids to food tolerance
(3) History of special diets
(4) Knowledge of diet restrictions
(5) Normal meal pattern

b. Objective
(1) Diet order (Na^+; K^+; protein)

7. Elimination
a. Subjective
(1) Bowel pattern
(2) Laxative use
(3) Nocturia
(4) Symptoms of urinary tract infection
b. Objective
(1) Urinalysis
(2) Urine culture
(3) Serum creatinine
(4) Serum urea nitrogen
(5) Stool guaiac

8. Skin and hygiene habits
a. Subjective
(1) Bathing pattern
(2) History of dental care
b. Objective
(1) Lesions (skin, mucous membranes)
(2) Moisture (skin, mucous membranes)
(3) Parotitis
(4) Condition of teeth

9. Comfort; rest; sleep
a. Subjective
(1) Pruritus (extent, relief measures)
(2) Sleep pattern (adequacy of rest)
(3) Pain (nature, extent, etc)
(4) Breath odor (control measures)
b. Objective
(1) Scratching
(2) Sleeping during day
(3) Nonverbal signs of pain
(4) Fever

10. Mobility; functional ability
a. Subjective
(1) Fatigue (extent; recovery with rest)
(2) Weakness of an extremity
(3) Numbness; tingling
b. Objective
(1) Balance
(2) Gait
(3) Muscle tone
(4) Decreased sensation

11. Sexuality
a. Subjective
(1) Menses (pattern)
(2) Concerns regarding sexual function and reproduction
b. Objective
(1) Behavior when with significant others

Palpation of the kidney

Palpation of the kidney is performed while assessing the organs of the abdomen. Normally the left kidney is not palpable; occasionally the lower pole of the right kidney can be felt. To examine the kidney the individual lies in a supine position with the examiner on the right side of the examining table or bed. Each kidney is examined in the following manner: (1) the flank is elevated anteriorly with one hand; (2) the kidney is palpated lightly with the palmar surface of the hand; and (3) the individual is asked to inspire during palpation. Sometimes the lower pole of the right kidney can be felt as a rounded smooth mass that descends with inspiration.

An enlarged spleen can be mistaken for an enlarged left kidney. To differentiate between the two, percussion is necessary. An enlarged spleen has a dull percussive note, while resonance is heard over the kidney.

■ DIAGNOSTIC STUDIES

Special examinations of the urinary system are performed to identify the location and nature of existing disease. The accuracy of findings in many of the following tests is dependent on the assistance of the person in restricting or augmenting intake of fluids or in collecting specimens at designated time intervals. The person is given clear, precise directions, and written instructions are a valuable supplement to verbal directions. Some examinations are performed under sedation. If the person is to return home after such a procedure, prior discussion includes making arrangements for someone to accompany the person home following the procedure.

□ Examination of the urine

Urinalysis

In identifying disease of the urinary tract, one of the first tests performed is the urinalysis. This test yields information about probable locations and causes of urinary disease, and some information as to the extent of the illness. Urinalysis is a test that assists in establishing tentative diagnoses and predicting additional tests and observations required to make precise diagnoses. Urinalysis also indicates abnormalities of nonrenal and nonurologic origin (for example, diabetes mellitus). Table 56-1 indicates possible normal and abnormal findings.

Ideally the urine specimen is collected from the first voiding of the day. This sample is preferable because it is concentrated and abnormal constituents are more likely to be present. The person is given a clean container in which to catch urine. Cleansing the meatus prior to col-

Table 56-1. Urine constituents identified on a urinalysis test: normal and abnormal findings

Test	Normal	Abnormal
Color	Amber-yellow	Red indicates hematuria (possible urinary obstruction, renal calculi, tumor, renal failure)
Clarity	Clear	Cloudy: debris, bacterial sediment (urinary infection)
pH	4.6 to 8.0 (average 6.0)	Alkaline upon standing or with urinary tract infection Increased acidity with renal tubular acidosis
Specific gravity	1.003 to 1.035	Usually reflects fluid intake, the less the fluid intake, the higher the specific gravity If specific gravity remains low (1.010 to 1.014), renal disease is suspected
Protein	0 to 8 mg/100 ml	Proteinuria may occur with high protein diet and exercise (particularly prolonged) Seen in renal disease
Sugar	0	Glycosuria occurs after a high intake of sugar or with diabetes mellitus
Ketones	0	Ketonuria occurs with starvation and diabetic ketoacidosis
Red blood cells	0 to 4	Injury to kidney tissue (see hematuria)
White blood cells	0 to 5	Urinary tract infection (UTI)
Casts	0	UTI, renal disease

lection of the specimen decreases likelihood of external contamination; mild soap followed by water or a special cleansing solution may be used. At least 50 to 100 ml of urine is collected for the test to ensure a sufficient amount to determine specific gravity in addition to microscopic analysis. If analysis of the urine cannot be performed immediately, the specimen must be refrigerated to retard bacterial growth.

Multiple-glass test

The multiple-glass test is performed on a man when infection of the lower urinary tract is to be evaluated. A full bladder is required for this test as a number of samples will be taken during a single voiding. The man cleanses the area about the meatus with an antiseptic solution prior to specimen collection, with care being taken throughout the procedure to avoid introducing new bacteria into the specimens. The man is asked to void about 100 ml into a container; this sample contains organisms and sediment "washed" from the urethra. Without interrupting the urinary stream, another 100 ml of urine is voided into a second container. This urine contains organisms and sediment representative of that in the bladder and kidney. The man is then instructed to stop voiding and the physician gently massages the prostate; a third specimen, which contains secretions from the prostate gland is then collected.

Composite specimens

A specimen of all the urine excreted over a specific period of time is often required for the urologic diagnosis. The duration of urine collections may vary from 2 to 24 hours. Specimens are examined for sugar, protein, sediment (blood cells and casts), 17-ketosteroids, electrolytes, catecholamines, and breakdown products of protein metabolism. These tests provide information regarding (1) the ability of the kidneys to excrete and conserve various solutes; (2) the production in the body of excessive hormones that are excreted in the urine; (3) changes in the body's regulation of glucose metabolism; and (4) identification of organisms difficult to recognize through routine urine cultures.

The accuracy of findings in this type of test is in most instances entirely dependent on cooperation of the patient. Whether the specimen is to be obtained in the hospital or in the home, the person needs to be told exactly how to collect it as follows:

1. The bladder is emptied and the urine *discarded* at the appointed time to start the test.
2. Urine from *all* subsequent voidings is saved.
3. Some specimens need to be kept cold during the collection period; some need preservatives added; some need no special care.
4. The person should void into a separate receptacle

before defecation to prevent contamination of the specimen.

5. The bladder is emptied and the urine *added* to the collection at the appointed time to end the test.
6. The designated amount is sent to the laboratory properly labeled.
7. If an aliquot (5 to 10 ml sample of the total specimen) is the designated amount, the total amount collected is (1) measured and recorded on the specimen requisition and (2) mixed well before the aliquot is selected.

Composite urine tests may also involve collecting urine from multiple sources from the body. For instance, the person may pass urine from his urethra and also have a nephrostomy tube from which urine drains. Ureteral catheters may also be in place, with urine being collected from each kidney separately. Depending upon the function of the test, whether the purpose is to measure the identified element in the urine as a whole or to measure separately the excretion of this element from each kidney, the urine collected from each source might be combined into one specimen container or collected into separate well-labeled containers.

Urine culture

Urine cultures are obtained to confirm suspected infections and identify causative organisms for appropriate antimicrobial therapy. Cultures are also obtained for periodic screening of urine when the threat of urinary tract infection persists.

Urine in a properly collected and stored sample is considered to be normal if it contains 10,000 or fewer organisms per milliliter. Organisms of this count magnitude are the result of normal urethral flora and do not signify urinary tract infection. A urinary tract infection is diagnosed when bacterial counts in a properly collected and stored sample reach 100,000 or greater organisms per milliliter and the organisms are of one or very largely one bacterial type.[16] Contamination of the urine specimen during collection is most likely when bacterial counts include predominant colonies of *Staphylococcus*, *Streptococcus*, and diphtheroids, when two or more organisms contribute significantly to the total bacterial count, or when repeated cultures yield differing results. All of these results are indications of a need to repeat the culture, paying particular attention to the collection of the specimen and to its handling.

Specimens for urine culture may be obtained either by catheterization or voiding. It should be made clear, however, that urethral catheterization should never be used routinely in collecting urine for culture because of the risk of introducing additional bacteria into the bladder. Catheterization may be necessary to obtain a sterile urine specimen when the person is unable to void even after being adequately hydrated or if the person is incontinent of urine. When a catheter is passed, meticulous attention is given to nontraumatic aseptic technique. After urine flow from the catheter is established, 5 to 10 ml of urine should be collected directly into a sterile specimen container. Care must be taken to ensure that the rim and the inside of the container are not touched by the catheter or by the hands. If a culture tube with a cotton plug is used as specimen container, care must be taken to keep the tube upright to prevent moistening the cotton and thereby contaminating the specimen. Cultures may also be ordered on the urine taken from the renal pelvis during ureteral catheterization or when ureterostomy or nephrostomy tubes are in place.

In collecting a voided specimen for culture, the nurse must decide if the patient is capable of independently obtaining the specimen or if nursing or medical personnel will need to collect the specimen. Most persons who are ambulatory and are given precise and unhurried direction will be able to collect their own midstream urine specimen (see boxed material below).

The first voided specimen of the day should be used whenever possible because bacteria will be more numerous. If the specimen is not cultured immediately, refrigeration is mandatory to prevent growth of organisms in the specimen.

DIRECTIONS FOR COLLECTING A MIDSTREAM URINE SPECIMEN

Equipment needed

Sterile container for the urine
3 sponges (cotton or gauze) saturated with cleansing solution

General directions

Only outside of collecting container is touched
Urine is collected in container well after urinary stream is started

Special directions

Female

Labia are kept separated throughout procedure
Meatus is cleansed with one front-to-back motion with each of the three cleansing sponges

Male

Foreskin is retracted if man is uncircumcised
Glans is cleansed with each of the three cleansing sponges

Evaluating bladder function

Measurement of residual urine

Normally the bladder contains little or no urine after voiding; however, certain disease states inhibit the bladder from emptying completely. Some common conditions in which incomplete emptying of the bladder occurs are benign prostatic hypertrophy, urethral strictures, and interruptions in bladder innervation. Urine left in the bladder after voiding is called *residual urine*.

One way to determine the amount of residual urine is to *catheterize* the person immediately after voiding. This may be ordered by the physician on a one-time or on a serial basis. Prior to catheterizing the person, the physician is consulted regarding the plan for establishing urinary drainage. If a large residual urine is suspected, the physician may wish the catheter to be left in place in the bladder. Residual urine volumes of 50 ml or less indicate near-normal or returning bladder function.

To avoid passing a catheter to measure residual urine volumes, roentgenographic examination of retained urine may be performed. In this procedure a radiopaque substance excreted by the kidneys is injected intravenously. As the dye is excreted in the urine, it passes into the bladder. A sufficient amount of urine containing the radiopaque material is allowed to accumulate in the bladder before the person is instructed to void. Immediately after voiding a roentgenogram is taken. Any urine retained in the bladder will be visualized on the roentgenogram.

Cystometrograms

Cystometric examination is performed to evaluate bladder tone. In general, the examination is indicated when incontinence is present or when there is evidence or suspicion of neurologic dysfunction of the bladder. The cystometrogram provides data on (1) the presence of a spastic or flaccid muscular tone, (2) the presence of fullness and urgency sensations, (3) the effect of drug therapy in establishing or changing bladder tone, (4) the rate of change in bladder tone with a progressive illness, such as multiple sclerosis, (5) the person's ability to generate sufficient pressure to expel urine using Credé or Valsalva maneuver, (6) the intactness and innervation of the urinary sphincter, and (7) the residual urine volume. This data assists in diagnosis and in planning effective management of the dysfunction.

A Foley catheter is inserted prior to the examination. After the patient assumes a supine position, a liter bottle of normal saline or sterile distilled water and a cystometer are connected to the catheter. Fluid is instilled at a constant and specified rate; measurements of the pressure exerted on the fluid by the bladder musculature are taken and recorded after the instillation of every 50 ml of fluid. The patient is asked to report feelings of fullness, the need to void, and any urgency or discomfort. Fluid is instilled until urgency occurs, or is discontinued after determining that sensation is absent. During cystometric examination, bethanechol chloride (Urecholine) may be administered to determine its effect on enhancing the tone of a flaccid bladder, or an anticholingergic medication may be given to assess relaxation in a hyperactive bladder. There is no specific care required by person after cystometric examination.

Electromyography (p. 831) may be used to evaluate sphincter tone and intactness of nerve pathways.

Evaluating renal functioning

Tests of renal function are carried out when findings in the general physical evaluation of the person or in the urinalysis suggest renal disease. The best overview of the person's clinical condition is obtained when the results of a number of tests are compared.

Clearance tests

When renal disease is suspected, the physician will want to determine the amount of damage, if any, that has already occurred. The most practical and efficient way to identify losses in renal function is by means of clearance tests. These tests measure the amount of blood that an individual's kidneys can "clear" of a substance in a given amount of time. When the person's values are compared to normal values, changes in renal function become apparent. Clearance tests are also used to monitor the direction of change and the rate of change in renal function over time.

The *creatinine clearance* test is the most practical and widely used of all clearance tests. Creatinine is a substance that results from the breakdown of muscle tissue. It is produced at a relatively fixed and uniform rate throughout the day, it can be measured readily in the blood, and it is not influenced by dietary intake. Creatinine is excreted through the kidneys; it is filtered in the glomerulus and passes practically unchanged through the renal tubules. It is an ideal naturally occurring substance that, when blood and urine values are compared, allows one to estimate changes in glomerular filtration rates and overall kidney function. The creatinine clearance value for an individual is expressed in terms of milliliters per minute and is determined according to the following equation:

$$\text{Creatinine clearance (ml/min)} = \frac{\text{Urine volume (ml/min)} \times \text{Urine creatinine concentration (mg/ml)}}{\text{Plasma creatinine concentration (mg/ml)}}$$

For this test, a morning-to-morning 24-hour urine collection is obtained. (Refer to collection of composite urine specimens on p. 1234). Immediately after the final urine specimen is collected, a blood specimen is drawn to determine the serum creatinine level. Both blood and urine specimens are sent together for analysis. Analysis of the total urine volume for the test period is essential for accurate determination of renal function. If one voiding is accidentally discarded, the test must be repeated. A shorter period of time may be used in instances when collection of accurate urine collections over a 24-hour period are next to impossible.

Normal clearance values for creatinine are approximately 95 to 140 ml/min for men and 85 to 125 ml/min for women. In individuals with depressed renal function these values will be decreased.

The *urea* clearance test is seldom used, as it is influenced by urine flow and is less accurate than the creatinine clearance test.

The sodium excretion test measures tubular function. Specifically, this test provides information as to the kidneys' ability to appropriately excrete or conserve this electrolyte; in chronic renal failure either inappropriate retention or excretion of sodium can occur. Knowledge of urinary excretion of this electrolyte is helpful in calculating sodium intake requirements of the patient. In order to determine change in direction and degree of tubular functions, comparison of current and past sodium excretion studies should be made. The test is performed by analyzing the sodium content of a 24-hour urine collection.

Blood chemistry tests

A major function of the kidney is excretion of byproducts of metabolism. The two most commonly ordered tests of renal function, *serum creatinine* and *blood urea nitrogen* (BUN) tests, are measures of the kidneys' ability to excrete metabolic wastes. Specifically, these tests measure serum concentrations of nitrogenous products derived from protein breakdown. In health, serum creatinine concentration approximates 0.9 to 1.5 mg/100 ml, and blood urea nitrogen ranges from 10 to 20 mg/100 ml. In the later stages of renal insufficiency, nitrogen products are retained and serum values are markedly elevated. No special preparation is required for these tests. In interpreting test results, however, it should be remembered that high-protein diets; rapid cellular destruction from trauma, infection, and fever; and strenuous, prolonged muscular activity increase nitrogen waste levels. Abnormally high laboratory values of urea nitrogen occur in these states and may not reflect the person's true level of renal function.

Since the kidneys are also responsible for regulating the *concentration of electrolytes* in the extracellular fluid compartment, analysis of the levels of these electrolytes yields information about kidney function. The electrolytes most frequently evaluated include potassium (3.5 to 5.0 mEq/liter of blood), sodium (138 to 148 mEq/liter), calcium (9.0 to 11.0 mg/100 ml), chloride (100 to 106 mEq/liter), and phosphorus (3.0 to 4.5 mg/100 ml). Levels of serum electrolytes in persons with renal disease are dependent on the location and severity of pathologic conditions of the kidneys and hence can be quite varied from person to person.

In kidney disease involving the glomeruli, loss of *plasma proteins* may occur. It has been demonstrated that various types of glomerular lesions exist and that these lesions allow passage of different amounts and types of plasma proteins into the glomerular filtrate. Serum determinations of plasma protein fractions and total protein content can assist in evaluating the nature and extent of the renal disease.

Fishberg concentration test

The Fishberg concentration test involves a controlled effort to determine the ability of the kidneys to conserve fluid. Clinically the test is useful in making a differential diagnosis between diabetes insipidus (p. 570) and psychogenic polydipsia. The test involves a period of dehydration for the person (usually 8 to 12 hours overnight). During the test no fluid is taken. Morning specimens ensure maximum concentrations of substances in the urine. Three hourly urine specimens are collected to determine volume, specific gravity, and osmolality. The person is carefully observed for signs of vascular collapse, indicating severe dehydration.

□ Visualization of the urinary tract

Visualization tests measure both structure and function of organs and tissues in the urinary system. They are used both in initially diagnosing and in evaluating response to treatment over a period of time.

Several of these tests are dependent on roentgenograms for visualization of the urinary tract. Since the kidneys lie retroperitoneally, any accumulation of flatus or feces in the intestines could obstruct the view of the kidneys on a roentgenogram. To assure visualization, emptying of the bowel is carried out prior to examination. The person's age and state of health are considered in determining the extensiveness of the bowel preparation.

Infants, young children, elderly people, and physically debilitated individuals should not be subjected to vigorous bowel preparation as dehydration and serious electrolyte disturbances may ensue. Some instances of preexisting conditions in which bowel cleansing is especially hazardous are severe nutritional deficiencies, colitis, presence of an ileostomy, fluid and electrolyte disturbances, and renal insufficiency or failure. Bowel preparation for individuals with any of these conditions should be discussed with the patient's physician or the radiologist.

Preparation usually includes a cathartic such as 60 ml of castor oil or bisacodyl (Dulcolax) tablets the night before the test and nothing by mouth after midnight. If bowel evacuation has been ineffective, a bisacodyl suppository or enema may be given in the morning. Ineffectiveness of these efforts is communicated to the physician and the radiology department well before the time scheduled for examination.

Physical safety of the person must be assured when vigorous cathartics are employed. Urgency, fatigue, and weakness are common following bowel cleansing; falls and accidents easily occur in these states. Sedation, which slows reaction time and further unsteadies gait, should be withheld. Prior to sleep the person should become familiar with his surroundings and with the location of his call light. Close observation is provided throughout the night, with assistance provided as indicated.

Roentgenograms of the urinary tract may be ordered in conjunction with other abdominal studies. Problems may arise in visualizing the urinary system if barium studies have been recently carried out. This problem is prevented by scheduling tests so that examination of the urinary tract precedes barium swallows, gastrointestinal series, and barium enemas. They may be done on the same day, however, as long as the urogram is done first.

Radiologic examination of the abdomen (KUB)

A flat plate film of the abdomen can reveal gross structural changes in the kidneys and urinary system. The size, shape, and placement of the kidneys can be determined, and calcifications or stones located in a kidney, pelvis, or ureter can be visualized. Bowel preparations may or may not be ordered for this examination.

Intravenous pyelography (excretory urogram)

In the intravenous pyelogram (IVP) a roentgenogram can demonstrate the size and location of the kidneys, cysts or tumors within the kidneys, filling of the renal pelves, and the outline of the ureters and bladder. This is accomplished through the excretion by the kidneys of a radiopaque dye that has been injected intravenously. The IVP tests kidney excretory function and the patency of the urinary tract. This test may be performed in a clinic or hospital setting.

Preparation for the examination includes bowel cleansing usually with 60 ml of castor oil, and withholding of fluids for up to 8 hours prior to testing to produce slight dehydration and greater concentration of dye in the kidneys and urinary system.

Before examination an attempt is made to learn whether the person is sensitive to iodine, as the radiopaque material injected intravenously contains this substance. The test should not be performed on individuals with known sensitivity to iodine because anaphylaxis can result. At times it is difficult to determine sensitivity prior to use. Two precautions are taken to prevent serious reactions to the dye during IVP examination: (1) most dye preparations have antihistamine added as a precautionary measure and (2) emergency drugs such as epinephrine are immediately available in the examination area.

For the roentgenogram the person is placed on an x-ray table. A roentgenogram of the abdomen (KUB film) is taken first to identify size and position of the kidneys, the amount of gas in the bowel, and any radiopaque stones in the urinary tract. After this film is read, the radiopaque dye (Hypaque, Renografin) is given intravenously. The patient is informed that he may experience a feeling of warmth, a flushing of the face, and a salty taste in the mouth as the physician slowly injects the dye. These sensations should abate within a few minutes; some relief may be obtained by taking deep breaths. The person is closely observed for any signs of respiratory distress, sudden diaphoresis and clamminess, urticaria, instability in vital signs, or any unusual sensation; any of these may indicate a reaction to the contrast medium. Tripelennamine (Pyribenzamine), diphenhydramine hydrochloride (Benadryl), epinephrine (Adrenalin), oxygen, and cardiopulmonary resuscitation equipment should be available for immediate use.

Sometimes a large plastic ball is strapped firmly on the abdomen to prevent dye from passing freely down the ureters until after roentgenograms of the kidneys have been taken. Roentgenograms are usually taken at 3, 5, 10, and 20 minutes after the dye has been injected. If obstruction or poor renal function is present, additional films may be taken 1 and 2 hours later.

Body section roentgenography

Body section roentgenography consists of roentgenograms of a section of the body taken with a rotating x-ray tube. One type of body section roentgenography is *tomography* in which the x-ray tube is moved in the direction of an arc. A *nephrotomogram* is a tomogram taken after intravenous injection of a radiopaque dye. After the person is placed on an x-ray table, a circulation time study (p. 925) is done to guide the timing of the series to be taken. A radiopaque dye such as sodium acetrizoate (Pyelokon R), with dehydrocholic acid (Decholin) added, is then given intravenously. The patient is instructed to indicate the moment that he tastes the dehydrocholic acid and the films are then taken. Physical preparation of the patient is the same as that for intravenous pyelography. He should be instructed to expect the same sensations when the dye is given, and he should be observed for the same drug reactions. Since the regulation of the time interval is dependent on

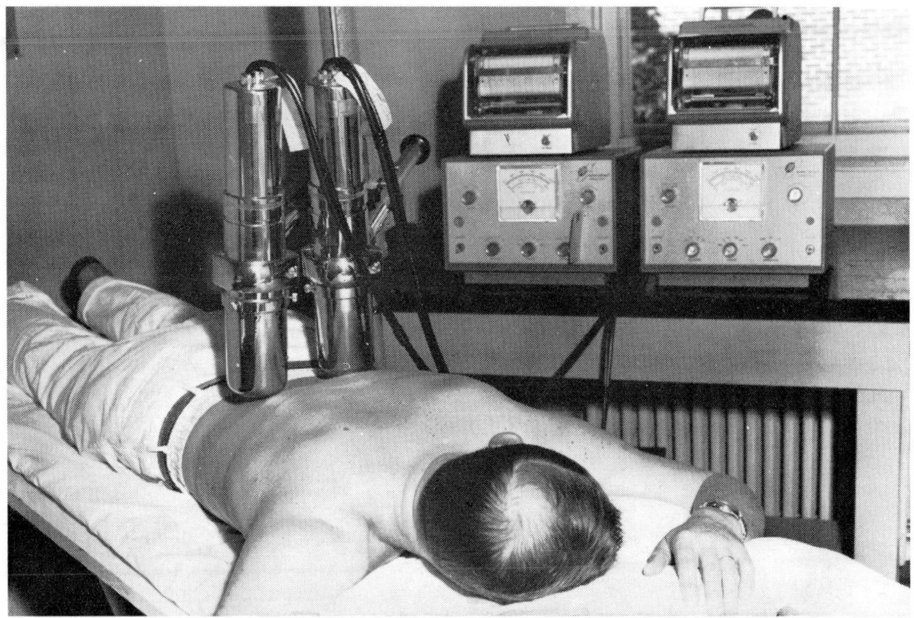

Fig. 56-6. Radiorenography. Scintillation probes are in place over both kidneys. (Courtesy Veterans Administration Center, Martinsburg, W. Va.; from Abt, A. F., and Balkus, V. A.: J. Urol. **85:**95, 1961.)

the person's cooperation, it is important that he understand his role in the procedure.

Radiorenography

Radiorenography tests involve scintillation scanning or photography techniques in visualizing the urinary tract. Diagnostically these tests can measure renal blood flow and renal tubular or excretory function. Therefore they are useful tests in (1) detecting obstructions in the upper urinary tract, (2) detecting renal vascular disease in hypertensive patients, (3) detecting acute renal failure within 48 hours of onset of oliguria, (4) monitoring the function of transplanted kidneys and detecting early signs of rejection, and (5) general follow-up of patients with renal disease and evaluation of the effectiveness of their treatment.

In radiorenography a preparation containing a radioactive isotope such as iodohippurate sodium tagged with ^{131}I or ^{125}I (Hippuran) is injected intravenously. No precautions need be taken against radioactivity, as only tracer doses of the isotope are used. When iodine isotopes are used, Lugol's solution need not be given prior to examination to prevent thyroid damage because the isotopes used are bound to large molecules that prevent their uptake by the thyroid gland. There are no dietary or activity restrictions prior to testing. The test lasts only minutes and can be repeated a number of times.

In performing the test the patient is placed on an x-ray table and scintillating probes are placed over the kidney(s) being examined (Fig. 56-6). The radioisotope is injected and scanning or photographic recording is begun. The patient should feel no pain or discomfort as the test is being carried out.

Renal angiography

The renal angiogram provides an outline of the vascularization of the kidneys. The examination is particularly useful in attempting to evaluate the possibility of renal artery stenosis as a causative factor in hypertension and in demonstrating renal neoplasms and abnormal renal vessels.

Preparation of the individual is similar to that for the IVP. In addition, sedation of the patient is often carried out using secobarbital or similar medication. When sedation is used, attention must be given to safety of the person.

In performing the test, a contrast material similar to that used in intravenous pyelography is injected. Precautions should be taken against iodine sensitivity reactions. As the dye is injected and passes into the renal vasculature, roentgenograms are taken in rapid succession. The dye may be injected intravenously, and circulation time is calculated to ensure proper timing in taking the roentgenograms, or it may be injected intraarterially. The latter technique is more widely performed and is termed aortography. In *translumbar aortography* the radiopaque dye is injected into the aorta by way of a long needle inserted through the soft tissue in the lumbar region. If a *femoral percutaneous aortogram* is performed, a catheter is threaded from a puncture of the femoral artery upward to the level of the renal arteries; dye is then injected through this catheter. After the roentgenograms have been taken and the catheter or needle removed, a pressure dressing is applied to the puncture site.

Care after the procedure includes observing the site for bleeding, especially within the first 4 hours after the procedure. The dressing is observed for fresh bleeding, the puncture area is checked for swelling and increasing tenderness, vital signs are monitored frequently, and distal pulses are taken if femoral percutaneous aortography has been performed. Bed rest is indicated for at least 8 hours after the test, and the pressure dressing is left in place until the following morning.

Venocavography

Venocavography determines patency in the venous system and can detect masses in the renal veins. A contrast medium is injected into the inferior vena cava via the femoral vein, and roentgenograms are taken. Preparation of the patient and precautions observed during and after the test are similar to those for angiography.

Retroperitoneal pneumography

The retroperitoneal pneumogram is an x-ray examination performed to diagnose adrenal or retroperitoneal tumors not visible on a flat plate examination. In this test the patient is placed in a side-lying position, and 400 to 800 ml of gas is injected in the retroperitoneal space as a contrast medium. Carbon dioxide is the gas most commonly used as it is rapidly absorbed into the bloodstream.

Preparation for this examination is similar to that carried out for the IVP. The patient is sedated, as discomfort, abdominal cramping, and nausea and vomiting may occur as the gas is injected. Following this test the patient should be kept in bed for a few hours and comfort maintained. Bleeding should not be precipitated by this procedure.

Cystoscopy and retrograde pyelography

Cystoscopy is the examination of the inside of the bladder through an instrument called a cystoscope (Fig. 56-7). The instrument is connected to an illuminating source, thus enabling direct visualization of the bladder wall. Cystoscopic examination may be performed as part of a series of diagnostic tests or as an emergency measure in locating the source of and controlling heavy bleeding.

Most hospitals require a signed permit prior to cystoscopy after the person is given an explanation of what is to occur. Fluids are usually forced for several hours before the procedure. This ensures a continuous flow of urine in the event specimens need to be collected and aids in preventing multiplication of bacteria that may be introduced during the procedure. If general anesthesia is to be used, fluids may be administered intravenously. If roentgenograms are to be taken during the procedure, bowel preparation may be ordered.

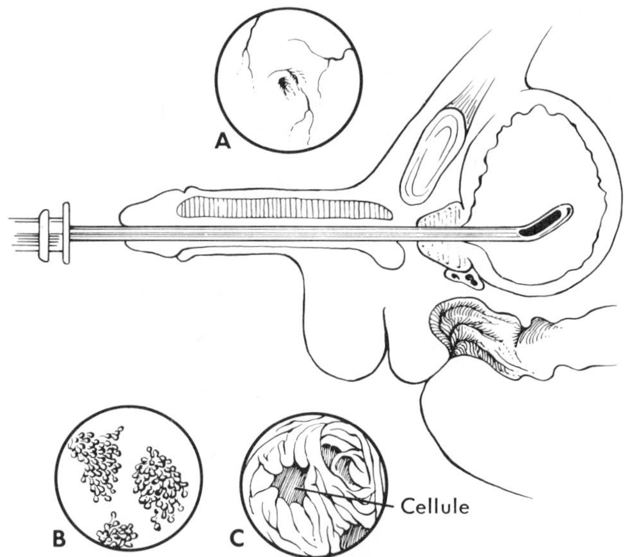

Fig. 56-7. Cystoscope inserted for examination of bladder. **A,** Appearance of normal ureteral orifice as seen through cystoscope. **B,** Appearance of papillomas of bladder as seen through cystoscope. **C,** Appearance of trabeculated bladder as seen through cystoscope. Note formation of cellules.

The cystoscopic examination may be performed with or without anesthesia. General anesthesia is required for cystoscopy when the person is quite apprehensive or when much manipulation is anticipated. In these instances, anesthesia reduces the possibility of trauma to the urethra or perforation of the bladder caused by sudden vigorous movement by the patient during the examination. Children are usually given a general anesthetic for this procedure. Much of the discomfort felt during this procedure is the result of contraction or spasm of the bladder sphincters; this can be decreased through deep-breathing exercises and general relaxation on the part of the patient. A sedative such as diazepam (Valium) and a narcotic such as morphine or meperidine hydrochloride (Demerol) are usually given an hour prior to the examination.

If the patient is relatively comfortable, the cystoscope should be passed with little pain, provided there is no obstruction in the urethra. A local anesthetic such as procaine (usually 4%) may be instilled into the urethra prior to insertion of the cystoscope.

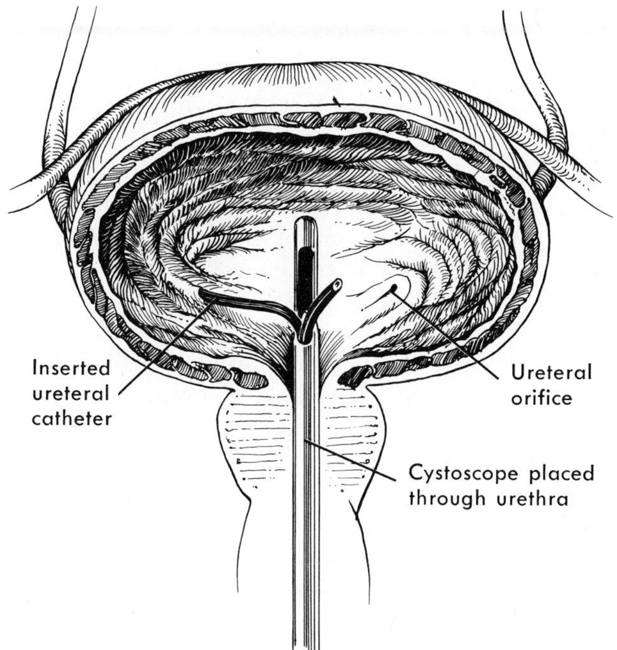

Fig. 56-8. Ureteral catheterization through cystoscope. Note ureteral catheter inserted into right orifice. Left ureteral catheter is ready to be inserted.

When the patient is awake, passing the instrument will be followed immediately by a strong desire to void. This occurs as a result of the pressure the instrument exerts against the internal sphincter. During the examination the bladder is distended with distilled water to make visualization more effective. As the bladder becomes increasingly distended, the urge to void will increase.

During cystoscopy a number of tests may be performed on the urinary system. Cystography involves the injection of a radiopaque dye (Skiodan) or air as a contrast medium to visualize the bladder and determine its size, shape, and any irregularities. Bladder capacity may be measured through instillation of distilled water. A *voiding cystourethrogram* can reveal reflux of urine into the ureters on voiding, a bladder malfunction that can lead to pyelonephritis.

Ureteral catheterization (with a nylon, radiopaque, size 4 to 6 Fr catheter) can be performed through the cystoscope. The catheter is inserted into the ureteral opening in the bladder, into the ureter, and into the renal pelvis (Fig. 56-8). This procedure may involve one or both ureters. It is performed (1) when culture and analysis of urine from individual kidneys is required, (2) when tests of renal function are to be performed on the kidneys separately, and (3) when visualization of the urinary tract is desired and IVP visualization has been inadequate, obstruction is present, or sensitivity to intravenous radiopaque material is noted.

Visualization of the urinary tract through ureteral catheterization is termed *retrograde pyelography*. This involves injecting 4 to 8 ml of radiopaque material (Hypaque, Renografin) gently into the ureteral catheter. While the solution is being injected, the patient who is awake may feel slight discomfort in the kidney region. Pain should not be experienced unless too much of the solution is injected, and the renal pelvis becomes overdistended. Roentgenograms are taken and demonstrate filling of the renal collecting structures. As the catheter is withdrawn, more of the contrast medium is injected, filling the ureter. Immediately another roentgenogram is made to outline the ureteral structure.

Urethrography involves instilling 20 ml of radiopaque water-soluble lubricant into the urethra in order to visualize urethral irregularities of size and shape.

Care should be taken that the person does not stand or walk alone immediately after cystoscopy. Blood that has drained from the legs while in the lithotomy position will flow back into the vessels of the feet and legs as standing is assumed. Accidents caused by dizziness and fainting can occur from the sudden change in distribution of blood.

Three complications of cystoscopy that need to be monitored are bleeding, perforation of the bladder, and spread of infection throughout the urinary tract or into the bloodstream. Observation for frank bleeding (pink-tinged urine is normal) is necessary. Urine output and voiding pattern are monitored to detect obstruction, and fluid intake is increased to prevent stasis. Mild analgesics are given for discomfort, and warmth is provided if the patient complains of being chilly. Vital signs are checked as necessary.

Ultrasound

Ultrasound is a noninvasive procedure that involves passing sound waves into internal body structures and recreating images of these structures. This is accomplished through a computer that interprets tissue density based upon sound waves and displays this information in picture form. The procedure is painless and requires no preparation other than explanation. Ultrasound can be used to identify masses, obstructions, and malformations of structures in the urinary tract. It cannot be used when structures to be examined lie behind bony tissue, as this prevents passage of the sound waves to deeper structures.

□ Renal biopsy

Renal biopsy is potentially the most accurate diagnostic test for determining both the type and the stage of progression of renal pathologic conditions. Specifically, this test aids in differentiating diagnoses, in following the progression of disease, in choosing therapy most beneficial to the patient, and in determining prognosis of the illness. The biopsy can be performed either through a skin puncture (closed biopsy) or through an incision (open biopsy).

Inherent in biopsy of this vascular tissue is a potential threat of hemorrhage. Throughout the procedure, care is given to prevent and to detect early any loss of blood. Before biopsy is performed, a thorough medical evaluation with particular attention being given to detection of any abnormality in bleeding or coagulation time is carried out. The patient's blood is usually typed and cross matched with 2 units of blood; the blood is held for the patient until any threat of bleeding has passed.

An open biopsy carries less risk of hemorrhage and provides better visualization of the kidney; however, the risk of infection is increased, and a longer period of recovery is required.

Preparation of the patient prior to biopsy also includes discussing the procedure with him, covering the necessity for the examination, the procedure itself, and care to be anticipated and identifying his concerns. The preparation of the patient is shared by the physician and the nurse. In most institutions it is necessary to have the patient sign a special permit prior to having the biopsy performed. The biopsy is carried out in the patient's room, in the radiology department, or in the operating room.

The procedure for percutaneous (closed) biopsy is as follows: Prior to biopsy, the patient is taken to the radiology department for localization of the kidney. This is accomplished with a plain film, a dye contrast film, or fluroscopic location. The position of the kidney in relation to body landmarks is marked on the skin in ink. The lower pole of the kidney is located, this being the site for biopsy, since it contains the fewest number of large vessels, The patient is then transported to the area where the biopsy will be performed. Sedation is usually not required except for children or adults who are restless and unable to relax sufficiently to follow necessary instructions during the test. The patient is placed prone over a sandbag or firm pillow and an additional soft pillow. The body should be bent at the level of the diaphragm, with the shoulders on the bed and the spine in straight alignment. Blood pressure and pulse rate are determined at this point and are recorded. Preparation of the skin is carried out to remove as many surface contaminants as possible. The physician identifies the location for biopsy, and a local anesthetic agent is injected. As the biopsy is being taken, the patient is instructed to hold his breath. Pain may be felt in the kidney region as the tissue sample is taken. The needle is withdrawn immediately, and pressure is applied to the site for 20 minutes. A pressure bandage is then applied, and the patient is turned onto his back; he is kept flat (one small pillow may be used under the head) and motionless for the next 4 hours. Coughing and any activity that increases abdominal venous pressure is to be avoided during this time. Blood pressure and pulse should be taken each 15 minutes for 1 hour, every 30 minutes during the next hour, and every hour for an additional 2 to 3 hours. The patient should remain in bed for at least 24 hours. All urine is observed for hematuria, and bed rest is maintained until the urine is clear. Initially the patient's urine is likely to demonstrate blood, but this rarely continues after a 24-hour period. Once out of bed, the patient should be cautioned against any heavy lifting for a period of 10 days.

REFERENCES AND SELECTED READINGS

1. Black, D.A.K.: The measure of renal function, Am. Heart J. **85:**147-152, 1973.
2. *Fennell, S.: Percutaneous renal biopsy, Am. J. Nurs. **75:**1292-1294, 1975.
3. French, R.: Guide to diagnostic procedures, ed. 4, New York, 1975, McGraw-Hill Book Co.
4. Garb, S.: Laboratory tests in common use, ed. 6, New York, 1976, Springer Publishing Co., Inc.
5. *Goldberger, E.: A primer of water, electrolyte, and acid-base syndromes, ed. 5, Philadelphia, 1975, W. B. Saunders Co.
6. Hamburger, J., et al.: Structure and function of the kidney, Philadelphia, 1971, W. B. Saunders Co.
7. Jaenike, J.: Fluid and electrolyte abnormalities associated with advanced renal disease. In Hansen, G., editor: Caring for patients with chronic renal disease, Rochester, N.Y., 1972, Rochester Regional Med. Prog.
8. Kellerman, E.: Ultrasonic echography in renal disease, Hosp. Pract. **11:**109-116, 1976.
9. *Kelly, A. E., and Gensini, G. G.: Renal arteriography, Am. J. Nurs. **64:**97-99, 1964.
10. McCann, W., and Jude, J.: The synthesis of glucose by the kidney, Bull. Johns Hopkins Hosp. **103:**77, 1958.
11. Papper, S.: The effects of age in reducing renal function, Geriatrics **28:**83-87, 1973.
12. *Pillay, V.: Clinical testing of renal function, Med. Clin. North Am. **55:**231-241, 1971.
13. Pitts, R.: Physiology of the kidney and body fluids, ed. 3, Chicago, 1974, Year Book Medical Publishers, Inc.
14. *Steele, B. W.: Interpretation of renal function tests, Geriatrics **29:**63-66, and 69-71, 1974.
15. *Stroot, V., et al.: Fluids and electrolytes: a practical approach, ed. 2, Philadelphia, 1977, F. A. Davis Co.
16. U.S. Department of Health, Education, and Welfare, Center for Disease Control: Outline for surveillance and control of nosocomial infections, 1973, Atlanta.

AUDIOVISUAL RESOURCE

Infections of the kidney and the urinary tract, Atlanta, 1974, National Medical Audiovisual Center (cassette tape, filmstrip, guide, workbook).

---

*References preceded by an asterisk are particularly well suited for student reading.

57

Management of the person with impaired elimination

JOAN NIVINSKI
NANCY DURHAM
PAULA LAMBRECHT MILLER

The normal pattern of elimination is frequently altered within the bowel or bladder. The deviation results in an altered nutritional state as well as an alteration in the absorptive, secretory, or storage function of the particular organ.

The underlying pathology presents a mosaic pattern of symptoms varying from ill-defined and vague complaints, such as dysuria or abdominal fullness, to the more overt signs of bleeding or diarrhea. Although many of the symptoms are transitory, such as with bowel problems following dietary indiscretions, and respond to medical therapy, it is important to remember that the symptoms may mask more extensive problems that require corrective surgery. Surgical deviation of the urinary or fecal stream is one method of corrective surgery. Some of the problems may become chronic in that the person will require supportive care for his lifetime through the use of a urinary drainage catheter or through bladder or bowel retraining for continued urinary or rectal incontinence.

■ FACILITATION OF NORMAL BOWEL ELIMINATION

□ Factors promoting normal bowel elimination

The mechanisms involved in normal elimination are discussed in Chapter 55. There are a number of factors that promote the normal elimination of feces from the gastrointestinal tract.

Bowel habits

One of the primary interferences with normal elimination is poor bowel habits. The defecation reflex can be inhibited at will unless it is excessively strong, and persons learn to control evacuation in this way. The defecation reflex is stronger when natural impulses are followed, especially during the periods of mass movements (p. 1218). Persons who delay defecation as part of their natural patterns often become constipated; as the stool remains in the tract, additional water is reabsorbed, resulting in a hard stool.

Foods

Certain foods contain cellulose, which is indigestable and which leaves a residue that is propelled through the gastrointestinal tract. The residue acts as an irritant to stimulate normal peristaltic movements and the defecation reflex. Examples of bulk or roughage foods are the skin and fibers of fruits and vegetables, and the coverings of grains found in bran and whole wheat flours and cereals. Some foods such as prune juice promote increased peristalsis.

Fluids

An adequate fluid intake is necessary for maintenance of normal stool consistency. If the body lacks fluid (dehydration), the colon will reabsorb an increased amount of fluid from the chyme. The result will be a hardened stool.

Activity

Physical activity enhances normal peristaltic movements. Persons who are inactive have a higher incidence of constipation.

Emotional equilibrium

Stress affects gastrointestinal activity; therefore maintenance of normal bowel elimination includes taking measures to decrease stress. Stimulation of the sympathetic nervous system inhibits gastrointestinal activity, slowing peristalsis yet as the same time stimulating the internal anal sphincter. During a stressful situation, movement is temporarily halted but incontinence can occur. Long-term stress effects are influenced by the parasympathetic system, which increases peristaltic activity, causing diarrhea. Thus stress can cause incontinence, constipation, or diarrhea.

□ Common bowel dysfunctions

General dysfunction of bowel elimination includes slow passage of the fecal matter through the colon, resulting in a hard stool usually passed infrequently (constipation) or rapid passage of chyme through the intestinal tract resulting in a watery stool (diarrhea). The causes of these dysfunctions are varied and may or may not be associated with pathology (Table 57-1). It can be noted in the Table that many causes of constipation are related to secondary factors that can be prevented, while most causes of diarrhea have a pathologic basis.

Measures to increase peristalsis

Occasional constipation per se is not detrimental to health, although it can cause a feeling of general discomfort or abdominal fullness, anorexia, and anxiety in some persons. Intractable constipation is termed *obstipation*. Habitual constipation leads to decreased intestinal muscle tone, increased use of the Valsalva maneuver as the person bears down in the attempt to pass the hardened stool, and an increased incidence of hemorrhoids. If the stool is permitted to remain in the colon until it becomes exceedingly hard, a *fecal impaction* occurs. The impaction blocks the rectum and must be removed. If it cannot be softened and removed by oil and cleansing enemas, digital removal with a gloved finger may be necessary. This is a very uncomfortable experience for the patient and preventive measures must be instituted for all persons at high risk of developing impaction, including persons on prolonged bed rest, nutritionally depleted, dehydrated, or those receiving constipating medications or undergoing barium studies. Preventive measures include identification and assessment of high-risk persons and carrying out measures to increase peristalsis.

Health teaching is one of the most important measures for prevention of constipation, since it is the individual who will need to carry out the suggested measures for the rest of his life. For the person who has been assessed as having poor bowel habits, an explanation is needed of the mechanisms underlying the need for a consistent time for defecation in order to maximize natural responses (after meals, especially breakfast). Travel, work schedules, or altered sleep patterns con-

Table 57-1. Comparison of causes of diarrhea or constipation

Specific pathology	Secondary factors	Medications
Diarrhea	Fecal impaction	Cathartics
Infections caused by pathogens and parasites	Food or fluids that promote hyperperistalsis	Cardiotonic drugs
Viral enteritis	Electrolyte imbalances	Antibiotics
Amebiasis		Antacids
Cathartic habituation		Other systemic medications
Gastrocolonic fistulas		
Malignant tumors		
Ulcerative colitis		
Malabsorption problems		
Pancreatic insufficiency		
Biliary tract disorders		
Diabetic neuropathy		
Tabes dorsalis		
Hyperthyroidism		
Extensive pelvic pathology		
Constipation	Inadequate fluid intake	Belladonna and derivatives
Colonic or rectal lesions	Low residue or starvation diets	Narcotics (codeine)
Hypometabolism	Physical inactivity	Diuretics
Neuroses	Prolonged bed rest	Salts of bismuth, calcium, and iron
Intestinal obstruction	Fecal impaction	Aluminum hydroxide or aluminum phosphate gels
	Barium ingestion	

tribute to poor bowel habits. The effects of inadequate food, fluids, and activity on normal bowel elimination are included in the teaching plan.

The daily use of enemas and laxatives or cathartics is to be avoided, as these decrease the muscular tone and mucus production of the rectum and may result in water and electrolyte imbalances. They also become habit forming as the weakened muscle tone adds to the inability to expel the fecal contents, which then leads to the continued taking of enemas and laxatives. If the person experiencing bowel dysfunction is unsuccessful in his initial attempts to regain normal function, he needs encouragement to continue his efforts, as considerable time may be needed to change a long standing condition.

For the person who is hospitalized and experiencing constipation, data analysis will identify potential causes. If the therapeutic diet is a contributing factor, consultation with the dietitian may be helpful. Measures to improve the intake of food (Chapter 53) and fluids (Chapter 20) are carried out as indicated. A constipating antacid may be exchanged with one that has a laxative effect. Ambulation is encouraged for all hospitalized patients as permitted. Privacy for bowel evacuation must be provided. Additional stimulation may be needed to increase peristalsis. For those persons who lack innervation of the rectum (paraplegics), digital stimulation of evacuation may be necessary. Various medications such as stool softeners or laxatives are frequently ordered, but efforts are made to promote normal bowel elimination.

Measures to decrease peristalsis

Diarrhea, or the passage of watery or loosely formed stools, may result from disturbances in either the small or large intestines. The definition is based upon the consistency of the stool and not the number expelled per day. The stools are often accompanied by pain in the periumbilical region and lower quadrant, flatulence, borborygmi, and abdominal distention. Bodily water losses from diarrhea can be extensive, leading to dehydration, hyponatremia, hypokalemia, and metabolic alkalosis (Chapter 20). Diarrhea can be distressing to the patient because it reflects loss of control of body function, interferes with other activities, and may lead to skin breakdown.

Measures to slow peristalsis include determination of the underlying cause, change in dietary intake to allow the bowel to "rest" during its inflamed state, and restriction of fruit juices that stimulate peristalsis. A high-protein low-fat diet is usually recommended with increased fluid intake (no iced or carbonated fluids) to counterbalance the excessive losses. Antidiarrheal drugs such as diphenoxylate hydrochloride with atropine (Lomotil) and tincture of opium (paregoric) may be ordered. Kaolin and pectate appear to be of limited value in the control of diarrhea. Comfort measures include periods of rest, an environment conducive to privacy and free of odors, and provision for personal hygiene after *each* loose stool.

Outcome criteria for the person with bowel dysfunction

The patient or significant others can:

1. Explain the relationship of dietary and fluid intake to the formation of a normal stool.
2. Describe the relationship of activity to normal bowel evacuation.
3. Describe a plan incorporating good bowel habits.
4. Describe the effect of prescribed medications on bowel function.
5. State what to do when diarrhea or constipation occurs.

■ DECOMPRESSION OF THE INTESTINAL TRACT

□ Purpose

Decompression, or deflation, of the intestinal tract is accomplished by attaching a tube passed by way of the nose or mouth into the intestine to the suction apparatus. This procedure is used to drain fluids and gas that accumulate above the mechanical intestinal obstruction, to deflate the intestines during paralytic ileus, and to deflate the bowel before or after intestinal surgery.

□ Types of intestinal tubes

The tubes most often used for intestinal decompression are the Miller-Abbott tube and the Cantor tube. The length of these tubes permits their passage through the entire intestinal tract. There is a small balloon on the tip of each, which, when inflated with air or injected with water or mercury, acts like a bolus of food. This balloon stimulates peristalsis, which advances it along the intestinal tract. If peristalsis is absent, the weight of the mercury in the balloon will usually carry it forward. When a Miller-Abbott tube is used, the mercury is inserted into the balloon of the tube after the tube is passed.

The choice of tube depends on the physician's preference. The Miller-Abbott tube is a double-lumen tube. One lumen leads to the balloon and the other has openings along its course, permitting drainage of intestinal contents and irrigation. The external end of the tube contains a metal adapter with two openings—one for drainage of secretions and the other for inflating the balloon. (See Fig. 57-1.) In irrigating this tube, the nurse must be careful that the correct opening is used—the one marked "suction." The other opening is for inflating or deflating the balloon. It should be clamped off and labeled "do not touch."

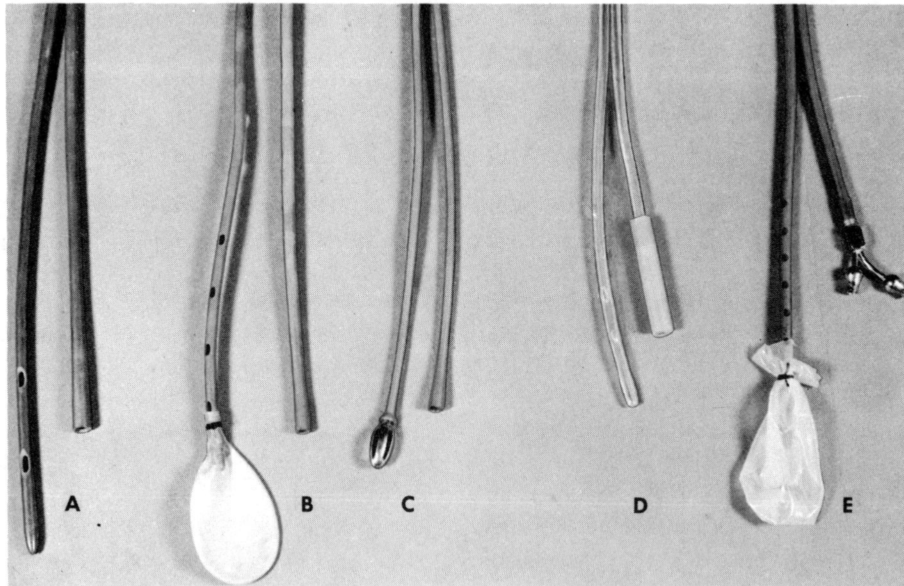

Fig. 57-1. Tips and ends to be attached to suction for various types of tubes used for gastrointestinal intubation. **A,** Rubber nasogastric tube. **B,** Cantor tube. **C,** Rehfuss tube for duodenal drainage. **D,** Plastic nasogastric tube. **E,** Miller-Abbott tube.

The Cantor tube is a single tube with only one opening, which is used for drainage. Before the tube is inserted, the balloon is injected with mercury with a needle and syringe. The needle opening is so small that the globules of mercury cannot escape through it. The mercury can be pushed about so that the balloon is elongated for easy insertion.

Another intestinal tube, the Harris tube, is a single tube also and similar to the Cantor tube except that there is a metal tip on the end of the tube, which is followed by the small bag containing the mercury.

□ Insertion of tubes

Intestinal tubes are passed in the manner described under gastric analysis (p. 1164). The addition of the balloon on the tip of the tube makes its insertion through the nose doubly difficult for the patient. The tube can be mechanically inserted only into the stomach. Its passage along the remainder of the gastrointestinal tract is dependent on gravity and peristalsis. The weight of the mercury in the balloon helps propel the tube through the intestines. After the tube reaches the stomach, its passage through the pylorus and into the duodenum can be facilitated in many ways. Position and activity aid in its passage. After passage of the tube, the patient is usually encouraged to lie on his right side for 2 hours, on his back in a Fowler's position for 2 hours, and then on his left side for 2 hours. Passage of the tube through the pylorus is usually ascertained by roentgenographic or fluoroscopic examination. After the tube has passed the pylorus, the patient may be encouraged to walk about to increase peristalsis and to speed the advancement of the tube through the intestines with the help of gravity. During this time the physician or the nurse advances the tube 7 to 10 cm (3 to 4 inches) through the nose or mouth at specified intervals. The intestinal tube should not be secured to the face until it has reached the desired point in the intestines, since taping the tube will prevent it from advancing with peristalsis. The pull of the mercury on the end of the tube may move the bowel along with the tube and cause telescoping of the bowel. This results in *intussusception*, which is a serious complication. The tube should be monitored carefully by roentgenographic examination at least once daily to assure that coiling of the tube or telescoping of the bowel has not occurred. Extra tubing should be coiled on the bed or, if the patient is up, pinned to his clothing.

Decompression is accomplished by attaching a suction apparatus to the tube either as the tube advances or after it has reached the obstructed portion of the bowel.

□ Care of the patient with an intestinal tube

Drainage is measured every 24 hours and the fluid and electrolytes lost are replaced by the parenteral routes. If the tip of the tube is far down in the intestine and if the patient is not nauseated or vomiting, he may be permitted light foods such as clear or cream soups, custards, gelatins, milk, or fruit juice, all of which can be absorbed in the upper part of the small intestine.

The tube may require irrigation with normal saline

to check its patency. Because the fluid has a longer distance to travel than in a nasogastric tube, it is difficult to aspirate the solution used. If no return flow can be obtained, only a small amount of fluid is used and the amount instilled is recorded.

Nasal and pharyngeal discomfort usually is pronounced, and the nursing measures described under gastric intubation are employed (p. 1211). Signs of the return of peristalsis (bowel sounds, passage of flatus rectally, or spontaneous bowel movement) are reported to the physician, since they usually indicate that the tube is no longer needed.

□ Removal of intestinal tubes

The intestinal tube is usually left in the intestine longer than the nasogastric tube remains in the stomach. It is always removed gradually several centimeters at a time. Some resistance may be felt as it is withdrawn because of the pull against peristalsis. The patient may feel a tugging sensation and become nauseated. When the tip of the tube reaches the posterior nasopharynx, it may be brought out through the mouth so that the balloon and mercury can be detached. The tube is then pulled through the nose. Since the tube usually has a fecal odor and may cause nausea, the tubing should be removed from sight at once and the patient is given oral care as soon as it is removed. For several days after removal of an intestinal tube, the patient's throat may be sore and he may be hoarse. Gargles and lozenges can be continued until these symptoms subside.

Occasionally the balloon of an intestinal tube may extrude from the anus. If this occurs, the upper end of the tube is disconnected from suction and removed through the rectum. Removal is usually done slowly and with the help of peristaltic action.

■ MANAGEMENT OF STOMAS FOR FECAL DIVERSION

Temporary or permanent diversion of the fecal stream is performed to permit escape of feces when there is an obstruction of the bowel or a known lesion such as cancer that requires removal of the distal portion of the bowel. It may also be done to permit healing of the distal intestine after an infection, perforation, or traumatic injury, since it diverts the fecal stream from the affected area. It is sometimes performed as a palliative measure in the treatment of an obstruction caused by an inoperable growth. The site of the diversion may be the ilium (ileostomy) or colon (colostomy) (Fig. 57-2, *A* and *B*).

During surgery, the stomal opening is formed by bringing the end of the intestine up through a small abdominal incision. The intestinal tissue is folded upon itself like a cuff, supported slightly above the abdominal wall and sutured into place. The remaining distal intestinal tissue is generally removed in a permanent colostomy as the incidence of malignant changes is high. A variation of this technique occurs when a temporary stomal opening is formed (Fig. 57-2, *C*). A loop of intestine is brought up through a small abdominal incision and supported on the abdominal wall by a glass or rubber rod. In this variation there is a proximal and a distal loop of intestine. The distal loop remains as the connection with the rectum; the proximal loop is in direct connection with the remainder of the bowel and small intestine.

The actual location of the stoma on the abdominal wall is guided by two principles: (1) the extent of the surgery and the length of bowel remaining and (2) appreciation for the fit of the appliance. The person marking the site for the stoma should look for a smooth area where there are less wrinkles or rolls of fat, and a site where the person can reach the stoma easily. The site should also be selected with the view toward usual clothing worn by the person; for example, if a belt is usually worn, the beltline is not suitable for a stoma.

At the close of the operation, some type of protective appliance is placed over the stomal opening. In most instances this will be a temporary disposable bag, although many surgeons will apply the permanent appliance. Application of a bag serves three main functions: (1) it prevents possible contamination of the main surgical incision; (2) it provides immediate feedback to the patient regarding the "feel" or sensation of the appliance; and (3) it provides accurate observation, assessment, and measurement of the stomal drainage.

□ Preoperative care

When the physician first tells the person of the probable need for a colostomy, the immediate reaction is likely to be one of shock and disbelief. Whether the colostomy is to be temporary or permanent, it is very difficult for most people to accept. Knowledge that it is a lifesaving measure, confidence in the surgeon, and sometimes explanation and acceptance of the proposed operation by significant others may assist in the decision to have the operation. It is not unusual for the patient to be sad, withdrawn, and depressed upon learning of the need for a colostomy.

The nurse should know what the patient has been told by the physician and be prepared to supplement information and assess how much information to give the patient preoperatively on care of the colostomy. Some patients definitely benefit from discussing the care, reading materials, seeing equipment, and talking to persons who are living normal lives following a colostomy. Others find this approach upsetting. The patient should, however, have a simple explanation of the anatomy of the colon, how surgery will alter the normal bowel function, and how the colostomy can be managed as a routine part

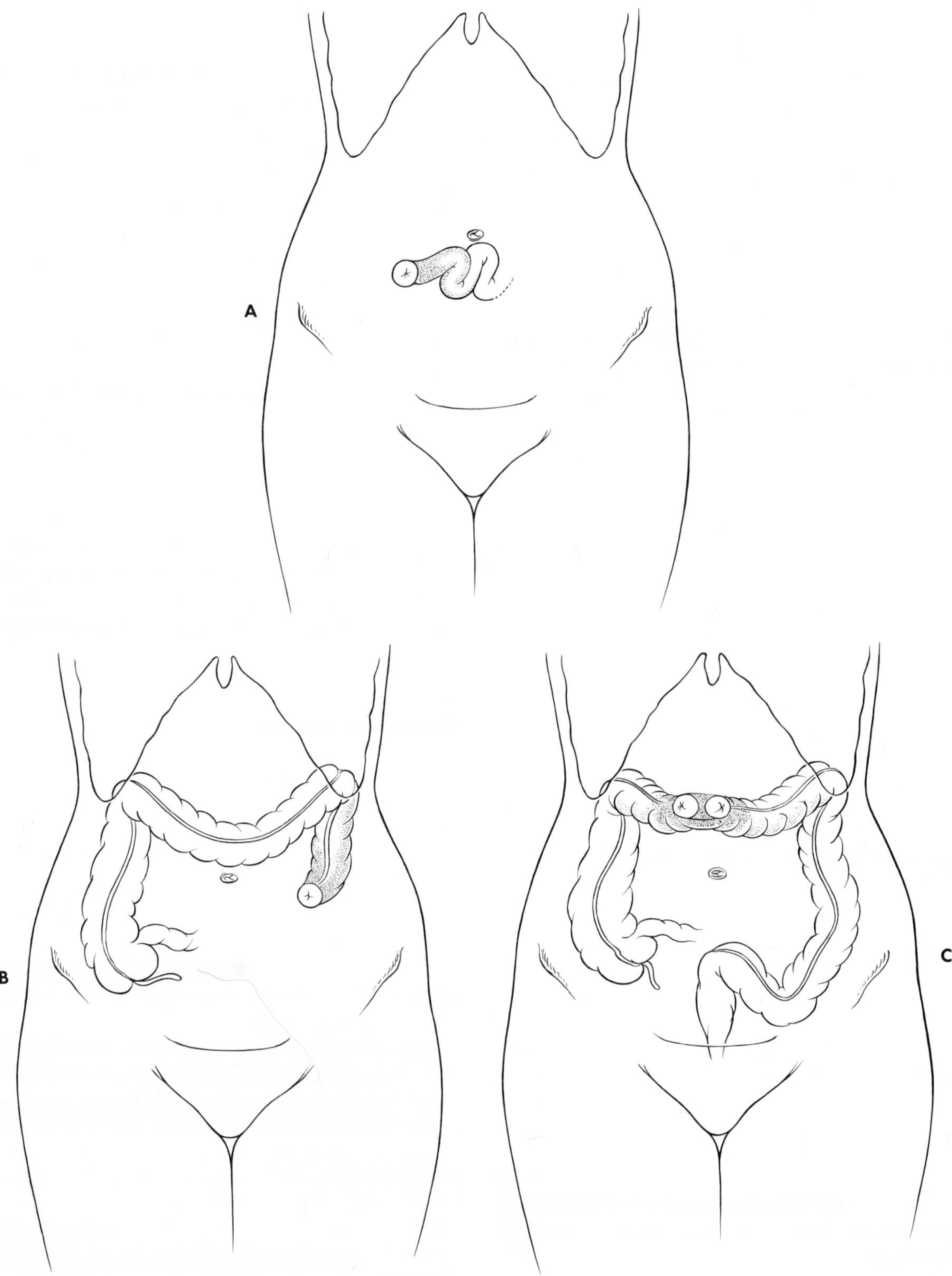

Fig. 57-2. A, Ileostomy. **B,** Permanent colostomy. **C,** Transverse colostomy.

of his daily activities. The nurse needs to assess the patient's readiness for this kind of learning and plan accordingly.

Some hospitals have printed materials for patients who have had a colostomy. Booklets on colostomy care also may be packaged with colostomy bags and equipment sold commercially. If printed material is used, it should be carefully discussed with the patient before it is left with him. After he has reviewed it, the nurse should plan to spend additional time answering any questions he may have. One of the advantages of printed material is that the patient has a reference available after his discharge from the hospital. It adds to his security in caring for himself.

During the preoperative period, effort should be made to augment the patient's confidence in the members of the medical and nursing staff, since the patient who has complete confidence in the persons who will treat and care for him is more likely to accept his situation postoperatively and be more willing to start to learn self-care. The patient watches every facial expression or gesture of the nurses and is extremely sensitive to evidence of distaste. If other persons accept the colostomy as not unusual, it helps the patient to feel that it is not a calamity that has happened to him alone.

The importance of significant others in the total planning with the patient cannot be forgotten. They must be encouraged and given the opportunity to discuss freely their own feelings and reactions to the surgery. They are given an opportunity to grieve for the patient's alteration and then are gently guided to recognize those areas in which they may provide support to the patient. The nurse gathers data at this time to anticipate how to include the significant others in the total care program, plan for specific transmission of information, plan the opportunity for ongoing discussion of feelings, and identify those areas in which the significant others may not be able to contribute. Significant others who provide sup-

Table 57-2. Comparative aspects of ileostomy and colostomy in preparation for teaching

Skin care	Stoma functioning	Usual drainage	Appliance	Control	Complications
Ileostomy Immediate protection of surrounding skin to prevent autodigestion (appliance to fit within 3 mm [1/8 inch] of stoma) Skin care to include: Wash and dry area well Use "barrier" between appliance and skin	Within 48 hours mucus produced Within 3 weeks stoma size shrinks to allow for fit of permanent appliance	Continuous liquid fecal stream	Will require a permanent set	Essentially none Control may *not* be achieved with irrigations	Excessive loss of water and electrolytes Stricture or inversion of stoma Skin excoriation and autodigestion Bleeding from decrease of vitamin K Undernutrition
Permanent colostomy Immediate protection of surrounding skin to prevent excoriation (appliance to fit within 6 mm [1/4 inch] of stoma) Skin care to include: Wash and dry area well Use "barrier" between appliance and skin	Same as ileostomy	Sigmoid colostomy: formed stool Transverse colostomy: semiliquid to semiformed stool Ascending (right colon) colostomy: liquid fecal stream	Temporary set until control is achieved Use of a permanent set will depend upon stool formation Permanent set is generally necessary	Irrigations and modifications in diet Modifications in diet (irrigations may assist in control) Same as ileostomy	Stricture or inversion of stoma Skin excoriation (*Candida*) Dehydration if water loss excessive

port, acceptance, and reassurance will enhance the direct acceptance of the alteration by the patient.

□ Postoperative care

The immediate postoperative care for colostomy patients follows the guidelines for the care of any major surgery patient (Chapter 23). Hemorrhage through or around the stoma is rare and, if it occurs, is reported immediately. The stoma will begin to secrete mucus within 48 hours, and fecal drainage should begin within 72 hours.

The *temporary,* or loop, colostomy must be opened to allow for mucus and fecal drainage. Generally in 72 hours the surgeon makes an opening in both the proximal and distal loops using a cautery needle. The patient is reassured that there will be no feeling of pain although a distinctive odor will be present. Adequate ventilation of the patient's room during and following this procedure is essential. The supporting rod will be removed 5 to 7 days after the surgery. The loop of intestine will continue to be supported on the abdominal wall because of the healing process of the wound and its sutures.

Attention to fluid balance is of extreme importance, especially for the patient with an ileostomy (Table 57-2). This individual no longer has a large bowel for reabsorption of water, and excessive loss of fluids through the stoma will precipitate rapid dehydration. Loss of fluids through the colostomy stoma is usually not excessive and is replaceable by oral intake.

Skin care

Attention to the maintenance of skin integrity around the stoma begins in the initial postoperative period. If no appliance has been placed over the stoma, the nurse ascertains from the surgeon when this may be done. In the meantime the skin around the stoma must be kept clean and dry at all times. This will require ingenuity on the part of the nurse regarding how to apply the dressing most effectively. It also requires a planned program of dressing changes at specific intervals rather than waiting until the dressing is thoroughly saturated. Fecal drainage onto the skin surface will cause excoriation and eventual breakdown of tissue. Drainage of small intestinal contents (ileostomy), which contain lytic enzymes, will autodigest the skin surface. For this reason, all attempts are made to prevent the initial breakdown. There are many commercial products available (Karaya powder or shields, silicone sprays, pastes, creams, solutions, and so on) that are reported to protect the skin surrounding the stoma. Whichever product is chosen, it must meet three criteria: (1) be acceptable to the patient and increase his comfort, (2) be affordable, and (3) allow for proper adherence of the appliance over the stoma. Because many individuals are sensitive to the compounds within these commercial products, material should be tested on a normal area of skin (thigh) for possible reaction prior to using it around the stoma.

One effective means of protecting the skin surface is the use of Maalox, compound tincture of benzoin, and Karaya powder. The skin surface is washed and dried thoroughly. A thin layer of Maalox is applied and allowed to dry to a chalky white. A heat lamp (25-watt bulb) assists in the rapid drying process. A thin layer of the compound tincture of benzoin is applied and allowed to dry until if feels "sticky." A layer of Karaya powder is sprinkled on next and the excess is brushed off. At least three more layers of Maalox, benzoin and Karaya powder are applied in the above order, finishing with a layer of benzoin. After the skin preparation dries to a sticky consistency, the appliance is placed over the stoma. This is a fairly time-consuming procedure, and any drainage through the stoma must be dried immediately before it can dampen the skin surface. This layered application will allow the appliance to be removed without disturbing the skin protection. The skin around the stoma is washed with warm, soapy water in 72 hours so that assessment of skin healing can be made. The protective skin preparation is then reapplied.

At times a secondary infection caused by bacteria or fungi may develop around the stoma. In this situation the nurse would avoid the use of alkaline products on the skin surface, as bacteria and fungi growth will increase in an alkaline media.

Teaching

Teaching the patient regarding anticipated independent care of the stoma begins in the immediate postoperative phase. Each time the dressing and appliance are changed the patient is informed of the state of skin and the incision healing as well as a description of the stoma. A concise explanation of each step in the procedure provides information to the patient. The nursing care plan includes detailed information regarding the approaches and techniques used so that consistency of approach is used by all nurses caring for the patient.

The nurse observes the patient's personal reaction to the information being shared and decides whether to continue with this approach or modify it until the patient indicates more readiness for learning. The word "stoma" is used consistently by the nurse when talking with the patient. This familiarizes the patient with the correct terminology and assists in the acceptance of the altered body part into the person's self-concept, thus decreasing distortion or fantasy.

Patient feelings

Not only will the nurse describe what is being observed during the appliance and dressing change, but the nurse may also reflect back to the patient what he may be feeling (apathy, interest, disgust, avoidance). This provides an opportunity for the patient to begin to verbalize and explore his feeling early in the postoperative course.

Removal of any part of the body involves a sense of loss; therefore the patient may experience grief and mourning over the lost part, including shock, denial, anger, and depression. (See Chapter 19 for a discussion of these reactions.) In addition, because the surgery results in fecal contents being expelled through an unnatural opening in the abdomen, the patient will experience changes in body image and may have feelings of guilt, shame, disgust, and withdrawal. (These are discussed in Chapter 28.) Usually the formation of a stoma is viewed as mutilating surgery, but for some individuals the surgery may be a relief or release from coping with chronic pain, diarrhea, or debility. No matter what reaction is expressed, the patient will need time and support of others to work through his feelings.

Most persons do not wish to look at the stoma immediately, and if they are in the shock-denial phase of grieving, they will not hear what is being described about it. The patient is not pushed to look at the stoma but is gently encouraged to look at it as he evidences interest in doing so. Some patients will look at the stoma if left alone. The nurse can deliberately leave the room for a minute, leaving the stoma exposed, being ready upon return to provide emotional support to the patient. A patient who still will not look at the stoma or show any interest in his care after 2 to 3 weeks may need more extensive counseling, and a consultation with a psychiatric nurse specialist may be helpful.

If it is acceptable to both the significant other and the patient, the significant other is included as an observer as the nurse implements care throughout the entire teaching program.

Self-care

Encouragement should be given to the patient to participate in his own care. Techniques used to accomplish this include having the patient hand supplies or equipment to the nurse and having the patient handle the appliance prior to giving it to the nurse. Continual feedback from the patient is necessary as the nurse asks him to describe the steps of the procedure.

Questions regarding whether the individual will achieve his former bowel evacuation pattern must be answered honestly. For example, the patient with an ileostomy may be able to control the volume of the liquid fecal stream by diet and fluid intake, while the patient with a sigmoid colostomy will generally be able to achieve evacuation of a normally formed stool (Table 57-2).

As the patient assumes increased responsibility for cleansing the skin and placing the appliance over the stoma, the nurse assists in deciding which position (lying, sitting, or standing) is best assumed before giving self-care. The upright position has the advantage of providing better visualization of the stoma itself.

Permanent appliance

Initially the stoma is reddened and edematous, and within 2 to 3 weeks it shrinks and achieves its permanent appearance. Once this has been accomplished, the permanent appliance is obtained. Prior to this time the patient is shown a variety of appropriate commercial appliances, is given an explanation of the advantages, disadvantages, and cost of each, and is assisted in choosing one for purchase.

Measurement of the stoma is necessary before the appliance ring (base) is ordered. A scale for stoma measurement is available from each manufacturer and is specifically sized for that product. Ileostomy rings should be no larger than 3 mm (1/8 inch) of the stoma circumference. Colostomy rings should be no larger than 6 mm (1/4 inch) of the stoma circumference. If the stoma should shrink to an irregular shape or invert slightly below the abdominal wall, special commercial appliances are available.

It should be stressed to the patient and significant others that the appliances are not generally noticeable under clothing. The prevention of odor may be accomplished in several ways, the most important of which is thorough cleansing of the permanent bag or changing of the disposable bag at regular intervals. Proper fit of the appliance also decreases the possibility of odor leakage. Many commercial deodorizers are available, and they are sprayed inside the bag and not on the skin surface. Small bits of charcoal, sodium bicarbonate, oil of peppermint, or spice may also be used to reduce odor. Avoidance of excessive amounts of gas-forming foods or fluids will also decrease possible odor. These would be the same foods or fluids that produced gas in the person prior to surgery.

It is recommended that the patient or significant other purchase the needed equipment prior to discharge from the hospital. If the patient has chosen disposable bags (Fig. 57-3), he should have a sufficient number to last for a least a week. If he has chosen a permanent appliance, two complete sets are purchased so that one can be cleansed and dried while the other is worn.

The permanent bags and rings are made of soft rubber or a flexible plastic compound and will deteriorate if a harsh cleansing substance is used. Thoroughly washing the equipment in a mild soap and warm water, rinsing it well under warm running water, and drying it thoroughly is generally sufficient. It is recommended

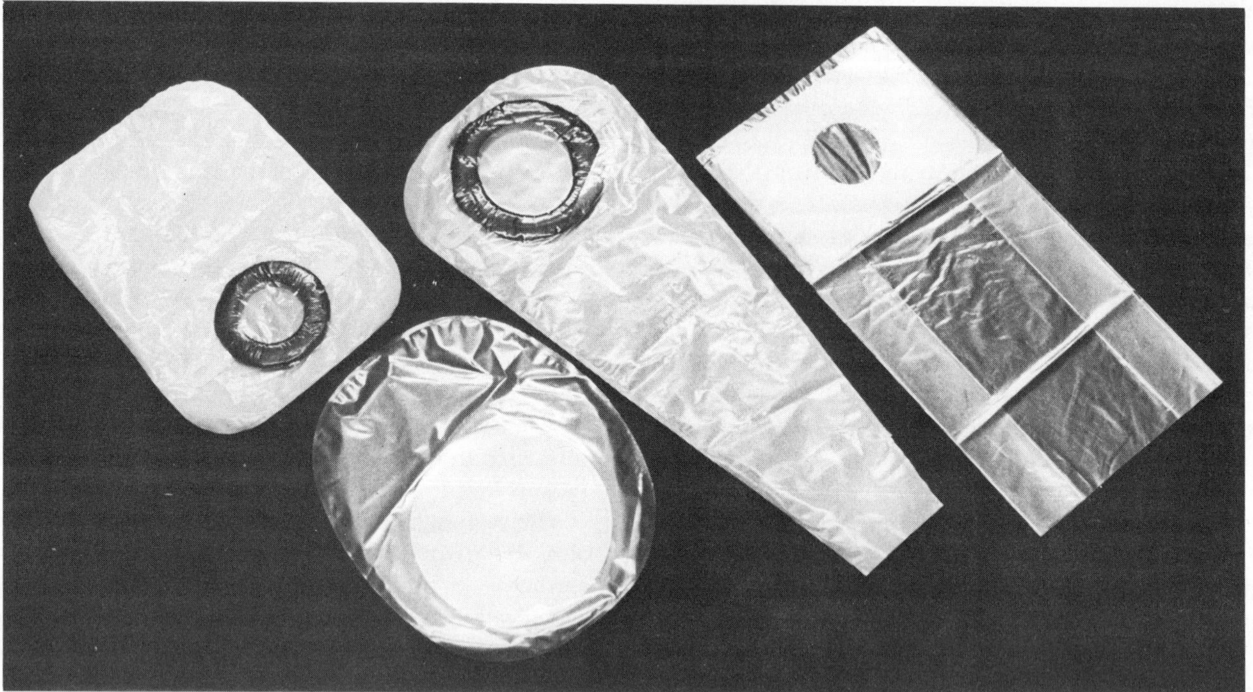

Fig. 57-3. Examples of disposable colostomy bags. Two bags with dark rings have Karaya seal; other two bags use adhesive seal.

that the ring (base) be removed once a week for cleaning and thorough inspection of the skin and stoma. Ideally the patient and significant other will be comfortable in utilizing the patient's own equipment prior to discharge.

Colostomy irrigation

Irrigation of the bowel may be ordered after a colostomy. There is some controversy among surgeons regarding the benefits of irrigation. In theory, the daily irrigations "retrain" the bowel for normal evacuation through the stoma. The individuals who respond least favorably to irrigation are those whose fecal stream is liquid or semisoft, who respond to stress with diarrhea, or whose presurgery bowel evacuation was irregular. It is not unusual for some individuals to achieve satisfactory bowel evacuation with a proper balance of diet, fluids, and exercise alone.

When irrigation is ordered, it is begun between the fifth and seventh postoperative day. To assess if the stoma opening is unobstructed, the nurse, wearing a fingercot or glove, inserts the well-lubricated little finger of the examining hand very gently into the stoma. There may be an initial "sphincterlike" tightening, which will relax within a few seconds. Inserting the finger to its depth and gently rotating it will determine if the opening is patent and will accept the irrigating tip. This maneuver will also indicate the correct *direction* for insertion of the catheter to avoid trauma to the walls of the mucosa.

Various types of commercial irrigation sets are available, but the principles for irrigation are the same. The cup that fits over the opening has a small hole in the center through which to insert a catheter, or there may be a cone tip as part of the set. The cup is usually plastic so that returns can be seen readily. It is held snugly in place against the abdominal wall with elasticized straps. Outlet tubing attached to the cup allows drainage of the fecal material into the toilet. The irrigating method is described in the boxed material on p. 1253.

As soon as the patient is ambulatory, the irrigation should be performed with the patient sitting on a commode or toilet. Since the procedure may be time-consuming, the patient should be comfortably supported. If during the insertion of the fluid the patient has abdominal cramps, the inflow is clamped for several minutes. Excessive cramping may be caused by the pressure or rate of fluid flow, or to a solution that is too warm or too cold. Marked increase in peristalsis will occur and may hamper passage of fecal material through the intestine.

If elimination has been regulated, only a small dress-

COLOSTOMY IRRIGATION

Equipment

Irrigating bag with 500 to 750 ml warm tap water
Tubing with air released and clamped
Catheter or cone lubricated with petroleum jelly
Paper bag for dressings (if applicable)

Method

1. Remove appliance or dressing.
2. Cleanse area around colostomy with tissue as necessary.
3. Insert cone tip 2 cm (1 inch) or catheter 7 to 8 cm (3 inches) in direction of remaining colon.
4. Fasten cup snugly to abdomen; let outlet tubing drain into bowl.
5. Release clamp and allow fluid to flow gently.
6. Close clamp and hold catheter or cone in place for 2 to 3 minutes to retain solution in colon.
7. Remove catheter or cone and allow solution to drain.
8. If returns are slow, ask patient to change position (lean forward or move side to side) to help expel fluid.
9. Apply clean pouch or dressing.

ing such as a piece of gauze or tissue needs to be worn over the colostomy. Plastic-covered gauze dressings are available for this purpose. This dressing prevents the clothing from being stained with the small amount of mucus that may drain from the opening. When elimination is well regulated, it is preferable that the person *not* wear a colostomy bag, thus obviating any possibility of odors. Some persons, however, worry lest they have drainage, and can become regulated only when a bag is worn.

A permanent colostomy may need to be dilated because of narrowing of the opening due to shrinkage during and after healing. If the ostomate has difficulty inserting the irrigation tube, this should be reported to the surgeon immediately. In an effort to avoid stoma stricture, the surgeon may advise the ostomate to insert a well-lubricated finger into the colostomy opening about once a week, or daily if necessary.

The person who has a temporary loop colostomy will not be retraining the bowel for evacuation. He irrigates the distal loop (mucus fistula) by order of the physician. This irrigation cleanses the lower bowel, enhances healing, and instills topical medication, if needed. The patient will need to be taught to identify the distal opening and to learn that the solution will be expelled through the rectum. The actual time spent for the irrigation is less than that experienced by the person with a permanent colostomy.

Diet

Dietary modifications include avoiding excessive gas-forming foods and those known to cause diarrhea. An adequate amount of fluid is necessary to promote a stool that is easily evacuated from a permanent colostomy. For those individuals whose fecal stream will remain semisoft or of liquid consistency, a plan is devised that balances sufficient fluid intake to meet body needs and to avoid excessive fecal losses that result in water and electrolyte imbalance.

Activity

For most persons whose condition warrants it, optimal recovery is achieved within 3 months, and they can return to their normal activities including returning to work. The person may participate in sports, although it is advisable to avoid direct contact sports such as football. Swimming, traveling, playing tennis, and participating in planned exercise programs are all possible. The ostomate is encouraged to resocialize and continue those activities that resulted in satisfaction prior to the surgery. Only then can the person learn which activities are too tiring and will need to be modified.

Sexuality

The opportunity for the ostomate and significant other to ask questions regarding the return to normal sexual functioning needs to be provided. It is most often the nurse who hears cues such as "I guess I'll never be able . . ." or "I wonder what my wife. . . ." The nurse takes this opportunity to clarify this concern with the person. Arrangements can be made, if desired by the patient, for the significant other to be present when a frank discussion of sexual functioning is carried out by the nurse or physician. Many persons will not verbalize their concerns about sexuality so that a deliberate opening must be planned to facilitate expression of these concerns. A pamphlet *Sex and the Ostomate* is available from the United Ostomy Association.*

Community resources

During hospitalization there are additional resources available to the patient and significant others to assist in adaptation and coping with the colostomy. A representative from the local "Ostomy Club" who has been through the same experience may be helpful during both the preoperative as well as the postoperative period and will visit the patient if requested to do so. Social worker, clinical nurse specialist, dietitian, and clergy may all be consulted as the needs are presented.

The patient and significant others should also be in-

*United Ostomy Association, Inc., 1111 Wilshire Blvd., Los Angeles, Calif. 90017.

formed of the United Ostomy Association* to which the ostomate may become a member and through group sharing learn how others in his local community are dealing with and effectively handling their alteration. The American Cancer Society will also provide assistance with home supplies, medications, transportation, and so on.

Teaching before discharge should include knowledge of common complications that should be reported directly to the health care provider. The more common complications include persistent diarrhea, constipation, or stricture of the stoma. Less common complications include bleeding from or around the stoma, prolapse or inversion of the stoma, and leakage of fluid around the appliance.

Closure of the colostomy

If the colostomy was performed to relieve obstruction or to divert the fecal stream to permit healing of a portion of the bowel, the person will be readmitted to the hospital at a later date for a further examination and for possible resection of the diseased portion of the bowel. The opening may subsequently be closed.

In preparation for a resection of the bowel and closure of the colostomy the physician may order irrigations of the distal loop. Fluid, usually normal saline solution, is instilled into the distal loop through a catheter attached to a funnel or Asepto syringe. For this irrigation the patient should sit on the bedpan or on the toilet, since unless there is complete obstruction, the solution may be expelled rectally. Mucus and shreds of necrotic tissue may be passed. The returns should be inspected before they are discarded. A nonabsorbable sulfonamide derivative such as phthalylsulfathiazole dissolved in a small amount of water may be slowly instilled into the distal loop and rectum after the irrigation. The patient should retain this solution as long as possible, since the antibiotic lowers the bacterial count of the bowel contents and lessens the risk of postoperative infection.

□ Outcome criteria for the person with a surgical diversion of the fecal stream

The patient or significant others can:

1. Describe the relationship of adequate dietary and fluid intake to the formation of a normal stool.
2. Describe the relationship of activity to normal bowel evacuation.
3. Demonstrate the correct use of stomal appliance: removal, cleansing of stoma, inspection of skin, application of appliance, cleansing of equipment, and ordering of new equipment.
4. Demonstrate, if needed, the correct technique for irrigation of the remaining segment of bowel.
5. Determine a specific time of day for anticipated normal evacuation.
6. Determine modifications in routine for particular home situation, work situation, and anticipated travel.
7. State how to obtain available professional and community resources.
8. Utilize a resource person with whom they may share their thoughts and feelings regarding the alteration and its impact on the future.
9. State plans for regular follow-up care and symptoms that necessitate physician or nurse clinician contact:
   a. Changes in configuration, color, consistency, or odor of stool.
   b. Bleeding through stoma or rectum.
   c. Persistent diarrhea or lack of stool evacuation despite medications, treatment, fluids, diet, and exercise program.
   d. Increasing difficulty in digital dilatation of the stoma.
   e. Persistent skin excoriation despite treatment and fluid and diet alterations.
   f. Changes in contour of the stoma (prolapse, inversion) or signs of infection.
   g. Persistent leakage around the appliance.

■ FACILITATION OF URINARY ELIMINATION

Normal urinary output varies depending on a number of factors, such as the amount of fluid intake, the amount of fluid loss from sources other than the kidney (p. 208), the amount of solutes excreted in the urine, or the action of antidiuretic hormone. An adequate amount of urine must be produced daily in order for the kidney to carry out its functions. A urine output of 100 to 400 ml/day is termed *oliguria;* less than 100 ml/day is termed *anuria.*

Under normal conditions the person eating an adequate diet has a urine output essentially equal to fluid input. Inadequate urine output may occur because of two major reasons, either the kidney is not producing urine *(urinary suppresion)* or the flow of urine is blocked between the kidneys and the urethral opening *(urinary retention).* Disease conditions influencing production of urine are discussed in Chapter 59. Measures that can be taken when inadequate fluid intake (dehydration) is present can be found in Chapter 20.

Causes of urinary retention may be categorized as either mechanical or functional. Mechanical obstruction refers to an anatomic blockage of urine flow at any level in the urinary tract. Such mechanical obstructions may be congenital (urethral stricture) or acquired (calculus, inflammation, injury, tumor or hyperplasia, pregnancy).

*United Ostomy Association, Inc., 1111 Wilshire Blvd., Los Angeles, Calif. 90017.

Functional obstruction refers to the impairment of urine flow in the absence of mechanical obstruction, such as neurogenic bladder dysfunction, ureterovesical reflux, or decreased peristaltic activity of the ureter. For assessment of inability to void, see p. 1231.

Interventions for urinary retention are aimed at reestablishment of urine flow. Some mechanical obstructions must be corrected by surgical intervention; others, such as that caused by an enlarged prostate, may require temporary urethral catheter drainage. If the person is having difficulty eliminating urine from the bladder in the absence of mechanical obstruction, measures that encourage voiding are attempted before catheterization is instituted. These measures may include assuring a position that facilitates voiding (positional stimuli), running water or blowing bubbles in water (auditory stimuli), or pouring water over the perineum or placing the hands in water (tactile stimuli). Sitting in lukewarm water may help relax the urinary sphincters. Bethanechol chloride (Urecholine) may be given to initiate voiding by stimulation of the detrusor muscle of the bladder. Persons having long-term problems may be taught to carry out intermittent catheterization rather than maintaining an indwelling catheter.

□ Assisted urinary drainage

Assisted urinary drainage is utilized in a variety of clinical situations in both acute and chronic care. Following are major reasons for catheter drainage of some part of the urinary system:

1. Relieve temporary anatomic or physiologic obstruction
2. Permit healing of various parts of the urinary system postoperatively
3. Permit accurate measurement of urinary output in severely ill patients
4. Relieve inability to void
5. Achieve continence
6. Prevent urinary tract infections in certain persons with neurogenic bladder dysfunction
7. Irrigate the bladder

Reestablishment of the flow of urine is an immediate treatment goal. The type of catheter used to provide drainage in the presence of obstruction will depend upon the location of the blockage.

Catheters are used in urinary tract surgery to facilitate healing of some portion of the urinary tract by diverting urine from above the operative site, or by "splinting" a narrow portion of the tract to prevent stricture until healing occurs. In critical care settings where hourly fluid balance assessments are necessary, urethral catheter drainage may be employed until the patient's condition has stabilized.

Temporary inability to void accompanies spinal cord injury, and postoperative patients may also experience temporary urinary retention and may require one or two urethral catheterizations until their usual voiding pattern is resumed. Persons who have urogenital surgery and some women following childbirth may have urinary retention secondary to edema of surrounding tissues.

In certain circumstances urethral catheterization may be used to control urinary incontinence. Incontinence itself is not adquate reason for continuous catheter drainage unless urine retention is present or the integrity of the skin is threatened despite all possible nursing measures to manage the incontinence. Generally the dangers of catheterization (infection) outweigh the advantages. Intermittent catheterization, however, is utilized as a means of continence for certain persons with neurogenic bladder dysfunction associated with birth defects, chronic illness, and spinal cord trauma. Not only can it offer continence to these persons, but it also can decrease urinary tract infections in persons who otherwise retain large amounts of residual urine in the bladder.

Urethral catheterization may be performed in order to provide irrigation of the bladder with a medicated solution when infection is present or to prevent excessive clot formation in the presence of bleeding. Irrigation may be ordered intermittently. If irrigation is required continuously or more often than every 3 hours, a special closed irrigation system should be used.

Types of catheters

Catheters are hollow tubes made of rubber, nylon, silk, plastic, metal, or glass. The circumference measurement is used to designate the size of the catheters and is specified in French units. One French (Fr) unit is equal to 1 mm in circumference. The size of the catheter to be used depends upon the purpose for which it is used as well as the size and age of the patient. Appropriate urethral catheter sizes for adult males are 16 to 22 Fr, and for females, 14 to 20 Fr. Adult ureters are generally intubated with sizes 4 to 6 Fr.

Straight catheters include the following: (1) the *Robinson* catheter, which is made of rubber or plastic, has a hollow tip with two or more openings, and is the catheter most frequently used for intermittent catheterizations (Fig. 57-4, *B*); (2) the *coudé* catheter, which has a curved tip and is used for older men or when hypertrophy of the prostate is suspected in order to avoid trauma to the gland (Fig. 57-4, *D*); (3) the *whistle-tip* catheter, which has a whistle-shaped opening at the tip that is ideal for use when hematuria and blood clots are present (Fig. 57-4, A); and (4) the *filiform* catheter, which is a stiff catheter used when a urethral stricture is present.

Self-retaining, or indwelling, catheters are employed when continuous drainage is required and are usually

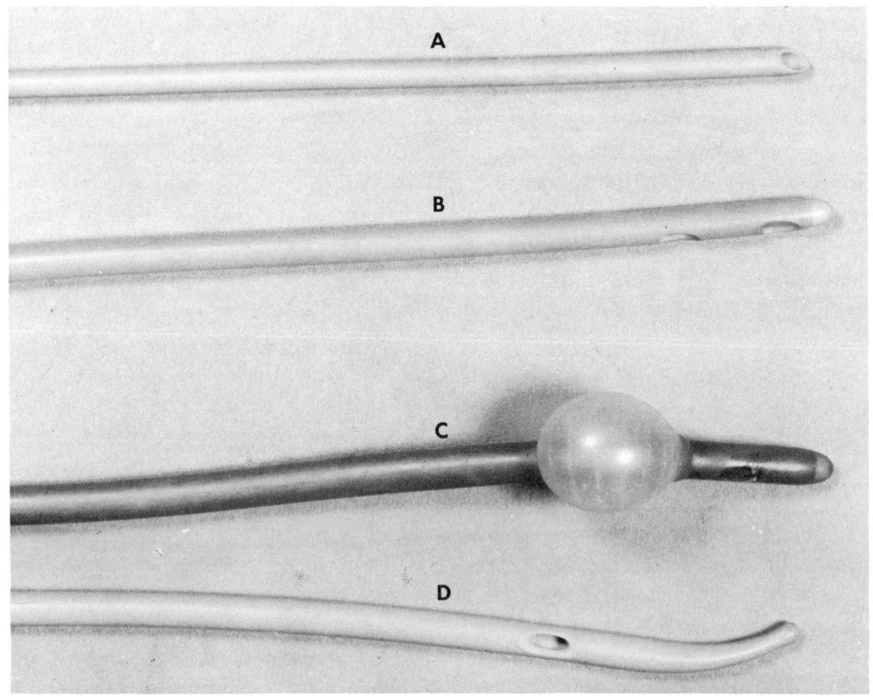

Fig. 57-4. Urethral catheters. **A,** Whistle-tip catheter. **B,** Many-eyed Robinson catheter. **C,** Foley catheter. **D,** Coudé catheter.

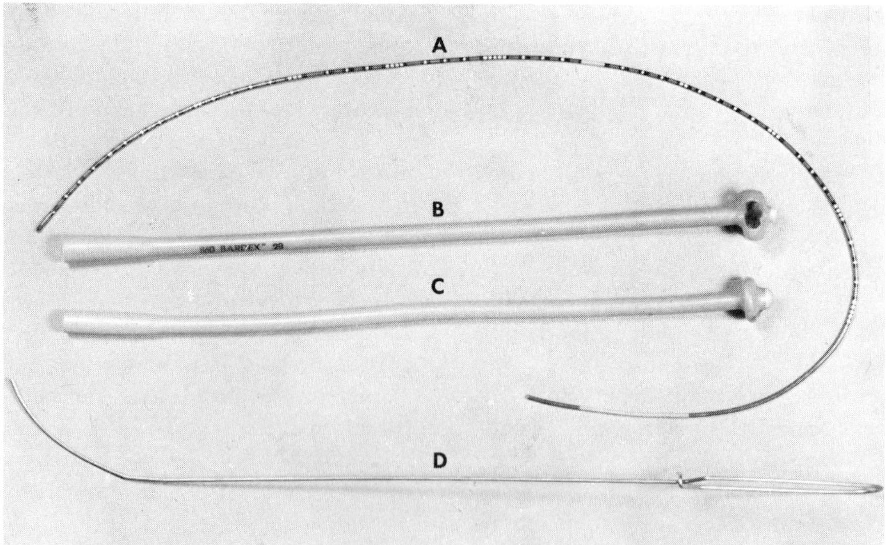

Fig. 57-5. A to **C,** Catheters used to drain renal pelvis. **A,** Ureteral catheters. **B,** Malecot (bat-wing) catheter. **C,** Pezzer (mushroom) catheter. **D,** Stylet used to insert urethral catheter into male patient.

made of latex rubber because this material is more flexible and less irritating to the tissues than the red rubber catheters. Self-retaining catheters include the following:

1. The *Foley* catheter, the most frequently used, has a double lumen with an inflatable balloon near its tip. The balloon is inflated with either normal saline or sterile water after it has been placed well within the bladder (Fig. 57-4, *C*). These catheters are constructed with either a 5 ml balloon (for routine use) or a 30 ml balloon (for use when hemostasis is required) and may have one or two openings. They may be straight or have a curved tip (coudé-shaped) and may have a short or long tip. A three-way Foley catheter has a third lumen that is used for the inflow of irrigating fluids. A disadvantage of the Foley catheter is the small lumen of its outlet channel compared to its external diameter.

2. The *Malecot* catheter (Fig. 57-5, *B*), made of rubber or plastic, has a large single channel, and its tip is in the shape of two or four rings that collapse into the shape of a tube when traction is applied as during its removal.

3. The *Pezzer*, or *mushroom*, catheter is similar to the Malecot except that its tip forms a noncollapsible mushroom shape (Fig. 57-5, *C*).

Ureteral catheters are much smaller and longer than urethral catheters (Fig. 57-5, *A*) and are made of nylon, polyethylene, Teflon, Dacron, silicone, woven silk, or rubber.

Drainage systems

Catheters that have been placed in the urinary system are usually allowed to drain by gravity. The procedure of connecting a catheter to a collecting device and

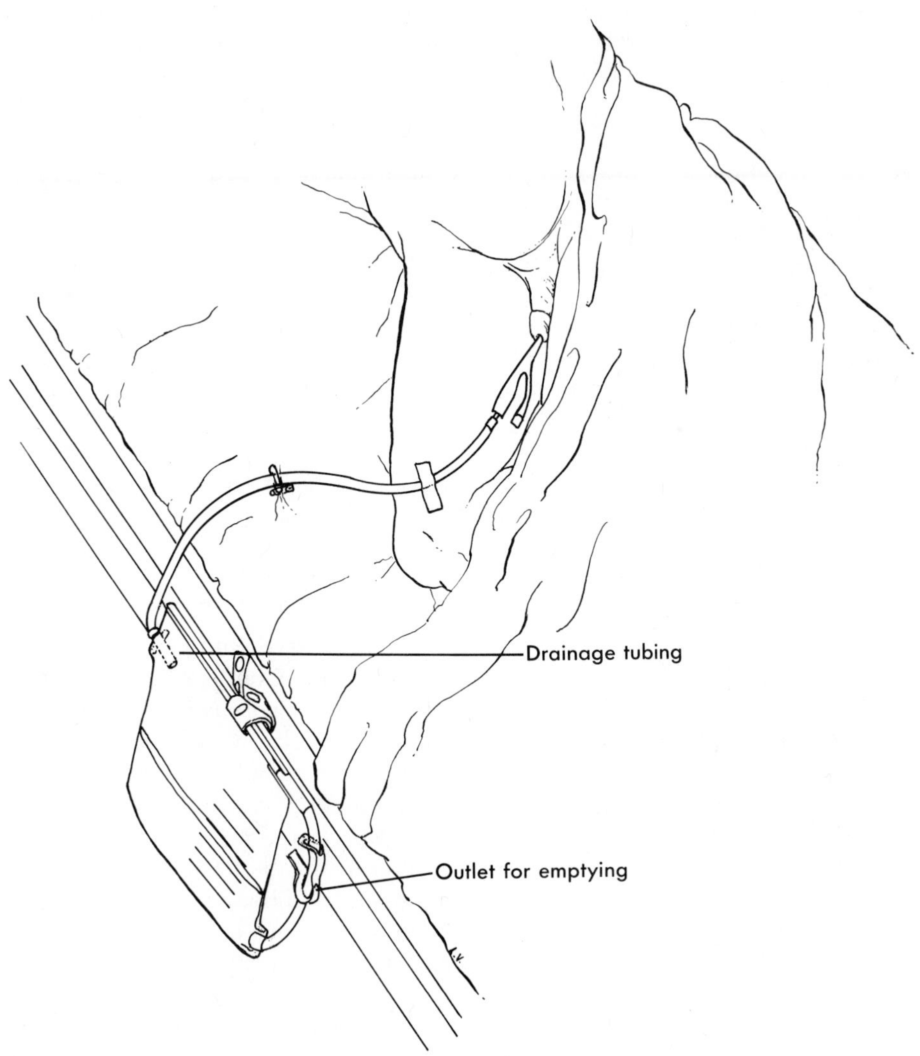

Fig. 57-6. Disposable closed urinary drainage system. Tubing is attached at top of interior of drainage bag.

allowing drainage to flow by gravitational force is called *straight drainage*. *Closed drainage* refers to the design of the collection set-up and indicates that the drainage tube is sealed to the collection container; this lessens the chance for contamination of the set-up and decreases the risk of urinary tract infection. For drainage to occur in a system that is closed to the outside, some air must be introduced to break the vacuum that would otherwise exist. In the closed system, an air vent that is filtered to lessen the danger of infection is provided. Most closed urinary drainage systems employ disposable plastic drainage bags and tubing (Fig. 57-6).

Proper maintenance of the drainage system is a nursing function. Attention to the following points will help to maintain drainage and decrease the entry of organisms into the system: (1) Once the catheter has been connected to the drainage system it should not be disconnected except if necessary when performing ordered irrigations. Samples of urine should be obtained by inserting a small-bore needle at a slant directly into the catheter at a point immediately above the connection with the drainage tubing (Fig. 57-7). (2) The drainage bag must not be elevated above the level of the patient's bladder or cavity being drained as reflux of urine will occur. Drainage bags should be suspended from the bed frame when the patient is recumbent, suspended from the frame of the cart when a patient is being transported, and from below the knee level when the patient is ambulatory. (3) Drainage bags and tubing should not be allowed to rest on the floor. (4) Kinks or loops of tubing below the level of the drainage container should be avoided; to prevent interference with flow of urine, excess tubing may be clipped and coiled on the bed. The patency of all tubes should be checked each time a patient is repositioned. (5) The drainage bag should not be allowed to become completely filled with urine as this leads to stasis of urine in the drainage tubing and wetting of the air filter in the drainage container. (6) The drainage container should not be held upside down when being emptied as this causes reflux of urine into the drainage tubing and bladder. (7) Cultures of the urine should be taken at frequent intervals when a patient has an indwelling drainage tube. (8) The collecting system should be checked daily for signs of sediment and leaks. Any of these findings indicates the need for a new collection system.

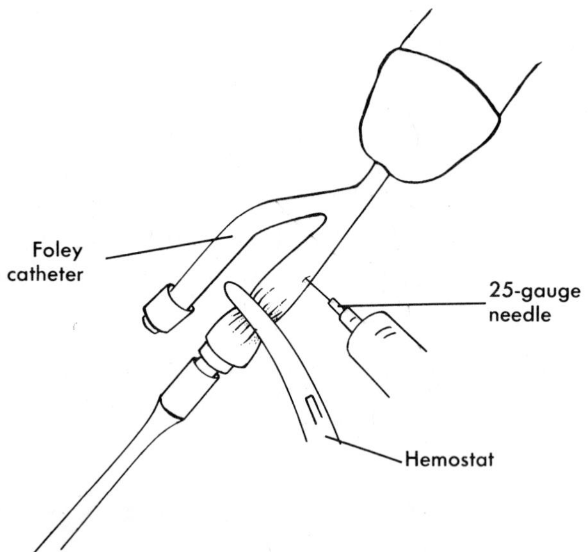

Fig. 57-7. Needle and syringe are used to remove sterile specimen from Foley catheter in closed drainage system.

Since the purpose of the catheter is to promote drainage of urine, *patency* of the system must be assured. The flow of urine from a catheter is checked hourly when urine is bloody and at least every 2 hours when there is no evidence of disturbance in drainage. Common causes of obstruction of urine flow may be internal or external. Hemorrhage leads to formation of clots that may plug a catheter, and infection increases sediment in the urine that may clog the drainage system. Any evidence of bleeding or change in the amount of bleeding is reported to the physician. To detect the buildup of sediment in the drainage system, the catheter may be rolled between the fingers to detect any gritty accumulation, and drainage tubing is visually inspected. External causes of obstruction in urine flow include kinking and dependent loops in the tubing. If correction of these problems fails to restore the flow of urine, irrigation, if ordered, may be done. In the event that none of these measures restores the flow of urine, the physician is notified.

Catheter irrigation

Catheters should not be irrigated without a physician's order. Gentleness is mandatory in any irrigation procedure. Vigorous instillation of fluid into the kidney or bladder is likely to damage these organs and spread or initiate infections. All equipment used must be sterile, and attention to asepsis must be maintained throughout the procedure. Sterile normal saline solution is usually ordered for catheter irrigation because it is nonirritating to tissues and because its clarity makes for easy observation of abnormal constitutents in the urine. Acetic acid, for its acidifying effect, and neomycin solutions may also be ordered as irrigating substances.

When a catheter is to be irrigated, the size of the cavity into which the fluid is being instilled should be considered. *The renal pelvis of an adult should never be irrigated with more than 4 to 6 ml of fluid.* Commonly 30 to 60 ml of fluid is used to irrigate an adult urethral catheter. The quantity, frequency, and type of irrigating solution should be specified by the physician.

After instillation, the irrigating fluid should be allowed to return by gravity. If fluid can be easily instilled but fails to return, a clot or small plug may be acting as a valve over the catheter opening. If this occurs, the nurse should not continue to add fluid, but instead may try to dislodge a possible obstruction by "milking" the tubing. If after a 10- to 15-minute period the catheter is not draining properly, the physician is notified.

When frequent irrigation of a urethral catheter appears necessary, intermittent irrigation should be considered. This involves alternately instilling fluid from a reservoir (usually suspended above patient level) into the bladder through the catheter and allowing the solution to return freely to the collecting bag. Intermittent irrigation is not recommended for irrigation of the kidney because control of inflow in 4 to 6 ml amounts is difficult and instillation of larger amounts into the renal pelvis may lead to tissue damage.

Another variation in bladder irrigation involves the use of a three-way Foley catheter. Constant irrigation involves continuous and simultaneous inflow and outflow of irrigating solution for the bladder. The system is used more frequently after surgery of the bladder or prostate when bleeding is expected and clot formation with obstruction of the bladder outlet is a threat.

In calculating the patient's output when either intermittent or continuous irrigation of the bladder is employed, the amount of irrigating fluid is subtracted from the total volume of urinary drainage obtained in the same time period. The difference between these two values is the patient's actual urinary output.

Several catheters may be used at one time for some postoperative patients. The nurse must know where each is inserted in order to determine how much drainage may be epxected from each. In most instances it is necessary to record drainage separately when noting urine output.

Drainage of the kidney, pelvis, and ureters

If a ureter becomes obstructed, a catheter must be placed directly into the renal pelvis. This prevents renal damage that otherwise would occur as pressure in the kidney increases because of continued urine formation. When there is complete obstruction of a ureter, a *nephrostomy* or *pyelostomy* tube may be inserted surgically into the renal pelvis. The surgical incision is located laterally and posteriorly in the kidney region. Catheters used as nephrostomy or pyelostomy tubes are usually of the Pezzer (mushroom) or Malecot (batwing) types (Fig. 57-5). An alternate form of drainage for a ureteral obstruction is the surgical placement of a ureterostomy tube (a whistle-tip or many-eyed Robinson catheter, size 6 or 8 Fr) that is passed through an incision in the upper outer quadrant of the abdomen into the ureter above the obstruction. The catheter is then passed through the ureter to the renal pelvis.

If the ureter is unobstructed or partially obstructed, the renal pelvis may be drained by a ureteral catheter, which is passed up the ureter to the renal pelvis by means of a cystoscope. Ureteral catheterization is performed prior to gynecologic and lower abdominal surgery when there is danger of not recognizing and accidentally injuring the ureter during the operation. Ureteral catheterization is also used after surgery involving the ureters in order to prevent stricture as the ureter heals. This is referred to as a *splinting catheter* when used for this purpose (Fig. 57-8). Whether it is expected to drain urine will depend upon its relation to other catheters used.

Adequate anchorage of *nephrostomy* and *ureteral* catheters must be provided to prevent accidental dislodgement and trauma to the tissues in which they lie. The openings made for these tubes are essentially fistulas that rapidly decrease in size on removal of the catheter. Even 30 minutes after removal of this type of catheter it is often impossible to reinsert a similar-sized tube. When a catheter is inserted during surgery, it is usually sutured in place. In this case, additional anchorage consists of affixing the tube to the skin with adhesive tape after the skin has been cleansed. When the tube is not sutured in place, it should be anchored to the skin at *two points* using adhesive—with some slack in the tubing between the anchor points.

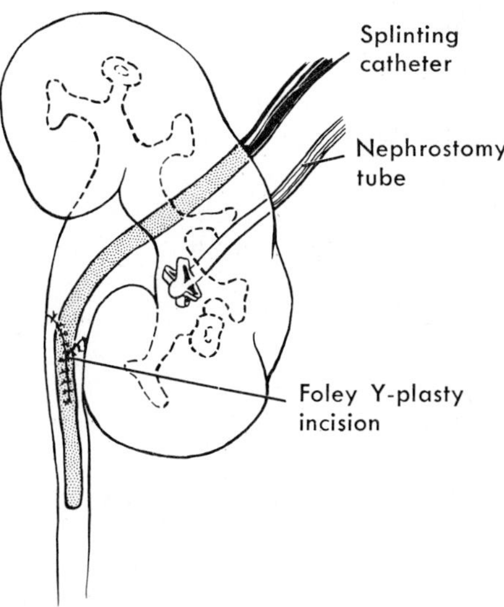

Fig. 57-8. Placement of splinting catheter after repair of ureteropelvic stricture. Note use of nephrostomy tube from drainage of urine during healing of anastomosis.

Free drainage of catheters leading to the renal pelvis is the utmost importance. Since the normal renal pelvis has only a 5 to 8 ml capacity, great pressure can be exerted on renal structures even when these catheters are obstructed for only a few minutes. Care must be taken to prevent kinking of the tubes while the patient is in the side-lying position in bed.

In some cases nephrostomy tubes may be left in place for several months, with the patient returning to the hospital later for its removal. Occasionally the nephrostomy tube serves as a form of urinary diversion for long-term use. The person at home with a catheter draining the kidney pelvis must know how to obtain medical assistance quickly should the catheter obstruct or become dislodged.

Drainage of the bladder

When obstruction occurs below the bladder, constant drainage must be provided to prevent renal damage, which may occur because of inadequate emptying of the lower urinary system. One means of providing drainage is by the use of a *cystostomy* tube (usually a Foley, Malecot, or Pezzer catheter), which is placed directly into the bladder through a suprapubic incision. This method is usually used when the urethra is completely obstructed or when the prolonged use of a urethral catheter is to be avoided in a male patient. During some operative procedures both a cystostomy tube and a small urethral catheter will be inserted to drain the bladder. Both catheters must be monitored for patency. If patency is assured, it is not necessary to record the output from each catheter separately, since both tubes drain the bladder. The catheters will not necessarily drain equal amounts of urine. As is true with nephrostomy and ureteral catheters, secure anchorage of these catheters is also necessary.

Urethral catheterization is the most common means of draining the bladder, and insertion of this type of catheter is a nursing responsibility in many settings. The Foley catheter is most frequently used for this purpose.

Catheterization is a major cause of urinary tract infections, and strict asepsis should be practiced by anyone carrying out this procedure or assembling the drainage equipment. The need for urethral catheterization must be carefully evaluated; use of urethral catheter drainage only for nursing convenience is not appropriate. Institutional policies differ in regard to whether female nursing personnel may catheterize male patients; however, catheterization of a patient of either sex may be performed by a health care professional of either sex in the same professional manner as he or she would perform any other aspect of the patient's nursing care—competently and with respect for the patient's possible feelings of embarrassment.

When a female patient is catheterized, the supine or lateral position may be used; the male patient should be supine. The patient should have thorough explanation of the procedure prior to the catheterization. Privacy is maintained in order to help the patient feel less embarrassed and more relaxed. The patient is encouraged to take deep breaths during insertion of the catheter in order to divert attention from the procedure and to increase relaxation of the bladder sphincters, making the procedure less uncomfortable.

If the nurse finds it difficult to pass the catheter, the procedure is discontinued and the physician notified. Traumatic catheterization predisposes to urinary tract infection and formation of urethral strictures. In patients who have urethral disorders, it is not unusual to be unable to pass a standard catheter; special equipment such as catheter directors, filiform catheters, or sounds may be needed. The introduction of such equipment into the urinary tract is not a nursing procedure; neither is catheterization of a patient in the immediate postoperative period following surgery of the urethra or bladder. (For specific information on the catheterization procedure refer to a fundamentals of nursing or urologic nursing text.)

In addition to the previously discussed basic principles of catheter drainage maintenance, the meatal-catheter junction is cleansed twice a day with soap and water in order to prevent urinary tract infections. Vigorous cleaning is avoided, as this predisposes to infection by causing irritation and by removing protective microorganisms. Irrigation of the catheter may be necessary when urine flow is sluggish, but is not recommended on a routine basis.

The urethral catheter is anchored securely, not only for patient comfort, but also to prevent complications. For the female the catheter is taped to the inner thigh, allowing sufficient slack to prevent tension at the bladder neck. For the male the catheter should be taped on either side between the groin and iliac crest, or on the lower abdomen, so that the penile-scrotal angle is straightened. This avoids pressure and friction that can lead to necrosis of tissue and the formation of urethral ulceration and fistulas.

The urethral catheter is changed when it is in danger of becoming obstructed by encrustations within its lumen. The person who will have an indwelling urethral catheter at home will either have to be able to learn to change his own catheter or have a plan for assistance to do this when needed.

Home care for the person with urinary catheter drainage

The person who requires catheter drainage at home on a temporary or permanent basis must be able to safely maintain his urinary drainage system. If the person is incapable of this because of physical or mental status, another person must be instructed in all necessary care. Written instructions are provided to supplement and reinforce the information. The services of a community health nurse may be indicated. The following areas must be included in homegoing preparation of any person with indwelling catheter drainage: maintaining catheter patency, preventing urinary tract infection, maintaining activity, dealing with catheter problems, obtaining supplies, and continuing with urologic surveillance.

Maintenance of patency of the catheter. The person (or care provider) must know how to check for kinks in the tubing and should be aware of the most appropriate way to secure the catheter to prevent kinking. An adequate fluid intake of 2 to 3 liters (quarts) of fluid per day should be encouraged unless contraindicated by the person's condition. Persons who will be irrigating their own catheters at home should practice this under supervision several times before discharge.

Prevention of urinary tract infection. The person (or care provider) must be helped to understand the importance of cleanliness as a means of preventing complications. Instruction includes cleansing the meatal-catheter junction with soap and water twice daily. Any drainage system should be a closed one; however, change of the collecting system (from leg bag to night drainage, for example) will be necessary. The person is taught to wipe the catheter and tubing with 70% alcohol prior to disconnection and reconnection and to protect the disconnected ends with sterile gauze or with a premade connector cap.

When equipment must be sterilized at home, instruction is given in how to do this properly. Prior to use, the equipment, which has been washed with soap and water, is boiled for a full 10 minutes in a pan of water. Other parts of the system such as collection bags and tubing should be kept as clean as possible by daily washing with soap and water, followed by 15 minutes of soaking in a solution of equal parts of vinegar and water (half-strength vinegar). Teaching also includes the need to keep the drainage collection receptacle at a level lower than the cavity being drained.

Activity. The patient needs to be well informed about the mechanics of adapting his urinary drainage system to his optimal level of activity. He should be informed that adaptations can be made to accommodate travel and that he should seek advice about this if he is planning a trip. A shower or tub bath with a catheter in place is generally permitted unless there is an unhealed surgical incision. Adhesive tape will need to be replaced afterward. There is no need for either man or woman to remove an indwelling catheter prior to intercourse—a question the patient may be hesitant to voice (p. 1475). The patient should be encouraged to ask any questions he has relating to his return to his usual life style.

Dealing with catheter problems. The patient (or care provider) should be informed about how to handle problems such as obstruction of the catheter or displacement of the catheter. He should know whether he is to contact his physician or to seek help through a clinic or emergency room. The amount of time he can safely wait before obtaining help will depend upon the type of catheter and its location.

Obtaining supplies. At discharge the patient should be provided with adequate supplies for at least a few days. He should be given a list of names, addresses, and phone numbers of where additional supplies may be obtained and what resources are available to assist with payment if necessary. A written list of the specific supplies needed by the patient should be provided to aid the patient who is likely to be confused by the many products available.

Ongoing care. The person with a urinary catheter of any type will need continued urologic surveillance. Instruction includes the need to contact the physician if back pain, fever, or other urinary tract symptoms are present and to plan for regular examination by the physician as well.

Management of the patient after removal of a catheter

It is normal to note some dribbling of urine for a few hours after a urethral catheter has been removed because of dilation of the sphincter muscles by the catheter. Dribbling or urine that persists longer than a few hours should be reported to the physician; this symptom may indicate damage to the sphincters. In determining the type of intervention necessary to reestablish bladder control, information about the nature of the incontinency is gathered. Incontinence is described as complete (constant dribbling) or occurring only on urgency or stress. It should also be observed whether incontinence is present in all positions (lying, sitting, standing). If muscular weakness of the sphincters is the major problem, incontinence is least likely to occur when the person is in a prone position and most likely to be a problem when the person stands or walks. Perineal exercises (p. 1273) may help to regain control of voiding.

Another problem that may arise after removal of a catheter is inability to void. No patient with an adequate intake should go longer than 6 to 8 hours without voiding. It is not uncommon for a patient with edema of the bladder neck to require temporary reinsertion of a catheter to facilitate urinary output. It is the nurse's responsibility to accurately determine and record all spontaneous voiding of the patient until adequacy of output has been well established.

Color and consistency of the urine is noted. *Cystitis* (inflammation of the bladder) may develop after catheter removal because of incomplete emptying of the bladder as muscle tone is being reestablished. Any abnormalities in color, odor, or sediment are reported.

Education of the patient about signs and symptoms of urinary retention, changes in the color and consistency of the urine, and incontinence and dysuria are undertaken when bladder drainage is discontinued. Often the first indicators of dysfunction are subjective judgments that the patient offers about himself. This information greatly increases the ability to detect early recurrence of urinary drainage problems and should be sought and clearly recorded.

Outcome criteria for the person with an indwelling catheter

The patient:

1. Maintains free flow of urine through the catheter.
2. Does not acquire a urinary tract infection.

The patient or significant others can:

1. Explain the purpose and expected duration of the catheter.
2. Demonstrate aseptic technique in care of the catheter.
3. State how to arrange for reestablishment of urine flow should failure of adequate flow occur.
4. State where to obtain needed supplies.
5. Describe signs and symptoms of urinary tract infection requiring medical attention.
6. State plans for follow-up care.

□ Intermittent catheter drainage

Intermittent catheterization of the urinary bladder is being used with increasing frequency in the treatment of neurogenic bladder dysfunction secondary to spinal cord trauma, birth defects, urinary retention, and some chronic diseases. Originally it was carried out only as a sterile procedure used in hospital settings. More recently, a clean, unsterile technique has been adapted by some urologists that facilitates home use of this method.[30]

Because periodic complete emptying of the bladder eliminates residual urine (an excellent culture medium for multiplication of bacteria) and maintains a good blood supply to the bladder wall by avoiding high intrabladder pressures, infections are often decreased, even when only a clean technique is used.

Individuals are evaluated for their appropriateness for this form of management by the urologist. Potential for success with this form of therapy should be further evaluated, utilizing input from the nurse clinician, psychologist, social worker, and other involved health care professionals. Teaching, however, is generally a nursing responsibility in either an inpatient or outpatient setting. Before a teaching plan can be made, the nurse must know whether a clean or sterile technique is to be taught and the frequency with which it is to be used. Knowledge of the person's physical, mental, and emotional status as well as usual life style must also be utilized in planning a program suitable for each person.

The hospitalized patient previously on an established intermittent catheterization program at home may require catheterization by nursing personnel during illness, but may be encouraged to continue self-care as able.

The goals of intermittent catheterization may vary from patient to patient but are generally to prevent urinary retention and its sequelae (urinary tract infection and renal damage) and to achieve continence. The patient should know exactly what is expected of his treatment plan to elicit his full cooperation.

Intervention

The hospitalized patient with intermittent catheter drainage of the bladder may be one for whom the treatment is temporary (as in the early phases of spinal cord trauma), one who is learning the technique for home use, or one who has been using intermittent catheterization prior to admission. Even though the clean technique is suitable for home use, sterile technique is necessary during hospitalization to decrease the possibility of hospital-acquired infection when the catheterization is performed by hospital personnel. When hospitalized, the patient who customarily performs self-catheterization may continue to use clean technique if this method is used at home, but preferably a sterile catheter will be used each time or special precautions are taken to store the reusable catheter in a closed container. Specimens for culture must be obtained by the usual sterile catheterization technique to avoid contamination of the specimen. The patient is informed about the reasons why sterile precautions are necessary in the hospital setting.

A size 14 Fr Robinson catheter is generally used for an adult. The volume of urine obtained with each catheterization is recorded to assure that schedule adjustments can be made if necessary. The adult bladder should not be permitted to hold more than 300 ml at any time, since greater amounts lead to overdistention of the bladder with greater susceptibility to infection. The usual frequency of catheterization is every 3 to 4 hours during the waking hours. Persons may also have to catheterize themselves once or twice at night if they have a large output of urine at night. It is important to realize that the person who normally does not perform self-catheterization at night at home may need to do so during periods where the fluid intake is greater than usual, as with intravenous fluid administration.

In some instances the physician will prescribe the frequency of catheterizations; in other instances, adjustment of the schedule may be a nursing judgment. If the nurse notes that excess volumes of urine are being obtained with a prescribed schedule, the physician is consulted about the need to alter the schedule.

Color, clarity, and odor of the urine are noted and any symptoms of urinary tract infection reported. Periodic urine specimens are obtained and sent for culture and sensitivity. Some individuals are maintained on long-term antibiotic therapy prophylactically.

The person is helped to understand the rationale for intermittent catheter drainage, and the regularity of bladder emptying must be stressed. Basic anatomy of the genitalia and urinary tract is pointed out to aid the person to understand where the catheter is inserted and to alleviate fears of causing damage by misplacement of the catheter.

In most cases, clean (not sterile) catheterization technique is prescribed for home use. Hand washing is advised prior to each catheterization, and the meatal area is cleansed with soap and water. After inserting the catheter and draining the bladder, the catheter is removed and washed with soap and water before being stored in a clean, closed container for the next use. The catheter is reused until it becomes either too soft or too hard to be directed properly.

Most individuals require much support during the actual teaching, but very quickly become comfortable with the procedure. Initially a mirror is used to teach women where to place the catheter. The woman should learn to catheterize while sitting on the commode, using palpation to locate the urethral meatus. Men may sit or stand to catheterize themselves. It is important that they use generous amounts of lubricant to avoid urethral irritation; women generally do not require lubrication of the catheter.

If the person, because of age or physical limitations, is unable to catheterize himself, a care provider may be instructed in the technique. The individual or care provider must know where additional catheters may be obtained.

If sterile catheterization technique is needed for home use, more time and practice will be required in order to learn good sterile technique. Careful explanation of sterilization of equipment must be provided, and planning for adapting sterile intermittent self-catheterization to the individual's usual life style must be worked out with the person.

If teaching of self-catheterization is performed on an outpatient basis or if hospitalization is short, follow-up for adjustment of schedule and other concerns of adaptation to home routine should be provided. This may be done by the primary nurse, the physician, or by referral to a visiting nurse. Ongoing urologic care with periodic urine cultures is essential.

Outcome criteria for the person who is using the intermittent catheter drainage technique

The person can:

1. Explain the reason for the intermittent catheter drainage.
2. State the need for regular, periodic, complete emptying of the bladder.
3. Demonstrate self-catheterization using clean technique unless sterile technique is prescribed.
4. Describe how to adapt the catheterization routine to the individual life style.
5. State how to obtain needed supplies.
6. Describe symptoms of urinary tract infection requiring medical care.
7. State plans for ongoing urologic care.

■ MANAGEMENT OF FLUID BALANCE WITH URINARY PROBLEMS

Management of fluid balance is a fundamental and common problem for persons requiring urologic procedures and nephrology care. Maintaining normal fluid balance helps to (1) preserve renal function in individuals having ongoing kidney insufficiency or failure, (2) prevent the development of acute renal failure caused by fluid depletion, (3) prevent inadequate tissue perfusion and shock from depletion of blood volume, (4) provide continuous urine formation to help alleviate stasis of urine and bacterial growth, and (5) prevent fluid overload with increased cardiac work and formation of peripheral and cerebral edema. The potential for altered states of fluid balance for urologic and renal patients thus commonly involves both abnormal losses and gains of fluid.

Accurate assessment of a patient's hydration state depends upon a thorough physical examination and carefully kept records of fluid losses and gains. Most often fluid balance records and patient observations are obtained by nursing personnel. The following information should provide some direction to nurses regarding crucial observations to be made and data to be recorded, and specific instances in urologic and nephrology nursing where problems of fluid balance are likely to arise. For general information on fluid and electrolyte balance the reader is referred to Chapter 20; for common electrolyte problems accompanying renal disease the reader is referred to Chapter 59.

□ Prevention

In order to prevent the occurrence of fluid imbalance, three considerations are important to nursing practice. First, persons prone to developing fluid imbalances and the specific nature of their potential fluid problems require identification. Individuals predisposed to developing *fluid overload* include (1) those with acute renal failure where kidney shutdown and oliguria are the rule; (2) those with bilateral obstructive disease attributed to strictures, tumors, or calculi, who present with anuria or severely decreased urine output; and (3) those with chronic renal failure characterized by a limited and fixed ability to excrete fluid through the kidneys. The common defect in fluid handling in the above situations is an inability to excrete more than a low and fixed volume of urine per day, regardless of fluid intake.

Individuals susceptible to *fluid depletion* or dehydration include (1) those recovering from acute renal failure and in a phase of the illness where the kidneys do not appropriately conserve body fluid; (2) those with chronic renal failure whose urine output per day is fixed at a high volume (200 ml/day or greater) and who are unable to obtain or retain fluids sufficient to replace those lost through the kidneys; and (3) persons on diuretic therapy whose oral intake does not keep up with renal and other body fluid losses. The kidneys of these persons are unable to conserve fluid when intake is low or when extrarenal losses are high. Such situations occur, for example, when there is vomiting or diarrhea over prolonged periods, when fluids are restricted for several diagnostic tests in succession, when there is sudden sodium restriction or loss, which decrease thirst, or when individuals become weak and unable to replace fluid losses on their own.

In addition, certain urologic situations make it very difficult to measure fluid output accurately. These include copious wound drainage or continuous bladder irrigation following urologic surgery, ill-fitting urinary appliances, and incontinence.

A second consideration in preventing fluid imbalances involves collecting appropriate baseline data and continuing to monitor the patient who is at risk of developing fluid problems. Such data will assist both in diagnosing imbalances and in the ongoing management of these problems. For example, when the diagnosis is chronic renal failure, the nurse would wish to obtain information regarding the ability to excrete fluid. Fluid intake and output measurements along with daily weights will help to identify the ability of the person to regulate body fluid balance.

Prevention of fluid imbalances is also achieved through efforts to educate individuals about potential problems they may have in handling fluids. Persons with chronic renal failure and those on diuretic therapy in particular will need to be given guidelines about current goals for fluid management, potential problems with fluid balance, signs and symptoms indicating a problem, and mechanisms for correcting fluid problems or in receiving assistance when they cannot manage the problems on their own.

□ Outcome criteria for the person having fluid imbalance with urinary problems

The patient will:

1. Exhibit no signs of abnormal fluid loss or gain:
   a. No peripheral edema.
   b. No orthostatic hypotension.
   c. Blood pressure stable and within normal range.

The patient or significant others can:

1. Explain any dietary (sodium) and fluid intake restrictions.
2. Explain how these restrictions will be met.

■ MANAGEMENT OF STOMAS FOR URINARY DIVERSION

Urinary diversion procedures are required to treat malignancies of the urinary tract, birth defects, neurogenic bladder dysfunction, chronic progressive pyelonephritis, and irreparable trauma to the urinary tract. Cutaneous ureterostomy and ureteroileocutaneous anastomosis (ileal conduit) are currently the most frequently performed urinary diversions that result in an external stoma. The colonic conduit (or sigmoid loop) is also being performed with increasing frequency.

Cutaneous ureterostomy is often employed when the physical condition prohibits more extensive surgical procedures or when the diversion is expected to be a temporary measure. One or both ureters are excised from the bladder and brought out through the skin either at the flank or the anterior abdominal wall to create a small stoma. When both ureters are involved, each may be brought out to the skin surface separately, resulting in two stomas, or they may be joined at some point and brought out through the abdominal wall to form only one stoma. Ureterostomy stomas tend to be small and prone to stenosis or stricture.

The *ureteroileocutaneous anastomosis* (also called an *ileal conduit, ileal loop,* or Bricker procedure) is the most common form of permanent urinary diversion. During the surgical procedure, the ureters are excised from the bladder and transplanted into one end of a 15 to 20 cm (6- to 8-inch) segment of ileum that has been resected from the intestinal tract with its mesentery, which contains the blood supply. The remaining intestinal segments are anastomosed, and gastrointestinal function is expected to return to its normal preoperative state after healing. The end of the resected ileum into which the ureters are connected is sutured closed and the other

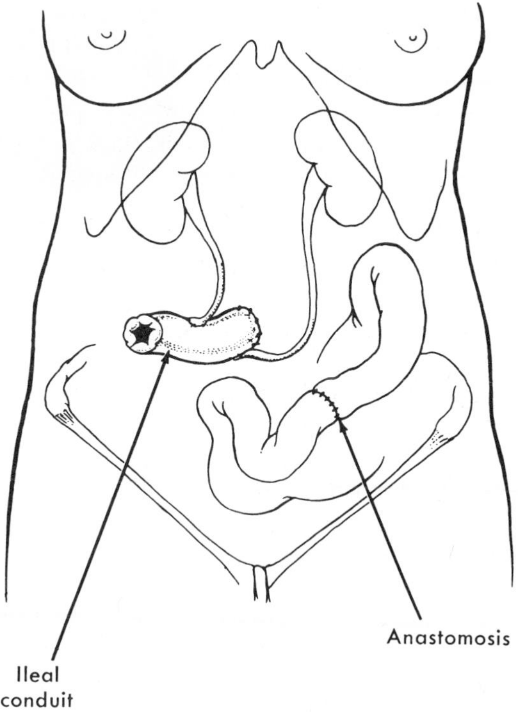

Fig. 57-9. Ileal conduit or ileal loop.

end is brought through the abdominal wall to the skin surface to create a stoma. The urinary bladder may be resected or may be left intact, depending upon the reason for the diversion (Fig. 57-9).

The ileal segment is intended to serve as a passageway for urinary flow rather than as a reservoir; therefore urine flow is continuous from an ileal conduit. Electrolyte imbalance caused by reabsorption of waste products from the urine in the ileal segment is generally not a problem in a well-functioning ileal conduit.

The *colonic loop* (sigmoid loop) is basically performed like an ileal conduit except that a segment of colon instead of ileum acts as the conduit for the passage of urine. Preoperative and postoperative nursing care and ongoing management are the same as that for ileal conduit surgery.

Any procedure for diversion of urine that results in an external stoma leads to a significant change in the person's body image. Reactions may vary depending upon the reason for the procedure, but virtually every person will require time and much nursing support while adapting to his altered means of urine elimination. It is vital that the nurse understand why and how the decision regarding urinary diversion was made in order to understand and support the person's adjustment and acceptance. For example, the person who has elected urinary diversion to achieve continence when all other methods have failed will be likely to react much differently than the person who had a urinary diversion performed suddenly following the diagnosis of bladder carcinoma.

□ Intervention

Preoperative preparation

Much of the basis for successful adjustment of the person undergoing urinary diversion can be provided in the preoperative period. Persons who have been well informed about the surgical procedure as well as the postoperative period and long-term management goals are generally better able to adjust to the entire experience than those who do not receive such preparation. As soon as a person learns that a urinary diversion is contemplated, many questions arise, and it is important that accurate answers be given at this time. The well-informed nurse in any setting recognizes that concerns are present and encourages verbalization of them. The nurse in the outpatient urology clinic, for example, can begin preoperative preparation even prior to hospital admission.

The preoperative preparation of every person scheduled for urinary diversion needs to include certain basic information. It must be recognized, however, that some of the information will not be retained because of factors such as poor physical status, fear, or anxiety, and that reinforcement of the information at a later time will be necessary. Psychologic preparation should begin with an assessment of the individual's understanding about what is to be done, misconceptions, and urgent concerns. The person who is fearful about sexual abilities may be unable to attend to a discussion of urinary appliances until there has been an opportunity to have this concern addressed. The timing and manner in which the necessary information is presented is based upon the person's questions, intellectual and emotional status, and understanding of the type of diversion to be performed.

There must be preparation for the appearance of the stoma. Preoperatively a photograph showing a stoma with and without an appliance is included with the description of the appearance, color, and location of the stoma.

Basic long-term management principles should also be mentioned preoperatively. Details of long-term management are probably best reserved for those persons who request them preoperatively. At a minimum, the person is shown an appliance and there is a discussion of how it is adhered to the body. He should also be assured that he will be assisted to master his stomal management before he is discharged.

Physical preparation for surgery for ureterostomy is similar to that for any abdominal surgery. Prior to an ileal or colonic conduit diversion there is usually a complete cleansing of the bowel to reduce the possibility of fecal contamination when the bowel is resected. The cleansing routine generally consists of a clear liquid diet for about 3 days, followed by nothing by mouth for at least 8 hours before surgery. Cleansing enemas are usually ordered until returns are clear, and an intestinal antibiotic such as neomycin is administered by mouth or by enema. If surgery is delayed for any reason, the surgeon needs to be consulted before continuing with the regimen, since vitamin B and K deficiencies may result, and fungus infection may occur.

The stoma is usually constructed on the right side of the abdomen below the waist. Determination of the exact placement for the stoma site is ideally made prior to surgery and should include evaluation of the person's body when in the lying, sitting, and standing positions. Since a smooth, even skin surface surrounding the stoma is important for optimal adherence of an applicance, it is important that the site selected be free from scars, skin folds, and bony prominences.

Postoperative care

Following a cutaneous ureterostomy, the person generally returns from surgery with catheters inserted through the ureters to drain the renal pelves. These are usually left in place for 7 to 14 days. Patency of the catheters must be maintained because hydronephrosis can rapidly ensue if obstruction occurs.

Following an ileal or colonic conduit procedure there may or may not be splinting catheters in place in the stoma for the first few days postoperatively. A nasogastric tube with gastric suction will be used for 5 to 7 days to allow for the return of effective intestinal peristalsis and the healing of the intestinal anastomosis site. Adequate drainage through the nasogastric tube is maintained to prevent pressure on the intestinal anastomosis. Nothing by mouth is permitted until peristalsis has resumed; then a normal diet is gradually resumed, beginning with small amounts of water. Intravenous fluids are continued until an adequate diet is possible. A regular diet is resumed in simple ureterostomies, since the procedure does not involve the intestinal tract.

Skin care. In any type of urinary diversion, care must be taken to prevent urine leakage onto the surrounding skin. If all the urine is draining from the catheters in the stoma, skin care should present little problem for the first few days, since the catheter will be connected to constant drainage.

If there is urine drainage around the catheters, if no catheters were used, or when catheters have been re-

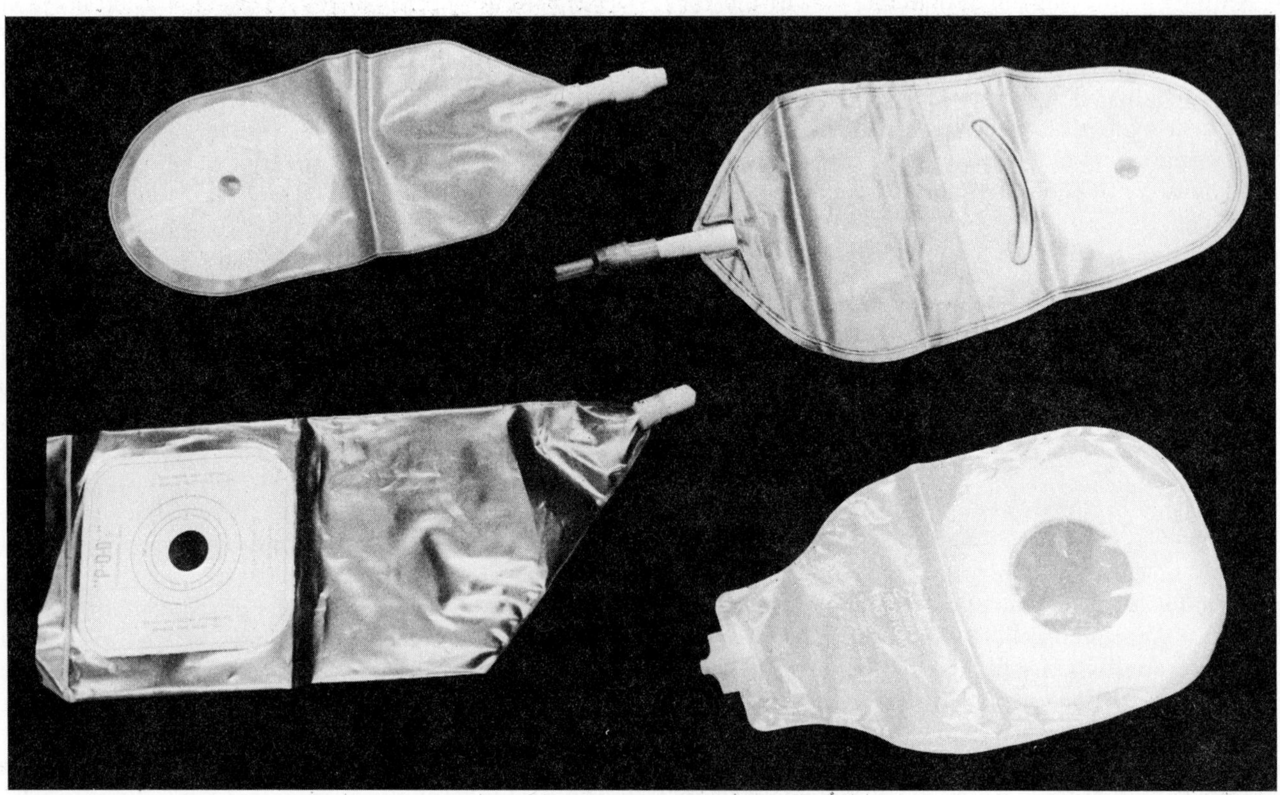

Fig. 57-10. Examples of postoperative drainage bags for urinary stoma.

moved, a temporary postoperative drainage bag is applied over the stoma to collect the continuous urine drainage. An appropriate bag has an opening hole cut not larger than 3 mm (⅛ inch) all around the stoma and has an end that can be attached to drainage tubing (Fig. 57-10). For skin protection and better adherence of the bag, a skin barrier, *Stomahesive*, is particularly useful. Directions for its use are included with the product. Tincture of benzoin, also useful for skin protection and better bag adherence, should be used with caution because it can cause severe skin reactions in some individuals when used under an adhesive. Temporary appliances with Karaya rings are generally not acceptable for use with urinary stomas because urine usually erodes the Karaya, causing leakage.

The bag is changed periodically. If the stoma can be well visualized through the bag and if the bag is adhering well to the body, changing the bag every 2 to 3 days is generally adequate. Clean, unsterile technique is used to change the bag. Following is the method for changing a temporary urostomy bag:

1. Have all supplies ready before bag is removed.
2. Cut an opening in new bag's adhesive backing about 3 mm (⅛ inch) larger than stoma. Make certain that opening is not overly large so that exposure of peristomal skin to urine is prevented. Remove adhesive backing and set aside.
3. Gently remove old bag from skin.
4. Cleanse peristomal skin thoroughly with soap and water. Mucus secretions should be washed off stoma gently.
5. Hold a rolled piece of gauze or cotton balls over stomal opening to absorb draining urine while surrounding skin is being cared for.
6. When skin is *completely* dry, apply skin barrier as directed.
7. Apply bag around stoma, keeping adhesive area free of wrinkles or creases. Press gently but firmly in place completely around stoma. In early postoperative period, bag is placed so that it drains to side of bed, facilitating drainage while the person is lying in bed.
8. Attach end of bag to drainage tubing, adapting ends as necessary for a leakproof connection.

During each bag change procedure, the condition of the stoma and peristomal skin is assessed. The stoma should be bright pink or red—any evidence of gray or black discoloration is reported to the surgeon, since this may indicate necrosis of the stoma. Careful checking of the stoma that is in contact with a catheter is imperative, since improper positioning of the catheter may exert pressure on the stomal tissue, leading to necrosis. The normal stoma may either protrude or be flush with the skin, and edema is common in the early postoperative period. The peristomal skin must be checked for signs of irritation that may be caused by urine leakage, too large a bag opening surrounding the stoma, or allergy to the adhesive backing or tape.

Urine output. Following any type of urinary diversion, urine output must be carefully monitored in the postoperative phase. Edema of the stoma or of the ureteral anastomosis site may cause failure of adequate urine drainage that may lead to hydronephrosis or to a break in the anastomosis. Other complications that may first be detected by a decreased urine output include dehydration, obstruction of the ureters, ileal loop ileus, or compromised renal function.

Decreased urine output associated with symptoms of peritonitis (fever, abdominal distention, and pain) should alert the nurse to the possibility of intraperitoneal leakage caused by a leak at either the intestinal or ureterointestinal anastomosis. If this occurs, emergency surgery is required to repair the leak.

The color and nature of the urine output is also noted. Blood in the urine is expected in the early postoperative period with gradual clearing. Mucus, a normal discharge from the intestinal segment, is normally secreted from an ileal or colonic conduit. Mucus threads in the urine from an ureterostomy, however, is abnormal and may indicate the presence of an infection.

The abdominal incision is observed *at least daily* for healing of the suture line. Care of this incision is sometimes complicated by the possibility of urine leakage onto it. An appropriate postoperative drainage bag will minimize this problem.

Body image. Persons with urinary stomas experience some of the same feelings regarding change in body image as do persons with fecal stomas (p. 1250). They need time and opportunity to explore their feelings and to learn to cope effectively with the changes. Competent physical nursing care is also important, since the person who experiences frequent urine leakage or skin excoriation from poor nursing care will most likely feel all the more discouraged and depressed about the surgical procedure and the inability to urinate normally.

Self-care. As soon as the person feels able to do so, he is encouraged to begin to participate in his own stomal care with adequate supervision and support. During the bag changing procedures and related nursing care, the nurse can explain important aspects of his ongoing management. This all cannot be accomplished in a day or two prior to discharge! If possible, one nurse should coordinate the care and teaching. Having one well-informed person responsible for nursing care assists in the development of a trusting relationship that allows the person to feel free to discuss any concerns.

Appliances. Measurement for a permanent ap-

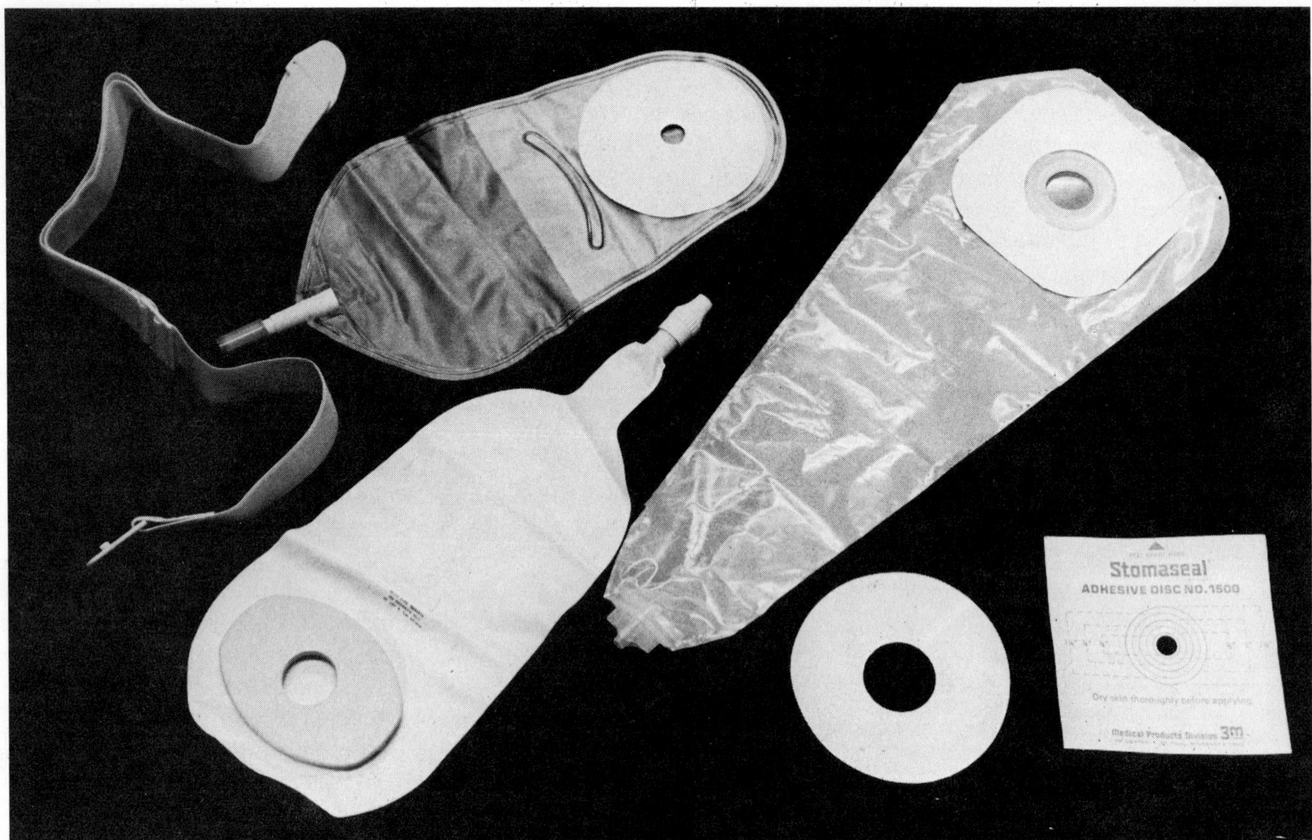

Fig. 57-11. Some examples of urinary appliances used by persons for long-term management of urinary tract diversion. Adhesive tape disks and belt are also shown.

pliance occurs about 7 days after surgery when the major edema has subsided. Continued shrinkage of the stoma will probably occur in the following 6 to 8 weeks, so that a check for appropriate fit is required at that time. Several manufacturers provide measuring cards with various-sized holes that can be placed around the stoma to determine the size that will allow 1.5 to 3 mm of skin to show around the stoma. An alternative method is to measure the diameter of the stoma and add 3 to 6 mm to the measurement to obtain the proper size for ordering. Too large an opening size will permit excoriation of exposed skin while an opening size that is too small may restrict circulation or cause trauma to the stoma.

Several types of appliances are available (Fig. 57-11). All have two things in common—a pouch to collect the urine and an outlet at the bottom for easy emptying every 3 or 4 hours. The basic types of bags are (1) permanent appliances that can be washed and reused, (2) semidisposable bags that fit onto a permanent disk, and (3) one-piece disposable appliances that are discarded after use. All are adhered to the body with some form of adhesive to form a watertight seal. The type of appliance used depends upon the individual's preference, body build, and special needs, such as physical or visual impairment. The person is informed of the choices available, but much direction and guidance in selecting the most appropriate appliance may be required. Cost comparisons for the various types of appliances can be made by comparing the expected life of the bag with the current price.

The individual (or care provider) must learn how to manage the assembly, application, emptying, cleaning, and changing of whatever appliance is chosen. The permanent appliance is obtained prior to discharge so that the person can demonstrate the ability to assemble and apply the appliance. A family member or friend is included in the teaching to provide support at home, but the individual, unless limited physically, is encouraged to be responsible for self-care.

The permanent appliance should be one that will remain in place and free of leakage for a least 24 hours.

Most persons can wear an appliance for 3 to 5 days between changes: an interval longer than 5 days should be discouraged because of potential odor and crystallization problems. An appropriate schedule that eliminates leakage problems will need to be determined. For example, if the bag tends to leak on the fourth day, it will need to be changed every 3 days, *before* leakage occurs.

Following is the *method for changing a permanent urostomy appliance:*

1. Remove bag from abdomen.
2. Prepare appliance to be applied by applying skin cement or a double adhesive tape disk to clean faceplate. (For a disposable bag, peel off protective paper from tape portion of appliance.)
3. Wash stoma and surrounding skin with soap and water. Rinse well. Pat dry. Hold a cotton ball or gauze pad over stoma to prevent urine leakage onto clean, dry skin.
4. Apply a skin barrier product (Stomahesive, Skin-Prep) if being used.
5. Apply sticky part of appliance to clean, dry skin (or onto skin barrier), centering faceplate over stoma. (If using skin cement instead of adhesive disks, a thin layer is required on skin as well as on faceplate.)
6. Press firmly but gently completely around stoma to assure a good seal. Attach belt if desired.

Proper cleaning of reusable equipment is essential for odor control, general hygiene, and prevention of stomal complications. Manufacturers include cleaning instructions with their equipment. Following are the principles for proper cleaning of reusable urinary appliances:

1. Clean equipment promptly.
2. Use adhesive remover as necessary to remove residue from faceplate.
3. Wash both faceplate and bag in soap and water.
4. Avoid soaking equipment for prolonged periods of time (20 to 30 minutes in soap and water is sufficient). Longer soaking speeds deterioration of many appliances.
5. For odor problems, soak appliance in half-strength vinegar water for an additional 20 to 30 minutes.

Problems. *Odor* problems are generally caused by urinary infection, inadequate cleansing of equipment, and urine leakage. In the absence of these problems, odor is generally not a problem. For those desiring additional assurance, commercial deodorant products are available. Full- or half-strength white vinegar, 30 to 60 ml, or one or two crushed aspirin tablets placed through the bottom of the bag can help to reduce urine odor by acidifying the urine in the bag.

Peristomal skin problems may be caused by urine leakage, adhesive allergy, improper appliance fit, or pressure. Treatment of skin problems requires finding and eliminating the cause of the problem. A light dusting of Karaya gum powder or the application of a skin barrier such as Stomahesive under the adhesive will permit healing of minor skin irritations. Yeast infections may require the use of an antifungal spray or powder under the adhesive. Proper appliance fit is essential to protect peristomal skin from irritation by urine. Pressure caused by the faceplate may require obtaining a smaller faceplate or trimming of the faceplate to relieve any pressure areas. Persons subject to skin allergies from adhesives should have any new adhesive tested on another site on the abdomen before it is applied to the peristomal area. An area that shows a reaction is more easily healed if it is exposed to air rather than being covered.

Stomal problems include bleeding and alkaline crusting. A small amount of bleeding from the stoma is not unusual, especially after bag changes or after the stoma has been slightly traumatized. Such minor bleeding should subside within 1 to 2 hours. If bleeding persists or is unusually severe, the physician is notified. The blood may be originating from the urinary tract and may be related to complications such as infection or calculi. Alkaline deposits may be observed on the stoma and the peristomal skin when the urine is alkaline. Persistence of this problem can lead to tissue hyperkeratosis and eventual stomal stenosis or occlusion. Such deposits also lead to stomal irritation and bleeding. Treatment of the problem involves good hygiene and the acidification of the urine by internal or external means. Ascorbic acid is prescribed, and the acidity of the urine may be tested with Nitrazine paper so that the appropriate dosage to achieve acidification may be determined. Externally, half-strength white vinegar soaks may be prescribed four times a day or 30 to 60 ml of full- or half-strength vinegar may be inserted into the bottom of the bag and allowed to bathe the stoma for at least 15 minutes four times a day.

Discharge plans. Before discharge from the hospital the nurse must be certain that the individual can manage the urinary drainage and can detect any deviations from normal. At least one return visit or an opportunity for telephone contact with the primary nurse involved in the teaching is extremely helpful so that questions that arise after returning home can be discussed. Visiting nurse assistance may be required for a period of time. Ongoing urologic care will be required, including urine cultures, which are correctly obtained by catheter from the ileal or sigmoid loop stoma. A specimen taken from the bag is likely to be contaminated. Catheterization of a ureterostomy stoma is generally done by the physician unless nurses have been instructed in the procedure.

□ Outcome criteria for the person with a urinary stoma

The patient or significant others can:

1. Explain rationale for urinary diversion and describe anatomic variation created by diversion.
2. Describe any necessary activity restrictions and duration of limits (avoidance of heavy lifting).
3. Recognize normal stomal and peristomal skin conditions, and state changes requiring medical assistance:
   a. Keep stoma pink, moist, patent, clean, and free of infection.
   b. Keep peristoma skin intact and free of infection.
4. Describe potential for return to preoperative sexual performance and fertility.
5. Demonstrate care of appliance:
   a. Change and empty appliance.
   b. State how often to empty and change appliance.
   c. Describe principles of care of appliance including cleaning and maintenance.
   d. Describe types of appliances available and where to seek help in selecting appropriate appliances.
   e. State where and how to order appropriate appliances and supplies.
   f. Describe how to measure stoma for optimal appliance fit.
6. State plans for follow-up care and continued urologic surveillance.

■ MANAGEMENT OF THE INCONTINENT PERSON

Urinary or fecal incontinence, the involuntary expulsion of urine or feces, may be encountered in a number of temporary and permanent conditions in a variety of settings. Inability to control elimination is a problem that frequently leads to emotional distress and can seriously

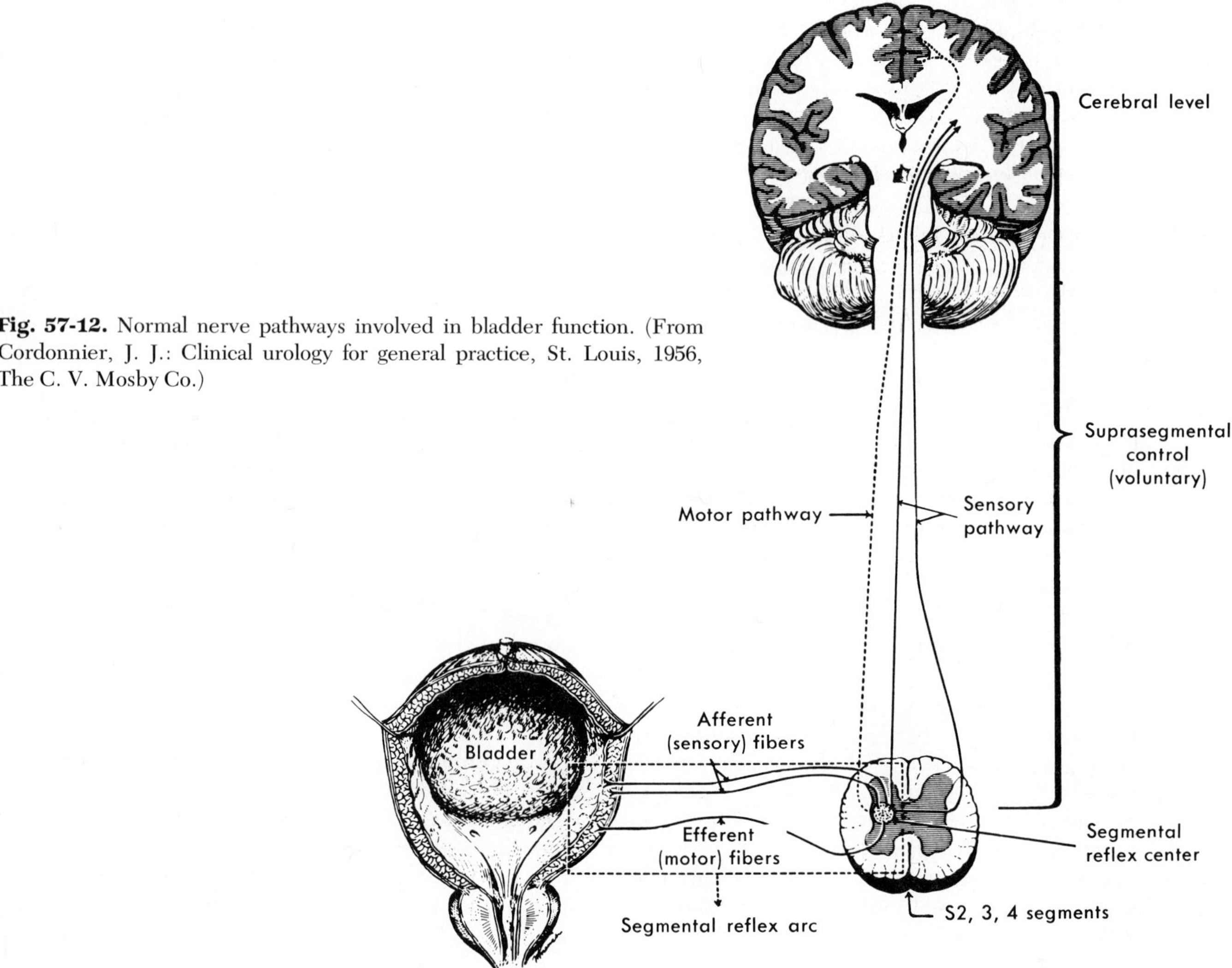

Fig. 57-12. Normal nerve pathways involved in bladder function. (From Cordonnier, J. J.: Clinical urology for general practice, St. Louis, 1956, The C. V. Mosby Co.)

impair an individual's socialization patterns if not managed in a suitable manner. Persons may feel that incontinence is dirty, disgraceful, and childlike. Whether temporary or permanent, incontinence must be managed either by the person or by others in a way that makes the person feel physically and emotionally comfortable and socially acceptable.

Persons with incontinence often present baffling management problems. Solutions require that the nurse understand the physiologic basis of incontinence.

□ Urinary incontinence

Bladder sphincter control is necessary to have urinary continence. Such control requires normal voluntary and involuntary muscle action coordinated by a normal urethrobladder reflex. Understanding this coordinated sequence of nerve stimuli and muscle action will help the nurse understand how continence is maintained.

As bladder filling occurs, the pressure within the bladder gradually increases. The detrusor muscle (the three-layered bladder wall) responds by relaxing to accommodate the greater volume. When a certain point of filling is reached, usually 150 to 200 ml of urine, the parasympathetic stretch receptors located in the bladder wall are stimulated. The stimuli are transmitted through the afferent fibers of the reflex arc to the reflex center for micturition. This reflex center is located in the S2 to S4 segments of the spinal cord (Fig. 57-12). Impulses are then carried through the efferent fibers of the reflex arc to the bladder, causing reflex contraction of the detrusor muscle. The internal sphincter, which is normally closed, reciprocally opens and the urine enters the posterior urethra. Relaxation of the external sphincter and perineal muscles follows, and the bladder content is released. Completion of this reflex act can be interrupted and voiding postponed through release of inhibitory impulses from the cortical center, which results in voluntary contraction of the external sphincter. If any part of this complex function is upset, there is apt to be incontinence of urine.

Etiology

The five major causes of urinary incontinence and the nature of the incontinence they cause are outlined in Table 57-3.

Cerebral clouding is most common in the aged. In many instances the very elderly person is incontinent because of a lack of awareness of the need to empty the bladder. This type of incontinence is often not associated with any definite pathology at the cerebral level. Cere-

Table 57-3. Major causes of urinary incontinence

	Factors involved				
Cause of urinary incontinence	**Awareness of need to void**	**Cortical ability to inhibit voiding**	**Reflex arc**	**Bladder response to filling**	**Result**
Cerebral clouding	Impaired	Impaired	Intact	Normal	Uncontrolled voiding due to reflex response
Infection	Intact	Intact, but overcome by strong reflex response	Abnormally stimulated	Heightened	Voiding due to strong reflex response (urgency)
Disturbance of CNS pathways (cortical lesions)	Diminished	Impaired	Intact	Heightened	Voiding due to reflex response
Disturbance of urethrobladder reflex					
Upper motor neuron lesion	Destroyed	Destroyed	Intact but deranged	Heightened	Voiding due to reflex response
Lower motor neuron lesion	Destroyed	Destroyed	Destroyed or impaired	Diminished to absent	Distension or incomplete emptying
Tissue damage	Intact	Intact, but not functional due to poor muscle response	Intact	Normal	Loss of control of voiding due to muscular impairment

bral clouding also occurs in acutely ill persons, who may be so ill that cerebration is dulled. They may not be able to think, or may not have the energy to exercise voluntary control. Likewise a person who is comatose is incontinent because of loss of the ability to control voluntarily the opening of the external sphincter. As soon as urine is released into the posterior urethra, the bladder contracts and empties. This is the reason why voiding sometimes occurs under anesthesia.

Infection anywhere in the urinary tract may lead to incontinence, since bacteria in the urine cause irritation of the mucosa of the bladder and stimulate the urethrobladder reflex abnormally.

Disturbance of the central nervous system pathways may occur in diseases such as cerebral embolus, cerebral hemorrhage, brain tumor, meningitis, or traumatic injury of the brain. Adequate voluntary (cortical or cerebral) control of bladder function is prevented in these situations. Urgency incontinence may be present as a result of the inability to inhibit completion of the urethrobladder reflex by the higher centers.

Disturbance of the urethrobladder reflex may result from lesions of the spinal cord or damage to peripheral nerves of the bladder. This form of incontinence may be seen in persons with spinal cord malformations, injuries, or tumors, and those with compression of the cord caused by fractures of the vertebrae, herniated disc, metastatic tumor, or postoperative edema of the spinal cord. This type of difficulty can result in two types of responses known as "neurogenic bladder." The person with a neurogenic bladder has no way of knowing when voiding is occurring.

Lesions above the S2 level of the spinal cord or impairment of the cerebrocortical centers do not destroy the reflex arc for voiding, although they may derange it. Such lesions destroy the potential for cortical control to inhibit the reflex. The result is an "upper motor neuron" or "automatic" bladder. The bladder is hypertonic and has a small capacity (less than 150 ml). The increased detrusor tone and increased sensitivity to small amounts of urine present in the bladder result in precipitous voiding and the potential for vesicoureteral reflux.

Damage to nerves in the cauda equina or sacral segments of the spinal cord may cause destruction of the reflex arc by interruption of its afferent, efferent, or central components. The result is a "lower motor neuron" or "flaccid" bladder. The bladder is hypotonic with capacities of 500 ml or more. Overflow incontinence, retention of residual urine, and the potential for vesicoureteral reflux are problems imposed by a hypotonic bladder.

Overflow incontinence is considered to be caused by pressure exerted on the distended bladder by the abdominal muscles. Residual urine, urine remaining in the bladder after incomplete emptying, provides a medium for the growth of bacteria, and urinary tract infections are common.

Tissue damage to the sphincters of the bladder from instrumentation, surgery, or accidents, scarring following urethral infections, lesions involving the sphincter, or relaxation of the perineal structures may cause urinary incontinence. The latter cause of incontinence is seen occasionally following childbirth. The problem is local in nature and does not involve the nervous system.

Assessment

Until the cause of a patient's urinary incontinence is understood, the question of whether rehabilitation of the bladder is possible cannot be answered. The nurse's role in the assessment includes accurate recording of intake and output, amount and frequency of voiding, symptoms of urgency, indications of the state of awareness of the need to void, and the appearance of the urine. In the assessment the nurse must also include general data concerning the person's condition, ability to follow directions, and any other factors that may predispose to or directly cause urinary incontinence.

After all available data concerning incontinence have been collected and a reasonable cause for the incontinence determined, a program of appropriate management may be instituted. If the incontinence has been a long-standing problem well managed by the person or the family, continuation of usual methods of management is facilitated. In these instances, particularly in a hospital or other institutional setting, the nurse should ascertain the method used by the person and provide whatever equipment or assistance is needed during the stay. Although the person may be managing well, additional suggestions may be offered by the nurse concerning newer equipment available, less costly equipment, and so on as appropriate. The patient may wish to try alternative methods even after discharge from the setting.

No program of bladder retraining or management of uncontrolled incontinence is likely to be successful without the cooperation of the individual involved. The probable outcomes of the management program should be included in planning for implementation of the program.

Control of urinary incontinence is largely dependent upon its cause. Measures include treatment of associated conditions, programs of bladder retraining, surgical procedures, or the use of internal or external drainage devices. Both the person and nurse need to know that rehabilitation may take weeks or months to accomplish. The person often becomes dicouraged by recurring accidental voiding and needs a great deal of encouragement. It is often helpful to teach the physiology of voiding so that there is better understanding of the problem. Consistency in carrying out any plan for bladder control is often the key to success.

Interventions related to cause

Sphincter dysfunction. Repair of a sphincter that has been cut is almost impossible. When the *external* sphincter has been damaged, the person will be incontinent on urgency. A voiding schedule can be planned so that voiding occurs before the bladder is full enough to exert sufficient pressure to open the internal sphincter involuntarily. When the *internal* sphincter is damaged, there may be no acute feeling of the need to void. Here the problem is not one of incontinence but of retention. To assure regular emptying of the bladder, a regular voiding schedule is necessary. If both sphincters are damaged, there will be total incontinence.

Stress incontinence. Urinary incontinence that occurs during coughing, straining, or heavy lifting is termed stress incontinence. It is seen primarily in women who have relaxed pelvic musculature, but it may also occur in men following prostatectomy. When bladder pressure is suddenly increased, urine enters the proximal third of the urethra then returns to the bladder when the pressure is decreased after exertion. Some of the urine escapes through the ureter. The person is continent at night because bladder pressure is decreased in the recumbent position. A woman who has a cystocele (p. 1423) may not be aware of the problem until after the cystocele is repaired.[28]

Perineal exercises are helpful in controlling mild stress incontinence. The exercises consist in tightening and relaxing perineal and gluteal muscles and can be performed in a number of ways. Much of the problem of incontinence cause by a relaxed perineum in women can be prevented if perineal exercises are taught before and following childbirth. These exercises also may be included as part of the health teaching of any woman. Following are different methods for performing perineal exercises:

1. Tighten the perineal muscles as if to prevent voiding. Hold for 3 seconds, then relax.
2. Inhale through pursed lips while tightening perineal muscles.
3. Bear down as if to have a bowel movement. Relax then tighten perineal muscles.
4. Hold a pencil in the fold between the buttock and thigh.
5. Sit on the toilet with knees held wide apart. Start and stop the urinary stream.

Surgery may be indicated for severe stress incontinence. A *vesicourethropexy* (Marshall-Marchetti operation) consists of fixation of the urethra to the fascia of the rectus muscle of the abdomen with support given to the neck of the bladder. A suprapubic incision is usually made, but a transvaginal repair may be carried out if there is scar tissue around the urethra from vaginal surgery. A urethral catheter is inserted postoperatively and maintained for 4 to 5 days. The urine may be pink, but the urethral catheter is not irrigated as a rule. It is not uncommon for difficulty in voiding to be experienced immediately after the indwelling catheter is removed. The woman is observed for signs of vaginal bleeding. Straining and use of the Valsalva maneuver should be avoided until healing has occurred, and mild laxatives may be given to prevent straining from constipation. Surgeons differ in the amount of activity permitted in the early postoperative period.

Urgency. Incontinence caused by urinary tract infection is generally temporary, responding to treatment of the infection by systemic antibiotics. Specific causes of infection such as obstruction must be identified and corrected where possible. Provision must be made for adequate fluid intake of 3,000 ml or more per day unless contraindicated by the person's medical condition. Because of heightened bladder sensitivity to even small amounts of urine, urgency to void demands rapid response by the nurse to the request for help to void. Persons who are aware of the need to void, but who experience urgency, become irritable and embarrassed if their calls for assistance are not answered quickly enough to prevent incontinence.

The person who has a brain tumor, meningitis, or traumatic injury to the brain that prevents adequate voluntary control of bladder function and causes urgency incontinence by inhibiting cortical control over the urethrobladder reflex may also respond to a bladder retraining program. If the person's condition or response prohibits such a program, an internal or external drainage device may be used.

Neurogenic dysfunction. Persons with injuries of the spinal cord experience a transitory period of "spinal shock" in which urinary retention occurs. This is treated with continuous or intermittent catheter drainage that aims to prevent urinary tract infection and overdistention of the bladder. Following this acute stage, further management depends upon the exact nature of any residual neurogenic bladder dysfunction. Persons with a lesion above the sacral segments and who have an intact urethrobladder reflex may initiate voiding by pinching or stroking trigger areas of the thighs or suprapubic area. In a hypotonic bladder, the use of the Credé method, which consists of exerting manual pressure over the bladder, may be ordered to provide for more complete bladder emptying. The appropriateness of this technique must be determined by the physician based upon the person's complete urologic status. An increasing number of persons with neurogenic bladder dysfunction are being taught intermittent self-catheterization using clean technique to prevent infection and manage incontinence (p. 1262). Maintenance of a regular schedule is stressed, and the frequency is determined on an individual basis.

Certain medications are sometimes utilized alone or in conjunction with an intermittent catheterization program in the management of incontinence related to neurogenic bladder dysfunction. Alpha adrenergic drugs such as ephedrine sulfate are used to increase urethral resistance. Anticholinergic drugs such as propantheline (Pro-Banthine) are prescribed to control the reflex bladder activity.

General interventions

Bladder retraining. When incontinence is caused by dulled cerebration in the elderly, confusion, or acute illness, control can usually be established if a persistent retraining schedule is carried out. A voiding schedule is developed and strictly adhered to until the person gradually relearns to recognize and react appropriately to the feeling of having to void. A successful program of this type, leading to complete rehabilitation, or continence, requires mental competence of the individual. Otherwise someone else must always remind the person to follow the schedule.

People ordinarily void on awakening, before retiring, and before or after meals. If a diuretic such as coffee has been taken it is usually necessary to void about 30 minutes later. Using this knowledge, the nurse can begin to set up a schedule for placing the person on a bedpan or taking the person to the toilet. Then, if a record is kept for a few days of the times the person voids involuntarily, it is usually possible to determine the normal voiding pattern. If the schedule based on the pattern of incontinence is not successful, toileting every 1 to 2 hours should be carried out on a 24-hour basis.

During the retraining program, *mobilization* of the individual, attention to the *position* assumed for voiding, and adequate *fluid* intake contribute to reduction of the possiblity of infection. Complete emptying of the bladder eliminates the possibility of residual urine acting as a medium for bacterial growth, while a high fluid intake provides for internal bladder irrigation.

Elderly persons isolated from their families and familiar surroundings, confused by institutionalization, or suffering feelings of loss of self-esteem frequently respond well to mobilization in bladder retraining programs. Their circulation is enhanced by the imposed mobility, their awareness is increased, and they respond to the attention given them. In instances where nurses believe that it is easier to change bed linen than it is to establish an appropriate bladder retraining program, a disservice is done to the individual and more work is actually created for the nurse. The person becomes subject to urinary tract infection and skin breakdown, and feelings of worthlessness are increased. For those who can be continent, incontinence is an indignity.

When it is possible, toileting should be carried out in surroundings that will remind the person of the voiding function; that is, the person should be taken to the bathroom where the toilet can be used. If this is not possible, a bedside commode can be an adequate substitute. Many men can void into a urinal more easily if allowed to stand at the bedside. The use of a bedpan is unfamiliar and distasteful to most persons, but in instances where women must remain in bed, voiding into a bedpan can be facilitated if the head of the bed is rolled up as high as allowed. This kind of positioning is more consistent with the position normally assumed for voiding and facilitates complete emptying of the bladder. Few persons can void adequately in the supine position.

Providing adequate amounts of fluids, a minimum of 3,000 ml per day, is necessary to ensure that there will be adequate amounts of urine produced and present in the bladder to stimulate the voiding reflex at the proper times. Fluids may be given at scheduled times, the largest portion being given during the day before 4:00 PM to decrease the frequency of voiding through the night. Persons on fluid restriction because of medical problems should, of course, receive no more fluids than the amount prescribed.

External urinary drainage. Occasionally there are justifications for the use of an indwelling catheter for the incontinent patient. Such reasons include the need to protect a surgical incision or to permit healing of a decubitus ulcer in the area. Indwelling catheterization, however, presents many potential dangers such as urinary tract infection, urethritis, epididymitis, and urethral fistulas. All other means to manage the incontinence should be tried before resorting to catheterization. (Refer to p. 1255 for details of catheter management.)

For the man, external drainage can be easily accomplished by applying a watertight apparatus to the penis. The following is a satisfactory method. Select a condom of the correct size. Puncture a hole in the closed end of the condom with an applicator stick. Attach the punctured end of the condom to a firm rubber or plastic drainage tube with either a 3 mm (1/8 inch) piece of rubber tubing or a strip of adhesive tape (Fig. 57-13). Before applying the condom, clean and dry the penis thoroughly and check it for edema, skin breaks, or discoloration. Invert the condom and roll it onto the penis. There should be no roll at the top that could cause constriction. At least 2.5 cm (1 inch) of the condom should remain between the meatus and drainage tube to allow for penile erection. There should not be so much slack as to cause twisting and subsequent interference with drainage. Elastoplast is then applied over the condom

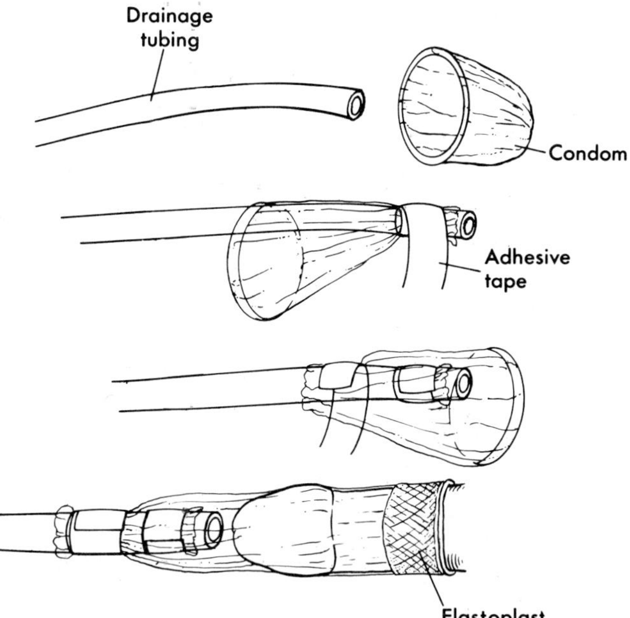

Fig. 57-13. One method of making an external drainage apparatus.

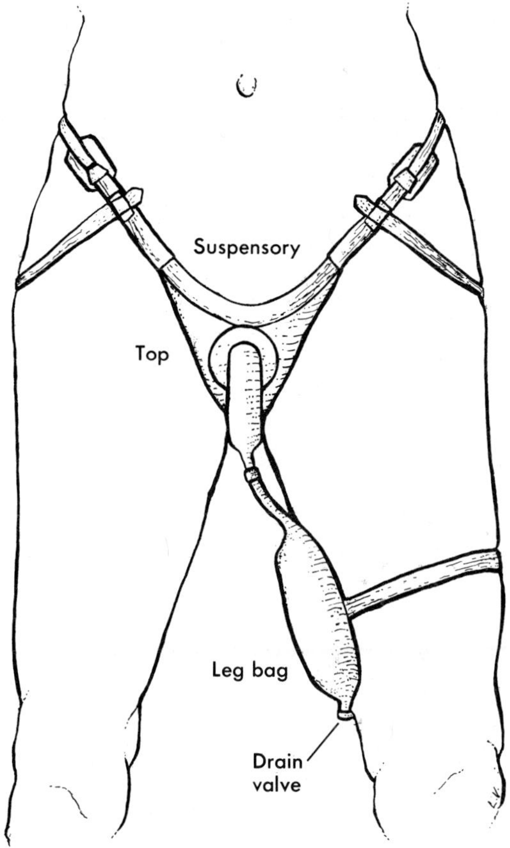

Fig. 57-14. Rubber urinary appliance. Note that it is supported by strap around waist and under buttock and is connected to drainage bag strapped to leg. Drain valve at bottom of bag is removed for emptying.

and around the penis (never touching the skin). *Under no circumstances should adhesive tape be used.* The Elastoplast must not be constricting.

External catheters are also available commercially. Many of these, however, are manufacured of a stiff material that cannot be made to conform to the penis as well as the catheters that are made from condoms.

The external catheter must be removed daily and the skin washed and checked. Frequent checking is necessary to determine whether edema or irritation is present and to ensure proper drainage. This is especially important in men with loss of sensation. The external device is attached to straight drainage or to a leg bag. Some men may be embarrassed to have a female nurse apply an external drainage apparatus. If a man is particularly anxious, it may be advisable to have a male nurse apply this device. Female nurses can provide this aspect of a man's care in a professional manner with respect for his feelings.

For persons who need external catheter drainage indefinitely, a rubber urinary appliance (sometimes called an incontinence urinal) may be used (Fig. 57-14). There are several models available, and the one best suited to the person's needs is selected. The appliance may cause skin irritation, however, since the rubber sheath fits snugly. Two appliances are required to allow for cleaning and drying. They must be washed in mild soap, turned inside out, and thoroughly dried before application.

Most persons prefer to manage their own incontinence if they are at all able to do so. The nurse supports and encourages this, offering assistance as necessary and instruction in basic principles of skin care, equipment selection, and maintenance. The choice of management method should take into account the person's ability to manage as independently as is possible.

Artificial sphincter. A relatively new surgical procedure, implantation of an artificial urinary sphincter, can be utilized to achieve continence when other methods have failed. In this procedure a hydraulically activated sphincter mechanism is placed around the urethra or bladder neck. The sphincter is made to open and close at will by squeezing one of two bulbs implanted under the skin of the labia or scrotum (Fig. 57-15). Postoperative nursing care of the person with such an implant includes observation for and reporting of fever or pain on inflation of the device, swelling of the genitalia, and recurrence of incontinence. Complications of the procedure include erosion of the urethra, abscess, cellulitis, and mechanical malfunctions in the system.

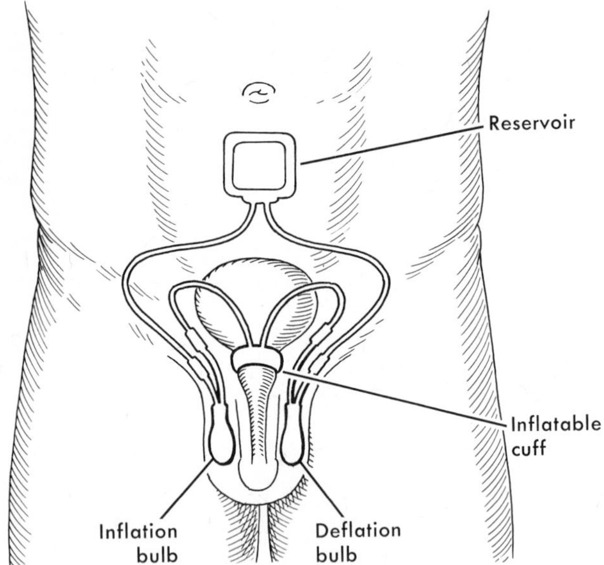

Fig. 57-15. Artificial bladder sphincter. Compression and release of inflation pump bulb inflates cuff surrounding urethra stopping urine flow. Compression and release of deflation pump bulb deflates inflatable cuff, returning fluid to storage reservoir. This releases urethral constriction, permitting urine to flow.

□ Fecal incontinence

As with urinary incontinence, the problem of fecal incontinence may be better understood if there is first an understanding of fecal continence. Normally the contents of the bowel are moved by mass movements to the rectum. The rectum then stores this material until defecation occurs. Defecation may occur reflexly because of distention of the rectal musculature, or it may be inhibited voluntarily. Voluntary emptying of the rectum occurs when the anal sphincter (under voluntary control) is relaxed and the abdominal and pelvic muscles contract.

Fecal continence is not so subject to neurologic impairment as is urinary continence. The musculature of the bowel contains its own nerve centers within the wall of the intestine and is not greatly affected by upper or lower motor neuron lesions. Peristalsis persists or can be stimulated even when there is somatic paralysis.

Fecal incontinence is as disturbing as urinary incontinence. It is, however, more readily managed.

Etiology

There are several causes of fecal incontinence. The anal sphincter may be relaxed, the voluntary control of defecation may be interrupted in the central nervous system, or messages may not be transmitted to the brain because of a lesion within the cord or external pressure on the cord. The disorders causing breakdown of conscious control are identical to those affecting the bladder. Perineal relaxation and actual damage of the anal sphincter are often caused by injury during childbirth or during perineal operations. Relaxation usually increases with the general loss of muscle tone in aging. Perineal exercises similar to those used in urinary incontinence may help some patients.

Assessment

Records are kept concerning the normal bowel habits, the frequency of defecations, the nature of the stool, the awareness of the need to defecate, the degree of sphincter control, and the ability to produce intraabdominal pressure to aid in expelling the feces. The person's general condition is also considered, as is willingness of the person and the significant others to be involved in a bowel control program. In establishing a bowel control program the nurse must bear in mind that feces may be expelled from the rectum by peristalsis so long as the stool is kept soft.

Intervention

If fecal incontinence is to be prevented, bowel training or a regular routine of stimulation of peristalsis and of going to the toilet should be carried out. Ordinarily the bowel is trained to empty at regular intervals. Once a day or every other day after breakfast is common. Food and fluids increase peristalsis, which may stimulate defecation. The taking of certain food or fluids may be associated with the accustomed time for defecation. For example, coffee or orange juice may provide the stimulus for some people. Most persons will be more relaxed and thus more likely to have a bowel movement if placed in as near the normal position as possible and if they have privacy. Glycerin suppositories (usually two are needed) help stimulate evacuation of the bowel; they should be inserted about 2 hours before the usual time of defecation. They are lubricated with petrolatum and pushed well into the rectum against the mucosa with a gloved finger. If the person is unconscious or has disease of the spinal cord, it may be necessary to use the laxative suppository bisacodyl (Dulcolax). Suppositories are most effective if given following a meal because the gastrocolic reflex will provide additional stimulus.

Results from bisacodyl usually occur within a half hour. Care must be taken not to insert the suppository into a bolus of stool, since it is then ineffective.

Routine enemas and laxatives are to be avoided because they cause dependence, decrease the normal production of mucus, increase the possibility of trauma or perforation, and become less effective with prolonged use. At times, enemas may be necessary for the person with spinal cord injury; if so, no more than 500 ml of a

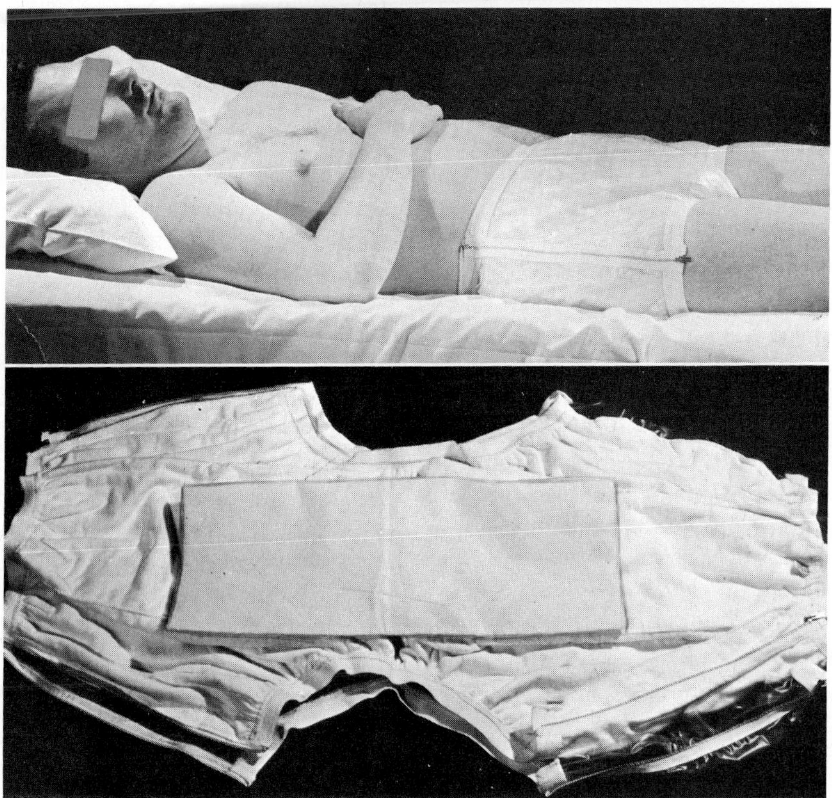

Fig. 57-16. Protective pants for incontinent patient. Protective pads may be disposable or washable. Cotton jersey liner must be worn under plastic pants to prevent excoriation of skin, which must have special care. (Courtesy Ferguson Manufacturing Co., Grand Rapids, Mich.)

nonirritating fluid is sufficient. Lying on the left side assists in retaining fluid. It may be necessary to pinch the buttocks together securely around the rectal tube to retain the fluid in the bowel. An indwelling catheter with a balloon may be used to prevent the fluid from being expelled until a sufficient amount has been instilled.

It is possible for persons with cord lesions to develop *automatic* defecation. Suppositories are given every day at the same time. If these person are able to sit up, they should sit on the toilet. In addition to using suppositories, they may have to take stool softeners to keep the stool from becoming hard and causing an impaction. A diet that provides adequate bulk and a minimum of 3,000 ml of fluids daily is a necessary part of the program. Massaging the abdomen toward the sigmoid area and digital rectal stimulation are additional measures that may be necessary to aid in evacuation. In order to have an effective bowel program it must be consistent, and it requires cooperation and diligence on the part of the staff as well as the individual and significant others. It is necessary to keep a daily record to determine whether the program is producing the desired results. If results are obtained within an hour and impaction and incontinence do not occur, the program can be changed to every other day.

When establishing a bowel program, the person and a significant other are included in the planning. They can help determine whether a morning or evening program is best. The individual's previous habits and current and future activities are considered in the planning. The general welfare of the person is benefited so much by automatic defecation that the time and energy expended to accomplish it are well spent. If "accidents" occur during the bowel training program, the person and significant other are reassured that these are temporary and do not indicate that the program is a failure.

Diarrhea, which occurs in incontinent persons, may be a symptom of *fecal impaction*. Impaction is frequently a problem of the elderly. A rectal examination will identify the presence of an impaction in the rectum. The impaction is broken up through digital manipulation as necessary, and then an oil enema followed by a cleansing enema is given. If the leakage continues despite enemas and is liquid in consistency, a rectal tube (28 or 30 Fr) may be inserted into the rectum and anchored in the fold under the buttock with adhesive tape and attached to straight drainage. Fecal impaction may also cause urinary incontinence by creating pressure on the bladder. Such urinary incontinence will cease when the fecal impaction is removed. If the diarrhea is not caused by an impaction, other possible causes will need to be ascertained (p. 1244).

□ Uncontrolled urinary and fecal incontinence

In some instances, none of the above measures are appropriate or successful. Therefore nursing goals of assisting the person to remain clean, free of odor, and free of decubiti may require external urinary protection; the type varies with the sex, functional status, and physical status of the person.

Those who are incapacitated by critical illness or unconsciousness are dependent upon the nursing staff to manage their incontinence by protective pants or external catheter drainage. Others may be capable of some or all of their own management. Men and women may wear protective plastic pants that are lined by disposable or washable absorbent pads (Fig. 57-16). A resourceful person may be able to improvise equipment that is as comfortable and is less costly than commercially prepared pants. Zippers, Velcro, elastic, and a variety of waterproof materials may be used. Bedding and furniture can be protected with waterproof materials such as the squares of absorbent cellucotton backed with light plastic that are commercially available.

Whatever the type of padding, liners, or pants used, frequent changing is required for skin protection and comfort. The perineal and genital areas are thoroughly washed with soap and water and dried well at each changing. If possible, the person should be bathed in a tub of warm water at least once a day. Periodic exposure of the perineal area to the air is beneficial. Zinc oxide powder can be applied to lessen irritation. Excess amounts of powder are avoided, as this will cake on the skin, causing irritation. Deodorant sprays for use on dressings and liners are valuable. The individual and significant other are cautioned that deodorant sprays may cause skin irritation caused by hypersensitivity. Deodorant room fresheners may be helpful if the odor is strong.

Special bed arrangements are helpful for persons who are confined to bed for long periods of time. A *Bradford frame* with an opening under which a pan or urinal can be placed is helpful for a person who is incontinent. A similar arrangement can be improvised by building the bed up with padding so that there is a depressed area in which a receptacle for drainage can be placed. This arrangement should be made so that the receptacle does not come in contact with the patient's skin. Sometimes, if the problem is expected to go on for years, a circular hole can be cut in the mattress, the edges padded, and a funnel and collection bottle placed beneath the opening. A *Stryker frame, Foster bed,* or *CircOlectric bed* also can be modified to accommodate the incontinent person.

If the person can be up, his favorite chair can be equipped with a commode seat. Special commode wheelchairs are also available, making it possible for the person to be more comfortable and to mingle socially with others.

□ Outcome criteria for the incontinent patient

1. The patient is free of perineal skin excoriation.
2. The patient is free of urinary odor.
3. The patient or significant others can:
   a. Describe the relationship of adequate hygiene to the maintenance of skin integrity.
   b. Describe the relationship of adequate food and fluid intake to facilitate bladder and bowel training.
   c. Describe a bowel/bladder training plan.
   d. Describe how to care for minor skin problems if they occur.
   e. State how to obtain professional and community resources:
      (1) Agencies that are available when necessary.
      (2) How to obtain and maintain any needed supplies and equipment (drainage systems, commodes, protective padding, special beds).
      (3) Where and when to seek assistance if problems are encountered.
   f. State plans for follow-up care.

REFERENCES AND SELECTED READINGS

1. American Cancer Society, Inc.: Colostomy, ileostomy and ureterostomy care: a guide of practical information for nurses, New York, 1971, The Society.
2. Anderson, H. C.: Newton's geriatric nursing, ed. 5, St. Louis, 1971, The C. V. Mosby Co.
3. *Beaumont, E.: Urinary drainage system, Nurs. 74 **4**:52-60, Jan. 1974.
4. Birum, L., and Zimmerman, D.: Catheter plugs as a source of infection, Am. J. Nurs. **71**:2150-2152, 1971.
5. *Champion, V: Clean technique for intermittent self-catheterization, Nurs. Res. **25**:13-18, 1976.
6. *Chezem, J.: Urinary diversion: select aspects of nursing management. Nurs. Clin. North Am. **11**:445-456, 1976.
7. *Cleland, V., Cox, F., Berggren, H., et al.: Prevention of bacteruria in female patients with indwelling catheters, Nurs. Res. **20**:309-318, 1971.
8. *De Groot, J.: Catheter-induced urinary tract infections: how can we prevent them? Nurs. 76 **6**:34-37, March 1976.
9. De Groot, J., and Kunin, C.: Indwelling catheters, Am. J. Nurs. **75**:448-449, 1975.
10. Dericks, V.: The psychological hurdles of new ostomates: helping them up and over, Nurs. 74 **4**:52-55, Oct. 1974.

*References preceded by an asterisk are particularly well suited for student reading.

11. Diokno, A., and Taub, M.: Experience with the artificial urinary sphincter at Michigan, J. Urol. **116**:496-500, 1976.
12. *Dlin, B., Pulman, A., and Rhinegold, E.: Psychosexual responses to ileostomy and colostomy, Am. Oper. Rm. Nurs. J. **69**:77-84, Nov. 1969.
13. *Dobbins, J., and Aliet, C.: Experience with the lateral position for catheterization, Nurs. Clin. North Am. **6**:373-379, 1971.
14. Donovan, C., and Lenneberg, E.: Guidelines for the rehabilitation of ostomy patients, Glenville, Ill., 1975, International Association of Enterostomal Therapy, Inc.
15. Gallagher, A. M.: Body image changes in the patient with a colostomy, Nurs. Clin. North Am. **7**:669-676, 1972.
16. *Garner, J.: Urinary catheter care, Nurs. 74 **4**:54-56, Feb. 1974.
17. Gibbs, G. E., and White, M.: Stomal care, Am. J. Nurs. **72**:268-271, 1972.
18. Grant, M., and Kubo, W.: Assessing a patient's hydration status, Am. J. Nurs. **75**:1306-1311, 1975.
19. Gross, P. A., Harkauy, L. M., Barden, G. E., et al.: The fallacy of cultures of the tips of Foley catheters, Surg. Gynecol. Obstet. **139**:597-598, 1974.
20. Gutowski, F.: Ostomy procedure: nursing care before and after, Am. J. Nurs. **72**:262-267, 1972.
21. Harrower, H. W.: Management of colostomy, ileostomy and ileal conduit, Surg. Clin. North Am. **48**:941-953, 1968.
22. Holliday, J.: Bowel programs of patients with spinal cord injury: a clinical study, Nurs. Res. **67**:4-15, 1967.
23. *Jensen, V.: Better techniques for bagging stomas. Pt. I. Urinary ostomies, Nurs. 74 **4**:60-64, July 1974.
24. Katona, E. A.: Learning colostomy control, Am. J. Nurs. **67**:534-541, 1967.
25. Keuhnelian, J., and Sanders, V.: Urologic nursing, New York, 1970, Macmillan Publishing Co., Inc.
26. *Kunin, C.: Detection, prevention and management of urinary tract infections, ed. 2, Philadelphia, 1974, Lea & Febiger.
27. Langford, T.: Nursing problem: bacteruria and indwelling catheter, Am. J. Nurs. **72**:113-115, 1972.
28. Lapides, J.: Fundamentals of urology, Philadelphia, 1976, W. B. Saunders Co.
29. Lapides, J, Diokno, A. C., Gould, F. R., et al.: Further observations on self-catheterization, J. Urol. **116**:169-171, 1976.
30. Lapides, J., Diokno, A. C., Silber, S. J., et al.: Clean, intermittent self-catheterization in the treatment of urinary tract disease, Trans. Am. Assoc. Genitourin. Surg. **63**:92-95, 1971.
31. Licht, S., editor: Rehabilitation and medicine, New Haven, Conn., 1968, Elizabeth Licht Publishing Co.
32. *Lyons, A. S., and Brockmeier, M. J.: Mechanical management of the ileostomy stoma, Surg. Clin. North Am. **52**:979-990, 1972.
32a. Mahoney, J. M.: Guide to ostomy care, Boston, 1976, Little, Brown & Co.
33. *Murray, B. S., Elmore, J., and Sawyer, J. R.: The patient has an ileal conduit, Am. J. Nurs. **71**:1560-1565, 1971.
34. Patterson, D., and Schuster, P. A.: Artificial urinary sphincter, Can. Nurs. **4**:27-31, 1975.
35. *Rush, A.: Cancer and the ostomy patient, Nurs. Clin. North Am. **11**:405-415, 1976.
36. Rusk, H. A.: Rehabilitation medicine: a textbook on physical medicine and rehabilitation, ed. 4, St. Louis, 1977, The C. V. Mosby Co.
37. Scott, F. B., Bradley, W. E., and Timm, G. W.: Treatment of urinary incontinence by an implanted urinary sphincter, J. Urol. **112**:75-82, 1974.
38. *Secor, S. M.: Colostomy rehabilitation, Am. J. Nurs. **70**:2400-2401, 1970.
39. *Shapbell, N. J., and Sweigart, J. E.: A urinary device for patients with problem stomas, Nurs. Clin. North Am. **9**:383-386, 1974.
40. *Sill, A. R.: Bulb-syringe technique for colonic stoma irrigation, Am. J. Nurs. **70**:536-537, 1970.
41. Spraggon, E.: Urinary diversion stomas: a guide for patients and nurses, ed. 2, Edinburgh, 1975, Churchill Livingstone.
42. Stamm, W.: Guidelines for prevention of catheter-associated urinary tract infections, Ann. Intern. Med. **82**:386-390, 1975.
43. *United Ostomy Association, Inc.: Sex, courtship, and the single ostomate, Los Angeles, 1973, The Association.
43a. *United Ostomy Association, Inc.: Sex and the male ostomate, Los Angeles, 1973, The Association.
43b. *United Ostomy Association, Inc.: Sex, pregnancy, and the female ostomate, Los Angeles, 1972, The Association.
44. *Vukovich, V., and Grubb, R. D.: Care of the ostomy patient, St. Louis, ed. 2, 1977, The C. V. Mosby Co.
45. *Watson, P. G., Woods, R. Y., Wechsler, N. L., et al.: Comprehensive care of the ileostomy patient, Nurs. Clin. North Am. **11**:427-444, 1976.
46. *Watt, R.: Irrigation—yes or no? Am. J. Nurs. **77**:442-444, 1977.
47. *Watt, R.: Ostomies: why, how and where—an overview, Nurs. Clin. North Am. **11**:393-404, 1976.
48. *Watt, R.: Urinary diversion, Am. J. Nurs. **74**:1806-1811, 1974.
49. *Wentworth, A., and Cox, B.: Nursing management of the patient with a continent ileostomy, Am. J. Nurs. **77**:1424-1428, 1976.
50. Whitehead, S.: Nursing care of the adult urology patient, New York, 1970, Appleton-Century-Crofts.
51. Whyte, J., and Thistle, N.: Male incontinence: the inside story on external collection, Nurs. 76 **6**:66-67, Sept. 1976.
52. Winter, C. C., and Morel, A.: Nursing care of the patients with urologic diseases, ed. 4, St. Louis, 1977, The C. V. Mosby Co.
53. Wyker, A., and Gillenwater, J.: Method of urology, Baltimore, 1975, The Williams & Wilkins Co.
54. Yahle, M.: An ostomy information clinic, Nurs. Clin. North Am. **11**:457-467, 1976.

AUDIOVISUAL RESOURCE

Bowel and bladder retraining, Garden Grove, Calif., 1967, Trainex (filmstrip, cassette, script).

58

Problems of the lower gastrointestinal tract

NANCY DURHAM

Problems that affect the lower gastrointestinal tract present a mosaic of symptoms in the individual. Some of these result in temporary dysfunction and as such may require no specific intervention from health personnel (diarrhea, for example). The symptoms may be ignored by the person through choice or through lack of understanding of their possible significance. Other problems may present no particular symptoms until the disease has become one of extensive alteration in function. Whatever the alteration may be, it will in one way or another alter the normal absorptive function of the gastrointestinal tract and in this way alter nutrition, elimination, and fluid and electrolyte balance.

Prevention of problems of the lower gastrointestinal tract is not always possible as the cause of many of the particular diseases is unknown. Of increasing emphasis in prevention is the ongoing research related to cancer of the colon and rectum. Although the overall incidence rates have changed little over the last few years, there does appear to be an increase in the rate among nonwhite males.

The relationship of diet to carcinoma has been studied in terms of dietary influences on the flora of the gastrointestinal tract and for the effect of diet on bile acids and cholesterol metabolism. The consumption of simple sugars and high amounts of animal protein, fat, and cholesterol may account for an increased incidence of bowel cancer, since the incidence is lower among populations where a vegetarian diet is typical.

Prevention of bowel problems is important not only in relation to mortality but also to work productivity. "Intestinal flu," diarrhea, and recuperation from bowel surgery account for an increasingly higher percentage of work time lost. Intensive health education beginning in childhood should assist in reducing the incidence of some of the more common problems of the lower gastrointestinal tract.

■ BOWEL SURGERY

Surgical intervention in the large or small intestine generally consists of removal of a portion of the bowel (resection) and then joining the remaining ends together (anastomosis) to reestablish bowel continuity. The term "ostomy" is used to refer to an *opening*. Within the intestinal tract this opening is surgically constructed in two distinctly different ways.

In the first method a loop or end of a portion of bowel is joined to another existing organ. For example, a gastrojejunostomy is the joining of the jejunum to a portion of the stomach; an esophagojejunostomy is the joining of the jejunum to the end of the esophagus (see Fig. 54-7). This method maintains continuity of the intestinal tract in a nearly normal manner.

In the second method a loop or end of the bowel is brought out onto the abdominal surface and provides for drainage of intestinal contents directly to the outside of the body through the "stomal" opening. This method interrupts the normal continuity of the intestine but does allow maintenance of function. For example, an ileostomy is an opening into the ileum of the small intestine; a colostomy is an opening into the large intestine (colon).

□ Resection and anastomosis of the bowel

Preoperative care

Preoperative preparation of the person who is to have surgery of the bowel varies in some respects from that of preparation for other abdominal surgery.

Diet. During the preoperative period a low-residue diet is given so that the bowel will contain little or no stool at the time of surgery. Bowel-cleansing methods plus the inability of the bowel to absorb vitamins require the administration of Vitamins K and C. Parenteral fluids and electrolytes are given to replace losses from the bowel preparation, from the restricted food and oral fluid intake, and from the bowel absorptive failure. In the debilitated person intravenous hyperalimentation may be used to administer fluid, electrolytes, and proteins and to prevent negative nitrogen balance in preparation for surgery (p. 362). Twenty-four hours prior to surgery a clear-liquid diet may be given if tolerated. The reasons for the diet restriction as well as for the intravenous fluids are explained to the individual and family.

Prevention of infection. Antibiotics specific for organisms found in the bowel may be administered 3 to 5 days before surgery in an attempt to decrease the bacterial count of bowel contents, which helps to decrease the incidence of postoperative wound infection. Oral antibiotics used to "sterilize" the bowel include succinylsulfathiazole (Sulfasuxidine), phthalylsulfathiazole (Sulfathalidine), and neomycin. These drugs are poorly absorbed from the gastrointestinal tract and thus their concentration in the bloodstream is low. A cathartic such as magnesium sulfate may be given before they are administered, and then the drugs are given in large doses every 4 hours until the operation is performed. A daily cathartic or enemas followed by instillation of phthalylsulfathiazole into the bowel may be prescribed.

Some surgeons do not prescribe oral antibiotics because they do not believe the bowel can be sterilized and because use of antibiotics may cause *pseudomembranous enterocolitis*, an infrequent but serious disease of the colon.

Still others believe intestinal antibiotics are of little value without significant reduction of stool mass. Rigorous purging and diet reduction may be poorly tolerated by the elderly or the acutely ill person. Therefore the general physical state of the individual is carefully assessed as well as the degree of bowel obstruction in order to modify preoperative preparation.

Intubation. A nasogastric or intestinal tube is inserted before the operation. Since the passage of a tube into the intestines may take as long as 24 hours, intestinal intubation is usually started the day before surgery. As the tube passes through the small intestine, the bowel becomes "threaded" on it and thus is compactly held together and shortened while the operation is performed. Before and after surgery, the intestinal tube is usually attached to a suction apparatus for the aspiration of intestinal contents. This prevents the accumulation of gas and intestinal fluid around the suture line. If a nasogastric tube is used, it is inserted the morning the operation is scheduled.

Postoperative care

Extensive handling of the gastrointestinal organs during surgery causes a marked inhibition of peristalsis, either cessation of movement *(paralytic ileus)* or weak ineffectual movements *(adynamic ileus)*. Care during the early postoperative period is therefore directed at preventing the buildup of gas or fluid in the gastrointestinal tract, which can cause excessive fluid and electrolyte disturbances, pressure on the suture line, or inhibition of respiration by elevation of the diaphragm. The length of time required for peristalsis to return depends on the extent of bowel manipulation. Presence of bowel sounds or passage of gas signals the return of function.

Fluid and electrolyte balance. Until peristalsis returns and the anastomosis is partially healed, the nasogastric or intestinal tube is used, and special attention is given to keeping the tube draining and to maintaining fluid and electrolyte balance. The surgeon carefully checks the amount of fluid needed and reviews the daily output from voiding and from gastric drainage. Recording of these fluids must be accurate. Electrolytes lost through the gastric drainage are replaced with the parenteral fluids.

Until the intestinal tube is removed nothing is given by mouth. The patient needs frequent mouth care. If an intestinal tube is used, an antibiotic solution may be ordered for mouth care, since colon bacteria may travel up the tube by capillary action. After the tube is removed, foods are added gradually until a full diet is resumed. Occasionally, bland foods may be ordered for some time following surgery.

Elimination. Because there may be some difficulty in voiding after bowel surgery, all available nursing measures are instituted to prevent urinary retention. If these fail a Foley catheter may be used (p. 1257). Pain in the incision may be severe and may interfere with full respiratory excursion. Narcotics are administered as necessary for pain, and the patient is encouraged to cough and to breathe deeply and to change position every hour to two. Encouragement and assistance are often necessary in doing so during the first day or two postoperatively.

A rectal tube can be inserted to facilitate the passage of flatus. Drugs to stimulate expulsion of flatus such as dexpanthenol (Ilopan) or neostigmine (Prostigmin) may be administered. Since ambulation is of great assistance in starting peristalsis, the patient is assisted out of bed a day or two after surgery, even while the nasogastric or intestinal tube is still in use. The passage of gas or stool rectally should be reported to the surgeon at once, since it usually indicates the return of peristalsis and means that oral intake can be resumed and that the intestinal tube can be removed.

It is not unusual after a resection of the bowel for diarrhea to occur after peristalsis returns. Usually it is temporary and soon disappears. When the stool becomes normal, the patient is advised to avoid becoming constipated because a hard stool and straining to expel it could possibly injure the anastomosis, depending on its location. Persons who have a tendency to develop constipation postoperatively are advised to try drinking fruit juice and water before breakfast or to take a glass of prune juice daily. They should not take laxatives without medical approval. Stool softeners or a mild bulk cathartic such as psyllium (Metamucil) is prescribed frequently.

□ Temporary cecostomy

Although the treatment of choice for growths in the ascending colon is a resection and anastomosis or a transverse colostomy, a temporary cecostomy is occasionally performed to relieve obstruction when major surgery would be too dangerous. With the use of local anesthetic to control pain, an opening is made into the cecum through a small incision in the right lower quadrant of the abdomen, and a catheter is inserted into the bowel. The catheter is sutured to the skin and provides an outlet for feces, which is still fluid in the ascending colon. Tubing is attached to the catheter, which is attached to a container that is capped to control odors but that is provided with an air vent so that drainage can occur. The tubing should be long enough so that persons can move about freely. In order to keep the tube open, it is usually irrigated every 4 hours with a physiologic solution of sodium chloride. The fluid is allowed to run in by gravity and flows out by inverting the syringe or funnel or by aspiration.

The dressings around the tube are changed as frequently as necessary, and the skin is kept clean and dry. After the tube is removed, skin care and changes of dressing are continued until all drainage ceases. Occasionally an ileostomy bag is used to keep drainage off the skin. A water-soluble chlorophyll derivative (Chloresium) may be applied for its soothing, anti-pruritic, and deodorizing effects.

□ Abdominoperineal resection of the bowel

Most malignant growths in the rectum are removed by an operation known as an abdominoperineal resection of the bowel. The operation is performed through two incisions: a low midline incision of the abdomen and a wide circular incision about the anus. Through the abdominal incision the sigmoid colon is divided and the lower portion is freed from its attachments and temporarily left beneath the peritoneum of the pelivc floor. The proximal end of the sigmoid is then brought out through a small stab wound on the abdominal wall and becomes the permanent colostomy. Through the perineal incision the anus and rectum are freed from the perineal muscles, and the anus, the rectum containing the growth, and the distal portion of sigmoid are removed. The perineal wound may be closed around Penrose drains, or it may be left wide open and packed with gauze and a rubber dam to cause it to heal slowly from the inside outward.

Preoperative care

Preoperative nursing care is similar to that for other intestinal surgery. Some surgeons pass ureteral catheters preoperatively so that the ureters are not inadvertently tied off during surgery. A Foley catheter is inserted into the bladder and attached to a straight drainage system to keep the bladder empty during surgery and thus prevent operative injury. In addition to the preoperative teaching about the stoma (p. 1247), the patient will need to know about the perineal incision. This will heal by secondary intention (p. 399) and therefore will take much longer to heal than a usual incision.

Postoperative care

Shock. Postoperative shock is a frequent occurrence because of the large amount of tissue removed at the time of surgery. Measures to monitor and treat shock are therefore instituted (p. 216).

Wound care. In the immediate postoperative period, rectal dressings are watched carefully for signs of excessive bleeding. The usual drainage is serosanguineous and profuse, and the dressing may have to be reinforced during the first few hours postoperatively. Disposable pads are placed under the hips and are changed frequently.

If the perineal wound has been packed, the packing is removed gradually. If a drainage tube or drain has been sutured in the perineal wound, it usually is removed by the second or third postoperative day. After it is removed the wound is usually irrigated once or twice a day to remove secretions and tissue debris, to prevent abcesses from forming in the dead space that may be left, and to help ensure healing of the wound from the inside outward. If a catheter is to be inserted into the wound for the irrigation, the nurse should ascertain from the surgeon how deep it can be inserted and in what direction to insert it. Precise directions as to how to do the irrigation should be recorded on the nursing care plan.

Normal saline solution or diluted hydrogen peroxide is frequently used as the irrigating solution. When the patient is permitted out of bed, sitz baths may be substituted for the irrigations, and as drainage from the wound decreases, a perineal pad may be substituted for the dressing. A rubber ring should be used during the sitz bath so that water can flow freely around the incision. The response in healing is often quite remarkable when this is done. Since the patient is usually ready to leave the hospital before the perineal wound has completely closed, arrangements must be made to continue with the sitz baths at home. If a bathtub is not available, a large basin may be used. Portable sitz baths are available and may be rented from hospital supply firms. They may be more comfortable to use than a regular tub.

After the surgeon has changed the first dressing (usually 24 hours postoperatively), the dressing is changed by the nurse as necessary. Since the dressing requires frequent changing, a T binder is used to hold the dressing in place and to give support without causing skin irritation. Care of the colostomy is described on p. 1250.

Many patients complain of phantom rectal sensations and of feeling the necessity to defecate.[42] An explanation of cortical perception and transmission of nerve impulses often helps the patient cope with these sensations.

Urinary elimination. The Foley catheter usually is left in the bladder postoperatively to prevent the bladder from becoming distended and from pressing against the repaired pelvic floor until it heals. Its use also eliminates the need for women to use the bedpan to void (a very painful procedure after this operation) and prevents contamination of the wound and dressings with urine. After the catheter is removed, the patient may be unable to void or may void inadequately. It may then have to be reinserted for several more days, or the patient may be catheterized at specified intervals as necessary until able to void normally. Occasionally following this operation the male patient requires a prostatectomy for benign prostatic hypertrophy. Antibiotics and large amounts of fluid are given when an indwelling catheter is used. Special care should be taken that the catheter drains constantly so that residual urine does not remain in the bladder.

Pain. A narcotic for pain is usually required at regular intervals for the first 2 to 3 days postoperatively.

Activity. Most patients prefer a side-lying position because of severe discomfort in the supine position. A soft foam pad may relieve pressure on the perineal area when the patient does lie on his back. Frequent turning is encouraged, and considerable assistance may be necessary during the early postoperative period because of the incisional pain. Isometric exercises and quadriceps drills (p. 373) are encouraged. The potential for the development of postoperative thrombophlebitis is very high.

Convalescence after an abdominal perineal resection is prolonged and may require many months. During this time the individual should remain under close supervision.

□ Surgical bypass procedure for massive obesity

In recent decades it has been clearly recognized that obese individuals have a shortened life span.[7] Statistics of insurance companies have shown a substantial increase in mortality from arteriosclerotic cardiovascular disease and cirrhosis of the liver in those who are considered morbidly obese. Massively obese persons have an increased predisposition for diabetes, hypertension, bronchitis, osteoarthritis, and other serious ailments.

Since medical treatment in the form of dietary restriction, medications for appetite control, as well as hypnosis and psychiatric therapy often is unsuccessful, surgical procedures have been tried in an attempt to alleviate the problem of obesity. Various surgical procedures have evolved in an effort to "shunt" or bypass a portion of the small intestine and limit the area available for absorption of fats and carbohydrates. The most recent procedure is the jejunoileal bypass in which approximately 14 inches of the jejunum and 4 inches of the ileum are preserved for the bypass anastomosis.[27] The 14 inches of the proximal jejunum is anastomosed to the side of the ileum 4 inches from the ileocecal valve. The retention of the ileocecal area is an important factor in retarding the intestinal transit time and thus permitting longer contact of the chyme to the intestinal mucosa. The long length of bypassed jejunoileum is anastomosed with the ileal end to the transverse colon or sigmoid colon.

Persons selected for surgery are carefully evaluated physically and mentally. Studies are carried out with special attention being given to the cardiopulmonary and endocrine status as well as the gastrointestinal assessment of the stomach, small bowel, and colon function. Preoperative measurements of serum calcium, potassium, magnesium, and other electrolytes plus assessment of vitamins A, B_{12}, and C and folic acid are made. *Psychologic evaluation* is considered essential by most physicians in determining the individual's response to weight loss and change in body image and acceptance of the close surveillance of metabolic changes that may occur postoperatively.[27] Despite the careful selection, many patients and their significant others experience long-range psychologic problems and difficulties in adjustments of life style.

The majority of the patients have an uneventful recovery. In some, hypokalemia and hypocalcemia may occur and supplementation may be necessary. Malabsorption of the fat-soluble vitamins A, D, E, and K and particularly vitamin B_{12} may cause a deficiency and require replacement therapy. Some may have diarrhea as a result of diminished fat digestion and absorption. They are taught to avoid excessive liquid intake and excessive fat intake as a means of controlling bowel function. Occasionally medication may be necessary to control persistent diarrhea.[33]

Weekly follow-up is essential in the immediate postoperative period, and periodic clinical evaluation in the subsequent years must be impressed on the person. After discharge, rehabilitation and desired loss of weight is achieved by the physician's long-range metabolic and nutritional follow-up[7,10,27]

□ Outcome criteria for the person who has had intestinal surgery

The patient or significant others can:

1. Describe any medication or treatment program to be followed at home:
   a. State dosage, frequency, action, and side effects of medications (antibiotics, stool softeners).
   b. Demonstrate correct technique for cleansing of incisional area (if drainage or stoma is present) and the application of a dressing or appliance.
2. Describe a plan for any dietary modifications needed:
   a. State means of meeting fluid and nutrient requirements.
   b. List specific foods to be avoided if applicable (high roughage).
3. Describe the health maintenance or follow-up program:
   a. Explain the basic pathologic condition and overall treatment program in his own words.
   b. Explain the rationale for avoidance of situations that lead to an increase in intraabdominal pressure (chronic or acute cough, constipation.)
   c. State whom to contact if additional symptoms occur (red, edematous, or draining incision; constipation; signs of systemic infection; abdominal pain).
   d. State plans for regular follow-up care.
   e. State how to obtain any necessary or desired community resources.

■ INFLAMMATION OR INFECTION OF THE INTESTINAL TRACT

The mucous membrane of the intestinal tract responds to the process of inflammation in a manner similar to that of other tissues. The mucosa becomes reddened and edematous, has an increased temperature, is painful to touch, and loses some of its functional ability. As the surface of the mucosal membrane alters, the cells are exposed to an environment that includes lytic enzymes, pathogens, and trauma from food particles. This may cause further cellular damage. If pathogenic microorganisms or parasites are present, infection may occur.

At times pathogens or particles of feces will become lodged within small areas of the mucosa, multiply, and break down resulting in fistulous tracts as seen in diverticulitis. These tracts or passageways may connect from one area of the gastrointestinal tract to another, to another organ, or to the outside of the body.

As the inflammation or infectious process resolves, the mucosal layer heals and muscular damage is replaced with scar tissue. This scarring will often draw the surrounding tissue closer together and shorten the length of the tract. Since scar tissue loses its secretory and absorptive properties, some function is lost, and the tissue is more easily traumatized leading to local areas of bleeding. This scarring and bleeding is seen in *ulcerative colitis* and *Crohn's disease*.

□ Acute inflammations

Appendicitis

Appendicitis is an inflammatory lesion of the vermiform appendix. It is more common among males, and it occurs most frequently between the ages of 10 and 30 years, although it may occur at any age. Although there is no certain cause of the disease, occlusion of the lumen of the appendix by hardened feces (fecaliths), by foreign objects, or by kinking of the appendix may impair the circulation and lower resistance to organisms within the body such as the colon bacilli or the streptococcus organisms. A small part of the appendix may be edematous or necrotic, or the entire appendix may be involved. An abscess may develop in the appendiceal wall or in the surrounding tissue. The serious danger is that the appendix will rupture and cause generalized peritonitis.

Prevention. In the United States there are still some deaths each year from appendicitis. If symptoms had not been neglected or if the individual had not been given a cathartic, some of these deaths might have been prevented. It is important therefore that the nurse continue to help teach the public that symptoms of right lower quadrant or periumbilical pain accompanied by loss of appetite, elevation of temperature, and possibly nausea, vomiting, and diarrhea should be reported to a physician. Persons with these symptoms should not be treated at home by local heat, enemas, or cathartics.

Clinical picture. The typical symptoms of acute appendicitis are pain about the umbilicus and throughout the abdomen (which may soon become localized at a point known as *McBurney's point* exactly halfway between the umbilicus and the crest of the right ilium) and nausea, anorexia, and vomiting. Light palpation of the abdomen will elicit pain in the right lower quadrant. Rebound tenderness is a common finding. The abdominal musculature overlying the area may feel tense due to voluntary rigidity. Rigidity noted over the entire abdomen is generally an indication of rupture of the appendix with resultant peritonitis. The person will often be noted to be lying on his side or on his back with his knees flexed in an attempt to decrease muscular strain on the abdominal wall.

Acute appendicitis is remarkable for the suddenness of its onset. The person may have felt quite well an hour or two before the onset of severe pain. Approximately 90% of these persons will have a white cell count above 10,000/cu mm, and approximately three fourths will have a neutrophil count above 75%. The temperature usually is irregularly elevated about 2° to 4° above normal and is accompanied by an increase in pulse.

These symptoms are present in about 60% of those with acute appendicitis.[31]

There will be an area of hyperesthetic skin over the inflamed appendix prior to perforation. The nurse may elicit this response by stroking the skin surface over the right lower quadrant with the point of a pin or by lightly grasping the skin over the right lower quadrant between the thumb and forefinger and gently pulling the fold upward. Both measures will elicit a verbal or facial pain response.

Other persons have less well-defined local symptoms because of the location of the appendix. It may be retrocecal, or it may lie adjacent to the ureter. If the symptoms are questionable urinalysis and an intravenous pyelogram may be performed to rule out acute pyelitis or a ureteral stone. Many other diseases produce symptoms similar to appendicitis, and they sometimes need to be ruled out before a positive diagnosis can be made. Some of these are acute salpingitis, regional ileitis, mesenteric lymphadenitis, and biliary colic.

The older person with acute appendicitis may experience only dull pain. Children who develop appendicitis may have only slight abdominal pain, although usually they vomit. Because the abdominal omentum is not well developed in children, if the appendix perforates, peritonitis can develop easily because the infection cannot be walled off so quickly. It is recommended therefore that the ill child who refuses food and who vomits be taken to a physician for diagnosis and treatment. A cathartic should *never* be given for these complaints.

Intervention. When appendicitis is suspected, the person usually is hospitalized at once and placed on bed rest for observation and the necessary diagnostic procedures that must be performed. Since an operation may be performed shortly after admission nothing is given by mouth while reports of the blood count are awaited. Sometimes a nasogastric tube is passed and attached to suction. Parenteral fluids may be given during this time. Narcotics are not given until the cause of the pain has been determined, since they would mask signs or symptoms. An ice bag to the abdomen may be ordered to help relieve pain. A rectal examination combined with abdominal palpation will confirm the diagnosis by specifying the exact location of the pain over McBurney's point as well as pain experienced by the digital examination.

An appendectomy is usually scheduled as an emergency operation. A general or regional anesthetic is used, and the appendix is removed through a small incision over McBurney's point or through a right paramedial incision. The incision usually heals with no drainage. Drains are used when an abscess is discovered, when the appendix has ruptured and peritonitis has developed, and sometimes when the appendix was edematous and ready to rupture and was surrounded by clear fluid.

Bowel function is usually normal soon after surgery. Nausea and vomiting disappear with surgical treatment, and the patient is permitted food as tolerated. Convalescence is usually short.

Peritonitis

Peritonitis is an inflammatory involvement of the peritoneum caused by trauma or by rupture of an organ containing bacteria, which are then introduced into the abdominal cavity. Some of the organisms found are *Escherichia coli*, streptococci (both aerobic and anaerobic), staphylococci, pneumococci, and gonococci. Peritonitis also can be caused by chemical response to irritating substances such as might occur following rupture of the fallopian tube in an ectopic pregnancy, perforation of a gastric ulcer, or traumatic rupture of the spleen or liver. Inflammation due to chemical causes, however, is so closely followed by invasion of blood-borne bacteria that it is only a few hours before organisms may be isolated from most fluids that accumulate in peritonitis.

Natural barriers are used in the body's attempt to control the inflammation. Adhesions quickly form in an attempt to wall off the infection, and the omentum helps to enclose areas of inflammation. These processes may result in involvement of only part of the abdominal cavity and may finally narrow the infected area to a small, enclosed one (abscess). As healing occurs, fibrous adhesions may shrink and disappear entirely so that no trace of infection can be found on surgical exploration of the abdomen at a much later date, or they may persist as constrictions that may permanently bind the involved structures together. Sometimes they cause an intestinal obstruction by occluding the lumen of the bowel. If abscesses form, they are usually in the lower abdomen. They may, however, be walled off elsewhere. For example, abscess formation following a ruptured appendix may develop under the diaphragm (see Fig. 20-1) and may even perforate that structure and cause empyema.

Clinical picture. Local reactions of the peritoneum include redness, inflammation, and the production of large amounts of fluid containing electrolytes and proteins. Hypovolemia, electrolyte imbalance, dehydration, and finally shock develop due to the loss of the fluid, electrolytes, and proteins into the peritoneal cavity. The fluid usually becomes purulent as the condition progresses and as bacteria become more numerous. Peristalsis is halted by the severe peritoneal infection, and all the symptoms of acute intestinal obstruction (p. 1293) may occur. Nausea, vomiting, pain in the abdomen on palpation, severe distention with absence of bowel sounds, rigidity of the abdomen and failure to pass anything rec-

a fatty apron like membrane hanging down from the stomach + transverse colon in the abdominal cavity tally occur. Peritonitis also causes serious systemic symptoms including high temperature, high white blood cell count, tachycardia, weakness, diaphoresis, pallor, and all other signs of severe systemic reaction and shock. Peritonitis is a very serious condition that had an extremely high mortality before antimicrobial and bacteriostatic drugs and other modern treatment became available.

Intervention. Management usually consists of emergency measures to combat infection, restore intestinal motility, and supply lost electrolytes and fluids. Massive doses of antibiotics are administered parenterally. Intestinal or gastric intubation (p. 1211) is usually ordered at once, the tubes are attached to suction, and a rectal tube is inserted. Fluids and electrolytes are given intravenously. Nothing is given orally, and narcotics and sedatives are given for severe pain and apprehension as soon as the diagnosis is confirmed and there is no danger of masking symptoms.

The patient who has acute peritonitis needs constant nursing care, since extreme apprehension is common. Mouth care is given, and protection is needed to prevent drying and cracking of the lips, since dehydration is usually marked. Usually the person is placed in a semi-Fowler position so that gravity may help localize pus in the lower abdomen or the pelvis. Also in this position deeper breaths can be taken with less pain, which helps to prevent respiratory complications.

If the peritonitis is caused by a perforation which is releasing irritating or infected material into the abdominal cavity, surgery is performed as soon as the patient's condition permits. However, if the patient is in shock it may be several hours before shock can be relieved and before surgery can be safely performed. The operation usually consists of closure of the abnormal opening into the abdominal cavity and removal of the fluid that has accumulated.

□ Chronic inflammations

Crohn's disease: regional enterocolitis

Crohn's disease is a nonspecific inflammation that can affect any area of the small or large intestine. The most commonly involved areas are the terminal ileum, cecum, and ascending colon. The disease may occur in several segments separated by normal mucosa. Regional enterocolitis is characterized by cobblestone ulcerations along the mucosa, a thickening of the intestinal wall, and the formation of scar tissue. The ulcers are likely to perforate and form fistulas that connect with the abdominal wall or with any hollow viscus such as the bladder, colon, or vagina. Scar tissue may form as the ulcers heal, preventing the normal absorption of food, and strictures may form causing intestinal obstruction. Mesenteric lymph nodes are enlarged and firm. Differences between Crohn's disease and ulcerative colitis are illustrated in Table 58-1.

Table 58-1. Comparison of Crohn's disease and ulcerative colitis

	Crohn's disease	Ulcerative colitis
General appearance	Usually normal	May feel and look ill
Age	Bimodal: 20 to 30 years and 40 to 50 years	Mostly young adults
Area affected	Mainly the terminal ileum, cecum, and ascending colon (right side)	Colon only, primarily the descending colon (left side)
Extent of involvement	Segmental areas of involvement	Continuous, diffuse areas of involvement
Inflammation	Mostly submucosal	Mostly mucosal
Mucosal appearance	Cobblestone effect, granulomas	Ulcerations
Cancer potential	Normal incidence	Increased incidence
Character of stools	No blood; may have some fat; three to four semisoft per day	Blood present; no fat; frequent liquid stools
Reasons for surgery	Fistulas; intestinal obstruction	Poor response to medical therapy; hemorrhage, perforation
Complications	Fistulas; perianal disease; strictures, vitamin and iron deficiencies; perforation, fistulas to other organs	Pseudopolyps; hemorrhage; toxic megacolon; cachexia; perforation less often, causes peritonitis

Crohn's disease occurs most frequently in the young adult between the ages of 20 and 30 years. The incidence peaks again between 40 and 50 years of age. There is a high rate of recurrence, and the mortality is 5% to 18%.[4] There is a high incidence among the English and a low incidence in the nonemergent societies. The incidence rate appears to be increasing in American blacks and in emergent societies, indicating the possible relationship of stress to the onset of symptoms.

The cause of Crohn's disease is unclear. There is conflicting data relating to environmental or genetic factors as etiologic factors.[4] No specific causative agents have been found. Some evidence suggests a transmissible agent with a long latent period as a possible causative factor in susceptible persons.[4]

Clinical picture. The person with *acute* regional enterocolitis usually has severe abdominal pain or cramps localized in the right lower quadrant, malaise, moderate fever, and mild diarrhea. The white blood cell count is elevated. Often the disease is diagnosed as acute appendicitis, but on exploratory surgery a normal appendix but an inflamed ileum is found.

Chronic regional enterocolitis is characterized by a long history of diarrhea, abdominal pain, loss of weight, anemia, fistula formation, and finally intestinal obstruction. Weight loss and anemia result from chronic persistent inflammation of the bowel, decreased food intake, and malabsorption. The diarrhea may consist of three or four semisolid stools daily containing mucus and pus but no blood. Steatorrhea may also be present if the ulceration extends high in the small intestine. The abdominal colicky pain is relieved with a bowel movement. A mass sometimes can be felt in the area of the appendix or cecum. Perineal suppuration and strictures at the anus and rectosigmoid junction may be noted on sigmoidoscopy.

Radiographs of the small and large intestine confirm the diagnosis. Ureteral calculi and hydronephrosis may occur as a result of obstruction at the ureterovesicle junction from the inflammatory mass. Intravenous pyelography may be used to identify the presence of these complications.

Intervention. There is no specific therapy for Crohn's disease, and treatment is mainly supportive care. Activity may be somewhat restricted with rest periods suggested to conserve energy.

Diet. A well-balanced, high-calorie, high-protein diet is encouraged. Fats or high-fiber foods may be poorly tolerated by some persons, and their diets will need appropriate modifications. Fad diets are to be avoided. If food intake is decreased, vitamin supplements are added. Replacement vitamin B_{12} is given when there is a marked loss of ileum. When anemia is present, iron-dextran (Imferon) is given by Z-track injection, since oral intake of iron is ineffective because of the intestinal ulceration.

Medications. Analgesic and anticholinergic drugs may be given on a temporary basis to decrease abdominal pain and intestinal motility. Intestinal antibiotics such as phthalylsulfathiazole (Sulfathalidine) may be administered orally to treat local suppurative infections. Sulfasalazine (Azulfidine) is a popular but less effective microbial agent used to treat regional enterocolitis.[4] Steroids have not demonstrated any long-term influence in the course of the disease, although they may be helpful in an acute episode. Azathioprine (Imuran), an immunosuppresive agent, has been effective in decreasing diarrhea in some persons.

Surgery. If intestinal obstruction occurs or if there are fistulas, especially to the bladder, surgery is indicated. The involved portion of the intestines is removed and the proximal portion is anastomosed to the remaining colon (ileoascending or ileotransverse colostomy). Unfortunately the recurrence rate of the disease is high (30% at 3 years, 60% at 10 years).[4] Surgery may be helpful in young persons in the hope that they will be among the 40% in whom recurrence does not occur. A diversionary temporary ileostomy procedure to permit rest of the inflamed portion of the intestinal tract is no longer being performed.

Ulcerative colitis

Ulcerative colitis is an inflammatory disease of the colon. The cause is unknown, and the numerous theories that have been suggested have not been proved. Recent investigative studies are pursuing the autoimmune phenomenon as a significant causative factor.[15] The effect of stress on the precipitation of symptoms has been noted for many years. Although no "ulcerative colitis personality" has been demonstrated to occur in all persons with this disease, the personality makeup of many of these persons seems to be such that they accept the disease stoically but have difficulty conforming to a prescribed regimen. Many demonstrate a behavior pattern of anger and frustration. They often are very sensitive and fastidious and demand structured perfection in their life activities. The picture presented by the individual is one of being very independent and attempting to be in control of the situation, while in reality the person has a dependent personality that requires that needs be anticipated and met by the nurse.

Ulcerative colitis may occur at any age in either sex, but it is found most often in adolescents and young adults. In 75% of those with ulcerative colitis the onset occurred between the ages of 15 and 49 years. When seen in the elderly the condition is attributed to ischemic disease of the bowel. The disease varies in severity, and the person may be symptom free between periods of acute distress. A severe attack may be brought on by an acute infection, an emotional upset, or unknown factors.

In the early stages of ulcerative colitis only the rectum or rectosigmoid colon is affected, with the rectal mucosa containing many superficial bleeding points. As the diseases progresses, advancing up the colon, the bowel mucosa becomes edematous and thickened. The superficial bleeding points gradually enlarge and become ulcerated. The ulcers may bleed or perforate, causing abscess formation or peritonitis. The edematous mucosa may undergo changes and form pseudopolyps, which may become cancerous. The continuous healing process, with formation of scar tissue between the frequent relapses, may cause the colon to lose its normal elasticity and its absorptive capability. Normal mucosa is replaced by scar tissue, and the colon becomes thickened, rigid, and pipelike.

Clinical picture. The diagnosis of ulcerative colitis is based on the history and symptoms and on results obtained from barium enemas, from proctoscopic and sigmoidoscopic examinations, and on failure to find any causative organisms in the stools.

The main symptom of an acute attack of the disease is diarrhea. There may be as many as 15 or 20 liquid stools a day containing blood, mucus, and pus. Abdominal cramps may or may not occur before the bowel movement. As the scarring within the bowel progresses, the feeling of the urge to defecate is lost leading to involuntary leakage of stool. There may be loss of appetite, low-grade fever, and occasionally nausea and vomiting. With the persistence of these symptoms as well as the marked depression of colonic absorption, weakness, dehydration, debility and cachexia occur. Hypokalemia and hypoproteinemia are common. A distended abdomen is suggestive of *toxic megacolon*, a marked dilation of the colon that may result in rupture of the colon.

Intervention. The person with ulcerative colitis may be admitted to the hospital for immediate supportive treatment during an acute exacerbation of the disease or for preparation for surgery during a remission. Medical treatment for ulcerative colitis is directed toward restoring nutrition, combating infection, reducing the motility of the inflamed bowel, and treating the psychogenic factors that may be involved.

Emotional support. If the disease is of long duration the patient is usually thin, nervous, and apprehensive and is inclined to be preoccupied with his physical condition. These qualities, which are caused by the illness, are superimposed on the basic personality pattern of many persons with this disease—sensitivity, insecurity, and dependence. This makes it hard for the nurse to get to know and understand the patient. Sometimes specialized medical and nursing consultation is indicated. All members of the nursing staff should use the same approach to the patient. Although the patient may accept treatment and nursing care, depression is common. Hostility may also be a form of behavior exhibited by the patient. The nurse needs to see this as the patient's way of testing the environment and the professional staff and in effect is a way of asking, "Do you really care for me and want to help me?" Acceptance of behavior, together with gentle, intelligent nursing care, will help the nurse gradually gain the patient's confidence and will increase the patient's ability to accept certain essentials of treatment such as the diet regimen.

All procedures and treatments must be carefully explained to the patient. For example, explaining that that medication is available for controlling bowel movements sometimes reduces apprehension. The nurse should listen carefully to the patient's own report of things that seem to stimulate peristalsis and cause frequency of bowel movements. If the patient believes that certain foods or combinations of foods cause diarrhea, this fact should be noted on the nursing care plan and reported to the dietitian. Other information such as the best time for bathing, whether soon after a meal (to permit a long rest period afterward) or later (when food is partially digested), is included in the nursing care plan.

Comfort and rest. Bed rest may be prescribed for the acutely ill patient, and care must be taken for thin persons that bony prominences are protected by an alternating-pressure mattress, foam pad, or sheepskin. Measures to ensure rest are explored with the patient. Sedatives or tranquilizers are often prescribed to alleviate nervous tension.

The environment is kept warm, and drafts and chilling must be avoided. Extra covers should be provided so that the patient may use them as he wishes. Heat in the room and covers should provide enough warmth and protection to permit regular airing of the room to help remove odors and to supply fresh air.

Diet. A high-protein, high-caloric, high-vitamin diet is usually urged to help the person regain nutritional losses and to foster healing. Because there is no conclusive evidence that the diet affects the condition, often any desired food is permitted.

Elimination. It is crucial that a record be kept of the number, amount, and character of the stools and that specimens of stool are sent to the laboratory as requested. Antispasmodic drugs such as belladonna preparations are given to slow peristalsis. Medications such as kaolin and bismuth (bismuth subcarbonate) may be used to help coat and protect the irritated intestinal mucosa and to give better consistency to the stools, and paregoric or diphenoxylate (Lomotil) may be used to lessen the frequency of stools.

Although each bowel movement may be very small, the commode or bedpan should be emptied as often as it is used. The patient wants the bedpan accessible at all times and may even insist on keeping it in bed. Room deodorizers are sometimes used to dispel unpleasant odors. Patients who brace themselves on the bedpan by leaning on their elbows, thereby causing pressure areas, will need these areas massaged frequently with a lubricant. If the patient spends much time on the bedpan, it can be padded with foam rubber, or a fracture pan can be used. If the commode is used it can also be protected with a piece of foam rubber or with a rubber ring. Linen is kept fresh, and the patient's perineum, buttocks, and anal region are washed thoroughly several times a day. Dibucaine (Nupercaine) or other prescribed ointment may be applied to the anus to relieve discomfort. Sitz baths are beneficial to the skin and circulation and are often permitted two or three times a day.

Medications. Antibiotics may be ordered to prevent or to treat secondary infection. Sulfasalazine (Azulfidine) is now widely used in the treatment of ulcerative colitis, and many physicians consider it the drug of choice. Like all sulfa drugs, sulfasalazine can cause serious side effects; therefore the nurse may wish to review these when administering this drug. The side effects of oliguria and crystalluria are particularly apt to be a problem in patients with ulcerative colitis unless they maintain a liberal fluid intake.

ACTH and the adrenal steroids such as prednisone may be prescribed in the treatment of ulcerative colitis. They often produce dramatic results in severe cases of the disease by decreasing the toxemia and fever; diminishing diarrhea, bleeding, and rectal urgency; and promoting a sense of well-being. It should be understood, however, that while corticotropin and the corticosteroids suppress the inflammation associated with ulcerative colitis, they do not cure the disease. A relapse rate as high as 80% has been reported when patients were withdrawn from steroid therapy.[4] Nevertheless many patients' lives have been saved since these drugs became available. (For nursing care of patients receiving steroid therapy, see p. 850.) Since some experts believe that ulcerative colitis may be caused by an autoimmune reaction, azathioprine (Imuran) may be prescribed in addition to steroids.

Surgery. About 20% of patients with ulcerative colitis require surgery because of complications such as hemorrhage or perforation.[4] An ileostomy and a subtotal colectomy may be performed in an attempt to cure the condition when the disease is so incapacitating that it makes an invalid of the patient or when no improvement has been obtained from medical treatment over a period of time. Choice of surgery depends on the individual patient and on the physician. It is recognized that surgery does not remove the basic condition that led to development of the disease. Many patients, however, seem to recover almost completely following a total colectomy and are able to lead normal, useful lives.

One of three surgical procedures is usually chosen in the treatment of a particular patient: an *ileostomy* and a *partial colectomy* may be performed, leaving a rectal stump, which may be anastomosed to the ileum at a later date; a *total proctocolectomy* through an abdominal perineal incision may be done, leaving the patient with a permanent ileostomy; or the large bowel may be resected and the ileum anastomosed to the remaining segment of colon at the time of the surgery.

A different type of surgical approach is the "continent ileostomy," or "Kock's pouch." An intraabdominal reservoir is fashioned and a "nipple valve" is formed by intussusception of the distal ileum to provide continence. The capacity of the pouch increases slowly over 6 months until it can hold approximately 500 ml. Contents of the pouch are removed several times a day by catheterization. Difficulties have occurred with valve failure and in keeping the ileal contents from becoming too thick and plugging up the stoma. This procedure eliminates the need for wearing an external ileostomy bag.

After a partial colectomy the patient returns from the operating room with two openings, or stomas, on the abdominal wall. The proximal opening, which is usually on the right side, is the ileostomy from which liquid stool will flow. The distal opening, usually on the left side, leads to the remnant of lower bowel that has not yet been removed. If a total colectomy was performed, the patient will have only an ileostomy, since the large bowel and rectum are removed.

When a partial colectomy was performed the patient may be readmitted to the hospital later to have the ileum anastomosed to the rectum or to have the rectum removed. For the care of the patient with an ileostomy, refer to Chapter 57.

Long-term care. During the patient's convalescence the nurse is alert for any emerging problems. Because the physical causes of this condition are unknown, and because the condition itself is not cured but only alleviated by the variety of treatments available, effort is made to learn of and control the emotional components of the disease. The social worker may be asked to talk to the patient and attempt to learn of social, economic, or other problems that are of concern. The community health nurse may make a home visit before the patient leaves the hospital to determine whether care can be given properly at home and to report any other pertinent information. The family is instructed in ways to help the patient, such as preparing food and thus helping to maintain nutrition, and understanding and accepting the disease and the patient's behavior. The patient needs careful follow-up on an outpatient basis.

Diverticulosis and diverticulitis

A diverticulum of the colon is an outpouching of mucosa (through a weak point in the muscular layer of the bowel wall) resulting from persistent and abnormally high intracolonic pressure. The presence of many diverticula in the sigmoid and the descending colon is called *diverticulosis.* If diverticula become inflamed, the term *diverticulitis* is used. The cause of diverticula in unknown. Studies in the past few years suggest that the removal of indigestible fiber from the diet may contribute to the development of the disease.[8] At least 10% of the total population in the United States has this condition, which is much more common in middle-aged and elderly persons than in the young. Some experts have described it as the most common disease of the colon.[8] In itself a diverticulum is a benign condition usually causing no symptoms. It may, however, become impacted with feces and become irritated, inflamed, and infected. Diverticulitis may sometimes be prevented by care in selection of food and avoidance of constipation.

Clinical picture. The patient with diverticulitis complains of general discomfort or pain in the left lower quadrant. There may be local tenderness, leukocytosis, and fever. Hemorrhage occurs in about 10% to 20% of all persons and may be chronic and mild or severe.

Intervention. The traditional diet for diverticulosis used to be a low-residue diet, but this approach is now questioned. It is believed that a high-fiber diet, by increasing the bulk of the stool, permits an easier flow of feces through the bowel and less straining at stool.[22,26,28] The eating of whole bran daily is commonly advised by physicians.

The cramplike (colic) pains of diverticulitis can be eased by medication. When medication is necessary meperidine hydrochloride (Demerol) is preferred over morphine as meperidine decreases colonic pressure and rests the bowel.[25] Antispasmodics may also be ordered. Metamucil or other bland bulk laxatives help to keep the feces moving and decrease pain. Antibiotics are given when there are signs of infection. Bleeding diverticula are usually treated by rest and sedation.

A possible complication of diverticulitis is perforation, with resultant abscess formation or generalized peritonitis. The inflammatory process may also cause bowel obstruction. Surgery may be required for treatment of these conditions, and occasionally surgery is performed to remove a portion of the seriously involved bowel. A colostomy is sometimes necessary.

Anal fissure

An anal fissure is a slitlike ulcer resembling a crack in the lining of the anal canal at or below the anorectal line. Usually it is the result of trauma caused by passage of hard-formed stool that overstretches the anal lining. The ulcer does not heal readily. Defecation initiates spasm of the anal sphincter causing severe pain that lasts for some time. Slight bleeding may occur, and constipation is usually caused by restraining of bowel movements to avoid pain.

Anal examination causes muscle spasm of the sphincter. Since spasm results in pain, the fissure must be examined with the patient under anesthesia. Treatment usually consists of digital dilation of the sphincter, or the anal ulcer may be surgically excised.

Local pain and spasm sometimes can be relieved by warm compresses, sitz baths, and use of analgesic ointments. Colace is usually ordered to lubricate the canal and to soften the stool. Postoperatively the care is similar to that given following a hemorrhoidectomy (p. 1296).

Anal abscess

An anal abscess is located in tissues around the anus. It is caused by infection from the anal canal and may follow an anal fissure. If the abscess involves the anal, para-anal, or perineal tissues, there is throbbing local pain caused by pressure on the somatic sensory nerves in the perineum and local signs of inflammation. The person finds it difficult to sit or lie on the area. In fact, any position is uncomfortable because reflected pain is common.

If the abscess is located deep in the ischiorectal tissues, however, the person is aware only of vague discomfort until the disease spreads into an area where there are nerve fibers. The person with an *ischiorectal abscess* is usually very ill. Fever, chills, and malaise are present, and the abscess must be incised and drained.

Postoperative care. Postoperatively patients usually prefer to lie on their side or abdomen. Because some difficulty in voiding is common, nursing measures should be initiated to prevent bladder distention.

There is usually a large amount of seropurulent drainage from the wound, and the physician may order that the dressings be changed as necessary. The wound is usually packed with gauze, and the nurse may be asked to wet the pack with warm normal saline solution or to repack the wound with warm normal saline dressings at specified intervals. The packs should be inserted into the bottom of the wound, since it is important that it heal from the inside outward. The skin around the wound is protected with petroleum jelly to prevent irritation from drainage. The wet dressing is covered with oiled silk or plastic material to prevent wick contamination and to prevent wetting the bed. The dressing can be held in place by Montgomery straps or a T binder.

As healing progresses, sitz baths are usually ordered. If the wound is located near the anus the patient is advised to cleanse the area carefully after defecation and to take a sitz bath after each defecation. Until healing is complete and all drainage disappears, a small dressing is worn over the wound. A stool softener may be given to prevent or to treat constipation. Antibiotics usually are administered.

The patient is often discharged from the hospital before the wound has completely healed. Sitz baths are continued at home. If any difficulties are encountered they should be reported to the physician.

Anal fistula

An anal fistula is an inflammatory sinus or tract with a primary opening in an anal crypt and with a secondary opening on the anal, paraanal, or perineal skin or in the rectal mucous membrane. It results from the rupture or drainage of an anal abscess. The individual has a periodic drainage that stains underclothing. An anal fistula is usually a chronic condition, and unfortunately many persons attempt to treat themselves with over-the-counter remedies before they seek competent medical care. The person is encouraged to have a gastrointestinal tract examination to rule out regional enteritis or other colon diseases.

The treatment for an anal fistula is a *fistulectomy* or a *fistulotomy.* A fistulectomy consists of an excision of the entire fistulous tract. The overhanging edges, if any, are trimmed away to leave an open, saucer-shaped wound. This procedure is usually performed when the fistula is quite straight and somewhat superficial. When a fistulotomy is performed the entire tract is laid open and the overlying skin margins are excised to leave a wide, saucer-shaped wound. The membranous lining of the remaining half of the fistulous tract quickly acquires a covering of granulation tissue. This procedure is usually used when a deep fistulous tract exists.

Postoperatively with both procedures warm, wet dressings are usually applied. A stool softener or mild laxative may be given orally daily until the first bowel movement occurs, and sitz baths are prescribed to keep the area clean and to relieve discomfort. The patient who has had an operation for a fistula is more comfortable sitting on a protected pillow or a piece of very thick foam rubber rather than on a rubber ring.

Outcome criteria for the person with a chronic inflammatory disease of the lower gastrointestinal tract

The patient or significant others can:

1. Describe the dietary modifications needed after discharge:
   a. Plan a diet that includes adequate protein, calories, and vitamins.
   b. List any specific foods to be avoided (high roughage, fats).
2. Explain any medication program to be followed at home:
   a. State action, dosage, frequency, and side effects of medications (antibiotics, antidiarrheals, antispasmodics).
   b. Describe the use of medications to be taken as needed for discomfort.
3. Describe the health maintenance follow-up program:
   a. Explain in own words the basic pathologic condition and overall treatment program.
   b. Describe the need to avoid infectious agents in the environment.
   c. List signs requiring immediate contact with health care provider (abdominal pain or distention, increasing diarrhea, presence of blood or pus in the stool, signs and symptoms of systemic infection, constipation).
   d. State plans for regular follow-up care.
4. Describe measures for supportive care:
   a. Verbalize the relationship between compliance with therapy and optimal health.
   b. Identify a source for an ongoing supportive relationship.
   c. Verbalize awareness of potential surgery.

☐ Parasitic infections

Amebiasis

Amebiasis is caused by the protozoan parasite *Entamoeba histolytica,* which primarily invades the large intestine and secondarily invades the liver. The active, motile form of the protozoa, the trophozoite, is not infectious and if ingested is easily destroyed by digestive enzymes. The inactive form, or cyst, however, is highly resistant to extremes in temperature, most chemicals, and the digestive juices. When the cyst is swallowed in fecally contaminated food or water, it easily passes into the intestines, where the active trophozoite is released and enters the intestinal wall. Here it feeds on the mucosal cells, causing ulceration of the intestinal mucosa.

Prevention. It is estimated that at least 10% of the population of the United States have amebiasis in the acute, chronic, or asymptomatic stages.[4] Although the disease exists chiefly in tropical countries, it also prevails wherever sanitation is poor. The cyst, which is the infectious agent, can survive for long periods outside the body, and it is transmitted by direct contact from person to person, by insects, and by contaminated water, milk, and other foods. For this reason persons traveling in tropical countries should drink only boiled water and eat only cooked foods. The most infectious agent is the "carrier," who, although having few or no symptoms of the disease, passes the cysts in his stools. If his hygienic habits are poor and if he is a food handler, he can easily transmit the cysts to the food he prepares for consumption by others.

Clinical picture. Although the disease varies in severity, the onset is usually acute with symptoms developing within 2 to 4 days of exposure. Weakness, prostration, nausea, vomiting, a gripping pain in the right lower quadrant of the abdomen, and tenesmus usually occur. Each day the person has numerous semifluid, foul-smelling stools containing mucus and pus.

If either the trophozoite or the cyst can be found in the stool, a positive diagnosis of amebiasis can be made and definitive treatment started. It is easier to find the parasite in the stool during the acute stage of the disease than later. Immediately after defecation a warm stool should be sent to the laboratory for examination. Several stool specimens from successive bowel movements may be requested. If the laboratory is at a distance, the specimen container should be transported on a hot-water bottle or in a pan of warm water. When special laboratory facilities are required, a fresh stool can be placed in a preservative and sent to the Center for Disease Control, Atlanta, for diagnosis.

Intervention. The person with a mild or asymptomatic form of amebiasis is treated on an outpatient basis; 90% of all persons usually respond to a course of amebicidal therapy. If the halogenated hydroquinolines such as diiodohydroxyquin (Diodoquin) are given, the person may have some diarrhea. Neurotoxicity to this agent has been reported. The drug is administered in a dose of 650 mg three times a day for 20 days. Tetracycline may be prescribed alone or in combination with diiodohydroxyquin. The maximum daily dose of tetracycline is 2 g daily for 7 days.

Emetine hydrochloride may be used for severe disease, especially when liver abscess is present. The patient receiving emetine hydrochloride is placed on strict bed rest, and pulse rate and blood pressure are watched carefully because the drug is very toxic. Some of the many signs of toxicity to this drug include nausea, vomiting, diarrhea, generalized weakness, cardiac irregularity, fall in blood pressure, neuritis, desquamation of the skin, loss of the sense of taste, and mental depression. Emetine hydrochloride usually is given for 7 to 10 days. Injections can cause tissue necrosis; therefore injection sites are carefully rotated. Metronidazole is used along with emetine hydrochloride to treat liver abscess. It is administered two to three times daily for 7 days.

Amebiasis is a disease with remissions and exacerbations, and it may persist for years. During acute exacerbations the person may become dehydrated, exhausted, or anemic and require hospitalization. Infusions and blood transfusions are often necessary. A bland low-residue diet is commonly prescribed, and the person may be advised to avoid alcohol and tobacco.

A careful record of intake and output is kept, and generous amounts of oral fluids are encouraged. The number and character of the stools should be described. Excretion precautions are observed, and the bedpan is sterilized after each use. In handling the bedpan precautions are taken because some cysts are usually passed. Cleanliness should be stressed, and patients should know why it is so important to wash their hands after bowel movements. Particular emphasis is placed on careful washing of hands before meals to avoid reinfection.

Persons known to be exposed to amebiasis should have stool examinations weekly for 3 weeks. If infected they will be treated as described for the asymptomatic form of the disease.[1]

Trichinosis (trichinellosis, trichiniasis)

Trichinosis is caused by the larvae of a species of roundworm, *Trichinella spiralis*, which become encysted in the striated muscles of humans, hogs, and other animals, particularly those (such as rodents) that consume infected pork in garbage. Trichinosis is found worldwide with the highest incidence occurring in Europe and the United States. Autopsy reports show that at least 5% of the population of the United States is affected with trichinosis. It occurs much more often in hogs that have been fed garbage than in those fed on grain. The larvae do not form cysts in pork. Therefore they are not visible to the naked eye and cannot be seen by food inspectors.

Trichinosis is transmitted through inadequately cooked food. Pork is the most common source of infection. When infected food is eaten, live encysted larvae develop within the intestine of the host; they mate and produce eggs that hatch in the uterus of the female worm. The larvae are discharged in huge numbers (approximately 1,500 per worm) into the lymphatics and lacteals of the host's small intestine at the rate of about two an hour for about 6 weeks. They pass to the muscles of the host, where they become encysted by the reaction of the host's body and may remain for 10 years or longer.

Prevention. No immunization is available, yet the disease could be eradicated with the knowledge that we now possess.[4] Basic scientific facts necessary for the complete prevention of the disease in human beings have been known for years. Trichinae can be killed by cooking at a temperature of 60 C (140 F) for 30 minutes per pound of meat and by freezing at a temperature of −18 C (0 F) for 24 hours. They are not killed by smoking, pickling, or other methods of processing. Sausage and other infected pork products carelessly prepared are a common source of infection in humans. Other meats ground in the same machine without thorough cleaning or cut on the same meat block may also cause infection. There is a need for thorough cooking of all pork products consumed at home regardless of how sanitary the local meat market may appear to be. A safe rule to follow is to never eat pork products in a restaurant but only at home where adequate cooking can be assured, and to never eat any ground meat without thoroughly cooking it.

Clinical picture. Signs and symptoms of trichinosis are varied. Although the reason is unknown, edema appears as puffiness about the eyes, particularly involving the upper lids. If a very large number of larvae have been ingested, nausea, vomiting, and diarrhea due to intestinal irritation usually occur about 4 days after the infected food has been eaten. On about the seventh day, when the larvae migrate throughout the body to the muscles, there are usually muscle stiffness, weakness, and remittent fever. The extent of these symptoms depends on the number of larvae present and the resistance of the host. There may be pain in the back, the muscles of the eyeballs, the muscles of chewing, and elsewhere in the body. Muscles of the diaphragm are often affected, causing pain on breathing. The diagnosis is confirmed by finding larvae in a biopsy taken from the deltoid or gastrocnemius muscle in the fourth week of infection. An increase in the eosinophil count is a characteristic finding in trichinosis and persists for several weeks after the onset of acute symptoms. Persistent fever may also be present.

Intervention. Treatment is symptomatic. Usually the person is confined to bed and placed on a high-caloric, high-protein diet. Analgesics are given for muscle pain and prednisolone, 5 mg, three times daily, may relieve fever, edema, and muscle pain.[4] Symptoms may also be relieved by thiabendazole, 25 mg/kg for 5 to 7 days.

In the acutely ill person circulatory collapse can occur if hypoproteinemia is present. Trichinosis can cause death, which usually occurs from pneumonia or cachexia from 4 to 6 weeks following the onset of symptoms. Death may also occur from paralysis of the respiratory muscles.

Outcome criteria for the person with a parasitic infection of the gastrointestinal tract

The patient or significant others can:

1. Describe specific substances to be avoided (alcohol, tobacco).
2. Describe the health maintenance and follow-up program:
   a. Demonstrate correct hand-washing technique.
   b. State the basis for proper disposal of stool.
   c. Describe the basis for ongoing periodic stool examination and method of providing the specimen.
   d. State plans for follow-up care.
   e. Identify other family members who may require medical examination.

INTESTINAL OBSTRUCTION

Intestinal obstruction is an extremely serious condition that if not treated promptly, can cause death within a few hours. Intestinal obstruction develops when intestinal contents cannot pass through the lumen of the bowel. It may be due to mechanical causes, neurogenic causes (paralytic ileus), or vascular abnormalities (Fig. 58-1). *Mechanical obstruction* is most often caused by strangulated hernias and adhesions, although cancer of the large bowel accounts for the majority of cases of mechanical obstruction in the colon. Other mechanical causes are *volvulus* (a twisting of the bowel) and *intussusception* (telescoping of a segment of the bowel within itself, most common in emaciated infants and small children). Volvulus occurs most often in elderly persons, and the sigmoid loop of the large bowel is usually affected. Bands, strictures, and adhesions that cause obstruction of the bowel lumen may be congenital but usually result from previous abdominal surgery or peritonitis.

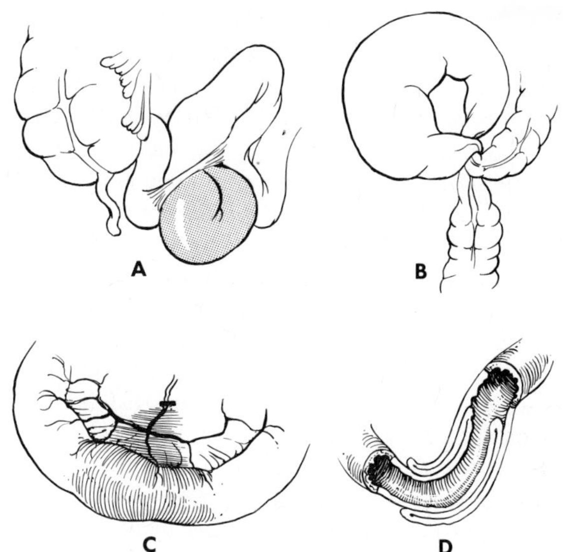

Fig. 58-1. Some causes of intestinal obstruction. **A,** Constriction by adhesions. **B,** Volvulus. **C,** Mesenteric thrombosis. **D,** Intussusception.

In *neurogenic obstruction* there is interference with the innervation of the bowel, which causes peristalsis to cease or to be markedly retarded. Paralytic ileus may be a complication of peritonitis, acute medical illness such as pneumonia, a reaction to severe pain, or changes in circulatory supply to the bowel. Other causes of paralytic ileus include handling of the bowel during surgery, spinal cord lesions, electrolyte imbalance (hypokalemia), or toxic conditions such as uremia.

Obstruction due to vascular disease is relatively rare and usually occurs in persons who have evidence of other vascular disease. Occlusion commonly occurs in the superior mesenteric vessels, cutting off the blood supply to a large segment of the bowel. When the affected portion of the bowel is unable to perform its muscular function, peristalsis ceases and the bowel becomes distended with fluid, gas, and food residue and rapidly becomes gangrenous.

Clinical picture. The symptoms of intestinal obstruction vary according to the degree and site of obstruction. In general, sudden acute mechanical occlusions located high in the intestinal tract produce more intense and earlier symptoms than those occurring lower in the system. When the lumen of the bowel first becomes obstructed, there is an increase in peristalsis above the occlusion in an attempt to move intestinal contents past the obstruction. Auscultation will reveal loud, frequent peristaltic sounds (borborygmi). As the peristaltic waves become more forceful they cause sharp intermittent or cramping abdominal pain. The increased peristaltic activity also injures the intestinal wall, causing edema around the obstructed area, and the intestine proximal to the obstruction becomes distended. Normally most of the fluid in the intestinal tract is absorbed through the intestinal wall, helping to maintain fluid and electrolyte balance. When the intestine is obstructed, however, the normal absorptive power of the intestinal mucosa is lacking because of irritation from hyperactivity or impairment of circulation. Most of the gas consists of swallowed air that contains about 79% nitrogen and is slowly absorbed from the intestinal tract. The combined presence of fluid and this gas in the bowel causes increased tension and may occlude the blood supply, resulting in leakage of bacteria through the walls of the tract and eventual gangrene. The bowel distal to the obstruction remains empty and constricted so that there is no passage of gas or stool rectally.

Vomiting occurring with intestinal obstruction may be frequent, abrupt in onset, copious, often spontaneous, and foul in odor (often fecal). Such vomiting is caused by reverse peristalsis, as the intestinal contents are regurgitated into the stomach, from which they are ejected. In general, the higher the obstruction, the earlier and more severe is the vomiting. If the obstruction is in the large bowel, vomiting may not occur as the ileocecal valve permits fluid to enter the colon but prevents its passage back into the ileum.

Failure of the normal absorptive powers of the intestinal wall to continue and the loss of fluid through vomiting cause severe fluid and electrolyte imbalance. Bacteria and toxins escaping through the affected bowel may cause toxemia and peritonitis. Signs of shock develop, and immediate treatment for shock is required.

Intervention. The treatment for intestinal obstruction is intestinal intubation, the administration of fluids and electrolytes by infusion, and the relief of mechanical and vascular obstruction by surgery. Paralytic ileus is not treated surgically unless gangrene of a portion of the bowel has occurred. The operative procedure varies with the cause and the location of the obstruction and the general condition of the patient. If constricting bands or adhesions are found, they are cut, and it may be necessary to resect the occluded bowel and to anastomose the remaining segments. It may be necessary to do a temporary cecostomy or colostomy, and later when the patient is in better physical condition a resection and anastomosis of the bowel may be performed.

Nursing interventions include maintaining intestinal decompression and keeping an accurate record of all intake and output. Intravenous fluids are ordered to maintain fluid and electrolyte balance. Any increase in temperature may indicate more obstruction or peritonitis and is reported. Good supportive care is necessary. Pain and vomiting often leave the patient physically and emotionally exhausted. Assistance in simple activities such as turning in bed may be necessary, and encouragement and assurance that the intubation and other treatments usually result in lessening of symptoms within a short time are helpful. Skin and mouth care are essential. Any vomitus is immediately removed from the bedside, since its foul odor may increase nausea.

Pulmonary ventilation should receive the nurse's careful attention. Since intestinal distention may cause respiratory distress, Fowler's position is usually more comfortable for the patient, who is encouraged to breathe through the nose and not to swallow air because it increases the distention and discomfort. A rectal tube may be used to provide relief from lower abdominal distention. Enemas or colonic irrigations may be ordered, and the results of these treatments are carefully observed and recorded.

The nurse assesses the return of peristalsis by listening for bowel sounds and evaluates the resolution of abdominal distention by measuring the abdominal girth. Passage of flatus or any abnormal substances such as blood or mucus is reported to the physician. Urinary retention due to pressure on the bladder may occur, and the patient is monitored for the amount of urine at each voiding. A total 24-hour urinary output below 500 ml is reported to the physician.

■ VASCULAR OCCLUSIONS

□ Mesentric vascular occlusion

Mesenteric vascular occlusion is common, occurring frequently in persons with heart disease resulting in emboli to the intestines. Often the patient is elderly. It also may occur in patients who are recovering from recent abdominal surgery. Thrombosis of the mesenteric vein may occur as a complication of cirrhosis of the liver, following splenectomy, or as a result of an extension of a thrombophlebitic process in the ileocolic veins. The superior mesenteric arteries usually are occluded. Causes other than atherosclerosis or intravascular thromboses of the mesenteric vessels include polycythemia, sickle cell disease, other blood dyscrasias, and pancreatic disorders.

The blood supply to the lower part of the jejunum and ileum is usually interrupted by a mesenteric vascular occlusion. The walls of the intestine become thickened and edematous, then reddened, and finally black and gangrenous. Infarction of the small bowel may develop over a period of several weeks or may appear suddenly.

Clinical picture. In partial blockage of the superior mesenteric artery by an atherosclerotic plaque, pain is crampy and colicky in nature and may last for several hours after a meal. The pain is associated with the demand for oxygen needed for the increased intestinal muscular activity. In the event of sudden occlusion, the patient complains of an acute onset of sharp abdominal pain between the zyphoid process and umbilicus and nausea and vomiting. There is disturbed bowel function. The white blood cell count is elevated. Occasionally a tender mass may be palpable in the epigastrium. The abdomen may be distended, and there will be an absence of bowel sounds. If there has been hemorrhage into the peritoneal cavity, generalized abdominal rigidity will be noted. The patient may be in shock when first seen, even when the condition is reported at the onset of symptoms.

Intervention. Immediate hospitalization is required. Nothing is given orally, and a nasogastric tube is inserted and attached to suction. Parenteral fluids are started. Treatment depends on the suddenness and cause of the occlusion. If a clot can be found and removed after opening the superior mesenteric artery, the blood flow will be restored. If necessary, damaged bowel tissue is removed surgically. Chronic occlusion may be corrected by endarterectomy or a bypass procedure.

The patient who has surgery for vascular occlusion usually is given heparin and bishydroxycoumarin (Dicumarol) or sodium warfarin (Coumadin). Antispasmodic drugs such as papaverine hydrochloride may also be given. The patient may be very ill both preoperatively and postoperatively and may need constant nursing care. The mortality from mesenteric vascular occlusion is high, particularly among elderly persons.

□ Hemorrhoids

Hemorrhoids are one of the most common afflictions of humans, and they cause an enormous amount of pain and discomfort. Congestion occurs in the veins of the hemorrhoidal plexus and leads to varicosities within the lower rectum and the anus. The cause for the development of this condition is not definitely known, but many factors seem to be involved. Heredity, occupations requiring long periods of standing or sitting, the erect posture assumed by human beings, structural absence of valves in the hemorrhoidal veins, increase of intraabdominal pressure caused by constipation, straining at defecation, and pregnancy all are factors predisposing to development of hemorrhoids.

Clinical picture. *Internal hemorrhoids* appear above the internal sphincter and are not apparent to the individual unless they become so large that they protrude through the anus, where they may become constricted and painful. Internal hemorrhoids often bleed on defecation, and although the amount of blood lost may be small, continuous oozing over a long period of time may cause iron-deficiency anemia. *External hemorrhoids* appear outside the anal sphincter. They bleed relatively rarely and seldom cause pain unless a hemorrhoidal vein ruptures and a so-called thrombosis occurs. If this occurs the hemorrhoid becomes inflamed and extremely painful.

Many persons have both internal and external hemorrhoids. Constipation often predisposes to the development of hemorrhoids and usually becomes worse after they occur because the person tries to restrain bowel movements that produce pain or bleeding. Other people resort to laxatives without competent medical supervision. Although hemorrhoids rarely undergo malignant degeneration, constipation and bleeding are symptoms of cancer of the rectum. For this reason all persons with these symptoms should have a medical examination to rule out cancer. The nurse is often in a position to advise persons who have what they assume to be painless bleeding hemorrhoids of long duration to visit their physician.

Intervention. The treatment of hemorrhoids consists of local treatment, sclerosing by injection, ligation, or surgery.

Local treatment. The local application of ice, warm compresses, or analgesic ointments such as dibucaine (Nupercaine) gives temporary relief from pain and reduces the edema around external hemorrhoids or prolapsed internal ones. Sitz baths are also extremely helpful in relieving pain. The physician may prescribe agents to soften the stool. Thrombosed external hemorrhoids usually respond to this treatment with lessening of pain and absorption of the confined blood. Finally only a painless skin tag remains, and it is not removed surgically unless it causes strictures or its presence interferes with cleanliness enough to cause serious aggravation. If a thrombosed external hemorrhoid does not respond to medical treatment, it may be incised to release the encased blood. This procedure usually is performed in a physician's office and results in immediate relief of pain.

Injection. Injection is used in the treatment of moderate-sized internal hemorrhoids that cause bleeding or are protruding. A sclerosing solution such as 5% phenol in oil is injected carefully into the submucous areolar tissue in which the hemorrhoidal veins lie to produce an inflammatory reaction. Fibrous induration, which surrounds and constricts the veins, occurs at the site of the injection in 2 or 3 weeks. Bleeding from the hemorrhoids usually stops within 24 to 48 hours. There is some local pain at the time of the injection but there usually is no limitation of activity following this treatment.

Ligation. Internal hemorrhoids may be treated by ligating them with rubber bands. The hemorrhoid is grasped with a forceps and pulled down into a special instrument which, when the trigger handle is pressed, slips an elastic band over it. The rubber band constricts the circulation and causes necrosis. The destroyed tissue usually sloughs off within a week. An enema is given prior to the treatment to prevent a bowel movement for 24 hours so that there is no straining that would cause the rubber band to break or slip off. No anesthesia is required, and the procedure usually is performed in the physician's office. Local discomfort is minimal and usually is relieved by aspirin or Darvon.

Surgery. Surgical excision with ligation *(hemorrhoidectomy)* is the treatment used most often for all external hemorrhoids and for internal ones that do not respond well to sclerosing or ligation. There are several methods by which a hemorrhoidectomy may be performed. However, the classic procedure involves excising each hemorrhoid and tying the pedicle with a ligature. The raw areas in the anus then heal by secondary intention.

Preoperatively the patient may be given a laxative and is encouraged to eat a full, normal diet until a few hours before the anesthetic is given. Stool softeners are often given to soften the stool and facilitate its passage through the rectum postoperatively, and a bulk laxative such as psyllium (Metamucil) may be given to increase the bulk of the stool.

Postoperatively the patient's vital signs are monitored to rule out internal bleeding. During the first 24 hours after surgery a ligature on one of the pedicles may slip off, causing a hemorrhage that may go undetected because blood will gather in the anal canal and not be expelled immediately. This can also occur during the seventh to tenth day after surgery when the suture may slough off and separate from the pedicle. If hemorrhage does occur, a Foley catheter may be inserted into the *rectum* and the balloon inflated to put pressure on the bleeding areas.[25]

Comfort. Because the operation is usually considered minor and dressings may not be used, there may be a tendency to minimize this operative procedure. In reality it can cause more discomfort than some more serious operations, and the patient assumes a position of least discomfort. When lying supine a support such as a flotation pad under the buttocks will help to distribute the pressure and relieve discomfort. Ice packs, warm wet compresses, analgesic ointments, and narcotics may be given. The patient is usually permitted out of bed the evening of surgery or the day after, and sitz baths usually are ordered to be taken at least twice a day for relief of pain and discomfort. The patient is monitored frequently during the initial sitz baths as hypotension may occur secondary to dilation of the pelvic blood vessels in the early postoperative period.

Elimination. The patient often has difficulty voiding after a hemorrhoidectomy. This difficulty can usually be overcome by getting the patient out of bed to urinate. Sitz baths also stimulate voiding.

Stool softeners are continued as preoperatively, and the patient is encouraged to have a bowel movement as soon as the inclination occurs. Passing a stool of normal consistency as soon as possible after surgery prevents the formation of strictures and preserves the normal lumen of the anus. The incidence of wound infection is slight after rectal surgery due to local tissue resistance to the bacteria normally present in the rectum. It is most likely to occur if bowel action has been delayed and healing tissues have become adherent. If the patient complains of much pain about the area and is fearful of having a bowel movement, the surgeon often orders medication such as dextropropoxyphene hydrochloride (Darvon) or Darvon Compound (32 to 65 mg) to be taken a short time before a bowel movement is attempted. The patient needs careful nursing attention when attempting the first bowel movement, since it may cause dizziness and even fainting.

If a spontaneous bowel movement does not occur within 2 or 3 days postoperatively, laxatives are increased and an oil-retention enema followed by a cleansing enema may be given through a small rectal tube. The patient is advised to take a sitz bath after each bowel movement to keep the operative area clean and to relieve local irritation. This practice should be continued until a return visit to the physician (usually within 1 or 2 weeks).

Following a hemorrhoidectomy the patient is advised to avoid constipation by eating a diet containing adequate fruit and roughage, exercising moderately, drinking plenty of fluids, and establishing a regular time for daily bowel movements. Stool softeners or a mild laxative may be prescribed to be taken daily or every other day for some time.

Outcome criteria for the person who has had rectal surgery

The patient or significant others can:

1. Describe a plan to enhance evacuation of a soft stool including sufficient fluids, bulk-producing foods, and regular exercise.
2. Explain the rationale for thorough cleansing of the rectal area after each stool evacuation until healing has occurred.
3. State symptoms requiring medical follow-up (rectal

bleeding, continued pain on defecation, constipation, suppurative drainage on dressings).
4. State plans for regular follow-up care.

■ CANCER OF THE BOWEL

Malignant tumors of the large bowel and rectum are the most common forms of cancer in the United States. Approximately one fourth of all gastrointestinal tract cancers arise in the colon. Each year approximately 70,000 Americans are found to have cancer of the bowel, and there are approximately 39,000 deaths. The number of cases is thought to be increasing in frequency because of the increase in the life span. Although the cause of cancer of the colon is unknown, various carcinogens have been suggested such as food additives, bacteria, and stool bulk (roughage) as well as bowel transit time (bowel stasis). In addition isolated polyps are known to undergo malignant changes.[11] *Familial polyposis* therefore may predispose to the development of cancer of the lower bowel. Because in the early stages symptoms of cancer of the colon are vague and may be absent, it is now recommended that the yearly physical examination of persons over 40 years of age include a rectal examination for the presence of this disease. Since carcinoma of the lower bowel is more common in men than in women, it has also been recommended that all men over 40 years of age have this examination. In some cancer detection clinics, proctoscopic examinations are performed routinely on all men past 35 years of age. Seventy-five percent of the cancers of the lower bowel occur in the rectum and sigmoid colon.[30]

Early discovery of the growth and its immediate removal offer a fairly good chance for cure. In the beginning stage of the cancer growth the tumor is confined to the intestinal mucosa, gradually extending around the bowel to form a stricture and causing early symptoms of bowel obstruction. Eventually the cancer penetrates the wall of the colon and spreads either directly into the peritoneum or into abdominal organs or indirectly through the lymphatics into the surrounding lymph nodes and through the blood vessels to the liver and other structures.

Cancer of the rectum metastasizes slowly, since the tumor extends by direct extension through the rectal wall to surrounding tissues before metastasis through the lymphatic and venous systems occurs.

Anyone who develops a change in bowel patterns such as constipation, diarrhea, or alternating constipation and diarrhea, a change in the shape of the stool, or the passing of blood should consult a physician.

Clinical picture. Symptoms of cancer of the colon vary with the location of the growth. Carcinoma of the colon on the right side *(ascending colon)* usually is a large cauliflower-like growth. It causes severe anemia, nausea, vomiting, and alternating constipation and diarrhea. A mass is usually palpable on the right side of the abdomen. There are no symptoms of obstruction as a rule because the fecal contents in this portion of the colon are still liquid and able to flow past the growth.

Carcinoma of the colon on the left side *(descending colon)* often produces symptoms of partial obstruction because the stool is harder on that side. Although tumors in this area are usually smaller than those found in the colon on the right side, they proliferate fibrous tissue which, as it contracts, causes narrowing of the lumen of the bowel. Because the stool in the bowel on the left side is formed, it has difficulty passing by the tumor and through the stenosed area. Progressive constipation occurs, and the stool may be small or flattened, "pencil shaped," or "ribbon-shaped." Blood, mucus, and pus may be passed with the bowel movement. The abdomen may become distended, and rumbling of flatus and fluid may be heard.

The most common symptoms of cancer of the sigmoid colon and rectum are the passage of small amounts of bright red blood in the stool and an alteration in bowel habits. Either constipation or diarrhea may occur, or these two conditions may alternate. Pain does not occur until the disease is far advanced.

Carcinoma of the colon may cause a complete obstruction, and the acute symptoms of obstruction may be the first indication that anything is wrong. Occasionally the tumor perforates into the peritoneal cavity and peritonitis occurs before any other signs of illness have been noticed by the individual (p. 1285).

Diagnosis of cancer of the colon is made by physical examination, sigmoidoscopy, and barium enema examination. Cancer of the rectum can be accurately diagnosed by pathologic examination of a biopsy of the lesion taken during a proctoscopic examination.

Intervention. The treatment of cancer of the colon is always surgical, and the tumor, surrounding colon, and lymph nodes are resected. If possible the remaining portions of the bowel are anastomosed. If cancer of the ascending colon is found, the colon on the right side is entirely removed *(right colectomy)*, and the ileum is anastomosed to the transverse colon *(ileotransverse colostomy)*. Growths of the descending colon or upper sigmoid are removed by a *left colectomy*, and the remaining sigmoid is anastomosed to the transverse colon (p. 1280). Usually growths in the middle and lower third of the rectum require removal of the entire rectum (abdominoperineal resection, p. 1282), leaving the patient with a permanent colostomy. For growths in the upper third of the rectum it may be possible to resect that portion containing the tumor and then anastomose the remaining segments so that the anal sphincter is maintained and normal bowel evacuation is possible.

If the cancerous growth is such that it is not resectable, or if the growth has caused an obstruction with accompanying inflammation, an opening may be made into the cecum *(cecostomy)* or into the transverse colon *(transverse colostomy,* p. 1247) as a palliative measure to permit the escape of fecal contents. When the edema and the inflammation around the tumor subside, the growth is resected, the bowel sections are anastomosed, and the cecostomy or colostomy usually is closed.

■ HERNIA

A hernia is a protrusion of an organ or structure from its normal cavity through a congenital or acquired defect. Depending on its location, the hernia may contain peritoneal fat, a loop of bowel, a section of bladder, or a portion of the stomach. If the protruding structure of the organ can be returned by manipulation to its own cavity, it is called a *reducible* hernia. If it cannot, it is called an *irreducible* or an *incarcerated* hernia. The size of the defect through which the structure or organ passes (the neck of the hernia) determines largely whether the hernia can be reduced. When the blood supply to the structure within the hernia becomes occluded, the hernia is said to be *strangulated.*

□ Types of hernias

An *indirect inguinal hernia* is one in which a loop of intestine passes through the abdominal ring and follows the course of the spermatic cord into the inguinal canal (Fig. 58-2). The descent of the hernia may end in the inguinal canal, or it may proceed into the scrotum (and occasionally into the labia). It is caused by the intestines being forced by increased intraabdominal pressure into a congenital defect resulting from failure of the processus vaginalis to close after the descent of the testes in the male and after fixation of the ovaries in the female. Indirect hernias are much more common in men than in women. This higher incidence in men may be explained in part by their participation in more vigorous exercise and by the size of the testes, which must pass through the inguinal ring during fetal life.

A *direct inguinal hernia* is one that passes through the posterior inguinal wall. It is caused by increased intraabdominal pressure against a congenitally weak posterior inguinal wall. These hernias are more common in men. They are the most difficult to repair and are likely to recur after surgery.

A *femoral hernia* is one in which a loop of intestine passes through the femoral ring and down the femoral canal. It appears as a round bulge below the inguinal ligament and is thought to be due to a congenital weakness in the femoral ring. Increased intraabdominal pressure due to pregnancy or obesity probably causes the herniation through weakened muscle. Femoral hernias are more common in women than in men, and the incidence of strangulated hernia is high. This is thought to be because of the inclination of the female pelvis.

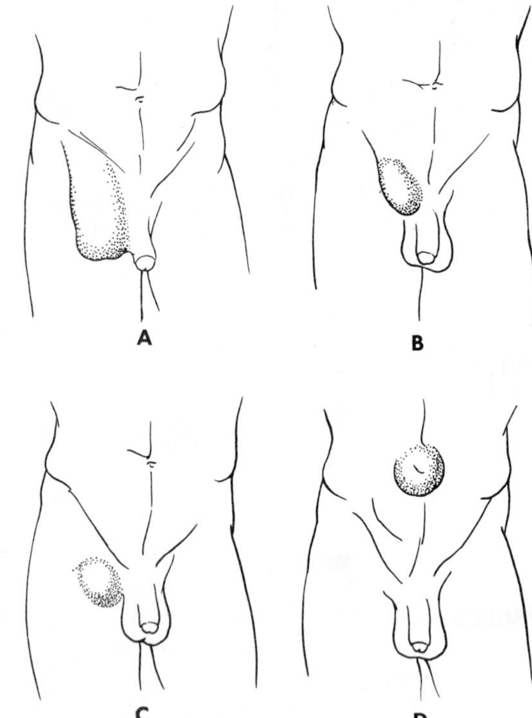

Fig. 58-2. Types of hernias. **A,** Large indirect inguinal hernia. **B,** Direct inguinal hernia. **C,** Femoral hernia. **D,** Umbilical hernia.

An *umbilical hernia* is one in which a loop of intestine passes through the umbilical ring. It is caused either by the failure of the umbilicus to close at birth or by a congenital defect in the umbilical scar, which opens in adult life when there is increased intraabdominal pressure such as occurs in pregnancy, intestinal obstruction, chronic cough, or chronic obstructive pulmonary disease (COPD). Infantile umbilical hernias occur frequently in nonwhite babies. Umbilical hernias that occur in adults are seen most often in elderly, obese women.

An *incisional hernia* is one that occurs through an old surgical incision. It is caused by the failure of the resected and approximated muscles and fascial tissues to heal properly because of wound infections, drains, or poor physical condition. As a result of increased intraabdominal pressure a portion of the intestine or other organs and tissues may protrude through the weakened scar.

Assessment. The person with a hernia complains of a lump in the groin, around the umbilicus, or protruding from an old surgical incision. The swelling may have always been present or it may have appeared suddenly after coughing, straining, lifting, or other vigorous exertion.

Palpation of the herniated area will reveal the contents of the sac as soft and nodular (omentum) or smooth and fluctuant (bowel). Fingertip palpation is utilized to feel the edges of the ring and its contents by inserting the examining fingertip into the ring and feeling for the impulse as the person coughs. At no time should the nurse attempt to replace (reduce) the sac in the ring, as the result may be the rupture of the strangulated contents or a reduction in the mass without relief of strangulation.

A femoral hernia may be palpated by placing the index finger over the femoral artery. The middle finger will then overlie the femoral vein and the ring finger overlies the femoral canal. As the person coughs, the nurse's fingertips will feel the sensation if the herniated sac is in the canal area.

A hernia may cause no symptoms except swelling that disappears when the person lies down and reappears on standing or coughing. If pain is present it may be due to local irritation of the parietal peritoneum or to traction on the omentum. An incarcerated hernia may become strangulated, causing severe pain and symptoms of intestinal obstruction such as nausea, vomiting, and distention. These complications require emergency surgery, and a portion of bowel may have to be resected if it has become gangrenous from impairment of its circulation.

Intervention. The person can very often reduce the hernia (return it to its normal postion) by lying down with the feet elevated or by lying in a tub of warm water and pushing the mass gently back toward the abdominal cavity. If the person's physical condition does not permit surgery, the physician sometimes advocates the use of a *truss* to keep the hernia reduced. However, this device is not a cure, and its use is somewhat rare today. A truss is a pad made of firm material that is placed over the opening through which the hernia protrudes and is held in place with a belt. The truss should be applied before getting out of bed and after the hernia has been reduced. If the hernia cannot be reduced, the truss should not be applied, and medical treatment should be sought.

The only cure for a hernia is surgical treatment. The herniating tissues are returned to the abdominal cavity, and the defect in the fascia or muscle is closed with sutures *(herniorrhaphy)*. To prevent recurrence of the hernia and to facilitate closure of the defect, a *hernioplasty* may be performed using fascia, filigree wire, tantalum mesh, stainless steel mesh, or a variety of plastic materials to strengthen the muscle wall.

The *preoperative* preparation for a hernia repair includes examination to detect any diseases of the respiratory system that might cause increased intraabdominal pressure postoperatively. A chronic cough due to excessive smoking or other causes or excessive sneezing due to an allergy might cause weakening of the repair before the incision has completely healed. The operation is postponed until the respiratory disorder is under control. The nurse should report to the surgeon any signs of incipient upper respiratory infection, since such an infection may occur after the patient has been examined.

In addition to good general *postoperative* care, the nurse who in caring for the patient who has had an operation for a hernia should prevent tension on the newly repaired tissues. Postoperatively the nurse is alert for signs of respiratory infection. If a cough occurs, medications are usually prescribed to depress the cough reflex. They are given as ordered to prevent paroxysms of coughing and subsequent strain on the repair. The patient is instructed to hold his hand firmly over the operative area when coughing or sneezing.

Since urinary retention may occur after a herniorrhaphy, appropriate nursing measures are taken to prevent the bladder from becoming overdistended. Catheterization is sometimes necessary. The patient is usually permitted to get out of bed to void on the operative day, and full ambulatory privileges are granted after the first postoperative day.

The person who has elective surgery for a hernia usually is permitted a full diet as soon as it is tolerated. If a spinal anesthetic is used and the abdominal cavity is not entered, there is usually no loss of peristalsis, and the patient is able to eat normally at once. If a general anesthetic is used, fluid and food are restricted until peristalsis returns. When an umbilical or a large incisional hernia has been repaired, a nasogastric tube attached to suction may be used to prevent postoperative vomiting and distention with subsequent strain on the suture line. Fluids are given parenterally, and food and fluids by mouth are restricted. Abdominal distention following a hernia repair is reported at one. A nasogastric tube may be passed or a rectal tube inserted. Mild cathartics may be prescribed, since straining during defecation increases intraabdominal pressure and should be avoided.

Because of postoperative inflammation, edema, and hemorrhage, swelling of the scrotum often occurs after repair of an indirect inguinal hernia. This complication is extremely painful, and any movement of the patient causes discomfort. It is difficult to turn, to get into or out of bed, and to walk. Ice bags help to relieve pain. The scrotum is usually supported with a suspensory or is elevated on a rolled towel. Narcotics may sometimes be necessary for pain, and antibiotics may be administered to prevent the development of epididymitis. When a patient has a swollen scrotum, the nurse must check his voiding carefully. He may delay voiding because moving about increases pain and discomfort. Ecchymosis of the lower abdominal wall or upper thigh may occur after extensive manipulation during surgery. The patient can be reassured that this will fade in a few days. Sexual functioning is not affected.

Wound infection occurs occasionally. It interferes with healing, and if it is not recognized early and treated adequately, the surgical repair may weaken. Infections are treated with antibiotics systemically and with dressings or packs locally.

The patient who has had elective surgery for a hernia is restricted from strenuous activity for at least 3 weeks and will need to consult the surgeon about returning to work. If the work entails lifting, the physician needs to know this, and good body mechanics are reviewed with the patient before discharge.

REFERENCES AND SELECTED READINGS

1. American Academy of Pediatrics: Report of the Committee on Infectious Diseases, ed. 17, Evanston, Ill., 1974, The Academy.
2. American Cancer Society, Inc.: 1977 Cancer facts and figures, New York, 1977, The Society.
3. Beahrs, O. H., and Adson, M. A.: Ileal pouch with ileostomy rather than ileostomy alone, Am. J. Surg. **125**:154-158, 1973
4. Beeson, P. B., and McDermott, W., editors: Textbook of medicine, ed. 14, Philadelphia, 1975, W. B. Saunders Co.
5. Binder, S. C., and Katz, B.: Regional enteritis: a review of the literature, Ohio State Med. J. **73**:661-666, 1977.
6. Bockus, H. L.: Gastroenterology, ed. 3, vol. 1, Philadelphia, 1974, W. B. Saunders Co.
7. Braasch, J. W.: The surgical treatment of obesity, Surg. Clin. North Am. **51**:667-672, 1971.
8. Burkitt, D. P., Walker, A. R. P., and Painter, N. S.: Dietary fiber and diseases, J.A.M.A. **229**:1068-1073, 1974.
9. Byrne, J. J., and Hennessy, V. L.: Diverticulitis of the colon, Surg. Clin. North Am. **52**:991-999, 1972.
10. *Chandler, J. G.: Surgical treatment of massive obesity, Postgrad. Med. **56**:124-132, 1974.
11. Cole, J. W.: Carcinogens and carcinogenesis in the colon, Hosp. Practice **8**:123-130, 1973.
12. *Cole, W. H.: Cancer of the colon and rectum, Surg. Clin. North Am. **52**:871-881, 1972.
13. Cole, W. H., and Zollinger, R. M.: Textbook of surgery, ed. 9, New York, 1970, Appleton-Century-Crofts.
14. *deLuca, J.: The ulcerative colitis personality, Nurs. Clin. North Am. **5**:22-23, 1970.
15. Dworken, H. J.: The alimentary tract, Philadelphia, 1974, W. B. Saunders Co.
16. *Edwards, H.: Crohns' disease, Nurs. Mirror **70**:24-31, 1970.
17. Ferguson, J. H.: Acute intestinal obstruction, Practitioner **209**:164-169, 1972.
18. Gianella, R. A., Broitman, S. A., and Zamcheck, N.: Salmonella enteritis. I. Role of reduced gastric secretion in pathogenesis. II. Fulminant diarrhea in and effects on the small intestine, Am. J. Dig. Dis. **16**:1000-1013, 1971.
19. *Given, B., Simmons, S.: Gastroenterology in clinical nursing, ed. 2, St. Louis, 1975, The C. V. Mosby Co.
20. Herter, F. P.: Preparation of the bowel for surgery, Surg. Clin. North Am. **52**:859-869, 1972.
21. *Heydman, A.: Intestinal bypass for obesity, Am. J. Nurs. **74**:1102-1104, 1974.
22. High fiber diets and colonic disease, Am. J. Nurs. **77**:255, 1977.
23. Krupp, M., and Chatton, M.: Current medical diagnosis and treatment, Los Altos, Calif., 1976, Lange Medical Publications.
24. Matt, R., and Nundy, S.: Rectal carcinoma, abdominoperineal and anterior resection, Surg. Clin. North Am. **54**:741-749, July 1974.
25. Nankin, P., Jacobson, M., and Evans, R.: Hiatus hernia, Surg. Clin. North Am. **51**:1347-1353, 1971.
26. Painter, N.: Diverticular disease of the colon: a bane of the elderly, Geriatrics **31**:89-94, 1976.
27. Payne, J. H., DeWinda, L., Schwab, C. E., et al.: Surgical treatment of morbid obesity: sixteen years of experience: Arch. Surg. **106**:432-437, 1973.
28. *Plumley, P. F., and Francis, B.: Dietary management of diverticular disease, J. Am. Diet. Assoc. **63**:527-530, 1973
29. Rhoads, J. E.: The control of large bowel cancer, Cancer **36**:2314-2318, 1975.
30. Robinson, C.: Normal and therapeutic nutrition, ed. 15, New York, 1974, Macmillan, Inc.
31. Sabiston, D. C., editor: Christopher's textbook of surgery, ed. 11, Philadelphia, 1977, W. B. Saunders Co.
32. Schwartz, A. I., et al.: Principles of surgery, ed. 2, New York, 1974, McGraw-Hill Book Co.
33. Scott, H. W., Jr., Dean, R., Shull, H. J., et al.: Considerations in use of jejunoileal bypass in patients with morbid obesity, Ann. Surg. **177**:723-735, 1973.
34. Sheridan, J. L.: Obstructions of the intestinal tract, Nurs. Clin. North Am. **10**:147-155, 1975.
35. Sleisenger, M. H., and Fordtran, J. S.: Gastrointestinal diseases: pathology-diagnosis-management, ed. 2, Philadelphia, 1978, W. B. Saunders Co.
36. Smith, A., ed.: Diverticular disease, Clin. Gastroenterol. **4**: 3-219, Jan. 1975.
37. Spiro, H. M.: Clinical gastroenterology, ed. 2, New York, 1977, Macmillan, Inc.
38. *Werrin, M., and Kronick, D.: Salmonella control in hospitals, Am. J. Nurs. **66**:528-531, 1966.
39. Williams, S. R.: Nutrition and diet therapy, ed. 3, St. Louis, 1977, The C. V. Mosby Co.
40. Wintrobe, M. M., et al., editors: Harrison's principles of internal medicine, ed. 8, New York, 1977, McGraw-Hill Book Co.
41. Wright, B.: Physical disability, New York, 1960, Harper & Row, Publishers.
42. *Yahle, M.: An ostomy information clinic, a community resource, Nurs. Clin. North Am. **11**:457-468, 1976.
43. Zimmerman, W. J., and Zinter, D. E.: The prevalence of trichiniasis in swine in the United States, 1966-1970, HSMHA Health Rep. **86**:937-945, 1971.

*References preceded by an asterisk are particularly well suited for student reading.

59

Problems of the urinary system

PAULA LAMBRECHT MILLER

Disease of the urinary system is a major cause of morbidity and a significant cause of mortality in the United States. In 1975 disease of the urinary system was reported as a causative factor in approximately 43,000 deaths, of these 38% were from malignancy, 19% from nephritis and nephrosis, 11% from kidney infections, and 3% from hypertrophy of the prostate gland. These figures indicate that mortality from disease of the urinary system is generally associated with destruction of renal tissue. When disease involves the kidneys, renal function is directly threatened. When disease occurs in the lower urinary tract, it not only affects tissue locally but can threaten renal function through spread of infection and obstruction of urine flow. The primary objective for treatment of disease in any part of the urinary tract should be early detection and adequate therapy directed toward preserving or improving renal function, for without renal function life can continue for only a few days.

During the past decade some of the most striking developments in treatment of individuals with disease of the urinary system have been in the area of prolonging life after renal function has ceased. Dialysis and transplantation have given hundreds of people each year a continued, though somewhat uncertain, life expectancy. Technical, physical, and psychosocial components of the new life style of these individuals demand the nurse's attention.

Nurses can assist in significantly reducing the morbidity of the urinary system. This can be achieved through increasing public awareness of preventive measures, assisting in early detection of signs and symptoms of disease, and providing long-term care to the growing population of chronically ill individuals with urinary tract disease. This chapter defines common problems of the person with disease of the urinary system and identifies requirements for nursing care prior to and during the acute and chronic phases of illness.

INFECTION OF URINARY TRACT

Urinary tract infections are a significant source of morbidity in the United States. These infections contribute to illness during the acute infection and also are significant in the development of chronic renal failure. Infection occurs in both acute and chronic stages in all portions of the urinary tract.

Table 59-1 summarizes factors contributing to infection of the urinary tract. Although the great majority of noncomplicated urinary infections are asymptomatic and clear spontaneously, there remains a portion significant enough to warrant consideration as a health problem. There is no controversy among those practicing preventive health care regarding the question of the need for screening of asymptomatic infections; however, there exists difficulty in identifying the specific risk groups in which the detection and treatment of these infections yield significant improvement in the person's health. As the health care of our population becomes more oriented toward prevention of health problems, specific target populations will be better defined and the number of screening programs for asymptomatic urinary tract infection will increase.

Females seem more predisposed to urinary tract infections than males. Factors postulated in their higher infection rates include a shorter urethra with a close proximity to the rectum and the lack of prostatic fluid protection present in the male. Infection rates for females approximate 1% of schoolaged girls and 4% of women through childbearing years.[38] Incidence of infection in females increases directly with sexual activity and aging. Pregnancy does not seem to increase infection rates, although spontaneous clearing of infections is decreased during pregnancy and there is higher incidence of acute kidney infections progressing from the lower urinary tract.[70]

Structural and functional abnormalities of the urinary tract, obstruction to the flow of urine, and impaired bladder innervation promote infection of the urinary tract. Mechanisms involved include stasis of urine, which provides a culture medium for bacteria; reflux of infected urine higher into the urinary tract; and increasing hydrostatic pressure.

Certain chronic health problems predispose to uri-

Table 59-1. Risk factors associated with development of urinary tract infection

Risk factor	Common examples
Female population	
Structural abnormality	Strictures Incompetent ureterovesicle junction anomalies
Obstruction	Tumors Prostatic hypertrophy Calculi Iatrogenic causes
Impaired bladder innervation	Congenital spinal cord malformation Spinal cord injury Multiple sclerosis
Chronic disease	Gout Diabetes mellitus Hypertension Sickle cell disease Chronic renal disease
Instrumentation	Catheterization Diagnostic procedures

nary tract infection through changing the metabolism of tissues, creating extrarenal obstructions, and altering the function and structure of kidney tissue. Common among these health problems are diabetes mellitus, gout, hypertension, polycystic kidney disease, and glomerulonephritis.

Instrumentation of the urinary tract is associated with high rates of infection. Catheterization, even when performed without break in asepsis, results in significant infection of the bladder. Nosocomial infections account for a sizable percentage of all urinary tract infections. Prevention and control of all urinary tract infections can be most significantly influenced through a lowering of this nosocomial infection rate.

Infections of the lower urinary tract involve the urinary bladder (cystitis) and the urethra (urethritis). In the upper urinary tract infection involves the kidney (pyelonephritis). The etiologic factors and general preventive and management principles are the same for infection anywhere in the urinary tract. Pyelonephritis is discussed in greater detail on p. 1319.

Prevention. Three considerations are important in preventing infection of the lower urinary tract: (1) preventing or minimizing morbidity that can accompany these infections, (2) preventing recurrence of the infection, and (3) preventing renal damage from untreated, inadequately treated, or ascending infection. Since individuals with lower urinary tract infections seek medical attention as a result of symptoms or are identified through routine urinalysis or screening of populations at high risk, both education of the public and community health case finding assist in decreasing urinary tract infection and its complications. Public education should center on (1) the need for prompt medical attention for symptoms, (2) the need to continue with drug therapy even though symptoms abate, (3) the importance of follow-up care and repeated urine cultures, and (4) maintenance of fluid intake of 3 to 4 liters per day if the person's health permits.

Clinical picture. The symptoms that bring the person to medical attention typically include urgency, burning on urination (dysuria), and slight to gross hematuria. Most persons, however, are asymptomatic or minimally symptomatic, the infection being identified only on routine examination of the urine. Bacteriuria and positive urine cultures serve as the basis for diagnosing lower urinary tract infections. Growth of a single pathogen in excess of 1×10^5 organisms/ml of urine in a properly obtained and stored midstream specimen (p. 1325) indicates infection. The organisms most frequently infecting the urinary tract are those normally inhabiting the intestine; these include *Escherichia coli*, *Proteus*, and *Enterobacter*. Drug-resistant strains of *Staphylococcus* and *Pseudomonas*, along with various other organisms commonly found in hospitals, are frequently those involved in nosocomial urinary tract infections.

Intervention. Treatment goals for lower urinary tract infections include sterilizing the urine and identifying any illness or urinary tract abnormality that may be contributing to the infection. After culture and sensitivity studies a 10- to 14-day course of drug therapy is instituted. It is crucial that urine culture be obtained prior to initiating drug therapy to ensure appropriateness of antimicrobial medication and to decrease the development of resistant strains of organisms. The urine should be recultured every few months during the following year to reconfirm urine sterility.

Even with the first documented urinary tract infection in a male or a child, it has been recommended that a urologic workup including an intravenous pyelogram and voiding cystogram be performed. This workup should be performed on a woman with the second documented urinary tract infection or when infection cannot be cleared.[50] This recommendation is based on the premise that urinary tract infections are not common in males and children and that a significant portion of infections in these populations and in women with infections that do not clear with drug therapy involve abnormality of the urinary tract.

Medications commonly used in the treatment of urinary tract infection include urinary antiseptics such as sulfisoxazole (Gantrisin) or nitrofurantoin (Furadantin) and systemic antibiotics. Sulfonamides are widely used; they are usually effective against the organisms causing a large percentage of urinary tract infections, are safe, and are less likely than most systemic antibiotics to contribute to growth of resistant organisms. Urinary antiseptics that contain analgesic properties may be prescribed for the patient when burning is a problem.

Additional treatment includes increasing fluid intake to 3 to 4 liters per day unless contraindicated. Increased fluids help to dilute the urine, which lessens irritations and burning, and provide a continual flow of urine to discourage stasis and multiplication of bacteria in the urinary tract. Sitz baths may provide comfort for individuals with urethritis. Patient education concerning the problem, the requirements for drug therapy, and follow-up care should facilitate early identification of recurrence and completion of drug regimens for eradication of bacteria. Success in both of these areas is directly dependent on patient follow-through and comprise the means by which the patient is able to assist in overcoming this health problem.

For individuals with chronic bacteriuria, urine acidifying agents may be prescribed. The effect of these medications is to provide a less suitable environment for bacterial growth and to enhance the effectiveness of antibiotic and urinary antiseptics. When bacteriuria becomes constant, prophylaxis may be undertaken with antimicrobial drugs.

Outcome criteria for the person with urinary tract infection

The patient will:

1. Have relief of symptoms.
2. Show no damage in kidney function; current damage is arrested.
3. Have sterile urine or bacterial urine count of less than 1,000 organisms/ml.
4. Have identified or corrected any disease or abnormality that would contribute to reinfection or relapse.

The patient or significant other can:

1. State signs and symptoms of lower urinary tract infection.
2. Explain when and how to take prescribed medication.
3. State plan for follow-up urine cultures.
4. State rationale and means of increasing fluid intake to 3 to 4 liters/day.

■ CONGENITAL MALFORMATIONS OF URINARY TRACT

Variation from the normal anatomic structure of the urinary tract occurs in about 10% to 15% of the population.[44] These deviations range in severity from minor, easily correctable anomalies to those incompatible with life.

The following congenital malformations are included in this text because of their potential influence on urinary tract function in adult life. The reader is referred to other specialty texts for information about additional defects that can be repaired in early life without expected residual urologic sequelae or those that result in death before adulthood.[59,61]

Partial or complete duplication of the ureters is a relatively common anomaly of the urinary tract. Unilateral duplication occurs in about one of 200 births, while bilateral duplication occurs in about one in 1,200 births.[44] This defect includes duplication of the renal pelvis as well as the ureters. A *complete duplication* refers to the occurrence of two separate ureters from one kidney. More common is a *partial duplication* in which the duplicate ureters unite at some point between the kidney and bladder. The clinical significance of duplication of the ureter is dependent on the presence of obstruction or reflux. Obstruction at the point where the two ureters join or reflux from one ureter into the other in a partial duplication may lead to dilation of the ureter, hydronephrosis, and persistent or recurrent urinary tract infections. In the case of complete duplication the ureter draining the upper pole of the kidney may open either into the bladder or into the vulva, urethra, or seminal vesicle. If the ureter drains ectopically (outside the bladder), incontinence and obstruction are generally present. Surgical intervention when necessitated by obstruction or reflux may include reimplantation of an ectopic ureter into the bladder, resection of the duplicated ureter, resection of the hydronephrotic portion of the kidney, or nephrectomy if severe renal damage has occurred. *Triplication of the ureters* occurs infrequently, and management is the same as for duplication.

Horseshoe kidney refers to fusion of the kidneys, usually at their lower poles. The incidence varies between one in 600 and one in 1,800 births.[44] Potential problems that may arise because of anterior angulation of the ureters include stasis, hydronephrosis, and possible calculus formation. Surgical treatment when indicated because of obstruction consists of division of the fused part. Cases uncomplicated by obstruction or calculi are generally not treated surgically.

Hydroureter, dilation of the ureter, may result from obstruction in the lower urinary tract, from vesicoureteral reflux, or from an atonic lower ureteral segment, all of which may be congenital. In some cases of severe ureteral dilation peristalsis in the lower ureter is decreased secondary to atony. Urinary diversion for a time may allow the ureter to become amenable to future repair and reimplantation into the bladder. If such attempts fail, urinary diversion is permanent. Congenital deficiency of abdominal musculature, or prune belly syndrome, is rare and includes extreme hydronephrosis

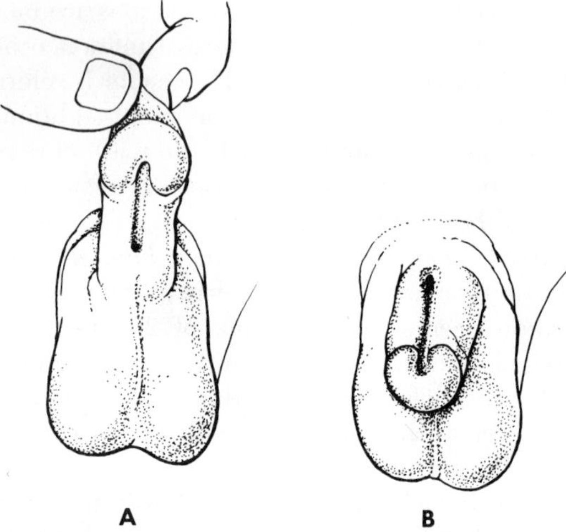

Fig. 59-1. A, Hypospadias. **B,** Epispadias.

and dilated ureters. Treatment usually necessitates permanent urinary diversion.

Exstrophy of the bladder and *epispadias* are developmental anomalies that often occur together. They result from failure of the midline to close adequately during fetal development and may vary a great deal in their severity.

Epispadias is a failure of closure on the dorsal surface of the penis and may extend from the glans to the perineum (Fig. 59-1, *B*). The defect often extends to the urinary sphincter, causing incontinence. If surgical correction involving the urinary sphincter is not successful, urinary diversion may be performed.

Exstrophy of the bladder, which occurs in approximately one in 40,000 births, may consist only of a small fistula leading to the surface of the abdominal wall that drains urine, or it may be so extensive that most of the interior of the bladder is everted on the outer abdominal wall. Usually the sphincter muscles of the urethra are faulty and epispadias is present. The muscles below the umbilicus are separated and the pubic rami are not joined. Operations for exstrophy of the bladder may include attempts to reconstruct sphincter muscles of the urethra and to close the bladder and abdominal walls. If satisfactory repair cannot be made, as is frequently the case in complete exstrophy, permanent urinary diversion may be necessary. If untreated the bladder wall undergoes squamous metaplastic changes that predispose the patient to adenocarcinoma in later life.

Hypospadias is a common anomaly in which the urethra opens in the male at any ventral point on the penis between the glans and perineum (Fig. 59-2, *A*). It is almost always accompanied by *chordee,* fibrous bands causing curvature of the penis. In the female the urethra opens into the vagina. Very slight anomalies require no intervention; when treatment is indicated, surgical reconstruction of the urethra (and release of chordee in the male) are done. Postoperative strictures may occur, which require further treatment.

Congenital malformations of the spinal cord such as myelomeningocele and sacral agenesis frequently cause bladder dysfunction due to disturbances of innervation (neurogenic bladder). Complications arising from neurogenic bladder dysfunction include infection, hydronephrosis and calculus formation. Treatment is aimed at controlling incontinence and preserving renal function and may include such methods as credé of the bladder, intermittent catheterization, systemic medications, or urinary diversion or other forms of surgical treatment.

For details in the care of the person having surgical treatment for the above malformations, see specialized nursing texts.[74]

TRAUMA TO URINARY TRACT

Assessing intactness of urinary tract structures must be part of the evaluation of any person with traumatic injury to the lower trunk. Injuries particularly related to urinary tract damage include fractures of the pelvis and sharp blows to the body. Pelvic fractures may result in *bladder perforation* and *ureteral* and *urethral tearing.* Following these injuries urinary output may be scant or absent, the urine may be bloody, and symptoms of peritonitis may appear. Treatment is directed toward stabilizing the patient and surgically repairing the perforation or laceration. Prior to stabilizing the patient, a cystotomy may be performed to provide urinary drainage when injury involves the bladder or urethra.

A sharp blow to the body, particularly to the lower back, may result in *contusion, tearing,* or *rupture of a kidney.* Signs and symptoms include hematuria and pain and tenderness of the upper abdominal quadrant and flank on the involved side. Signs of shock may be present or absent depending on the extent of hemorrhage. Treatment includes control of bleeding, prevention of shock, and promoting drainage of the urinary tract. Vital signs, fluid balance records, and hematocrit level are monitored to assess hemostasis. Complaints of pain may indicate developing ureteral colic, likely signifying obstruction of the ureter by a clot. Surgical intervention is required to control severe hemorrhage. Spontaneous healing of the kidney is otherwise permitted. Bed rest is maintained until gross hematuria clears; thereafter activity is progressed according to continued absence of hematuria.

OBSTRUCTION OF URINARY SYSTEM

Obstruction of any part of the urinary system from the kidney to the urethra will generate pressure that may cause functional and anatomic damage to the renal parenchyma. When any part of the urinary tract is obstructed, urine collects behind the obstruction producing a dilation of the structure. Muscles of the affected area contract in an effort to push the urine around the obstruction. Partial obstruction may produce slow dilation of structures above the obstruction without functional impairment. As the obstruction increases, however, pressure builds up in the tubular system behind the obstruction causing a backflow of urine. The urine backup eventually reaches the kidney causing dilation of the kidney pelvis *(hydronephrosis)*. Pressure buildup in the renal pelvis leads to destruction of kidney tissue and eventual renal failure.

With obstruction urine flow is decreased even to the point of stagnation. This stagnant urine provides a good culture medium for bacterial growth, and rarely is obstruction seen without some infection. The specific effects that occur with obstruction will depend on the location of the obstruction, the extent of obstruction (partial or complete), and the duration. Obstruction in the *lower* urinary tract causes bladder distention. If this is prolonged, muscle fibers become hypertrophied and *diverticuli* (herniated sacs of bladder mucosa) develop between the hypertrophied muscle bands. Since the diverticulum holds stagnant urine, infection often occurs, and bladder stones may form. Causes of obstruction of the lower urinary tract include bladder neoplasms, urethral stricture, calculi, tumors, or benign prostatic hypertrophy (BPH).

Obstruction of the *upper* urinary tract leads even more quickly to hydronephrosis because of the small size of the ureters and kidney pelvis. Increased pressure causes partial ischemia of arteries between the renal cortex and medulla and dilation of the renal tubules leading to tubular damage. Stasis of urine in the dilated pelvis predisposes to infection and calculi, which add to the renal damage. Some urine can backflow up the renal tubule into the veins and lymphatics as a compensatory mechanism to prevent kidney damage. The unaffected kidney then takes on increased elimination of waste products. With prolonged obstruction the unaffected kidney hypertrophies and may function as effectively alone as both kidneys did before the obstruction. Obstruction of both kidneys leads to renal failure (p. 1327).

Causes of ureteral obstruction include calculi, trauma, nephroptosis ("floating" or "dropped" kidney), an enlarged lymph node (as in lymphosarcoma, reticulum cell sarcoma, or Hodgkin's disease), or a congenital anomaly. Obstruction in the kidney can occur at the tubule level (in the form of casts or inflammation) or in the pelvis from calculi, ptosis, or polycystic disease.

Clinical picture. Hydronephrosis can occur without any symptoms as long as kidney function is adequate and urine can drain. An acute upper urinary tract obstruction will cause pain, nausea, vomiting, local tenderness, spasm of the abdominal muscles, and a mass in the kidney region. The pain is caused by the stretching of the tissues and by hyperperistalsis. Since the amount of pain is proportionate to the rate of stretching, a slowly developing hydronephrosis may cause only a dull flank pain, whereas a sudden blockage of the ureter such as may occur from a stone causes a severe stabbing (colicky) pain in the flank or abdomen. The pain may radiate to the genitalia and thigh and is caused by the increased peristaltic action of the smooth muscle of the ureter in an effort to dislodge the obstruction and force urine past it.

The nausea and vomiting frequently associated with acute ureteral obstruction are caused by a reflex reaction to the pain and will usually be relieved as soon as pain is relieved. A markedly dilated kidney, however, may press on the stomach causing continued gastrointestinal symptoms. If the renal function has been seriously impaired, nausea and vomiting may be symptoms of impending uremia. (See p. 1328 for discussion of uremia and renal failure.)

When the bladder is distended from lower urinary tract obstruction, the person will experience lower abdominal discomfort and a feeling of the need to void although he or she is unable to do so. The bladder may be palpated above the symphysis pubis. With partial obstruction such as by benign prostatic hypertrophy the man first complains of increasing urinary frequency because the bladder fails to empty completely at each voiding and therefore refills more quickly to the amount that causes the urge to void (usually 250 to 500 ml). Nocturia may also be present.

Diagnostic examinations may include cystoscopy and retrograde pyelography (p. 1240) to identify the source of the obstruction. Selection of other diagnostic tests will depend on the probable cause.

Intervention. When obstruction occurs the treatment consists of reestablishing adequate drainage from the urinary system. This may be temporarily accomplished by placing a catheter above the point of obstruction. Sometimes surgery must be performed to insert a catheter (nephrostomy, ureterostomy, suprapubic cystostomy). Later, definitive treatment is dependent on the cause. The infection is treated with antibiotics, fluids, and rest. Urinary antiseptics may also be given.

The person with a sudden obstruction is frequently acutely ill and may have severe colic but will not be able to remain in bed until the pain has been relieved. It is not unusual to see a person with acute renal colic walking the floor "doubled up" and vomiting. Narcotics such as morphine and meperidine and antispasmodic drugs such as propantheline bromide (Pro-Banthine) and belladonna preparations are usually necessary to relieve severe colicky pain. After narcotics have been given, the patient will be dizzy and must be protected from injury. As the pain eases the patient can usually be made relatively comfortable in bed. As soon as the nausea subsides large amounts of fluids are urged.

Care of the patient requiring urologic surgery. The basic needs of the patient requiring urologic surgery are the same as those of any other surgical patient. Special emphasis must be placed on promotion of ventilation and adequate urinary output, prevention of distention and hemorrhage, and attention to drainage tubes and dressings.

Ventilation. Surgery of the kidney or upper ureters usually involves a flank incision that can influence respiratory status. Because the incision is directly below the diaphragm, deep breathing is painful and the patient is reluctant to take deep breaths or to move about. Splinting of the chest is common and therefore atelectasis or other respiratory complications must be guarded against. In addition, because of the placement of the incision there is a greater incisional pull every time the person moves, as compared with an abdominal incision. The patient is often reluctant to turn in bed or to get up to ambulate. Most patients will be more comfortable turning themselves if they are given time, side rails to hold onto, and encouragement. Incisional pain usually requires a narcotic every 3 to 4 hours for 24 to 48 hours after surgery, and turning, ambulation, and breathing exercises can be planned to maximize the effect of the analgesics. Patients may lie on the affected side unless a nephrostomy tube is in place. Even then they can be tilted to the affected side with pillows placed at the back for support. It must be ascertained that the tube is not kinked and that there is no traction on it.

Urinary output. The urinary output is monitored carefully for several days postoperatively to ascertain adequate renal functioning and drainage. The output should be at least 50 ml/hour, preferably greater in order to prevent urinary stasis and subsequent infection. A urinary output of 20 to 30 ml/hour in a patient with satisfactory fluid intake (at least 1,200 ml/day) and in the absence of signs of urinary retention is reported immediately to the physician. Urinary output includes drainage from nephrostomy or cystostomy tubes, urethral or ureteral catheters, and an estimate from urine-soaked dressings. Daily weights are compared with the preoperative weight and with each other to identify fluid retention.

Distention. Following kidney surgery most patients have some abdominal distention that may be due in part to pressure on the stomach and intestinal tract during surgery. Patients who have had renal colic prior to surgery frequently develop paralytic ileus postoperatively. This condition may be related to the reflex gastrointestinal tract symptoms caused by postoperative pain. Because of the problem of abdominal distention following renal surgery, food and fluids by mouth are often restricted for 24 to 48 hours postoperatively. By the fourth postoperative day most patients tolerate a regular diet. Fluids are usually forced to 3,000 ml/day.

Hemorrhage. Hemorrhage may follow such operative procedures as prostatectomy, nephrolithotomy, or nephrectomy. It occurs most often when the highly vascular parenchyma of the kidney has been incised. The bleeding may occur on the day of surgery, or it may occur 8 to 12 days postoperatively, during the period when tissue sloughing normally occurs with healing. The presence of bright red blood on the dressing or in the urine is reported immediately to the physician. The patient is observed for signs of shock. Since many patients with urologic disease have hypertension, the blood pressure may be relatively high but still represent a marked drop for the individual. Comparisons should therefore be made with baseline data.

If hemorrhage occurs, a pressure dressing is applied over the incision while awaiting the physician's arrival. Measures to prevent shock are instituted (p. 214). Several liters of sterile physiologic saline solution for irrigation should be available.

Dressings. There may be large amounts of urinary drainage following urologic surgery except after nephrectomy. The drainage may be pink or dark red but should not be bright red. If the surgery involves a flank incision, drainage is usually the heaviest on the posterior edge of the dressing because of gravity flow. It is important therefore to turn the patient on the side opposite the surgery to examine the posterior edge of the dressing. When a suprapubic incision is present, drainage is heaviest on the side and in the inguinal region.

The dressings are usually held in place by Montgomery straps and must be changed frequently. Urinary drainage irritates the skin, has an unpleasant odor, and leads to discomfort. If a drain is present, the end of the drain should be placed over dressings, then covered with additional dressings to absorb the drainage. If a drainage tube is present, presence of large amounts of drainage on the dressing with little drainage coming from the tube indicates blockage of the tube. If a large amount of drainage is present, a disposable drainage bag used for urinary stomas (p. 1266) may be applied over the drainage site.

Drainage tubes. A catheter is usually inserted during surgery to drain urine from the operative area and permit healing to occur. Different types of drainage tubes may be inserted, and each tube is connected to a sepa-

If the stone has passed to the lower third of the ureter, it can sometimes be removed by *manipulation*. Special catheters with corkscrew tips, expanding baskets, and loops are passed through the cystoscope, and an attempt is made to "snare" the stone. This procedure is performed with the patient under anesthesia. The aftercare of a patient on whom manipulation has been carried out is the same as that following cystoscopy. Any signs suggestive of peritonitis or a decreased urinary output are carefully watched for, since the ureter occasionally is perforated during manipulation.

Surgery. Surgical intervention is indicated when a large stone (greater than 1 cm) is producing pain, obstruction, or infection. The operation for removal of a stone from the ureter is a *ureterolithotomy.* A radiograph is taken immediately preceding surgery, since the stone may have moved, and it is desirable to make the incision into the ureter directly over the stone. If the stone is in the lower third of the ureter a rectus incision is made. If it is in the upper two thirds a flank approach is used. If the patient has a ureteral stricture that causes stones to form, a plastic operation to relieve the stricture may be carried out as part of the operation.

Removal of a stone through or from the renal pelvis is known as a *pyelolithotomy.* Removal of a stone through the parenchyma is a *nephrolithotomy* (Fig. 59-2). Occasionally the kidney may have to be split from end to end (a kidney split) to remove the stone. Patients in whom such a split is done may have severe hemorrhage following surgery.

Bladder stones may be removed through a suprapubic incision, or they may be crushed with a lithotrite (stone crusher) that is passed transurethrally. This procedure is known as a *litholapaxy.* Following bladder stone removal, the bladder may be irrigated (intermittently or constantly) with an acid solution such as magnesium and sodium citrate (G solution) or Renacidin to counteract the alkalinity caused by the infection and to help wash out the remaining particles of stone. If there has been a suprapubic incision, the care of the incision is similar to that following a suprapubic prostatectomy. (See p. 1306 for care of the patient requiring urologic surgery.)

Long-term care. Persons who have recurrent renal calculi benefit from ongoing prophylactic therapy, which is determined by the type of stone being produced. *All* persons with recurrent renal stones should drink fluids in sufficient quantity to produce very dilute urine and nocturia. This may amount to a daily intake of up to 4 to 5 liters of fluid.[58] The purpose of the increased fluid intake is to rinse away any precipitates that can serve as a nidus for stone formation.

Any underlying identifiable cause of calciuria is treated to prevent recurrence of *calcium* stones. Hydrochlorothiazide (HCTZ) in doses of 50 mg/twice a day may be prescribed for persons with hypercalciuria to decrease urinary excretion of calcium. Persons receiving HCTZ therapy must be monitored carefully for signs of electrolyte imbalances.

As previously stated, more than 50% of calcium stones are idiopathic. Foods high in calcium are sometimes restricted, but a very-low-calcium diet is usually unsatisfactory because it is unpalatable. The solubility of oxalate salts is not pH dependent; therefore manipulation of pH is not useful. Sodium or potassium phosphate, 1.5 to 2.0 g/day, may be prescribed to decrease urinary calcium.

Phosphatic calculi develop in alkaline urine; therefore their prevention depends on keeping the urine acid and preventing urinary tract infection. Medications such as ascorbic acid or ammonium chloride may be given for a time to increase urine acidity.

The Shorr regimen has given beneficial results in the prevention of phosphatic calculi. A diet containing only 1,300 mg of phosphorus daily is prescribed, and 40 ml of aluminum hydroxide gel are taken after meals and at bedtime. The aluminum combines with the excess phosphorus, causing it to be excreted through the bowel instead of through the kidney, thus decreasing the possibility of stone formation. Constipation frequently results from this regimen.

Prophylaxis for *uric acid* stones consists in alkalinizing the urine by the administration of sodium bicarbonate and acetazolamide (Diamox) sufficient to maintain a urine pH of 6.0 to 6.5. Allopurinol (Zyloprim) may be prescribed to inhibit synthesis of uric acid.

Outcome criteria for the person with recurrent renal calculi

The person or significant others can:

1. Describe a plan to achieve a daily fluid intake of 4 to 5 liters, sufficient to maintain a dilute urine.
2. Describe the need to be as active as possible and prevent long periods of immobilization.
3. Plan menus to include any dietary restrictions.
4. State name, dosage, desired action, and side effects of medications prescribed to acidify or alkalinize the urine.
5. State plans for follow-up care:
   a. Describe signs of recurrence of calculi (pain in costovertebral angle or radiating anteriorly to external genitalia).
   b. Describe assessment and prevention of urinary tract infection.

□ Tumors of the kidney

Malignant renal tumors, primarily adenocarcinomas, account for 3% of all cancers. Small benign renal tumors (adenomas) may occur without causing significant damage or symptoms. Renal cell carcinomas rarely occur before the age of 30 years, are more commonly seen in the 50- to 70-year age range, and occur twice as often in men as in women. The tumor is usually large at the time of diagnosis and may invade the ureters or renal vein and metastasize to the lungs and bones.

Clinical picture. Hematuria is the most frequent symptom of renal cell carcinoma. Unfortunately the hematuria is often intermittent, lessening the person's concern and causing procrastination in seeking medical care. Any person with hematuria should have a complete urologic examination, since it is only by immediate investigation of the first signs of hematuria that there is any hope of cure. Other symptoms may include dull flank pain, flank mass, weight loss, fever, and polycythemia. Hypertension may result from stimulation of the renin-angiotensin system.

An intravenous pyelogram may show a distortion of renal outline suggesting a kidney tumor. Small tumors in the parenchyma may not be apparent on a routine pyelogram but may be identified by nephrotomography (p. 1238). Renal cell carcinoma may be differentiated from a renal cyst by a nephrotomograph. Renal scanning or angiography may also be performed to differentiate a cyst from a tumor.

Intervention. Unless the person is a poor surgical risk or has extensive metastases, the diseased kidney is removed *(nephrectomy)* through a transabdominal, thoracoabdominal, or retroperitoneal approach. The first two approaches are preferred in order to secure the renal artery and vein and prevent any spread of malignant cells.[58] (See p. 1306 for care of the person requiring urologic surgery.)

Following surgery for a malignant tumor that is radiosensitive, the patient is usually given a course of x-ray therapy. Hospitalization is not always necessary during this time. Radiation may also be used over the metastatic sites as palliative treatment for the person with an inoperable tumor. Chemotherapy has not yet proved of value in the treatment of renal cell carcinomas. The survival rate after therapy depends on the extent of metastasis. The 10-year survival rate is very low, especially since many persons do not seek initial treatment until the disease is far advanced.

Wilms' tumor

Children under the age of 7 years may develop an embryonal type of highly malignant renal growth called Wilms' tumor. It metastasizes early. A mass in the abdomen may be the first sign, and later hematuria and anemia may occur. Excellent therapeutic results have been obtained by a combination of nephrectomy, radiation, and chemotherapy.

□ Tumors of the bladder

The most common site of cancer in the urinary tract is the bladder. Cancer of the bladder occurs three times more often in males than in females and multiple tumors are common, with about 25% of patients having more than one lesion at the time of diagnosis. This figure increases to about 50% in patients with papilloma, grade I carcinoma, over a 5-year period. Approximately 40% of the tumors involve the trigone, and an additional 45% involve the posterior and lateral bladder walls. Known factors predisposing to bladder cancer are exposure to the chemicals beta-naphthylamine and xenylamine, infestation with *Schistoma haematobium,* and smoking. The tumor is a transitional cell epithelioma or carcinoma, and usually starts as a benign papilloma or leukoplakia.

Clinical picture. Painless hematuria is the first symptom in the majority of bladder tumors. It is usually intermittent, and the individual may fail to seek treatment. Painless hematuria occurs also in nonmalignant urinary tract disease and in cancer of the kidney; therefore any hematuria should be investigated. Cystitis (p. 1302) may be the first symptom of a bladder tumor, since the tumor may act as a foreign body in the bladder. Renal failure due to obstruction of the ureters sometimes is the reason given for seeking medical care. Vesicovaginal fistulas may occur before other symptoms develop. The last two conditions indicate a poor prognosis because usually the tumor has infiltrated widely.

Cytologic examination of the urine may identify malignant cells before the lesion can be visualized by cystoscopy. The diagnosis is established by cystoscopic visualization of the bladder with biopsy. Clinical determination of the invasiveness of the tumor is important in establishing a therapeutic regimen and in predicting the prognosis, especially since some bladder tumors are more malignant than indicated by the grading of the biopsy. Any person who has had a papilloma removed should have a cystoscopic examination every 3 months for 2 years and then at less frequent intervals if there is no evidence of a new lesion. Repeated cystoscopies may seem unacceptable to patients who dread them. The necessity for frequent examination should be fully explained by the urologist and the explanation reinforced by the nurse. Emphasis should be placed on the necessity for repeated cystoscopies, since papillomas tend to recur without symptoms until they are far-advanced tumors.

Intervention. The treatment is dependent on the size of the lesion and the depth of the tissue involvement. Small tumors with minimal tissue layer involvement may be adequately treated with *transurethral fulguration* or excision. A Foley catheter may or may not be inserted after surgery. The urine may be pink tinged, but gross bleeding is unusual. Burning on urination may be relieved by forcing fluids and applying heat over the bladder region by means of a heating pad or a sitz bath. The patient is discharged within a few days after surgery.

Segmental resection. If the tumor involves the dome of the bladder, a segmental resection of the bladder may be carried out. Over half of the bladder may be resected, and although the patient may have a capacity of no more than 60 ml immediately postoperatively, the elastic tissue of the bladder will regenerate so that the patient is able to retain from 200 to 400 ml of urine within several months.

The decreased size of the bladder, however, is of major importance in the postoperative period. The patient will return from surgery with catheters draining the bladder both from a cystostomy opening and from the urethra. This is to obviate the possibility of obstruction of drainage, since it would take only a very short time for the bladder to become distended and there would be danger of disrupting the suture line on the bladder. Because the bladder capacity is limited, the catheters usually cause severe bladder spasm.

As soon as the urethral catheter is removed, the patient becomes acutely aware of the small capacity of the bladder. Most patients will need to void at least every 20 minutes, and they need to be reassured that the bladder capacity will gradually increase. Meanwhile they should be urged to force fluids to 3,000 ml but should be advised to space the fluids so that time spent in the bathroom is not an inconvenience. They also should take large quantities of fluids at one time, limit fluids for several hours before planning to go out, and take no fluids after 6 PM.

Cystectomy. A cystectomy, or complete removal of the bladder, usually is performed only when the disease appears curable. Complete removal of the bladder requires permanent urinary diversion, which may be accomplished by various methods. The most common methods used at present are ureterosigmoidostomy and ileal conduit.

In *ureterosigmoidostomy* (ureterointestinal anastomosis) the ureters are transplanted into the intact bowel and urine drains from the rectum. Although this is a more socially acceptable method than the ileal conduit, hydronephrosis, renal infection, and electrolyte imbalances frequently occur. The kidneys may empty poorly because the rectum normally has a higher pressure than the bladder due to fecal contents and peristalsis. As the ureters and renal pelvis dilate from the increased pressure, bacteria easily move into the area and an infection develops. The intestinal tract also has absorptive powers, and chloride from the urine may be reabsorbed causing hyperchloremic acidosis.

Preoperative preparation for a ureterosigmoidostomy is similar to that for bowel surgery (p. 1281). Postoperatively an indwelling catheter may be place in the *rectum* until peristalsis returns, to promote drainage of urine and prevent backflow of urine to the kidneys. The tube is secured to the gluteal fold with a double flap of adhesive tape. The urine output is monitored closely for signs of urinary obstruction.

When oral intake is permitted, fluids are forced and a low-chloride, high-potassium diet is given. Chloride is avoided because of the potential for hyperchloremic acidosis. Potassium is needed to replace that lost during acidosis. The patient is encouraged to avoid gas-forming foods and activities that lead to swallowing of air such as gum chewing or drinking of carbonated beverages. Passing of flatus leads to incontinence of urine mixed with stool, which has an offensive odor.[68]

Increased pressure within the rectum, such as occurs with the Valsalva maneuver, should be avoided to prevent reflux of urine. The patient should empty the rectum whenever there is a sense of pressure or fullness, about every 2 to 3 hours or more often if necessary. During the night a catheter connected to gravity drainage may be inserted in the rectum to facilitate drainage and permit a good night's sleep. The patient is not given enemas, rectal suppositories, or strong cathartics that can increase rectal pressure. Since the stool is usually soft from the presence of urine, these measures are rarely needed.

The patient is monitored for signs of postoperative complications. Fever, hematuria, or flank pain may indicate *urinary tract infection* or *calculi.* If an *obstruction* of the ureter at the site of the anastomosis occurs, there will be fever, abdominal and flank pain, and decreased urinary output. Symptoms of *electrolyte imbalance* include nausea, vomiting, and muscle weakness. If urea is being reabsorbed by the intestinal mucosa the patient may have increased thirst, headache, increased urinary output, and lethargy due to the osmotic properties of the urea.

The *ileoureterocutaneous anastomosis,* or *ileal conduit,* is the most common urinary diversion. Urine will drain from a stoma in the abdominal wall following this procedure. (See p. 1264 for further information about ileal conduit and management of the person with a urinary stoma.) Immediately after the cystectomy the patient is usually acutely ill. Since not only the bladder but also large amounts of surrounding tissue are removed (the male patient also has a radical perineal prostatectomy), the patient may have a circulatory disturbance. This may be surgical shock, thrombosis, or cardiac decompensation. There is a long vertical or transverse abdominal incision, and there may be a perineal incision. The patient may be given nothing by mouth for several days, and a nasogastric tube may be inserted. The nursing care is the same as that given any patient after major abdominal surgery plus the routine care for a perineal wound and the care of the diverted urinary drainage.

Radiation therapy. External radiation with supervoltage x-rays or cobalt teletherapy may be used when a large tumor is present or metastasis has occurred. Unless the urinary stream has been diverted prior to radiation, contraction of the bladder and serious cystitis often occur. If a urinary diversion procedure has been performed, however, radiation of the bladder may decrease bleeding from the tumor and relieve pain.

Internal radiation may be used for small localized tumors on the bladder wall. *Radioisotopes* contained in a balloon of a Foley catheter may be inserted into the bladder. The catheter is attached to drainage, and all urine must be saved and sent to the radioisotope department for monitoring prior to disposal. Severe cystitis and proctitis usually result from this treatment, and the patient may be very uncomfortable for several days or weeks. Forcing fluids gives some relief from the symptoms, and urinary antiseptics and antispasmodic drugs are usually ordered. A low-residue diet and mineral oil may be ordered to keep the stools soft and lessen rectal discomfort.

A less common method of internal radiation therapy is the implantation of *radon seeds* around the base of a bladder tumor. This usually is done through a cystotomy but may also be done transurethrally through a cystoscope. If a cystostomy has been performed the patient may have a cystotomy tube inserted, but more often a urethral catheter will be used, and the cystotomy incision will be completely closed. (See p. 472 for precautions that should be taken when radiation treatment is used.) Radiation treatment usually causes a rather severe cystitis, which is treated by sedatives, antispasmodic drugs, fluids, and heat locally.

Chemotherapy. The use of chemotherapeutic agents is primarily palliative. 5-Fluorouracil (5-FU) and doxorubicin hydrochloride (Adriamycin) are the more commonly used agents. Thio-TEPA may be given by a topical administration. The patient is dehydrated for 8 to 12 hours prior to treatment. The Thio-TEPA is then instilled in the bladder by catheter and is retained for 2 hours. This treatment may be repeated once a week for up to 4 weeks.

□ Benign prostatic hypertrophy

Benign prostatic hypertrophy or hyperplasia (BPH) is an adenomatous enlargement of the prostate gland. The prostate is an encapsulated gland weighing about 20 g that encircles the male urethra below the bladder neck. When the middle lobe of the gland enlarges, it causes narrowing of the urethra. More than half of all men over 50 years of age and 75% of men over 70 have some symptoms of prostatic enlargement. The cause is not known but appears to be related to the presence of male hormones.

Clinical picture. One of the early symptoms of benign prostatic hypertrophy is *nocturia* (awakening at night to void) due to irritability of the bladder trigone (base of the bladder).[58] The man notices that the urinary stream is smaller and more difficult to start *(hesitancy)*. The bladder muscle must contract more forcibly to push the urine past the partial obstruction, and the overworked muscles hypertrophy. Stagnant urine is held in trabeculae, or cellules, formed by sagging of the atonic mucous membranes between hypertrophied muscle bands. The bladder will not empty completely at each voiding *(residual urine)*; this urine becomes alkaline from stasis and is a fertile medium for bacterial growth. The man will then complain of symptoms of cystitis (frequency, urgency), and bladder stones may occur. Some men develop hematuria from rupture of blood vessels that have become overstretched. Destruction of renal function can eventually occur from backpressure up the ureter to the kidney.

Enlargement of the lateral lobes of the prostate gland may be palpated by digital rectal examination. Enlargement of the middle lobe is diagnosed by signs of partial obstruction of the urethra and visualization of the obstruction and bladder trabeculae by cystoscopy.

Intervention. Surgery is the primary treatment for benign prostatic hypertrophy when the symptoms are causing discomfort or urinary retention, recurrent urinary tract infections, damage to the bladder outlet, or decreased kidney function. During surgery the capsule of the prostate gland is left intact, while the adenomatous soft tissue is removed by one of four surgical routes: transurethral, suprapubic, retropubic, or perineal. See Table 59-3 for a comparison of the different approaches.

Transurethral resection (TUR) of the prostate gland is the most common approach. A resectoscope (an instrument similar to a cystoscope but equipped with a cutting and cauterization loop attached to electric current) is passed through the urethra. The bladder is irrigated continuously during the procedure. The patient is grounded against electric shocks by a lubricated metal plate placed under his hips. Tiny pieces of tissue are cut away, and the bleeding points are sealed by cauterization (Fig. 59-3). A transurethral prostatectomy may be performed with the patient under general or spinal anesthesia.

Postoperatively the bladder is constantly irrigated with normal saline solution or another solution prescribed by the surgeon. This is accomplished by attaching one opening of the Foley catheter to tubing connected to a bottle of irrigating solution hung on an intravenous pole. The other opening of the Foley catheter is attached to a collection receptacle. The purpose of con-

Table 59-3. Comparison of types of prostatic surgery

	Transurethral resection	Suprapubic resection	Retropubic resection	Perineal resection	Radical perineal resection
Reason for surgery	Enlargement of medial lobe surrounding urethra	Extremely large mass of obstructing tissue	Large mass located high in pelvic area	Large mass located low in pelvic area	Cancer of prostate gland
Location of incision	No incision; removal by way of urethra	Low midline abdominal incision through bladder to prostate gland	Low midline abdominal incision into prostate gland (bladder not incised)	Incision between scrotum and rectum	Large perineal incision between scrotum and rectum
Drainage tubes	Three-way Foley catheter with 30-ml bag in urethra, constant irrigation for 24 hours	Cystotomy tube or drain through incision; Foley catheter with 30-ml bag in urethra	Foley catheter with 30-ml bag in urethra	Foley catheter with 30-ml bag in urethra	Foley catheter with 30-ml bag in urethra; drain in incision
Bladder spasms	Yes	Yes	Few	Few	Few
Dressing	No dressing	Abdominal dressing easily soaked with urinary drainage	Abdominal dressing; no urinary drainage	Perineal dressing; no urinary drainage	Perineal dressing; urinary drainage
Complications	Hemorrhage, water intoxication, incontinence	Hemorrhage, wound infection	Hemorrhage, wound infection	Hemorrhage, wound infection	Urinary incontinence, wound infection, impotence, sterility

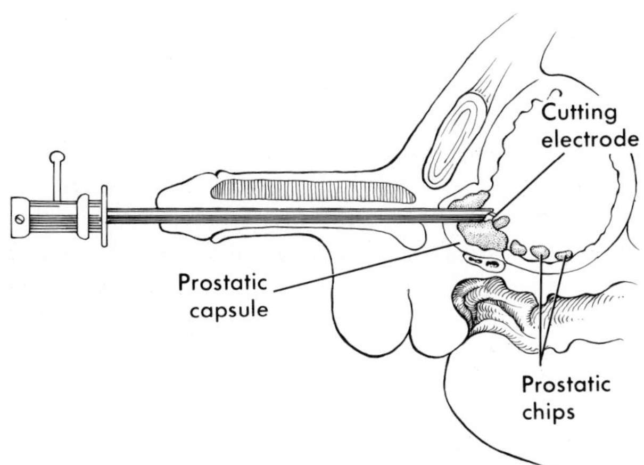

Fig. 59-3. Transurethral resection of prostate gland by means of resectoscope. Note cutting and cauterizing loop of instrument, enlarged prostate gland surrounding urethra, and tiny pieces of prostatic tissue that have been cut away.

stant irrigation is to keep the bladder free of clots. Constant irrigation is usually discontinued in 24 hours if there are no clots draining from the bladder. Manual irrigation is usually required during straight gravity drainage to keep the catheter draining. The urine will be a darker red after the constant irrigation is discontinued because it will not be diluted by the irrigating fluid. The urine will become progressively lighter in color as healing occurs.

The catheter may be removed in 2 to 5 days after transurethral resection, depending on the extent of the resection. The patient may not be able to void on removal of the catheter because of urethral edema. If he cannot void, the catheter may be reinserted for another day or two. Incontinence and dribbling from loss of sphincter tone frequently occur and can be very distressing to the patient. He should be warned that this is a common problem. Sphincter tone can be strengthened by perineal exercises (p. 1273). The total amount of urine passed with each voiding will be small initially. It takes up to 2 months for the bladder to return to its normal capacity.

Water intoxication may result from excessive irrigating solution being absorbed into the venous sinusoids

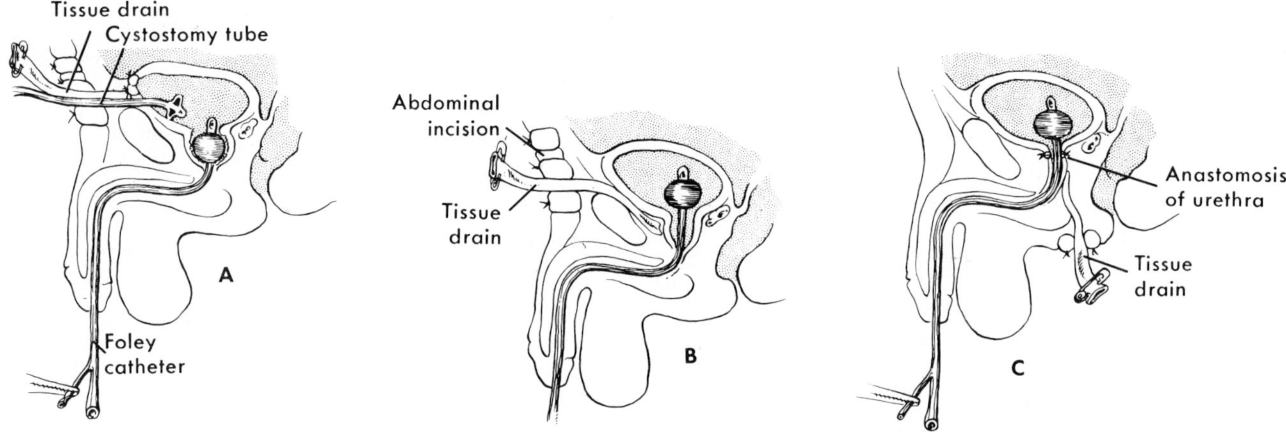

Fig. 59-4. Three methods of surgical removal of prostate gland. **A,** Suprapubic prostatectomy. Note placement of tissue drain, cystostomy tube, and inflated Foley catheter in prostatic fossa. **B,** Retropubic prostatectomy. Note intact bladder, placement of tissue drain, and retention catheter. **C,** Radical perineal prostatectomy. Note placement of tissue drain in incision between scrotum and rectum and anastomosis of urethra made necessary by excision of prostate gland and its capsule.

during surgery. The patient is observed closely for signs of cerebral edema (restlessness, confusion, change in behavior). (For additional information on water intoxication, see p. 301).

The alternate methods of prostatectomy are open operations. In the *suprapubic* resection the prostate gland is removed from the urethra by way of the bladder. Bleeding may continue into the postoperative period because the points of bleeding are not well visualized during surgery.[58] The usual method of draining urine following surgery is illustrated in Fig. 59-4, *A*. In some instances only the Foley catheter or the cystostomy tube is used. In the latter situation the prostatic fossa is packed for hemostasis. The dressings become saturated and need frequent changing. Urine is present in the drainage because of the bladder incision and will decrease as healing takes place. The Foley catheter must be kept open and draining; if blockage occurs there will be an increase in urinary drainage through the cystostomy tube. Good aseptic technique is imperative as cystostomy wounds easily become infected, as evidenced by a light bluish-green drainage. The cystostomy tube is usually removed 3 to 4 days postoperatively, but the urethral catheter may not be removed until the suprapubic wound is well healed.

In a *retropubic* prostatectomy the bladder is retracted but not incised, and the adenomatous prostatic tissue is removed through an incision into the anterior prostatic capsule. A drain is inserted (Fig. 59-4, *B*), but there should be no urinary drainage. If urinary or purulent drainage, fever, or pain on walking occurs, the surgeon is notified, since such symptoms may be due to deep wound infection or pelvic abscess. This may occur after the patient has been discharged from the hospital. Bleeding is less than occurs with suprapubic prostatectomy. The Foley catheter is usually removed in 3 to 5 days, and the patient rarely has difficulty in initiating voiding.

The *perineal* prostatectomy is performed more rarely. The incision is made between the scrotum and the rectum (Fig. 59-4, *C*). The posterior capsule of the prostate gland is incised, and all the adenomatous tissue is removed. The *radical* perineal prostatectomy is performed when cancer of the prostate gland is present (p. 1441).

Bladder spasms occur primarily following transurethral or suprapubic prostatectomy because of irritation of the bladder mucosa. Drinking large amounts of fluids helps assure constant passage of fluid over the bladder mucosa, decreasing irritation. The 30-ml inflation bag on the Foley catheter puts pressure on the internal sphincter, giving the patient a continual feeling of having to void. If the catheter is draining properly, this sensation usually passes momentarily. Trying to void around the catheter causes the bladder muscles to contract, resulting in painful bladder spasms. If the patient is aware of the purpose of the catheter, he may resist trying to void and thus decrease some of the bladder spasms. Belladonna and opium (B & O) suppositories are frequently prescribed to relieve bladder spasms and are usually quite effective. As the nerve endings become fatigued, the frequency and severity of the spasms will decrease.

The length of time required for spasm to lessen varies. Most patients have less spasm by the end of 24 to 48 hours.

Hemorrhage may result if the catheter becomes displaced. A Foley catheter with a 30-ml inflation bag (in place of the usual 5-ml bag) is used in prostatic surgery in order to provide hemostasis. The larger bag provides counterpressure on the bleeding vessels in the prostatic fossa. Slight traction on the catheter may decrease the bleeding. The patient should not strain to have a bowel movement because straining may cause prostatic hemorrhage. Stool softeners are usually prescribed, and when necessary a laxative is given. Enemas are not given, and rectal tubes and rectal thermometers are not used for about 1 week postoperatively, since they exert pressure on the resected prostatic capsule. Prolonged sitting is avoided as it increases abdominal pressure and fosters bleeding.

Surgery of the prostate gland may invoke *concerns* regarding sexual functioning or the ability to be continent of urine. The nurse may need to provide openings during interactions with the patient in order to promote expressions of these concerns by the patient. Impotence occurs physiologically only when the perineal nerves are cut during a radical perineal prostatectomy and not with the other types of prostatectomies. If the man believes that the surgery will or may produce impotence, however, this may occur because of psychologic influences. Urinary incontinence frequently follows radical perineal prostatectomy and only occasionally after transurethral prostatectomy. If the man has some difficulty after any type of prostatectomy, he may fear permanent incontinence even though this is unlikely. He should be given an opportunity to discuss these concerns, be given information about the probability of the return of continence, and encouraged to carry out perineal exercises.

The patient should not exercise vigorously or do any heavy lifting for about 3 weeks after discharge from the hospital. He usually is also advised not to drive a car. A stool softener or mild cathartic may be ordered for about 6 weeks to obviate straining. Fluids should be taken freely for at least 3 weeks after discharge. After healing is complete, dilation of the urethra may be necessary because urethral mucosa in the prostatic area is destroyed by the operation, and strictures may have formed with healing.

Outcome criteria for the man following prostatectomy

The patient or significant other can:

1. Explain care of the catheter if discharged with an indwelling catheter.
2. Describe perineal exercises if mild incontinence is present.
3. State measures to prevent constipation.
4. Describe signs of wound infection, urinary retention, or excessive bleeding requiring medical intervention.
5. State plans for medical follow-up.
6. State activities to be avoided because of possible bleeding (sexual intercourse, heavy lifting, straining at stool) until medical permission to perform them is given (about 2 to 4 weeks).

■ RENAL DISEASE

Although kidney disease is often equated with a severe life-threatening illness without reversibility, this picture is seen in only a very small percentage of individuals in whom kidney disease has been diagnosed. Renal problems are extremely varied (1) in cause and potential for a cure as compared with control of the illness, (2) in the signs and symptoms the patient shows that reflect differences in the kidney structures involved and the functions impaired, (3) in the event or progression of the illness and the "sickness" of the patient, and (4) in the onset of the problem, which can be sudden, occur gradually, or be entirely unknown to the person.

The overall goal for managing renal problems is to preserve renal function. This must be achieved through prompt recognition of the illness, cure of those problems that can be eradicated, and control of those problems that cannot be reversed.

The National Kidney Foundation,* through state and

*116 East 27th Street, New York, N.Y. 10016.

Table 59-4. Effect of kidney disease on structure and function

Site of disease	Renal process affected	Effect on function
Glomeruli	Alters filtration process in capillary tufts	Loss of large amounts of protein and RBCs
Tubules	Destroys ability to modify fluid	Interferes with conservation of electrolytes and elimination of waste materials
Vascular bed	Decreased blood supply to glomeruli and tubules	Decreased function depending on structure affected
Interstitial tissue	Destroys kidney tissue by pressure as cysts fill and scar tissue forms	Decreased function depending on structure affected

local offices, provides assistance to those concerned with kidney disease. Services of this organization include direct service to patients, public education, and funding for research.

□ Classification of renal disease

Renal disease usually alters the functional ability of one of the major structural parts of the kidney: the glomeruli, the tubules, the vascular bed, or the interstitial tissue (Table 59-4). When disease is persistent or severe in nature, all of the kidney structures may become affected and the kidney becomes nonfunctional. In the following section on common diseases of the kidney an illness involving each of the major renal structures is discussed.

Illness can occur that influences renal function without directly involving kidney tissue. Problems of this nature are seen when urinary output decreases and the clearance of materials normally excreted by the kidneys falls. Problems commonly involve either a reduction in blood supply to the kidneys (prerenal disease) or an obstruction in the flow of urine within the urinary tract (postrenal disease). The signs and symptoms of renal failure that these conditions precipitate may disappear as the underlying extrarenal problems are resolved. The classification of renal disease is given in Table 59-5.

Within the broad area of kidney disease, certain illnesses are more amenable than others to prevention, as follows:

Glomerular disease
Acute poststreptococcal glomerulonephritis
Infective endocarditis
Toxemia of pregnancy

Vascular disease
Nephrosclerosis
Hypersensitivity angiitis

Tubular disease
Acute tubular insufficiency
Hypokalemic nephropathy
Hypercalcemic nephropathy
Obstructive nephropathy

Interstitial disease
Pyelonephritis
Drug and heavy-metal poisoning
Urate nephropathy[51]

□ Acute glomerulonephritis

Glomerulonephritis is a disease that affects the glomeruli of both kidneys. Etiologic factors are many and varied; they include immunologic reactions (lupus erythematosus, streptococcal infection), vascular injury (hypertension), metabolic disease (diabetes mellitus), and disseminated intravascular coagulation (DIC). Glomerulonephritis exists in acute, latent, and chronic forms.

The most common form of *acute glomerulonephritis*

Table 59-5. Classification of renal disease

Prerenal (poor kidney perfusion)	Renal (primary kidney pathology)	Postrenal (obstructive disorders)
Hypovolemia	Glomerular	Calculi
Blood or plasma loss	Nephritis: acute and chronic	Tumor
Sodium or water loss	Diabetic sclerosis	Benign prostatic hypertrophy
Cardiac failure	Lupus erythematosus	Cancer
Myocardial infarct	Nephrotic syndrome	Strictures or stenosis
Congestive failure	Vascular	
Arrhythmias	Nephrosclerosis	
Septic shock	Vasculitis	
	Tubular	
	Toxins or poisons	
	Ischemic injury	
	Congenital dysfunction	
	Interstitial	
	Pyelonephritis	
	Tuberculosis	
	Analgesic or heavy-metal toxicity	
	Tumors or cysts	
	Polycystic disease	
	Benign or malignant tumors	

occurs after a streptococcal infection. The illness is a result of an antigen-antibody complex reaction with glomerular tissue that produces swelling and death of capillary cells. Strains of beta-hemolytic streptococci are involved in mediating this antigen-antibody reaction. Common sites of infection include the throat (tonsillitis, strep throat) and the skin (impetigo). Children of preschool and grade-school age are most likely to develop the illness. Of all individuals developing acute poststreptococcal glomerulonephritis, approximately 1% to 2% will develop end-stage renal failure in which dialysis or transplantation is required to maintain life. Approximately 90% of children and 50% of adults with acute glomerulonephritis attain full recovery from illness, although recovery may require up to 2 years.[51] Little inference regarding prognosis can be made on the severity of the acute episode. Persons with mild illness may develop chronic disease, and those with severe illness may completely recover and have no recurrence of the illness.

Prevention. Prevention of poststreptococcal acute glomerulonephritis involves prompt medical treatment of sore throat and upper respiratory tract infections. Cultures should be obtained, and when indicated appropriate antibiotics are prescribed.

Clinical picture. Common complaints are shortness of breath, mild headache, weakness, and anorexia. Usual signs include proteinuria, hematuria, increased urine specific gravity, dependent edema, and an elevated antistreptolysin O titer. Additionally signs of elevation in blood pressure, decreased urine output, and elevation in serum urea nitrogen and creatine levels may be present. Signs and symptoms reflect damage to the glomeruli with leaking of protein and red cells into the urine, varying degrees of decreased glomerular filtration with retention of wastes, and fluid overloading of varying severity.

Intervention

Control of infection. Persistent infection is treated promptly to help further decrease antigen-antibody complex formation. Persons with poststreptococcal glomerulonephritis are given a prophylactic antibiotic; the drug of choice is penicillin. Rationale for this therapy is based on preventing further infections that could reactivate the nephritis. Prophylactic therapy may be continued for months after the acute phase of illness. Exposure to any infection must be avoided, since even mild infections may reactivate nephritis.

Activity. Bed rest is instituted until clinical signs disappear; this may involve a period of several months. Ambulation is begun when blood sedimentation rates and blood pressure are normal and edema abates. If ambulation causes an increase in proteinuria or hematuria, bed rest is reinstituted. Since the period of bed rest may be long and the person usually does not feel ill, the nurse may need to continue reinforcing the importance of bed rest and assist in planning diversionary activities and the constructive use of time. For small children this can present no small problem. When bed rest is reinstituted after periods of ambulation, the person may become depressed. Helping the person to express concerns and feelings can serve as a basis for helping make realistic plans about the illness and its sequelae.

Maintenance of fluid balance. Edema and fluid overloading are anticipated and treated initially with dietary sodium restrictions. The amount of restriction depends on the severity of fluid retention, and it is maintained until dependent edema and circulatory overload are no longer a problem. Diuretics are generally reserved for managing severe fluid overload and pulmonary edema. The nurse is constantly alert for signs of fluid overload (p. 303). Blood pressure elevation is treated with antihypertensive drugs only after fluid control has proved unsuccessful in controlling hypertension. Dietary protein is reduced only when blood urea nitrogen and creatinine levels are elevated. The diet should contain sufficient carbohydrate to prevent protein being used for energy. This helps maintain nitrogen balance.

Long-term care. Up to 2 years may be required for resolution of the illness. During this time proteinuria, hematuria, and cellular debris may exist microscopically. The person generally shows little to no change from normal in renal function. At this point normal activities may be continued, although fatigue, trauma, and infection need to be avoided as they exacerbate illness. Good general health measures are stressed. Since these persons usually feel well, they often must be convinced of the need to continue prescribed treatment and to return for routine follow-up health care. They should understand which signs and symptoms are significant and indicate a need for medical attention. They need to be encouraged to pursue care even though they were thoroughly examined only a short time previously.

□ Chronic glomerulonephritis

Although chronic glomerulonephritis may follow the acute disease, the majority of persons give no history of the disease. In most instances no evidence of predisposing infection can be found. The course of chronic glomerulonephritis is extremely varied. Some persons with minimal impairment in renal function continue to feel well and show little progression of disease. With other individuals the progression of renal deterioration may be slow but steady and end in renal failure. In still other individuals the progression of disease is rapid.

Clinical picture. Various symptoms of failing renal function, none of which may seem severe, may lead the person to seek health care. There may be a slow onset of recurrent dependent edema, or there may be mild headache, especially in the morning. Dyspnea on exertion or difficulty sleeping in a flat position may be noted. Blurring of vision may lead the person to an ophthalmologist, who may be the first to suspect chronic renal disease based on ocular vascular changes. Nocturia is a common complaint. Occasionally chronic nephritis is discovered during routine physical examination or may be discovered by a school nurse who observes marked visual changes and lassitude in a student. Weakness, fatigue, and weight loss are common but nonspecific symptoms of chronic glomerulonephritis. Early in the disease urinalysis shows the presence of albumin, casts, and blood. At this point renal function tests may be normal. The ability of the kidneys to regulate the internal environment will begin to decrease as more and more glomeruli become scarred and the amount of functional renal tissue is reduced. Finally, when few intact nephrons remain, hematuria and proteinuria decrease, the specific gravity of the urine becomes fixed, and the nonprotein nitrogen level in the blood is increased.

Intervention. No specific therapy exists to arrest or reverse the disease process. With some forms of chronic glomerulonephritis steroid therapy may be attempted, although results of this therapy in arresting disease are not well documented. Care involves teaching the person to live healthfully: to avoid infections, to eat a balanced diet within modifications of sodium intake if prescribed, to appropriately administer medications, and to maintain follow-up health care visits and report to the physician any exacerbations in signs and symptoms. Treatment of renal failure (p. 1327) begins when the illness destroys so much kidney tissue that the individual is no longer able to independently control his or her internal environment.

With any exacerbation of hematuria, hypertension, and edema, the person is put to bed, and treatment similar to that for acute glomerulonephritis is instituted. Signs of pulmonary edema and congestive failure are monitored for when caring for these persons. Treatment is symptomatic and supportive.

Women with chronic glomerulonephritis who become pregnant appear to be susceptible to toxemia and to spontaneous abortion. The woman who has had nephritis of any nature should be urged to see a physician if she plans on pregnancy. When pregnancy does occur, she should remain under close health supervision.

Outcome criteria for the person with glomerulonephritis

The patient or significant others can:

1. Explain the rationale for therapy (prolongation of bed rest, maintenance of fluid balance).
2. Explain dietary changes (decreased sodium intake, adequate caloric intake, controlled protein intake if prescribed).
3. Explain medication program to be followed at home (prophylactic penicillin therapy).
4. Explain health maintenance program:
   a. Measures to prevent further infection.
   b. Signs that require immediate medical attention (hematuria, hypertension, edema, headaches).
   c. Plans for continued follow-up health care.

□ Nephrotic syndrome (nephrosis)

Nephrotic syndrome is a condition involving damage to the glomeruli where quantities of protein are lost in the urine. This condition has been associated with allergic reactions (insect bites, pollen, acute glomerulonephritis), infections (herpes zoster), systemic disease (diabetes mellitus, sickle cell disease), circulatory problems (severe congestive heart failure, chronic constrictive pericarditis), and pregnancy. Known glomerular disease is the most common precipitating event in adults; in children the syndrome appears frequently with no evidence of a causative factor. In approximately 25% of children and 50% to 75% of adults who develop nephrosis the disease progresses to renal failure within 5 years.[9] In other individuals (particularly children) there may be remissions, or nephrosis may exist in a chronic form. Other than treating underlying illness, little can be done to prevent the occurrence or recurrence of nephrosis.

Clinical picture. Characteristic manifestations of the nephrotic syndrome include severe generalized edema that is particularly noticeable in dependent areas, pronounced proteinuria that contains albumin and globulin protein fractions, and hypoalbuminemia. Serum lipids are often elevated; hypertension and hematuria occur when glomerulonephritis is the underlying disease. Urine volumes and renal function may be either normal or markedly altered. Altered renal function and development of renal failure occur as a result of progressing glomerulonephritis.

Loss of appetite and fatigue are common. Women usually have amenorrhea or other disturbances in their reproductive cycle.

Intervention. Treatment of nephrotic syndrome is directed toward reducing albuminuria, controlling edema, and promoting general health. Corticosteroids may be useful in controlling the illness, but the response to them will vary from remission of nephrosis to no response. Prednisone is the steroid preparation most frequently prescribed. The diet should contain normal to increased amounts of protein (1 g/kg body weight per day) and be high in calories. Periodic determination of proteinuria and measures of renal function provide the physician with data for monitoring response to treatment and level of kidney function.

To control edema, sodium intake is reduced and diuretics are employed to increase excretion of fluid. When diuretics are administered over prolonged periods, hypokalemia usually results (p. 308). Potassium may be supplemented through dietary intake; medication supplements should be initiated only after attempts to increase serum potassium through dietary means have failed. Bed rest is usually ordered when edema is severe; however, immobility is contraindicated for prolonged periods.

Persons with nephrosis need to direct particular attention toward preventing infection, since body defenses are impaired by urinary protein losses and edematous tissues are particularly susceptible to injury. When infection is suspected it is important to give immediate attention to the problem. Culture and sensitivity studies are done and appropriate antibiotics are prescribed. The person is informed of the importance of prescribed medication and diet therapy and of the need for follow-up health care.

Outcome criteria for the person with nephrotic syndrome

1. Independence in activities of daily living is maintained.
2. The person remains free of infection.
3. Edema and blood pressure are controlled; pulmonary edema and congestive heart failure do not occur.

The patient or significant others can:

1. Describe measures to prevent infection.
2. State name, dosage, frequency, and side effects of prescribed medications (steroids, diuretics).
3. State dietary prescription (increased calories, adequate protein, decreased sodium) and plan appropriate meals.
4. State plans requiring immediate attention (increase in edema, fatigue, headache, presence of infection).
5. State plans for follow-up health care.

□ Pyelonephritis

Pyelonephritis refers to bacterial infection of kidney tissue. This infection usually begins in the lower urinary tract and ascends into the kidneys. Lower urinary tract infection may be asymptomatic, and kidney involvement may be the first indication of lower (urinary) tract disease. Often the diagnostic workup of a person with pyelonephritis reveals previously unknown urinary tract obstruction or the presence of other chronic kidney disease. *Escherichia coli* is the most common organism identified in pyelonephritis, and resistance to antibiotic therapy rarely results. Pyelonephritis is most commonly associated with (1) pregnancy, (2) obstruction, instrumentation or trauma of the urinary tract, and (3) chronic health problems including diabetes, analgesic abuse, polycystic kidney disease, and hypertensive kidney disease.

Infection of the kidney occurs in both acute and chronic forms. Although acute pyelonephritis may temporarily affect renal function, rarely does this progress to a level of renal failure. Chronic pyelonephritis destroys renal tissue permanently through repeated inflammation and scarring. The process of developing chronic renal failure from repeated kidney infection occurs over a number of years or after several extensive and fulminant infections. It is estimated that pyelonephritis represents the original diagnosis in one third of all persons with chronic renal disease.[65]

The most significant efforts in preventing pyelonephritis are through detection and adequate treatment of lower urinary tract infections.

Clinical picture. Signs and symptoms of pyelonephritis usually include those associated with lower urinary tract infection, along with fever, chills, malaise, costovertebral tenderness, and leukocytosis. The urine shows white blood cells, white blood cell casts, and bacteria. Signs and symptoms of renal failure may be present when nephron damage has been significant (p. 1322).

Intervention. Optimal treatment includes early detection of the illness, antibacterial therapy based on urine cultures, and correction and treatment of any underlying systemic disease or urinary tract abnormality. Anyone with symptoms of dysuria, cloudy urine, or frequent small voidings should be examined for urinary tract infection and appropriately treated. Persons complaining of fever and costovertebral tenderness should be encouraged to seek medical attention.

The course of antibiotic therapy may extend over weeks, and the person may need to be reminded of the necessity to continue taking the medication even when symptoms disappear and he or she begins to feel better. Continuing drug therapy to eradicate all infection and prevent development of resistant strains of organisms is stressed. Follow-up urine cultures are done again 2 weeks after drug therapy has been discontinued and every month thereafter for the next several months. Increasing fluid intake to 3 liters/day in persons capable of excreting this amount of fluid is desirable to prevent stasis of urine and further bacterial growth. Should infection become chronic, the person may be placed on drug therapy indefinitely; the goal is to reduce and control the bacterial population of the urinary tract so that renal damage is prevented. Urine cultures should be repeated periodically and the person should be instructed in the signs and symptoms indicating reactivation of infection and the need for medical attention.

Outcome criteria for the person with pyelonephritis

The patient or significant others can:

1. State name, dosage, frequency, and side effects of antibiotic therapy.
2. Explain rationale for continued antibiotic therapy even when symptoms are no longer present.
3. State rationale and method for increasing fluid intake.
4. State signs and symptoms of kidney infection and need to seek health care when symptoms recur.
5. State plan for follow-up urine cultures and health care.

□ Tuberculosis of the kidney

Renal tuberculosis is an example of a kidney infection that is secondary to an infection in a different site (pulmonary tuberculosis). It is acquired by hematogenous spread and is most common in men between 20 and 40 years of age. Treatment is primarily medical and consists of antituberculosis medication therapy coupled with rest and good nutrition. Respiratory isolation is not necessary.

□ Hypertensive renal disease (nephrosclerosis)

Hypertension is a major precipitating factor of renal damage. It is estimated that approximately 10% of individuals with essential hypertension develop severe renal damage, and approximately 1% will develop end-stage renal failure and die unless supportive care is provided.[51] Regardless of origin (essential or renal), hypertension that is untreated over a period of time leads to the sclerosing of renal arterioles. The blood supply to glomeruli, tubules, and interstitium gradually decreases. Scarring and death of kidney tissue occurs, and signs of renal insufficiency develop when damage to the kidneys has become extensive. *Nephrosclerosis* is the term given to this destructive process.

Prevention. Preventive care includes greater screening efforts to detect persons with elevated blood pressure, adequate treatment and follow-up for those with hypertension, and education regarding the nature of the illness, the diet and medications, and the importance of periodic follow-up health care. Yearly blood pressure monitoring of persons with elevated blood pressure is a minimum preventive care measure.

Clinical picture. By the time the person develops signs and symptoms indicating kidney involvement, the disease has progressed to an extreme point. Deterioration in renal function progresses gradually unless an acute or malignant phase of hypertension (p. 1048) occurs to accelerate the process. Signs and symptoms are those of chronic renal failure (p. 1327).

Intervention. Treatment of nephrosclerosis is directed toward early detection and treatment of hypertension. Causative factors are sought, and treatment to lower blood pressure is begun (p. 1051). When significant renal damage exists, stabilizing the person's current level of function or slowing deterioration of kidney tissue is the goal. Control of hypertension is continued, and management of end-stage disease and uremic symptoms provides for comfort and increased independence in daily living, although renal function may not improve.

□ Polycystic kidney disease

Polycystic kidney disease is an inherited defect that involves the kidneys bilaterally. Cysts develop that compress and destroy functional renal tissue. Polycystic disease occurs primarily in two distinct age groups, infancy and middle age. Infants developing this illness typically die within a few months. Adults in the 40- to 50-year range generally become symptomatic and develop end-stage disease 10 to 15 years after symptoms arise. Males and females seem equally affected.

There is no preventive care for the illness. Early detection and medical care that prevents and controls infection retards the development of renal failure.

Clinical picture. Signs and symptoms include discomfort and pain in the flank; the awareness of a "mass," which is the enlarged cystic kidney; fever, chills, and malaise when infection occurs; and hematuria with rupturing of cysts. Colicky pain may be experienced when clots are passed down the ureter. Signs and symptoms of uremia occur when renal function deteriorates to the point of the end-stage renal disease. When the diagnosis of polycystic kidney disease is made, tests of renal function are obtained. These serve to evaluate current renal status and provide a baseline for detecting future changes in kidney function.

Intervention. Management of the person with polycystic disease centers largely on preventing infection or bleeding and on dealing with the emotional impact of having a genetically determined illness. Infection is difficult to eradicate in polycystic kidneys and when uncontrolled leads to further destruction of kidney tissue. Frequent culture of the urine is performed, and instrumentation of the urinary tract is avoided whenever possible. Bleeding occurs with rupture of cysts and varies from miscroscopic to gross hematuria. Bed rest is instituted when bleeding is sufficient to turn the urine from pink to red. Nephrectomy may be required to control continuing, severe bleeding. Treatment for renal failure is instituted when signs and symptoms of uremia appear.

The emotional overtones of this illness can be severely disrupting to the individual and the family. Challenge exists in helping a person deal with an illness on an individual basis when relatives have died of the same disease and children have not yet developed symptoms. Counseling regarding family health care and the person's role in passing on a potentially fatal disease to children will at some time be required.

Outcome criteria for the person with polycystic kidney disease

The person or significant others can:

1. State signs and symptoms of infection and blood loss requiring medical attention.
2. State plans for follow-up health care.
3. Describe appropriate health screening and follow-up care for children.

■ RENAL FAILURE

Renal failure indicates a state of total or nearly total loss of the kidney's ability to excrete waste products and to maintain fluid and electrolyte balance. Laboratory tests reflect the changes in the internal environment, and the person appears clinically ill. The person in renal failure cannot independently sustain life. Renal failure may be acute in onset or may develop slowly and progressively over a course of several years. When renal failure occurs suddenly, as within a few days, biochemical changes are often dramatic, and the person has little time to adjust to these changes. The person becomes very ill and hospitalization, frequently involving placement in a critical care area, becomes necessary.

When renal failure occurs as the end result of a chronic kidney illness where kidney tissue is destroyed progressively over the course of several months or years, control of symptoms and preservation of functional abilities are achievable goals. Dietary adjustment, medications, and attention to preventing additional illnesses compensate for loss of kidney function in early stages of progressing renal failure. As renal function continues to deteriorate, dialysis or transplantation additionally becomes necessary to support life.

Renal insufficiency designates significant loss of renal function but with enough function remaining to maintain an internal environment consistent with life, providing no additional stresses to health occur. The individual may appear and feel well although laboratory data reflect a deterioration in renal function. Renal insufficiency occurs as a phase in gradually and chronically progressive renal disease.

□ Acute renal failure

Acute renal failure occurs as a sudden and frequently reversible decrease or cessation of kidney function. It generally follows an identifiable trauma of either toxic or ischemic nature. The health of the individual prior to the insult is usually good to adequate. Renal *ischemia* occurs when blood flow to the kidneys is reduced due to trauma or disease (see box below). The response of the normal kidney is vasoconstriction, which compounds the problem of reduced renal blood flow and increases renal ischemia. Perfusion problems affect both kidneys. When ischemia is prolonged, renal tubular tissue dies and frank renal failure develops.

A variety of substances are *toxic* to the cells of the renal tubules (see box below). The kidney with its large blood flow, ability to concentrate solute inside the tubules, and ability to concentrate fluid in the medullary portion of the kidney (where the tubules are located) creates conditions where exposure of tubular cells to toxins is maximized. The kidneys are affected bilaterally.

Additionally other conditions can precipitate acute renal failure: (1) acute glomerular disease, (2) acute severe infection of kidney tissue, (3) bilateral occlusion of the renal arteries, (4) mechanical obstructions in the urinary tract, and (5) hemoglobinemia and myoglobinemia. All of these conditions lead to massive and rapid destruction of kidney tissue.

Prognosis. Recovery from an episode of acute renal failure depends on the underlying illness, the condition of the patient, and the careful, supportive management given during the period of kidney shutdown. Mortality associated with acute tubular necrosis approaches 40%;

CONDITIONS AND SUBSTANCES THAT PRODUCE ISCHEMIC OR NEPHROTOXIC INJURY TO THE KIDNEY

Ischemic (inadequate perfusion of the kidney)
- Hypovolemia
- Blood loss (surgery, trauma)
- Plasma loss (burns, surgery, acute pancreatitis)
- Sodium and water loss (prolonged diarrhea or vomiting, gastrointestinal tract drainage, sustained high fever)
- Cardiac failure
- Myocardial infarction
- Cardiac arrhythmias
- Congestive heart failure
- Septic shock

Toxic (injury to kidney cells)
- Solvents (carbon tetrachloride, methanol, ethylene glycol)
- Heavy metals (lead, arsenic, mercury)
- Antibiotics (kanamycin, gentamicin, polymyxin B, amphotericin B, colistin, neomycin, phenazopyridine)
- Pesticides
- Mushrooms

these statistics largely reflect the deaths of severely ill persons in whom renal failure is a sequela to extensive underlying illness. Owing to the more widespread availability of dialysis, deaths directly attributable to decreased renal function from potassium intoxication, fluid overload, and acidosis have become less prevalent. The potential for recovery of renal function for those who survive the acute episode of tubular insufficiency is good. Although recovery statistics indicate that kidney tissue may regenerate more completely after toxic injury in comparison with ischemic injury, follow-up studies of persons years after episodes of acute tubular insufficiency show normal to near normal renal function.[51]

For those in whom acute renal failure has been caused by glomerular disease or severe infection of kidney tissue, the prognosis may not be as favorable. Return of renal function is determined by the extent of scarring and obliteration of functional renal tissue that has occurred during the acute episode of kidney failure. A significant number of adults who develop acute glomerulonephritis show some decrease in renal function, which may remain at a level not producing biochemical abnormalities or may progress to a chronic form of renal failure.

Prevention. The incidence of acute renal failure can be reduced through identification and observation of populations at risk and identification and control of environmental risk factors. The greatest incidence of acute renal failure occurs in persons who have undergone major trauma, extensive burns, aortic surgery, massive blood loss, or severe myocardial infarction with or without associated arrhythmia. Acute renal failure also frequently occurs in patients with sepsis and in those having abnormal intravascular coagulation, since these acutely ill persons are prime candidates for inadequate kidney perfusion. Frequent monitoring of urinary output and detection of excessive losses of body fluid will help to identify instances of inadequate renal perfusion prior to development of actual renal failure.

Significant factors in preventive care for the general population include control of nephrotoxic drugs, increased medical supervision of persons with sore throat and upper respiratory tract infection, and increased case finding and treatment of individuals with bacteriuria and obstructive disease of the urinary system. Attempts to control the distribution and identification of nephrotoxic drugs and chemicals is largely accomplished through the Federal Drug Administration (FDA). Identification of nephrotoxic drugs and chemicals, enforced labeling of these substances, and drug dispensing by prescription only are examples of this agency's attempts to promote the public health. Proper labeling and storage of potentially toxic drugs and chemicals in the home can reduce further the number of accidental ingestions of nephrotoxic substances.

Clinical picture. Signs and symptoms indicating the onset of acute renal failure appear rapidly and are a direct result of retention of fluids, electrolytes, and waste materials. Typically the person is acutely ill; in addition to the renal failure frequently being superimposed on an already severely compromised individual, biochemical changes occur rapidly and give the person little time to adjust to the altered internal environment. Either *oliguria* (urine output below 400 ml/day) or *anuria* (urine output below 100 ml/day) may be present, although oliguria is more frequent. Classically the patient in acute renal failure shows a fall in urinary output within 1 to 2 days to between 50 and 400 ml/day. The specific gravity of the urine is low (1.01), and the osmolality of the urine approaches that of the person's serum (280 mOsm to 320 mOsm). Specific gravity and urine osmolality remain within this fixed range and reflect tubular damage with loss of concentrating ability. Additionally the urine may show a higher concentration of sodium than would be expected in the case of dehydration or low circulating blood volume. This finding reflects the damaged kidneys' inability to conserve sodium ions and is an important consideration in diagnosing the existence of acute renal failure.

Fluid intake in excess of the diminished urine output and insensible losses is retained in the body, resulting in edema. When fluid overload is excessive, signs of congestive failure and pulmonary edema are present. Hypertension accompanies acute renal failure when the person is hypervolemic, although this is usually not a finding when fluid balance is controlled.

Retention of electrolytes and waste materials from cellular metabolism produce typical signs and symptoms often referred to as the development of *uremia.* Serum potassium, urea nitrogen, and creatinine values rise sharply. In the person who has already sustained illness and trauma, urea nitrogen values may increase at a rate of 30 mg/100 ml/day. As urinary excretion of the acid end products of metabolism decreases, acidosis occurs, carbon dioxide values decline to 15 mEq/liter or less, and Kussmaul's breathing occurs (p. 328). Symptoms attributable to retained wastes and altered electrolyte balance include nausea, vomiting, drowsiness, fatigue, and shortness of breath with fluid overloading. Signs produced by these internal changes include confusion, convulsions, coma, gastrointestinal tract bleeding, and asterixis (p. 612).

Additional problems that frequently beset the person with acute renal failure include pericarditis and infection. Pericarditis is thought to develop as a result of pericardial irritation from accumulated metabolic wastes. It is diagnosed by the presence of a cardiac friction rub and pleuriticlike pain over the precordium. Fever often accompanies pericarditis. When fluid accumulates in the pericardial sac, the rub becomes less intense or absent and pulsus paradoxus (pulse weaker during inspiration) is likely to be present. Pericardial effusion can be confirmed by echocardiography. Infection frequently develops in response to lowered host resistance, multiple trauma, and immobility during the course of the illness.

When oliguria or rising creatinine and urea nitrogen values are noted, the physician must determine whether the decreased output and decreased renal function are the results of inadequate renal perfusion or of frank renal failure. This distinction directs treatment. In instances of poor kidney perfusion, restoring circulating volume by adding fluids and otherwise increasing cardiac output prevents death of kidney tissue and subsequent renal failure. In contrast the treatment of true renal failure is supportive and is based on careful balance of input and output of fluid, electrolytes, and wastes. In addition to the urine sodium concentration as a diagnostic sign, the physician may wish to challenge the patient's ability to excrete fluid. The poorly perfused but intact kidney will respond to this challenge with increased urine flow; the kidney in acute failure will not produce more urine. In attempting to produce a greater urine flow, the physician may give mannitol, 25 to 50 g, intravenously as an osmotic diuretic, or furosemide, 40 to 80 mg. The test may be repeated again if there is no response to the initial trial, although subsequent attempts to produce urine in this manner are contraindicated.

When the cause of a sudden acute decline in renal function cannot be identified, particularly when anuria is present, cystoscopy and retrograde pyelography may be used to detect the presence of any obstructive urinary tract disease.

The course of acute renal failure is usually characterized by an initial oliguric phase followed in a number of days to a few weeks by a diuretic period. Major patient care problems during the oliguric phase of illness include (1) inability to excrete metabolic wastes, (2) inability to regulate electrolytes, (3) inability to excrete fluid loads, (4) difficulty maintaining adequate nutrition, (5) increased potential for injury, and (6) discomfort. Major patient care problems arising during the diuretic portion of the illness include (1) inability to appropriately conserve fluid and (2) inability to appropriately conserve electrolytes.

Intervention: oliguric phase. During the oliguric phase of acute renal failure, development of hyperkalemia, severe acidosis, severe fluid overload and pulmonary edema, infection, convulsions, or pericarditis connotes some urgency for control or resolution. Included among these problems are the major causes of death resulting from acute kidney failure. These conditions and their management are discussed in the following section.

Control and excretion of metabolic waste buildup. Because the patient's ability to excrete metabolic wastes (nonprotein nitrogen products and acids) cannot keep pace with production of these substances, alternative routes of excretion and control over production of these materials must be found. Means available to accomplish this include providing carbohydrate to spare protein stores, preventing additional tissue trauma, and increasing excretion of wastes through the lungs and through renal dialysis. Of these dialysis is by far the most efficient and is the only true means available for controlling the internal environment of the severely ill hypercatabolic person. Daily laboratory tests will determine blood nonprotein nitrogens and bicarbonate levels, which serve a guide for determining the frequency of dialysis (p. 1333).

Decreasing the production of metabolic wastes can be influenced through dietary means. Calories in the form of carbohydrates and fats provide energy and spare body protein stores, thus decreasing nonprotein nitrogen production. The body recycles urea to synthesize amino acids for protein building so that some regeneration of tissues can occur even though protein intake is curtailed.

Preventing infections and tissue breakdown decreases production of metabolic wastes. Aseptic technique should be rigorously pursued in all treatments performed on the patient. Indwelling catheters are a common source of infection and are to be avoided. The patient should be isolated from anyone with an infection, including other patients, health care personnel, and visitors. Detecting existent infections early so that treatment can be instituted promptly decreases tissue breakdown. When the patient is extremely weak and immobile, frequent turning and repositioning to prevent decubiti must be performed. Skin care in patients with edematous tissues should include observation and prevention of pressure and trauma; these tissues are particularly prone to breakdown.

Acidosis develops when hydrogen ion secretion and bicarbonate ion production diminish in the tubular cells. The pH of the blood decreases, the carbon dioxide content decreases, and central nervous system symptoms of drowsiness progressing to stupor and coma may appear. Although the lungs are unable to compensate totally for the increasing acid load, they help determine the rate at which acidosis develops and the frequency or need for dialysis. In compensating for increased metabolic acid loads, the lungs attempt to excrete more carbon dioxide

(p. 325). To maximize this pathway for acid excretion, pulmonary hygiene should be carried out. Preventing atelectasis and maintaining maximal lung expansion are goals of nursing care.

Regulation of electrolytes. Some common electrolyte disturbances occurring in acute renal failure are hyperkalemia, hyponatremia (usually indicative of overhydration), and increased body sodium content. The rate of accumulation of electrolytes varies greatly in acute renal failure; each patient must be managed individually. Daily or more frequent assessment of laboratory data and clinical signs and symptoms is needed to determine current electrolyte abnormalities and need for treatment.

HYPERKALEMIA. Patients in renal failure with extensive tissue trauma, infection, or bleeding are at a high risk of developing hyperkalemia. In the normal individual the potassium ion is exchanged in the distal convoluted tubule of the nephron for either sodium or hydrogen ions; for the healthy person there is no mechanism in the body to conserve the potassium ion. However, in the individual with acute renal failure in whom a large number of tubular cells are no longer functional, there exists no mechanism to remove potassium from the body. Hyperkalemia is said to exist when the serum concentration of this ion reaches a level of 5.5 mEq/liter or higher. Serum concentrations of 7 to 10 mEq/liter can be quickly reached in acute renal failure and are incompatible with normal cardiac function and life.

In monitoring for signs of potassium toxicity, electrocardiography and laboratory determinations of serum potassium are the most reliable indicators. Rarely does the patient become symptomatic, and pulse changes must not be relied on to indicate the degree of rise of potassium in the patient's system.

Interventions to control the rise of serum potassium and prevent cardiac arrest include those that (1) decrease the intake of potassium, (2) decrease the liberation of potassium from body tissues, and (3) assist in removal of potassium from the body by nonrenal means.

Decreasing the intake of potassium is achieved by administering intravenous feedings or a diet in which potassium content is very low or absent. All fluids and drugs that the patient receives intravenously should be checked for potassium content. Some medications (for example, most penicillin preparations) contain large amounts of this ion. *Controlling the breakdown of body tissues* is extremely important in preventing a rapid rise in serum potassium. Prevention of pressure sores, trauma, bleeding, and infections should be major goals for nursing care. To *promote the excretion of potassium* from the body when the kidneys are nonfunctional, an exchange resin such as polystyrene sodium sulfonate (Kayexalate) is likely to be ordered for the patient. This drug reduces serum potassium by exchanging sodium for potassium ions in the intestinal tract. It can be administered orally, through a nasogastric tube, or by enema. The medication is given orally when the patient's condition permits; oral daily doses range from 15 to 60 g/day. When sodium sulfonate is administered in enema form, the usual dose is 50 g of exchange resin for each enema; it may be repeated daily or as necessary to lower serum potassium. The medication is a powder that when mixed becomes a thick paste within a few seconds; therefore preparation should take place at the bedside just prior to administration. Often mannitol is used to mix the powdered sodium sulfonate, since it induces an osmotic shift of fluid into the bowel producing diarrhea, which helps to expel the medication and additional fluid from the hypervolemic patient. If spontaneous bowel movements do not occur, a cathartic or cleansing enema can be given to ensure the elimination of potassium from the bowel.

HYPONATREMIA. Hyponatremia in acute renal failure most commonly develops with overhydration of the patient. The oliguric patient cannot excrete large volumes of urine; when the administration of sodium-free or low-sodium intravenous or oral fluids continues in such an individual, the serum is diluted and the serum concentration of sodium falls. Signs and symptoms of hyponatremia include warm, moist, flushed skin, muscle weakness, muscle twitching, and behavioral changes involving confusion, delirium, coma, and convulsions. Serum sodium concentrations will be below 130 mEq/liter. The hematocrit value suddenly falls without evidence of bleeding; this is caused by hemodilution.

INCREASED BODY SODIUM CONTENT. Increases in total body content of sodium also occur in acute renal failure. Commonly this occurs when the patient is receiving medications high in sodium content and excess sodium in the diet. Edema and increasing blood pressure indicate retention of sodium and fluids even though the serum sodium concentration is normal or below normal.

Control of fluids. The oliguric or anuric patient is unable to excrete more than minimal amounts of fluid. Nursing care is directed toward three broad objectives: (1) monitoring for signs of fluid overload (p. 1302), (2) maintaining the patient's energy expenditure at a level compatible with his state of health, and (3) controlling or helping the patient to control fluid intake.

All observations regarding the patient's state of hydration need to prominently recorded so that hour-to-hour and day-to-day comparisons can be made. Any finding indicating retention of fluids is reported to the physician. Edema can first be noted in dependent areas such as the feet and legs, in the presacral area, and around the eyes. The patient is observed carefully for signs of pulmonary edema (p. 1009) and congestive heart failure (p. 1003). Central venous or arterial monitoring lines will help to provide data for short-term comparisons in managing the fluid balance of the critically ill person. Accurate recording of intake and output is extremely important as are daily weight records.

The patient in renal failure is unable to excrete fluid loads, and much energy is expended just to maintain current functional status. Positioning and activity are determined daily based on assessment of the energy level and ability to ventilate adequately.

Controlling fluid intake is essential when the ability to excrete fluid is limited. All fluid (parenteral and oral) must total only slightly more than daily output if severe overhydration is to be avoided. When the patient is neither to gain nor lose additional body fluid, the physician will calculate the patient's fluid replacement using the following as a guide: intake will approximate 500 ml/day plus urine output and adjustments for additional fluid lost through fever, diarrhea, and wound drainage. Thirst is a problem that can defy control of fluid intake. Fortunately when sodium intake is controlled, extreme thirst does not develop.

Devices that allow 50 to 150 ml of fluid to be isolated from the main intravenous solution container and drip chambers that allow precise control of fluids through administration of smaller drops of fluid are added safety measures when giving fluids parenterally to anuric or oliguric individuals. Accuracy in fluid balance records is essential. For the patient who is unable to take medications with small amounts of fluid, medications may be given in soft foods such as applesauce.

Maintenance of adequate nutrition. Most persons in acute renal failure are too ill to tolerate oral feedings either initially or for sustained periods of time. Some patients who are able to tolerate fluids orally find that eating food compounds the nausea they experience as a result of an altered biochemical environment and accompanying gastrointestinal tract irritation. Intravenous hypertonic glucose in amounts of 100 g/day or more provides a temporary source of energy that slows the burning of the body's own protein stores. For patients who are severely ill or nauseated, maintaining positive nitrogen balance is not feasible. It is suggested that glucose solutions not be administered in concentrations greater than 10% and that these be administered into large veins to prevent sclerosing of veins.[51] The amount of fluid that can be given within a 24-hour period will influence the total caloric intake provided to the patient. The patient receiving 100 g of intravenous glucose a day will burn approximately 225 g (8 oz) of body tissue per day.[66]

If the patient is able to tolerate oral feedings, dietary protein and potassium are avoided unless dialysis has been initiated. In this case modest amounts of protein and potassium are allowed, thus increasing protein available for tissue building and increasing the palatibility of the diet. Foods high in carbohydrate and fat content are encouraged. A total intake of 2,000 caloies per day is desired although often not achieved due to anorexia and nausea.

Prevention of injury. Monitoring safety is a major nursing responsibility. Specific care for the person with acute renal failure should include preventing falls and physical trauma, preventing infection, and assisting with prevention of drug toxicity by monitoring medication therapy.

The person in acute renal failure is weak, may be confused, and may have visual changes. The amount of supervision required during daily care must be assessed continually. Falls from bed, chair, and during transfer can be prevented by judicious assessment of the person's behavior and capabilities. Convulsions may be precipitated by dialysis, occur as the result of metabolic and electrolyte imbalances, or be the result of coexisting central nervous system disease.

Infection is a leading cause of mortality in persons with acute renal failure. Nosocomial infections (p. 331) are readily contracted by patients whose ability to resist invading organisms is low. Protective isolation is used in some medical centers, while in others this is not thought necessary. Strict attention to aseptic technique must be maintained.

Monitoring prescribed medications is a shared nursing and medical responsibility. The route of excretion and signs of toxicity should be known for all medications that the patient receives. The potential for drug toxicity exists when medications normally excreted by the kidneys are retained in the body as a result of renal damage. Commonly used drugs that fall into this category include antibiotics, cardiac glycosides, and analgesics.[6] Drugs should also be monitored for potassium and sodium content; large increases in daily intake of these ions can result from medication.

Promotion of comfort. Major discomforts that the alert patient commonly experiences include nausea, pain, and thirst. Nausea is generally a result of the renal failure through disturbances in the body's internal environment. The only truly effective treatment is control of uremia with dialysis and good supportive care, which involves correction of electrolyte abnormalities, nonprotein nitrogen levels, and acid-base imbalance. Antiemetic medications at best seem to provide only partial and short-lived relief of nausea and may be contraindicated for patients with liver disease in addition to renal failure.

Pain is a common experience for most acutely ill patients with renal failure. The origins of pain are not related to the renal failure itself but to the trauma, surgery, and insertion of multiple tubes and lines that most of these acutely ill patients undergo. Pain can be controlled safely through the use of narcotic and synthetic narcotic medications. When giving these medications, a judgment needs to be made regarding existing level of central nervous system depression, a common finding in acute acidotic uremia. Medication within "normal" drug dosages can bring about severe respiratory depression, unconsciousness, and death due to the synergistic effects of the person's metabolic state and the actions of the analgesic. It is always safer to determine the patient's tolerance to medication by starting with smaller doses of the medication, which can then be augmented. The respiratory rate and level of awareness provide data as to the patient's tolerance of the analgesic.

Thirst becomes a problem for the alert patient when oral intake is dramatically reduced and the majority of fluid intake is parenteral. Thirst does not become as great a problem when sodium intake is controlled, although for the person who is mouth breathing it is still a discomfort. Fluid that is allowed may be given as ice chips and spaced throughout the day. Meticulous oral care should provide additional relief.

Integrating the emotional aspects of the acute illness. During the acute phase of the illness, biochemical aberrations will generally cause alterations in both the level of awareness and personality of the patient. The family members and occasionally the patient will be aware of these changes such as faltering memory or an inability to think clearly. The biochemical changes may be extensive enough to cause coma. When the patient is sufficiently alert to begin relating to the environment, it should be anticipated that the confusion contributed by the altered internal environment will increase the patient's difficulty in processing information about his condition and surroundings. Simple conversations that attempt to structure the environment and the situation are useful in assisting the person to maintain orientation. These conversations with the patient may require frequent repetition. The patient who perceives a decreased memory or ability to think clearly is assisted to express these concerns and is given reassurance that mental capacities will return with recovery of physical health.

Belligerent, vocal, angry behavior may be seen in previously docile patients. Often this is a source of embarrassment to the family; the patient is generally quite ill and probably unaware of the behavior. Reassurance may be provided, indicating that personalities return to previous states when biochemical alterations are corrected.

Outcome criteria for the person in renal failure during the oliguric phase. The patient demonstrates control of internal environment through:

1. Absence of pulmonary edema.
2. Absence or control of peripheral edema.
3. Control of blood pressure (range between 170/100 and 100/60 mm Hg).
4. Restored or maintained mental alertness.
5. Control of electrolyte balance:
   a. Sodium range 125 to 145 mEq/liter.
   b. Potassium range 3.0 to 6.0 mEq/liter.
   c. Bicarbonate above 14 mEq/liter.
6. Control of protein catabolism:
   a. Urea nitrogen below 100 mg/100 ml.
   b. Creatinine below 12 mg/100 ml.
   c. Absence of skin breakdown.
7. Absence of bleeding.

The patient is free of:

1. Infection.
2. Injury resulting from decreased level of awareness and strength.
3. Toxicity from inadequately excreted medication.

Intercurrent illness is resolved or controlled (congestive heart failure, shock).

Intervention: diuretic phase. After a period of oliguria or anuria, which may last a few days to a week, patients recovering renal function pass into another distinct phase of illness characterized by increased urinary output. Increased output indicates that the damaged nephrons are healing and are able to begin excreting urine. At first daily urine volume increases slowly, although within 1 to 2 days diuresis up to or exceeding 4 to 5 liters/day may occur. Although fluid can be excreted, the kidneys are not yet healed. Often there is inability to excrete proportional amounts of waste materials, and serum concentrations of urea nitrogen may rise or remain elevated as urine volume increases. At times excessive excretion of sodium and potassium occurs during diuresis. Complete recovery of renal function is slow and requires anywhere from days to a few weeks. Return of the renal function to normal or near normal levels is evidenced when the kidney can both conserve and dilute urine and when serum electrolytes and nonprotein nitrogen levels become normal.

Nursing care during the diuretic phase is directed toward detecting fluid losses and electrolyte imbalances. Much of the fluid excreted during diuresis in excess of an amount proportional to the patient's intake may be fluid that has accumulated in the body during the oliguric phase of illness. However, serious fluid and electrolyte depletion can occur. In addition to detecting fluid and electrolyte imbalances, several nursing care objectives established during the oliguric phase should be continued. These include maintaining nutritional intake, maintaining safety of the patient, and preventing infection.

Nursing observations and recording needed in judging the adequacy of hydration and serum sodium of the patient include (1) changes in mental awareness and activity, (2) degree of thirst, (3) moistness of mucous membranes, (4) development of skin turgor, (5) development of tachycardia and postural hypotension, and (6) accurate daily weight, fluid balance, and vital signs.

Outcome criteria for the person with renal failure during the diuretic phase. The patient or significant others can:

1. State extent of recovery of kidney function.
2. Identify any preventable environmental or health factor involved in generating the illness.
3. Plan a diet to maintain positive nitrogen balance and sufficient caloric intake.
4. Identify signs and symptoms of dehydration and sodium and potassium loss.
5. Describe plans for prevention of infection.
6. State plans for follow-up health care.

□ Chronic renal failure

Chronic renal failure exists when the kidneys are no longer capable of maintaining an internal environment consistent with life and when return of function is not anticipated. For the majority of individuals the transition from health to a state of chronic or permanent disease is a slow one extending over a number of years. Recurrent infections and exacerbations of nephritis, obstruction of the urinary tract, and destruction of vessels from diabetes and longstanding hypertension lead to scarring of kidney tissue and progressive loss of renal function. Some individuals, however, develop total irreversible loss of renal function acutely; such loss of renal function usually develops in a matter of a few hours or days and follows a direct traumatic insult to the kidneys.

Chronic renal failure exists as a major health problem in the United States. Approximately 8 million individuals now have chronic kidney disease; approximately 60,000 persons die each year as the result of renal failure.[65]

Prognosis. The individual with chronic renal failure can to some extent control and manage the symptoms of the disease. Although renal function that has been lost due to destruction of kidney tissue cannot be recovered, the life of the person can be maintained by limiting the intake of substances that require excretion and by providing alternative routes of excretion from the body for waste and electrolytes. By adhering to a prescribed management routine, albeit quite strict and demanding, life may be sustained. For some individuals medication and diet therapy alone may control uremic symptoms; other individuals may require in addition dialysis or transplantation to control the symptoms of their disease.

Prevention. Obstruction and infection of the urinary tract and hypertensive disease are common and often asymptomatic causes of renal damage and renal failure. A significant reduction in the incidence of renal failure can be effected through increasing attention to general health promotion. Yearly physical examinations in which blood pressure is determined, urinalysis is performed, and the patient is questioned about dysuria or pain in the urinary tract assist in early detection of disease that may lead to renal failure.

General health maintenance can reduce the number of individuals progressing from renal insufficiency into frank renal failure. Care is aimed toward adequately treating medical problems and closely supervising the person's health status in times of stress (infection, pregnancy).

Clinical picture. Although the clinical course of chronic renal disease varies from individual to individual, there are common features of the illness. Signs and symptoms result from disordered fluid and electrolyte balance, alterations in regulatory functions of the body, and retention of solutes. *Azotemia* (excess nitrogenous products in the blood), *anemia*, and *acidosis* are always present. Potassium and hydrogen ion excretion is impaired. Fluid and sodium balance is abnormal and may involve either abnormal retention or secretion of sodium and water; thus urinary volume can be decreased, normal, or increased. With end-stage renal disease, hyperuricemia is a common finding, although the varied serum levels of uric acid seem to have no definite relationship to the exact level of kidney function.[51] Increased levels of serum phosphate are characteristic, and calcium levels may be low or normal. These findings result from decreased renal excretions of phosphate and simultaneous reduction in ionized serum calcium. Through increased production of parathormone the body may reestablish a normal serum calcium level, although this is accomplished at the expense of the individual's bone matrix.

Hypertension may or may not be present. Often with the development of end-stage renal disease blood pressure is elevated and seems to be the result of increased total body water, a renally released vasopressor, or an inadequately secreted vasodepressor.[9] Glucose intolerance may be seen although usually not of sufficient severity to warrant treatment. The rising blood sugar level appears to be the result of an altered biochemical environment produced by the failing kidneys and does not signify the development of diabetes mellitus. As renal failure progresses the patient develops increased pigmentation of the skin, the skin becomes sallow or brownish in tone. Wtih more advanced and insufficiently treated renal failure the patient may develop muscular twitching, numbness in the feet and legs, pericarditis, and pleuritis. These signs will disappear with restabilization of the patient with diet and medication or with the additional assistance of dialysis.

The symptoms of uremia usually develop so slowly

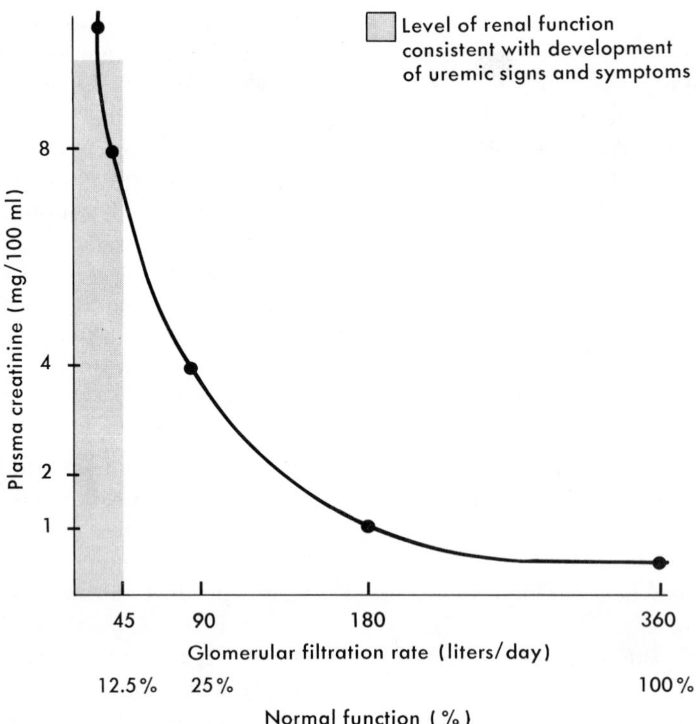

Fig. 59-5. Glomerular filtration and plasma creatinine level.

that the patient and his family often do not recall the time of onset of the illness. Symptoms generally noticed as uremia develops include lethargy, headaches, physical and mental fatigue, weight loss, irritability, and depression. Anorexia, persistent nausea and vomiting, shortness of breath on either mild or no exertion, and pitting edema are symptomatic of severe loss of renal function. Pruritus may be absent, mild, or severe.

The point at which the patient becomes obviously symptomatic and displays signs typical of renal failure occurs when approximately 80% to 90% of renal function has been lost (Fig. 59-5). At this level of renal function creatinine clearance values will fall to 15 ml/minute or less.

Alterations in fertility. As end-stage renal failure develops, most women note changes in their menstrual cycle. Bleeding may occur at more widely spaced intervals, may be heavier or lighter in flow than normal, or may cease all together. This obvious change in reproductive cycle is usually accompanied by changes in fertility. Ovulation may occur normally or may occur only a few times a year. Pregnancy in uremic women is of much lower incidence than in normal population. In men impotence may occur as chronic renal failure progresses toward endstage disease. Dialysis or more vigorous treatment of uremia is indicated to return or maximize reproductive function. It should be stressed that sexual activity of some persons with chronic renal failure may remain quite normal even though changes in reproductive ability are present.

Intervention. Major problems for the patient in chronic renal failure include (1) inability to appropriately control fluid balance, (2) inability to regulate electrolyte balance, (3) inability to excrete metabolic wastes, (4) inability to transport oxygen to cells, (5) inability to maintain normal rest and sleep patterns, (6) difficulty in maintaining adequate nutrition, (7) increased potential for physical injury, (8) discomfort, (9) alterations in fertility, and (10) changes in life style, group membership, and feelings regarding the self.

Treatment goals for the person with chronic renal failure are as follows:

1. Stabilization of the internal environment as demonstrated by:
   a. Mental alertness, attention span, and appropriate interaction with the environment.
   b. Absence or control of peripheral edema, absence of pulmonary edema.
   c. Control of electrolyte balance:
      Sodium 125 to 145 mEq/liter
      Potassium 3 to 6 mEq/liter

Bicarbonate	> 15 mEq/liter
Calcium	9 to 11 mg/100 ml
Phosphate	3 to 5 mg/100 ml

d. Serum albumin > 2 g/100 ml.

e. Control of protein catabolism and protein breakdown products:

Urea nitrogen	< 100 mg/100 ml
Creatinine	< 15 mg/100 ml
Uric acid	< 12 mg/100 ml

f. Absence of joint inflammation and pain.

2. Infection and abnormal bleeding are not present.
3. Blood pressure is controlled at less than 160/100 mm Hg sitting and less than 30 mm Hg postural change on standing.
4. Anorexia, nausea, and pruritus are absent or controlled.
5. Intercurrent illness is resolved or controlled (heart failure, infection, dehydration).
6. There is no toxicity from inadequately excreted medication.
7. Nutrient intake is sufficient to maintain positive nitrogen balance.

Control of fluid balance. The ability to excrete sodium and water in the urine varies considerably in chronic renal failure. Although volume problems for most patients with chronic end-stage renal failure involve *hypervolemia* resulting from a marked inability to excrete sodium in water, some patients are unable to conserve these substances and are subject to *hypovolemic* states. With either marked inability to excrete or conserve body fluid, the patient can develop severe fluid imbalances in a relatively short period of time. Care is directed toward identifying fluid imbalances and in providing an intake of sodium and water equivalent to the amounts of these substances excreted. The desired effect of this care is to maintain the patient in a normotensive, normovolemic state. (For further information on assessment and intervention of hypervolemia and hypovolemia, see Chapter 20.)

Controlling sodium intake can be an extremely challenging problem for both the nurse and the patient. Any sudden increase in weight indicates accumulating fluid, and the source of this fluid must be sought with the patient. Often when the person is not acutely ill and is responsible for control of his intake, the problem can be traced to excess sodium ingestion, which produces thirst. In helping to avoid this cycle of thirst leading to increased fluid ingestion and overhydration, the patient is carefully taught the allowances of sodium and fluid in the diet and what restrictions are to be observed in purchasing commercially prepared foods. The words "sodium" and "salt" should be sought on food labels when the person is on a severely sodium-restricted diet, and these foods should be avoided. At times the person is unable to offer an explanation for increasing thirst and sodium ingestion. At this point the question of home self-medication (for example, sodium bicarbonate for indigestion) should be raised. After failure to uncover increased intake of either sodium or fluid to explain hypervolemia, the person is asked to list for a period of 3 consecutive days all foods and fluids ingested. This list can then be reviewed with the individual and used not only to uncover instances of dietary indiscretion but also as a teaching tool.

Regulation of electrolyte balance. Potassium and phosphorus retention occur in chronic renal failure. Nursing care is aimed toward identifying signs and symptoms of *hyperkalemia* and *hyperphosphatemia* and toward reducing intake and providing alternative routes of excretion for these substances from the body.

Signs of potassium intoxication and the role of cation exchange resins in utilizing the intestinal tract as an alternative route of excretion are discussed on p. 1324. Serum potassium can be at least partially controlled in chronic renal failure by decreasing dietary and drug intake. Thorough diet teaching of the patient and all persons responsible for food preparation is essential. This teaching should help the patient identify the foods that are high in potassium and the methods of cooking that can reduce the potassium content of the diet. *Salt substitutes should be avoided by all patients with chronic renal disease as they contain large amounts of potassium.* Medications that are prescribed for the patient should be reviewed for potassium content.

Significant rises in serum potassium can be averted by preventing tissue breakdown. Potassium is largely an intracellular cation, and extensive tissue damage can liberate a lethal amount of this ion into the system of the patient with chronic renal failure. Patients should be advised to seek medical attention when symptoms of infection or other problems first appear.

When the kidneys fail, the ability to excrete phosphorus decreases. A vicious cycle of ionized serum calcium depletion and bone demineralization can begin. The problem is identified by laboratory determinations of serum calcium and phosphorus levels and through radiographs of the hands, feet, and skull to show demineralized areas of bone. Treatment involves administering an aluminum hydroxide preparation. This medication binds phosphorus in the intestinal tract, thus providing an alternative route for phosphorus excretion. Usual doses of aluminum hydroxide range from 1 to 5 g/day.

Prevention of metabolic waste buildup. Azotemia and *acidosis* occur in all patients with chronic renal failure, although the severity of the problems and the degree to which the person has developed tolerance to his altered internal environment vary considerably. Nursing care should be directed toward (1) decreasing the production of metabolic wastes, (2) promoting excretion of volatile acids by the lungs, and (3) detecting increasing acidosis and its clinical effect on the patient.

Metabolic waste production can be significantly reduced by controlling dietary protein intake and by preventing catabolism of existing protein stores. The amount of protein allowed in the diet for the person with chronic renal failure can vary from 20 to 80 g/day. The specific level of protein intake prescribed depends on the presence of some means for clearing the products of protein breakdown from the patient's system. Dietary protein intake is more liberal for persons who have some ability to excrete wastes in their urine and for those being treated with dialysis. When restricting dietary protein, the quality of that allowed must be high. The persons must be taught to select foods that contain all of the essential amino acids. When calories are provided in the form of carbohydrate and fat for immediate energy needs, smaller amounts of protein can suffice for cellular growth and repair. Catabolism of existing protein stores liberates nitrogenous wastes. For this reason sources of potential infection such as indwelling catheters are avoided, and when infection is noted it is immediately treated.

In chronic renal failure the kidneys are unable to excrete hydrogen ions and to manufacture bicarbonate. Metabolic acidosis results. On the basis of laboratory data acidosis may appear to be severe; however, persons with chronic renal failure adjust to lowered serum bicarbonate levels and often do not become acutely symptomatic even when bicarbonate levels reach values of 15 to 16 mEq/liter. Because of this adjustment, treatment with bicarbonate is often not carried out. The lungs assume a prominent role in regulating acid-base balance, and helping the individual to maintain pulmonary function becomes an important objective for nursing care.

Determining patient tolerance of a state of acidosis that can fluctuate from moderate to critical levels (as additional stresses such as infection and blood loss occur) is important in the nursing care given the patient. Severe acidosis results in central nervous system depression (p. 328).

Maintenance of oxygen transport to cells. Anemia universally accompanies chronic disease. Hematocrit values of 16% to 22% are not abnormal for these individuals. Anemia results from both a decreased production of red blood cells and a decrease in longevity of the cells in circulation. Although oral iron supplements may be tried, iron is not well absorbed by the gastrointestinal tract in chronic renal failure, and in some individuals it may cause nausea and vomiting. Since dietary sources of folate (folic acid) may be restricted in chronic renal failure, and food preparation may further decrease the amount of folate ingested, this vitamin may be given as a medication. A sufficient dose is 1 mg/day. Transfusions are not generally given unless the hematocrit level becomes extremely low. The reason for this is that when transfusions are given frequently the patient's own stimulus to red cell production is decreased.

The severely anemic person complains of extreme fatigue and shortness of breath. Because of a lack of red cells there is inability to transport sufficient oxygen to cells for energy production. Milder complaints of the anemic person include an inability to work or play without extended rest periods. Nursing activities can be directed toward helping identify activities essential to daily living and helping the person to modify these activities according to existing energy level. Preventing the accumulation of excess fluid in a person with a very low hematocrit level allows energy to be used for activities of daily living rather than for carrying extra fluid. Other important nursing activities include helping the person to control blood losses. A soft toothbrush is recommended for oral care. Antacids taken at regular and frequent intervals can reduce gastrointestinal tract bleeding. The person is instructed to observe for melena and to report this finding to the physician without delay.

Some degree of peripheral neuropathy occurs in almost all persons with chronic renal failure. Numbness, tingling, and burning of the extremities are common complaints. Treatment that is effective in controlling these symptoms consists of more intensive management of the uremic state.

Promotion of comfort, rest, and sleep. Rarely does the person with chronic renal failure have acute sharp pain; however, these individuals are subject to a wide variety of chronic discomforts. Most commonly these discomforts include pruritus, muscle cramping, numbness and tingling in the hands and feet, thirst, headaches, and irritation of the eyes. Most persons with end-stage renal disease develop pruritus. Patients relate that itching is of a deep sensation. A variety of theories have been postulated as to the origin of the itching. However, the exact cause of this problem has not yet been identified. Factors that seem to exacerbate the itching include increasing levels of serum phosphorus, dry skin, warm moist heat, and emotional stress. Itching is largely symptomatic, and measures that are effective in controlling it vary from individual to individual. Reducing levels of serum phosphorus with aluminum hydroxide preparations decreases itching for most patients. Keeping the skin moist and supple through use of lotions and bath oils, controlling the room temperature during sleep to prevent excessive warmth, emollient baths, and bathing with a vinegar solution are measures alone or in combination that may provide some relief from itching. Medications such as trimeprazine tartrate (Temaril) are also prescribed as necessary and for some individuals provide much relief from itching. Since emotional stress seems to increase the itching, helping the person verbalize feelings may provide for some resolution of conflict and help decrease these manifestations of psychologic stress. The urge to scratch the skin is acute in some persons. Because scratching is often vigorous, injury to the skin with subsequent infection can result. Fingernails are trimmed closely. In preference to fingernails, a soft cloth should be used to scratch the skin.

Muscle cramping in the lower extremities and the hands is common in renal failure. Often cramping can be correlated with sodium depletion. Primary treatment for muscle cramping involves controlling the state of uremia and fluid and electrolyte balance. Temporary measures of heat and massage are effective for some persons.

Headaches in chronic renal failure result from a variety of causes. These include increasing blood pressure, progressing uremia, and rapid changes in osmotic gradients between cellular, interstitial, and intravascular compartments. Treatment of these problems has been discussed previously.

Ocular irritation in chronic renal failure is caused by calcium deposits in the conjunctiva that cause burning and watering of the eyes. Treatment involves controlling the plasma phosphate level through administration of oral aluminum hydroxide preparations. "Artificial tears" (methylcellulose) placed in the conjunctival sac every few hours also help to reduce irritation.

Insomnia and chronic daytime fatigue are common complaints of persons with chronic renal failure. This reversal of normal sleep patterns has been attributed to a variety of causes. These include (1) recurring occupation with thoughts concerning the disease state and changes in life style required by the illness, (2) pruritus, and (3) the state of uremia itself. Reduction of high serum levels of urea nitrogen and creatinine through decreasing dietary intake of protein or dialysis may bring sleep patterns more toward normal. When control of uremia fails to cure insomnia, mild central nervous system depressants may be ordered.

General comfort at bedtime is needed to induce sleep at any time and is especially important whenever sleeping problems arise. Comfort measures can include warm baths, pursuing quiet activities an hour or two before bedtime, controlling itching, or anything the patient finds calming and soothing.

The individual who is awake a significant portion of the night may need to plan for rest periods during the day. These rest periods should be taken far enough ahead of bedtime to prevent compounding sleeplessness.

Maintenance of adequate nutrition. Maintaining a good nutritional intake can be difficult for persons with chronic renal failure. Anorexia, nausea, and vomiting frequently occur, and diets can be so severely restricted that they bear little resemblance to the normal dietary patterns. In uremia disturbances in fluid, electrolyte, and waste composition of body fluids occur and produce changes in osmotic gradients in all cells. When these changes occur in the cells of the gastrointestinal tract and the central nervous system, anorexia, nausea, and vomiting result. Persons with uremia are prone to bleeding of the gastrointestinal tract and the oral cavity. Urea is broken down to ammonia by the action of intestinal bacteria. Since ammonia is a mucosal irritant, ulceration and bleeding can occur. In addition to the gastrointestinal tract problems that lead to nausea and vomiting, there is a decreased salivary flow in persons with chronic renal disease. An ammonia smell and taste can accumulate in the mouth quickly and can further compound anorexia. Treatment includes administering antacids every 2 to 4 hours to decrease gastrointestinal irritation. Dietary control of uremia, perhaps augmented by dialysis, should help to control disturbances in fluid, electrolyte, and waste composition of body fluids and thus help to control nausea and vomiting. Oral hygiene, especially before meals, is important to combat anorexia.

Modifying the diet as possible to the preferences of the individual can also help to maintain intake of food. Dietary teaching and meal planning can be approached according to an exchange system similar to that used for individuals with diabetes. With this approach there is greater ability to modify the diet according to personal preferences. The pattern of meals during the day is also a matter of personal preference. Some individuals prefer two or three meals a day. When eating patterns are known and used in dietary instruction and meal planning, intake of food is likely to increase.

Actual eating of prepared food can be promoted through attempting to decrease emotional tension at the dinner table. Periods other than mealtime should be used to discuss family and individual problems. Food that is attractively arranged and well flavored is likely to be more acceptable to the patient. Spices and other flavorings can add variety to foods that are prepared without sodium. It is interesting that most persons relate that their taste for salt disappears once they have adhered to a low-sodium diet for a few weeks. When the gastrointestinal tract is ulcerated, bland foods may be tried in an attempt to increase ingestion of food.

Promotion of safety. Common injuries to the person in chronic renal failure include infection, accidents due to decrease in mental and visual awareness of the environment, and improper usage of medications. In chronic renal failure resistance to infection is decreased. Control of infection is essentially similar to that described in the section on care of the patient in acute renal failure. In addition the person is counseled to avoid exposure to individuals with known infections and to avoid extreme fatigue, which lowers body resistance.

The buildup of osmotically active particles and fluid in the body that occurs in uremia produces changes in the cells of the brain that may lead to confusion and impairment in decision-making ability. In some instances convulsions and coma may result from the changed internal environment. Fluid accumulation and hypertension can produce visual changes. Nursing care should involve assessing and helping the family to assess the safety of the decisions that the patient makes and his awareness of the environment. At times the person may need to be helped in limiting activities to a level commensurate with his mental processes and level of awareness. For instance, blurred vision and delayed reaction time contraindicate driving an automobile. Convulsions and coma may result from severe fluid, electrolyte, and waste imbalances. In most instances when the person is subject to developing these complications hospitalization is necessary. Individuals caring for the patient need to be aware of the possibility of seizure activity and take appropriate precautions. Correcting abnormal body chemistry is the most important measure for preventing coma or convulsions.

Education about medications is carried out with the person in the areas of both medications that have been prescribed for him and over-the-counter or folk medicines. The use of common popular medications that are sold without prescription must be discouraged. All medications should be prescribed by the physician. Aspirin is dangerous because it is normally excreted by the kidneys and may rapidly build to toxic levels and it prolongs bleeding time. Ingestion of sodium bicarbonate (baking soda) to treat indigestion can result in extremely large intakes of sodium. Many cold preparations also contain large amounts of sodium. Remembering to take prescribed medications can be a problem for the person who may have to take over 2 dozen pills each day. Correlating pill-taking times with major activities of the day is often helpful. Medications that are frequently given to those with chronic renal failure are identified as follows:

1. Drugs that increase intake of essential substances:
   a. Vitamins
   b. Folic acid
   c. Calcium
   d. Bicarbonate
   e. Iron
2. Drugs that promote excretion of nonessential or excessive substances
   a. Diuretics (sodium and water)
   b. Phosphate binders
   c. Exchange resins (potassium)
   d. Allopurinol (uric acid)
3. Drugs that regulate body processes
   a. Antihypertensives (↓ BP)
   b. Cardiac glycosides (↑ rate; ↓ arrthymias)
   c. Steroids (↓ inflammatory response)
   d. Laxatives or stool softeners (↓ constipation)
   e. Androgens (↑ RBC production)
4. Drugs that promote comfort and rest
   a. Mild analgesics (without aspirin)
   b. Trimeprazine (Temaril)
   c. Diazepam (Valium)
   d. Mild hypnotics

Coping with changes in life style, group membership, and feelings regarding self. Numerous alterations in life style, group membership, and membership, and feelings regarding the self occur for the person with chronic renal failure. The numerous physical changes that occur often make it difficult to carry on activities that were once normally pursued. Chronic fatigue may make it impossible for the person to continue to be employed. Because the patient is often tired and not feeling well, it may be difficult to plan in advance for social events. The former roles of the sick member of the family must often be taken on by another. When roles cannot easily be changed or additionally assumed by other members of the family, serious threats to the organization of the family group occur. Physical appearance also changes and is of much concern to most persons. As uremia progresses, the individual often becomes thin and weaker and appears sallow. Thoughts concerning death and the quality of this changed life are common.

Denial often becomes a chief defense mechanism for the patient. With it the individual can periodically forget the constant threat to life. The use of this mental mechanism for the person with chronic renal failure can be quite appropriate as long as it is not manifested by maladaptive or harmful behavior. Inappropriate uses of denial involve continuous dietary indiscretion and failure to take prescribed medications.

The patient with chronic renal failure needs the hope and encouragement that with treatment he will be able to live with a lessening of discomfort and will have a continued existence to pursue what seems most productive and important to him. Hope should not be focused on cure but on learning to manage a new style of life. In managing the changes that occur as a result of chronic renal failure, the patient should be encouraged to be as independent and as active as possible. He should be taught to manage his treatment and should be given the responsibility of doing so. Nursing care should be provided as part of the team approach that assists the patient in identifying problems and resources and helps the patient and his family adjust to the changing style of life.

Outcome criteria for the person with chronic renal failure

The patient or significant others can:

1. Explain the dietary program:
   a. State means of identifying content of foods.
   b. Explain use of small frequent feedings to maintain nutrient intake when anorexic or nauseated.
   c. State fluid prescription and identify sources of fluid in diet.
2. Demonstrate measurement of fluid intake and output and accurate recording of intake and output.
3. State name, dosage, frequency, purpose and side effects of medications.
4. Describe measures useful in controlling common discomforts (pruritus, insomnia).
5. Describe preventive health care measures (good oral hygiene, prevention of infection, avoidance of bleeding).
6. Relate a plan for gradual increase in physical activity including need for rest periods and measures to conserve energy.
7. Describe plan for health care follow-up:
   a. State signs and symptoms of progressing disease that require immediate medical attention.
   b. Explain the goals of health care.
   c. Explain plans for continued management of other chronic health problems and relate changes in management required as a result of kidney failure.

□ Management of the person dying of renal failure

At times nursing care must be provided for the patient who is dying from renal failure. Major objectives should be maintaining the comfort and the safety of the patient and providing opportunity for the patient and his family to vent feelings and arrive at some degree of emotional comfort. In providing physical comfort to the patient, diets may be liberalized. Frequent turning and repositioning are necessary to prevent skin excoriation and breakdown. Oral care is extremely important, since sores in the mouth, once developed, are almost impossible to cure. Mineral oil is an acceptable protective lubricant for the alert patient. A water-soluble lubricant with a vegetable base (such as K-Y jelly) is preferable for the stuporous patient. Hydrogen peroxide is helpful in removing blood from the mouth and the nose.

As death approaches, the patient often becomes severely confused or comatose. As his level of awareness and ability to control the environment decrease, it becomes the responsibility of the nursing staff to provide safety for the patient. The specific care required for the unconscious patient is described in Chapter 27.

Providing an opportunity for the patient and family to ventilate feelings is one of the more important aspects of nursing care for a patient with either acute or chronic onset of uremia. Thoughts concerning death and alarm over treatments produce considerable anxiety. The wishes of the patient and family regarding spiritual counseling should be determined. Through demonstrating interest in the patient's needs and attending to his comfort, the nurse can do a great deal to help the patient and his family accept the patient's ultimate death.

□ Dialysis

Dialysis involves the movement of fluid and particles across a semipermeable membrane. It is a treatment that can help restore normal fluid and electrolyte balance, control acid-base balance, and remove waste and toxic material from the body. It is a treatment that can sustain life successfully in both acute and chronic situations where substitution for or augmentation of normal renal function is needed. Specifically dialysis is used to remove excessive amounts of drugs and toxins in poisonings of both an intentional and accidental nature, to correct serious electrolyte and acid-base imbalances, to maintain kidney function when renal shutdown occurs as a result of transusion reactions, to temporarily replace renal function in person with acute renal failure of various origins, and to permanently substitute for loss of renal function in persons with chronic end-stage kidney disease.

Dialysis is based on three principles: diffusion, osmosis, and ultrafiltration (Fig. 59-6). *Diffusion* involves the movement of particles from an area of greater to an area of lesser concentration. In the body this usually occurs across a semipermeable membrane. Diffusion is involved in the clearance of solute from the patient's body in both hemodialysis and peritoneal dialysis. Diffusion results in the movement of urea, creatinine, and uric acid from the patient's blood into the dialysate solution. This solution contains fewer particles to be removed from the bloodstream and higher concentrations of particles to be added to the blood (Fig. 59-7). Since the dialysate contains no protein waste products, the concentration of these substances in the blood will decrease due to random movement of the particles across the semipermeable membrane into the dialysate. The same principle applies to the movement of potassium ions. Although the concentration of red blood cells and protein is high in blood, these molecules are quite large and do not diffuse through the membrane pores; hence they are not lost from the blood.

Osmosis involves the movement of fluid across a semipermeable membrane from an area of lesser to an area of greater concentration of particles. Osmosis is responsible for movement of extra fluid from the patient, particularly in peritoneal dialysis. Fig. 59-7 shows that glucose has been added to the dialysate to make its parti-

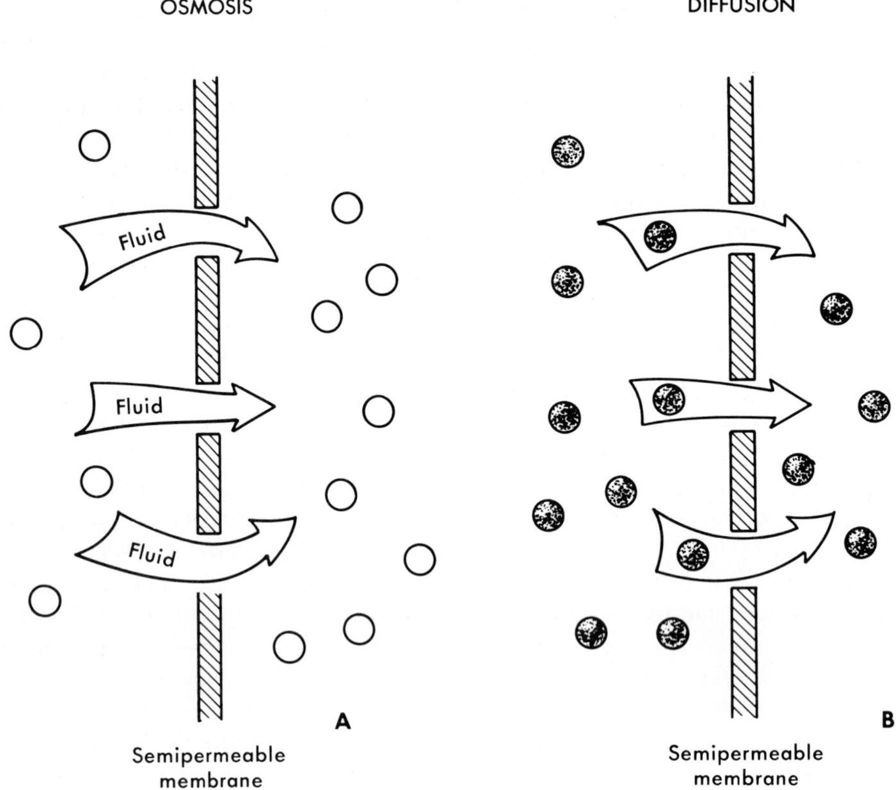

Fig. 59-6. A, Process of osmosis. **B,** Process of diffusion.

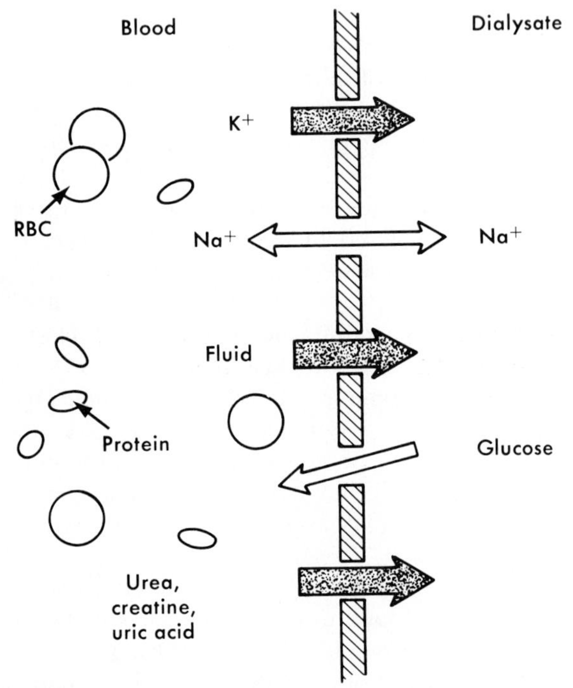

Fig. 59-7. Osmosis and diffusion in dialysis. Net movement of major particles and fluid is illustrated.

cle concentration greater than that of the patient's blood. Fluid will then move through the pores of the membrane from the patient's blood to the dialysate.

Ultrafiltration involves the movement of fluid across a semipermeable membrane as a result of an artificially created pressure gradient. Ultrafiltration is more efficient than osmosis for removal of fluid and is used in hemodialysis for this purpose. During dialysis osmosis and diffusion or ultrafiltration and diffusion occur simultaneously.

Hemodialysis

Procedure. Hemodialysis has been a practical lifesaving treatment for persons with impaired renal function for over 15 years. The major limitations in providing this treatment to all individuals who could benefit from it are initial case finding, expense of the equipment, and the necessity of highly trained personnel. The availability of hemodialysis, especially for the chronically ill person, now lags little behind need due to the impetus given the development of a nationwide end-stage renal disease program by the federal government. Home dialysis, once a mandatory move for those seeking dialysis care, is now largely a personal choice of the person and the family.

Hemodialysis involves shunting the patient's blood from the body through a machine in which diffusion and ultrafiltration occur and back into the patient's circulation. In order to perform hemodialysis there must be an access to the patient's blood, a mechanism to transport the blood to and from the dialyzer, and a dialyzer (area in which the exchange of fluid electrolytes and waste products occurs).

Presently two major means exist for gaining access to the patient's bloodstream. These are the external shunt and arteriovenous fistula. The external shunt (Fig. 59-8, *A*) is constructed by placing two cannulas through a skin incision into a large vein and a large artery that lie close to each other. When dialysis is not occurring, the cannulas are connected to each other so that blood continually flows through the tubes and patency of the system is maintained. For dialysis the cannulas are separated. The arterial cannula is connected to a line that delivers the patient's blood to the dialyzer; the venous cannula is attached to a line that returns blood to the patient's body. Infection, clotting of the shunt, and erosion of the skin around the insertion area of the cannulae are problems that occur with enough frequency to limit general use of the external shunt to situations that are acute and temporary.

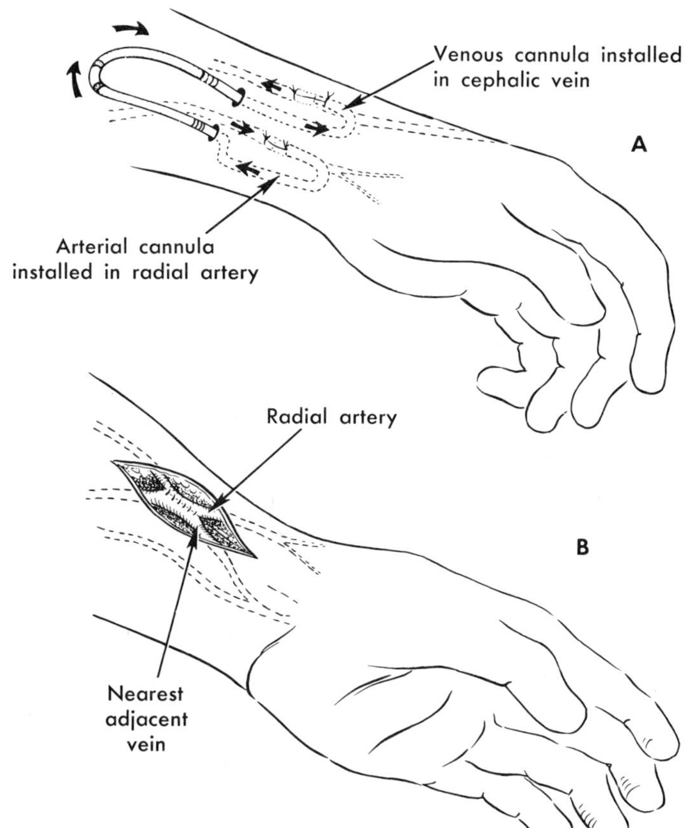

Fig. 59-8. Two common forms of venous access for hemodialysis. **A,** External shunt, **B,** Arteriovenous fistula.

The other common method of access to the patient's blood supply is the arteriovenous fistula (Fig. 59-8, *B*). This procedure increases blood flow into superficial veins, making the patient's blood easily accessible for dialysis. Direct access to the patient's blood is established by inserting needles of large diameter into the superficial veins "fed" by the fistula. The fistula, like the shunt, is generally located in an upper extremity, although the legs may also be used.

Precautions must be taken to maintain the patency of a shunt or fistula. During the patient's hospitalization it is the nurse who is the most consistent observer of the shunt or fistula and the individual most able to see that precautionary measures are followed by all individuals dealing with the patient. To ensure proper maintenance of the shunt or fistula in the home, the same care that the nurse provides in the hospital must be taught to the patient or his family.

Decreasing the flow of blood through the shunt or fistula for even short periods can result in clotting. Decreased blood flow results from (1) systemic hypotension, (2) infection of the shunt or fistula, (3) compression of the shunt or fistula, (4) tight bandages or restrictive clothing, (5) phlebitis from punctures of the involved veins, and (6) prolonged inflation of the blood pressure cuff when taking the blood pressure. All of these must be avoided.

Because the external shunt involves a break in the surface of the skin, special attention is given to preventing infection. A dry, sterile dressing that is changed daily should cover the shunt. The cannula insertion sites should be observed for any signs of infection. Any redness, tenderness, swelling, or excessive warmth of the skin in these areas is reported to the physician.

Clotting of the shunt or fistula can be detected by an absence of the palpable or audible *bruit* along the venous portion of the shunt or fistula. Since blood can be observed as it flows through a shunt, clotting may also be detected by the presence of dark or separated blood in the tubing. When it is suspected that a shunt has clotted, the physician should be notified immediately as it may be possible to clear the shunt.

Several types of hemodialyzers are currently in use (Fig. 59-9). Although quite different in appearance, all artificial kidneys function similarly.

Pretreatment care. Prior to the procedure patients should have an opportunity to become familiar with the dialysis unit. They should be given an explanation of what will happen and what will be expected of them during the treatment. Patients often want to know (1) what types of pain will be experienced during the treatment, (2) how long and how often the dialysis will be, (3) what they should feel like after the treatment, (4) what they will be allowed to do and to eat during dialysis, and (5) if family members may be present during the therapy.

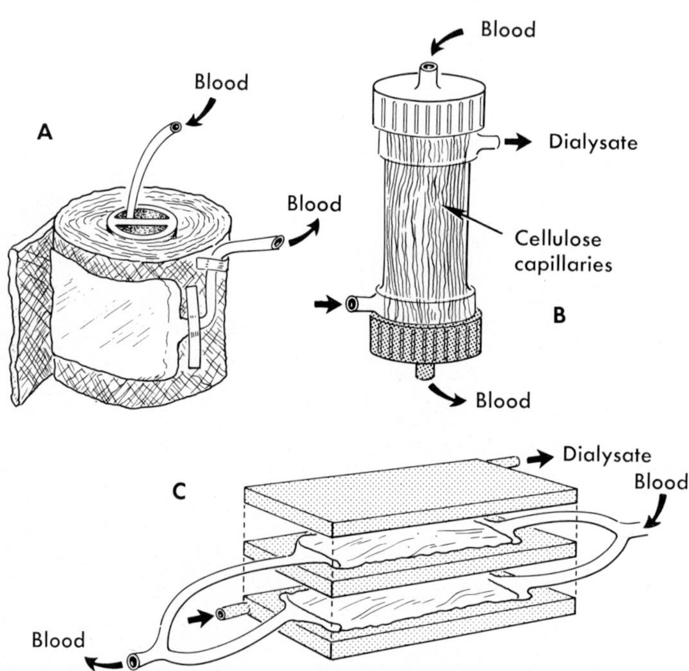

Fig. 59-9. Examples of dialyzers. **A,** Coil dialyzer. **B,** Hollow fiber dialyzer. **C,** Kill (flat plate) dialyzer, which is being used less frequently.

When the patient has an external shunt, no pain should be experienced during initiation to dialysis. However, pain of a moderate degree may be present when venipuncture is performed in an arteriovenous fistula. A local anesthetic is used in most dialysis centers prior to insertion of the needles.

Patients should be told that they may experience some headache and nausea during the treatment and for a few hours afterward. Headache and nausea result from changes in fluid, acid-base, and waste balance during dialysis. The symptoms should never be extreme, and relief should be attained from rest and sleep, mild analgesics, or antiemetics. Postural hypotension may also occur following dialysis; it is transitory in nature and due to a relative depletion of intravascular volume secondary to fluid removal. The hypotension may produce dizziness and faintness. Relief should be obtained within a few hours with rest. The patient is assured that all of these symptoms will abate and that frequent monitoring during the procedure will help to control the degree of change that occurs during dialysis and the development of these symptoms.

A dialysis treatment lasts from 3 to 6 hours, depending on the type of dialyzer used and the time necessary to correct the fluid, electrolyte, acid-base, and waste problems that are present. Dialysis for an acute problem may be carried out daily or as often as the condition of the patient warrants. Hemodialysis for chronic renal failure is usually performed two or three times a week.

Many persons expect to leave the dialysis treatment with a feeling of well-being. Few persons feel this way; most experience some minor discomfort that diminishes a few hours after dialysis. The greatest feeling of well-being seems to occur the day after dialysis.

Eating and activity during dialysis are largely a matter of individual preference. Some persons sleep throughout their treatment; others may read and carry on various activities. The person's ability to eat during dialysis must be individually determined. Some individuals may become quite hungry, while for others the smell of food causes nausea. Patients may ask that they be allowed to eat foods not generally allowed during dialysis. Practice indicates that either allowing or discouraging eating freely during dialysis is a matter of individual unit philosophy.

Prior to dialysis the patient is weighed, vital signs are taken, a sample of blood is drawn to determine the level of serum electrolytes and waste products, and the patient's physical status is assessed.

Care during dialysis. Nursing care of the patient during hemodialysis should center around (1) monitoring the physical status of the patient prior to and during dialysis for evidence of physiologic imbalance and change, (2) comfort and safety needs of the patient, and (3) helping the patient to understand and adjust to the care and changes in life style. This latter objective involves educating the person as to the specifics of the treatment program (diet and medications in particular) and how these relate to altered kidney function. The person is encouraged to express concerns and feelings, and attempts must be made to help the individual work through these feelings (Fig. 59-10).

Physiologic imbalances. Most physical problems that occur during dialysis are related to hypotension

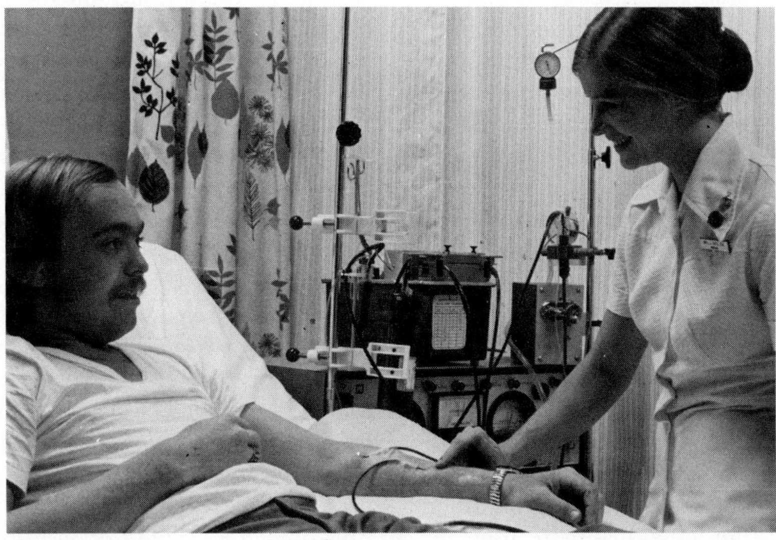

Fig. 59-10. Professional nurse must provide physical and emotional support to patient receiving hemodialysis.

from excessive removal of fluid, disequilibrium from a rapid reduction in extracellular electrolytes and wastes, and bleeding due to the heparinization needed to prevent blood from clotting while passing through the dialyzer. *Hypovolemia* and *shock* can occur during dialysis as a result of rapid removal of fluid from the intravascular compartment. Since this can occur faster than reequilibration of intracellular and intravascular volume relationships, the person may appear edematous and yet exhibit signs of shock. Signs and symptoms that indicate that the intravascular volume is being rapidly depleted are anxiety, restlessness, dizziness, nausea and vomiting, diaphoresis, tachycardia, and hypotension.

To avoid depleting the intravascular space and producing shock, the blood pressure and pulse rate are checked every 30 to 60 minutes, more frequently when the patient shows any of the previously mentioned signs and symptoms. Blood pressure readings should show only a slight gradual drop during the course of dialysis. Because the rate and pressure at which blood flows through the dialyzer are proportional to the rate and amount of fluid removed, blood flow and dialyzer pressure settings are carefully monitored. (A flow rate of 200 to 250 ml of blood per minute is a reasonable rate.) Unless the individual is severely hypertensive, rapid-acting antihypertensive medications are usually withheld the morning of dialysis until after the treatment has been completed. Additionally all sedating drugs (analgesics, tranquilizers, hypnotics) and those primarily affecting the vasculature (nitroglycerine) will predispose the patient to hypotensive episodes. Self-medication with these agents prior to and during dialysis must be carefully reviewed with each patient.

In treating a patient who shows signs of hypovolemia, inital nursing measures include determing the blood pressure and pulse, placing the head of the bed in a flat position, and raising the patient's feet. Administration of normal saline solution may be necessary to restore blood pressure. Throughout a hypotensive episode vital signs, level of consciousness, and any complaints offered are closely monitored. It is important for the nurse to know that vomiting frequently accompanies hypotension. Because an upper extremity must be maintained fairly immobile during the dialysis, it may be awkward for the patient to clear the mouth if vomiting should occur. The patient is helped to a safe position so that aspiration is avoided.

The patient is weighed before and after dialysis to determine the amount of fluid loss during treatment. When the weight losses of several dialysis treatments are correlated with the patient's blood pressure, pulse, and other indications of hypovolemia, an individual pattern of the patient's tolerance to fluid removal can be determined. This trend or pattern can be used to help adjust the rate and overall effect of the dialysis in keeping with the patient's physiologic tolerance.

A *disequilibrium phenomenon* occurs for many dialysis patients. This syndrome occurs toward the end of or after dialysis. It results when fluid and wastes are cleared from the blood and concentration gradients are created between intravascular and intracellular compartments, particularly within the central nervous system. Intracellular pH changes and cerebral edema occur. Signs and symptoms of disequilibrium include headache, restlessness, mental confusion, and nausea and vomiting. Severe disequilibrium may result in convulsions, especially in children when blood urea nitrogen levels exceed the concentration of 100 mg/ml.

Treatment includes keeping the patient quiet, reducing environmental discomfort such as temperature extremes and bright lights, and remaining with the patient to ensure physical safety. Mild analgesics may help to relieve headache. If disequilibrium becomes severe and the patient is still on dialysis, the therapy may be discontinued. Disequilibrium reactions are more likely to occur during the first few dialysis treatments.

Care of the patient on dialysis should also include preventing *blood loss*. To prevent the patient's blood from clotting as it flows through the dialyzer, heparin is administered. Protamine sulfate may or may not be given to the patient to counteract the effect of heparin. The patient is watched for signs of bleeding anywhere in the body. At the end of the treatment when dialysis needles are removed from the fistula, pressure dressings are applied to the puncture sites. They are observed at frequent intervals to detect hemorrhage. During and shortly after dialysis, treatments that cause tissue trauma should not be performed. These commonly include venipuncture and intramuscular infections. The patient who has had recent surgery, dental extractions, or recent trauma to soft tissues will be given protamine sufate during dialysis to prevent hemorrhage. These patients need to be closely observed for signs of bleeding.

Comfort. Nursing care should also include measures to increase the patient's physical comfort. Lying relatively immobile for a period of 4 to 8 hours can produce pressure over bony prominences and general restlessness. Changing the patient's position increases tolerance to limited movement. Mouth care is required if the patient is nauseated and vomiting. Because an upper extremity is generally kept immobile during dialysis, the patient may need help at mealtimes and with recreational and other activities requiring the use of two hands.

Changes in the life style. Much has been written in the literature concerning the changing style of life of the person receiving dialysis treatment and adaptation patterns that commonly arise for coping with required adjustments. The literature also contains much regarding nursing measures most helpful in assisting persons to incorporate their treatment into their style of living. The reader is referred to references 1, 12, 47, 57, 59.

Peritoneal dialysis

In peritoneal dialysis the dialyzing fluid is instilled into the peritoneal cavity and the peritoneum becomes the dialyzing membrane (Fig. 59-11). In comparison with hemodialysis treatments, which last 3 to 6 hours, peritoneal dialysis is maintained continuously for up to 36 hours. The procedure, once instituted, becomes largely a nursing responsibility. Peritoneal dialysis is used in treating acute and chronic renal failure. It is used as an alternative to hemodialysis for home dialysis.

Procedure. Access to the peritoneum is gained through introduction of a catheter into the peritoneal space. For acutely ill patients and those who are chronically ill and require sporadic dialysis, a sterile catheter is inserted for each procedure. For the chronically ill person treated on a routine basis, a special catheter is placed into the peritoneal space; the catheter remains until it malfunctions or another form of treatment is selected for the patient. These catheters present a continued potential entrance for organisms into the peritoneum. Each patient must be thoroughly instructed in the care of the catheter and the signs and symptoms that could indicate local or peritoneal infection and that should be reported to the physician.

For all patients weight, blood pressure, and pulse are recorded prior to initiating the procedure. These values serve as baseline information for use in assessing changes in the patient's condition. For persons undergoing insertion of a peritoneal catheter prior to dialysis, assessment should be made of their knowledge regarding the procedure and of their anxiety level. A mild sedative may help the severely anxious person to better tolerate the insertion of the catheter. It is important that these patients void just prior to initiation of dialysis; this will decompress the bladder and prevent accidental puncture during catheter placement.

In inserting a peritoneal catheter the physician

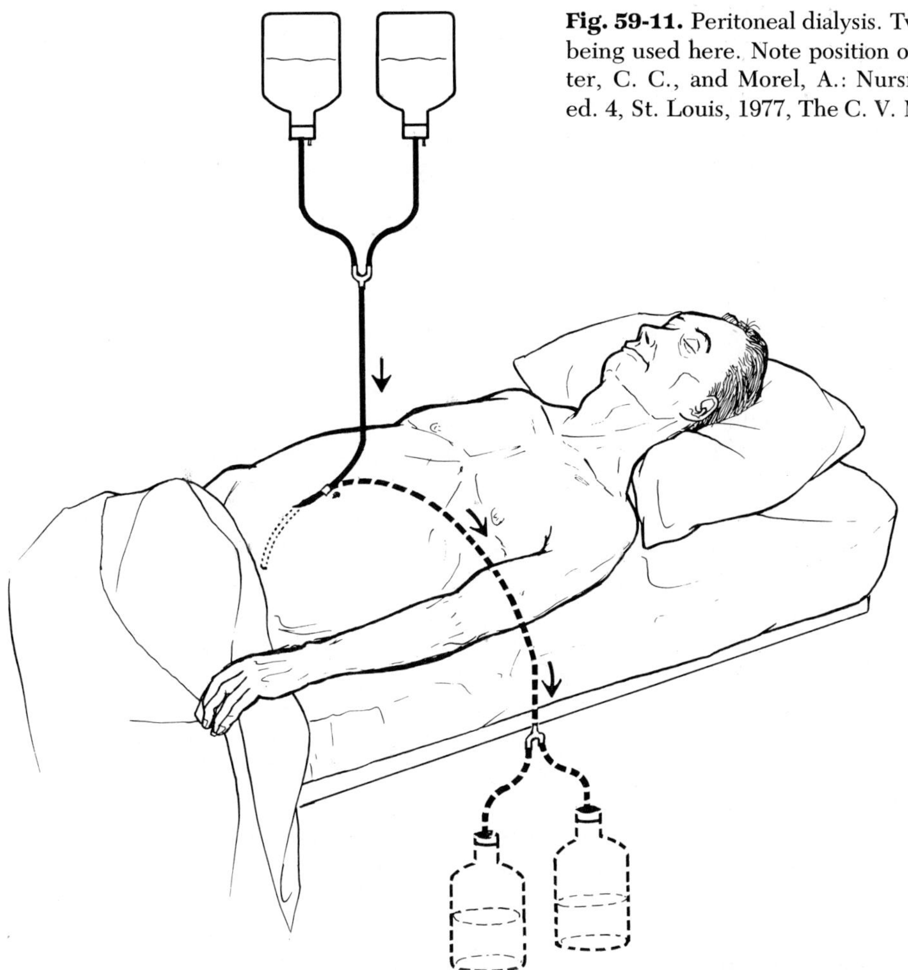

Fig. 59-11. Peritoneal dialysis. Two 1,000-ml bottles of dialysate solution are being used here. Note position of catheter in peritoneal cavity. (From Winter, C. C., and Morel, A.: Nursing care of patients with urologic diseases, ed. 4, St. Louis, 1977, The C. V. Mosby Co.)

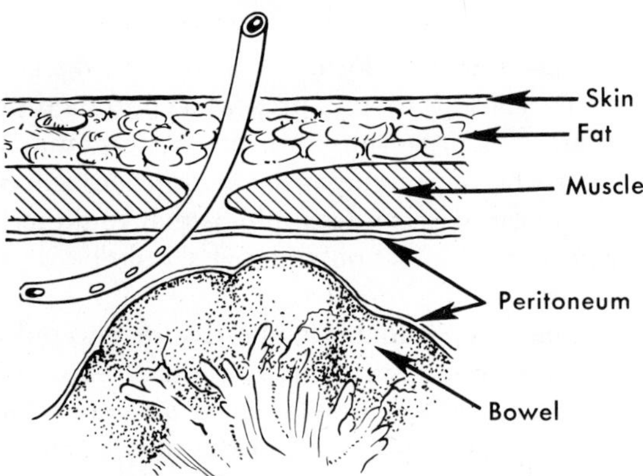

Fig. 59-12. Catheter in place in peritoneal cavity.

cleanses the abdomen and anesthetizes a small area in the midline of the abdomen below the umbilicus. A small incision is made, and the many-eyed nylon catheter is inserted into the peritoneal cavity (Fig. 59-12). A dressing is placed around the protruding catheter. Dialysis is initiated for the person with a permanent catheter by carefully cleansing the catheter and surrounding skin with a bacteriocidal agent. Approximately 2 liters of sterile dialysate warmed to body temperature are attached by tubing to the catheter and allowed to run into the peritoneal cavity as rapidly as possible. This usually takes about 10 minutes. The tubing is then clamped, and 10 to 30 minutes are allowed for osmosis of fluid and diffusion of particles into the dialyzing solution. At the end of the dwell time the tubing is unclamped and the fluid is allowed to flow freely from the abdomen. Fluid should drain in a steady stream. Drainage time should average about 10 to 15 minutes. The first drainage may be pink tinged as a result of the trauma of catheter insertion; however, this should clear with the second or third drainage. At no time should fluid draining from the abdomen appear grossly bloody. After fluid has drained from the abdomen, another cycle is started immediately. After the dialysis has been completed, the permanent catheter is again cleansed and a sterile cap is applied to the tip, the temporary catheter is removed, and the incision is covered with a dry sterile dressing. The small abdominal wound from the catheter should heal completely in 1 to 2 days.

Care during peritoneal dialysis. Complications most commonly associated with peritoneal dialysis include hypotension and hypovolemia, inadequate drainage of fluid from the peritoneal space, pain, atelectasis, respiratory distress, and peritonitis. As with hemodialysis, *hypotension* is most likely to result from rapid removal of fluid from the intravascular space. In addition to checking vital signs and observing the patient's behavior, records of fluid balance are crucial in determining the amount of fluid that has been removed. The net gain or loss of fluid from the abdomen should be determined at the completion of each cycle. To decrease the amount of fluid that is being removed from the vascular space, the physician may decrease the hypertonicity of the dialysate and may increase the rate at which fluid is running through an intravenous line.

Drainage of fluid from the abdomen can be slow or impossible to start. Generally this problem results when the tip of the catheter has become lodged against abdominal tissues. It may also result from plugging of the catheter with blood or fibrin that has accumulated as a result of tissue trauma. A small amount of heparin may be added to the dialysate to decrease the chance of a clot forming in the catheter. When the dialysate does not drain freely from the abdomen, the patient should be turned from side to side in an attempt to reposition the catheter in the peritoneal cavity. In addition firm pressure may be applied to the abdomen with both hands and the head of the bed may be raised. If the flow of the dialysate does not increase, the physician is called to irrigate or alter the position of the catheter.

Severe pain should not be experienced during peritoneal dialysis. Moderate levels of pain are often experienced as fluid is instilled and withdrawn from the peritoneal cavity. Procaine hydrochloride may be instilled with the dialysate in an attempt to control the patient's discomfort. Mild analgesics may be ordered for administration at 3- to 4-hour intervals during the procedure.

When the patient is markedly overhydrated and shows evidence of congestive failure and pulmonary edema, *respiratory difficulty* may be encountered as the dialyzing fluid infuses. The quality and rate of respiration should be closely observed. The head of the bed can be raised to decrease the pressure of the dialysate on the diaphragm. The patient, although encouraged to eat while being dialyzed, may find that this increases respiratory difficulty. To help overcome additional pressure created by a full stomach, frequent small meals may be provided. The amount of dialyzing fluid used for each cycle may be decreased when respiratory distress becomes prolonged and severe.

Peritonitis is an ever present threat during peritoneal dialysis. Aseptic technique must be rigidly maintained during insertion of the catheter and throughout the procedure. Care should be taken to avoid contaminating the solution or the tubing when new bottles of dialysate are hung. Cultures of the dialysate fluid are performed routinely to ensure continued attention to asepsis and to identify organisms if peritonitis should develop subsequently. The patient should be observed for signs of peritonitis. These include an elevated temperature and tenderness or pain of the abdomen.

Although the patient is confined to bed for the length of the dialysis, comfort and diversion can be provided. The patient may turn from side to side and move about in bed as he wishes as long as the catheter remains undisturbed. The patient may be provided assistance with oral care and bathing as needed. Visiting and other diversional activity should be encouraged when the patient's physical condition permits.

In the future it is probable that conventional peritoneal dialysis will be used increasingly in both home and in-center dialysis settings. Advances in the management of patients with chronic end-stage renal disease will likely reflect greater emphasis on home and self-dialysis. Continuous ambulatory peritoneal dialysis (CAPD)[55a,56a] is one new development that should make self-dialysis increasingly useful and practical. Basically CAPD involves continuous contact of dialysate and peritoneal membrane. Two liters of dialysate are maintained intraperitoneally and exchanged by the patient through a permanent peritoneal catheter four to five times each day. Major advantages of this treatment form include (1) steady state of blood chemistry values, (2) reduction in cost of dialysis, (3) patient can dialyze alone in any location without need for machinery and continuous technical supervision, (4) shorter patient training period, and (5) fewer restrictions on life style.

Though peritonitis is the major problem associated with continuous ambulatory peritoneal dialysis, refinement in techniques during exchange of dialysate should reduce the incidence of this problem and make CAPD a practical home procedure.

Outcome criteria for the person experiencing dialysis

The patient or significant others can:

1. Explain the process of dialysis and relate work of dialysis to own body needs.
2. State observations required of the shunt or fistula for hemodialysis regarding infection and clotting and state means of obtaining care when these occur.
3. State observation indicating infection of the peritoneal cavity or catheter and state means of obtaining care when these occur.
4. Demonstrate appropriate care of venous access or permanent peritoneal catheter.
5. Relate common side effects of treatment, means for controlling mild symptoms, and means of obtaining medical attention for severe or persisting complications.
6. Explain changes in medication schedule required before and after dialysis.
7. Plan a work and activity schedule as physical capabilities permit with minimum interference from scheduled dialysis time.

□ Kidney transplantation

Kidney transplants are being performed with increasing frequency in an effort to prolong the lives of persons with chronic renal failure. At present the ability to completely overcome the body's tendency to reject the grafted kidney has not been achieved. Persons undergoing kidney transplantation in essence exchange a program of chronic hemodialysis and its limitations for a new problem. Unless the kidney has been donated by an identical twin, the body senses the graft as a foreign tissue and attempts to destroy it. Immunosuppressive medications such as azathioprine (Imuran) and prednisone are given to suppress rejection. They are continued for as long as the kidney is viable.

Preoperative care. Nursing care of the patient in the preoperative phase includes physical and emotional preparation for the surgery. The patient and family should understand the outcomes expected from the surgery and the follow-up care that will be required. They should be prepared for the possibility of the kidney not functioning after transplantation. The nature of the surgery and location of the kidney, the possible need for postoperative dialysis, the use of immunosuppressive drugs, and the need for infection prevention after surgery must be explained to them. As any surgical patient, the individual should know of any drainage tubes that will be inserted during surgery, that medication will be given for relief of pain, and that after only a few hours moving about, coughing, and deep breathing will be necessary.

Throughout the period from the patient's acceptance as a transplant candidate to the time of surgery, the concerns and anxieties of the patient and family regarding transplantation need to be identified. As appropriate, the nurse and other members of the health team are called to help in dealing with these concerns and anxieties.

The patient must be in optimal physical condition for transplantation. Dialysis may be required prior to transplantation to assure optimal fluid and electrolyte balance, acid-base balance, and removal of wastes from the patient. The integrity of the fistula or shunt must be maintained. Prior to surgery the extremity containing the fistula or shunt may be wrapped to draw attention to it and identify it as containing a fistula or shunt. This identification will help all individuals caring for the person to avoid using the affected extremity for blood pressure determinations, drawing of blood, or an intravenous infusion.

Surgery. During surgery the transplanted kidney is placed in the iliac fossa (Fig. 59-13). Generally the

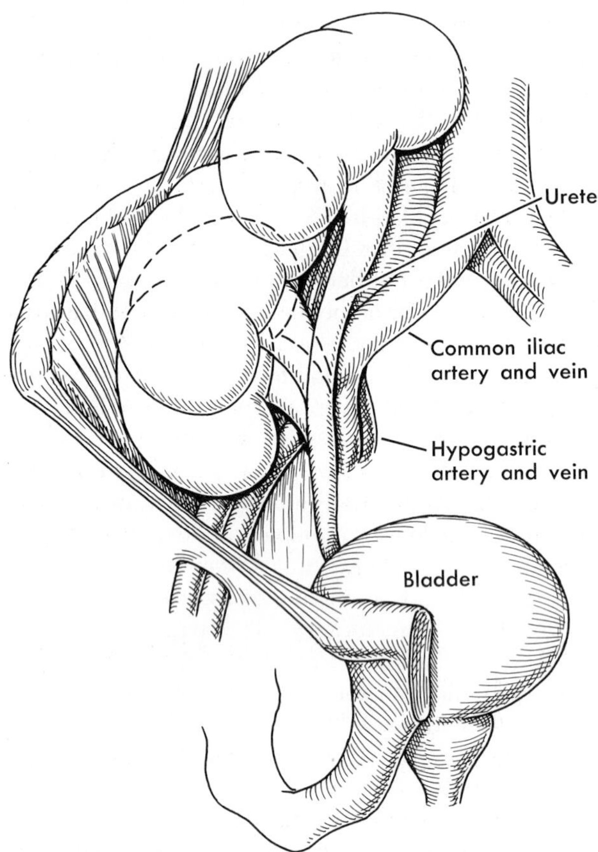

Fig. 59-13. Various positions for placement of homografted kidney. (Redrawn from Starzl, T. E., et al.: Techniques of renal homotransplantation, Arch. Surg. **89:**87, 1964. Copyright 1964, American Medical Association.)

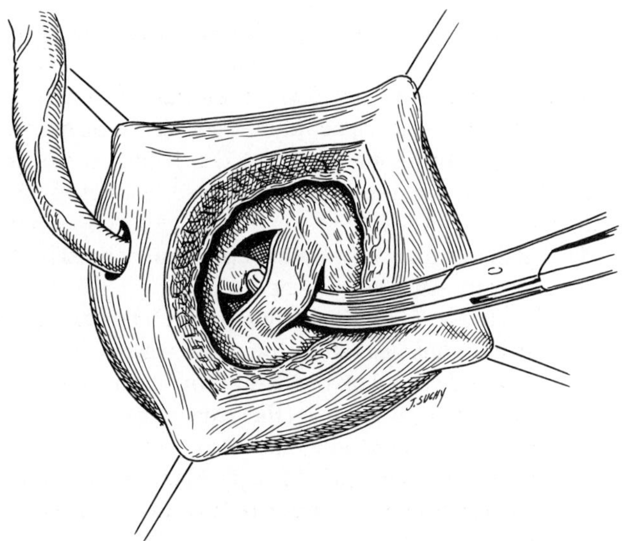

Fig. 59-14. Extraction of intravesical ureter through preformed submucosal tunnel. (Redrawn from Starzl, T. E., et al.: Techniques of renal homotransplantation, Arch. Surg. **89:**87, 1964. Copyright 1964, American Medical Association.)

peritoneal cavity is not entered. The patient's own kidneys may not be disturbed unless they are infected or are the cause of significant hypertension. The donor ureter is used to the extent that is possible. If long enough it is connected to the bladder in such a way as to prevent reflux of urine (Fig. 59-14). If the ureter is short, a ureteroureterostomy may be performed. A catheter is placed in the wound to promote drainage of accumulating fluid.

Postoperative care. Immediate postoperative care includes maintaining drainage of the urinary bladder, assessing the adequacy of fluid and electrolyte balance, protecting the patient from infection, observing for signs and symptoms of rejection, and identifying the effects of medications that have been administrered throughout the entire care cycle. A free flow of communication must be maintained with the patient and family regarding the individual's progress.

During surgery a Foley catheter is inserted into the bladder to promote drainage of urine and to prevent bladder distention and pressure on the newly anastomosed ureter. If gross hematuria or clots are noted in the drainage system, the physician should be notified immediately.

As with any surgical patient, the possibility of hemorrhage and hypovolemia exits. Blood pressure and pulse are determined frequently. Because the patient may have little or no urinary output for a number of hours to weeks after transplantation, fluid and electrolyte balance must be monitored carefully. Parameters indicating disturbed fluid and electrolyte balance are listed in the discussion of care of the patient with chronic renal failure (p. 1328). Any drainage from dressing or tubes should be carefully calculated into the patient's fluid balance record.

Rejection, the leading cause of graft failure, may occur as a hyperacute event (difficulty as the new kidney is anastomosed into the renal function), as an acute event, or as a slow and progressive decline in renal function. Signs and symptoms indicating rejection include rising serum creatine level; decreasing renal clearance of creatinine; decreasing urine output; fever, pain, or tenderness over the kidney; and malaise. Treatment of rejection involves increasing steroid doses. Depending on the severity of the rejection episode, oral or a combination of oral and intravenous steroids are used. Most rejection episodes are suppressed, although two or three events in succession indicate a poor prognosis for the new kidney. Most patients receiving cadaveric grafts undergo one rejection within the first 3 months after transplantation and commonly experience rejection episodes up through a year after surgery. The rate for rejection episodes for kidneys received from living relatives is substantially lower than for cadaver kidneys, although rejection occurs with frequency in this group also. The person should be helped to feel that although rejection is always a serious medical event, it should not be equated with unequivocable loss of the graft.

Since the person is *immunosuppressed,* it is imperative that protection from infection be provided. Reverse isolation is now not commonly practiced in most institutions. A system of closed drainage is meticulously maintained for the catheter draining the bladder. Cleansing of the perineum is performed once every 8 hours to help prevent bacteria entering the meatus and bladder. Good pulmonary hygiene to prevent pulmonary infection is important.

Side effects of therapy with immunosuppressive medication include leukopenia, facial and body changes, increased appetite, gastrointestinal tract irritation and bleeding, hepatotoxicity, decreased wound healing, depression, and personality changes. Any of these effects can be noted within the first few weeks of administration. Depression of white cell count is the goal of therapy; however, severe depression with white cell counts below 3,000 cells/cu mm is likely to increase significantly the risk of infection with the potential of death. Facial and body changes secondary to steroid therapy are disturbing to all patients. Support during the time of acute change in body appearance and reassurance that these changes will be minimized as steroid doses are gradually reduced are important. Gastrointestinal tract irritation occurs as gastric acid secretion increases and gastric mucus production decreases in response to steroids. Antacids taken between meals can reduce this irritation. Hepatotoxicity with symptoms of hepatitis may result from azathioprine (Imuran) administration and requires a change in immunosuppressive medication. Anxiety and fear of losing control may occur as the person perceives changes in behavior. It is helpful for the patient to know that steroids are capable of producing these changes. Psychiatric intervention may be required should behavior become maladaptive; steroid dosage is gradually reduced to the lowest level compatible with preservation of renal function and body metabolism, as is done with all patients receiving transplants.

Early in the postoperative course the patient should begin to become involved in learning to manage self-care. By the time the patient is discharged from the hospital, the following should be understood: (1) dietary limitation, (2) medications, their dosage, and effects, (3) how to care for the incision, (4) any precautions necessary in regard to activity and preventing trauma to the graft site, (5) how to measure own intake and output and record daily weights, (6) how to take his or her temperature, (7) how to collect a 24-hour urine specimen, (8) signs and symptoms of rejection, and (9) means of contacting health care personnel. The importance of regular follow-up visits and close medical supervision cannot be overemphasized. Subsequent health visits should include physiologic evaluation of the person and opportunity to raise questions regarding present life style and new health concerns. These visits should also include continuation of patient education concerning transplantation. Overall goals for ambulatory care include physiologic stabilization of the patient as evidenced by stabilized or improving renal function, stability in mental function and emotional state, control of side effects of immunosuppressive medication, hematocrit and hemoglobin levels progressively increased toward normal, and the patient free of severe morbidity as a result of graft rejection. Emphasis is placed on promoting maximal patient control over the health and life situation.

Outcome criteria for the person having a kidney transplantation

The patient or significant others can:

1. Explain the prescribed diet and how it will be achieved.
2. Describe the medication plan:
   a. State name, dosage, frequency, rationale, and side effects of prescribed medications (immunosuppressives, antacids).
   b. State method of obtaining medications.
3. Demonstrate accurate taking and recording of oral temperature, 24-hour urine specimens, weight, fluid intake, and urine output.
4. Explain recommended preventive health care measures:
   a. State measures useful in preventing infection.
   b. State plan for dental and gynecologic health care.
   c. State need to avoid immunization with live-virus vaccines.
5. Relate a program for continued health supervision:
   a. Explain concept of immunosuppression and relate this to health care needs.
   b. Describe signs and symptoms requiring immediate medical attention.
   c. Relate appropriate information regarding sexual functioning and family planning.
   d. State need to preserve dialysis access.
   e. State resources available for assistance with illness and rehabilitative concerns and means of contact with resources.
   f. Explain specific plans for follow-up health care.

REFERENCES AND SELECTED READINGS

1. *Abram, H.: The psychiatrist, the treatment of CRF and the prolongation of life. II. Am. J. Psychiatry **126**:157-167, 1969.
2. Abram, H., Hester, L. R., Sheridan, W. F., et al.: Sexual functioning in patients with chronic renal disease, J. Nerv. Ment. Dis. **160**:220-226, 1975.
3. Anderson, C. F., Nelson, R. A., Margie, J. D., et al.: Nutritional therapy for adults with renal disease, J.A.M.A. **223**:68-72, 1973.
4. Asscher, A.: The detection and natural history of urinary infection. In Blandy, J., editor: Urology, London, 1976, Blackwell Scientific Publications.
5. Bailey, G., editor: Hemodialysis: principles and practice, New York, 1972, Academic Press, Inc.
6. *Bennett, W. M., Singer, I., and Coggins, C. J.: A guide to drug therapy in renal failure, J.A.M.A. **230**:1544-1553, 1974.
7. Bergersen, B.: Pharmacology in nursing, ed. 14, St. Louis, 1979, The C. V. Mosby Co.
8. *Bernbeck, L.: Conservative care of patients with renal failure. In Schlotter, L., editor: Nursing and the nephrology patient, Flushing, N.Y., 1973, Medical Examination Publishing Co.
9. Black, D. A. K., editor: Renal disease, ed. 2, Philadelphia, 1972, F. A. Davis Co.
10. *Blount, M., and Kinney, A.: Chronic steroid therapy, Am. J. Nurs. **74**:1626-1631, 1974.
11. Bois, M. S., Barfield, N. B., Taylor, C. E., et al.: Nursing care of patients having renal transplants, Am. J. Nurs. **68**:1238-1239, 1968.
12. Brundage, D.: Nursing management of renal problems, St. Louis, 1976, The C. V. Mosby Co.
13. *Burton, B.: Current concepts of nutrition and diet in diseases of the kidney, J. Am. Diet. Assoc. **65**:623-633, 1974.
14. Campbell, M., and Harrison, J., editors: Urology, ed. 3, vols. 1-3, Philadelphia, 1970, W. B. Saunders Co.
15. Castelnuovo-Tedesco, P., editor: Psychiatric aspects of organ transplantation, New York, 1971, Grune and Stratton, Inc.
16. Chapman, W., et al.: editors: The urinary system, Philadelphia, 1973, W. B. Saunders Co.
17. Cimino, J.: Diagnosis and management of urinary tract infection, Hosp. Med. **10**:59-62, 1974.
18. Cooper, H., and Robinson, E.: Treatment of genitourinary tuberculosis: report after 24 years, J. Urol. **108**:136-142, 1972.
19. *deGreco, F., and Krumlovsky, F.: Chronic renal failure: clinical and therapeutic considerations, Postgrad. Med. **52**:176-183, 1972.
20. Dolan, P., and Greene, H.: Renal failure and peritoneal dialysis, Nurs. '75 **5**:40-49, 1975.
21. Fearing, M.: Osteodystrophy in patients with chronic renal failure, Nurs. Clin. North Am. **10**:461-468, 1975.
22. *Fellows, B., and Blagg, C.: Acute renal failure and renal dialysis. In Meltzer, L., Abdellah, F., and Kitchell, J., editors: Concepts and practices of intensive care for nurse specialists, ed. 2, Philadelphia, 1976, The Charles Press, Publishers.
23. Flamenbaum, W.: Pathophysiology of acute renal failure, Arch. Intern. Med. **131**:911-928, 1973.
24. Ford, C.: Open forum: cadaver transplantation, Dialysis and Transplantation **4**:8-32, 1975.
25. Fox, R., and Swazey, J.: The courage to fail: a social view of organ transplants and dialysis, Chicago, 1974, University of Chicago Press.
26. Freedman, P.: Acute renal failure, Heart Lung **4**:873-878, 1975.
27. Gault, M. H., Rudwal, T. C., Engles, W. D., et al.: Syndrome associated with the abuse of analgesics, Ann. Int. Med. **68**:906-923, 1968.
28. *Gault, P.: The prostate: coping with dangerous and distressing complications, Nurs. '77 **7**:34-38, 1977.
29. Goldberger, E.: A primer of water, electrolyte and acid-base syndromes, ed. 5, Philadelphia, 1975, Lea & Febiger.
30. Goodman, L., and Gilman, A., editors: The pharmacological basis of therapeutics, ed. 5, New York, 1975, Macmillan, Inc.
31. Goodwin, N. J., Valenti, C., Hall, J. E., et al.: Effects of uremia and chronic hemodialysis on the reproductive cycle, Am. J. Obstet. Gynecol. **100**:528-535, 1968.
32. Gutch, C., and Stoner, M.: Review of hemodialysis for nurses and dialysis personnel, ed. 2, St. Louis, 1975, The C. V. Mosby Co.
33. Hansen, F.: Caring for patients with chronic renal disease, Philadelphia, 1974, J. B. Lippincott Co.
34. Harrison, T., et al.: editors: Principles of internal medicine, ed. 7, New York, 1977, McGraw-Hill Book Co.
35. *Hickman, B. W.: All about sex . . . despite dialysis, Am. J. Nurs. **77**:606-607, 1977.
36. Johnson, K., et al.: Nursing care of the patient with acute renal failure, Nurs. Clin. North Am. **10**:421-430, 1975.
37. Kark, R.: Symposium on diseases of the kidney, Med. Clin. North Am. **55**:1-241, 1971.
38. Kass, E. H., et al.: Significance of bacteriuria in preventive medicine. In Kass, E. H., editor: Progress in pyelonephritis, Philadelphia, 1965, F. A. Davis Co.
39. *Katz, A.: Kidney transplantation: patient selection and management, Med. Clin. North Am. **54**:75-94, 1970.
40. Keuhnelian, J., and Saunders, V.: Urologic nursing, New York, 1970, Macmillan, Inc.
41. *Kobrzycki, P.: Renal transplant-complications, Am. J. Nurs. **77**:641-643, 1977.
42. Kunin, C.: Detection, prevention and management of urinary tract infections, ed. 2, Philadelphia, 1974, Lea & Febiger.
43. Lang, G., and Levin, S.: Diagnosis and treatment of urinary tract infections, Med. Clin. North Am. **55**:1439-1456, 1971.
44. Lapides, J.: Fundamentals of urology, Philadelphia, 1976, W. B. Saunders Co.
45. Lazarus, J.: Hepatitis and hemodialysis. In Bailey, G., editor: Hemodialysis: principles and practice, New York, 1972, Academic Press, Inc.
46. Lennon, E.: The surgical dialysis patient, Nurs. Clin. North Am. **4**:443-450, 1969.
47. Levy, N.: Living or dying: adaptation to hemodialysis, Springfield, Ill., 1974, Charles C Thomas, Publisher.
48. Lowrie, E. G., Lazarus, J. M., Mocelin, A. J., et al.: Survival of patients undergoing chronic hemodialysis and renal transplantation, N. Engl. J. Med. **288**:863-867, 1973.
49. *Miller, R., and Tassistro, C.: Peritoneal dialysis, N. Engl. J. Med. **281**:945 .949, 1969.
50. *O'Neil, M., editor: Symposium on care of the patient with renal disease, Nurs. Clin. North Am. **10**:411-516, 1975.
51. Papper, S.: Clinical nephrology, Boston, 1971, Little, Brown and Co.
52. Papper, S.: Renal failure, Med. Clin. North Am. **55**:335-357, 1971.
53. Paulson, D.: Carcinoma of the bladder and urethra, Hosp. Med. **11**:63-68, 1975.
54. Penn. I., Markowski, E., Droegemueller, W., et al.: Parenthood in renal homograft recipients, J.A.M.A. **216**:1755-1761, 1971.
55. Pollak, V., and Mendoza, N.: Rapidly progressive glomerulonephritis, Med. Clin. North Am. **55**:1397-1416, 1971.

55a. *Popovitch, R. P., Monterief, J. W., Nolfe, K. D., et al.: Contin-

*References preceded by an asterisk are particularly well suited for student reading.

uous ambulatory peritoneal dialysis, Ann. Intern. Med. **88:** 449-456, 1978.
56. *Pullman, T., and Coe, F.: Chronic renal failure, Clin. Symp. **25:**1-32, 1973.
56a. *Robson, M. D., and Oreopoulos, D. G.: Continuous ambulatory peritoneal dialysis: a revolution in the treatment of chronic renal failure, Dialysis and Transplantation **7:**999-1003, 1978.
57. *Rodriguez, D.: Moral issues in hemodialysis and renal transplantation, Nurs. Forum **10:**210-220, 1971.
58. Rous, S. N.: Urology in primary care, St. Louis, 1976, The C. V. Mosby Co.
59. Schlotter, L., editor: Nursing and the nephrology patient: a symposium on current trends and issues, Flushing, N.Y., 1973, Medical Examination Publishing Co., Inc.
60. *Schumann, D.: The renal donor, Am. J. Nurs. **74:**105-110, 1974.
61. Scott, R., et al.: Urology illustrated, New York, 1975, Churchill Livingstone.
62. Smith, D.: General urology, Canada, 1975, Lange Medical Publications.
63. Smith, R. B., and Skinner, D. G., editors: Complications of urologic surgery: prevention and management, Philadelphia, 1976, W. B. Saunders Co.
64. Strauss, M., and Welt, C., editors: Diseases of the kidney, ed. 2, Boston, 1971, Little, Brown and Co.
65. U.S. Department of Health, Education and Welfare: Outline for surveillance and control of nosocomial infections, Atlanta, 1974, Center for Disease Control, Bureau of Epidemiology.
66. U.S. Department of Health, Education and Welfare: Monthly vital statistics report, Provisional statistics, Annual summary for U.S., 1976, vol. 26, #13, Washington, D.C., 1977, U.S. Government Printing Office.
67. U.S. National Institutes of Allergy and Infectious Disease, Transplantation and Immunology Branch, U.S. kidney transplant fact book, Bethesda, Md., 1972, ACS/NIH Registry.
68. *Watt, R. C.: Urinary diversion, Am. J. Nurs. **74:**1806-1811, 1974.
69. Whalley, R.: Bacteriuria of pregnancy, Am. J. Obstet. Gynecol. **97:**723-728, 1967.
70. Whelan, J., et al.: Urologic nursing procedures, New York, 1970, Institute of Rehabilitation Medicine.
71. Whitehead, S.: Nursing care of the adult urology patient, New York, 1970, Appleton-Century-Croft.
72. Williams, H.: Nephrolithiasis, N. Engl. J. Med. **290:**33-38, 1974.
73. Williams, S.: Nutrition and diet therapy, ed. 3, St. Louis, 1977, The C. V. Mosby Co.
73a. *Wineman, R. J.: End-stage renal disease, Dialysis and Transplantation **7:**1034-1037, 1064, 1978.
74. Winter, C. C., and Morel, A.: Nursing care of patients with urologic diseases, ed. 4, St. Louis, 1977, The C. V. Mosby Co.
75. Wolf, Z. R.: What patients awaiting kidney transplant want to know, Am. J. Nurs. **76:**92-94, 1976.
76. Woodrow, M., Wilsey, G., and Wiley, N.: Suprapubic catheters. Part I. A direct line to better drainage, Nurs. '76 **6:**40-45, 1976. Part II. **6:**40-42, 1976.

AUDIOVISUAL RESOURCES

1. Immunologic aspects of organ transplantation, Upjohn, 1965. (Movie, 8 mm.)
2. Infections of the kidney and the urinary tract, Atlanta, 1974, National Medical Audiovisual Center. (Cassette tape, slides, script.)
3. Principles of hemodialysis, Garden Grove, Calif., 1971, Trainex. (Cassette tape, filmstrip, guide, workbook.)
4. Vidt, D.: Peritoneal dialysis: a bedside procedure, 1971, Abbott Laboratories. (Film.)

UNIT X

Problems related to sexuality and reproduction

Sexuality and reproductive concerns are being presented to nurses with increasing frequency. Persons are becoming more aware of their sexual and reproductive health and are more comfortable about discussing sexual and reproductive issues. It is becoming increasingly necessary for nurses to provide counseling and education to persons with concerns related to family planning, sexuality, venereal diseases, malignancies of the reproductive system, and the changes in sexual and reproductive experiences throughout the life cycle.

Assessment of the reproductive and sexual systems is described first in this unit. Common approaches to *management of the person with a reproductive or sexual problem* follows. A discussion of *reproductive problems*, *problems of sexuality*, and *problems of the breast* concludes the unit.

60

Assessment of the reproductive and sexual systems

ELLA CINKOTA
NANCY FUGATE WOODS

Conditions affecting healthful functioning of the reproductive systems of men and women take a high toll in terms of loss of life and acute and chronic physical and emotional stress. The nurse has a responsibility to assist in general health education, to refer patients to good medical care, and to understand the treatment available and the nursing care needed when disease develops. A sound knowledge of the structure and functions of the reproductive system is essential to the assessment process.

■ ANATOMY AND PHYSIOLOGY

□ Pelvis

The bones of the pelvis are shown in Fig. 60-1. Anteriorly the pubic bones join at the symphysis pubis. The inferior borders of the pubic bones and symphysis form an inverted V, called the pubic arch. The sacrum and coccyx come together at the sacrococcygeal joint, which is movable. The sacral hiatus is the site of administration of caudal anesthetics.

The pelvis is divided into two parts, the true and the false pelvis, by a bony ridge called the pelvic brim. The false pelvis is the broad, expanded portion above the pelvic brim. The narrow part below the pelvic brim is the true pelvis. The true pelvis is further described as having an inlet and an outlet. The inlet is located at the pelvic brim, and the outlet is at the base of the pelvis. The iliac spines mark the midpoint between the inlet and the outlet. The distances between the bones of the true pelvis have special significance during childbirth, since it is through this bony canal that the baby must pass to be born.

Like other bones of the skeletal system, the pelvic bones undergo changes during periods of growth and development until maturity is reached. The major differences between the pelves of men and women are in the contour of the pelvis and thickness of the bones. While variations are seen in both sexes, the female pelvis is more delicate because the bones are thinner and lighter in weight. In females the pelvis is wider and more shallow due to the flaring of the iliac bones; the male pelvis tends to be narrow and deep. In women the sacrum is shorter, wider, and less curved, and the coccyx is more movable. The pubic arch is wider and more rounded in women, and the ischial spines are less prominent. The typical architecture of the female pelvis is especially suited for childbirth.

□ Female genital system

External structures

Fig. 60-2 shows the external genitalia of a female. Collectively the external genitalia are often referred to as the vulva. The mons pubis is the rounded area in front of the symphysis pubis. It consists of a collection of fatty tissue beneath the skin and is covered with hair after puberty.

The labia majora are two prominent, longitudinal folds of tissue extending back from the mons pubis. These labia are thicker in front, gradually become thinner as they extend back, and appear to flatten out as they merge with the adjacent tissues in the area of the perineum. The labia majora have two surfaces. The outer surface is covered by a thin layer of skin containing hair follicles and sebaceous and sweat glands. The inner surfaces are smooth, lack hair, and are supplied with a large number of sebaceous follicles.

The labia minora are two smaller folds of tissue that run parallel to the labia majora and are sometimes concealed between the folds of the labia majora. In sexually active women and in women who have borne children, the labia minora may project beyond the labia majora. The labia minora join near the clitoris, extend backward

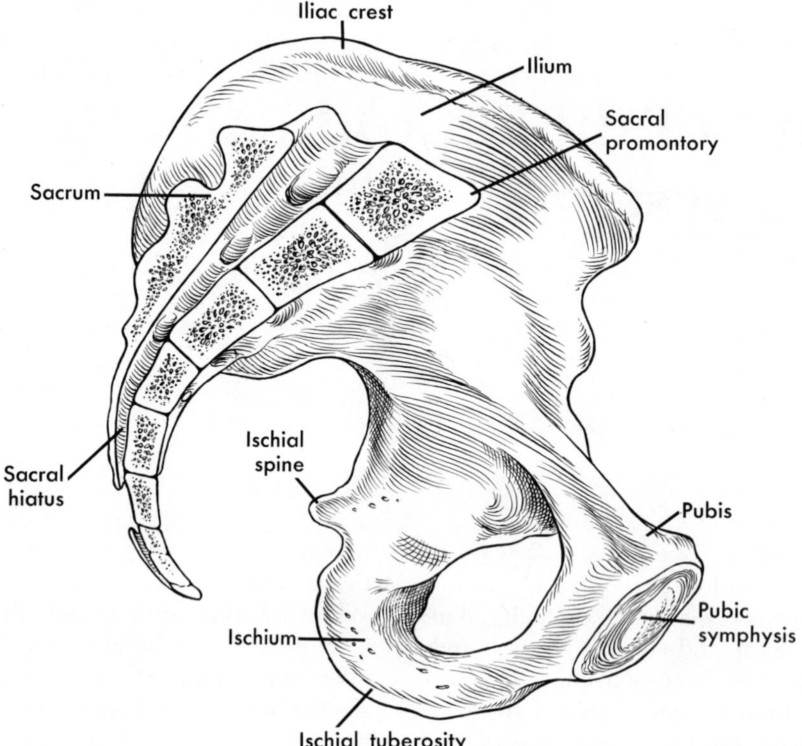

Fig. 60-1. Three major pelvic bones.

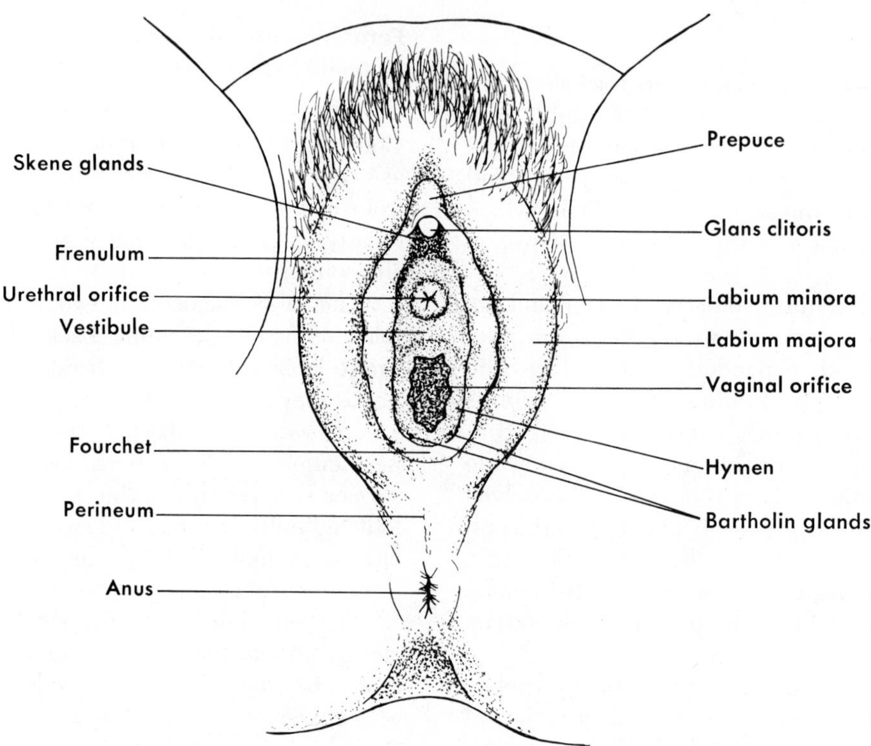

Fig. 60-2. External female genitalia.

to enclose the urethral and vaginal openings, and merge with the labia majora in the perineum. The labia minora are made up of connective and elastic tissue and contain little fatty tissue. Sweat glands and hair follicles are absent from the labia minora, but sebaceous glands are present.

The clitoris is situated near the anterior folds of the labia minora. The glans of the clitoris is a small, rounded area consisting of erectile tissue enclosed in a layer of fibrous membrane. Although it is often compared with or said to be homologous to the penis in males, the clitoris is unique in that its sole physiologic functions are initiation and elevation of sexual tension levels. The clitoris serves as both receptor and transformer of sexual stimuli. Sexual stimulation initiates a process whereby the clitoris becomes enlarged, erect, and very sensitive to sexual stimuli. Female orgasm can occur from stimulation of the clitoris but also results from stimulation of other sites; in fact, female orgasm has been documented in instances where the clitoris had been surgically removed.

The hymen is an irregular membranous fold of varying thickness that partially covers the vaginal orifice. The hymen may be avulsed (broken) by coitus, digital examination, vigorous exercise, or surgery. Absence of the hymen does not denote lack of virginity. Remnants of the hymen usually persist after avulsion and form an irregular border around the vaginal opening.

The location of Skene's (periurethral) glands and Bartholin's glands should be noted because they are common sites of infection. Skene's glands are located on each side of the urethral meatus. Bartholin's glands are situated at each side of the vaginal opening near the bases of the labia. Since both Skene's and Bartholin's glands are very small, their openings are just visible. They may not be palpable unless the women is very thin or unless the glands are enlarged because of infection.

The appearance of the vulvar structures varies with age. Before puberty the external genitalia are characterized by absence of pubic hair, and the labia minora are more prominent than the labia majora. With deposit of body fat and hormone effects during puberty, the labia majora increase in thickness and pubic hair appears. With the onset of the menopause and gradual withdrawal of hormones, the external genitalia again becomes less prominent, and the pubic hair begins to thin. In elderly

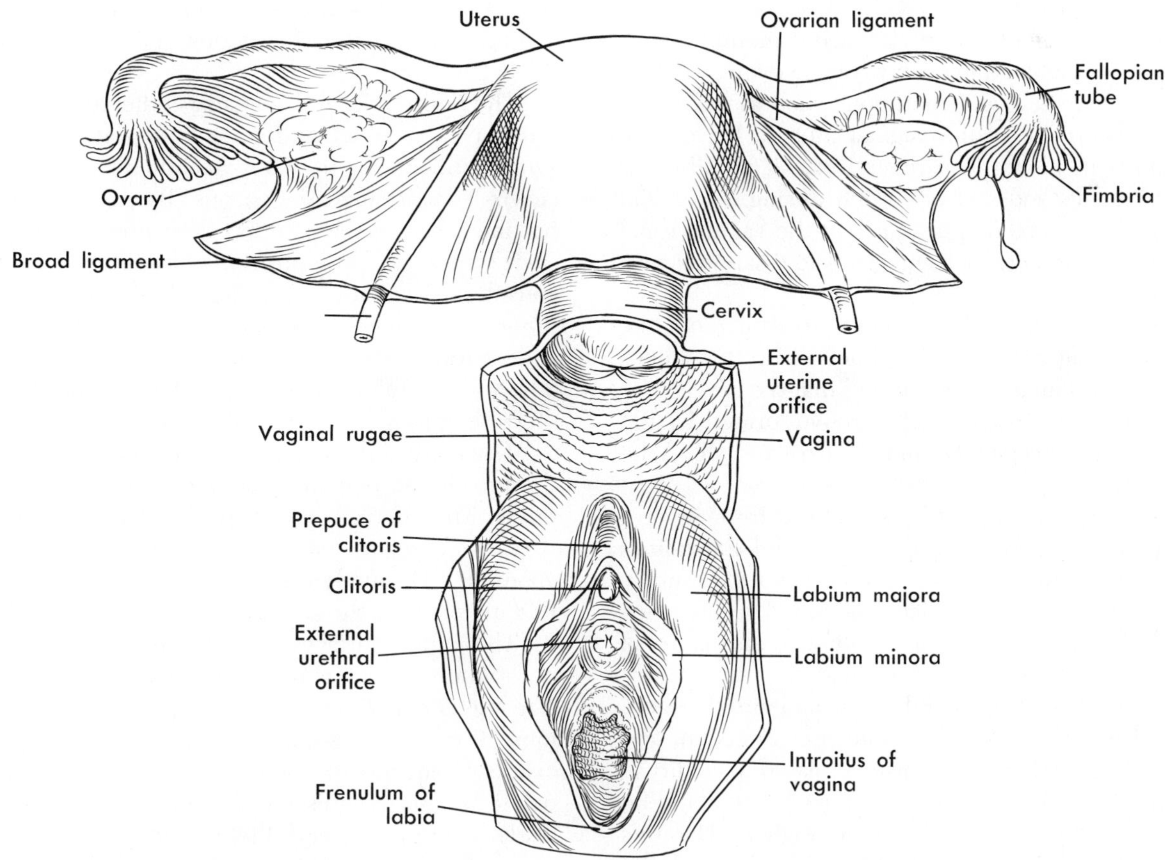

Fig. 60-3. Female internal organs of reproduction. Major ligaments are shown.

women the vulva may appear wrinkled, shrunken, and almost flat. During the life span congenital defects, childbirth, infection or other diseases, and surgery may alter the structure and appearance of the external genitalia.

Internal organs

The female internal reproductive organs are shown in Fig. 60-3. In relation to the skeletal system, the internal reproductive organs are located in the true pelvis. Unless their size is increased by a disease process or by pregnancy, the internal organs of reproduction remain within the cavity of the true pelvis. An exception is noted during sexual response when the uterus elevates into the false pelvis.

The vaginal orifice serves as the boundary between the external structures and the internal organs. The functions of the vagina are to receive the penis during intercourse, allow for birth of a baby, and permit discharge of the menstrual flow. The vagina is located between the rectum and urethra and is a soft, tubular structure that extends upward and back from the vaginal opening.

The length of the vaginal canal varies, and the posterior wall is longer than the anterior wall. The anterior wall averages 6 to 8 cm in length, while the posterior wall averages 8 to 9 cm.

The vagina is lined with pink mucous membrane arranged in folds called *rugae*. Physiologic events such as pregnancy and pathologic conditions such as infections often alter the color of the vaginal mucosa because of congestion with blood. The rugae make it possible for the vagina to distend and to stretch during coitus and childbirth. The rugated appearance of the vaginal canal is prominent in adolescence and tends to disappear with multiparity.

The vaginal walls end in a blind pouch *around* the cervix. Note that the vaginal epithelium is continuous with the epithelium of the cervix and that the cervix projects into the upper vagina. The groove formed by the termination of the vagina around the cervix is called the vaginal vault.

The vagina is lubricated by secretions from its own cells and by secretions from the cervix and Bartholin's glands. The combined vaginal secretions are normally acid during the years of ovarian function. The presence of Döderlein bacilli and estrogen influence the acidity of the vagina. When adequate estrogen stimulation is present, the cells of the vagina and cervix contain glycogen. Lactic acid is produced by breakdown of glycogen, and the degree of glycogen breakdown is related to acidity of the vagina. Prior to puberty the vaginal pH tends to be neutral. With the onset of puberty the vaginal pH varies between 4.0 and 5.0 depending on the phase of the menstrual cycle and the level of estrogen. The pH is lowest at the time of ovulation and just before menstruation. During pregnancy a pH of 4.0 or less is common. Neutral or alkaline values are normally found in postmenopausal women. The importance of vaginal acidity is demonstrated by the fact that most pathogenic bacteria produce signs of vaginal infection when the pH falls below 4.0 or rises above 5.0.

Until puberty the vaginal epithelium is thin. The epithelium thickens at the time of puberty, and this state persists through the reproductive years until the menopause, when the epithelium again thins. The thickness of the vaginal epithelium is closely related to estrogen levels.

The natural barriers to infection (thickness of the vaginal epithelium and acidity of the vagina) are minimal before puberty and after menopause, predisposing females in these age groups to vaginal infections and trauma of the vaginal mucosa.

The uterus is a hollow, muscular organ located between the urinary bladder and rectum. It consists of two portions, the corpus (body) and the cervix. The upper, rounded area of the corpus is called the fundus. The lowest, constricted portion is the cervix. The size of the uterus decreases from the fundus to the cervix, giving the contour of the uterus a triangular appearance. Although the size of the uterus varies among women, its average size is 7 to 7.5 cm. long, 4.5 to 5 cm wide, and 2.5 to 3 cm thick.

The position, shape, and size of the uterus vary at different periods of life and under different circumstances. During infancy the uterus is an abdominal organ, and the cervix is larger than the corpus. By puberty the uterus has increased in size and has descended into the pelvic cavity. In women the position of the uterus is subject to considerable variation (see Fig. 62-2). During pregnancy the uterus changes remarkably in size, shape, structure, and position and returns to its prepregnancy state within 6 to 8 weeks following delivery. During menopause the uterus begins to hypertrophy and decreases in size.

The body of the uterus is normally bent forward over the bladder so that the fundus is behind the symphysis pubis. The cervix curves forward. The relationship between the corpus and the cervix produces an angle of about 90°. The angle is decreased as the urinary bladder fills and elevates the corpus.

The outer surfaces of the uterus are covered by peritoneum, which is reflected from the abdominal wall. The anterior and posterior reflections of the peritoneum join at the sides to enclose the fallopian tubes and ovaries. Reflection of the peritoneum over the top of the pelvic organs creates spaces between the uterus and bladder anteriorly and the uterus and rectum posteriorly. The posterior space is known as the cul-de-sac of Douglas and is clinically important in that the peritoneal cavity can be entered through the posterior vaginal wall with little risk of damaging adjacent organs or structures.

The uterus is lined with mucous-membrane-type tissue called endometrium. The cavity of the uterus is continuous with the cervical canal and has an average capacity of 3 to 8 ml. Near the fundus the uterus opens into the lumen of the fallopian tubes. Thus there is a direct route from the vagina through the cervix, uterus, and fallopian tubes to the peritoneum. This is important in prevention of infection and its spread by continuity of tissue.

The cervix is firm, smooth, and round. Its color is usually lighter pink than that of the vagina. The lower portion of the cervix protrudes into the vagina, and in the center of the vaginal portion of the cervix is the external os. Extending upward from the external os is the cervical canal, which averages 2 to 3 cm in length. The cervical canal terminates as it joins the corpus, and the junction of the cervical canal and the corpus is termed the internal cervical os. The functions of the cervix are to secrete mucus to facilitate transport of sperm, to dilate during labor, and to provide a channel for discharge of the menstrual flow.

Changes in the physical properties and in the pH of the cervical mucus are significant in the treatment of infertility and in fertility control. At the time of ovulation the cervical mucus becomes thinner and more elastic. These changes enhance penetration of the cervical mucus by sperm. The viscosity of the cervical mucus can be determined by studies of mucus flow and elasticity. The term *spinnbarkeit* is applied to describe the characteristic ability of the cervical mucus to stretch and recoil.

The fallopian tubes are two narrow, muscular canals averaging 12 cm in length. They extend outward from the corpus near the fundus and are enclosed in the folds of the broad ligaments.

The walls of the fallopian tubes contain smooth muscles possessing peristaltic properties. Mucous membrane containing cilia lines the fallopian tubes. At the time of ovulation peristaltic and ciliary action increase, and it is likely that these combined actions provide the mechanism for ovum transport.

The functions of the fallopian tubes are to serve as a site for union of the sperm and ovum and to transport the ovum to the uterus. Fertilization of the ovum occurs in the distal third of the fallopian tube. If a stricture of the fallopian tube exists in the proximal portion, the fertilized ovum may not be able to pass the point of obstruction, and an ectopic (tubal) pregnancy may result.

The ovaries are endocrine glands as well as reproductive organs. There are normally two ovaries, each lying near the fimbriae of the fallopian tubes. They are partly enclosed by the broad ligaments. The functions of the ovaries are to produce mature ova and to secrete estrogen and progesterone. Ovarian functions are readily disturbed by acute and chronic diseases. The functions can also be altered or interrupted by surgery, radiation, and the ingestion of drugs such as oral contraceptives.

The ovaries undergo histologic changes due to endocrine stimulation as well as physical changes in position, size, and shape during the life span. At birth the ovaries are very small, round, smooth, and light pink and are located in false pelvis. Between infancy and puberty the ovaries increase in size, become more flattened, assume a grayish color, and descend into the true pelvis. During the childbearing years the ovaries appear long and flat, have a nodular surface due to the presence of follicles, and lie close to the pelvic walls. During pregnancy the ovaries are lifted out of the pelvis by the enlarging uterus but descend into the pelvis after childbirth. After menopause the ovaries undergo rapid regressive changes. They decrease in size, their surfaces become wrinkled, and the color fades from gray to white. In most postmenopausal women the ovaries are so small that they cannot be palpated during vaginal examination.

After puberty the surfaces of the ovaries are covered by connective tissue fibers that form a layer called the *tunica albuginea.* Immediately below the connective tissue is the ovarian cortex containing a large number of minute vesicles, the primordial follicles. Each primordial follicle contains an undeveloped ovum having the capacity to respond to stimulation by pituitary hormones. It is estimated that each ovary contains 500,000 primordial follicles at the time of birth. Many of the primordial follicles disintegrate before puberty, and the process of disintegration continues throughout the childbearing years. Consequently, few if any primordial follicles are found in the ovaries after menopause.

Unlike sperm, which are produced constantly by males, only one ovum matures at a time, and the process of ovum maturation requires an average of 28 days. When the ovum reaches maturity, it leaves the ovary by the process of ovulation.

□ Male genital system

The male reproductive organs and associated structures are shown in Fig. 60-4. In males the reproductive organs produce sperm, suspend the sperm in a liquid, and deliver the sperm into the vagina to fertilize an ovum. Another important function is secretion of male hormones, the androgens. The male genitalia include the testes, vas deferens, seminal vesicles, ejaculatory ducts, and penis, along with the prostate and bulbourethral glands, which are accessory structures.

The testes produce the sperm. During fetal life the testes are located in the abdominal cavity behind the peritoneum. Prior to birth the testes descend through the inguinal canals and inguinal rings into the scrotum and are suspended in position by the spermatic cords.

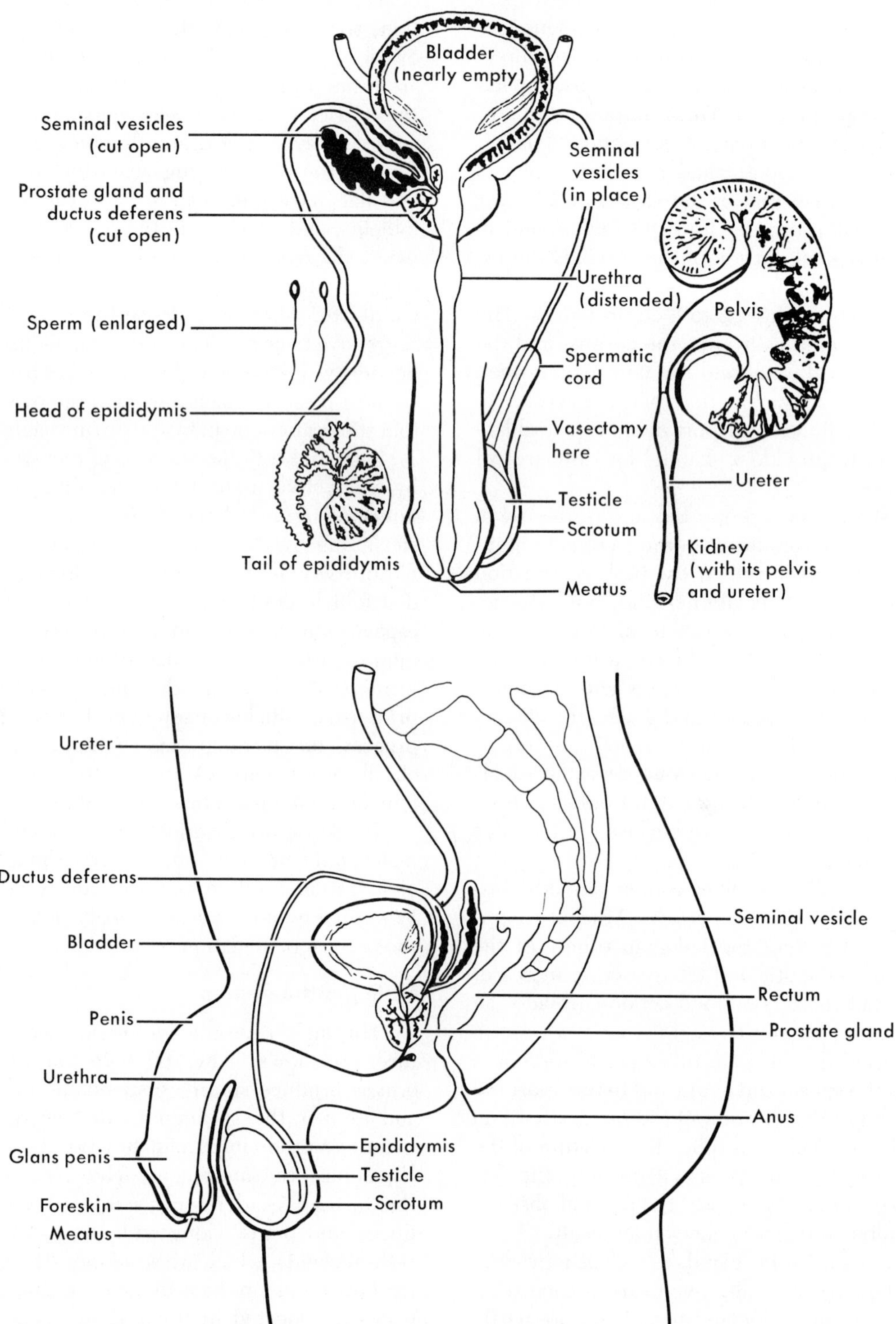

Fig. 60-4. Male organs of reproduction. Note relatively large size of seminal vesicle as compared with testicle.

The testes are oval. The spermatic cords are attached to the posterior borders of the testes. At the lateral edge of each spermatic cord is the epididymis, which appears as a narrow, flattened structure.

The testes are composed of glandular tissue covered by fibrous tissue. The glandular tissue is composed of many lobules differing in size according to their location. The lobules consist of small convoluted structures, the seminiferous tubules. The seminiferous tubules produce the sperm, and spermatozoa in different stages of development can be seen along the cells of the tubules.

After puberty the lining of the seminiferous tubules continually forms millions of sperm. Approximately 74 days are required for conversion of immature sperm to mature sperm. Each mature sperm has a whiplike tail making it possible for the sperm to move freely in the proper environment. Due to the environment of the testes, the sperm are passive. Some of the sperm are moved by peristaltic action in the epididymis and vas deferens to the prostate gland. The seminal vesicles and prostate gland produce most of the fluid in which the sperm can be suspended and made motile.

In addition to producing sperm, the testes function as an endocrine gland. The male hormone, testosterone, is produced by the testes and is responsible for development of the genitalia during puberty and for maintaining the genitalia in a functional state during life. Androgenic hormones are also responsible for the development of secondary sex characteristics including growth of body hair and thickening of the vocal cords.

The spermatic cords extend from the deep inguinal rings and consist of arteries, veins, lymphatics, nerves, and the excretory duct of the testes held together by the spermatic fascia. At the deep inguinal rings the structures of the spermatic cords converge with the structures of the testes. The spermatic cords then pass through the inguinal canals, emerge through the superficial inguinal rings, and pass downward into the scrotum.

The scrotum is a cutaneous pouch that covers and protects the testes and spermatic cords. Because the testes are surrounded by serous membrane and are suspended in the cavity of the scrotum, the testes are capable of being moved about readily. The ease of movement of the testes within the scrotum protects the testes against injury.

The skin of the scrotum is thin, brownish, very elastic because it contains rugae, and contains sebaceous follicles. Thinly scattered hairs cover the skin. Because of the rugae, the skin of the scrotum is capable of great distention, and the scrotum may become greatly enlarged when edema is present. The surface of the scrotum is divided into two halves by a ridge (raphe) that extends anteriorly to the undersurface of the penis and posteriorly along the midline of the perineum to the anus. The left side of the scrotum normally hangs lower than the right side due to the greater length of the left spermatic cord.

The external appearance of the scrotum varies under different conditions. In warm temperatures and in older or debilitated men, the scrotum becomes elongated and flat. In young, healthy men and in cool temperatures, the scrotum appears short, more wrinkled, and closely applied to the testes. In some newborn boys exposed to chilling the scrotum may appear empty because the spermatic cords tend to contract. This pulls the testes into the inguinal canal when the inguinal rings are not closed.

The epididymis is located at the lateral edge of the posterior segment of the testes and is continuous with the vas deferens. The vas deferens serves as the excretory duct of the testes, is a constituent of the spermatic cord, and separates from the spermatic cord at the inguinal ring. After taking a complex path through the pelvis, the vas deferens descends, enters the base of the prostate gland, becomes greatly narrowed, and joins the ducts of the seminal vesicles to form the ejaculatory duct.

The seminal vesicles are two membranous pouches located between the bladder and the rectum. They are lobulated in structure and secrete fluid to be added to the secretions of the testes. The lower end of each seminal vesicle becomes constricted into a straight duct and joins the vas deferens to form the ejaculatory duct. The ejaculatory duct begins at the base of the prostate gland, runs posteriorly and downward, and enters the prostate gland in the midline. In the prostate gland the ejaculatory duct opens into the prostatic portion of the urethra.

The penis is attached to the front and sides of the pubic arch. When flaccid the penis is cylindrical in shape; when erect it assumes a triangular shape with rounded angles. The penis consists of three masses of cavernous tissue held together by fibrous tissue. The greatest part of the urethra extends through the center of the penis.

The skin covering the penis is dark in color, contains no fat, and is loosely applied to the underlying tissues. At the pubis the skin is covered with hair in a characteristic triangular distribution. At the neck of the penis the skin is folded upon itself to form the prepuce (foreskin). The prepuce covers a variable amount of the glans at the tip of the penis; the prepuce may be retracted, exposing the glans in the uncircumcized male. The glans is covered by a membranous tissue that is continous with the mucous membrane of the urethra. Small, sensitive papillae are located on the surface of the glans, the inner surface of the prepuce, and the neck of the penis. These papillae secrete a sebaceous substance having a characteristic odor. When mixed with epithelial cells, the combined discharge is called *smegma* and is similar to the deposits found between the labial folds in women.

The penis is enclosed in a strong capsule of fascia. Numerous cords are given off from the inner surface of the capsule, cross in all directions, and divide the penis into compartments. This gives the entire inner structure of the penis a spongy appearance. Within the structure of muscle fibers and fibrous and elastic tissue are the numerous blood vessels and nerves of the penis.

When the male is sexually aroused, erection of the penis occurs involuntarily. Since the penis consists largely of spaces in which blood can collect, the mechanism of erection involves the blood vessels. Each space in the penis is supplied by a vein having a small sphincter at its outlet. When erection begins, the walls of the vascular spaces relax, while the outlet sphincters contract. At the same time the arteries bring an increased flow of blood to the penis. This results in collection of blood within the cavernous spaces of the penis, hardening of the penis, and erection. During erection enough blood passes through the sphincters of the veins to maintain circulation but not enough to empty the spaces. The erection is normally maintained until repeated stimulation results in reflex, involuntary ejaculation.

Ejaculation, the male orgasm, involves contractions of the muscular walls of the epididymis and vas deferens. These contractions force the passive sperm upward to the prostate gland. The seminal vesicles, which also have muscular walls, contract and force their contents into the urethra with the sperm. The fluid secreted by the seminal vesicles makes up most of the volume of the ejaculate. In the seminal fluid the sperm become motile and begin to move about actively. As the seminal fluid moves into the prostatic portion of the urethra, the urethra walls begin peristaltic movement. The semen is thus forced down the urethra and through the urinary meatus in short series of spurts, called ejaculation. Shortly following ejaculation, erection of the penis begins to subside. The vascular spaces relax, causing the blood to flow freely from the spaces within the penis. The walls of the vascular spaces contract as they empty of blood, and the body of the penis returns to its flaccid state.

The prostate gland is located below the internal urethral orifice, behind the symphysis pubis, and close to the rectal wall. It is so situated that it extends around the beginning of the urethra. The prostate gland averages 4 cm in width at its base, 3 cm from top to bottom, 2 cm from front to back, and 20 g in weight.

The prostate gland is enveloped in a firm, adherent capsule. Internally the prostate gland is partly muscular and partly glandular. The glandular substance of the prostate gland consists of numerous follicular pouches that open into long canals. These canals join to form from 12 to 20 small excretory ducts. The prostatic ducts open into the prostatic portion of the urethra, thereby adding the prostatic secretion to the seminal fluid.

Clinically the prostate gland is important because of its affinity for congestive, inflammatory, hyperplastic, and malignant diseases. Since the prostate gland is close to the rectal wall, it is easily palpable by rectal examination, and this makes diagnosis of problems at an early stage possible. Because of the anatomic relationship of the prostate gland to the urethra, most prostatic diseases present urinary tract symptoms.

The bulbourethral (Cowper's) glands are two small, round bodies located at the sides and to the back of the membranous portion of the urethra. They are enclosed by the transverse fibers of the sphincter muscles of the urethra. Each gland has an excretory duct that opens into the urethra. The main excretory duct of a Cowper gland represents the joining of many ducts from the internal glandular tissue substance.

□ Pelvic ligaments and muscles

The internal and external reproductive structures are maintained in their positions by groups of ligaments and muscles (Fig. 60-3). In the female the broad ligaments, consisting of peritoneum, extend from the surfaces of the uterus to the sides of the pelvis and support the uterus in a horizontal position. The free margins of the broad ligament enclose and support the fallopian tubes and ovaries. The ovaries are suspended from the broad ligament by means of the ovarian ligaments.

The round ligaments extend laterally from the anterior surface of the uterine fundus. They pass through the abdominal wall, inguinal canals, and inguinal rings and terminate by dissemination of their fibers in the labia majora and surrounding tissues, holding the corpus forward over the urinary bladder. These ligaments are capable of stretching to allow for increase in size and alteration of position of the uterus during pregnancy.

The uterosacral ligaments originate from the posterior surface of the uterus at the level of the internal os. They arch posteriorly and are inserted into the sacrum at the level of the second and third sacral vertebrae. Because the uterosacral ligaments exert backward tension on the cervix, they maintain the cervix and vagina at right angles to each other. The uterosacral ligaments thus prevent prolapse of the uterus by preventing the corpus from taking a position in line with the vagina.

The cardinal ligaments arise from the base of the broad ligaments. They integrate with the uterosacral ligaments and with the pelvic fascia and fan outward around the base of the uterus. The cardinal ligaments

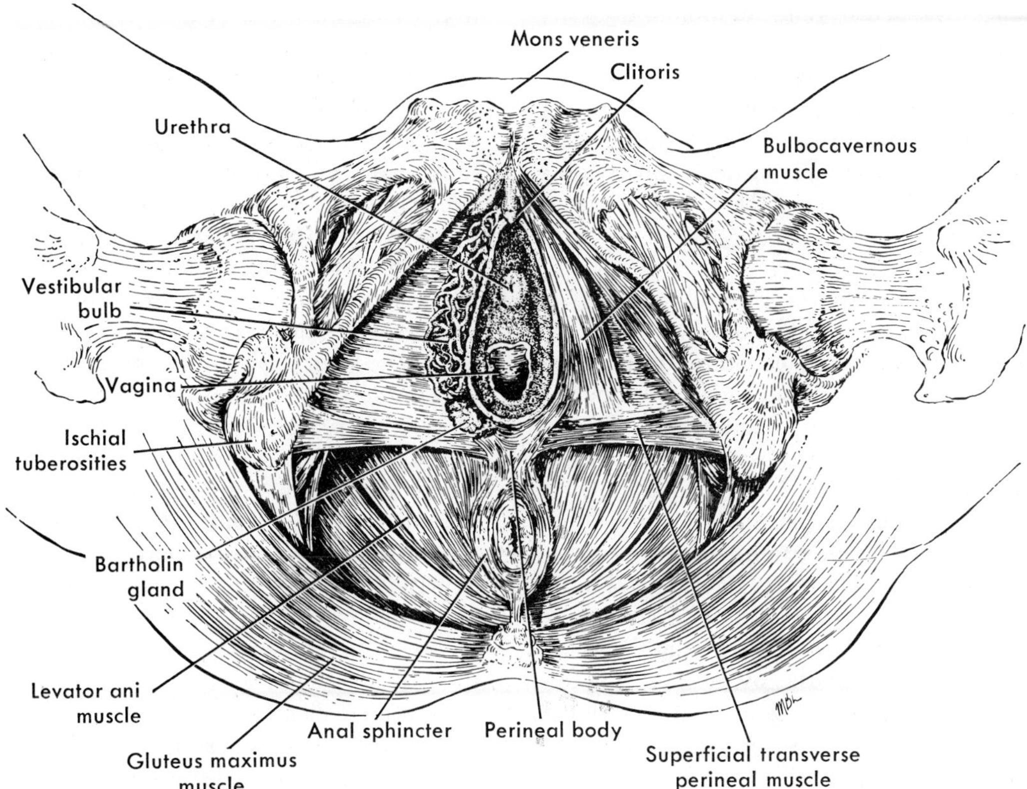

Fig. 60-5. Female pelvic floor in dissection from below. Coccygeus muscle is obscured by gluteus maximus muscle. (From Ingalls, A. J., and Salerno, C.: Maternal and child health nursing, ed. 3, St. Louis, 1975, The C. V. Mosby Co.)

provide the chief support for the cervix and upper vagina, preventing descent of these structures.

The muscles of the pelvic floor are shown in Fig. 60-5. The pelvic diaphragm consists of the levator ani and coccygeus muscles together with the pelvic fascia and stretches across the bottom of the pelvic cavity. The anal cavity, the urethra, and in females the vagina, pierce the pelvic diaphragm.

The muscles of the perineum, commonly called the perineal body or perineal center, reinforce the support provided by the levator ani and coccygeus muscles. The perineal body consists of a mass of several muscles extending across the center of the pelvic outlet. It is located between the anus and bulb in males and between the anus and vagina in females. Together the pelvic diaphragm and perineum support the pelvic organs and external genitalia from below.

In females the perineum is wider and thicker than it is in males. The muscles of the perineal body are the means of approach to the bladder and prostate gland in males, and they are the site of perineal incisions and lacerations during childbirth.

□ Blood, lymph, and nerve supply

In males and females the organs of reproduction are supplied with blood from the aorta as it branches downward and divides into the internal iliac (hypogastric) artery.

The ovarian and uterine arteries anastomose to furnish the ovaries with blood. The venous drainage is similar to the arterial supply to the reproductive organs, with the blood vessels emptying into the vena cava.

In males blood is similarly supplied to and drained from the reproductive organs. The pudendal branches of the aorta divide into the testicular arteries, and arteries supplying the seminal vesicles are derived from the inferior vesical and middle rectal arteries. Most of the blood to the penis is furnished through the internal pudendal artery. Venous return is similar to the arterial supply. Blood from the penis, testes, and prostate gland is returned to the internal iliac vein and then to the vena cava.

In both males and females lymphatic drainage of the external and internal organs of reproduction is extensive. Both superficial and deep lymphatics empty into the external iliac, internal iliac, and preaortic lymph nodes. Nerve supply is derived from sympathetic and parasympathetic fibers.

□ Endocrine functions

The major hormones produced by the ovaries are estrogen and progesterone. Estrogen is the hormone responsible for the development of secondary sex characteristics at the time of puberty. After puberty the primary function of estrogen is to cause development of the endometrium in preparation for implantation of a fertilized ovum. Progesterone enhances the preceding action of estrogen on the endometrium.

Like production of a mature ovum, secretion of ovarian hormones occurs in a cyclic fashion, with each cycle requiring an average of 28 days. Unless stimulated by pituitary hormones, however, the ovaries do not fulfill their hormone-secreting and ovum-producing functions.

In describing the ovarian-pituitary-uterine cycles, it is common to relate the events occurring to phases of the menstrual cycle. Hormonal control of the menstrual cycle shown in Fig. 60-6. The first day of the menstrual flow is the first day of the menstrual cycle.

During the menstrual phase of the cycle, (menstruation), the endometrium breaks down and is shed. Withdrawal of estrogen and progesterone prior to the onset of menstrual flow results in rupture of uterine capillaries and necrosis of endometrial tissue. The menstrual phase of the cycle lasts an average of 4 days. When menstruation ceases, the postmenstrual phase begins and extends over the next 14 days, ending with ovulation.

During the postmenstrual phase the pituitary gland secretes increasing amounts of follicle-stimulating hormone (FSH). Of the pituitary hormones, FSH is probably the most important for ovarian function because it stimulates a primordial follicle to develop into a mature graafian follicle containing a mature ovum. Since the graafian follicle produces estrogen, FSH is essential for estrogen production.

As the graafian follicle matures it secretes increasing amounts of estrogen, resulting in proliferation of endometrial cells. The endometrium becomes thicker and softer as preparation for implantation of a fertilized ovum begins. While increasing in size, the graafian follicle moves toward the surface of the ovary, where it appears as a blisterlike structure. Finally the graafian follicle ruptures (ovulation), allowing the ovum and follicular fluid to escape. The ovum enters the fallopian tube and is carried in the direction of the uterus. With ovulation the postmenstrual phase ends and the premenstrual phase begins. The premenstrual phase lasts for approximately 10 to 14 days.

Prior to ovulation estrogen exerts still other effects. It influences the cervical epithelium in such a way that the cervical mucus increases in quantity and attains a clear, elastic state. This permits the sperm to more readily enter the cervix. The high level of estrogen prior to ovulation suppresses pituitary release of FSH and triggers release of luteinizing hormone (LH).

As the level of FSH is falling and the level of estrogen is rising in the postmenstrual phase, the pituitary gland secretes increasing amounts of LH. There is a sharp rise in LH levels 12 to 24 hours before ovulation, followed by a peak level about 8 hours after ovulation. This change in hormone levels is reflected in the basal body temperature, which drops just before ovulation and rises after ovulation.

Ovulation marks the beginning of the premenstrual phase of the menstrual cycle. Under the influence of LH the corpus luteum forms in the ovary at the site of the ruptured graafian follicle. The hormone produced by the corpus luteum is progesterone. Progesterone further alters the endometrium by stimulating growth of cells and circulation of blood to the uterus. With these additional endometrial changes, the uterine environment is prepared for implantation of a fertilized ovum.

If pregnancy occurs, the corpus luteum remains active for about 6 months. By that time the placenta is developed and assumes the function of secreting progesterone to maintain the endometrium. If pregnancy does not occur, the corpus luteum degenerates in about 10 days, progesterone secretion drops markedly, and the endometrium degenerates. Menstruation results, and the cycle begins again.

On the day of ovulation about 25% of women experience pain in the lower abdomen on the side of ovulation. This pain is referred to as *mittelschmerz* and is probably a result of peritoneal irritation from follicular fluid or blood released from the ovary with the ovum. This sign rarely occurs with every cycle and is therefore an unreliable indicator of ovulation. If the pain occurs on the right side and is severe, it may be mistaken for appendicitis.

In males secretion of the androgenic hormones increases at puberty, resulting in appearance of secondary sex characteristics and production of mature sperm. Of the androgens, testosterone is most closely related to reproduction, since it specifically stimulates maturation of sperm and is responsible for maintaining the reproductive organs in a functional state. Testosterone secretion is closely related to pituitary gland function. The rate of secretion of testosterone is determined by levels of LH in the blood.

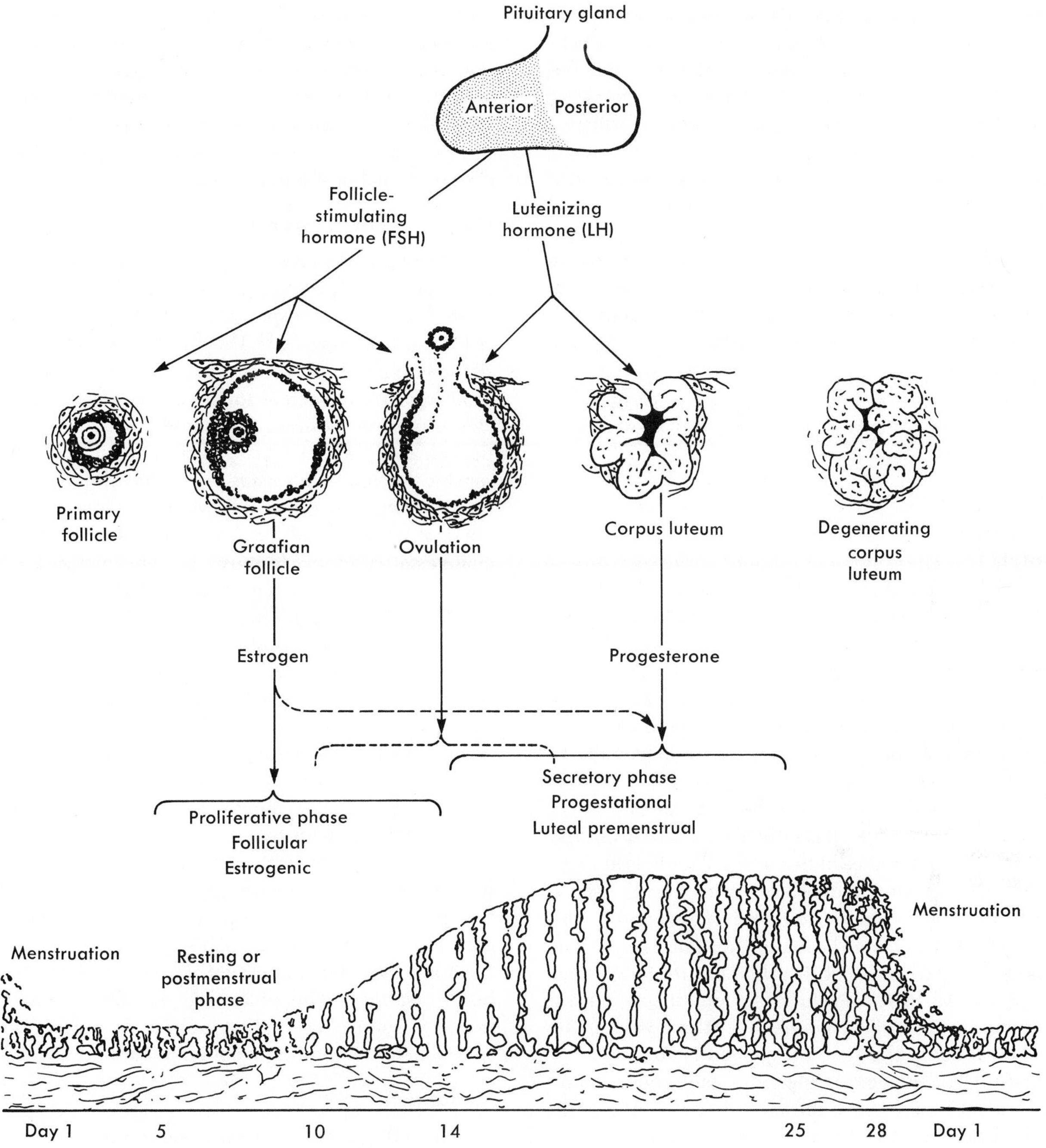

Fig. 60-6. Hormone control of menstrual cycle.

■ SEXUALITY AND HEALTH

□ Definition of sexuality

Human sexuality is not merely a biologic phenomenon. Rather, sexuality pervades the total person and involves a complex interplay of biologic, psychologic, and sociocultural variables.

Healthy sexual function is an elusive concept, its definition involving a person's unique combination of feelings, attitudes, and values that shape what is "healthy" at a given moment and in specific social situations. There are, however, commonalities found among definitions of sexual health. First there is usually congruence between biologic sex, gender identity, and gender role; that is, a person of female biologic sex usually sees herself as a woman (gender identity) and behaves in a feminine manner (gender role).[41] Next, in most societies an expectation exists about performance of proscribed roles that are congruent with biologic sex.[17] Finally, the presence of adequate circulatory and neurologic structures and function, the appropriate hormonal milieu, and intact genitalia provide the capacity to initiate and respond to sexual stimuli in a manner integrating the physiologic with the psychosocial experience. This concept of sexual health is consistent with the definition accepted by the World Health Organization:

> Sexual health is the integration of the somatic, emotional, intellectual, and social aspects of sexual being, in ways that are positively enriching and that enhance personality, communication, and love.[15]

□ Evolution of gender identity

The evolution of gender identity and gender roles illustrates how each component influences the sexuality of the very young child and ultimately the adult. Money and Ehrhardt's description of psychosexual differentiation indicates that the X or Y chromosome from the paternal sperm sets in motion a process analogous to a relay race; that is, each component has control of the process for a time, eventually yielding control to another.[41] The chromosomes tag the undifferentiated fetal gonads as male or female, thus setting in motion another process by which hormonal secretions of the testis in turn affect the appearance of the genitals as well as pathways in the brain. It is the appearance of the infant's genitals at birth that sets in motion another series of events, those primarily dependent on socialization of the child. The behavior of other persons during infancy and early childhood and the appearance of the child's external genitals are instrumental in the evolution of childhood gender identity and role. In fact, gender identity seems to be well established by the time the person is 18 months of age. At puberty biologic influences again come to the fore as hormones influence the morphology of the genitals and eroticism.

Thus from conception we are all sexual beings, subject to multiple influences throughout life. If the processes described above proceed without interference, the person's biologic sex (female or male) will be congruent with gender identity (person sees herself or himself as a woman or a man) and gender role (outward manifestations of masculinity or femininity). (Consequences of lack of congruence between sex, gender identity, and gender role are explored briefly in Chapter 63.)

This complex set of biologic and psychosocial variables set in motion by the event of conception has a pervasive influence on the remainder of our lives. The biologic component of sexuality, sexual function or expression, constantly interacts with the psychologic components of gender identity, cognition, and affect as well as with social factors such as sanctioned roles and mores and folkways regulating sexual expression. Such complexity mandates a holistic approach to conceptualizing clients' sexual problems and concerns.

□ Human sexual response

Masters and Johnson, pioneers in the scientific study of the physiologic aspects of sexual behavior, demonstrated that sexual response is a cyclic phenomenon consisting of four phases.[37] The *excitement phase,* the initial component of the cycle, develops from sexually arousing stimuli such as touch; an increase in sexual tension is observed during this phase. Next, a consolidation period, the *plateau phase,* occurs, during which sexual tension becomes intensified. The involuntary climax of sexual tension, *orgasm,* follows and involves only a small portion of the sexual response cycle. During this period changes attributable to muscular tension and congestion of blood vessels reach a peak and begin to dissipate. During the *resolution phase,* an involutionary period, the changes involving the blood vessels, sexual organs, and muscular tension are reversed. Women may at this time begin another sexual response cycle immediately; men must observe an obligatory period during which they cannot be restimulated to higher levels of sexual tension.[37]

The physiologic changes seen during human sexual response depend on two main principles: myotonia and vasocongestion. It is through the congestion of pelvic blood vessels and involuntary muscular contractions in the pelvic organs and other parts of the body that changes supportive or orgastic experience are attained. It should also be noted that sexual response is a total body response. The phase-specific descriptions of the sexual response cycle that follow illustrate the widespread involvement in this phenomenon.

Excitement

The hallmark of sexual arousal in the woman is vaginal lubrication. Believed to result from transudation of a mucoidlike substance across the vaginal mucosa, lubrication appears within seconds of sexual stimulation. The vaginal barrel becomes longer and wider as the uterus begins to elevate in the pelvis. Vasocongestive changes may also be seen in the external genitalia: the clitoris becomes longer and wider, and the labia minora flatten and separate from the vaginal opening. As the labia minora become vasocongested, they actually extend outward, lengthening the vaginal barrel. The man's penis rapidly becomes erect, tensing of the scrotal sac is noted, and the testes begin to rise toward the perineum.[37]

Extragenital changes are also seen with sexual excitement: the woman's nipples become erect, the areolae become engorged, venous patterns in the breast become more evident, and breast size actually increases. The sex flush, which looks like a red, maculopapular rash, appears over the chest in some persons. The man's nipples may also become erect. An increase in both the heart rate and blood pressure is evident, paralleling the level of sexual excitement.[37]

Plateau

During the plateau phase the clitoris retracts upward beneath the clitoral hood. Clitoral stimulation may still occur indirectly as the penis exerts traction on the labia while moving in and out of the vagina. The orgasmic platform, the extremely vascular tissue at the outer portion of the vagina and the labia minora, becomes increasingly congested. The uterus continues to elevate in the pelvis, which creates a tenting effect in the innermost portion of the vagina. Externally the labia majora become more congested, and the labia minora deepen in color as a result of vasocongestion. A few drops of mucoidlike material are secreted from Bartholin glands, probably to assist with the lubrication of the outermost portion of the vagina. The diameter of the penis continues to increase, especially at the coronal ridge, and the testes increase in size to 50% over their unstimulated state as they elevate closer to the perineum. A few drops of mucoid material are secreted from Cowper's glands.

The woman's areolae are now so engorged that it is difficult to see the erect nipple. The sex flush continues to spread, sometimes involving the neck, face, and arms. Hyperventilation occurs in both sexes, along with heart rates of 100 to 175 beats per minute. There is elevation of systolic blood pressure (20 to 60 mm Hg for women, 20 to 80 for men) and diastolic blood pressure (10 to 20 mm Hg for women, 10 to 40 mm Hg for men).

Orgasm

Orgasm involves the climactic release of sexual tension and is evident in contractions throughout the body. The woman's orgasmic platform contracts rapidly, and expulsive contractions along the entire male urethra propel semen from the vas out through the penis. During orgasm the internal bladder sphincter in the male contracts, thus preventing semen from being propelled backward into the bladder. Uterine contractions are also noted in the female with orgasm, much like those characteristic of labor. The rectal sphincter also contracts rapidly in both men and women during orgasm.

Resolution

During this phase vasocongestion is gradually lost from the clitoris and breasts but rapidly from the orgasmic platform. The clitoris quickly returns to its usual position from under the clitoral hood. Vasocongestion of the labia dissipates, nipple erection recedes, and the uterus descends to its usual position in the pelvis. Cardiovascular and respiratory rates quickly return to normal. In the man there is initially a rapid loss of erection to 1 to 1.5 times the size of the penis in its unstimulated state. Later there is a slower resolution of vasocongestion until the penis returns to prestimulation size. The scrotum and testes lose their vasocongestive changes, and the testes rapidly descend into the scrotum. Occasionally a thin film of perspiration may appear over the entire body.

Requirements for healthy sexual response

The requirements for the sexual response described above include intact sexual organs, adequate vasculature to support the vasocongestive changes, functional innervation of the genital organs, and the appropriate hormonal milieu.[29] The sexual experience depends on the two responses discussed earlier: myotonia and vasocongestion. These changes are thought to be mediated by the autonomic nervous system. Perception of the sexual experience at cortical levels requires intact sensory pathways from the genitalia and other peripheral structures to the cortex. The capacity to stimulate oneself or a partner sexually depends on the presence of intact motor pathways from higher centers to the effector muscles involved. It should also be noted that thought and feelings or visual, auditory, and olfactory-gustatory stimuli alone may result in arousal to orgasmic experience even in the absence of tactile perception. Adequate hormonal milieu, with appropriate hormonal release, influences both the structure and function of the genitalia; for example, the decreased estrogen levels during menopause are believed to be responsible for a decreased amount of vaginal lubrication in the woman.[37] Finally, the presence of intact genital structures is usually thought to be a requisite for sexual response, but substitution of prosthetic devices for sexual organs is an option beginning to be explored.

□ Assessment

Subjective data

Men and women who present themselves for a checkup or with a complaint related to the genital tract should have a complete history taken. Some persons who at first appear to have no symptoms indicating involvement of the reproductive organs may be found to have a problem of the genital system. Careful eliciting of information will help define the problem(s) so that immediate attention can be directed to relieving the cause of complaint or preventing problems from occurring.

Many of the problems that individuals bring to the attention of nurses and physicians concern subjects or body areas that they are hesitant to discuss. Careful, tactful questioning can assist them to feel more at ease, and often they are relieved that the topic has been raised by someone else. Sympathy and understanding, along with respect for personal feelings, are essential in obtaining information that individuals might omit because of fear, tension, or embarrassment. Listening with attention and interest are reassuring to the individuals and assist them to be more open and free in expression.

Past medical history. The person's history of previous illnesses is carefully recorded and includes any previous treatment for conditions that might influence functioning of the reproductive organs.

Males are questioned about their past history concerning pain or swelling of the scrotum or testes, sores on the penis, discharges from the urethra, urinary tract problems, ability to achieve and maintain an erection, and previous surgery or treatments for problems of the genitourinary tract. Both males and females should be questioned about a history of syphilis, gonorrhea, or other venereal diseases.

Family history. The incidence of such diseases as diabetes, hypertension, coronary occlusion, and cancer should be obtained and recorded. Some chronic diseases that tend to recur in families influence functioning of the reproductive organs.

Gynecologic-obstetric history. In securing information for the gynecologic history, as with other aspects of the history, it is important to assess the person's level of understanding and to use words that are readily understood. Many persons are hesitant to give information because they lack knowledge of medical terms and are embarrassed because of this lack. Questions should be clearly stated so that accurate answers will be given. For example, few women can answer questions about the menarche, but most could answer the question, "How old were you when your periods began?"

When taking the history is is usual to begin with previous illnesses or surgery related to the reproductive organs. The gynecologic-obstetric history is outlined in the box above.

Because countless women are using some form of contraception and since some of the contraceptives in use may affect the state of reproductive health, a complete contraceptive history should be taken. Information includes types of contraceptives used in the past and at present, how long each type was used, why a specific method was discontinued and another substituted, and any problems that occurred during the use of contraception.

Patient's complaint. The patient's complaint should be recorded in the patient's own languare in order to direct the questioning and to assess the urgency of any problem. The data should include location of the symptoms, duration, severity, treatment by a physician, and attempts the patient has made to relieve the problem.

Once a general statement or description of the patient's chief complaint is obtained, more specific questioning can follow. If pain is a complaint, the patient should be asked to describe it in clear terms, for example, sharp, dull, cramping, steady, intermittent. The site of the pain can usually be determined by asking the patient to show where it is. Identification of events or activities that increase or decrease the pain is important. Such facts as the use of heat or cold, self-medication, alterations in position, coughing, or having intercourse and their influence on the pain should be obtained.

When the patient complains of bleeding, as much specific information should be obtained as possible. If a woman complains of bleeding, vague statements such as "irregular periods" or "intermittent bleeding" are inadequate. Data about the last two menstrual periods should be obtained. If the menstrual periods are irregular, the range of the cycles and duration of flow are recorded. Bleeding between menstrual periods is described in terms of number of days before or after a menstrual period and duration of bleeding at these times. In addition characteristics of the blood lost are obtained and recorded.

In men complaints of bleeding are often related to the presence of blood in the urine, and other symptoms such as pain on voiding may be present. Frank bleeding may be present in the form of bright or dark blood on the

GYNECOLOGIC-OBSTETRIC HISTORY

- Previous illness or surgery involving the reproductive organs
- Menstrual history
  - Age at menarche
  - Interval and duration of menstrual periods
  - Pain with menstruation, including days of cycle on which it occurs, duration, and factors that intensify or alleviate it
  - Amount of flow (number of tampons or pads)
  - Presence of clots, their size, and dates on which they appear
  - Dates of onset of last two menstrual periods and duration of flow
- Obstetric history
  - Pregnancies (dates, length of gestation, type of delivery, birth weight, complications during or after pregnancy)
  - Abortions, miscarriages

underwear, and the patient is questioned about this. Associated symptoms of other types of discharge, burning or itching of the genitalia, and ability to initiate urination are determined.

In a similar way specific descriptions of complaints of a tumor, mass, swelling, sore on the genitalia, discharges other than bleeding, and symptoms related to the bladder and rectum are obtained by questioning the patient.

Since the reproductive tract is sensitive to endocrine functioning and the use of medications, all patients are questioned about these. In women it is especially important to determine whether hormones or contraceptive pills are being taken.

Sexual history. Many health care providers may not be experienced in eliciting a sexual history and may be uneasy when doing so (at first). No doubt this uneasiness is conditioned by social prohibitions about discussing intimate matters such as sexual experiences or behavior. However, health professionals are expected to be informed, willing to discuss sexual matters openly with clients, and prepared to educate and counsel clients appropriately. Nurses who are hesitant to deal with sexual matters with clients will be helped by working through their own feelings about sex and sexual matters. Seeking counsel from other nurses or health professionals who are comfortable with the topic is often helpful. Recently special courses and workshops on sexuality for nurses have become available, and some nurses may find it helpful to attend one of these. During the past decade the public has been exposed to explicit portrayal of sex and sexuality. Although sometimes criticized, this candor has had salutory effects: more people are willing and able to discuss their sexual concerns. As a result health professionals are increasingly expected to be informed, willing to discuss these concerns, and able to educate and counsel clients.

Although there is no single approach to taking a sexual history, application of certain principles will facilitate both the client's and the practitioner's comfort. Absolute requirements for history taking include provision of privacy, such as in a closed room; an atmosphere of trust between client and practitioner, such as assurance of confidentiality for the client; and comfort on the part of the practitioner with her or his own sexuality.

Some principles for promoting client-practitioner comfort follow. First, obtaining the sexual history early in the therapeutic relationship conveys to the client that sexuality is a legitimate component of health and that it is normal and usual for it to be examined in the context of a physical examination or health history. Next, the sexual history itself may be therapeutic. Within the context of obtaining the data the practitioner can provide permission for the client to discuss her or his concerns, provide limited information or suggestions, or validate the normalcy and acceptability of the client's concerns and practices. Avoiding overreaction such as shock and horror to the information related by the client, as well as underreaction such as boredom, facilitates truthful history giving on the part of the client. Use of language that the client understands and with which the practitioner is comfortable will also facilitate obtaining an adequate picture of the client's concerns. It may be necessary for both the client and the practioner to define their terms; street language may be unfamiliar to the nurse, and highly technical language may be confusing to the client. The nurse may need to become familiar with some commonly used street language in order to be sure what the client is reporting.[35,57] The technique of moving from less sensitive to more sensitive areas paves the way for both the client and practitioner. For example, the nurse may explore a woman's sexual role before discussing her ability to have orgasm, her menstrual history before her experience with sexual variations, and her personal experiences with sex education before her actual sexual experiences.

"Unloading the question" is another technique useful in obtaining a sexual history. This consists of prefacing the question with a statement referring to the known variation in or prevalence of a specific behavior. For example, the question related to frequency of intercourse may be asked in the following fashion: "Some women have intercourse several times a week, some a few times a week, and still others not at all. On the average, how often do you have intercourse?" This approach conveys to the client that no matter what her practices, they fit into the framework of known behavioral patterns.

Referring to the ubiquity of sexual practices is another useful strategy. This consists of asking clients "how" or "when" they began certain sexual practices as opposed to the more threatening "did you ever?" approach. Prefacing an inquiry by a statement such as "Many people experience. . . . " conveys to the client that his or her practices or experiences are not too unusual to relate.

Following the life cycle chronology is another useful technique inasmuch as it provides for a logical unfolding of events. Finally, terminating the sexual history by inquiring whether the client has additional questions or issues to discuss conveys a willingness on the part of the practitioner to further explore sexual matters.

Brief sexual assessment. A brief assessment can be incorporated in the nursing history by means of three questions. The first of these deals with the person's *role,* the next with the *affective-cognitional elements* of sexuality, and the last with *biologic aspects* of sexual function. These questions may be modified to deal with illness, hospitalization, life events, or any other relevant entity that may influence or interfere with sexual health.

Has your (illness, pregnancy, hospitalization) interfered with your being a (husband, wife, father, mother)? Has your (abortion, heart attack) changed the way you see yourself as a (woman, man)? Has your (colostomy, hysterectomy) changed your ability to function sexually (or your sex life)? These questions may also be adapted to elicit the client's expectations of changes resulting from procedures or hospitalization that he or she is about to experience. Similar questions may be found in the format for the nursing history described by McPhetridge.[40] These brief items invite the client to explore sexual concerns. Often it is unnecessary for the practitioner to ask the second and third questions, as many clients proceed to state their concerns about masculinity, femininity, and sexual functioning without further prompting.

Sexual problem history. The sexual problem history may be used in conjunction with the brief history described above or alone in the context of sexual counseling or therapy. Although the parameters explored in a sexual problem history will vary with the theoretical framework guiding the nurses' practice, there are commonalities to be explored regardless of the approach to therapy. The approach described below has been suggested by Annon.[4]

The first component of the sexual problem history is a *description,* in the client's terms, of the current problem or concern. Next, the *onset and course* of the problem are explored. The practitioner may wish to inquire about the age of the client when the problem began, whether it had an insidious onset or occurred suddenly, whether the client can identify any precipitating events, and whether there are other life events associated with the sexual problem. The course of the sexual problem can be described in terms of its fluctuations over time, such as with the changing intensity of a disease process, and whether the problem has any functional relationships to phenomena such as medication or alcohol use.

Of great importance is the *client's conception of the cause and persistence of the problem.* This data will enable the nurse to respond directly to the client's concerns rather than dealing with them indirectly.

Past attempts at treatment and their results may be explored, including evaluations by other health practitioners such as physicians, the use of other professional help such as professional counselors, and finally the attempts that the client has made to cope with the problem.

The last component of the sexual problem history includes an examination of the *client's current expectations and the goals* identified for treatment. A woman complaining of inability to have orgasm may have the expectations of having orgasm with intercourse rather than by self-stimulation. If her expectations are not stated precisely, the practitioner may inappropriately treat her with the latter goal in mind or refer her to a practitioner whose approach to therapy would not be congruent with her goals.

Alternative approaches. Although the two approaches to obtaining sexual history data described above are probably most appropriate for nurses, several alternatives exist. For further information about these alternatives the reader is referred to references 4, 29, 33, 36, and 49.

Objective data

Physical examination. When patients present themselves for a checkup or because of a problem of the genital tract, a complete physical examination should be done. Men should have a rectal examination, and woman should have a pelvic examination and thorough examination of the breasts.

Both men and women may put off medical examination of the reproductive tract, since this type of examination may cause intense emotional reactions. Fear, embarrassment, and cultural mores play an important part in this emotional distress. In our culture people frequently fear that their anxieties concerning carcinoma, venereal disease, sterility, or the climacteric will be verified. Many are embarrassed by the required exposure of the external genitalia during examination. Many patients also may be fearful that some condition will be discovered that will require surgery resulting in sterility or impotence. The nurse who is sensitive to the many thoughts and fears that may trouble patients will be better prepared to help them accept the necessary examination.

Men should be encouraged to have a yearly rectal examination to detect early prostatic disease. The positive aspects of such an examination should be pointed out. It is customary in some areas for male practitioners to request a female "chaperone's" presence during the female patients' pelvic examination. However, it is customary for males to be examined without the presence of a chaperone.

Preparation. Whether the physical examination is to be performed by a nurse or a physician, it is a function of the nurse to prepare the patient for the examination. Preparation includes informing the patient of what is to be done, by whom and why, what the patient needs to do in preparation for the examination and why, what the patient can do to feel more relaxed and comfortable during the examination, and when the patient will be informed of findings of the examination.

For female patients the use of visual aids are useful when a pelvic examination is to be done. Models of the pelvic organs, pamphlets, and films such as *The*

*Gynecologic Examination** assist with presentation of information about the purposes of the examination, what is done, and what to expect.

Women who are scheduled ahead of time for physical examination should be advised to avoid douching and application of any vaginal preparations (medicinal or deodorant) for at least 24 hours prior to examination. Patients should void immediately before examination, since an empty bladder makes palpation of the pelvic organs easier, decreases patient discomfort, eliminates possible distortion of the position of pelvic organs caused by a full bladder, and obviates the danger of incontinence during examination.

Abdominal examination. Information related to the reproductive organs is obtained by inspection, palpation, percussion, and auscultation of the lower abdomen. The abdomen is inspected for the presence of scars and for size and contour. If scars are noted, the patient should be questioned about these even though information may have been obtained during the history taking. Any localized areas of prominence should be noted, since these may indicate enlargement of the reproductive organs or adjacent structures. The skin of the abdomen and pubic area is inspected for amount, distribution, and character of hair, abnormal pigmentation, and lesions. Abdominal muscle tone is assessed by having the patient cough or raise the head. Such actions reveal muscle weakness by producing bulging around the umbilicus, inguinal region, or in the midline between the rectus muscles. Women who have been pregnant are more likely to have diastasis recti. In men hernias most often are evident in the inguinal areas.

Abdominal palpation follows inspection. Since the reproductive organs are normally situated in the pelvic cavity, they are usually not palpable through the abdominal wall. Therefore abdominal palpation is done for the purposes of ruling out or discovering abnormalities. Palpation should be light at first, then followed by deep palpation (p. 1222). An estimate of the amount of pressure needed to palpate can be obtained by gently picking up the skin in either lower quadrant to estimate the thickness of the abdominal wall.

If the patient has complained of pain, the site of pain should never be palpated first. Instead palpation is started in the farthest removed quadrants, and the area of pain is gradually and gently approached. Observation of the patient for responses indicating pain or tenderness on palpation is necessary. For patients who are nonreactive, it is advisable to seek verbal confirmation of the absence of pain or tenderness. The site and degree of any pain or tenderness should be recorded.

Enlargement of the uterus is detected by palpating in the midline of the lower abdomen. Palpation is started just below the umbilicus and continued in the direction of the symphysis pubis. In contrast to a full bladder, which feels soft, an enlarged uterus feels firm and may be round or asymmetric. During pregnancy the uterus is not palpable as an abdominal organ until about the end of the third month. A firm, isolated area of enlargement may be due to the presence of a tumor of the uterus. In males a distended bladder after voiding requires further evaluation, as does bulging in either or both inguinal areas.

Enlargment of the fallopian tubes and ovaries may be detected by palpation of the right and left lower quadrants. Even when enlarged, these organs are not always palpable through the abdominal wall. However, enlargement is often associated with pain or tenderness on palpation of the lower quadrants. The round ligaments are often palpable in the lower quadrants, stretching from the iliac crests to the pubic bones, and they should not be confused with the fallopian tubes.

Percussion of the lower abdomen is directed chiefly to the organs or masses that are palpable. A tumor such as an ovarian cyst or fibroid tumor of the uterus produces dullness, or a flat note, over the area, while a uterus enlarged because of pregnancy usually produces a hollow note.

Auscultation is used to determine the presence and quality of peristaltic movement. During pregnancy it is possible to hear the fetal heartbeat through the abdominal wall by the twentieth week if an ordinary stethoscope is used. If devices with doppler signals and amplification are used, the fetal heartbeat may be heard several weeks earlier.

Pelvic examination. Following abdominal examination a pelvic examination is performed. The following equipment may be necessary:

1. Bivalve vaginal specula (various sizes)
2. Uterine tenaculum forceps
3. Sponge forceps
4. Biopsy forceps (sterile)
5. Cautery unit with tips
6. Uterine sounds and probes (sterile)
7. Gloves (disposable rubber or plastic)
8. Lubricant (water soluble, vegetable base)
9. Aspirator or wooden blade for Pap smear
10. Cotton applicators
11. Cotton balls
12. Gauze sponges
13. Topical antiseptic solution
14. Specimen bottles with fixative solution

*Your Health, Educational Division, 5841 S. Maryland Ave., Chicago, Illinois 60637.

15. Glass microscope slides
16. Test tubes and culture tubes

Good lighting is important for a pelvic examination. Probably the best lighting is obtained with a head mirror.

A lighted speculum can be used for the pelvic examination. A mirror used by the examiner enables the woman to visualize her genitalia, often correcting myths about the vagina and other structures. This educational approach to the pelvic examination may provide many women with their first opportunity to view and identify their genitalia.

Several positions may be used for the pelvic examination. Arthritis and other conditions that limit the woman's mobility may preclude some of these positions. Furthermore, some positions such as the knee-chest position are both uncomfortable and embarrassing for women of almost any age or physical condition. Nurses can interpret the necessity for such positions.

In *Sims's position (used for rectal examination)* (Fig. 60-7, *A*) the woman is placed on her left side with her left arm and hand behind her. The left thigh is only slightly flexed, and the right knee is flexed sharply on the abdomen. The woman is draped so that only the perineum is exposed.

For the *dorsal recumbent position (lithotomy position)* (Fig. 60-7, *B*) the lower leaf of the examining table should be dropped before the woman gets onto the table, since dropping it may be frightening to her after her feet have been placed in the stirrups. There should be a footstool handy so that she can be guided to step on the stool, sit down on the edge of the table, and then lie back. Most women are able to place their own legs in the stirrups; they should be told to raise both legs and put them in the stirrups simultaneously. When a woman needs help, two persons may assist, with one on each side of the patient so that both can hold one leg and simultaneously place them in position without abruptly lifting the lower extremities. Gentleness and gradual positioning are essential to prevent strain or twisting of the hip joint. Metal stirrups are the most satisfactory. However, if they are used the patient should wear her shoes because the heels help to hold the feet in the stirrups.

Care must be taken to see that there is no pressure on the legs when sling stirrups are used, since nerve damage and impairment of circulation can occur. The buttocks need to be moved down so that they are even with the end of the table. The pillow under the head is pulled down at the same time to assure comfort for the patient. The woman is then draped in such a manner that only the perineum is exposed. The triangular drape is most often used, since it provides a flap that can be brought down for privacy if a few moments should intervene between draping and examination.

The pelvic examination can be done with the woman

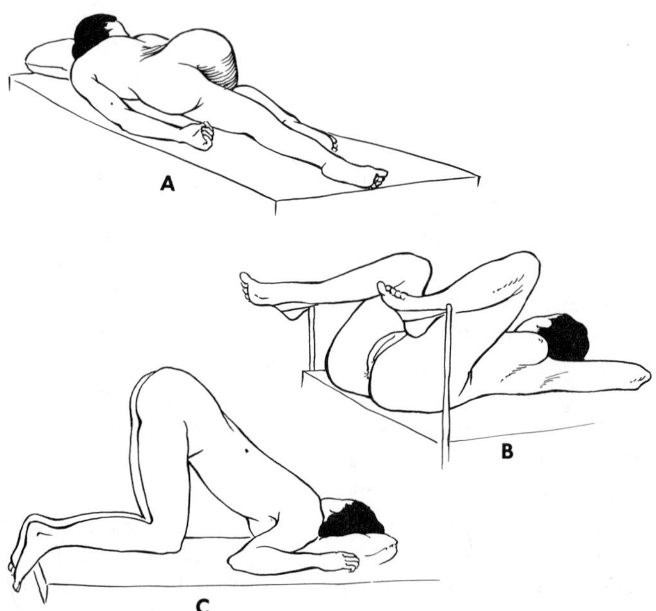

Fig. 60-7. Various positions that can be assumed for examination of rectum and vagina. **A,** Sims's (lateral) position; note position of left arm and right leg. **B,** Lithotomy position; note position of buttocks on edge of examining table and support of feet. **C,** Knee-chest (genupectoral) position; note placement of shoulders and head.

in bed it if is inadvisable for her to be moved to an examining table. The woman can be helped to assume a position across the bed, and her feet can be supported on the seats of two straight chairs. Some practitioners find this a useful adaptation when the pelvic examination is done at home.

For the *knee-chest position* (Fig. 60-7, *C*), first drop the lower end of the examination table, then help the woman get on her hands and knees on the table. Her buttocks will be uppermost, and her thighs will be sharply flexed on her trunk. The woman's head is turned to one side and rests on the table. Her arms are flexed and resting well forward (often above her head), and her knees are apart. Her feet extend over the lower edge of the table to prevent pressure on her toes. Drapes expose only her perineum. This examination can also be done by positioning the woman crosswise on the bed.

INSPECTION AND PALPATION OF FEMALE EXTERNAL GENITALIA. This portion of the pelvic examination is done before internal examination. Protective gloves are usually worn throughout the examination.

The external genitalia are first inspected for gross deviations from normal. The size and contour of the labia, presence and distribution of pubic hair, tone of the perineum, presence of vaginal discharge or lesions, and presence of hemorrhoids are all noted. The opening of the vagina and the tissues around the vaginal opening are inspected for contour and symmetry. If the structures appear distorted or if the vaginal opening appears asymmetric, the tissues should be palpated. Most often irregularity or distortion of tissues in this area is due to scars from lacerations, an ulcer just inside the vagina, or infections and cysts in the location of Skene's or Bartholin's glands. The skin of the entire vulvar area is observed for signs of inflammation, and if there is a vaginal discharge that causes itching, the skin may be broken due to scratching. Any type of rash or lesion of the skin is significant and should be reported to the physician.

Inspection of the tissues and structures within the labial folds is important. To expose the area adequately, the labia minora are separated using two fingers as when a catheterization is being performed. This maneuver makes the clitoris, urinary meatus, vaginal opening, and tissues around these structures more readily visible. The tissues are inspected for signs of inflammation, cysts, nodules, papules, and ulcerations. Especially important is the presence of a spontaneous purulent discharge from the meatus. If there is reason to suspect a urethral infection without evidence of urethral discharge, the urethra may be "stripped." This is done by placing the forefinger into the vagina for about half the finger's length. The finger is then bent so that its tip touches the anterior wall of the vagina in the midline behind the urethra. While exerting gentle pressure, the finger is then slowly withdrawn. This maneuver forces any accumulation of discharge out through the meatus. A culture should be taken whenever a purulent discharge from the urethra is present.

Skene's and Bartholin's glands are closely inspected and palpated. These are common sites of infection, especially due to the gonococcus organisms. If there is a purulent discharge from either of these glands, a smear or culture should be taken. Bartholin's glands are palpated by placing one finger inside the base of the vagina and a thumb on the outside of the labia majora near the perineum. Pressure is made by bringing the finger and thumb together. To palpate Skene's glands a finger is placed over the site of the glands, and gentle, inward pressure is applied. Usually these glands can be palpated only in thin women. Therefore if they are enlarged, and especially if they are enlarged and tender, this usually indicates cystic formation, infection, or an abscess.

The vaginal opening and perineum are further inspected and palpated for loss of muscle tone. The patient is asked to bear down, and the vaginal opening is inspected for prolapse of tissue into the vagina and visibility of the cervix. When the patient is asked to bear down, only a slight bulging of the entire vulva is normally seen. It may be observed that the vagina seems to gape either with or without straining, particularly in women who are multiparous. If this is so, it should be determined by palpation with one finger in the vagina whether (1) the anterior vaginal wall appears as the bladder pushes downward in the front, (2) the posterior vaginal wall appears as the rectum is pushed foreward from the back, or (3) both the anterior and posterior vaginal walls protrude into the vagina.

Perineal muscle tone is further tested by inserting two fingers into the vagina and asking the patient to tighten her muscles. The muscles can be felt to contract around the fingers if there is normal muscle tone but not if the muscles are weakened. Still an additional estimate of muscle tone can be made by placing two fingers inside the vagina. The fingers are slightly spread, and traction is applied against the tissues by pressing toward the examiner. If the muscles tone is normal, the tissues cannot be displaced more than a finger's breadth. If the muscles of the perineum are weak, the tissues can be readily depressed.

INSPECTION AND PALPATION OF INTERNAL ORGANS. It is now considered good practice to first perform a speculum examination of the vagina and cervix before introducing lubricated fingers to palpate. It has been shown that some lubricants in common use prevent securing of adequate specimens from the cervix and might alter laboratory findings.[25] Methods for obtaining cervical and vaginal specimens are discussed later in this chapter.

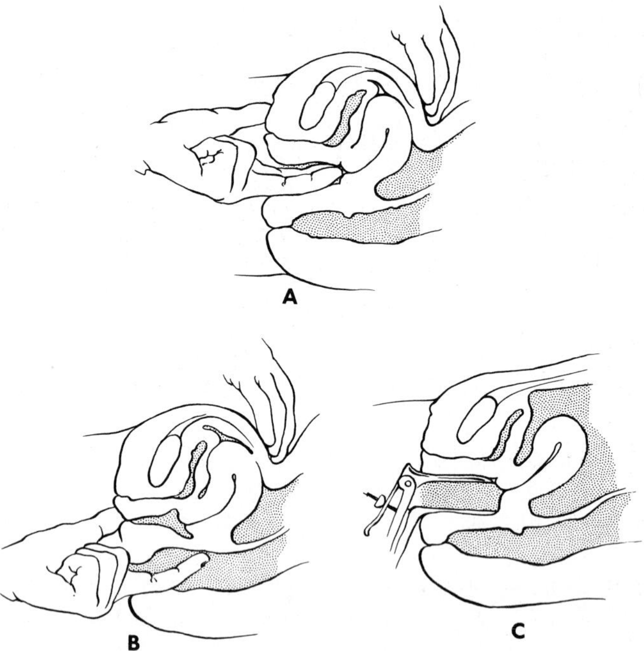

Fig. 60-8. Methods of pelvic examination. **A,** Digital examination of vagina with abdominal palpation to determine size and position of uterus. **B,** Digital rectal examination with abdominal palpation. **C,** Examination of vagina and cervix using bivalve vaginal speculum.

In order to provide for inspection of the vagina and cervix, it is necessary to select the size speculum that provides the best exposure without producing undue discomfort for the woman (Fig. 60-8). In general the smallest size is used when examining children and elderly women; the medium size is used for adult, nulliparous women; and the large size is used for women who have had children.

The speculum is lubricated with warm water. The labia minora are separated and held in this position with one hand while the speculum is introduced with the other hand. The speculum is held so that the blades are firmly closed to avoid pinching of tissues and so that the blades are verticle with the handles of the speculum to one side. This position of the speculum allows the instrument to fit better the contour of the vagina. (Some examiners contend that inserting and subsequently turning the speculum creates discomfort. They recommend inserting the speculum with the blades parallel to the examination table.)

The speculum is advanced into the vagina close to the rectal wall while slight downward pressure is exerted on the posterior vaginal wall. When the speculum blades are about three fourths their length inside the vagina, the speculum is turned so that the handle is downward within the palm of the hand. The lever is pressed to open the blades, and an attempt is made to visualize the cervix. The cervix is almost immediately visible, and the external os can readily be seen. If the cervix is not visualized, the speculum is withdrawn slightly until the cervix comes into view.

The screw on the speculum is tightened to hold the blades in the open position. Cervical specimens are collected at this point. The cervix is next inspected for color, contour, and shape of the external os. In nulliparous women the external os appears as a round depressed area (Fig. 60-9). In multiparous women the cervical os usually appears as a transverse slit in the center of the cervix. The surface of the cervix is inspected to determine whether it is smooth, irregular, or raw and whether there is any purulent or other type of discharge from the os. It is not uncommon to see a red, somewhat raw appearing area (an erosion) on the surface of the cervix. There may be scars appearing as white or reddened slits radiating from the cervical os. These are lacerations of the cervix and are often present in women who have borne children (Fig. 60-9). Occasionally a stalked polyp may be seen extending through the cervical os as a bright or dark red mass. These polyps frequently cause bleeding and require further study.

After inspection of the cervix, the screw on the speculum is loosened and the speculum is slowly withdrawn. Pressure on the lever is maintained to make inspection of the vagina possible. As the speculum is with-

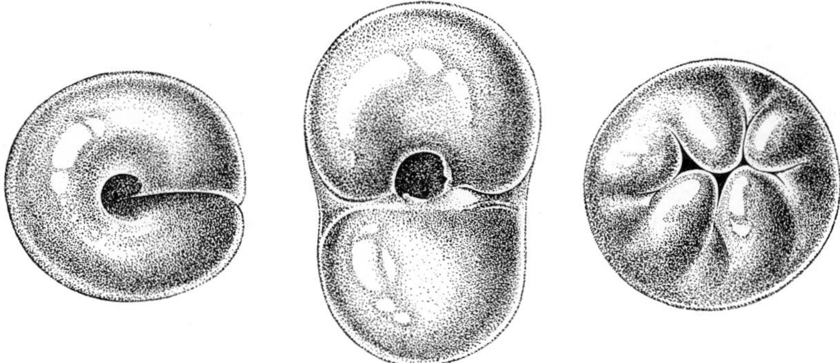

Fig. 60-9. Nulliparous cervix and laceration of cervix. (From Malasanos, L., Barkauskas, V., Moss, M., and Stoltenberg-Allen, K.: Health assessment, St. Louis, 1977, The C. V. Mosby Co.)

drawn, the cervix is checked to see whether contact with the cervix has caused bleeding. Slight spotting from collection of cervical specimens may be present. However, frank bleeding that ceases only with application of pressure is significant. The walls of the vagina are inspected as the speculum is withdrawn. The color of the vaginal walls, normally pink, is noted, as is the presence or absence of rugae. Discharges from the walls of the vagina and lesions of any type are also noted.

Palpation of the internal reproductive organs follows speculum examination. Lubricant should be used on the first and middle fingers of the examining hand. The hand is held so that the first and middle fingers are straight and close together. The thumb is stretched straight up, and the ring and small fingers are curled into the palm of the hand. Throughout the examination, the examiner's wrist is held in a rigid, straight line.

The labia minora are separated, and the first and middle fingers are slowly but firmly introduced into the vaginal canal. As the fingers are advanced, the elbow is raised slightly so that the fingers can follow the normal curve of the posterior vaginal wall. The fingers are advanced until the cervix is felt. Usually the cervix is located with ease. In nonpregnant women the cervix normally has a consistency similar to the tip of the nose. It feels smooth and round, is about 2.54 cm in diameter, and under normal circumstances moves easily in all directions. Normally the cervix is situated in the midline.

The cervix is palpated for consistency and contour. It is noted whether the cervix feels softer or harder than normal and whether the surface and shape feel regular or irregular. Areas of irregularity and abnormal tension should be carefully noted in terms of site. For example, abnormalities can be described as being in position 12 o'clock, 6 o'clock, 9 o'clock.

An attempt is made to insert a finger into the cervical os to detect masses, but excessive force should not be used. In nulliparous women the cervix is usually closed. In multiparous women the cervix may admit one or two fingers. Movability of the cervix in all directions is checked, and any restrictions of movement are noted. The vaginal vault is palpated for areas of tenderness and presence of masses. Feces in the rectum may be palpated, and this can later be verified by rectal examination.

Bimanual palpation (Fig. 60-8) follows palpation of the cervix. The gloved fingers are placed behind the cervix, and the ungloved hand is placed palm down on the abdomen with the fingertips just below the umbilicus. The wrist is bent, and the fingers are pressed into the abdominal wall. The hand is then pulled toward the examiner so that the uterus is forced against the fingers inside the vagina. Usually the fundus can be felt anterior to the cervix between the two hands. If not, the uterus may lie posteriorly and be palpated through the posterior vaginal vault. The size, shape, and regularity of the uterine surface is palpated. Normally the uterus feels firm and the fundus is round. Localized areas of enlargement are noted and the approximate size and shape of masses are determined. Because the uterus is normally movable and easy to displace, loss of movability is readily detected. This, too, is noted and recorded.

The areas around the fallopian tubes and ovaries require deep palpation. Normally the fallopian tubes are not palpable, and therefore any enlargement is significant. An enlarged fallopian tube resembles an enlarged ovary to a great extent, and it may not be possible to distinguish between the two.

On bimanual examination the ovaries are normally slightly tender to palpation and are not always palpable, especially in obese women. When palpable, the ovaries feel smooth and oval in shape if no pathologic condition exists. Any readily palpable mass in the areas of the fallopian tubes and ovaries that feels irregular, round, or very firm indicates a possible deviation from normal. Because the ovaries atrophy during the menopause, any mass felt in the areas of the ovaries in postmenopausal women is usually a sign of a problem.

Rectal examination is usually done when masses are palpated in the rectum (p. 1223). If it is necessary for any reason to repeat any part of the examination requiring insertion of fingers into the vagina, the glove is changed following rectal examination.

Following the pelvic examination a woman may need assistance with removing lubricating jelly or discharge that may be on her genitalia, removing her legs from the stirrups, and getting down from the table. Some women may also require assistance with dressing. Elderly women merit careful assistance following the pelvic examination, since unnatural positions such as the knee-chest and lithotomy positions may alter the normal circulation of blood sufficiently to cause faintness.

Equipment is rinsed with cold water, washed well with soap and water, rinsed, and sterilized. The linen or other protective covering on the table is changed. Disposable protective sheets are now available to facilitate easy preparation of the examining table for the next patient and also to prevent cross contamination of linen.

While some nurses perform pelvic examinations as part of their practices, in some instances the nurse's involvement includes acting as a chaperone during the examination when it is performed by a man, encouraging the woman to relax and providing assistance as necessary. The nurse assisting with a pelvic examination has an ideal opportunity to create an educational atmosphere, encouraging the woman to learn more about her body and to explore concerns about her body, its functions, and her sexuality. Following the examination, nurses can reinforce findings, discuss treatment plans, or provide necessary health education.

EXAMINATION OF INFANTS AND GIRLS. At birth, female infants should be examined for evidence of any abnormalities detectable by inspection of the external genitalia. The clitoris, urinary meatus, and labia minora normally protrude beyond the labia majora. A mucus discharge, sometimes lightly tinged with blood (pseudomenstruation), is normal and indicates withdrawal of hormones present in the intrauterine milieu. Hospital and community health nurses should be certain that mothers know what is normal. Girls born to mothers who have taken diethylstilbestrol (DES) during pregnancy should be observed with particular care, since large doses of this hormone have been associated with vaginal and cervical cancer in the offspring. (A national registry for vaginal adenocarcinoma was established in 1973.) Without alarming the mother, the nurse can advise her to bring any abnormality observed in the child to the physician's attention, particularly abnormal perimenarchial bleeding.

Unless there are definite indications making examination necessary, detailed examination of the internal reproductive organs is usually delayed until after puberty. When examination is necessary, it may be done with the child under anesthesia. A urethroscope may be used to visualize the cervix when a speculum cannot be used.

EXAMINATION OF MALES. As with women, men should have an examination of the genital system during physical examination. Examination of the male genitourinary system includes inspection and palpation of the lower abdomen, inspection and palpation of the external genitalia, and palpation of the prostate gland by rectal examination.

Most often male patients are requested not to void until they are seen by the physician. This allows the physician to evaluate ability to start and maintain a stream and to assess characteristics of the urinary stream by observing the patient during voiding.

The abdomen is palpated above the symphysis pubis to determine whether the bladder is distended. If so, as evidenced by a soft, palpable mass, the patient is questioned regarding the time of last voiding. If the man has recently voided or if he is unable to void, the physician orders catheterization.

The inguinal area is inspected for areas of bulging due to hernias. The man is requested to raise his head or to cough in order to make presence of herniation more evident. The inguinal lymph nodes are palpated for enlargement, pain, or tenderness. The amount and distribution of pubic hair is noted.

The penis is inspected for abnormalities of the prepuce, glans, and urethral meatus and for visible evidence of infection and masses. The prepuce is retracted to determine the presence and degree of phimosis, an elongation of the foreskin such that it constricts the urethral orifice and cannot be retracted. It is important to note whether the urethra is centrally located or whether it opens on the upper or lower surface of the glans. The urinary meatus is inspected for lesions, periurethral abscess, and purulent or bloody discharge. The skin along the shaft of the penis is checked for lesions of any type and for general color.

The scrotum is observed for color of the skin, tension of the skin surfaces, size, symmetry, and the presence of lesions on the skin surfaces. Unilateral or bilateral enlargement usually indicates presence of a mass or edema. Palpation of the scrotum is necessary to distinguish between enlargement due to a mass and swelling due to collection of fluid. The size, location, and consistency of any mass is carefully noted.

The prostate gland is palpated by means of a rectal

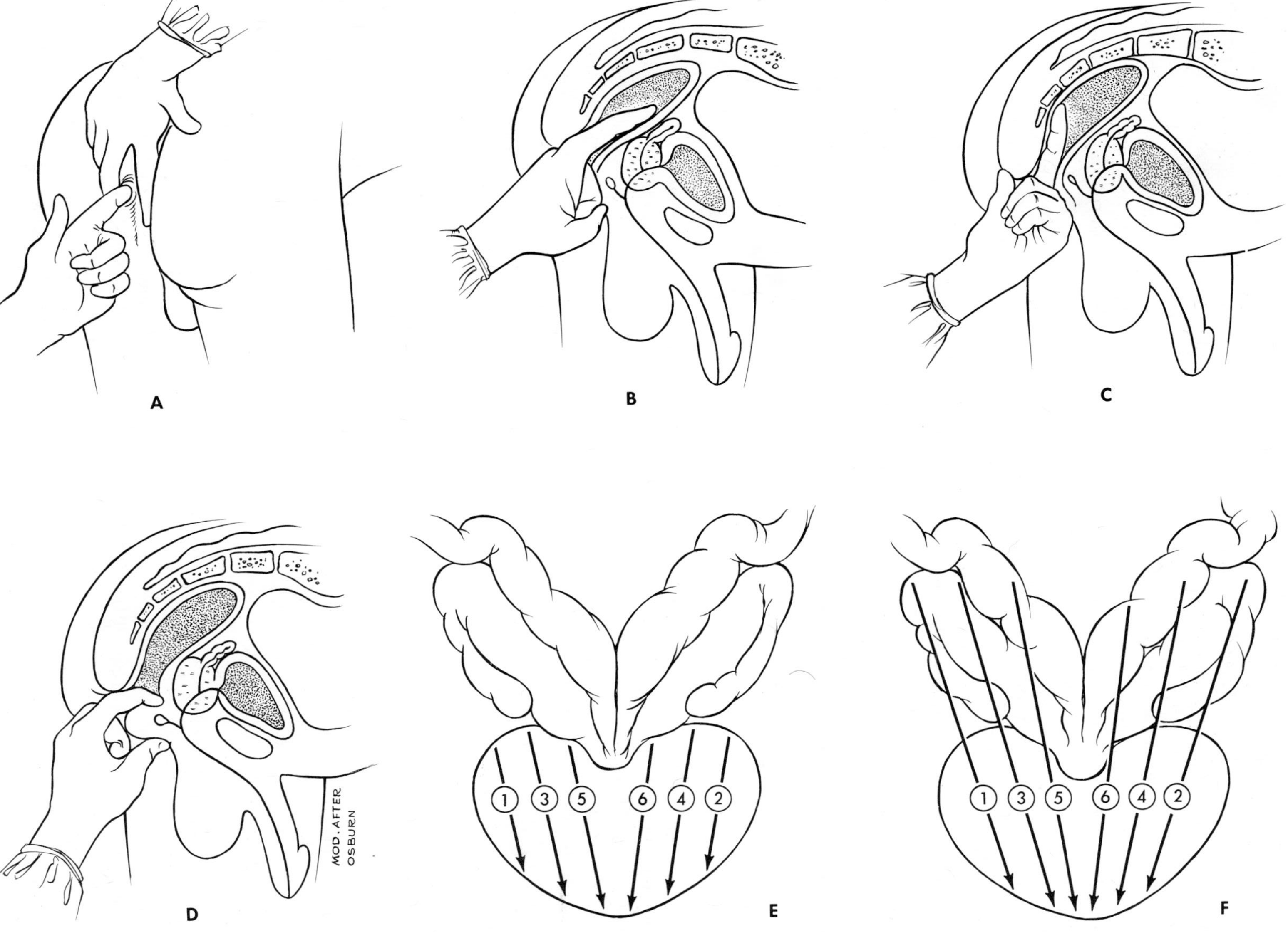

Fig. 60-10. Rectal examination. **A,** Introduction of protected, well-lubricated finger. **B,** Palpation of prostate gland and seminal vesicles, lateral view. **C,** Palpation of anterior surface of sacrum and coccyx. **D,** Palpation of Cowper's glands. **E,** Massage of prostate gland for specimen collection or treatment; order of strokes is indicated by gradually working toward center (verumontanum). **F,** Massage of seminal vesicles and prostate gland. (From Campbell, M. F., and Harrison, J. H.: Urology, vol. 1, ed. 3, Philadelphia, 1970, W. B. Saunders Co.)

examination (Fig. 60-10). Rectal examination on a regular basis is the most important step in the diagnosis of prostatic disease, especially carcinoma. Cancer of the prostate gland may start as a localized, hard nodule, palpable by rectal examination, before proceeding to an advanced, inoperable or incurable stage. For this reason it is recommended that all men, especially those over the age of 50 years, have a rectal examination at least once a year.[43]

All newborn male infants should be examined shortly after birth for visible evidence of problems related to the urogenital system. The prepuce of most infants extends beyond the glans, and the excess is frequently removed by circumcision. Mothers are instructed in care of the circumcised area to prevent infection. The infant is closely observed for voiding. If the urethral opening is on the upper or lower surface of the glans and if the prepuce is long, the infant may be unable to void and will develop a distended bladder. The scrotum is palpated to determine whether the testes have descended. If the scrotal sac appears collapsed or feels empty, the infant may have become chilled. He should be warmed and the scrotum reassessed at a later time.

Other data in assessment of sexual problems

Laboratory data useful in the determination of cause of sexual dysfunction include blood work, such as complete blood counts, thyroid function tests, glucose tolerance tests, and chemistry determinations. Vaginal cytology, endocrine workups, electrocardiograms, and chest films may reveal underlying abnormalities responsible for sexual problems. A number of conditions that affect sexuality directly or indirectly are discussed in Chapter 63.

Diagnostic studies. In addition to routine urinalysis and blood count, some specific studies requiring samples of blood or urine may be done.

Tests for syphilis. Serologic testing is used for detecting syphilis. The tests in common use require a sample of venous blood. Two types of tests, treponemal and nontreponemal, are presently available. The tests differ in the type of antibody measured and in the antigen used to detect antibodies.

The nontreponemal tests, commonly called serologic tests for syphilis (STS), measure an antibodylike substance called reagin. The Venereal Disease Research Laboratory (VDRL) test is the most frequently used serologic test for syphilis and is the test used most often for routine premarital and prenatal screening.

Syphilitic reagin is thought to form from tissue breakdown products resulting from the interaction of the organism and body tissues. STS are usually reported as nonreactive, weakly reactive, or reactive. If any degree of reactivity is found, a quantitative test is done by diluting the serum progressively until an end point of reactivity is reached. Quantitiative reactions are reported in ratios and reflect the *highest dilution* at which the serum reacts. For example, a reaction reported as 1:16 means that the person's serum was diluted 16 times and still produced reaction but that no reaction occurred when the serum was diluted more than 16 times.

A reactive STS is usually confirmed by alternate serologic tests. For this purpose the Fluorescent Treponemal Antibody-Absorption Test (FTA-ABS) is most often used, since it is the most sensitive and specific test for syphilis available.

Because antibodies are not present in the serum of the infected person until the organism gains entry into the circulation, serologic tests for syphilis may be negative and the individual may still be infected. Once antibodies are present, they do not completely disappear from the serum. Even though treated and noninfected, the person may have a positive serology test for an indefinite period of time. If successful therapy is given before antibodies develop, these tests may never be positive unless the person again becomes infected and develops antibodies. Therefore serologic tests in use today do not always indicate an active syphilitic infection and only detect the presence of antibodies. There is presently an urgent need for specific, rapid method of detecting infection due to syphilis, and these are being studied. Until new tests are developed, the the patient's history, clinical symptoms if any, and serologic testing are the means most often used to make a diagnosis of syphilis.

Pregnancy tests. Testing for pregnancy is very commonly employed so that management can be started as soon as possible. This is true whether a woman intends to deliver her baby or elects to have an abortion or whether the physician suspects an ectopic pregnancy. Most of the commonly used pregnancy tests are based on two facts. First, human chorionic gonadotropin (HCG) is present in the serum of pregnant women within 10 to 14 days after the first missed menstrual period. Second, HCG produces antisera. Currently available methods of pregnancy testing fall into four groups: biologic, immunologic, radioimmunoassay, and radioreceptorassay tests.

Biologic tests for pregnancy have been in use since the mid-1920s. Among the better known biologic tests are the *Ascheim-Zondek* test, the *Friedman* test, and the *Hogben* test. These tests require that an early morning voided urine specimen from the woman be injected into a laboratory animal. If human chorionic gonadotropin is present in the urine, the test is positive as indicated by rapid maturational changes in the ovaries of the laboratory animal. Biologic tests for pregnancy are 95% accurate after 2 weeks following the first missed menstrual period. They require 48 hours to obtain a result. The degree of accuracy is considered to be an advantage of biologic tests. The length of time required for a report is considered a disadvantage.

Since the early 1960s a number of commercial immunologic tests for pregnancy have become available (Ortho, Hyland, Roche). Depending on the specific test, blood or urine specimens are required from the woman. Results are obtained within 2 minutes to 2 hours depending on the test used. The short period for obtaining results is an advantage of immunologic tests. However, these tests are not as sensitive in detecting pregnancy as are other tests. When used in women in whom menstruation is delayed for up to 2 weeks, they show positive results 53.3% of the time.[30] Immunologic pregnancy tests are valuable in screening women who are possibly pregnant. It is generally believed that women with negative immunologic tests should have further examination for pregnancy.

In 1972 the radioimmunoassay test for pregnancy became available. This test requires a sample of blood from the woman and detects human chorionic gonadotropin as early as 7 to 9 days following ovulation. However, the test requires 72 hours for reliable results, a greater period of time than is needed for any other test. For this reason the radioimmunoassay test has not gained popularity.

The radioreceptorassay test for pregnancy was developed in 1974 and is reported to be a rapid and reliable test for pregnancy.[48] The test can be performed in 1 hour and is 99% accurate by 6 to 8 days following ovulation.[39] A sample of blood from the finger is used in performing the test. This test is relatively new and has not as yet enjoyed wide use.

Recently, "do-it-yourself" pregnancy tests have been made available to women through department and drug stores. One such test has been evaluated and found to be 50% reliable.[5] Although a self-performed early pregnancy test is of utility in detecting one's pregnancy shortly after a missed period, tests of this type need to be improved to provide a greater degree of accuracy and reliability.

Two conditions, *hydatidiform mole* and *choriocarcinoma,* produce false-positive pregnancy tests. In both of these conditions trophoblastic tissue secretes chorionic gonadotropin in abundance.

Vaginal and cervical smears and cultures. Smears and cultures taken from the vagina and cervix are commonly used in gynecology for screening and diagnosis. Perhaps the best known of the smears is the Papanicolaou test (Pap smear).

The Pap smear is performed by microscopic examination of cells collected from the cervix. Samples of cells can be obtained by using a vaginal pipette with a rubber tip, an applicator, or a specially designed wooden spatula. Secretions containing exfoliated cells are preferably obtained from the cervix or external os. Glass slides should be labeled and ready for use. A solution of 95% alcohol and ether in a wide-mouthed jar is used because rapid fixation of the smear is essential. The secretions are collected, smeared on the glass slide, and immediately placed in the fixative solution. Very little material is needed, but there should be enough to make a distinct blur on the slide. Some experts believe that two samples should be taken to increase the chances of detecting abnormal cells.[50]

It should be noted that the Pap test makes it possible to detect abnormal cells, not all of which are cancerous. However, the Pap smear has made it possible through routine use to detect precancerous conditions and cancer of the cervix early enough to make treatment of these conditions almost 100% successful.[51] For detection of atypical cells, the Pap smear is 95% accurate.

When the Pap smear is positive, additional tissue studies are indicated. The woman should understand that the Pap smear is not necessarily conclusive and that biopsy or even surgery may be necessary to verify the diagnosis of premalignancy or malignancy.

Many women are familiar with the Pap test because of the vast amount of publicity it has received. Securing the specimen does not cause pain. Since the procedure can be used to obtain cell samples for study in cases of infertility or when women are taking estrogen preparations, the woman may be required to learn how to take the smear herself. It is imperative that the woman be taught how to insert the aspirator or spatula deeply enought to reach the cervix, how to prepare the slide, and how to place the slide in the fixative (Fig. 60-11).

Pap tests of a do-it-yourself variety are available. These can be used by women who are reluctant or unable to visit a physician for examination. The same instruction is required for an adequate specimen to be obtained. The Pap test alone is not a substitute for the more complete history and examination necessary for preventive care, and women should be encouraged to have a yearly pelvic examination.

To ensure that an adequate and reliable specimen is taken, certain precautions must be observed. These precautions apply to all Pap smears, whether they are taken by a physician, a nurse, or the patient. The smear should not be taken if the woman is menstruating. A tub bath or douche of any type should not be taken for at least 48 hours before the Pap test. Cauterization of the cervix produces distortion of the cells of the cervix, and this may persist for 6 weeks. Radiation produces distortion of cells for a much longer period. The Pap smear should be delayed for at least 1 month after use of topical antibiotics because they produce rapid, heavy shedding of cells.

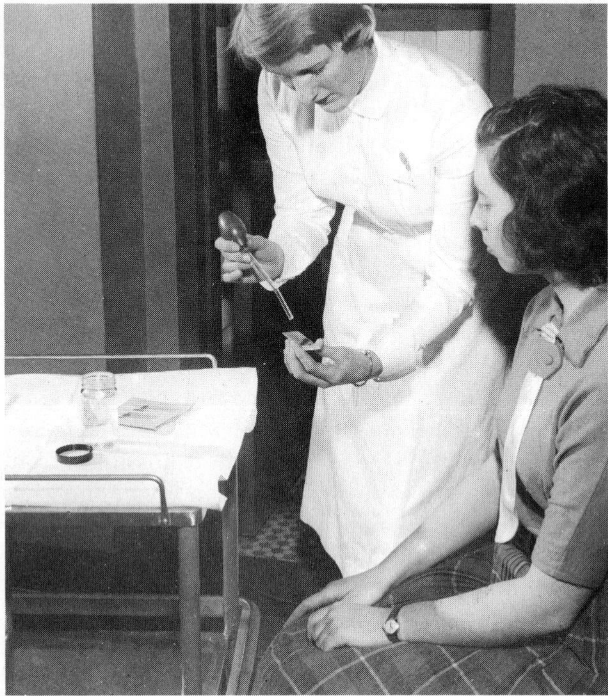

Fig. 60-11. Nurse shows patient how to fix slide after taking vaginal smear, a necessary procedure if patient must take daily smears at home.

Systemic antibiotics do not produce this effect. If two specimens are taken, one from the cervix and one from the vagina, each must be carefully labeled for site and placed in the solution so that the unsmeared sides are back to back. This prevents mixing of vaginal and cervical secretions and assists the pathologist or cytologist in determining the source of abnormal cells if they are found.

Many women experience some vaginal bleeding in the form of spotting after a Pap smear has been taken. They should be advised that this is expected and normal, but that any bleeding in excess of spotting is abnormal and should be reported to the health care provider.

Smears or cultures are also taken from various sites when symptoms of infection are present. Most infectious diseases of the reproductive tract produce a purulent discharge. In men the most common site of purulent discharge is the urinary meatus. The cervix, urethra, Skene's glands, and Bartholin's glands are the most common sites of infection in women. Smears or cultures of the discharge are usually successful in identification of the organism responsible for the infection. The venereally transmitted diseases require a number of different diagnostic studies, and these are discussed in Chapter 62.

Schiller's test. This simple test helps the physician to decide whether other diagnostic procedures should be performed when cervical disease is suspected. For example, Schiller's test assists with identifying the area from which a cervical biopsy should be taken.

Schiller's test reveals the presence of atypical cervical cells. A solution of 3.5% iodine or Lugol's solution is applied to the cervix. Atypical cells, both malignant and benign, do not contain glycogen and will fail to stain. Early cancerous lesions and also benign lesions such as cervicitis may appear as glistening areas of a lighter color than surrounding tissue. The tissue having lighter color indicates, for example, the site from which a biopsy should be taken.

Cervical biopsy. In the event that the physician wishes to send a piece of cervical tissue to the laboratory for pathologic examination, a cervical biopsy is taken. This procedure usually can be performed safely on an outpatient basis. The biopsy procedure should be scheduled for a week after the end of a menstrual period, since the cervix is more vascular before and after menstruation. The woman should know what is to be done and why. She should be told that there may be momentary discomfort, but that an anesthetic will not be required.

In addition to the equipment needed for a pelvic examination, the following items should be available:

1. Biopsy forceps
2. Uterine tenaculum forceps
3. Specimen bottle containing 10% formalin or, if specimen can be delivered to pathology laboratory immediately following procedure, wet saline sponge and waxed paper (specimens should be labeled with woman's name, date, source of specimen, and physician's name)
4. Cautery unit and cautery tips
5. Silver nitrate sticks
6. Gauze packing, tampon, oxidized cellulose (Oxycel)

A cervical biopsy can be secured by using a scalpel, but most often a special punch-biopsy forceps is used. A speculum is used to expose the cervix, and a small piece of the cervix is excised. Bleeding is minimal following a punch biopsy but is usually checked by use of electric cautery, silver nitrate, or vaginal packing.

Following the procedure the nurse ascertains that the woman understands the physician's instructions. Sometimes the main points are written out. Instructions will vary, but they usually include the following:

1. Rest more than usual for the next 24 hours. Avoid lifting and marked exertion.
2. Leave the tampon or packing in place as long as the physician advises (usually 8 to 24 hours).
3. Report to the hospital or physician's office if

bleeding is excessive. Usually more than occurs during normal menses is considered excessive.

4. Do not use an internal douche or have sexual relations until the next visit to the physician unless specific instructions have been given as to when intercourse can be safely resumed.

Conization of cervix. If more than one area of the cervix requires tissue examination or if the suspected cervical lesion is widespread, conization of the cervix is performed. This method of obtaining tissue from the cervix is also preferred when cancer of the cervix is suspected. Conization of the cervix is sometimes performed as a therapeutic measures in cases of chronic cervical infections in which the inflammatory process has involved the deep tissues of the cervix.

Women are often hospitalized for a conization procedure. A local or general anesthetic is administered. A cone-shaped portion of the cervix containing the suspected malignant or infected tissue is removed. Bleeding from the site of conization is greater than that occurring from punch biopsy. If the bleeding is excessive or if hemorrhage seems liekly, the cervix is sutured on each side to control blood loss. Oozing is controlled by cauterization, application of a hemostatic substance, or packing. The nursing care is the same as that required after a dilation and curettage.

Semen analysis. Analysis of the semen is indicated in evaluation of male and female infertility, following male sterilization by vasectomy, and in cases of rape.

Multiple semen examinations are done to determine the presence, number, maturity, shape, and motility of sperm. The man may be instructed to secure a specimen of semen at home by masturbation, but because of rapid deterioration of sperm, most physicians prefer a fresh sample collected in the physician's office or in the laboratory. If collected at home the specimen of semen should be taken to the office or laboratory within 2 to 3 hours.

The semen is usually collected following a 3-day period of continence. The specimen is ejaculated into a clean, wide-mouthed jar supplied by the laboratory or physician. The dates of the last emission and of the current specimen should be recorded.

A gross examination of the semen for its physical properties is first carried out. Semen is normally a highly viscous, opaque, grayish-white fluid that spontaneously liquefies within 10 to 20 minutes after ejaculation. After this time the semen appears translucent, turbid, and viscous. Semen is normally slightly alkaline, with a pH of about 7.7. The normal volume in an ejaculation of semen averages 3.5 ml.

After the semen liquefies, a sperm count is taken. The normal mean sperm count is 100 million sperm per milliliter of semen, with a normal range of 60 million to 150 million/ml. The sperm are also examined for motility and presence and number of abnormal forms. It is generally accepted that normal semen contains more than 70% motile sperm and fewer than 30% abnormal forms. A sperm count of less than 20 million/ml of semen, sperm motility under 40%, and over 25% abnormal sperm forms are known to lower the chance of fertilization of an ovum. Also, men who are infertile may have an increased, rather than a decreased, volume of semen, and the increased volume of semen is often associated with a significantly decreased sperm count.

The *postcoital test* involves examination of the cervical mucus of women following intercourse to measure both the ability of sperm to penetrate the mucus and remain active and the quality of the cervical mucus. This test is valuable in evaluation of infertility. Similar tests are done in cases of rape, where secretions from the vagina and cervix are examined for the presence of sperm.

For the postcoital test, mucus is aspirated from the cervical canal and examined for the presence and number of sperm. Characteristics of the cervical mucus (spinnbarkeit) are also studied. At the time of ovulation under normal circumstances, the amount of cervical mucus is maximum, but the viscosity is decreased. This facilitates penetration of the cervical mucus by the sperm. If the cervical mucus lacks the characteristics normally associated with ovulation and large numbers of sperm are found in the cervix, it indicates that the sperm are unable to enter the cervix in the number required for an ovum to be fertilized.

The woman who is to have a postcoital test is advised to see the physician within 1 hour after intercourse. She is instructed not to void, douche, or bathe between intercourse and the examination and to use a perineal pad while traveling to the physician's office. The woman should be informed of how the specimen is to be collected for examination. After the examination the woman should be instructed in additional studies to be done or measures to be taken at home.

Following vasectomy (p. 1398) it is essential to examine the semen for gradual reduction in sperm count and eventual disappearance of sperm to validate effectiveness of the surgery.

Prostatic smears and biopsies. When the prostate gland is enlarged or when a suspect prostatic lesion is palpated by rectal examination, a biopsy of the prostate gland or smear of the prostatic secretions may be done.

For a *prostatic smear* the physician first massages the prostate gland (Fig. 60-10). The next voided urine specimen is collected, and a smear is prepared in the laboratory. It is possible to detect some cases of cancer and tuberculosis of the prostate gland by this method.

Most often biopsies of the prostate gland are used for

diagnosis. Various methods are used to obtain tissue specimens from the prostate gland.

For a *perineal needle biopsy* the patient is placed in the lithotomy position (Fig. 60-7, *B*) and a finger is inserted into the rectum to identify the area from which the biopsy is to be taken. The biopsy needle is inserted through the perineum into the prostate gland, and a core of tissue is removed. This technique is considered a minor procedure and can be done on an outpatient basis. The specimen of tissue obtained by perineal needle biopsy is very small and is about 95% accurate for obtaining cells adequate for study.[16]

A *transrectal needle biopsy* is performed in a manner similar to a perineal needle biopsy. The major difference is that the biopsy needle is inserted through the rectal wall into the prostate gland. Because the needle can be inserted more directly into the prostate gland, this method is slightly more accurate in obtaining tissue specimens than is the perineal needle biopsy method.

When a *transurethral biopsy* is done, the biopsy needle is inserted through the urethra toward the prostate gland. This method is used least and is usually confined to cases where the prostatic lesion is producing bladder obstruction. Of all the methods, transurethral biopsy is the least adequate for obtaining specimens.

To obtain a specimen of tissue by *open perineal biopsy*, a small incision is made in the perineum between the anus and the scrotum. This technique gives the greatest accuracy, since the suspect lesion can be clearly identified and multiple specimens can be taken from the prostate gland.

The needle techniques may or may not be done as inpatient procedures. A local or general anethetic is most often given. Dressings are not required when needle biopsies are taken. Patients should be cautioned to watch for bright red bleeding and to report the occurrence to the physician.

A dressing is required following open perineal biopsy and can be held in place for about 24 hours with a two-tailed binder. The patient is instructed not to contaminate the incision while cleansing himself following defecation by wiping from front to back. Cleansing by perineal irrigation is sometimes advised for both cleanliness and comfort. Unless the physician prescribes a solution, warm water poured from front to back over the incision can be used. A heat lamp with a 60-W bulb placed 30 cm from the perineum is often used two or three times a day to encourage healing and for comfort. The man must be in a position in which the scrotum is elevated so that the heat strikes the incision. One method is to allow the scrotum to rest on a wide piece of adhesive tape extending from thigh to thigh. Alternately, an exaggerated Sims position (Fig. 60-7, *A*) gives satisfactory wound exposure. After sutures are removed, sitz baths may be used instead of the heat lamp, and they add a great deal to the general comfort of the patient. The man usually remains hospitalized after an open perineal biopsy until the laboratory findings are reported. If he is not hospitalized, he requires instruction in self-care, including signs to report, prevention of infection of the incision, use of heat lamp, and sitz baths.

Testicular smears and biopsies. Biopsies or smears from the testes can be obtained by the needle method or by an incision made through the scrotum. Most often an incision is used. After a local or general anesthetic has been administered, a small incision about 2.5 cm long is made, and a small piece of the testis is removed. A dressing is applied, and postoperative management is similar to that after open perineal prostatic biopsy. Testicular biopsies are sometimes used in evaluation of fertility. If sperm are present in the biopsied tissue but are absent from the semen, absence of the sperm is most often due to stricture of tubal systems beyond the testes.

Enzyme values. Enzyme values play a role in diagnosis of cancer of the prostate gland. The enzyme tests of most value are phosphatase levels. The phosphatases are secreted in the serum of the tumor mass in the prostate gland and are reflected in changes in the blood chemistry. The phosphatases are labeled as acid or alkaline, depending on the optimal pH. Acid phosphatase usually has a pH of 4.0 to 6.0, while alkaline phosphatase usually ranges between pH 8.5 to 9.5.[43] A rise in phosphatase value is indicative of cancer of the prostate gland but is not conclusively diagnostic. Usually the phosphatase values are repeated for reliability, since such events as rectal examination or recent episodes of fever may cause either an elevation or drop in phosphatase level. Additional studies such as prostatic biopsy are done to confirm the diagnosis.

Screening for endometrial cancer. With the decline of mortality due to cervical cancer, greater attention has been directed toward developing mass screening techniques to detect early cancer of the endometrium (uterus). An ideal method for mass screening has not yet been developed, but continued refinement of available methods and development of new methods will probably make it possible for screening for uterine cancer to become part of every woman's health care program. Since women over the age of 50 years are more likely to develop cancer of the uterus, screening of postmenopausal women assumes greater significance.

A variety of methods for screening and diagnosis of uterine cancer are now in use. It is generally agreed that the Pap smear is inadequate for detecting uterine cancer. Reports of accuracy of the Pap smear range from 45% to 75%.[45] Variation in the reported rates of accuracy is probably due to a combination of factors, including the site from which samples are taken, clinical grade of the

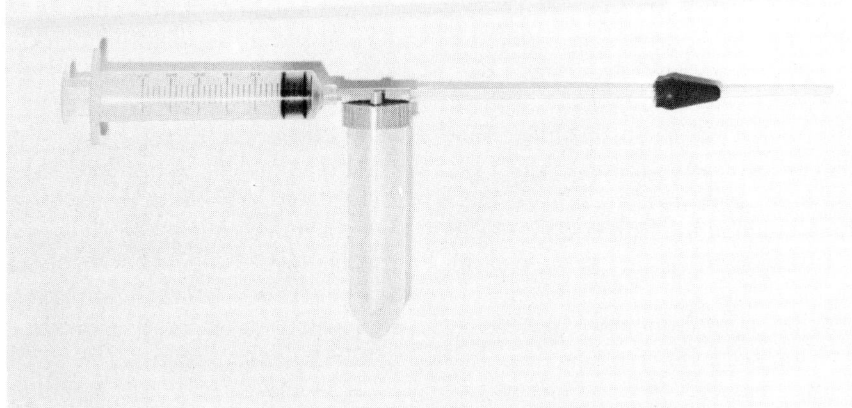

Fig. 60-12. Gravlee Jet Washer used to obtain endometrial cells for microscopic study by irrigation of uterine cavity. (Courtesy The Upjohn Co., Kalamazoo, Mich.)

uterine malignancy, and care exercised in obtaining specimens. Studies indicate that less than one half of women with uterine cancer have an abnormal Pap smear at the time of routine screening.[27,44] Probably the main reason the Pap smear is inadequate is that cells rarely exfoliate from the endometrium in the early stages of uterine cancer.

Endometrial cells obtained by *aspiration smear* show malignant changes between 75% and 92% of the time when uterine cancer exists.[9] The aspiration method is popular because of its simplicity. In this method a small cannula is inserted through the cervix into the uterine cavity and suction is applied by means of a syringe attached to the cannula. The specimen obtained is prepared as for a Pap smear.

The *endometrial biopsy* is similar to a cervical biopsy in that small samples of tissue are obtained with a biopsy forceps. The specimens are taken from several sites of the uterine cavity to increase the chances of obtaining malignant cells. For diagnosis of endometrial cancer, the biopsy method is reported to be 90.6% accurate.[11]

Obtaining endometrial cells by *jet washings* of the uterine cavity is one of the newer methods for screening and diagnosing cancer of the uterus. The device used in this method is shown in Fig. 60-12. The irrigating device is inserted into the uterus, and the uterine cavity is irrigated with about 30 ml of normal saline solution. The normal saline solution containing cells from the uterine cavity is returned by suction into a collecting chamber. The cells are then centrifuged out, stained, and examined microscopically. Studies indicate that washing of the uterine cavity results in obtaining malignant cells in 91.5% of the cases.[11]

Vacuum curettage of the endometrium is still another method used in screening and diagnosis. The procedure and apparatus used are similar to those used in suction curettage for performing an abortion. The cervix is dilated, and the suction tip is inserted through the cervix into the uterus. Suction is applied, and the entire uterine cavity is suctioned to secure specimens. The literature reports small numbers of patients studied using this method, and further study is needed before conclusions can be reached regarding its accuracy as a diagnostic method for cancer.

Dilation and curettage. The most prevalent and preferred method of obtaining endometrial cells for study is dilation and curettage (D and C). Since the entire uterine cavity is "scraped," a large tissue sample is obtained. This makes the likelihood of missing malignant cells minimal. In addition to suspected malignancy, endometrial tissue may be studied for influence of ovarian hormones on the endometrial cells. D and C is sometimes used for the treatment of excessive or prolonged uterine bleeding. This procedure is often carried out to induce abortion and is frequently used following a spontaneous abortion to reduce the chances of hemorrhage. Occasionally dilation alone is done to treat dysmenorrhea or to correct a stricture or stenosis of the cervical canal. Most of the precedures used for screening and diagnosis of endometrial cancer require some dilation of the cervix in order to introduce instruments into the uterus.

For a D and C, metal dilators of graduated sizes are inserted into the cervical canal. Once the cervix is dilated, curettes having a sharp surface are used to remove endometrial tissue. The major complications of a D and C are hemorrhage and perforation of the uterus. Perforation is a greater risk during pregnancy because the uterus is much softer than in the nonpregnant state. Preoperative care includes informing the woman what will be done and why and preparing her for anesthesia. She may or may not have a perineal shave done in preparation for the procedure. Many physicians now believe that shaving is not necessary and that the discomfort due to regrowth of pubic hair can be avoided.

Following a D and C the woman is observed for excessive bleeding. A perineal pad is placed over the perineum. To ensure that all blood loss will be absorbed by the pad and to add to the woman's comfort, the pad is anchored with a sanitary belt. The amount of bleeding is checked at least every 15 minutes for 2 hours. Thereafter blood loss is assessed as indicated by the woman's condition, and such observations may need to be made every hour for about 8 hours if active bleeding continues. The blood loss should always be recorded in estimated milliliters. A blood loss of at least 60 ml is required to saturate a perineal pad. It is important to record each pad change as well as blood loss. Any excessive bleeding should be reported to the physician.

The woman having a D and C may experience mild cramping postoperatively. Mild analgesics such as codeine sulfate and acetylsalicylic acid are usually ordered to relieve pain. Abdominal pain that is continuous, sharp, and is not relieved by analgesics should be reported at once, since this type of pain may indicate perforation of the uterus.

After a D and C, women are observed for voiding, usually no problems are experienced. Most women are permitted to ambulate as soon as they recover from anesthesia and vital signs are stable; most are discharged on the day following surgery, and some are discharged on the day of surgery. These women can resume most of their normal daily activities, increasing to normal activity in about a week. The degree of activity permitted is partly dependent on the reason for the D and C. Vigorous exercising is discouraged, and the woman is usually told to abstain from intercourse until her return visit to the physician, at which time she is advised as to when intercourse can safely be resumed. The menstrual cycle usually is not upset by a D and C. All vaginal bleeding should disappear in a week to 10 days. Women should be advised to report recurrence of bright red blood or the development of a vaginal discharge with an unpleasant odor.

Rubin test. The Rubin test (uterotubal insufflation) is done to determine whether the fallopian tubes are patent, and this test may be part of the study done in cases of infertility. The procedure is considered highly safe and is most often done on an outpatient basis.

Various devices and instruments for the test are available. The majority of these require a constant source of carbon dioxide, a flow meter and pressure gauge, and an apparatus to record the degree of tubal peristaltic action and resistance. The woman is prepared as for a pelvic examination, and under sterile technique carbon dioxide is forced into the uterus. The woman usually feels pain under the scapula if the fallopian tubes are open.

With normal tubal patency the pressure of gas flow rises to a height ranging between 60 to 120 mm Hg and then falls to a constant level. If tubal obstruction is present, there is a steady rise of gas pressure to 200 mm Hg. The fallopian tubes are considered to be patent if the flow of carbon dioxide is within normal limits and if gas is demonstrated under the diaphragm, as indicated by shoulder pain or visualization by radiograph.

It is important that the Rubin test be scheduled to avoid ovulation so that fertilization of an ovum is not prevented by the test. The optimal time for performing the test is 3 to 4 days following the last day of a menstrual period. Since the test is usually done on an outpatient basis, instruction of the woman in preparation for the test is important. She is usually advised to take a laxative the night before the test. On the morning of the test, the woman is given an enema or bisacodyl (Dulcolax) suppository. Prior to the test the procedure should be explained, and the woman should be told what she can expect to feel. When the cervix is dilated the woman may experience pain, and if gas passes through the fallopian tubes pain in the shoulder usually occurs.

Visualization of pelvic structures. Several methods of visualizing the pelvic organs and other structures are in use. *Radiographs* of the pelvis are taken during pregnancy to determine the size and shape of the pelvis. Since it is important to determine the relationship between the size of the mother's pelvis and the size of the fetal head, radiograph pelvimetry is not usually done until after the thirty-sixth week of pregnancy.

The pelvic organs can be seen when a contrast medium is used, as in a *hysterogram* or *hysterosalpingogram.* A sterile, opaque, aqueous contrast medium is injected through the cervix into the uterus for a hysterogram. For a hysterosalpingogram, the dye is also injected into the fallopian tubes. Radiographs are then taken to observe the structure of the uterus and fallopian tubes. As with the Rubin test, these studies are preferably done 3 or 4 days after the end of a menstrual period to avoid interfering with ovum transport. Preparation for these studies is similar to preparation for a Rubin test.

In addition the pelvic organs and surrounding tissues can be visualized without the use of radiographs or contrast media. The procedures by which this can be accomplished are culdoscopy, hysteroscopy, and peritoneoscopy (laparoscopy). Depending on the organs and structures inspected, these methods are valuable for determining the cause of abnormal bleeding, in evaluating the stage of malignancies, and for inspecting organs for size, shape, and position.

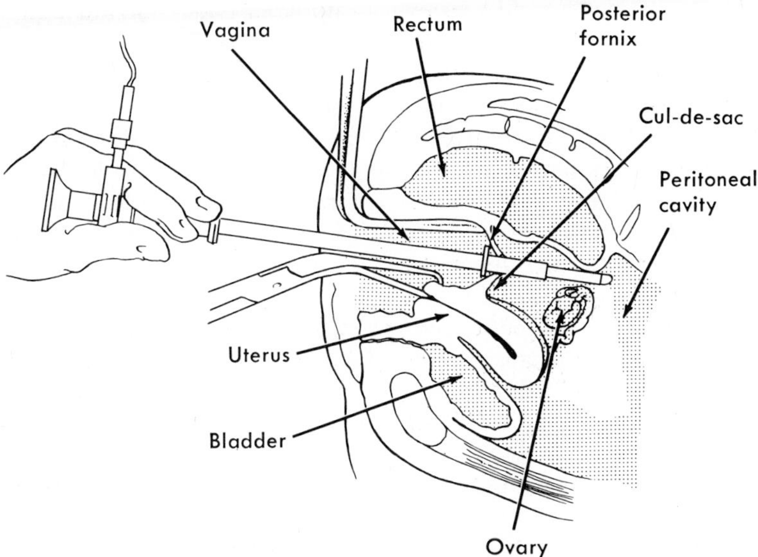

Fig. 60-13. With patient in knee-chest position, culdoscope is inserted through posterior fornix of vagina into cul-de-sac of Douglas. Note that ovaries can be seen.

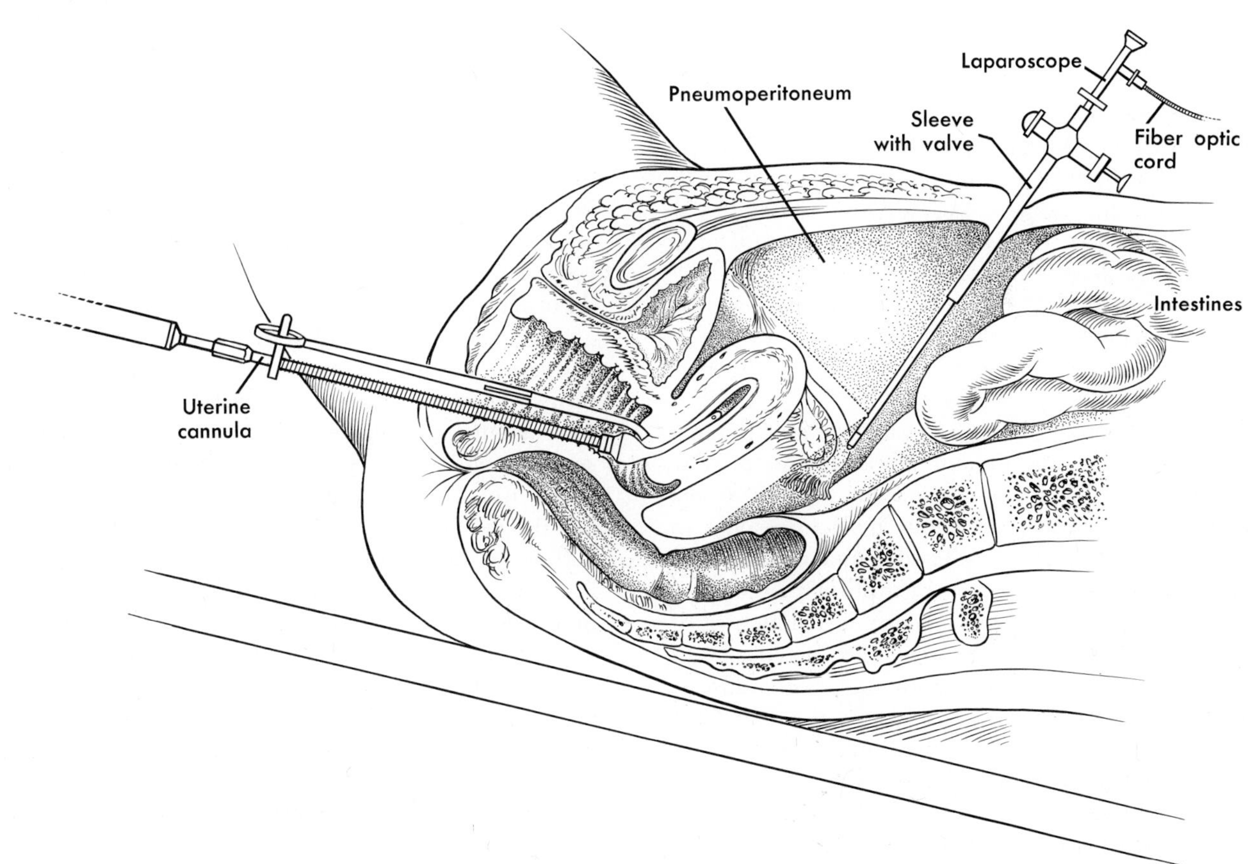

Fig. 60-14. Schema of gynecologic laparoscopy. (From Cohen, M. R.: Laparoscopy, culdoscopy and gynecography: techniques and atlas, vol. 1, Philadelphia, 1970, W. B. Saunders Co.)

Culdoscopy is an examination in which a culdoscopy is inserted through the posterior vaginal vault into the cul-de-sac of Douglas (Fig. 60-13). The fallopian tubes and ovaries can be seen as well as the presence of pus, blood, or other abnormal fluids in the cul-de-sac. If such fluids are observed, the physician may perform a *culdocentesis* by inserting a needle into the site and aspirating a specimen for laboratory study.

Laparoscopy is a procedure by which the pelvic organs are studied by insertion of a laparoscope through the abdominal wall (Fig. 60-14). A local anesthetic is injected prior to insertion of the instrument. Laparoscopy is useful in inspecting the outer surfaces of the uterus, the fallopian tubes, and the ovaries for appearance. For example, a tubal pregnancy can be seen. In addition to inspection of the pelvic structures, the laparoscope is used for sterilization by tubal ligation.

Hysteroscopy is the procedure used to inspect the inside of the uterus. The hysteroscope is inserted through the cervix rather than the abdomen. This procedure is contraindicated whenever a pregnancy is suspected.

Most of the procedures used for visualizing the pelvic organs can be performed as outpatient procedures. Since direct inspection by hysteroscopy and laparoscopy are relatively new procedures in gynecology, many patients are hospitalized for the procedure. Maintaining asepsis throughout any of these procedures is important in preventing infection. During the procedures, air may enter the abdominal cavity and cause discomfort. Placing the woman in a prone position with a pillow under the abdomen may decrease discomfort. Douching and intercourse should be avoided for about 1 week following a culdoscopy. Complications such as hemorrhage and infection are rare following these procedures, but women should be cautioned to report fever or pain in the lower abdomen.

Methods most often used for visualization of the male reproductive organs and related structures include cystoscopy and visualization of the seminal vesicles. *Cystoscopic examination* allows the physician to inspect the condition of the urethral and bladder mucosa and to detect prostatic encroachment on the urethra (p. 1240).

Radiographs are used to diagnose obstruction of the seminal vesicles. Two techniques are in use. One method utilizes a specially designed panendoscope through which catheters are passed into the ejaculatory ducts. The second method requires surgical exposure of the vas through an incision in the scrotum and introduction of small plastic catheters into the vas. For both methods, radiographs are taken to inspect the positions of the catheters.

Endocrine studies. Because the endocrine system is so closely related to reproductive function, almost any study for endocrine function may be ordered, for example, thyroid function tests. In women having menstrual problems and in cases of infertility, ovarian function is often studied.

Endocrine studies include determination of estrogen secretion and estrogen levels in women. Secretion of estrogen in the secretory phase of the menstrual cycle can be estimated by study of the elasticity of the cervical mucus. Quantitative determinations of estriol levels is accomplished by measuring the amount of estriol in a 24-hour collection of urine. The same studies are done during pregnancy to measure indirectly the placental secretion of hormones. All of the urine voided in a 24-hour period is collected in one container and kept cold until it is sent to the laboratory. If the woman is to collect the urine at home, she is provided with a container, told to save all her urine for 24 hours, instructed to keep the urine cold by refrigeration or by surrounding the urine container with ice in a basin, and to bring the urine specimen to the laboratory when the 24 hours elapse.

In addition to infertility, estrogen level determination is valuable in discovering whether amenorrhea is due to pituitary, ovarian, or uterine failure of function. With pituitary or ovarian problems the estrogen level is low; with uterine problems the estrogen level is normal. A combination of urinary estriol levels with endometrial tissue studies helps to pinpoint failure of the uterus to respond to estrogen stimulation.

Determination of male hormone levels is sometimes helpful in treating fertility problems. The levels of 17-ketosteroids, pituitary gonadotropins, and corticosteroids may be determined. A 24-hour sample of urine is required, and the procedure for collection is the same as for urinary estriols.

Frequently men and women show signs of anxiety and depression following diagnostic studies and procedures that necessitate waiting for pathology reports. Fear about the findings and the possible ways in which sexuality and fertility might be affected is common. Many times patients are poorly informed and worry needlessly. Nurses can reduce the distress associated with many of these procedures by providing factual information and avoiding hedging. Collaboration with the physician may facilitate patients being informed quickly, thus avoiding unnecessary waiting and anxiety.

REFERENCES AND SELECTED READINGS

1. Alfonso, J. F.: Value of the Gravlee Jet Washer in the diagnosis of endometrial cancer, Obstet. Gynecol. **46**:141-146, 1975.
2. American Cancer Society, Inc.: 1976 Cancer facts and figures, New York, 1976, The Society.
3. American Cancer Society, Inc.: Close-up standard breast examination, CA **24**:291-293, 1974.
4. Annon, J.: The behavioral treatment of sexual problems, Honolulu, 1974, Enaoling Systems, Inc.

5. Baker, L. D., Yert, L. W., Chase, M. C., et al.: Evaluation of a "do-it-yourself" pregnancy test, Am. J. Public Health **66:** 166-167, 1976.
6. Bloom, M., and VanDongan, L.: Clinical gynecology: integration of structure and function, Philadelphia, 1972, J. B. Lippincott Co.
7. Campbell, M. F., and Harrison, J. H., editors: Urology, ed. 3, vols. 1 and 2, Philadelphia, 1970, W. B. Saunders Co.
8. Cibilia, L. A.: Gynecologic laparoscopy: diagnostic and operatory, Philadelphia, 1976, Lea & Febiger.
9. Cohen, C. J., and Gusberg, S. B.: Screening for endometrial cancer, Clin. Obstet. Gynecol. **18:**27-39, 1975.
10. Cohen, M. R.: Laparoscopy, culdoscopy, and gynecography: techniques and atlas, vol. 1, Philadelphia, 1970, W. B. Saunders Co.
11. Creasman, W. T., and Weed, J. C.: Screening techniques in endometrial cancer, Cancer **38**(Suppl.):436-440, 1976.
12. Curnow, R. N.: The use of additional information in estimating disease risks from family histories, Biometrics **30:**655-665, 1974.
13. Denis, R., Jr., Barnett, J. M., and Forbes, S. E.: Diagnostic suction curettage, Obstet. Gynecol. **42:**301-303, 1973.
14. DePetrillo, A. D., et al.:. Gravlee Jet Washer effectiveness as performed by obstetric-gynecologic paramedical personnel, Am. J. Obstet. Gynecol. **117:**371-374, 1974.
15. Education and treatment in human sexuality: the training of health professionals: Report of a WHO meeting, Geneva, 1975, World Health Organization.
16. Flocks, R. H., and Culp, D. A.: Surgical urology, ed. 4, Chicago, 1975, Year Book Medical Publishers, Inc.
17. Friedl, E.: Women and men: an anthropologist's view, New York, 1975, Holt, Rinehart and Winston, Inc.
18. Galask, R. P., Larsen, B., and Ohm, M. J.: Vaginal flora and its role in disease entities, Clin. Obstet. Gynecol. **19:**61-81, 1976.
19. *Gillies, D. A., and Alyn, I. B.: Patient assessment and management by the nurse practitioner, Philadelphia, 1976, W. B. Saunders Co.
20. Green, R.: Taking a sexual history. In Green, R., editor: Human sexuality: a health practitioner's test, Baltimore, 1975, The Williams and Wilkins Co.
21. Greenhill, J. P.: The nonsurgical management of vaginal relaxation, Clin. Obstet. Gynecol. **15:**1083-1097, 1972.
22. Greenhill, J. P.: Surgical gynecology, ed. 4, Chicago, 1969, Year Book Medical Publishers, Inc.
23. Hammond, C. B., and Lewis, J. L.: Gestational trophoblastic neoplasms. In Davis' gynecology and obstetrics, New York, 1972, Harper & Row, Publishers.
24. Herbert, P., et al.: Colposcopy: what is it? JOGN Nurs. **5:**29-32, 1976.
25. Hobson, L. B.: Examination of the patient, New York, 1975, McGraw-Hill Book Co.
26. Hofmeister, F. J.: Endometrial biopsy: another look, Am. J. Obstet. Gynecol. **118:**773-777, 1974.
27. Jones, W. E., Kanner, H. M., Kanner, H. H., et al.: Adenocarcinoma of the endometrium: twenty-five years' experience in private practice: Am. J. Obstet. Gynecol. **113:**549-557, 1972.
28. *Kaiser, B. L., and Kaiser, I. H.: The challenge of women's movement to American gynecology, Am. J. Obstet. Gynecol. **120:**652-665, 1974.
29. Kaplan, H. S.: The new sex therapy, New York, 1974, Brunner-Mazel, Inc.
30. Landesmann, R., and Saxena, B. B.: Results of the first 1,000 radioreceptor assays for the determination of human chorionic gonadatropin: a new, rapid, reliable and sensitive pregnancy test, Fertil. Steril. **27:**357-368, 1976.
31. Lindemann, H. J., and Mohr, J.: CO_2 hysteroscopy: diagnosis and treatment, Am. J. Obstet. Gynecol. **124:**129-133, 1976.
32. Lindemann, H. J., Siegler, A. M., and Mohr, J.: The hysteroflator 1000S, J. Reprod. Med. **16:**145-146, 1976.
33. LoPiccolo, J., and Steger, J.: The sexual interaction inventory: a new instrument for assessment of sexual dysfunction, Arch. Sex. Behav. 3:585-593, 1974.
34. *Lytle, N.: Nursing of women in the age of liberation, Dubuque, Ia., 1977, William C. Brown Co., Publishers.
35. Mandetta, A., and Gustaveson, P.: Abortion to zoophilia, Chapel Hill, N.C., 1976, Carolina Population Center.
36. Masters, W., and Johnson, V.: Human sexual inadequacy, Boston, 1970, Little, Brown and Co.
37. Masters, W., and Johnson, V.: Human sexual response, Boston, 1966, Little, Brown and Co.
38. McGowan, L.: Cytologic methods for the detection of endometrial carcinoma, Gynecol. Oncol. **2:**272-278, 1974.
39. McNally, L. K., and Galeener, J. T.: Current practice in obstetric and gynecologic nursing, vol. 1, St. Louis, 1976, The C. V. Mosby Co.
40. McPhetridge, L. M.: Nursing history: one means to personalize care, Am. J. Nurs. **68:**68-75, 1968.
41. Money, J., and Ehrahardt, A.: Man, woman, boy, girl, Baltimore, 1972, The Johns Hopkins University Press.
42. Moniff, G. R. J.: Infectious diseases in obstetrics and gynecology, New York, 1974, Harper & Row, Publishers.
43. Murphy, G. P.: The diagnosis of prostatic cancer, Cancer **37** (Suppl.):589-596, 1976.
44. Nahlos, W. A., Lund, C. J., and Rudolph, J. H.: Cancer of the corpus uteri, Obstet. Gynecol. **38:**564-570, 1971.
45. Ng, A. B., and Reagan, J. W.: Incidence and prognosis of endometrial carcinoma by histologic grade and extent, Obstet. Gynecol. **35:**437-443, 1970.
46. Novak, E. R., Jones, G. S., and Jones, H. W., Jr.: Novak's textbook of gynecology, ed. 9, Baltimore, 1975, The Williams & Wilkins Co.
47. Phillips, J. M.: The impact of laparoxcopy, hysteroscopy, fetoscopy and culdoscopy of gynecologic practice, J. Reprod. Med. **16:**187-190, 1976.
48. Radioreceptor assay: a new pregnancy test: Am. J. Nurs. **76:**1281, 1976.
49. Schiller, P.: Creative approach to sex education and counseling, New York, 1974, ssociation Press.
50. Schulman, J. J., Hontz, A., Sedlis, A., et al.: The Pap smear: take two, Am. J. Obstet. Gynecol. **121:**1024-1028, 1975.
51. Silverberg, E., and Holleb, A. I.: Major trends in cancer: 25 year survey, CA **25:**2-7, 1975.
52. Skydel, B., and Crowder, A. S.: Diagnostic procedures: a reference for health practitioners and a guide for patient counseling, Boston, 1975, Little, Brown and Co.
53. Strand, M. M., and Elmer, L. A.: Clinical laboratory tests: a manual for nurses, St. Louis, 1976, The C. V. Mosby Co.
54. Tovell, H. M.: Cone biopsy of the cervix, Clin. Obstet. Gynecol. **19:**2-15, 1976.
55. Villee, D. B.: Human endocrinology: a developmental approach, Philadelphia, 1975, W. B. Saunders Co.
56. Webb, M. J., and Gaffey, T. A.: Outpatient diagnostic aspiration curettage, Obstet. Gynecol. **47:**239-242, 1976.
57. Wilson R.: Introduction to sexual counseling, Chapel Hill, N.C., 1974, Carolina Population Center.

*References preceded by an asterisk are particulary well suited for student reading.

AUDIOVISUAL RESOURCES

1. Controversies in laparoscopy. Audiotape and slides, module no. 5, Audio-Digest Foundation, 1250 South Glendale Ave., Glendale, Calif., 91205.
2. Laparoscopy—what's new. Audiotape and slides, module no. 15, Audio-Digest Foundation, 1250 South Glendale Ave., Glendale, Calif. 91205.
3. Operative laparoscopy in gynecology. Film, Materials Utilization Branch, National Medical Audiovisual Center (Annex), Station K, Atlanta, Ga. 33024.
4. Ovulation. Audiotape and slides, module no. 4, Audio-Digest Foundation, 1250 South Glendale Ave., Glendale, Calif., 91205.
5. Physical assessment of the well adult: abdomen. Audiotape and slides, module V, Wiley Biomedical, John Wiley & Sons, Inc., 605 Third Ave., New York, N.Y. 10016.
6. Physical assessment of the well adult: rectum and genitalia. Audiotape and slides, Module VI, Wiley Biomedical, John Wiley & Sons, Inc., 605 Third Ave., New York, N.Y. 10016.
7. Sex in today's world. Film, The American Journal of Nursing Co., Educational Services Division, 10 Columbus Circle, New York, N.Y. 10019.

61

Management of the person with a reproductive or sexual problem

ELLA CINKOTA
NANCY FUGATE WOODS

Although present day society in general is much more open than in the past regarding discussion of reproductive and sexual matters, many people still find it difficult to ask questions about the reproductive organs and sex. When this occurs, people often act on the basis of incomplete information or misinformation received from uninformed sources. This means that many reproductive or sexual problems may be disregarded or treatment may be delayed.

Nurses are in a strategic position to give information based on sound knowledge and can give cues to people indicating willingness to discuss sexual and reproductive matters with them. By listening to people express their thoughts, ideas, beliefs, and attitudes, nurses can assess the extent of their knowledge, can recognize deviations from normal, and can determine needs for help. By treating the topics of sexuality and reproduction is a serious, objective way, nurses can put people at ease and can encourage a climate in which questioning is encouraged.

In some instances people are more comfortable discussing matters related to reproduction and sexuality with someone of their own sex. The woman's movement in particular has emphasized the need for women to better understand their own bodies and has raised questions about the insensitivity of some male physicians to female problems.[7] For this reason female nurses and physicians may be preferred sources of information and other help for some women's groups. Obtaining factual information at an early age may prevent physical, emotional, reproductive, and sexual problems in later years.

■ PREPARATION FOR PUBERTY

□ Sex education

Sex education begins when a child is born. From that moment on the infant begins to experience the self as a sexual being, responding to and absorbing the attitudes of those in the environment. From the way he is touched and handled, the infant senses the importance of all parts of his body. He touches himself and feels and learns from his own exploration and from the responses of other to his exploration. The infant learns from the way he is bathed. Therefore the genitalia should be bathed as carefully and tenderly as the rest of the body, for bathing is perhaps the most important introduction to sex education that the infant receives.

Sex education involves more than teaching the facts of life, for sexuality is the sum total of the self and the experiences of the self. Thus sex education teaches one how to be a responsible human being. As a child grows, he experiences attitudes and relationships and begins to interact with those around him and with his environment. During these early years the child quite naturally incorporates the attitudes of those who surround him and starts to behave like them. Since parents are usually the most influential persons to the very young child, it is necessary that they have healthy attitudes to accompany the facts that are needed for teaching children how to live.

Parents often ask nurses questions about sex, and frequently they want to know how and what to teach their children. Nurses not only can help parents understand the anatomy and physiology of the reproductive system but also can help them see the importance of their own attitudes and the importance of how they behave toward each other and how they relate to their children. For example, parents need to understand that young children do not want lengthy explanations, but that they do need direct and truthful answers to specific questions.

Although many schools have added sex education to their curricula, the subject has aroused much controversy among parents and educators. It is hoped that careful planning with parents about course content will avoid misunderstandings, and it may help parents to learn facts that they need to know before they can teach children themselves. Thus in addition to teaching parents individually, nurses can work with various community groups. The school nurse and the public health nurse are most likely to have this opportunity, but in small communities any nurse may be asked to help with sex education. Nurses may participate in parent-teacher programs and by using drawings, filmstrips, and films can explain anatomy and the reproductive processes. Church groups as well as organizations such as the Girl Scouts that include courses in sex education and personal hygiene as a part of their programs provide nurses with opportunities to participate in community programs. The school nurse may be asked to help physical education teachers cover course content and sometimes teach or help teach classes in hygiene for children.

Nurses can evaluate articles in daily papers and popular magazines in order to advise parents on the use of this information. Often books for parents can be recommended to help them answer children's questions about sex. Books specifically for children can also be recommended. There are many pamphlets and books on sex education, but only a few can be mentioned here. Most state departments of health supply material. *When Children Ask About Sex** and *Your Child and Sex: A Guide for Parents*† are useful references for parents in answering questions about sex and reproduction commonly asked by children. For people contemplating marriage and for adults, *Reproduction, Sex, and Preparation for Marriage*‡ and *Sex Questions and Answers*§ offers accurate information.

□ Sexual activity

In most social organizations the family is the basic unit of society. The family continues to serve the same basic human needs although its structure may vary across cultures and between generations.

Like the family, the institution of marriage is timeless and complex. Traditional monogamous marriages remain the norm, although different forms of marriage and family life styles are practiced by some people. The communal living group in which people pool their resources and share the responsibilities of family life is one example. Single couples living together as husband and wife is another. Still a different notion is that of renewable marriages in which marriage is on a limited-term contract with an option to renew the contract by mutual consent at the end of a specified time.

Single young people are experiencing a new sense of sexual freedom, and this has led to frequent sexual intercourse for its own sake rather than in association with love and marriage. While studies indicate that sexual behavior patterns are changing, they also show that the behavior is not in the direction of increased promiscuity.[35] An increasing number of unmarried couples no longer consider marriage as a prerequisite for sexual relationships. There is, among these couples, however, a mutual commitment to a love relationship before sexual intercourse. Among many of them there is also contemplation of marriage.

It is advisable for couples planning sexual relationships, marriage, and childbearing to have complete physical examinations, including a serologic test for syphilis (now compulsory in all except five states). Women should have a pelvic examination. At this time a tight hymenal ring, which could make intercourse difficult, can be dilated or incised, provided this procedure is psychologically and culturally acceptable to both the woman and her prospective husband.

Prior to marriage the couple can talk freely with their physician, their religious adviser, and particularly with each other concerning the physical, psychologic, and religious implications of sex. It is important that cultural differences be considered and that questions or differences about intercourse and size and spacing of the prospective family be discussed at this time.

Women often ask female nurses about intercourse. Tremendous variation exists is the sexual activity of married couples. With adequate knowledge, patience, and understanding, a couple can usually work out a plan that is satisfactory to both. Frequency of intercourse may vary from one or more times a day to once a month or less. The frequency normally drops considerably after the first year or two of marriage.

From 25% to 50% of married couples have some difficulty in intercourse, often due to worry or guilt feelings related to sex, inability to meet cultural standards for satisfactory intercourse, or fear of an unplanned or unwanted pregnancy. This may result in inability to experience orgasm in women and impotence in men. The couple can discuss these problems frankly with a health professional or spiritual adviser, since reassurance and additional sex education may relieve the situation. A few persons may need psychiatric help.

Absence of menstruation (amenorrhea) in the sexually active female who is not practicing effective conception prevention and who has a history of normal menstrual cycles usually indicates pregnancy. It is important to note that conception occurs approximately 14 to 16 days *before* a woman misses her first period. By

*Child Study Association of America, New York, 1974, Child Study Association.

†Pomeroy, W. B.: New York, 1974, Delacorte Press.

‡Crawley, L. T.: Englewood Cliffs, N.J., 1973, Prentice-Hall, Inc.

§Brown, F., and Kempton, R. T.: New York, 1970, McGraw-Hill Book Co.

this time the fertilized ovum has become implanted in the uterus. From the standpoint of healthful embryonic development and the changing health needs of the pregnant woman, it is essential that women become knowledgeable about the importance of health care as soon as pregnancy is suspected. Regardless of the cause of amenorrhea, assistance from a health professional should be sought at once.

Some women may have a slight vaginal discharge following intercourse. If it is irritating, a douche with plain water or with 15 ml of white vinegar to a liter of water may be used from 1 to 3 hours after intercourse. For marked discharge not alleviated by this means, further advice should be sought. Normally douches are not needed for cleanliness, and it is inadvisable to douche routinely because excessive douching alters the pH of the vagina and predisposes to acute and chronic infections. Some normal women have troublesome odor, especially in warm weather and following the menstrual period, which can be relieved by an occasional douche with warm water or vinegar in water. Also vaginal deodorants in powder, spray, and suppository forms have become increasingly popular and are available without prescription.

■ MENSTRUATION

□ Puberty and menarche

The onset of menstruation in young girls in properly called the *menarche*. The average age of the menarche has gradually decreased over the past 100 years, and this is attributed to improved nutrition. In the northern hemisphere the average age of the menarche is 13 years, with the normal range between 10 and 17 years. The onset of menstruation occurs at an earlier age in the southern hemisphere.

It is not possible to predict the exact time at which the first menstrual period will occur. In general most girls experience beginning breast development, broadening of the hips, and growth of axillary and pubic hair several months before the menarche. Some irregularity in duration of menstrual cycles and in the amount of flow is normal for the first few years. By the age of 18 to 20 years the menstrual cycle usually assumes a rhythmic pattern with minor variations. Theoretically, conception is possible with the menarche, but anovulatory cycles are common during the early years of menstruation.

□ Normal menstruation

There is normal variation among women in the intervals between menstrual periods. Menstruation occurs on an average of every 28 days, but most cycles occur within a normal range of 26 to 34 days. The cycles of an individual woman may normally vary by 1 to 3 days. The menstrual flow usually lasts for 3 to 7 days, with an average of 4 days. The flow is light at first, increases toward the middle of the period, gradually tapers off, and finally stops.

Some women have heavier flows than others. Normally there is a loss of from 30 to 180 ml of menstrual fluid during the period. One half to three fourths of the fluid is blood, and the remainder is mucus, fragments of endometrial cells, and desquamated vaginal epithelium. The average woman needs approximately one dozen pads or one dozen tampons for the entire period; however, this is highly variable in relation to both the amount of flow and esthetic concern. Normally menstrual fluid does not clot unless it is retained in the uterus or vagina for a prolonged time. It is believed that the endometrium produces an anticoagulant that prevents clotting of blood in the uterus. An occasional very small "clot" may occur, and this is probably a particle of endometrial tissue.

During pregnancy menstruation ceases, then returns within 6 to 8 weeks following delivery, although lactation suppresses the menses for varying periods of time. Unless disease occurs, the menstrual periods recur during adult life until the woman reaches menopause. The pattern of the menstrual cycle may be upset by such things as changes in climate, changes in working hours, emotional trauma, fatigue, and acute or chronic illness. Any of these factors may alter the life style temporarily and produce change in the menstrual cycle by way of the nerve centers of the hypothalamus that influence the rate and timing of pituitary stimulation of the ovaries. A period that is missed, earlier or later than expected, or shorter or longer than usual is not significant if it occurs for only 1 month. If any of these irregularities continue, a health professional should be consulted.

Before and during menstruation a variety of discomforts may be present, and these are considered normal. Slight aching in the lower back, legs, and pelvis, especially on the day of onset of the flow, occurs frequently. A slight tendency toward fatigue during the menses is common, and many women experience a spurt of energy a few days before the period begins. Breast changes are also often noticed. These changes are usually noticed before the menses begin and last for 1 to 2 days after the flow starts. They include sensations of tingling, fullness, tenderness, and increase in size of the breasts. Breast changes associated with menstruation reflect the influence of estrogen during the ovarian cycle. Some women note mood changes premenstrually. The exact role of cultural expectations in the cause of premenstrual tension is being explored.

Lower abdominal cramps are often associated with menstruation and may or may not be normal. Painful menstruation, called dysmenorrhea, is discussed later in this chapter.

□ Promoting positive attitudes

Menstruation is a manifestation of normal body function and should be treated as such. The "period" and "monthly period" are sensible and accurate terms to use if the individual does not wish to say, "I am menstruating." Because of the negative connotations engendered by such terms as "being sick" or "having the curse," girls and women can be encouraged to avoid using them and to use appropriate terms instead. Some women consider the menstrual periods a time of great inconvenience, perhaps because of inadequate knowledge of the physiology of menstruation, inadequate information about how it is possible to maintain usual physical, mental, and social activities, or because of sociocultural conditioning.

□ Health teaching

Before engaging in any discussion of menstruation, the nurse can first assess the individual's knowledge and level of understanding. Once this is done, a teaching plan can be designed to meet the specific learning needs of the person. All information can be given in an open, factual manner, but latitude must be allowed for individuals to express their feelings, thoughts, beliefs, and concerns.

Girls and women often want and need information about menstruation. Their understanding may be limited or inaccurate because of word-of-mouth information passed along by peers, parents, and others who are poorly informed. On the other hand nurses may find women who know about the entire menstrual cycle but have difficulty in accepting it as a normal process. Women need to know the facts concerning the physiology of menstruation. They also need to know what discomforts are normally associated with the menstrual period and what measures can be taken to relieve them. They need to know what signs indicate deviations from normal and what actions to take regarding possible problems.

Nurses are often questioned about methods of sanitary protection during menstruation. Either pads or tampons can be used, depending on which is most comfortable and acceptable. If tampons are of the correct size and are properly inserted, there should be no discomfort when they are worn. If the tampons are not easily inserted or if they produce pain when in place, a health professional should be consulted.

In order to increase knowledge and to reduce fear and anxiety, women can be informed of the events that may temporarily alter the menstrual cycle. However, they also need to be informed of symptoms indicating potential problems so that medical attention can be sought. In order to become knowledgeable about the patterns of their menstrual cycles, women can be encouraged to keep a written record. Establishing this habit makes it possible to predict the onset of the next menstrual period and to determine the range of cycles and duration of flow. Should it be necessary to seek the attention of a health professional for any reason, the date of onset of the last menstrual period (LMP) would be known.

Some women have marked discomfort during menstruation and take a variety of medications to relieve the symptoms. Women can be advised to treat minor discomforts with rest, warmth, and small amounts of acetylsalicylic acid. Use of patent medications and other nonprescribed remedies is discouraged, and women should be urged to seek medical evaluation if discomfort is incapacitating.

Daily bathing and frequent changing of sanitary devices add greatly to comfort and hygiene during menstruation. A warm tub bath often relieves slight pelvic discomfort, although many women prefer to take showers during the menstrual period. Cold baths and showers may increase discomfort, but many women use tampons and go swimming during their periods with no ill effects.

Daily activities may be continued for both physical and mental health. If fatigue is associated with menstruation, exercise may need to be modified to provide for additional rest. Fatigue should be avoided, and exercises or activities that are more vigorous than usually practiced can be postponed until after menstruation.

The diets of women of childbearing age are often inadequate, and after reviewing their diets with them, suggestions can be made about ways to make their diets more adequate. Most women experience some fluid retention preceding menstruation, and many notice weight gain that may be controlled to some extent by restricting the intake of salt and other foods high in sodium. Edema from other causes can be ruled out by having the woman observe her weight on a daily basis. If edema is present at times other than the premenstrual and menstrual periods, the woman should be advised to consult a physician. The preceding statements about health counseling in relation to menstruation apply not only to women but to young girls as well, since many of them can benefit from accurate and useful information.

□ Outcome criteria

As a result of instruction, women can:

1. Gather information about their menstrual cycles.
2. Judge whether their menstrual cycles are normal.
3. Distinguish between occasional irregularity in the menstrual cycle and symptoms indicating problems.
4. If a problem exists:
   a. Seek health care.

b. Give well-informed answers to questions about their problems.
5. Exercise judgment regarding self-medication and practices of folk medicine.

□ Investigation of major complaints

Problems related to the menstrual cycle are common. They comprise a variety of symptoms directly or indirectly related to the pelvic organs and may be due to any one or a combination of causes.

Women who seek care because of absence of menstruation *(amenorrhea)*, irregular periods, excessive flow, or *dysmenorrhea* should have a complete history taken and a physical examination done. Close questioning about the menstrual periods and sexual activity is important (p. 1360). The history should include use of medication including tranquilizers and hormones, since these often disrupt the menstrual cycle.

A pelvic examination to assess the state of the reproductive organs is essential. If a sexually active woman complains of amenorrhea, a pregnancy test is usually done. Urinalysis, complete blood count, study of cervical and endometrial tissue, hormone assays, or visualization of the pelvic organs may be indicated to determine the cause of the problem.

Dilation and curettage (D and C) is often the method selected for obtaining endometrial tissue for study. In many cases, a D and C is temporarily therapeutic because it removes hypertrophied endometrium. Unless the direct cause of the menstrual problem is found, however, and unless treatment for the cause is instituted, symptoms tend to recur. Women having a D and C should understand the purpose of the procedure and should be urged to remain under medical care even though the D and C has helped the problem (p. 1375).

Dysmenorrhea

Uterine pain with menstruation, commonly called "menstrual cramps," is properly termed *dysmenorrhea*. Although estimates vary, it is generally believed that at least one third of all women have some degree of dysmenorrhea. Studies in industry have shown dysmenorrhea to be one of the most common causes of absenteeism. Dysmenorrhea is probably a common reason for abseentism among girls attending school.

Dysmenorrhea is commonly described as a cramping pain in the lower abdomen. Backache is also commonly present. The pain may occur before the menstrual flow begins or during the first 2 days of the period. Most often the pain begins to subside with the onset of the flow. Dysmenorrhea has most often been attributed to contractions of the uterus, although other factors may be involved. Hormone dysfunctions, infections, displacements of the uterus, endometriosis, stricture of the cervical canal, and constipation are associated with dysmenorrhea. Women who have poor posture, take little exercise, and have poor eating habits have a higher incidence of dysmenorrhea.

Prevention. Knowledge of predisposing factors resulting in dysmenorrhea is limited. Pathologic conditions resulting in dysmenorrhea cannot always be prevented. Advising women at an early age to maintain good posture, to exercise, and to practice good nutrition may or may not reduce the incidence of dysmenorrhea; this area requires study. Prevention of pressure on the uterus from a full bladder or constipation can be corrected by teaching.

Theoretically it should be possible to discover some hormone dysfunctions, uterine displacements, and cervical strictures if women practiced the habit of having a yearly physical examination. Infections can be discovered and treated early before the uterus becomes involved in the process. Positive attitudes can be encouraged, since a woman who regards menstruation as normal is less likely to experience it as an illness. Recent studies suggest a possible link between prostaglandin activity and dysmenorrhea. Women who are consistently unable to engage in usual activities because of pain associated with menstruation should be urged to seek health care.

Assessment. Since the degree of pain perceived by individual women is subjective, dysmenorrhea is open to wide interpretation by patients, nurses, and physicians. Some women have minor cramping that they barely notice. Others require use of comfort measures such as decreased activity, local applications of heat, and mild analgesia. Still others are incapacitated and are unable to carry out their usual activities.

Nurses are often asked for practical suggestions to relieve dysmenorrhea. In helping with the immediate problem, an assessment is made to determine whether menstrual periods are in any way abnormal and to discover the degree of pain. If the periods are normal and pain is not severe, counseling the woman about nutrition, exercise, and rest is appropriate.

Intervention. If no cause of dysmenorrhea can be found, the woman is advised to try such measures as rest, moderate exercise, good nutrition, and avoidance of constipation. Local application of heat and mild analgesics are usually prescribed. Nurses can also explore the utility of nonpharmacologic measures such as systematic relaxation, exercise, and some of the techniques used to cope with discomfort during childbirth. There are currently several investigations in progress to explore the utility of biofeedback and autogenic training in the treatment of dysmenorrhea.[26] Medication with flufenamic acids is also being explored.[61]

If the uterus is found to be in an abnormal position

and can be manually returned to a normal position, a pessary may be inserted for a trial period to learn whether malposition is the cause of dysmenorrhea (Fig. 62-4). Dilation of the cervical canal is done when a cervical stricture is found and thought to be the cause of dysmenorrhea. Hormone therapy using estrogens is based on laboratory analysis of hormone levels and may be used in cases of hyperplasia of the endometrium.

Outcome criteria for the woman with dysmenorrhea. The woman can:

1. Examine her daily activities and evaluate them for necessary modifications.
2. Identify activities that relieve or aggravate dysmenorrhea.
3. Carry out prescribed care.
4. Explain the rationale for therapy, its expected and side effects, and actions to deal with side effects.
5. Evaluate the effectiveness of therapy.
6. Explain the effects on the reproductive functions of any necessary surgery and carry out prescribed self-care both pre- and postoperatively.

Amenorrhea

Amenorrhea is the term used when menstruation is absent. Temporary amenorrhea, in which one period is missed, may be normal in the event of emotional stress, sudden changes of climate, or acute episodes of illness. Its causes are summarized in the box below.

Aside from menopause, the most common cause of amenorrhea is pregnancy. In breast-feeding mothers amenorrhea may persist through lactation, leading to the common misconception that breast-feeding is a safe method of contraception.

CAUSES AND DURATION OF AMENORRHEA

Causes	Duration
Pregnancy	Up to 9 months, although some women may continue to menstruate while pregnant
Postpartum	6 to 8 weeks
Lactation	Variable; may be suppressed during the entire time the woman is lactating
Following contraceptive use	Up to 6 months
Following hysterectomy or bilateral oophorectomy	Permanent

Women who take oral contraceptives may have amenorrhea for up to 6 months after discontinuing the pill. Amenorrhea is a consequence of removal of the uterus or removal of both ovaries. Frequently amenorrhea is a symptom of a problem in the reproductive system such as congenital defects, dysfunction of the ovaries, and other endocrine disorders. Nutritional anemia, wasting chronic illness such as tuberculosis, and psychogenic factors such as fear of pregnancy or desire for pregnancy may be associated with amenorrhea.

Instruction of girls and women of all ages can do much to encourage them to seek prompt health care in the event of amenorrhea. Knowledge of the conditions under which amenorrhea is normal and abnormal assists women to make better informed judgments about the need for health care.

Assessment. Early diagnosis and prompt management are necessary if reproductive and genital problems of a more serious nature are to be prevented. Sexually active women need to be urged to see a physician as soon as a menstrual period is missed, since maintaining health during pregnancy is vital for both the mother and the fetus. For those women who do not wish to remain pregnant early diagnosis is important if the least traumatic methods are to be used in terminating pregnancy. Women who suspect their amenorrhea is due to menopause can be examined to confirm their suspicions. A Pap smear and endometrial tissue studies are necessary if premalignant and malignant conditions are to be diagnosed early.

Intervention. When a woman complains of amenorrhea, the usual complete history is taken and a physical examination is done. It is important to know whether menstruation has ever occurred, especially in young girls. The number of periods missed and whether amenorrhea was present previously are important. Recent use of medications and drugs needs to be determined. Women who have recently discontinued oral contraceptives and heroin users[13] often have menstrual abnormalities, of which amenorrhea is common. Girls over 14 years of age who have not started to menstruate usually have a pelvic examination to rule out congenital deformity such as absence of reproductive organs or imperforate hymen.

Treatment of amenorrhea is dependent on the cause. If a pregnancy is not present, hormone therapy may be required except in women who have recently used oral contraceptives. Cystic disease of the ovaries, ovarian cysts, and ovarian tumors are usually treated surgically, but few congenital defects can be surgically managed. Nutritional habits may need to be corrected and thyroid hormones may need to be supplemented.

Outcome criteria for the woman with amenorrhea. The woman can:

1. State the health team's plan for determining its cause.
2. State what preparations for laboratory tests and clinical studies are necessary and carry out these preparations.
3. Make a decision about treatment when presented with its alternatives, consequences, and risks.
4. Participate in evaluating the effectiveness of treatment.

Abnormal menstruation

Abnormal bleeding from the vagina requires immediate medical attention. There are two type: *menorrhagia,* or prolonged profuse menstrual flow during the regular period, and *metrorrhagia,* or bleeding between periods.

Menorrhagia in an adolescent girl may be due to a blood dyscrasia or to an endocrine disturbance. This is called *functional bleeding.* Menorrhagia in adult women is likely to be a symptom of an ovarian tumor, a uterine myoma, or pelvic inflammatory disease.

Any bleeding, even slight spotting, between periods is significant. Metrorrhagia may be a symptom of many disorders, including benign or malignant uterine tumors; pelvic inflammatory disease; abnormal conditions of pregnancy such as a threatened abortion, ectopic pregnancy, or hydatid mole; blood dyscrasias; senile vaginitis; and bleeding at ovulation caused by the withdrawal of estrogen. The wide use of combined ovarian hormones such as norethindrone to suppress ovulation sometimes causes bleeding at irregular times. When metrorrhagia is present, however, prompt medical examination is indicated even though the cause may not be serious. The cause, not the symptom, must be treated, and nurses have a responsibility to help disseminate this information to all women. Early diagnosis and treatment increase the possibility of cure even when the cause is a malignancy.

REPRODUCTIVE SYSTEM AND AGING PROCESS

As compared with other topics, little new scientific knowledge concerning the reproductive system and the aging process has evolved. Much of what is known about cessation of reproductive ability and menstruation, especially the psychologic aspects, is based on studies carried out many years ago. With social change and with the emergence of many different life sytles, these areas are in need of current study.

Women reach the *climacteric* between the ages of 40 and 50 years. During this time, which usually lasts for 1 year to 18 months, there is a gradual decline in ovarian function. The ovaries gradually cease to produce ova and estrogen, and as a result the menses become scanty, irregular, and spaced farther apart. Finally the menstrual periods stop altogether, and the *menopause* occurs. Men also have a climacteric, but it is usually less noticeable and occurs at a much older age; some men may never experience the climacteric.

With the climacteric and menopause there is a gradual reduction in fertility. However, the menopause does not mark the end of active sexual life. Since sexual function is not dependent on the release of ova or hormones, women can enjoy sexual activity during the climacteric and after the menopause. Men, too, often continue a fairly active sex life after many signs of normal aging such as hypertrophy of the prostate gland have occurred. Atrophy is a normal process in the postmenopausal period and varies greatly among women. Changes are most striking in the vagina, in which the loss of estrogen results in a thinned, easily traumatized epithelium. Vulvar changes also occur as evidenced by flattening of the labia and thinning of pubic hair.

During the climacteric most women experience hot flashes (flushes), which are felt as waves of warmth accompanied by flushing of the skin, especially the face, and perspiration. These hot flashes last seconds to minutes. They may be so mild as to be hardly noticed or so severe that they produce distress. Many women go through the climacteric with little awareness of its occurrence.

The menopause may be artificially induced by such procedures as irradiation of the ovaries, surgical removal of both ovaries, or hysterectomy. Each of these have one common consequence, namely, cessation of menstruation. Beyond this, however, differences occur. Since the menopause is induced by cessation of ovarian function, surgical removal of both ovaries results in menopause with all its physiologic changes. When the uterus is removed but the ovaries are left in place, menstruation ceases, but the ovaries continue to function provided the age of climacteric has not been reached.

Most women have heard of the "change of life." Depending on the climate in which they were reared and on their own changes in attitude toward normal functions of the reproductive organs, women may feel more or less free to discuss the menopause and their feelings and concerns during this period of life. Since many problems related to the reproductive organs occur in this age group, and since it is important for mental health that women be helped to make the menopause as comfortable as possible, it is important for nurses to identify women who can profit from interventions.

Education regarding the menopause should precede its onset. Understanding human behavior and the emotional impact cessation of reproductive ability may have and skill is using direct and indirect approaches assist in establishing a climate that permits open, honest discussion. Many women appreciate openings made by nurses to discuss the menopause. Women approaching the menopause, regardless of whether it is an event of normal aging or is artificially induced, need to know what the menopause is, why it occurs, the effects menopause has on reproductive and sexual ability, what can be done to make the menopause more comfortable, and what symptoms require medical attention. Anatomic teaching aids are usually useful. Pamphlets that the patient can read may be very helpful and include *Changing Years, The Menopause,* Male "Menopause" Crisis in the Middle Years,*† and *Sex Life After Sixty.*‡

Women who have led varied lives and have had many interests outside of homemaking probably experience less emotional distress during the menopause. Those who have primarily been homemakers and whose children are emancipated may need to be encouraged to develop new interests and social contacts to maintain feelings of being worthwhile.

Some women feel they are less attractive than before. Moderate exercise to maintain muscle tone is beneficial to both health and physical appearance. Advice regarding diet to control weight is appreciated by many women. Reassuring women that feelings of depression and uselessness are common can do much to alleviate fears. Men sometimes have feelings of depression and uselessness if they perceive a decline in sexual ability. They require the same explanation as women regarding what is happening to them and what they can do to maintain a healthful attitude and productive life.

Many men and women have heard of "change of life babies" and fear they may become pregnant during the menopause. When counseling menopausal women about contraception, it is important to remember that the menstrual cycles and ovulation are irregular and that if pregnancy is to be prevented a highly reliable contraceptive method is necessary. The rhythm method is unreliable during the menopause. The diaphragm, condom, or intrauterine device give adequate protection. There are some advantages to oral contraceptives during the menopause. They give excellent protection against pregnancy at an age when pregnancy is usually not desired, when pregnancy is more dangerous to the woman from an obstetric viewpoint, and when fetal anomalies of some types are more likely to occur. On the other hand, greater mortality due to thromboembolus and a higher incidence of cancer have been linked to the use of oral contraceptives. Therefore, when counseling about a contraceptive method it is necessary to assess the chances of pregnancy occurring, the risks pregnancy might carry, alternatives should pregnancy occur, and the chances of a woman being able to successfully use an alternate method.

Because the incidences of cancer of the uterus and cancer of the prostate gland is higher in menopausal men and women, they should be urged to have physical examinations including screening for cancer at least once a year. All women should be advised that bleeding after the menopause, menstrual periods that become increasingly heavy, and contact bleeding noted after douching or intercourse require the attention of a health professional.

Intervention. Approximately 10% of women have pronounced symptoms during the menopause. Vasomotor reactions producing hot flashes and excessive perspiration may occur and are caused by lack of estrogen. Although other symptoms may occur, only the atrophy of the vaginal mucosa and vasomotor spasms can be linked directly to hormonal change.

Women may have pain during intercourse (dyspareunia) because of atrophy of the vaginal canal. This condition is most often treated with estrogen replacement. Vaginal infections are common among women experiencing the menopause due to alteration in the physical and chemical properties of the vaginal mucosa. Thus women need to know the signs of infection of the vagina and when to consult a physician. Such vaginal infections are treated according to the causative organsim but frequently respond to vinegar douching.

Among the physiologic effects of the menopause is change in the skeletal system. About 25% of postmenopausal women develop osteoporosis.[4] As with other menopausal problems, this is usually treated with estrogen. In addition to the usual physical examination and history, the menopausal woman should have a Pap smear. Screening for endometrial cancer is also desirable. As previously mentioned, counseling regarding activities of daily living is appropriate.

Estrogen therapy during the menopause has long been in use, and over the years there has been much debate over the advantages and disadvantages of this therapy. Recent reports suggest that administration of estrogens to postmenopausal women is associated with an increased risk of endometrial cancer.[39,65]

Most often estrogen is prescribed for the relief of hot flashes. In considering the benefits and risks of estrogen therapy, certain information is valuable. A study investigating the extent of estrogen use during the menopause suggests that estrogens are sometimes prescribed for trivial reasons and that estrogens are likely to be used by women for an extended time.[68] Only 26% of the

---

*Gray, M.: New York, 1970, New Academy Press.

†Public Affairs Committee, Inc. 381 Park Ave., New York, N.Y. 10016.

‡Butler, R. N., and Lewis M. I.: New York, 1976, Harper & Row, Publishers.

women studied reported problems with hot flashes before therapy, yet 51% had taken estrogen for more than 3 months; the median period of estrogen use was 10 years.

The latent effects of estrogen therapy have caused some concern about the association of estrogen and uterine cancer.[55] Use of estrogens for treatment of the menopause became popular in the early 1960s. The latency period for human carcinogens is generally accepted to be about a decade. It is therefore possible that the results of years of estrogen treatment of the menopause are just beginning to emerge.

Whether estrogen should be used for prevention and management of osteoporosis in postmenopausal women is also being debated. It is believed that estrogens may retard bone resorption temporarily,[45] but that later reverses in bone formation may negate or reverse gains made by estrogen therapy.[56]

The evidence to date suggests a causal relationship of some type between menopausal estrogen therapy and uterine cancer in some women. There is cause for concern and vigilance. It has been suggested that when estrogen is used for relief of menopausal symptoms it should be administered in a cyclic manner, with the woman taking estrogen for 3 weeks, then abstaining from medication for 1 week.[55] In general it is desirable to use the lowest dose possible to relieve symptoms, with the eventual goal of gradual and complete withdrawal of medication. During estrogen therapy women should be seen at least every 6 months for examination and for review of menopausal symptoms. The examination should include the breasts and reproductive organs, Pap smear, and blood pressure.

Women undergoing treatment for the menopause may be required to take douches, especially if vaginal infections are present. Douches are also commonly prescribed for application of heat and medications and for cleansing in the pre- and postoperative periods when pelvic surgery is done. Some women use douches for contraception. In any of these cases the nurse can ensure that the woman knows how to douche.

If possible, the best results are achieved from douching while lying in a bathtub (Fig. 61-1) rather than while sitting on the toilet seat. When a vinegar douche is to be used, 30 ml of white vinegar are diluted in 2 liters of water. The temperature should be about 40 C (105 F) unless otherwise ordered. The douche tip is inserted upward and backward and moved about to prevent fluid from being forced into the cervix and to ensure flushing of the posterior vaginal vault. If a medicated or hot douche is to be used, the labia are held together for a few minutes to allow the vagina to fill and thus benefit all areas. Douches prescribed for local heat are continued for about 30 minutes. Petroleum jelly may be used to prevent burning the labia. Following douching, the tub is cleansed well with soap and water.

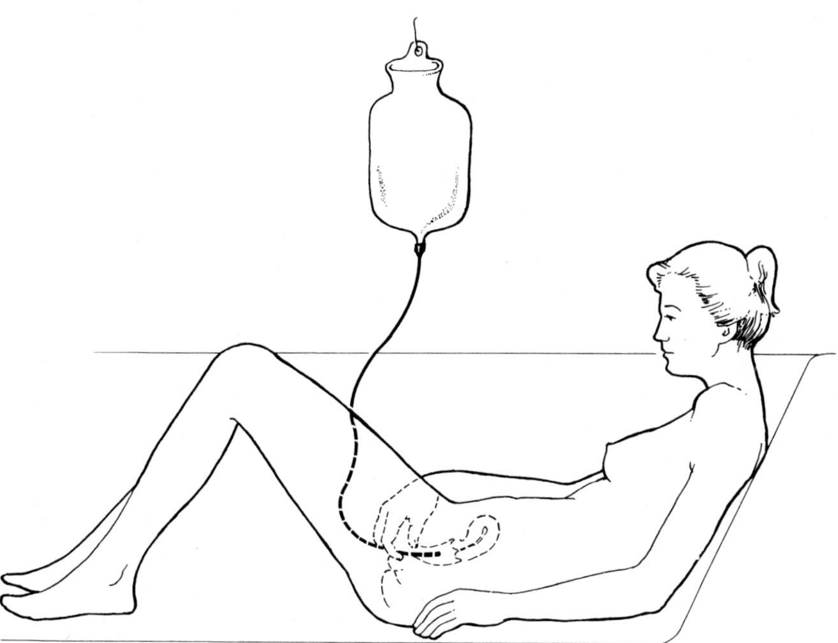

Fig. 61-1. Vaginal douche should be taken while lying in bathtub. Douche pan may be placed under patient in tub if desired.

Outcome criteria for the person experiencing menopause

As a consequence of health management during menopause, men and women can:

1. Make informed decisions about birth control.
2. Consider the possible consequences and alternatives should pregnancy occur.
3. State the signs of menopause and self-care actions to safely maximize their comfort.
4. In the event that a health practitioner is consulted regarding problems of menopause, state the treatment regimen, its purpose, and anticipated results.

FAMILY PLANNING AND CONTRACEPTION

Overpopulation has become a worldwide problem of such magnitude that it affects every living being. Ecologic insights force us to look at life and our environment in a different way than in previous decades. We now know that we have few choices left if we are to survive on this planet. Beyond the question of survival are questions of quality of life. Thus birth control and family planning become not only matters of personal concern but take into consideration the rights of others.

For the first time in the history of humankind it is now possible to regulate conception with a high degree of reliability. During the past 20 to 30 years there has been a sharp decline in the birth rate in the United States and similarly developed nations. This drop is attributed to widespread use of highly effective fertility and birth control methods including oral contraceptives, intrauterine devices, and new techniques for performing abortions and sterilizations.

Contraception remains a controversial issue. The incentives and imperatives for separating sexual and reproductive functions have been widely discussed from the standpoint of medical care, sociology, psychology, demography, economics, theology, and the law. Prevention of the birth of unwanted children and prevention of illness are two of the themes addressed pro and con in the literature.

Regardless of the personal and global issues involved, individuals and couples are required more than ever before to examine the consequences of their actions and to select from among the various alternatives the one most consistent with their beliefs, needs, and sense of responsibility. Bound into these issues and pressures for individual responsibility are controversies surrounding the use of particular methods of conception prevention, advantages and disadvantages of methods available for birth control, and the problems incurred by the use of individual methods of preventing pregnancy.

Mortality associated with the use of various methods of birth control has received much attention through the years. Reports continue to be made indicating that very low rates of mortality are associated with all *reversible* methods of fertility control as compared with mortality associated with pregnancy and childbirth.[70] Mortality reported for tubal ligation and hysterectomy for sterilization of women is higher than for any other form of birth control. However, these rates are still lower than mortality during pregnancy and childbirth. The mortality due to hysterectomy is considerably higher than that for tubal sterilization, yet increasing numbers of women are having hysterectomies to prevent pregnancy. No mortality due to vasectomy is reported in the literature.

Counseling of individuals and couples

People choose a method of preventing pregnancy for reasons other than risk to health or life. These reasons include effectiveness, convenience, reversibility, ethical considerations, cost, life style, and noninterference with enjoyment of sexual intercourse. Much of the literature is devoted to the concerns of risk to health and life and very little to other factors, including risks attended by reproduction.

In order for people to make a fully meaningful and responsible choice, they need to be informed of all of the advantages and disadvantages of all methods or combination of methods available for preventing pregnancy. With the flood of publicity in the media, especially regarding congressional hearings and actions, considerable anxiety and confusion on the part of the public has resulted. Usually the publicity is directed toward one aspect of health risks associated with one method of conception control, and the risks are not presented in comparison with risks associated with pregnancy and childbirth. In addition certain biases are inherent in the lay literature regarding which forms of contraception are most desirable. Thus health professionals are given the task of fitting pieces of information together to form a whole picture with meaning and perspective and of presenting the total block of information to persons seeking information, advice, and help.

Individuals who use a reversible method of birth control and then decide to change have two alternatives: they can choose an alternate method or not use any method of birth control. When the second alternative is chosen, pregnancy is very likely. Pregnancy then may lead to either an abortion or continuation of the pregnancy resulting in the birth of an unwanted child. It is therefore important that information be fully given, including risks to health and life and risks of pregnancy. Only in this way can people make an intelligent judgment of the risks they are willing to take and assume responsibility for their actions.

One of the greatest responsibilities of nurses is to assist sexually active people in making decisions regarding contraception, childbearing, and pregnancy spacing in a well-informed manner. Experience has shown that, on an individual basis, the best method of contraception is one that is acceptable to both sexual partners, readily available, convenient and easy to use, effective and safe, and inexpensive and does not interfere with the enjoyment of the sex act. These factors should be explored with persons seeking assistance with birth control.

In many clinics nurses take an active role in managing birth control programs. The nurse's role includes history taking, physical examination, counseling, and evaluating the effectiveness of various methods of birth control during follow-up visits. In some settings nurses in extended roles prescribe the method of birth control. Outside of these settings nurses have many opportunities to seek out individuals and couples in need of birth control information.

Counseling individuals or couples regarding birth control goes beyond teaching them how to use a method correctly. If couples are to accept responsibility for conception control, the nurse needs to assess the extent to

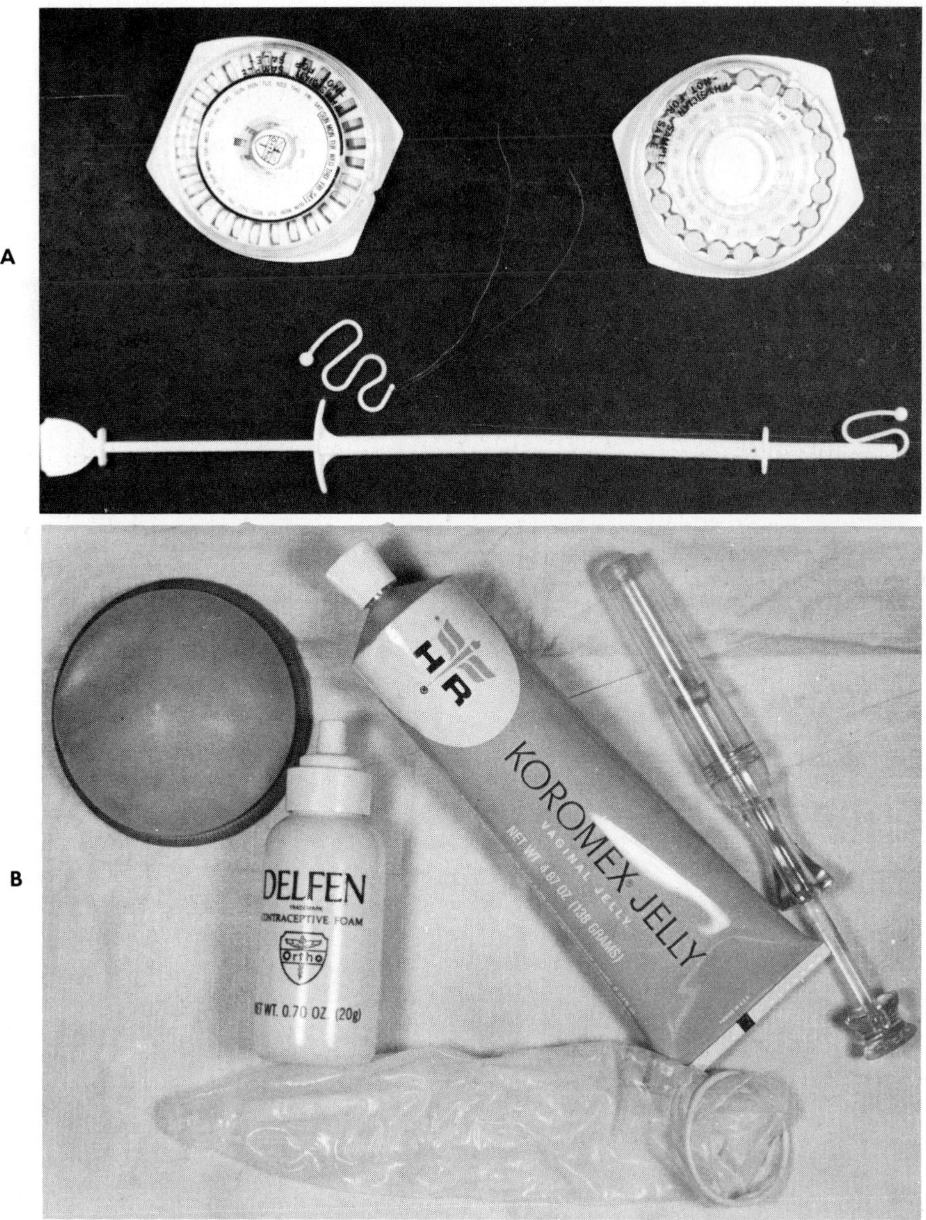

Fig. 61-2. A, Two types of oral contraceptives and Lippes loop with applicator. **B** *(left to right),* Diaphragm, contraceptive foam for vaginal application, contraceptive jelly and vaginal applicator, and condom.

Table 61-1. Summary of methods of conception control

Method	Action	Safety-effectiveness	Effects	Contraindications
Oral contraceptive ("The Pill") Combination pill: each pill contains progestin and estrogen; schedule: one pill daily for 21 days, then discontinue for 7 days; placebo may be advised for last 7 days; pill cycle started and repeated on fifth day after onset of menstrual flow	Inhibit ovulation by suppression of pituitary gonadotropin Produce cervical mucus that is hostile to sperm Modify tubal transport of ovum May have effect on endometrium to make implantation unlikely	100% effective if taken accurately Failure results from failure to take pill regularly If woman forgets to take pill one day, she can "make up" by taking two pills next day Chances of pregnancy increased if pill is missed for 2 days or more Highly acceptable to users; easy to take Linked with mortality due to thromboembolus phenomena Does not alter fertility	Useful Relief of dysmenorrhea in 60% to 90% of cases Relief of premenstrual tension Regulation of menstrual cycles Relief of acne in 80% to 90% of cases Improved feeling of well-being Minor (side effects usually decrease after third cycle) Weight gain Breast tenderness Headaches Corneal edema Nausea Breakthrough bleeding Hypertension Major side effects Thromboembolus disorders May also decrease lactation in breast-feeding women	Undiagnosed vaginal bleeding Breast or pelvic cancer Liver disease Cardiovascular disease Renal disease Thyroid disease Diabetes Uterine fibroid tumors Use with caution if history of: Epilepsy Multiple sclerosis Porphyria Otosclerosis Asthma
Intrauterine contraceptive device (IUD or IUCD) Small objects of various shapes made of plastic, nylon, or steel inserted into uterus; most have nylon string attached that protrudes from cervix into vagina; inserted using aseptic technique; follow-up visits in 1 month, then individualized EXAMPLES Lippes loop Saf-T-Coil Birnberg bow Margulies coil Hall-Stone ring Copper T Copper seven	Unknown Probably modifies endometrium or myometrium to prevent inflammation Probably hastens tubal transport of ovum	Easily inserted, highly effective: 97% to 99% Can be inserted any time during cycle; presence of menstrual flow rules out early pregnancy Can be inserted immediately postpartum, but expulsion rate is higher Can be left in place indefinitely Effectiveness highly dependent on knowing IUD remains in place; women need to be taught to feel for string after each period Spontaneous expulsion occurs most often during menstruation (expulsion rates: 10% to 20%)	Uterine cramping Heavy menstrual flow Irregular menses NOTE: Usually disappear in 2 to 3 months Problems Infection: usually minor and occurs soon after insertion Perforation of uterus: varies with types of device; highest rates in first 6 weeks postpartum; usually occurs at time of insertion	Current infection of reproductive tract Uterine fibroids Undiagnosed vaginal bleeding

Table 61-1. Summary of methods of conception control—cont'd

Method	Action	Safety-effectiveness	Effects	Contraindications
Intrauterine contraceptive device—cont'd		Failure rate (pregnancy) 1.5% to 3% during first year of use; rate declines thereafter Does not alter fertility		
Diaphragm (with spermicidal foam, cream, jelly) Rubber dome attached to flexible metal ring; inserted into vagina to cover cervix; available in various sizes (require careful fitting); self-inserted by user; inner surface of diaphragm coated with spermicide before insertion; inserted at least 2 hours before intercourse and left in place at least 6 hours after intercourse	Provides mechanical barrier to sperm Spermicidal preparation destroys large number of sperm	97% to 98% effective if fitted properly and used correctly Requires sustained motivation for repeated insertion and removal Refitting necessary after childbirth, abortion, surgery of cervix and vagina, or weight change of 10 lb or more	None	Severe uterine prolapse
Condom ("rubber," "safes," "prophylactics") Thin, flexible plastic worn over penis; available without prescription; does not require medical supervision	Provides mechanical barrier to prevent sperm from entering vagina Prevents spread of venereal diseases	Effectiveness increased with use of diaphragm by woman Effectiveness decreased by tearing or slipping of condom during intercourse Failure rate 10% to 15%	None	None
Rhythm ("safe period") Periodic abstinence from intercourse during fertile periods of menstrual cycle; days 12 to 16 before expected date of menstruation are possible ovulating days; since sperm can survive up to 48 hours, days 11, 17, and 18 added to fertile period	Sexual abstinence around time of ovulation	Safe 65% to 85% effective Fertile period varies; precise time of ovulation not known Effectiveness increased with calculation of fertile period, high motivation to prevent pregnancy, determination of basal body temperature	Frustration Lack of sexual gratification during period of abstinence	Irregular menstrual cycles Medical contraindications to pregnancy
Chemical contraceptive (jellies, creams, foams, suppositories) Applied inside vagina by means of plunger-type applicator or aerosol spray	Contains spermicidal ingredients Partial barrier to entrance of sperm into cervix	Effectiveness increased when used with diaphragm or condom Easily available without prescription Effectiveness depends on dispersion of substance within vagina	None	None

Continued

Table 61-1. Summary of methods of conception control—cont'd

Method	Action	Safety-effectiveness	Effects	Contraindications
Chemical contraceptive —cont'd		Low effectiveness rate: 20% failure rate for foams, creams, jellies; 30% failure rate for suppositories		
Postcoital douche	Removes sperm from vagina by washing	Safe 30% to 35% failure rate Some sperm have entered uterus 1 to 10 minutes after ejaculation	None	None unless douching is medically contraindicated

which misunderstanding, superstition, and fear exist and to take action by presenting facts about reproduction as well as facts about contraceptive methods. For example, lay people sometimes confuse contraception, which is temporary and reversible, with sterilization, and the differences need to be pointed to them.

People may have many questions about contraception, and the nurse can anticipate some that are frequently asked:

1. What methods are most effective in preventing pregnancy?
2. How safe are the available methods? Will they harm the couple, the individual, or a future child?
3. Will contraception interfere with sexual intercourse in any way?
4. Do the methods hamper or prevent later desired pregnancies?
5. How convenient are the different methods?
6. What do the different methods cost?

Often nurses must initiate the discussion of conception control, although this is now a commonly expressed concern of clients. In many instances women who are hesitant to pose questions about birth control are relieved when nurses indicate that this is an acceptable concern.

Direct or indirect questions may be used to initiate discussions. Questions may be more direct; that is, "Would you like help in planning your family?" "Do you want help in preventing pregnancy before you are ready for another child?" "Do you want information about birth control?"

Also questions can be posed more indirectly and individualized for the pateints' circumstances. For example, new mothers and fathers often respond to the childbirth experience by remarking, "I don't want to go through that again for a while." This provides an opportunity for the nurse to raise the question of how they plan to prevent pregnancy until they are ready for another child. Another opportunity may arise when nurses are in contact with parents of an acute or chronically ill child. A statement such as, "Your child is going to keep you busy for some time; how will you manage if a baby comes along?" can provoke discussion of contraception. A couple or family having economic problems might welcome a comment such as, "I've noticed you are having a hard time. How will things be if you find you are expecting a child?"

Pamphlets can be placed where patients have access to them, and this often gives the nurse a cue to the patient's interest. To verify this the nurse might say, "I noticed you looking at this pamphlet. What information or help can I give you?"

The various methods of contraception, their actions, advantages, and disadvantages are summarized in Table 61-1. The data in Table 61-2 may be helpful in counseling women who are utilizing the rhythm method. In order for the rhythm method to be used with reliability, however, the woman must be certain of the length of her menstrual cycles and the shortest and longest ranges of her cycles. Nurses need to discuss with individuals or couples their contemplated or usual sexual activity. For example, a woman who engages in sexual intercourse only occasionally is not necessarily a good candidate for birth control pills. For her, an alternative method may be more suitable.

Explaining some of the methods requiring insertion or application (Fig. 61-2) may be valuable. Audiovisual materials such as *Family Planning Series** are very useful in giving individuals and couples information about methods of birth control.

The records of hospitalized patients are a source of in-

*Milner Fenwick, Inc., 3800 Liberty Heights Ave., Baltimore, Md. 21215.

Table 61-2. Ovulation and the menstrual cycle

Shortest cycle (in days)	First unsafe day	Longest cycle (in days)	Last unsafe day
20	2nd	20	9th
21	3rd	21	10th
22	4th	22	11th
23	5th	23	12th
24	6th	24	13th
25	7th	25	14th
26	8th	26	15th
27	9th	27	16th
28*	10th*	28	17th
29	11th	29	18th
30	12th	30*	19th*
31	13th	31	20th
32	14th	32	21st
33	15th	33	22nd
34	16th	34	23rd
35	17th	35	24th
36	18th	36	25th

*Example: A woman whose cycles range from 28 to 30 days has her first "unsafe" day on the tenth day after the start of any period and her last "unsafe" day on the nineteenth day after the start of any period.

formation regarding the patient's history, physical condition, and reason for current hospitalization. The medical and nursing records should be reviewed before the nurse offers assistance with birth control and family planning.

During the interview and physical examination, the patient's reliability should be assessed. Ability to recall facts or to give information readily may give clues as to the most reliable method for the patient. For example, a woman who states she is taking vitamins but often forgets them, or a woman who when questioned about self-medication states she hates taking pills or does not believe in medicines, may not be the best candidate for oral contraceptives. Although judgment about reliability needs to be reserved until follow-up visits reveal a repeated pattern of missed pills, the initial interview will alert the nurse to question the woman carefully during future visits.

Physical examination is directed toward discovering conditions that indicate which methods of contraception should not be used and why. During the examination opportunities for health teaching arise, and the nurse can take advantage of these. All women seeking assistance for conception prevention should have a Pap test done and should be encouraged to have an annual physical examination. In addition serology and cervical smears and cultures are usually taken to detect infections, and individuals can be instructed at this time about how to prevent infection, how to recognize infection, and the need for medical care when infection occurs.

Finally it is especially important that the woman's value system is respected even though it may not be congruent with that of the health provider. The decisions regarding family size need to be made by the woman, not by the health professional.

□ Intervention

When assisting people to select a method of birth control, personal beliefs and biases must be avoided. The nurse's personal opinions about preferred methods may be dangerous to the patient's health and may force the patient to follow a practice not really desired, and this in turn may result in the pregnancy the patient wishes to avoid. Information should be given about each method, how the method works, the degree of protection against pregnancy provided by the method, self-care requirements, side effects of the method, contraindications to use, and the need for follow-up care. Information is repeated in the same way for each method. Once the patient has selected a method, information about that method is reviewed again.

□ Methods

Oral contraceptives

It has been estimated that over 20 million women worldwide are using oral contraceptives (the Pill) and that in the United States about 20% of women of childbearing age are using this method to prevent conception.[33] Many individuals and couples are apprehensive about the safety of the Pill because of reports linking the use of oral contraceptives to cancer and thromboembolic disease.[27,34,38,64] Although apprehensive, many women using the Pill are incorrectly or poorly informed about the correct use and side effects of the drug. According to a study of women using oral contraceptives, most of them read the labeling and package insert and found the information useful, but after reading this information some women were still inadequately informed about correct usage and side effects.[14] When questioned, these women preferred information about oral contraceptives from health professionals. This information indicates that merely handing printed information to those taking oral contraceptives and telling them to read it is inadequate. Such a procedure should be accompanied by verbal information and questioning to determine the accuracy and degree of knowledge about oral contraceptives. The printed information can then be utilized by the patient for future reference.

Women taking oral contraceptives require close supervision. To ensure that they will return for periodic examination, they are given a prescription or supply of pills for only 1 to 3 months. The advantages of returning for checkups should be emphasized. When an oral contraceptive is prescribed, the woman should be told when

Table 61-3. Symptoms that may be associated with use of oral contraceptives

Due to hormone excess		Due to hormone deficiency	
Estrogen	**Progestogen**	**Estrogen**	**Progestogen**
Nausea, vomiting Headache Edema Vertigo Uterine cramps Breast changes, mastalgia Cervical erosion Cervical mucorrhea Vein complications (eg., thrombosis, phlebitis) Chloasma Increase in size of myoma (if present)	Increased appetite, weight gain Fatigue Decrease in libido Depression Absence of withdrawal bleeding Headache* Breast fullness* Cholestatic jaundice Increased tendency to thromboembolism Hirsutism Loss of scalp hair Acneform rash	Breakthrough bleeding early in cycle Absence of withdrawal bleeding Hot flashes, nervousness Candidal vaginitis	Breakthrough bleeding late in cycle Menorrhagia with clotting Delay of withdrawal bleeding

(From Effler, S. B.: Gynecologic aspects of the "routine" checkup, Postgrad. Med. **59:**164-170, 1976.)
*During medication-free period.

to take it and what to do if she misses a day. One or two pills can be made up by taking them as soon as the woman realizes she has missed them. If three or more pills are missed, the woman should discard the pills remaining for that cycle and begin a new cycle 7 days from the day she took the last pill. During this time an alternate method of contraception should be employed.

Unfortunately "making up" pills can increase the risk of pregnancy. Low levels of estrogen and progestogen resulting from missed pills may stimulate the pituitary gland to release FSH and LH, resulting in the development of a graafian follicle. If the woman takes two or three pills at one time, this causes a sharp rise in estrogen level and may trigger ovulation.

Women should also be advised about storing pills used for contraception. Not only are they dangerous if ingested by children, but they are affected by extremes in temperature. High humidity may soften the pills and cause them to disintegrate, while extreme heat may decrease their potency.

During interim care the woman should be closely observed for side effects and emerging problems. Table 61-3 shows symptoms associated with oral contraceptives. This information can be used for instructing patients about problems to report and as a guide for screening for problems during follow-up visits. The incidence of vaginal infections is higher among women using oral contraceptives. If infections occur and persist, a different oral contraceptive or an entirely different method of birth control may be necessary.

Intrauterine devices

At the present time the intrauterine devices (IUD) that seem to be most widely used are the Lippes loop, Saf-T-Coil, copper T, and copper Seven. Pregnancy rates for IUD users range from less than 1% for copper devices and the Lippes loop to 18% for noncopper devices.[32] It is well known that women using intrauterine devices have menstrual periods that are heavier and that they more often have intermenstrual spotting than do women using other methods of contraception. The bleeding experienced by women using an IUD may be due to spontaneous abortion. A recent report indicates that 12% to 19% of women using a copper-type IUD demonstrated human chorionic gonadotropin in their blood.[33] This adds to the evidence that the IUD probably interferes with pregnancy by producing degeneration of a fertilized ovum, that fertilization of the ovum can and does occur, and that tubal pregnancy occurs more often in women using the IUD.

Women using an interuterine device are required to feel for the string on the device to be sure it is still in place. Many women fear the device will get lost inside them. Showing them a model of the pelvis and how the device is situated when in place helps them overcome this fear. Informing the woman that the string becomes soft with body heat and that her sexual partner probably will not be aware of it during intercourse is usually reassuring. Many women also welcome hearing that tampons can be used during the menstrual period when an IUD is in place.

Other methods

Other methods of birth control may be preferred by people whose religious beliefs conflict with the use of some forms of birth control, those who question the long-term effects of hormone use, and those who believe in avoiding additives to their bodies. Table 61-2 may be helpful in counseling women who wish to use the rhythm method. To be reliable, this method requires that the woman be certain of the length of the menstrual cycles and the shortest and longest ranges of her cycles. Recently the "ovulation method" of birth control has been described,[71] and in conjunction with the basal body temperature may make the rhythm method more reliable. The ovulation method is based on changes in cervical mucus and sensations of wetness and dryness perceived by the woman. Secretion of a thick, yellowish, or cloudy mucus indicates that ovulation is beginning and is accompanied by a sensation of increased wetness. As ovulation occurs the mucus becomes more clear and watery but has the ability to stretch *(spinnbarkeit)*. At this time the sensation of wetness increases still more. Even though not menstruating regularly, menopausal women note these same changes in mucus and can become aware of a fertile period. Intercourse is avoided on the days when sensations of wetness are present. If a discharge due to infection is present, this may interfere with the woman's ability to make reliable observations and increases the risk of conception.

□ Counseling

When counseling couples regarding birth control, it is important to make notations about their plans for having children and their desired family size. In this way couples can be advised about the appropriate time for discontinuing contraception. Removal of an intrauterine device restores fertility within 1 to 2 months. After long-term use of oral contraceptives, about 75% of women are able to become pregnant within 2 months after discontinuing the Pill.[9] With all other temporary methods, fertility is restored immediately after the method is discontinued.

It is generally accepted that, for preservation of health, pregnancies and childbirth should be spaced to avoid the consequences of stress of the body. Most experts believe that an interval of at least 2 years between pregnancies is desirable. In the years between pregnancies, every effort needs to be made to improve and maintain health so that when pregnancy does occur the woman is more likely to face fewer risks and the fetus is more likely to have a better chance for growth and development in a healthful environment. To these ends nurses can make a valuable contribution to the health of women and children.

The availability of systemic contraceptives for men has lagged behind the development of safe and effective contraceptives for women. Considerable study has been devoted to correcting this deficiency, and some beginning achievements have resulted.

Study of newer, safer contraceptives for women continues. The postcoital (morning after) pill has enjoyed publicity but is not widely prescribed. These preparations, taken by the woman after she has had intercourse, contain potent synthetic estrogens that probably prevent implantation of the ovum. Nausea commonly accompanies such high doses of estrogen. Long-term preparations that can be administered orally or by injection are being investigated.

□ Outcome criteria for family planning

Persons who have participated in family planning or birth control counseling can:

1. Select a method (or no method) that is most acceptable to them.
2. Use the selected method consistently.
3. Describe how the method prevents conception and necessary actions to make the method reliable.
4. Compare the risks associated with the method with risks of pregnancy.
5. State the side effects of the method.
6. State the complications of the method that require the attention of a health professional.
7. Describe self-care actions to relieve minor, common discomforts associated with the method.
8. State the optimum time for a pregnancy.
9. If a pregnancy is desired, discontinue the birth control method.
10. If an alternative method is necessary, explain why this is desirable.
11. Describe the effects of temporary or permanent methods of fertility control on reproductive ability.

■ STERILIZATION

In addition to the conception control methods mentioned above, voluntary sterilization has become increasingly acceptable to both men and women as a method of preventing pregnancy. It has been estimated that 1,500,000 American women have already been sterilized and that every year approximately 100,000 American women elect surgical sterilization.[23] In addition each year between 500,000 and 1,000,000 American men have vasectomies.[67]

A profile of men and women seeking sterilization indicates they come from all strata of society, are between 25 and 50 years of age, are married, have large families, and are likely to be white and of the Protestant faith. The primary reason given by both men and women for wishing sterilization is a desire to limit family size.[22] Other reasons include financial inability to support a large family, concern over population growth, problems with other methods of contraception, and age, with some couples preferring personal freedom over risk of childbearing with advancing age.[22] More frequently than women, men give as an important reason for sterilization their wish for an effective contraceptive that does not interfere with sexual pleasure.[1] Also men express concern over the health of their sex partners. Almost 83% of men whose sexual partners (including wives) used or were currently using oral contraceptives felt that the Pill was actually or potentially harmful to the woman.[1]

Medical indications for sterilization broadly include any condition or situation in which pregnancy would be attended by risks to health or life of the woman or her infant. Included in this category are severe heart disease and diabetes and probable genetic defects in the infant.

The laws governing sterilization vary from state to state; some states have laws that are unclear, while other states have no laws at all. In general if the surgery does not violate specific state provisions and if written, informed consent is given by a man or woman legally capable of giving permission, the surgery can be performed by a physician. The need for medical consultation may be regulated, however, by hospital policy.

□ Methods

The most common surgical procedure for elective sterilization of women is tubal sterilization. Hysterectomy is being performed more often for this purpose. Bilateral salpingectomy, bilateral oophorectomy, and pelvic radiation in large doses also bring about cessation of childbearing, although the primary purposes of these procedures is not sterilization.

Tubal sterilization can be accomplished by different surgical techniques. One method requires a small incision through the abdominal wall, usually in the midline. The fallopian tubes are located, and a loop of the midportion is elevated. The loop is then ligated at the base. Most often a bilateral salpingectomy is done to produce greater effectiveness. If this is the case, a small piece of each fallopian tube is excised. Hospitalization for 2 to 4 days is required and includes the usual preoperative and postoperative care. A local or general anesthetic is given.

The increased demand for tubal sterilization, along with refinement of techniques to simplify procedures used, has given rise to the use of culdoscopic and laparoscopic methods of tubal ligation. The culdoscopic method does not require an abdominal incision, since the surgery is performed by way of the cul-de-sac of Douglas, approached through the vagina. The fallopian tubes are coagulated by means of an electric current. A local anesthetic is usually used. The culdoscopic method results in little postoperative pain and a short period of hospitalization.

Laparoscopic tubal sterilization requires only a very small incision for the purpose of introducing the laparoscope through the abdominal wall. A segment of each tube is grasped with forceps, and an electric current is passed through the forceps to bring about coagulation of the tissues. A local or general anesthetic may be used, and postoperative pain is minimal. Both culdoscopic and laparoscopic tubal sterilization have been advocated as outpatient procedures. Postoperative complications are low for both of these procedures, although there is a slightly higher incidence of pelvic infection and pelvic abscess if the culdoscopic method is used.[31]

Tubal sterilization using one of the abdominal approaches is often performed in the early postpartum period or at the time of cesarean section, since the fallopian tubes have not descended into the pelvis and are more readily accessible at this time.

Successful sterilization (conception prevented) seems partly dependent on the technique used. The main causes of failure are recanalization of the fallopian tube, erroneous ligation, and pregnancy resulting from tuboperitoneal fistula. The failure rates reported vary from 1 in 57 to 1 in 340 women having tubal sterilization.[63]

Bilateral vasectomy (Fig. 61-3) is the surgical procedure for accomplishing sterilization of men. At least eleven techniques are described to accomplish what is generally considered to be a safe, simple procedure. Two reasons probably account for the variety of techniques developed. The first is the tendency of the vas deferens to spontaneously rejoin, a distressing long-term complication. The second reason centers around developing techniques having potential reversibility.

Bilateral partial vasectomy is the surgical method most often used. Because of its safety and simplicity, the procedure is most often performed on an outpatient basis in a clinic or a physician's office using a local anesthetic. A small incision is made in the scrotum to expose the sheath of the vas. The sheath is opened, the vas deferens is exposed, and a segment measuring 0.63 to 1.27 cm is removed. The segmented ends of the vas are then ligated. Some physicians prefer to coagulate the severed ends of the vas to ensure sterility. The incision is then closed by suturing.

Complications following vasectomy are rare and of a minor nature when they do occur. Bruising, mild edema, and mild discomfort are common and usually subside without treatment. Infection of the wound occurs in about 3% of patients.[22] Hematoma formation may occur. The incidence of failure due to recanalization is reported to be between 0% and 6%.[22] The cause of spontaneous recanalization (reanastomosis) is unknown, but duplication of the vas has occasionally been noted. The literature does not report any occurences of mortality due to vasectomy.

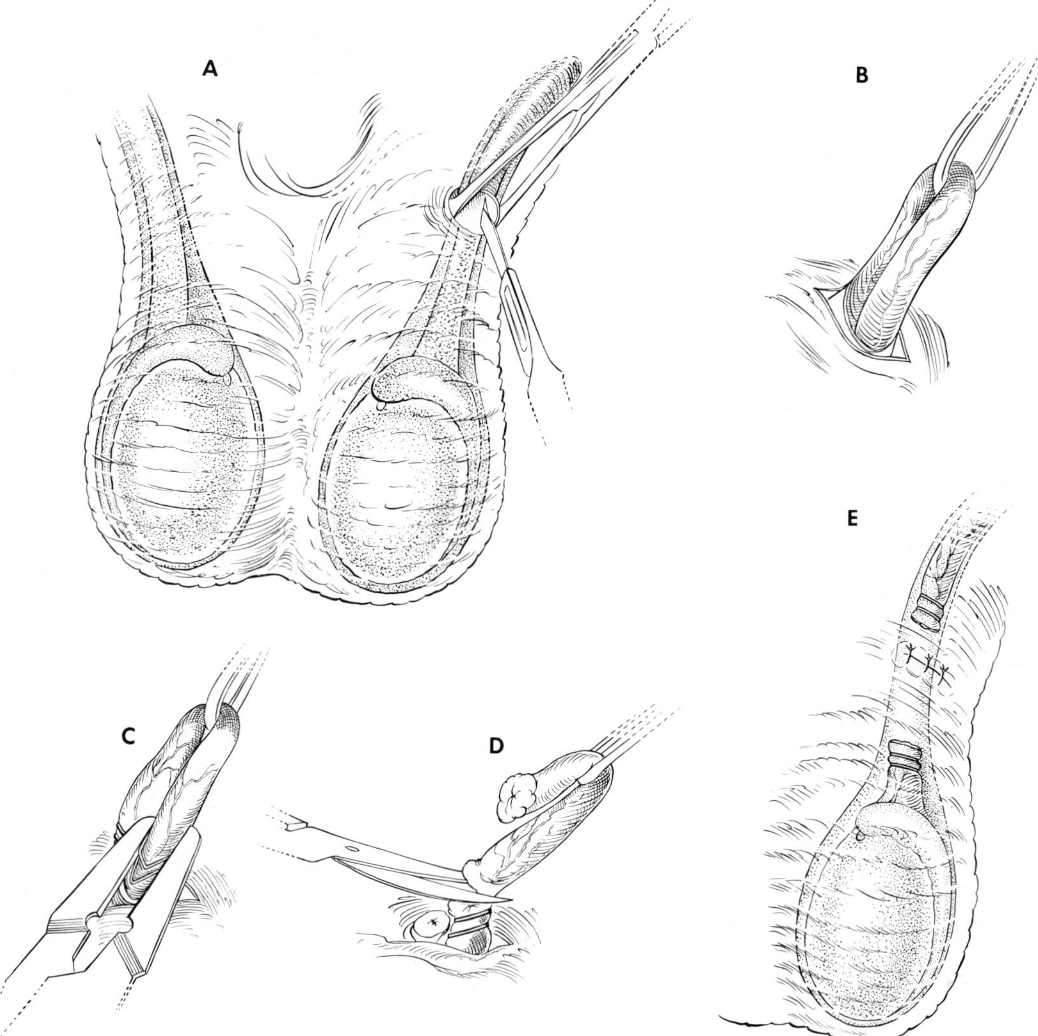

Fig. 61-3. Vasectomy procedure. **A,** Bilateral incision used to expose sheath. **B** and **C,** Vas exposed and occluded. **D,** Segment is excised. **E,** Vas is replaced in sheath and skin sutured. (Modified from Davis, J. E.,: Am. J. Nurs. **72:**510, 1972.)

□ Physiologic effects

While tubal sterilization terminates a woman's ability to bear children, ovarian hormones and menstrual functioning are not altered and an artificial menopause is not induced. Ability to derive satisfaction from sexual intercourse is not impaired, and some women may experience greater enjoyment from intercourse with the removal of fear of pregnancy.

Since vasectomy interrupts the continuity of the vas deferens, sperm are prevented from being ejaculated with other components of the semen. However, sperm are still produced. Residual fertility lasting for a variable period is present because of sperm in the semen beyond the point of occlusion of the vas. Sperm *gradually* disappear from the ejaculate; thus conception is possible in the immediate postoperative period.

Requests for reversal of previous sterilizations may be made because of divorce and remarriage, loss of children through death, or change in economic status, as well as for other reasons. For both men and women the chances of reversing the effects of sterilization are very small.

Attempts at reconstruction of the fallopian tubes to restore fertility have been made for many years. The surgery performed primarily involves an end-to-end anastomosis of the ligated and dissected tubes with or without insertion of plastic lumen. Tissue reactions due to rejection of plastic materials are common. The success

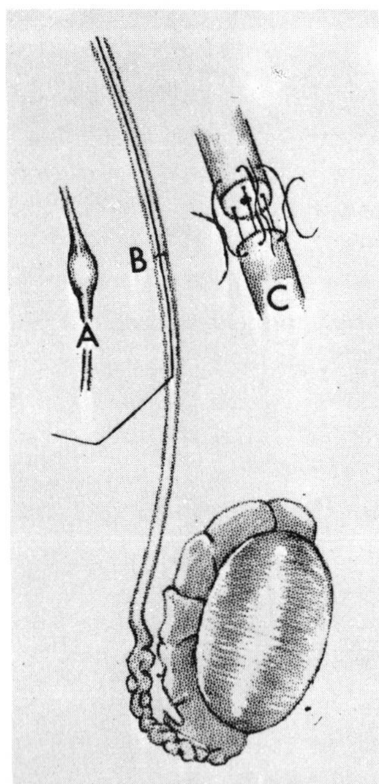

Fig. 61-4. Technique of vasovasostomy. A, Nodule of scar tissue at point of vasectomy. B, Reanastomosis over nylon splint. C, Magnified illustration of anastomosis. (From Hackett, R. E., and Waterhouse, K.: Am. J. Obstet. Gynecol. 116:438-455, 1973.)

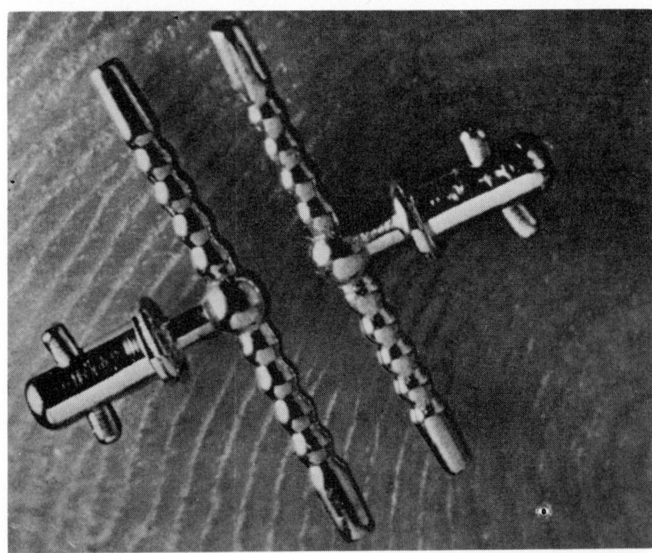

Fig. 61-5. Vas valve (Bionyx Control). (From Hackett, R. E., and Waterhouse, K.: Am. J. Obstet. Gynecol. 116:438-455, 1973.)

of restoring tubal function is partly dependent on the original surgery performed, especially regarding the amount of the tubal portion excised. Ligation of the tubes produces adhesions that must be dissected away to the point of tubal patency, and this reduces the amount of remaining tubal structure. Also the length of the fallopian tube remaining after reconstruction may play a role in permitting adequate time for a fertilized ovum to undergo maturational changes in preparation for implantation. Some of these changes occur within the fallopian tube. Success in rendering the fallopian tubes functional after sterilization is usually measured in terms of pregnancy rate following reconstruction. Reports of success range from 50%[73] to 69%.[41]

A surgical attempt to restore male fertility following vasectomy is called a *vasovasostomy* (Fig. 61-4). An attempt is made to rejoin the severed ends of the vas deferens. Success is measured by the presence of sperm in semen specimens following reconstruction. Reports of success in restoring fertility range from 37% to 90%.[22] A notable point is that although sperm reappear in the semen, the pregnancy rate following vasovasostomy is low, and the reason for this is unknown. Only 20% to 25% of vasovasostomies result in pregnancy.[11]

Considerable research is now in progress for the development of a reversible vasectomy device. One such device is shown in Fig. 61-5. Other devices include the vas plug, intravas device, and the vas clips. Ideally, reversible vasectomy devices would effectively block the vas deferens, would permit simple and safe insertion and removal of the device, could be turned on and off to provide for timing of conception, would not cause discomfort when in place, and would not cause complications. The ideal vasectomy device has not been developed, and the incidence of pain and tissue reaction is high with the devices now available.

Following a vasectomy it is important for the man to report for semen analysis as advised. Disappearance of the sperm from the semen and methods of determining this are described on p. 1373.

□ Psychologic aspects

Men and women who elect sterilization seem to have little or no regret after the surgery. One study reports that over 90% of women having tubal sterilization expressed no regret but that some women were disturbed emotionally by having been sterilized.[36] The method of elective sterilization seems to make little difference to women regarding their emotional responses. Depression, loss of self-esteem, physical complaints, feelings of guilt, and difficulty in sexual adjustment after surgery are reported to be some of the psychologic responses of women to sterilization even when the surgery is elective.[24] From psychologic studies it is suggested that women who regretted having been sterilized had preexisting emotional problems.[54]

Women who were dissatisfied after sterilization describe themselves as having feelings of inferiority, weakness, emptiness, being torn up inside, being a damaged and changed person, and having less desire for and gratification from sexual intercourse. These emotional reactions are less likely to occur if a woman requests sterilization and it is done for reasons of family size rather than for organic disease.[69]

Studies indicate that 95% to 99% of men are satisfied with the results of vasectomy and that, like women, some men have increased emotional difficulties after sterilization.[11] In a follow-up study of men who had vasectomies it was found that 70% percent were happier than before the surgery and that frequency of intercourse had increased.[15]

There is a need to recognize that tubal sterilization affects men as well as women and that vasectomies affect women as well as men when there is mutual caring and concern between them. This concern may be best illustrated by a woman who described her feelings when she and her husband selected vasectomy as their method of contraception: "The worst part of the experience was that I had not anticipated the range of my reactions. Now it seems that these transitions may have been natural. Perhaps if I had known the experiences of others, I would have passed more easily through these feelings. We try to prepare husbands for childbirth; we should recognize the need to prepare wives for vasectomy."[26]

□ Intervention

Preoperative counseling and care

The findings of studies regarding the psychologic aspects of sterilization indicate a need to identify men and women prior to surgery who may later have strong regrets and emotional problems. One aim of counseling prior to surgery is to confirm that the decision for sterilization is made as objectively as possible. Asking hypothetical questions about the possibility of divorce, loss of the spouse, or loss of a child can assist in estimating whether the decision to be sterilized has been treated as a serious step.

Previous experience with other methods of contraception can be explored and reasons for dissatisfaction with the methods determined. It may be that an individual or couple lacks knowledge about contraceptive methods and with adequate information might choose something other than sterilization. Care must be taken, however, that persons who are knowledgeable and have made a firm, objective decision are not made to feel that their decision is a poor one or is unacceptable.

The nature and consequences of the surgery must be explained to the patient. It is important to emphasize that the sterilization procedure does nothing to increase or decrease sexual performance or enjoyment but simply removes the chance of pregnancy. It is common for lay people to equate sterilization with castration and loss of femininity or masculinity. Even those patients who know the difference need reassurance.

Visual aids and models can be of great value in giving explanations about the surgery to patients. Use of films such as *Freedom from Pregnancy,** *Sterilization by Laparoscopy,*† and *Tubal Ligation*† and pamphlets such as *Voluntary Sterilization for Men and Women*‡ are useful in increasing patients' understanding.

The facts of reversibility, including current success rates, are discussed. In the case of vasectomy the chance of recanalization with return of fertility should be pointed out. The man or couple also must be informed of progressive rather than immediate sterility following vasectomy, and alternate methods of protection until sterility results should be discussed.

For men having vasectomies, a preoperative specimen of semen is examined to serve as a baseline for interpreting sperm disappearance following surgery. The patient is instructed to shave the scrotal hair and to take a shower the night before surgery. He is advised to bring briefs-type underpants with him on the day of surgery to hold the postoperative dressing in place.

Postoperative care

Most women having tubal sterilization can be discharged when effects of the general anesthetic have disappeared and when vital signs are stable. Exceptions are women who have recently delivered a baby and those having tubal sterilization by other than the laparoscopic abdominal method. All women need to be advised of the signs of infection and the need to report persistent pain in the lower abdomen or pelvis. Women having culdoscopic sterilization probably should be advised to abstain from intercourse for about a week to reduce the chances of infection and trauma. Those having abdominal tubal sterilization may resume intercourse when healing has taken place and when pain does not prevent it. All patients need to be adivsed when to report to the physician for follow-up examination.

Following vasectomy men are advised to expect slight swelling of the scrotum and minor pain. They should be advised to report bleeding, increased swell-

---

*Allend'or Productions, Inc., 3449 Cahuenga West, Hollywood, Calif. 90068.

†Milner Fenwick, Inc., 3800 Liberty Heights Ave., Baltimore, Md. 21215.

‡Planned Parenthood World Population, 810 Seventh Ave., New York, N.Y. 10019.

ing, hematoma, or persistent pain immediately. A day of reduced activity is usually desirable following vasectomy, and intercourse can be resumed in 2 to 3 days. The man should be reminded of the need for an alternate method of conception prevention until the physician reports that the semen no longer contains sperm.

Disappearance of sperm from the ejaculate following vasectomy and the methods for determining when sterility actually occurs have been studied extensively. The standard procedure has been to take a sperm count 4 weeks following vasectomy. Some experts believe that at least two consecutive sperm-free specimens must be found before the man can be considered sterile.[22] Others utilize the number of ejaculations required to render the semen free of sperm in establishing guidelines for sterility following vasectomy. It has been noted that after 12 ejaculations 65.5% of men become aspermatic, after 24 ejaculations 97.5% of men become aspermatic, and after 36 ejaculations all men (except those with spontaneous reanastomosis of the vas) become aspermatic.[41] Reanastomosis is suspected if sperm fail to disappear from the ejaculate despite an adequate number of ejaculations, if there is an increase in sperm in the semen after two successive sperm counts, if motile sperm are found in the semen beyond 3 months following vasectomy, and if, of course, pregnancy occurs.

In the postoperative period both men and women need opportunities to express their feelings about having been sterilized. Information previously given regarding sexual performance may need to be repeated. If the patient expresses feelings of regret or guilt, a review of the reasons for the sterilization may be of assistance in recognizing that the decision was made as objectively as possible.

□ Outcome criteria for persons who elect sterilization

The person can:

1. Describe the physiologic effects of sterilization and the small chances of reversing sterility.
2. Carry out self-care activities consistent with the surgery performed.
3. Describe how activities of daily living need to be modified during the postoperative period.
4. State the signs of complications of surgery.
5. If complications of surgery occur, seek help from a clinician.

■ INFERTILITY

It has been estimated that 10% to 15% of married couples in the United States are unwillingly childless. Although infertility is most often attributed to women, about 40% of infertile marriages result from sterility of men.

Married couples wishing to have children and who find themselves unable to do so experience immeasurable emotional distress. Feelings of inadequacy are common, as are anger and guilt. Couples who are informed that they will never be able to have children experience a life crisis with all of its ramifications and have a strong need to grieve. For those who are told they are a normal, fertile couple and for whom pregnancy does not result despite months or years of tests, studies, examinations, and advice, feelings of frustration alternating with hope are high. All of these couples require emotional support, including encouragement to grieve, to express their anger and other feelings in order to regain objectivity, and to avoid premature decisions and actions about alternatives. The urgent need for such support is reflected in the emergence of support groups organized by infertile individuals and couples.*

It is important that couples who wish to have children and are unsuccessful after about a year of trying to achieve pregnancy seek medical advice. Infertility evaluation often requires a long time. Sometimes sterility cannot be treated successfully, and alternatives such as adoption are considered. Because of legalized abortion fewer babies are available for adoption, and the infertile couple may face further frustration as they attempt to find a child to adopt.

□ Prevention

There are many causes of infertility in men and women. Some of these are preventable, while others are not. Some cause of infertility can be corrected, while other causes do not respond to any form of treatment.

Infertility in women may be due to diseases of the cervix and uterus that inhibit passage of active sperm, obstructions of the fallopian tubes that interfere with transport of ova, ovarian and other endocrine gland disturbances that inhibit release of ova, and hormonal problems that leave the endometrium unprepared for implantation.

One of the most common, preventable causes of infertility in women is infection of the pelvic organs, especially those due to gonorrhea, which cause obstruction of fallopian tubes. An estimated 17% of women have symptoms of salpingitis as the first sign of gonorrheal infection, and during the course of treatment about 4.5% are surgically sterilized.[74] Such serious consequences are preventable through prophylactic use of penicillin for women exposed to gonorrhea and through early diagnosis and treatment of all vaginal and cervical infections.

Many of the ovarian and hormonal problems that cause infertility produce symptoms such as menstrual irregularities and ill health before a problem with concep-

*RESOLVE, Inc., P.O. Box 474, Belmont, Mass. 02178.

tion is ever recognized. Many of these problems can be managed with hormone therapy, provided women seek help for such problems at an early age or as soon as deviations are noticed.

In men infertility may be caused by obstruction of the vas deferens, destruction of the testicular tissue by disease, undescended testes, and hormonal deficiencies. Bilateral undescended testes (cryptorchism) should be corrected surgically prior to puberty. In later life cryptorchism may produce sterility because of failure of the testes to develop their sperm-producing function, even if the condition is surgically corrected. Destruction of testicular tissue by infectious processes can be prevented through prompt treatment when symptoms first appear.

☐ Assessment and intervention

Attempts to correct infertility are based on data obtained through a detailed history and physical examination as well as data obtained from laboratory tests and clinical studies. A sexual history is taken and sexual practices are reviewed. Advice about sexual intercourse is given if this seems to be the problem.

Most physicians prefer to carry out examination of the man first, as it is more easily accomplished and less time consuming. The first special test done is multiple semen examinations (p. 1373) to determine the presence, number, maturity, and motility of sperm. Normal findings indicate fertility.

Absence of sperm in the semen may indicate a stricture along the vas deferens. A biopsy of the testes is done, and if sperm are being produced, there is a stricture. The stricture can sometimes be successfully repaired by plastic surgery (vasovasostomy).

If the sperm count and motility rate of sperm are low, thyroid extract and vitamins may be prescribed, along with a well-balanced diet, rest, and moderate exercise. A lack of vitamins A and E in the diet may cause some atrophy of the sperm-producing structures. The couple should be advised to have frequent intercourse during the fertile period (usually 14 to 16 days after the beginning of a menstrual period). Several days of continence should be practiced just before the period of fertility. When the man is completely aspermatic, conception is impossible, and the couple should be counseled regarding the alternatives open to them.

If the man is found to be fertile, examination of the woman is carried out. A complete history and physical examination are done. If there is an infection of the reproductive tract, it is treated. A systematic check is then made of each organ that might affect the woman's reproductive ability.

If menstruation occurs regularly, this usually indicates that the ovaries are producing hormones. To determine whether ovulation is occurring, the woman is instructed to keep a basal body temperature chart to help determine the presence and time of ovulation. In the interim, cervical secretions are examined for pH and spinnbarkeit. A postcoital test is usually done. If sperm are being destroyed by vaginal and cervical secretions, smears from these sites are studied. If the secretions are too acid or too alkaline, medicated douches may be prescribed. A douche using sodium bicarbonate (15 ml to 1 liter of water) taken just before intercourse has been found to increase the motility of sperm in many cases.

If a question remains regarding ovulation, endometrial biopsies, urinary estriol levels, and thyroid function tests may be done. Laparoscopic inspection of the ovaries may be carried out to determine if ovulation has, in fact, occurred. If an obstruction of the fallopian tubes is suspected, tubal patency studies are indicated. Tubal strictures or obstructions are sometimes repaired by plastic surgery, but the rates of success in restoring tubal function are very low. If ovulation is occurring, the couple may require advice concerning timing of intercourse and ovulation.

Couples who are found to be infertile are confronted with the need to make choices from among available alternatives. Remaining childless or adopting a child are the usual alternatives from which they must select. The couple needs objective guidance when making a decision, and they need to help in making a sound decision to prevent regret stemming from premature and hastily made decisions.

The couple first needs time to cope with the crisis of being told they are infertile, and they need to be permitted to handle their grief (see Chapter 19). Once the initial crisis is dealt with, the couple is better prepared to discuss alternatives. Couples who elect to remain childless need to be informed that with advancing age there is increased difficulty in adopting children, should they change their minds at a later time, but this must be done in such a way that they will not feel guilty about not wanting to adopt a child. Those couples deciding on adoption need to be presented with the facts concerning their chances of success in locating the child of their choice and the need to undergo still another long process before obtaining a child. These couples need information about reliable adoption agencies and may need help in dealing with frustration during adoption procedures. Some couples will not be successful in their attempts to adopt a child and will need help in coping with still another crisis.

Artificial insemination is an alternative in some cases of infertility. This is a highly controversial topic, surrounded by deep personal feelings, and must be approached with tact. However, infertile couples should know about this alternative and should have an opportunity to make their own decision.

Medically the procedure of aritficial insemination is simple, safe, inexpensive, and highly successful. A few drops of semen are injected into the upper portion of the cervical canal as close to the time of ovulation as possible. The major indication for artificial insemination is male infertility. Loss of children because of Rh or ABO incompatability and severe hereditary defects transmitted by the man are other indications. Therefore artificial insemination is not reserved only for infertile couples.

Artificial insemination is *homologous* when the husband's semen is used and *heterologous* when donor semen is used. Honologous insemination may be employed in cases where functional problems exist, such as failure to maintain an erection, premature ejaculation, and structural defects such as hypospadias. Heterologous insemination may be indicated in male infertility and when there is a history of hereditary disorders and blood incompatability.

Donor selection in heterologous insemination is a very important part of the procedure. Criteria for donor selection is based on semen analysis as well as on a complete history and physical examination. Donor candidates with venereal disease, diabetes, blood diseases, prostatic infection, and a family history of hereditary disorders are excluded. Fertility of donors must be proved by semen analysis. The semen should show a sperm count of over 100 million/ml, have a predominance of normal sperm forms, and have a greater than 70% sperm motility.[19]

Artificial insemination has not been widely practiced or publicized. Many people are poorly informed about it, and some people find the topic highly distressing or distasteful and refuse to discuss it. Others may not have considered artificial insemination, wish to have additional information, and welcome opportunities to discuss the subject.

■ MANAGEMENT OF SEXUAL PROBLEMS

Health practitioners have demonstrated an increased awareness of their responsibilities for providing sex education and counseling to individuals as evidenced by the recent increase of nursing literature dealing with sexual issues. Even though the literature is beginning to reflect nursing's acknowledgement of the validity of these roles, many professional education programs have not yet emphasized sexual health to the same extent as other components of health. Consequently many professionals feel unprepared for assuming the role of sex educator or counselor.

□ Scope of services for sexual health care

The report of a recent World Health Organization meeting dealing with education and treatment in human sexuality acknowledges that a variety of sexual health services are needed, ranging from education or dissemination of information to the community to intensive therapy for complex sexual dysfunctions. Participants in the conference recommended that sexual health education of the community and of other health practitioners receive first priority, as it would reach the largest number of people. Further it was indicated that sex education was not only a part of preventive medicine but also an important component in assisting persons with sexual problems. Next the group recommended that health professionals including nurses and other practitioners be able to provide counseling for individuals and couples with sexual problems. Finally, provision for sex therapy by professionals with special preparation was seen as an essential health service for those person with complex problems.

□ Prerequisites for intervention

With the scope of sexual health services in mind, it is easy to see that each level of intervention requires a slightly different professional preparation. However, three prerequisites are common to each level of intervention. First, a knowledge base is required, including an understanding of sexual response, knowledge of the variety of sexual behaviors that exist in our society and their prevalence, an understanding of the types of sexual dysfunctions, and an awareness of the relationship between age, life events, pathologic conditions, behavioral problems, pharmaceutical agents, and sexual function. Without such a knowledge base the practitioner has no basis for discriminating between normal and abnormal responses or the interruption of client's concerns, and thus no basis for education or counseling.

Although a knowledge base is essential to effective intervention, an awareness of the professional's own value system, including the biases and beliefs about appropriate and inappropriate sexual behavior, are also important. Unless the professional can accept her or his own sexuality and is comfortable with her or his own behavior, it will be difficult to convey comfort to others. Self-acceptance is seen as prerequisite to the development of a nonjudgmental and tolerant approach. Just as individuals have belief systems related to sexual phenomena, so do professionals. This does not imply that the sex educator or counselor must condone every variety of sexual activity. Rather, it is essential that they be aware of their own feelings and values and attempt to keep them in perspective by acknowledging them. This will assist them to maintain a supportive climate that encourages sharing of feeling by clients and simultaneously permits professionals to acknowledge the validity of their own beliefs.[75]

Furthermore there are some issues about which the professional has such strong beliefs that his or her own value system would interfere with effective intervention. An example encountered in practice is the health professional whose basic conviction is that homosexuality is an illness or deviation, despite the acceptance of the American Psychiatric Association that homosexuality is but one variation in sexual expression or orientation. No matter how extensive the professional's training, knowledge base, and therapy skills, such a strong basic belief is likely to greatly interfere with the ability to relate objectively to a homosexual's sexual problems. Often professionals need to acknowledge their inability to deal with sexual problems because of their own value systems. Topics likely to elicit bias among health professionals include abortion, alternative life styles such as mate swapping, and other sexual variations.

Finally, the professional needs to be able to communicate genuinely and therapeutically with clients. Often this involves using the client's own language, which may be quite different from that of the health professional. Without the ability to interact accurately and empathetically with individuals, the most sophisticated knowledge base and objective attitudes are of little benefit. A framework for developing skills supportive of sex education and counseling includes the progression from active listening techniques to sophisticated psychotherapeutic skills.

□ Prevention of sexual problems

Nurses may prevent sexual problems among client populations through three strategies: education of client groups likely to have sexual concerns, provision of anticipatory guidance throughout the life cycle, and promotion of a milieu conducive to sexual health.

Education of client populations implies more than mere dissemination of information. As in the case of educating nurses to provide sex education, clients may also need assistance in exploring the attitudes and values that shape their sexual behavior and in developing the ability to communicate comfortably about sexual phenomena. Thus providing accurate knowledge about sex and sexuality is not synonymous with education for a healthy sexuality.

Nurses are often in strategic positions to provide *anticipatory guidance* at sensitive points in the life cycle. Adolescence and middle age are two life periods during which anxiety about sexuality is likely to surface. By informing individuals about the usual changes experienced at these points (e.g., nocturnal emissions or concerns about masturbation in adolescents and worry about effects of menopause on the ability to function sexually among middle-aged persons), nurses can assist individuals to cope realistically with major changes in their bodies. Adults with young children can also benefit from anticipatory guidance regarding their childrens' sexuality.

Finally, nurses can assist individuals to *provide a milieu conducive to sexual health.* Some approaches useful in developing such a milieu include minimizing guilt experienced in conjunction with sexual thoughts, feelings, and behavior. This may be accomplished by assisting persons to examine objectively the consequences of their activities within a reality-oriented framework. Reduction of performance anxiety, that is, concern about how well one is able to function, can be facilitated by helping individuals to understand the relationship between being attentive to their own performance at the expense of losing touch with their sexual feelings. "Spectatoring" refers to the habit of watching oneself or a partner perform. Just as in athletics, one cannot be both spectator and performer without minimizing the effectiveness of the performance.

Often individuals need to be advised to modify their environments to reduce competing stimuli. Use of anxiety-provoking settings or those prone to interruption can help to establish dysfunctional patterns. (The relationship between anxiety and orgasmic dysfunction and premature ejaculation has been well established.)

Finally, maintenance of good general health facilitates optimum sexual functioning. Fatigue, pain, and malaise are stimuli that compete with sexual pleasure.

■ PROMOTION OF SEXUAL HEALTH

□ Principles for promoting sexual health

Mims[48] cites some basic principles involved in the promotion of sexual health. The first of these acknowledges that there is no single set of appropriate sexual values in our society; rather, the professional needs to accept that major conflicts of values exist. A second principle basic to promotion of sexual health is that education, that is, provision of accurate and adequate information, is more helpful than indoctrination. Although it is often tempting to impose one's own solutions to sexual concerns or a values conflict on others, growth of the individual is more likely to be fostered by guidance rather than by indoctrination. Finally, it is suggested that individuals be assisted to make their own informed choices rather than conform to guidelines established by a professional or an agency. It is the individuals, and not the health professional, who will have to cope with the consequences of their choices.

□ Levels of intervention

Annon[2] presents an extremely useful distinction between the various levels of intervention possible for persons with sexual concerns or problems. He terms these levels *permission, limited information, specific suggestions, and intensive therapy.* These are listed in order of sophistication, with permission giving requiring the most basic preparation and intensive therapy requiring specific educational preparation in sex therapy theory and techniques. Annon's contention is that sexual problems may be resolved on a variety of levels and do not always require counseling or intensive therapy.

Permission

Often individuals merely want to know that they are normal, acceptable, and not "perverted," and they seek out the health professional for validation of their sexual normalcy. Permission is not merely a therapeutic measure but also a preventive one. It can be applied in a variety of settings in the community and at social gatherings as well as in the hospital. This type of intervention requires minimal preparation on the part of the professional. Permission may be applied to thoughts, fantasies, dreams, and feelings as well as to overt sexual behaviors. At times nurses will be asked to provide individuals with permission *not* to engage in certain sexual behaviors if this is their choice. This may relieve individuals from feeling pressured to conform to someone else's standards for sexual behavior that are not necessarily their own.

Persons with disabling diseases that interfere with their usual forms of sexual expression may seek permission to discuss alternative approaches to sexual pleasure. For example, cord-injured persons may welcome the permission from staff members to discuss alternatives to penis-vagina intercourse. Women who do not experience orgasm with every act of intercourse may be seeking permission *not* to do so, even though some of their friends insist that "normal women do." The adolescent who is comparing his sexual prowess with that of peers may seek permission *not* to be sexually active. A common concern among young married couples is the normalcy of oral-genital sex. Often these couples merely seek reassurance that this variation is not perverted, or on the contrary that it is not mandatory to engage in this practice unless both partners are comfortable with it.

In summary, permission giving can help individuals break associations between behaviors, thoughts, fantasies, dreams, and labels. Usually these labels bear negative connotations such as "dirty," "perverted," or "abnormal."[2] Even though most sexual acts could be considered normal in some sense (e.g., statistically or phylogenetically), individuals do need to be aware of the consequences of their behavior. These consequences may include legal prosecution or social ostracism, and such concerns need to be explored with the individual before the counselor gives blanket permission to engage in such practices.

Limited information

The next level of intervention can also be therapeutic as well as preventive. It involves providing information to individuals that is directly relevant to their particular problems or concerns. Rather than condoning the individual's behavior, this approach may result in a change of behavior on the basis of an informed decision. Some common areas of sexual concern that may require only limited information include worry over breast and genital shape, configuration, and size; masturbation; sexual intercourse during menstruation; oral-genital sex. The counselor familiar with famous myths associated with each of these topics can appreciate that providing individuals with basic factual information regarding any of these concerns may be responsible for the resolution of their sexual worries.

A common concern among adolescent and young adult men is penis size. Giving the information that the smaller flaccid penis becomes about as large when erect as larger flaccid penises may be sufficient to relieve anxieties that interfere with sexual function. A woman who is about to have a hysterectomy is often concerned that she will no longer be able to have intercourse or that she will have no more sexual desire. Informing the woman in advance of the surgery that this is not true may remove unnecessary barriers from the resumption of sexual activity. Similar information would be helpful to a man about to undergo a prostatectomy. Even though the man having a transurethral resection is likely to experience retrograde ejaculation, he may still have an erection and enjoy intercourse. Having this bit of information prior to surgery may avert dysfunctional sex later.

In sum, providing limited information can free the individual from anxieties connected with sexual performance or assumptions about negative effects of health-illness conditions on sexual activity. Combating popular mythology with this approach is often a sufficient preventive or therapeutic measure.

Specific suggestions

Prior to giving individuals specific suggestions regarding direct attempts to help them change their behavior in order to reach a designated goal, it is essential to obtain a sexual problem history. This approach presupposes a brief approach to counseling individuals, with the understanding that if results are not achieved within a limited period referral to someone prepared to provide intensive sexual therapy will be made. Again specific suggestions may be preventive as well as therapeutic. Some specific suggestions may relate to the conditions conducive to optimum sexual functioning, specific approaches to use given certain illnesses or surgeries, and directives for coping with some sexual dysfunctions.

One specific suggestion often incorporated in sexual

EXAMPLES OF SPECIFIC SUGGESTIONS FOR PERSONS RECOVERING FROM MYOCARDIAL INFARCTION

To minimize cardiac workload:

Avoid having intercourse in either very hot or very cold rooms.

Wait about 3 hours after eating a meal or drinking alcoholic beverages.

Allow plenty of time to rest afterwards.

Explore positions that do not require you to support your own or your partner's full body weight, such as lying on your side or sitting in a chair.

Consult your health care provider if:

You have chest pain during or after intercourse.

You feel extremely tired after having intercourse.

You feel your heart beating very loudly for more than a few minutes after intercourse.

counseling is that a couple having difficulties with intercourse abstain from it for a specified period. This admonition is designed to reduce the "pressure to perform" perceived by a member of the dysfunctional couple.

The counseling approach applied to persons who have just had a myocardial infarction is outlined in the box above. These suggestions are designed to minimize the effects of cardiovascular problems during intercourse. Similar specific suggestions can be given to cord-injured persons, including positions most likely to be comfortable, care of the Foley catheter before and during intercourse, and techniques available to stimulate the noninjured partner. Use of imagery (fantasy) can also be incorporated as a specific suggestion. Ostomy patients often have concerns about accidents involving their appliances during intercourse. Specific suggestions might include emptying the appliance before initiating sexual activity, employing cosmetic covers for the stoma bag, or avoiding excess pressure over the stoma site until the ostomy incision is well healed.

Finally, nurses can offer some rather simple directives for coping with specific sexual dysfunctions. The man who is a premature ejaculator can be taught to use the "squeeze technique" (p. 1481), or the partner may learn to apply it. Women who have inadequate lubrication and experience painful intercourse as a consequence of steroid starvation during the postpartum or menopause may benefit from the use of a water-soluble lubricant such as K-Y jelly.

Intensive sexual therapy

This approach combines techniques and concepts of psychotherapy with special appraoches to intervention with individuals or couples having sexual problems. Usually the problems involved are one or more of the sexual dysfunctions discussed in Chapter 64. Since a discussion of the many approaches to intensive therapy is beyond the scope of this text, interested readers are referred to references 2, 28, 36, 42, 46. These forms of therapy usually require intensive preparation beyond that provided in most schools of nursing. However, an awareness of the sexual dysfunctions discussed in Chapter 64 will enable nurses to refer clients with complex problems to trained therapists.

□ Modalities for intervention

Several modalities exist for intervening on behalf of individuals with sexual concerns or problems. The first context in which nurses may intervene is the one-to-one relationship. Individuals may initiate questions about their sexual concerns or problems that do not require intervention with both partners. Others may not have a current partner, or a partner may be unwilling to be involved in counseling.

Often sexual issues may arise in the course of dealing with family problems. Some sexual issues may be appropriately addressed in the context of family therapy.[59] Sexual issues also may be addressed in group therapy settings where peer consultation and support are available to the individual.

Finally, sexual issues are thought to be most profitably addressed in the context of the dyad. The assumption here is that there is never an uninvolved partner in a relationship where sexual problems exist.[42]

REFERENCES AND SELECTED READINGS

1. *Ager, J. W., Werley, H. H., Allen, D. V., et al.: Vasectomy: who gets one and why, Am. J. Public Health, **64**:680-686, 1974.
2. Annon, J.: The behavioral treatment of sexual problems, Honolulu, 1974, Enabling Systems, Inc.
3. Bai, J., Greenwald, E., Caterini, H., et al.: Drug-related menstrual aberrations, Obstet. Gynecol. **44**:713-719, 1974.
4. Banner, E. A.: The menopause and thereafter, Postgrad. Med. **59**:174-178, 1976.
5. Behrman, S. J., and Kistner, R. W., editors: Progress in infertility, ed. 2, Boston, 1975, Little, Brown and Co.
6. Bernard, J.: The future of marriage, New York, 1972, World Publishing Co.
7. Boston Women's Health Book Collective: Our bodies, ourselves: a book by and for women, Boston, 1973, Simon & Shuster, Inc.
8. Bremner, W. J., and deKrester, D. M.: The prospects for new, reversible male contraception, N. Engl. J. Med. **295**:1111-1115, 1976.
9. *Cowart, M., and Newton, D. W.: Oral contraceptives: how best to explain their effects to patients, Nursing '76 **6**:44-48, 1976.
10. Cramer, D. E., Cutler, S. J., and Christine, B.: Trends in the in-

*References preceded by an asterisk are particularly well suited for student reading.

cidence of endometrial cancer in the United States, Gynecol. Oncol. **2**:130-143, 1974.

11. Davis, J. E.: Vasectomy, Am. J. Nurs. **72**:509-513, 1972.
12. Duvall, E. M.: Family development, ed. 4, Philadelphia, 1971, J. B. Lippincott Co.
13. *Effer, S.: Gynecologic aspects of the "routine" checkup, Postgrad. Med. **59**:164-170, 1976.
14. *Faulkner, W. L., and Ory, H. W.: Intrauterine devices and acute pelvic inflammatory disease, J.A.M.A. **235**:1851-1853, 1976.
15. Ferber, A. S., Tietze, C., and Lewit, C.: Men with vasectomies: a study of medical, sexual and psycho-social changes, Psychosom. Med. **29**:354-366, 1967.
16. Fleckenstein, L., Joubert, P., Lawrence, R., et al.: Oral contraceptive patient information: a questionnaire study of attitudes, knowledge and preferred information sources, J.A.M.A. **235**:1331-1336, 1976.
17. *Fleischauer, M. L.: A modified Lamaze approach in the treatment of primary dysmenorrhea, J. Am. Coll. Health Assoc. **25**:273-275, 1977.
18. Foreman, J.: Vasectomy clinic, Am. J. Nurs. **73**:819-821, 1973.
19. Garcia, C. R., and Rosenfeld, D.: Family planning, Philadelphia, 1976, F. A. Davis Co.
20. *Gilbert, S.: Artificial insemination, Am. J. Nurs. **76**:259-260, 1976.
21. Greenhill, J. P., Surgical gynecology, ed. 4, Chicago, 1969, Year Book Medical Publishers, Inc.
22. Guillebaud, J., Bonner, J., Morehead, J., et al.: Menstrual blood loss with intrauterine devices, Lancet **1**:387-390, 1976.
23. Hackett, R. E., and Waterhouse, K.: Vasectomy reviewed, Am. J. Abstet. Gynecol. **116**:438-455, 1973.
24. Hall, R. E.: The Supreme Court decision on abortion, Am. J. Obstet. Gynecol. **116**:1-8, 1973.
25. Hampton, P. T., and Tarnasky, W. G.: Hysterectomy and tubal ligation: a comparison of the psychological aftermath, Am. J. Obstet. Gynecol. **119**:949-952, 1974.
26. Heczey, M. D.: Effects of biofeedback and autogenic training on dysmenorrhea. Presented at The Menstrual Cycle: An Interdisciplinary Conference, University of Illinois, Chicago, June 27-28, 1977.
27. Houghton, B.: Vasectomies affect women, too, Am. J. Nurs. **73**:821, 1973.
28. Hulka, J. F., and Davis, J. W.: Vasectomy and reversible vasocclusion, Fertil. Steril. **23**:683-696, 1972.
29. Kaplan, H. S.: The new sex therapy, New York, 1974, Brunner/Mazel, Inc.
30. Kaufman, R. H., Reeves, K. O., and Dougherty, C. M.: Severe atypical endometrical changes and sequential contraceptive use, J.A.M.A. **236**:923-926, 1976.
31. Koetsawang, S., Bhiraleus, P., Rachawat, D., et al.: Comparison of culdoscopic and laparoscopic tubal sterilization, Am. J. Obstet. Gynecol. **124**:601-606, 1976.
32. Landesman, R., Couthino, E. M., and Saxena, B. B.: Detection of human chorionic gonadotropin in blood of regularly bleeding women using copper intrauterine contraceptive devices, Fertil. Steril. **27**:1062-1066, 1976.
33. Landesman, R., and Saxena, B. B.: Results of the first 1,000 radioreceptor assays for the determination of human chorionic gonadotropin: a new, rapid, reliable and sensitive pregnancy test, Fertil. Steril. **27**:357-368, 1976.
34. *Langer, A., Devanesan, M., Pelosi, M. A., et al.: Choice of an oral contraceptive, Am. J. Obstet, Gynecol. **126**:153-157, 1976.
35. Lindemann, C. A.: Birth control and unmarried young women, New York, 1974, Springer Publishing Co., Inc.
36. LoPiccolo, J., and Steger, J.: The sexual interaction inventory: a new instrument for assessment of sexual dysfunction, Arch. Sex. Behav. **3**:585-593, 1974.
37. Lu, T., and Chun, D.: A long-term follow-up of 1,055 cases of postpartum tubal ligation, J. Obstet. Gynecol. Br. Commonw. **74**:875-880, 1967.
38. Lyon, F. A.: The development of adenocarcinoma of the endometrium in young women receiving long-term sequential oral contraception: report of four cases, Am. J. Obstet. Gynecol. **123**:229-301, 1975.
39. Mack, T. M., Pike, M. C., Henderson, B. E., et al.: Estrogens and endometrial cancer in a retirement community, N. Engl. J. Med. **294**:1262-1267, 1976.
40. Marik, J. J., Friedman, S., and Tyler, E. T.: A simple technique of laparoscopic tubal sterilization, J. Reprod. Med. **15**:109-113, 1975.
41. Marshall, S., and Lyon, R. P.: Variablility of sperm disappearance from the ejaculate following vasectomy, J. Urol. **107**:815-817, 1972.
42. Masters, W., and Johnson, V.: Human sexual inadequacy, Boston, 1970, Little, Brown and Co.
43. McCalister, D. V., Thiessen, V., and McDermott, M.: Readings in family planning: a challenge to the health professions, St. Louis, 1973, The C. V. Mosby Co.
44. McCormick, W., and Torres, J.: A method of Pomeroy tubal ligation reanastomosis, Obstet. Gynecol. **47**:623-625, 1976.
45. Meema, H. E., and Meema, S.: Involutional (physiologic) bone loss in women and the feasibility of preventing structural failure, J. Am. Geriatr. Soc. **22**:443-452, 1974.
46. Menning, B. E.: RESOLVE: a support group for infertile couples, Am. J. Nurs. **76**:258-259, 1976.
47. Meyer, J. K., editor: Clinical management of sexual disorders, Baltimore, 1976, The Williams & Wilkins Co.
48. Mims, F.: Sexual health education and counseling, Nurs. Clin. North Am. **10**:519-528, 1975.
49. Moss, W. M.: Sutureless technique for bilateral partial vasectomy, Fertil. Steril. **23**:33-37, 1972.
50. Nathanson, C. A.: Illness and the feminine role: a theoretical review, Soc. Sci. Med. **9**:57-62, 1975.
51. Novak, E. R., and Woodruff, J. D.: Novak's gynecologic and obstetric pathology with clinical and endocrine relations, ed. 7, Philadelphia, 1974, W. B. Saunders Co.
52. Novak, E. R., Jones, G. S., and Jones, H. W., Jr.: Novak's textbook of gynecology, ed. 9, Baltimore, 1975, The Williams & Wilkins Co.
53. Ory, H., Naib, Z., Conger, S. B., et al.: Contraceptive choice and prevalence of cervical dysplasia and carcinoma in situ, Am. J. Obstet. Gynecol. **124**:573-577, 1976.
54. Peel, J., and Potts, M.: Textbook of contraceptive practice, New York, 1969, Cambridge University Press.
55. Proudfit, C. M.: Estrogens and menopause, J.A.M.A. **236**:939-940, 1976.
56. Riggs, B. L., Jowsey, J., Goldsmith, R. S., et al.: Short- and long-term effects of estrogen and synthetic anabolic hormones in postmenopausal osteoporosis, J. Clin. Invest. **51**:1659-1663, 1972.
57. Robins, J.: Failures of contraceptive practice, N.Y. State J. Med. **76**:361-365, 1976.
58. Rudel, H., et al.: Birth control: contraception and abortion, New York, 1973, Macmillan, Inc.
59. Satir, V.: Conjoint family therapy, rev. ed., Palo Alto, 1967, Science and Behavior Books, Inc.
60. Schenker, J. G., Eyal, F., and Polishuk, W. J.: Fertility after tubal pregnancy, Surg. Gynecol. Obstet. **135**:74-76, 1972.
61. Schwarta, A., Zor, U., Lindner, H., and Naor, S.: Primary

dysmenorrhea: alleviation by an inhibitor of prostaglandin synthesis and action, Obstet. Gynecol. **44**:709-712, 1974.
62. *Siegel, E., and Morris, N. M.: Family planning: its health rationale, Nurs. Digest **3**:55-57, 1975.
63. *Siegler, A. M.: Tubal sterilization, Am. J. Nurs. **72**:1624-1629, 1972.
64. Silverberg, S., and Makowski, E.: Endometrial carcinoma in young women taking oral contraceptive agents, Obstet. Gynecol. **46**:503, 505, 506, 1975.
65. Smith, D. C., Prentice, R., Thompson, D. J., et al.: Association estrogen and endometrial carcinoma, N. Engl. J. Med. **293**:1164-1167, 1975.
66. Sorensen, R.: Adolescent sexuality in contemporary America, New York, 1975, World Publishers Co.
67. Squires, J. W., Barb, M. W., and Pinch, L. W.: The morbidity of vasectomy, Surg. Gynecol. Obstet. **143**:237-240, 1976.
68. Stadel, B. V., and Weiss, N.: Characteristics of menopausal women: a survey of King and Pierce counties in Washington, 1973-1974, Am. J. Epidemiol. **102**:209-216, 1975.
69. Thompson, B., and Baird, D.: Follow-up of 186 sterilized women, Lancet **1**:1023-1027, 1968.
70. Tietze, C., Bongaarts, J., and Schearer, B.: Mortality associated with the control of fertility, Fam. Plann. Perspect. **8**:6-14, 1976.
71. *Timby, B. K.: Ovulation method of birth control, Am. J. Nurs. **76**:928-929, 1976.
72. Ulfelder, H.: The stilbestrol-adenosis-carcinoma syndrome, Cancer **38** (Suppl.):426-431, July 1976.
73. Umezaki, C., Katayama, K. P., and Jones, H. W., Jr.: Pregnancy rates after reconstructive surgery on the fallopian tubes, Obstet. Gynecol. **43**:418-424, 1974.
74. U.S. Department of Health, Education and Welfare, Public Health Service: VD fact sheet, ed. 32, DHEW No. (CDC) 76-8195, Atlanta, Center for Disease Control.
75. Woods, J. S.: Drug effects on human sexual behavior. In Woods, N. F.: Human sexuality in health and illness, ed. 2, St. Louis, 1979, The C. V. Mosby Co.

AUDIOVISUAL RESOURCES

1. Communicating family planning: speak, they are listening. Motion picture, Media Resources Branch, National Medical Ausiovisual Center (Annex), Station K, Atlanta, Ga. 30324.
2. Infertility and sterility. Motion picture or audiotape and slides, The American Journal of Nursing Co., Educational Services Division, 10 Columbus Circle, New York, N.Y. 10019.
3. The nurse's role in family planning. Film strip, The American Journal of Nursing Co., Educational Services Division, 10 Columbus Circle, New York, N.Y. 10019.

62

Reproductive problems

ELLA CINKOTA

Although men and women are better informed today about matters relating to reproductive health, they still tend to neglect preventive aspects, and some seek assistance only when signs of illness appear. As professionals and lay people become more enlightened about prevention of problems of the genital tract, there is heightened awareness of the importance of illness prevention and health promotion throughout the life span.

In spite of advances in medicine, science, and technology, diseases and disorders of the genital system continue to threaten the lives and the physical and emotional health of men and women. Many of these problems are preventable. Many of them can be treated and cured. Some are neither preventable nor curable. Nurses occupy a unique position in that their daily contacts with men and women provide opportunities to actively seek out persons in need of information and other forms of help. Assisting people to find answers to their questions, to seek solutions to their problems, and to increase their awareness of health-promoting measures are within the province of nursing.

■ INFECTIONS OF THE VULVA AND VAGINA

□ Epidemiology

Although the vulva and vagina are considered to be relatively resistant to infection, inflammation and localized infection are quite common. Many organisms play a causative role, including streptococci, staphylococci, *Pseudomonas, Escherichia coli, Candida albicans, Trichomonas vaginalis, Treponema pallidum,* and *Neisseria gonorrhoeae.* Normally the vagina is protected from infection by its acidity and the presence of Döderlein's bacilli. If the vaginal pH is elevated, the invading organisms are numerous, or the woman's resistance is decreased by aging, malnutrition, disease, emotional disturbances, or the use of drugs that alter properties of the tissues, infection may result.

Organisms causing infection of the vulva and vagina are most often introduced from outside sources such as clothing, hands, douche nozzles or other contaminated articles, or during intercourse. In sexually active women, reinfection may occur following treatment unless the sex partner is also treated.

Nonspecific vaginitis

Nonspecific vaginitis is a superficial vaginal infection variously referred to as *Haemophilus vaginalis* or *Corynebacterium vaginale.* The final determination of the name of the causative organism has not been made. The possible venereal transmission of this type of vaginitis is currently under study.

Corynebacterium vaginale is characterized by a small amount of homogenous gray or grayish-white discharge. The discharge usually has a disagreeable odor, and since it is less irritating than discharges caused by other organisms, pruritus is mild or absent. On inspection, the vaginal walls are slightly reddened and the discharge appears to adhere to the mucosal lining. Diagnosis is confirmed by microscopic examination of a smear or culture of the vaginal discharge. Treatment consists of oral ampicillin given 4 times a day for 7 to 10 days and is usually effective. Sulfonamide vaginal tablets or creams may be prescribed and are said to be "possibly effective."[75] Some physicians recommend treating the patient's sexual partner at the same time.

Senile vaginitis

Also called atrophic vaginitis, senile vaginitis most often occurs in women of menopausal and postmenopausal ages. Pyogenic bacterial invasion of the thin, atrophied vaginal mucosa produces symptoms of burning, pruritus, and leukorrhea. Senile vaginitis usually treated with warm douches of a weak acid solution such as vinegar (15 ml [1 tablespoon] to 1 liter [1 quart] of water). Estrogenic preparations, given orally or applied intravaginally as an ointment, may help to restore the vaginal epithelium to a normal state.

Bartholinitis

Invasion of Bartholin's glands by streptococci, staphylococci, gonococci, or *E. coli* may result in infection. The infection is usually unilateral but may be bilateral. With infection the duct from the gland becomes partially or completely obstructed, resulting in severe redness, enlargement of the gland, and edema of the surrounding tissues. The area becomes tender, and even walking may become difficult because of the pain. Sometimes the abscess that forms ruptures and affords almost immediate relief of pain. Most often, however, this is followed by recurrence of symptoms. The usual course of the infectious process results in an abscess that does not rupture and requires surgical incision and drainage. A smear or culture is usually taken to identify the causative organism, and an appropriate antibiotic is prescribed.

Occasionally acute bartholinitis subsides, leaving fibrotic or scar tissue. When this occurs a Bartholin's cyst develops. The cyst may vary in size from a few centimeters in diameter to the size of a hen's egg, is mobile, and is not tender. If the cyst grows to be of sufficient size as to interfere with walking or intercourse, or if it shows signs of inflammation, it may be excised surgically.

Skene's glands are less often infected than are Bartholin's glands. When infection does occur, the local symptoms include redness, enlargement of the gland, tenderness, and accumulation of pus. These also may spontaneously rupture or require incision and drainage. Identification of the causative organism by smear or culture is important in determining the need for antibiotic therapy. Infections proven to be or strongly suspected of being sexually transmitted are discussed in the section on venereal diseases.

□ Prevention

Recognition of predisposing factors is important in the prevention of vulvar and vaginal infections. Following are risk factors associated with vulvar and vaginal infections:

1. Pregnancy
2. Premenarchal age
3. Menopausal and postmenopausal status
4. Allergies
5. Diabetes
6. Oral contraceptives
    a. Inadequate hygiene
    b. Excessive douching or use of vaginal inserts
    c. Intercourse with an infected partner

Those in whom the natural barriers to infection (low estrogen levels, thinness of the vaginal epithelium, or reduced acidity of the vagina) are at a minimum are at greatest risk.

Some women may require instruction in daily health and hygiene practices. Women also may need to know the characteristics of normal vaginal discharges and how to distinguish between these and abnormal discharges. They need to be informed of the other signs of vaginal and vulvar infections and the particular significance of lesions on the vulva. Sexually active women may require information about how to recognize signs of infection in their partners and the importance of seeking medical attention when they suspect the partner is infected. Pregnant and diabetic women need to know about their predisposition to infections and how to prevent infection from occurring, and they need to be urged to seek professional help as soon as signs of infection develop.

□ Clinical picture

The patient is asked to give a detailed account of her symptoms, including duration and what she has done to relieve them. The history should include sexual practices and information about signs of infection in the sex partner. The history and physical examination may reveal predisposing factors, patterns of repeated infections, or evidence of concurrent problems. In such cases, further examination, laboratory tests, or clinical studies may be indicated.

The vulva and vagina are inspected and palpated (Chapter 60). A smear or culture is taken from the vagina, and a Pap smear may also be taken. Palpation of the internal organs of reproduction will determine whether upward extension of infection has occurred.

The common signs of infection of the vulva and vagina are inflammation of the tissues, abnormal discharge from the vagina, urethra, or Bartholin's glands, and itching (pruritus). The discharge may be purulent, white, and curdlike, or grayish white. *Leukorrhea*, a white vaginal discharge, is a symptom of vaginal infections, but it is also associated with erosions of the cervix. This discharge differs from the normal vaginal discharge occurring just before menstruation in that it is more abundant, thicker, and is associated with inflammation and pruritus. Pruritus is a symptom rather than a disease. In addition to infection, severe itching may be present because of menopausal changes in the epithelium, vitamin A deficiency, irritation from chronic discharge, high urinary sugar content as in diabetes mellitus, pediculosis pubis, scabies, allergies, and cancer of the vulva. With severe pruritus there are usually excoriations of the skin caused by scratching and secondary infection may result.

Lesions of various types may be seen on the vulva, between the labial folds, or inside the vagina. These may appear as macules, papules, boils, abscesses, or eroded areas. Skene's or Bartholin's glands may be enlarged because of accumulation of pus.

□ Intervention

Since most women having vulvar and vaginal infections are treated on an outpatient basis, it is imperative that they be actively involved in decisions and plans related to therapy.

A variety of methods are available for management

and treatment of vulvar and vaginal infections. The major goals are to cure the infection, prevent reinfection, and prevent complications associated with infections of the reproductive tract.

Abscesses require incision and drainage, and this is usually done at the time the woman first seeks medical attention. Antibiotics may be given if gonorrhea or systemic effects of another infection are present. The woman needs to be advised to expect a small amount of purulent drainage that may be slightly tinged with blood and to report any active, bright red bleeding promptly. Relief from pain occurs almost immediately following incision and drainage. The woman may experience soreness or mild pain for about a day. Perineal irrigations serve the purposes of cleansing and giving comfort. Nurses can suggest that women use warm water to cleanse the the involved area after each voiding or bowel movement.

Douching (p. 1389) is frequently prescribed for treatment of vaginal infections, but is contraindicated in pregnancy. Local applications in the form of vaginal suppositories, ointments, or creams are commonly employed when vaginal infection occurs. A model of the pelvis is of great value in showing women how to use these preparations. The woman is advised of the importance of handwashing before and after each application. Because the substances used melt with body heat, the patient is advised to lie down after insertion to facilitate distribution of the medication in the vaginal canal and to prevent loss of medication from the vagina.

Most of the suppositories, creams, and ointments used contain an antibiotic or a drug specific to the causative organism. Estrogenic preparations are sometimes prescribed. All of these medications are considered safe and rarely produce side effects or local reactions. The patient is cautioned, however, to report aggravation of any symptoms or appearance of symptoms not previously noted.

Heat increases circulation, promotes healing, and provides comfort. Applications of heat may be prescribed in the form of hot soaks, douches, perineal irrigations, or sitz baths. The patient may require instruction in any of these procedures. If both heat and local applications of medications are prescribed, the patient is instructed to use the medication after application of heat.

Most women with vaginal infections are advised to abstain from intercourse during the period of treatment. The extent to which abstinence is possible should be explored, and if this is not feasible for the woman, use of a condom by the male partner until symptoms of infection disappear can be suggested.

Women taking oral contraceptives should be carefully screened and examined during interim visits for signs of vaginal infection. If repeated episodes of infection occur, it may be necessary for the patient to try an alternate brand of the Pill. If infections continue, it usually becomes necessary for the woman to use an entirely different method of birth control.

When pruritus is present, the patient needs to know that any irritation such as scratching can aggravate the itching and predispose to secondary infection. Frequent bathing, sitz baths, and careful cleansing are essential for comfort as well as prevention of complcations. Soothing lotions are sometimes prescribed to relieve itching. If the pruritus is severe enough to interfere with sleep, the physician may prescribe a mild sedative.

All patients need to know when to return for follow-up and what steps to take in preparation for examination at the time of the return visit (Chapter 60).

Women need to know what observations to make regarding success of treatment and what signs to report indicating problems.

☐ Outcome criteria for the woman with a vulvar or vaginal infection

The woman can:

1. Demonstrate an increase in knowledge about her body and promoting her health.
2. Practice habits that improve or promote her health.
3. Describe how infections occur and are spread.
4. Identify ways to prevent reinfection.
5. State how changes in daily practices influence control of infection.

When the women must employ therapies at home, she should be able to:

1. State the limitations imposed by the infection and self-care activities.
2. Describe a realistic schedule of therapy and necessary modifications of daily living.
3. Cite alternative ways in which the needs of family members can be met.

When women who have vulvar or vaginal infections are presented with alternatives of therapy, they will be able to:

1. State reasons for their choice of therapy.
2. Describe the rationale and expected results of the treatment.
3. Describe use and methods of cleaning and storing special equipment, if such is required.

■ CERVICITIS

Infection of the cervix is known as cervicitis. The gonococcus, streptococcus, staphylococcus, and a variety of other aerobic and anaerobic organisms may be responsible for the infection. There are two forms of cervicitis: acute and chronic. *Chronic cervicitis* is the most frequent of all the pathologic conditions of the cervix.[65] Cervicitis usually progresses from the acute to the chronic form if not treated, and it may go undetected for a long period of time. This condition presents few symptoms, and those symptoms occurring do not ordinarily lead women to seek medical attention. Leukorrhea may be the only sign, and if it is small in amount, the woman may not become concerned. Pain does not usually occur unless the infection extends upward, involving the uterus or adjacent pelvic structures. A long history of leukorrhea may lead the nurse or physician to suspect cervicitis.

Cervicitis may follow childbirth or abortion, or it may be caused by infection of a cervical laceration or erosion. In untreated cervicitis the tissues are constantly irritated, and there is some evidence that this irritation predisposes to cancer.[44]

□ Prevention

If the practice of careful examination 6 weeks postpartum were adhered to, and if women presented themselves for yearly examination, much acute and chronic cervicitis could be prevented.

During childbirth the cervix is frequently lacerated as it stretches and thins to allow the baby to pass through the birth canal. These torn surfaces do not always heal properly and thus serve as foci for infection. At the examination made 6 weeks following delivery, improperly healed lacerations of the cervix and cervical erosions can be easily detected and treated.

Prompt detection and treatment of infections of the vulva and vagina can prevent upward spread of infection resulting in cervicitis. The preventive aspects discussed under infection of the vulva and vagina are applicable to prevention of cervical infections. Opportunities similarly arise for teaching women about desirable health habits and prescribed therapy.

□ Clinical picture

Acute cervicitis may be present without subjective symptoms. When inspected, however, the cervix is grossly erythematous and edematous, and the mucosa around the external os is everted. There is usually a mucoid, purulent discharge from the cervix; but the amount may be so small it is not noticed by the patient. A smear or culture of the discharge is taken to determine the causative organism.

Chronic cervicitis is a common cause of leukorrhea. On examination, a laceration or eversion of the cervix may be seen. Purulent discharge from the cervix is common, and erythema and hypertrophy of the cervix are usually present. Inclusion cysts, appearing as gray or white vesicles, may be seen on the surface of the cervix. A reddened, irritated area (an erosion) may or may not be present.

A Pap smear or cervical biopsy is frequently taken when patients have cervicitis. This is usually done as a precautionary measure to rule out malignancy.

□ Intervention

Acute cervicitis can usually be adequately treated with hot douches and local antibiotics. Antibiotics may be given orally or parenterally. In chronic cervicitis the infection has extended deeper into the tissues, and the patient must be hospitalized for at least one day for conization of the cervix (Chapter 60).

When cervical lacerations or erosions are present, the area is usually cauterized. Silver nitrate sticks may be used for very small lesions. For larger areas requiring cauterization, an electric cautery unit is used. The patient is informed that a small, lubricated sheet of lead will be placed against the skin under the lumbar areas as a safety device for grounding electrical charges and that there will be slight bleeding, which will be controlled by a tampon or packing that will be inserted by the physician. The odor of burning tissue when a cautery is used is distressing to some patients. They should be told to expect an odor but that the odor is insignificant and that the procedure is over quickly.

Following cauterization the nurse can ascertain that the patient understands instructions for follow-up care. Directions will vary, but they usually include the following:

1. Leave the tampon or packing in place as long as the physician advises (usually 8 to 24 hours).
2. Report to the hospital or physician's office if bleeding is excessive. (More than occurs during a normal menses is considered excessive.)
3. Do not use a douche or have sexual relations until the next visit to the physician unless specific instructions have been given as to when intercourse can be safely resumed.
4. An unpleasant discharge caused by sloughing of destroyed cells may appear 4 to 5 days following cauterization. A warm bath several times a day will help this condition, which should not last more than a few days.

Additional opportunities for teaching and counseling may arise during the course of treatment for cervicitis.

■ PELVIC INFLAMMATORY DISEASE

Pelvic inflammatory disease (PID) is an infectious process involving the fallopian tubes, ovaries, pelvic peritoneum, pelvis veins or pelvic connective tissue. The infection may be confined to one structure or it may be widespread and involve all of the pelvic structures. Inflammation of the fallopian tube is known as *salpingitis* and inflammation of the ovary is known as *oophoritis.*

The routes of pelvic infection are shown in Fig. 62-1. Despite advances in venereal disease control, detection,

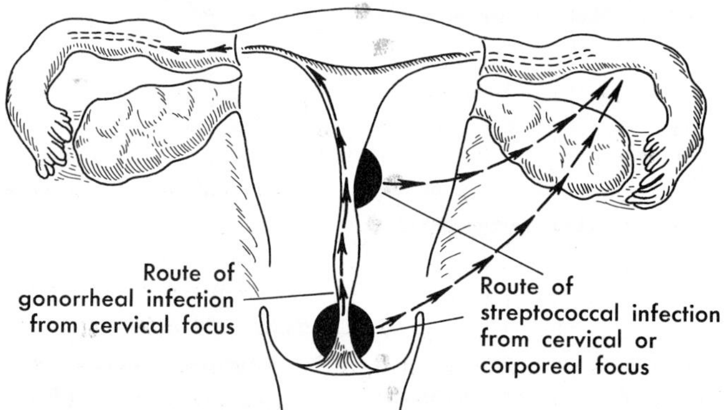

Fig. 62-1. Two chief routes of pelvic infection. (From Novak, E. R., Jones, G. J., and Jones, H. W., Jr.: Novak's textbook of gynecology, ed. 9, © 1975 The Williams & Wilkins Co., Baltimore.)

and treatment, the gonococcus remains the most common causative organism. In addition to sexual intercourse, pathogens may invade the pelvic organs during childbirth or the postpartum period, or when an abortion is done. The rupture of any adjacent structure may spill organisms into the pelvic cavity, producing secondary infection. For example, when the appendix perforates, pelvic peritonitis may follow. Pelvic inflammatory disease is reported to occur five times more often among women using intrauterine devices for birth control than among women using other methods.[25]

Pathogenic organisms are usually introduced from the outside and pass up the cervical canal into the uterus. They seem to cause little trouble in the uterus but pass into the pelvis by way of the fallopian tubes, through thrombosed uterine veins, or through the lymphatics of the uterus. The structures invaded become involved in an acute or chronic inflammatory process. Many of the pathogens causing PID lodge in the fallopian tubes. Purulent material collects in the tubes, adhesions form, strictures may occur, and sterility is a frequent result. Infertility is one of the most serious consequences of PID. Obstruction of the fallopian tubes because of the results of inflammation may be complete or partial. Complete obstruction of the tubes makes conception impossible. Partial tubal obstruction predisposes the woman to ectopic pregnancy, since the fertilized ovum cannot reach the uterus even though the sperm has been able to pass the stricture and produce conception. Adhesions resulting from inflammation may cause such distress that complete removal of the uterus, fallopian tubes, and ovaries may be necessary. Although generalized peritonitis can occur, the infection usually remains confined to the lower abdomen and pelvis. An abscess in the cul-de-sac of Douglas is common.

Women using oral contraceptives are predisposed to vaginal infections, and those using intrauterine devices are at higher risk of developing PID. These women need to be urged to present themselves for regular checkups for signs of infection as well as other problems. Instruction in prevention of infection and signs of infection is important.

□ Prevention

The potential destructive effects of PID on the reproductive organs, coupled with the prevalence of gonorrhea, should mobilize every nurse to engage in case finding for the purpose of education. To prevent PID and its serious consequences it is important to prevent infections of the vulva, vagina, and cervix, and to treat these infections promptly when they do occur. Knowing the factors that predispose women to PID is important in identification of the population at risk.

Hospitalized women usually have decreased resistance and need protection against infection. Gynecologic disorders of long duration are especially debilitating. Surgery of the reproductive tract, childbearing, and abortion lower resistance and provide portals of entry for organisms. Cleanliness and asepsis are important in giving care to these women, and every attempt should be made to prevent introduction of organsims into the reproductive tract.

Every sexually active woman having a physical examination should have a routine cervical smear or culture taken to screen for gonorrhea. Women need to be informed of methods of preventing infection, how to recognize infection in their sexual partners, and what to do when they suspect infection has occurred.

□ Clinical picture

Signs and symptoms of acute PID include severe abdominal pain, pelvic pain, malaise, nausea and vomiting, and fever with leukocytosis. There may be a foul-smelling purulent vaginal discharge. These symptoms last for a variable period of time. If they are mild and the woman ignores them, the symptoms may temporarily subside. Some cases of acute PID never reach the attention of a nurse or physician.

Chronic pelvic inflammatory disease is generally considered to be a result of undiagnosed, inadequately treated, or neglected acute PID. This type of pelvic inflammation is characterized by chronic, dull, aching pain in the lower abdomen, backache, constipation, malaise, low-grade fever, and disturbances of menstruation. During periods of exacerbation, acute symptoms return. Occasionally a patient may be considered neurotic because of the repeated, nonspecific nature of her complaints. The diagnosis of PID may be made when the patient seeks medical care for another problem, such as menstrual irregularity or infertility.

Abdominal palpation usually reveals the presence of pain and tenderness in the lower abdomen and lower quadrants. Most often, *both* lower quadrants are painful on palpation. On vaginal examination, the pain and tenderness increase because of movability of the pelvic organs. Masses may be felt in either one or both quadrants, indicating enlargement of the fallopian tubes or ovaries or an abscess. A mass may be palpated in the cul-de-sac of Douglas when abscess formation occurs in this site. If adhesions are present, the pelvic organs may be less movable than is normal.

Smears and cultures taken from the vagina, cervix, or cul-de-sac of Douglas may aid in identification of the causative organism and its sensitivity to antibiotics. Culdoscopy is usually done when an abscess in the cul-de-sac is suspected. If an abscess is seen, a specimen is secured by aspiration. Laparoscopy has gained popularity in diagnosis of PID, since it permits visualization of the reproductive organs and adjacent tissues.

□ Intervention

Patients having PID are usually hospitalized because of the intensive antibiotic therapy required. They are placed on bed rest in mid-Fowler's position to provide dependent drainage so that abscesses will not form high in the abdomen, where they might rupture and cause generalized peritonitis. Antibiotics are the drugs of choice in treating pelvic inflammatory disease. Intravenous fluids may be indicated.

Heat applied to the abdomen, either a hot water bottle or electric heating pad, may be ordered to improve circulation and provide comfort. Analgesics may be necessary for pain. During hospitalization the patient should be observed for increase or decrease in pain and change in the amount, color, consistency, and odor of any vaginal discharge. The temperature is taken every 4 hours until fever subsides.

Salpingectomy may be necessary in the event of tubal abscess, and all of the reproductive organs may require removal in severe cases of chronic inflammation. Surgery of the reproductive organs is discussed later in this chapter (p. 1435).

□ Outcome criteria for the woman with early pelvic inflammatory disease

The woman can:

1. Describe the potentially undesirable effects of such infections on her general health and functioning of the reproductive organs.
2. Participate in the program of care by carrying out prescribed self-care measures.
3. Describe how organisms gain entry to the reproductive organs and how infection can spread by continuity of tissue.
4. State the signs indicating improvement or lack of response to therapy.
5. Seek health care when problems of care and therapy arise.
6. If treated on an outpatient basis, the woman should be able to:
   a. Order her activities based on priorities.
   b. Present plans for modification in daily activities to provide for self-care requirements.

■ PUERPERAL INFECTION

Puerperal (postpartum) infection refers to infections of the reproductive organs and pelvic tissues that occur following childbirth or a spontaneous or induced abortion. Most often the uterus (as in endometritis) is the organ involved. Infection is most often caused by streptococci. The usual route for infection is through the vagina and cervix, but patients delivered by cesarean section also develop puerperal infection.

With improved obstetrics and availability of antibiotics, deaths from puerperal infection have declined markedly during this century. However, despite these advances, the incidence of puerperal infection has not decreased during the past 20 years. Because of the varying criteria used to diagnose puerperal infection, the reported incidence ranges between 1% and 8% of all deliveries.[32] Postpartum infections continue to rank among the three leading causes of mortality in obstetrics.

□ Prevention

Prevention of infection has become a major goal in the management of pregnant and newly delivered women. Women at risk for postpartum infection include those who have poor nutrition, develop obstetric complications during the childbearing cycle, have prolonged labor, have premature rupture of the membranes, are delivered by cesarean section, have chronic diseases, have preexisting infection of the reproductive tract, and who are delivered without the benefit of aseptic technique. In addition to good nutrition, adequate rest and exercise, and treatment of preexisting infection, antibiotics are given to prevent infection in women who are at risk.

□ Clinical picture

Fever, cramping or dull pain in the lower abdomen, pain and tenderness on palpation of the abdomen over the uterus, foul-smelling vaginal discharge (lochia), and malaise are characteristic signs of puerperal infection.

□ Intervention

When signs of infection appear, the woman is placed on bed rest, fluids are urged, infusions may be given, and antibiotic therapy is instituted. It is still common practice in many hospitals to separate infected mothers from other patients and from the newborn infant to prevent spread of infection. The psychologic aspect of mother-infant adaptation and the effects of separating mothers and newborn infants are discussed in specialized texts.

Because of short hospitalization following delivery and abortion, signs of infection may not appear until after the patient is discharged. Therefore patients need to be informed of the signs indicating puerperal infection, and they should be advised to contact the physician if such signs appear. To prevent infection following discharge, women should be instructed in self-care, including perineal irrigation, expected changes in the lochia, rest, nutrition, and exercise, and the importance of having an examination in the postpartum period.

■ ABORTION

The obstetric and legal definition of abortion is termination of a pregnancy before the twenty-eighth week of gestation (viability). There is consensus that viability means that a state of development exists that, theoretically, is compatible with survival outside of the uterus. Argument continues, however, as to when viability actually occurs. The definition used in reporting perinatal statistics is that fetal weight of 400 g or less constitutes an abortion.

There are several types of abortion, which are usually classified as follows:

1. Spontaneous abortions
   a. Threatened abortion
   b. Inevitable abortion
   c. Incomplete abortion
   d. Complete abortion
   e. Missed abortion
   f. Habitual abortion
2. Induced abortions
   a. Therapeutic (legal) abortion
   b. Criminal abortion

□ Spontaneous abortions

Spontaneous abortions result from "natural" causes, that is, without the aid of mechanical or medicinal intervention. Estimates of the incidence of spontaneous abortions range from 10% to 20% of all pregnancies. The wide range of estimate is partially due to the belief that many women may experience an abortion without ever being aware conception had occurred. These women probably have very minor symptoms that they do not recognize as signs of an abortion and that do not require hospitalization.

It is known that a large number of embryos spontaneously aborted in the first 12 weeks of gestation are abnormal. In addition to defective embryos, an intrauterine environment that is not adequate for sustaining embryonic and fetal development may result from inadequate nutrition, injuries and anomalies of the reproductive tract, endocrine disorders, and acute and chronic illnesses. For the past 30 years the incompetent cervix has been considered a cause of abortions occurring during the second trimester of pregnancy, usually between 14 and 16 weeks. The etiology of diminished resistance of the internal cervical os to the increasing weight of the embryo is unknown. Both congenital and tramatic causes have been implicated. There is increasing evidence that women having repeated induced abortions are predisposed to incompetent cervix with future pregnancies.[7,99]

Spontaneous abortions are classified according to a sequence of progression of severity of symptoms. Medical or surgical intervention at any point in the sequence may alter the progression. In threatened abortion the process has presumably started, as evidenced by vaginal bleeding or spotting, minor cramping from uterine contractions, and mild backache. The cervix has not started to dilate, and the process may or may not respond to treatment. Management consists of bed rest and evaluation of the effects of blood loss. Mild sedatives and progesterone may be prescribed in an attempt to conserve the pregnancy.

In an inevitable abortion the process has progressed so far that it is impossible to salvage the pregnancy. The symptoms include copious vaginal bleeding, rupture of the amniotic sac, severe abdominal cramping, and dilatation of the cervix. Supportive treatment consists of bed rest, monitoring for effects of blood loss, blood transfusion as indicated, and medications for relief of pain. Medical intervention may take a variety of forms, depending on the patient's general condition. The process may be permitted to terminate spontaneously and be followed by a dilatation and curettage. Oxytocin may be administered to hasten the process and to decrease blood loss, and this may be followed by a dilatation and curettage, or a dilatation and curettage may be performed first with oxytocin administered concomitantly.

An incomplete abortion is one in which part of the products of conception (usually the embryo) is expelled and part is retained. There is abdominal pain from uterine contractions. Vaginal bleeding is usually moderate to heavy and continues until all the retained products are passed spontaneously or are removed by dilatation and curettage. Oxytocic drugs are administered to control blood loss, and transfusion may be required.

When all of the products of conception are expelled spontaneously, a complete abortion has occurred. Bleeding is usually minimal, but oxytocic drugs may be given and a dilatation and curettage performed as precautionary management.

A missed abortion is one in which the products of conception are not spontaneously expelled after embryonic death occurs. The term is usually applied when at least 2 months elapse between embryonic death and expulsion. The uterus fails to increase in size, and the changes anticipated with advancing pregnancy do not appear. There is some difference of opinion regarding management of the patient when the diagnosis is made. Some physicians feel that it is better to wait for spontaneous abortion to follow. Infection and hemorrhage are rare, but the idea of "carrying a dead baby" is distressing to many women. Occasionally hypofibrinogenemia may occur as a consequence of entry into the maternal circulation of thromboplastin from the uterus and placenta. For this reason as well as for the resulting emotional stress, many physicians believe the uterus should be evacuated as soon as possible. This may be accomplished by different methods, depending on the period of gestation reached when embryonic death occurs. If it is less than 12 weeks, a dilatation and curettage may be performed, or the abortion process may be induced with oxytocin. Induction with oxytocin may be carried out after the twelfth week.

Habitual abortion refers to a condition in which spontaneous abortion occurs in three or more consecutive pregnancies. The causes are similar to those stated for spontaneous abortion. Treatment is dependent on the point in the abortive process reached and on determining the causative factors.

Prevention

Application of knowledge of the factors predisposing women to spontaneous abortion and educating women at an early age regarding desirable health habits can assist in preventing spontaneous abortions. Establishing a healthful intrauterine environment and maintaining such an environment must begin in the years before childbearing is undertaken. Good nutrition, prevention of illness and disease, prompt prenatal care, and remaining under supervision during pregnancy all increase the chance of successful childbearing.

Assisting couples to select a method of contraception other than abortion after two or more abortions have been done may decrease the changes of development of incompetent cervix.

During the prenatal period, it is important for women to seek prompt prenatal care, remain under care of a nurse or physician, and to follow advice about self-care. Women need to be advised of the signs of abortion and the need to contact the physician immediately. Hospitalization is necessary if attempts are to be made to conserve the pregnancy.

Women having three or more consecutive spontaneous abortions should be carefully screened and followed during subsequent pregnancies to establish a diagnosis of incompetent cervix. At the present time, most experts agree that a positive diagnosis is best made by the finding of progressive, painless cervical dilatation with bulging of the membranes through the cervix after the twelfth week of pregnancy in a woman with a history of repeated abortions. In some cases the diagnosis is confirmed at a time when cervical dilatation has progressed to the extent that it is not possible to prevent abortion. Once the diagnosis is made, however, surgical intervention is highly successful in preventing future spontaneous abortions.

The surgery consists of closing the internal os of the cervix by suturing in a purse-string (drawstring) fashion. Shirodkar's procedure, MacDonald's procedure, and Barker's procedure refer to the surgery performed; the techniques used are similar to each other. Timing of the surgery is debated, and there are proponents[48] of the interim repair (repair of the cervix between pregnancies) and proponents[4] of the more usual repair during pregnancy.

There is a need for standardization in selecting patients for surgery and for evaluating the results of surgery performed at different times. A scoring system using five criteria for cervical cerclage has been suggested.[7] To apply the scoring system, a value of 1 is given for each criterion met by the patient. The patient receives a total score of between 1 and 5. It is reported that as the total score increases, the average number of weeks between surgery and delivery increases; that is, the higher the score the better are the chances of successful surgery. The scoring system also has prognostic value in predicting the outcome of future pregnancies.

Clinical picture

In order to determine treatment required, it is necessary to determine the extent to which the abortive process has progressed. A menstrual history is taken to estimate the duration of pregnancy. The time of onset of symptoms, the amount and type of vaginal discharge, and the degree, duration, and site of pain are assessed. If clots are passed, they should be saved for examination to determine whether they contain embryonic or placental tissue. The vital signs are taken to estimate effects of blood loss. A vaginal examination may or may not be done to determine the extent of cervical dilatation. In general , the greater the blood loss, pain, and cervical dilatation, the less chance there is of salvaging the pregnancy.

The patient's psychologic response must also be assessed in order that emotional support can be given. Many women, especially those experiencing repeated disappointments because of spontaneous abortion and those highly motivated to have a baby, experience feelings of guilt and tend to associate the abortion with some forbidden event or act. They require factual information about the causes of abortion. During the abortion process, women are more concerned with the present rather than the future and their ability to bear children. Therefore emphasis should be placed on what is happening and what the woman can do to help herself at the present time.

Intervention

The treatments for various types of spontaneous abortion have been discussed previously. In general, the earlier in the process the woman is treated, the better are the chances of conserving the pregnancy. Assisting women to cope with the crisis of loss of a pregnancy is important for their emotional health. Opportunities for counseling individuals and couples about family planning and desirable health practices often arise.

Outcome criteria for the woman having a spontaneous abortion

1. The woman treated on an outpatient basis can:
   a. Identify how her usual activities will need to be modified in order to follow advice and instructions.
   b. Determine alternatives for meeting the needs of other family members when necessary.
2. The woman treated at home can state and recognize the signs of progression or regression of the abortion process and give information related to the signs.
3. The woman hospitalized for spontaneous abortion can:
   a. Explain the medical and nursing plans of care.
   b. Take measures to restrict activity and reduce stress.
   c. State the chances for successful treatment and alternatives necessary if treatment is not successful.
4. The woman who has completed the abortion process will recognize her loss and her need to grieve. She will:
   a. Identify supportive persons in her environment.
   b. Seek help from appropriate people.
   c. Be able to discuss how the abortion came about.
   d. Begin to resolve any feelings of guilt.
   e. Decide when she wishes to undertake another pregnancy.
   f. Select a method of preventing pregnancy until the desired time for conception.
5. Upon discharge from the hospital the woman can:
   a. State what modifications in activities and health practices are required, the signs of complications, and the need to report them.
   b. State when she is expected to return for a follow-up visit and the purposes of such visits.

□ Induced abortions

The topics of therapeutic and criminal abortion have received great attention for hundreds of years. Volumes have been written about these types of abortions, ranging from medical aspects to legal, sociologic, psychologic, moral, and economic aspects.

Criminal abortion refers to termination of pregnancy without legal justification. Usually such abortions are either self-induced or performed by nonprofessionals outside of hospitals and clinics. Estimates of the number of criminal abortions range from 500,000 to 1,500,000 per year. The availability of elective abortion services seems to have reduced the use of illegal abortions. This is partly reflected by the decreased numbers of women being admitted to hospitals with symptoms of sepsis resulting from criminally induced abortions.[39]

Attempts to bring about a criminal abortion are generally made by ingestion of quinine, douching with soap and water, or inserting lye or potassium permanganate crystals into the vagina. These rarely act as abortifacients. Instead, they can cause serious toxicity, local trauma, and may even result in death. Insertion of foreign bodies such as catheters, knitting needles, and metal coat hangers into the uterus is another common method by which abortions are attemtped. While these are more effective, they are attended by highly serious consequences including perforation of the uterus, hemorrhage, infection, permanent infertility resulting from infection, and death from blood loss or infection.

Whether induced abortions should or could be prevented remains a question open to personal opinion and considerable debate. In the United States the legality of abortions and the circumstances under which they might be justifiably performed by physicians became a major area of controversy by 1968, and by 1972 the legality and morality of abortions had assumed extremely unclear aspects. On January 22, 1973, the United States Supreme Court, in an unprecedented action, reached a decision regarding legalization of abortions. It ruled that a state could not intervene in the abortion decision between a woman and her physician during the first 12 weeks of pregnancy.[81] Although the Supreme Court did not take the position that a woman has an absolute right to abortion regardless of period of gestation or individual circumstances, its decision regarding the first trimester renders all previous original and reform laws unconstitutional.

The major ground for the Supreme Court decision is based on personal liberty provided by the Fourteenth Amendment to the Constitution. In essence this means the woman has a right to privacy and includes the right to decide whether to terminate her pregnancy.

Not all the issues, however, were settled by the Supreme Court's action. After the end of the first trimester, the states reserve rights to enact legislation and other regulations to protect maternal health. The states are now required to adopt statutes specifying the circumstances under which abortions can be legally performed.

Despite the Supreme Court ruling, arguments continue. Many states have not revised laws to provide for second- and third-trimester abortions, and the laws vary greatly. Various attitudes, beliefs, and values are evident in the variety of terms used today. "Therapeutic" abortion no longer simply means an abortion performed by a physician when the mother's life is threatened by serious physiopathologic conditions. The term has gradually been broadened to include threats to health, both physical and emotional. However, some state laws have not clearly defined what constitutes a threat to health. "Abortion on demand," "legalized abortion," "abortion on request," "elective abortion," and "social abortion" are some of the terms in common use.

Therapeutic abortions for purely medical reasons (the presence of serious physiopathologic conditions) have become more rare as the science of obstetrics has developed. Severe heart disease, pulmonary hypertension, pulmonary tuberculosis, chronic nephritis, diabetes, and malignancy are listed as medically sound reasons for terminating pregnancy by abortion. With increased effectiveness of conception control and availability of sterilization, fewer women who are at risk of developing life-threatening conditions during pregnancy are becoming pregnant.

Today many induced abortions are performed for "social" reasons. Social and economic pressures for small families are strong. There is an increased tendency among people to see abortion as an alternative method of birth control. Despite advances in the effectiveness of methods available for conception control, the continued demand for elective abortion indicates that many women see abortion as a means of birth control and possibly that deficiencies in knowledge, motivation, or availability of contraceptive services continues to be a problem.[76]

Table 62-1. Comparison of mortality rates

Causes of mortality	Mortality rate
Maternal mortality from childbirth	20/100,000 pregnancies
Criminal abortion	100/100,000 abortions
Legal abortion	3/100,000 abortions
Thromboembolic disorders from use of oral contraceptives	3/100,000 users

"Medically sound" reasons for performing abortions have been expanded to include such aspects as the fate of the unwanted child after birth, psychologic stress, history of genetic abnormalities, the effects of teratogens (agents causing embryonic defects), maternal and fetal blood incompatibility, rape, and incest.

The continued liberalization and acceptance of induced abortion as a means of birth control has raised concern over the effects of repeated induced abortions on women electing this method. There is growing concern over the late sequelae of repeat induced abortion including cervical incompetence,[99] ectopic pregnancy,[68] secondary sterility,[69] and Rh immunization.[74] Women utilizing abortion as a means of birth control need to be informed of these possible consequences in order to make informed choices.

Almost universally, when abortion is liberalized and legalized and made available, the maternal mortality rate drops and the incidence of septic and incomplete abortions decreases.[39] Statistics document that mortality with legal abortions induced in the first trimester has dropped to such low levels that the risk of having an abortion is much less than the risk of carrying a pregnancy to full term. To point out the low risk to maternal life associated with induced abortions, comparisons have been made with other causes of mortality (Table 62-1).

Both the physical and psychologic long-term effects of induced abortions require continued study. Psychologic studies indicate that adverse reactions to an abortion experience are influenced by legal, moral, and social antiabortion climates in that such a climate is punitive to the woman. Cultural attitudes have a pervasive effect and are likely to influence the way a woman reacts to an abortion. Attitudes of health care professionals influence the woman's feeling about herself and the abortion experience. The nurse's feelings and values about abortions, and identification with the roles of women, can influence the patient's response to abortion and perceptions of herself as a woman.[12]

Counseling

Counseling women regarding abortion is an appropriate function for nurses to assume, provided the nurse has the knowledge, skills, and abilities to assist individual women to cope with a situation that may have both immediate and long-term effects.

Preabortion counseling includes assisting the woman to make a decision regarding her state of pregnancy. This requires that the patient be helped with identifying the alternatives available to her, the consequences of the various alternatives, and selecting the alternative that is best for her in her circumstances. If this process is employed, the woman is more likely to arrive at a decision she feels is the best one she could make and less likely to experience excessive emotional distress. Therefore it is important in the counseling process to avoid telling the woman what to do or expressing opinions about what is best for her. For those women who seem unable to reach a decision, the nurse may arrange for referral to a counselor or social worker for further assistance.

For patients who decide to have an abortion, it is necessary that the nurse be able to explain the methods that will most likely be used, where an abortion may be obtained, and what will be required in terms of finances and time. It may be important that other health team members become involved in assisting the woman with planning. Preabortion counseling may also involve beginning explorations about conception control and family planning. Depending on her readiness to pursue these topics, the woman may be given information about the availability of services and methods. Otherwise she can be reassured the topic can be discussed at a later time.

In counseling the nurse will usually find that an objective approach, utilizing facts and terms the woman can understand, and conveying an attitude of willingness and readiness to assist her will encourage the woman to remain as objective as possible. Continuity in care seems to be particularly important to people in stressful situations, and it may be helpful to inform the woman about the personnel she is likely to encounter. Nursing care plans should be available to other nurses who will be participating in the patient's care whenever this is possible.

When hospitalized for an abortion, patients feel some degree of anxiety, and their behaviors must be interpreted with great care. If a patient begins to ask questions or verbalize feelings, it does not necessarily mean she has "changed her mind." It might mean that, under anxiety, she cannot recall what she was told would be done and needs to have this information repeated. Nurses cannot assume that the patient was not informed of the procedure and its consequences or that the patient has made a poor decision. Those patients who seem to be expressing "second thoughts" or seem to be doubtful about whether their decision should be carried out usually find it helpful to review how they initially reached the decision.

In the postabortion period a variety of emotional responses may be seen. Relief that the problem has been solved might be mingled with some minor feelings of guilt. Those women who express regret and guilt can be helped by again reviewing with them their decision-making process. They may need to be aware that such feelings may recur from time to time and that remembering how and why they reached the decision to have an abortion may help. Postabortion patients are candidates for conception control information. Many of these patients wish to learn more about reproduction and prevention of pregnancy. The approaches and methods described previously will be of assistance to the nurse engaged in counseling about conception control.

The date of the last menstrual period is important to ascertain, since the method selected for inducing abortion is partly determined by the period of gestation reached. The woman's physical and emotional states are also important. Although the methods for inducing abortion are generally considered very safe, some methods require greater physical and emotional energy.

A pregnancy test (p. 1370) is usually done to confirm pregnancy and to rule out other causes of amenorrhea. A vaginal or cervical smear should be done to detect infection, and a pelvic examination is usually done to confirm the length of gestation and to rule out diseases of the reproductive tract. A routine urinalysis and complete blood count are done.

The extent to which patients are able to handle the crisis of having a pregnancy terminated by induced abortion is partially dependent on the timing and quality of medical and nursing interventions. Women seeking abortion will engage in problem solving and select from the various alternatives available to them that alternative which is most advantageous to them in terms of physical, emotional, social, and economic resources. The decision made will be based on factual information, and patients will be better able to make an objective choice. Women having an induced abortion will understand the procedure to be used, length of hospitalization required, cost, and effects on physical and emotional health. They will realize that deep feelings are involved regardless of the degree of objectivity involved in the decision to have an abortion. Knowing this, women will be better prepared to handle such feelings when they do arise. They will identify supportive persons with whom they can discuss their feelings following discharge from the hospital or clinic.

Intervention

Several methods are available for inducing abortion. The particular method selected for a patient is highly dependent on the length of gestation at the time a woman seeks an abortion. As the pregnancy progresses, the methods required to be effective increase in complexity, are attended by greater risks to the woman, are more time-consuming in terms of length of hospitalization, are more expensive, and are perhaps more emotionally traumatic.

In the first trimester, abortion is performed in special clinics as an outpatient procedure or in acute-care settings. Many special abortion clinics have opened as a result of the demand for abortion in the early weeks of pregnancy. Some clinics provide counseling and referral services; others have facilities in which abortions can be performed. If admitted to an acute care setting, the woman may be admitted and discharged on the same day or remain only one night.

Vacuum aspiration. Vacuum aspiration (suction curettage) has increased in popularity because of its ease and safety in bringing about termination of pregnancy in the first few weeks. It has become the method of choice for inducing abortions in clinics and hospitals providing abortions for large numbers of patients.

Vacuum aspiration can be performed as soon as pregnancy is suspected, and very brief hospitalization is required. The equipment used is similar to that used for suction curettage. The cervix is dilated and the uterus is evacuated by means of a vacuum suction machine. When vacuum aspiration is employed immediately after the first menses is missed, a soft catheter of 5 to 6 mm in diameter is used, and very little cervical dilatation is required. *Menstrual extraction* and *minisuction* are terms also used when vacuum aspiration is done following the first missed menstrual period.

The procedure can be performed under either local or general anesthesia. The patient is observed for excess bleeding and pain immediately following the procedure, and can be discharged as soon as the vital signs are stable and effects of anesthesia have subsided. There is a low incidence of complications of vacuum aspiration. An incidence of 1.4% major complications, including uterine perforation, fever lasting 3 days or more, and retained tissue, is reported.[38]

Dilatation and curettage. Dilatation and curettage is an alternative method for accomplishing abortion in the first 12 to 14 weeks. The products of conception and superficial layer of the endometrium are scraped from the walls of the uterus. A paracervical block or general anesthesia is used. Oxytocin is usually administered intramuscularly or in an intravenous infusion after the procedure is completed. Blood loss is usually minimal, and physical care is similar to that for any patient having a dilatation and curettage (p. 1375).

Intraamniotic injection. Intraamniotic injection (saline injection, "salting out") is the method most often used after the sixteenth week of gestation. Occasionally it may be attempted as early as the fourteenth week, but the chances of failure are greater, since the amniotic sac is not well distended.

Since the woman must be responsive to detect adverse effects, general anesthesia is not used. Sedatives, analgesics, and tranquilizing agents are usually administered prior to the procedure, and a local anesthetic is used. The procedure is performed under aseptic conditions. The local anesthetic is injected into the skin and abdominal wall in the midline below the umbilicus. A 17- or 18-gauge spinal length needle is introduced through the abdominal and uterine walls into the amniotic sac. The stylet is removed and the physician observes for the flow of amniotic fluid from the needle. When the amniotic fluid appears, a syringe is attached to the needle and the amniotic fluid is aspirated. An alternative method of using a size 14 trocar and cannula to which a short length of rubber or plastic tubing is attached may be preferred by the physician. The total amount of amniotic fluid aspirated averages 200 ml for this period of gestation but may vary by about 50 ml. The amniotic fluid is replaced by 20% sodium chloride solution, and the amount injected is at least equivalent to the amount of amniotic fluid aspirated. Some physicians prefer to inject an additional 50 ml over the amount of amniotic fluid withdrawn, since there is some evidence that the additional fluid injected has a distending effect on the uterus. Most physicians elect to alternately withdraw and inject 15 to 20 ml of fluid and sodium chloride solution to prevent collapse of the amniotic sac that might result from withdrawal of all of the amniotic fluid.

During introduction of the needle the injection is made slowly, and care is taken to avoid insertion into the placenta or a blood vessel. The patient is closely observed during the procedure and for at least 1 hour afterward for untoward effects. These include shocklike symptoms or vascular collapse and abdominal pain resulting from injection into a blood vessel or the placenta.

The action of hypertonic solutions in inducing labor is not completely clear. The hypertonic solution disrupts the placenta, and this result alone produces an intrauterine environment incompatible with life. Disruption of the placenta may also release the progesterone block, causing uterine contractions to result. The volume of fluid in the uterus may be significant in that the body attempts to balance the effects of the hypertonic solution. In doing so the volume of intraamniotic fluid is increased. This expands the uterus beyond its normal size for gestation and probably triggers stretch receptors and pacemakers within the uterus.

The abortive process (labor) begins 12 to 36 hours after the injection of sodium chloride solution. The patient is hospitalized throughout this time and observed for late untoward effects as well as the onset of abortion. The products of conception are most often expelled as in a spontaneous, complete abortion. Once the symptoms of abortion appear (abdominal pain, vaginal bleeding, rupture of the amniotic sac), oxytocin may be administered by infusion to hasten the process and minimize blood loss. A dilatation and curettage may be performed after the abortion is completed as a precaution against excessive blood loss. If labor does not ensue within 36 to 48 hours following the injection, oxytocin by infusion is usually administered to initiate contractions of the uterus.

The thirteenth to sixteenth weeks of pregnancy pose difficulties for patients seeking an abortion. Most physicians consider this time to be too late for safe curettage and too early for intraamniotic injection.

Hysterotomy. An abortion may also be performed by hysterotomy. This method is usually selected for terminating pregnancies that have advanced to 16 weeks or more, or when a tubal sterilization is to be carried out at the same time. Hysterotomy involves incision through the abdominal wall and uterus to remove the products of conception. A general or spinal anesthesia is administered, and the patient has a longer period of hospitalization because of the surgical procedure. The postoperative complications that might occur are similar to those occurring after any abdominal surgery.

Experimental drugs. While an abortion pill, systemic abortion injection, or uterine insert to produce an abortion have not been developed as yet, it is quite likely that much simpler methods of inducing abortion will evolve if the current trend of increasing demand for elective abortion continues.

One group of drugs, the prostaglandins, is currently undergoing study. Intraamniotic injection of prostaglandins has been associated with a high incidence of complications, including fall in hematocrit, failure to abort within 48 hours after injection, infection requiring antibiotic therapy, cervical lacerations, and uterine rupture.[22] There is additional concern that with intraamniotic injection of prostaglandins, as with intraamniotic injection of saline, cervical incompetence may develop in future pregnancies because of atypical cervical dilatation.

Intravaginal administration of prostaglandins is also being studied and is reported to have a high success rate of inducing abortion within 12 hours and a low complication rate.[49] Complications are less serious with intravaginal administration of prostaglandins, but are distressing to the patient, and include fever, nausea and vomiting, and diarrhea during administration. In some instances fetuses with signs of viability are expelled, thus creating serious ethical conflicts for health professionals.

Outcome criteria for the woman experiencing an induced abortion

The woman can:

1. Describe methods of limiting family size other than abortion.
2. Have literature about these methods available for her use at home.
3. State her needs for health care follow-up:
   a. List signs of complications that need to be reported.
   b. State method of obtaining nursing or medical assistance.
   c. State the appropriate time to report for her follow-up examination and counseling.
4. Describe available community resources for family planning.

■ ECTOPIC PREGNANCY

An ectopic pregnancy is one in which the fertilized ovum becomes embedded outside the body of the uterus. Since it is almost always located in the fallopian tube, the term "tubal pregnancy" is often used.

Ectopic pregnancy is an increasing problem in gynecology. The incidence of tubal pregnancy has risen since 1970.[90] Factors contributing to ectopic pregnancy include presence of an intrauterine device, pelvic infection, oral contraceptives containing only progesterone, induced abortion, and tubal surgery including sterilization.

This condition occurs frequently in women who have a narrowed fallopian tube caused either by inflammation or by a congenital stricture. The sperm may be small enough to pass through the stricture, but the larger fertilized ovum may be unable to do so. The ovum may then attach itself to the tubal wall and develop into an embryo. As the embryo grows, the fallopian tube stretches and finally ruptures. This rupture usually occurs within the first 6 weeks of pregnancy.

□ Clinical picture

The woman experiences a sudden severe pain on one side of the abdomen in conjunction with a history of amenorrhea and often of suspected pregnancy. She may go into shock quickly after the onset of pain because of massive hemorrhage into the peritoneal cavity.

Because of its frequency, ruptured tubal pregnancy is one of the most common surgical emergencies in women. Laparoscopy may be performed to make the diagnosis. The radioreceptorassay test for pregnancy may have some value in diagnosing pregnancy. It has been noted that women are usually operated on within 2 hours following admission to the hospital.[82] Because the radioreceptorassay can be performed in 1 hour, pregnancy can be quickly confirmed. The test, however, does not reveal the site of pregnancy, and the patient's history and complaints on admission are important.

□ Intervention

Emergency treatment for shock and hemorrhage is given. Early treatment of a ruptured ectopic pregnancy is imperative to prevent death from hemorrhage. Immediately on diagnosis the woman is prepared for a salpingectomy. The primary purpose of surgery for tubal pregnancy is saving of the woman's life. The surgery also affects the woman's future fertility and her risk of future ectopic pregnancy. Estimates of impaired infertility following tubal surgery for ectopic pregnancy range from 33%[90] to 60%.[83]

If there has been prolonged bleeding preoperatively, the postoperative course may be complicated by peritonitis, since the blood in the abdomen becomes infected with organisms.

The nursing care combines the aspects of emergency treatment of a patient who has sustained a severe hemorrhage, general care of a patient who has had major abdominal surgery and who may have peritonitis, and care of a woman whose pregnancy has been terminated prematurely.

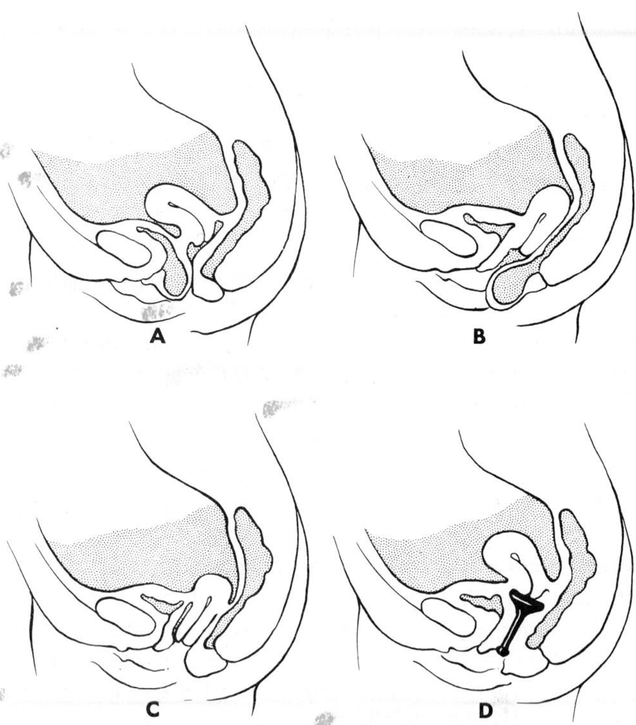

Fig. 62-2. Abnormalities of vagina. **A,** Cystocele: downward displacement of bladder toward vaginal orifice. **B,** Rectocele: pouching of rectum into posterior wall of vagina. **C,** Prolapse of uterus into vaginal canal. **D,** Stem pessary in place to maintain normal anatomic position of uterus.

■ UTERINE DISPLACEMENT

Displacement of the uterus, bladder, and rectum can be congenital or acquired because of stretching of the ligaments supporting the uterus and stretching of the muscles of the perineal floor. Acquired displacement of these structures usually results from unrepaired lacerations during childbirth and ill-advised bearing down during labor. Repeated, close pregnancies especially predispose to loss of muscle tone and displacement of the uterus and other pelvic structures.

With better obstetric care, use of episiotomies to prevent tearing of the pelvic muscles, immediate repair of all tears, and the trend toward fewer pregnancies and births per woman, fewer women should require vaginal wall repairs late in life. Perineal exercises practiced following delivery help to prevent relaxation. Apparently relaxation may also be caused by a congenital weakness of the muscles of the pelvis because it occurs occasionally in women who have had no children.

As the uterus begins to drop, the vaginal walls become relaxed, and a fold of vaginal mucosa may protrude outside the vaginal orifice. This is known as a colpocele. With the relaxation of the vaginal walls, the bladder may herniate into the vagina (a cystocele), or the rectal wall may herniate into the vagina (a rectocele) (Fig. 62-2). Both conditions may occur simultaneously.

Older women may have suffered from these conditions for years and yet may not have sought medical attention. They may remember that their mothers had a similar condition and think that it is to be expected in women who have borne children. Since they are not incapacitated, some decide not to spend money to have reparative surgery that they know is available. Some delay seeking treatment because they dread surgery. However, untreated displacements of the uterus may cause complications such as cervical ulceration and infection, cystitis, and hemorrhoids.

□ Clinical picture

A sign of relaxation of the pelvic musculature is a dragging pain in the back and in the pelvis. It is made worse by standing or walking. The woman who has a cystocele may complain of urinary incontinence accompanying activity that increases intraabdominal pressure such as coughing, laughing, walking, or lifting (stress incontinence). The cystocele may become so pronounced that in order for the patient to void the bladder must be pushed back into place by holding the finger against the anterior vaginal wall. If the patient has a rectocele, she may complain of constipation and resultant hemorrhoids.

□ Intervention

Cystoceles and rectoceles are treated by plastic operations designed to tighten the vaginal wall. The operation is done through the vagina. The repair for a cystocele is called an anterior colporrhaphy; that for a rectocele, a posterior colporrhaphy. Old tears of the pelvic floor, usually caused by childbearing, may also be repaired. Such repair is called a perinorrhaphy.

As part of the preoperative preparation, a cleansing douche is frequently ordered the morning of surgery. When surgery involving the vagina is performed, postoperative nursing care includes prevention of pressure on the vaginal suture line and prevention of wound infection. Perineal dressings are seldom used.

Perineal care is given at least twice a day and after each voiding or defecation. Sterile cotton balls moistened with benzalkonium chloride, bichloride of mercury, or normal saline solution may be used, or the patient may be placed on a douche pan and the solution poured over the perineum. Cleansing is always done away from the vagina toward the rectum so that contamination is avoided. An indwelling catheter may be inserted and attached to continuous drainage for 24 to 48 hours. After removal, the usual methods to encourage voiding can be employed.

A heat lamp may be used for 15 to 20 minutes two or three times a day to encourage healing of the perineum. The heat lamp should be used after perineal care to help dry the area and thereby prevent sloughing of tissue. If the patient complains of perineal discomfort, an ice pack applied locally helps to reduce swelling and give relief. A plastic bag or disposable glove filled with ice, firmly tied and covered, makes an adaptable pack. When sutures have been removed, sitz baths are usually ordered.

Beginning on the tenth postoperative day, a daily vaginal douche with normal saline solution is usually prescribed. Occasionally douches are ordered during the immediate postoperative period. Sterile equipment and sterile solution should then be used. The douche nozzle should be very gently inserted and very carefully rotated.

After discharge the woman who has had a vaginal repair should continue to take a daily douche and a daily tub bath. A laxative may be prescribed to be taken each night to prevent constipation and excessive stress on the surgical site. When she returns to the clinic or to the physician's office, the woman is told when to discontinue the douches and laxative and when it is safe for her to resume sexual intercourse. Women who have had vaginal repair procedures, like other patients having gynecologic surgery, need to avoid jarring activities and heavy lifting for at least 6 weeks postoperatively.

If a *posterior colporrhaphy* is scheduled, a cathartic may be given approximately 24 hours before surgery, and several enemas usually are given preoperatively to help assure an empty bowel at the time of surgery and immediately thereafter. Up to 24 hours preoperatively the patient may be permitted only clear liquids orally to further reduce bowel contents. Postoperatively the patient may be kept flat in bed or in a low Fowler's position to prevent increased intraabdominal pressure or strain on the wound. Special attention must be given to exercise for the patient's legs, to having her turn frequently, and to having her cough deeply. For 5 days only liquids are permitted orally, and camphorated tincture of opium (paregoric) is also given to inhibit bowel function. At the end of this time, mineral oil is given each night, and an oil retention enema is given the morning after the first laxative is given. Only a soft rectal tube and small amount of oil (200 ml) should be used. Straining to produce a bowel movement is discouraged. Enemas for relieving flatus and for cleansing the bowel usually are not given until at least a week postoperatively.

After an *anterior colporrhaphy* an indwelling catheter is usually left in the bladder for about 4 days. The catheter should keep the bladder completely empty. If a catheter is not used and if the patient is taking sufficient fluid, voiding should be checked at least every 4 hours. No more than 150 ml of urine should be allowed to accumulate in the bladder. It is usually very difficult to catheterize a patient following a vaginal repair, since the urethral orifice may be distorted and edematous. Having the patient take deep breaths may help in locating the orifice because it dilates slightly with each breath. A soft rubber catheter should be used. Ambulation is begun immediately after surgery. A regular diet is given, and mineral oil is taken each night to lessen the need to strain on defecation.

Sometimes a vaginal plastic procedure does not relieve the *stress incontinence* caused by a cystocele and by general relaxation of the pelvic floor. When this happens, the ligaments about the bladder neck may be shortened in such a way that the bladder drops less easily into the vagina. The degree of incontinence may be tested by filling the bladder to various levels with sterile normal saline solution and then having the pateint cough or strain while standing. If the incontinence is marked, the patient may be placed in a lithotomy position while the physician fills the bladder with normal saline solution and supports the bladder neck with a finger or with a clamp in the vagina to test the effectiveness of the bladder with this support. If the patient can cough and strain down without being incontinent, she is considered a good candidate for the operation. The surgery is done through a suprapubic incision, and it is usually combined with further vaginal repair. A urethral catheter is inserted, and the nursing care is similar to that following a vaginal repair. If the catheter does not drain freely or if the patient without a catheter does not void within 4 to 6 hours, the physician should be notified. Pressure from a full bladder may disrupt the repair.

PROLAPSE OF THE UTERUS

Prolapse of the uterus, or procidentia uteri, is a marked downward displacement of the uterus. The severity of the displacement is designated as first, second, or third degree. In a first-degree prolapse the cervix is still within the vagina. In a second-degree prolapse the cervix protrudes from the vaginal orifice. In a third-degree prolapse the entire uterus, suspended by its stretched ligaments, hangs below the vaginal orifice. In both second-degree and third-degree prolapses the cervix becomes irritated from clothing, the circulation becomes impaired, and ulceration often follows.

Clinical picture

Displacement of the uterus may cause dysmenorrhea, although many women with known displacements have no difficulty. Some women with displacement complain of chronic backache, pelvic pressure, easy fatigue, and leukorrhea in addition to painful menstruation.

Common kinds of displacement are *anteflexion, retroflexion,* and *retroversion* of the uterus caused by congenitally weak uterine ligaments, adhesions following infections or surgery in the pelvic region, or the strain of pregnancy on the ligaments. A space-filling lesion in this region or even a full bladder or rectum may also displace the uterus enough to cause symptoms. Normally the body of the uterus flexes forward at a 45° angle at the cervix. In retroflexion this angle is increased. In anteflexion it is decreased. In retroversion the whole uterus is tipped backward (Fig. 62-3).

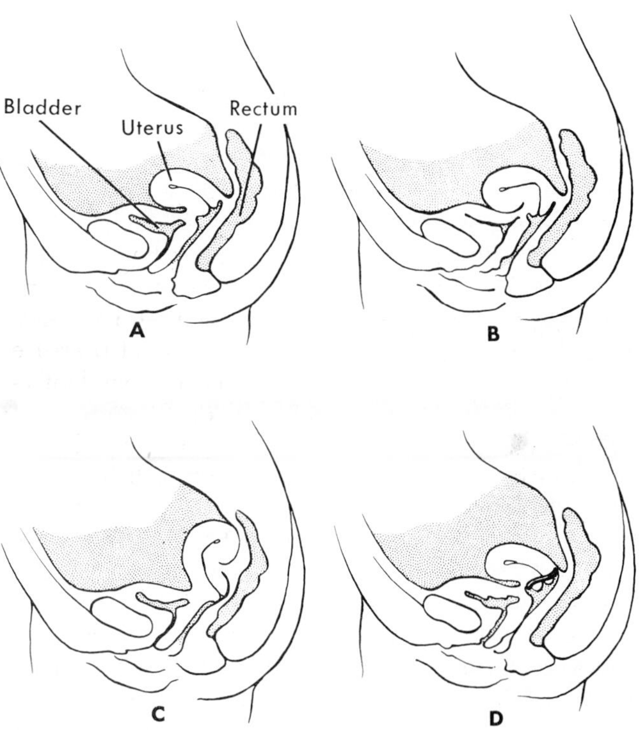

Fig. 62-3. Normal and abnormal positions of uterus. **A,** Normal anatomic position of uterus in relation to adjacent structures. **B,** Anterior displacement of uterus. **C,** Retroversion or backward displacement of uterus. **D,** Normal anatomic position of uterus maintained by use of rubber S-shaped pessary.

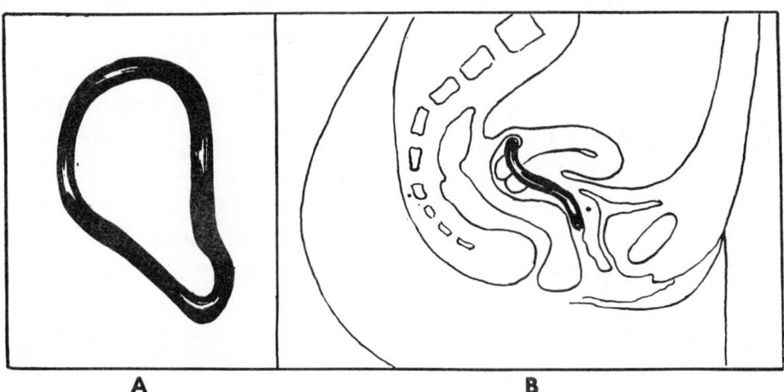

Fig. 62-4. A, Albert Smith pessary. **B,** Pessary in place to hold posterior vaginal fornix, and with it attached cervix, well backward and upward in pelvis. (From Beacham, D. W., and Beacham, W. D.: Synopsis of gynecology, ed. 9, St. Louis, 1977, The C. V. Mosby Co.)

□ Intervention

If the displacement is not caused by some coexistent pelvic disease, various pelvic exercises may be recommended in an attempt to return the uterus to a normal position. These exercises, employing the principles of gravity, stretch or strengthen the uterine ligaments. Some exercises used are knee-chest exercises, the monkey trot, lying on the abdomen 2 hours a day, and premenstrual exercises. Corrective exercises for poor posture may also be prescribed.

In doing knee-chest exercises, the woman in instructed to assume a knee-chest position (Fig. 60-7) and to separate the labia to allow air to enter the vagina, since this helps to produce normal positioning of the uterus. This position should be maintained for 5 minutes two or three times a day.

In doing the monkey trot, the woman is instructed to walk about on her hands and feet, keeping the knees straight. This should be done for 5 minutes two or three times a day.

The usual treatment for a uterine prolapse is hysterectomy. This procedure may sometimes be done by the vaginal route. If any operation is contraindicated because of the age or general condition of the patient, a pessary may be inserted to hold the uterus up in the pelvis (Fig. 62-4). A string should be attached to the pessary, and after its insertion the woman pins the string to her underclothing. This type of pessary occasionally becomes displaced and might cause the patient embarrassment.

■ FISTULAS

Fistulas can occur in several locations (Fig. 62-5). They may occur when a malignant lesion has spread or when radiation treatment has been used for a malignancy, or they may be caused by trauma at surgery.

Most women with vesicovaginal and rectovaginal fistulas tend to become withdrawn. Occasionally, however, a woman becomes immune to the odors, and this presents a serious problem to her family. It puts a strain on family relationships at a time when she is desperately in need of approval and acceptance. Often it is better for the physician or nurse to bring the problem to the woman's attention than to have it mentioned by a member of the family. Nurses then help the woman devise a means of caring for herself so that she can be assured that she is free of odor. Chlorine solution (for example, 5 ml [1 teaspoon] of chlorine household bleach to 1 liter [1 quart] of water) makes a satisfactory deodorizing douche, and this solution is also excellent for external perineal irrigation. Sitz baths and thorough cleansing of the surrounding skin with mild soap and water are helpful. Deodorizing powders such as sodium borate can be used. Care is time-consuming and must be repeated at regular intervals to ensure cleanliness. Protective pants can be worn. Some large department stores now stock plastic pants that button at the side to avoid bulkiness (Fig. 62-6). A protective apron worn backward under other clothing or a petticoat with a posterior lining of plastic waterproof material also protects the woman from

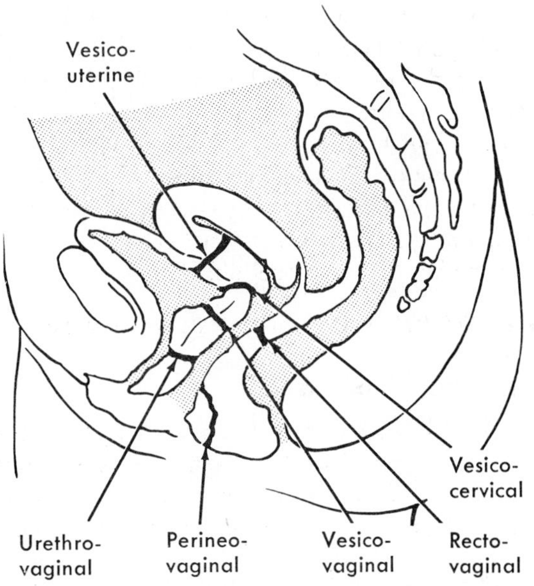

Vesico-uterine
Vesico-cervical
Urethro-vaginal
Perineo-vaginal
Vesico-vaginal
Recto-vaginal

Fig. 62-5. Types of fistulas that may develop in vagina and uterus.

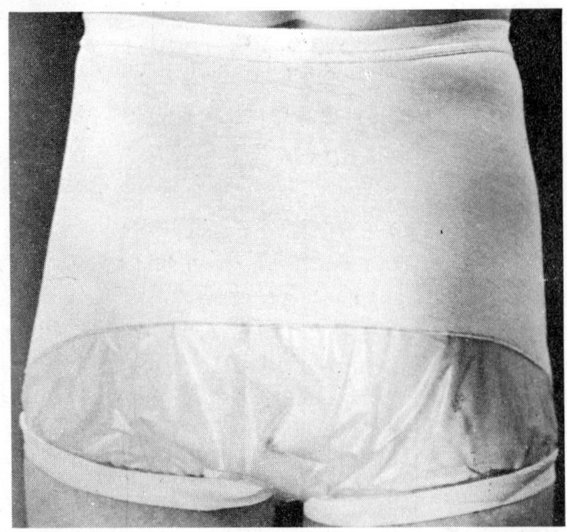

Fig. 62-6. Pants with plastic reinforcement of crotch. They usually give adequate protection to woman with stress incontinence. (Courtesy Ferguson Manufacturing Co., Grand Rapids, Mich.)

embarrassment of soiling clothing or furniture when she is seated.

The patient needs encouragement from the medical and nursing staff, and she needs assurance that they understand her problem. When fistulas persist, couples have special problems that require patience and understanding. Husband and wife should be encouraged to communicate with one another regarding interference with their sexual relationship.

□ Ureterovaginal fistulas

Ureterovaginal fistulas complicate gynecologic treatment rather frequently. In treating cancer of the uterus, either by radiation or surgery, or occasionally when a hysterectomy is done, the blood supply to the ureter may be impaired or other damage may occur. The ureteral wall sloughs, and a fistula opens from the ureter to the vagina. This causes a constant drip of urine through the vagina. A ureterovaginal fistula usually heals spontaneously after a period of time. If it does not, repair procedures may be attempted, and occasionally an ileobladder must be made (p. 1264).

□ Vesicovaginal fistulas

Vesicovaginal fistulas, or fistulas between the bladder and the vagina, and urethrovaginal fistulas, between the urethra and the vagina, may follow radiation of the cervix, gynecologic surgery, or trauma during delivery. It is impossible to perform surgery to repair the fistula until the inflammation and induration have subsided. This may take 3 to 4 months. A suprapubic incision is made into the bladder, the fistula tract is dissected out, and the defect is closed by primary closure or by using a graft from the bladder or adjacent mucosal wall.

Postoperatively usually both a suprapubic tube and a urethral catheter are inserted to drain the bladder. These tubes are sometimes attached to a "bubble" suction drainage apparatus in order to assure that the bladder is kept empty. Bladder drainage is maintained for about 3 weeks or until the wound is completely healed. The catheters should not be irrigated unless it is absolutely necessary, and only very gentle pressure should be used when irrigating them. Signs of urinary drainage from the vagina should be noted. There is normally a small amount of serosanguineous drainage from the vagina for a few days postoperatively. Vaginal douches may be ordered and should be given gently and with very little pressure from the fluid. The patient is kept in bed for several days and then is usually allowed to sit at the side of the bed. She will need to remain in her room beside her bed if bubble suction is being used. Such confinement is tiring, and visitors, television, radio, reading materials, and a variety of occupational therapy activities may help to pass the time satisfactorily.

The results of repair operations for fistulas are not always successful. The patient must sometimes have several operations, and each successive hospitalization increases her anxiety about the outcome of surgery and lessens her ability to accept the discomforts and inconveniences entailed. All possible nursing measures should be taken to prevent infection and to be certain that free drainage of urine is assured. Obstruction of drainage tubes may place pressure against the newly repaired vesicovaginal wall and cause healing tissue to break down, resulting in return of the fistula.

□ Rectovaginal fistulas

Rectovaginal fistulas are less common than vesicovaginal fistulas. The constant escape of flatus and fecal material through the vagina is particularly distressing to the patient, especially so because rectovaginal fistulas are quite resistant to satisfactory surgical treatment. They may be due to the same causes as vesicovaginal fistulas. Surgical repair is usually done through the rectum. It may not be satisfactory, and operations may have to be repeated. The nursing care is similar to that needed by patients following surgery for other types of rectal fistulas (p. 1291). In addition, the patient will need sympathetic understanding and encouragement, since the emotional reactions are much more severe.

If there is dribbling of fecal material into the vagina, it may be temporarily lessened by giving a high enema, and the woman at home is encouraged to do this before going out. (After surgery, of course, enemas are never permitted until healing is complete). They may be given during the preoperative period. A soft rubber catheter should be used and should be directed carefully on the side of the rectum opposite the fistula. The catheter must go beyond the fistulous opening, or the fluid will return through the vagina and no benefit will be derived from the treatment. While a constipating diet will temporarily prevent fecal material from going into the vagina, it eventually will cause pressure and may aggravate the condition and increase the size of the fistula. The woman therefore is advised against restricting diet and fluids in an effort to control action.

■ BENIGN TUMORS OF THE FEMALE GENITAL TRACT

□ Ovarian tumors and cysts

There are a vast variety of nonmalignant tumors of the female reproductive tract. Tumors of the ovaries alone represent a long list of forms, and their classification according to type can be obtained from specialized texts.

Approximately 30% of women have no symptoms of ovarian tumors at the time the growth is detected, and about 80% of them are discovered at the time of routine

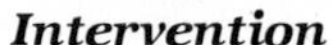

pelvic examination.[36] Women between the ages of 45 and 60 are at greatest risk for developing ovarian tumors.

Clinical picture

Symptoms are usually nonspecific. With rapidly growing cysts or tumors of the ovary, the first symptom may be increase in abdominal size. Complaints of fatigue and sensations of weight, fullness, or pressure in the pelvis are common. Pain is an unusual symptom in the absence of acute complications such as twisting of an ovarian cyst on its pedicle. Increase in the size of the tumor may cause pressure symptoms such as urinary frequency and constipation, and backache may be present. Ovarian tumors and cysts are a frequent cause of menstrual irregularities.

Palpation of reproductive organs during pelvic examination usually reveals a mass or enlargement of the ovary. One or both ovaries normally atrophy and become nonpalpable after the menopause; any mass palpated in the area of the ovaries requires further evaluation. Laparoscopy or exploratory laparotomy are usually done to confirm the diagnosis.

Intervention

Ovarian tumors and cysts are treated surgically, and most often an oophorectomy is performed.

Fibroid tumors

It has been estimated that 20% to 25% of women over 30 years of age develop uterine fibroid tumors (myoma).[65] Uterine myomas are more common in black women and in women who have never been pregnant. They rarely become malignant. Because their growth is stimulated by ovarian hormones, fibroid tumors of the uterus tend to disappear spontaneously with the advent of the menopause.

Clinical picture

Menorrhagia is the most common symptom of myomas. If the tumor is very large, it may cause pelvic circulatory congestion and may press on surrounding viscera. The woman may complain of low abdominal pressure, backache, constipation, or dysmenorrhea. If a ureter is compressed by the tumor, there may be signs and symptoms of ureteral obstruction. Sometimes the pedicle on which a myoma is growing becomes twisted, causing severe pain. Large tumors growing into the opening of the fallopian tubes may cause sterility, those in the body of the uterus may cause spontaneous abortions, and those near the cervical opening may make the delivery of a baby difficult and may contribute to hemorrhage postpartally.

Intervention

The treatment of fibroid tumors depends on the symptoms and the age of the patient, on whether more children are desired, and how near she is to the menopause. If the symptoms are not severe, the woman may simply need close health supervision. If the tumor is near the outer wall of the uterus, a *myomectomy* (surgical removal of the tumor) may be performed. This operation leaves the muscle walls of the uterus relatively intact. If there is severe bleeding or obstruction, a hysterectomy is usually necessary. Occasionally, if surgery is contraindicated or if the woman is approaching the menopause, x-ray therapy or radiation is used to reduce the size of the tumor and to stop vaginal bleeding.

Endometriosis

Endometriosis is a condition in which endometrial cells that normally line the uterus are seeded throughout the pelvis and occasionally extend to as distant a location as the umbilicus (Fig. 62-7). The disease appears to be increasing, although the increased incidence may be a result of better diagnosis and recognition of the condition. It is not known how endometriosis first develops. Theories include congenital presence of endometrial cells out of their normal location, their transfer by means of blood vessels or the lymphatic system, and reflux of menstrual fluid containing endometrial cells up the fallopian tubes and into the pelvic cavity. None of these theories has been proved. With each menstrual period, the endometrial cells are stimulated by the ovarian hormones and bleed into the surrounding areas, causing an inflammation. Subsequent adhesions may be so severe that pelvic organs may become fused together, occasionally causing a stricture of the bowel or interference with bladder function. Encased blood may lead to palpable tumor masses, which often occur on the ovary and are known as *chocolate cysts*. Occasionally these cysts rupture and spread endometrial cells still farther throughout the pelvis.

Clinical picture

Usually endometriosis progresses very gradually and does not produce symptoms until the age of 30 to 40. Occasionally, however, symptoms appear when the woman is in her teens. The characteristic symptom of endometriosis is pain and general discomfort accompanying menstruation that becomes progressively worse and that was not present at the onset of the menses. This one characteristic feature should alert the nurse to urge that the woman see a gynecologist at once. Many women with severe pain related to menstruation have been judged to be neurotic when in reality they were suffering from endometriosis. Other symptoms of endometriosis

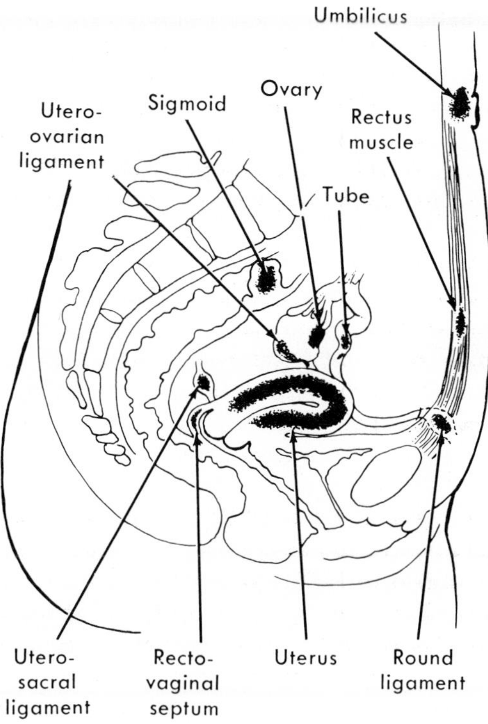

Fig. 62-7. Sites of endometrial implants.

are a feeling of fullness in the lower abdomen, dyspareunia, and general poor health. Sometimes the disease is far advanced and yet has caused no symptoms at all. Approximately 40% to 50% of women are infertile, and endometriosis is sometimes first detected when a woman presents herself with the complaint of inability to conceive.

Intervention

Although a great deal of study of endometriosis is under way at present, its response to treatment is still variable and poorly understood. For this reason treatment is highly individualized. If the woman is young and wants to have children, the treatment for endometriosis is usually as conservative as possible. Pregnancy is beneficial because menstruation ceases during this time. If a young woman has endometriosis, she and her husband usually are advised to have their family without delay because the fertility rate is low, sterility caused by adhesions may occur, and a hysterectomy may have to be done within a reasonable period of time. Nursing the infant is also recommended because it delays the onset of menstruation following delivery.

Because they imitate the state of pregnancy by inducing the ovaries to become anovulatory, antiovulatory drugs are frequently prescribed. Oral progestational drugs used over a period of 4 to 6 months are not uncommon. The starting dose is usually 5 to 10 mg daily and the dose is increased by 10 mg every 2 weeks until a therapeutic level is reached or until the maximum dose of 40 mg/day is reached. This dosage produces a situation known as pseudopregnancy and causes the errant endometrial cells to be temporarily quiescent. The disadvantages of this treatment are that irregular bleeding may occur and that the symptoms of early pregnancy, including nausea, vomiting, depression, and fatigue, may be troublesome.

Drugs having reversible antigonadotropic action by suppressing ovarian activity (Danazol) have recently become available.[21] These drugs are given in a dose of 200 mg twice a day for 3 to 6 months. Treatment can be extended up to 9 months if necessary, or it can be reinstituted if symptoms recur. Antigonadotropic drugs are contraindicated if the woman has undiagnosed abnormal vaginal bleeding, impaired hepatic, renal, or cardiac function, is pregnant, or is breast-feeding an infant.

When the involvement is severe and does not respond to hormonal treatment, surgery may be necessary. A total hysterectomy, oophorectomy, and salpingectomy may be done. Removal of the ovaries prevents further bleeding of endometrial implants that cannot be removed. If the woman is premenopausal and the ovaries must be removed, she may be given very small amounts of estrogen to preserve secondary sexual characteristics and permit more normal living. The menopause stops the progress of this condition.

□ Cervical polyps

Cervical polyps form when an area of the cervical mucosa proliferates. These growths are usually visible at the cervical os as bright red, vascular, fragile areas. They are most often pedunculated and appear to protrude from the cervical canal. Polyps may occur singly or in clusters.

Because of the vascularity of the polyp, bleeding is a common symptom. Generally no other symptom is present. The characteristics of the bleeding associated with polyps closely resemble the signs of early cancer of the cervix. The bleeding is small in amount and occurs between menstrual periods. Especially characteristic is the contact bleeding produced by coitus, douching, or by vaginal examination.

The pedicle by which the polyp is attached is usually quite small so that the polyp can easily be removed by twisting the pedicle at its base or by use of a biopsy forceps or sharp curette.[65] Tissue examination of removed polyps is essential, since epidermoid cancer arises from cervical polyps in a small percentage of cases.

■ CARCINOMA OF THE FEMALE GENITAL TRACT

□ Epidemiology

Cancer between the ages of 20 and 40 is three times more common in women than in men.[85] The major sites of cancer in women are the skin, breasts, colon and rectum, and the uterus including the cervix. Of these, cancer of the uterus ranks third in frequency. Since 1950, mortality caused by uterine cancer has declined, more so among white than black women. Reduction in deaths from cancer of the uterus is attributed to a sharp drop in deaths from cervical cancer because of early detection with the Pap smear, which is widely used.

Cancer of the uterus accounts for about 14% of all female cancers. Invasive cancer of the cervix occurs in about 6%, and cancer of the corpus in about 8% of cancers among women.[16] Uterine cancer is reported to be more than twice as common among nonwhites than whites and is one of the leading causes of cancer deaths in females of all ages over 25 years.[94]

Most often, cancer of the uterus occurs between the ages of 45 and 69 and is more prevalent among women who do not have regular examinations or Pap smears. Cervical cancer has its highest frequency between the ages of 40 and 49. Cancer of the cervix is seen more often in women who come from low socioeconomic backgrounds, marry at an early age, are young at the time of first coitus, have coitus with uncircumcised male partners, and who are infected with herpesvirus type 2.[44,86]

Puerto Rican immigrants develop cervical cancer about four times more often than do mainland women, leading to the suspicion that environmental factors of urbanization have a causative role.[86] Cleanliness may play a role in protection against cancer. This had led some investigators to consider the possible venereal transmission of etiologic viruses.[59,73] Herpes genitalis seems to fit the viral model of carcinogens in that the disease is sexually transmitted, is prevalent around the world, and is found in a large number of women having cancer of the cervix.

The ovaries are the sixth leading site of cancer in women and account for about 5% of all female cancers.[86] There is a sharp increase in the incidence of ovarian cancer after the age of 35, with the greatest number of cases discovered between the ages of 50 and 59.[85] The risk of developing cancer of the ovary is higher if a close relative has had a cancer in this site. A number of epidemiologic factors are suspected of being linked with ovarian cancer including nulliparity, infertility, endometriosis, irradiation of the pelvic organs, group A type blood, and chemical carcinogens such as asbestos and talc.[86]

In comparison to other sites, cancer of the vulva and vagina occur rarely. Cancer of the vulva occurs 0.7% and cancer of the vagina 0.2% of the time in cancers in women.[85] Pregnancy history, racial differences, and marital status do not seem to have an etiologic relationship to cancer of the vulva. Some skin conditions associated with chronic irritation such as exposure to coal tar derivatives, x-ray treatment of benign lesions, chronic leukoplakia, and chronic pruritus have been implicated as predisposers to vulvar cancer.

Parity, family history, and race do not appear to be related etiologically to vaginal cancer. Chronic irritation resulting from prolonged use of pessaries, prolapse of the uterus, leukorrhea, and use of chemicals and hormones have been suspected of predisposing to cancer of the vagina. In recent years reports of vaginal and cervical cancer among teenagers have appeared in the literature. When studied, the case histories revealed that their mothers had been treated during pregnancy with diethylstilbestrol (DES).[91] There is now enough evidence accumulated to recommend that synthetic estrogens not be used during pregnancy. Daughters of mothers who received DES are urged to have frequent pelvic examinations and to remain under close medical supervision.

□ Prevention

Dramatic decreases in deaths due to cancer are associated with early detection and treatment. The decline in deaths, for example, from cervical cancer is primarily because of increased use of the Pap smear for mass screening combined with more frequent and more thorough gynecologic examination.

To salvage more lives through diagnosis and treatment, it is important to first determine the population at risk and then to provide them with the means by which frequent, inexpensive screening can be accomplished. The risk factors associated with genital cancer have been given above. Application of this knowledge in practice assists with identification of specific individuals at risk for cancer. For example, a strong family history of cancer, industrial occupations exposing individuals to chemicals, or a history of long-standing local tissue irritation should alert nurses to advise women with such histories to have frequent examinations for the appearance of cancer.

Uterine cancer deaths could be greatly reduced if every adult woman had an annual physical examination including Pap smear and if postmenopausal women and those approaching menopausal age had abnormal bleeding checked by their physician. Many older women have not had a physical examination since their childbearing years, especially those in rural areas.[86] There is a need to persuade older women to have periodic examinations and to see a physician if they have abnormal vaginal bleeding. Instructing women in the signs of infection and to report them when they occur can assist the prompt diagnosis and management of conditions causing irritation of tissues, and can especially be of value in discovering and treating genital herpes.

With a decrease in mortality due to cancer of the cervix, screening and diagnostic techniques for endometrial cancer have assumed greater importance. The methods currently used are discussed in Chapter 60. Since no single procedure has been universally successful in screening, a combination of methods probably affords the best chances for detecting cancer of the uterus. Screening and its potential for the future takes on greater significance, since precursors to cancer can be detected in the uterine cavity before advanced, invasive cancer develops.[13]

Endometrial sampling of all women in the high-risk age group remains a goal. In the meantime, every effort needs to be made to take advantage of contacts with women for the purposes of teaching, recording histories, and performing physical examinations as well as endometrial sampling. The American Cancer Society has recommended that every woman at the time of menopause should have a pelvic examination and that those who are at risk for uterine cancer should also have a sample of the endometrium examined for cancer and percursors to cancer.[86]

One of the most important functions of nurses is to participate actively in programs of preventive health care. For women, this includes encouragement to have a yearly pelvic examination, including a Pap smear, and to be aware of the warning signs of cancer of the cervix and uterus. Assisting women to become better informed about gynecologic examinations can assist them to handle their fears of such examinations (Chapter 60). It is important to seek out candidates for education regarding cancer of the reproductive tract and to offer them information. Hospitalized women, women in ambulatory care settings, and women seen in their homes provide opportunities for nurses to inform women about cancer detection and to teach them the warning signs of cancer. Pamphlets such as *Cancer Facts for Women* and *Stay Healthy, Learn About Uterine Cancer* are available from the American Cancer Society or your local affiliate and are appropriate for educating people.

□ Assessment and treatment of specific cancers by site

Cancer of the cervix

Cervical cancer is second only to cancer of the breast in its frequency of occurrence. It is a disease of young women, occurring most often in the 30- to 50-year age group. If detected in the preinvasive stage, cancer of the cervix is 100% curable.

In 1929 the Cancer Committee of the League of Nations developed for statistical study an international classification originally ranged from stages I to IV. However, since the discovery of the Pap smear technique, stage O has been added. If there is early diagnosis, the prognosis is excellent because the preclinical state (stage O) of cancer frequently exists 5 to 10 years before the visible stage I lesion appears. In the early stages the symptoms are a slight watery vaginal discharge, lengthening of the menstrual period, or occasional spotting of blood between periods. Spotting is often noticed following intercourse, after taking a douche, after defecating, or after heavy lifting (Table 62-2).

Treatment of cancer of the cervix depends on the stage of the tumor, the woman's age and general health, and the presence of complications. Treatment of carcinoma in situ may consist of an excisional conization of the cervix (or cryosurgery in some institutions) if the woman is young, wishes to have more children, and invasive cancer has been ruled out. In other women, simple hysterectomy is preferred to radiotherapy, particularly for those in whom preservation of ovarian function is desirable. Invasive cancer of the cervix can be treated by means of surgery or radiotherapy. Usually the tumors above stage I and II are treated with radiotherapy. Surgery for stage I and II disease may be reserved in some institutions for those women desiring preservation of ovarian function. Comparable cure rates are obtained with either surgery or radiotherapy. However, the morbidity associated with both approaches is considered in light of the individual woman and her problem.

If treatment is not instituted, the disease will advance progressively, with the vaginal discharge becoming dark, bloody, and foul smelling because of infection

Table 62-2. Cancer of the cervix

Stage	0	I	II	III	IV
Involvement	Confined within epithelium of cervix	Completely confined to cervix	Extends outside cervix but does not involve pelvic wall or lower third of uterus	Involves pelvic wall and lower third of vagina	Extends beyond stage III; involves (1) bladder or (2) rectum or (3) metastatic spread

and necrosis of tissue. Bladder or rectal symptoms such as fistulas or symptoms of pressure may appear. As lymph glands anterior to the sacrum become involved, back and leg pains occur from pressure on the nerves. Emaciation, anemia, and irregular fever, secondary to the local infection and tissue necrosis, may then follow. The woman with untreated cancer of the cervix has a life expectancy of from 2 to 4 years following the appearance of the cervical lesion.

Cancer of the corpus

The major sites and types of cancer of the uterus are shown in Fig. 62-8. Cancer of the endometrium is a slow-growing form of cancer and is very amenable to treatment if detected early.

The early signs of endometrial cancer are unexpected or irregular vaginal bleeding. If these signs are heeded and medical attention is sought, the chance for cure is good. Since these tumors often arise from a polyp, anyone who has uterine polyps or who has had polyps removed from the uterus should have periodic pelvic examinations.

Cancer of the corpus may be treated by total hysterectomy (excision of the uterus including the cervix) or by irradiation therapy (intrauterine radiation and deep x-ray therapy to the pelvis). Often intrauterine irradiation is used preoperatively to shrink the tumor and to decrease the amount of local infection so that the operation will be safer and more easily performed. Since tumors of the fundus of the uterus occur later in life, the surgical course is frequently complicated by other conditions commonly seen in geriatric patients such as hypertension, diabetes mellitus, poor circulation, and malnutrition.

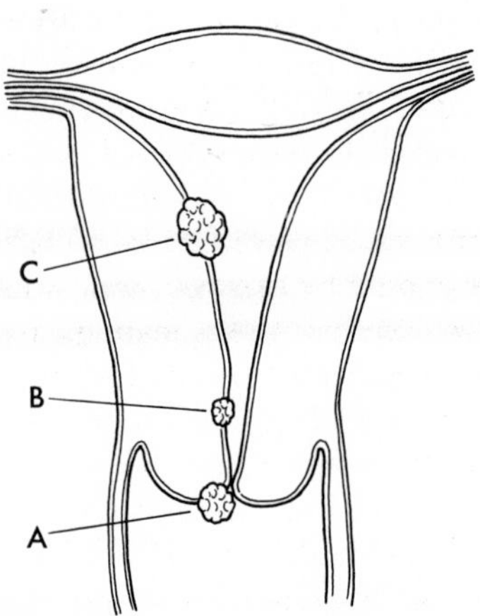

Fig. 62-8. Types and locations of carcinoma of uterus. **A,** Epidermoid carcinoma of cervix. **B,** Adenocarcinoma of cervix. **C,** Adenocarcinoma of corpus uteri. (From Novak, E. R., Jones, G. J., and Jones, H. W., Jr.: Novak's textbook of gynecology, ed. 9, © 1975 The Williams & Wilkins Co., Baltimore.)

Cancer of the ovary

Cancer of the ovary appears to be increasing in the United States, and so far it has defied all attempts at early diagnosis. Over one-half of all patients having this condition are inoperable when the disease is discovered, and the 5-year survival rate is only 15% to 20%.[85] Most gynecologists believe that the only hope for the patient lies in early and vigorous treatment of the ovarian cysts, which may be precursors of malignant disease. They believe that all patients suspected of having tumors of the ovary should have an exploratory abdominal operation because malignant tumors of the ovary usually give no symptoms until local metastasis occurs and there is ascites from increased pressure within the portal system, edema of the legs from pressure on veins passing through the pelvic cavity, or pain in the back or the legs from pressure on nerves, or until there are symptoms of distant metastasis. The silent onset and growth of ovarian tumors almost surely doom the woman in whom diagnosis is not made prior to onset of symptoms. The only effective means of assuring early diagnosis is a pelvic examination every 6 months, including careful ovarian palpation, and surgical exploration of any questionable ovarian growth. If possible, the ovary and the tumor are completely removed at operation. If the tumor is malignant, the operation is followed by deep x-ray therapy. Chemotherapy has prolonged the lives of some patients; nitrogen mustard and TEM are drugs often used, and the alkylating agent chlorambucil has been found to produce a favorable response in approximately 25% of all patients. (For the nursing care of patients receiving these drugs, see p. 475.)

Hydatidiform mole

A hydatidiform mole is a tumor mass of chorionic cells in the uterus that masquerades as a pregnancy. The cause is unknown. The uterus rapidly increases in size because of enlargement of the ovarian follicles. There is also an increase in the level of chorionic gonadotropin in the blood and urine. Treatment consists of the administration of Syntocinon (synthetic oxytocin), which causes evacuation of the mole from the uterus. After the mole is expelled, curettage is done. On rare occasions hysterectomy may be necessary. Bleeding following curettage is often quite extensive, and several units of whole blood replacement may be necessary.

Because approximately 10% to 15% of hydatidiform moles are malignant, it is recommended that a chemotherapeutic drug be given before or immediately following the evacuation of the uterus. The chorionic gonadotropin levels should be checked periodically (usually biweekly). Levels that fail to return to normal indicate that there may be a malignant component, which will need to be vigorously treated. Since some spontaneous abortions actually may be the expulsion of hydatidiform moles, all aborted tissue should be sent for pathologic examination.

Chorioepithelioma (choriocarcinoma)

Chorioepithelioma is a highly malignant neoplasm derived from chorionic epithelium. It may occur after a full-term delivery, miscarriage, or hydatidiform mole, although the previous pregnancy is not always recognized. The tumor appears as a dark, hemorrhagic grumose mass either on the uterine wall or in the substance of the uterine wall (the intramural cavity). The surface of the wall later becomes extremely ulcerated, and there is spreading and penetration of the uterine musculature. The chief symptom is bleeding with offensive odor and profuse discharge. There may be early metastases involving the lung, brain, liver, bone, and even the skin as well as the vagina and vulva. Cough or hemoptysis is a sign indicative of pulmonary involvement, and such involvement should be ruled out by x-ray examination.

As the disease advances, there is increasing emaciation and weakness with anemia from frequent, profuse hemorrhage. Treatment may be medical or surgical. Surgical removal of the involved organs such as a lobectomy (removal of a lobe of the lung) may be done.

A successful treatment is the use of the folic acid antagonist, methotrexate (Amethopterin), which is patently toxic to the decidua. A 15 to 25 mg dose is administered intramuscularly each day for 5 days, and a similar course of therapy is repeated a week later. Complications of this drug (stomatitis, nausea, vomiting) sometimes interfere with the patient's treatment. Actinomycin D may also be used for tumors that do not respond to methotrexate[36] (p. 477).

Cancer of the vulva

Cancer of the vulva is usually seen in older women, beyond the age of 65. A form of vulvitis known as *leukoplakia* often precedes cancer of the vulva. Pruritus, either as a symptom of another disease or of cancer, is frequently present in the woman's history. The symptoms of leukoplakia and cancer of the vulva are very similar, and the diagnosis is confirmed by biopsy. If leukoplakia does not respond to conservative treatment, some physicians recommend a *vulvectomy* (surgical excision of the vulva) to prevent the development of cancer. If cancer is already present, the treatment may be radical vulvectomy. This involves dissection of bilateral inguinal lymph nodes, excision of the vulva, excision of the mons pubis and terminal portion of the urethra and vagina, and excision of portions of the round ligaments and saphenous veins. In some instances much less radical surgery is performed. Patients with cancer of the vulva are often poor surgical risks because of concurrent physical disease or problems related to age.

The woman requiring a vulvectomy has some special nursing needs in addition to routine preoperative and postoperative care. Preoperatively she is given enemas, and postoperatively she is given a low-residue diet. These measures obviate the need for straining to defecate and help prevent contamination of the vulval wound. A Foley catheter usually is employed to provide urinary drainage. When the catheter is removed, the patient may be unable to void because of difficulty in relaxing the perineum. Sitz baths may help. If the inguinal nodes have been dissected, a heat lamp may be directed to the groins. After all the sutures are removed, sitz baths may be substituted for the heat lamp. Large amounts of tissues are removed from the vulva and the groins during the operation, and the sutures are usually quite taut, leading to severe discomfort. The patient will usually need analgesic medication at frequent intervals during the 2 or 3 weeks before sutures can be removed. Following an inguinal node dissection, pillows need to be arranged to prevent undue pulling on the taut inguinal sutures when the patient moves. If the patient is lying on her side, she will be more comfortable if her upper leg is supported by a pillow. If she is lying on her back, a low Fowler's position puts less tension on the sutures. Wound hemorrhage is a possible complication.

The vulval wound is frequently left exposed, but if a dressing is used, it is held in place with a T binder. The wound is cleansed twice a day with solutions such as hydrogen peroxide, normal saline solution, benzalkonium chloride, or other antiseptic solutions. Following this, a heat lamp is used to dry the area. The heat also improves local circulation, thus stimulating healing.

The wounds following a vulvectomy or an inguinal node dissection also heal slowly, and the woman may become quite discouraged. Diversional activities and socializing with other patients may help her to pass the time. Privacy should be assured, and women should be encouraged to express their feelings concerning this disfiguring surgery. Some women feel that their femininity has been irreparably damaged or that the disfigurement may end their sexual life. Actually, by the time of discharge the wounds are usually healed, and the convalescence will be similar to that following any surgical procedure. Sexual intercourse can usually be resumed.

□ Management of the woman with a gynecologic malignancy

Management of the woman who has a gynecologic malignancy may include surgery, radiation therapy, or both modalities.

Radiation therapy

Internal radiation is used to treat cancer of the cervix and cancer of the body of the uterus because of the accessibility of these body parts and because of their generally favorable response to this form of treatment. The radioactive materials most often used are radium and cobalt 60 (or iridium 192), which has been made radioactive by artificial means. (For discussion of radiation treatment and the general nursing care and precautions involved, see p. 467.)

It is important that all normal tissues remain in their natural position and do not come nearer to the radioactive substance than is anticipated and provided for by the protective materials used. Before treatment begins, a cleansing enema and a low-residue diet are given to prevent distention of the bowel. A catheter may be inserted to prevent distention of the bladder. Gauze packing is usually inserted into the vagina to push both the rectum and the bladder away from the area being irradiated. Cleansing enemas are not given during the treatment. To prevent any displacement of the radioactive substance, the patient is kept flat in bed and is allowed to turn only from side to side. A roentgenogram is taken after the radioactive substance is inserted to determine its exact location.

The colpostat and tandem incorporating radioactive cobalt and intrauterine applicators or needles containing radium or radioactive iridium are most often used (Fig. 62-9). The amount of radioactive substance used and the number of hours it is left in place are determined by the amount of radiation needed to kill the less resistant cancer cells withouth damaging normal cells. Radioactive materials used for internal treatment must be removed at exactly the indicated time, and the nurse is often responsible for reminding the physician to do this. If possible, the time of insertion should be planned so that removal will be at a convenient hour; for example, not in the middle of the night or during visiting hours.

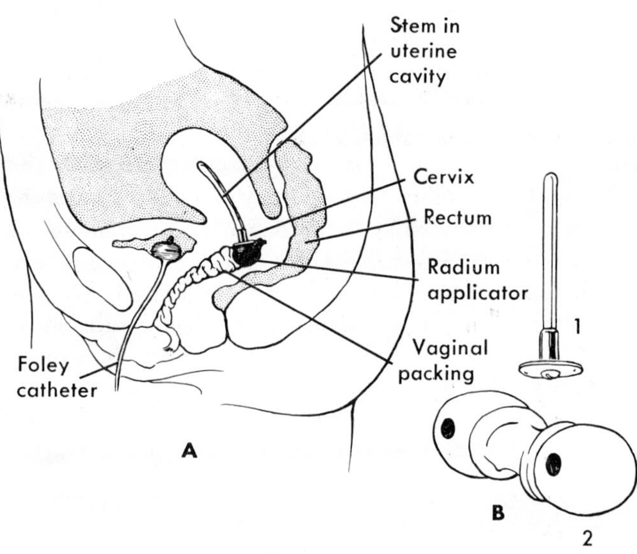

Fig. 62-9. A, Radium applicator in place in uterus. Note Foley catheter to decompress bladder and vaginal packing used. **B,** *1,* Intrauterine applicator. *2,* Colpostat.

Since the presence of anything in the cervix stimulates uterine contractions, the woman who has a colpostat or intrauterine applicator in place may have severe uterine contractions as a result of dilation of the cervix. She should know that they will occur. Often a narcotic is given at regular intervals while the applicator is in place. There will be foul-smelling vaginal discharge from destruction of cells. Good perineal care is essential, and it must be remembered that since the patient must lie on her back, she will need assistance. A deodorizer is helpful.

Patients may develop radiation sickness, with nausea, vomiting, diarrhea, malaise, and fever. This probably is a systemic reaction to the breakdown and reabsorption of cell proteins. (See p. 433 for discussion of care.) Local reaction may include cystitis and proctitis. Camphorated tincture of opium (paregoric) helps relieve the diarrhea. If it is severe, a cornstarch enema (15 ml [1 tablespoon] of cornstarch to 250 ml [1 cup] of lukewarm water) may be ordered. Oil retention enemas are also sometimes given. The woman is urged to drink at least 3 liters of fluid a day to help relieve any irritation of the urinary system.

Since the woman who is receiving radiation treatment usually either knows or suspects the diagnosis, she is likely to be depressed. Nurses can spend some time talking with her but should remain at a safe distance (p. 474). The reason for this precaution should be explained to the patient. Close members of the family should be encouraged to visit when it is considered safe for them to do so.

Following removal of the radioactive agent, the catheter is removed, a cleansing enema is given, and the woman is allowed out of bed. Vaginal discharge will continue for some time, and the patient may need to take douches for as long as the odor and vaginal discharge persist. Usually douches are ordered twice a day. The woman who is returning home needs detailed instruction in how to give herself douches and what solutions to use. Some vaginal bleeding may occur for 1 to 3 months after irradiation of the cervix or the body of the uterus. The woman who is at home should report persistent rectal irritation to the physician. Emollient enemas may be prescribed to be taken at home. The woman is usually discharged from the hospital within a day or two after the applicators are removed but may return for another course of radiation.

Complications to watch for following radiation of the uterus are vesicovaginal fistulas, ureterovaginal fistulas, cystitis, phlebitis, and hemorrhage. Each is caused by irritation and destruction of adjacent tissue either by the radiation or by extension of the disease process. The patient is urged to report even minor symptoms or complaints to her physician.

If the patient is treated by x-ray therapy for a lesion of the reproductive system, the care is the same as that given a patient receiving this treatment elsewhere in the body (p. 470). However, one important point should be emphasized: she should always void immediately before the treatment to prevent damage to the bladder.

Surgery

Psychologic responses. Surgery such as a bilateral oophorectomy or a hysterectomy upsets many women emotionally. Some women worry about the effect it will have on their femininity and wonder about possible changes in secondary sex characteristics. Young women may feel bitterly disappointed because they can no longer have children. Others may be relieved from the fear of becoming pregnant. Some women worry about gaining weight, although weight gain is more often caused by overeating than to hormonal changes. It is true that the childbearing function will be terminated, but usually the vagina is intact so that several weeks following surgery women can resume normal sexual intercourse.

Older women may be less upset by the prospects of surgery of this kind than are those who have not reached the menopause. Postoperatively, however, almost all patients feel depressed for several days. This apparently is because of a change in hormonal balance and of psychologic reaction. The patient often is unable to explain why she is depressed and crying. Grieflike responses to loss of a body part may appear as they do following surgery in other cases. Feelings of guilt, shame, and remorse are not uncommon. Encouraging the woman to continue activities associated with being female such as using makeup, arranging her hair, and wearing her own clothing often helps the woman to regain her perspective of being feminine. During this period she needs understanding and sympathetic care. Families need to be

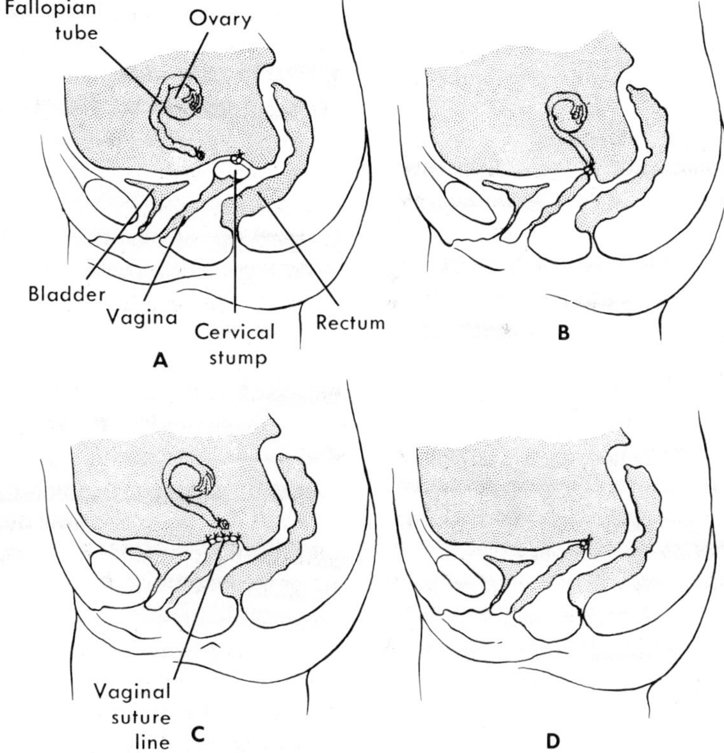

Fig. 62-10. A, Cross-section of subtotal hysterectomy. Note that cervical stump, fallopian tubes, and ovaries remain. **B,** Cross-section of total hysterectomy. Note that fallopian tubes and ovaries remain. **C,** Cross-section of vaginal hysterectomy. Note that fallopian tubes and ovaries remain. **D,** Total hysterectomy, salpingectomy, and oophorectomy. Note that uterus, fallopian tubes, and ovaries are completely removed.

helped to accept these responses calmly, and a husband may need help in understanding her need for reassurance of his continued love and affection.

Hysterectomy. If a hysterectomy is to be performed, the preoperative physical preparation is the same as that for any other abdominal surgery, except that the perineum is completely shaved. A vaginal douche may be given. Postoperatively the patient has an abdominal dressing and wears a perineal pad. If a vaginal hysterectomy is performed, there will be no abdominal incision, but sterile perineal pads will need changing frequently. The dressings should be observed for any sign of bleeding every 15 minutes for 2 hours and then at least every hour for 8 hours. There is normally a moderate amount of serosanguineous drainage. A supportive binder can be applied to the abdomen, especially if there has been a *radical hysterectomy* (removal of the ovaries, tubes, uterus with the cervix, and parametrial tissue) and extensive node dissection (Fig. 62-10).

Following a hysterectomy, especially one in which there has been extensive node and parametrial resection, the bladder may be temporarily atonic as a result of nerve trauma, and a Foley catheter is used to maintain constant drainage of the bladder. If no catheter is used and if the woman is unable to void within 8 hours, she is usually catheterized. The catheter (if used) is removed on the third or fourth postoperative day, and the woman may be catheterized if abnormal residual urine is suspected.

Abdominal distention may complicate a hysterectomy. It is caused by nerve damage, by handling of the viscera during operation, or by sudden release of pressure on the intestines such as occurs on removal of a large myoma. Some physicians insert a nasogastric tube prophylactically following surgery, and most physicians restrict food and fluids orally for 24 to 48 hours. There is usually an order for a rectal tube and for a heating pad to the abdomen to be used as necessary. If the surgery has been extensive, a soft rectal tube should be selected to prevent trauma to the bowel. A Fleet's enema is usually given on the second or third postoperative day. When peristalsis returns, fluids and food are started gradually.

There may be interference with *circulation* during hysterectomy, and thrombophlebitis of the vessels of the pelvis and upper thigh is a rather common complication. The patient should *never* rest with the knees bent or with the thighs sharply flexed. The knee gatch should not be used, and the bed should not be raised at the head to more than a mid-Fowler's position. The woman should exercise her feet and legs every hour, and she should move about in bed, turning from her side to her back and to a partial face-lying position. A pillow can be used to support the abdominal wound. The head of the bed should be put completely flat for a short time every 2 hours during the first 24 hours postoperatively and then at least every 4 hours until the patient is ambulatory. These precautions help prevent stasis of blood in the pelvic vessels. If the woman has varicosities, the physician may order elevation of the legs for a few minutes every 2 or 3 hours to permit blood to drain from the legs. Nurses need to be sure that there is no undue pressure on the calves of the legs, that the elevation is uniform, and that there is no flexing at the popliteal region in order to lessen the possibility of thrombus formation. Antiembolic stockings or Ace bandages may be applied from the toes to just below the knee, excluding the popliteal region. Recent research on thrombophlebitis has indicated that improperly applied Ace bandages are a major cause of postoperative thrombus formation. The bandages should be reapplied twice a day to assure a snug, even pressure. The woman often is permitted out of bed the day following surgery.

Other nursing care is the same as that following any abdominal surgery. Special attention should be given to any complaint of low back pain or to lessened urinary output, since it is possible that a ureter could have been accidentally ligated. Occasionally the ureter, the bladder, or the rectum is traumatized.

The woman should know what surgery has been done, what changes in herself she should expect, and what care she needs when she leaves the hospital. If a *total hysterectomy* has been done, the premenopausal patient will not menstruate. A *subtotal hysterectomy*, however, permits menses to continue, since a portion of the uterus with its endometrial lining is left. She can resume sexual intercourse after the wound is healed. Most patients are more comfortable if they wear a girdle. Heavy lifting should be avoided for about 2 months. Activities such as riding over rough roads, walking swiftly, and dancing tend to cause congestion of blood in the pelvis and should be avoided for several months. Physical activity that does not cause strain, such as swimming, may be engaged in because it is helpful both for physical and mental well-being.

Unilateral salpingectomy and oophorectomy. The woman who has a unilateral salpingectomy (removal of one fallopian tube) or a unilateral oophorectomy (removal of one ovary) usually requires postoperative nursing care similar to that given any patient having abdominal surgery. If the surgery is done to remove a large ovarian cyst, however, there may be considerable abdominal distention because of the sudden release of pressure on the intestines. The care is similar to that given for distention following a hysterectomy. If the surgery is done to remove a tumor that has caused changes in sex characteristics, the patient usually needs much understanding and encouragement from the nurse. She may shun others prior to surgery, and it is wise to let her have privacy if she so desires. She may be reassured that following surgery the abnormal sexual changes will gradually disappear.

Bilateral oophorectomy and radiation of the ovaries. If the ovaries are removed by surgery or are rendered inactive by radiation, the woman will have symptoms of the climacteric. When the menopause is artificially induced, the symptoms are often more severe than in the normal climacteric. Therefore at least a portion of an ovary is left unless this is detrimental to the patient's prognosis. Estrogens relieve the symptoms and may be given to most patients unless surgery has been done for a malignancy. A bilateral oophorectomy may have been done primarily to remove the hormonal supply. This procedure is sometimes used in conjunction with radical mastectomy for cancer of the breast. The period of adjustment after a bilateral oophorectomy is long and is often trying not only for the patient but also for her family.

Pelvic exenteration. In a pelvic exenteration all reproductive organs and adjacent tissues are removed. Nursing care includes the care given the patient having a hysterectomy, the care given the patient having an abdominal perineal resection of the bowel, and the care given the patient having an ileobladder with transplantation of the ureters. Since this operation includes a radical hysterectomy, pelvic node dissection, cystectomy, vaginectomy, and a rectal resection, it requires unusual physical, social, and emotional adjustments on the part of the woman.

After a pelvic exenteration, both urine and feces pass from the body through openings in the abdominal wall. The woman cannot contemplate having children, cannot have vaginal intercourse, and will have symptoms of the menopause. Until she is able to accept her situation realistically, her rehabilitation will progress very slowly. This acceptance cannot be forced, but the patient must be encouraged gradually to resume self-care. She will undoubtedly have recurring periods of depression and discouragement. She should be helped to express her feelings about the radical changes in her body. The family should understand what the surgery will entail, and they too need encouragement. Acceptance of the situation by the patient's husband is a very important factor in giving her the reassurance and courage necessary to face her future, and he may need to talk about his feelings with the nurse or others.

□ Care of the woman with incurable disease of the female reproductive system

The women with incurable disease of the reproductive system frequently has a lingering terminal illness. Most carcinomas of the female reproductive system do not metastasize to vital areas such as the liver. By direct spread they eventually cause death from carcinomatosis and from kidney failure that results from obstruction of both ureters by the tumor.

The nursing care is the same as for any patient with a terminal cancer elsewhere (p. 486), but there are some special measures that help to make the patient more comfortable. Frequent changes of position help relieve abdominal and pelvic pressure, and alternate hot and cold applications to the abdomen may bring some relief from pain. A chordotomy is sometimes done to relieve severe pain (p. 354).

As cells die and are expelled, vaginal discharge may be profuse and have a foul odor. This is upsetting to the woman, her family, and her friends. The most effective means of decreasing the odor is to give the patient perineal care every 4 hours and to give a cleansing douche at least twice daily. Copious amounts of water should be used. Solutions containing chlorine are useful in destroying odors, and aromatic preparations added to the water may make the patient feel cleaner and more acceptable.

Meticulous care must be given to the skin, since the woman is usually emaciated and may develop pitting edema. If the woman has ascites, she may rest better if the head of the bed is elevated.

■ DISEASES OF THE MALE REPRODUCTIVE SYSTEM

The female nurse must be particularly sensitive to the reactions and feelings of male patients who have disease of the reproductive system. The patient may feel more comfortable discussing his problems with a male nurse or male physician.

□ Infections

Nonspecific pyogenic organisms as well as specific organisms such as gonococci and tubercle bacilli may cause stubborn infections of the male reproductive system. Urethritis, prostatitis, seminal vesiculitis, and epididymitis are the most common infections. Infecting organisms may reach the genital organs by direct spread through the urethra, or they may be borne by blood or lymph.

Because urethral infection spreads so readily to the genital organs, men should not be catheterized unless it is absolutely necessary. Every means should be used to help them void normally. They are often allowed to stand to void even when they are to be on bed rest otherwise. Because of the length and curvature of the male urethra, some trauma to the urethral mucosa is likely to accompany catheterization or the passage of instruments such as a cystoscope. The distal part of the urethra is not sterile, and trauma makes the area susceptible to attack from the bacteria present. Fluids should be given liberally following passage of instruments through the urethra.

Nonspecific urethritis

Nonspecific urethritis is an inflammation of the urethra caused by such organisms as staphylococci, *Escherichia coli, Pseudomonas,* and streptococci. Although the symptoms and complications are essentially the same as those of gonorrheal urethritis, this infection is rarely caused by sexual contact. The patient complains of urgency, frequency, and burning on urination. There may be a purulent urethral discharge. (See p. 1447 for discussion of gonorrheal urethritis.)

Treatment of nonspecific urethritis consists of antibiotics and chemotherapy, hot sitz baths, and increased fluid intake. To drain periurethral glands, the urethra may be dilated with sounds (Fig. 62-11). Dilation is followed by the instillation of a mild antiseptic such as 1:10,000 silver nitrate solution. Physical rest, improvement of general health, and decreased sexual activity are usually suggested. Nonspecific urethritis is difficult to cure and may become a chronic problem that ultimately results in chronic prostatitis.

Prostatitis

The patient with prostatitis usually has acute symptoms of urinary obstruction. He suddenly has difficulty in voiding, perineal tenderness and pain, and elevation of temperature. There may be hematuria. Treatment is usually conservative, consisting of antibiotics and chemotherapy, forcing fluids, physical rest, and local application of heat by sitz baths or lower rectal irrigations or both.

Before having a rectal irrigation, the patient should have a cleansing enema. Then, by means of a Y connector on the rectal tube, tap water is allowed to flow alternately in and out of the rectum. The use of 2 liters of water 46 C (115 F) and the insertion of the tube only 7.5 to 10 cm (3 to 4 inches) into the rectum will concentrate heat in the area of the prostate gland.

Prompt treatment of prostatitis may obviate the need for an indwelling catheter by preventing edema of the prostate and resultant obstruction of the urethra. Occasionally *prostatic abscesses* complicate the clinical course and may have to be drained surgically. Recurrent episodes of acute prostatitis may cause fibrotic tissue to form, and a prostatectomy may be necessary to relieve the resultant obstruction (p. 1312).

Epididymitis

Epididymitis, one of the most common infections of the male reproductive system, may be caused by any pyogenic organism, but it frequently is a complication of gonorrhea or of tuberculosis of the urinary system. Since bilateral epididymitis usually causes sterility, special attention is given to the prevention of this infection. Untreated epididymitis leads rather rapidly to necrosis of testicular tissue and septicemia. When bladder drainage over a long period of time is necessary, a cystotomy is done so that a urethral catheter is avoided. An older patient who must have surgery of the prostate, such as transurethral resection that will require leaving a urethral catheter in place for a long time, may be advised to have a *bilateral vasectomy* to prevent any infection from descending via the ductus deferens to the epididymis. Often the operation is done prior to any cystoscopic

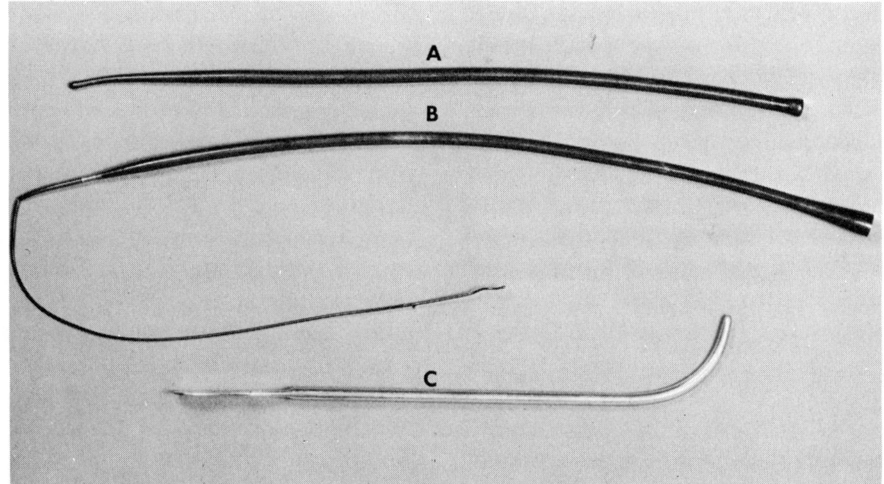

Fig. 62-11. A, Bougie for urethral dilation. **B,** Filiform. Note long, fine, flexible tip. **C,** Metal sound for urethral dilation.

examination. Since bilateral vasectomy causes sterility, permission must be granted by the patient. The vasectomies are done through two very small incisions in the scrotum or in the groins. Local anesthesia is used. Postoperatively the patient should still be watched for symptoms of epididymitis, since the organisms may have invaded the epididymis prior to the vasectomy. The man complains of severe tenderness, pain, and swelling of the scrotum, which is hot to the touch. His temperature may be markedly elevated, and he has general malaise. He often walks with a characteristic "duck waddle" in an attempt to protect the affected part. This walk may first disclose difficulty in the patient who is too embarrassed to describe his trouble.

The patient with epididymitis is usually put to bed and the scrotum elevated either on towel rolls or with adhesive strapping known as a Bellevue bridge (Fig. 62-12). Ice is used to help reduce the swelling and to relieve the pain and discomfort. Heat is usually contraindicated because the normal temperature of the scrotal contents is below normal body temperature, and excessive exposure to heat may cause destruction of sperm cells. If an ice cap is used, it should be placed under the scrotum and should be removed for short intervals every hour to prevent ice burns. Antibiotic therapy is given. At least 3 liters of fluid should be taken daily. When the patient is allowed out of bed, he should wear a scrotal support.

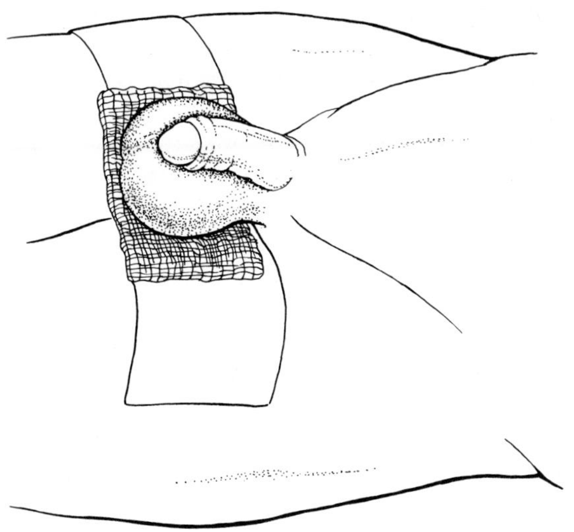

Fig. 62-12. Bellevue bridge.

Paraphimosis

Paraphimosis is a condition in which the prepuce is retracted over the glans and forms a constriction that is sometimes impossible to reduce as edema develops in the glans (Fig. 62-13). Cool compresses are applied to the penis, and it is elevated for a short time before a gentle attempt is made to reduce the prepuce. If this measure fails, emergency surgery must be done. A dorsal slit is made in the prepuce to prevent necrosis of the glans caused by impairment of its blood supply. A circumcision usually is done later to prevent recurrences.

Circumcision, or surgical excision of the prepuce, is widely recommended for all male infants in the immediate newborn period. The reasons are that it makes cleansing of the area so much simpler and that cancer of the glans penis is almost unknown among men who were circumcised soon after birth. If the operation is performed a few days after birth, no general anesthetic is needed. Older patients, even if they need anesthesia, are not hospitalized for more than a few hours for this operation. The wound is covered with gauze generously impregnated with petrolatum. Bleeding usually is controlled by applying a pressure dressing that may be bulky and that

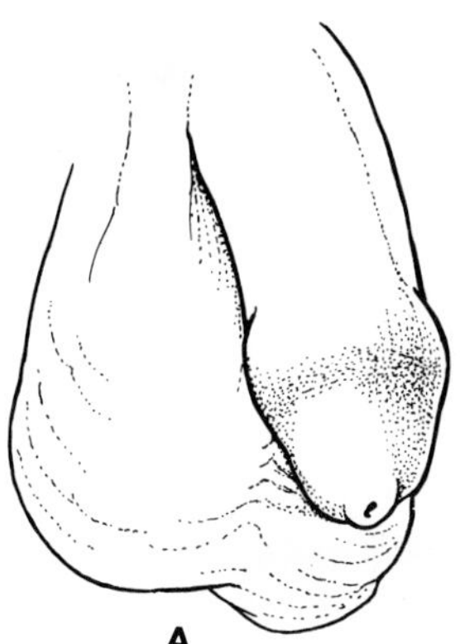

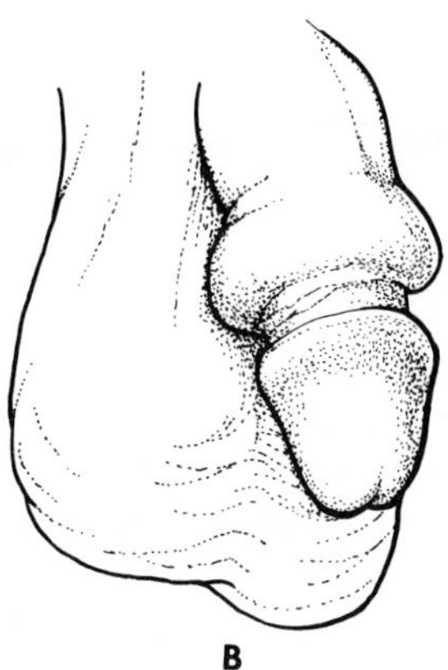

Fig. 62-13. A, Phimosis. Note pinpoint opening of foreskin. **B,** Paraphimosis. Note foreskin is retracted but has become constricting band around penis.

sometimes must be removed before the patient can void. It should be removed cautiously and replaced after voiding with a petrolatum dressing. If the patient goes home, he or his mother, if the patient is a child, is taught to change the dressing at each voiding for a few days and to try, if possible to avoid fecal contamination of the area. Instruction is also given to be alert for signs of bleeding. If severe bleeding occurs, a firm dressing should be applied to the penis and the patient should go at once to the physician's office or the hospital emergency room. Very occasionally, if bleeding persists, it is necessary to resuture the wound. An estrogen preparation may be prescribed for adult patients for several days after surgery to prevent penile erections, which are painful.

Orchitis

An infection of the testicle is known as orchitis. It may be caused by pyogenic bacteria, the gonococcus, or the tubercle bacillus, or it may be a complication of mumps contracted after puberty. Although the latter occurs in a relatively small percentage of cases, if bilateral, it usually causes sterility. Any boy after puberty or man who is exposed to mumps usually is given gamma globulin immediately unless he has already had the disease. If there is any doubt, globulin usually is given. Although it may not prevent mumps, the disease is likely to be less severe with less likelihood of complications.

The symptoms and the treatment of orchitis are the same as those of epididymitis. Stilbestrol, which inhibits normal function, cortisone, and antibiotics may be given. Sometimes the tunica albuginea must be excised surgically to improve circulation to the testicle.

□ Scrotal and testicular enlargement

Immediate medical attention should be sought for any swelling of the scrotum or the testicles within it. Scrotal enlargements should be diagnosed—not treated symptomatically with suspensories, which give relief and encourage procrastination.

Hydrocele

A hydrocele is a benign, painless collection of fluid within the tunica vaginalis that leads to swelling of the scrotum. It occurs fairly often in infant boys as well as in adults. The cause is usually unknown. Occasionally hydrocele is treated by aspirating the fluid and injecting a sclerosing drug such as urea hydrochloride into the scrotal sac, but excision of the tunica vaginalis (hydrocelectomy) is the preferred treatment. Postoperatively a pressure dressing is applied on the scrotum, which is elevated. The patient should be observed carefully for any symptoms of hemorrhage. Bleeding may not be external. The patient needs a scrotal support when he is up and about and may still require one after he is discharged from the hospital. He should have two scrotal suspensories, since they should be washed each day. Immediately after surgery or following an infection, most patients require an extra large suspensory or perhaps an athletic support (jockstrap).

Testicular neoplasm

Cancer of the testicle is usually painless, but it may be accompanied by an aching or dragging sensation in the groin and by swelling of the testicle. The swelling is frequently first discovered by men following trauma, but it usually is not caused by the trauma. Testicular swelling should always make one suspicious of neoplasm of the testicle. This condition is usually seen in men between 25 and 35 years of age, and it accounts for about 3% of all malignant tumors of the male reproductive system.[11]

An *undescended testicle* is much more likely to become malignant than one that is in the scrotum at birth or descends shortly thereafter. This is an important reason for encouraging parents to consent to surgical intervention to bring the undescended testicle of a young boy to a normal position. This does not eliminate the possibility of a neoplasm developing, but the testicle is located in a position where it may be examined carefully and regularly.

Clinical picture. Men with suspicious testicular swelling are asked to collect a first-voided morning urine specimen. This is sent for an Aschheim-Zondek test, the same test used to detect pregnancy in women. One type of testicular tumor, the one with the poorest prognosis, gives a positive Aschheim-Zondek reaction. For all types of testicular tumors the testicle is removed surgically (orchiectomy) and the adjacent area is explored for metastatic node involvement. Metastasis often has occurred before the initial lesion is discovered.

Intervention. Cancer of the testicle is usually treated with a course of radiation therapy, and a *radical node dissection* may be done. This dissection may be unilateral or bilateral.

Following a radical node dissection, there is danger of hemorrhage. Active movement may be contraindicated, since nodes may have been resected from around many large abdominal vessels, but gentle passive turning and leg and arm movement are essential to prevent postoperative pneumonia and thrombosis. Deep breathing should be encouraged at hourly intervals. A turning sheet and a chest support are usually helpful. The patient is extremely uncomfortable and needs frequent and large doses of narcotics and sedative drugs.

When a radical node dissection is performed, the patient may be placed in a Trendelenburg position for 2 weeks to allow the kidney to become fixed in place, since frequently all the fatty tissue supporting it must be removed. The patient may need to be fed and bathed during this period. He may have difficulty voiding in this position. For defecation, permission from the physician may have to be obtained to lower the foot of the bed. Occupational and diversional therapy should be provided. Since many patients find it impossible even to read in the Trendelenburg position, they may appreciate being read to, having the use of books that can be projected on the ceiling, or having access to "talking books" used by blind persons.

Since radiation therapy often is begun the day after surgery, the man may develop radiation sickness during his hospital stay or during continued treatment as an outpatient. Hormones and chemotherapy are not effective in slowing the progress of cancer in this organ.

Patients and their families are extremely upset by the diagnosis of neoplasm of the testicle. The physician frequently is quite frank with the family and with the patient because he believes the man needs to be able to make necessary arrangements to provide for his family. The patient's prognosis may be measured in only months or in several years. Some men are openly depressed. Others may seem to be taking the news too well. Nurses can listen carefully to both the patient and his family and sometimes suggest that help be obtained from others such as the social worker or the spiritual adviser. (For further discussion see p. 466).

Spermatocele

A spermatocele is a nontender cystic mass containing sperm. It is attached to the epididymis. Since the lesion is benign and usually there are few symptoms, excision is rarely necessary. If the patient if uncomfortable, he is usually advised to wear a scrotal support to prevent undue discomfort until after he has a family. Large masses may then be excised.

Varicocele

A varicocele is a dilation of the spermatic vein and is commonly seen on the left side only, probably because the left spermatic vein is much longer than the right. A varicocele on the right side only is suggestive of an abdominal tumor. The use of a scrotal support is usually all that is necessary to relieve any dragging sensation, but the spermatic vein may be ligated.

Torsion of the testicle

Torsion of the testicle or kinking of the spermatic artery causes severe pain, tenderness, and swelling of the testicle. It often follows activity that puts a sudden pull on the cremasteric muscle such as may occur from jumping into cold water. Operative intervention may be indicated and must be done within a few hours because interruption of blood supply to the testicle causes necrosis of the organ.

□ Cancer of the prostate gland

Epidemiology

The prostate gland is the second most common site of cancer among men, occurring in 17% of all cancers; it is responsible for 9% of all deaths due to cancer in men.[86] Prostatic cancer rarely occurs before the age of 50, and there is an increased familial risk. Its incidence has increased by more than 20% since 1940.[86] The increased incidence may reflect greater attention on the need for early diagnosis, improved diagnostic methods, and the fact that men are better informed about cancer than in past.

No classification system for the stages of prostatic cancer has been accepted. However, the following represents a sampling of classification systems most often used.[19]

Stage I: Microscopic lesions found in the prostate removed because of benign hypertrophy

Stage II: Nodules confined to the prostate gland; no capsular adherence or urethral involvement; normal serum acid phosphatase level

Stage III: Carcinoma involving prostatic capsule, seminal vesicles, urethra, bladder, and pelvic lymph nodes, or a malignant tumor of less extent with an elevated serum acid phosphatase level

Stage IV: Findings in stage III, plus evidence of extrapelvic lesions or osseous involvement

Cancer of the prostate may start as a discrete, localized, hard nodule palpable in the prostate before progressing to an advanced, inoperable, and incurable stage. For this reason there is agreement that all men near and over the age of 50 should have an annual rectal examination.

Clinical picture

Cancer of the prostate gland is most often diagnosed when the man seeks medical advice because of symptoms of urethral obstruction or because of sciatica (low back, hip, and leg pain). The pain is caused by metastasis of the cancer to the bones. This form of cancer frequently occurs concurrently with benign prostatic hypertrophy that causes the urethral obstruction. However, the cancer itself may be so far advanced as to cause obstruction.

Most carcinomas of the prostate gland are adjacent to the rectal wall and can be detected by rectal examination before symptoms appear.

Intervention

In patients in whom a diagnosis is made prior to local extension of the cancer or distant metastasis, a radical resection of the prostate gland usually is curative. The entire prostate gland, including the capsule and the adjacent tissue, is removed. The remaining urethra is then anastomosed to the bladder neck. Since the internal and external sphincters of the bladder lie in close approximation to the prostate gland, it is not unusual for the patient to have urinary incontinence following this type of surgery. He also will be both impotent and sterile. The perineal approach is most often used, but the procedure may be accomplished by the retropubic route (Fig. 59-4, *B* and *C*).

If the patient is to have a perineal approach in surgery, he is given a bowel preparation, which includes enemas, cathartics, and phthalylsulfathiazole (Sulfathalidine) or neomycin preoperatively and only clear fluids the day before surgery to prevent fecal contamination of the operative site. Postoperatively he may be permitted nothing orally, or clear liquids or a low-residue diet may be given until wound healing is well advanced. He may also be given camphorated tincture of opium to inhibit bowel action. If the retropubic approach is used, the preoperative care is similar to that of any patient having major surgery.

Regardless of the surgical approach, the patient returns from surgery with a urethral catheter inserted. A large amount of urinary drainage on the dressing for a number of hours is not unusual. It should decrease rapidly, however. There should not be the amount of bleeding that follows other prostatic surgery, and since the catheter is not being used for hemostasis, the patient usually has little bladder spasm. The catheter is used both for urinary drainage and as a splint for the urethral anastomosis. Therefore care should be taken that it does not become dislodged or blocked. The catheter is usually left in the bladder for 2 or 3 weeks.

The care of the perineal wound is the same as that following a perineal biopsy except that healing is usually slower. If there has been a retropubic surgical approach, the wound and possible wound complications are the same as for a simple retropubic prostatectomy (p. 1314).

Since perineal surgery causes relaxation of the perineal musculature, the patient may suddenly have fecal incontinence. It is disturbing to the patient and sometimes can be avoided by starting perineal exercises within a day or two after surgery. Control of the rectal sphincter usually returns readily. Perineal exercises should be continued even after rectal sphincter control returns, since they also strengthen the bladder sphincters, and unless the bladder sphincters have been permanently damaged, the patient will regain urinary control more readily on removal of the catheter. (See p. 1273 for perineal exercises.)

The patient with carcinoma of the prostate gland is often very depressed after surgery because he suddenly realizes the implications of being impotent and perhaps permanently incontinent. He usually has been told by the physician before the operation that these consequences are possible, but he may not have fully comprehended their meaning. He needs to be encouraged, and provision should be made to keep him dry so that he will feel able to be up and to socialize with others without fear of having obvious incontinence. (See p. 1274 for ways to manage incontinence.) Until the physician has ascertained that return of urinary sphincter control is unlikely, a method that gives only partial protection, such as the use of a bathing cap, is preferable since the patient is more likely to attempt to regain voluntary control.

When cancer of the prostate gland is inoperable, or when signs of metastasis occur following surgery, medical treatment is given. Relief from conservative treatment is quite dramatic in many patients and may last for 10 years or more in some instances. Usually the response is quite good for about a year and then the patient's condition begins to deteriorate.

The Huggins treatment may be used for inoperable cancer of the prostate gland to cause atrophy of the local lesion, control metastases, and relieve pain. It is based on the elimination of androgens by removal of the testicles or the giving of estrogenic hormones or both. The estrogen given is usually stilbestrol 3 mg/day for 1 to 2 weeks. The dosage is then reduced to 1.5 to 3 mg/day. This measure frequently will relieve the pain. Stilbestrol causes engorgement and tenderness of the male breasts. It may also cause nausea. Severe side effects should be reported to the physician so that the dosage or type of estrogenic preparation may be adjusted. If a large tumor does not diminish in size with this treatment, some of the prostate gland may be resected to relieve obstruction. This procedure is most often done transurethrally (p. 1312).

When symptoms begin to recur, or if the patient is very uncomfortable and needs immediate relief when the diagnosis of cancer is first made, a *bilateral orchiectomy (castration)* may be done. This operative procedure is technically minor and is often done under local anesthesia, but it may cause the patient considerable psychologic distress. The man's permission for sterilization must be obtained. If he is married, he is usually urged to discuss the operation with his wife. This surgery eliminates the testicular source of male hormones and seems to cause regression or at least slows the cancer growth. Very occasionally a hypophysectomy may be done to further reduce hormonal stimulation.

□ Lesions of the external genitalia

Any lesion of the external genitalia requires medical attention, and no ulcer of the genitalia should be treated by the patient before seeing a physician lest the diagnosis be obscured. Although lesions are present in a wide variety of conditions, they should always be considered infectious until proved otherwise, since each

 impotence: inability to have and maintain an erection

of the venereal diseases, with the exception of gonorrhea, produces a genital lesion or ulceration. These lesions will be discussed in the section to follow, which deals with the venereal diseases.

Cancer of the penis

Cancer of the penis is far less common than formerly, but it still accounts for almost 3% of all cancers in men. Apparently it could be eliminated completely, since carcinoma practically never develops in men who have been circumcised as infants. Usually the patient is over 50 years of age, but the condition has developed in men in their twenties. Most often the glans is the site of the initial malignant lesion.

Treatment for carcinoma of the penis is surgery with partial or total amputation of the penis. Removal of adjacent tissues and inguinal lymph nodes may be necessary, and this treatment may be followed by radiation therapy. Occasionally radiation therapy is used before surgery is done. Radiation therapy may be given externally, or needles, seeds, or plaques containing radioactive substances may be used. The physical nursing care is similar to that needed by women who have had a vulvectomy with inguinal node dissection (p. 1443). Since the treatment causes such serious changes in a man's total life, the emotional reactions are profound, and very specialized care is needed. For further discussion of the treatment and the nursing care involved, see specialized nursing texts.

■ VENEREAL DISEASE

□ Epidemiology

Venereal disease (VD) is the most common communicable disease in the United States today. Although syphilis and gonorrhea have received greatest attention, there are other infections that are transmitted by sexual contact. These include chancroid, granuloma inguinale, lymphogranuloma venereum, herpes genitalis, trachomoniasis, and candidiasis. In most of the literature, trichomoniasis and candidiasis are not addressed as venereally transmitted diseases and are generally held to be insignificant infections. Chancroid, granuloma inguinale, and lymphogranuloma venereum are frequently referred to as the "minor" venereal diseases, perhaps because of their low frequency in the United States. In some regions of the world, however, the so-called "minor" venereal infections are epidemic or near epidemic. The sexually transmissible diseases will probably lose their distinction as "major" and "minor" eventually. From reports of their prevalence and effects on general and reproductive health,[54,75] the minor venereal diseases require greater attention than they have so far been given.

All states require that each case of syphilis and gonorrhea be reported to the state or local health officer. Chancroid, granuloma inguinale, and lymphogranuloma venereum are reportable in most states. Herpes genitalis, trichomoniasis, and candidiasis are not reportable in any state. Therefore the true incidence of venereal diseases is not known.

The importance of sexually transmitted diseases continues to increase. Gonorrhea ranks first and syphilis ranks third among the reportable communicable diseases.[93] The reported number of cases of gonorrhea and syphilis since 1941 is shown in Fig. 62-14. Gonorrhea has continually increased since 1963. Note that although the *total number* of cases of syphilis has decreased steadily since about 1963, the number of reported cases of primary and secondary syphilis has *increased* since 1970. The number of early latent cases of syphilis reported seems to have leveled off since about 1973. The current statistics for late syphilis indicate a decrease of 12.6% between 1974 and 1975.[93] This decrease partly reflects control programs in effect between 1955 and 1965 and therefore a decrease in the late consequences of syphilis.

Intensive screening of pregnant women and increased prenatal care have resulted in dramatic decreases in the incidence of congenital syphilis. A decrease of 23.2% in the incidence of congenital syphilis occurred between 1974 and 1975. It is felt that of all the methods by which syphilis can be acquired, congenital syphilis is the most preventable, yet 1,024 cases were reported in 1975.[93]

The greatest percentage of cases of syphilis is believed to be unreported. It has been estimated that close to 100,000 new cases of syphilis actually occurred in 1973 than are reflected in the statistics.[77]

Gonorrhea has become so prevalent in the United States that the greatest number ever to be reported since the Public Health Service began keeping records was reported in 1974.[3] As with syphilis, the number of reported cases does not reflect the true incidence. This is thought to be because of the failure of physicians to report cases of gonorrhea, but may also be because of the fact that women present little or no evidence of infection so that underdiagnosis may occur. It is estimated that at least 2,600,000 cases of gonorrhea actually occurred in the United States in 1975 as compared to the 938,778 cases reported.[93]

The magnitude of the problem of gonorrhea can be better understood in terms of its effects on the health of a population. Reported gonorrhea rose by 6.5% among males and 8.8% among females between 1974 and 1975, with both sexes at greatest risk during the reproductive ages.[92] Pelvic inflammatory disease occurred in 17% of all women known to have gonorrhea, and this translates into 220,000 cases of PID per year.[93] Because of necessary treatment for PID, about 4.5% of women are surgically sterilized annually, reflecting a total number of

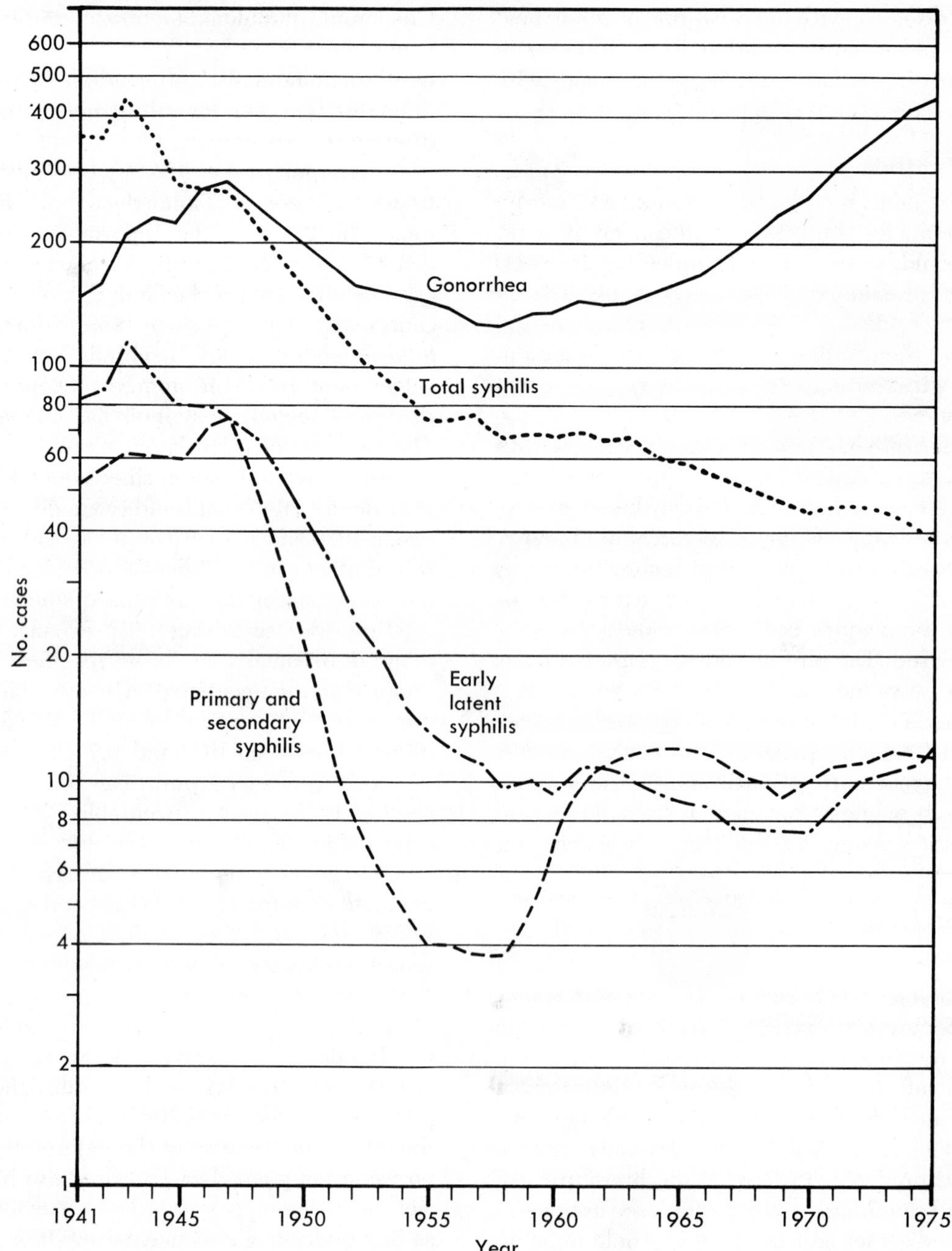

Fig. 62-14. Reported cases of syphilis and gonorrhea per 100,000 population in United States: 1941 to 1975.

9,900 sterilizations per year.[92] About 5,750 girls are absent from school each *day* because of gonorrhea.[3]

Lymphogranuloma venereum (LGV) occurs with relative infrequency in the United States, but it is prevalent in Southeast Asia. It is thought to be endemic among blacks in the United States,[75] but epidemiologic studies are needed to determine its true incidence. Reports of the incidence of LGV vary from 828 cases reported in 1972[54] to 600 cases in 1973[75] to 374 cases in 1974.[92] The symptoms of LGV resemble those of other venereal diseases, and its reported incidence may be influenced by this.

Chancroid infection occurs more frequently than LGV in the United States but is still considered one of the minor venereal diseases. Reports of its incidence indicate that in 1971 there were 1,320 cases[54] and in 1974 there were 1,064 cases in the United States.[92] Although it is found worldwide, chancroid is most prevalent in tropical and semitropical areas. The disease occurs more often in men than in women, and more often among nonwhite than white people. However, repeated references to the relationship between chancroid and the poor, socially deprived, and unhygienic can be misleading. In American troops in Korea the incidence of chancroid was as great as that of syphilis, and in troops in Vietnam chancroid ranked second to the incidence of gonorrhea.[92] It is possible that returning military personnel may have introduced the disease into areas where it did not previously exist.

Granuloma inguinale (donovanosis) is common in tropical and subtropical areas and rarely occurs in the United States. It is very common in New Guinea, India, and the Caribbean. The role of sexual transmission has been debated because there is a reported incidence of 12.1% infection rate among married couples having steady sexual partners. The disease, however, is mildly contagious and probably requires repeated exposures for spread of infection. Predisposing factors are poorly understood. Most experts believe that donovanosis is transmitted by sexual contact. Under 100 cases were reported in the United States each year between 1972 and 1974. The disease is more common in men than women and is especially common among homosexual men.[75]

Genital herpes (herpesvirus hominis type 2) is not a reportable disease, and therefore its true incidence is not known. Major interest in the causative virus has been generated because of its probable etiologic significance to cervical cancer rather than because of its significance as a venereal disease. There is general agreement that the virus is spread by sexual contact, since the age of infected persons parallels the age of patients with other sexually transmitted diseases. Genital herpes is often found concurrently with one or more of the other venereal diseases and is believed to be prevalent among prostitutes.[54] It has been estimated that 300,000 cases of genital herpes occur yearly in the United States.[93]

There is disagreement about whether yeast infections such as candidiasis should be classed as venereal. The organism is commonly found on mucous membrane surfaces in women who have no symptoms of infection. The greatest incidence of candidiasis occurs during the ages of maximum sexual activity. The causative organism is frequently cultured from the urethra of regular male sex partners, and urethritis and balanitis (inflammation of the glans penis) occur in up to 10% of men who engage in sexual activity with infected women.[54] Women who respond to therapy and become reinfected are usually married women having one sex partner.[75] *Candida albicans,* the causative organism, is found in the mouth, gastrointestinal tract, and vagina of 25% to 50% of women.[54] Differentiation between colonization and true infection may be difficult in some cases. Colonization rate and the chance of true infection increases in diabetic persons, during pregnancy, and with diseases or therapies that impair body defenses (use of broad-spectrum antibiotics, corticosteroids, and oral contraceptives).

Trichomoniasis may well be the most frequently acquired sexually transmitted disease in the United States, with an estimated incidence of 3 million cases occurring annually.[93] The causative organism, *Trichomonas vaginalis,* is found in 3% to 15% of women under the care of private physicans, 13% to 23% of women attending gynecologic clinics,[75] and in 50% of women who have gonorrhea.[54] There is no documentation of the rate at which asymptomatic carriers become symptomatic.

Trichomoniasis is frequently viewed as an innocuous infection, yet there are serious implications for health. During the postpartum period in women who have trichomoniasis, the rate of persistent fever, prolonged vaginal discharge, and endometritis is twice as high than in women who do not harbor the organism.[75] About 90% of patients with trichomoniasis have cervical erosions and leukorrhea, and it has been suggested that chronic irritation may predispose to cervical cancer.[65] Interpretation of cervical cytology, as in the Pap smear, is unreliable in the presence of trichomoniasis, since the infection produces atypical cervical cells.[75] Unless repeated cervical smears are taken, cancer of the cervix may be missed. Trichomoniasis results in prostatis in men 40% of the time, and, finally, reversible sterility can occur as a result of inhibition of sperm motility by toxins produced by the organism.[75]

□ Social factors

In explaining the trends of reported cases of venereal diseases in the United States, three changes occurring in recent years are often referred to in the literature. The first of these concerns use of antibiotics and changes in the antibiotic susceptibility of pathogenic organisms. The widespread, perhaps indiscriminate, use of penicillin and other antibiotics between the late 1940s and early 1950s parallels the decline in both syphilis and gonorrhea. It is said that the organisms developed a greater resistance to antibiotics over time and that they have therefore become less effective than previously. There is no firm evidence to indicate a decrease in effectiveness of penicillin against syphilis.[8] However, the gonococcus tends to develop resistance to antibiotics.[17]

A second explanation for the rise in incidence of venereal diseases is that they are more likely to occur if a social system is permissive. During times of war and other catastrophes it is easier for agencies to control interpersonal behavior, while in times of peace and absence of national crisis, civil liberties tend to flourish. The incidence curve of syphilis and gonorrhea (Fig. 62-14) during the years of World War II seems to support this thesis.

The third explanation centers around sexual behavior patterns and includes permissiveness. Concern has been particularly expressed about the prevalence of gonorrhea among adolescents who are considered to be promiscuous. Age-wise, in fact, rates for gonorrhea show young adults age 20 to 24 years to be at greatest risk for acquiring gonorrhea, with the second highest risk group being teenagers age 15 to 19.[8] The incidence of syphilis according to age indicates young adults to be at greatest risk, but that teenagers are the fourth highest risk group by age.[93]

The above discussion makes an assumption of sexual promiscuity, and in doing so, requires acknowledgement of advances in contraceptive technology, especially the Pill. These social changes are often termed the three *P*s (permissiveness, promiscuity, and the Pill).[18] The underlying idea is that, with the advent of antibiotics and the Pill, people began to lose fear of untreated venereal disease and pregnancy, and that sexual promiscuity increased significantly, leading to increased exposure to infection.

If the definition of promiscuity is that sexual relations are not restricted to one partner, studies show that patients diagnosed in clinics as having venereal disease are not promiscuous. In one study 66.4% of patients having a venereal disease named only one sexual contact.[18] It must be realized, however, that persons may hesitate to admit to having more than one sex partner for any number of reasons.

In the past, prostitution has been considered a major force in the transmission of venereal diseases. Prior to World War II it was estimated that approximately 75% of all venereal diseases could be traced to prostitutes, and that at least 10% of all prostitutes had contracted a venereal disease at least once. Today less than 5% of patients with syphilis can be classed as prostitutes.[8] Also, most persons with gonorrhea are single and under 25 years of age, and most clients of prostitutes are usually older, married men.[8]

Prior to 1960, homosexuals were rarely mentioned in the literature as carriers of venereal disease. By 1972, however, it was noted that about 14.4% of all syphilitic infections are spread by persons who name only sexual partners of the same sex.[3] In 1975, two instances of outbreaks of gonorrhea were reported.[3] One of these occurred in a large county jail, where 10 cases of gonorrhea were traced to an infected homosexual inmate.

The condom was the main method of contraception used prior to the advent of antibiotics and oral contraceptives. The use of the condom may have discouraged spread of the venereal diseases by providing a mechanical barrier to the organism. The Pill has almost revolutionized contraception practices, and it has been noted that neutralization of the vaginal and cervical environment by estrogenic substances predisposes to infection. Women who use oral contraceptives do seem to have more than one sex partner.[18] It would appear that individual characteristics of persons engaging in sexual activity need to be more closely studied before any conclusions about permissiveness, promiscuity, and use of the Pill can be made.

□ Education

Reluctance to permit teaching about human sexuality and venereal diseases in the school is in conflict with our highly sex-oriented society. Those who are in a position to present facts and information may hesitate to do so for a variety of reasons. Parental disapproval seems to stem from beliefs that children are too young and innocent to learn about such things as sexuality and venereal disease. Another belief seems to be that to teach facts or give information about these topics implies approval and encouragement of premarital sex at an early age. There seems to be fear that giving information increases curiosity and experimentation, and this might be a risk if facts are not presented completely and consequences are not included.

Sex education can be separated to some extent from venereal disease education by including venereal disease in general health courses. Even so, educators might remain hesitant. Inadequate instruction and inappropriate approaches can have highly negative consequences. If dealt with too lightly, young people may feel that venereal disease is no more serious than any other infection and that it is easily and simply cured by a shot of penicillin. They may not become aware of the immediate problems of infecting others or of the long-term effects of repeated or chronic infections. If presented in such a way that shame is associated with sexual activity and venereal disease, young people may be ashamed or afraid to admit they have venereal disease and may delay seeking health care.

□ Sexual transmission

The venereal diseases are contagious diseases spread almost exclusively by contact during sexual intercourse, that is, when mucous membrane surfaces come in contact during genital, oral, or anal sexual activity. Since the causative organisms survive only very briefly outside a warm, moist environment, there is almost no way to contract venereal disease from toilet seats, towels, or bed linens. There are some notable exceptions to sexual transmission. During pregnancy the fetus may become infected in utero by placental transmission, and the infant may acquire congenital syphilis or be stillborn. Development of syphilis after accidental inoculation or following blood transfusion from infected individuals occurs extremely rarely. Infants of mothers with gonorrhea may contract infections of the eyes (ophthalmia neonatorum) during birth, and unless treated, this can lead to permanent blindness.

☐ Gonorrhea

Gonorrhea, often referred to as "GC" or "the clap" by lay people, is caused by *Neisseria gonorrhoeae*. Gonorrhea is of great concern because of its epidemic rise, high reinfection rate, and seriousness of residual effects. The incubation period is 3 to 5 days.

In men, the gonococcus is introduced into the anterior urethra during sexual activity. In about 90% of infected men, urethritis is the first symptom to appear.[8] Other symptoms quickly follow and include purulent discharge from the urethra, dysuria, swelling of the penis, and balanitis. Because of the distress produced by the symptoms, men usually present themselves for examination early in the disease. As a result, diagnosis is made and treatment instituted early, and complications and residual effects of gonorrhea are uncommon among men. Sterility from orchitis or epididymitis can occur as a residual effect, but this is rare.

The incidence of men with asymptomatic gonorrhea is believed to be low; however, there is an increasing awareness of the importance of men with asymptomatic infection in the transmission of gonorrhea. Some men have been found to have no symptoms of infection despite positive tests for gonorrhea 2 weeks after exposure.[3]

In contrast to men, women rarely have early, distressing symptoms of gonorrhea. The early signs include a slight purulent discharge, a vague feeling of fullness in the pelvis, and discomfort or aching in the abdomen. Since these signs are not perceived as severe, women may disregard them. If the bladder is involved, there is burning, frequency, and urgency of urination, and women are more likely to seek medical assistance because of discomfort. Bartholin's glands may become infected, resulting in distention and swelling that makes it painful for the woman to walk or sit. These symptoms may also lead the woman to see a physician.

Gonorrhea in women most often begins as asymptomatic cervicitis, and the infection can be present for extended periods without causing noticeable signs. A high number of infected, asymptomatic women is the result. These women do not receive treatment unless gonorrhea is diagnosed through screening or unless the woman is identified by the sexual partner and presents herself for treatment. Frequently, complications are the first indicators of gonorrhea in women. *Salpingitis* is the most common complication, with an estimated 17% of women presenting themselves with symptoms of salpingitis as the first sign of infection.[93] During the course of treatment for salpingitis, many women are surgically sterilized. In cases of untreated gonorrhea, the residual effects of chronic PID, infertility, and ectopic pregnancy are well known.

Other complications of untreated gonorrhea in both men and women include dermatitis, carditis, meningitis, and arthritis. The incidence of these complications is higher among women because of the prolonged period of infection without symptoms.

Clinical picture

Gonorrheal infection may be suspected on the basis of history, symptoms, and clinical evidence obtained by physical examination. However, identification of the organism is necessary to confirm the diagnosis and to rule out other problems. In men the diagnosis is confirmed by gram-stained smear of the discharge from the penis. Culture of the discharge from the penis is usually reserved for those whose smears are negative in the presence of strong clinical evidence.

Gram-stained cervical smears are inadequate for diagnosing gonorrhea in women. These smears are negative in about 50% of women having gonorrhea, and are falsely positive in a significant number of cases.[8] Therefore cultures from the cervix, urethra, and anus are usually taken. Fluorescent-tagged antibody methods are usually used to identify the gonococcus. Because of the greater length of time required to obtain reports of cultures, treatment is usually instituted on a presumptive basis.

Intervention

Therapy for gonorrhea presents a greater problem than that for syphilis because the gonococcus tends to develop resistance to antibiotics. It also is believed that inadequate therapy is common in the United States.[8] Several drug regimens are in use with emphasis on single-dose treatment to avoid problems in followup and patient cooperation. Aqueous penicillin has been the antibiotic of choice in the treatment of gonorrhea. It is now recommended, for both men and women, that a dose of 4.8 million units of aqueous penicillin be given intramuscularly in combination with 1 g of oral probenecid. Spectinomycin in an intramuscualr injection of 2 g for men and 4 g for women has also been effective.

The most common and clinically significant reactions to penicillin are allergic reactions, of which urticaria is the most common. Before initiating treatment it is important to screen for a history of previous reaction to penicillin. Symptoms of life-threatening reactions such as anaphylaxis most often occur within 30 minutes after injection, and although such reactions are rare, it may be advisable to detain patients for this period of time after parenteral administration of penicillin.[78]

Syphilis

Syphilis is caused by a spirochete, *Treponema pallidum*, that gains entry into the body through either the mucous membrane or skin during intercourse. The organism is readily destroyed by physical and chemical agents including heat, drying, and mild disinfectants such as soap and water.

The incubation period for syphilis is usually 3 weeks. However, symptoms can appear as early as 9 days or as long as 3 months after exposure. If untreated, the disease progresses through four identifiable states (Table 62-3).

Clinical picture

Syphilis is most often diagnosed by standard serologic tests (Chapter 60). Massive screening programs have made serologic diagnosis of syphilis very common. Darkfield microscopic examination of tissue scraping from lesions or material obtained by aspiration of regional lymph nodes also reveal the presence of the spirochete, especially during the primary and secondary stages. A presumptive diagnosis is made on the basis of suspicious lesions, positive serology, known exposure to infection, and involvement of regional lymph nodes. False-positive serologic reactions are common among persons previously treated for syphilis. Infectious mononucleosis, hepatitis, pregnancy, viral pneumonia, malaria, chickenpox, measles and smallpox vaccination, narcotic addiction, and terminal malignancy have also been associated with false-positive serology.[77]

Intervention

Syphilis can be successfully treated at any stage of the disease, although treatment may have to be more prolonged in latent and late syphilis. While syphilis can be cured in late stages, the damage to the body is much less easily managed.

No change has been demonstrated in the effectiveness of penicillin in the treatment of syphilis,[77,84] and for this reason penicillin remains the drug of choice. All types of penicillin are effective, but penicillin G benzathine and penicillin aluminum monosterate are preferred because they are long acting and can be given in a limited number of injections.

Patients with primary, secondary, and latent syphilis (and their contacts) are usually given 2.4 million units of penicillin intramuscularly in both buttocks. Patients with late syphilis are generally given 2.4 million units intramuscularly at 7-day intervals until a total of 7.2 to 9.6 million units have been given. When the use of penicillin is contraindicated because of drug sensitivity, tetracycline in a total dosage of 30 g over a period of 10 days is effective.

Pregnant women with penicillin sensitivity pose problems for treatment. In the large dosage required to treat syphilis, tetracycline produces mottling and staining of fetal dentition, and possible abnormal bone forma-

Table 62-3. Stages of syphilis

Primary	Secondary	Latent	Late
Duration 2 to 8 weeks	Appears 2 to 4 weeks after chancre appears; extends over 2 to 4 years	5 to 20 years	Terminal if not treated
Clinical signs Hard sore or pimple on vulva or penis that breaks and forms painless, draining chancre; may be a single chancre or groups of more than one; may be present also on lips, tongue, hands, rectum, or nipples; chancre heals leaving almost invisible scar	Depends on site; low-grade fever, headache, anorexia, weight loss, anemia, sore throat, hoarseness, reddened and sore eyes, jaundice with or without hepatitis, aching of joints, muscles, long bones; sores on body or generalized fine rash; condylomata lata (venereal warts) on rectum or genitalia	No clinical signs	Tumorlike masses, gumma, on any area of body; damage to heart valves and blood vessels; meningitis, paralysis, lack of coordination, paresis, insomnia, confusion, delusions, impaired judgment, slurred speech
Communicability Exudates from lesions and chancre are highly contagious	Exudates from lesions highly contagious; blood contains organisms	Contagious for about 2 years; not contagious to others after that; blood contains organisms	Noncontagious; spinal fluid may contain organisms

tion may occur.[53] If given in the usual adult dose, inadequate placental transfer of tetracycline is likely and congenital syphilis would probably develop. Erythromycin in a dose of 30 g over a period of 10 days seems to be the best alternative treatment for pregnant women with syphilis.

□ Chancroid

Chancroid is a sexually transmitted disease caused by a gram-negative bacillus, *Haemophilus ducreyi.* Although it rarely occurs in the United States, there is a need for surveillance to determine increase in incidence. The infection is more prevalent in men.

The incubation period varies from 1 to 14 days and averages 4 to 5 days. The primary lesion appears as an inflamed macule that rapidly progresses to vesicle and pustule stages. By the time the patient seeks medical care the lesions have usually become ulcerated. Multiple lesions in various stages of progression may be seen and are caused by rupture of vesicles and pustules and autoinnoculation. There may be single or multiple ulcers.

Clinical picture

In women, the lesions of chancroid are most often found on the labia, anus, clitoris, vagina, and cervix. A few women do not have any lesions but may present signs of mild vaginitis. In men the lesions appear on the prepuce, glans, or shaft of the penis.

The ulcers found in chancroid are typically ragged and irregular. They appear excavated, have a granulating, purulent surface, and are painful. Often, edema of the surrounding tissues is present. Involvement of the inguinal lymph nodes occurs in about 50% of all cases of chancroid within 2 weeks after appearance of the primary lesion.[75] The enlarged lymph nodes, called *buboes,* are most often unilateral, painful, and spherical in shape. The skin over the buboes is inflamed. The buboes tend to become softer as abscesses form. These abscesses in turn may suppurate and rupture, further spreading the infection. Generalized symptoms of infection usually appear when inguinal abscesses form.

Diagnosis of chancroid depends on demonstration of the organism. A specimen is collected by aspiration of a vesicle, pustule, or lymph node, or from the margin of an ulcer. A gram-stained smear is prepared and visualized by microscope.

Intervention

Treatment consists of oral sulfonamides given in doses of 1 g every 6 hours for 10 to 14 days. For persons having allergies to sulfonamides, kanamycin or streptomycin may be used.

Local therapy for chancroid is beneficial for comfort and prevention of complications. Cleansing the lesions with a debriding solution three times a day aids in removing necrotic tissue and provides comfort as well. In men having ulcers of the glans or prepuce, the prepuce should be retracted during treatment unless there is edema of the prepuce. This site of ulceration may lead to phimosis, requiring circumcision once the lesions are healed. Cleanliness is essential for prevention of secondary infection.

□ Donovanosis

Donovanosis, commonly called *granuloma inguinale* or *granuloma venereum,* is believed to be most often transmitted by sexual contact. The infection is caused by a gram-negative bacillus, *Calymmatobacterium (Donovania) granulomatis,* widely referred to as Donovan bacillus. The incubation period is unknown but is estimated to be 8 to 12 weeks.[75]

Clinical picture

Lesions appear on the genitalia and in the perianal area. The most common sites of lesions are the prepuce and glans in men and the vagina and labia in women. The infection first appears with development of subcutaneous nodules. These elevated areas eventually ulcerate, producing sharply defined, painless lesions. The ulcers enlarge slowly and bleed on contact. With ulceration, the infection tends to spread along the pubic region. Involvement of the lymph nodes is uncommon but can occur and produce occlusion of the lymphatics, resulting in elephantiasis.

Smears of exudates taken from the lesions do not always demonstrate the causative organism, even when donovanosis is present. Therefore a sample of tissue is taken from the lesion, is crushed between two slides, and is stained. The specimen is examined for the presence of Donovan bodies, which represent the intracellular stage of the causative organism. Examination of a tissue sample also makes it possible to differentiate between donovanosis and cancer.

Intervention

Penicillin is of limited value in the treatment of donovanosis.[75] Tetracyclines are sometimes effective when given in doses of 500 mg orally four times a day for 2 weeks. Resistance to these drugs, however, may develop. If the infection does not respond to tetracyclines, gentamicin 40 mg daily for 2 weeks or chloramphenicol 500 mg three times a day for 2 weeks is usually effective. If an antibiotic is effective, clinical response is usually evident in a week.

□ Lymphogranuloma venereum

Lymphogranuloma venereum (LGV) is a systemic, sexually transmitted disease caused by members of a group of organisms called *Chlamydia*. Other members of this group are the causative organisms of trachoma and psittacosis. The disease is contracted by vaginal, anal, or oral intercourse, and primary innoculation with the organism may occur at any site involved in close contact. The incubation period is 7 to 12 days. Lymphadenitis of regional lymph nodes draining the site of primary infection occurs, and the disease spreads by way of the lymphatic system.

Clinical picture

There are three clinical phases of infection in LGV: (1) innoculation and appearance of the primary lesion, (2) lymphatic spread and generalized symptoms, and (3) late complications. In individual cases any one of the phases may be absent or go unnoticed.

The primary lesion, which is transient, appears as a papule, small erosion, or vesicle. The most common sites of the primary lesion are the prepuce and glans in men and the vagina and cervix in women. Since it is painless, the primary lesion may go unnoticed, especially in women. Localized edema may be present. If the rectum is infected, there is a bloody discharge followed by a mucopurulent discharge, diarrhea, and cramping.

Involvement of the lymphatics follows appearance of primary lesions in 1 to 4 weeks. If the primary lesion is on the penis, anal margin, clitoris, or upper vulva, the superficial inguinal lymph nodes are involved. Infection of the vagina or cervix as the primary sites produces involvement of the deep iliac and anorectal lymph nodes. The buboes that appear are firm and lobular. The skin over the superficial nodes is bluish-red and adheres to the nodes. The first indications of infection in most patients is a feeling of stiffness and aching in the groin followed by swelling in the inguinal area. Constitutional symptoms of infection may or may not appear at this time. The involved lymph nodes may suppurate, causing extensive scarring. Obstruction of the lymphatics may result, leading to chronic edema and ulceration. Lymphatic spread of the infection is accompanied by generalized symptoms that vary. Mild to severe fever, malaise, nausea, and vomiting may occur. Abdominal pain, symptoms of cystitis, and urinary retention are common when pelvic lymph nodes are involved.

Among the most severe complications of LGV are development of perianal abscesses, rectovaginal or rectovesical fistulas, and rectal strictures. In the last clinical phase, generalized infection is indicated by blood values showing anemia, leukocytosis, and elevated sedimentation rate.

The Frei test has been widely used in the diagnosis of LGV. This is a skin test that gives a positive reaction within 6 weeks following infection. However, the Frei test is not specific for LGV and is less than 70% sensitive.[92] Persons infected with any chlamydial organism may have a positive Frei test. The LGV complement-fixation test (LGV-CFT) requires that the organism be isolated in tissue culture and has gained increased use because it is 90% to 95% sensitive.[75] It is also a nonspecific test, but it can be titrated, and a rising titer over several weeks is of diagnostic value. Specific tests for LGV, including immunofluorescence and neutralization tests, have been developed, but they are not widely available and have had only limited evaluation for accuracy in diagnosis. A positive Frei or LGV-CFT test along with careful history and physical examination affords the best chances for diagnosing LGV.

Intervention

Early antibiotic therapy is essential for controlling and reducing morbidity due to LGV, and it is generally agreed that treatment should not be delayed until diagnostic test results are obtained. Tetracycline in a dosage of 500 mg four times a day for at least 3 weeks is the treatment of choice. If drug sensitivity or pregnancy precludes use of tetracycline, sulfasoxazole 4 mg orally followed by 500 mg every 6 hours for 3 weeks is usually effective. Flocculent lymph nodes may be aspirated to prevent scarring and destruction of lymphatic channels. This is usually done in conjunction with antibiotic therapy. Surgical removal of the lymph nodes is not advised, since this may increase lymphedema and elephantiasis.[75]

If rectal stricture supervenes, rectal dilatation at 2-week intervals may be attempted. Development of fistulae is especially distressing and requires that surgical repair be accomplished. LGV is a disease characterized by remissions and exacerbations, and thorough surveillance is important. Antibiotic therapy should be reinstituted as soon as symptoms of reactivation occur. Biopsy of lesions and lymph nodes is advised in chronic cases of LGV, since cancer may develop in the ulcerative lesions and may be overlooked as a result of similarity in appearance.[65]

□ Herpes genitalis

Herpes genitalis (genital herpes, HVH-2) is caused by infection by herpesvirus hominis type 2 (HVH-2). It is now generally accepted that HVH-2 is spread by sexual contact. Recent interest in herpes genitalis has been generated because of the contagious, debilitating nature of the disease and because of its association with cancer.[45,70]

The incubation period is 3 to 7 days. The primary lesion appears as a vesicle on the external genitalia in men and women or on the vagina or cervix in women. These lesions often ulcerate, especially when located on moist surfaces. Primary infections are associated with local inflammation, pain, enlargement of the inguinal lymph nodes, and generalized signs of infection. These symptoms usually lead the individual to seek medical attention.

Clinical picture

Vaginal discharge is common among women, and discharge from the urethra is usual in men having primary infections. Urinary tract involvement may occur and is reflected in symptoms of dysuria or urinary retention. The lesions can cause severe pain, requiring hospitalization for parenteral analgesia. Subclinical infections in which patients are unaware of any problem occur in only about 10% of the cases of genital herpes.[61]

Recurrent infections are usually milder and of shorter duration than primary infections, and usually produce local rather than systemic reaction. The patient experiencing a recurrent infection often has prodromal signs of paresthesia and burning at the site where the lesion will erupt. Factors known to predispose to recurrent infection include fever, emotional upsets, premenstrual tension, and overexposure to heat and sunshine.[61] While the mode of recurrent infection is not clear, it has been theorized that during primary infection the virus ascends sensory nerve sheaths, localizing in corresponding nerve ganglia,[31] and that when the environment becomes favorable, the virus is reactivated.[45] Lesions of recurrent infections usually occur in the site of primary infection.

Diagnosis of herpes genitalis is made by isolation of the virus from specimens obtained from lesions. Pap smears or fluid from the vesicles collected in transport medium demonstrate cellular characteristics of viruses.

Intervention

Treatment for genital herpes has most often been symptomatic, since there is presently no known cure for the disease. A therapeutic approach now being used involves photodynamic inactivation of the virus. That the inherent photosensitivity of HVH-2 could be increased by the use of dye was demonstrated in 1969.[95] The treatment, called dye-light therapy, consists of application of 0.1% aqueous neutral red or proflavine dye, followed by exposure to a 15-watt fluorescent light for 15 minutes at a distance of 6 inches.[26] The application of dye with light seems to disrupt the structure of the viral DNA strand, inhibiting replication and causing the virus to become noninfectious.[29] The therapy is not applicable if lesions are located where light cannot be applied, as in the vagina. Local preparations such as analgesic ointment, Burow's solution compresses, corticosteroid creams, and iodoxuridine liquifilm may afford relief from discomfort but do not affect the course of the disease.

Recent literature demonstrates concern about methods of therapy that alter DNA, such as the use of neutral red and light treatment. Instead of a controversial therapy that damages the nucleic acid of these viruses, thus possibly contributing to their oncogenic potential, topical application of ethyl ether is suggested. Although controlled clinical trials are needed, early evidence suggests that after the inital discomfort associated with the ether applications, the lesions heal in 1 to 2 days.[79]

□ Trichomoniasis

A protozoan, *Trichomonas vaginalis*, is the causative organism of trichomoniasis. Evidence suggests that the incubation period ranges between 4 to 28 days.[75] The sexual transmission of trichomoniasis is well established.

Clinical picture

Only 25% of women harboring the organism are asymptomatic.[75] Pruritus of the vulva and vagina is the predominant symptom among women. The itching may be so severe as to awaken the patient, and excoriation from scratching is common. Secondary infection of the broken skin may result.

Classically, the symptoms of trichomoniasis in women are a copious, frothy, green or greenish-yellow vaginal discharge, inflammation of the labia minora and lower vagina, and a red-speckled appearance of the vaginal canal and cervix. A small number of patients present this classic picture, usually presented in texts.[54] Most patients have a vaginal discharge, but it is small in amount and yellow, and there is some inflammation of the labia and vagina.[54] Itching is almost universally present, however, and dyspareunia, dysuria, and urinary frequency may also occur.

In men, urethritis and its symptoms of purulent discharge, itching, burning, and inflammation are the signs of trichomoniasis most often seen. Prostatitis, epididymitis, and urethral stricture may occur as complications among men. However, study of these consequences of trichomoniasis have not been extensive and are not well documented.

Diagnosis of trichomoniasis is most often made by preparing a hanging drop slide containing a specimen of the discharge and observing the motile organism under the microscope. Serologic and skin tests are currently being investigated but lack reliability so far. Because of the high incidence of coexisting gonorrhea, smears or cultures for gonococci should also be taken.

Intervention

The treatment of choice for trichomoniasis is metronidazole (Flaygl) 250 mg orally three times a day for 7 to 10 days. Vaginal inserts of metronidazole are less effective but are the alternative therapy for pregnant women. The drug is known to cross the placental barrier, but the effects of metronidazole on the fetus have not been established.

The sexual partners of women are variously treated. Some men are treated with a course of metronidazole; some are treated only if they present symptoms of active infection, and some are treated only if the woman fails to respond to treatment or has recurrent episodes of infection.[54] Differences in opinion as to whether asymptomatic patients and all sex partners of infected patients should be treated might be resolved with scientific investigations of the natural history of trichomoniasis.

□ Candidiasis

Candidiasis, commonly called monilial infection or monilial vaginitis, is an infection caused by a yeast form, *Candida albicans*. The overall incidence of candidiasis in the United States is unknown. Whether the infection is sexually transmitted is debated. Superinfection results following prolonged antibiotic therapy, such as by tetracycline.

Clinical picture

Women having symptoms of candidiasis most often complain of pruritus of the vulva. A vaginal discharge that is thick, white, and curdlike is characteristic. The vulva appears inflamed and edematous, and excoriations from scratching are often present. White patches that appear to adhere to the mucosal surfaces are often seen in the vagina. Similar white, curdlike patches appear on the mucous membrane surfaces and tongue in newborn infants infected by the organism, causing a condition known as *thrush*.

Little is known about candidiasis occurring among men. Symptoms of balanitis may be present.[75] Asymptomatic urethritis occurs in up to 10% of infected men.[75]

Diagnosis may be suspected from the patient's history of predisposing factors and symptoms, but it is usually made by microscopic examination of a smear of the discharge. Therapy consists of nystatin (Mycostatin) vaginal suppositories inserted twice a day for 10 to 14 days. Men with balanitis should be treated with nystatin ointment applied to the glans several times a day. A solution of 1% gentian violet applied to the vagina, or gentian violet suppositories, has been popular for several years because of its effectiveness. However, because it stains clothing, gentian violet lacks patient acceptance and may not be effective if the patient does not use it as directed.

□ Prevention and control of venereal diseases

Prevention and control measures currently used for syphilis and gonorrhea can serve as the model for prevention and control of all of the sexually transmitted diseases. These measures include identification and treatment of exposed persons who are asymptomatic, interviewing patients with infection for identification of contacts, examination and preventive treatment of contacts, educational programs for the public, and active involvement of professionals in programs of control.

Nursing role

The nurse's first responsibility in venereal disease control is to educate patients who have a sexually transmitted infection. To act in a responsible manner, nurses must be knowledgeable about the venereal diseases most prevalent, signs and symptoms of venereal diseases, methods used in diagnosis, treatments used, and where individuals can obtain help and information. Nurses also can influence the knowledge and attitudes of their colleagues and peers toward venereal disease and its control. Nurses can exert influence in the community by taking an active role in programs of education.

Before nurses can be effective in working with patients who have venereal diseases, they must confront their own feelings and attitudes about venereal diseases. The patient is often young, fearful of pain, and unaccustomed to surroundings in a clinic or physician's office. Young patients especially fear that their families and friends may learn they have a venereal disease.

Many patients focus on how the venereal diseases are spread rather than on the consequences of having an infection. For single persons, contracting a venereal disease and securing help means they must admit to having sexual relations, and this means some of them at least may feel guilty about their sexual activity. Patients with a venereal disease have not only a physical but a social, emotional, and perhaps economic problem as well. They need constructive and comprehensive help. The nurse who is successful in working with persons having a venereal disease is one who can create an atmosphere of trust in which the person feels free to discuss all aspects of the problem.

Persons who seek help recognize they have a problem; they want to get better and stay well. Because of this they are highly motivated to do what is necessary, are receptive to information and advice, and are attentive when advice is given. Nurses can take advantage of the patient's readiness to learn and motivation to improve and maintain health.

A careful history and physical examination are important. Previous episodes of genital infection, chronic health problems, and factors predisposing to venereal diseases may be revealed. Careful documentation of the person's present problem aids in the diagnosis, treatment, and follow-up. Pelvic examination is necessary for determining the extent of the infection. The person should be informed of the purposes and importance of the history, examination, and laboratory tests so that greater cooperation, especially in giving information, can be obtained.

Once the diagnosis, tentative or conclusive, is made, focus should first be placed on obtaining a cure and preventing complications and reinfection. Many lay people know the treatment for syphilis and gonorrhea is penicillin but they may not be fully informed about this and other aspects of treatment. Because some of the venereal diseases respond to penicillin or other antibiotics, many people believe that all genital infections can be cured simply, and this is not so. Some people believe that antibiotics not only cure an infection, but that they produce immunity against reinfection as well. Persons receiving an antibiotic or other medications for sexually transmitted diseases must be informed of the action of the drug, its duration of effectiveness, side effects, chances of cure, and the need for follow-up. They need to be advised that treatment failures do occur and that reinfection rates are high. Return visits should be encouraged whenever possible, since adequacy of treatment of all of the sexually transmitted diseases is evaluated best by laboratory analysis for the specific organism.

Persons treated for sexually transmitted infections need information about self-care. To understand their therapy and to responsibly engage in self-care, they must be informed about the venereal nature of the infection, how it is transmitted, and the possibility of reinfection and infection of their sexual partner or partners. The patient needs to know that it is important for sexual partners to be checked for signs of infection, to be advised of what the signs are, and to seek health care if signs or symptoms are present or appear. Patients should be advised to abstain from intercourse until cured. If sexual intercourse cannot be avoided, a condom should be used by the man to prevent infection or reinfection.

Education of patients regarding hygiene and personal health practices is beneficial for reducing the chances of secondary infection, recurrence, and infections of various types in the future. Frequent bathing and hand washing are indicated. It is known that many of the organisms causing venereal diseases are destroyed by soap and water. For women, douching is contraindicated unless prescribed for the purpose of applying heat or medication. All women should be informed that, for personal cleanliness, frequent douching at any time is not advisable, since this may disturb the vaginal and cervical environments and predispose to infection. If douching is prescribed, the patient should be instructed in the procedure (p. 1389).

If lesions are present on body surfaces, the patient should be instructed in their care. Unless contraindicated, a hot bath is taken two to three times a day, and lesions are kept as dry as possible between bathings. Both men and women should be advised to wear cotton underwear, and women should be advised to avoid using pantyhose, since they tend to trap moisture and prevent circulation of air. Unless specifically prescribed as local medications, the patient should not apply any lotion, cream, or ointment to any of the lesions.

Opportunities to engage in instruction regarding diet, exercise, nutrition, contraception, and reproduction often arise when persons are being treated for a venereal disease. Nurses can pursue any of these opportunities.

Opportunities for promoting healthy attitudes about sexual activity and sexually transmitted diseases also frequently arise. These topics are approached tactfully and with consideration of the patient's feelings. Adolescents especially require an approach that indicates understanding balanced with ability to help them set limits. Developmental tasks of adolescence require that young people find means of sexual gratification within the context of meaningful sexual relationships. In their search, adolescents need to be reassured that mutually rewarding relationships involving sexual gratification can be fulfilling. However, within this context, adolescents need to recognize that consequences of their behavior may include unwanted pregnancy and venereal disease. Nurses may not always feel comfortable in exploring the meaning of sexual experiences with adolescents who they know are, or suspect of being, sexually active. Despite this, nurses do have an obligation to provide patients with information about venereal disease prevention.

Many films are available from local and state health departments including *How to Keep from Catching VD,* which is especially good for teenagers; *Look What's Going Around,* intended to increase patient cooperation in bringing contacts to treatment; and *VD Prevention,* which explains how venereal diseases can be prevented.

Contact investigation

In the prevention and control of venereal diseases, especially gonorrhea, emphasis is placed on interviewing for information regarding their sexual contacts. The named contacts are then sought out for examination and treatment. Lay people knowledgeable about the required reporting to the local health department of some of the venereal diseases may be very hesitant to name their sexual contacts. Young people often fear that their parents and the parents of the sexual partner will find out about their infection. Minors need to know that they can probably obtain treatment without parental consent. Presently, 35 states permit physicians to treat minors for venereal disease without obtaining parental consent, and several states are proposing changes in existing legislation restricting treatment of minors.[3] Lay people also may perceive reporting of venereal diseases as a threat from an official agency, and may hesitate to name their contacts out of a sense of protection if they do not know that no punishment is involved.

Interviewing the patient for contacts is done at the time of the initial visit, in the event that the patient does not return for follow-up. This interview is probably best done after the patient is examined, the type of infection is determined, and treatment is prescribed. If assessment is accompanied by information giving, the patient should be better informed about venereal diseases and how they are treated after the examination is over. Hopefully the patient will be less concerned about self, and more willing and able to give information about sexual contacts.

Interviewing for contacts involves two aspects. The patient is first asked to name sexual contacts. Second, the patient is interviewed for "cluster suspects" who are friends or acquaintances, who may have been exposed to the same contacts, or who have symptoms of a venereal disease. Since one focus of venereal disease control is on increasing self-referrals, the patient is asked to advise known contacts and cluster suspects to present themselves for examination and preventive treatment. There is reason to believe that patients do not name all their contacts at the time of the first interview and that a reinterview, after the patient has reflected, will usually result in additional names of contacts. [3]

Whenever possible, the contacts of the infected person are located and advised to have an examination and tests as soon as possible. If the sexual contacts do not have symptoms of infection at the time of the first examination, treatment is instituted to abort infection. Giving preventive treatment to named contacts who have no clinical evidence of infection has gained popularity and acceptance in the United States, and indications are present that this same approach is being used more often in management of patients having the "minor" venereal diseases.

☐ Current and future needs

The epidemic nature of gonorrhea makes it evident that measures for control of spread need to be even more vigorously applied and that new measures may be necessary to check the spread of infection. Efforts to implement mass education and screening programs need to be continued. Program efforts are directed toward creating public awareness of the problem of sexually transmitted diseases and their control methods, and to inform the public of the possible serious consequences of these diseases. There also is a need to expand screening, contact tracing, and diagnostic and treatment programs.

Little is known about some of the sexually transmitted diseases. Surveillance over some of them is inadequate, so that even the true incidence of several sexually transmitted infections is not known. Treatment of several of these diseases is poorly understood because knowledge of the natural history of the causative organisms is inadequate. Such knowledge is necessary to understand the epidemiology of the spread of these diseases so that treatment and prevention can be better directed than is now possible. Diagnostic methods need to be improved so that they are more reliable and can be carried out inexpensively for large numbers of people. Alternative therapies for prophylaxis require development of agents to be used specifically and with discretion for treatment or exposed individuals, for treatment of persons sensitive to specific drugs, and for the management of pregnant women.

In order to better understand the modes of transmission and circumstances surrounding spread of the venereal diseases, knowledge of human behavior is required. Considerable research has been done in recent years regarding sexual behavior patterns, contraceptive practices, and permissiveness. While these have been helpful, there is little consensus about whether these variables influence the incidence and spread of venereal diseases. Further study will add to the pool of knowledge, which can be applied in programs of detection, treatment and prevention.

Development of prophylactic vaccines, especially for gonorrhea and syphilis, needs to be given high priority. To accomplish this, techniques for growing the organisms need to be developed, and this in turn requires knowledge of the natural history and evolution of specific organsims, including viruses.

History has revealed that treatment alone has never conquered any of the major communicable diseases, but that programs through which the public becomes better informed and demands services, as well as the development of protective vaccines, have been almost always universally successful in preventing disease.

REFERENCES AND SELECTED READINGS

1. Alkhateeb, W., Lukeroth, C. J., and Riggs, M.: A comparison of three educational techniques used in a venereal disease clinic, Public Health Rep. **90:**159-164, 1975.
2. American Cancer Society: Cancer facts and figures, New York, 1976, The Society.
3. American Social Health Association: Today's VD control program, New York, 1975, The Association.
4. Baden, M. F., and Baden, E. E.: Cervical incompetence: repair during pregnancy, Am. J. Obstet. Gynecol. **74:**241-245, 1975.
5. Baird, D.: Induced abortion: epidemiologic aspects, J. Med. Ethics **1:**122-126, 1975.
6. Blaustein, A.: Pathology of the female genital tract, New York, 1976, Springer-Verlag New York, Inc.
7. Block, M. F., and Rahhal, D. K.: Cervical incompetence: a diagnostic and prognostic scoring system, Obstet. Gynecol. **47:**279-281, 1976.
8. *Blount, J. H., Darrow, W. W., and Johnson, R. E.: Venereal

*References preceded by an asterisk are particularly well suited for student reading.

disease in adolescents, Pediatr. Clin. North Am. **20:**1021-1033, 1973.

9. Bolognese, R. J., and Corson, S. L.: Interruption of pregnancy: a total patient approach, Baltimore, 1975, The Williams & Wilkins Co.
10. *Bouchard, R., and Owens, N. F.: Nursing care of the cancer patient, St. Louis, 1976, The C.V. Mosby Co.
11. Campbell, M. F., and Harrison, J. H., editors: Urology, ed. 3, vols. 1 and 2, Philadelphia, 1970, W. B. Saunders Co.
12. *Char, W. J.: Abortion and acute identity crisis in nurses, Am. J. Psychiatry **128:**66-71, 1972.
13. Cohen, C. J. and Gusberg, S. B.: Screening for endometrial cancer, Clin. Obstet. Gynecol. **18:**27-39, 1975.
14. Creasman, W. T., and Weed, J. C.: Screening techniques in endometrial cancer, Cancer **38**(suppl.):436-440, 1976.
15. *Cronenwett, L. R., and Choyce, J. M.: Saline abortion, Am. J. Nurs. **71:**1754-1757, 1971.
16. Cutler, S. J., and Young, J., Jr.: Third national cancer survey: incidence data, National Cancer Institute monograph no. 41, DHEW publ. no. (NIH) 75-787, Washington, D.C., 1975, U.S. Government Printing Office.
17. *Darrow, W. W.: Approaches to the problem of venereal disease prevention, Prev. Med. **5:**165-175, 1976.
18. *Darrow, W. W.: Changes in sexual behavior and venereal diseases, Clin. Obstet. Gynecol. **18:**255-267, 1975.
19. del Regato, J. A.: Cancer of the prostate, J.A.M.A. **235:**1727-1730, 1976.
20. *Dewhurst, J. E., and Weeks, A. R.: Occult manifestations of septic abortion, Nurs. Mirror **142:**62-63, 1976.
21. Dimowski, W. P., and Cohen, M. R.: Treatment of endometriosis with an antigonadotropin, Danazol: a laparoscopic and histologic evaluation, Obstet. Gynecol **46:**147-154, 1975.
22. Duenholter, J. H., and Gant, N. F.: Complications following prostaglandin F_2a-induced midtrimester abortion, Obstet. Gynecol. **46:**247-250, 1975.
23. Editorial: Herpesvirus and cancer of the uterine cervix, Br. Med. J. **1:**671-672, 1976.
24. Effer, S.: Gynecologic aspects of the "routine" checkup, Postgrad. Med. **59:**164-170, 1976.
25. *Faulkner, W. L., and Ory, H. W.: Intrauterine devices and acute pelvic inflammatory disease, J.A.M.A. **235:**1851-1853, 1976.
26. Felber, T., et al.: Photodynamic inactivation of herpes simplex, J.A.M.A. **223:**289-292, 1973.
27. Flocks, R. H., and Culp, D. A.: Surgical urology, ed. 4, Chicago, 1975, Year Book Medical Publishers, Inc.
28. Friedman, C. M., Greenspan, R., and Mittleman, F.: The decision-making process and the outcome of therapeutic abortion, Am. J. Psychiatry **131:**1332-1337, 1974.
29. Friedrich, E.: Relief for herpes vulvitis, Obstet. Gynecol. **41:**74-77, 1973.
30. Galask, R. P., Larsen, B., and Ohm, M. J.: Vaginal flora and its role in disease entities, Clin. Obstet. Gynecol. **19:**61-81, 1976.
31. Gardner, H. L., and Kaufman, R. H.: Herpes genitalis: clinical features, Clin. Obstet. Gynecol. **15:**896-911, 1972.
32. Gibbs, R. S., and Weinstein, A. J.: Puerperal infection in the antibiotic era, Am. J. Obstet. Gynecol. **124:**769-787, 1976.
33. Gordon, G. S., and Greenberg, B. G.: Exogenous estrogens and endometrial cancer, Postgrad. Med. **59:**66-77, 1976.
34. Greenhill, J. P.: The nonsurgical management of vaginal relaxation, Clin. Obstet. Gynecol. **15:**1083-1097, 1972.
35. Greenhill, J. P.: Surgical gynecology, ed. 4, Chicago, 1969, Year Book Medical Publishers, Inc.
36. Greenwald, E. F.: Ovarian tumors, Clin. Obstet. Gynecol. **18:**61-86, 1975.

36a. Hammond, C. B., and Lewis, J. L.: Gestational trophoblastic neoplasms. In Davis' gynecology and obstetrics, Hagerstown, Md., 1972, Harper & Row, Publishers, Inc.

37. *Hall, R. E.: The Supreme Court decision on abortion, Am. J. Obstet. Gynecol. **116:**1-8, 1973.
38. Hodgson, J. E., and Portmann, K. C.: Complications of 10,453 consecutive first-trimester abortions: a prospective study, Am. J. Obstet. Gynecol. **120:**802-807, 1974.
39. Kahan, R. S., Baker, L. D., and Freeman, M. G.: The effect of legalized abortion on morbidity resulting from criminal abortion, Am. J. Obstet. Gynecol. **121:**114-116, 1975.
40. *Kaiser, B. L., and Kaiser, I. H.: The challenge of the woman's movement to American gynecology, Am. J. Obstet. Gynecol. **120:**652-665, 1974.
41. *Kane, F. J., Jr., et. al.: Motivational factors in abortion patients, Am. J. Psychiatry **130:**290-293, 1973.
42. Kaufman, R. H., Reeves, K. O., and Dougherty, C. M.: Severe atypical endometrial changes and sequential contraceptive use, J.A.M.A. **236:**923-926, 1976.
43. Kessler, I. I.: Perspectives on the epidemiology of cervical cancer with special reference to the herpesvirus hypothesis, Clin. Orthop. **99:**1091-1110, 1974.
44. Kessler, I. I., and Aurelian, L.: Uterine cervix cancer. In Schottenfeld, D.: Cancer epidemology and prevention: current concepts, Springfield, Ill., 1975, Charles C Thomas, Publisher.
45. Kibrick, S.: Herpes simplex. In Charles, D., and Finland, M.: Obstetric and perinatal infections, Philadelphia, 1973, Lea & Febiger.
46. Kraus, S. J.: Complications of gonococcal infection, Med. Clin. North Am. **56:**1115-1125, 1972.
47. *Lasagna, L.: The VD epidemic: how it started, where it's going, and what to do about it, Philadelphia, 1975, Temple University Press.
48. Lash, A. F., and Lash, S. R.: Habitual abortion: the incompetent internal os of the cervix, Am. J. Obstet. Gynecol. **59:**68-76, 1950.
49. Laurensen, N. H., Secher, N. J., and Wilson, K. H.: Midtrimester abortion induced by intravaginal administration of prostaglandin E_2 suppositories, Am. J. Obstet. Gynecol. **122:**947-954, 1975.
50. Lyon, F. A.: The development of adenocarcinoma of the endometrium in young women receiving long-term sequential oral contraception: a report of four cases, Am. J. Obstet. Gynecol. **123:**299-301, 1975.
51. Mack, T. M., Pike, M. C., Henderson, B. E., et al.: Estrogens and endometrial cancer in a retirement community, N. Engl. J. Med. **294:**1262-1267, 1976.
52. MacMahon, B.: Risk factors for endometrial cancer, Gynecol. Oncol. **2:**122-129, 1974.
53. Mamunes, P., Cave, V. G., Budell, J. W., et al.: Early diagnosis of neonatal syphilis: evaluation of a gamma M-fluorescent treponemal antibody test, Am. J. Dis. Child. **120:**17-21, 1970.
54. McCormack, W. M.: Sexually transmissible conditions other than gonorrhea and syphilis, In Practice of Medicine, vol. 3, 1974.
55. McGowan, L.: Cytologic methods for the detection of endometrial carcinoma, Gynecol. Oncol. **2:**272-278, 1974.
56. *Morton, B. M.: VD: a guide for nurses and counselors, Boston, 1976, Little, Brown & Co.
57. Murphy, G. P.: The diagnosis of prostatic cancer, Cancer **37** (1 suppl.): 589-596, 1976.
58. Murphy, G. P.: Prostatic malignancy. In Conn, H. F., and Conn, R. B., Jr., editors: Current diagnosis, vol. 4, Philadelphia, 1974, W. B. Saunders Co.
59. Nahmias, A. J., Naib, Z. M., and Josey, W. E.: Epidemiological

studies relating genital herpetic infection to cervical carcinoma, Clin. Orthop. **99:**1111-1117, 1974.

60. *Nathanson, C. S.: Illness and the feminine role: a theoretical review, Soc. Sci. Med. **9:**57-62, 1975.
61. *Neeson, J. D.: Herpes genitalis: a nursing perspective, Nurs. Clin. North Am. **124:**599-607, 1975.
62. Neighbor, R. M., and Newman, R. L.: Incidence of cervical cancer in perimenopausal women detected by Papanicolaou smears, Am. J. Obstet. Gynecol. **124:**348-351, 1976.
63. New studies tighten link between herpes virus, cervical cancer: J.A.M.A. **234:**1101-1103, 1975.
64. Ng. A. B.: The cellular detection of endometrial carcinoma and its precursors, Gynecol. Oncol. **2:**162-179, 1974.
65. Novak, E. R. and Woodruff, J. D.: Novak's gynecologic and obstetric pathology with clinical and endocrine relations, ed. 7, Philadelphia, 1974, W. B. Saunders Co.
66. Novak, E. R., Jones, G. S., and Jones, H. W., Jr.: Novak's textbook of gynecology, ed. 9, Baltimore, 1975, The Williams & Wilkins Co.
67. Ory, H., Naib, Z., Conger, S. B., et al.: Contraceptive choice and prevalence of cervical dysplasia and carcinoma in situ. Am. J. Obstet. Gynecol. **124:**573-577, 1976.
68. Panayotou, P. P., Induced abortion and ectopic pregnancy, Am. J. Obstet. Gynecol. **114:**507-510, 1972.
69. Pantelakis, S. N., Stefanos, C. G., and Doxiadis, S. A.: Influence of induced and spontaneous abortions on the outcome of subsequent pregnancies, Am. J. Obstet. Gynecol. **116:**799-805, 1973.
70. Poste, G., Hawkins, D. F., and Thomlinson, J.: Herpes hominis infection of the female genital tract, Obstet. Gynecol. **40:**871-875, 1972.
71. Prout, C. R., Jr.: Diagnosis and staging of prostatic carcinoma, Cancer **32:**1096-1103, 1973.
72. Rawls, W. E., Gardner, E., and Herman, L.: Herpes genitalis: venereal aspects, Clin. Obstet. Gynecol. **15:**913-917, 1972.
73. Rawls, W. E., Gardner, H. L., and Kaufman, R. L.: Antibodies to genital herpes virus in patients with carcinoma of the cervix, Am. J. Obstet. Gynecol. **107:**710-716, 1970.
74. Reid, E. P.: Rh sensitization following abortion, Can. Med. Assoc. J. **111:**1182, 1974.
75. Rein, M. F., and Chapel, T. A.: Trichomoniasis, candidiasis, and the other minor venereal diseases, Clin. Obstet. Gynecol. **18:**73-88, 1975.
76. *Robins, J.: Failures of contraceptive practice, N.Y. State J. Med. **76:**361-365, 1976.
77. Rudolph, A. H., and Duncan, W. C.: Syphilis—diagnosis and treatment, Clin. Obstet. Gynecol. **18:**163-182, 1975.
78. Rudolph, A. H., and Price, E. V.: Penicillin reactions among patients in venereal disease clinics: a national survey, J.A.M.A. **223:**499-501, 1973.
79. Sabin, A. B.: Editorial: Misery of recurrent herpes: what to do? N. Engl. J. Med. **293:**986-988, 1975.
80. Sandberg, E. C.: Benign cervical and vaginal changes associated with exposure to stilbestrol in utero, Am. J. Obstet. Gynecol. **125:**777-779, 1976.
81. Sarvis, B., and Rodman, H.: The abortion controversy, New York, 1973, Columbia University Press.
82. Saxena, B. B., and Landesman, R.: The use of radioreceptor assay of human chorionic gonadotropin for the diagnosis and management of ectopic pregnancy. Fertil. Steril. **26:**397-404, 1975.
83. Schenker, J. G., Eyal, F., and Polishuk, E. J.: Fertility after tubal pregnancy, Surg. Gynecol. Obstet. **135:**74-76, 1972.
84. Schroeter, A. L., Lucas, J. B., Price, E. V., et al.: Treatment for early syphilis and reactivity of serologic tests, J.A.M.A. **221:**471-476, 1972.
85. Silverberg, E.: Gynecologic cancer: statistical and epidemiological information, New York, 1973, The American Cancer Society, Inc.
86. Silverberg, E., and Holleb, A.: Cancer statistics 1975, Cancer **25:**8-21, 1975.
87. Silverberg, S., and Makowski, E.: Endometrial carcinoma in young women taking oral contraceptive agents, Obstet. Gynecol. **46:**503, 505, 506, 1975.
88. Tobias, J. S., and Griffiths, C. T.: Management of ovarian carcinoma: current concepts and future prospects, N. Engl. J. Med. **294:**877-882, 1976.
89. Tomkinson, J. S.: Carcinoma of the vulva, Nurs. Times **72:**854-855, 1976.
90. Tubal pregnancy and surgery, Br. Med. J. **1:**607-608, 1976.
91. Ulfelder, H.: The stilbestrol-adenosis-carcinoma syndrome, Cancer **38**(suppl.):426-431, 1976.
92. U.S. Department of Health, Education, and Welfare, Public Health Service: Chancroid, donovanosis, lymphogranuloma venereum, DHEW publ. no. (CDC) 75-8302, Atlanta, 1975, Center for Disease Control.
93. U.S. Department of Health, Education, and Welfare, Public Health Service: VD fact sheet 1975, DHEW publ. no. (CDC) 76-8195, Atlanta, 1975, Center for Disease Control.
94. U.S. Public Health Service, National Vital Statistics Division: Vital statistics of the United States, annual, 1930-1973, Washington, D.C., 1975, U.S. Government Printing Office.
95. Wallis, C., Trulock, S., and Melnick, J. L.: Inherent photosensitivity of herpes virus and other enveloped viruses, J. Gen. Virol. **5:**53-61, 1969.
96. *West, J.: Venereal disease contact tracing, Nurs. Mirror, **142:**60-61, 1976.
96. *Williamson, J.: Carcinoma of the body of the uterus, Nurs. Times, **72:**822-823, 1976.
98. Winick, C., and Kinsie, P. M.: The lively commerce, Chicago, 1971, Triangle Press.
99. Wright, C. S., Campbell, S., and Beazley, J.: Second-trimester abortion after vaginal termination of pregnancy, Lancet **1:**1278-1279, 1972.
100. Zeligman, I.: An atlas of nonvenereal genital lesions, Consultant **16:**91-95, 1976.
101. Ziel, H. K., and Finkle, W. D.: Increased risk of endometrial carcinoma among users of conjugated estrogens, N. Engl. J. Med. **293:**1167-1170, 1975.

AUDIOVISUAL RESOURCES

1. Current legal and medical aspects of abortion, audiotape, module no. 11, 1973, Audio-Digest Foundation, 1250 South Glendale Ave., Glendale, Calif. 91205.
2. Current practice in managing ovarian neoplasia, audiotape, module no. 17, 1976, Audio-Digest Foundation, 1250 South Glendale Ave., Glendale, Calif. 91205.
3. Lymph node spread from cancer of the uterine cervix, motion picture (T-2104-X), 1970, Media Resources Branch, National Medical Audiovisual Center (Annex), Station K, Atlanta, Ga. 30324.
4. Pelvic infection and venereal disease, audiotape, module no. 8, 1974, Audio-Digest Foundation, 1250 South Glendale Ave., Glendale, Calif. 91205.
5. Vaginitis and vulvitis, audiotape, module no. 21, 1973, Audio-Digest Foundation, 1250 South Glendale Ave., Glendale, Calif. 91205.

63

Problems of the breast

BARBARA C. LONG

The breasts are associated functionally with the reproductive system as an organ for milk production in the postpartum woman. The female sex hormones influence the development of the breasts and the production of milk. The breasts are also associated with feelings of sexuality and are an integral component of sexual behavior. The development of the breasts in the adolescent indicates to her the approach of womanhood and emphasizes her femininity. The breasts, especially the nipples, which are erectile tissue, are erogenous areas in sexual activity. The advertising media stresses the desirability of the female breast; femininity is typified by the model's curved breasts, while maleness is typified by the flat expansive chest of the lifeguard. Diseases of the breast, therefore, evoke varied feelings and cause fears and concerns that can influence self-examination or the seeking of diagnostic and therapeutic care.

The most common diseases of the breast are dysplasia (fibrocystic disease), carcinoma, fibroadenoma, and infections. Although these diseases occur primarily in women, *they can also occur in men.* Carcinoma requires the most extensive nursing care and is discussed in greater detail.

■ CARCINOMA OF THE BREAST

Nurses play a vital role in regard to carcinoma of the breast. Their responsibilities include (1) educating women so that breast cancer may be discovered and treated early, (2) caring for the patient who has had a breast removed because of cancer, (3) assisting the patient with physical and emotional rehabilitation, and (4) assisting the patient when metastasis has occurred and chemotherapy or irradiation is needed.

□ Epidemiology

Carcinoma of the breast is the most common malignancy in women and is also the leading cause of cancer death in women over 35. It is the leading cause of death in women aged 40 to 50. It is estimated that 1 out of 13 women in the United States will develop cancer of the breast, with the probability increasing with age.[3] The American Cancer Society estimates that 90,000 new cases will be discovered yearly and that one-third of these will die from the disease. The mortality rate for cancer of the breast in the United States has remained about the same for the past 35 years, with the rate fixed at 24 to 25 per 100,000. [3] Unfortunately the present 5-year survival rate for all patients with cancer of the breast, whether treated or untreated, is approximately 50%. This low survival rate is due in part to the frequent failure to detect the lesion before regional involvement occurs and failure to seek medical treatment as soon as a lesion is discovered. Studies show that approximately 83% of all women treated when the lesion appears localized have a 5-year life expectancy, compared with 52% for those with obvious regional involvement at the time of treatment. Survival at the end of 5 years, however, cannot be considered synonymous with cure. Many women who are treated before regional involvement is apparent die of the disease after 5 years, and the 10-year survival rate for these patients is only 33.4%.[56]

Breast cancer occurs in both premenopausal and postmenopausal women, with peak incidences at ages 45 to 49 and 65. The premenopausal incidence is thought to be related to ovarian hormonal function and the postmenopausal to adrenal function.[29] Many tumors of the breast in women past the menopause are malignant, whereas benign fibroadenomas occur largely in younger women.

Causes of carcinoma of the breast are not known but appear to include a number of factors rather than just one (multifocal). The boxed material on p. 1458 identifies the major factors that increase the possibility that breast cancer will occur. Among other potential risk factors are a prolonged menstrual activity (early menarche and late menopause) and the presence of cancer elsewhere in the body. Whites have a higher incidence of breast cancer than blacks, especially United States–born Jewish women of high socioeconomic class. The obese, hypertensive, diabetic person also appears to have a higher risk.[29]

MAJOR RISK FACTORS ASSOCIATED WITH BREAST CANCER

Sex:	Female
Age:	Over 35
Familial history:	Mother/sister with premenopausal or bilateral breast cancer
Pregnancy:	None (nullipara)

Breast feeding or a single breast injury does *not* influence the incidence of breast cancer. Often a lump is discovered after a minor injury because the woman feels her breast at the time of injury and may note a mass that was already present. Preparations of estrogen for menopausal symptoms do not increase the potential for the development of breast cancer but can accelerate preexisting cancer.[29]

□ Prognosis

Prognosis in carcinoma of the breast depends to a great extent on early diagnosis, the type of cancer present (slow or fast growing), genetic determination, and complete surgical removal of all tissues containing malignant cells before metastasis occurs. It is estimated that approximately 40% of all patients who seek medical attention for cancer of the breast are incurable at the time of the initial examination. Since the disease develops in a relatively accessible part of the body, it is unfortunate that early diagnosis is not made more often so that more lives might be saved. At the present time the American Cancer Society still recommends removal of the entire breast (radical or modified radical mastectomy) as the surgical treatment for operable breast cancer.[3] The Society also believes that surgical procedures that remove less than the entire breast have not been scientifically proved to be as effective as mastectomy, owing to the multifocal aspect of breast cancer.

□ Prevention

Although measures to prevent breast cancer are not known, *mortality* from breast cancer can be prevented in many instances through early diagnosis and treatment. All women should have a complete medical examination that includes palpation of the breasts at least once a year, and women over 30 years of age with a familial history of breast cancer should have an examination at least twice a year. A Gallup survey conducted for the American Cancer Society in late 1973 indicated that about one-half of the female population does not have an annual breast examination by a physician and that the lack of examination is more prevalent among older women, poorly educated, low income, and black women.[3]

Women should be taught that the prognosis for cancer of the breast is likely to be much better *if the cancer is discovered early and treatment instituted immediately*. Although 95% of all breast cancers are discovered by self-examination, many are not reported for several months. Fear of mutilation or of death are the two main reasons why some women delay seeking medical advice and treatment and hesitate to risk confirmation of their fears when a tumor is discovered. National statistics on deaths from cancer of the breast are widely publicized, and as a result, many women fear the disease and delay seeking medical help. Also, some women have had a relative or a friend who died from the disease, which causes the fear to be even more acute. Unfortunately the average woman may tell only her closest friends when a breast has been successfully removed for cancer. As a result, deaths from the disease are much better known than cures by surgery with no recurrence. Some women wish to avoid the expense or embarrassment of an examination, or they rationalize that their trouble would appear trivial to the busy physician. Sometimes they seek the advice of nurses. It then becomes the responsibility of the nurse to stress the urgency of getting medical advice at once. The publicized mastectomies of prominent women in recent years has encouraged other women to obtain breast examinations.

In an attempt to improve and assess the relative effectiveness of early detection of breast cancer, the National Cancer Institute and the American Cancer Society in 1973 jointly funded 27 screening centers around the country to provide free diagnostic services. A decision was made in 1977 to continue the nationwide screening project despite the controversy over the use of roentgenographic examinations used in the screening process (p. 1461). The screening centers during the first 3 years of the project detected 1,800 breast cancers in 280,000 women examined.[48] Another new approach is the sponsoring of a breast health clinic by nurses with the primary purpose of teaching breast self-examination.*

Breast self-examination

All women, beginning with the high school age, should know how to carry out breast self-examination and should practice this regularly as a health habit. The 1973 Gallup survey reported that only 18% of the 1,000 women sampled carried out monthly breast examinations. This was attributed to lack of knowledge of the importance of and the method for doing breast self-examination and fears concerning possible findings.[18]

*Breast Health Clinic, University Hospital, Seattle, Washington.

Nurses working in the hospital or community settings have the responsibility of teaching women how to examine their breasts and of explaining why it is necessary. When working with groups of women, arrangements can be made with the American Cancer Society in large cities or through the local health departments in small communities for showing movies developed for the general public describing one method of self-examination. The nurse follows through by teaching the women the breast self-examination and by answering questions. The woman then practices palpation of lumps on models of the breast.

Self-examination of the breasts should be done regularly *each month*. The best time is at the conclusion of, or a few days following, the menstrual period. Some women have engorgement of the breast premenstrually, and the breasts may have a lumpy consistency at that time. This condition usually disappears a few days after the onset of menstruation, although occasionally lumpiness and tenderness may extend throughout the menstrual cycle. Because of this possible change, it is important that the breasts be examined at the same time each month in relation to the menstrual cycle. Women who have passed the menopause should examine their breasts on the same day each month.

There are several approaches that can be followed when carrying out breast self-examination. All of these approaches follow these general guidelines: (1) the approach used is systematic; (2) the entire breast tissue is examined, including the tail (Fig. 63-1) and the nipple; (3) examination is carried out in both the horizontal and vertical body positions; and (4) the pads of the fingertips are used for palpation.

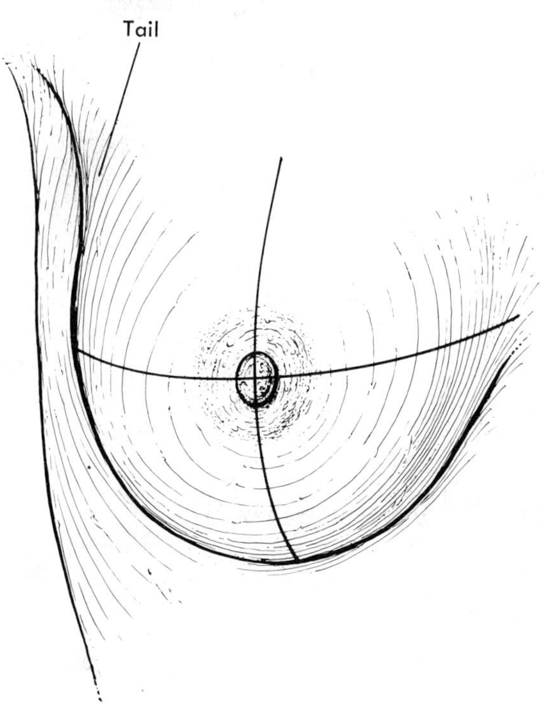

Fig. 63-1. Breast mass includes "tail" that extends from upper, outer quadrant toward axilla. (From Malasanos, L., Barkauskas, V., Moss, M., and Stoltenberg-Allen, K.: Health assessment, St. Louis, 1977, The C. V. Mosby Co.)

There are essentially three different approaches that are most commonly employed for breast palpation: (1) dividing the breast into quadrants and examining the area in each quadrant from the outer perimeter towards the nipple; (2) palpating the inner half then the outer half of the breast; or (3) palpating in concentric circles beginning at the outer rim of breast tissue and moving toward the nipple (Fig. 63-2). The method of approach suggested by the American Cancer Society is described in Fig. 63-2.

Some women need help in learning self-examination; they may, for example, feel a rib when examining the lower half of the breast and become alarmed. However, most women learn quite readily. If a lump of any kind is discovered, it should not be rubbed or touched excessively. It should be left alone, and the advice of a physician should be sought at once.

It will be interesting to see if women will be less reluctant to perform self-examination of their breasts and seek medical advice concerning lumps in the breast now that carcinoma of the breast has received such widespread publicity in the United States and now that the women's movement stresses "self-health" and awareness of one's body.

□ Assessment

Subjective data

If the woman is a high-risk candidate for potential development of breast cancer (see boxed material on p. 1458), it is important to ascertain her knowledge of risk factors, breast self-examination practices, and feelings concerning the potential for breast cancer. This data provides a base for health teaching and exploring of feelings. All women should be questioned concerning their knowledge and practices related to breast self-examination.

If the client has been diagnosed as having a breast tumor that is or may be malignant, the following additional data is obtained as a baseline for planning care:

1. Identification of family relationships and the existence and availability of support persons
2. Usual coping mechanisms
3. Feelings and thoughts about own sexuality and the relationship of the breast to these feelings
4. Thoughts about feelings of sex partner (if appropriate) concerning forthcoming diagnostic procedures or potential surgery

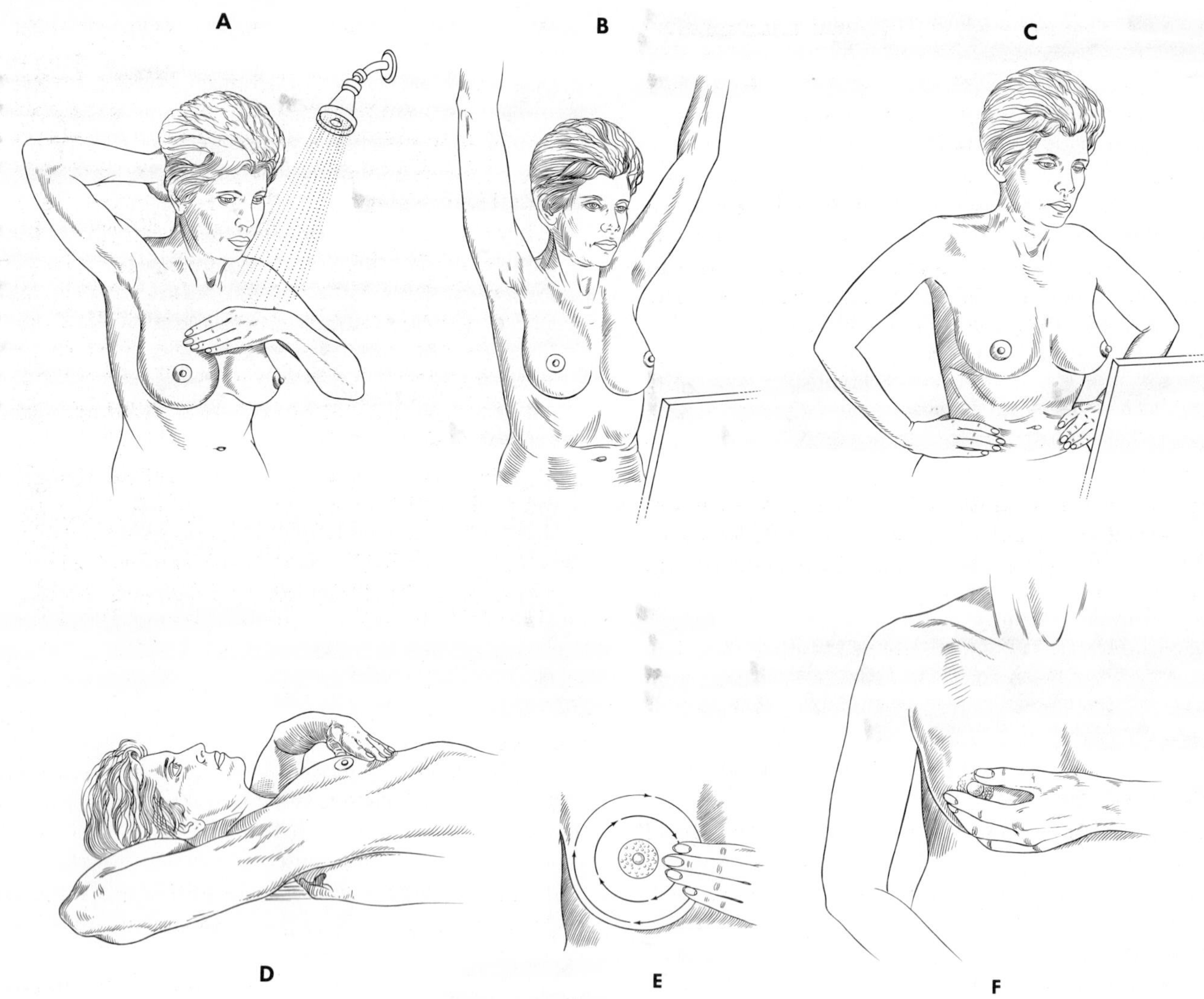

Fig. 63-2. Breast self-examination. **A,** Examine breasts during bath or shower as hands glide easier over wet skin. Use right hand to examine left breast and vice versa. **B,** Sit before a mirror. Inspect breasts with hands at sides then raised overhead. Look for changes in contour or dimpling of skin. **C,** Place hands on hips and press down firmly to flex chest muscles. **D,** Lie down with one hand under head and pillow or folded towel under that shoulder. **E,** Palpate that breast with other hand using concentric circle method. It usually takes three circles to cover all breast tissue. Repeat with other breast. **F,** End with squeezing nipple to check for discharge.

If possible, data is obtained from the sex partner (if appropriate) regarding his feelings of the forthcoming surgery. This identifies possible conflicts in perceptions, the degree of support that can be anticipated from the sex partner, and the potential effects of the partner's feelings on the client's adaptation.

Objective data

The woman's breasts are inspected to determine size and symmetry, contour, and appearance of the skin. Although there is often some difference in breast size, that is, the left breast may be smaller than the right, they usually are relatively symmetrical. Variations in breast contour may include the presence of masses, dimpling, or flattening. The color of the skin, presence of thickened areas, and abnormalities of the venous pattern may be indicative of pathologic processes. The nipple may be inverted; this is usually not pathologic, but the direction in which the nipples are pointing may provide clues to masses. Discharge from the nipple may be indicative of pathologies, may merely vary in certain women with the hormonal fluctuation, or may appear only in response to breast manipulation. Ulcerated areas and other lesions of the nipple require further exploration.

The only early sign of carcinoma of the breast is a small palpable mass. Pain is seldom a symptom of early cancer. Dimpling of the skin (sometimes referred to as *peau d'orange* because of its orange rind appearance) over a hard lump, puckering of the skin, changes in the color of the skin over the lesion, alteration of contour of the breast, distortion of the nipple, serous or bloody discharge from the nipple, and unusual scaling or inversion of the nipple are signs that the lesion is well established and has invaded surrounding tissues. In the advanced phases of neglected cases there may be ulceration of the skin, with subsequent infection of necrotic tissue. Spread to the axillary lymph nodes occurs early. Because of the distribution of the lymph vessels and because there are no lymph nodes between the two breasts to delay spread of malignant cells, these carcinomatous cells may spread rapidly through the lymph vessels with metastasis occurring in the opposite breast and in the mediastinum. Sometimes discovery of enlarged lymph nodes or pain in the ribs or vertebrae is the first indication to the patient that anything is wrong, particularly when the lesion is deep in the breast tissue and routine palpation of the breast has not been carried out.

Diagnostic tests

Mammography is an x-ray technique used to detect lesions before they are palpable (Fig. 63-3). Early cancers are often easily seen on the developed films as small densities with stippled calcifications within. It is about 80% to 97% accurate in detecting early breast carcinoma. Mammography has limitations, particularly in the penetration of dense and heavy breasts.[41]

Considerable controversy exists concerning the use of mammography as a screening device. The routine screening of women under age 50 by mammography is not recommended by some authorities including the National Cancer Institute because of the increased hazard of radiation carcinogenesis.[54] The American Cancer Society, however, asserts that improved mammography techniques have decreased radiation dosage to low levels and that the potential for diagnosing breast cancer is considerably greater than the inherent risk. Mammography is recommended by this group for women in whom breast cancer is suspected and those who are high-risk candidates regardless of age.[3]

Xeroradiography (Fig. 63-4) is a newer technique that is becoming more widely used. In xeroradiography an aluminum plate with an electrically charged selenium layer is used in the place of x-ray film and is exposed in the usual manner using special mammoradiographic equipment. This technique, which is also known as xeromammography, is recommended for women who have large breasts, a family history of breast cancer or questionable physical findings, or those who have had a mastectomy in the other breast.

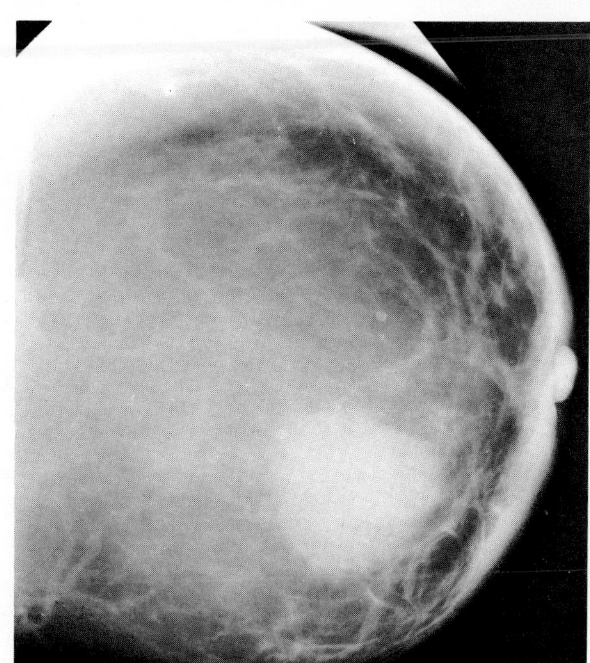

Fig. 63-3. Mammogram of patient with area of density indicating carcinoma. (From Cramer, L. M., and Lapayowker, M. S.: Applied anatomy of the female breast: surgical, radiographic, and thermographic. In Masters, F. W., and Lewis, J. R., Jr., editors: Symposium on aesthetic surgery of the face, eyelid, and breast, vol. 4, St. Louis, 1972, The C. V. Mosby Co.)

An additional less valuable screening device is *thermography*. In this procedure an infrared scanner is used to measure the heat emissions coming from the breast. Abnormal variations in an area because of increased vascularization may indicate the presence of a neoplasm. Early detection of breast masses by using sound waves, *sonography*, is also being explored.

Biopsy. The only way to determine conclusively whether a tumor is benign or malignant is by microscopic examination of a section of the tumor obtained by biopsy (p. 465). When axillary lymph nodes can be felt, the diagnosis of malignancy can be made with relative certainty before the operation, and an axillary node may be excised for microscopic study. Most surgeons believe that if there is the slightest possibility of cancer, it is safer to remove the entire mass rather than risk permitting a malignant tumor to remain. Pieces of a tumor are seldom removed surgically because there is danger of releasing malignant cells into the blood and lymphatic systems at the time of the operation.

Until recently the most common approach has been to remove the tumor and examine a frozen section of the

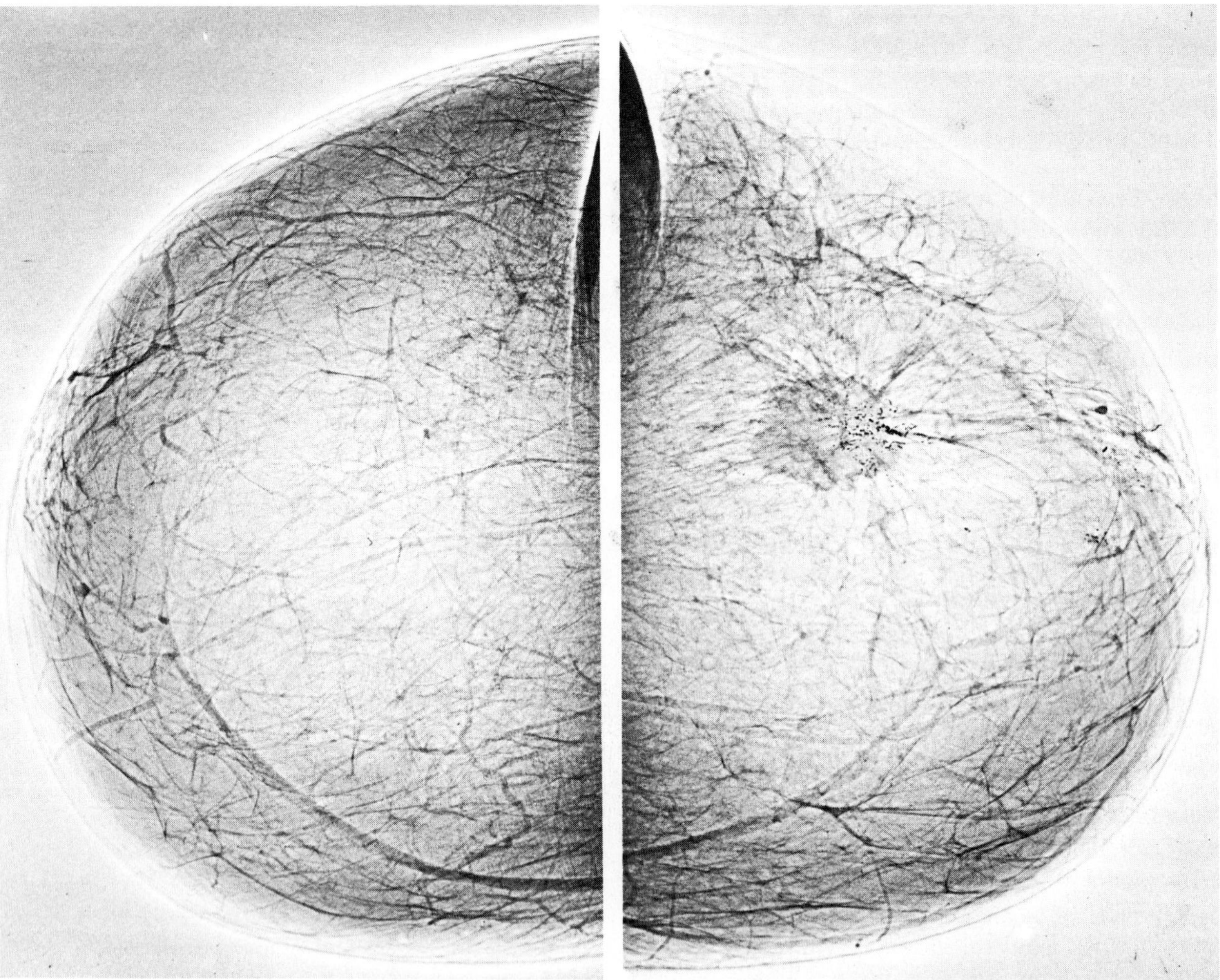

Fig. 63-4. Xeroradiographs. **A,** Normal left breast, **B,** Right breast shows mass with spiculated margins characteristic of neoplasm. (Courtesy University Hospitals of Cleveland, Cleveland, Ohio.)

tissue under the microscope. If the tumor is found to be malignant, the first incision is closed, the surgical set-up is completely changed, and the more extensive operation is then performed. In this approach to surgery, when the patient goes for a biopsy, she does not know in advance whether the breast will be removed or the extent of surgery that will be performed.

An increasing number of surgeons are now scheduling the patient for a biopsy alone. The patient then goes home and awaits the biopsy results. She thus has time to make decisions about and prepare herself psychologically for the more extensive surgery if a malignancy is found. The disadvantage of this approach is the stress of waiting for the diagnostic results and then facing the prospect of a repeat hospital admission and a second surgical procedure. In the Gallup survey cited earlier, 47% of the women indicated they would prefer to sign the consent for surgery early (the first approach described above), while 48% would prefer the second approach in order to get other opinions (20%) or to discuss the situation after diagnosis (28%).[18]

In either of the above approaches, after excision of the tumor masses the pathologist usually will send cancer tissue to a special laboratory for determination of estrogen receptors. Such studies are helpful in future management of the patient. The hormone assay test identifies those breast cancers that are hormone dependent; that is, their growth is stimulated by steroid hormones, especially estrogen. Postmenopausal women have a higher incidence of hormone-dependent breast cancers.[52] Treatment such as removal of the ovaries or endocrine chemotherapy (Chapter 25) removes the source of estrogen and thereby can retard growth and spread of these malignant cells. A negative hormone assay test indicates that the breast cancer is not hormone dependent and therefore oophorectomy or endocrine chemotherapy will not be effective.

□ Interventions

Surgery

Surgery is the treatment of choice unless extensive metastasis has occurred and the tumor is very large, ulcerated, and inoperable.

Types of surgery. Following are different types of surgeries that can be performed to remove a breast mass:

1. *Lumpectomy:* simple removal of a lump or tumor mass
2. *Partial mastectomy:* removal of tumor mass and 2.5 to 7.5 cm (1 to 3 inches) of surrounding tissue
3. *Subcutaneous mastectomy (adenomammectomy):* removal of all breast tissue, leaving skin, areola, and nipple intact
4. *Simple mastectomy:* removal of entire breast but not lymph nodes
5. *Modified radical mastectomy:* complete removal of breast and part of lymph nodes (pectoralis minor but not pectoralis major may also be removed)
6. *Radical mastectomy:* complete removal of breast, axillary lymph nodes, pectoral muscles, and adjacent fat and fascia
7. *Extended radical mastectomy (supraradical):* same as radical mastectomy plus removal of parasternal lymph nodes

Recently there has been considerable discussion in lay periodicals and in medical journals about the surgical treatment of carcinoma of the breast. In some articles it is suggested that a lumpectomy is sufficient to treat some carcinomas of the breast and that a mastectomy is not necessary. This approach, however, is *not* recommended by the majority of authorities. At this time there have been no controlled clinical studies to prove that one method is better than another, and there appears to be no dramatic difference among the mastectomy procedures on a 5-year survival rate.[30] The determination of the best procedure should consider a 10-year survival rate,[30] however, and the American Cancer Society's position as of 1977 is that removal of the entire breast, most often the modified radical or radical, is the recommended treatment of operable breast cancer.

A *modified* radical mastectomy is often performed for early, well-localized, small lesions of the breast, and it appears to be as curative as the classic radical mastectomy. In the *radical* mastectomy the judgment of the surgeon regarding the amount of overlying skin that can safely be left to cover the defect determines whether a skin graft will be necessary. Preoperatively the surgeon may order the skin of the anterior surface of a thigh shaved and prepared surgically in case need for a graft should arise. If the lesion is located in the medial quadrant of the breast, particularly the upper medial quadrant, an *extended* radical mastectomy may be performed, as lesions of the medial quadrant tend to metastasize to the internal mammary chain of lymph nodes. A *simple* mastectomy sometimes is performed if cancer is believed to be limited to the breast or as a palliative measure to remove an ulcerated carcinoma of the breast in disease that is known to be advanced.

Preoperative care. Since much emphasis is placed on the breast as a symbol of attractiveness, the thought of losing a breast becomes almost intolerable to many women. This is particularly true of those who depend largely on physical attractiveness to hold the esteem of others and to secure gratification of their emotional needs. Psychologists have pointed out that there is a symbolic connection between the breasts and motherhood that is severely threatened when a breast must be removed.[44] It is understandable that women may be seriously threatened emotionally by the loss of a part of the body that is so closely associated with sexual attractiveness and motherliness. Carcinoma of the breast often occurs at the menopause or soon after when some women feel that they have lost much of their sexual attractiveness. Surgical removal of the breast may save a woman's life, but it also may cause her to feel less feminine.

Although she may try to conceal fear, any woman who is hospitalized for removal of a breast tumor is always anxious, and some may be in a state of near panic. Most of the fears are related to sexual acceptance, social isolation, disfigurement, recurrence, and death. Many of these women have been unable to discuss their worries and feelings with their significant others, including their spouse. The nurse can help the patient to express feelings and can help her to understand what breast surgery means to her as a person. The woman who is having breast surgery has a special need to feel understood and accepted by all persons who are giving preoperative care.

Simple explanations may decrease the patient's fear of the unknown. The surgeon usually discusses the diagnosis and treatment with the patient and significant other. If it seems that the patient does not fully comprehend the surgeon's explanation, the nurse reports this to the surgeon, who in turn can talk with the patient again and clarify any misconceptions, hopefully alleviating needless anxiety. Since perception is limited when anxiety levels are high, it is helpful if the nurse can be present when information is given to the patient. The nurse can then reinforce or clarify given information.

The American Cancer Society sponsors a volunteer program, Reach to Recovery, in which the patient has an opportunity to visit with a woman who has had a mastectomy. This encourages the patient, and she will receive practical help from someone who has made a satisfactory adjustment to the same operation. Although most of the patient visits by the volunteer from Reach to Recovery occur during the postoperative period, preoperative visits may be very helpful to some women.

Additional testing may be done. If a diagnosis of a malignancy is almost a certainty, x-ray examinations such as a bone survey and liver function studies may be ordered to rule out the possibility of metastases to these areas of the body. Preparing the patient for procedures that will take place before and after surgery is of utmost importance in allaying her fears as well as in setting the stage for successful rehabilitation.

Preoperative teaching should include the following information if a mastectomy is planned. A dressing may or may not be applied to the incision and a catheter attached to suction may be used. With more extensive surgery, the arm will be elevated and movement will be restricted initially. If the breast is removed, there will be a tendency for the shoulder to droop on the opposite side because of the inequality of weight, but this can be prevented by close attention to posture. Poor posture may give more evidence that a breast has been removed than will a slight inequality in the breast contours. While padding and prosthetic devices are used to take the place of the breast and restore normal contours to the upper body, stooped, awkward posture cannot be hidden. Exercises will be taught postoperatively to help improve posture and to strengthen muscles. Telling the patient about the exercises helps to give her the feeling that there is something in the situation that she can control and contribute to, and thus aids in a positive attitude toward rehabilitation.

Postoperative care

Wound care. Following removal of the breast and adjacent tissue, a stab wound may be made near the axilla and a catheter inserted and attached to a low constant suction, such as that provided by a Hemovac (Fig. 23-10) or an Emerson suction. The purpose of the catheter is to remove blood and serum that may collect under the skin flaps, preventing healing and predisposing to infection. The Hemovac must be checked frequently and emptied to maintain suction on the catheter and prevent buildup of fluid under the skin flaps. There is usually very little drainage from around the incision when a catheter is draining properly. The catheter may be clamped for short periods of ambulation and is usually removed within 3 to 5 days when the amount of drainage is less than 100 ml in 24 hours.

At one time pressure dressings rather than a catheter were used to prevent the accumulation of fluid under the skin. Many surgeons now believe that the use of a catheter and a smaller dressing is preferable to the use of a large pressure dressing.

The wound or the dressing is checked often for the first few hours to detect hemorrhage or excessive serous oozing. The bedclothes under the patient must be examined for blood that may flow from the axillary region backward. Any evidence of bleeding is reported to the surgeon. If the wound is not covered with a dressing, a cradle may be used to protect it from the bed covers. When pressure dressings are used, they are checked to be certain they do not hamper circulation. Signs of circulatory obstruction such as swelling and numbness of the lower arm or inability to move the fingers must be reported at once. The nurse, however, should never loosen dressings without specific instruction from the surgeon.

If a graft has been taken from the thigh, this area may be covered with a firm pressure dressing, or fine mesh gauze may be used and the wound exposed to the air. The patient may complain of severe discomfort in this donor site as soon as she reacts from anesthesia.

If dressings are applied over the breast area, they usually are not changed for several days after the operation. The skin sutures closing the breast and axillary incision are often removed on the sixth to the eighth postoperative day.

Comfort. Incisional pain occurs from the trauma to the tissues and tension on the suture line. Pain may be referred to the affected arm or shoulder, and numbness and tingling may occur. The patient may complain of a feeling of constriction over the chest that is painful, causing her to take short, shallow breaths. Measures to promote ventilation of the lungs are therefore instituted (p. 950).

When the patient recovers from the effects of anesthesia, she is usually more comfortable lying on her back with her head elevated. If the operated arm is not incorporated in the dressing, the arm is elevated to prevent muscle strain and edema. The pillows are arranged so that the hand is higher than the arm, and the arm is above the level of the right atrium. *No blood pressure readings, injections, or blood testing* should be done on the *affected* arm because of potential circulatory impairment or infection. The patient may be more comfortable sitting up straight during back care, since turning toward the affected side may be exceedingly painful. An overhead frame and trapeze are useful in facilitating turning and sitting up in bed.

Activity and exercise. Exercises are essential to

prevent shortening of muscles and contracture of joints and to preserve muscle tone so that the affected arm can be used without limitations. To prevent additional deformities, exercises should be bilateral ones with the patient using both arms simultaneously. The surgeon decides when specific postoperative exercises should be started. This will depend on the extent of the operation and whether skin grafting has been necessary.

Slings are to be avoided whenever possible as they encourage immobility. Gentle exercises started early in the postoperative course help decrease muscle tension as well as regain muscle function more quickly.[49] The patient is encouraged under close supervision to exercise to the limits of incisional pulling and pain. A specific exercise schedule planned by nurse and patient together has a greater chance of success. Usually the patient is encouraged to flex and extend her fingers immediately on return to her room. She should also be encouraged to pronate and supinate her forearm; simply turning the palm up and down will do this. Squeezing a rubber ball is often started on the first postoperative day, and brushing the teeth and hair are encouraged as soon as can be tolerated.

Additional exercises are begun as permitted. (See boxed material opposite for suggested exercises.) With proper exercise, full range of motion will return; that is, both arms can be extended equally high above the head. This will not be achieved before the patient leaves the hospital; therefore the patient must be encouraged to continue exercises begun in the hospital on a regular basis. Following radical mastectomy, full muscle power of the arm may not return, and there may be a limitation of strength, especially with horizontal adduction.[49]

Participation in classes with others who have undergone the same operation usually stimulates the patient to learn the prescribed exercises. As soon as possible, normal activities should take the place of exercises, provided the patient understands how particular exercises can be accomplished by specific tasks. The patient must know what motion is intended in each exercise. It is not enough simply to ask her to comb her own hair or to wash her own back. For example, the patient may brush her hair with the arm on the affected side, but she may lower her head and hunch her shoulders in such a way that she does not get normal use of the shoulder joint and attached muscles. The whole intent of the exercise may therefore be lost. A small handbook entitled *Reach to Recovery** is available for use by nurses in teaching patients and distribution to patients.

Swimming is excellent exercise for the patient who has had a mastectomy. Bathing suits are designed that cover up scarring and can be fitted so that the loss of a breast is not obvious.

Fatigue is a common complaint during the restorative period, and exercise is planned to avoid excess fatigue. Discharge planning should also include planned rest periods.

Emotional support. If the patient has had the breast removed immediately following a frozen section, she is told by the surgeon that the breast was removed when she has recovered from the effects of anesthesia. It usually is her first question, and she will try to determine the fact by feeling the dressing. Reactions such as crying, withdrawal, or anger are to be expected, and the patient needs considerable understanding and support.

Loss of a breast involves two major concepts: change in body image and mourning over loss. In addition to

*Published by the American Cancer Society, Inc.; available from local chapters of the society.[28]

POSTMASTECTOMY ARM EXERCISES

Exercise: Climbing the wall

1. Stand facing wall with toes close to wall.
2. Bend elbows and place palms of hands against wall at shoulder level.
3. Move both hands parallel to each other up the wall as far as possible until incisional pull or pain occur.
4. Move both hands down to starting position.
5. Goal: complete extension with elbow straight.
6. Activities that utilize the same action: reaching top shelves, hanging out clothes, washing windows, hanging curtains, setting hair.

Exercise: Arm swinging

1. Bend forward from waist, permitting both arms to relax and hang naturally.
2. Swing arms together left to right (motion comes from shoulder).
3. Swing arms in circles parallel to floor, clockwise and counterclockwise.
4. Stand up slowly.

Exercise: Rope pull

1. Attach a rope over a shower rod or hook.
2. Grasp each end of rope, alternately pulling on each end, raising affected arm to a point of incisional pull or pain.
3. Shorten rope over time until affected arm is raised almost directly overhead.

Exercise: Elbow spread

1. Clasp hands behind neck.
2. Raise elbows to chin level, holding head erect. Move slowly and rest when incisional pull or pain occur.
3. Gradually spread elbows apart. Rest when pull or pain occur.

these losses, the patient is trying to cope with the fear of cancer and its potential spread and death. Removal of a breast for cancer is therefore an extremely stressful situation. The initial response is usually shock. Denial may take the form of the woman speaking about the "cancer" and the "mastectomy" but never dealing with the loss or her fears on a feeling level. The impact of the loss then occurs at a later date when support systems may not be as available.

Avoidance of looking at the dressing or incision can be expected initially. The incision is large and the feeling experienced by most women is that of mutilation. Postponing looking at the incision delays the impact that the breast is indeed gone. Preparing the woman in advance concerning the size of the incision is helpful, but she still needs considerable support when viewing the incision. She is encouraged to look at the incision several times before discharge from the hospital, while health professionals are available for support.

Feelings of anger and resentment occur and are frequently projected on the staff. Families also express anger and may complain about the care the patient is receiving. Feelings of decreased self-worth and self-esteem on the part of the patient plus increased dependency needs often produce depression. (For more detailed discussion on mourning and body image, see Chapters 19 and 28.) The feeling of being isolated and alone during this experience can be helped by interaction with others who have had the same experience, such as a visitor from the "Reach to Recovery" program (p. 1464).

Phantom symptoms of the missing breast occur in about one-third of women having a mastectomy, and there is a greater incidence in premenopausal women. Phantom breast symptoms can be very distressing to the woman who is trying to cope with the absence of the breast.

After the patient is discharged, she will usually experience periods of depression, especially when extensive surgery has been performed and recovery is slow. She may have difficulty sleeping or concentrating on

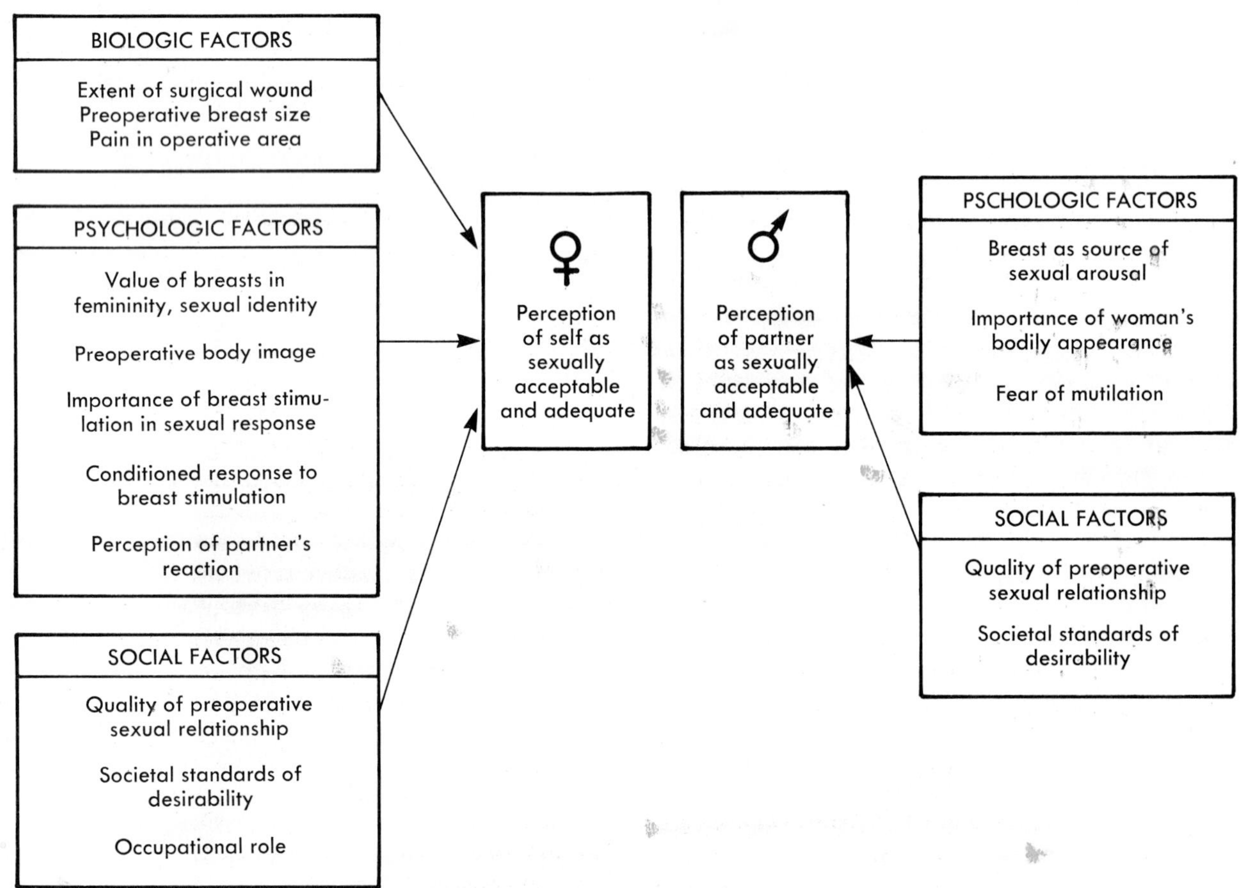

Fig. 63-5. Factors influencing a couple's sexual adaptation to mastectomy. (From Woods, N. F.: J. Obstet. Gynecol. Neonatal Nurs. **4:**34, 1975).

tasks. Awareness of this by the patient and significant others facilitates family support when this occurs. Some patients remain at home, avoid their friends, hesitate to engage in social activities, and thus make life unhappy for themselves and their families. The reasons for withdrawal from social participation include fear of rejection by others because of loss of body intactness. Healing of the incision so that she is able to wear a fitted brassiere usually reassures the woman and encourages her to participate in home and social activities.

Sexual adaptation. Woods has identified a number of factors that can influence sexual adaptation following mastectomy[66] (Fig. 63-5). Women with very small or very large breasts may have unresolved feelings about breast size and may also experience more difficulty in obtaining a satisfactory breast prosthesis. The woman who perceives the surgery as mutilating may withdraw from the sexual relationship, fearing rejection from her partner.[66] Women who felt sexually inadequate prior to surgery may find these feelings enhanced postoperatively and use the surgery as a reason for withdrawing from sexual relationships. Sexual and marital counseling are helpful for couples who are unable to communicate their feelings openly with each other.

Breast prostheses and clothing. Information about breast prostheses is given to the patient whenever she asks about it or appears interested; this may occur preoperatively as well as postoperatively. The volunteer from "Reach to Recovery" can provide information and suggestions concerning prostheses or special clothing. The volunteer is often of great assistance in helping the patient with selection of an artificial breast, since her recommendations are based on personal experience and the experience of other women who have had a mastectomy.

Until the incision is well healed, the woman is advised to wear one of her own brassieres, which can be lightly padded with a soft, fluffy filling (Fig. 63-6). Plain cotton can be covered with gauze and lightly tacked to the inside of the brassiere. The patient will probably want to wear a hospital gown until she has obtained a nightgown that covers the surgical area. Opaque, high-neck, loose-hanging gowns are usually most acceptable to the patient. Both gown and robe should have wide arm holes to prevent constriction of the underarm. When the woman goes home, loose-fitting, front-fastened shirts with wide armholes are suggested.

Breast prostheses are not fitted until at least 6 weeks postoperatively. Choosing and being fitted for a prosthesis has been reported by many women as being a time of trauma, confusion, and disappointment.[62] The woman should therefore take her time and explore the various types before making a final decision. (A listing of places where postmastectomy clothes and breast prostheses can

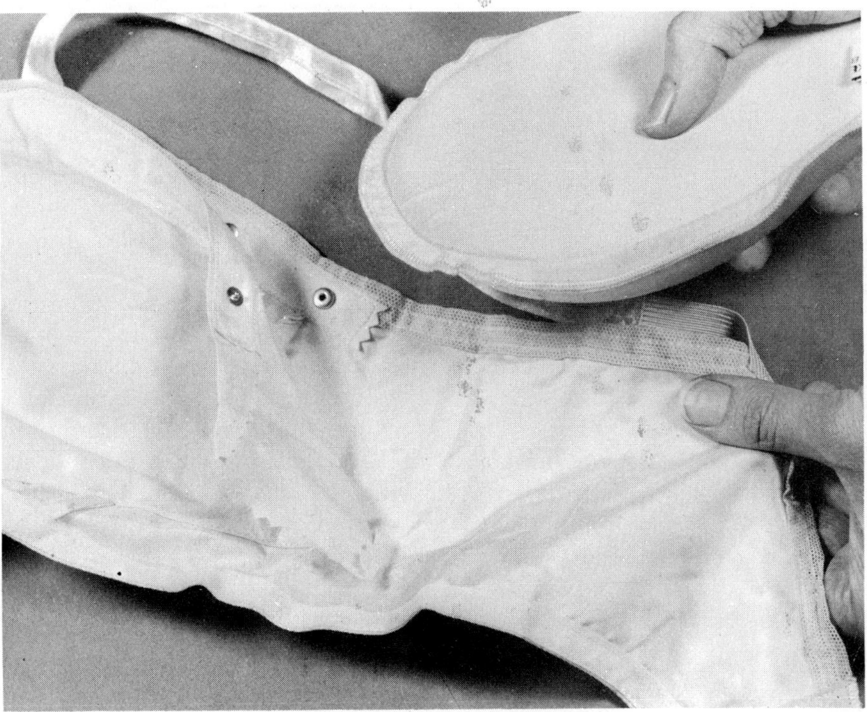

Fig. 63-6. Inner pocket that will hold padding or prosthesis securely can be made in patient's own brassiere. Note snaps that simplify removal of padding.

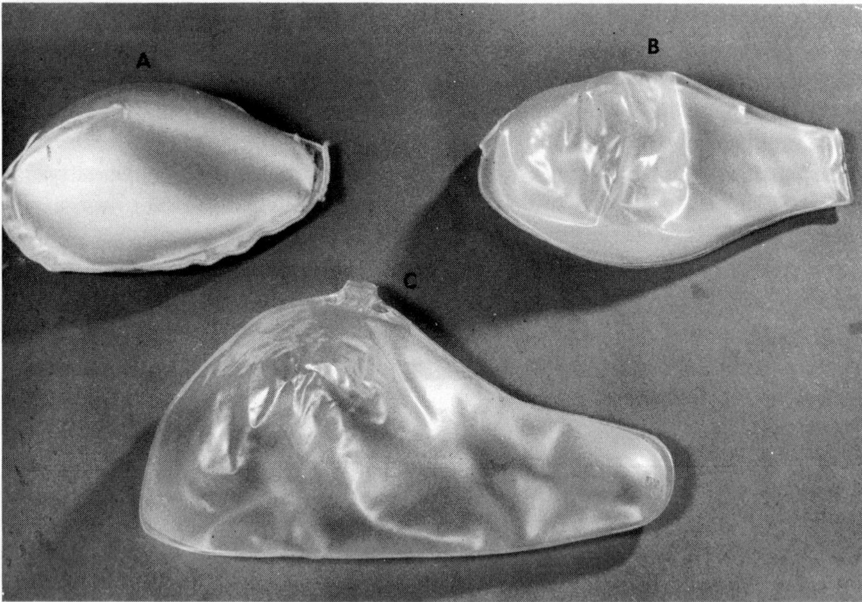

Fig. 63-7. Several types of breast prostheses are available. **A,** Foam rubber prosthesis. **B,** Prosthesis containing fluid. **C,** Prosthesis containing air.

be purchased as well as general guidelines for purchase can be found in the references.[2,62,63])

Breast prostheses vary in price, type, and weight. The most popular form is a liquid- or silicone-filled type[62] (Fig. 63-7). Cheap foam types may be worn by small-breasted women who have had less extensive surgery, but this type is unweighted and more difficult to keep in place. A large-breasted woman needs a heavier-weighted prosthesis. Firm molded types have a disadvantage of remaining elevated when the woman is lying supine, whereas fluid types have a more natural look. Thin brassiere straps should be avoided following extensive surgery.[62]

Lymphedema. Many patients develop a slight edema of the upper arm that disappears within a week. A few patients, however, develop a severe edema that persists, may become permanent, and that is caused by surgical interruption of lymph channels and nodes. The incidence is greater in persons who are obese, develop infections, or are subjected to irradiation. Some surgeons order an elastic sleeve that gives additional support to the vessels in the arm. This should extend from the wrist to the shoulder. It is similar to an elastic support stocking and usually may be removed when the patient is in bed. A diuretic such as chlorothiazide (Diuril) may be ordered to help relieve the edema.

Special care must be taken to prevent minor infections of the hands and arms in patients with lymphedema, and if they do occur, medical treatment should be sought at once, since the infection spreads quickly because of the improperly functioning lymph system. The patient is advised to use cuticle cream instead of cuticle scissors, to wear rubber gloves when using harsh household products, and to wear canvas gloves when gardening. The axillae should be kept clean with soap and water, deodorants used sparingly, and an electric razor used for shaving. Care is advised to prevent burns of the affected arm and hand. Injections, blood pressure measurements, and constricting clothing are to be avoided on the affected arm.

Long-term adaptation. During the recovery period at home, many women experience varied symptoms that may last for several years. In a study of 49 women in North Carolina interviewed 4 years following a mastectomy, 53% reported one or more of the following symptoms still existing: swelling, weakness, stiffness, trouble moving and numbness of the arm, poor healing, and pain.[67] About three-fourths of the sample experienced symptoms immediately following surgery, especially weakness and stiffness of the arm. The study also reported that women with a high number of physical symptoms were more likely to have a high number of symptoms of depression. Measures that can be taken to prevent the symptoms from developing may assist the woman in her adaptation to the loss of the breast. She also needs to be prepared for potential occurrence of these symptoms.

Outcome criteria for the woman who has had a mastectomy. The patient or significant others can:

1. Identify feelings related to loss of the breast.

2. Describe and demonstrate exercises to be continued until full range of motion to the affected shoulder returns.
3. State types of breast prostheses available and where these may be obtained.
4. Describe types of clothing to be avoided (constricting of arm).
5. Describe plans for return to social activities as carried out before surgery.
6. Describe plans for avoidance of fatigue.
7. Describe health maintenance or follow-up program.
   a. State symptoms indicating need for immediate medical attention (edema of affected arm, redness or infection within or surrounding the scar, mass in unaffected breast).
   b. Describe measures to prevent infection and compression of affected arm.
   c. State plans for regular medical follow-up.
   d. Demonstrate self-examination of remaining breast tissue and state plans for monthly self-examination.

Breast reconstruction

Reconstruction mammaplasty is a possibility for some women following a mastectomy. Extensive physical and psychologic assessment is indicated before the procedure is considered.[60] The procedure is an additional stressor for the woman and is expensive, but may be attractive to women experiencing discomfort from external prostheses or from muscle strain from uneven chest weight. It is contraindicated when there is a probability that metastasis will occur or when there is a concern about adequate healing.[60]

The surgery consists of an implant placed under the subcutaneous tissue. If a radical mastectomy has been done, a more extensive procedure is necessary to provide a base for the implant. A dermal fat graft from the gluteal fold will be done first with the implant inserted at a later date.[60] A nipple can be reconstructed if necessary from labial tissue. Drains are usually inserted in order to prevent a hematoma. The reconstructed breast will not be symmetrical with the existing breast.

A brassiere is worn postoperatively in order to maintain implant position and alignment. Vigorous activity is avoided immediately postoperatively, but the patient is encouraged to move her arms slowly. Pain medications are discouraged, as the degree of discomfort serves as an index to the degree of movement that can be tolerated without disrupting the reconstruction.

Radiotherapy

Radiotherapy is often used in conjunction with surgery; it may also be used instead of surgery when the tumor is large, ulcerated, and inoperable. It tends to decrease bleeding, stimulate healing, and may diminish the size of the tumor. Treatment can be started as soon as the day after surgery and may be continued on an ambulatory basis after the patient leaves the hospital. (For details of care of patients receiving radiation treatment, see p. 470.) Radiotherapy is also used to treat painful metastatic bone lesions, which occur in the spine, ribs, hips, and pelvis of about 30% of all patients who develop metastasis from carcinoma of the breast, and to treat lesions in the brain, which occur in about 10% of all cases of metastasis.

Pelvic irradiation may be given to reduce estrogenic activity. This is most likely to be used in women over age 40 who have not entered the menopause. The effectiveness of pelvic irradiation can be determined by examining vaginal smears for loss of estrogenic effect.

Therapy when metastasis occurs

In advanced carcinoma of the breast the treatment is palliative; that is, it affords relief but does not effect a cure. Although some of the procedures may seem radical, they produce temporary regression of the tumor, lessen pain, and permit the patient to remain active. The treatments are used only when the lesion and symptoms are no longer amenable to surgery or radiation therapy. They are often used in specific sequence and only after recurrence of symptoms of metastasis. The choice of procedure depends on the patient and whether she has experienced the menopause.

Since estrogens are believed to enhance the growth of malignant cells in women who are not past the menopause, several operative procedures are now used to remove the estrogen supply in persons with positive hormone assay tests (p. 1462). Surgeries include bilateral oophorectomy (p. 1437) and bilateral adrenalectomy (p. 581), performed when the effect of the oophorectomy has subsided, or a hypophysectomy, which suppresses the function of both ovaries and the adrenal glands by removal of the pituitary gland (p. 569).

Premenopausal women who do not respond to oophorectomy or pelvic irradiation are usually treated with corticosteroids and chemotherapeutic agents. On the other hand, women who respond to induction of the menopause and who later have a metastasis of their disease are treated with bilateral adrenalectomy or hypophysectomy.

If the patient is more than 1 year past the menopause, she is treated with either estrogens or androgens. At this age, these hormones seem to produce a regression of the tumor in some persons. The reason they do so is not known, although hormonal therapy does prevent physiologic secretion of estrogen from the adrenal gland. Testosterone propionate is the androgen most often used and may be given in doses of 50 mg (3/4 grain) intramuscularly twice a week for an indefinite period. Much larger doses may also be given. Treatment with testosterone will cause secondary changes that are distressing to the patient. These include deepening of the voice, coarsening of the skin, and appearance of hair on the face and the rest of the body. The patient usually gains weight. She should be warned that these changes may occur, and she may need to pay greater attention to details of personal grooming than formerly was necessary.

Diethylstilbestrol (stilbestrol) is the estrogen commonly used. It may be given in oral doses of 15 mg (1/4 grain) daily. The drug is better tolerated if the entire dose is given at bedtime. Occasionally uterine bleeding occurs and is often felt to be a withdrawal effect caused by failure of the patient to take the drug regularly. Increasing the dosage of the estrogen for several days often controls the bleeding. The corticosteroids may produce regression of the tumor in some patients. However, the use of these hormones may cause undesirable side effects. New drugs such as nafoxidine and tamoxifen (antiestrogens) are now being used in certain patients with metastatic disease. If the patient does not respond to estrogenic therapy, *chemotherapy* (p. 475) and *immunotherapy* (p. 484) are used for treatment. Both of these therapies are being used more widely and are discussed in depth in Chapter 25.

■ NONMALIGNANT DISEASE OF THE BREAST

□ Dysplasia

Dysplasia *(fibrocystic disease)* is characterized by thickened nodular areas in the breast that usually become painful during or prior to menstruation. The process is almost always bilateral. It occurs mostly in women between 30 years of age and menopause. A variety of changes take place in the breast tissue, which in some cases includes the formation of cysts. The condition is thought to be caused by hormonal imbalance. There is failure of normal involution following the reaction of the breasts to the cyclic activity of the female sex hormones. The nodules or cysts may be singular or multiple, may increase in size, or remain the same. They are usually fairly soft and tender on palpation and are movable, sliding under the examining fingers.

The woman who discovers such a mass (or masses) in her breast should seek the advice of a physician, who will decide whether the lesion should be measured and checked at frequent intervals, whether hormones should be administered, or whether aspiration of the cyst should be considered. There is little evidence that dysplasia predisposes to the development of malignancy, but the presence of nodules in the breast makes the early detection of malignant lesions much more difficult. For this reason, some physicians suggest periodic mammography or xeroradiography of the breast to detect any changes.

□ Fibroadenoma

Fibroadenomas are tumors of fibroblastic and epithelial origin that are thought to be caused by hyperestrinism. They are usually firm, round, freely movable, nontender, and encapsulated. They occur most often in women under 25 years of age.

The woman who discovers such a mass should not delay in seeking medical consultation. Usually the tumor will be removed under local anesthesia and will be examined microscopically to be sure it is not malignant. Although the hospital stay for excision of an adenoma is short and the patient returns to the surgeon's office or clinic for the sutures to be removed, she needs thoughtful nursing care, since she usually is extremely fearful of cancer.

□ Infections

Infection of the nipple. Infection usually follows cracks in the nipple during lactation. This condition is less common than previously, since women are taught to "toughen" the nipple during pregnancy so that cracking during breast-feeding is less likely to occur.

Infection of the breast. An infection can occur in the breast by direct spread from cracked or infected nipples and following congestion or "caking" during lactation when a portion of the breast becomes engorged from blockage of gland ducts. Manual expression of excess milk and hormone treatment for women who are not going to nurse their infants have reduced the incidence of infections of the breast. The microorganisms causing the infection may be transmitted to the mother's breast from the nasopharynx of the newborn infant who has been exposed to infected infants and hospital personnel or from the hands of the patient or those of hospital personnel. Staphylococcal infections are the most common. Infections in the breast can also occur with no specific cause and perhaps follow infections elsewhere in the body. These infections can occur at times other than during pregnancy or lactation.

Infections of the breast cause pain, redness, swelling, and elevation of temperature. The treatment is usually conservative. Antibiotics are usually given systemically. Sometimes local heat is used, and at other times ice packs may be prescribed. If the condition does not subside with conservative treatment and becomes localized to form an abscess, surgical drainage is necessary. To help prevent infections of the breast from occurring, there is a continued need for strict aseptic technique in nurseries for newborn infants. This includes preventing infected persons (carriers) from coming in contact with mothers and babies.

☐ Gynecomastia

Gynecomastia is a hyperplasia (overdevelopment) of the stroma and ducts in the mammary glands in the male. It occurs during puberty and after the age of 40, and is also seen in patients with liver disease. Most are idiopathic, however, and the cause is thought to be an abnormally large estrogen secretion. It also frequently is seen following estrogen therapy for carcinoma of the prostate. Gynecomastia is a nonmalignant lesion, but physicians may suggest removal and biopsy of the breast, since older men occasionally develop carcinoma of the breast.

REFERENCES AND SELECTED READINGS

1. Ackerman, L. V., del Regato, J. A., and Spjut, H. J.: Cancer—diagnosis, treatment, and prognosis, ed. 5, St. Louis, 1977, The C. V. Mosby Co.
2. *After mastectomy: finding the right prosthesis, Consumer Reports **40**:652-654, 1975.
3. *American Cancer Society, Inc.: 1977 cancer facts and figures, New York, 1977, The Society.
4. American Cancer Society, Inc.: Close-up standard breast examination, CA **24**:291-293, 1974.
5. Anderson, D. E.: A high-risk group for breast cancer, Cancer Bull. **25**:23-25, 1973.
6. Bouchard, R., and Owens, N.: Nursing care of the cancer patient, ed. 3, St. Louis, 1976, The C. V. Mosby Co.
7. Cady, B.: Modern management of breast cancer: a point of view, Arch. Surg. **104**:270-275, 1972.
8. Cancer Advisory Committee: Optimal criteria for care of patients with cancer, J.A.M.A. **227**:57-63, 1974.
9. Carter, S. K.: Single and combination nonhormonal chemotherapy in breast cancer, Cancer **30**:1543-1555, 1972.
10. Cowles, J. K.: Informed consent, New York, 1976, Coward, McCann & Geoghegan, Inc.
11. Crile, G., Jr.: Conservative treatment of advanced breast cancer, Am J. Surg. **126**:343-344, 1973.
12. Crile, G., Jr., Esselstyn, C. B., Jr., Hermann, R. E., et al.: Partial mastectomy for carcinoma of the breast, Surg. Gynecol. Obstet. **136**:929-933, 1973.
13. Dao, T. L.: Ablation therapy for hormone-dependent tumors, Ann. Rev. Med. **23**:1-18, 1972.
14. Donegan, W. L.: Mastectomy in the primary management of invasive mammary carcinoma, Adv. Surg. **6**:1-101, 1972.
15. Egan, R. L.: Contributions of mammography in the detection of early breast cancer, Cancer **28**:1555-15557, 1971.
16. *Farabee, J. M.: Mammography, chemography offer optimism for breast cancer diagnosis, A.O.R.N.J. **19**:837-842, 1974.
17. Freudlich, I. M.: Thermography, N. Engl. J. Med. **287**:880-881, 1972.
18. *Gallup polls women on attitudes on breast cancer, Am. J. Nurs. **74**:124, 1974.
19. *Gribbons, C. A., and Aliapoulios, M. A.: Treatment for advanced breast carcinoma, Am. J. Nurs. **72**:678-682, 1972.
20. Haagensen, C. D.: Diseases of the breast, ed. 2, Philadelphia, 1971, W. B. Saunders Co.
21. *Harrell, H. C.: To lose a breast, Am. J. Nurs. **72**:676-677, 1972.
22. *Harley, I. D., and Brandt, E. M.: Control and prevention of lymphedema following radical mastectomy, Nurs. Res. **67**:333-336, 1967.
23. Healey, J. E., Jr.: Role of rehabilitation medicine in the care of the patient with breast cancer, Cancer **28**:1666-1671, 1971.
24. Kaufman, S., and Goldstein, M.: Combination chemotherapy in disseminated carcinoma of the breast, Surg. Gynecol. Obstet. **137**:83-86, July 1973.
25. Kelley, R. M.: Hormones and chemotherapy in breast cancer, Cancer **28**:1686-1691, 1971.
26. Ketchem, A. S.: Predictable categories of increased risk to breast cancer, A.O.R.N.J. **19**:852-858, 1974.
27. *Kushner, R.: Breast cancer: a personal history and an investigative report, New York, 1975, Harcourt Brace Jovanovich, Inc.
28. Lasser, T., and Clark, W. K.: Reach to recovery, New York, 1972, Simon & Schuster, Inc.
29. *Leis, H.: Risk factors in breast cancer, A.O.R.N.J. **22**:723-732, 1975.
30. *Leis, H. P., and Pelnik, S.: Breast cancer: a therapeutic dilemma, A.O.R.N.J. **19**:813-820, 1974.
31. Lesnick, G. J.: Detection of breast cancer in young women, J.A.M.A. **237**:967-969, 1977.
32. *Levene, M. B.: A new role for radiation therapy, Am. J. Nurs. **77**:1443-1444, 1977.
33. *Levene, M. B., Harris, J. R., and Hellman, S.: Treatment of carcinoma of the breast by radiation therapy, Cancer **39**(suppl.): 2840-2845, 1977.
34. *Mamaril, A. P.: Preventing complications after radical mastectomy, Am. J. Nurs. **74**:2000-2003, 1974.
35. Markel, W. M.: The American Cancer Society's program for the rehabilitation of the breast cancer patient. Cancer **28**:1676-1680, 1971.
36. Mayo, P., and Wilkey, N. L.: Prevention of cancer of the breast and cervix, Nurs. Clin. North Am. **3**:229-241, 1968.
37. *McCorkle, M. R.: Coping with physical symptoms in metastatic breast cancer, Am. J. Nurs. **73**:1034-1038, 1973.
38. McLaughlin, C. W., Jr., and Coe, J. D.: Cancer of the breast, Am. J. Surg. **125**:734-737, 1973.
39. *Owen, M. L.: Special care for the patient who has a breast biopsy or mastectomy, Nurs. Clin. North Am. **7**:373-382, 1973.
40. *Perras, C.: Subcutaneous mastectomy, Am. J. Nurs. **73**:1568-1570, 1973.
41. *Phillips, C. W., et al.: Xeroradiology of the breast, Nurs. Digest **2**:89-92, 1974.
42. *Poliby, J.: Psychological effects of radical mastectomy, Public Health Rev. **4**:279-295, 1975.
43. *Quint, J. C.: The impact of mastectomy, Am. J. Nurs. **63**:88-92, 1963.
44. *Rennecker, R., and Cutler, M.: Psychological problems of adjustment to cancer of the breast, J.A.M.A. **148**:833-838, 1952.
45. Rosemond, F. P.: Newer concepts in the management of patients with breast cancer, Cancer **28**:1372-1375, 1971.
46. *Rothenberg, R. E.: The complete book of breast care, New York, 1975, Crown Publishers, Inc.
47. Sabiston, D. C., editor: Christopher's textbook of surgery, ed. 11, Philadelphia, 1977, W. B. Saunders Co.
48. Sayler, C., Egan, J. F., Raines, J. R., et al.: Mammographic screening: value in diagnosis of early breast cancer, J.A.M.A. **238**:872-873, 1977.
49. *Schmid, W. L., Kiss, M., and Hibert, L.: The team approach to rehabilitation after mastectomy, A.O.R.N. J. **19**:821-836, 1974.
50. Schurman, D. J., and Amstutz, H. C.: Orthopedic management of patients with carcinoma of the breast, Surg. Gynecol. Obstet. **137**:831-836, 1973.
51. Schwartz, G. F.: Evaluation of the patient with a breast tumor, Surg. Clin. North Am. **53**:717-734, 1973.
52. Schwartz, M. K.: Hormone receptor assay, Am. J. Nurs. **77**:1445-1446, 1977.

*References preceded by an asterisk are particularly well suited for student reading.

53. Segaloff, A.: Hormonal therapy of breast cancer, Cancer **30:**1541-1542, 1972.
54. *Simon, N., and Silverstone, S.: Radiation as a cause of breast cancer, Bull. N.Y. Acad. Med. **52:**741-751, 1976.
55. Snyderman, R. K., editor: Symposium on problems of the female breast as related to neoplasm and reconstruction, St. Louis, 1973, The C. V. Mosby Co.
56. Southwick, H. W., Slaughter, D. P., and Humphrey, L. J.: Surgery of the breast, Chicago, 1968, Year Book Medical Publishers, Inc.
57. *Stillman, M. J.: Women's health beliefs about breast cancer and breast self-examination, Nurs. Res. **26:**121-127, 1977.
58. Strax, P.: New techniques in mass screening for breast cancer, Cancer **28:**1563-1568, 1971.
59. Swartz, H. M., and Reichling, B. A.: Risks of mammoplasty, J.A.M.A. **237:**965-966, 1977.
60. *Thomas, S. G., and Yates, M. M.: Breast reconstruction after mastectomy, Am. J. Nurs. **77:**1438-1442, 1977.
61. Todd, A.: Prophylactic mastectomy, Am. J. Nurs. **77:**1447-1449, 1977.
62. *Winkler, W. A.: Choosing the prosthesis and clothing, Am. J. Nurs. **77:**1433-1436, 1977.
63. *Winkler, W. A.: Post-mastectomy: a personal guide to physical and emotional recovery, New York, 1976, Hawthorn Books, Inc.
64. Women's attitudes regarding breast cancer, Occup. Health Nurs. **22:**20-23, 1974.
65. *Woods, N. F.: Psychologic aspects of breast cancer: review of literature, J. Gynecol. Nurs. **4:**15-22, 1975.
66. *Woods, N. F.: Influences on sexual adaptation to mastectomy, J. Obstet. Gynecol. Neonatal Nurs. **4:**33-37, 1975.
67. *Woods, N. F., and Earpe, J. A.: Women with cured breast cancer: a description of women's experiences four years after mastectomy (unpublished manuscript).
68. Zeisller, R. H., Rose, G. B., and Nelson, P. A.: Postmastectomy lymphedema: late results of treatment in 385 patients, Arch. Phys. Med. Rehab. **53:**159-166, 1972.

64

Problems of sexuality

NANCY FUGATE WOODS

This chapter will examine the common etiologies of sexual problems, present a nursing practice framework for identifying clients likely to experience concerns or problems related to their sexuality, and describe the most common sexual concerns or problems encountered in medical-surgical nursing practice. It will also present a brief overview of sexual problems requiring intensive therapy and statement of outcome criteria for intervention with clients experiencing sexual problems.

■ ETIOLOGIES OF SEXUAL PROBLEMS

Just as most diseases, which were once viewed from a monoetiologic framework, are now recognized to be determined by a multiplicity of factors, so it is also recognized that sexual problems have multiple etiologies. Three classes of etiologic variables to be explored here are the biologic, behavioral, and socioenvironmental.

□ Biologic determinants

Biologic determinants of sexual problems may relate to illness, use of pharmacologic agents, and the aging process. Although these variables may negatively influence an individual's sexual function, it should be kept in mind that even given optimum health, sexual response remains vulnerable to interference from behavioral and socioenvironmental factors. Kaplan[5] estimates that the number of sexually dysfunctional patients whose dysfunction is purely organic ranges from 3% to 20%.

Interferences with the processes of vasocongestion and myotonia may be a direct result of diseases affecting the nervous system or circulatory system, as well as of pharmacologic agents that act in a similar fashion. Additionally, pathologic or pharmacologically induced processes that reduce the individual's androgen level interfere with libido in both sexes and impair male erection. Next, any entity that causes painful sensations with either stimulation or intercourse can interfere with sexual function. Although aging often leads to concerns about sexual response, experts agree that there need not be a decrease in interest in sex or in sexual activity.

□ Behavioral determinants

There are a number of theories to explain the psychologic origins of sexual dysfunction. While there is no agreement regarding the nature of the behavioral factors involved, there is general agreement that the majority of sexual difficulties are attributable to experiential factors. Psychoanalysts believe that unconscious conflicts resulting from childhood experiences are the roots of sexual problems, whereas systems theorists attribute sexual dysfunction to unhealthy transactions between sexual partners. The learning theorists and behavioral school accord the blame for such problems to conditioning.[5] Thus guilt, anxiety, and other emotions can interfere with sexual response.

□ Socioenvironmental determinants

Several schools of sex therapy focus primarily on interpersonal components of sexual problems, treating both partners or the relationship as the client. Their approach is based on the assumption that neither partner is uninvolved in the etiology and treatment of the dysfunction. This dyadic approach to therapy recognizes the power of social stimuli to create and maintain a sexually dysfunctional relationship.[7]

Environmental stimuli may lead to sexual problems or inability to express oneself sexually; these may include the presence of stimuli that compete with sexual sensation, the absence of a partner, or obstacles to interacting sexually with a partner. An example of the former is competing environmental noises, the latter, institutionalization.[16]

Thus while sexual concerns and problems may result from any one of these variables, it is likely that a combination of these contribute to the problems of an individual.

■ NURSING PRACTICE FRAMEWORK FOR IDENTIFYING PERSONS AT RISK OF SEXUAL CONCERNS OR PROBLEMS

Although many persons themselves will identify their sexual concerns and problems, in many instances nurses need to initiate discussion of issues of potential concern to the individual. In the context of clinical nursing practice, many persons are "at risk" of experiencing sexual concerns or problems. A framework for identifying these persons will be described briefly, and illustrative examples given. It should be pointed out that while some will be affected by several of these entities, others may have only one.

Potential threats to sexual health include anatomic disruptions, physiologic interferences, body image distortion, environmentally induced problems, and behavioral problems.[16] Superimposed on these may be variations in life events and changes throughout the life cycle.

Anatomic disruptions are probably best exemplified by the spinal cord–injured person who has sustained irreversible damage to neural pathways and consequently has interference with usual methods of sexual function. *Physiologic derangements,* such as those assoicated with diabetes and circulatory insufficiency, probably alter the individual's ability to respond to sexual stimuli by interfering with the processes of vasocongestion and sensorimotor conduction essential to sexual response. *Pharmacologic* agents are capable of inducing sexual problems by interfering with hormonal, neurologic, and circulatory mechanisms. *Body image distortion* may accompany surgery or traumatic injury. Having an altered image of oneself may interfere with sexual expression and alter the person's current sexual relationship. *Environmental restrictions* may minimize sexual opportunity or accessibility of a partner. *Life events,* such as pregnancy, although not pathologic entities in themselves, require adaptation to changes in biology as well as emotional response. Certain parts of the *life cycle* bring sexual issues to the forefront, for example, adolescence and middlescence. Finally, *behavioral problems* such as inability to form a relationship with another person may result in inappropriate sexual expression or thwart the client's attempts at sexual expression. Those problems most likely to be encountered in medical-surgical nursing practice will be explored in more detail.

■ COMMON SEXUAL PROBLEMS AND CONCERNS

□ Anatomic disruption

The person with a spinal cord injury best exemplifies the sexual consequences of anatomic disruption. Other conditions resulting in sexual problems or concerns as a result of anatomic disruption are listed in Table 64-1.

Table 64-1. Anatomic disruptions and their hypothesized interferences with sexual health*

System	Hypothesized mechanism of interference
Central and peripheral nervous systems	
Spinal cord injury	Disrupts integrity of peripheral nerves and spinal cord reflexes involved in sexual response (e.g., erection)
Spinal cord tumors	
Herniated disc	
Multiple sclerosis	
Spina bifida	
Amyotrophic lateral sclerosis	
Tumors of frontal or temporal lobes	May interfere with function of centers controlling sexual drive
Cerebrovascular accident	
Trauma to frontal or temporal lobes	
Cardiovascular system	
Thrombus formation in vessels of penis	May interfere with blood supply to penis, thus interfering with erection
Leriche syndrome	
Sickle cell disorders	
Leukemia	
Trauma to vasculature supplying sexual organs	
Genital system	
Prostatectomy, radical perineal	May destroy nerve supply, interfering with sensory and motor aspects of sexual response
Abdominal perineal resection	
Lumbar sympathectomy	May result in disturbed ejaculation
Rhizotomy	May result in impotence as well as disturbed ejaculation
Absence of penis or penile injury	Precludes or discourages intromission
Imperforate hymen	
Congenital absence of vagina	
Obstetrical trauma or poor episiotomy	Leaves gaping vaginal opening or painful scarring, thus discouraging intercourse
Damage to pubococcygeus muscle	

*Adapted from Kaplan, H. S.: The new sex therapy, New York, 1974, Quadrangle Press.

The literature on sexual function following cord injury confirms that men and women alike are anxious to know about the future of their sexuality. Shortly after cord injury, it may be difficult to determine the extent to which sexual activity will return. However, after spinal shock subsides, many men regain their ability to have an erection.

One major difference between sexual response in spinal cord–injured persons and those who are not disabled in this manner is that genital sexual functioning and cerebral or cognitional eroticism become separated. In those persons who have complete transections of the cord, an erection may not be perceived unless the person can visualize it or feel it with a nonaffected appendage.

Often questions are raised about the likelihood of any form of sexual function among cord-injured persons. In general, the higher the lesion, the more likely the person is to be able to experience an erection. Men with cervical lesions are able to achieve erections in a greater percentage of cases than those with lumbar or sacral lesions. In fact, if there is injury to the sacral cord, the nerves supplying the pelvis and involved in the reflex arc permitting erection are likely to be damaged, and thus reflexogenic erections often are not possible. When the lower motor neuron is damaged, there is sometimes the potential for psychogenically induced erections. In this case, thoughts or feelings perceived at higher levels of the cortex may trigger erections.

The major complication of cord injury is the decreased likelihood of experiencing ejaculation. Generally, ejaculation is infrequent, and is much less frequent in men with complete transections than those with partial lesions.

Thus a person's sexual function after cord injury is dependent on two biologic variables: the number of fibers that were severed (complete versus incomplete lesions) and the level of the injury (cervical, thoracic, lumbar, or sacral). Erection can occur in response to local stimulation, which produces it reflexly, or in response to psychogenic stimuli. In the latter case, impulses from the brain can sometimes bypass the injured portion of the cord via the autonomic nervous system. Indeed, some men with complete denervation of the genitals report experiencing erection and orgasm. Usually psychogenic erections are much less common than reflexogenic erections. Ejaculation usually cannot occur.[1]

Because of the sensory losses associated with cord injury, the experience of orgasm as it occurred prior to injury is usually impossible. However, there are many cord-injured persons who report what is an orgasm-like experience in other parts of their bodies. This sensation is commonly referred to the breasts in women. Additionally, recent work with imagery or fantasy seems promising. In this technique the person's thoughts and feelings are channeled to produce a psychic experience similar to orgasm.[2]

Sexual options available to the cord-injured person depend on numerous factors, including their sexual value systems, muscle strength in the upper extremities, presence of hip flexors and extensors, the presence of appliances, and access to a partner. The first of these, the individual's sexual value system, in conjunction with a partner's, determines what range of behaviors is acceptable. For example, oral genital stimulation is a viable means for a cord-injured man to stimulate his partner, but this may be prohibited within the couple's sexual value system. The muscle strength of the arms will determine to what extent the person can support the body weight, thus determining the variety of positions that can be used. The ability to flex and extend the hips may enable the man or woman to take a more active role in intercourse by thrusting the pelvis. Weakness in these muscles can be compensated by use of a water bed, which amplifies movement (and also decreases skin problems). The presence of a urinary appliance may not be a problem. Condom catheters and leg bags can be removed prior to intercourse, Foley catheters can be taped in place and left in the bladder, or the urinary collection system can be positioned in such a way that it is not likely to become clamped off or ruptured by the partner's weight. If the patient has an indwelling catheter, the woman with adequate vaginal lubrication usually does not have trouble accommodating the catheter in her vagina.[10]

With orgasmic release, some cord-injured persons experience violent muscle spasms. These can sometimes be managed with medication, but there is a trade-off involved—some antispasmodics precipitate sexual dysfunction.

For those cord-injured men who cannot obtain a full erection, the "stuffing" technique may be a useful approach. The penis is literally stuffed in the partner's vagina. By then contracting her pubococcygeus muscle, the woman can experience sexual sensations similar to those previously associated with penile thrusting.[10]

Though not much has been written about adaptation of homosexuals to cord injury, probably similar concerns and options are appropriate. For those not currently involved in a relationship, opportunity is likely to be a problem just as it is for heterosexuals.

Perhaps one of the greatest assets the cord-injured persons can have is the presence of a caring partner. Those partners who are not involved in a caring relationship at the time of their injuries are faced with the problems of developing new relationships as well as experimenting with "what works" sexually.

Fertility is usually unimpaired in cord-injured wom-

Table 64-2. Physiologic interferences with sexual health*

Physiologic interferences	Hypothesized mechanism of action
Systemic diseases	
Pulmonary disease Renal disease Malignancies Infections Degenerative diseases Some cardiovascular diseases	Debility, pain, and depression probably interfere with sexual libido as well as expression.
Metabolic disruptions	
Cirrhosis Mononucleosis Hepatitis	Hepatic problems in the man result in estrogen buildup due to inability of the liver to conjugate estrogens; similar processes occur in the woman along with general debility.
Hypothyroidism Addison's disease Hypogonadism Hypopituitarism Acromegaly Feminizing tumors Cushing's disease Diabetes mellitus	By depression of CNS function, general debilitation, and depression, libido may be decreased, and impaired arousal in the woman and impaired erectile abilities in the man may result.
Diseases of the genitalia	
Priapism Peyronie's disease Balanitis Phimosis Genital herpes Trauma to penis Vaginal infections Senile vaginitis Vulvitis Leukoplakia Bartholin's cyst Allergic response to vaginal sprays and deodorants Vaginitis following radiation therapy Pelvic inflammatory disease Fibroadenomas Endometriosis Uterine prolapse Anal fissures, hemorrhoids Pelvis masses Ovarian cysts	Each of these problems involves damage to genital organs, which may result in painful intercourse.
Prostatitis Urethritis	Local irritability, damage to genitals, and consequent interference with reflex mechanisms involved in erection and ejaculation.
Medical or surgical castration	
Orchiectomy Radiation therapy Oophorectomy, adrenalectomy	Lowered androgen levels depress libido and lead to impotence, retarded ejaculation, or impaired sexual responsiveness.

*Adapted from Kaplan, H. S.: The new sex therapy, New York, 1974, Quadrangle Press.

en, but because of a number of factors, sperm may not be viable in cord-injured men. Use of artificial insemination (either with the man's own or a donor's semen) is a possibility for those who want children. Normal pregnancy is possible for women with cord injuries. Careful health monitoring is essential as the incidence of urinary tract infections may be greater in cord-injured women during pregnancy, they may fail to perceive the beginnings of labor because of loss of sensation, and in a few instances cesarean section may be necessitated.

Although in the past much emphasis has been placed on the cord-injured person's ability to help the partner achieve sexual gratification, new techniques, such as imagery, actively seek to help the disabled person adapt to the sexual changes experienced. Nurses as health professionals may be involved in long-term relationships with these persons and have an excellent opportunity to assess their sexual concerns and intervene by teaching or counseling.

Hearing nothing about sexuality constitutes a rather potent message. Sex is often absent from conversations with staff, although activities such as dressing, bathing, grooming, bowel and bladder control, and mobility are constantly stressed. In the past, many individuals—patients and health professionals alike—assumed that sexual function was no longer an issue.

□ Physiologic interference with sexual health

Many illnesses alter physiologic processes essential to the sexual response, including nervous transmission, vasocongestion, hormonal metabolism, myotonia, and perception of pleasurable sensation. Pharmacologic agents that interfere with these basic physiologic activities have the potential to affect sexual drive as well as performance. Table 64-2 illustrates some illnesses and Table 64-3 some drugs that have the potential to interfere with sexual response and the hypothesized mechanism by which they limit sexual response.

In general, it appears that the extent of a physiologic disorder and its chronicity determine relative frequency of sexual problems. For example, frequency of sexual dysfunction among women with diabetes increases with the duration of the disease, although no correlation exists between sexual dysfunction and actual complications of the disease.[6] This relationship between chronicity and dysfunction is also observed in men with diabetes.[14] A high incidence of impotence is found among diabetic men during the first year after diagnosis. It is believed that in this instance the lack of diabetic control (physiologic derangement) is responsible for the sexual dysfunction.[13]

For chronic illnesses as a group, it is easy to hypothesize a relationship between perception of health status, degree of fatigue, metabolic derangements, altered roles, fear of dying, and the demands of a chronic illness on the partner and changes in the sexual relationship.

The relationship between extent of physiologic derangement and degree of sexual dysfunction is also demonstrated by pharmacologically induced changes. For example, alcohol induces transiently positive changes; in small doses it initially promotes relaxation and release of inhibitions as do other psychoactive drugs. However, in larger doses alcohol has negative effects on sexual function, leading to central nervous system depression and interference with motor activity.[14]

Several categories of drugs have demonstrable negative effects on sexual function. These include antihypertensives, antidepressants, antihistamines, antispasmodics, sedatives and tranquilizers, ethyl alcohol, some sex hormone preparations, and some narcotics and psychoactive drugs. Examples of these drugs are listed in Table 64-3.

Although some medical-surgical conditions do not interfere directly with sexual function, their perceived seriousness or the presence of symptoms discourages persons from engaging in their usual sexual practices. One very common example is associated with cardiac disease, more specifically myocardial infarction. Although marital coitus probably does not demand a great energy expenditure, many persons are fearful of attempting intercourse after having a heart attack. One study of married men who had had myocardial infarctions demonstrated that heart rates with orgasm were much lower in this group (about 117 beats per minute on the average) than among the younger group studied by Masters and Johnson.[4] An active physical conditioning program did produce significant improvements in the frequency and quality of sexual activity for men who had had a myocardial infarction. The energy expenditure associated with sex seemed to be better tolerated by those who exercised regularly.

In general, the literature indicates that the post-myocardial infarction patient may return to regular sexual activity provided there are no symptoms of congestive heart failure. However, certain conditions that increase energy expenditure during coitus are to be avoided. These include having intercourse shortly after a meal or soon after alcohol consumption, as both increase the heart rate and metabolic demands, and avoiding extremes in temperatures and anxiety-provoking or secretive situations. Positions that require the person who has had a myocardial infarction to support the entire body weight of the partner or self are to be avoided if possible.[4] (Sample instructions for cardiac patients appear in the boxed material on p. 1407.)

Table 64-3. Pharmacologic interferences by drug or drug category*

Drug	Mechanism of action
Antihypertensives	
Guanethidine (Ismelin)	Peripheral blockade of nervous innervation of sex glands
Reserpine (Serpasil)	
Mecamylamine (Inversine)	
Trimethaphan (Arfonad)	
Spironolactone (Aldactone)	
Antidepressants	
Imipramine (Tofranil)	Central depression; peripheral blockade of nervous innervation of sex glands
Desipramine (Norpramin, Pertofrane)	
Amitriptyline (Elavil)	
Nortriptyline (Aventyl)	
Protriptyline (Vivactil)	
Phenelzine sulfate (Nardil)	
Tranylcypromine sulfate (Parnate)	
Pargyline (Eutonyl)	
Antihistamines	
Diphenhydramine (Benadryl)	Blockade of parasympathetic nervous innervation of sex glands
Promethazine (Phenergan)	
Chlorpheniramine (Chlor-trimeton)	
Antispasmodics	
Methantheline (Banthine)	Ganglionic blockage of nervous innervation of sex glands
Glycopyrrolate (Robinul)	
Hexocyclium (Tral)	
Poldine (Nacton)	
Sedatives and tranquilizers	
Chlorpromazine (Thorazine, Megaphen)	Central sedation; blockade of autunomic innervation of sex glands; suppression of hypothalamic and pituitary fuction; tranquilization and relaxation
Prochlorperazine (Compazine)	
Thioridazine (Mellaril)	
Mesoridazine (Serentil)	
Chlordiazepoxide (Librium)	
Diazepam (Valium)	
Benperidol	
Phenoxybenzamine (Dibenzyline)	
Chlorprothixene (Taractan)	
Ethyl alcohol	Central depression; suppression of motor activity; diuresis; release of inhibitions; relaxation
Sex hormone preparations	
Cyproterone acetate	Antiandrogenic effects on sexual function; loss of libido; decreased potency
Methandrostenolone (Dianabol)	
Nandrolone phenpropionate (Durabolin)	
Norethandrolone (Nilevar)	
Narcotics and psychoactive drugs	
Morphine	Central depression; decreased libido and impaired potency
Heroin	
Cocaine	Release of inhibitions; increased suggestibility; relaxation; improvement of well-being
Marijuana	
LSD	
Amphetamines	
Barbiturates	
Amytal	General depressant effects on all nervous tissues
Nembutal	
Seconal	
Pentothal	
Methadone	Can impair fertility by reducing size and secretory activity of secondary sex organs, resulting in extremely low ejaculate volume and low sperm motility

*Adapted from Woods, J. S.: Drug effects on human sexual behavior. In Woods, N. F.: Human sexuality in health and illness, ed. 2, St. Louis, 1979, the C. V. Mosby Co.

Table 64-4. Some health problems resulting in body image changes that may raise sexual concerns

Surgically induced	Traumatically induced	Others
Mastectomy Ostomy Hysterectomy Amputation of limb(s)	Burns Lacerations, scarring Amputations	Dermatologic disorders Obesity Congenital anomalies of sexual organs (e.g., absence of penis, hypospadias) Unusual breast size, including immaturity or hypertrophy

□ Body image changes

The extent to which distortion of body image influences sexuality often depends on the perceptions of two persons: oneself and a significant other. Multiple variables may influence the body image of a woman who has had a mastectomy. Among these are biologic factors such as size of the incision and pain in the operative area. Psychologic factors such as the value she assigns to her breasts, her preoperative body image, and social factors such as the quality of her preoperative sexual relationship are also influential. A sexual partner's reaction may be similarly affected.[16]

The *visibility* of a defect plays an important role in sexual adaptation. Goffman refers to individuals with "spoiled identities" whose interactions with others are marked by disgrace and rejection, and who may elicit withdrawal on the part of others.[3] Visibility of a disability seems to be just as disruptive of marital and family relations as it is of other social relationships.[18]

Finally, the *meaning* and *significance* one attaches to a changed body part may interfere with sexual behavior. The amputee who views his loss as castration, the woman who sees her hysterectomy as a neutering surgery, and the person who equates an ostomy with loss of adult control are likely to experience problems with self-image and, in turn, sexual adjustment. Thus both society's perception of the person and the individual's concept of self can interfere with sexual health. Some common health problems resulting in body image change are listed in Table 64-4.

□ Environmental restrictions

Enviromental factors such as privacy, competing stimuli, and segregation interfere with sexual expression. Institionalization rarely affords sufficient privacy for sexual expression. As indicated by Masters' and Johnson's work, the presence of incongruous stimuli is capable of interfering with the progression of sexual arousal.[8] Finally, many institutions segregate persons on the basis of sex. For whatever reason this may be done, the act of segregation may elicit a range of adaptation including masturbation, homosexual activity, or withdrawal[10] from human warmth. Often these adaptive behaviors are punished, and those who resort to them are stigmatized. In some institutions staff members may assume an in loco parentis stance, treating even aging persons as if they required protection from their sexual inclinations.

□ Aging process

Changes in sexual function become accentuated during middle age, although their onset is gradual and they probably begin long before they are perceived. Men need more time to attain an erection, and once attained, it is likely to be less full than in earlier years. The testes elevate more slowly with sexual excitement, and vasocongestive changes in the scrotum and testes are less noticeable. With prolongation of the plateau phase of the sexual response cycle, the middle-aged man actually achieves much better control over ejaculation than he had as a young adult.[8]

Orgasm is perceived as happening more quickly and feelings of ejaculatory inevitability may disappear entirely. Resolution of sexual tension becomes more rapid with age, and the obligatory refractory period (a period during which the men cannot be restimulated to orgasm) becomes longer. With aging, men actually gain better control of ejaculation, and because of reduced ejaculatory demand, they may be satisfied not to ejaculate with each intercourse.[8]

Menopausal changes ensue in women: the vagina atrophies, resulting in a delay in production of vagina lubrication and diminished expansion of the vaginal barrel. Atrophic changes in external genitalia as well as the breasts are apparent. The woman's orgasmic experience becomes shorter and resolution occurs more rapidly.[8]

Studies of healthy aging individuals indicate that a decline in overall interest and activity is seen with age. However, men from each age range tend to report greater interest and activity than women in each respective age range. For men, past sexual experience, age, objective and subjective health factors, and social class influence sexual interest and activity. For women, the most important factors were marital status, age, and the enjoyment they derived from sex during younger years. Level of sexual activity in youth appears to be related to that in older years.[11]

As men age, an interest-activity gap appears. That is, they desire more sexual activity than they are able to experience. This gap grows as men age; however, it remains small for women. It is suggested that women without a socially acceptable partner adaptively inhibit their sexual interest.[12] Other social factors, such as the role loss associated with children leaving the parents' home and retirement are likely to influence the aging person's sexual interests.

□ Gender disorders

Although many gender disorders exist, they are encountered less often in medical-surgical practice than the problems discussed earlier. Recently the media have called attention to one gender identity problem, transsexualism, which may be encountered in many medical-surgical services.

Transsexualism refers to the condition of people who are convinced that they are "trapped in the body of the wrong sex." These persons believe that they belong to the opposite sex and desire the body, appearance, and social status of the opposite sex. Many actually live in the role of the opposite sex prior to treatment. Male-to-female transsexuals are usually treated initially with hormonal therapy, and later surgical revision of their genitals is performed. The surgery involves removal of the male genitalia and revision of the scrotal and neighboring tissue to resemble the female genitals. Usually the surgery is cosmetically successful, and an artificial but functional vagina can be created. These women are, of course, sterile, since they have neither ovaries nor uteri.

The female-to-male transsexual has a less cosmetically effective and functional surgical transformation. In a series of procedures, the breasts and the vulva are revised and a phallus is created. Hormonal therapy is also used to effect the transformation. Often the creation of the penis requires extensive grafting and surgical revision, and the female-to-male transformation is consequently more difficult and usually less satisfactory. After the transformation these men are also sterile.

Both men and women electing transsexual surgery require considerable emotional support. Usually they have careful psychologic assessments prior to and following the surgery. Because of their cultural conditioning, nurses sometimes find it difficult to relate appropriately to the transsexual. Often it is necessary to analyze one's attitudes and values carefully in order to be accepting of these patients.

Transsexualism should not be confused with transvestism, the act of dressing in the clothing of the opposite sex. Additionally, transsexuals are not to be assumed to be homosexuals.

Hermaphroditism is a congenital condition in which the reproductive structures appear ambiguous. Early life experiences seem to have profound impact on our gender identities. Therefore it is important that sexual assignment be correctly established very early in life to prevent gender confusion later on.

■ SEXUAL PROBLEMS REQUIRING INTENSIVE THERAPY

Although nurses educate and counsel persons with a variety of sexual concerns and problems, some individuals experience complex dysfunctions that may require referral to a sex therapist or psychotherapist. (These therapists may well be nurses who have advanced preparation in sex therapy or psychotherapy skills.) Some of the sexual dysfunctions that require intensive therapy will be described here, since nurses in medical-surgical practice may diagnose them from the sexual history and wish to make appropriate referrals.

□ Female sexual dysfunctions

Five types of sexual dysfunction have been identified in females: general sexual dysfunction, orgasmic dysfunction, vaginismus, sexual anesthesia, and dyspareunia.

General sexual dysfunction refers to a condition in which inhibition of sexual arousal occurs. There may be a lack of erotic feeling, lack of vaginal lubrication or expansion, or no formation of the orgasmic platform. *Primary orgasmic dysfunction* occurs in the woman who has not experienced orgasm with sexual activity, including intercourse or masturbation. *Secondary orgasmic dysfunction* is characterized by inability to experience orgasm under certain conditions. The woman with secondary orgasmic dysfunction has experienced orgasmic sensations with one form of stimulation at some point in her life. This problem does not preclude the woman from experiencing sexual arousal and its physiologic accompaniments. Rather, only the orgasmic portion of the sexual response cycle seems impaired. *Vaginismus* is a relatively rare sexual problem characterized by an involuntary, conditioned spasm of the vaginal outlet, thus causing it to shut tightly. This problem precludes sexual intercourse, but vaginismic women may be orgasmic with alternative methods of sexual stimulation. *Sexual anesthesia* is characterized by feeling nothing in response to sexual stimulation. This absence of sensation is thought to be a neurotic manifestation.[7] *Dyspareunia*, painful intercourse, may be attributable to a number of factors, ranging from a full lower bowel to feelings of aversion toward sexual intercourse. It is sometimes experienced by women with steroid starvation, for example, the postpartum mother and the postmenopausal woman.

□ Male sexual dysfunctions

Three types of sexual dysfunction can be experienced by men. These include erectile dysfunction, premature ejaculation, and retarded ejaculation. *Erectile dysfunction*, impotence, probably affects most men at least once

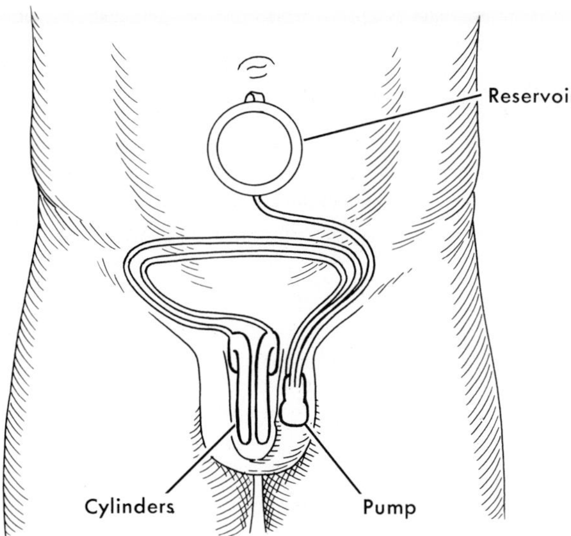

Fig. 64-1. Inflatable penile prosthetic implant. Reservoir is implanted under abdominal muscles, inflatable cylinders in each corpus cavernosum, and pump inside scrotum. Man can compress pump to fill cylinders from reservoir, producing penile erection. Small release valve in lower portion of pump bulb releases fluid to return the penis to flaccid state.

in their lifetimes, and transient episodes of impotence are estimated to occur in half of all men. Thus these fleeting episodes are considered within the range of normal. Impotence occurs in varying degrees: some men experience total inability to attain erection, others are merely bothered by an inability to attain an erection of sufficient hardness. This frustrating, humiliating condition may lead to decreased self-esteem and consequent depression. Impotence is described as primary if the man has never been able to achieve or maintain an erection that would permit intercourse. Secondary impotence, a more common phenomenon, occurs situationally and is likely to be the variety seen in conjunction with pathophysiologically and pharmacologically induced states. The penile prosthetic implant has recently been devised as a method of treatment for organic impotence in men. There are two types of penile prostheses. The older type consists of the implantation of two sponge-filled silicone rods in the corpora cavernosa. This maintains the penis in a constant semierect position. The newer and more acceptable method for many men is the inflatable penile prosthesis (Fig. 64-1). Both types of prostheses are implanted surgically and do not interfere with normal urinary elimination. The silicone implants are inserted through perineal or penile incisions and the inflatable prostheses through perineal and abdominal incisions. Penile edema is minimal, but scrotal edema may occur with the inflatable type. Pain may be severe during the first week, and mild pain may continue for several weeks after surgery. *Premature ejaculation* occurs when the man cannot inhibit his ejaculation for a long enough period of time to permit his partner to experience orgasm in at least half of their attempts at intercourse. This is thought likely to be a conditioned response to hurried circumstances and is treated quite successfully by means of the "squeeze technique." This technique requires the man or his partner to place the thumb and second and third fingers at the coronal ridge of the glans, exerting enough pressure over this area for 3 or 4 seconds to relieve the feeling of ejaculatory inevitability. *Retarded ejaculation*, also known as ejaculatory incompetence, implies that despite the amount and quality of stimulation of the penis, intravaginal ejaculation either does not occur or is so delayed that the couple experiences pelvic irritation and fatigue as a result.

■ OUTCOME CRITERIA FOR PERSONS EXPERIENCING SEXUAL CONCERNS OR PROBLEMS

The persons can:

1. Express sexuality in a manner comfortable and rewarding to both partners.
2. Identify erotically pleasing stimuli that facilitate sexual arousal.
3. Maintain, with cooperation of the partner, a relationship conducive to sexual functioning.
4. Express sexual feelings in a manner consistent with personal values and beliefs.
5. Relate knowledge of venereal disease prevention and family planning to personal sexual relationships.
6. Accurately describe how medical or surgical problems or treatment are likely or not likely to interfere with sexual functioning.
7. Explore with the partner any adaptations in sexual behavior necessitated by illness, hospitalization, or medication.

The first four criteria are applicable to persons of all ages and health statuses. The last three are particularly relevant to those persons hospitalized for medical-surgical problems.

REFERENCES AND SELECTED READINGS

1. Bors, E., and Comarr, A. E.: Neurological disturbances of sexual function, with special reference to 529 patients with spinal cord injury, Urol. Surv. **10**:191-222, 1960.
2. Cole, T.: Sexuality and the spinal cord injury. In Green, M.: Human sexuality: a health practitioner's text, Baltimore, 1975, The Williams & Wilkins Co.
3. *Goffman, E.: Stigma: notes on the management of a spoiled identity, Englewood Cliffs, N.J., 1963, Prentice-Hall, Inc.

*References preceded by an asterisk are particularly well suited for student reading.

4. *Hellerstein, H., and Friedman, E. H.: Sexual activity and the post-coronary patient, Arch. Intern. Med. **125**:987-999, 1970.
5. Kaplan, H. S.: The new sex therapy, New York, 1974, Brunner/Mazel, Inc.
6. Kolodny, R. C.: Sexual dysfunction in diabetic females, Diabetes **20**:557-559, 1971.
7. Masters, W., and Johnson, V.: Human sexual inadequacy, Boston, 1970, Little, Brown & Co.
8. Masters, W., and Johnson, V.: Human sexual response, Boston, 1966, Little, Brown & Co.
9. Money, J., and Ehrhardt, A.: Man and woman, boy and girl, Baltimore, 1972, The Johns Hopkins University Press.
10. *Mooney, T., Cole, T., and Chilgren, R.: Sexual options for paraplegics and quadriplegics, Boston, 1975, Little, Brown & Co.
11. Pfeiffer, E., and Davis, G. C.: Determinants of sexual behavior in middle and old age, J. Am. Geriatr. Soc. **20**:151-158, 1972.
12. Pfeiffer, E., Verwoerdt, A., and Wang, H. S.: The natural history of sexual behavior in a biologically advantaged group of aged individuals, J. Gerontol. **24**:193-198, 1969.
13. *Rubin, A., and Babbott, D.: Impotence and diabetes mellitus, J.A.M.A. **168**:498-500, 1958.
14. Schoffling, K., Federlin, K., Ditschueit, H., and Pfeiffer, E. F.: Disorders of sexual function in the male diabetes, Diabetes **12**:519-527, 1963.
14a. Wood, R. Y., and Rose, K.: Penile implants for impotence, Am. J. Nurs. **78**:234-238, 1978.
15. *Woods, J. S.: Drug effects on human sexual behavior. In Woods, N. F.: Human sexuality in health and illness, ed. 2, St. Louis, 1979, The C. V. Mosby Co.
16. *Woods, N. F.: Human sexuality in health and illness, ed. 2, St. Louis, 1979, The C. V. Mosby Co.
17. *Woods, N. F.: Influences on sexual adaptation to mastectomy, J. Obstet. Gynecol. Neonatal Nurs. **4**:33-37, 1975.
18. Zahn, M. A.: Incapacity, impotence, and invisible impairment: their effects upon interpersonal relations, J. Health Soc. Behav. **14**:115-123, 1973.

UNIT XI

Problems related to impaired protective mechanisms

Protection from the environment involves an intact integument and an ability to defend oneself from foreign matter that has the potential to harm the outer skin barrier. The skin is a visible organ and can be assessed without the use of involved or invasive equipment. Assessment of the skin provides the nurse and other health personnel with additional data concerning other functions of the body such as nutrition (including fluid hydration) and elimination.

Persons with problems of the integument or immune system are at risk with the environment. Many of the skin conditions have been known for many years because of the obvious evidence presented to the naked eye. Because of the overtness of skin lesions, including burns, persons afflicted with these problems may experience psychologic problems. Nurses need to be cognizant of the problems to assist the person with coping and adaptation. The underlying bases of problems of the immune system is relatively new and more complex, although the symptoms of conditions such as allergies have been known for many years. Lives are now being saved through a better understanding of the bases of immunodeficiency diseases.

This unit begins with *assessment* of the integument and immune status. The next two chapters discuss the *general nursing care* requirements of the person with a *dermatologic* problem or with *burns*. The last two chapters deal with specific *problems of the integument and immune response*.

65

Assessment of the integument and immune status

BARBARA C. LONG

The integument, or skin, is the largest organ of the body. It is exposed to the external environment and provides the first line of defense of the body; yet at the same time it is affected by changes in the internal environment. Assessment of the integument and immune response provides data about how the person is affected by and is coping with both external and internal environments. Data obtained in the assessment provide the bases for identification of nursing problems related to the skin, potential for infection, fluid and electrolyte imbalances, nutritional imbalances, or inadequate oxygenation of tissues. Baseline observations are useful for identifying changes that may occur.

■ ANATOMY AND PHYSIOLOGY OF THE SKIN

□ Structure of the skin

The skin is composed of two main layers, the epidermis and the dermis (Fig. 65-1). The *epidermis* is composed of two parts, a thin layer of closely packed dead squamous cells covering a second layer of cells containing melanin, which gives skin its color. The dead cells are constantly being shed and replaced by deeper cells. Blood vessels do not reach into the epidermis.

The second main layer, the *dermis* or corium, is connected to the epidermis by a convoluted layer of cells that produce new cells for the epidermis. The dermis is composed of bundles of collagen fibers that act to support the epidermis. It is well supplied with nerves and blood vessels and contains the sweat glands, sebaceous glands, and hair follicles.

Thickness of the skin varies over different areas of the body. Exposed areas such as the hands and face are usually thicker. The skin on the inner aspect of the arms is thinner and therefore more sensitive to heat.

Sweat glands excrete directly to the surface of the skin and are under control of the sympathetic nervous system. There are two types of sweat glands, *eccrine* and *apocrine*. The eccrine glands are distributed throughout the body and are more abundant in the forehead, palms, and soles of the feet. Eccrine glands assist in the heat-regulating mechanisms of the body. The aprocrine glands are found mainly in the axillary and genital regions. Some of the protoplasm of these secretory cells is secreted with the fluid, and it is bacterial decomposition of the sweat from these glands that is responsible for body odor.[2] Sweat glands of the axilla, palms, and soles are mostly under psychic control.

Sebaceous glands secrete an oily, odorless fluid *(sebum)* into the hair follicles. Ear wax is sebum from glands in the external ear canal. Sebum protects the hair follicle from infection and lubricates the skin.

Beneath the skin is the subcutaneous tissue composed of loose connective tissue filled with fat cells. Fat conducts heat only one-fourth as rapidly as do other tissues and thus serves as the heat insulator of the body.[5]

□ Functions of the skin

Protection. An intact skin is the first line of defense against bacterial and foreign substance invasion, slight physical trauma, heat, or rays. Bacteria present on the skin are usually nonpathogenic. Bacteria that penetrate hair follicles are usually removed by the sebum.

Heat regulation. Body temperature is controlled by *radiation* of heat from the surface of the skin, *conduction* of heat from skin to other objects or air, removal of heat by air currents on the skin *(convection)*, or *evaporation* of water from skin surfaces. Insensible water evaporation from the skin and lungs occurs at a rate of 600 to 1,000 ml per day. On a hot day the only way the body can lose heat is by evaporation, and anything that restricts evaporation under these conditons will increase body temperature. Blood vessels of the skin assist in control of body temperature by constriction in cold environments to promote conservation of heat, and dilation in warm environments to promote loss of heat by radiation. These mechanisms help maintain a constant internal body temperature.

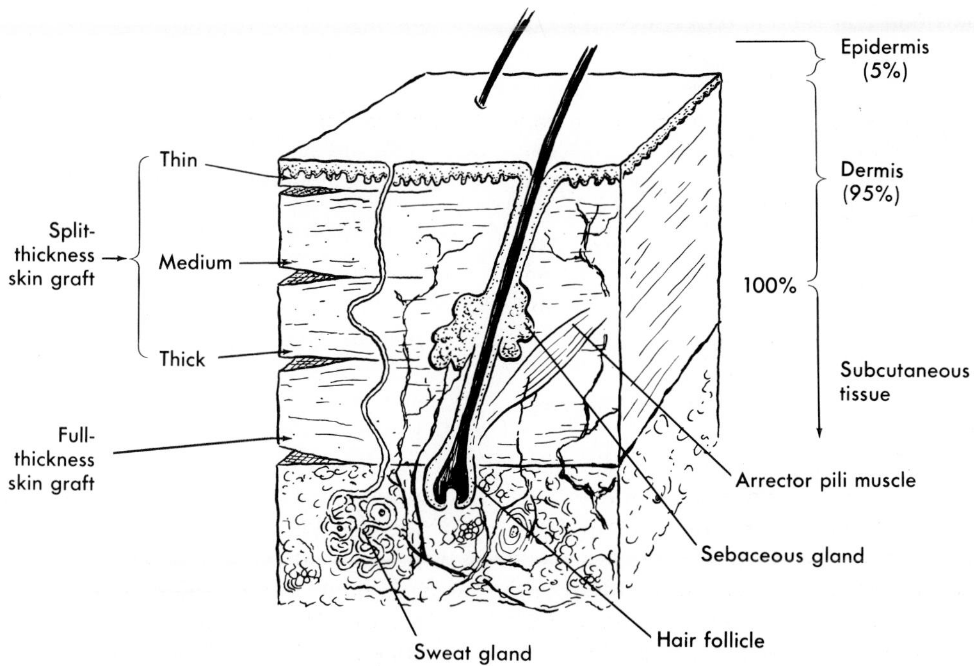

Fig. 65-1. Layers of skin involved in various types of skin grafts. Thickness of epidermis and dermis pictured here is typical of that found on lateral thigh of adult. (Redrawn from Graab, W. S., and Smith, J. W.: Plastic surgery, Boston, 1968, Little, Brown & Co.)

Sensory perception. Receptors for pain, touch, heat, and cold are present in the skin.

Excretion. Water lost through the skin is a factor in maintaining water balance in the body. Salt is lost through excessive sweating in addition to water. A person can become acclimatized to a continuous hot environment, however, and the amount of salt lost decreases over time.

Vitamin D production. Synthesis of vitamin D takes place in the skin by the effect of sunlight (ultraviolet rays). Vitamin D is necessary in the metabolism of calcium and phosphorus (p. 211).

Expression. Since the skin is the part of the body that is visible to others, it serves as a means of communicating feelings. Also because of its visibility, skin is largely involved in a person's feelings of *body image*. Individuals become concerned when there is fear of or presence of disfigurement. (The reader is referred to Chapter 28 for a discussion of body image.)

■ SUBJECTIVE DATA

Data to be obtained from a person on an initial health history are of two types: (1) information to identify a potential dermatologic or allergic problem and (2) information specific to a skin condition or allergy that is already present.

□ General information

1. History of dermatologic disease: identification of any skin conditions that may be familial or that may recur (allergy).
2. Occupation: contact with potential skin irritants such as arsenic, lead, chromium, strong acids or bases (contact dermatitis); abnormal heat or unhygienic environment (infections, insect infestations); hands constantly in water (dermatitis).
3. Seasonal factors: exposure to excessive sun (burn, skin cancer) or cold (frostbite); pollens (allergies, hay fever).
4. Recreational activities such as painting, camping, yard work: exposure to paint compounds, poison ivy, poison oak, or sumac (dermatitis venenata).
5. Travel to foreign countries: exposure to contagious disease.
6. Drugs: steroids (glucocorticoids) are antiinflammatory and may produce false-negative response to skin testing; antimetabolites may depress bone marrow, resulting in thrombocytopenia (potential for hemmorhage) or leukopenia (potential for infection).

□ Specific information

1. Onset of the problem: initial sites; when were changes first noticed; skin appearance at onset; any

other symptoms noted at time of onset such as pain, itching, sneezing, rhinitis; any specific known cause such as contact with poison ivy, exposure to a known allergen, stress.
2. Changes since onset: changes in location of lesions; changes in appearance; new symptoms such as pain or itching.
3. If cause is unknown: recent exposure to sensitizing substances such as metals, toxic inhalants, animal dander, foods, poisonous plants, pollens (depending on symptoms), new drug prescriptions such as penicillin.
4. Alleviating factors: physician-prescribed or self-prescribed treatment.
5. If cause is an allergen: previous history including pattern and sequence of symptoms and signs, preventive or desensitization measures, medical follow-up (continual or symptomatic).
6. Psychologic reaction to problem: withdrawal from social activities, cosmetics for cover-up, feelings concerning self in view of the problem (body image).

■ OBJECTIVE DATA

□ Methods of assessment

The skin is an organ that can be examined by *direct inspection* and *observation* with no tools but a good light. *Palpation* is also used in gathering data related to certain types of lesions.

Considerable data can be obtained from physical assessment of the skin, not only concerning dermatologic problems, but also concerning the health status of the individual. A systematic head-to-toe skin assessment is usually carried out while gathering other significant data in the initial interview and physical assessment of the person. Specific areas of the skin are reassessed as potential or existing problems are identified.

□ Guidelines for skin assessment

1. Be prepared: have a good light available. If the lighting is inadequate, lesions may be missed or described inaccurately.
2. Be systematic: if only some parts of the skin are inspected, an important parameter may be omitted or a lesion missed.
3. Be thorough: look at all areas carefully. If the person is lying down, be sure to examine the back, especially the sacral area. Lift folds of tissue, such as under the breasts or gluteal folds. Embarrassment by the examiner or anticipated embarrassment of the examinee may result in inadequate data.
4. Be specific: when lesions are identified, describe the lesions using the metric system and established parameters (e.g., color, size, shape).
5. Compare right side with left side: when observing changes in skin color or tissue shape, always compare one side of the body with the other to differentiate structural from pathologic changes.
6. Record the data: unrecorded data is lost data. Baseline observations indicating normality or abnormality are needed for comparison with subsequent

Table 65-1. Skin color changes

Color	Physiology	Conditions
Redness	Vasodilatation: more rapid blood flow, more oxygenated blood giving a reddish hue (erythema)	Blushing, heat, inflammation, fever, alcohol ingestion, extreme cold (below 15 C)[5], hot flushes
Whiteness (pallor)	Vasoconstriction: slower blood flow, less blood in capillaries	Cold, fear, shock
	Partially obstructed blood flow: less blood in capillaries	Vasospasm, thrombus, narrowed vessels
	Fluid between blood vessels and skin surface	Edema
	Decreased oxygenation of blood due to decreased hemoglobin	Anemia
	Loss of melanin	Vitiligo
Bluish	Deoxygenated hemoglobin (cyanosis) seen in ear lobes, lips, mucous membranes of mouth, nail beds	Heart or lung disease, inadequate respiration, peripheral blood vessel obstruction
Yellow	Increased bile pigment in blood eventually distributed to skin and mucous membranes, and to sclera of eye	Liver disease, obstruction of bile ducts, chronic uremia, rapid hemolysis
Brown	Increased melanin deposits: normal in brown-black races	Aging, sunburn
Dullness	Vasoconstriction in dark skin	Cold, fear, shock

findings. Changes need to be recorded to determine progress toward achieving desired outcomes.

□ Parameters of general skin assessment

The objective data to be collected when examining the skin for general health status include skin color, temperature, moisture, elasticity, turgor, texture, and odor.

Color

Changes in skin color are best observed in the lips, mucous membranes of the mouth, ear lobes, finger and toe nails, and the extremities. The lips show rapid color changes.[10]

Color of the skin varies with the amount of *melanin* in the cells and with the *blood supply* (Table 65-1). Variations of general pigmentation are seen within one individual; an increase in pigmentation is usually seen on exposed surfaces and in the areola of the nipples. Albinos have a congenital inability to produce melanin. Elderly light-skinned persons may normally develop irregular brown patches (Fig. 65-2). Severe trauma can destroy cells producing melanin and result in hypopigmentation; scar tissue is hypopigmented tissue. Some healthy persons develop a condition called *vitiligo* in which there is a failure of melanin formation in certain areas, producing sharply demarcated white patches. Vitiligo can also occur with hyperthyroidism, pernicious anemia, and adrenal cortical insufficiency.[3] A normal finding in most persons is pigmented moles or *nevi.* Changes in color of moles, especially to black or greenish-black, should be reported to a physician at once for determination of possible malignancy or *melanoma* (p. 1534).

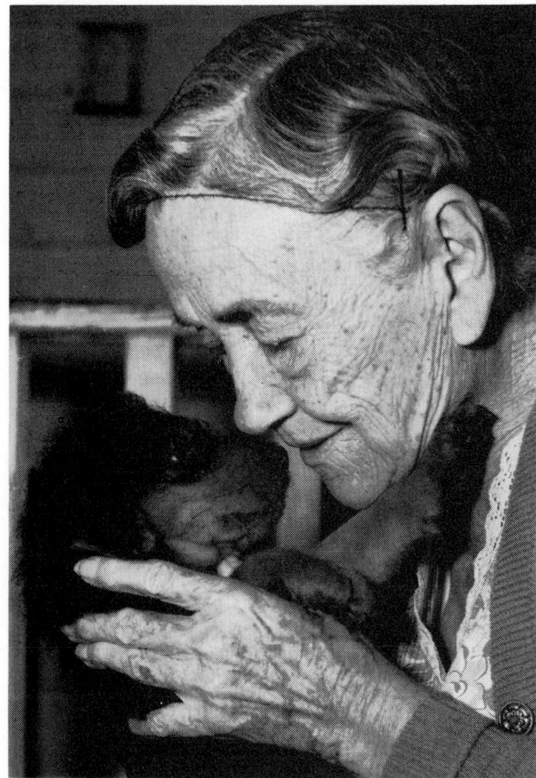

Fig. 65-2. Elderly patients have skin changes. Note discolored spots on skin and tiny raised area on this woman's eyelid. (VanDerMeid from Monkmeyer Press Photo Service.)

The degree of blood supplied to the skin produces color changes. The rate of blood flow through the skin is highly variable because of its function in heat control. The blood vessels are innervated by the sympathetic nervous system, thus vasoconstriction occurs with the stress response. With vasoconstriction, smaller amounts of blood pass through the vessels, producing decreased redness; a dark skin becomes duller and a light skin whiter (pallor). Vasodilatation increases the amount of oxygenated blood flow, and the skin acquires a reddish color (erythema). Vascular flush areas of the body are the "butterfly" band from cheek to cheek across the nose, the neck, upper chest, flexor surfaces of the extremities, and genital areas.[6]

Changes in blood composition can also alter skin color. Excess deoxygenated hemoglobin gives a bluish tint *(cyanosis)* to the skin and mucous membranes. An excess of bile pigment results in a yellowish tint to the skin and sclera of the eyes.

Temperature

The temperature of the skin is regulated by vasoconstriction or vasodilatation. If an excess amount of heat is being produced within the body such as with fever or exercise, or if the external environment increases, the sympathetic centers in the hypothalamus are inhibited and vasodilatation occurs. An increase in the amount of blood flow creates a sensation of warmth on the skin. A local inflammation of the skin or underlying tissue also produces vasodilatation; this is part of the inflammatory response (p. 178). Cold skin is caused by vasoconstriction as a result of sympathetic stimulation. To assess the temperature of the skin, the backs of the fingers, which are more sensitive than the finger tips, should be used.

Moisture

Skin is assessed as being *dry, moist,* or *oily.* Dry skin is frequently seen in the elderly person because of decreased activity of the sebaceous glands. Dry skin and mucous membranes are also seen in persons who are dehydrated as water moves from the cells into the intravascular compartments. Persons with hypothyroidism have thick, dry, leathery skin.

Moist skin is caused by the presence of water or sweat on the surface. Overheating produces sweating. Persons with hyperthyroidism have moist, smooth skin. Some persons have more effective sweat mechanisms than others. Stress, shock, or any situation that stimulates the sympathetic nervous system will cause increased fluid loss through the sweat glands. Since vasoconstriction is also occurring with stimulation of the sympathetic nervous system, the skin is cold and wet (clammy).

Oily skin is frequently seen in the adolescent. An excess amount of sebum formation by the sebaceous glands may lead to blocking of the follicular orifices, resulting in blackheads *(comedo)*, acne, or sebaceous cysts.

Elasticity, mobility, and turgor

The skin is very elastic and moves freely over most areas. It loses its mobility when it becomes stretched; this occurs with edema when the interstitial spaces become filled with fluid and swelling occurs. Skin becomes rigid in the person with scleroderma, a collagen disease, as a result of collagenous fibrosis of the tissue. *Turgor* is the speed of skin return to normal position of fullness after it has been stretched. Decreased turgor indicates dehydration of the tissue. To assess elasticity and turgor, a portion of skin over the sternum is picked up (elasticity) and the speed of return to normal is assessed (turgor). Skin that has decreased turgor will remain for a few seconds in a fold before returning slowly to normal (Fig. 65-3).

Texture

Roughness may occur normally on exposed areas, especially elbows and the soles of the feet. The skin of an infant is usually soft and smooth, while that of an elderly person may be rough and lack underlying tissue substance (atrophy). Roughness may occur with hypothyroidism.

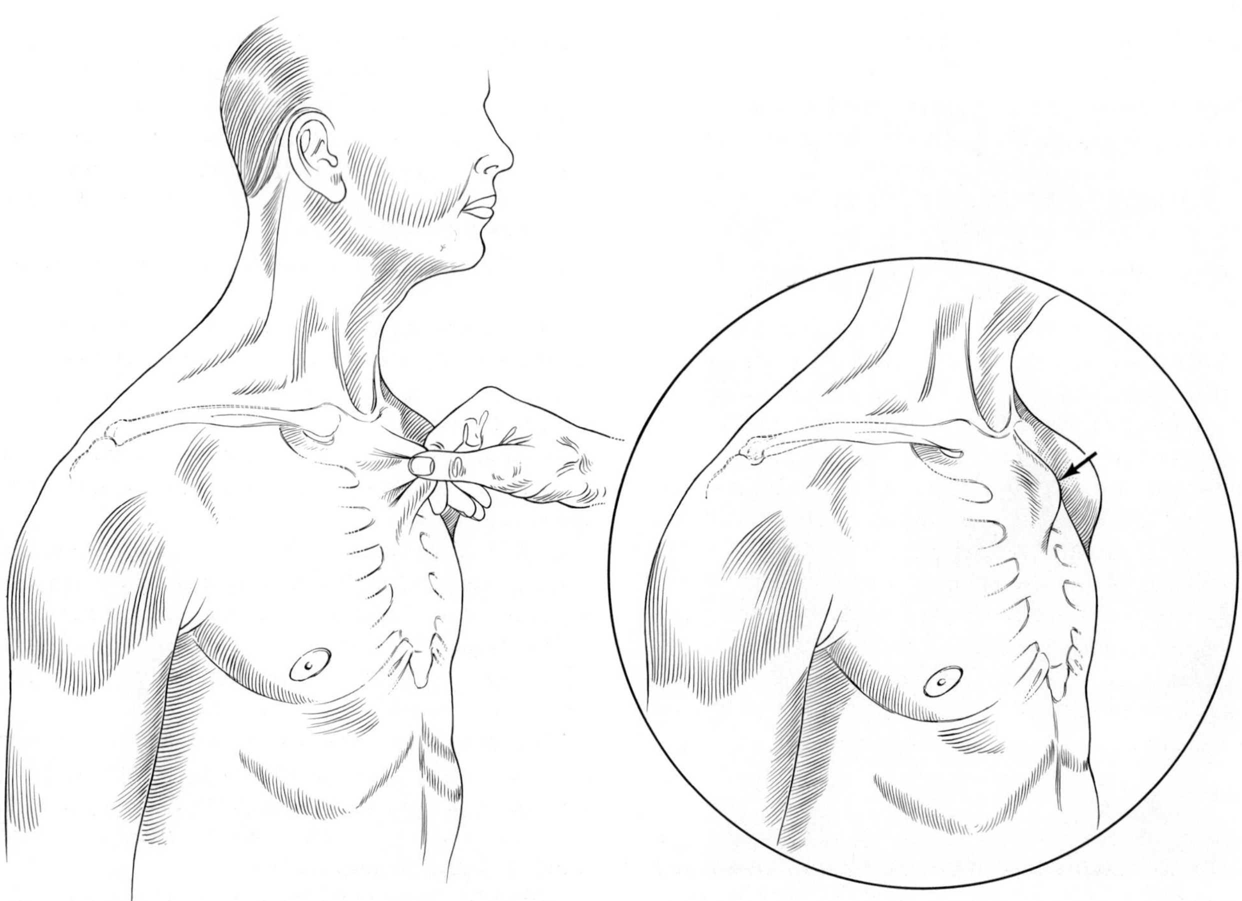

Fig. 65-3. Examination of skin turgor. When skin over sternum is picked up, a fold of skin remains for a few seconds when poor turgor is present.

Odor

Normal clean skin is usually free of odor except for areas containing apocrine sweat glands. Odor occurs because of bacterial decomposition of protein matter. Some draining skin lesions may produce an odor.

□ Accessory structures

Hair

If the person is wearing a wig or other hairpiece, this should be removed temporarily for inspection of the hair and scalp. It is easy to miss lesions on the scalp, and the person can assist by indicating areas of itching, pain, or roughness.

Hair growth, pattern, and distribution are indicators of the general state of health of an individual.[5] Excessive hair growth *(hirsutism)* is usually related to hormonal changes. Hair loss *(alopecia)* occurs normally with age, especially in some men. Abnormal hair loss may be caused by hormonal imbalance, general ill health, infections of the scalp, typhoid fever, chronic liver disease, stress, or drugs (antimetabolites). Changes in hair distribution on the body may be caused by hormonal changes. Hair loss on the dorsum of the toes may be indicative of decreased arterial circulation.

Hair should also be free of lice or nits. Nits are the eggs of the lice and are usually found imbedded on hair strands behind the ears. They are observed as small, glistening, greyish specks along the hairshaft near the scalp.

Nails

The appearance of the nails change with age and with ill health. Changes in hardness, brittleness, roughness, or shape may be indicative of some metabolic diseases, nutritional imbalances including vitamin dificiencies, or digestive disturbances. Pale nail beds and poor capillary return (slow return to normal color after the nail is pinched) may indicate hypoxia or anemia. Clubbing of the nails refers to the elimination of the small concave portion at the base of the nail by soft tissue growth; this occurs with certain pulmonary diseases (Fig. 65-4).

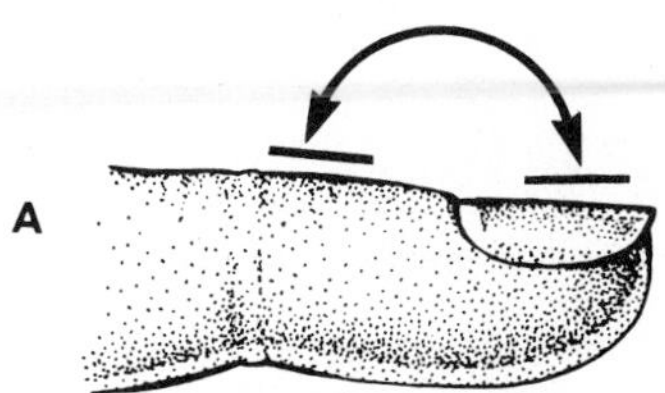

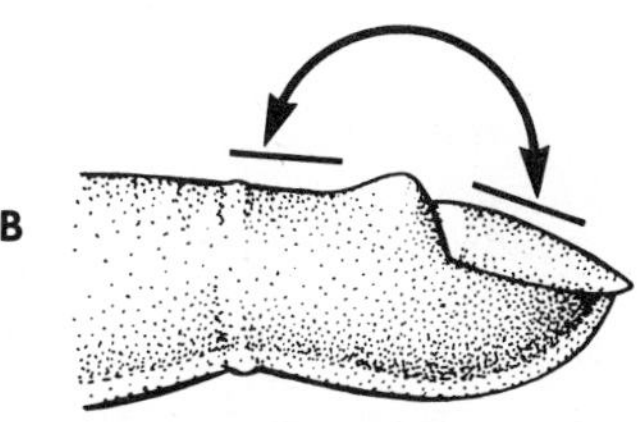

Fig. 65-4. Diagram showing clubbing of finger. **A,** Normal angle of nail. **B,** Abnormal angle of nail seen in late clubbing. (From Malasanos, L., Barkauskas, V., Moss, M., and Stoltenberg-Allen, K.: Health assessment, St. Louis, 1977, The C. V. Mosby Co.)

Infections of the tissue around the nail may occur *(paronychia)* characterized by red, shiny skin and painful swelling around the edge of the nail. The infection may result from trauma or from certain diseases such as psoriasis or dermatitis. If the nail is lost, it will usually grow back unless the nail bed has been injured.

□ Lesions

When lesions are observed, the following parameters are used for description: type, color, size, shape and configuration, texture, effect of pressure, distribution, arrangement, and variety.

Type. Use of medical terminology facilitates communication (Table 65-2). For example, use of the term "vesicle" will immediately establish the lesion as a clear, fluid-filled lesion smaller than 1 cm.

Size. The metric system is used for descriptions. A helpful hint is to measure a portion of one's own fingers, such as the distance from the tip of the right thumb to the first joint, or the width of the nail on the right little finger. This can then be used as a gauge for estimating the size of a lesion.

Shape and configuration. Shape can be described as round, oval, and so on. *Configuration* refers to the sharpness of demarcation of the lesion; that is, is it discrete or diffuse.

Texture. The lesion is described as rough or smooth, dry or moist, on the surface or deeply penetrating into the tissue.

Effect of pressure. Some vascular lesions blanch when pressure is applied and then return to their original color. Other lesions remain the same with pressure.

Arrangement. Some lesions occur in patches while others occur diffusely over the body. This is an important parameter when describing rashes.

Distribution. Some lesions occur in certain parts of the body, such as on exposed areas as with contact dermatitis, or on main body areas as in chickenpox. The lesions may follow the area of distribution of one of the spinal nerves as in herpes zoster.

Variety. In some diseases, such as smallpox, the lesions may all occur at the same time, whereas in chickenpox the lesions occur in crops so that there may be

Table 65-2. Types of skin lesions

Observed skin changes	Differentiation	Term	Example
Change in color or texture			
Spot	Circumscribed, flat, color change	Macule	Freckle
Discoloration, (reddish-purple)	Bleeding beneath the surface, injury to tissue	Contusion	Bruise
Soft whitening	Caused by repeated wetting of skin	Maceration	Between toes after soaking
Flake	Dry cells of surface	Scale	Dandruff, psoriasis
Roughness from dried fluid	Dry exudate over lesions	Crust	Eczema, impetigo
Roughness from cells	Leathery thickening of outer skin layer	Lichenification	Callus on foot
Change in shape			
Fluid-filled lesions	Less than 1 cm, clear fluid	Vesicle	Blister, chickenpox
	Greater than 1 cm, clear fluid	Bulla	Large blister, pemphigus
	Small, thick yellowish fluid (pus)	Pustule	Acne
	Semisolid	Cyst	Sebaceous cyst
Solid mass, *cellular* growth	Less than 5 mm	Papule	Small mole, raised rash
	5 mm to 2 cm	Nodule	Enlarged lymph node
	Greater than 2 cm	Tumor	Benign or malignant tumor
	Excess connective tissue over scar	Keloid	Overgrown scar
Swelling of tissue	Generalized swelling: fluid between cells	Edema	Inflammation, swelling of feet
	Circumscribed surface edema, transient, some itching	Wheal	Allergic reaction
Breaks in skin surfaces			
Oozing, scraped surface	Loss of superficial surface of skin	Abrasion	"Floor burn," scrape
Scooped-out depression	Loss of deeper layers of skin	Ulcer	Decubitus, stasis ulcer
Superficial linear skin breaks	Scratch marks, frequently by finger nails	Excoriations	Scratching
Linear crack or cleft	Slit or splitting of skin layers	Fissure	Athlete's foot
Jagged cut	Tearing of skin surface	Laceration	Accidental cut by blunt object
Linear cut, edges approximated	Cutting by sharp instrument	Incision	Knife cut
Vascular lesions			
Small, flat, round, purplish-red spot	Intradermal or submucous hemorrhage	Petechia	Bleeding tendency, vitamin C deficiency
Spiderlike, red, small	Dilatation of capillaries, arterioles, or venules	Telangiectasis	Liver disease, vitamin B deficiency
Discoloration, reddish-purple	Escape of blood into tissue	Ecchymosis	Trauma to blood vessels

lesions at different stages of development occurring at the same time.

DIAGNOSTIC TESTS

Culture

If a lesion is draining and there are symptoms of infection, a culture may be taken to identify the causative organism. If the causative factor is believed to be a fungus, a potassium hydroxide (KOH) examination may be carried out. The lesion is scraped with a knife blade, and the scraping placed on a slide and put into a KOH solution for microscopic analysis.[6]

Wood's light

In order to assist in the diagnoses of certain conditions, such as tinea of the scalp, a fungal infection, the hair is illuminated by a special filter (Wood's light) attached to an ultraviolet lamp. The infected hairs fluoresce or appear luminous under the light.

Allergy tests

Intracutaneous test. Small amounts of extracts of various allergenic substances to which sensitivity is suspected are injected intradermally at spaced intervals, usually on the forearm or in the scapular region. Control tests with the diluent alone are carried out concurrently. The test is positive if a wheal with surrounding erythema appears in 15 to 30 minutes but not in the control test. The test is begun with highly diluted solutions and then repeated with stronger extracts if the results are negative, in order to avoid a systemic reaction. The person should be observed for signs of anaphylactic shock.

Scratch test. The scratch test is less sensitive than the intradermal test, but the person is less likely to sustain a systemic reaction. The extract is placed on the skin and the skin is lightly scratched. The test is positive if erythema occurs in 30 minutes.

Patch test. This is the simplest of the skin tests. The sensitizing substance is applied to a 2.5 cm (1 inch) square piece of soft cotton, covered with a piece of occlusive tape, and left in place for 48 hours. The patches must remain dry and clean. The test is read 20 to 30 minutes after the patch is removed. Positive results are read as follows:

+	Erythema only
++	Erythema and papules
+++	Erythema, papules and small vessicles
++++	All the above plus bullae and at times ulceration[1]

Positive reactions may take several weeks to subside.

Conjunctival test. Occasionally one drop of test extract is instilled in the eye to test for sensitivity. Redness of the conjunctiva and tearing will appear within 5 to 15 minutes in an allergic person.

Use test. Substances such as foods, cosmetics, or fabrics to which a person is suspected of being allergic are eliminated from use and then added individually according to a set schedule. Reaction to the use test may be immediate or over a period of time. Some persons become discouraged during the testing and may need encouragement to adhere to the testing schedule.

REFERENCES AND SELECTED READINGS

1. Arndt, K.: Manual of dermatologic therapeutics, Boston, 1974, Little, Brown & Co.
2. *Bates, B.: A guide to physical examination, Philadelphia, 1974, J. B. Lippincott Co.
3. Beeson, P., and McDermott, W., editors: Textbook of medicine, ed. 14, Philadelphia, 1975, W. B. Saunders Co.
4. Brown, M. S., and Alexander, M.: Physical examination. Pt. 3. Examining the skin, Nurs. 73 3:39-43, 1973.
5. Guyton, A.: Textbook of medical physiology, ed. 5, Philadelphia, 1977, W. B. Saunders Co.
6. Judge, R., and Zuidema, G.: Physical diagnosis: a physiological approach to the clinical examination, ed. 2, Boston, 1963, Little, Brown & Co.
7. Kram, J. A., Bourne, H. R., Maibach, H. I., et al.: Cutaneous immediate hypersensitivity in man: effects of systemically administered adrenergic drugs, J. Allergy Clin. Immunol. **56**:387-392, 1975.
8. *Malasanos, L., Barkauskas, V., Moss, M., and Allen, K. S.: Health assessment, St. Louis, 1977, The C. V. Mosby Co.
9. *Roach, L.: Color changes in dark skin, Nurs. 72 **2**:19-22, 1972.
10. *Roberts, S.: Skin assessment for color and temperature, Am. J. Nurs. **75**:610-613, 1975.
11. Sana, J., and Judge, R.: Physical appraisal methods in nursing practice, Boston, 1975, Little, Brown & Co.
12. Sherman, J., and Fields, S.: Guide to patient evaluation, Flushing, N. Y., 1974, Medical Examination Publishing Co., Inc.

---

*References preceded by an asterisk are particularly well suited for student reading.

66

Management of the person with a dermatologic problem

ROSEMARY CRAYCROFT YEGANEF
BARBARA C. LONG

The specific management of persons with dermatologic problems varies with each disease entity. There are general principles, however, that the nurse should follow in the care of these individuals.

Defining and removing the cause of the disorder is the first step in restoring the structure and function of the skin. Nursing care should be directed toward prevention of the disease by instruction in proper hygienic measures, emphasizing the importance of seeking medical advice for changing skin conditions, and education in proper maintenance therapy. Other considerations in nursing care are relief of patient discomfort, prevention of infection after lesions occur, and encouraging healing of the lesions.

■ PREVENTION OF DERMATOLOGIC DISORDERS

□ Avoidance of causative agents

The first step in prevention of dermatologic conditions may be directed toward avoidance of the causative agent. This may be a specific antigen, contact irritant, microorganisms, trauma, or insect. Instructing the person to avoid a known causative agent is preventive medicine; however, it may not be that simple. Many dermatologic diseases have no known cause or are hereditary, or once the mechanism of the disease is known, it is not always possible to remove the trigger factors. Finally, symptoms may persist long after the agent is removed. Therefore the nurse's responsibility is one of educating the patient about good skin care, the importance of rest and avoidance of emotional stress, good nutrition, and, lastly, close observation to determine changes in skin conditions.

□ Cleansing

The outer layer of skin cells and the perspiration are acid in reaction, and their presence inhibits the life and growth of bacteria. Strong soaps that are alkaline in reaction may neutralize this protective acid condition of the skin. They may also remove the oily secretion of the sebaceous glands, which lubricate the outer skin layers and contribute to their health. It is sometimes necessary to remove excess oil and scale or debris. This facilitates the absorption of medication, promotes healing, and enhances the appearance of the skin. In psoriasis, for example, removal of scale by mechanical means and slowing of skin metabolism are prime objectives.

Normal skin should be washed often enough to remove excess oils and excretions and to prevent odor. Care must be taken not to cause drying or irritation. Maintaining a proper degree of hydration in the skin will prevent dryness and itching, which may lead to scratching, excoriation, and further trauma. Hydrating the stratum corneum, or outer layer of skin, may be accomplished by soaking in a tub of water for 20 to 30 minutes and then immediately applying a lubricating lotion or cream. This application of a cream prevents the rapid loss of water from the skin surface.

□ Nutrition

Good diet and nutrition play an important role in preventing the occurrence of skin lesions. Some skin lesions may be directly associated with dietary intake. Excessive dryness of the skin and thickening of the stratum corneum at the hair follicle openings may be caused by nutritional deficiencies. Elevated blood lipids secondary to hyperlipoproteinemia may take the form of xanthomas on the skin surface. Restriction of sodium in patients who are on steroids may lessen or prevent edema as a side effect.

Hypersensitive individuals may be placed on restrictive diets to exclude intake of known causative agents or as a diagnostic tool to identify causative agents. Persons who are allergic to penicillin are placed on a mold-free or penicillin-free diet and are instructed to avoid consuming milk and its by-products. Milk is frequently contaminated with penicillin when penicillin is given to the animals for bovine mastitis.

Whatever the product or food additive the hypersensitive person is to avoid, he should read labels carefully. It also may be necessary to request information from the manufacturer if questions about food additives arise. Upon discharge from the hospital, the patient should know the type of diet he is to follow at home. This would include knowledge of any restrictions, methods of preparing these foods, if necessary, and the duration of the prescribed diet.

□ Rest

Rest and relief from emotional stress may prevent exacerbations of existing diseases. *Alopecia areata*, which is a circumscribed patch of hair loss, has frequently been seen to follow several weeks after a real or threatened loss of a loved one. The direct relationship of emotional stress has not been explained.

Persons should be made aware that lack of rest or emotional tension can be a trigger factor in the development of skin conditions. For example, the person will be able to cite the fact that she was tense from the recent preparation for her daughter's wedding, and that this may have precipitated flare-up of her psoriasis.

□ Observations of changes

Care of normal skin should include regular observation of pigmented skin areas, moles, or other apparently minor skin lesions. Any change in size, color, or general appearance should be reported to a physician at once, since a change in moles or new skin growths is one of the danger signals of cancer. Ultraviolet irradiation seems to be the most common, least disputed exogenous factor in the cause of skin cancer. Basal cell carcinoma has been found to occur more frequently in sunny climates, in fair-skinned persons, in older people, and in those who work outdoors.

Patients should be instructed to avoid the sun if they have been diagnosed as having a skin condition that is aggravated by ultraviolet light. This is accomplished by the use of sunscreen lotions when outside, covering exposed skin surfaces by use of long sleeves and a hat, and most important, by regular medical follow-up.

□ Dangers of self-treatment

People should be urged to seek competent medical help when skin conditions develop. Although skin diseases rarely cause death, they may be reflections of serious systemic illness and can account for much human discomfort and for serious interruption of work and other activities. Many persons are inclined to rely on the advice of friends or the local druggist, or on medications they may have on hand. Each individual's skin reacts differently to treatment, and the skin that is already irritated or diseased may respond violently to inexpert treatment. Because of changes in the skin, medications prescribed even for a similar skin ailment in the same patient some time previously may not produce a favorable response. Medications may deteriorate, and for this reason old medications are not safe. The person may be spared much discomfort and expense if he turns to a specialist when symptoms first develop and before a mild skin condition becomes a real problem.

■ PSYCHOLOGIC EFFECTS OF DERMATOLOGIC PROBLEMS

There is a certain degree of "beauty orientation" in Western culture. Beauty pageants are popular, advertisements in the media use beautiful models to attract the reader, and in public groups, heads turn as a good-looking person walks by. Cosmetics to enhance good looks are extensively used, by men as well as women. It is no wonder, therefore, that skin diseases or physical defects that detract from "good looks" produce psychologic reactions.

A person's emotional reaction to a deformity or defect must not be underestimated. One's pride in himself, his ability to think well of himself, and to regard himself favorably in comparison with others are essential to the development and maintenance of a well-integrated personality. Every person who has a defect or a handicap, particularly if it is conspicuous to others suffers from some threat to his emotional security. The extent of the emotional reaction and the amount of maladjustment that follows depend on the individual's makeup and his ability to cope with emotional insults. Disfigurements almost invariably lead to disturbing experiences. The child who has webbed fingers may be ridiculed at school; the adolescent girl who has acne scars may be self-conscious and avoid social situations; and the young man with a posttraumatic scar on his face may be refused a salesman's job. Under any of these circumstances it is not unusual for the individual to withdraw from a society that is unkind. The defect may be used to justify failure to assume responsibility or to justify striking out against an unkind society by such reactions as becoming a "problem child" or, in some extreme cases, a criminal.

Skin diseases that produce marked disfigurement of visible body surfaces can therefore effect alterations in body image, as described in Chapter 28. Feelings of decreased worth by persons with large draining lesions or with severe disfigurement are reinforced during interactions with others. Some people are repelled when viewing persons with severe skin diseases, or they may experience a threat to their own body integrity and physically withdraw to avoid interaction. Persons may also frequently experience nonverbal messages of disgust when others view them for the first time. This is markedly poignant when those nonverbal messages are sent by significant others or by health professionals.

The person with severe facial disfigurement may also experience job discrimination. One woman was moved sequentially from a large office to a smaller office to a single office and finally to the evening hours in a lonely room so that co-workers could avoid looking at her. She lived alone and was increasingly deprived of social contacts with others. It was only after her eyesight failed and she was encouraged to attend groups for the blind that she was able to develop meaningful relationships again.

In working with the person with severe skin disease, the nurse first examines his or her own feelings that could be expressed nonverbally in a negative manner. Measures to assist the patient and family to deal with and cope with their feelings are described in Chapters 16 and 28.

■ GENERAL INTERVENTION

□ Relief of pruritus

Pruritus or itching is a cutaneous symptom that provokes the desire to scratch. Recent studies indicate pruritus arises as a result of the stimulation of the subepidermal nerve network by proteolytic enzymes. Proteinase is released from the epidermis as a result of either primary irritation or allergic sensitization reactions. Other causes of pruritus include blood and cellular infiltrates as well as superficial bacterial and fungal flora.

The pruritus found in association with many dermatoses and allergic reactions is caused by the release of chemical mediators in the skin. It may appear, however, without clinical signs, as in metabolic and endocrine disorders of diabetes, obstructive biliary disease, and uremia.

Pruritus may be caused by infestations such as hookworm, neoplasms, especially Hodgkin's disease, or subclinical hypersensitivity reactions to drugs. Acute and chronic emotional stress may be precipitating factors. The most common cause of itching is dry skin. Whatever the cause, pruritus ranges from an annoyance to a severe, distressing, or exhausting symptom.

A major step in treating pruritus is to attempt to remove the itch stimuli and break the itch-scratch cycle. Cold causes vasoconstriction and will provide some relief. Hydration in a tepid bath followed by the application of an emollient lotion is helpful. Topical anesthetics dull the itch sensation and topical corticosteroids decrease inflammation. In some persons antihistamines are of some value as are tranquilizers.

The awareness of pruritus may be more acute during the night because of a decrease in diverting stimuli. Cool, light, nonrestrictive bed clothing may help allay itching. Soft, old sheets should be used on the bed, and sometimes "neutral" linen is necessary. It is prepared by rinsing the linen in a mild acid solution, which counteracts the excess alkaline of ordinary laundry soap or detergent. A tablespoon (15 ml) of vinegar to a quart (liter) of water may be used in the home.

Excessive drying of the skin caused by high room temperature and low humidity can also increase pruritus. It occurs readily in the elderly person who already has a dry skin. Usually a room temperature of 20 C (68 to 70 F) and humidity of 30% to 40% are best for the person with pruritus.

□ Temperature control

The individual who has a generalized flush, or erythema, and the one who has an extensive exfoliative dermatitis may be losing body heat at an abnormally increased rate and may need a room temperature of 32.2 C (90 F) or more to maintain normal body temperature. Care must be taken to avoid chilling, particularly after baths, when compresses are used, or when parts of the body are exposed.

□ Hygienic measures: baths and soaks

The patient with skin disease should not bathe until he has been examined by a physician. Clothing, dressings, and the lesions themselves with crusts or exudates should be left undisturbed unless a definite order has been given for their care. Exudate may be removed upon order of a physician, and a specific method of removal should be prescribed. Hard crust or thickened exudates often are soaked with physiologic solution of sodium chloride, peroxide, pHisoHex in water, or a mild solution of tincture of green soap in warm water. Clean techniques should be used unless sterile technique is indicated. Care should be taken to avoid reinfection from soiled outer dressings or other sources.

Tub baths are a frequent means of cleansing the body and are part of the treatment in many dermatologic conditions. Depending on the skin condition being treated, the additives to bath water will vary. Many times persons with psoriasis who are using crude coal tar are permitted to wash with pHisoHex or Dial soap while in the tub. This will help prevent folliculitis because of the antibacterial properties within the soap. Special attention should be paid to intertriginous areas (areas between skin surfaces such as between fingers or toes) where creams and topical medications may collect. Tub baths or soaks to a specific body part are soothing and antipruritic. Baths are an effective means of rehydrating the skin. The tub soak should last 20 to 30 minutes with a water temperature between 32 to 38 C (90 to 100 F). If creams or ointments are to be applied after a bath, it should be done immediately, as this lessens itching, retains moisture, and prevents "drying out" of the outer layer of skin. Patients should be assisted in and out of the tub. A rubber mat should be used and special attention given to the potential for slipping when oils are used.

Many persons with arthropathic psoriasis find it difficult to use a tub because of their limited mobility. If a lift is not available to lower the patient into the tub or if the lift is too difficult to maneuver in the bathroom, sitting on a chair under a gentle shower is the next best alternative. After a bath the skin should be patted dry; vigorous rubbing is avoided.

Substances may be added to the bath for specific therapeutic effects. *Oatmeal, soybean* powder, and soluble *cornstarch* may be added to lessen pruritus or when soap is contraindicated. Directions for preparation of a colloidal bath are as follows:

1. Add 0.45 kg (2 cups) of cereal (oatmeal, soybean, or bran) to 480 ml (2 cups) of boiling water.
2. Stir cereal while boiling for 5 minutes.
3. Fill tub three-fourths full with *tepid* water (35 C [95 F])
4. Pour the cooked cereal into a mesh or gauze bag and stir the bag through the bath for a few minutes until the water becomes opalescent.
5. The bag may also be used as a mop to gently pat the skin to remove crusts and debris.

Potassium permanganate ($KMNO_4$) is used in a bath or soak to deodorize and dry lesions for such conditions as pyoderma gangrenosum or slow-healing ulcers, and to help prevent infection in pemphigus lesions. The dilution is ordered by the physician, usually at a 1:32,000 or 1:16,000 dilution. If tablets of $KMNO_4$ are used in preparing the solution, the mix should be strained through gauze to filter out any undissolved particles that may cause irritation.

Sulfur acts as an antibacterial agent for such conditions as acne or hidradenitis suppurativa. If a sulfur bath suspension is used, it is important to rinse the body with tepid water to remove any residual particles of sulfur.

Tar baths are used frequently prior to ultraviolet light therapy in persons with psoriasis. Balnetar Bath Oil and Polytar Bath are two popular brand names used for this purpose. Tar residual is thought to enhance the effect the ultraviolet light has on the skin.

The tub used for a medicated bath should be disinfected after each use by pouring 240 ml (1 cup) of bleach into the used tub water, letting it stand for 5 minutes, then wiping the sides and bottom of the tub. The tub is then drained and cleaned in the usual fashion. If the bath is to be taken at home, the person should know how to prepare any treatment tub bath prescribed by the physician. This would include gathering supplies, mixing solutions if necessary, and special precautions to be followed with the specific treatment.

□ Topical medications

Application of medications to the skin surface may take many forms. Wet dressings, creams, pastes, ointments, or lotion can be used. The nurse should know the purpose for which a local application is ordered, the drug (or drugs) contained in the preparation, and any toxic signs that may occur from its use.

Wet dermatologic dressings

Wet dressings are used over various skin lesions to provide an antipruritic, antifungal, and astringent effect. Scales and exudate are loosened and removal is facilitated. The temperature of the solution for soaking the dressings should be lukewarm (32 to 38 C [90 to 100 F]).

Solutions for wet dressings that have an astringent effect include physiologic saline (0.9%), aluminum subacetate 0.25%, and aluminum acetate 1:20 or 1:40 solution (Burow's solution). Silver nitrate solution at 1:1,000 or 1:10,000 dilution has an antibacterial effect and is frequently used with extensive burns (p. 1519). Since silver nitrate causes staining, gloves should be worn for application.

Wet tap-water dressings are sometimes used over corticosteroid creams covering a severely inflamed psoriasis lesion. The action of the wet dressing in conjunction with the steroid hastens the reduction of inflammation and eases the patient's discomfort. This type of total body dressing is employed for 24 to 48 hours and is changed every 3 to 6 hours as ordered. It is important to remember that occlusion of a moist dressing may cause excessive maceration of the skin. Covering the area with plastic wrap, oiled silk, wax paper, or a "chux" pad should be avoided unless specifically ordered by the physician.

The type of dressing material used for a wet dressing should be one without cotton filling, since cotton leaves particles and a residue on the skin, which may cause irritation. Several layers of fine-mesh gauze is ideal, and roller gauze is excellent for extremities. A mask for the face may be designed by cutting out openings for the eyes, nose, and mouth from several thicknesses of gauze. To prepare the wet dressing, the prescribed solution is placed in a basin with the dressings. The excess moisture is squeezed out of the dressing and the dressing is then applied to the body. A flannel covering is placed over the dressing and secured in place. The flannel prevents rapid evaporation of water and chilling of the patient.

If the lesions are infected, the dressings should be placed in plastic bags before being discarded in the appropriate container. If the lesions are closed, the dressings may be used repeatedly for 24 hours.

Wet-to-dry dressings are used to *debride* wounds or ulcerations. A fine mesh gauze is moistened with the prescribed solution, placed over the lesion, and allowed to dry. The crust and debris is removed as the dressing is pulled off dry. This process is usually repeated every 4 to 8 hours. Half-strength Dakin's solution is frequently used for this purpose.

A small area of skin is often tested to determine if the person will tolerate the cream or lotion over the entire body. The topical medication is applied to a small area (silver-dollar size) on the person's forearm. The time and the exact location of the trial are recorded, and the skin response to the trial medication is read 24 hours later. Crude coal tar is frequently tested in this manner.

Vehicles for topical medication

Topical medications can be prepared in a variety of bases (Table 66-1). *Powders* are effective in reducing friction and moisture in intertriginous areas. *Lotions* must be shaken well, as the insoluble powder may settle out. The addition of alcohol increases the cooling effect of a lotion. *Ointments* do not usually leave an oily residue on the skin unless they have a petrolatum base. A nonporous covering such as plastic should not be used over an ointment unless so prescribed, as the heat retention may increase percutaneous absorption of the medication.

Application of topical medications

Lotions with a water or alcohol base should be applied by patting gently. A gauze pledget should be used for extremely thin lotions. Lotions with an oily base are applied thinly and evenly with the palm of the hand.

Powders should first be sprinkled into the hand, then applied to the skin to avoid getting excess powder into the air and thus causing irritation to the mucous membrane. Powders should be used sparingly to prevent caking.

Ointments may be applied with gloved hands or with the bare palm, depending on the type of ointment used. If a dressing is to be applied, the ointment may be spread on the dressing with a tongue blade before application to the skin. Anthralin may be caustic to normal skin, so gloves should be worn. Crude coal tar is always applied in firm, long, downward strokes to prevent folliculitis, since tar is an irritant. Creams, as opposed to ointments, may be rubbed in.

Many times some topical medications such as crude coal tar are removed prior to other treatment. Crude coal tar must be removed in the morning prior to ultraviolet light therapy (following the Goeckerman regimen). This is done by applying corn oil in long downward strokes over the skin surface, then wiping with gauze pledgets, leaving only a thin film of tar. A general rule to remember is to remove only the excess ointment or ointments having a consistency of cold cream, prior to a bath or wet dressing. Cottonseed oil may be used to remove caked, oily-based lotions, using a gauze pledget.

Table 66-1. Comparison of vehicles for topical medications

Type	Base	Effect
Powder	Dry	Drying by absorbing moisture; cooling by evaporating moisture
Lotion	Powder suspended in water or oil	Protective, cleansing, cooling, antipruritic effect depending on drug and base used
Creams and ointments	Emulsions of oil and water	Occlusive covering over skin to prolong contact of medication with skin—good skin penetration; warming effect
Paste	50% or more powder in ointment base	Holds medication for longer period of time with slower skin penetration

□ Teaching of self-help skills

Many persons with skin disease are not hospitalized. In the home and in the clinic the nurse must be specific in instructions to the person or to the family member who will be responsible for his care. It is best to write out instructions specifically. A common mistake that some persons make when at home is to believe that if some is good, more is better. While a skin ailment may respond to an ointment rubbed on very gently and lightly, trauma from vigorous rubbing may counteract all benefit and may even make the condition worse. The individual, in his eagerness to cure the condition, may not realize how vigorous his own administrations are. The nurse can help the patient to improvise equipment that he needs.

The nurse should always assume initial responsibility for the application of topical medications and various treatments. At some point in the patient's hospitalization these responsibilities should be transferred to the patient. There may be a need for a visiting nurse to assist the person at home, and this should be determined prior to discharge.

Many times the person may use old linen such as napkins, pillowcases, and socks for dressings. A plastic shower cap may be used on the scalp as an occlusive covering at night. The person may have a plastic occlusion suit to wear at bedtime. These are usually worn over a steroid cream. Instructions for the care of this suit should include daily washing to prevent the caking of creams and collection of scales and exudate.

□ Outcome criteria for the person with a dermatologic condition

The person or significant others can:

1. Explain the rationale for the prescribed treatments.
2. Demonstrate prescribed baths, soaks, or medicated dressings.
3. Describe any special precautions to be observed during treatments, including:
   a. Avoidance of nonporous coverings over dressings unless so ordered.
   b. Complete dissolving of tablets or crystals in baths or soaks.
   c. Avoidance of excessive rubbing of medications over lesions.
   d. Application of thin layers of lotions or powders.
4. Describe the prescribed medication routine: route of administration, vehicle to be used, dosage, frequency, duration of topical application, side effects, and where supplies can be obtained.
5. Describe plans for socialization with others.

■ PLASTIC SURGERY

Plastic surgery is surgery that is performed to improve the appearance or function of the visual parts of the body. Plastic surgery has been attempted for centuries. Surgery of this kind was performed prior to the era of the Roman Empire. Hindu records describe some good results from efforts to alter deformities caused by disease or other misfortune. In the sixteenth century, Italian surgeons did remarkable work in plastic surgery, and there was interest in the emotional aspects of facial deformities. The discovery of anesthetics and of the cause of infection enabled surgeons to make strides in this field. Disfigurements resulting from World Wars I and II challenged the imagination of surgeons so that new techniques were developed.

□ Purposes of plastic surgery

The main purposes of such surgery are to restore function, prevent further loss of function, and cosmetically improve the defects caused by deformities present at birth, from disease, or from trauma. Plastic surgery such as skin grafting may be performed as an emergency measure in severe burns. It is also performed for aesthetic improvement.

Although medical science has made progress in learning the causes of some developmental anomalies (for example, it has been learned that German measles contracted during the first trimester of pregnancy may cause anomalies in the infant), it is not possible at the present time to prevent the occurrence of many defects at birth. Many birth defects such as cleft lip and cleft palate require plastic surgery. The cause of cancer is still unknown, and extensive surgery will continue to be used until a better method of treatment is discovered. Following surgical treatment for this disease, plastic surgery often is necessary. Trauma such as that sustained in automobile accidents often necessitates plastic surgery, and it seems likely that the number of people requiring such treatment will increase. Plastic surgery is often needed following loss of skin and scarring from burns. *Keloid tissue,* the thick, weltlike masses of overgrowth of scar tissue, which most commonly occur in dark-skinned persons, will often require plastic surgery. Posttraumatic scars in which subcutaneous tissues are separated from, or are adherent to, underlying structures such as bone may be corrected by plastic surgery.

The two aspects of plastic surgery, *reconstruction* and *correction,* are evident in most plastic surgical treatment. Often several medical specialists care for patients needing reconstructive and corrective surgery. The dental surgeon, the ear, nose, and throat specialist, and the plastic surgeon may all work together, for example, in treatment of the child who has a cleft lip and a cleft palate.

□ Directing the person in seeking appropriate care

Many people do not know that it is possible to correct a congenital defect. Some parents may delay seeking medical care for a child with a defect caused by a congenital anomaly because of their own guilt feelings. They may hope that somehow, miraculously, the child will "outgrow" the condition. Often they do not realize that the normal development of the child depends on the early treatment of some conditions. A defect may interfere with the use of a part of the body so that normal growth does not take place. This result follows the principle that form follows function; for instance, a child's deformed and therefore unused hand does not grow at the same rate as the hand that is used normally. Contractures of joints and atrophy of muscles occur with disuse, thus increasing the defect and handicap; for example, facial asymmetry can result from contractures in the neck that prevent uniform action of the muscles of both sides of the face even though the muscles themselves are not affected.

Parents need to know that healthy emotional development in the child is dependent on normal physical appearance. When a defect is allowed to persist, there may be emotional maladjustment that will affect the child's entire life. For example, conspicuous patches of brightly discolored skin present at birth and known as birthmarks or portwine stains are quite common. These stains, particularly if they are on the face or neck, cause the child great emotional distress and sometimes lead to serious personality maladjustment. Yet many people do not know that they may sometimes be effectively treated by tattooing.

Plastic surgery may require repeated and long hospitalizations that may place serious financial strain on the patient and his family if they must assume responsibility for the major part of the expense. Clinic nurses, community health nurses, social workers, and welfare agency personnel can help in preparing the patient for this problem and in helping him to meet it. If the patient is an adult, leaves from employment, financial support while undergoing treatment, and plans for convalescent care and rehabilitation are examples of problems that must be faced in many instances. The person should be encouraged to discuss his problems freely, since their solution does affect his medical treatment.

Many parents do not know that financial resources are available to cover costs of plastic surgery for children. Every state in the country has a plan for medical care of crippled children. This program is partially supported by matching funds from the federal government, administered by the Office of Child Development (formerly the Children's Bureau) of the Department of Health, Education, and Welfare, which was created soon after the first White House Conference on Child Care, held in Washington, D.C., in 1909. Children and adolescents up to 21 years of age with defects requiring plastic surgery are eligible for care under this plan. If the nurse encounters a child who might benefit from medical treatment, the family can be encouraged to discuss this with their physician. If the family has no personal physician, the local hospital may conduct a clinic or may recommend a physician designated to care for eligible children in the area or the state. Small community hospitals may not have clinics of their own but may refer patients to larger hospitals or special clinics in nearby cities. In larger communities the school nurse is usually well informed about available resources.

□ Corrective surgery

Implants and transplants

In plastic surgery the surgeon may use, in addition to the patient's own tissues, inert materials and tissues from other human beings. Inert substances must meet several criteria. They must not be irritating or contribute to the development of cancer, they should be an appropriate consistency for their intended use, and they should not deteriorate or change their shape and form with time. A large variety of substances has been used in the past, including wax, metal, ivory, and bone that has been rendered inert by boiling. In recent years materials such as Teflon and silicone have been used extensively, since they appear to be nonirritating and they retain their form indefinitely.

For many years reconstructive procedures have been attempted in which the tissues of other human beings are used. Whenever these tissues are used, however, there is the potential of rejection of the tissue because of the body's immune response (p. 198). The least difficulty is encountered with tissues such as the cornea of the eye that have a very limited blood supply.

Grafts. The most common procedure used in plastic surgery is grafting, or the transplantation of skin and other tissue from one part of the body to another part, or from a donor.

Graft sources. An *autograft* is skin, bone, cartilage, fat, fascia, muscle, or nerves that are moved from one part of the body to another.

Tissue transplanted from another person is called a *homograft (allograft).* It can be obtained from living persons, or it can be taken from persons shortly after death. Tissue taken under the latter circumstances can be used only if cancer or an infectious disease was not present. The use of homografts may be necessary when the patient's condition is poor and autografting is impossible. For example, the patient may be in shock but require the covering of large burned areas by grafted skin. The survival time of homografts varies from a few days to a number of weeks. Depending on the tissue used and the recipient site, the transplanted tissue will then die and slough or be absorbed and replaced by the host's own developing tissues. They are used only as temporary grafts.

Heterografts (xenografts) consist of tissue from another species. They are rejected by the recipient and are used only in special cases. For example, if tissue in banks is not readily available, it may be more feasible to use heterografts to cover the open wounds of patients with massive burns. The transplant acts as an antigen, and the body forms antibodies against it that prevent growth and function of the graft. When bone, cartilage, or blood vessels are obtained from sources other than the patient, they do not become part of the patient's body but act as a framework around which the body usually lays down cells of its own. The graft is then gradually absorbed over a period of time.

Grafting procedures. Plastic surgery may be performed by means of free grafting—cutting tissue from one part of the body and moving it directly to another part. It may also be done by leaving one end of the graft attached to the body to provide a blood supply for the graft until blood vessels form at the new place of attachment. The surgeon selects skin for grafting that is similar in texture and thickness to that which has been lost. He studies the normal lines of the skin and its elasticity to avoid noticeable scars. Scar tissue contracts with time, and in normal circumstances this process is good because it produces a complete closure of the line of injury. However, in some cases scar tissue may contract in such a way that surrounding tissues are pulled out of normal contour, and distortion may result. The plastic surgeon is an artist as well as a surgeon, and he studies cosmetic and many other aspects of the patient's problem before he decides on the type of graft or plastic procedure that will be most effective.

Free grafts. Free grafts are those that are lifted completely from one site and placed at another site. There are several types of free grafts, each with its advantages and limitations. Split-thickness grafts consist of the epidermis and varying thicknesses of the dermis. Full-thickness grafts include the entire dermis and epidermis (Fig. 65-1).

Thin split-thickness grafts (Ollier-Thiersch grafts), which have only a very thin layer of the dermis, are of limited use because they contract easily, often become shiny and discolored, and have poor wearing qualities. They are often used to replace mucous membrane in reconstructive surgery of such areas as the mouth and vagina. Appropriate means to prevent excessive contraction of the graft as it heals must be taken. Thin split-thickness homografts may be used to cover large burned areas to reduce the loss of body fluids. Within a few weeks the grafts can be removed and replaced with intermediate or thick split-thickness autografts.

Intermediate and *thick split-thickness grafts* are widely used. These grafts have a thicker layer of dermis attached to the epidermis and do not wrinkle, contract, or become discolored as easily as the thin split-thickness graft. The donor site is able to reepithelialize completely, since the deeper layers of the dermis have been left intact. These split-thickness grafts can be used to cover almost any part of the body. They can be cut into large pieces with a dermatome set to ensure a uniform thickness of the graft, and these can then be cut into smaller pieces to correspond to the size of the area to be grafted.

Full-thickness grafts (Wolfe's grafts) are used primarily to cover small areas where matching skin color and texture are important, such as on the face. One disadvantage of the full-thickness graft is that only a moderate-sized piece of full-thickness skin can survive as a free graft under the best circumstances because the blood supply cannot become established quickly enough to provide essential nutrition. For nourishment these grafts depend entirely on existing lymph until their own blood supply can be established. It takes at least 2 weeks for blood supply to become established, although it is usually possible to tell within a week whether the graft is going to survive. If the graft dies, the skin is irretrievably lost to the body, since regeneration of skin at the donor site is not possible. If possible, the surrounding skin at the donor site is usually undermined so that the skin edges can be brought together, and grafting of the donor site is not necessary. This means that full advantage may have been taken of the elastic quality of the skin, and another graft probably cannot be taken from the same place for some time.

Pedicle flap. When a large and deep defect is to be covered, a skin flap or pedicle flap may be used. "Sliding," "rotating," or "tubed" are some of the terms used to identify various types of grafts that are never completely removed from the body at any one time, thereby maintaining a direct vascular supply for nourishment of the tissue. Skin flap grafts may include skin and subcutaneous tissue and sometimes fat and cartilage or bone. Depending on the relative locations of the donor and the recipient sites, the skin graft may be released from the donor site on three sides. For example, it may be slid sideways directly over the recipient site and sutured in place, or it may be lifted and sutured to another area of the body such as a skin flap from the abdomen being sutured to the hand or arm. This type of grafting is called *primary grafting.* If the skin graft is to be moved a considerable distance, and primary grafting is not feasible, the edges of the graft are often sutured together to form a tube. This graft is known as a *tubed pedicle* or *suitcase handle graft* (Fig. 66-1). This modification lessens the

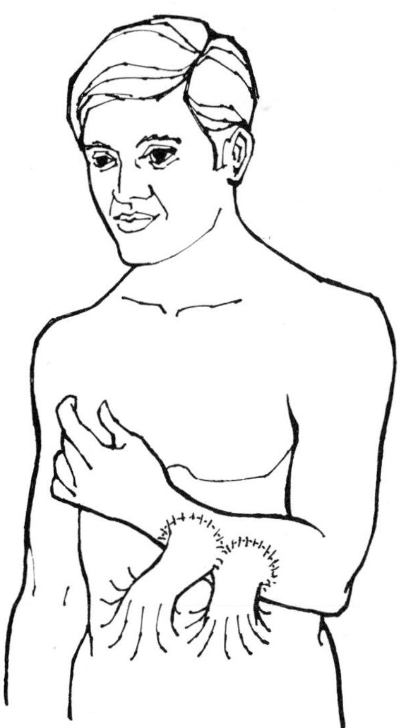

Fig. 66-1. Bilateral tubed pedicle flaps from abdomen to forearm. At later operation they will be detached from forearm and spread to cover burned areas on trunk.

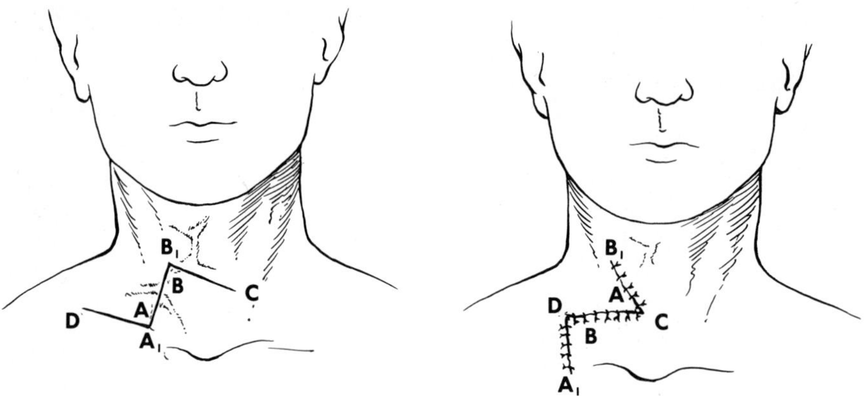

Fig. 66-2. By means of Z-plasty operations, scar tissue can be removed and defects can be covered without need to transplant skin.

danger of the flap becoming infected and permits tissues such as fat or cartilage to be easily transferred. This type of graft may be used to cover a defect on the back of the neck with skin from the abdomen. For example, the piece of skin taken from the abdomen may be grafted to the wrist. Then, when circulation is safely established there, the attachment on the abdomen may be released and attached to its final location on the neck. The attachment on the wrist is maintained until circulation is established in the neck, at which time the graft is freed from the wrist and the tube opened and sutured into place to cover the defect. Circulation from the new attachment is often tested by putting a rubber-covered clamp or tourniquet about the pedicle close to its oldest attachment and noting the color and warmth of the pedicle at intervals of 10 to 15 minutes. Usually it takes 3 to 6 weeks for new blood vessels to become established. These grafts are less likely to die than are free grafts, but strangulation can occur from pressure, and tissue can be lost from infection. Tubed pedicle grafts are often taken from the abdomen, where fat and subcutaneous tissue are available, to support skin areas of the body that are subject to pressure such as the heel, the sole of the foot, and the palm of the hand. The piece of skin taken is fairly narrow, and adjacent skin is undermined so that edges can be sutured together. When this wound has healed, a small gauze dressing is usually placed between the tubed pedicle and the suture line to keep the area dry and free from the accumulation of dead skin.

Procedures for contractures

Plastic surgeons make excellent use of the natural elastic quality of normal skin. Operations known as Z-*plasty* and Y-*plasty* are often performed. Scar tissue can often be removed, and the Z- or Y-shaped incision enables the surgeon to undermine adjacent skin, draw the edges together, and cover the defect without using skin from another part of the body (Fig. 66-2). These procedures are naturally limited by the size of the scar and its location, since elasticity of skin varies in different parts of the body. Z-plasty and Y-plasty procedures are suitable for such locations as the axilla, the inner aspects of the elbow, and the neck and throat. They are not so useful in treating defects on the back or on the palmar surfaces of the hand because the skin in these areas cannot be undermined and stretched.

Dermabrasion

Pockmarks, scars from acne, and certain other disfiguring marks may be removed from the skin by abrasive action. The variable results depend on the type and extent of the condition, but there is usually noticeable improvement in the patient's appearance (Fig. 66-3). Preoperatively the patient is prepared by the surgeon for the degree of improvement to be expected so that his expectations are realistic. He is also informed about the face bandage he may wear, postoperative swelling, discomfort, crusting, and the erythema, which may persist for several weeks. The procedure is performed under local or general anesthesia, depending on the size of the area to be treated, the individual patient, and the preference of the surgeon. It may be done in the clinic, the surgeon's office, or the hospital, again depending on the extent of the procedure and the preference of the physician. Hospitalization is necessary if a general anesthetic is used.

The skin is washed with germicidal soap for several days prior to surgery, and then a nonirritating aqueous antiseptic such as benzalkonium chloride is used to prepare the skin in the operating room. Ethyl chloride or

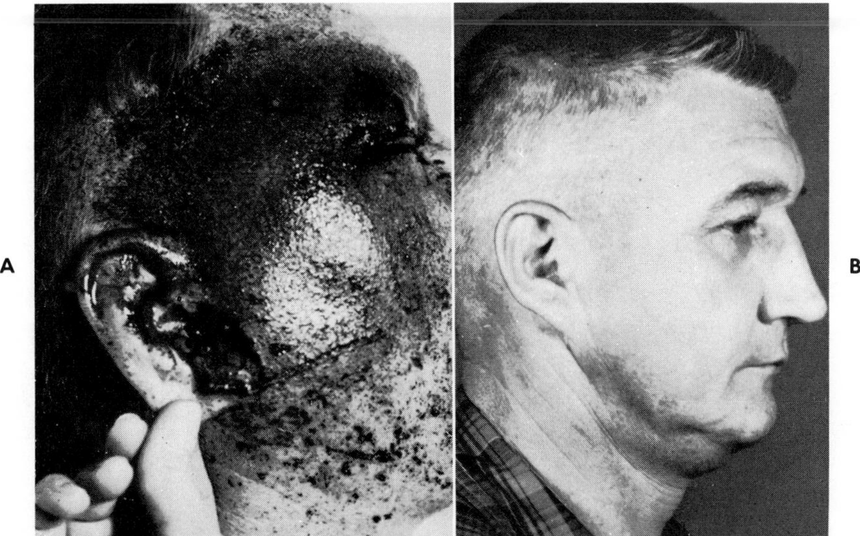

Fig. 66-3. A, Meticulous cleansing and dermabrasion were required to remove impregnated bits of galvanized metal. **B,** Postoperative view of patient 17 years after dermabrasion. (From Havener, W. H., Saunders, W. H., Keith C. F., and Prescott, A. W.: Nursing care in eye, ear, nose, and throat disorders, ed. 3, St. Louis, 1974, The C. V. Mosby Co.)

other less flammable spray anesthetics such as Frigiderm are used most often for local anesthesia. After the skin preparation has been completed, the skin is stretched and its superficial layers are removed either by sandpapering or by using an abrasive machine (Dermabrader). If the procedure has not been extensive and oozing is slight, the area may be left uncovered. Usually it is covered either with an ointment or by compresses moistened with an antiseptic solution such as benzalkonium chloride and then by a pressure dressing that covers the entire face except for the eyes, nose, and mouth. Prepared dressings that adhere less readily to the skin surface, such as Telfa dressings, are also used. Dermabrasion may be done in stages. At least 2 weeks and often longer may intervene between treatments.

Chemical peeling

Chemical peeling is a newer approach to changing the condition of the skin. There are specific indications for dermabrasion and for chemical peeling and some indications overlap. Chemical peeling is particularly suited for removing fine wrinkles of the face. A special chemical solution is applied to the skin, and then a waterproof tape mask is applied to the area. As the solution is applied, the patient experiences a brief burning sensation. Later, after the mask is applied, the burning pain returns and medication for relief of the pain is frequently necessary. When the mask is removed, the skin is edematous and weeping. A crust develops that separates spontaneously as the skin underneath leaks. Following the procedure, the skin of the person is sensitive to direct and indirect sunlight for a period of 3 to 6 months.[1]

Tattooing

Tattooing has been found useful in plastic surgery for changing the color of grafted skin so that it more closely resembles the surrounding skin. This treatment is usually given on an ambulatory basis. Pigment is carefully selected and blended with the normal skin coloring by a skilled technician who then impregnates the grafted skin, using a tattooing needle. The procedure is painful, since no anesthetic is used. Sometimes the patient is given a sedative such as phenobarbital or is instructed to take such medication approximately 1 hour before coming to the clinic or the physician's office. Prior to the tattooing, the skin is cleansed with a gauze sponge moistened with alcohol or normal saline solution. There may be a slight serous oozing from the skin after the treatment and it should be left to dry and crust. Sometimes a piece of sterile gauze can be placed over the tattooed area, and an ice bag may be applied if severe discomfort follows the treatment.

Tattooing is usually done in several stages. The amount done at one time depends on individual circumstances such as the location of the part treated and the emotional reactions of the patient. For example, treatment of the skin close to the eye is often quite painful and is extremely trying for the patient. Therefore

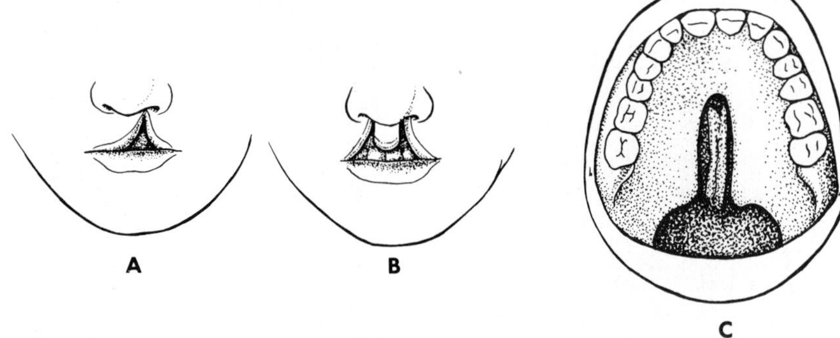

Fig. 66-4. Cleft lip and palate. **A,** Single cleft of lip. **B,** Double cleft of lip. **C,** Cleft of posterior palate.

usually only a small amount of tattooing is done at one time. Children may be given a general anesthetic for treatment around the eyes. Grafted skin may change in color with time, so tattooing done for the purpose of changing the color of grafted skin may have to be repeated.

Portwine stains that are too large to treat by excision and grafting have also responded to this method of treatment with excellent results. The whole area may be treated at one time and the treatments repeated so that the color changes slowly. This is a tedious procedure if the stain is large and dark but, finally, in some cases the stain is barely apparent to the casual observer.

□ Reconstructive surgery

Reconstructive surgery is carried out to correct birth defects, repair tissues destroyed by trauma or disease, or replace tissue removed by other surgeries.

Birth defects

Birth defects can occur in any part of the body. Providing they are treated at the proper time in the child's life, most of them can be improved a great deal by reconstructive procedures and some can be corrected entirely. Among the more common defects are cleft lip and cleft palate, urogenital anomalies (p. 1303), and musculoskeletal defects. (Musculoskeletal anomalies are discussed fully in orthopedic nursing texts.)

Cleft lip. *Cleft lip* (Figs. 66-4 and 66-5) usually is repaired surgically soon after birth. Some surgeons repair the defect in the first few days of life before the baby leaves the hospital. In some cases the repair is done when the infant is 6 to 8 weeks old and there is more tissue available for the repair. A second operation often is necessary but does not imply that the first one was not successful. A *cleft palate* is a much more difficult defect to treat than a cleft lip. It is repaired as early as possible,

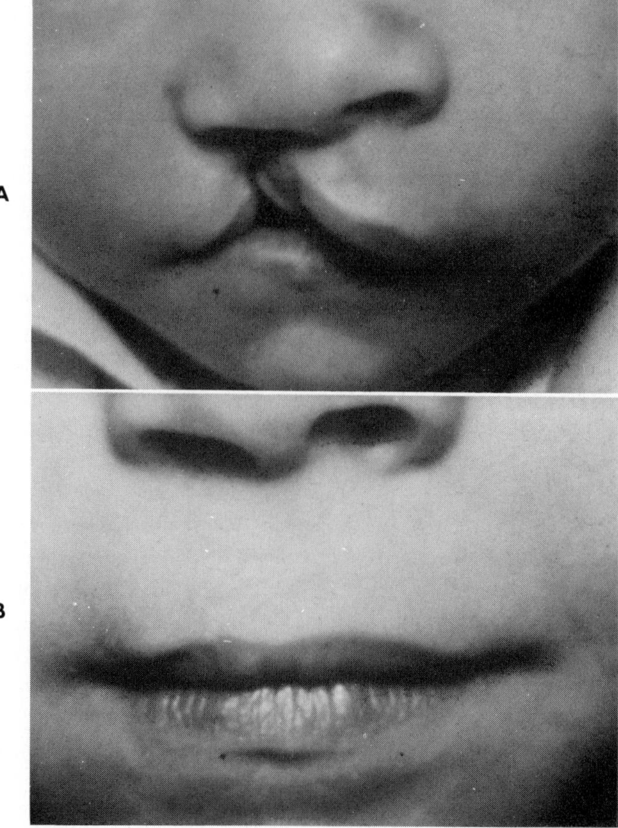

Fig. 66-5. A, Patient with almost complete cleft lip. **B,** Three years after surgery. (From Brauer, R. O.: Repair of the unilateral cleft lip. In Georgiade, N. G., editor: Symposium on management of cleft lip and palate and associated deformities, vol. 8, St. Louis, 1974, The C. V. Mosby Co.)

depending on the extent of the defect and the condition of the child. Most specialists believe that it should always be repaired by the time speech is attempted. The many nursing problems that are encountered in teaching mothers to feed and care for an infant with this defect and that the nurse needs to know to care for a child who has had a cleft lip or cleft palate repaired are included in pediatric nursing texts and current periodicals and will not be included here.

Maxillofacial surgery

Maxillofacial surgery is a specialty requiring a surgeon with unusual preparation and nurses with special knowledge and experience. Maxillofacial surgery received impetus as a result of the injuries sustained in World War II and the increase in radical surgery for malignancies of the head and neck (p. 1105). The surgeon works closely with the dental surgeon and with the specialist in problems of the nose and throat. When damage has been so great that reconstruction with living tissue is impossible, it is sometimes possible to construct prosthetic parts of the face that are so true to natural color and contour that they are not easily detectable. For example, a side of the nose may be replaced by a prosthetic part that is colored to match the patient's skin and disguised with marking to resemble skin.

Rhinoplasty. Reconstructive surgery of the nose can be done either to correct an anatomic problem (p. 1091) or for cosmetic reasons. Bone and cartilage may be removed from the nose if it is irregular, or they may be inserted if a defect such as a saddle nose is being corrected (Fig. 66-6). A local anesthetic is often used for these procedures unless it will interfere with a study of contours during the operation. In this case an intravenous or a rectal anesthetic may be used. The incision is usually made at the end of the nose inside the nostril so that it is not conspicuous. A nasal splint made of plaster, tongue blades, or crinoline may be used for protection. Immediately after surgery there will be ecchymosis and swelling around the eyes and nose. Ice compresses and an ice bag may be used to help prevent these reactions. The patient must anticipate waiting several weeks before evaluating the final result of the surgery.

Otoplasty. Another common operation, usually for purely cosmetic reasons, is the removal of some of the cartilage from the ears in order to flatten them against the head. This procedure is relatively simple and requires only a short hospitalization.

Rhytidoplasty. "Face-lifting" is also performed primarily for cosmetic reasons. An incision is made at the hairline, and excess skin is separated from its underlying tissue and removed. The remaining skin is pulled up and sutured at the hairline, thus removing wrinkles and giving firmness and smoothness to the face. A gentle pressure dressing is then applied and left in place for 24 to 48 hours. The patient is often discharged at this time and sutures are removed later in the surgeon's office. The patient frequently needs medication for pain in the postoperative period because of the extent to which the tissue has been undermined.

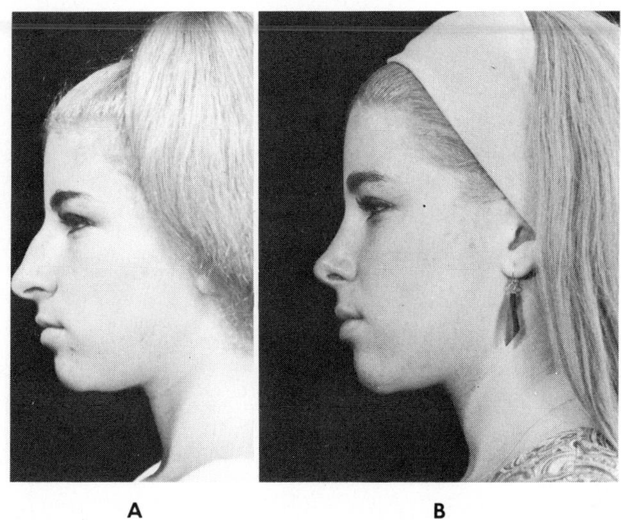

Fig. 66-6. A, Preoperative appearance of 16-year-old girl. **B,** Postoperative appearance 1 year after rhinoplasty. (From Peck, G. C.: Surgery of the nasal tip. In Masters, F. W., and Lewis, J. R., Jr., editors: Symposium on aesthetic surgery of the nose, ears, and chin, vol. 6, St. Louis, 1973, The C. V. Mosby Co.)

Mammaplasty

Reconstructive breast surgery may be done to replace breast tissue removed by surgery (p. 1469) or to improve the appearance of a woman's breasts. Some women develop conspicuously large and pendulous breasts that they wish to have reduced in size. Large breasts are embarrassing to some women and make it difficult for them to participate in sports, maintain good posture, and buy clothes that fit. Such women often respond to reconstructive surgery remarkably well (Fig. 66-7). Cosmetic surgery of the breast may also be done to make unusually small breasts larger (Fig. 66-8). A variety of plastic materials may be used for this procedure.

Reconstructive surgery of the breast is usually a major procedure and requires the use of general anesthesia. A variety of dressings are used postoperatively, and some of them restrict arm motion. The woman must be instructed not to use her arms to lift herself, since this strain on the pectoral girdle must be avoided. The nipples should be checked frequently for signs of vascular insufficiency, and either pallor or venous congestion of the nipples should be reported at once. The woman is advised to wear a firm, supporting brassiere both night

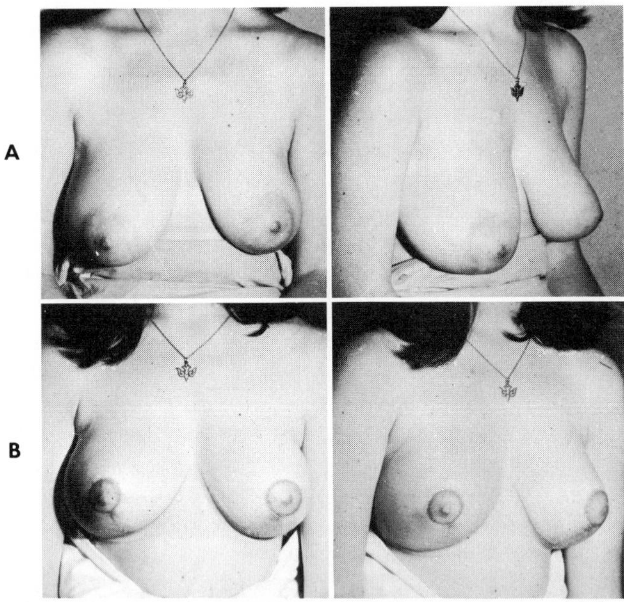

Fig. 66-7. Surgical correction of moderate degree of hypertrophy and ptosis in 20-year-old patient via nipple transposition procedure. **A,** Preoperative views. **B,** Postoperative views. (From Wise, R. J.: Surgical management of the hypertrophic breast. In Masters, F. W., and Lewis, J. R., Jr., editors: Symposium on aesthetic surgery of the face, eyelid, and breast, vol. 4, St. Louis, 1972, The C. V. Mosby Co.)

and day for several months after surgery. It is important that the fit be such that firm, constant support is provided when the patient is in the prone position. If the woman cannot make necessary adjustment in brassieres she already owns or cannot buy satisfactory ready-made brassieres, she may need to have some specially made. Large department stores usually provide this service.

□ General management of the person experiencing plastic surgery

Preoperative care

Emotional factors related to surgery. It is believed that any plastic surgery for an obvious defect is justified if it helps the person to feel he has a better chance for recognition among other persons. The plastic surgeon may reshape a nose or repair a deformed hand so that an emotionally stable person will have more assurance among others. However, it is foolish to assume that reconstructive surgery alone will correct a basic personality problem. Some people blame an apparently trivial physical defect for a long series of failures in their lives when the major defect lies within their personalities. Because of this possibility, the person is usually carefully studied before surgery is planned. It is necessary to know what the person expects the surgery to accomplish before the physician can decide whether such expectations are realistic and if surgery should be performed.

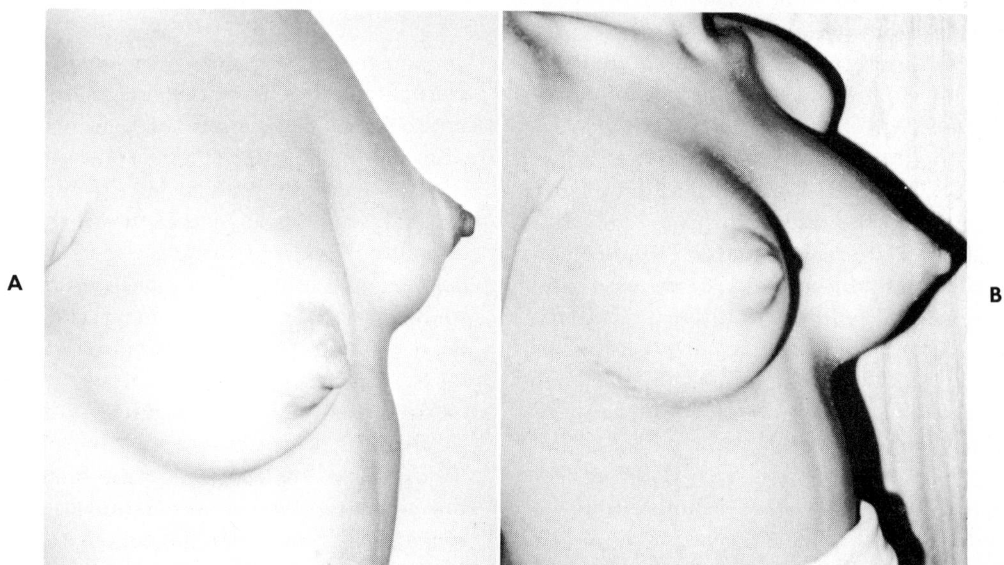

Fig. 66-8. A, Preoperative appearance of patient. **B,** Early postoperative appearance following augmentation with Silastic mammary prosthesis, new seamless design, medium size. (From Gerow, F. J.: Surgical management of micromastia. In Masters, F. W., and Lewis, J. R., Jr., editors: Symposium on aesthetic surgery of the face, eyelid, and breast, vol. 4, St. Louis, 1972, The C. V. Mosby Co.)

It is also necessary to learn about the social standards and cultural mores of the community in which the person lives and his adjustment to them. His economic contribution as a citizen and as a member of a family, his characteristic pattern in interpersonal relationships, and whether he has previously sought medical treatment for the particular problem should be assessed. The nurse and the social worker are often called on to assist the surgeon in his efforts to learn as much as possible about the patient. By observing and recording the patient's behavior at home, in school, in the clinic, on arrival at the hospital, and during preparation for surgery, the nurse can assist the surgeon in his study of the patient. Sometimes the help of specialists in psychology and psychiatry is sought.

Before surgery the surgeon will tell the patient what probably can be done and what changes are possible. It is important that the nurse know what the patient has been told so that misunderstandings and misinterpretations can be avoided. It must be repeatedly explained to him that the immediate results may not meet his expectations. The patient may become alarmed and discouraged if he has not been prepared for the normal appearance of skin grafts and reconstructed tissue immediately after surgery. Postoperative tissue reaction may distort normal contours, suture lines may be reddened, and the color of the newly transplanted skin may differ somewhat from that of surrounding skin. The appearance of the surgical area changes as the edema decreases and the suture line becomes less reddened and indurated. Six months after surgery the scar will be less noticeable than at 6 days or 6 weeks postoperatively.

The patient who is admitted to the hospital for plastic surgery may have extensive scarring and deformity and may be exceedingly sensitive to scrutiny by the people he encounters. On the other hand, the patient may have little apparent deformity, and it may be difficult to understand why the patient wishes to have surgery. The nurse cannot possibly know what the disfigurement means to the individual patient and should avoid judging whether surgery is necessary. Nurses may be inclined to concentrate their efforts on the more physically ill patients. Yet it is important for nurses to learn about each patient who is to have plastic surgery and to assure him of their interest.

Diet. The patient should be in the best possible physical condition before plastic surgery. A diet high in protein and vitamins prior to elective surgery is thought to help in the "take" or healing of a graft. Hemoglobin and clotting times are usually determined, and the blood protein level is assayed because a normal blood protein level has been found necessary for satisfactory growth of grafted tissue.

Care of operative site. The wound that is to receive the graft must be free from infections that would delay healing, lead to more scar tissue formation, or cause death of the graft. Infection is treated by the administration of antibiotics and by the use of warm soaks and compresses. A sterile physiologic solution of sodium chloride is the solution most often used. Before skin grafting is attempted, any dead tissue that is adherent to the wound is removed by debridement; otherwise this tissue will interfere with the graft's healing.

The *donor site* (the area from which skin is to be taken) is washed with a germicidal soap the evening before surgery, and this cleansing may be repeated the morning of operation. Frequently the site is shaved in the operating room after the patient is anesthetized so that the damage of cutting the skin is minimized. Strong antiseptics are avoided because they may irritate the skin. If the *recipient site* (the area that is to receive the graft) is not an open wound, it is cleansed in the same way.

Postoperative care

In addition to general supportive care of any patient who has had surgery, the nurse has special responsibilities necessary to assure the success of the plastic surgery procedure. Maintaining pressure dressings as requested, preventing infection of grafted areas, and applying compresses to stimulate circulation to the graft all require meticulous nursing attention.

Care of the wound (recipient site). A graft must be in constant contact with the underlying tissue in order to attach itself and to grow. Anything that comes between the undersurface of the graft and the recipient area such as a discharge caused by infection, excess serous fluid, or blood will float the graft away from close contact and may cause it to die. To prevent floating, some surgeons insert the drains at strategic spots along the edges of the graft, or a small catheter is inserted on the edge of the graft under the recipient skin and attached to suction to remove the fluid.

If the recipient site is a clean wound with no infection, the graft usually is sutured with many fine sutures to hold it in place and in contact with the normal skin adjacent to it. If the recipient site is known to be infected, only a few scattered sutures, if any, may be used, and the grafted site may not be dressed. The area is inspected frequently to see if the skin is adhering to the underlying tissue. If fluid collects under the skin graft, it is removed by aspiration with a sterile needle and syringe or the fluid is rolled to the wound edge with a sterile applicator.

A wide variety of materials are used as dressings. The choice depends on the kind of graft and the surgeon's preference. Petrolatum, Furacin, Adaptic gauze, or Telfa dressings are often selected. Silver foil may also be used. Often the graft is covered with a piece of coarse-mesh gauze that is anchored to the adjacent skin edges

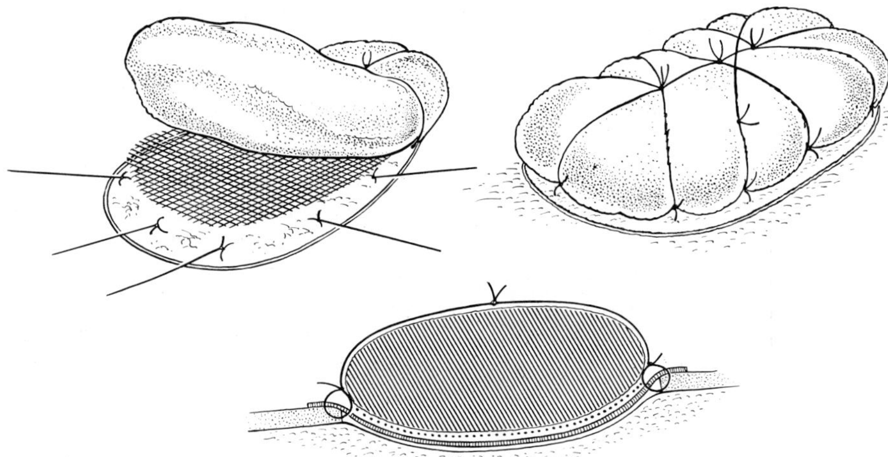

Fig. 66-9. Tieover dressing used as pressure dressing on skin graft. (Modified from McGregor, I. A.: Fundamental techniques of plastic surgery and their surgical applications, ed. 4, Baltimore, 1969, The Williams & Wilkins Co.)

with an elastic bandage (Elastoplast) to give firm, gentle pressure and to immobilize the area. The first dressing may be covered with a compress of sterile normal saline solution. Because the compress is moist, it fits the contour of the wound better. Continuous pressure is necessary to keep the graft adherent to the recipient bed, but pressure should not be so firm as to cause death of the graft. Marine sponges, rubber sponges, cotton pads, and mechanic's waste may be applied as outer dressings by the surgeon to provide the desired amount of pressure. Occasionally the sutures anchoring the graft at the skin edges are left uncut and brought over a pressure dressing to hold it firmly against the graft (Fig. 66-9). The graft site is elevated when possible and protected from pressure and motion. The nurse should be certain that dressings do not become loosened so that pressure is reduced and that the patient *does not lie on these dressings* or in any other way increase the pressure on them. When flap grafts are used, slings and casts may assure immobilization and help to keep parts of the body in the correct relationship for healing (Fig. 66-10).

Some surgeons believe that grafts are stimulated in their effort to establish blood supply by the use of *warm, moist compresses*, and sterile normal saline solution is usually ordered for this purpose. The greatest care must be taken that infection is not introduced when compresses are being changed and moistened. Hands must be washed before dressings are handled or compresses changed. Meticulous technique is followed so that infection does not occur. Care is taken so that the newly grafted skin is not traumatized. The temperature of the compress solution should not be over 40.5 C (105 F), and compresses should be applied with sterile forceps. Com-

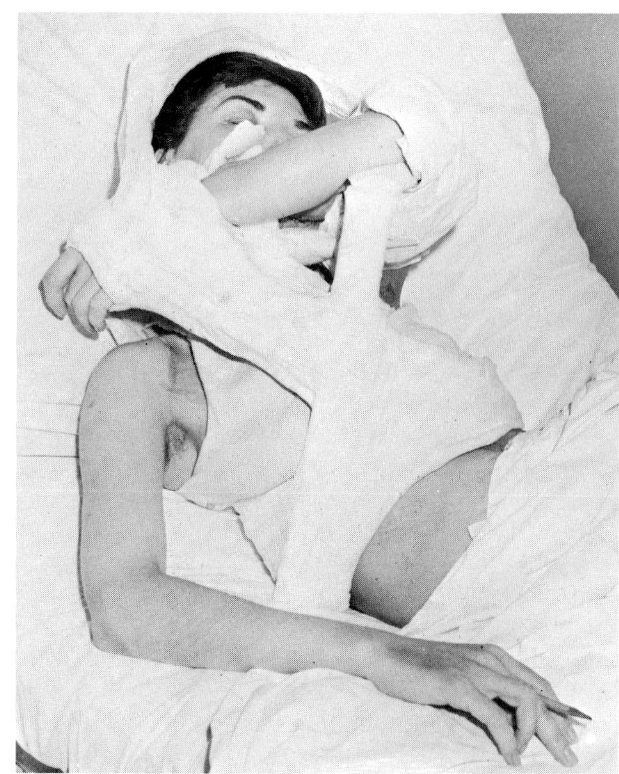

Fig. 66-10. Plastic operations sometimes require patient to be in extremely awkward positions. Eating, mouth hygiene, and communicating with others are problems in caring for this patient. Note pencil used for communicating.

presses may sometimes be covered with a sterile petroleum jelly dressing and moistened by gently directing fluid from a sterile Asepto syringe under the edge of the dressings. Sterile tubes with tiny openings (Dakin's tubes) may also be placed through the outer compresses to provide a means of moistening the inner dressings without disturbing them and without introducing infection.

The patient may be placed on an oscillating bed in order to improve circulation to the graft as well as to help prevent circulatory complications such as thrombophlebitis. Some physicians prescribe vasodilating drugs such as tolazoline hydrochloride (Priscolin), nicotinic acid, papaverine hydrochloride, and alcohol in a further attempt to produce vasodilation at the recipient site.

The patient frequently needs support when he sees the operative site for the first time. The nurse is present when dressings are removed and assesses the reaction of the patient so that immediate and future nursing intervention can be planned and implemented. If it is not possible to remove all mirrors to prevent the patient from inspecting the results of facial surgery, dressings may be left on longer than necessary to cover wounds. Members of the patient's family should also know what to expect so that they will not be unduly worried and so that they can give support to the patient if apprehension occurs.

Inner dressings on the recipient site are changed by the surgeon 1 to 2 days after surgery, and it is usually possible to know then whether the result of the operation is satisfactory. Sutures may be removed at this time. When a dressing is no longer necessary, lanolin or cold cream may be applied to the donor site to relieve dryness and discomfort.

Care of the donor site. When split-thickness grafts have been used, the donor site (often the anterior surface of the thigh) may be a greater source of discomfort to the patient than the recipient site. A Telfa dressing or Furacin petrolatum gauze may be applied to the area and then protected by a firm outer dressing, which is anchored with an Elastoplast bandage that does not encircle the thigh lest it hamper circulation. Or the dressing is secured by wrapping the leg with Kerlix or an elastic bandage. Some plastic surgeons remove the outer dressing in 2 days and others wait 2 weeks. The patient has intense pain for a short period when the outer dressing is removed from the donor site.

Another method of treatment is to cover the area with one firm layer of gauze anchored firmly at the edges and leave it exposed to the air. It is believed by some surgeons that healing occurs faster with this method and that there is less danger of death of the deeper skin layer, which must develop the new outer skin layer. If this open method is used, the patient must be supervised carefully so that he does not injure the donor site, since this will cause severe pain. A heat lamp may be used to hasten drying of the donor site. A bed cradle is used to prevent pressure from bedclothes and to allow the donor site to be exposed to the air. Analgesic drugs such as dextropropoxyphene hydrochloride (Darvon), acetylsalicylic acid (aspirin), meperidine hydrochloride (Demerol), and pentazocine (Talwin) may be needed for pain and should not be withheld during the first few days postoperatively.

Cast care after plastic surgery. The general care of the patient with a cast is similar to that of patients with casts following other types of surgery (p. 857). The cast is applied in this case to support a graft. Immediately after application and frequently thereafter the cast must be examined for cracks or breaks that will interfere with support for the graft, and it must be carefully checked to make certain that no excessive pressure is being exerted. Pillows can be used to give support and to lessen strain on body parts.

One major difference in cast care following plastic surgery is that the patient is sometimes placed in very awkward positions, especially after pedicle flap surgery (Fig. 66-1). Arrangements should be made for the patient to see what goes on around him. Sometimes this is made possible by changing his position in bed or the position of the bed in the room. In some instances putting the patient "head to foot" in the bed is helpful. A mirror may be attached to the bed and arranged at such an angle that the patient can see at least a part of the room if his head, neck, and shoulder movements are restricted by a cast.

Care after dermabrasion. If the patient has had a general anesthetic, he must be turned to his side to prevent the dressing from becoming wet or contaminated in the event of vomiting or excessive salivation. The dressing is checked for signs of bleeding, and the patient must be observed for signs of respiratory embarrassment, which may be caused by pressure from the dressing. A pressure dressing usually is removed after 48 hours, and the patient is discharged to return to the physician's office or the clinic. Washing the face and shaving are seldom permitted until all the crusts have fallen away, but some physicians permit the person to wash his face gently with a mild soap as soon as the dressing has been removed. If the person's face feels dry after healing has occurred, gentle lubrication with substances such as cold cream usually is advised.

Long-term care

Persons requiring successive surgeries or prolonged inactivity need support to continue the planned therapies and preventive measures to ensure normal muscle and joint function (Chapter 41).

Outcome criteria for the person having plastic surgery

The patient or significant others can:

1. Explain the treatment program:
   a. Care of the wound and donor site.
   b. Care of the cast (if applicable).
2. Describe the need for follow-up care.

REFERENCES AND SELECTED READINGS

1. Baker, T. J., and Garden, H. L.: Chemical face peeling and dermabrasion, Surg. Clin. North Am. **51**:387-402, 1971.
2. Bergersen, B. S.: Pharmacology in nursing, ed. 13, St. Louis, 1976, The C. V. Mosby Co.
3. Converse, J. M., editor: Reconstruction plastic surgery: principles and procedures in correction, reconstruction and transplantation, ed. 2, Philadelphia, 1977, W. B. Saunders Co.
4. Cronin, T. D., and Brauer, R. O.: Augmentation mammoplasty, Surg. Clin. North Am. **51**:441-452, 1971.
5. Dison, N.: Clinical nursing techniques, ed. 3, St. Louis, 1975, The C. V. Mosby Co.
6. Fitzpatrick, T. B., et al.: Dermatology in general medicine, New York, 1971, McGraw-Hill Book Co.
7. Griesmer, R.: How emotional trauma causes skin problems, Medical Insights, Dec. 1971.
8. Griesmer, R.: How skin problems cause emotional complications, Medical Insights, Nov. 1971.
9. Grossman, A. R.: Augmentation mammaplasty, Springfield, Ill., 1976, Charles C Thomas, Publisher.
10. Hardy, J. D., editor: Textbook of surgery: principles and practice, ed. 5, Philadelphia, 1977, J. B. Lippincott Co.
11. Hurwitz, A.: About faces, Am. J. Nurs. **71**:2168-2171, 1971.
12. Jones, F. A.: The skin—a mirror of the gut, Geriatrics **28**:75-81, 1973.
13. *Kinmont, P. D.: Pruritus as a dermatological problem, Practitioner **208**:622-632, 1972.
14. Korting, G. W.: Diseases of the skin in children and adolescents, Philadelphia, 1970, W. B. Saunders Co.
15. Leider, M.: Some principles of dermatologic nursing, RN **35**:48-53, 1972.
16. Lewis, G. M., and Clayton, E. W.: Practical dermatology, ed. 3, Philadelphia, 1967, W. B. Saunders Co.
17. *Macgregor, F. C.: Selection of cosmetic surgery patients, Surg. Clin. North Am. **51**:289-298, 1971.
18. *Management of common skin problems, Postgrad. Med. **52**:63-194, 1972.
19. Marlow, D. R.: Textbook of pediatric nursing, ed. 5, Philadelphia, 1977, W. B. Saunders Co.
20. Mathews, K. P.: A current view of urticaria, Med. Clin. North Am. **58**:185-205, 1974.
21. McGregor, I. A.: Fundamental techniques of plastic surgery, ed. 6, Baltimore, 1975, The Williams & Wilkins Co.
22. *Miller, S. H.: Breast reconstruction following mastectomy, A.O.R.N. J. **25**:945-952, 1977.
23. Parrish, J.: Dermatology and skin care, New York, 1975, McGraw-Hill Book Co.
24. Pillsbury, D. M.: A manual of dermatology, Philadelphia, 1971, W. B. Saunders Co.
25. Rees, T. D., editor: Cosmetic surgery, Surg. Clin. North Am. **51**:265-531, 1971.
26. Rees, T. D., and Wood-Smith, D.: Cosmetic facial surgery, Philadelphia, 1973, W. B. Saunders Co.
27. Rhoads, J. E., et al.: Surgery: principles and practice, ed. 5, Philadelphia, 1977, J. B. Lippincott Co.
28. Robin, M.: How emotions affect skin problems in school children, J. Sch. Heath **43**:370-373, 1973.
29. *Rosillo, R. H. Welty, M. J., and Graham, W. P. III: The patient with maxillofacial cancer: psychological aspects, Nurs. Clin. North Am. **8**:153-158, 1973.
30. Rowell, N.: Urticaria, Practitioner **208**:614-621, 1972.
31. *Ruppe, J. P.: Skin infections: their role in health today, J. Sch. Health **43**:373-380, 1973.
32. Sabiston, D. C, editor: Davis-Christopher textbook of surgery, ed. 11, Philadelphia, 1977, W. B. Saunders Co.
33. Saitoh, M., Uzuka, M., and Sakamoto, M.: Human hair cycle, J. Invest. Dermatol. **54**:65-61, 1970.
34. Sauer, G. C.: Manual of skin diseases, ed. 3, Philadelphia, 1973, J. B. Lippincott Co.
35. *Shapiro, C. S., Johnson, J., Vincent, M., et al.: Nursing care of the cleft-lip/cleft-palate child, RN **36**:46-60, 1973.
36. Shelley, W. B.: Consultations in dermatology, Philadelphia, 1972, W. B. Saunders Co.
37. *Tierney, E. A.: Accepting disfigurement when death is the alternative, Am. J. Nurs. **75**:2149-2150, 1975.
38. *Welty, M. J., Graham, W. P. III, and Rosillo, R. H.: The patient with maxillofacial cancer: surgical treatment and nursing care, Nurs. Clin. North Am. **8**:137-151, 1973.
39. Williams, S. R.: Nutrition and diet therapy, ed. 3, St. Louis, 1977, The C. V. Mosby Co.
40. Wood-Smith, D., and Porowski, P. C., editors: Nursing care of the plastic surgery patient, St. Louis, 1967, The C. V. Mosby Co.
41. Woods, J. E., and Payne, W. S.: Contour restoration following simple or modified radical mastectomy, J.A.M.A. **235**:1588-1589, 1976.

*References preceded by an asterisk are particularly well suited for student reading.

67

Management of the person with burns

CATHERINE O'MALLEY

Burns are wounds caused by excessive exposure of the body to heat. The most common cause of burns is fire, which kills 12,000 and scars and injures 300,000 Americans each year, including 50,000 persons who must be hospitalized for periods of 6 weeks to 2 years. Many of these deaths could have been prevented. Other causes of burns include scalding water, electricity, chemicals, radiation, and other rays such as x-rays. Knowledge, patience, and understanding are needed in the nursing care of severely burned persons during the acute and the long-term recovery phases. Principles of burn care remain the same regardless of etiology.

■ CLASSIFICATION OF BURNS

Burns are classified as first, second, and third degree, depending on their depth. First- and second-degree burns are classified are *partial-thickness* burns, whereas third-degree burns are *full-thickness* burns (Fig. 67-1). A *first-degree* burn is one in which the outer layer of skin is injured and reddened without blister formation; mild sunburn is a good example. A *second-degree* burn injures all of the epidermis and much of the corium. Blister formation is characteristic, and there is usually considerable subcutaneous edema. The deeper layers of the corium are not destroyed and regeneration can occur. First-degree and second-degree burns are likely to be painful because nerve endings have been injured and exposed. During the healing phase the person experiences dryness and itching caused by increased vascularization, destruction of sebaceous glands, and decreased perspiration.

A *third-degree* burn is one in which all layers of skin are destroyed, thus making regeneration impossible. Nerves, muscles, bone, and blood supply also may be injured or destroyed in third-degree burns. Nerves are destroyed, resulting in a painless wound. The destroyed tissue will be unable to epithelialize; therefore these areas must be covered either by skin growing from normal skin around the edges of the burned area, by scar tissue, or by skin grafts. Skin grafting is preferred for its aesthetic advantages.

■ PHYSIOLOGIC CHANGES OCCURRING IN SEVERE BURNS

As a result of burns, normal skin function is diminished, resulting in physiologic alterations. These include (1) loss of protective barriers against infection, (2) escape of body fluids, (3) lack of temperature control, (4) destroyed sweat and sebaceous glands, and (5) a diminished number of sensory receptors. The severity of these alterations will depend on the extent of the burn and the depth to which damage has occurred.

Increased knowledge of the physiologic changes that occur during severe burns has led to the saving of many lives. There are three stages that occur following *severe* burns: the immediate hypovolemic stage, the diuretic stage, and the long-term rehabilitative stage.

□ Hypovolemic stage

The hypovolemic stage begins from the time of the burn and lasts for the first 48 to 72 hours. It is characterized by a rapid *shift of fluid* from the vascular compartments into the interstitial spaces. When tissues are burned, vasodilation, increased capillary permeability, and changes in the permeability of tissue cells in and around the burn area occur. As a result, abnormally large amounts of extracellular fluid, sodium chloride, and protein pass into the burned area to cause blister formation and local edema or escape through the open wound. Visible fluid loss makes up only a small part of the fluid lost from the circulating blood and other essential fluid compartments. Most of the fluid loss occurs deep in the wound, where the fluid extravasates into the deeper tissues. Burns of areas such as highly vascular muscle tissue or the face are believed to cause greater fluid shift than comparable burns of other parts of the body. Fully one-

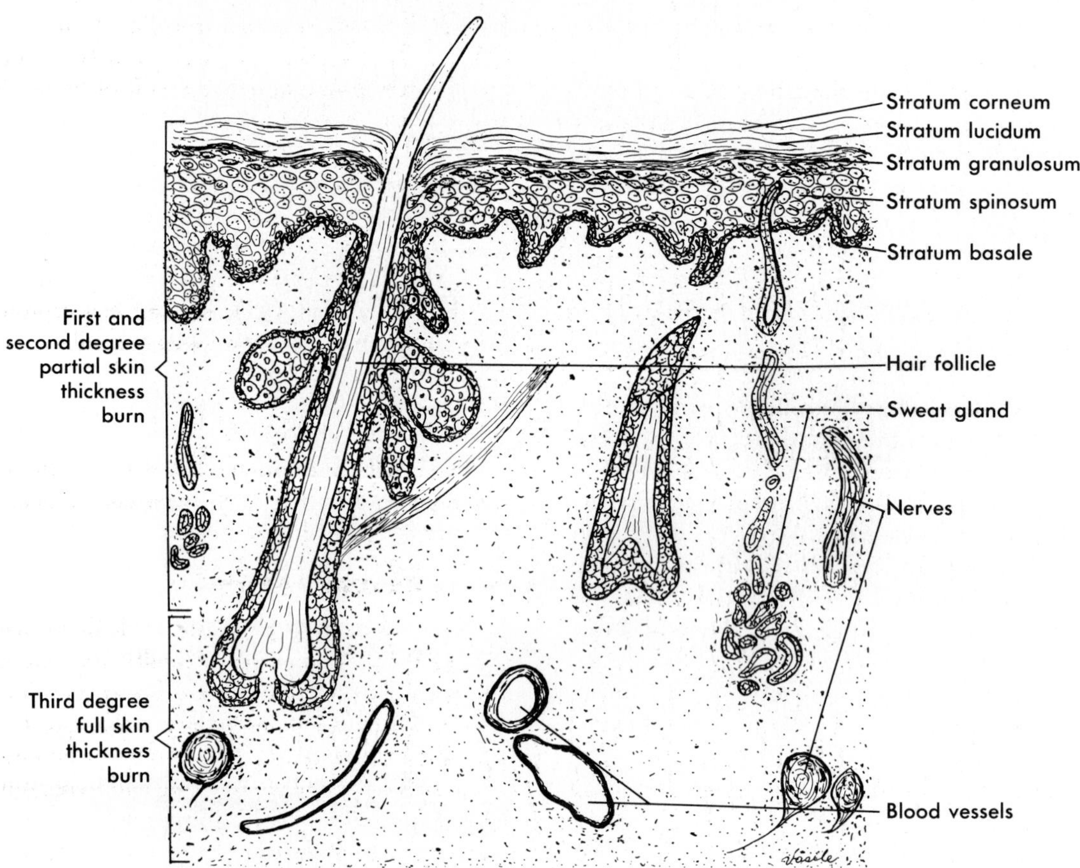

Fig. 67-1. Levels of human skin involved in burns.

half of the extracellular fluid of the body can shift from its normal distribution to the site of a severe burn. The extracellular fluid constitutes about 20% of the body weight. Three-fourths of it surrounds the cells, and one-fourth is found in blood plasma (see Table 67-1). For a person weighing 68 kg (150 pounds), this means that from 4.5 to 6.5 kg or from 5 to 7.5 liters of fluids may be removed from the interstitial spaces and bloodstream. Hypovolemic shock occurs, resulting in a tremendous drop in blood pressure and inadequate blood flow through the kidneys, which in turn leads to further shock anuria, and death within a short time if treatment is not given promptly or is inadequate.

Dehydration of the nondamaged tissue cells may result. More fluids and sodium are lost initially from the capillaries than is protein. This increases the capillary osmotic pressure, leading to dehydration even though edema is present in the burned area. As protein continues to be lost into the burned area because of the increased capillary permeability, *hypoproteinemia* results. The increased amount of protein in the tissue spaces is a further contributing factor to edema formation. Proteins may be lost through the open wound and nitrogen is lost through the kidney from catabolism, leading to a significant negative nitrogen balance. The blood urea nitrogen (BUN) is elevated when oliguria is present.

Table 67-1. Approximate division of total body fluid into compartments*

Body fluid compartments	Liters of fluid	
	Lean adult weighing 45 kg	Lean adult weighing 68 kg
Intravascular (plasma)	2.8	4.2
Interstitial	8.4	12.5
Intracellular	22.3	33.3
TOTAL	33.5	50.0

*Note that the smaller the individual, the less fluid he has in each compartment and that plasma is reduced most markedly with decrease in size. The normal size and body type of the individual are considered when fluid replacement is ordered.

With loss of fluid from the vascular system,

hemoconcentration occurs and the hematocrit rises. Blood flow becomes sluggish in the burned area and cellular nutrition decreases. Large numbers of red blood cells become trapped in the burned area and are hemolyzed. Renal damage and hematuria may occur as a result of reduced blood volume and passage of the end products of the hemolyzed cells through the glomeruli. The decreased renal blood flow leads to *oliguria*.

Electrolyte imbalances also occur. *Hyperkalemia* (excessive serum potassium) results from injury to the tissue cells and red blood cells, and from the diminished urinary output, and may lead to heart block and ventricular failure. Potassium may be encouraged to move back into the cells by the administration of insulin, since potassium is transported back into the cells along with glucose. Sodium is retained by the body as a result of the endocrine response to stress. Aldosterone is increased, leading to sodium reabsorption by the kidney. This sodium, however, quickly passes into the interstitial spaces of the burn area with the fluid shift; therefore despite the increased amount of sodium in the body, most of the sodium is trapped in the edema fluid, and a *sodium deficit* occurs. Inadequate tissue perfusion results in anaerobic metabolism and the acid end products are retained because of the decreased kidney function. *Metabolic acidosis* may then occur.

Respiratory distress may result from burns of the airway or from the effects of hypovolemic shock. Most airway burns are of the upper airway, since this is where incoming air is normally cooled and humidified.[19]

□ Diuretic stage

The diuretic stage begins about 48 to 72 hours after the person was burned, and the changes may occur rapidly. A *fluid shift* occurs in the opposite direction from the initial stage, and the edema fluid returns to the vascular system. Blood volume increases, leading to increased renal blood flow and diuresis unless renal damage has occurred. Serum electrolyte and hematocrit levels will be decreased because of the *hemodilution*. Fluid overload may occur if fluids from intravenous therapy and fluids returning from the interstitial spaces exceed urine production. In some persons, however, fluid lost in the urine is greater than the fluids being returned to the vascular system, and *dehydration* may result. Sodium is lost with diuresis, and a *sodium deficit* may occur. *Hypokalemia* results from potassium moving back into the cells or being excreted in the urine. Protein continues to be lost from the wounds. *Metabolic acidosis* remains a possibility because of the loss of sodium bicarbonate in the urine and the increased fat metabolism secondary to a decreased carbohydrate intake.

Following the period of fluid shifts, the patient remains acutely ill. This period is characterized by anemia and malnutrition. *Anemia* develops from the loss of red blood cells. *Negative nitrogen balance* begins at the onset of the burn and is the result of tissue destruction, protein loss, and the stress response. It continues throughout the acute period and is secondary to continued loss of protein from the wound, from tissue catabolism resulting from immobility, and from decreased protein intake. *Hypovitaminosis* may also occur from the decreased intake of vitamins. Increased metabolism from loss of water and heat from the wound, loss of fluid during diuresis, and catabolism during tissue breakdown lead to *weight loss*.

□ Rehabilitative stage

The rehabilitative stage begins when the burned area is reduced to less than 20% of the body surface. The person is now in an anabolic phase.

■ PREVENTION OF BURNS

Nurses can help prevent accidental burns from occurring by participating in health education programs that stress fire prevention and the consequences of fires such as burns, deformities, and death, and by promoting legislation that would control some of people's thoughtless practices and make working and living environments safer. Community health nurses are in an unusually advantageous position to recognize unsafe practices in the home and to help families develop safe habits of living.

Approximately 80% of accidental burns occur in the home and primarily are caused by ignorance, carelessness, and curiosity of children. Infants and children are the most common victims of fires in and about the home. Young children should be supervised in their play and should never be left at home alone. Children should be taught at an early age about the hazards of fire. Parents must carefully check play areas for all fire hazards such as live extension wires, matches, and unprotected floor heaters and should remove them. Serious burns to children often result from pot handles that project beyond the stove top, or appliance cords within the reach of toddlers. A large number of children have been burned to death or permanently disabled or disfigured by fireworks. Legislation in many states now prohibits the sale of fireworks, but violations of the law and accidents still occur.

A high incidence of burn injuries affecting adults are related to accidents while cooking or smoking or otherwise using matches. Burns commonly occur when the person is distracted while cooking or falls asleep while smoking. Elimination of smoking completely may provide a safer as well as more healthful society. Activities persons were engaged in when they caught on fire in their homes are shown in Table 67-2.

Each year brings increased demand for careful in-

Table 67-2. Activity of persons burned by fire*

Playing with matches/lighter	175	11.3†
Smoking	152	10.0
Using matches/lighter	116	7.5
Fell asleep while smoking	100	6.4
Reaching across stove	86	5.5
Sleeping	77	5.0
Standing too close to stove	64	4.1
Leaning against stove	47	3.0

*From Flammable fabric investigations, Washington, D.C., 1973, Department of Health, Education, and Welfare, Food and Drug Administration, Bureau of Product Safety, FY66-FY72.
†Percent based on 1,554 cases in which activity is known.

spection and regulation of places in which the ill and infirm are housed. Aged persons frequently are housed in old and poorly equipped structures, and many of them have been burned to death. Nurses can bring necessary pressures to bear to ensure adequate protection and planned evacuation should a fire occur. Attention is being focused on places where large numbers of people congregate. Laws require that doors in public buildings be hinged to swing outward, that draperies and decorations be fireproof, and that stairways with special fire doors be used in new apartment buildings and hotels. Nurses working in institutions need to encourage and participate in fire prevention programs.

Rigid enforcement of laws requiring that industrial products be labeled when known to be flammable and that new products be tested carefully for their flammable qualities before being placed on the market is further evidence of government effort to protect the public from accident by fire. Industry can be made safer by constant vigilance by management in cooperation with fire safety officers and health care professionals to identify hazards and implement a safety program. All chemicals should be labeled, and antidotes identified and available. A core of every work force should be versed in emergency treatment of all types of burns for the protection of every employee.

Sunburn should be cautioned against, as even a relatively mild first-degree burn of a large part of the body can cause change of fluid distribution and kidney damage. Camp nurses should keep this in mind in their educational programs for children and camp counselors.

■ INTERVENTION

□ Comprehensive team approach

Comprehensive care of the burn patient can best be provided by a multidisciplinary team approach. This is a desirable method designed to meet the complex and varied needs of the patient. The nurse's role in the team is to coordinate the interactions of the various disciplines and to incorporate the team's suggestions and approaches into an effective plan of care. Because this type of care is most likely to be available in specialized burn units and centers, patients are frequently moved to these units when it is safe to transport them. When such specialized care is not available, the nurse may be able to serve as a catalyst and suggest the active involvement of as many disciplines as are available in the care of the patient.

□ Immediate care

Prehospitalization emergency care

If flame is involved and clothing is on fire, the victim's first reaction is to run, which only fans the flame. Rolling the burning person in a blanket on the ground to exclude oxygen, thereby putting out the fire, is one of the best procedures. The person whose clothing is aflame should never stand, since this increases the danger of inhalation burns in which heat and smoke are drawn into the lungs.

Once all flame is extinguished, it is important that the burning agent be removed and the wound cooled. Clothing and gross debris are carefully removed, avoiding the removal of any clothing that adheres to the burned area. Tepid water (or saline if available) is used in copious amounts until the wound is cool to the touch. Once the wound is cooled, the victim may be wrapped for transport to a medical facility.

Chemicals should be identified, and unless the action of the chemical is enhanced by water, excessive flushing with water is initiated. As much as 20 to 30 minutes of continuous flushing may be necessary to assure complete removal of the destructive agent. Burns occurring about the eyes should also be lavaged with copious amounts of cool, clean water, and if the burn was caused by acids, the procedure should be repeated in 10 to 15 minutes.

Persons who are burned on the face and neck or those who have inhaled flame, steam, or smoke should be observed closely for signs of laryngeal edema and airway obstruction. Data indicating potential or existing airway burns include singed nasal hair, burns of the mouth or throat, brassy-sounding or sooty cough, and respiratory distress. Immediate arrangements should be made to transport these patients to a hospital or burn center if one is available (see Table 67-3 for a list of burn centers). Often burns are more severe than they first appear to be. Thus all persons with burns, even if the burns appear to be superficial, should be seen by a physician. The hospital or burn center should be notified, so that preparations can be made for the arrival of the patient, since a well-prepared and well-equipped team of personnel is needed to care for the severely burned person.

While awaiting transportation to a medical facility,

Table 67-3. Burn units and centers in the United States*

Location	Physician(s) in charge	Hospital(s)	Bed capacity (no.)	Annual admissions (no.)
Chicago, Ill.	John Boswick, M.D.; Nelson Stone, M.D.	Cook County Hospital	35	425
San Antonio, Tex.	Basil Pruitt, Col. M.C.	U.S. Army Surgical Research Unit, Brooke Army Medical Center	60	390
Cincinnati, Ohio	Bruce MacMillan, M.D.; Robert Hummel, M.D.	Shrine Burns Institute, Cincinnati General Hospital	55	325
Los Angeles, Calif.	John Winkley, M.D.	Los Angeles County General Hospital	30	325
Galveston, Tex.	Duane Larson, M.D.; Stephen Lewis, M.D.	Shrine Burns Insitute, John Sealey Hospital	30	300
Boston, Mass.	Oliver Cope, M.D.	Shrine Burns Institute, Massachusetts General Hospital	30	225
Milwaukee, Wis.	George Collentine, M.D.	St. Mary's Hospital	30	225
Richmond, Va.	B. W. Haynes, M.D.	Medical College of Virginia Hospital	36	220
Dallas, Tex.	Charles Baxter, M.D.	Parkland Memorial Hospital	12	200
Atlanta, Ga.	H. Harlan Stone, M.D.	Grady Memorial Hospital, Emory University Hospital	25	180
Brooklyn, N.Y.	I. C. Song, M.D.; Bertram Bromberg, M.D.	King's County Hospital	6	175
Ann Arbor, Mich.	Irving Feller, M.D.	University of Michigan Medical Center, St. Joseph Mercy Hospital	14	150
Mobile, Ala.	John Crosby, M.D.; Byron Green, M.D.	Mobile General Hospital	8	150
St. Paul, Minn.	James Lafeve, M.D.	St. Paul Ramsey Hospital	10	150
Akron, Ohio	Clifford Boeckman, M.D.	Children's Hospital of Akron	14	140
Houston, Tex.	Melvin Spira, M.D.	Ben Taub General Hospital	12	140
Columbus, Ohio	E. Thomas Boles, M.D.	Children's Hospital	20	125
Orange, Calif.	Irving Rappaport, M.D.	Orange County Medical Center	8	125
Tulsa, Okla.	Frank Clingan, M.D.	Hillcrest Medical Center	10	125
Albany, N.Y.	Mark Wong, M.D.	Albany Medical Center	10	120
Detroit, Mich.	James Lloyd, M.D.	Children's Hospital	11	120
Cleveland, Ohio	Richard Fratianne, M.D.	Cleveland Metropolitan General Hospital	15	115
New York, N.Y.	Ronald Ollstein, M.D.; George Crikelair, M.D.	Harlem Hospital Center	20	100
Phoenix, Ariz.	William Price, M.D.	Maricopa County General Hospital	9	100

*Modified from Feller, I., and Crane, C. H.: J.A.M.A. **215**:463-464, 1971.

the burned person should be kept quiet and lying down. Exposed burned surfaces should be covered with sterile dressings or with the cleanest material available, such as clean sheets. These coverings may be soaked in cool water to ease the pain, reduce the edema, and prevent evaporation of body water. Ice should be avoided because sudden vasoconstriction causes severe shifting of fluid. *Oils, salves, and ointments should not be used on burns*, since these materials hamper treatment. Pain in extensive burns is best controlled by gentle and minimal handling and by the application of dressings to exclude air from the burned skin surfaces. Occasionally deep, third-degree burns are almost painless, since nerve endings have been destroyed, and for the first few minutes the person may appear not too badly affected. A burn should never be underestimated. In most cases, however, first- and second-degree burns will accompany third-degree burns, causing discomfort to the person.

Since the extent of the burn is extremely difficult to determine, if there is any question, no fluids should be given until a medical estimate can be made. For obviously small burns, fluids may be given with caution.

Large burns are frequently accompanied by sluggish peristalsis. To prevent aspiration, nothing should be given by mouth if the person is nauseated or vomiting.

Inpatient immediate care

Assessment. On arrival at the hospital, any of the remaining clothes of the patient are removed and the patient's condition is assessed. Respiratory status is evaluated first and immediate treatment initiated as indicated. Vital signs are taken for baseline data and for identification of hypovolemic shock. *The patient should be weighed.* This measurement will be used to determine fluid therapy and to evaluate progress. Venous and arterial blood samples are taken to determine protein, electrolyte, red blood cell, pH, and blood gas levels.

Determination of the severity of the burn, its treatment, and the prognosis of the patient is dependent on (1) the presence of preexisting conditions such as cardiac, pulmonary, renal, and hepatic disease, and injuries sustained during burn trauma such as fractures or internal injuries; (2) the area of the body that is burned (burns of the hands, feet, face, neck, and most joint surfaces may produce the most serious loss of function and the most conspicuous disfigurement); and (3) the degree and depth of tissue injury.

The severity of the burn is assessed by the percentage of body surface involved and the depth of the burn wound. For adults, the "rule of nines" is used (Fig. 67-2). These calculations are modified for infants and children under 10 years of age because of their relatively larger heads and smaller extremities. (See pediatric textbooks for these figures.) The age of the patient is important in estimating the severity of the burn. Infants tolerate burns poorly, and the mortality in this group is high, even with small burns. In burns involving up to 30% of the body surface in older children and in adults under the age of 50, the mortality rate is quite low. As the age of the patient increases beyond 50, the mortality rate rises even in burns of less than 30%.[2]

Immediate treatment. Rapid and efficient care can be provided by anticipation of patient needs and supplying organized admission areas to treat burns. If any respiratory distress is present, an airway should be established. Prophylactic intubation should be initiated if any heat or smoke has been inhaled, or if the head, neck, or face are involved (Fig. 67-3). Inhalation injuries are best managed with controlled ventilation as swelling of the upper airway can progress to obstruction. Endotracheal intubation is preferred over a tracheostomy because edema of the respiratory passages frequently subsides within a few days and avoidance of surgical trauma is desired. Depending on the severity of symptoms, emergency treatment may include oxygen, suctioning, and postural drainage.

Oral fluids should be withheld and a nasogastric tube is usually inserted as fluids via this method help to prevent paralytic ileus. A Foley catheter is also inserted so that there can be accurate monitoring of urinary output. A central venous line will be required to permit fluid

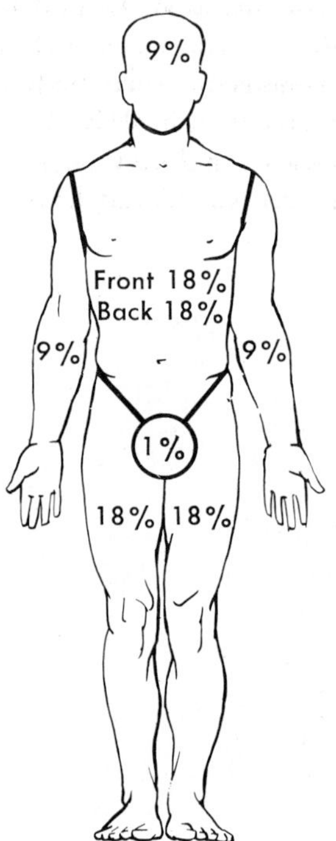

Fig. 67-2. "Rule of nines" is used to estimate amount of skin surface burned.

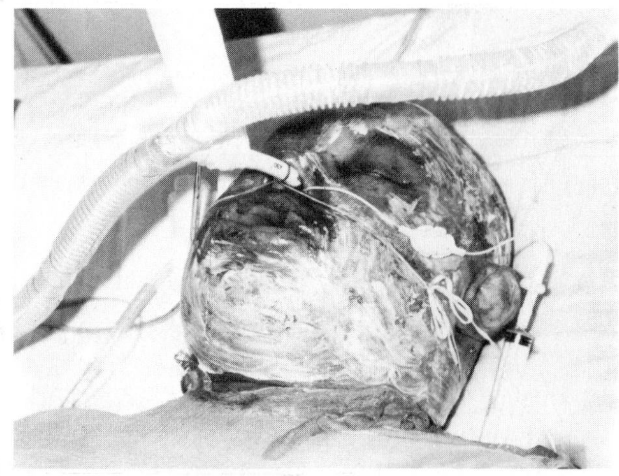

Fig. 67-3. Patient with severe edema 5 hours after burn occurred. Airway was managed with endotracheal intubation. Edema subsided and patient was extubated 4 days after admission. (Courtesy Burn Center, Cleveland Metropolitan General Hospital, Cleveland, Ohio.)

replacement and monitoring of fluid volume. Morphine sulfate or meperidine hydrochloride is often given intravenously to the patient with an extensive burn. The intravenous route is used because of inadequate absorption at peripheral sites. Large doses of sedatives and analgesics are avoided because of the danger of respiratory depression and because they may mask other symptoms.

All debris and loose skin is removed from the burn wound, and the area is cleansed with a solution of 1 liter saline, 250 ml hydrogen peroxide, and 15 ml Dreft detergent. Dressings with the selected topical preparation are applied. An *escharotomy* (linear incision of constricting eschar) may be necessary when constriction of circulation or respiration is evident (Figs. 67-4 and 67-5). *Eschar* (a crust formed on the burn wound) from third-degree burns rapidly contracts, causing restriction to soft tissues, vessels, and underlying organs. Frequent observations of chest excursion in addition to respiratory rate are necessary to determine respiratory restriction. Pulses must be checked every 15 minutes to assure uninterrupted vascular flow to all extremities. Particular caution is necessary with the presence of a circumferential burn.

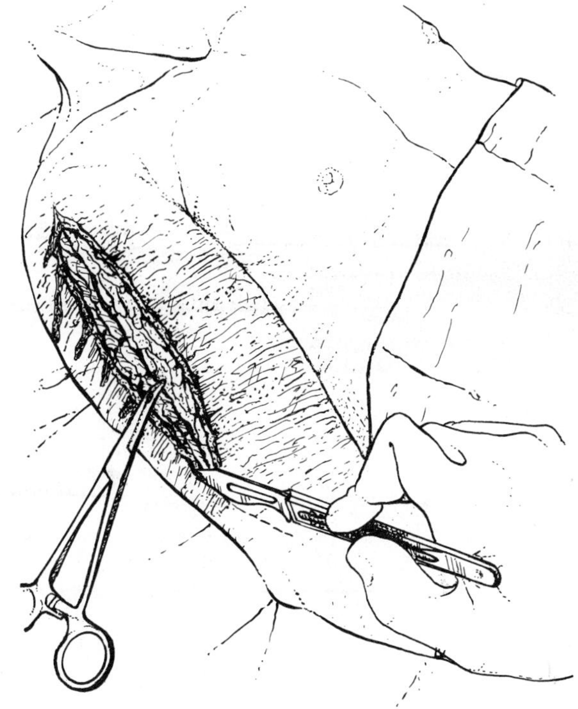

Fig. 67-4. Escharotomy surgically performed for circumferential burn of upper arm.

□ Inability to regulate body fluids

Replacement of fluids and electrolytes is an essential part of the treatment and is instituted as soon as the extent of the burn and the patient's condition have been determined. Ideally, fluid therapy is started within an hour following a severe burn. Insertion of a central venous line permits the rapid administration of fluids and electrolytes.

Three types of fluid are considered in calculating the needs of the patient:(1) colloids, including plasma and plasma expanders such as dextran, (2) electrolytes such as physiologic solution of sodium chloride, Ringer's solution, Hartmann's solution, and Tyrode's solution, and (3) nonelectrolyte fluids such as distilled water with 5% glucose. Medical authorities do not agree as to the proportion of colloid and electrolyte fluids needed. Several formulas are described in the medical literature to guide physicians in determining the type and amount of fluids to be administered, based on the patient's weight and age and the percentage of the body burned.[19,23] The present trend is to administer balanced salt solutions (such as Ringer's), water, and plasma, and to use whole blood only if a large number of red cells are destroyed or if anemia develops.

Fluids administered during the first 48 hours are given to maintain circulating blood volume. Additional fluids and electrolytes are added to replace losses from vomiting or from nasogastric drainage. The amount of fluid replacement required during the first 48 hours is determined by assessment of several factors; these include urinary output, serum electrolyte levels, blood gas findings, central venous pressure, body weight, desire to maintain the hematocrit at slightly above normal levels, level of consciousness, and vital signs. Fluid needs for the first 24 hours are calculated from the time of the

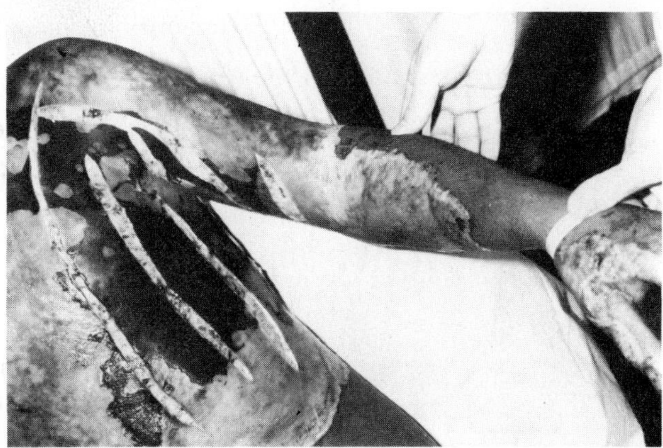

Fig. 67-5. Escharotomy used to alleviate circulatory and pulmonary constriction. (Courtesy Burn Center, Cleveland Metropolitan General Hospital, Cleveland, Ohio.)

burn. Usually the patient receives *one-half the total amount in the first 8 hours,* one-fourth in the second 8 hours, and one-fourth in the third 8 hours. One-half of the total amount given on the first day is given in the second 24 hours.

Patients complain of moderate to severe thirst. If oral fluids are permitted, accurate recording of ingested fluids is important. Unlimited oral intake and failure to measure it may result in too much fluid in the circulating blood, resulting in water intoxication. A Swan-Ganz catheter may be inserted to monitor pulmonary arterial and capillary wedge pressure (p. 923) in the severely burned patient for identification of hypovolemia or hypervolemia.

The rate of urinary output is probably the most reliable measure of determining the adequacy of fluid therapy during the first 48 hours. Hourly checking and measuring of urinary output is one of the most important responsibilities of the nurse. Usually a retention catheter is inserted and drained into a calibrated container. The amount of urine is measured and recorded every hour. The care of the patient with an indwelling catheter is discussed on p. 1260. The urine should be observed for color and analyzed for a positive hematocrit level. The physician is notified if hematuria or a positive Hemastix reaction is present. A urine flow of 30 to 50 ml/hour is adequate for an adult. The urine flow should be at least 15 ml/hour for infants and 25 ml/hour for older children. If the urinary output rises above or falls below these figures, the physician is notified immediately. Fluid therapy will need to be adjusted accordingly. Lack of urinary output may indicate insufficient fluids or acute tubular necrosis. All efforts must be taken to provide sufficient fluid to protect vital organs.

After the first 48 to 72 hours the urinary output is no longer a reliable guide to fluid needs, since water deprivation may occur even when the urinary output for adults is 1,000 ml/day or more. Severely burned patients require a large fluid intake to compensate for the loss of fluid into the tissues and from the wound. Fluid needs then are determined by measuring serum electrolyte levels. Fluid replacement during the diuretic stage is based on individual assessment. Parenteral fluids may be discontinued if serum electrolytes return to normal. If dehydration occurs from the diuresis, fluid replacement therapy may be continued until blood volume is stabilized. The patient is observed closely for signs of water intoxication (p. 301) or pulmonary edema (p. 1009).

The hyperkalemia of the first stage can change to hypokalemia within a very few hours during diuresis or as the potassium moves back into cells. The serum levels of potassium are monitored closely, and potassium is replaced parenterally when hypokalemia results. Adequate kidney function must be present.

□ Break in skin integrity

Infection control

A major principle in the care of the burned person is the prevention of infection. Local and systemic infections (septicemia) are the most common complications of burns and are a major cause of death, particularly in burns covering more than 25% of the body. Autogenous sources are the primary sources of infection initially, although the wound is highly susceptible to infection from exogenous sources. The person's own bacteria become trapped under the eschar, and aggressive wound management is necessary. Daily tubbings and mechanical debridement must be done to remove wound exudate and debris from the wound. Washing and friction removes build-up of debris and supports healthy tissue regeneration. Topical agents are more effective in preventing local infection because impairment of the vasculature in the burn area prevents the systemic antibiotics reaching the wound. Antibiotics may be given prophylactically, or they may be withheld until an infection does occur.

The organisms that usually infect burn wounds are *Staphylococcus aureus, Pseudomonas aeruginosa,* and the coliform bacilli. In the past few years there has been a high incidence of fungal infections resulting from the use of broad-spectrum antibiotics. *Candida albicans,* which normally is found in the gastrointestinal tract, accounts for the majority of the fungal infections. Cultures of the patient's nose, throat, wound, and unburned skin, and a punch biopsy may be taken on admission and at biweekly intervals to determine the bacteria present and their sensitivity to antibiotics.

All persons who approach the patient should wear gowns and masks to prevent the introduction of their organisms into the wound. Persons with upper respiratory infections should not be permitted near the patient. Good aseptic surgical techniques and sterile gloves are used when applying dressings. Hydrotherapy tanks used for aggressive cleansing of burn wounds need particular attention to prevent infection of burn wounds when the tanks are used by different patients.

The extent of local cleansing depends of the severity of the burn and the judgment of the physician. Detergents or antiseptic preparations, such as povidone-iodine (Betadine), are effective cleansing agents. A rather extensive debridement may be carried out at the initial cleansing. The wounds are then treated by the open or closed methods. Tetanus toxoid or antitoxin is usually given to the person who has received extensive burns. Hair on skin areas adjacent to burn tissue is shaved once a week.

Care of severely burned persons in special burn units can contribute to decreased infection because the environment is specifically geared to infection control. If the patient is cared for on a general hospital unit, a private room is preferable, and all equipment needed by the patient should remain in his room. Reverse isolation precautions are usually carried out.

Methods of treatment

There are several methods of treating the burned area, depending on the location of the burn, its size and depth, the facilities available, and the patient's response to the therapy. One method may be started and then replaced with another during the course of treatment. Only those commonly used today are described here.

Open or exposure method of treatment. The exposure method of treatment was accidentally discovered to be effective in 1888 when, during a serious steamboat fire on the Mississippi, those in attendance ran out of bandages and later observed that the neglected persons fared better than those who received more intensive local treatment.[14] Today, the exposure method is used most often in the treatment of burns involving the face, neck, perineum, and broad areas of the trunk. The burned area is cleansed and exposed to the air (Fig. 67-6). The exudate of a partial-thickness burn dries in 48 to 72 hours and forms a hard crust that protects the

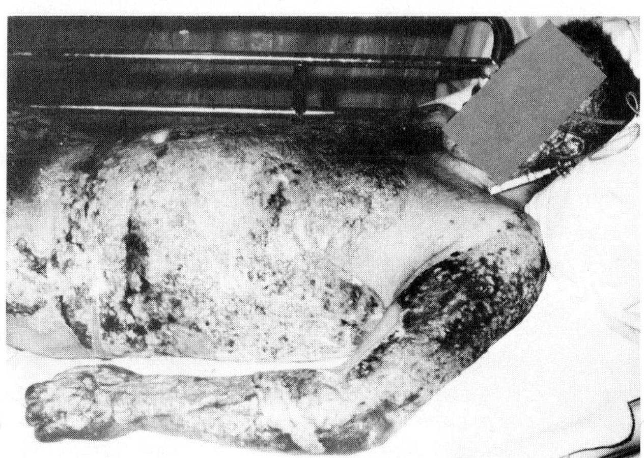

Fig. 67-6. Severely burned man being treated by open method. (Courtesy Burn Center, Cleveland Metropolitan General Hospital, Cleveland, Ohio.)

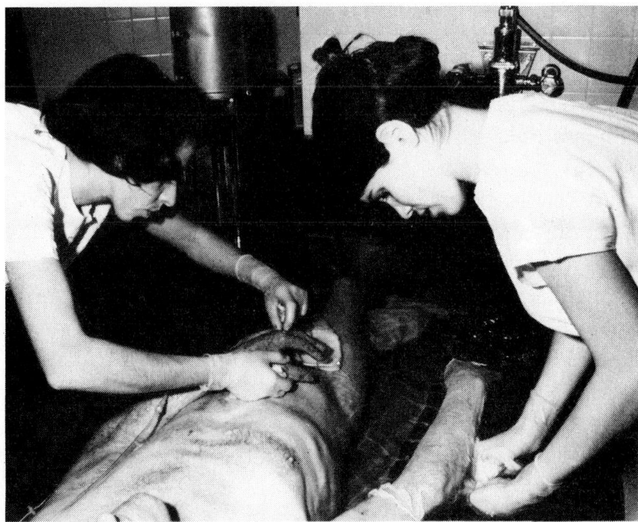

Fig. 67-7. Nurses debriding patient in hydrotherapy bath. (Courtesy Burn Center, Cleveland Metropolitan General Hospital, Cleveland, Ohio.)

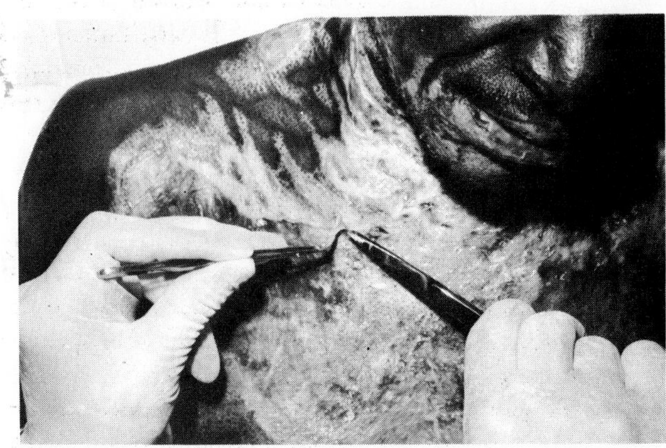

Fig. 67-8. Nurse's role in burn centers may include debridement of patient's eschar. (Courtesy Burn Unit, Cook County Hospital, Chicago, Ill.)

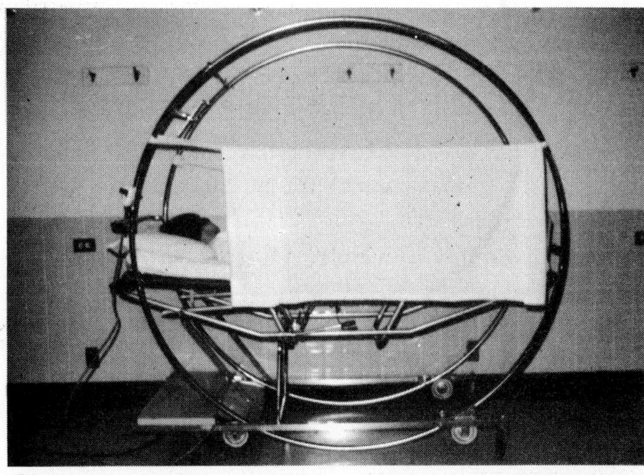

Fig. 67-9. Another exposure method of treating burns. A sheet is draped over CircOlectric bed so that burned areas are not touched. (Courtesy Burn Unit, Cook County Hospital, Chicago, Ill.)

wound. Epithelialization occurs beneath this crust and may be complete in 14 to 21 days. The crust then falls off spontaneously, leaving a healed, unscarred surface. The dead skin of a full-thickness burn is dehydrated and converted to an eschar (black, leathery dead tissue covering) in 48 to 72 hours. Loose eschar may be gradually removed through the use of whirlpool baths or debridement (Figs. 67-7 and 67-8). Uninfected eschar acts as a protective covering. The danger of infection exists as bacteria proliferate beneath the eschar. Spontaneous separation, produced by bacterial action, occurs unless surgical debridement is performed.

Isolation technique is essential when the exposure method is used. The nurse caring for the patient should wear a sterile gown and mask, and sterile linen may be used on the patient's bed. Infants may need to have their hands restrained to prevent them from picking off crusts. Until the wounds are healed, children's toys need to be sterilized to prevent them from causing infection.

A cradle may be used on the bed since no clothing or bedclothes are allowed directly over burned areas. If the burn is extensive, a CircOlectric bed draped with a sheet is an ideal way to care for the patient (Fig. 67-9). The burned person can be kept from embarrassing exposure by wearing a halter and loin cloth. Lights or heat lamps may be used with caution to provide warmth and the patient has maximum freedom to move about and perform exercises for the prevention of contracture and the improvement of circulation.

Patients having exposure treatment complain of pain and chilling. Pain may be controlled by administering morphine sulfate, meperidine hydrochloride (Demerol), barbiturates, or propoxyphene hydrochloride (Darvon) as ordered. Discomfort can be decreased if drafts are avoided and the temperature of the room is kept at 24.4 C (85 F). Patients lose more heat from burned surfaces than from the normal skin surfaces, since there is no vascular bed to contract and retain heat in the body. The humidity of the room also should be controlled. A humidity of 40% to 50% usually is considered satisfactory. Portable electric humidifiers and dehumidifiers can be used to achieve and maintain this level.

Closed method of treatment. In the closed method of burn treatment the wounds are washed and dressings are changed at least once each day and frequently twice. Commonly the dressing consists of gauze impregnated with topical ointments and a gauze wrap. When a dressing is in place, nursing observation should include checking for signs of impaired circulation such as numbness, pain, and tingling and being alert for signs of infection (odor on dressings and elevated temperature and pulse rate).

Hydrotherapy

Hydrotherapy is a valuable adjunct to therapy and should be used when available in the care of the burned person. It is a more painless method for removal of dressings, aids in the cleansing of the wound by removal of loose eschar and other debris, and facilitates range-of-motion exercises with minimum energy expenditure and discomfort. Tubbing is usually performed once or twice daily for 20 to 30 minutes and is started after the patient's vital signs and fluid balance have stabilized. The patient must receive careful personal care before being placed in the tub so that fecal contamination is minimal. Those in attendance should wear gowns and gloves until the wounds are healed. The patient is never left unattended during the procedure because fainting and injury may occur.

Topical applications

The application of topical agents to the burned area has helped to decrease infection and hasten healing. There are a number of agents currently being used, each having certain advantages and disadvantages. The ideal agent has not yet been developed.

Mafenide (Sulfamylon). Mafenide is a white cream containing sulfonamide. It diffuses through devascularized areas and is an effective bacteriostatic agent against many gram-negative as well as gram-positive microorganisms. The cream is applied with a sterile gloved hand in a thin layer just enough to cover the burn completely. The wound is usually left open to the air. Washing of the wound and reapplication of the cream is necessary when the wound is no longer covered with ointment. Metabolic acidosis may result when impaired renal function is present because of inhibition of carbonic anhydrase. Side effects include pain and allergic manifestations. Treatment is usually continued until healing is occurring or the wound is ready for grafting.

Silver sulfadiazine (Silvadene). Silver sulfadiazine is a white cream with bactericidal action against many gram-negative and gram-positive bacteria, as well as against *Candida albicans*. It does not result in metabolic acidosis, but some persons develop sensitivity reactions. The patient is observed for side effects common with sulfonamide drugs. The wound may develop a slimy, greyish appearance simulating an infection, despite negative cultures.[27] The ointment is applied in a thin layer with a sterile gloved hand to cover the burn after wound cleansings. The wound may be covered or left exposed.

Povidone-iodine (Betadine). Povidone-iodine ointment is a reddish brown germicidal preparation of 10% povidone-iodine (1% available iodine) with broad-spectrum microbicidal action. It kills gram-positive and gram-negative bacteria, fungi, yeasts, viruses, and protozoa. It is nonirritating and nonsensitizing and permits air to reach the site after application. It is applied at least three times daily. The methods of application are (1) "buttering"—using the gloved hand, a 1/4-inch thick layer is spread on burned surfaces and (2) the modified closed technique—single-thickness povidone-iodine-impregnated gauze is applied to the affected areas, and additional ointment is spread on top of the gauze layer.

Silver nitrate treatment. Although silver nitrate is being used less often than in the past, some physicians still prescribe it. In this treatment, thick gauze dressings are saturated with a 0.5% solution of silver nitrate, and the dressings are kept wet so that the solution remains in constant contact with burned surfaces. The purpose of these dressings is to retain moisture and heat and to reduce evaporation. The proponents of this method of treatment believe that it reduces mortality, lessens pain, eliminates odors, and has a bacteriostatic effect.[23] The dressings are removed every 12 to 24 hours, and the patient may be placed in a bath of salt solution with the temperature carefully maintained at the same level as the body. When skin grafts are applied, silver nitrate dressings are placed over the graft and donor sites on the first postoperative day. Because the silver nitrate solution is hypotonic, electrolytes are lost into the wound. Therefore throughout treatment, frequent determinations of blood sodium levels are necessary, and sodium that is lost may need to be replaced.

Isolation technique is not required when the burn is treated with silver nitrate dressings, but clean dressings and sterile gloves and instruments are used. Because everything that comes in contact with the silver nitrate solution is stained black, the nurse wears a gown and gloves when applying the solution to protect skin, nails, and clothing. Although linen can be specially treated to remove stains, great care must be taken to prevent splashing the solution on the furniture, walls, and floors.

Other applications. *Furazoleum* is a research drug that can be applied either directly to the wound or gauze rolls may be saturated with it. It is a bright saffron-colored cream that is very soluble in water and is heat stable. At high concentrations it is bactericidal to all organisms with the exception of *Proteus* and yeasts.

Neomycin is a bactericidal agent that causes miscoding in the messenger RNA of bacterial cells. It is effective against most organisms but has a serious toxic effect and can cause irreversible hearing loss or kidney failure when used over a long period of time.

In addition to ointments, two other solutions are used frequently in burn care. These are sodium chloride solution and a mixture of equal parts of acetic acid, peroxide, and normal saline solution, commonly referred to as "thirds." *Normal* or balanced *saline* solutions are applied to clean granulation tissue or to new grafts to maintain moisture or are used with fine mesh gauze to provide for slight debridement. The *"thirds" solution* has limited antimicrobial action and is most effective against organisms that are affected by changes in pH. It is also used to clean dirty granulation tissue.

Wound coverings

The burn wound may be covered with dressings or grafts.

Dressings. Large bulky dressings are rarely used today for large-scale burns except in selected instances, as infection control is more difficult and partial thickness burns may develop into full-thickness wounds.[19] The purposes of applying some type of light covering include prevention of infection from exogenous sources, facilitation of debridement, maximum contact by topical agents, and prevention of fluid evaporation with loss of body heat. The type of dressing that is usually applied consists of a single layer of fine-mesh gauze held in place by a wrapping of a coarse gauze such as Kerlix.

The dressing change may be a painful procedure, and if analgesics are required, they should be given 30 minutes before the procedure for maximum effectiveness. Most dressing changes are performed after tubbing, as this facilitates dressing removal and is less painful. Additional debridement of eschar and dead tissue may be performed before the new dressing is applied.

Wet dressings may be used such as with silver nitrate or normal saline applications. A single layer of fine-mesh gauze is usually placed over the wound, covered with thick gauze pads to maintain moisture, and held in place with a gauze wrapping. The dressings must be kept wet. Plastic wrap should *not* be used to cover the dressings, as this prevents any fluid evaporation, causing increased heat at the wound site and resulting in patient discomfort and increased tissue destruction and infection.

Skin grafts. Skin grafts are applied to cover the burn wound and speed healing, to prevent contractures from occurring, and to shorten convalescence. Successful grafting reduces the patient's vulnerability to infection and prevents the loss of body heat and water vapor from the open wound or eschar. Most skin grafts are applied between the fifth and twenty-first day after the initial injury, depending on the depth and extent of the burn and the condition of the base. Small areas of third-degree burns such as those that occur on the dorsum of the hand may be excised and skin grafted during the first 24 to 48 hours to hasten healing and to help restore function more quickly. The wound is prepared for the graft as described on p. 1505.

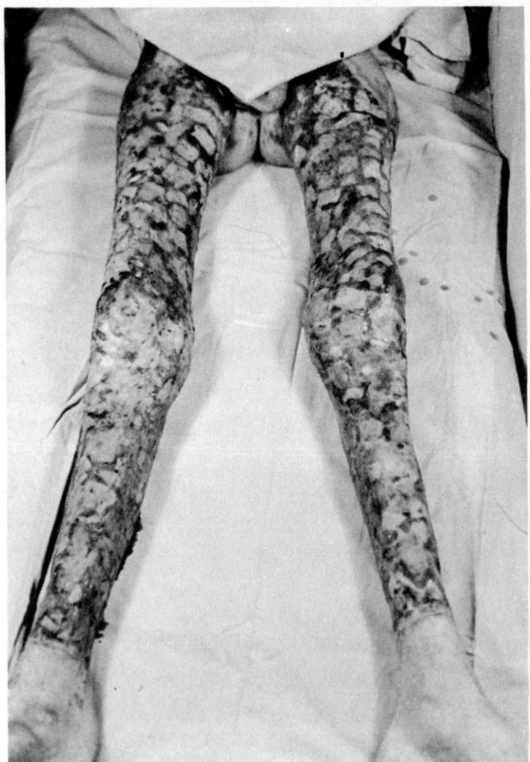

Fig. 67-10. Postage stamp grafts have been cut from split-thickness graft and have been used to partially cover large burned areas on lower limbs. (From Artz, C. P., and Reiss, E.: The treatment of burns, Philadelphia, 1957, W. B. Saunders Co.)

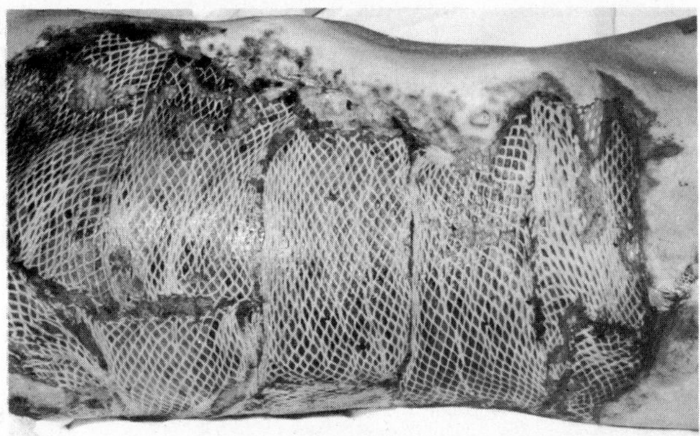

Fig. 67-11. Mesh graft covering full-thickness burn. (Courtesy Burn Unit, Cook County Hospital, Chicago, Ill.)

Split-thickness grafts usually are used. These grafts include the upper layer of the skin and part of the under layer but are not taken so deep as to prevent regeneration of the skin at the site from which they are taken (donor site). They grow as normal skin on the burned areas (recipient sites). These grafts are removed with a dermatome from almost any unburned part of the body. They may be removed in strips or small squares (postage stamps) (Fig. 67-10). Another type of split-thickness graft is the *mesh graft,* which is used when few donor sites are available and there are large areas of burned body surface to be covered. The graft is removed with a dermatome and then meshed with a special instrument. The meshing of the graft makes it more distensible and thus it can be used to cover wider areas of the body surface (Fig. 67-11). Grafts may be laid on the burn wounds and held in place with dressings or sutured into place and left exposed. Pressure dressings may be applied to secure the graft, provide even compression, and act as a splint. If the loss of skin is so great that life is threatened, the skin of other persons, that of recently deceased persons, or stored postmortem skin is taken to cover burned surfaces (homografts). The use of homografts helps to limit infection and loss of water, electrolytes, and protein and helps to reduce pain in the burn wound. Homografts may survive 4 to 5 weeks before being rejected, but they usually are needed only about 10 days if applied to cover a large granulating wound.[2]

The donor site, which presents an oozing, painful surface, may be covered with sterile gauze and a pressure dressing or it may be covered with a fine-mesh gauze and left exposed to the air. The drainage from the wound dries and serves as a protective covering. The wound usually heals within 2 weeks. Many patients complain of quite severe pain in the donor site, and the nurse should not hesitate to give medications that are ordered for pain. The pain should subside within a day or two. Sometimes an odor develops from the dead tissue at either the donor site or the recipient site, which is distressing to the patient and should be reported to the physician. If infection has developed, antibiotics may be administered and the wound treated with wet dressings.

Heterografts of materials such as pigskin or a synthetic substitute are being used commonly to provide temporary protection to wounds, reduce pain, promote granulation, and reduce surface bacterial count.

□ Increased nutritional requirements

Metabolism is increased following moderate to severe burns as a result of stress, fluid loss, fever, infection, hypercatabolism, and immobility. Uninjured cells have increased metabolic activity initially as a result of decreased oxygenation from the hypovolemia. The catabolic phase may last for 30 to 40 days in persons with extensive injury.[19]

The protein and caloric needs of the burned person

are highly variable, depending on the extent and depth of injury and on the person's age and preburn nutritional state. The daily *protein* requirement is greater than normal because of the negative nitrogen balance that is present following burns (p. 1511). The normal daily protein requirement is 0.8 g/kg of body weight for adults, whereas the recommended daily intake for the burned person is 2 to 4 g/kg. The daily *caloric* requirement increases from a normal of 1,700 to 3,000 calories to 3,500 to 5,000 calories. The caloric requirement for children varies from 90 to 100 calories per kilogram of body weight for children under 3 years of age to 70 calories per kilogram of body weight for children between 4 and 12 years of age.

Supplemental vitamins are needed. Vitamin C promotes healing (p. 401), and the daily requirement in the burn patient increases from a normal of 45 mg to 1 to 2 g. The B-complex vitamins are necessary for the metabolism of the increased protein and carbohydrate intake. Sodium chloride, potassium, and calcium preparations also may be administered intravenously or orally, depending on the extent of the burned area and serum electrolyte levels. Iron preparations are required for persons who become anemic.

Weight loss and gain are monitored for evaluation of nutritional status of the severely burned person. Weight gain occurs initially because of the fluid retention. Following diuresis there is a marked loss of weight caused by loss of fluid and negative nitrogen balance. The weight curve will level out at a point below the preburn weight, and weight gain does not begin until the wounds are nearly all grafted.[19]

The person with large-scale burns may develop paralytic ileus because of the neuroendocrine response to stress, or may have nausea and vomiting to such an extent that nutrition must be provided entirely by the parenteral route. Intravenous fluids are given during the hypovolemic stage (p. 1515). When fluid balance is achieved, efforts are directed to meet the increased nutritional requirements. If the person is unable to eat the quantities of necessary nutrients, total parenteral nutrition (TPN) (p. 321) or tube feedings may be necessary. If nausea is present, a chilled solution containing 3 to 4 g ($1\frac{1}{2}$ teaspoons) of table salt and 1.5 to 2 g ($\frac{1}{2}$ teaspoon) of sodium bicarbonate in 1 liter (quart) of water flavored with lemon juice (Haldane's solution) can often be retained while supplying needed electrolytes. Carbonated beverages are also an acceptable means of supplying some necessary electrolytes as well as sugar. Salty solutions such as meat broths often are given to help replace sodium chloride that is lost into the tissues and in wound exudate, but broths or fruit juices that contain potassium are withheld for 48 hours or until the serum potassium levels go down.

If the patient is able to feed himself, appetite may improve. It is important that painful and disagreeable changes of dressings and other treatments be timed so that they do not immediately precede meals.

The high-protein powdered milk preparations are valuable in increasing the amount of protein taken and often seem to leave the patient with less of a feeling of oversatiation than may result from large servings of meats that are often high in fat.

The diet is advanced as quickly as possible to a regular one, but because of the patient's poor appetite, the utmost imagination and ingenuity on the part of the dietitian and the nurse are needed to motivate the patient to eat what he needs. Sometimes relatives are helpful in suggesting favorite foods. Milkshakes supply large amounts of nourishment. They are also valuable because very ill patients can take fluids more easily than they can chew and swallow solid foods.

Bulk foods and fruit juices must be stressed in the diet of the severely burned patient because they aid in elimination. Fecal impaction is a common problem for burn patients. Bulk-forming laxatives such as preparations of the psyllium seed (Metamucil) may be given, or a fecal softener such as dioctyl sodium sulfosuccinate (Colace) may be ordered.

□ Limitation of mobility

Contractures are among the most serious long-term complications of burns. Two major types of contractures occur—those caused by muscle and joint stiffening and those occurring after skin grafting. Many patients must undergo painful reconstructive surgery that would not have been necessary if those in attendance had been alert to the prevention of contractures. A large responsibility for the prevention of contractures rests with the nurse, who is with the patient more than anyone else. Nursing care should be planned so that the patient's position is changed regularly during the day and night. Early skin grafting prevents many contractures by mobilizing the patient sometimes months earlier than would otherwise be possible.

Burned patients often have severe pain as healing progresses. They are anemic, debilitated, and very often is a state of depression. The nurse must never let sympathy interfere with concern for the patient's ultimate good. The patient must be helped to maintain range of joint motion and thus prevent scars from healing in positions that will result in deformity. It is important that patients understand why ambulation or motion is necessary even though it may be painful. Constant encouragement can be provided by setting short-term achievable goals. Since normal skin and normal tissues grow while scar tissue shrinks, children are more likely to develop deformities than adults, and what begins as a minor deformity in childhood may become a major one with increased growth.

For a definite interval of time each day, patients with burns should lie prone and also flat on their backs with no pillow or elevation of the head of the bed. This can be accomplished more easily if the patient is placed on a Stryker frame, a Foster bed, or a CircOlectric bed. These beds facilitate the use of the bedpan and urinal, permit change of position with a minimum of handling, and permit larger skin surfaces to remain free from body pressure than is possible when the patient lies in bed. These special beds are particularly useful when both back and front of the trunk, thighs, and legs have been burned. They allow turning of the patient with a minimum of handling and thus help decrease pain.

Prolonged rest in a semi-Fowler's position or with the pillow pushing the head forward must be avoided. Many patients like this position because it enables them to see about the room better. The bed can often be turned so that the patient can look about without having to assume positions that may lead to the formation of contractures. It is often advisable to change the bedside table from one side of the bed to the other at intervals. Mirrors help these patients keep in better touch with their environment, provided that the patient is able to cope with his appearance.

If burns have been sustained about the neck, chin, and face, the patient should always lie in a position of hyperextension of the neck for most of each day. A pillow may be placed under his shoulders and the bed lowered to a level position. Facial exercises are encouraged to prevent scars from tightening as they form. Chewing gum and blowing balloons provide exercise that helps to prevent facial contractures.

Burns of the hand can easily result in contractures. Differences of opinion exist about methods of positioning that best preserve function and prevent contractures, therefore consultation with the physiatrist (rehabilitation specialist) and physician is recommended. Burns on the dorsal surfaces of the hand are frequently positioned in a flexed position of function, whereas the hand with burns of the palmar surface may be positioned in hyperextension. Total hand burns are splinted as for dorsal burns.[19] Various types of splints (p. 847) may be used. Some physicians prefer to use the open method of treatment, providing for frequent exercise to prevent contractures.

Exercises for prevention and correction of contractures are begun as soon as the patient's vital signs are stable. Supervision by a physical therapist is desirable. When burns are completely covered (by healing or graft), exercises may be performed more easily in an occupational therapy or physical therapy department where the patient also may benefit from a change in environment. In the department of physical medicine, exercises often are done in water. A Hubbard tank may be used for this purpose. The occupational therapist may help the patient to improve range of motion in a satisfying and efficient fashion by teaching functional activities of daily living and crafts suitable for particular needs such as typing, weaving, or a host of other activities. The nurse must know what the patient is being taught by the physical therapist and the occupational therapist so that progress can be continued on the nursing unit.

The patient who is not hospitalized and the one who returns home early because of skin grafting need instruction in how to prevent contractures from developing. Contracture clinics are available for burn patients and are associated with some burn centers. If community health nursing services are available, a physical therapist or occupational therapist may be called on to assist the patient at home. If this service is not available, the nurse in the hospital or the community health nurse may have to take responsibility for teaching the patient how to prevent contractures from developing.

□ Threats to integrity and body image

The emotional impact of severe burns is enormous and reality based. During the first few days the patient is too ill to fully comprehend what has happened. Patients fear that they may not survive, and the fear of death is a major concern. Other fears include pain and suffering, disfigurement, prolonged hospitalization, and disruption of life style. Patients who are severely burned usually are exhausted and often demoralized by the pain, treatment, and frequent dressing changes. Many defense mechanisms may be evident as the patient attempts to control pain. Care givers need to be supportive, although they may find the patient's behavior unacceptable. Support and understanding will allow the patient to develop more acceptable means of coping with the stressful situation. Diazepam (Valium) may be helpful in decreasing anxiety and providing muscle relaxation. The pain can be minimized by clear explanations that gain the patient's cooperation, planned use of analgesics, careful sterile technique, gentle handling, and permitting the patient to participate in the treatment whenever possible. Depending on the age of the patient and the extent of the pain, distracting activities may be helpful.

After the initial period comes the long healing period and the realization of endless implications. Patients' reactions are determined by their personality makeup, by their degree of total adjustment to life, and by the extent and location of the burns. Burns on the face make adjustment particularly difficult. All kinds of fears arise to harrass the patient. "Will my spouse still care for me? Can I ever let my children see me?" To the adolescent, the thought of being different or conspicuous may be unbearable. Fears about not being taken back on the job often haunt the wage earner who is badly burned. If possible, the patient should see facial burns only after being prepared for the experience. Support and understanding will be needed in order for the patient to cope with what will be seen in the mirror. The patient will exhibit readiness by asking to look in the mirror. Interaction with other burned patients who are further along in their healing process may help the patient feel that recovery is possible. In some instances the recovery is incredible, and although differences in skin pigmentation remain, the redness that accompanies burns and newly healed skin often fades considerably within a few months. Pigmentation problems are more acute for persons with brown or black skin. Their skin may be a different shade, freckled, or whitish in color.

Clinical observation indicates that the burned individual experiences concern about changes in appearance and its effect on others. Since the skin, peripheral blood vessels, and lymph vessels are damaged, the burned patient's sense of body boundary probably is altered. Patients undergoing debridement following loosening of burn eschar describe sensations of having their skin torn away from them. It has been asserted that persons who perceive their body boundaries as being well-defined tend to be more confident and have a higher goal and task completion drives. It is therefore possible that those who lose a part of that sense of definiteness will tend to take a more languid approach to life with less successful interactions with others.[50]

The patient should have an opportunity to talk about any problems and fears. Some patients may discuss these with the nurse when they cannot express them to relatives, and the nurse must be prepared to listen and help the individual accept necessary changes in life style. (See current literature for further discussion.[50,51]) Almost every burned patient and his family needs the help of the social worker. The nurse should recognize this need and initiate the referral. Visiting hours can be used to talk with relatives who may be able to give information that will clarify the patient's needs and resources. This time also provides opportunity for the nurse to help relatives and friends accept their loved one's change in appearance and to help them plan for the return of the loved one to the community.

□ Teaching needs

Patients have a great need for education so that they may take increasing responsibility for their own care. They need to learn (1) care of the healed burn wound, (2) nutritional needs, (3) prevention of injury, (4) recognition of signs and symptoms of complications, and (5) methods of coping with resocialization. Complete and comprehensive instructions followed by return demonstrations contribute to learning the necessary skills to be independent and prudent in self-care activities after discharge. Patients should not be discharged from the hospital until they can care for themselves physically and are prepared to meet the stresses involved in return to their former living patterns. Accentuation of strengths of the individual and focus on effective coping mechanisms will overshadow the limitations the person may be experiencing.

■ REHABILITATION

Complete recovery and rehabilitation of the severely burned patient is a long and costly process. Many industries have compensation insurance to cover part of the cost, and the patient should be encouraged to discuss financial problems with the physician and with the social worker if one is available. Patients under 21 years of age are eligible for care financed in part by the Office of Child Development (formerly the Children's Bureau) through its aid to states for their programs for crippled children. This care will cover surgical procedures and care, special rehabilitative services, and social service.

Patients who have been burned should have medical checkups at regular intervals indefinitely and should be advised to report any unusual change in the burn scar at once. There is a fairly high frequency of malignant degeneration of scar tissue following burns. This is particularly true when the burn is caused by electricity or by x-rays.

■ OUTCOME CRITERIA FOR THE PERSON WITH BURNS

1. Following the acute phase the patient will:
   a. Be in a state of homeostasis (normal blood volume, normal serum electrolytes, vital signs at preburn levels).
   b. Be in a state of positive nitrogen balance.
   c. Be free of infection.
   d. Have intact integumentation.
   e. Be free of contractures.
   f. Be mobile and independent in self-care.
2. At discharge the patient or significant others can:
   a. Demonstrate care of the burn wound.
   b. State name, dosage, frequency, desired effect, and side effects of topical or systemic antibiotics.
   c. Demonstrate range-of-motion exercises to prevent contractures.
   d. Plan a diet high in protein, calories, vitamins, and minerals.
   e. Describe injuries that can occur to the healing wound or graft and methods of prevention of injury.
   f. Describe plans for return to former activities (work, social activities).
   g. Describe plans for follow-up health care:

1. State signs and symptoms requiring intervention (wound infection, loss of weight, contractures, changes in scar tissue).
2. State plans for continued medical care until wounds are fully healed.

REFERENCES AND SELECTED READINGS

1. *Andreasen, N. J., Noyes, R., Jr., Hartford, C. E., et al.: Management of emotional reactions in seriously burned adults, N. Engl. J. Med. **286**:65-69, 1972.
2. Artz, C. P., and Moncrief, J. A.: The treatment of burns, ed. 2, Philadelphia, 1969, W. B. Saunders.
3. Artz, C. P., and Yarbourgh, D. R. III: Major body burn, J.A.M.A. **223**:1355-1357, 1973.
4. Beal, J. M., and Echenhoff, J. E.: Intensive and recovery room care, London, 1969, Macmillan Publishing Co., Inc.
5. Bell, J. G.: Bitsy was so little . . . and her problems so big. Nurs. 77 **7**:35-37, June 1977.
6. Boswick, J. A.: Symposium on surgery of burns, Surg. Clin. North Am. **50**:1191-1446, 1970.
7. Boswick, J. A., and Stone, N. H.: The planning of patient care in a hospital burn unit, Surg. Clin. North Am. **50**:275-283, 1970.
8. Boswick, J. A., and Stone, N. H.: Methods and materials in managing the severely burned patient, Surg. Clin. North Am. **48**:177-190, 1968.
9. Bowden, M. L., and Feller, I.: Family reaction to a severe burn, Am. J. Nurs. **73**:316-319, 1973.
10. Brentano, L., Gravens, D. L., Moyer, C. A., et al.: Bacteriology of large human burns treated with silver nitrate, Arch. Surg. **93**:456-466, 1966.
11. Burned children: infection, and nursing care, Nurs. Clin. North Am. **5**:131-142, 1970.
12. Campbell, L.: Special behavioral problems of the burned child, Am. J. Nurs. **76**:220-224, 1976.
13. Castillo, J.: Treatment of thermal injuries, Surg. Clin. North Am. **53**:627-637, 1973.
14. Cockshott, W. P.: The history of the treatment of burns, Surg. Gynecol. Obstet. **102**:116-124, 1956.
15. Current nursing care of the burned patient, Nurs. Clin. North Am. **5**:563-575, 1970.
16. Curreri, P. W., Richmond, D., Marvin, J., et al.: Dietary requirements of patients with major burns, J. Am. Diet Assoc. **65**:415-417, 1974.
17. *de Tornay, R., and Doswell, W. M.: Nursing decisions: experiences in clinical problem solving, series 2, no. 7: Karen A., a patient with burns, RN **40**:59-68, May 1977.
18. *Emig, E., and Lloyd, J. R.: How to get burned children home sooner, RN **40**:37-39, July 1977.
19. *Feller, I., and Archanbeault, C.: Nursing the burned patient, Ann Arbor, Mich., 1973, Institute for Burn Medicine Press.
20. Fox, C. L., Rappole, B. W., and Stanford, W.: Control of *Pseudomonas* infection in burns by silver sulfadiazine, Surg. Gynecol. Obstet. **128**:1021-1026, 1969.
21. *Hadley, R. D.: Knowledge, understanding: keys to burn patient care, Am. Nurse **9**:9-10, Dec. 15, 1977.
22. Hamburg, D. A., Hamburg, B., and deGoza, S., et al.: Clinical importance of emotional problems in care of patients with burns, N. Engl. J. Med. **248**:355-359, 1953.
23. Hardy, J. D., editor: Textbook of surgery: principles and practice, ed. 5, Philadelphia, 1977, Lippincott Co.
24. Hartford, C. E.: The early treatment of burns, Nurs. Clin. North Am. **8**:447-455, 1973.
25. Hummel, R. P., MacMillan, B. G., and Altemeier, W. A.: Topical and systemic antibacterial agents in the treatments of burns, Ann. Surg. **172**:370-383, 1970.
26. Jacoby, F. G.: Individualized burn wound dressings, Nurs. 77 **7**:62-63, June 1977.
27. *Jacoby, F. G.: Nursing care of the patient with burns, ed. 2, St. Louis, 1976, The C. V. Mosby Co.
28. *Jones, C. S., and Feller, I.: Burns: what to do during the first crucial hours, Nurs. 77 **7**:22-31, March 1977.
29. Kavanagh, C.: The severely burned child: a portrait of need and giving, Mat. Child Nurs. **2**:223, 1977.
30. Korloff, B.: Social and economic consequences of deep burns. In Wallace, A. B., and Wilkinson, A. W., editors: Second international congress on research in burns, Edinburgh, 1966, E. & S. Livingstone.
31. *Kunsman, J.: Nursing care after primary excision, RN **37**:25-26, Aug. 1974.
32. *Minckley, B. B.: Expert nursing care for burned patients, Am. J. Nurs. **70**:1888-1893, 1970.
33. *Moncrief, J. A.: Burns, N. Engl. J. Med. **288**:444-454, 1973.
34. Nelson, W. E.: Textbook of pediatrics, ed. 10, Philadelphia, 1975, W. B. Saunders Co.
35. Noonan, J., and Noonan, L.: Two burned patients in flotation therapy, Am. J. Nurs. **68**:316-319, 1968.
36. Polk, H., and Stone, H. H., editors: Contemporary burn management, Boston, 1971, Little, Brown & Co.
37. *Quinly, S., et al.: Identity problems and the adaptation of nurses to severely burned children, Am. J. Psychiatry **128**:58-63, 1971.
38. Reyes, M., et al.: Burns. In Meltzer, L. E., Abdellah, F. G., and Kitchell, J. R., editors: Concepts and practices of intensive care for nurse specialists, ed. 2, Bowie, Md., 1976, The Charles Press Publishers, Inc.
39. *Rogenes, P. R., and Moylan, J.: Restoring fluid balance in the patient with severe burns, Am. J. Nurs. **76**:1952-1957, 1976.
40. Sabiston, D. C., editor: Davis-Christopher textbook of surgery, ed. 11, Philadelphia, 1977, W. B. Saunders Co.
41. *Savedra, M.: Coping with pain: strategies of severely burned children, Mat. Child Nurs. J. **5**:197-203, 1976.
42. *Septic shock in a burn patient, nursing grand rounds, Nurs. 76 **6**:39-43, 1976.
43. *Sheehy, E.: Primary excision: innovation in pediatric burn care, RN **37**:21-25, Aug. 1974.
44. Silver, H. K., et al.: Handbook of pediatrics, ed. 12, Los Altos, Calif., 1977, Lange Medical Publications.
45. Singletary, Y.: More than skin deep, J. Psychiatr. Nurs. **15**:7-13, Feb. 1977.
46. Smith, C. A., editor: Profiles of burn management, Miami, 1969, Industrial Medicine Publishing Co., Inc. (Reprinted from Industrial Medicine and Surgery, Aug.-Dec. 1968.)
47. *Tichy, A. M.: Stress of hospitalization: perspectives of burn care, Commun. Nurs. Res. **9**:23-39, April 1977.
48. *Wagner, M.: Emergency care of the burned patient, Am. J. Nurs. **77**:1788-1791, 1977.
49. *Williams, B. P.: The burned patient's need for teaching, Nurs. Clin. North Am. **6**:615-639, 1971.
50. Williams, B. P.: The problems and life-style of a severely burned man. In Bergersen, B., Anderson, E. H., Duffy, M., Lohr, M., and Rose, M. H., editors: Current concepts in clinical nursing, vol. 2, St. Louis, 1969, The C. V. Mosby Co.
51. *Williams, B. P.: Life-styles of severely burned men. In ANA clinical sessions, New York, 1969, Appleton-Century Crofts.
52. Williams, S. R.: Nutrition and diet therapy, ed. 3, St. Louis, 1977, The C. V. Mosby Co.

*References preceded by an asterisk are particularly well suited for student reading.

68

Problems of the integument

ROSEMARY CRAYCROFT YEGANEF

Problems affecting the skin are a result of various causes. There may be parasitic infestations, fungal, bacterial, or viral infections, reactions to substances encountered externally or taken internally, or new growths. Many of the skin manifestations have no known cause, while others are hereditary. This chapter provides an overview of the more common determatologic disorders the nurse is likely to encounter.

■ PARASITIC INFESTATIONS

□ Pediculosis

Pediculi (lice) are most often found among individuals who have poor personal hygiene habits. Lice are not restricted to low-income urban populations, however, and many children get head lice from their classmates or from people on crowded buses. Control and treatment of pediculosis (lice infestation) in middle- or upper-income populations can be hampered by refusal of parents to admit that their children have pediculosis.

Lice obtain their nutrition by sucking blood from the skin. They leave their eggs on the skin surface attached to hair shafts, and this results in the transference from person to person.

There are three types of lice that infest humans: the head louse, the body louse, and the pubic louse. The head louse *(Pediculosis capitis)* attaches itself to the hair shaft, laying about eight eggs a day. The eggs or *nits* are firmly attached to the hair or threads of clothing. They may be viewed with a hand lens and appear as grayish, glistening oval bodies. Intense itching is caused from the bite of the insect with contamination from saliva, head parts, and feces of the lice. Scratching may lead to further trauma with the possibility of secondary infection and enlarged cervical lymph nodes. The head louse is usually confined to the scalp and beard.

The body louse *(Pediculosis corporis)* resides chiefly in the seams of clothing around the neck, waist, and thighs. The bite causes minute hemorrhagic points and severe itching. Transmission is by direct contact or by way of clothing, bedding, and towels.

The pubic louse *(Phthirus pubis)* differs slightly from the head and body louse. It resembles a tiny crab, having clawlike pincers that attach firmly to the pubic hair. Nits are visible in the pubic hair. *P. pubis* is transmitted by sexual contact, bed clothing, towels, and occasionally by toilet seats.

Assessment. Diagnosis is made by finding nits or lice on a person who also has pinpoint erythema, raised macules, and a complaint of pruritus.

Intervention. Treatment is topical, and the effective agents are gamma benzene hexachloride (Kwell) or benzyl benzoate. Kwell comes in shampoo, lotion or cream. There may be a need to repeat treatment in severe cases. Treatment of head lice consists of shampooing vigorously with the medication. A fine-toothed comb may be used to remove remaining nits. The hair may be shampooed with regular shampoo in 24 hours. Treatment of body lice consists in an initial cleansing bath followed by application of a thin layer of lotion or cream. After 24 hours the person bathes and redresses in clean clothes. If eyelashes are infested, the nits are removed and a local application of 0.25% physostigmine (Eserine) is used.

Clothing, linen, and towels should be washed in very hot water or dry cleaned. Garments that have been stored for 1 month will not be infested.

□ Scabies

Scabies is caused by the female itch mite *(Sarcoptes scabiei)* that penetrates the stratum corneum and burrows into the skin. Scabies is acquired through intimate contact, or may be transmitted by way of clothing, linen, or towels. It is not always associated with poor hygiene.

Assessment. Eggs are laid by the female as she travels through the skin, setting up an allergic reaction causing redness, swelling, and vesiculation. The burrows have a wavy, brownish, threadlike appearance. They are found in the interdigital webs, the flexor surface of the wrist, nipples, penis, axillary folds, and buttocks. Secondary reactions from *S. scabiei* include papules, pustules, excoriations, and bacterial infections.

Norwegian scabies is a rare variant found to produce less pruritus but extensive hyperkeratosis and inflammation. The person is found to be infested with thousands of organisms.

Intervention. Treatment is topical with benzyl benzoate and gamma benzene hexachloride (Kwell). Medication should be left on the skin for 24 hours. Clothing and linen should be washed in very hot water or dry cleaned.

□ Bed bugs

The bite of *Cimex lectularius* produces purpuric spots often occurring in clusters of four or more. Itching and burning are experienced over the ankle and lower leg, the most frequent site of the bite. The presence of bedbugs often can be detected if the bedcovers are thrown back at night in a lighted room and can be seen most frequently at the foot of the bed. They may also be found along the seams of mattresses and in cracks in the bed frame. Spraying with benzene hexachloride over the mattress, floor, and walls is usually sufficient for control of bed bugs.

□ Outcome criteria for the person with a parasitic infestation

The person or significant others can:

1. Describe preventive hygiene measures.
2. Explain method of transmission of the parasite.
3. Describe care of clothing and linens (washing in hot water or dry cleaning).
4. Explain medication and treatment program: desired effect of drug, areas of application, number of applications.

■ FUNGAL INFECTIONS

Fungi are larger and more complex than bacteria. They may be unicellular, such as yeasts, or multicellular, such as molds. Many types are pathogenic to humans, causing common skin disorders or serious systemic diseases such as blastomycosis. Certain types of fungi cause few symptoms, while others produce inflammatory or hypersensitivity reactions.

□ Candidiasis (moniliasis)

Candida albicans, a yeastlike fungus, normally inhabits the gastrointestinal tract, mouth, and vagina, but not usually the skin. The inflammation associated with the organism's overgrowth on the skin is caused by the toxins that are released. Some predisposing factors causing an overgrowth of *C. albicans* are pregnancy, use of birth control pills, poor nutrition, antibiotic therapy, and hematopoietic disease. Yeast thrives in a warm, moist environment such as the perineum and intertriginous areas.

Assessment. *Thrush* is candidiasis of the mucous membrane. The lesions are small white spots on the buccal mucosa and may extend down the esophagus. Vaginal thrush causes intense itching with a cheesy vaginal discharge. Skin lesions appear as pruritic, eroded, moist, inflamed areas with vesicles and pustules. Diagnosis of moniliasis at any site is made by clinical appearance and microscopic examination.

Intervention. Treatment is aimed at the precipitating factors. Other measures include keeping the skin dry to avoid maceration, wearing loose, absorbent clothing, and using topical medications such as powders that help to keep the skin dry. Nystatin (Mycostatin), an antibiotic available in tablets, powder, or vaginal suppositories, is very effective against yeast infections.

□ Dermatophytoses (tinea)

One form of superficial fungus infections, or dermatophytoses, is ringworm, which is not caused by a worm, nor are the lesions always round. *Tinea capitis*, or ringworm of the scalp, has worldwide distribution, especially among prepubertal children. Over 90% of tinea capitis in the United States is caused by the *Microsporum* fungus. The characteristic lesion is round, and erythema, a slight scaling, and some pustules may appear at the edge of the lesion. Hair loss occurs, with the hair shaft broken off at skin level. The hair loss is only temporary, since the lesions usually heal without scarring. *Tinea barbae*, or ringworm of the beard, may be more severe, causing folliculitis, lymph node enlargement, marked redness, and scar formation with hair loss.

Tinea corporis (body ringworm) is most common in children and involves the nonhairy skin. Typical lesions appear flat with an erythematous scaling border and clearing center. *Tinea cruris*, or ringworm of the groin area (commonly referred to as "jock itch"), is found in warm, moist areas of friction. It is seen most often in men, especially those who have tinea pedis.

Tinea pedis, or athlete's foot, is a relatively common dermatophytosis. The lesions are pruritic, scaly, erythematous rashes on the soles of the feet and interdigital webs. The toes may become affected, resulting in distorted, brittle, discolored, white or yellow toe nails. When the fungus infects the nails, it is called *onychomycosis*.

Assessment. Diagnosis of tinea is made by observation of the characteristic lesion and by microscopic examination of the scales or hairs. A Wood's light (p. 1491) can be used to identify fungus on hairs.

Intervention. In treating the area involved, it should be remembered that fungi flourish in warm, moist regions. Treatment is aimed at keeping skin sur-

folliculitis: inflammation of hair follicles of the skin. forms small reddish raised areas.

faces clean and dry. Shower shoes should be worn in public showers. Powders may be helpful on the feet and intertriginous areas. A change of socks and shoes during the day is helpful in tinea pedis.

Griseofulvin is an antifungal antibiotic that, after oral ingestion, concentrates in the horny layer of the skin. Tinea corporis and tinea pedis that are extensive respond well to systemic therapy of griseofulvin in 3 to 4 weeks. It is the only effective treatment of onychomycosis. Griseofulvin reduces the effectiveness of anticoagulants; therefore adjustments in dosages may have to be made. It has also been noted that phenobarbital given concomitantly with griseofulvin may decrease the antifungal properties.

Application of ointments may be preceded by soaks in potassium permanganate 1:10,000, an old and effective method of treatment. Ammoniated mercury ointment, benzoic and salicylic acid ointment (Whitfield's), and tolnaftate (Tinactin) are also used.

In tinea capitis it is important to instruct the person to have a separate comb and brush to prevent the spread of the fungus. In all fungus infections, linen, clothing, and towels should be laundered frequently in hot water. Hygiene is important, but it is not possible to avoid total contact with pathogenic fungi.

□ Outcome criteria for the person with a fungal infection

The person or significant others can:

1. Describe drug name, dosage, route, desired effect, frequency, and duration of treatment.
2. Describe proper foot care, avoidance of moisture and heat, use of own toilet articles, and care of linen and clothes.
3. Describe plans for medical follow-up for severe infections.

■ BACTERIAL INFECTIONS

□ Furuncles and carbuncles

Furuncles (boils) are purulent lesions of the skin involving sebaceous glands and hair follicles. They often occur in crops (furunculosis) and are caused in most instances by staphylococci. *Carbuncles* are also caused by staphylococci but differ from furuncles in that they are much larger and involve not only the skin but also the subcutaneous tissues. Furuncles are likely to occur on the face, neck, forearms, groin, and legs, whereas carbuncles are usually limited to the nape of the neck and the back. Both occur most often in poorly nourished, fatigued, or otherwise susceptible persons whose hygiene may be poor, in debilitated elderly people, and in persons who have inadequately treated diabetes mellitus.

Assessment. A furuncle usually begins as a small pustule at the base of a hair follicle; a carbuncle develops at the base of several hair follicles. Local swelling and redness soon occur, and there is severe local pain, which is decreased by moving the involved part as little as possible. Within 3 to 5 days the lesion becomes elevated or "points up," the surrounding skin becomes shiny, and the center or "core" turns yellow (p. 179). A carbuncle has several cores. The boil will usually rupture spontaneously, but it may be surgically incised and drained. As drainage occurs, the pain is immediately relieved. The drainage soon changes from a yellow purulent material to a serosanguineous discharge. All drainage usually subsides within a few hours to a few days; the redness and swelling subside gradually.

Intervention. Hot, wet dressings are used to help bring the boil to a head, but these dressings are discontinued as soon as drainage occurs in order to prevent skin maceration and spread of infection. As the boil drains, care must be taken to keep the infected drainage off the surrounding skin, as organisms may be harbored in hair follicles and furunculosis may recur. The person is cautioned to keep his hands away from the drainage to prevent spread of infection.

If the person is hospitalized, wound isolation procedures are followed until the drainage subsides lest the organism be carried to others. Health personnel should wash their hands thoroughly after caring for the patient and should avoid getting the drainage on their own skin.

The person who is at home must be taught to be scrupulously careful in hygiene practices to prevent accidentally passing the organisms to others in the family or to persons at work. It is not uncommon for entire families to have some type of staphylococcal infection after one member has had a boil.

Furuncles and carbuncles tend to recur in susceptible individuals, and the staphylococci causing them often are resistent to local treatment and to antibiotics. Sunshine, autogenous vaccine, and pHisoHex to cleanse the skin are used, although their benefits are uncertain.

□ Acne vulgaris

Acne vulgaris is one of the most troublesome and most common skin conditions of adolescence. Lack of cleanliness is often blamed for the development of the condition by the person or his family. In reality, cleanliness plays no part in the *initial* development of the condition.

Acne vulgaris is definitely known to have a relationship to hormonal activity. It usually makes its appearance at puberty, and in girls its activity can be clearly related to gonadal activity during different parts of the menstrual cycle. Hormonal activity produces hyperkeratosis of the follicular orifices, which leads to blocking of the secretions (sebum) and the formation of discolored fatty plugs or blackheads (comedones). After the blackhead forms there is hypertrophy of the sebaceous glands, and secondary infection occurs. Sometimes cysts and nodules then form, and unsightly scars result despite the best treatment.

Intervention. Acne will not be cured but can be controlled during adolescence. It is important, especially among boys, to stress that controlling the acne is their responsibility; it is up to them to maintain the prescribed treatments.

Although there is no cure for acne vulgaris, a wide variety of treatments are utilized with varying success. The face should be kept clean by washing with a mild soap or antibacterial solution. A blackhead may be safely removed by a nurse or physician with the use of a specially designed instrument. The person should never squeeze his skin to express comedones or to break a pustule. He should be taught to avoid touching his face with his hands, since this may cause more infection by grinding dirt and organisms into open pores.

Systemic antibiotics such as tetracycline or erythromycin may be used in the treatment of acne vulgaris. Topical agents with antiseptic as well as drying and desquamation effects include salicylic acid and sulfur soaps (SAStid), and gels or lotions containing benzoyl peroxide (Pan Oxyl 10%). Retin-A is also used to peel and dry the skin surface. Vleminckx (sulfurated lime) hot packs may be used on the face for the same purpose. Persons with acne who have large cysts may need interlesional injection of triamcinolone. The cysts usually resolve in 1 to 2 weeks.

Diet as a factor in acne is thought by some persons to be overrated. If a person knows certain foods cause a flare-up, these should be eliminated from the diet. Fad diets should be avoided. Usually face washing at morning and night with a drying soap is adequate. Women should avoid oil-based cosmetics for they may be occlusive and contribute to the plugging of the hair follicles.

After the acne is under control, dermabrasion (p. 1500) may be used to lessen the pitting and scarring; the effectiveness is approximately 50%. Some complications of dermabrasion are hyperpigmentation, infection, and persistent erythema. A technique of injecting fibrin into areas of pitting may help minimize the defect.

□ Acne rosacea

Acne rosacea is a skin condition that usually affects people over 25 years of age. The actual cause is unknown. Over the years many causative factors have been suggested including bacteria, vitamin deficiency, hormonal imbalance, alcohol, caffeine, psychic factors, and heredity. Acne rosacea begins with redness over the cheeks and nose, followed by papules, pustules, and enlargement of superficial blood vessels. Years of acne rosacea lead to an irregular, bulbous thickening of the skin of the distal part of the nose (rhinophyma), with a red-purple discoloration and dilated follicles.

There is no specific treatment for acne rosacea. Some persons respond to tetracycline and topical peeling agents, but there is no specific treatment for the vascular component. Avoiding stimuli that cause vasodilatation seems appropriate. Rhinophyma may be treated by plastic surgery.

□ Impetigo contagiosa

Impetigo contagiosa is a superficial skin disease produced by a form of streptococci often in association with staphylococci. It is largely a disease of children and may be endemic in nurseries unless special precautions are taken. The disease begins as a vesicle usually in the area of the mouth or nostrils, although it can be anywhere on the body. It becomes pustular and dries to form a honey-colored crust that comes off as the lesion heals. Scarring does not result unless superimposed infection or trauma occurs. Greatest care must be taken to isolate the patient and to prevent reinfection with fingers and clothing. Treatment usually consists of systemic antibiotics such as penicillin. Gentle mechanical washings or soaks may remove crusts.

□ Erysipelas

Erysipelas is an acute febrile disease caused by the hemolytic streptococcus and characterized by localized inflammation and swelling of the skin and subcutaneous tissues, usually of the face. A bright, sharp line separates the diseased skin from the normal skin. Elderly people with poor resistance are most often affected. Erysipelas was a serious disease before the advent of antibiotics; penicillin is the drug of choice.

□ Outcome criteria for the person with a bacterial skin infection

The patient or significant others can:

1. Describe measures to avoid bacterial spread by:
   a. Avoidance of contamination from drainage.
   b. Cleansing practices.
   c. Disposal of contaminated articles.
2. Describe the medical treatment program:
   a. Demonstrate use of hot packs, if appropriate.
   b. State name of drug, dosage, purpose, route, frequency, and side effects.
   c. State plans for health care follow-up.

■ VIRAL DISEASES

□ Verrucae

Verrucae (warts) are caused by a virus that may be transmitted from one person to another. Warts should be removed to prevent crops of them from developing. Electrodesiccation (drying by electric current) is one of the better methods of treatment; it is safer than the use of acids such as nitric acid, which may injure normal tissue. Warts sometimes disappear spontaneously, and this unexplained characteristic leads to the many tales of their being charmed by a variety of means. Warts may grow inward on the soles of the feet (plantar warts) and cause severe pain and incapacity. Plantar warts may be treated with x-ray therapy, frozen with liquid hydrogen (the most common), or peeled with salicylic acid.

□ Herpes simplex

One of the most common viruses found in humans is the herpes simplex virus (HSV). It occurs as two similar yet serologically different strains, type 1 and type 2. The type 1 virus is found primarily in lesions of the face and mouth (fever blister, cold sore), eye (keratitis), and brain (encephalitis). Type 2 is associated with a lesion of the genitalia that can be transmitted by sexual contact. HSV has a DNA-containing core surrounded by a phospholipid covering.

Assessment. Most persons experience the initial contact with HSV as a young child. The HSV remains in the cells of the sensory nerves that supply the affected areas and cause recurrent lesions when the person is subjected to stresses. The appearance of vesicles is preceded by several hours by a sensation of burning or itching. A cluster of vesicles appear at the mucocutaneous junctions of the lips or nose, or as an inflammation of the cornea of one eye with photophobia and tearing. The type 2 virus lesions occur in the vagina or cervix of the woman or on the penile skin of the man. The lesions are painful and frequently crack open. A crust gradually forms, and the lesions heal in about 10 days.

Intervention. There is no safe, effective, systemic approach at this time to treatment of recurrent herpes simplex of the face or genitalia. Local treatment is the most effective if given *early* to prevent the virus from multiplying and thus hasten healing for general comfort. The vesicles on the face can be opened and 70% alcohol applied every 1 to 2 hours to break down the fat-soluble covering of the virus, thus inactivating it. Ether has also been used as a solvent. The drug 5-iodo-2-deoxyuridine (idoxuridine) that inhibits viral DNA is effective in the treatment of HSV-induced keratitis. Disagreement exists of the effectiveness of idoxuridine for skin manifestations, but some positive results have been achieved with early hourly applications.[43]

Another controversial method of treatment is photoinactivation. A heterocyclic dye (neutral red, proflavine, methylene blue) is applied to vesicles that have been opened, and the area is then subjected to exposure to an ordinary fluorescent light for 15 minutes. The light exposure is repeated for 30 minutes at 8 hours and again at 36 hours after dye application.[43] The dye binds to the viral nucleic acid in the presence of light, thus destroying it. Controversy over use of photoinactivation centers on the potential oncogenicity of the dyes.

After the initial phase of vesicle eruption, the goal of therapy is promotion of comfort. Pain may be relieved by analgesics such as aspirin or by application of warm, moist compresses. Spirits of camphor applied as a liquid or in small tubes of camphorated lip ice may be helpful.

□ Herpes zoster

Herpes zoster, or shingles, is caused by the same virus (V-Z) that causes varicella (chickenpox). Varicella is believed to be the primary infection in a nonimmune host, while herpes zoster is thought to be the response in a partially immune host. Although herpes zoster is far less communicable than chickenpox, persons who have not had chickenpox may develop it after exposure to the vesicular lesions of persons with herpes zoster. For this reason, susceptible persons should not care for patients with herpes zoster.

Herpes zoster can be a serious condition in any adult and may even lead to death from exhaustion in elderly debilitated individuals. It is one of the most drawn out and exasperating conditions found in elderly patients and leads to discouragement and demoralization. Contrary to popular thought, one episode of herpes zoster does *not* provide immunity, and the disease may recur.[2] Herpes zoster often occurs in persons with Hodgkin's disease and in those with lymphoid and some bone cancers because of reduced cell-mediated immunity.

Assessment. In herpes zoster, clusters of small vesicles usually form in a line. They follow the course of the peripheral sensory nerves and often are unilateral. Since they follow nerve pathways, the lesions never cross the midline of the body. Nerves on both sides of the body, however, can be involved. Two-thirds of persons with herpes zoster develop lesions over thoracic dermatomes, and the remainder show involvement of the trigeminal nerve with lesions on the face, eye, and scalp. The rash develops first as macules but progresses rapidly to vesicles. The fluid becomes turbid, and crusts develop and drop off in about 10 days.

Malaise, fever, itching, and pain over the involved area may precede the eruption of the lesions. Discomfort from pain and itching is the major problem with herpes zoster. The pain may vary from a light burning sensation to a deep visceral type pain, and may be intermittent or constant. It usually persists for up to 4 weeks. In approximately 30% of persons over age 40, the pain may last for months or years, especially in the elderly.[2] Enlargement of the lymph nodes may also occur with the rash.

Intervention. There is no specific therapy for the

treatment of herpes zoster, and the care is primarily symptomatic. If discomfort is severe, the person may benefit from a short period of rest, especially if malaise and fever have occurred. Loose clothing is suggested to minimize contact with the affected area. Pruritus may be relieved by the application of calamine lotion or collodion over the vesicular area. Analgesics are usually necessary. Corticosteroids such as methylprednisolone (Medrol) may be given to shorten the period of acute pain, but they have no effect on healing of the skin lesions.

Postherpetic neuralgia presents difficulties in obtaining relief of pain because of limited results from the usual analgesics. Narcotics should be avoided because of the persistency of the pain and potential for addiction. Medications that have proved useful for some persons include carbamazepine (Tegretol), phenothiazines such as chlorpromazine (Thorazine), or sedatives. The cooling effect of ethyl chloride spray may provide some temporary relief.

□ Outcome criteria for the person with a herpes infection

The person or significant others can:

1. Describe the nature of the condition and the probability of recurrence.
2. Describe measures that can be taken to decrease discomfort (alcohol, camphor, or moist compresses over lesions of herpes simplex; calamine lotion or collodion over lesions of herpes zoster; analgesics).

■ DERMATITIS (ECZEMA)

Dermatitis is an inflammation of the skin that usually proceeds through the stages of redness or erythema, vesicle formation with oozing, crusting, scaling, and thickening of the skin. Eczema may be caused by external factors in the environment (contact dermatitis) or to endogenous factors (atopic eczema). *Atopic eczema* occurs primarily in children although it may occur in adults. Infantile eczema occurs after 2 months of age and is characterized by pruritic, weeping papules that merge to form plaques. In children past infancy the lesions are drier and more lichenified. Infantile eczema may be outgrown only to be replaced by asthma or hay fever. The tendency to develop these conditions is inherited. Persons with atopic dermatitis are very susceptible to superimposed herpes simplex or vaccinia infections.[7]

Contact dermatitis is caused by environmental factors. There are two types of contact dermatitis, primary irritant dermatitis and allergic contact dermatitis. *Irritant dermatitis* is caused by the effect of environmental irritants such as acids, solvents, or detergents, and they affect all persons having sufficient exposure. The dermatitis usually occurs on exposed areas such as the hands. People whose work demands constant wetting of the skin often develop irritant dermatitis. The *allergic contact dermatitis* is a cell-mediated immune reaction and requires a length of exposure to an antigen such as oils of plants *(dermatitis venenata)*, cosmetics, synthetics, chemicals, jewelry, or biologic substances. Nurses and physicians have been known to become so sensitive to penicillin and streptomycin that they must wear gloves when handling these medications. The symptoms of contact dermatitis may develop within a few hours or after several days following contact. The symptoms vary from redness with itching and burning to vesicle formation and severe edema followed by secondary infection.

Prevention. Dermatitis venenata is largely preventable. Everyone should be taught to recognize the leaves of poisonous plants such as poison ivy, poison oak, or sumac found in his part of the country. Sensitivity to poisonous resins varies with individuals. Almost all people, however, are sensitive to some extent, and everyone should wear clothing that protects his skin if he is knowingly in contact with poisonous plants. Some persons are so sensitive that minute particles of the irritating oil carried in smoke or borne in the air after someone has crushed the plant are sufficient to cause a severe skin reaction. Pets may carry the irritating resin to their owners. The resins can remain on clothing for several days.

The person who develops a sensitivity to materials encountered in his daily work may need to change his mode of employment permanently. Known allergens should be avoided. Gloves may be worn when working with harsh irritants. Persons with a sensitivity to detergents may need to carry their own nondetergent soap for use at all times. Clothing and linen may need to be washed in a mild soap such as Ivory for persons sensitive to washing detergents.

Intervention. If there has been known contact with the oleoresin of a poisonous plant, the skin is washed thoroughly with alkaline laundry soap or detergent and then rinsed with alcohol, preferably within 10 minutes of exposure. The greatest care must be taken not to involve new areas by contact with exudate from active lesions. Although the condition usually does not last over a week, it may persist in some sensitive individuals for weeks and even months. Secondary infections may occur.

Acute dermatitis regardless of cause usually responds rapidly to wet dressings with Burow's solution (aluminum acetate in a 1:40 dilution). Crusts and scales are not removed but are allowed to drop off naturally as the skin heals. Topical medications such as benzocaine, antihistamines, nitrofurazone, or neomycin sulfate should be avoided.[7] If pruritus is intense, colloidal baths may be soothing and relieve the itching. Aspirin or Vistaril may also ease some of the discomfort from pruritus.

Systemic corticosteroids are usually avoided except for extensive acute exacerbations. *Topical* corticosteroids, such as hydrocortisone 1%, are effective and can be used safely over a period of time. They seem to hasten the drying of lesions and limit the progress of the condition. Dermatitis of the hands can be treated by covering the areas with a topical corticosteroid, then encasing the hands in gloves or plastic bags overnight. Superimposed infections are treated by *systemic* antibiotics such as erythromycin.

□ Other types of dermatitis

Neurodermatitis

Neurodermatitis, lichen simplex chronicus, is an inflammation of the skin of neural origin. There is usually no lesion of the skin but only redness. Pruritus is often severe. Thickening and hardening (lichenification) of the skin occurs. The person is often a tense, nervous person who has developed a neurotic habit of rubbing and scratching his skin. Local applications of corticosteroid creams or ointments usually produce improvement in most persons.

Dermatitis medicamentosa

Dermatitis medicamentosa is the name used to designate reactions of the skin to drugs taken internally. Bromides, penicillin and other antibiotics, iodides, barbiturates, and sulfonamides frequently cause skin eruptions. Skin lesions vary from some that are highly colored and sharply defined to others that may resemble urticaria, with large, flat wheals covering almost the entire body. The treatment for drug sensitivity consists of finding and discontinuing the offending medication. Patch testing may be necessary.

Exfoliative dermatitis

Exfoliative dermatitis is usually caused by drugs containing heavy metals such as mercury, bismuth, or arsenic, and is seen less often since the antibiotics and the bacteriostatic drugs have largely replaced drugs containing the heavy metals. Signs include redness, edema, and massive desquamation (shedding of epidermal cells). The person may lose the entire outer layer of skin from the soles of his feet and the palms of his hands. Colloidal baths help allay the itching and make the erythema and desquamation less conspicuous. The skin loss does not cause scarring. Persons with known sensitivities should avoid taking drugs containing heavy metals.

□ Outcome criteria for the person with dermatitis

The person or significant others can:

1. State causative agents (if known), source of the agent, and method of contact.
2. Describe measures to prevent further contacts.
3. Describe problems of self-treatment and the need for medical follow-up.
4. Describe medical treatment program:
   a. State name of medication, purpose, dosage, route and frequency, and side effects.
   b. Demonstrate treatment measures to be carried out at home.

■ OTHER TOXIC SKIN REACTIONS

Erythema multiforme is a skin condition believed to occur secondary to an underlying systemic disease such as an infection. The skin eruption is characterized by red to purple macules, papules, and vesicles. Most often the lesions occur on the wrists, back of the hands, ankles, tops of the feet, knees, elbows, face, palms, and soles of the feet; the entire body may be involved. The skin eruption may be preceded by fever, chest pain, and arthralgia. The treatment is to seek out the underlying cause and eliminate it if possible. Other treatment is supportive, and corticosteroids are often used. Local treatment includes baths, soaks, and dressings. Fluids are forced, and the person is encouraged to eat a high-calorie diet. If lesions appear in the mouth, special mouth care is indicated, including irrigations with warm salt solution.

Communicable diseases such as measles, chickenpox, smallpox, scarlet fever, and typhoid fever produce skin reactions (Table 68-1). Nodes and hemorrhagic spots in the skin also accompany severe acute rheumatic fever.

■ DERMATOSES

□ Psoriasis

Psoriasis is a genetically determined, chronic, epidermal proliferative disease. It is not infectious or contagious and is not a nervous disorder. Approximately 2% to 4% of the population of the United States has psoriasis; 5% of this group have associated inflammatory arthritis. The average age of occurrence in men is about 20 years, but it affects both sexes in all age groups.

Assessment. The turnover time for normal skin is 28 days. After the basal cell divides, it normally takes 14 days to reach the stratum corneum, and an additional 14 days for this cell to be sloughed off. In psoriasis the time is accelerated to 4 to 7 days.

The lesions of psoriasis are elevated, erythematous, sharply circumscribed, scaling plaques. The primary lesion is a papule; these papules then join to form plaques. In the black person the plaques may appear to be purple. Lesions may occur over the entire body, but are found more commonly on the scalp, elbows, shins, and trunk. Beefy red lesions may be observed in an acute flare-up. The nails of persons with psoriasis have characteristic involvement; there may be pitting of the nails, yellowish

Table 68-1. Skin reactions of some communicable diseases

Disease	Cause	Incubation period (days)	Place of rash origin	Skin lesions
Measles (rubeola)	Rubeola virus	11 (8 to 14)	Face	Pink macular-papular rash; lesions coalesce
German measles; 3-day measles (rubella)	Rubella virus	14 to 21	Face	Pink macular-papular rash; lesions usually discrete, may coalesce
Scarlet fever (scarlatina)	Hemolytic streptococcus	1 to 3	Neck, chest	Bright red (scarlet) macules (pinpoint)
Chickenpox (varicella)	V-Z virus	14 to 21	Back, chest	Macule, papule, vesicle, crust, lesions at different stages
Smallpox (variola)	Variola virus	12 (7 to 21)	Face	Macule, papule, vesicle, crust, lesions all at same stage
Typhoid fever	*Salmonella typhosa*	14 (7 to 21)	Abdomen	Macular rash

discoloration, and onycholysis (separation of the nail from the nail bed).

Psoriasis takes many forms. *Arthropathic psoriasis* is one of the cruelest forms and may produce crippling. The nails are always involved and show denting and pitting. *Pustular psoriasis* (von Zumbusch) may present with fever, tenderness of the skin, and sterile pustules.

Intervention. Because of the overproduction of skin in psoriasis, treatment is based on slowing mitotic activity. Initially the lesions may be treated with topical steroids and wet dressings to decrease inflammation. Topical medications such as crude coal tar, anthralin, and related compounds are frequently used as they appear to have a keratolytic effect. The combination of tar and ultravioliet light known as the Goeckerman regimen (see boxed material) is one of the oldest forms of therapy for psoriasis that is quite effective and still widely used today in modified forms. Anthralin, a distillate of crude coal tar, is used over stubborn plaques of psoriasis. Gloves should be worn during application because of its irritating effect.

Methotrexate, an antimetabolite, is reserved for those cases of psoriasis that are resistant to topical treatment. When used appropriately, it has shown a good to excellent clearing of lesions in 80% of the patients. The person on methotrexate should be monitored closely. An initial liver biopsy and creatinine clearance level is done initially and repeated at intervals to determine liver and renal function. Hematologic toxicity is a side effect that can be monitored by periodic blood counts.

A recently developed treatment in psoriasis is the combination of orally administered methoxsalen (Psoralen) and long-wave ultraviolet light (UVA), hence the name PUVA therapy. Methoxsalen is a photosensitizing agent and does not produce systemic toxicity as may occur with methotrexate. The results of PUVA therapy in one study show complete clearing of lesions in 90% of the patients.[48] Some side effects of PUVA therapy include pruritus, erythema, localized blistering, a moderate flare-up of psoriasis (Koebner phenomenon), and transient nausea. The dosage schedules vary and are calculated according to body weight. The person is exposed to long-wave ultraviolet light (320 to 400 nm) 2 hours after ingestion of the methoxsalen. Photochemotherapy in psoriasis causes inhibition of increased DNA synthesis within the psoriatic lesion. Since the skin remains photosensitive until methoxsalen is excreted, persons receiv-

GOECKERMAN REGIMEN

1. Apply crude coal tar two to three times a day over all affected areas.
2. Remove tar with corn oil prior to ultraviolet therapy, leaving a thin film on skin.
3. Give ultraviolet light therapy.
4. Give tub bath with soap and oil. Shampoo scalp.
5. Reapply tar to skin and lotion to scalp.
6. Have person wear pajamas for 3 days to act as a dressing.

ing this treatment are warned to avoid exposure to the sun at least 8 hours after ingestion of the medication.[48]

Since the lesions of psoriasis are commonly found in visible skin areas, the person is faced with a socially disabling disease. He may need help in identifying and coping with his feelings and with changes that may occur in his life style (see Chapter 28).

Lesions may fade with treatment, only to recur eventually in the same area or elsewhere. The disease is not curable and may wax and wane continuously. If the person is not aware of this, he may lose confidence in his physician and may seek a quick cure. Because psoriasis is so common and so stubborn in response to treatment, manufacturers of patent remedies find a lucrative field for their products among persons who have the disease. Anyone who reads the daily newspapers or watches television regularly has seen numerous promises of cure. The person with psoriasis should be warned lest he take these advertisements seriously and waste his money.

Outcome criteria for the person with psoriasis. The person or significant others can:

1. Describe the nature of the condition (noncurable, recurrence of symptoms).
2. Describe the prescribed treatment program.
3. State the problems of self-medication.
4. Describe plans for medical follow-up.
5. Describe plans for socialization with others.

☐ Pemphigus

Pemphigus is a skin condition characterized by enormous bullae that appear all over the body and on the mucous membranes. The lesions break and are followed by crusts that heal and leave scars. The disease is characterized histologically by acantholysis (cells slip past one another and fluid accumulates between the cells). By placing the thumb firmly on the skin and exerting lateral sliding pressure, the upper epidermis can be dislodged, resulting in erosion or blister (Nikolsky's sign).

The cause of pemphigus is unknown, but recent studies and immunofluorescent techniques demonstrate that pemphigus may be a type of autoimmune disease. It usually manifests itself in middle age. In more than one-half the patients the first lesion appears in the mouth, and pain from oral lesions may prevent adequate food intake. The treatment of choice for severe pemphigus is systemic corticosteroid therapy.

Nursing care of a person with pemphigus is very difficult. Foster or Stryker frames may be used in an effort to move the patient as painlessly as possible and prevent weight bearing on raw surfaces. Dakin's solution compresses may be applied to oozing lesions to help control odors and infection. Reverse isolation may be indicated. Special mouth care is usually necessary, and bland diets are more easily tolerated.

Emotional support and encouragement of both the patient and his family are extremely important. The patient may fear that he is so repulsive that no one will take care of him, and he needs constant reassurance and evidence of continued interest in him by the staff. Family and friends should be prepared for the patient's appearance before they visit him if they have not seen him recently. The family are encouraged to visit often and to behave as normally as they possibly can.

☐ Dermatitis herpetiformis

Dermatitis herpetiformis is a chronic skin condition usually seen in men. The lesion is a vesicular, papular, pruritic eruption of unknown cause. There is a characteristic distribution of lesions, usually symmetrical, bilateral, and appearing over the surfaces of the limbs, on the buttocks, and on the scalp. Scarring and hyperpigmentation may occur after the lesions heal. Some persons have associated atrophy of the villi of the small intestine that may or may not be accompanied by signs of malabsorption. Treatment is with systemic sulfones, and the response is often diagnostic because of the improvement. Antipruritic medications may or may not relieve the intense pruritus.

■ CHANGES IN SKIN

The skin gradually changes as one grows older. Collagen becomes less flexible and more mature. The aging of skin is greatly influenced by sun exposure habits. The decline in sex hormones causes some atrophy of the skin. In the elderly, skin tags, seborrheic keratoses, and lentigines (brown spots on light skin) are common.

☐ Benign lesions

Seborrheic keratoses. Seborrheic keratoses occur most often in persons past middle age. The lesions resemble large, darkened, greasy warts and are often found around the trunk, on the back, and under the breasts. They seldom become malignant but should be observed at intervals for any change. They often can be removed easily with dichloracetic acid or carbon dioxide snow.

Stasis dermatitis. Stasis dermatitis is a common skin condition of the lower extremities in older persons. It is usually preceded by varicosities and poor circulation. With the reduction in venous return from the legs, substances normally carried away by the circulation remain in the tissues and irritate them. The skin is often reddened and edematous. Pruritus may be quite severe. Breaks in the skin are often caused by scratching, and infection then is introduced by the hands, clothing, and other sources.

The most important treatment for stasis dermatitis is prevention by careful attention to the treatment of peripheral vascular conditions and preventing the constriction of the circulation to the extremities.

Angiomas. Angiomas are tufts of blood vessels that may occur spontaneously either as tiny bright red lesions or as purplish vascular lesions. The lesions should be watched closely, for although they do not usually become malignant, they may suddenly develop extensive vascular channels that may be difficult or impossible to remove surgically.

Corns and calluses. Corns are thickened skin lesions with a center core that thickens inwardly and causes acute pain on pressure. They are often caused by the pressure of ill-fitting shoes and occur on the toes. A corn is best treated by correction of shoes and by placing a small felt pad with a hole in the center over it to relieve pressure. Popular corn remedies seldom produce a cure, since their active ingredient is usually salicylic acid, which only dissolves the outer layer of skin. As soon as the medicated pad is removed, a new layer of skin forms unless pressure is relieved.

Calluses, or thickening of circumscribed areas of the horny layer of the skin, often appear on the plantar surface of the foot when the metatarsal arch has fallen and there is constant pressure against the sole of the shoe. They are often successfully treated by relief of the pressure and by regular massage with softening lotions and creams.

□ Malignant and premalignant lesions

Malignancies of the skin are more accessible to treatment than are those in any other part of the body. Education of the person in reporting suspicious lesions and prompt action by nurses and physicians when such lesions are reported should make malignancies of the skin a largely controllable disease. By far the best treatment is early and complete surgical removal of the lesion.

Leukoplakia. Leukoplakia occurs as raised, even shiny areas of various sizes on the mucous membrane of the mouth and also the genitalia in women. Surgical removal is the treatment of choice. If the lesions are too extensive to be removed by surgery, radiotherapy or electrodesiccation may be used. In the early stages, leukoplakia of oral mucosa may be controlled by careful mouth hygiene. The patient who smokes should stop smoking as smoking is definitely known to aggravate the condition. Any loose or jagged teeth are removed, periodontal treatment is given if necessary, and frequent mouth irrigations with an alkaline solution are advised.

Senile keratoses. Senile keratoses usually begin as scaly, raised lesions in exposed parts of the body. The lesion is firm to pressure, and there is usually an elevated surface or border that bleeds easily. Senile keratoses require prompt surgical treatment because they may undergo malignant degeneration and become squamous cell carcinoma.

Basal cell carcinoma. Basal cell carcinoma is usually seen in fair-skinned persons who are frequently exposed to the sun. The lesion usually appears on the sun-exposed surfaces of the skin. The tumors grow slowly and rarely metastasize, but may become locally invasive. A typical form known as a rodent ulcer often develops from senile keratoses.

Basal cell carcinomas should be removed. This may be done through cryosurgery, chemosurgery, or electrosurgery as well as the conventional incisional surgery. The cure rate (95%) is good with the above therapies.

Squamous cell carcinoma. This type of lesion becomes invasive into local tissue. If untreated, metastasis to regional nodes developes. The lesion may appear with central ulceration but more commonly, abnormal keratinization results in the lesion being covered with scale. Early surgical excision is the treatment of choice.

All persons with skin cancer should be instructed to avoid direct exposure to the sun. Sunscreen lotions and creams along with protective clothing should be employed. Skin should be examined at regular intervals.

Pigmented moles—malignant melanomas. Pigmented moles may be precancerous. These skin lesions may be present at birth or may appear at any time of life. The blue or greenish-black type (melanotic nevus) is the most dangerous of all. Yellow and brownish moles are less likely to become malignant. Blue or black moles should be removed even if they are not raised above the normal skin surface. Most physicians agree that any mole that shows signs of growth or that is in a part of the body where it is traumatized by clothing should be removed at once. The malignant melanoma, deriving its name from the melanin, or pigment, in the basal layer in the skin, is the most dangerous of all cancerous skin lesions. The mortality is extremely high, and often wide metastasis has occurred before the lesion is noticed.

There are three signs of malignancy of pigmented lesions: (1) varigated color, including red, white or blue, (2) irregular border, and (3) irregular surface. Skin biopsy is diagnostic. Treatment of malignant melanoma is complete, wide, and full-thickness excision. A skin graft may be necessary to cover the defect.

Sarcoma and fibrosarcoma. Sarcoma and fibrosarcoma are lesions that may develop quite suddenly from seemingly innocuous nodules somewhere in the skin. Unfortunately metastasis often occurs before the original node shows much change. For this reason any nodule in the skin should be reported to a physician at once.

Mycosis fungoides. Mycosis fungoides is one of the most dreaded of all skin diseases. It begins as an itching, thickened lesion in the skin and progresses to a tumor stage that finally breaks down and destroys the skin. A large, soft, mushy vegetative lesion develops that destroys all the normal adjacent structures. Lesions may break out in several parts of the body. While the patient lives, all resemblance to his normal self is lost, and the disease, which lasts an average of 7 years from the date of onset of symptoms, is invariably fatal.[2] X-ray therapy is sometimes used to allay itching in the early stages, and nitrogen mustard is sometimes given intravenously. Corticosteroids delay the process somewhat but do not affect the final outcome. The nursing care for mycosis fungoides in late stages is similar to that required for pemphigus. Electron-beam irradiation has been helpful because it can be applied to the total skin surface; the rays are adjusted so that deep tissues are not affected.[36]

REFERENCES AND SELECTED READINGS

1. Barnowe, K., et al.: Round table discussion: skin diseases in a rural practice, Nurse Pract. **1**:11-14, 1976.
2. Beeson, P. B., and McDermott, W., editors: Textbook of medicine, ed. 14, Philadelphia, 1975, W. B. Saunders Co.
3. Bergersen, B. S.: Pharmacology in nursing, ed. 14, St. Louis, 1979, The C. V. Mosby Co.
4. Bergstresser, P. R., Schreiber, S. H., and Weinstein, G. D.: Systemic chemotherapy for psoriasis, Arch. Dermatol. **112**:977-981, 1976.
5. *Bowden, L.: Current trends in treating malignant melanoma, A.O.R.N. J. **17**:84-91, 1973.
6. Criep, L. H.: Dermatologic allergy: immunology, diagnosis, management, Philadelphia, 1970, W. B. Saunders Co.
7. *Dobson, R. L.: Diagnosis and treatment of eczema, J.A.M.A. **235**:2228-2229, 1976.
8. Felber, T. D., et al.: Photodynamic inactivation of herpes simplex, J.A.M.A. **223**:289-292, 1973.
9. Fisher, A. A.: Contact dermatitis, ed. 2, Philadelphia, 1973, Lea & Febiger.
10. Fitzpatrick, T. B., et al.: Dermatology in general medicine, New York, 1971, McGraw-Hill Book Co.
11. Goodwin, P., Hamilton, S., and Fry, L.: The cell cycle in psoriasis, Br. J. Dermatol. **90**:517-521, 1974.
12. Hanifin, J. M., and Lobitz, W. C.: Newer concepts of atopic dermatitis, Arch. Dermatol. **113**:663-669, 1977.
13. *Kimmig, J., and Janner, M.: Frieboes/Schonfeld color atlas of dermatology, Am. ed. trans. and rev. by H. Goldschmidt and D. M. Pillsbury, Philadelphia, 1966, W. B. Saunders Co.
14. Kligman, A. M., Mills, O. H., Jr., and Leyden, J. J.: Acne vulgaris: a treatable disease, Postgrad. Med. **55**:99-105, 1974.
15. Korting, G. W.: Diseases of the skin in children and adolescents, Philadelphia, 1970, W. B. Saunders Co.
16. Levine, G. M., and Calvan, C. D.: Color atlas of dermatology, Chicago, 1973, Year Book Medical Publishers, Inc.
17. Lewis, G. M., and Clayton, E. W.: Practical dermatology, ed. 3, Philadelphia, 1967, W. B. Saunders Co.
18. Management of common skin problems, Postgrad. Med. **52**:63-194, 1972.
19. Marisco, A. R.: Ultraviolet light and tar in the Goeckerman treatment of psoriasis, Arch. Dermatol. **112**:1249-1250, 1976.
20. Marlow, D. R.: Textbook of pediatric nursing, ed. 5, Philadelphia, 1977, W. B. Saunders Co.
21. Mathews, K. P.: A current view of urticaria, Med. Clin. North Am. **58**:185-205, 1974.
22. Michaëlsson, G., Pettersson, L., and Juhlin, L.: Purpura caused by food and drug additives, Arch. Dermatol. **109**:49-52, 1974.
23. Mihm, M. C., Jr., Early detection of primary cutaneous malignant melanoma: a color atlas, N. Engl. J. Med. **289**:989-996, 1973.
24. Millikan, L. E.: Superficial and cutaneous fungal infections: diagnosis and treatment, Postgrad. Med. **60**:52-58, 1976.
25. Mitchell, D. M.: Eczema, Practitioner **208**:597-606, 1972.
26. Myers, M. C., Photodynamic inactivation in recurrent infections with herpes simplex virus, J. Infect. Dis. **133**(suppl.):A145-A150, 1976.
27. Nahmias, A. J., and Roizman, B.: Infection with herpes-simplex viruses 1 and 2, N. Engl. J. Med. **289**:667-674, 719-725, and 781-789, 1973.
28. Nelson, W. E., editor: Textbook of pediatrics, ed. 10, Philadelphia, 1975, W. B. Saunders Co.
29. North, C., and Weinstein, G.: Treatment of psoriasis, Am. J. Nurs. **76**:410-412, 1976.
30. Orkin, M.: Resurgence of scabies, J.A.M.A. **217**:593-597, 1971.
31. Parrish, J. H.: Dermatology and skin care, New York, 1975, McGraw-Hill Book Co.
32. Parrish, J. H., Fitzpatrick, T. B., Tannenbaum, L., et al.: Photochemotherapy of psoriasis with oral methoxsalen and longwave ultraviolet light, N. Engl. J. Med. **291**:1207-1213, 1974.
33. *Pearson, L. B.: Acne: a common clinical entity for the nurse practitioner, Nurse Pract. **2**:28-29, 1977.
34. Pegum, J. S.: Advances in the treatment of diseases of the skin, Practitioner **209**:453-459, 1972.
35. Pillsbury, D. M.: A manual of dermatology, Philadelphia, 1971, W. B. Saunders Co.
36. Pol, M. L.: Mycosis fungoides and electron beam therapy: the nursing concepts and related care of these patients, In ANA clinical sessions, New York, 1967, Appleton-Century-Crofts.
37. Reisner, R. M.: Acne vulgaris, Pediatr. Clin. North Am. **21**:851-864, 1973.
38. Robin, M.: How emotions affect skin problems in school children, J. Sch. Health **43**:370-373, 1973.
39. Rowel, N.: Urticaria, Practitioner **208**:614-621, 1972.
40. *Ruppe, J. P.: Skin infections: their role in health today, J. Sch. Health **43**:373-380, 1973.
41. Sauer, G. C.: Manual of skin diseases, ed. 3, Philadelphia, 1973, J. B. Lippincott Co.
42. Shelley, W. B.: Consultations in dermatology II, Philadelphia, 1974, W. B. Saunders Co.
43. Smith, E. B.: Management of herpes simplex infections of the skin, J.A.M.A. **235**:1731-1733, 1976.
44. Soter, N. A., Wilkinson, D. S., and Fitzpatrick, T. B.: Clinical dermatology. N. Engl. J. Med. **289**:189-195, 242-249, 296-302, 1973.
45. Spangler, A. S.: Treatment of depressed scars with fibrin foam —seventeen year study, J. Dermatol. Surg. **4**:65-69, 1975.
46. Systemic antibiotics for treatment of acne vulgaris, Arch. Dermatol. **111**:1630-1636, 1975.
47. Wexler, L.: Gamma benzene hexachloride in treatment of pediculosis and scabies, Am. J. Nurs. **69**:565-566, 1969.
48. Wolf, K., et al.: Photochemotherapy for psoriasis with orally administered methoxsalen, Arch. Dermatol. **112**:943-950, 1976.
49. Weinstein, G. D.: Managing psoriasis, Postgrad. Med. **52**:190-194, 1972.

*References preceded by an asterisk are particularly well suited for student reading.

69

Problems associated with impaired immune response

BARBARA C. LONG
WILMA J. PHIPPS

The knowledge concerning problems associated with impaired immune responses has expanded rapidly in recent years, and identification and treatment of persons with immunodeficiencies have improved markedly. Organ transplantations have achieved greater success as a result of increased knowledge concerning foreign-tissue rejection. Early progress has been made in trying to stimulate the body's immunologic response to cancers in order to prevent further malignant growth. Discoveries concerning immunoglobulins have given a better understanding of hypersensitivity (allergic) reactions.

The immune response of the body is discussed in detail in Chapter 14, including the immunologic bases of (1) immunodeficiencies, (2) gammopathies (abnormal production of immunoglobulins), (3) hypersensitivities, and (4) autoimmunities. This chapter discusses the care of persons with immunodeficiency disease and those receiving immunosuppressive therapy, persons with allergies (type I hypersensitivity), and persons experiencing blood transfusion reactions (type II hypersensitivity). Information on anaphylactic shock and other types of hypersensitivities is presented in Chapter 14. Delayed hypersensitivities are usually manifested as skin conditions, primarily allergic contact dermatitis. Additional information on some of the gammopathies and autoimmune diseases can be found in other sections of the text.

IMMUNODEFICIENCY AND IMMUNOSUPPRESSION

Protection of the host depends on an intact immune system. Deficiencies may result from improper development (primary immunodeficiencies) or as a secondary result of some interference with the immune system (secondary immunodeficiencies). The primary immunodeficiencies are mainly disorders occurring in children; a brief introduction to primary immunodeficiencies can be found on p. 192.

Some immunoglobulin deficiencies may not become evident until the person is an adult, and these are termed common variable immunodeficiencies (CVI). The deficiencies differ among persons having CVI; these deficiencies are primarily IgA or IgM, although most persons have sufficient IgA. They develop recurrent virulent infections and display a high incidence of malignancies, hematologic disorders, and autoimmune diseases.[2] Gamma globulin may be given during acute episodes, but recurrent pulmonary infections often lead to death from pulmonary insufficiency.[2] (References at the end of the chapter contain selected immunology texts for the reader desiring further information on primary immunodeficiencies.)

Secondary immunodeficiencies are present to one degree or another in most of the major disease conditions experienced by humans in addition to the normal response to aging. Thus when caring for any person beyond the age of 60 years or with any acute disease condition, the concepts of immunodeficiency must be considered. Situations in which immunodeficiency plays a major role include malnutrition, infections (especially viral), autoimmune diseases, lymphomas (including Hodgkin's disease), neoplasia, allergies, trauma, and transplantations. Major stress of any type can affect the immune response due to the increase in corticosteroid production and alterations in protein metabolism. Suppression of the immune system may result from medical therapies, including irradiation and drug therapy.

Nutrition and immunity

Malnutrition leads to an increased susceptibility to infection, and conversely infection leads to increased nutritional requirements. *Protein calorie malnutrition* is associated with thymic atrophy and reduction in lymphoid tissue. Primary immune responses and delayed hypersensitivity responses are affected. Persons experiencing large-scale burns or other trauma develop protein deficiency, which affects their immune response. Attention to the nutritional requirements of all acutely ill persons can help to prevent acquired immunologic abnormalities.[2] Vitamin deficiencies can also affect the immune response. Vitamin B_6 (pyridoxine) and pantothenic acid deficiencies depress antibody formation and cause delayed hypersensitivity reactions. Vitamin C influences infection primarily by its effect in the healing process.

□ Irradiation

Both primary and secondary immune responses (p. 186) may be suppressed by irradiation, but suppression of primary sensitization is more effective than suppression of immunologic memory. Irradiation destroys lymphocytes, either directly or through depletion of the precursor stem cells (p. 1059). It may be directed at local areas or at the total body. Local irradiation of allografts has been attempted with poor success in preventing graft rejection. The effect of total body irradiation depends on the size of the radiation dose. The hematopoietic, gastrointestinal, and central nervous systems are affected in that order as the dosage is increased.[12] Unfortunately the hematopoietic system is affected at the same dosage level as the lymphoid tissues; hence a sufficient dosage to decrease lymphoid activity will create problems in the hematopoietic system. To achieve sufficient immunosuppression by irradiation, such as prior to organ transplantation, bone marrow atrophy leading to pancytopenia usually results.[12]

□ Drug immunosuppression

A number of drugs affect the immune system (Table 69-1). Antimetabolites are frequently given in combination with steroids for immunosuppression therapy in order to decrease the dosage of both antimetabolites and steroids, thereby decreasing serious side effects. Azathioprine is the antimetabolite of choice for persons receiving kidney transplantation.

Corticosteroids are given for therapy in a large number of diseases. If infections are present, the severity of the infection may increase despite the minimizing

Table 69-1. Effect of selected drugs on the immune system

Drug	Immune system impairment	Indications for immunosuppressive therapy
Corticosteroids	Impairment of T-cell function Catabolism of immunoglobulins (decreased IgG) Lymphocytopenia Type I hypersensitivity: vasoconstriction, eosinopenia Type III hypersensitivity: decreased vascular permeability Type IV hypersensitivity: decreased macrophage function	Diseases where immune disorder is unknown Tissue and organ transplantation Autoimmune diseases
Antimetabolites (azathioprine)	Interference with RNA, DNA, and protein synthesis Depression of bone marrow and antibody reproduction Decreased primary immune response	Autoimmune diseases Tissue transplantation Dermatologic disease (pemphigus, psoriasis) Neoplasia
Alkylating agents (cyclophosphamide)	Interference with DNA, RNA, and protein synthesis Lymphocytolytic effect Suppression of primary immune response	Autoimmune disease Tissue transplantation Inflammatory disease of unknown cause
Antilymphocytic serum (ALS, ALG)	Inhibition of lymphocyte stimulation by specific antigens Inhibition of lymphocyte mobility Agglutination and lysis of lymphocytes in the presence of complement	Renal transplantation Bone marrow transplantation Autoimmune disease
Antibiotics (actinomycin D, chloramphenicol, tetracycline)	Interference with DNA-directed RNA synthesis Suppression of primary immune response Inhibition of protein synthesis	None

of symptoms, due to the antiinflammatory effects of the steroids. Persons receiving corticosteroid therapy are highly susceptible to superimposed infections.

□ Assessment

Persons with recurrent infections or who are suspected of having an immunodeficiency should receive a thorough medical evaluation. The type of recurrent infection may give a clue as to the type of deficiency. Recurrent viral or fungal infections are suggestive of T-cell-mediated deficiencies. Lymphopenia is often present. Delayed-type hypersensitivity skin tests such as PPD or *Candida* antigen or node biopsy may help to establish the diagnosis of a T-cell deficiency. Persons with recurrent bacterial infections may have an underlying B-cell (humoral) deficiency. Tests for the presence of B-cell deficiency include measurement of serum immunoglobulin levels, skin tests with inactivated vaccines (DPT, Schick), and bone marrow studies. Persons concerned about the skin tests can be told that the tests indicate the ability of the body to react to the foreign proteins and that the specific diseases are not thought to be present.

□ Intervention

Treatment of secondary immunodeficiencies consists primarily in treatment of the underlying condition that has affected the immune response. Specific replacement therapy may be given for primary immunodeficiencies. When the humoral (B-cell) deficiency is present, gamma globulin or fresh-frozen plasma free of HB_sAg (hepatitis antigen) may be given. *Gamma globulin* is a purified concentrated solution of antibodies found in normal plasma. It can be given as a prophylactic measure against viral diseases such as measles, German measles, poliomyelitis, mumps, and hepatitis. A dose of 0.01 ml/lb body weight is injected *intramuscularly*. Some localized reaction (tenderness, erythema) may be experienced. For the treatment of immunodeficiency much larger doses must be given (0.25 to 0.45 ml/lb body weight), and these large volumes are more painful and less well tolerated. When giving gamma globulin intramuscularly a large-bore (18 to 20) needle is recommended, and the solution should be injected slowly. Large amounts need to be divided and given at separate sites. *Plasma therapy* is better tolerated by the individual than large doses of gamma globulin, and all five immunoglobulins are included in the plasma. Homologous serum hepatitis and transfusion reactions, however, are potential risks with plasma therapy.

Replacement therapy for T-cell-mediated immune deficiencies is more complex. *Transfer factor* extracted from the lymphocytes of humans who have demonstrated delayed hypersensitivity reactions has benefitted some persons. Repeated injections are required. *Thymosin*, a thymic hormone, has been effective in some instances in which the T-cell precursors are already present. Bone marrow transplants have also been used. Immunotherapy for neoplasia is discussed on p. 484.

The most important factor in the care of the immunodeficient or immunosuppressed person is *protection from infection*. If the degree of immunosuppression is minimal, careful medical asepsis techniques may be the only requirements. This involves good hygiene practices, careful handwashing before touching body areas, and avoidance by the person of other individuals with infections. The person should learn to avoid bumping or breaking the skin, and even very minor skin breaks should receive meticulous cleaning and protection. Medical attention should be sought for small skin lesions that do not heal quickly or for larger skin lesions. Skin areas must be examined daily for signs of symptom-free lesions. Injections should be avoided as much as possible as this involves penetration of the protective skin barrier. Nutrition must be maintained at an optimum level with special emphasis on adequate protein, vitamin, and mineral intake. Fluid intake should also be adequate to prevent tissue dehydration or low urine output that can lead to skin or urinary tract infections.

Hospitalized patients with moderate immunosuppression who demonstrate leukopenia or lymphopenia are sometimes placed in *reverse* (protective) isolation, although there is question about the effectiveness of this system. The person is placed in a single room with the door closed, and all who enter wear mask and gown and carry out isolation technique. If the person is acutely ill, good mouth care, perineal care, and pulmonary hygiene are important for prevention of infection.

Persons with severe immunodeficiency require the highest degree of protection from infection. *Life islands* consist of plastic tents that completely surround the patient's bed. Sterile objects are passed through portholes irradiated by ultraviolet light. Patient care is given by special arm gloves built into the plastic wall. Life islands are more confining for the patient and are used less frequently since the advent of the *laminar air flow units* (see Fig. 25-11). Air flow across the unit is laminar (in layers) to decrease microorganisms moving toward the patient, and the air is filtered continuously through microfilters. Persons who remain downstream from the patient need not wear protection, but anyone approaching or giving care to the patient wears cap, mask, and gown. All equipment is sterilized prior to entry to the room. It is imperative that measures be carried out to prevent social isolation of the patient. Infants born with severe immunodeficiency disease have been maintained in laminar air flow units for long periods until therapy is successful so that they may survive in the normal environment.

■ ALLERGY (TYPE I HYPERSENSITIVITY)

The body's mechanism for dealing with foreign proteins (the antigen-antibody response, p. 181) is not reserved only for pathogenic organisms. It also comes into action against other foreign substances such as pollens, food, animal serum, and dander as well as a variety of other material such as house dust, cosmetics, synthetic products, and drugs. Some people also develop allergic response (hypersensitivity) to bacteria.

The factors involved in causing an antigen-antibody reaction in hypersensitivity states are described in Chapter 14. The following discussion concerns some problems encountered by persons who are allergic. Allergy refers to a state of altered reactivity in which certain substances are allergens that cause a hypersensitivity reaction.

□ Epidemiology

About 20% of the population react to allergens that are not antigens for the remainder of the population. These individuals are referred to as being "atopic." This tendency to become hypersensitive is inherited genetically as a dominant trait. If both parents are atopic, all the children will be atopic. What these individuals become hypersensitive to, however, will be determined by the allergens to which they are exposed. Three factors are helpful in understanding atopy: (1) atopic individuals will not form antibodies unless exposed to a substance that is antigenic for them; (2) an atopic child is like a blank sheet; that is, the child does not inherit a specific allergy such as hay fever or asthma, but the allergy will manifest itself in response to the allergen(s) to which the child is exposed; and (3) atopic allergies are the most common form of allergy. The most common allergens for the atopic person are:

1. Foods, primarily a problem from birth to 2 years of age and manifested primarily as infantile eczema. Between 80% to 85% of these allergies disappear by age 2 years.
2. Environmental inhalants such as house dust and animal dander, which are primarily a problem from age 2 to 6 years.
3. Seasonal inhalants such as tree and grass pollens and fungus spores, which mainly affect those over age 6 years.

Children who develop eczema from food allergy are highly allergic individuals, and the majority of them (80% to 85%) will develop hay fever or asthma before the age of 6 years.

Environmental and seasonal inhalants are about equally important allergens, but environmental inhalants are easier to control by providing a controlled environment in the home (discussed later in this section).

In order to determine if seasonal inhalants are the cause of an allergic response, one needs to know when trees, grasses, and molds are pollenating in that geographic area. One also needs to know which trees and grasses are insect pollenated and therefore cannot cause an allergic response.

There are several facts about allergens which it is helpful for the nurse to understand:

1. Persons who believe they have "rose fever" are really allergic to pollenating grasses, and persons who believe they are allergic to goldenrod are really allergic to ragweed, since both roses and goldenrod are insect pollenated.
2. Persons may be allergic to the pollen of one tree and not another; therefore there is need to know which tree is pollenating at the time symptoms appear.
3. Persons who are allergic to pollenating grasses will have the same symptoms no matter which grass is pollenating. If they move from one geographic area to another they will become sensitized to whatever grasses are present in that area. For example, *ragweed* is a grass that causes an allergic response in many persons. It is not present in all parts of the United States, but atopic individuals moving into the ragweed belt of the Great Lakes Basin will become sensitized to it. If these persons later move to an area of the country such as the Pacific Northwest where there is no ragweed, they will become sensitized to another type of pollenating grass.
4. Persons may be allergic to spores of molds and not realize it. A careful history detailing where molds are most likely to be found may be helpful, including (1) inside the home: basements that are warm and damp or, when there is no basment, in crawl spaces under the house; (2) outside the house: leaves of certain trees, wheat, corn, and so on. Molds do not grow in sunshine and require increased humidity for growth. Thus in the northeastern and midwestern regions of the United States they are a more common problem in the fall of the year. For both pollens and spores the highest counts (amounts in the air) occur between 12 midnight and 8 AM.

When a person who has a tendency to become allergic first comes in contact with the specific allergen to which he or she is sensitive, antibodies are formed. These antibodies are *fixed*, in contrast to circulating antibodies, and are located close to the shock organ affected. Thus the antibodies may be fixed in the nose in hayfever, in the chest in asthma, and in the skin in hives and urticaria. These fixed antibodies are activated when

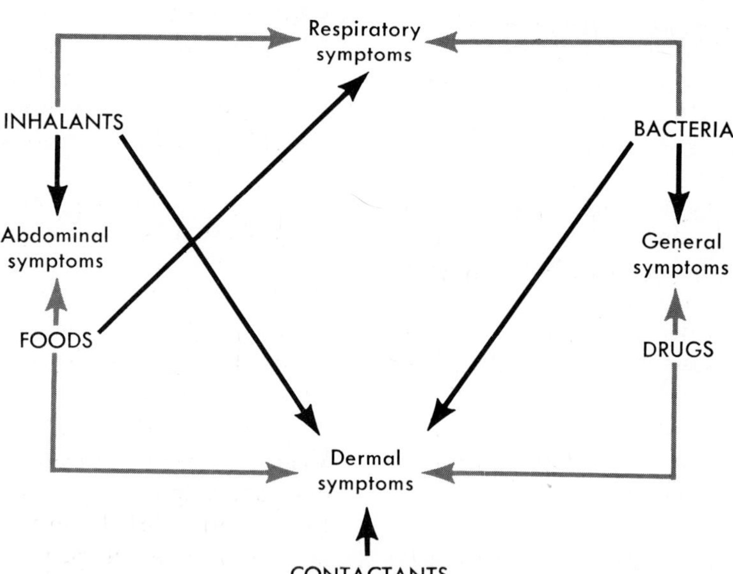

Fig. 69-1. Causes of allergic responses and symptoms produced.

the individual next comes in contact with the allergen. This results in an antigen-antibody reaction causing tissue damage, which liberates histamine or a histamine-like substance.

Histamine has three main effects: (1) it constricts smooth muscle such as in the bronchi, resulting in bronchospasm and constriction of conducting airways; (2) it increases vascular permeability, resulting in such conditions as hives or mucosal edema in asthma; and (3) it increases mucous gland secretions, resulting in increased mucus production as occurs in hayfever and asthma. Factors influencing an allergic response are summarized in the box opposite.

FACTORS THAT INFLUENCE AN ALLERGIC RESPONSE (AMOUNT OF REACTION)

Allergen: amount and type

Antibodies: number

Histamine: amount liberated

Tissue: adequacy in preventing histamine from reaching sites

Response: tissue to histamine

□ Clinical picture

The symptoms seen in the person with an allergic reaction will be determined by the organ affected. The person with hay fever will have sneezing, tearing of the eyes, and watery discharge from the nose; the individual who has asthma will wheeze when the bronchial muscles are constricted; and the person with a skin allergy will have hives, urticaria, and skin rash. Nausea, vomiting, and diarrhea may also be allergic reactions (Fig. 69-1).

□ Assessment

History

It usually is possible to determine the specific allergens to which a person is hypersensitive by taking a detailed history and then testing for sensitivity.

Skin testing

Skin tests are often used to determine whether a person has a sensitivity to certain substances in the external environment. Several methods of testing are used. Small amounts of extracts of various allergenic substances to which the person is suspected to have a sensitivity may be injected intradermally at spaced intervals, usually on the outer surface of the upper arm, on the forearm, or in the scapular region. The extract also may be placed on the skin and the skin scratched lightly *(scratch test)*. These two methods are used most often to test for sensitivity to pollen, feathers, dander, and dust. They also may be used to test for sensitivity to foods, but the results are often inaccurate. When clothing or other material is the suspected allergen, a small piece of it may be put against the skin under an airtight patch for 48 to 72 hours *(patch test)*. Sensitivity to soaps and other cleaning agents such as detergents is often tested in this way. An infant may be tested indirectly by injecting his blood serum at spaced intervals under the skin of a nonallergic person. Twenty-four hours later the extract of the suspected allergenic substance is injected at these sites. Tests for allergenic substances usually are done in series; for example, pollens from trees are tested first, then pollens from grasses, and so on. Positive reactions to allergens are indicated by the appearance of a *wheal* or redness at the test site. Occasionally one drop of a test extract is instilled into the eye to test for sensitivity *(conjunctival test)*. Redness of the conjunctiva and tearing will appear within 5 to 15 minutes in an allergic person.

Food diary

A person with a food allergy is asked to keep a food diary for at least a week. On the basis of this diary, suspect foods such as milk, wheat products, and eggs may be removed from the diet (elimination diet) until symptoms subside and then added one at a time in an attempt to identify the offending foods. Babies on this diet often must be given a special nonmilk formula made of products such as soybeans or barley. The mothers need instructions in preparing the formula. A similar elimination process may be used to test for allergy to other substances such as cosmetics or fabrics.

Special hospital rooms

Some hospitals now have environmentally controlled rooms that may be used to remove a highly allergic person from the usual environment and thus facilitate the search for the substances to which the individual is sensitive. The room is kept free from substances most likely to be allergenic and is air conditioned to prevent inflow of pollens through open windows. The rooms may also be used for treatment. When the symptoms have subsided, various articles used at home may be introduced one at a time to see if they cause symptoms. Only a limited number of staff members are allowed to enter the room, and they may be requested to avoid the use of cosmetics and to wear special gowns.

The nurse may be helpful by providing encouragement to the person who may have to undergo tests that may last for weeks or months. By suggesting common allergenic substances, the nurse may help the person give a more complete history. Nurses are often called on to help the person plan for elimination testing.

□ Intervention

The best treatment for an allergy is to prevent the person from coming in contact with the allergen or allergens to which he or she is sensitive. If the allergen is a *food*, it should be eliminated from the diet. Often infants who have food allergies outgrow them by 2 years of age. Infants who could not tolerate cow's milk can often drink it as they grow older. Persons who are sensitive to environmental or seasonal inhalants should be taught how to control exposure to these allergens. This is most often accomplished by having a controlled room (usually the bedroom) in which the individual can spend much of his or her time when at home.

Preparing an environmentally controlled room

A properly prepared room is especially important for atopic children, since they are apt to be hypersensitive to a variety of allergens.

Persons whose allergies are due to *environmental* inhalants will need a room free of house dust, animal dander, fungus spores, and other allergens. Because 90% of the air-borne particles in the house (such as house dust) are 5 μm or less in size, an electrostatic filter will be necessary. An electrostatic filter attracts particles by means of highly charged metal plates, which can be removed for cleaning. These filters come in portable models for room use or can be attached to the central heating system.

The room should also have wooden floors or be covered with linoleum or plastic tile. No rugs other than cotton throw rugs that can be washed frequently should be used, since carpets trap materials that produce house dust. Closet doors should be rendered airtight by applying weather stripping around the door. It is also recommended that clothes be placed in plastic bags. The closet should be cleaned frequently to prevent accumulation of house dust. Atopic children and adults are often allergic to animal dander, and most allergists will not allow them to have any fur-bearing pets. Goldfish may be a suitable substitute pet. Persons who are allergic to animal dander must also avoid feather pillows and other inanimate articles that may contain animal dander. Only cotton curtains that are made of smooth material and can be easily washed should be used. The bed should have a mattress made from an allergen-free material such as foam rubber or be completely encased in an allergenproof cover. Pillows should be made of a nonallergenic substance such as foam rubber, Dacron, or Acrilan. A room air conditioner may add to the comfort of the individual and is often prescribed by the physician. *Daily damp dusting* of the room should be done to lessen the amount of dust in the air.

The person who is sensitive to *seasonal* inhalants (tree and grass pollens and fungus spores) will benefit from eliminating all outside air from the bedroom. This can be achieved by sealing the windows and installing an air conditioner or an electrostatic window filter. The cost of electrostatic filters and air conditioners prescribed by a physician is an income-tax-deductible medical expense.

Avoidance of allergens

In addition some persons with allergies such as that caused by ragweed may be advised to vacation outside of the ragweed area during the peak of the pollenating season. This is quite possible for many persons and prevents them from having seasonal attacks of hay fever or asthma.

Usually the individual with hay fever will find relief from symptoms after about 1/2 hour in an environmentally controlled room. However, the symptoms of the individual with asthma will not be relieved until all antigenic inhalants are removed from the environment. This may take days or weeks to accomplish. Experience has shown that individuals who understand what they are hypersensitive to can remain symptom free for years as long as they avoid these allergens. Since the antibodies to the allergens are always present in the body, the individual will have symptoms if he or she comes in contact with the offending allergen. This is especially true of animal dander, and parents should understand that atopic children can probably never have a fur-bearing pet.

Desensitization

Sometimes an attempt is made to slowly desensitize a patient by injecting small but increasingly larger doses of the allergen at regular intervals (usually 1 to 4 weeks) over a long period. This treatment may take years or it may have to be continued indefinitely. It is about 80% effective against hay fever but less effective in asthma and dermatitis. It is essential that the individual, or the parents if the patient is a child, understand that desensitization is of little value until the environment is controlled; otherwise the constant exposure to allergens will only increase antibody response.

When a person has been desensitized to a particular food, the food may be resumed, but only small amounts should be taken at first. If any symptoms develop, the food is stopped and the physician is notified.

Specific care of the patient with asthma is discussed on p. 1126; care for the patient with allergic dermatitis is discussed on p. 1530.

Medications

Persons who are allergic may take maintenance medications to prevent an allergic attack or will require medication during an attack. Medications used to prevent an attack include preparations such as ephedrine, aerosolizide bronchodilating agents, and cromolyn sodium (Aarane). All of these drugs may be prescribed for persons with asthma. Cromolyn sodium has been found to be effective in the treatment of patients with chronic asthma. It works by partially or completely preventing the immediate allergic response to the offending allergen. *It should not be used to treat an acute asthmatic attack.*

Antihistamines are commonly used to prevent and treat hay fever. They have a tendency to produce drowsiness and should be scheduled at times when alertness is not essential. Persons taking antihistamines should not drive motor vehicles or operate machinery.

During an acute allergic reaction epinephrine (Adrenalin) is commonly administered. The corticosteroids also may be given. They are believed to be effective in tightening up the tissues so that histamine is prevented from reaching mucous glands and other sites. When corticosteroids are prescribed the person should be tuberculin tested first, and if results are positive should be placed on isoniazid therapy (see p. 1117 for discussion of this precaution).

□ Outcome criteria for the person with atopic allergy

The person or significant others can:

1. Explain what substances are allergens and must be avoided.
2. Describe in detail how to prepare an environmentally controlled room.
3. Describe measures to be taken during periods of high pollen counts (restrict periods out of doors, remain in environment that is air conditioned).
4. Describe dietary restriction, if any. Relate how daily nutritional needs will be met.
5. Explain each medication prescribed in terms of expected action, route and frequency of administration, expected side effects, and precautions to be observed when taking medications.
6. List signs and symptoms that require immediate medical intervention (asthma attack not relieved by usual means).
7. Describe plans for ongoing health care.

■ BLOOD TRANSFUSION REACTIONS (TYPE II HYPERSENSITIVITY)

Blood replacement therapy is used when there has been excessive blood loss (whole blood or blood components), in treatment of diseases of the hematopoietic system, or in open-heart surgery. Blood transfusions are not without dangers to the recipient; therefore the transfusion of one unit (500 ml) of blood for minor therapy is not usually recommended. Replacement therapy may be whole blood or one or more of the blood components (Table 69-2).

Blood transfusion is an example of a successful allograft. Successful transfusions became possible after the discovery of the major blood groups (ABO) and of an-

Table 69-2. Types of blood replacement

Component	Indications
Whole blood	Loss of blood volume (trauma, surgery)
Packed red cells	Anemias Liver and kidney disease
Washed red cells	Febrile reaction after receiving leukocyte-poor red cells
Leukocyte-poor red cells	Febrile transfusion reactions
Frozen red cells (leukocyte free)	Prospective transplant recipients
Platelet concentrate	Thrombocytopenia
Cryoprecipitate (antihemophelic factor)	Hemophilia
Gamma globulin	Prophylaxis for certain virus diseases Immunodeficiency disease
Plasma	Shock
Fresh-frozen plasma	Immunodeficiency disease

tigenic subgroups. (The reader is referred to a physiology text for further information on the various blood groups and subgroups.) The serious reaction to blood transfusion (type II hypersensitivity) occurs as a result of naturally occurring antibodies to the red blood cell antigens of the blood groups of the donor blood (p. 197).

Prevention of reactions

The frequency of blood transfusion reactions is unknown but is estimated to be 2% to 3%. Approximately 8 million units of blood are administered in the United States annually; therefore over 160,000 transfusion reactions can be expected yearly.[4] Measures to prevent reactions thus assume major importance, since acute hemolytic reactions can be fatal.

Donor prescreening

Prescreening of potential blood donors is essential. Blood received from volunteer donors through the American Red Cross Blood Service or hospital blood banks is preferable to that of paid donors, as paid donors may be less apt to report present or previous diseases that may affect the recipient. Requirements have been delineated that include guidelines for persons with heart, lung, liver, or kidney disease. Persons who are not accepted as donors include those with a history of (1) infectious diseases such as hepatitis, tuberculosis, syphilis, or malaria, (2) malignant disease, (3) allergies or asthma, and (4) polycythemia vera or abnormal bleeding tendencies. Temporary deferments include pregnancy, recent major surgery, hypotension, and anemia. The donor's hemoglobin level is tested prior to giving blood, and the hemoglobin acceptance level should be above 13.5 g/100 ml for men and 12.5 g/100 ml for women.[9] Temperature, pulse, and blood pressure should be within normal ranges. Children and elderly persons are also excluded in order to protect the donor from adverse effects of blood loss. Donors should wait at least 8 weeks between blood donations and should not give blood more than five times a year.

After the blood has been collected, the blood group and subgroups including Rh typing are identified and the blood is tested for syphilis and hepatitis. The blood *must* be cross-matched with blood from the recipient in order to determine compatibility to prevent an acute hemolytic reaction.

Administration safeguards

Some of the serious reactions that have occurred during transfusions have been due to human error. Cross-matching and testing in the laboratory must be accurate. Blood must be kept cold until ready to use. If blood has remained at room temperature for over 30 minutes, it should not be returned to refrigeration and then reissued, as this contributes to growth of gram-negative organisms that can produce serious septicemia.[14] Blood being administered to the patient should be given within a 4-hour period. The unit of blood must be labeled with the name of the person for whom it is intended, and this label must be checked against the patient's wristband before the blood is administered. The patient must be monitored throughout the administration of the blood. All blood products should be administered through filters.

Complications of blood transfusions

Immunologic transfusion reactions

Several immunologic reactions can occur with the administration of blood; these reactions are listed in Table 69-3. The most serious reaction is the acute hemolytic reaction, which occurs during the first 50 ml of blood transfusion. If symptoms appear, the blood flow is stopped immediately, but an intravenous line is kept open with normal saline in the event that shock occurs. Shock, disseminated intravascular coagulation (DIC) (p. 1070), and renal shutdown are treated as they occur. Since fever is a sign of both acute hemolytic reaction and the less serious pyrogenic reaction, the transfusion is stopped until the diagnosis is made. If an allergic reaction is present, the transfusion is usually continued with concomitant therapy (antihistamines, epinephrine).

Symptoms of transfusion reactions are nonspecific; therefore errors may be made in diagnosis. Persons receiving blood transfusions are usually seriously ill, and many of the symptoms may be due to the underlying

Table 69-3. Immunologic reactions to blood transfusions

Reaction	Cause	Mechanism	Symptoms	Occurrence	Action
Acute hemolytic	Recipient has antibody with which transfused red cells are incompatible	Red cells agglutinate, rapid hemolysis Capillary plugging	Headache Lumbar pain Constriction of chest Nausea, vomiting Chills, fever Hemoglobinuria Signs of shock, DIC, renal shutdown	Shortly after initiation of transfusion	Transfusion stopped Saline continued IV Blood unit and blood sample from patient sent to lab for immediate testing Treat for shock, DIC, renal shutdown as they occur
Delayed hemolytic	Anamnestic immune response	Slow hemolysis	Jaundice Anemia	Days to weeks after transfusion	Monitor adequacy of urinary output and degree of anemia
Allergic	Transfer of an antigen or a reaginic antibody from donor to recipient	Immune sensitivity to foreign serum protein (type I hypersensitivity)	Urticaria Wheezing Dyspnea Bronchospasm	Within 30 min after initiation of transfusion	Mild: give antihistamine, continue transfusion Severe: give aqueous epinephrine (0.5 ml of 1:1,000 IM)
Pyrogenic	Reaction of antigen other than on RBC (WBC, platelets) Bacterial contamination	Leukocyte agglutination Bacterial pyrogens	Fever, chills Flushing Palpitations Tachycardia	Within 30 to 90 min after initiation of transfusion	Stop transfusion Treat symptomatically (antipyretics) after ascertaining that acute hemolytic reaction is not occurring Transfuse with leukocyte-poor blood or washed RBC

medical condition. Persons are monitored carefully for any changes in existing symptoms, and these are reported immediately to the physician.

Nonimmunologic reaction

Complications other than of immunologic origin may also occur. *Fluid volume overload* (p. 303) is one of the more frequent reactions, especially in children, in the elderly, in persons with congestive heart failure, or in persons who are severely anemic (less than 4 to 5 g/100 ml).[4] Fluid overload may be prevented by the use of packed cells in place of whole blood. If symptoms of hypervolemia occur, the rate of the infusion is slowed or stopped depending on the severity of symptoms.

Air embolism may result when blood is administered under air pressure following severe blood loss. If an embolus should occur, the transfusion is stopped immediately, and the patient is positioned on a left side-lying Trendenlenburg position to divert the air away from the pulmonary artery. *Disease transmission* of hepatitis, malaria, syphilis, and cytomegalovirus disease may also result from blood transfusions.

Complications of massive blood replacement

When blood is administered in large amounts over a short period of time (exchange of one blood volume within 24 hours),[14] additional problems may occur. Platelets deteriorate rapidly in stored blood, and *throm-*

bocytopenia with abnormal bleeding may result. Infusions of cold blood may stimulate *cardiac arrythmias;* therefore large amounts of blood given rapidly should be warmed during administration. Blood-warming equipment consisting of coils that warm the blood can be used, or the blood may be warmed by placing part of the transfusion tubing in a water bath warmed to body temperature (37 C [98.6 F]).

Electrolyte imbalances may also result from transfusion of large amounts of stored blood preserved by the addition of acid citrate dextrose (ACD). Increased potassium that results from the breakdown of red blood cells can be a severe problem in the person with renal insufficiency. *Hypocalcemia* may result from the bindings of the sodium citrate with serum calcium ions. This can be aggravated by preexisting liver disease or by hypothermia.[14]

□ Pheresis therapy

A newer therapy (pheresis) involves the separation and removal of selected blood components from an individual's blood.[19] Persons may experience overproduction or malfunction of one or more blood components. Blood may be removed, centrifuged to remove selected components, and then returned to the person. This can be done manually, removing not more than 500 ml at one time, or by means of a continuous-flow centrifuge machine (blood cell separator). The continuous-flow centrifuge machine pumps blood from the patient's arm, through the centrifuge machine, then back into the opposite arm.[19] The patient is monitored for signs of hemorrhage, pyrogenic reaction, hypovolemia or hypervolemia, and electrolyte imbalance.

REFERENCES AND SELECTED READINGS

1. Aisner, J.: Platelet transfusion therapy, Med. Clin. North Am. **61**:1133-1145, 1977.
2. Alexander, J. W., and Good, R. A.: Fundamentals of clinical immunology, Philadelphia, 1977, W. B. Saunders Co.
3. Barber, H. K.: Immunology for the clinician, New York, 1977, John Wiley & Sons, Inc.
4. Beeson, P. B., editor: Textbook of medicine, ed. 14, Philadelphia, 1975, W. B. Saunders Co.
5. Bridgewater, S. C., Voignier, R. R., and Smith, C. S.: Allergies in children: recognition, Am. J. Nurs. **78**:614-616, 1978.
6. Buckley, R. H.: Plasma therapy in immunodeficiency disease, Birth Defects **11**:347-349, 1975.
7. *Child, J., Collins, D., and Collins, J.: Blood transfusions, Am. J. Nurs. **72**:1602-1605, 1972.
8. Creep, L. H.: Allergy and clinical immunology, New York, 1976, Grune & Stratton, Inc.
9. Davidsohn, I., and Henry, J. B.: Todd-Sanford clinical diagnosis by laboratory methods, ed. 15, Philadelphia, 1974, W. B. Saunders Co.
10. Dharan, M.: Immunoglobulin abnormalities, Am. J. Nurs. **76**:1626-1628, 1976.
11. *Donley, D. L.: Nursing the patient who is immunosuppressed, Am. J. Nurs. **76**:1619-1625, 1976.
12. Freedman, S. O., and Gold, P.: Clinical immunology, ed. 2, Hagerstown, Md., 1976, Harper & Row, Publishers, Inc.
13. Glaser, R. S.: The body is the hero, New York, 1976, Random House.
14. Grindon, A. J.: Untoward reactions to blood transfusion. In Conn, H. F.: Current therapy, Philadelphia, 1978, W. B. Saunders Co.
15. Harris, J., editor: Symposium on clinical immunology, Med. Clin. North Am. **56**:1-575, 1972.
16. Hitzig, W. H., and Muntener, V.: Conventional immunoglobin therapy, Birth Defects **11**:339-342, 1975.
17. McPhaul, J. J., Jr.: IgA-associated glomerulonephritis, Ann. Rev. Med. **28**:37-42, 1977.
18. Old, L. S.: Cancer immunology, Sci. Am. **236**:62-79, 1977.
19. *Rossman, M., Slavin, R., and Taft, E. G.: Pheresis therapy: patient care, Am. J. Nurs. **77**:1135-1141, 1977.
20. Samter, M., editor: Symposium on immunotherapy in malignant disease, Med. Clin. North Am. **60**:1-648, 1976.
21. Sell, S.: Immunology, immunopathology and immunity, ed. 2, Hagerstown, Md., 1975, Harper & Row, Publishers, Inc.
22. Stiller, C. R., Russell, A. S., and Dosseter, J. B.: Autoimmunity: present concepts, Ann. Intern. Med. **82**:405-410, 1975.
23. Tarnawski, A., and Balko, B.: Antibiotics and immune processes, Lancet **1**:674-675, 1973.
24. *Tenczynski, J.: Leukapheresis: the process, Am. J. Nurs. **77**:1133-1134, 1977.
25. Terry, W. D., editor: Symposium on immunotherapy in malignant disease, Med. Clin. North Am. **60**:1-648, 1976.
26. Thaler, M. S., Klausner, R. D., and Cohen, H. S.: Medical immunology, Philadelphia, 1977, J. B. Lippincott Co.
27. *Voignier, R. R., and Bridgewater, S. C.: Allergies in children: testing and treating, Am. J. Nurs. **78**:617-619, 1978.

*References preceded by an asterisk are particularly well suited for student reading.

UNIT XII

Critical care nursing

Critical illness occurs when problems that individually may not be intense enough to culminate in crises interact to cause major disturbances in a person's physiologic equilibrium. The complex interrelationship among these problems leads to disturbances or failure of several systems, and in turn this multisystem failure aggravates the complexity of the problems. Critical illness usually is a life-threatening event that endangers or involves the respiratory, cardiovascular, renal, and central nervous systems as well as each person's self-concept.

A critically ill person is in crisis or at a turning point with potentially negative outcomes. Multiple physiologic, psychologic, and social stressors impinge on critically ill patients and their significant others. Whether a critical illness experience will culminate in a crisis for the patient and the significant others depends on their perceptions of the event, the support systems available to them, and their previous coping skills.

The stressors imposed by critical illness threaten the equilibrium of both the patient and the significant others because of sudden actual or potential losses that disrupt the individuals current life style. Patients may face loss of life, loss of biologic function and body integrity, and loss of independence and control over their bodily functions as well as their immediate destinies. They also face potential loss of identity and feelings of self-worth as life-threatening physiologic problems assume the priority and attention of the health care team. In addition they may lose financial security and the potential to retain or to regain their premorbid life style. Significant others lose the ability to change or alter the events that present hazards to the well-being of loved ones and are faced with the very real threat of permanent loss through death. Within a systems perspective these stressors become input that influence the patient's and significant others' behavior and their ability to cope with the losses threatened by critical illness.

The nurse caring for a person who is critically ill is in a position to reestablish a state of equilibrium through use of crisis and systems theories integrated with refined decision-making skills. The essence of critical care nursing lies in the decision-making process and the willingness of the nurse to act on the decisions. The decision-making process is founded on highly developed and integrated assessment and management skills that (1) reduce the impact of losses and subsequent stressors experienced by a critically ill patient and significant others, (2) promote realistic perceptions of the illness experience for the individual and the significant others, (3) identify support systems, (4) provide support to previously learned coping behaviors, and (5) foster the learning of new coping skills.

The following chapters discuss the assessment and management of critically ill patients as physiologic, psychologic, and social beings. The first chapter presents a framework for data collection and recording and guidelines *for assessment.* The second chapter discusses *managing patients who are critically ill* in terms of preventive, supportive, and restorative interventions directed toward alleviation of physiologic, psychologic, and social stressors. In the third and final chapter assessment and management principles are applied to an actual *case study of a patient who suffers multisystem failure.*

70

Assessment of the critically ill patient

MARY K. KIRKPATRICK

The assessment process for the critically ill differs from the assessment of other patients in terms of the number of supportive devices available to assist in data collection, the constantly changing data from laboratory parameters, the constant and sometimes rapidly changing physiologic status of the patient, the complexity and the magnitude of interrelated problems, and the time constraint within which the nurse collects data and makes decisions. One of the distinguishing features of the assessment of the critically ill stems from the predicament of the patient who may be in a potential life-death situation. Even when a life-death situation is not present, other limitations may be imposed on nursing assessment. For example, the patient's diminished mental status or the presence of an endotracheal or tracheostomy tube may preclude verbal communication. The assessment of critically ill patients is often limited by their close proximity to other patients, the shorter amount of time available to the nurse to elicit information, and the presence of machines and other devices that may hamper the assessment process. The numerous pieces of equipment and the use of invasive monitoring techniques such as pressure devices also contribute to the crisis environment that surrounds the critically ill. Another significant aspect of these patients is the constant change in priorities that results from changes in their biologic status. Often the physiologic assessment takes precedence over the psychologic assessment because of the critical state of the patient.

While eliciting the patient's collaboration in the assessment process is imperative in all settings, the nature of the critically ill patient's physiologic and psychologic status often prohibits subjective input. Due to the patient's condition, nurses may first elicit input from the significant others. Nevertheless, this in no way negates the advantages of eliciting subjective data from the patient when feasible.

■ BASELINE ASSESSMENT

After receiving a detailed report of the patient's current physical and emotional status and any interventions that were instituted and their effects, the nurse proceeds to the patient's bedside to make a firsthand assessment of the patient. Using the flow sheet to record the routine measurements and observations (chart pp. 1550-1551) and the narrative notes to summarize the patient's status at the beginning and at the end of each shift, the nurse documents (1) the patient's vital signs; (2) a head-to-toe assessment (see Chapter 8); (3) physiologic measurements such as central venous pressure and intraarterial blood pressure; (4) color, amount, and consistency of drainage and secretions; and (5) observations about mental status. Physiologic measurements such as vital signs are obtained periodically throughout a 24-hour period, while other observations are recorded only if they represent a change from the initial baseline assessment. For example, hourly central venous pressure readings may be recorded, while the patient's behavior will not be recorded unless there is a marked change.

Nursing notes will depict pertinent changes in the patient's status, significant interventions, and observations about the reactions of significant others. Changes in a patient's condition are often reflected in several parameters over time. An isolated observation has limited usefulness for accurately predicting or validating a problem. For example, a sudden and moderate fall in a patient's blood pressure can result from the effects of a narcotic, a change of position, or circulating blood volume. The change in blood pressure along with an increasing pulse rate, falling central venous pressure, diminishing urine output, and deterioration of the patient's mental status is a more accurate predictor of a low circulating blood volume than any one measure alone.

At the conclusion of the nurse's workday, a summary is written about the patient's status as depicted in the data collected over time. Interpretative statements as well as evaluative remarks regarding the effectiveness of interventions during the shift are made; for example, "Mr. Jones shows progressive signs of congestive heart failure: increased peripheral edema, decreased urine output, jugular vein distention." Documentation is a continuous process when caring for the critically ill patient.

APPROACH TO BEDSIDE

The nurse caring for a critically ill patient is in a unique position to correlate the bedside assessment of a patient's signs and symptoms with data from the monitors. *It is imperative to note the danger of complete dependency on a monitor. This may cause adequate and reliable data obtained directly from the patient to be missed.*

The nurse approaching the bedside of a critically ill patient is able to inspect him and his surroundings in order to elicit significant data. Critical illness always endangers and involves the ventilatory, circulatory, renal, and neurologic subsystems as well as the self-esteem of the person. Therefore the nurse needs to be alert to changes in these subsystems. For example, cardiac or respiratory distress can be assessed by the position a patient assumes in bed or the number of pillows requested in order for the patient to gain maximal function of his ventilatory system. The patient who is short of breath will sit up, or if already sitting up will lean forward in order to facilitate breathing. Facial expressions are also helpful in assessing the patient. The patient who is in pain may grimace or grit his teeth. The patient's expression may reveal fright, sadness, or other feelings.

In addition specific input from supportive or monitoring devices contributes significant data to the assessment of the critically ill patient. An example of specific input from the ventilator elicited while the nurse is enroute to the bedside is the flashing of the yellow light on the MA-1 respirator, indicating the patient's capability to assist the ventilator, or the flashing red light accompanied by a constant noise that is indicative of obstruction in the airway.

Cardiac monitors, intracranial pressure monitors, and intraarterial blood pressure devices are commonly used for continuous surveillance of the patient's status. While monitors are not to be completely relied on for accuracy, the electrocardiogram, intracranial pressure monitors, arterial pressure monitors, and other devices afford the nurse a moment-to-moment assessment of vital signs or subsystem parameter readings. Listening to the sounds of the monitor as well as viewing the oscilloscope provides constant data to the nurse.

Another clue is the presence of an odor. The nurse may smell the acetone breath of the unconscious patient who is in ketosis or the aroma of alcohol from an accident victim. The odor from a tracheostomy tube or an incision may sometimes be the first clue to an infection.

ASSESSMENT OF VITAL FUNCTIONS

Assessment priorities for the critically ill involve the vital functions of ventilatory, circulatory, neurologic, and renal subsystems. While standard techniques may be used to obtain data, the data collection is focused on early signs and symptoms of multisystem complications. These are likely to be evident in data obtained from vital signs, records of fluid intake and output, blood gas analyses, and other physiologic indices.

Because nursing and medical interventions occur so frequently, observations of their impact on vital functions are made at frequent intervals. The effects of interventions may be monitored by responses in the physiologic parameters already noted.

□ Ventilatory subsystems

Constant observation of ventilatory function as well as the effectiveness of ventilatory supports is essential. Data used to measure ventilatory function include changing mental status, pulmonary rate and rhythm, quality of breath sounds, skin color, and changing circulatory status.

Changes in the person's mental status may provide early cues to hypoxia, cyanosis being one of the last changes to occur with hypoxia. Hypoxia resulting from ventilatory impairment may be further aggravated by a low hemoglobin level. Tachycardia and other cardiac arrhythmias are often prominent symptoms of hypoxia. The importance of respiratory rate and rhythm has been addressed elsewhere (p. 931). The quality of breath sounds may indicate the presence of atelectasis as well as the effectiveness of pulmonary toilet. Adventitious sounds may indicate the need for devices such as blow bottles or three-ball inspirometry. Laboratory data such as arterial blood gas values, chest radiographs, or tidal volume measurements are used to validate observations.

The patient often requires ventilatory support such as a respirator attached to an endotracheal or tracheostomy tube. These supports mandate observations of the equipment itself as well as the impact of the support on the patient's status. The effectiveness of ventilatory equipment is usually monitored by periodic blood gas analyses. For example, the use of PEEP (positive end-expiratory pressure) should increase the oxygen content of the patient's blood. When chest tubes are present, nurses ascertain their patency, the color and amount of drainage, absence or presence of bubbling of the fluid in the collection bottle, and presence of crepitus around the tube site (see p. 971 for discussion of care of patients with chest tubes). When a mechanical ventilator is used nurses must be alert to potential complications such as pneumothorax, infection, atelectasis, decreased cardiac output, and gastrointestinal tract bleeding from a stress ulcer. Therefore changes in vital signs and in breath and bowel sounds must be constantly monitored. The presence of occult blood in the stool or nasogastric drainage may indicate gastrointestinal tract bleeding. Thus ventilatory assessment implies much more than observation of pulmonary status alone.

SURGICAL INTENSIVE CARE UNIT FLOW SHEET

Surgical procedure: ______________________ **7 AM weight:** ______ **kg**

	Vital signs										Set FI_{O_2}	Blood gases				
Date / Time	T	P	R	BP	CVP	MAP	PAP	MPAP	Wedge	CO	Meas. FI_{O_2}	pH	PCO_2	PO_2	HCO_3	Base / Sat.
8-hour total: 3 PM																
8-hour total: 11 PM																
8-hour total: 7 AM																
24-hour total																

Pulmonary function								Ventilator parameters		
Time	TV	$\dot{V}$	VC	Qs/Qt	Vd/Vt	FRC	NIF	TV	$\dot{V}$	Infla. pres.

Intake						Output					Chest tube			
CVP line		Periph. IV					SP. GR.							
Type	Amt.	Type	Amt.	Oral	Amt.	Urine	SPOT.				In	Out	Bal.	Patient notes

Total intake: **Total output:**

□ Cardiovascular subsystems

The critical care nurse may use a format for cardiovascular assessment similar to that described in Chapters 8 and 43. However, observations are made at frequent intervals, and particular attention is devoted to the assessment of arrhythmias. In addition cardiovascular pressures are frequently monitored.

The cardioscope can be used to validate data obtained by palpation or auscultation. For example, the skipped beat in a patient's apical pulse may be depicted as a premature ventricular contraction on the monitor. Data obtained from the cardioscope should include the basic rhythm, the type of cardiac arrhythmia, and its frequency and duration. The cardioscope can also be used to evaluate the person's electrolyte status (potassium level) as well as the effects of certain medications such as sympathomimetic agents such as isoproterenol (Isuprel). The cardioscope may also provide data about the effectiveness of an internal pacemaker.

Data other than that obtained with the cardioscope are crucial in the evaluation of an arrhythmia. The blood pressure, level of consciousness, renal output, electrolyte levels, and blood levels of drugs may provide cues to cause as well as the effects of the arrhythmia.

Along with observing the cardioscope, the nurse measures various pressures to evaluate the circulatory status. While the central venous pressure reflects the functioning of the right atrium and vascular volume, the pulmonary capillary wedge pressure obtained through the use of a Swan-Ganz catheter more readily indicates left ventricular function (Fig. 43-7). Measurement of the intraarterial blood pressure enables the nurse to assess vascular volume, a *pulsus alternans* reflecting ventricular failure, or a *pulsus paradoxus* reflecting cardiac tamponade. The measurement of cardiac output also provides important data about the pumping function of the heart.

What is "normal" for one patient may not be normal for another; therefore serial readings of these values must be observed to evaluate a patient's status. In addition to the level of these pressures, nurses consider the position of the patient when the measurements were made, the previous pressure readings as well as the normal range, the amount and type of intravenous infusions, the underlying cardiovascular dysfunction, the type of medications the patient is receiving, and the functioning of the vascular lines.[35]

Other parameters to assess in evaluating the cardiovascular subsystem are urine output; blood loss from chest tubes; the difference between the arterial and venous oxygen saturation; hemoglobin and the hemotocrit levels; enzyme levels, especially CPK, LDH, and SGOT; and electrolytes including calcium, sodium, and potassium.

□ Renal subsystems

The guidelines for assessing the renal subsystem are noted in Chapters 8 and 56. Laboratory findings as well as other patient data are used to monitor renal function. The monitoring of hourly urine output is often accompanied by determination of specific gravity of the urine. Serum and urine osmolality, blood urea nitrogen, creatinine levels, and sodium and potassium levels are commonly used as indices of renal function. Changes in renal status often precipitate changes in the patient's weight and mental status. Signs and symptoms of renal dysfunction may also include cardiovascular changes such as edema, distention of neck veins, adventitious chest sounds, gallop rhythm, and changes in pulse and blood pressure.[16]

The nurse also assesses the inputs likely to influence renal parameters. These include the type and amount of additives in intravenous fluids as well as irrigating solutions. The urinary output is obviously influenced by fluid input as well as by many medications such as digitalis and diuretics.

Other subsystem dysfunctions such as dehydration, hypervolemia or hypovolemia, ADH changes, or osmotic diuresis induced by total parenteral nutrition (hyperalimentation) may alter renal output, since they influence the renal function of the critically ill person.

A final mediating factor is the presence of an indwelling urinary catheter. While its function is supposedly facilitating, inattention to its patency or urinary tract infection may interfere with the accurate assessment of renal outputs.

□ Neurologic subsystems

Clues are elicited while assessing other subsystems to provide information regarding the critically ill patient's orientation to time, place, and person and the appropriateness of responses to either verbal or tactile stimuli. Determining the intactness of the cranial nerves as well as the functional status of the musculoskeletal system, which is dependent on innervation, is essentially the same as for other patients (see Chapters 8 and 40).

While determining the presence or absence of a neurologic sign remains significant, it is the returning or the diminishing of a sign that is often more relevant in critical care settings. Subtle and slight changes such as the return of reflexes following anesthesia or trauma or even a slight decrease in the level of consciousness may be extremely significant.

In addition to recognizing and interpreting neurologic changes, the evaluation of parameters that alter the patient's neurologic status becomes imperative. While assessing the appropriate or inappropriate behavioral response to stimuli continues to be important, assessing the types of posturing or ventilatory pattern provides valuable information with respect to the physiologic basis of the neurologic dysfunction. For example, metabolic changes resulting from vital subsystem dysfunction, as in the case of ventilatory insufficiency, may alter the patient's level of consciousness. Therefore the integration of data from the assessment of other subsystems is paramount.

For the critically ill patient the assessment of the neurologic subsystem is complicated by the environment as well as by the use of medications. Due to the lack of sensory input, such as absence of a clock or an overload of sensory input such as constant interruptions, a patient's disorientation may not necessarily reflect a neurologic deficit. Drugs can alter a patient's thought processes as well as perceptions, gait, and responsiveness. In no other part of the assessment can concomitant clues provide such essential information. Often it is necessary to continuously arouse the patient to his highest level of consciousness, and a painful stimulus may be the only way to elicit a response.

The late signs and symptoms of increased intracranial pressure are apt to be more readily encountered among critically ill patients. In addition to the vital signs and the neurologic assessment, data regarding intracranial pressure can be obtained by means of the subarachnoid screw, which directly measures changes in the intracranial pressure.

It is not enough merely to assess the neurologic status in relation to the other subsystems, but communicating the observations by recording them is imperative. Establishing a data base, following the sequence of events frequently, and recognizing subtle and concomitant clues are of great significance in the care of the critically ill patient.

■ ASSESSMENT OF OTHER PHYSIOLOGIC PARAMETERS

□ Integumentary and musculoskeletal status

The importance of assessing the integument, which protects the body from the external environment, is intensified in the care of the critically ill where there is often inadequate circulation, oxygenation, and nutrition along with long periods of immobility. Factors that enhance physiologic inadequacies and immobility must be considered, including pain and the presence of monitoring devices or equipment that necessitates that a patient lie in a supine position or that interferes with position change. Also prevalent in the critical care setting are factors that intensify the hazards of immobility such as the use of vasoconstricting drugs, which predispose a patient to skin breakdown. The length of time the critically ill person is confined to bed, his state of debilitation, inadequate hydration, effects of medications, and changes in ingestion and digestion patterns predispose the individual to contractures and skin breakdown.

Assessing the range of motion and muscle tone of all extremities for any bedridden patient is imperative. However, in the critically ill complications of procedures themselves often affect the musculoskeletal and integumentary systems. For example, the insertion of a transvenous pacemaker can result in a "frozen" or stiff shoulder if appropriate range of motion is not maintained. In addition the restraints on or contraindications to moving a patient, such as the placement of tubes or catheters in the femoral area, impose barriers to movement. Restrictions often increase with the amount of equipment and are unrelated to the patient's mental status. When immobility is not required, the usual assessment of activity tolerance as reflected in the patient's pulse, fatigue, shortness of breath, and other symptoms guides the nurse.

□ Fluid and electrolyte balance

Disturbances of fluid and electrolyte balance are common to the critically ill and are secondary to a dysfunctional subsystem, therapeutic regimens such as nasogastric suction, the presence of pain, and prolonged periods of stress. While assessment of the functional capacity of the renal subsystem provides a major part of the data regarding fluid and electrolyte balance, it is imperative to recognize the interrelatedness of electrolyte balance with other subsystems. For example, renal dysfunction changes the level of circulating potassium, and in turn this electrolyte potentiates cardiovascular dysfunction. Electrolyte balance is even more crucial due to an already weakened subsystem. Because therapeutic regimens may entail a number of devices such as a nasogastric tube and the use of medications that deplete the body of fluids and electrolytes, fluid and electrolyte disturbances may be compounded. For example, the loss of potassium through the nasogastric tube as well as its excretion in response to certain diuretics may potentiate electrolyte disturbances, thus necessitating frequent and constant monitoring. While critically ill patients usually receive intravenous fluids that contain electrolyte supplements such as potassium, elevated or lowered electrolyte levels must be carefully monitored. This is especially so since electrolytes such as potassium are known to be depleted during surgery and other periods of stress. The signs and symptoms of the "hypo" and "hyper" electrolyte states, urine and serum levels of electrolytes, and electrocardiographic changes due to electrolyte disturbance provide diagnostic cues (see Chapter 20). Because of the complexity of the critically ill patient's problems, physical signs and symptoms may be masked or difficult to determine. Therefore validation of electrolyte imbalance by the use of laboratory values is necessary. Electrolytes most commonly assessed because of their importance and their continually changing levels are potassium, sodium, and chloride.

Often critically ill patients have multiple intravenous infusions simultaneously. In addition to the usual assessment of type and amount of fluid and the additives being infused, the signs and symptoms of overhydration and dehydration as reflected by integumentary signs, weight changes, and subsystem changes are noted. Hourly measurements of intake and output are mandated by the critical state of the patient. Although weighing patients daily provides the most accurate data about fluid balance, it is essential that weight changes be examined in light of any variation in the weighing procedure required by the presence of life-support equipment.

□ Nutritional and elimination status

During the time that the nutritional demands for repair of the debilitated state are greatly increased, the critically ill patient commonly is unable to take nutritional supplements orally because of illness or therapy. With increasing complications the caloric, nitrogen, and fluid requirements are proportionately higher, and intravenous nutritional supplementation is required. The patient's catabolic state mandates that special attention be given to protein and caloric intake.

To assess the nutritional status of the critically ill person it is necessary to determine (1) his present condition, (2) the length of time nutritional status has been impaired or is expected to be impaired, (3) daily vitamin and caloric needs, (4) nitrogen balance, (5) changes in body weight, and (6) the means by which the nutritional status is maintained (gastrostomy or intravenous routes). Complications of these nutritional supplements as well as changes in subsystems that may cause a supplement to become a potential hazard necessitate constant surveillance.

With increased excretion of solute or in the presence of a potential osmotic diuretic state, assessment of the patient's tolerance of amino acids, presence of hyperglycemia manifested by glycosuria, or potential hypoglycemic reaction is essential. Often these nursing assessments may indicate the need for immediate cessation of the prescribed therapy. In addition careful observation of the hydration status is essential for patients receiving nutritional supplements parenterally.

Inspection of the oral cavity is of particular significance. The presence of nasogastric and endotracheal tubes hampers oral hygiene. The use of medications such as anticoagulants and some chemotherapeutic agents predispose patients to oral problems such as bleeding gums. Other factors to assess with respect to the nutritional status of the critically ill include abdominal distention, the presence or absence of bowel sounds, pain that inhibits the patient's desire for food, tolerance and preference for food, and the patient's elimination status.

A gastrointestinal tract complication well known to the nurse in the critical care area is bleeding resulting from intense and prolonged stress. While the observation of the patient's pale color and fatigued appearance increases the nurse's level of suspicion, the objective assessment of occult blood in stools or gastrointestinal tract drainage, the drop in hematocrit and hemoglobin levels, and the presence of abdominal pain validate this suspicion. Predisposition of patients to stress ulcers can be assessed from past history as well as current use of anticoagulant agents including aspirin, warfarin sodium (Coumadin), or heparin and the prolonged use of mechanical ventilators. An antacid regimen is commonly prescribed to prevent or treat this complication.

While bowel elimination often receives less attention than other vital functions, it may precipitate major complications. Not only is the patient's elimination pattern disrupted as a result of a medical or surgical procedure or prohibited intake of food, but the common use of medications such as meperidine (Demerol) or codeine, which predispose the patient to constipation, and the long periods of immobility, the effect of continued stress, and fluid and electrolyte disturbances exacerbate elimination problems. Use of the bedpan or bedside commode, with only a curtain serving as a means of separation from the patient in the next bed, decreases the amount of privacy available to the patient. In addition to assessing the effects of the previously mentioned factors on a patient's elimination status, it is important to determine the most effective position for elimination, the optimum time for elimination, and the utility of a regimen to facilitate a normal bowel movement. When appliances are used for elimination such as with a colostomy, it is imperative that the nurse monitor complications from such appliances, such as skin breakdown under the colostomy bag. The patient's tolerance of energy expenditure while using a bedpan or a bedside commode can also be assessed. Helping the patient learn positions that facilitate elimination as well as breathing techniques that minimize the Valsalva maneuver are especially significant in the care of patients who are vulnerable to the negative effects of straining when attempting to have a bowel movement.

■ ASSESSING THE IMPACT OF THE CRITICAL CARE ENVIRONMENT

□ Environment

The environment of most critical care units is considerably different from the environment in general care units. Not only is the critically ill patient forced into a state of dependency, he is also maintained in an environment conducive to both sensory deprivation and sensory overload (see Chapter 26). The openness of some critical care areas and close proximity of patients reduces privacy, while the number of procedures and almost constant presence of artificial light in addition to the noise in critical care areas demand constant assessment of the type and amount of sensory input. Eliciting input regarding a patient's usual routine and how the routine can be altered to maintain his individual preferences and foster his normal body rhythms is very significant. For example, critically ill persons may have time lapses of from days to weeks during which they are not aware of the date, the time, or the place. It is imperative that the nurse daily assess the patient's orientation and the situations that enhance meaningful stimulation. Varying the time or amount of visiting hours for the family may increase patterned input.

The amount of sensory overload and sensory deprivation increases relative to the severity of illness and the needs of the patient. Consequently, constant observation for signs and symptoms of delirium or postoperative psychosis is essential. It is not enough to identify the signs and symptoms of these disorders. Steps should be taken to determine the factors casuing the disorders. These include therapeutic and idiosyncratic causes as well as environmental factors. The effects of medications, constant interventions by personnel, the individual's own emotional state, and his age as well as the status of the critical subsystems may all contribute to altered behavioral states.

A factor common to the critical care environment is the noise level. The nurse assesses the noise with respect to the equipment, staff, and patients' input as well as to extraneous sources such as a radio. Critical analysis of the source, the amount, and the level of stimuli is essential, for what may be advantageous for one patient is often disadvantageous for another. Means by which to individualize such input requires constant attention.

☐ Complications of therapy

Infection is an ever present problem. The critically ill patient's debilitated state increases vulnerability to infection. In addition invasive procedures, exposure to many personnel, and the administration of steroids all increase the risk of infection. At the same time, steroids and prophylactic antibiotics may mask the presence of an infection. For these reasons personnel in critical care units must be particularly vigilant in maintaining sterile and nontraumatic technique, especially when suctioning tubes or inserting or irrigating catheters.

Careful assessment is made of the skin surrounding each tube or catheter entrance for increased tenderness and warmth. An increase in the white blood cell count or the growth of organisms from cultures of secretions validates the presence of an infection. When an infection occurs, nurses investigate the potential causes of the infection such as inadequate aseptic technique or cross-contamination through shared equipment, and appropriate steps are taken to prevent such hazards from occurring in the future.

☐ Comfort

Because of the many lifesaving measures that must be instituted when patients are in an intensive care unit, comfort of the patient may not be a major priority. Yet patients in these areas are extremely vulnerable because of their dependent states and the numerous factors that can predispose them to discomfort and unsafe situations for long periods.

Hygiene

Because the patient cannot meet his own hygienic needs, this responsibility is assumed by the nurse. Meticulous and frequent mouth care is important, especially for patients who have nasogastric tubes. The presence of an indwelling catheter requires careful perineal care. A recent study suggests that the care of the perineum should not be too vigorous as such practice may increase rather than decrease urinary tract infections.[21] The position of urinary catheters and means for maintaining the position are ascertained in order to provide comfort and to prevent complications.[22]

Body alignment

Due to the patient's condition, the nurse must monitor his body alignment and changes in position. A critically ill person requires more frequent turning to prevent complications such as skin breakdown and atelectasis. It is the nurse's responsibility to assess the patient's capability to turn, to determine the frequency of position change, contraindications to turning (such as possible malfunctioning of a monitor when a patient turns), effects of a position on the patient's physical state, and need for passive and active range of motion. Preventive care must begin in the critical care setting.

Pain

The critically ill patient may have multiple painful sites. When the patient is unable to talk, the cause of pain must be determined without benefit of the patient's description. Pharmacologic agents to relieve the pain may be administered more frequently to the critically ill than to those less ill. Pain medications are commonly given intravenously; this necessitates astute observation of the effects of the medications, since they act very rapidly and can lead to dangerous side effects. To avoid potentiating the effects of anesthesia or previously administered medications, the time that anesthesia or other medications were given is noted before an analgesic is administered. Identifying factors that influence pain such as treatments, body position, fatigue, or annoying sounds from machinery is as essential as noting the effectiveness of pain medications. Immediate feedback about the presence of pain may be elicited from the monitors, which indicate an elevated blood pressure or pulse rate in the presence of pain.

Safety

Many factors in the critical care setting make this environment potentially hazardous. Frequently the patient is confused or his sensorium is depressed from medications, anesthesia, and so on. The patient who is confused may be resistive to therapy and may attempt to remove catheters and other tubes. This often necessitates confining the patient with soft restraints. The effects of restraints on the circulation, nerve functioning, and the patient's behavior are assessed to assure that protective devices are not creating further problems.

Most critical care areas are air conditioned, and the cool room temperature may impede an already poor circulation, in turn causing the patient to receive diminished effects of medications or to slow down their excretion. The critically ill patient may have few bedcovers due to an already elevated body temperature, and he should be observed for chilling, which would result in undesirable demands on his already taxed metabolism.

Another major hazard is the presence of much electrical equipment. Considerable information is available about electrical hazards and safety, and it is a nursing responsibility to assure that hazards are recognized, that equipment is in good working order, that safety practices are observed, and that all equipment is properly grounded to reduce the possibility of electrical shock.

■ ASSESSMENT OF PSYCHOLOGIC STATUS

The admission of a patient who is critically ill produces anxiety or fear in the patient and significant others. The patient may be threatened with a number of losses: life itself; impairment, if not severance, of the functional capacity of a subsystem; insult to body integrity due to the state of disability or helplessness; and loss of comfort due to pain. His predicament becomes that of forced dependency, immobilization, and lack of control in an unfamiliar, if not frightening, environment that may depersonalize and insult his person while affording few, if any, means for him to respond to this crisis. No longer can his significant others afford him support by their physical presence. He is usually isolated and removed from familiar faces except for brief periods. Even in the short visits with significant others, the patient may be deprived of his usual means of communication because he is intubated.

The patient's response to critical illness will be determined by factors that influence behavior. These include *basic personality, perceptions* of the illness and what is happening to him, his usual mode of *coping,* cultural background, the reaction of significant others, and the openness or closedness of the critical care unit.

□ Perceptions

It is imperative to assess the patient's perception of the situation and its meaning to him. The critical care setting is an intense one with respect to the pace of activity as well as the person's physical condition. The potentially fatal outcome of critical illness compounds this. Consequently the patient's emotional responses may be more intense than that observed in less ill patients. He may react with greater anger or hostility, or he may experience prolonged periods of depression, shock, and disbelief.

Culture influences perceptions of the critical care environment. The dramatization of emergency or life-threatening situations in the mass media may cause the patient to perceive his situation as more serious than it really is. Previous illnesses and hospitalizations also influence the patient's perceptions. For individuals who have no experience with illness or hospitalization the anxiety may be even greater, since they have no idea of what to expect from the environment or the personnel caring for them.

The assessment of the patient's perception is made by observing, listening, and eliciting from him or others how he views or feels about what is occurring. When a patient is unable to communicate verbally, assessment is restricted to nonverbal clues such as facial expressions, hand gestures, body movements, and muscle tone. If physical status does not permit the patient to communicate, the input of significant others is imperative. Because the environmental stimuli are so numerous, it is often difficult to differentiate between a patient's perception of his physical status and his perception of his environment or therapeutic regimen.

□ Coping behaviors

In addition to assessing the general regulators of behavior, it is necessary to assess three main characteristics of response of the critically ill: the *emotional,* the *behavioral,* and the *physiologic.* These apply to both the patient and his significant others. An *emotional response* to either a psychologic or social loss may be similar to the adaptation to illness. The nurse's assessment of a patient's emotional response should include possible explanations for the feelings of anxiety or depression. Anxiety due to a fear of dying may be intensified by pain or dyspnea or by nursing and medical measures. A critically ill person and his significant others may also experience helplessness, hopelessness, and powerlessness intensified by their isolation.[30]

Behavioral responses that indicate anxiety and a fear of dying may include unwillingness to participate in personal care when able to do so, withdrawal from interactions with others, and facial or postural expressions of no longer caring, or giving up. The nurse can validate inferences about these responses by urging the patient or his family to ventilate their feelings.

The behavioral modes of dissipating excess energy or discharging stress are greatly limited by the patient's health status as well as by the environment.[28] Consequently excess energy may be evidenced by hyperactive, anxious, angry, or talkative states, while energy deficits are manifested by fatigue, depression, or withdrawal.

Determining whether a response is physiologic or behavioral is often difficult because of the confounding variables of the environment, the patient's physical state, and the effects of medication. For example, a patient may be lethargic and unresponsive to a procedure because of a hypoxic or medicated state, or he may be hyperactive and overresponsive to the same procedure because of sensory overload from his environment.

It is imperative in judging whether behavior is adaptive or maladaptive to consider both the appropriateness of the behavior relative to the situation and the previous behavior patterns of the individual. For example, a patient may experience confusion or loss of sense of time when the natural body rhythms are disrupted. This is a common experience of patients in intensive care areas who are kept awake day and night by constant noise, bright lights, and frequent procedures. An analogy is the "jet lag" experienced by travelers.

Altered *physiologic responses*, including those of the autonomic nervous system such as increased or abnormal heart rate, dilated pupils, increased respirations, and dizziness, may also denote the adaptation to crisis (see Chapter 12). Other physiologic responses may include weight loss, constipation, and insomnia.

□ Communication problems

Nurses need to assess the patient's and significant others' desire to talk and to express feelings. Input from significant others will assist the nurse in interpreting what the critical illness means to them and to the patient and their usual means of coping with crisis.

If the patient's usual modes of communication are altered, it is necessary to assess the utility of alternative ways to communicate such as writing, using sign language or alphabet charts, and lipreading. It is also necessary for the nurse to assess the effect of alternate means of communication on the patient who becomes upset over the amount of the time required for the interpretation of sign language.

□ Knowledge assessment

In addition to identifying the patient's and significant others' reaction to the illness, it is necessary to assess the effect that the environment has on each of them. Determining what each of them knows about monitors, machines, tubes, and procedures as well as their readiness to learn about the equipment, the rationales for the regimens, and information about objectives of care guides the amount of consumer education that is given. It is necessary to assess the patient's mental status to determine how often information needs to be repeated. Repetition is often necessary because pain, physical status, and the psychologic adjustment of the patient may interfere with learning. Recognizing that the patient may not retain data, the nurse continually observes the effect that information has on him and whether it relieves or increases his anxiety. The need for information sharing with the critically ill patient has been documented.[7]

The observance of the patient's rights is just as important in a critical care setting as in other hospital areas. These rights are the right to be informed, right to have interpretations, right to have someone listen, right to question, right to family, and right to deny. The guiding principle is prefacing each nursing action with an explanation to facilitate the patient's rights.[32]

The perceptions of a patient and significant others depend on the information that they have or are given about the patient's physical status, the procedures and routines of the critical care environment, the objectives of care, and the prognosis. Often the frequency of nursing tasks and the pace of the unit limit the amount of communication with the patient and significant others. The nurse needs to determine that the perceptions of the patient and significant others are accurate, since often they misinterpret the patient's condition, the purpose of equipment, and so on. In addition the nurse needs to constantly assess the readiness of the patient and significant others for additional information and should plan a time to meet with them.

■ ASSESSMENT OF SOCIOLOGIC STRESSORS

While the assessment of the social systems is the same for the critically ill as for any other patient, certain aspects may not take precedence until after physiologic stability is achieved. Often in a life-threatening situation the patient or significant others may request the presence and support of the hospital chaplain or another clergyman. The presence of a clergyman who can give support to the patient and significant others is especially important, since the efforts of physicians and nurses are directed toward maintaining the patient's life.

Another aspect of the social system to be assessed is the interaction and continuity of the relationship between the patient and significant others. Those characteristics that make the assessment different are the imposed restrictions (sometimes unnecessarily placed) on the visiting privileges of significant others, the specialized areas (often behind closed doors) that serve to separate the critically ill from other patients as well as from significant others, and the lack of involvement of significant others in the care of the patient. It is necessary to assess the frequency and the quality of interactions between the client and significant others, the strengths and limitations of the significant others, the availability of significant others, and the state of stress or crisis in which the significant others find themselves. The impact of the crisis and the continued stress on the significant others can be assessed by observing their facial expressions, their attentiveness or lack of it, and their coping behaviors. It is necessary for the nurse to identify factors that increase or decrease the stress of the significant others. For example, lack of information regarding a patient's status, inability to visit frequently, and the general emotional climate in the waiting room may increase the significant others' discomfort. Family members commonly spend the night in the waiting rooms or sleep in the hospital lobby, since they desire to be present if anything adverse happens to the patient. Consequently they may be exhausted at a time when continuously high levels of energy are demanded.

It is also important to assess the problem-solving ability of the significant others in the midst of stress. The identification of the coping mechanisms on which significant others rely as well as their ability to begin to act and to make decisions regarding changed roles, life styles, and responsibilities is imperative. The prescribed role of the patient, such as head of the family, often must be assumed by another family member. The nurse can be instrumental in assessing the willingness of the significant others to identify and utilize other resources and support systems. For example, the critical illness of a small child may require unlimited time of one or both parents, requiring that a grandparent or another adult assume the parental role in the home.

The nurse obtains much of the data about the strengths and limitations of the family through observation of their emotional and behavioral responses to the situation as well as by talking to other family members. The assessment of the family with respect to mental status, communication patterns, emotional stability, physical status, affection and cohesion among family members, and socialization with each other is similar to an assessment of a family in another situation. However, the duration of stress associated with having a critically ill family member, the abrupt change in family roles, and isolation from the loved one creates additional stressors for the family. The reality of a change in life style for the patient and its effect on the life style of the significant others must be assessed from the beginning to prepare them for the anticipated outcomes.

□ Discharge from the unit

Discharge from a critical care unit can be a time of emotional unrest for patients, particularly if the transfer is made abruptly without advanced notice and proper preparation of the patient. In order to assure a smooth discharge from the unit, it is necessary that the nurse assess the patient's perception of what is to occur; how he feels about the transfer, especially with respect to the anxiety he may experience in being separated from constant surveillance by machines and nurses; and what his transfer means to him personally. If a patient views the transfer as positive progression, his response will be considerably different than if he believes he is being moved simply to make a bed available for another patient. Unfortunately the latter situation does occur, and in such a situation the patient requires considerable support during and after the transfer. Often the patient, his significant others, and the intensive care nurses are upset by his sudden transfer. Nurses need to be careful not to convey their dismay or concern about the transfer to the patient who is already very upset by his sudden move from the intensive care setting.

The significant others must be informed about the reasons for the transfer and reassured that the patient will be safe in the new environment and that the nurses there are competent to meet his needs. This is more difficult for the intensive care nurses if the patient is transferred abruptly, but it is essential that an effort be made to reassure the significant others so that they can support and reassure the patient rather than contributing to or increasing his anxiety. If the patient and significant others do not believe that his physical condition is stable enough for him to leave the critical care unit, a crisis in confidence may occur.

In summary, the principles that govern the assessment of any patient are applicable to the assessment of the critically ill person. The collaboration with the patient and his family, the explanation of each nursing activity, and the recognition of increased psychophysiologic vulnerability because of the severity of the illness may provide the opportunity for growth for all concerned. The interaction that takes place during this period of crisis may strengthen relationships between the patient and his significant others and may also determine their ability to cope with future crises.

REFERENCES AND SELECTED READINGS

1. *Abbey, J. C.: Nursing observations of fluid imbalance, Nurs. Clin. North Am. **3**:77-86, 1968.
2. Aguilera, D. C., and Messick, J. M.: Crisis intervention: theory and methodology, ed. 3, St. Louis, 1978, The C. V. Mosby Co.
3. Auger, J. R.: Behavioral systems and nursing behavioral assessment and nursing, New Jersey, 1976, Prentice-Hall Inc., pp. 145-170.
4. *Bolin, R. H.: Sensory deprivation: an overview, Nurs. Forum **13**:241-258, 1974.
5. Byrne, M. L., and Thompson, L. F.: Key concepts for the study and practice of nursing, ed. 2, St. Louis, 1978, The C. V. Mosby Co.
6. Caplan, G.: Concepts of mental health and consultation, Washington, D.C., U.S. Department of Health, Education and Welfare, pp. 183-206.
7. *Cassem, N. H., Hackett, T., and Bascon, C.: Reactions of coronary patients to the C.C.U. nurse, Am. J. Nurs. **70**:312-319, 1970.
8. *Codd, J., and Grohar, M. E.: Postoperative pulmonary complications, Nurs. Clin. North Am. **10**:5-15, 1975.
9. *Corbell, M.: Nursing process for a patient with a body image disturbance, Nurs. Clin. North Am. **6**:155-163, 1971.
10. Davis, M. Z.: Socioemotional components of coronary care, Am. J. Nurs. **72**:705-709, 1972.

10a. *Dodd, M. J.: Assessing mental status, Am. J. Nurs. **78**:1500-1503, 1978.

11. Downs, F. S.: Bedrest and sensory disturbances, Am. J. Nurs. **74**:434-438, 1974.
12. Fitzgerald, L. M.: Mechanical ventilation, Heart Lung **5**:945-949, 1976.
13. *Garrett, J. J.: Oliguria in postoperative patients, Nurs. Clin. North Am. **10**:59-67, 1975.
14. *Gordon, M.: Assessing activity tolerance, Am. J. Nurs. **76**:72-75, 1975.
15. Hamilton, W. P.: Common cardiovascular problems in the postoperative period, Nurs. Clin. North Am. **10**:27-41, 1975.
16. *Heath, J. K.: A conceptual basis for assessing body water status, Nurs. Clin. North Am. **6**:189-198, 1971.
17. Hudak, C. M., Gallo, B. M., and Lohr, T.: Critical care nursing, Philadelphia, 1973, J. P. Lippincott Co.
18. Kiely, W. R.: Psychiatric aspects of critical care. In Zschoche, D. A.: Mosby's comprehensive review of critical care, St. Louis, 1976, The C. V. Mosby Co.
19. Klein, R., Kliner, W., and Lipos, D.: Transfer from a coronary care unit: some adverse responses, Arch. Int. Med. **122**:104-108, 1968.
20. Kuenzi, S. H., and Fenton, M. V.: Crisis intervention in acute care areas, Am. J. Nurs. **75**:830-834, 1975.
21. Kumin, C. M.: Detection, prevention and management of urinary tract infections, ed. 2, Philadelphia, 1974, Lea & Febiger.
22. Lawson, B. N.: Clinical assessment of cardiac patients in acute care facilities, Nurs. Clin. North Am. **7**:431-434, 1972.
23. Laycock, J.: Nursing the patient on the ventilator, Nurs. Clin. North Am. **10**:17-25, 1975.
24. Lewis, L.: Systematic assessment: what it can do for the hospitalized patient, Med. Arts Sci. **27**:39-50, 1973.
25. *Maykoski, K., and Fabre, D.: Nursing assessment of the surgical intensive care patient, Nurs. Clin. North Am. **10**:83-106, 1975.
26. McVan, B.: Odors: what the nose knows, Nurs. '77 **7**:46-49, 1977.
27. Methery, N. A.: Water and electrolyte balance in the postoperative patient, Nurs. Clin. North Am. **10**:49-57, 1975.
28. Murray, R. L. E.: Assessment of psychological status in the surgical I.C.U. patients, Nurs. Clin. North Am. **10**:69-81, 1975.
29. Obier, K., and Haywood, L. J.: Enhancing therapeutic communication with acutely ill patients, Heart Lung **2**:49-53, 1973.
30. Roberts, S. L.: Behavioral concepts and the critically ill patients, New Jersey, 1976, Prentice-Hall, Inc.
31. Roberts, S. L.: Systems approach in assessing behavioral problems of critical care patients, Heart Lung **4**:593-598, 1975.

31a. *Smith, R. N.: Invasive pressure monitoring, Am. J. Nurs. **78**:1514-1521, 1978.

32. Storlie, F.: Patient teaching in critical care, New York, 1975, Appleton-Century-Crofts.
33. Strauss, A.: The intensive care unit: its characteristics and social relationships, Nurs. Clin. North Am. **3**:7-15, 1968.
34. Woods, N. F., and Falk, S. A.: Noise stimuli in the acute care area, Nurs. Res. **23**:144-150, 1974.
35. Woods, S. L.: Monitoring PA pressures, Am. J. Nurs. **76**:1765-1771, 1976.
36. Zetterland, J. D.: An evaluation of visiting policies for intensive and coronary care units. In Duffey, M., Anderson, E. H., Bergersen, B. S., Lohr, M., and Rose, M. H.: Current concepts in clinical nursing, vol. 3, St. Louis, 1971, The C. V. Mosby Co.

*References preceded by an asterisk are particularly well suited for student reading.

71

Management of the critically ill patient

SALLY SCHAFER

The nursing process is the same in critical care situations as it is in any other patient care setting. Management of critically ill patients requires establishing a data base, identifying problems and potential problems, delineating priorities, defining outcome criteria, determining goals for intervention, carrying out the planned interventions, evaluating the effects of intervention, and modifying goals and plans as necessary. Management of critically ill patients differs from management of other patients because of an ever changing data base; a larger number of complex, interrelated problems; frequent reordering of priorities, and time limitations imposed by the rapidity with which the data base changes.

Nurses in critical care settings are called on to make decisions rapidly and to act on those decisions based on discriminating observations, understanding of the interrelationship among phenomena observed, and a current and comprehensive assessment of the situation. It is essential to keep pace with the constant input of new data in order to identify new problems as they arise, make predictions about potential problems that might occur, and intervene according to appropriate priorities and goals.

The ultimate goal of nursing intervention for any patient, regardless of the nature of his illness, is to promote, sustain, and restore optimum level of physiologic, psychologic, and social functioning. However, in a critical care setting the immediate goal of ensuring a patient's survival initially determines the priorities for intervention. Once the question of a patient's survival has been determined, priorities are reordered and other problems can be addressed.

The life-threatening and potentially life-threatening events that are a part of critical illness require constant vigilance by members of the critical care team in order to maintain a patient in a homeokinetic state, to prevent complications, and to restore optimum function. Since nurses are in 24-hour attendance of a patient, they are the first to recognize changes in his condition. In most critical care units there is one nurse for every one to three patients, depending on each patient's physiologic stability, numbers of personnel available, and care requirements.

When assuming responsibility for the care of a critically ill patient, the nurse receives a detailed report of significant changes that have occurred, interventions that were instituted and their effects, and a summary of the patient's current physical and emotional status. A well-organized comprehensive report will highlight problems and priorities and will help the nurse establish initial goals for intervention.

Having received this report, the nurse proceeds to the patient's bedside, where introductions are made either by the nurse or by the nurse who has been with the patient during the previous shift. The patient is engaged in discussion as to his concerns and his perceptions of his condition. This approach to the patient can accomplish several purposes. It reinforces to the patient that he is seen first as a worthwhile person and second as a patient who is critically ill.

There are advantages in having the nurse who has been with the patient and the nurse who is new to the situation go through the initial interaction with the patient together. First, the patient is not only aware that an exchange of information has taken place, but he participates in the exchange. He can see that the new nurse is familiar with and understands his problems and concerns, which in turn allays his anxieties and helps develop trust in the new nurse. Second, the new nurse can validate initial observations with the nurse who is more familiar with the patient's condition. And finally, the nurse leaving the setting can orient the new nurse to procedures and equipment at the bedside that may be new or unfamiliar.

Several factors inherent in critical care situations may require altering the approach described. The nurse who has been caring for the patient may be unavailable, the patient may be intubated or have a tracheostomy making communication more difficult, the patient may be disoriented or his level of consciousness may hamper or preclude his interacting effectively, or there may be a change in the patient's condition requiring immediate action. Nevertheless, whenever possible the nurse entering the critical care setting considers an approach to the patient that will convey respect for him as a worthwhile human being, recognize his need for input and some control over his care, foster feelings of security and trust in the nurse, and give the nurse an opportunity to make meaningful observations about the patient.

Following the initial interaction the nurse continues to collect data for a baseline assessment. This includes making a complete assessment of the patient's physical condition, psychologic status, and immediate environment and comparing these findings with those already reported. The nurse reviews medical and nursing orders and the most recent progress notes, observes the frequency of routines and treatments, and notes pertinent laboratory data and test results. From this assessment appropriate priorities for patient care are established. The frequency of routines, observations, and treatments as ordered by physicians and other nurses provides input but does not determine priorities. The critically ill patient's condition changes rapidly, and the therapeutic regimen must be altered to meet those changing needs. Taking vital signs every hour may not be sufficient if a patient has a labile blood pressure but may be too often if the patient's condition is stable and he needs rest. In many instances nursing judgment will determine the appropriate frequency of routines and treatments, such as the patient's readiness for ambulation, change in diet, or the need for tranquilizers, sedatives, or analgesics.

Problems that initially require the most attention are usually physiologic in nature. However, when a patient's survival is not in immediate jeopardy, that is, when his condition is stable either from a return in function of his own homeokinetic mechanisms or from support of medical and nursing therapies, problems of a psychosocial nature may assume equal if not primary emphasis.

With problems identified and priorities established, the nurse reviews the data pertinent to each problem and determines the desired outcomes of interventions. Despite varying pathologic conditions the commonalities among critically ill patients helps to identify desired behaviors for patients and their significant others. These behaviors become the criteria by which the effectiveness of patient care is evaluated. In order to reach the desired outcomes, specific interventions are determined for each problem. The following outcome criteria and goals for intervention are relevant for all critically ill patients; however, the emphasis and priority each receives will be determined by the nature and number of physiologic, psychologic, and social stressors in each patient situation.

■ ALLEVIATION AND PREVENTION OF PHYSIOLOGIC AND PHYSICAL STRESSORS

□ Patient outcomes

1. Show improvement of signs and symptoms from the primary insult.
2. Show no signs or symptoms indicative of severe physiologic reaction to stress or to the therapeutic regimen such as hyperglycemia, stress ulcer, colitis, paralytic ileus, hypertension, myocardial infarction, cerebral vascular accident, infection, injuries, altered neurologic function, renal failure, extreme fatigue.
3. Be free of complications from prolonged immobility or restricted activity.
4. Experience maintenance and improvement in all vital functions such as respiratory, circulatory, neurologic, and renal.
5. Maintain an adequate nutritional status.
6. Be free of extreme physical discomfort.

□ Goals of intervention

Restore and support vital functions

Of primary concern is the patient's cardiovascular, respiratory, renal, and neurologic function. Among interventions receiving major emphasis are those directed toward preventing hypoxia by maintaining a patent airway and supporting respiratory function, preventing circulatory collapse and supporting cardiac output and peripheral perfusion, maintaining adequate glomerular filtration, and preventing renal failure.

One of the most important nursing responsibilities is monitoring of vital functions by means of direct observation and by direct and indirect measurement of physiologic parameters. Ongoing physical assessment, measurement of vital signs, determination of cardiac and respiratory function, precise recording of intake and output, and collection of specimens of urine, blood, secretions, and drainage for analysis are routine nursing functions in critical care areas. In most instances critical care is primarily preventive care accomplished through intensive physical and mechanical monitoring, astute observations, and early intervention by nurses.

Promote physical comfort and protect from personal injury

Critical illness leaves many patients dependent and unable to take care of their basic physical needs. They are also vulnerable to actual and potential danger in the environment. The patient's comfort is primarily the responsibility of the nurse, and care will include attention to personal hygiene and grooming, frequent repositioning, maintaining proper body alignment, appropriate use of analgesics, sedatives, and tranquilizers, and emphasis on all measures to promote rest. Critically ill patients are bombarded with routine monitoring procedures, tests, treatments, and interactions with many different members of the health care team, all of which may be important to the patient's well-being but allow little time for rest. When setting priorities the nurse plans direct care activities and coordinates activities and services of other health care workers to provide the patient with uninterrupted periods of rest. The nurse's attention to comfort measures not only adds to a patient's feelings of well-being but also conveys to him and significant others the nurse's concern and respect for him as a human being, thereby engendering a sense of trust.

Ensuring a patient's safety requires adequate numbers of personnel to meet a patient's needs for observation, monitoring, and prompt intervention. Safety measures also include assuring that electrical equipment is safe and functioning properly. It is not unusual for critically ill patients to be disoriented or confused as a result of physiologic or psychologic disturbances or from effects of analgesics, sedatives, and tranquilizers. Side rails need to be in place when a patient is unattended, and measures need to be taken to ensure a patient's safety when he is out of bed.

Critically ill patients frequently receive vasopressor, cardiotonic, and antiarrhythmic medications to support their faltering homeokinetic mechanisms. The dosages of these medications have a small margin of safety and even when administered within that safety range can cause severe side effects. Accurate administration, validation of dosages with colleagues, and close observation for untoward effects of medications is necessary. The fluid balance of the patient whose conditions is critical is often tenuous and requires constant attention. The amount of fluid administered must be balanced with output in order to prevent fluid overload or dehydration.

Infection is a potential problem in the critically ill. In addition to being debilitated, many patients receive a variety of antibiotics that potentially may allow resistant organisms to multiply. In addition some patients receive steroids that make them more vulnerable to infection and also mask signs and symptoms of infection, which then may go untreated. Invasive procedures and disruption of skin integrity as with the insertion of intravenous catheters increase the risk of infection. Because of the openness of many critical care units and the close proximity of patients, it is especially important that there be adequate air exchange in the unit. In order to prevent infection, stringent handwashing policies and strict sterile technique in all procedures including suctioning of tubes and irrigation of catheters is required. In addition the patient is observed carefully for signs or symptoms of infection such as an elevated white blood cell count, elevated temperature, or change in amount, consistency, or odor of body secretions or drainage.

Preserve and maintain musculoskeletal function

Most critically ill patients are confined to bed for varying lengths of time and are hampered further in movements by pain, presence of tubing, and connection to equipment such as a respirator. Preserving function of weight-bearing muscles, maintaining joint mobility, and preventing skin breakdown is a real challenge to nurses caring for these patients. All of the preventive and supportive nursing care techniques used for any bedridden patient are appropriate in this situation (see Chapter 29). A primary nursing responsibility is to help determine a patient's readiness for increased activity. This decision is based on an assessment of his ability to tolerate activity without undue stress on his cardiovascular and respiratory systems and not on the nature or number of tubes and pieces of equipment surrounding the patient. If vital signs and blood pressure are stable, the patient is conscious, and it is not contrary to medical therapy, he will benefit both physiologically and psychologically from being out of bed. Physical support from several staff members may be required at first, but every effort needs to be made to help the patient bear some, if not all, of his weight, since *lifting* him from bed to a chair will *not* exercise weight-bearing muscles or prevent decalcification of bones.

Promote and maintain fluid and electrolyte balance

Critically ill patients are very vulnerable to fluid and electrolyte alterations. Pain and apprehension aggravate the body's physiologic response to stress, resulting in sodium and chloride retention, potassium excretion, and decreased urinary output. Many patients have temporary or permanent alterations in ingestion, elimination, and metabolism caused by renal failure or insufficiency, ostomies, injuries to the digestive tract, paralytic ileus, nausea, vomiting, diarrhea, or increased insensible water loss, all of which compound existing fluid and electrolyte disturbances. Disturbances in fluid and electrolyte balance secondary to medical and nursing interventions and therapies such as surgery, nasogastric suction, irrigations, and diuretics are also common occurrences.

To prevent potential disturbances and to promote fluid and electrolyte balance the nurse monitors several parameters. Meticulous intake and output records are kept, including fluids received by all routes (oral, intravenous, arterial line, irrigations, nasogastric) and drainage from all sources (bladder, bowel, ostomy, surgical drains). The patient is weighed daily, and the specific gravity of urine is measured at least every 4 hours. Vital signs and central venous pressure (CVP) are monitored, and the patient is observed for specific signs and symptoms of dehydration or fluid overload. All laboratory data reporting fluid and electrolyte status are reviewed as soon as they are available.

In addition to collecting this data, the nurse administers fluids and supplemental electrolytes as ordered. When the patient has several sources of intake, it is a nursing responsibility to maintain ordered fluid intake. Fluid orders are often written in relationship to output, and the nurse must adjust intravenous intake in accord with urine output.

Maintain adequate nutritional status and normal bowel function

Critically ill patients are subject to nutritional deficits due to alterations in amount and type of nutrients ingested; disturbances in ingestion, digestion, absorption, and elimination; and the increased demand for energy than many aspects of critical illness impose. Patients are often not allowed anything by mouth or are anorexic. Their caloric and nutritional requirements may be partially or totally supplied depending on the type of intravenous fluids prescribed. Concurrently immobility-induced catabolism causes negative nitrogen balance at a time when many patients need extra protein to rebuild cells broken down by surgery, injuries, or disease. The energy required to cope physically with multisystem failure makes extraordinary demands on the body. Severely burned patients experience high energy demands with decreased mobility, enormous tissue damage and cellular breakdown, loss of protein, and alterations in ingestion imposed by the injury or by medical therapy. Critically ill patients with respiratory insufficiency and secondary respiratory infection who require frequent and vigorous pulmonary care to mobilize secretions also experience extreme weakness and fatigue and need high-protein, high-caloric nutrition.

To maintain positive nitrogen balance nursing interventions may include supplying patients who are able to eat with high-protein, high-calorie foods in frequent small amounts. In order to combat anorexia, these meals need to reflect the patient's food preferences. Vitamin supplements are ordered routinely in intravenous solutions. The nurse may be responsible for administering total parenteral nutrition (hyperalimentation) intravenously or prepared formulas given through nasogastric or gastrostomy tubes for patients unable to take food by mouth. Observing and monitoring for the side effects and complications of total parenteral nutrition becomes part of the nurse's routine patient assessment. (See Chapter 20 for more information on fluids and electrolytes).

Bowel dysfunction may be caused by disruption in integrity of the gastrointestinal tract from disease, surgery, injury, immobility, altered dietary patterns, and lack of privacy or the opportunity to use regular bathroom facilities. Except for patients with loss of integrity in the gastrointestinal tract, normal bowel function can be promoted by assuring adequate fluid intake and giving stool softeners or laxatives. These medications combat constipation and impaction resulting from loss of muscle tone and the defecation reflex. Providing as much privacy as possible and helping the patient to assume the most normal position for defecation are simple but important nursing actions. If the patient is able to be out of bed, the bedside commode can be used while the patient is up.

Alleviation and prevention of physiologic and environmental stressors by disease, trauma, and the therapeutic regimen initially may be the major although not exclusive emphasis in the care of the critically ill. When vital functions are stable, the outcome of a critical illness is determined largely by preventive and restorative nursing interventions that have as their goal the preservation and maintenance of optimum functional status. Since physiologic and psychosocial stressors conjointly influence the attainment of their optimum level of functioning by the critically ill patient and his significant others, it is essential that nursing intervention be directed toward all these stressors concurrently.

■ ALLEVIATION AND PREVENTION OF PSYCHOLOGIC STRESSORS FOR THE PATIENT AND SIGNIFICANT OTHERS

□ Patient outcomes

1. Show no signs or symptoms indicative of severe psychologic reactions to stress (i.e., inappropriate affect, distortion of reality).
2. Experience no disturbances in sensation or perception related to the environment.
3. Be able to state plans for medical and nursing care.
4. Be able to state plans for transfer from the critical care unit.

□ Goals of intervention

Determine patient's or significant other's perceptions of the illness and therapeutic regimen

Psychologic response to illness or injury experienced by a patient and significant others will be determined by their perception of the situation and its meaning to them. Their perception depends on their premorbid personalities, current psychologic status, and adequacy of coping mechanisms.

Misperception or misinterpretation of elements in the environment such as the presence of a cardiac monitor often results in adding unnecessary stressors. Because it is the *perception* of the event or element that in part determines the degree of stress caused, not merely the event or element itself, nurses need to frequently determine the perception of the patient and significant others about what is happening.

Another major determinant of when and if a crisis will ensue is the ability of the patient and significant others to cope with the perceived stressor. The patient's perceptions and the ability to cope with stressors are assessed through psychologic as well as physiologic monitoring.

Psychologic monitoring entails eliciting information from the patient and significant others about how he is perceiving the environment, his physical condition, and the procedures and routines being performed on and for him. Techniques used to elicit this information might include asking open-ended questions such as, "How are things going for you today?" or, to the significant others, "How does he(she) seem to you today?"; recognizing and following up on nonverbal cues: "You look worried (uncomfortable, nervous)"; and interpreting the patient's or significant others' behavior such as anger, withdrawal, uncooperativeness, or passiveness as clues to their psychologic states. Awareness of popular public and cultural misconceptions about hospitals, specific diseases, and treatments aids in understanding the patient's misperceptions and misconceptions.

Acknowledge, accept, and encourage patient and significant others to ventilate their feelings

The psychologic impact of critical illness is a major influence on a patient's immediate and eventual survival and a crucial factor in defining his optimum level of wellness. The critically ill person is partially or totally isolated from the usual support system, is alienated from familiar surroundings and daily living patterns, and is dependent on others to meet basic needs, not the least of which is survival itself. A critically ill person has limited alternatives with which to cope with these stressors, and depending on past experiences may have few appropriate coping behaviors in his repertoire. Feelings of helplessness, powerlessness, loneliness, and depersonalization and disturbances in body image are common. Modes of dissipating the frustration, anger, hostility, depression, and anxiety generated by these feelings are circumscribed by physical limitations and the therapeutic regimen.

Health care providers can provide many of these patients with means of coping with multiple stressors by maintaining an atmosphere of openness and acceptance that encourages them to talk about their feelings. A basic need of these patients is to share difficult experiences with others and to identify problems.[23] Talking with patients openly and honestly decreases feelings of depersonalization and anxiety and prevents isolation and alienation. Expressing emotionally laden material in an atmosphere of acceptance discharges stress while maintaining the patient's self-esteem. Recognizing that anger and hostility are often indicative of fear and anxiety and that depression and withdrawal may be signs of hopelessness, loneliness, powerlessness, or loss assist the nurse in accepting these feelings as normal and expected in this situation. The nurse who encourages the patient to talk about how he feels provides an avenue for relieving tension and promotes psychologic well-being. Encouraging the patient to express his feelings helps him to identify why he is feeling and behaving in a manner that may be unusual and anxiety provoking for him; at the same time it gives him permission to feel and act that way. Using cognitive feedback such as, "It's normal in this situation for you to be angry," invites an expression of feelings. Health team members who are helping a patient to talk about his feelings need to be ready to accept whatever emotionally laden material may be expressed.[17] Often a hospital chaplain or clergyman from the community can help health care providers develop the ability to handle this aspect of patient care comfortably.

Patients who are intubated are unable to express their feelings even though they are alert and oriented, and therefore they are particularly vulnerable to psychologic stressors. To help prevent feelings of isolation and alienation in the person who is unable to communicate verbally, paper and pencil or a magic slate are placed within easy reach. However, writing about concerns, anxieties, and feelings is time consuming and cumbersome. Not all patients are willing to write out their feelings, either because it requires more energy than they have or they are unsure about how to express their feelings in writing. Nurses need to be particularly sensitive to stressors in the environment, to recognize behavior as clues to a patient's psychologic state, and to verbalize feelings for the patient that are common to most patients in similar situations and thus validate with the patient that he too is experiencing some of these feelings. Being empathetic with the patient conveys acceptance and understanding and counteracts feelings of depersonalization, isolation, loneliness, and powerlessness.

Provide information and clarify misconceptions about physical status and plans and goals of treatment

As already mentioned, the patient's *perception* of stress and not the stress itself determines his reaction to his illness and the intensive care environment. Failure to give simple explanations and adequate information result in the patient perceiving his condition and the rationale for procedures and treatments as far more threatening than actually may be the case. Care given without explanations and communication may falsely impress the patient and significant others with the severity of illness and the patient's total dependence on lifesaving equipment. The cardiac monitor may be believed to keep the heart beating rather than monitoring the heartbeat. Administering blood as a precautionary measure may be perceived as a lifesaving intervention for what is thought to be a deteriorating condition.

Much of what a patient learns about his health problems and their relation to his self-image depends on what is taught directly and indirectly by the health care team.[23] Patient teaching in critical care requires short-term goals. Pain, discomfort, weakness, anxiety, noise, and confusion are some of the obstacles to learning experienced by these patients. Despite such obstacles, patients and significant others need explanations of procedures and purposes of treatments. A patient may not believe what he is told the first time or may be coping with the situation by denying the problems. In either case there needs to be reinterpretation and reiteration of previous explanations regarding diagnosis, prognosis, and current physical status. Keeping the patient and significant others apprised of his condition and treatment plans helps them perceive the situation accurately, enhances their ability to cope realistically and effectively, and promotes their cooperation by making them members of the health care team.

Encourage and support involvement of patient and significant others in decision making and care

The essence of crisis intervention is to help people cope with a major life crisis such as a critical illness. The patient is assisted to formulate his own goals and is helped to reach them. When the patient and significant others are knowledgeable about goals and the rationale for treatments and understand the patient's current physical status and prognosis, they can be involved in many aspects of his care and can make decisions and set goals consistent with the treatment regimen. Involving the significant others in care and decision making serves at least two purposes. First, involvement decreases feelings of helplessness, powerlessness, and anxiety. Second, when significant others understand treatment goals and support them and are involved in the patient's care, they are able to continue this behavior after the patient is transfered from the intensive care unit. Significant others can make valuable contributions in the care of the patient in a variety of ways. Even when a patient is unconscious, visits by significant others who talk to him and touch him may be supportive to the patient and help decrease the helpless feelings of the significant others.

An alert patient can be involved in making a schedule for his activities and treatments throughout the day. If he is taking food by mouth, he and his significant others can help make choices in planning his menu. Significant others can assist a patient at mealtime if help is needed. They can encourage a postoperative patient to deep breathe and help support his incision as he coughs, and they can remind him of his fluid limit or offer him fluids frequently depending on the goals of therapy. Significant others can be very helpful as they reiterate and reinforce explanations about physical status, prognosis, and treatments.

Promote and maintain a sensory-regulated environment

The environment of critical care units is a major stressor with which patients must cope. Most critical care units are designed so that patients are in direct view of the staff and are in close proximity to each other so they can be observed at all times and action can be taken immediately to avert a crisis. Some critical care units consist of one room with adjacent patient units separated only by curtains; other units have adjacent patient units separated by glass or partial glass partitions; and still others have private rooms for each patient, some with glass partitions for easy visibility.

The open ward design exposes the patient not only to the activity related to his own care but also to the activities of other patients' care. Bright lights, monotonous noises, equipment alarms, crises with other patients, and noise generated by personnel culminate in sensory monotony and overload for the patient. Research indicates that noise generated by operation of equipment commonly found in critical care areas (bed scales, IPPB outflow valve, two cardiac monitors operating simultaneously) reached a level that could easily awaken patients.[34] Also implicated in generating high noise levels were conversation and non-patient-related activities of personnel. The bustling and noisy atmosphere of critical care areas is perceived as highly emotionally charged by patients and interferes with their relaxation, rest, and sleep.

Providing a sensory-regulated environment requires attention to the lack of meaningful stimulation to the patient as well as to overstimulation by disruptive activities and noise. Environmental stressors contribute to a patient's experiencing sensory deprivation or emotional touch deprivation. The spatially confined environment and limited mobility of the patient are among factors common to all critically ill patients. Limited mobility reduces the quantity and quality of sensory input. The alert patient has decreased interactions with his environment, and this causes disturbances in time, pattern, form, and temperature perception and discrimination.

The technical environment and language further reduces the meaningfulness of stimulation. In some instances there is reduction in the intensity of stimulation, as with patients with hearing loss, patients without glasses who have poor sight, patients who cannot eat or who are on bland, monotonous diets that do not stimulate the sense of taste, or patients who are not stimulated by their own voices because they are intubated and cannot speak.

Reducing the amount of disturbing sensory bombardment and providing meaningful sensory input for patients is crucial to promoting rest and preventing disturbances in patients' reality orientations. Not all disruptive input can be eliminated, but actions can be taken to limit the amount of input, thus reducing the intensity of environmental stressors. Bedside conversations that exclude patient participation should be limited to essential interactions. Spacing patients as far apart as possible and placing alert, stable patients in the most quiet area of an open unit helps reduce noise generated by the care of other patients. Limiting the frequency of taking vital signs and disruptive observations, particularly at night, and planning care to provide for the least disturbance of the patient encourages rest. One study suggests (1) reducing the noise level by using tactile stimuli in arousing patients rather than calling their names; (2) turning the surface of a bedside monitor with the amplifier away from the patient and turning the sound off if the oscilloscope is easily visible to staff; (3) positioning an MA-1 respirator with bellows away from the patient's ear; (4) refraining from using bedpan washers and hoppers at night; (5) using carpet and draperies to absorb sound in utility areas and nursing stations; and (6) placing staff lounges away from patient care areas.[34] If someone is always present in the nursing station, a telephone with a flashing light instead of a bell can be used to limit noise.

To provide meaningful sensory input that will help maintain orientation, wall clocks and calendars that are large enough to be seen easily by patients are essential. If surroundings permit, keeping familiar objects at the bedside, listening to a radio over earphones, displaying cards from friends, or being in a bed near a window also help to maintain a patient's reality orientation.

Frequent orientation of a patient to person, place, time, and physical status has been shown to diminish the sensory distortion that leads to delirium in postoperative cardiac patients.[4] Patients with tracheostomies need to be encouraged to talk whenever the cuff of the tracheostomy tube is deflated so they can hear their own voices. Patients need to be engaged in self-care when possible in order to keep them involved purposefully with themselves and their environment. Visits from significant others who bring news about family, friends, and current events keep the patient in touch with social realities and need to be emphasized as important contributions to the patient's total care.

Promote and maintain the patient's reality orientation

Despite attempts to control stress-producing environmental factors and to provide a sensory-regulated environment, some patients will exhibit disturbed thought processes, indicated by confusion, impaired judgment, delusions and phobias, and perceptual disturbances such as illusions, hallucinations, and paresthesia. Factors other than environmental that contribute to these problems are certain medications, premorbid psychologic status and physical condition, metabolic state as indicated by blood chemistries and blood gases, and age. Patients receiving narcotics and barbiturates, highly anxious patients, patients with multiple, interrelated, debilitating physical problems, patients with disturbed metabolic and respiratory function, patients deprived of sleep, and older patients are most prone to disturbed thought processes and perceptual distortions.

Some patients are aware of intermittent breaks from reality and disturbances in thought processes but are reluctant to share these with the health care team. Being aware of possible attempts by patients to conceal thought and perceptual distortions, nurses need to assess patients' behavior for clues that these are occurring. Patients who seem indifferent to people and events, who are unusually preoccupied, who sleep poorly, whose conversation is disjointed, whose attention span is brief, and whose affect seems inappropriate may be experiencing reality disturbances.

Patients affected by reality disturbances and their significant others need to be reassured that these disturbances are transient and are not unusual in such circumstances. Significant others can be involved in providing meaningful sensory input by orienting and reorienting the patient to person, time, place, and physical status and events occurring around him and physical characteristics of the environment. Changing medications, correcting disturbed metabolic phenomena, and permitting uninterrupted sleep when possible are other actions to be taken to help resolve the problem and minimize deleterious effects.

Prepare patient or significant others for transfer from critical care unit

For many patients and their significant others transfer from the critical care area is a time of considerable psychologic stress. The critical care area with its sophisticated electronic equipment and attentive, knowledgeable, and highly skilled personnel connotes security and protection. Discharge from this area to an area with less nursing personnel per patient, less frequent interaction with staff, and where the patient is expected to be more independent often seems premature to the patient and significant others, particularly if they have misconceptions regarding the patient's physical status and care requirements. The anxiety precipitated by the transfer can be prevented or reduced if the patient or significant others are taught to interpret the meaning of particular signs and symptoms and helped to understand the purpose of equipment and routines. Signs that indicate progress need to be pointed out continuously. Informing the patient and significant others of plans for transfer as soon as such plans begin to be discussed (not waiting until the day of transfer) helps them adjust to the idea gradually and gives them time to plan for it. They need to know the projected date of transfer, what to expect on the new unit, and what will be expected of them. Ideally a nurse from the receiving unit is introduced to the patient and significant others prior to transfer. After transfer, visits from members of the critical care unit staff are helpful in conveying continued concern for the patient's welfare and in promoting trust in the nursing staff in the new setting. This is accomplished by validating with the patient that he is receiving attention and care appropriate to his improved status.

■ ALLEVIATION AND PREVENTION OF SOCIAL STRESSORS FOR THE PATIENT AND SIGNIFICANT OTHERS

□ Patient outcomes

1. Maintain continuity in their relationship.
2. Make knowledgeable decisions for instituting changes in therapy, life style, established family roles, and relationships.

□ Goals of intervention

Promote continuity in relationship between the patient and significant others

As mentioned previously, in the critical care setting a patient's physiologic needs often assume priority over his psychologic needs, and the patient's social being is marginally recognized and less seldom addressed. Limited visiting hours and the strange technical environment and language of the critical care unit isolate patients from their significant others and prevent them from assuming their usual social roles. For the most part, a person who is critically ill is approached exclusively in the context of his role as patient. Efforts need to be made to retain a link between the patient and significant others while he is physically removed from them.

Some of the same techniques described above that involve significant others with the patient's care serve to promote continuity in their relationship. The patient is able to maintain identity with roles other than that of patient when significant others are involved in supporting the therapeutic regimen, explaining and reinterpreting information about his physical status and progress, and keeping him informed about people and events in his premorbid social environment. Including significant others when teaching the patient promotes consistency of the information given and prevents misunderstandings and misinterpretations between the patient, significant others, and staff. Relaying messages between patients and significant others by telephone helps maintain contact.

One of the most effective and important ways to prevent disruption in relationships is to prepare significant others for their first visit with the patient in the critical care unit. Before the significant others enter the area, the patient's physical appearance and the environment should be described to them. They need to know the patient's level of consciousness, his ability to communicate, and his ability to understand their communication. They need to realize the importance of their presence to the patient and his need for their support. When the significant others approach the bedside, a staff member should stay with them and facilitate the initial interaction between them and the patient. At each subsequent visit the nurse responsible for the patient's care should meet with the significant others to answer questions and apprise them of his status and progress.

Support changes in roles and relationships between the patient and significant others

While efforts need to be made to help a patient maintain identity with his premorbid social roles, he cannot fulfill the obligations and responsibilities of those roles during illness. Roles of parent, spouse, breadwinner, sexual partner, decision maker, employer or employee, and leader may be altered, reversed, or eliminated. The responsibilities of the patient need to be assumed by family and friends. Depending on the length of the illness and period of recovery, it may be some time, if ever, before a patient can function fully in those roles. Dwindling or absent financial resources may result in changes in social status, social mobility, and life style.

During the critical phase of illness the significant others will be attempting to cope with precipitous role changes and may need help working through problems that arise as family members and friends assume or fail to assume additional responsibilities. When disintegration among significant others occurs and no one assumes the role formerly held by the patient, members of the health care team may need to be directive in helping the family to reorganize themselves and their resources. The most stable family member may be designated as the decision maker or the one to be called first in case of emergency. The family may need help in planning visiting schedules that will be least disruptive to their daily lives and still meet their needs and those of the patient. They may also need assistance in identifying supportive figures within and without the immediate family who can be called on for assistance.

DOCUMENTATION OF PATIENT CARE

An integral part of all nursing intervention is reporting and recording of pertinent data about the patient's physical, physiologic, and emotional status, his response to medical and nursing therapies, and plans for changing or continuing with nursing interventions. Written and verbal communication promotes continuity and consistency in patient care in any setting; however, in critical care settings where the variety and intensity of physiologic and psychosocial stressors interact to produce multiple problems and frequently changing priorities, reporting of new data and documentation of the effect of interventions on a patient's condition is crucial. Because of the large amount of data collected and the time available for recording, most critical care areas use a flow sheet as an efficient and organized means of reporting information (see p. 1550).

At the conclusion of each shift a summary is written that highlights the patient's primary problems as reflected by the pattern of data collected throughout the shift. Included in the summary are a range of the patient's vital signs and other physiologic measurements, intake and output totals, the patient's response to treatments and procedures, plans for further observations and interventions, and comments about the patient's reaction to and interactions during visits from significant others.

Although the evaluation *process* is the same in the critical care unit as it is in other patient care areas, multisystem embarrassment, constant fluctuation in the data base, rapidly changing priorities, and shorter periods between interventions impose constraints that influence the nature of evaluation.

A general systems perspective negates a cause-effect relationship because of the number of intervening variables introduced by suprasystems and subsystems. When a patient suffers multisystem failure, interventions directed at one system have direct as well as indirect effects on other systems. As a result an outcome is obtained that may be different from one that the same interventions might have produced in isolation. Decisions about modifying a plan of action based on generalizations about the impact of a single intervention are usually inappropriate and unwise.

Goals for intervention in critical care areas are short term and fluctuate according to the patient's changing condition. Evaluation of those goals likewise is short term and often narrowed to specific interventions. For example, the outcome of an IPPB treatment is evaluated in terms of its immediate effect on breath sounds, ability to mobilize secretions, and general ventilatory status. Due to the instability of a patient's condition, an intervention that is effective at one time may not bring about the desired outcome at another time. For example, if a patient's ventilatory status deteriorates, an IPPB treatment may not be effective, and more aggressive therapy may be needed to maintain ventilatory function. In order to keep pace with the continuous reassessment and reordering of priorities, the frequency of evaluation in critical care areas is increased, resulting in less time between evaluation and modification of interventions. Many times the opportunity to repeat the intervention and to observe for the same or different outcomes is limited. Because of sophisticated monitoring devices, decisions can be made based on a data base that is larger and collected in a shorter time.

In most critical care areas nurses have more flexibility and autonomy in decision making and intervention than do nurses on general care divisions. This increased latitude in role functions coexists with the responsibility and accountability for making sound decisions based on accurate interpretation of the data base and the changes in a patient's physiologic and emotional behavior.

REFERENCES AND SELECTED READINGS

1. *Adams, M., Hanson, R., Korkool, D., Beaulieu, A., Bellville, E., and Morss, K.: Psychological response in critical care units, Am. J. Nurs. **78**:1504-1512, 1978.

1a. Aguilera, D. C., and Messick, J. M.: Crisis intervention: theory and methodology, ed. 3, 1978, St. Louis, The C. V. Mosby Co.

2. *Black, Sister K.: Social isolation and the nursing process, Nurs. Clin. North Am. **8**:575-586, 1973.

3. *Bolin, R. H.: Sensory deprivation: an overview, Nurs. Forum **13**:240-258, 1974.

3a. *Borgen, L.: Total parenteral nutrition in adults, Am. J. Nurs. **78**:224-228, 1978.

3b. *Breu, C., and Dracup, K.: Helping the spouses of critically ill patients, Am. J. Nurs. **78**:50-53, 1978.

4. *Budd, S., and Brown, W.: Effect of reorientation technique on postcardiotomy delirium, Nurs. Res. **23**:341-348, 1974.

5. Byrne, M. L., and Thompson, L. F.: Key concepts for the study and practice of nursing, ed. 2, 1978, St. Louis, The C. V. Mosby Co.

6. *Codd, J., and Grohar, M. E.: Postoperative pulmonary complications, Nurs. Clin. North Am. **10**:5-15, 1975.

7. *Davis, M. Z.: Socioemotional components of coronary care, Am. J. Nurs. **72**:705-709, 1972.

8. Downs, F. A.: Bed rest and sensory disturbances, Am. J. Nurs. **74**:434-438, 1974.

9. *Ellis, R.: Unusual sensory and thought disturbances after cardiac surgery, Am. J. Nurs. **72**:2021-2025, 1972.

10. *Garrett, J. J.: Oliguria in postoperative patients, Nurs. Clin. North Am. **10**:59-67, 1975.

11. *Gentry, W. D., Musante, G., and Haney, T.: Anxiety and urinary sodium/potassium as stress indicators on admission to coronary-care unit, Heat Lung **2**:875-877, 1973.

*References preceded by an asterisk are particularly well suited for student reading.

12. *Hamilton, W. P.: Common cardiovascular problems in the postoperative period, Nurs. Clin. North Am. **10**:27-41, 1975.
12a. *Haughey, B.: CVP lines: monitoring and maintaining, Am. J. Nurs. **78**:635-638, 1978.
13. Hudak, C. M., Gallo, B. M., and Lohr, T.: Critical care nursing, Philadelphia, 1973, J. B. Lippincott Co.
14. Janis, I. L.: Psychological stress, New York, 1958, John Wiley & Sons, Inc.
15. Kiely, W. F.: Psychiatric aspects of critical care. In Zschoche, D. A., editor: Mosby's comprehensive review of critical care. St. Louis, 1976, The C. V. Mosby Co.
16. *Kiely, W. F.: Critical care psychiatric syndromes, Heart Lung **2**:54-57, 1973.
17. *Kuenzi, S. H., and Fenton, M. V.: Crisis intervention in acute care areas, Am. J. Nurs. **75**:830-834, 1975.
18. *Lambertsen, E. C.: The nature and objectives of intensive care nursing, Nurs. Clin. North Am. **3**:3-6, 1968.
19. Leavell, H. R., and Clark, E. G.: Preventive medicine for the doctor in his community, New York, 1965, McGraw-Hill Book Co., Inc.
20. Meltzer, L. E., Abdellah, F. G., and Kitchen, J. R.: Concepts and practices of intensive care for nurse specialists, ed. 2, Bowie, Md., 1976, Publishers, Charles Press Inc.
21. *Metheny, N. A.: Water and electrolyte balance in the postoperative patient, Nurs. Clinc. North Am. **10**:49-57, 1975.
22. *Murray, R. L. E.: Assessment of psychological status in the surgical ICU patient, Nurs. Clin. North Am. **10**:69-81, 1975.
23. *Obier, K., and Haywood, L. J.: Enhancing therapeutic communication with acutely ill patients, Heart Lung **2**:49-53, 1973.
24. Olson, E. V.: The impact of serious illness on the family system, Postgrad. Med. **47**:169-174, 1970.
25. *Olson, E. V.: Hazards of immobility, Am. J. Nurs. **67**:779-796, 1967.
26. Roberts, S. L.: Behavioral concepts and the critically ill patient, New Jersey, 1976, Prentice-Hall, Inc.
27. *Roberts, S. L.: Systems approach in assessing behavioral problems of critical care patients, Heart Lung **4**:593-598, 1975.
28. Selye, H.: The stress of life, New York, 1958, John Wiley & Sons, Inc.
29. *Sobel, S.: Personalization on the coronary-care unit, Am. J. Nurs. **69**:1439-1442, 1969.
30. *Spicer, M. R.: What about the patient? Patient-centered management in an intensive care area, Nurs. Clin. North Am. **7**:313-322, 1972.
31. *Stephenson, C. A.: Stress in the critically ill patient, Am. J. Nurs. **77**:1806-1809, 1977.
32. Storlie, F.: Patient teaching in critical care, New York, 1975, Appleton-Century-Crofts.
32a. *Trockman, G.: Caring for the confused or delirious patient, Am. J. Nurs. **78**:1495-1499, 1978.
33. Waisbren, B. A.: Critical care manual: a systems approach method, New York, 1972, Medical Examination Publishing Co., Inc.
34. Walker, B. J.: Nursing care to assess and prevent common cardiovascular problems, Nurs. Clin. North Am. **10**:43-48, 1975.
35. *Woods, N. F., and Falk, S. A.: Noise stimuli in the acute care area, Nurs. Res. **23**:144-150, 1974.
36. Zimmer, M. J.: Guidelines for development of outcome criteria, Nurs. Clin. North Am. **9**:317-321, 1974.

72

Case study of a critically ill patient

SALLY SCHAFER
MARY K. KIRKPATRICK

This chapter presents a case study of a young girl who suffered multiple-system trauma as a result of an automobile accident. The format follows the systems approach. Changing priorities and emphases in care as the patient progresses along the recovery continuum are presented. Nursing diagnosis of patient stressors is identified at two phases in her hospitalization: on admission and prior to transfer from the critical care unit. Appropriate patient outcomes and nursing orders are given or presented for each nursing diagnosis.

□ Admission note

Sandy J. is an 18-year-old, single student who was admitted following an automobile accident. She was transferred from a rural hospital to a medical center approximately 100 miles away after she developed respiratory insufficiency. This is her first hospitalization. Her father and older brother accompanied her to the medical center.

Sandy sustained multisystem trauma including circulatory instability with possible ruptured spleen, pulmonary contusions with bilateral and partial pneumothorax, head trauma with facial lacerations and contusions, and fractures of the right ilium and left femur, tibia, and fibula. Immediate medical intervention included a tracheostomy, closed reduction of all fractures with application of a left long leg cast and traction, and suturing of facial lacerations.

On admission to the critical care unit, Sandy is in respiratory distress (rate 32, Po_2 43, Pco_2 46, HCO_3 30, pH 7.32). She is hypotensive (BP 80-90/50) and has tachycardia (pulse 120, regular). She also is oliguric (10 ml of urine last hour), febrile (38.2 C), and is alternately agitated and somnolent. She has a cuffed tracheostomy tube, a urinary retention catheter, nasogastric tube, central venous pressure catheter, intravenous infusions including a dopamine drip, and a long leg cast with balanced traction on her left leg.

□ Assessment data

Physiologic

Further nursing assessment reveals that Sandy's pupils are equal and reactive to light. She moves all extremities spontaneously, follows simple commands and responds appropriately to verbal and painful stimulation when fully aroused, and becomes less agitated when verbal reassurance is offered and contact is maintained through touching her, as when holding her hand. Her general color is pale including her lips and nailbeds. Her facial lacerations are dry and well approximated. Without ventilatory assistance her respirations are slightly labored at rest with the head of the bed elevated 30°. Her respiratory rate increases and substernal and intercostal retractions are apparent when she is agitated. Her chest movement is symmetrical, and breath sounds are equal but diminished in the lower lobes with diffuse rales throughout all lobes. A moderate amount of thick white secretions is suctioned through the tracheostomy. Sandy tolerates suctioning without arrhythmias or significant change in color. She is receiving ventilatory assistance from a volume ventilator (patient triggered, 50% oxygen with 12 cm positive end-expiratory pressure [PEEP] 20 cm of water pressure, 800 ml volume). Her apical pulse is regular without extra heart sounds, and the cardiac monitor shows a sinus tachycardia. Occasionally bowel sounds are auscultated, and her abdomen is firm and moderately distended with diffuse tenderness on palpation. Her abdominal girth is 81.2 cm. Her peripheral pulses are equally palpable bilaterally but weak, and her extremities are cool to touch, pale in color, with good movement and sensation. Skin surrounding the cast and intravenous infusion sites is dry without evidence of inflammation. The nasogastric tube is draining a moderate amount of green-brown fluid (200 ml since leaving the previous hospital) and irrigates freely. Urninary drainage is clear yellow with a specific gravity of 1.022; the catheter irrigates freely. Central venous pressure

(CVP) reads 5 cm of water. A solution of 5% dextrose in water is infusing through the CVP line at 60 drops/ minute. An IV solution of 500 D5W with 400 mg dopamine at 15 cm/hour is currently maintaining a systolic pressure of greater than 100 mm Hg (3 μg/kg/min).

Laboratory values on admission were K^+ 3.7, Na^+ 142, Cl^-99, BUN 24, Hgb 10.1, Hct 34, CO_2 33 mEq/liter, glucose 150.

Behavioral

Sandy makes no attempt to communicate verbally. Her facial expression is strained and sad, and her wide eyes stare at each movement of the health team members. She is confused regarding the date and time but nonverbally confirms the admission to the medical center by nodding her head when explanations are given. She is restless and agitated when aroused, but this subsides with explanations and reassurance. Family interaction appears warm and reassuring and elicits her increased cooperation.

Sociocultural background

Sandy is 18 years old. Her mother died in childbirth, and she has been reared primarily by her father with assistance from an aunt. She lives with her father and brother on a farm in a small rural town in the South. She has been reared in the Protestant faith. Her father had adequate insurance coverage.

Upon Sandy's admission her father and brother stood in the doorway of the waiting room adjacent to the critical care unit quietly watching the activities of the health care team members who were caring for Sandy.

The immediate admitting patient care orders are shown in the box opposite.

The nursing diagnoses, patient outcomes, nursing goals, and orders shown in Table 72-1 were developed from the admission nursing assessment.

■ OUTPUT

□ Progress note (actual outcome)

Four weeks following admission Sandy's vital functions are self-sustaining and her recovery has progressed to where she will be transferred from the critical care unit within the next several days.

Sandy is alert and oriented. Her vital signs are stable and within normal limits except for a low-grade fever (37.5 C). Her respirations are easy without ventilatory support or oxygen therapy (arterial blood gases: pH 7.41, Pco_2 38, Po_2 90, HCO_3 24, saturation 96%, Hct 40, Hgb 14). She receives continuous humidification to her tracheostomy, IPPB treatments every 4 hours, and clapping and modified postural drainage every 4 hours by the physical therapist. Her secretions are thick, yellow, and moderate in amount. Cultures reveal a *Pseudomonas* in-

ADMITTING ORDERS

NPO
NG to intermittent low Gomco suction
Measure abdominal girth q1h
Vital signs q15 min, temperature q4h
CVP q30 min
Hourly I & O with specific gravity (24 hr totals)
Foley catheter to straight drainage
Circulation checks q15 min until stable, then q$^1/_2$h
Neurologic checks q15 min
Volume ventilator with 50% O_2 with 12 cm PEEP
Suction q1h prn with tracheostomy care
Passive range of motion (ROM) q4h
Cardiac monitor: mount ECG strip
Bed rails up at all times
Left leg to balanced suspension traction with Thomas splint

Laboratory
Arterial blood gases q1h
Hct q2h, monitor WBC, creatinine clearance
Coagulation studies (PTT, APTT) stat, then every morning
Electrolytes stat, chem. 6 q4h × 2, then every morning
Type and cross match two units of blood
CBC
X-ray (portable) stat, ECG stat

Intravenous fluids
D5W 500 ml with 400 mg dopamine to keep systolic BP above 100 mm Hg and free of signs and symptoms of extreme peripheral vasoconstriction
Replace NG drainage ml/ml with D5 $^1/_2$ NS (each bottle with 20 mEq KCL)
CVP line with 1,000 D5W to keep open (TKO)
5% Dextrose in Ringer's lactate 1,000 ml q8h alternating with 1,000 ml D5 $^1/_2$ NS (each bottle with 20 mEq KCL)
Dextran 70 500 ml/day

Medications
Lasix 40 mg IV stat and q6h unless K^+ falls below 3.5 mEq/liter
Ancef 1 g q8h
Tylenol 1.2 g per rectum now and q4h for temp 38.2 C
Solu-Medrol 80 mg IV q6h
Valium 5 mg IM q2-3h prn for agitation
Riopan 60 ml q2h via NG tube and clamp for 15 min
Morphine sulfate 1-3 mg IV push q2-3hr prn
Garamycin 60 mg IV tid

fection. She is able to clear most secretions from her tracheostomy with vigorous coughing, requiring suctioning more frequently after IPPB treatments and on awakening in the morning. Her breath sounds are equal bilaterally, audible with scattered rales and rhonchi in all lobes, which clear with coughing or suctioning. Her apical pulse is regular; peripheral pulses are equal and strong bilaterally. Bowel sounds are audible, and her abdomen is soft. She had a splenectomy the day after admission. Her abdominal incision is dry and well approximated without sutures. She has not had a bowel movement for several days. The nasogastric tube has been discontinued, and she is eating a regular diet, although due to anorexia she eats very little solid food. She has lost 6.8 kg (15 lb) since admission. All intravenous infusions and the arterial line have been discontinued. The condition of her skin is good without areas of disruption. Healed facial lacerations are without sutures, but suture lines are visible with ecchymotic areas remaining. She is voiding in sufficient quantities; her urine is clear yellow, and specific gravities are within the normal range.

Sandy's behavior indicates a labile psychologic status with intermittent periods of withdrawal, crying, and anger. She communicates by writing and mouthing words but at times becomes very frustrated with these procedures and withdraws. Some days she is interested and involved in her care and is able to assume increasing responsibility for self-care. She has been told that the current medical treatment emphasis is to clear up her pneumonia, and it is important that accumulated secretions not be retained in her lungs. She consistently requests to be suctioned if she is unable to clear her respiratory tract by coughing. She has also been told that she can further assist in her recovery process by improving her strength through increasing her daily activity and eating high-caloric, high-protein foods. She is hesitant to get out of bed due to discomfort with movement, and requests to return to bed because of fatigue after sitting in a chair for a brief period. Sandy will agree to transfer to a chair after receiving medication for pain and has remained out of bed for increasing lengths of time each day. Her oral intake remains very poor, consisting primarily of clear liquids.

Having asked for a mirror several days ago and inspected her face, Sandy has become more withdrawn, irritable, passive, and less cooperative in her care. She denies that viewing her face bothers her and refuses to discuss the expected changes.

Information gained during periods when Sandy communicates more freely indicates that she has been a typical teenager with average academic and social pursuits. A recent high-school graduate, Sandy planned to attend a nearby community college in the fall and has a full-time summer job to help absorb the burden of that expense. Recently Sandy has realized that classes begin in 1 month and that she will be unable physically and financially to attend.

Sandy's father, brother, and aunt visit every other weekend now that her condition is stable. She is most communicative and interested in her care immediately before, during, and after their visits.

At the time of this progress note, the patient care orders are shown in the box above.

The nursing diagnoses, patient outcomes, nursing goals and orders at the time of transfer from the critical care unit are shown in Table 72-2.

PATIENT CARE ORDERS

Vital signs q4h except when asleep (temperature q4h 37-38.5 C; q2h 38.5 C; q1h > 39 C)
Discontinue IV
Regular diet (high protein, high caloric) with supplemental feedings
Advance activity as tolerated
IPPB q4h
Physical therapist for percussion q4h
Digital occlusion intermittently of tracheostomy for communication
Colace 100 mg at HS
Tylenol 100 mg for temperature above 38.5 C
Keflex 250 mg PO q6h
Multivitamin with iron every day
Chest x-ray examination every AM
WBC daily
Sputum culture daily

□ Evaluation

Comparing the *actual* outcomes of Sandy's medical and nursing interventions since admission with those *predicted* on admission reveals that Sandy experienced both improvement of signs and symptoms from the primary insult (automobile accident) and restoration and maintenance of vital functions. She developed no signs or symptoms indicative of severe physiologic stress (GI tract bleeding, diabetes). Laboratory values and physical assessment indicate fluid and electrolyte balance. She is generally free of physical discomfort, complaining of pain only when transferring between bed and chair. She has had neither prolonged nor severe psychologic reactions to stress nor displayed any thought disturbances, hallucinations, or delusions that would indicate disturbances in sensation or perception. A respiratory infection (low-grade fever and positive sputum cultures) is not surprising in light of her general debility and the presence of a tracheostomy tube.

Text continued on p. 1582.

Table 72-1. Nursing plan on admission

Input	Throughput	
Nursing diagnosis of stressors	**Predicted patient outcomes**	**Nursing orders**
1. Effects of primary insult	1. Improvement in signs and symptoms of the primary insult (head trauma)	**Goal:** *Restore and support vital functions*
a. Altered level of consciousness and agitation related to head trauma, ventilatory insufficiency, or anxiety	a. Alert and oriented Moves all uninjured extremities Quiet when undisturbed; easily aroused	a. Neurologic checks q15min, arouse to highest level of consciousness Orient to surroundings and events Monitor pulse pressure Monitor vital signs Maintain unobstructed airway Provide reassurance; explain procedures; use touch to enhance verbal communication
b. Shock related to possible internal hemorrhage	b. Vital signs stable: pulse 80/120, BP 100 systolic, RR 12-20 CVP > 5 cm H_2O pressure Hct and Hgb within normal limits Color pink Skin warm, dry Peripheral pulses present Urine output 30 ml/hr No increase in abdominal girth	b. Monitor vital signs q15min Monitor CVP q1h Measure and monitor abdominal girth q30min Measure urine output with specific gravity q1h Titrate dopamine infusion to keep systolic BP 100 mm Hg Monitor Hct and Hgb
c. Ventilatory insufficiency related to lung contusions, pneumothorax, and head trauma	c. Maintains open airway Maintains arterial blood gases within normal range Maintains pulmonary function parameters within normal range (shunt, dead space, inspiratory force, tidal and minute volumes)	c. Suction tracheostomy q1h and prn Auscultate breath sounds before and after suctioning and cuff deflation Monitor central and peripheral color continuously Note characteristics and changes in respiratory pattern, increases in tracheal secretions Monitor arterial blood gases (ABG) Measure pulmonary function q shift: tidal volume (TV) and minute volume (MV)
d. Oliguria related to trauma or decreased circulatory volume	d. Maintains urine output > 30 ml/hr	d. Measure urine output q1h, note color and characteristics Test specific gravity q1h Maintain IV infusion rates as ordered Titrate dopamine infusion to keep systolic BP > 100 mm Hg
2. Effects of critical illness Potential physiologic reactions (hyperglycemia, gastrointestinal ulcer) related to stress secondary to multisystem failure	2. No signs or symptoms of severe physiologic reactions to stress Free of signs and symptoms of diabetes mellitus Free of signs and symptoms of gastrointestinal ulcer	**Goal:** *Restore and support vital functions* Monitor urine for sugar and acetone Monitor amount of urine output (O > I may indicate hyperglycemic osmotic diuresis) Monitor nasogastric drainage and stools for frank and occult blood Monitor Hct Check for abdominal distention Administer antacid (Riopan) as ordered

Continued.

Table 72-1. Nursing plan on admission—cont'd

Input	Throughput	
Nursing diagnosis of stressors	**Predicted patient outcomes**	**Nursing orders**
3. Untoward effects of treatment	3. No signs or symptoms of toxic or untoward physiologic reactions to therapy	**Goal:** *Protect from injury*
a. Potential untoward effects related to medications	a. Tolerates medications and is free of signs and symptoms of side effects from: Dextran 70 Morphine sulfate 1-3 mg q2-3h or prn until free of pain Solu-Medrol 80 mg IV q6h Garamycin 60 mg	a. Maintain dextran infusion at consistent rate to prevent interstitial-to-plasma fluid shift Morphine sulfate: monitor respirations Solu-Medrol: give Riopan as ordered; continue psychologic assessment Garamycin: monitor BUN, creatinine clearance; note and record allergic response
b. Potential circulatory impairment and skin irritation related to long leg cast	b. Maintains adequate circulation to immobilized extremity Free of skin excoriation, disruption, and inflammation surrounding cast	b. Circulation checks q2h Adhesive tape to rough cast edges Protection of cast and surrounding skin from moisture and drainage
c. Potential infection related to invasive procedures	c. Maintains normal body temperature Maintains WBC within normal range Free of purulent drainage	c. Check temperature q4h; if 38.5 C (R), check q2h; if 39 C (R), check check q1h Check WBC daily Note consistency, color, odor, and amounts of all drainage Anchor catheter securely to prevent movement Change IV tubing q24h Change IV dressing q24h
d. Potential stress ulcer related to ventilatory assistance	d. See Outcomes 2	d. See Orders 2
e. Potential tracheal erosion related to cuff pressure of tracheostomy tube	e. Maintains closed airway system with consistent cuff volume	e. Use minimal inflating volume necessary to maintain seal Check cuff volume and pressure every shift Record cuff volume and pressure every shift Use swivel adapter on endotracheal tube to prevent traction or pull on tubes
4. Problems related to fractures	4. Free of complications of immobility-restricted activity	**Goal:** *Preserve and maintain musculoskeletal function*
a. Potential emboli related to thrombus formation or fracture	a. Free of sudden, sharp chest pain Maintains adequate ventilation Free of signs and symptoms of local inflammation of extremities Absence of pink frothy secretions	a. Check for signs and symptoms of phlebitis Check for pink frothy secretions Assess ventilatory status including signs and symptoms of hypoxia Do passive range of motion q4h Give dextran as ordered

Table 72-1. Nursing plan on admission—cont'd

Input	Throughput	
Nursing diagnosis of stressors	**Predicted patient outcomes**	**Nursing orders**
4. Problems related to fractures —cont'd b. Potential skin breakdown related to immobility	b. Skin integrity maintained without signs of circulatory impairment (redness, tenderness) over bony prominences	b. Keep skin dry Use alternating-air-pressure mattress Tilt, prop with pillows q2h Massage bony prominences and apply lubricating lotions liberally each shift
5. Nutritional deficits Catabolism and negative nitrogen balance related to trauma, immobility, increased metabolic rate	5. Maintains nutritional status Stable weight	**Goal:** *Maintain adequate nutritional status* a. Decrease negative effects of immobility: (1) Exercises: active-passive ROM and resistive exercises q4h to decrease loss of calcium from bone (2) Scrupulous hygienic care and prevention of skin disruption to decrease tissue breakdown b. Control increase in metabolic rate: Controlled environmental temperature and appropriate use of covers to prevent increased body temperature Use of antipyretics prn Careful handwashing and strict aseptic technique to decrease infection risk c. Vitamin supplements per IV or NG d. Weight daily
6. Fluid and electrolyte imbalance Potential fluid and electrolyte imbalance related to NG drainage, stress reaction, increased insensible H_2O loss per ventilatory system	6. Maintains fluid and electrolyte balance Intake equals output Na^+, K^+, Cl^- within normal limits Weight stable Skin turgor normal Moist mucous membranes Respiratory rate within normal limits Absence of ECG changes related to electrolyte imbalance Absence of muscular cramps	**Goal:** *Promote and maintain fluid and electrolyte balance* Replace NG drainage ml/ml with 5% dextrose in 0.25 NS Monitor electrolyte lab values Weigh daily Assess skin turgor and mucous membranes Monitor respiratory rate Check specific gravity q4h Check signs and symptoms of fluid overload and dehydration Monitor ECG
7. Pain Pain at sites of injuries	7. Free of extreme physical discomfort a. With use of analgesics and progressive relaxation techniques is able to tolerate position changes and procedures involved in the therapeutic regimen	**Goal:** *Promote physical comfort and protect from personal injury* Move slowly when positioning Maintain body alignment Assess need and effectiveness of analgesic Assist her using progressive relaxation techniques to control pain

Continued.

Table 72-1. Nursing plan on admission—cont'd

Input	Throughput	
Nursing diagnosis of stressors	**Predicted patient outcomes**	**Nursing orders**
7. Pain—cont'd	b. Rests quietly when undisturbed	Check traction for alignment and free movement Assess environment for potential dangers to safety and discomfort Give medication for pain prior to procedures such as bed change, bath
8. Impairment of vital functions	8. Maintenance and improvement of vital functions	**Goal:** *Restore and support vital functions*
a. Potential CNS disturbances related to head trauma	a. Remains alert and oriented to person, place, time Maintains stable vital signs	a. Neurologic checks q1h including signs and symptoms of increased intracranial pressure Vital signs q1h
b. Potential systemic infection related to debilitation, iatrogenic factors	b. Maintains normal body temperature Maintains WBC within normal range Cultures remain negative	b. Check temp q4h if 38.5 C (R); if 39 C (R) check q1h Check WBC daily Prevent skin disruptions Use sterile suctioning techniques Avoid cross-contamination from other patients Inspect IV sites, apply Betadine and maintain sterile dressings every day Do foley care every shift Give Garamycin
9. Psychologic response to illness and therapy	9. Shows no signs or symptoms of severe psychologic reactions to stress	**Goal:** *Promote and maintain reality orientation, minimize anxiety*
a. Potential disorientation related to medication effects and trauma	a. Oriented to person, time, place, surroundings, activities	a. Use open-ended questions Recognize nonverbal cues Observe behavior
b. Anxiety related to unfamiliar environment and procedures	b. Rests quietly when undisturbed Is able to cooperate and follow directions	b. Recognize nonverbal cues and behavior as indicative of perception Use cognitive feedback Provide reassurance Explain all procedures before doing them Identify self and other care givers Enlist her cooperation in care (e.g., turning, taking deep breaths and coughing, lying quietly for procedures) Remain with her when physical care or monitoring is not required Use touch at times other than for purposes of physical care (e.g., when talking with her)

Table 72-1. Nursing plan on admission—cont'd

Input	Throughput	
Nursing diagnosis of stressors	**Predicted patient outcomes**	**Nursing orders**
9. Psychologic response to illness and therapy—cont'd		
c. Inability to communicate verbally due to tracheostomy	c. Shows no signs or symptoms of severe psychologic reaction to stress Communicates effectively (i.e., gets basic needs met through means other than speech)	c. Anticipate needs Provide pad and pencil, magic slate, alphabet chart, pictures Ask questions to be answered yes or no Speak slowly Reassure that her inability to talk is temporary (i.e., there is nothing wrong with her voice)
d. Potential delusions/hallucinations related to inappropriate environmental stimulation and extreme fatigue	d. Experiences no disturbances in sensation or perception related to the environment Oriented to reality Communicates coherently Cooperates with care Follows directions	d. Reduce sensory overload Provide meaningful sensory input Orient to person, place, time, surroundings, activities When possible, try not to awaken if she's sleeping (after frequent neurologic checks are no longer needed)
10. Family's response to crisis		**Goal:** *Determine father's and brother's perceptions of the situation*
a. Father's and brother's lack of knowledge related to unfamiliar environment and confusion about Sandy's condition	a. Significant others able to state plans for medical and nursing care State all of Sandy's current major problems (e.g., respiratory, neurologic, orthopedic injuries, shock) Describe nursing and medical care emphasis State rationale for potential surgery	Recognized nonverbal and verbal cues as indications of their perceptions Determine their previous experience with similar situations **Goal:** *Provide information and clarify misconceptions* Discuss Sandy's condition with significant others in terms of nursing priorities and interventions (i.e., major nursing care emphases at this time are to monitor her condition, facilitate optimum ventilation, regulate medication to keep her blood pressure stable, promote optimum comfort, and decrease her fear and anxiety) Facilitate a meeting with the physician to clarify medical problems and treatment Sandy's major medical problem is difficulty breathing as a result of lung damage from the accident and low blood pressure from possible bleeding in her abdomen

Continued.

Table 72-1. Nursing plan on admission—cont'd

Input	Throughput	
Nursing diagnosis of stressors	**Predicted patient outcomes**	**Nursing orders**
10. Family's response to crisis—cont'd		Major medical interventions will be to assist her breathing until she can breathe on her own and to support her vital functions Drowsiness and confusion are not unusual for patients in Sandy's situation and will be temporary Explain purposes of equipment in the environment
b. Anxiety of father and brother related to unfamiliar environment and confusion about Sandy's condition	b. Significant others able to discuss feelings and fears with members of the health care team Demonstrate behaviors indicative of lowered anxiety (e.g., sit quietly between visits with Sandy, demonstrates more relaxed facial expression and body posture) Demonstrate constructive means for dealing with anxiety, (e.g., take walks between visits, talk with chaplain, eat meals regularly, communicate with relatives about Sandy's condition)	**Goal:** *Acknowledge, accept, and encourage ventilation of feelings by father and brother* Anticipate feelings of helplessness, powerlessness, frustration Identify behaviors indicative of the grieving process (shock, disbelief, anger) Use therapeutic means of communication to facilitate verbalization of feelings Identify need for chaplain referral Allow flexibility in length and frequency of visiting periods
c. Separation from significant others	c. Maintains continuity in relationship with significant others Acknowledges significant others' presence during visiting periods Attempts to communicate by touching significant others	**Goal:** *Promote continuity in relationship between Sandy and significant others* Inform Sandy that father and brother are in waiting room Provide flexibility in length and frequency of visiting periods Continually reassure that family are nearby Facilitate interactions between Sandy and family during visiting periods
d. Family stress related to indecision about immediate changes in daily living patterns	d. Make knowledgeable decisions for instituting changes in therapy, life style, established family roles and relationships Make realistic decisions consistent with Sandy's condition (e.g., stay in nearby motel at least for first 24 hours; father makes arrangements for assistance on the farm for several days)	**Goal:** *Support decisions for temporary life style changes* Explore viable options regarding the assumption of responsibility for the care of the farm, making sleeping and eating arrangements, acquisition of personal belongings
		Goal: *Provide information and clarify misconceptions* See diagnosis 10a

Table 72-2. Nursing plan at time of transfer from critical care unit

Input	Throughput	
Nursing diagnosis of stressors	**Predicted patient outcomes**	**Nursing orders**
1. Respiratory infection related to invasive procedures, restricted activity, and debilitation.	1. Without signs and symptoms of physiologic reaction to therapy Sputum culture free of pathogenic organisms Clear breath sounds Temperature normal	**Goal:** *Promote physical comfort; protect from personal injury* Administer tracheostomy care q4h Adhere to sterile suctioning technique Monitor amount, consistency, and odor of secretions Collect secretions for culture and sensitivity every AM Avoid cross-contamination from other patients (do not exchange IPPB machine with other patients) Avoid assigning personnel with URI to care for Sandy Ensure as much uninterrupted rest as possible **Goal:** *Restore and maintain vital functions* Deep-breathing exercises with percussion q4h Change position q2h OOB to chair 4 times a day **Goal:** *Promote adequate nutritional status* Determine food preferences of high-caloric, high-protein content
2. Muscle weakness related to restricted activity	2. Free of complications of immobility-restricted activity Assumes responsibility for increasing number of self-care activities Tolerates sitting in a chair for increasing periods of time	**Goal:** *Preserve and maintain musculoskeletal function* Continue active ROM q4h Assess activity tolerance Promote independence in self-care activities
3. Inadequate nutritional intake related to anorexia, increased metabolic demands (infection, trauma), immobility	3. Maintains nutritional status Maintains or gains weight Increases caloric and protein intake	**Goal:** *Maintain adequate nutritional status* Determine food preferences Monitor calories daily **Goal:** *Promote physical comfort* Give oral hygiene before and after meals Provide aesthetic environment Control environmental temperature and administer Tylenol as ordered to decrease metabolic demands

Continued.

Table 72-2. Nursing plan at time of transfer from critical care unit—cont'd

Input	Throughput	
Nursing diagnosis of stressors	**Predicted patient outcomes**	**Nursing orders**
3. Inadequate nutritional intake —cont'd		**Goal:** *Preserve and maintain musculoskeletal functions* Assist to bed, OOB 4 times a day Continue active ROM exercises q4h
4. Constipation related to low-roughage diet, decreased activity, difficulty using bedpan	4. Maintains normal bowel function Has stool of normal frequency, color, and consistency every other day Soft, nontender abdomen	4. **Goal:** *Promote normal elimination* Offer warm beverage, offer bedpan in 20 minutes Push fluids to 3,000 ml/day Determine food preferences of high roughage content **Goal:** *Preserve and maintain musculoskeletal function* Continue exercise regimen **Goal:** *Promote physical comfort* Ensure privacy when using bedpan Use room deodorizer after use of bedpan Hygienic measures after bowel movement Position patient to facilitate elimination
5. Pain in fracture sites related to movement and therapeutic regimen	5. Free from extreme physical discomfort Tolerates increasing activity without change in vital signs Tolerates increasing activity with decreasing amounts of analgesics Tolerates activity with assistance of progressive relaxation techniques	5. **Goal:** *Promote physical comfort and protect from personal injury* Give analgesic prior to movement and procedures Clarify reasons for pain and acknowledge as normal Reassess effectiveness of analgesic Differentiate types of pain Assist Sandy in learning progressive relaxation techniques to control pain
6. Altered body image related to injuries and tracheostomy	6. Sandy will show no indication of negative reaction to change in appearance Discusses feelings with supportive person	6. **Goal:** *Acknowledge, accept, and encourage ventilation of feelings by Sandy* Determine perception and explore with Sandy extent of physical limitations now and in the future Provide information and clarify misconceptions

Table 72-2. Nursing plan at time of transfer from critical care unit—cont'd

Input	Throughput	
Nursing diagnosis of stressors	**Predicted patient outcomes**	**Nursing orders**
7. Potential anxiety and intensified feelings of loss related to transfer from critical care unit	7. Sandy able to state plans for transfer from CCU States day of anticipated transfer States name of receiving unit Describes differences in routines between CCU and receiving unit Recognizes staff members from receiving unit Discusses fears with supportive person Free from signs and symptoms of severe physiologic or psychologic reaction to stress	7. **Goal:** *Prepare Sandy and significant others for her transfer* Support Sandy's involvement in decision making regarding transfer, private or semiprivate room, means of transportation for transfer (e.g., wheelchair, stretcher) Introduce Sandy to at least one staff member from receiving unit prior to transfer Inform Sandy on initial consideration for transfer Promote independence in self-care **Goal:** *Acknowledge, accept, and encourage ventilation of feelings* Point out improvement in condition and impending transfer as signs of recovery Emphasize positive aspects of transfer (e.g., increased privacy, less disruption of rest and sleep, more flexible visiting hours, indicates improvement in physical condition See Orders 6
8. Depression related to loneliness (loss of significant other's support), lack of diversion (boredom), hopelessness (discouraged about slow recovery)	8a. Patient able to discuss feelings and fears with members of health care team Demonstrates behaviors reflective of decreased withdrawal, increased involvement in self-care b. Patient and significant others maintain continuity in relationships Communicates with family weekly by telephone or letter with assistance from nurse	8. **Goal:** *Acknowledge, accept, and encourage ventilation of feelings by Sandy and significant others* Suggest sending of cards by family and friends Explore types of diversional activities of interest to Sandy Promote continuity in relationship between patient and significant others (father, brother, aunt, cousins) Flexible family visiting hours Facilitate continuity in relationships with peer group (e.g., ask family to bring news of friends, explore possibility of including friends in family visit)

Increased catabolism from restricted activity and increased metabolic demands from a low-grade fever along with anorexia led to weight loss and concern about her nutritional status. Bed rest and an essentially liquid diet contributed to mild constipation. Restricted activity and prolonged immobility resulted in some loss of muscle tone and muscle weakness despite active and passive exercises.

Frustration from cumbersome alternatives to verbal communication and withdrawal secondary to depression made it impossible for Sandy to verbalize her feelings and her fears about her physical appearance, prolonged recovery, and changes in her life style.

Prior to her depression and increasing withdrawal, Sandy seemed to understand the medical and nursing treatment goals and rationale for her care, as was evidenced by her cooperation in her pulmonary care and other daily activities.

As she became less withdrawn her spirits improved around the time of her family's visits. Unfortunately they are able to visit only every other weekend, and during their absence she experiences loneliness from separation, which compounds her depression.

SUMMARY

For the patient and significant others, critical illness is a time of crisis, usually involving severe physiologic, psychologic, and social stressors. The foregoing patient study illustrates that the initial focus of the critical care team is on patient survival and support of significant others in their attempt to cope with the situation. The case study also illustrates the changes in priorities as the patient progresses toward recovery. The emphasis of the health care team then changes to assist the patient and significant others in adjusting to temporary and permanent life style changes and in making knowledgeable decisions and plans in order to progress to maximal recovery. Progression toward recovery means that the patient and significant others must cope with other aspects of illness such as rehabilitation and the adjustment to temporary and permanent changes in life style. The emphasis of health professionals also changes as they assist the patient and significant others to make knowledgeable decisions and plans for the future.

REFERENCES AND SELECTED READINGS

1. *Aspinall, M. J.: Nursing diagnosis: the weak link, Nurs. Outlook **24**:433-437, 1976.
2. *Gebbie, K., and Lavin, M. A.: Classifying nursing diagnosis, Am. J. Nurs. **74**:250-253, 1974.
3. *Gordon, M.: Nursing diagnosis and the diagnostic process, Am. J. Nurs. **76**:1298-1300, 1976.
4. *Mundinger, M. O., and Jauron, G. D.: Developing a nursing diagnosis, Nurs. Outlook **75**:94-98, 1975.

*References preceded by an asterisk are particularly well suited for student reading.

Index

E

J